powered by unbound MEDICINE

DAVIS'S DRUGGUIDE.COM

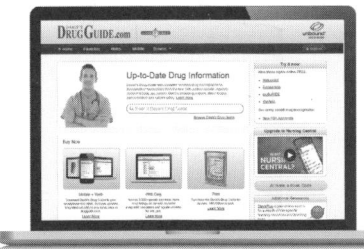

The **Access Code** below unlocks a FREE, 1-year subscription to

www.DRUGGUIDE.com

- Search the complete 5,000-drug database and appendices quickly and efficiently.
- Build your knowledge with extensively cross-referenced drugs.
- Keep up to date with FDA drug news.

BONUS! Access 1,700 monographs from your desktop, laptop, or any mobile device with a web browser.

1. Scratch off the shiny surface below to reveal your unique Access Code
2. Go to **www.DrugGuide.com**
3. Enter your code

SCRATCH OFF
shiny surface with care!

Book cannot be returned for a refund once this code is scratched off.

Each Drug Guide Online code may only be redeemed one time. If your code has already been used, visit DrugGuide.com to purchase access.

HOW TO USE YOUR DRUG GUIDE

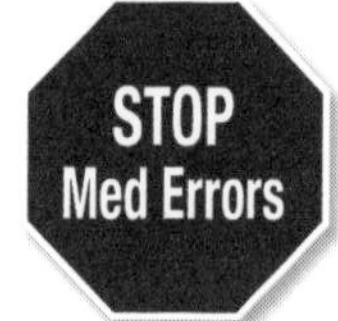

REMS

traZODone (traz-oh-done)
~~Desyrel~~, ✤Oleptro, ✤Trazorel

Classification
Therapeutic: antidepressants

Pregnancy Category C

Risk Evaluation and Mitigation Strategies (REMS) Icon

Active and Discontinued Drug Trade Names

RED tab for High Alert medications

Icon for pharmacogenomic content

Life-threatening side effects in **RED**, CAPITALIZED letters

Drug-drug, drug-food, and drug-natural product interactions

Adult & pediatric dosages, with pharmacogenomic content, when applicable

warfarin **1273**

HIGH ALERT

warfarin (war-fa-rin)
Coumadin, Jantoven

Classification
Therapeutic: anticoagulants
Pharmacologic: coumarins

Pregnancy Category X

Indications
Prophylaxis and treatment of: Venous thrombosis, Pulmonary embolism, Atrial fibrillation with embolization. Management of myocardial infarction: Decreases risk of death, Decreases risk of subsequent MI, Decreases risk of future thromboembolic events. Prevention of thrombus formation and embolization after prosthetic valve placement.

Action
Interferes with hepatic synthesis of vitamin K-dependent clotting factors (II, VII, IX, and X). **Therapeutic Effects:** Prevention of thromboembolic events.

Pharmacokinetics
Absorption: Well absorbed from the GI tract after oral administration.
Distribution: Crosses the placenta but does not enter breast milk.
Protein Binding: 99%.
Metabolism and Excretion: Metabolized by the liver.
Half-life: 42 hr.

TIME/ACTION PROFILE (effects on coagulation tests)

ROUTE	ONSET	PEAK	DURATION
PO, IV	36–72 hr	5–7 days†	2–5 days‡

† At a constant dose
‡ After discontinuation

Contraindications/Precautions
Contraindicated in: Uncontrolled bleeding; Open wounds; Active ulcer disease; Recent brain, eye, or spinal cord injury or surgery; Severe liver or kidney disease; Uncontrolled hypertension; **OB:** Crosses placenta and may cause fatal hemorrhage in the fetus. May also cause congenital malformation.
Use Cautiously in: Malignancy; Patients with history of ulcer or liver disease; History of poor compliance; Women with childbearing potential; ⧖ Asian patients or those who carry the CYP2C9*2 allele and/or the CYP2C9*3 allele, or with the VKORC1 AA genotype (↑ risk of bleeding with standard dosing; lower initial doses should be considered); **Pedi:** Has been used safely but may require more frequent PT/INR assessments; **Geri:** Due to greater than expected anticoagulant response, initiate and maintain at lower doses.

Adverse Reactions/Side Effects
GI: cramps, nausea. **Derm:** dermal necrosis. **Hemat:** BLEEDING. **Misc:** fever.

Interactions
Drug-Drug: Abciximab, androgens, capecitabine, cefotetan, chloramphenicol, clopidogrel, disulfiram, fluconazole, fluoroquinolones, itraconazole, metronidazole (including vaginal use), **thrombolytics, eptifibatide, tirofiban, ticlopidine, sulfonamides, quinidine, quinine, NSAIDs, valproates,** and **aspirin** may ↑ the response to warfarin and ↑ the risk of bleeding. Chronic use of **acetaminophen** may ↑ the risk of bleeding. Chronic **alcohol** ingestion may ↓ action of warfarin; if chronic **alcohol** abuse results in significant liver damage, action of warfarin may be ↑ due to ↓ production of clotting factor. Acute **alcohol** ingestion may ↑ action of warfarin. **Barbiturates, carbamazepine, rifampin,** and **hormonal contraceptives containing estrogen** may ↓ the anticoagulant response to warfarin. **Many other drugs** may affect the activity of warfarin.
Drug-Natural Products: St. John's wort ↓ effect. ↑ bleeding risk with **anise, arnica, chamomile, clove, dong quai, fenugreek, feverfew, garlic, ginger, ginkgo, Panax ginseng, licorice,** and others.
Drug-Food: Ingestion of large quantities of **foods high in vitamin K content** (see list in Appendix M) may antagonize the anticoagulant effect of warfarin.

Route/Dosage
⧖ **PO, IV (Adults):** 2–5 mg/day for 2–4 days; then adjust daily dose by results of INR. Initiate therapy with lower doses in geriatric or debilitated patients or in Asian patients or those with CYP2C9*2 and/or CYP2C9*3 alleles or VKORC1 AA genotype.
PO, IV (Children >1 mo): *Initial loading dose*—0.2 mg/kg (maximum dose: 10 mg) for 2–4 days then adjust daily dose by results of INR, use 0.1 mg/kg if liver dysfunction is present. *Maintenance dose range*—0.05–0.34 mg/kg/day.

Availability (generic available)
Tablets: 1 mg, 2 mg, 2.5 mg, 3 mg, 4 mg, 5 mg, 6 mg, 7.5 mg, 10 mg. **Cost:** *Generic*—1 mg $10.83/100, 2 mg $10.83/100, 2.5 mg $10.83/100, 3 mg $10.83/100, 4 mg $10.83/100, 5 mg $8.52/100, 6 mg $10.64/100, 7.5 mg $10.83/100, 10 mg $10.83/100. **Powder for injection:** 5 mg/vial.

W

✤ = Canadian drug name. ⧖ = Genetic implication. ~~Strikethrough~~ = Discontinued.
*CAPITALS indicates life-threatening; underlines indicate most frequent.

New Heading

REP heading detailing information on the use of drugs in males and females of reproductive age

NURSING IMPLICATIONS

All 5 steps of the nursing process

Assessment

- Assess for signs of bleeding and hemorrhage (bleeding gums; nosebleed; unusual bruising; tarry, black stools; hematuria; fall in hematocrit or BP; guaiac-positive stools, urine, or nasogastric aspirate).
- Assess for evidence of additional or increased thrombosis. Symptoms depend on area of involvement.
- Geri: Patients over 60 yr exhibit greater than expected PT/INR response. Monitor for side effects at lower therapeutic ranges.
- Pedi: Achieving and maintaining therapeutic PT/INR ranges may be more difficult in pediatric patients. Assess PT/INR levels more frequently.
- ***Lab Test Considerations:*** Monitor PT, INR and other clotting factors frequently during therapy. Therapeutic PT ranges 1.3–1.5 times greater than control; however, the INR, a standardized system that provides a common basis for communicating and interpreting PT results, is usually referenced. Normal INR (not on anticoagulants) is 0.8–1.2. An INR of 2.5–3.5 is recommended for patients at very high risk of embolization (for example, patients with mitral valve replacement and ventricular hypertrophy). Lower levels are acceptable when risk is lower. Heparin may affect the PT/INR; draw blood for PT/INR in patients receiving both heparin and warfarin at least 5 hr after the IV bolus dose, 4 hr after cessation of IV infusion, or 24 hr after subcut heparin injection. Asian patients and those who carry the CYP2C9*2 allele and/or the CYP2C9*3 allele, or those with VKORC1 AA genotype may require more frequent monitoring and lower doses.
- Monitor hepatic function and CBC before and periodically throughout therapy.
- Monitor stool and urine for occult blood before and periodically during therapy.
- ***Toxicity and Overdose:*** Withholding 1 or more doses of warfarin is usually sufficient if INR is excessively elevated or if minor bleeding occurs. If overdose occurs or anticoagulation needs to be immediately reversed, the antidote is vitamin K (phytonadione, AquaMEPHYTON). Administration of whole blood or plasma also may be required in severe bleeding because of the delayed onset of vitamin K.

Potential Nursing Diagnoses

Ineffective tissue perfusion (Indications)
Risk for injury (Side Effects)

Implementation

- ***High Alert:*** Medication errors involving anticoagulants have resulted in serious harm or death from internal or intracranial bleeding. Before administering, evaluate recent INR or PT results and have second practitioner independently check original order.
- Do not confuse Coumadin (warfarin) with Avandia (rosiglitazone) or Cardura (doxazosin). Do not confuse Jantoven (warfarin) with Janumet (sitagliptin/metformin) or Januvia (sitagliptin).
- Because of the large number of medications capable of significantly altering warfarin's effects, careful monitoring is recommended when new agents are started or other agents are discontinued. Interactive potential should be evaluated for all new medications (Rx, OTC, and natural products).
- **PO:** Administer medication at same time each day. Medication requires 3–5 days to reach effective levels; usually begun while patient is still on heparin.
- Do not interchange brands; potencies may not be equivalent.

IV Administration

- **Direct IV:** Reconstitute each 5-mg vial with 2.7 mL of sterile water for injection. Reconstituted solution is stable for 4 hr at room temperature. ***Diluent:*** No further dilution needed before administration. ***Concentration:*** 2 mg/mL. ***Rate:*** Administer over 1–2 min.
- **Y-Site Compatibility:** amikacin, ascorbic acid, bivalrudin, cefazolin, ceftriaxone, dopamine, epinephrine, heparin, lidocaine, morphine, nitroglycerin, oxytocin, potassium chloride, ranitidine.
- **Y-Site Incompatibility:** aminophylline, ceftazidime, ciprofloxacin, dobutamine, esmolol, gentamicin, labetalol, promazine.

Subhead for IV administration in the Nursing Implications section, as well as subheads for Diluent, Concentration, and Rate

Patient/Family Teaching

- Instruct patient to take medication as directed. Take missed doses as soon as remembered that day; do not double doses. Inform health care professional of missed doses at time of checkup or lab tests. Inform patients that anticoagulant effect may persist for 2–5 days following discontinuation. Advise patient to read *Medication Guide* before starting therapy and with each Rx refill.
- Review foods high in vitamin K (see Appendix M). Patient should have consistent limited intake of these foods, as vitamin K is the antidote for warfarin, and alternating intake of these foods will cause PT levels to fluctuate. Advise patient to avoid cranberry juice or products during therapy.
- Caution patient to avoid IM injections and activities leading to injury. Instruct patient to use a soft toothbrush, not to floss, and to shave with an electric razor during warfarin therapy. Advise patient that venipunctures and injection sites require application of pressure to prevent bleeding or hematoma formation.

More patient safety information than any other drug guide

= Canadian drug name. = Genetic implication. ~~Strikethrough~~ = Discontinued.
*CAPITALS indicates life-threatening; underlines indicate most frequent.

Find enhanced Canadian content throughout—in the monographs, appendices, and index.

Davis's DRUG GUIDE FOR NURSES®

FIFTHTEENTH EDITION

APRIL HAZARD VALLERAND, PhD, RN, FAAN
College of Nursing Alumni Endowed Professor of Nursing
Wayne State University
College of Nursing
Detroit, Michigan

CYNTHIA A. SANOSKI, BS, PharmD, FCCP, BCPS
Chair, Department of Pharmacy Practice
Thomas Jefferson University
Jefferson School of Pharmacy
Philadelphia, Pennsylvania

JUDITH HOPFER DEGLIN, PharmD
Consultant Pharmacist
Hospice of Southeastern Connecticut
Norwich, Connecticut

Contributing Editor:

Holly G. Mansell, BSP, PharmD
Assistant Professor of Pharmacy
College of Pharmacy and Nutrition
University of Saskatchewan
Saskatoon, SK, Canada

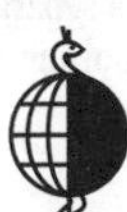

F. A. DAVIS COMPANY • Philadelphia

F. A. Davis Company
1915 Arch Street
Philadelphia, PA 19103
www.fadavis.com

Printed in China

Last digit indicates print number 10 9 8 7 6 5 4 3 2 1
Editor-in-Chief, Nursing: Jean Rodenberger
Acquisitions Editor: Megan Klim
Content Project Manager: Christina L. Snyder
Director of Production: Michael W. Bailey

NOTE: As new scientific information becomes available through basic and clinical research, recommended treatments and drug therapies undergo changes. The authors and publisher have done everything possible to make this book accurate, up to date, and in accord with accepted standards at the time of publication. However, the reader is advised always to check product information (package inserts) for changes and new information regarding dose and contraindications before administering any drug. Caution is especially urged when using new or infrequently ordered drugs.

Library of Congress Cataloging-in-Publication Data

Names: Vallerand, April Hazard, author. | Sanoski, Cynthia A., author. |
Deglin, Judith Hopfer, 1950 , author.
Title: Davis's drug guide for nurses / April Hazard Vallerand, Cynthia A.
Sanoski, Judith Hopfer Deglin.
Other titles: Drug guide for nurses
Description: Fifteenth edition. | Philadelphia : F.A. Davis Company, [2017] |
Includes bibliographical references and index.
Identifiers: LCCN 2016001572| ISBN 9780803657052 (US pbk.) | ISBN
9780803657069 (Canadian pbk.)
Subjects: | MESH: Pharmaceutical Preparations--administration & dosage | Drug
Therapy--nursing | Pharmacology, Clinical--methods | Handbooks | Nurses'
Instruction
Classification: LCC RM301.12 | NLM QV 735 | DDC 615.102/4613--dc23 LC record available at
http://lccn.loc.gov/2016001572

DEDICATION

To my son, Ben, whose sensitivity and sense of humor make even the toughest day easier.
To my daughter, Katharine, whose dedication and passion in seeking her goals I admire.
Watching you both grow to become wonderful young adults gives me such pride and joy. Your support of my work inspires me. Thank you for sharing so much of your lives with me. I love you.

AHV

To my wonderful mother, Geraldine, who has provided her continual love, support, and wisdom as I continue to pursue all of my personal and professional goals.

CAS

In loving memory of my older children, Samantha Ann and Randy Eli, both struck and killed by a drinking driver on January 9, 1997. They remain forever in our hearts. The wonder and joy they brought to our lives continues to inspire us.

To Stu, for his continued support and love.

To my daughter Hanna, whose hard work, talent, and grace never cease to amaze me.
To my son Reuben, whose smile warms my heart and whose energy is boundless.
To my parents, who always inspired me.

JHD

ACKNOWLEDGMENTS

We offer our thanks to the students and nurses who have used our book for almost 30 years. We hope our book provides you with the current knowledge of pharmacotherapeutics you need to continue to give quality care in our rapidly changing health-care environment.

April, Cindy, and Judi

CONSULTANTS

Michelle Farkas, PMHNP-BC
Private Practice
Dearborn, MI

Jamie Crawley, PhD, RN
Assistant Professor
University of Windsor
Faculty of Nursing
Windsor, ON, Canada

Lisa E. Davis, PharmD, FCCP, BCPS, BCOP
Associate Professor of Clinical Pharmacy
University of the Sciences in Philadelphia
Philadelphia College of Pharmacy
Philadelphia, PA

Wanda Edwards, PMHCNS-BC, NP
Instructor (Clinical)
Wayne State University
College of Nursing
Detroit, MI

Deborah A. Ennis, RN, MSN, CCRN
Harrisburg Area Community College
Harrisburg, PA

Linda Felver, PhD, RN
Associate Professor
Oregon Health & Science University
School of Nursing
Portland, OR

Charlene C. Gyurko, PhD, RN, CNE
Assistant Professor
Purdue University, North Central
School of Nursing
Westville, IN

Althea DuBose Hayes, RD
Renal Dietitian
Greenfield Health System,
a division of Henry Ford Health System
Southfield, MI

Therese Jamison, MSN, APRN-BC, ACNP
Associate Professor
Madonna University
School of Nursing
Livonia, MI

Janeen Kidd, RN, BN
Instructor/School Placement Project Coordinator
University of Victoria
School of Nursing
Victoria, BC, Canada

Norma Perez, BSN, RN
Nursing Faculty & Clinical Coordinator
Ivy Tech Community College
School of Nursing
Valparaiso, IN

Kim Subasic, MSN, RN
The University of Scranton
Scranton, PA

Gladdi Tomlinson, RN, MSN
Professor of Nursing
Harrisburg Area Community College
Harrisburg, PA

Linda S. Weglicki, PhD, RN, MSN
Program Director
National Institute of Nursing Research
Office of Extramural Programs
Bethesda, MD

Marcella Williams, RN, MS, AOCN®
Adjunct Faculty
Lansing Community Hospital
Staff Nurse, Sparrow Health System
Lansing, MI

F. A. DAVIS PHARMACOLOGIC PUBLICATIONS ADVISORY BOARD

F.A. Davis Canadian Advisory Board

Anan Ahmed, BSP
Pharmacist, Shopper's Drug Market
MSC Candidate, University of Saskatchewan
Saskatoon, Saskatchewan

Andrea M. Brandt, BScN, MS
Pharmacology Instructor, Lead Faculty, Nursing
Georgian College
Barrie, Ontario

Melanie Deveau, MN-ANP, RN, NP
Nurse Practitioner, Cardiovascular Program
Adjunct Lecturer
Dalhousie University - Yarmouth Site
Yarmouth, Nova Scotia

Lisa Keeping-Burke, RN, PhD. (McGill)
Assistant Professor, Department of Nursing and Health Sciences, UNB
Adjunct Assistant Professor, School of Nursing, Queen's University
Saint John, New Brunswick

Duncan (Stewart) MacLennan, MN, NP
Faculty Lecturer, Faculty of Nursing
University of Alberta
Edmonton, Alberta

Kerry Mansell, BSP, PharmD
Assistant Dean and Associate Professor of Pharmacy
University of Saskatchewan
Saskatoon, Saskatchewan

Craig Miller
Instructor - PN
Assiniboine Community College
Brandon, Manitoba

Wendy Neander, PhD (c), MN, BScN, BScv
Assistant Teaching Professor, School of Nursing
University of Victoria
Nanaimo, British Columbia

Aroha Page, RN, BA, BScN, Grad.Dip Health Sci, M.Phil(N), PhD(UCSF)FRCNA
Associate Professor, School of Nursing
Nipissing University
Faculty of Applied & Professional Studies
North Bay, Ontario

Vincent Salyers, Ed. D, MSN, BA
Associate Dean, Faculty of Health & Community Studies
Mount Royal University
Calgary, Alberta

Michael Scarcello, RN, HBScN, MA
Clinical Nurse Specialist Program Coordinator, Practical Nursing Program
Confederation College
Thunder Bay, Ontario

Jeff Taylor, BSP, MSc, PhD
Professor of Pharmacy
University of Saskatchewan
Saskatoon, Saskatchewan

Jim Wohlgemuth, RN, MN, CTN-B
Instructor, Nursing Education & Health Studies
Grande Prairie Regional College
Grande Prairie, Alberta

CONTENTS

HOW TO USE *DAVIS'S DRUG GUIDE FOR NURSES*

Davis's Drug Guide for Nurses provides comprehensive, up-to-date drug information in well-organized, nursing-focused monographs. It also includes extensive supplemental material in 16 appendices, thoroughly addresses the issue of safe medication administration, and educates the reader about 50 different therapeutic classes of drugs. In this 15th edition, we have continued the tradition of focusing on safe medication administration by including a **Medication Safety Tools** and even more information about health care's most vulnerable patients: children, the elderly, pregnant women, and breast feeding mothers. Look for more Pedi, Geri, OB, and Lactation headings throughout the monographs. In addition, we've included information relevant to Canadian students and nurses. You'll find an appendix comparing Canadian and U.S. pharmaceutical practices, more Canada-only combination drugs in the Combination Drugs appendix, and additional Canadian brand names in the drug monographs. To help you find this information quickly, we've also added a maple leaf icon (✱) in the index next to each Canadian entry. We have added pharmacogenomic information throughout numerous monographs to guide the nurse in selecting and monitoring various drug therapies. To help you find this information quickly, we've added a double helix icon (🧬) to denote this information as it applies to specific drugs. Use this book to enhance your competence in implementing and evaluating medication therapies. The following sections describe the organization of *Davis's Drug Guide for Nurses* and explain how to quickly find the information you need.

Safe Medication Use Articles

"Medication Errors: Improving Practices and Patient Safety", "Detecting and Managing Adverse Drug Reactions", "Overview of Risk Evaluation and Mitigation Systems (REMS)", "Special Dosing Considerations", and "Educating Patients About Safe Medication Use" comprise the safe medication use articles and provide an overview of the medication safety issues that confront practitioners and patients. Leading off this series, the medication errors article familiarizes you with the systems issues and clinical situations repeatedly implicated in medication errors and suggests practical means to avoid them. It also teaches you about *high alert* medications, which have a greater potential to cause patient harm than other medications. "Detecting and Managing Adverse Drug Reactions" explains the different types of adverse reactions and provides guidance on how to detect and manage them. "Risk Evaluation and Mitigation Strategies (REMS)" explains strategies developed by the pharmaceutical industry and required by the Food and Drug Administration (FDA) to minimize adverse drug reactions from potentially dangerous drugs. We have highlighted the drugs that currently have approved REMS programs associated with their use by adding a REMS label at the top of applicable drug monographs. "Special Dosing Considerations" identifies the patient populations, such as neonates and patients with renal impairment, who require careful dose adjustments to ensure optimal therapeutic outcomes. "Educating Patients About Medication Use" reviews the most important teaching points for nurses to discuss with their patients and their families. In addition to these safety articles, other critical information is highlighted in red throughout the drug monographs. This allows the reader to quickly identify important information and to see how nursing practice, including assessment, implementation, and patient teaching, relates to it.

Classifications Profile

Medications in the same therapeutic class often share similar mechanisms of action, assessment guidelines, precautions, and interactions. The Classifications Profile provides summaries of the major therapeutic classifications used in *Davis's Drug Guide for Nurses*. It also provides patient teaching information common to all agents within the class and a list of drugs within each class.

Medication Safety Tools

Updated for this edition is a section with tables and charts that nurses can use for a quick but thorough reference to information that will help them avoid making medication errors. It includes lists of drugs that are associated with adverse reactions and falls in the elderly; proper dosing for pediatric intravenous medications; confused drug names; FDA-approved Tall Man letters and more.

Drug Monographs

Drug monographs are organized in the following manner:

High Alert Status: Some medications, such as chemotherapeutic agents, anticoagulants, and insulins, have a greater potential for harm than others. These medications have been identified by the *Institute for Safe Medication Practices* as **high alert drugs**. *Davis's Drug Guide for Nurses* includes a high alert tab in the upper right corner of the monograph header in appropriate medications to alert the nurse to the medication's risk. The term "high alert" is used in other parts of the monograph as well, to help the nurse administer these medications safely. See the article "Medication Errors: Improving Practices and Patient Safety" for a complete list of high alert medications in *Davis's Drug Guide for Nurses*. Refer to ISMP.org for all solutions, groups, and individual high alert drugs.

Generic/Brand Name: The generic name appears first, with a pronunciation key, followed by an alphabetical list of trade names. Canadian trade names are preceded by a maple leaf (✱). Brand names that have been discontinued have a slash through them (~~Decadron~~). Common names, abbreviations, and selected foreign names are also included.

Classification: The therapeutic classification, which categorizes drugs by the disease state they are used to treat, appears first, followed by the pharmacologic classification, which is based on the drug's mechanism of action.

Controlled Substance Schedule: All drugs regulated by federal law are placed into one of five schedules, based on the drug's medicinal value, harmfulness, and potential for abuse or addiction. Schedule I drugs, the most dangerous and having no medicinal value, are not included in *Davis's Drug Guide for Nurses*. (See Appendix H for a description of the Schedule of Controlled Substances.)

Pregnancy Category: Pregnancy categories (A, B, C, D, and X) provide a basis for determining a drug's potential for fetal harm and are included in each monograph. The designation UK is used when the pregnancy category is unknown. (See Appendix G for more information.)

Indications: Medications are approved by the FDA for specific disease states. This section identifies the diseases or conditions for which the drug is commonly used and includes significant unlabeled uses as well.

Action: This section contains a concise description of how the drug produces the desired therapeutic effect.

Pharmacokinetics: Pharmacokinetics refers to the way the body processes a medication by absorption, distribution, metabolism, and excretion. This section also includes information on the drug's half-life.

Absorption: Absorption describes the process that follows drug administration and its subsequent delivery to systemic circulation. If only a small fraction is absorbed following oral administration (diminished bioavailability), then the oral dose must be much greater than the parenteral dose. Absorption into systemic circulation also follows other routes of administration such as topical, transdermal, intramuscular, subcutaneous, rectal, and ophthalmic routes. Drugs administered intravenously are 100% bioavailable.

Distribution: This section comments on the drug's distribution in body tissues and fluids. Distribution becomes important in choosing one drug over another, as in selecting an antibiotic that will penetrate the central nervous system to treat meningitis or in avoiding drugs that cross the placenta or concentrate in breast milk. Information on protein binding is included for drugs that are >95% bound to plasma proteins, which has implications for drug-drug interactions.

Metabolism and Excretion: Drugs are primarily eliminated from the body either by hepatic conversion to active or inactive compounds (metabolism or biotransformation) and subsequent excretion by the kidneys, or by renal elimination of unchanged drug. Therefore, drug metabolism and excretion information is important in determining dosage regimens and intervals for patients with impaired renal or hepatic function. The creatinine clearance (CCr) helps quantify renal function and guides dosage adjustments. Formulas to estimate CCr are included in Appendix E.

Half-Life: The half-life of a drug is the amount of time it takes for the drug concentration to decrease by 50% and roughly correlates with the drug's duration of action. Half-lives are given for drugs assuming the patient has normal renal or hepatic function. Conditions that alter the half-life are noted.

Time/Action Profile: The time/action profile table provides the drug's onset of action, peak effect, and duration of activity. This information can aid in planning administration schedules and allows the reader to appreciate differences in choosing one route over another.

Contraindications and Precautions: Situations in which drug use should be avoided are listed as contraindications. In general, most drugs are contraindicated in pregnancy or lactation, unless the potential benefits outweigh the possible risks to the mother or baby (e.g., anticonvulsants, antihypertensives, and antiretrovirals). Contraindications may be absolute (i.e., the drug in question should be avoided completely) or relative, in which certain clinical situations may allow cautious use of the drug. The precautions portion includes disease states or clinical situations in which drug use involves particular risks or in which dosage modification may be necessary. Extreme cautions are noted separately to draw attention to conditions under which use of the drug results in serious, potentially life-threatening consequences.

Adverse Reactions and Side Effects: Although it is not possible to include all reported reactions, major side effects for all drugs are included. Life-threatening adverse reactions or side effects are **CAPITALIZED**, and the most frequent side effects are underlined. Those underlined generally have an incidence of 10% or greater. Those not underlined occur in fewer than 10% but more than 1% of patients. Although life-threatening reactions may be rare (fewer than 1%), they are included because of their significance. The following abbreviations are used for body systems:

CNS: central nervous system
EENT: eye, ear, nose, and throat
Resp: respiratory
CV: cardiovascular
GI: gastrointestinal
GU: genitourinary
Derm: dermatologic
Endo: endocrinologic
F and E: fluid and electrolyte
Hemat: hematologic
Local: local
Metab: metabolic
MS: musculoskeletal
Neuro: neurologic
Misc: miscellaneous
Rep: reproductive

Interactions: Drug interactions are a significant risk for patients. As the number of medications a patient receives increases, so does the likelihood of drug-drug interactions. This section provides the most important drug-drug interactions and their physiological effects. Significant drug-food and drug-natural product interactions are also noted as are recommendations for avoiding or minimizing these interactions.

Route and Dosage: Routes of administration are grouped together and include recommended doses for adults, children, and other more specific age groups (such as geriatric patients). Dosage units are expressed in the terms in which they are usually prescribed. For example, penicillin G dosage is given in units rather than in milligrams. Dosing intervals also are provided in the manner in which they are frequently ordered. If a specific clinical situation (indication) requires a different dose or interval, this is listed separately for clarity. Specific dosing regimens for hepatic or renal impairment are also included.

Availability: This section lists the strengths and concentrations of available dose forms. Such information is useful in planning more convenient regimens (fewer tablets/capsules, less injection volume) and in determining whether certain dosage forms are available (suppositories, oral concentrates, sustained- or extended-release forms). Flavors of oral liquids and chewable tablets have been included to improve compliance and adherence in pediatric patients. General availability and average wholesale prices of commonly prescribed drugs have also been added as an aid to nurses with prescriptive authority.

Nursing Implications: This section helps the nurse apply the nursing process to pharmacotherapeutics. The subsections provide a step-by-step guide to clinical assessment, implementation (drug administration), and evaluation of the outcomes of pharmacologic therapy.

Assessment: This section includes guidelines for assessing patient history and physical data before and during drug therapy. Assessments specific to the drug's various indications are also included. The **Lab Test Considerations** section provides the nurse with information regarding which laboratory tests to monitor and how the results may be affected by the medication. **Toxicity and Overdose** alerts the nurse to therapeutic serum drug concentrations that must be monitored and signs and symptoms of toxicity. The antidote and treatment for toxicity or overdose of appropriate medications also are included.

Potential Nursing Diagnoses: The two or three most pertinent North American Nursing Diagnoses Association (NANDA) diagnoses that potentially apply to a patient receiving the medication are listed. Each diagnosis includes the pharmacologic effect from which the diagnosis has been derived. For instance, the patient receiving immunosuppressant drugs should be diagnosed with Risk for Infection. The diagnosis is followed by the term Side Effects in parentheses. Since patient education is fundamental to all nurse-patient interactions, the diagnosis Deficient Knowledge should be assumed to be a nursing diagnosis applicable to all drugs.

Implementation: Guidelines specific for medication administration are discussed in this subsection. **High Alert** information, i.e., information that directly relates to preventing medication errors with inherently dangerous drugs, is included first if applicable. Sound-alike look-alike name confusion alerts are also included here. Other headings in this section provide data regarding routes of administration. **PO** describes when and how to administer the drug, whether tablets may be crushed or capsules opened, and when to administer the medication in relation to food. The **IV** section includes specific information about administering the medication intravenously. This section has been thoroughly updated and contains a prominent IV Administration heading that introduces this section. **pH and medication administration:** Medications with a pH less than 7 are acidic; those with a pH greater than 7 are basic or alkaline. This number can help you determine if a drug or solution is acidic or alkaline. Chemical phlebitis may occur when infusing medications or solutions intravenously that are irritating to the vein wall. Acidic medications are irritating to the vessel walls. A wrong diluent can greatly affect the pH of the resulting IV solution. Incompatible solutions can also alter pH. To prevent tissue damage, burning, pain and irritation, it is imperative that the body's pH not be altered. Nurses should also be aware that any additive to a solution may increase or decrease the pH. Bold, red headings are included to highlight the recommended **diluents** and **concentrations**. These headings complement the **rate** heading and make this critical information easy to find. Several subsections comprise the IV Administration section. The first section, **IV Push**, which refers to administering medications from a syringe directly into a saline lock, Y-site of IV tubing, or a 3-way stopcock, provides details for reconstitution, concentration, dilution, and rate. **Rate** is also included in both other methods of IV administration, direct or intermittent infusion. **Intermittent Infusion** and **Continuous Infusion** specify standard dilution solutions and amounts, stability information, and rates. In addition, a quick reference for information about dilution amounts in neonates and infants, who are extremely sensitive to excess fluids, is contained in the new **Medication Safety Tools** section. **Y-Site Compatibility/Incompatibility** identifies medications compatible or incompatible with each drug when administered via Y-site injection or 3-way stopcock in IV tubing. **Additive Compatibility/Incompatibility** identifies medications compatible or incompatible when admixed in solution. Compatibility of diluted medications administered through a Y-site for continuous or intermittent infusion is usually limited to 24 hours. **Solution Compatibility/ Incompatibility** identifies compatible or incompatible solutions for dilution for administration purposes. Compatibility information is compiled from Trissel's *Handbook of Injectable Drugs*, 17th ed and *Micromedex*. Compatibility and incompatibility information is also located in charts found on DavisPlus (http://davisplus.fadavis.com, keyword drug guide).

Patient/Family Teaching: This section includes information that should be taught to patients and/or families of patients. Side effects that should be reported, information on minimizing and managing side effects, details on administration, and follow-up requirements are presented. The nurse also should refer to the **Implementation** section for specific information to teach to the patient and family about taking the medication. **Home Care Issues** discusses aspects to be considered for medications taken in the home setting.

Evaluation: Outcome criteria for determination of the effectiveness of the medication are provided.

REFERENCES

1. *International Journal of Comprehensive Pharmacy: A Guide on Intravenous Drug Compatibilities Based on their pH.* Vilma Loubnan and Soumana C Nasser Vol. 01, Issue 05, 2010.
2. Phillips, Lynn D, and Gorski, Lisa A. *Manual of I.V. Therapeutics.* 6th Edition. F.A. Davis Company: Philadelphia, 2014.

EVIDENCE-BASED PRACTICE AND PHARMACOTHERAPEUTICS: Implications for Nurses

Note: The content below is an excerpt from an article written exclusively for the 12th edition of **Davis's Drug Guide for Nurses**. To access the full article, visit **DavisPlus**, F.A. Davis's online center for student and instructor ancillaries, at http://davisplus.fadavis.com.

The purpose of evidence-based practice is to improve the outcomes of treatment for patients. How pharmacologic agents affect patients is often the subject of research; such research is required by the Food and Drug Administration (FDA) before and after drug approval. Any medication can be the subject of an evidence-based clinical review article. But what does "evidence-based" mean and how does it relate to nursing?

According to Ingersoll, "Evidence-based nursing practice is the conscientious, explicit, and judicious use of theory-derived, research-based information in making decisions about care delivery to individuals or groups of patients and in consideration of individual needs and preferences" (2000, p. 152). Still subject to debate are questions about the sufficiency and quality of evidence. For example, what kind of evidence is needed? How much evidence is necessary to support, modify, or change clinical practice? And, were the studies reviewed of "good" quality and are their results valid?

In general, clinicians use **hierarchy of evidence** schemas to rank types of research reports from the most valuable and scientifically rigorous to the least useful. The hierarchy makes clear that some level of evidence about the effect of a particular treatment or condition exists, even if the evidence is considered weak. Figure 1 illustrates a hierarchy of evidence pyramid with widely accepted rankings: the most scientifically rigorous at the top, the least scientifically rigorous at the bottom. Practitioners and clinicians should look for the highest level of available evidence to answer their clinical questions. However, it is important that clinicians also apply the second fundamental principle of EBP, which is that evidence alone is not sufficient to make clinical decisions. Decision makers must always trade off the benefits and risks, and the costs associated with alternative treatment options, and by doing so, consider the patients' values and preferences.

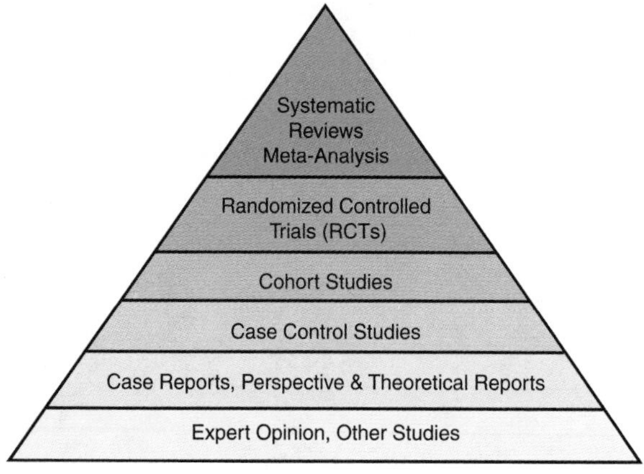

Figure 1: Hierarchy of Scientific Evidence Pyramid

Evidence-Based Practice and Its Importance in Pharmacology

Evidence-based practices in pharmacology generally are derived from well-designed randomized controlled trials (RCTs) or other experimental designs that investigate drugs' therapeutic and non-therapeutic effects. However, although FDA-approved pharmacologic agents have undergone rigorous testing through RCTs, nurses have the responsibility to evaluate the findings for the best scientific evidence available and to determine the most appropriate, safest, and efficacious drugs for their patients.

While numerous databases are available through Internet searches, two valuable and quickly accessible resources for evaluating the current highest level of pharmacologic evidence are 1) the Cochrane Database of Systematic Reviews and the Central Register of Controlled Trials and 2) the National Guidelines Clearinghouse (NGC), supported by the Agency for Healthcare Research and Quality (AHRQ). The Cochrane library and databases provide full text of high-quality, regularly updated systematic reviews, protocols, and clinical trials. The Web address is http://www.cochrane.org/reviews.clibintro.htm.

AHRQ's Evidence-Based Practice Centers (EPCs) provide evidence reports and technology assessments that can assist nurses in their efforts to provide the highest quality and safest pharmacologic health care available. The EPCs systematically review the relevant scientific literature, conduct additional analyses (when appropriate) prior to developing their reports and assessments, and provide guideline comparisons. The Web address is http://www.guideline.gov.

Evidence-based systematic reports and guidelines provide nurses with instantaneous access to the most current knowledge, enabling them to critically appraise the scientific evidence and its appropriateness to their patient population. This is especially important given the need for nurses to keep abreast of the rapidly changing pharmacologic agents in use. New drugs are approved each month, compelling nurses to know these drugs' intended uses, therapeutic effects, interactions, and adverse effects.

Evidence-based practice requires a shift from the traditional paradigm of clinical practice—grounded in intuition, clinical experience, and pathophysiologic rationale—to a paradigm in which nurses must combine clinical expertise, patient values and preferences, and clinical circumstances with the integration of the best scientific evidence in order to make conscientious, well-informed, research-based decisions that affect nursing patient care.

***

Linda S. Weglicki, PhD, RN, MSN
Health Scientist Administrator
Office of Extramural Programs
National Institute of Nursing Research
National Institutes of Health
Bethesda, Maryland

REFERENCES

1. DiCenso, A., Guyatt, G., & Ciliska, D. (2005). *Evidence-based nursing: A guide to clinical practice*. St. Louis, MO: Elsevier Mosby.
2. Guyatt, G., & Rennie, D. (2002). *Users' guide to the medical literature: Essentials of evidence-based clinical practice*. Chicago, IL: American Medical Association Press.

3. Ingersoll, G.L. (2000). "Evidence-based nursing: What it is and what it isn't." *Nursing Outlook*. 48(4), 151-152.
4. Institute of Medicine (IOM). (2001). *Crossing the quality chasm: A new health system for the 21st century*. Washington, DC: National Academy Press.
5. Leavitt, S.B. (2003). Evidence-based addiction medicine for practitioners: Evaluating and using research evidence in clinical practice. Addiction Treatment Forum, March. Retrieved May, 2007, from http://www.atforum.com/SiteRoot/pages/addiction_resources/EBAM_16_Pager.pdf
6. Melnyk, B.M., & Fineout-Overholt, E. (2005). *Evidence-based practice in nursing & healthcare: A guide to best practice*. Philadelphia, PA: Lippincott Williams & Wilkins.
7. Mitchell, G.J. (1999). "Evidence-based practice: Critique and alternative view." *Nursing Science Quarterly*. 12, 30-35.
8. Polit, D.F., & Beck, C.T. (2008). *Nursing research: Generating and assessing evidence for practice*. (8th ed). Philadelphia, PA: Lippincott Williams & Wilkins.
9. Sackett, D., Rosenberg, W., Gray, J., Haynes, R., & Richardson, W. (1996). "Evidence-based medicine: What it is and what it isn't." *British Medical Journal*. 312, 71-72.

PHARMACOGENOMICS

Introduction

Multiple variables influence the selection and optimization of drug therapy for each individual patient. Pharmacogenomics, the study of the influence of individual genetic variations on drug response in patients, may yield additional information to further enhance safe and effective medication use. Whereas the field originally focused on the effects of specific variants within individual genes on drug response (i.e., pharmacogenetics), efforts increasingly examine the role of multiple variants across the genome and their potential relationship to drug therapy outcomes.

As our understanding of pharmacogenomics and the biological relevance of specific genetic variants in individuals' drug metabolizing enzymes, drug transporter proteins, and drug target receptors to certain drug responses has increased, we have learned that multiple variations across the genome can contribute to significant and relatively predictable treatment outcomes. Virtually every therapeutic area involving medication use includes a drug for which documented genetic variability has the potential to affect drug response. Some of this information is included in the FDA-approved package insert prescribing information. For some agents, the suitability of a specific drug or the determination of an appropriate initial dose for an individual patient based on pharmacogenetic information has been incorporated into dosing algorithms and patient care. As such, it is essential that health care professionals can interpret and utilize this information to facilitate safer and more effective use of medications for individual patients.

Genetic Variation within the Human Genome

The human genome is comprised of approximately 3 billion nucleotide base pair sequences that encode for molecular DNA with, except for identical twins, each individual having his/her own unique human genome sequence. Four nucleotide bases (adenine, guanine, cytosine, and thymine) are responsible for constituting the sequence of each single strand of DNA. Variations in nucleotide sequences can occur, and contribute to alterations in the expression and activities of certain genes. The location of these variations within a DNA sequence on a particular chromosome can have a profound impact on the ultimate biological activity or characteristic of that gene or lead to little or unknown consequences.

Proteins are involved in most enzymatic, structural, and biologic functions associated with drug disposition and effects. The processes involved in DNA replication, RNA transcription, and translation to synthesized proteins are complex. Each of these processes is potentially susceptible to consequences of DNA sequence variations.

Genetic variations can take many forms, including single nucleotide base substitutions (e.g., a cytosine substituted for an adenine), insertions or deletions of a nucleotide base within a sequence, and deletions or extra copies of entire DNA sequences. Variations in DNA that occur at a frequency of greater than 1% in the population are called polymorphisms. The most common genetic variations in humans are referred to as single nucleotide polymorphisms (SNPs) and result from the substitution of one nucleotide base for another. The specific location of a SNP within a gene is important. As mentioned previously, genetic variations can be of unknown or no clinical consequence or they can lead to a truncated, dysfunctional, or complete lack of protein product that is associated with an alteration in drug response.

Clinical Significance of Genetic Polymorphisms

SNPs and other genetic variations influence drug response at different levels through alterations in the activities of enzymes or proteins involved in drug absorption, transport, metabolism, elimination, or at the drug target receptor (site of drug action). Clinically relevant polymorphisms have been identified for genes that encode for most of the common enzymes involved in drug metabolism. Most enzymes are localized intracellularly throughout a wide variety of tissues in the body, including the enterocytes that line the intestine and within hepatocytes. Variants that cause diminished or absent enzyme activity decrease drug metabolism processes. In this case, if the drug is metabolized to an inactive product, then the prolonged persistence of the parent drug in the body could result in excessive pharmacologic effects and potential toxicities may occur. If the drug requires enzymatic conversion to a pharmacologically active metabolite, drug response may be reduced or absent. In contrast, if the variation is due to extra copies of a gene that results in increased enzymatic activity, opposite effects on drug metabolism and response can occur.

Similar outcomes can be associated with polymorphisms in genes that encode for membrane transporter proteins that are responsible for drug transport into cells (influx), as well as proteins that participate in energy-dependent processes that export drugs out of cells (efflux transporters). Polymorphisms in drug transport proteins can influence drug response by altering drug gastrointestinal absorption, uptake and distribution in tissues, exposure to intracellular drug metabolizing enzymes, and elimination via the bile or urine. Finally, some genes that encode for certain drug receptors are highly polymorphic, resulting in attenuated or exaggerated drug responses. The number of polymorphic genes responsible for variations in drug response at drug receptors is relatively small compared to those associated with drug metabolizing enzymes or transport proteins; however, this area has undergone the least amount of study to date.

Incorporating Pharmacogenomic Information into Clinical Practice

Most drugs are initiated in individual patients based on knowledge about their safety and effectiveness within the general population. Information regarding patient characteristics (e.g., age, ethnicity, renal/hepatic function, concomitant disease, etc.) known to contribute to variability in drug response, when available, is considered at this time. Currently, there are more than 50 drugs with pharmacogenomic information included in the package insert. For selected agents, dosing recommendations based on an individual's genetic information (i.e., genotype) for specific drugs and drug classes are also considered. Genomic biomarkers can play an important role in identifying responders and non-responders, avoiding drug toxicity, and adjusting the dose of drugs to optimize their efficacy and safety. However, the typical strategy for most drug therapy is to monitor the patient's response to treatment and modify regimens as necessary. Patients who develop exaggerated pharmacologic responses or elicit no pharmacologic effect may be expressing a phenotype suggestive of altered drug disposition or target receptor effect that could be associated with an underlying genetic polymorphism. As we continue to learn more about these associations and can incorporate pharmacogenomic information into decisions regarding drug therapy for individual patients, the ultimate goal is to improve therapeutic outcomes by limiting drug exposure to patients that are most likely to derive no therapeutic benefit and/or experience toxic drug effects.

For example, some genetic variants are associated with hypersensitivity reactions to a specific drug. A prescriber who is contemplating initiating that drug for a patient may determine whether the patient possesses that variant in his or her DNA. If that specific variant is present, the prescriber might select an alternate agent, thereby avoiding a potentially life-threatening hypersensitivity reaction. In another example, patients who are determined to have a genetic variant that results in an inactive metabolizing enzyme would not be appropriate candidates for an analgesic drug that requires that enzyme to convert the drug to the active analgesia-producing form. On the other hand, if that metabolizing enzyme is responsible for conversion of an active parent drug to an inactive metabolite, the starting dose of the drug may be reduced or perhaps an alternate drug might be selected.

Several Clinical Laboratory Improvement Amendment (CLIA)-approved laboratories offer pharmacogenetic testing to identify relevant genetic polymorphisms that predict drug response and can be used to initiate appropriate drugs and dosing regimens for individual patients. Some of these tests, while recommended in drug prescribing information, are costly and may not be covered by insurance. Patients may not fully understand the utility of undergoing genetic testing and providing a specimen for DNA analysis, which is typically performed on a blood, saliva, buccal swab, or other tissue collection. On the other hand, patients who are engaged in their medical care may be familiar with the concept of "personalized medicine" and seek information about available tests to "individualize" their own drug therapy. Currently, four drugs are required to have pharmacogenetic testing performed before they are prescribed: cetuximab, trastuzumab, maraviroc, and dasatinib. Other drugs have labeling that include "test recommended" or "for information only". Health care professionals will need to be familiar with pharmacogenetic tests that are recommended for specific drug therapies, how to interpret the results of those tests, and how to incorporate pharmacogenetic data with other clinical information to optimize patient drug therapy and health care outcomes.

***

Lisa E. Davis, PharmD, ACCP, BCPS, BCOP
Associate Professor of Clinical Pharmacy
Philadelphia College of Pharmacy
University of the Sciences in Philadelphia
Philadelphia, PA

Pertinent Resources:

Aquilante CL, Zineh I, Beitelshees AL, Langaee TY. Common laboratory methods in pharmacogenomics studies. *Am J Health-Syst Pharm* 2006;63:2101-10.

Court MH. A pharmacogenomics primer. *J Clin Pharmacol* 2007;47:1087-1103.

Evans WE, McLeod HL. Pharmacogenomics – drug disposition, drug targets, and side effects. *N Engl J Med* 2003;348:538-49.

Evans WE, Relling MV. Moving towards individualized medicine with pharmacogenomics. *Nature* 2004;429:464-8.

NCBI Genetics Primer: http://www.ncbi.nlm.nih.gov/pmc/articles/PMC3860415/pdf/arcr-34-3-270.pdf

Roden DM, Altman RB, Benowitz NL, et al. Pharmacogenomics: challenges and opportunities. *Ann Intern Med* 2006;145:749-57.

Shin J, Kayser SR, Langaee TY. Pharmacogenetics: from discovery to patient care. *Am J Health-Syst Pharm* 2009;66:625-37.

Weiss ST, McLeod HL, Flockhart DA, et al. Creating and evaluating genetic tests predictive of drug response. *Nat Rev Drug Disc* 2008;7:568-74.

Wilkinson GR. Drug metabolism and variability among patients in drug response. *N Engl J Med* 2005; 352:2211-21.

MEDICATION ERRORS: Improving Practices and Patient Safety

It is widely acknowledged that medication errors result in thousands of adverse drug events, preventable reactions, and deaths per year. Nurses, physicians, pharmacists, patient safety organizations, the Food and Drug Administration, the pharmaceutical industry, Health Canada, and other parties share in the responsibility for determining how medication errors occur and designing strategies to reduce error.

One impediment to understanding the scope and nature of the problem has been the reactive "blaming, shaming, training" culture that singled out one individual as the cause of the error. Also historically, medication errors that did not result in patient harm—near-miss situations in which an error could have but didn't happen—or errors that did not result in serious harm were not reported. In contrast, serious errors often instigated a powerful punitive response in which one or a few persons were deemed to be at fault and, as a result, lost their jobs and sometimes their licenses.

In 1999, the Institute of Medicine (IOM) published *To Err Is Human: Building a Safer Health System*, which drew attention to the problem of medication errors. It pointed out that excellent health care providers do make medication errors, that many of the traditional processes involved in the medication-use system were error-prone, and that other factors, notably drug labeling and packaging, contributed to error. Furthermore, the IOM report, in conjunction with other groups such as the United States Pharmacopeia (USP) and the Institute for Safe Medication Practices (ISMP), called for the redesign of error-prone systems to include processes that anticipated the fallibility of humans working within the system. This initiative is helping shift the way the health care industry addresses medication errors from a single person/bad apple cause to a systems issue.[1]

The National Coordinating Council for Medication Error Reporting and Prevention (NCC-MERP) developed the definition of a medication error that reflects this shift and captures the scope and breadth of the issue:

> "A medication error is any preventable event that may cause or lead to inappropriate medication use or patient harm while the medication is in the control of the health care professional, patient, or consumer. Such events may be related to professional practice, health care products, procedures, and systems, including prescribing; order communication; product labeling, packaging, and nomenclature; compounding; dispensing; distribution; administration; education; monitoring; and use."[2]

Inherent in this definition's mention of related factors are the human factors that are part of the medication use system. For example, a nurse or pharmacist may automatically reach into the bin where dobutamine is usually kept, see "do" and "amine" but select dopamine instead of dobutamine. Working amidst distractions, working long hours or shorthanded, and working in a culture where perfection is expected and questioning is discouraged are other examples of the human factors and environmental conditions that contribute to error.

The goal for the design of any individual or hospital-wide medication use system is to determine where systems are likely to fail and to build in safeguards that minimize the potential for error. One way to begin that process is to become familiar with medications or practices that have historically been shown to be involved in serious errors.

High Alert Medications

Some medications, because of a narrow therapeutic range or inherent toxic nature, have a high risk of causing devastating injury or death if improperly ordered, prepared, stocked, dispensed, administered, or monitored. Although these medications may not be involved in more errors, they require special attention due to the potential for serious, possibly fatal consequences. These have been termed **high-alert medications**, to communicate the need for extra care and safeguards. Many of these drugs are used commonly in the general population or are used frequently in urgent clinical situations. The Joint Commission (TJC) monitors the use of frequently prescribed high-alert medications, which include insulin, opiates and narcotics, injectable potassium chloride (or phosphate) concentrate, intravenous anticoagulants (such as heparin), sodium chloride solutions above 0.9 percent, and others. See the High Alert Drugs table in the **Medication Safety Tools** section, and Table 1 in this article for a complete list of the high alert meds found in *Davis's Drug Guide for Nurses*. (Visit the Institute for Safe Medication Practices at www.ismp.org for more information on high alert drugs.)

Causes of Medication Errors

Many contributing factors and discrete causes of error have been identified, including failed communication, poor drug distribution practices, dose miscalculations, drug packaging and drug-device related problems, incorrect drug administration, and lack of patient education.[3]

Failed Communication: Failed communication covers many of the errors made in the ordering phase, and although ordering is performed by the prescriber, the nurse, the clerk, and the pharmacist who interpret that order are also involved in the communication process.

- ***Poorly handwritten or verbal orders.*** Handwriting is a major source of error and has led to inaccurate interpretations of the drug intended, the route of administration, the frequency, and dose. Telephone and verbal orders are likewise prone to misinterpretation.
- ***Drugs with similar-sounding or similar-looking names.*** Similar sounding names, or names that look similar when handwritten, are frequently confused. Amiodarone and amrinone (now renamed inamrinone to help prevent confusion), or Zebeta® and Diabeta® are two examples. The USP has identified over 700 "sound-alike, look-alike" drugs. Mix-ups are more likely when each drug has similar dose ranges and frequencies.

Several of the sound-alike/look-alike drugs were targeted for labeling intervention by the FDA, which requested manufacturers of 33 drugs with look-alike names to voluntarily revise the appearance of the established names. The revision visually differentiates the drug names by using "tall man" letters (capitals) to highlight distinguishing syllables (ex.: acetoHEXAMIDE versus acetaZOLAMIDE or buPROPrion versus busPIRone. See the TALL MAN Lettering table in the **Medication Safety Tools** section for the list of the pairs of drugs that are commonly confused, often with serious consequences.

- ***Misuse of zeroes in decimal numbers.*** Massive, ten-fold overdoses are traceable to not using a leading zero (.2 mg instead of 0.2 mg) or adding an unnecessary trailing zero (2.0 mg instead of 2 mg) in decimal expressions of dose. Similar overdosages are found in decimal expressions in which the decimal point is obscured by poor handwriting, stray marks, or lined orders sheets (e.g., reading 3.1 grams as 31 grams). Under-dosing also may occur by the same mechanism and prevent a desired, perhaps life-saving effect.
- ***Use of apothecary measures (grains, drams) or package units (amps, vials, tablets) instead of metric measures (grams, milligrams, milliequivalents).*** Apothecary measurements are poorly understood and their abbreviations are easily confused with other units of measurement. Use of such measures should be abandoned. Errors also occur when dosage units are used instead of metric weight. For example, orders for 2 tablets, 1 1/2 vials, or 2 ampules can result in overdose or underdose when the medications ordered come in various strengths.
- ***Misinterpreted abbreviations.*** Abbreviations can be misinterpreted or, when used in the dosage part of the order, can result in incorrect dosage of the correct medication. For example, lower or uppercase "U" for units has been read as a zero, making 10 u of insulin look like 100 units when handwritten. The Latin abbreviation "QOD" for every other day has been misinterpreted as QID (4 times per day). See Table 2 for a list of confusing abbreviations and safer alternatives.
- ***Ambiguous or incomplete orders.*** Orders that do not clearly specify dose, route, frequency, or indication do not communicate complete information and are open to misinterpretation.

Poor Distribution Practices: Poor distribution includes error-prone storing practices such as keeping similar-looking products next to each other. Dispensing multidose floor stock vials of potentially dangerous drugs instead of unit doses is also associated with error as is allowing non-pharmacists to dispense medications in the absence of the pharmacist.

Dose Miscalculations: Dose miscalculations are a prime source of medication error. Also, many medications need to be dose-adjusted for renal or hepatic impairment, age, height and weight, and body composition (i.e., correct for obesity). Complicated dosing formulas provide many opportunities to introduce error. Often vulnerable populations, such as premature infants, children, the elderly, and those with serious underlying illnesses, are at greatest risk.

Drug Packaging and Drug Delivery Systems: Similar packaging or poorly designed packaging encourages error. Drug companies may use the same design for different formulations, or fail to highlight information about concentration or strength. Lettering, type size, color, and packaging methods can either help or hinder drug identification.

Drug delivery systems include infusion pumps and rate controllers. Some models do not prevent free flow of medication, leading to sudden high dose infusion of potent and dangerous medications. The lack of safeguards preventing free flow and programming errors are among the problems encountered with infusion control devices.

Incorrect Drug Administration: Incorrect drug administration covers many problems. Misidentification of a patient, incorrect route of administration, missed doses, or improper drug preparation are types of errors that occur during the administration phase.

Lack of Patient Education: Safe medication use is enhanced in the hospital and the home when the patient is well informed. The knowledgeable patient can recognize when something has changed in his or her medication regimen and can question the health care provider. At the same time, many issues related to medication errors, such as ambiguous directions, unfamiliarity with a drug, and confusing packaging, affect the patient as well as the health care provider, underscoring the need for careful education. Patient education also enhances adherence, which is a factor in proper medication use.

Prevention Strategies

Since medication use systems are complex and involve many steps and people, they are error-prone. On an individual basis, nurses can help reduce the incidence of error by implementing the following strategies:

- Clarify any order that is not obviously and clearly legible. Ask the prescriber to print orders using block style letters.
- Do not accept orders with the abbreviation "u" or "IU" for units. Clarify the dosage and ask the prescriber to write out the word units.
- Clarify any abbreviated drug name or the abbreviated dosing frequencies q.d., QD, q.o.d., QOD, and q.i.d or QID. Suggest abandoning Latin abbreviations in favor of spelling out dosing frequency.
- Do not accept doses expressed in package units or volume instead of metric weight. Clarify any order written for number of ampules, vials, or tablets (e.g., calcium chloride, 1 ampule or epinephrine, 1 Bristojet).
- Decimal point errors can be hard to see. Suspect a missed decimal point and clarify any order if the dose requires more than 3 dosing units.
- If dose ordered requires use of multiple dosage units or very small fractions of a dose unit, review the dose, have another health care provider check the original order and recalculate formulas, and confirm the dose with the prescriber.
- If taking a verbal order, ask prescriber to spell out the drug name and dosage to avoid sound-alike confusion (e.g., hearing Cerebyx for Celebrex, or fifty for fifteen). Read back the order to the prescriber after you have written it in the chart. Confirm and document the indication to further enhance accurate communication.
- Clarify any order that does not include metric weight, dosing frequency, or route of administration.
- Check the nurse's/clerk's transcription against the original order. Make sure stray marks or initials do not obscure the original order.

- Do not start a patient on new medication by borrowing medications from another patient. This action bypasses the double check provided by the pharmacist's review of the order.
- Always check the patient's name band before administering medications. Verbally addressing a patient by name does not provide sufficient identification.
- Use the facility's standard drug administration times to reduce the chance of an omission error.
- Be sure to fully understand any drug administration device before using it. This includes infusion pumps, inhalers, and transdermal patches.
- Have a second practitioner independently check original order, dosage calculations, and infusion pump settings for high alert medications.
- Realize that the printing on packaging boxes, vials, ampoules, prefilled syringes, or any container in which a medication is stored can be misleading. Be sure to differentiate clearly the medication and the number of milligrams per milliliter versus the total number of milligrams contained within. Massive overdoses have been administered by assuming that the number of milligrams per ml is all that is contained within the vial or ampule. Read the label when obtaining the medication, before preparing or pouring the medication, and after preparing or pouring the medication.
- Educate patients about the medications they take. Provide verbal and written instructions and ask the patient to restate important points. Refer to Educating Patients about Safe Medication Use on page 29 for recommendations on what patients should understand about their medications.

As stated previously, errors are a result of problems within the medication use system and cannot be eliminated by the vigilance of any one group of health care providers. System redesign involves strong leadership from administration and all involved departments. Health care facilities should consider the following when addressing the issue of medication errors:

- Do not provide unit stock of critical, high alert medications. If eliminating these medications from floor stock is not feasible, consider reducing the number available and standardizing the concentrations or forms in which the medication is available.
- Create committees that address safety issues.
- Install a computer physician order entry (CPOE) system to help reduce prescribing orders. Link order entry to pertinent lab, allergy, and medication data.
- Implement bar code technology to ensure the right drug reaches the right patient.
- Develop policies that discourage error-prone prescribing practices such as inappropriate use of verbal orders, use of confusing dosing symbols, and use of abbreviations.
- Develop policies that encourage better communication of medication information such as requiring block-style printing of medications, including indication in prescription, and using both the trade and generic name in prescriptions.
- Ensure a reasonable workload for pharmacists and nurses, and provide a well-designed work area.
- Limit the availability of varying concentrations of high alert medications.
- Provide standard concentrations and infusion rate tables.
- Supply pharmacy and patient care areas with current reference material.
- Cultivate a culture that does not assign blame when medication errors occur but looks for root causes instead.
- Encourage staff to participate in the USP-ISMP-MERP error reporting program.

REFERENCES

1. Kohn, L.T., Corrigan, J.M., and Donaldson, M.S. (eds). *To Err Is Human: Building a Safer Health System.* National Academy Press, Washington, DC (1999).
2. National Coordinating Council for Medication Error Reporting and Prevention. http://www.nccmerp.org/aboutMedErrors.html
3. Cohen, M.R. *Medication Errors.* American Pharmacists Association, Washington DC (2007).
4. Branowicki, P., et al. "Improving complex medication systems: an interdisciplinary approach." *J Nurs Adm.* (2003) Apr; 33(4):199-200.

5. Burke, K.G. "Executive summary: the state of the science on safe medication administration symposium." *J Infus Nurs.* (2005). Mar-Apr; 28(2 Suppl):4-9.
6. McPhillips, H.A., et al. "Potential medication dosing errors in outpatient pediatrics." *J Pediatr.* (2005) Dec; 147(6):727-8.
7. ISMP. "What's in a name? Ways to prevent dispensing errors linked to name confusion." *ISMP Medication Safety Alert!* 7(12) June 12, 2002. http://www.ismp.org/Newsletters/acutecare/archives/Jun02.asp
8. Santell, J.P., Cousins, D.D., "Medication Errors Related to Product Names." *Joint Commission J Qual Pt. Safety* (2005); 31:649-54.

Table 1: High Alert Medications in Davis's Drug Guide for Nurses

aldesleukin	erlotinib	mitoxantrone
alemtuzumab	esmolol	morphine
alitretinoin	etoposides	nalbuphine
amiodarone	fentanyl (buccal, transmucosal)	nateglinide
amphotericin B cholesteryl sulfate/ lipid complex/liposome	fentanyl (parenteral)	nesiritide
argatroban	fentanyl (transdermal)	nilotinib
arsenic trioxide	fludarabine	nitroprusside
asparaginase	fluorouracil	norepinephrine
azacitidine	fondaparinux	oxaliplatin
bendamustine	gefitinib	oxycodone compound
bevacizumab	gemcitabine	oxymorphone
bivalirudin	gemtuzumab ozogamicin	oxytocin
bleomycin	heparin	paclitaxel
bortezomib	heparins (low molecular weight)	pancuronium
buprenorphine	hydrocodone	panitumumab
busulfan	hydromorphone	pazopanib
butorphanol	hydroxyurea	pegaspargase
capecitabine	hypoglycemic agents, oral	pemetrexed
carboplatin	idarubicin	pentazocine
carmustine	ifosfamide	potassium phosphates
cetuximab	imatinib	potassium supplements
chloralhydrate	insulin mixtures	pramlintide
chlorambucil	insulins (intermediate-acting)	procarbazine
cisplatin	insulins (long-acting)	promethazine (IV)
cladribine	insulins (rapid-acting)	propofol
clofarabine	insulins (short-acting)	propranolol
codeine	irinotecan	repaglinide
colchicine (IV)	ixabepilone	rituximab
cyclophosphamide	labetalol	sodium chloride (hypertonic)
cytarabine	lapatinib	sunitinib
dacarbazine	lepirudin	temsirolimus
DAUNOrubicin hydrochloride	lidocaine	thalidomide
decitabine	magnesium sulfate (IV, parenteral)	thioguanine
digoxin	mechlorethamine	thrombolytic agents
DOBUTamine	melphalan	tirofiban
docetaxel	meperidine	topotecan
DOPamine	methadone	trastuzumab
DOXOrubicin hydrochloride	methotrexate	vinBLAStine
DOXOrubicin hydrochloride liposome	metoprolol	vinCRIStine
epinephrine	midazolam	vinorelbine
epirubicin	milrinone	warfarin
eptifibatide	mitomycin	

Table 2: Abbreviations and Symbols Associated with Medication Errors

Abbreviation/Symbol	Intended Meaning	Mistaken For	Recommendation
AZT	Zidovudine	Azathioprine	Use full drug name
CPZ	Compazine (prochlorperazine)	Thorazine (chlorpromazine)	Use full drug name
HCl	Hydrochloric acid	KCl (potassium chloride)	Use full drug name
HCT	Hydrocortisone	Hydrochlorothiazide	Use full drug name
HCTZ	Hydrochlorothiazide	Hydrocortisone	Use full drug name
$MgSO_4$*	Magnesium sulfate	Morphine sulfate	Use full drug name
MS, MSO_4*	Morphine sulfate	Magnesium sulfate	Use full drug name
MTX	Methotrexate	Mitoxantrone	Use full drug name
Nitro drip	Nitroglycerin	Nitroprusside	Use full drug name
Norflox	Norfloxacin	Norflex (orphenadrine)	Use full drug name
PCA	Procainamide	Patient controlled analgesia	Use full drug name
PIT	Pitocin (oxytocin)	Pitressin (vasopressin)	Use full drug name
SSRI	Sliding scale regular insulin	Selective serotonin reuptake inhibitor	Spell out "sliding scale regular insulin"
μg†	Microgram	Mg (milligram)	Use mcg
/ (slash mark)	"per"	"1" (numeral one)	Spell out "per"
HS or hs	Half strength or hour of sleep (at bedtime)	One mistaken for the other	Spell out "half strength" or "bedtime"
D/C	Discharge or discontinue	One mistaken for the other	Spell out "discharge" or "discontinue"
+	Plus sign	"4" (numeral four)	Spell out "and"
Zero **after** a decimal point (e.g., 1.0 mg)*	1 mg	10 mg	DO NOT USE zero after a decimal point
No zero **before** a decimal point (e.g., .1 mg)*	.1 mg	1 mg	ALWAYS USE zero before a decimal point
u or U*	units	0 (zero), 4 (four) or cc	Spell out "units"
I.U.*	International Units	IV or 10	Spell out "units"
q.d. or QD*	Every day	q.i.d. (4 times per day)	Write out "daily"
q.o.d. or QOD*	Every other day	q.i.d. (4 times per day) or qd (daily)	Write out "every other day"
TIW	3 times a week	3 times a day or twice a week	Spell out "3 times weekly"
IN	Intranasal	IM or IV	Spell out "intranasal" or use "NAS"
SC, SQ, sub q	Subcutaneously	SC mistaken as SL (sublingual), SQ as "5 every" or "every"	Use subcut or write out "subcutaneously"
AD, AS, AU	Right ear, left ear, each ear	OD, OS, OU (right eye, left eye, each eye)	Spell out "right ear", "left ear", "each ear"
OD, OS, OU	Right eye, left eye, each eye	AD, AS, AU (right ear, left ear, each ear)	Spell out "right eye", "left eye", "each eye"
Cc†	cubic centimeters	u (units)	Use ml
@†	At	2	Use "at"
>†	Greater than	7 or <	Spell out "greater than"
<†	Less than	L or >	Spell out "less than"
&	And	2	Use "and"
°	Hour	Zero (q 1° seen as q 10)	Use "hr", "h", or "hour"
Drug name and dose run together. Example: Inderal 40 mg	Inderal 40 mg	Inderal 140 mg	Leave space between drug name, dose, and unit of measure
Numerical dose and unit of measure run together. Example: 10 mg	10 mg	100 mg	Leave space between drug dose and unit of measure

*Appears on TJC's "Do Not Use" list of abbreviations.

†May be considered by TJC for possible inclusion in the "Do Not Use" list in the future.

Modified from ISMP's List of Error-Prone Abbreviations, Symbols, and Dose Designations, 2011.

DETECTING AND MANAGING ADVERSE DRUG REACTIONS

An *adverse drug reaction* (ADR) is any unexpected, undesired, or excessive response to a medication that results in:

- temporary or permanent serious harm or disability
- admission to a hospital, transfer to a higher level of care, or prolonged stay
- death.

Adverse drug reactions are distinguished from adverse drug events, in which causality is uncertain, and side effects, which may be bothersome to the patient and necessitate a change in therapy but are not considered serious.[1] Although some ADRs are the result of medication errors, many are not.

Types of ADRs

The Food and Drug Administration (FDA) classifies ADRs into 2 broad categories: Type A and Type B.[2] Type A reactions are predictable reactions based on the primary or secondary pharmacologic effect of the drug. Dose-related reactions and drug-drug interactions are examples of Type A reactions. Type B reactions are unpredictable, are not related to dose, and are not the result of the drug's primary or secondary pharmacologic effect. Idiosyncratic and hypersensitivity reactions are examples of Type B reactions.

Dose-Related Reactions (Toxic Reactions): In dose related reactions, the dose prescribed for the patient is excessive. Although a variety of mechanisms may interact, reasons for this type of reaction include:

- renal or hepatic impairment
- extremes in age (neonates and frail elderly)
- drug-drug or drug-food interactions
- underlying illness.

Dose-related reactions are often the result of preventable errors in prescribing in which physiologic factors such as age, renal impairment, and weight were not considered sufficiently, or in inadequate therapeutic monitoring. Medications with narrow therapeutic ranges (digoxin, aminoglycosides, antiepileptic drugs) and those that require careful monitoring or laboratory testing (anticoagulants, nephrotoxic drugs) are most frequently implicated in dose-related reactions.[34] Dose-related reactions usually are managed successfully by temporarily discontinuing the drug and then reducing the dose or increasing the dosing interval. In some instances, the toxic effects need to be treated with another agent (e.g., Digibind for digoxin toxicity or Kayexalate for drug-induced hyperkalemia). Appropriately timed therapeutic drug level monitoring, review of new drugs added to an existing regimen that may affect the drug level, and frequent assessment of relevant laboratory values are critical to safe medical management and prevention of dose-related reactions.

Drug-Drug Interactions: Drug-drug interactions occur when the pharmacokinetic or pharmacodynamic properties of an individual drug affect another drug. Pharmacokinetics refers to the way the body processes a medication (absorption, distribution, metabolism, and elimination). In a drug-drug interaction, the pharmacokinetic properties of one drug can cause a change in drug concentration of another drug and an altered response. For example, one drug may block enzymes that metabolize a second drug. The concentration of the second drug is then increased and may become toxic or cause adverse reactions. Pharmacodynamic drug-drug interactions involve the known effects and side-effects of the drugs. For example, two drugs with similar therapeutic effects may act together in a synergistic way. The increased anticoagulant effects that occur when warfarin and aspirin are taken together, or the increased central nervous system (CNS) depression that results when two drugs with CNS depressant effects potentiate each other, are examples of pharmacodynamic drug-drug interactions. Certain classes of drugs are more likely to result in serious drug-drug interactions, and patients receiving these agents should be monitored carefully. The medication classes include anticoagulants, oral hypoglycemic agents, nonsteroidal anti-inflammatory agents, monoamine oxidase inhibitors, antihypertensives, antiepileptics, and antiretrovirals. In addition, specific drugs such as theophylline, cimetidine, lithium, and digoxin may result in serious ADRs.

Idiosyncratic Reactions: Idiosyncratic reactions occur without relation to dose and are unpredictable and sporadic. Reactions of this type may manifest in many different ways, including fever, blood dyscrasias, cardiovascular effects, or mental status changes. The time frame between the occurrence of a problem and initiation of therapy is sometimes the only clue linking drug to symptom. Some idiosyncratic reactions may be explained by genetic differences in drug-metabolizing enzymes.

Hypersensitivity Reactions: Hypersensitivity reactions are usually allergic responses. Manifestations of hypersensitivity reactions range from mild rashes, to nephritis, pneumonitis, hemolytic anemia, and anaphylaxis. Protein drugs (vaccines, enzymes) are frequently associated with hypersensitivity reactions. In most instances, antibody formation is involved in the process and therefore cross-sensitivity may occur. An example of this is hypersensitivity to penicillin and cross-sensitivity with other penicillins and/or cephalosporins. Documenting drugs to which the patient is allergic and the specific hypersensitivity reaction is very important. If the reaction to an agent is anaphylaxis the nurse should monitor the patient during administration of a cross-hypersensitive agent, especially during the initial dose, and ensure ready access to emergency resuscitative equipment.

Recognizing an ADR

Adverse drug reactions should be suspected whenever there is a negative change in a patient's condition, particularly when a new drug has been introduced. Strategies that can enhance recognition include knowing the side effect/adverse reaction profile of medications. Nurses should be familiar with a drug's most commonly encountered side effects and adverse reactions before administering it. (In *Davis's Drug Guide for Nurses*, side effects are underlined, and adverse reactions are CAPITALIZED and appear in second color in the **Adverse Reactions and Side Effects** section.) As always, monitoring the patient's response to a medication and ongoing assessment are key nursing actions. Learn to recognize patient findings that suggest an ADR has occurred. These include:

- rash
- change in respiratory rate, heart rate, blood pressure, or mental state
- seizure
- anaphylaxis
- diarrhea
- fever.

Any of these findings can suggest an ADR and should be reported and documented promptly so that appropriate interventions, including discontinuation of suspect medications, can occur. Prompt intervention can prevent a mild adverse reaction from escalating into a serious health problem. Other steps taken by the health care team when identifying and treating an ADR include:

1. Determining that the drug ordered was the drug given and intended.
2. Determining that the drug was given in the correct dosage by the correct route.
3. Establishing the chronology of events: time drug was taken and onset of symptoms.
4. Stopping the drug and monitoring patient status for improvement (dechallenge).
5. Restarting the drug, if appropriate, and monitoring closely for adverse reactions (rechallenge).[2]

Prevention

Health care organizations have responded to consumer, regulator, and insurer pressures by developing programs that aim to eliminate preventable ADRs. In the inpatient setting, computer systems can display the patient's age, height, weight, and creatinine clearance or serum creatinine concentration and send an alert to the clinician if a prescribed dose is out of range for any of the displayed parameters. Allergy alerts and drug-drug interactions can be presented to the clinician at the time an order is entered.

In the outpatient setting, strategies that increase the patient's knowledge base and access to pharmacists and nurses may help prevent adverse reactions.[5] Outpatient pharmacy computer systems that are linked within a chain of pharmacies may allow the pharmacist to view the patient's profile if the patient is filling a prescription in a pharmacy other than the usual one. Many pharmacy computers have dose limits and drug-drug reaction verification to assist pharmacists filling orders.

Such strategies are a valuable auxiliary to, but cannot replace, conscientious history taking, careful patient assessment, and ongoing monitoring. A thorough medication history including all prescription and nonprescription drugs, all side effects and adverse reactions encountered, allergies, and all pertinent physical data should be available to the prescriber. The prescriber is responsible for reviewing this data, along with current medications, laboratory values, and any other variable that affects drug response.

It is not expected that practitioners will remember all relevant information when prescribing. In fact, reliance on memory is error-fraught, and clinicians need to use available resources to verify drug interactions whenever adding a new drug to the regimen. Setting expectations that clinicians use evidence-based information rather than their memories when prescribing, dispensing, administering or monitoring patients has the potential to reduce the incidence of preventable ADRs.

Reporting Adverse Drug Reactions in the U.S.:

Food and Drug Administration MedWatch Program: To monitor and assess the incidence of adverse reactions, the FDA sponsors MedWatch, a program that allows health care practitioners and consumers the opportunity to report serious adverse reactions or product defects encountered from medications, medical devices, special nutritional products, or other FDA-regulated items. The FDA considers serious those reactions that result in death, life-threatening illness or injury, hospitalization, disability, congenital anomaly, or those that require medical/surgical intervention.

In addition to reporting serious adverse reactions, health care providers should also report problems related to suspected contamination, questionable stability, defective components, or poor packaging/labeling. Reports should be submitted even if there is some uncertainty about the cause/effect relationship or if some details are missing. This reporting form may be accessed at www.fda.gov/medwatch/report/hcp.htm. Reports also may be faxed to the FDA (1-800-FDA-0178). Reactions to vaccines should be reported to the Vaccine Adverse Event Reporting System (VAERS; 1-800-822-7967). Nurses share with other health care providers an obligation to report adverse reactions to the MedWatch program so that all significant data can be analyzed for opportunities to improve patient care.

Reporting Adverse Drug Reactions in Canada:

The Marketed Health Products Directorate of Health Canada coordinates adverse reaction reporting activities, and analyzes reports submitted from regional centers in each province. MedEffect Canada encourages health professionals, patients and regulatory authorities to report adverse reactions as they occur, either by email, mail or the Health Canada website.[10] Health care professionals reporting adverse reactions are required to supply information regarding patient characteristics, details about the reaction(s), current treatment, and outcomes. Information identifying the patient or health care provider remains confidential.

Adverse reaction reports are analyzed to investigate any associations with the health product. Based on the outcome, regulatory bodies decide on a course of action, which may include performing additional post-marketing studies, re-assessment of the risk versus benefit of the product, packaging modification, addition of warnings in patient information leaflets, or issuing public alerts or market withdrawals. Updates regarding adverse reactions are published in the Canadian Adverse Reaction Newsletter every 3 months.

Access the following link for the Consumer Side Effect Reporting Form: http://www.hc-sc.gc.ca/dhp-mps/alt_formats/pdf/medeff/report-declaration/ar-ei_cons_form-eng.pdf
Access the following link for the health professional Canada Vigilance Adverse Reaction Reporting Form: http://www.hc-sc.gc.ca/dhp-mps/alt_formats/pdf/medeff/report-declaration/ar-ei_form-eng.pdf

REFERENCES

1. Lehmann, J. "Adverse Events - Adverse Reactions." *Drug Intel* (2002-2003) http://www.drugintel.com/public/medwatch/adverse_drug_events.htm (accessed 10 July 2003).
2. Goldman, S., Kennedy, D., Lieberman, R., "Clinical Therapeutics and the Recognition of Drug-Induced Disease." FDA MEDWATCH Continuing Education Article (1995) http://www.fda.gov/medwatch/articles/dig/rcontent.htm#toc (accessed 10 July 2003).
3. Daniels, C., Calis, K., "Clinical Analysis of Adverse Drug Reactions." Pharmacy Update National Institutes of Health. Sept-Oct 2001. http://www.cc.nih.gov/phar/updates/septoct01/01sept-oct.html (accessed 10 July 2003).
4. Winterstein, A., et. al. "Identifying Clinically Significant Preventable Adverse Drug Events Through a Hospital's Database of Adverse Drug Reaction Reports." *Am J Health-Syst Pharm* 59(18):1742-1749, 2002.
5. Ghandi, T., Weingart, S., Borus, J., et. al. "Adverse Drug Events in Ambulatory Care." *New England Journal of Medicine.* Volume 348:1556-1564. Number 16. April 17, 2003.
6. Bennett, CL, et al. "The Research on Adverse Drug Events and Reports (RADAR) project." *JAMA.* 2005 May 4;293(17):2131-40.
7. Field, TS, et al. "The costs associated with adverse drug events among older adults in the ambulatory setting." *Med Care.* 2005 Dec;43(12):1171-6.
8. Petrone, K, Katz, P. "Approaches to appropriate drug prescribing for the older adult." *Prim Care.* 2005 Sep;32(3):755-75.
9. Pezalla, E. "Preventing adverse drug reactions in the general population." *Manag Care Interface.* 2005 Oct;18(10):49-52.
10. "Adverse Reaction Information." *MedEffect Canada.* October 2012. http://www.hc-sc.gc.ca/dhp-mps/medeff/advers-react-neg/index-eng.php#a5 (accessed 16 April, 2014).

OVERVIEW OF RISK EVALUATION AND MITIGATION SYSTEMS (REMS)

Over the past several decades, the Food and Drug Administration (FDA) has employed a number of "risk management" programs designed to detect, evaluate, prevent, and mitigate drug adverse events for drugs with the potential for serious adverse drug reactions. Some of the risk management plans used by the FDA over the years have included the use of patient package inserts, medication guides, restricted access programs, and classification of drugs as controlled substances. These programs were acknowledged by the FDA as Risk Minimization Action Plans (RiskMAPS) in 2005. With these programs, the FDA only had the authority to mandate postmarketing commitments from drug manufacturers before the drug was approved; however, these requirements could not be enforced after the drug was approved.

The Food and Drug Administration Amendments Act of 2007 has given the FDA the authority to subject drugs to new risk identification and communication strategies in the postmarketing period. These new strategies, called Risk Evaluation and Mitigation Strategies (REMS), can be required for any drug or drug class that is associated with serious risks. The FDA can require a REMS if it believes that this program is necessary to ensure that the benefits outweigh the potential risks of the drug. The FDA can require a REMS either as part of the drug approval process or during the postmarketing period if new information becomes available regarding potentially harmful effects that are associated with the use of the drug.

Components of the REMS may include a medication guide, a patient package insert, a communication plan, other elements to ensure safe use, and/or an implementation system. A REMS for New Drug Applications or Biologics License Applications requires a timetable for submission of assessment of the REMS. A variety of elements to ensure safe use of drugs can be required as part of the REMS if it is believed that a medication guide, patient package insert, or communication plan are not adequate to mitigate the serious risks associated with a particular drug. These elements may include the following:

- Health care providers who prescribe the drug are specifically trained and/or certified.
- Pharmacies, practitioners, or health care settings that dispense the drug are specifically trained and/or certified.
- The drug is dispensed to patients only in certain health care settings, such as hospitals, or physicians' offices.
- The drug is dispensed only to patients with evidence or other documentation of safe-use conditions, such as laboratory test results.
- Patients using the drug are subject to certain monitoring.
- Patients using the drug are enrolled in a registry.

The FDA maintains an updated list of these REMS programs at http://www.fda.gov/Drugs/DrugSafety/PostmarketDrugSafetyInformationforPatientsandProviders/ucm111350.htm. A REMS tag has been added at the top of the monographs of drugs associated with these programs.

SPECIAL DOSING CONSIDERATIONS

For many patients the average dose range for a given drug can be toxic. The purpose of this section is to describe vulnerable patient populations for which special dosing considerations must be made to protect the patient and improve clinical outcomes.

The Pediatric Patient

Most drugs prescribed to children are not approved by the Food and Drug Administration (FDA) for use in pediatric populations. This does not mean it's wrong to prescribe these drugs to children, rather it means that the medications were not tested in children. The lack of pediatric drug information can result in patient harm or death, such as what occurred with the drug chloramphenicol. When given to very young children, chloramphenicol caused toxicity and multiple deaths. Referred to as "gray baby syndrome," this toxic reaction was eventually found to be dose dependent. The FDA now requires that new drugs that may be used in children include information for safe pediatric use. For this edition of *Davis's Drug Guide for Nurses*, we have had the pediatric dosing for the top 100 drugs used in children revised and updated by a pediatric pharmacist with a Doctor of Pharmacy (PharmD) degree.

The main reason for adjusting dosages in pediatric patients is body size, which is measured by body weight or body surface area (BSA). Weight-based pediatric drug dosages are expressed in number of milligrams per kilogram of body weight (mg/kg) while dosages calculated on BSA are expressed in number of milligrams per meter squared (mg/m^2). BSA is determined using a BSA nomogram or calculated by using formulas (Appendix E).

The neonate and the premature infant require additional adjustments secondary to immature function of body systems. For example, absorption may be incomplete or altered secondary to differences in gastric pH or motility. Distribution may be altered because of varying amounts of total body water, and metabolism and excretion can be delayed due to immature liver and kidney function. Furthermore, rapid weight changes and progressive maturation of hepatic and renal function require frequent monitoring and careful dosage adjustments. Gestational age, as well as weight, may be needed to properly dose some drugs in the neonate.

The Geriatric Patient

Absorption, distribution, metabolism, and excretion are altered in adults over 65 years of age, putting the older patient at risk for toxic reactions. Pharmacokinetic properties in the older patient are affected by

- diminished gastrointestinal (GI) motility and blood flow, which delays absorption
- percentage of body fat, lean muscle mass, and total body water, which alters distribution
- decreased plasma proteins, especially in the malnourished patient, which alters distribution by allowing a larger proportion of free or unbound drug to circulate and exert effects
- diminshed hepatic function, which slows metabolism.
- diminished renal function, which delays excretion

Older patients should be prescribed the lowest possible effective dose at the initiation of therapy followed by careful titration of doses as needed. Just as importantly, they should be monitored very carefully for signs and symptoms of adverse drug reactions.

Another concern is that many elderly patients are prescribed multiple drugs and are at risk for polypharmacy. As the number of medications a patient takes increases, so does the risk for an adverse drug reaction. One drug may negate or potentiate the effects of another drug (drug-drug interaction). This situation is compounded by concurrent use of nonprescription drugs and natural products. In general, doses of most medications (especially digoxin, sedative/hypnotics, anticoagulants, nonsteroidal anti-inflammatory agents, antibiotics, and antihypertensives) should be decreased in the geriatric population. The Beers List/Criteria, which appears in the *Medication Safety Tools section*, is a list of drugs to be used with caution in the elderly, and is based on these concerns.

The Patient of Reproductive Age

Generally, pregnant women should avoid medications, except when absolutely necessary. Both the mother and the fetus must be considered. The placenta protects the fetus only from extremely large molecules. The fetus is particularly vulnerable during the first and the last trimesters of pregnancy. During the first trimester, vital organs are forming and ingestion of teratogenic drugs may lead to fetal malformation or miscarriage. Unfortunately, this is the time when a woman is least likely to know that she is pregnant. In the third trimester, drugs administered to the mother and transferred to the fetus may not be safely metabolized and excreted by the fetus. This is especially true of drugs administered near term. After the infant is delivered, he or she no longer has the placenta to help with drug excretion, and drugs administered before delivery may result in toxicity.

Of course, many conditions, such as asthma, diabetes, gastrointestinal disorders, and mental illness affect pregnant women and require long-term medication use. When the medications are used, whether over-the-counter or prescription, prescribing the lowest effective dose for the shortest period of time necessary is the rule.

The possibility of a medication altering sperm quality and quantity in a potential father also is an area of concern. Male patients should be informed of this risk when taking any medications known to have this potential.

Renal Disease

The kidneys are the major organ of drug elimination. Failure to account for decreased renal function is a preventable source of adverse drug reactions. Renal function is measured by the creatinine clearance (CCr), which can be approximated in the absence of a 24-hour urine collection (Appendix E). In addition, dosages in the renally impaired patient can be optimized by measuring blood levels of certain drugs (e.g., digoxin, aminoglycosides).

Patients with underlying renal disease, premature infants with immature renal function, and elderly patients with an age-related decrease in renal function require careful dose adjustments. Renal function may fluctuate over time and should be re-assessed periodically.

Liver Disease

The liver is the major organ of drug metabolism. It changes a drug from a relatively fat-soluble compound to a more water-soluble substance, which means that the drug can then be excreted by the kidneys. Liver function is not as easily quantified as renal function, and it therefore is difficult to predict the correct dosage for a patient with liver dysfunction based on laboratory tests.

A patient who is severely jaundiced or who has very low serum proteins (particularly albumin) can be expected to have some problems metabolizing drugs. In advanced liver disease, portal vascular congestion also impairs drug absorption. Examples of drugs that should be carefully dosed in patients with liver disease include theophylline, diuretics, phenytoin, and sedatives. Some drugs (e.g., enalapril, carisoprodol) must be activated in the liver to exert their effect and are known as prodrugs. In patients with liver dysfunction, these drugs may not be converted to the active component, thereby resulting in decreased efficacy.

Heart Failure

Heart failure results in passive congestion of blood vessels in the gastrointestinal tract, which impairs drug absorption. Heart failure also slows drug delivery to the liver, delaying metabolism. Renal function is frequently compromised as well, adding to delayed elimination and prolonged drug action. Dosages of drugs metabolized mainly by the liver or excreted mainly by the kidneys should be decreased in patients with congestive heart failure.

Body Size

Drug dosing is often based on total body weight. However, some drugs selectively penetrate fatty tissues. If the drug does not penetrate fatty tissues (e.g., digoxin, gentamicin), dosages for the obese patient should be determined by ideal body weight or estimated lean body mass. Ideal body weight may be determined from tables of desirable weights or may be estimated using formulas for lean body mass when the patient's height and weight are known (Appendix E). If such adjustments are not made, considerable toxicity can result.

Body size is also a factor in patients who are grossly underweight. Elderly patients, chronic alcoholics, patients with acquired immune deficiency, and patients who are terminally ill from cancer or other debilitating illnesses need careful attention to dosing. Patients who have had a limb amputated also need to have this change in body size taken into account.

Drug Interactions

Use of multiple drugs, especially those known to interact with other drugs, may necessitate dosage adjustments. Drugs highly bound to plasma proteins, such as warfarin and phenytoin, may be displaced by other highly protein-bound drugs. When this phenomenon occurs, the drug that has been displaced exhibits an increase in its activity because the free or unbound drug is active.

Some drugs decrease the liver's ability to metabolize other drugs. Drugs capable of doing this include cimetidine and ketoconazole. Concurrently administered drugs that are also highly metabolized by the liver may need to be administered in decreased dosages. Other agents such as phenobarbital, other barbiturates, and rifampin are capable of stimulating the liver to metabolize drugs more rapidly, requiring larger doses to be administered. Concurrently administered drugs that are also highly metabolized by the liver may need to be administered in higher dosages.

Drugs that significantly alter urine pH can affect excretion of drugs for which the excretory process is pH dependent. Alkalinizing the urine will hasten the excretion of acidic drugs. An example of this is administering sodium bicarbonate in cases of aspirin overdose to promote the renal excretion of aspirin. Alkalinizing the urine will increase reabsorption of alkaline drugs, which prolongs and enhances drug action. Acidification of the urine will hasten the excretion of alkaline drugs. Acidification of the urine will also enhance reabsorption of acidic drugs, prolonging and enhancing drug action.

Some drugs compete for enzyme systems with other drugs. Allopurinol inhibits the enzyme involved in uric acid production, but it also inhibits metabolism (inactivation) of 6-mercaptopurine, greatly increasing its toxicity. The dosage of mercaptopurine needs to be significantly reduced when coadministered with allopurinol.

The same potential for interactions exists for some foods. Dietary calcium, found in high concentrations in dairy products, combines with tetracycline or fluoroquinolones and prevents their absorption. Foods high in pyridoxine (vitamin B_6) can negate the anti-Parkinson effect of levodopa. Grapefruit juice inhibits the enzyme that breaks down some drugs, and concurrent ingestion may significantly increase drug levels and the risk for toxicity.

Many commonly taken natural products interact with pharmaceutical drugs. St. John's wort, garlic, ephedra, and other natural products can interact with medications and cause known or unpredictable reactions.

Nurses and prescribers should consult drug references and remember that the average dosing range for drugs is intended for an average patient. However, every patient is an individual with specific drug-handling capabilities. Taking these special dosing considerations into account allows for an individualized drug regimen that promotes the desired therapeutic outcome and minimizes the risk of toxicity.

The Cytochrome P450 System: What Is It and Why Should I Care?[1]

Looking beyond the obvious takes time, energy, insight, and fortitude; yet this is what we are called to do. We are nurses—tireless care providers. Yet, when the subject of the liver's enzyme system, also called the cytochrome P450 system, is discussed, we feel the urge to run the other way . . . or better yet, to just ignore the conversation. Yet, can we do this as the tireless care provider? The answer to this question is clear and simple: no, we cannot. This is because numerous medications, nutrients, and herbal therapies are metabolized through the cytochrome P450 (CYP450) enzyme system. This system can be inhibited or induced by drugs, and once altered can be clinically significant in the development of drug-drug interactions that may cause unanticipated adverse reactions or therapeutic failures. This article will review the basic concepts of the CYP450 system and relate these concepts to clinically significant altered responses.

The CYP450 enzymes are essential for the production of numerous agents including cholesterol and steroids. Additionally, these enzymes are necessary for the detoxification of foreign chemicals and the metabolism of drugs. CYP450 enzymes are so named because they are bound to membranes within a cell (cyto) and contain a heme pigment (chrome and P) that absorbs light at a wavelength of 450 nm when exposed to carbon monoxide.[2] There are more than 50 CYP450 enzymes, but the CYP1A2, CYP2C19, CYP2D6, CYP1A2, CYP3A4, and CYP3A5 enzymes are responsible for metabolizing 45% of drug metabolism. The CYP2D6 (20–30%), the CYP2C9 (10%) and the CYP2E1 and CYP1A2 (5%) complete this enzyme system.[3]

Drugs that cause CYP450 drug interactions are referred to as either inhibitors or inducers. An inducing agent can increase the rate of another drug's metabolism by as much as two- to threefold that develops over a period of a week. When an inducing agent is prescribed with another medication, the dosage of the other medication may need to be adjusted since the rate of metabolism is increased and the effect of the medication reduced. This can lead to a therapeutic failure of the medication. Conversely, if a medication is taken with an agent that inhibits its metabolism, then the drug level can rise and possibly result in a harmful or adverse effect. Information regarding a drug's CYP450 metabolism and its potential for inhibition or induction can be found on the drug label and accessed through the U.S. Food and Drug Administration (FDA) or manufacturer's websites.[2]

When we assess our patients and provide management modalities, these are implemented within a framework of the patient's heritage, race, and culture. This is also true in pharmacology as well (i.e., "pharmacogenetics"). This concept is important to examine since we know that there exists genetic variability, which may influence a patient's response to commonly prescribed drug classes. This genetic variability can be defined as polymorphism. Seven percent of Caucasians and 2–7% of African Americans are poor metabolizers of drugs dependent on CYP2D6, which metabolizes many beta blockers, antidepressants, and opioids. This is because the drug's metabolism via CYP450 enzymes exhibits genetic variability.[2]

Recently, researchers have studied the genetic variability in metabolism among women who were prescribed tamoxifen and medications that inhibit the CYP2D6 enzyme. To review, tamoxifen is biotransformed to the potent antiestrogen, endoxifen, by this enzyme. CYP2D6 genetic variation (individuals considered extensive metabolizers versus poor metabolizers) and inhibitors of the enzyme markedly reduce endoxifen plasma concentrations in tamoxifen-treated patients.

The researchers concluded that CYP2D6 metabolism is an "independent predictor of breast cancer outcome in post-menopausal women receiving tamoxifen for early breast cancer. Determination of CYP2D6 genotype may be of value in selecting adjuvant hormonal therapy and it appears CYP2D6 inhibitors should be avoided in tamoxifen-treated women."[4] Do oncology patients come to us with only their cancer and its treatment? No, they come with multifaceted dimensions and co-morbid conditions such as hypertension, dyslipidemia, depression, seizure disorders, etc. For example, several antidepressants (paroxetine [Paxil] and fluoxetine [Prozac]) are inhibitors of metabolism when given with drugs metabolized through the CYP2D6 enzyme, such as haloperidol (Haldol), metoprolol (Lopressor), and hydrocodone. Thus, the therapeutic response can be accentuated. Medications that inhibit the CYP3A4 enzyme such as amiodarone and antifungals, can affect the therapeutic response of fentanyl, alprazolam (Xanax), and numerous statins; as a result, the effect of these drugs can be enhanced leading to potential toxic levels.[5]

At times, these CYP450 inducers and inhibitors are commonly ingested items such as grapefruit juice and tobacco. In the case of grapefruit juice, there are numerous medications known to interact with grapefruit juice including statins, antiarrhythmic agents, immunosuppressive agents, and calcium channel blockers. Furthermore, the inhibition of the enzyme system seems to be dose dependent; thus, the more a patient drinks, the more the inhibition that occurs. Additionally, the effects can last for several days if grapefruit juice is consumed on a regular basis. Luckily, the effect of this is not seen with other citrus juices.

Hopefully, this brief review has opened the door to your inquisitive nature on how the liver's enzyme system is affected by numerous medications and why some patients experience clinically significant unanticipated adverse reactions or therapeutic failures.

CYP1A2

Substrates	Inhibitors	Inducers
alosetron, amitriptyline, clozapine, cyclobenzaprine, desipramine, diazepam, duloxetine, fluvoxamine, imipramine, mexiletine, mirtazapine, olanzapine, propranolol, ropinirole, theophylline, (R)-warfarin	cimetidine, ciprofloxacin, fluvoxamine, ketoconazole, lidocaine, mexiletine	carbamazepine, cigarette smoke, phenobarbital, rifampin

CYP2C9

Substrates	Inhibitors	Inducers
celecoxib, glimepiride, glipizide, losartan, montelukast, nateglinide, phenytoin, sulfamethoxazole, voriconazole, (S)-warfarin	amiodarone, efavirenz, fluconazole, fluvastatin, ketoconazole, sulfamethoxazole, zafirlukast	carbamazepine, phenobarbital, phenytoin, rifampin

CYP2C19

Substrates	Inhibitors	Inducers
citalopram, diazepam, escitalopram, esomeprazole, imipramine, lansoprazole, nelfinavir, omeprazole, pantoprazole, phenytoin, rabeprazole, voriconazole	efavirenz, esomeprazole, fluoxetine, fluvoxamine, lansoprazole, omeprazole, rabeprazole, sertraline, ticlopidine	carbamazepine, phenytoin, rifampin

CYP2D6

Substrates	Inhibitors	Inducers
amitriptyline, aripiprazole, atomoxetine, codeine, desipramine, dextromethorphan, duloxetine, flecainide, fluoxetine, haloperidol, imipramine, lidocaine, metoprolol, mexiletine, mirtazapine, nefazodone, nortriptyline, oxycodone, paroxetine, propafenone, propranolol, risperidone, ritonavir, tramadol, venlafaxine	amiodarone, cimetidine, clozapine, desipramine, duloxetine, fluoxetine, haloperidol, lidocaine, methadone, paroxetine, pimozide, quinidine, ritonavir, sertraline, ticlopidine	None

CYP3A

Substrates	Inhibitors	Inducers
alprazolam, amiodarone, aprepitant, aripiprazole, atorvastatin, boceprevir, buspirone, calcium channel blockers, carbamazepine, cilostazol, citalopram, clarithromycin, clonazepam, cyclosporine, dapsone, diazepam, disopyramide, efavirenz, ergot derivatives, erlotinib, erythromycin, escitalopram, estrogens, fentanyl, gefitinib, glucocorticoids, imatinib, indinavir, irinotecan, itraconazole, ketoconazole, lansoprazole, lidocaine, losartan, lovastatin, methadone, midazolam, mirtazapine, montelukast, nateglinide, nefazodone, nelfinavir, nevirapine, ondansetron, paclitaxel, pimozide, protease inhibitors, quetiapine, quinidine, repaglinide, rifabutin, sildenafil, simvastatin, sirolimus, sorafenib, sunitinib, tacrolimus, tadalafil, tamoxifen, telaprevir, theophylline, tiagabine, ticlopidine, vardenafil, (R)-warfarin, zolpidem, zonisamide	amiodarone, aprepitant, cimetidine, clarithromycin, cyclosporine, diltiazem, efavirenz, erythromycin, fluconazole, grapefruit juice, imatinib, indinavir, itraconazole, ketoconazole, metronidazole, nefazodone, nelfinavir, quinidine, ritonavir, saquinavir, sertraline, verapamil, voriconazole	carbamazepine, efavirenz, nevirapine, phenobarbital, phenytoin, rifabutin, rifampin, St. John's wort

REFERENCES

1. Jamison, T. (Winter 2008). Oncology Nursing Society, Metro Detroit Chapter Newsletter, Volume XXIII, Issue 1.
2. Lynch, T. & Price, A (2007). The effect of P450 metabolism on drug response, interactions, and adverse effects. American Family Physician, 76(3), 391–397.
3. Arcangelo, V. P. & Peterson, A. M. (2006). Pharmacotherapeutics for Advanced Practice: A Practical Approach. (2nd ed). Philadelphia: Lippincott Williams and Wilkins.
4. Goetz, M., Knox, S, Suman, V., & Rae, J. (2007). The impact of cytochrome P450 2D6 metabolism in women receiving adjuvant tamoxifen. Breast Cancer Research and Treatment. 101(1), 113–122.
5. Lehne, R. (2007). Pharmacology: for Nursing Care (6th edition). St Louis, MO: Saunders, Elsevier.

EDUCATING PATIENTS ABOUT SAFE MEDICATION USE

Research has shown that patients need information about several medication-related topics, no matter what the medication. A well-informed patient and/or family can help prevent medication errors by hospital staff and is less likely to make medication errors at home. Adherence to the medication regimen is another goal achieved through patient education.

Before beginning any teaching, however, always assess the patient's current knowledge by asking if he or she is familiar with the medication, how it is taken at home, what precautions or follow-up care is required, and other questions specific to each drug. Based on the patient's current knowledge level and taking into consideration factors such as readiness to learn, environmental and social barriers to learning or adherence, and cultural factors, discuss the following:

1. **Generic and brand names of the medication.** Patients should know both the brand and generic names of each medication for two reasons. It helps them identify their medications when a generic equivalent is substituted for a brand name version, and it prevents patients or health care providers from making sound-alike confusion errors when giving or documenting a medication history. An example of this is saying Celebrex but meaning or hearing Cerebyx.

2. **Purpose of the medication.** Patients have a right to know what the therapeutic benefit of the medication will be but also should be told the consequences of not taking the prescribed medication. This may enhance adherence. For example, a patient may be more likely to take blood pressure medication if told lowering high blood pressure will prevent heart attack, kidney disease, or stroke, rather than saying only that it will lower blood pressure.

3. **Dosage and how to take the medication.** To derive benefit and avoid adverse reactions or other poor outcomes, the patient must know how much of the medication to take and when to take it. Refer to dosages in metric weight (i.e., milligram, gram) rather than dosage unit (tablet) or volume (1 teaspoon). The patient must also be informed of the best time to take the medication, for example, on an empty or a full stomach, before bedtime, or with or without other medications. If possible, help the patient fit the medication schedule into his or her own schedule, so that taking the medication is not difficult or forgotten.

4. **What to do if a dose is missed.** Always explain to patients what to do if a dose is missed. Patients have been reported to take a double dose of medications when a missed dose occurs, putting themselves at risk for side effects and adverse reactions.

5. **Duration of therapy.** It is not uncommon for patients to stop taking a medication when they feel better or to discontinue a medication when they cannot perceive a benefit. For very long term, even lifelong therapy, the patient may need to be reminded that the medication helps maintain the current level of wellness. Patients may need to be reminded to finish short-term courses of medications even though they frequently will feel much better before the prescription runs out. Some medications cannot be discontinued abruptly and patients should be warned to consult a health care professional before discontinuing such agents. Patients will need to know to refill prescriptions several days before running out or to take extra medication if traveling.

6. **Minor side effects and what to do if they occur.** Inform the patient that all medications have potential side effects. Explain the most common side effects associated with the medication and how to avoid or manage them if they occur. An informed patient is less likely to stop taking a medication because of a minor and potentially avoidable side effect.

7. **Serious side effects and what to do if they occur.** Inform the patient of the possibility of serious side effects. Describe signs and symptoms associated with serious side effects, and tell the

patient to immediately inform a physician or nurse should they occur. Tell the patient to call before the next dose of the medication is scheduled and to not assume that the medication is the source of the symptom and prematurely discontinue it.

8. **Medications to avoid.** Drug-drug interactions can dampen drug effects, enhance drug effects, or cause life-threatening adverse events such as cardiac dysrhythmias, hepatitis, renal failure, or internal bleeding. The patient and family need to know which other medications, including which over-the-counter medications, to avoid.

9. **Foods to avoid and other precautions.** Food-drug interactions are not uncommon and can have effects similar to drug-drug interactions. Excessive sun exposure resulting in severe dermal reactions is not uncommon and represents an environmental-drug interaction. Likewise, the patient should be informed of what activities to avoid, in case the medication affects alertness or coordination, for example.

10. **How to store the medication:** Medications must be stored properly to maintain potency. Most medications should not be stored in the bathroom medicine cabinet because of excess heat and humidity. In addition, thoughtful storage practices, such as separating two family members' medications, can prevent mix-ups and inadvertent accessibility by children (or pets). Review storage with patients and ask about current methods for storing medications.

11. **Follow-up care.** Anyone taking medication requires ongoing care to assess effectiveness and appropriateness of medications. Many medications require invasive and noninvasive testing to monitor blood levels; hematopoietic, hepatic, or renal function; or other effects on other body systems. Ongoing medical evaluation may result in dosage adjustments, change in medication, or discontinuation of medication.

12. **What not to take.** Inform patients not to take expired medications or someone else's medication. Warn them not to self-medicate with older, no-longer-used prescriptions even if the remaining supply is not expired. Tell patients to keep a current record of all medications taken and to ask health care providers if new medications are meant to replace a current medication.

As you teach, encourage the patient and the family to ask questions. Providing feedback about medication questions will increase their understanding and help you identify areas that need reinforcement. Also, ask patients to repeat what you have said and return to demonstrate application or administration techniques.

Stress the importance of concurrent therapies. Medications often are only a part of a recommended therapy. Review with the patient and family other measures that will enhance or maintain health. Always consider the cultural context in which health information is provided and plan accordingly. This might include obtaining a same-gender translator or adjusting dosing times to avoid conflict with traditional rituals.

Finally, provide written instructions in a simple and easy-to-read format. Keep in mind that most health care information is written at a 10th grade reading level, while many patients read at a 5th grade level. Tell patients to keep the written instructions, so that they can be reviewed at home, when stress levels are lower and practical difficulties in maintaining the medication plan are known.

• ANTI-ALZHEIMER'S AGENTS

PHARMACOLOGIC PROFILE

General Use
Management of Alzheimer's dementia.

General Action and Information
All agents act by ↑ the amount of acetylcholine in the CNS by inhibiting cholinesterase. No agents to date can slow the progression of Alzheimer's dementia. Current agents may temporarily improve cognitive function and therefore improve quality of life.

Contraindications
Hypersensitivity.

Precautions
Use cautiously in patients with a history of "sick sinus syndrome" or other supraventricular cardiac conduction abnormalities (may cause bradycardia). Cholingeric effects may result in adverse GI effects (nausea, vomiting, diarrhea, weight loss) and may also ↑ gastric acid secretion resulting in GI bleeding, especially during concurrent NSAID therapy. Other cholinergic effects may include urinary tract obstruction, seizures, or bronchospasm.

Interactions
Additive effects with other drugs having cholinergic properties. May exaggerate the effects of succinylcholine-type muscle relaxation during anesthesia. May ↓ therapeutic effects of anticholinergics.

NURSING IMPLICATIONS

Assessment
- Assess cognitive function (memory, attention, reasoning, language, ability to perform simple tasks) throughout therapy.
- Monitor nausea, vomiting, anorexia, and weight loss. Notify health care professional if these side effects occur.

Potential Nursing Diagnoses
- Disturbed thought process (Indications).
- Imbalanced nutrition: less than body requirements.
- Deficient knowledge, related to disease process and medication regimen (Patient/Family Teaching).

Implementation

Patient/Family Teaching
- Instruct patient and caregiver that medication should be taken as directed.
- Advise patient and caregiver to notify health care professional if nausea, vomiting, anorexia, and weight loss occur.

Evaluation/Desired Outcomes
- Temporary improvement in cognitive function (memory, attention, reasoning, language, ability to perform simple tasks) in patients with Alzheimer's disease.

• ANTIANEMICS

PHARMACOLOGIC PROFILE

General Use

Prevention and treatment of anemias.

General Action and Information

Iron (ferrous fumarate, ferrous gluconate, ferrous sulfate, iron dextran, iron sucrose, polysaccharide-iron complex, sodium ferric gluconate complex) is required for production of hemoglobin, which is necessary for oxygen transport to cells. Cyanocobalamin and hydroxocobalamin (vitamin B_{12}) and folic acid are water-soluble vitamins that are required for red blood cell production. Darbepoetin, epoetin, and peginesatide stimulate production of red blood cells.

Contraindications

Undiagnosed anemias. Hemochromatosis, hemosiderosis, hemolytic anemia (Iron). Uncontrolled hypertension (darbepoetin, epoetin, and peginesatide).

Precautions

Use parenteral iron (iron dextran, iron sucrose, sodium ferric gluconate complex) cautiously in patients with a history of allergy or hypersensitivity reactions.

Interactions

Oral iron can ↓ the absorption of tetracyclines, fluoroquinolones, or penicillamine. Vitamin E may impair the therapeutic response to iron. Phenytoin and other anticonvulsants may ↓ the absorption of folic acid. Darbepoetin, epoetin, and peginesatide may ↑ the requirement for heparin during hemodialysis.

NURSING IMPLICATIONS

Assessment

- Assess patient's nutritional status and dietary history to determine possible causes for anemia and need for patient teaching.

Potential Nursing Diagnoses

- Activity intolerance (Indications).
- Imbalanced nutrition: less than body requirements (Indications).
- Deficient knowledge, related to disease process and medication regimen (Patient/Family Teaching).

Implementation

- Available in combination with many vitamins and minerals (see Appendix B).

Patient/Family Teaching

- Encourage patients to comply with diet recommendations of health care professional. Explain that the best source of vitamins and minerals is a well-balanced diet with foods from the four basic food groups.
- Patients self-medicating with vitamin and mineral supplements should be cautioned not to exceed RDA. The effectiveness of mega doses for treatment of various medical conditions is unproven and may cause side effects.

Evaluation/Desired Outcomes

- Resolution of anemia.

• ANTIANGINALS

PHARMACOLOGIC PROFILE

General Use

Nitrates are used to treat and prevent attacks of angina. Only nitrates (sublingual, lingual spray, or intravenous) may be used in the acute treatment of attacks of angina pectoris. Calcium channel blockers, beta blockers, and ranolazine are used prophylactically in long-term management of angina.

General Action and Information

Several different groups of medications are used in the treatment of angina pectoris. The nitrates (isosorbide dinitrate, isosorbide mononitrate, and nitroglycerin) are available as a lingual spray, sublingual tablets, parenterals, transdermal systems, and sustained-release oral dosage forms. Nitrates dilate coronary arteries and cause systemic vasodilation (↓ preload). Calcium channel blockers dilate coronary arteries (some also slow heart rate). Beta blockers ↓ myocardial oxygen consumption via a ↓ in heart rate. Ranolazine ↓ myocardial oxygen consumption. Therapy may be combined if selection is designed to minimize side effects or adverse reactions.

Contraindications

Hypersensitivity. Avoid use of beta blockers or calcium channel blockers in advanced heart block, cardiogenic shock, or untreated HF.

Precautions

Beta blockers should be used cautiously in patients with diabetes mellitus, pulmonary disease, or hypothyroidism.

Interactions

Nitrates, calcium channel blockers, and beta blockers may cause hypotension with other antihypertensives or acute ingestion of alcohol. Verapamil, diltiazem, and beta blockers may have additive myocardial depressant effects when used with other agents that affect cardiac function. Verapamil and ranolazine have a number of other significant drug-drug interactions.

NURSING IMPLICATIONS

Assessment

- Assess location, duration, intensity, and precipitating factors of patient's anginal pain.
- Monitor BP and pulse periodically throughout therapy.

Potential Nursing Diagnoses

- Acute pain (Indications).
- Ineffective tissue perfusion (Indications).
- Deficient knowledge, related to disease process and medication regimen (Patient/Family Teaching).

Implementation

- Available in various dose forms. See specific drugs for information on administration.

Patient/Family Teaching

- Instruct patient on concurrent nitrate therapy and prophylactic antianginals to continue taking both medications as ordered and to use SL nitroglycerin as needed for anginal attacks.
- Advise patient to contact health care professional immediately if chest pain does not improve; worsens after therapy; is accompanied by diaphoresis or shortness of breath; or if severe, persistent headache occurs.
- Caution patient to make position changes slowly to minimize orthostatic hypotension.
- Advise patient to avoid concurrent use of alcohol with these medications.

Evaluation/Desired Outcomes

- Decrease in frequency and severity of anginal attacks.
- Increase in activity tolerance.

• ANTIANXIETY AGENTS

PHARMACOLOGIC PROFILE

General Use

Antianxiety agents are used in the management of various forms of anxiety, including generalized anxiety disorder (GAD). Some agents are more suitable for intermittent or short-term use (benzodiazepines) while others are more useful long-term (buspirone, doxepin, fluoxetine, paroxetine, sertraline, venlafaxine).

General Action and Information

Most agents cause generalized CNS depression. Benzodiazepines may produce tolerance with long-term use and have potential for psychological or physical dependence. These agents have NO analgesic properties.

Contraindications

Hypersensitivity. Should not be used in comatose patients or in those with pre-existing CNS depression. Should not be used in patients with uncontrolled severe pain. Avoid use during pregnancy or lactation.

Precautions

Use cautiously in patients with hepatic dysfunction, severe renal impairment, or severe underlying pulmonary disease (benzodiazepines only). Use with caution in patients who may be suicidal or who may have had previous drug addictions. Patients may be more sensitive to CNS depressant effects; dosage ↓ may be required.

Interactions

Mainly for benzodiazepines; additive CNS depression with alcohol, antihistamines, some antidepressants, opioid analgesics, or phenothiazines may occur. Most agents should not be used with MAO inhibitors.

NURSING IMPLICATIONS

Assessment

- Monitor BP, pulse, and respiratory status frequently throughout IV administration.
- Prolonged high-dose therapy may lead to psychological or physical dependence. Restrict the amount of drug available to patient, especially if patient is depressed, suicidal, or has a history of addiction.
- **Anxiety:** Assess degree of anxiety and level of sedation (ataxia, dizziness, slurred speech) before and periodically throughout therapy.

Potential Nursing Diagnoses

- Risk for injury (Side Effects).
- Deficient knowledge, related to disease process and medication regimen (Patient/Family Teaching).

Implementation

- Patients changing to buspirone from other antianxiety agents should receive gradually ↓ doses. Buspirone will not prevent withdrawal symptoms.

Patient/Family Teaching

- May cause daytime drowsiness. Caution patient to avoid driving and other activities requiring alertness until response to medication is known.

- Advise patient to avoid the use of alcohol and other CNS depressants concurrently with these medications.
- Advise patient to inform health care professional if pregnancy is planned or suspected.

Evaluation/Desired Outcomes

- Decrease in anxiety level.

• ANTIARRHYTHMICS

PHARMACOLOGIC PROFILE

General Use

Suppression of cardiac arrhythmias.

General Action and Information

Correct cardiac arrhythmias by a variety of mechanisms, depending on the group used. The therapeutic goal is ↓ symptomatology and ↑ hemodynamic performance. Choice of agent depends on etiology of arrhythmia and individual patient characteristics. Treatable causes of arrhythmias should be corrected before therapy is initiated (e.g., electrolyte disturbances, other drugs). Antiarrhythmics are generally classified by their effects on cardiac conduction tissue (see the following table). Adenosine, atropine, and digoxin are also used as antiarrhythmics.

MECHANISM OF ACTION OF MAJOR ANTIARRHYTHMIC DRUGS

CLASS	DRUGS	MECHANISM
IA	quinidine, procainamide, disopyramide	Na channel blockers, ↑ APD and ERP, ↓ membrane responsiveness
IB	lidocaine, phenytoin, mexiletine	Na channel blockers, ↓ APD and ERP
IC	flecainide, propafenone	Profound slowing of conduction by blocking Na channels, markedly depress phase 0
II	esmolol, propranolol, metoprolol	Beta-blockers; ↓ AV nodal conduction, ↓ automaticity
III	amiodarone, dofetilide, dronedarone, ibutilide, sotalol	K channel blockers; amiodarone and dronedarone also have Na channel, beta-receptor, and Ca-channel blocking properties
IV	diltiazem, verapamil	Non-dihydropyridine Ca channel blockers; ↓ AV nodal conduction

APD = action-potential duration; AV = atrioventricular; Ca = calcium; ERP = effective refractory period; K = potassium; Na = sodium.

Contraindications

Differ greatly among various agents. See individual drugs.

Precautions

Differ greatly among agents used. Appropriate dosage adjustments should be made in elderly patients and those with renal or hepatic impairment, depending on agent chosen. Correctable causes (electrolyte abnormalities, drug toxicity) should be evaluated. See individual drugs.

Interactions

Differ greatly among agents used. See individual drugs.

NURSING IMPLICATIONS

Assessment

- Monitor ECG, pulse, and BP continuously throughout IV administration and periodically throughout oral administration.

CLASSIFICATIONS

Potential Nursing Diagnoses
- Decreased cardiac output (Indications).
- Deficient knowledge, related to disease process and medication regimen (Patient/Family Teaching).

Implementation
- Take apical pulse before administration of oral doses. Withhold dose and notify physician or other health care professional if heart rate is <50 bpm.
- Administer oral doses with a full glass of water. Most sustained-release preparations should be swallowed whole. Do not crush, break, or chew tablets or open capsules, unless specifically instructed.

Patient/Family Teaching
- Instruct patient to take oral doses around the clock, as directed, even if feeling better.
- Instruct patient or family member on how to take pulse. Advise patient to report changes in pulse rate or rhythm to health care professional.
- Caution patient to avoid taking OTC medications without consulting health care professional.
- Advise patient to carry identification describing disease process and medication regimen at all times.
- Emphasize the importance of follow-up exams to monitor progress.

Evaluation/Desired Outcomes
- Resolution of cardiac arrhythmias without detrimental side effects.

• ANTIASTHMATICS

PHARMACOLOGIC PROFILE

General Use
Management of acute and chronic episodes of reversible bronchoconstriction. Goal of therapy is to treat acute attacks (short-term control) and to ↓ incidence and intensity of future attacks (long-term control). The choice of modalities depends on the continued requirement for short term control agents.

General Action and Information
Adrenergic bronchodilators and phosphodiesterase inhibitors both work by ↑ intracellular levels of cyclic-3', 5'-adenosine monophsphate (cAMP); adrenergics by ↑ production and phosphodiesterase inhibitors by ↓ breakdown. ↑ levels of cAMP produce bronchodilation. Corticosteroids act by ↓ airway inflammation. Anticholinergics (ipratropium) produce bronchodilation by ↓ intracellular levels of cyclic guanosine monophosphate (cGMP). Leukotriene receptor antagonists and mast cell stabilizers ↓ the release of substances that can contribute to bronchospasm.

Contraindications
Inhaled corticosteroids, long-acting adrenergic agents, and mast cell stabilizers should not be used during acute attacks of asthma.

Precautions
Adrenergic bronchodilators and anticholinergics should be used cautiously in patients with cardiovascular disease. Chronic use of systemic corticosteroids should be avoided in children or during pregnancy or lactation. Patients with diabetes may experience loss of glycemic control during corticosteroid therapy. Corticosteroids should never be abruptly discontinued.

Interactions
Adrenergic bronchodilators and phosphodiesterase inhibitors may have additive CNS and cardiovascular effects with other adrenergic agents. Cimetidine ↑ theophylline levels and the risk

of toxicity. Corticosteroids may ↓ the effectiveness of antidiabetics. Corticosteroids may cause hypokalemia which may be additive with potassium-losing diuretics and may also ↑ the risk of digoxin toxicity.

NURSING IMPLICATIONS

Assessment

- Assess lung sounds and respiratory function prior to and periodically throughout therapy.
- Assess cardiovascular status of patients taking adrenergic bronchodilators or anticholinergics. Monitor for ECG changes and chest pain.

Potential Nursing Diagnoses

- Ineffective airway clearance (Indications).
- Deficient knowledge, related to disease process and medication regimen (Patient/Family Teaching).
- Noncompliance (Patient/Family Teaching).

Implementation

- **PO:** Administer oral doses of glycopyrrolate, propantheline, or scopolamine 30 min before meals.
- Scopolamine transdermal patch should be applied at least 4 hr before travel.

Patient/Family Teaching

- Instruct patient to take antiasthmatics as directed. Do not take more than prescribed or discontinue without discussing with health care professional.
- Advise patient to avoid smoking and other respiratory irritants.
- Instruct patient in correct use of metered-dose inhaler or other administration devices (see Appendix D).
- Advise patient to contact health care professional promptly if the usual dose of medication fails to produce the desired results, if symptoms worsen after treatment, or if toxic effects occur.
- Patients using inhalation medications and bronchodilators should be advised to use the bronchodilator first and allow 5 minutes to elapse before administering other medications, unless otherwise directed by health care professional.

Evaluation/Desired Outcomes

- Prevention of and reduction in symptoms of asthma.

• ANTICHOLINERGICS

PHARMACOLOGIC PROFILE

General Use

Atropine—Bradyarrhythmias. **Ipratropium**—bronchospasm (inhalation) and rhinorrhea (intranasal). **Scopolamine**—Nausea and vomiting related to motion sickness and vertigo. **Propantheline and glycopyrrolate**— ↓ gastric secretory activity and ↑ esophageal sphincter tone. Atropine and scopolamine are also used as ophthalmic mydriatics. Benztropine, biperidin, and trihexyphenidyl are used in the management of Parkinson's disease. Oxybutynin and tolterodine are used as urinary tract spasmodics.

General Action and Information

Competitively inhibit the action of acetylcholine. In addition, atropine, glycopyrrolate, propantheline, and scopolamine are antimuscarinic in that they inhibit the action of acetylcholine at sites innervated by postganglionic cholinergic nerves.

Contraindications

Hypersensitivity, narrow-angle glaucoma, severe hemorrhage, tachycardia (due to thyrotoxicosis or cardiac insufficiency), or myasthenia gravis.

Precautions
Geriatric and pediatric patients are more susceptible to adverse effects. Use cautiously in patients with urinary tract pathology; those at risk for GI obstruction; and those with chronic renal, hepatic, pulmonary, or cardiac disease.

Interactions
Additive anticholinergic effects (dry mouth, dry eyes, blurred vision, constipation) with other agents possessing anticholinergic activity, including antihistamines, antidepressants, quinidine, and disopyramide. May alter GI absorption of other drugs by inhibiting GI motility and ↑ transit time. Antacids may ↓ absorption of orally administered anticholinergics.

NURSING IMPLICATIONS

Assessment
- Assess vital signs and ECG frequently during IV drug therapy. Report any significant changes in heart rate or BP or increase in ventricular ectopy or angina promptly.
- Monitor intake and output ratios in elderly or surgical patients; may cause urinary retention.
- Assess patient regularly for abdominal distention and auscultate for bowel sounds. Constipation may become a problem. Increasing fluids and adding bulk to the diet may help alleviate constipation.

Potential Nursing Diagnoses
- Decreased cardiac output (Indications).
- Impaired oral mucous membrane (Side Effects).
- Constipation (Side Effects).

Implementation
- **PO:** Administer oral doses of glycopyrrolate, propantheline, or scopolamine 30 min before meals.
- Scopolamine transdermal patch should be applied at least 4 hr before travel.

Patient/Family Teaching
- Instruct patient that frequent rinses, sugarless gum or candy, and good oral hygiene may help relieve dry mouth.
- May cause drowsiness. Caution patient to avoid driving or other activities requiring alertness until response to medication is known.
- **Ophth:** Advise patients that ophthalmic preparations may temporarily blur vision and impair ability to judge distances. Dark glasses may be needed to protect eyes from bright light.

Evaluation/Desired Outcomes
- Increase in heart rate.
- Decrease in nausea and vomiting related to motion sickness or vertigo.
- Dryness of mouth.
- Dilation of pupils.
- Decrease in GI motility.
- Resolution of signs and symptoms of Parkinson's disease.

• ANTICOAGULANTS

PHARMACOLOGIC PROFILE

General Use
Prevention and treatment of thromboembolic disorders including deep vein thrombosis, pulmonary embolism, and atrial fibrillation with embolization. Also used in the management of myocardial infarction (MI) sequentially or in combination with thrombolytics and/or antiplatelet agents.

General Action and Information

Anticoagulants are used to prevent clot extension and formation. They do not dissolve clots. The two types of anticoagulants in common use are parenteral heparins and oral warfarin. Therapy is usually initiated with heparin or a heparin-like agent because of rapid onset of action, while maintenance therapy consists of warfarin. Warfarin takes several days to produce therapeutic anticoagulation. In serious or severe thromboembolic events, heparin therapy may be preceded by thrombolytic therapy. Low doses of heparin or heparin-like compounds and fondaparinux are mostly used to prevent deep vein thrombosis after certain surgical procedures and in similar situations in which prolonged bedrest increases the risk of thromboembolism. Argatroban is used as anticoagulation in patients who have developed thrombocytopenia during heparin therapy.

Contraindications

Underlying coagulation disorders, ulcer disease, malignancy, recent surgery, or active bleeding.

Precautions

Anticoagulation should be undertaken cautiously in any patient with a potential site for bleeding. Pregnant or lactating patients should not receive warfarin. Heparin does not cross the placenta. Heparin and heparin-like agents should be used cautiously in patients receiving epidural analgesia.

Interactions

Warfarin is highly protein bound and may displace or be displaced by other highly protein-bound drugs. The resultant interactions depend on which drug is displaced. Bleeding may be potentiated by aspirin or large doses of penicillins or penicillin-like drugs, cefotetan, cefoperazone, valproic acid, or NSAIDs.

NURSING IMPLICATIONS

Assessment

- Assess patient taking anticoagulants for signs of bleeding and hemorrhage (bleeding gums; nosebleed; unusual bruising; tarry, black stools; hematuria; fall in hematocrit or BP; guaiac-positive stools; urine; or NG aspirate).
- Assess patient for evidence of additional or increased thrombosis. Symptoms will depend on area of involvement.
- **Lab Test Considerations:** Monitor prothrombin time (PT) or international normalized ratio (INR) with warfarin therapy, activated partial thromboplastin time (aPTT) with full-dose heparin therapy and hematocrit, and other clotting factors frequently during therapy.
- Monitor bleeding time throughout antiplatelet therapy. Prolonged bleeding time, which is time and dose dependent, is expected.
- **Toxicity and Overdose:** If overdose occurs or anticoagulation needs to be immediately reversed, the antidote for heparins is protamine sulfate; for warfarin, the antidote is vitamin K (phytonadione [AquaMEPHYTON]). Administration of whole blood or plasma may also be required in severe bleeding due to warfarin because of the delayed onset of vitamin K.

Potential Nursing Diagnoses

- Ineffective tissue perfusion (Indications).
- Risk for injury (Side Effects).
- Deficient knowledge, related to disease process and medication regimen (Patient/Family Teaching).

Implementation

- Inform all health care professionals caring for patient of anticoagulant therapy. Venipunctures and injection sites require application of pressure to prevent bleeding or hematoma formation.
- Use an infusion pump with continuous infusions to ensure accurate dosage.

Patient/Family Teaching

- Caution patient to avoid activities leading to injury, to use a soft toothbrush and electric razor, and to report any symptoms of unusual bleeding or bruising to health care professional immediately.
- Instruct patient not to take OTC medications, especially those containing aspirin, NSAIDs, or alcohol, without advice of health care professional.
- Review foods high in vitamin K (see Appendix J) with patients on warfarin. Patient should have consistent limited intake of these foods, as vitamin K is the antidote for warfarin and greatly alternating intake of these foods will cause PT levels to fluctuate.
- Emphasize the importance of frequent lab tests to monitor coagulation factors.
- Instruct patient to carry identification describing medication regimen at all times and to inform all health care professionals caring for patient of anticoagulant therapy before laboratory tests, treatment, or surgery.

Evaluation/Desired Outcomes

- Prevention of undesired clotting and its sequelae without signs of hemorrhage. Prevention of stroke, MI, and death in patients at risk.

• ANTICONVULSANTS

PHARMACOLOGIC PROFILE

General Use

Anticonvulsants are used to ↓ the incidence and severity of seizures due to various etiologies. Some anticonvulsants are used parenterally in the immediate treatment of seizures. It is not uncommon for patients to require more than one anticonvulsant to control seizures on a long-term basis. Many regimens are evaluated with serum level monitoring. Several anticonvulsants also are used to treat neuropathic pain.

General Action and Information

Anticonvulsants include a variety of agents, all capable of depressing abnormal neuronal discharges in the CNS that may result in seizures. They may work by preventing the spread of seizure activity, depressing the motor cortex, raising seizure threshold, or altering levels of neurotransmitters, depending on the group. See individual drugs.

Contraindications

Previous hypersensitivity.

Precautions

Use cautiously in patients with severe hepatic or renal disease; dose adjustment may be required. Choose agents carefully in pregnant and lactating women. Fetal hydantoin syndrome may occur in offspring of patients who receive phenytoin during pregnancy.

Interactions

Barbiturates stimulate the metabolism of other drugs that are metabolized by the liver, ↓ their effectiveness. Hydantoins are highly protein-bound and may displace or be displaced by other highly protein-bound drugs. Lamotrigine, tiagabine, and topiramate are capable of interacting with several other anticonvulsants. For more specific interactions, see individual drugs. Many drugs are capable of lowering seizure threshold and may ↓ the effectiveness of anticonvulsants, including tricyclic antidepressants and phenothiazines.

NURSING IMPLICATIONS

Assessment

- Assess location, duration, and characteristics of seizure activity.
- **Toxicity and Overdose:** Monitor serum drug levels routinely throughout anticonvulsant therapy, especially when adding or discontinuing other agents.

Potential Nursing Diagnoses

- Risk for injury (Indications) (Side Effects).
- Deficient knowledge, related to disease process and medication regimen (Patient/Family Teaching).

Implementation

- Administer anticonvulsants around the clock. Abrupt discontinuation may precipitate status epilepticus.
- Implement seizure precautions.

Patient/Family Teaching

- Instruct patient to take medication every day, exactly as directed.
- May cause drowsiness. Caution patient to avoid driving or other activities requiring alertness until response to medication is known. Do not resume driving until physician gives clearance based on control of seizures.
- Advise patient to avoid taking alcohol or other CNS depressants concurrently with these medications.
- Advise patient to carry identification describing disease process and medication regimen at all times.

Evaluation/Desired Outcomes

- Decrease or cessation of seizures without excessive sedation.

• ANTIDEPRESSANTS

PHARMACOLOGIC PROFILE

General Use

Used in the treatment of various forms of endogenous depression, often in conjunction with psychotherapy. Other uses include: Treatment of anxiety (doxepin, duloxetine, fluoxetine, paroxetine, sertraline, venlafaxine); Enuresis (imipramine); Chronic pain syndromes (amitriptyline, doxepin, duloxetine, imipramine, nortriptyline); Smoking cessation (bupropion); Bulimia (fluoxetine); Obsessive-compulsive disorder (fluoxetine, fluvoxamine, paroxetine, sertraline); Social anxiety disorder (paroxetine, sertraline, venlafaxine).

General Action and Information

Antidepressant activity is most likely due to preventing the reuptake of dopamine, norepinephrine, and serotonin by presynaptic neurons, resulting in accumulation of these neurotransmitters. The major classes of antidepressants are the tricyclic antidepressants, the selective serotonin reuptake inhibitors (SSRIs), and the serotonin/norepinephrine reuptake inhibitors (SNRIs). Most tricyclic agents possess significant anticholinergic and sedative properties, which explains many of their side effects (amitriptyline, amoxapine, doxepin, imipramine, nortriptyline). The SSRIs are more likely to cause insomnia (fluoxetine, fluvoxamine, paroxetine, sertraline). The SNRIs include desvenlafaxine, duloxetine, levomilnacipran, and venlafaxine.

Contraindications

Hypersensitivity. Should not be used in narrow-angle glaucoma. Should not be used in pregnancy or lactation or immediately after MI.

Precautions

Use cautiously in older patients and those with pre-existing cardiovascular disease. Elderly men with prostatic enlargement may be more susceptible to urinary retention. Anticholinergic side effects of tricyclic antidepressants (dry eyes, dry mouth, blurred vision, and constipation) may require dosage modification or drug discontinuation. Dosage requires slow titration; onset of therapeutic response may be 2–4 wk. May ↓ seizure threshold, especially bupropion.

Interactions

Tricyclic antidepressants—May cause hypertension, tachycardia, and convulsions when used with MAO inhibitors. May prevent therapeutic response to some antihypertensives. Additive CNS depression with other CNS depressants. Sympathomimetic activity may be enhanced when used with other sympathomimetics. Additive anticholinergic effects with other drugs possessing anticholinergic properties. **MAO inhibitors**—Hypertensive crisis may occur with concurrent use of MAO inhibitors and amphetamines, methyldopa, levodopa, dopamine, epinephrine, norepinephrine, desipramine, imipramine, reserpine, vasoconstrictors, or ingestion of tyramine-containing foods. Hypertension or hypotension, coma, convulsions, and death may occur with meperidine or other opioid analgesics and MAO inhibitors. Additive hypotension with antihypertensives or spinal anesthesia and MAO inhibitors. Additive hypoglycemia with insulin or oral hypoglycemic agents and MAO inhibitors. SSRIs, bupropion, or venlafaxine should not be used in combination with or within weeks of MAO inhibitors (see individual monographs). Risk of adverse reactions may be ↑ by almotriptan, frovatriptan, rizatriptan, naratriptan, sumatriptan, or zolmitriptan.

NURSING IMPLICATIONS

Assessment

- Monitor mental status and affect. Assess for suicidal tendencies, especially during early therapy. Restrict amount of drug available to patient.
- **Toxicity and Overdose:** Concurrent ingestion of MAO inhibitors and tyramine-containing foods may lead to hypertensive crisis. Symptoms include chest pain, severe headache, nuchal rigidity, nausea and vomiting, photosensitivity, and enlarged pupils. Treatment includes IV phentolamine.

Potential Nursing Diagnoses

- Ineffective coping (Indications).
- Risk for injury (Side Effects).
- Deficient knowledge, related to disease process and medication regimen (Patient/Family Teaching).

Implementation

- Administer drugs that are sedating at bedtime to avoid excessive drowsiness during waking hours, and administer drugs that cause insomnia (fluoxetine, fluvoxamine, paroxetine, sertraline, MAO inhibitors) in the morning.

Patient/Family Teaching

- Caution patient to avoid alcohol and other CNS depressants. Patients receiving MAO inhibitors should also avoid OTC drugs and foods or beverages containing tyramine (see Appendix J) during and for at least 2 wk after therapy has been discontinued, as they may precipitate a hypertensive crisis. Health care professional should be contacted immediately if symptoms of hypertensive crisis develop.
- Inform patient that dizziness or drowsiness may occur. Caution patient to avoid driving and other activities requiring alertness until response to the drug is known.
- Caution patient to make position changes slowly to minimize orthostatic hypotension.

- Advise patient to notify health care professional if dry mouth, urinary retention, or constipation occurs. Frequent rinses, good oral hygiene, and sugarless candy or gum may diminish dry mouth. An increase in fluid intake, fiber, and exercise may prevent constipation.
- Advise patient to notify health care professional of medication regimen and any herbal alternative therapies before treatment or surgery. MAO inhibitor therapy usually needs to be withdrawn at least 2 wk before use of anesthetic agents.
- Emphasize the importance of participation in psychotherapy and follow-up exams to evaluate progress.

Evaluation/Desired Outcomes

- Resolution of depression.
- Decrease in anxiety.
- Control of bedwetting in children over 6 yr of age.
- Management of chronic neurogenic pain.

• ANTIDIABETICS

PHARMACOLOGIC PROFILE

General Use

Insulin is used in the management of type 1 diabetes mellitus. It may also be used in type 2 diabetes mellitus when diet and/or oral medications fail to adequately control blood sugar. The choice of insulin preparation (rapid-acting, intermediate-acting, long-acting) depends on the degree of control desired, daily blood glucose fluctuations, and history of previous reactions. Oral agents are used primarily in type 2 diabetes mellitus. Oral agents are used when diet therapy alone fails to control blood glucose or symptoms or when patients are not amenable to using insulin. Some oral agents may be used with insulin.

General Action and Information

Insulin, a hormone produced by the pancreas, lowers blood glucose by ↑ transport of glucose into cells and promotes the conversion of glucose to glycogen. It also promotes the conversion of amino acids to proteins in muscle, stimulates triglyceride formation, and inhibits the release of free fatty acids. Sulfonylureas, nateglinide, repaglinide, the dipeptidyl peptidase IV inhibitors (e.g. sitagliptin), and the glucagon-like peptide-1 receptor agonists (e.g. exenatide) ↓ blood glucose by stimulating endogenous insulin secretion by beta cells of the pancreas and by ↑ sensitivity to insulin at intracellular receptor sites. Intact pancreatic function is required. Miglitol delays digestion of ingested carbohydrates, thus lowering blood glucose, especially after meals. It may be combined with sulfonylureas. Pioglitazone, rosiglitazone, and metformin ↑ insulin sensitivity.

Contraindications

Insulin—Hypoglycemia. **Oral hypoglycemic agents**—Hypersensitivity (cross-sensitivity with other sulfonylureas and sulfonamides may exist). Hypoglycemia. Type 1 diabetes. Avoid use in patients with severe kidney, liver, thyroid, and other endocrine dysfunction. Should not be used in pregnancy or lactation.

Precautions

Insulin—Infection, stress, or changes in diet may alter requirements. **Oral hypoglycemic agents**—Use cautiously in geriatric patients. Dose ↓ may be necessary. Infection, stress, or changes in diet may alter requirements. Use with sulfonylureas with caution in patients with a history of cardiovascular disease. Metformin may cause lactic acidosis.

Interactions

Insulin—Additive hypoglycemic effects with oral hypoglycemic agents. **Oral hypoglycemic agents**—Ingestion of alcohol may result in disulfiram-like reaction with some agents. Alcohol, corticosteroids, rifampin, glucagon, and thiazide diuretics may ↓ effectiveness. Anabolic steroids, chloramphenicol, MAO inhibitors, most NSAIDs, salicylates, sulfonamides, and warfarin may ↑ hypoglycemic effect. Beta blockers may produce hypoglycemia and mask signs and symptoms.

NURSING IMPLICATIONS

Assessment

- Observe patient for signs and symptoms of hypoglycemic reactions.
- Acarbose, miglitol, and pioglitazone do not cause hypoglycemia when taken alone but may ↑ the hypoglycemic effect of other hypoglycemic agents.
- Patients who have been well controlled on metformin but develop illness or laboratory abnormalities should be assessed for ketoacidosis or lactic acidosis. Assess serum electrolytes, ketones, glucose, and, if indicated, blood pH, lactate, pyruvate, and metformin levels. If either form of acidosis is present, discontinue metformin immediately and treat acidosis.
- **Lab Test Considerations:** Serum glucose and glycosylated hemoglobin should be monitored periodically throughout therapy to evaluate effectiveness of treatment.

Potential Nursing Diagnoses

- Imbalanced nutrition: more than body requirements (Indications).
- Deficient knowledge, related to medication regimen (Patient/Family Teaching).
- Noncompliance (Patient/Family Teaching).

Implementation

- Patients stabilized on a diabetic regimen who are exposed to stress, fever, trauma, infection, or surgery may require sliding scale insulin. Withhold oral hypoglycemic agents and reinstitute after resolution of acute episode.
- Patients switching from daily insulin dose may require gradual conversion to oral hypoglycemics.
- **Insulin:** Available in different types and strengths and from different species. Check type, species, source, dose, and expiration date with another licensed nurse. Do not interchange insulins without physician's order. Use only insulin syringes to draw up dose. Use only U100 syringes to draw up insulin lispro dose.

Patient/Family Teaching

- Explain to patient that medication controls hyperglycemia but does not cure diabetes. Therapy is long-term.
- Review signs of hypoglycemia and hyperglycemia with patient. If hypoglycemia occurs, advise patient to take a glass of orange juice or 2–3 tsp of sugar, honey, or corn syrup dissolved in water (glucose, not table sugar, if taking miglitol), and notify health care professional.
- Encourage patient to follow prescribed diet, medication, and exercise regimen to prevent hypoglycemic or hyperglycemic episodes.
- Instruct patient in proper testing of serum glucose and ketones.
- Advise patient to notify health care professional if nausea, vomiting, or fever develops; if unable to eat usual diet; or if blood glucose levels are not controlled.
- Advise patient to carry sugar or a form of glucose and identification describing medication regimen at all times.
- Insulin is the recommended method of controlling blood glucose during pregnancy. Counsel female patients to use a form of contraception other than oral contraceptives and to notify health care professional promptly if pregnancy is planned or suspected.
- **Insulin:** Instruct patient on proper technique for administration; include type of insulin, equipment (syringe and cartridge pens), storage, and syringe disposal. Discuss the importance of not changing brands of insulin or syringes, selection and rotation of injection sites, and compliance with therapeutic regimen.
- **Sulfonylureas:** Advise patient that concurrent use of alcohol may cause a disulfiram-like reaction (abdominal cramps, nausea, flushing, headache, and hypoglycemia).

- **Metformin:** Explain to patient the risk of lactic acidosis and the potential need for discontinuation of metformin therapy if a severe infection, dehydration, or severe or continuing diarrhea occurs or if medical tests or surgery is required.

Evaluation/Desired Outcomes

- Control of blood glucose levels without the appearance of hypoglycemic or hyperglycemic episodes.

• ANTIDIARRHEALS

PHARMACOLOGIC PROFILE

General Use

For the control and symptomatic relief of acute and chronic nonspecific diarrhea.

General Action and Information

Diphenoxylate/atropine, difenoxin/atropine, and loperamide slow intestinal motility and propulsion. Bismuth subsalicylate affects fluid content of the stool. Bismuth subsalicylate is also used as part of the management of ulcer disease due to *Helicobacter pylori*. Polycarbophil acts as an antidiarrheal by taking on water within the bowel lumen to create a formed stool. Polycarbophil may also be used to treat constipation. Octreotide is used specifically for diarrhea associated with GI endocrine tumors.

Contraindications

Previous hypersensitivity. Severe abdominal pain of unknown cause, especially when associated with fever.

Precautions

Use cautiously in patients with severe liver disease or inflammatory bowel disease. Safety in pregnancy and lactation not established (diphenoxylate/atropine and loperamide). Octreotide may aggravate gallbladder disease.

Interactions

Polycarbophil ↓ the absorption of tetracycline. Octreotide may alter the response to insulin or oral hypoglycemic agents.

NURSING IMPLICATIONS

Assessment

- Assess the frequency and consistency of stools and bowel sounds before and throughout therapy.
- Assess patient's fluid and electrolyte status and skin turgor for dehydration.

Potential Nursing Diagnoses

- Diarrhea (Indications).
- Constipation (Side Effects).
- Deficient knowledge, related to disease process and medication regimen (Patient/Family Teaching).

Implementation

- Shake liquid preparations before administration.

Patient/Family Teaching

- Instruct patient to notify health care professional if diarrhea persists; or if fever, abdominal pain, or palpitations occur.

Evaluation/Desired Outcomes
- Decrease in diarrhea.

• ANTIEMETICS

PHARMACOLOGIC PROFILE

General Use
Phenothiazines, dolasetron, granisetron, metoclopramide, ondansetron, and palonosetron are used to manage nausea and vomiting of many causes, including surgery, anesthesia, and antineoplastic and radiation therapy. Aprepitant is used specifically with emetogenic chemotherapy. Dimenhydrinate, scopolamine, and meclizine are used almost exclusively to prevent motion sickness.

General Action and Information
Phenothiazines act on the chemoreceptor trigger zone to inhibit nausea and vomiting. Dimenhydrinate, scopolamine, and meclizine act as antiemetics mainly by diminishing motion sickness. Metoclopramide ↓ nausea and vomiting by its effects on gastric emptying. Dolasetron, granisetron, palonosetron, and ondansetron block the effects of serotonin at 5-HT_3 receptor sites. Aprepitant acts as a selective antagonist at substance P/neurokinin 1 receptors in the brain.

Contraindications
Previous hypersensitivity.

Precautions
Use phenothiazines cautiously in children who may have viral illnesses. Choose agents carefully in pregnant patients (no agents are approved for safe use).

Interactions
Additive CNS depression with other CNS depressants including antidepressants, antihistamines, opioid analgesics, and sedative/hypnotics. Phenothiazines may produce hypotension when used with antihypertensives, nitrates, or acute ingestion of alcohol.

NURSING IMPLICATIONS

Assessment
- Assess nausea, vomiting, bowel sounds, and abdominal pain before and following administration.
- Monitor hydration status and intake and output. Patients with severe nausea and vomiting may require IV fluids in addition to antiemetics.

Potential Nursing Diagnoses
- Deficient fluid volume (Indications).
- Imbalanced nutrition: less than body requirements (Indications).
- Risk for injury (Side Effects).

Implementation
- For prophylactic administration, follow directions for specific drugs so that peak effect corresponds to time of anticipated nausea.
- Phenothiazines should be discontinued 48 hr before and not resumed for 24 hr following myelography, as they lower seizure threshold.

Patient/Family Teaching
- Advise patient and family to use general measures to decrease nausea (begin with sips of liquids and small, nongreasy meals; provide oral hygiene; and remove noxious stimuli from environment).

- May cause drowsiness. Advise patient to call for assistance when ambulating and to avoid driving or other activities requiring alertness until response to medication is known.
- Advise patient to make position changes slowly to minimize orthostatic hypotension.

Evaluation/Desired Outcomes

- Prevention of, or decrease in, nausea and vomiting.

• ANTIFUNGALS

PHARMACOLOGIC PROFILE

General Use

Treatment of fungal infections. Infections of skin or mucous membranes may be treated with topical or vaginal preparations. Deep-seated or systemic infections require oral or parenteral therapy. New parenteral formulations of amphotericin employ lipid encapsulation technology designed to decrease toxicity.

General Action and Information

Kill (fungicidal) or stop growth of (fungistatic) susceptible fungi by affecting the permeability of the fungal cell membrane or protein synthesis within the fungal cell itself.

Contraindications

Previous hypersensitivity.

Precautions

Because most systemic antifungals may have adverse effects on bone marrow function, use cautiously in patients with depressed bone marrow reserve. Amphotericin B commonly causes renal impairment. Fluconazole requires dosage adjustment in the presence of renal impairment. Adverse reactions to fluconazole may be more severe in HIV-positive patients.

Interactions

Differ greatly among various agents. See individual drugs.

NURSING IMPLICATIONS

Assessment

- Assess patient for signs of infection and assess involved areas of skin and mucous membranes before and throughout therapy. Increased skin irritation may indicate need to discontinue medication.

Potential Nursing Diagnoses

- Risk for infection (Indications).
- Impaired skin integrity (Indications).
- Deficient knowledge, related to disease process and medication regimen (Patient/Family Teaching).

Implementation

- Available in various dosage forms. Refer to specific drugs for directions for administration..
- **Topical:** Consult physician or other health care professional for cleansing technique before applying medication. Wear gloves during application. Do not use occlusive dressings unless specified by physician or other health care professional.

Patient/Family Teaching

- Instruct patient on proper use of medication form.
- Instruct patient to continue medication as directed for full course of therapy, even if feeling better.

- Advise patient to report increased skin irritation or lack of therapeutic response to health care professional.

Evaluation/Desired Outcomes

- Resolution of signs and symptoms of infection. Length of time for complete resolution depends on organism and site of infection. Deep-seated fungal infections may require prolonged therapy (weeks–months). Recurrent fungal infections may be a sign of serious systemic illness.

• ANTIHISTAMINES

PHARMACOLOGIC PROFILE

General Use

Relief of symptoms associated with allergies, including rhinitis, urticaria, and angioedema, and as adjunctive therapy in anaphylactic reactions. Some antihistamines are used to treat motion sickness (dimenhydrinate and meclizine), insomnia (diphenhydramine), Parkinson-like reactions (diphenhydramine), and other nonallergic conditions.

General Action and Information

Antihistamines block the effects of histamine at the H_1 receptor. They do not block histamine release, antibody production, or antigen-antibody reactions. Most antihistamines have anticholinergic properties and may cause constipation, dry eyes, dry mouth, and blurred vision. In addition, many antihistamines cause sedation. Some phenothiazines have strong antihistaminic properties (hydroxyzine and promethazine).

Contraindications

Hypersensitivity and angle-closure glaucoma. Should not be used in premature or newborn infants.

Precautions

Elderly patients may be more susceptible to adverse anticholinergic effects of antihistamines. Use cautiously in patients with pyloric obstruction, prostatic hypertrophy, hyperthyroidism, cardiovascular disease, or severe liver disease. Use cautiously in pregnancy and lactation.

Interactions

Additive sedation when used with other CNS depressants, including alcohol, antidepressants, opioid analgesics, and sedative/hypnotics. MAO inhibitors prolong and intensify the anticholinergic properties of antihistamines.

NURSING IMPLICATIONS

Assessment

- Assess allergy symptoms (rhinitis, conjunctivitis, hives) before and periodically throughout therapy.
- Monitor pulse and BP before initiating and throughout IV therapy.
- Assess lung sounds and character of bronchial secretions. Maintain fluid intake of 1500–2000 mL/day to decrease viscosity of secretions.
- **Nausea and Vomiting:** Assess degree of nausea and frequency and amount of emesis when administering for nausea and vomiting.
- **Anxiety:** Assess mental status, mood, and behavior when administering for anxiety.
- **Pruritus:** Observe the character, location, and size of affected area when administering for pruritic skin conditions.

Potential Nursing Diagnoses

- Ineffective airway clearance (Indications).
- Risk for injury (Adverse Reactions).
- Deficient knowledge, related to disease process and medication regimen (Patient/Family Teaching).

Implementation

- When used for prophylaxis of motion sickness, administer at least 30 min and preferably 1–2 hr before exposure to conditions that may precipitate motion sickness.
- When administering concurrently with opioid analgesics (hydroxyzine, promethazine), supervise ambulation closely to prevent injury secondary to increased sedation.

Patient/Family Teaching

- Inform patient that drowsiness may occur. Avoid driving or other activities requiring alertness until response to drug is known.
- Caution patient to avoid using concurrent alcohol or CNS depressants.
- Advise patient that good oral hygiene, frequent rinsing of mouth with water, and sugarless gum or candy may help relieve dryness of mouth.
- Instruct patient to contact health care professional if symptoms persist.

Evaluation/Desired Outcomes

- Decrease in allergic symptoms.
- Prevention or decreased severity of nausea and vomiting.
- Decrease in anxiety.
- Relief of pruritus.
- Sedation when used as a hypnotic.

• ANTIHYPERTENSIVES

PHARMACOLOGIC PROFILE

General Use

Treatment of hypertension of many causes, most commonly essential hypertension. Parenteral products are used in the treatment of hypertensive emergencies. Oral treatment should be initiated as soon as possible and individualized to ensure adherence and compliance for long-term therapy. Therapy is initiated with agents having minimal side effects. When such therapy fails, more potent drugs with different side effects are added in an effort to control BP while causing minimal patient discomfort.

General Action and Information

As a group, the antihypertensives are used to lower BP to a normal level (<130–140 systolic and <80–90 mm Hg diastolic) or to the lowest level tolerated. The goal of antihypertensive therapy is prevention of end-organ damage. Antihypertensives are classified into groups according to their site of action. These include alpha-1 receptor antagonists, centrally-acting alpha-adrenergic agonists; beta blockers; vasodilators; ACE inhibitors; angiotensin II receptor antagonists; calcium channel blockers; aliskiren; and diuretics. Hypertensive emergencies may be managed with parenteral agents, such as enalaprilat or fenoldopam.

Contraindications

Hypersensitivity to individual agents.

Precautions

Choose agents carefully in pregnancy and during lactation. ACE inhibitors, angiotensin II receptor antagonists, and aliskiren should be avoided during pregnancy. Centrally acting alpha-adrenergic agonists and beta blockers should be used only in patients who will comply, because abrupt discontinuation of these agents may result in rapid and excessive rise in BP (rebound phenomenon). Thiazide diuretics may ↑ the requirement for treatment of patients with diabetes. Vasodilators may cause tachycardia if used alone and are commonly used in combination with beta blockers. Some antihypertensives cause sodium and water retention and are usually combined with a diuretic.

Interactions

Many drugs can negate the therapeutic effectiveness of antihypertensives, including NSAIDs, sympathomimetics, decongestants, appetite suppressants, antidepressants, and MAO inhibitors. Hypokalemia from diuretics may ↑ the risk of digoxin toxicity. Potassium supplements and potassium-sparing diuretics may cause hyperkalemia when used with ACE inhibitors, angiotensin II receptor antagonists, or aliskiren.

NURSING IMPLICATIONS

Assessment

- Monitor BP and pulse frequently during dosage adjustment and periodically throughout therapy.
- Monitor intake and output ratios and daily weight.
- Monitor frequency of prescription refills to determine compliance.

Potential Nursing Diagnoses

- Ineffective tissue perfusion (Indications).
- Deficient knowledge, related to disease process and medication regimen (Patient/Family Teaching).
- Noncompliance (Patient/Family Teaching).

Implementation

- Many antihypertensives are available as combination products to enhance compliance (see Appendix B).

Patient/Family Teaching

- Instruct patient to continue taking medication, even if feeling well. Abrupt withdrawal may cause rebound hypertension. Medication controls, but does not cure, hypertension.
- Encourage patient to comply with additional interventions for hypertension (weight reduction, low-sodium diet, regular exercise, discontinuation of smoking, moderation of alcohol consumption, and stress management).
- Instruct patient and family on proper technique for monitoring BP. Advise them to check BP weekly and report significant changes.
- Caution patient to make position changes slowly to minimize orthostatic hypotension. Advise patient that exercise or hot weather may enhance hypotensive effects.
- Advise patient to consult health care professional before taking any OTC medications, especially cold remedies.
- Advise patient to inform health care professional of medication regimen before treatment or surgery.
- Patients taking ACE inhibitors, angiotensin II antagonists, or aliskiren should notify health care professional if pregnancy is planned or suspected.
- Emphasize the importance of follow-up exams to monitor progress.

Evaluation/Desired Outcomes

- Decrease in BP.

• ANTI-INFECTIVES

PHARMACOLOGIC PROFILE

General Use
Treatment and prophylaxis of various bacterial infections. See specific drugs for spectrum and indications. Some infections may require additional surgical intervention and supportive therapy.

General Action and Information
Kill (bactericidal) or inhibit the growth of (bacteriostatic) susceptible pathogenic bacteria. Not active against viruses or fungi. Anti-infectives are subdivided into categories depending on chemical similarities and antimicrobial spectrum.

Contraindications
Known hypersensitivity to individual agents. Cross-sensitivity among related agents may occur.

Precautions
Culture and susceptibility testing are desirable to optimize therapy. Dosage modification may be required in patients with hepatic or renal insufficiency. Use cautiously in pregnant and lactating women. Prolonged inappropriate use of broad spectrum anti-infective agents may lead to superinfection with fungi or resistant bacteria.

Interactions
Penicillins and aminoglycosides chemically inactivate each other and should not be physically admixed. Erythromycin and clarithromycin may ↓ hepatic metabolism of other drugs. Probenecid ↑ serum levels of penicillins and related compounds. Highly protein-bound anti-infectives such as sulfonamides may displace or be displaced by other highly bound drugs. See individual drugs. Extended-spectrum penicillins (ticarcillin, piperacillin) and some cephalosporins (cefoperazone, cefotetan) may ↑ the risk of bleeding with anticoagulants, thrombolytic agents, antiplatelet agents, or NSAIDs. Fluoroquinolone absorption may be ↓ by antacids, bismuth subsalicylate, calcium, iron salts, sucralfate, and zinc salts.

NURSING IMPLICATIONS

Assessment
- Assess patient for signs and symptoms of infection prior to and throughout therapy.
- Determine previous hypersensitivities in patients receiving penicillins or cephalosporins.
- Obtain specimens for culture and sensitivity prior to initiating therapy. First dose may be given before receiving results.

Potential Nursing Diagnoses
- Risk for infection (Indications).
- Deficient knowledge, related to disease process and medication regimen (Patient/Family Teaching).
- Noncompliance (Patient/Family Teaching).

Implementation
- Most anti-infectives should be administered around the clock to maintain therapeutic serum drug levels.

Patient/Family Teaching
- Instruct patient to continue taking medication around the clock until finished completely, even if feeling better.
- Advise patient to report the signs of superinfection (black, furry overgrowth on the tongue; vaginal itching or discharge; loose or foul-smelling stools) and allergy to health care professional.

- Instruct patient to notify health care professional if fever and diarrhea develop, especially if stool contains pus, blood, or mucus. Advise patient not to treat diarrhea without consulting health care professional.
- Instruct patient to notify health care professional if symptoms do not improve.

Evaluation/Desired Outcomes

- Resolution of the signs and symptoms of infection. Length of time for complete resolution depends on organism and site of infection.

• ANTINEOPLASTICS

PHARMACOLOGIC PROFILE

General Use

Used in the treatment of various solid tumors, lymphomas, and leukemias. Also used in some autoimmune disorders such as rheumatoid arthritis (cyclophosphamide, methotrexate). Often used in combinations to minimize individual toxicities and ↑ response. Chemotherapy may be combined with other treatment modalities such as surgery and radiation therapy. Dosages vary greatly, depending on extent of disease, other agents used, and patient's condition. Some agents (daunorubicin, doxorubicin) are available in lipid-based formulations that have less toxicity with greater efficacy.

General Action and Information

Act by many different mechanisms (see the following table). Many affect DNA synthesis or function; others alter immune function or affect hormonal status of sensitive tumors. Action may not be limited to neoplastic cells.

MECHANISM OF ACTION OF VARIOUS ANTINEOPLASTICS

MECHANISM OF ACTION	AGENT	EFFECTS ON CELL CYCLE
ALKYLATING AGENTS Cause cross-linking of DNA	busulfan carboplatin chlorambucil cisplatin cyclophosphamide ifosfamide mechlorethamine melphalan procarbazine temozolamide	Cell cycle–nonspecific
ANTHRACYCLINES Interfere with DNA and RNA synthesis	daunorubicin doxorubicin epirubicin idarubicin	Cell cycle–nonspecific
ANTITUMOR ANTIBIOTIC	bleomycin	Cell cycle–nonspecific (except bleomycin)
Interfere with DNA and RNA synthesis	mitomycin mitoxantrone	
ANTIMETABOLITES	cytarabine	Cell cycle–specific, work mostly in S phase (DNA synthesis)
Take the place of normal proteins	fluorouracil hydroxyurea methotrexate	
ENZYMES Deplete asparagine	asparaginase pegaspargase	Cell-cycle phase–specific
ENZYME INHIBITORS Inhibits topoisomerase	irinotecan topotecan	Cell-cycle phase–specific
Inhibits kinase	imatinib	Unknown
HORMONAL AGENTS	bicalutamide	Unknown

(continued) MECHANISM OF ACTION OF VARIOUS ANTINEOPLASTICS

MECHANISM OF ACTION	AGENT	EFFECTS ON CELL CYCLE
Alter hormonal status in tumors that are sensitive	estramustine	
	flutamide	
	leuprolide	
	megestrol	
	nilutamide	
	tamoxifen	
	testosterone (androgens)	
	triptorelin	
HORMONAL AGENTS—AROMATASE INHIBITORS	anastrazole	Unknown
Inhibit enzyme responsible for activating estrogen	letrozole	
IMMUNE MODULATORS	aldesleukin	Unknown
	alemtuzumab	
	gemtuzumab	
	toremifene	
	trastuzumab	
PODOPHYLLOTOXIN DERIVATIVES	etoposide	Cell-cycle phase–specific
Damages DNA before mitosis		
TAXOIDS	docetaxel	Cell-cycle phase–specific
Interupt interphase and mitosis	paclitaxel	
VINCA ALKALOIDS	vinblastine	Cell cycle–specific, work during M phase (mitosis)
Interfere with mitosis	vinCRIStine	
	vinorelbine	
MISCELLANEOUS	aldesleukin	Unknown
	altretamine	Unknown

Contraindications

Previous bone marrow depression or hypersensitivity. Contraindicated in pregnancy and lactation.

Precautions

Use cautiously in patients with active infections, ↓ bone marrow reserve, radiation therapy, or other debilitating illnesses. Use cautiously in patients with childbearing potential.

Interactions

Allopurinol ↓ metabolism of mercaptopurine. Toxicity from methotrexate may be ↑ by other nephrotoxic drugs or larger doses of aspirin or NSAIDs. Bone marrow depression is additive. See individual drugs.

NURSING IMPLICATIONS

Assessment

- Monitor for bone marrow depression. Assess for bleeding (bleeding gums, bruising, petechiae, guaiac stools, urine, and emesis) and avoid IM injections and rectal temperatures if platelet count is low. Apply pressure to venipuncture sites for 10 min. Assess for signs of infection during neutropenia. Anemia may occur. Monitor for ↑ fatigue, dyspnea, and orthostatic hypotension.
- Monitor intake and output ratios, appetite, and nutritional intake. Prophylactic antiemetics may be used. Adjusting diet as tolerated may help maintain fluid and electrolyte balance and nutritional status.
- Monitor IV site carefully and ensure patency. Discontinue infusion immediately if discomfort, erythema along vein, or infiltration occurs. Tissue ulceration and necrosis may result from infiltration.
- Monitor for symptoms of gout (↑ uric acid, joint pain, and edema). Encourage patient to drink at least 2 L of fluid each day. Allopurinol may be given to ↓ uric acid levels. Alkalinization of urine may be ordered to ↑ excretion of uric acid.

Potential Nursing Diagnoses

- Risk for infection (Side Effects).
- Imbalanced nutrition: less than body requirements (Adverse Reactions).
- Deficient knowledge, related to disease process and medication regimen (Patient/Family Teaching).

Implementation

- Solutions for injection should be prepared in a biologic cabinet. Wear gloves, gown, and mask while handling medication. Discard equipment in designated containers.
- Check dose carefully. Fatalities have resulted from dosing errors.

Patient/Family Teaching

- Caution patient to avoid crowds and persons with known infections. Health care professional should be informed immediately if symptoms of infection occur.
- Instruct patient to report unusual bleeding. Advise patient of thrombocytopenia precautions.
- These drugs may cause gonadal suppression; however, patient should still use birth control, as most antineoplastics are teratogenic. Advise patient to inform health care professional immediately if pregnancy is suspected.
- Discuss with patient the possibility of hair loss. Explore methods of coping.
- Instruct patient to inspect oral mucosa for erythema and ulceration. If ulceration occurs, advise patient to use sponge brush and to rinse mouth with water after eating and drinking. Topical agents may be used if mouth pain interferes with eating. Stomatitis pain may require treatment with opioid analgesics.
- Instruct patient not to receive any vaccinations without advice of health care professional. Antineoplastics may ↓ antibody response and ↑ risk of adverse reactions.
- Advise patient of need for medical follow-up and frequent lab tests.

Evaluation/Desired Outcomes

- Decrease in size and spread of tumor.
- Improvement in hematologic status in patients with leukemia.

• ANTIPARKINSON AGENTS

PHARMACOLOGIC PROFILE

General Use

Used in the treatment of Parkinson's disease.

General Action and Information

Drugs used in the treatment of Parkinson's disease and other dyskinesias are aimed at restoring the natural balance of two major neurotransmitters in the CNS: acetylcholine and dopamine. The imbalance is a deficiency in dopamine that results in excessive cholinergic activity. Drugs used are either anticholinergics (benztropine, biperiden, and trihexyphenidyl) or dopaminergic agonists (bromocriptine, levodopa/carbidopa, pramipexole, ropinirole). Entacapone and tolcapone inhibit the enzyme that breaks down levodopa, thereby enhancing its effects.

Contraindications

Anticholinergics should be avoided in patients with angle-closure glaucoma.

Precautions

Use cautiously in patients with severe cardiac disease, pyloric obstruction, or prostatic enlargement.

Interactions

Pyridoxine, MAO inhibitors, benzodiazepines, phenytoin, phenothiazines, and haloperidol may antagonize the effects of levodopa. Agents that antagonize dopamine (phenothiazines, metoclopramide) may ↓ effectiveness of dopamine agonists.

NURSING IMPLICATIONS

Assessment

- Assess parkinsonian and extrapyramidal symptoms (akinesia, rigidity, tremors, pill rolling, mask facies, shuffling gait, muscle spasms, twisting motions, and drooling) before and throughout course of therapy. On-off phenomenon may cause symptoms to appear or improve suddenly.
- Monitor BP frequently during therapy. Instruct patient to remain supine during and for several hours after first dose of bromocriptine, as severe hypotension may occur.

Potential Nursing Diagnoses

- Impaired physical mobility (Indications).
- Risk for injury (Indications).
- Deficient knowledge, related to disease process and medication regimen (Patient/Family Teaching).

Implementation

- In the carbidopa/levodopa combination, the number following the drug name represents the milligram of each respective drug.

Patient/Family Teaching

- May cause drowsiness or dizziness. Advise patient to avoid driving or other activities that require alertness until response to medication is known.
- Caution patient to make position changes slowly to minimize orthostatic hypotension.
- Instruct patient that frequent rinsing of mouth, good oral hygiene, and sugarless gum or candy may decrease dry mouth. Patient should notify health care professional if dryness persists (saliva substitutes may be used). Also notify the dentist if dryness interferes with use of dentures.
- Advise patient to confer with health care professional before taking OTC medications, especially cold remedies, or drinking alcoholic beverages. Patients receiving levodopa should avoid multivitamins. Vitamin B_6 (pyridoxine) may interfere with levodopa's action.
- Caution patient that decreased perspiration may occur. Overheating may occur during hot weather. Patients should remain indoors in an air-conditioned environment during hot weather.
- Advise patient to increase activity, bulk, and fluid in diet to minimize constipating effects of medication.
- Advise patient to notify health care professional if confusion, rash, urinary retention, severe constipation, visual changes, or worsening of parkinsonian symptoms occur.

Evaluation/Desired Outcomes

- Resolution of parkinsonian signs and symptoms
- Resolution of drug-induced extrapyramidal symptoms.

• ANTIPLATELET AGENTS

PHARMACOLOGIC PROFILE

General Use

Antiplatelet agents are used to treat and prevent thromboembolic events such as stroke and MI.

General Action and Information
Inhibit platelet aggregation, prolong bleeding time, and are used to prevent MI or stroke (aspirin, clopidogrel, dipyridamole, ticlopidine, prasugrel, ticagrelor). Eptifibatide, abciximab, and tirofiban are used in the management of acute coronary syndromes. These agents are often used concurrently/sequentially with anticoagulants and thrombolytics.

Contraindications
Hypersensitivity, ulcer disease, active bleeding, and recent surgery.

Precautions
Use cautiously in patients at risk for bleeding (trauma, surgery). History of GI bleeding or ulcer disease. Safety not established in pregnancy, lactation, or children.

Interactions
Concurrent use with NSAIDs, heparin, thrombolytics, or warfarin may ↑ the risk of bleeding.

NURSING IMPLICATIONS

Assessment
- Assess patient for evidence of additional or ↑ thrombosis. Symptoms will depend on area of involvement.
- Assess patient taking antiplatelet agents for symptoms of stroke, peripheral vascular disease, or MI periodically throughout therapy.
- **Lab Test Considerations:** Monitor bleeding time throughout antiplatelet therapy. Prolonged bleeding time, which is time- and dose-dependent, is expected.

Potential Nursing Diagnoses
- Ineffective tissue perfusion (Indications).
- Risk for injury (Side Effects).
- Deficient knowledge, related to disease process and medication regimen (Patient/Family Teaching).

Implementation
- Use an infusion pump with continuous infusions to ensure accurate dosage.

Patient/Family Teaching
- Instruct patient to notify health care professional immediately if any bleeding is noted.

Evaluation/Desired Outcomes
- Prevention of stroke, MI, and vascular death in patients at risk.

• ANTIPSYCHOTICS

PHARMACOLOGIC PROFILE

General Use
Treatment of acute and chronic psychoses, particularly when accompanied by ↑ psychomotor activity. Use of clozapine is limited to schizophrenia unresponsive to conventional therapy. Selected agents are also used as antihistamines or antiemetics. Chlorpromazine is also used in the treatment of intractable hiccups.

General Action and Information
Block dopamine receptors in the brain; also alter dopamine release and turnover. Peripheral effects include anticholinergic properties and alpha-adrenergic blockade. Most antipsychotics are phenothiazines except for haloperidol, which is a butyrophenone, and clozapine, which is a miscellaneous compound. Newer "atypical" agents such as olanzapine, quetiapine, risperidone, and ari-

piprazole may have fewer adverse reactions. Phenothiazines differ in their ability to produce sedation (greatest with chlorpromazine and thioridazine), extrapyramidal reactions (greatest with prochlorperazine and trifluoperazine), and anticholinergic effects (greatest with chlorpromazine).

Contraindications

Hypersensitivity. Cross-sensitivity may exist among phenothiazines. Should not be used in angle-closure glaucoma. Should not be used in patients who have CNS depression.

Precautions

Safety in pregnancy and lactation not established. Use cautiously in patients with symptomatic cardiac disease. Avoid exposure to extremes in temperature. Use cautiously in severely ill or debilitated patients and patients with respiratory insufficiency, diabetes, prostatic hypertrophy, or intestinal obstruction. May ↓ seizure threshold. Clozapine may cause agranulocytosis. Most agents are capable of causing neuroleptic malignant syndrome. Should not be used routinely for anxiety or agitation not related to psychoses.

Interactions

Additive hypotension with acute ingestion of alcohol, antihypertensives, or nitrates. Antacids may ↓ absorption. Phenobarbital may ↑ metabolism and ↓ effectiveness. Additive CNS depression with other CNS depressants, including alcohol, antihistamines, antidepressants, opioid analgesics, or sedative/hypnotics. Lithium may ↓ blood levels and effectiveness of phenothiazines. May ↓ the therapeutic response to levodopa. May ↑ the risk of agranulocytosis with antithyroid agents.

NURSING IMPLICATIONS

Assessment

- Assess patient's mental status (orientation, mood, behavior) before and periodically throughout therapy.
- Monitor BP (sitting, standing, lying), pulse, and respiratory rate before and frequently during the period of dosage adjustment.
- Observe patient carefully when administering medication to ensure medication is actually taken and not hoarded.
- Monitor patient for onset of *akathisia*—restlessness or desire to keep moving—and extrapyramidal side effects; *parkinsonian*—difficulty speaking or swallowing, loss of balance control, pill rolling, mask-like face, shuffling gait, rigidity, tremors; and *dystonia*—muscle spasms, twisting motions, twitching, inability to move eyes, weakness of arms or legs—every 2 mo during therapy and 8–12 wk after therapy has been discontinued. Parkinsonian effects are more common in geriatric patients and dystonias are more common in younger patients. Notify health care professional if these symptoms occur, as ↓ in dosage or discontinuation of medication may be necessary. Trihexyphenidyl, benztropine, or diphenhydramine may be used to control these symptoms.
- Monitor for *tardive dyskinesia*—uncontrolled rhythmic movement of mouth, face, and extremities; lip smacking or puckering; puffing of cheeks; uncontrolled chewing; rapid or worm-like movements of tongue. Notify health care professional immediately if these symptoms occur; these side effects may be irreversible.
- Monitor for development of *neuroleptic malignant syndrome*—fever, respiratory distress, tachycardia, convulsions, diaphoresis, hypertension or hypotension, pallor, tiredness, severe muscle stiffness, loss of bladder control. Notify health care professional immediately if these symptoms occur.

Potential Nursing Diagnoses

- Disturbed thought process (Indications).
- Deficient knowledge, related to disease process and medication regimen (Patient/Family Teaching).
- Noncompliance (Patient/Family Teaching).

Implementation

- Keep patient recumbent for at least 30 min following parenteral administration to minimize hypotensive effects.
- Phenothiazines should be discontinued 48 hr before and not resumed for 24 hr following myelography, as they ↓ the seizure threshold.
- **PO:** Administer with **food**, **milk**, or a full glass of **water** to minimize gastric irritation.
- Dilute most concentrates in 120 mL of distilled or acidified tap water or **fruit juice** just before administration.

Patient/Family Teaching

- Advise patient to take medication exactly as directed and not to skip doses or double up on missed doses. Abrupt withdrawal may lead to gastritis, nausea, vomiting, dizziness, headache, tachycardia, and insomnia.
- Advise patient to make position changes slowly to minimize orthostatic hypotension.
- Medication may cause drowsiness. Caution patient to avoid driving or other activities requiring alertness until response to the medication is known.
- Caution patient to avoid taking alcohol or other CNS depressants concurrently with this medication.
- Advise patient to use sunscreen and protective clothing when exposed to the sun to prevent photosensitivity reactions. Extremes of temperature should also be avoided, as these drugs impair body temperature regulation.
- Advise patient that ↑ activity, bulk, and fluids in the diet helps minimize the constipating effects of this medication.
- Instruct patient to use frequent mouth rinses, good oral hygiene, and sugarless gum or candy to minimize dry mouth.
- Advise patient to notify health care professional of medication regimen before treatment or surgery.
- Emphasize the importance of routine follow-up exams and continued participation in psychotherapy as indicated.

Evaluation/Desired Outcomes

- Decrease in excitable, paranoic, or withdrawn behavior. Relief of nausea and vomiting. Relief of intractable hiccups.

• ANTIPYRETICS

PHARMACOLOGIC PROFILE

General Use

Used to lower fever of many causes (infection and inflammation).

General Action and Information

Antipyretics lower fever by affecting thermoregulation in the CNS and by inhibiting the action of prostaglandins peripherally. Many antipyretics affect platelet function; of these, aspirin has the most profound effect as compared with other salicylates, ibuprofen, or ketoprofen.

Contraindications

Avoid aspirin, ibuprofen, or ketoprofen in patients with bleeding disorders (risk of bleeding is less with other salicylates). Aspirin and other salicylates should be avoided in children and adolescents.

Precautions

Use aspirin, ibuprofen, or ketoprofen cautiously in patients with ulcer disease. Avoid chronic use of large doses of acetaminophen.

Interactions

Large doses of aspirin may displace other highly protein-bound drugs. Additive GI irritation with aspirin, ibuprofen, ketoprofen, and other NSAIDs or corticosteroids. Aspirin, ibuprofen, ketoprofen, or naproxen may ↑ the risk of bleeding with other agents affecting hemostasis (anticoagulants, thrombolytic agents, antiplatelets, and antineoplastics).

NURSING IMPLICATIONS

Assessment

- Assess fever; note presence of associated symptoms (diaphoresis, tachycardia, and malaise).

Potential Nursing Diagnoses

- Risk for imbalanced body temperature (Indications).
- Deficient knowledge, related to disease process and medication regimen (Patient/Family Teaching).

Implementation

- Administration with food or antacids may minimize GI irritation.
- Available in oral and rectal dosage forms and in combination with other drugs.

Patient/Family Teaching

- Advise patient to consult health care professional if fever is not relieved by routine doses or if greater than 39.5°C (103°F) or lasts longer than 3 days.
- Centers for Disease Control and Prevention warns against giving aspirin to children or adolescents with varicella (chickenpox) or influenza-like or viral illnesses because of a possible association with Reye's syndrome.

Evaluation/Desired Outcomes

- Reduction of fever.

• ANTIRETROVIRALS

PHARMACOLOGIC PROFILE

General Use

The goal of antiretroviral therapy in the management of HIV infection is to improve CD4 cell counts and ↓ viral load. If accomplished, this generally results in slowed progression of the disease, improved quality of life, and ↓ opportunistic infections. Perinatal use of agents also prevents transmission of the virus to the fetus. Post-exposure prophylaxis with antiretrovirals is also recommended.

General Action and Information

Because of the rapid emergence of resistance and toxicities of individual agents, HIV infection is almost always managed by a combination of agents. Selections and doses are based on individual toxicities, underlying organ system disease, concurrent drug therapy, and severity of illness. Various combinations are used; up to 4 agents may be used simultaneously.

Contraindications

Hypersensitivity. Because of highly varying toxicities among agents, see individual monographs for more specific information.

Precautions

Many agents require modification for renal impairment. Protease inhibitors may cause hyperglycemia and should be used cautiously in patients with diabetes. Hemophiliacs may also be at risk of bleeding when taking protease inhibitors. See individual monographs for specific information.

Interactions

There are many significant and potentially serious drug-drug interactions among the antiretrovirals. They are affected by drugs that alter metabolism; some agents themselves affect metabolism. See individual agents.

NURSING IMPLICATIONS

Assessment

- Assess patient for change in severity of symptoms of HIV and for symptoms of opportunistic infections throughout therapy.
- **Lab Test Considerations:** Monitor viral load and CD4 counts prior to and periodically during therapy.

Potential Nursing Diagnoses

- Risk for infection (Indications).
- Deficient knowledge, related to disease process and medication regimen (Patient/Family Teaching).
- Noncompliance (Patient/Family Teaching).

Implementation

- Administer doses around the clock.

Patient/Family Teaching

- Instruct patient to take medication exactly as directed, around the clock, even if sleep is interrupted. Emphasize the importance of complying with therapy, not taking more than prescribed amount, and not discontinuing without consulting health care professional. Missed doses should be taken as soon as remembered unless almost time for next dose; patient should not double doses. Inform patient that long-term effects are unknown at this time.
- Instruct patient that antiretrovirals should not be shared with others.
- Inform patient that antiretroviral therapy does not cure HIV and does not ↓ the risk of transmission of HIV to others through sexual contact or blood contamination. Caution patient to use a condom during sexual contact and to avoid sharing needles or donating blood to prevent spreading the AIDS virus to others.
- Advise patient to avoid taking any Rx, OTC, or herbal products without consulting health care professional.
- Emphasize the importance of regular follow-up exams and blood counts to determine progress and to monitor for side effects.

Evaluation/Desired Outcomes

- Decrease in viral load and increase in CD4 counts in patients with HIV.

• ANTIRHEUMATICS

PHARMACOLOGIC PROFILE

General Use

Antirheumatics are used to manage symptoms of rheumatoid arthritis (pain, swelling) and in more severe cases to slow down joint destruction and preserve joint function. NSAIDs, aspirin, and other salicylates are used to manage symptoms such as pain and swelling, allowing continued motility and improved quality of life. Corticosteroids are reserved for more advanced swelling and discomfort, primarily because of their ↑ side effects, especially with chronic use. They can be used to control acute flares of disease. Neither NSAIDs nor corticosteroids prevent disease progression or joint destruction. Disease-modifying antirheumatics drugs (DMARDs) slow the progression of rheumatoid arthritis and delay joint destruction. DMARDs are reserved for severe cases because of their toxicity. Several months of therapy may be required before benefit is noted and maintained. Serious and frequent adverse reactions may require discontinuation of therapy, despite initial benefit.

General Action and Information

Both NSAIDs and corticosteroids have potent anti-inflammatory properties. DMARDs work by a variety of mechanisms. See individual agents, but most work by suppressing the autoimmune response thought to be responsible for joint destruction.

Contraindications

Hypersensitivity. Patients who are allergic to aspirin should not receive other NSAIDs. Corticosteroids should not be used in patients with active untreated infections.

Precautions

NSAIDs and corticosteroids should be used cautiously in patients with a history of GI bleeding. Corticosteroids should be used with caution in patients with diabetes. Many DMARDs have immunosuppressive properties and should be avoided in patients for whom immunosuppression poses a serious risk, including patients with active infections, underlying malignancy, and transplant recipients.

Interactions

NSAIDs may diminish the response to diuretics and antihypertensives. Corticosteroids may augment hypokalemia from other medications and ↑ the risk of digoxin toxicity. DMARDs ↑ the risk of serious immunosuppression with other immunosuppressants.

NURSING IMPLICATIONS

Assessment

- Assess patient monthly for pain, swelling, and range of motion.

Potential Nursing Diagnoses

- Chronic pain (Indications).
- Deficient knowledge, related to disease process and medication regimen.

Implementation

- Most agents require regular administration to obtain maximum effects.

Patient/Family Teaching

- Instruct patient to contact health care professional if no improvement is noticed within a few days.

Evaluation/Desired Outcomes

- Improvement in signs and symptoms of rheumatoid arthritis.

• ANTITUBERCULARS

PHARMACOLOGIC PROFILE

General Use

Used in the treatment and prevention of tuberculosis. Combinations are used in the treatment of active disease tuberculosis to rapidly ↓ the infectious state and delay or prevent the emergence of resistant strains. In selected situations, intermittent (twice weekly) regimens may be employed. Streptomycin is also used as an antitubercular. Rifampin is used in the prevention of meningococcal meningitis and *Haemophilus influenzae* type b disease.

General Action and Information
Kill (tuberculocidal) or inhibit the growth of (tuberculostatic) mycobacteria responsible for causing tuberculosis. Combination therapy with two or more agents is required, unless used as prophylaxis (isoniazid alone).

Contraindications
Hypersensitivity. Severe liver disease.

Precautions
Use cautiously in patients with a history of liver disease or in elderly or debilitated patients. Ethambutol requires ophthalmologic follow-up. Safety in pregnancy and lactation not established, although selected agents have been used without adverse effects on the fetus. Compliance is required for optimal response.

Interactions
Isoniazid inhibits the metabolism of phenytoin. Rifampin significantly ↓ levels of many drugs.

NURSING IMPLICATIONS

Assessment
- Mycobacterial studies and susceptibility tests should be performed prior to and periodically throughout therapy to detect possible resistance.
- Assess lung sounds and character and amount of sputum periodically throughout therapy.

Potential Nursing Diagnoses
- Risk for infection (Indications).
- Deficient knowledge, related to disease process and medication regimen (Patient/Family Teaching).
- Noncompliance (Patient/Family Teaching).

Implementation
- Most medications can be administered with food if GI irritation occurs.

Patient/Family Teaching
- Advise patient of the importance of continuing therapy even after symptoms have subsided.
- Emphasize the importance of regular follow-up exams to monitor progress and check for side effects.
- Inform patients taking rifampin that saliva, sputum, sweat, tears, urine, and feces may become red-orange to red-brown and that soft contact lenses may become permanently discolored.

Evaluation/Desired Outcomes
- Resolution of the signs and symptoms of tuberculosis. Negative sputum cultures.

• ANTIULCER AGENTS

PHARMACOLOGIC PROFILE

General Use
Treatment and prophylaxis of peptic ulcer and gastric hypersecretory conditions such as Zollinger-Ellison syndrome. Histamine H_2-receptor antagonists (blockers) and proton pump inhibitors are also used in the management of gastroesophageal reflux disease (GERD).

General Action and Information
Because a great majority of peptic ulcer disease may be traced to GI infection with the organism *Helicobacter pylori*, eradication of the organism ↓ symptomatology and recurrence. Anti-infectives with significant activity against the organism include amoxicillin, clarithromycin, metro-

nidazole, and tetracycline. Bismuth also has anti-infective activity against *H. pylori*. Regimens usually include: a histamine H_2-receptor antagonist, or a proton pump inhibitor, and 2 anti-infectives with or without bismuth subsalicylate for 10–14 days.. Other medications used in the management of gastric/duodenal ulcer disease are aimed at neutralizing gastric acid (antacids), ↓ acid secretion (histamine H_2 antagonists, proton pump inhibitors, misoprostol), or protecting the ulcer surface from further damage (misoprostol, sucralfate). Histamine H_2-receptor antagonists competitively inhibit the action of histamine at the H_2 receptor, located primarily in gastric parietal cells, resulting in inhibition of gastric acid secretion. Misoprostol ↓ gastric acid secretion and ↑ production of protective mucus. Proton pump inhibitors prevent the transport of hydrogen ions into the gastric lumen.

Contraindications
Hypersensitivity. Pregnancy.

Precautions
Most histamine H_2 antagonists require dose reduction in renal impairment and in elderly patients. Magnesium-containing antacids should be used cautiously in patients with renal impairment. Misoprostol should be used cautiously in women with childbearing potential.

Interactions
Calcium- and magnesium-containing antacids ↓ the absorption of tetracycline and fluoroquinolones. Cimetidine inhibits the ability of the liver to metabolize several drugs, ↑ the risk of toxicity from warfarin, tricyclic antidepressants, theophylline, metoprolol, phenytoin, propranolol, and lidocaine. Omeprazole ↓ metabolism of phenytoin, diazepam, and warfarin. All agents that ↑ gastric pH will ↓ the absorption of ketoconazole and some of the protease inhibitors (e.g. atazanavir).

NURSING IMPLICATIONS

Assessment
- Assess patient routinely for epigastric or abdominal pain and frank or occult blood in the stool, emesis, or gastric aspirate.
- **Antacids:** Assess for heartburn and indigestion as well as the location, duration, character, and precipitating factors of gastric pain.
- **Histamine H_2 Antagonists:** Assess elderly and severely ill patients for confusion routinely. Notify health care professional promptly should this occur.
- **Misoprostol:** Assess women of childbearing age for pregnancy. Medication is usually begun on 2nd or 3rd day of menstrual period following a negative serum pregnancy test within 2 wk of beginning therapy.
- **Lab Test Considerations:** Histamine H_2 antagonists antagonize the effects of pentagastrin and histamine during gastric acid secretion test. Avoid administration during the 24 hr preceding the test.
- May cause false-negative results in skin tests using allergen extracts. These drugs should be discontinued 24 hr prior to the test.

Potential Nursing Diagnoses
- Acute pain (Indications).
- Deficient knowledge, related to disease process and medication regimen (Patient/Family Teaching).

Implementation
- **Antacids:** Antacids cause premature dissolution and absorption of enteric-coated tablets and may interfere with absorption of other oral medications. Separate administration of antacids and other oral medications by at least 1 hr.

- Shake liquid preparations well before pouring. Follow administration with water to ensure passage to stomach. Liquid and powder dosage forms are considered to be more effective than chewable tablets.
- Chewable tablets must be chewed thoroughly before swallowing. Follow with half a glass of water.
- Administer 1 and 3 hr after meals and at bedtime for maximum antacid effect.
- **Misoprostol:** Administer with meals and at bedtime to reduce the severity of diarrhea.
- **Proton Pump Inhibitors:** Administer before meals, preferably in the morning. Capsules should be swallowed whole; do not open, crush, or chew.
- May be administered concurrently with antacids.
- **Sucralfate:** Administer on an empty stomach 1 hr before meals and at bedtime. Do not crush or chew tablets. Shake suspension well prior to administration. If nasogastric administration is required, consult pharmacist, as protein-binding properties of sucralfate have resulted in formation of a bezoar when administered with enteral feedings and other medications.

Patient/Family Teaching

- Instruct patient to take medication as directed for the full course of therapy, even if feeling better. If a dose is missed, it should be taken as soon as remembered but not if almost time for next dose. Do not double doses.
- Advise patient to avoid alcohol, products containing aspirin, NSAIDs, and foods that may cause an ↑ in GI irritation.
- Advise patient to report onset of black, tarry stools to health care professional promptly.
- Inform patient that cessation of smoking may help prevent the recurrence of duodenal ulcers.
- **Antacids:** Caution patient to consult health care professional before taking antacids for more than 2 wk or if problem is recurring. Advise patient to consult health care professional if relief is not obtained or if symptoms of gastric bleeding (black, tarry stools; coffee-ground emesis) occur.
- **Misoprostol:** Emphasize that sharing of this medication may be dangerous.
- Inform patient that misoprostol may cause spontaneous abortion. Women of childbearing age must be informed of this effect through verbal and written information and must use contraception throughout therapy. If pregnancy is suspected, the woman should stop taking misoprostol and immediately notify her health care professional.
- **Sucralfate:** Advise patient to continue with course of therapy for 4–8 wk, even if feeling better, to ensure ulcer healing.
- Advise patient that an ↑ in fluid intake, dietary bulk, and exercise may prevent drug-induced constipation.

Evaluation/Desired Outcomes

- Decrease in GI pain and irritation. Prevention of gastric irritation and bleeding. Healing of duodenal ulcers can be seen by x-rays or endoscopy. Therapy with histamine H_2 antagonists is continued for at least 6 wk after initial episode. Decreased symptoms of GERD. Increase in the pH of gastric secretions (antacids). Prevention of gastric ulcers in patients receiving chronic NSAID therapy (misoprostol only).

• ANTIVIRALS

PHARMACOLOGIC PROFILE

General Use

Acyclovir, famciclovir, and valacyclovir are used in the management of herpes virus infections. Acyclovir and valacyclovir are also used in the management of chickenpox. Oseltamivir and zanamivir are used primarily in the prevention of influenza infections. Cidofovir, ganciclovir, valganciclovir, and foscarnet are used in the treatment of cytomegalovirus (CMV) retinitis. Vidarabine is used only to treat ophthalmic viral infections. Penciclovir, famciclovir, valacyclovir, and docosanol are used in the treatment and prevention of oral-facial herpes simplex.

General Action and Information
Most agents inhibit viral replication.

Contraindications
Previous hypersensitivity.

Precautions
All except zanamivir require dose adjustment in renal impairment. Acyclovir may cause renal impairment. Acyclovir may cause CNS toxicity. Foscarnet ↑ risk of seizures.

Interactions
Acyclovir may have additive CNS and nephrotoxicity with drugs causing similar adverse reactions.

NURSING IMPLICATIONS

Assessment
- Assess patient for signs and symptoms of infection before and throughout therapy.
- **Ophth:** Assess eye lesions before and daily during therapy.
- **Topical:** Assess lesions before and daily during therapy.

Potential Nursing Diagnoses
- Risk for infection (Indications).
- Impaired skin integrity (Indications).
- Deficient knowledge, related to disease process and medication regimen (Patient/Family Teaching).

Implementation
- Most systemic antiviral agents should be administered around the clock to maintain therapeutic serum drug levels.

Patient/Family Teaching
- Instruct patient to continue taking medication around the clock for full course of therapy, even if feeling better.
- Advise patient that antivirals and antiretrovirals do not prevent transmission to others. Precautions should be taken to prevent spread of virus.
- Instruct patient in correct technique for topical or ophthalmic preparations.
- Instruct patient to notify health care professional if symptoms do not improve.

Evaluation/Desired Outcomes
- Prevention or resolution of the signs and symptoms of viral infection. Length of time for complete resolution depends on organism and site of infection.

• BETA BLOCKERS

PHARMACOLOGIC PROFILE

General Use
Management of hypertension, angina pectoris, tachyarrhythmias, migraine headache (prophylaxis), MI (prevention), glaucoma (ophthalmic use), heart failure (HF) (bisoprolol, carvedilol and sustained-release metoprolol only) and hyperthyroidism (management of symptoms only).

General Action and Information
Beta blockers compete with adrenergic (sympathetic) neurotransmitters (epinephrine and norepinephrine) for adrenergic receptor sites. Beta$_1$-adrenergic receptor sites are located chiefly in

the heart where stimulation results in increased heart rate, contractility, and AV conduction. $Beta_2$-adrenergic receptors are found mainly in bronchial and vascular smooth muscle and the uterus. Stimulation of $beta_2$-adrenergic receptors produces vasodilation, bronchodilation, and uterine relaxation. Blockade of these receptors antagonizes the effects of the neurotransmitters. Beta blockers may be relatively selective for $beta_1$-adrenergic receptors (acebutolol, atenolol, betaxolol, bisoprolol, esmolol, and metoprolol) or nonselective (carvedilol, labetalol, nadolol, penbutolol, pindolol, propranolol, and timolol) blocking both $beta_1$- and $beta_2$-adrenergic receptors. Carvedilol and labetalol have additional alpha-adrenergic blocking properties. Ophthalmic beta blockers ↓ production of aqueous humor.

Contraindications

Uncompensated HF (most beta blockers), acute bronchospasm, some forms of valvular heart disease, bradyarrhythmias, and heart block.

Precautions

Use cautiously in pregnant and lactating women (may cause fetal bradycardia and hypoglycemia). Use cautiously in any form of lung disease. Use with caution in patients with diabetes or severe liver disease. Beta blockers should not be abruptly discontinued in patients with cardiovascular disease.

Interactions

May cause additive myocardial depression and bradycardia when used with other agents having these effects (digoxin, diltiazem, verapamil, and clonidine). May antagonize the therapeutic effects of bronchodilators. May alter the requirements for insulin or hypoglyemic agents in patients with diabetes. Cimetidine may ↓ the metabolism and ↑ the effects of some beta blockers.

NURSING IMPLICATIONS

Assessment

- Monitor BP and pulse frequently during dosage adjustment and periodically throughout therapy.
- Monitor intake and output ratios and daily weight. Assess patient routinely for signs and symptoms of HF (dyspnea, rales/crackles, weight gain, peripheral edema, jugular venous distention).
- **Angina:** Assess frequency and severity of episodes of chest pain periodically throughout therapy.
- **Migraine Prophylaxis:** Assess frequency and severity of migraine headaches periodically throughout therapy.

Potential Nursing Diagnoses

- Ineffective tissue perfusion (Indications).
- Deficient knowledge, related to disease process and medication regimen (Patient/Family Teaching).
- Noncompliance (Patient/Family Teaching).

Implementation

- Take apical pulse prior to administering. If heart rate is <50 bpm or if arrhythmias occur, hold medication and notify health care professional.
- Many beta blockers are available in combination products to enhance compliance (see Appendix B).

Patient/Family Teaching

- Instruct patient to continue taking medication, even if feeling well. Abrupt withdrawal may cause life-threatening arrhythmias, hypertension, or myocardial ischemia. Medication controls, but does not cure, hypertension.
- Encourage patient to comply with additional interventions for hypertension (weight reduction, low-sodium diet, regular exercise, smoking cessation, moderation of alcohol consumption, and stress management).

- Instruct patient and family on proper technique for monitoring BP. Advise them to check BP weekly and report significant changes to health care professional.
- Caution patient to make position changes slowly to minimize orthostatic hypotension. Advise patient that exercising or hot weather may enhance hypotensive effects.
- Advise patient to consult health care professional before taking any OTC medications or herbal/alternative therapies, especially cold remedies.
- Caution patient that these medications may cause ↑ sensitivity to cold.
- Patients with diabetes should monitor blood glucose closely, especially if weakness, malaise, irritability, or fatigue occurs.
- Advise patient to advise health care professional of medication regimen prior to treatment or surgery.
- Advise patient to carry identification describing disease process and medication regimen at all times.
- Emphasize the importance of follow-up exams to monitor progress.
- **Ophth:** Instruct patient in correct technique for administration of ophthalmic preparations.

Evaluation/Desired Outcomes

- Decrease in BP.
- Decrease in frequency and severity of anginal attacks.
- Control of arrhythmias.
- Prevention of myocardial reinfarction.
- Prevention of migraine headaches.
- Decrease in tremors.
- Lowering of intraocular pressure.

• BONE RESORPTION INHIBITORS

PHARMACOLOGIC PROFILE

General Use

Bone resorption inhibitors are primarily used to treat and prevent osteoporosis in postmenopausal women. Other uses include treatment of osteoporosis due to other causes, including corticosteroid therapy, treatment of Paget's disease of the bone, and management of hypercalcemia.

General Action and Information

Biphosphonates (alendronate, etidronate, ibandronate, pamidronate, risedronate, tiludronate, and zoledronic acid) inhibit resorption of bone by inhibiting hydroxyapatite crystal dissolution and osteoclast activity. Raloxifene binds to estrogen receptors, producing estrogen-like effects on bone including ↓ bone resorption and ↓ bone turnover.

Contraindications

Hypersensitivity. Biphosphonates should not be used in patients with hypocalcemia. Raloxifene should not be used in women with childbearing potential or a history of thromboembolic disease.

Precautions

Use cautiously in patients with renal impairment; some agents should be avoided in moderate to severe renal impairment.

Interactions

Calcium supplements ↓ absorption of biphosphonates. Tilundronate's effects may be altered by aspirin or other NSAIDs. Aspirin may ↑ GI adverse reactions with bisphosphonates. Cholestyramine ↓ absorption of raloxifene (concurrent use is contraindicated).

C L A S S I F I C A T I O N S

NURSING IMPLICATIONS

Assessment

- Assess patients for low bone density before and periodically during therapy.
- Assess for symptoms of Paget's disease (bone pain, headache, decreased visual and auditory acuity, ↑ skull size).
- **Lab Test Considerations:** Monitor serum calcium in patients with osteoporosis. Monitor alkaline phosphatase in patients with Paget's disease.

Potential Nursing Diagnoses

- Risk for injury (Indications).
- Deficient knowledge, related to disease process and medication regimen (Patient/Family Teaching).

Implementation

Patient/Family Teaching

- Instruct patient to take medication exactly as directed.
- Encourage patient to participate in regular exercise and to modify behaviors that ↑ the risk of osteoporosis.

Evaluation/Desired Outcomes

- Prevention of, or decrease in, the progression of osteoporosis in postmenopausal women. Decrease in the progression of Paget's disease.

• BRONCHODILATORS

PHARMACOLOGIC PROFILE

General Use

Used in the treatment of reversible airway obstruction due to asthma or chronic obstructive pulmonary disease (COPD). Recommendations for management of asthma recommend that rapid-acting inhaled beta-agonist bronchodilators (not salmeterol) be reserved as acute relievers of bronchospasm; repeated or chronic use indicates the need for additional long-term control agents, including inhaled corticosteroids, mast cell stabilizers, long-acting bronchodilators (oral theophylline or beta-agonists), and leukotriene modifiers (montelukast, zafirlukast).

General Action and Information

Beta-adrenergic agonists (albuterol, arformoterol, epinephrine, formoterol, indacaterol, levalbuterol, metaproterenol, pirbuterol, salmeterol, and terbutaline) produce bronchodilation by stimulating the production of cyclic adenosine monophosphate (cAMP). Onset of action allows use in management of acute attacks except for arformoterol, formoterol, indacaterol, and salmeterol, which have delayed onset. Phosphodiesterase inhibitors (aminophylline and theophylline) inhibit the breakdown of cAMP. Ipratropium and tiotropium are anticholinergic compounds that produce bronchodilation by blocking the action of acetylcholine in the respiratory tract.

Contraindications

Hypersensitivity to agents or preservatives (bisulfites) used in their formulation. Avoid use in uncontrolled cardiac arrhythmias.

Precautions

Use cautiously in patients with diabetes, cardiovascular disease, or hyperthyroidism.

Interactions
Therapeutic effectiveness may be antagonized by concurrent use of beta blockers. Additive sympathomimetic effects with other adrenergic (sympathetic) drugs, including vasopressors and decongestants. Cardiovascular effects may be potentiated by antidepressants and MAO inhibitors.

NURSING IMPLICATIONS

Assessment
- Assess BP, pulse, respiration, lung sounds, and character of secretions before and throughout therapy.
- Patients with a history of cardiovascular problems should be monitored for ECG changes and chest pain.

Potential Nursing Diagnoses
- Ineffective airway clearance (Indications).
- Activity intolerance (Indications).
- Deficient knowledge, related to disease process and medication regimen (Patient/Family Teaching).

Implementation
- Administer around the clock to maintain therapeutic plasma levels.

Patient/Family Teaching
- Emphasize the importance of taking only the prescribed dose at the prescribed time intervals.
- Encourage the patient to drink adequate liquids (2000 mL/day minimum) to ↓ the viscosity of the airway secretions.
- Advise patient to avoid OTC cough, cold, or breathing preparations without consulting health care professional and to minimize intake of xanthine-containing foods or beverages (colas, coffee, and chocolate), as these may ↑ side effects and cause arrhythmias.
- Caution patient to avoid smoking and other respiratory irritants.
- Instruct patient on proper use of metered-dose inhaler (see Appendix D).
- Advise patient to contact health care professional promptly if the usual dose of medication fails to produce the desired results, symptoms worsen after treatment, or toxic effects occur.
- Patients using other inhalation medications and bronchodilators should be advised to use bronchodilator first and allow 5 min to elapse before administering the other medication, unless otherwise directed by health care professional.

Evaluation/Desired Outcomes
- Decreased bronchospasm. Increased ease of breathing.

• CALCIUM CHANNEL BLOCKERS

PHARMACOLOGIC PROFILE

General Use
Used in the treatment of hypertension (amlodipine, diltiazem, felodipine, isradipine, nicardipine, nifedipine, nisoldipine, verapamil) or in the treatment and prophylaxis of angina pectoris or coronary artery spasm (amlodipine, diltiazem, felodipine, nicardipine, verapamil). Verapamil and diltiazem are also used as antiarrhythmics. Nimodipine is used to prevent neurologic damage due to certain types of cerebral vasospasm.

General Action and Information
Block calcium entry into cells of vascular smooth muscle and myocardium. Dilate coronary arteries in both normal and ischemic myocardium and inhibit coronary artery spasm. Diltiazem

and verapamil ↓ AV nodal conduction. Nimodipine has a relatively selective effect on cerebral blood vessels.

Contraindications

Hypersensitivity. Contraindicated in bradycardia, 2nd- or 3rd-degree heart block, or uncompensated HF (all except for amlodipine and felodipine).

Precautions

Safety in pregnancy and lactation not established. Use cautiously in patients with liver disease or uncontrolled arrhythmias.

Interactions

May cause additive bradycardia when used with other agents having these effects (beta blockers, digoxin, and clonidine). Effectiveness may be ↓ by phenobarbital or phenytoin and ↑ by propranolol or cimetidine. Verapamil and diltiazem may ↑ serum digoxin levels and cause toxicity.

NURSING IMPLICATIONS

Assessment

- Monitor BP and pulse frequently during dosage adjustment and periodically throughout therapy.
- Monitor intake and output ratios and daily weight. Assess patient routinely for signs and symptoms of HF (dyspnea, rales/crackles, weight gain, peripheral edema, jugular venous distention).
- **Angina:** Assess frequency and severity of episodes of chest pain periodically throughout therapy.
- **Arrhythmias:** ECG should be monitored continuously during IV therapy and periodically during long-term therapy with verapamil or diltiazem.
- **Cerebral Vasospasm:** Assess patient's neurological status (level of consciousness, movement) before and periodically during therapy with nimodipine.

Potential Nursing Diagnoses

- Ineffective tissue perfusion (Indications).
- Acute pain (Indications).
- Deficient knowledge, related to disease process and medication regimen (Patient/Family Teaching).

Implementation

- May be administered without regard to meals.
- Do not open, crush, or chew sustained-release capsules.

Patient/Family Teaching

- Instruct patient to continue taking medication, even if feeling well.
- Caution patient to make position changes slowly to minimize orthostatic hypotension. Advise patient that exercising or hot weather may enhance hypotensive effects.
- Instruct patient on the importance of maintaining good dental hygiene and seeing dentist frequently for teeth cleaning to prevent tenderness, bleeding, and gingival hyperplasia (gum enlargement).
- Advise patient to consult health care professional before taking any OTC medications or herbal/alternative therapies, especially cold remedies.
- Advise patient to advise health care professional of medication regimen prior to treatment or surgery.
- Advise patient to carry identification describing disease process and medication regimen at all times.
- Emphasize the importance of follow-up exams to monitor progress.

- **Angina:** Instruct patients on concurrent nitrate therapy to continue taking both medications as directed and using SL nitroglycerin as needed for anginal attacks. Advise patient to contact health care professional if chest pain worsens or does not improve after therapy, or is accompanied by diaphoresis or shortness of breath, or if severe, persistent headache occurs. Caution patient to discuss exercise precautions with health care professional prior to exertion.
- **Hypertension:** Encourage patient to comply with additional interventions for hypertension (weight reduction, low-sodium diet, regular exercise, smoking cessation, moderation of alcohol consumption, and stress management). Medication controls, but does not cure, hypertension.
- Instruct patient and family on proper technique for monitoring BP. Advise them to check BP weekly and report significant changes to health care professional.

Evaluation/Desired Outcomes

- Decrease in BP.
- Decrease in frequency and severity of anginal attacks.
- Decrease need for nitrate therapy.
- Increase in activity tolerance and sense of well-being.
- Suppression and prevention of supraventricular tachyarrhythmias.
- Improvement in neurological deficits due to vasospasm following subarachnoid hemorrhage.

• CENTRAL NERVOUS SYSTEM STIMULANTS

PHARMACOLOGIC PROFILE

General Use

Used in the treatment of narcolepsy and as adjunctive treatment in the management of attention deficit hyperactivity disorder (ADHD).

General Action and Information

Produce CNS stimulation by ↑ levels of neurotransmitters in the CNS. Produce CNS and respiratory stimulation, dilated pupils, ↑ motor activity and mental alertness, and a diminished sense of fatigue. In children with ADHD, these agents ↓ restlessness and ↑ attention span.

Contraindications

Hypersensitivity. Should not be used in pregnant or lactating women. Should not be used in hyperexcitable states. Avoid using in patients with psychotic personalities or suicidal/homicidal tendencies. Contraindicated in glaucoma and severe cardiovascular disease.

Precautions

Use cautiously in patients with a history of cardiovascular disease, hypertension, diabetes mellitus, or in elderly or debilitated patients. Continual use may result in psychological dependence or addiction.

Interactions

Additive sympathomimetic (adrenergic) effects. Use with MAO inhibitors can result in hypertensive crises. Alkalinizing the urine (sodium bicarbonate, acetazolamide) ↓ excretion and enhances effects of amphetamines. Acidification of the urine (ammonium chloride, large doses of ascorbic acid) ↓ effect of amphetamines. Phenothiazines may also ↓ effects. Methylphenidate may ↓ the metabolism and ↑ effects of other drugs (warfarin, anticonvulsants, tricyclic antidepressants).

NURSING IMPLICATIONS

Assessment

- Monitor BP, pulse, and respiration before administering and periodically during therapy.
- Monitor weight biweekly and inform health care professional of significant weight loss.

- Monitor height periodically in children; inform health care professional if growth inhibition occurs.
- May produce false sense of euphoria and well-being. Provide frequent rest periods and observe patient for rebound depression after the effects of the medication have worn off.
- **ADHD:** Assess attention span, impulse control, and interactions with others in children. Therapy may be interrupted at intervals to determine if symptoms are sufficient to warrant continued therapy.
- **Narcolepsy:** Observe and document frequency of episodes.

Potential Nursing Diagnoses

- Disturbed thought process (Side Effects).
- Deficient knowledge, related to disease process and medication regimen (Patient/Family Teaching).

Implementation

Patient/Family Teaching

- Instruct patient not to alter dose without consulting health care professional. These medications have high dependence and abuse potential. Abrupt cessation with high doses may cause extreme fatigue and mental depression.
- Advise patient to avoid intake of large amounts of caffeine.
- Medication may impair judgment. Caution patient to avoid driving or other activities requiring judgment until response to medication is known.
- Inform patient that periodic holidays from the drug may be used to assess progress and decrease dependence.

Evaluation/Desired Outcomes

- Decreased frequency of narcoleptic episodes.
- Improved attention span and social interactions.

• CORTICOSTEROIDS

PHARMACOLOGIC PROFILE

General Use

Used in replacement doses (20 mg of hydrocortisone or equivalent) systemically to treat adrenocortical insufficiency. Larger doses are usually used for their anti-inflammatory, immunosuppressive, or antineoplastic activity. Used adjunctively in many other situations, including hypercalcemia and autoimmune diseases. Topical corticosteroids are used in a variety of inflammatory and allergic conditions. Inhalant corticosteroids are used in the chronic management of reversible airway disease (asthma); intranasal and ophthalmic corticosteroids are used in the management of chronic allergic and inflammatory conditions.

General Action and Information

Produce profound and varied metabolic effects, in addition to modifying the normal immune response and suppressing inflammation. Available in a variety of dosage forms, including oral, injectable, topical, and inhalation. Prolonged used of large amounts of topical or inhaled agent may result in systemic absorption and/or adrenal suppression.

Contraindications

Serious infections (except for certain forms of meningitis). Do not administer live vaccines to patients on larger doses.

Precautions

Prolonged treatment will result in adrenal suppression. Do not discontinue abruptly. Additional doses may be needed during stress (surgery and infection). Safety in pregnancy and lactation not established. Long-term use in children will result in ↓ growth. May mask signs of infection. Use lowest dose possible for shortest time possible. Alternate-day therapy is preferable during long-term treatment.

Interactions

Additive hypokalemia with amphotericin B and potassium-losing diuretics. Hypokalemia may ↑ the risk of digoxin toxicity. May ↑ requirements for insulin or oral hypoglycemic agents. Phenytoin, phenobarbital, and rifampin stimulate metabolism and may ↓ effectiveness. Oral contraceptives may block metabolism. Cholestyramine and colestipol may ↓ absorption.

NURSING IMPLICATIONS

Assessment

- These drugs are indicated for many conditions. Assess involved systems prior to and periodically throughout course of therapy.
- Assess patient for signs of adrenal insufficiency (hypotension, weight loss, weakness, nausea, vomiting, anorexia, lethargy, confusion, restlessness) prior to and periodically throughout course of therapy.
- Children should have periodic evaluations of growth.

Potential Nursing Diagnoses

- Risk for infection (Side Effects).
- Deficient knowledge, related to disease process and medication regimen (Patient/Family Teaching).
- Disturbed body image (Side Effects).

Implementation

- If dose is ordered daily or every other day, administer in the morning to coincide with the body's normal secretion of cortisol..
- **PO:** Administer with meals to minimize gastric irritation.

Patient/Family Teaching

- Emphasize need to take medication exactly as directed. Review symptoms of adrenal insufficiency that may occur when stopping the medication and that may be life-threatening.
- Encourage patients on long-term therapy to eat a diet high in protein, calcium, and potassium and low in sodium and carbohydrates.
- These drugs cause immunosuppression and may mask symptoms of infection. Instruct patient to avoid people with known contagious illnesses and to report possible infections. Advise patient to consult health care professional before receiving any vaccinations.
- Discuss possible effects on body image. Explore coping mechanisms.
- Advise patient to carry identification in the event of an emergency in which patient cannot relate medical history.

Evaluation/Desired Outcomes

- Suppression of the inflammatory and immune responses in autoimmune disorders, allergic reactions, and organ transplants.
- Replacement therapy in adrenal insufficiency.
- Resolution of skin inflammation, pruritus, or other dermatologic conditions.

• DIURETICS

PHARMACOLOGIC PROFILE

General Use

Thiazide diuretics and loop diuretics are used alone or in combination in the treatment of hypertension or edema due to HF or other causes. Potassium-sparing diuretics have weak diuretic and antihypertensive properties and are used mainly to conserve potassium in patients receiving thiazide or loop diuretics. Osmotic diuretics are often used in the management of cerebral edema.

General Action and Information

Enhance the selective excretion of various electrolytes and water by affecting renal mechanisms for tubular secretion and reabsorption. Groups commonly used are thiazide diuretics and thiazide-like diuretics (chlorothiazide, chlorthalidone, hydrochlorothiazide, indapamide, and metolazone), loop diuretics (bumetanide, furosemide, and torsemide), potassium-sparing diuretics (amiloride, spironolactone, and triamterene), and osmotic diuretics (mannitol). Mechanisms vary, depending on agent.

Contraindications

Hypersensitivity. Thiazide and loop diuretics may exhibit cross-sensitivity with other sulfonamides.

Precautions

Use with caution in patients with renal or hepatic disease. Safety in pregnancy and lactation not established.

Interactions

Additive hypokalemia with corticosteroids and amphotericin B, piperacillin. Hypokalemia may ↑ the risk of digoxin toxicity. Potassium-losing diuretics ↓ lithium excretion and may cause toxicity. Additive hypotension with other antihypertensives or nitrates. Potassium-sparing diuretics may cause hyperkalemia when used with potassium supplements, ACE inhibitors, angiotensin II receptor antagonists, and aliskiren.

NURSING IMPLICATIONS

Assessment

- Assess fluid status throughout therapy. Monitor daily weight, intake and output ratios, amount and location of edema, lung sounds, skin turgor, and mucous membranes.
- Assess patient for anorexia, muscle weakness, numbness, tingling, paresthesia, confusion, and excessive thirst. Notify health care professional promptly if these signs of electrolyte imbalance occur.
- **Hypertension:** Monitor BP and pulse before and during administration. Monitor frequency of prescription refills to determine compliance in patients treated for hypertension.
- **Increased Intracranial Pressure:** Monitor neurologic status and intracranial pressure readings in patients receiving osmotic diuretics to decrease cerebral edema.
- **Increased Intraocular Pressure:** Monitor for persistent or increased eye pain or decreased visual acuity.
- **Lab Test Considerations:** Monitor electrolytes (especially potassium), blood glucose, BUN, and serum uric acid levels before and periodically throughout course of therapy.
- Thiazide and loop diuretics may cause ↑ serum cholesterol, low-density lipoprotein (LDL) cholesterol, and triglyceride concentrations.

Potential Nursing Diagnoses

- Excess fluid volume (Indications).
- Deficient knowledge, related to disease process and medication regimen (Patient/Family Teaching).

Implementation

- Administer oral diuretics in the morning to prevent disruption of sleep cycle.
- Many diuretics are available in combination with other antihypertensives or potassium-sparing diuretics.

Patient/Family Teaching

- Instruct patient to take medication exactly as directed. Advise patients on antihypertensive regimen to continue taking medication, even if feeling better. Medication controls, but does not cure, hypertension.
- Caution patient to make position changes slowly to minimize orthostatic hypotension. Caution patient that the use of alcohol, exercise during hot weather, or standing for long periods during therapy may enhance orthostatic hypotension.
- Instruct patient to consult health care professional regarding dietary potassium guidelines.
- Instruct patient to monitor weight weekly and report significant changes.
- Caution patient to use sunscreen and protective clothing to prevent photosensitivity reactions.
- Advise patient to consult health care professional before taking OTC medication concurrently with this therapy.
- Instruct patient to notify health care professional of medication regimen before treatment or surgery.
- Advise patient to contact health care professional immediately if muscle weakness, cramps, nausea, dizziness, or numbness or tingling of extremities occurs.
- Emphasize the importance of routine follow-up.
- **Hypertension:** Reinforce the need to continue additional therapies for hypertension (weight loss, regular exercise, restricted sodium intake, stress reduction, moderation of alcohol consumption, and cessation of smoking).
- Instruct patients with hypertension in the correct technique for monitoring weekly BP.

Evaluation/Desired Outcomes

- Decreased BP.
- Increased urine output.
- Decreased edema.
- Reduced intracranial pressure.
- Prevention of hypokalemia in patients taking diuretics.
- Treatment of hyperaldosteronism.

• HORMONES

PHARMACOLOGIC PROFILE

General Use

Used in the treatment of deficiency states including diabetes mellitus (insulin), diabetes insipidus (desmopressin), hypothyroidism (thyroid hormones), and menopause (estrogens or estrogens/progestins). Estrogenic and progestational hormones are used as contraceptive agents in various combinations and sequences. Hormones may be used to treat hormonally sensitive tumors (androgens, estrogens) and in other selected situations. See individual drugs.

General Action and Information

Natural or synthetic substances that have a specific effect on target tissue. Differ greatly in their effects, depending on individual agent and function of target tissue.

Contraindications

Differ greatly among individual agents; see individual entries.

Precautions

Differ greatly among individual agents; see individual entries.

Interactions

Differ greatly among individual agents; see individual entries.

NURSING IMPLICATIONS

Assessment

- Monitor patient for symptoms of hormonal excess or insufficiency.
- **Sex Hormones:** BP and hepatic function tests should be monitored periodically throughout therapy.

Potential Nursing Diagnoses

- Sexual dysfunction (Indications).
- Disturbed body image (Indications) (Side Effects).
- Deficient knowledge, related to disease process and medication regimen (Patient/Family Teaching).

Implementation

- **Sex Hormones:** During hospitalization, continue to administer according to schedule followed prior to hospitalization.

Patient/Family Teaching

- Explain dose schedule (and withdrawal bleeding with female sex hormones).
- Emphasize the importance of follow-up exams to monitor effectiveness of therapy and to ensure proper development of children and early detection of possible side effects.
- **Female Sex Hormones:** Advise patient to report signs and symptoms of fluid retention, thromboembolic disorders, mental depression, or hepatic dysfunction to health care professional.

Evaluation/Desired Outcomes

- Resolution of clinical symptoms of hormone imbalance including menopause symptoms and contraception.
- Correction of fluid and electrolyte imbalances.
- Control of the spread of advanced metastatic breast or prostate cancer.
- Slowed progression of postmenopausal osteoporosis.

• IMMUNOSUPPRESSANTS

PHARMACOLOGIC PROFILE

General Use

Azathioprine, basiliximab, cyclosporine, everolimus, mycophenolate, sirolimus, and tacrolimus are used with corticosteroids in the prevention of transplantation rejection reactions. Muromonab-CD3 is used to manage rejection reactions not controlled by other agents. Azathioprine, cyclophosphamide, and methotrexate are used in the management of selected autoimmune diseases (nephrotic syndrome of childhood and severe rheumatoid arthritis).

General Action and Information

Inhibit cell-mediated immune responses by different mechanisms. In addition to azathioprine and cyclosporine, which are used primarily for their immunomodulating properties, cyclophosphamide and methotrexate are used to suppress the immune responses in certain disease states (nephrotic syndrome of childhood and severe rheumatoid arthritis). Muromonab-CD3 is a recombinant immunoglobulin antibody that alters T-cell function. Basiliximab is a monoclonal antibody.

Contraindications

Hypersensitivity to drug or vehicle.

Precautions

Use cautiously in patients with infections. Safety in pregnancy and lactation not established.

Interactions

Allopurinol inhibits the metabolism of azathioprine. Drugs that alter liver-metabolizing processes may change the effect of cyclosporine, tacrolimus, or sirolimus. The risk to toxicity of methotrexate may be ↑ by other nephrotoxic drugs, large doses of aspirin, or NSAIDs. Muromonab-CD3 has additive immunosuppressive properties; concurrent immunosuppressive doses should be ↓ or eliminated.

NURSING IMPLICATIONS

Assessment

- Monitor for infection (vital signs, sputum, urine, stool, WBC). Notify physician or other health care professional immediately if symptoms occur.
- **Organ Transplant:** Assess for symptoms of organ rejection throughout therapy.
- **Lab Test Consideration:** Monitor CBC and differential throughout therapy.

Potential Nursing Diagnoses

- Risk for infection (Side Effects).
- Deficient knowledge, related to disease process and medication regimen (Patient/Family Teaching).

Implementation

- Protect transplant patients from staff and visitors who may carry infection.
- Maintain protective isolation as indicated.

Patient/Family Teaching

- Reinforce the need for lifelong therapy to prevent transplant rejection. Review symptoms of rejection for transplanted organ and stress the need for patient to notify health care professional immediately if they occur.
- Advise patient to avoid contact with contagious persons. Patients should not receive vaccinations without first consulting with health care professional.
- Emphasize the importance of follow-up exams and lab tests.

Evaluation/Desired Outcomes

- Prevention or reversal of rejection of organ transplants or decrease in symptoms of autoimmune disorders.

• LAXATIVES

PHARMACOLOGIC PROFILE

General Use

Used to treat or prevent constipation or to prepare the bowel for radiologic or endoscopic procedures.

General Action and Information

Induce one or more bowel movements per day. Groups include stimulants (bisacodyl, sennosides), saline laxatives (magnesium salts and phosphates), stool softeners (docusate), bulk-forming agents (polycarbophil and psyllium), and osmotic cathartics (lactulose, polyethylene glycol/electrolyte). ↑ fluid intake, exercising, and adding more dietary fiber are also useful in the management of chronic constipation.

Contraindications

Hypersensitivity. Contraindicated in persistent abdominal pain, nausea, or vomiting of unknown cause, especially if accompanied by fever or other signs of an acute abdomen.

Precautions
Excessive or prolonged use may lead to dependence. Should not be used in children unless advised by a physician or other health care professional.

Interactions
Theoretically may ↓ the absorption of other orally administered drugs by ↓ transit time.

NURSING IMPLICATIONS

Assessment
- Assess patient for abdominal distention, presence of bowel sounds, and usual pattern of bowel function.
- Assess color, consistency, and amount of stool produced.

Potential Nursing Diagnoses
- Constipation (Indications).
- Deficient knowledge, related to disease process and medication regimen (Patient/Family Teaching).

Implementation
- May be administered at bedtime for morning results.
- Taking oral doses on an empty stomach will usually produce more rapid results.
- Do not crush or chew enteric-coated tablets. Take with a full glass of water or juice.
- Stool softeners and bulk laxatives may take several days for results.

Patient/Family Teaching
- Advise patients, other than those with spinal cord injuries, that laxatives should be used only for short-term therapy. Long-term therapy may cause electrolyte imbalance and dependence.
- Advise patient to ↑ fluid intake to a minimum of 1500–2000 mL/day during therapy to prevent dehydration.
- Encourage patients to use other forms of bowel regulation: ↑ bulk in the diet, ↑ fluid intake, and ↑ mobility. Normal bowel habits are individualized and may vary from 3 times/day to 3 times/wk.
- Instruct patients with cardiac disease to avoid straining during bowel movements (Valsalva maneuver).
- Advise patient that laxatives should not be used when constipation is accompanied by abdominal pain, fever, nausea, or vomiting.

Evaluation/Desired Outcomes
- A soft, formed bowel movement.
- Evacuation of the colon.

• LIPID-LOWERING AGENTS

PHARMACOLOGIC PROFILE

General Use
Used as a part of a total plan including diet and exercise to ↓ blood lipids in an effort to ↓ the morbidity and mortality of atherosclerotic cardiovascular disease and its sequelae.

General Action and Information
HMG-CoA reductase inhibitors (atorvastatin, fluvastatin, lovastatin, pitavastatin, pravastatin, rosuvastatin simvastatin) inhibit an enzyme involved in cholesterol synthesis. Bile acid sequestrants (cholestyramine, colestipol, colesevelam) bind cholesterol in the GI tract. Ezetimibe inhibits the

absorption of cholesterol in the small intestine. Fenofibrate, gemfibrozil, and niacin act by other mechanisms (see individual monographs).

Contraindications

Hypersensitivity. HMG-CoA reductase inhibitors are contraindicated in pregnancy.

Precautions

Safety of other drugs in pregnancy, lactation, and children not established. See individual drugs. Dietary therapy should be given a 2–3 mo trial before drug therapy is initiated.

Interactions

Bile acid sequestrants (cholestyramine and colestipol) may bind lipid-soluble vitamins (A, D, E, and K) and other concurrently administered drugs in the GI tract. The risk of myopathy from HMG-CoA reductase inhibitors is ↑ by niacin, erythromycin, gemfibrozil, and cyclosporine.

NURSING IMPLICATIONS

Assessment

- Obtain a diet history, especially in regard to **fat** and alcohol consumption.
- **Lab Test Considerations:** Serum cholesterol and triglyceride levels should be evaluated before initiating and periodically throughout therapy. Medication should be discontinued if paradoxical increase in cholesterol level occurs.
- Liver function tests should be assessed before and periodically throughout therapy. May cause an ↑ in levels.

Potential Nursing Diagnoses

- Deficient knowledge, related to disease process and medication regimen (Patient/Family Teaching).
- Noncompliance (Patient/Family Teaching).

Implementation

- See specific medications to determine timing of doses in relation to meals.

Patient/Family Teaching

- Advise patient that these medications should be used in conjunction with diet restrictions (**fat**, **cholesterol**, **carbohydrates**, and alcohol), exercise, and cessation of smoking.

Evaluation/Desired Outcomes

- Decreased serum triglyceride and LDL **cholesterol** levels and improved HDL cholesterol ratios. Therapy is usually discontinued if the clinical response is not evident after 3 mo of therapy.

• MINERALS/ELECTROLYTES/pH MODIFIERS

PHARMACOLOGIC PROFILE

General Use

Prevention and treatment of deficiencies or excesses of electrolytes and maintenance of optimal acid/base balance for homeostasis. Acidifiers and alkalinizers are also used to promote urinary excretion of substances that accumulate in certain disease states (kidney stones, uric acid).

General Action and Information

Electrolytes and minerals are necessary for many body processes. Maintenance of electrolyte levels within normal limits is required for many physiological processes such as cardiac, nerve, and muscle function; bone growth and stability; and a number of other activities. Minerals and electrolytes may also serve as catalysts in many enzymatic reactions. Acid/base balance allows for normal transfer of substances at the cellular and intracellular level.

Contraindications
Contraindicated in situations in which replacement would cause excess or when risk factors for retention are present.

Precautions
Use cautiously in disease states in which electrolyte imbalances are common such as significant hepatic or renal disease, adrenal or pituitary disorders.

Interactions
Depend on individual agents. Alkalinizers and acidifiers can alter the excretion of drugs for which elimination is pH dependent. See specific entries.

NURSING IMPLICATIONS

Assessment
- Observe patient carefully for evidence of electrolyte excess or insufficiency. Monitor lab values before and periodically throughout therapy.

Potential Nursing Diagnoses
- Imbalanced nutrition: less than body requirements (Indications).
- Deficient knowledge, related to medication regimen (Patient/Family Teaching).

Implementation
- **Potassium Chloride:** Do not administer potassium chloride undiluted.

Patient/Family Teaching
- Review diet modifications with patients with chronic electrolyte disturbances.

Evaluation/Desired Outcomes
- Return to normal serum electrolyte concentrations and resolution of clinical symptoms of electrolyte imbalance.
- Changes in pH or composition of urine, which prevent formation of renal calculi.

• NATURAL/HERBAL PRODUCTS

PHARMACOLOGIC PROFILE

General Use
These remedies are used for a wide variety of conditions. Prescriptions are not required and consumers have the choice of many products.

General Action and Information
Use of these agents is based on historical and sometimes anecdotal evidence. The FDA has little control over these agents, so currently there is little standardization among products.

Contraindications
Hypersensitivity. Most products are plant extracts that may contain a variety of impurities.

Precautions
Elderly, pediatric, and pregnant or lactating patients should be aware that these agents carry many of the same risks as prescription medications. Patients with serious chronic medical conditions should consult their health care professional before use.

Interactions

These agents have the ability to interact with prescription medications and may prevent or augment a desired therapeutic outcome. St. John's wort and kava-kava have the greatest risk for serious interactions.

NURSING IMPLICATIONS

Assessment

- Assess the condition for which the patient is taking the product.

Potential Nursing Diagnoses

- Deficient knowledge, related to disease process and medication regimen (Patient/Family Teaching).

Implementation

- **PO:** Administer salicylates and NSAIDs after meals or with food to minimize gastric irritation.

Patient/Family Teaching

- Discuss with patient the reason for using the product. Encourage patient to choose products with USP label, if possible, to guarantee content and purity of medication.
- Inform patient of known side effects and interactions with other medications.

Evaluation/Desired Outcomes

- Improvement in condition for which medication was taken.

• NONOPIOID ANALGESICS

PHARMACOLOGIC PROFILE

General Use

Used to control mild to moderate pain and/or fever. Phenazopyridine is used only to treat urinary tract pain, and capsaicin is used topically for a variety of painful syndromes.

General Action and Information

Most nonopioid analgesics inhibit prostaglandin synthesis peripherally for analgesic effect and centrally for antipyretic effect. Tramadol is a centrally acting agent.

Contraindications

Hypersensitivity and cross-sensitivity among NSAIDs may occur.

Precautions

Use cautiously in patients with severe hepatic or renal disease, chronic alcohol use/abuse, or malnutrition. Tramadol has CNS depressant properties.

Interactions

Long-term use of acetaminophen with NSAIDs may ↑ the risk of adverse renal effects. Prolonged high-dose acetaminophen may ↑ the risk of bleeding with warfarin. Hepatotoxicity may be additive with other hepatotoxic agents, including alcohol. NSAIDs ↑ the risk of bleeding with warfarin, thrombolytic agents, antiplatelet agents, some cephalosporins, and valproates (effect is greatest with aspirin). NSAIDs may also ↓ the effectiveness of diuretics and antihypertensives. The risk of CNS depression with tramadol is ↑ by concurrent use of other CNS depressants, including alcohol, antihistamines, sedative/hypnotics, and some antidepressants.

NURSING IMPLICATIONS

Assessment

- Patients who have asthma, allergies, and nasal polyps or who are allergic to tartrazine are at an ↑ risk for developing hypersensitivity reactions.

- **Pain:** Assess pain and limitation of movement; note type, location, and intensity prior to and at the peak (see Time/Action Profile) following administration.
- **Fever:** Assess fever and note associated signs (diaphoresis, tachycardia, malaise, chills).
- **Lab Test Considerations:** Hepatic, hematologic, and renal function should be evaluated periodically throughout prolonged high-dose therapy. Aspirin and most NSAIDs prolong bleeding time due to suppressed platelet aggregation and, in large doses, may cause prolonged prothrombin time. Monitor hematocrit periodically in prolonged high-dose therapy to assess for GI blood loss.

Potential Nursing Diagnoses

- Acute pain (Indications).
- Risk for imbalanced body temperature (Indications).
- Deficient knowledge, related to disease process and medication regimen (Patient/Family Teaching).

Implementation

- **PO:** Administer salicylates and NSAIDs after meals or with food to minimize gastric irritation.

Patient/Family Teaching

- Instruct patient to take salicylates and NSAIDs with a full glass of water and to remain in an upright position for 15–30 min after administration.
- Adults should not take acetaminophen longer than 10 days and children not longer than 5 days unless directed by health care professional. Short-term doses of acetaminophen with salicylates or NSAIDs should not exceed the recommended daily dose of either drug alone.
- Caution patient to avoid concurrent use of alcohol with this medication to minimize possible gastric irritation; 3 or more glasses of alcohol per day may ↑ the risk of GI bleeding with salicylates or NSAIDs. Caution patient to avoid taking acetaminophen, salicylates, or NSAIDs concurrently for more than a few days, unless directed by health care professional to prevent analgesic nephropathy.
- Advise patients on long-term therapy to inform health care professional of medication regimen prior to surgery. Aspirin, salicylates, and NSAIDs may need to be withheld prior to surgery.

Evaluation/Desired Outcomes

- Relief of mild to moderate discomfort.
- Reduction of fever.

• NONSTEROIDAL ANTI-INFLAMMATORY AGENTS

PHARMACOLOGIC PROFILE

General Use

NSAIDs are used to control mild to moderate pain, fever, and various inflammatory conditions, such as rheumatoid arthritis and osteoarthritis. Ophthalmic NSAIDs are used to ↓ postoperative ocular inflammation, to inhibit perioperative miosis, and to ↓ inflammation due to allergies.

General Action and Information

NSAIDs have analgesic, antipyretic, and anti-inflammatory properties. Analgesic and anti-inflammatory effects are due to inhibition of prostaglandin synthesis. Antipyretic action is due to vasodilation and inhibition of prostaglandin synthesis in the CNS. COX-2 inhibitors (celecoxib) may cause less GI bleeding.

Contraindications

Hypersensitivity to aspirin is a contraindication for the whole group of NSAIDs. Cross-sensitivity may occur.

Precautions

Use cautiously in patients with a history of bleeding disorders, GI bleeding, and severe hepatic, renal, or cardiovascular disease. Safe use in pregnancy is not established and, in general, should be avoided during the second half of pregnancy.

Interactions

NSAIDs prolong bleeding time and potentiate the effect of warfarin, thrombolytic agents, some cephalosporins, antiplatelet agents, and valproates. Prolonged use with aspirin may result in ↑ GI side effects and ↓ effectiveness. NSAIDs may also ↓ response to diuretics or antihypertensive therapy. COX-2 inhibitors do not negate the cardioprotective effect of low-dose aspirin.

NURSING IMPLICATIONS

Assessment

- Patients who have asthma, allergies, and nasal polyps or who are allergic to tartrazine are at an ↑ risk for developing hypersensitivity reactions.
- **Pain:** Assess pain and limitation of movement; note type, location, and intensity prior to and at the peak (see Time/Action Profile) following administration.
- **Fever:** Assess fever and note associated signs (diaphoresis, tachycardia, malaise, chills).
- **Lab Test Considerations:** Most NSAIDs prolong bleeding time due to suppressed platelet aggregation and, in large doses, may cause prolonged PT. Monitor periodically in prolonged high-dose therapy to assess for GI blood loss.

Potential Nursing Diagnoses

- Acute pain (Indications).
- Risk for imbalanced body temperature (Indications).
- Deficient knowledge, related to disease process and medication regimen (Patient/Family Teaching).

Implementation

- **PO:** Administer NSAIDs after meals or with food to minimize gastric irritation.

Patient/Family Teaching

- Instruct patient to take NSAIDs with a full glass of water and to remain in an upright position for 15–30 min after administration.
- Caution patient to avoid concurrent use of alcohol with this medication to minimize possible gastric irritation; 3 or more glasses of alcohol per day may ↑ the risk of GI bleeding with salicylates or NSAIDs. Caution patient to avoid taking acetaminophen, salicylates, or NSAIDs concurrently for more than a few days, unless directed by health care professional to prevent analgesic nephropathy.
- Advise patient on long-term therapy to inform health care professional of medication regimen prior to surgery. NSAIDs may need to be withheld prior to surgery.

Evaluation/Desired Outcomes

- Relief of mild to moderate discomfort
- Reduction of fever.

CLASSIFICATIONS

• OPIOID ANALGESICS

PHARMACOLOGIC PROFILE

General Use

Management of moderate to severe pain. Fentanyl is also used as a general anesthetic adjunct.

General Action and Information

Opioids bind to opiate receptors in the CNS, where they act as agonists of endogenously occurring opioid peptides (eukephalins and endorphins). The result is alteration to the perception of and response to pain.

Contraindications

Hypersensitivity to individual agents.

Precautions

Use cautiously in patients with undiagnosed abdominal pain, head trauma or pathology, liver disease, or history of addiction to opioids. Use smaller doses initially in the elderly and those with respiratory diseases. Prolonged use may result in tolerance and the need for larger doses to relieve pain. Psychological or physical dependence may occur.

Interactions

↑ the CNS depressant properties of other drugs, including alcohol, antihistamines, antidepressants, sedative/hypnotics, phenothiazines, and MAO inhibitors. Use of partial-antagonist opioid analgesics (buprenorphine, butorphanol, nalbuphine, and pentazocine) may precipitate opioid withdrawal in physically dependent patients. Use with MAO inhibitors or procarbazine may result in severe paradoxical reactions (especially with meperidine). Nalbuphine or pentazocine may ↓ the analgesic effects of other concurrently administered opioid analgesics.

NURSING IMPLICATIONS

Assessment

- Assess type, location, and intensity of pain prior to and at peak following administration. When titrating opioid doses, ↑ of 25–50% should be administered until there is either a 50% ↓ in the patient's pain rating on a numerical or visual analogue scale or the patient reports satisfactory pain relief. A repeat dose can be safely administered at the time of the peak if previous dose is ineffective and side effects are minimal. Patients requiring higher doses of opioid agonist-antagonists should be converted to an opioid agonist.
- Opioid agonist-antagonists are not recommended for prolonged use or as first-line therapy for acute or cancer pain.
- An equianalgesic chart (see Appendix I) should be used when changing routes or when changing from one opioid to another.
- Assess BP, pulse, and respirations before and periodically during administration. If respiratory rate is <10/min, assess level of sedation. Physical stimulation may be sufficient to prevent significant hypoventilation. Dose may need to be ↓ by 25–50%. Initial drowsiness will diminish with continued use.
- Assess prior analgesic history. Antagonistic properties of agonist-antagonists may induce withdrawal symptoms (vomiting, restlessness, abdominal cramps, and ↑ BP and temperature) in patients physically dependent on opioids.
- Prolonged use may lead to physical and psychological dependence and tolerance. This should not prevent patient from receiving adequate analgesia. Most patients who receive opioid analgesics for pain do not develop psychological dependence. Progressively higher doses may be required to relieve pain with chronic therapy.
- Assess bowel function routinely. Prevention of constipation should be instituted with ↑ intake of fluids and bulk, stool softeners, and laxatives to minimize constipating effects. Stimu-

lant laxatives should be administered routinely if opioid use exceeds 2–3 days, unless contraindicated.
- Monitor intake and output ratios. If significant discrepancies occur, assess for urinary retention and inform physician or other health care professional.
- **Toxicity and Overdose:** If an opioid antagonist is required to reverse respiratory depression or coma, naloxone is the antidote. Dilute the 0.4-mg ampule of naloxone in 10 mL of 0.9% NaCl and administer 0.5 mL (0.02 mg) by IV push every 2 min. For children and patients weighing <40 kg, dilute 0.1 mg of naloxone in 10 mL of 0.9% NaCl for a concentration of 10 mcg/mL and administer 0.5 mcg/kg every 1–2 min. Titrate dose to avoid withdrawal, seizures, and severe pain.

Potential Nursing Diagnoses
- Acute pain (Indications).
- Disturbed sensory perception (auditory, visual) (Side Effects).
- Risk for injury (Side Effects).
- Deficient knowledge, related to disease process and medication regimen (Patient/Family Teaching).

Implementation
- Do not confuse morphine with hydromorphone or meperidine; errors have resulted in fatalities.
- Explain therapeutic value of medication before administration to enhance the analgesic effect.
- Regularly administered doses may be more effective than prn administration. Analgesic is more effective if given before pain becomes severe.
- Coadministration with nonopioid analgesics may have additive analgesic effects and may permit lower doses.
- Medication should be discontinued gradually after long-term use to prevent withdrawal symptoms.

Patient/Family Teaching
- Instruct patient on how and when to ask for pain medication.
- Medication may cause drowsiness or dizziness. Caution patient to call for assistance when ambulating or smoking and to avoid driving or other activities requiring alertness until response to medication is known.
- Advise patient to make position changes slowly to minimize orthostatic hypotension.
- Caution patient to avoid concurrent use of alcohol or other CNS depressants with this medication.
- Encourage patient to turn, cough, and breathe deeply every 2 hr to prevent atelectasis.

Evaluation/Desired Outcomes
- Decreased severity of pain without a significant alteration in level of consciousness or respiratory status.

• SEDATIVE/HYPNOTICS

PHARMACOLOGIC PROFILE

General Use
Sedatives are used to provide sedation, usually prior to procedures. Hypnotics are used to manage insomnia. Selected agents are useful as anticonvulsants (clorazepate, diazepam, phenobarbital), skeletal muscle relaxants (diazepam), adjuncts in the management of alcohol withdrawal syndrome (chlordiazepoxide, diazepam, oxazepam), adjuncts in general anesthesia (droperidol), or as amnestics (midazolam, diazepam).

General Action and Information
Cause generalized CNS depression. May produce tolerance with chronic use and have potential for psychological or physical dependence. These agents have NO analgesic properties.

Contraindications
Hypersensitivity. Should not be used in comatose patients or in those with pre-existing CNS depression. Should not be used in patients with uncontrolled severe pain. Avoid use during pregnancy or lactation.

Precautions
Use cautiously in patients with hepatic dysfunction, severe renal impairment, or severe underlying pulmonary disease. Use with caution in patients who may be suicidal or who may have had previous drug addictions. Hypnotic use should be short-term. Geriatric patients may be more sensitive to CNS depressant effects; dosage ↓ may be required.

Interactions
Additive CNS depression with alcohol, antihistamines, some antidepressants, opioid analgesics, or phenothiazines. Barbiturates induce hepatic drug-metabolizing enzymes and can ↓ the effectiveness of drugs metabolized by the liver, including oral contraceptives. Should not be used with MAO inhibitors.

NURSING IMPLICATIONS

Assessment
- Monitor BP, pulse, and respiratory status frequently throughout IV administration. Prolonged high-dose therapy may lead to psychological or physical dependence. Restrict the amount of drug available to patient, especially if patient is depressed, suicidal, or has a history of addiction.
- **Insomnia:** Assess sleep patterns before and periodically throughout course of therapy.
- **Seizures:** Observe and record intensity, duration, and characteristics of seizure activity. Institute seizure precautions.
- **Muscle Spasms:** Assess muscle spasms, associated pain, and limitation of movement before and throughout therapy.
- **Alcohol Withdrawal:** Assess patient experiencing alcohol withdrawal for tremors, agitation, delirium, and hallucinations. Protect patient from injury.

Potential Nursing Diagnoses
- Insomnia (Indications).
- Risk for injury (Side Effects).
- Deficient knowledge, related to disease process and medication regimen (Patient/Family Teaching).

Implementation
- Supervise ambulation and transfer of patients following administration of hypnotic doses. Remove cigarettes. Side rails should be raised and call bell within reach at all times. Keep bed in low position.

Patient/Family Teaching
- Discuss the importance of preparing the environment for sleep (dark room, quiet, avoidance of nicotine and caffeine). If less effective after a few weeks, consult health care professional; do not ↑ dose. Gradual withdrawal may be required to prevent reactions following prolonged therapy.
- May cause daytime drowsiness. Caution patient to avoid driving and other activities requiring alertness until response to medication is known.
- Advise patient to avoid the use of alcohol and other CNS depressants concurrently with these medications.
- Advise patient to inform health care professional if pregnancy is planned or suspected.

Evaluation/Desired Outcomes

- Improvement in sleep patterns.
- Control of seizures.
- Decrease in muscle spasms.
- Decreased tremulousness.
- More rational ideation when used for alcohol withdrawal.

• SKELETAL MUSCLE RELAXANTS

PHARMACOLOGIC PROFILE

General Use

Two major uses are spasticity associated with spinal cord diseases or lesions (baclofen and dantrolene) or adjunctive therapy in the symptomatic relief of acute painful musculoskeletal conditions (cyclobenzaprine, diazepam, and methocarbamol). IV dantrolene is also used to treat and prevent malignant hyperthermia.

General Action and Information

Act either centrally (baclofen, carisoprodol, cyclobenzaprine, diazepam, and methocarbamol) or directly (dantrolene).

Contraindications

Baclofen and oral dantrolene should not be used in patients in whom spasticity is used to maintain posture and balance.

Precautions

Safety in pregnancy and lactation not established. Use cautiously in patients with a history of previous liver disease.

Interactions

Additive CNS depression with other CNS depressants, including alcohol, antihistamines, antidepressants, opioid analgesics, and sedative/hypnotics.

NURSING IMPLICATIONS

Assessment

- Assess patient for pain, muscle stiffness, and range of motion before and periodically throughout therapy.

Potential Nursing Diagnoses

- Acute pain (Indications).
- Impaired physical mobility (Indications).
- Risk for injury (Side Effects).

Implementation

- Provide safety measures as indicated. Supervise ambulation and transfer of patients.

Patient/Family Teaching

- Encourage patient to comply with additional therapies prescribed for muscle spasm (rest, physical therapy, heat).
- Medication may cause drowsiness. Caution patient to avoid driving or other activities requiring alertness until response to drug is known.
- Advise patient to avoid concurrent use of alcohol or other CNS depressants with these medications.

Evaluation/Desired Outcomes

- Decreased musculoskeletal pain
- Decreased muscle spasticity
- Increased range of motion
- Prevention or decrease in temperature and skeletal rigidity in malignant hyperthermia.

• THROMBOLYTICS

PHARMACOLOGIC PROFILE

General Use

Acute management of ST-segment-elevation MI. Alteplase is also used in the management of acute pulmonary embolism and acute ischemic stroke.

General Action and Information

Converts plasminogen to plasmin, which then degrades fibrin in clots. Alteplase, reteplase, and tenecteplase directly activate plasminogen. Results in lysis of blood clots.

Contraindications

Hypersensitivity. Active internal bleeding, history of cerebrovascular accident, recent CNS trauma or surgery, neoplasm, or arteriovenous malformation, severe uncontrolled hypertension, and known bleeding tendencies.

Precautions

Recent (within 10 days) major surgery, trauma, GI or GU bleeding. Severe hepatic or renal disease. Subacute bacterial endocarditis or acute pericarditis. Use cautiously in geriatric patients. Safety not established in pregnancy, lactation, or children.

Interactions

Concurrent use with antiplatelet agents, NSAIDs, warfarin, or heparins may ↑ the risk of bleeding, although these agents are frequently used together or in sequence. Risk of bleeding may also be ↑ by concurrent use with cefotetan, cefoperazone, and valproic acid.

NURSING IMPLICATIONS

Assessment

- Begin therapy as soon as possible after the onset of symptoms.
- Monitor vital signs, including temperature, continuously for coronary thrombosis and at least every 4 hr during therapy for other indications. Do not use lower extremities to monitor BP.
- Assess patient carefully for bleeding every 15 min during the 1st hr of therapy, every 15–30 min during the next 8 hr, and at least every 4 hr for the duration of therapy. Frank bleeding may occur from sites of invasive procedures or from body orifices. Internal bleeding may also occur (↓ neurologic status; abdominal pain with coffee-ground emesis or black, tarry stools; hematuria; joint pain). If uncontrolled bleeding occurs, stop medication and notify physician immediately.
- Assess neurologic status throughout therapy.
- Altered sensorium or neurologic changes may be indicative of intracranial bleeding.
- **Coronary Thrombosis:** Monitor ECG continuously. Notify physician if significant arrhythmias occur. IV lidocaine or procainamide may be ordered prophylactically. Cardiac enzymes should be monitored. Coronary angiography may be ordered following therapy to monitor effectiveness of therapy.
- Monitor heart sounds and breath sounds frequently. Inform physician if signs of HF occur (rales/crackles, dyspnea, S3 heart sound, jugular venous distention).
- **Pulmonary Embolism:** Monitor pulse, BP, hemodynamics, and respiratory status (rate, degree of dyspnea, arterial blood gases).

- **Cannula/Catheter Occlusion:** Monitor ability to aspirate blood as indicator of patency. Ensure that patient exhales and holds breath when connecting and disconnecting IV syringe to prevent air embolism.
- **Acute Ischemic Stroke:** Assess neurologic status. Determine time of onset of stroke symptoms. Alteplase must be administered within 3–4.5 hr of onset (within 3 hr in patients >80 years, those taking oral anticoagulants, those with a baseline National Institutes of Health Stroke Scale score >25, or those with both a history of stroke and diabetes).
- **Lab Test Considerations:** Hematocrit, hemoglobin, platelet count, fibrin/fibrin degradation product (FDP/fdp) titer, fibrinogen concentration, prothrombin time, thrombin time, and activated partial thromboplastin time may be evaluated prior to and frequently throughout therapy. Bleeding time may be assessed prior to therapy if patient has received platelet aggregation inhibitors. Obtain type and cross match and have blood available at all times in case of hemorrhage. Stools should be tested for occult blood loss and urine for hematuria periodically during therapy.
- **Toxicity and Overdose:** If local bleeding occurs, apply pressure to site. If severe or internal bleeding occurs, discontinue infusion. Clotting factors and/or blood volume may be restored through infusions of whole blood, packed RBCs, fresh frozen plasma, or cryoprecipitate. Do not administer dextran, as it has antiplatelet activity. Aminocaproic acid may be used as an antidote.

Potential Nursing Diagnoses

- Ineffective tissue perfusion (Indications).
- Risk for injury (Side Effects).
- Deficient knowledge, related to disease process and medication regimen (Patient/Family Teaching).

Implementation

- This medication should be used only in settings in which hematologic function and clinical response can be adequately monitored.
- Starting two IV lines prior to therapy is recommended: one for the thrombolytic agent, the other for any additional infusions.
- Avoid invasive procedures, such as IM injections or arterial punctures, with this therapy. If such procedures must be performed, apply pressure to all arterial and venous puncture sites for at least 30 min. Avoid venipunctures at noncompressible sites (jugular vein, subclavian site).
- Systemic anticoagulation with heparin is usually begun several hours after the completion of thrombolytic therapy.
- Acetaminophen may be ordered to control fever.

Patient/Family Teaching

- Explain purpose of medication and the need for close monitoring to patient and family. Instruct patient to report hypersensitivity reactions (rash, dyspnea) and bleeding or bruising.
- Explain need for bedrest and minimal handling during therapy to avoid injury. Avoid all unnecessary procedures such as shaving and vigorous tooth brushing.

Evaluation/Desired Outcomes

- Lysis of thrombi and restoration of blood flow
- Prevention of neurologic sequelae in acute ischemic stroke
- Cannula or catheter patency.

• VACCINES/IMMUNIZING AGENTS

PHARMACOLOGIC PROFILE

General Use

Immune globulins provide passive immunization to infectious diseases by providing antibodies. Immunization with vaccines and toxoids containing bacterial or viral antigenic material results in endogenous production of antibodies.

General Action and Information

Immunity from immune globulins is rapid, but short-lived (up to 3 months). Active immunization with vaccine or toxoids produces prolonged immunity (years).

Contraindications

Hypersensitivity to product, preservatives, or other additives. Some products contain thimerisol, neomycin, and/or **egg protein**.

Precautions

Severe bleeding problems (IM injections).

Interactions

↓ antibody response to vaccine/toxoids and ↑ risk of adverse reactions in patients receiving concurrent antineoplastic, immunosuppressive, or radiation therapy.

NURSING IMPLICATIONS

Assessment

- Assess previous immunization history and history of hypersensitivity.

Potential Nursing Diagnoses

- Risk for infection (Indications).
- Deficient knowledge, related to disease process and medication regimen (Patient/Family Teaching).

Implementation

- Measles, mumps, and rubella vaccine, trivalent oral polio virus vaccine, and diphtheria toxoid, tetanus toxoid, and pertussis vaccine may be given concurrently.
- Administer each immunization by appropriate route.

Patient/Family Teaching

- Inform patient/parent of potential and reportable side effects of immunization. Health care professional should be notified if patient develops fever over 39.4°C (103°F); difficulty breathing; hives; itching; swelling of the eyes, face, or inside of nose; sudden severe tiredness or weakness; or convulsions occur.
- Review next scheduled immunization with parent. Emphasize the importance of keeping a record of immunizations and dates given.

Evaluation/Desired Outcomes

- Prevention of diseases through active immunity.

• VASCULAR HEADACHE SUPPRESSANTS

PHARMACOLOGIC PROFILE

General Use

Used for acute treatment of vascular headaches (migraine, cluster headaches, migraine variants). Other agents such as some beta blockers and some calcium channel blockers are used for suppression of frequently occurring vascular headaches.

General Action and Information

Ergot derivatives (ergotamine, dihydroergotamine) directly stimulate alpha-adrenergic and serotonergic receptors, producing vascular smooth muscle vasoconstriction. Almotriptan, eletriptan, frovatriptan, naratriptan, rizatriptan, sumatriptan, and zolmitriptan produce vasoconstriction by acting as serotonin (5-HT_1) agonists.

Contraindications

Avoid using these agents in patients with ischemic cardiovascular disease.

Precautions

Use cautiously in patients who have a history of, or at risk for, cardiovascular disease.

Interactions

Avoid concurrent use of ergot derivative agents with serotonin agonist agents; see also individual agents.

NURSING IMPLICATIONS

Assessment

- Assess pain location, intensity, duration, and associated symptoms (photophobia, phonophobia, nausea, vomiting) during migraine attack and frequency of attacks.

Potential Nursing Diagnoses

- Acute pain (Indications).
- Deficient knowledge, related to disease process and medication regimen (Patient/Family Teaching).

Implementation

- Medication should be administered at the first sign of a headache.

Patient/Family Teaching

- Inform patient that medication should be used only during a migraine attack. It is meant to be used for relief of migraine attacks but not to prevent or reduce the number of attacks.
- Advise patient that lying down in a darkened room following medication administration may further help relieve headache.
- May cause dizziness or drowsiness. Caution patient to avoid driving or other activities requiring alertness until response to medication is known.
- Advise patient to avoid alcohol, which aggravates headaches.

Evaluation/Desired Outcomes

- Relief of migraine attack.

• VITAMINS

PHARMACOLOGIC PROFILE

General Use

Used in the prevention and treatment of vitamin deficiencies and as supplements in various metabolic disorders.

General Action and Information

Serve as components of enzyme systems that catalyze numerous varied metabolic reactions. Necessary for homeostasis. Water-soluble vitamins (B-vitamins and vitamin C) rarely cause toxicity. Fat-soluble vitamins (vitamins D and E) may accumulate and cause toxicity.

Contraindications

Hypersensitivity to additives, preservatives, or colorants.

Precautions

Dose should be adjusted to avoid toxicity, especially for fat-soluble vitamins.

Interactions

Pyridoxine in large amounts may interfere with the effectiveness of levodopa. Cholestyramine, colestipol, and mineral oil ↓ absorption of fat-soluble vitamins.

NURSING IMPLICATIONS

Assessment

- Assess patient for signs of vitamin deficiency before and periodically throughout therapy.
- Assess nutritional status through 24-hr diet recall. Determine frequency of consumption of vitamin-rich foods.

Potential Nursing Diagnoses

- Imbalanced nutrition: less than body requirements (Indications).
- Deficient knowledge, related to disease process and medication regimen (Patient/Family Teaching).

Implementation

- Because of infrequency of single vitamin deficiencies, combinations are commonly administered.

Patient/Family Teaching

- Encourage patients to comply with diet recommendations of physician or other health care professional. Explain that the best source of vitamins is a well-balanced diet with foods from the four basic food groups.
- Patients self-medicating with vitamin supplements should be cautioned not to exceed RDAs. The effectiveness of megadoses for treatment of various medical conditions is unproved and may cause side effects and toxicity.

Evaluation/Desired Outcomes

- Prevention of, or decrease in, the symptoms of vitamin deficiencies.

• WEIGHT CONTROL AGENTS

PHARMACOLOGIC PROFILE

General Use

These agents are used in the management of exogenous obesity as part of a regimen including a reduced-calorie diet. They are especially useful in the presence of other risk factors including hypertension, diabetes, or dyslipidemias.

General Action and Information

Phentermine is an anorexiant designed to ↓ appetite via its action in the CNS. Orlistat is a lipase inhibitor that ↓ absorption of dietary fat.

Contraindications

None of these agents should be used during pregnancy or lactation. Phentermine should not be used in patients with severe hepatic or renal disease, uncontrolled hypertension, known HF, or cardiovascular disease. Orlistat should not be used in patients with chronic malabsorption.

Precautions

Phentermine should be used cautiously in patients with a history of seizures, or angle-closure glaucoma and in geriatric patients.

Interactions

Phentermine may have additive, adverse effects with CNS stimulants, some vascular headache suppressants, MAO inhibitors, and some opioids (concurrent use should be avoided). Orlistat ↓ absorption of some fat-soluble vitamins and beta-carotene.

NURSING IMPLICATIONS

Assessment

- Monitor weight and dietary intake prior to and periodically during therapy. Adjust concurrent medications (antihypertensives, antidiabetics, lipid-lowering agents) as needed.

Potential Nursing Diagnoses

- Disturbed body image (Indications).
- Imbalanced nutrition: more than body requirements (Indications).
- Deficient knowledge, related to medication regimen (Patient/Family Teaching).

Implementation

Patient/Family Teaching

- Advise patient that regular physical activity, approved by healthcare professional, should be used in conjunction with medication and diet.

Evaluation/Desired Outcomes

- Slow, consistent weight loss when combined with a reduced-calorie diet.

abacavir (ah-**back**-ah-veer)

Ziagen

Classification

Therapeutic: antiretrovirals

Pharmacologic: nucleoside reverse transcriptase inhibitors

Pregnancy Category C

Indications

Management of HIV infection (AIDS) in combination with other antiretrovirals (not with lamivudine and/or tenofovir).

Action

Converted inside cells to carbovir triphosphate, its active metabolite. Carbovir triphosphate inhibits the activity of HIV-1 reverse transcriptase, which in turn terminates viral DNA growth. **Therapeutic Effects:** Slows the progression of HIV infection and decreases the occurrence of its sequelae. Increases CD4 cell counts and decreases viral load.

Pharmacokinetics

Absorption: Rapidly and extensively (83%) absorbed.

Distribution: Distributes into extravascular space and readily distributes into erythrocytes.

Metabolism and Excretion: Mostly metabolized by the liver; 1.2% excreted unchanged in urine.

Half-life: 1.5 hr.

TIME/ACTION PROFILE (blood levels)

ROUTE	ONSET	PEAK	DURATION
PO	unknown	unknown	unknown

Contraindications/Precautions

Contraindicated in: Hypersensitivity (rechallenge may be fatal); Concurrent use of antiretroviral combination products containing abacavir; Lactation: Breast feeding not recommended for HIV-infected patients.

Use Cautiously in: Coronary heart disease; OB: Safety not established; Pedi: Children <3 mo (safety not established).

Exercise Extreme Caution in: Patients positive for HLA-B*5701 allele (unless exceptional circumstances exist where benefits clearly outweigh the risks).

Adverse Reactions/Side Effects

CNS: headache, insomnia. **CV:** MYOCARDIAL INFARCTION. **GI:** HEPATOMEGALY (WITH STEATOSIS), diarrhea, nausea, vomiting, anorexia. **Derm:** rashes. **F and E:** LACTIC ACIDOSIS. **Misc:** HYPERSENSITIVITY REACTIONS, fat redistribution, immune reconstitution syndrome.

Interactions

Drug-Drug: Alcohol ↑ blood levels. May ↑ **methadone** metabolism in some patients; slight ↑ in **methadone** dosing may be needed.

Route/Dosage

PO (Adults): 300 mg twice daily.

PO (Children ≥3 mo): *Oral solution*—8 mg/kg twice daily *or* 16 mg/kg once daily (not to exceed 600 mg/day); *Tablets*—14–19 kg: 150 mg twice daily *or* 300 mg once daily; 20–24 kg: 150 mg in AM and 300 mg in PM *or* 450 mg once daily; ≥25 kg: 300 mg twice daily *or* 600 mg once daily.

Availability (generic available)

Tablets: 300 mg. **Oral solution (strawberry/banana flavor):** 20 mg/mL. ***In combination with:*** lamivudine (Epzicom); lamivudine and zidovudine (Trizivir); lamivudine and dolutegravir (Triumeq). See Appendix B.

NURSING IMPLICATIONS

Assessment

- Assess patient for change in severity of HIV symptoms and for symptoms of opportunistic infections throughout therapy.
- Assess for signs of hypersensitivity reactions (fever; rash; gastrointestinal—nausea, vomiting, diarrhea, abdominal pain; constitutional—malaise, fatigue, achiness; respiratory—dyspnea, cough, pharyngitis). May also cause elevated liver function tests, increased creatine phosphokinase or creatinine, and lymphopenia. Patients who carry the HLA-B*5701 allele are at high risk for hypersensitivity reaction. Discontinue promptly if hypersensitivity reaction is suspected. Regardless of HLA-B*5701 status, permanently discontinue abacavir if hypersensitivity cannot be ruled out, even when other diagnoses are possible. Following a hypersensitivity reaction, never restart abacavir or abacavir-containing products. More severe symptoms may occur within hours and may include life-threatening hypotension and death. Symptoms usually resolve upon discontinuation.
- May cause lactic acidosis and severe hepatomegaly with steatosis. Monitor patient for signs (↑ serum lactate levels, ↑ liver enzymes, liver enlargement on palpation). Therapy should be suspended if clinical or laboratory signs occur.
- ***Lab Test Considerations:*** Monitor viral load and CD4 cell count regularly during therapy.
- Screen for HLA-B*5701 allele prior to initiation of therapy to decrease risk of hypersensitivity reaction. Screening is also recommended prior to reinitiation of abacavir in patients of unknown HLA-B*5701 status who have previously tolerated abacavir.
- Monitor liver function. May cause ↑ levels of AST, ALT, and alkaline phosphatase, which usually re-

solve after interruption of therapy. Lactic acidosis may occur with hepatic toxicity, causing hepatic steatosis; may be fatal, especially in women.

- May cause ↑ serum glucose and triglyceride levels.

Potential Nursing Diagnoses

Risk for infection (Indications)
Noncompliance (Patient/Family Teaching)

Implementation

- **PO:** May be administered with or without food. Oral solution is clear to opalescent and yellow, may be stored at room temperature or refrigerated; do not freeze. Tablet may be used with children if able to swallow and dose is correctly calculated.

Patient/Family Teaching

- Emphasize the importance of taking abacavir as directed. Must always be used in combination with other antiretroviral drugs. Do not take more than prescribed amount, and do not stop taking without consulting health care professional. Take missed doses as soon as remembered; do not double doses. Advise patient to read the *Medication Guide* prior to starting therapy and with each Rx refill in case of changes.
- Instruct patient not to share abacavir with others.
- Inform patient that abacavir does not cure AIDS or prevent associated or opportunistic infections. Abacavir does not reduce risk of transmission of HIV to others through sexual contact or blood contamination. Caution patient to use a condom, and avoid sharing needles or donating blood to prevent spreading the AIDS virus to others. Advise patient that long-term effects of abacavir are unknown.
- Advise patient of potential for hypersensitivity reactions that may result in death. Instruct patient to discontinue abacavir and notify health care professional immediately if symptoms of hypersensitivity or signs of Immune Reconstitution Syndrome (signs and symptoms of an infection) occur. Advise patient to read *Medication Guide* thoroughly with each refill in case of changes. A warning card summarizing symptoms of abacavir hypersensitivity is provided with each prescription; instruct patient to carry card at all times.
- Instruct patient to notify health care professional immediately if symptoms of lactic acidosis (tiredness or weakness, unusual muscle pain, trouble breathing, stomach pain with nausea and vomiting, cold especially in arms or legs, dizziness, fast or irregular heartbeat) or if signs of hepatotoxicity (yellow skin or whites of eyes, dark urine, light-colored stools, lack of appetite for several days or longer, nausea, abdominal pain) occur. These symptoms may occur more frequently in patients that are female, obese, or have been taking medications like abacavir for a long time.
- Inform patient that redistribution and accumulation of body fat may occur, causing central obesity, dorsocervical fat enlargement (buffalo hump), peripheral wasting, breast enlargement, and cushingoid appearance. The cause and long-term effects are not known.
- Advise patient to notify health care professional of all Rx or OTC medications, vitamins, or herbal products being taken and to consult with health care professional before taking other medications, especially methadone and other antiretrovirals.
- Advise female patients to avoid breast feeding and to notify health care professional if pregnancy is planned or suspected. Encourage women who become pregnant while taking abacavir to enroll in the Antiretroviral Pregnancy Registry by calling 1-800-258-4263.
- Emphasize the importance of regular follow-up exams and blood counts to determine progress and monitor for side effects.

Evaluation/Desired Outcomes

- Delayed progression of AIDS, and decreased opportunistic infections in patients with HIV.
- Decrease in viral load and increase in CD4 cell counts.

abacavir/dolutegravir/lamivudine

(ah-**back**-ah-veer/doe-loo-**teg**-ra-vir/la-**mi**-vyoo-deen)
Triumeq

Classification
Therapeutic: antiretrovirals (combination)
Pharmacologic: integrase strand transfer inhibitors (INSTI) (dolutegravir), nucleoside reverse transcriptase inhibitors (abacavir, lamivudine)

Pregnancy Category C

Indications

Treatment of HIV-1 infection.

Action

Abacavir—Converted inside cells to carbovir triphosphate, its active metabolite. Carbovir triphosphate inhibits the activity of HIV-1 reverse transcriptase, which in turn terminates viral DNA growth. *Dolutegravir*—Inhibits HIV-1 integrase, which is required for viral replication. *Lamuvudine*—After intracellular conversion to its active form (lamivudine-5-triphosphate), inhibits viral DNA synthesis by inhibiting the enzyme reverse transcriptase. **Therapeutic Effects:** Evidence of decreased viral replication and reduced viral load with slowed progression of HIV and its sequelae.

Pharmacokinetics

Abacavir

Absorption: Rapidly and extensively (83%) absorbed.

Distribution: Distributes into extravascular space and readily distributes into erythrocytes.
Metabolism and Excretion: Mostly metabolized by the liver; 1.2% excreted unchanged in urine.
Half-life: 1.5 hr.
Dolutegravir
Absorption: Absorption follows oral administration; bioavailability is unknown.
Distribution: Enters CSF.
Protein Binding: >98.9%.
Metabolism and Excretion: Metabolized primarily by the UGT1A1 enzyme system with some metabolism by CYP3A4. 53% excreted unchanged in feces. Metabolites are renally excreted, minimal renal elimination of unchanged drug. ⧖ Poor metabolizers of dolutegravir have ↑ levels and ↓ clearance.
Half-life: 14 hr.
Lamivudine
Absorption: Well absorbed after oral administration (86% in adults, 66% in infants and children).
Distribution: Distributes into the extravascular space. Some penetration into CSF; remainder of distribution unknown.
Metabolism and Excretion: Mostly excreted unchanged in urine; <5% metabolized by the liver.
Half-life: *Adults*—3.7 hr; *children*—2 hr.

TIME/ACTION PROFILE (blood levels)

ROUTE	ONSET	PEAK	DURATION
PO	unknown	unknown	24 hr

Contraindications/Precautions
Contraindicated in: Hypersensitivity to any component (especially abacavir, rechallenge may be fatal); Resistance to any component; Presence of HLA-B*5701 allele; Concurrent use of dofetilide; Concurrent administration of lamivudine or abacavir alone or in other combination antiretroviral dose forms; Lactation: Breast feeding not recommended for HIV-infected patients; Moderate to severe liver impairment; CCr <50 mL/min.
Use Cautiously in: Underlying hepatitis B or C (may worsen liver function); Patients with HIV-1/HCV coinfection receiving interferon alfa with/without ribavirin (may be at risk for hepatic decompensation, dose alteration or discontinuation of interferon and/or ribavirin may be necessary); Mild hepatic impairment (if dose ↓ of abacavir is necessary, combination should be given as individual components); Underlying cardiovascular disease, including history of hypertension, hyperlipidema, smoking history or diabetes mellitus; OB: Use only if potential benefit justifies potential risk to the fetus; Pedi: Safety and effectiveness not established.

Adverse Reactions/Side Effects
Abacavir/dolutegravir/lamivudine.
CNS: fatigue, headache, insomnia. **CV:** MYOCARDIAL INFARCTION. **GI:** HEPATOMEGALY (WITH STEATOSIS), HEPATOTOXICITY (↑ WITH HEPATITIS B OR C), exacerbation of Hepatitis B. **F and E:** LACTIC ACIDOSIS. **Misc:** HYPERSENSITIVITY REACTIONS, immune reconstitution syndrome, redistribution/accumulation of body fat.

Interactions
Drug-Drug: Abacavir: Alcohol ↑ blood levels. May ↑ **methadone** metabolism in some patients; slight ↑ in **methadone** dosing may be needed. **Dolutegravir:** May ↑ blood levels and toxicity from **dofetilide**; concurrent use contraindicated. Blood levels and effectiveness are ↓ by **etravirine** (should not be used concurrently without atazanavir/ritonavir, darunavir/ritonavir or lopinavir/ritonavir). Blood levels and effectiveness are ↓ by **efavirenz**, **fosamprenavir/ritonavir**, **tipranavir/ritonavir**, **carbamazepine**, and **rifampin**; ↑ dosage of dolutegravir recommended. Blood levels and effectiveness may be↓ by **nevirapine**; avoid concurrent use. May ↑ blood levels and toxicity from **metformin**; do not exceed metformin dose of 1000 mg/day. Blood levels and effectiveness may be ↓ by other **metabolic inducers** including **oxcarbazepine**, **phenobarbital**, and **phenytoin**; avoid concurrent use. Absorption and effectiveness may be ↓ by cation-containing **antacids**, **buffered medications**, oral **calcium supplements**, oral **iron supplements**, **laxatives**, or **sucralfate**; dolutegravir should be taken 2 hr before or 6 hr after; may also take dolutegravir and calcium or iron supplements with food. **Lamivudine: Trimethoprim/sulfamethoxazole** ↑ levels (dose alteration may be necessary in renal impairment). ↑ risk of pancreatitis with concurrent use of other **drugs causing pancreatitis**. ↑ risk of neuropathy with concurrent use of other **drugs causing neuropathy**. Combination therapy with **tenofovir** and **abacavir** may lead to virologic nonresponse; avoid use.
Drug-Natural Products: Blood levels and effectiveness may be ↓ **St. John's wort**; avoid concurrent use.

Route/Dosage
PO (Adults): One tablet (abacavir 600 mg/dolutegravir 50 mg/lamivudine 300 mg) daily; *Concurrent efavirenz, fosamprenavir/ritonavir, tipranavir/ritonavir, carbamazepine or rifampin*—additional 50–mg dose of dolutegravir is required separated by 12 hr.

Availability
Tablets: abacavir 600 mg/dolutegravir 50 mg/lamivudine 300 mg per tablet.

NURSING IMPLICATIONS

Assessment

- Assess patient for change in severity of HIV symptoms and for symptoms of opportunistic infections throughout therapy.
- Assess for signs of hypersensitivity reactions (fever; rash; gastrointestinal—nausea, vomiting, diarrhea, abdominal pain; constitutional—malaise, fatigue, achiness; respiratory—dyspnea, cough, pharyngitis). May also cause elevated liver function tests, increased creatine phosphokinase or creatinine, and lymphopenia. ⧖ Patients who carry the HLA-B*5701 allele are at high risk for hypersensitivity reaction. Discontinue promptly if hypersensitivity reaction is suspected. Regardless of HLA-B*5701 status, permanently discontinue if hypersensitivity cannot be ruled out, even when other diagnoses are possible. Following a hypersensitivity reaction, never restart abacavir-containing products. More severe symptoms may occur within hr and may include life-threatening hypotension and death. Symptoms usually resolve upon discontinuation.
- May cause lactic acidosis and severe hepatomegaly with steatosis. Monitor patient for signs (↑ serum lactate levels, ↑ liver enzymes, liver enlargement on palpation). Therapy should be suspended if clinical or laboratory signs occur.
- Assess patient, especially pediatric patients, for signs of pancreatitis (nausea, vomiting, abdominal pain) periodically during therapy. May require discontinuation of therapy.
- Monitor patient for signs and symptoms of peripheral neuropathy (tingling, burning, numbness, or pain in hands or feet); may be difficult to differentiate from peripheral neuropathy of severe HIV disease. May require discontinuation of therapy.
- ***Lab Test Considerations:*** Monitor viral load and CD4 cell count regularly during therapy.
- ⧖ Screen for HLA-B*5701 allele prior to initiation of therapy to decrease risk of hypersensitivity reaction. Screening is also recommended prior to reinitiation of abacavir in patients of unknown HLA-B*5701 status who have previously tolerated abacavir.
- Monitor liver function periodically. May cause ↑ levels of AST, ALT, and alkaline phosphatase, which usually resolve after interruption of therapy. Patients with concurrent Hepatitis B or C should be followed for at least several mo after stopping therapy. Lactic acidosis may occur with hepatic toxicity, causing hepatic steatosis; may be fatal, especially in women.
- May cause ↑ serum glucose, lipase, and triglyceride levels.

Potential Nursing Diagnoses

Risk for infection (Indications)
Noncompliance (Patient/Family Teaching)

Implementation

- **PO:** Administer without regard to food.
- Take *Triumeq* 2 hr before or 6 hr after antacids, laxatives, other medications containing aluminum, magnesium, sucralfate, or buffering agents, calcium, or iron. Supplements containing calcium or iron can be taken with *Triumeq* if taken with food.

Patient/Family Teaching

- Emphasize the importance of taking abacavir as directed. Must always be used in combination with other antiretroviral drugs. Do not take more than prescribed amount, and do not stop taking without consulting health care professional. Take missed doses as soon as remembered until 4 hr of time of next dose; do not double doses. Advise patient to read the *Medication Guide* prior to starting therapy and with each Rx refill in case of changes.
- Instruct patient not to share medication with others.
- Inform patient that medication does not cure AIDS or prevent associated or opportunistic infections. Medication does not reduce the risk of transmission of HIV to others through sexual contact or blood contamination. Caution patient to use a condom, and avoid sharing needles or donating blood to prevent spreading the AIDS virus to others. Advise patient that the long-term effects of medication are unknown at this time.
- Advise patient of potential for hypersensitivity reactions that may result in death. Instruct patient to discontinue medication and notify health care professional immediately if symptoms of hypersensitivity or signs of Immune Reconstitution Syndrome (signs and symptoms of inflammation from previous infections) occur. A warning card summarizing symptoms of hypersensitivity is provided with each prescription; instruct patient to carry card at all times.
- Instruct patient to notify health care professional immediately if symptoms of lactic acidosis (tiredness or weakness, unusual muscle pain, trouble breathing, stomach pain with nausea and vomiting, cold especially in arms or legs, dizziness, fast or irregular heartbeat) or if signs of hepatotoxicity (yellow skin or whites of eyes, dark urine, light-colored stools, lack of appetite for several days or longer, nausea, abdominal pain) occur. These symptoms may occur more frequently in patients that are female, obese, or have been taking medications for a long time.
- Instruct patient to notify health care professional promptly if signs of peripheral neuropathy or pancreatitis occur.
- Inform patient that redistribution and accumulation of body fat may occur, causing central obesity, dorsocervical fat enlargement (buffalo hump), peripheral wasting, breast enlargement, and cushingoid appearance. The cause and long-term effects are not known.
- Advise patient to notify health care professional of all Rx or OTC medications, vitamins, or herbal products

being taken and to consult with health care professional before taking other medications, especially methadone, St. John's Wort, and other antiretrovirals.

- Advise female patients to avoid breast feeding and to notify health care professional if pregnancy is planned or suspected. Breast feeding should be avoided during therapy. Pregnant patients should be encouraged to enroll in the Antiretroviral Pregnancy Registry by calling 1-800-258-4263.
- Emphasize the importance of regular follow-up exams and blood counts to determine progress and monitor for side effects.

Evaluation/Desired Outcomes

- Delayed progression of AIDS, and decreased opportunistic infections in patients with HIV.
- Decrease in viral load and increase in CD4 cell counts.

abiraterone (a-bi-**ra**-te-rone)

Zytiga

Classification

Therapeutic: antineoplastics

Pharmacologic: enzyme inhibitors

Pregnancy Category X

Indications

With prednisone in the treatment of metastatic castration-resistant prostate cancer.

Action

Inhibits the enzyme 17α-hydroxylase/C17,20–lyase, which is required for androgen production. May also result in increased mineralocortocoid production.
Therapeutic Effects: Decreased androgen production with decreased spread of androgen-sensitive prostate cancer.

Pharmacokinetics

Absorption: Hydrolyzed to its active compound following oral administration.
Distribution: Unknown.
Protein Binding: >99%.
Metabolism and Excretion: Metabolized by esterases to inactive compounds; eliminated primarily in feces as unchanged drug and metabolites; 5% excreted in urine.
Half-life: 12 hr.

TIME/ACTION PROFILE (blood level)

ROUTE	ONSET	PEAK	DURATION
PO	unknown	2 hr	12 hr

Contraindications/Precautions

Contraindicated in: Severe hepatic impairment (Child-Pugh Class C); OB: Pregnancy or potential to become pregnant (may cause fetal harm); Lactation: Lactation.
Use Cautiously in: Cardiovascular disease (safety not established if LVEF <50% or NYHA Class III or IV heart failure; Recent myocardial infarction; Ventricular arrhythmias; Electrolyte abnormalities or hypertension (correct/treat prior to initiation); Pre-existing liver disease (dose modification required for Child-Pugh Class B); Stress, infection, trauma, acute disease process (may result in adrenocortical insufficiency requiring additional corticosteroids).

Adverse Reactions/Side Effects

Noted for combination treatment with prednisone.
Resp: cough. **CV:** arrhythmia, edema, hypertension. **GI:** HEPATOTOXICITY, diarrhea, dyspepsia. **Derm:** hot flush. **Endo:** adrenocortical insufficiency (due to concurrent prednisone). **F and E:** hypokalemia. **GU:** nocturia, urinary frequency. **MS:** fracture, joint pain/discomfort.

Interactions

Drug-Drug: Acts as an inhibitor of the CYP2D6 and CYP2C8 enzyme system; avoid concurrent use with agents that are substrates of CYP2D6, especially those with narrow therapeutic indices, including **thioridazine** and **dextromethorphan** (CYP2D6 substrates) as well as **pioglitazone** (CYP2C8 substrate); if concurrent use is necessary, dose ↓ of substrate may be required. Abiraterone is a substrate of the CYP3A4 enzyme system. Concurrent use of strong CYP3A4 inducers including **carbamazepine**, **phenobarbital**, **phenytoin**, **rifabutin**, **rifapentine**, or **rifampin** should be avoided or undertaken with caution.

Route/Dosage

PO (Adults): 1000 mg once daily used in combination with 5 mg prednisone twice daily; *Concurrent use of strong CYP3A4 inducer*— 1000 mg twice daily.

Hepatic Impairment

PO (Adults): *Child-Pugh Class B*— 250 mg once daily with 5 mg prednisone twice daily.

Availability

Tablets: 250 mg.

NURSING IMPLICATIONS

Assessment

- Monitor BP and assess for fluid retention at least monthly. Control hypertension during therapy.
- Monitor for signs and symptoms of adrenocortical insufficiency (hypotension, weight loss, weakness, nausea, vomiting, anorexia, lethargy, confusion, restlessness), especially in patients under stress or

who are withdrawn from or have decreased prednisone dose. Symptoms may be masked by abiraterone.

- ***Lab Test Considerations:*** Monitor AST, ALT, and bilirubin prior to, every 2 wks for 3 mo, and monthly thereafter. If AST and/or ALT ↑ >5 times upper limit of normal or bilirubin ↑ >3 times upper limit of normal in patients with baseline moderate hepatic impairment, interrupt abiraterone. Following return of liver function to baseline or AST and ALT ↑ >2.5 times upper limit of normal or bilirubin ↑ >1.5 times upper limit of normal may re-start at a reduced dose of 750 mg once daily. Monitor serum transaminases and bilirubin every 2 wks for 3 mo and monthly thereafter. If hepatotoxicity recurs, may restart at 500 mg once daily following return to baseline or AST and ALT ↑ >2.5 times upper limit of normal or bilirubin ↑ >1.5 times upper limit of normal. If hepatotoxicity recurs at 500 mg dose, discontinue therapy.
- Monitor serum potassium and sodium at least monthly during therapy. May cause hypokalemia; control during therapy.
- May cause ↑ triglycerides and ↓ phosphorous.

Potential Nursing Diagnoses

Deficient knowledge, related to medication regimen (Patient/Family Teaching)

Implementation

- Control hypertension and correct hypokalemia prior to starting therapy.
- **PO:** Administer once daily with twice daily prednisone on an empty stomach at least 1 hr before or 2 hrs after meals; food increases absorption. Swallow tablets whole with water; do not crush, break, or chew.

Patient/Family Teaching

- Instruct patient to take medication as directed and not to stop abiraterone or prednisone without consulting health care professional. If a dose is missed, take the following day. If more than 1 dose is missed, consult health care professional. Do not share medication with others, even if they have the same symptoms; may be dangerous.
- Instruct patient to notify health care professional of all Rx or OTC medications, vitamins, or herbal products being taken and to consult with health care professional before taking other medications.
- Advise patient to notify health care professional of side effects that are bothersome or persistent.
- Rep: Advise female patient to use effective contraception during therapy and for 1 wk after therapy and to notify health care professional immediately of pregnancy is suspected or if breast feeding. Male patients should use a condom and another form of contraception during sex with a women of child-bearing potential during and for 1 wk after therapy. Pregnant women should not touch tablets without wearing gloves.
- Explain need for continued follow-up exams and lab tests to assess possible side effects.

Evaluation/Desired Outcomes

- Decreased spread of androgen-sensitive prostate cancer.

acetaminophen (oral, rectal)

(a-seet-a-**min**-oh-fen)

✱Abenol, Acephen, ✱Acet, ✱Children Feverhalt, ✱Fortolin, Infant's Feverall, ✱Pediaphen, ✱Pediatrix, ✱Taminol, ✱Tempra, Tylenol

acetaminophen (intravenous)

Ofirmev

Classification

Therapeutic: antipyretics, nonopioid analgesics

Pregnancy Category B (oral, rectal), C (intravenous)

Indications

PO, Rect: Treatment of: Mild pain, Fever. **IV:** Treatment of: Mild to moderate pain, Moderate to severe pain with opioid analgesics, Fever.

Action

Inhibits synthesis of prostaglandins that may serve as mediators of pain and fever, primarily in the CNS. Has no significant anti-inflammatory properties or GI toxicity. **Therapeutic Effects:** Analgesia. Antipyresis.

Pharmacokinetics

Absorption: Well absorbed following oral administration. Rectal absorption is variable. Intravenous administration results in complete bioavailability.

Distribution: Widely distributed. Crosses the placenta; enters breast milk in low concentrations.

Metabolism and Excretion: 85–95% metabolized by the liver (CYP2E1 enzyme system). Metabolites may be toxic in overdose situation. Metabolites excreted by the kidneys.

Half-life: Neonates: 7 hr; Infants and Children: 3–4 hr; Adults: 1–3 hr.

TIME/ACTION PROFILE (analgesia and antipyresis)

ROUTE	ONSET	PEAK	DURATION
PO	0.5–1 hr	1–3 hr	3–8 hr†
Rect	0.5–1 hr	1–3 hr	3–4 hr
IV‡	within 30 min	30 min	4–6 hr

†Depends on dose.

‡Antipyretic effects.

Contraindications/Precautions

Contraindicated in: Previous hypersensitivity; Products containing alcohol, aspartame, saccharin, sugar, or tartrazine (FDC yellow dye #5) should be avoided in patients who have hypersensitivity or intolerance to these compounds; Severe hepatic impairment/active liver disease.

Use Cautiously in: Hepatic disease/renal disease (lower chronic doses recommended); Alcoholism, chronic malnutrition, severe hypovolemia or severe renal impairment (CCr <30 mL/min, ↑ dosing interval and ↓ daily dose may be necessary); Chronic alcohol use/abuse; Malnutrition; OB: Use in pregnancy only if clearly needed (for IV); Lactation: Use cautiously (for IV); Pedi: Neonates (safety and effectiveness not established) (for IV).

Adverse Reactions/Side Effects

CNS: agitation (↑ in children) (IV), anxiety (IV), headache (IV), fatigue (IV), insomnia (IV). **Resp:** atelectasis (↑ in children) (IV), dyspnea (IV). **CV:** hypertension (IV), hypotension (IV). **GI:** HEPATOTOXICITY (↑ DOSES), constipation (↑ in children) (IV), ↑ liver enzymes, nausea (IV), vomiting (IV). **F and E:** hypokalemia (IV). **GU:** renal failure (high doses/chronic use). **Hemat:** neutropenia, pancytopenia. **MS:** muscle spasms (IV), trismus (IV). **Derm:** ACUTE GENERALIZED EXANTHEMATOUS PUSTULOSIS, STEVENS-JOHNSON SYNDROME, TOXIC EPIDERMAL NECROLYSIS, rash, urticaria.

Interactions

Drug-Drug: Chronic high-dose acetaminophen (>2 g/day) may ↑ risk of bleeding with **warfarin** (INR should not exceed 4). Hepatotoxicity is additive with other **hepatotoxic substances**, including **alcohol**. Concurrent use of **isoniazid**, **rifampin**, **rifabutin**, **phenytoin**, **barbiturates**, and **carbamazepine** may ↑ the risk of acetaminophen-induced liver damage (limit self-medication); these agents will also ↓ therapeutic effects of acetaminophen. Concurrent use of **NSAIDs** may ↑ the risk of adverse renal effects (avoid chronic concurrent use). **Propranolol** ↓ metabolism and may ↑ effects. May ↓ effects of **lamotrigine** and **zidovudine**.

Route/Dosage

Children ≤12 yr should not receive >5 PO or rectal doses/24 hr without notifying physician or other health care professional. No dose adjustment needed when converting between IV and PO acetaminophen in adults and children ≥50 kg.

PO (Adults and Children >12 yr): 325–650 mg q 6 hr or 1 g 3–4 times daily or 1300 mg q 8 hr (not to exceed 3 g or 2 g/24 hr in patients with hepatic/renal impairment).

PO (Children 1–12 yr): 10–15 mg/kg/dose q 6 hr as needed (not to exceed 5 doses/24 hr).

PO (Infants): 10–15 mg/kg/dose q 6 hr as needed (not to exceed 5 doses/24 hr).

PO (Neonates): 10–15 mg/kg/dose q 6–8 hr as needed.

IV (Adults and Children ≥13 yr and ≥50 kg): 1000 mg q 6 hr or 650 mg q 4 hr (not to exceed 1000 mg/dose, 4 g/day, and less than 4 hr dosing interval).

IV (Adults and Children ≥13 yr and <50 kg): 15 mg/kg q 6 hr or 12.5 mg/kg q 4 hr (not to exceed 15 mg/kg/dose, 75 mg/kg/day, and less than 4 hr dosing interval).

IV (Children 2–12 yr): 15 mg/kg q 6 hr or 12.5 mg/kg q 4 hr (not to exceed 15 mg/kg/dose, 75 mg/kg/day, and less than 4 hr dosing interval).

Rect (Adults and Children >12 yr): 325–650 mg q 4–6 hr as needed or 1 g 3–4 times/day (not to exceed 4 g/24 hr).

Rect (Children 1–12 yr): 10–20 mg/kg/dose q 4–6 hr as needed.

Rect (Infants): 10–20 mg/kg/dose q 4–6 hr as needed.

Rect (Neonates): 10–15 mg/kg/dose q 6–8 hr as needed.

Availability (generic available)

Chewable tablets (fruit, bubblegum, or grape flavor): 80 mg^OTC^, 160 mg^OTC^. **Tablets:** 160 mg^OTC^, 325 mg^OTC^. **Caplets:** 325 mg^OTC^. **Solution (berry, fruit, and grape flavor):** 100 mg/mL^OTC^. **Liquid (mint):** 160 mg/5 mL^OTC^. **Elixir (grape and cherry flavor):** 160 mg/5 mL^OTC^. **Drops:** 160 mg/ 5 mL ^OTC^. **Suspension:** ✱ 100 mg/mL^OTC^, ✱ 160 mg/5 mL^OTC^. **Syrup:** 160 mg/5 mL^OTC^. **Suppositories:** 80 mg^OTC^, 120 mg^OTC^, 325 mg^OTC^. **Solution for intravenous infusion:** 1000 mg/100 mL in 100-mL vials. ***In combination with:*** many other medications. See Appendix B.

NURSING IMPLICATIONS

Assessment

- Assess overall health status and alcohol usage before administering acetaminophen. Patients who are malnourished or chronically abuse alcohol are at higher risk of developing hepatotoxicity with chronic use of usual doses of this drug.
- Assess amount, frequency, and type of drugs taken in patients self-medicating, especially with OTC drugs. Prolonged use of acetaminophen increases risk of adverse hepatic and renal effects. For short-term use, combined doses of acetaminophen and salicylates should not exceed the recommended dose of either drug given alone. Do not exceed maximum daily dose of acetaminophen when considering all routes of administration and all combination products containing acetaminophen.
- Assess for rash periodically during therapy. May cause Stevens-Johnson syndrome. Discontinue ther-

apy if rash (reddening of skin, blisters, and detachment of upper surface of skin peeling) or if accompanied with fever, general malaise, fatigue, muscle or joint aches, blisters, oral lesions, conjunctivitis, hepatitis and/or eosinophilia.

- **Pain:** Assess type, location, and intensity prior to and 30–60 min following administration.
- **Fever:** Assess fever; note presence of associated signs (diaphoresis, tachycardia, and malaise).
- ***Lab Test Considerations:*** Evaluate hepatic, hematologic, and renal function periodically during prolonged, high-dose therapy.
- May alter results of blood glucose monitoring. May cause falsely ↓ values when measured with glucose oxidase/peroxidase method, but probably not with hexokinase/G6PD method. May also cause falsely ↑ values with certain instruments; see manufacturer's instruction manual.
- Increased serum bilirubin, LDH, AST, ALT, and prothrombin time may indicate hepatotoxicity.
- ***Toxicity and Overdose:*** If overdose occurs, **acetylcysteine** (Acetadote) is the antidote.

Potential Nursing Diagnoses

Acute pain (Indications)
Risk for imbalanced body temperature (Indications)

Implementation

- Do not confuse Tylenol with Tylenol PM.
- To prevent fatal medication errors ensure dose in milligrams (mg) and milliliters (mL) is not confused; dosing is based on weight for patients under 50 kg; programming of infusion pump is accurate; and total daily dose of acetaminophen from all sources does not exceed maximum daily limits.
- When combined with opioids do not exceed the maximum recommended daily dose of acetaminophen.
- **PO:** Administer with a full glass of water.
- May be taken with food or on an empty stomach.

IV Administration

- **Intermittent Infusion:** *For 1000 mg dose*, insert vented IV set through septum of 100 mL vial; may be administered without further dilution. *For doses <1000 mg*, withdraw appropriate dose from vial place in a separate empty, sterile container for IV infusion. Place small volume pediatric doses up to 60 mL in a syringe and administer via syringe pump. Solution is clear and colorless; do not administer solutions that are discolored of contain particulate matter. Administer within 6 hrs of breaking vial seal. ***Rate:*** Infuse over 15 min. Monitor end of infusion in order to prevent air embolism, especially if acetaminophen is primary infusion.
- **Y-Site Compatibility:** buprenorphine, butorphanol, cefoxitin, ceftriaxone, clindamycin, D5W, dexamethasone, D10W, D5/LR, D5/0.9% NaCl, diphenhydramine, dolasetron, droperidol, fentanyl, granisetron, heparin, hydrocortisone, hydromorphone, ketorolac, LR, lidocaine, lorazepam, mannitol, meperidine, methylprednisolone, metoclopramide, midazolam, morphine, nalbuphine, 0.9% NaCl, ondansetron, piperacillin/tazobactam, potassium chloride, prochlorperazine, ranitidine, sufentanil, vancomycin.
- **Y-Site Incompatibility:** acyclovir, chlorpromazine, diazepam.
- **Additive Incompatibility:** Do not mix with other medications.

Patient/Family Teaching

- Advise patient to take medication exactly as directed and not to take more than the recommended amount. Chronic excessive use of >4 g/day (2 g in chronic alcoholics) may lead to hepatotoxicity, renal or cardiac damage. Adults should not take acetaminophen longer than 10 days and children not longer than 5 days unless directed by health care professional. Short-term doses of acetaminophen with salicylates or NSAIDs should not exceed recommended daily dose of either drug alone.
- Advise patient to avoid alcohol (3 or more glasses per day increase the risk of liver damage) if taking more than an occasional 1–2 doses and to avoid taking concurrently with salicylates or NSAIDs for more than a few days, unless directed by health care professional.
- Advise patient to discontinue acetaminophen and notify health care professional if rash occurs.
- Inform patients with diabetes that acetaminophen may alter results of blood glucose monitoring. Advise patient to notify health care professional if changes are noted.
- Caution patient to check labels on all OTC products. Advise patients to avoid taking more than one product containing acetaminophen at a time to prevent toxicity.
- Advise patient to consult health care professional if discomfort or fever is not relieved by routine doses of this drug or if fever is greater than 39.5°C (103°F) or lasts longer than 3 days.
- Pedi: Advise parents or caregivers to check concentrations of liquid preparations. All OTC single ingredient acetaminophen liquid products now come in a single concentration of 160 mg/5 mL. Errors have resulted in serious liver damage. Have parents or caregivers determine the correct formulation and dose for their child (based on the child's age/weight), and demonstrate how to measure it using an appropriate measuring device.

Evaluation/Desired Outcomes

- Relief of mild to moderate pain.
- Reduction of fever.

acetaZOLAMIDE
(a-seet-a-**zole**-a-mide)
✱Acetazolam, Diamox, Diamox Sequels

Classification
Therapeutic: anticonvulsants, antiglaucoma agents, diuretics, ocular hypotensive agent
Pharmacologic: carbonic anhydrase inhibitors

Pregnancy Category C

Indications
Lowering of intraocular pressure in the treatment of glaucoma. Management of acute altitude sickness. Edema due to HF. Adjunct to the treatment of refractory seizures. **Unlabeled Use:** Reduce cerebrospinal fluid production in hydrocephalus. Prevention of renal calculi composed of uric acid or cystine.

Action
Inhibition of carbonic anhydrase in the eye results in decreased secretion of aqueous humor. Inhibition of renal carbonic anhydrase, resulting in self-limiting urinary excretion of sodium, potassium, bicarbonate, and water. CNS inhibition of carbonic anhydrase and resultant diuresis may ↓ abnormal neuronal firing. Alkaline diuresis prevents precipitation of uric acid or cystine in the urinary tract. **Therapeutic Effects:** Lowering of intraocular pressure. Control of some types of seizures. Prevention and treatment of acute altitude sickness. Diuresis and subsequent mobilization of excess fluid. Prevention of uric acid or cystine renal calculi.

Pharmacokinetics
Absorption: Dose dependent; erratic with doses >10 m g/kg/day.
Distribution: Crosses the placenta and blood-brain barrier; enters breast milk.
Protein Binding: 95%.
Metabolism and Excretion: Excreted mostly unchanged in urine.
Half-life: 2.4–5.8 hr.

TIME/ACTION PROFILE (lowering of intraocular pressure)

ROUTE	ONSET	PEAK	DURATION
PO	1–1.5 hr	2–4 hr	8–12 hr
PO-ER	2 hr	8–18 hr	18–24 hr
IV	2 min	15 min	4–5 hr

Contraindications/Precautions
Contraindicated in: Hypersensitivity or cross-sensitivity with sulfonamides may occur; Hepatic disease or insufficiency; Concurrent use with ophthalmic carbonic anhydrase inhibitors (brinzolamide, dorzolamide) is not recommended; OB: Avoid during first trimester of pregnancy.
Use Cautiously in: Chronic respiratory disease; Electrolyte abnormalities; Gout; Renal disease (dosage ↓ necessary for CCr <50 mL/min); Diabetes mellitus; OB: Use with caution during second or third trimester of pregnancy; Lactation: Safety not established.

Adverse Reactions/Side Effects
CNS: depression, fatigue, weakness, drowsiness. **EENT:** transient nearsightedness. **GI:** anorexia, metallic taste, nausea, vomiting, melena. **GU:** crystalluria, renal calculi. **Derm:** STEVENS-JOHNSON SYNDROME, rashes. **Endo:** hyperglycemia. **F and E:** hyperchloremic acidosis, hypokalemia, growth retardation (in children receiving chronic therapy). **Hemat:** APLASTIC ANEMIA, HEMOLYTIC ANEMIA, LEUKOPENIA. **Metab:** weight loss, hyperuricemia. **Neuro:** paresthesias. **Misc:** allergic reactions including ANAPHYLAXIS.

Interactions
Drug-Drug: Excretion of **barbiturates**, **aspirin**, and **lithium** is ↑ and may lead to ↓ effectiveness. Excretion of **amphetamine**, **quinidine**, **procainamide**, and possibly **tricyclic antidepressants** is ↓ and may lead to toxicity. May ↑ **cyclosporine** levels.

Route/Dosage
PO (Adults): *Glaucoma (open angle)*—250–1000 mg/day in 1–4 divided doses (up to 250 mg q 4 hr) or 500-mg extended-release capsules twice daily. *Epilepsy*—4–16 mg/kg/day in 1–4 divided doses (maximum 30 mg/kg/day or 1 g/day). *Altitude sickness*—250 mg 2–4 times daily started 24–48 hr before ascent, continued for 48 hr or longer to control symptoms. *Antiurolithic*—250 mg at bedtime. *Edema*—250–375 mg/day. *Urine alkalinization*—5 mg/kg/dose repeated 2–3 times over 24 hr.
PO (Children): *Glaucoma*—8–30 mg/kg (300–900 mg/m²/day) in 3 divided doses (usual range 10–15 mg/kg/day). *Edema*—5 mg/kg/dose once daily. *Epilepsy*—4–16 mg/kg/day in 1–4 divided doses (maximum 30 mg/kg/day or 1 g/day).
PO (Neonates): *Hydrocephalus*—5 mg/kg/dose q 6 hr ↑ by 25 mg/kg/day up to a maximum of 100 mg/kg/day.
IV (Adults): *Glaucoma (closed angle)*—250–500 mg, may repeat in 2–4 hr to a maximum of 1 g/day. *Edema*—250–375 mg/day.
IV (Children): *Glaucoma*—5–10 mg/kg q 6 hr, not to exceed 1 g/day. *Edema*—5 mg/kg/dose once daily.
IV (Neonates): *Hydrocephalus*—5 mg/kg/dose q 6 hr ↑ by 25 mg/kg/day up to a maximum of 100 mg/kg/day.

Availability (generic available)

Tablets: 125 mg, 250 mg. **Extended-release capsules:** 500 mg. **Powder for injection:** 500 mg/vial.

NURSING IMPLICATIONS

Assessment

- Observe for signs of hypokalemia (muscle weakness, malaise, fatigue, ECG changes, vomiting).
- Assess for allergy to sulfonamides.
- **Intraocular Pressure:** Assess for eye discomfort or decrease in visual acuity.
- **Seizures:** Monitor neurologic status in patients receiving acetazolamide for seizures. Initiate seizure precautions.
- **Altitude Sickness:** Monitor for decrease in severity of symptoms (headache, nausea, vomiting, fatigue, dizziness, drowsiness, shortness of breath). Notify health care professional immediately if neurologic symptoms worsen or if patient becomes more dyspneic and rales or crackles develop.
- **Edema:** Monitor intake and output ratios and daily weight during therapy.
- ***Lab Test Considerations:*** Serum electrolytes, complete blood counts, and platelet counts should be evaluated initially and periodically during prolonged therapy. May cause ↓ potassium, bicarbonate, WBCs, and RBCs. May cause ↑ serum chloride.
- May cause ↑ in serum and urine glucose; monitor serum and urine glucose carefully in diabetic patients.
- May cause false-positive results for urine protein and 17-hydroxysteroid tests.
- May cause ↑ blood ammonia, bilirubin, uric acid, urine urobilinogen, and calcium. May ↓ urine citrate.

Potential Nursing Diagnoses

Disturbed sensory perception (visual) (Indications)

Implementation

- Do not confuse Diamox with Diabinese.
- Encourage fluids to 2000–3000 mL/day, unless contraindicated, to prevent crystalluria and stone formation.
- A potassium supplement without chloride should be administered concurrently with acetazolamide.
- **PO:** Give with food to minimize GI irritation. Tablets may be crushed and mixed with fruit-flavored syrup to minimize bitter taste for patients with difficulty swallowing. Extended-release capsules may be opened and sprinkled on soft food, but do not crush, chew, or swallow contents dry. Extended-release capsules are only indicated for glaucoma and altitude sickness; do not use for epilepsy or diuresis.
- **IM:** Extremely painful; avoid if possible.

IV Administration

- **IV Push:** Reconstitute 500 mg of acetazolamide in at least 5 mL of sterile water for injection. Use reconstituted solution within 24 hr. ***Concentration:*** 100 mg/mL. ***Rate:*** Not to exceed 500 mg/min.
- **Intermittent Infusion:** ***Diluent:*** Further dilute in 50–100 mL of D5W, D10W, 0.45% NaCl, 0.9% NaCl, LR, or combinations of dextrose and saline or dextrose and LR solution. ***Concentration:*** 5–10 mg/mL. ***Rate:*** Infuse over 15–30 min.

Patient/Family Teaching

- Instruct patient to take as directed. Take missed doses as soon as possible unless almost time for next dose. Do not double doses. Patients on anticonvulsant therapy may need to gradually withdraw medication.
- Advise patient to report numbness or tingling of extremities, weakness, rash, sore throat, unusual bleeding or bruising, fever, or signs/symptoms of a sulfonamide adverse reaction (Stevens-Johnson syndrome [flu-like symptoms, spreading red rash, or skin/mucous membrane blistering], toxic epidermal necrolysis [widespread peeling/blistering of skin]) to health care professional. If hematopoietic reactions, fever, rash, hepatic, or renal problems occur, acetazolamide should be discontinued.
- May occasionally cause drowsiness. Caution patient to avoid driving and other activities that require alertness until response to the drug is known.
- Caution patient to use sunscreen and wear protective clothing to prevent photosensitivity reactions.
- Advise patient to notify health care professional of all Rx or OTC medications, vitamins, or herbal products being taken and to consult with health care professional before taking other medications.
- **Intraocular Pressure:** Advise patient of the need for periodic ophthalmologic exams; loss of vision may be gradual and painless.

Evaluation/Desired Outcomes

- Decrease in intraocular pressure when used for glaucoma. If therapy is not effective or patient is unable to tolerate one carbonic anhydrase inhibitor, using another may be effective and more tolerable.
- Decrease in the frequency of seizures.
- Reduction of edema.
- Prevention of altitude sickness.
- Prevention of uric acid or cystine stones in the urinary tract.

acetylcysteine

(a-se-teel-**sis**-teen)

Acetadote, ✤Mucomyst, ✤Parvolex

Classification

Therapeutic: antidotes (for acetaminophen toxicity), mucolytic

Pregnancy Category B

Indications

PO: Antidote for the management of potentially hepatotoxic overdose of acetaminophen (administer within 8–10 hours [IV] or 24 hours [PO] of ingestion). **Inhaln:** Mucolytic in the management of conditions associated with thick viscid mucous secretions. **Unlabeled Use:** Prevention of radiocontrast-induced renal dysfunction (oral).

Action

PO: Decreases the buildup of a hepatotoxic metabolite in acetaminophen overdosage. **IV:** Decreases the buildup of a hepatotoxic metabolite in acetaminophen overdosage. **Inhaln:** Degrades mucus, allowing easier mobilization and expectoration. **Therapeutic Effects: PO:** Prevention or lessening of liver damage following acetaminophen overdose. **Inhaln:** Lowers the viscosity of mucus.

Pharmacokinetics

Absorption: Absorbed from the GI tract following oral administration. Action is local following inhalation; remainder may be absorbed from pulmonary epithelium.

Distribution: Crosses the placenta; 0.47 L/kg.

Protein Binding: 83% bound to plasma proteins.

Metabolism and Excretion: Partially metabolized by the liver, 22% excreted renally.

Half-life: *Adults*—5.6 hr (↑ in hepatic impairment) *newborns*—11 hr.

TIME/ACTION PROFILE

ROUTE	ONSET	PEAK	DURATION
PO (antidote)	unknown	30–60 min	4 hr
Inhaln (mucolytic)	1 min	5–10 min	short

Contraindications/Precautions

Contraindicated in: Hypersensitivity.

Use Cautiously in: Severe respiratory insufficiency, asthma, or history of bronchospasm; History of GI bleeding (oral only); OB, Lactation: Safety not established.

Adverse Reactions/Side Effects

CNS: drowsiness. **CV:** vasodilation, tachycardia, hypotension. **EENT:** rhinorrhea. **Resp:** <u>bronchospasm</u>, bronchial/tracheal irritation, chest tightness, ↑ secretions. **GI:** <u>nausea</u>, <u>vomiting</u>, stomatitis. **Derm:** <u>rash</u>, clamminess, pruritus, urticaria. **Misc:** allergic reactions (primarily with IV), including ANAPHYLAXIS, ANGIOEDEMA, chills, fever.

Interactions

Drug-Drug: Activated charcoal may adsorb orally administered acetylcysteine and ↓ its effectiveness as an antidote.

Route/Dosage

Acetaminophen Overdose

PO (Adults and Children): 140 mg/kg initially, followed by 70 mg/kg q 4 hr for 17 additional doses.

IV (Adults and Children): *Loading dose*—150 mg/kg (maximum: 15 g) over 60 min initially followed by *First maintenance dose*—50 mg/kg (maximum: 5 g) over 4 hr, then *second maintenance dose*—100 mg/kg (maximum: 10 g) over 16 hr.

Mucolytic

Inhaln (Adults and Children 1–12 yrs): *Nebulization via face mask*—3–5 mL of 20% solution or 6–10 mL of the 10% solution 3–4 times daily; *nebulization via tent or croupette*—volume of 10–20% solution required to maintain heavy mist; *direct instillation*—1–2 mL of 10–20% solution q 1–4 hr; *intratracheal instillation via tracheostomy*—1–2 mL of 10–20% solution q 1–4 hr (up to 2–5 mL of 20% solution via tracheal catheter into particular segments of the bronchopulmonary tree).

Inhaln (Infants): *Nebulization*—1–2 ml of 20% solution or 2–4 mL of 10% solution 3–4 times daily.

Prevention of Radiocontrast-Induced Renal Dysfunction

PO (Adults): 600 mg twice daily for 2 days, beginning the day before the procedure.

Availability (generic available)

Solution for inhalation: 10% (100 mg/mL), 20% (200 mg/mL). **Solution for injection:** 20% (200 mg/mL).

NURSING IMPLICATIONS

Assessment

- **Antidote in Acetaminophen Overdose:** Assess type, amount, and time of acetaminophen ingestion. Assess plasma acetaminophen levels. Initial levels are drawn at least 4 hr after ingestion of acetaminophen. Plasma level determinations may be difficult to interpret following ingestion of extended-release preparations. Do not wait for results to administer dose.
- *IV:* Assess for anaphylaxis. Erythema and flushing are common, usually occurring 30–60 min after initiating infusion, and may resolve with continued administration. If rash, hypotension, wheezing, or dyspnea occur, initiate treatment for anaphylaxis (antihistamine and epinephrine). Interrupt acetylcysteine infusion until symptoms resolve and restart carefully. If anaphylaxis recurs, discontinue acetylcysteine and use alternative form of treatment.
- Assess patient for nausea, vomiting, and urticaria. Notify health care professional if these occur.
- **Mucolytic:** Assess respiratory function (lung sounds, dyspnea) and color, amount, and consist-

ency of secretions before and immediately following treatment to determine effectiveness of therapy.

- ***Lab Test Considerations:*** Monitor AST, ALT, and bilirubin levels along with prothrombin time every 24 hr for 96 hr in patients with plasma acetaminophen levels indicating potential hepatotoxicity.
- Monitor cardiac and renal function (creatinine, BUN), serum glucose, and electrolytes. Maintain fluid and electrolyte balance, correct hypoglycemia, and administer vitamin K or fresh frozen plasma or clotting factor concentrate if prothrombin time ratio exceeds 1.5 or 3, respectively.

Potential Nursing Diagnoses

Risk for self-directed violence (Indications)
Ineffective airway clearance (Indications)
Deficient knowledge, related to medication regimen (Patient/Family Teaching)

Implementation

- Do not confuse Mucomyst with Mucinex.
- After opening, solution for inhalation may turn light purple; does not alter potency. Refrigerate open vials and discard after 96 hr.
- Drug reacts with rubber and metals (iron, nickel, copper); avoid contact.
- **PO:** Dilute 20% solution with cola, water, or juice to a final concentration of 1:3 for patients weighing up to 20 kg or with enough diluent to make a 5% solution for patients weighing more than 20 kg, to increase palatability. May be administered by duodenal tube if patient is unable to swallow. If patient vomits loading dose or maintenance doses within 1 hr of administration, readminister dose.
- **Acetaminophen Overdose**—Empty stomach contents by inducing emesis or lavage prior to administration.

IV Administration

- **Intermittent Infusion:** Most effective if administered within 8 hr of acetaminophen ingestion. ***Diluent:*** Dilute in D5W. ***Concentration:*** **For loading dose:** *For patients 5–20 kg:* Dilute 150 mg in 3 mL/kg of diluent. *For patients 21–40 kg:* Dilute 150 mg/kg in 100 mL. *For patients 41–100 kg:* Dilute 150 mg/kg in 200 mL. **For Second Dose:** *For patients 5–20 kg:* Dilute 50 mg/kg in 7 mL/kg of diluent. *For patients 21–40 kg:* Dilute 50 mg/kg in 250 mL of diluent. *For patients 41–100 kg:* Dilute 50 mg/kg in 500 mL. **For Third Dose:** *For patients 5–20 kg:* Dilute 100 mg/kg in 14 mL/kg of diluent. *For patients 21–40 kg:* 100 mg/kg diluted in 500 mL of diluent. *For patients 41–100 kg:* Dilute 100 mg/kg in 1000 mL. Adjust fluid volume for patients requiring fluid restriction. Vials are single-use. Discard after using. Reconstituted solution is stable for 24 hr at room temperature. ***Rate:*** Administer **Loading Dose** over 1 hr.
- Administer **For Second Dose:** over 4 hr.
- Administer **For Third Dose:** over 16 hr.
- **Inhaln: Mucolytic**—Encourage adequate fluid intake (2000–3000 mL/day) to decrease viscosity of secretions.
- For nebulization, the 20% solution may be diluted with 0.9% NaCl for injection or inhalation or sterile water for injection or inhalation. May use 10% solution undiluted. May be administered by nebulization, or 1–2 mL may be instilled directly into airway. During administration, when 25% of medication remains in nebulizer, dilute with equal amount of 0.9% NaCl or sterile water.
- An increased volume of liquefied bronchial secretions may occur following administration. Have suction equipment available for patients unable to effectively clear airways.
- If bronchospasm occurs during treatment, discontinue and consult health care professional regarding possible addition of bronchodilator to therapy. Patients with asthma or hyperactive airway disease should be given a bronchodilator prior to acetylcysteine to prevent bronchospasm.
- Rinse patient's mouth and wash face following treatment, as drug leaves a sticky residue.

Patient/Family Teaching

- **Acetaminophen Overdose:** Explain purpose of medication to patient.
- **Inhaln:** Instruct patient to clear airway by coughing deeply before taking aerosol treatment.
- Inform patient that unpleasant odor of this drug becomes less noticeable as treatment progresses and medicine dissipates.

Evaluation/Desired Outcomes

- Decreased acetaminophen levels.
- No further increase in hepatic damage during acetaminophen overdose therapy.
- Decreased dyspnea and clearing of lung sounds when used as a mucolytic.
- Prevention of radiocontrast-induced renal dysfunction.

aclidinium (a-kli-**din**-ee-um)

✱Tudorza Genuair, Tudorza Pressair

Classification
Therapeutic: COPD agents
Pharmacologic: anticholinergics

Pregnancy Category C

Indications

Long-term maintenance treatment of bronchospasm associated with COPD, including chronic bronchitis and emphysema. Not for acute (rescue) use.

Action

Acts as an anticholinergic by inhibiting the M_3 receptor in bronchial smooth muscle. **Therapeutic Effects:** Bronchodilation with lessened symptoms of COPD.

A

Pharmacokinetics

Absorption: 6% systemically absorbed following inhalation.

Distribution: Unknown.

Metabolism and Excretion: Rapidly hydrolyzed; metabolites are not pharmacologically active. Metabolites are eliminated in urine (54–65%) and feces (20–33%). 1% excreted unchanged in urine.

Half-life: 5–8 hr.

TIME/ACTION PROFILE (improvement in FEV_1)

ROUTE	ONSET	PEAK	DURATION
Inhaln	within 1 hr	2–4 hr	12 hr

Contraindications/Precautions

Contraindicated in: None noted.

Use Cautiously in: Narrow-angle glaucoma; Prostatic hyperplasia or bladder neck obstruction; Severe hypersensitivity to milk proteins; History of hypersensitivity to atropine (cross-sensitivity may occur); OB: Use only if potential benefit justifies potential risk to the fetus; Lactation: Use cautiously; Pedi: Safety and effectiveness not established.

Adverse Reactions/Side Effects

CNS: headache. **EENT:** worsening of narrow-angle glaucoma. **Resp:** paradoxical bronchospasm. **GU:** urinary retention. **Misc:** immediate hypersensitivity reactions including ANAPHYLAXIS, ANGIOEDEMA, and URTICARIA.

Interactions

Drug-Drug: ↑ risk of anticholinergic effects with other **anticholingerics**.

Route/Dosage

Inhaln (Adults): One inhalation (400 mcg) twice daily.

Availability

Dry powder metered-dose inhaler: 400 mcg/actuation.

NURSING IMPLICATIONS

Assessment

- **Inhaln:** Assess respiratory status (rate, breath sounds, degree of dyspnea, pulse) before administration and at peak of medication. Consult health care professional about alternative medication if severe bronchospasm is present; onset of action is too slow for patients in acute distress. If paradoxical bronchospasm (wheezing) occurs, withhold medication and notify health care professional immediately.
- Monitor for signs and symptoms of hypersensitivity reactions (angioedema [swelling of the lips, tongue, or throat], bronchospasm, urticaria, rash, itching, anaphylaxis) during therapy, especially in patients with a history of hypersensitivity reactions to atropine or milk products. Discontinue aclidinium if symptoms occur.

Potential Nursing Diagnoses

Ineffective airway clearance (Indications)
Activity intolerance (Indications)

Implementation

- **Inhaln:** Administer every 12 hr. See Appendix D for administration of inhalation medications.
- When aclidinium is administered concurrently with other inhalation medications, administer adrenergic bronchodilators first, followed by aclidinium, then corticosteroids. Wait 5 min between medications.

Patient/Family Teaching

- Instruct patient in proper use of inhaler and to take medication as directed. Omit missed doses and take next dose at the usual time; do not double doses. Advise patient to read *Medication Guide* before beginning therapy and with each Rx refill in case of changes.
- Advise patient to have a rapid-acting bronchodilator available for use at all times to treat sudden symptoms. Notify health care professional immediately if sudden shortness of breath occurs immediately after using aclidinium inhaler, if breathing becomes worse, if rescue inhaler is needed more often than usual, or if rescue inhaler does not work as well at relieving symptoms.
- Caution patient to avoid getting powder into eyes.
- Advise patient to inform health care professional if symptoms of new or worsened increased eye pressure (eye pain or discomfort, nausea or vomiting, blurred visions, seeing halos or bright colors around lights, red eyes), new or worsened urinary retention (difficulty urinating, painful urination, urinating frequently, urination in a weak stream or drips), or allergic reactions (rash, hives, swelling of the face, mouth, and tongue, breathing problems) occur.
- Advise patient to consult health care professional before taking any Rx, OTC, or herbal products or alcohol concurrently with this therapy. Caution patient also to avoid smoking and other respiratory irritants.
- Advise patient to notify health care professional if pregnancy is planned or suspected, or if breast feeding.
- Explain need for pulmonary function tests prior to and periodically during therapy to determine effectiveness of medication.

Evaluation/Desired Outcomes

- Decreased dyspnea.
- Improved breath sounds.

acyclovir (ay-sye-kloe-veer)

Sitavig, ✤Xerese, Zovirax

Classification

Therapeutic: antivirals

Pharmacologic: purine analogues

Pregnancy Category B (PO, buccal, IV), C (topical)

Indications

PO: Recurrent genital herpes infections. Localized cutaneous herpes zoster infections (shingles) and chickenpox (varicella). **Buccal:** Recurrent herpes labialis (cold sores) in nonimmunosuppressed patients. **IV:** Severe initial episodes of genital herpes in nonimmunosuppressed patients. Mucosal or cutaneous herpes simplex infections or herpes zoster infections (shingles) in immunosuppressed patients. Herpes simplex encephalitis. **Topical:** *Cream*—Recurrent herpes labialis (cold sores). *Ointment*—Treatment of limited non–life-threatening herpes simplex infections in immunocompromised patients (systemic treatment is preferred).

Action

Interferes with viral DNA synthesis. **Therapeutic Effects:** Inhibition of viral replication, decreased viral shedding, and reduced time for healing of lesions.

Pharmacokinetics

Absorption: Despite poor absorption (15–30%), therapeutic blood levels are achieved.

Distribution: Widely distributed. CSF concentrations are 50% of plasma. Crosses placenta; enters breast milk.

Protein Binding: <30%.

Metabolism and Excretion: >90% eliminated unchanged by kidneys; remainder metabolized by liver.

Half-life: Neonates: 4 hr; Children 1–12 yr: 2–3 hr; Adults: 2–3.5 hr (↑ in renal failure).

TIME/ACTION PROFILE (antiviral blood levels)

ROUTE	ONSET	PEAK	DURATION
PO	unknown	1.5–2.5 hr	4 hr
IV	prompt	end of infusion	8 hr

Contraindications/Precautions

Contraindicated in: Hypersensitivity to acyclovir or valacyclovir; Hypersensitivity to milk protein concentrate (buccal only).

Use Cautiously in: Pre-existing serious neurologic, hepatic, pulmonary, or fluid and electrolyte abnormalities; Renal impairment (dose alteration recommended if CCr <50 mL/min); Geri: Due to age related ↓ in renal function; Obese patients (dose should be based on ideal body weight); Patients with hypoxia; OB, Lactation: Safety not established.

Adverse Reactions/Side Effects

CNS: SEIZURES, dizziness, headache, hallucinations, trembling. **GI:** diarrhea, nausea, vomiting, ↑ liver enzymes, hyperbilirubinemia, abdominal pain, anorexia. **GU:** RENAL FAILURE, crystalluria, hematuria, renal pain. **Derm:** STEVENS-JOHNSON SYNDROME, acne, hives, rash, unusual sweating. **Endo:** changes in menstrual cycle. **Hemat:** THROMBOTIC THROMBOCYTOPENIC PURPURA/HEMOLYTIC UREMIC SYNDROME (high doses in immunosuppressed patients). **Local:** pain, phlebitis, local irritation. **MS:** joint pain. **Misc:** polydipsia.

Interactions

Drug-Drug: Probenecid ↑ blood levels of acyclovir. ↑ blood levels and risk of toxicity from **theophylline**; dose adjustment may be necessary. ↓ blood levels and may ↓ effectiveness of **valproic acid** or **phenytoin**. Concurrent use of other **nephrotoxic drugs** ↑ risk of adverse renal effects. **Zidovudine** and IT **methotrexate** may ↑ risk of CNS side effects.

Route/Dosage

Initial Genital Herpes

PO (Adults and Children): 200 mg q 4 hr while awake (5 times/day) for 7–10 days or 400 mg q 8 hr for 7–10 days; maximum dose in children: 80 mg/kg/day in 3–5 divided doses.

IV (Adults and Children): 5 mg/kg q 8 hr or 750 mg/m²/day divided q 8 hr for 5–7 days.

Chronic Suppressive Therapy for Recurrent Genital Herpes

PO (Adults and Children): 400 mg twice daily or 200 mg 3–5 times/day for up to 12 mo. Maximum dose in children: 80 mg/kg/day in 2–5 divided doses.

Intermittent Therapy for Recurrent Genital Herpes

PO (Adults and Children): 200 mg q 4 hr while awake (5 times/day) or 400 mg q 8hr or 800 mg q 12 hr for 5 days, start at first sign of symptoms. Maximum dose in children: 80 mg/kg/day in 2–5 divided doses.

Acute Treatment of Herpes Zoster in Immunosuppressed Patients

PO (Adults): 800 mg q 4 hr while awake (5 times/day) for 7–10 days. *Prophylaxis*—400 mg 5 times/day.

PO (Children): 250–600 mg/m²/dose 4–5 times/day.

Herpes Zoster in Immunocompetent Patients

PO (Adults and Children): 4000 mg/day in 5 divided doses for 5–7 days, maximum dose in children: 80 mg/kg/day in 5 divided doses.

Chickenpox

PO (Adults and Children): 20 mg/kg (not to exceed 800 mg/dose) qid for 5 days. Start within 24 hr of rash onset.

Mucosal and Cutaneous Herpes Simplex Infections in Immunosuppressed Patients

IV (Adults and Children >12 yr): 5 mg/kg q 8 hr for 7 days.
IV (Children <12 yr): 10 mg/kg q 8 hr for 7 days.
Topical (Adults): 0.5 in. ribbon of 5% *ointment* for every 4-square-in. area q 3 hr (6 times/day) for 7 days.

Herpes Simplex Encephalitis

IV (Adults): 10 mg/kg q 8 hr for 14–21 days.
IV (Children 3 mo–12 yr): 10 mg/kg q 8 hr for 14–21 days.
IV (Children birth–3 mo): 20 mg/kg q 8 hr for 14–21 days.
IV (Neonates , premature): 10 mg/kg q 12 hr for 14–21 days.

Varicella Zoster Infections in Immunosuppressed Patients

IV (Adults): 10 mg/kg q 8 hr for 7–10 days.
IV (Children <12 yr): 10 mg/kg q 8 hr for 7–10 days.

Renal Impairment

PO, IV (Adults and Children): *CCr >50 mL/min/1.73 m²*—no dosage adjustment needed; *CCr 25 –50 mL/min/1.73 m²*—administer normal dose q 12 hr; *CCr 10–25 mL/min/1.73 m²*—administer normal dose q 24 hr; *CCr 0–10 mL/min/1.73 m²*—50% of dose q 24 hr.
IV (Neonates): *SCr 0.8–1.1 mg/dL:* Administer 20 mg/kg/dose q 12 hr; *SCr 1.2–1.5 mg/dL:* Administer 20 mg/kg/dose q 24 hr; *SCr >1.5 m g/dL:* Administer 10 mg/kg/dose q 24 hr.

Herpes labialis

Topical (Adults and Children >12 yr): Apply 5 times/day for 4 days; start at first symptoms.
Buccal (Adults): Apply one 50–mg buccal tablet to the upper gum region within 1 hr of onset of prodromal symptoms (but before appearance of any lesions).

Availability (generic available)

Capsules: 200 mg. **Cost:** *Generic*—$97.70/100. **Tablets:** 400 mg, 800 mg. **Cost:** *Generic*—400 mg $6.99/30, 800 mg $17.91/30. **Buccal tablets:** 50 mg. **Suspension (banana flavor):** 200 mg/5 mL. **Cost:** *Generic*—$137.70/473 mL. **Powder for injection:** 500 mg/vial, 1000 mg/vial. **Solution for injection:** 25 mg/mL, 50 mg/mL. **Cream:** 5%. **Cost:** $565.24/5 g. **Ointment:** 5%. **Cost:** *Generic*—$797.59/30 g. ***In combination with:*** hydrocortisone (Xerese). See Appendix B.

NURSING IMPLICATIONS

Assessment

- Assess lesions before and daily during therapy.
- Assess frequency of recurrences.
- Monitor neurologic status in patients with herpes encephalitis.
- ***Lab Test Considerations:*** Monitor BUN, serum creatinine, and CCr before and during therapy. ↑ BUN and serum creatinine levels or ↓ CCr may indicate renal failure.

Potential Nursing Diagnoses

Risk for impaired skin integrity (Indications)
Risk for infection (Patient/Family Teaching)

Implementation

- Do not confuse Zovirax with Doribax, Zyvox, or Zostrix.
- Start acyclovir treatment as soon as possible after herpes simplex symptoms appear and within 24 hr of a herpes zoster outbreak.
- **PO:** Acyclovir may be administered with food or on an empty stomach, with a full glass of water.
- Shake oral suspension well before administration.
- **Buccal:** Apply tablet with a dry finger immediately after taking out of blister to upper gum just above canine. Hold in place with pressure on lip for 30 seconds to ensure adhesion. May be more comfortable to apply rounded side of tablet to gum surface. Apply on same side as herpes labialis symptoms within 1 hr of onset of symptoms, before appearance of herpes labialis lesions. Once applied, stays in position and dissolves slowly during day; do not crush, suck, chew, or swallow. May eat and drink while tablet is in place; avoid interfering with adhesion of tablet (chewing gum, touching, or pressing tablet after placement, wearing upper denture, brushing teeth). If the teeth need to be cleaned while tablet is in place, rinse mouth gently. Drink plenty of liquids to prevent dry mouth.

IV Administration

- **IV:** Maintain adequate hydration (2000–3000 mL/day), especially during first 2 hr after IV infusion, to prevent crystalluria.
- Observe infusion site for phlebitis. Rotate infusion site to prevent phlebitis.
- Do not administer acyclovir injectable topically, IM, subcut, PO, or in the eye.
- **Intermittent Infusion:** Reconstitute 500-mg or 1-g vial with 10 mL or 20 mL, respectively, of sterile water for injection. Do not reconstitute with bacteriostatic water with benzyl alcohol or parabens. Shake well to dissolve completely. ***Diluent:*** Dilute in at least 100 mL of D5W, 0.9% NaCl, dextrose/saline combinations or LR. ***Concentration:*** 7 mg/mL. Patients requiring fluid restriction: 10 mg/mL. ***Rate:***

Administer via infusion pump over 1 hr to minimize renal tubular damage.

- Use reconstituted solution within 12 hr. Once diluted for infusion, the solution should be used within 24 hr. Refrigeration results in precipitation, which dissolves at room temperature.
- **Y-Site Compatibility:** alemtuzumab, alfentanil, allopurinol, amikacin, aminophylline, amphotericin B cholesteryl, amphotericin B lipid complex, amphotericin B liposome, ampicillin, anidulafungin, argatroban, atracurium, azithromycin, bivalirudin, bleomycin, bumetanide, buprenorphine, busulfan, butorphanol, calcium chloride, calcium gluconate, carboplatin, carmustine, cefazolin, cefotaxime, cefoxitin, ceftaroline, ceftazidime, ceftriaxone, cefuroxime, chloramphenicol, cisplatin, clindamycin, cyclophosphamide, cytarabine, dactinomycin, dantrolene, dexamethasone, dexmedetomidine, digoxin, dimenhydrinate, diphenhydramine, docetaxel, doripenem, doxacurium, doxorubicin liposome, doxycycline, enalaprilat, ephedrine, ertapenem, erythromycin lactobionate, etoposide, etoposide phosphate, famotidine, fentanyl, filgrastim, fluconazole, fluorouracil, furosemide, glycopyrrolate, heparin, hetastarch, hydrocortisone, hydromorphone, ifosfamide, imipenem/cilastatin, insulin, isoproterenol, leucovorin calcium, linezolid, lorazepam, magnesium sulfate, mannitol, mechlorethamine, melphalan, methohexital, methotrexate, methylprednisolone, metoprolol, metronidazole, milrinone, mitoxantrone, multivitamin infusion, nafcillin, naloxone, nesiritide, nitroglycerin, octreotide, oxacillin, oxytocin, paclitaxel, pamidronate, pancuronium, pantoprazole, pemetrexed, penicillin G potassium, pentobarbital, perphenazine, phenobarbital, potassium acetate, potassium chloride, propofol, propranolol, ranitidine, remifentanil, rituximab, rocuronium, sodium acetate, sodium bicarbonate, succinylcholine, sufentanil, teniposide, theophylline, thiopental, thiotepa, tigecycline, tirofiban, tobramycin, trastuzumab, trimethoprim/sulfamethoxazole, vancomycin, vasopressin, vinblastine, vincristine, voriconazole, zidovudine, zoledronic acid.
- **Y-Site Incompatibility:** amifostine, amphotericin B colloidal, ampicillin/sulbactam, amsacrine, aztreonam, cefepime, chlorpromazine, ciprofloxacin, daptomycin, dexrazoxane, diazepam, dobutamine, dolasetron, dopamine, doxorubicin hydrochloride, epinephrine, epirubicin, eptifibatide, esmolol, fenoldopam, fludarabine, foscarnet, gemcitabine, haloperidol, hydralazine, hydroxyzine, idarubicin, irinotecan, ketamine, ketorolac, labetalol, levofloxacin, lidocaine, methyldopate, midazolam, mycophenolate, nicardipine, nitroprusside, ondansetron, palonosetron, pentamidine, phenylephrine, phenytoin, piperacillin/tazobactam, potassium phosphates, procainamide, prochlorperazine, promethazine, quinupristin/dalfopristin, sargramostim, sodium phosphates, streptozocin, tacrolimus, vecuronium, verapamil, vinorelbine.
- **Topical:** Apply to skin lesions only; do not use in the eye.

Patient/Family Teaching

- Instruct patient to take medication as directed for the full course of therapy. Take missed doses as soon as possible but not just before next dose is due; do not double doses. Acyclovir should not be used more frequently or longer than prescribed.
- Advise patients that the additional use of OTC creams, lotions, and ointments may delay healing and may cause spreading of lesions.
- Inform patient that acyclovir is not a cure. The virus lies dormant in the ganglia, and acyclovir will not prevent the spread of infection to others.
- Advise patient that condoms should be used during sexual contact and that no sexual contact should be made while lesions are present.
- Patient should consult health care professional if symptoms are not relieved after 7 days of topical therapy or if oral acyclovir does not decrease the frequency and severity of recurrences. Immunocompromised patients may require a longer time, usually 2 weeks, for crusting over of lesions.
- Instruct women with genital herpes to have yearly Papanicolaou smears because they may be more likely to develop cervical cancer.
- **Topical:** Instruct patient to apply ointment in sufficient quantity to cover all lesions every 3 hr, 6 times/day for 7 days. 0.5-in. ribbon of ointment covers approximately 4 square in. Use a finger cot or glove when applying to prevent inoculation of other areas or spread to other people. Keep affected areas clean and dry. Loose-fitting clothing should be worn to prevent irritation.
- Avoid drug contact in or around eyes. Report any unexplained eye symptoms to health care professional immediately; ocular herpetic infection can lead to blindness.
- **Buccal:** Instruct patient on correct application and use of buccal tablet. If buccal tablet does not adhere or falls off within first 6 hours, reposition immediately with same tablet. If tablet cannot be repositioned, apply new tablet. If swallowed within first 6 hours, advise patient to drink a glass of water and apply a new tablet. Do not reapply if tablet falls out after 6 hrs.

Evaluation/Desired Outcomes

- Crusting over and healing of skin lesions.
- Decrease in frequency and severity of recurrences.
- Acceleration of complete healing and cessation of pain in herpes zoster.
- Decrease in intensity of chickenpox.

A

adalimumab (a-da-li-**mu**-mab)
Humira

Classification
Therapeutic: antirheumatics
Pharmacologic: DMARDs, monoclonal antibodies

Pregnancy Category B

Indications

Moderately to severely active rheumatoid arthritis (may be used alone or with methotrexate or other DMARDs). Psoriatic arthritis (may be used alone or with other DMARDs). Active ankylosing spondylitis. Moderately to severely active Crohn's disease in patients who have responded inadequately to conventional therapy. Moderately to severely active ulcerative colitis in patients who have responded inadequately to immunosuppressants such as corticosteroids, azathioprine, or 6–mercaptopurine. Moderate to severely active polyarticular juvenile idiopathic arthritis (to be used as monotherapy or with methotrexate). Moderate to severe chronic plaque psoriasis in patients who are candidates for systemic therapy or phototherapy and when other systemic therapies are deemed inappropriate. Moderate to severe hidradenitis suppurativa.

Action

Neutralizes and prevents the action of tumor necrosis factor (TNF), resulting in anti-inflammatory and antiproliferative activity. **Therapeutic Effects:** Decreased pain and swelling with decreased rate of joint destruction in patients with rheumatoid arthritis, psoriatic arthritis, juvenile idiopathic arthritis, and ankylosing spondylitis. Reduced signs and symptoms and maintenance of clinical remission of Crohn's disease. Induction and maintenance of clinical remission of ulcerative colitis. Reduced severity of plaques. Reduced number of abscesses and inflammatory nodules.

Pharmacokinetics

Absorption: 64% absorbed after subcut administration.

Distribution: Synovial fluid concentrations are 31–96% of serum.

Metabolism and Excretion: Unknown.

Half-life: 14 days (range 10–20 days).

TIME/ACTION PROFILE (improvement)

ROUTE	ONSET	PEAK	DURATION
Subcut	8–26 wk	131 hr*	2 wk†

*Blood level.
†Following discontinuation.

Contraindications/Precautions

Contraindicated in: Hypersensitivity; Concurrent use of anakinra or abatacept; Active infection (including localized); Lactation: Potential for serious side effects in the infant; discontinue drug or provide formula.

Use Cautiously in: History of chronic or recurrent infection or underlying illness/treatment predisposing to infection; History of exposure to tuberculosis; History of opportunistic infection; Patients residing, or who have resided, where tuberculosis, histoplasmosis, coccidioidomycoses, or blastomycosis is endemic; Preexisting or recent-onset CNS demyelinating disorders; History of lymphoma; Geri: ↑ risk of infection/malignancy; OB: Use only if clearly needed; Pedi: Children <2 yr (safety not established); ↑ risk of lymphoma (including hepatosplenic T-cell lymphoma [HSTCL] in patients with Crohn's disease or ulcerative colitis), leukemia, and other malignancies.

Adverse Reactions/Side Effects

CNS: headache, Guillain-Barre syndrome, multiple sclerosis. **CV:** hypertension. **EENT:** optic neuritis. **GI:** abdominal pain, nausea. **GU:** hematuria. **Derm:** rash, psoriasis. **Hemat:** neutropenia, thrombocytopenia. **Local:** injection site reactions. **Metab:** hypercholesterolemia, hyperlipidemia. **MS:** back pain. **Misc:** allergic reactions including ANAPHYLAXIS, ANGIOEDEMA, INFECTIONS (including reactivation tuberculosis and other opportunistic infections due to bacterial, invasive fungal, viral, mycobacterial, and parasitic pathogens), MALIGNANCY (including lymphoma, HSTCL, leukemia, and skin cancer), fever.

Interactions

Drug-Drug: Concurrent use with **anakinra**, **abatacept**, or other **TNF blocking agents** ↑ risk of serious infections and is contraindicated. Concurrent use with **azathioprine** and/or **methotrexate** may ↑ risk of HSTCL. **Live vaccinations** should not be given concurrently.

Route/Dosage

Rheumatoid Arthritis, Ankylosing Spondylitis, and Psoriatic Arthritis

Subcut (Adults): 40 mg every other week; patients not receiving concurrent methotrexate may receive additional benefit by increasing dose to 40 mg once weekly.

Crohn's Disease

Subcut (Adults): 160 mg initially on Day 1 (given as four 40-mg injections in one day or as two 40-mg injections given in two consecutive days), followed by 80 mg 2 wk later on Day 15. Two wk later (Day 29), begin maintenance dose of 40 mg every other wk. Aminosalicylates, corticosteroids, and/or immunomodulatory agents (e.g. azathioprine, 6–mercaptopurine, methotrexate) may be continued during therapy.

Subcut (Children ≥6 yr and ≥40 kg): 160 mg initially on Day 1 (given as four 40-mg injections in one day or as two 40-mg injections given in two consecutive days), followed by 80 mg 2 wk later on Day 15 (given as two 40-mg injections in one day). Two wk later (Day 29), begin maintenance dose of 40 mg every other wk. Aminosalicylates, corticosteroids, and/or immunomodulatory agents (e.g. azathioprine, 6–mercaptopurine, methotrexate) may be continued during therapy.
Subcut (Children ≥6 yr and 17–<40 kg): 80 mg initially on Day 1 (given as two 40-mg injections in one day), followed by 40 mg 2 wk later on Day 15. Two wk later (Day 29), begin maintenance dose of 20 mg every other wk. Aminosalicylates, corticosteroids, and/or immunomodulatory agents (e.g. azathioprine, 6–mercaptopurine, methotrexate) may be continued during therapy.

Ulcerative Colitis

Subcut (Adults): 160 mg initially on Day 1 (given as four 40-mg injections in one day or as two 40-mg injections given in two consecutive days), followed by 80 mg 2 wk later on Day 15. Two wk later (Day 29), begin maintenance dose of 40 mg every other wk. Aminosalicylates, corticosteroids, and/or immunomodulatory agents (e.g. azathioprine, 6–mercaptopurine, methotrexate) may be continued during therapy.

Juvenile Idiopathic Arthritis

Subcut (Children 2–17 yr): *10–<15 kg*—10 mg every other wk; *15–<30 kg*—20 mg every other wk; *≥30 kg*—40 mg every other wk.

Plaque Psoriasis

Subcut (Adults): 80 mg initially, then in 1 wk, begin regimen of 40 mg every other wk.

Hidradenitis Suppurativa

Subcut (Adults): 160 mg initially (given as four 40-mg injections on Day 1 or as two 40-mg injections per day on Days 1 and 2), followed by 80 mg 2 wk later on Day 15. Two wk later (Day 29), begin maintenance dose of 40 mg every wk.

Availability

Solution for subcutaneous injection (prefilled syringes): 10 mg/0.2 mL, 20 mg/0.4 mL, 40 mg/0.8 mL. **Solution for subcutaneous injection (vials):** 40 mg/0.8 mL. **Prefilled pen:** 40 mg/0.8 mL.

NURSING IMPLICATIONS

Assessment

- Assess for signs of infection (fever, dyspnea, flu-like symptoms, frequent or painful urination, redness or swelling at the site of a wound), including tuberculosis and Hepatitis B virus (HBV), prior to and periodically during therapy. Adalimumab is contraindicated in patients with active infection. New infections should be monitored closely; most common are upper respiratory tract infections, bronchitis, and urinary tract infections. Infections may be fatal, especially in patients taking immunosuppressive therapy.
- Monitor for injection site reactions (redness and/or itching, rash, hemorrhage, bruising, pain, or swelling). Rash will usually disappear within a few days. Application of a towel soaked in cold water may relieve pain or swelling.
- Assess patient for latex allergy. Needle cover of syringe contains latex and should not be handled by persons sensitive to latex.
- Monitor patient for signs of anaphylaxis (urticaria, dyspnea, facial edema) following injection. Medications (antihistamines, corticosteroids, epinephrine) and equipment should be readily available in the event of a severe reaction. Discontinue adalimumab immediately if anaphylaxis or other severe allergic reaction occurs.
- Assess patient for latent tuberculosis with a tuberculin skin test prior to initiation of therapy. Treatment of latent tuberculosis should be started before therapy with adalimumab.
- Assess for signs and symptoms of systemic fungal infections (fever, malaise, weight loss, sweats, cough, dypsnea, pulmonary infiltrates, serious systemic illness with or without concomitant shock). Ascertain if patient lives in or has traveled to areas of endemic mycoses. Consider empiric antifungal treatment for patients at risk of histoplasmosis and other invasive fungal infections until pathogens are identified. Consult with an infectious diseases specialist. Consider stopping adalimumab until infection has been diagnosed and adequately treated.
- **Arthritis:** Assess pain and range of motion before and periodically during therapy.
- **Crohn's Disease or Ulcerative Colitis:** Monitor frequency and consistency of bowel movements periodically during therapy.
- **Plaque Psoriasis:** Assess skin lesions periodically during therapy.
- **Hidradenitis Suppurativa:** Monitor skin lesions (abscesses, inflammatory nodules, draining fistulas) during therapy.
- ***Lab Test Considerations:*** May cause agranulocytosis, granulocytopenia, leukopenia, pancytopenia, and polycythemia.
- Monitor CBC with differential periodically during therapy. May cause leukopenia, neutropenia, thrombocytopenia, and pancytopenia. Discontinue adalimumab if symptoms of blood dyscrasias (persistent fever) occur.
- Monitor for HBV blood tests before starting during, and for several months after therapy is completed.

Potential Nursing Diagnoses

Acute pain (Indications)
Risk for infection (Side Effects)

Implementation

- Administer a tuberculin skin test prior to administration of adalimumab. Patients with active latent TB should be treated for TB prior to therapy.
- Immunizations should be current prior to initiating therapy. Patients on adalimumab may receive concurrent vaccinations, except for live vaccines.
- Administer initial injection under supervision of a health care professional.
- Vial is for institutional use only. With training, patient may use pen and pre-filled syringes at home.
- Do not administer solutions that are discolored or contain particulate matter. Discard unused solution.
- Other DMARDs should be continued during adalimumab therapy.
- **Subcut:** Vial may be left at room temperature for 15–30 min before injecting. Administer at a 45° angle in upper thighs or abdomen, avoiding the 2 inches around the navel. Put pressure on injection site for 10 sec, do not rub. Rotate injection sites; avoid areas that are tender, bruised, hard, or red. Refrigerate prefilled syringes and pens.

Patient/Family Teaching

- Instruct patient on the correct technique for administering adalimumab. Review *Medication Guide*, preparation of dose, administration sites and technique, and disposal of equipment into a puncture-resistant container.
- Advise patient to use calendar stickers provided by manufacturer to assist in remembering when dose is due. If a dose is missed, instruct patient to administer as soon as possible, then take next dose according to regular schedule. If more than prescribed dose is taken, caution patient to consult health care professional or the HUMIRA Patient Resource Center at 1-800-4HUMIRA (448-6472).
- Caution patient to notify health care professional immediately if signs of infection, HBV (muscle aches, clay-colored bowel movements, feeling very tired, fever, dark urine, chills, skin or eyes look yellow, stomach discomfort, little or no appetite, skin rash, vomiting), severe rash, swollen face, or difficulty breathing occurs or if nervous system problems (numbness or tingling, problems vision, weakness in arms or legs, dizziness) occur while taking adalimumab.
- Advise patient to notify health care professional of all Rx or OTC medications, vitamins, or herbal products being taken and to consult with health care professional before taking other medications.
- Instruct patient to notify health care professional of medication regimen prior to treatment or surgery.
- Advise female patients to notify health care professional if pregnancy is planned or suspected or if breast feeding. Encourage patient to contact the pregnancy registry by calling 1-877-311-8972 if pregnant.
- **Pen:** Clean area for injection with alcohol swab. Hold pen with gray cap pointing up. Check solution through window; if discolored, cloudy, or contains flakes, discard solution. Turn pen over and point cap down to make sure solution reaches fill line; if not, do not use and contact pharmacist. Remove gray cap exposing the needle and the plum cap exposing the button; removing the plum cap activates the pen. Pinch skin and place pen, with window visible, against skin at a 90° angle and press button until a click is heard. Hold pen in place until all solution is injected (10 seconds) and yellow marker is visible in window and has stopped moving. Continue to pinch skin throughout injection. Remove needle and press with a gauze pad or cotton ball for 10 seconds. Do not rub injection site. Dispose of pen into a puncture-resistant container.

Evaluation/Desired Outcomes

- Decreased pain and swelling with decreased rate of joint destruction in patients with rheumatoid arthritis.
- Decreased signs and symptoms, slowed progression of joint destruction, and improved physical function in patients with psoriatic arthritis.
- Reduced signs and symptoms of ankylosing spondylitis.
- Decreased signs and symptoms, and maintenance of remission, in patients with Crohn's disease or ulcerative colitis.
- Reduced pain and swelling in patients moderate to severe polyarticular juvenile idiopathic arthritis (JIA) in children 2 yr of age and older.
- Reduced severity of plaques in patients with severe chronic plaque psoriasis.
- Improvement in skin lesions in patients with hidradenitis suppurativa.

adenosine (a-**den**-oh-seen)

Adenocard, Adenoscan

Classification

Therapeutic: antiarrhythmics

Pregnancy Category C

Indications

Conversion of paroxysmal supraventricular tachycardia (PSVT) to normal sinus rhythm when vagal maneuvers are unsuccessful. As a diagnostic agent (with noninvasive techniques) to assess myocardial perfusion defects occurring as a consequence of coronary artery disease.

Action

Restores normal sinus rhythm by interrupting re-entrant pathways in the AV node. Slows conduction time through the AV node. Also produces coronary artery vasodilation. **Therapeutic Effects:** Restoration of normal sinus rhythm.

Pharmacokinetics

Absorption: Following IV administration, absorption is complete.
Distribution: Taken up by erythrocytes and vascular endothelium.
Metabolism and Excretion: Rapidly converted to inosine and adenosine monophosphate.
Half-life: <10 sec.

TIME/ACTION PROFILE (antiarrhythmic effect)

ROUTE	ONSET	PEAK	DURATION
IV	immediate	unknown	1–2 min

Contraindications/Precautions

Contraindicated in: Hypersensitivity; 2nd- or 3rd-degree AV block or sick sinus syndrome, unless a functional artificial pacemaker is present; Myocardial ischemia/infarction (only Adenoscan).
Use Cautiously in: Patients with a history of asthma (may induce bronchospasm); Unstable angina; OB, Lactation: Safety not established.

Adverse Reactions/Side Effects

CNS: SEIZURES (only with Adenoscan), STROKE (only with Adenoscan), apprehension, dizziness, headache, head pressure, lightheadedness. **EENT:** blurred vision, throat tightness. **Resp:** shortness of breath, chest pressure, hyperventilation. **CV:** MI, VENTRICULAR TACHYCARDIA, facial flushing, transient arrhythmias, chest pain, hypotension, palpitations. **GI:** metallic taste, nausea. **Derm:** burning sensation, facial flushing, sweating. **MS:** neck and back pain. **Neuro:** numbness, tingling. **Misc:** HYPERSENSITIVITY REACTIONS, heaviness in arms, pressure sensation in groin.

Interactions

Drug-Drug: Carbamazepine may ↑ risk of progressive heart block. **Dipyridamole** ↑ effects of adenosine (dose ↓ of adenosine recommended). Effects of adenosine ↓ by **theophylline** or **caffeine** (↑ doses of adenosine may be required). Concurrent use with **digoxin** may ↑ risk of ventricular fibrillation.

Route/Dosage

IV (Adults and Children >50 kg): *Antiarrhythmic (Adenocard)*—6 mg by rapid IV bolus; if no results, repeat 1–2 min later as 12-mg rapid bolus. This dose may be repeated (single dose not to exceed 12 mg). *Diagnostic use (Adenoscan)*—140 mcg/kg/min for 6 min (0.84 mg/kg total).
IV (Children <50 kg): *Antiarrhythmic*—0.05–0.1 mg/kg as a rapid bolus, may repeat in 1–2 min; if response is inadequate, may increase by 0.05–0.1 mg/kg until sinus rhythm is established or maximum dose of 0.3 mg/kg is used.

Availability (generic available)

Injection: 3 mg/mL in 2–mL vial (Adenocard), 3 mg/mL in 20–mL and 30-mL vials (Adenoscan).

NURSING IMPLICATIONS

Assessment

- Monitor heart rate frequently (every 15–30 sec) and ECG continuously during therapy. A short, transient period of 1st-, 2nd-, or 3rd-degree heart block or asystole may occur following injection; usually resolves quickly due to short duration of adenosine. Once conversion to normal sinus rhythm is achieved, transient arrhythmias (premature ventricular contractions, atrial premature contractions, sinus tachycardia, sinus bradycardia, skipped beats, AV nodal block) may occur, but generally last a few seconds.
- Monitor BP during therapy.
- Assess respiratory status (breath sounds, rate) following administration. Patients with history of asthma may experience bronchospasm.

Potential Nursing Diagnoses

Decreased cardiac output (Indications)

Implementation

IV Administration

- **IV:** Crystals may occur if adenosine is refrigerated. Warm to room temperature to dissolve crystals. Solution must be clear before use. Do not administer solutions that are discolored or contain particulate matter. Discard unused portions.
- **IV Push:** ***Diluent:*** Administer undiluted. ***Concentration:*** 3 mg/mL. ***Rate:*** Administer over 1–2 seconds via peripheral IV as proximal as possible to trunk. Slow administration may cause increased heart rate in response to vasodilation. Follow each dose with 20 mL rapid saline flush to ensure injection reaches systemic circulation.
- **Intermittent Infusion(for use in diagnostic testing):** ***Diluent:*** Administer 30-mL vial undiluted. ***Concentration:*** 3 mg/mL. ***Rate:*** Administer at a rate of 140 mcg/kg/min over 6 min for a total dose of 0.84 mg/kg. Thallium-201 should be injected as close to the venous access as possible at the midpoint (after 3 min) of the infusion.

Patient/Family Teaching

- Caution patient to change positions slowly to minimize orthostatic hypotension. Doses >12 mg decrease BP by decreasing peripheral vascular resistance.
- Instruct patient to report facial flushing, shortness of breath, or dizziness.
- Advise patient to avoid products containing methylxanthines (caffeinated coffee, tea, carbonated drinks or drugs such as aminophylline or theophylline) prior to myocardial perfusion imaging study.

Evaluation/Desired Outcomes
- Conversion of supraventricular tachycardia to normal sinus rhythm.
- Diagnosis of myocardial perfusion defects.

ado-trastuzumab
(ado tras-**tooz**-doo-mab-)
Kadcyla

Classification
Therapeutic: antineoplastics
Pharmacologic: drug-antibody conjugates

Pregnancy Category D

Indications
HER2-positive metastatic breast cancer previously treated with trastuzumab and a taxane.

Action
A HER2-targeted antibody and microtubule inhibitor conjugate. Trastuzumab, the antibody, attaches to receptors and is taken into the cell, where the microtubule inhibitor, DM1, causes cell cycle arrest and death. **Therapeutic Effects:** Decreased spread of metastatic breast cancer, with improved progression-free survival.

Pharmacokinetics
Absorption: IV administration results in complete bioavailability.
Distribution: Unknown.
Metabolism and Excretion: DM1 is metabolized by CYP3A4/5.
Half-life: 4 days.

TIME/ACTION PROFILE (comparative improvement in progression-free survival)

ROUTE	ONSET	PEAK	DURATION
IV	4–6 mos	10–12 mos	2 yr

Contraindications/Precautions
Contraindicated in: Interstitial lung disease or pneumonitis; Concurrent use of strong CYP3A4 inhibitors; Lactation: Breast feeding should be avoided; OB: May cause fetal harm.
Use Cautiously in: Underlying cardiovascular or pulmonary disease, including dyspnea at rest; Rep: Women with childbearing potential (contraception required during and for 7 mo following treatment); Pedi: Safety and effectiveness not established.

Adverse Reactions/Side Effects
CNS: fatigue, headache, dizziness, insomnia, weakness. **Resp:** PULMONARY TOXICITY, cough. **EENT:** blurred vision, conjuncitivitis, dry eyes, ↑ lacrimation. **CV:** LEFT VENTRICULAR DYSFUNCTION, hypertension, peripheral edema. **GI:** HEPATOTOXICITY, constipation, ↑ liver enzymes, nausea, altered taste, diarrhea, dry mouth, dyspepsia, stomatitis, vomiting. **Derm:** pruritus, rash. **F and E:** hypokalemia. **Hemat:** HEMORRHAGE, THROMBOCYTOPENIA, anemia, neutropenia. **MS:** musculoskeletal pain, arthralgia, myalgia. **Neuro:** peripheral neuropathy. **Misc:** HYPERSENSITIVITY REACTIONS, chills, infusion-related reactions, fever.

Interactions
Drug-Drug: Blood levels and risk of toxicity may be ↑ by concurrent use of **strong inhibitors of CYP3A4** including **atazanavir**, **clarithromycin**, **indinavir**, **itraconazole**, **ketoconazole**, **nefazodone**, **nelfinavir**, **ritonavir**, **saquinavir**, **telithromycin**, and **voriconazole**, and should be avoided, waiting 3 half-lives of inhibitor to start treatment. Concurrent use of **anticoagulants**, or **antiplatelet agents**, especially during the first cycle, may ↑ risk of bleeding.

Route/Dosage
IV (Adults): 3.6 mg/kg once every 3 wk continued until disease progresses or unacceptable toxicity occurs. Dose modifications (↓ or temporary discontinuation) required for ↑ transaminases, hyperbilirubinemia, left ventricular dysfunction, peripheral neuropathy or thrombocytopenia.

Availability
Lyophilized powder for intravenous injection (requires reconstitution): 100 mg/vial, 160 mg/vial.

NURSING IMPLICATIONS
Assessment
- Evaluate left ventricular function in all patients prior to and every 3 months during therapy. *If symptomatic HF:* discontinue ado-trastuzumab. *If left ventricular ejection fraction (LVEF) <40%:* Hold dose. Repeat LVSF assessment within 3 wks. If LVEF <40% is confirmed, discontinue therapy. *If LVEF 40% to ≤45% and decrease is ≥10% points from baseline:* Hold dose. Repeat LVEF within 3 wks. If LVEF has not recovered to within 10% points from baseline, discontinue therapy. *If LVEF 40% to ≤45% and decrease is <10% points from baseline:* Continue therapy with ado-trastuzumab. Repeat LVEF within 3 wks. *If LVEF >45%:* Continue therapy.
- Monitor infusion site closely for infiltration and extravasation closely. Within 24 hrs erythema, tenderness, skin irritation, pain, or swelling at infusion site is seen if extravasation occurs.
- Assess for signs and symptoms of infusion reactions (fever, chills, flushing, dyspnea, hypotension, wheezing, bronchospasm, tachycardia). Interrupt therapy if symptoms are severe. Observe closely during first infusion. Permanently discontinue for life-threatening reactions.

- Monitor neurologic status before and during treatment. Assess for paresthesia (numbness, tingling, pain, burning sensation), loss of deep tendon reflexes (Achilles reflex is usually first involved), weakness (wrist drop or footdrop, gait disturbances), cranial nerve palsies (jaw pain, hoarseness, ptosis, visual changes), arthralgia, myalgia, muscle spasm, autonomic dysfunction (ileus, difficulty voiding, orthostatic hypotension, impaired sweating), and CNS dysfunction (decreased level of consciousness, agitation, hallucinations). Temporarily discontinue therapy in patients with Grade 3 or 4 peripheral neuropathy (severe symptoms; limiting self-care activities of daily living (ADL) until resolution to ≤ Grade 2 (moderate symptoms; limiting instrumental ADL) neuropathy.
- Monitor for signs and symptoms of pulmonary toxicity (dyspnea, cough, fatigue, pulmonary infiltrates). Permanently discontinue therapy if interstitial lung disease or pneumonitis develops.
- Monitor for hemorrhage (central nervous system, respiratory, gastrointestinal hemorrhage) during therapy, especially in patients receiving anticoagulants, antiplatelet therapy, or who have thrombocytopenia.
- ***Lab Test Considerations:*** HER2 protein overexpression is used to determine whether treatment with ado-trastuzumab is indicated. HER2 protein overexpression should be determined by labs with proficiency in specific technology used.
- Monitor serum transaminases and bilirubin prior to starting therapy and before each dose. *If AST /ALT is Grade 2 (>2.5 to ≤5 × upper limit of normal):* Treat at same dose. *If AST/ALT is Grade 3 (>5 to ≤20 × upper limit of normal):* Do not administer ado-trastuzumab until AST/ALT recovers to Grade ≤2, and then reduce 1 dose level. *If AST/ALT is Grade 4 (>20 × upper limit of normal):* Permanently discontinue ado-trastuzumab. *If serum bilirubin is Grade 2 (>1.5 to ≤3 × upper limit of normal)*: Hold dose until bilirubin recovers to Grade ≤1, then treat at same dose level. *If bilirubin is Grade 3 (>3 to ≤10 × upper limit of normal):* Hold dose until bilirubin recovers to Grade ≤1, then reduce 1 dose level. *If bilirubin is Grade 4 (>10 × upper limit of normal):* Permanently discontinue ado-trastuzumab. Permanently discontinue ado-trastuzumab in patients with AST/ALT >3 × upper limit of normal and concomitant total bilirubin >2 × upper limit of normal.
- Monitor platelet count prior to starting therapy and before each dose. Nadir of thrombocytopenia occurs by Day 8 and generally improves to Grade 0 or 1 by next scheduled dose. *If thrombocytopenia is Grade 3 (PLT 25,000/mm^3 to <50,000/mm^3:* Hold dose until platelet count recovers to ≤Grade 1 (≥75,000/mm^3), then treat at same dose level. *If thrombocytopenia is Grade 4 (PLT <25,000/mm$_3$):* Hold dose until platelet count recovers to ≤Grade 1, then reduce 1 dose level.
- May cause ↓ hemoglobin, neutrophils, and serum potassium.

Potential Nursing Diagnoses

Deficient knowledge, related to medication regimen (Patient/Family Teaching)

Implementation

- ***High Alert:*** Do not confuse ado-trastuzumab (Kadcyla) with trastuzumab (Herceptin). Double check names. Trade name of administered product should be clearly recorded in patient file to improve traceability.
- ***High Alert:*** Fatalities have occurred with chemotherapeutic agents. Before administering, clarify all ambiguous orders; double check single, daily, and course-of-therapy dose limits; have second practitioner independently double check original order, dose calculations and infusion pump settings.
- Solution should be prepared in a biologic cabinet. Wear gloves, gown, and mask while handling medication. Discard IV equipment in specially designated containers.

IV Administration

- **Intermittent Infusion:** Reconstitute by slowly inject 5 or 8 mL of Sterile Water for Injection into 100 or 160 mg vial of ado-trastuzumab respectively, for a solution of 20 mg/mL. Swirl gently until dissolved; do not shake. Solution is clear, colorless to pale brown, and slightly opalescent; do not administer solutions that are discolored or contain particulate matter. Use reconstituted vials immediately or store in refrigerator up to 4 hr; then discard. Do not freeze. Calculate amount of solution needed. ***Diluent:*** Withdraw from vial and add to infusion bag containing 250 mL of 0.9% NaCl; do not use dextrose solutions. Gently invert bag to mix without foaming. Use diluted solution immediately; may be stored in refrigerator up to 24 hrs prior to use, then discard; do not freeze or shake. Administer every 3 wks (21–day cycle); if cycle is delayed, administer as soon as possible. Do not wait until next planned cycle; maintain 3-wk interval between doses. ***Rate:*** Infuse through a 0.2 or 0.22 micron in-line non-protein adsorptive polyethersulfone (PES) filter. Do not administer as IV push or bolus. *First infusion:* Infuse over 90 min; observe for infusion related reaction. *Subsequent infusions:* Infuse over 30 min if prior infusions were well tolerated. Observe patient during infusion and for at least 90 min after infusion.
- Management of increased serum transaminases, hyperbilirubinemia, left ventricular dysfunction, thrombocytopenia, pulmonary toxicity, or peripheral neuropathy may require temporary interruption, dose reduction, or discontinuation.
- Dose reduction schedule is: *Starting dose*—3.6 mg/kg; *First dose reduction*—3 mg/kg; *Second*

dose reduction—2.4 mg/kg; *Requirement for further dose reduction*—discontinue therapy.
- **Y-Site Incompatibility:** Do not mix or administer with other medications.

Patient/Family Teaching
- Explain purpose of medication to patient.
- Inform patient of potential liver injury and HF. Advise patient to notify health care professional immediately if signs and symptoms of liver injury (nausea, vomiting, abdominal pain, jaundice, dark urine, pruritus, anorexia) or HF (new onset or worsening shortness of breath, cough, swelling of ankles/legs, palpitations, weight gain of >5 lbs in 24 hrs, dizziness, loss of consciousness) occur.
- Advise patient to notify health care professional if signs of peripheral neuropathy (burning, numbness, pain in hands and feet/legs) occur.
- Rep: Ado-trastuzumab can cause fetal harm. Advise male and female patient to use a highly effective method (IUD, hormonal contraceptive, tubal ligation, partner's vasectomy) of contraception during and for at least 7 months after last dose. Instruct patient to notify health care professional promptly if pregnancy is suspected or if breast feeding. Encourage women who have been exposed to ado-trastuzumab either directly or through seminal fluid, to enroll in the MotHER Pregnancy Registry by contacting 1-800-690-6720 and to immediately report exposure to Genentech Adverse Event Line at 1-888-835-2555.

Evaluation/Desired Outcomes
- Decreased spread of metastatic breast cancer.

afatinib (a-fa-ti-nib)
Gilotrif

Classification
Therapeutic: antineoplastics
Pharmacologic: kinase inhibitors

Pregnancy Category D

Indications
First-line treatment of metastatic non-small cell lung cancer (NSCLC) where the tumor has a specific epidermal growth factor receptor (EGFR) deletion or substitution mutation detectable by an FDA-approved test.

Action
Inhibits tyrosine kinases which results in slowed proliferation of specific tumor cell lines. **Therapeutic Effects:** Decreased spread of NSCLC.

Pharmacokinetics
Absorption: Well abosrbed (92%) following oral administration; absorption is decreased by high fat meal.
Distribution: Unknown.
Metabolism and Excretion: Metabolites occur partly as protein-bound products. Excretion is primarily fecal (85%) as parent drug; 4% excreted in urine.
Half-life: 37 hr.

TIME/ACTION PROFILE (improved progression-free survival)

ROUTE	ONSET	PEAK	DURATION
PO	3 mos	12 mos	20 mos

Contraindications/Precautions
Contraindicated in: Lactation: Discontinue drug or discontinue breast feeding; OB: May cause fetal harm.
Use Cautiously in: Moderate-severe renal or hepatic impairment (dose adjustment may be necessary); Asian ethnicity (may be ↑ susceptible to interstitial lung disease); OB: Patients with child-bearing potential (highly effective contraception should be used during and for at least 2 wks after last dose); Pedi: Safe and effective use in children has not been established.

Adverse Reactions/Side Effects
EENT: keratitis. **Resp:** INTERSTITIAL LUNG DISEASE. **GI:** HEPATIC TOXICITY, diarrhea, ↓ appetite, stomatitis. **Derm:** cutaneous reactions (including bullous/blistering/exfoliating reactions, acneiform eruptions and palmar-plantar erythrodysesthesia), dry skin, pruritus, paronychia, rash. **F and E:** hypokalemia.

Interactions
Drug-Drug: Concurrent use of **P-gp inhibitors** including **amiodarone**, **cyclosporine**, **erythromycin**, **itraconazole**, **ketoconazole**, **quinidine ritonavir**, **saquinavir**, **tacrolimus**, or **verapamil** ↑ blood levels and the risk of toxicity; dosage adjustment may be necessary (ritonavir may be given concurrently or 6 hr after). Concurrent use of **P-gp inducers** including **carbamazepine**, **phenobarbital**, **phenytoin rifampicin** or **rifampin** ↓ blood levels and may ↓ effectiveness; dosage adjustment may be necessary.

Route/Dosage
PO (Adults): 40 mg/day; *concurrent use of P-gp inhibitors*—reduce dose by 10 mg/day if necessary; *concurrent use of P-gp inducers*—increase dose by 10 mg/day if necessary. Dose reductions recommended for various toxicities. Continue until disease progression or occurrence of unacceptable toxicity.

Availability
Tablets: 20 mg, 30 mg, 40 mg.

NURSING IMPLICATIONS
Assessment
- Monitor for diarrhea; occurs frequently. Provide patient with an antidiarrheal agent (loperamide) at the

onset of diarrhea and until diarrhea ceases for 12 hrs. If diarrhea is severe and lasts more than 48 hr despite use of antidiarrheal agent (Grade 2 or higher), withhold afatinib until diarrhea resolves to Grade 1 or less, then resume with reduced dose of 10 mg/day.

- Assess for cutaneous reactions (bullous, blistering, exfoliative lesions; rash, erythema, acneiform rash) periodically during therapy. Discontinue afatinib if life-threatening lesions or prolonged Grade 2 cutaneous lesions lasting ≥7 days, intolerable Grade 2, or Grade 3 cutaneous reactions occur. Withhold afatinib until reaction resolves to Grade 1 or less and resume at 10 mg/day.
- Monitor for signs and symptoms of interstitial lung disease (lung infiltration, pneumonitis, acute respiratory distress syndrome, allergic alveolitis; may occur more commonly in patients of Asian ethnicity. Withhold afatinib if symptoms occur; discontinue if interstitial lung disease is confirmed.
- ***Lab Test Considerations:*** Monitor liver function tests periodically during therapy. If severe decline in liver function occurs, discontinue afatinib. May cause ↑ AST and ALT.
- May cause hypokalemia.

Potential Nursing Diagnoses

Diarrhea (Side Effects)

Implementation

- **PO:** Administer once daily on an empty stomach, at least 1 hr before or 2 hrs after meals.

Patient/Family Teaching

- Instruct patient to take afatinib as directed. Take missed dose as soon as remembered unless within 12 hrs of next dose, then omit and take next dose at scheduled time; do not double doses.
- Caution patient to notify health care professional if signs and symptoms of keratitis (acute or worsening eye inflammation, lacrimation, light sensitivity, blurred vision, eye pain, and/or red eye) occur. Withhold if symptoms occur; if ulcerative keratitis is confirmed, discontinue afatinib. Advise patient that use of contact lenses is also a risk factor.
- Advise patient to wear sunscreen and protective clothing during therapy to minimize risk of skin disorders.
- Inform patient that diarrhea occurs in most patients and may cause dehydration and renal impairment. Notify health care professional if diarrhea is severe or persistent, if new or worsening lung symptoms (difficulty breathing, shortness of breath, cough, fever), symptoms of liver problems (yellow skin or whites of eyes, dark brown urine, pain on right side of abdomen, unusual bleeding or bruising, lethargy) or if symptoms of left ventricular dysfunction (shortness of breath, exercise intolerance, cough, fatigue, swelling or ankles or feet, palpitations, sudden weight gain) occur.
- Advise patient to notify health care professional of all Rx or OTC medications, vitamins, or herbal products being taken and to consult with health care professional before taking other medications.
- Advise female patients to use highly effective contraception during and for at least 2 wks after last dose and to avoid breast feeding. If pregnancy occurs, instruct patient to notify health care professional immediately.

Evaluation/Desired Outcomes

- Decreased spread of non-small cell lung cancer.

REMS

albiglutide (al-bi-gloo-tide)

Tanzeum

Classification

Therapeutic: antidiabetics

Pharmacologic: glucagon-like peptide-1 (GLP-1) receptor agonists

Pregnancy Category C

Indications

Adjunct to diet and exercise in the treatment of type 2 diabetes mellitus (not recommended as first-line therapy).

Action

Acts as an agonist at the glucagon-like peptide-1 (GLP-1) receptor resulting in augmented glucose-dependent insulin secretion. Bound to a molecule of human albumin which results in prolonged duration of action. **Therapeutic Effects:** Improved glycemic control.

Pharmacokinetics

Absorption: Bioavailability following subcutaneous injection unknown.

Distribution: Unknown.

Metabolism and Excretion: Degraded by proteolytic enzymes; albumin portion is broken down by vascular endothelium.

Half-life: 5 days.

TIME/ACTION PROFILE (effect on HbA1c)

ROUTE	ONSET	PEAK	DURATION
subcut	within 4 wk	12 wk†	throughout treatment

† Steady-state levels achieved in 4–5 wk.

Contraindications/Precautions

Contraindicated in: Hypersensitivity; History of pancreatitis; Personal or family history of medullary thyroid carcinoma; Multiple Endocrine Neoplasia syndrome type 2; History of severe gastrointestinal disease; Lactation: Discontinue albiglutide or discontinue breast feeding.

Use Cautiously in: Renal impairment (monitor renal function during initiation and dose escalation);

Geri: May be more sensitive to drug effects; OB: Avoid use during pregnancy (taper and discontinue at least 1 mo prior to planned pregnancy; Pedi: Safety and effectiveness not established.

Adverse Reactions/Side Effects

GI: PANCREATITIS, diarrhea, nausea, delayed gastric emptying, dyspepsia, reflux. **GU:** renal impairment (in association with nausea, vomiting, dehydration).
Endo: THYROID C-CELL TUMORS, hypoglycemia (↑ with insulin/sulfonylureas), ↑ risk of thyroid C-cell tumors.
Local: injection site reactions. **Misc:** hypersensitivity reactions.

Interactions

Drug-Drug: ↑ risk of hypoglycemia with other **antidiabetic agents**, especially **insulin** and **sulfonylureas** (dose reduction of insulin or sulfonylureas may be warranted). May alter the absorption of concurrently administered **oral medications**.

Route/Dosage

Subcut (Adults): 30 mg once weekly, may ↑ to 50 mg once weekly if needed.

Availability

Lypohilized powder for subcutaneous injection (requires reconstitution): 30 mg/single-use Pen, 50 mg/single-use Pen.

NURSING IMPLICATIONS

Assessment

- Observe patient taking concurrent insulin for signs and symptoms of hypoglycemic reactions (sweating, hunger, weakness, dizziness, tremor, tachycardia, anxiety).
- If thyroid nodules or elevated serum calcitonin are noted, patient should be referred to an endocrinologist.
- Monitor for signs and symptoms of hypersensitivity reactions (pruritus, rash, dyspnea). If signs and symptoms occur, discontinue therapy and treat symptomatically.
- Monitor for pancreatitis (persistent severe abdominal pain, sometimes radiating to the back, with or without vomiting). If pancreatitis is suspected, discontinue albiglutide; if confirmed, do not restart albiglutide.
- ***Lab Test Considerations:*** Monitor serum HbA1c periodically during therapy to evaluate effectiveness.

Potential Nursing Diagnoses

Imbalanced nutrition: more than body requirements (Indications)
Noncompliance (Patient/Family Teaching)

Implementation

- Patients stabilized on a diabetic regimen who are exposed to stress, fever, trauma, infection, or surgery may require administration of insulin.
- Albiglutide is not indicated to patients with diabetes type I or for diabetic ketoacidosis.
- **Subcut:** Administer once weekly at any time of the day, without regard to food. Day of the week may be changed as long as last dose was administered 4 or more days before. Inject into abdomen, thigh, or upper arm. Solution should be clear and colorless; do not administer solutions that are discolored or contain particulate matter.
- Consider decreasing dose of concurrently administered insulin secretagogues (e.g. sulfonylureas) or insulin to reduce risk of hypoglycemia.
- Follow manufacturer's instructions carefully regarding use of pen for administration. Use within 8 hrs of reconstitution.

Patient/Family Teaching

- Instruct patient on use of *Tanzeum* pen and to take albiglutide as directed. Pen should never be shared between patients, even if needle is changed. Store pen in refrigerator; do not freeze. After initial use, pen may be stored at room temperature or refrigerated up to 30 days. Keep pen cap on when not in use. Protect from excessive heat and sunlight. Remove and safely discard needle after each injection and store pen without needle attached. Advise patient to read the *Patient Medication Guide* before starting albiglutide and with each Rx refill.
- If a dose is missed take as soon as possible within 3 days of missed dose. If longer than 3 days are missed, instruct patient to wait and take next dose at usual weekly time.
- Inform patient that nausea is the most common side effect, but usually decreases over time.
- Explain to patient that this medication controls hyperglycemia but does not cure diabetes. Therapy is long-term.
- Review signs of hypoglycemia and hyperglycemia with patient. If hypoglycemia occurs, advise patient to take a glass of orange juice or 2–3 tsp of sugar, honey, or corn syrup dissolved in water and notify health care professional.
- Encourage patient to follow prescribed diet, medication, and exercise regimen to prevent hypoglycemic or hyperglycemic episodes.
- Instruct patient in proper testing of serum glucose and ketones. These tests should be closely monitored during periods of stress or illness, and health care professional should be notified if significant changes occur.
- Advise patient to tell health care professional what medications they are taking and to avoid taking new

Rx, OTC, vitamins, or herbal products without consulting health care professional.

- Advise patient to discontinue albiglutide and notify health care professional immediately if signs of pancreatitis (nausea, vomiting, abdominal pain) occur.
- Advise patient to carry a form of sugar (sugar packets, candy) and identification describing disease process and medication regimen at all times.
- Advise patient to inform health care professional of medication regimen before treatment or surgery.
- Inform patient of risk of benign and malignant thyroid C-cell tumors. Advise patient to notify health care professional if symptoms of thyroid tumors (lump in neck, hoarseness, trouble swallowing, shortness of breath) or if signs of allergic reaction (swelling of face, lips, tongue, or throat; fainting or feeling dizzy; very rapid heartbeat; problems breathing or swallowing; severe rash or itching) occur.
- If pregnancy is planned, consider stopping albiglutide at least 1 mo before a planned pregnancy. Insulin is the preferred method of controlling blood glucose during pregnancy. Counsel female patients to notify health care professional if pregnancy is planned or suspected or if breast feeding.
- Emphasize the importance of routine follow-up exams.

Evaluation/Desired Outcomes

- Improved glycemic control.

albuterol (al-byoo-ter-ole)

Accuneb, ✤Airomir, Proair HFA, Proair Respiclick, Proventil HFA, ✤Salbutamol, Ventolin HFA, ✤Ventolin Diskus, ✤Ventolin Nebules, VoSpire ER

Classification

Therapeutic: bronchodilators

Pharmacologic: adrenergics

Pregnancy Category C

Indications

Used as a bronchodilator to control and prevent reversible airway obstruction caused by asthma or COPD. **Inhaln:** Used as a quick-relief agent for acute bronchospasm and for prevention of exercise-induced bronchospasm. **PO:** Used as a long-term control agent in patients with chronic/persistent bronchospasm.

Action

Binds to $beta_2$-adrenergic receptors in airway smooth muscle, leading to activation of adenyl cyclase and increased levels of cyclic-3′, 5′-adenosine monophosphate (cAMP). Increases in cAMP activate kinases, which inhibit the phosphorylation of myosin and decrease intracellular calcium. Decreased intracellular calcium relaxes smooth muscle airways. Relaxation of airway smooth muscle with subsequent bronchodilation. Relatively selective for $beta_2$ (pulmonary) receptors. **Therapeutic Effects:** Bronchodilation.

Pharmacokinetics

Absorption: Well absorbed after oral administration but rapidly undergoes extensive metabolism.

Distribution: Small amounts appear in breast milk.

Metabolism and Excretion: Extensively metabolized by the liver and other tissues.

Half-life: Oral 2.7–5 hr; Inhalation: 3.8 hr.

TIME/ACTION PROFILE (bronchodilation)

ROUTE	ONSET	PEAK	DURATION
PO	15–30 min	2–3 hr	4–6 hr or more
PO–ER	30 min	2–3 hr	12 hr
Inhaln	5–15 min	60–90 min	3–6 hr

Contraindications/Precautions

Contraindicated in: Hypersensitivity to adrenergic amines.

Use Cautiously in: Cardiac disease; Hypertension; Hyperthyroidism; Diabetes; Glaucoma; Seizure disorders; Excess inhaler use may lead to tolerance and paradoxical bronchospasm; **OB, Lactation, Pedi:** Safety not established for pregnant women near term, breast-feeding women, and children <2 yr; **Geri:** ↑ risk of adverse reactions; may require dose ↓.

Adverse Reactions/Side Effects

CNS: nervousness, restlessness, tremor, headache, insomnia (**Pedi:** occurs more frequently in young children than adults), hyperactivity in children. **Resp:** PARADOXICAL BRONCHOSPASM (excessive use of inhalers). **CV:** chest pain, palpitations, angina, arrhythmias, hypertension. **GI:** nausea, vomiting. **Endo:** hyperglycemia. **F and E:** hypokalemia. **Neuro:** tremor.

Interactions

Drug-Drug: Concurrent use with other **adrenergic agents** will have ↑ adrenergic side effects. Use with **MAO inhibitors** may lead to hypertensive crisis. **Beta blockers** may negate therapeutic effect. May ↓ serum **digoxin** levels. Cardiovascular effects are potentiated in patients receiving **tricyclic antidepressants**. Risk of hypokalemia ↑ concurrent use of **potassium-losing diuretics**. Hypokalemia ↑ the risk of **digoxin** toxicity.

Drug-Natural Products: Use with caffeine-containing herbs (**cola nut, guarana, tea, coffee**) ↑ stimulant effect.

Route/Dosage

PO (Adults and Children ≥12 yr): 2–4 mg 3–4 times daily (not to exceed 32 mg/day) or 4–8 mg of extended-release tablets twice daily.

PO (Geriatric Patients): Initial dose should not

exceed 2 mg 3–4 times daily, may be ↑ carefully (up to 32 mg/day).

PO (Children 6–12 yr): 2 mg 3–4 times daily or 0.3–0.6 mg/kg/day as extended-release tablets divided twice daily; may be carefully ↑ as needed (not to exceed 8 mg/day).

PO (Children 2–6 yr): 0.1 mg/kg 3 times daily (not to exceed 2 mg 3 times daily initially); may be carefully ↑ to 0.2 mg/kg 3 times daily (not to exceed 4 mg 3 times daily).

Inhaln (Adults and Children ≥4 yr): *Via metered-dose inhaler*—2 inhalations q 4–6 hr or 2 inhalations 15 min before exercise (90 mcg/spray); some patients may respond to 1 inhalation. *NIH Guidelines for acute asthma exacerbation: Children*—4–8 puffs q 20 min for 3 doses then q 1–4 hr; *Adults*—4–8 puffs q 20 min for up to 4 hr then q 1–4 hr prn.

Inhaln (Adults and Children >12 yr): *Via dry powder inhaler*—2 inhalations q 4–6 hr or 2 inhalations 15–30 min before exercise (90 mcg/spray); some patients may respond to 1 inhalation q 4 hr.

Inhaln (Adults and Children >12 yr): *NIH Guidelines for acute asthma exacerbation via nebulization or IPPB*—2.5–5 mg q 20 min for 3 doses then 2.5–10 mg q 1–4 hr prn; *Continuous nebulization*—10–15 mg/hr.

Inhaln (Children 2–12 yr): *NIH Guidelines for acute asthma exacerbation via nebulization or IPPB*—0.15 mg/kg/dose (minimum dose 2.5 mg) q 20 min for 3 doses then 0.15–0.3 mg/kg (not to exceed 10 mg) q 1–4 hr prn *or* 1.25 mg 3–4 times daily for children 10–15 kg *or* 2.5 mg 3–4 times daily for children >15 kg; *Continuous nebulization*—0.5–3 mg/kg/hr.

Inhaln (Neonates): 1.25 mg/dose q 8 hr via nebulization or 1–2 puffs via MDI into the ventilator circuit q 6 hrs.

Availability (generic available)

Tablets: 2 mg, 4 mg. **Cost:** *Generic*—4 mg $565.87/100. **Extended-release tablets:** 4 mg, 8 mg. **Oral syrup (strawberry-flavored):** 2 mg/5 mL. **Metered-dose aerosol:** 90 mcg/inhalation in 6.7-g, 8-g, 8.5-g, and 18-g canisters (200 metered inhalations), ✱100 mcg/spray. **Cost:** *Proair HFA*—$52.53/8.5-g canister; *Proventil HFA*—$62.62/6.7-g canister; *Ventolin HFA*—$19.08/8-g canister. **Inhalation solution:** 0.63 mg/3 mL (0.021%), 1.25 mg/3 mL (0.042%), 2.5 mg/3 mL (0.083%), ✱1 mg/mL, ✱2 mg/mL, 5 mg/mL (0.5%). **Cost:** *Generic*—2.5 mg/3 mL $40.82/90 mL, 5 mg/mL $51.02/60 mL. **Powder for inhalation (Proair Respiclick):** 90 mcg/inhalation (200 metered inhalations). **Powder for inhalation (Ventolin Diskus):** ✱200 mcg. ***In combination with:*** ipratropium (Combivent, DuoNeb). See Appendix B.

NURSING IMPLICATIONS

Assessment

- Assess lung sounds, pulse, and BP before administration and during peak of medication. Note amount, color, and character of sputum produced.
- Monitor pulmonary function tests before initiating therapy and periodically during therapy.
- Observe for paradoxical bronchospasm (wheezing). If condition occurs, withhold medication and notify health care professional immediately.
- ***Lab Test Considerations:*** May cause transient ↓ in serum potassium concentrations with nebulization or higher-than-recommended doses.

Potential Nursing Diagnoses

Ineffective airway clearance (Indications)

Implementation

- **PO:** Administer oral medication with meals to minimize gastric irritation.
- Extended-release tablets should be swallowed whole; do not break, crush, or chew.
- **Inhaln:** Shake inhaler well, and allow at least 1 min between inhalations of aerosol medication. Prime the inhaler before first use by releasing 4 test sprays into the air away from the face. *Proair Respiclick* does not require priming. **Pedi:** Use spacer for children < 8 yr of age.
- For nebulization or IPPB, the 0.5-, 0.83-, 1-, and 2-mg/mL solutions do not require dilution before administration. The 5 mg/mL (0.5%) solution must be diluted with 1–2.5 mL of 0.9% NaCl for inhalation. Diluted solutions are stable for 24 hr at room temperature or 48 hr if refrigerated.
- For nebulizer, compressed air or oxygen flow should be 6–10 L/min; a single treatment of 3 mL lasts about 10 min.
- IPPB usually lasts 5–20 min.

Patient/Family Teaching

- Instruct patient to take albuterol as directed. If on a scheduled dosing regimen, take missed dose as soon as remembered, spacing remaining doses at regular intervals. Do not double doses or increase the dose or frequency of doses. Caution patient not to exceed recommended dose; may cause adverse effects, paradoxical bronchospasm (more likely with first dose from new canister), or loss of effectiveness of medication.
- Instruct patient to contact health care professional immediately if shortness of breath is not relieved by medication or is accompanied by diaphoresis, dizziness, palpitations, or chest pain.
- Instruct patient to prime unit with 4 sprays before using and to discard canister after 200 sprays. Actuators should not be changed among products.

- Inform patient that these products contain hydrofluoralkane (HFA) and the propellant and are described as non-CFC or CFC-free (contain no chlorofluorocarbons).
- Instruct patient to notify health care professional of all Rx or OTC medications, vitamins, or herbal products being taken and to consult health care professional before taking any OTC medications or alcoholic beverages concurrently with this therapy. Caution patient also to avoid smoking and other respiratory irritants.
- Inform patient that albuterol may cause an unusual or bad taste.
- **Inhaln:** Instruct patient in the proper use of the metered-dose inhaler or nebulizer (see Appendix D).
- Advise patients to use albuterol first if using other inhalation medications and allow 5 min to elapse before administering other inhalant medications unless otherwise directed.
- Advise patient to rinse mouth with water after each inhalation dose to minimize dry mouth and clean the mouthpiece with water at least once a week.
- Instruct patient to notify health care professional if there is no response to the usual dose or if contents of one canister are used in less than 2 wk. Asthma and treatment regimen should be re-evaluated and corticosteroids should be considered. Need for increased use to treat symptoms indicates decrease in asthma control and need to re-evaluate patient's therapy.

Evaluation/Desired Outcomes

- Prevention or relief of bronchospasm.

alclometasone, See CORTICOSTEROIDS (TOPICAL/LOCAL).

alendronate (a-len-drone-ate)

Binosto, Fosamax

Classification

Therapeutic: bone resorption inhibitors

Pharmacologic: biphosphonates

Pregnancy Category C

Indications

Treatment and prevention of postmenopausal osteoporosis. Treatment of osteoporosis in men. Treatment of Paget's disease of the bone. Treatment of corticosteroid-induced osteoporosis in patients (men and women) who are receiving ≥7.5 mg of prednisone/day (or equivalent) with evidence of decreased bone mineral density.

Action

Inhibits resorption of bone by inhibiting osteoclast activity. **Therapeutic Effects:** Reversal of the progression of osteoporosis with decreased fractures. Decreased progression of Paget's disease.

Pharmacokinetics

Absorption: Poorly absorbed (0.6–0.8%) after oral administration.

Distribution: Transiently distributes to soft tissue, then distributes to bone.

Metabolism and Excretion: Excreted in urine.

Half-life: 10 yr (reflects release of drug from skeleton).

TIME/ACTION PROFILE (inhibition of bone resorption)

ROUTE	ONSET	PEAK	DURATION
PO	1 mo	3–6 mo	3 wk–7 mo†

†After discontinuation of alendronate.

Contraindications/Precautions

Contraindicated in: Abnormalities of the esophagus which delay esophageal emptying (i.e. strictures, achalasia); Inability to stand/sit upright for at least 30 min; Renal insufficiency (CCr <35 mL/min); **OB, Lactation:** Safety not established.

Use Cautiously in: History of upper GI disorders; Pre-existing hypocalcemia or vitamin D deficiency; Invasive dental procedures, cancer, receiving chemotherapy, corticosteroids, or angiogenesis inhibitors, poor oral hygiene, periodontal disease, dental disease, anemia, coagulopathy, infection, or poorly-fitting dentures (may ↑ risk of jaw osteonecrosis).

Adverse Reactions/Side Effects

CNS: headache. **EENT:** blurred vision, conjunctivitis, eye pain/inflammation. **CV:** atrial fibrillation. **GI:** abdominal distention, abdominal pain, acid regurgitation, constipation, diarrhea, dyspepsia, dysphagia, esophageal cancer, esophageal ulcer, esophagitis, flatulence, gastritis, nausea, taste perversion, vomiting. **Derm:** erythema, photosensitivity, rash. **MS:** musculoskeletal pain, femur fractures, osteonecrosis (primarily of jaw). **Resp:** asthma exacerbation.

Interactions

Drug-Drug: Calcium supplements, **antacids**, and **levothyroxine** may ↓ the absorption of alendronate. Doses >10 mg/day ↑ risk of adverse GI events when used with **NSAIDs**. IV **ranitidine** ↑ blood levels.

Drug-Food: Food significantly ↓ absorption. **Caffeine (coffee, tea, cola)**, **mineral water**, and **orange juice** also ↓ absorption.

Route/Dosage

PO (Adults): *Treatment of osteoporosis*— 10 mg once daily or 70 mg once weekly. *Prevention of osteoporosis*—5 mg once daily or 35 mg once weekly. *Paget's disease*—40 mg once daily for 6 mo. Retreatment may be considered for patients who relapse. *Treatment of corticosteroid-induced osteoporosis in men and premenopausal women*—5 mg once daily.

Treatment of corticosteroid-induced osteoporosis in postmenopausal women not receiving estrogen— 10 mg once daily.

Availability (generic available)

Tablets: 5 mg, 10 mg, 35 mg, 40 mg, 70 mg. **Cost:** *Generic*— 10 mg $20.94/100, 35 mg $6.99/4, 70 mg $8.22/4. **Oral solution (raspberry flavor):** 70 mg/ 75 mL. **Cost:** *Generic*— $23.44/75 mL. **Effervescent tablets (strawberry flavor):** 70 mg. **Cost:** $168.00/ 4. ***In combination with:*** Cholecalciferol (Fosamax plus D) See Appendix B.

NURSING IMPLICATIONS

Assessment

- **Osteoporosis:** Assess patients for low bone mass before and periodically during therapy.
- **Paget's Disease:** Assess for symptoms of Paget's disease (bone pain, headache, decreased visual and auditory acuity, increased skull size).
- ***Lab Test Considerations:*** *Osteoporosis:* Assess serum calcium before and periodically during therapy. Hypocalcemia and vitamin D deficiency should be treated before initiating alendronate therapy. May cause mild, transient ↑ of calcium and phosphate.
- **Paget's Disease:** Monitor alkaline phosphatase before and periodically during therapy. Alendronate is indicated for patients with alkaline phosphatase twice the upper limit of normal.

Potential Nursing Diagnoses

Risk for injury (Indications)

Implementation

- **PO:** Administer first thing in the morning with 6–8 oz plain water 30 min before other medications, beverages, or food. Oral solution should be followed by at least 2 ounces of water. Swallow tablets whole; do not crush, break, or chew.
- For *effervescent tablets* dissolve 1 tablet in half a glass (4 oz) of plain room temperature water (not mineral water or flavored water). Wait at least 5 minutes after the effervescence stops, stir the solution for approximately 10 seconds and drink contents.

Patient/Family Teaching

- Instruct patient on the importance of taking exactly as directed, first thing in the morning, 30 min before other medications, beverages, or food. Waiting longer than 30 min will improve absorption. Alendronate should be taken with 6–8 oz plain water (mineral water, orange juice, coffee, and other beverages decrease absorption). If a dose is missed, skip dose and resume the next morning; do not double doses or take later in the day. If a weekly dose is missed, take the morning after remembered and resume the following week on the chosen day. Do not take 2 tablets on the same day. Do not discontinue without consulting health care professional.
- Caution patient to remain upright for 30 min following dose to facilitate passage to stomach and minimize risk of esophageal irritation. Advise patient to discontinue alendronate and notify health care provider if pain or difficulty swallowing, retrosternal pain, or new/worsening heartburn occur.
- Advise patient to eat a balanced diet and consult health care professional about the need for supplemental calcium and vitamin D.
- Encourage patient to participate in regular exercise and to modify behaviors that increase the risk of osteoporosis (stop smoking, reduce alcohol consumption).
- Advise patient to inform health care professional of alendronate therapy prior to dental surgery.
- Caution patient to use sunscreen and protective clothing to prevent photosensitivity reactions.
- Advise patient to notify health care professional if blurred vision, eye pain, or inflammation occur.
- Advise female patient to notify health care professional if pregnancy is planned or suspected or if breast feeding.

Evaluation/Desired Outcomes

- Prevention of or decrease in the progression of osteoporosis in postmenopausal women. Reassess need for medication periodically. Consider discontinuation of alendronate after 3–5 years in patients with low-risk of fractures. If discontinued, reassess fracture risk periodically.
- Treatment of osteoporosis in men.
- Decrease in the progression of Paget's disease.
- Treatment of corticosteroid-induced osteoporosis.

alfuzosin (al-fyoo-zo-sin)

Uroxatral, ✱Xatral

Classification

Therapeutic: urinary tract antispasmodics

Pharmacologic: peripherally acting antiadrenergics

Pregnancy Category B

Indications

Management of symptomatic benign prostatic hyperplasia (BPH).

Action

Selectively blocks $alpha_1$- adrenergic receptors in the lower urinary tract to relax smooth muscle in the bladder neck and prostate. **Therapeutic Effects:** Increased urine flow and decreased symptoms of BPH.

Pharmacokinetics

Absorption: 49% absorbed following oral administration; food enhances absorption.

Distribution: Unknown.

Metabolism and Excretion: Mostly metabolized by the liver (CYP3A4 enzyme system); 11% excreted unchanged in urine.

Half-life: 10 hr.

TIME/ACTION PROFILE

ROUTE	ONSET	PEAK	DURATION
PO-ER	within hr	8 hr	24 hr

Contraindications/Precautions

Contraindicated in: Hypersensitivity; Moderate to severe hepatic impairment; Potent inhibitors of the CYP3A4 enzyme system; Concurrent use of other alpha-adrenergic blocking agents; Severe renal impairment; Pedi: Children.

Use Cautiously in: Congenital or acquired QTc prolongation or concurrent use of other drugs known to prolong QTc; Mild hepatic impairment; Symptomatic hypotension; Concurrent use of antihypertensive agents, phosphodiesterase type 5 inhibitors, or nitrates (↑ risk of postural hypotension); Previous hypotensive episode with other medications; Geri: Consider age-related changes in body mass and cardiac, renal, and hepatic function when prescribing.

Adverse Reactions/Side Effects

CNS: dizziness, fatigue, headache. **EENT:** intraoperative floppy iris syndrome. **Derm:** TOXIC EPIDERMAL NECROLYSIS. **Resp:** bronchitis, sinusitis, pharyngitis. **CV:** postural hypotension. **GI:** abdominal pain, constipation, dyspepsia, nausea. **GU:** erectile dysfunction, priapism. **Hemat:** thrombocytopenia.

Interactions

Drug-Drug: Ketoconazole, **itraconazole**, and **ritonavir** ↓ metabolism and significantly ↑ levels and effects (concurrent use contraindicated). Levels are ↑ by **cimetidine**, **atenolol**, and **diltiazem**. May ↑ levels and effects of **atenolol** and **diltiazem** (monitor BP and heart rate). ↑ risk of hypotension with **antihypertensives**, **nitrates**, **phosphodiesterase type 5 inhibitors** (including **sildenafil**, **tadalafil**, and **vardenafil**) and acute ingestion of **alcohol**.

Route/Dosage

PO (Adults): 10 mg once daily.

Availability (generic available)

Extended-release tablets: 10 mg.

NURSING IMPLICATIONS

Assessment

- Assess for symptoms of benign prostatic hyperplasia (urinary hesitancy, feeling of incomplete bladder emptying, interruption of urinary stream, impairment of size and force of urinary stream, terminal urinary dribbling, straining to start flow, dysuria, urgency) before and periodically during therapy.
- Assess for orthostatic reaction and syncope. Monitor BP (lying and standing) and pulse frequently during initial dose adjustment and periodically thereafter. May occur within a few hr after initial doses and occasionally thereafter.
- Rule out prostatic carcinoma before therapy; symptoms are similar.

Potential Nursing Diagnoses

Risk for injury (Side Effects)
Noncompliance (Patient/Family Teaching)

Implementation

- **PO:** Administer with food at the same meal each day. Tablets must be swallowed whole; do not crush, break, or chew.

Patient/Family Teaching

- Instruct patient to take medication with the same meal each day. Take missed doses as soon as remembered. If not remembered until next day, omit; do not double doses.
- May cause dizziness or drowsiness. Advise patient to avoid driving or other activities requiring alertness until response to the medication is known.
- Caution patient to avoid sudden changes in position to decrease orthostatic hypotension.
- Advise patient to consult health care professional before taking any cough, cold, or allergy remedies.
- Instruct patient to notify health care professional of medication regimen before any surgery, especially cataract surgery.
- Advise patient to notify health care professional if priapism, angina, frequent dizziness, rash, or fainting occurs.
- Emphasize the importance of follow-up exams to evaluate effectiveness of medication.
- Geri: Assess risk for falls; implement fall prevention program and instruct patient and family in preventing falls at home.

Evaluation/Desired Outcomes

- Decreased symptoms of benign prostatic hyperplasia.

alirocumab (a-li-**roe**-kyoo-mab)

Praluent

Classification
Therapeutic: lipid-lowering agents
Pharmacologic: proprotein convertase subtilisin kexin type 9 (PCSK9) inhibitor antibodies

Indications

Lowering of low density lipoprotein cholesterol (LDL-C) as an adjunct to diet and maximally tolerated statin (HMG CoA reductase inhibitor) therapy in patients with heterozygous familial hypercholesterolemia (HeFH) or cardiovascular disease who require supplemental agents.

Action

A human monoclonal immunoglobulin (IgG1) produced in genetically engineered Chinese hamster ovary cells that binds to PSCSK9 inhibiting its binding to the low density lipoprotein receptor (LDLR) resulting in ↑ number of LDLRs available to clear LDL from blood.

Therapeutic Effects: ↓ LDL-C.

Pharmacokinetics

Absorption: Well absorbed (85%) following subcut administration.

Distribution: Mostly distributed in the circulatory system; crosses the placenta.

Metabolism and Excretion: Eliminated by binding to PCSK9 and by proteolytic degradation.

Half-life: 17–20 days.

TIME/ACTION PROFILE (effect circulating unbound PCSK9)

ROUTE	ONSET	PEAK	DURATION
subcut	rapid	4–8 hr	2 wk

Contraindications/Precautions

Contraindicated in: History of serious hypersensitivity to alirocumab.

Use Cautiously in: Severe renal/hepatic impairment; Geri: Elderly patients may be more sensitive to drug effects; OB: Crosses the placenta, consider fetal risks; Lactation: Consider benefits of breast feeding against possible risk to infant; Pedi: Safe and effective use in children has not been established.

Adverse Reactions/Side Effects

CNS: confusion. **Local:** injection site reactions.

Misc: serious allergic reactions including VASCULITIS.

Interactions

Drug-Drug: None noted.

Route/Dosage

Subcut (Adults): 75 mg every two weeks, if desired LDL-C has not been achieved, dose may be ↑ to 150 mg every two weeks.

Availability

Solution for subcutaneous injection: 75 mg/mL in prefilled pen, 75 mg/mL in prefilled syringe, 150 mg/mL in prefilled pen, 150 mg/mL in prefilled syringe.

NURSING IMPLICATIONS

Assessment

- Obtain a diet history, especially with regard to fat consumption.
- Monitor for signs and symptoms of hypersensitivity reactions (pruritus, rash, urticaria, hypersensitivity vasculitis and hypersensitivity reactions requiring hospitalization) during therapy. If severe symptoms occur, discontinue alirocumab.
- ***Lab Test Considerations:*** Assess LDL-C levels within 4 to 8 weeks of initiating or titrating alirocumab, to assess response and adjust dose, if needed.

Potential Nursing Diagnoses

Noncompliance, related to diet and medication regimen (Patient/Family Teaching)

Implementation

- **Subcut:** Administer every 2 wks. Allow solution to warm to room temperature for 30–40 min before injecting. Do not use if at room temperature for ≥24 hrs. Solution is clear and colorless to pale yellow; do not administer solutions that are cloudy or contain particulate matter. Do not shake. Inject into thigh, abdomen, or upper arm. Rotate sites with each injection. Do not inject into areas with skin disease or injury (sunburns, rashes, inflammation, skin infections). Do not reuse pre-filled pen or syringe. Do not administer other injectable drugs at same site. Store in refrigerator; do not freeze.

Patient/Family Teaching

- Instruct patient in correct technique for self-injection, care and disposal of equipment. Administer missed doses within 7 days, then resume original schedule. If not administered within 7 days, wait until next dose on original schedule. Advise patient to read *Patient Information* before starting therapy and with each Rx refill in case of changes.
- Advise patient that this medication should be used in conjunction with diet restrictions (fat, cholesterol, carbohydrates, alcohol), exercise, and cessation of smoking.
- Instruct patient to notify health care professional of all Rx or OTC medications, vitamins, or herbal products being taken and to consult health care professional before taking any other Rx, OTC, or herbal products.
- Advise patient to notify health care professional of medication regimen prior to treatment or surgery.
- Advise patient to notify health care professional if pregnancy is planned or suspected or if breast feeding.

Evaluation/Desired Outcomes

- ↓ LDL-C levels.

allopurinol (al-oh-**pure**-i-nole)

Aloprim, Lopurin, Zyloprim

Classification

Therapeutic: antigout agents, antihyperuricemics

Pharmacologic: xanthine oxidase inhibitors

Pregnancy Category C

Indications

PO: Prevention of attack of gouty arthritis and nephropathy. **PO, IV:** Treatment of secondary hyperuricemia, which may occur during treatment of tumors or leukemias.

Action

Inhibits the production of uric acid by inhibiting the action of xanthine oxidase. **Therapeutic Effects:** Lowering of serum uric acid levels.

Pharmacokinetics

Absorption: Well absorbed (80%) following oral administration.

Distribution: Widely distributed in tissue and breast milk.

Protein Binding: <1%.

Metabolism and Excretion: Metabolized to oxypurinol, an active compound with a long half-life. 12% excreted unchanged, 76% excreted as oxypurinol.

Half-life: 1–3 hr (oxypurinol 18–30 hr).

TIME/ACTION PROFILE (hypouricemic effect)

ROUTE	ONSET	PEAK	DURATION
PO, IV	1–2 days	1–2 wk	1–3 wk†

†Duration after discontinuation of allopurinol.

Contraindications/Precautions

Contraindicated in: Hypersensitivity.

Use Cautiously in: Acute attacks of gout; Renal insufficiency (dose ↓ required if CCr <20 mL/min); Dehydration (adequate hydration necessary); OB, Lactation: Rarely used; Geri: Begin at lower end of dosage range.

Adverse Reactions/Side Effects

CV: hypotension, flushing, hypertension, bradycardia, and heart failure (reported with IV administration). **CNS:** drowsiness. **GI:** diarrhea, hepatitis, nausea, vomiting. **GU:** renal failure, hematuria. **Derm:** rash (discontinue drug at first sign of rash), urticaria. **Hemat:** bone marrow depression. **Misc:** hypersensitivity reactions.

Interactions

Drug-Drug: Use with **mercaptopurine** and **azathioprine** ↑ bone marrow depressant properties—doses of these drugs should be ↓. Use with **ampicillin** or **amoxicillin** ↑ risk of rash. Use with **oral hypoglycemic agents** and **warfarin** ↑ effects of these drugs. Use with **thiazide diuretics** or **ACE inhibitors** ↑ risk of hypersensitivity reactions. Large doses of allopurinol may ↑ risk of **theophylline** toxicity. May ↑ **cyclosporine** levels.

Route/Dosage

Management of Gout

PO (Adults and Children >10 yr): *Initially*—100 mg/day; ↑ at weekly intervals based on serum uric acid (not to exceed 800 mg/day). Doses >300 mg/day should be given in divided doses; *Maintenance dose*—100–200 mg 2–3 times daily. Doses of ≤300 mg may be given as a single daily dose.

Management of Secondary Hyperuricemia

PO (Adults and Children >10 yr): 600–800 mg/day in 2–3 divided doses starting 1–2 days before chemotherapy or radiation.

PO (Children 6–10 yr): 10 mg/kg/day in 2–3 divided doses (maximum 800 mg/day) or 300 mg daily in 2–3 divided doses.

PO (Children <6 yr): 10 mg/kg/day in 2–3 divided doses (maximum 800 mg/day) or 150 mg daily in 3 divided doses.

IV (Adults and Children >10 yr): 200–400 mg/m²/day (up to 600 mg/day) as a single daily dose or in divided doses q 8–24 hr.

IV (Children <10 yr): 200 mg/m²/day initially as a single daily dose or in divided doses q 8–24 hr (maximum dose 600 mg/day).

Renal Impairment

(Adults and Children): *CCr 10–50 mL/min*—↓ dose to 50% of recommended; *CCr <10 mL/min*—↓ dosage to 30% of recommended.

Availability (generic available)

Tablets: 100 mg, ✱200 mg, 300 mg. **Cost:** *Generic*—100 mg $10.83/100, 300 mg $10.83/100. **Powder for injection:** 500 mg/vial.

NURSING IMPLICATIONS

Assessment

- Monitor intake and output ratios. Decreased kidney function can cause drug accumulation and toxic effects. Ensure that patient maintains adequate fluid intake (minimum 2500–3000 mL/day) to minimize risk of kidney stone formation.
- Assess patient for rash or more severe hypersensitivity reactions. Discontinue allopurinol immediately if rash occurs. Therapy should be discontinued permanently if reaction is severe. Therapy may be reinstated after a mild reaction has subsided, at a lower dose (50 mg/day with very gradual titration). If skin rash recurs, discontinue permanently.
- **Gout:** Monitor for joint pain and swelling. Addition of colchicine or NSAIDs may be necessary for acute

attacks. Prophylactic doses of colchicine or an NSAID should be administered concurrently during first 3–6 mo of therapy because of an increased frequency of acute attacks of gouty arthritis during early therapy.

- ***Lab Test Considerations:*** Serum and urine uric acid levels usually begin to ↓ 2–3 days after initiation of oral therapy.
- Monitor blood glucose in patients receiving oral hypoglycemic agents. May cause hypoglycemia.
- Monitor hematologic, renal, and liver function tests before and periodically during therapy, especially during the first few mo. May cause ↑ serum alkaline phosphatase, bilirubin, AST, and ALT levels. ↓ CBC and platelets may indicate bone marrow depression. ↑ BUN, serum creatinine, and CCr may indicate nephrotoxicity. These are usually reversed with discontinuation of therapy.

Potential Nursing Diagnoses

Acute pain (Indications)

Implementation

- Do not confuse Zyloprim with zolpidem.
- **PO:** May be administered after milk or meals to minimize gastric irritation; give with plenty of fluid. May be crushed and given with fluid or mixed with food for patients who have difficulty swallowing.

IV Administration

- **Intermittent Infusion:** Reconstitute each 500 mg vial with 25 mL of sterile water for injection. Solution should be clear and almost colorless with only slight opalescence. ***Diluent:*** Dilute to desired concentration with 0.9% NaCl or D5W. Administer within 10 hr of reconstitution; do not refrigerate. Do not administer solutions that are discolored or contain particulate matter. ***Concentration:*** Not >6 mg/mL. ***Rate:*** Infusion should be initiated 24–48 hr before start of chemotherapy known to cause tumor cell lysis. Rate of infusion depends on volume of infusate (100–300 mg doses may be infused over 30 minutes). May be administered as a single infusion or equally divided infusions at 6-, 8-, or 12-hr intervals.
- **Y-Site Compatibility:** acyclovir, aminophylline, amphotericin B lipid complex, anidulafungin, argatroban, aztreonam, bivalirudin, bleomycin, bumetanide, buprenorphine, butorphanol, calcium gluconate, carboplatin, caspofungin, cefazolin, cefotetan, ceftazidime, ceftriaxone, cefuroxime, cisplatin, cyclophosphamide, dactinomycin, dexamethasone sodium phosphate, dexmedetomidine, docetaxel, doxorubicin liposome, enalaprilat, etoposide, famotidine, fenoldopam, filgrastim, fluconazole, fludarabine, fluorouracil, fosphenytoin, furosemide, ganciclovir, gemcitabine, granisetron, heparin, hetastarch, hydrocortisone, hydromorphone, ifosfamide, leucovorin calcium, linezolid, lorazepam, mannitol, mesna, methotrexate, metronidazole, milrinone, mitoxantrone, morphine, nesiritide, octreotide, oxytocin, paclitaxel, pamidronate, pantoprazole, pemetrexed, piperacillin/tazobactam, potassium chloride, ranitidine, sodium acetate, teniposide, thiotepa, tigecycline, tirofiban, trimethoprim/sulfamethoxazole, vancomycin, vasopressin, vinblastine, vincristine, voriconazole, zidovudine, zoledronic acid.
- **Y-Site Incompatibility:** alemtuzumab, amikacin, amiodarone, carmustine, cefotaxime, chlorpromazine, clindamycin, cytarabine, dacarbazine, daptomycin, daunorubicin, dexrazoxane, diltiazem, diphenhydramine, doxorubicin, doxycycline, droperidol, epirubicin, ertapenem, etoposide phosphate, floxuridine, foscarnet, gentamicin, haloperidol, hydroxyzine, idarubicin, imipenem/cilastatin, irinotecan, mechlorethamine, meperidine, methylprednisolone sodium succinate, metoprolol, moxifloxacin, mycophenolate, nalbuphine, ondansetron, palonosetron, pancuronium, potassium acetate, prochlorperazine, promethazine, sodium bicarbonate, streptozocin, tacrolimus, tobramycin, topotecan, vecuronium, vinorelbine.

Patient/Family Teaching

- Instruct patient to take allopurinol as directed. Take missed doses as soon as remembered. If dosing schedule is once daily, do not take if remembered the next day. If dosing schedule is more than once a day, take up to 300 mg for next dose.
- Instruct patient to continue taking allopurinol along with an NSAID or colchicine during an acute attack of gout. Allopurinol helps prevent, but does not relieve, acute gout attacks.
- Alkaline diet may be ordered. Urinary acidification with large doses of vitamin C or other acids may increase kidney stone formation (see Appendix J). Advise patient of need for increased fluid intake.
- May occasionally cause drowsiness. Caution patient to avoid driving or other activities requiring alertness until response to drug is known.
- Instruct patient to report skin rash, blood in urine, or influenza symptoms (chills, fever, muscle aches and pains, nausea, or vomiting) to health care professional immediately; skin rash may indicate hypersensitivity.
- Advise patient that large amounts of alcohol increase uric acid concentrations and may decrease the effectiveness of allopurinol.
- Emphasize the importance of follow-up exams to monitor effectiveness and side effects.

Evaluation/Desired Outcomes

- Decreased serum and urinary uric acid levels. May take 2–6 wk to observe clinical improvement in patients treated for gout.

almotriptan (al-moe-**trip**-tan)

Axert

Classification

Therapeutic: vascular headache suppressants

Pharmacologic: 5-HT_1 agonists

Pregnancy Category C

Indications

Acute treatment of migraine headache (for adolescents, migraines should be ≥4 hr in duration).

Action

Acts as an agonist at specific 5-HT_1 receptor sites in intracranial blood vessels and sensory trigeminal nerves. **Therapeutic Effects:** Cranial vessel vasoconstriction with associated decrease in release of neuropetides and resultant decrease in migraine headache.

Pharmacokinetics

Absorption: Well absorbed following oral administration (70%).

Distribution: Unknown.

Metabolism and Excretion: 40% excreted unchanged in urine; 27% metabolized by monoamine oxidase-A (MAO-A); 12% metabolized by cytochrome P450 hepatic enzymes (3A4 and 2D6); 13% excreted in feces as unchanged and metabolized drug.

Half-life: 3–4 hr.

TIME/ACTION PROFILE (Blood levels)

ROUTE	ONSET	PEAK	DURATION
PO	unknown	1–3 hr	unknown

Contraindications/Precautions

Contraindicated in: Hypersensitivity; Ischemic cardiovascular, cerebrovascular, or peripheral vascular syndromes (including ischemic bowel disease); History of significant cardiovascular disease; Uncontrolled hypertension; Should not be used within 24 hr of other 5-HT_1 agonists or ergot-type compounds (dihydroergotamine); Basilar or hemiplegic migraine; Concurrent MAO-A inhibitor therapy or within 2 wk of discontinuing MAO-A inhibitor therapy.

Use Cautiously in: Cardiovascular risk factors (hypertension, hypercholesterolemia, cigarette smoking, obesity, diabetes, strong family history, menopausal women or men >40 yr); use only if cardiovascular status has been evaluated and determined to be safe and first dose is administered under supervision; Impaired hepatic or renal function; Hypersensitivity to sulfonamides (cross-sensitivity may occur); OB, Lactation: Safety not established; Pedi: Children <12 yr (safety not established).

Adverse Reactions/Side Effects

CNS: drowsiness, headache. **CV:** CORONARY ARTERY VASOSPASM, MI, VENTRICULAR ARRHYTHMIAS, myocardial ischemia. **GI:** dry mouth, nausea. **Neuro:** paresthesia.

Interactions

Drug-Drug: Concurrent use with **MAO-A inhibitors** ↑ blood levels and the risk of adverse reactions (concurrent use or use within 2 wk or MAO inhibitor is contraindicated). Concurrent use with other **5-HT_1 agonists** or **ergot-type compounds (dihydroergotamine)** may result in additive vasoactive properties (avoid use within 24 hr of each other). ↑ serotonin levels and serotonin syndrome may occur when used concurrently with **SSRI and SNRI antidepressants.** Blood levels and effects may be ↑ by **ketoconazole, itraconazole, ritonavir,** and **erythromycin** (inhibitors of CYP3A4 enzymes).

Route/Dosage

PO (Adults and Children ≥12 yr): 6.25–12.5 mg initially, may repeat in 2 hr; not to exceed 2 doses per 24-hr period.

Hepatic/Renal Impairment

PO (Adults): 6.25 mg initially, may repeat in 2 hr; not to exceed 2 doses per 24-hr period.

Availability (generic available)

Tablets: 6.25 mg, 12.5 mg.

NURSING IMPLICATIONS

Assessment

- Assess pain location, character, intensity, and duration and associated symptoms (photophobia, phonophobia, nausea, vomiting) during migraine attack.
- Assess for serotonin syndrome (mental changes [agitation, hallucinations, coma], autonomic instability [tachycardia, labile BP, hyperthermia], neuromuscular aberations [hyperreflexia, incoordination], and/or GI symptoms [nausea, vomiting, diarrhea]), especially in patients taking other serotonergic drugs (SSRIs, SNRIs).

Potential Nursing Diagnoses

Acute pain (Indications)

Implementation

- Do not confuse Axert with Antivert.
- **PO:** Tablets should be swallowed whole with liquid.

Patient/Family Teaching

- Inform patient that almotriptan should only be used during a migraine attack. It is meant to be used for relief of migraine attacks but not to prevent or reduce the number of attacks.
- Instruct patient to administer almotriptan as soon as symptoms of a migraine attack appear, but it may be administered any time during an attack. If migraine symptoms return, a second dose may be used. Allow at least 2 hr between doses, and do not use more than 2 doses in any 24-hr period.

- If first dose does not relieve headache, additional almotriptan doses are not likely to be effective; notify health care professional.
- Caution patient not to take almotriptan within 24 hr of another vascular headache suppressant.
- Advise patient that lying down in a darkened room following almotriptan administration may further help relieve headache.
- Advise patient that overuse (use more than 10 days/month) may lead to exacerbation of headache (migraine-like daily headaches, or as a marked increase in frequency of migraine attacks). May require gradual withdrawal of almotriptan and treatment of symptoms (transient worsening of headache).
- Advise patient to notify health care professional prior to next dose of almotriptan if pain or tightness in the chest occurs during use. If pain is severe or does not subside, notify health care professional immediately. If feelings of tingling, heat, flushing, heaviness, pressure, drowsiness, dizziness, tiredness, or sickness develop discuss with health care professional at next visit.
- May cause dizziness or drowsiness. Caution patient to avoid driving or other activities requiring alertness until response to medication is known.
- Advise patient to avoid alcohol, which aggravates headaches, during almotriptan use.
- Advise patient to notify health care professional of all Rx or OTC medications, vitamins, or herbal products being taken and to consult with health care professional before taking other medications.
- Advise patient to notify health care professional immediately if signs or symptoms of serotonin syndrome occur.
- Caution patient not to use almotriptan if pregnant, suspects pregnancy, plans to become pregnant, or is breast feeding. Adequate contraception should be used during therapy.

Evaluation/Desired Outcomes

- Relief of migraine attack.

alogliptin (al-oh-**glip**-tin)

Nesina

Classification

Therapeutic: antidiabetics

Pharmacologic: dipeptidyl peptidase-4 (DDP-4) inhibitors

Pregnancy Category B

Indications

Adjunct with diet and exercise to improve glycemic control in adults with type 2 diabetes mellitus.

Action

Acts as a competitive inhibitor of dipeptidyl peptidase-4 (DDP-4) which slows the inactivation of incretin hormones, thereby increasing their concentrations and reducing fasting and postprandial glucose concentrations. **Therapeutic Effects:** Improved control of blood glucose.

Pharmacokinetics

Absorption: Completely absorbed following oral administration (100%).

Distribution: Well distributed into tissues.

Metabolism and Excretion: Not extensively metabolized, 76% excreted unchanged in urine.

Half-life: 21 hr.

TIME/ACTION PROFILE (inhibition of DDP-4)

ROUTE	ONSET	PEAK†	DURATION
PO	unknown	1–2 hr	24 hr

†Multiple dosing.

Contraindications/Precautions

Contraindicated in: Type 1 diabetes; Diabetic ketoacidosis; Previous severe hypersensitivity reactions.

Use Cautiously in: Liver disease; Geri: May have ↑ sensitivity to effects; Lactation: Use cautiously; OB: Use during pregnancy only if clearly needed; Pedi: Safety and effectiveness not established.

Adverse Reactions/Side Effects

CNS: headache. **Derm:** STEVENS-JOHNSON SYNDROME. **GI:** HEPATOTOXICITY, PANCREATITIS, ↑ liver enzymes. **MS:** arthralgia. **Misc:** hypersensitivity reactions including ANAPHYLAXIS, ANGIOEDEMA.

Interactions

Drug-Drug: ↑ risk of hypoglycemia with **sulfonylureas** and **insulin**; dose adjustments may be necessary.

Route/Dosage

PO (Adults): 25 mg once daily.

Renal Impairment

PO (Adults): *CCr ≥30 mL/min– <60 mL/min*—12.5 mg once daily; *CCr <30 mL/min*–6.25 mg once daily.

Availability

Tablets: 6.25 mg, 12.5 mg, 25 mg. ***In combination with:*** metformin (Kazano), pioglitazone (Oseni).

NURSING IMPLICATIONS

Assessment

- Observe for signs and symptoms of hypoglycemic reactions (abdominal pain, sweating, hunger, weakness, dizziness, headache, tremor, tachycardia, anxiety).

- Monitor for signs of pancreatitis (nausea, vomiting, anorexia, persistent severe abdominal pain, sometimes radiating to the back) during therapy. If pancreatitis occurs, discontinue alogliptin and monitor serum and urine amylase, amylase/creatinine clearance ratio, electrolytes, serum calcium, glucose, and lipase.
- Assess for rash periodically during therapy. May cause Stevens-Johnson syndrome. Discontinue therapy if severe or if accompanied with fever, general malaise, fatigue, muscle or joint aches, blisters, oral lesions, conjunctivitis, hepatitis and/or eosinophilia.
- ***Lab Test Considerations:*** Monitor hemoglobin A1C prior to and periodically during therapy.
- Monitor renal function prior to and periodically during therapy.

Potential Nursing Diagnoses

Imbalanced nutrition: more than body requirements (Indications)
Noncompliance (Patient/Family Teaching)

Implementation

- Patients stabilized on a diabetic regimen who are exposed to stress, fever, trauma, infection, or surgery may require administration of insulin.
- **PO:** May be administered without regard to food.

Patient/Family Teaching

- Instruct patient to take alogliptin as directed. Take missed doses as soon as remembered, unless it is almost time for next dose; do not double doses. Advise patient to read *Medication Guide* before starting and with each Rx refill in case of changes.
- Explain to patient that alogliptin helps control hyperglycemia but does not cure diabetes. Therapy is usually long term.
- Instruct patient not to share this medication with others, even if they have the same symptoms; it may harm them.
- Encourage patient to follow prescribed diet, medication, and exercise regimen to prevent hyperglycemic or hypoglycemic episodes.
- Review signs of hypoglycemia and hyperglycemia with patient. If hypoglycemia occurs, advise patient to take a glass of orange juice or 2–3 tsp of sugar, honey, or corn syrup dissolved in water, and notify health care professional.
- Instruct patient in proper testing of blood glucose and urine ketones. These tests should be monitored closely during periods of stress or illness and health care professional notified if significant changes occur.
- Advise patient to stop taking alogliptin and notify health care professional promptly if symptoms of hypersensitivity reactions (rash; hives; swelling of face, lips, tongue, and throat; difficulty in breathing or swallowing) or pancreatitis occur.
- Advise patient to notify health care professional of all Rx or OTC medications, vitamins, or herbal products being taken and to consult with health care professional before taking other medications.
- Advise patient to notify health care professional if pregnancy is planned or suspected or if breast feeding.

Evaluation/Desired Outcomes

- Improved hemoglobin A1C, fasting plasma glucose and 2-hr post-prandial glucose levels.

ALPRAZolam (al-pray-zoe-lam)

Xanax, Xanax XR

Classification
Therapeutic: antianxiety agents
Pharmacologic: benzodiazepines

Schedule IV

Pregnancy Category D

Indications

Generalized anxiety disorder (GAD). Panic disorder. Anxiety associated with depression. **Unlabeled Use:** Management of symptoms of premenstrual syndrome (PMS) and premenstrual dysphoric disorder. Insomnia, irritable bowel syndrome (IBS) and other somatic symptoms associated with anxiety. Used as an adjunct with acute mania, acute psychosis.

Action

Acts at many levels in the CNS to produce anxiolytic effect. May produce CNS depression. Effects may be mediated by GABA, an inhibitory neurotransmitter. **Therapeutic Effects:** Relief of anxiety.

Pharmacokinetics

Absorption: Well absorbed (90%) from the GI tract; absorption is slower with extended-release tablets.
Distribution: Widely distributed, crosses blood-brain barrier. Probably crosses the placenta and enters breast milk. Accumulation is minimal.
Metabolism and Excretion: Metabolized by the liver (CYP3A4 enzyme system) to an active compound that is subsequently rapidly metabolized.
Half-life: 12–15 hr.

TIME/ACTION PROFILE (sedation)

ROUTE	ONSET	PEAK	DURATION
PO	1–2 hr	1–2 hr	up to 24 hr

Contraindications/Precautions

Contraindicated in: Hypersensitivity; Cross-sensitivity with other benzodiazepines may exist; Pre-existing CNS depression; Severe uncontrolled pain; Angle-closure glaucoma; Obstructive sleep apnea or pulmonary disease; Concurrent use with itraconazole or ketoconazole; OB, Lactation: Use in pregnancy or lactation may cause CNS depression, flaccidity, feeding difficulties, and seizures in infant.
Use Cautiously in: Renal impairment (↓ dose required); Hepatic impairment (↓ dose required); Con-

current use with nefazodone, fluvoxamine, cimetidine, fluoxetine, hormonal contraceptives, diltiazem, isoniazid, erythromycin, clarithromycin, or grapefruit juice (↓ dose may be necessary); History of suicide attempt or alcohol/drug dependence, debilitated patients (↓ dose required); Pedi: Safety and efficacy not established; ↓ dosage and frequent monitoring required; Geri: Appears on Beers list. Elderly patients have ↑ sensitivity to benzodiazepines; associated with ↑ risk of falls and excessive CNS effects (↓ dose required).

Adverse Reactions/Side Effects

CNS: dizziness, drowsiness, lethargy, confusion, hangover, headache, mental depression, paradoxical excitation. **EENT:** blurred vision. **GI:** constipation, diarrhea, nausea, vomiting, weight gain. **Derm:** rash. **Misc:** physical dependence, psychological dependence, tolerance.

Interactions

Drug-Drug: Alcohol, **antidepressants**, other **benzodiazepines**, **antihistamines**, and **opioid analgesics**—concurrent use results in ↑ CNS depression. **Hormonal contraceptives**, **disulfiram**, **fluoxetine**, **isoniazid**, **metoprolol**, **propranolol**, **valproic acid**, **CYP3A4 inhibitors** (**erythromycin**, **ketoconazole**, **itraconazole**, **fluvoxamine**, **cimetidine**, **nefazodone**) ↑ levels and effects; dose adjustments may be necessary; concurrent use with ketoconazole and itraconazole contraindicated. May ↓ efficacy of **levodopa**. **CYP3A4 inducers** (**rifampin**, **carbamazepine**, or **barbiturates**) ↓ levels and effects. Sedative effects may be ↓ by **theophylline**. **Cigarette smoking** ↓ levels and effects.
Drug-Natural Products: Kava-kava, **valerian**, or **chamomile** can ↑ CNS depression.
Drug-Food: Concurrent ingestion of **grapefruit juice** ↑ levels and effects.

Route/Dosage

Anxiety

PO (Adults): 0.25–0.5 mg 2–3 times daily (not to exceed 4 mg/day).
PO (Geriatric Patients): Begin with 0.25 mg 2–3 times daily.

Panic Attacks

PO (Adults): 0.5 mg 3 times daily; may be ↑ by 1 mg or less every 3–4 days as needed (not to exceed 10 mg/day). *Extended-release tablets*—0.5–1 mg once daily in the morning, may be ↑ every 3–4 days by not more than 1 mg/day; up to 10 mg/day (usual range 3–6 mg/day).

Availability (generic available)

Tablets: 0.25 mg, 0.5 mg, 1 mg, 2 mg. **Cost:** *Generic*—0.25 mg $10.59/100, 0.5 mg $5.25/100, 1 mg $10.41/100, 2 mg $15.13/100. **Extended-release tablets:** 0.5 mg, 1 mg, 2 mg, 3 mg. **Cost:** *Generic*—1 mg $54.05/180, 2 mg $86.76/180, 3 mg $319.38/60. **Orally disintegrating tablets (orange-flavor):** 0.25 mg, 0.5 mg, 1 mg, 2 mg. **Cost:** *Generic*—0.25 mg $151.73/100, 0.5 mg $189.04/100, 1 mg $252.22/100, 2 mg $428.86/100. **Oral solution (concentrate):** 1 mg/mL. **Cost:** *Generic*—$81.10/30 mL.

NURSING IMPLICATIONS

Assessment

- Assess degree and manifestations of anxiety and mental status (orientation, mood, behavior) prior to and periodically during therapy.
- Assess patient for drowsiness, light-headedness, and dizziness. These symptoms usually disappear as therapy progresses. Dose should be reduced if these symptoms persist.
- Geri: Assess CNS effects and risk of falls. Institute falls prevention strategies.
- Prolonged high-dose therapy may lead to psychological or physical dependence. Risk is greater in patients taking >4 mg/day. Restrict the amount of drug available to patient. Assess regularly for continued need for treatment.
- ***Lab Test Considerations:*** Monitor CBC and liver and renal function periodically during long-term therapy. May cause ↓ hematocrit and neutropenia.
- ***Toxicity and Overdose:*** Flumazenil is the antidote for alprazolam toxicity or overdose. (Flumazenil may induce seizures in patients with a history of seizures disorder or who are taking tricyclic antidepressants).

Potential Nursing Diagnoses

Anxiety (Indications)
Risk for injury (Side Effects)
Risk for falls (Side Effects)

Implementation

- Do not confuse Xanax (alprazolam) with Zantac (ranitidine), Fanapt (iloperidone), or Tenex (guanfacine).
- Do not confuse alprazolam with lorazepam.
- If early morning anxiety or anxiety between doses occurs, same total daily dose should be divided into more frequent intervals.
- **PO:** May be administered with food if GI upset occurs. Administer greatest dose at bedtime to avoid daytime sedation.
- Tablets may be crushed and taken with food or fluids if patient has difficulty swallowing. Do not crush, break, or chew extended-release tablets.
- Taper by 0.5 mg every 3 days to prevent withdrawal. Some patients may require longer tapering period (months).

- For *orally disintegrating tablets:* Remove tablet from bottle with dry hands just prior to taking medication. Place tablet on tongue. Tablet will dissolve with saliva; may also be taken with water. Remove cotton from bottle and reseal tightly to prevent moisture from entering bottle. If only 1/2 tablet taken, discard unused portion immediately; may not remain stable.

Patient/Family Teaching

- Instruct patient to take medication as directed; do not skip or double up on missed doses. If a dose is missed, take within 1 hr; otherwise, skip the dose and return to regular schedule. If medication is less effective after a few weeks, check with health care professional; do not increase dose. Abrupt withdrawal may cause sweating, vomiting, muscle cramps, tremors, and seizures.
- May cause drowsiness or dizziness. Caution patient to avoid driving and other activities requiring alertness until response to the medication is known. Geri: Instruct patient and family how to reduce falls risk at home.
- Advise patient to avoid drinking grapefruit juice during therapy.
- Advise patient to avoid the use of alcohol or other CNS depressants concurrently with alprazolam. Instruct patient to consult health care professional before taking Rx, OTC, or herbal products concurrently with this medication.
- Inform patient that benzodiazepines are usually prescribed for short-term use and do not cure underlying problems.
- Teach other methods to decrease anxiety (exercise, support group, relaxation techniques).
- Advise patient to not share medication with anyone.

Evaluation/Desired Outcomes

- Decreased sense of anxiety without CNS side effects.
- Decreased frequency and severity of panic attacks.
- Decreased symptoms of premenstrual syndrome.

alteplase, See THROMBOLYTIC AGENTS.

aluminum hydroxide

AlternaGEL, Alu-Cap, ✤Alugel, Aluminet, Alu-Tab, Amphojel, Basalgel, Dialume

Classification

Therapeutic: antiulcer agents, hypophosphatemics

Pharmacologic: antacids, phosphate binders

Pregnancy Category UK

Indications

Lowering of phosphate levels in patients with chronic renal failure. Adjunctive therapy in the treatment of peptic, duodenal, and gastric ulcers. Hyperacidity, indigestion, reflux esophagitis.

Action

Binds phosphate in the GI tract. Neutralizes gastric acid and inactivates pepsin. **Therapeutic Effects:** Lowering of serum phosphate levels. Healing of ulcers and decreased pain associated with ulcers or gastric hyperacidity. Constipation limits use alone in the treatment of ulcer disease. Frequently found in combination with magnesium-containing compounds.

Pharmacokinetics

Absorption: With chronic use, small amounts of aluminum are systemically absorbed.

Distribution: If absorbed, aluminum distributes widely, crosses the placenta, and enters breast milk. Concentrates in the CNS with chronic use.

Metabolism and Excretion: Mostly excreted in feces. Small amounts absorbed are excreted by the kidneys.

Half-life: Unknown.

TIME/ACTION PROFILE

ROUTE	ONSET	PEAK	DURATION
PO†	hr–days	days–wk	days
PO‡	15–30 min	30 min	30 min–3 hr

†Hypophosphatemic effect.

‡Antacid effect.

Contraindications/Precautions

Contraindicated in: Severe abdominal pain of unknown cause.

Use Cautiously in: Hypercalcemia; Hypophosphatemia; OB: Generally considered safe; chronic high-dose therapy should be avoided.

Adverse Reactions/Side Effects

GI: constipation. **F and E:** hypophosphatemia.

Interactions

Drug-Drug: Absorption of **tetracyclines**, **chlorpromazine**, **iron salts**, **isoniazid**, **digoxin**, or **fluoroquinolones** may be decreased. **Salicylate** blood levels may be decreased. **Quinidine**, **mexiletine**, and **amphetamine** levels may be increased if enough antacid is ingested such that urine pH is increased.

Route/Dosage

Hypophosphatemia

PO (Adults): 1.9–4.8 g (30–40 mL of regular suspension or 15–20 mL of concentrated suspension) 3–4 times daily.

PO (Children): 50–150 mg/kg/24 hr in 4–6 divided doses; titrate to normal serum phosphate levels.

Antacid

PO (Adults): 500–1500 mg (5–30 mL) 3–6 times daily.

Availability (generic available)

Capsules: 475 mg^{OTC}, 500 mg^{OTC}. **Tablets:** 300 mg^{OTC}, 500 mg^{OTC}, 600 mg^{OTC}. **Suspension:** 320 mg/5 mL^{OTC}, 450 mg/5 mL^{OTC}, 600 mg/5 mL^{OTC}, 675 mg/5 mL^{OTC}. ***In combination with:*** magnesium carbonate, calcium carbonate, simethicone, and mineral oil. See Appendix B.

NURSING IMPLICATIONS

Assessment

- Assess location, duration, character, and precipitating factors of gastric pain.
- ***Lab Test Considerations:*** Monitor serum phosphate and calcium levels periodically during chronic use of aluminum hydroxide.
- May cause increased serum gastrin and decreased serum phosphate concentrations.
- In treatment of severe ulcer disease, guaiac stools, and emesis, monitor pH of gastric secretions.

Potential Nursing Diagnoses

Acute pain (Indications)
Constipation (Side Effects)

Implementation

- Antacids cause premature dissolution and absorption of enteric-coated tablets and may interfere with absorption of other oral medications. Separate administration of aluminum hydroxide and oral medications by at least 1–2 hr.
- Tablets must be chewed thoroughly before swallowing to prevent their entering small intestine in undissolved form. Follow with a glass of water.
- Shake liquid preparations well before pouring. Follow administration with water to ensure passage into stomach.
- Liquid dosage forms are considered more effective than tablets.
- **Hypophosphatemic:** For phosphate lowering, follow dose with full glass of water or fruit juice.
- **Antacid:** May be given in conjunction with magnesium-containing antacids to minimize constipation, except in patients with renal failure. Administer 1 and 3 hr after meals and at bedtime for maximum antacid effect.
- For treatment of peptic ulcer, aluminum hydroxide may be administered every 1–2 hr while the patient is awake or diluted with 2–3 parts water and administered intragastrically every 30 min for 12 or more hr per day. Physician may order NG tube clamped after administration.
- For reflux esophagitis, administer 15 mL 20–40 min after meals and at bedtime.

Patient/Family Teaching

- Instruct patient to take aluminum hydroxide exactly as directed. If on a regular dosing schedule and a dose is missed, take as soon as remembered if not almost time for next dose; do not double doses.
- Advise patient not to take aluminum hydroxide within 1–2 hr of other medications without consulting health care professional.
- Advise patients to check label for sodium content. Patients with HF or hypertension, or those on sodium restriction, should use low-sodium preparations.
- Inform patients of potential for constipation from aluminum hydroxide.
- **Hypophosphatemia:** Patients taking aluminum hydroxide for hyperphosphatemia should be taught the importance of a low-phosphate diet.
- **Antacid:** Caution patient to consult health care professional before taking antacids for more than 2 wk if problem is recurring, if taking other medications, if relief is not obtained, or if symptoms of gastric bleeding (black tarry stools, coffee-ground emesis) occur.

Evaluation/Desired Outcomes

- Decrease in serum phosphate levels.
- Decrease in GI pain and irritation.
- Increase in the pH of gastric secretions. In treatment of peptic ulcer, antacid therapy should be continued for at least 4–6 wk after symptoms have disappeared because there is no correlation between disappearance of symptoms and healing of ulcers.

amcinonide, See CORTICOSTEROIDS (TOPICAL/LOCAL).

amifostine (a-mi-fos-teen)

Ethyol

Classification
Therapeutic: cytoprotective agents

Pregnancy Category C

Indications

Reduces renal toxicity from cisplatin. Reduces the incidence of moderate to severe xerostomia from postoperative radiation for head and neck cancer in which the radiation port includes a large portion of the parotid glands.

Action

Converted by alkaline phosphatase in tissue to a free thiol compound that binds and detoxifies damaging metabolites of cisplatin and reactive oxygen species generated by radiation. **Therapeutic Effects:** Decreased renal damage from cisplatin. Decreased severity of xerostomia following radiation for head and neck cancer.

Pharmacokinetics

Absorption: IV administration results in complete bioavailability.
Distribution: Unknown.
Metabolism and Excretion: Rapidly cleared from plasma; converted to cytoprotective compounds by alkaline phosphatase in tissues.
Half-life: 8 min.

TIME/ACTION PROFILE

ROUTE	ONSET	PEAK	DURATION
IV	unknown	unknown	unknown

Contraindications/Precautions

Contraindicated in: Known sensitivity to aminothiol compounds; Hypotension or dehydration; Lactation: Use an alternative to breast milk; Concurrent antineoplastic therapy for other tumors (especially malignancies of germ cell origin).
Use Cautiously in: OB, Pedi: Safety not established; Geri: Geriatric patients or patients with cardiovascular disease have ↑ risk of adverse reactions.

Adverse Reactions/Side Effects

CNS: dizziness, somnolence. **EENT:** sneezing. **CV:** hypotension. **GI:** hiccups, nausea, vomiting. **Derm:** flushing. **F and E:** hypocalcemia. **Misc:** allergic reactions including ANAPHYLAXIS, STEVENS-JOHNSON SYNDROME, TOXIC EPIDERMAL NECROLYSIS, TOXODERMA, ERYTHEMA MULTIFORMA, EXFOLIATIVE DERMATITIS (↑ when used as a radioprotectant), chills.

Interactions

Drug-Drug: Concurrent use of **antihypertensives** ↑ risk of hypotension.

Route/Dosage

Reduction of Renal Damage with Cisplatin

IV (Adults): 910 mg/m² once daily, within 30 min before chemotherapy; if full dose is poorly tolerated, subsequent doses should be ↓ to 740 mg/m².

Reduction of Xerostomia from Radiation

IV (Adults): 200 mg/m² once daily, as a 3-minute infusion starting 15–30 min before standard fraction radiation therapy.

Availability (generic available)

Powder for injection: 500 mg/vial.

NURSING IMPLICATIONS

Assessment

- Monitor BP before and every 5 min during infusion. Discontinue antihypertensives 24 hr prior to treatment. If significant hypotension requiring interruption of therapy occurs, place patient in Trendelenburg position and administer an infusion of 0.9% NaCl using a separate IV line. If BP returns to normal in 5 min and patient is asymptomatic, infusion may be resumed so that full dose may be given.
- Assess fluid status before administration. Correct dehydration before instituting therapy. Nausea and vomiting are frequent and may be severe. Administer prophylactic antiemetics including dexamethasone 20 mg IV and a serotonin-antagonist antiemetic (dolasetron, granisetron, ondansetron, palonosetron) before and during infusion. Monitor fluid status closely.
- Observe patient for signs and symptoms of anaphylaxis (rash, pruritus, laryngeal edema, wheezing). Discontinue the drug and notify physician or other health care professional immediately if these problems occur. Keep epinephrine, an antihistamine, and resuscitation equipment close by in case of an anaphylactic reaction.
- **Xerostomia:** Assess patient for dry mouth and mouth sores periodically during therapy.
- Monitor patient for skin reactions before, during, and after amifostine administration; reactions may be delayed by several weeks after initiation of therapy. Permanently discontinue amifostine in patients who experience serious or severe cutaneous reactions or cutaneous reactions associated with fever or other symptoms of unknown cause. Withhold therapy and obtain dermatologic consultation and biopsy for cutaneous reactions or mucosal lesions of unknown cause appearing outside of injection site or radiation port, and for erythematous, edematous, or bullous lesions on the palms of the hand or soles of the feet.
- ***Lab Test Considerations:*** Monitor serum calcium concentrations before and periodically during therapy. May cause hypocalcemia. Calcium supplements may be necessary.

Potential Nursing Diagnoses

Risk for injury (Indications)

Implementation

IV Administration

- **Intermittent Infusion:** ***Diluent:*** Reconstitute with 9.7 mL of sterile 0.9% NaCl. Dilute further with 0.9% NaCl. Do not administer solutions that are discolored or contain particulate matter. Solution is stable for 5 hr at room temperature or 24 hr if refrigerated. ***Concentration:*** Adults: dilute dose to a final volume of 50 mL; Children: 5–40 mg/mL. ***Rate:*** *For renal toxicity:* Administer over 15 min within 30 min before chemotherapy administration. Longer infusion times are not as well tolerated. *For xerostomia:* Administer over 3 min starting 15–30 min prior to radiation therapy.
- **Y-Site Compatibility:** amikacin, aminophylline, amphotericin B liposome, ampicillin, ampicillin/sul-

bactam, aztreonam, bivalirudin, bleomycin, bumetanide, buprenorphine, butorphanol, calcium gluconate, carboplatin, carmustine, caspofungin, cefazolin, cefotaxime, cefotetan, cefoxitin, ceftazidime, ceftriaxone, cefuroxime, cimetidine, ciprofloxacin, clindamycin, cyclophosphamide, cytarabine, dacarbazine, dactinomycin, daptomycin, daunorubicin hydrochloride, dexamethasone, dexmedetomidine, diltiazem, diphenhydramine, dobutamine, docetaxel, dopamine, doxorubicin hydrochloride, doxycycline, droperidol, enalaprilat, epirubicin, ertapenem, etoposide, etoposide phosphate, famotidine, fenoldopam, floxuridine, fluconazole, fludarabine, fluorouracil, furosemide, gemcitabine, gentamicin, granisetron, haloperidol, heparin, hydrocortisone, hydromorphone, idarubicin, ifosfamide, imipenem/cilastatin, leucovorin, levofloxacin, linezolid, lorazepam, magnesium sulfate, mannitol, mechlorethamine, meperidine, mesna, methotrexate, methylprednisolone, metoclopramide, metronidazole, milrinone, mitomycin, morphine, nalbuphine, nesiritide, octreotide, ondansetron, oxaliplatin, paclitaxel, palonosetron, pantoprazole, pemetrexed, piperacillin/tazobactam, potassium chloride, promethazine, ranitidine, rituximab, sodium acetate, sodium bicarbonate, streptozocin, tacrolimus, teniposide, thiotepa, tigecycline, tirofiban, tobramycin, trastuzumab, trimethoprim/sulfamethoxazole, vancomycin, vasopressin, vecuronium, vinblastine, vincristine, vinorelbine, voriconazole, zidovudine.

- **Y-Site Incompatibility:** acyclovir, amphotericin B colloidal, cisplatin, ganciclovir, hydroxyzine, minocycline, prochlorperazine, quinupristin/dalfopristin.
- **Additive Incompatibility:** Do not mix with other solutions or medications.

Patient/Family Teaching

- Explain the purpose of amifostine infusion to patient.
- Inform patient that amifostine may cause hypotension, nausea, vomiting, flushing, chills, dizziness, somnolence, hiccups, and sneezing.
- Advise patient to notify health care professional if skin reactions occur.

Evaluation/Desired Outcomes

- Prevention of renal toxicity associated with repeated administration of cisplatin in patients with ovarian cancer.
- Decreased severity of xerostomia from radiation treatment of head and neck cancer.

amikacin, See AMINOGLYCOSIDES.

aMILoride, See DIURETICS (POTASSIUM-SPARING).

aminocaproic acid

(a-mee-noe-ka-**pro**-ik **a**-sid)

Amicar

Classification

Therapeutic: hemostatic agents

Pharmacologic: fibrinolysis inhibitors

Pregnancy Category C

Indications

Management of acute, life-threatening hemorrhage due to systemic hyperfibrinolysis or urinary fibrinolysis. **Unlabeled Use:** Prevention of recurrent subarachnoid hemorrhage. Prevention of bleeding following oral surgery in hemophiliacs. Management of severe hemorrhage caused by thrombolytic agents.

Action

Inhibits activation of plasminogen. **Therapeutic Effects:** Inhibition of fibrinolysis. Stabilization of clot formation.

Pharmacokinetics

Absorption: Rapidly absorbed following oral administration.

Distribution: Widely distributed.

Metabolism and Excretion: Mostly eliminated unchanged by the kidneys.

Half-life: Unknown.

TIME/ACTION PROFILE (peak blood levels)

ROUTE	ONSET	PEAK	DURATION
PO	unknown	2 hr	N/A
IV	unknown	2 hr	N/A

Contraindications/Precautions

Contraindicated in: Active intravascular clotting.

Use Cautiously in: Upper urinary tract bleeding; Cardiac, renal, or liver disease (dosage reduction may be required); Disseminated intravascular coagulation (should be used concurrently with heparin); OB, Lactation: Safety not established; Pedi: Do not use products containing benzyl alcohol with neonates.

Adverse Reactions/Side Effects

CNS: dizziness, malaise. **EENT:** nasal stuffiness, tinnitus. **CV:** arrhythmias, hypotension (IV only). **GI:** anorexia, bloating, cramping, diarrhea, nausea. **GU:** diuresis, renal failure. **MS:** myopathy.

Interactions

Drug-Drug: Concurrent use with **estrogens, conjugated** may result in a hypercoagulable state. Concurrent use with **clotting factors** may ↑ risk of thromboses.

Route/Dosage

Acute Bleeding Syndromes due to Elevated Fibrinolytic Activity

PO (Adults): 5 g 1st hr, followed by 1–1.25 g q hr for 8 hr or until hemorrhage is controlled; or 6 g over 24 hr after prostate surgery (not >30 g/day).
IV (Adults): 4–5 g over 1st hr, followed by 1 g/hr for 8 hr or until hemorrhage is controlled; or 6 g over 24 hr after prostate surgery (not >30 g/day).
PO, IV (Children): 100 mg/kg or 3 g/m^2 over 1st hr, followed by continuous infusion of 33.3 mg/kg/hr; or 1 $g/m^2/hr$ (total dose not >18 $g/m^2/24$ hr).

Subarachnoid Hemorrhage

PO (Adults): *To follow IV*—3 g q 2 hr (36 g/day). If no surgery is performed, continue for 21 days after bleeding stops, then decrease to 2 g q 2 hr (24 g/day) for 3 days, then 1 g q 2 hr (12 g/day) for 3 days.
IV (Adults): 36 g/day for 10 days followed by PO.

Prevention of Bleeding Following Oral Surgery in Hemophiliacs

PO (Adults): 75 mg/kg (up to 6 g) immediately after procedure, then q 6 hr for 7–10 days; syrup may also be used as an oral rinse of 1.25 g (5 mL) 4 times a day for 7–10 days.
IV, PO (Children): *Also for epistaxis*—50–100 mg/kg/dose administered IV every 6 hr for 2–3 days starting 4 hr before the procedure. After completion of IV therapy, aminocaproic acid should be given as 50–100 mg/kg/dose orally every 6 hr for 5–7 days.

Availability

Tablets: 500 mg, 1000 mg. **Syrup (raspberry flavor):** 1.25 g/5 mL. **Injection:** 250 mg/mL.

NURSING IMPLICATIONS

Assessment

- Monitor BP, pulse, and respiratory status as indicated by severity of bleeding.
- Monitor for overt bleeding every 15–30 min.
- Monitor neurologic status (pupils, level of consciousness, motor activity) in patients with subarachnoid hemorrhage.
- Monitor intake and output ratios frequently; notify physician if significant discrepancies occur.
- Assess for thromboembolic complications (especially in patients with history). Notify health care professional of positive Homans' sign, leg pain and edema, hemoptysis, dyspnea, or chest pain.
- ***Lab Test Considerations:*** Monitor platelet count and clotting factors prior to and periodically throughout therapy in patients with systemic fibrinolysis.
- ↑ CPK, AST, and serum aldolase may indicate myopathy.
- May ↑ serum potassium.

Potential Nursing Diagnoses

Ineffective tissue perfusion (Indications)
Risk for injury (Indications, Side Effects)

Implementation

- **PO:** Syrup may be used as an oral rinse, swished for 30 sec 4 times/day for 7–10 days for the control of bleeding during dental and oral surgery in hemophilic patients. Small amounts may be swallowed, except during 1st and 2nd trimesters of pregnancy. Syrup may be applied with an applicator in children or unconscious patients.

IV Administration

- **IV:** Stabilize IV catheter to minimize thrombophlebitis. Monitor site closely.
- **Intermittent Infusion: *Diluent:*** Do not administer undiluted. Dilute initial 4–5 g dose in 250 mL of sterile water for injection, 0.9% NaCl, D5W, or LR. Do not dilute with sterile water in patients with subarachnoid hemorrhage. ***Concentration:*** 20 mg/mL. ***Rate:*** Single doses: Administer over 1 hr. Rapid infusion rate may cause hypotension, bradycardia, or other arrhythmias.
- **Continuous Infusion:** Administer IV solution using infusion pump to ensure accurate dose. Administer via slow IV infusion.
- ***Rate:*** Initial dose may be followed by a continuous infusion of 1–1.25 g/hr in adults or 33.3 mg/kg/hr in children.
- **Y-Site Compatibility:** alemtuzumab, alfentanil, amikacin, aminophylline, amphotericin B colloidal, amphotericin B lipid complex, amphotericin B liposome, ampicillin, ampicillin/sulbactam, anidulafungin, argatroban, atracurium, azithromycin, aztreonam, bivalirudin, bleomycin, bumetanide, buprenorphine, butorphanol, calcium chloride, calcium gluconate, carboplatin, carmustine, cefazolin, cefepime, cefotaxime, cefotetan, ceftazidime, ceftriaxone, cefuroxime, cisatracurium, clindamycin, cyclophosphamide, cyclosporine, cytarabine, daptomycin, dexamethasone, dexmedetomidine, digoxin, diltiazem, diphenhydramine, dobutamine, docetaxel, dopamine, doxacurium, droperidol, enalaprilat, ephedrine, epinephrine, epirubicin, ertapenem, erythromycin, esmolol, etoposide, etoposide phosphate, famotidine, fenoldopam, fentanyl, fluconazole, fludarabine, foscarnet, fosphenytoin, furosemide, gemcitabine, gentamicin, granisetron, haloperidol, heparin, hydrocortisone, hydromorphone, idarubicin, ifosfamide, imipenem/cilastatin, irinotecan, isoproterenol, ketorolac, labetalol, levofloxacin, levorphanol, lidocaine, linezolid, lorazepam, magnesium sulfate, mannitol, mechloreth-

amine, meperidine, meropenem, methohexital, methylprednisolone, metoclopramide, metoprolol, metronidazole, milrinone, mitoxantrone, morphine, nalbuphine, naloxone, nesiritide, nitroglycerin, nitroprusside, octreotide, ondansetron, oxaliplatin, oxytocin, palonosetron, pamidronate, pantoprazole, pamidronate, pancuronium, pantoprazole, pemetrexed, pentamidine, pentobarbital, phenobarbital, phenylephrine, piperacillin/tazobactam, potassium acetate, potassium chloride, potassium phosphates, procainamide, promethazine, propranolol, ranitidine, remifentanil, rocuronium, sargramostim, sodium bicarbonate, sodium phosphates, succinylcholine, sufentanil, tacrolimus, teniposide, theophylline, thiotepa, tigecycline, tirofiban, tobramycin, trimethoprim/sulfamethoxazole, vancomycin, vasopressin, vecuronium, verapamil, vincristine, voriconazole, zidovudine, zoledronic acid.

- **Y-Site Incompatibility:** acyclovir, amiodarone, caspofungin, chlorpromazine, ciprofloxacin, diazepam, dolasetron, doxycycline, filgrastim, ganciclovir, midazolam, mycophenolate, nicardipine, phenytoin, prochlorperazine, quinupristin/dalfopristin, thiopental.
- **Additive Incompatibility:** Do not admix with other medications.

Patient/Family Teaching

- Instruct patient to notify the nurse immediately if bleeding recurs or if thromboembolic symptoms develop.
- **IV:** Caution patient to make position changes slowly to avoid orthostatic hypotension.

Evaluation/Desired Outcomes

- Cessation of bleeding.
- Prevention of rebleeding in subarachnoid hemorrhage without occurrence of undesired clotting.

AMINOGLYCOSIDES

amikacin (am-i-**kay**-sin)
~~Amikin~~

gentamicin† (jen-ta-**mye**-sin)
~~Garamycin~~

neomycin (neo-oh-**mye**-sin)

streptomycin (strep-toe-**mye**-sin)

tobramycin† (toe-bra-**mye**-sin)
Bethkis, Kitabis Pak, TOBI, TOBI Podhaler

Classification
Therapeutic: anti-infectives
Pharmacologic: aminoglycosides

Pregnancy Category C (gentamicin, topical use of others), D (amikacin, neomycin, streptomycin, tobramycin)

†See Appendix C for ophthalmic use

Indications

Amikacin, gentamicin, and tobramycin: Treatment of serious gram-negative bacterial infections and infections caused by staphylococci when penicillins or other less toxic drugs are contraindicated. **Streptomycin:** In combination with other agents in the management of active tuberculosis. **Neomycin:** Used orally to prepare the GI tract for surgery, to decrease the number of ammonia-producing bacteria in the gut as part of the management of hepatic encephalopathy, and to treat diarrhea caused by *Escherichia coli*. **Tobramycin by inhalation:** Management of *Pseudomonas aeruginosa* in cystic fibrosis patients. **Gentamicin, streptomycin:** In combination with other agents in the management of serious enterococcal infections. **Gentamicin IV:** Prevention of infective endocarditis. **Gentamicin (topical):** Treatment of localized infections caused by susceptible organisms. **Unlabeled Use:** Amikacin: In combination with other agents in the management of *Mycobacterium avium* complex infections.

Action

Inhibits protein synthesis in bacteria at level of 30S ribosome. **Therapeutic Effects:** Bactericidal action. **Spectrum:** Most aminoglycosides notable for activity against: *P. aeruginosa*, *Klebsiella pneumoniae*, *E.coli*, *Proteus*, *Serratia*, *Acinetobacter*, *Staphylococcus aureus*. In treatment of enterococcal infections, synergy with a penicillin is required. Streptomycin and amikacin also active against *Mycobacterium*.

Pharmacokinetics

Absorption: Well absorbed after IM administration. IV administration results in complete bioavailability. Some absorption follows administration by other routes. Minimal systemic absorption with neomycin (may accumulate in patients with renal failure).
Distribution: Widely distributed throughout extracellular fluid; cross the placenta; small amounts enter breast milk. Poor penetration into CSF (↑ when meninges are inflammed).
Metabolism and Excretion: Excretion is >90% renal.
Half-life: 2–4 hr (↑ in renal impairment).

TIME/ACTION PROFILE (blood levels*)

ROUTE	ONSET	PEAK	DURATION
PO (neomycin)	rapid	1–4 hr	N/A
IM	rapid	30–90 min	6–24 hr
IV	rapid	15–30 min†	6–24 hr

*All parenterally administered aminoglycosides.
†Postdistribution peak occurs 30 min after the end of a 30-min infusion and 15 min after the end of a 1-hr infusion.

Contraindications/Precautions

Contraindicated in: Hypersensitivity to aminoglycosides; Most parenteral products contain bisulfites and should be avoided in patients with known intolerance; Pedi: Products containing benzyl alcohol should be avoided in neonates; Intestinal obstruction (neomycin only).
Use Cautiously in: Renal impairment (dose adjustments necessary; blood level monitoring useful in preventing ototoxicity and nephrotoxicity); Hearing impairment; Neuromuscular diseases such as myasthenia gravis; Obese patients (dose should be based on ideal body weight); OB: Tobramycin and streptomycin may cause congenital deafness; Lactation: Safety not established; Pedi: Neonates have ↑ risk of neuromuscular blockade; difficulty in assessing auditory and vestibular function and immature renal function; Geri: Difficulty in assessing auditory and vestibular function and age-related renal impairment.

Adverse Reactions/Side Effects

CNS: ataxia, vertigo. **EENT:** ototoxicity (vestibular and cochlear). **GU:** nephrotoxicity. **GI:** *Neomycin*—diarrhea, nausea, vomiting. **F and E:** hypomagnesemia. **MS:** muscle paralysis (high parenteral doses). **Neuro:** ↑ neuromuscular blockade. **Resp:** apnea; *Tobramycin, Inhaln only*, bronchospasm, wheezing. **Misc:** hypersensitivity reactions.

Interactions

Drug-Drug: Inactivated by **penicillins** and **cephalosporins** when coadministered to patients with renal insufficiency. Possible respiratory paralysis after **inhalation anesthetics** or **neuromuscular blocking agents**. ↑ incidence of ototoxicity with **loop diuretics** or **mannitol (IV)**. ↑ incidence of nephrotoxicity with other **nephrotoxic drugs**. Neomycin may ↑ anticoagulant effects of **warfarin**. Neomycin may ↓ absorption of **digoxin** and **methotrexate**.

Route/Dosage

Amikacin

IM, IV (Adults and Children): 5 mg/kg q 8 hr or 7.5 mg/kg q 12 hr (not to exceed 1.5 g/day). *Mycobacterium avium complex*—7.5–15 mg/kg/day divided q 12–24 hr.
IM, IV (Neonates): *Loading dose*—10 mg/kg; *Maintenance dose*—7.5 mg/kg q 12 hr.

Renal Impairment

IM, IV (Adults): *Loading dose*—7.5 mg/kg, further dosing based on blood level monitoring and renal function assessment.

Gentamicin

Many regimens are used; most involve dosing adjusted on the basis of blood level monitoring and assessment of renal function.
IM, IV (Adults): 1–2 mg/kg q 8 hr (up to 6 mg/kg/day in 3 divided doses); *Once-daily dosing (unlabeled)*—4–7 mg/kg q 24 hr.
IM, IV (Children >5 yr): 2–2.5 mg/kg/dose q 8 hr; *Once daily*—5–7.5 mg/kg/dose q 24 hr; *Cystic fibrosis*—2.5–3.3 mg/kg/dose q 6–8 hr; *Hemodialysis*—1.25–1.75 mg/kg/dose postdialysis.
IM, IV (Children 1 mo–5 yr): 2.5 mg/kg/dose q 8 hr; *Once daily*—5–7.5 mg/kg/dose q 24 hr; *Cystic fibrosis*—2.5–3.3 mg/kg/dose q 6–8 hr; *Hemodialysis*—1.25–1.75 mg/kg/dose postdialysis.
IM, IV (Neonates full term and/or >1 wk): *Weight <1200 g*—2.5 mg/kg/dose q 18–24 hr; *Weight 1200–2000 g*—2.5 mg/kg/dose q 8–12 hr; *Weight >2000 g*—2.5 mg/kg/dose q 8 hr; *ECMO*—2.5 mg/kg/dose q 18 hr, subsequent doses based on serum concentrations; *Once daily*—3.5–5 mg/kg/dose q 24 hr.
IM, IV (Neonates premature and/or ≤1 wk): *Weight <1000 g*—3.5 mg/kg/dose q 24 hr; *Weight 1000–1200 g*—2.5 mg/kg/dose q 18–24 hr; *Weight >1200 g*—2.5 mg/kg/dose q 12 hr; *Once daily*—3.5–4 mg/kg/dose q 24 hr.
IT (Adults): 4–8 mg/day.
IT (Infants >3 mo and Children): 1–2 mg/day.
IT (Neonates): 1 mg/day.
Topical (Adults and Children >1 mo): Apply cream or ointment 3–4 times daily.

Renal Impairment

IM, IV (Adults): Initial dose of 2 mg/kg. Subsequent doses/intervals based on blood level monitoring and renal function assessment.

Neomycin

PO (Adults): *Preoperative intestinal antisepsis*—1 g q hr for 4 doses, then 1 g q 4 hr for 5 doses *or* 1 g at 1 PM, 2 PM, and 11 PM on day before surgery; *Hepatic encephalopathy*—1–3 g q 6 hr for 5–6 days; may be followed by 4 g/day chronically.
PO (Children): *Preoperative intestinal antisepsis*—15 mg/kg q 4 hr for 2 days *or* 25 mg/kg at 1 PM, 2 PM, and 11 PM on day before surgery; *Hepatic encephalopathy*—12.5–25 mg/kg q 6 hr for 5–6 days (maximum dose = 12 g/day).

Streptomycin

IM (Adults): *Tuberculosis*—1 g/day initially, decreased to 1 g 2–3 times weekly; *Other infections*—250 mg–1 g q 6 hr *or* 500 mg–2 g q 12 hr.

IM (Children): *Tuberculosis*—20 mg/kg/day (not to exceed 1 g/day); *Other infections*—5–10 mg/kg q 6 hr *or* 10–20 mg/kg q 12 hr.

Renal Impairment

IM (Adults): 1 g initially, further dosing determined by blood level monitoring and assessment of renal function.

Tobramycin

IM, IV (Adults): 1–2 mg/kg q 8 hr *or* 4–6.6 mg/kg/day q 24 hr.
IM, IV (Adults): 3–6 mg/kg/day in 3 divided doses, or 4–6.6 mg/kg once daily.
IM, IV (Children >5 yr): 6–7.5 mg/kg/day divided q 8 hr, up to 13 mg/kg/day divided q 6–8 hr in cystic fibrosis patients (dosing interval may vary from q 6 hr–q 24 hr, depending on clinical situation).
IM, IV (Children 1 mo–5 yr): 7.5 mg/kg/day divided q 8 hr, up to 13 mg/kg/day divided q 6–8 hr in cystic fibrosis.
IM, IV (Neonates): *Preterm <1000 g*—3.5 mg/kg/dose q 24 hr; *0–4 weeks, <1200 g*—2.5 mg/kg/dose q 18 hr; *Postnatal age <7 days*—2.5 mg/kg/dose q 12 hr; *Postnatal age >7200 days,1200–2000 g*—2.5 mg/kg/dose q 8–12 hr; *Postnatal age >7200 days, >2000 g*—2.5 mg/kg/dose q 8 hr.
Inhaln (Adults and Children ≥6 yr): *Nebulizer solution*—300 mg twice daily for 28 days, then off for 28 days, then repeat cycle; *powder for inhalation*—Inhale contents of four 28-mg capsules twice daily for 28 days, then off for 28 days, then repeat cycle.

Renal Impairment

IM, IV (Adults): 1 mg/kg initially, further dosing determined by blood level monitoring and assessment of renal function.

Availability

Amikacin (generic available)

Injection: 50 mg/mL, 250 mg/mL.

Gentamicin (generic available)

Injection: 10 mg/mL, 40 mg/mL. **Premixed injection:** 40 mg/50 mL, 60 mg/50 mL, 60 mg/100 mL, 70 mg/50 mL, 80 mg/50 mL, 80 mg/100 mL, 90 mg/100 mL, 100 mg/50 mL, 100 mg/100 mL, 120 mg/100 mL. **Topical cream:** 0.1%. **Topical ointment:** 0.1%.

Neomycin (generic available)

Tablets: 500 mg. ***In combination with:*** other topical antibiotics or anti-inflammatory agents for skin, ear, and eye infections. See Appendix B.

Streptomycin (generic available)

Injection: 1 g.

Tobramycin (generic available)

Injection: 10 mg/mL, 40 mg/mL. **Nebulizer solution (TOBI, Kitabis Pak):** 300 mg/5 mL. **Nebulizer solution (Bethkis):** 300 mg/4 mL. **Powder for inhalation (TOBI Podhaler):** 28 mg/capsule. **Powder for injection (requires reconstitution):** 1200 mg/vial. **Premixed injection:** 80 mg/100 mL.

NURSING IMPLICATIONS

Assessment

- Assess for infection (vital signs, wound appearance, sputum, urine, stool, WBC) at beginning of and throughout therapy.
- Obtain specimens for culture and sensitivity before initiating therapy. First dose may be given before receiving results.
- Evaluate eighth cranial nerve function by audiometry before and throughout therapy. Hearing loss is usually in high-frequency range. Prompt recognition and intervention are essential in preventing permanent damage. Monitor for vestibular dysfunction (vertigo, ataxia, nausea, vomiting). Eighth cranial nerve dysfunction is associated with persistently elevated peak aminoglycoside levels. Discontinue aminoglycosides if tinnitus or subjective hearing loss occurs.
- Monitor intake and output and daily weight to assess hydration status and renal function.
- Assess for signs of superinfection (fever, upper respiratory infection, vaginal itching or discharge, increasing malaise, diarrhea).
- **Hepatic Encephalopathy:** Monitor neurologic status. Before administering oral medication, assess patient's ability to swallow.
- ***Lab Test Considerations:*** Monitor renal function by urinalysis, specific gravity, BUN, creatinine, and CCr before and during therapy.
- May cause ↑ BUN, AST, ALT, serum alkaline phosphatase, bilirubin, creatinine, and LDH concentrations.
- May cause ↓ serum calcium, magnesium, potassium, and sodium concentrations (streptomycin and tobramycin).
- ***Toxicity and Overdose:*** Monitor blood levels periodically during therapy. Timing of blood levels is important in interpreting results. Draw blood for peak levels 1 hr after IM injection and 30 min after a 30-min IV infusion is completed. Draw trough levels just before next dose. Peak level for **amikacin** is 20–30 mcg/mL; trough level should be <10 mcg/mL. Peak level for **gentamicin** and **tobramycin** should not exceed 10 mcg/mL; trough level should not exceed 2 mcg/mL. Peak level for **streptomycin** should not exceed 25 mcg/mL.

Potential Nursing Diagnoses

Risk for infection (Indications)
Disturbed sensory perception (auditory) (Side Effects)

Implementation

Keep patient well hydrated (1500–2000 mL/day) during therapy.

- **Preoperative Bowel Prep:** Neomycin is usually used in conjunction with erythromycin, a low-residue diet, and a cathartic or enema.
- **PO:** Neomycin may be administered without regard to meals.
- **IM:** IM administration should be deep into a well-developed muscle. Alternate injection sites.
- **IV:** If aminoglycosides and penicillins or cephalosporins must be administered concurrently, administer in separate sites, at least 1 hr apart.

Amikacin

IV Administration

- **Intermittent Infusion:** ***Diluent:*** Dilute with D5W, D10W, 0.9% NaCl, dextrose/saline combinations, or LR. Solution may be pale yellow without decreased potency. Stable for 24 hr at room temperature. ***Concentration:*** 10 mg/mL. ***Rate:*** Infuse over 30–60 min for adults and children and over 1–2 hr in infants.
- **Y-Site Compatibility:** acyclovir, aldesleukin, alemtuzumab, alfentanil, amifostine, aminophylline, amiodarone, anidulafungin, argatroban, ascorbic acid, atropine, aztreonam, benztropine, bivalirudin, bleomycin, bumetanide, buprenorphine, butorphanol, calcium chloride, calcium gluconate, cangrelor, carboplatin, carmustine, caspofungin, chloramphenicol, chlorpromazine, cisatracurium, cisplatin, clindamycin, cyanocobalamin, cyclophosphamide, cyclosporine, cytarabine, dactinomycin, daptomycin, dexamethasone, dexmedetomidine, dexrazoxane, digoxin, diltiazem, diphenhydramine, dobutamine, docetaxel, dolasetron, dopamine, doripenem, doxorubicin hydrochloride, doxycycline, enalaprilat, ephedrine, epinephrine, epirubicin, epoetin alfa, eptifibatide, ertapenem, erythromycin, esmolol, etoposide, etoposide phosphate, famotidine, fentanyl, filgrastim, fluconazole, fludarabine, fluorouracil, foscarnet, fosphenytoin, furosemide, gemcitabine, gentamicin, glycopyrrolate, granisetron, hydrocortisone, hydromorphone, idarubicin, ifosfamide, imipenem/cilastatin, irinotecan, isoproterenol, ketamine, ketorolac, labetalol, leucovorin, levofloxacin, lidocaine, linezolid, lorazepam, magnesium sulfate, mannitol, mechlorethamine, melphalan, meperidine, mesna, methotrexate, methylprednisolone, metoclopramide, metoprolol, metronidazole, midazolam, milrinone, mitoxantrone, morphine, multivitamins, mycophenolate, nalbuphine, naloxone, nicardipine, nitroglycerin, nitroprusside, norepinephrine, octreotide, ondansetron, oxaliplatin, oxytocin, paclitaxel, palonosetron, pamidronate, pancuronium, papaverine, pemetrexed, pentazocine, perphenazine, phenobarbital, phenylephrine, phytonadione, posaconazole, potassium acetate, potassium chloride, procainamide, prochlorperazine, promethazine, propranolol, protamine, pyridoxime, quinupristin/dalfopristin, ranitidine, remifentanil, rituximab, rocuronium, sargramostim, sodium acetate, sodium bicarbonate, streptokinase, succinylcholine, sufentanil, tacrolimus, teniposide, theophylline, thiamine, thiotepa, tigecycline, tirofiban, tobramycin, tolazoline, topotecan, vancomycin, vasopressin, vecuronium, verapamil, vinblastine, vincristine, vinorelbine, voriconazole, warfarin, zidovudine, zoledronic acid.
- **Y-Site Incompatibility:** allopurinol, amphotericin B cholesteryl, amphotericin B colloidal, amphotericin B lipid complex, amphotericin B liposome, azathioprine, dacarbazine, dantrolene, diazepam, diazoxide, folic acid, ganciclovir, ibuprofen lysine, indomethacin, mitomycin, pentamidine, pentobarbital, phenytoin, propofol, trastuzumab, trimethoprim/sulfamethoxazole.

Gentamicin

IV Administration

- **Intermittent Infusion:** ***Diluent:*** Dilute each dose with D5W, 0.9% NaCl, or LR. Do not use solutions that are discolored or that contain a precipitate. ***Concentration:*** 10 mg/mL. ***Rate:*** Infuse slowly over 30 min–2 hr.
- **Y-Site Compatibility:** aldesleukin, alemtuzumab, alfentanil, alprostadil, amifostine, amikacin, aminophylline, amiodarone, anidulafungin, argatroban, ascorbic acid, atropine, aztreonam, benztropine, bivalirudin, bleomycin, bumetanide, buprenorphine, butorphanol, calcium chloride, calcium gluconate, carboplatin, carmustine, caspofungin, chlorpromazine, ciprofloxacin, cisatracurium, cisplatin, clindamycin, cyanocobalamin, cyclophosphamide, cyclosporine, cytarabine, dactinomycin, daptomycin, dexmedetomidine, dexrazoxane, digoxin, diltiazem, dimenhydrinate, diphenhydramine, dobutamine, docetaxel, dolasetron, dopamine, doripenem, doxapram, doxorubicin hydrochloride, doxorubicin liposome, doxycycline, enalaprilat, ephedrine, epinephrine, epirubicin, epoetin alfa, eptifibatide, ertapenem, erythromycin, esmolol, etoposide, etoposide phosphate, famotidine, fenoldopam, fentanyl, fluconazole, fludarabine, fluorouracil, foscarnet, fosphenytoin, gemcitabine, glycopyrrolate, granisetron, hydromorphone, ifosfamide, imipenem/cilastatin, irinotecan, isoproterenol, ketamine, ketorolac, labetalol, leucovorin, levofloxacin , lidocaine, linezolid, lorazepam, magnesium sulfate, mannitol, mechlorethamine, melphalan, meperidine, meropenem, mesna, metaraminol, methylprednisolone, metoclorpamide, metoprolol, metronidazole, midazolam, milrinone, mitoxantrone, morphine, multivitamins, mycophenolate, nalbuphine, naloxone, nicardipine, nitroglycerin, nitroprusside, norepinephrine, octreotide, ondansetron, oxaliplatin,

oxytocin, paclitaxel, palonosetron, pamidronate, pancuronium, papaverine, pentazocine, perphenazine, phenobarbital, phenylephrine, phytonadione, posaconazole, potassium acetate, potassium chloride, procainamide, prochlorperazine, promethazine, propranolol, protamine, pyridoxine, ranitidine, remifentanil, rituximab, rocuronium, sargramostim, sodium acetate, sodium bicarbonate, streptokinase, succinylcholine, sufentanil, tacrolimus, telavancin, teniposide, theophylline, thiamine, thiotepa, tigecycline, tirofiban, tobramycin, topotecan, trastuzumab, trimetaphan, vancomycin, vasopressin, vecuronium, verapamil, vinblastine, vincristine, vinorelbine, vitamin B complex with C, voriconazole, zidovudine, zoledronic acid.

- **Y-Site Incompatibility:** allopurinol, amphotericin B chloesteryl, amphotericin B colloidal, amphotericin B lipid complex, amphotericin B liposome, azathioprine, cangrelor, cefotetan, dacarbazine, dantrolene, diazepam, diazoxide, folic acid, ganciclovir, idarubicin, indomethacin, methotrexate, pemetrexed, pentamidine, pentobarbital, phenytoin, propofol, trimethoprim/sulfamethoxazole, warfarin.

Tobramycin

IV Administration

- **Intermittent Infusion:** ***Diluent:*** Dilute each dose of tobramycin in 50–100 mL of D5W, D10W, D5/0.9% NaCl, 0.9% NaCl, Ringer's or lactated Ringer's solution. ***Concentration:*** not >10 m g/mL. Pediatric doses may be diluted in proportionately smaller amounts. Stable for 24 hr at room temperature, 96 hr if refrigerated. ***Rate:*** Infuse slowly over 30–60 min in both adult and pediatric patients.
- **Y-Site Compatibility:** acyclovir, aldesleukin, alemtuzumab, alfentanil, alprostadil, alteplase, amifostine, aminophylline, amiodarone, anidulafungin, argatroban, ascorbic acid, atropine, aztreonam, benztropine, bivalirudin, bleomycin, bumetanide, buprenorphine, butorphanol, calcium chloride, calcium gluconate, carboplatin, carmustine, caspofungin, chloramphenicol, chlorpromazine, ciprofloxacin, cisatracurium, cisplatin, clindamycin, cyanocobalamin, cyclophosphamide, cyclosporine, cytarabine, dactinomycin, daptomycin, daunorubicin hydrochloride, dexmedetomidine, dexrazoxane, digoxin, diltiazem, dimenhydrinate, diphenhydramine, dobutamine, docetaxel, dolasetron, dopamine, doripenem, doxorubicin hydrochloride, doxorubicin liposome, doxycycline, enalaprilat, ephedrine, epinephrine, epirubicin, epoetin alfa, ertapenem, esmolol, etoposide, etoposide phosphate, famotidine, fenoldopam, fentanyl, filgrastim, fluconazole, fludarabine, fluorouracil, foscarnet, furosemide, gemcitabine, gentamicin, glycopyrrolate, granisetron, hydromorphone, idarubicin, ifosfamide, imipenem/cilastatin, irinotecan, isoproterenol, ketamine, ketorolac, labetalol, leucovorin, levofloxacin, lidocaine, linezolid, lorazepam, magnesium sulfate, mannitol, mechlorethamine, melphalan, meperidine, mesna, methotrexate, methylprednisolone, metoclopramide, metoprolol, metronidazole, midazolam, milrinone, minocycline, mitomycin, mitoxantrone, morphine, multivitamins, mycophenolate, nalbuphine, naloxone, nicardipine, nitroglycerin, nitroprusside, norepinephrine, octreotide, ondansetron, oxaliplatin, oxytocin, paclitaxel, palonosetron, pamidronate, pancuronium, papaverine, pentazocine, perphenazine, phenobarbital, phenylephrine, phytonadione, potassium acetate, potassium chloride, procainamide, prochlorperazine, promethazine, propranolol, protamine, pyridoxime, quinupristin/dalfopristin, ranitidine, remifentanil, rituximab, rocuronium, sodium acetate, sodium bicarbonate, streptokinase, succinylcholine, sufentanil, tacrolimus, telavancin, teniposide, theophylline, thiamine, thiotepa, tigecycline, tirofiban, tolazoline, topotecan, trastuzumab, vancomycin, vasopressin, vecuronium, verapamil, vinblastine, vincristine, vinorelbine, voriconazole, zidovudine, zoledronic acid.
- **Y-Site Incompatibility:** allopurinol, amphotericin B cholesteryl, amphotericin B colloidal, amphotericin B lipid complex, amphotericin B liposome, azathioprine, cangrelor, cefazolin, cefotetan, ceftriaxone, dacarbazine, dantrolene, dexamethasone, diazepam, diazoxide, folic acid, ganciclovir, hetastarch, indomethacin, oxacillin, pemetrexed, pentamidine, pentobarbital, phenytoin, piperacillin/tazobactam, propofol, sargramostim, trimethoprim/sulfamethoxazole.
- **Topical:** Cleanse skin before application. Wear gloves during application.
- **Inhaln:** Do not mix *TOBI* with dornase alpha in nebulizer.
- *TOBI Podhaler* capsules are not for oral use. Store capsules in blister until immediately before use. Use new Podhaler device provided with each weekly packet. Check to see capsule is empty after inhaling. If powder remains in capsule, repeat inhalation until capsule is empty.

Patient/Family Teaching

- Instruct patient to report signs of hypersensitivity, tinnitus, vertigo, hearing loss, rash, dizziness, or difficulty urinating.
- Advise patient of the importance of drinking plenty of liquids.
- Teach patients with a history of rheumatic heart disease or valve replacement the importance of using antimicrobial prophylaxis before invasive medical or dental procedures.

- Advise female patient to notify health care professional if pregnancy is planned or suspected or if breast feeding.
- **PO:** Instruct patient to take neomycin as directed for full course of therapy. Take missed doses as soon as possible if not almost time for next dose; do not take double doses.
- Caution patient that neomycin may cause nausea, vomiting, or diarrhea.
- **Topical:** Instruct patient to wash affected skin gently and pat dry. Apply a thin film of ointment. Apply occlusive dressing only if directed by health care professional. Patient should assess skin and inform health care professional if skin irritation develops or infection worsens.
- **Inhaln:** Instruct patient to take inhalation twice daily as close to 12 hr apart as possible; not <6 hr apart. Solution is colorless to pale yellow and may darken with age without effecting quality. Administer over 15 min period using a hand-held PARI LC PLUS reusable nebulizer with a *PARI VIOS (for Bethkis) or DeVibiss Pulmo Aide (for TOBI)* compressor. Instruct patient on multiple therapies to take others first and use *tobramycin* last. Tobramycin-induced bronchospasm may be reduced if tobramycin is administered after bronchodilators. Instruct patient to sit or stand upright during inhalation and breathe normally through mouthpiece of nebulizer. Nose clips may help patient breath through mouth. Store at room temperature for up to 28 days. Advise patient to disinfect the nebulizer parts (except tubing) by boiling them in water for a full 10 minutes every other treatment day.
- Instruct patient in correct technique for use of *TOBI Podhaler*. Wipe mouthpiece with clean, dry cloth after use; do not wash with water.

Evaluation/Desired Outcomes

- Resolution of the signs and symptoms of infection. If no response is seen within 3–5 days, new cultures should be taken.
- Prevention of infection in intestinal surgery (neomycin).
- Improved neurologic status in hepatic encephalopathy (neomycin).
- Endocarditis prophylaxis (gentamicin).

HIGH ALERT

amiodarone

(am-ee-**oh**-da-rone)

✤Cordarone, Nexterone, Pacerone

Classification

Therapeutic: antiarrhythmics (class III)

Pregnancy Category D

Indications

Life-threatening ventricular arrhythmias unresponsive to less toxic agents. **Unlabeled Use: PO:** Management of supraventricular tachyarrhythmias. **IV:** As part of the Advanced Cardiac Life Support (ACLS) and Pediatric Advanced Life Support (PALS) guidelines for the management of ventricular fibrillation (VF)/pulseless ventricular tachycardia (VT) after cardiopulmonary resuscitation and defibrillation have failed; also for other life-threatening tachyarrhythmias.

Action

Prolongs action potential and refractory period. Inhibits adrenergic stimulation. Slows the sinus rate, increases PR and QT intervals, and decreases peripheral vascular resistance (vasodilation). **Therapeutic Effects:** Suppression of arrhythmias.

Pharmacokinetics

Absorption: Slowly and variably absorbed from the GI tract (35–65%). IV administration results in complete bioavailability.
Distribution: Distributed to and accumulates slowly in body tissues. Reaches high levels in fat, muscle, liver, lungs, and spleen. Crosses the placenta and enters breast milk.
Protein Binding: 96% bound to plasma proteins.
Metabolism and Excretion: Metabolized by the liver, excreted into bile. Minimal renal excretion. One metabolite has antiarrhythmic activity.
Half-life: 13–107 days.

TIME/ACTION PROFILE (suppression of ventricular arrhythmias)

ROUTE	ONSET	PEAK	DURATION
PO	2–3 days (up to 2–3 mo)	3–7 hr	wk–mos
IV	2 hr	3–7 hr	unknown

Contraindications/Precautions

Contraindicated in: Patients with cardiogenic shock; Severe sinus node dysfunction; 2nd- and 3rd-degree AV block; Bradycardia (has caused syncope unless a pacemaker is in place); Hypersensitivity to amiodarone or iodine; OB: Can cause fetal hypo- or hyperthyroidism; Lactation: Enters breast milk and can cause harm to the neonate; use an alternative to breast milk; Pedi: Safety not established; products containing benzyl alcohol should not be used in neonates.
Use Cautiously in: History of HF; Thyroid disorders; Corneal refractive laser surgery; Severe pulmonary or liver disease; Geri: Initiate therapy at the low end of the dosing range due to ↓ hepatic, renal, or cardiac function; comorbid disease; or other drug therapy.

Adverse Reactions/Side Effects

CNS: confusional states, disorientation, hallucinations, dizziness, fatigue, malaise, headache, insomnia. **EENT:** corneal microdeposits, abnormal sense of smell, dry eyes, optic neuritis, optic neuropathy, photophobia. **Resp:** ADULT RESPIRATORY DISTRESS SYNDROME (ARDS), PULMONARY FIBROSIS, PULMONARY TOXICITY. **CV:** CHF,

WORSENING OF ARRHYTHMIAS, QT INTERVAL PROLONGATION, bradycardia, hypotension. **GI:** anorexia, constipation, nausea, vomiting, abdominal pain, abnormal sense of taste, ↑ liver enzymes. **GU:** ↓ libido, epididymitis. **Derm:** TOXIC EPIDERMAL NECROLYSIS (rare), photosensitivity, blue discoloration. **Endo:** hypothyroidism, hyperthyroidism. **Neuro:** ataxia, involuntary movement, paresthesia, peripheral neuropathy, poor coordination, tremor.

Interactions

Drug-Drug: ↑ risk of QT prolongation with **fluoroquinolones**, **macrolides**, and **azole antifungals** (undertake concurrent use with caution). ↑ levels of **digoxin** (↓ dose of digoxin by 50%). ↑ levels of **class I antiarrhythmics** (**quinidine**, **mexiletine**, **lidocaine**, or **flecainide**— ↓ doses of other drugs by 30–50%). ↑ levels of **cyclosporine**, **dextromethorphan**, **methotrexate**, **phenytoin**, **carvedilol**, and **theophylline**. **Phenytoin** ↓ amiodarone levels. ↑ activity of **warfarin** (↓ dose of warfarin by 33–50%). ↑ risk of bradyarrhythmias, sinus arrest, or AV heart block with **beta blockers** or **calcium channel blockers**. **Cholestyramine** may ↓ amiodarone levels. **Cimetidine** and **ritonavir** ↑ amiodarone levels. Risk of myocardial depression is ↑ by **volatile anesthetics**. ↑ risk of myopathy with **lovastatin** and **simvastatin** (do not exceed 40 mg/day of lovastatin or 20 mg/day of simvastatin).

Drug-Natural Products: St. John's wort induces enzymes that metabolize amiodarone; may ↓ levels and effectiveness. Avoid concurrent use.

Drug-Food: Grapefruit juice inhibits enzymes in the GI tract that metabolize amiodarone resulting in ↑ levels and risk of toxicity; avoid concurrent use.

Route/Dosage

Ventricular Arrhythmias

PO (Adults): 800–1600 mg/day in 1–2 doses for 1–3 wk, then 600–800 mg/day in 1–2 doses for 1 mo, then 400 mg/day maintenance dose.

PO (Children): 10 mg/kg/day (800 mg/1.72 m^2/day) for 10 days or until response or adverse reaction occurs, then 5 mg/kg/day (400 mg/1.72 m^2/day) for several weeks, then ↓ to 2.5 mg/kg/day (200 mg/1.72 m^2/day) or lowest effective maintenance dose.

IV (Adults): 150 mg over 10 min, followed by 360 mg over the next 6 hr and then 540 mg over the next 18 hr. Continue infusion at 0.5 mg/min until oral therapy is initiated. If arrhythmia recurs, a small loading infusion of 150 mg over 10 min should be given; in addition, the rate of the maintenance infusion may be ↑. *Conversion to initial oral therapy*—If duration of IV infusion was <1 wk, oral dose should be 800–1600 mg/day; if IV infusion was 1–3 wk, oral dose should be 600–800 mg/day; if IV infusion was >3 wk, oral dose should be 400 mg/day. *ACLS guidelines for pulseless VF/VT*—300 mg IV push, may repeat once after 3–5 min with 150 mg IV push (maximum cumulative dose 2.2 g/24 hr; unlabeled).

IV: Intraosseous (Children and infants): *PALS guidelines for pulseless VF/VT*—5 mg/kg as a bolus; *Perfusion tachycardia*—5 mg/kg loading dose over 20–60 min (maximum of 15 mg/kg/day; unlabeled).

Supraventricular Tachycardia

PO (Adults): 600–800 mg/day for 1 wk or until desired response occurs or side effects develop, then ↓ to 400 mg/day for 3 wk, then maintenance dose of 200–400 mg/day.

PO (Children): 10 mg/kg/day (800 mg/1.72 m^2/day) for 10 days or until response or side effects occur, then 5 mg/kg/day (400 mg/1.72 m^2/day) for several weeks, then ↓ to 2.5 mg/kg/day (200 mg/1.72 m^2/day) or lowest effective maintenance dose.

Availability (generic available)

Tablets: 100 mg, 200 mg, 400 mg. **Injection:** 50 mg/mL. **Premixed infusion (Nexterone):** 150 mg/100 mL D5W (does not contain polysorbate 80 or benzyl alcohol), 360 mg/200 mL D5W (does not contain polysorbate 80 or benzyl alcohol).

NURSING IMPLICATIONS

Assessment

- Monitor ECG continuously during IV therapy or initiation of oral therapy. Monitor heart rate and rhythm throughout therapy; PR prolongation, slight QRS widening, T-wave amplitude reduction with T-wave widening and bifurcation, and U waves may occur. QT prolongation may be associated with worsening of arrhythmias; monitor closely during IV therapy. Report bradycardia or increase in arrhythmias promptly; patients receiving IV therapy may require slowing rate, discontinuing infusion, or inserting a temporary pacemaker.
- Assess pacing and defibrillation threshold in patients with pacemakers and implanted defibrillators at beginning and periodically during therapy.
- Assess for signs of pulmonary toxicity (rales/crackles, decreased breath sounds, pleuritic friction rub, fatigue, dyspnea, cough, wheezing, pleuritic pain, fever, hemoptysis, hypoxia). Chest x-ray and pulmonary function tests are recommended before therapy. Monitor chest x-ray every 3–6 mo during therapy to detect diffuse interstitial changes or alveolar infiltrates. Bronchoscopy or gallium radionuclide scan may also be used for diagnosis. Usually reversible after withdrawal, but fatalities have occurred.
- **IV:** Assess for signs and symptoms of ARDS throughout therapy. Report dyspnea, tachypnea, or rales/crackles promptly. Bilateral, diffuse pulmonary infiltrates are seen on chest x-ray.

- Monitor BP frequently. Hypotension usually occurs during first several hours of therapy and is related to rate of infusion. If hypotension occurs, slow rate.
- **PO:** Assess for neurotoxicity (ataxia, proximal muscle weakness, tingling or numbness in fingers or toes, uncontrolled movements, tremors); common during initial therapy, but may occur within 1 wk to several mo of initiation of therapy and may persist for more than 1 yr after withdrawal. Dose reduction is recommended. Assist patient during ambulation to prevent falls.
- Ophthalmic exams should be performed before and regularly during therapy and whenever visual changes (photophobia, halos around lights, decreased acuity) occur. May cause permanent loss of vision.
- Assess for signs of thyroid dysfunction, especially during initial therapy. Lethargy; weight gain; edema of the hands, feet, and periorbital region; and cool, pale skin suggest hypothyroidism and may require decrease in dose or discontinuation of therapy and thyroid supplementation. Tachycardia; weight loss; nervousness; sensitivity to heat; insomnia; and warm, flushed, moist skin suggest hyperthyroidism and may require discontinuation of therapy and treatment with antithyroid agents.
- ***Lab Test Considerations:*** Monitor liver and thyroid functions before and every 6 mo during therapy. Drug effects persist long after discontinuation. Thyroid function abnormalities are common, but clinical thyroid dysfunction is uncommon.
- Monitor AST, ALT, and alkaline phosphatase at regular intervals during therapy, especially in patients receiving high maintenance dose. If liver function studies are 3 times normal or double in patients with elevated baseline levels or if hepatomegaly occurs, dose should be reduced.
- May cause asymptomatic ↑ in ANA titer concentrations.
- Monitor serum potassium, calcium, and magnesium prior to starting and periodically during therapy. Hypokalemia, hypocalcemia, and/or hypomagnesemia may ↓ effectiveness or cause additional arrhythmias; correct levels before beginning therapy. Monitor closely when converting from IV to oral therapy, especially in geriatric patients.

Potential Nursing Diagnoses

Decreased cardiac output (Indications)
Impaired gas exchange (Side Effects)

Implementation

- ***High Alert:*** IV vasoactive medications are inherently dangerous; fatalities have occurred from medication errors involving amiodarone. Before administering, have second practitioner check original order, dose calculations, and infusion pump settings. Patients should be hospitalized and monitored closely during IV therapy and initiation of oral therapy. IV therapy should be administered only by physicians experienced in treating life-threatening arrhythmias.
- Do not confuse amiodarone with amantadine.
- **PO:** May be administered with meals and in divided doses if GI intolerance occurs or if daily dose exceeds 1000 mg.

IV Administration

- **IV:** Administer via volumetric pump; drop size may be reduced, causing altered dosing with drop counter infusion sets.
- Administer through an in-line filter.
- Infusions exceeding 2 hr must be administered in glass or polyolefin bottles to prevent adsorption. However, polyvinyl chloride (PVC) tubing must be used during administration because concentrations and infusion rate recommendations have been based on PVC tubing.
- **IV Push: *Diluent:*** Administer undiluted. May also be diluted in 20–30 mL of D5W or 0.9% NaCl. ***Concentration:*** 50 mg/mL. ***Rate:*** Administer IV push.
- **Intermittent Infusion: *Diluent:*** Dilute 150 mg of amiodarone in 100 mL of D5W. Infusion stable for 2 hr in PVC bag, or use pre-mixed bags. ***Concentration:*** 1.5 mg/mL. ***Rate:*** Infuse over 10 min. Do not administer IV push.
- **Continuous Infusion: *Diluent:*** Dilute 900 mg (18 mL) of amiodarone in 500 mL of D5W. Infusion stable for 24 hr in glass or polyolefin bottle. ***Concentration:*** 1.8 mg/mL. Concentration may range from 1–6 mg/mL (concentrations >2 m g/mL must be administered via central venous catheter). ***Rate:*** Infuse at a rate of 1 mg/min for the first 6 hr, then decrease infusion rate to 0.5 mg/min and continue until oral therapy initiated.
- **Y-Site Compatibility:** alemtuzumab, alfentanil, amikacin, amphotericin B lipid complex, anidulafungin, atracurium, atropine, bleomycin, buprenorphine, busulfan, butorphanol, calcium chloride, cangrelor, carboplatin, carmustine, caspofungin, ceftaroline, chlorpromazine, ciprofloxacin, cisatracurium, cisplatin, clindamycin, cyclophosphamide, dacarbazine, dactinomycin, daptomycin, daunorubicin, dexmedetomidine, dexrazoxane, diltiazem, diphenhydramine, docetaxel, dolasetron, dopamine, doripenem, doxycycline, droperidol, enalaprilat, ephedrine, epinephrine, erythromycin lactobionate, esmolol, etoposide, etoposide phosphate, famotidine, fenoldopam, fluconazole, gemcitabine, gentamicin, glycopyrrolate, granisetron, haloperidol, hydralazine, hydromorphone, idarubicin, ifosfamide, irinotecan, isoproterenol, ketamine, labetalol, lidocaine, linezolid, lorazepam, mannitol, meperidine, mesna, metoclopramide, metoprolol, metronidazole, midazolam, milrinone, mitoxantrone, morphine, moxifloxacin, mycophenolate, nafcillin, nalbuphine, naloxone, nesiritide, nicardipine, nitroglycerin, octreotide, ondansetron, oxaliplatin, palonosetron, pancuronium, pemetrexed, penicillin

G potassium, pentamidine, pentazocine, phenylephrine, procainamide, prochlorperazine, promethazine, propranolol, quinupristin/dalfopristin, remifentanil, rifampin, rocuronium, streptozocin, succinylcholine, sufentanil, tacrolimus, teniposide, theophylline, tirofiban, tobramycin, topotecan, vancomycin, vasopressin, vecuronium, vinblastine, vincristine, vinorelbine, voriconazole, zoledronic acid.

- **Y-Site Incompatibility:** acyclovir, allopurinol, amifostine, aminocaproic acid, aminophylline, ampicillin, ampicillin/sulbactam, azithromycin, bivalirudin, cefotaxime, cefotetan, ceftazidime, chloramphenicol, cytarabine, dantrolene, dexamethasone, diazepam, digoxin, doxorubicin, ertapenem, fludarabine, fluorouracil, foscarnet, fosphenytoin, ganciclovir, heparin, hydrocortisone, imipenem-cilastatin, ketorolac, leucovorin, levofloxacin, mechlorethamine, melphalan, meropenem, methotrexate, micafungin, mitomycin, paclitaxel, pentobarbital, phenobarbital, phenytoin, piperacillin/tazobactam, potassium acetate, potassium phosphates, ranitidine, sodium acetate, sodium bicarbonate, sodium phosphates, thiopental, thiotepa, tigecycline, trimethoprim/sulfamethoxazole, verapamil.

Patient/Family Teaching

- Instruct patient to take amiodarone as directed. If a dose is missed, do not take at all. Consult health care professional if more than two doses are missed. Advise patient to read the *Medication Guide* prior to first dose and with each Rx refill in case of changes.
- Advise patient to avoid drinking grapefruit juice during therapy.
- Inform patient that side effects may not appear until several days, weeks, or yr after initiation of therapy and may persist for several mo after withdrawal.
- Teach patients to monitor pulse daily and report abnormalities.
- Advise patients that photosensitivity reactions may occur through window glass, thin clothing, and sunscreens. Protective clothing and sunblock are recommended during and for 4 mo after therapy. If photosensitivity occurs, dose reduction may be useful.
- Inform patients that bluish discoloration of the face, neck, and arms is a possible side effect of this drug after prolonged use. This is usually reversible and will fade over several mo. Notify health care professional if this occurs.
- Instruct male patients to notify health care professional if signs of epididymitis (pain and swelling in scrotum) occur. May require reduction in dose.
- Advise patient to notify health care professional of all Rx or OTC medications, vitamins, or herbal products being taken and to consult with health care professional before taking other medications, especially St. John's wort.
- Instruct patient to notify health care professional of medication regimen before treatment or surgery.
- Advise patient to notify health care professional if signs and symptoms of thyroid dysfunction occur.
- Advise female patient to notify health care professional if pregnancy is planned or suspected and to avoid breast feeding during therapy.
- Emphasize the importance of follow-up exams, including chest x-ray and pulmonary function tests every 3–6 mo and ophthalmic exams after 6 mo of therapy, and then annually.

Evaluation/Desired Outcomes

- Cessation of life-threatening ventricular arrhythmias. Adverse effects may take up to 4 mo to resolve.

amitriptyline

(a-mee-**trip**-ti-leen)

✤Elavil, ✤Levate

Classification

Therapeutic: antidepressants

Pharmacologic: tricyclic antidepressants

Pregnancy Category C

Indications

Depression. **Unlabeled Use:** Anxiety, insomnia, treatment-resistant depression. Chronic pain syndromes (i.e., fibromyalgia, neuropathic pain/chronic pain, headache, low back pain).

Action

Potentiates the effect of serotonin and norepinephrine in the CNS. Has significant anticholinergic properties. **Therapeutic Effects:** Antidepressant action.

Pharmacokinetics

Absorption: Well absorbed from the GI tract.

Distribution: Widely distributed.

Protein Binding: 95% bound to plasma proteins.

Metabolism and Excretion: Extensively metabolized by the liver. Some metabolites have antidepressant activity. Undergoes enterohepatic recirculation and secretion into gastric juices. Probably crosses the placenta and enters breast milk.

Half-life: 10–50 hr.

TIME/ACTION PROFILE (antidepressant effect)

ROUTE	ONSET	PEAK	DURATION
PO	2–3 wk (up to 30 days)	2–6 wk	days–wk

Contraindications/Precautions

Contraindicated in: Angle-closure glaucoma; Known history of QTc interval prolongation, recent MI, or heart failure.

Use Cautiously in: May ↑ risk of suicide attempt/ideation especially during dose early treatment or dose adjustment; risk may be greater in children or adolescents; Patients with pre-existing cardiovascular disease; Prostatic hyperplasia (↑ risk of urinary retention); History of seizures (threshold may be ↓); OB: Use only if clearly needed and maternal benefits outweigh risk to fetus; Lactation: May cause sedation in infant; Pedi: Children <12 yr (safety not established); Geri: Appears on Beers list. ↑ risk of adverse reactions including falls secondary to sedative and anticholinergic effects.

Adverse Reactions/Side Effects

CNS: SUICIDAL THOUGHTS, lethargy, sedation. **EENT:** blurred vision, dry eyes, dry mouth. **CV:** ARRHYTHMIAS, TORSADE DE POINTES, hypotension, ECG changes, QT interval prolongation. **GI:** constipation, hepatitis, paralytic ileus, ↑ appetite, weight gain. **GU:** urinary retention, ↓ libido. **Derm:** photosensitivity. **Endo:** changes in blood glucose, gynecomastia. **Hemat:** blood dyscrasias.

Interactions

Drug-Drug: Amitriptyline is metabolized in the liver by the cytochrome P450 2D6 enzyme, and its action may be affected by drugs that compete for metabolism by this enzyme, including other **antidepressants**, **phenothiazines**, **carbamazepine**, **class 1C antiarrhythmics** including **propafenone**, and **flecainide**; when these drugs are used concurrently with amitriptyline, dosage ↓ of one or the other or both may be necessary. Concurrent use of other drugs that inhibit the activity of the enzyme, including **cimetidine**, **quinidine**, **amiodarone**, and **ritonavir**, may result in ↑ effects of amitriptyline. May cause hypotension, tachycardia, and potentially fatal reactions when used with **MAO inhibitors** (avoid concurrent use—discontinue 2 wk before starting amitriptyline). Concurrent use with **SSRI antidepressants** may result in ↑ toxicity and should be avoided (**fluoxetine** should be stopped 5 wk before starting amitriptyline). Concurrent use with **clonidine** may result in hypertensive crisis and should be avoided. Concurrent use with **levodopa** may result in delayed or ↓ absorption of levodopa or hypertension. Blood levels and effects may be ↓ by **rifampin**, **rifapentine**, and **rifabutin**. Concurrent use with **moxifloxacin** ↑ risk of adverse cardiovascular reactions. ↑ CNS depression with other **CNS depressants** including **alcohol**, **antihistamines**, **clonidine**, **opioids**, and **sedative/hypnotics**. **Barbiturates** may alter blood levels and effects. **Adrenergic** and **anticholinergic** side effects may be ↑ with other agents having **anticholinergic** properties. **Phenothiazines** or **oral contraceptives** ↑ levels and may cause toxicity. **Nicotine** may ↑ metabolism and alter effects.

Drug-Natural Products: **St. John's wort** may ↓ serum concentrations and efficacy. Concomitant use of **kava-kava**, **valerian**, or **chamomile** can ↑ CNS depression. ↑ anticholinergic effects with **jimson weed** and **scopolia**.

Route/Dosage

PO (Adults): 75 mg/day in divided doses; may be ↑ up to 150 mg/day *or* 50–100 mg at bedtime, may ↑ by 25–50 mg up to 150 mg (in hospitalized patients, may initiate with 100 mg/day, and ↑ total daily dose up to 300 mg).

PO (Geriatric Patients): 10–25 mg at bedtime; may ↑ by 10–25 mg weekly if tolerated (usual dose range = 25–150 mg/day).

Availability (generic available)

Tablets: 10 mg, 25 mg, 50 mg, 75 mg, 100 mg, 150 mg. **Cost:** *Generic*—25 mg $9.33/100, 75 mg $9.83/100.

NURSING IMPLICATIONS

Assessment

- Obtain weight and BMI initially and periodically during treatment.
- Assess fasting glucose and cholesterol levels in overweight/obese individuals.
- Monitor BP and pulse before and during initial therapy. Notify health care professional of decreases in BP (10–20 mm Hg) or sudden increase in pulse rate. Patients taking high doses or with a history of cardiovascular disease should have ECG monitored before and periodically during therapy.
- **Depression:** Monitor mental status (orientation, mood behavior) frequently. Assess for suicidal tendencies, especially during early therapy. Restrict amount of drug available to patient.
- Assess for suicidal tendencies, especially during early therapy. Restrict amount of drug available to patient. Risk may be increased in children, adolescents, and adults ≤24 yrs. After starting therapy, children, adolescents, and young adults should be seen by health care professional at least weekly for 4 wk, every 3 wk for next 4 wk, and on advice of health care professional thereafter.
- **Pain:** Assess intensity, quality, and location of pain periodically during therapy. May require several weeks for effects to be seen. Use pain scale to monitor effectiveness of medication. Assess for sexual dysfunction (decreased libido; erectile dysfunction). Geri: Geriatric patients started on amitriptyline may be at an increased risk for falls; start with low dose and monitor closely. Assess for anticholinergic effects (weakness and sedation).
- ***Lab Test Considerations:*** Assess leukocyte and differential blood counts, liver function, and serum glucose before and periodically during therapy. May cause an ↑ serum bilirubin and alkaline phosphatase. May cause bone marrow depression. Serum glucose may be ↑ or ↓.

Potential Nursing Diagnoses

Ineffective coping (Indications)
Chronic pain (Indications)
Risk for injury (Side Effects)

Implementation

- Dose increases should be made at bedtime because of sedation. Dose titration is a slow process; may take weeks to months. May give entire dose at bedtime. Sedative effect may be apparent before antidepressant effect is noted. May require tapering to avoid withdrawal effects.
- **PO:** Administer medication with or immediately after a meal to minimize gastric upset. Tablet may be crushed and given with food or fluids.

Patient/Family Teaching

- Instruct patient to take medication as directed. If a dose is missed, take as soon as possible unless almost time for next dose; if regimen is a single dose at bedtime, do not take in the morning because of side effects. Advise patient that drug effects may not be noticed for at least 2 wk. Abrupt discontinuation may cause nausea, vomiting, diarrhea, headache, trouble sleeping with vivid dreams, and irritability.
- May cause drowsiness and blurred vision. Caution patient to avoid driving and other activities requiring alertness until response to drug is known.
- Orthostatic hypotension, sedation, and confusion are common during early therapy, especially in geriatric patients. Protect patient from falls and advise patient to make position changes slowly. Institute fall precautions. Advise patient to make position changes slowly. Refer as appropriate for nutrition/weight management and medical management.
- Advise patient to avoid alcohol or other CNS depressant drugs during and for 3–7 days after therapy has been discontinued.
- Advise patient, family and caregivers to look for suicidality, especially during early therapy or dose changes. Notify health care professional immediately if thoughts about suicide or dying, attempts to commit suicide, new or worse depression or anxiety, agitation or restlessness, panic attacks, insomnia, new or worse irritability, aggressiveness, acting on dangerous impulses, mania, or other changes in mood or behavior occur.
- Instruct patient to notify health care professional if urinary retention, dry mouth, or constipation persists. Sugarless candy or gum may diminish dry mouth, and an increase in fluid intake or bulk may prevent constipation. If symptoms persist, dose reduction or discontinuation may be necessary. Consult health care professional if dry mouth persists for >2 wk.
- Caution patient to use sunscreen and protective clothing to prevent photosensitivity reactions. Alert patient that medication may turn urine blue-green in color.
- Inform patient of need to monitor dietary intake. Increase in appetite may lead to undesired weight gain.
- Advise patient to notify health care professional of medication regimen before treatment or surgery. Medication should be discontinued as long as possible before surgery.
- Advise patient to notify health care professional if pregnancy is planned or suspected or if breast feeding.
- Therapy for depression is usually prolonged and should be continued for at least 3 mo to prevent relapse. Emphasize the importance of follow-up exams to monitor effectiveness, side effects, and improved coping skills. Advise patient and family that treatment is not a cure and symptoms can recur after discontinuation of medication.

Evaluation/Desired Outcomes

- Increased sense of well-being.
- Renewed interest in surroundings.
- Increased appetite.
- Improved energy level.
- Improved sleep.
- Decrease in chronic pain symptoms.
- Full therapeutic effects may be seen 2–6 wk after initiating therapy.

amLODIPine (am-loe-di-peen)

Norvasc

Classification

Therapeutic: antihypertensives

Pharmacologic: calcium channel blockers

Pregnancy Category C

Indications

Alone or with other agents in the management of hypertension, angina pectoris, and vasospastic (Prinzmetal's) angina.

Action

Inhibits the transport of calcium into myocardial and vascular smooth muscle cells, resulting in inhibition of excitation-contraction coupling and subsequent contraction. **Therapeutic Effects:** Systemic vasodilation resulting in decreased BP. Coronary vasodilation resulting in decreased frequency and severity of attacks of angina.

Pharmacokinetics

Absorption: Well absorbed after oral administration (64–90%).

Distribution: Probably crosses the placenta.

Protein Binding: 95–98%.

Metabolism and Excretion: Mostly metabolized by the liver.

Half-life: 30–50 hr (↑ in geriatric patients and patients with hepatic impairment).

TIME/ACTION PROFILE (cardiovascular effects)

ROUTE	ONSET	PEAK	DURATION
PO	unknown	6–9	24 hr

Contraindications/Precautions

Contraindicated in: Hypersensitivity; Systolic BP <90 mm Hg.

Use Cautiously in: Severe hepatic impairment (dose reduction recommended); Aortic stenosis; History of HF; OB, Lactation, Pedi: Children <6 yr (safety not established); Geri: Dose reduction recommended; ↑ risk of hypotension.

Adverse Reactions/Side Effects

CNS: dizziness, fatigue. **CV:** peripheral edema, angina, bradycardia, hypotension, palpitations. **GI:** gingival hyperplasia, nausea. **Derm:** flushing.

Interactions

Drug-Drug: Strong CYP3A4 inhibitors, including **ketoconazole**, **itraconazole**, **clarithromycin**, and **ritonavir** may ↑ levels. Additive hypotension may occur when used concurrently with **fentanyl**, other **antihypertensives**, **nitrates**, acute ingestion of **alcohol**, or **quinidine**. Antihypertensive effects may be ↓ by concurrent use of **nonsteroidal anti-inflammatory agents**. May ↑ risk of neurotoxicity with **lithium**. ↑ risk of myopathy with **simvastatin** (do not exceed 20 mg/day of simvastatin). May ↑ **cyclosporine** and **tacrolimus** levels.

Route/Dosage

PO (Adults): 5–10 mg once daily; *antihypertensive in fragile or small patients or patients already receiving other antihypertensives*—initiate at 2.5 mg/day, ↑ as required/tolerated (up to 10 mg/day) as an antihypertensive therapy with 2.5 mg/day in patients with hepatic insufficiency.

PO (Geriatric Patients): *Antihypertensive*—Initiate therapy at 2.5 mg/day, ↑ as required/tolerated (up to 10 mg/day); *antianginal*—initiate therapy at 5 mg/day, ↑ as required/tolerated (up to 10 mg/day).

PO (Children 6–17 yr): 2.5–5 mg once daily.

Hepatic Impairment

PO (Adults): *Antihypertensive*—Initiate therapy at 2.5 mg/day, ↑ as required/tolerated (up to 10 mg/day); *antianginal*—initiate therapy at 5 mg/day, ↑ as required/tolerated (up to 10 mg/day).

Availability (generic available)

Tablets: 2.5 mg, 5 mg, 10 mg. **Cost:** *Generic*—2.5 mg $11.35/100, 5 mg $12.86/100, 10 mg $8.42/100. ***In combination with:*** aliskiren/hydrochlorothiazide (Amturnide), atorvastatin (Caduet), benazepril (Lotrel), olmesartan (Azor), perindopril (Prestalia), telmisartan (Twynsta), valsartan (Exforge), olmesartan/hydrochlorothiazide (Tribenzor), and valsartan/hydrochlorothiazide (Exforge HCT). See Appendix B.

NURSING IMPLICATIONS

Assessment

- Monitor BP and pulse before therapy, during dose titration, and periodically during therapy. Monitor ECG periodically during prolonged therapy.
- Monitor intake and output ratios and daily weight. Assess for signs of HF (peripheral edema, rales/crackles, dyspnea, weight gain, jugular venous distention).
- Monitor frequency of prescription refills to determine adherence.
- **Angina:** Assess location, duration, intensity, and precipitating factors of patient's anginal pain.
- ***Lab Test Considerations:*** Total serum calcium concentrations are not affected by calcium channel blockers.

Potential Nursing Diagnoses

Ineffective tissue perfusion (Indications)
Acute pain (Indications)

Implementation

- **Do not confuse amlodipine with amiloride. Do not confuse Norvasc with Navane.**
- **PO:** May be administered without regard to meals.

Patient/Family Teaching

- Advise patient to take medication as directed, even if feeling well. Take missed doses as soon as possible within 12 hrs of missed dose. If >12 hrs since missed dose, skip dose and take next dose at scheduled time; do not double doses. May need to be discontinued gradually.
- Instruct patient on correct technique for monitoring pulse. Instruct patient to contact health care professional if heart rate is <50 bpm.
- Caution patient to change positions slowly to minimize orthostatic hypotension.
- May cause drowsiness or dizziness. Advise patient to avoid driving or other activities requiring alertness until response to the medication is known.
- Instruct patient on importance of maintaining good dental hygiene and seeing dentist frequently for teeth cleaning to prevent tenderness, bleeding, and gingival hyperplasia (gum enlargement).
- Instruct patient to notify health care professional of all Rx or OTC medications, vitamins, or herbal products being taken, to avoid alcohol, and to consult health care professional before taking any new medications, especially cold preparations.
- Advise patient to notify health care professional if irregular heartbeats, dyspnea, swelling of hands and feet, pronounced dizziness, nausea, constipation, or hypotension occurs or if headache is severe or persistent.
- Caution patient to wear protective clothing and use sunscreen to prevent photosensitivity reactions.
- Advise patient to inform health care professional of medication regimen before treatment or surgery.

- Instruct female patient to notify health care professional if pregnancy is planned or suspected or if breast feeding.
- **Angina:** Instruct patient on concurrent nitrate or beta-blocker therapy to continue taking both medications as directed and to use SL nitroglycerin as needed for anginal attacks.
- Advise patient to contact health care professional if chest pain does not improve or worsens after therapy, if it occurs with diaphoresis, if shortness of breath occurs, or if severe, persistent headache occurs.
- Caution patient to discuss exercise restrictions with health care professional before exertion.
- **Hypertension:** Encourage patient to comply with other interventions for hypertension (weight reduction, low-sodium diet, smoking cessation, moderation of alcohol consumption, regular exercise, and stress management). Medication controls but does not cure hypertension.
- Instruct patient and family in proper technique for monitoring BP. Advise patient to take BP weekly and to report significant changes to health care professional.

Evaluation/Desired Outcomes

- Decrease in BP.
- Decrease in frequency and severity of anginal attacks.
- Decrease in need for nitrate therapy.
- Increase in activity tolerance and sense of well-being.

amoxicillin (a-mox-i-**sill**-in)

~~Amoxil~~, Moxatag, ✱Novamoxin, ~~Trimox~~

Classification
Therapeutic: anti-infectives, antiulcer agents
Pharmacologic: aminopenicillins

Pregnancy Category B

Indications

Treatment of: Skin and skin structure infections, Otitis media, Sinusitis, Respiratory infections, Genitourinary infections. Endocarditis prophylaxis. Postexposure inhalational anthrax prophylaxis. Management of ulcer disease due to *Helicobacter pylori*. **Unlabeled Use:** Lyme disease in children <8 yr.

Action

Binds to bacterial cell wall, causing cell death. **Therapeutic Effects:** Bactericidal action; spectrum is broader than penicillins. **Spectrum:** Active against: Streptococci, Pneumococci, Enterococci, *Haemophilus influenzae*, *Escherichia coli*, *Proteus mirabilis*, *Neisseria meningitidis*, *N. gonorrhoeae*, *Shigella*, *Chlamydia trachomatis*, *Salmonella*, *Borrelia burgdorferi*, *H. pylori*.

Pharmacokinetics

Absorption: Well absorbed from duodenum (75–90%). More resistant to acid inactivation than other penicillins.
Distribution: Diffuses readily into most body tissues and fluids. CSF penetration increased when meninges are inflamed. Crosses placenta; enters breast milk in small amounts.
Metabolism and Excretion: 70% excreted unchanged in the urine; 30% metabolized by the liver.
Half-life: Neonates: 3.7 hr; Infants and Children: 1–2 hr; Adults: 0.7–1.4 hr.

TIME/ACTION PROFILE (blood levels)

ROUTE	ONSET	PEAK	DURATION
PO	30 min	1–2 hr	8–12 hr

Contraindications/Precautions

Contraindicated in: Hypersensitivity to penicillins (cross-sensitivity exists to cephalosporins and other beta-lactams).
Use Cautiously in: Severe renal insufficiency (↓ dose if CCr <30 mL/min); Infectious mononucleosis, acute lymphocytic leukemia, or cytomegalovirus infection (↑ risk of rash); **OB, Lactation:** Has been used safely.

Adverse Reactions/Side Effects

CNS: SEIZURES (high doses). **GI:** CLOSTRIDIUM DIFFICILE-ASSOCIATED DIARRHEA (CDAD), diarrhea, nausea, vomiting, ↑ liver enzymes. **Derm:** rash, urticaria. **Hemat:** blood dyscrasias. **Misc:** allergic reactions including ANAPHYLAXIS, SERUM SICKNESS, superinfection.

Interactions

Drug-Drug: Probenecid ↓ renal excretion and ↑ blood levels of amoxicillin—therapy may be combined for this purpose. May ↑ effect of **warfarin**. May ↓ effectiveness of **oral contraceptives**. **Allopurinol** may ↑ frequency of rash.

Route/Dosage

Most Infections

PO (Adults): 250–500 mg q 8 hr *or* 500–875 mg q 12 hr (not to exceed 2–3 g/day).
PO (Adults and Children ≥12 yr): *Extended-release tablets (for Strep throat)*—775 mg once daily for 10 days.
PO (Children >3 mo): 25–50 mg/kg/day in divided doses q 8 hr *or* 25–50 mg/kg/day individual doses q 12 hr; *Acute otitis media due to highly resistant strains of S. pneumoniae*—80–90 mg/kg/day divided q 12 hr; *Postexposure inhalational anthrax*

prophylaxis—<40 kg: 45 mg/kg/day in divided doses q 8 hr; >40 k g: 500 mg q 8 hr.
PO (Infants ≤3 mo and neonates): 20–30 mg/kg/day in divided doses q 12 hr.

H. Pylori

PO (Adults): *Triple therapy*—1000 mg amoxicillin twice daily with lansoprazole 30 mg twice daily and clarithromycin 500 mg twice daily for 14 days *or* 1000 mg amoxicillin twice daily with omeprazole 20 mg twice daily and clarithromycin 500 mg twice daily for 14 days *or* amoxicillin 1000 mg twice daily with esomeprazole 40 mg daily and clarithromycin 500 mg twice daily for 10 days. *Dual therapy*—1000 mg amoxicillin three times daily with lansoprazole 30 mg three times daily for 14 days.

Endocarditis Prophylaxis

PO (Adults): 2 g 1 hr prior to procedure.
PO (Children): 50 mg/kg 1 hr prior to procedure (not to exceed adult dose).

Gonorrhea

PO (Adults and Children ≥40 kg): single 3 g dose.
PO (Children >2 yr and <40 kg): 50 mg/kg with probenecid 25 mg/kg as a single dose.

Renal Impairment

PO (Adults CCr 10–30 mL/min): 250–500 mg q 12 hr.

Renal Impairment

PO (Adults CCr <10 mL/min): 250–500 mg q 24 hr.

Availability (generic available)

Chewable tablets (cherry, banana, peppermint flavors): 125 mg, 200 mg, 250 mg, 400 mg. **Cost:** *Generic*—250 mg $15.89/30. **Tablets:** 500 mg, 875 mg. **Cost:** *Generic*—875 mg $9.53/30. **Extended-release tablets:** 775 mg. **Cost:** $524.90/30. **Capsules:** 250 mg, 500 mg. **Cost:** *Generic*—250 mg $5.90/30, 500 mg $5.90/30. **Suspension (pediatric drops) (bubblegum flavor):** 50 mg/mL. **Powder for oral suspension (strawberry [125 mg/5 mL] and bubblegum [200 mg/5 mL, 250 mg/5 mL, 400 mg/5 mL] flavors):** 125 mg/5 mL, 200 mg/5 mL, 250 mg/5 mL, 400 mg/5 mL. **Cost:** *Generic*—125 mg/5 mL $4.11/150 mL, 200 mg/5 mL $6.84/75 mL, 250 mg/5 mL $6.09/100 mL, 400 mg/5 mL $7.33/75 mL. ***In combination with:*** clarithromycin and lansoprazole in a compliance package (Prevpac). See Appendix B.

NURSING IMPLICATIONS

Assessment

- Assess for infection (vital signs; appearance of wound, sputum, urine, and stool; WBC) at beginning of and throughout therapy.
- Obtain a history before initiating therapy to determine previous use of and reactions to penicillins or cephalosporins. Persons with a negative history of penicillin sensitivity may still have an allergic response.
- Observe for signs and symptoms of anaphylaxis (rash, pruritus, laryngeal edema, wheezing). Notify health care professional immediately if these occur.
- Obtain specimens for culture and sensitivity prior to therapy. First dose may be given before receiving results.
- Monitor bowel function. Diarrhea, abdominal cramping, fever, and bloody stools should be reported to health care professional promptly as a sign of Clostridium difficile-associated diarrhea (CDAD). May begin up to several weeks following cessation of therapy.
- ***Lab Test Considerations:*** May cause ↑ serum alkaline phosphatase, LDH, AST, and ALT concentrations.
- May cause false-positive direct Coombs' test result.

Potential Nursing Diagnoses

Risk for infection (Indications, Side Effects)
Noncompliance (Patient/Family Teaching)

Implementation

- **PO:** Administer around the clock. May be given without regard to meals or with meals to decrease GI side effects. Capsule contents may be emptied and swallowed with liquids. Extended-release tablets should be swallowed whole; do not crush, break, or chew. Chewable tablets should be crushed or chewed before swallowing with liquids.
- Shake oral suspension before administering. Suspension may be given straight or mixed in formula, milk, fruit juice, water, or ginger ale. Administer immediately after mixing. Discard refrigerated reconstituted suspension after 10 days.

Patient/Family Teaching

- Instruct patients to take medication around the clock and to finish the drug completely as directed, even if feeling better. Advise patients that sharing of this medication may be dangerous.
- Pedi: Teach parents or caregivers to calculate and measure doses accurately. Reinforce importance of using measuring device supplied by pharmacy or with product, not household items.
- Advise patient to report the signs of superinfection (furry overgrowth on the tongue, vaginal itching or discharge, loose or foul-smelling stools) and allergy.
- Instruct patient to notify health care professional immediately if diarrhea, abdominal cramping, fever, or bloody stools occur and not to treat with antidiarrheals without consulting health care professional.
- Instruct the patient to notify health care professional if symptoms do not improve.
- Teach patients with a history of rheumatic heart disease or valve replacement the importance of using antimicrobial prophylaxis before invasive medical or dental procedures.
- Instruct female patients taking oral contraceptives to use an alternate or additional nonhormonal method

of contraception during therapy with amoxicillin and until next menstrual period.

Evaluation/Desired Outcomes

- Resolution of the signs and symptoms of infection. Length of time for complete resolution depends on the organism and site of infection.
- Endocarditis prophylaxis.
- Eradication of *H. pylori* with resolution of ulcer symptoms.
- Prevention of inhalational anthrax (postexposure).

amoxicillin/clavulanate

(a-mox-i-**sill**-in/klav-yoo-**lan** -ate)

Augmentin, Augmentin ES, Augmentin XR, ✱Clavulin

Classification

Therapeutic: anti-infectives

Pharmacologic: aminopenicillins/beta lactamase inhibitors

Pregnancy Category B

Indications

Treatment of a variety of infections including: Skin and skin structure infections, Otitis media, Sinusitis, Respiratory tract infections, Genitourinary tract infections.

Action

Binds to bacterial cell wall, causing cell death; spectrum of amoxicillin is broader than penicillin. Clavulanate resists action of beta-lactamase, an enzyme produced by bacteria that is capable of inactivating some penicillins. **Therapeutic Effects:** Bactericidal action against susceptible bacteria. **Spectrum:** Active against: Streptococci, Pneumococci, Enterococci, *Haemophilus influenzae*, *Escherichia coli*, *Proteus mirabilis*, *Neisseria meningitidis*, *N. gonorrhoeae*, *Staphylococcus aureus*, *Klebsiella pneumoniae*, *Shigella*, *Salmonella*, *Moraxella catarrhalis*.

Pharmacokinetics

Absorption: Well absorbed from the duodenum (75–90%). More resistant to acid inactivation than other penicillins.

Distribution: Diffuses readily into most body tissues and fluids. Does not readily enter brain/CSF; CSF penetration is ↑ in the presence of inflamed meninges. Crosses the placenta and enters breast milk in small amounts.

Metabolism and Excretion: 70% excreted unchanged in the urine; 30% metabolized by the liver.

Half-life: 1–1.3 hr.

TIME/ACTION PROFILE (peak blood levels)

ROUTE	ONSET	PEAK	DURATION
PO	30 min	1–2 hr	8–12 hr

Contraindications/Precautions

Contraindicated in: Hypersensitivity to penicillins or clavulanate; Suspension and chewable tablets contain aspartame and should be avoided in phenylketonurics; History of amoxicillin/clavulanate-associated cholestatic jaundice.

Use Cautiously in: Severe renal insufficiency (dose ↓ necessary); Infectious mononucleosis (↑ risk of rash); Hepatic impairment (dose cautiously, monitor liver function).

Adverse Reactions/Side Effects

CNS: SEIZURES (high doses). **GI:** CLOSTRIDIUM DIFFICILE-ASSOCIATED DIARRHEA (CDAD), diarrhea, hepatic dysfunction, nausea, vomiting. **GU:** vaginal candidiasis. **Derm:** rash, urticaria. **Hemat:** blood dyscrasias. **Misc:** allergic reactions including ANAPHYLAXIS and SERUM SICKNESS, superinfection.

Interactions

Drug-Drug: Probenecid ↓ renal excretion and ↑ blood levels of amoxicillin—therapy may be combined for this purpose. May ↑ the effect of **warfarin**. Concurrent **allopurinol** therapy ↑ risk of rash. May ↓ the effectiveness of **hormonal contraceptives**.

Drug-Food: Clavulanate absorption is ↓ by a **high fat** meal.

Route/Dosage

Most Infections (Dosing based on amoxicillin component)

PO (Adults and Children >40 kg): 250 mg q 8 hr or 500 mg q 12 hr.

Serious Infections and Respiratory Tract Infections

PO (Adults and Children >40 kg): 875 mg q 12 hr *or* 500 mg q 8 hr; *Acute bacterial sinusitis*—2000 mg q 12 hr for 10 days as extended release (XR) product; *Community-acquired pneumonia*—2000 mg every 12 hr for 7–10 days as extended release (XR) product.

Recurrent/persistent acute otitis media due to Multidrug-resistant *Streptococcus pneumonia*, *H. influenzae*, or *M. catarrhalis*

PO (Children <40 kg): 80–90 mg/kg/day in divided doses q 12 hr for 10 days (as ES formulation only).

Renal Impairment

PO (Adults): *CCr 10–30 mL/min*—250–500 mg q 12 hr (do not use 875 mg tablet); *CCr <10 mL/min*—250–500 mg q 24 hr.

Otitis Media, Sinusitis, Lower Respiratory Tract Infections, Serious Infections

PO (Children ≥3 mo): *200 mg/5 mL or 400 mg/5 mL suspension*—45 mg/kg/day divided q 12 hr; *125 mg/5 mL or 250 mg/5 mL suspension*—40 mg/kg/day divided q 8 hr.

Less Serious Infections

PO (Children ≥3 mo): *200 mg/5 mL or 400 mg/5 mL suspension*—25 mg/kg/day divided q 12 hr *or* 20 mg/kg/day divided q 8 hr (as 125 mg/5 mL or 250 mg/5 mL suspension).

PO (Children <3 mo): 15 mg/kg q 12 hr (125 mg/mL suspension recommended).

Availability (generic available)

Tablets: 250 mg amoxicillin with 125 mg clavulanate, 500 mg amoxicillin with 125 mg clavulanate, 875 mg amoxicillin with 125 mg clavulanate. **Cost:** *Generic*—500 mg $18.98/20, 875 mg $23.46/30. **Chewable tablets (cherry-banana flavor):** 200 mg amoxicillin with 28.5 mg clavulanate, 400 mg amoxicillin with 57 mg clavulanate. **Cost:** *Generic*—200 mg $36.17/20, 400 mg $68.93/20. **Extended-release tablets (scored):** 1000 mg amoxicillin with 62.5 mg clavulanate. **Cost:** *Generic*—$108.62/28. **Powder for oral suspension (125 mg/5 mL is banana flavor; 200 mg/5ml is fruit flavor; 250 mg/5 mL is orange flavor; 400 mg/5 mL is fruit flavor; 600 mg/5 mL is orange or strawberry-creme flavor):** 125 mg amoxicillin with 31.25 mg clavulanate/5 mL, 200 mg amoxicillin with 28.5 mg clavulanate/5 mL, 250 mg amoxicillin with 62.5 mg clavulanate/5 mL, 400 mg amoxicillin with 57 mg clavulanate/5 mL, 600 mg amoxicillin with 42.9 mg clavulanate/5 mL (ES formulation). **Cost:** *Generic*—200 mg $36.17/100 mL, 250 mg $86.43/100 mL, 400 mg $68.93/100 mL, 600 mg $83.03/125 mL.

NURSING IMPLICATIONS

Assessment

- Assess for infection (vital signs; appearance of wound, sputum, urine, and stool; WBC) at beginning of and throughout therapy.
- Obtain a history before initiating therapy to determine previous use of and reactions to penicillins or cephalosporins. Persons with a negative history of penicillin sensitivity may still have an allergic response.
- Observe for signs and symptoms of anaphylaxis (rash, pruritus, laryngeal edema, wheezing). Notify health care professional immediately if these occur.
- Obtain specimens for culture and sensitivity prior to therapy. First dose may be given before receiving results.
- Monitor bowel function. Diarrhea, abdominal cramping, fever, and bloody stools should be reported to health care professional promptly as a sign of Clostridium difficile-associated diarrhea (CDAD). May begin up to several weeks following cessation of therapy.
- ***Lab Test Considerations:*** May cause ↑ serum alkaline phosphatase, LDH, AST, and ALT concentrations. Elderly men and patients receiving prolonged treatment are at ↑ risk for hepatic dysfunction.
- May cause false-positive direct Coombs' test result.

Potential Nursing Diagnoses

Risk for infection (Indications, Side Effects)
Noncompliance (Patient/Family Teaching)

Implementation

- **PO:** Administer around the clock. Administer at the start of a meal to enhance absorption and to decrease GI side effects. Do not administer with high fat meals; clavulanate absorption is decreased. XR tablet is scored and can be broken for ease of administration. Capsule contents may be emptied and swallowed with liquids. Chewable tablets should be crushed or chewed before swallowing with liquids. Shake oral suspension before administering. Refrigerated reconstituted suspension should be discarded after 10 days.
- Two 250-mg tablets are not bioequivalent to one 500-mg tablet; 250-mg tablets and 250-mg chewable tablets are also not interchangeable. Two 500-mg tablets are not interchangeable with one 1000-mg XR tablet; amounts of clavulanic acid and durations of action are different. Augmentin ES 600 (600 mg/5 mL) does not contain the same amount of clavulanic acid as any of the other Augmentin suspensions. Suspensions are not interchangeable.
- Pedi: Do not administer 250-mg chewable tablets to children <40 kg due to clavulanate content. Children <3 mo should receive the 125-mg/5 mL oral solution.

Patient/Family Teaching

- Instruct patients to take medication around the clock and to finish the drug completely as directed, even if feeling better. Advise patients that sharing of this medication may be dangerous.
- Pedi: Teach parents or caregivers to calculate and measure doses accurately. Reinforce importance of using measuring device supplied by pharmacy or with product, not household items.
- Advise patient to report the signs of superinfection (furry overgrowth on the tongue, vaginal itching or discharge, loose or foul-smelling stools) and allergy.
- Instruct patient to notify health care professional immediately if diarrhea, abdominal cramping, fever, or bloody stools occur and not to treat with antidiarrheals without consulting health care professionals.

A

- Instruct the patient to notify health care professional if symptoms do not improve or if nausea or diarrhea persists when drug is administered with food.
- Instruct female patients taking oral contraceptives to use an alternate or additional method of contraception during therapy and until next menstrual period; may decrease effectiveness of hormonal contraceptives.

Evaluation/Desired Outcomes

- Resolution of the signs and symptoms of infection. Length of time for complete resolution depends on the organism and site of infection.

amphetamine mixtures

(am-**fet**-a-meen)

Amphetamine Salt, ~~Adderall~~, Adderall XR

Classification

Therapeutic: central nervous system stimulants

Schedule II

Pregnancy Category C

Indications

ADHD. Narcolepsy.

Action

Causes release of norepinephrine from nerve endings. Pharmacologic effects are: CNS and respiratory stimulation, Vasoconstriction, Mydriasis (pupillary dilation). **Therapeutic Effects:** Increased motor activity, mental alertness, and decreased fatigue in narcoleptic patients. Increased attention span in ADHD.

Pharmacokinetics

Absorption: Well absorbed after oral administration.
Distribution: Widely distributed in body tissues, with high concentrations in the brain and CSF. Crosses placenta and enters breast milk.
Metabolism and Excretion: Some metabolism by the liver. Urinary excretion is pH-dependent. Alkaline urine promotes reabsorption and prolongs action.
Half-life: Children 6–12 yrs: 9–11 hr; Adults: 10–13 hr (depends on urine pH).

TIME/ACTION PROFILE (CNS stimulation)

ROUTE	ONSET	PEAK	DURATION
PO	tablet: 0.5–1 hr	tablet: 3 hr capsule: 7 hr	4–6 hr

Contraindications/Precautions

Contraindicated in: Hyperexcitable states including hyperthyroidism; Psychotic personalities; Suicidal or homicidal tendencies; Chemical dependence; Glaucoma; Structural cardiac abnormalities (may ↑ the risk of sudden death); OB: Potentially embryotoxic.
Use Cautiously in: Cardiovascular disease (sudden death has occurred in children with structural cardiac abnormalities or other serious heart problems); History of substance use disorder (misuse may result in serious cardiovascular events/sudden death); Hypertension; Diabetes mellitus; Tourette's syndrome (may exacerbate tics); Geri: Geriatric or debilitated patients may be more susceptible to side effects.

Adverse Reactions/Side Effects

CNS: hyperactivity, insomnia, restlessness, tremor, aggression, anger, behavioral disturbances, dizziness, hallucinations, headache, mania, irritability, skin picking, talkativeness, thought disorder, tics. **EENT:** blurred vision, mydriasis. **CV:** SUDDEN DEATH, palpitations, tachycardia, cardiomyopathy (increased with prolonged use, high doses), hypertension, hypotension, peripheral vasculopathy. **GI:** anorexia, constipation, cramps, diarrhea, dry mouth, metallic taste, nausea, vomiting. **GU:** erectile dysfunction, libido changes, priapism. **Derm:** alopecia, urticaria. **Endo:** growth inhibition (with long term use in children). **MS:** RHABDOMYOLYSIS. **Neuro:** paresthesia. **Misc:** psychological dependence.

Interactions

Drug-Drug: Use with **MAO inhibitors** or **meperidine** can result in hypertensive crisis. ↑ adrenergic effects with other **adrenergics** or **thyroid preparations**. **Drugs that alkalinize urine (sodium bicarbonate, acetazolamide)** ↓ excretion, ↑ effects. **Drugs that acidify urine (ammonium chloride,** large doses of **ascorbic acid)** ↑ excretion, ↓ effects. ↑ risk of hypertension and bradycardia with **beta blockers**. ↑ risk of arrhythmias with **digoxin**. **Tricyclic antidepressants** may ↑ effect of amphetamine but may ↑ risk of arrhythmias, hypertension, or hyperpyrexia. **Proton pump inhibitors** may ↑ effects.
Drug-Natural Products: Use with **St. John's wort** may ↑ serious side effects (avoid concurrent use).
Drug-Food: Foods that alkalinize the urine (fruit juices) can ↑ effect of amphetamine.

Route/Dosage

Dose is expressed in total amphetamine content (amphetamine + dextroamphetamine).

ADHD

PO (Children ≥6 yr): 5 mg/day 1–2 times daily; ↑ daily dose by 5 mg at weekly intervals. Sustained-release capsules can be given once daily, tablets every 8–12 hr. If starting therapy with extended-release capsules, start with 10 mg once daily and ↑ by 10 mg/day at weekly intervals (up to 40 mg/day).

PO (Adults): 20 mg/day initially (as extended-release product).
PO (Children 3–5 yr): 2.5 mg/day in the morning; ↑ daily dose by 2.5 mg at weekly intervals not to exceed 40 mg/day.

Narcolepsy

PO (Adults and Children ≥12 yr): 10–60 mg/day in divided doses; start with 10 mg/day, ↑ by 10 mg/day at weekly intervals. Sustained-release capsules can be given once daily, tablets every 8–12 hr.
PO (Children 6–12 yr): 5 mg once daily; may ↑ by 5 mg/day at weekly intervals to a maximum of 60 mg/day.

Availability (generic available)

Amount is expressed in total amphetamine content (amphetamine + dextroamphetamine).
Tablets: 5 mg, 7.5 mg, 10 mg, 12.5 mg, 15 mg, 20 mg, 30 mg. **Cost:** *Generic*—All strengths $171.40/100.
Extended-release capsules: 5 mg, 10 mg, 15 mg, 20 mg, 25 mg, 30 mg. **Cost:** *Generic*—All strengths $613.15/100.

NURSING IMPLICATIONS

Assessment

- Monitor BP, pulse, and respiration before and periodically during therapy. Obtain a history (including assessment of family history of sudden death or ventricular arrhythmia), physical exam to assess for cardiac disease, and further evaluation (ECG and echocardiogram), if indicated. If exertional chest pain, unexplained syncope, or other cardiac symptoms occur, evaluate promptly.
- May produce a false sense of euphoria and well-being. Provide frequent rest periods and observe patient for rebound depression after the effects of the medication have worn off.
- Monitor closely for behavior change.
- Has high dependence and abuse potential. Tolerance to medication occurs rapidly; do not increase dose.
- **ADHD:** Monitor weight biweekly and height periodically and inform health care professional of significant loss.
- Assess child's attention span, impulse control, and interactions with others. Therapy may be interrupted at intervals to determine whether symptoms are sufficient to continue therapy.
- **Narcolepsy:** Observe and document frequency of narcoleptic episodes.
- ***Lab Test Considerations:*** May interfere with urinary steroid determinations.
- May cause ↑ plasma corticosteroid concentrations; greatest in evening.

Potential Nursing Diagnoses

Disturbed thought process (Side Effects)

Implementation

- Do not confuse Adderall with Inderal or Adderall XR.
- **PO:** Use the lowest effective dose.
- May be taken without regard to food. Administer short acting doses 4–6 hrs apart.
- Extended-release capsules may be swallowed whole or opened and sprinkled on applesauce; swallow contents without chewing. Applesauce should be swallowed immediately; do not store. Do not divide contents of capsule; entire contents of capsule should be taken.
- **ADHD:** Pedi: When symptoms are controlled, dose reduction or interruption of therapy may be possible during summer months or may be given on each of the 5 school days, with medication-free weekends and holidays.

Patient/Family Teaching

- Instruct patient to take medication at least 6 hr before bedtime to avoid sleep disturbances. Missed doses should be taken as soon as remembered up to 6 hr before bedtime. With extended release capsule, avoid afternoon doses to prevent insomnia. Do not double doses. Advise patient and parents to read the *Medication Guide* prior to starting therapy and with each Rx refill in case of changes. Instruct patient not to alter dose without consulting health care professional. Abrupt cessation of high doses may cause extreme fatigue and mental depression.
- Inform patient that sharing this medication may be dangerous.
- Inform patient that the effects of drug-induced dry mouth can be minimized by rinsing frequently with water or chewing sugarless gum or candies.
- Advise patient to limit caffeine intake.
- May impair judgment. Advise patient to use caution when driving or during other activities requiring alertness until response to medication is known.
- Inform patient that periodic holidays from the drug may be used to assess progress and decrease dependence. Pedi: Children should be given a drug-free holiday each year to reassess symptoms and treatment. Doses will change as children age due to pharmacokinetic changes such as slower hepatic metabolism.
- Advise patient and/or parents to notify health care professional of behavioral changes (new or worse behavior and thought problems, bipolar illness, or aggressive behavior or hostility; new psychotic symptoms such as hearing voices, believing things that are not true, are suspicious, or new manic symptoms).
- Advise patient to notify health care professional if symptoms of heart problems (chest pain, shortness of breath, fainting), nervousness, restlessness, insomnia, dizziness, anorexia, or dry mouth becomes severe. Pedi: If reduced appetite and weight loss occur, advise parents to provide high calorie meals when drug levels are low (at breakfast and or bedtime).
- Inform patients of risk of peripheral vasculopathy. Instruct patients to notify health care professional of any new numbness; pain; skin color change from

pale, to blue, to red; or coolness or sensitivity to temperature in fingers or toes, and call if unexplained wounds appear on fingers or toes.

- Caution patients to inform health care professional if they have ever abused or been dependent on alcohol or drugs, or if they are now abusing or dependent on alcohol or drugs.
- Advise patient to notify health care professional of all Rx or OTC medications, vitamins, or herbal products being taken and to consult with health care professional before taking other medications.
- Advise patient to notify health care professional if pregnancy is planned or suspected, or if breast feeding.
- Emphasize the importance of routine follow-up exams to monitor progress.
- **Home Care Issues:** Advise parents to notify school nurse of medication regimen.

Evaluation/Desired Outcomes

- Improved attention span.
- Decrease in narcoleptic symptoms.

HIGH ALERT

amphotericin B deoxycholate

(am-foe-**ter**-i-sin)

✤Fungizone

amphotericin B lipid complex

Abelcet

amphotericin B liposome

AmBisome

Classification

Therapeutic: antifungals

Pregnancy Category B

Indications

IV: Treatment of progressive, potentially fatal fungal infections. The lipid complex, and liposome formulations should be considered for patients who are intolerant (e.g., renal dysfunction) or refractory to amphotericin B dexycholate. **Amphotericin B liposome:** Management of suspected fungal infections in febrile neutropenic patients: Treatment of visceral leishmaniasis, Treatment of cryptococcal meningitis in HIV patients.

Action

Binds to fungal cell membrane, allowing leakage of cellular contents. Toxicity (especially acute infusion reactions and nephrotoxicity) is less with lipid formulations. **Therapeutic Effects:** Can be fungistatic or fungicidal (depends on concentration achieved and susceptibility of organism). **Spectrum:** Active against: Aspergillosis, Blastomycosis, Candidiasis, Coccidioidomycosis, Cryptococcosis, Histoplasmosis, Leishmaniasis (liposomal formulation only), Mucormycosis.

Pharmacokinetics

Absorption: IV administration results in complete bioavailability.

Distribution: Extensively distributed to body tissues and fluids. Poor penetration into CSF.

Metabolism and Excretion: Elimination is very prolonged. Detectable in urine up to 7 wk after discontinuation.

Half-life: Biphasic—initial phase, 24–48 hr; terminal phase, 15 days. *Cholesteryl sulfate*—28 hr. *Lipid complex*—174 hr. *Liposomal*—100–153 hr.

TIME/ACTION PROFILE (blood levels)

ROUTE	ONSET	PEAK	DURATION
IV	rapid	end of infusion	24 hr

Contraindications/Precautions

Contraindicated in: Hypersensitivity; Lactation: Potential for distribution into breast milk and toxicity in infant; discontinue nursing.

Use Cautiously in: Renal impairment or electrolyte abnormalities; Patients receiving concurrent leukocyte transfusions (↑ risk of pulmonary toxicity); OB: Has been used safely.

Adverse Reactions/Side Effects

CNS: anxiety, confusion, headache, insomnia. **Resp:** dyspnea, hypoxia, wheezing. **CV:** chest pain, hypotension, tachycardia, edema, hypertension. **GI:** diarrhea, hyperbilirubinemia, ↑ liver enzymes, nausea, vomiting, abdominal pain. **GU:** nephrotoxicity, hematuria. **F and E:** hyperglycemia, hypocalcemia, hypokalemia, hypomagnesemia. **Hemat:** anemia, leukopenia, thrombocytopenia. **Derm:** pruritis, rashes. **Local:** phlebitis. **MS:** arthralgia, myalgia. **Misc:** HYPERSENSITIVITY REACTIONS, chills, fever, acute infusion reactions.

Interactions

Drug-Drug: ↑ risk of nephrotoxicity, bronchospasm, and hypotension with **antineoplastics**. Concurrent use with **corticosteroids** ↑ risk of hypokalemia. Concurrent use with **zidovudine** may ↑ the risk of myelotoxicity and nephrotoxicity. Concurrent use with **flucytosine** ↑ antifungal activity but may ↑ the risk of toxicity from flucytosine. Combined use with **azole antifungals** may induce fungal resistance. ↑ risk of nephrotoxicity with other **nephrotoxic agents** such as **aminoglycosides**, **cyclosporine**, or **tacrolimus**. Hypokalemia from amphotericin ↑ the risk of **digoxin** toxicity. Hypokalemia may enhance the curariform effects of **neuromuscular blocking agents**.

Route/Dosage

Specific dosage and duration of therapy depend on nature of infection being treated.

Amphotericin Deoxycholate

IV (Adults): Give test dose of 1 mg. If test dose tolerated, initiate therapy with 0.25 mg/kg/day (doses up to 1.5 mg/kg/day may be used, depending on type of infection) (alternate-day dosing may also be used); *Bladder irrigation*—Instill 50 mcg/mL solution into bladder daily for 5–10 days.
IV (Infants and Children): Give test dose of 0.1 mg/kg (maximum dose 1 mg) or may administer initial dose of 0.25–1 mg/kg/day over 6 hr (without test dose) (some infections may require 1.5 mg/kg/day; alternate-day dosing may be used).
IT (Adults): 25–300 mcg q 48–72 hr, ↑ to 500 mcg–1 mg as tolerated (maximum total dose = 15 mg).
IT (Children): 25–100 mcg q 48–72 hr; ↑ to 500 mcg as tolerated.

Amphotericin B Lipid Complex (Abelcet)

IV (Adults and Children): 2.5–5 mg/kg q 24 hr (no test dose needed).

Amphotericin B Liposome (AmBisome)

IV (Adults and Children): *Empiric therapy*—3 mg/kg q 24 hr; *Documented infections*—3–5 mg/kg q 24 hr; *Visceral leishmaniasis (immunocompetent patients)*—3 mg/kg q 24 hr on days 1–5, then 3 mg/kg q 24 hr on days 14 and 21; *Visceral leishmaniasis (immunosuppressed patients)*—4 mg/kg q 24 hr on days 1–5, then 4 mg/kg q 24 hr on days 10, 17, 24, 31, and 38; *Cryptococcal meningitis in HIV patients*—6 mg/kg q 24 hr.

Availability (generic available)

Amphotericin Deoxycholate

Powder for injection: 50 mg/vial.

Amphotericin B Lipid Complex

Suspension for injection: 5 mg/mL.

Amphotericin B Liposome

Powder for injection: 50 mg/vial.

NURSING IMPLICATIONS

Assessment

- Monitor patient closely during test dose and the first 1–2 hr of each dose for fever, chills, headache, anorexia, nausea, or vomiting. Premedicating with antipyretics, corticosteroids, antihistamines, meperidine, and antiemetics may decrease these reactions. Febrile reaction usually subsides within 4 hr after the infusion is completed.
- Assess injection site frequently for thrombophlebitis or leakage. Drug is very irritating to tissues.
- Monitor vital signs every 15 min during test dose and every 30 min for 2–4 hr after administration. Meperidine and dantrolene have been used to prevent and treat rigors. Assess respiratory status (lung sounds, dyspnea) daily. If respiratory distress occurs, discontinue infusion immediately; anaphylaxis may occur. Equipment for cardiopulmonary resuscitation should be readily available.
- Monitor intake and output and weigh daily. Adequate hydration (2000–3000 mL/day) and maintaining sodium balance may minimize nephrotoxicity.
- ***Lab Test Considerations:*** Monitor CBC, BUN and serum creatinine, and potassium and magnesium levels daily. If BUN and serum creatinine ↑ significantly, may need to discontinue or consider switching to lipid complex, or liposomal formulation.

Potential Nursing Diagnoses

Risk for infection (Indications)

Implementation

- Do not confuse amphotericin deoxycholate with amphotericin B lipid complex (Abelcet), or amphotericin B liposome (AmBisome); they are not interchangeable.
- This drug should be administered IV only to hospitalized patients or those under close supervision. Diagnosis should be confirmed before administration.

Amphotericin B Deoxycholate

IV Administration

- **Test dose:** Reconstitute 50-mg vial with 10 mL of sterile water for injection to achieve a concentration of 5 mg/mL. Reconstituted vial stable for 24 hr at room temperature or 1 wk if refrigerated. ***Diluent:*** Further dilute with 500 mL of D5W. May be diluted in 250 mL of D5W if being administered via a central venous catheter. Protect infusion from light. Infusion stable for 24 hr at room temperature or 2 days if refrigerated. To obtain test dose, withdraw 1 mg (10 mL) from 500 mL infusion and further dilute with D5W to a total volume of 20 mL. ***Concentration:*** 0.05 mg/mL. ***Rate:*** Infuse over 10–30 min to determine patient tolerance. Pedi: Infuse over 30–60 min.
- **Intermittent Infusion: *Diluent:*** Reconstitute and dilute 50-mg vial as per the directions above. ***Concentration:*** Final concentration of infusion should not exceed 0.1 mg/mL for peripheral infusion or 0.25 mg/mL for central line administration. ***Rate:*** Infuse slowly over 4–6 hr.
- **Y-Site Compatibility:** aldesleukin, aminocaproic acid, argatroban, carmustine, dactinomycin, diltiazem, etoposide, hydromorphone, ifosfamide, lorazepam, nesiritide, octreotide, oxaliplatin, tacrolimus, teniposide, thiotepa, zidovudine, zoledronic acid.
- **Y-Site Incompatibility:** acyclovir, alemtuzumab, alfentanil, allopurinol, amifostine, amikacin, ampi-

cillin, ampicillin/sulbactam, anidulafungin, atropine, azithromycin, aztreonam, benztropine, bivalirudin, bleomycin, bumetanide, butorphanol, calcium chloride, calcium gluconate, cangrelor, carboplatin, caspofungin, cefepime, cefotetan, ceftaroline, chloramphenicol, chlorpromazine, cisplatin, clindamycin, cyanocobalamin, cyclophosphamide, cytarabine, dacarbazine, dantrolene, daptomycin, daunorubicin, dexamethasone, dexmedetomidine, dexrazoxane, diazepam, digoxin, diphenhydramine, dobutamine, docetaxel, dolasetron, dopamine, doxorubicin, doxorubicin liposome, doxycycline, ephedrine, epinephrine, epirubicin, epoetin alfa, eptifibatide, ertapenem, erythromycin, esmolol, etoposide phosphate, famotidine, fenoldopam, filgrastim, fluconazole, fludarabine, fluorouracil, foscarnet, fosphenytoin, ganciclovir, gemcitabine, gentamicin, glycopyrrolate, granisetron, haloperidol, hetastarch, hydralazine, hydrocortisone, hydroxyzine, idarubicin, irinotecan, isoproterenol, ketorolac, labetalol, leucovorin, levofloxacin, lidocaine, linezolid, melphalan, meperidine, mechlorethamine, meropenem, mesna, methotrexate, methylprednisolone, metoclopramide, metoprolol, metronidazole, midazolam, milrinone, mitomycin, mitoxantrone, morphine, mycophenolate, nafcillin, nalbuphine, nicardipine, nitroprusside, norepinephrine, ondansetron, oxacillin, paclitaxel, palonosetron, pamidronate, pancuronium, pantoprazole, papaverine, pemetrexed, penicillin G, pentamidine, pentazocine, phenylephrine, phenytoin, piperacillin/tazobactam, potassium acetate, potassium chloride, prochlorperazine, promethazine, propofol, propranolol, protamine, pyridoxine, quinupristin/dalfopristin, rituximab, rocuronium, sodium acetate, sodium bicarbonate, succinylcholine, telavancin, thiamine, tigecycline, tirofiban, tobramycin, topotecan, trastuzumab, trimethoprim/sulfamethoxazole, vancomycin, vasopressin, vecuronium, verapamil, vinblastine, vincristine, vinorelbine, voriconazole.

- **Solution Incompatibility:** LR injection, saline solutions.

Amphotericin B Lipid Complex

IV Administration

- **Intermittent Infusion:** ***Diluent:*** Shake vial gently until yellow sediment at bottom has dissolved. Withdraw dose from required number of vials with 18-gauge needle. Replace needle from syringe filled with amphotericin B lipid complex with 5-micron filter needle. Each filter needle may be used to filter the contents of no more than 4 vials. Insert filter needle of syringe into IV bag of D5W and empty contents of syringe into bag. Protect from light. Infusion is stable for 6 hr at room temperature or 48 hr if refrigerated. ***Concentration:*** Final concentration of infusion should be 1 mg/mL; a concentration of 2 mg/mL can be used for pediatric patients or patients who cannot tolerate large volumes of fluid. ***Rate:*** Do not use an in-line filter. Infuse at a rate of 2.5 mg/kg/hr via infusion pump. If infusion exceeds 2 hr, mix contents by shaking infusion bag every 2 hr. If administering through an existing line, flush line with D5W before infusion or use a separate line.
- **Y-Site Compatibility:** acyclovir, allopurinol, aminocaproic acid, aminophylline, amiodarone, anidulafungin, argatroban, azithromycin, aztreonam, bumetanide, buprenorphine, busulfan, butorphanol, carboplatin, carmustine, cefazolin, cefepime, cefotaxime, cefotetan, cefoxitin, ceftazidime, ceftriaxone, cefuroxime, chloramphenicol, chlorpromazine, cisatracurium, clindamycin, cyclophosphamide, cyclosporine, cytatabine, dactimomycin, dexamethasone, digoxin, diphenhydramine, docetaxel, doxorubicin liposome, enalaprilat, ephedrine, epinephrine, eptifibatide, ertapenem, etoposide, famotidine, fentanyl, fludarabine, fluorouracil, fosphenytoin, furosemide, ganciclovir, granisetron, heparin, hydrocortisone, hydromorphone, ifosfamide, insulin, ketorolac, lidocaine, linezolid, lorazepam, mannitol, melphalan, meperidine, methotrexate, methylprednisolone, metoclopramide, mitomycin, nafcillin, nesiritide, nitroglycerin, nitroprusside, octreotide, oxaliplatin, paclitaxel, pamidronate, pantoprazole, pemetrexed, pentazocine, pentobarbital, phenobarbital, piperacillin/tazobactam, procainamide, ranitidine, succinylcholine, sufentanil, tacrolimus, telavancin, teniposide, theophylline, thiopental, thiotepa, verapamil, vinblastine, vincristine, zidovudine, zoledronic acid.
- **Y-Site Incompatibility:** alemtuzumab, alfentanil, amifostine, amikacin, ampicillin, ampicillin/sulbactam, bivalirudin, bleomycin, calcium chloride, calcium gluconate, caspofungin, ciprofloxacin, cisplatin, dacarbazine, dantrolene, daptomycin, daunorubicin, dexmedetomidine, dexrazoxane, diazepam, diltiazem, dobutamine, dolasetron, dopamine, doxorubicin, doxycycline, droperidol, epirubicin, erythromycin, esmolol, etoposide phosphate, fenoldopam, fluconazole, foscarnet, gemcitabine, gentamicin, glycopyrrolate, haloperidol, hydralazine, hydroxyzine, idarubicin, imipenem/cilastatin, irinotecan, isoproterenol, labetalol, leucovorin, levofloxacin, magnesium sulfate, mechlorethamine, meropenem, mesna, metoprolol, metronidazole, midazolam, milrinone, mitoxantrone, morphine, moxifloxacin, mycophenolate, nalbuphine, naloxone, nicardipine, norepinephrine, ondansetron, pancuronium, pentamidine, phenylephrine, phenytoin, potassium acetate, potassium phosphates, prochlorperazine, promethazine, propranolol, quinupristin/dalfopristin, remifentanil, rocuronium, sodium acetate, sodium bicarbonate, sodium phos-

phates, streptozocin, tirofiban, tobramycin, topotecan, trimethoprim/sulfamethoxazole, vancomycin, vasopressin, vecuronium, vinorelbine, voriconazole.

- **Solution Incompatibility:** saline solutions.

Amphotericin B Liposome

IV Administration

- **Intermittent Infusion:** ***Diluent:*** Reconstitute each 50–mg vial with 12 mL of sterile water for injection to achieve concentration of 4 mg/mL. Immediately shake vial vigorously for at least 30 seconds until all particulate matter is completely dispersed. Reconstituted vials are stable for 24 hr if refrigerated. Withdraw appropriate volume for dilution into a syringe. Attach the 5-micron filter to the syringe and inject syringe contents into an appropriate volume of D5W. Infusion should be administered within 6 hr of dilution. ***Concentration:*** Final concentration of infusion should be 1–2 mg/mL; a lower concentration (0.2–0.5 mg/mL) may be used for infants and small children. ***Rate:*** Infuse over 2 hr. Infusion time may be shortened to 1 hr if patient tolerates infusion without any adverse reactions. If discomfort occurs during infusion, duration of infusion may be increased. May be administered through an in-line filter with pore diameter of at least 1 micron. If administering through an existing line, flush line with D5W before infusion or use a separate line.
- **Y-Site Compatibility:** acyclovir, amifostine, aminocaproic acid, aminophylline, anidulafungin, argatroban, atropine, azithromycin, bivalirudin, bumetanide, buprenorphine, busulfan, butorphanol, carboplatin, carmustine, cefazolin, cefoxitin, ceftriaxone, cefuroxime, clindamycin, cyclophosphamide, cytarabine, dactinomycin, daptomycin, dexamethasone, dexmedetomidine, diphenhydramine, doxorubicin liposomal, enalaprilat, ephedrine, epinephrine, eptifibatide, ertapenem, esmolol, etoposide, famotidine, fenoldopam, fentanyl, fludarabine, fluorouracil, foscarnet, fosphenytoin, furosemide, granisetron, haloperidol, heparin, hydrocortisone, hydromorphone, ifosfamide, isoproterenol, ketorolac, lidocaine, linezolid, mesna, methotrexate, methylprednisolone, metoprolol, milrinone, mitomycin, nesiritide, nitroglycerin, nitroprusside, octreotide, oxaliplatin, oxytocin, palonosetron, pamidronate, pancuronium, pantoprazole, pemetrexed, pentobarbital, phenobarbital, phenylephrine, piperacillin/tazobactam, potassium acetate, potassium chloride, procainamide, ranitidine, sufentanil, tacrolimus, theophylline, thiopental, thiotepa, tigecycline, trimethoprim/sulfamethoxazole, vasopressin, vincristine, voriconazole, zidovudine, zoledronic acid.
- **Y-Site Incompatibility:** alemtuzumab, alfentanil, amikacin, ampicillin, ampicillin/sulbactam, aztreonam, bleomycin, calcium chloride, calcium gluconate, caspofungin, cefepime, cefotaxime, cefotetan, ceftazidime, chlorpromazine, ciprofloxacin, cisplatin, cyclosporine, dacarbazine, daunorubicin, dexrazoxane, diazepam, digoxin, diltiazem, dobutamine, docetaxel, dolasetron, dopamine, doxorubicin, doxycycline, droperidol, epirubicin, erythromycin, etoposide phosphate, gemcitabine, gentamicin, hetastarch, hydroxyzine, idarubicin, imipenem/cilastatin, irinotecan, labetalol, leucovorin, levofloxacin, lorazepam, magnesium sulfate, mannitol, mechlorethamine, meperidine, meropenem, metoclopramide, metronidazole, midazolam, mitoxantrone, morphine, mycophenolate, nalbuphine, naloxone, nicardipine, ondansetron, paclitaxel, pentamidine, phenytoin, potassium phosphates, prochlorperazine, promethazine, propranolol, quinupristin/dalfopristin, sodium bicarbonate, sodium phosphates, telavancin, teniposide, tobramycin, vancomycin, vecuronium, verapamil, vinblastine, vinorelbine.
- **Solution Incompatibility:** Do not dilute or admix with saline solutions, other medications, or solutions containing a bacteriostatic agent.

Patient/Family Teaching

- Explain need for long duration of IV or topical therapy.
- **IV:** Inform patient of potential side effects and discomfort at IV site. Advise patient to notify health care professional if side effects occur.
- **Home Care Issue:** Instruct family or caregiver on dilution, rate, and administration of drug and proper care of IV equipment.

Evaluation/Desired Outcomes

- Resolution of signs and symptoms of infection. Several weeks to months of therapy may be required to prevent relapse.

ampicillin (am-pi-**sil**-in)

Classification
Therapeutic: anti-infectives
Pharmacologic: aminopenicillins

Pregnancy Category B

Indications

Treatment of the following infections: Skin and skin structure infections, Soft-tissue infections, Otitis media, Sinusitis, Respiratory infections, Genitourinary infections, Meningitis, Septicemia. Endocarditis prophylaxis. **Unlabeled Use:** Prevention of infection in certain high-risk patients undergoing cesarean section.

Action

Binds to bacterial cell wall, resulting in cell death. **Therapeutic Effects:** Bactericidal action; spectrum is broader than penicillin. **Spectrum:** Active against: Streptococci, nonpenicillinase-producing staphylococci, *Listeria*, Pneumococci, Enterococci, *Haemophilus influenzae*, *Escherichia coli*, *Enterobacter*, *Klebsiella*, *Proteus mirabilis*, *Neisseria meningitidis*, *N. gonorrhoeae*, *Shigella*, *Salmonella*.

Pharmacokinetics

Absorption: Moderately absorbed from the duodenum (30–50%).

Distribution: Diffuses readily into body tissues and fluids. CSF penetration is ↑ in the presence of inflamed meninges. Crosses the placenta; enters breast milk in small amounts.

Metabolism and Excretion: Variably metabolized by the liver (12–50%). Renal excretion is variable (25–60% after oral dosing; 50–85% after IM administration).

Half-life: Neonates: 1.7–4 hr; Children and Adults: 1–1.5 hr (↑ in renal impairment).

TIME/ACTION PROFILE (blood levels)

ROUTE	ONSET	PEAK	DURATION
PO	rapid	1.5–2 hr	4–6 hr
IM	rapid	1 hr	4–6 hr
IV	rapid	end of infusion	4–6 hr

Contraindications/Precautions

Contraindicated in: Hypersensitivity to penicillins.

Use Cautiously in: Severe renal insufficiency (dose ↓ required if CCr <10 mL/min); Infectious mononucleosis, acute lymphocytic leukemia or cytomegalovirus infection (↑ incidence of rash); Patients allergic to cephalosporins; OB: Has been used during pregnancy; Lactation: Distributed into breast milk. Can cause rash, diarrhea, and sensitization in the infant.

Adverse Reactions/Side Effects

CNS: SEIZURES (high doses). **GI:** CLOSTRIDIUM DIFFICILE-ASSOCIATED DIARRHEA (CDAD), diarrhea, nausea, vomiting. **Derm:** rash, urticaria. **Hemat:** blood dyscrasias. **Misc:** allergic reactions including ANAPHYLAXIS and SERUM SICKNESS, superinfection.

Interactions

Drug-Drug: Probenecid ↓ renal excretion and ↑ blood levels of ampicillin—therapy may be combined for this purpose. Large doses may ↑ the risk of bleeding with **warfarin**. ↑ risk of with concurrent **allopurinol** therapy. May ↓ the effectiveness of oral **hormonal contraceptives**.

Route/Dosage

Respiratory and Soft-Tissue Infections

PO (Adults and Children ≥20 kg): 250–500 mg q 6 hr.

PO (Children <20 kg): 50–100 mg/kg/day in divided doses q 6–8 hr (not to exceed 2–3 g/day).

IM, IV (Adults and Children ≥40 kg): 500 mg to 3 g q 6 hr (not to exceed 14 g/day).

IM, IV (Children <40 kg): 100–200 mg/kg/day in divided doses q 6–8 hr (not to exceed 12 g/day).

Bacterial Meningitis Caused by *H. influenzae, Streptococcus pneumoniae,* Group B streptococcus or *N. meningitidis* or Septicemia

IM, IV (Adults): 500 mg to 3 g q 6 hr (not to exceed 14 g/day).

IM, IV (Children >1 mo): 200–400 mg/kg/day in divided doses q 6 hr (not to exceed 12 g/day).

IM, IV (Neonates ≤7 days): 200 mg/kg/day divided q 8 hr.

IM, IV (Neonates >7 days): 300 mg/kg/day divided q 6 hr.

GI/GU Infections other than *N. gonorrhoeae*

PO (Adults and Children >20 kg): 250–500 mg q 6 hr (larger doses for more serious/chronic infections).

PO (Children ≤20 kg): 50–100 mg/kg/day in divided doses q 6 hr.

N. gonorrhoeae

PO (Adults): 3 g with 1 g probenecid.

IM, IV (Adults and Children ≥40 kg): 500 mg q 6 hr.

IM, IV (Children <40 kg): 100–200 mg/kg/day in divided doses q 6–8 hr.

Urethritis Caused by *N. gonorrhoeae* in Men

IM, IV (Adults and Children ≥40 kg): 500 mg, repeated 8–12 hr later; additional doses may be necessary for more complicated infections (prostatitis, epididymitis).

Prevention of Bacterial Endocarditis

IM, IV (Adults): 2 g 30 min before procedure (gentamicin may be added for high-risk patients); additional 1 g may be given 6 hr later for high-risk patients.

IM, IV (Children): 50 mg/kg (not to exceed 2 g) 30 min before procedure (gentamicin may be added for high-risk patients); additional 25 mg/kg may be given 6 hr later for high-risk patients.

Renal Impairment

(Adults and Children): *CCr ≤10 mL/min*—↑ dosing interval to q 12 hr.

Availability (generic available)

Capsules: 250 mg, 500 mg. **Suspension (wild cherry flavor):** 125 mg/5 mL, 250 mg/5 mL. **Powder for injection:** 125 mg/vial, 250 mg/vial, 500 mg/vial, 1 g/vial, 2 g/vial, 10 g/vial.

NURSING IMPLICATIONS

Assessment

- Assess patient for infection (vital signs, wound appearance, sputum, urine, stool, and WBC) at beginning of and throughout therapy.
- Obtain a history before initiating therapy to determine previous use and reactions to penicillins or cephalosporins. Persons with a negative history of penicillin sensitivity may still have an allergic response.
- Obtain specimens for culture and sensitivity before therapy. First dose may be given before receiving results.
- Observe patient for signs and symptoms of anaphylaxis (rash, pruritus, laryngeal edema, wheezing). Discontinue the drug and notify health care professional immediately if these occur. Keep epinephrine, an antihistamine, and resuscitation equipment close by in the event of an anaphylactic reaction.
- Monitor bowel function. Diarrhea, abdominal cramping, fever, and bloody stools should be reported to health care professional promptly as a sign of Clostridium difficile-associated diarrhea (CDAD). May begin up to several weeks following cessation of therapy.
- Assess skin for "ampicillin rash," a nonallergic, dull red, macular or maculopapular, mildly pruritic rash.
- ***Lab Test Considerations:*** May cause ↑ AST and ALT.
- May cause transient ↓ estradiol, total conjugated estriol, estriol-glucuronide, or conjugated estrone in pregnant women.
- May cause a false-positive direct Coombs' test result.
- May cause a false-positive urinary glucose.

Potential Nursing Diagnoses

Risk for infection (Indications, Side Effects)
Noncompliance (Patient/Family Teaching)

Implementation

- Reserve IM or IV route for moderately severe or severe infections or patients unable to take oral medication. Change to PO as soon as possible.
- **PO:** Administer around the clock on an empty stomach at least 1 hr before or 2 hr after meals with a full glass of water. Capsules may be opened and mixed with water. Reconstituted oral suspensions retain potency for 7 days at room temperature and 14 days if refrigerated. Combination with probenecid should be used immediately after reconstitution.
- **IM:** Reconstitute for IM or IV use by adding sterile water for injection 0.9–1.2 mL to the 125-mg vial, 0.9–1.9 mL to the 250-mg vial, 1.2–1.8 mL to the 500-mg vial, 2.4–7.4 mL to the 1-g vial, and 6.8 mL to the 2-g vial.

IV Administration

- **IV Push:** Add 5 mL of sterile water for injection to each 125-, 250-, or 500-mg vial or at least 7.4–10 mL of diluent to each 1- or 2-g vial. Solution should be used within 1 hr of reconstitution. ***Rate:*** Doses of 125–500 mg may be given over 3–5 min (not to exceed 100 mg/min). Rapid administration may cause seizures.
- **Intermittent Infusion: *Diluent:*** Reconstitute vials as per the directions above. Further dilute in 50 mL or more of 0.9% NaCl, D5W, D5/0.45% NaCl, or LR. Administer within 4 hr (more stable in NaCl). ***Concentration:*** Not to exceed 30 mg/mL. ***Rate:*** Infuse over 10–15 min.
- **Y-Site Compatibility:** acyclovir, alemtuzumab, alprostadil, amifostine, anidulafungin, argatroban, bivalirudin, bleomycin, carboplatin, carmustine, cisplatin, cyclophosphamide, cytarabine, dactinomycin, daptomycin, dexmedetomidine, docetaxel, doxacurium, doxapram, doxorubicin liposome, eptifibatide, etoposide, etoposide phosphate, filgrastim, fludarabine, fluorouracil, foscarnet, gemcitabine, granisetron, hetastarch, ifosfamide, irinotecan, levofloxacin, linezolid, mechlorethamine, melphalan, methotrexate, metronidazole, milrinone, octreotide, oxaliplatin, paclitaxel, palonosetron, pamidronate, pancuronium, pantoprazole, pemetrexed, perphenazine, potassium acetate, propofol, remifentanil, rituximab, rocuronium, sodium acetate, teniposide, thiotepa, tigecycline, tirofiban, trastuzumab, vecuronium, vincristine, vitamin B complex with C, voriconazole, zoledronic acid.
- **Y-Site Incompatibility:** If aminoglycosides and penicillins must be administered concurrently, administer in separate sites at least 1 hr apart, aminophylline, amphotericin B cholesterol, amphotericin B colloidal, amphotericin B lipid complex, amphotericin B liposome, buprenorphine, caspofungin, chlorpromazine, dantrolene, diazepam, diazoxide, diphenhydramine, dobutamine, dopamine, doxorubicin hydrochloride, doxycycline, epirubicin, fenoldopam, fluconazole, ganciclovir, haloperidol, hydroxyzine, idarubicin, ketamine, lorazepam, midazolam, mitoxantrone, mycophenolate, nafcillin, nesiritide, nicardipine, nitroprusside, ondansetron, papaverine, penicillin G potassium, pentamidine, pentazocine, pentobarbital, phenobarbital, phenytoin, prochlorperazine, promethazine, protamine, quinupristin/dalfopristin, sargramostim, sodium bicarbonate, tranexamic acid, trimethoprim/sulfamethoxazole, verapamil, vinorelbine.

Patient/Family Teaching

- Instruct patient to take medication around the clock and to finish the drug completely as directed, even if feeling better. Advise patients that sharing of this medication can be dangerous.
- Advise patient to report the signs of superinfection (furry overgrowth on the tongue, vaginal itching or discharge, loose or foul-smelling stools) and allergy.
- Caution patient to notify health care professional if fever and diarrhea occur, especially if stool contains

blood, pus, or mucus. Advise patient not to treat diarrhea without consulting health care professional. May occur up to several weeks after discontinuation of medication.

- Instruct the patient to notify health care professional if symptoms do not improve.
- Patients with a history of rheumatic heart disease or valve replacement need to be taught the importance of using antimicrobial prophylaxis before invasive medical or dental procedures.
- Advise patients taking oral contraceptives to use an alternate or additional nonhormonal method of contraception while taking ampicillin and until next menstrual period.
- Advise female patient to notify health care professional if breast feeding.

Evaluation/Desired Outcomes

- Resolution of the signs and symptoms of infection. Length of time for complete resolution depends on the organism and site of infection.
- Endocarditis prophylaxis.

ampicillin/sulbactam

(am-pi-**sil**-in/sul-**bak**-tam)

Unasyn

Classification

Therapeutic: anti-infectives

Pharmacologic: aminopenicillins/beta lactamase inhibitors

Pregnancy Category B

Indications

Treatment of the following infections: Skin and skin structure infections, soft-tissue infections, Otitis media, Intra-abdominal infections, Sinusitis, Respiratory infections, Genitourinary infections, Meningitis, Septicemia.

Action

Binds to bacterial cell wall, resulting in cell death; spectrum is broader than that of penicillin. Addition of sulbactam increases resistance to beta-lactamases, enzymes produced by bacteria that may inactivate ampicillin. **Therapeutic Effects:** Bactericidal action. **Spectrum:** Active against: Streptococci, Pneumococci, Enterococci, *Haemophilus influenzae*, *Escherichia coli*, *Proteus mirabilis*, *Neisseria meningitidis*, *N. gonorrhoeae*, *Shigella*, *Salmonella*, *Bacteroides fragilis*, *Moraxella catarrhalis*. Use should be reserved for infections caused by beta-lactamase–producing strains.

Pharmacokinetics

Absorption: Well absorbed from IM sites.

Distribution: Ampicillin diffuses readily into bile, blister and tissue fluids. Poor CSF penetration unless meninges are inflamed. Crosses the placenta; enters breast milk in small amounts.

Metabolism and Excretion: Ampicillin is variably metabolized by the liver (12–50%). Renal excretion is also variable. Sulbactam is eliminated unchanged in urine.

Protein Binding: *Ampicillin*—28%; *sulbactam*—38%.

Half-life: *Ampicillin*—1–1.8 hr; *sulbactam*—1–1.3 hr.

TIME/ACTION PROFILE (blood levels)

ROUTE	ONSET	PEAK	DURATION
IM	rapid	1 hr	6–8 hr
IV	immediate	end of infusion	6–8 hr

Contraindications/Precautions

Contraindicated in: Hypersensitivity to penicillins or sulbactam; History of cholestatic jaundice or hepatic dysfunction with ampicillin/sulbactam.

Use Cautiously in: Severe renal insufficiency (dosage ↓ required if CCr <30 mL/min); Epstein-Barr virus infection, acute lymphocytic leukemia, or cytomegalovirus infection (↑ risk of rash).

Adverse Reactions/Side Effects

CNS: SEIZURES (high doses). **GI:** HEPATOTOXICITY, CLOSTRIDIUM DIFFICILE-ASSOCIATED DIARRHEA (CDAD), diarrhea, cholestasis, nausea, vomiting. **Derm:** rash, urticaria. **Hemat:** blood dyscrasias. **Local:** pain at IM site, pain at IV site. **Misc:** allergic reactions including ANAPHYLAXIS and SERUM SICKNESS, phlebitis, superinfection, ↑liver enzymes.

Interactions

Drug-Drug: Probenecid ↓ renal excretion and ↑ levels of ampicillin—therapy may be combined for this purpose. May potentiate the effect of **warfarin**. Concurrent **allopurinol** therapy (↑ risk of rash). May ↓ levels and effectiveness of **hormonal contraceptives**.

Route/Dosage

Dosage based on ampicillin component.

IM, IV (Adults and Children ≥40 kg): 1–2 g ampicillin q 6–8 hr (not to exceed 12 g ampicillin/day).

IM, IV (Children ≥1 yr): 100–200 mg ampicillin/kg/day divided q 6 hr; *Meningitis*—200–400 mg ampicillin/kg/day divided every 6 hr; maximum dose: 8 g ampicillin/day.

IM, IV (Infants >1 mo): 100–150 mg ampicillin/kg/day divided q 6 hr.

Renal Impairment

IM, IV (Adults, Children, and Infants): *CCr 15–29 mL/min*—Administer q 12 hr; *CCr 5–14*—Administer q 24 hr.

Availability (generic available)

Powder for injection: 1.5 g/vial (1 g ampicillin with 500 mg sulbactam), 3 g/vial (2 g ampicillin with 1 g sulbactam), 15 g/vial (10 g ampicillin with 5 g sulbactam).

NURSING IMPLICATIONS

Assessment

- Assess patient for infection (vital signs, wound appearance, sputum, urine, stool, and WBCs) at beginning and throughout therapy.
- Obtain a history before initiating therapy to determine previous use of, and reactions to, penicillins or cephalosporins. Persons with a negative history of penicillin sensitivity may still have an allergic response.
- Obtain specimens for culture and sensitivity before therapy. First dose may be given before receiving results.
- Observe patient for signs and symptoms of anaphylaxis (rash, pruritus, laryngeal edema, wheezing). Discontinue the drug and notify the physician or other health care professional immediately if these occur. Keep epinephrine, an antihistamine, and resuscitation equipment close by in the event of an anaphylactic reaction.
- Monitor bowel function. Diarrhea, abdominal cramping, fever, and bloody stools should be reported to health care professional promptly as a sign of CDAD. May begin up to several months following cessation of therapy.
- ***Lab Test Considerations:*** Monitor hepatic function periodically during therapy. May cause ↑ AST, ALT, LDH, bilirubin, alkaline phosphatase, BUN, and creatinine.
- May cause ↓ hemoglobin, hematocrit, RBC, WBC, neutrophils, and lymphocytes.
- May cause transient ↓ estradiol, total conjugated estriol, estriol-glucuronide, or conjugated estrone in pregnant women.
- May cause a false-positive Coombs' test result.

Potential Nursing Diagnoses

Risk for infection (Indications, Side Effects)

Implementation

- **IM:** Reconstitute for IM use by adding 3.2 mL of sterile water or 0.5% or 2% lidocaine HCl to the 1.5-g vial or 6.4 mL to the 3-g vial. Administer within 1 hr of preparation, deep IM into well-developed muscle.

IV Administration

- **IV Push:** ***Diluent:*** Reconstitute 1.5-g vial with 3.2 mL of sterile water for injection and the 3-g vial with 6.4 mL. ***Concentration:*** 375 mg ampicillin/sulbactam per mL. ***Rate:*** Administer over at least 10–15 min within 1 hr of reconstitution. More rapid administration may cause seizures.
- **Intermittent Infusion:** Reconstitute vials as per directions above. ***Diluent:*** Further dilute in 50–100 mL of 0.9% NaCl, D5W, D5/0.45% NaCl, or LR. Stability of solution varies from 2–8 hr at room temperature or 3–72 hr if refrigerated, depending on concentration and diluent. ***Concentration:*** Final concentration of infusion should be 3–45 mg of ampicillin/sulbactam per mL. ***Rate:*** Infuse over 15–30 min.
- **Y-Site Compatibility:** alemtuzumab, amifostine, aminocaproic acid, anidulafungin, argatroban, azithromycin, bivalirudin, bleomycin, cangrelor, carboplatin, carmustine, cisplatin, cyclophosphamide, cytarabine, dactinomycin, daptomycin, dexmedetomidine, dexrazoxane, docetaxel, doxorubicin liposomal, eptifibatide, etoposide, etoposide phosphate, fenoldopam, filgrastim, fludarabine, fluorouracil, foscarnet, fosphenytoin, granisetron, hydromorphone, ifosfamide, irinotecan, leucovorin, levofloxacin, linezolid, mesna, methotrexate, metronidazole, milrinone, mitomycin, octreotide, oxaliplatin, paclitaxel, palonosetron, pamidronate, pancuronium, pantoprazole, pemetrexed, potassium acetate, remifentanil, rituximab, rocuronium, sodium acetate, televancin, teniposide, thiotepa, tigecycline, tirofiban, trastuzumab, vecuronium, vinblastine, vincristine, voriconazole, zoledronic acid.
- **Y-Site Incompatibility:** acyclovir, amiodarone, amphotericin B colloidal, amphotericin B lipid complex, amphotericin B liposome, azathioprine, caspofungin, chlorpromazine, ciprofloxacin, dacarbazine, dantrolene, daunorubicin, diazepam, diazoxide, dobutamine, dolasetron, doxorubicin, doxycycline, epirubicin, ganciclovir, haloperidol, hydralazine, hydrocortisone sodium succinate, hydroxyzine, idarubicin, lansoprazole, lorazepam, mechlorethamine, methylprednisolone sodium succinate, midazolam, mitoxantrone, mycophenolate, nesiritide, nicardipine, ondansetron, papaverine, pentamidine, pentazocine, phenytoin, prochlorperazine, promethazine, protamine, quinupristin/dalfopristin, sargramostim, topotecan, tranexamic acid, trimethoprim/sulfamethoxazole, verapamil, vinorelbine. If aminoglycosides and penicillins must be given concurrently, administer in separate sites at least 1 hr apart.

Patient/Family Teaching

- Advise patient to report signs of superinfection (furry overgrowth on the tongue, vaginal itching or discharge, loose or foul-smelling stools) and allergy.
- Caution patient to notify health care professional if fever and diarrhea occur, especially if stool contains blood, pus, or mucus. Advise patient not to treat diarrhea without consulting health care professional. May occur up to several weeks after discontinuation of medication.
- Rep: Advise patients taking oral contraceptives to use an alternative or additional nonhormonal method of

contraception while taking ampicillin/sulbactam and until next menstrual period.

- Instruct the patient to notify health care professional if symptoms do not improve.

Evaluation/Desired Outcomes

- Resolution of signs and symptoms of infection. Length of time for complete resolution depends on the organism and site of infection.

anastrozole (a-nass-troe-zole)

Arimidex

Classification

Therapeutic: antineoplastics

Pharmacologic: aromatase inhibitors

Pregnancy Category X

Indications

Adjuvant treatment of postmenopausal hormone receptor-positive early breast cancer. Initial therapy in women with postmenopausal hormone receptor-positive or hormone receptor unknown, locally advanced, or metastatic breast cancer. Advanced postmenopausal breast cancer in women with disease progression despite tamoxifen therapy.

Action

Inhibits the enzyme aromatase, which is partially responsible for conversion of precursors to estrogen. **Therapeutic Effects:** Lowers levels of circulating estrogen, which may halt progression of estrogen-sensitive breast cancer.

Pharmacokinetics

Absorption: 83–85% absorbed following oral administration.

Distribution: Unknown.

Metabolism and Excretion: 85% metabolized by the liver; 11% excreted renally.

Half-life: 50 hr.

TIME/ACTION PROFILE (lowering of serum estradiol)

ROUTE	ONSET	PEAK	DURATION
PO	within 24 hr	14 days	6 days†

†Following cessation of therapy.

Contraindications/Precautions

Contraindicated in: OB: Potential harm to fetus or spontaneous abortion.

Use Cautiously in: Women with childbearing potential; Ischemic heart disease; Lactation, Pedi: Safety not established.

Adverse Reactions/Side Effects

CNS: headache, weakness, dizziness. **EENT:** pharyngitis. **Resp:** cough, dyspnea. **CV:** MYOCARDIAL INFARCTION, angina, peripheral edema. **F and E:** hypercalcemia. **GI:** nausea, abdominal pain, anorexia, constipation, diarrhea, dry mouth, vomiting. **GU:** pelvic pain, vaginal bleeding, vaginal dryness. **Derm:** rash, sweating. **Metab:** hypercholesterolemia, weight gain. **MS:** back pain, arthritis, bone pain, carpal tunnel syndrome, fracture, myalgia. **Neuro:** paresthesia. **Misc:** allergic reactions including ANGIOEDEMA, URTICARIA, ANAPHYLAXIS, hot flashes, pain.

Interactions

Drug-Drug: None significant.

Route/Dosage

PO (Adults): 1 mg daily.

Availability (generic available)

Tablets: 1 mg.

NURSING IMPLICATIONS

Assessment

- Assess patient for pain and other side effects periodically during therapy.
- ***Lab Test Considerations:*** May cause ↑ GGT, AST, ALT, alkaline phosphatase, total cholesterol, and LDL cholesterol levels.

Potential Nursing Diagnoses

Acute pain (Side Effects)

Implementation

- **PO:** Take medication consistently with regard to food.

Patient/Family Teaching

- Instruct patient to take medication as directed. Take missed doses as soon as remembered unless it is almost time for next dose. Do not double doses. Advise patient to read the *Patient Information* leaflet before starting and with each Rx refill; changes may occur.
- Inform patient of potential for adverse reactions, and advise patient to notify health care professional immediately if allergic reactions (swelling of the face, lips, tongue, and/or throat, difficulty in swallowing and/or breathing), liver problems (general feeling of not being well, yellowing of skin or whites of eyes, pain on the right side of abdomen), skin reactions (lesions, ulcers, or blisters), or chest pain occurs.
- Advise patient that vaginal bleeding may occur during first few weeks after changing over from other hormonal therapy. Continued bleeding should be evaluated.
- Teach patient to report increase in pain so treatment can be initiated.

- Advise patient to notify health care professional immediately if pregnancy is planned or suspected, or if breast feeding.

Evaluation/Desired Outcomes

- Slowing of disease progression in women with advanced breast cancer.

ANGIOTENSIN-CONVERTING ENZYME (ACE) INHIBITORS

benazepril (ben-**aye**-ze-pril)
Lotensin

captopril (**kap**-toe-pril)
~~Capoten~~

enalapril/enalaprilat
(e-**nal**-a-pril/e-**nal**-a-pril-at)
Epaned, Vasotec, 🍁Vasotec IV

fosinopril (foe-**sin**-oh-pril)
~~Monopril~~

lisinopril (lyse-**in**-oh-pril)
Prinivil, Zestril

moexipril (moe-**eks**-i-pril)
Univasc

perindopril (pe-**rin**-do-pril)
Aceon, 🍁Coversyl

quinapril (**kwin**-a-pril)
Accupril

ramipril (ra-**mi**-pril)
Altace

trandolapril (tran-**doe**-la-pril)
Mavik

Classification
Therapeutic: antihypertensives
Pharmacologic: ACE inhibitors

Pregnancy Category D

Indications

Alone or with other agents in the management of hypertension. **Captopril, enalapril, fosinopril, lisinopril, quinapril, ramipril, trandolapril:** Management of HF. **Captopril, lisinopril, ramipril, trandolapril:** Reduction of risk of death or development of HF following MI. **Enalapril:** Slowed progression of left ventricular dysfunction into overt heart failure. **Ramipril:** Reduction of the risk of MI, stroke, and death from cardiovascular disease in patients at risk (>55 yr old with a history of CAD, stroke, peripheral vascular disease, or diabetes with another cardiovascular risk factor). **Captopril:** ↓ progression of diabetic nephropathy. **Perindopril:** Reduction of risk of death from cardiovascular causes or nonfatal MI in patients with stable CAD.

Action

ACE inhibitors block the conversion of angiotensin I to the vasoconstrictor angiotensin II. ACE inhibitors also prevent the degradation of bradykinin and other vasodilatory prostaglandins. ACE inhibitors also ↑ plasma renin levels and ↓ aldosterone levels. Net result is systemic vasodilation. **Therapeutic Effects:** Lowering of BP in hypertensive patients. Improved symptoms in patients with HF (selected agents only). ↓ development of overt heart failure (enalapril only). Improved survival and ↓ development of overt HF after MI (selected agents only). ↓ risk of death from cardiovascular causes or MI in patients with stable CAD (perindopril only). ↓ risk of MI, stroke or death from cardiovascular causes in high-risk patients (ramipril only). ↓ progression of diabetic nephropathy (captopril only).

Pharmacokinetics

Absorption: *Benazepril*—37% absorbed after oral administration. *Captopril*—60–75% absorbed after oral administration (↓ by food). *Enalapril*—55–75% absorbed after oral administration. *Enalaprilat*—IV administration results in complete bioavailability. *Fosinopril*—36% absorbed after oral administration. *Lisinopril*—25% absorbed after oral administration (much variability). *Moexipril*—13% bioavailability as moexiprilat after oral administration (↓ by food). *Perindopril*—25% bioavailability as perindoprilat after oral administration. *Quinapril*—60% absorbed after oral administration (high-fat meal may ↓ absorption). *Ramipril*—50–60% absorbed after oral administration. *Trandolapril*—70% bioavailability as trandolapril at after oral administration.
Distribution: All ACE inhibitors cross the placenta. *Benazepril, captopril, enalapril, fosinopril, quinapril,* and *trandolapril*—Enter breast milk. *Lisinopril*—Minimal penetration of CNS. *Ramipril*—Probably does not enter breast milk. *Trandolapril*—Enters breast milk.
Protein Binding: *Benazepril*—95%, *Fosinopril*—99.4%, *Moexipril*—90%, *Quinapril*—97%.
Metabolism and Excretion: *Benazepril*—Converted by the liver to benazeprilat, the active metabolite. 20% excreted by kidneys; 11–12% nonrenal (biliary elimination). *Captopril*—50% metabolized by the liver to inactive compounds, 50% excreted unchanged by the kidneys. *Enalapril, enalaprilat*—Enalapril is converted by the liver to enalaprilat, the active metabolite; primarily eliminated by the kidneys. *Fosinopril*—Converted by the liver and GI mucosa to fosinoprilat, the active metabolite—50% excreted in urine, 50% in feces. *Lisinopril*—100% eliminated by the kidneys. *Moexipril*—Converted by liver and GI mucosa to moexiprilat, the active metabolite; 13% excreted in urine, 53% in feces. *Perindopril*—Converted by the liver to perindoprilat, the active metabolite; primarily

excreted in urine. *Quinapril*—Converted by the liver, GI mucosa, and tissue to quinaprilat, the active metabolite: 96% eliminated by the kidneys. *Ramipril*—Converted by the liver to ramiprilat, the active metabolite; 60% excreted in urine, 40% in feces. *Trandolapril*—Converted by the liver to trandolaprilat, the active metabolite; 33% excreted in urine, 66% in feces.

Half-life: *Benazeprilat*—10–11 hr. *Captopril*—2 hr (↑ in renal impairment). *Enalapril-* 2 hr (↑ in renal impairment). *Enalaprilat*—35–38 hr (↑ in renal impairment). *Fosinoprilat*—12 hr. *Lisinopril*—12 hr (↑ in renal impairment). *Moexiprilat*—2–9 hr (↑ in renal impairment). *Perindoprilat*—3–10 hr (↑ in renal impairment). *Quinaprilat*—3 hr (↑ in renal impairment). *Ramiprilat*—13–17 hr (↑ in renal impairment). *Trandolaprilat*—22.5 hr (↑ in renal impairment).

TIME/ACTION PROFILE (effect on BP—single dose†)

ROUTE	ONSET	PEAK	DURATION
Benazepril	within 1 hr	2–4 hr	24 hr
Captopril	15–60 min	60–90 min	6–12 hr
Enalapril PO	1 hr	4–8 hr	12–24 hr
Enalapril IV	15 min	1–4 hr	4–6 hr
Fosinopril	within 1 hr	2–6 hr	24 hr
Lisinopril	1 hr	6 hr	24 hr
Moexipril	within 1 hr	3–6 hr	up to 24 hr
Perindoprilat	within 1–2 hr	3–7 hr	up to 24 hr
Quinapril	within 1 hr	2–4 hr	up to 24 hr
Ramipril	within 1–2 hr	3–6 hr	24 hr
Trandolapril	within 1–2 hr	4–10 hr	up to 24 hr

†Full effects may not be noted for several wks.

Contraindications/Precautions

Contraindicated in: Hypersensitivity; History of angioedema with previous use of ACE inhibitors (also in absence of previous use of ACE inhibitors for benazepril); Concurrent use with aliskiren in patients with diabetes or moderate-to-severe renal impairment (CCr <60 mL/min); OB: Can cause injury or death of fetus—if pregnancy occurs, discontinue immediately; Lactation: Certain ACE inhibitors appear in breast milk; discontinue drug or use formula.

Use Cautiously in: Renal impairment, hepatic impairment, hypovolemia, hyponatremia, concurrent diuretic therapy; ⧖ Black patients with hypertension (monotherapy less effective, may require additional therapy; ↑ risk of angioedema); Women of childbearing potential; Surgery/anesthesia (hypotension may be exaggerated); Pedi: Safety not established for most agents; benazepril, fosinopril, and lisinopril may be used in children ≥6 yr (captopril and enalapril may be used in children of all ages); Geri: Initial dose ↓ recommended for most agents due to age-related ↓ in renal function.

Exercise Extreme Caution in: Family history of angioedema.

Adverse Reactions/Side Effects

CNS: dizziness, drowsiness, fatigue, headache, insomnia, vertigo, weakness. **Resp:** <u>cough</u>, dyspnea. **CV:** <u>hypotension</u>, chest pain, edema, tachycardia. **Endo:** hyperuricemia. **GI:** <u>taste disturbances</u>, abdominal pain, anorexia, constipation, diarrhea, nausea, vomiting. **GU:** erectile dysfunction, proteinuria, renal dysfunction, renal failure. **Derm:** flushing, pruritis, rashes. **F and E:** hyperkalemia. **Hemat:** AGRANULOCYTOSIS, neutropenia (captopril only). **MS:** back pain, muscle cramps, myalgia. **Misc:** ANGIOEDEMA, fever.

Interactions

Drug-Drug: Excessive hypotension may occur with concurrent use of **diuretics** and other **antihypertensives.** ↑ risk of hyperkalemia with concurrent use of **potassium supplements, potassium-sparing diuretics,** or **potassium-containing salt substitutes.** ↑ risk of hyperkalemia, renal dysfunction, hypotension, and syncope with concurrent use of **angiotensin II receptor blockers** or **aliskiren**; avoid concurrent use with aliskiren in patients with diabetes or CCr <60 mL/min; avoid concurrent use with angiotensin II receptor blockers. **NSAIDs** and selective **COX-2 inhibitors** may blunt the antihypertensive effect and ↑ the risk of renal dysfunction. Absorption of fosinopril may be ↓ by **antacids** (separate administration by 1–2 hr). ↑ levels and may ↑ risk of **lithium** toxicity. Quinapril may ↓ absorption of **tetracycline, doxycycline,** and **fluoroquinolones** (because of magnesium in tablets). ↑ risk of angioedema with **temsirolimus, sirolimus,** or **everolimus.**

Drug-Food: Food significantly ↓ absorption of captopril and moexipril (administer drugs 1 hr before meals).

Route/Dosage

Benazepril

⧖ **PO (Adults):** 10 mg once daily, ↑ gradually to maintenance dose of 20–40 mg/day in 1–2 divided doses (begin with 5 mg/day in patients receiving diuretics).

PO (Children ≥6 yr): 0.2 mg/kg once daily; may be titrated up to 0.6 mg/kg/day (or 40 mg/day).

Renal Impairment

PO (Adults): *CCr <30 mL/min*—Initiate therapy with 5 mg once daily.

Renal Impairment

PO (Children ≥6 yr): *CCr <30 mL/min*—Contraindicated.

Captopril

PO (Adults): *Hypertension*—12.5–25 mg 2–3 times daily, may be ↑ at 1–2 wk intervals up to 150 mg 3 times daily (begin with 6.25–12.5 mg 2–3 times daily in patients receiving diuretics) (maximum dose

= 450 mg/day); *HF*—25 mg 3 times daily (6.25–12.5 mg 3 times daily in patients who have been vigorously diuresed); titrated up to target dose of 50 mg 3 times daily; *Post-MI*—6.25-mg test dose, followed by 12.5 mg 3 times daily, may be ↑ up to 50 mg 3 times daily; *Diabetic nephropathy*—25 mg 3 times daily.
PO (Children): *HF*—0.3 mg/kg–0.5 mg/kg/dose 3 times daily, titrate up to a maximum of 6 mg/kg/day in 2–4 divided doses; *Older Children*—6.25–12.5 mg/dose q 12–24 hr, titrate up to a maximum of 6 mg/kg/day in 2–4 divided doses.
PO (Infants): *HF*—0.15–0.3 mg/kg/dose, titrate up to a maximum of 6 mg/kg/day in 1–4 divided doses.
PO (Neonates): *HF*—0.05–0.1 mg/kg/dose q 8–24 hr, may ↑ as needed up to 0.5 mg/kg q 6–24 hr; *Premature neonates*—0.01 mg/kg/dose q 8–12 hr.

Renal Impairment

PO (Adults): *CCr 10–50 mL/min*—Administer 75% of dose; *CCr <10 mL/min*—Administer 50% of dose.

Enalapril/Enalaprilat

PO (Adults): *Hypertension*—2.5–5 mg once daily, ↑ as required up to 40 mg/day in 1–2 divided doses (initiate therapy at 2.5 mg once daily in patients receiving diuretics); *HF*—2.5 mg 1–2 times daily, titrated up to target dose of 10 mg twice daily; begin with 2.5 mg once daily in patients with hyponatremia (serum sodium <130 mEq/L); *Asymptomatic left ventricular dysfunction*—2.5 mg twice daily, titrated up to a target dose of 10 mg twice daily.
PO (Children >1 mo): *Hypertension*—0.08 mg/kg once daily; may be slowly titrated up to a maximum of 0.58 mg/kg/day.
IV (Adults): *Hypertension*—0.625–1.25 mg (0.625 mg if receiving diuretics) q 6 hr; can be titrated up to 5 mg q 6 hr.
IV (Children >1 mo): *Hypertension*—5–10 mcg/kg/dose given q 8–24 hr.

Renal Impairment

PO, IV (Adults): *Hypertension CCr 10–50 mL/min*—Administer 75% of dose; *CCr <10 mL/min*—Administer 50% of dose.

Renal Impairment

PO, IV (Children >1 mo): *CCr <30 mL/min*—Contraindicated.

Fosinopril

PO (Adults): *Hypertension*—10 mg once daily, may be ↑ as required up to 80 mg/day. *HF*—10 mg once daily (5 mg once daily in patients who have been vigorously diuresed), may be ↑ over several weeks up to 40 mg/day.
PO (Children ≥6 yr and >50 kg): *Hypertension*—5–10 mg once daily.

Lisinopril

PO (Adults): *Hypertension*—10 mg once daily, can be ↑ up to 20–40 mg/day (initiate therapy at 5 mg/day in patients receiving diuretics); *HF*—5 mg once daily; may be titrated every 2 wk up to 40 mg/day; begin with 2.5 mg once daily in patients with hyponatremia (serum sodium <130 mEq/L); *Post-MI*—5 mg once daily for 2 days, then 10 mg daily.
PO (Children ≥6 yr): *Hypertension*—0.07 mg/kg once daily (up to 5 mg/day), may be titrated every 1–2 wk up to 0.6 mg/kg/day (or 40 mg/day).

Renal Impairment

PO (Adults): *CCr 10–30 mL/min*—Begin with 5 mg once daily; may be slowly titrated up to 40 mg/day; *CCr <10 ml/min*—Begin with 2.5 mg once daily; may be slowly titrated up to 40 mg/day.

Renal Impairment

(Children ≥6 yr): *CCr <30 mL/min*—Contraindicated.

Moexipril

PO (Adults): 7.5 mg once daily, may be ↑ up to 30 mg/day in 1–2 divided doses (begin with 3.75 mg/day in patients receiving diuretics).

Renal Impairment

PO (Adults): *CCr ≤40 mL/min*—Initiate therapy at 3.75 mg once daily, may be titrated upward carefully to 15 mg/day.

Perindopril

PO (Adults): *Hypertension*—4 mg once daily, may be slowly titrated up to 16 mg/day in 1–2 divided doses (should not exceed 8 mg/day in elderly patients) (begin with 2–4 mg/day in 1–2 divided doses in patients receiving diuretics); *Stable CAD*—4 mg once daily for 2 weeks, may be ↑, if tolerated, to 8 mg once daily; for elderly patients, begin with 2 mg once daily for 1 week (may be ↑, if tolerated, to 4 mg once daily for 1 week, then, ↑ as tolerated to 8 mg once daily).

Renal Impairment

PO (Adults): *CCr 30–60 mL/min*—2 mg/day initially, may be slowly titrated up to 8 mg/day in 1–2 divided doses.

Quinapril

PO (Adults): *Hypertension*—10–20 mg once daily initially, may be titrated q 2 wk up to 80 mg/day in 1–2 divided doses (initiate therapy at 5 mg/day in patients receiving diuretics); *HF*—5 mg twice daily initially, may be titrated at weekly intervals up to 20 mg twice daily.

Renal Impairment

PO (Adults): *CCr >60 mL/min*—Initiate therapy at 10 mg/day; *CCr 30–60 mL/min*—Initiate therapy at 5 mg/day; *CCr 10–30 mL/min*—Initiate therapy at 2.5 mg/day.

Ramipril

PO (Adults): *Hypertension*—2.5 mg once daily, may be ↑ slowly up to 20 mg/day in 1–2 divided doses (initiate therapy at 1.25 mg/day in patients receiving diuretics). *HF post-MI*— 1.25–2.5 mg twice daily initially, may be ↑ slowly up to 5 mg twice daily. *Reduction in risk of MI, stroke, and death from cardiovascular causes*— 2.5 mg once daily for 1 wk, then 5 mg once daily for 3 wk, then ↑ as tolerated to 10 mg once daily (can also be given in 2 divided doses).

Renal Impairment

PO (Adults): *CCr <40 mL/min*— Initiate therapy at 1.25 mg once daily, may be slowly titrated up to 5 mg/day in 1–2 divided doses.

Trandolapril

🧬 **PO (Adults):** *Hypertension*— 1 mg once daily (2 mg once daily in black patients); *HF post-MI*— Initiate therapy at 1 mg once daily, titrate up to 4 mg once daily if possible.

Renal Impairment

PO (Adults): *CCr <30 mL/min*— Initiate therapy at 0.5 mg once daily, may be slowly titrated upward (maximum dose = 4 mg/day).

Hepatic Impairment

PO (Adults): Initiate therapy at 0.5 mg once daily, may be slowly titrated upward (maximum dose = 4 mg/day).

Availability

Benazepril (generic available)

Tablets: 5 mg, 10 mg, 20 mg, 40 mg. **Cost:** *Generic*— All strengths $10.83/100. ***In combination with:*** amlodipine (Lotrel) and hydrochlorothiazide (Lotensin HCT). See Appendix B.

Captopril (generic available)

Tablets: 12.5 mg, 25 mg, 50 mg, 100 mg. **Cost:** *Generic*— 12.5 mg $77.18/100, 25 mg $83.44/100, 50 mg $143.08/100, 100 mg $190.54/100. ***In combination with:*** hydrochlorothiazide (Capozide). See Appendix B.

Enalapril (generic available)

Tablets: 2.5 mg, 5 mg, 10 mg, 20 mg. **Cost:** *Generic*— 2.5 mg $88.33/100, 5 mg $106.37/100, 10 mg $117.81/100, 20 mg $167.64/100. **Powder for oral solution (requires reconstitution):** 1 mg/mL. ***In combination with:*** hydrochlorothiazide (Vaseretic). See Appendix B.

Enalaprilat (generic available)

Injection: 1.25 mg/mL.

Fosinopril (generic available)

Tablets: 10 mg, 20 mg, 40 mg. **Cost:** *Generic*— All strengths $107.08/90. ***In combination with:*** hydrochlorothiazide. See Appendix B.

Lisinopril (generic available)

Tablets: 2.5 mg, 5 mg, 10 mg, 20 mg, 30 mg, 40 mg. **Cost:** *Generic*— 2.5 mg $9.63/100, 5 mg $10.83/100, 10 mg $6.99/100, 20 mg $9.14/100, 30 mg $10.83/100, 40 mg $7.41/100. ***In combination with:*** hydrochlorothiazide (Prinzide, Zestoretic). See Appendix B.

Moexipril (generic available)

Tablets: 7.5 mg, 15 mg. **Cost:** *Generic*— 7.5 mg $138.92/100, 15 mg $145.54/100. ***In combination with:*** hydrochlorothiazide (Uniretic).

Perindopril (generic available)

Tablets: 2 mg, 4 mg, 8 mg. **Cost:** *Generic*— 2 mg $189.77/100, 4 mg $221.27/100, 8 mg $268.76/100. ***In combination with:*** amlodipine (Prestalia). See Appendix B.

Quinapril (generic available)

Tablets: 5 mg, 10 mg, 20 mg, 40 mg. **Cost:** *Generic*— 5 mg $27.20/100, 10 mg $39.19/100, 20 mg $21.04/100, 40 mg $27.50/100. ***In combination with:*** hydrochlorothiazide (Accuretic, Quinaretic). See Appendix B.

Ramipril (generic available)

Capsules: 1.25 mg, 2.5 mg, 5 mg, 10 mg. **Cost:** *Generic*— 1.25 mg $153.01/100, 2.5 mg $180.61/100, 5 mg $189.49/100, 10 mg $221.72/100.

Trandolapril (generic available)

Tablets: 1 mg, 2 mg, 4 mg. **Cost:** *Generic*— All strengths $123.93/100. ***In combination with:*** verapamil (Tarka). See Appendix B.

NURSING IMPLICATIONS

Assessment

- **Hypertension:** Monitor BP and pulse frequently during initial dose adjustment and periodically during therapy. Notify health care professional of significant changes.
- Monitor frequency of prescription refills to determine adherence.
- Assess patient for signs of angioedema (swelling of face, extremities, eyes, lips, tongue, difficulty in swallowing or breathing); may occur at any time during therapy. Discontinue medication and provide supportive care.
- **HF:** Monitor weight and assess patient routinely for resolution of fluid overload (peripheral edema, rales/crackles, dyspnea, weight gain, jugular venous distention).
- ***Lab Test Considerations:*** Monitor BUN, creatinine, and electrolyte levels periodically. Serum potassium, BUN and creatinine may be ↑, whereas sodium levels may be ↓. If ↑ BUN or serum creatinine concentrations occur, dose reduction or withdrawal may be required.

- Monitor CBC periodically during therapy. Certain drugs may rarely cause slight ↓ in hemoglobin and hematocrit, leukopenia, and eosinophilia.
- May cause ↑ AST, ALT, alkaline phosphatase, serum bilirubin, uric acid, and glucose.
- Assess urine protein prior to and periodically during therapy for up to 1 yr in patients with renal impairment or those receiving >150 m g/day of captopril. If excessive or ↑ proteinuria occurs, re-evaluate ACE inhibitor therapy.
- *Captopril:* May cause positive ANA titer.
- *Captopril:* May cause false-positive test results for urine acetone.
- *Captopril:* Monitor CBC with differential prior to initiation of therapy, every 2 wk for first 3 mo, and periodically for up to 1 yr in patients at risk for neutropenia (patients with renal impairment or collagen-vascular disease) or at first sign of infection. Discontinue therapy if neutrophil count is <1000/mm^3.

Potential Nursing Diagnoses

Decreased cardiac output (Indications, Side Effects)
Noncompliance (Patient/Family Teaching)

Implementation

- Do not confuse Accupril with Aciphex. Do not confuse benazepril with Benadryl. Do not confuse captopril with carvedilol. Do not confuse Zestril with Zegerid, Zetia, or Zyprexa.
- Correct volume depletion, if possible, before initiation of therapy.
- **PO:** Precipitous drop in BP during first 1–3 hr after first dose may require volume expansion with normal saline but is not normally considered an indication for stopping therapy. Discontinuing diuretic therapy or cautiously increasing salt intake 2–3 days before initiation may ↓ risk of hypotension. Monitor closely for at least 1 hr after BP has stabilized. Resume diuretics if BP is not controlled.

Benazepril

- **PO:** For patients with difficulty swallowing tablets, pharmacist may compound oral suspension; stable for 30 days if refrigerated. Shake suspension before each use.

Captopril

- **PO:** Administer 1 hr before or 2 hr after meals. May be crushed if patient has difficulty swallowing. Tablets may have a sulfurous odor.
- An oral solution may be prepared by crushing a 25-mg tablet and dissolving it in 25–100 mL of water. Shake for at least 5 min and administer within 30 min.

Enalapril

- **PO:** For patients with difficulty swallowing tablets, pharmacist may prepare oral solution. Shake solution before each use. Solution is stable at controlled room temperature for 60 days.

Enalaprilat

IV Administration

- **IV Push:** ***Diluent:*** May be administered undiluted. ***Concentration:*** 1.25 mg/mL. ***Rate:*** Administer over at least 5 min.
- **Intermittent Infusion:** ***Diluent:*** Dilute in up to 50 mL of D5W, 0.9% NaCl, D5/0.9% NaCl, or D5/LR. Diluted solution is stable for 24 hr. ***Rate:*** Administer as a slow infusion over at least 5 min.
- **Y-Site Compatibility:** acyclovir, alemtuzumab, alfentanil, allopurinol, amifostine, amikacin, aminocaproic acid, aminophylline, amiodarone, amphotericin B lipid complex, amphotericin B liposome, anidulafungin, argatroban, ascorbic acid, atracurium, atropine, azathioprine, azithromycin, aztreonam, benztropine, bivalirudin, bleomycin, bumetanide, buprenorphine, butorphanol, calcium chloride, calcium gluconate, cangrelor, carboplatin, carmustine, cefazolin, cefotaxime, cefotetan, cefoxitin, ceftaroline, ceftazidime, ceftriaxone, cefuroxime, chloramphenicol, chlorpromazine, cisatracurium, cisplatin, cladribine, clindamycin, cyanocobalamin, cyclophosphamide, cyclosporine, cytarabine, dacarbazine, dactinomycin, daptomycin, daunorubicin, dexamethasone , dexmedetomidine, dexrazoxane, digoxin, diltiazem, diphenhydramine, dobutamine, docetaxel, dolasetron, dopamine, doripenem, doxacurium, doxorubicin, doxorubicin liposome, doxycycline, ephedrine, epinephrine, epirubicin, epoetin, eptifibatide, ertapenem, erythromycin, esmolol, etoposide, etoposide phosphate, famotidine, fenoldopam, fentanyl, filgrastim, fluconazole, fludarabine, fluorouracil, folic acid, foscarnet, fosphenytoin, furosemide, ganciclovir, gemcitabine, gentamicin, glycopyrrolate, granisetron, heparin, hetastarch, hydrocortisone sodium succinate, hydromorphone, idarubicin, ifosfamide, imipenem/cilastatin, indomethacin, insulin, irinotecan, isoproterenol, ketorolac, labetalol, leucovorin, levofloxacin, lidocaine, linezolid, lorazepam, magnesium sulfate, mannitol, mechlorethamine, melphalan, meperidine, meropenem, mesna, methotrexate, methylprednisolone, metoclopramide, metoprolol, metronidazole, midazolam, milrinone, mitomycin, mitoxantrone, morphine, moxifloxacin, multivitamins, mycophenolate, nafcillin, nalbuphine, naloxone, nicardipine, nitroglycerin, nitroprusside, norepinephrine, octreotide, ondansetron, oxacillin, oxaliplatin, oxytocin, paclitaxel, palonosetron, pamidronate, pancuronium, papaverine, pemetrexed, penicillin G, pentamidine, pentazocine, pentobarbital, phenobarbital, phenylephrine, phytonadione, piperacillin/tazobactam, potassium acetate, potassium chloride, potassium phosphates, procainamide, prochlorperazine, promethazine, propofol, propranolol, protamine, pyridoxine, quinupristin/dalfopristin, ranitidine, remifentanil, rituximab, rocuronium, sodium acetate, sodium bicarbonate, streptokinase,

succinylcholine, sufentanil, tacrolimus, teniposide, tetracycline, theophylline, thiamine, thiotepa, tigecycline, tirofiban, tobramycin, topotecan, trastuzumab, vancomycin, vasopressin, vecuronium, verapamil, vinblastine, vincristine, vinorelbine, voriconazole, zoledronic acid.

- **Y-Site Incompatibility:** amphotericin B colloidal, caspofungin, cefepime, dantrolene, diazepam, diazoxide, phenytoin.

Lisinopril

- **PO:** For patients with difficulty swallowing tablets, pharmacist may compound oral suspension; stable at room temperature for 4 wk. Shake suspension before each use.

Moexipril

- **PO:** Administer moexipril on an empty stomach, 1 hr before a meal.

Ramipril

- **PO:** Capsules may be opened and sprinkled on applesauce, or dissolved in 4 oz water or apple juice for patients with difficulty swallowing. Effectiveness is same as capsule. Prepared mixtures can be stored for up to 24 hr at room temperature or up to 48 hr if refrigerated.

Trandolapril

- **PO:** May be taken with or without food.

Patient/Family Teaching

- Instruct patient to take medication as directed at the same time each day, even if feeling well. Take missed doses as soon as possible but not if almost time for next dose. Do not double doses. Warn patient not to discontinue ACE inhibitor therapy unless directed by health care professional.
- Caution patient to avoid salt substitutes or foods containing high levels of potassium or sodium unless directed by health care professional (see Appendix J).
- Caution patient to change positions slowly to minimize hypotension. Use of alcohol, standing for long periods, exercising, and hot weather may ↑ orthostatic hypotension.Instruct patient to notify health care professional of all Rx or OTC medications, vitamins, or herbal products being taken and consult health care professional before taking any new medications, especially cough, cold, or allergy remedies.
- May cause dizziness. Caution patient to avoid driving and other activities requiring alertness until response to medication is known.
- Advise patient to inform health care professional of medication regimen prior to treatment or surgery.
- Advise patient that medication may cause impairment of taste that generally resolves within 8–12 wk, even with continued therapy.
- Instruct patient to notify health care professional immediately if rash; mouth sores; sore throat; fever; swelling of hands or feet; irregular heart beat; chest pain; dry cough; hoarseness; swelling of face, eyes, lips, or tongue; difficulty swallowing or breathing occur; or if taste impairment or skin rash persists. Persistent dry cough may occur and may not subside until medication is discontinued. Consult health care professional if cough becomes bothersome. Also notify health care professional if nausea, vomiting, or diarrhea occurs and continues.
- Advise diabetic patients to monitor blood glucose closely, especially during first month of therapy; may cause hypoglycemia.
- Advise women of childbearing age to use contraception and notify health care professional if pregnancy is planned or suspected. If pregnancy is detected, discontinue medication as soon as possible.
- Emphasize the importance of follow-up examinations to monitor progress.
- **Hypertension:** Encourage patient to comply with additional interventions for hypertension (weight reduction, low sodium diet, discontinuation of smoking, moderation of alcohol consumption, regular exercise, and stress management). Medication controls but does not cure hypertension.
- Instruct patient and family on correct technique for monitoring BP. Advise them to check BP at least weekly and to report significant changes to health care professional.

Evaluation/Desired Outcomes

- Decrease in BP without appearance of excessive side effects.
- Decrease in signs and symptoms of HF (some drugs may also improve survival).
- Decrease in development of overt HF (enalapril).
- Reduction of risk of death or development of HF following MI.
- Reduction of risk of death from cardiovascular causes and MI in patients with stable CAD (perindopril).
- Reduction of risk of MI, stroke, or death from cardiovascular causes in patients at high-risk for these events (ramipril).
- Decrease in progression of diabetic nephropathy (captopril).

ANGIOTENSIN II RECEPTOR ANTAGONISTS

azilsartan (a-zill-**sar**-tan)
Edarbi

candesartan (can-de-**sar**-tan)
Atacand

eprosartan (ep-roe-**sar**-tan)
Teveten

irbesartan (ir-be-**sar**-tan)
Avapro

losartan (loe-**sar**-tan)
Cozaar

olmesartan (ole-me-**sar**-tan)
Benicar, ✱Olmetec

telmisartan (tel-mi-**sar**-tan)
Micardis

valsartan (val-**sar**-tan)
Diovan

Classification
Therapeutic: antihypertensives
Pharmacologic: angiotensin II receptor antagonists

Pregnancy Category D

Indications

Alone or with other agents in the management of hypertension. Treatment of diabetic nephropathy in patients with type 2 diabetes and hypertension (irbesartan and losartan only). Management of HF (New York Heart Association class II-IV) in patients who cannot tolerate ACE inhibitors (candesartan and valsartan only) or in combination with an ACE inhibitor and beta-blocker (candesartan only). Prevention of stroke in patients with hypertension and left ventricular hypertrophy (losartan only). Reduction of risk of death from cardiovascular causes in patients with left ventricular systolic dysfunction after MI (valsartan only). Reduction of risk of myocardial infarction, stroke, or cardiovascular death in patients ≥55 yr who are at high risk for cardiovascular events and are unable to take ACE inhibitors (telmisartan only).

Action

Blocks vasoconstrictor and aldosterone-producing effects of angiotensin II at receptor sites, including vascular smooth muscle and the adrenal glands. **Therapeutic Effects:** Lowering of BP. Slowed progression of diabetic nephropathy (irbesartan and losartan only). Reduced cardiovascular death and hospitalizations due to HF in patients with HF (candesartan and valsartan only). Decreased risk of cardiovascular death in patients with left ventricular systolic dysfunction who are post-MI (valsartan only). Decreased risk of stroke in patients with hypertension and left ventricular hypertrophy (effect may be less in black patients) (losartan only).

Pharmacokinetics

Absorption: *Azilsartan*—Azilsartan medoxomil is converted to azilsartan, the active component. 60% absorbed; *Candesartan*—Candesartan cilexetil is converted to candesartan, the active component; 15% bioavailability of candesartan; *Eprosartan*—13% absorbed after oral administration; *Irbesartan*—60–80% absorbed after oral administration; *Losartan*—well absorbed, with extensive first-pass hepatic metabolism, resulting in 33% bioavailability; *Olmesartan*—Olmesartan medoxomil is converted to olmesartan, the active component; 26% bioavailability of olmesartan; *Telmisartan*—42–58% absorbed following oral administration (bioavailability ↑ in patients with hepatic impairment); *Valsartan*—10–35% absorbed following oral administration.

Distribution: All angiotensin receptor blockers (ARBs) cross the placenta; *Candesartan*—enters breast milk.

Protein Binding: All ARBs are >90% protein-bound.

Metabolism and Excretion: *Azilsartan*—50% metabolized by the liver, primarily by the CYP2C9 enzyme system. 55% eliminated in feces, 42% in urine (15% as unchanged drug); *Candesartan*—Minor metabolism by the liver; 33% excreted in urine, 67% in feces (via bile); *Eprosartan*—Excreted primarily unchanged in feces via biliary excretion; *Irbesartan*—Some hepatic metabolism; 20% excreted in urine, 80% in feces; *Losartan*—Undergoes extensive first-pass hepatic metabolism; 14% is converted to an active metabolite. 4% excreted unchanged in urine; 6% excreted in urine as active metabolite; some biliary elimination; *Olmesartan*—30–50% excreted unchanged in urine, remainder eliminated in feces via bile; *Telmisartan*—Excreted mostly unchanged in feces via biliary excretion; *Valsartan*—Minor metabolism by the liver; 13% excreted in urine, 83% in feces.

Half-life: *Azilsartan*—11 hr; *Candesartan*—9 hr; *Eprosartan*—20 hr; *Irbesartan*—11–15 hr; *Losartan*—2 hr (6–9 hr for metabolite); *Olmesartan*—13 hr; *Telmisartan*—24 hr; *Valsartan*—6 hr.

TIME/ACTION PROFILE (antihypertensive effect with chronic dosing)

DRUG	ONSET	PEAK	DURATION
Azilsartan	within 2 hr	18 hr	24 hr
Candesartan	2–4 hr	4 wk	24 hr
Eprosartan	1–2 hr	2–3 wk	12–24 hr
Irbesartan	within 2 hr	2 wk	24 hr
Losartan	6 hr	3–6 wk	24 hr
Olmesartan	within 1 wk	2 wk	24 hr
Telmisartan	within 3 hr	4 wk	24 hr
Valsartan	within 2 hr	4 wk	24 hr

Contraindications/Precautions

Contraindicated in: Hypersensitivity; Concurrent use with aliskiren in patients with diabetes or moderate-to-severe renal impairment (CCr <60 mL/min); Severe hepatic impairment (candesartan); OB: Can cause injury or death of fetus—if pregnancy occurs, discontinue immediately; Lactation: Discontinue drug or use formula.

Use Cautiously in: HF (may result in azotemia, oliguria, acute renal failure and/or death); Volume- or salt-depleted patients or patients receiving high doses of diuretics (correct deficits before initiating therapy or initiate at lower doses); ⧖ Black patients (may not be effective); Impaired renal function due to primary renal disease or HF (may worsen renal function); Obstructive biliary disorders (telmisartan) or hepatic impairment (losartan, or telmisartan); Women of childbearing potential; Pedi: Safety not established in children <18 yr (<6 yr for losartan, olmesartan, and valsartan).

Adverse Reactions/Side Effects

CNS: dizziness, anxiety, depression, fatigue, headache, insomnia, weakness. **CV:** hypotension, chest pain, edema, tachycardia. **Derm:** rashes. **EENT:** nasal congestion, pharyngitis, rhinitis, sinusitis. **GI:** abdominal pain, diarrhea, drug-induced hepatitis, dyspepsia, nausea, vomiting. **GU:** impaired renal function. **F and E:** hyperkalemia. **MS:** arthralgia, back pain, myalgia. **Misc:** ANGIOEDEMA.

Interactions

Drug-Drug: **NSAIDs** and selective **COX-2 inhibitors** may blunt the antihypertensive effect and ↑ the risk of renal dysfunction. ↑ antihypertensive effects with other **antihypertensives** and **diuretics**. Telmisartan may ↑ serum **digoxin** levels. Concurrent use of **potassium-sparing diuretics**, **potassium-containing salt substitutes**, or **potassium supplements** may ↑ risk of hyperkalemia. ↑ risk of hyperkalemia, renal dysfunction, hypotension, and syncope with concurrent use of **ACE inhibitors** or **aliskiren**; avoid concurrent use with aliskiren in patients with diabetes or CCr <60 mL/min; avoid concurrent use with ACE inhibitors. Candesartan, valsartan, and irbesartan may ↑ **lithium** levels. Irbesartan and losartan may ↑ effects of **amiodarone**, **fluoxetine**, **glimepiride**, **glipizide**, **phenytoin**, **rosiglitazone**, and **warfarin**. **Rifampin** may ↓ effects of losartan. ↑ risk of renal dysfunction when telmisartan used with **ramipril** (concurrent use not recommended). **Colesevelam** may ↓ olmesartan levels; administer olmesartan ≥4 hr before colesevelam.

Route/Dosage

Azilsartan

PO (Adults): 80 mg once daily, initial dose may be ↓ to 40 mg once daily if high doses of diuretics are used concurrently.

Candesartan

PO (Adults): *Hypertension*—16 mg once daily; may be ↑ up to 32 mg/day in 1–2 divided doses (begin therapy at a lower dose in patients who are receiving diuretics or are volume depleted). *HF*—4 mg once daily initially, dose may be doubled at 2 wk intervals up to target dose of 32 mg once daily.

PO (Children 6–16 yr and >50 k g): 8–16 mg/day (in 1–2 divided doses); may be ↑ up to 32 mg/day (in 1–2 divided doses).

PO (Children 6–16 yr and <50 kg): 4–8 mg/day (in 1–2 divided doses); may be ↑ up to 16 mg/day (in 1–2 divided doses).

PO (Children 1–5 yr): 0.20 mg/kg/day (in 1–2 divided doses); may be ↑ up to 0.4 mg/kg/day (in 1–2 divided doses).

Hepatic Impairment

PO (Adults): *Moderate hepatic impairment*—Initiate at 8 mg once daily.

Eprosartan

PO (Adults): 600 mg once daily; may be ↑ to 800 mg/day (in 1–2 divided doses) (usual range 400–800 mg/day).

Renal Impairment

PO (Adults): *CCr <60 mL/min*—Do not exceed 600 mg/day.

Irbesartan

PO (Adults): *Hypertension*—150 mg once daily; may be ↑ to 300 mg once daily. Initiate therapy at 75 mg once daily in patients who are receiving diuretics or are volume depleted. *Type 2 diabetic nephropathy*—300 mg once daily.

Losartan

PO (Adults): *Hypertension*—50 mg once daily initially (range 25–100 mg/day as a single daily dose or 2 divided doses) (initiate therapy at 25 mg once daily in patients who are receiving diuretics or are volume depleted). *Prevention of stroke in patients with hypertension and left ventricular hypertrophy*—50 mg once daily initially; hydrochlorothiazide 12.5 mg once daily should be added and/or dose of losartan ↑ to 100 mg once daily followed by an ↑ in hydrochlorothiazide to 25 mg once daily based on BP response. *Type 2 diabetic nephropathy*—50 mg once daily, may ↑ to 100 mg once daily depending on BP response.

Hepatic Impairment

PO (Adults): 25 mg once daily initially; may be ↑ as tolerated.

PO (Children > 6 yr): *Hypertension*—0.7 mg/kg once daily (up to 50 mg/day), may be titrated up to 1.4 mg/kg/day (or 100 mg/day).

Renal Impairment

PO (Children > 6 yr): *CCr <30 mL/min*—Contraindicated.

Olmesartan

PO (Adults): 20 mg once daily; may be ↑ up to 40 mg once daily (patients who are receiving diuretics or are volume-depleted should be started on lower doses).
PO (Children 6–16 yr): *≥35 kg*—20 mg once daily; may be ↑ after 2 wk up to 40 mg once daily; *20–34.9 kg*—10 mg once daily; may be ↑ after 2 wk up to 20 mg once daily.

Telmisartan

PO (Adults): *Hypertension*—40 mg once daily (volume-depleted patients should start with 20 mg once daily); may be titrated up to 80 mg/day; *Cardiovascular risk reduction*—80 mg once daily.

Valsartan

PO (Adults): *Hypertension*—80 mg or 160 mg once daily initially in patients who are not volume-depleted; may be ↑ to 320 mg once daily; *HF*—40 mg twice daily, may be titrated up to target dose of 160 mg twice daily as tolerated; *Post-MI*—20 mg twice daily (may be initiated ≥ 12 hr after MI); dose may be titrated up to target dose of 160 mg twice daily, as tolerated.
PO (Children 6–16 yr): *Hypertension*—1.3 mg/kg once daily (maximum dose = 40 mg/day); may be ↑ up to 2.7 mg/kg once daily (maximum dose = 160 mg/day).

Availability

Azilsartan

Tablets: 40 mg, 80 mg. **Cost:** All strengths $113.23/30. ***In combination with:*** chlorthalidone (Edarbyclor); see Appendix B.

Candesartan (generic available)

Tablets: 4 mg, 8 mg, 16 mg, 32 mg. **Cost:** *Generic*—4 mg $99.16/30, 8 mg $99.16/30, 16 mg $285.56/30, 32 mg $386.60/30. ***In combination with:*** hydrochlorothiazide (Atacand HCT); see Appendix B.

Eprosartan (generic available)

Tablets: 400 mg, 600 mg. **Cost:** *Generic*—600 mg $102.78/30. ***In combination with:*** hydrochlorothiazide (Teveten HCT); see Appendix B.

Irbesartan (generic available)

Tablets: 75 mg, 150 mg, 300 mg. **Cost:** *Generic*—75 mg $10.44/90, 150 mg $279.97/90, 300 mg $31.13/90. ***In combination with:*** hydrochlorothiazide (Avalide); see Appendix B.

Losartan (generic available)

Tablets: 25 mg, 50 mg, 100 mg. **Cost:** *Generic*—25 mg $151.43/90, 50 mg $67.88/30, 100 mg $277.36/90. ***In combination with:*** hydrochlorothiazide (Hyzaar); see Appendix B.

Olmesartan

Tablets: 5 mg, 20 mg, 40 mg. **Cost:** 5 mg $288.15/90, 20 mg $358.41/90, 40 mg $543.45/100. ***In combination with:*** hydrochlorothiazide (Benicar HCT); amlodipine (Azor); see Appendix B.

Telmisartan (generic available)

Tablets: 20 mg, 40 mg, 80 mg. **Cost:** 20 mg $445.33/90, 40 mg $441.19/90, 80 mg $441.19/90. ***In combination with:*** hydrochlorothiazide (Micardis HCT); amlodipine (Twynsta); see Appendix B).

Valsartan (generic available)

Tablets: 40 mg, 80 mg, 160 mg, 320 mg. **Cost:** 40 mg $330.05/90, 80 mg $428.25/90, 160 mg $469.86/90, 320 mg $581.92/90. ***In combination with:*** amlodipine (Exforge); hydrochlorothiazide (Diovan HCT); amlodipine and hydrochlorothiazide (Exforge HCT); see Appendix B.

NURSING IMPLICATIONS

Assessment

- Assess BP (lying, sitting, standing) and pulse periodically during therapy. Notify health care professional of significant changes.
- Monitor frequency of prescription refills to determine adherence.
- Assess patient for signs of angioedema (dyspnea, facial swelling). May rarely cause angioedema.
- **HF:** Monitor daily weight and assess patient routinely for resolution of fluid overload (peripheral edema, rales/crackles, dyspnea, weight gain, jugular venous distention).
- ***Lab Test Considerations:*** Monitor renal function and electrolyte levels periodically. Serum potassium, BUN, and serum creatinine may be ↑.
- May cause ↑ AST, ALT, and serum bilirubin (candesartan and olmesartan only).
- May cause ↑ uric acid, slight ↓ in hemoglobin and hematocrit, neutropenia, and thrombocytopenia.

Potential Nursing Diagnoses

Risk for injury (Adverse Reactions)
Noncompliance (Patient/Family Teaching)

Implementation

- Do not confuse Benicar with Mevacor. Do not confuse Diovan with Zyban.
- Correct volume depletion, if possible, prior to initiation of therapy.
- **PO:** May be administered without regard to meals.

Losartan

- **PO:** For patients with difficulty swallowing tablets, pharmacist can compound oral suspension; stable for 4 wk if refrigerated. Shake suspension before each use.

Patient/Family Teaching

- Emphasize the importance of continuing to take as directed, even if feeling well. Take missed doses as soon as remembered if not almost time for next dose; do not double doses. Instruct patient to take medication at the same time each day. Warn patient not to discontinue therapy unless directed by health care professional.

- Caution patient to avoid salt substitutes containing potassium or food containing high levels of potassium or sodium unless directed by health care professional. See Appendix J.
- Caution patient to avoid sudden changes in position to decrease orthostatic hypotension. Use of alcohol, standing for long periods, exercising, and hot weather may increase orthostatic hypotension.
- May cause dizziness. Caution patient to avoid driving or other activities requiring alertness until response to medication is known.
- Instruct patient to notify health care professional of all Rx or OTC medications, vitamins, or herbal products being taken and consult health care professional before taking any new medications, especially NSAIDs and cough, cold, or allergy remedies.
- Instruct patient to notify health care professional of medication regimen prior to treatment or surgery.
- Instruct patient to notify health care professional if swelling of face, eyes, lips, or tongue occurs, or if difficulty swallowing or breathing occurs.
- Advise women of childbearing age to use contraception and notify health care professional if pregnancy is suspected or planned, or if breast feeding. If pregnancy is detected, discontinue medication as soon as possible.
- Emphasize the importance of follow-up exams to evaluate effectiveness of medication.
- **Hypertension:** Encourage patient to comply with additional interventions for hypertension (weight reduction, low-sodium diet, discontinuation of smoking, moderation of alcohol consumption, regular exercise, stress management). Medication controls but dose not cure hypertension.
- Instruct patient and family on proper technique for monitoring BP. Advise them to check BP at least weekly and to report significant changes.

Evaluation/Desired Outcomes

- Decrease in BP without appearance of excessive side effects.
- Slowed progression of diabetic nephropathy (irbesartan, losartan).
- Decreased cardiovascular death and HF-related hospitalizations in patients with HF (candesartan).
- Decreased hospitalizations in patients with HF (valsartan).
- Decreased risk of cardiovascular death in patients with left ventricular systolic dysfunction after MI (valsartan).
- Reduced risk of stroke in patients with hypertension and left ventricular hypertrophy (losartan).
- Reduction of risk of myocardial infarction, stroke, or cardiovascular death (telmisartan).

anidulafungin

(a-**ni**-du-la-fun-gin)

Eraxis

Classification

Therapeutic: antifungals

Pharmacologic: echinocandins

Pregnancy Category C

Indications

Candidemia and other serious candidal infections including intra-abdominal abscess, peritonitis. Esophageal candidiasis.

Action

Inhibits the synthesis of fungal cell wall. **Therapeutic Effects:** Death of susceptible fungi. **Spectrum:** Active against *Candida albicans*, *C. glabrata*, *C. parapsilosis*, and *C. tropicalis*.

Pharmacokinetics

Absorption: IV administration results in complete bioavailability.

Distribution: Crosses the placenta.

Metabolism and Excretion: Undergoes chemical degradation without hepatic metabolism; <1% excreted in urine.

Half-life: 40–50 hr.

TIME/ACTION PROFILE (blood levels)

ROUTE	ONSET	PEAK	DURATION
IV	rapid	end of infusion	24 hr

Contraindications/Precautions

Contraindicated in: Hypersensitivity.

Use Cautiously in: Underlying liver disease (may worsen); OB, Lactation: Pregnancy or lactation; Pedi: Safety not established.

Adverse Reactions/Side Effects

Resp: bronchospasm, dyspnea. **CV:** hypotension. **GI:** diarrhea, ↑ liver enzymes. **Derm:** flushing, rash, urticaria. **F and E:** hypokalemia. **Misc:** ANAPHYLAXIS, infusion reaction.

Interactions

Drug-Drug: None noted.

Route/Dosage

IV (Adults): *Esophageal candidiasis*— 100 mg loading dose on day 1, then 50 mg daily. *Candidemia and other candidal infections*— 200 mg loading dose on day 1, then 100 mg daily.

Availability

Lyophilized powder for IV use (requires reconstitution): 50 mg/vial.

NURSING IMPLICATIONS

Assessment

- Assess infected area and monitor cultures before and periodically during therapy.
- Specimens for culture should be taken before instituting therapy. Therapy may be started before results are obtained.
- Monitor for signs and symptoms of anaphylaxis (rash, urticaria, flushing, pruritus, bronchospasm, dyspnea, hypotension); usually related to histamine release. To decrease risk, do not exceed a rate of infusion of 1.1 mg/minute.
- ***Lab Test Considerations:*** May cause ↑ ALT, AST, alkaline phosphatase, and hepatic enzymes.
- May cause hypokalemia.
- May cause neutropenia and leukopenia.

Potential Nursing Diagnoses

Risk for infection (Indications)

Implementation

IV Administration

- **Intermittent Infusion:** Reconstitute each 50 mg vial with 15 mL or the 100 mg vial with 30 mL of Sterile Water for Injection for a concentration of 3.33 mg/mL. May be stored in refrigerator for up to 1 hr. ***Diluent:*** Further dilute within 24 hr by transferring contents of reconstituted vial into IV bag of D5W or 0.9% NaCl. For the 50 mg dose, dilute with 85 mL for an infusion volume of 100 mL. For the 100 mg dose, dilute with 170 mL for an infusion volume of 200 mL. For the 200 mg dose, dilute with 340 mL for a total infusion volume of 400 mL. ***Concentration:*** Final concentration should not exceed 0.5 mg/mL. Do not administer solutions that are discolored or contain particulate matter. Store reconstituted solution in refrigerator; do not freeze. Administer within 24 hr. ***Rate:*** Administer at a rate not to exceed 1.1 mg/min (1.4 mL/min or 84 mL/hr).
- **Y-Site Compatibility:** acyclovir, alemtuzumab, alfentanil, allopurinol, amifostine, amikacin, aminophylline, amiodarone, amphotericin B lipid complex, amphotericin B liposome, ampicillin, ampicillin/sulbactam, argatroban, aresnic trioxide, atracurium, azithromycin, aztreonam, bivalirudin, bleomycin, bumetanide, buprenorphine, bulsulfan, butorphanol, calcium chloride, calcium gluconate, carboplatin, carmustine, caspofungin, cefazolin, cefepime, cefotaxime, cefotetan, cefoxitin, ceftazidime, ceftriaxone, cefuroxime, chloramphenicol, ciprofloxacin, cisatracurium, cisplatin, clindamycin, cyclophosphamide, cyclosporine, cytarabine, dacarbazine, dactinomycin, daunorubicin hydrochloride, dexamethasone, dexmedetomidine, digoxin, diltiazem, diphenhydramine, dobutamine, docetaxel, dolasetron, dopamine, doripenem, doxacurium, doxorubicin hydrochloride, doxorubicin liposome, doxycycline, droperidol, enalaprilat, ephedrine, epinephrine, epirubicin, eptifibatide, erythromycin, esmolol, etoposide, etoposide phosphate, famotidine, fenoldopam, fentanyl, fluconazole, fludarabine, fluorouracil, foscarnet, fosphenytoin, furosemide, ganciclovir, gemcitabine, gentamicin, glycopyrrolate, granisetron, haloperidol, heparin, hydralazine, hydrocortisone, hydromorphone, idarubicin, ifosfamide, imipenem/cilastatin, insulin, irinotecan, isoproterenol, ketorolac, labetalol, leucovorin, levofloxacin, linezolid, lorazepam, mannitol, mechlorethamine, melphalan, meperidine, meropenem, mesna, metaraminol, methotrexate, methyldopate, methylprednisolone, metoclopramide, metoprolol, metronidazole, midazolam, milrinone, mitomycin, mitoxantrone, morphine, mycophenolate, nafcillin, naloxone, nesiritide, nicardipine, nitroglycerin, nitroprusside, norepinephrine, octreotide, ondansetron, oxaliplatin, oxytocin, paclitaxel, palonosetron, pamidronate, pancuronium, pantoprazole, pentamidine, pentazocine, pentobarbital, phenobarbital, phentolamine, phenylephrine, piperacillin/tazobactam, potassium acetate, potassium chloride, procainamide, prochlorperazine, promethazine, propranolol, quinupristin/dalfopristin, ranitidine, remifentanil, rocuronium, sodium acetate, streptozocin, succinylcholine, sufentanil, tacrolimus, teniposide, theophylline, thiopental, thiotepa, tirofiban, tobramycin, topotecan, trimethoprim/sulfamethoxazole, vancomycin, vasopressin, vecuronium, verapamil, vinblastine, vincristine, vinorelbine, voriconazole, zidovudine, zoledronic acid.
- **Y-Site Incompatibility:** amphotericin B colloidal, dantrolene, diazepam, ertapenem, magnesium sulfate, nalbuphine, pemetrexed, phenytoin, potassium phosphates, sodium bicarbonate, sodium phosphates.

Patient/Family Teaching

- Explain purpose of medication to patient.
- Instruct patient to notify health care professional if signs and symptoms of anaphylaxis occur or if diarrhea becomes pronounced.

Evaluation/Desired Outcomes

- Resolution of clinical and laboratory indications of fungal infections. Duration of therapy should be based on the patients clinical response. Therapy should be continued for at least 14 days after the last positive culture. For esophageal candidiasis, treatment should continue for at least 7 days following resolution of symptoms.

ANTIFUNGALS (TOPICAL)

butenafine (byoo-**ten**-a-feen)
Lotrimin Ultra, Mentax

ciclopirox (sye-kloe-**peer**-ox)
Loprox, Penlac, ✱Stieprox

A

clotrimazole (kloe-**trye**-ma-zole)
✱Canesten, ✱Clotrimaderm, Lotrimin AF, Mycelex

econazole (ee-**kon**-a-zole)
Ecoza

ketoconazole
(kee-toe-**koe**-na-zole)
Extina, ✱Ketoderm, Nizoral, Nizoral A-D, Xolegel

miconazole (mye-**kon**-a-zole)
Fungoid, Lotrimin AF, Micatin, ✱Micozole, Zeasorb-AF

naftifine (**naff**-ti-feen)
Naftin

nystatin (nye-**stat**-in)
~~Mycostatin~~, ✱Nyaderm, Nystop

oxiconazole (ox-i-**kon**-a-zole)
Oxistat

sulconazole (sul-**kon**-a-zole)
Exelderm

terbinafine (ter-**bin**-a-feen)
Lamisil AT

tolnaftate (tol-**naff**-tate)
✱Absorbine Jr, ✱Flexitol, ✱Fungicure, Lamisil AF, ✱Pitrex, Podactin, ✱Proclearz, Tinactin

Classification
Therapeutic: antifungals (topical)

Pregnancy Category B (butenafine, ciclopirox, clotrimazole, naftifine, oxiconazole, terbinafine), C (econazole, ketoconazole, miconazole, sulconazole, tolnaftate), UK (nystatin)

Indications
Treatment of a variety of cutaneous fungal infections, including cutaneous candidiasis, tinea pedis (athlete's foot), tinea cruris (jock itch), tinea corporis (ringworm), tinea versicolor, seborrheic dermatitis, dandruff, and onychomycosis of fingernails and toes.

Action
Butenafine, nystatin, clotrimazole, econazole, ketoconazole, miconazole, naftifine, oxiconazole, sulconazole, and terbinafine affect the synthesis of the fungal cell wall, allowing leakage of cellular contents. Tolnaftate distorts the hyphae and stunts mycelial growth in fungi. Ciclopirox inhibits the transport of essential elements in the fungal cell, disrupting the synthesis of DNA, RNA, and protein. **Therapeutic Effects:** Decrease in symptoms of fungal infection.

Pharmacokinetics
Absorption: Absorption through intact skin is minimal.
Distribution: Distribution after topical administration is primarily local.
Metabolism and Excretion: Metabolism and excretion not known following local application.
Half-life: *Butenafine*—35 hr; *Ciclopirox*—5.5 hr (gel); *Terbinafine*—21 hr.

TIME/ACTION PROFILE (resolution of symptoms/lesions†)

ROUTE	ONSET	PEAK	DURATION
Butenafine	unknown	up to 4 wk	unknown
Tolnaftate	24–72 hr	unknown	unknown

† Only the drugs with known information included in this table.

Contraindications/Precautions
Contraindicated in: Hypersensitivity to active ingredients, additives, preservatives, or bases; Some products contain alcohol or bisulfites and should be avoided in patients with known intolerance.
Use Cautiously in: Nail and scalp infections (may require additional systemic therapy); OB, Lactation: Safety not established.

Adverse Reactions/Side Effects
Local: burning, itching, local hypersensitivity reactions, redness, stinging.

Interactions
Drug-Drug: Econazole may ↑ levels of and risk of bleeding from **warfarin**.

Route/Dosage
Butenafine
Topical (Adults and Children >12 yr): Apply once daily for 2 wk for tinea corporis, tinea cruris, or tinea versicolor. Apply once daily for 4 wk or once daily for 7 days for tinea pedis.

Ciclopirox
Topical (Adults and Children >10 yr): *Cream/lotion*—Apply twice daily for 2–4 wk; *Topical solution (nail lacquer)*—Apply to nails at bedtime or 8 hr prior to bathing for up to 48 wk. Each daily application should be made over the previous coat and then removed with alcohol every 7 days; *Gel*—Apply twice daily for 4 wk; *Shampoo*—5–10 mL applied to scalp, lather and leave on for 3 min, rinse; repeat twice weekly for 4 wk (at least 3 days between applications).

Clotrimazole

Topical (Adults and Children >3 yr): Apply twice daily for 1–4 wk.

Econazole

Topical (Adults and Children): Apply once daily for tinea pedis (for 4 wk), tinea cruris (for 2 wk), tinea corporis (for 2 wk), or tinea versicolor (for 2 wk). Apply twice daily for cutaneous candidiasis (for 2 wk).

Ketoconazole

Topical (Adults): Apply cream once daily for cutaneous candidiasis (for 2 wk), tinea corporis (for 2 wk), tinea cruris (for 2 wk), tinea pedis (for 6 wk), or tinea versicolor (for 2 wk). Apply cream twice daily for seborrheic dermatitis (for 4 wk). For dandruff, use shampoo twice weekly (wait 3–4 days between treatments) for 4 wk, then intermittently.

Miconazole

Topical (Adults and Children >2 yr): Apply twice daily. Treat tinea cruris for 2 wk and tinea pedis or tinea corporis for 4 wk.

Naftifine

Topical (Adults and Children 12–17 yr): Apply cream once daily for 2 wk. Apply gel twice daily for up to 4 wk.

Nystatin

Topical (Adults and Children): Apply 2–3 times daily until healing is complete.

Oxiconazole

Topical (Adults and Children): Apply cream or lotion 1–2 times daily for tinea pedis (for 4 wk), tinea corporis (for 2 wk), or tinea cruris (for 2 wk). Apply cream once daily for tinea versicolor (for 2 wk).

Sulconazole

Topical (Adults): Apply 1–2 times daily (twice daily for tinea pedis). Treat tinea corporis, tinea cruris, or tinea versicolor for 3 wk, and tinea pedis for 4 wk.

Terbinafine

Topical (Adults): Apply twice daily for tinea pedis (for 1 wk) or daily for tinea cruris or tinea corporis for 1 wk.

Tolnaftate

Topical (Adults): Apply twice daily for tinea cruris (for 2 wk), tinea pedis (for 4 wk), or tinea corporis (for 4 wk).

Availability

Butenafine

Cream: 1%[Rx, OTC].

Ciclopirox (generic available)

Cream: 0.77%. **Gel:** 0.77%. **Lotion:** 0.77%. **Nail lacquer:** 8%. **Shampoo:** 1%, ✱1.5%.

Clotrimazole (generic available)

Cream: 1%[OTC]. **Solution:** 1%[OTC]. ***In combination with:*** betamethasone (Lotrisone). See Appendix B.

Econazole (generic available)

Cream: 1%.

Ketoconazole (generic available)

Cream: 2%. **Shampoo:** 1%[OTC], 2%. **Foam:** 2%. **Gel:** 2%.

Miconazole (generic available)

Cream: 2%[Rx, OTC]. **Lotion powder:** 2%[OTC]. **Ointment:** 2%[OTC]. **Powder:** 2%[OTC]. **Spray powder:** 2%[OTC]. **Spray liquid:** 2%[OTC]. **Solution:** 2%[OTC]. **Tincture:** 2%[OTC]. ***In combination with:*** zinc oxide (Vusion). See Appendix B.

Naftifine

Cream: 1%, 2%. **Gel:** 2%.

Nystatin (generic available)

Cream: 100,000 units/g[Rx, OTC]. **Ointment:** 100,000 units/g[Rx, OTC]. **Powder:** 100,000 units/g[Rx, OTC]. ***In combination with:*** triamcinolone. See Appendix B.

Oxiconazole

Cream: 1%. **Lotion:** 1%.

Sulconazole

Cream: 1%. **Solution:** 1%.

Terbinafine (generic available)

Cream: 1%[OTC]. **Gel:** 1%[OTC]. **Spray liquid:** 1%[OTC].

Tolnaftate (generic available)

Cream: 1%[OTC]. **Solution:** 1%[OTC]. **Powder:** 1%[OTC]. **Spray powder:** 1%[OTC]. **Spray liquid:** 1%[OTC].

NURSING IMPLICATIONS

Assessment

- Inspect involved areas of skin and mucous membranes before and frequently during therapy. Increased skin irritation may indicate need to discontinue medication.

Potential Nursing Diagnoses

Risk for impaired skin integrity (Indications)
Risk for infection (Indications)

Implementation

- Consult health care professional for proper cleansing technique before applying medication.
- Choice of vehicle is based on use. Ointments, creams, and liquids are used as primary therapy. Lotion is usually preferred in intertriginous areas; if cream is used, apply sparingly to avoid maceration. Powders are usually used as adjunctive therapy but may be used as primary therapy for mild conditions (especially for moist lesions).
- **Topical:** Apply small amount to cover affected area completely. Avoid use of occlusive wrappings or dressings unless directed by health care professional.

- **Nail lacquer:** Avoid contact with skin other than skin immediately surrounding treated nail. Avoid contact with eyes or mucous membranes. Removal of unattached, infected nail, as frequently as monthly, by health care professional is needed with use of this medication. Up to 48 wk of daily application and professional removal may be required to achieve clear or almost clear nail. 6 mo of treatment may be required before results are noticed.
- **Ciclopirox or Ketoconazole shampoo:** Moisten hair and scalp thoroughly with water. Apply sufficient shampoo to produce enough lather to wash scalp and hair and gently massage it over the entire scalp area for approximately 1 min. Rinse hair thoroughly with warm water. Repeat process, leaving shampoo on hair for an additional 3 min. After the 2nd shampoo, rinse and dry hair with towel or warm air flow. Shampoo twice a week for 4 wk with at least 3 days between each shampooing and then intermittently as needed to maintain control.
- **Ketoconazole foam:** Hold container upright and dispense foam into cap of can or other smooth surface; dispensing directly on to hand is not recommended as the foam begins to melt immediately on contact with warm skin. Pick up small amounts with fingertips and gently massage into affected areas until absorbed. Move hair to allow direct application to skin.

Patient/Family Teaching

- Instruct patient to apply medication as directed for full course of therapy, even if feeling better. Emphasize the importance of avoiding the eyes.
- Caution patient that some products may stain fabric, skin, or hair. Check label information. Fabrics stained from cream or lotion can usually be cleaned by hand washing with soap and warm water; stains from ointments can usually be removed with standard cleaning fluids.
- Patients with athlete's foot should be taught to wear well-fitting, ventilated shoes, to wash affected areas thoroughly, and to change shoes and socks at least once a day.
- Advise patient to report increased skin irritation or lack of response to therapy to health care professional.
- **Nail lacquer:** File away loose nail and trim nails every 7 days after solution is removed with alcohol. Do not use nail polish on treated nails. Inform health care professional if patient has diabetes mellitus before using.

Evaluation/Desired Outcomes

- Decrease in skin irritation and resolution of infection. Early relief of symptoms may be seen in 2–3 days. For *Candida,* tinea cruris, and tinea corporis, 2 wk are needed, and for tinea pedis, therapeutic response may take 3–4 wk. Recurrent fungal infections may be a sign of systemic illness.

ANTIFUNGALS (VAGINAL)

butoconazole
(byoo-toe-**kon**-a-zole)
Gynezole-1, Mycelex-3

clotrimazole (kloe-**trye**-ma-zole)
✱Canesten, ✱Clotrimaderm, Gyne-Lotrimin-3, Mycelex-7

miconazole (mye-**kon**-a-zole)
Monistat-1, Monistat-3, Monistat-7, Vagistat-3

terconazole (ter-**kon**-a-zole)
Terazol-3, Terazol-7

tioconazole (tye-oh-**kon**-a-zole)
1–Day, Monistat-1Day, Vagistat-1

Classification
Therapeutic: antifungals (vaginal)

Pregnancy Category B (clotrimazole), C (butoconazole, miconazole, terconazole, tioconazole)

Indications

Treatment of vulvovaginal candidiasis.

Action

Affects the permeability of the fungal cell wall, allowing leakage of cellular contents. Not active against bacteria. **Therapeutic Effects:** Inhibited growth and death of susceptible *Candida*, with decrease in accompanying symptoms of vulvovaginitis (vaginal burning, itching, discharge).

Pharmacokinetics

Absorption: Absorption through intact skin is minimal.
Distribution: Unknown. Action is primarily local.
Metabolism and Excretion: Negligible with local application.
Half-life: Not applicable.

TIME/ACTION PROFILE

ROUTE	ONSET	PEAK	DURATION
All agents	rapid	unknown	24 hr

Contraindications/Precautions

Contraindicated in: Hypersensitivity to active ingredients, additives, or preservatives; OB: Safety not established; Lactation: Safety not established.
Use Cautiously in: None noted.

Adverse Reactions/Side Effects

Derm: *terconazole*—TOXIC EPIDERMAL NECROLYSIS.
GU: itching, pelvic pain, vulvovaginal burning. **Misc:** *terconazole*—ANAPHYLAXIS.

Interactions

Drug-Drug: Concurrent use of vaginal miconazole with **warfarin** ↑ risk of bleeding/bruising (appropriate monitoring recommended).

Route/Dosage

Butoconazole

Vag (Adults and Children ≥12 yr): 1 applicatorful (5 g) at bedtime for 3 days (Mycelex-3) *or* one applicatorful single dose (Gynezole-1).

Clotrimazole

Vag (Adults and Children >12 yr): *Vaginal tablets*—100 mg at bedtime for 7 nights (preferred regimen for pregnancy) *or* 200 mg at bedtime for 3 nights. *Vaginal cream*—1 applicatorful (5 g) of 1% cream at bedtime for 7 days *or* 1 applicatorful (5 g) of 2% cream at bedtime for 3 days.

Miconazole

Vag (Adults and Children ≥12 yr): *Vaginal suppositories*—one 100-mg suppository at bedtime for 7 days *or* one 200-mg suppository at bedtime for 3 days *or* one 1200-mg suppository as a single dose. *Vaginal cream*—1 applicatorful of 2% cream at bedtime for 7 days *or* 1 applicatorful of 4% cream at bedtime for 3 days. *Combination packages*—contain a cream or suppositories as well as an external vaginal cream (may be used twice daily for up to 7 days, as needed, for symptomatic management of itching).

Terconazole

Vag (Adults): *Vaginal cream*—1 applicatorful (5 g) of 0.4% cream at bedtime for 7 days *or* 1 applicatorful (5 g) of 0.8% cream at bedtime for 3 days. *Vaginal suppositories*—1 suppository (80 mg) at bedtime for 3 days.

Tioconazole

Vag (Adults and Children ≥12 yr): 1 applicatorful (4.6 g) at bedtime as a single dose.

Availability

Butoconazole

Vaginal cream: 2%$^{Rx, OTC}$.

Clotrimazole (generic available)

Vaginal tablets: 100 mg^{OTC}, 200 mg^{OTC}. **Vaginal cream:** 1%^{OTC}, 2%^{OTC}.

Miconazole (generic available)

Vaginal cream: 2%^{OTC}, 4%^{OTC}. **Vaginal suppositories:** 100 mg^{OTC}, 200 mg$^{Rx, OTC}$. ***In combination with:*** combination package of three 200-mg suppositories and 2% external cream^{OTC}; one 1200-mg suppository and 2% external cream^{OTC}; 4% vaginal cream and 2% external cream^{OTC}; seven 100-mg suppositories and 2% external cream^{OTC}; 2% vaginal cream and 2% external cream^{OTC}.

Terconazole (generic available)

Vaginal cream: 0.4%, 0.8%. **Vaginal suppositories:** 80 mg.

Tioconazole

Vaginal ointment: 6.5%^{OTC}.

NURSING IMPLICATIONS

Assessment

- Inspect involved areas of skin and mucous membranes before and frequently during therapy. Increased skin irritation may indicate need to discontinue medication.

Potential Nursing Diagnoses

Risk for infection (Indications)
Risk for impaired skin integrity (Indications)

Implementation

- Consult health care professional for proper cleansing technique before applying medication.
- **Vag:** Applicators are supplied for vaginal administration.

Patient/Family Teaching

- Instruct patient to apply medication as directed for full course of therapy, even if feeling better. Therapy should be continued during menstrual period.
- Instruct patient on proper use of vaginal applicator. Medication should be inserted high into the vagina at bedtime. Instruct patient to remain recumbent for at least 30 min after insertion. Advise use of sanitary napkins to prevent staining of clothing or bedding.
- Advise patient to avoid using tampons while using this product.
- Advise patient to consult health care professional regarding intercourse during therapy. Vaginal medication may cause minor skin irritation in sexual partner. Advise patient to refrain from sexual contact during therapy or have male partner wear a condom. Some products may weaken latex contraceptive devices. Another method of contraception should be used during treatment.
- Advise patient to report to health care professional increased skin irritation or lack of response to therapy. A second course may be necessary if symptoms persist.
- Instruct patient to stop using medication and notify health care professional if rash or signs and symptoms of anaphylaxis (wheezing, rash, hives, shortness of breath) occur.
- Advise patient to dispose of applicator after each use (except for terconazole).

Evaluation/Desired Outcomes

- Decrease in skin irritation and vaginal discomfort. Therapeutic response is usually seen after 1 wk. Diagnosis should be reconfirmed with smears or cultures before a second course of therapy to rule out other pathogens associated with vulvovaginitis. Recurrent vaginal infections may be a sign of systemic illness.

REMS

apixaban (a-pix-a-ban)

Eliquis

Classification

Therapeutic: anticoagulants

Pharmacologic: factor Xa inhibitors

Pregnancy Category B

Indications

Decreases risk of stroke/systemic embolism associated with nonvalvular atrial fibrillation. Prevention of deep vein thrombosis that may lead to pulmonary embolism following knee or hip replacement surgery. Treatment of and reduction in risk of recurrence of deep vein thrombosis (DVT) or pulmonary embolism (PE).

Action

Acts as a selective, reversible site inhibitor of factor Xa, inhibiting both free and bound factor. Does not affect platelet aggregation directly, but does inhibit thrombin-induced platelet aggregation. Decreases thrombin generation and thrombus development. **Therapeutic Effects:** Treatment and prevention of thromboembolic events.

Pharmacokinetics

Absorption: 50% absorbed following oral administration.

Distribution: Unknown.

Metabolism and Excretion: 25% metabolized (mostly by CYP3A4) and excreted in urine and feces. Biliary and direct intestinal excretion account for fecal elimination.

Half-life: 6 hr (12 hr after repeated dosing due to prolonged absorption).

TIME/ACTION PROFILE (effect on hemostasis)

ROUTE	ONSET	PEAK	DURATION
PO	unknown	3–4 hr†	24 hr

†Blood levels.

Contraindications/Precautions

Contraindicated in: Previous severe hypersensitivity reactions; Active pathological bleeding; Severe hepatic impairment; Not recommended for use in patients with prosthetic heart valves; Concurrent use of strong dual inducers of CYP3A4 and P-gp; PE with hemodynamic instability or requiring thrombolysis or pulmonary embolectomy; Lactation: Should not be used.

Use Cautiously in: Neuroaxial spinal anesthesia or spinal puncture, especially if concurrent with an indwelling epidural catheter, drugs affecting hemostasis, history of traumatic/repeated spinal puncture or spinal deformity (↑ risk of spinal hematoma); Discontinuation ↑ risk of thromboses; Surgery; Renal impairment (dose ↓ may be required; Moderate hepatic impairment (↑ risk of bleeding); Concurrent use of strong dual inhibitors of CYP3A4 and P-gp systems (dose ↓ required); OB: Use during pregnancy only if potential benefit outweighs possible risks to mother and fetus; Pedi: Safety and effectiveness not established.

Adverse Reactions/Side Effects

Hemat: <u>BLEEDING</u>. **Misc:** hypersensitivity reactions including ANAPHYLAXIS.

Interactions

Drug-Drug: ↑ risk of bleeding with other **anticoagulants**, **fibrinolytics**, **heparins**, **NSAIDs**, **SNRIs**, **SSRIs**, or **thrombolytics**. Concurrent use of strong inhibitors of both the CYP3A4 and P-gP enzyme systems (including **clarithromycin**, **itraconazole**, **ketoconazole**, and **ritonavir**) ↑ levels and bleeding risk; dosage of apixaban should be ↓ to 2.5 mg twice daily. If other reasons for ↓ dose exist, apixaban should be avoided. Inducers of the CYP3A4 enzyme system and the P-gp system including **carbamazepine**, **phenytoin**, **rifampin** will ↓ levels and may ↑ risk of thromboses; avoid concomitant use.

Drug-Natural Products: Concurrent use **St. John's wort**, a strong dual inducer of the CYP3A4 and P-gp enzyme systems can ↓ levels and ↑risk of thromboses and should be avoided.

Route/Dosage

Reduction in Risk of Stroke/Systemic Embolism in Nonvalvular Atrial Fibrillation

PO (Adults): 5 mg twice daily; *Any 2 of the following: age ≥80 yr, weight ≤60 kg, serum creatinine ≥1.5mg/dL*—2.5 mg twice daily; *Concurrent use of strong inhibitors of both CYP3A4 and P-gp*—2.5 mg twice daily; if patient already taking 2.5 mg twice daily, avoid concomitant use.

Renal Impairment

PO (Adults): *HD*—5 mg twice daily; *HD and either age ≥80 yr or weight ≤60 kg*—2.5 mg twice daily.

Prevention of Deep Vein Thrombosis Following Knee or Hip Replacement Surgery

PO (Adults): 2.5 mg twice daily, initiated 12–24 hr post-operatively (when hemostasis is achieved) continued for 35 days after hip replacement or 12 days after knee replacement.

Treatment of DVT or PE

PO (Adults): 10 mg twice daily for 7 days, then 5 mg twice daily.

Reduction is Risk of Recurrence of DVT or PE

PO (Adults): 2.5 mg twice daily after ≥6 mo of treatment of DVT or PE.

Availability

Tablets: 2.5 mg, 5 mg.

NURSING IMPLICATIONS

Assessment

- Assess patient for symptoms of stroke, DVT, PE, or peripheral vascular disease periodically during therapy.

Potential Nursing Diagnoses

Ineffective tissue perfusion (Indications)
Risk for injury (Adverse Reactions)

Implementation

- When *converting from warfarin*, discontinue warfarin and start apixaban when INR is <2.0.
- When *converting from apixaban to warfarin*, apixaban affects INR, so INR measurements may not be useful for determining appropriate dose of warfarin. If continuous anticoagulation is necessary, discontinue apixaban and begin both a parenteral anticoagulant and warfarin at time of next dose of apixaban, dicontinue parenteral anticoagulant when INR reaches acceptable range.
- When *switching between apixaban and anticoagulants other than warfarin*, discontinue one being taken and begin the other at the next scheduled dose.
- *For surgery*, discontinue apixaban at least 48 hrs before invasive or surgical procedures with a moderate or high risk of unacceptable or clinically significant bleeding or at least 24 hrs prior to procedures with a low risk of bleeding or where the bleeding would be non-critical in location and easily controlled.
- **PO:** Administer twice daily without regard to food.
- For patients who cannot swallow tablet, 5 mg and 2.5 mg tablets can be crushed, suspended in 60 mL of D5W, and administered immediately through a nasogastric tube; do not administer crushed tablets by oral route.

Patient/Family Teaching

- Instruct patient to take apixaban as directed. Take missed doses as soon as remembered on the same day and resume twice daily administration; do not double doses. Do not discontinue without consulting health care professional; may increase risk of having a stroke, DVT, or PE. If temporarily discontinued, restart as soon as possible. Store apixaban at room temperature. Advise patient to read *Medication Guide* before beginning therapy and with each Rx refill in case of changes.
- Inform patient that they may bruise and bleed more easily or longer than usual. Advise patient to notify health care professional immediately if signs of bleeding (unusual bruising, pink or brown urine, red or black, tarry stools, coughing up blood, vomiting blood, pain or swelling in a joint, headache, dizziness, weakness, recurring nose bleeds, unusual bleeding from gums, heavier than normal menstrual bleeding, dyspepsia, abdominal pain, epigastric pain) occurs or if injury occurs, especially head injury.
- Caution patient to notify health care professional if skin rash or signs of severe allergic reaction (chest pain or tightness, swelling of face or tongue, trouble breathing or wheezing, feeling dizzy or faint) occur.
- Advise patient to notify health care professional of medication regimen prior to treatment or surgery.
- Instruct patient to notify health care professional of all Rx or OTC medications, vitamins, or herbal products being taken and consult health care professional before taking any new medications. Risk of bleeding is increased with aspirin, NSAIDs, warfarin, heparin, SSRIs or SNRIs.
- Inform patient having had neuraxial anesthesia or spinal puncture to watch for signs and symptoms of spinal or epidural hematomas (numbness or weakness of legs, bowel or bladder dysfunction). Notify health care professional immediately if symptoms occur.
- Advise female patient to notify health care professional if pregnancy is planned or suspected or if breast feeding.

Evaluation/Desired Outcomes

- Reduction in the risk and treatment of stroke and systemic embolism.

aprepitant (oral)

(a-**prep**-i-tant)
Emend

fosaprepitant (injection)

(fos-a-**prep**-i-tant)
Emend

Classification
Therapeutic: antiemetics
Pharmacologic: neurokinin antagonists

Pregnancy Category B

Indications

PO, IV: Prevention of: Acute and delayed nausea and vomiting associated with initial and repeat courses of highly emetogenic chemotherapy, Nausea and vomiting associated with initial and repeat courses of moderately emetogenic chemotherapy. **PO:** Prevention of postoperative nausea and vomiting.

Action

Acts as a selective antagonist at substance P/neurokinin 1 (NK_1) receptors in the brain. **Therapeutic Effects:** Decreased nausea and vomiting associated with chemotherapy. Augments the antiemetic effects of dexamethasone and 5-HT_3 antagonists (ondansetron).

Pharmacokinetics

Absorption: 60–65% absorbed following oral administration. Following IV administration, fosaprepitant is rapidly converted to aprepitant, the active component.

Distribution: Crosses the blood brain barrier; remainder of distribution unknown.

Metabolism and Excretion: Mostly metabolized by the liver (CYP3A4 enzyme system); not renally excreted.

Half-life: *Aprepitant*—9–13 hr.

TIME/ACTION PROFILE (antiemetic effect)

ROUTE	ONSET	PEAK	DURATION
PO	1 hr	4 hr*	24 hr
IV	rapid	end of infusion*	24 hr

*Blood level.

Contraindications/Precautions

Contraindicated in: Hypersensitivity; Concurrent use with pimozide (risk of life-threatening adverse cardiovascular reactions); Lactation: May cause unwanted effects in nursing infants.

Use Cautiously in: Concurrent use with any agents metabolized by CYP3A4; OB: Use only if clearly needed; Children <18 yr (IV) and <6 mo (PO) (safety and effectiveness not established).

Adverse Reactions/Side Effects

CV: dizziness, fatigue, weakness. **Derm:** STEVENS-JOHNSON SYNDROME. **GI:** diarrhea. **Misc:** hiccups, hypersensitivity reaction (flushing, erythema, dyspnea) (IV).

Interactions

Drug-Drug: Aprepitant inhibits, induces, and is metabolized by the CYP3A4 enzyme system; it also induces the CYP2C9 system. Concurrent use with other medications that are metabolized by CYP3A4 may result in ↑ toxicity from these agents including **docetaxel, paclitaxel, etoposide, irinotecan, ifosfamide, imatinib, vinorelbine, vinblastine, vincristine, midazolam, triazolam,** and **alprazolam**; concurrent use should be undertaken with caution. Concurrent use with **drugs that significantly inhibit the CYP3A4 enzyme system** including (**ketoconazole, itraconazole, nefazodone, clarithromycin, ritonavir, nelfinavir,** and **diltiazem**) may ↑ blood levels and effects of aprepitant. Concurrent use with **drugs that induce the CYP3A4 enzyme system** including **rifampin, carbamazepine,** and **phenytoin** may ↓ blood levels and effects of aprepitant. ↑ blood levels and effects of **dexamethasone** (regimen reflects a 50% dose reduction); a similar effect occurs with **methylprednisolone** (↓ IV dose by 25%, ↓ PO dose by 50% when used concurrently). May ↓ the effects of **warfarin** (careful monitoring for 2 wk recommended), **oral contraceptives** (use alternate method), and **phenytoin**.

Route/Dosage

Prevention of Nausea and Vomiting Associated with Highly Emetogenic Chemotherapy

PO (Adults): 125 mg given 1 hr prior to chemotherapy (Day 1) (with dexamethasone 12 mg PO given 30 min prior to chemotherapy and a 5-HT_3 antagonist given prior to chemotherapy), then 80 mg once daily for 2 days (Days 2 and 3) (with dexamethasone 8 mg once daily for 3 days [Days 2–4]).

IV (Adults): *Single-dose regimen*—150 mg given 30 min prior to chemotherapy (Day 1) (with dexamethasone 12 mg PO given 30 min prior to chemotherapy and a 5-HT_3 antagonist given prior to chemotherapy). Continue dexamethasone on Days 2–4 (8 mg PO on Day 2, 8 mg twice daily on Days 3 and 4); *3-day regimen*—115 mg given 30 min prior to chemotherapy (Day 1) (with dexamethasone 12 mg PO given 30 min prior to chemotherapy and a 5-HT_3 antagonist given prior to chemotherapy), then 80 mg PO once daily for 2 days (Days 2 and 3) (with dexamethasone 8 mg once daily for 3 days [Days 2–4]).

PO (Children ≥12 yr): 125 mg given 1 hr prior to chemotherapy (Day 1) (with PO dexamethasone at 50% of recommended dose given 30 min prior to chemotherapy and a 5-HT_3 antagonist given prior to chemotherapy), then 80 mg once daily for 2 days (Days 2 and 3) (with PO dexamethasone at 50% of recommended dose once daily for 3 days [Days 2–4]).

PO (Children <12 yr and ≥30 kg): 125 mg given 1 hr prior to chemotherapy (Day 1) (with PO dexamethasone at 50% of recommended dose given 30 min prior to chemotherapy and a 5-HT_3 antagonist given prior to chemotherapy), then 80 mg once daily for 2 days (Days 2 and 3) (with PO dexamethasone at 50% of recommended dose once daily for 3 days [Days 2–4]).

Prevention of Nausea and Vomiting Associated with Moderately Emetogenic Chemotherapy

PO (Adults): 125 mg given 1 hr prior to chemotherapy (Day 1) (with dexamethasone 12 mg PO given 30 min prior to chemotherapy and a 5-HT_3 antagonist), then 80 mg once daily for 2 days (Days 2 and 3).

IV (Adults): 115 mg given 30 min prior to chemotherapy on Day 1 (with dexamethasone 12 mg PO given 30

min prior to chemotherapy and a 5-HT_3 antagonist), then 80 mg PO once daily for 2 days (Days 2 and 3).
PO (Children ≥12 yr): 125 mg given 1 hr prior to chemotherapy (Day 1) (with PO dexamethasone at 50% of recommended dose given 30 min prior to chemotherapy and a 5-HT_3 antagonist), then 80 mg once daily for 2 days (Days 2 and 3).
PO (Children <12 yr and ≥30 kg): 125 mg given 1 hr prior to chemotherapy (Day 1) (with PO dexamethasone at 50% of recommended dose given 30 min prior to chemotherapy and a 5-HT_3 antagonist), then 80 mg once daily for 2 days (Days 2 and 3).

Prevention of Postoperative Nausea and Vomiting

PO (Adults): 40 mg given within 3 hr prior to induction of anesthesia.

Availability

Capsules: 40 mg, 80 mg, 125 mg. **Lyophilized solid (requires reconsititution prior to injection):** 115 mg/vial, 150 mg/vial.

NURSING IMPLICATIONS

Assessment

- Assess nausea, vomiting, appetite, bowel sounds, and abdominal pain prior to and following administration.
- Monitor hydration, nutritional status, and intake and output. Patients with severe nausea and vomiting may require IV fluids in addition to antiemetics.
- Assess for rash periodically during therapy. May cause Stevens-Johnson syndrome. Discontinue therapy if severe rash or if accompanied with fever, general malaise, fatigue, muscle or joint aches, blisters, skin peeling, sores, oral lesions, conjunctivitis, hepatitis and/or eosinophilia.
- Monitor for signs and symptoms of infusion site reaction (erythema, edema, pain, thrombophlebitis). Treat symptomatically.
- ***Lab Test Considerations:*** Monitor clotting status closely during the 2 wk period, especially at 7–10 days, following aprepitant therapy in patients on chronic warfarin therapy.
- May cause mild, transient ↑ in alkaline phosphatase, AST, ALT, and BUN.
- May cause proteinuria, erythrocyturia, leukocyturia, hyperglycemia, hyponatremia, and ↑ leukocytes.
- May cause ↓ hemoglobin and WBC.

Potential Nursing Diagnoses

Risk for deficient fluid volume (Indications)
Imbalanced nutrition: less than body requirements (Indications)

Implementation

- For chemotherapy, aprepitant is given as part of a regimen that includes a corticosteroid and a 5-HT_3 antagonist (see Route/Dosage).
- **PO:** Administer daily for 3 days. *Day 1*—administer 125 mg 1 hr prior to chemotherapy. *Days 2 and 3*—administer 80 mg once in the morning. May be administered without regard to food.

IV Administration

- **Single-Dose Regimen: Intermittent Infusion:** Inject 5 mL of 0.9% NaCl for Injection into vial. Swirl gently; avoid shaking or jetting saline into vial. ***Diluent:*** Prepare an infusion bag of 145 mL 0.9% NaCl. Withdraw entire volume from vial, and transfer to infusion bag for a total volume of 150 mL. ***Concentration:*** 1 mg/mL. Gently invert bag 2–3 times. Solution is stable for 24 hr at room temperature. Inspect solution for particulate matter. Do not administer solutions that are discolored or contain particulate matter. ***Rate:*** Infuse over 20–30 min.
- **3-Day Regimen: Intermittent Infusion:** Inject 5 mL of 0.9% NaCl for Injection into vial. Swirl gently; avoid shaking or jetting saline into vial. ***Diluent:*** Prepare an infusion bag of 110 mL 0.9% NaCl. Withdraw entire volume from vial, and transfer to infusion bag for a total volume of 115 mL. ***Concentration:*** 1 mg/mL. Gently invert bag 2–3 times. Solution is stable for 24 hr at room temperature. Inspect solution for particulate matter. Do not administer solutions that are discolored or contain particulate matter. ***Rate:*** Administer over 15 min.
- **Y-Site Compatibility:** dexamethasone, granisetron, methylprednisolone, ondansetron, palonosetron.
- **Solution Incompatibility:** Incompatible with solutions containing divalent cations (calcium, magnesium) including LR and Hartmann's solution.

Patient/Family Teaching

- Instruct patient to take aprepitant as directed. Direct patient to read the *Patient Package Insert* before starting therapy and each time Rx renewed in case of changes.
- Instruct patient to notify health care professional if nausea and vomiting occur prior to administration.
- Advise patient to notify health care professional immediately if symptoms of hypersensitivity reaction (hives, rash, itching, redness of the face/skin, difficulty in breathing or swallowing) occur.
- Instruct patient to notify health care professional of all Rx or OTC medications, vitamins, or herbal products being taken and consult health care professional before taking any new medications.
- Advise patient and family to use general measures to decrease nausea (begin with sips of liquids and small, nongreasy meals; provide oral hygiene; remove noxious stimuli from environment).
- Rep: Caution patient that aprepitant and fosaprepitant may decrease effectiveness of oral contraceptives. Advise patient to use alternate nonhormonal methods of contraception during and for 1 mo following treatment. Advise patient to notify health care professional if pregnancy is planned or suspected or if breast feeding.

Evaluation/Desired Outcomes

- Decreased nausea and vomiting associated with chemotherapy.
- Prevention of postoperative nausea and vomiting.

HIGH ALERT

argatroban (ar-**gat**-tro-ban)

Classification
Therapeutic: anticoagulants
Pharmacologic: thrombin inhibitors

Pregnancy Category B

Indications

Prophylaxis or treatment of thrombosis in patients with heparin-induced thrombocytopenia. As an anticoagulant in patients with or at risk for heparin-induced thrombocytopenia who are undergoing percutaneous coronary intervention (PCI).

Action

Inhibits thrombin by binding to its receptor sites. Inhibition of thrombin prevents activation of factors V, VIII, and XII; the conversion of fibrinogen to fibrin; platelet adhesion and aggregation. **Therapeutic Effects:** Decreased thrombus formation and extension with decreased sequelae of thrombosis (emboli, postphlebotic syndromes).

Pharmacokinetics

Absorption: IV administration results in complete bioavailability.
Distribution: Unknown.
Metabolism and Excretion: Mostly metabolized by the liver; excreted primarily in feces via biliary excretion. 16% excreted unchanged in urine, 14% excreted unchanged in feces.
Half-life: 39–51 min (↑ in hepatic impairment).

TIME/ACTION PROFILE (anticoagulant effect)

ROUTE	ONSET	PEAK	DURATION
IV	immediate	1–3 hr	2–4 hr

Contraindications/Precautions

Contraindicated in: Major bleeding; Hypersensitivity; Lactation: Lactation.
Use Cautiously in: Hepatic impairment (↓ initial infusion rate recommended); OB: Use only if clearly needed; Pedi: Safety not established.

Adverse Reactions/Side Effects

CV: hypotension. **GI:** diarrhea, nausea, vomiting. **Hemat:** BLEEDING. **Misc:** allergic reactions including ANAPHYLAXIS, fever.

Interactions

Drug-Drug: Risk of bleeding may be ↑ by concurrent use of **antiplatelet agents**, **thrombolytic agents**, or **other anticoagulants**.
Drug-Natural Products: ↑ bleeding risk with **anise**, **arnica**, **chamomile**, **clove**, **feverfew**, **garlic**, **ginger**, **ginkgo**, **Panax ginseng**, and others.

Route/Dosage

IV (Adults): 2 mcg/kg/min as a continuous infusion; adjust infusion rate on the basis of activated partial thromboplastin time (aPTT). *Patients undergoing PCI*—350 mcg/kg bolus followed by infusion at 25 mcg/kg/min, activated clotting time (ACT) should be assessed 5–10 min later. If ACT is 300–450 sec, procedure may be started. If ACT <300 sec, give additional bolus of 150 mcg/kg and ↑ infusion rate to 30 mcg/kg/min. If ACT is >450 sec infusion rate should be ↓ to 15 mcg/kg/min and ACT rechecked after 5–10 min. If thrombotic complications occur or ACT drops to <300 sec, an additional bolus of 150 mcg/kg may be given and the infusion rate ↑ to 40 mcg/kg/min followed by ACT monitoring. If anticoagulation is required after surgery, lower infusion rates should be used.

Hepatic Impairment

IV (Adults): 0.5 mcg/kg/min as a continuous infusion; adjust infusion rate on the basis of aPTT.

Availability (generic available)

Solution for injection: 100 mg/mL. **Premixed infusion:** 50 mg/50 mL, 125 mg/125 mL, 250 mg/250 mL.

NURSING IMPLICATIONS

Assessment

- Monitor vital signs periodically during therapy. Unexplained decreases in BP may indicate hemorrhage. Assess patient for bleeding. Arterial and venous punctures, IM injections, and use of urinary catheters, nasotracheal intubation, and nasogastric tubes should be minimized. Noncompressible sites for IV access should be avoided. Monitor for blood in urine, lower back pain, pain or burning on urination. If bleeding cannot be controlled with pressure, decrease dose or discontinue argatroban immediately.
- Monitor for signs of anaphylaxis (rash, coughing, dyspnea) throughout therapy.
- ***Lab Test Considerations:*** Monitor aPTT prior to initiation of continuous infusion, 2 hours after initiation of therapy, and periodically during therapy to confirm aPTT is within desired therapeutic range.
- For patients undergoing PCI, monitor ACT as described in Route and Dose section.
- Assess hemoglobin, hematocrit, and platelet count prior to, and periodically during, argatroban ther-

apy. May cause ↓ hemoglobin and hematocrit. Unexplained ↓ hematocrit may indicate hemorrhage.

- Use of argatroban concurrently with multiple doses of warfarin will result in more prolonged prothrombin time and international normalized ratio (INR) (although there is not an ↑ in vitamin K-dependent factor X_a activity) than when warfarin is used alone. Monitor INR daily during concomitant therapy. Repeat INR 4–6 hr after argatroban is discontinued. If repeat value is below desired therapeutic value for warfarin alone, restart argatroban therapy and continue until desired therapeutic range for warfarin alone is reached. To obtain the INR for warfarin alone when dose of argatroban is >2 mcg/kg/min, temporarily reduce argatroban dose to 2 mcg/kg/min; INR for combined therapy may then be obtained 4–6 hr after argatroban dose was reduced.
- ***Toxicity and Overdose:*** There is no specific antidote for argatroban. If overdose occurs, discontinue argatroban. Anticoagulation parameters usually return to baseline within 2–4 hr after discontinuation.

Potential Nursing Diagnoses

Ineffective tissue perfusion (Indications)

Implementation

- Do not confuse argatroban with Aggrastat.
- All parenteral anticoagulants should be discontinued before argatroban therapy is initiated. Oral anticoagulation may be initiated with maintenance dose of warfarin; do not administer loading dose. Discontinue argatroban therapy when INR for combined therapy is >4.

IV Administration

- **IV:** Do not administer solutions that are cloudy or contain particulate matter. Discard unused portion.
- **IV Push:** ***Diluent:*** Bolus dose of 350 mcg/kg should be given prior to continuous infusion in patients undergoing PCI. For Diluent information, see Continuous Infusion section below. ***Rate:*** Administer bolus over 3–5 min.
- **Continuous Infusion:** ***Diluent:*** Dilute each 100 mg/mL in 0.9% NaCl, D5W, or LR. Mix by repeated inversion for 1 min. Diluted solution is slightly viscous, clear, and colorless to pale yellow and may show a slight haziness that disappears upon mixing; solution must be clear before use. Solution is stable at controlled room temperature and ambient light for 24 hrs, or for 96 hrs at controlled room temperature or refrigerated and protected from light; do not expose to direct sunlight. Pre-mixed solutions are clear and colorless. Store at room temperature, do not refrigerate or freeze. ***Concentration:*** 1 mg/mL. ***Rate:*** Based on patient's weight (See Route/Dosage section). Dose adjustment may be made 2 hr after starting infusion or changing dose until steady-state aPTT is 1.5–3 times the initial baseline value (not to exceed 100 sec).
- **Y-Site Compatibility:** acyclovir, alemtuzumab, alfentanil, allopurinol, amifostine, amikacin, aminocaproic acid, aminophylline, amphotericin B lipid complex, amphotericin B liposome, ampicillin, ampicillin/sulbactam, anidulafungin, atropine, azithromycin, aztreonam, bivalirudin, bleomycin, buprenorphine, busulfan, butorphanol, calcium acetate, calcium chloride, calcium gluconate, carboplatin, carmustine, caspofungin, cefazolin, cefotaxime, cefotetan, cefoxitin, ceftazidime, ceftriaxone, cefuroxime, chloramphenicol, chlorpromazine, ciprofloxacin, cisatracurium, cisplatin, clindamycin, cyclophosphamide, cyclosporine, cytarabine, dacarbazine, dactinomycin, daptomycin, daunorubicin, dexamethasone, dexmedetomidine, dexrazoxane, digoxin, diltiazem, diphenhydramine, dobutamine, docetaxel, dolasetron, dopamine, doxacurium, doxacurium, doxorubicin, doxorubicin liposomal, doxycycline, droperidol, enalaprilat, ephedrine, epinephrine, epirubicin, eptifibatide, ertapenem, erythromycin, esmolol, etoposide, etoposide phosphate, famotidine, fenoldopam, fentanyl, fluconazole, fludarabine, fluorouracil, foscarnet, fosphenytoin, furosemide, ganciclovir, gemcitabine, gentamicin, glycopyrrolate, granisetron, haloperidol, heparin, hydralazine, hydrocortisone, hydromorphone, ibutilide, idarubicin, ifosfamide, imipenem/cilastatin, insulin, irinotecan, isoproterenol, ketorolac, labetalol, leucovorin, levofloxacin, lidocaine, linezolid, lorazepam, magnesium sulfate, mannitol, mechlorethamine, melphalan, meperidine, meropenem, mesna, methotrexate, methylprednisolone, metoclopramide, metoprolol, metronidazole, midazolam, milrinone, mitomycin, mitoxantrone, morphine, moxifloxacin, mycophenolate, nafcillin, nalbuphine, naloxone, nesiritide, nicardipine, nitroglycerin, nitroprusside, norepinephrine, octreotide, ondansetron, oxaliplatin, oxytocin, paclitaxel, palonosetron, pamidronate, pancuronium, pantoprazole, pentamidine, pentazocine, pentobarbital, phenobarbital, phenylephrine, piperacillin/tazobactam, potassium acetate, potassium chloride, potassium phosphates, procainamide, prochlorperazine, promethazine, propranolol, quinupristin/dalfopristin, ranitidine, remifentanil, rocuronium, sodium acetate, sodium bicarbonate, sodium phosphates, streptozocin, succinylcholine, sufentanil, tacrolimus, teniposide, theophylline, thiopental, thiotepa, tigecycline, tirofiban, tobramycin, topotecan, trimethoprim/sulfamethoxazole, vancomycin, vasopressin, vecuronium, verapamil, vinblastine, vincristine, vinorelbine, voriconazole, zidovudine, zoledronic acid.
- **Y-Site Incompatibility:** cefepime, dantrolene, diazepam, phenytoin.

Patient/Family Teaching

- Inform patient of the purpose of argatroban.
- Instruct patient to notify health care professional immediately if any bleeding is noted.

Evaluation/Desired Outcomes

- Decreased thrombus formation and extension.
- Decreased sequelae of thrombosis (emboli, postphlebitic syndromes).

ARIPiprazole (a-ri-**pip**-ra-zole)

Abilify, Abilify Maintena

Classification

Therapeutic: antipsychotics, mood stabilizers

Pharmacologic: serotonin-dopamine activity modulators (SDAM)

Pregnancy Category C

Indications

Schizophrenia (Abilify and Abilify Maintena). Acute and maintenance therapy of manic and mixed episodes associated with bipolar disorder (as monotherapy or with lithium or valproate) (Abilify only). Adjunctive treatment of depression in adults (Abilify only). Agitation associated with schizophrenia or bipolar disorder (Abilify only). Irritability associated with autism spectrum disorder in children (Abilify only). Tourette's disorder.

Action

Psychotropic activity may be due to agonist activity at dopamine D_2 and serotonin 5-HT_{1A} receptors and antagonist activity at the 5-HT_{2A} receptor. Also has $alpha_1$ adrenergic blocking activity. **Therapeutic Effects:** Decreased manifestations of schizophrenia. Decreased mania in bipolar patients. Decreased symptoms of depression. Decreased agitation associated with schizophrenia or bipolar disorder. Decreased emotional and behavioral symptoms of irritability. Decreased incidence of tics.

Pharmacokinetics

Absorption: Well absorbed (87%) following oral administration; 100% following IM injection.

Distribution: Extensive extravascular distribution.

Protein Binding: *aripiprazole and dehydro-aripiprazole*—>99%.

Metabolism and Excretion: Mostly metabolized by the liver (CYP3A4 and CYP2D6 isoenzymes); the CYP2D6 enzyme system exhibits genetic polymorphism; ~7% of population may be poor metabolizers (PMs) and may have significantly ↑ aripiprazole concentrations and an ↑ risk of adverse effects (↓ dose by 50% in PMs); one metabolite (dehydro-aripiprazole) has antipsychotic activity. 18% excreted unchanged in feces; <1% excreted unchanged in urine.

Half-life: *Aripiprazole*—75 hr; *dehydro-aripiprazole—94 hr*; ER injectable suspension: 30–46 days.

TIME/ACTION PROFILE (antipsychotic effect)

ROUTE	ONSET	PEAK	DURATION
PO	unknown	2 wk	unknown
ER-IM	unknown	unknown	unknown

Contraindications/Precautions

Contraindicated in: Hypersensitivity; Lactation: Excreted in breast milk; discontinue drug or bottle feed.

Use Cautiously in: Known cardiovascular or cerebrovascular disease; Conditions which cause hypotension (dehydration, treatment with antihypertensives or diuretics); Diabetes (may ↑ risk of hyperglycemia); Seizure disorders; Patients at risk for aspiration pneumonia; Concurrent ketoconazole or other potential CYP3A4 inhibitors (↓ aripiprazole dose by 50%); Concurrent quinidine, fluoxetine, paroxetine, or other potential CYP2D6 inhibitors; Concurrent carbamazepine or other potential CYP3A4 inducers; OB: Neonates at ↑ risk for extrapyramidal symptoms and withdrawal after delivery when exposed during the 3rd trimester; use only if maternal benefit outweighs risk to fetus; Pedi: May ↑ risk of suicide attempt/ideation especially during dose early treatment or dose adjustment; risk may be greater in children, adolescents, and young adults taking antidepressants (safe use in children/adolescents not established); Geri: ↑ risk of mortality in elderly patients treated for psychosis related to dementia/neurocognitive disorders.

Adverse Reactions/Side Effects

CNS: SUICIDAL THOUGHTS, drowsiness, extrapyramidal reactions, akathisia, confusion, depression, fatigue, hostility, insomnia, lightheadedness, manic reactions, impaired cognitive function, nervousness, restlessness, seizures, tardive dyskinesia. **Resp:** dyspnea. **CV:** bradycardia, chest pain, edema, hypertension, orthostatic hypotension, tachycardia. **EENT:** blurred vision, conjunctivitis, ear pain. **GI:** constipation, anorexia, ↑ salivation, nausea, vomiting, weight gain, weight loss. **GU:** urinary incontinence. **Hemat:** AGRANULOCYTOSIS, anemia, leukopenia, neutropenia. **Derm:** dry skin, ecchymosis, skin ulcer, sweating. **MS:** muscle cramps, neck pain. **Metab:** dyslipidemia, hyperglycemia. **Neuro:** abnormal gait, tremor. **Misc:** HYPERSENSITIVITY REACTIONS, NEUROLEPTIC MALIGNANT SYNDROME, ↓ heat regulation.

Interactions

Drug-Drug: Ketoconazole, **clarithromycin**, or other **strong CYP3A4 inhibitors** ↓ metabolism and ↑ effects (↓ aripiprazole dose by 50%). **Quinidine**, **fluoxetine**, **paroxetine**, or **other strong CYP2D6 inhibitors** ↓ metabolism and ↑ effects (↓ aripiprazole dose by at least 50%). Concurrent **carbamazepine** or **other potential CYP3A4 inducers** ↑ metabolism and ↓ effects (double aripiprazole dose).

Route/Dosage

If used concurrently with combination of strong, moderate, or weak CYP3A4 and CYP2D6 inhibitors, ↓ oral aripiprazole dose by 75%. Aripiprazole dose should be ↓ by 75% in CYP2D6 PMs who are concomitantly receiving a strong CYP3A4 inhibitor.

Schizophrenia

PO (Adults): 10 or 15 mg once daily; doses up to 30 mg/day have been used; increments in dosing should not be made before 2 wk at a given dose.
PO (Children 13–17 yr): 2 mg once daily; ↑ to 5 mg once daily after 2 days, and then to target dose of 10 mg once daily after another 2 days; may further ↑ dose in 5-mg increments if needed (max: 30 mg/day).
IM (Adults): 400 mg every month; after 1st injection, continue treatment with oral aripiprazole (10–20 mg/day) for 14 days; if no adverse reactions to 400 mg/month dose, may ↓ dose to 300 mg every month. *CYP2D6 PMs*—↓ dose to 300 mg monthly; *CYP2D6 PMs concomitantly receiving strong CYP3A4 inhibitor*—↓ dose to 200 mg monthly; *Concomitant therapy with strong CYP2D6 or CYP3A4 inhibitor*—↓ dose to 300 mg monthly (if originally receiving 400 mg monthly) or 200 mg monthly (if originally receiving 300 mg monthly); *Concomitant therapy with strong CYP2D6 and CYP3A4 inhibitor*—↓ dose to 200 mg monthly (if originally receiving 400 mg monthly) or 160 mg monthly (if originally receiving 300 mg monthly); *Concomitant therapy with CYP3A4 inducer*—Avoid use.

Acute Manic or Mixed Episodes Associated with Bipolar I Disorder

PO (Adults): 15 mg once daily as monotherapy or 10–15 mg once daily with lithium or valproate; target dose is 15 mg once daily; may ↑ to 30 mg once daily, if needed.
PO (Children 10–17 yr): 2 mg once daily; ↑ to 5 mg once daily after 2 days, and then to target dose of 10 mg once daily after another 2 days; may further ↑ dose in 5-mg increments if needed (max: 30 mg/day).

Maintenance Treatment of Bipolar I Disorder

PO (Adults): Continue same dose needed to stabilize patient during acute treatment.
PO (Children 10–17 yr): Continue same dose needed to stabilize patient during acute treatment.

Depression

PO (Adults): 2–5 mg once daily, may titrate upward at 1-wk intervals to 5–10 mg once daily (max: 15 mg/day).

Irritability Associated with Autistic Disorder

PO (Children 6–17 yr): 2 mg once daily; ↑ to 5 mg once daily after at least 1 wk; may further ↑ dose in 5-mg increments if needed at ≥1-wk intervals (max: 15 mg/day).

Tourette's Disorder

PO (Children 6–18 yr and ≥50 kg): 2 mg once daily; ↑ to target dose of 5 mg once daily after 2 days; may further ↑ dose if needed at ≥1-wk intervals (max: 10 mg/day).
PO (Children 6–18 yr and <50 kg): 2 mg once daily; ↑ to 5 mg once daily after 2 days, and then to target dose of 10 mg once daily after 5 days; may further ↑ dose in 5-mg increments if needed at ≥1-wk intervals (max: 20 mg/day).

Availability (generic available)

Tablets: 2 mg, 5 mg, 10 mg, 15 mg, 20 mg, 30 mg. **Cost:** 2 mg $2,208.52/90, 5 mg $2,208.52/90, 10 mg $2,208.52/90, 15 mg $2,208.52/90, 20 mg $3,107.38/90, 30 mg $3,107.38/90. **Orally disintegrating tablets (vanilla flavor):** 10 mg, 15 mg. **Cost:** All strengths $955.82/30. **Extended-release injectable suspension:** 300 mg/vial or prefilled syringe, 400 mg/vial or prefilled syringe. **Oral solution (orange cream):** 1 mg/mL.

NURSING IMPLICATIONS

Assessment

- Assess mental status (orientation, mood, behavior) before and periodically during therapy. Assess for suicidal tendencies, especially during early therapy for depression. Restrict amount of drug available to patient. Risk may be increased in children, adolescents, and adults ≤24 yrs.
- Assess weight and BMI initially and throughout therapy. Compare weight of children and adolescents with that expected during normal growth.
- Obtain fasting blood glucose and cholesterol levels initially and periodically during therapy.
- Monitor BP (sitting, standing, lying), pulse, and respiratory rate before and periodically during therapy.
- Observe patient carefully when administering medication to ensure that medication is actually taken and not hoarded or cheeked.
- Monitor patient for onset of akathisia (restlessness or desire to keep moving) and extrapyramidal side effects (*parkinsonian*—difficulty speaking or swallowing, loss of balance control, pill rolling of hands, masklike face, shuffling gait, rigidity, tremors; and *dystonic*—muscle spasms, twisting motions, twitching, inability to move eyes, weakness of arms or legs) periodically throughout therapy. Report these symptoms.
- Monitor for tardive dyskinesia (uncontrolled rhythmic movement of mouth, face, and extremities; lip smacking or puckering; puffing of cheeks; uncontrolled chewing; rapid or worm-like movements of tongue). Notify health care professional immediately if these symptoms occur, as these side effects may be irreversible.

- Monitor for development of neuroleptic malignant syndrome (fever, muscle rigidity, altered mental status, respiratory distress, tachycardia, seizures, diaphoresis, hypertension or hypotension, pallor, tiredness, loss of bladder control). Notify health care professional immediately if these symptoms occur.
- ***Lab Test Considerations:*** May cause ↑ creatinine phosphokinase.
- Monitor CBC frequently during initial months of therapy in patients with pre-existing or history of low WBC. May cause leukopenia, neutropenia, or agranulocytosis. Discontinue therapy if this occurs.
- Monitor blood glucose and cholesterol levels initially and periodically during therapy.

Potential Nursing Diagnoses

Disturbed thought process (Indications)
Imbalanced nutrition: risk for more than body requirements (Side Effects)

Implementation

- Do not confuse aripiprazole with rabeprazole.
- **PO:** Administer once daily without regard to meals.
- *Orally disintegrating tablets:* Do not open blister until ready to administer. For single tablet removal, open package and peel back foil on blister to expose tablet. Do not push tablet through foil; may damage tablet. Immediately upon opening blister, using dry hands, remove tablet and place entire orally disintegrating tablet on tongue. Tablet disintegration occurs rapidly in saliva. Take tablet without liquid; but if needed, it can be taken with liquid. Do not attempt to split tablet.
- **Extended-Release IM:** Available in vials or dual chamber prefilled syringes. *For vials,* reconstitute 300 mg dose with 1.5 mL and 400 mg dose with 1.9 mL of Sterile Water for Injection; discard extra sterile water. Withdraw air to equalize pressure in vial. Shake vial vigorously for 30 seconds until suspension is uniform; suspension is opaque and milky white. If injection is not given immediately, shake vial vigorously to re-suspend prior to injection. Do not store suspension in syringe. Determine volume needed for dose: from 400 mg vial: 400 mg = 2 mL, 300 mg = 1.5 mL, 200 mg = 1.0, and 160 mg = 0.8 mL. From 300 mg vial: 300 mg = 1.5 mL, 200 mg = 1 mL, and 160 mg =0.8 mL. *For prefilled syringes,* push plunger rod slightly to engage threads. Rotate plunger rod until rod stops rotating to release diluent; middle stopper will be at indicator line. Vertically shake syringe vigorously for 20 seconds until drug is uniformly milky-white. *For deltoid site,* use 23 gauge needle, 1 inch in length for non-obese patients and 22 gauge 1.5 inch for obese patients. *For gluteal site,* use 22 gauge needle, 1.5 inches in length for non-obese patients and and 22 gauge, 2 inch for obese patients. Inject deep into deltoid or gluteal site; do not massage. Continue oral dosing of aripiprazole for 2 wks after first dose of *Abilify Maintena.*
- If second or third doses of *Abilify Maintena* are missed and > 4 weeks and < 5 weeks since last injection, administer injection as soon as possible. If > 5 weeks since last injection, restart concomitant oral aripiprazole for 14 days with next administered injection. If fourth or subsequent doses are missed and >4 weeks and <6 weeks since last injection, administer injection as soon as possible. If >6 weeks since last injection, restart concomitant oral aripiprazole for 14 days with next administered injection.

Patient/Family Teaching

- Advise patient to take medication as directed and not to skip doses or double up on missed doses. Take missed doses as soon as remembered unless almost time for the next dose. Emphasize importance of maintaining regular scheduled injections when taking *Abilify Maintena.*
- Inform patient of possibility of extrapyramidal symptoms and tardive dyskinesia. Instruct patient to report these symptoms immediately.
- Advise patient to make position changes slowly to minimize orthostatic hypotension.
- Medication may cause drowsiness and lightheadedness. Caution patient to avoid driving or other activities requiring alertness until response to medication is known.
- Advise patient and family to notify health care professional if thoughts about suicide or dying, attempts to commit suicide; new or worse depression; new or worse anxiety; feeling very agitated or restless; panic attacks; trouble sleeping; new or worse irritability; acting aggressive; being angry or violent; acting on dangerous impulses; an extreme increase in activity and talking; other unusual changes in behavior or mood occur.
- Inform patient that aripiprazole may cause weight gain. Advise patient to monitor weight periodically. Notify health care professional of significant weight gain.
- Instruct patient to notify health care professional of all Rx or OTC medications, vitamins, or herbal products being taken and to consult health care professional before taking any new medications. Caution patient to avoid taking alcohol or other CNS depressants concurrently with this medication.
- Advise patient that extremes in temperature should be avoided, because this drug impairs body temperature regulation.
- Advise patient to notify health care professional of medication regimen prior to treatment or surgery.
- Advise female patients to notify health care professional if pregnancy is planned or suspected and to

avoid breast feeding during therapy. Encourage pregnant patients to enroll in registry by contacting National Pregnancy Registry for Atypical Antipsychotics at 1-866-961-2388 or visit http://womensmentalhealth.org/clinical-and-research-programs/pregnancyregistry/.

- Emphasize the importance of routine follow-up exams and continued participation in psychotherapy as indicated.

Evaluation/Desired Outcomes

- Decrease in excitable, paranoic, or withdrawn behavior.
- Decrease incidence of mood swings in patients with bipolar disorders.
- Increased sense of well-being in patients with depression.
- Decreased agitation associated with schizophrenia or bipolar disorder.
- Decreased emotional and behavioral symptoms of irritability.
- Decrease in tics.

asenapine (a-**sen**-a-peen)

Saphris

Classification

Therapeutic: antipsychotics, mood stabilizers

Pharmacologic: dibenzo-oxepino pyrroles

Pregnancy Category C

Indications

Schizophrenia. Acute treatment of manic/mixed episodes associated with bipolar I disorder (as monotherapy or with lithium or valproate).

Action

May act through combined antagonism of dopaminergic (D_2) and 5-HT_{2A} receptors. **Therapeutic Effects:** Decreased symptoms of acute schizophrenia and mania/mixed episodes of bipolar I disorder.

Pharmacokinetics

Absorption: 35% absorbed following SL administration.

Distribution: Rapidly distributed throughout the body. Vd is approximately 20–25 L/kg; 95% bound to plasma proteins.

Metabolism and Excretion: Highly metabolized; primarily by CYP1A2 and UGTA14 enzyme systems 50% excreted in urine, 40% in feces, primarily as metabolites.

Half-life: 24 hr.

TIME/ACTION PROFILE (antipsychotic effect)

ROUTE	ONSET	PEAK	DURATION
SL	unknown	0.5–1.5 hr†	12–24 hr

† Blood levels.

Contraindications/Precautions

Contraindicated in: Hypersensitivity; Dementia-related psychoses; Severe hepatic impairment; Lactation: Avoid use.

Use Cautiously in: History of cardiac arrhythmias, congenital QT prolongation, electrolyte abnormalities (especially hypomagnesemia or hypokalemia; correct prior to use) or concurrent use of medications known to prolong the QTc interval (may ↑ risk of life-threatening arrhythmias); History of seizures or conditions/medications known to ↓ seizure threshhold; History of leukopenia/neutropenia; Strenuous exercise, exposure to extreme heat, concurrent medications with anticholinergic activity, or risk of dehydration; History of suicide attempt; Geri: ↑ risk of adverse reactions; consider age-related ↓ in hepatic function, cardiovascular status, and concurrent medications; Geri: ↑ risk of mortality and stroke/TIA in elderly patients treated for dementia-related psychosis; OB: Neonates at ↑ risk for extrapyramidal symptoms and withdrawal after delivery when exposed during the 3rd trimester; use only if benefit outweighs risk to fetus; Pedi: Children <10 yr (safety and effectiveness not established).

Adverse Reactions/Side Effects

CNS: NEUROLEPTIC MALIGNANT SYNDROME, SEIZURES, SUICIDAL THOUGHTS, akathisia, dizziness, drowsiness, extrapyramidal symptoms, anxiety, fatigue, syncope, tardive dyskinesia. **CV:** QT INTERVAL PROLONGATION, bradycardia, orthostatic hypotension, tachycardia. **GI:** oral hypoesthesia, dry mouth, dyspepsia, dysphagia, oral blisters, oral inflammation, oral peeling/sloughing, oral ulcers. **Endo:** dyslipidemia, hyperglycemia, hyperprolactinemia. **Hemat:** AGRANULOCYTOSIS, leukopenia, neutropenia. **Metab:** weight gain, ↑ appetite. **Misc:** HYPERSENSITIVITY (including anaphylaxis, angioedema, hypotension, tachycardia, dyspnea, wheezing, and rash), ANGIOEDEMA.

Interactions

Drug-Drug: Concurrent use of **QTc interval prolonging drugs** including **Class 1A antiarrhythmics** such as **quinidine** and **procainamide** or **Class 3 antiarrhythmics** including **amiodarone** and **sotalol** or other **antipsychotics** including **ziprasidone**, **chlorpromazine** or **thioridazine** or certain **antibiotics** such as **moxifloxacin**; may ↑ risk of torsade de pointes and/or sudden death. Concurrent use should be avoided. **Fluvoxamine**, a strong inhibitor of CYP1A2, ↑ levels and risk of toxicity; use cautiously. Similar effects may occur with **paroxetine**, a CYP2D6 substrate and inhibitor. Drugs having similar properties (**substrates/inhibitors of CYP2D6**) should also be used cautiously with asenapine. ↑ risk of CNS depression with other **CNS depressants** including **antihistamines**, some **antidepressants**, **sedative/hypnotics**, and **alcohol**.

Route/Dosage

Schizophrenia

SL (Adults): 5 mg twice daily; may ↑ to 10 mg twice daily after 1 wk.

Acute Manic/Mixed Episodes Associated with Bipolar I Disorder

SL (Adults): *Monotherapy*—10 mg twice daily; may ↓ to 5 mg twice daily if tolerated poorly; *Adjunctive therapy with lithium or valproate*—5 mg twice daily; may ↑ to 10 mg twice daily.
SL (Children 10–17 yr): *Monotherapy*—2.5 mg twice daily; may ↑ to 5 mg twice daily after 3 days; may ↑ to 10 mg twice daily after another 3 days.

Availability

Sublingual tablets (black cherry flavor): 2.5 mg, 5 mg, 10 mg.

NURSING IMPLICATIONS

Assessment

- Assess mental status (orientation, mood, behavior) before and periodically during therapy. Assess for suicidal tendencies. Restrict amount of drug available to patient. Risk may be increased in children, adolescents, and adults ≤24 yrs.
- Assess weight and BMI initially and throughout therapy.
- Monitor BP (sitting, standing, lying) and pulse before and periodically during therapy.
- Observe patient carefully when administering medication to ensure that medication is actually taken and not hoarded or cheeked.
- Monitor patient for onset of akathisia (restlessness or desire to keep moving) and extrapyramidal side effects (*parkinsonian*—difficulty speaking or swallowing, loss of balance control, pill rolling of hands, masklike face, shuffling gait, rigidity, tremors; and *dystonic*—muscle spasms, twisting motions, twitching, inability to move eyes, weakness of arms or legs) periodically throughout therapy. Report these symptoms.
- Monitor for tardive dyskinesia (uncontrolled rhythmic movement of mouth, face, and extremities; lip smacking or puckering; puffing of cheeks; uncontrolled chewing; rapid or worm-like movements of tongue). Notify health care professional immediately if these symptoms occur, as these side effects may be irreversible.
- Monitor for development of neuroleptic malignant syndrome (fever, muscle rigidity, altered mental status, respiratory distress, tachycardia, seizures, diaphoresis, hypertension or hypotension, pallor, tiredness, loss of bladder control). Discontinue asenapine and notify health care professional immediately if these symptoms occur.
- Monitor for symptoms related to hyperprolactinemia (menstrual abnormalities, galactorrhea, sexual dysfunction).
- Assess patient for signs and symptoms of hypersensitivity reactions, including anaphylaxis, angioedema, hypotension, tachycardia, swollen tongue, dyspnea, wheezing and rash.
- ***Lab Test Considerations:*** Obtain fasting blood glucose and cholesterol levels initially and periodically during therapy.
- Monitor CBC frequently during initial months of therapy in patients with pre-existing or history of low WBC. May cause leukopenia, neutropenia, or agranulocytosis. Monitor patients with neutropenia for fever or other symptoms of infection and treat promptly. Discontinue therapy if ANC <1000/mm^3 occurs.
- May cause transient ↑ in serum ALT.

Potential Nursing Diagnoses

Disturbed thought process (Indications)

Implementation

- **SL:** Open packet immediately before use by firmly pressing thumb button and pulling out tablet pack. Do not push tablet through or cut or tear tablet pack. Peel back colored tab and gently remove tablet. Place tablet under tongue and allow to dissolve completely; dissolves in saliva within seconds. Do not split, crush, chew, or swallow tablets. Avoid eating or drinking for 10 min after administration. Slide tablet pack back into case until it clicks.

Patient/Family Teaching

- Advise patient to take medication as directed and not to skip doses or double up on missed doses. Take missed doses as soon as remembered unless almost time for the next dose.
- Inform patient of possibility of extrapyramidal symptoms and tardive dyskinesia. Instruct patient to report these symptoms immediately.
- Advise patient to make position changes slowly to minimize orthostatic hypotension.
- Medication may cause drowsiness and dizziness. Caution patient to avoid driving or other activities requiring alertness until response to medication is known.
- Advise patient and family to notify health care professional if thoughts about suicide or dying, attempts to commit suicide; new or worse depression; new or worse anxiety; feeling very agitated or restless; panic attacks; trouble sleeping; new or worse irritability; acting aggressive; being angry or violent; acting on dangerous impulses; an extreme increase in activity and talking; other unusual changes in behavior or mood or if signs and symptoms of hypersensitivity reactions (difficulty breathing, itching, swelling of

the face, tongue or throat, feeling lightheaded) occur.

- Inform patient that oral ulcers, blisters, peeling/sloughing, and inflammation may occur at application site. Advise patient to notify health care professional if these occur, may require discontinuation. Inform patient that numbness or tingling of mouth or throat may occur shortly after administration of asenapine; usually resolves within 1 hr.
- Instruct patient to notify health care professional of all Rx or OTC medications, vitamins, or herbal products being taken, to avoid alcohol, and to consult health care professional before taking any new medications and to avoid taking alcohol or other CNS depressants concurrently with this medication.
- Advise patient that extremes in temperature should be avoided, because this drug impairs body temperature regulation.
- Advise patient to notify health care professional of medication regimen prior to treatment or surgery.
- Advise female patients to notify health care professional if pregnancy is planned or suspected and to avoid breast feeding during therapy. Encourage pregnant patients to enroll in registry by contacting National Pregnancy Registry for Atypical Antipsychotics at 1-866-961-2388 or visit http://womensmentalhealth.org/clinical-and-research-programs/pregnancyregistry/.
- Emphasize the importance of routine follow-up exams and continued participation in psychotherapy as indicated.

Evaluation/Desired Outcomes

- Decrease in excitable, paranoic, or withdrawn behavior.
- Decrease incidence of mood swings in patients with bipolar disorders.
- Decreased agitation associated with schizophrenia or bipolar disorder.

HIGH ALERT

asparaginase *Erwinia chrysanthemi*

(a-**spare**-a-ji-nase)

Erwinaze

Classification

Therapeutic: antineoplastics

Pharmacologic: enzymes

Pregnancy Category C

Indications

Part of combination chemotherapy in the treatment of acute lymphocytic leukemia (ALL) in patients who developed hypersensitivity to *E. coli*-derived asparaginase.

Action

Catalyst in the conversion of asparagine (an amino acid) to aspartic acid and ammonia. Depletes asparagine in leukemic cells. **Therapeutic Effects:** Death of leukemic cells.

Pharmacokinetics

Absorption: Bioavailability after IM administration unknown; IV administration results in complete bioavailability.

Distribution: Remains in the intravascular space. Poor penetration into the CSF.

Metabolism and Excretion: Slowly sequestered in the reticuloendothelial system.

Half-life: IV: 8–30 hr; IM: 39–49 hr.

TIME/ACTION PROFILE

ROUTE	ONSET	PEAK†	DURATION
IM	unknown	unknown	unknown
IV	unknown	unknown	unknown

Contraindications/Precautions

Contraindicated in: Previous hypersensitivity; History of pancreatitis with prior L-asparaginase; History of serious thrombosis or hemorrhagic events with prior L-asparaginase; Lactation: Lactation.

Use Cautiously in: OB: Use only if the potential benefit justifies the potential risk to the fetus.

Adverse Reactions/Side Effects

GI: PANCREATITIS, ↑ liver function tests, nausea, vomiting. **Endo:** hyperglycemia. **Hemat:** hemorrhage, thromboembolic events. **Misc:** hypersensitivity reactions including ANAPHYLAXIS, fever.

Interactions

Drug-Drug: None known.

Route/Dosage

IM, IV (Adults and Children): *Substitution for E.coli-derived asparaginase*—25,000 International Units/m² substituted for each dose of *E.coli*-derived asparaginase; *Substitution for pegasparagase*—25,000 International Units/m² 3 times a wk (Mon/Wed/Fri) for 6 doses substituted for each dose of pegasparagase.

Availability

Powder for injection: 10,000 International Units/vial.

NURSING IMPLICATIONS

Assessment

- Monitor vital signs before and periodically during therapy; may cause fever.
- Monitor for signs and symptoms of pancreatitis (abdominal pain, nausea, vomiting, ↑ serum amylase) during therapy. If abdominal pain >72 hrs and serum amylase ↑ ≥2.0 x upper limit of normal occur, discontinue therapy. If mild pancreatitis occurs, withhold asparaginase *Erwinia chrysanthemi* until symptoms and serum amylase return to normal; then restart.
- Monitor for hypersensitivity reaction (urticaria, diaphoresis, facial swelling, joint pain, hypotension,

bronchospasm). Epinephrine and resuscitation equipment should be readily available.

- ***Lab Test Considerations:*** Monitor CBC and coagulation studies before and periodically throughout therapy. May ↓ fibrinogen, protein C activity, protein S activity, and anti-thrombin III. If thrombotic or hemorrhagic event occurs, withhold asparaginase *Erwinia chrysanthemi* until symptoms resolve; then resume therapy.
- Hepatotoxicity may be manifested by ↑ AST, ALT, bilirubin, or cholesterol. Liver function test results usually return to normal after therapy. May cause pancreatitis; monitor frequently for ↑ amylase or glucose.
- Monitor blood glucose prior to and periodically during therapy. May cause hyperglycemia treatable with fluids and insulin.
- *For IV doses,* monitoring pre-dose nadir serum asparaginase activity (NSAA) levels and switch to IM administration if desired NSAA levels are not achieved.

Potential Nursing Diagnoses

Deficient knowledge, related to medication regimen (Patient/Family Teaching)

Implementation

- ***High Alert:*** Fatalities have occurred with chemotherapeutic agents. Before administering, clarify all ambiguous orders; double-check single, daily, and course-of-therapy dose limits; have second practitioner independently double check original order and dose calculations.
- Solution should be prepared in a biologic cabinet. Wear gloves, gown, and mask while handling medication. Discard equipment in specially designated containers.
- Reconstitute by adding 1 or 2 mL of 0.9% NaCl for injection (without preservatives) against inner wall of the 10,000-IU vial. Swirl vial gently; do not shake or invert. Administer no more than 2 mL per injection site. ***Concentration:*** Reconstitution with 1 mL = 10,000 IU/mL; with 2 mL = 5,000 IU/mL. Solution is clear and colorless; do not administer solutions that are discolored or contain a precipitate. Withdraw dose needed into a polypropylene syringe and administer within 15 min of reconstitution. Do not refrigerate or freeze; administer within 4 hrs or discard. Inject IM with no >2 mL/site. Do not save unused portions; discard.
- **IM:** Limit volume to 2 mL at each injection site. If volume >2 mL, use multiple injection sites.

IV Administration

- **Intermittent Infusion:** For IV use, slowly inject reconstituted solution into 100 mL 0.9% NaCl at room temperature; do not shake or squeeze IV bag. ***Rate:*** Infuse over 1 hr.
- **Y-Site Incompatibility:** Do not infuse other IV drugs through same IV line.

Patient/Family Teaching

- Instruct patient to notify health care professional if signs and symptoms of hypersensitivity reaction, pancreatitis, thrombosis or hemorrhage (headache, arm or leg swelling, shortness of breath, chest pain) or hyperglycemia (excess thirst or increase in frequency or volume of urination), occur.
- Advise female patients to notify health care professional if pregnancy is planned or suspected, or if breast feeding.
- Emphasize need for periodic lab tests to monitor for side effects.

Evaluation/Desired Outcomes

- Improvement of hematologic status in patients with leukemia.

aspirin, See SALICYLATES.

atazanavir (a-ta-**zan**-a-veer)

Reyataz

Classification
Therapeutic: antiretrovirals
Pharmacologic: protease inhibitors

Pregnancy Category B

Indications

HIV infection (with other antiretrovirals).

Action

Inhibits the action of HIV protease, preventing maturation of virions. **Therapeutic Effects:** ↑ CD4 cell counts and ↓ viral load with subsequent slowed progression of HIV and its sequelae.

Pharmacokinetics

Absorption: Rapidly absorbed (↑ by food).
Distribution: Enters cerebrospinal fluid and semen.
Metabolism and Excretion: 80% metabolized (CYP3A); 13% excreted unchanged in urine.
Half-life: 7 hr.

TIME/ACTION PROFILE (blood levels)

ROUTE	ONSET	PEAK	DURATION
PO	rapid	2.5 hr	24 hr

Contraindications/Precautions

Contraindicated in: Hypersensitivity; Severe hepatic impairment; Concurrent use of ergot derivatives, midazolam (PO), pimozide, triazolam, alfuzosin, sildenafil (Revatio), rifampin, irinotecan, lovastatin, simvastatin, indinavir, nevirapine, or St. John's wort; Pedi: ↑ risk of kernicterus in infants <3 mo.

Use Cautiously in: Mild to moderate hepatic impairment; Pre-existing conduction system disease (marked first-degree AV block or second- or third-degree AV block) or concurrent use of other drugs that increase the PR interval (especially those metabolized by CYP3A4, including verapamil or diltiazem); Diabetes mellitus; Hemophilia (↑ risk of bleeding); Phenylketonuria (oral powder contains aspartame); OB: Use only if clearly needed; Breast feeding is not recommended if HIV-infected.

Adverse Reactions/Side Effects

When used in combination with other antiretrovirals.
CNS: headache, depression, dizziness, insomnia. **CV:** ↑ PR interval, heart block. **GI:** HEPATOTOXICITY, nausea, abdominal pain, ↑ bilirubin, cholelithiasis, diarrhea, jaundice, ↑ liver enzymes, vomiting. **Derm:** DRESS SYNDROME, ERYTHEMA MULTIFORME, STEVENS-JOHNSON SYNDROME, rash. **Endo:** hyperglycemia. **GU:** nephrolithiasis. **Metab:** fat redistribution. **MS:** myalgia. **Misc:** ANGIOEDEMA, fever, immune reconstitution syndrome.

Interactions

Drug-Drug: Atazanavir is an inhibitor of CYP3A and UGT1A1 enzyme systems. It is also a substrate of CYP3A. ↑ blood levels and risk of toxicity from **ergot derivatives (ergotamine, dihydroergotamine, methylergonovine)**, **midazolam (PO)**, **pimozide**, **triazolam**, **lovastatin**, **simvastatin**, **sildenafil (Revatio)**, **alfuzosin**, and **irinotecan**; concurrent use is contraindicated. Concurrent use with **indinavir** may ↑ risk of hyperbilirubinemia; concurrent use is contraindicated. Levels are significantly ↓ by **rifampin** and **nevirapine**; may promote viral resistance; concurrent use is contraindicated. Combination therapy with **tenofovir** may lead to ↓ virologic response and possible resistance (100 mg **ritonavir** should be added to boost blood levels and dose of atazanavir ↓ to 300 mg/day). Levels are significantly ↓ by **omeprazole**; do not exceed omeprazole dose of 20 mg/day when used with atazanavir and ritonavir in treatment-naive patients (should be taken at least 12 hr before atazanavir and ritonavir); should not be used in treatment-experienced patients. Concurrent use with **didanosine** buffered tablets will ↓ absorption and levels; give atazanavir with food 2 hr before or 1 hr after **didanosine**. **Efavirenz** ↓ levels and may promote viral resistance; 600 mg efavirenz should be given with atazanavir 400 mg/day and ritonavir 100 mg/day to counteract this effect in treatment-naive patients (should not be used with atazanavir in treatment-experienced patients). ↑ **saquinavir** levels. Levels are ↑ by **ritonavir**; ↓ atazanavir dose to 300 mg/day. **Nevirapine** may ↓ levels and atazanavir may ↑ **nevirapine** levels; avoid concurrent use. **Antacids** or **buffered medications** will ↓ absorption; atazanavir should be given 2 hr before or 1 hr after. ↑ levels of **lidocaine**, **amiodarone**, or **quinidine**; blood level monitoring is recommended. ↑ risk of bleeding with **warfarin**. ↑ of **tricyclic antidepressants**; blood level monitoring is recommended. ↑ levels of **rifabutin**; ↓ rifabutin dose by 75% (150 mg every other day or 3 times weekly). ↑ levels of **diltiazem** and its active metabolite; ↓ diltiazem dose by 50% and ECG monitoring recommended. Similar precautions may be needed with **felodipine**, **nifedipine**, **nicardipine**, and **verapamil**. ↑ levels of **fluticasone**; consider alternative therapy; should not be used when atazanavir used with ritonavir. ↓ levels of **voriconazole** when atazanavir is used with ritonavir; avoid concurrent use. **Voriconazole** may also ↑ levels of atazanavir (when used without ritonavir). ↑ levels of **ketoconazole** or **itraconazole** when atazanavir is used with ritonavir. ↑ levels of **trazodone**; ↓ dose of trazodone. ↑ levels of **sildenafil**, **vardenafil**, and **tadalafil**; ↓ **sildenafil** dose to 25 mg every 48 hr; ↓ **vardenafil** dose to 2.5 mg every 72 hr (when atazanavir used with ritonavir) or 2.5 mg every 24 hr (when atazanavir used alone); ↓ **tadalafil** dose to 10 mg every 72 hr. Exercise caution and monitor for hypertension, visual changes, and priapism. ↑ levels and risk of myopathy from **atorvastatin** or **rosuvastatin**; use lowest possible dose of statin; do not exceed rosuvastatin dose of 10 mg/day. Levels may be ↓ by **histamine H_2 antagonists**, promoting viral resistance; separate doses by at least 10 hr. ↑ levels of **cyclosporine**, **sirolimus**, and **tacrolimus**; monitor immunosuppressant blood levels. ↑ levels of **clarithromycin**; ↓ clarithromycin dose by 50% or consider alternative therapy. May ↓ levels of some **estrogens** found in **hormonal contraceptives**; use alternative nonhormonal method of contraception. May ↑ levels of **buprenorphine**; consider ↓ dose of buprenorphine. Concurrent use of other **drugs known to ↑ PR interval** may ↑ risk of heart block. May ↑ risk of adverse effects with **salmeterol**; concurrent use not recommended. May ↑ **bosentan** levels; initiate bosentan at 62.5 mg once daily or every other day; if patient already receiving bosentan, discontinue bosentan at least 36 hr before initiation of atazanavir and then restart bosentan at least 10 days later at 62.5 mg once daily or every other day; do not use with atazanavir alone (should be used with atazanavir and ritonavir). May ↑ **tadalafil (Adcirca)** levels; initiate tadalafil (Adcirca) at 20 mg once daily; if patient already receiving tadalfil (Adcirca), discontinue tadalafil (Adcirca) at least 24 hr before initiation of atazanavir and then restart tadalafil (Adcirca) at least 7 days later at 20 mg once daily. May ↑ **colchicine** levels; ↓ dose of colchicine; do not administer colchicine if patients have renal or hepatic impairment. Concurrent use of **boceprevir** with atazanavir and ritonavir results in ↓ atazanavir and ritonavir levels; concurrent use not recommended. **Carbamazepine**, **phenytoin**, and **phenobarbiral** may ↓ levels; do not give concurrently with atazanvir without using ritonavir. Concurrent use of **lamotrigine** with atazanavir and ritonavir results in ↓ lamotrigine levels; concurrent use not recommended. Concurrent use of **voriconazole** with atazanavir and ritonavir may result in either ↓ or ↑ voriconazole levels; concurrent use not recommended. May ↑ **quetiapine** levels; ↓ quetiapine dose to 1/6 of current dose.

Drug-Natural Products: St. John's wort significantly ↓ blood levels; concurrent use is contraindicated.

Route/Dosage

PO (Adults): *Therapy-naive*—400 mg once daily *or* 300 mg once daily with ritonavir 100 mg once daily (must be used with ritonavir in pregnancy); should be used at a dose of 300 mg once daily with ritonavir 100 mg once daily if used concomitantly with tenofovir, H_2 receptor antagonist, or proton pump inhibitor; should be used at a dose of 400 mg once daily with ritonavir 100 mg once daily if used concomitantly with efavirenz. *Therapy-experienced*—300 mg once daily with ritonavir 100 mg once daily; should be used at dose of 400 mg once daily with ritonavir 100 mg once daily if used with tenofovir *and* a H_2 receptor antagonist; in pregnant patients in 2nd or 3rd trimester, should be used at a dose of 400 mg once daily with ritonavir 100 mg once daily if used with tenofovir *or* a H_2 receptor antagonist.

PO(Capsules) (Children ≥6 yr): *Therapy–naïve or therapy–experienced (15–19 kg)*—150 mg once daily with ritonavir 100 mg once daily; *Therapy–naïve or therapy–experienced (20–39 kg)*—200 mg once daily with ritonavir 100 mg once daily; *Therapy–naïve or therapy–experienced (≥40 kg)*—300 mg once daily with ritonavir 100 mg once daily; *Therapy–naïve, ≥13 yr, ≥40 kg and unable to tolerate ritonavir*—400 mg once daily;.

PO(Oral Powder) (Children ≥3 mo and 10–24.9 kg): *Therapy–naïve or therapy–experienced (10–14.9 kg)*—200 mg once daily with ritonavir 80 mg once daily; *Therapy–naïve or therapy–experienced (15–24.9 kg)*—250 mg once daily with ritonavir 80 mg once daily.

Renal Impairment

PO (Adults): *Therapy-naive and HD*—300 mg once daily with ritonavir 100 mg once daily; *Therapy-experienced and HD*—contraindicated.

Hepatic Impairment

PO (Adults): *Moderate hepatic impairment*—300 mg once daily (do not use with ritonavir).

Availability (generic available)

Capsules: 150 mg, 200 mg, 300 mg. **Oral powder:** 50 mg/packet. ***In combination with:*** cobicistat (Evotaz). See Appendix B.

NURSING IMPLICATIONS

Assessment

- Assess for change in severity of HIV symptoms and for symptoms of opportunistic infections throughout therapy.
- Assess for rash which can occur within initial 8 wk of therapy. Usually resolves within 2 weeks without altering therapy. Discontinue therapy if rash becomes severe.
- ***Lab Test Considerations:*** Monitor viral load and CD4 cell count regularly during therapy.
- May cause ↑ serum amylase, lipase and hyperglycemia.
- May ↑ liver enzymes.
- May ↑ creatine kinase.
- May cause ↓ hemoglobin, neutrophils, and platelets.
- May cause ↑ in unconjugated bilirubin; reversible on discontinuation.

Potential Nursing Diagnoses

Risk for infection (Indications)
Noncompliance (Patient/Family Teaching)

Implementation

- **PO:** Administer daily with food to enhance absorption. Capsules should be swallowed whole; do not open.
- For oral powder, mix oral powder with applesauce or yogurt or a beverage (milk, infant formula, or water) for infants who can drink from a cup. For infants (less than 6 months) who cannot eat solid food or drink from a cup, mix oral powder with infant formula and administer using an oral dosing syringe. Administration in infant formula using an infant bottle is not recommended because full dose may not be delivered. Administer entire dose within 1 hr. *If mixed with food,* add an additional spoonful of food to container, mix, and administer residual mixture. *If mixed with liquid,* mix packet contents into 30 mL of liquid and give to child to drink. Add an additional 15 mL more of beverage to drinking cup, mix, and have the child drink the residual mixture. If water is used, food should also be taken at the same time. *If mixing with infant formula,* mix in 10 mL of formula, draw up and administer in left or right cheek of infant. Pour another 10 mL of formula into medicine cup to rinse off remaining oral powder in cup. Draw up residual mixture into syringe and administer into either right or left inner cheek of infant. Additional food may be given after consumption of the entire mixture. Administer ritonavir immediately following oral powder administration.

Patient/Family Teaching

- Emphasize the importance of taking atazanavir with food as directed. Advise patient to read the *Patient Information* before taking and with each Rx refill;

may be updated. Atazanavir must always be used in combination with other antiretroviral drugs. Do not take more than prescribed amount and do not stop taking without consulting health care professional. Take missed doses as soon as remembered, then return to regular dose schedule. If within 6 hr of next dose, omit dose and take next dose at regular time. Do not double doses.

- Instruct patient that atazanavir should not be shared with others.
- Inform patient that atazanavir does not cure HIV or prevent associated or opportunistic infections. Atazanavir does not reduce the risk of transmission of HIV to others through sexual contact or blood contamination. Caution patient to use a condom and to avoid sharing needles or donating blood to prevent spreading the HIV virus to others.
- Instruct patient to notify health care professional of all Rx or OTC medications, vitamins, or herbal products being taken and consult health care professional before taking any new medications, especially St. John's wort; interactions may be fatal.
- May cause dizziness. Caution patient to notify health care professional if this occurs and to avoid driving and other activities requiring alertness until response to medication is known.
- Instruct patient to notify health care professional immediately if signs and symptoms of hepatitis (flu-like symptoms, tiredness, nausea, lack of appetite, yellow skin or eyes, dark urine, pale stools, pain or sensitivity to touch on right side below ribs), skin reactions with symptoms (flu-like symptoms, fever, muscle aches, conjunctivitis, blisters, mouth sores, swelling of face, tiredness), gallbladder disorder (right or middle upper stomach pain, fever, nausea, vomiting, or yellowing of skin and whites of eyes), kidney stones (side pain, blood in urine, pain upon urination), change in heart rhythm, high blood sugar, or signs of immune reconstitution syndrome (signs and symptoms of an infection) occur.
- Inform patient that redistribution and accumulation of body fat may occur, causing central obesity, dorsocervical fat enlargement (buffalo hump), peripheral wasting, breast enlargement, and cushingoid appearance. The cause and long-term effects are not known.
- Instruct females using hormonal contraceptives to use an alternative nonhormonal method of contraception. Advise patient to notify health care professional if pregnancy is planned or suspected and to avoid breast feeding. If pregnant patient is exposed to atazanavir, register patient in *Antiretroviral Pregnancy Registry* by calling 1-800-258-4263.
- Emphasize the importance of regular follow-up exams and blood counts to determine progress and monitor for side effects.

Evaluation/Desired Outcomes

- Delayed progression of HIV and decreased opportunistic infections in patients with HIV.
- Decrease in viral load and increase in CD4 cell counts.

atenolol (a-ten-oh-lole)

Tenormin

Classification

Therapeutic: antianginals, antihypertensives
Pharmacologic: beta blockers

Pregnancy Category D

Indications

Management of hypertension. Management of angina pectoris. Prevention of MI.

Action

Blocks stimulation of $beta_1$ (myocardial)-adrenergic receptors. Does not usually affect $beta_2$ (pulmonary, vascular, uterine)-receptor sites. **Therapeutic Effects:** Decreased BP and heart rate. Decreased frequency of attacks of angina pectoris. Prevention of MI.

Pharmacokinetics

Absorption: 50–60% absorbed after oral administration.
Distribution: Minimal penetration of CNS. Crosses the placenta and enters breast milk.
Metabolism and Excretion: 40–50% excreted unchanged by the kidneys; remainder excreted in feces as unabsorbed drug.
Half-life: 6–9 hr.

TIME/ACTION PROFILE (cardiovascular effects)

ROUTE	ONSET	PEAK	DURATION
PO	1 hr	2–4 hr	24 hr

Contraindications/Precautions

Contraindicated in: Uncompensated HF; Pulmonary edema; Cardiogenic shock; Bradycardia or heart block.
Use Cautiously in: Renal impairment (dosage ↓ recommended if CCr ≤35 mL/min); Hepatic impairment; Geriatric patients (↑ sensitivity to beta blockers; initial dosage ↓ recommended); Pulmonary disease (including asthma; beta selectivity may be lost at higher doses); Diabetes mellitus (may mask signs of hypoglycemia); Thyrotoxicosis (may mask symptoms); Patients with a history of severe allergic reactions (intensity of reactions may be ↑); OB: Crosses the placenta and may cause fetal/neonatal bradycardia, hypotension, hypoglycemia, or respiratory depression; Lactation, Pedi: Safety not established.

Adverse Reactions/Side Effects

CNS: fatigue, weakness, anxiety, depression, dizziness, drowsiness, insomnia, memory loss, mental status changes, nervousness, nightmares. **EENT:** blurred vision, stuffy nose. **Resp:** bronchospasm, wheezing. **CV:** BRADYCARDIA, HF, PULMONARY EDEMA, hypotension, peripheral vasoconstriction. **GI:** constipation, diarrhea, ↑ liver enzymes, nausea, vomiting. **GU:** erectile dysfunction, ↓ libido, urinary frequency. **Derm:** rashes. **Endo:** hyperglycemia, hypoglycemia. **MS:** arthralgia, back pain, joint pain. **Misc:** drug-induced lupus syndrome.

Interactions

Drug-Drug: General anesthesia, **IV phenytoin**, and **verapamil** may cause additive myocardial depression. Additive bradycardia may occur with **digoxin**. Additive hypotension may occur with other **antihypertensives**, acute ingestion of **alcohol**, or **nitrates**. Concurrent use with **amphetamine**, **cocaine**, **ephedrine**, **epinephrine**, **norepinephrine**, **phenylephrine**, or **pseudoephedrine** may result in unopposed alpha-adrenergic stimulation (excessive hypertension, bradycardia). Concurrent **thyroid** administration may ↓ effectiveness. May alter the effectiveness of **insulins** or **oral hypoglycemic agents** (dosage adjustments may be necessary). May ↓ the effectiveness of **theophylline**. May ↓ the beneficial beta_1-cardiovascular effects of **dopamine** or **dobutamine**. Use cautiously within 14 days of **MAO inhibitor** therapy (may result in hypertension).

Route/Dosage

PO (Adults): *Antianginal*—50 mg once daily; may be ↑ after 1 wk to 100 mg/day (up to 200 mg/day). *Antihypertensive*—25–50 mg once daily; may be ↑ after 2 wk to 50–100 mg once daily. *MI*—50 mg, then 50 mg 12 hr later, then 100 mg/day as a single dose or in 2 divided doses for 6–9 days or until hospital discharge.

Renal Impairment

PO (Adults): *CCr 15–35 mL/min*—dosage should not exceed 50 mg/day; *CCr <15 mL/min*—dosage should not exceed 50 mg every other day.

Availability (generic available)

Tablets: 25 mg, 50 mg, 100 mg. **Cost:** *Generic*—All strengths $10.83/100. ***In combination with:*** chlorthalidone (Tenoretic). See Appendix B.

NURSING IMPLICATIONS

Assessment

- Monitor BP, ECG, and pulse frequently during dosage adjustment period and periodically throughout therapy.
- Monitor intake and output ratios and daily weights. Assess routinely for HF (dyspnea, rales/crackles, weight gain, peripheral edema, jugular venous distention).
- Monitor frequency of prescription refills to determine adherence.
- **Angina:** Assess frequency and characteristics of angina periodically throughout therapy.
- ***Lab Test Considerations:*** May cause ↑ BUN, serum lipoprotein, potassium, triglyceride, and uric acid levels.
- May cause ↑ ANA titers.
- May cause ↑ in blood glucose levels.
- ***Toxicity and Overdose:*** Monitor patients receiving beta blockers for signs of overdose (bradycardia, severe dizziness or fainting, severe drowsiness, dyspnea, bluish fingernails or palms, seizures). Notify physician immediately if these signs occur.

Potential Nursing Diagnoses

Decreased cardiac output (Side Effects)
Noncompliance (Patient/Family Teaching)

Implementation

- **PO:** Take apical pulse before administering drug. If <50 bpm or if arrhythmia occurs, withhold medication and notify physician or other health care professional.

Patient/Family Teaching

- Instruct patient to take atenolol as directed at the same time each day, even if feeling well; do not skip or double up on missed doses. Take missed doses as soon as possible up to 8 hr before next dose. Abrupt withdrawal may cause life-threatening arrhythmias, hypertension, or myocardial ischemia.
- Advise patient to make sure enough medication is available for weekends, holidays, and vacations. A written prescription may be kept in wallet in case of emergency.
- Teach patient and family how to check pulse and BP. Instruct them to check pulse daily and BP biweekly and to report significant changes.
- May cause drowsiness or dizziness. Caution patients to avoid driving or other activities that require alertness until response to the drug is known.
- Advise patients to change positions slowly to minimize orthostatic hypotension.
- Caution patient that atenolol may increase sensitivity to cold.
- Instruct patient to notify health care professional of all Rx or OTC medications, vitamins, or herbal products being taken, to avoid alcohol, and to consult health care professional before taking any new medications, especially cold preparations.
- Patients with diabetes should closely monitor blood glucose, especially if weakness, malaise, irritability, or fatigue occurs. Medication does not block sweating as a sign of hypoglycemia.

- Advise patient to notify health care professional if slow pulse, difficulty breathing, wheezing, cold hands and feet, dizziness, light-headedness, confusion, depression, rash, fever, sore throat, unusual bleeding, or bruising occurs.
- Instruct patient to inform health care professional of medication regimen before treatment or surgery.
- Advise female patient to notify health care professional if pregnancy is planned or suspected, or if breast feeding.
- Advise patient to carry identification describing disease process and medication regimen at all times.
- **Hypertension:** Reinforce the need to continue additional therapies for hypertension (weight loss, sodium restriction, stress reduction, regular exercise, moderation of alcohol consumption, and smoking cessation). Medication controls but does not cure hypertension.

Evaluation/Desired Outcomes

- Decrease in BP.
- Reduction in frequency of angina.
- Increase in activity tolerance.
- Prevention of MI.

atomoxetine

(a-to-**mox**-e-teen)

Strattera

Classification

Therapeutic: agents for attention deficit disorder

Pharmacologic: selective norepinephrine reuptake inhibitors

Pregnancy Category C

Indications

Attention-Deficit/Hyperactivity Disorder (ADHD).

Action

Selectively inhibits the presynaptic transporter of norepinephrine. **Therapeutic Effects:** Increased attention span.

Pharmacokinetics

Absorption: Well absorbed following oral administration.

Distribution: Unknown.

Protein Binding: 98%.

Metabolism and Excretion: Mostly metabolized by the liver (CYP2D6 enzyme pathway). A small percentage of the population are poor metabolizers and will have higher blood levels with ↑ effects.

Half-life: 5 hr.

TIME/ACTION PROFILE

ROUTE	ONSET	PEAK	DURATION
PO	unknown	1–2 hr	12–24 hr

Contraindications/Precautions

Contraindicated in: Hypersensitivity; Concurrent or within 2 wk therapy with MAO inhibitors; Angle-closure glaucoma; Pheochromocytoma; Hypertension, tachycardia, cardiovascular or cerebrovascular disease.

Use Cautiously in: Pre-existing psychiatric illness; Pedi: May ↑ risk of suicide attempt/ideation especially during dose early treatment or dose adjustment; risk may be greater in children or adolescents; Concurrent albuterol or vasopressors (↑ risk of adverse cardiovascular reactions); OB: Use only if benefits outweigh risks to fetus; Lactation, Pedi: Safety not established.

Adverse Reactions/Side Effects

CNS: SUICIDAL THOUGHTS, dizziness, fatigue, mood swings, behavioral disturbances, hallucinations, hostility, mania, thought disorder; *Adults*, insomnia. **CV:** hypertension, orthostatic hypotension, QT interval prolongation, syncope, tachycardia. **GI:** HEPATOTOXICITY, dyspepsia, nausea, vomiting; *Adults*, dry mouth, constipation. **Derm:** rash, urticaria. **GU:** *Adults*—dysmenorrhea, ejaculatory problems, erectile dysfunction, libido changes, priapism, urinary hesitation, urinary retention. **Metab:** ↓ appetite, weight/growth loss. **MS:** RHABDOMYOLYSIS. **Neuro:** *Adults*—paresthesia. **Misc:** allergic reactions including ANGIONEUROTIC EDEMA and ANAPHYLAXIS.

Interactions

Drug-Drug: Concurrent use with **MAO inhibitors** may result in serious, potentially fatal reactions (do not use within 2 wk of each other). ↑ risk of cardiovascular effects with **albuterol** or **vasopressors** (use cautiously). **Drugs which inhibit the CYP2D6 enzyme pathway (quinidine, fluoxetine, paroxetine)** will increase blood levels and effects, dose ↓ recommended.

Route/Dosage

PO (Children and adolescents <70 kg): 0.5 mg/kg/day initially, may be ↑ every 3 days to a daily target dose of 1.2 mg/kg, given as a single dose in the morning or evenly divided doses in the morning and late afternoon/early evening (not to exceed 1.4 mg/kg/day or 100 mg/day whichever is less). *If taking concurrent CYP2D6 inhibitor (quinidine, fluoxetine, paroxetine)*—0.5 mg/kg/day initially, may ↑ if needed to 1.2 mg/kg/day after 4 wk.

PO (Adults, adolescents, and children >70 kg): 40 mg/day initially, may be ↑ every 3 days to a daily target dose of 80 mg/day given as a single dose in the morning or evenly divided doses in the morning and late afternoon/early evening; may be further ↑ after 2–4 wk up to 100 mg/day. *If taking concurrent CYP2D6 inhibitor (quinidine, fluoxetine, paroxetine)*—40 mg/day initially, may ↑ if needed to 80 mg/day after 4 wk.

Hepatic Impairment

PO (Adults and Children): *Moderate hepatic impairment (Child-Pugh Class B)*—↓ initial and target dose by 50%; *Severe hepatic impairment (Child-*

Pugh Class C)—↓ initial and target dose to 25% of normal.

Availability (generic available)

Capsules: 10 mg, 18 mg, 25 mg, 40 mg, 60 mg, 80 mg, 100 mg.

NURSING IMPLICATIONS

Assessment

- Assess attention span, impulse control, and interactions with others.
- Monitor BP and pulse periodically during therapy. Obtain a history (including assessment of family history of sudden death or ventricular arrhythmia), physical exam to assess for cardiac disease, and further evaluation (ECG and echocardiogram), if indicated. If exertional chest pain, unexplained syncope, or other cardiac symptoms occur, evaluate promptly.
- Monitor growth, body height, and weight in children.
- Assess for signs of liver injury (pruritus, dark urine, jaundice, right upper quadrant tenderness, unexplained "flu-like" symptoms) during therapy. Monitor liver function tests at first sign of liver injury. Discontinue and do not restart atomoxetine in patients with jaundice or laboratory evidence of liver injury.
- Monitor closely for notable changes in behavior that could indicate the emergence or worsening of suicidal thoughts or behavior or depression.

Potential Nursing Diagnoses

Disturbed thought process (Indications)
Impaired social interaction (Indications)

Implementation

- Do not confuse atomoxetine with atorvastatin.
- **PO:** Administer without regard to food. Capsules should be swallowed whole; do not open, crush, or chew. Doses may be discontinued without tapering.

Patient/Family Teaching

- Instruct patient to take medication as directed. Take missed doses as soon as possible, but should not take more than the total daily amount in any 24-hr period. Advise patient and parents to read the *Medication Guide* prior to starting therapy and with each Rx refill.
- Inform patient that sharing this medication may be dangerous.
- Advise patient and family to notify health care professional if thoughts about suicide or dying, attempts to commit suicide; new or worse depression; new or worse anxiety; feeling very agitated or restless; panic attacks; trouble sleeping; new or worse irritability; acting aggressive or hostile; being angry or violent; acting on dangerous impulses; an extreme increase in activity and talking; other unusual changes in behavior or mood occur or if signs and symptoms of severe liver injury (pruritus, dark urine, jaundice, right upper quadrant tenderness, or unexplained "flu-like" symptoms) occur.
- Instruct patient to notify health care professional of all Rx or OTC medications, vitamins, or herbal products being taken and consult health care professional before taking any new medications.
- May cause dizziness. Caution patient to avoid driving or other activities requiring alertness until response to medication is known.
- Advise female patients to notify health care professional if pregnancy is planned or suspected or if they are breast feeding.
- Pedi: Advise parents to notify school nurse of medication regimen.

Evaluation/Desired Outcomes

- Improved attention span and social interactions in ADHD.

atorvastatin, See HMG-CoA REDUCTASE INHIBITORS (statins).

atovaquone (a-toe-va-kwone)

Mepron

Classification
Therapeutic: anti-infectives

Pregnancy Category C

Indications

Treatment of mild to moderate *Pneumocystis jirovecii* pneumonia (PJP) in patients who are unable to tolerate trimethoprim/sulfamethoxazole. Prophylaxis of *PJP*.

Action

Inhibits the action of enzymes necessary to nucleic acid and ATP synthesis. **Therapeutic Effects:** Active against *P. jirovecii*.

Pharmacokinetics

Absorption: Absorption is poor but is increased by food, particularly fat.
Distribution: Enters CSF in very low concentrations (<1% of plasma levels).
Protein Binding: >99.9%.
Metabolism and Excretion: Undergoes enterohepatic recycling; elimination occurs in feces.
Half-life: 2.2–2.9 days.

TIME/ACTION PROFILE (blood levels)

ROUTE	ONSET	PEAK	DURATION
PO	unknown	1–8 hr; 24–96 hr†	12 hr

†Two peaks are due to enterohepatic recycling.

Contraindications/Precautions

Contraindicated in: Hypersensitivity; Lactation: May appear in breast milk.

Use Cautiously in: ↓ hepatic, renal, or cardiac function (dose modification may be necessary); GI disorders (absorption may be limited); OB: Safety not established; Pedi: Safety not established.

Adverse Reactions/Side Effects

CNS: headache, insomnia. **Resp:** cough. **GI:** diarrhea, nausea, vomiting. **Derm:** rash. **Misc:** fever.

Interactions

Drug-Drug: May interact with **drugs that are highly bound to plasma proteins** (does not appear to interact with phenytoin).

Drug-Food: Food ↑ absorption.

Route/Dosage

Treatment

PO (Adults): 750 mg twice daily for 21 days.

PO (Children): 40 mg/kg/day (unlabeled).

Prevention

PO (Adults and Adolescents 13–16 yr): 1500 mg once daily.

Availability (generic available)

Suspension: 750 mg/5 mL. ***In combination with:*** proguanil (Malarone). See Appendix B.

NURSING IMPLICATIONS

Assessment

- Assess patient for signs of infection (vital signs, lung sounds, sputum, WBCs) at beginning of and throughout therapy.
- Obtain specimens prior to initiating therapy. First dose may be given before receiving results.
- ***Lab Test Considerations:*** Monitor hematologic and hepatic functions. May cause mild, transient anemia and neutropenia. May also cause ↑ serum amylase, AST, ALT, and alkaline phosphatase.
- Monitor electrolytes. May cause hyponatremia.

Potential Nursing Diagnoses

Risk for infection (Indications, Side Effects)

Deficient knowledge, related to medication regimen (Patient/Family Teaching)

Implementation

- **PO:** Administer with food twice daily for 21 days for treatment and once daily for prevention.
- Shake suspension gently prior to administration.

Patient/Family Teaching

- Instruct patient to take atovaquone as directed around the clock for full course of therapy, even if feeling better. Emphasize the importance of taking atovaquone with food, especially foods high in fat; taking without food may decrease plasma concentrations and effectiveness.
- Advise patient to notify health care professional if rash occurs.
- Advise female patient to notify health care professional if pregnancy is planned or suspected or if breast feeding.

Evaluation/Desired Outcomes

- Resolution of the signs and symptoms of infection.

atropine† (at-ro-peen)

Atro-Pen

Classification

Therapeutic: antiarrhythmics

Pharmacologic: anticholinergics, antimuscarinics

Pregnancy Category C

†See Appendix C for ophthalmic use

Indications

IM: Given preoperatively to decrease oral and respiratory secretions. **IV:** Treatment of sinus bradycardia and heart block. **IV:** Reversal of adverse muscarinic effects of anticholinesterase agents (neostigmine, physostigmine, or pyridostigmine). **IM, IV:** Treatment of anticholinesterase (organophosphate pesticide) poisoning. **Inhaln:** Treatment of exercise-induced bronchospasm.

Action

Inhibits the action of acetylcholine at postganglionic sites located in: Smooth muscle, Secretory glands, CNS (antimuscarinic activity). Low doses decrease: Sweating, Salivation, Respiratory secretions. Intermediate doses result in: Mydriasis (pupillary dilation), Cycloplegia (loss of visual accommodation), Increased heart rate. GI and GU tract motility are decreased at larger doses. **Therapeutic Effects:** Increased heart rate. Decreased GI and respiratory secretions. Reversal of muscarinic effects. May have a spasmolytic action on the biliary and genitourinary tracts.

Pharmacokinetics

Absorption: Well absorbed following subcut or IM administration.

Distribution: Readily crosses the blood-brain barrier. Crosses the placenta and enters breast milk.

Metabolism and Excretion: Mostly metabolized by the liver; 30–50% excreted unchanged by the kidneys.

Half-life: Children <2 yr: 4–10 hr; Children >2 yr: 1.5–3.5 hr; Adults: 4–5 hr.

TIME/ACTION PROFILE (inhibition of salivation)

ROUTE	ONSET	PEAK	DURATION
IM, subcut	rapid	15–50 min	4–6 hr
IV	immediate	2–4 min	4–6 hr

Contraindications/Precautions

Contraindicated in: Hypersensitivity; Angle-closure glaucoma; Acute hemorrhage; Tachycardia secondary to cardiac insufficiency or thyrotoxicosis; Obstructive disease of the GI tract.

Use Cautiously in: Intra-abdominal infections; Prostatic hyperplasia; Chronic renal, hepatic, pulmonary, or cardiac disease; OB, Lactation: Safety not established; IV administration may produce fetal tachycardia; Pedi: Infants with Down syndrome have increased sensitivity to cardiac effects and mydriasis. Children may have increased susceptibility to adverse reactions. Exercise care when prescribing to children with spastic paralysis or brain damage; Geri: Increased susceptibility to adverse reactions.

Adverse Reactions/Side Effects

CNS: drowsiness, confusion, hyperpyrexia. **EENT:** blurred vision, cycloplegia, photophobia, dry eyes, mydriasis. **CV:** tachycardia, palpitations, arrhythmias. **GI:** dry mouth, constipation, impaired GI motility. **GU:** urinary hesitancy, retention, impotency. **Resp:** tachypnea, pulmonary edema. **Misc:** flushing, decreased sweating.

Interactions

Drug-Drug: ↑ anticholinergic effects with other **anticholinergics**, including **antihistamines**, **tricyclic antidepressants**, **quinidine**, and **disopyramide**. Anticholinergics may alter the absorption of other **orally administered drugs** by slowing motility of the GI tract. **Antacids** ↓ absorption of **anticholinergics**. May ↑ GI mucosal lesions in patients taking oral **potassium chloride** tablets. May alter response to **beta-blockers**.

Route/Dosage

Preanesthesia (To Decrease Salivation/Secretions)

IM, IV, Subcut (Adults): 0.4–0.6 mg 30–60 min pre-op.
IM, IV, Subcut (Children >5 kg): 0.01–0.02 mg/kg/dose 30–60 min preop to a maximum of 0.4 mg/dose; minimum: 0.1 mg/dose.
IM, IV, Subcut (Children <5 kg): 0.02 mg/kg/dose 30–60 min preop then q 4–6 hr as needed.

Bradycardia

IV (Adults): 0.5–1 mg; may repeat as needed q 5 min, not to exceed a total of 2 mg (q 3–5 min in Advanced Cardiac Life Support guidelines) or 0.04 mg/kg (total vagolytic dose).
IV (Children): 0.02 mg/kg (maximum single dose is 0.5 mg in children and 1 mg in adolescents); may repeat q 5 min up to a total dose of 1 mg in children (2 mg in adolescents).
Endotracheal (Children): use the IV dose and dilute before administration.

Reversal of Adverse Muscarinic Effects of Anticholinesterases

IV (Adults): 0.6–12 mg for each 0.5–2.5 mg of neostigmine methylsulfate or 10–20 mg of pyridostigmine bromide concurrently with anticholinesterase.

Organophosphate Poisoning

IM (Adults): 2 mg initially, then 2 mg q 10 min as needed up to 3 times total.
IV (Adults): 1–2 mg/dose q 10–20 min until atropinic effects observed then q 1–4 hr for 24 hr; up to 50 mg in first 24 hr and 2 g over several days may be given in severe intoxication.
IM (Children >10 yr >90 lbs): 2 mg.
IM (Children 4–10 yr 40–90 lbs): 1 mg.
IM (Children 6 mo–4 yr 15–40 lbs): 0.5 mg.
IV (Children): 0.02–0.05 mg/kg q 10–20 min until atropinic effects observed then q 1–4 hr for 24 hr.

Bronchospasm

Inhaln (Adults): 0.025–0.05 mg/kg/dose q 4–6 hr as needed; maximum 2.5 mg/dose.
Inhaln (Children): 0.03–0.05 mg/kg/dose 3–4 times/day; maximum 2.5 mg/dose.

Availability (generic available)

Injection: 0.05 mg/mL, 0.1 mg/mL, 0.4 mg/mL, 1 mg/mL, 0.5 mg/0.7 mL Auto-injector, 1 mg/0.7 mL Auto-injector, 2 mg/0.7 mL Auto-injector.

NURSING IMPLICATIONS

Assessment

- Assess vital signs and ECG tracings frequently during IV drug therapy. Report any significant changes in heart rate or BP, or increased ventricular ectopy or angina to health care professional promptly.
- Monitor intake and output ratios in elderly or surgical patients because atropine may cause urinary retention.
- Assess patients routinely for abdominal distention and auscultate for bowel sounds. If constipation becomes a problem, increasing fluids and adding bulk to the diet may help alleviate constipation.
- ***Toxicity and Overdose:*** If overdose occurs, physostigmine is the antidote.

Potential Nursing Diagnoses

Decreased cardiac output (Indications)
Impaired oral mucous membrane (Side Effects)
Constipation (Side Effects)

Implementation

- **IM:** Intense flushing of the face and trunk may occur 15–20 min following IM administration. In children, this response is called "atropine flush" and is not harmful.

IV Administration

- **IV Push:** ***Diluent:*** Administer undiluted. ***Rate:*** Administer over 1 min; more rapid administration may be used during cardiac resuscitation (follow with 20 mL saline flush). Slow administration (over >1 min) may cause a paradoxical bradycardia (usually resolved in approximately 2 min).
- **Y-Site Compatibility:** abciximab, alfentanyl, amikacin, aminophylline, amiodarone, argatroban, ascorbic acid, azathioprine, aztreonam, benztropine, bivalirudin, bumetanide, buprenorphine, butorphanol, calcium chloride, calcium gluconate, cefazolin, cefotaxime, cefotetan, cefoxitin, ceftazidime, ceftriaxone, cefuroxime, chloramphenicol, chlorpromazine, clindamycin, cyanocobalamin, cyclosporine, dexamethasone, dexmedetomidine, digoxin, diphenhydramine, dobutamine, dopamine, doripenem, doxycycline, enalaprilat, ephedrine, epinephrine, epoetin alfa, eptifibatide, erythromycin, esmolol, etomidate, famotidine, fenoldopam, fentanyl, fluconazole, folic acid, furosemide, ganciclovir, gentamicin, glycopyrrolate, heparin, hydrocortisone sodium succinate, hydromorphone, imipenem/cilastatin, indomethacin, insulin, isoproterenol, ketamine, ketorolac, labetalol, lidocaine, magnesium sulfate, mannitol, meperidine, meropenem, methadone, methyldopate, methylprednisolone, metoclopramide, metoprolol, midazolam, morphine, multivitamins, nafcillin, nalbuphine, naloxone, nitroglycerin, nitroprusside, norepinephrine, ondansetron, oxacillin, oxytocin, palonosetron, papaverine, penicillin G, pentamidine, pentazocine, pentobarbital, phenobarbital, phentolamine, phenylephrine, phytonadione, potassium chloride, procainamide, prochlorperazine, promethazine, propranolol, protamine, pyridoxime, ranitidine, sodium bicarbonate, streptokinase, succinylcholine, sufentanil, theophylline, thiamine, tirofiban, tobramycin, tolazoline, vancomycin, vasopressin, verapamil, vitamin B complex with C.
- **Y-Site Incompatibility:** amphotericin B colloidal, dantrolene, diazepam, diazoxide, pantoprazole, phenytoin, trimethoprim/sulfamethoxazole, thiopental.
- **Endotracheal:** Dilute with 5–10 mL of 0.9% NaCl.
- ***Rate:*** Inject directly into the endotracheal tube followed by several positive pressure ventilations.

Patient/Family Teaching

- May cause drowsiness. Caution patients to avoid driving or other activities requiring alertness until response to medication is known.
- Instruct patient that oral rinses, sugarless gum or candy, and frequent oral hygiene may help relieve dry mouth.
- Caution patients that atropine impairs heat regulation. Strenuous activity in a hot environment may cause heat stroke. Advise patient to notify health care professional of all Rx or OTC medications, vitamins, or herbal products being taken and to consult with health care professional before taking other medications.
- Pedi: Instruct parents or caregivers that medication may cause fever and to notify health care professional before administering to a febrile child.
- Geri: Inform male patients with benign prostatic hyperplasia that atropine may cause urinary hesitancy and retention. Changes in urinary stream should be reported to health care professional.

Evaluation/Desired Outcomes

- Increase in heart rate.
- Dryness of mouth.
- Reversal of muscarinic effects.

avanafil (av-an-a-fil)

Stendra

Classification

Therapeutic: erectile dysfunction agents

Pharmacologic: phosphodiesterase type 5 inhibitors

Pregnancy Category C

Indications

Treatment of erectile dysfunction.

Action

Enhances effects of nitric oxide released during sexual stimulation. Nitric oxide activates guanylate cyclase, which produces ↑ levels of cyclic guanosine monophosphate (cGMP). cGMP produces smooth muscle relaxation of the corpus cavernosum, which promotes ↑ blood flow and subsequent erection. Inhibits the enzyme phosphodiesterase type 5 (PDE5), PDE5 inactivates cGMP. **Therapeutic Effects:** Enhanced blood flow to the corpus cavernosum and erection sufficient to allow sexual intercourse. Requires sexual stimulation.

Pharmacokinetics

Absorption: Rapidly absorbed following oral administration.

Distribution: Minimal amounts enter semen.

Protein Binding: 99%.

Metabolism and Excretion: Mostly metabolized by the liver (primarily by the CYP3A4 enzyme system), metabolites excreted in feces (62%) and urine (21%). One metabolite had inhibitory activity on PDE5.

Half-life: 5 hr.

TIME/ACTION PROFILE (effect on BP)

ROUTE	ONSET	PEAK	DURATION
PO	within 1 hr	1–2 hr	unknown

A

Contraindications/Precautions

Contraindicated in: Hypersensitivity; Concurrent use of nitrates; Severe renal or hepatic impairment; Concurrent use of strong CYP3A4 inhibitors; Serious underlying cardiovascular disease (including history of MI, stroke, or serious arrhythmia within 6 mo), cardiac failure, or coronary artery disease with unstable angina, angina with sexual intercourse; History of HF, coronary artery disease, uncontrolled hypertension (BP >170/110 mm Hg) or hypotension (BP <90/50 mm Hg), dehydration, autonomic dysfunction, or severe left ventricular outflow obstruction; Hereditary degenerative retinal disorders; Women.

Use Cautiously in: Serious underlying cardiovascular disease or conditions in which sexual activity is not advised; History of sudden severe vision loss or non-arteritic ischemic optic neuropathy (NAION); may ↑ risk of recurrence; Low cup to disk ratio, age >50 yr, diabetes, hypertension, coronary artery disease, hyperlipidemia, or smoking (↑ risk of NAION); Alpha adrenergic blockers (patients should be on stable dose of alpha blockers before treatment, initiate with 50 mg dose); Anatomic penile deformity (angulation, cavernosal fibrosis, Peyronie disease); Conditions associated with priapism (sickle cell anemia, multiple myeloma, leukemia); Concurrent use of moderate CYP3A4 inhibitors (initiate with 50 mg dose); History of hearing loss; Bleeding disorders or peptic ulceration; Geri: Elderly may be more sensitive to drug effects; Pedi: Safety not established.

Adverse Reactions/Side Effects

CNS: headache, dizziness. **EENT:** nasal congestion, nasopharyngitis, sudden hearing/vision loss. **GU:** priapism. **Derm:** flushing. **MS:** back pain.

Interactions

Drug-Drug: Blood levels and effects may be ↑ by **CYP3A4 inhibitors**, concurrent use of **strong CYP3A4 inhibitors** including **atazanavir**, **clarithromycin**, **indinavir**, **itraconazole**, **ketoconazole**, **nefazodone**, **nelfinavir**, **saquinavir**, and **telithromycin** is contraindicated. A similar but lesser effect is expected with **moderate CYP3A4 inhibitors** including **erythromycin**, **aprepitant**, **diltiaziem**, **fluconazole**, **fosamprenavir**, **ritonavir** and **verapamil**; initial dose should not exceed 50 mg/24 hr. ↑ risk of hypotension with **nitrates**, **alpha-adrenergic blockers**, **antihypertensives** and **alcohol**(more than 3 units); concurrent use with **nitrates** is contraindicated, dosage adjustments may be necessary with others. If **nitrates** are medically necessary, at 12 hr should pass following avanafil administration.

Route/Dosage

PO (Adults): 100 mg 15 min prior to sexual activity, not to exceed once daily (range 50–200 mg, use lowest effective dose); *Concurrent alpha-blockers or moderate CYP3A4 inhibitors*—50 mg, not to exceed once daily.

Availability

Tablets: 50 mg, 100 mg, 200 mg.

NURSING IMPLICATIONS

Assessment

- Determine ED before administration. Avanafil has no effect in the absence of sexual stimulation.

Potential Nursing Diagnoses

Sexual dysfunction (Indications)
Ineffective tissue perfusion (Adverse Reactions)

Implementation

- **PO:** Administer dose as needed for ED at least 15 min prior to sexual activity.
- May be administered without regard to food.

Patient/Family Teaching

- Instruct patient to take avanafil as needed for ED at least 15 min before sexual activity and not more than once per day. Inform patient that sexual stimulation is required for an erection to occur after taking avanafil.
- Advise patient that avanafil is not indicated for use in women.
- Caution patient not to take avanafil concurrently with alpha adrenergic blockers (unless on a stable dose) or nitrates. If chest pain occurs after taking avanafil, instruct patient to seek immediate medical attention.
- Advise patient to avoid excess alcohol intake (≥3 units) in combination with avanafil; may increase risk of orthostatic hypotension, increased heart rate, decreased standing BP, dizziness, headache.
- Instruct patient to notify health care professional promptly if erection lasts longer than 4 hr, if they are not satisfied with their sexual performance, develop unwanted side effects or if they experience sudden or decreased vision loss in one or both eyes or loss or decrease in hearing, ringing in the ears, or dizziness.
- Advise patient to notify health care professional of all Rx or OTC medications, vitamins, or herbal products being taken and to consult with health care professional before taking other medications that may interact with avanafil.
- Inform patient that avanafil offers no protection against sexually transmitted diseases. Counsel patient that protection against sexually transmitted diseases and HIV infection should be considered.

Evaluation/Desired Outcomes

- Male erection sufficient to allow intercourse.

azaTHIOprine

(ay-za-**thye**-oh-preen)

Azasan, Imuran

Classification

Therapeutic: immunosuppressants

Pharmacologic: purine antagonists

Pregnancy Category D

Indications

Prevention of renal transplant rejection (with corticosteroids, local radiation, or other cytotoxic agents). Treatment of severe, active, erosive rheumatoid arthritis unresponsive to more conventional therapy. **Unlabeled Use:** Management of Crohn's disease or ulcerative colitis.

Action

Antagonizes purine metabolism with subsequent inhibition of DNA and RNA synthesis. **Therapeutic Effects:** Suppression of cell-mediated immunity and altered antibody formation.

Pharmacokinetics

Absorption: Readily absorbed after oral administration.

Distribution: Crosses the placenta. Enters breast milk in low concentrations.

Metabolism and Excretion: Metabolized to mercaptopurine, which is further metabolized (one route is by thiopurine methyltransferase [TPMT] to form an inactive metabolite). Minimal renal excretion of unchanged drug.

Half-life: 3 hr.

TIME/ACTION PROFILE

ROUTE	ONSET	PEAK	DURATION
PO (anti-inflammatory)	6–8 wk	12 wk	unknown

Contraindications/Precautions

Contraindicated in: Hypersensitivity; Concurrent use of mycophenolate; OB: Has been shown to cause fetal harm; Lactation: Appears in breast milk .

Use Cautiously in: Infection; Malignancies; ↓ bone marrow reserve; Previous or concurrent radiation therapy; Other chronic debilitating illnesses; Severe renal impairment/oliguria (↑ sensitivity); Patients with TPMT enzyme deficiency (substantial dose ↓ are required to avoid hematologic adverse events); OB: Patients with childbearing potential; Pedi: ↑ risk of hepatosplenic T-cell lymphoma [HSTCL] in patients with inflammatory bowel disease.

Adverse Reactions/Side Effects

CNS: PROGRESSIVE MULTIFOCAL LEUKOENCEPHALOPATHY. **EENT:** retinopathy. **Resp:** pulmonary edema. **GI:** anorexia, hepatotoxicity, nausea, vomiting, diarrhea, mucositis, pancreatitis. **Derm:** alopecia, rash. **Hemat:** anemia, leukopenia, pancytopenia, thrombocytopenia. **MS:** arthralgia. **Misc:** MALIGNANCY (including post-transplant lymphoma, HSTCL, and skin cancer), SERUM SICKNESS, chills, fever, Raynaud's phenomenon, retinopathy.

Interactions

Drug-Drug: Additive myelosuppression with **antineoplastics**, **cyclosporine**, and **myelosuppressive agents**. **Allopurinol** inhibits the metabolism of azathioprine, increasing toxicity. Dose of azathioprine should be ↓ to 25–33% of the usual dose when used with allopurinol. May ↓ antibody response to **live-virus vaccines** and ↑ the risk of adverse reactions.

Drug-Natural Products: Concommitant use with **echinacea** and **melatonin** may interfere with immunosuppression.

Route/Dosage

Renal Allograft Rejection Prevention

PO (Adults and Children): 3–5 mg/kg/day initially; maintenance dose 1–3 mg/kg/day.

Rheumatoid Arthritis

PO (Adults and Children): 1 mg/kg/day for 6–8 wk, ↑ by 0.5 mg/kg/day q 4 wk until response or up to 2.5 mg/kg/day, then ↓ by 0.5 mg/kg/day q 4–8 wk to minimal effective dose.

Inflammatory Bowel Disease (Crohn's Disease or Ulcerative Colitis) (unlabeled use)

PO (Adults and Children): 50 mg once daily; may ↑ by 25 mg/day every 1–2 wk as tolerated to target dose of 2–3 mg/kg/day.

Availability (generic available)

Tablets: 50 mg, 75 mg, 100 mg.

NURSING IMPLICATIONS

Assessment

- Assess for infection (vital signs, sputum, urine, stool, WBC) during therapy.
- Monitor intake and output and daily weight. Decreased urine output may lead to toxicity with this medication.
- **Rheumatoid Arthritis:** Assess range of motion; degree of swelling, pain, and strength in affected joints; and ability to perform activities of daily living before and periodically during therapy.
- ***Lab Test Considerations:*** Monitor renal, hepatic, and hematologic functions before beginning therapy, weekly during the 1st mo, bimonthly for the next 2–3 mo, and monthly thereafter.
- Leukocyte count of <3000 or platelet count of <100,000/mm^3 may necessitate a reduction in dose or temporary discontinuation.

- ↓ in hemoglobin may indicate bone marrow suppression.
- Hepatotoxicity may be manifested by ↑ alkaline phosphatase, bilirubin, AST, ALT, and amylase concentrations. Usually occurs within 6 mo of transplant, rarely with rheumatoid arthritis, and is reversible on discontinuation of azathioprine.
- May ↓ serum and urine uric acid and plasma albumin.

Potential Nursing Diagnoses

Risk for infection (Indications)

Implementation

- Do not confuse azaTHIOprine with azaCITIDine.
- Protect transplant patients from staff members and visitors who may carry infection. Maintain protective isolation as indicated.
- **PO:** May be administered with or after meals or in divided doses to minimize nausea.

Patient/Family Teaching

- Instruct patient to take azathioprine as directed. If a dose is missed on a once-daily regimen, omit dose; if on several-times-a-day dosing, take as soon as possible or double next dose. Consult health care professional if more than 1 dose is missed or if vomiting occurs shortly after dose is taken. Do not discontinue without consulting health care professional.
- Advise patient to report unusual tiredness or weakness; cough or hoarseness; fever or chills; lower back or side pain; painful or difficult urination; severe diarrhea; black, tarry stools; blood in urine; or transplant rejection to health care professional immediately.
- Reinforce the need for lifelong therapy to prevent transplant rejection.
- Instruct patient to notify health care professional of all Rx or OTC medications, vitamins, or herbal products being taken and consult health care professional before taking any new medications or receiving any vaccinations while taking this medication.
- Advise patient to avoid contact with persons with contagious diseases and persons who have recently taken oral poliovirus vaccine or other live viruses.
- Rep: This drug may have teratogenic properties. Advise patient to use contraception during and for at least 4 mo after therapy is completed.
- Emphasize the importance of follow-up exams and lab tests.
- **Rheumatoid Arthritis:** Concurrent therapy with salicylates, NSAIDs, or corticosteroids may be necessary. Patient should continue physical therapy and adequate rest. Explain that joint damage will not be reversed; goal is to slow or stop disease process.

Evaluation/Desired Outcomes

- Prevention of transplant rejection.
- Decreased stiffness, pain, and swelling in affected joints in 6–8 wk in rheumatoid arthritis. Therapy is discontinued if no improvement in 12 wk.

azilsartan, See ANGIOTENSIN II RECEPTOR ANTAGONISTS.

azithromycin

(aye-**zith**-roe-mye-sin)

Zithromax, Zmax

Classification

Therapeutic: agents for atypical mycobacterium, anti-infectives

Pharmacologic: macrolides

Pregnancy Category B

Indications

Treatment of the following infections due to susceptible organisms: Upper respiratory tract infections, including streptococcal pharyngitis, acute bacterial exacerbations of chronic bronchitis and tonsillitis, Lower respiratory tract infections, including bronchitis and pneumonia, Acute otitis media, Skin and skin structure infections, Nongonococcal urethritis, cervicitis, gonorrhea, and chancroid. Prevention of disseminated *Mycobacterium avium* complex (MAC) infection in patients with advanced HIV infection. *Extended-release suspension (ZMax)* Acute bacterial sinusitis and community-acquired pneumonia in adults. **Unlabeled Use:** Prevention of bacterial endocarditis. Treatment of cystic fibrosis lung disease. Treatment and post-exposure prophylaxis of pertussis in infants.

Action

Inhibits protein synthesis at the level of the 50S bacterial ribosome. **Therapeutic Effects:** Bacteriostatic action against susceptible bacteria. **Spectrum:** Active against the following gram-positive aerobic bacteria: *Staphylococcus aureus*, *Streptococcus pneumoniae*, *S. pyogenes* (group A strep). Active against these gram-negative aerobic bacteria: *Haemophilus influenzae*, *Moraxella catarrhalis*, *Neisseria gonorrhoeae*. Also active against: *Bordetella pertussis*, *Mycoplasma*, *Legionella*, *Chlamydia pneumoniae*, *Ureaplasma urealyticum*, *Borrelia burgdorferi*, *M. avium*. Not active against methicillin-resistant *S. aureus*.

Pharmacokinetics

Absorption: Rapidly absorbed (40%) after oral administration. IV administration results in complete bioavailability.

Distribution: Widely distributed to body tissues and fluids. Intracellular and tissue levels exceed those in serum; low CSF levels.
Protein Binding: 7–51%.
Metabolism and Excretion: Mostly excreted unchanged in bile; 4.5% excreted unchanged in urine.
Half-life: 11–14 hr after single dose; 2–4 days after several doses; 59 hr after extended release suspension.

TIME/ACTION PROFILE (serum)

ROUTE	ONSET	PEAK	DURATION
PO	rapid	2.5–3.2 hr	24 hr
IV	rapid	end of infusion	24 hr

Contraindications/Precautions

Contraindicated in: Hypersensitivity to azithromycin, erythromycin, or other macrolide anti-infectives; History of cholestatic jaundice or hepatic dysfunction with prior use of azithromycin; QT interval prolongation, hypokalemia, hypomagnesemia, or bradycardia; Concurrent use of quinidine, procainamide, dofetilide, amiodarone, or sotalol.
Use Cautiously in: Severe liver impairment (dose adjustment may be required); Severe renal impairment (CCr <10 mL/min); Myasthenia gravis (may worsen symptoms); Geri: May have ↑ risk of QT interval prolongation; OB, Lactation: Safety not established.

Adverse Reactions/Side Effects

CNS: dizziness, seizures, drowsiness, fatigue, headache. **CV:** TORSADES DE POINTES, chest pain, hypotension, palpitations, QT interval prolongation. **GI:** HEPATOTOXICITY, CLOSTRIDIUM DIFFICILE-ASSOCIATED DIARRHEA (CDAD), abdominal pain, diarrhea, nausea, cholestatic jaundice, ↑ liver enzymes, dyspepsia, flatulence, melena, oral candidiasis, pyloric stenosis. **GU:** nephritis, vaginitis. **Hemat:** anemia, leukopenia, thrombocytopenia. **Derm:** STEVENS-JOHNSON SYNDROME, TOXIC EPIDERMAL NECROLYSIS, photosensitivity, rash. **EENT:** ototoxicity. **F and E:** hyperkalemia. **Misc:** ANGIOEDEMA.

Interactions

Drug-Drug: Quinidine, procainamide, dofetilide, sotalol, and **amiodarone** may ↑ risk of QT interval prolongation; concurrent use should be avoided. **Aluminum-** and **magnesium-containing antacids** ↓ peak levels. **Nelfinavir** ↑ levels (monitor carefully); azithromycin also ↓ nelfinavir levels. **Efavirenz** ↑ levels. May ↑ the effects and risk of toxicity of **warfarin** and **zidovudine**. Other macrolide anti-infectives have been known to ↑ levels and effects of **digoxin, theophylline, ergotamine, dihydroergotamine, triazolam, carbamazepine, cyclosporine, tacrolimus,** and **phenytoin**; careful monitoring of concurrent use is recommended.

Route/Dosage

Most Respiratory and Skin Infections

PO (Adults): 500 mg on 1st day, then 250 mg/day for 4 more days (total dose of 1.5 g); *Acute bacterial sinusitis*—500 mg once daily for 3 days or single 2-g dose of extended-release suspension (Zmax).
PO (Children ≥ 6 mo): *Pneumonia/Pertussis*—10 mg/kg (not >500 m g/dose) on 1st day, then 5 mg/kg (not >250 m g/dose) for 4 more days. *Pharyngitis/tonsilitis*—12 mg/kg once daily for 5 days (not >500 m g/dose); *Acute bacterial sinusitis*—10 mg/kg/day for three days.
PO (Neonates): *Pertussis, treatment and post-exposure prophylaxis*—10 mg/kg/dose once daily for 5 days.

Otitis Media

PO (Children ≥6 mo): 30 mg/kg single dose (not >1500 mg/dose) *or* 10 mg/kg/day as a single dose (not >500 m g/dose) for 3 days *or* 10 mg/kg as a single dose (not >500 m g/dose) on 1st day, then 5 mg/kg as a single dose (not >250 m g/dose) daily for 4 more days.

Acute Bacterial Exacerbations of Chronic Bronchitis

PO (Adults): 500 mg on 1st day, then 250 mg/day for 4 more days (total dose of 1.5 g) *or* 500 mg daily for 3 days.

Community-Acquired Pneumonia

IV, PO (Adults): *More severe*—500 mg IV q 24 hr for at least 2 doses, then 500 mg PO q 24 hr for a total of 7–10 days; *less severe*—500 mg PO, then 250 mg/day PO for 4 more days or 2 g single dose as extended-release suspension (Zmax).
PO (Children >6 mo): 10 mg/kg on 1st day, then 5 mg/kg for 4 more days.

Pelvic Inflammatory Disease

IV, PO (Adults): 500 mg IV q 24 hr for 1–2 days, then 250 mg PO q 24 hr for a total of 7 days.

Endocarditis Prophylaxis

PO (Adults): 500 mg 1 hr before procedure.
PO (Children): 15 mg/kg 1 hr before procedure.

Nongonococcal Urethritis, Cervicitis, Chancroid, Chlamydia

PO (Adults): Single 1-g dose.
PO (Children): *Chancroid:* Single 20-mg/kg dose (not >1000 mg/dose). *Urethritis or cervicitis:* Single 10-mg/kg dose (not >1000 mg/dose).

Gonorrhea

PO (Adults): Single 2-g dose.

Prevention of Disseminated MAC Infection

PO (Adults): 1.2 g once weekly (alone or with rifabutin).
PO (Children): 5 mg/kg once daily (not >250 mg/dose) or 20 mg/kg (not >1200 mg/dose) once weekly (alone or with rifabutin).

Cystic Fibrosis

PO (Children ≥6 yrs, weight ≥25 kg to <40 kg): 250 mg q MWF. ≥40 kg: 500 mg q MWF.

Availability (generic available)

Tablets: 250 mg, 500 mg, 600 mg. **Cost:** *Generic*—250 mg \$8.82/6, 500 mg \$10.03/3, 600 mg \$104.62/30. **Powder for oral suspension (cherry, creme de vanilla, and banana flavor):** 1 g/pkt. **Cost:** *Generic*—\$72.45/3 pkts. **Powder for oral suspension (cherry, creme de vanilla, and banana flavor):** 100 mg/5 mL, 200 mg/5 mL. **Cost:** *Generic*—100 mg/5 mL \$34.88/15 mL, 200 mg/5 mL \$34.88/22.5 mL. **Extended-release oral suspension (ZMax) (cherry-banana):** 2-g single-dose bottle. **Cost:** \$128.36/1 bottle. **Powder for injection:** 500 mg/vial.

NURSING IMPLICATIONS

Assessment

- Assess patient for infection (vital signs; appearance of wound, sputum, urine, and stool; WBC) at beginning of and throughout therapy.
- Obtain specimens for culture and sensitivity before initiating therapy. First dose may be given before receiving results.
- Observe for signs and symptoms of anaphylaxis (rash, pruritus, laryngeal edema, wheezing). Notify health care professional immediately if these occur.
- Assess patient for skin rash frequently during therapy. Discontinue azithromycin at first sign of rash; may be life-threatening. Stevens-Johnson syndrome or toxic epidermal necrolysis may develop. Treat symptomatically; may recur once treatment is stopped.
- ***Lab Test Considerations:*** May cause ↑ serum bilirubin, AST, ALT, LDH, and alkaline phosphatase concentrations.
- May cause ↑ creatine phosphokinase, potassium, prothrombin time, BUN, serum creatinine, and blood glucose concentrations.
- May occasionally cause ↓ WBC and platelet count.

Potential Nursing Diagnoses

Risk for infection (Indications, Side Effects)
Noncompliance (Patient/Family Teaching)

Implementation

- *Zmax extended release oral suspension* is not bioequivalent or interchangeable with azithromycin oral suspension.
- **PO:** Administer 1 hr before or 2 hr after meals.
- For administration of single 1-g packet, thoroughly mix entire contents of packet with 2 oz (60 mL) of water. Drink entire contents immediately; add an additional 2 oz of water, mix and drink to assure complete consumption of dose. Do not use the single packet to administer doses other than 1000 mg of azithromycin. Pedi: 1-g packet is not for pediatric use.
- For *Zmax*, shake suspension well and drink entire contents of bottle. Use within 12 hr of reconstitution. If patient vomits within 1 hr of administration, contact prescriber for instructions. *Zmax* may be taken without regard to antacids containing magnesium or aluminum hydroxide.

IV Administration

- **Intermittent Infusion:** ***Diluent:*** Reconstitute each 500-mg vial with 4.8 mL of sterile water for injection to achieve a concentration of 100 mg/mL. Reconstituted solution is stable for 24 hr at room temperature. Further dilute the 500-mg dose in 250 mL or 500 mL of 0.9% NaCl, 0.45% NaCl, D5W, LR, D5/0.45% NaCl, or D5/LR. Infusion is stable for 24 hr at room temperature or for 7 days if refrigerated. ***Concentration:*** Final concentration of infusion is 1–2 mg/mL. ***Rate:*** Administer the 1-mg/mL solution over 3 hr or the 2-mg/mL solution over 1 hr. Do not administer as a bolus.
- **Y-Site Compatibility:** acyclovir, alemtuzumab, alfentanil, aminophylline, amphotericin B lipid complex, amphotericin B liposome, ampicillin/sulbactam, anidulafungin, argatroban, atracurium, bivalirudin, bleomycin, bumetanide, buprenorphine, butorphanol, calcium chloride, calcium gluconate, carboplatin, carmustine, cefazolin, cefepime, cefotetan, cefoxitin, ceftaroline, ceftazidime, cisatracurium, cisplatin, cyclophosphamide, cyclosporine, cytarabine, daptomycin, dedxamethasone, dexmedetomidine, dexrazoxane, digoxin, diltiazem, diphenhydramine, dobutamine, docetaxel, dopamine, doripenem, doxacurium, doxycycline, droperidol, enalaprilat, ephedrine, epinephrine, eptifibatide, ertapenem, esmolol, etoposide, etoposide phosphate, fenoldopam, fluconazole, fluorouracil, foscarnet, fosphenytoin, ganciclovir, gemcitabine, granisetron, haloperidol, heparin, hetastarch, hydrocortisone, hydromorphone, idarubicin, ifosfamide, irinotecan, isoproterenol, leucovorin, levorphanol, lidocaine, linezolid, lorazepam, magnesium sulfate, mannitol, mechlorethamine, meperidine, meropenem, mesna, methohexital, methotrexate, methylprednisolone, metoclopramide, metronidazole, milrinone, nalbuphine, naloxone, nesiritide, nitroglycerin, nitroprusside, octreotide, ondansetron, oxaliplatin, oxytocin, paclitaxel, palonosetron, pamidronate, pancuro-

nium, pantoprazole, pemetrexed, pentobarbital, phenobarbital, phenylephrine, potassium acetate, potassium phosphates, procainamide, prochlorperazine, promethazine, propranolol, ranitidine, remifentanil, rocuronium, sodium acetate, sodium bicarbonate, sodium phosphates, succinylcholine, sufentanil, tacrolimus, telavancin, teniposide, thiotepa, tigecycline, tirofiban, trimethoprim/sulfamethoxazole, vancomycin, vasopressin, vecuronium, verapamil, vincristine, voriconazole, zidovudine, zoledronic acid.

- **Y-Site Incompatibility:** amiodarone, amphotericin B colloidal, chlorpromazine, diazepam, doxorubicin, epirubicin, midazolam, mitoxantrone, mycophenolate, nicardipine, pentamidine, piperacillin-tazobactam, potassium chloride, quinupristin/dalfopristin, thiopental.

Patient/Family Teaching

- Instruct patients to take medication as directed and to finish the drug completely, even if they are feeling better. Take missed doses as soon as possible unless almost time for next dose; do not double doses. Advise patients that sharing of this medication may be dangerous.
- Instruct patient not to take azithromycin with food or antacids.
- May cause drowsiness and dizziness. Caution patient to avoid driving or other activities requiring alertness until response to medication is known.
- Advise patient to use sunscreen and protective clothing to prevent photosensitivity reactions.
- Advise patient to report symptoms of chest pain, palpitations, yellowing of skin or eyes, or signs of superinfection (black, furry overgrowth on the tongue; vaginal itching or discharge; loose or foul-smelling stools) or rash.
- Instruct patient to notify health care professional if fever and diarrhea develop, especially if stool contains blood, pus, or mucus. Advise patient not to treat diarrhea without advice of health care professional.
- Advise patients being treated for nongonococcal urethritis or cervicitis that sexual partners should also be treated.
- Instruct parents, caregivers, or patient to notify health care professional if symptoms do not improve.
- Pedi: Tell parents or caregivers that medication is generally well tolerated in children. Most common side effects in children are mild diarrhea and rash. Tell parents to notify health care practitioner if these occur.

Evaluation/Desired Outcomes

- Resolution of the signs and symptoms of infection. Length of time for complete resolution depends on the organism and site of infection.

aztreonam (az-tree-oh-nam)

Azactam, Cayston

Classification
Therapeutic: anti-infectives
Pharmacologic: monobactams

Pregnancy Category B

Indications

Treatment of serious gram-negative infections including: Septicemia, Skin and skin structure infections, Intra-abdominal infections, Gynecologic infections, Respiratory tract infections, Urinary tract infections. Useful for treatment of multi-resistant strains of some bacteria including aerobic gram-negative pathogens. **Inhaln:** To improve respiratory symptoms in cystic fibrosis (CF) patients with *Pseudomonas aeruginosa.*

Action

Binds to the bacterial cell wall membrane, causing cell death. **Therapeutic Effects:** Bactericidal action against susceptible bacteria. **Spectrum:** Displays significant activity against gram-negative aerobic organisms only: *Escherichia coli*, *Serratia*, *Klebsiella oxytoca or pneumoniae*, *Citrobacter*, *Proteus mirabilis*, *Pseudomonas aeruginosa*, *Enterobacter*, *Haemophilus influenzae*. Not active against: *Staphylococcus aureus*, *Enterococcus*, *Bacteroides fragilis*, *Streptococci*.

Pharmacokinetics

Absorption: Well absorbed following IM administration. Low absorption follows administration by inhalation.

Distribution: Widely distributed. Crosses the placenta and enters breast milk in low concentrations. High concentrations achieved in sputum with inhalation.

Protein Binding: 56%.

Metabolism and Excretion: 60–70% excreted unchanged by the kidneys. 10% of inhaled dose excreted unchanged in urine. Small amounts metabolized by the liver.

Half-life: Adults: 1.5–2 hr; Children: 1.7 hr; Neonates: 2.4–9 hr(↑ in renal impairment).

TIME/ACTION PROFILE (blood levels)

ROUTE	ONSET	PEAK	DURATION
IM	rapid	60 min	6–8 hr
IV	rapid	end of infusion	6–8 hr
Inhaln	rapid	unknown	Several hours

Contraindications/Precautions

Contraindicated in: Hypersensitivity.

Use Cautiously in: Renal impairment (dosage ↓ required if CCr 30 mL/min or less); Cross-sensitivity with penicillins or cephalosporins may occur rarely. Has been used safely in patients with a history of penicillin or cephalosporin allergy; Patients with FEV_1 <25% or >75% predicted, or patients colonized with *Burkholderia cepacia* (safety and effectiveness not established); OB, Lactation: Safety not established; Pedi: Children <7 yr (inhalation) (safety and effectiveness not established); Geri: Consider age-related ↓ in renal function.

Adverse Reactions/Side Effects

CNS: SEIZURES. **EENT:** nasal congestion (inhalation), nasopharyngeal pain (inhalation). **CV:** chest discomfort (inhalation). **GI:** CLOSTRIDIUM DIFFICILE-ASSOCIATED DIARRHEA (CDAD), abdominal pain (inhalation), altered taste, diarrhea, nausea, vomiting. **Resp:** cough (inhalation), wheezing (inhalation), bronchospasm (inhalation). **Derm:** rash. **Local:** pain at IM site, phlebitis at IV site. **Misc:** allergic reactions including ANAPHYLAXIS, fever (inhalation), superinfection.

Interactions

Drug-Drug: Serum levels may be ↑ by **furosemide** or **probenecid**.

Route/Dosage

IM, IV (Adults): *Moderately severe infections*—1–2 g q 8–12 hr; *severe or life-threatening infections (including those due to Pseudomonas aeruginosa)*—2 g q 6–8 hr; *urinary tract infections*—0.5–1 g q 8–12 hr.
IV (Children 1 mo–16 yr): *Mild to moderate infections infections*—30 mg/kg q 8 hr; *moderate to severe infections infections*—30 mg/kg q 6–8 hr; *cystic fibrosis*—50 mg/kg q 6–8 hr.
IV (Neonates > 2 kg): 30 mg/kg q 6–8 hr.
IV (Neonates ≤ 2 kg): 30 mg/kg q 8–12 hr.
Inhaln (Adults and Children >7 yr): 75 mg three times daily for 28 days.

Renal Impairment

IV (Adults): *CCr 10–30 mL/min*—1–2 g initially, then 50% of usual dosage at usual interval; *CCr <10 mL/min*—500 mg–2 g initially, then 25% of usual dosage at usual interval (1/8 of initial dose should also be given after each hemodialysis session).

Availability (generic available)

Injection: 500 mg/vial, 1 g/vial, 2 g vial. **Premixed containers:** 1 g/50 mL, 2 g/50 mL. **Lyphilized powder for use with diluent provided in Altera Nebulizer System only (Cayston):** 75 mg/vial with 1 mL ampule of diluent (0.17% sodium chloride).

NURSING IMPLICATIONS

Assessment

- Assess for infection (vital signs; wound appearance, sputum, urine, and stool; WBC) at beginning of and throughout therapy.
- Obtain a history before initiating therapy to determine previous use of and reactions to penicillins and cephalosporins. Patients allergic to these drugs may exhibit hypersensitivity reactions to aztreonam. However, aztreonam can often be used in these patients.
- Obtain specimens for culture and sensitivity before initiating therapy. First dose may be given before receiving results.
- Assess respiratory status prior to and following inhalation therapy.
- Observe for signs and symptoms of anaphylaxis (rash, pruritus, laryngeal edema, wheezing). Notify the health care professional immediately if these occur.
- Monitor bowel function. Report diarrhea, abdominal cramping, fever, and bloody stools to health care professional promptly as a sign of Clostridium difficile-associated diarrhea (CDAD). May begin up to several weeks following cessation of therapy.
- ***Lab Test Considerations:*** May cause ↑ in AST, ALT, alkaline phosphatase, LDH, and serum creatinine. May cause ↑ prothrombin and partial thromboplastin times, and positive Coombs' test.

Potential Nursing Diagnoses

Risk for infection (Indications)
Ineffective airway clearance (Indications)

Implementation

- After adding diluent to vial, shake immediately and vigorously. Not for multidose use; discard unused solution. IV route is recommended if single dose >1 g or for severe or life-threatening infection.
- **IM:** Use 15-mL vial and dilute each gram of aztreonam with at least 3 mL of 0.9% NaCl, or sterile or bacteriostatic water for injection. Stable at room temperature for 48 hr or 7 days if refrigerated.
- Administer into large, well-developed muscle.

IV Administration

- **IV Push:** Reconstitute 15 mL vial with 6–10 mL of sterile water for injection. ***Rate:*** Administer slowly over 3–5 min by direct injection or into tubing of a compatible solution.
- **Intermittent Infusion:** Reconstitute 15 mL vial with at 3 mL of Sterile Water for Injection. ***Diluent:*** Dilute further with 0.9% NaCl, Ringer's or LR, D5W, D10W, D5/0.9% NaCl, D5/0.45% NaCl, D5/0.2% NaCl, D5/LR, or sodium lactate. ***Concentration:*** Do not exceed 50 mg/mL. Solution is stable for 48 hr at room temperature and 7 days if refrigerated. Solutions range from colorless to light, straw yellow or may develop a pink tint upon standing; this does not affect potency. ***Rate:*** Infuse over 20–60 min.
- **Y-Site Compatibility:** alemtuzumab, alfentanil, allopurinol, amifostine, amikacin, aminophylline, amphotericin B lipid complex, anidulafungin, argatroban, ascorbic acid, atracurium, atropine, benztropine, bivalirudin, bleomycin, bumetanide,

buprenorphine, butorphanol, calcium chloride, calcium gluconate, carboplatin, carmustine, caspofungin, cefazolin, cefepime, cefotaxime, cefotetan, cefoxitin, ceftazidime, ceftriaxone, cefuroxime, chloramphenicol, ciprofloxacin, cisatracurium, cisplatin, clindamycin, cyanocobalamin, cyclophosphamide, cyclosporine, cytarabine, dacarbazine, dactinomycin, daptomycin, dexamethasone sodium phosphate, dexmedetomidine, digoxin, diltiazem, dobutamine, docetaxel, dopamine, doxacurium, doxorubicin hydrochloride, doxorubicin liposome, doxycycline, droperidol, enalaprilat, ephedrine, epinephrine, epirubicin, epoetin alfa, eptifibatide, ertapenem, esmolol, etoposide, etoposide phosphate, famotidine, fenoldopam, fentanyl, filgrastim, floxuridine, fluconazole, fludarabine, fluorouracil, folic acid, foscarnet, furosemide, gemcitabine, gentamicin, glycopyrrolate, granisetron, heparin, hetastarch, hydrocortisone, hydromorphone, idarubicin, ifosfamide, insulin, irinotecan, isoproterenol, ketorolac, labetalol, leucovorin, levofloxacin, lidocaine, linezolid, magnesium sulfate, mannitol, mechlorethamine, melphalan, meperidine, mesna, metaraminol, methotrexate, methoxamine, methyldopate, methylprednisolone sodium succinate, metoclopramide, metoprolol, midazolam, milrinone, morphine, multivitamins, nafcillin, nalbuphine, naloxone, nesiritide, nicardipine, nitroglycerin, nitroprusside, norepinephrine, octreotide, ondansetron, oxacillin, oxaliplatin, oxytocin, paclitaxel, palonosetron, pamidronate, pancuronium, pemetrexed, penicillin G, phenobarbital, phentolamine, phenylephrine, phytonadione, piperacillin/tazobactam, potassium acetate, potassium chloride, procainamide, propofol, propranolol, protamine, pyridoxime, ranitidine, remifentanil, rituximab, rocuronium, sargramostim, sodium acetate, sodium bicarbonate, streptokinase, succinylcholine, sufentanil, tacrolimus, teniposide, theophylline, thiamine, thiotepa, tigecycline, tirofiban, tobramycin, tolazoline, trimetaphan, vasopressin, vecuronium, verapamil, vinblastine, vincristine, vinorelbine, voriconazole, zidovudine, zoledronic acid.

- **Y-Site Incompatibility:** acyclovir, amphotericin B cholesteryl, amphotericin B colloidal, amphotericin B liposome, amsacrine, azathioprine, azithromycin, chlorpromazine, dantrolene, daunorubicin hydrochloride, diazepam, diazoxide, erythromycin, ganciclovir, indomethacin, lorazepam, metronidazole, mitomycin, mitoxantrone, mycophenolate, pantoprazole, papaverine, pentamidine, pentazocine, pentobarbital, phenytoin, prochlorperazine, streptozocin, trastuzumab.
- **Inhaln:** Open glass aztreonam vial by removing metal ring and pulling tab, and removing gray rubber stopper. Twist tip of diluent ampule and squeeze contents into glass aztreonam vial. Replace rubber stopper and swirl gently until contents are completely dissolved. Administer immediately after reconstitution using *Altera Nebulizer System*. Pour reconstituted solution into handset of nebulizer. Turn unit on. Place mouthpiece into mouth and breathe normally only through mouth. Administration takes 2–3 min. Do not use other nebulizers or mix with other medications. Do not administer IV or IM. Refrigerate azotreonam and diluent; may be stored at room temperature for up to 28 days. Protect from light.
- Administer short-acting bronchodilator between 15 min and 4 hr or long-acting bronchodilator between 30 min and 12 hr prior to treatment. If taking multiple inhaled therapies, administer in the following order: bronchodilator, mucolytic, and lastly, aztreonam.

Patient/Family Teaching

- Advise patient to report the signs of superinfection (furry overgrowth on the tongue, vaginal itching or discharge, loose or foul-smelling stools) and allergy.
- Instruct patient to notify health care professional if fever and diarrhea develop, especially if stool contains blood, pus, or mucus. Advise patient not to treat diarrhea without consulting health care professional.
- Advise patient to notify health care professional if new or worsening symptoms or signs of anaphylaxis occur.
- **Inhaln:** Instruct patient to use aztreonam as directed for the full 28–day course, even if feeling better. If a dose is missed, take all 3 daily doses, as long as doses are at least 4 hrs apart. Skipping doses or not completing full course of therapy may decrease effectiveness and increase likelihood of bacterial resistance not treatable in the future. Inform patient of the importance of using a bronchodilator prior to treatment and in use and cleaning or nebulizer.

Evaluation/Desired Outcomes

- Resolution of signs and symptoms of infection. Length of time for complete resolution depends on the organism and site of infection.
- Improvement in respiratory symptoms in patients with cystic fibrosis.

B

baclofen (**bak**-loe-fen)
Gablofen, Lioresal

Classification
Therapeutic: antispasticity agents, skeletal muscle relaxants (centrally acting)

Pregnancy Category C

Indications
PO: Treatment of reversible spasticity due to multiple sclerosis or spinal cord lesions. **IT:** Treatment of severe spasticity of cerebral or spinal origin (should be reserved for patients who do not respond or are intolerant to oral baclofen) (should wait at least one year in patients with traumatic brain injury before considering therapy). **Unlabeled Use:** Management of pain in trigeminal neuralgia.

Action
Inhibits reflexes at the spinal level. **Therapeutic Effects:** Decreased muscle spasticity; bowel and bladder function may also be improved.

Pharmacokinetics
Absorption: Well absorbed after oral administration.
Distribution: Widely distributed; crosses the placenta.
Protein Binding: 30%.
Metabolism and Excretion: 70–80% eliminated unchanged by the kidneys.
Half-life: 2.5–4 hr.

TIME/ACTION PROFILE (effects on spasticity)

ROUTE	ONSET	PEAK	DURATION
PO	hr–wk	unknown	unknown
IT	0.5–1 hr	4 hr	4–8 hr

Contraindications/Precautions
Contraindicated in: Hypersensitivity.
Use Cautiously in: Patients in whom spasticity maintains posture and balance; Patients with epilepsy (may ↓ seizure threshold); Renal impairment (↓ dose may be required); OB, Lactation: Safety not established; Pedi: Children <4 yr (intrathecal) (safety not established); Geri: ↑ risk of CNS side effects.

Adverse Reactions/Side Effects
CNS: SEIZURES (IT), dizziness, drowsiness, fatigue, weakness, confusion, depression, headache, insomnia. **EENT:** nasal congestion, tinnitus. **CV:** edema, hypotension. **GI:** nausea, constipation. **GU:** frequency. **Derm:** pruritus, rash. **Metab:** hyperglycemia, weight gain. **Neuro:** ataxia. **Misc:** hypersensitivity reactions, sweating.

Interactions
Drug-Drug: ↑ CNS depression with other **CNS depressants** including **alcohol**, **antihistamines**, **opioid analgesics**, and **sedative/hypnotics**. Use with **MAO inhibitors** may lead to ↑ CNS depression or hypotension.
Drug-Natural Products: Concomitant use of **kava-kava**, **valerian**, or **chamomile** can ↑ CNS depression.

Route/Dosage
PO (Adults): 5 mg 3 times daily. May increase q 3 days by 5 mg/dose up to 80 mg/day (some patients may have a better response to 4 divided doses).
PO (Children ≥8 yr): 30–40 mg daily divided q 8 hr; titrate to a maximum of 120 mg/day.
PO (Children 2–7 yr): 20–30 mg daily divided q 8 hr; titrate to a maximum of 60 mg/day.
PO (Children <2 yr): 10–20 mg daily divided q 8 hr; titrate to a maximum of 40 mg/day.
IT (Adults): 100–800 mcg/day infusion; dose is determined by response during screening phase.
IT (Children ≥4 yr): 25–1200 mcg/day infusion (average 275 mcg/day); dose is determined by response during screening phase.

Availability (generic available)
Tablets: 10 mg, 20 mg. **Cost:** *Generic*—10 mg $10.83/100, 20 mg $11.04/100. **Intrathecal injection:** 50 mcg/mL, 500 mcg/mL, 1000 mcg/mL, 2000 mcg/mL.

NURSING IMPLICATIONS

Assessment
- Assess muscle spasticity before and periodically during therapy.
- Observe patient for drowsiness, dizziness, or ataxia. May be alleviated by a change in dose.
- **IT:** Monitor patient closely during test dose and titration. Resuscitative equipment should be immediately available for life-threatening or intolerable side effects.
- ***Lab Test Considerations:*** May cause ↑ in serum glucose, alkaline phosphatase, AST, and ALT levels.

Potential Nursing Diagnoses
Impaired wheelchair mobility (Indications)
Risk for injury (Adverse Reactions)

Implementation
- **PO:** Administer with milk or food to minimize gastric irritation.
- **IT:** For *screening phase,* dilute for a concentration of 50 mcg/mL with sterile preservative-free NaCl for injection. Test dose should be administered over at least 1 min. Observe patient for a significant decrease in muscle tone or frequency or severity of

spasm. If response is inadequate, 2 additional test doses, each 24 hr apart, 75 mcg/1.5 mL and 100 mcg/2 mL respectively, may be administered. Patients with an inadequate response should not receive chronic IT therapy. Avoid use of prefilled syringes for filling reservoir of pump; prefilled syringes are not sterile.

- Dose titration for implantable IT pumps is based on patient response. If no substantive response after dose increase, check pump function and catheter patency.

Patient/Family Teaching

- Instruct patient to take baclofen as directed. Take a missed dose within 1 hr; do not double doses. Caution patient to avoid abrupt withdrawal of this medication because it may precipitate an acute withdrawal reaction (hallucinations, increased spasticity, seizures, mental changes, restlessness). Discontinue baclofen gradually over 2 wk or more.
- May cause dizziness and drowsiness. Advise patient to avoid driving or other activities requiring alertness until response to drug is known.
- Instruct patient to change positions slowly to minimize orthostatic hypotension.
- Advise patient to avoid concurrent use of alcohol or other CNS depressants while taking this medication.
- Instruct patient to notify health care professional if frequent urge to urinate or painful urination, constipation, nausea, headache, insomnia, tinnitus, depression, or confusion persists.
- Advise patient to report signs and symptoms of hypersensitivity (rash, itching) promptly.
- **IT:** Caution patient and caregiver not to discontinue IT therapy abruptly. May result in fever, mental status changes, exaggerated rebound spasticity, and muscle rigidity. Advise patient not to miss scheduled refill appointments and to notify health care professional promptly if signs of withdrawal occur.

Evaluation/Desired Outcomes

- Decrease in muscle spasticity and associated musculoskeletal pain with an increased ability to perform activities of daily living.
- Decreased pain in patients with trigeminal neuralgia. May take weeks to obtain optimal effect.

basiliximab (ba-sil-**ix**-i-mab)

Simulect

Classification

Therapeutic: immunosuppressants

Pharmacologic: monoclonal antibodies

Pregnancy Category B

Indications

Prevention of acute organ rejection in patients undergoing renal transplantation; used with corticosteroids and cyclosporine.

Action

Binds to and blocks specific interleukin-2 (IL-2) receptor sites on activated T lymphocytes. **Therapeutic Effects:** Prevention of acute organ rejection following renal transplantation.

Pharmacokinetics

Absorption: IV administration results in complete bioavailability.

Distribution: Unknown.

Metabolism and Excretion: Unknown.

Half-life: 7.2 days.

TIME/ACTION PROFILE (effect on immune function)

ROUTE	ONSET	PEAK	DURATION
IV	2 hr	unknown	36 days

Contraindications/Precautions

Contraindicated in: Hypersensitivity; OB: May affect fetal developing immune system; Lactation: May enter breast milk.

Use Cautiously in: Women with childbearing potential; Geri: Due to greater incidence of infection.

Adverse Reactions/Side Effects

Noted for patients receiving corticosteroids and cyclosporine in addition to basiliximab.

CNS: dizziness, headache, insomnia, weakness. **EENT:** abnormal vision, cataracts. **Resp:** coughing. **CV:** HEART FAILURE, edema, hypertension, angina, arrhythmias, hypotension. **GI:** abdominal pain, constipation, diarrhea, dyspepsia, moniliasis, nausea, vomiting, GI bleeding, gingival hyperplasia, stomatitis. **Derm:** acne, wound complications, hypertrichosis, pruritus. **Endo:** hyperglycemia, hypoglycemia. **F and E:** acidosis, hypercholesterolemia, hyperkalemia, hyperuricemia, hypocalcemia, hypokalemia, hypophosphatemia. **Hemat:** bleeding, coagulation abnormalities. **MS:** back pain, leg pain. **Neuro:** tremor, neuropathy, paresthesia. **Misc:** hypersensitivity reactions including ANAPHYLAXIS, infection, weight gain, chills.

Interactions

Drug-Drug: Immunosuppression may be ↑ with other **immunosuppressants**.

Drug-Natural Products: Concommitant use with **echinacea** and **melatonin** may interfere with immunosuppression.

Route/Dosage

IV (Adults and Children ≥35 kg): 20 mg given 2 hr before transplantation; repeated 4 days after transplantation. Second dose should be withheld if complications or graft loss occurs.

IV (Children <35 kg): 10 mg given 2 hr before transplantation; repeated 4 days after transplantation. Second dose should be withheld if complication or graft loss occurs.

Availability
Powder for reconstitution: 20 mg/vial, 10 mg/vial.

NURSING IMPLICATIONS

Assessment
- Monitor for signs of anaphylactic or hypersensitivity reactions (hypotension, tachycardia, cardiac failure, dyspnea, wheezing, bronchospasm, pulmonary edema, respiratory failure, urticaria, rash, pruritus, sneezing) at each dose. Onset of symptoms is usually within 24 hr. Resuscitation equipment and medications for treatment of severe hypersensitivity should be readily available. If a severe hypersensitivity reaction occurs, basiliximab therapy should be permanently discontinued. Patients who have previously received basiliximab should only receive subsequent therapy with extreme caution.
- Monitor for infection (fever, chills, rash, sore throat, purulent discharge, dysuria). Notify physician immediately if these symptoms occur; may necessitate discontinuation of therapy.
- ***Lab Test Considerations:*** May cause ↑ or ↓ hemoglobin, hematocrit, serum glucose, potassium, and calcium concentrations.
- May cause ↑ serum cholesterol levels.
- May cause ↑ BUN, serum creatinine, and uric acid concentrations.
- May cause ↓ serum magnesium, phosphate, and platelet levels.

Potential Nursing Diagnoses
Risk for infection (Side Effects)

Implementation

IV Administration

- Basiliximab is usually administered concurrently with cyclosporine and corticosteroids.
- Reconstitute with 2.5 mL or 5 mL of sterile water for injection for the 10 mg or 20 mg vial, respectively. Shake gently to dissolve powder.
- **IV Push:** ***Diluent:*** May be administered undiluted. Bolus administration may be associated with nausea, vomiting, and local reactions (pain). ***Concentration:*** 4 mg/mL. ***Rate:*** Administer over 20–30 min via peripheral or central line.
- **Intermittent Infusion:** ***Diluent:*** Dilute further with 25–50 mL of 0.9% NaCl or D5W. Gently invert bag to mix; do not shake, to avoid foaming. Solution is clear to opalescent and colorless; do not administer solutions that are discolored or contain particulate matter. Discard unused portion. Administer within 4 hr or may be refrigerated for up to 24 hr. Discard after 24 hr. ***Concentration:*** 0.08–0.16 mg/mL. ***Rate:*** Administer over 20–30 min via peripheral or central line.
- **Additive Incompatibility:** Do not admix; do not administer in IV line containing other medications.

Patient/Family Teaching
- Explain purpose of medication to patient. Explain that patient will need to resume lifelong therapy with other immunosuppressive drugs after completion of basiliximab course.
- May cause dizziness. Caution patient to avoid driving or other activities requiring alertness until response is known.
- Instruct patient to continue to avoid crowds and persons with known infections, because basiliximab also suppresses the immune system.

Evaluation/Desired Outcomes
- Prevention of acute organ rejection in patients receiving renal transplantation.

becaplermin (be-**kap**-lerm-in)
Regranex

Classification
Therapeutic: wound/ulcer/decubiti healing agent
Pharmacologic: platelet-derived growth factors

Pregnancy Category C

Indications
Treatment of lower extremity diabetic neuropathic ulcers extending to subcut tissue or beyond and having adequate blood supply.

Action
Promotes chemotaxis of cells involved in wound repair and enhances formation of granulation tissue. **Therapeutic Effects:** Improved healing.

Pharmacokinetics
Absorption: Minimal absorption (<3%).
Distribution: Action is primarily local.
Metabolism and Excretion: Unknown.
Half-life: Unknown.

TIME/ACTION PROFILE (improvement in ulcer healing)

ROUTE	ONSET	PEAK	DURATION
Topical	within 10 wk	unknown	unknown

Contraindications/Precautions
Contraindicated in: Known hypersensitivity to becaplermin or parabens; Known neoplasm at site of application; Wounds that close by primary intention.
Use Cautiously in: Known malignancy; OB, Lactation, Pedi: Safety not established.

Adverse Reactions/Side Effects

Derm: erythematous rash at application site. **Misc:** MALIGNANCY (MAY LEAD TO ↑ MORTALITY, ESPECIALLY WITH USE OF ≥3 TUBES).

Interactions

Drug-Drug: None known.

Route/Dosage

Topical (Adults): Length of gel *in inches* from 15- or 7.5-g tube = length × width of ulcer area × 0.6; from the 2-g tube = length × width of ulcer area × 1.3. Length of gel *in centimeters* from 15- or 7.5-g tube = length × width of ulcer area ÷ 4; from the 2-g tube = length × width of ulcer area ÷ 2; for 12 hr each day.

Availability

Gel: 100 mcg/g (0.01%) in 2-, 7.5-, and 15-g tubes.

NURSING IMPLICATIONS

Assessment

- Assess size, color, drainage, and skin surrounding wound at weekly or biweekly intervals. Amount of gel to be applied is recalculated based on wound size.

Potential Nursing Diagnoses

Impaired tissue integrity (Indications)
Deficient knowledge, related to medication regimen (Patient/Family Teaching)

Implementation

- **Topical:** Calculated amount is applied as a thin layer (1/16-in. thick) and covered with a moist saline dressing for 12 hr; dressing is removed, ulcer rinsed and redressed with moist dressing without becaplermin for rest of day. Process is repeated daily.
- Store gel in refrigerator; do not freeze. Do not use beyond expiration date on crimped end of tube.

Patient/Family Teaching

- Instruct patient on proper technique for application. Wash hands before applying gel and use cotton swab or tongue depressor to aid in application. Tip of tube should not come in contact with ulcer or any other surface; recap tightly after each use. Squeeze calculated amount of gel onto a clean, firm, nonabsorbable surface (wax paper). Spread gel with swab or tongue depressor over the ulcer surface in an even layer to the thickness of a dime. Cover with a saline-moistened gauze dressing.
- Do not apply more than calculated amount; has not been shown to be beneficial. If a dose is missed, apply as soon as remembered. If not remembered until next day, skip dose and return to regular dosing schedule. Do not double doses.
- After 12 hr, rinse ulcer gently with saline or water to remove residual gel and cover with saline-moistened gauze.
- Emphasize the importance of strict wound care and non–weight-bearing program.

Evaluation/Desired Outcomes

- Improved healing of ulcers. If the ulcer does not decrease in size by 30% within 10 wk or if complete healing has not occurred within 20 wk, continuation of therapy should be reassessed.

beclomethasone, See CORTICOSTEROIDS (INHALATION) and CORTICOSTEROIDS (NASAL).

REMS

belatacept (be-lat-a-sept)

Nulojix

Classification
Therapeutic: immunosuppressants
Pharmacologic: fusion proteins

Pregnancy Category C

Indications

Prevention of organ rejection following kidney transplant in adult patients; in combination with basiliximab induction, mycophenolate and corticosteroids.

Action

Binds to CD80 and CD86 sites, thereby blocking T-cell costimulation; result is inhibition of T-lymphocyte proliferation and cytokine production. **Therapeutic Effects:** Prolonged graft survival with decreased production of anti-donor antibodies following kidney transplantation.

Pharmacokinetics

Absorption: IV administration results in complete bioavailability.
Distribution: Unknown.
Metabolism and Excretion: Unknown.
Half-life: 9.8 days.

TIME/ACTION PROFILE

ROUTE	ONSET	PEAK	DURATION
IV	unknown	end of infusion	up to 4 wk

Contraindications/Precautions

Contraindicated in: Ebstein-Barr virus (EBV) seronegativity or unknown EBV serostatus; Liver transplantation; Lactation: Avoid breast feeding.
Use Cautiously in: Cytomegalovirus (CMV) infection/T-cell depleting therapy (↑ risk of post-transplant lymphoproliferative disorder [PTLD]), CMV prophylaxis recommended for 3 mos following transplant; Change in body weight >10% (dose adjustment recommended); Unknown tuberculosis status (latent infection should be treated prior to use); Evidence of polyoma virus-associated nephropathy (PVAN), ↓ immunosuppression may be necessary; OB: Use only if

potential benefit to mother outweighs potential risk to fetus; Pedi: Safety and effectiveness not established.

Adverse Reactions/Side Effects

CNS: PROGRESSIVE MULTIFOCAL LEUKOENCEPHALOPATHY (PML), headache. **Resp:** cough. **CV:** hypertension, peripheral edema. **GI:** constipation, diarrhea, nausea, vomiting. **GU:** proteinuria. **Endo:** new-onset diabetes mellitus. **F and E:** hyperkalemia, hypokalemia. **Hemat:** anemia, leukopenia. **Misc:** POST-TRANSPLANT LYMPHOPROLIFERATIVE DISORDER (PTLD), ↑ RISK OF MALIGNANCY, SERIOUS INFECTIONS, fever, graft dysfunction.

Interactions

Drug-Drug: May ↓ antibody response to and ↑ risk of adverse reactions from live virus vaccines; avoid use during treatment. May ↑ blood levels, effects and toxicity of **mycophenolic acid**.

Route/Dosage

Prescribed dose must be evenly divisible by 12.5 to ensure accurate preparation.

IV (Adults): *Initial phase*—10 mg/kg on day of transplant/prior to implantation, day 5 (96 hr after day 1 dose), end of week 2, 4, 8, and 12 post transplantation; *Maintenance phase*—10 mg/kg end of week 16 and every four weeks (±3 days) thereafter.

Availability

Lyophilized powder for injection (requires reconstitution): 250 mg/vial.

NURSING IMPLICATIONS

Assessment

- Assess for symptoms of organ rejection throughout therapy.
- Assess for signs of progressive multifocal leukoencephalopathy (hemiparesis, apathy, confusion, cognitive deficiencies, and ataxia) periodically during therapy.
- Monitor for signs and symptoms of infection (fever, dyspnea) periodically during therapy.
- Assess for signs and symptoms of post-transplant lymphoproliferative disorder (changes in mood or usual behavior, confusion, problems thinking, loss of memory, changes in walking or talking, decreased strength or weakness on one side of the body, changes in vision) during and for at least 36 mo post-transplant.
- Monitor for infusion reactions (hypotension, hypertension) during therapy.
- ***Lab Test Considerations:*** May cause hyperkalemia, hypokalemia, hypophosphatemia, hyperglycemia, hypocalcemia, hypercholesterolemia, hypomagnesemia, and hyperuricemia.

Potential Nursing Diagnoses

Risk for infection (Adverse Reactions)

Implementation

- Pre-medication is not required.
- Cortisone doses should be consistent with clinical trials experience. Cortisone doses were tapered to between 10–20 mg/day by first 6 wks after transplant, then remained at 10 mg (5–10 mg) per day for first 6 months after transplant.
- Treat patient for latent tuberculosis prior to therapy.
- Prophylaxis for *Pneumocystis jiroveci* is recommended after transplant.

IV Administration

- **Intermittent Infusion:** Calculate number if vials required for total infusion dose. Reconstitute contents of each vial with 10.5 mL of 0.9% NaCl or D5W using the silicone-free disposable syringe provided and an 18–21 gauge needle for a concentration of 25 mg/mL. Direct stream of diluent to wall of vial. Rotate and invert vial gently; do not shake to avoid foaming. Solution is clear to slightly opalescent and colorless to pale yellow; do not use of opaque particles, discoloration, or other particles are present. Calculate total volume needed for infusion dose. ***Diluent:*** Dilute further with 0.9% NaCl or D5W if reconstituted with sterile water for injection, 0.9% NaCl if reconstituted with 0.9% NaCl, or with D5W if reconstituted with D5W. ***Concentration:*** 2 mg/mL. Withdraw amount of diluent from infusion container equal to volume of infusion dose. Using same silicone-free disposable syringe used for reconstitution, withdraw required amount of belatacept solution from vial, inject into infusion container, and rotate gently to mix. Typical infusion volume is 100 mL, but may range from 50–250 mL. Transfer from vial to infusion container immediately; infusion must be completed within 24 hr of reconstitution. May be refrigerated and protected from light for 24 hr. Do not administer solutions that are discolored or contain particulate matter. Discard unused solution in vials. ***Rate:*** Infuse over 30 min using a non-pyrogenic, low-protein-binding filter with 0.2–1.2 micron pore size.
- **Y-Site Incompatibility:** Do not mix or infuse in same line with other agents.

Patient/Family Teaching

- Reinforce the need for lifelong therapy to prevent transplant rejection. Review symptoms of rejection for the transplanted organ, and stress need to notify health care professional immediately if signs of rejection or infection occur.
- Advise patient to avoid contact with persons with contagious diseases.
- Inform patient of the increased risk of skin cancer and other malignancies. Advise patient to use sun-

screen with a high protection factor and wear protective clothing to decrease risk of skin cancer.

- Advise patient to notify health care professional of all Rx or OTC medications, vitamins, or herbal products being taken and to consult with health care professional before taking other medications.
- Advise patient to notify health care professional immediately if signs or symptoms of infection, post-transplant lymphoproliferative disorder or progressive multifocal leukoencephalopathy occur.
- Advise patients to avoid live vaccines during therapy.
- Rep: Advise female patients to notify health care professional if pregnancy is planned or suspected or if breast feeding. Encourage patients who become pregnant or whose partners have received belatacept to register with the National Transplant Pregnancy Registry (NTPR) by calling 1-877-955-6877.
- Emphasize the importance of routine follow-up laboratory tests.

Evaluation/Desired Outcomes

- Prevention of rejection of transplanted kidneys.

belimumab (be-li-moo-mab)

Benlysta

Classification
Therapeutic: immunosuppressants
Pharmacologic: monoclonal antibodies

Pregnancy Category C

Indications

Treatment of active autoantibody-positive systemic lupus erythematosus (SLE) in patients currently receiving standard therapy.

Action

A monoclonal antibody produced by recombinant DNA technique that specifically binds to B-lymphocyte stimulator protein (BLyS), thereby inactivating it. **Therapeutic Effects:** ↓ survival of B cells, including auroreactive ones and ↓ differentiation into immunoglobulin-producing plasma cells. Result is ↓ disease activity with lessened damage/improvement in mucocutaneous, musculoskeletal and immunologic manifestations of SLE.

Pharmacokinetics

Absorption: IV administration results in complete bioavailability.
Distribution: Unknown.
Metabolism and Excretion: Unknown.
Half-life: 19.4 days.

TIME/ACTION PROFILE (reduction in activated B cells)

ROUTE	ONSET	PEAK	DURATION
IV	8 wk	unknown	52 wk†

†With continuous treatment.

Contraindications/Precautions

Contraindicated in: Hypersensitivity; Concurrent use of other biologicals or cyclophosphamide; Concurrent use of live vaccines; Lactation: Not recommended.
Use Cautiously in: Infections (consider temporary withdrawal for acute infections, treat aggressively); Previous history of depression or suicidal ideation (may worsen); Geri: May be more sensitive to drug effects, consider age-related changes in renal, hepatic and cardiac function, concurrent drug therapy and chronic disease states; OB: Use during pregnancy only if potential maternal benefit outweighs potential fetal risk.; Rep: Women with childbearing potential should use adequate contraception during and for 4 mo following treatment

Adverse Reactions/Side Effects

CNS: PROGRESSIVE MULTIFOCAL LEUKOENCEPHALOPATHY (PML), depression, insomnia, migraine, fatigue. **GI:** nausea, diarrhea. **GU:** cystitis. **Hemat:** leukopenia. **MS:** extremity pain, myalgia. **Derm:** rash. **Misc:** allergic reactions including ANAPHYLAXIS, INFECTION, infusion reactions, fever, facial edema.

Interactions

Drug-Drug: ↑ risk of adverse reactions and ↓ immune response to **live vaccines**; should not be given concurrently.

Route/Dosage

PO (Adults): 10 mg/kg every 2 wk for 3 doses, then every 4 wk.

Availability

Lyophilized powder for IV administration (requires reconstitution and dilution): 120 mg/vial, 400 mg/vial.

NURSING IMPLICATIONS

Assessment

- Monitor patient for signs of anaphylaxis (hypotension, angioedema, urticaria, rash, pruritus, wheezing, dyspnea, facial edema) during and following injection. Medications (antihistamines, corticosteroids, epinephrine) and equipment should be readily available in the event of a severe reaction. Discontinue belimumab immediately if anaphylaxis or other severe allergic reaction occurs.
- Monitor for infusion reactions (headache, nausea, skin reactions, bradycardia, myalgia, headache, rash, urticaria, hypotension). There is insufficient evidence to determine whether premedication diminishes frequency or severity. Infusion rate may be slowed or interrupted if an infusion reaction occurs.

- Assess for signs of infection (fever, dyspnea, flu-like symptoms, frequent or painful urination, redness or swelling at the site of a wound), including tuberculosis, prior to injection. Belimumab is contraindicated in patients with active infection. New infections should be monitored closely; most common are upper respiratory tract infections, bronchitis, and urinary tract infections. Signs and symptoms of inflammation may be lessened due to suppression from belimumab. Infections may be fatal, especially in patients taking immunosuppressive therapy. If patient develops a serious infection, consider discontinuing belimumab until infection is controlled.
- Assess mental status and mood changes. Inform health care professional if patient demonstrates significant ↑ in depressed mood, anxiety, nervousness, or insomnia.
- Assess for signs of progressive multifocal leukoencephalopathy (hemiparesis, apathy, confusion, cognitive deficiencies, and ataxia) periodically during therapy.

Potential Nursing Diagnoses

Risk for infection (Adverse Reactions)

Implementation

- Consider premedication for prophylaxis against infusion reactions and hypersensitivity reactions.

IV Administration

- **Intermittent Infusion:** Remove belimumab from refrigerator and allow to stand 10–15 min to reach room temperature. Reconstitute 120 mg vial with 1.5 mL and 400 mg vial with 4.8 mL of Sterile Water for Injection by directing stream toward side if vial to minimize foaming. Swirl gently for 60 seconds. Allow vial to sit at room temperature during reconstitution, swirling gently for 60 seconds every 5 min until powder is dissolved. Do not shake. Reconstitution usually takes 10–15 min, but may take up to 30 min. Protect from sunlight. Solution is opalescent and colorless to pale yellow and without particles. Small bubbles are expected and acceptable. ***Concentration:*** 80 mg/mL. ***Diluent:*** 0.9% NaCL. Remove volume of patient's dose from a 250 mL infusion bag and discard. Replace with required amount of reconstituted solution. Gently invert bag to mix. Do not administer solutions that are discolored or contain particulate matter. Discard unused solution in vial. If not used immediately, refrigerate and protect from light. Solution is stable for 8 hrs. ***Rate:*** Infuse over 1 hr; may slow or interrupt rate if patient develops an infusion reaction.
- **Y-Site Incompatibility:** Do not administer with dextrose solutions or other solutions or medications.

Patient/Family Teaching

- Instruct patient to read *Medication Guide* prior to each treatment session in case of changes.
- Caution patient to notify health care professional immediately if signs of infection (fever, sweating, chills, muscle aches, cough, shortness of breath, blood in phlegm, weight loss, warm, red or painful skin or sores, diarrhea or stomach pain, burning on urination, urinary frequency, feeling tired), progressive multifocal leukoencephalopathy, severe rash, swollen face, or difficulty breathing occurs while taking.
- Advise patient, family, and caregivers to look for depression and suicidality, especially during early therapy or dose changes. Notify health care professional immediately if thoughts about suicide or dying, attempts to commit suicide; new or worse depression or anxiety; agitation or restlessness; panic attacks; insomnia; new or worse irritability; aggressiveness; acting on dangerous impulses, mania, or other changes in mood or behavior or if symptoms of serotonin syndrome occur.
- Caution patient to avoid receiving live vaccines for 30 days before and during belimumab therapy.
- Rep: Advise women of childbearing potential to use adequate contraception and to avoid breast feeding during and for at least 4 mo after final treatment.

Evaluation/Desired Outcomes

- Improvement in mucocutaneous, musculoskeletal, and immunologic disease activity in patients with SLE.

benazepril, See ANGIOTENSIN-CONVERTING ENZYME (ACE) INHIBITORS.

benzathine penicillin G, See PENICILLINS.

benztropine (benz-troe-peen)

Cogentin

Classification

Therapeutic: antiparkinson agents
Pharmacologic: anticholinergics

Pregnancy Category C

Indications

Adjunctive treatment of all forms of Parkinson's disease, including drug-induced extrapyramidal effects and acute dystonic reactions.

Action

Blocks cholinergic activity in the CNS, which is partially responsible for the symptoms of Parkinson's disease. Restores the natural balance of neurotransmitters in the CNS. **Therapeutic Effects:** Reduction of rigidity and tremors.

Pharmacokinetics

Absorption: Well absorbed following PO and IM administration.
Distribution: Unknown.
Metabolism and Excretion: Unknown.
Half-life: Unknown.

TIME/ACTION PROFILE (antidyskinetic activity)

ROUTE	ONSET	PEAK	DURATION
PO	1–2 hr	several days	24 hr
IM, IV	within min	unknown	24 hr

Contraindications/Precautions

Contraindicated in: Hypersensitivity; Children <3 yr; Angle-closure glaucoma; Tardive dyskinesia.
Use Cautiously in: Prostatic hyperplasia; Seizure disorders; Cardiac arrhythmias; OB, Lactation: Safety not established; Geri: ↑ risk of adverse reactions.

Adverse Reactions/Side Effects

CNS: confusion, depression, dizziness, hallucinations, headache, sedation, weakness. **EENT:** blurred vision, dry eyes, mydriasis. **CV:** arrhythmias, hypotension, palpitations, tachycardia. **GI:** constipation, dry mouth, ileus, nausea. **GU:** hesitancy, urinary retention. **Misc:** decreased sweating.

Interactions

Drug-Drug: Additive anticholinergic effects with **drugs sharing anticholinergic properties**, such as **antihistamines**, **phenothiazines**, **quinidine**, **disopyramide**, and **tricyclic antidepressants**. Counteracts the cholinergic effects of **bethanechol**. **Antacids** and **antidiarrheals** may ↓ absorption.
Drug-Natural Products: ↑ anticholinergic effect with **angel's trumpet**, **jimson weed**, and **scopolia**.

Route/Dosage

Parkinsonism

PO (Adults): 1–2 mg/day in 1–2 divided doses (range 0.5–6 mg/day).

Acute Dystonic Reactions

IM, IV (Adults): 1–2 mg, then 1–2 mg PO twice daily.

Drug-Induced Extrapyramidal Reactions

PO, IM, IV (Adults): 1–4 mg given once or twice daily (1–2 mg 2–3 times daily may also be used PO).

Availability (generic available)

Tablets: 0.5 mg, 1 mg, 2 mg. **Cost:** *Generic*—0.5 mg $26.07/100, 1 mg $25.74/100, 2 mg $51.86/100. **Injection:** 1 mg/mL.

NURSING IMPLICATIONS

Assessment

- Assess parkinsonian and extrapyramidal symptoms (restlessness or desire to keep moving, rigidity, tremors, pill rolling, masklike face, shuffling gait, muscle spasms, twisting motions, difficulty speaking or swallowing, loss of balance control) before and throughout therapy.
- Assess bowel function daily. Monitor for constipation, abdominal pain, distention, or absence of bowel sounds.
- Monitor intake and output ratios and assess patient for urinary retention (dysuria, distended abdomen, infrequent voiding of small amounts, overflow incontinence).
- Patients with mental illness are at risk of developing exaggerated symptoms of their disorder during early therapy with benztropine. Withhold drug and notify physician or other health care professional if significant behavioral changes occur.
- **IM/IV:** Monitor pulse and BP closely and maintain bedrest for 1 hr after administration. Advise patients to change positions slowly to minimize orthostatic hypotension.

Potential Nursing Diagnoses

Impaired physical mobility (Indications)
Risk for injury (Indications)

Implementation

- **PO:** Administer with food or immediately after meals to minimize gastric irritation. May be crushed and administered with food if patient has difficulty swallowing.
- **IM:** Parenteral route is used only for dystonic reactions.

IV Administration

- **IV Push:** IV route is rarely used because onset is same as with IM route. ***Rate:*** Administer at a rate of 1 mg over 1 min.
- **Y-Site Compatibility:** alfentanil, amikacin, aminophylline, ascorbic acid, atracurium, atropine, azathioprine, aztreonam, bumetanide, buprenorphine, butorphanol, calcium chloride, calcium gluconate, cefazolin, cefotaxime, cefotetan, cefoxitin, ceftazidime, ceftriaxone, cefuroxime, chlorpromazine, clindamycin, cyanocobalamin, cyclosporine, dexamethasone, digoxin, diphenhydramine, dobutamine, dopamine, doxycycline, enalaprilat, ephedrine, epinephrine, epoetin alfa, erythromycin, esmolol, famotidine, fentanyl, fluconazole, folic acid, gentamicin, glycopyrrolate, heparin, hydrocortisone, imipenem/cilastatin, insulin, isoproterenol, ketorolac, labetalol, lidocaine, magnesium sulfate, mannitol, meperi-

dine, metaraminol, methyldopate, methylprednisolone, metoclopramide, metoprolol, midazolam, morphine, multivitamins, nafcillin, nalbuphine, naloxone, nitroglycerin, nitroprusside, norepinephrine, ondansetron, oxacillin, oxytocin, papaverine, penicillin G, pentamidine, pentazocine, phenobarbital, phentolamine, phenylephrine, phytonadione, potassium chloride, procainamide, prochlorperazine, promethazine, propranolol, protamine, pyridoxime, ranitidine, sodium bicarbonate, streptokinase, succinylcholine, sufentanil, tacrolimus, theophylline, thiamine, tobramycin, tolazoline, vancomycin, vasopressin, verapamil.

- **Y-Site Incompatibility:** amphotericin B colloidal, chloramphenicol, dantrolene, diazepam, diazoxide, furosemide, ganciclovir, indomethacin, pentobarbital, phenytoin, sulfamethoxazole/trimethoprim.

Patient/Family Teaching

- Encourage patient to take benztropine as directed. Take missed doses as soon as possible, up to 2 hr before the next dose. Taper gradually when discontinuing or a withdrawal reaction may occur (anxiety, tachycardia, insomnia, return of parkinsonian or extrapyramidal symptoms).
- May cause drowsiness or dizziness. Advise patient to avoid driving or other activities that require alertness until response to the drug is known.
- Instruct patient that frequent rinsing of mouth, good oral hygiene, and sugarless gum or candy may decrease dry mouth. Patient should notify health care professional if dryness persists (saliva substitutes may be used). Also, notify the dentist if dryness interferes with use of dentures.
- Caution patient to change positions slowly to minimize orthostatic hypotension.
- Instruct patient to notify health care professional if difficulty with urination, constipation, abdominal discomfort, rapid or pounding heartbeat, confusion, eye pain, or rash occurs.
- Advise patient to confer with health care professional before taking OTC medications, especially cold remedies, or drinking alcoholic beverages.
- Caution patient that this medication decreases perspiration. Overheating may occur during hot weather. Patient should notify health care professional if unable to remain indoors in an air-conditioned environment during hot weather.
- Advise patient to avoid taking antacids or antidiarrheals within 1–2 hr of this medication.
- Emphasize the importance of routine follow-up exams.

Evaluation/Desired Outcomes

- Decrease in tremors and rigidity and an improvement in gait and balance. Therapeutic effects are usually seen 2–3 days after the initiation of therapy.

betamethasone, **See CORTICOSTEROIDS (SYSTEMIC) and CORTICOSTEROIDS (TOPICAL/LOCAL).**

bevacizumab

(be-va-**kiz**-oo-mab)

Avastin

Classification

Therapeutic: antineoplastics

Pharmacologic: monoclonal antibodies

Pregnancy Category C

Indications

First- or second-line treatment of metastatic colon or rectal carcinoma (with IV 5–fluorouracil-based chemotherapy for first-line therapy; with fluoropyrimidine-irinotecan- or fluoropyrimidine-oxaliplatin-based chemotherapy for second-line therapy. First line treatment of patients with unresectable, locally advanced, recurrent or metastatic non-squamous, non-small cell lung cancer with carboplatin and paclitaxel. Patients with progressive glioblastoma following prior therapy. Metastatic renal cell carcinoma (with interferon alfa). Persistent, recurrent, or metastatic cervical carcinoma (with paclitaxel and cisplatin or paclitaxel and topotecan). Platinum-resistant recurrent epithelial ovarian, fallopian tube, or primary peritoneal cancer (with paclitaxel, pegylated liposomal doxorubicin, or topotecan).

Action

A monoclonal antibody that binds to vascular endothelial growth factor (VEGF), preventing its attachment to binding sites on vascular endothelium, thereby inhibiting growth of new blood vessels (angiogenesis). **Therapeutic Effects:** Decreased metastatic disease progression and microvascular growth.

Pharmacokinetics

Absorption: IV administration results in complete bioavailability.

Distribution: Unknown.

Metabolism and Excretion: Unknown.

Half-life: 20 days (range 11–50 days).

TIME/ACTION PROFILE

ROUTE	ONSET	PEAK	DURATION
IV	rapid	end of infusion	14 days

Contraindications/Precautions

Contraindicated in: Hypersensitivity; Recent hemoptysis or other serious recent bleeding episode; First

28 days after major surgery; OB: Pregnancy (can cause fetal harm); Lactation: Discontinue nursing during treatment and, due to long half-life, for several weeks following treatment.

Use Cautiously in: Cardiovascular disease; Diabetes (↑ risk of arterial thromboembolic events); OB: Women with childbearing potential; Pedi: Safety not established; Geri: ↑ risk of serious adverse reactions including arterial thromboembolic events.

Adverse Reactions/Side Effects

CNS: REVERSIBLE POSTERIOR LEUKOENCEPHALOPATHY SYNDROME (RPLS). **CV:** HF, THROMBOEMBOLIC EVENTS, hypertension, hypotension. **Resp:** HEMOPTYSIS, non-gastrointestinal fistulas, nasal septum perforation. **GI:** GI PERFORATION. **GU:** nephrotic syndrome, ovarian failure, proteinuria. **Hemat:** BLEEDING. **Derm:** NECROTIZING FASCIITIS. **Misc:** WOUND DEHISCENCE, impaired wound healing, infusion reactions.

Interactions

Drug-Drug: ↑ blood levels of SN 38 (the active metabolite of **irinotecan**); significance is not known. ↑ risk of microangiopathic hemolytic anemia when used with **sunitinib**; concurrent use should be avoided.

Route/Dosage

Colorectal Cancer

IV (Adults): 5 mg/kg every 14 days when used in combination with bolus-IFL chemotherapy regimen; 10 mg/kg every 14 days when used with FOLFOX4 chemotherapy regimen 5 mg/kg every 14 days or 7.5 mg/kg every 21 days when used in combination with a fluoropyrimidine-irinotecan or fluoropyrimidine-oxaliplatin based chemotherapy regimen.

Lung Cancer

IV (Adults): 15 mg/kg every 3 wk.

Glioblastoma

IV (Adults): 10 mg/kg every 14 days.

Renal Cell Carcinoma

IV (Adults): 10 mg/kg every 14 days.

Cervical Carcinoma

IV (Adults): 15 mg/kg every 3 wk.

Epithelial Ovarian, Fallopian Tube, or Primary Peritoneal Cancer

IV (Adults): 10 mg/kg every 2 wk when given with paclitaxel, pegylated liposomal doxorubicin, or topotecan (weekly) *or* 15 mg/kg every 3 wk when given with topotecan (every 3 wk).

Availability

Solution for injection (requires dilution): 25 mg/mL.

NURSING IMPLICATIONS

Assessment

- Assess for signs of GI perforation (abdominal pain associated with constipation, fever, nausea, and vomiting), fistula formation, and wound dehiscence during therapy; discontinue therapy if this occurs.
- Assess for signs of hemorrhage (epistaxis, hemoptysis, bleeding) and thromboembolic events (stroke, MI, deep vein thrombosis, pulmonary embolus) during therapy; may require discontinuation. Do not administer to patients with recent history of hemoptysis of ≥1/2 teaspoon of red blood.
- Monitor BP every 2–3 wk during therapy. Temporarily suspend therapy during severe hypertension not controlled with medical management; permanently discontinue if hypertensive crisis occurs.
- Assess for infusion reactions (stridor, wheezing) during therapy.
- Assess for signs of HF (dyspnea, peripheral edema, rales/crackles, jugular venous distension) during therapy.
- Monitor for signs of RPLS (headache, seizure, lethargy, confusion, blindness). Hypertension may or may not be present. May occur with in 16 hr to 1 yr of initiation of therapy. Treat hypertension if present and discontinue bevacizumab therapy. Symptoms usually resolve within days.
- ***Lab Test Considerations:*** Monitor serial urinalysis for proteinuria during therapy. Patients with a 2+ or greater urine dipstick require further testing with a 24-hr urine collection. Suspend therapy for ≥2 grams of proteinuria/24 hours and resume when proteinuria is <2 gm/24 hours. Discontinue therapy in patients with nephrotic syndrome.
- May cause leukopenia, thrombocytopenia, hypokalemia, and bilirubinemia.

Potential Nursing Diagnoses

Ineffective tissue perfusion (Adverse Reactions)

Implementation

- Avoid administration for at least 28 days following major surgery; surgical incision should be fully healed due to potential for impaired wound healing.

IV Administration

- **Intermittent Infusion:** ***Diluent:*** Dilute prescribed dose in 100 mL of 0.9% NaCl. Do not shake. Discard unused portions. Do not administer solution that is discolored or contains particulate matter. Stable if refrigerated for up to 8 hr. ***Rate:*** Administer initial dose over 90 min. If well tolerated, second infusion may be administered over 60 min. If well tolerated, all subsequent infusions may be administered over 30 min. **Do not administer as an IV push or bolus.**
- **Additive Incompatibility:** Do not mix or administer with dextrose solutions.

B

Patient/Family Teaching
- Inform patient of purpose of medication.
- Advise patient of the need for monitoring BP periodically during therapy; notify health care professional if BP is elevated.
- Advise patient to report any signs of bleeding, unusual bleeding, high fever, rigors, sudden onset of worsening neurological function, or persistent or severe abdominal pain, severe constipation, or vomiting immediately to health care professional.
- Inform patient of increased risk of wound healing complications and arterial thromboembolic events.
- Rep: Bevacizumab is teratogenic. Advise female patients to use effective contraception during and for at least 6 mo after last dose. Inform female patient of risk of ovarian failure that may lead to sterility following therapy.

Evaluation/Desired Outcomes
- Decreased metastatic disease progression and microvascular growth.

bicalutamide
(bye-ka-**loot**-a-mide)
Casodex

Classification
Therapeutic: antineoplastics
Pharmacologic: antiandrogens

Pregnancy Category X

Indications
Treatment of metastatic prostate carcinoma in conjunction with luteinizing hormone–releasing hormone (LHRH) analogs (goserelin, leuprolide).

Action
Antagonizes the effects of androgen at the cellular level. **Therapeutic Effects:** Decreased spread of prostate carcinoma.

Pharmacokinetics
Absorption: Well absorbed after oral administration.
Distribution: Unknown.
Protein Binding: 96%.
Metabolism and Excretion: Mostly metabolized by the liver.
Half-life: 5.8 days.

TIME/ACTION PROFILE (blood levels)

ROUTE	ONSET	PEAK	DURATION
PO	unknown	31.3 hr	unknown

Contraindications/Precautions
Contraindicated in: Hypersensitivity; Women.
Use Cautiously in: Moderate to severe liver impairment; Pedi: Safety not established.

Adverse Reactions/Side Effects
CNS: weakness, dizziness, headache, insomnia. **Resp:** dyspnea. **CV:** chest pain, hypertension, peripheral edema. **GI:** HEPATOTOXICITY, constipation, diarrhea, nausea, abdominal pain, ↑ liver enzymes, vomiting. **GU:** hematuria, erectile dysfunction, incontinence, nocturia, urinary tract infections. **Derm:** alopecia, photosensitivity, rash, sweating. **Endo:** breast pain, gynecomastia. **Hemat:** anemia. **Metab:** hyperglycemia, weight loss. **MS:** back pain, pelvic pain, bone pain. **Neuro:** paresthesia. **Misc:** generalized pain, hot flashes, flu-like syndrome, infection.

Interactions
Drug-Drug: May ↑ the effect of **warfarin**.

Route/Dosage
PO (Adults): 50 mg once daily (must be given concurrently with LHRH analog).

Availability (generic available)
Tablets: 50 mg.

NURSING IMPLICATIONS
Assessment
- Assess patient for adverse GI effects. Diarrhea is the most common cause of discontinuation of therapy.
- ***Lab Test Considerations:*** Monitor serum prostate-specific antigen (PSA) periodically to determine response to therapy. If levels rise, assess patient for disease progression. May require periodic LHRH analogue administration without bicalutamide.
- Monitor serum transaminases before, regularly during first 4 mo of therapy, and periodically during therapy. May cause ↑ serum alkaline phosphatase, AST, ALT, and bilirubin concentrations. If patient is jaundice or if transaminases ↑2 times normal, discontinue bicalutamide; levels usually return to normal after discontinuation.
- May cause ↑ BUN and serum creatinine, and ↓ hemoglobin and WBCs.
- May cause ↓ glucose tolerance in males taking LHRH agonists concurrently; monitor blood glucose in patients receiving bicalutamide in combination with LHRH agonists.

Potential Nursing Diagnoses
Diarrhea (Adverse Reactions)

Implementation
- Start treatment with bicalutamide at the same time as LHRH analogue.
- **PO:** May be administered in the morning or evening, without regard to food.

Patient/Family Teaching

- Instruct patient to take bicalutamide along with the LHRH analog as directed at the same time each day. If a dose is missed, omit and take the next dose at regular time; do not double doses. Do not discontinue without consulting health care professional. Advise patient to read *Patient Information* prior to starting and with each Rx refill in case of changes.
- May cause dizziness. Caution patient to avoid driving or other activities requiring alertness until response to medication is known.
- Advise patient to stop taking bicalutamide and notify health care professional immediately of symptoms of liver dysfunction (nausea, vomiting, abdominal pain, fatigue, anorexia, "flu-like" symptoms, dark urine, jaundice, or right upper quadrant tenderness) or interstitial lung disease (trouble breathing with or without a cough or fever).
- Advise patient to notify health care professional of all Rx or OTC medications, vitamins, or herbal products being taken and to consult health care professional before taking any new medications.
- Instruct patient to report severe or persistent diarrhea.
- Discuss with patient the possibility of hair loss. Explore methods of coping.
- Advise patient to use sunscreen, avoid sunlight or sunlamps and tanning beds, and wear protective clothing to prevent photosensitivity reactions.
- Emphasize the importance of regular follow-up exams and blood tests to determine progress; monitor for side effects.

Evaluation/Desired Outcomes

- Decreased spread of prostate carcinoma.

bisacodyl (bis-a-**koe**-dill)

Bisac-Evac, ✱Bisacolax, Biscolax, ✱Carter's Little Pills, ✱Codulax, Correctol, Dacodyl, Doxidan, Dulcolax, Ex-Lax Ultra, Femilax, Fleet Laxative, ✱Soflax-Ex

Classification
Therapeutic: laxatives
Pharmacologic: stimulant laxatives

Pregnancy Category C

Indications

Treatment of constipation. Evacuation of the bowel before radiologic studies or surgery. Part of a bowel regimen in spinal cord injury patients.

Action

Stimulates peristalsis. Alters fluid and electrolyte transport, producing fluid accumulation in the colon. **Therapeutic Effects:** Evacuation of the colon.

Pharmacokinetics

Absorption: Variable absorption follows oral administration; rectal absorption is minimal; action is local in the colon.
Distribution: Small amounts of metabolites excreted in breast milk.
Metabolism and Excretion: Small amounts absorbed are metabolized by the liver.
Half-life: Unknown.

TIME/ACTION PROFILE (evacuation of bowel)

ROUTE	ONSET	PEAK	DURATION
PO	6–12 hr	unknown	unknown
Rectal	15–60 min	unknown	unknown

Contraindications/Precautions

Contraindicated in: Hypersensitivity; Abdominal pain; Obstruction; Nausea or vomiting (especially with fever or other signs of an acute abdomen).
Use Cautiously in: Severe cardiovascular disease; Anal or rectal fissures; Excess or prolonged use (may result in dependence); OB, Lactation: May be used during pregnancy and lactation.

Adverse Reactions/Side Effects

GI: abdominal cramps, nausea, diarrhea, rectal burning. **F and E:** hypokalemia (with chronic use). **MS:** muscle weakness (with chronic use). **Misc:** protein-losing enteropathy, tetany (with chronic use).

Interactions

Drug-Drug: Antacids, histamine H_2-receptor antagonists, and **gastric acid–pump inhibitors** may remove enteric coating of tablets resulting in gastric irritation/dyspepsia. May ↓ the absorption of other **orally administered drugs** because of ↑ motility and ↓ transit time.
Drug-Food: Milk may remove enteric coating of tablets, resulting in gastric irritation/dyspepsia.

Route/Dosage

PO (Adults and Children ≥12 yr): 5–15 mg/day (up to 30 mg/day) as a single dose.
PO (Children 3–11 yr): 5–10 mg/day (0.3 mg/kg) as a single dose.
Rect (Adults and Children ≥12 yr): 10 mg/day single dose.
Rect (Children 2–11 yr): 5–10 mg/day single dose.
Rect (Children <2 yr): 5 mg/day single dose.

Availability (generic available)

Enteric-coated tablets: 5 mg[OTC]. **Enteric coated and delayed release:** 5 mg[OTC]. **Suppositories:** 10 mg[OTC]. **Rectal solution:** 10 mg/30 mL[OTC]. ***In combination with:*** In Bowel Preparation kits with Magnesium citrate (Evac-Q-Kwik[OTC], EZ-EM Prep Kit[OTC], LiquiPrep Bowel Evacuant[OTC], Tridate Bowel Cleansing Kit[OTC]), Phosphate/biphosphate (Fleet Prep Kit. No. 1[OTC], Fleet Prep Kit No.2[OTC], Fleet Prep Kit No.3[OTC]), sennosides (X-Prep Bowel Evacuant Kit #1[OTC]), sennosides, magnesium citrate, magnesium sulfate (X-Prep Bowel Evacuant Kit #2[OTC]). See Appendix B.

NURSING IMPLICATIONS

Assessment

- Assess patient for abdominal distention, presence of bowel sounds, and usual pattern of bowel function.
- Assess color, consistency, and amount of stool produced.

Potential Nursing Diagnoses

Constipation (Indications)

Implementation

- Do not confuse Dulcolax (bisacodyl) with Dulcolax (docusate sodium).
- May be administered at bedtime for morning results.
- **PO:** Taking on an empty stomach will produce more rapid results.
- Do not crush or chew enteric-coated tablets. Take with a full glass of water or juice.
- Do not administer oral doses within 1 hr of milk or antacids; this may lead to premature dissolution of tablet and gastric or duodenal irritation.
- **Rect:** Suppository or enema can be given at the time a bowel movement is desired. Lubricate suppositories with water or water-soluble lubricant before insertion. Encourage patient to retain the suppository or enema 15–30 min before expelling.

Patient/Family Teaching

- Advise patients, other than those with spinal cord injuries, that laxatives should be used only for short-term therapy. Prolonged therapy may cause electrolyte imbalance and dependence.
- Advise patient to increase fluid intake to at least 1500–2000 mL/day during therapy to prevent dehydration.
- Encourage patients to use other forms of bowel regulation (increasing bulk in the diet, increasing fluid intake, or increasing mobility). Normal bowel habits may vary from 3 times/day to 3 times/wk.
- Instruct patients with cardiac disease to avoid straining during bowel movements (Valsalva maneuver).
- Advise patient that bisacodyl should not be used when constipation is accompanied by abdominal pain, fever, nausea, or vomiting.

Evaluation/Desired Outcomes

- Soft, formed bowel movement when used for constipation.
- Evacuation of colon before surgery or radiologic studies, or for patients with spinal cord injuries.

bismuth subsalicylate

(**biz**-muth sub-sa-**lis**-i-late)

Bismatrol, Kaopectate, Kao-Tin, Kapectolin, Peptic Relief, Pepto-Bismol

Classification

Therapeutic: antidiarrheals, antiulcer agents

Pharmacologic: adsorbents

Pregnancy Category C

Indications

Mild to moderate diarrhea. Nausea, abdominal cramping, heartburn, and indigestion that may accompany diarrheal illnesses. Treatment of ulcer disease associated with *Helicobacter pylori* (with anti-infectives). Treatment/prevention of traveler's (enterotoxigenic *Escherichia coli*) diarrhea. **Unlabeled Use:** Chronic infantile diarrhea.

Action

Promotes intestinal adsorption of fluids and electrolytes. Decreases synthesis of intestinal prostaglandins. **Therapeutic Effects:** Relief of diarrhea. Eradication of *H. pylori* with decreased recurrence of ulcer disease (with other agents).

Pharmacokinetics

Absorption: Bismuth is not absorbed; salicylate split from parent compound is >90% absorbed from the small intestine. Salicylate is highly bound to albumin.

Distribution: Salicylate crosses the placenta and enters breast milk.

Metabolism and Excretion: Bismuth is excreted unchanged in the feces. Salicylate undergoes extensive hepatic metabolism.

Half-life: Salicylate—2–3 hr for low doses; 15–30 hr with larger doses.

TIME/ACTION PROFILE (relief of diarrhea and other GI symptoms)

ROUTE	ONSET	PEAK	DURATION
PO	within 24 hr	unknown	unknown

Contraindications/Precautions

Contraindicated in: Aspirin hypersensitivity; cross-sensitivity with NSAIDs or oil of wintergreen may occur. Pedi: During or after recovery from chickenpox or flu-like illness (contains salicylate, which can cause Reye's syndrome); Geri: Geriatric patients who may have fecal impaction.

Use Cautiously in: Patients undergoing radiologic examination of the GI tract (bismuth is radiopaque); Diabetes mellitus; Gout; OB, Lactation: Safety not established; avoid chronic use of large doses; Pedi, Geri: Potential for impaction.

Adverse Reactions/Side Effects

GI: constipation, gray-black stools, impaction (infants, debilitated patients).

Interactions

Drug-Drug: If taken with **aspirin**, may ↑ the risk of salicylate toxicity. May ↓ absorption of **tetracycline** or **fluoroquinolones** (separate administration by 2–4 hr). May ↓ effectiveness of **probenecid** (large doses).

Route/Dosage

PO (Adults): *Antidiarrheal*—2 tablets or 30 mL (15 mL of extra/maximum strength) q 30 min *or* 2 tablets q 60 min as needed (not to exceed 4.2 g/24 hr). *Antiulcer*—524 mg 4 times daily (as 2 tablets, 30 mL of regular strength suspension or 15 mL of extra/maximum strength).

PO (Children 9–12 yr): 1 tablet or 15 mL (7.5 mL of extra/maximum strength) q 30–60 min (not to exceed 2.1 g/24 hr).

PO (Children 6–9 yr): 10 mL (5 mL of extra/maximum strength) q 30–60 min (not to exceed 1.4 g/24 hr).

PO (Children 3–6 yr): 5 mL (2.5 mL of extra/maximum strength) q 30–60 min (not to exceed 704 mg/24 hr).

Availability (generic available)

Tablets: 262 mg^OTC^. **Chewable tablets (cherry and other flavors):** 262 mg^OTC^, ✱300 mg^OTC^. **Liquid (cherry, caramel, peppermint, and other flavors):** 262 mg/15 mL^OTC^, ✱264 mg/15 mL^OTC^, 525 mg/15 mL^OTC^. ***In combination with:*** metronidazole and tetracycline (Pylera—combination capsule). See Appendix B.

NURSING IMPLICATIONS

Assessment

- **Diarrhea:** Assess the frequency and consistency of stools, presence of nausea and indigestion, and bowel sounds before and during therapy.
- Assess fluid and electrolyte balance and skin turgor for dehydration if diarrhea is prolonged.
- **Ulcers:** Assess for epigastric or abdominal pain and frank or occult blood in the stool, emesis, or gastric aspirate.
- ***Lab Test Considerations:*** Chronic high doses may cause falsely ↑ uric acid levels with colorimetric assay.
- May interfere with radiologic examination of the GI tract.
- May cause abnormal results with alkaline phosphatase, AST, and ALT tests.
- May cause ↓ potassium levels and serum T_3 and T_4 concentrations.
- Large doses of salicylates may also cause prolonged prothrombin time (PT).
- For additional lab test considerations related to salicylate content, see salicylates monograph.

Potential Nursing Diagnoses

Diarrhea (Indications)
Constipation (Side Effects)

Implementation

- Do not confuse Kaopectate (bismuth subsalicylate) with Kaopectate Stool Softener (docusate calcium).
- **PO:** Shake liquid before using. Chewable tablets may be chewed or allowed to dissolve before swallowing.

Patient/Family Teaching

- Instruct patient to take medication exactly as directed.
- Inform patient that medication may temporarily cause stools and tongue to appear gray-black.
- Instruct patient that this medication contains aspirin. Advise patient taking concurrent aspirin products to discontinue bismuth subsalicylate if tinnitus, ringing in the ears, occurs.
- **Diarrhea:** Instruct patient to notify health care professional if diarrhea persists for more than 2 days or if accompanied by a high fever.
- U.S. Centers for Disease Control and Prevention warn against giving salicylates to children or adolescents with varicella (chickenpox) or influenza-like or viral illnesses because of a possible association with Reye's syndrome.
- **Ulcers:** Advise patient to consult health care professional before taking other OTC ulcer remedies concurrently with bismuth subsalicylate.

Evaluation/Desired Outcomes

- Decrease in diarrhea.
- Decrease in symptoms of indigestion.
- Prevention of traveler's diarrhea.
- Treatment of ulcers.

bisoprolol (bis-oh-proe-lol)

Zebeta

Classification
Therapeutic: antihypertensives
Pharmacologic: beta blockers

Pregnancy Category C

Indications

Management of hypertension.

Action

Blocks stimulation of $beta_1$ (myocardial)-adrenergic receptors. Does not usually affect $beta_2$ (pulmonary, vascular, uterine)-receptor sites. **Therapeutic Effects:** Decreased BP and heart rate.

Pharmacokinetics

Absorption: Well absorbed after oral administration, but 20% undergoes first-pass hepatic metabolism.

Distribution: Unknown.

Metabolism and Excretion: 50% excreted unchanged by the kidneys; remainder renally excreted as metabolites; 2% excreted in feces.

Half-life: 9–12 hr.

TIME/ACTION PROFILE (antihypertensive effect)

ROUTE	ONSET	PEAK	DURATION
PO	unknown	1–4 hr	24 hr

Contraindications/Precautions

Contraindicated in: Uncompensated HF; Pulmonary edema; Cardiogenic shock; Bradycardia or heart block.

Use Cautiously in: Renal impairment (dosage ↓ recommended); Hepatic impairment (dosage ↓ recommended); Pulmonary disease (including asthma; $beta_1$ selectivity may be lost at higher doses); avoid use if possible; Diabetes mellitus (may mask signs of hypoglycemia); Thyrotoxicosis (may mask symptoms); Patients with a history of severe allergic reactions (intensity of reactions may be ↑); OB, Lactation, Pedi: Safety not established; crosses the placenta and may cause fetal/neonatal bradycardia, hypotension, hypoglycemia, or respiratory depression; Geri: ↑ sensitivity to beta blockers; initial dosage ↓ recommended.

Adverse Reactions/Side Effects

CNS: fatigue, weakness, anxiety, depression, dizziness, drowsiness, insomnia, memory loss, mental status changes, nervousness, nightmares. **EENT:** blurred vision, stuffy nose. **Resp:** bronchospasm, wheezing. **CV:** BRADYCARDIA, HF, PULMONARY EDEMA, hypotension, peripheral vasoconstriction. **GI:** constipation, diarrhea, ↑ liver function tests, nausea, vomiting. **GU:** erectile dysfunction, ↓ libido, urinary frequency. **Derm:** rash. **Endo:** hyperglycemia, hypoglycemia. **MS:** arthralgia, back pain, joint pain. **Misc:** drug-induced lupus syndrome.

Interactions

Drug-Drug: General anesthetics, **IV phenytoin**, and **verapamil** may cause additive myocardial depression. Additive bradycardia may occur with **digoxin**, **diltiazem**, **verapamil**, or **clonidine**. Additive hypotension may occur with other **antihypertensives**, acute ingestion of **alcohol**, or **nitrates**. Concurrent use with **amphetamine**, **cocaine**, **ephedrine**, **epinephrine**, **norepinephrine**, **phenylephrine**, or **pseudoephedrine** may result in unopposed alpha-adrenergic stimulation (excessive hypertension, bradycardia). Concurrent thyroid preparation administration may ↓ effectiveness. May alter the effectiveness of **insulins** or **oral hypoglycemic agents** (dose adjustments may be necessary). May ↓ the effectiveness of **theophylline**. May ↓ the $beta_1$-cardiovascular effects of **dopamine** or **dobutamine**. Use cautiously within 14 days of **MAO inhibitor** therapy (may result in hypertension).

Route/Dosage

PO (Adults): 5 mg once daily, may be ↑ to 10 mg once daily (range 2.5–20 mg/day).

Renal Impairment

Hepatic Impairment

PO (Adults): *CCr <40 mL/min*—Initiate therapy with 2.5 mg/day, titrate cautiously.

Availability (generic available)

Tablets: 5 mg, 10 mg. ***In combination with:*** hydrochlorothiazide (Ziac). See Appendix B.

NURSING IMPLICATIONS

Assessment

- Monitor BP, ECG, and pulse frequently during dosage adjustment period and periodically throughout therapy.
- Monitor intake and output ratios and daily weights. Assess routinely for signs and symptoms of HF (dyspnea, rales/crackles, weight gain, peripheral edema, jugular venous distention).
- Monitor frequency of prescription refills to determine adherence.
- ***Lab Test Considerations:*** May cause increased BUN, serum lipoprotein, potassium, triglyceride, and uric acid levels.
- May cause increased ANA titers.
- May cause increase in blood glucose levels.

Potential Nursing Diagnoses

Decreased cardiac output (Side Effects)
Noncompliance (Patient/Family Teaching)

Implementation

- Do not confuse Zebeta with Diabeta or Zetia.
- **PO:** Take apical pulse before administering. If <50 bpm or if arrhythmia occurs, withhold medication and notify physician or other health care professional.
- May be administered without regard to meals.

Patient/Family Teaching

- Instruct patient to take medication exactly as directed, at the same time each day, even if feeling well; do not skip or double up on missed doses. If a dose is missed, it should be taken as soon as possible up to 4 hr before next dose. Abrupt withdrawal may precipitate life-threatening arrhythmias, hypertension, or myocardial ischemia.
- Teach patient and family how to check pulse and BP. Instruct them to check pulse daily and BP biweekly and to report significant changes to health care professional.
- May cause drowsiness. Caution patients to avoid driving or other activities that require alertness until response to the drug is known.

- Advise patients to change positions slowly to minimize orthostatic hypotension.
- Caution patient that this medication may increase sensitivity to cold.
- Instruct patient to notify health care professional of all Rx or OTC medications, vitamins, or herbal products being taken and to consult health care professional before taking any Rx, OTC, or herbal products, especially cold preparations, concurrently with this medication. Patients on antihypertensive therapy should also avoid excessive amounts of coffee, tea, and cola.
- Diabetics should closely monitor blood glucose, especially if weakness, malaise, irritability, or fatigue occurs. Medication does not block dizziness or sweating as signs of hypoglycemia.
- Advise patient to notify health care professional if slow pulse, difficulty breathing, wheezing, cold hands and feet, dizziness, light-headedness, confusion, depression, rash, fever, sore throat, unusual bleeding, or bruising occurs.
- Instruct patient to inform health care professional of medication regimen before treatment or surgery.
- Advise patient to carry identification describing disease process and medication regimen at all times.
- **Hypertension:** Reinforce the need to continue additional therapies for hypertension (weight loss, sodium restriction, stress reduction, regular exercise, moderation of alcohol consumption, and smoking cessation). Medication controls but does not cure hypertension.

Evaluation/Desired Outcomes

- Decrease in BP.

HIGH ALERT

bivalirudin (bi-val-i-**roo**-din)

Angiomax

Classification

Therapeutic: anticoagulants

Pharmacologic: thrombin inhibitors

Pregnancy Category B

Indications

Used in conjunction with aspirin to reduce the risk of acute ischemic complications in patients with unstable angina who are undergoing percutaneous transluminal angioplasty (PCTA) or percutaneous coronary intervention (PCI). Patients with or at risk of heparin-induced thrombocytopenia (HIT) and thrombosis syndrome (HITTS) who are undergoing PCI.

Action

Specifically and reversibly inhibits thrombin by binding to its receptor sites. Inhibition of thrombin prevents activation of factors V, VIII, and XII; the conversion of fibrinogen to fibrin; platelet adhesion and aggregation. **Therapeutic Effects:** Decreased acute ischemic complications in patients with unstable angina (death, MI, or the urgent need for revascularization procedures).

Pharmacokinetics

Absorption: IV administration results in complete bioavailability.

Distribution: Unknown.

Metabolism and Excretion: Cleared from plasma by a combination of renal mechanisms and proteolytic breakdown.

Half-life: 25 min (↑ in renal impairment).

TIME/ACTION PROFILE (anticoagulant effect)

ROUTE	ONSET	PEAK	DURATION
IV	immediate	unknown	1–2 hr

Contraindications/Precautions

Contraindicated in: Active major bleeding; Hypersensitivity.

Use Cautiously in: Any disease state associated with an ↑ risk of bleeding; Heparin-induced thrombocytopenia or heparin-induced thrombocytopenia-thrombosis syndrome; Patients with unstable angina not undergoing PTCA; Patients with other acute coronary syndromes; Concurrent use with other platelet aggregation inhibitors (safety not established); Renal impairment (↓ infusion rate if GFR <30 mL/min); Lactation, Pedi: Safety not established; OB: Use only if clearly needed.

Adverse Reactions/Side Effects

CNS: headache, anxiety, insomnia, nervousness. **CV:** hypotension, bradycardia, hypertension. **GI:** nausea, abdominal pain, dyspepsia, vomiting. **Hemat:** BLEEDING. **Local:** injection site pain. **MS:** back pain. **Misc:** pain, fever, pelvic pain.

Interactions

Drug-Drug: Risk of bleeding may be ↑ by concurrent use of **abciximab**, **heparin**, **low molecular weight heparins**, **clopidogrel**, **thrombolytics**, or any other **drugs that inhibit coagulation**.

Drug-Natural Products: ↑ risk of bleeding with **arnica**, **chamomile**, **clove**, **dong quai**, **feverfew**, **garlic**, **ginger**, **gingko**, **Panax ginseng**, and others.

Route/Dosage

IV (Adults): 0.75 mg/kg as a bolus injection, followed by an infusion at a rate of 1.75 mg/kg/hr for the duration of the PCI procedure. An activated clotting time (ACT) should be performed 5 min after bolus dose and an additional bolus dose of 0.3 mg/kg may be administered if needed. Continuation of the infusion (at a rate of 1.75 mg/kg/hr) for up to 4 hr post-procedure is optional. If needed, the infusion may be continued beyond this initial 4 hr at a rate of 0.2 mg/kg/hr for up to 20 hr. Therapy should be initiated prior to the procedure and given in conjunction with aspirin.

B

Renal Impairment

IV (Adults): No ↓ in the bolus dose is needed in any patient with renal impairment. *GFR 10–29 mL/min*—↓ infusion rate to 1 mg/kg/hr; *Dialysis-dependent patients (off dialysis)*—↓ infusion rate to 0.25 mg/kg/hr. ACT should be monitored in all patients with renal impairment.

Availability (generic available)

Powder for injection: 250 mg/vial.

NURSING IMPLICATIONS

Assessment

- Assess for bleeding. Most common is oozing from the arterial access site for cardiac catheterization. Arterial and venous punctures, IM injections, and use of urinary catheters, nasotracheal intubation, and nasogastric tubes should be minimized. Noncompressible sites for IV access should be avoided. If bleeding cannot be controlled with pressure, discontinue bivalirudin immediately.
- Monitor vital signs. May cause bradycardia, hypertension, or hypotension. An unexplained decrease in BP may indicate hemorrhage.
- ***Lab Test Considerations:*** Assess hemoglobin, hematocrit, and platelet count prior to bivalirudin therapy and periodically during therapy. May cause ↓ hemoglobin and hematocrit. An unexplained ↓ in hematocrit may indicate hemorrhage.
- Monitor ACT periodically in patients with renal dysfunction.

Potential Nursing Diagnoses

Ineffective tissue perfusion (Indications)

Implementation

- Administer IV just prior to PTCA, in conjunction with aspirin 300 mg to 325 mg/day. Do not administer IM.

IV Administration

- **IV Push:** (for bolus dose) Reconstitute each 250-mg vial with 5 mL of sterile water for injection. Reconstituted vials are stable for 24 hr if refrigerated. ***Diluent:*** Further dilute in 50 mL of D5W or 0.9% NaCl. Withdraw bolus dose out of bag. Infusion is stable for 24 hr at room temperature. ***Concentration:*** Final concentration of infusion is 5 mg/mL. ***Rate:*** Administer as a bolus injection.
- **Intermittent Infusion:** Reconstitute each 250-mg vial as per the above directions. ***Diluent:*** Further dilute in 50 mL of D5W or 0.9% NaCl. If infusion is to be continued after 4 hr (at a rate of 0.2 mg/kg/hr), reconstituted vial should be diluted in 500 mL of D5W or 0.9% NaCl. Infusion is stable for 24 hr at room temperature. ***Concentration:*** 5 mg/mL (for infusion rate of 1.75 mg/kg/hr); 0.5 mg/mL (for infusion rate of 0.2 mg/kg/hr). ***Rate:*** Based on patient's weight (see Route/Dosage section).
- **Y-Site Compatibility:** acyclovir, alfentanil, allopurinol, amifostine, amikacin, aminocaproic acid, aminophylline, amphotericin B liposome, ampicillin, ampicillin-sulbactam, anidulafungin, argatroban, arsenic trioxide, atropine, azithromycin, aztreonam, bleomycin, bumetanide, buprenorphine, busulfan, butorphanol, calcium chloride, calcium gluconate, cangrelor, carboplatin, carmustine, cefazolin, cefepime, cefotaxime, cefotetan, cefoxitin, ceftazidime, ceftriaxone, cefuroxime, chloramphenicol, ciprofloxacin, cisatracurium, cisplatin, clindamycin, cyclophosphamide, cyclosporine, cytarabine, dacarbazine, dactinomycin, daptomycin, daunorubicin, dexamethasone, dexmedetomidine, dexrazoxane, digoxin, diltiazem, diphenhydramine, docetaxel, dolasetron, dopamine, doxorubicin, doxorubicin liposome, doxycycline, droperidol, enalaprilat, ephedrine, epinephrine, epirubicin, epoprostenol, eptifibatide, ertapenem, erythromycin, esmolol, etoposide, etoposide phosphate, famotidine, fenoldopam, fentanyl, fluconazole, fludarabine, fluorouracil, foscarnet, fosphenytoin, furosemide, ganciclovir, gemcitabine, gentamicin, glycopyrrolate, granisetron, heparin, hydralazine, hydrocortisone, hydromorphone, idarubicin, ifosfamide, imipenem/cilastatin, insulin, irinotecan, isoproterenol, ketorolac, leucovorin, levofloxacin, lidocaine, linezolid, magnesium sulfate, mannitol, mechlorethamine, melaphalan, meperidine, meropenem, mesna, methohexital, methotrexate, methylprednisolone, metoclopramide, metoprolol, metronidazole, midazolam, milrinone, mitomycin, mitoxantrone, morphine, moxifloxacin, mycophenolate, nafcillin, nalbuphine, naloxone, nesiritide, nicardipine, nitroglycerin, nitroprusside, norepinephrine, octreotide, ondansetron, oxaliplatin, oxytocin, paclitaxel, palonosetron, pamidronate, pancuronium, pemetrexed, pentobarbital, phenobarbital, phenylephrine, piperacillin-tazobactam, potassium acetate, potassium chloride, potassium phosphates, procainamide, propranolol, ranitidine, remifentanil, rocuronium, sodium acetate, sodium bicarbonate, sodium phosphates, streptozocin, succinylcholine, sufentanil, tacrolimus, teniposide, theophylline, thiopental, thiotepa, tigecycline, tirofiban, tobramycin, topotecan, trimethoprim/sulfamethoxazole, vasopressin, vecuronium, verapamil, vinblastine, vincristine, vinorelbine, voriconazole, warfarin, zidovudine, zoledronic acid.
- **Y-Site Incompatibility:** alteplase, amiodarone, amphotericin B colloidal, amphotericin B lipid complex, caspofungin, chlorpromazine, dantrolene, diazepam, pentamidine, pentazocine, phenytoin, pro-

chlorperazine, quinupristin/dalfopristin, reteplase, streptokinase, vancomycin.

Patient/Family Teaching

- Inform patient of the purpose of bivalirudin.
- Instruct patient to notify health care professional immediately if any bleeding or bruising is noted.
- Instruct patient to notify health care professional of all Rx or OTC medications, vitamins, or herbal products being taken and consult health care professional before taking any new medications.

Evaluation/Desired Outcomes

- Decreased acute ischemic complications in patients with unstable angina (death, MI or the urgent need for revascularization procedures).

HIGH ALERT

bleomycin (blee-oh-mye-sin)

Blenoxane

Classification

Therapeutic: antineoplastics

Pharmacologic: antitumor antibiotics

Pregnancy Category D

Indications

Treatment of: Lymphomas, Squamous cell carcinoma, Testicular embryonal cell carcinoma, Choriocarcinoma, Teratocarcinoma. Intrapleural administration to prevent the reaccumulation of malignant effusions.

Action

Inhibits DNA and RNA synthesis. **Therapeutic Effects:** Death of rapidly replicating cells, particularly malignant ones.

Pharmacokinetics

Absorption: Well absorbed from IM and subcut sites. Absorption follows intrapleural and intraperitoneal administration.

Distribution: Widely distributed, concentrates in skin, lungs, peritoneum, kidneys, and lymphatics.

Metabolism and Excretion: 60–70% excreted unchanged by the kidneys.

Half-life: 2 hr (↑ in renal impairment).

TIME/ACTION PROFILE (tumor response)

ROUTE	ONSET	PEAK	DURATION
IV, IM, Subcut	2–3 wk	unknown	unknown

Contraindications/Precautions

Contraindicated in: Hypersensitivity; OB, Lactation: Potential for fetal, infant harm.

Use Cautiously in: Renal impairment (dose ↓ required if CCr <35 mL/min); Pulmonary impairment; Nonmalignant chronic debilitating illness; Patients with childbearing potential; Geri: ↑ risk of pulmonary toxicity and reduction in renal function.

Adverse Reactions/Side Effects

CNS: aggressive behavior, disorientation, weakness. **Resp:** PULMONARY FIBROSIS, pneumonitis. **CV:** hypotension, peripheral vasoconstriction. **GI:** anorexia, nausea, stomatitis, vomiting. **Derm:** hyperpigmentation, mucocutaneous toxicity, alopecia, erythema, rashes, urticaria, vesiculation. **Hemat:** anemia, leukopenia, thrombocytopenia. **Local:** pain at tumor site, phlebitis at IV site. **Metab:** weight loss. **Misc:** ANAPHYLACTOID REACTIONS, chills, fever.

Interactions

Drug-Drug: Hematologic toxicity ↑ with concurrent use of **radiation therapy** and other **antineoplastics**. Concurrent use with **cisplatin** ↓ elimination of bleomycin and may ↑ toxicity. ↑ risk of pulmonary toxicity with other **antineoplastics** or thoracic **radiation therapy**. **General anesthesia** ↑ the risk of pulmonary toxicity. ↑ risk of Raynaud's phenomenon when used with **vinblastine**.

Route/Dosage

Lymphoma patients should receive initial test doses of 2 units or less for the first 2 doses.

IV, IM, Subcut (Adults and Children): 0.25–0.5 unit/kg (10–20 units/m^2) weekly or twice weekly initially. If favorable response, lower maintenance doses given (1 unit/day or 5 units/wk IM or IV). May also be given as continuous IV infusion at 0.25 unit/kg or 15 units/m^2/day for 4–5 days.

Intrapleural (Adults): 15–20 units instilled for 4 hr, then removed.

Availability (generic available)

Injection: 15 units/vial, 30 units/vial.

NURSING IMPLICATIONS

Assessment

- Monitor vital signs before and frequently during therapy.
- Assess for fever and chills. May occur 3–6 hr after administration and last 4–12 hr.
- Monitor for anaphylactic (fever, chills, hypotension, wheezing) and idiosyncratic (confusion, hypotension, fever, chills, wheezing) reactions. Keep resuscitation equipment and medications on hand. Lymphoma patients are at particular risk for idiosyncratic reactions that may occur immediately or several hours after therapy, usually after the first or second dose.
- Assess respiratory status for dyspnea and rales/crackles. Monitor chest x-ray before and periodically during therapy. Pulmonary toxicity occurs primarily in geriatric patients (age 70 or older) who have received 400 or more units or at lower doses in patients who received other antineoplastics or thoracic radiation. May occur 4–10 wk after therapy. Discontinue and do not resume bleomycin if pulmonary toxicity occurs.

- Assess nausea, vomiting, and appetite. Weigh weekly. Modify diet as tolerated. Antiemetics may be given before administration.
- ***Lab Test Considerations:*** Monitor CBC before and periodically during therapy. May cause thrombocytopenia and leukopenia (nadir occurs in 12 days and usually returns to pretreatment levels by day 17).
- Monitor baseline and periodic renal and hepatic function.

Potential Nursing Diagnoses

Risk for injury (Side Effects)
Disturbed body image (Side Effects)

Implementation

- ***High Alert:*** Fatalities have occurred with chemotherapeutic agents. Before administering, clarify all ambiguous orders; double-check single, daily, and course-of-therapy dose limits; have second practitioner independently double-check original order and dose calculations.
- Prepare solution in a biologic cabinet. Wear gloves, gown, and mask while handling medication. Discard equipment in specially designated containers.
- Lymphoma patients should receive a 1- or 2-unit test dose 2–4 hr before initiation of therapy. Monitor closely for anaphylactic reaction. May not detect reactors.
- Premedication with acetaminophen, corticosteroids, and diphenhydramine may reduce drug fever and risk of anaphylaxis.
- Reconstituted solution is stable for 24 hr at room temperature and for 14 days if refrigerated.
- **IM, Subcut:** Reconstitute vial with 1–5 mL of sterile water for injection, 0.9% NaCl, or bacteriostatic water for injection. Do not reconstitute with diluents containing benzyl alcohol when used for neonates.

IV Administration

- **Intermittent Infusion:** Prepare IV doses by diluting 15-unit vial with at least 5 mL of 0.9% NaCl. ***Diluent:*** Further dilute dose in 50 to 1000 mL of D5W or 0.9% NaCl. ***Rate:*** Administer slowly over 10 min.
- **Y-Site Compatibility:** allopurinol, amifostine, aminocaproic acid, aminophylline, amiodarone, anidulafungin, atracurium, aztreonam, bivalirudin, bumetanide, busulfan, calcium chloride, calcium gluconate, carboplatin, carmustine, caspofungin, cefepime, chlorpromazine, cimetidine, cisatracurium, cisplatin, codeine, cyclophosphamide, cyclosporine, cytarabine, dacarbazine, dactinomycin, daptomycin, daunorubicin, dexamethasone, dexmedetomidine, dexrazoxane, digoxin, diltiazem, diphenhydramine, dobutamine, docetaxel, dopamine, doxacurium, doxorubicin, doxorubicin liposome, droperidol, enalaprilat, epinephrine, epirubicin, ertapenem, esmolol, etoposide, etoposide phosphate, famotidine, fenoldopam, filgrastim, fludarabine, fluorouracil, fosphenytoin, furosemide, gemcitabine, glycopyrrolate, granisetron, haloperidol, heparin, hetastarch, hydralazine, hydrocortisone, idarubicin, ifosfamide, insulin, isoproterenol, ketorolac, labetalol, leucovorin calcium, levofloxacin, lidocaine, magnesium sulfate, mannitol, mechlorethamine, melphalan, meperidine, mesna, metaraminol, methotrexate, methyldopate, methylprednisolone, metoclopramide, metoprolol, milrinone, mitomycin, mitoxantrone, naloxone, nesiritide, nicardipine, nitroglycerin, norepinephrine, octreotide, ondansetron, oxaliplatin, paclitaxel, palonosetron, pancuronium, pantoprazole, pemetrexed, phentolamine, phenylephrine, piperacillin/tazobactam, potassium chloride, potassium phosphates, procainamide, quinupristin/dalfopristin, rituximab, sargramostim, sodium acetate, teniposide, thiotepa, tirofiban, trastuzumab, vinblastine, vincristine, vinorelbine, voriconazole.
- **Y-Site Incompatibility:** amphotericin B liposome, dantrolene, phenytoin, tigecycline.
- **Intrapleural:** Dissolve 60 units in 50–100 mL of 0.9% NaCl.
- May be administered through thoracotomy tube. Position patient as directed.

Patient/Family Teaching

- Instruct patient to notify health care professional if fever, chills, wheezing, faintness, diaphoresis, shortness of breath, prolonged nausea and vomiting, or mouth sores occur.
- Encourage patient not to smoke because this may worsen pulmonary toxicity.
- Explain to the patient that skin toxicity may manifest itself as skin sensitivity, hyperpigmentation (especially at skin folds and points of skin irritation), and skin rashes and thickening.
- Instruct patient to inspect oral mucosa for erythema and ulceration. If ulceration occurs, advise patient to use sponge brush and rinse mouth with water after eating and drinking. Opioid analgesics may be required if pain interferes with eating.
- Discuss with patient the possibility of hair loss. Explore coping strategies.
- Advise patient of the need for contraception during therapy.
- Instruct patient not to receive any vaccinations without advice of health care professional.
- Emphasize need for periodic lab tests to monitor for side effects.

Evaluation/Desired Outcomes

- Decrease in tumor size without evidence of hypersensitivity or pulmonary toxicity.

bortezomib (bor-tez-o-mib)

Velcade

Classification

Therapeutic: antineoplastics

Pharmacologic: proteasome inhibitors

Pregnancy Category D

Indications

Multiple myeloma (as initial therapy or after progression); with melphalan and prednisone. Mantle cell lymphoma.

Action

Inhibits proteasome, a regulator of intracellular protein catabolism, resulting in disruption of various intracellular processes. Cytotoxic to a variety of cancerous cells. **Therapeutic Effects:** Death of rapidly replicating cells, particularly malignant ones.

Pharmacokinetics

Absorption: IV administration results in complete bioavailability.

Distribution: Unknown.

Metabolism and Excretion: Mostly metabolized by the liver (P450 enzymes); excretion is unknown.

Half-life: 9–15 hr.

TIME/ACTION PROFILE

ROUTE	ONSET	PEAK	DURATION
IV	unknown	38 days*	unknown

*Median time to response based on clinical parameters.

Contraindications/Precautions

Contraindicated in: Hypersensitivity to bortezomib, boron, or mannitol; Intrathecal administration (may cause death); OB: Potential fetal harm; Lactation: Potential for serious adverse reaction in nursing infants.

Use Cautiously in: OB: Women with childbearing potential; Moderate to severe hepatic impairment (may ↑ levels, risk of toxicity); History of or risk factors for HF; Pedi: Safety not established.

Adverse Reactions/Side Effects

CNS: PROGRESSIVE MULTIFOCAL LEUKOENCEPHALOPATHY (PML), REVERSIBLE POSTERIOR LEUKOENCEPHALOPATHY SYNDROME (RPLS), fatigue, malaise, weakness, dizziness, syncope. **EENT:** blurred vision, diplopia. **CV:** hypotension, HF. **Resp:** pneumonia. **GI:** LIVER FAILURE, anorexia, constipation, diarrhea, nausea, vomiting. **Hemat:** BLEEDING, anemia, neutropenia, thrombocytopenia. **Neuro:** peripheral neuropathy. **Misc:** fever, tumor lysis syndrome.

Interactions

Drug-Drug: Concurrent neurotoxic medications including **amiodarone**, some **antivirals**, **nitrofurantoin**, **isoniazid**, or **HMG-CoA reductase inhibitors** may ↑ risk of peripheral neuropathy.

Route/Dosage

Previously Untreated Multiple Myeloma

IV, Subcut (Adults): 1.3 mg/m² twice weekly for Cycles 1–4 (days 1, 4, 8, 11, 22, 25, 29, and 32; no treatment during cycle 3), then once weekly for Cycles 5–9 (days 1, 8, 22, and 29; no treatment during Cycle 7); further cycles/doses depend on response and toxicity.

Previously Untreated Mantle Cell Lymphoma

IV, Subcut (Adults): 1.3 mg/m² twice weekly on days 1, 4, 8, and 11, followed by a 10–day rest (days 12–21); repeat for 5 additional cycles; further cycles/doses depend on response and toxicity.

Relapsed Multiple Myeloma and Mantle Cell Lymphoma

IV, Subcut (Adults): 1.3 mg/m² twice weekly for 2 wk (days 1, 4, 8, and 11), followed by a 10–day rest; further cycles/doses depend on response and toxicity. For patients with multiple myeloma who have previously responded to bortezomib therapy and who have relapsed ≥6 mo after prior bortezomib therapy can be started on their last tolerated dose; dose should be given twice weekly (days 1, 4, 8, and 11) q 3 wk for a maximum of 8 cycles.

Hepatic Impairment

IV (Adults): *Moderate or severe hepatic impairment*—0.7 mg/m² per injection for the first cycle, then may ↑ to 1 mg/m² per injection or ↓ further to 0.5 mg/m² per injection, based on tolerability.

Availability

Lyophilized powder for injection (requires reconstitution): 3.5 mg/vial.

NURSING IMPLICATIONS

Assessment

- Monitor vital signs frequently during therapy. May cause fever and orthostatic hypotension requiring adjustment of antihypertensives, hydration, or administration of mineralocorticoids.
- Monitor for GI adverse effects. May require antidiarrheals, antiemetics, and fluid and electrolyte replacement to prevent dehydration. Weigh weekly; modify diet as tolerated.
- Monitor for signs and symptoms of tumor lysis syndrome (tachypnea, tachycardia, hypotension, pulmonary edema). Patients with high tumor burden prior to treatment are at increased risk.
- Monitor for signs of RPLS (headache, seizure, lethargy, confusion, blindness). Hypertension may or may not be present. May occur with in 16 hr to 1 yr of initiation of therapy. Treat hypertension if present and discontinue bortezomib therapy. Symptoms usually resolve within days.

- Assess for any new signs or symptoms that may be suggestive of PML, an opportunistic infection of the brain caused by the JC virus, that leads to death or severe disability; withhold dose and notify health care professional promptly. PML symptoms may begin gradually but usually worsen rapidly. Symptoms vary depending on which part of brain is infected (mental function declines rapidly and progressively, causing dementia; speaking becomes increasingly difficult; partial blindness; difficulty walking; rarely, headaches and seizures occur). Diagnosis is usually made via gadolinium-enhanced MRI and CSF analysis. Risk of PML increases with the number of infusions. Withhold bortezomib at first sign of PML.
- ***Lab Test Considerations:*** Monitor CBC frequently during therapy. Assess platelet count before each dose. Dose modifications for hematologic toxicity are made based on indication and concurrent drug therapy; see manufacturer's recommendations. The nadir of thrombocytopenia is day 11 and recovery is usually by next cycle. Occurs more commonly in cycles 1 and 2, but may occur throughout therapy. May require discontinuation of therapy.
- Monitor blood glucose levels closely in patients taking oral hypoglycemic agents; may require adjustment of antidiabetic agent dose.

Potential Nursing Diagnoses

Risk for injury (Adverse Reactions)

Implementation

- Should be administered under the supervision of a physician experienced in the use of antineoplastic therapy.
- Solution should be prepared in a biologic cabinet. Wear gloves, gown, and mask while handling medication. Discard IV equipment in specially designated containers.

IV Administration

- **Subcut:** Reconstitute each vial with 1.4 mL of 0.9% NaCl. ***Concentration:*** 2.5 mg/mL. Solution should be clear and colorless; do not administer solutions that are discolored or contain particulate matter. May inject into thigh or abdomen; rotate injection sites. Inject into sites at least 1 inch from other sites and avoid tender, bruised, erythematous, or indurated sites. If local injection site reactions occur, may inject a less concentrated (1 mg/mL) solution.
- **IV Push:** Reconstitute each vial with 3.5 mL of 0.9% NaCl. Solution should be clear and colorless; do not administer solutions that are discolored or contain particulate matter. ***Concentration:*** 1 mg/mL. Administer reconstituted solution within 8 hr at room temperature; 3 of the 8 hr may be stored in a syringe. ***Rate:*** Administer as a 3–5 second bolus injection twice weekly for 2 wk followed by a 10-day rest period. At least 72 hr should elapse between consecutive doses.
- *If peripheral neuropathy is Grade 1 (paresthesia or loss of reflexes without pain or loss of function)* continue prescribed dose. *If paresthesia is Grade 1 with pain or Grade 2 (interfering with function but not with daily activities)* reduce dose to 1.0 mg/m^2. *If peripheral neuropathy is Grade 2 with pain or Grade 3 (interfering with activities of daily living)* withhold dose until toxicity resolves, then re-initiate with a reduced dose of 0.7 mg/m^2 and decrease frequency to once/wk. *If peripheral neuropathy is Grade 4 (permanent sensory loss that interferes with daily function)* discontinue bortezomib.

Patient/Family Teaching

- Caution the patient that dehydration may occur with vomiting or diarrhea. Advise patient to maintain fluid intake and to notify health care professional if dizziness or fainting occurs.
- Instruct patient to contact health care professional if they experience new or worsening signs of peripheral neuropathy (tingling, numbness, pain, burning feeling in the feet or hands, weakness in the arms or legs), PML (progressive weakness on one side of the body or clumsiness of limbs; disturbance of vision; changes in thinking, memory, and orientation leading to confusion and personality changes), or if symptoms of dehydration (dizziness, fainting) due to vomiting or diarrhea; rash; shortness of breath; cough; swelling of feet, ankles, or legs; convulsions; persistent headache; reduced eyesight; increase in BP or blurred vision occur.
- May cause dizziness and blurred vision. Caution patient to avoid driving or other activities requiring alertness until response to medication is known.
- Advise patient to notify health care professional of all Rx or OTC medications, vitamins, or herbal products being taken and consult health care professional before taking Rx, OTC, or herbal products, especially St. John's Wort.
- Advise diabetic patients taking oral hypoglycemic agents to monitor blood glucose frequently and notify health care professional of changes in blood sugar.
- Advise patient of the need for contraception and to avoid breast feeding during therapy. Patient should notify health care professional immediately if pregnancy is suspected.

Evaluation/Desired Outcomes

- Decrease in serum and urine myeloma protein.
- Decrease in size and spread of malignancy.

brentuximab
(bren-**tux**-i-mab)
Adcetris

Classification
Therapeutic: antineoplastics
Pharmacologic: drug-antibody conjugates

Pregnancy Category D

Indications
Treatment of Hodgkin's lymphoma in patients who have failed autologous hematopoietic stem cell transplant (auto-HSCT) or who have failed two prior multi-agent chemotherapies and are not candidates for auto-HSCT. Treatment of Hodgkin's lymphoma in patients who are at high risk of relapse or progression as post-auto-HSCT consolidation. Treatment of systemic anaplastic large cell lymphoma after failure of at least one multi-agent chemotherapy regimen.

Action
An antibody-drug conjugate (ADC) made up three parts: an antibody specific for human CD30 (cAC10, a cell membrane protein of the tumor necrosis factor receptor), a microtubule disrupting agent monomethyl auristatin (MMAE) and a protease-cleavable linker that attaches MMAE covalently to cAC10. The combination disrupts the intracellular microtubule network causing cell-cycle arrest and apoptotic cellular death. **Therapeutic Effects:** Decreased spread of lymphoma.

Pharmacokinetics
Absorption: IV administration results in complete bioavailability.
Distribution: Unknown.
Metabolism and Excretion: Small amounts of MMAE that are released are metabolized by the liver and eliminated mostly by the kidneys.
Half-life: *ADC*—4–6 days.

TIME/ACTION PROFILE (blood levels)

ROUTE	ONSET	PEAK	DURATION
IV (ADC)	unk	end of infusion	3 wk
IV (MMAE)	unk	1–3 days	3 wk

Contraindications/Precautions
Contraindicated in: Concurrent use of bleomycin (↑ risk of pulmonary toxicity); OB: Pregnancy; Severe renal impairment (CCr <30 mL/min); Moderate or severe hepatic impairment; Lactation: Breast feeding should be avoided.
Use Cautiously in: Geri: Safety and effectiveness not established; Pedi: Safety and effectiveness not established.

Adverse Reactions/Side Effects
CNS: PROGRESSIVE MULTIFOCAL LEUKOENCEPHALOPATHY (PML), anxiety, dizziness, fatigue, headache, insomia. **Resp:** ACUTE RESPIRATORY DISTRESS SYNDROME, INTERSTITIAL LUNG DISEASE, cough, dyspnea, oropharyngeal pain. **CV:** peripheral edema. **GI:** HEPATOTOXICITY, abdominal pain, constipation, ↓ appetite, diarrhea, nausea, vomiting. **Derm:** STEVENS-JOHNSON SYNDROME, TOXIC EPIDERMAL NECROLYSIS, alopecia, night sweats, pruritus, rash, dry skin. **Hemat:** NEUTROPENIA, THROMBOCYTOPENIA, anemia. **MS:** arthralgia, back pain, extremity pain, myalgia, muscle spasm. **Metab:** weight loss. **Neuro:** peripheral neuropathy. **Misc:** infusion reactions including ANAPHYLAXIS, TUMOR LYSIS SYNDROME, fever, lymphadenopathy, chills.

Interactions
Drug-Drug: MMAE is both a substrate and inhibitor of the CYP3A4/5 enyzyme system. **Bleomycin** may ↑ risk of pulmonary toxicity; concurrent use contraindicated. **Strong CYP3A4 inhibitors**, including **ketoconazole** may ↑ levels and risk of adverse reactions. **Strong CYP3A4 inducers**, including **rifampin**, may ↓ levels and effectiveness.

Route/Dosage
IV (Adults): 1.8 mg/kg (max dose = 180 mg) every 3 weeks until disease progression or unacceptable toxicity. For Hodgkin's lymphoma post-auto-HSCT consolidation treatment, initiate therapy within 4–6 wk post-auto-HSCT or upon recovery of auto-HSCT; treatment should be continued for a maximum of 16 cycles or until disease progression or unacceptable toxicity.

Renal Impairment
IV (Adults): *CCr <30 mL/min*—Avoid use.

Hepatic Impairment
IV (Adults): *Mild (Child-Pugh A)*—1.2 mg/kg (max dose = 120 mg) every 3 weeks until disease progression or unacceptable toxicity; *Moderate (Child-Pugh B) or severe (Child-Pugh C)*—Avoid use.

Availability
Lyophilized powder for IV injection (requires reconstitution): 50 mg/vial.

NURSING IMPLICATIONS

Assessment
- Monitor for signs and symptoms of peripheral neuropathy (hypoesthesia, hyperesthesia, paresthesia, discomfort, burning, neuropathic pain, weakness). For new or worsening neuropathy Grade 2 or 3, delay next dose until neuropathy improves to Grade 1 or baseline, then restart at 1.2 mg/kg.

- Assess for signs and symptoms of infusion-related reaction, including anaphylaxis (rash, pruritus, dyspnea, swelling of face and neck). If anaphylaxis occurs, discontinue infusion immediately; do not restart. Treat other infusion-related reactions by stopping and treating symptoms. Premedicate patient prior to subsequent infusions with acetaminophen, an antihistamine, and a corticosteroid.
- Monitor patient for tumor lysis syndrome due to rapid reduction in tumor volume (acute renal failure, hyperkalemia, hypocalcemia, hyperuricemia, or hypophosphatemia). Risks are higher in patients with greater tumor burden and rapidly proliferating tumors; may be fatal. Correct electrolyte abnormalities, monitor renal function and fluid balance, and administer supportive care, including dialysis, as indicated.
- Assess patient for skin rash frequently during therapy. Discontinue at first sign of rash; may be life-threatening. Stevens-Johnson syndrome may develop. Treat symptomatically; may recur once treatment is stopped.
- Assess for any new signs or symptoms that may be suggestive of PML, an opportunistic infection of the brain caused by the JC virus, that leads to death or severe disability; withhold dose and notify health care professional promptly. PML symptoms may begin gradually but usually worsen rapidly. Symptoms vary depending on which part of brain is infected (mental function declines rapidly and progressively, causing dementia; speaking becomes increasingly difficult; partial blindness; difficulty walking; rarely, headaches and seizures occur). Diagnosis is usually made via gadolinium-enhanced MRI and CSF analysis. Risk of PML increases with the number of infusions. Withhold brentuximab at first sign of PML.
- Monitor for signs and symptoms of pulmonary toxicity (cough, dyspnea) during therapy. If new or worsening pulmonary symptoms occur, hold brentuximab during assessment and until symptoms improve.
- ***Lab Test Considerations:*** Monitor CBC prior to each dose and more frequently in patients with Grade 3 or 4 neutropenia. Prolonged (≥1 wk) severe neutropenia may occur. Hold dose of brentuximab for Grade 3 or 4 neutropenia until resolution to baseline or Grade 2 or lower. Consider growth factor support for subsequent cycles for patients who developed Grade 3 or 4 neutropenia. Discontinue brentuximab or reduce dose to 1.2 mg/kg in patients with recurrent Grade 4 neutropenia despite use of growth factors.
- Monitor liver enzymes and bilirubin periodically during therapy. Signs of new, worsening, or recurrent hepatotoxicity may require decrease in dose, or interruption or discontinuation of therapy.

Potential Nursing Diagnoses

Risk for infection (Adverse Reactions)

Implementation

IV Administration

- **Intermittent Infusion:** Calculate dose and number of brentuximab vials needed. Calculate for 100 kg for patients weighing >100 kg. Reconstitute each 50 mg vial with 10.5 mL of Sterile Water for Injection for a concentration of 5 mg/mL. Direct stream to side of vial. Swirl gently; do not shake. Solution should be clear to slightly opalescent, and colorless. Do not administer solutions that are discolored or contain a precipitate. Withdraw volume of brentuximab dose from infusion bag of at least 100 mL. ***Diluent:*** 0.9% NaCl, D5W, or LR. Invert bag gently to mix. Dilute immediately into infusion bag or store solution in refrigerator; use within 24 hrs of reconstitution. Do not freeze. ***Rate:*** Infuse over 30 min. Do not administer as IV push or bolus.
- **Y-Site Incompatibility:** Do not administer with other products.

Patient/Family Teaching

- Instruct patient to notify health care professional of any numbness or tingling of hands or feet or any muscle weakness.
- Advise patient to notify health care professional immediately signs and symptoms of infection (fever of ≥100.5 F°, chills, cough, pain on urination), hepatotoxicity (fatigue, anorexia, right upper abdominal discomfort, dark urine, jaundice), PML (changes in mood or usual behavior, confusion, thinking problems, loss of memory, changes in vision, speech, or walking, decreased strength or weakness on one side of body), pulmonary toxicity, abdominal pain, or infusion reactions (fever, chills, rash, breathing problems within 24 hr of infusion) occur.
- Caution female of childbearing age to use effective contraception during therapy. Avoid pregnancy and breast feeding. If pregnancy is suspected, notify health care professional promptly.

Evaluation/Desired Outcomes

- Decreases spread of lymphoma.

brexpiprazole

(brex-**pip**-ra-zole)

Rexulti

Classification

Therapeutic: none assigned, antipsychotics, antidepressants

Pharmacologic: serotonin-dopamine activity modulators (SDAM)

Indications

Treatment of schizophrenia. Adjunctive treatment of major depressive disorder.

Action

Psychotropic activity may be due to partial agonist activity at dopamine D_2 and serotonin 5-HT_{1A} receptors and antagonist activity at the 5-HT_{2A} receptor. **Therapeutic Effects:** Decreased manifestations of schizophrenia including excitable, paranoic, or withdrawn behavior. Improvement in symptoms of depression with increased sense of wellbeing.

Pharmacokinetics

Absorption: Well absorbed (95%) following oral administration.
Distribution: Displays extravascular distribution.
Protein Binding: >99%.
Metabolism and Excretion: Metabolized by CYP3A4 and CYP2D6; 25% excreted in urine (<1% unchanged), 46% in feces (14% unchanged).
Half-life: 91 hr.

TIME/ACTION PROFILE (improvement in symptoms)

ROUTE	ONSET	PEAK	DURATION
PO (schizophrenia)	within 1–2 wk	4–6 wk	unknown
PO (depression)	within 1 wk	5 wk	unknown

Contraindications/Precautions

Contraindicated in: Hypersensitivity.
Use Cautiously in: History of seizures, concurrent use of medications that may ↓ seizure threshold; Pre-existing cardiovascular disease, dehydration, hypotension, concurrent antihypertensives, diuretics, electrolyte imbalance (↑ risk of orthostatic hypotension, correct deficits before treatment); Pre-existing low WBC (may ↑ risk of leukopenia/neutropenia; History of diabetes, metabolic syndrome or dyslipidemia (may exacerbate); Patients <24 yr (may ↑ suicidal ideation/behaviors, monitor carefully); Geri: Elderly patients with dementia-induced psychoses (↑ risk of serious adverse cardiovascular reactions and death), consider age, concurrent medical conditions and medications, renal/hepatic/cardiac function; Poor CYP2D6 metabolizers (PM), dose ↓ required; OB: Safe use in pregnancy has not been established, use during third trimester may result in extrapyramidal/withdrawal symptoms in infant; Lactation: Consider health benefits against risk of adverse effects in infant; Pedi: Safe and effective use in children has not been established (may ↑ suicidal ideation/behaviors).

Adverse Reactions/Side Effects

CNS: SEIZURES, abnormal dreams, dizziness, drowsiness, headache, restlessness. **EENT:** blurred vision. **CV:** cerebrovascular adverse reactions (↑ in elderly patients with dementia-related psychoses), orthostatic hyptension/syncope. **GI:** abdominal pain, constipation, diarrhea, dry mouth, dysphagia, excess salivation, flatulence. **Hemat:** agranulocytosis, leukopenia, neutropenia. **Metab:** ↑ appetite, ↑ weight, hyperglycemia/diabetes, dyslipidemia. **Neuro:** akathisia, dystonia, extrapyramidal symptoms, tardive dyskinesia, tremor. **Misc:** NEUROLEPTIC MALIGNANT SYNDROME, allergic reactions including ANAPHYLAXIS, body temperature dysregulation.

Interactions

Drug-Drug: Concurrent use with strong CYP3A4 inhibitors including **clarithromycin**, **itraconazole** or **ketoconazole**↑ blood levels, effects and risk of adverse reactions; ↓ dose of brexpiprazole required. Concurrent use with strong CYP2D6 inhibitors including **fluoxetine**, **paroxetine** or **quindine**↑ blood levels, effects and risk of adverse reactions; ↓ dose of brexpiprazole required. Combined use of **strong or moderate CYP3A4 inhibitors with strong or moderate CYP2D6 inhibitors** in addition to brexpiprazole including the following combinations **itraconazole + quinidine**, **fluconazole + paroxetine**, **itraconazole + duloxetine** or **fluconazole + duloxetine**↑ blood levels, effects and risk of toxicity; ↓ dose of brexpiprazole required. Concurrent use of **strong inducers of CYP3A4** including **rifampin**↓ blood levels and effectiveness; ↑ dose of brexpiprazole required. Concurrent use of **anithypertensives** or **diuretics** (↑ risk of hypotension). Concurrent use of **medications that may ↓ seizure threshhold** (↑ risk of seizures).
Drug-Natural Products: Concurrent use of **St. John's wort**↓ blood levels and effectiveness; ↑ dose of brexpiprazole required.

Route/Dosage

PO (Adults): *Schizophrenia*—1 mg daily initially, may be increased to 2–4 mg daily (not to exceed 4 mg daily); *Major depressive disorder*—0.5 or 1 mg daily initially, may be increased to 2 mg daily (not to exceed 3 mg daily); *known CYP2D6 poor metabolizers*—decrease usual dose by half. *Concurrent use of strong CYP2D6 inhibitors (schizophrenia only) or CYP3A4 inhibitors*—50% of the usual dose; *Concurrent use with strong/moderate CYP2D6 with strong/moderate CYP3A4 inhibitors*—25% of the usual dose; *Known CYP2D6 poor metabolizer taking concurrent strong/moderate CYP3A4 inhibitors*—25% of the usual dose; *Concurrent use of strong CCYP3A4 inducers*—double usual dose, titrate by clinical response.

Hepatic Impairment

PO (Adults): *Moderate to severe hepatic impairment [Child-Pugh score ≥7]*—maximum daily dose should not exceed 3 mg for schizophrenia or 2 mg for major depressive disorder.

Renal Impairment

PO (Adults): *Moderate/severe/end-stage renal impairment [CCr < 60 mL/min]*—maximum daily dose should not exceed 3 mg for schizophrenia or 2 mg for major depressive disorder.

Availability

Tablets: 0.25 mg, 0.25 mg, 0.5 mg, 1 mg, 2 mg, 3 mg, 4 mg.

NURSING IMPLICATIONS

Assessment

- Assess mental status (orientation, mood, behavior) before and periodically during therapy. Assess for suicidal tendencies, especially during early therapy for depression. Restrict amount of drug available to patient. Risk may be increased in children, adolescents, and adults ≤24 yrs.
- Assess weight and BMI initially and throughout therapy.
- Obtain fasting blood glucose and cholesterol levels initially and periodically during therapy.
- Monitor BP (sitting, standing, lying), pulse, and respiratory rate before and periodically during therapy.
- Observe patient carefully when administering medication to ensure that medication is actually taken and not hoarded or cheeked.
- Monitor patient for onset of akathisia (restlessness or desire to keep moving) and extrapyramidal side effects (*parkinsonian*—difficulty speaking or swallowing, loss of balance control, pill rolling of hands, masklike face, shuffling gait, rigidity, tremors; and *dystonic*—muscle spasms, twisting motions, twitching, inability to move eyes, weakness of arms or legs) periodically throughout therapy. Report these symptoms.
- Monitor for tardive dyskinesia (uncontrolled rhythmic movement of mouth, face, and extremities; lip smacking or puckering; puffing of cheeks; uncontrolled chewing; rapid or worm-like movements of tongue). Notify health care professional immediately if these symptoms occur, as these side effects may be irreversible.
- Monitor for development of neuroleptic malignant syndrome (fever, muscle rigidity, altered mental status, respiratory distress, tachycardia, seizures, diaphoresis, hypertension or hypotension, pallor, tiredness, loss of bladder control). Notify health care professional immediately if these symptoms occur.
- ***Lab Test Considerations:*** Monitor CBC frequently during initial months of therapy in patients with pre-existing or history of low WBC. May cause leukopenia, neutropenia, or agranulocytosis. Discontinue therapy if severe neutropenia (ANC <1000 mm^3 occurs).
- Monitor blood glucose and cholesterol levels initially and periodically during therapy.

Potential Nursing Diagnoses

Disturbed thought process (Indications)
Imbalanced nutrition: risk for more than body requirements (Side Effects)

Implementation

- **PO:** Administer once daily without regard to meals.

Patient/Family Teaching

- Advise patient to take medication as directed and not to skip doses or double up on missed doses. Take missed doses as soon as remembered unless almost time for the next dose. Do not stop taking brexpiprazole without consulting health care professional. Advise patient to read *Medication Guide* before starting and with each Rx refill in case of changes.
- Inform patient of possibility of extrapyramidal symptoms and tardive dyskinesia. Instruct patient to report these symptoms immediately.
- Advise patient to make position changes slowly to minimize orthostatic hypotension.
- Medication may cause drowsiness and lightheadedness. Caution patient to avoid driving or other activities requiring alertness until response to medication is known.
- Advise patient and family to notify health care professional if thoughts about suicide or dying, attempts to commit suicide; new or worse depression; new or worse anxiety; feeling very agitated or restless; panic attacks; trouble sleeping; new or worse irritability; acting aggressive; being angry or violent; acting on dangerous impulses; an extreme increase in activity and talking; other unusual changes in behavior or mood occur.
- Inform patient that brexipiprazole may cause weight gain. Advise patient to monitor weight periodically. Notify health care professional of significant weight gain.
- Instruct patient to notify health care professional of all Rx or OTC medications, vitamins, or herbal products being taken and to consult health care professional before taking any new medications. Caution patient to avoid taking alcohol or other CNS depressants concurrently with this medication.
- Advise patient that extremes in temperature should be avoided, because this drug impairs body temperature regulation.
- Advise patient to notify health care professional of medication regimen prior to treatment or surgery.
- Advise female patients to notify health care professional if pregnancy is planned or suspected and to avoid breast feeding during therapy. Encourage

pregnant patients to enroll in registry by contacting National Pregnancy Registry for Atypical Antipsychotics at 1-866-961-2388 or visit http://womensmentalhealth.org/clinical-and-research-programs/pregnancyregistry/.

- Emphasize the importance of routine follow-up exams and continued participation in psychotherapy as indicated.

Evaluation/Desired Outcomes

- Decrease in excitable, paranoic, or withdrawn behavior.
- Increased sense of wellbeing in patients with depression.

budesonide, See CORTICOSTEROIDS (INHALATION), CORTICOSTEROIDS (NASAL), and CORTICOSTEROIDS (SYSTEMIC).

bumetanide (byoo-**met**-a-nide)

~~Bumex~~, ✱Burinex

Classification
Therapeutic: diuretics
Pharmacologic: loop diuretics

Pregnancy Category C

Indications

Edema due to heart failure, hepatic disease, or renal impairment. **Unlabeled Use:** Reversal of oliguria in preterm neonates.

Action

Inhibits the reabsorption of sodium and chloride from the loop of Henle and distal renal tubule. Increases renal excretion of water, sodium chloride, magnesium, potassium, and calcium. Effectiveness persists in impaired renal function. **Therapeutic Effects:** Diuresis and subsequent mobilization of excess fluid (edema, pleural effusions).

Pharmacokinetics

Absorption: Well absorbed after oral or IM administration.

Distribution: Widely distributed.

Protein Binding: 72–96%.

Metabolism and Excretion: Partially metabolized by liver; 50% eliminated unchanged by kidneys and 20% excreted in feces.

Half-life: 60–90 min (6 hr in neonates).

TIME/ACTION PROFILE (diuretic effect)

ROUTE	ONSET	PEAK	DURATION
PO	30–60 min	1–2 hr	4–6 hr
IM	30–60 min	1–2 hr	4–6 hr
IV	2–3min	15–45 min	2–3 hr

Contraindications/Precautions

Contraindicated in: Hypersensitivity; Cross-sensitivity with thiazides and sulfonamides may occur; Hepatic coma or anuria.

Use Cautiously in: Severe liver disease (may precipitate hepatic coma; concurrent use with potassium-sparing diuretics may be necessary); Electrolyte depletion; Diabetes mellitus; Increasing azotemia; Lactation, Pedi: Safety not established; bumetanide is a potent displacer of bilirubin and should be used cautiously in critically ill or jaundiced neonates because of risk of kernicterus. Injection contains benzyl alcohol, which may cause gasping syndrome in neonates; Geri: May have ↑ risk of side effects, especially hypotension and electrolyte imbalance, at usual doses.

Adverse Reactions/Side Effects

CNS: dizziness, encephalopathy, headache. **EENT:** hearing loss, tinnitus. **CV:** hypotension. **GI:** diarrhea, dry mouth, nausea, vomiting. **GU:** ↑ BUN, excessive urination. **Derm:** STEVENS-JOHNSON SYNDROME, TOXIC EPIDERMAL NECROLYSIS, photosensitivity, pruritis, rash. **Endo:** hyperglycemia, hyperuricemia. **F and E:** dehydration, hypocalcemia, hypochloremia, hypokalemia, hypomagnesemia, hyponatremia, hypovolemia, metabolic alkalosis. **MS:** arthralgia, muscle cramps, myalgia.

Interactions

Drug-Drug: ↑ risk of hypotension with **antihypertensives**, **nitrates**, or acute ingestion of **alcohol**. ↑ risk of hypokalemia with other **diuretics**, **amphotericin B**, **stimulant laxatives**, and **corticosteroids**. Hypokalemia may ↑ risk of **digoxin** toxicity. ↓ **lithium** excretion, may cause **lithium** toxicity. ↑ risk of ototoxicity with **aminoglycosides**. **NSAIDS**↓ effects of bumetanide.

Route/Dosage

PO (Adults): 0.5–2 mg/day given in 1–2 doses; titrate to desired response (maximum daily dose = 10 mg/day).

PO (Infants and Children): 0.015–0.1 mg/kg/dose every 6–24 hrs (maximum: 10 mg/day).

PO (Neonates): 0.01–0.05 mg/kg/dose every 12–24 in term neonates or every 24–48 hrs in preterm neonates.

IM, IV (Adults): 0.5–1 mg/dose, may repeat q 2–3 hr as needed (up to 10 mg/day).

IM, IV (Infants and Children): 0.015–0.1 mg/kg/dose every 6–24 hrs (maximum: 10 mg/day).

IM, IV (Neonates): 0.01–0.05 mg/kg/dose every 12–24 in term neonates or every 24–48 hrs in preterm neonates.

Availability (generic available)

Tablets: 0.5 mg, 1 mg, 2 mg, ✱5 mg. **Cost:** *Generic*—0.5 mg $30.20/100, 1 mg $44.52/100, 2 mg $75.18/100. **Injection:** 0.25 mg/mL.

NURSING IMPLICATIONS

Assessment

- Assess fluid status during therapy. Monitor daily weight, intake and output ratios, amount and location of edema, lung sounds, skin turgor, and mucous membranes. Notify health care professional if thirst, dry mouth, lethargy, weakness, hypotension, or oliguria occurs.
- Monitor BP and pulse before and during administration. Monitor frequency of prescription refills to determine compliance.
- Assess patients receiving digoxin for anorexia, nausea, vomiting, muscle cramps, paresthesia, and confusion; ↑ risk of digoxin toxicity due to potassium-depleting effect of diuretic. Potassium supplements or potassium-sparing diuretics may be used concurrently to prevent hypokalemia.
- Assess patient for tinnitus and hearing loss. Audiometry is recommended for patients receiving prolonged high-dose IV therapy. Hearing loss is most common after rapid or high-dose IV administration in patients with decreased renal function or those taking other ototoxic drugs.
- Assess for allergy to sulfonamides.
- Assess patient for skin rash frequently during therapy. Discontinue bumetanide at first sign of rash; may be life-threatening. Stevens-Johnson syndrome or toxic epidermal necrolysis may develop. Treat symptomatically; may recur once treatment is stopped.
- Geri: Diuretic use is associated with increased risk for falls in older adults. Assess falls risk and implement fall prevention strategies.
- ***Lab Test Considerations:*** Monitor electrolytes, renal and hepatic function, serum glucose, and uric acid levels before and periodically during therapy. May cause ↓ serum sodium, potassium, calcium, and magnesium concentrations. May also cause ↑ BUN, serum glucose, creatinine, and uric acid levels.

Potential Nursing Diagnoses

Excess fluid volume (Indications)
Risk for deficient fluid volume (Side Effects)

Implementation

- If administering twice daily, give last dose no later than 5 PM to minimize disruption of sleep cycle.
- IV is preferred over IM for parenteral administration.
- **PO:** May be taken with food to minimize gastric irritation.

IV Administration

- **IV Push:** ***Diluent:*** Administer undiluted. ***Concentration:*** 0.25 mg/mL. ***Rate:*** Administer slowly over 1–2 min.
- **Continuous Infusion:** ***Diluent:*** May dilute in D5W or 0.9% NaCl. May also administer as undiluted drug. Protect from light. ***Concentration:*** Not to exceed 0.25 mg/mL. ***Rate:*** Infuse over 5 min. May be administered over 12 hr for patients with renal impairment.
- **Y-Site Compatibility:** acyclovir, alfentanil, allopurinol, amifostine, amikacin, aminocaproic acid, aminophylline, amiodarone, amphotericin B lipid complex, amphotericin B liposome, anidulafungin, argatroban, ascorbic acid, atropine, azithromycin, aztreonam, benztropine, bivalirudin, bleomycin, buprenorphine, butorphanol, calcium chloride, calcium gluconate, carboplatin, carmustine, caspofungin, cefazolin, cefepime, cefotaxime, cefoxitin, ceftaroline, ceftazidime, ceftriaxone, cefuroxime, chloramphenicol, cisatracurium, cisplatin, cladribine, clindamycin, cyanocobalamin, cyclophosphamide, cyclosporine, cytarabine, dactinomycin, daptomycin, dexamethasone, dexmedetomidine, dexrazoxane, digoxin, diltiazem, diphenhydramine, dobutamine, docetaxel, dopamine, doripenem, doxorubicin, doxorubicin liposomal, doxycycline, enalaprilat, ephedrine, epinephrine, epirubicin, epoetin alfa, eptifibatide, ertapenem, erythromycin, esmolol, etoposide, etoposide phosphate, famotidine, fentanyl, filgrastim, fluconazole, fludarabine, fluorouracil, folic acid, furosemide, gemcitabine, gentamicin, glycopyrrolate, granisetron, heparin, hetastarch, hydrocortisone sodium succinate, hydromorphone, idarubicin, ifosfamide, imipenem/cilastatin, indomethacin, insulin, irinotecan, isoproterenol, ketorolac, labetalol, leucovorin calcium, levofloxacin, lidocaine, linezolid, lorazepam, magnesium sulfate, mannitol, mechlorethamine, melphalan, meperidine, methotrexate, methyldopate, methylprednisolone sodium succinate, metoclopramide, metoprolol, metronidazole, micafungin, milrinone, mitoxantrone, morphine, moxifloxacin, multivitamins, mycophenolate, nafcillin, nalbuphine, naloxone, nitroglycerin, nitroprusside, norepinephrine, octreotide, ondansetron, oxacillin, oxaliplatin, oxytocin, paclitaxcel, palonosetron, pamidronate, pancuronium, pantoprazole, pemetrexed, penicillin G, pentazocine, pentobarbital, phenobarbital, phentolamine, phenylephrine, phytonadione, piperacillin/tazobactam, potassium acetate, potassium chloride, procainamide, promethazine, propofol, propranolol, protamine, pyridoxime, ranitidine, remifentanil, rifampin, rituximab, rocuronium, sodium acetate, sodium bicarbonate, streptokinase, succinylcholine, sufentanil, tacrolimus, teniposide, theophylline, thiamine, thiotepa, tigecycline, tirofiban, tobramycin, tolazoline, trastuzumab, vancomycin, vasopressin, vecuronium, verapamil, vinblastine, vincristine, vinorelbine, voriconazole, zoledronic acid.

- **Y-Site Incompatibility:** alemtuzumab, amphotericin B colloidal, azathioprine, chlorpromazine, dantrolene, diazepam, diazoxide, fenoldopam, ganciclovir, haloperidol, papaverine, pentamidine, phenytoin, quinupristin/dalfopristin, trimethoprim/sulfamethoxazole.

Patient/Family Teaching

- Instruct patient to take bumetanide as directed. Take missed doses as soon as possible; do not double doses.
- Caution patient to change positions slowly to minimize orthostatic hypotension. Caution patient that drinking alcohol, exercising during hot weather, or standing for long periods may enhance orthostatic hypotension.
- Instruct patient to consult health care professional regarding a diet high in potassium. See Appendix J.
- Advise patient to contact health care professional of gain more than 3 lbs in one day.
- Instruct patient to notify health care professional of all Rx or OTC medications, vitamins, or herbal products being taken and to consult health care professional before taking any OTC medications concurrently with this therapy.
- Instruct patient to notify health care professional of medication regimen before treatment or surgery.
- Caution patient to use sunscreen and protective clothing to prevent photosensitivity reactions.
- Advise patient to contact health care professional immediately if rash, muscle weakness, cramps, nausea, dizziness, numbness, or tingling of extremities occurs.
- Advise patients with diabetes to monitor blood glucose closely; may cause increased levels.
- Emphasize the importance of routine follow-up examinations.
- Geri: Caution older patients or their caregivers about increased risk for falls. Suggest strategies for fall prevention.

Evaluation/Desired Outcomes

- Decrease in edema.
- Decrease in abdominal girth and weight.
- Increase in urinary output.

bupivacaine, See EPIDURAL LOCAL ANESTHETICS.

bupivacaine liposome (injection)

(byoo-**pi**-vi-kane **lye**-poe-some)

Exparel

Classification

Therapeutic: anesthetics (topical/local)

Pharmacologic: amides

Pregnancy Category C

Indications

Postoperative single-use infiltration of surgical sites.

Action

Local anesthetics inhibit initiation and conduction of sensory nerve impulses by altering the influx of sodium and efflux of potassium in neurons, slowing or stopping pain transmission. Liposome formulation prolongs the duration of action. **Therapeutic Effects:** Lessened postoperative pain.

Pharmacokinetics

Absorption: Depends on amount injected and vascularity of administration site. Some systemic absorption occurs; however action is primarily local.

Distribution: Widely distributed following release from liposomes, high concentrations in highly perfused organs (heart, lungs, liver, brain). Crosses the placenta.

Protein Binding: 95%.

Metabolism and Excretion: Mostly metabolized by the liver, metabolites are primarily renally excreted; 6% excreted unchanged in urine.

Half-life: *Following bunionectomy*—34.1 hr; *following hemorrhoidectomy*—23.8 hr.

TIME/ACTION PROFILE (blood levels)

ROUTE	ONSET	PEAK	DURATION
infiltration	unknown	0.5–2 hr	96 hr†

† Pain relief lasted for 24 hr.

Contraindications/Precautions

Contraindicated in: Hypersensitivity; cross-sensitivity with other amide local anesthetics (ropivacaine, lidocaine, mepivacaine, prilocaine) may occur; OB: Obstetrical paracervical block anesthesia (may cause fetal bradycardia/death).

Use Cautiously in: Impaired cardiovascular function; Hepatic disease (blood levels ↑ in severe hepatic impairment); Renal impairment (risk of toxic reactions may be ↑); OB, Lactation, Pedi: Pregnancy, lactation, and children<18 yr (safety not established).

Adverse Reactions/Side Effects

CNS: CENTRAL NERVOUS SYSTEM TOXICITY, dizziness, drowsiness, headache, insomnia. **CV:** peripheral edema, prolonged AV conduction, tachycardia. **GI:** constipation, nausea, vomiting. **Derm:** pruritus.

Hemat: anemia. **MS:** back pain, muscle spasm. **Misc:** hypersensitivity reactions including ANAPHYLACTOID-LIKE REACTIONS and LARYNGEAL EDEMA, fever, procedural pain.

Interactions

Drug-Drug: Should not be administered concurrently with local **lidocaine**, wait at least 20 minutes before infiltration with bupivacaine liposome. Should not be admixed with **other local anesthetics**. Should not be used within 96 hr of **other formulations of bupivacaine**; overall exposure and risk of toxicity/adverse reactions will be ↑.

Route/Dosage

Infiltration (Adults): *Bunionectomy*—106 mg (8 mL) given as 7 mL into osteotomy and 1 mL into subcutaneous tissue; *Hemorrhoidectomy*—266 mg (20 mL) diluted to a volume of 30 mL and given as six 5 mL aliquots.

Availability

Liposome injectable suspension (for infiltration only): 13.3 mg/mL.

NURSING IMPLICATIONS

Assessment

- Assess infiltrated area for pain following administration and periodically during therapy.
- Monitor cardiovascular and respiratory status (vital signs, level of consciousness) constantly following infiltration. Notify health care professional immediately if signs of cardiac toxicity (atrioventricular block, ventricular arrhythmias, cardiac arrest) occur.
- Monitor for central nervous system toxicity. Notify health care professional promptly if they occur. Early signs of central nervous system toxicity include (restlessness, anxiety, incoherent speech, lightheadedness, numbness and tingling of the mouth and lips, metallic taste, tinnitus, dizziness, blurred vision, tremors, twitching, depression or drowsiness).
- Monitor for signs and symptoms of allergic reactions (urticaria, pruritus, erythema, angioneurotic edema, laryngeal edema, tachycardia, sneezing, nausea, vomiting, syncope, excessive sweating, elevated temperature, severe hypotension). Have resuscitative equipment available.

Potential Nursing Diagnoses

Acute pain (Indications)

Implementation

- Do not confuse with propofol. In a syringe suspension is milky white and may be mistaken for other medications. Label syringe to ensure dose is not administered IV.
- **Infiltration:** May be administered undiluted or diluted with 0.9% NaCl or Lactated Ringers solution up to 0.89 mg/mL. Invert vial multiple times to re-suspend particles immediately prior to withdrawal from vial. Injected with a 25 gauge or larger bore needle slowly into soft tissues of surgical site with frequent aspiration to check for blood and minimize risk of intravascular injection. Use diluted suspension within 4 hrs of preparation in a syringe. Vials are for single dose; discard unused portions. May be stored in refrigerator for up to 30 days prior to opening. Do not use if solution is discolored or has been frozen or exposed to high temperatures for extended period.
- Do not administer in an area with povidone iodine until dry. If administered with other non-bupivacaine local anesthetics, administer other agents first and wait at least 20 min before infiltrating with bupivacaine liposome. Do not administer other forms of bupivacaine within 96 hr of bupivacaine liposome.

Patient/Family Teaching

- Inform patient that infiltration may cause temporary loss of sensation or motor activity in infiltrated area.
- Instruct patient to notify health care professional of pregnancy is known or suspected or if breast feeding.

Evaluation/Desired Outcomes

- Prolongation of postoperative analgesia.

REMS HIGH ALERT

buprenorphine

(byoo-pre-**nor**-feen)
Buprenex, Butrans, ~~Subutex~~

Classification
Therapeutic: opioid analgesics
Pharmacologic: opioid agonists/antagonists

Schedule III

Pregnancy Category C

Indications

IM, IV: Management of moderate to severe acute pain. **Transdermal:** Moderate to severe chronic pain in opioid-tolerant patients requiring use of daily, around-the-clock long-term opioid treatment and for which alternative treatment options are inadequate (extended-release). **SL:** Treatment of opioid dependence (preferred for induction only); suppresses withdrawal symptoms in opioid detoxification.

Action

Binds to opiate receptors in the CNS. Alters the perception of and response to painful stimuli while producing generalized CNS depression. Has partial antagonist properties that may result in opioid withdrawal in physically dependent patients when used as an analgesic.

Therapeutic Effects: IM, IV, Transdermal: Decreased severity of pain. **SL:** Suppression of withdrawal symptoms during detoxification and maintenance from heroin or other opioids. Produces a relatively mild withdrawal compared to other agents.

Pharmacokinetics

Absorption: Well absorbed after IM and SL use; 15% of transdermal dose absorbed through skin; IV administration results in complete bioavailability.

Distribution: Crosses the placenta; enters breast milk. CNS concentration is 15–25% of plasma.

Protein Binding: 96%.

Metabolism and Excretion: Mostly metabolized by the liver mostly via the CYP3A4 enzyme system; one metabolite is active; 70% excreted in feces; 27% excreted in urine.

Half-life: 2–3 hr (parenteral); 26 hr (transdermal).

TIME/ACTION PROFILE (analgesia)

ROUTE	ONSET	PEAK	DURATION
IM	15 min	60 min	6 hr†
IV	rapid	less than 60 min	6 hr†
SL	unknown	unknown	unknown
Transdermal	unknown	unknown	7 days

†4–5 hr in children.

Contraindications/Precautions

Contraindicated in: Hypersensitivity; Significant respiratory depression (transdermal); Acute or severe bronchial asthma (transdermal); Paralytic ileus (transdermal); Acute, mild, intermittent, or postoperative pain (transdermal); Long QT syndrome (transdermal); Concurrent use of class I or III antiarrhythmics (transdermal); Lactation: Enters breast milk; avoid use or discontinue nursing.

Use Cautiously in: ↑ intracranial pressure; Severe renal or pulmonary disease; Moderate or severe hepatic disease (dose ↓ needed for severe impairment); Hypothyroidism; Seizure disorders; Adrenal insufficiency; Alcoholism; Biliary tract disease; Acute pancreatitis; Debilitated patients (dose ↓ required); Undiagnosed abdominal pain; Prostatic hyperplasia; OB: Safety not established; prolonged use of extended-release or SL buprenorphine during pregnancy can result in neonatal opioid withdrawal syndrome; Pedi: Safety not established in children (sublingual and transdermal) or children <2 yr (parenteral); Geri: ↑ risk of respiratory depression (dose ↓ required).

Adverse Reactions/Side Effects

CNS: confusion, dysphoria, hallucinations, sedation, dizziness, euphoria, floating feeling, headache, unusual dreams. **EENT:** blurred vision, diplopia, miosis (high doses). **Resp:** RESPIRATORY DEPRESSION. **CV:** hypertension, hypotension, palpitations, QT interval prolongation (transdermal). **GI:** HEPATOTOXICITY, nausea, constipation, dry mouth, ileus, vomiting. **GU:** urinary retention. **Derm:** sweating, clammy feeling, erythema, pruritis, rash. **Misc:** ANAPHYLAXIS, physical dependence, psychological dependence, tolerance.

Interactions

Drug-Drug: Use of high-dose transdermal buprenorphine with **class I antiarrhythmics** or **class I antiarrhythmics** may ↑ risk of QT interval prolongation; avoid concurrent use. Use with extreme caution in patients receiving **MAO inhibitors** (↑ CNS and respiratory depression and hypotension—↓ buprenorphine dose by 50%; may need to ↓ **MAO inhibitor** dose; do not use transdermal formulation within 14 days of **MAO inhibitor**). ↑ CNS depression with **alcohol**, **antihistamines**, **antidepressants**, and **sedative/hypnotics**. May ↓ effectiveness of other **opioid analgesics**. Inhibitors of the CYP3A4 enzyme system including **itraconazole**, **ketoconazole**, **erythromycin**, **ritonavir**, **indinavir**, **saquinavir**, **atazanavir**, or **fosamprenavir** may ↑ blood levels and effects; may need to ↓ buprenorphine dose. Inducers of the CYP3A4 enzyme system including **carbamazepine**, **rifampin**, or **phenytoin** may ↓ blood levels and effects; buprenorphine dose modification may be necessary during concurrent use. Concurrent abuse of buprenorphine and **benzodiazepines** may result in coma and death.

Drug-Natural Products: Concomitant use of **kava-kava**, **valerian**, **chamomile**, or **hops** can ↑ CNS depression.

Route/Dosage

Analgesia

IM, IV (Adults): 0.3 mg q 4–6 hr as needed. May repeat initial dose after 30 min (up to 0.3 mg q 4 hr or 0.6 mg q 6 hr); 0.6-mg doses should be given only IM.

IM, IV (Children 2–12 yr): 2–6 mcg (0.002–0.006 mg)/kg q 4–6 hr.

Transdermal (Adults): *Opioid-naive*—Transdermal system delivering 5–20 mcg/hr applied every 7 days. Initiate with 5 mcg/hr system; each dose titration may occur after 72 hr; do not exceed dose of 20 mcg/hr (due to ↑ risk of QT interval prolongation); *Previously taking <30 mg/day of morphine or equivalent*—Initiate with 5 mcg/hr system; each dose titration may occur after 72 hr; do not exceed dose of 20 mcg/hr (due to ↑ risk of QT interval prolongation); apply patch every 7 days; *Previously taking 30–80 mg/day of morphine or equivalent*—Initiate with 10 mcg/hr system; each dose titration may occur after 72 hr; do not exceed dose of 20 mcg/hr (due to ↑ risk of QT interval prolongation); apply patch every 7 days; *Previously taking >80 m g/day of morphine or equivalent*—Consider use of alternate analgesic.

Hepatic Impairment

Transdermal (Adults): *Mild to moderate hepatic impairment*—Initiate with 5 mcg/hr system.

Treatment of opioid dependence

SL (Adults): *Induction*—8 mg once daily on Day 1, then 16 mg once daily on Day 2–4; *Maintenance*—Patients should preferably be transitioned to Suboxone; if patient cannot tolerate naloxone, then can use Subutex (dose can be ↑ or ↓ by 2–4 mg, as needed to prevent signs/symptoms of opioid withdrawal).

Hepatic Impairment

SL (Adults): *Severe hepatic impairment*— ↓initial dose and adjustment dose by 50%.

Availability (generic available)

Sublingual tablets: 2 mg, 8 mg. **Injection (Buprenex):** 300 mcg (0.3 mg)/mL. **Transdermal system (Butrans):** 5 mcg/hr, 7.5 mcg/hr, 10 mcg/hr, 15 mcg/hr, 20 mcg/hr. ***In combination with:*** naloxone (Bunavail, Suboxone, Zubsolv). See Appendix B.

NURSING IMPLICATIONS

Assessment

- **Pain:** Assess type, location, and intensity of pain before and 1 hr after IM and 5 min (peak) after IV administration. When titrating opioid doses, increases of 25–50% should be administered until there is either a 50% reduction in the patient's pain rating on a numerical or visual analogue scale or the patient reports satisfactory pain relief. A repeat dose can be safely administered at the time of the peak if previous dose is ineffective and side effects are minimal. Single doses of 600 mcg (0.6 mg) should be administered IM. Patients requiring doses higher than 600 mcg (0.6 mg) should be converted to an opioid agonist. Buprenorphine is not recommended for prolonged use (except transdermal) or as first-line therapy for acute or cancer pain. SL formulation (Subutex) should not be used to relieve pain.
- An equianalgesic chart (see Appendix I) should be used when changing routes or when changing from one opioid to another.
- Assess level of consciousness, BP, pulse, and respirations before and periodically during administration. If respiratory rate is <10/min, assess level of sedation. Dose may need to be decreased by 25–50%. Buprenorphine 0.3–0.4 mg has approximately equal analgesic and respiratory depressant effects to morphine 10 mg.
- Assess previous analgesic history. Antagonistic properties may induce withdrawal symptoms (vomiting, restlessness, abdominal cramps, increased BP and temperature) in patients who are physically dependent on opioid agonists. Symptoms may occur up to 15 days after discontinuation and persist for 1–2 wk.
- Buprenorphine has a lower potential for dependence than other opioids; however, prolonged use may lead to physical and psychological dependence and tolerance. This should not prevent patient from receiving adequate analgesia. Most patients receiving buprenorphine for pain do not develop psychological dependence. If tolerance develops, changing to an opioid agonist may be required to relieve pain.
- Assess bowel function routinely. Prevent constipation with increased intake of fluids and bulk, and laxatives to minimize constipating effects. Administer stimulant laxatives routinely if opioid use exceeds 2–3 days, unless contraindicated.
- **Transdermal:** Assess risk for opioid addiction, abuse, or misuse prior to administration. Monitor for respiratory depression, especially during initiation or following dose increase; serious, life-threatening, or fatal respiratory depression may occur. Misuse or abuse of *Butrans* by chewing, swallowing, snorting or injecting buprenorphine extracted from transdermal system will result in the uncontrolled delivery of buprenorphine and risk of overdose and death.
- Maintain frequent contact during periods of changing analgesic requirements, including initial titration, between the prescriber, other members of the healthcare team, the patient, and the caregiver/family.
- **Treatment of Opioid Dependence:** Assess patient for signs and symptoms of opioid withdrawal before and during therapy.
- ***Lab Test Considerations:*** May cause ↑ serum amylase and lipase levels.
- Monitor liver function tests prior to and periodically during therapy for opioid dependence.
- ***Toxicity and Overdose:*** If an opioid antagonist is required to reverse respiratory depression or coma, naloxone (Narcan) is the antidote. Dilute the 0.4-mg ampule of naloxone in 10 mL of 0.9% NaCl and administer 0.5 mL (0.02 mg) by IV push every 2 min. For children and patients weighing <40 kg, dilute 0.1 mg of naloxone in 10 mL of 0.9% NaCl for a concentration of 10 mcg/mL and administer 0.5 mcg/kg every 1–2 min. Titrate dose to avoid withdrawal, seizures, and severe pain. Naloxone may not completely reverse respiratory depressant effects of buprenorphine; may require mechanical ventilation, oxygen, IV fluids, and vasopressors.

Potential Nursing Diagnoses

Acute pain (Indications)
Risk for injury (Side Effects)
Ineffective coping (Indications)

Implementation

- **Pain:** Explain therapeutic value of medication before administration to enhance the analgesic effect.

- Regularly administered doses may be more effective than prn administration. Analgesic is more effective if given before pain becomes severe.
- Coadministration with nonopioid analgesics has additive effects and may permit lower opioid doses.
- **SL:** Administer sublingually. Usually takes 2–10 min for tablets to dissolve. If more than one tablet is prescribed, place multiple tablets under the tongue or 2 at a time until all tablets are dissolved. Do not chew or swallow; decreases amount of medication absorbed. Not used for analgesia; may cause death in opioid naïve patients.
- **IM:** Administer IM injections deep into well-developed muscle. Rotate sites of injections.

IV Administration

- **IV Push:** May give IV undiluted. ***High Alert:*** Administer slowly. Rapid administration may cause respiratory depression, hypotension, and cardiac arrest. ***Rate:*** Give over at least 2 minutes.
- **Y-Site Compatibility:** acetaminophen, acyclovir, alfentanil, allopurinol, amifostine, amikacin, aminocaproic acid, amphotericin B lipid complex, amphotericin B liposome, anidulafungin, argatroban, ascorbic acid, atropine, azithromycin, aztreonam, benztropine, bivalirudin, bleomycin, bumetanide, butorphanol, calcium chloride, calcium gluconate, carboplatin, carmustine, cefazolin, cefepime, cefotaxime, cefotetan, cefoxitin, ceftazidime, ceftriaxone, cefuroxime, chloramphenicol, chlorpromazine, cisatracurium, cisplatin, cladribine, clindamycin, cyanocobalamin, cyclophosphamide, cyclosporine, cytarabine, dactinomycin, daptomycin, dexamethasone, dexmedetomidine, dexrazoxane, digoxin, diltiazem, diphenhydramine, dobutamine, docetaxel, dolasetron, dopamine, doxorubicin, doxycycline, enalaprilat, ephedrine, epinephrine, epirubicin, epoetin alfa, eptifibatide, ertapenem, erythromycin, esmolol, etoposide, etoposide phosphate, famotidine, fenoldopam, fentanyl, filgrastim, fluconazole, fludarabine, foscarnet, gemcitabine, gentamicin, glycopyrrolate, granisetron, heparin, hetastarch, hydrocortisone, idarubicin, ifosfamide, imipenem/cilastatin, insulin, irinotecan, isoproterenol, ketorolac, labetalol, leucovorin, levofloxacin, lidocaine, linezolid, lorazepam, magnesium sulfate, mannitol, mechlorethamine, melphalan, meperidine, methotrexate, methyldopate, methylprednisolone, metoclopramide, metoprolol, metronidazole, midazolam, milrinone, mitoxantrone, morphine, multivitamins, mycophenolate, nafcillin, nalbuphine, naloxone, nesiritide, nicardipine, nitroglycerin, nitroprusside, norepinephrine, octreotide, ondansetron, oxacillin, oxaliplatin, oxytocin, paclitaxel, palonosetron, pamidronate, pancuronium, papaverine, pemetrexed, penicillin G, pentamidine, pentazocine, phenylephrine, phytonadione, piperacillin/tazobactam, potassium acetate, potassium chloride, procainamide, prochlorperazine, promethazine, propofol, propranolol, protamine, pyridoxine, quinupristin/dalfopristin, ranitidine, remifentanil, rituximab, rocuronium, sodium acetate, streptokinase, succinylcholine, sufentanil, tacrolimus, teniposide, theophylline, thiamine, thiotepa, tigecycline, tirofiban, tobramycin, trastuzumab, vancomycin, vasopressin, vecuronium, verapamil, vinblastine, vincristine, vinorelbine, voriconazole, zoledronic acid.
- **Y-Site Incompatibility:** alemtuzumab, aminophylline, amphotericin B cholesteryl, ampicillin, dantrolene, diazepam, diazoxide, doxorubicin liposome, fluorouracil, indomethacin, pantoprazole, pentobarbital, phenobarbital, phenytoin, sodium bicarbonate, trimethoprim/sulfamethoxazole.
- **Transdermal:** Buprenorphine may cause withdrawal in patients who are already taking opioids. For conversion from other opioids to buprenorphine transdermal, taper current around-the-clock opioids for up to 7 days to no more than 30 mg of morphine or equivalent per day before beginning treatment with buprenorphine transdermal. May use short-acting analgesics as needed until analgesic efficacy with buprenorphine transdermal is attained. Buprenorphine transdermal may not provide adequate analgesia for patients requiring greater than 80 mg/day oral morphine equivalents.
- Apply system to flat, hairless, nonirritated, and nonirradiated site on the upper outer arm, upper chest, upper back or the side of the chest. If skin preparation is necessary, use clear water and clip, do not shave, hair. Allow skin to dry completely before application. Apply immediately after removing from package. Do not alter the system (i.e., cut) in any way before application. Remove liner from adhesive layer and press firmly in place with palm of hand for 30 sec, especially around the edges, to make sure contact is complete. Remove used system and fold so that adhesive edges are together. Flush system down toilet immediately on removal or follow the institutional policy. Apply new system to a different site. After removal, wait a minimum of 3 weeks before applying to the same site. If patch falls off during 7-day dosing interval, dispose of patch and place a new patch on at a different site.
- May be titrated no less than every 72 hrs. Dose adjustments in 5 mcg/hr, 7.5 mcg/hr, or 10 mcg/hr increments may be used by using no more than two patches.
- To discontinue, taper dose gradually to prevent signs and symptoms of withdrawal; consider introduction of immediate-release opioid medication.
- **Treatment of Opioid Dependence:** Must be prescribed by health care professional with special training. Induction is usually started with buprenorphine SL over 3–4 days. Initial dose should be administered at least 4 hr after last opioid dose and preferably when early signs of opioid withdrawal appear. Once patient is on a stable dose, maintenance

therapy with buprenorphine/naloxone (Suboxone) is preferred for continued, unsupervised treatment.

Patient/Family Teaching

- Medication may cause drowsiness or dizziness. Advise patient to call for assistance when ambulating and to avoid driving or other activities requiring alertness until response to medication is known.
- Advise patient to avoid concurrent use of alcohol or other CNS depressants.
- Instruct patient to notify health care professional of all Rx or OTC medications, vitamins, or herbal products being taken and to consult health care professional before taking any OTC medications concurrently with this therapy.
- Advise patient to notify health care professional if pregnancy is planned or suspected, or if breast feeding.
- **Pain:** Instruct patient on how and when to ask for pain medication.
- Encourage patients on bedrest to turn, cough, and deep-breathe every 2 hr to prevent atelectasis.
- Instruct patient to change positions slowly to minimize orthostatic hypotension.
- Advise patient that good oral hygiene, frequent mouth rinses, and sugarless gum or candy may decrease dry mouth.
- **Transdermal:** Instruct patient in correct method for application, removal, storage, and disposal of transdermal system. Wear patches for 7 days. May be worn while bathing, showering, or swimming. Do not discontinue or change dose without consulting health care professional. Instruct patient to read the *Medication Guide* prior to starting and with each Rx refill.
- Advise patients and caregivers/family members of the potential side effects. Instruct patient to notify health care professional if pain is not controlled or if bothersome side effects occur. Contact immediately if difficulty or changes in breathing, unusual deep "sighing" breathing slow or shallow breathing, new or unusual snoring, slow heartbeat, severe sleepiness, cold, clammy skin, feeling faint, dizzy, confused, or cannot think, walk, or talk normally, or if swelling or blistering around patch occurs.
- Advise patient that fever, electric blankets, heating pads, saunas, hot tubs, and heated water beds increase release of buprenorphine from patch.
- Advise patient referred for MRI test to discuss patch with referring health care professional and MRI facility to determine if removal of patch is necessary prior to test and for directions for replacing patch.
- **Opioid Dependence:** Instruct patient in correct use of medication; directions for use must be followed exactly. Medication must be used regularly, not occasionally. Take missed doses as soon as remembered; if almost time for next dose, skip missed dose and return to regular dosing schedule. Do not take 2 doses at once unless directed by health care professional. Do not discontinue use without consulting health care professional; abrupt discontinuation may cause withdrawal symptoms. If medication is discontinued, flush unused tablets down the toilet.
- Caution patient that buprenorphine may be a target for people who abuse drugs; store medications in a safe place to protect them from theft. Selling or giving this medication to others is against the law.
- Caution patient that injection of *Suboxone* can lead to severe withdrawal symptoms.
- Advise patient if admitted to the emergency room to inform treating physician and emergency room staff of physical dependence on opioids and of treatment regimen.
- Advise patient to notify health care professional promptly if faintness, dizziness, confusion, slowed breathing, skin or whites of eyes turn yellow, urine turns dark, light-colored stools, decreased appetite, nausea, or abdominal pain occur.

Evaluation/Desired Outcomes

- Decrease in severity of pain without a significant alteration in level of consciousness or respiratory status.
- Suppression of withdrawal symptoms during detoxification and maintenance from heroin or other opioids.

REMS

buPROPion (byoo-proe-pee-on)

Aplenzin, Forfivo XL, Wellbutrin, Wellbutrin SR, Wellbutrin XL, Zyban

Classification

Therapeutic: antidepressants, smoking deterrents

Pharmacologic: aminoketones

Pregnancy Category C

Indications

Treatment of depression (with psychotherapy). Depression with seasonal affective disorder (Aplenzin and Wellbutrin XL only). Smoking cessation (Zyban only). **Unlabeled Use:** Treatment of ADHD in adults (SR only). To increase sexual desire in women.

Action

Decreases neuronal reuptake of dopamine in the CNS. Diminished neuronal uptake of serotonin and norepinephrine (less than tricyclic antidepressants). **Therapeutic Effects:** Diminished depression. Decreased craving for cigarettes.

Pharmacokinetics

Absorption: Although well absorbed, rapidly and extensively metabolized by the liver.

Distribution: Unknown.

Metabolism and Excretion: Extensively metabolized by the liver into 3 active metabolites (CYP2B6 involved in formation of one of the active metabolites).

Half-life: 14 hr (active metabolites may have longer half-lives).

TIME/ACTION PROFILE (antidepressant effect)

ROUTE	ONSET	PEAK	DURATION
PO	1–3 wk	unknown	unknown

Contraindications/Precautions

Contraindicated in: Hypersensitivity; Concurrent use of MAO inhibitors or MAO-like drugs (linezolid or methylene blue); Concurrent use of ritonavir; Seizure disorders; Arteriovenous malformation, severe head injury, CNS tumor, CNS infection, severe stroke, anorexia nervosa, bulimia, or abrupt discontinuation of alcohol, benzodiazepines, barbiturates, or antiepileptic drugs (↑ risk of seizures); Lactation: Potential for serious adverse reactions in nursing infants.

Use Cautiously in: Renal/hepatic impairment (↓ dose recommended) (Forfivo XL not recommended in patients with renal or hepatic impairment); Recent history of MI; History of suicide attempt; Unstable cardiovascular status; May ↑ risk of suicide attempt/ideation especially during early treatment or dose adjustment; this risk appears to be greater in adolescents or children; Angle-closure glaucoma; OB: Use only if benefit to patient outweighs potential risk to fetus; Geri: ↑ risk of drug accumulation; ↑ sensitivity to effects.

Exercise Extreme Caution in: Severe hepatic cirrhosis (↓ dose required); Pedi: ↑ risk of suicidal thinking and behavior. Observe carefully, especially at initiation of therapy and during ↑ or ↓ in dose.

Adverse Reactions/Side Effects

CNS: SEIZURES, SUICIDAL THOUGHTS/BEHAVIOR, agitation, headache, aggression, anxiety, delusions, depression, hallucinations, hostility, insomnia, mania, panic, paranoia, psychoses. **CV:** hypertension. **GI:** dry mouth, nausea, vomiting, change in appetite, weight gain, weight loss. **Derm:** photosensitivity. **Endo:** hyperglycemia, hypoglycemia, syndrome of inappropriate ADH secretion. **Neuro:** tremor.

Interactions

Drug-Drug: Concurrent use with **MAO-inhibitors** may ↑ risk of hypertensive reactions; concurrent use contraindicated; at least 14 days should elapse between discontinuation of MAO inhibitor and initiation of bupropion (or visa versa). Concurrent use with **MAO-inhibitor like drugs**, such as **linezolid** or **methylene blue** may ↑ risk of hypertensive reactions; concurrent use contraindicated; do not start therapy in patients receiving **linezolid** or **methylene blue**; if **linezolid** or **methylene blue** need to be started in a patient receiving bupropion, immediately discontinue bupropion and monitor for 2 wk or until 24 hr after last dose of linezolid or methylene blue, whichever comes first (may resume bupropion therapy 24 hr after last dose of linezolid or methylene blue). ↑ risk of adverse reactions when used with **amantadine**, or **levodopa**. ↑ risk of seizures with **phenothiazines**, **antidepressants**, **theophylline**, **corticosteroids**, **OTC stimulants/anorectics**, or cessation of **alcohol** or **benzodiazepines** (avoid or minimize alcohol use). **Ritonavir**, **lopinavir/ritonavir**, and **efavirenz** may ↓ levels; may need to ↑ bupropion dose. May ↑ **citalopram** levels. **Carbamazepine** may ↓ blood levels and effectiveness. Concurrent use with **nicotine** replacement may cause hypertension. ↑ risk of bleeding with **warfarin**. Bupropion and one of its metabolites inhibit the CYP2D6 enzyme system and may ↑ levels and risk of toxicity from **antidepressants** (SSRIs and tricyclic), **haloperidol**, **risperidone**, **thioridazine**, **haloperidol**, **beta blockers**, **flecainide**, and **propafenone**. May ↓ levels and efficacy of **tamoxifen**. May ↓ the efficacy of **tamoxifen**.

Route/Dosage

Depression

PO (Adults): *Immediate-release*—100 mg twice daily initially; after 3 days may ↑ to 100 mg 3 times daily; after at least 4 wk of therapy, may ↑ up to 450 mg/day in divided doses (not to exceed 150 mg/dose; wait at least 6 hr between doses at the 300 mg/day dose or at least 4 hr between doses at the 450-mg/day dose). *Sustained-release*—150 mg once daily in the morning; after 3 days, may ↑ to 150 mg twice daily with at least 8 hr between doses; after at least 4 wk of therapy, may ↑ to a maximum daily dose of 400 mg given as 200 mg twice daily. *Extended-release (Wellbutrin XL)*—150 mg once daily in the morning, may be ↑ after 4 days to 300 mg once daily; some patients may require up to 450 mg/day as a single daily dose. *Extended-release (Aplenzin)*—174 mg once daily in the morning, may be ↑ after 4 days to 348 mg once daily; some patients may require up to 522 mg/day as a single daily dose. *Extended-release (Forfivo XL)*—450 mg once daily (should NOT be used as initial therapy; it should only be used in patients who have been receiving 300 mg/day of another bupropion formulation for at least 2 wk and require titration up to 450 mg/day or in those patients receiving 450 mg/day of another bupropion formulation).

Hepatic Impairment

PO (Adults): *Moderate-to-severe hepatic impairment (Aplenzin)*—Max dose: 174 mg every other day.

Seasonal Affective Disorder

PO (Adults): *Extended-release (Wellbutrin XL)*—150 mg/day in the morning; if dose is well tolerated, ↑

to 300 mg/day in one wk. Doses should be tapered to 150 mg/day for 2 wk before discontinuing; *Extended-release (Aplenzin)*—174 mg once daily in the morning, may be ↑ after 7 days to 348 mg once daily.

Hepatic Impairment

PO (Adults): *Moderate-to-severe hepatic impairment (Aplenzin)*—Max dose: 174 mg every other day.

Smoking cessation

PO (Adults): *Zyban*—150 mg once daily for 3 days, then 150 mg twice daily for 7–12 wk (doses should be at least 8 hr apart).

Availability (generic available)

Tablets: 75 mg, 100 mg. **Cost:** *Generic*—75 mg $79.43/100, 100 mg $106.01/100. **Sustained-release tablets:** 100 mg, 150 mg, 200 mg. **Cost:** *Generic*—100 mg $51.12/180, 150 mg $59.60/180, 200 mg $52.33/180. **Extended-release tablets (Wellbutrin XL):** 150 mg, 300 mg. **Cost:** *Generic*—150 mg $74.84/90, 300 mg $63.94/90. **Extended-release tablets (Aplenzin):** 174 mg, 348 mg, 522 mg. **Cost:** 174 mg $359.09/30, 348 mg $473.36/30, 522 mg $1,077.23/30. **Extended-release tablets (Forfivo XL):** 450 mg. **Cost:** $176.40/30.

NURSING IMPLICATIONS

Assessment

- Monitor mood changes. Inform health care professional if patient demonstrates significant increase in anxiety, nervousness, or insomnia.
- Assess mental status and mood changes, especially during initial few months of therapy and during dose changes. Risk may be increased in children, adolescents, and adults ≤24 yrs. Inform health care professional if patient demonstrates significant increase in signs of depression (depressed mood, loss of interest in usual activities, significant change in weight and/or appetite, insomnia or hypersomnia, psychomotor agitation or retardation, increased fatigue, feelings of guilt or worthlessness, slowed thinking or impaired concentration, suicide attempt or suicidal ideation). Restrict amount of drug available to patient.
- ***Lab Test Considerations:*** Monitor hepatic and renal function closely in patients with kidney or liver impairment to prevent ↑ serum and tissue bupropion concentrations.
- May cause false-positive urine test for amphetamines.

Potential Nursing Diagnoses

Ineffective coping (Indications)

Implementation

- Do not confuse bupropion with buspirone. Do not confuse Wellbutrin SR with Wellbutrin XL. Do not confuse Zyban with Diovan. Do not administer bupropion (Wellbutrin) with Zyban, which contain the same ingredients.
- Administer doses in equally spaced time increments during the day to minimize the risk of seizures. Risk of seizures increases fourfold in doses greater than 450 mg per day.
- May be initially administered concurrently with sedatives to minimize agitation. This is not usually required after the 1st wk of therapy.
- Insomnia may be decreased by avoiding bedtime doses. May require treatment during 1st wk of therapy.
- Nicotine patches, gum, inhalers, and spray may be used concurrently with bupropion.
- When converting from other brands of bupropion to *Aplenzin* 522 mg/day *Aplenzin* is equivalent to 450 mg/day bupropion HCl, 348 mg/day *Aplenzin* is equivalent to 300 mg/day bupropion HCl and 174 mg/day *Aplenzin* is equivalent to 150 mg/day bupropion HCl.
- **PO:** Swallow sustained-release or extended-release tablets whole; do not break, crush, or chew.
- May be administered with food to lessen GI irritation.
- **Seasonal Affective Disorder:** Begin administration in autumn prior to the onset of depressive symptoms. Continue therapy through winter and begin to taper and discontinue in early spring.

Patient/Family Teaching

- Instruct patient to take bupropion as directed. Take missed doses as soon as possible and space day's remaining doses evenly at not less than 4-hr intervals. Missed doses for smoking cessation should be omitted. Do not double doses or take more than prescribed. May require 4 wk or longer for full effects. Do not discontinue without consulting health care professional. May require gradual reduction before discontinuation.
- May impair judgment or motor and cognitive skills. Caution patient to avoid driving and other activities requiring alertness until response to medication is known.
- Advise patient, family, and caregivers to look for suicidality, especially during early therapy or dose changes. Notify health care professional immediately if thoughts about suicide or dying, attempts to commit suicide, new or worse depression or anxiety, agitation or restlessness, panic attacks, insomnia, new or worse irritability, aggressiveness, acting on dangerous impulses, mania, or other changes in mood or behavior occur.
- Instruct patient to notify health care professional of all Rx or OTC medications, vitamins, or herbal products being taken, to avoid alcohol during therapy

and to consult with health care professional before taking other medications with bupropion, such as Zyban.

- Inform patient that frequent mouth rinses, good oral hygiene, and sugarless gum or candy may minimize dry mouth. If dry mouth persists for more than 2 wk, consult health care professional regarding use of saliva substitute.
- Advise patient to notify health care professional if rash or other troublesome side effects occur.
- Inform patient that unused shell of XL tablets may appear in stool; this is normal.
- Advise patient to use sunscreen and protective clothing to prevent photosensitivity reactions.
- Advise patient to notify health care professional of medication regimen before treatment or surgery.
- Instruct female patients to inform health care professional if pregnancy is planned or suspected or if breast feeding or planning to breast feed.
- Emphasize the importance of follow-up exams to monitor progress. Encourage patient participation in psychotherapy.
- **Smoking Cessation:** Smoking should be stopped during the 2nd week of therapy to allow for the onset of bupropion and to maximize the chances of quitting.
- Advise patient to stop taking bupropion and contact a health care professional immediately if agitation, depressed mood, and any changes in behavior that are not typical of nicotine withdrawal, or if suicidal thoughts or behavior occur.

Evaluation/Desired Outcomes

- Increased sense of well-being.
- Renewed interest in surroundings. Acute episodes of depression may require several months of treatment.
- Cessation of smoking.

bupropion/naltrexone

(byoo-**proe**-pee-on nal-**trex**-one)

Contrave

Classification

Therapeutic: weight control agents

Pharmacologic: aminoketones, opioid antagonists

Pregnancy Category X

Indications

Adjunct to calorie-reduced diet and increased physical activity for chronic weight management in obese patients (BMI $\geq$30 kg/m^2) or overweight patients (BMI $\geq$27 kg/m^2) with at least one other comorbidity (hypertension, type 2 diabetes or dyslipidemia).

Action

Bupropion—an antidepressant that acts as a weak inhibitor of neuronal reuptake of dopamine and norepinephrine. *Naltrexone*—acts as an opioid antagonist. In combination they effect two different brain areas involved in food intake: the hypothalamic appetite regulatory center and mesolimbic dopamine circuit reward system. **Therapeutic Effects:** Decreased appetite with associated weight loss.

Pharmacokinetics

Bupropion

Absorption: Well absorbed but rapidly metabolized by the liver. Absorption is enhanced by a high-fat meal.

Distribution: Parent drug and metabolites enter breast milk.

Metabolism and Excretion: Extensively metabolized; three metabolites are pharmacologically active. Excretion is mostly renal as metabolites, minimal renal excretion of unchanged drug.

Half-life: 21 hr (longer for some metabolites).

Naltrexone

Absorption: Well absorbed orally, undergoes extensive first pass hepatic metabolism resulting in 5–40% bioavailability. Absorption is enhanced by a high-fat meal.

Distribution: Parent drug and metabolites enter breast milk.

Metabolism and Excretion: Metabolized to 6–beta-naltrexol. Both parent drug and metabolite are pharmacologically active. Excretion is mostly renal as metabolite, less than 2% as unchanged drug.

Half-life: *naltrexone*—5 hr; *6–beta-naltrexol*—13 hr.

TIME/ACTION PROFILE (weight loss)

ROUTE	ONSET	PEAK	DURATION
PO	within 4 wk	6 mos	unknown

Contraindications/Precautions

Contraindicated in: Known hypersensitivity to bupropion or naltrexone; Uncontrolled hypertension; End-stage renal disease; Seizure disorders; Anorexia or bulimia; During withdrawal from or discontinuation of alcohol, benzodiazepines, barbiturates or antiepileptics; Chronic opioid/opiate agonist or partial agonist use or acute opiate withdrawal; During/within 14 days of MAOIs; Concurrent use of CYP2B6 inducers; Concurrent use of other bupropion-containing medications; OB: Pregnancy (may cause fetal harm); Lactation: Discontinue bupropion/naltrexone or discontinue breast feeding; Pedi: Not recommended for use in children.

Use Cautiously in: History of suicidal behavior/ideation; History of seizure risk (avoid administration with a high-fat meal, adhere to recommended dose); History of cardiac/cerebrovascular disease; History of angle-closure glaucoma; Diabetes mellitus (weight loss may result in hypoglycemia if treatment is not adjusted); Concurrent use of drugs that ↓ seizure threshold; Moderate to severe renal impairment (use lower dose); Hepatic impairment (use lower dose); Geri: Elderly may be ↑ sensitive to adverse CNS reactions and ↓ renal eliminination; Concurrent ingestion of alcohol (avoid or reduce consumption).

Adverse Reactions/Side Effects

CNS: SUICIDAL THOUGHTS/BEHAVIOR, headache, anxiety, dizziness, insomnia, neuropsychiatric reactions. **CV:** hypertension, tachycardia. **EENT:** angle-closure glaucoma (bupropion), tinnitus. **GI:** nausea, constipation, vomiting, abdominal pain, diarrhea, dry mouth, dysgeusia, hepatotoxicity (naltrexone). **Derm:** hot flush, sweating. **Neuro:** tremor. **Misc:** allergic reactions including ANAPHYLAXIS/ANAPHYLACTOID REACTIONS.

Interactions

Drug-Drug: Concurrent or use within 14 days with **MAOIs** ↑ risk of hypertensive reactions. Bupropion inhibits the CYP2D6 enzyme system and can ↑ blood levels and risk of adverse reactions from **antidepressants** including **SSRIs** and many **tricyclic antidepressants**, **antipsychotics** including **haloperidol**, **risperidone** and **thioridazine**, **beta-blockers** including **metoprolol**, and **Type 1C antiarrhythmics** including **flecanide** and **propafenone**. Dose adjustments may be necessary. Blood levels and effectiveness may be ↓ by**CYP2B6 inducers** including **carbamazepine**, **efavirenz**, **ritonavir**, **lopinavir**, **phenobarbital** and **phenytoin**; concurrent use should be avoided. Blood levels and risk of toxicity of bupropion may be ↑ by **CYP2B6 inhibitors** including **clopidogrel** (dose should not exceed one tablet twice daily). Concurrent use of **drugs that ↓ seizure threshold** may ↑ risk of seizures. **Dopaminergic drugs** including **amantadine** and **levodopa** may ↑ risk of CNS toxicity. Concurrent use with **opioids** may ↑ risk of overdose. Concurrent ingestion of **alcohol** may ↑ risk of neuropsychiatric reactions (reduce consumption or avoid). May ↓ renal excretion of and ↑ blood levels/risk of toxicity from **amantadine**, **amiloride**, **cimetidine**, **dopamine**, **famotidine**, **memantine**, **metformin**, **pindolol**, **procainamide**, **ranitidine**, **varenicline**, and **oxaliplatin** (careful monitoring is recommended). May ↑ sensitivity to **opioids**.

Route/Dosage

PO (Adults): *Week 1*—one tablet in the morning; *week 2*—one tablet in the morning and one tablet in the evening; *week 3*—two tablets in the morning and one tablet in the evening; *week 4 and onward*—two tablets in the morning and two tablets in the evening; *concurrent use of CYP2B6 inhibitors*—dose should not exceed one tablet twice daily.

Renal Impairment

PO (Adults): *Moderate to severe renal impairment*—dose should not exceed one tablet in the morning and one tablet in the evening.

Hepatic Impairment

PO (Adults): Dose should not exceed one tablet in the morning.

Availability

Extended-release tablets: 90 mg bupropion/8 mg naltrexone.

NURSING IMPLICATIONS

Assessment

- Monitor patients for weight loss and adjust concurrent medications (antihypertensives, antidiabetics, lipid-lowering agents) as needed.
- Assess mental status and mood changes, especially during initial few mo of therapy. Risk may be increased in children, adolescents, and adults ≤24 yrs. Inform health care professional if patient demonstrates significant increase in signs of depression (depressed mood, loss of interest in usual activities, insomnia or hypersomnia, psychomotor agitation or retardation, increased fatigue, feelings of guilt or worthlessness, slowed thinking or impaired concentration, suicide attempt or suicidal ideation). Restrict amount of drug available to patient.
- Monitor BP and heart rate periodically during therapy, especially in patient with hypertension.
- Monitor for signs and symptoms of anaphylactic reactions (pruritus, urticaria, hives, angioedema, dyspnea). Discontinue therapy and treat symptomatically.
- ***Lab Test Considerations:*** Monitor blood glucose prior to and during therapy in patients with type 2 diabetes; may cause hypoglycemia.
- May cause false-positive urine test for amphetamines.

Potential Nursing Diagnoses

Disturbed body image (Indications)
Imbalanced nutrition: more than body requirements (Indications)

Implementation

- **PO:** Administer in the morning and evening according to dose escalation schedule. Swallow tablets whole; do not break, crush, or chew.
- Do not administer with a high-fat meal; may increase risk of seizures.

Patient/Family Teaching

- Instruct patient to take medication as directed, following the dose escalation schedule. If a dose is missed, omit and wait until next scheduled dose; do not double doses. Advise patient to read *Medication Guide* before starting therapy and with each Rx refill in case of changes.
- Instruct patient to adhere to a reduced-calorie diet and increased physical activity.

- Advise patient, family, and caregivers to look for suicidality, especially during early therapy. Notify health care professional immediately if thoughts about suicide or dying, attempts to commit suicide, new or worse depression or anxiety, agitation or restlessness, panic attacks, insomnia, new or worse irritability, aggressiveness, acting on dangerous impulses, mania, or other changes in mood or behavior occur.
- Advise patient to notify health care professional if signs and symptoms of liver damage (stomach pain lasting more than a few days, dark urine, yellowing of skin and whites of eyes, tiredness) occurs.
- Advise patients they may be more sensitive to opioids, even at lower doses, during therapy. Patients physically dependant on opioid analgesics should wait at least 7–10 days without opioids, or 2 wks without methadone, before beginning bupropion/naltrexone.
- Advise patient to notify health care professional of all Rx or OTC medications, vitamins, or herbal products being taken and to consult with health care professional before taking other medications and to minimize or avoid alcohol during therapy.
- Instruct female patients to inform health care professional if pregnancy is planned or suspected or if breast feeding.

Evaluation/Desired Outcomes

- Decreased appetite with associated weight loss. Evaluate therapy after 12 wks at maintenance dose. If patient has not lost 5% of baseline body weight discontinue medication; clinically meaningful weight loss is unlikely.

busPIRone (byoo-**spye**-rone)

BuSpar, ✱Bustab

Classification

Therapeutic: antianxiety agents

Pregnancy Category B

Indications

Management of anxiety.

Action

Binds to serotonin and dopamine receptors in the brain. Increases norepinephrine metabolism in the brain. **Therapeutic Effects:** Relief of anxiety.

Pharmacokinetics

Absorption: Rapidly absorbed.

Distribution: Unknown.

Protein Binding: 95% bound to plasma proteins.

Metabolism and Excretion: Extensively metabolized by the liver (CYP3A4 enzyme system); 20–40% excreted in feces.

Half-life: 2–3 hr.

TIME/ACTION PROFILE (relief of anxiety)

ROUTE	ONSET	PEAK	DURATION
PO	7–10 days	3–4 wk	unknown

Contraindications/Precautions

Contraindicated in: Hypersensitivity; Severe hepatic or renal impairment; Concurrent use of MAO inhibitors; Ingestion of large amounts of grapefruit juice.

Use Cautiously in: Patients receiving other antianxiety agents (other agents should be slowly withdrawn to prevent withdrawal or rebound phenomenon); Patients receiving other psychotropics; Lactation, OB, Pedi: Safety not established.

Adverse Reactions/Side Effects

CNS: dizziness, drowsiness, excitement, fatigue, headache, insomnia, nervousness, weakness, personality changes. **EENT:** blurred vision, nasal congestion, sore throat, tinnitus, altered taste or smell, conjunctivitis. **Resp:** chest congestion, hyperventilation, shortness of breath. **CV:** chest pain, palpitations, tachycardia, hypertension, hypotension, syncope. **GI:** nausea, abdominal pain, constipation, diarrhea, dry mouth, vomiting. **GU:** changes in libido, dysuria, urinary frequency, urinary hesitancy. **Derm:** rashes, alopecia, blisters, dry skin, easy bruising, edema, flushing, pruritus. **Endo:** irregular menses. **MS:** myalgia. **Neuro:** incoordination, numbness, paresthesia, tremor. **Misc:** clamminess, sweating, fever.

Interactions

Drug-Drug: Use with **MAO inhibitors** may result in hypertension and is not recommended. **Erythromycin**, **nefazodone**, **ketoconazole**, **itraconazole**, **ritonavir**, and other **inhibitors of CYP3A4** ↑ blood levels and effects of buspirone; dose reduction is recommended (↓ to 2.5 mg twice daily with erythromycin; ↓ to 2.5 mg once daily with nefazodone). **Rifampin**, **dexamethasone**, **phenytoin**, **phenobarbital**, **carbamazepine**, and other **inducers of CYP3A4** ↓ blood levels and effects of buspirone; dose adjustment may be necessary. Avoid concurrent use with **alcohol**.

Drug-Natural Products: Concomitant use of **kava-kava**, **valerian**, or **chamomile** can ↑ CNS depression.

Drug-Food: Grapefruit juice ↑ serum levels and effect; ingestion of large amounts of grapefruit juice is not recommended.

Route/Dosage

PO (Adults): 7.5 mg twice daily; ↑ by 5 mg/day q 2–4 days as needed (not to exceed 60 mg/day). Usual dose is 20–30 mg/day (in 2 divided doses).

Availability (generic available)

Tablets: 5 mg, 7.5 mg, 10 mg, 15 mg, 30 mg. **Cost:** *Generic*—5 mg $77.12/100, 7.5 mg $109.08/100, 10 mg $134.50/100, 15 mg $201.92/100, 30 mg $218.10/100.

NURSING IMPLICATIONS

Assessment

- Assess degree and manifestations of anxiety before and periodically during therapy.
- Buspirone does not appear to cause physical or psychological dependence or tolerance. However, patients with a history of substance use disorder should be assessed for tolerance or impaired control. Restrict amount of drug available to these patients.

Potential Nursing Diagnoses

Anxiety (Indications)
Risk for injury (Side Effects)

Implementation

- Do not confuse buspirone with bupropion.
- Patients changing from other antianxiety agents should receive gradually decreasing doses. Buspirone will not prevent withdrawal symptoms.
- **PO:** May be administered with food to minimize gastric irritation. Food slows but does not alter extent of absorption.

Patient/Family Teaching

- Instruct patient to take buspirone exactly as directed. Take missed doses as soon as possible if not just before next dose; do not double doses. Do not take more than amount prescribed.
- May cause dizziness or drowsiness. Caution patient to avoid driving or other activities requiring alertness until response to the medication is known.
- Advise patient to avoid concurrent use of alcohol or other CNS depressants.
- Instruct patient to notify health care professional of all Rx or OTC medications, vitamins, or herbal products being taken and to consult health care professional before taking any Rx, OTC, or herbal products.
- Instruct patient to notify health care professional if any chronic abnormal movements occur (dystonia, motor restlessness, involuntary movements of facial or cervical muscles) or if pregnancy is suspected.
- Emphasize the importance of follow-up exams to determine effectiveness of medication.

Evaluation/Desired Outcomes

- Increase in sense of well-being.
- Decrease in subjective feelings of anxiety. Some improvement may be seen in 7–10 days. Optimal results take 3–4 wk of therapy. Buspirone is usually used for short-term therapy (3–4 wk). If prescribed for long-term therapy, efficacy should be periodically assessed.

HIGH ALERT

B

busulfan (byoo-**sul**-fan)

Busulfex, Myleran

Classification
Therapeutic: antineoplastics
Pharmacologic: alkylating agents

Pregnancy Category D

Indications

PO: Treatment of chronic myelogenous leukemia (CML) and bone marrow disorders. **IV:** With cyclophosphamide as a conditioning regimen before allogenic hematopoietic progenitor cell transplantation for CML.

Action

Disrupts nucleic acid function and protein synthesis (cell-cycle phase–nonspecific). **Therapeutic Effects:** Death of rapidly growing cells, especially malignant ones.

Pharmacokinetics

Absorption: Rapidly absorbed from the GI tract.
Distribution: Unknown.
Metabolism and Excretion: Extensively metabolized by the liver.
Half-life: 2.5 hr.

TIME/ACTION PROFILE (effects on blood counts)

ROUTE	ONSET	PEAK	DURATION
PO	1–2 wk	weeks	up to 1 mo†
IV	unknown	unknown	13 days‡

†Complete recovery may take up to 20 mo.
‡After administration of last dose.

Contraindications/Precautions

Contraindicated in: Hypersensitivity; Failure to respond to previous courses; OB, Lactation: Potential for serious side effects in fetus or infant.
Use Cautiously in: Active infections; ↓ bone marrow reserve; Obese patients (base dose on ideal body weight); Other chronic debilitating diseases; Patients with childbearing potential; Geri: Begin therapy at lower end of dose range due to ↑ frequency of impaired cardiac, hepatic, or renal function.

Adverse Reactions/Side Effects

Incidence and severity of adverse reactions and side effects are increased with IV use.
CNS: *IV*—SEIZURES, CEREBRAL HEMORRHAGE/COMA, anxiety, confusion, depression, dizziness, headache, encephalopathy, mental status changes, weakness.
EENT: *PO*—cataracts; *IV*, epistaxis, pharyngitis, ear

✱ = Canadian drug name. ⚕ = Genetic implication. ~~Strikethrough~~ = Discontinued.
*CAPITALS indicates life-threatening; underlines indicate most frequent.

disorders. **CV:** hepatic veno-oclusive disease (↑ allogenic transplantation). **Resp:** *PO*— PULMONARY FIBROSIS; *IV*, alveolar hemorrhage, asthma, atelectasis, cough, hemoptysis, hypoxia, pleural effusion, pneumonia, rhinitis, sinusitis. **CV:** *PO*— CARDIAC TAMPONADE (WITH HIGH-DOSE CYCLOPHOSPHAMIDE); *IV*, chest pain, hypotension, tachycardia, thrombosis, arrhythmias, atrial fibrillation, cardiomegaly, ECG changes, edema, heart block, heart failure, hypertension, pericardial effusion, ventricular extrasystoles. **GI:** *PO*—drug-induced hepatitis, nausea, vomiting; *IV*, abdominal enlargement, anorexia, constipation, diarrhea, dry mouth, hematemesis, nausea, rectal discomfort, vomiting, abdominal pain, dyspepsia, hepatomegaly, pancreatitis, stomatitis. **GU:** oliguria, dysuria, hematuria. **Derm:** *PO*—itching, rashes, acne, alopecia, erythema nodosum, exfoliative dermatitis, hyperpigmentation. **Endo:** *PO*—sterility, gynecomastia. **F and E:** hypokalemia, hypomagnesemia, hypophosphatemia. **Hemat:** BONE MARROW DEPRESSION. **Local:** inflammation/pain at injection site. **Metab:** *PO and IV*—hyperuricemia; *IV*, hyperglycemia. **MS:** arthralgia, myalgia, back pain. **Misc:** allergic reactions, chills, fever, infection.

Interactions

Drug-Drug: Concurrent or previous (within 72 hr) use of **acetaminophen** may ↓ elimination and ↑ toxicity. Concurrent use with high-dose **cyclophosphamide** in patients with thalassemia may result in cardiac tamponade. Concurrent use with **itraconazole** or **phenytoin** ↓ blood level effectiveness. Long-term continuous therapy with **thioguanine** may ↑ risk of hepatic toxicity. ↑ bone marrow suppression with other **antineoplastics** or **radiation therapy**. May ↓ the antibody response to and ↑risk of adverse reactions from **live-virus vaccines**.

Route/Dosage

Many other regimens are used. See current protocols for up-to-date dosage.

PO (Adults): *Induction*—1.8 mg/m²/day or 60 mcg (0.06 mg)/kg/day until WBCs <15,000/mm³. Usual dose is 4–8 mg/day (range 1–12 mg/day). *Maintenance*—1–3 mg/day.

PO (Children): 0.06–0.12 mg/kg/day or 1.8–4.6 mg/m²/day initially. Titrate dose to maintain WBC of approximately 20,000/mm³.

IV (Adults): 0.8 mg/kg q 6 hr (dose based on ideal body weight or actual weight, whichever is less; in obese patients, dosage should be based on adjusted ideal body weight) for 4 days (total of 16 doses); given in combination with cyclophosphamide.

Availability

Tablets: 2 mg. **Solution for injection:** 6 mg/mL.

NURSING IMPLICATIONS

Assessment

- ***High Alert:*** Monitor for bone marrow depression. Assess for bleeding (bleeding gums, bruising, petechiae, guaiac stools, urine, emesis) and avoid IM injections and taking rectal temperatures. Apply pressure to venipuncture sites for at least 10 min. Assess for signs of infection (fever, chills, sore throat, cough, hoarseness, lower back or side pain, difficult or painful urination) during neutropenia. Anemia may occur. Monitor for increased fatigue, dyspnea, and orthostatic hypotension. Notify health care professional if these symptoms occur.
- Monitor intake and output ratios and daily weights. Report significant changes in totals.
- Monitor for symptoms of gout (increased uric acid, joint pain, lower back or side pain, swelling of feet or lower legs). Encourage patient to drink at least 2 L of fluid each day. Allopurinol may be given to decrease uric acid levels. Alkalinization of urine may be ordered to increase excretion of uric acid.
- Assess for pulmonary fibrosis (fever, cough, shortness of breath) periodically during and after therapy. Discontinue therapy at the first sign of pulmonary fibrosis. Usually occurs 8 mo–10 yr (average 4 yr) after initiation of therapy.
- **IV:** Premedicate patient with phenytoin before IV administration to minimize the risk of seizures.
- Administer antiemetics before IV administration and on a fixed schedule throughout IV administration.
- ***Lab Test Considerations:*** Monitor CBC with differential and platelet count before and weekly during therapy. The nadir of leukopenia occurs within 10–15 days and the nadir of WBC at 11–30 days. Recovery usually occurs within 12–20 wk. Notify health care professional if WBC is <15,000/mm³ or if a precipitous drop occurs. Institute thrombocytopenia precautions if platelet count is <150,000/mm³. Bone marrow depression may be severe and progressive, with recovery taking 1 mo–2 yr after discontinuation of therapy.
- Monitor serum ALT, bilirubin, alkaline phosphatase, and uric acid before and periodically during therapy. May cause ↑ uric acid levels.
- May cause false-positive cytology results of breast, bladder, cervix, and lung tissues.

Potential Nursing Diagnoses

Disturbed body image (Side Effects)
Risk for injury (Side Effects)
Risk for infection (Side Effects)

Implementation

- ***High Alert:*** Fatalities have occurred with chemotherapeutic agents. Before administering, clarify all ambiguous orders; double check single, daily, and course-of-therapy dose limits; have second practitioner independently double check original order, calculations, and infusion pump settings.

B

- ***High Alert:*** Do not confuse Myleran with Alkeran or Leukeran.
- **PO:** Administer at the same time each day. Administer on an empty stomach to decrease nausea and vomiting.

IV Administration

- **IV:** Prepare solution in a biologic cabinet. Wear gloves, gown, and mask while handling IV medication. Discard IV equipment in specially designated containers.
- **Intermittent Infusion:** ***Diluent:*** Dilute with 10 times the volume of busulfan using 0.9% NaCl or D5W. ***Concentration:*** ≥0.5 mg/mL. When drawing busulfan from vial, use needle with 5-micron nylon filter provided, remove calculated volume from vial, remove needle and filter, replace needle and inject busulfan into diluent. Do not use polycarbonate syringes with busulfan. Only use filters provided with busulfan. Always add busulfan to diluent, not diluent to busulfan. Solution diluted with 0.9% NaCl or D5W is stable for 8 hr at room temperature and solution diluted with 0.9% NaCl is stable for 12 hr if refrigerated. Administration must be completed during this time. Solution is clear and colorless; do not administer solutions that are discolored or contain a precipitate. ***Rate:*** Administer via central venous catheter over 2 hr every 6 hr for 4 days for a total of 16 doses. Use infusion pump to administer entire dose over 2 hr.
- **Y-Site Compatibility:** acyclovir, amphotericin B lipid complex, amphotericin B liposome, anidulafungin, argatroban, bivalirudin, bleomycin, caspofungin, daptomycin, dexmedetomidine, diltiazem, docetaxel, ertapenem, fenoldopam, granisetron, hetastarch, hydromorphone, levofloxacin, linezolid, lorazepam, meperidine, metronidazole, milrinone, nesiritide, octreotide, ondansetron, paclitaxel, palonosetron, pancuronium, piperacillin/tazobactam, potassium acetate, quinupristin/dalfopristin, rituximab, sodium acetate, tacrolimus, tigecycline, tirofiban, trastuzumab, vasopressin, zoledronic acid.
- **Y-Site Incompatibility:** idarubicin, thiotepa, vecuronium, voriconazole.

Patient/Family Teaching

- Instruct patient to take medication as directed, at the same time each day, even if nausea and vomiting are a problem. Consult health care professional if vomiting occurs shortly after dose is taken. If a dose is missed, do not take at all; do not double doses.
- Advise patient to notify health care professional if fever; sore throat; signs of infection; lower back or side pain; difficult or painful urination; sores in the mouth or on the lips; chills; dyspnea; persistent cough; bleeding gums; bruising; petechiae; or blood in urine, stool, or emesis occurs. Instruct patient to use soft toothbrush and electric razor. Caution patient not to drink alcoholic beverages or take products containing aspirin or NSAIDs.
- Caution patient to avoid crowds and persons with known infections. Health care professional should be informed immediately if symptoms of infection occur.
- Discuss with patient the possibility of hair loss. Explore methods of coping.
- Instruct patient not to receive any vaccinations without advice of health care professional.
- Advise patient to notify health care professional if unusual bleeding; bruising; or flank, stomach, or joint pain occurs. Advise patients on long-term therapy to notify health care professional immediately if cough, shortness of breath, and fever occur or if darkening of skin, diarrhea, dizziness, fatigue, anorexia, confusion, or nausea and vomiting become pronounced.
- Inform patient of increased risk of a second malignancy with busulfan.
- Review with patient the need for contraception during therapy. Women need to use contraception even if amenorrhea occurs.

Evaluation/Desired Outcomes

- Decrease in leukocyte count to within normal limits.
- Decreased night sweats.
- Increase in appetite.
- Increased sense of well-being. Therapy is resumed when leukocyte count reaches 50,000/mm³.

BUTALBITAL COMPOUND
(byoo-**tal**-bi-tal)

butalbital, acetaminophen†
Axocet, Bucet, Bupap, Butex Forte, Dolgic, Marten-Tab, Phrenilin, Phrenilin Forte, Repap CF, Sedapap, Tencon, Triaprin

butalbital, acetaminophen, caffeine†
Endolor, Esgic, Esgic-Plus, Fioricet, Margesic, Medigesic, Repan, Triad

butalbital, aspirin, caffeine‡
Fiorinal, Fiortal, ✱Tecnal

Classification
Therapeutic: nonopioid analgesics (combination with barbiturate)
Pharmacologic: barbiturates

Schedule III (products with aspirin only)

Pregnancy Category D

†For information on acetaminophen component in formulation, see acetaminophen monograph

‡For information on aspirin component in formulation, see salicylates monograph

Indications
Management of mild to moderate pain.

Action
Contain an analgesic (aspirin or acetaminophen) for relief of pain, a barbiturate (butalbital) for its sedative effect, and some contain caffeine, which may be of benefit in vascular headaches. **Therapeutic Effects:** Decreased severity of pain with some sedation.

Pharmacokinetics
Absorption: Well absorbed.
Distribution: Widely distributed; cross the placenta and enter breast milk.
Metabolism and Excretion: Mostly metabolized by the liver.
Half-life: 35 hr.

TIME/ACTION PROFILE

ROUTE	ONSET	PEAK	DURATION
PO	15–30 min	1–2 hr	2–6 hr

Contraindications/Precautions
Contraindicated in: Hypersensitivity to individual components; Cross-sensitivity may occur; Comatose patients or those with pre-existing CNS depression; Uncontrolled severe pain; Aspirin should be avoided in patients with bleeding disorders or thrombocytopenia; Acetaminophen should be avoided in patients with severe hepatic or renal disease; Caffeine should be avoided in patients with severe cardiovascular disease; Pregnancy or lactation; Porphyria.
Use Cautiously in: History of suicide attempt or drug addiction; Chronic alcohol use/abuse (for aspirin and acetaminophen content); Geri: Appears on Beers list. Geriatric patients are at increased risk for side effects (dosage reduction recommended); Use should be short-term only; Children (safety not established).

Adverse Reactions/Side Effects
CNS: *caffeine*—drowsiness, hangover, delirium, depression, excitation, headache (with chronic use), insomnia, irritability, lethargy, nervousness, vertigo. **Resp:** respiratory depression. **CV:** *caffeine*—palpitations, tachycardia. **GI:** *caffeine*—constipation, diarrhea, epigastric distress, heartburn, nausea, vomiting. **Derm:** dermatitis, rash. **Misc:** hypersensitivity reactions including ANGIOEDEMA and SERUM SICKNESS, physical dependence, psychological dependence, tolerance.

Interactions
Drug-Drug: Additive CNS depression with other **CNS depressants**, including **alcohol**, **antihistamines**, **antidepressants**, **opioid analgesics**, and **sedative/hypnotics**. May increase the liver metabolism and decrease the effectiveness of other drugs including **hormonal contraceptives**, **chloramphenicol**, **acebutolol**, **propranolol**, **metoprolol**, **timolol**, **doxycycline**, **corticosteroids**, **tricyclic antidepressants**, **phenothiazines**, **phenylbutazone**, and **quinidine**. **MAO inhibitors**, **primidone**, and **valproic acid** may prevent metabolism and increase the effectiveness of butalbital. May enhance the hematologic toxicity of **cyclophosphamide**.
Drug-Natural Products: **St. John's wort** may decrease barbiturate effect. Concurrent use of **kava-kava**, **valerian**, **skullcap**, **chamomile**, or **hops** can increase CNS depression.

Route/Dosage
PO (Adults): 1–2 capsules or tablets (50–100 mg butalbital) every 4 hr as needed for pain (not to exceed 4 g acetaminophen or aspirin/24 hr).

Availability (generic available)
Tablets and capsules: 50 mg. ***In combination with:*** aspirin, acetaminophen, caffeine, and codeine Rx. See Appendix B.

NURSING IMPLICATIONS

Assessment
- Assess type, location, and intensity of pain before and 60 min following administration.
- Prolonged use may lead to physical and psychological dependence and tolerance. This should not prevent patient from receiving adequate analgesia. Most patients who receive butalbital compound for pain do not develop psychological dependence.
- Assess frequency of use. Frequent, chronic use may lead to daily headaches in headache-prone individuals because of physical dependence on caffeine and other components. Chronic headaches from overmedication are difficult to treat and may require hospitalization for treatment and prophylaxis.

Potential Nursing Diagnoses
Acute pain (Indications)
Risk for injury (Side Effects)

Implementation
- Do not confuse Fiorinal with Fioricet.
- Explain therapeutic value of medication before administration to enhance the analgesic effect.
- Regularly administered doses may be more effective than prn administration. Analgesic is more effective if given before pain becomes severe.

- Medication should be discontinued gradually after long-term use to prevent withdrawal symptoms.
- **PO:** Oral doses should be administered with food, milk, or a full glass of water to minimize GI irritation.

Patient/Family Teaching

- Instruct patient to take medication exactly as directed. Do not increase dose because of the habit-forming potential of butalbital. If medication appears less effective after a few weeks, consult health care professional. Doses of acetaminophen or aspirin should not exceed the maximum recommended daily dose. Chronic excessive use of >4 g/day (2 g in chronic alcoholism) may lead to hepatotoxicity, renal or cardiac damage.
- Advise patients with vascular headaches to take medication at first sign of headache. Lying down in a quiet, dark room may also be helpful. Medications taken for prophylaxis should be continued.
- May cause drowsiness or dizziness. Advise patient to avoid driving and other activities requiring alertness until response to medication is known.
- Caution patient to avoid concurrent use of alcohol or other CNS depressants.
- Advise patient to use an additional nonhormonal method of contraception while taking butalbital compound.

Evaluation/Desired Outcomes

- Decrease in severity of pain without a significant alteration in level of consciousness.

B

butenafine, See ANTIFUNGALS (TOPICAL).

butoconazole, See ANTIFUNGALS (VAGINAL).

HIGH ALERT

cabazitaxel (ka-ba-zi-**tax**-el)
Jevtana

Classification
Therapeutic: antineoplastics
Pharmacologic: taxoids

Pregnancy Category D

Indications

Hormone-refractory metastatic prostate cancer previously treated with a regimen including docetaxel (used in combination with prednisone).

Action

Binds to intracellular tubulin and promotes its assembly into microtubules while inhibiting disassembly. Result is inhibition of mitotis and interphase. **Therapeutic Effects:** Death of rapidly replicating cells, particularly malignant ones, with ↓ spread of metastatic prostate cancer.

Pharmacokinetics

Absorption: IV administration results in complete bioavailability.
Distribution: Equally distributed between blood and plasma.
Metabolism and Excretion: Extensively (>95%) metabolized by the liver, 80–90% by CYP3A4/5 enzyme system. Metabolites are excreted in urine and feces. Minimal renal excretion.
Half-life: *Terminal elimination*—95 hr.

TIME/ACTION PROFILE (blood levels)

ROUTE	ONSET	PEAK	DURATION
IV	rapid	end of infusion	unknown

Contraindications/Precautions

Contraindicated in: Severe hypersensitivity to cabazitaxel or polysorbate 80; Neutrophils ≤1,500/mm³; Hepatic impairment (total bilirubin ≥3x upper limit of normal [ULN]); Concurrent use of strong CYP3A4 inhibitors or inducers; OB: Avoid use during pregnancy (may cause fetal harm); Lactation: Breast feeding should be avoided.
Use Cautiously in: Concurrent use of moderate CYP3A4 inhibitors; Patients with neutropenia or a history of pelvic radiation, adhesions, ulceration, or GI bleeding (↑ risk of GI adverse reactions); Concomitant use of steroids, NSAIDs, or antithrombotics (↑ risk of GI adverse reactions); Severe renal impairment (CCr <30 mL/min) or end-stage renal disease; Hemoglobin <10 g/dL; Mild or moderate hepatic impairment (dose ↓ required); OB: Patients with childbearing potential (pregnancy should be avoided); Geri: ↑ risk of adverse reactions; Pedi: Safety and effectiveness not established.

Adverse Reactions/Side Effects

CNS: weakness, fatigue. **Resp:** dyspnea. **CV:** arrhythmias, hypotension. **GI:** DIARRHEA, ENTEROCOLITIS, GI BLEED, GI PERFORATION, ILEUS, abdominal pain, abnormal taste, anorexia, constipation, nausea, vomiting, dyspepsia. **GU:** RENAL FAILURE, hematuria. **Derm:** alopecia. **F and E:** electrolyte imbalance. **Hemat:** NEUTROPENIA, THROMBOCYTOPENIA, anemia, leukopenia. **MS:** arthralgia, back pain, muscle spasms. **Neuro:** peripheral neuropathy. **Misc:** allergic reactions including ANAPHYLAXIS, fever.

Interactions

Drug-Drug: Strong CYP3A inhibitors including **ketoconazole**, **itraconazole**, **clarithromycin**, **atazanavir**, **indinavir**, **nefazodone**, **nelfinavir**, **ritonavir**, **saquinavir**, **telithromycin** and **voriconazole** ↑ levels and risk of toxicity; concomitant use contraindicated. **Strong CYP3A inducers** including **phenytoin**, **carbamazepine**, **rifampin**, **rifabutin**, **rifapentin**, and **phenobarbital** may ↓ levels and effectiveness; concomitant use contraindicated.
Drug-Natural Products: St. John's wort may ↓ levels and effectiveness; concomitant use contraindicated.

Route/Dosage

PO (Adults): 25 mg/m² every 3 wk (with prednisone 10 mg PO daily).

Hepatic Impairment

PO (Adults): *Mild hepatic impairment (total bilirubin >1x to ≤1.5x ULN or AST >1.5x ULN)*—20 mg/m² every 3 wk (with prednisone 10 mg PO daily); *Moderate hepatic impairment (total bilirubin >1.5x to ≤3x ULN)*—15 mg/m² every 3 wk (with prednisone 10 mg PO daily); *Severe hepatic impairment (total bilirubin >3x ULN)*—Contraindicated.

Availability

Viscous solution for injection (requires two dilutions prior to IV administration): 40 mg/mL (contains polysorbate 80) comes with diluent (5.7 mL of 13% [w/w] ethanol in water for injection).

NURSING IMPLICATIONS

Assessment

- Assess for hypersensitivity reactions (generalized rash/erythema, hypotension, bronchospasm, swelling of face). May occur within minutes following initiation of infusion. If severe reactions occur, discontinue infusion immediately and provide supportive therapy.
- Assess for signs and symptoms of GI toxicity (abdominal pain and tenderness, fever, persistent con-

stipation, nausea, vomiting, severe diarrhea); may result in death due to electrolyte imbalance. Premedication is recommended. Treat with rehydration, anti-diarrheal, or antiemetic therapy as needed. If Grade ≥3 diarrhea or persisting diarrhea occurs despite appropriate medication, fluid and electrolyte replacement, delay treatment until improvement or resolution, then reduce dose to 20 mg/mL.

- Assess for signs and symptoms of peripheral neuropathy (pain, burning, numbness in hands, feet, or legs) during therapy. *If Grade 2 occurs,* withhold until improvement or resolution, then reduce dose to 20 mg/mL. *If ≥Grade 3 occurs,* discontinue therapy.
- ***Lab Test Considerations:*** Monitor CBC weekly during cycle 1 and before each treatment cycle thereafter. Do not administer if neutrophils ≤1500/mm^3. If prolonged grade 3 neutropenia (>1 wk) despite appropriate medication including filgrastim, delay treatment until neutrophil count is >1500 mm^3, then reduce dose to 20 mg/m^2. Use filgrastim for secondary prophylaxis.
- If febrile neutropenia occurs, delay therapy until improvement or resolution and neutrophil count is >1500/mm^3, then reduce dose to 20 mg/m^2. Use filgrastim for secondary prophylaxis.
- Discontinue cabazitaxel if prolonged Grade 3 neutropenia, febrile neutropenia, or Grade 3 diarrhea occur at the 20 mg/m^2 dose.
- May cause hematuria.
- May cause Grade 3–4 ↑ AST, ↑ ALT, and ↑ bilirubin.

Potential Nursing Diagnoses

Risk for infection (Adverse Reactions)

Implementation

- ***High Alert:*** Fatalities have occurred with chemotherapeutic agents. Before administering, clarify all ambiguous orders; double check single, daily, and course-of-therapy dose limits; have second practitioner independently double check original order and dose calculations.
- Prepare solution in a biologic cabinet. Wear gloves, gown, and mask while handling medication. Discard equipment in specially designated containers. If solution comes in contact with skin or mucosa, wash with soap and water immediately.
- Premedicate at least 30 min before each dose with antihistamine (diphenhydramine 25 mg or equivalent), corticosteroid (dexamethasone 8 mg or equivalent), and H_2 antagonist (ranitidine 50 mg or equivalent). Antiemetic prophylaxis, PO or IV, is recommended.

IV Administration

- Two dilutions are required. Do not use PVC infusion containers or polyurethane infusion sets for preparation or infusion.
- **First Dilution: *Diluent:*** Mix vial with entire contents of supplied diluent. Direct needle to inside wall id vial and inject slowly to avoid foaming. Mix gently by repeated inversions for at least 45 sec; do not shake. Let stand for a few minutes to allow foam to dissipate. ***Concentration:*** 10 mg/mL. **Second Dilution:** . ***Diluent:*** Withdraw recommended dose from cabazitaxel solution and dilute further into a setrile 250 mL PVC-free container of 0.9% NaCl or D5W. If dose >65 mg is required, use a larger volume of infusion vehicle so concentration does not exceed 0.26 mg/mL. Gently invert container to mix. ***Concentration:*** 0.10–0.26 mg/mL. Stable for 8 hr (including 1 hr infusion) at room temperature or 24 hr if refrigerated. May crystalize over time. Do not use if crystalized, discolored, or contains particulate matter; discard. ***Rate:*** Infuse over 1 hr at room temperature through a 0.22 micrometer nominal pore size filter.
- **Y-Site Incompatibility:** Do not mix with other medication.

Patient/Family Teaching

- Instruct patient to take oral prednisone as prescribed and to notify health care professional if a dose is missed or not taken in time.
- Advise patient to notify health care professional immediately if signs or symptoms of hypersensitivity reactions; fever; sore throat; signs of infection; lower back or side pain; difficult or painful urination; sores on the mouth or on the lips; bleeding gums; bruising; petechiae; blood in urine, stool, or emesis; unusual swelling occurs. Caution patient to avoid crowds and persons with known infections. Instruct patient to use soft toothbrush and electric razor and to avoid falls. Patient should also be cautioned not to drink alcoholic beverages or to take products containing aspirin or NSAIDs; may precipitate GI hemorrhage.
- Instruct patient to notify health care professional of all Rx or OTC medications, vitamins, or herbal products being taken and consult health care professional before taking any new medications, especially St. John's Wort.
- May cause dizziness. Caution patient to avoid driving or other activities requiring alertness until response to medication is known.
- Advise female patients of the need for contraception and to avoid breast feeding during therapy.
- Instruct patient not to receive any vaccinations without advice of health care professional.
- Emphasize need for periodic lab tests to monitor for side effects. Advise patient to monitor temperature frequently.

Evaluation/Desired Outcomes

- ↓ in size and spread of metastatic prostate cancer.

C

cabergoline (ka-ber-goe-leen)

~~Dostinex~~

Classification
Therapeutic: antihyperprolactinemic
Pharmacologic: dopamine agonists

Pregnancy Category B

Indications
Treatment of hyperprolactinemia (idiopathic or pituitary in origin).

Action
Inhibits secretion of prolactin by acting as a dopamine agonist. **Therapeutic Effects:** Decreased secretion of prolactin in hyperprolactinemia.

Pharmacokinetics
Absorption: Well absorbed but undergoes extensive first-pass hepatic metabolism.
Distribution: Widely distributed; concentrates in pituitary.
Metabolism and Excretion: Extensively metabolized by the liver; <4% excreted unchanged in urine.
Protein Binding: 40–42%.
Half-life: 63–69 hr.

TIME/ACTION PROFILE (effect on serum prolactin levels)

ROUTE	ONSET	PEAK	DURATION
PO	unknown	2–3 hr	unknown

Contraindications/Precautions
Contraindicated in: Hypersensitivity to cabergoline or ergot alkaloids; Uncontrolled hypertension; History of pulmonary, pericardial, or retroperitoneal fibrotic disorders; History of cardiac valvular disease; Lactation: Has been associated with hypertension, stroke, and seizures. Not to be used for suppression of physiologic lactation.
Use Cautiously in: Hepatic impairment; Patients who have received medications associated with valvular disorders; OB: Use only if clearly needed; Pedi: Safety not established.

Adverse Reactions/Side Effects
CNS: dizziness, headache, depression, drowsiness, fatigue, impulse control disorders (gambling, sexual), nervousness, vertigo, weakness. **Resp:** PULMONARY FIBROSIS, pleural effusion. **EENT:** abnormal vision. **CV:** PERICARDIAL FIBROSIS, VALVULAR DISORDERS, postural hypotension, hot flashes. **GI:** RETROPERITONEAL FIBROSIS, constipation, nausea, abdominal pain, dyspepsia, vomiting. **GU:** dysmenorrhea. **Endo:** breast pain. **Neuro:** paresthesia.

Interactions
Drug-Drug: ↑ risk of hypotension with **antihypertensives**. May ↑ the effects of **SSRIs** and other **serotonin agonists** (induces serotonin syndrome). Effectiveness may be ↓ by **phenothiazines**, **butyrophenones (haloperidol)**, **thioxanthenes**, or **metoclopramide** (avoid concurrent use).

Route/Dosage
PO (Adults): 0.25 mg twice weekly; may be ↑ at 4-wk intervals up to 1 mg twice weekly.

Availability (generic available)
Tablets: 0.5 mg.

NURSING IMPLICATIONS

Assessment
- Monitor BP before and frequently during initial therapy. Initial doses >1 m g may cause orthostatic hypotension. Use with caution when administering concurrently with other medications that lower BP. Supervise ambulation and transfer during initial dosing to prevent injury from hypotension.
- Evaluate the cardiac status and monitor echocardiography at baseline and every 6–12 mo after initiation of therapy or as indicated clinically by signs and symptoms of valvular disease (dyspnea, edema, HF, new cardiac murmur). Use lowest dose and reassess need for therapy periodically.
- Monitor for signs and symptoms of pulmonary fibrosis (dyspnea, persistent coughing, difficulty with breathing while lying down, peripheral edema) periodically during therapy. Obtain chest x-ray prior to therapy and chest x-ray and CT scan periodically during therapy to assess for pulmonary fibrosis.
- ***Lab Test Considerations:*** Monitor serum prolactin concentrations monthly until normalized (<20 mcg/L in women and <15 mcg/L in men).
- Monitor erythrocyte sedimentation rate (ESR) and creatinine at baseline and as needed during therapy.

Potential Nursing Diagnoses
Risk for injury (Side Effects)
Impaired physical mobility (Indications)

Implementation
- **PO:** May be taken without regard to food.

Patient/Family Teaching
- Instruct patient to take medication as directed. Take missed doses as soon as possible within 1 or 2 days. If not remembered until time of next dose, double dose. If nausea occurs, discuss with health care professional.
- May cause drowsiness and dizziness. Caution patient to avoid driving and other activities requiring alertness until response to medication is known.
- Advise patient to change positions slowly to minimize orthostatic hypotension.

- Caution patient to avoid concurrent use of alcohol during therapy.
- Instruct patients taking cabergoline for pituitary tumors to inform health care professional immediately if signs of tumor enlargement occur (blurred vision, sudden headache, severe nausea, and vomiting).
- Advise patient to notify health care professional if signs of valvular disorders (shortness of breath, swelling in extremities) occurs.
- Advise patient to notify health care professional if new or increased gambling, sexual, or other impulse control disorders occur.
- Advise women to consult with health care professional regarding a nonhormonal method of birth control. Women should contact health care professional promptly if pregnancy is planned or suspected.
- Emphasize the importance of regular follow-up exams to determine effectiveness and monitor side effects.

Evaluation/Desired Outcomes

- Decrease in galactorrhea in patients with hyperprolactinemia.
- After a normal serum prolactin level has been maintained for more than 6 mo, cabergoline may be discontinued. Serum prolactin levels should be monitored periodically to determine necessity of reinstituting cabergoline.

CALCITONIN

calcitonin (salmon)
(kal-si-**toe**-nin)
✱Calcimar, Miacalcin

calcitonin (rDNA)
Fortical

Classification
Therapeutic: hypocalcemics
Pharmacologic: hormones

Pregnancy Category C

Indications

IM, Subcut: Treatment of Paget's disease of bone. Adjunctive therapy for hypercalcemia. **IM, Subcut, Intranasal:** Management of postmenopausal osteoporosis.

Action

Inhibits osteoclastic bone resorption and promotes renal excretion of calcium. **Therapeutic Effects:** Decreased rate of bone turnover. Lowering of serum calcium.

Pharmacokinetics

Absorption: Completely absorbed from IM and subcut sites. Rapidly absorbed from nasal mucosa; absorption is 3% compared with parenteral administration.

Distribution: Unknown.

Metabolism and Excretion: Rapidly metabolized in kidneys, blood, and tissues.

Half-life: 40–90 min.

TIME/ACTION PROFILE

ROUTE	ONSET	PEAK	DURATION
IM, subcut†	unknown	2 hr	6–8 hr
Intranasal‡	rapid	31–39 min	unknown

†Effects on serum calcium; effects on serum alkaline phosphates and urinary hydroxyproline in Paget's disease may require 6–24 mo of continuous treatment.

‡Serum levels of administered calcitonin.

Contraindications/Precautions

Contraindicated in: Hypersensitivity to calcitonin, salmon protein or gelatin diluent (in some products); OB, Lactation: Use not recommended.

Use Cautiously in: Pedi: Safety not established.

Adverse Reactions/Side Effects

CNS: *nasal only*—headaches. **EENT:** *nasal only*—rhinitis, epistaxis, nasal irritation. **GI:** *IM, subcut*—nausea, vomiting. **GU:** *IM, subcut*—urinary frequency. **Derm:** rash. **Local:** injection site reactions. **MS:** *nasal*—arthralgia, back pain. **Misc:** MALIGNANCY, allergic reactions including ANAPHYLAXIS, facial flushing, swelling.

Interactions

Drug-Drug: Previous bisphosphonate therapy, including **alendronate**, **risedronate**, **etidronate**, **ibandronate**, or **pamidronate**, may ↓ response to calcitonin. May ↓ **lithium** levels.

Route/Dosage

Postmenopausal osteoporosis

IM, Subcut (Adults): 100 units every other day.
Intranasal (Adults): 1 spray (200 units)/day in alternating nostrils.

Paget's disease

IM, Subcut (Adults): 100 units/day initially, after titration, maintenance dose is usually 50 units/day or every other day.

Hypercalcemia

IM, Subcut (Adults): 4 units/kg q 12 hr; if adequate response not achieved, may ↑ dose after 1–2 days to 8 units/kg q 12 hr, and if necessary after 2 more days may be ↑ to 8 units/kg q 6 hr.

Availability (generic available)

Injection: 200 units/mL. **Nasal spray:** 200 units/actuation.

NURSING IMPLICATIONS

Assessment

- Observe patient for signs of hypersensitivity (skin rash, fever, hives, anaphylaxis, serum sickness).

Keep epinephrine, antihistamines, and oxygen nearby in the event of a reaction.

- Assess patient for signs of hypocalcemic tetany (nervousness, irritability, paresthesia, muscle twitching, tetanic spasms, seizures) during the first several doses of calcitonin. Parenteral calcium, such as calcium gluconate, should be available in case of this event.
- **Intranasal:** Assess nasal mucosa, septum, turbinates, and mucosal blood vessels periodically during therapy. If severe ulceration occurs, drug should be discontinued.
- ***Lab Test Considerations:*** Monitor serum calcium and alkaline phosphatase periodically during therapy. Levels should normalize within a few months of initiation of therapy.
- Urine hydroxyproline (24 hr) may be monitored periodically in patients with Paget's disease.

Potential Nursing Diagnoses

Acute pain (Indications)
Risk for injury (Indications, Side Effects)

Implementation

- Do not confuse Fortical with Foradil.
- In patients with suspected sensitivity to calcitonin, skin test should be considered before starting therapy. Test dose is prepared in a dilution of 10 units/mL by withdrawing 0.05 mL in a tuberculin syringe and filling to 1 mL with 0.9% NaCl for injection. Mix well and discard 0.9 mL. Administer 0.1 mL intradermally on inner aspect on forearm and observe site for 15 min. More than mild erythema or wheal constitutes positive response.
- Store injection and unopened nasal spray bottle in refrigerator. Nasal spray bottle in use can be stored at room temperature.
- **IM, Subcut:** Inspect injection site for the appearance of redness, swelling, or pain. Rotate injection sites. Subcut is the preferred route. Use IM route if dose exceeds 2 mL in volume. Use multiple sites to minimize inflammatory reaction.

Patient/Family Teaching

- Advise patient to take calcitonin as directed. If dose is missed and medication is scheduled for twice a day, take only if possible within 2 hr of correct time. If scheduled for daily dose, take only if remembered that day. If scheduled for every other day, take when remembered and restart alternate day schedule. If taking 1 dose 3 times weekly (Mon, Wed, Fri), take missed dose the next day and set each injection back 1 day; resume regular schedule the following week. Do not double doses.
- Instruct patient in the proper method of self-injection and care and disposal of equipment.
- Advise patient to report signs of hypercalcemic relapse (deep bone or flank pain, renal calculi, anorexia, nausea, vomiting, thirst, lethargy) or allergic response promptly.
- Reassure patient that flushing and warmth following injection are transient and usually last about 1 hr.
- Explain that nausea following injection tends to decrease even with continued therapy.
- Instruct patient to follow low-calcium diet if recommended by health care professional (see Appendix J). Women with postmenopausal osteoporosis should adhere to a diet high in calcium and vitamin D.
- Inform patient of increased risk of malignancy.
- **Osteoporosis:** Advise patients receiving calcitonin for the treatment of osteoporosis that exercise has been found to arrest and reverse bone loss. The patient should discuss any exercise limitations with health care professional before beginning program.
- **Intranasal:** Instruct patient on correct use of nasal spray. Demonstrate procedure for use. Before first use, activate pump by holding upright and depressing white side arms down toward bottle 5 times until a full spray is emitted. Following activation, place nozzle firmly in nostril with head in an upright position and depress the pump toward the bottle. The pump should NOT be primed before each daily use. Discard bottle 30 days after first use.
- Advise patient to notify health care professional if significant nasal irritation occurs.

Evaluation/Desired Outcomes

- Lowered serum calcium levels.
- Decreased bone pain.
- Slowed progression of postmenopausal osteoporosis. Significant increases in bone marrow density may be seen as early as 6 mo after initiation of therapy.

calcitriol, See VITAMIN D COMPOUNDS.

HIGH ALERT

CALCIUM SALTS

calcium acetate (25% Ca or 12.6 mEq/g)
(**kal**-see-um **ass**-e-tate)
Eliphos, PhosLo, Phoslyra

calcium carbonate (40% Ca or 20 mEq/g)
(**kal**-see-um **kar**-bo-nate)
Alka-Mints, Amitone, ✤Apo-Cal, BioCal, Calcarb, Calci-Chew, Calciday, Calcilac, Calci-Mix, ✤Calcite,

✱Calglycine, Cal-Plus, ✱Calsan, Caltrate, Chooz, Dicarbosil, Equilet, Gencalc, Liqui-Cal, Liquid Cal-600, Maalox Antacid Caplets, Mallamint, ✱Mylanta Lozenges, Nephro-Calci, ✱Nu-Cal, Os-Cal, Oysco, Oyst-Cal, Oystercal, Rolaids Calcium Rich, Surpass, Surpass Extra Strength, Titralac, Tums, Tums E-X

calcium chloride (27% Ca or 13.6 mEq/g)
(**kal**-see-um **kloh**-ride)

calcium citrate (21% Ca or 12 mEq/g) (**kal**-see-um **si**-trate)
Cal-Citrate 250, Citrical, Citrical Liquitab

calcium gluconate (9% Ca or 4.5 mEq/g)
(**kal**-see-um **gloo**-koh-nate)
Kalcinate

calcium lactate (13% Ca or 6.5 mEq/g) (**kal**-see-um **lak**-tate)
Cal-Lac

tricalcium phosphate (39% Ca or 19.5 mEq/g)
(tri-**kal**-see-um **foss**-fate)
Posture

Classification
Therapeutic: mineral and electrolyte replacements/supplements
Pharmacologic: antacids

Pregnancy Category C (calcium acetate, calcium chloride, calcium gluconate injections), UK (calcium carbonate, calcium citrate, calcium lactate, tricalcium phosphate)

Indications

PO, IV: Treatment and prevention of hypocalcemia. **PO:** Adjunct in the prevention of postmenopausal osteoporosis. **IV:** Emergency treatment of hyperkalemia and hypermagnesemia and adjunct in cardiac arrest or calcium channel blocking agent toxicity (calcium chloride, calcium gluconate). **Calcium carbonate:** May be used as an antacid. **Calcium acetate:** Control of hyperphosphatemia in end-stage renal disease.

Action

Essential for nervous, muscular, and skeletal systems. Maintain cell membrane and capillary permeability. Act as an activator in the transmission of nerve impulses and contraction of cardiac, skeletal, and smooth muscle. Essential for bone formation and blood coagulation. Binds to dietary phosphate to form an insoluble calcium phosphate complex, which is excreted in the feces, resulting in decreased serum phosphorus concentrations (calcium acetate). **Therapeutic Effects:** Replacement of calcium in deficiency states. Control of hyperphosphatemia in end-stage renal disease without promoting aluminum absorption (calcium acetate).

Pharmacokinetics

Absorption: Absorption from the GI tract requires vitamin D. IV administration results in complete bioavailability.
Distribution: Readily enters extracellular fluid. Crosses the placenta and enters breast milk.
Metabolism and Excretion: Excreted mostly in the feces; 20% eliminated by the kidneys.
Half-life: Unknown.

TIME/ACTION PROFILE (effects on serum calcium)

ROUTE	ONSET	PEAK	DURATION
PO	unknown	unknown	unknown
IV	immediate	immediate	0.5–2 hr

Contraindications/Precautions

Contraindicated in: Hypercalcemia; Renal calculi; Ventricular fibrillation; Concurrent use of calcium supplements (calcium acetate).
Use Cautiously in: Patients receiving digitalis glycosides; Severe respiratory insufficiency; Renal disease; Cardiac disease; OB: Hypercalcemia may ↑ risk of maternal and fetal complications; Lactation: Breast feeding not expected to harm infant provided that serum calcium levels monitored.

Adverse Reactions/Side Effects

CNS: syncope (IV only), tingling. **CV:** CARDIAC ARREST (IV only), arrhythmias, bradycardia. **F and E:** hypercalcemia. **GI:** constipation, diarrhea (oral solution only), nausea, vomiting. **GU:** calculi, hypercalciuria. **Local:** phlebitis (IV only).

Interactions

Drug-Drug: Hypercalcemia ↑ the risk of **digoxin** toxicity. Chronic use with **antacids** in renal insufficiency may lead to milk-alkali syndrome. **Calcium supplements**, including calcium-containing antacids, may ↑ risk of hypercalcemia; avoid concurrent use. Ingestion by mouth ↓ the absorption of orally administered **phenytoin** and **iron salts**; take 1 hr before or 3 hr after oral calcium supplements. Excessive amounts may ↓ the effects of **calcium channel blockers**. Calcium acetate may ↓ absorption of orally administered **tetracyclines**; take ≥1 hr before calcium acetate. Calcium acetate may ↓ absorption of orally administered **fluoroquinolones**; take ≥2 hr before or 6 hr after calcium acetate. Calcium acetate may ↓ absorption of orally administered **levothyroxine**; take ≥4 hr before or 4 hr after calcium acetate. ↓ absorption of **etidronate** and **risedronate** (do not take within 2 hr of calcium supplements). Concurrent use with **diuretics (thiazide)** may result in hypercalcemia. May ↓ the ability of **sodium polystyrene sulfonate** to decrease serum potassium.

Drug-Food: Cereals, **spinach**, or **rhubarb** may ↓ the absorption of calcium supplements.

Route/Dosage

Doses are expressed in mg, g, or mEq of calcium.

PO (Adults): *Prevention of hypocalcemia, treatment of depletion, osteoporosis*—1–2 g/day. *Antacid*—0.5–1.5 g as needed (calcium carbonate only). *Hyperphosphatemia in end-stage renal disease (calcium acetate only)*—1334 mg with each meal, may ↑ gradually (in absence of hypercalcemia) to achieve target serum phosphate levels (usual dose = 2001–2668 mg with each meal).

PO (Children): *Supplementation*—45–65 mg/kg/day.

PO (Infants): *Neonatal hypocalcemia*—50–150 mg/kg (not to exceed 1 g).

IV (Adults): *Emergency treatment of hypocalcemia, cardiac standstill*—7–14 mEq. *Hypocalcemic tetany*—4.5–16 mEq; repeat until symptoms are controlled. *Hyperkalemia with cardiac toxicity*—2.25–14 mEq; may repeat in 1–2 min. *Hypermagnesemia*—7 mEq.

IV (Children): *Emergency treatment of hypocalcemia*—1–7 mEq. *Hypocalcemic tetany*—0.5–0.7 mEq/kg 3–4 times daily.

IV (Infants): *Emergency treatment of hypocalcemia*—<1 mEq. *Hypocalcemic tetany*—2.4 mEq/kg/day in divided doses.

Availability (generic available)

Calcium Acetate

Gelcaps: 667 mg (169 mg elemental Ca). **Tablets:** 667 mg (169 mg elemental Ca). **Oral solution:** 667 mg (169 mg elemental Ca)/5 mL.

Calcium Carbonate

Tablets: 500 mg (200 mg Ca)^{OTC}, 600 mg (240 mg Ca)^{OTC}, 650 mg (260 mg Ca)^{OTC}, 667 mg (266.8 mg Ca)^{OTC}, 1 g (400 mg Ca)^{OTC}, 1.25 g (500 mg Ca)^{OTC}, 1.5 g (600 mg Ca)^{OTC}. **Chewable tablets:** 350 mg (300 mg Ca)^{OTC}, 420 mg (168 mg Ca)^{OTC}, 450 mg ^{OTC}, 500 mg (200 mg Ca)^{OTC}, 750 mg (300 mg Ca)^{OTC}, 1 g (400 mg Ca)^{OTC}, 1.25 g (500 mg Ca)^{OTC}. **Gum tablets:** 300 mg ^{OTC}, 450 mg ^{OTC}, 500 mg (200 mg Ca)^{OTC}. **Capsules:** 1.25 g (500 mg Ca)^{OTC}. **Lozenges:** 600 mg (240 mg Ca)^{OTC}. **Oral suspension:** 1.25 g (500 mg Ca)/5 mL^{OTC}. **Powder:** 6.5 g (2400 mg Ca)/packet^{OTC}.

Calcium Chloride

Injection: 10% (1.36 mEq/mL).

Calcium Citrate

Tablets: 250 mg^{OTC}.

Calcium Gluconate

Tablets: 500 mg (45 mg Ca)^{OTC}, 650 mg (58.5 mg Ca)^{OTC}, 975 mg (87.75 mg Ca)^{OTC}, 1 g (90 mg Ca)^{OTC}. **Injection:** 10% (0.45 mEq/mL).

Calcium Lactate

Tablets: 325 mg (42.45 mg Ca)^{OTC}, 500 mg ^{OTC}, 650 mg (84.5 mg Ca)^{OTC}.

Tricalcium Phosphate

Tablets: 600 mg (234 mg Ca)^{OTC}.

NURSING IMPLICATIONS

Assessment

- **Calcium Supplement/Replacement:** Observe patient closely for symptoms of hypocalcemia (paresthesia, muscle twitching, laryngospasm, colic, cardiac arrhythmias, Chvostek's or Trousseau's sign). Notify health care professional if these occur. Protect symptomatic patients by elevating and padding siderails and keeping bed in low position.
- Monitor BP, pulse, and ECG frequently throughout parenteral therapy. May cause vasodilation with resulting hypotension, bradycardia, arrhythmias, and cardiac arrest. Transient increases in BP may occur during IV administration, especially in geriatric patients or in patients with hypertension.
- Assess IV site for patency. Extravasation may cause cellulitis, necrosis, and sloughing.
- Monitor patient on digoxin for signs of toxicity.
- **Antacid:** When used as an antacid, assess for heartburn, indigestion, and abdominal pain. Inspect abdomen; auscultate bowel sounds.
- ***Lab Test Considerations:*** Monitor serum calcium or ionized calcium, chloride, sodium, potassium, magnesium, albumin, and parathyroid hormone (PTH) concentrations before and periodically during therapy for treatment of hypocalcemia.
- *For patients with hyperphosphatemia*: Monitor serum calcium twice weekly during adjustment phase. If serum calcium level is >12 mg/dL, discontinue therapy and start hemodialysis as needed; lower dose or temporarily stop therapy for calcium level between 10.5 and 11.9 mg/dL.
- May cause ↓ serum phosphate concentrations with excessive and prolonged use. When used to treat hyperphosphatemia in renal failure patients, monitor phosphate levels.
- ***Toxicity and Overdose:*** Assess patient for nausea, vomiting, anorexia, thirst, severe constipation, paralytic ileus, and bradycardia. Contact health care professional immediately if these signs of hypercalcemia occur.

Potential Nursing Diagnoses

Imbalanced nutrition: less than body requirements (Indications)

Risk for injury related to osteoporosis or electrolyte imbalance (Indications)

Implementation

- ***High Alert:*** Errors with IV calcium gluconate and chloride have occurred secondary to confusion over which salt is ordered. Clarify incomplete orders. Confusion has occurred with milligram doses of calcium chloride and calcium gluconate, which are not equal. Chloride and gluconate forms are routinely available on most hospital crash carts; specify form of calcium desired. Doses should be expressed in mEq.
- Do not confuse Os-Cal (calcium carbonate) with Asacol (mesalamine).
- In arrest situations, the use of calcium chloride is now limited to patients with hyperkalemia, hypocalcemia, and calcium channel blocker toxicity.
- **PO:** Administer calcium carbonate or phosphate 1–1.5 hr after meals and at bedtime. Chewable tablets should be well chewed before swallowing. Dissolve effervescent tablets in glass of water. Follow oral doses with a full glass of water, except when using calcium carbonate as a phosphate binder in renal dialysis. Administer on an empty stomach before meals to optimize effectiveness in patients with hyperphosphatemia.
- **IM:** IM administration of calcium salts can cause severe necrosis and tissue sloughing. Do not administer IM.

IV Administration

- **IV:** IV solution should be warmed to body temperature and given through a small-bore needle in a large vein to minimize phlebitis. Do not administer through a scalp vein. May cause cutaneous burning sensation, peripheral vasodilation, and drop in BP. Patient should remain recumbent for 30–60 min after IV administration.
- If infiltration occurs, discontinue IV. May be treated with application of heat, elevation, and local infiltration of normal saline, 1% procaine HCl, or hyaluronidase.
- ***High Alert:*** Administer slowly. High concentrations may cause cardiac arrest. Rapid administration may cause tingling, sensation of warmth, and a metallic taste. Halt infusion if these symptoms occur, and resume infusion at a slower rate when they subside.
- Do not administer solutions that are not clear or that contain a precipitate.

Calcium Chloride

IV Administration

- **IV Push:** May be administered undiluted by IV push.
- **Intermittent/Continuous Infusion:** May be diluted with D5W, D10W, 0.9% NaCl, D5/0.25% NaCl, D5/0.45% NaCl, D5/0.9% NaCl, or D5/LR.
- ***Rate:*** Maximum rate for adults is 0.7–1.4 mEq/min (0.5–1 mL of 10% solution); for children, 0.5 mL/min.
- **Y-Site Compatibility:** acyclovir, alemtuzumab, alfentanil, amikacin, aminocaproic acid, aminophylline, amiodarone, anidulafungin, argatroban, ascorbic acid, atropine, azithromycin, aztreonam, benztropine, bivalirudin, bleomycin, bumetanide, buprenorphine, butorphanol, calcium gluconate, carboplatin, carmustine, caspofungin, cefotaxime, cefotetan, cefoxitin, ceftaroline, chloramphenicol, chlorpromazine, cisplatin, clindamycin, cyanocobalamin, cyclophosphamide, cyclosporine, cytarabine, dacarbazine, dactinomycin, daptomycin, dexmedetomidine, dexrazoxane, digoxin, diltiazem, diphenhydramine, dobutamine, docetaxel, dopamine, doxorubicin, doxycycline, enalaprilat, ephedrine, epinephrine, epirubicin, epoetin alfa, eptifibatide, ertapenem, erythromycin, esmolol, etoposide, etoposide phosphate, famotidine, fenoldopam, fentanyl, fluconazole, fludarabine, furosemide, ganciclovir, gemcitabine, gentamicin, glycopyrrolate, granisetron, heparin, hetastarch, hydromorphone, idarubicin, ifosfamide, insulin, irinotecan, isoproterenol, labetalol, leucovorin, lidocaine, linezolid, lorazepam, mannitol, mechlorethamine, meperidine, mesna, methotrexate, metoclopramide, metoprolol, metronidazole, micafungin, midazolam, milrinone, mitomycin, mitoxantrone, morphine, moxifloxacin, multivitamin, mycophenolate, nafcillin, nalbuphine, naloxone, nesiritide, nicardipine, nitroglycerin, nitroprusside, norepinephrine, octreotide, ondansetron, oxaliplatin, oxytocin, paclitaxel, palonosetron, pancuronium, papaverine, penicillin G, pentazocine, pentobarbital, phenobarbital, phenylephrine, phytonadione, piperacillin/tazobactam, potassium acetate, potassium chloride, procainamide, promethazine, propranolol, protamine, pyridoxine, ranitidine, rocuronium, streptokinase, succinylcholine, sufentanil, tacrolimus, teniposide, theophylline, thiamine, thiotepa, tigecycline, tirofiban, tobramycin, topotecan, vancomycin, vasopressin, vecuronium, verapamil, vinblastine, vincristine, vinorelbine, voriconazole.
- **Y-Site Incompatibility:** amphotericin B colloidal, amphotericin B lipid complex, amphotericin B liposome, azathioprine, cefazolin, ceftazidime, ceftriaxone, cefuroxime, dantrolene, diazepam, diazoxide, doxorubicin liposomal, fluorouracil, folic acid, foscarnet, fosphenytoin, haloperidol, indomethacin, ketorolac, magnesium sulfate, methylprednisolone, pantoprazole, pemetrexed, phenytoin, potassium phosphates, prochlorperazine, propofol, quinupristin/dalfopristin, sodium bicarbonate, sodium phosphates, trimethoprim/sulfamethoxazole.

Calcium Gluconate

IV Administration

- **IV Push:** Administer slowly by IV push. ***Rate:*** Maximum administration rate for adults is 1.5–2 mL/min.
- **Continuous Infusion:** May be further diluted in 1000 mL of D5W, D10W, D20W, D5/0.9% NaCl, 0.9% NaCl, D5/LR, or LR.
- ***Rate:*** Administer at a rate not to exceed 200 mg/min over 12–24 hr.
- **Y-Site Compatibility:** acyclovir, aldesleukin, alemtuzumab, alfentanil, allopurinol, amifostine, amikacin, aminocaproic acid, aminophylline, anidulafungin, ascorbic acid, atropine, azathioprine, azithromycin, aztreonam, benztropine, bivalirudin, bleomycin, bumetanide, buprenorphine, butorphanol, calcium chloride, carboplatin, carmustine, caspofungin, cefazolin, cefepime, cefotaxime, cefotetan, cefoxitin, ceftazidime, cefuroxime, chloramphenicol, chlorpromazine, ciprofloxacin, cisatracurium, cisplatin, cladribine, clindamycin, cyanocobalamin, cyclophosphamide, cyclosporine, cytarabine, dacarbazine, dactinomycin, daptomycin, daunorubicin, dexmedetomidine, dexrazoxane, digoxin, diltiazem, dimenhydrinate, diphenhydramine, dobutamine, docetaxel, dolasetron, dopamine, doripenem, doxorubicin, doxorubicin liposome, doxycycline, enalaprilat, ephedrine, epinephrine, epirubicin, epoetin alfa, eptifibatide, ertapenem, erythromycin, esmolol, etoposide, etoposide phosphate, famotidine, fenoldopam, fentanyl, filgrastim, fludarabine, fluorouracil, folic acid, furosemide, ganciclovir, gemcitabine, gentamicin, glycopyrrolate, granisetron, heparin, hetastarch, hydromorphone, idarubicin, ifosfamide, insulin, irinotecan, isoproterenol, ketamine, labetalol, leucovorin, levofloxacin, lidocaine, linezolid, lorazepem, magnesium sulfate, mannitol, mechlorethamine, melphalan, meperidine, metaraminol, methotrexate, metoclopramide, metoprolol, metronidazole, micafungin, midazolam, milrinone, mitoxantrone, morphine, moxifloxacin, multivitamins, nafcillin, nalbuphine, naloxone, nesiritide, nicardipine, nitroglycerin, nitroprusside, norepinephrine, octreotide, ondansetron, oxaliplatin, oxytocin, paclitaxel, palonosetron, pancuronium, pantoprazole, papaverine, penicillin G, pentamidine, pentazocine, pentobarbital, phenobarbital, phenylephrine, phytonadione, piperacillin/tazobactam, potassium acetate, potassium chloride, procainamide, prochlorperazine, promethazine, propofol, propranolol, protamine, pyridoxine, ranitidine, remifentanil, rituximab, rocuronium, sargramostim, sodium acetate, streptokinase, succinylcholine, sufentanil, tacrolimus, telavancin, teniposide, theophylline, thiamine, thiotepa, tigecycline, tirofiban, tobramycin, trastuzumab, vancomycin, vasopressin, vecuronium, verapamil, vinblastine, vincristine, vinorelbine, vitamin B complex with C, voriconazole.
- **Y-Site Incompatibility:** amphotericin B colloidal, amphotericin B lipid complex, amphotericin B liposome, cangrelor, ceftriaxone, dantrolene, diazepam, diazoxide, foscarnet, fosphenytoin, indomethacin, methylprednisolone, mycophenolate, oxacillin, pemetrexed, phenytoin, potassium phosphates, quinupristin/dalfopristin, sodium bicarbonate, sodium phosphates, topotecan, trimethoprim/sulfamethoxazole.

Patient/Family Teaching

- Instruct patient not to take enteric-coated tablets within 1 hr of calcium carbonate; this will result in premature dissolution of the tablets.
- Do not administer concurrently with foods containing large amounts of oxalic acid (spinach, rhubarb), phytic acid (brans, cereals), or phosphorus (milk or dairy products). Administration with milk products may lead to milk-alkali syndrome (nausea, vomiting, confusion, headache). Do not take within 1–2 hr of other medications if possible.
- Instruct patients on a regular schedule to take missed doses as soon as possible, then go back to regular schedule.
- Advise patient that calcium carbonate may cause constipation. Review methods of preventing constipation (increasing bulk in diet, increasing fluid intake, increasing mobility) and using laxatives. Severe constipation may indicate toxicity.
- Advise patient to avoid excessive use of tobacco or beverages containing alcohol or caffeine.
- **Calcium Supplement:** Encourage patients to maintain a diet adequate in vitamin D (see Appendix J).
- **Osteoporosis:** Advise patients that exercise has been found to arrest and reverse bone loss. Patient should discuss any exercise limitations with health care professional before beginning program.
- **Hyperphosphatemia:** Advise patient to notify health care professional promptly if signs and symptoms of hypercalcemia (constipation, anorexia, nausea, vomiting, confusion, stupor) occur.
- Advise patient to avoid taking calcium-containing supplements, including calcium-based antacids during therapy.

Evaluation/Desired Outcomes

- Increase in serum calcium levels.
- Decrease in the signs and symptoms of hypocalcemia.
- Resolution of indigestion.
- Control of hyperphosphatemia in patients with renal failure (calcium acetate only).

canagliflozin
(kan-a-gli-**floe**-zin)
Invokana

Classification
Therapeutic: antidiabetics
Pharmacologic: sodium-glucose co-transporter 2 (SGLT2) inhibitors

Pregnancy Category C

Indications
Adjunct to diet and exercise in the management of type 2 diabetes mellitus. May be used with other antidiabetic agents.

Action
Inhibits proximal renal tubular sodium-glucose co-transporter 2 (SGLT2), which determines reabsorption of glucose from the tubular lumen. Inhibits reabsorption of glucose, lowers renal threshold for glucose, and increases excretion of glucose in urine. **Therapeutic Effects:** Improved glycemic control.

Pharmacokinetics
Absorption: Well absorbed (65%) following oral administration.
Distribution: Extensive tissue distribution.
Protein Binding: 99%.
Metabolism and Excretion: Mostly metabolized by UDP-glucuronyl transferases (UGT) to inactive metabolites, minimal metabolism by CYP3A4 (7%). 50% excreted in feces as parent drug and metabolites, 33% as metabolites in urine, <1% excreted in urine as unchanged drug.
Half-life: 10.6 hr.

TIME/ACTION PROFILE (effects on HbA1C)

ROUTE	ONSET	PEAK	DURATION
PO	unknown	unknown	24 hr

Contraindications/Precautions
Contraindicated in: Hypersensitivity; Severe renal impairment (eGFR <45 mL/min/1.73 m^2), end-stage renal disease or on dialysis; Severe hepatic impairment; Lactation: Avoid use, discontinue breast feeding or discontinue canagliflozin.
Use Cautiously in: eGFR <60 mL/min/1.73 m^2 (monitor frequently), ↑ risk of adverse reactions related to ↓ intravascular volume; Geri: ↑ risk of adverse reactions related to ↓ intravascular volume; Hypotension (correct prior to treatment, especially if eGFR 30–60 mL/min, age >75 yr, or concurrent use of loop diuretics, ACE inhibitors, or ARBs; OB: Use during pregnancy only if potential maternal benefit justifies potential fetal risk; Pedi: Safety and effectiveness not established.

Adverse Reactions/Side Effects
CV: hypotension. **GI:** abdominal pain, constipation, nausea. **GU:** female mycotic infections, glucosuria, male mycotic infections, ↓ renal function, urinary tract infection, ↑ urination, vulvovaginal pruritus. **Endo:** HYPOGLYCEMIA (WITH OTHER MEDICATIONS). **F and E:** hyperkalemia, hypermagnesemia, hyperphosphatemia, thirst. **Metab:** hyperlipidemia. **MS:** bone fractures. **Misc:** hypersensitivity reactions, including generalized urticaria.

Interactions
Drug-Drug: Blood levels are ↓ by **UGT inducers** including **phenobarbital**, **phenytoin**, **rifampin**, and **ritonavir**; ↑dose may be required. ↑ risk of hypoglycemia with **insulin** or **insulin secretagogues**; dose adjustments may be required. May ↑ blood levels and effects of **digoxin**; levels should be monitored. ↑ risk of hyperkalemia with **potassium-sparing diuretics** or **medications that interfere with the renin-angiotensin-aldosterone system**.

Route/Dosage
PO (Adults): *eGFR ≥ 60 mL/min/1.73 m^2*— 100 mg once daily initially, may be increased to 300 mg once daily; *Concurrent use of UGT inducers (phenobarbital, phenytoin, rifampin, ritonavir)*—if maintenance dose is 100 mg daily, may require increase to 300 mg daily.

Renal Impairment
PO (Adults): *eGFR 45–60 mL/min/1.73 m^2*— 100 mg once daily.

Availability
Tablets: 100 mg, 300 mg. ***In combination with:*** metformin (Invokamet). See Appendix B.

NURSING IMPLICATIONS
Assessment
- Observe patient for signs and symptoms of hypoglycemic reactions (abdominal pain, sweating, hunger, weakness, dizziness, headache, tremor, tachycardia, anxiety).
- Monitor for signs and symptoms of volume depletion (dizziness, feeling faint, weakness, orthostatic hypotension) after initiating therapy.
- ***Lab Test Considerations:*** Monitor hemoglobin A1C prior to and periodically during therapy.
- May cause ↑ uric acid levels.
- May ↑ serum creatinine and ↓ eGFR. Monitor renal function, especially in patients with eGFR <60 mL/min/1.73 m^2.
- May cause ↑ serum potassium, magnesium, and phosphate levels. Monitor electrolytes periodically during therapy.
- May cause ↑ LDL-C. Monitor serum lipid levels periodically during therapy.

Potential Nursing Diagnoses

Imbalanced nutrition: more than body requirements (Indications)
Noncompliance (Patient/Family Teaching)

Implementation

- Patients stabilized on a diabetic regimen who are exposed to stress, fever, trauma, infection, or surgery may require administration of insulin.
- Correct volume depletion prior to beginning therapy with canagliflozin.
- **PO:** Administer before the first meal of the day.

Patient/Family Teaching

- Instruct patient to take canagliflozin as directed. Take missed doses as soon as remembered, unless it is almost time for next dose; do not double doses. Advise patient to read the *Medication Guide* before starting and with each Rx refillin case of changes.
- Explain to patient that canagliflozin helps control hyperglycemia but does not cure diabetes. Therapy is usually long term.
- Instruct patient not to share this medication with others, even if they have the same symptoms; it may harm them.
- Encourage patient to follow prescribed diet, medication, and exercise regimen to prevent hyperglycemic or hypoglycemic episodes.
- Review signs of hypoglycemia and hyperglycemia with patient. If hypoglycemia occurs, advise patient to take a glass of orange juice or 2–3 tsp of sugar, honey, or corn syrup dissolved in water, and notify health care professional.
- Instruct patient in proper testing of blood glucose and urine ketones. Inform patient that canagliflozin will cause a positive test result when testing for urine glucose. These tests should be monitored closely during periods of stress or illness and health care professional notified if significant changes occur.
- Inform patient that canagliflozin may cause yeast infections. Women may have signs and symptoms of a vaginal yeast infection (vaginal odor, white or yellow vaginal discharge [may be lumpy or look like cottage cheese], vaginal itching). Men may have signs and symptoms of a yeast infection of the penis (redness, itching, or swelling of penis; rash on penis; foul smelling discharge from penis; pain in skin around penis). Advise patient to notify health care professional if yeast infection occurs.
- Advise patient to notify health care professional promptly if rash; hives; or swelling of face, lips, or throat occur.
- Inform patient of increased risk for bone fractures and discuss factors that may increase risk.
- Advise patient to notify health care professional of all Rx or OTC medications, vitamins, or herbal products being taken and to consult with health care professional before taking other medications, especially other oral hypoglycemic medications.
- Advise patient to notify health care professional if pregnancy is planned or suspected or if breast feeding.

Evaluation/Desired Outcomes

- Improved hemoglobin A1C and glycemic control in adults with Type II diabetes.

---

candesartan, See ANGIOTENSIN II RECEPTOR ANTAGONISTS.

---

cangrelor (kan-**grel**-or)

Kengreal

Classification
Therapeutic: antiplatelet agents
Pharmacologic: platelet aggregation inhibitors

Pregnancy Category C

Indications

Adjunct to percutaneous coronary intervention (PCI) to ↓ risk of periprocedural MI, repeat coronary revascularization or stent thrombosis in patients not currently receiving a $P2Y_{12}$ platelet inhibitor and are not receiving a glycoprotein IIb/IIIa inhibitor.

Action

Inhibits platelet aggregation by reversibly interacting with platelet $P2Y_{12}$ADP-receptors, preventing signal transduction and platelet activation. **Therapeutic Effects:** ↓ risk of periprocedural MI, repeat coronary revascularization or stent thrombosis associated with PCI.

Pharmacokinetics

Absorption: IV administration results in complete bioavailability.
Distribution: Unk.
Protein Binding: 97–98%.
Metabolism and Excretion: Metabolized rapidly in the blood stream; metabolites do not have antiplatelet activity. 58% excreted by kidneys, 35% in feces.
Half-life: 3–6 min.

TIME/ACTION PROFILE (antiplatelet effect)

ROUTE	ONSET	PEAK	DURATION
IV	rapid	2 min	1 hr†

† following discontinuation.

Contraindications/Precautions

Contraindicated in: Hypersensitivity; Significant severe bleeding.

Use Cautiously in: CCr < 30 mL/min (↑ risk of further decline in renal function); OB: Consider potential maternal benefits and fetal risks; Pedi: Safe and effective use in children has not been established.

Adverse Reactions/Side Effects

Resp: dyspnea. **Hemat:** bleeding. **Misc:** allergic reactions including ANAPHYLAXIS.

Interactions

Drug-Drug: Concurrent use of other **$P2Y_{12}$ inhibitors** including **clopidogrel**, **prasugrel**, or **tigagrelor** ↑ risk of bleeding. Blocks antiplatelet effects of concurrently administered **clopidogrel** or **prasugrel**.

Route/Dosage

IV (Adults): 30 mcg/kg bolus prior to PCI, then 4 mcg/kg/min infusion for 2 hr or duration of procedure, whichever is longer; should be followed by initiation of an oral $P2Y_{12}$platelet inhibitor.

Availability

Lyophilized powder for IV injection (requires reconstitution): 50 mg/vial.

NURSING IMPLICATIONS

Assessment

- Monitor for signs and symptoms of bleeding during and following infusion.
- Monitor for signs and symptoms of hypersensitivity reaction (bronchospasm, angioedema, stridor) during therapy. Discontinue therapy and treat symptomatically.

Potential Nursing Diagnoses

Ineffective tissue perfusion (Indications)

Implementation

- **IV Push:** Reconstitute each 50 mg vial with 5 mL of Sterile Water for injection. Swirl gently until dissolved; avoid vigorous mixing. Allow foam to settle. Solution is clear and colorless to pale yellow; do not administer solutions that are discolored or contain particulate matter. ***Diluent:*** Withdraw reconstituted solution and add to 250 mL of 0.9% NaCl or D5W. Dilute immediately. Stable for 12 hrs if diluted with D5W or 24 hrs if diluted with 0.9% NaCl at room temperature. Discard unused portion. ***Concentration:*** 200 mcg/mL. Patients >100 kg will require at least 2 bags. ***Rate:*** Administer rapidly over <1 min from diluted bag via IV push or pump. Ensure bolus completely administered before beginning infusion.
- **Intermittent Infusion:** Start infusion immediately after administration of bolus. ***Rate:*** 4 mcg/kg/min for at least 2 hrs or duration of PCI, whichever is longer.
- **Y-Site Incompatibility:** Infusion requires a dedicated line.
- To maintain platelet inhibition, administer either ticagrelor 180 mg PO at any time during or immediately after discontinuation, or prasugrel 60 mg PO or clopidogrel 600 mg PO immediately after discontinuation of infusion; do not administer prasugrel or clopidogrel prior to discontinuation of infusion.

Patient/Family Teaching

- Caution patient to notify health care professional if bleeding occurs.
- Advise female patient to notify health care professional if pregnancy is suspected or if breast feeding.

Evaluation/Desired Outcomes

- ↓ risk of periprocedural MI, repeat coronary revascularization or stent thrombosis associated with PCI.

HIGH ALERT

capecitabine

(kap-pe-**site**-a-been)

Xeloda

Classification

Therapeutic: antineoplastics

Pharmacologic: antimetabolites

Pregnancy Category D

Indications

Metastatic colorectal cancer. Adjuvant treatment for Dukes' C colon cancer following primary resection. Metastatic breast cancer that has worsened despite prior therapy with anthracycline (daunorubicin, doxorubicin, idarubicin) (to be used in combination with docetaxel). Metastatic breast cancer that is resistant to both paclitaxel and an anthracycline (daunorubicin, doxorubicin, idarubicin) or is resistant to paclitaxel and further anthracycline therapy is contraindicated.

Action

Converted in tissue to 5-fluorouracil (5-FU), which inhibits DNA and RNA synthesis by preventing thymidine production. The enzyme responsible for the final step in the conversion to 5-FU may be found in higher concentrations in some tumors. **Therapeutic Effects:** Death of rapidly replicating cells, particularly malignant ones.

Pharmacokinetics

Absorption: Well absorbed after oral administration.

Distribution: Unknown.

Metabolism and Excretion: Metabolized mostly in tissue and by the liver to 5-FU; 5-FU is metabolized by dihydropyrimidine dehydrogenase to a less toxic compound; inactive metabolites are excreted primarily in urine.

Half-life: 45 min.

TIME/ACTION PROFILE (blood levels)

ROUTE	ONSET	PEAK	DURATION
PO	unknown†	1.5 hr (2 hr for 5-FU)‡	unknown

†Onset of antineoplastic effect is 6 wk.

‡Peak 5-FU levels occur at 2 hr.

Contraindications/Precautions

Contraindicated in: Hypersensitivity to capecitabine or 5-FU; Severe renal impairment (CCr <30 mL/min); OB: Potential for fetal harm or death; Lactation: Potential for serious adverse effects in nursing infants.

Use Cautiously in: Dihydropyrimidine dehydrogenase deficiency (patients at ↑ risk of 5-FU toxicity); Mild-moderate renal impairment (↓ starting dose to 75% in patients with CCr 30–50 mL/min); Hepatic dysfunction; Coronary artery disease; Pedi: Safety not established; Geri: ↑ risk of severe diarrhea in patients ≥80 yr.

Adverse Reactions/Side Effects

CNS: fatigue, headache, dizziness, insomnia. **EENT:** eye irritation, epistaxis, rhinorrhea. **CV:** edema, chest pain. **GI:** DIARRHEA, NECROTIZING ENTEROCOLITIS, abdominal pain, anorexia, constipation, dysgeusia, hyperbilirubinemia, nausea, stomatitis, vomiting, dyspepsia, xerostomia. **Derm:** STEVENS-JOHNSON SYNDROME, TOXIC EPIDERMAL NECROLYSIS, dermatitis, hand-and-foot syndrome, nail disorder, alopecia, erythema, rashes. **F and E:** dehydration. **GU:** acute renal failure. **Hemat:** anemia, leukopenia, thrombocytopenia. **MS:** arthralgia, myalgia. **Neuro:** peripheral neuropathy. **Resp:** cough, dyspnea. **Misc:** fever.

Interactions

Drug-Drug: May ↑ risk of bleeding with **warfarin** (frequent monitoring of PT/INR recommended). Toxicity ↑ by concurrent **leucovorin**. **Antacids** may ↑ absorption. May ↑ blood levels and risk of toxicity from **phenytoin** (may need to ↓ phenytoin dose). ↑ incidence of acute renal failure with other **nephrotoxic drugs**.

Drug-Food: Food ↑ absorption, although capecitabine should be given within 30 min after a meal.

Route/Dosage

PO (Adults): 1250 mg/m^2 twice daily for 14 days, followed by 7-day rest period; given in 3-wk cycles.

Renal Impairment

PO (Adults): *CCr 30–50 mL/min*—↓ initial dose to 75% of usual.

Availability (generic available)

Tablets: 150 mg, 500 mg.

NURSING IMPLICATIONS

Assessment

- Assess mucous membranes, number and consistency of stools, and frequency of vomiting. Assess for signs of infection (fever, chills, sore throat, cough, hoarseness, pain in lower back or side, difficult or painful urination). Assess for bleeding (bleeding gums; bruising; petechiae; and guaiac-test stools, urine, and emesis). Avoid IM injections and taking rectal temperatures. Apply pressure to venipuncture sites for 10 min. Anemia may occur. Monitor for increased fatigue, dyspnea, and orthostatic hypotension.
- Notify health care professional if symptoms of toxicity (stomatitis, uncontrollable vomiting, diarrhea, fever) occur; drug may need to be discontinued or dose decreased. Patients with severe diarrhea should be monitored carefully, administered antidiarrheal agents (loperamide) and given fluid and electrolyte replacements if they become dehydrated. Grade 2 diarrhea (4 to 6 stools/day or nocturnal stools), Grade 3 (7 to 9 stools/day or incontinence and malabsorption), Grade 4 (≥10 stools/day or grossly bloody diarrhea or need for parenteral support). If grade 2, 3 or 4 diarrhea occurs, immediately stop therapy until diarrhea resolves or decreases in intensity to Grade 1. Grade 3 or 4 diarrhea usually lasts 5 days.
- Assess patient for mucocutaneous and dermatologic toxicity (Stevens-Johnson syndrome, toxic epidermal necrolysis, hand-and-foot syndrome). Grade 1 (numbness, dysesthesia/paresthesia, tingling, painless swelling or erythema of hands and/or feet and/or discomfort which does not disrupt normal activities). Grade 2 (painful erythema and swelling of hands and/or feet and/or discomfort affecting the patient's activities of daily living). Grade 3 (moist desquamation, ulceration, blistering or severe pain of hands and/or feet and/or severe discomfort causing patient to be unable to work or perform activities of daily living). *If Grade 2 or 3 occurs,* interrupt therapy until Grade 1. Decrease doses following Grade 3.
- ***Lab Test Considerations:*** Monitor hepatic (serum alkaline phosphatase, AST, ALT, and bilirubin), renal, and hematologic (hematocrit, hemoglobin, leukocyte, platelet count) function before and periodically during therapy. May cause leukopenia, anemia, and thrombocytopenia. Leukopenia may require discontinuation of therapy. Therapy should be interrupted if serum bilirubin ↑ to 1.5 times normal or greater; may be reinstituted after bilirubin returns to normal.
- Monitor PT or INR frequently in patients receiving warfarin and capecitabine to adjust warfarin dose. May cause ↑ bleeding within a few days to several months of initiation of therapy to 1 mo following discontinuation of therapy. Risk is greater in patients over 60 yr.

Potential Nursing Diagnoses

Risk for infection (Side Effects)
Imbalanced nutrition: less than body requirements (Side Effects)

Implementation

- ***High Alert:*** Fatalities have occurred with chemotherapeutic agents. Before administering, clarify all ambiguous orders; double-check single, daily, and course-of-therapy dose limits; have second practitioner independently double-check original order and dose calculations. Do not confuse capecitabine (Xeloda) with orlistat (Xenical).
- Dose modifications are based on degree of toxicity encountered. Once a dose has been reduced because of toxicity, it should not be increased at a later time. See manufacturer's recommendations.
- **PO:** Administer every 12 hr for 2 wk, followed by a 1-wk rest period. Swallow tablets whole; do not crush or cut. Tablets should be taken with water within 30 min after a meal.

Patient/Family Teaching

- Instruct patient to take medication every 12 hr with water within 30 min after a meal. Missed doses should be omitted; continue regular schedule. Do not double dose. Advise patient to read *Patient Package Insert* before starting and with each Rx refill in case of changes.
- Inform patient of the most common side effects. Instruct patient to notify health care provider immediately if any of the following occur: diarrhea (>4 bowel movements in a day or any diarrhea at night), vomiting (more than once in 24 hr), nausea (loss of appetite and significant decrease in daily food intake), stomatitis (pain, redness, swelling, or sore in mouth), hand-and-foot syndrome (pain, swelling, or redness of hands and/or feet), fever, or infection (temperature of ≥100.5° F or other signs of infection).
- Instruct patient to notify health care professional if he or she is taking folic acid.
- Instruct patient to notify health care professional if fever; chills; sore throat; signs of infection; yellowing of skin or eyes; abdominal pain; joint or flank pain; swelling of feet or legs; bleeding gums; bruising; petechiae; or blood in urine, stool, or emesis occurs. Caution patient to avoid crowds and persons with known infections. Instruct patient to use soft toothbrush and electric razor. Patients should be cautioned not to drink alcoholic beverages or take products containing aspirin or NSAIDs.
- Advise patient to rinse mouth with clear water after eating and drinking and to avoid flossing to minimize stomatitis. Viscous lidocaine may be used if mouth pain interferes with eating. Stomatitis pain may require treatment with opioid analgesics.
- Advise patient to notify health care professional of all Rx or OTC medications, vitamins, or herbal products being taken and to consult with health care professional before taking other medications.
- Rep: Review with both female and male patients the need for contraception during therapy. Advise female patient to notify health care professional immediately if pregnancy is suspected or if breast feeding.
- Emphasize the importance of routine follow-up lab tests to monitor progress and to check for side effects.

Evaluation/Desired Outcomes

- Tumor regression.

capsaicin (kap-**say**-sin)

Capzasin-HP, Capzasin-P, DiabetAid Pain and Tingling Relief, Qutenza, Salonpas Hot, Zostrix Diabetic Foot Pain, Zostrix, Zostrix-HP

Classification

Therapeutic: nonopioid analgesics (topical)

Pregnancy Category UK

Indications

Temporary management of pain due to rheumatoid arthritis and osteoarthritis. Treatment of pain associated with postherpetic neuralgia (topical and transdermal) or diabetic neuropathy. **Unlabeled Use:** Treatment of postmastectomy pain syndrome. Treatment of complex regional pain syndrome.

Action

Topical: May deplete and prevent the reaccumulation of a chemical (substance P) responsible for transmitting painful impulses from peripheral sites to the CNS. **Transdermal**: Initially stimulates the transient receptor potential vanilloid 1 (TRPV1) receptors on nociceptive nerve fibers in the skin; this is followed by pain relief thought to be due to a reduction in TRPV1–expressing nociceptive nerve endings. **Therapeutic Effects:** Relief of discomfort associated with painful peripheral syndromes.

Pharmacokinetics

Absorption: Unknown.
Distribution: Unknown.
Metabolism and Excretion: Unknown.
Half-life: Unknown.

TIME/ACTION PROFILE

ROUTE	ONSET	PEAK	DURATION
topical	1–2 wk	2–4 wk†	unknown
transdermal	unknown	unknown	unknown

†May take up to 6 wk for head and neck neuralgias.

Contraindications/Precautions

Contraindicated in: Hypersensitivity to capsaicin or hot peppers; Not for use near eyes or on open or broken skin.

Use Cautiously in: OB, Lactation: Safety not established; Pedi: Safety not established in children <18 yr (transdermal) or <2 yr (topical).

Adverse Reactions/Side Effects

CV: *Patch*—↑ BP. **Resp:** cough. **Derm:** pain (after application of patch), transient burning.

Interactions

Drug-Drug: None significant.

Route/Dosage

Topical (Adults and Children ≥2 yr): Apply to affected areas 3–4 times daily.

Transdermal (Adults): Apply up to 4 patches for 60 min (single use); may be repeated q 3 mo, as needed based on pain (should not be used more frequently than q 3 mo).

Availability (generic available)

Cream: 0.1%OTC, 0.025%OTC, 0.035%OTC, 0.075%OTC. **Gel:** 0.025%OTC. **Lotion:** 0.025%OTC. **Topical liquid:** 0.15%OTC. **Transdermal patch (Qutenza):** 0.025%/patch, 8% (179 mg)/patch. ***In combination with:*** methylsalicylate (ZiksOTC). See Appendix B.

NURSING IMPLICATIONS

Assessment

- Assess pain intensity and location before and periodically throughout therapy.
- **Transdermal:** Monitor BP periodically during application.

Potential Nursing Diagnoses

Chronic pain (Indications)
Noncompliance (Patient/Family Teaching)

Implementation

- Do not confuse Zostrix with Zovirax.
- **Topical:** Apply to affected area not more than 3–4 times daily. Avoid getting medication into eyes or on broken or irritated skin. Do not bandage tightly.
- Topical lidocaine may be applied during the first 1–2 wk of treatment to reduce initial discomfort.
- **Transdermal:** Identify treatment area (painful area including areas of hypersensitivity and allodynia) and mark on the skin. If needed, clip hair (do not shave) in and around treatment area to promote patch adherence. Cut patch to size and shape of treatment area. Gently wash area with mild soap and water and dry thoroughly. Apply topical anesthetic to the entire treatment area and surrounding 1–2 cm and keep the local anesthetic in place until skin is anesthetized prior to the application of patch. Remove the topical anesthetic with a dry wipe. Gently wash treatment area with mild soap and water and dry. Use only nitrile gloves when handling capsaicin and cleaning capsaicin residue from skin; latex gloves do not provide adequate protection. Apply patch to dry, intact skin. Apply patch within 2 hr of opening pouch. Tear pouch open along the three dashed lines and remove patch. Inspect patch and identify the outer surface backing layer with the printing on one side and the capsaicin-containing adhesive on the other side. Adhesive side of the patch is covered by a clear, unprinted, diagonally cut release liner. Cut patch before removing protective release liner. Peel a small section of the release liner back and place adhesive side of patch on treatment area. While slowly peeling back release liner from under patch with one hand, use other hand to smooth the patch down on to skin. Once patch is applied, leave in place for 60 min. To ensure patch maintains contact with treatment area, a dressing, such as rolled gauze, may be used. Instruct the patient not to touch the patch or treatment area.
- Even following use of a local anesthetic prior to administration of capsaicin, patients may experience substantial procedural pain. Prepare to treat acute pain during and following application with local cooling (such as an ice pack) and/or appropriate analgesic medication (opioids).
- Remove patches by gently and slowly rolling inward. After removal, generously apply *Cleansing Gel* to treatment area and leave on for at least 1 min. Remove *Cleansing Gel* with a dry wipe and gently wash area with mild soap and water and dry thoroughly. Aerosolization of capsaicin can occur upon rapid removal of patches. Remove patches gently and slowly by rolling adhesive side inward. If irritation of eyes or airways occurs, remove affected individual from the vicinity. Flush eyes and mucous membranes with cool water. Inhalation of airborne capsaicin can result in coughing or sneezing. Provide supportive care if shortness of breath develops. If skin not intended to be treated comes in contact with capsaicin, apply *Cleansing Gel* for 1 min and wipe off with dry gauze. After *Cleansing Gel* has been wiped off, wash area with soap and water.

Patient/Family Teaching

- **Topical:** Instruct patient on the correct method for application of capsaicin. Rub cream into affected area well so that little or no cream is left on the surface. Gloves should be worn during application or hands should be washed immediately after application. If application is to hands for arthritis, do not wash hands for at least 30 min after application.
- Advise patient to apply missed doses as soon as possible unless almost time for next dose. Pain relief lasts only as long as capsaicin is used regularly.
- Advise patient that transient burning may occur with application, especially if applied fewer than 3–4 times daily. Burning usually disappears after the first few days but may continue for 2–4 wk or longer. Burning is increased by heat, sweating, bathing in warm water, humidity, and clothing. Burning usually decreases in frequency and intensity the longer capsaicin is used. Decreasing number of daily doses will not lessen burning but may decrease amount of pain relief and may prolong period of burning.
- Caution patient to flush area with water if capsaicin gets into eyes and to wash with warm, but not hot,

soapy water if capsaicin gets on other sensitive areas of the body.

- Instruct patient with herpes zoster (shingles) not to apply capsaicin cream until lesions have healed completely.
- Advise patient to discontinue use and notify health care professional if pain persists longer than 1 mo, worsens, or if signs of infection are present.
- **Transdermal:** Inform patient that treated area may be sensitive for a few days to heat (e.g., hot showers or baths, direct sunlight, vigorous exercise).
- Advise patient that exposure of skin to capsaicin may result in transient erythema and burning sensation. Instruct patients not to touch patch and if they accidentally touch patch it may burn and/or sting.
- Instruct patient to notify health care professional immediately if irritation of eyes or airways occurs, or if any of the side effects become severe.
- If opioids are used to treat pain from patch, caution patient that opioids may cause drowsiness and to avoid driving or other activities requiring alertness until response to medication is known.
- May cause transient increases in BP. Instruct patients to inform health care professional if they have experienced any recent cardiovascular event.
- Instruct patients to notify health care professional if pregnancy is planned or suspected or if breast feeding.

Evaluation/Desired Outcomes

- Decrease in discomfort associated with:.
- Postherpetic neuropathy.
- Diabetic neuropathy.
- Rheumatoid arthritis.
- Osteoarthritis. Pain relief usually begins within 1–2 wk with arthritis, 2–4 wk with neuralgias, and 4–6 wk with neuralgias of the head and neck.

captopril, See ANGIOTENSIN-CONVERTING ENZYME (ACE) INHIBITORS.

carBAMazepine

(kar-ba-**maz**-e-peen)

Carbatrol, Epitol, Equetro, ✤Mazepine, TEGretol, ✤Tegretol CR, Tegretol-XR, Teril

Classification

Therapeutic: anticonvulsants, mood stabilizers

Pregnancy Category D

Indications

Treatment of tonic-clonic, mixed, and complex-partial seizures. Management of pain in trigeminal neuralgia or diabetic neuropathy. **Equetro only:** Acute mania and mixed mania. **Unlabeled Use:** Other forms of neurogenic pain.

Action

Decreases synaptic transmission in the CNS by affecting sodium channels in neurons. **Therapeutic Effects:** Prevention of seizures. Relief of pain in trigeminal neuralgia. Decreased mania.

Pharmacokinetics

Absorption: Absorption is slow but complete. Suspension produces earlier, higher peak, and lower trough levels.

Distribution: Widely distributed. Crosses the blood-brain barrier. Crosses the placenta rapidly and enters breast milk in high concentrations.

Protein Binding: *Carbamazepine*—75–90%; *epoxide*—50%.

Metabolism and Excretion: Extensively metabolized in the liver by cytochrome P450 3A4 to active epoxide metabolite; epoxide metabolite has anticonvulsant and antineuralgic activity.

Half-life: *Carbamazapine*—single dose—25–65 hr, chronic dosing—*Children*—8–14 hr; *Adults*—12–17 hr; *epoxide*—34±9 hr.

TIME/ACTION PROFILE (anticonvulsant activity)

ROUTE	ONSET	PEAK	DURATION
PO	up to 1 mo†	4–5 hr‡	6–12 hr
PO-ER	up to 1 mo†	2–3–12 hr‡	12 hr

†Onset of antineuralgic activity is 8–72 hr.

‡Listed for tablets; peak level occurs 1.5 hr after a chronic dose of suspension.

Contraindications/Precautions

Contraindicated in: Hypersensitivity; Bone marrow suppression; Concomitant use or use within 14 days of MAO inhibitors; Concurrent use of nefazodone; OB: Use only if potential benefits outweigh risks to the fetus; additional vitamin K during last weeks of pregnancy has been recommended; Lactation: Discontinue drug or bottle feed.

Use Cautiously in: All patients (may ↑ risk of suicidal thoughts/behaviors); Cardiac or hepatic disease; Renal failure (dosing adjustment required for CCr <10 mL/min; ↑ intraocular pressure; Geri: Older men with prostatic hyperplasia may be at ↑ risk for acute urinary retention or difficulty initiating stream.

Exercise Extreme Caution in: Patients positive for HLA-B*1502 or HLA-A*3101 alleles (unless benefits clearly outweigh the risks) (↑ risk of serious skin reactions).

Adverse Reactions/Side Effects

CNS: SUICIDAL THOUGHTS, ataxia, drowsiness, fatigue, psychosis, sedation, vertigo. **EENT:** blurred vision, corneal opacities, nystagmus. **Resp:** pneumonitis. **CV:**

HF, edema, hypertension, hypotension, syncope. **GI:** hepatitis, ↑ liver enzymes, pancreatitis, weight gain. **GU:** hesitancy, urinary retention. **Derm:** STEVENS-JOHNSON SYNDROME, TOXIC EPIDERMAL NECROLYSIS, nail shedding, photosensitivity, rash, urticaria. **F and E:** syndrome of inappropriate antidiuretic hormone (SIADH), hyponatremia. **Hemat:** AGRANULOCYTOSIS, APLASTIC ANEMIA, THROMBOCYTOPENIA, eosinophilia, leukopenia, lymphadenopathy. **Misc:** DRUG REACTION WITH EOSINOPHILIA AND SYSTEMIC SYMPTOMS (DRESS), chills, fever.

Interactions

Drug-Drug: May significantly ↓ levels of **nefazodone**; concurrent use contraindicated. May ↓ levels/effectiveness of **acetaminophen**, **alprazolam**, **aprepitant**, **buprenorphine**, **bupropion**, **calcium channel blockers**, **citalopram**, **clonazepam**, **corticosteroids**, **cyclosporine**, **doxycycline**, **estrogen-containing contraceptives**, **everolimus**, **haloperidol**, **imatinib**, **itraconazole**, **lamotrigine**, **levothyroxine**, **methadone**. **midazolam**, **olanzapine**, **paliperidone**, **phenytoin**, **protease inhibitors**, **risperidone**, **sertraline**, **sirolimus**, **tacrolimus**, **tadalafil**, **theophylline**, **tiagabine**, **topiramate**, **tramadol**, **trazodone**, **tricyclic antidepressants**, **valproic acid**, **warfarin**, **ziprasidone**, and **zonisamide**. May ↓ **aripiprazole** levels; double the aripiprazole dose. May ↓ **temsirolimus** and **lapatinib** levels; avoid concurrent use. Concurrent use (within 2 wk) of **MAO inhibitors** may result in hyperpyrexia, hypertension, seizures, and death. **Aprepitant**, **cimetidine**, **ciprofloxacin**, **clarithromycin**, **danazol**, **dantrolene**, **diltiazem**, **erythromycin**, **fluconazole**, **fluoxetine**, **fluvoxamine**, **isoniazid**, **itraconazole**, **ketoconazole**, **loratadine**, **olanzapine**, **omeprazole**, **oxybutynin**, **protease inhibitors**, **trazodone**, **voriconazole**, and **verapamil** may ↑ carbamazepine levels; may ↑ risk of toxicity. Enzyme inducers such as **rifampin**, **phenobarbital**, and **phenytoin** may ↓ levels. May ↑ risk of hepatotoxicity from **isoniazid**. May ↑ risk of CNS toxicity from **lithium**. May ↓ effects of **nondepolarizing neuromuscular blocking agents**. May ↑ risk of toxicity from **cyclophosphamide**.

Drug-Food: **Grapefruit juice** ↑ serum levels and oral bioavailability by 40% and therefore may ↑ effects.

Route/Dosage

PO (Adults): *Anticonvulsant*—200 mg twice daily (tablets) or 100 mg 4 times daily (suspension); ↑ by 200 mg/day q 7 days until therapeutic levels are achieved (range is 600–1200 mg/day) in divided doses q 6–8 hr; not to exceed 1 g/day in 12–15-yr-olds. Extended-release products are given twice daily (XR, CR). *Antineuralgic*—100 mg twice daily or 50 mg 4 times daily (suspension); ↑ by up to 200 mg/day until pain is relieved, then maintenance dose of 200–1200 mg/day in divided doses (usual range, 400–800 mg/day).

PO (Children 6–12 yr): 100 mg twice daily (tablets) or 50 mg 4 times daily (suspension). ↑ by 100 mg weekly until therapeutic levels are obtained (usual range 400–800 mg/day; not to exceed 1 g/day). Extended-release products (XR, CR) are given twice daily.

PO (Children <6 yr): 10–20 mg/kg/day in 2–3 divided doses; may be ↑ at weekly intervals until optimal response and therapeutic levels are acheived. Usual maintenance dose is 250–350 mg/day (not to exceed 35 mg/kg/day).

Availability (generic available)

Tablets: 200 mg. **Cost:** *Generic*—$7.18/100. **Chewable tablets:** 100 mg, ✤200 mg. **Cost:** *Generic*—$23.11/100. **Extended-release capsules:** 100 mg, 200 mg, 300 mg. **Cost:** *Generic*—All strengths $214.48/60. **Extended-release tablets:** 100 mg, 200 mg, 400 mg. **Cost:** *Generic*—200 mg $113.31/100, 400 mg $224.76/100. **Oral suspension (citrus/vanilla flavor):** 100 mg/5 mL. **Cost:** *Generic*—$74.77/450 mL.

NURSING IMPLICATIONS

Assessment

- Monitor closely for notable changes in behavior that could indicate the emergence or worsening of suicidal thoughts or behavior or depression.
- ⧖ Monitor for changes in skin condition in early therapy. Stevens-Johnson syndrome and toxic epidermal necrolysis are significantly more common in patients with a particular human leukocyte antigen (HLA) allele, HLA-B*1502 (occurs almost exclusively in patients with Asian ancestry, including South Asian Indians). Screen patients of Asian ancestry for the HLA-B*1502 allele before starting treatment with carbamazepine. If positive, carbamazepine should not be started unless the expected benefit outweighs increased risk of serious skin reactions. Patients who have been taking carbamazepine for more than a few months without developing skin reactions are at low risk of these events ever developing.
- Monitor for signs and symptoms of DRESS syndrome (fever, rash, and/or lymphadenopathy with organ system involvement, [hepatitis, nephritis, hematologic abnormalities, myocarditis, myositis] resembling an acute viral infection with eosinophilia. Discontinue carbamazepine if other cause not determined.
- **Seizures:** Assess frequency, location, duration, and characteristics of seizure activity.
- **Trigeminal Neuralgia:** Assess for facial pain (location, intensity, duration). Ask patient to identify stimuli that may precipitate facial pain (hot or cold foods, bedclothes, touching face).

- **Bipolar Disorder:** Assess mental status (mood, orientation, behavior) and cognitive abilities before and periodically during therapy.
- ***Lab Test Considerations:*** Monitor CBC, including platelet count, reticulocyte count, and serum iron, weekly during the first 2 mo and yearly thereafter for evidence of potentially fatal blood cell abnormalities. Medication should be discontinued if bone marrow depression occurs.
- ⧖ Perform genetic testing for the HLA-B*1502 allele in patients of Asian ancestry prior to beginning therapy.
- Liver function tests, urinalysis, and BUN should be routinely performed. May cause ↑ AST, ALT, serum alkaline phosphatase, bilirubin, BUN, urine protein, and urine glucose levels.
- Monitor serum ionized calcium levels every 6 mo or if seizure frequency increases. Thyroid function tests and ionized serum calcium concentrations may be ↓ hypocalcemia ↓ seizure threshold.
- Monitor ECG and serum electrolytes before and periodically during therapy. May cause hyponatremia.
- May occasionally cause ↑ serum cholesterol, high-density lipoprotein, and triglyceride concentrations.
- May cause false-negative pregnancy test results with tests that determine human chorionic gonadotropin.
- ***Toxicity and Overdose:*** Serum blood levels should be routinely monitored during therapy. Therapeutic levels range from 4–12 mcg/mL.

Potential Nursing Diagnoses

Risk for injury (Indications, Side Effects)
Chronic pain (Indications)
Disturbed thought process (Indications)

Implementation

- Do not confuse carbamazepine with oxcarbazepine. Do not confuse Tegretol with Trental or Tegretol XR.
- Implement seizure precautions as indicated.
- **PO:** Administer medication with food to minimize gastric irritation. May take at bedtime to reduce daytime sedation. Tablets may be crushed if patient has difficulty swallowing. Do not crush or chew extended-release tablets. Extended-release capsules may be opened and the contents sprinkled on applesauce or other similar foods.
- Do not administer suspension simultaneously with other liquid medications or diluents; mixture produces an orange rubbery mass.

Patient/Family Teaching

- Instruct patient to take carbamazepine around the clock, as directed. Take missed doses as soon as possible but not just before next dose; do not double doses. Notify health care professional if more than one dose is missed. Medication should be gradually discontinued to prevent seizures. Instruct patient to read the *Medication Guide* before starting and with each Rx refill; changes may occur.
- Advise patient to avoid grapefruit and grapefruit juice during therapy.
- Advise patient to notify health care professional of all Rx or OTC medications, vitamins, or herbal products being taken and to consult with health care professional before taking other medications.
- May cause dizziness or drowsiness. Advise patients to avoid driving or other activities requiring alertness until response to medication is known.
- Instruct patients that behavioral changes, skin rash, fever, sore throat, mouth ulcers, easy bruising, petechiae, unusual bleeding, abdominal pain, chills, rash, pale stools, dark urine, or jaundice should be reported to health care professional immediately. Advise patient and family to notify health care professional if thoughts about suicide or dying, attempts to commit suicide; new or worse depression; new or worse anxiety; feeling very agitated or restless; panic attacks; trouble sleeping; new or worse irritability; acting aggressive; being angry or violent; acting on dangerous impulses; an extreme increase in activity and talking, other unusual changes in behavior or mood occur.
- Inform patient that coating of *Tegretol XR* is not absorbed, but is excreted in feces and may be visible in stool.
- Advise patient not to take alcohol or other CNS depressants concurrently with this medication.
- Caution patients to use sunscreen and protective clothing to prevent photosensitivity reactions.
- Inform patient that frequent mouth rinses, good oral hygiene, and sugarless gum or candy may help reduce dry mouth. Saliva substitute may be used. Consult dentist if dry mouth persists >2 wk.
- Instruct patient to notify health care professional of medication regimen before treatment or surgery.
- Advise female patients to use a nonhormonal form of contraception while taking carbamazepine, to avoid breast feeding, and to notify health care professional if pregnancy is planned or suspected or if breast feeding.
- Emphasize the importance of follow-up lab tests and eye exams to monitor for side effects.
- **Seizures:** Advise patients to carry identification describing disease and medication regimen at all times.

Evaluation/Desired Outcomes

- Absence or reduction of seizure activity.
- Decrease in trigeminal neuralgia pain. Patients with trigeminal neuralgia who are pain-free should be reevaluated every 3 mo to determine minimum effective dose.
- Decreased mania and depressive symptoms in bipolar I disorder.

carbidopa/levodopa

(**kar**-bi-doe-pa/**lee**-voe-doe-pa)

Duopa, ✤Duodopa, Rytary, Sinemet, Sinemet CR

Classification
Therapeutic: antiparkinson agents
Pharmacologic: dopamine agonists

Pregnancy Category C (carbidopa/levodopa)

Indications

Parkinson's disease. Not useful for drug-induced extrapyramidal reactions.

Action

Levodopa is converted to dopamine in the CNS, where it serves as a neurotransmitter. Carbidopa, a decarboxylase inhibitor, prevents peripheral destruction of levodopa. **Therapeutic Effects:** Relief of tremor and rigidity in Parkinson's syndrome.

Pharmacokinetics

Absorption: Well absorbed following oral administration.
Distribution: Widely distributed. *Levodopa*— enters the CNS in small concentrations. *Carbidopa*— does not cross the blood-brain barrier but does cross the placenta. Both enter breast milk.
Metabolism and Excretion: *Levodopa*— mostly metabolized by the GI tract and liver. *Carbidopa*— 30% excreted unchanged by the kidneys.
Half-life: *Levodopa*— 1 hr; *carbidopa*— 1–2 hr.

TIME/ACTION PROFILE (antiparkinson effects)

ROUTE	ONSET	PEAK	DURATION
Carbidopa	unknown	unknown	5–24 hr
Levodopa	10–15 min	unknown	5–24 hr or more
Carbidopa/levodopa sustained release	unknown	2 hr	12 hr

Contraindications/Precautions

Contraindicated in: Hypersensitivity; Angle-closure glaucoma; Nonselective MAO inhibitor therapy; Malignant melanoma; Undiagnosed skin lesions; Some products contain tartrazine, phenylalanine, or aspartame and should be avoided in patients with known hypersensitivity.
Use Cautiously in: History of cardiac, psychiatric, or ulcer disease; OB, Pedi: Safety not established; Lactation: May ↓ serum prolactin; levodopa enters breast milk.

Adverse Reactions/Side Effects

CNS: depression, involuntary movements, anxiety, confusion, dizziness, drowsiness, hallucinations, memory loss, psychiatric problems, sudden sleep onset, urges (gambling, sexual). **CV:** orthostatic hypotension. **EENT:** blurred vision, mydriasis. **GI:** HEMORRHAGE (enteral suspension), GI PERFORATION (enteral suspension), PANCREATITIS (enteral suspension), constipation, nausea, vomiting, anorexia, bezoar (enteral suspension), dry mouth, hepatotoxicity, ileus (enteral suspension), peritonitis (enteral suspension). **Derm:** melanoma. **Hemat:** hemolytic anemia, leukopenia. **MS:** dyskinesias. **Neuro:** neuropathy. **Misc:** MELANOMA, darkening of urine or sweat.

Interactions

Drug-Drug: Use with **nonselective MAO inhibitors** may result in hypertensive reactions; concurrent use contraindicated (MAO inhibitor must be discontinued ≥2 wk before initiating carbidopa/levodopa). ↑ risk of arrhythmias with **inhalation hydrocarbon anesthetics** (especially **halothane**; if possible discontinue 6–8 hr before anesthesia). **Phenothiazines**, **haloperidol**, **papaverine**, **phenytoin**, and **reserpine** may ↓ effect of levodopa. Large doses of **pyridoxine** may ↓ beneficial effects of levodopa. Concurrent use with **methyldopa** may alter the effectiveness of levodopa and ↑ risk of CNS side effects. ↑ hypotension may result with concurrent **antihypertensives**. **Anticholinergics** may ↓ absorption of levodopa. ↑ risk of adverse reactions with **selegiline** or **cocaine**.
Drug-Natural Products: Kava-kava may ↓ levodopa effectiveness.
Drug-Food: Ingestion of foods containing large amounts of **pyridoxine** may ↓ effect of levodopa.

Route/Dosage

Carbidopa/Levodopa

PO (Adults): 25 mg carbidopa/100 mg levodopa 3 times daily; may be ↑ every 1–2 days until desired effect is achieved (max = 8 tablets of 25 mg carbidopa/100 mg levodopa/day).
Enteral (Adults): Patients must be converted to and be on stable dose of PO immediate-release carbidopa/levodopa tablets before initiation enteral suspension therapy. *Morning dose for Day 1 (mL) (to be administered over 10–30 min)* = (Amount of levodopa (in mg) in first dose of immediate-release carbidopa/levodopa taken by patient on previous day * 0.8)/20; *Continuous dose for Day 1 (mL) (to be administered over 16 hr)* = Determine amount of levodopa (in mg) patient received from immediate-release carbidopa/levodopa doses throughout 16 waking hours of previous day (do not include doses of immediate-release carbidopa/levodopa taken at night when calculating the levodopa amount). Then, subtract amount of first levodopa dose (in mg) taken by patient on previous day. Divide result by 20 to obtain the # of mL to be administered over 16 hr. Do not exceed dose of 2000 mg. At end of daily 16-hour infusion, patients will disconnect the pump from feeding tube and take their night-time dose of oral immediate-release carbidopa/levodopa tablets.

Total daily dose can be titrated after Day 1 based on patient response and tolerability.

Carbidopa/Levodopa Extended-Release (doses of Sinemet CR and Rytary are not interchangeable)

PO (Adults): *Patients not currently receiving levodopa (Sinemet CR)*—50 mg carbidopa/200 mg levodopa twice daily (minimum of 6 hr apart) initially. *Patients not currently receiving levodopa (Rytary)*—23.75 mg carbidopa/95 mg levodopa 3 times daily x 3 days, then 36.25 mg carbidopa/145 mg levodopa 3 times daily. May continue to ↑ dose as needed (max dose = 97.5 mg carbidopa/390 mg levodopa 3 times daily) May also ↑ frequency of administration up to 5 times daily (max dose = 612.5 mg carbidopa/2450 mg levodopa/day). *Conversion from immediate—release (IR) carbidopa/levodopa to Sinemet CR*—initiate therapy with at least 10% more levodopa content/day (may need up to 30% more) given at 4–8 hr intervals while awake. Allow 3 days between dosage changes; some patients may require larger doses and shorter dosing intervals. *Conversion from IR carbidopa/levodopa to Rytary*—If taking 400–549 mg/day of IR levodopa, give 3 capsules of Rytary 23.75 mg carbidopa/95 mg levodopa 3 times daily. If taking 550–749 mg/day of IR levodopa, give 4 capsules of Rytary 23.75 mg carbidopa/95 mg levodopa 3 times daily. If taking 750–949 mg/day of IR levodopa, give 3 capsules of Rytary 36.25 mg carbidopa/145 mg levodopa 3 times daily. If taking 950–1249 mg/day of IR levodopa, give 3 capsules of Rytary 48.75 mg carbidopa/195 mg levodopa 3 times daily. If taking ≥1250 mg/day of IR levodopa, give 4 capsules of Rytary 48.75 mg carbidopa/195 mg levodopa 3 times daily or 3 capsules of Rytary 61.25 mg carbidopa/245 mg levodopa 3 times daily.

Availability (generic available)

Tablets: 10 mg carbidopa/100 mg levodopa, 25 mg carbidopa/100 mg levodopa, 25 mg carbidopa/250 mg levodopa. **Cost:** *Generic*—10 mg/100 mg $25.28/100, 25 mg/100 mg $28.91/100, 25 mg/250 mg $19.22/100. **Orally disintegrating tablets (mint):** 10 mg carbidopa/100 mg levodopa, 25 mg carbidopa/100 mg levodopa, 25 mg carbidopa/250 mg levodopa. **Cost:** *Generic*—10 mg/100 mg $121.48/100, 25 mg/100 mg $137.18/100, 25 mg/250 mg $174.76/100. **Extended-release tablets (Sinemet CR):** 25 mg carbidopa/100 mg levodopa, 50 mg carbidopa/200 mg levodopa. **Cost:** *Generic*—25 mg/100 mg $93.90/100, 50 mg/200 mg $180.50/100. **Extended-release capsules (Rytary):** 23.75 mg carbidopa/95 mg levodopa, 36.25 mg carbidopa/145 mg levodopa, 48.75 mg carbidopa/195 mg levodopa, 61.25 mg carbidopa/245 mg levodopa. **Entereal suspension (Duopa):** 4.63 mg carbidopa/20 mg levodopa/mL in 100–mL single-use cassettes. ***In combination with:*** entacapone (Stalevo); see Appendix B.

NURSING IMPLICATIONS

Assessment

- Assess parkinsonian symptoms (akinesia, rigidity, tremors, pill rolling, shuffling gait, mask-like face, twisting motions, and drooling) during therapy. "On-off phenomenon" may cause symptoms to appear or improve suddenly.
- Assess BP and pulse frequently during period of dose adjustment.
- ***Lab Test Considerations:*** May cause false-positive test results in Coombs' test.
- May cause ↑ serum glucose. Dipstick for urine ketones may reveal false-positive results.
- Monitor hepatic and renal function and CBC periodically in patients on long-term therapy. May cause ↑ AST, ALT, bilirubin, alkaline phosphatase, LDH, and serum protein-bound iodine concentrations. May cause ↓ BUN, creatinine, and uric acid.
- May cause ↓ hemoglobin, ↓ hematocrit, agranulocytosis, hemolytic and nonhemolytic anemia, thrombocytopenia, leukopenia, and ↑ WBC.
- ***Toxicity and Overdose:*** Assess for signs of toxicity (involuntary muscle twitching, facial grimacing, spasmodic eye winking, exaggerated protrusion of tongue, behavioral changes). Consult health care professional if symptoms occur.

Potential Nursing Diagnoses

Impaired physical mobility (Indications)
Risk for injury (Indications)

Implementation

- Do not confuse Sinemet with Janumet.
- In the carbidopa/levodopa combination, the number following the drug name represents the milligrams of each respective drug.
- In preoperative patients or patients who are NPO, confer with health care professional about continuing medication administration.
- **PO:** Administer on a regular schedule. Hospitalized patients should be continued on same schedule as at home. Administer while awake, not around the clock to improve sleep and prevent side effects.
- Controlled-release tablets may be administered as whole or half tablets, but they should not be crushed or chewed.
- For *orally disintegrating tablets,* just prior to administration remove tablet from bottle with dry hands. Immediately place tablet on top of tongue. Tablet will dissolve in seconds, then swallow with saliva. Administration with liquid is not necessary.
- *For enteral administration,* administer *DUOPA* into the jejunum through a percutaneous endoscopic gastrostomy with jejunal tube (PEG-J) with CADD-Legacy 1400 portable infusion pump. Take suspension out of refrigerator 20 min prior to use; must be at room temperature for use. Administer over 16 hrs. If extra dose is needed, set function at 1 mL (20 mg of levodopa) when starting; may be adjusted in

0.2 mL increments. Limit to 1 extra dose every 2 hrs. Frequent extra doses may cause or worsen dyskinesias. Discontinue gradually; do not stop abruptly.
- *For extended-release capsules,* administer without regard to food. Swallow capsules whole; do not chew, divide, or crush. For patients with difficulty swallowing, open capsule and sprinkle entire contents on 1 to 2 tablespoons of applesauce; consume immediately. Do not store mixture for future use. Inform patients that first dose of day may be taken 1 to 2 hrs before eating, as a high fat, high calorie meal may delay the absorption of levodopa and onset of action by 2 to 3 hrs. Discontinue gradually; do not stop abruptly.

Patient/Family Teaching
- Instruct patient to take medication at regular intervals as directed. Do not change dose regimen or take additional antiparkinson drugs, including more carbidopa/levodopa, without consulting health care professional. Take missed doses as soon as remembered, unless next scheduled dose is within 2 hr; do not double doses.
- Explain that gastric irritation may be decreased by eating food shortly after taking medications but that high-protein meals may impair levodopa's effects. Dividing daily protein intake among all the meals may help ensure adequate protein intake and drug effectiveness. Do not drastically alter diet during carbidopa/levodopa therapy without consulting health care professional.
- May cause sudden onset of sleep, drowsiness, or dizziness. Advise patient to avoid driving and other activities that require alertness until response to drug is known.
- Caution patient to change positions slowly to minimize orthostatic hypotension. Health care professional should be notified if orthostatic hypotension occurs.
- Instruct patient that frequent rinsing of mouth, good oral hygiene, and sugarless gum or candy may decrease dry mouth.
- Caution patient to monitor skin lesions for any changes. Health care professional should be notified promptly because carbidopa/levodopa may activate malignant melanoma.
- Advise patient to notify health care professional of all Rx or OTC medications, vitamins, or herbal products being taken and to consult with health care professional before taking other medications, especially cold remedies. Large amounts of vitamin B_6 (pyridoxine) and iron may interfere with the action of levodopa.
- Inform patient that harmless darkening of saliva, urine, or sweat may occur.
- Advise patient to notify health care professional if palpitations, urinary retention, involuntary movements, behavioral changes, severe nausea and vomiting, new skin lesions, or new or increased gambling, sexual, or other intense urges occur. Dose reduction may be required.
- Inform patient that sometimes a "wearing-off" effect may occur at end of dosing interval. Notify health care professional if this poses a problem to lifestyle.
- Advise female patients to notify health care professional if pregnancy is planned or suspected or if breast feeding.

Evaluation/Desired Outcomes
- Resolution of parkinsonian signs and symptoms. Therapeutic effects usually become evident after 2–3 wk of therapy but may require up to 6 mo. Patients who take this medication for several yr may experience a decrease in the effectiveness of this drug.

carbonyl iron, See IRON SUPPLEMENTS.

HIGH ALERT

CARBOplatin (kar-boe-**pla**-tin)

~~Paraplatin~~

Classification

Therapeutic: antineoplastics

Pharmacologic: alkylating agents

Pregnancy Category D

Indications
Advanced ovarian carcinoma (with other agents). Palliative treatment of ovarian carcinoma unresponsive to other modalities.

Action
Inhibits DNA synthesis by producing cross-linking of parent DNA strands (cell-cycle phase–nonspecific). **Therapeutic Effects:** Death of rapidly replicating cells, particularly malignant ones.

Pharmacokinetics
Absorption: IV administration results in complete bioavailability.

Distribution: Unknown.

Protein Binding: Platinum is irreversibly bound to plasma proteins.

Metabolism and Excretion: Excreted mostly by the kidneys.

Half-life: *Carboplatin*—2.6–5.9 hr (increased in renal impairment); *platinum*—5 days.

TIME/ACTION PROFILE (effects on blood counts)

ROUTE	ONSET	PEAK	DURATION
IV	unknown	21 days	28 days

Contraindications/Precautions

Contraindicated in: Hypersensitivity to carboplatin, cisplatin, or mannitol; OB, Lactation: Pregnancy or lactation.

Use Cautiously in: Hearing loss; Electrolyte abnormalities; Renal impairment (dose ↓ recommended if CCr <60 mL/min); Active infections; Diminished bone marrow reserve (dose ↓ recommended); Other chronic debilitating illnesses; Geri: ↑ risk of thrombocytopenia, consider renal function in dose determination; Patients with childbearing potential; Pedi: Safety not established.

Adverse Reactions/Side Effects

CNS: weakness. **EENT:** ototoxicity. **GI:** abdominal pain, nausea, vomiting, constipation, diarrhea, hepatitis, stomatitis. **GU:** gonadal suppression, nephrotoxicity. **Derm:** alopecia, rash. **F and E:** hypocalcemia, hypokalemia, hypomagnesemia, hyponatremia. **Hemat:** ANEMIA, LEUKOPENIA, THROMBOCYTOPENIA. **Metab:** hyperuricemia. **Neuro:** peripheral neuropathy. **Misc:** hypersensitivity reactions including ANAPHYLACTIC-LIKE REACTIONS.

Interactions

Drug-Drug: ↑ nephrotoxicity and ototoxicity with other **nephrotoxic** and **ototoxic drugs (aminoglycosides, loop diuretics)**. ↑ bone marrow depression with other **bone marrow–depressing drugs** or **radiation therapy**. May ↓ antibody response to **live-virus vaccines** and ↑ risk of adverse reactions.

Route/Dosage

Other dosing formulas are used.

IV (Adults): *Initial treatment*—300 mg/m^2 with cyclophosphamide at 4-wk intervals. *Treatment of refractory tumors*—360 mg/m^2 as a single dose; may be repeated at 4-wk intervals, depending on response.

Renal Impairment

IV (Adults): *CCr 41–59 mL/min*—initial dose 250 mg/m^2; *CCr 16–40 mL/min*—initial dose 200 mg/m^2.

Availability (generic available)

Solution for injection: 10 mg/mL.

NURSING IMPLICATIONS

Assessment

- Assess for nausea and vomiting; often occur 6–12 hr after therapy (1–4 hr for aqueous solution) and may persist for 24 hr. Prophylactic antiemetics may be used. Adjust diet as tolerated to maintain fluid and electrolyte balance and ensure adequate nutritional intake. May require discontinuation of therapy.
- Monitor for bone marrow depression. Assess for bleeding (bleeding gums, bruising, petechiae, guaiac stools, urine, and emesis) and avoid IM injections and rectal temperatures if platelet count is low. Apply pressure to venipuncture sites for 10 min. Assess for signs of infection during neutropenia. Anemia may occur and may be cumulative; transfusions are frequently required. Monitor for increased fatigue, dyspnea, and orthostatic hypotension.
- Monitor for signs of anaphylaxis (rash, urticaria, pruritus, facial swelling, wheezing, tachycardia, hypotension). Discontinue medication immediately and notify physician if these occur. Epinephrine and resuscitation equipment should be readily available.
- Audiometry is recommended before initiation of therapy and subsequent doses. Ototoxicity manifests as tinnitus and unilateral or bilateral hearing loss in high frequencies and becomes more frequent and severe with repeated doses. Ototoxicity is more pronounced in children.
- ***Lab Test Considerations:*** Monitor CBC, differential, and clotting studies before and weekly during therapy. The nadirs of thrombocytopenia and leukopenia occur after 21 days and recover by 30 days after a dose. Nadir of granulocyte counts usually occurs after 21–28 days and recovers by day 35. Withhold subsequent doses until neutrophil count is >2000/mm^3 and platelet count is >100,000/mm^3.
- Monitor renal function and serum electrolytes before initiation of therapy and before each course of carboplatin.
- Monitor hepatic function before and periodically during therapy. May cause ↑ serum bilirubin, alkaline phosphatase, and AST concentrations.

Potential Nursing Diagnoses

Risk for infection (Adverse Reactions)
Risk for injury (Side Effects)

Implementation

- ***High Alert:*** Fatalities have occurred with chemotherapeutic agents. Before administering, clarify all ambiguous orders; double-check single, daily, and course-of-therapy dose limits; have second practitioner independently double-check original order, calculations, and infusion pump settings.
- ***High Alert:*** Do not confuse carboplatin with cisplatin. Do not confuse Paraplatin (carboplatin) with Platinol (cisplatin).
- ***High Alert:*** Carboplatin should be administered in a monitored setting under the supervision of a physician experienced in cancer chemotherapy.

IV Administration

- Solution should be prepared in a biologic cabinet. Wear gloves, gown, and mask while handling medication. Discard equipment in specially designated containers.
- Do not use aluminum needles or equipment during preparation or administration; aluminum reacts with the drug.

- **Intermittent Infusion:** ***Concentration:*** 0.5 mg/mL. Stable for 8 hr at room temperature. ***Rate:*** Infuse over 15–60 min.
- **Y-Site Compatibility:** acyclovir, alfentanil, amifostine, amikacin, aminocaproic acid, aminophylline, amiodarone, amphotericin B colloidal, amphotericin B lipid complex, amphotericin B liposome, ampicillin, ampicillin/sulbactam, anidulafungin, argatroban, atracurium, azithromycin, aztreonam, bivalirudin, bleomycin, bumetanide, buprenorphine, butorphanol, calcium acetate, calcium chloride, calcium gluconate, caspofungin, cefazolin, cefepime, defotaxime, cefotetan, cefoxitin, ceftazidime, ceftriaxone, cefuroxime, chloramphenicol, chlorpromazine, ciprofloxacin, cisatracurium, cisplatin, clindamycin, cyclophosphamide, cyclosporine, cytarabine, daptomycin, dexamethasone, dexmedetomidine, dextrazoxane, digoxin, diltiazem, diphenhydramine, decetaxel, dopamine, doxacurium, doxorubicin hydrochloride, doxycycline, droperidol, enalaprilat, ephedrine, ertapenem, erythromycin, esmolol, etoposide, etoposide phosphate, famotidine, fenoldopam, fentanyl, filgrastim, fluconazole, fludarabine, fluorouracil, foscarnet, fosphenytoin, furosemide, gemcitabine, gentamicin, glycopyrrolate, granisetron, haloperidol, heparin, hetastarch, hydralazine, hydrocortisone, hydromorphone, imipenem/cilastatin, insulin, isoproterenol, ketorolac, labetalol, leucovorin, levofloxacin, lidocaine, linezolid, lorazepam, magnesium sulfate, mannitol, melphalan, meperidine, meropenem, mesna, metaraminol, methotrexate, methyldopate, methylprednisolone, metoprolol, metronidazole, midazolam, milrinone, mintxantrone, morphine, nafcillin, nalbuphine, naloxone, nesiritide, nicardipine, nitroglycerine, nitroprusside, norepinephrine, octreotide, ondansetron, paclitaxel, palonosetron, pamidronate, pancuronium, pantoprazole, pemetrexed, pentamidine, pentazocine, pentobarbital, phenylephrine, piperacillin/tazobactam, potassium acetate, potassium chloride, potassium phosphates, prochlorperazine, propranolol, quinupristin/dalfopristin, ranitidine, remifentanil, rituximab, rocuronium, sargramostim, sodium acetate, sodium bicarbonate, sodium phosphates, succinylcholine, sufentanil, tacrolimus, teniposide, theophylline, thiotepa, tigecycline, tirofiban, tobramycin, trastuzumab, trimethoprim/sulfamethoxazole, vancomycin, vecuronium, verapamil, vincristine, vinorelbine, voriconazole, zidovudine, zoledronic acid.
- **Y-Site Incompatibility:** allopurinol, dantrolene, diazepam, dobutamine, epinephrine, metoclopramide, phenobarbital, phentolamine, phenytoin, procainamide, promethazine, thiopental.

Patient/Family Teaching

- Instruct patient to notify health care professional promptly if fever; chills; sore throat; signs of infection; lower back or side pain; difficult or painful urination; bleeding gums; bruising; pinpoint red spots on skin; blood in stools, urine, or emesis; increased fatigue, dyspnea, or orthostatic hypotension occurs.
- Caution patient to avoid crowds and persons with known infections. Instruct patient to use soft toothbrush and electric razor and to avoid falls. Caution patients not to drink alcoholic beverages or take medication containing aspirin or NSAIDs because they may precipitate gastric bleeding.
- Instruct patient to promptly report any numbness or tingling in extremities or face, decreased coordination, difficulty with hearing or ringing in the ears, unusual swelling, or weight gain to health care professional.
- Instruct patient not to receive any vaccinations without advice of health care professional and to avoid contact with persons who have received oral polio vaccine within the past several months.
- Advise patient of the need for contraception (if patient is not infertile as a result of surgical or radiation therapy).
- Instruct patient to inspect oral mucosa for erythema and ulceration. If ulceration occurs, advise patient to notify health care professional, rinse mouth with water after eating, and use sponge brush. Mouth pain may require treatment with opioids.
- Discuss with patient the possibility of hair loss. Explore methods of coping.
- Emphasize the need for periodic lab tests to monitor for side effects.

Evaluation/Desired Outcomes

- Decrease in size or spread of ovarian carcinoma.

cariprazine (kar-**ip**-ra-zeen)

Vraylar

Classification

Therapeutic: antipsychotics

Indications

Treatment of schizophrenia. Acute treatment of mania/mixed episodes due to bipolar I disorder.

Action

Acts as a partial agonist at dopamine D_2 receptors in the CNS and serotonin $5-HT_{1A}$; also acts an antogonist at $5-HT_{2A}$ receptors. **Therapeutic Effects:** Decreased incidence and severity of symptoms of schizophrenia. Decreased occurrence and severity of mania associated with bipolar 1 disorder.

Pharmacokinetics

Absorption: Well absorbed following oral administration.

Distribution: Unk.

Protein Binding: 91–97%.

Metabolism and Excretion: Two metabolites desmethyl cariprazine (DCAR) and didesmethyl cariprazine (DDCAR) are have antipsychotic activity. Metabolism occurs mostly via the CYP3A4 enzyme system, with further metabolism resulting in inactive metabolites; 21% excreted urine, 1.2% as unchanged drug.

Half-life: Cariprazine—2–4 days; *DDCAR*—1–3 weeks.

TIME/ACTION PROFILE (improvement in symptoms)

ROUTE	ONSET	PEAK	DURATION
PO (schizophrenia)	within 1–2 wk	4–6 wk	2 wk†
PO (mania due to bipolar 1 disorder)	within 5–7 days	2–3 wk	2 wk†

† Blood levels of drug and active metabolites following discontinuation.

Contraindications/Precautions

Contraindicated in: Hypersensitivity; Concurrent use of strong CYP3A4 inhibitors; Concurrent use of strong CYP3A4 inducers.

Use Cautiously in: Known cerebrovascular/cardiovascular disease, dehydration, concurrent use of diuretics/antihypertensives or syncope (↑ risk of orthostatic hypotension); Pre-existing ↓ WBC or ANC or history of drug-induced leukpenia/neutropenia; Geri: Elderly patients with dementia-related psychosis (↑ risk of adverse cardiovascular effects and death), consider age-related ↓ in renal/hepatic/cardiovascular function, concurrent disease states and medications (↓ initial dose recommended); Patients at risk of aspiration; OB: Neonates exposed in the third trimester may experience extrapyramidal symptoms/withdrawal; Lactation: Consider maternal and fetal benefits against possible adverse effects in infant; Pedi: Safe and effective use in children has not been established.

Adverse Reactions/Side Effects

EENT: blurred vision. **CNS:** drowsiness, headache, agitation, dizziness, fatigue, insomnia, restlessness. **Resp:** cough. **CV:** hyertension, orthostatic hypotension, tachycardia. **GI:** dyspepsia, nausea, ↓ appetite, constipation, diarrhea, dry mouth, dysphagia (↑aspiration risk), ↑ liver enzymes, vomiting. **Derm:** rash. **Hemat:** AGRANULOCYTOSIS, leukopenia, neutropenia. **Metab:** dyslipidemia, hyperglycemia/diabetes mellitus, weight gain. **MS:** arthralgia, back pain, extremity pain. **Neuro:** akathisia, extrapyramidal symptoms, tardive dyskinesia. **Misc:** NEUROLEPTIC MALIGNANT SYNDROME, body temperature dysregulation, late-occurring adverse reactions (consider long half-life of active drug).

Interactions

Drug-Drug: Blood levels, effects and risk of toxicity ↑ by concurrent use of**strong CYP3A4 inhibitors** including **itraconazole** and **ketoconazole**; concurrent use not recommended. Blood levels and effectiveness may be ↓ by concurrent use of**strong CYP3A4 inducers** including **carbamazepine** and **rifampin**; concurrent use not recommended. Concurrent use of **diuretics/antihypertensives** (↑ risk of orthostatic hypotension/syncope).

Route/Dosage

PO (Adults): *Schizophrenia*—1.5 mg/day initally, may be increased on second day to 3 mg, further increments of 1.5 mg or 3 mg may be made depending on response/tolerance up to maintenance dose of 1.5–6 mg/day; *Bipolar mania*—1.5 mg/day initially, may be increased on second day to 3 mg, further increments of 1.5 mg or 3 mg may be made depending on response/tolerance up to maintenance dose of 1.5–6 mg/day titrated up to 3–6 mg/day; *Concurrent use of strong CYP3A4 inhibitors*—decrease dose by 50%.

Availability

Caspules: 1.5 mg, 3 mg, 4.5 mg, 6 mg.

NURSING IMPLICATIONS

Assessment

- Assess mental status (orientation, mood, behavior) before and periodically during therapy.
- Assess weight and BMI initially and throughout therapy.
- Monitor BP (sitting, standing, lying), pulse, and respiratory rate before and periodically during therapy.
- Observe patient carefully when administering medication to ensure that medication is actually taken and not hoarded or cheeked.
- Monitor for adverse reactions and patient response for several weeks after starting therapy and after each dose increase. Due to long action, may not occur for several wks. Consider reducing dose or discontinuing drug if severe adverse reactions occur.
- Monitor patient for onset of akathisia (restlessness or desire to keep moving) and extrapyramidal side effects (*parkinsonian*—difficulty speaking or swallowing, loss of balance control, pill rolling of hands, masklike face, shuffling gait, rigidity, tremors; and *dystonic*—muscle spasms, twisting motions, twitching, inability to move eyes, weakness of arms or legs) periodically throughout therapy. Report these symptoms.
- Monitor for tardive dyskinesia (uncontrolled rhythmic movement of mouth, face, and extremities; lip smacking or puckering; puffing of cheeks; uncontrolled chewing; rapid or worm-like movements of tongue). Notify health care professional immediately

if these symptoms occur, as these side effects may be irreversible.

- Monitor for development of neuroleptic malignant syndrome (fever, muscle rigidity, altered mental status, respiratory distress, tachycardia, seizures, diaphoresis, hypertension or hypotension, pallor, tiredness, loss of bladder control). Notify health care professional immediately if these symptoms occur.
- ***Lab Test Considerations:*** Monitor CBC frequently during therapy in patients with pre-existing or history of low WBC. May cause leukopenia, neutropenia, or agranulocytosis. Discontinue therapy if severe neutropenia (ANC <1000 mm^3) occurs.
- Monitor fasting blood glucose and lipid profile initially and periodically during therapy.

Potential Nursing Diagnoses

Disturbed thought process (Indications)

Imbalanced nutrition: risk for more than body requirements (Side Effects)

Implementation

- **PO:** Administer once daily without regard to meals.

Patient/Family Teaching

- Advise patient to take medication as directed and not to skip doses or double up on missed doses. Take missed doses as soon as remembered unless almost time for the next dose. Do not stop taking cariprazine without consulting health care professional.
- Inform patient of possibility of extrapyramidal symptoms and tardive dyskinesia. Instruct patient to report these symptoms immediately.
- Advise patient to make position changes slowly to minimize orthostatic hypotension.
- Medication may cause drowsiness. Caution patient to avoid driving or other activities requiring alertness until response to medication is known.
- Advise patient and family to notify health care professional of new or worse depression; new or worse anxiety; feeling very agitated or restless; panic attacks; trouble sleeping; new or worse irritability; acting aggressive; being angry or violent; acting on dangerous impulses; an extreme increase in activity and talking; other unusual changes in behavior or mood occur.
- Inform patient that cariprazine may cause weight gain. Advise patient to monitor weight periodically. Notify health care professional of significant weight gain.
- Instruct patient to notify health care professional of all Rx or OTC medications, vitamins, or herbal products being taken and to consult health care professional before taking any new medications. Caution patient to avoid taking alcohol or other CNS depressants concurrently with this medication.
- Advise patient that extremes in temperature should be avoided, because this drug impairs body temperature regulation.
- Advise patient to notify health care professional of medication regimen prior to treatment or surgery.
- Advise female patients to notify health care professional if pregnancy is planned or suspected and to avoid breast feeding during therapy. Encourage pregnant patients to enroll in registry by contacting National Pregnancy Registry for Atypical Antipsychotics at 1-866-961-2388 or visit http://womensmentalhealth.org/clinical-and-research-programs/pregnancyregistry/.
- Emphasize the importance of routine follow-up exams and continued participation in psychotherapy as indicated.

Evaluation/Desired Outcomes

- Decrease in excitable, paranoic, or withdrawn behavior.
- Decreased occurrence and severity of mania associated with bipolar 1 disorder.

C

⧖ carisoprodol

(kar-i-**sop**-roe-dole)

Soma

Classification

Therapeutic: skeletal muscle relaxants (centrally acting)

Schedule IV

Pregnancy Category C

Indications

Adjunct to rest and physical therapy in the treatment of muscle spasm associated with acute painful musculoskeletal conditions.

Action

Skeletal muscle relaxation, probably due to CNS depression. **Therapeutic Effects:** Skeletal muscle relaxation.

Pharmacokinetics

Absorption: Well absorbed after oral administration.

Distribution: Crosses the placenta; high concentrations in breast milk.

Metabolism and Excretion: Mostly metabolized by the liver via CYP2C19 to meprobamate; ⧖ 2% of Whites, 4% of Blacks, and 14% of Asians have CYP2C19 genotype that results in reduced metabolism of carisoprodol (poor metabolizers) into its active metabolite (may result in ↑ sedation).

Half-life: 8 hr.

TIME/ACTION PROFILE (skeletal muscle relaxation)

ROUTE	ONSET	PEAK	DURATION
PO	30 min	unknown	4–6 hr

Contraindications/Precautions

Contraindicated in: Hypersensitivity to carisoprodol or to meprobamate; Porphyria or suspected porphyria.

Use Cautiously in: Severe liver or kidney disease; OB, Lactation, Pedi: Safety not established for pregnant women, breast feeding infants, or children <16 yr; Geri: Poorly tolerated due to anticholinergic effects. Appears on Beers list.

Adverse Reactions/Side Effects

CNS: dizziness, drowsiness, agitation, ataxia, depression, headache, insomnia, irritability, syncope. **Resp:** asthma attacks. **CV:** hypotension, tachycardia. **GI:** epigastric distress, hiccups, nausea, vomiting. **Derm:** flushing, rashes. **Hemat:** eosinophilia, leukopenia. **Misc:** ANAPHYLACTIC SHOCK, fever, psychological dependence, severe idiosyncratic reaction.

Interactions

Drug-Drug: Additive CNS depression with other **CNS depressants** including **alcohol**, **antihistamines**, **opioid analgesics**, and **sedative/hypnotics**.

Drug-Natural Products: Concomitant use of **kava-kava**, **valerian**, **skullcap**, **chamomile**, or **hops** can ↑ CNS depression.

Route/Dosage

PO (Adults ≥16 yr): 250–350 mg 4 times daily for no longer than 2–3 wk.

Availability (generic available)

Tablets: 250 mg, 350 mg. **Cost:** *Generic*—250 mg $330.59/100, 350 mg $59.62/100. ***In combination with:*** aspirin (Soma compound) and codeine. See Appendix B.

NURSING IMPLICATIONS

Assessment

- Assess patient for pain, muscle stiffness, and range of motion before and periodically throughout therapy.
- Observe patient for idiosyncratic symptoms that may appear within minutes or hours of administration during the first dose. Symptoms include extreme weakness, quadriplegia, dizziness, ataxia, dysarthria, visual disturbances, agitation, euphoria, confusion, and disorientation. Usually subsides over several hours.
- Geri: Assess geriatric patients for anticholinergic effects (sedation and weakness).

Potential Nursing Diagnoses

Acute pain (Indications)
Impaired bed mobility (Indications)
Risk for injury (Side Effects)

Implementation

- Should be used ONLY for acute treatment periods of no more than 2–3 wk.
- Provide safety measures as indicated. Supervise ambulation and transfer of patients.
- **PO:** Administer with food to minimize GI irritation. Give dose at bedtime.

Patient/Family Teaching

- Instruct patient to take medication as directed. Missed doses should be taken within 1 hr; if not, omit and return to regular dosing schedule. Do not double doses.
- Inform patient that use is limited to acute relief of musculoskeletal discomfort of 2–3 wk. Prolonged use may lead to dependence, withdrawal, and abuse. Encourage patient to comply with additional therapies prescribed for muscle spasm (rest, physical therapy, heat, etc). If musculoskeletal discomfort persists consult health care professional for further evaluation.
- May cause dizziness or drowsiness. Advise patient to avoid driving or other activities requiring alertness until response to drug is known.
- Instruct patient to change positions slowly to minimize orthostatic hypotension.
- Advise patient to avoid concurrent use of alcohol and other CNS depressants while taking this medication.
- Instruct patient to notify health care professional if signs of allergy (rash, hives, swelling of tongue or lips, dyspnea) or idiosyncratic reaction occur.

Evaluation/Desired Outcomes

- Decreased musculoskeletal pain and muscle spasticity.
- Increased range of motion.

carvedilol (kar-**ve**-di-lole)

Coreg, Coreg CR

Classification
Therapeutic: antihypertensives
Pharmacologic: beta blockers

Pregnancy Category C

Indications

Hypertension. HF (ischemic or cardiomyopathic) with digoxin, diuretics, and ACE inhibitors. Left ventricular dysfunction after myocardial infarction.

Action

Blocks stimulation of $beta_1$ (myocardial) and $beta_2$ (pulmonary, vascular, and uterine)-adrenergic receptor sites. Also has $alpha_1$ blocking activity, which may result in orthostatic hypotension. **Therapeutic Effects:** Decreased heart rate and BP. Improved cardiac output, slowing of the progression of HF and decreased risk of death.

Pharmacokinetics

Absorption: Well absorbed but rapidly undergoes extensive first-pass hepatic metabolism, resulting in 25–35% bioavailability. Food slows absorption.

Distribution: Unknown.

Protein Binding: 98%.

Metabolism and Excretion: Extensively metabolized (primarily by CYP2D6 and CYP2C9; the CYP2D6 enzyme system exhibits genetic polymorphism); ~7% of population may be poor metabolizers and may have significantly ↑ carvedilol concentrations and an ↑ risk of adverse effects); excreted in feces via bile, <2% excreted unchanged in urine.

Half-life: 7–10 hr.

TIME/ACTION PROFILE (cardiovascular effects)

ROUTE	ONSET	PEAK	DURATION
PO	within 1 hr	1–2 hr	12 hr
PO-CR	unknown	5 hr	24 hr

Contraindications/Precautions

Contraindicated in: History of serious hypersensitivity reaction (Stevens-Johnson syndrome, angioedema, anaphylaxis); Pulmonary edema; Cardiogenic shock; Bradycardia, heart block or sick sinus syndrome (unless a pacemaker is in place); Uncompensated HF requiring IV inotropic agents (wean before starting carvedilol); Severe hepatic impairment; Asthma or other bronchospastic disorders.

Use Cautiously in: HF (condition may deteriorate during initial therapy); Renal impairment; Hepatic impairment; Diabetes mellitus (may mask signs of hypoglycemia); Thyrotoxicosis (may mask symptoms); Peripheral vascular disease; History of severe allergic reactions (intensity of reactions may be increased); OB: Crosses placenta and may cause fetal/neonatal bradycardia, hypotension, hypoglycemia, or respiratory depression); Lactation, Pedi: Safety not established; Geri: ↑ sensitivity to beta blockers; initial dose reduction recommended.

Adverse Reactions/Side Effects

CNS: dizziness, fatigue, weakness, anxiety, depression, drowsiness, insomnia, memory loss, mental status changes, nervousness, nightmares. **EENT:** blurred vision, dry eyes, intraoperative floppy iris syndrome, nasal stuffiness. **Resp:** bronchospasm, wheezing. **CV:** BRADYCARDIA, HF, PULMONARY EDEMA. **GI:** diarrhea, constipation, nausea. **GU:** erectile dysfunction, ↓ libido. **Derm:** STEVENS-JOHNSON SYNDROME, TOXIC EPIDERMAL NECROLYSIS, itching, rashes, urticaria. **Endo:** hyperglycemia, hypoglycemia. **MS:** arthralgia, back pain, muscle cramps. **Neuro:** paresthesia. **Misc:** ANAPHYLAXIS, ANGIOEDEMA, drug-induced lupus syndrome.

Interactions

Drug-Drug: General anesthetics, **IV phenytoin**, **diltiazem**, and **verapamil** may cause ↑ myocardial depression. ↑ risk of bradycardia with **digoxin**. **Amiodarone** or **fluconazole** may ↑ levels. ↑ hypotension may occur with other **antihypertensives**, acute ingestion of **alcohol**, or **nitrates**. Concurrent use with **clonidine** ↑ hypotension and bradycardia. May ↑ withdrawal phenomenon from **clonidine** (discontinue carvedilol first). Concurrent administration of **thyroid preparations** may ↓ effectiveness. May alter the effectiveness of **insulins** or **oral hypoglycemic agents** (dose adjustments may be necessary). May ↓ effectiveness of **theophylline**. May ↓ beneficial beta$_1$-cardiovascular effects of **dopamine** or **dobutamine**. Use cautiously within 14 days of **MAO inhibitor** therapy (may result in hypotension/bradycardia). **Cimetidine** may ↑ toxicity from carvedilol. Concurrent **NSAIDs** may ↓ antihypertensive action. Effectiveness may be ↓ by **rifampin**. May ↑ serum **digoxin** levels. May ↑ blood levels of **cyclosporine** (monitor blood levels).

Route/Dosage

PO (Adults): *Hypertension*—6.25 mg twice daily, may be ↑ q 7–14 days up to 25 mg twice daily *or extended-release*—20 mg once daily, dose may be doubled every 7–14 days up to 80 mg once daily; *HF*—3.125 mg twice daily for 2 wk; may be ↑ to 6.25 mg twice daily. Dose may be doubled q 2 wk as tolerated (not to exceed 25 mg twice daily in patients <85 kg or 50 mg twice daily in patients >85 kg) *or extended-release*—10 mg once daily, dose may be doubled every 2 wk as tolerated up to 80 mg once daily; *Left ventricular dysfunction after MI*—6.25 mg twice daily, ↑ after 3–10 days to 12.5 twice daily then to target dose of 25 mg twice daily; some patients may require lower initial doses and slower titration *or extended-release*—20 mg once daily, dose may be doubled every 3–10 days up to 80 mg once daily.

Availability (generic available)

Tablets: 3.125 mg, 6.25 mg, 12.5 mg, 25 mg. **Cost:** *Generic*—All strengths $7.18/100. **Extended-release capsules:** 10 mg, 20 mg, 40 mg, 80 mg. **Cost:** all strengths $175.36/30.

NURSING IMPLICATIONS

Assessment

- Monitor BP and pulse frequently during dose adjustment period and periodically during therapy. Assess for orthostatic hypotension when assisting patient up from supine position.
- Monitor intake and output ratios and daily weight. Assess patient routinely for evidence of fluid overload (peripheral edema, dyspnea, rales/crackles, fatigue, weight gain, jugular venous distention). Pa-

tients may experience worsening of symptoms during initiation of therapy for HF.

- **Hypertension:** Check frequency of refills to determine adherence.
- ***Lab Test Considerations:*** May cause ↑ BUN, serum lipoprotein, potassium, triglyceride, and uric acid levels.
- May cause ↑ ANA titers.
- May cause ↑ in blood glucose levels.
- ***Toxicity and Overdose:*** Monitor patients receiving beta blockers for signs of overdose (bradycardia, severe dizziness or fainting, severe drowsiness, dyspnea, bluish fingernails or palms, seizures). Notify health care professional immediately if these signs occur.

Potential Nursing Diagnoses

Decreased cardiac output (Side Effects)
Noncompliance (Patient/Family Teaching)

Implementation

- Do not confuse carvedilol with captopril.
- Discontinuation of concurrent clonidine should be gradual, with carvedilol discontinued first over 1–2 wk with limitation of physical activity; then, after several days, discontinue clonidine.
- **PO:** Take apical pulse before administering. If <50 bpm or if arrhythmia occurs, withhold medication and notify health care professional.
- Administer with food to minimize orthostatic hypotension.
- Administer extended-release capsulesin the morning. Swallow whole; do not crush, break, or chew. Extended-release capsules may be opened and sprinkled on cold applesauce and taken immediately; do not store mixture.
- To convert from immediate-release to extended-release product, doses of 3.125 mg twice daily can be converted to 10 mg daily; doses of 6.25 mg twice daily can be converted to 20 mg daily; doses of 12.5 mg twice daily can be converted to 40 mg daily; and doses of 25 mg twice daily can be converted to 80 mg daily.

Patient/Family Teaching

- Instruct patient to take medication as directed, at the same time each day, even if feeling well. Do not skip or double up on missed doses. Take missed doses as soon as possible up to 4 hr before next dose. Abrupt withdrawal may precipitate life-threatening arrhythmias, hypertension, or myocardial ischemia.
- Advise patient to make sure enough medication is available for weekends, holidays, and vacations. A written prescription may be kept in wallet in case of emergency.
- Teach patient and family how to check pulse and BP. Instruct them to check pulse daily and BP biweekly. Advise patient to hold dose and contact health care professional if pulse is <50 bpm or BP changes significantly.
- May cause drowsiness or dizziness. Caution patients to avoid driving or other activities that require alertness until response to the drug is known.
- Advise patient to change positions slowly to minimize orthostatic hypotension, especially during initiation of therapy or when dose is increased.
- Caution patient that this medication may increase sensitivity to cold.
- Instruct patient to notify health care professional of all Rx or OTC medications, vitamins, or herbal products being taken and to consult health care professional before taking other Rx, OTC, or herbal products, especially cold preparations, concurrently with this medication.
- Patients with diabetes should closely monitor blood glucose, especially if weakness, malaise, irritability, or fatigue occurs. Medication may mask some signs of hypoglycemia, but dizziness and sweating may still occur.
- Advise patient to notify health care professional if slow pulse, difficulty breathing, wheezing, cold hands and feet, dizziness, confusion, depression, rash, fever, sore throat, unusual bleeding, or bruising occurs.
- Instruct patient to inform health care professional of medication regimen before treatment or surgery.
- Advise patient to carry identification describing disease process and medication regimen at all times.
- **Hypertension:** Reinforce the need to continue additional therapies for hypertension (weight loss, sodium restriction, stress reduction, regular exercise, moderation of alcohol consumption, and smoking cessation). Medication controls but does not cure hypertension.

Evaluation/Desired Outcomes

- Decrease in BP without appearance of detrimental side effects.
- Decrease in severity of HF.

caspofungin (kas-po-**fun**-gin)

Cancidas

Classification
Therapeutic: antifungals (systemic)
Pharmacologic: echinocandins

Pregnancy Category C

Indications

Invasive aspergillosis refractory to, or intolerant of, other therapies. Candidemia and associated serious infections (intra-abdominal abscesses, peritonitis, pleural space infections). Esophageal candidiasis. Suspected fungal infections in febrile neutropenic patients.

Action

Inhibits the synthesis of β (1, 3)-D-glucan, a necessary component of the fungal cell wall. **Therapeutic Effects:** Death of susceptible fungi.

Pharmacokinetics

Absorption: IV administration results in complete bioavailability.

Distribution: Widely distributed to tissues.

Protein Binding: 97%.

Metabolism and Excretion: Slowly and extensively metabolized; <1.5% excreted unchanged in urine.

Half-life: Polyphasic: *β phase*—9–11 hr; *γ phase*—40–50 hr.

TIME/ACTION PROFILE

ROUTE	ONSET	PEAK	DURATION
IV	unknown	end of infusion	24 hr

Contraindications/Precautions

Contraindicated in: Hypersensitivity; Concurrent use with cyclosporine.

Use Cautiously in: Moderate hepatic impairment (↓ maintenance dose recommended).

Adverse Reactions/Side Effects

CNS: headache, chills. **GI:** diarrhea, ↑ liver enzymes, nausea, vomiting. **Resp:** bronchospasm. **GU:** ↑ creatinine. **Derm:** flushing, pruritis, rash. **Local:** venous irritation at injection site. **Misc:** allergic reactions including ANAPHYLAXIS, ANGIOEDEMA, fever.

Interactions

Drug-Drug: Concurrent use with **cyclosporine** is not recommended due to ↑ risk of hepatic toxicity. May ↓ blood levels and effects of **tacrolimus**. Blood levels and effectiveness may be ↓ by **rifampin**; maintenance dose should be ↑ to 70 mg (in patients with normal liver function). Blood levels and effectiveness also may be ↓ by **efavirenz**, **nelfinavir**, **nevirapine**, **phenytoin**, **dexamethasone**, or **carbamazepine**; an ↑ in the maintenance dose to 70 mg should be considered in patients who are not clinically responding.

Route/Dosage

IV (Adults): 70 mg initially followed by 50 mg daily, duration determined by clinical situation and response; *Esophageal candidiasis*—50 mg daily, duration determined by clinical situation and response.

IV (Children ≥3 mo): 70 mg/m² (max: 70 mg) initially followed by 50 mg/m² daily (max: 70 mg/day), duration determined by clinical situation and response.

IV (Infants 1 to < 3 mo and Neonates): 25 mg/m²/dose once daily.

Hepatic Impairment

IV (Adults): *Moderate hepatic impairment*—70 mg initially followed by 35 mg daily, duration determined by clinical situation and response.

Availability

Powder for injection: 50 mg/vial, 70 mg/vial.

NURSING IMPLICATIONS

Assessment

- Assess patient for signs and symptoms of fungal infections prior to and periodically during therapy.
- Monitor patient for signs of anaphylaxis (rash, dyspnea, stridor) during therapy.
- ***Lab Test Considerations:*** May cause ↑ serum alkaline phosphatase, serum creatinine, AST, ALT, eosinophils, and urine protein and RBCs. May also cause ↓ serum potassium, hemoglobin, hematocrit, and WBCs.

Potential Nursing Diagnoses

Risk for infection (Indications)

Implementation

IV Administration

- **Intermittent Infusion:** ***Diluent:*** Allow refrigerated vial to reach room temperature. *For 70-mg or 50-mg dose*—Reconstitute vials with 10.8 mL of 0.9% NaCl, sterile water for injection, Bacteriostatic Water for Injection with methylparaben and propylparaben, or Bacteriostatic Water for Injection with 0.9% benzyl alcohol. Use preservative-free diluents for neonates. Do not dilute with dextrose solutions. Reconstituted solution is stable for 1 hr at room temperature. Withdraw 10 mL from vial and add to 250 mL of 0.9% NaCl, 0.45% NaCl, 0.225% NaCl, or LR. The 50-mg dose also can be diluted in 100 mL when volume restriction is necessary. Infusion is stable for 24 hr at room temperature or 48 hr if refrigerated. *For 35-mg dose*—Reconstitute a 50-mg or 70-mg vial as per the directions above. Remove the volume of drug equal to the calculated loading dose or calculated maintenance dose based on a concentration of 7 mg/mL (if reconstituted from the 70-mg vial) or a concentration of 5 mg/mL (if reconstituted from the 50-mg vial). White cake should dissolve completely. Mix gently until a clear solution is obtained. Do not use a solution that is cloudy, discolored, or contains precipitates. ***Concentration:*** 0.14–0.47 mg/mL. ***Rate:*** Infuse over 1 hr.
- **Y-Site Compatibility:** alfentanil, allopurinol, amifostine, amikacin, aminophylline, amiodarone, anidulafungin, atracurium, aztreonam, bleomycin, bumetanide, busulfan, butorphanol, calcium acetate, calcium chloride, calcium gluconate, carboplatin, carmustine, chlorpromazine, cimetidine, ciprofloxacin, cisatracurium, cisplatin, cyclophosphamide, cyclosporine, dacarbazine, dactinomycin, daptomycin, daunorubicin, dexmedetomidine, dexrazoxane, diltiazem, diphenhydramine, dobutamine, docetaxel, dolasetron, dopamine, dori-

penem, doxorubicin, doxycycline, droperidol, epinephrine, epirubicin, erythromycin, esmolol, etoposide, etoposide phosphate, famotidine, fenoldopam, fentanyl, fluconazole, fludarabine, ganciclovir, gemcitabine, gentamicin, glycopyrrolate, granisetron, haloperidol, hydrocortisone sodium succinate, hydromorphone, idarubicin, ifosfamide, imipenem/cilastatin, insulin, irinotecan, isoproterenol, labetalol, leucovorin, levofloxacin, linezolid, magnesium sulfate, mannitol, mechlorethamine, melphalan, meperidine, meropenem, mesna, metaraminol, methyldopate, metoclopramide, metoprolol, midazolam, milrinone, mitomycin, mitoxantrone, morphine, moxifloxacin, mycophenolate, nalbuphine, naloxone, nicardipine, nitroglycerin, norepinephrine, octreotide, ondansetron, oxaliplatin, oxytocin, paclitaxel, palonosetron, pentamidine, pentazocine, phentolamine, phenylephrine, potassium chloride, procainamide, prochlorperazine, promethazine, propranolol, quinupristin/dalfopristin, remifentanil, rocuronium, streptozocin, succinylcholine, sufentanil, tacrolimus, teniposide, theophylline, thiopental, thiotepa, tigecycline, tirofiban, tobramycin, topotecan, vancomycin, vasopressin, vecuronium, verapamil, vinblastine, vincristine, vinorelbine, voriconazole, zidovudine, zoledronic acid.

- **Y-Site Incompatibility:** amphotericin B colloidal, amphotericin B lipid complex, amphotericin B liposome, ampicillin, ampicillin/sulbactam, bivalirudin, cefazolin, cefepime, cefotaxime, cefotetan, cefoxitin, ceftazidime, ceftriaxone, cefuroxime, chloramphenicol, clindamycin, dantrolene, dexamethasone sodium phosphate, diazepam, digoxin, doxacurium, enalaprilat, ephedrine, ertapenem, fluorouracil, foscarnet, fosphenytoin, furosemide, heparin, ketorolac, lidocaine, methotrexate, methylprednisolone sodium succinate, nafcillin, nitroprusside, pamidronate, pancuronium, pemetrexed, pentobarbital, phenobarbital, phenytoin, piperacillin/tazobactam, potassium phosphates, ranitidine, sodium acetate, sodium bicarbonate, sodium phosphates, trimethoprim/sulfamethoxazole.
- **Solution Incompatibility:** Solutions containing dextrose.

Patient/Family Teaching

- Explain the purpose of caspofungin to patient and family.
- Advise patient to notify health care professional immediately if symptoms of allergic reactions (rash, facial swelling, pruritus, sensation of warmth, difficulty breathing) occur.

Evaluation/Desired Outcomes

- Decrease in signs and symptoms of fungal infections. Duration of therapy is determined based on severity of underlying disease, recovery from immunosuppression, and clinical response.

cefaclor, See CEPHALOSPORINS—SECOND GENERATION.

cefadroxil, See CEPHALOSPORINS—FIRST GENERATION.

ceFAZolin, See CEPHALOSPORINS—FIRST GENERATION.

cefdinir, See CEPHALOSPORINS—THIRD GENERATION.

cefditoren, See CEPHALOSPORINS—THIRD GENERATION.

cefepime (seff-e-peem)

Maxipime

Classification

Therapeutic: anti-infectives

Pharmacologic: fourth-generation cephalosporins

Pregnancy Category B

Indications

Treatment of the following infections caused by susceptible organisms: Uncomplicated skin and skin structure infections, Bone and joint infections, Uncomplicated and complicated urinary tract infections, Respiratory tract infections, Complicated intra-abdominal infections (with metronidazole), Septicemia. Empiric treatment of febrile neutropenic patients.

Action

Binds to the bacterial cell wall membrane, causing cell death. **Therapeutic Effects:** Bactericidal action against susceptible bacteria. **Spectrum:** Similar to that of second- and third-generation cephalosporins, but activity against staphylococci is less, whereas activity against gram-negative pathogens is greater, even for organisms resistant to first-, second-, and third-generation agents. Notable is increased action against: *Enterobacter*, *Haemophilus influenzae* (including β-lactamase-producing strains), *Escherichia coli*, *Klebsiella pneumoniae*, *Neisseria*, *Proteus*, *Providencia*, *Pseudomonas aeruginosa*, *Serratia*, *Moraxella catarrhalis*(including β-lactamase-producing strains). Not active against methicillin-resistant staphylococci or enterococci.

Pharmacokinetics

Absorption: Well absorbed after IM administration; IV administration results in complete bioavailability.

Distribution: Widely distributed. Crosses the placenta; enters breast milk in low concentrations. Some CSF penetration.
Protein Binding: 20%.
Metabolism and Excretion: 85% excreted unchanged in urine.
Half-life: *Adults*–2 hr (↑ in renal impairment); *Children 2 mo–6 yr*—1.7–1.9 hr.

TIME/ACTION PROFILE

ROUTE	ONSET	PEAK	DURATION
IM	rapid	1–2 hr	12 hr
IV	rapid	end of infusion	12 hr

Contraindications/Precautions
Contraindicated in: Hypersensitivity to cephalosporins; Serious hypersensitivity to penicillins.
Use Cautiously in: Renal impairment (↓ dosing/↑ dosing interval recommended if CCr ≤60 mL/min); History of GI disease, especially colitis; Patients with hepatic dysfunction or poor nutritional status (may be at ↑ risk of bleeding); Geriatric patients (dose adjustment due to age-related ↓ in renal function may be necessary); OB, Lactation: Pregnancy and lactation (safety not established).

Adverse Reactions/Side Effects
CNS: SEIZURES (↑ risk in renal impairment), encephalopathy, headache. **GI:** CLOSTRIDIUM DIFFICILE-ASSOCIATED DIARRHEA (CDAD), diarrhea, nausea, vomiting. **Derm:** rashes, pruritis, urticaria. **Hemat:** bleeding, eosinophilia, hemolytic anemia, neutropenia, thrombocytopenia. **Local:** pain at IM site, phlebitis at IV site. **Misc:** allergic reactions including ANAPHYLAXIS, superinfection, fever.

Interactions
Drug-Drug: Probenecid ↓ excretion and ↑ blood levels. Concurrent use of **loop diuretics** or **aminoglycosides** may ↑ risk of nephrotoxicity.

Route/Dosage
IM (Adults): *Mild-to-moderate uncomplicated or complicated urinary tract infections due to Escherichia coli*—0.5–1 g every 12 hr.
IV (Adults): *Moderate-to-severe pneumonia*—1–2 g every 12 hr. *Mild-to-moderate uncomplicated or complicated urinary tract infections*—0.5–1 g every 12 hr. *Severe uncomplicated or complicated urinary tract infections, moderate-to-severe uncomplicated skin and skin structure infections, complicated intra-abdominal infections*—2 g every 12 hr. *Empiric treatment of febrile neutropenia*—2 g every 8 hr.
IV (Children 1 mo–16 yr): *Uncomplicated and complicated urinary tract infections, uncomplicated skin and skin structure infections, pneumonia*—50 mg/kg every 12 hr (not to exceed 2 g/dose). *Febrile neutropenia*—50 mg/kg every 8 hr (not to exceed 2 g/dose).
IV (Neonates postnatal age ≥14 days): 50 mg/kg every 12 hr.
IV (Neonates postnatal age <14 days): 30 mg/kg every 12 hr; consider 50 mg/kg every 12 hr for *Pseudomonas* infections.

Renal Impairment
IM, IV (Adults): (See Manufacturer's specific recommendations) *CCr 30–60 mL/min*—0.5–1 g every 24 hr or 2 g every 12–24 hr; *CCr 11–29 mL/min*—0.5–2 g every 24 hr; *CCr <11 mL/min*—250 mg–1 g every 24 hr.

Availability (generic available)
Powder for injection: 500 mg, 1 g, 2 g. **Premixed containers:** 1 g/50 mL D5W, 2 g/100 mL D5W.

NURSING IMPLICATIONS
Assessment
- Assess patient for infection (vital signs; appearance of wound, sputum, urine, and stool; WBC) at beginning of and throughout therapy.
- Before initiating therapy, obtain a history to determine previous use of and reactions to penicillins or cephalosporins. Persons with a negative history of penicillin sensitivity may still have an allergic response.
- Obtain specimens for culture and sensitivity before initiating therapy. First dose may be given before receiving results.
- Observe patient for signs and symptoms of anaphylaxis (rash, pruritus, laryngeal edema, wheezing). Discontinue the drug and notify health care professional immediately if these symptoms occur. Keep epinephrine, an antihistamine, and resuscitation equipment close by in the event of an anaphylactic reaction.
- Monitor bowel function. Diarrhea, abdominal cramping, fever, and bloody stools should be reported to health care professional promptly as a sign of Clostridium difficile-associated diarrhea (CDAD). May begin up to several weeks following cessation of therapy.
- ***Lab Test Considerations:*** May cause positive results for Coombs' test in patients receiving high doses or in neonates whose mothers were given cephalosporins before delivery.
- May cause ↑ serum AST, ALT, bilirubin, BUN, and creatinine.
- May rarely cause leukopenia, neutropenia, thrombocytopenia, and eosinophilia.

Potential Nursing Diagnoses

Risk for infection (Indications, Side Effects)
Diarrhea (Adverse Reactions)
Deficient knowledge, related to medication regimen (Patient/Family Teaching)

Implementation

- **IM:** Reconstitute IM doses with sterile or bacteriostatic water for injection, 0.9% NaCl, or D5W. May be diluted with lidocaine to minimize injection discomfort.
- Inject deep into a well-developed muscle mass; massage well.
- IM route should only be used for treatment of mild-to-moderate uncomplicated or complicated urinary tract infections due to *Escherichia coli*.

IV Administration

- **IV:** Monitor injection site frequently for phlebitis (pain, redness, swelling). Change sites every 48–72 hr to prevent phlebitis.
- If aminoglycosides are administered concurrently, administer in separate sites, if possible, at least 1 hr apart. If second site is unavailable, flush lines between medications.
- **Intermittent Infusion:** Reconstitute with 5 mL sterile water, 0.9% NaCl, or D5W for the 500-mg vial, or 10 mL for the 1-g or 2-g vials. ***Diluent:*** Dilute further in 50–100 mL of D5W, 0.9% NaCl, D10W, D5/0.9% NaCl, or D5/LR. ***Concentration:*** Maximum 40 mg/mL.
- Solution is stable for 24 hr at room temperature and 7 days if refrigerated. ***Rate:*** Administer over 20–30 min.
- **Y-Site Compatibility:** amikacin, amphotericin B lipid complex, ampicillin-sulbactam, anidulafungin, azithromycin, aztreonam, bivalirudin, bleomycin, bumetanide, buprenorphine, butorphanol, calcium gluconate, carboplatin, carmustine, cyclophosphamide, cytarabine, dactinomycin, daptomycin, dexamethasone sodium phosphate, dexmedetomidine, docetaxel, doxacurium, doxorubicin liposome, eptifibatide, fenoldopam, fluconazole, fludarabine, fluorouracil, foscarnet, furosemide, gentamicin, granisetron, hetastarch, hydrocortisone sodium phosphate, hydrocortisone sodium succinate, hydromorphone, imipenem-cilastatin, insulin, ketamine, leucovorin, levofloxacin, linezolid, lorazepam, melphalan, mesna, methotrexate, methylprednisolone sodium succinate, metronidazole, milrinone, octreotide, oxytocin, paclitaxel, palonosetron, pamidronate, pancuronium, piperacillin-tazobactam, potassium acetate, ranitidine, remifentanil, rocuronium, sargramostim, sodium acetate, sodium bicarbonate, sufentanil, telavancin, thiotepa, ticarcillin-clavulanate, tigecycline, tirofiban, tobramycin, trimethoprim/sulfamethoxazole, vasopressin, zidovudine, zoledronic acid.
- **Y-Site Incompatibility:** acetylcysteine, acyclovir, alemtuzumab, amphotericin B cholesteryl, amphotericin B colloidal, amphotericin B liposome, argatroban, caspofungin, chlorpromazine, ciprofloxacin, cisplatin, dacarbazine, daunorubicin, dexrazoxane, diazepam, diltiazem, diphenhydramine, dolasetron, doxorubicin hydrochloride, droperidol, enalaprilat, epirubicin, erythromycin, etoposide, etoposide phosphate, famotidine, filgrastim, floxuridine, ganciclovir, gemcitabine, haloperidol, hydroxyzine, idarubicin, ifosfamide, irinotecan, magnesium sulfate, mannitol, mechlorethamine, meperidine, metoclopramide, midazolam, mitomycin, mitoxantrone, nalbuphine, nesiritide, ondansetron, oxaliplatin, pantoprazole, pemetrexed, phenytoin, prochlorperazine, promethazine, quinupristin/dalfopristin, streptozocin, tacrolimus, theophylline, vecuronium, vinblastine, vincristine, vinorelbine, voriconazole.

Patient/Family Teaching

- Advise patient to report signs of superinfection (furry overgrowth on the tongue, vaginal itching or discharge, loose or foul-smelling stools) and allergy.
- Instruct patient to notify health care professional if fever and diarrhea develop, especially if stool contains blood, pus, or mucus. Advise patient not to treat diarrhea without consulting health care professional.

Evaluation/Desired Outcomes

- Resolution of the signs and symptoms of infection. Length of time for complete resolution depends on the organism and site of infection.

---

cefixime, See CEPHALOSPORINS—THIRD GENERATION.

---

cefoperazone, See CEPHALOSPORINS—THIRD GENERATION.

---

cefotaxime, See CEPHALOSPORINS—THIRD GENERATION.

---

cefoTEtan, See CEPHALOSPORINS—SECOND GENERATION.

---

cefOXitin, See CEPHALOSPORINS—SECOND GENERATION.

---

cefpodoxime, See CEPHALOSPORINS—THIRD GENERATION.

cefprozil, See CEPHALOSPORINS—SECOND GENERATION.

ceftaroline (sef-tar-oh-leen)

Teflaro

Classification

Therapeutic: anti-infectives

Pharmacologic: cephalosporin derivatives

Pregnancy Category B

Indications

Treatment of acute bacterial skin/skin structure infections and community-acquired pneumonia.

Action

Binds to bacterial cell wall membrane, causing cell death. **Therapeutic Effects:** Bactericidal action against susceptible bacteria. **Spectrum:** *Treatment of skin/skin structure infections*—Active against *Staphylococcus aureus* (including methicillin-susceptible and -resistant strains), *Streptococcus pyogenes, Streptococcus agalactiae, Escherichia coli, Klebsiella pneumoniae*, and *Klebsiella oxytoca*; *Treatment of community acquired pneumonia—Streptococcus pneumoniae* (including pneumonia with bacteremia), *Staphylococcus aureus* (methicillin-susceptible strains only), *Haemophilus influenzae, Klebsiella pneumoniae, Klebsiella oxytoca*, and *Escherichia coli.*

Pharmacokinetics

Absorption: IV administration results in complete bioavailability of parent drug.

Distribution: Unknown.

Metabolism and Excretion: Ceftaroline fosamil is rapidly converted by plasma phosphatases to ceftaroline, the active metabolite; 88% excreted in urine, 6% in feces.

Half-life: 2.6 hr (after multiple doses).

TIME/ACTION PROFILE (blood levels)

ROUTE	ONSET	PEAK	DURATION
IV	rapid	end of infusion	12 hr

Contraindications/Precautions

Contraindicated in: Known serious hypersensitivity to cephalosporins.

Use Cautiously in: Known hypersensitivity to other beta-lactams; Renal impairment (dosage ↓ required for CCr ≤50 mL/min); Geri: Dose adjustment may be necessary for age-related ↓ in renal function; OB: Use only if potential benefit outweighs potential risk to fetus; Lactation: Use cautiously if breast feeding; Pedi: Safety and effectiveness not established.

Adverse Reactions/Side Effects

GI: CLOSTRIDIUM DIFFICILE-ASSOCIATED DIARRHEA (CDAD), diarrhea, nausea. **Derm:** rash. **Hemat:** hemolytic anemia. **Local:** phlebitis at injection site. **Misc:** hypersensitivity reactions including ANAPHYLAXIS.

Interactions

Drug-Drug: None noted.

Route/Dosage

IV (Adults 18 yr): *Skin/skin structure infections*—600 mg every 12 hr for 5–14 days; *Community-acquired pneumonia*—600 mg every 12 hr for 5–7 days.

Renal Impairment

IV (Adults >18 yr): *CCr >30 to ≤50 mL/min*—400 mg every 12 hr; *CCr ≥15 to ≤30 mL/min*—300 mg every 12 hr; *CCr <15 mL/min*—200 mg every 12 hr.

Availability

Powder for injection (requires reconstitution): 400 mg/vial, 600 mg/vial.

NURSING IMPLICATIONS

Assessment

- Assess for infection (vital signs; appearance of wound, sputum, urine, and stool; WBC) at beginning of and throughout therapy.
- Before initiating therapy, obtain a history to determine previous use of and reactions to penicillins, cephalosporins, or carbapenems. Persons with a negative history of sensitivity may still have an allergic response.
- Obtain specimens for culture and sensitivity before initiating therapy. First dose may be given before receiving results.
- Observe patient for signs and symptoms of anaphylaxis (rash, pruritus, laryngeal edema, wheezing). Discontinue the drug and notify health care professional immediately if these symptoms occur. Keep epinephrine, an antihistamine, and resuscitation equipment close by in the event of an anaphylactic reaction.
- Monitor bowel function. Diarrhea, abdominal cramping, fever, and bloody stools should be reported to health care professional promptly as a sign of Clostridium difficile-associated diarrhea (CDAD). May begin up to several mo following cessation of therapy.
- ***Lab Test Considerations:*** May cause seroconversion from a negative to a positive direct Coombs' test. If anemia develops during or after therapy, perform a direct Coombs' test. If drug-induced hemolytic anemia is suspected, discontinue ceftaroline and provide supportive care.

Potential Nursing Diagnoses

Risk for infection (Indications, Side Effects)
Diarrhea (Adverse Reactions)

Implementation

IV Administration

- **Intermittent Infusion:** Reconstitute with 20 mL of sterile water for injection, 0.9% NaCl, D5W, or LR. ***Diluent:*** Dilute further with 50–250 mL of same diluent unless reconstituted with Sterile Water for Injection, then use 0.9% NaCl, D5W, D2.5W, 0.45% NaCl, or LR. Mix gently to dissolve. Solution is clear to light or dark yellow; do not administer solutions that are discolored or contain particulate matter. Solution is stable for 6 hr at room temperature or 24 hr if refrigerated. ***Rate:*** Infuse over 5–60 min.
- **Y-Site Compatibility:** acyclovir, aminophylline, amiodarone, azithromycin, bumetanide, calcium chloride, calcium gluconate, ciprofloxacin, cisatracurium, clindamycin, cyclosporine, dexamethasone, digoxin, diltiazem, diphenhydramine, dopamine, doripenem, enalaprilat, esomeprazole, famotidine, fentanyl, fluconazole, furosemide, granisetron, haloperidol, heparin, hydrocortisone, hydromorphone, insulin, insulin lispro, levofloxacin, lidocaine, lorazepam, mannitol, meperidine, methylprednisolone, metoclopramide, metoprolol, metronidazole, midazolam, milrinone, morphine, moxifloxacin, multivitamins, norepinephrine, ondansetron, pantoprazole, potassium chloride, promethazine, propofol, ranitidine, remifentanil, sodium bicarbonate, trimethoprim/sulfamethoxazole, vasopressin, voriconazole.
- **Y-Site Incompatibility:** amphotericin B colloidal, caspofungin, diazepam, filgrastim, labetalol, potassium phosphates, sodium phosphates.

Patient/Family Teaching

- Explain the purpose of ceftaroline to patient. Emphasize the importance of completing therapy, even if feeling better.
- Instruct patient to notify health care professional if fever and diarrhea develop, especially if stool contains blood, pus, or mucus. Advise patient not to treat diarrhea without consulting health care professional.

Evaluation/Desired Outcomes

- Resolution of the signs and symptoms of infection. Length of time for complete resolution depends on the organism and site of infection.

cefTAZidime, See CEPHALOSPORINS—THIRD GENERATION.

ceftazidime/avibactam

(sef-**tay**-zi-deem / tay-zoe-**bak**-tam)
Avycaz

Classification
Therapeutic: anti-infectives
Pharmacologic: third-generation cephalosporins, beta lactamase inhibitors

Pregnancy Category B

Indications

With metronidazole in the treatment of complicated Intra-abdominal Infections (cIaIs). Treatment of complicated Urinary Tract Infections (cUTIs).

Action

Ceftazidime—Binds to the bacterial cell wall membrane, causing cell death. *Avibactam*—Inhibits beta-lactamase, an enzyme that destroys penicillins and cephosporins. **Therapeutic Effects:** Death of susceptible bacteria with resolution of infection. **Spectrum:** Active against *Escherichia coli, Klebsiella pneumoniae, Proteus mirabilis, Providencia stuartii, Enterobacter cloacae, Klebsiella oxytoca, Pseudomonas aeruginosa, Citrobacter koserii, Enterobacter aerogenes, Citrobacter freundii* and *Proteus* spp.

Pharmacokinetics

Absorption: IV administration results in complete bioavailability.
Distribution: *Ceftazidime*—Widely distributed, enters breast milk in low concentrations; *avibactam—widely distributed.*
Metabolism and Excretion: *ceftazidime*—minimally metabolized, 80–90% excreted unchanged in urine; *avibactam*—minimally metabolized, mainly excreted unchanged in urine.
Half-life: *Ceftazidime*—2.8–3.3hr (↑ in renal impairment); *avibactam*—2.2–2.7 hr.

TIME/ACTION PROFILE (blood levels)

ROUTE	ONSET	PEAK	DURATION
IV	rapid	end of infusion	8 hr (↑ in renal impairment)

Contraindications/Precautions

Contraindicated in: Known hypersensitivity to ceftazidime, other cephalosporins or avibactam-containing products; cross-sensitivity with other penicillins, carbapenems and cephalosporins may occur.
Use Cautiously in: CCr 30–50 mL/min (efficacy may be ↓, monitor renal function frequently and adjust dose if necessary); Geri: Consider age-related impairment of renal function; OB: Use during pregnancy only if clearly needed; Lactation: Use cautiously in breast-

feeding women; Pedi: Safe and effective use in children < 18 yr has not been established.

Adverse Reactions/Side Effects

CNS: SEIZURES (↑ in renal impairment), anxiety. **GI:** CLOSTRIDIUM DIFFICILE-ASSOCIATED DIARRHEA (CDAD), nausea, vomiting. **F and E:** hypokalemia. **Hemat:** eosinophilia, thrombocytopenia. **Misc:** hypersensitivity reactions including ANAPHYLAXIS and SERIOUS SKIN REACTIONS.

Interactions

Drug-Drug: Probenecid may ↓ renal excretion of avibactam; concurrent administration is not recommended;.

Route/Dosage

IV (Adults CCr >50 mL/min): 2.5 g (2 g ceftazidime/ 0.5 g avibactam) every 8 hr.

Renal Impairment

(Adults): *CCr 31–50 mL/min*—1.25 g (1 g ceftazidime/ 0.25 g avibactam) every 8 hr; *CCr 16–30 mL/ min*—0.94 g (0.75 g ceftazidime/0.19 g avibactam) every 12hr; *CCr 6–15 mL/min*—0.94 g (0.75 g ceftazidime/0.19 g avibactam) every 24 hr; *CCr 6–15 mL/ min*—0.94 g (0.75 g ceftazidime/0.19 g avibactam) every 48 hr: *hemodialysis*—Administer dose after or on day of hemodialysis.

Availability

Powder for IV injection (requires reconstitution): ceftazidime 2 g/avibactam 0.5 g in single-use vials.

NURSING IMPLICATIONS

Assessment

- Assess for infection (vital signs; appearance of wound, sputum, urine, and stool; WBC) at beginning of and throughout therapy.
- Before initiating therapy, obtain a history to determine previous use of and reactions to penicillins, cephalosporins or carbapenems. Persons with a negative history of sensitivity may still have an allergic response.
- Obtain specimens for culture and sensitivity before initiating therapy. First dose may be given before receiving results.
- Observe patient for signs and symptoms of anaphylaxis (rash, pruritus, laryngeal edema, wheezing). Discontinue the drug and notify health care professional immediately if these symptoms occur. Keep epinephrine, an antihistamine, and resuscitation equipment close by in the event of an anaphylactic reaction.
- Monitor bowel function. Diarrhea, abdominal cramping, fever, and bloody stools should be reported to health care professional promptly as a sign of Clostridium difficle associated diarrhea. May begin up to several months following cessation of therapy.
- Monitor for signs and symptoms of encephalopathy (disturbance of consciousness including confusion, hallucinations, stupor, coma), myoclonus, and seizures during and following therapy. May require immediate treatment, dose adjustment, or discontinuation of therapy.
- ***Lab Test Considerations:*** May cause seroconversion from a negative to a positive direct Coombs' test. If anemia develops during or after therapy, perform a direct Coombs' test.
- May cause a false-positive reaction for glucose in urine with certain methods; use enzymatic glucose oxidase reactions.

Potential Nursing Diagnoses

Risk for infection (Indications)
Diarrhea (Adverse Reactions)

Implementation

- Reconstitute with 10 mL of Sterile Water for injection. 0.9% NaCl, D5W, D5/0.9% NaCl, D5/0.45% NaCl, D2.5/0.9% NaCl, D2.5/0.45% NaCl, or LR. Mix gently. ***Diluent:*** Use same diluent used for reconstitution for a volume between 50 mL and 250 mL. ***Concentration:*** 40 and 10 mg/mL of ceftazidime and avibactam, respectively to 8 and 2 mg/mL of ceftazidime and avibactam, respectively.Solution ranges from clear to light yellow; do not administer solutions that are discolored or contain particulate matter. Solution is stable for 12 hrs at room temperature or 24 hrs if refrigerated. ***Rate:*** Infuse over 2 hrs.

Patient/Family Teaching

- Explain the purpose of ceftazidime/avibactam to patient.
- Instruct patient to notify health care professional if fever and diarrhea develop, especially if stool contains blood, pus, or mucus. Advise patient not to treat diarrhea without consulting health care professional.
- Advise patient to notify health care professional immediately if signs and symptoms of allergic reactions or nervous system reactions occur.
- Advise female patient to notify health care professional if pregnancy is planned or suspected or if breast feeding.

Evaluation/Desired Outcomes

- Resolution of the signs and symptoms of infection. Length of time for complete resolution depends on the organism and site of infection.

ceftibuten, See CEPHALOSPORINS—THIRD GENERATION.

ceftolozane/tazobactam
(sef-**tol**-o-zane/taz-oh-**bak**-tam)
Zerbaxa

Classification
Therapeutic: anti-infectives
Pharmacologic: cephalosporin derivatives, beta lactamase inhibitors

Pregnancy Category B

Indications
Treatment of complicated intra-abdominal infections (with metronidazole) and complicated urinary tract infections (including pyelonephritis).

Action
Ceftolozane: binds to bacterial cell wall membrane, causing cell death. Spectrum is extended compared with other penicillins. Tazobactam: Inhibits beta-lactamase, an enzyme that can destroy penicillins. **Therapeutic Effects:** Death of susceptible bacteria. **Spectrum:** Active against *Enterobacter cloacae*, *Escherichia coli*, *Klebsiella oxytoca*, *Klebsiella pneumniae*, *Proteus mirabilis*, *Pseudomonas aeruginosa*, *Bacteroides fragilis*, *Streptococcus anginosus*, *Streptococcus constellatus*, and *Streptococcus salivarius*.

Pharmacokinetics
Absorption: IV administration results in complete bioavailability.
Distribution: Unknown.
Metabolism and Excretion: *Ceftolozane*—minimal metabolism, excreted almost entirely (>95%) unchanged in urine; *tazobactam*—80% excreted unchanged in urine, some metablized to an inactive M1 metabolite which is excreted unchanged in urine.
Half-life: *Ceftolozane*—2.8 hr; *tazobactam*—0.9 hr.

TIME/ACTION PROFILE

ROUTE	ONSET	PEAK	DURATION
IV	rapid	end of infusion	8 hr

Contraindications/Precautions
Contraindicated in: Known serious hypersensitivity to ceftolozane/tazbactam, piperacillin/tazobactam or other beta-lactams.
Use Cautiously in: CCr 30–<50 mL/min (effectiveness may be ↓, adjust dose if necessary); CCr <50 mL/min (dose adjustment recommended); OB: Use during pregnancy only if potential benefit outweighs potential risks; Lactation: Use cautiously if breast feeding; Pedi: Safe and effective use in children has not been established.

Adverse Reactions/Side Effects
CNS: anxiety, dizziness, headache, insomnia. **CV:** atrial fibrillation, hypotension. **GI:** abdominal pain, constipation, diarrhea, CLOSTRIDIUM DIFFICILE-ASSOCIATED DIARRHEA (CDAD), nausea, vomiting. **Derm:** rash. **F and E:** hypokalemia. **Hemat:** anemia, thrombocytosis. **Misc:** hypersensitivity reactions including ANAPHYLAXIS.

Interactions
Drug-Drug: None noted.

Route/Dosage
IV (Adults): 1.5 g (1 g ceftolozane/0.5 g tazobactam) every 8 hr for 4–14 days for intra-abdominal infections or 7 days for urinary tract infections.

Renal Impairment
(Adults): *CCr 30–50 mL/min*—750 mg (500 mg ceftolozane/250 mg tazobactam) every 8 hr; *CCr 15–29 mL/min*—375 mg (250 mg ceftolozane/125 mg tazobactam) every 8 hr; *End-stage renal disease on hemodialysis*—Single loading dose of 750 mg (500 mg ceftolozane/250 mg tazobactam), then 150 mg (100 mg ceftolozane/50 mg tazobactam every 8 hr (on dialysis days administer as soon as possible after dialysis).

Availability
Powder for intravenous injection (requires reconstitution): 1 g ceftolozane/0.5 g tazobactam per vial.

NURSING IMPLICATIONS

Assessment
- Assess for infection (vital signs; appearance of wound, sputum, urine, and stool; WBC) at beginning of and throughout therapy.
- Before initiating therapy, obtain a history to determine previous use of and reactions to penicillins, cephalosporins, or other beta-lactams. Persons with a negative history of sensitivity may still have an allergic response.
- Obtain specimens for culture and sensitivity before initiating therapy. First dose may be given before receiving results.
- Observe patient for signs and symptoms of anaphylaxis (rash, pruritus, laryngeal edema, wheezing). Discontinue the drug and notify health care professional immediately if these symptoms occur. Keep epinephrine, an antihistamine, and resuscitation equipment close by in the event of an anaphylactic reaction.
- Monitor bowel function. Diarrhea, abdominal cramping, fever, and bloody stools should be reported to health care professional promptly as a sign of (CDAD). May begin up to several mo following cessation of therapy.

- ***Lab Test Considerations:*** Monitor creatinine clearance at least daily in patients with changing renal function and adjust dose accordingly.

Potential Nursing Diagnoses

Risk for infection (Indications, Side Effects)
Diarrhea (Adverse Reactions)

Implementation

IV Administration

- **Intermittent Infusion:** Reconstitute with 10 mL of sterile water for injection or 0.9% NaCl for injection; shake gently to dissolve for final volume of 11.4 mL. ***Diluent:*** Withdraw 11.4 mL for 1.5 g (1.0 g/0.5 g dose, 5.7 mL for 750 mg (500 mg/250 mg) dose, 2.9 mL for 375 mg (250 mg/125 mg) dose, or 1.2 mL for 150 mg (100 mg/50 mg) dose and add to 100 mL of 0.9% NaCl or D5W. Solution is clear, colorless to slightly yellow; do not administer solutions that are discolored or contain particulate matter. Solution is stable for 24 hr at room temperature or 7 days if refrigerated; do not freeze. ***Rate:*** Infuse over 1 hr.
- **Additive Incompatibility:** Do not mix with other drugs or solutions.

Patient/Family Teaching

- Explain the purpose of ceftolzane/tazobactam to patient.
- Instruct patient to notify health care professional if fever and diarrhea develop, especially if stool contains blood, pus, or mucus. Advise patient not to treat diarrhea without consulting health care professional.
- Advise female patient to notify health care professional if pregnancy is planned or suspected or if breast feeding.

Evaluation/Desired Outcomes

- Resolution of the signs and symptoms of infection. Length of time for complete resolution depends on the organism and site of infection.

cefTRIAXone, See CEPHALOSPORINS—THIRD GENERATION.

cefuroxime, See CEPHALOSPORINS—SECOND GENERATION.

ᛝ celecoxib (sel-e-**kox**-ib)

CeleBREX

Classification
Therapeutic: antirheumatics, nonsteroidal anti-inflammatory agents
Pharmacologic: COX-2 inhibitors

Pregnancy Category C

Indications

Relief of signs and symptoms of osteoarthritis, rheumatoid arthritis, ankylosing spondylitis, and juvenile rheumatoid arthritis. Management of acute pain including primary dysmenorrhea.

Action

Inhibits the enzyme COX-2. This enzyme is required for the synthesis of prostaglandins. Has analgesic, anti-inflammatory, and antipyretic properties. **Therapeutic Effects:** Decreased pain and inflammation caused by arthritis or spondylitis. Decreased pain.

Pharmacokinetics

Absorption: Bioavailability unknown.
Distribution: 97% bound to plasma proteins; extensive tissue distribution.
Metabolism and Excretion: Mostly metabolized by the hepatic CYP2C9 isoenzyme; ᛝ the CYP2C9 enzyme system exhibits genetic polymorphism; poor metabolizers may have significantly ↑ celecoxib concentrations and an ↑ risk of adverse effects; <3% excreted unchanged in urine and feces.
Half-life: 11 hr.

TIME/ACTION PROFILE (pain reduction)

ROUTE	ONSET	PEAK	DURATION
PO	24–48 hr	unknown	12–24 hr†

†After discontinuation.

Contraindications/Precautions

Contraindicated in: Hypersensitivity; Cross-sensitivity may exist with other NSAIDs, including aspirin; History of allergic-type reactions to sulfonamides; History of asthma, urticaria, or allergic-type reactions to aspirin or other NSAIDs, including the aspirin triad (asthma, nasal polyps, and severe hypersensitivity reactions to aspirin); Advanced renal disease; Severe hepatic dysfunction; Peri-operative pain from coronary artery bypass graft (CABG) surgery; OB: Should not be used in late pregnancy (may cause premature closure of the ductus arteriosus).
Use Cautiously in: Cardiovascular disease or risk factors for cardiovascular disease (may ↑ risk of serious cardiovascular thrombotic events, myocardial infarction, and stroke, especially with prolonged use or

use of higher doses); Pre-existing renal disease, heart failure, liver dysfunction, concurrent diuretic, or ACE inhibitor therapy (↑ risk of renal impairment); Hypertension or fluid retention; Renal insufficiency (may precipitate acute renal failure); Serious dehydration (correct deficits before administering); Patients who are known or suspected to be poor CYP2C9 metabolizers (↓ initial dose by 50%); Pre-existing asthma; Pedi: Safety not established in children <2 yr or for longer than 6 mo; Geri: Concurrent therapy with corticosteroids or anticoagulants, long duration of NSAID therapy, history of smoking, alcoholism, geriatric patients, or poor general health status (↑ risk of GI bleeding); Lactation: Lactation.

Exercise Extreme Caution in: History of ulcer disease or GI bleeding.

Adverse Reactions/Side Effects

CNS: dizziness, headache, insomnia. **CV:** HF, MYOCARDIAL INFARCTION, STROKE, THROMBOSIS, edema, hypertension. **GI:** GI BLEEDING, abdominal pain, diarrhea, dyspepsia, flatulence, nausea. **Derm:** EXFOLIATIVE DERMATITIS, STEVENS-JOHNSON SYNDROME, TOXIC EPIDERMAL NECROLYSIS, rash.

Interactions

Drug-Drug: CYP2C9 inhibitors may ↑ levels. May ↓ effectiveness of **ACE inhibitors**, **thiazide diuretics**, and **furosemide**. **Fluconazole** ↑ levels (use lowest recommended dosage). May ↑ risk of bleeding with **warfarin** and **aspirin**. May ↑ serum **lithium** levels. Does not inhibit the cardioprotective effect of low-dose **aspirin**.

Route/Dosage

PO (Adults): *Osteoarthritis*—200 mg once daily *or* 100 mg twice daily. *Rheumatoid arthritis*—100–200 mg twice daily. *Ankylosing spondylitis*—200 mg once daily *or* 100 mg twice daily; dose may be ↑ after 6 wk to 400 mg daily. *Acute pain, including dysmenorrhea*—400 mg initially, then a 200-mg dose if needed on the first day; then 200 mg twice daily as needed.

Hepatic Impairment

PO (Adults): *Moderate hepatic impairment (Child-Pugh Class B)*—↓ dose by 50%.

PO (Children ≥2 yr, ≥10 kg–≤25 kg): *Juvenile rheumatoid arthritis*—50 mg twice daily.

PO (Children ≥2 yr, ≥25 kg): *Juvenile rheumatoid arthritis*—100 mg twice daily.

Availability (generic available)

Capsules: 50 mg, 100 mg, 200 mg, 400 mg. **Cost:** 100 mg $387.18/100, 200 mg $621.67/100, 400 mg $1,576.25/180.

NURSING IMPLICATIONS

Assessment

- Assess range of motion, degree of swelling, and pain in affected joints before and periodically throughout therapy.
- Assess patient for allergy to sulfonamides, aspirin, or NSAIDs. Patients with these allergies should not receive celecoxib.
- Assess patient for skin rash frequently during therapy. Discontinue at first sign of rash; may be life-threatening. Stevens-Johnson syndrome may develop. Treat symptomatically; may recur once treatment is stopped.
- ***Lab Test Considerations:*** May cause ↑ AST and ALT levels.
- May cause hypophosphatemia and ↑ BUN.

Potential Nursing Diagnoses

Impaired physical mobility (Indications)
Acute pain (Indications)

Implementation

- Do not confuse with Celexa (citalopram) or Cerebyx (fosphenytoin).
- **PO:** May be administered without regard to meals. Capsules may be opened and sprinkled on applesauce and ingested immediately with water. Mixture may be stored in the refrigerator for up to 6 hr.

Patient/Family Teaching

- Instruct patient to take celecoxib exactly as directed. Do not take more than prescribed dose. Increasing doses does not appear to increase effectiveness. Use lowest effective dose for shortest period of time.
- Advise patient to notify health care professional promptly if signs or symptoms of GI toxicity (abdominal pain, black stools), skin rash, unexplained weight gain, edema, or chest pain occurs. Patients should discontinue celecoxib and notify health care professional if signs and symptoms of hepatotoxicity (nausea, fatigue, lethargy, pruritus, jaundice, upper right quadrant tenderness, flu-like symptoms) occur.
- Advise patient to notify health care professional if pregnancy is planned or suspected.

Evaluation/Desired Outcomes

- Reduction in joint pain in patients with osteoarthritis.
- Reduction in joint tenderness, pain, and joint swelling in patients with rheumatoid arthritis and juvenile rheumatoid arthritis.
- Decreased pain.
- Decreased pain with dysmenorrhea.

cephalexin, See CEPHALOSPORINS—FIRST GENERATION.

CEPHALOSPORINS—FIRST GENERATION

cefadroxil (sef-a-**drox**-ill)
~~Duricef~~

ceFAZolin (sef-**a**-zoe-lin)
~~Ancef~~

cephalexin (sef-a-**lex**-in)
Keflex

Classification
Therapeutic: anti-infectives
Pharmacologic: first-generation cephalosporins

Pregnancy Category B

Indications
Treatment of the following infections caused by susceptible organisms: Skin and skin structure infections (including burn wounds), Pneumonia, Urinary tract infections, Bone and joint infections, Septicemia. Not suitable for the treatment of meningitis. **Cefadroxil:** Pharyngitis and/or tonsillitis. **Cefazolin:** Perioperative prophylaxis, biliary tract infections, genital infections, bacterial endocarditis prophylaxis for dental and upper respiratory tract procedures. **Cephalexin:** Otitis media.

Action
Bind to bacterial cell wall membrane, causing cell death. **Therapeutic Effects:** Bactericidal action against susceptible bacteria. **Spectrum:** Active against many gram-positive cocci including: *Streptococcus pneumoniae*, Group A beta-hemolytic streptococci, Penicillinase-producing staphylococci. Not active against: Methicillin-resistant staphylococci, *Bacteroides fragilis*, *Enterococcus*. Active against some gram-negative rods including: *Klebsiella pneumoniae*, *Proteus mirabilis*, *Escherichia coli*.

Pharmacokinetics
Absorption: *Cefadroxil* and *cephalexin* are well absorbed following oral administration. *Cefazolin* is well absorbed following IM administration.
Distribution: Widely distributed. Cefazolin penetrates bone and synovial fluid well. All cross the placenta and enter breast milk in low concentrations. Minimal CSF penetration.
Metabolism and Excretion: Excreted almost entirely unchanged by the kidneys.
Half-life: *Cefadroxil*—60–120 min; *cefazolin*—90–150 min; *cephalexin*—50–80 min (all are ↑ in renal impairment).

TIME/ACTION PROFILE (blood levels)

ROUTE	ONSET	PEAK	DURATION
Cefadroxil PO	rapid	1.5–2 hr	12–24 hr
Cefazolin IM	rapid	0.5–2 hr	6–12 hr
Cefazolin IV	rapid	5 min	6–12 hr
Cephalexin PO	rapid	1 hr	6–12 hr

Contraindications/Precautions
Contraindicated in: Hypersensitivity to cephalosporins; Serious hypersensitivity to penicillins.
Use Cautiously in: Renal impairment (dosage ↓ and/or ↑ dosing interval recommended for: *cefadroxil* and *cephalexin*, if CCr ≤50 mL/min, and *cefazolin*, if CCr <30 mL/min; History of GI disease, especially colitis; Geri: Dose adjustment due to age-related ↓ in renal function may be necessary; OB, Lactation: Half-life is shorter and blood levels lower during pregnancy; have been used safely.

Adverse Reactions/Side Effects
CNS: SEIZURES (high doses). **GI:** CLOSTRIDIUM DIFFICILE-ASSOCIATED DIARRHEA (CDAD), diarrhea, nausea, vomiting, cramps. **Derm:** STEVENS-JOHNSON SYNDROME, rashes, pruritis, urticaria. **Hemat:** agranulocytosis, eosinophilia, hemolytic anemia, neutropenia, thrombocytopenia. **Local:** pain at IM site, phlebitis at IV site. **Misc:** allergic reactions including ANAPHYLAXIS and SERUM SICKNESS, superinfection.

Interactions
Drug-Drug: Probenecid ↓ excretion and ↑ blood levels of renally excreted cephalosporins. Concurrent use of **loop diuretics** or **aminoglycosides** may ↑ risk of renal toxicity.

Route/Dosage
Cefadroxil
PO (Adults): *Pharyngitis and tonsillitis*—500 mg q 12 hr or 1 g q 24 hr for 10 days. *Skin and soft-tissue infections*—500 mg q 12 hr or 1 g q 24 hr. *Urinary tract infections*—500 mg–1 g q 12 hr or 1–2 g q 24 hr.
PO (Children): *Pharyngitis, tonsillitis, or impetigo*—15 mg/kg q 12 hr or 30 mg/kg q 24 hr for 10 days. *Skin and soft-tissue infections*—15 mg/kg q 12 hr. *Urinary tract infections*—15 mg/kg q 12 hr.

Renal Impairment
PO (Adults): *CCr 25–50 mL/min*—500 mg q 12 hr; *CCr 10–25 mL/min*—500 mg q 24 hr; *CCr <10 mL/min*—500 mg q 36 hr.

Cefazolin

IM, IV (Adults): *Moderate to severe infections*—500 mg–2 g q 6–8 hr (maximum 12 g/day). *Mild infections with gram-positive cocci*—250–500 mg q 8 hr. *Uncomplicated urinary tract infections*—1 g q 12 hr. *Pneumococcal pneumonia*—500 mg q 12 hr. *Infective endocarditis or septicemia*—1–1.5 g q 6 hr. *Perioperative prophylaxis*—1 g given 30–60 min prior to incision. Additional 500 mg–1 g should be given for surgeries ≥2 hr. 500 mg–1 g should then be given for all surgeries q 6–8 hr for 24 hr postoperatively.

IM, IV (Children and Infants >1 mo): 16.7–33.3 mg/kg q 8 hr (maximum 6 g/day); *Bacterial endocarditis prophylaxis in penicillin-allergic patients:* 25 mg/kg 30 min prior to procedure (maximum dose = 1 g).

IM, IV (Neonates ≤7 days): 40 mg/kg/day divided q 12 hr.

IM, IV (Neonates >7 days and ≤2 kg): 40 mg/kg/day divided q 12 hr.

IM, IV (Neonates >7 days and >2 k g): 60 mg/kg/day divided q 8 hr.

Renal Impairment

IM, IV (Adults): *CCr 10–30 mL/min*—Administer q 12 hr; *CCr ≤10 mL/min*—Administer q 24 hr.

Cephalexin

PO (Adults): *Most infections*—250–500 mg q 6 hr. *Uncomplicated cystitis, skin and soft-tissue infections, streptococcal pharyngitis*—500 mg q 12 hr.

PO (Children): *Most infections*—25–50 mg/kg/day divided q 6–8 hr (can be administered q 12 hr in skin/skin structure infections or streptococcal pharyngitis). *Otitis media*—18.75–25 mg/kg q 6 hr (maximum = 4 g/day).

Renal Impairment

PO (Adults): *CCr 10–50 mL/min*—500 mg q 8–12 hr; *CCr <10 mL/min*—250–500 mg q 12–24 hr.

Availability

Cefadroxil (generic available)

Capsules: 500 mg. **Tablets:** 1 g. **Oral suspension (orange-pineapple flavor):** 250 mg/5 mL, 500 mg/5 mL.

Cefazolin (generic available)

Powder for injection: 500 mg/vial, 1 g/vial, 10 g/vial, 20 g/vial. **Premixed containers:** 1 g/50 mL D5W, 2 g/50 mL D5W.

Cephalexin (generic available)

Capsules: 250 mg, 500 mg, 750 mg. **Tablets:** 250 mg, 500 mg. **Oral suspension:** 125 mg/5 mL, 250 mg/5 mL.

NURSING IMPLICATIONS

Assessment

- Assess for infection (vital signs; appearance of wound, sputum, urine, and stool; WBC) at beginning and during therapy.
- Before initiating therapy, obtain a history to determine previous use of and reactions to penicillins or cephalosporins. Persons with a negative history of penicillin sensitivity may still have an allergic response.
- Obtain specimens for culture and sensitivity before initiating therapy. First dose may be given before receiving results.
- Observe patient for signs and symptoms of anaphylaxis (rash, pruritus, laryngeal edema, wheezing). Discontinue drug and notify health care professional immediately if these problems occur. Keep epinephrine, an antihistamine, and resuscitation equipment close by in case of an anaphylactic reaction.
- Monitor bowel function. Diarrhea, abdominal cramping, fever, and bloody stools should be reported to health care professional promptly as a sign of Clostridium difficile-associated diarrhea (CDAD). May begin up to several weeks following cessation of therapy.
- Assess patient for skin rash frequently during therapy. Discontinue cephalosporins at first sign of rash; may be life-threatening. Stevens-Johnson syndrome or toxic epidermal necrolysis may develop. Treat symptomatically; may recur once treatment is stopped.
- ***Lab Test Considerations:*** May cause positive results for Coombs' test in patients receiving high doses or in neonates whose mothers were given cephalosporins before delivery.
- May cause ↑ serum AST, ALT, alkaline phosphatase, bilirubin, LDH, BUN, creatinine.
- May rarely cause leukopenia, neutropenia, agranulocytosis, thrombocytopenia, or eosinophilia.

Potential Nursing Diagnoses

Risk for infection (Indications, Side Effects)
Diarrhea (Adverse Reactions)

Implementation

- Do not confuse cefazolin with cefotetan, cefoxitin, ceftazidime, or ceftriaxone. Do not confuse Keflex with Keppra.
- **PO:** Administer around the clock. May be administered on full or empty stomach. Administration with food may minimize GI irritation. Shake oral suspension well before administering. Use calibrated measuring device with liquid preparations. Refrigerate oral suspensions.

C

Cefazolin

- **IM:** Reconstitute IM doses with 2 mL or 2.5 mL of sterile water for injection to achieve a final concentration of 225–330 mg/mL.
- Inject deep into a well-developed muscle mass; massage well.

IV Administration

- **IV:** Monitor site frequently for thrombophlebitis (pain, redness, swelling). Change sites every 48–72 hr to prevent phlebitis.
- Do not use solutions that are cloudy or contain a precipitate.
- If aminoglycosides are administered concurrently, administer in separate sites, if possible, at least 1 hr apart. If second site is unavailable, flush line between medications.
- **IV Push:** ***Diluent:*** 0.9% NaCl, D5W, D10W, dextrose/saline combinations, D5/LR. ***Concentration:*** 100 mg/mL. May use up to 138 mg/mL in fluid-restricted patients. ***Rate:*** May administer over 3–5 min.
- **Intermittent Infusion:** ***Diluent:*** Reconstituted 500-mg or 1-g solution may be diluted in 50–100 mL of 0.9% NaCl, D5W, D10W, dextrose/saline combinations, D5/LR. Solution is stable for 24 hr at room temperature and 10 days if refrigerated. ***Concentration:*** 20 mg/mL. ***Rate:*** Administer over 10–60 min.
- **Y-Site Compatibility:** acyclovir, alfentanil, allopurinol, alprostadil, amifostine, aminocaproic acid, aminophylline, amphotericin B lipid complex, amphotericin B liposome, anidulafungin, argatroban, ascorbic acid, atracurium, atropine, azithromycin, aztreonam, benztropine, bivalirudin, bleomycin, bumetanide, buprenorphine, butorphanol, calcium gluconate, carboplatin, carmustine, cefotetan, cefoxitin, ceftazidime, ceftriaxone, cefuroxime, chlorampheniocol, cisplatin, clindamycin, cyanocobalamin, cyclophosphamide, cyclosporine, cytarabine, dactinomycin, daptomycin, dexamethasone, dexmedetomidine, digoxin, diltiazem, docetaxel, doxacurium, doxapram, doxorubicin liposome, enalaprilat, ephedrine, epinephrine, epirubicin, epoetin alfa, eptifibatide, esmolol, etoposide, etoposide phosphate, fenoldopam, fentanyl, filgrastim, fluconazole, fludarabine, fluorouracil, folic acid, foscarnet, furosemide, gemcitabine, glycopyrrolate, granisetron, heparin, hydrocortisone, ifosfamide, imipenem/cilastatin, indomethacin, insulin, irinotecan, isoproterenol, ketamine, ketorolac, leucovorin, lidocaine, linezolid, lorazepam, mannitol, mechlorethamine, melphalan, meperidine, metaraminol, methotrexate, methyldopate, methylprednisolone, metoclopramide, metoprolol, metronidazole, midazolam, milrinone, morphine, multivitamins, nafcillin, nalbuphine, naloxone, nesiritide, nicardipine, nitroglycerin, nitroprusside, norepinephrine, octreotide, ondansetron, oxacillin, oxaliplatin, oxytocin, paclitaxel, palonosetron, pamidronate, pancuronium, penicillin G, perphenazine, phenobarbital, phenylephrine, phytonadione, potassium acetate, potassium chloride, procainamide, propofol, propranolol, ranitidine, remifentanil, rituximab, sargramostim, sodium acetate, sodium bicarbonate, streptokinase, succinylcholine, sufentanil, tacrolimus, teniposide, theophylline, thiamine, thiotepa, tigecycline, tirofiban, tolazoline, trastuzumab, vasopressin, vecuronium, verapamil, vinblastine, vincristine, vitamin B complex with C, voriconazole, warfarin, zoledronic acid.
- **Y-Site Incompatibility:** alemtuzumab, amphotericin B cholesteryl, azathioprine, calcium chloride, caspofungin, cefotaxime, chlorpromazine, dantrolene, diazepam, diazoxide, diphenhydramine, dobutamine, dolasetron, dopamine, doxorubicin hydrochloride, doxycycline, erythromycin, ganciclovir, haloperidol, hydralazine, hydroxyzine, idarubicin, levofloxacin, mitoxantrone, mycophenolate, papaverine, pemetrexed, pentamidine, pentazocine, pentobarbital, phentolamine, phenytoin, prochlorperazine, promethazine, protamine, pyridoxime, quinupristin/dalfopristin, sodium citrate, tobramycin, trimethoprim/sulfamethoxazole, vinorelbine.

Patient/Family Teaching

- Instruct patient to take medication around the clock at evenly spaced times and to finish the medication completely as directed, even if feeling better. Take missed doses as soon as possible unless almost time for next dose; do not double doses. Instruct parents or caregivers to use calibrated measuring device with liquid preparations. Advise patient that sharing this medication may be dangerous.
- Advise patient to report signs of superinfection (furry overgrowth on the tongue, vaginal itching or discharge, loose or foul-smelling stools) and allergy.
- Instruct patient to notify health care professional if rash, or fever and diarrhea develop, especially if diarrhea contains blood, mucus, or pus. Advise patient not to treat diarrhea without consulting health care professional.

Evaluation/Desired Outcomes

- Resolution of signs and symptoms of infection. Length of time for complete resolution depends on the organism and site of infection.
- Decreased incidence of infection when used for prophylaxis.

CEPHALOSPORINS—SECOND GENERATION

cefaclor (**sef**-a-klor)
✱Ceclor

cefoTEtan (sef-oh-**tee**-tan)
~~Cefotan~~

cefOXitin (se-**fox**-i-tin)
Mefoxin

cefprozil (sef-**proe**-zil)
✱Cefzil

cefuroxime (se-fyoor-**ox**-eem)
Ceftin, Zinacef

Classification
Therapeutic: anti-infectives
Pharmacologic: second-generation cephalosporins

Pregnancy Category B

Indications

Treatment of the following infections caused by susceptible organisms: Respiratory tract infections, Skin and skin structure infections, Bone and joint infections (not cefaclor or cefprozil), Urinary tract infections (not cefprozil). **Cefotetan and cefoxitin:** Intra-abdominal and gynecologic infections. **Cefuroxime:** Meningitis, gynecologic infections, and Lyme disease. **Cefaclor, cefprozil, cefuroxime:** Otitis media. **Cefoxitin and cefuroxime:** Septicemia. **Cefotetan, cefoxitin, cefuroxime:** Perioperative prophylaxis.

Action

Bind to bacterial cell wall membrane, causing cell death. **Therapeutic Effects:** Bactericidal action against susceptible bacteria. **Spectrum:** Similar to that of first-generation cephalosporins but have ↑ activity against several other gram-negative pathogens including: *Haemophilus influenzae*, *Escherichia coli*, *Klebsiella pneumoniae*, *Morganella morganii*, *Neisseria gonorrhoeae* (including penicillinase-producing strains), *Proteus*, *Providencia*, *Serratia marcescens*, *Moraxella catarrhalis*. Not active against methicillin-resistant staphylococci or enterococci. **Cefuroxime:** Active against *Borrelia burgdorferi*. **Cefotetan and cefoxitin:** Active against *Bacteroides fragilis*.

Pharmacokinetics

Absorption: *Cefotetan, cefoxitin,* and *cefuroxime*—well absorbed following IM administration. *Cefaclor, cefprozil,* and *cefuroxime* —well absorbed following oral administration.

Distribution: Widely distributed. Penetration into CSF is poor, but adequate for cefuroxime (IV) to be used in treating meningitis. All cross the placenta and enter breast milk in low concentrations.

Metabolism and Excretion: Excreted primarily unchanged by the kidneys.

Half-life: *Cefaclor*—30–60 min; *cefotetan*—3–4.6 hr; *cefoxitin*—40–60 min; *cefprozil*—90 min; *cefuroxime*—60–120 min (all are ↑ in renal impairment).

TIME/ACTION PROFILE

ROUTE	ONSET	PEAK	DURATION
Cefaclor PO	rapid	30–60 min	6–12 hr
Cefaclor PO-CD	unknown	unknown	12 hr
Cefotetan IM	rapid	1–3 hr	12 hr
Cefotetan IV	rapid	end of infusion	12 hr
Cefoxitin IM	rapid	30 min	4–8 hr
Cefoxitin IV	rapid	end of infusion	4–8 hr
Cefprozil PO	unknown	1–2 hr	12–24 hr
Cefuroxime PO	unknown	2–3 hr	8–12 hr
Cefuroxime IM	rapid	15–60 min	6–12 hr
Cefuroxime IV	rapid	end of infusion	6–12 hr

Contraindications/Precautions

Contraindicated in: Hypersensitivity to cephalosporins; Serious hypersensitivity to penicillins.

Use Cautiously in: Renal impairment (↓ dose/↑ dosing interval recommended for: *cefotetan* if CCr ≤30 mL/min, *cefoxitin* if CCr ≤50 mL/min, *cefprozil* if CCr <30 mL/min, *cefuroxime* if CCr <30 mL/min); Patients with hepatic dysfunction, poor nutritional state, or cancer may be at ↑ risk for bleeding; History of GI disease, especially colitis; *Cefprozil (oral suspension)* contains aspartame and should be avoided in patients with phenylketonuria; Geri: Dose adjustment due to age-related ↓ in renal function may be necessary; may also be at ↑ risk for bleeding with *cefotetan* or *cefoxitin*; OB, Lactation: Have been used safely.

Adverse Reactions/Side Effects

CNS: SEIZURES (high doses). **GI:** CLOSTRIDIUM DIFFICILE-ASSOCIATED DIARRHEA (CDAD), diarrhea, cramps, nausea, vomiting. **Derm:** rashes, urticaria. **Hemat:** agranulocytosis, bleeding (↑ with cefotetan and cefoxitin), eosinophilia, hemolytic anemia, neutropenia, thrombocytopenia. **Local:** pain at IM site, phlebitis at IV site. **Misc:** allergic reactions including ANAPHYLAXIS and SERUM SICKNESS, superinfection.

Interactions

Drug-Drug: Probenecid ↓ excretion and ↑ blood levels. If **alcohol** is ingested within 48–72 hr of cefotetan, a disulfiram-like reaction may occur. Cefotetan may ↑ risk of bleeding with **anticoagulants**, **antiplatelet agents**, **thrombolytics**, and **NSAIDs**. **Antacids** ↓ absorption of cefaclor. Concurrent use of **aminoglycosides** or **loop diuretics** may ↑ risk of nephrotoxicity.

C

Route/Dosage

Cefaclor

PO (Adults): 250–500 mg q 8 hr or 375–500 mg q 12 hr as extended-release tablets.
PO (Children >1 mo): 6.7–13.4 mg/kg q 8 hr or 10–20 mg/kg q 12 hr (up to 1 g/day).

Cefotetan

IM, IV (Adults): *Most infections*—1–2 g q 12 hr. *Severe/life-threatening infections*—2–3 g q 12 hr. *Urinary tract infections*—500 mg–2 g q 12 hr *or* 1–2 g q 24 hr. *Perioperative prophylaxis*—1–2 g 30–60 min before initial incision (one-time dose).

Renal Impairment

IM, IV (Adults): *CCr 10–30 mL/min*—Usual adult dose q 24 hr *or* ½ usual adult dose q 12 hr; *<CCr 10 mL/min*—Usual adult dose q 48 hr *or* 1/4 usual adult dose q 12 hr.

Cefoxitin

IM, IV (Adults): *Most infections*—1 g q 6–8 hr. *Severe infections*—1 g q 4 hr *or* 2 g q 6–8 hr. *Life-threatening infections*—2 g q 4 hr *or* 3 g q 6 hr. *Perioperative prophylaxis*—2 g 30–60 min before initial incision, then 2 g q 6 hr for up to 24 hr.
IM, IV (Children and Infants >3 mo): *Most infections*—13.3–26.7 mg/kg q 4 hr *or* 20–40 mg/kg q 6 hr. *Perioperative prophylaxis*—30–40 mg/kg within 60 min of initial incision, then 30–40 mg/kg q 6 hr for up to 24 hr.

Renal Impairment

IM, IV (Adults): *CCr 30–50 mL/min*—1–2 g q 8–12 hr; *CCr 10–29 mL/min*—1–2 g q 12–24 hr; *CCr 5–9 mL/min*—0.5–1 g q 12–24 hr; *CCr <5 mL/min*—0.5–1 g q 24–48 hr.

Cefprozil

PO (Adults): *Most infections*—250–500 mg q 12 hr *or* 500 mg q 24 hr.
PO (Children 6 mo–12 yr): *Otitis media*—15 mg/kg q 12 hr. *Acute sinusitis*—7.5–15 mg/kg q 12 hr (higher dose should be used for moderate-to-severe infections).
PO (Children 2–12 yr): *Pharyngitis/tonsillitis*—7.5 mg/kg q 12 hr. *Skin/skin structure infections*—20 mg/kg q 24 hr.

Renal Impairment

PO (Adults and Children ≥6 mo): *CCr <30 mL/min*—½ of usual dose at normal dosing interval.

Cefuroxime

Cefuroxime oral tablets and oral suspension are not bioequivalent and are not substitutable on a mg-to-mg basis.
PO (Adults and Children >12 yr): *Pharyngitis/tonsillitis, maxillary sinusitis, uncomplicated UTIs*—250 mg q 12 hr. *Bronchitis, uncomplicated skin/skin structure infections*—250–500 mg q 12 hr. *Gonorrhea*—1 g (single dose). *Lyme disease*—500 mg q 12 hr for 20 days.
PO (Children 3 mo–12 yr): *Otitis media, acute bacterial maxillary sinusitis, impetigo*—15 mg/kg q 12 hr as oral suspension (not to exceed 1 g/day) *or* 250 mg q 12 hr as tablets. *Pharyngitis/tonsillitis*—10 mg/kg q 12 hr as oral suspension (not to exceed 500 mg/day).
IM, IV (Adults): *Uncomplicated urinary tract infections, skin/skin structure infections, disseminated gonococcal infections, uncomplicated pneumonia*—750 mg every 8 hr. *Bone/joint infections, severe or complicated infections*—1.5 g every 8 hr. *Life-threatening infections*—1.5 g every 6 hr. *Meningitis*—3 g every 8 hr. *Perioperative prophylaxis*—1.5 g IV 30–60 min before initial incision; 750 mg IM/IV every 8 hr can be given when procedure prolonged. *Prophylaxis during open-heart surgery*—1.5 g IV at induction of anesthesia and then every 12 hr for 3 additional doses. *Gonorrhea*—1.5 g IM (750 mg in two sites) with 1 g probenecid PO.
IM, IV (Children and Infants >3 mo): *Most infections*—12.5–25 mg/kg q 6 hr *or* 16.7–33.3 mg/kg q 8 hr (maximum dose = 6 g/day). *Bone and joint infections*—50 mg/kg q 8 hr (maximum dose = 6 g/day). *Bacterial meningitis*—50–60 mg/kg q 6 hr *or* 66.7–80 mg/kg q 8 hr.

Renal Impairment

IM, IV (Adults): *CCr 10–29 mL/min*—Give standard dose every 24 hr; *CCr <10 mL/min (no hemodialysis)*—Give standard dose every 48 hr; *Hemodialysis*—Give a an additional dose at end of each dialysis session.

Availability

Cefaclor (generic available)

Capsules: 250 mg, 500 mg. **Extended-release tablets (CD):** 375 mg, 500 mg. **Oral suspension (strawberry):** 125 mg/5 mL, 187 mg/5 mL, 250 mg/5 mL, 375 mg/5 mL.

Cefotetan (generic available)

Powder for injection: 1 g/vial, 2 g/vial, 10 g/vial. **Premixed containers:** 1 g/50 mL, 2 g/50 mL.

Cefoxitin (generic available)

Powder for injection: 1 g/vial, 2 g/vial, 10 g/vial. **Premixed containers:** 1 g/50 mL D5W, 2 g/50 mL D5W.

Cefprozil (generic available)

Tablets: 250 mg, 500 mg. **Oral suspension (bubblegum flavor):** 125 mg/5 mL, 250 mg/5 mL.

Cefuroxime (generic available)

Tablets: 250 mg, 500 mg. **Oral suspension (tutti-frutti flavor):** 125 mg/5 mL, 250 mg/5 mL. **Powder for injection:** 750 mg/vial, 1.5 g/vial, 7.5 g/vial. **Premixed containers:** 750 mg/50 mL, 1.5 g/50 mL.

NURSING IMPLICATIONS

Assessment

- Assess for infection (vital signs; appearance of wound, sputum, urine, and stool; WBC) at beginning and during therapy.
- Before initiating therapy, obtain a history to determine previous use of and reactions to penicillins or cephalosporins. Persons with a negative history of penicillin sensitivity may still have an allergic response.
- Obtain specimens for culture and sensitivity before initiating therapy. First dose may be given before receiving results.
- Observe patient for signs and symptoms of anaphylaxis (rash, pruritus, laryngeal edema, wheezing). Discontinue the drug immediately if these symptoms occur. Keep epinephrine, an antihistamine, and resuscitation equipment close by in the event of an anaphylactic reaction.
- Monitor bowel function. Diarrhea, abdominal cramping, fever, and bloody stools should be reported to health care professional promptly as a sign of Clostridium difficile-associated diarrhea (CDAD). May begin up to several weeks following cessation of therapy.
- ***Lab Test Considerations:*** May cause positive results for Coombs' test in patients receiving high doses or in neonates whose mothers were given cephalosporins before delivery.
- *Cefotetan*—monitor prothrombin time and assess patient for bleeding (guaiac stools; check for hematuria, bleeding gums, ecchymosis) daily in high-risk patients; may cause hypoprothrombinemia.
- May cause ↑ serum AST, ALT, alkaline phosphatase, bilirubin, LDH, BUN, and creatinine.
- *Cefoxitin* may cause falsely ↑ test results for serum and urine creatinine; do not obtain serum samples within 2 hr of administration.
- May rarely cause leukopenia, neutropenia, agranulocytosis, thrombocytopenia, and eosinophilia.

Potential Nursing Diagnoses

Risk for infection (Indications, Side Effects)
Diarrhea (Adverse Reactions)
Deficient knowledge, related to medication regimen (Patient/Family Teaching)

Implementation

- Do not confuse cefotetan with cefazolin, cefoxitin, ceftazidime, or ceftriaxone.
- **PO:** Administer around the clock. May be administered on full or empty stomach. Administration with food may minimize GI irritation. Shake oral suspension well before administering.
- Administer cefaclor extended-release tablets with food; do not crush, break, or chew.
- Do not administer *cefaclor* within 1 hr of antacids.
- *Cefuroxime* tablets should be swallowed whole, not crushed; crushed tablets have a strong, persistent bitter taste. Tablets may be taken without regard to meals. Suspension must be taken with food. Shake well each time before using. Tablets and suspension are not interchangeable.
- **IM:** Reconstitute IM doses with sterile or bacteriostatic water for injection or 0.9% NaCl for injection. May be diluted with lidocaine to minimize injection discomfort.
- Inject deep into a well-developed muscle mass; massage well.

IV Administration

- **IV:** Change sites every 48–72 hr to prevent phlebitis. Monitor site frequently for thrombophlebitis (pain, redness, swelling).
- If aminoglycosides are administered concurrently, administer in separate sites if possible, at least 1 hr apart. If second site is unavailable, flush line between medications.
- **IV Push:** Dilute each cephalosporin in at least 1 g/10 mL. Do not use preparations containing benzyl alcohol for neonates. ***Rate:*** Administer slowly over 3–5 min.

Cefotetan

- **Intermittent Infusion:** ***Diluent:*** Reconstituted solution may be further diluted in 50–100 mL of D5W or 0.9% NaCl. Solution may be colorless or yellow. Solution is stable for 24 hr at room temperature or 96 hr if refrigerated. ***Concentration:*** 10–40 mg/mL. ***Rate:*** Administer over 20–30 min.
- **Y-Site Compatibility:** acyclovir, alfentanil, allopurinol, amifostine, aminocaproic acid, aminophylline, amphotericin B lipid complex, anidulafungin, argatroban, ascorbic acid, atropine, azithromycin, aztreonam, benztropine, bivalirudin, bleomycin, bumetanide, buprenorphine, butorphanol, calcium chloride, calcium gluconate, carboplatin, carmustine, cefazolin, cefotaxime, cefoxitin, ceftriaxone, cefuroxime, chloramphenicol, cisplatin, clindamycin, cyanocobalamin, cyclophosphamide, cyclosporine, cytarabine, dacarbazine, dactinomycin, daptomycin, dexamethasone, dexmedetomidine, dexrazoxane, digoxin, diltiazem, docetaxel, dopamine, doxorubicin liposomal, enalaprilat, ephedrine, epinephrine, epoetin alfa, eptifibatide, etoposide, etoposide phosphate, fenoldopam, fentanyl, filgrastim, fluconazole, fludarabine, fluorouracil, folic acid, foscarnet, fosphenytoin, furosemide, gemcitabine, glycopyrrolate, granisetron, heparin, hetastarch, hydrocortisone, hydromorphone, ifosfamide, imipenem/cilastatin, irinotecan, isoproterenol, ketorolac, leucovorin, levofloxacin, lidocaine, linezolid, lorazepam, magnesium sulfate, mannitol, mechlorethamine, melphalan,

methotrexate, methylprednisolone, metoclopramide, metoprolol, metronidazole, milrinone, mitoxantrone, morphine, multivitamins, nafcillin, nalbuphine, naloxone, nesiritide, nitroglycerin, nitroprusside, norepinephrine, octreotide, oxacillin, oxaliplatin, oxytocin, paclitaxel, palonosetron, pamidronate, pancuronium, penicillin G, phenylephrine, phytonadione, potassium acetate, potassium chloride, procainamide, propofol, propranolol, pyridoxine, ranitidine, remifentanil, rituximab, rocuronium, sargramostim, sodium acetate, streptokinase, succinylcholine, sufentanil, tacrolimus, teniposide, theophylline, thiamine, thiotepa, tigecycline, tirofiban, topotecan, vasopressin, vecuronium, verapamil, vinblastine, vincristine, voriconazole, zoledronic acid.

- **Y-Site Incompatibility:** alemtuzumab, amiodarone, amphotericin B colloidal, amphotericin B liposome, azathioprine, caspofungin, chlorpromazine, dantrolene, daunorubicin hydrochloride, diazepam, diphenhydramine, dobutamine, dolasetron, doxorubicin hydrochloride, doxycycline, epirubicin, erythromycin, esmolol, ganciclovir, gentamicin, haloperidol, hydralazine, hydroxyzine, idarubicin, indomethacin, labetalol, mycophenolate, pantoprazole, papaverine, pemetrexed, pentamidine, pentazocine, pentobarbital, phenobarbital, phenytoin, prochlorperazine, promethazine, protamine, quinupristin/dalfopristin, sodium bicarbonate, tobramycin, trastuzumab, trimethoprim/sulfamethoxazole, vinorelbine.

Cefoxitin

- **Intermittent Infusion:** ***Diluent:*** Reconstituted solution may be further diluted in 50–100 mL of D5W, D10W, 0.9% NaCl, dextrose/saline combinations, D5/LR, Ringer's or LR. Stable for 24 hr at room temperature and 1 wk if refrigerated. Darkening of powder does not alter potency. ***Concentration:*** 40 mg/mL. ***Rate:*** Administer over 30–60 min.
- **Continuous Infusion:** May be diluted in 500–1000 mL for continuous infusion.
- **Y-Site Compatibility:** acetaminophen, acyclovir, alfentanil, amifostine, aminocaproic acid, aminophylline, amphotericin B lipid complex, amphotericin B liposome, anidulafungin, argatroban, ascorbic acid, atropine, azithromycin, aztreonam, benztropine, bivalirudin, bleomycin, bumetanide, buprenorphine, butorphanol, calcium chloride, calcium gluconate, cangrelor, carboplatin, carmustine, cefazolin, cefotaxime, cefotetan, ceftazidime, ceftriaxone, cefuroxime, chloramphenicol, cisplatin, clindamycin, cyanocobalamin, cyclophosphamide, cyclosporine, cytarabine, dacarbazine, dactinomycin, daptomycin, dexamethasone, dexmedetomidine, dexrazoxane, digoxin, diltiazem, docetaxel, dopamine, doxacurium, doxorubicin liposome, enalaprilat, ephedrine, epinephrine, epoetin alfa, eptifibatide, esmolol, etoposide, etoposide phosphate, fentanyl, fluconazole, fludarabine, fluorouracil, folic acid, foscarnet, furosemide, gemcitabine, glycopyrrolate, granisetron, heparin, hydrocortisone, hydromorphone, ifosfamide, imipenem/cilastatin, indomethacin, irinotecan, isoproterenol, ketorolac, leucovorin, lidocaine, linezolid, lorazepam, magnesium sulfate, mannitol, mechlorethamine, meperidine, methotrexate, metoclopramide, metoprolol, metronidazole, midazolam, milrinone, morphine, multivitamins, nafcillin, nalbuphine, naloxone, nesiritide, nitroglycerin, nitroprusside, norepinephrine, octreotide, ondansetron, oxacillin, oxaliplatin, oxytocin, paclitaxel, palonosetron, pamidronate, pantoprazole, penicillin G, perphenazine, phenylephrine, phytonadione, potassium acetate, potassium chloride, procainamide, propofol, propranolol, pyridoxine, ranitidine, remifentanil, rituximab, rocuronium, sodium acetate, streptokinase, succinylcholine, sufentanil, tacrolimus, teniposide, theophylline, thiamine, thiotepa, tigecycline, tirofiban, topotecan, vasopressin, vecuronium, verapamil, vinblastine, vincristine, voriconazole, zoledronic acid.
- **Y-Site Incompatibility:** alemtuzumab, azathioprine, caspofungin, chlorpromazine, dantrolene, daunorubicin hydrochloride, diazepam, diphenhydramine, dobutamine, dolasetron, doxorubicin hydrochloride, doxycycline, epirubicin, erythromycin, fenoldopam, filgrastim, ganciclovir, haloperidol, hydralazine, hydroxyzine, idarubicin, insulin, labetalol, levofloxacin, methylprednisolone, mitoxantrone, mycophenolate, papaverine, pemetrexed, pentamidine, pentazocine, pentobarbital, phenobarbital, phenytoin, prochlorperazine, promethazine, protamine, quinupristin/dalfopristin, sodium bicarbonate, trastuzumab, trimethoprim/sulfamethoxazole, vinorelbine.

Cefuroxime

- **Intermittent Infusion:** ***Diluent:*** Solution may be further diluted in 50–100 mL of 0.9% NaCl, D5W, D10W, or dextrose/saline combinations. Stable for 24 hr at room temperature and 48 hr if refrigerated. ***Concentration:*** 10–40 mg/mL. ***Rate:*** Administer over 15–60 min.
- **Continuous Infusion:** May also be diluted in 500–1000 mL for continuous infusion.
- **Y-Site Compatibility:** acyclovir, alfentanil, allopurinol, amifostine, aminocaproic acid, aminophylline, amphotericin B lipid complex, amphotericin B liposome, anidulafungin, argatroban, ascorbic acid, atropine, aztreonam, benztropine, bivalirudin, bleomycin, bumetanide, buprenorphine, butorphanol, calcium gluconate, cangrelor, carboplatin, carmus-

C

tine, cefazolin, cefotaxime, cefotetan, cefoxitin, ceftazidime, ceftriaxone, chloramphenicol, cisplatin, clindamycin, cyclophosphamide, cyanocobalamin, cyclophosphamide, cyclosporine, cytarabine, dactinomycin, daptomycin, dexmedetomidine, dexrazoxane, digoxin, diltiazem, dimenhydrinate, docetaxel, dopamine, doxorubicin liposomal, enalaprilat, ephedrine, epinephrine, epoetin alfa, eptifibatide, erythromycin, esmolol, etoposide, etoposide phosphate, famotidine, fenoldopam, fentanyl, fludarabine, fluorouracil, folic acid, foscarnet, fosphenytoin, furosemide, gemcitabine, glycopyrrolate, granisetron, heparin, hetastarch, hydrocortisone, hydromorphone, ifosfamide, imipenem/cilastatin, indomethacin, insulin, irinotecan, isoproterenol, ketamine, ketorolac, leucovorin, levofloxacin, lidocaine, linezolid, lorazepam, mannitol, mechlorethamine, melphalan, meperidine, methotrexate, methylprednisolone, metoclopramide, metoprolol, metronidazole, milrinone, morphine, multivitamins, nafcillin, nalbuphine, naloxone, nesiritide, nitroglycerin, nitroprusside, norepinephrine, octreotide, ondansetron, oxacillin, oxaliplatin, oxytocin, paclitaxel, palonosetron, pamidronate, pancuronium, pantoprazole, pemetrexed, penicillin G, perphenazine, phenylephrine, phytonadione, potassium acetate, potassium chloride, procainamide, propofol, propranolol, pyridoxine, ranitidine, remifentanil, rituximab, rocuronium, sargramostim, sodium acetate, streptokinase, succinylcholine, sufentanil, tacrolimus, teniposide, theophylline, thiamine, thiotepa, tigecycline, tirofiban, topotecan, trastuzumab, vasopressin, vecuronium, verapamil, vinblastine, vincristine, voriconazole, zoledronic acid.

- **Y-Site Incompatibility:** alemtuzumab, azathioprine, calcium chloride, caspofungin, chlorpromazine, dantrolene, daunorubicin hydrochloride, dexamethasone, diazepam, diphenhydramine, dobutamine, doxorubicin hydrochloride, doxycycline, epirubicin, filgrastim, ganciclovir, haloperidol, hydralazine, hydroxyzine, idarubicin, labetalol, magnesium sulfate, midazolam, mitoxantrone, mycophenolate, nicardipine, papaverine, pentamidine, pentazocine, pentobarbital, phenobarbital, phenytoin, prochlorperazine, promethazine, protamine, quinupristin/dalfopristin, sodium bicarbonate, trimethoprim/sulfamethoxazole, vinorelbine.

Patient/Family Teaching

- Instruct patient to take medication around the clock at evenly spaced times and to finish the medication completely, even if feeling better. Take missed doses as soon as possible unless almost time for next dose; do not double doses. Use calibrated measuring device with liquid preparations. Advise patient that sharing of this medication may be dangerous.
- Advise patient to report signs of superinfection (furry overgrowth on the tongue, vaginal itching or discharge, loose or foul-smelling stools) and allergy.
- Caution patients that concurrent use of alcohol with *cefotetan* may cause a disulfiram-like reaction (abdominal cramps, nausea, vomiting, headache, hypotension, palpitations, dyspnea, tachycardia, sweating, flushing). Alcohol and alcohol-containing medications should be avoided during and for several days after therapy.
- Instruct patient to notify health care professional if fever and diarrhea develop, especially if stool contains blood, pus, or mucus. Advise patient not to treat diarrhea without consulting health care professional.

Evaluation/Desired Outcomes

- Resolution of signs and symptoms of infection. Length of time for complete resolution depends on the organism and site of infection.
- Decreased incidence of infection when used for prophylaxis.

CEPHALOSPORINS—THIRD GENERATION

cefdinir (**sef**-di-nir)
~~Omnicef~~

cefditoren (sef-dye-**tor**-en)
Spectracef

cefixime (sef-**ik**-seem)
Suprax

cefotaxime (sef-oh-**taks**-eem)
Claforan

cefpodoxime (sef-poe-**dox**-eem)
✱Simplicef, ~~Vantin~~

cefTAZidime (sef-**tay**-zi-deem)
Fortaz, Tazicef

ceftibuten (sef-tye-**byoo**-ten)
Cedax

cefTRIAXone (sef-try-**ax**-one)
Rocephin

Classification
Therapeutic: anti-infectives
Pharmacologic: third-generation cephalosporins

Pregnancy Category B

Indications

Treatment of the following infections caused by susceptible organisms: Skin and skin structure infections (not cefixime), Urinary and gynecologic infections (not cefdinir, cefditoren, or ceftibuten), Respiratory tract infections (not cefdinir, cefditoren, or ceftibuten). **Cefotaxime, ceftazidime, ceftriaxone:** Meningitis and bone/joint infections. **Cefotaxime, ceftazidime, cef-**

triaxone: Intra-abdominal infections and septicemia. **Cefdinir, cefixime, cefpodoxime, ceftibuten, ceftriaxone:** Otitis media. **Cefotaxime, ceftriaxone:** Perioperative prophylaxis. **Ceftazidime:** Febrile neutropenia. **Cefotaxime, ceftriaxone:** Lyme disease.

Action

Bind to the bacterial cell wall membrane, causing cell death. **Therapeutic Effects:** Bactericidal action against susceptible bacteria. **Spectrum:** Similar to that of second-generation cephalosporins, but activity against staphylococci is less, whereas activity against gram-negative pathogens is greater, even for organisms resistant to first- and second-generation agents. Notable is increased action against: *Enterobacter*, *Haemophilus influenzae*, *Escherichia coli*, *Klebsiella pneumoniae*, *Neisseria gonorrhoeae*, *Citrobacter*, *Morganella*, *Proteus*, *Providencia*, *Serratia*, *Moraxella catarrhalis*, *Borrelia burgdorferi*. Some agents have activity against *N. meningitidis* (cefotaxime, ceftazidime, ceftriaxone). Some agents have enhanced activity against *Pseudomonas aeruginosa* (ceftazidime). Not active against methicillin-resistance staphylococci or enterococci. Some agents have activity against anaerobes, including *Bacteroides fragilis* (cefotaxime, ceftriaxone).

Pharmacokinetics

Absorption: *Cefotaxime, ceftazidime,* and *ceftriaxone* are well absorbed after IM administration. *Ceftibuten* is well absorbed after oral administration; *cefixime* 40–50% absorbed after oral administration (oral suspension); *cefdinir* 16–25% absorbed after oral administration. *Cefditoren pivoxil* and *cefpodoxime proxetil* are prodrugs that are converted to their active components in GI tract during absorption (*cefditoren*—14% absorbed [↑ by high-fat meal] *cefpodoxime*—50% absorbed).
Distribution: Widely distributed. Cross the placenta; enter breast milk in low concentrations. CSF penetration better than with first- and second-generation agents.
Protein Binding: *Ceftriaxone* ≥90%.
Metabolism and Excretion: *Cefdinir, ceftazidime,* and *cefditoren*—>85% excreted in urine. *Cefpodoxime*—30% excreted in urine. *Ceftibuten, ceftriaxone,* and *cefotaxime*—partly metabolized and partly excreted in the urine. *Cefixime*—50% excreted unchanged in urine, ≥10% in bile.
Half-life: *Cefdinir*—1.7 hr; *cefditoren*—1.6 hr; *cefixime*—3–4 hr; *cefotaxime*—1–1.5 hr; *cefpodoxime*—2–3 hr; *ceftazidime*—2 hr; *ceftibuten*—2 hr; *ceftriaxone*—6–9 hr (all except *ceftriaxone* are ↑ in renal impairment).

TIME/ACTION PROFILE

ROUTE	ONSET	PEAK	DURATION
Cefdinir PO	rapid	2–4 hr	12–24 hr
Cefditoren PO	rapid	1.5–3 hr	12 hr
Cefixime PO	rapid	2–6 hr	24 hr
Cefotaxime IM	rapid	0.5 hr	4–12 hr
Cefotaxime IV	rapid	end of infusion	4–12 hr
Cefpodoxime PO	unknown	2–3 hr	12 hr
Ceftazidime IM	rapid	1 hr	6–12 hr
Ceftazidime IV	rapid	end of infusion	6–12 hr
Ceftibuten PO	rapid	3 hr	24 hr
Ceftriaxone IM	rapid	1–2 hr	12–24 hr
Ceftriaxone IV	rapid	end of infusion	12–24 hr

Contraindications/Precautions

Contraindicated in: Hypersensitivity to cephalosporins; Serious hypersensitivity to penicillins; Pedi: Premature neonates up to a postmenstrual age of 41 wk (ceftriaxone only); Pedi: Hyperbilirubinemic neonates (may lead to bilirubin encephalopathy); Pedi: Neonates ≤28 days requiring calcium-containing IV solutions (↑ risk of precipitation formation); Carnitine deficiency or inborn errors of metabolism (cefditoren only); Hypersensitivity to milk protein (ceftidoren only; contains sodium caseinate).
Use Cautiously in: Renal impairment (↓ dosing/↑ dosing interval recommended for: *cefdinir* if CCr <30 mL/min, *cefixime* if CCr ≤60 mL/min, *cefotaxime* if CCr <20 mL/min, *cefpodoxime* if CCr <30 mL/min, *ceftazidime* if CCr ≤50 mL/min, *ceftibuten* and *cefditoren* if CCr <50 mL/min); Combined severe hepatic and renal impairment (dose reduction/↑ dosing interval recommended for *ceftriaxone*); Diabetes (*ceftibuten* and *cefdinir* suspension contain sucrose); History of GI disease, especially colitis; Geri: Dose adjustment due to age-related ↓ in renal function may be necessary; Pedi: ↑ risk of urolithiasis and acute renal failure (ceftriaxone only); OB, Lactation: Have been used safely.

Adverse Reactions/Side Effects

CNS: SEIZURES (high doses), headache. **GI:** *Clostridium difficile*-ASSOCIATED DIARRHEA, diarrhea, nausea, vomiting, cholelithiasis (ceftriaxone), cramps, pancreatitis (ceftriaxone). **Derm:** STEVENS-JOHNSON SYNDROME, rash, urticaria. **GU:** acute renal failure (ceftriaxone), urolithiasis (ceftriaxone). **Hemat:** agranulocytosis, bleeding, eosinophilia, hemolytic anemia, lymphocytosis, neutropenia, thrombocytopenia, thrombocytosis. **GU:** hematuria, vaginal moniliasis.

Local: pain at IM site, phlebitis at IV site. **Misc:** allergic reactions including ANAPHYLAXIS and SERUM SICKNESS, superinfection.

Interactions

Drug-Drug: Probenecid ↓ excretion and ↑ serum levels (cefdinir, cefditoren, cefixime, cefotaxime, cefpodoxime, ceftriaxone). Concurrent use of **loop diuretics**, **aminoglycosides**, or **NSAIDs** may ↑ risk of nephrotoxicity. **Antacids** ↓ absorption of cefdinir, cefditoren, and cefpodoxime. **Iron supplements** ↓ absorption of cefdinir. **H_2-receptor antagonists** ↓ absorption of cefditoren and cefpodoxime. Cefixime may ↑ **carbamazepine** levels. Ceftriaxone should not be administered concomitantly with any calcium-containing solutions. Ceftriaxone may ↑ risk of bleeding with **warfarin**.

Route/Dosage

Cefdinir

PO (Adults ≥13 yr): 300 mg q 12 hr *or* 600 mg q 24 hr (use q 12 hr dosing only for community-acquired pneumonia or skin and skin structure infections).
PO (Children 6 mo–12 yr): 7 mg/kg q 12 hr (use only for skin/skin structure infections) *or* 14 mg/kg q 24 hr; dose should not exceed 600 mg/day.

Renal Impairment

PO (Adults and Children ≥13 yr): *CCr <30 mL/min*—300 mg q 24 hr.

Renal Impairment

PO (Children 6 mo–12 yr): *CCr <30 mL/min*—7 mg/kg q 24 hr.

Cefditoren

PO (Adults and Children ≥12 yr): *Pharyngitis/tonsillitis, skin/skin structure infections*—200 mg twice daily; *Acute bacterial exacerbation of chronic bronchitis or community acquired pneumonia*—400 mg twice daily.

Renal Impairment

PO (Adults): *CCr 30–49 mL/min*—dose should not exceed 200 mg twice daily; *CCr <30 mL/min*—dose should not exceed 200 mg once daily.

Cefixime

PO (Adults and Children >12 yr or >50 kg): *Most infections*—400 mg once daily; *Gonorrhea*—400 mg single dose.
PO (Children): 8 mg/kg once daily *or* 4 mg/kg q 12h.

Renal Impairment

PO (Adults): *CCr 21–60 mL/min*—75% of standard dose once daily; *CCr ≤20 mL/min*—50% of standard dose once daily.

Cefotaxime

IM, IV (Adults and Children >12 yr): *Most uncomplicated infections*—1 g q 12 hr. *Moderate or severe infections*—1–2 g q 6–8 hr. *Life-threatening infections*—2 g q 4 hr (maximum dose = 12 g/day). *Gonococcal urethritis/cervicitis or rectal gonorrhea in females*—500 mg IM (single dose). *Rectal gonorrhea in males*—1 g IM (single dose). *Perioperative prophylaxis*—1 g 30–90 min before initial incision (one-time dose).
IM, IV (Children 1 mo–12 yr): *<50 kg*—100–200 mg/kg/day divided q 6–8 hr. *Meningitis*—200 mg/kg/day divided q 6 hr. *Invasive pneumococcal meningitis*—225–300 mg/kg/day divided q 6–8 hr. *≥50 kg*—see adult dosing.
IV (Neonates 1–4 wk): 50 mg/kg q 6–8 hr.
IV (Neonates ≤1 wk): 50 mg/kg q 8–12 hr.

Renal Impairment

(Adults): *CCr <20 mL/min*—↓ dose by 50%.

Cefpodoxime

PO (Adults): *Most infections*—200 mg q 12 hr. *Skin and skin structure infections*—400 mg q 12 hr. *Urinary tract infections/pharyngitis*—100 mg q 12 hr. *Gonorrhea*—200 mg single dose.
PO (Children 2 mo–12 yr): *Pharyngitis/tonsillitis/otitis media/acute maxillary sinusitis*—5 mg/kg q 12 hr (not to exceed 200 mg/dose).

Renal Impairment

PO (Adults): *CCr <30 mL/min*—↑ dosing interval to q 24 hr.

Ceftazidime

IM, IV (Adults and Children ≥12 yr): *Pneumonia and skin/skin structure infections*—500 mg–1 g q 8 hr. *Bone and joint infections*—2 g q 12 hr. *Severe and life-threatening infections*—2 g q 8 hr. *Complicated urinary tract infections*—500 mg q 8–12 hr. *Uncomplicated urinary tract infections*—250 mg q 12 hr. *Cystic fibrosis lung infection caused by* P. aeruginosa—30–50 mg/kg q 8 hr (maximum dose = 6 g/day).
IM, IV (Children 1 mo–12 yr): 33.3–50 mg/kg q 8 hr (maximum dose = 6 g/day).
IM, IV (Neonates ≤4 wk): 50 mg/kg q 8–12 hr.

Renal Impairment

IM, IV (Adults): *CCr 31–50 mL/min*—1 g q 12 hr; *CCr 16–30 mL/min*—1 g q 24 hr; *CCr 6–15 mL/min*—500 mg q 24 hr; *CCr <5 mL/min*—500 mg q 48 hr.

Ceftibuten

PO (Adults and Children ≥12 yr): 400 mg q 24 hr for 10 days.
PO (Children 6 mo–12 yr): 9 mg/kg q 24 hr for 10 days (maximum dose = 400 mg/day).

Renal Impairment

PO (Adults): *CCr 30–49 mL/min*—200 mg q 24 hr as capsules *or* 4.5 mg/kg q 24 hr as suspension; *CCr 5–29 mL/min*—100 mg q 24 hr as capsules *or* 2.25 mg/kg q 24 hr as suspension.

Ceftriaxone

IM, IV (Adults): *Most infections*—1–2 g q 12–24 hr. *Gonorrhea*—250 mg IM (single dose). *Meningitis*—2 g q 12 hr. *Perioperative prophylaxis*—1 g 30–120 min before initial incision (single dose).
IM, IV (Children): *Most infections*—25–37.5 mg/kg q 12 hr *or* 50–75 mg/kg q 24 hr; dose should not exceed 2 g/day. *Meningitis*—100 mg/kg q 24 hr *or* 50 mg/kg q 12 hr; dose should not exceed 4 g/day. *Acute otitis media*—50 mg/kg IM single dose; dose should not exceed 1 g. *Uncomplicated gonorrhea*—125 mg IM (single dose).

Availability

Cefdinir (generic available)

Oral suspension (strawberry): 125 mg/5 mL, 250 mg/5 mL. **Cost:** *Generic*—125 mg/5 mL $51.00/60 mL, 250 mg/5 mL $99.48/60 mL. **Capsules:** 300 mg.

Cefditoren (generic available)

Tablets: 200 mg, 400 mg. **Cost:** *Generic*—All strengths $294.81/20.

Cefixime

Oral suspension (strawberry): 100 mg/5 mL, 200 mg/5 mL, 500 mg/5 mL. **Cost:** 100 mg/5 mL $170.77/50 mL, 200 mg/5 mL $341.55/50 mL, 500 mg/5 mL $170.77/10 mL. **Tablets:** 400 mg. **Cost:** $1008.49/50. **Chewable tablets:** 100 mg, 150 mg, 200 mg. **Cost:** 100 mg $170.77/10, 200 mg $341.51/10.

Cefotaxime (generic available)

Powder for injection: 500 mg/vial, 1 g/vial, 2 g/vial, 10 g/vial, 20 g/vial. **Premixed containers:** 1 g/50 mL, 2 g/50 mL.

Cefpodoxime (generic available)

Tablets: 100 mg, 200 mg. **Cost:** *Generic*—100 mg $134.74/20, 200 mg $169.14/20. **Oral suspension (lemon creme):** 50 mg/5 mL, 100 mg/5 mL. **Cost:** *Generic*—50 mg/5 mL $35.28/50 mL, 100 mg/5 mL $86.17/50 mL.

Ceftazidime (generic available)

Powder for injection: 500 mg/vial, 1 g/vial, 2 g/vial, 6 g/vial. **Premixed containers:** 1 g/50 mL, 2 g/50 mL.

Ceftibuten

Capsules: 400 mg. **Cost:** $767.98/20. **Oral suspension (cherry):** 90 mg/5 mL. **Cost:** $179.83/90 mL.

Ceftriaxone (generic available)

Powder for injection: 250 mg/vial, 500 mg/vial, 1 g/vial, 2 g/vial, 10 g/vial. **Premixed containers:** 1 g/50 mL, 2 g/50 mL.

NURSING IMPLICATIONS

Assessment

- Assess for infection (vital signs; appearance of wound, sputum, urine, and stool; WBC) at beginning of and throughout therapy.
- Before initiating therapy, obtain a history to determine previous use of and reactions to penicillins or cephalosporins. Persons with a negative history of penicillin sensitivity may still have an allergic response.
- Obtain specimens for culture and sensitivity before initiating therapy. First dose may be given before receiving results.
- Observe for signs and symptoms of anaphylaxis (rash, pruritus, laryngeal edema, wheezing). Discontinue drug and notify health care professional immediately if these symptoms occur. Keep epinephrine, an antihistamine, and resuscitation equipment close by in the event of an anaphylactic reaction.
- Monitor bowel function. Diarrhea, abdominal cramping, fever, and bloody stools should be reported to health care professional promptly as a sign of Clostridium difficile-associated diarrhea (CDAD). May begin up to several weeks following cessation of therapy.
- Assess patient for skin rash frequently during therapy. Discontinue at first sign of rash; may be life-threatening. Stevens-Johnson syndrome may develop. Treat symptomatically; may recur once treatment is stopped.
- Pedi: Assess newborns for jaundice and hyperbilirubinemia before making decision to use ceftriaxone (should not be used in jaundiced or hyperbilirubinemic neonates).
- ***Lab Test Considerations:*** May cause positive results for Coombs' test in patients receiving high doses or in neonates whose mothers were given cephalosporins before delivery.
- Monitor prothrombin time and assess patient for bleeding (guaiac stools; check for hematuria, bleeding gums, ecchymosis) daily in patients receiving *cefditoren*, as this agentmay cause hypoprothrombinemia.
- May cause ↑ serum AST, ALT, alkaline phosphatase, bilirubin, LDH, BUN, and creatinine.
- May rarely cause leukopenia, neutropenia, agranulocytosis, thrombocytopenia, eosinophilia, lymphocytosis, and thrombocytosis.

Potential Nursing Diagnoses

Risk for infection (Indications, Side Effects)
Diarrhea (Adverse Reactions)
Deficient knowledge, related to medication regimen (Patient/Family Teaching)

Implementation

- Do not confuse ceftazidime with cefazolin, cefoxitin, cefotetan, or ceftriaxone.
- Cefditoren is not recommended for prolonged use since other piralate-containing compounds have caused clinical manifestations of carnitine deficiency when used over a period of months.
- **PO:** Administer around the clock. May be administered on full or empty stomach. Administration with food may minimize GI irritation. Shake oral suspension well before administering. Administer *cefditoren* with meals to enhance absorption. Administer *cefpodoxime tablets* with meals to enhance absorption (suspension may be administered without regard to meals. Administer *ceftibuten* at least 1 hr before or 2 hr after meals.
- *Cefixime oral suspension* should be used to treat otitis media (results in higher peak concentrations than tablets).
- Do not administer *cefdinir* or *cefpodoxime* within 2 hr before or after an antacid. Do not administer *cefpodoxime* within 2 hr before or after an H_2 receptor antagonist. Do not administer *cefdinir* within 2 hr before or after iron supplements. Do not administer *cefditoren* concomitantly with antacids.
- **IM:** Reconstitute IM doses with sterile or bacteriostatic water for injection or 0.9% NaCl for injection. May be diluted with lidocaine to minimize injection discomfort. Do not administer lidocaine-containing ceftriaxone IV.
- Inject deep into a well-developed muscle mass; massage well.

IV Administration

- **IV:** Monitor injection site frequently for phlebitis (pain, redness, swelling). Change sites every 48–72 hr to prevent phlebitis.
- If aminoglycosides are administered concurrently, administer in separate sites, if possible, at least 1 hr apart. If second site is unavailable, flush lines between medications.
- **IV Push:** Dilute cephalosporins in at least 1 g/10 mL. Avoid IV push administration of *ceftriaxone*. Do not use preparations containing benzyl alcohol for neonates. ***Rate:*** Administer slowly over 3–5 min.

Cefotaxime

- **Intermittent Infusion:** ***Diluent:*** Reconstituted solution may be further diluted in 50–100 mL of D5W, D10W, LR, dextrose/saline combinations, or 0.9% NaCl. Solution may appear light yellow to amber. Solution is stable for 24 hr at room temperature and 5 days if refrigerated. ***Concentration:*** 20–60 mg/mL. ***Rate:*** Administer over 20–30 min.
- **Y-Site Compatibility:** acyclovir, alfentanil, alprostadil, amifostine, aminophylline, aminocaproic acid, amphotericin B lipid complex, anidulafungin, argatroban, ascorbic acid, atropine, aztreonam, benztropine, bivalirudin, bleomycin, bumetanide, buprenorphine, butorphanol, calcium chloride, calcium gluconate, cangrelor, carboplatin, carmustine, cefotetan, cefoxitin, ceftriaxone, cefuroxime, cisplain, clindamycin, cyanocobalamin, cyclophosphamide, cyclosporine, cytarabine, dactinomycin, daptomycin, dexamethasone, dexmedetomidine, dexrazoxane, digoxin, diltiazem, dimenhydrinate, docetaxel, dopamine, doxorubicin liposomal, doxycycline, enalaprilat, ephedrine, epinephrine, epirubicin, epoetin alfa, eptifibatide, erythromycin, esmolol, etoposide, etoposide phosphate, famotidine, fenoldopam, fentanyl, fludarabine, fluorouracil, folic acid, foscarnet, fosphenytoin, furosemide, glycopyrrolate, granisetron, heparin, hetastarch, hydrocortisone, hydromorphone, ifosfamide, imipenem/cilastatin, indomethacin, insulin, isoproterenol, ketamine, ketorolac, leucovorin, lidocaine, linezolid, lorazepam, magnesium sulfate, mannitol, mechlorethamine, melphalan, meperidine, mesna, methotrexate, metoclopramide, metoprolol, metronidazole, midazolam, milrinone, morphine, multivitamins, nafcillin, nalbuphine, naloxone, nesiritide, nicardipine, nitroglycerin, nitroprusside, norepinephrine, octreotide, ondansetron, oxacillin, oxaliplatin, oxytocin, paclitaxel, palonosetron, pamidronate, pancuronium, penicillin G, perphenazine, phenylephrine, phytonadione, potassium acetate, potassium chloride, procainamide, propofol, propranolol, pyridoxime, ranitidine, remifentanil, rituximab, rocuronium, sargramostim, sodium acetate, streptokinase, succinylcholine, sufentanil, tacrolimus, teniposide, theophylline, thiamine, thiotepa, tigecycline, tirofiban, vasopressin, verapamil, vinblastine, vinorelbine, voriconazole, zoledronic acid.
- **Y-Site Incompatibility:** alemtuzumab, allopurinol, amiodarone, amphotericin B liposome, azathioprine, caspofungin, cefazolin, ceftazidime, chloramphenicol, chlorpromazine, dantrolene, daunorubicin hydrochloride, diazepam, diphenhydramine, dobutamine, dolasetron, doxorubicin hydrochloride, filgrastim, ganciclovir, gemcitabine, haloperidol, hydralazine, hydroxyzine, idarubicin, irinotecan, labetalol, methylprednisolone, mitoxantrone, mycophenolate, pantoprazole, papaverine, pemetrexed, pentamidine, pentazocine, pentobarbital, phenobarbital, phenytoin, prochlorperazine, promethazine, protamine, quinupristin/dalfopristin, sodium bicarbonate, trastuzumab, trimethoprim/sulfamethoxazole, vecuronium.

Ceftazidime

- **Intermittent Infusion:** ***Diluent:*** Reconstituted solution may be further diluted in at least 1 g/10 mL of 0.9% NaCl, D5W, D10W, dextrose/saline combinations, or LR. Dilution causes CO_2 to form inside vial, resulting in positive pressure; vial may require venting after dissolution to preserve sterility of vial. Not required with L-arginine formulation (Ceptaz). Solution may appear yellow to amber; darkening does not alter potency. Solution is stable for 18 hr at room temperature and 7 days if refrigerated. ***Concentration:*** 40 mg/mL. ***Rate:*** Administer over 15–30 min.

- **Y-Site Compatibility:** acyclovir, alfentanil, allopurinol, amifostine, aminocaproic acid, aminophylline, amphotericin B lipid complex, anakinra, anidulafungin, argatroban, atropine, aztreonam, benztropine, bivalirudin, bleomycin, bumetanide, buprenorphine, butorphanol, calcium gluconate, cangrelor, carboplatin, carmustine, cefazolin, cefotetan, cefoxitin, ceftriaxone, cefuroxime, ciprofloxacin, cisplatin, clindamycin, cyanocobalamin, cyclophosphamide, cyclosporine, cytarabine, dacarbazine, dactinomycin, daptomycin, dexamethasone, dexmedetomidine, dexrazoxane, digoxin, diltiazem, dimenhydrinate, docetaxel, dolasetron, dopamine, enalaprilat, ephedrine, epinephrine, epoetin alfa, eptifibatide, esmolol, etoposide, etoposide phosphate, famotidine, fenoldopam, fentanyl, filgrastim, fludarabine, fluorouracil, folic acid, foscarnet, fosphenytoin, furosemide, gemcitabine, glycopyrrolate, granisetron, heparin, hetastarch, hydrocortisone, hydromorphone, ibuprofen, ifosfamide, imipenem/cilastatin, indomethacin, insulin, irinotecan, isoproterenol, ketamine, ketorolac, labetalol, leucovorin calcium, levofloxacin, lidocaine, linezolid, lorazepam, magnesium sulfate, mannitol, mechlorethamine, melphalan, meperidine, mesna, methotrexate, methylprednisolone, metoclopramide, metoprolol, metronidazole, milrinone, mitomycin, morphine, multivitamins, nafcillin, nalbuphine, naloxone, nesiritide, nitroglycerin, norepinephrine, octreotide, oxacillin, oxaliplatin, oxytocin, paclitaxel, palonosetron, pamidronate, pancuronium, pantoprazole, penicillin G, phenobarbital, phenylephrine, phytonadione, potassium acetate, potassium chloride, procainamide, propranolol, pyridoxine, ranitidine, remifentanil, rituximab, rocuronium, sodium acetate, sodium bicarbonate, sodium citrate, streptokinase, succinylcholine, sufentanil, tacrolimus, telavancin, teniposide, thiotepa, tigecycline, tirofiban, trastuzumab, vasopressin, vecuronium, vinblastine, vincristine, vinorelbine, voriconazole, zidovudine, zoledronic acid.
- **Y-Site Incompatibility:** acetylcysteine, alemtuzumab, amiodarone, amphotericin B liposome, ascorbic acid, azathioprine, calcium chloride, caspofungin, cefotaxime, chloramphenicol, chlorpromazine, dantrolene, daunorubicin hydrochloride, diazepam, diphenhydramine, doxorubicin hydrochloride, doxorubicin liposome, doxycycline, epirubicin, ganciclovir, haloperidol, hydralazine, hydroxyzine, idarubicin, midazolam, mitoxantrone, mycophentolate, nitroprusside, papaverine, pemetrexed, pentamidine, pentazocine, phenytoin, prochlorperazine, promethazine, protamine, quinupristin/dalfopriatin, thiamine, topotecan, trimethoprim/sulfamethoxazole, verapamil, warfarin.

Ceftriaxone

- **Intermittent Infusion:** Reconstitute each 250-mg vial with 2.4 mL, each 500-mg vial with 4.8 mL, each 1-g vial with 9.6 mL, and each 2-g vial with 19.2 mL of sterile water for injection, 0.9% NaCl, or D5W for a concentration of 100 mg/mL. ***Diluent:*** Solution should be further diluted in 50–100 mL of 0.9% NaCl, D5W, D10W, D5/0.45% NaCl, or D5/0.9% NaCl. Solution may appear light yellow to amber. Solution is stable for 3 days at room temperature. ***Concentration:*** 40 mg/mL. ***Rate:*** Infuse over 30 min.
- **Y-Site Compatibility:** acetaminophen, acyclovir, alfentanil, allopurinol, amifostine, aminocaproic acid, aminophylline, amiodarone, amphotericin B lipid complex, amphotericin B liposome, anidulafungin, argatroban, atropine, aztreonam, benztropine, bivalirudin, bumetanide, buprenorphine, butorphanol, cangrelor, carboplatin, carmustine, cefazolin, cefotaxime, cefotetan, cefoxitin, ceftazidime, cefuroxime, cisatracurium, cisplatin, cyanocobalamin, cyclophosphamide, cyclosporine, cytarabine, dactinomycin, daptomycin, dexamethasone, dexmedetomidine, digoxin, diltiazem, docetaxel, dopamine, doxorubicin liposome, doxycycline, enalaprilat, ephedrine, epinephrine, epoetin alfa, epitifibatide, erythromycin, esmolol, etoposide, etoposide phosphate, fenoldopam, fentanyl, fludarabine, fluorouracil, folic acid, foscarnet, fosphenytoin, furosemide, gemcitabine, glycopyrrolate, granisetron, heparin, hetastarch, hydrocortisone, hydromorphone, ifosfamide, indomethacin, insulin, isoproterenol, ketorolac, levofloxacin, lidocaine, linezolid, lorazepam, mannitol, mechlorethamine, melphalan, meperidine, methotrexate, methylprednisolone, metoclopramide, metoprolol, metronidazole, midazolam, milrinone, morphine, multivitamins, nafcillin, nalbuphine, naloxone, nesiritide, nicardipine, nitroglycerin, nitroprusside, norepinephrine, octreotide, oxacillin, oxaliplatin, oxytocin, paclitaxel, palonosetron, pamidronate, pantoprazole, pemetrexed, penicillin G, phenobarbital, phenylephrine, phytonadione, potassium acetate, potassium chloride, procainamide, propranolol, pyridoxine, ranitidine, remifentanil, rituxumab, rocuronium, sargramostim, sodium acetate, sodium bicarbonate, streptokinase, succinylcholine, sufentanil, tacrolimus, telavancin, teniposide, theophylline, thiamine, thiotepa, tigecycline, tirofiban, topotecan, trastuzumab, vasopressin, vecuronium, verapamil, vinblastine, vincristine, voriconazole, warfarin, zidovudine, zoledronic acid.

- **Y-Site Incompatibility:** alemtuzumab, ascorbic acid, azathioprine, azithromycin, calcium chloride, calcium gluconate, caspofungin, chloramphenicol, chlorpromazine, clindamycin, dantrolene, daunorubicin hydrochloride, diazepam, diphenhydramine, dobutamine, doxorubicin hydrochloride, epirubicin, filgrastim, ganciclovir, haloperidol, hetastarch, hydralazine, hydroxyzine, idarubicin, imipenem/cilastatin, irinotecan, labetalol, leucovorin, magnesium sulfate, mitoxantrone, mycophenolate, papaverine, pentamidine, pentazocine, pentobarbital, phenytoin, prochlorperazine, promethazine, protamine, quinupristin/dalfopristin, tobramycin, trimethoprim/sulfamethoxazole, vinorelbine, Calcium-containing solutions, including parenteral nutrition, should not be mixed or co-administered, even via different infusion lines at different sites in patients <28 days old. In older patients, flush line thoroughly between infusions.

Patient/Family Teaching

- Instruct patient to take medication around the clock and to finish the medication completely, even if feeling better. Take missed doses as soon as possible unless almost time for next dose; do not double doses. Advise patient that sharing of this medication may be dangerous.
- Pedi: Instruct parents or caregivers to use calibrated measuring device with liquid preparations.
- Advise patient to report signs of superinfection (furry overgrowth on the tongue, vaginal itching or discharge, loose or foul-smelling stools) and allergy.
- Instruct patient to notify health care professional if rash, fever and diarrhea develop, especially if stool contains blood, pus, or mucus. Advise patient not to treat diarrhea without consulting health care professional.

Evaluation/Desired Outcomes

- Resolution of the signs and symptoms of infection. Length of time for complete resolution depends on the organism and site of infection.
- Decreased incidence of infection when used for prophylaxis.

ceritinib (se-ri-ti-nib)

Zykadia

Classification

Therapeutic: antineoplastics
Pharmacologic: kinase inhibitors

Pregnancy Category D

Indications

Treatment of anaplastic lymphoma kinase (ALK)-positive metastatic non-small cell lung cancer (NSCLC) that has progressed despite treatment with or intolerance to crizotinib.

Action

Acts as a tyrosine kinase inhibitor, inhibiting anaplastic lymphoma kinase as well as other kinases, resulting in decreased growth of certain malignant cell lines.
Therapeutic Effects: Slowed progression of metastatic NSCLC.

Pharmacokinetics

Absorption: Absorption follows oral administration; food significantly ↑ absorption and may ↑ risk of adverse reactions.
Distribution: Slight preference to distribute from plasma into red blood cells.
Metabolism and Excretion: Metabolized in the liver (mostly by CYP3A) and is a substrate of P-glucoprotein (P-gp); 68% eliminated unchanged in feces, 1.3% in urine.
Half-life: 41 hr.

TIME/ACTION PROFILE (clinical response)

ROUTE	ONSET	PEAK	DURATION
PO	unknown	4–6 hr (blood level)	7.1–7.4 mos

Contraindications/Precautions

Contraindicated in: OB: Pregnancy (may cause fetal harm); Lactation: Discontinue ceritinib or discontinue breast feeding.; Congenital long QT syndrome
Use Cautiously in: Females with reproductive potential (effective contraception required); Moderate to severe hepatic impairment/severe renal impairment (CCr <30 mL/min); HF, bradycardia, electrolyte abnormalities, or concurrent use of QT prolonging medications; Pedi: Safety and effectiveness not established.

Adverse Reactions/Side Effects

CNS: fatigue. **Resp:** INTERSTITIAL LUNG DISEASE/PNEUMONITIS. **CV:** QT INTERVAL PROLONGATION, bradycardia. **GI:** HEPATOTOXICITY, PANCREATITIS, abdominal pain, ↓ appetite, constipation, diarrhea, esophagitis/reflux/dysphagia, ↑ liver enzymes, nausea, vomiting, hepatotoxicity. **Derm:** rash. **Endo:** hyperglycemia. **F and E:** hypophosphatemia. **GU:** ↑ creatinine. **Hemat:** anemia. **Metab:** ↑ lipase.

Interactions

Drug-Drug: Concurrent use of strong **CYP3A inhibitors** including **ketoconazole**, **nefazodone**, and **telithromycin** ↑ blood levels and the risk of toxicities; avoid concurrent use; if unavoidable, ↓ ceritinib dose. Strong **CYP3A inducers** including **carbamazepine**, **phenytoin**, and **rifampin** may ↓ blood levels and effectiveness; avoid concurrent use. May ↑ blood levels and the risk of toxicity of CYP3A4 and CYP2C9 substrates, including **alfentanil**, **cyclosporine**, **dihyroergotamine**, **ergotamine**, **fentanyl**, **phenytoin**, **pimozide**, **quinidine**, **sirolimus**, **tacrolimus**, and **warfarin**; dose of these medications may need to be ↓.

Concurrent use of **QT interval prolonging medications** may ↑ risk of QT interval prolongation and torsade de pointes.

Drug-Food: Grapefruit/grapefruit juice ↑ blood levels and the risk of toxicity; concurrent ingestion should be avoided. **St. John's wort** ↓ blood levels and effectiveness; concurrent use should be avoided.

Route/Dosage

PO (Adults): 750 mg once daily; dose ↓/modification/discontinuation required for GI toxicity, ↑ liver enzymes, hyperglycemia, QT prolongation, or bradycardia; *Concurrent use of strong CYP3A inhibitors*—↓ dose by 1/3 rounded to the nearest 150 mg strength.

Availability

Capsules: 150 mg.

NURSING IMPLICATIONS

Assessment

- Assess for signs and symptoms of interstitial lung disease or pneumonitis (trouble breathing, shortness of breath, fever, cough with or without mucus, chest pain). If these symptoms occur, discontinue therapy permanently.
- Monitor ECG periodically during therapy. If QTc interval is >500 msec on at least 2 separate ECGs, withhold ceritinib until QTc interval <481 msec or recovery to baseline if QTc ≥481 msec, then resume ceritinib with a 150 mg dose reduction. If QTc interval prolongation occurs in combination with torsades de pointes or polymorphic ventricular tachycardia or signs and symptoms of serious arrhythmia, discontinue ceritinib permanently.
- If symptomatic bradycardia that is not life-threatening occurs, withhold ceritinib until recovery to asymptomatic bradycardia or a heart rate ≥ 60 bpm, evaluate concurrent medications causing bradycardia, and adjust dose of ceritinib. If clinically significant bradycardia requiring intervention or life-threatening bradycardia in patients taking concurrent medication known to cause bradycardia or a medication known to cause hypotension occurs, withhold ceritinib until recovery to asymptomatic bradycardia or a heart rate ≥60 bpm. If concurrent medication can be adjusted or discontinued, resume ceritinib with a 150 mg dose reduction and frequent monitoring. If life-threatening bradycardia occurs in patients not taking medications known to cause bradycardia or hypotension, discontinue ceritinib permanently.
- Assess for nausea, vomiting, diarrhea. If severe or intolerable nausea, vomiting, or diarrhea continue despite optimal antiemetic or antidiarrheal therapy, withhold ceritinib until improved; then resume with a 150 mg dose reduction.
- ***Lab Test Considerations:*** Monitor liver function tests at least monthly. If ALT or AST >5 times the upper limit of normal and total bilirubin is ≤2 times the upper limit of normal, withhold ceritinib until recovery to baseline or less than or equal to 3 times the upper limit of normal, then resume ceritinib with a 150 mg dose reduction. If ALT or AST >3 times the upper limit of normal and total bilirubin is >2 times the upper limit of normal in the absence of cholestasis or hemolysis, permanently discontinue ceritinib.
- Monitor fasting blood glucose prior to and periodically during therapy. If persistent hyperglycemia >250 m g/dL despite anti-hyperglycemic therapy, withhold ceritinib until hyperglycemia is adequately controlled, then resume with a 150 mg dose reduction. If adequate hyperglycemic control cannot be achieved, discontinue therapy.
- May cause ↓ hemoglobin and serum phosphate; ↑ creatinine.
- Monitor serum lipase and amylase prior to and periodically during therapy. May cause ↑ serum lipase and amylase. If ↑ lipase or amylase >2 x upper limit of normal, withhold ceritinib and monitor serum lipase and amylase. When recovery to <1.5 x upper limit of normal, resume with 150 mg dose.

Potential Nursing Diagnoses

Ineffective airway clearance (Indications)
Deficient knowledge, related to medication regimen (Patient/Family Teaching)

Implementation

- **PO:** Administer on an empty stomach, at least 2 hr before or after meals.

Patient/Family Teaching

- Instruct patient to take ceritinib as directed. Take missed doses as soon as remembered unless within 12 hrs of next dose. If vomiting occurs, do not administer additional dose, continue with next scheduled dose. Instruct patient to read *Patient Information* prior to starting therapy and with each Rx refill in case of changes.
- Inform patient to avoid consuming grapefruit and grapefruit juice during therapy.
- Advise patient to notify health care professional if nausea, vomiting, and diarrhea is severe or persistent; if signs and symptoms of hepatotoxicity (feeling tired, itchy skin, skin or whites of eyes turn yellow, nausea and vomiting, decreased appetite, pain on right side of stomach, dark or brown, tea-colored urine, bleed or bruise easily); pneumonitis; QTc interval prolongation or bradycardia (new chest pain, changes in heartbeat, palpitations, dizziness, fainting, or changes in or use of a new heart or BP medication); hyperglycemia (increased thirst, increased hunger, headaches, trouble thinking or concentra-

tion, urinating often, blurred vision, tiredness, breath smells like fruit).

- Rep: Advise female patient to use effective contraceptives during and for at least 2 wks following completion of therapy and to notify health care provider if pregnancy is planned or suspected or if breast feeding.

Evaluation/Desired Outcomes

- Slowed progression of metastatic NSCLC.

certolizumab pegol

(ser-toe-**liz**-u-mab pey-**gol**)

Cimzia

Classification

Therapeutic: gastrointestinal anti-inflammatories, antirheumatics

Pharmacologic: tumor necrosis factor blockers, DMARDs, monoclonal antibodies

Pregnancy Category B

Indications

Moderately-to-severely active Crohn's disease when response to conventional therapy has been inadequate. Moderately-to-severely active rheumatoid arthritis. Active psoriatic arthritis. Active ankylosing spondylitis.

Action

Neutralizes tumor necrosis factor (TNF), a prime mediator of inflammation; pegylation provides a long duration of action. **Therapeutic Effects:** Decreased signs/symptoms of Crohn's disease. Decreased pain and swelling, decreased rate of joint destruction and improved physical function in rheumatoid arthritis. Decreased joint swelling and pain in psoriatic arthritis. Decreased spinal pain and inflammation in ankylosing spondylitis.

Pharmacokinetics

Absorption: 80% absorbed following SC administration.

Distribution: Unknown.

Metabolism and Excretion: Unknown.

Half-life: 14 days.

TIME/ACTION PROFILE (blood levels)

ROUTE	ONSET	PEAK	DURATION
Subcut	unknown	50–120 hr	2–4 wk

Contraindications/Precautions

Contraindicated in: Active infection (including localized); Concurrent use of anakinra.

Use Cautiously in: History of chronic or recurrent infection or underlying illness/treatment predisposing to infection; History of exposure to tuberculosis; History of opportunistic infection; Patients residing, or who have resided, where tuberculosis, histoplasmosis, coccidioidomycoses, or blastomycosis is endemic; History of demyelinating disorders (may exacerbate); History of heart failure; Geri: May ↑ risk of infections; OB: Use in pregnancy only if clearly needed; avoid breast feeding; Pedi: Safety not established; ↑ risk of lymphoma (including hepatosplenic T-cell lymphoma [HSTCL] in patients with Crohn's disease), leukemia, and other malignancies.

Adverse Reactions/Side Effects

Derm: psoriasis, skin reactions (rarely severe). **Hemat:** hematologic reactions. **MS:** arthralgia. **Misc:** hypersensitivity reactions including ANAPHYLAXIS AND ANGIOEDEMA, INFECTIONS (including reactivation tuberculosis, hepatitis B reactivation, and other opportunistic infections due to bacterial, invasive fungal, viral, mycobacterial, and parasitic pathogens), MALIGNANCY (including lymphoma, HSTCL, leukemia, and skin cancer), lupus-like syndrome.

Interactions

Drug-Drug: Concurrent use with **anakinra** ↑ risk of serious infections (contraindicated). Concurrent use with **azathioprine** and/or **methotrexate** may ↑ risk of HSTCL. May ↓ antibody response to or ↑ risk of adverse reactions to **live vaccines** (contraindicated).

Route/Dosage

Crohn's Disease

Subcut (Adults): 400 mg initially, repeat 2 and 4 wk later; may be followed by maintenance dose of 400 mg every 4 wk.

Rheumatoid Arthritis, Psoriatic Arthritis, and Ankylosing Spondylitis

Subcut (Adults): 400 mg initially, repeat 2 and 4 wk later; then maintenance dose of 200 mg every 2 wk (400 mg every 4 wk may be used alternatively).

Availability

Lyophilized powder for subcutaneous injection (requires reconstitution): 200 mg/vial. **Prefilled syringe:** 200 mg/mL.

NURSING IMPLICATIONS

Assessment

- **Crohn's Disease:** Assess abdominal pain and frequency, quantity, and consistency of stools at beginning and during therapy.
- **Arthritis/Ankylosing Spondylitis:** Assess pain and range of motion before and periodically during therapy.
- Assess for signs of infection (fever, sore throat, dyspnea, WBC) prior to and during therapy. Monitor all patients for active TB during therapy, even if initial test was negative. Do not begin certolizumab during an active infection, including chronic or localized infections. If infection develops, monitor closely and discontinue certolizumab if infection becomes serious.

- Evaluate patients at risk for hepatitis B virus (HBV) infection for prior evidence of HBV infection before initiating therapy. Monitor carriers of HBV closely for clinical and lab signs of active HBV infection during and for several months following discontinuation of therapy. If HBV reactivation occurs, discontinue certolizumab and initiate antiviral therapy.
- Monitor for signs of hypersensitivity reactions (angioedema, dyspnea, hypotension, rash, serum sickness, urticaria). If reactions occur, discontinue certolizumab and treat symptomatically.
- Assess for signs and symptoms of systemic fungal infections (fever, malaise, weight loss, sweats, cough, dypsnea, pulmonary infiltrates, serious systemic illness with or without concomitant shock). Ascertain if patient lives in or has traveled to areas of endemic mycoses. Consider empiric antifungal treatment for patients at risk of histoplasmosis and other invasive fungal infections until the pathogens are identified. Consult with an infectious diseases specialist. Consider stopping certolizumab until the infection has been diagnosed and adequately treated.
- ***Lab Test Considerations:*** May cause anemia, leukopenia, pancytopenia, and thrombocytopenia.
- Monitor CBC with differential periodically during therapy. May cause leukopenia, neutropenia, thrombocytopenia, and pancytopenia. Discontinue certolizumab if symptoms of blood dyscrasias (persistent fever) occur.
- May cause ↑ liver enzymes.
- May cause erroneously ↑ aPTT.

Potential Nursing Diagnoses

Risk for infection (Side Effects)

Implementation

- Perform test for latent TB. If positive, begin treatment for TB prior to starting certolizumab therapy. Monitor for TB throughout therapy, even if latent TB test is negative.
- Bring medication to room temperature prior to reconstituting. Reconstitute 2 vials for each dose by adding 1 mL of Sterile Water for injection to each vial, using a 20-gauge needle, for a concentration of 200 mg/mL. Gently swirl so all powder comes into contact with sterile water; do not shake. Leave vials undisturbed for as long as 30 min to fully reconstitute. Solution is clear and colorless to pale yellow; do not administer solutions that are discolored or contain particulate matter. Do not leave reconstituted solution at room temperature for >2 hr prior to injection. May be refrigerated for up to 24 hr prior to injection; do not freeze.
- **Subcut:** Bring solution to room temperature prior to injection. Using a new 20-gauge needle for each vial, withdraw reconstituted solution into 2 separate syringes each containing 1 mL (200 mg/mL) of certolizumab. Switch each 20-gauge needle to a 23-gauge needle and inject the full contents of each syringe subcut into separate sides of the abdomen or thigh.

Patient/Family Teaching

- Advise patient of potential benefits and risks of certolizumab. Advise patient to read the *Medication Guide* prior to starting therapy.
- Inform patient of risk of infection. Advise patient to notify health care professional if symptoms of infection (fever, cough, flu-like symptoms, or open cuts or sores), including TB or reactivation of HBV infection, occur.
- Counsel patient about possible risk of lymphoma and other malignancies while receiving certolizumab.
- Advise patient to notify health care professional if signs of hypersensitivity reactions (rash, swollen face, difficulty breathing), or new or worsening medical conditions such as heart or neurological disease or autoimmune disorders occur and to report signs of bone marrow depression (bruising, bleeding, or persistent failure).
- Instruct patient to notify health care professional of all Rx or OTC medications, vitamins, or herbal products being taken and to consult health care professional prior to taking any Rx, OTC, vitamins, or herbal products.
- Advise patient to notify health care professional if pregnancy is planned or suspected or if breast feeding.

Evaluation/Desired Outcomes

- Decrease in signs and symptoms of Crohn's disease.
- Decreased pain and swelling with decreased rate of joint destruction in patients with rheumatoid arthritis.
- Decreased joint swelling and pain in psoriatic arthritis.
- Decreased spinal pain and inflammation in ankylosing spondylitis.

cetirizine (se-ti-ra-zeen)

✱Aller Relief, ✱Reactine, ZyrTEC

Classification

Therapeutic: allergy, cold, and cough remedies, antihistamines

Pharmacologic: piperazines (peripherally selective)

Pregnancy Category B

Indications

Relief of allergic symptoms caused by histamine release including: Seasonal and perennial allergic rhinitis, Chronic urticaria.

Action

Antagonizes the effects of histamine at H_1-receptor sites; does not bind to or inactivate histamine. Anticholinergic effects are minimal and sedation is dose related.

Therapeutic Effects: Decreased symptoms of histamine excess (sneezing, rhinorrhea, ocular tearing and redness, pruritus).

Pharmacokinetics

Absorption: Well absorbed following oral administration.

Distribution: Unknown.

Protein Binding: 93%.

Metabolism and Excretion: Excreted primarily unchanged by the kidneys.

Half-life: 7.4–9 hr (↓ in children to 6.2 hr, ↑ in renal impairment up to 19–21 hr).

TIME/ACTION PROFILE (antihistaminic effects)

ROUTE	ONSET	PEAK	DURATION
PO	30 min	4–8 hr	24 hr

Contraindications/Precautions

Contraindicated in: Hypersensitivity to cetirizine, hydroxyzine or any component; Lactation: Excreted in breast milk; not recommended for use.

Use Cautiously in: Patients with hepatic or renal impairment (dose ↓ recommended if CCr ≤31 mL/min or hepatic function is impaired); OB, Pedi: Safety not established for pregnant women or children <6 mo; Geri: Initiate at lower doses.

Adverse Reactions/Side Effects

CNS: dizziness, drowsiness (significant with doses >10 mg/day), fatigue. **EENT:** pharyngitis. **GI:** dry mouth.

Interactions

Drug-Drug: Additive CNS depression may occur with **alcohol, opioid analgesics**, or **sedative/hypnotics**. **Theophylline** may ↓ clearance and ↑ toxicity.

Route/Dosage

PO (Adults and children ≥6 yr): 5–10 mg given once or divided twice daily.

PO (Children 2–5 yr): 2.5 mg once daily initially, may be ↑ to 5 mg once daily or 2.5 mg every 12 hr.

PO (Children 1–2 yr): 2.5 mg once daily; may be ↑ to 2.5 mg every 12 hr.

PO (Children 6–12 mo): 2.5 once daily.

Hepatic/Renal Impairment

PO (Adults and Children ≥12 yr): *CCr ≤31 mL/min, hepatic impairment or hemodialysis*—5 mg once daily.

Hepatic/Renal Impairment

PO (Children 6–11 yr): start therapy at <2.5 mg/day.

Hepatic/Renal Impairment

PO (Children <6 yr): use not recommended.

Availability (generic available)

Tablets: 5 mg[OTC], 10 mg[OTC]. **Capsules:** 5 mg[OTC], 10 mg[OTC]. **Chewable tablets (grape):** 5 mg[OTC], 10 mg[OTC]. **Orally disintegrating tablets:** 10 mg. **Syrup (banana-grape and bubblegum flavors):** 1 mg/mL[OTC]. ***In combination with:*** pseudoephedrine (Zyrtec-D 12 hr) (See Appendix B).

NURSING IMPLICATIONS

Assessment

- Assess allergy symptoms (rhinitis, conjunctivitis, hives) before and periodically during therapy.
- Assess lung sounds and character of bronchial secretions. Maintain fluid intake of 1500–2000 mL/day to decrease viscosity of secretions.
- ***Lab Test Considerations:*** May cause false-negative result in allergy skin testing.

Potential Nursing Diagnoses

Ineffective airway clearance (Indications)
Risk for injury (Adverse Reactions)

Implementation

- Do not confuse cetirizine with sertraline or stavudine. Do not confuse Zyrtec (cetirizine) with Zerit (Stavudine), Lipitor (atorvastatin), Zantac (ranitidine), Zocor (simvastatin), Zyprexa (olanzapine), Zyrtec-D (cetirizine/pseudoephedrine), Zyrtec Itchy Eye Drops (ketotifen fumarate).
- **PO:** Administer once daily without regard to food.

Patient/Family Teaching

- Instruct patient to take medication as directed.
- May cause dizziness and drowsiness. Caution patient to avoid driving or other activities requiring alertness until response to medication is known.
- Advise patient to avoid taking alcohol or other CNS depressants concurrently with this drug.
- Advise patient that good oral hygiene, frequent rinsing of mouth with water, and sugarless gum or candy may minimize dry mouth. Patient should notify dentist if dry mouth persists >2 wk.
- Instruct patient to contact health care professional if dizziness occurs or if symptoms persist.

Evaluation/Desired Outcomes

- Decrease in allergic symptoms.

cetuximab (se-**tux**-i-mab)

Erbitux

Classification
Therapeutic: antineoplastics
Pharmacologic: monoclonal antibodies

Pregnancy Category C

Indications

Locally or regionally advanced squamous cell carcinoma of the head and neck with radiation. Recurrent or metastatic squamous cell carcinoma of the head and neck progressing after platinum-based therapy. Recurrent or metastatic squamous cell carcinoma of the head and neck in combination with platinum-based therapy with 5-fluorouracil. ⧛ *K-ras* wild-type, epidermal growth factor receptor (EGFR)-expressing metastatic colorectal cancer in patients who have not responded to irinotecan and oxaliplatin or are intolerant to irinotecan. ⧛ In combination with irinotecan in patients with *K-ras* wild-type, EGFR-expressing metastatic colorectal cancer who have not responded to irinotecan alone. ⧛ First-line treatment of *K-ras* wild-type, EGFR-expressing metastatic colorectal cancer in combination with irinotecan, 5-fluorouracil, and leucovorin (FOLFIRI).

Action

⧛ Binds specifically to EGFR, thereby preventing the binding of endogenous epidermal growth factor (EGF). This prevents cell growth and differentiation processes. Combination with irinotecan enhances antitumor effects of irinotecan. **Therapeutic Effects:** Decreased tumor growth and spread.

Pharmacokinetics

Absorption: IV administration results in complete bioavailability.
Distribution: Unknown.
Metabolism and Excretion: Unknown.
Half-life: 97–114 hr.

TIME/ACTION PROFILE

ROUTE	ONSET	PEAK	DURATION
IV	unknown	unknown	unknown

Contraindications/Precautions

Contraindicated in: Hypersensitivity to cetuximab or murine (mouse) proteins; ⧛ *RAS*-mutant metastatic colorectal cancer or unknown *RAS* mutation status (↑ mortality and tumor progression); OB, Lactation: Pregnancy or lactation.
Use Cautiously in: Exposure to sunlight (may exacerbate dermatologic toxicity); Pedi: Safety not established.

Adverse Reactions/Side Effects

Most adverse reactions reflect combination therapy with irinotecan.
CNS: malaise, depression, headache, insomnia. **EENT:** conjunctivitis, ulcerative keratitis. **Resp:** cough, dyspnea, interstitial lung disease. **CV:** CARDIOPULMONARY ARREST, PULMONARY EMBOLISM, SUDDEN CARDIAC DEATH. **GI:** abdominal pain, constipation, diarrhea, nausea, vomiting, anorexia, stomatitis. **GU:** renal failure. **Derm:** STEVENS-JOHNSON SYNDROME, TOXIC EPIDERMAL NECROLYSIS, acneform dermatitis, hypertrichosis, nail disorder, pruritus, skin desquamation, skin infection. **F and E:** dehydration, hypomagnesemia, peripheral edema. **Hemat:** anemia, leukopenia. **MS:** back pain. **Metab:** weight loss. **Misc:** INFUSION REACTIONS, fever, desquamation of mucosal epithelium.

Interactions

Drug-Drug: None noted.

Route/Dosage

Head & Neck Cancer with Radiation or in Combination with Platinum-Based Therapy with 5-Fluorouracil

IV (Adults): 400 mg/m² administered 1 wk prior to initiation of radiation therapy or on the day of initiation of platinum-based therapy with 5-fluorouracil (complete infusion 1 hr to prior to starting platinum-based therapy with 5-fluorouracil), followed by weekly maintenance doses of 250 mg/m² for the duration of radiation therapy or until disease progression or unacceptable toxicity with platinum-based therapy with 5-fluorouracil (complete infusion 1 hr prior to radiation therapy or platinum-based therapy with 5-fluorouracil). Dose modification recommended for dermatologic toxicity.

Head and Neck Cancer Monotherapy

IV (Adults): 400 mg/m² initial loading dose, followed by weekly maintenance doses of 250 mg/m² until disease progression or unacceptable toxicity; dose modification recommended for dermatologic toxicity.

Colorectal Cancer

IV (Adults): 400 mg/m² initial loading dose, followed by weekly maintenance doses of 250 mg/m² until disease progression or unacceptable toxicity; dose modification recommended for dermatologic toxicity.

Availability

Solution for injection: 2 mg/mL.

NURSING IMPLICATIONS

Assessment

- Assess for infusion reaction (rapid onset of airway obstruction [bronchospasm, stridor, hoarseness], urticaria, hypotension, loss of consciousness, myocardial infarction, cardiopulmonary arrest) for at least 1 hr following infusion. Longer observation periods may be required for those who experience infusion reactions. Most reactions occur during first dose, but may also occur in later doses. For severe reactions, immediately stop infusion and discontinue cetuximab permanently. Epinephrine, corticosteroids, IV antihistamines, bronchodilators, and oxygen should be available for reactions. Mild to moderate reactions (chills, fever, dyspnea) may be managed by slowing rate of infusion and administration of antihistamines.
- Assess for onset or worsening of pulmonary symptoms. Interrupt therapy to determine nature of symp-

toms. If interstitial lung disease is confirmed, discontinue cetuximab and treat appropriately.

- Assess for dermatologic toxicities (acneform rash, skin drying and fissuring, inflammatory and infectious sequelae [blepharitis, cheilitis, cellulitis, cyst]). Treat symptomatically. Acneform rash usually occurs within initial 2 wk of therapy and resolves following cessation, but may continue up to 28 days following therapy. *For 1st occurrence of acneform rash,* delay infusion 1–2 wks; if improvement, continue at 250 mg/m^2, if no improvement, discontinue cetuximab. *For 2nd occurrence,* delay infusion 1–2 wks; if improvement, reduce dose to 200 mg/m^2, if no improvement, discontinue cetuximab. *For 3rd occurrence,* delay infusion 1–2 wks; if improvement, reduce dose to 150 mg/m^2, if no improvement, discontinue cetuximab. *For 4th occurrence,* discontinue cetuximab.
- ***Lab Test Considerations:*** Determine Ras mutation and EGFR-expression status using FDA-approved tests prior to initiating treatment. Only patients whose tumors are K-Ras wild-type should receive cetuximab.
- ***Lab Test Considerations:*** May cause anemia and leukopenia.
- Monitor serum electrolytes, especially serum magnesium, potassium, and calcium, closely during and periodically for at least 8 wk following infusion. May cause hypomagnesemia, hypocalcemia, and hypokalemia; may occur from days to months after initiation of therapy. May require electrolyte replacement. May lead to cardiopulmonary arrest and sudden death.

Potential Nursing Diagnoses

Ineffective breathing pattern (Adverse Reactions)
Impaired skin integrity (Adverse Reactions)

Implementation

- Premedicate with histamine$_1$ antagonist (diphenhydramine 50 mg) 30–60 min prior to first dose; base subsequent administration on presence and severity of infusion reactions.
- Administer through a low protein binding 0.22-micrometer in-line filter placed as proximal to patient as possible. Solution should be clear and colorless and may contain a small amount of white amorphous cetuximab particles. Do not shake or dilute.
- Can be administered via infusion pump or syringe pump. Cetuximab should be piggybacked to the patient's infusion line.
- Observe patient for 1 hr following infusion.

IV Administration

- **Intermittent Infusion:** *For administration via infusion pump:* Draw up volume of a vial using vented spike needle or other transfer device. Transfer to a sterile evacuated container or bag. Repeat with new needle for each vial until calculated volume is in container. Affix infusion line and prime with cetuximab before starting infusion.
- *For administration via syringe pump:* Draw up volume of a vial using sterile syringe attached to an appropriate vented spike needle. Place syringe into syringe driver of a syringe pump and set rate. Connect infusion line and prime with cetuximab. Use a new needle and filter for each vial. ***Diluent:*** Do not dilute. ***Concentration:*** 2 mg/mL. ***Rate:*** Administer over 2 hr at a rate not to exceed 10 mg/min. Use 0.9% NaCl to flush line at end of infusion.
- Cetuximab infusion must be completed 1 hr prior to FOLFIRI (irinotecan, 5-fluoruracil, leucovorin) regimen. May infuse subsequent weekly infusions over 1 hr.

Patient/Family Teaching

- Explain purpose of cetuximab and potential side effects to patient.
- Advise patient to report dermatologic changes and signs and symptoms of infusion reactions (fever, chills, or breathing problems) promptly.
- Caution patient to wear sunscreen and hats and limit sun exposure during therapy during and for 2 mo following last dose of cetuximab.
- Rep: Advise both female and male patients to use adequate contraception during and for 6 mo following therapy and to avoid breast feeding during and for 2 mo following therapy.

Evaluation/Desired Outcomes

- Decreased tumor growth and spread.

chlorothiazide, See DIURETICS (THIAZIDE).

chlorproMAZINE

(klor-**proe**-ma-zeen)

~~Thorazine~~

Classification

Therapeutic: antiemetics, antipsychotics
Pharmacologic: phenothiazines

Pregnancy Category C

Indications

Second-line treatment for schizophrenia and psychoses after failure with atypical antipsychotics. Hyperexcitable, combative behavior in children. Nausea and vomiting. Intractable hiccups. Preoperative sedation. Acute intermittent porphyria. **Unlabeled Use:** Vascular headache. Bipolar disorder.

Action

Alters the effects of dopamine in the CNS. Has significant anticholinergic/alpha-adrenergic blocking activity. **Therapeutic Effects:** Diminished signs/symptoms of psychosis. Relief of nausea/vomiting/intractable hiccups. Decreased symptoms of porphyria.

C

Pharmacokinetics

Absorption: Variable absorption from tablets. Well absorbed following IM administration.

Distribution: Widely distributed; high CNS concentrations. Crosses the placenta; enters breast milk.

Protein Binding: ≥90%.

Metabolism and Excretion: Highly metabolized by the liver and GI mucosa. Some metabolites are active.

Half-life: 30 hr.

TIME/ACTION PROFILE (antipsychotic activity, antiemetic activity, sedation)

ROUTE	ONSET	PEAK	DURATION
PO	30–60 min	unknown	4–6 hr
IM	unknown	unknown	4–8 hr
IV	rapid	unknown	unknown

Contraindications/Precautions

Contraindicated in: Hypersensitivity; Hypersensitivity to sulfites (injectable); Cross-sensitivity with other phenothiazines may occur; Angle-closure glaucoma; Bone marrow depression; Severe liver/cardiovascular disease; Concurrent pimozide use.

Use Cautiously in: Diabetes; Respiratory disease; Prostatic hyperplasia; CNS tumors; Epilepsy; Intestinal obstruction; OB: Neonates at ↑ risk for extrapyramidal symptoms and withdrawal after delivery when exposed during the 3rd trimester; use only if benefit outweighs risk to fetus; Lactation: Discontinue drug or bottle feed; Pedi: Children with acute illnesses, infections, gastroenteritis, or dehydration (↑ risk of extrapyramidal reactions); Geri: ↑ risk of mortality in elderly patients treated for dementia-related psychosis; Geri: Geriatric/debilitated patients (↓ initial dose).

Adverse Reactions/Side Effects

CNS: NEUROLEPTIC MALIGNANT SYNDROME, sedation, extrapyramidal reactions, tardive dyskinesia. **EENT:** blurred vision, dry eyes, lens opacities. **CV:** hypotension (↑ with IM, IV), tachycardia. **GI:** constipation, dry mouth, anorexia, hepatitis, ileus, priapism. **GU:** urinary retention. **Derm:** photosensitivity, pigment changes, rash. **Endo:** galactorrhea, amenorrhea. **Hemat:** AGRANULOCYTOSIS, leukopenia. **Metab:** hyperthermia. **Misc:** allergic reactions.

Interactions

Drug-Drug: Pimozide ↑ the risk of potentially serious cardiovascular reactions; concurrent use contraindicated. May alter serum **phenytoin** levels. ↓ pressor effect of **norepinephrine** and eliminates bradycardia. Antagonizes peripheral vasoconstriction from **epinephrine** and may reverse some of its actions. May ↓ elimination and ↑ effects of **valproic acid**. May ↓ the pharmacologic effects of **amphetamine** and **related compounds**. May ↓ the effectiveness of **bromocriptine**. May ↑ blood levels and effects of **tricyclic antidepressants**. **Antacids** or **adsorbent antidiarrheals** may ↓ adsorption; administer 1 hr before or 2 hr after chlorpromazine. ↑ risk of anticholinergic effects with **antihistamines**, **tricyclic antidepressants**, **quinidine**, or **disopyramide**. Premedication with chlorpromazine ↑ the risk of neuromuscular excitation and hypotension when followed by **barbiturate** anesthesia. **Barbiturates** may ↑ metabolism and ↓ effectiveness. Chlorpromazine may ↓ **barbiturate** levels. Additive hypotension with **antihypertensives**. Additive CNS depression with **alcohol**, **antidepressants**, **antihistamines**, **MAO inhibitors**, **opioid analgesics**, **sedative/hypnotics**, or **general anesthetics**. Concurrent use with **lithium** may produce disorientation, unconsciousness, or extrapyramidal symptoms. Concurrent use with **meperidine** may produce excessive sedation and hypotension. Concurrent use with **propranolol** ↑ blood levels of both drugs.

Drug-Natural Products: Concomitant use of **kava-kava**, **valerian**, **chamomile**, or **hops** can ↑ CNS depression. ↑ anticholinergic effects with **angel's trumpet**, **jimson weed**, and **scopolia**.

Route/Dosage

PO (Adults): *Psychoses*—10–25 mg 2–4 times daily; may ↑ every 3–4 days (usual dose is 200 mg/day; up to 1 g/day). *Nausea and vomiting*—10–25 mg q 4 hr as needed. *Preoperative sedation*—25–50 mg 2–3 hr before surgery. *Hiccups/porphyria*—25–50 mg 3–4 times daily.

PO (Children): *Psychoses/nausea and vomiting*—0.55 mg/kg (15 mg/m²) q 4–6 hr as needed. *Preoperative sedation*—0.55 mg/kg (15 mg/m²) 2–3 hr before surgery.

IM (Adults): *Severe psychoses*—25–50 mg initially, may be repeated in 1 hr; ↑ to maximum of 400 mg q 3–12 hr if needed (up to 1 g/day). *Nausea/vomiting*—25 mg initially, may repeat with 25–50 mg q 3–4 hr as needed. *Nausea/vomiting during surgery*—12.5 mg, may be repeated in 30 min as needed. *Preoperative sedation*—12.5–25 mg 1–2 hr prior to surgery. *Hiccups/tetanus*—25–50 mg 3–4 times daily. *Porphyria*—25 mg q 6–8 hr until patient can take PO.

IM (Children 6 mo): *Psychoses/nausea and vomiting*—0.55 mg/kg (15 mg/m²) q 6–8 hr (not to exceed 40 mg/day in children 6 mo–5 yr, or 75 mg/day in children 5–12 yr). *Nausea/vomiting during surgery*—0.275 mg/kg, may repeat in 30 min as needed. *Preoperative sedation*—0.55 mg/kg 1–2 hr prior to surgery. *Tetanus*—0.55 mg/kg q 6–8 hr.

IV (Adults): *Nausea/vomiting during surgery*—up to 25 mg. *Hiccups/tetanus*—25–50 mg. *Porphyria*—25 mg q 8 hr.

IV (Children): *Nausea/vomiting during surgery*—0.275 mg/kg. *Tetanus*—0.55 mg/kg.

Availability (generic available)

Tablets: 10 mg, 25 mg, 50 mg, 100 mg, 200 mg. **Injection:** 25 mg/mL.

NURSING IMPLICATIONS

Assessment

- Assess mental status (orientation, mood, behavior) prior to and periodically during therapy.
- Assess weight and BMI initially and throughout therapy. Refer as appropriate for nutritional/weight and medical management.
- Assess positive (hallucinations, delusions, agitation) and negative (social withdrawal) symptoms of schizophrenia.
- Monitor BP (sitting, standing, lying), pulse, and respiratory rate prior to and frequently during the period of dose adjustment.
- Observe patient carefully when administering medication to ensure medication is actually taken and not hoarded.
- Assess fluid intake and bowel function. Increased bulk and fluids in the diet may help minimize constipation.
- Monitor patient for onset of akathisia (restlessness or desire to keep moving) and extrapyramidal side effects (*parkinsonian*—difficulty speaking or swallowing, loss of balance control, pill rolling of hands, mask-like face, shuffling gait, rigidity, tremors; and *dystonic*—muscle spasms, twisting motions, twitching, inability to move eyes, weakness of arms or legs) every 2 mo during therapy and 8–12 wk after therapy has been discontinued. Notify health care professional if these symptoms occur; reduction in dose or discontinuation may be necessary. Trihexyphenidyl, diphenhydramine, or benzotropine may be used to control these symptoms. Benzodiazepines may alleviate symptoms of akathisia.
- Monitor for tardive dyskinesia (uncontrolled rhythmic movement of mouth, face, and extremities; lip smacking or puckering; puffing of cheeks; uncontrolled chewing; rapid or worm-like movements of tongue, excessive eye blinking). Report these symptoms immediately; may be irreversible.
- Monitor for development of neuroleptic malignant syndrome (fever, respiratory distress, tachycardia, convulsions, diaphoresis, hypertension or hypotension, pallor, tiredness, severe muscle stiffness, loss of bladder control). Report these symptoms immediately.
- Monitor for symptoms related to hyperprolactinemia (menstrual abnormalities, galactorrhea, sexual dysfunction).
- **Preoperative Sedation:** Assess level of anxiety prior to and following administration.
- **Vascular Headache:** Assess type, location, intensity, and duration of pain and accompanying symptoms.
- ***Lab Test Considerations:*** Monitor CBC, liver function tests, and ocular exams periodically throughout therapy. May cause ↓ hematocrit, hemoglobin, leukocytes, granulocytes, platelets. May cause ↑ bilirubin, AST, ALT, and alkaline phosphatase. Agranulocytosis occurs 4–10 wk after initiation of therapy, with recovery 1–2 wk following discontinuation. May recur if medication is restarted. Liver function abnormalities may require discontinuation of therapy. May cause false-positive or false-negative pregnancy tests and false-positive urine bilirubin test results.
- Assess fasting blood glucose and cholesterol levels initially and periodically throughout therapy.
- May cause ↑ serum prolactin levels.

Potential Nursing Diagnoses

Disturbed thought process (Indications)
Imbalanced nutrition: risk for more than body requirements (Side Effects)

Implementation

- Do not confuse chlorpromazine with chlorpropamide, chlordiazepoxide, or prochlorperazine.
- Keep patient recumbent for at least 30 min following parenteral administration to minimize hypotensive effects.
- **Hiccups:** Initial treatment is with oral doses. If hiccups persist 2–3 days, IM injection may be used, followed by IV infusion.
- **PO:** Administer oral doses with food, milk, or a full glass of water to minimize gastric irritation. Tablets may be crushed.
- **IM:** Do not inject subcut. Inject slowly into deep, well-developed muscle. May be diluted with 0.9% NaCl or 2% procaine. Lemon-yellow color does not alter potency of solution. Do not administer solution that is markedly discolored or contains a precipitate.

IV Administration

- **IV Push:** ***Diluent:*** Dilute with 0.9% NaCl. ***Concentration:*** Do not exceed 1 mg/mL. ***Rate:*** Inject slowly at a rate of at least 1 mg/min for adults and 0.5 mg/min for children.
- **Continuous Infusion:** ***Diluent:*** May further dilute 25–50 mg in 500–1000 mL of D5W, D10W, 0.45% NaCl, 0.9% NaCl, Ringer's or lactated Ringer's injection, dextrose/Ringer's or dextrose/lactated Ringer's combinations.
- **Y-Site Compatibility:** alemtuzumab, alfentanyl, amikacin, amphotericin B lipid complex, amsacrine, anidulafungin, argatroban, ascorbic acid, atracurium, atropine, benztropine, bleomycin, buprenorphine, butorphanol, calcium chloride, calcium gluconate, carmustine, caspofungin, cisatracurium, cisplatin, cladribine, cyanocobalamin, cyclophosphamide, cyclosporine, cytarabine, dactinomycin, daptomycin, dexmedetomidine, digoxin, diltiazem, diphenhydramine, dobutamine, docetaxel, dopamine, doxacurium, doxorubicin, doxorubicin liposome, doxycycline, enalaprilat, ephedrine, epinephrine, epirubicin, erythromycin, esmolol, etoposide,

famotidine, fenoldopam, fentanyl, filgrastim, fluconazole, gemcitabine, gentamicin, glycopyrrolate, granisetron, hetastarch, hydrocortisone, hydromorphone, idarubicin, ifosfamide, isoproterenol, labetalol, levofloxacin, lidocaine, lorazepam, magnesium sulfate, mannitol, mechlorethamine, meperidine, methoxamine, methyldopate, methylprednisolone, metoclopramide, metoprolol, metronidazole, miconazole, midazolam, milrinone, mitoxantrone, morphine, multivitamins, mycophenolate, nafcillin, nalbuphine, naloxone, nitroglycerin, norepinephrine, octreotide, ondansetron, oxacillin, oxaliplatin, palonosetron, pamidronate, pancuronium, papaverine, penicillin G potassium, pentamidine, pentazocine, phentolamine, phytonadione, potassium acetate, potassium chloride, procainamide, prochlorperazine, promethazine, propofol, propranolol, protamine, pyridoxime, quinupristin/dalfopristin, ranitidine, rituximab, rocuronium, sodium acetate, succinylcholine, sufentanil, tacrolimus, teniposide, theophylline, thiamine, thiotepa, tirofiban, tolazoline, trimetaphan, vancomycin, vasopressin, vecuronium, verapamil, vincristine, vinorelbine, vitamin B complex with C, voriconazole, zoledronic acid.

- **Y-Site Incompatibility:** acetaminophen, acyclovir, allopurinol, amifostine, aminophylline, amphotericin B cholesteryl, amphotericin B colloidal, amphotericin B liposome, ampicillin, ampicillin/sulbactam, azathioprine, aztreonam, bivalirudin, bumetanide, carboplatin, cefazolin, cefepime, cefotaxime, cefotetan, cefoxitin, ceftriaxone, cefuroxime, chloramphenicol, clindamycin, dantrolene, dexamethasone, diazepam, diazoxide, epoetin alfa, eptifibatide, ertapenem, etoposide phosphate, fludarabine, fluorouracil, folic acid, furosemide, ganciclovir, hydralazine, imipenem/cilastatin, indomethacin, insulin, irinotecan, ketorolac, linezolid, melphalan, methotrexate, nitroprusside, paclitaxel, pantoprazole, pemetrexed, pentobarbital, phenobarbital, phenytoin, piperacillin/tazobactam, sargramostim, sodium bicarbonate, streptokinase, ticarcillin/clavulanate, tigecycline, trastuzumab, trimethoprim/sulfamethoxazole.

Patient/Family Teaching

- Advise patient to take medication as directed and not to skip doses or double up on missed doses. If a dose is missed, take within 1 hr or omit dose and return to regular schedule. Abrupt withdrawal may lead to gastritis, nausea, vomiting, dizziness, headache, tachycardia, and insomnia.
- Inform patient of possibility of extrapyramidal symptoms and tardive dyskinesia. Instruct patient to report these symptoms immediately to health care professional.
- Advise patient to change positions slowly to minimize orthostatic hypotension.
- May cause drowsiness. Caution patient to avoid driving or other activities requiring alertness until response to the medication is known.
- Caution patient to avoid taking alcohol or other CNS depressants concurrently with this medication.
- Advise patient to use sunscreen and protective clothing when exposed to the sun. Exposed surfaces may develop a temporary pigment change (ranging from yellow-brown to grayish purple). Extremes of temperature (exercise, hot weather, hot baths or showers) should also be avoided, because this drug impairs body temperature regulation.
- Instruct patient to use frequent mouth rinses, good oral hygiene, and sugarless gum or candy to minimize dry mouth. Consult health care professional if dry mouth continues for 2 wk.
- Advise patient not to take chlorpromazine within 2 hr of antacids or antidiarrheal medication.
- Inform patient that this medication may turn urine a pink-to-reddish-brown color.
- Advise patient to notify health care professional of medication regimen prior to treatment or surgery.
- Instruct patient to notify health care professional promptly if sore throat, fever, unusual bleeding or bruising, rash, weakness, tremors, visual disturbances, dark-colored urine, or clay-colored stools occur.
- Advise female patients to notify health care professional if pregnancy is planned or suspected or if breast feeding.
- Emphasize the importance of routine follow-up exams to monitor response to medication and detect side effects. Encourage continued participation in psychotherapy as indicated.
- Treatment is not a cure; symptoms may recur after discontinuation of medication.

Evaluation/Desired Outcomes

- Decrease in excitable, manic behavior. Therapeutic effects may not be seen for 7–8 wk.
- Relief of nausea and vomiting.
- Relief of hiccups.
- Preoperative sedation.
- Management of porphyria.
- Relief of vascular headache.
- Decrease in positive (hallucinations, delusions, agitation) symptoms of schizophrenia.

chlorthalidone, See DIURETICS (THIAZIDE).

cholecalciferol, See VITAMIN D COMPOUNDS.

choline and magnesium salicylates, See SALICYLATES.

ciclesonide, See CORTICOSTEROIDS (NASAL).

ciclopirox, See ANTIFUNGALS (TOPICAL).

cilostazol (sil-**os**-tah-zol)

Pletal

Classification

Therapeutic: antiplatelet agents

Pharmacologic: platelet aggregation inhibitors

Pregnancy Category C

Indications

Reduction of the symptoms of intermittent claudication as measured by increased walking distance.

Action

Inhibits the enzyme cyclic adenosine monophosphate (cAMP) phosphodiesterase III (PDE III), which results in increased cAMP in platelets and blood vessels, producing inhibition of platelet aggregation and vasodilation. **Therapeutic Effects:** Reduced symptoms of intermittent claudication with improved walking distance.

Pharmacokinetics

Absorption: Slowly absorbed after oral administration.

Distribution: Unknown.

Protein Binding: 95–98% bound to plasma proteins; one active metabolite is 97.4% bound, the other is 66% bound.

Metabolism and Excretion: Extensively metabolized by the liver, two metabolites have platelet aggregation inhibitory activity; metabolites are mostly excreted by the kidneys.

Half-life: *Cilostazol and its active metabolites*—11–13 hr.

TIME/ACTION PROFILE (symptom reduction)

ROUTE	ONSET	PEAK	DURATION
PO	2–4 wk	up to 12 wk	unknown

Contraindications/Precautions

Contraindicated in: Hypersensitivity; HF; OB: Potential for congenital defects, stillbirth, and low birth weight; Lactation: Potential risk to nursing infants; discontinue or bottle feed.

Use Cautiously in: Pedi: Safety not established.

Adverse Reactions/Side Effects

CNS: headache, dizziness. **CV:** hypotension, palpitations, tachycardia. **GI:** diarrhea.

Interactions

Drug-Drug: Concurrent administration of **ketoconazole**, **itraconazole**, **erythromycin**, **diltiazem**, **fluconazole**, **miconazole**, **fluvoxamine**, **fluoxetine**, **nefazodone**, **sertraline**, or **omeprazole** ↓ metabolism and ↑ levels and activity of cilostazol (use lower doses). Concurrent use with **aspirin** has additive effects on platelet function.

Drug-Food: Grapefruit juice inhibits metabolism and ↑ effects; concurrent use should be avoided.

Route/Dosage

PO (Adults): 100 mg twice daily (50 mg twice daily if receiving inhibitors of cilostazol metabolism).

Availability (generic available)

Tablets: 50 mg, 100 mg.

NURSING IMPLICATIONS

Assessment

- Assess patient for intermittent claudication before and periodically during therapy.
- ***Lab Test Considerations:*** May occasionally cause anemia, hyperlipemia, hyperuricemia, and albuminuria. May prolong bleeding time.

Potential Nursing Diagnoses

Activity intolerance (Indications)

Implementation

- **PO:** Administer on an empty stomach, 1 hr before or 2 hr after meals.

Patient/Family Teaching

- Instruct patient to take cilostazol on an empty stomach, exactly as directed.
- Advise patient to avoid grapefruit juice during therapy.
- May cause dizziness. Caution patient to avoid driving or other activities requiring alertness until response to medication is known.
- Advise patient to avoid smoking; nicotine constricts blood vessels.

Evaluation/Desired Outcomes

- Relief from cramping in calf muscles, buttocks, thighs, and feet during exercise.
- Improvement in walking endurance. Therapeutic effects may be seen in 2–4 wk.

cimetidine, See HISTAMINE H_2 ANTAGONISTS.

cinacalcet (sin-a-kal-set)

Sensipar

Classification

Therapeutic: hypocalcemics

Pharmacologic: calcimimetic agents

Pregnancy Category C

Indications

Secondary hyperparathyroidism in patients with chronic kidney disease (CKD) on dialysis. Hypercalcemia caused by parathyroid carcinoma. Severe hypercalcemia in patients with primary hyperparathyroidism in patients who are unable to undergo parathyroidectomy.

Action

Increases sensitivity of calcium-sensing receptors located on the surface of chief cells of parathyroid gland to levels of extracellular calcium. This decreases parathyroid hormone production with resultant decrease in serum calcium. **Therapeutic Effects:** Decreased bone turnover and fibrosis. Decreased serum calcium.

Pharmacokinetics

Absorption: Well absorbed following oral administration, absorption is enhanced by food and further enhanced by a high fat meal.

Distribution: Unknown.

Protein Binding: 93–97%.

Metabolism and Excretion: Highly metabolized by CYP3A4, CYP2D6, and CYP1A2 enzyme systems; 80% excreted in urine as metabolites, 15% in feces.

Half-life: 30–40 hr.

TIME/ACTION PROFILE (effect on PTH levels)

ROUTE	ONSET	PEAK	DURATION
PO	rapid	2–6 hr	6–12 hr

Contraindications/Precautions

Contraindicated in: Hypersensitivity; Hypocalcemia; Lactation: Discontinue drug or bottle-feed.

Use Cautiously in: History of seizure disorder (↑ risk of seizures with hypocalcemia); Chronic kidney disease patients who are not being dialyzed (↑ risk of hypocalcemia); Intact parathyroid hormone (iPTH) level <150 pg/mL (dose ↓ or discontinuation may be warranted); Moderate to severe hepatic impairment; OB: Use only if benefits justify risks to fetus; Pedi: Safety not established.

Adverse Reactions/Side Effects

CNS: seizures. **GI:** nausea, vomiting. **F and E:** hypocalcemia. **Metab:** adynamic bone disease.

Interactions

Drug-Drug: Inhibits CYP2D6 and may ↑ levels of **flecainide**, **vinblastine**, **thioridazine**, **metoprolol**, **carvedilol**, and most **tricyclic antidepressants**; dose adjustments may be necessary. Blood levels are ↑ by **strong CYP3A4 inhibitors** including **ketoconazole**, **itraconazole**, and **erythromycin**; monitoring and dose adjustment may be necessary.

Route/Dosage

PO (Adults): *Secondary hyperparathyroidism in CKD patients on dialysis*—30 mg once daily; may ↑ dose every 2–4 wk (dose range 30–180 mg once daily) based on iPTH levels; *Parathyroid carcinoma or primary hyperparathyroidism*—30 mg twice daily; may titrate every 2–4 wk up to 90 mg 3–4 times daily based on serum calcium levels.

Availability

Tablets: 30 mg, 60 mg, 90 mg.

NURSING IMPLICATIONS

Assessment

- Monitor for signs and symptoms of hypocalcemia (paresthesias, myalgias, cramping, tetany, convulsions) during therapy. If calcium levels decrease to below normal, serum calcium may be increased by adjusting dose (see Lab Test Considerations) and providing supplemental serum calcium, initiating or increasing dose of calcium-based phosphate binder or vitamin D.
- ***Lab Test Considerations:*** Monitor serum calcium and phosphorous levels within 1 wk after initiation of therapy or dose adjustment and monthly for patients with hyperparathyroidism or every 2 mo for patients with parathyroid carcinoma once maintenance dose has been established, especially in patients with a history of seizure disorder. Therapy should not be initiated in patients with serum calcium less than the lower limit of normal (8.4 mg/dL).
- If serum calcium ↓ below 8.4 mg/dL but remains above 7.5 mg/dL, or if symptoms of hypocalcemia occur, use calcium-containing phosphate binders and/or vitamin D sterols to ↑ serum calcium. If serum calcium ↓ below 7.5 mg/dL, or if symptoms of hypocalcemia persist and the dose of vitamin D cannot be ↑, withhold administration of cinacalcet until serum calcium levels reach 8.0 mg/dL, and/or symptoms of hypocalcemia resolve. Re-initiate therapy using next lowest dose of cinacalcet.
- Monitor serum iPTH levels 1 to 4 wk after initiation of therapy or dose adjustment, and every 1 to 3 mo

after maintenance dose has been established. If iPTH levels ↓ below 150–300 pg/mL, reduce dose or discontinue cinacalcet.

- Monitor liver function tests in patients with moderate to severe hepatic impairment during therapy.

Potential Nursing Diagnoses

Deficient knowledge, related to medication regimen (Patient/Family Teaching)

Implementation

- Cinacalcet may be used alone or in combination with vitamin D and/or phosphate binders.
- **PO:** Administer with food or shortly after a meal. Take tablets whole, do not crush, break or chew.

Patient/Family Teaching

- Instruct patient to take cinacalcet as directed.
- Advise patient to report signs and symptoms of hypocalcemia to health care professional promptly.
- Emphasize the importance of follow-up lab tests to monitor safely and efficacy.

Evaluation/Desired Outcomes

- Decreased serum calcium levels.

HIGH ALERT

CISplatin (sis-**pla**-tin)

~~Platinol~~

Classification
Therapeutic: antineoplastics
Pharmacologic: alkylating agents

Pregnancy Category D

Indications

Metastatic testicular and ovarian carcinoma. Advanced bladder cancer. Head and neck cancer. Cervical cancer. Lung cancer. Other tumors.

Action

Inhibits DNA synthesis by producing cross-linking of parent DNA strands (cell-cycle phase–nonspecific). **Therapeutic Effects:** Death of rapidly replicating cells, particularly malignant ones.

Pharmacokinetics

Absorption: IV administration results in complete bioavailability.
Distribution: Widely distributed; accumulates for months; enters breast milk.
Metabolism and Excretion: Excreted mainly by the kidneys.
Half-life: 30–100 hr.

TIME/ACTION PROFILE (effects on blood counts)

ROUTE	ONSET	PEAK	DURATION
IV	unknown	18–23 days	39 days

Contraindications/Precautions

Contraindicated in: Hypersensitivity; OB, Lactation: Pregnancy or lactation.
Use Cautiously in: Hearing loss; Renal impairment (dosage ↓ recommended); HF; Electrolyte abnormalities; Active infections; Bone marrow depression; Geri: ↑ risk of nephrotoxicity and peripheral neuropathy; Rep: Patients with childbearing potential.

Adverse Reactions/Side Effects

CNS: REVERSIBLE POSTERIOR LEUKOENCEPHALOPATHY SYNDROME (RPLS), SEIZURES, malaise, weakness. **EENT:** ototoxicity, tinnitus. **GI:** severe nausea, vomiting, diarrhea, hepatotoxicity. **GU:** nephrotoxicity, sterility. **Derm:** alopecia. **F and E:** hypocalcemia, hypokalemia, hypomagnesemia. **Hemat:** LEUKOPENIA, THROMBOCYTOPENIA, anemia. **Local:** phlebitis at IV site. **Metab:** hyperuricemia. **Neuro:** peripheral neuropathy. **Misc:** anaphylactoid reactions.

Interactions

Drug-Drug: ↑ risk of nephrotoxicity and ototoxicity with other **nephrotoxic** and **ototoxic drugs (aminoglycosides, loop diuretics)**. ↑ risk of hypokalemia and hypomagnesemia with **loop diuretics** and **amphotericin B**. May ↓ **phenytoin** levels. ↑ bone marrow depression with other **antineoplastics** or **radiation therapy**. May ↓ antibody response to **live-virus vaccines** and ↑ adverse reactions.

Route/Dosage

Other regimens are used.
IV (Adults): *Metastatic testicular tumors*—20 mg/m^2 daily for 5 days repeated q 3–4 wk. *Metastatic ovarian cancer*—75–100 mg/m^2, repeat q 4 wk in combination with cyclophosphamide *or* 100 mg/m^2 q 3 wk if used as a single agent. *Advanced bladder cancer*—50–70 mg/m^2 q 3–4 wk as a single agent.

Availability (generic available)

Powder for injection: 50 mg/vial. **Injection:** 1 mg/mL.

NURSING IMPLICATIONS

Assessment

- Monitor vital signs frequently during administration. Report significant changes.
- Monitor intake and output and specific gravity frequently during therapy. To reduce risk of nephrotoxicity, maintain urinary output of at least 100 mL/hr for 4 hr before initiating and for at least 24 hr after administration.
- Encourage patient to drink 2000–3000 mL/day of water to promote excretion of uric acid. Allopurinol and alkalinization of urine may be used to help prevent uric acid nephropathy.
- Assess patency of IV site frequently during therapy. Cisplatin may cause severe irritation and necrosis of tissue if extravasation occurs. If a large amount of highly concentrated cisplatin solution extravasates,

mix 4 mL of 10% sodium thiosulfate with 6 mL of sterile water or 1.6 mL of 25% sodium thiosulfate with 8.4 mL of sterile water and inject 1–4 mL (1 mL for each mL extravasated) through existing line or cannula. Inject subcut if needle has been removed. Sodium thiosulfate inactivates cisplatin.

- Severe and protracted nausea and vomiting usually occur 1–4 hr after a dose; vomiting may last for 24 hr. Administer parenteral antiemetic agents 30–45 min before therapy and routinely around the clock for the next 24 hr. Monitor amount of emesis and notify health care professional if emesis exceeds guidelines to prevent dehydration. Nausea and anorexia may persist for up to 1 wk.
- Monitor for bone marrow depression. Assess for bleeding (bleeding gums, bruising, petechiae, stools, urine, and emesis) and avoid IM injections and taking rectal temperatures if platelet count is low. Apply pressure to venipuncture sites for 10 min. Assess for signs of infection during neutropenia. Anemia may occur. Monitor for increased fatigue, dyspnea, and orthostatic hypotension.
- Monitor for signs of anaphylaxis (facial edema, wheezing, dizziness, fainting, tachycardia, hypotension). Discontinue medication immediately and report symptoms. Epinephrine and resuscitation equipment should be readily available.
- Medication may cause ototoxicity and neurotoxicity. Assess patient frequently for dizziness, tinnitus, hearing loss, loss of coordination, loss of taste, or numbness and tingling of extremities; may be irreversible. Notify health care professional promptly if these occur. Audiometry should be performed before initiation of therapy and before subsequent doses. Hearing loss is more frequent with children and usually occurs first with high frequencies and may be unilateral or bilateral.
- Monitor for inadvertent cisplatin overdose. Doses >100 m g/m^2/cycle once every 3–4 wk are rarely used. Differentiate daily doses from total dose/cycle. Symptoms of high cumulative doses include muscle cramps (localized, painful involuntary skeletal muscle contractions of sudden onset and short duration) and are usually associated with advanced stages of peripheral neuropathy.
- Monitor for signs of RPLS (headache, seizure, lethargy, confusion, blindness). Hypertension may or may not be present. May occur with in 16 hr to 1 yr of initiation of therapy. Treat hypertension if present and discontinue cisplatin therapy. Symptoms usually resolve within days.
- ***Lab Test Considerations:*** Monitor CBC with differential and platelet count before and routinely throughout therapy. The nadir of leukopenia, thrombocytopenia, and anemia occurs within 18–23 days and recovery 39 days after a dose. Withhold further doses until WBC is >4000/mm^3 and platelet count is >100,000/mm^3.
- Monitor BUN, serum creatinine, and CCr before initiation of therapy and before each course of cisplatin to detect nephrotoxicity. May cause ↑ BUN and creatinine and ↓ calcium, magnesium, phosphate, sodium, and potassium levels that usually occur 2nd wk after a dose. Do not administer additional doses until BUN is <25 mg/dL and serum creatinine is <1.5 mg/dL. May cause ↑ uric acid level, which usually peaks 3–5 days after a dose.
- May cause transiently ↑ serum bilirubin and AST concentrations.
- May cause positive Coombs' test result.

Potential Nursing Diagnoses

Risk for infection (Adverse Reactions)
Risk for injury (Side Effects)

Implementation

- ***High Alert:*** Fatalities have occurred with chemotherapeutic agents. Before administering, clarify all ambiguous orders; double-check single, daily, and course-of-therapy dose limits; have second practitioner independently double-check original order, calculations, and infusion pump settings.
- Do not confuse cisplatin with carboplatin. To prevent confusion, orders should include generic and brand names. Administer under supervision of a physician experienced in use of cancer chemotherapeutic agents.
- Solution should be prepared in a biologic cabinet. Wear gloves, gown, and mask while handling medication. If powder or solution comes in contact with skin or mucosa, wash thoroughly with soap and water. Discard equipment in specially designated containers.
- Hydrate patient with at least 1–2 L of IV fluid 8–12 hr before initiating therapy with cisplatin. Amifostine may be administered to minimize nephrotoxicity.
- Do not use aluminum needles or equipment during preparation or administration. Aluminum reacts with this drug, forms a black or brown precipitate, and renders the drug ineffective.
- Unopened vials of powder and constituted solution must not be refrigerated.

IV Administration

- **Intermittent Infusion:** Reconstitute 50-mg vial with 50 mL. Stable for 20 hr if reconstituted with sterile water, for 72 hr with bacteriostatic water. Do not refrigerate, because crystals will form. Solution should be clear and colorless; discard if turbid or if it contains precipitates.
- ***Diluent:*** Dilution in 2 L of 5% dextrose in 0.3% or 0.45% NaCl containing 37.5 g of mannitol is recommended. ***Concentration:*** Keep under 0.5 mg/mL

to prevent tissue necrosis. ***Rate:*** Variable. Administer over 6–8 hr. Maximum rate 1 mg/min.

- **Continuous Infusion:** Has been administered as continuous infusion over 24 hr to 5 days with resultant decrease in nausea and vomiting. ***High Alert:*** Clarify dose to ensure cumulative dose is not confused with daily dose; errors may be fatal.
- **Y-Site Compatibility:** acyclovir, alfentanil, allopurinol, amikacin, aminophylline, amiodarone, ampicillin, ampicillin/sulbactam, anidulafungin, argatroban, azithromycin, aztreonam, bivalirudin, bleomycin, bumetanide, buprenorphine, butorphanol, calcium chloride, calcium gluconate, carmustine, caspofungin, cefazolin, cefotaxime, cefotetan, ceftazidime, ceftriaxone, cefuroxime, chlorpromazine, ciprofloxacin, cisatracurium, cladribine, clindamycin, cyclophosphamide, cyclosporine, cytarabine, dactinomycin, daptomycin, daunorubicin hydrochloride, dexamethasone, dexmedetomidine, dexrazoxane, digoxin, diltiazem, diphenhydramine, dobutamine, docetaxel, dolasetron, dopamine, doripenem, doxacurium, doxorubicin, doxorubicin liposome, doxycycline, droperidol, enalaprilat, ephedrine, epinephrine, epirubicin, ertapenem, erythromycin, esmolol, etoposide, etoposide phosphate, famotidine, fenoldopam, fentanyl, filgrastim, fluconazole, fludarabine, fluorouracil, foscarnet, fosphenytoin, furosemide, ganciclovir, gemcitabine, gentamicin, glycopyrrolate, granisetron, haloperidol, heparin, hetastarch, hydrocortisone, hydromorphone, idarubicin, ifosfamide, imipenem/cilastatin, indomethacin, irinotecan, isoproterenol, ketorolac, labetalol, leucovorin calcium, levofloxacin, levorphanol, lidocaine, linezolid, lorazepam, magnesium sulfate, mannitol, melphalan, meperidine, meropenem, methotrexate, methylprednisolone, metoclopramide, metoprolol, metronidazole, midazolam, milrinone, mitomycin, mitoxantrone, moxifloxacin, nafcillin, naloxone, nesiritide, nicardipine, nitroglycerin, nitroprusside, norepinephrine, octreotide, ondansetron, oxaliplatin, paclitaxel, palonosetron, pamidronate, pancuronium, pemetrexed, pentamidine, pentazocine, pentobarbital, phenobarbital, phenylephrine, phenytoin, potassium acetate, potassium chloride, potassium phosphates, procainamide, prochlorperazine, promethazine, propofol, propranolol, quinupristin/dalfopristin, ranitidine, remifentanil, rituximab, sargramostim, sodium acetate, sodium bicarbonate, sodium phosphates, succinylcholine, sufentanil, tacrolimus, teniposide, theophylline, thiopental, tigecycline, tirofiban, tobramycin, topotecan, trastuzumab, vancomycin, vasopressin, vecuronium, verapamil, vinblastine, vincristine, vinorelbine, voriconazole, zidovudine, zoledronic acid.
- **Y-Site Incompatibility:** amifostine, amphotericin B cholesteryl sulfate, amphotericin B colloidal, amphotericin B lipid complex, amphotericin B liposome, cefepime, dantrolene, diazepam, insulin, pantoprazole, piperacillin/tazobactam, thiotepa.

Patient/Family Teaching

- Instruct patient to report pain at injection site immediately.
- Instruct patient to notify health care professional promptly if fever; chills; cough; hoarseness; sore throat; signs of infection; lower back or side pain; painful or difficult urination; bleeding gums; bruising; petechiae; blood in stools, urine, or emesis; increased fatigue; dyspnea; or orthostatic hypotension occurs. Caution patient to avoid crowds and persons with known infections. Instruct patient to use soft toothbrush and electric razor and to avoid falls. Caution patient not to drink alcoholic beverages or take medication containing aspirin or NSAIDs; may precipitate gastric bleeding.
- Instruct patient to report promptly any numbness or tingling in extremities or face, difficulty with hearing or tinnitus, unusual swelling, or joint pain.
- Instruct patient not to receive any vaccinations without advice of health care professional.
- Advise patient of the need for contraception, although cisplatin may cause infertility.
- Emphasize the need for periodic lab tests to monitor for side effects.

Evaluation/Desired Outcomes

- Decrease in size or spread of malignancies. Therapy should not be administered more frequently than every 3–4 wk, and only if lab values are within acceptable parameters and patient is not exhibiting signs of ototoxicity or other serious adverse effects.

citalopram (si-**tal**-oh-pram)

CeleXA

Classification

Therapeutic: antidepressants

Pharmacologic: selective serotonin reuptake inhibitors (SSRIs)

Pregnancy Category C

Indications

Depression. **Unlabeled Use:** Premenstrual dysphoric disorder (PMDD). Obsessive-compulsive disorder (OCD). Panic disorder. Generalized anxiety disorder (GAD). Posttraumatic stress disorder (PTSD). Social anxiety disorder (social phobia).

Action

Selectively inhibits the reuptake of serotonin in the CNS. **Therapeutic Effects:** Antidepressant action.

Pharmacokinetics

Absorption: 80% absorbed after oral administration.

Distribution: Enters breast milk.

Metabolism and Excretion: Mostly metabolized by the liver (10% by CYP3A4 and 2C19 enzymes); excreted unchanged in urine.
Half-life: 35 hr.

TIME/ACTION PROFILE (antidepressant effect)

ROUTE	ONSET	PEAK	DURATION
PO	1–4 wk	unknown	unknown

Contraindications/Precautions

Contraindicated in: Hypersensitivity; Concurrent use of MAO inhibitors or MAO-like drugs (linezolid or methylene blue); Concurrent use of pimozide; Congenital long QT syndrome, bradycardia, hypokalemia, hypomagnesemia, recent myocardial infarction, decompensated heart failure (↑ risk of QT interval prolongation); Concurrent use of QT interval prolonging drugs.
Use Cautiously in: History of mania; History of suicide attempt/ideation (↑ risk during early therapy and during dose adjustment); History of seizure disorder; Illnesses or conditions that are likely to result in altered metabolism or hemodynamic responses; Severe renal or hepatic impairment (maximum dose of 20 mg/day in patients with hepatic impairment); Poor metabolizers of CYP2C19 (↑ risk of QT interval prolongation) (maximum dose of 20 mg/day); Concurrent use of CYP2C19 inhibitors (↑ risk of QT interval prolongation) (maximum dose of 20 mg/day); Angle-closure glaucoma; OB: Use during third trimester may result in neonatal serotonin syndrome requiring prolonged hospitalization, respiratory and nutritional support; Lactation: Present in breast milk and may result in lethargy with ↓ feeding in infants; weigh risk/benefits; Pedi: May ↑ risk of suicide attempt/ideation especially during early treatment or dose adjustment in children/adolescents (unlabeled for pediatric use); Geri: ↓ doses recommended (maximum dose of 20 mg/day in patients >60 yr).

Adverse Reactions/Side Effects

CNS: NEUROLEPTIC MALIGNANT SYNDROME, SUICIDAL THOUGHTS, apathy, confusion, drowsiness, insomnia, weakness, agitation, amnesia, anxiety, ↓ libido, dizziness, fatigue, impaired concentration, ↑ depression, migraine headache. **EENT:** abnormal accommodation. **Resp:** cough. **CV:** TORSADE DE POINTES, postural hypotension, QT interval prolongation, tachycardia. **GI:** abdominal pain, anorexia, diarrhea, dry mouth, dyspepsia, flatulence, ↑ saliva, nausea, altered taste, ↑ appetite, vomiting. **GU:** amenorrhea, dysmenorrhea, ejaculatory delay, erectile dysfunction, polyuria. **Derm:** sweating, photosensitivity, pruritus, rash. **Metab:** weight loss, weight gain. **F and E:** hyponatremia. **MS:** arthralgia, myalgia. **Neuro:** tremor, paresthesia. **Misc:** SEROTONIN SYNDROME, fever, yawning.

Interactions

Drug-Drug: May cause serious, potentially fatal reactions when used with **MAO inhibitors**; concurrent use contraindicated; allow at least 14 days between citalopram and **MAO inhibitors**. Concurrent use with **MAO-inhibitor like drugs**, such as **linezolid** or **methylene blue**, may ↑ risk of serotonin syndrome; concurrent use contraindicated; do not start therapy in patients receiving **linezolid** or **methylene blue**; if **linezolid** or **methylene blue** need to be started in a patient receiving citalopram, immediately discontinue citalopram and monitor for signs/symptoms of serotonin syndrome for 2 wk or until 24 hr after last dose of linezolid or methylene blue, whichever comes first (may resume citalopram therapy 24 hr after last dose of linezolid or methylene blue). Concurrent use with **pimozide** may result in prolongation of the QTc interval and is contraindicated. **QT interval prolonging drugs** may ↑ the risk of QT interval prolongation and torsade de pointes (concurrent use should be avoided). **CYP2C19 inhibitors**, including **cimetidine** may ↑ levels and the risk of toxicity (maximum dose = 20 mg/day). Drugs that affect serotonergic neurotransmitter systems, including **tricyclic antidepressants**, **SNRIs**, **fentanyl**, **buspirone**, **tramadol** and **triptans** ↑ risk of serotonin syndrome. Use cautiously with other **centrally acting drugs** (including **alcohol**, **antihistamines**, **opioid analgesics**, and **sedative/hypnotics**; concurrent use with **alcohol** is not recommended). Serotonergic effects may be ↑ by **lithium** (concurrent use should be carefully monitored). **Ketoconazole**, **itraconazole**, **erythromycin**, and **omeprazole** may ↑ levels. **Carbamazepine** may ↓ blood levels. May ↑ levels of **metoprolol**. Use cautiously with **tricyclic antidepressants** due to unpredictable effects on serotonin and norepinephrine reuptake. ↑ risk of bleeding with **aspirin**, **NSAIDs**, **clopidogrel**, or **warfarin**.
Drug-Natural Products: ↑ risk of serotonergic side effects including serotonin syndrome with **St. John's wort** and **SAMe**.

Route/Dosage

PO (Adults): 20 mg once daily initially, may be ↑ in 1 wk to 40 mg/day (maximum dose); *Poor metabolizer of CYP2C19 or concurrent use of CYP2C19 inhibitor*—Do not exceed dose of 20 mg/day.
PO (Geriatric Patients): 20 mg once daily initially (do not exceed dose of 20 mg/day in patients >60 yr).

Hepatic Impairment

PO (Adults): 20 mg once daily (do not exceed dose of 20 mg/day).

Availability (generic available)

Tablets: 10 mg, 20 mg, 40 mg. **Cost:** *Generic*—10 mg $7.11/100, 20 mg $9.73/100, 40 mg $10.83/100.

Oral solution (peppermint flavor): 10 mg/5 mL. **Cost:** *Generic*—10 mg/5 mL $117.50/240 mL.

NURSING IMPLICATIONS

Assessment

- Monitor mood changes during therapy.
- Assess for suicidal tendencies, especially during early therapy and dose changes. Restrict amount of drug available to patient. Risk may be increased in children, adolescents, and adults ≤24 yr. After starting therapy, children, adolescents, and young adults should be seen by health care professional at least weekly for 4 wk, every 3 wk for the next 4 wk, and on advice of health care professional thereafter.
- Assess for sexual dysfunction (erectile dysfunction; decreased libido).
- Assess for serotonin syndrome (mental changes [agitation, hallucinations, coma], autonomic instability [tachycardia, labile BP, hyperthermia], neuromuscular aberrations [hyperreflexia, incoordination], and/or GI symptoms [nausea, vomiting, diarrhea]), especially in patients taking other serotonergic drugs (SSRIs, SNRIs, triptans).
- ***Lab Test Considerations:*** Monitor electrolytes (potassium and magnesium) in patients at risk for electrolyte imbalances prior to and periodically during therapy.

Potential Nursing Diagnoses

Ineffective coping (Indications)
Risk for injury (Side Effects)
Sexual dysfunction (Side Effects)

Implementation

- Do not confuse with Celebrex (celecoxib), Cerebyx (fosphenytoin), or Zyprexa (olanzapine).
- **PO:** Administer as a single dose in the morning or evening without regard to food.

Patient/Family Teaching

- Instruct patient to take citalopram as directed. Take missed doses as soon as remembered unless almost time for next dose; do not double doses. Do not stop abruptly; may cause anxiety, irritability, high or low mood, feeling restless or changes in sleep habits, headache, sweating, nausea, dizziness, electric shock-like sensations, shaking, and confusion. Advise patient to read the *Medication Guide* prior to starting therapy and with each refill in case of changes.
- May cause drowsiness, dizziness, impaired concentration, and blurred vision. Caution patient to avoid driving and other activities requiring alertness until response to the drug is known.
- Instruct patient to notify health care professional of all Rx or OTC medications, vitamins, or herbal products being taken and to consult health care professional before taking any other Rx, OTC, or herbal products, especially alcohol or other CNS depressants and St. John's Wort.
- Caution patient to change positions slowly to minimize dizziness.
- Advise patient, family, and caregivers to look for suicidality, especially during early therapy or dose changes. Notify health care professional immediately if thoughts about suicide or dying, attempts to commit suicide, new or worse depression or anxiety, agitation or restlessness, panic attacks, insomnia, new or worse irritability, aggressiveness, acting on dangerous impulses, mania, or other changes in mood or behavior or if symptoms of serotonin syndrome occur.
- Advise patient to use sunscreen and wear protective clothing to prevent photosensitivity reactions.
- Inform patient that frequent mouth rinses, good oral hygiene, and sugarless gum or candy may minimize dry mouth. If dry mouth persists for more than 2 wk, consult health care professional regarding use of saliva substitute.
- Instruct female patients to inform health care professional if pregnancy is planned or suspected, or if breast feeding. If used during pregnancy should be tapered during third trimester to avoid neonatal serotinin syndrome.
- Emphasize the importance of follow-up exams to monitor progress.

Evaluation/Desired Outcomes

- Increased sense of well-being.
- Renewed interest in surroundings. May require 1–4 wk of therapy to obtain antidepressant effects.

clarithromycin

(kla-**rith**-roe-mye-sin)
Biaxin, Biaxin XL

Classification
Therapeutic: agents for atypical mycobacterium, anti-infectives, antiulcer agents
Pharmacologic: macrolides

Pregnancy Category C

Indications

Respiratory tract infections including streptococcal pharyngitis, sinusitis, bronchitis, and pneumonia. Treatment (with ethambutol) and prevention of disseminated *Mycobacterium avium* complex (MAC). Treatment of following pediatric infections: Otitis media, Sinusitis, Pharyngitis, Skin/skin structure infections. Part of a combination regimen for ulcer disease due to *Helicobacter pylori*. Endocarditis prophylaxis.

Action

Inhibits protein synthesis at the level of the 50S bacterial ribosome. **Therapeutic Effects:** Bacteriostatic action. **Spectrum:** Active against these gram-positive aerobic bacteria: *Staphylococcus aureus*, *S. pneumoniae*, *S. pyogenes* (group A strep). Active against these gram-negative aerobic bacteria: *Haemophilus influen-*

zae, *Moraxella catarrhalis*. Also active against: *Mycoplasma*, *Legionella*, *H. pylori*, *M. avium*.

Pharmacokinetics

Absorption: Rapidly absorbed (50%) after oral administration.

Distribution: Widely distributed; tissue levels may exceed those in serum.

Protein Binding: 65–70%.

Metabolism and Excretion: 10–15% converted by the liver to 14-hydroxyclarithromycin, which has anti-infective activity; 20–30% excreted unchanged in urine. Metabolized by and also inhibits the CYP3A enzyme system.

Half-life: Dose-dependent and prolonged with renal dysfunction *250-mg dose*—3–4 hr; *500-mg dose*—5–7 hr.

TIME/ACTION PROFILE (serum levels)

ROUTE	ONSET	PEAK	DURATION
PO	unknown	2 hr	12 hr
PO-XL	unknown	4 hr	24 hr

Contraindications/Precautions

Contraindicated in: Hypersensitivity to clarithromycin, erythromycin, or other macrolide anti-infectives; History of cholestatic jaundice or hepatic dysfunction with clarithromycin; Concurrent use of pimozide, ergotamine, dihydroergotamine, lovastatin, simvastatin, quinidine, procainamide, dofetilide, amiodarone, or sotalol; Concurrent use of colchicine in patients with hepatic or renal impairment; QT interval prolongation, hypokalemia, hypomagnesemia, or bradycardia; OB: Avoid use during pregnancy unless no alternatives are available; Lactation: Not recommended for breast-feeding women.

Use Cautiously in: Severe liver or renal impairment (dose adjustment required if CCr <30 mL/min); Myasthenia gravis; Geri: May have ↑ risk of QT interval prolongation.

Adverse Reactions/Side Effects

CNS: headache. **CV:** TORSADES DE POINTES, QT interval prolongation. **Derm:** STEVENS-JOHNSON SYNDROME, pruritus, rash. **GI:** HEPATOTOXICITY, CLOSTRIDIUM DIFFICILE-ASSOCIATED DIARRHEA (CDAD), abdominal pain/discomfort, abnormal taste, diarrhea, dyspepsia, nausea. **Misc:** ANGIOEDEMA.

Interactions

Drug-Drug: Clarithromycin is an inhibitor of the CYP3A enzyme system. Concurrent use with other agents metabolized by this system can ↑ levels and risk of toxicity. May prolong the QT interval and ↑ risk of arrhythmias with **pimozide**; concurrent use contraindicated. May ↑ levels of **ergotamine** and **dihydroergotamine** and risk for acute ergot toxicity; concurrent use contraindicated. **Quinidine**, **procainamide**, **dofetilide**, **sotalol**, and **amiodarone** may ↑ risk of QT interval prolongation; concurrent use should be avoided. ↑ risk of rhabdomyolysis with **lovastatin** and **simvastatin**; concurrent use contraindicated. May ↑ serum levels and the risk of toxicity from **carbamazepine**, some **benzodiazepines (midazolam, triazolam, alprazolam)**, **cyclosporine**, **disopyramide**, **quinidine**, **ergot alkaloids**, **felodipine**, **omeprazole**, **tacrolimus**, **digoxin**, or **theophylline**. May ↑ levels and effects of **omeprazole**. **Ritonavir**↑ blood levels (↓ clarithromycin dose in patients with CCr <60 mL/min). ↑ levels and risk of myopathy from **atorvastatin** and **pravastatin**; use lowest dose of these agents; do not exceed atorvastatin dose of 20 mg/day or pravastatin dose of 40 mg/day. May ↑ or ↓ effects of **zidovudine**. Blood levels are ↑ by **delavirdine** and **fluconazole**. Blood levels may be ↓ by **rifampin**, **rifabutin**, **efavirenz**, and **nevirapine**. May ↑ levels and risk of toxicity from **colchicine**; ↓ colchicine dose in patients with normal renal and hepatic function; concurrent use is contraindicated in patients with renal or hepatic impairment. May ↑ **verapamil** levels and the risk for hypotension, bradycardia, and lactic acidosis. Concomitant use with **calcium channel blockers** metabolized by CYP3A4, including **verapamil**, **diltiazem**, **amlodipine**, and **nifedipine** may ↑ the risk of acute kidney injury, especially in patients older than 65 yr. May ↑ **warfarin** levels and the risk for bleeding. May ↑ blood levels and effects of **sildenafil**, **tadalafil**, and **vardenafil**; concurrent use not recommended. May ↑ levels of **tolterodine**. Concurrent use with **atazanavir** may ↑ clarithromycin and atazanavir levels; ↓ clarithromycin dose by 50%. Concurrent use with **itraconazole** may ↑ clarithromycin and itraconazole levels. Concurrent use with **saquinavir** may ↑ clarithromycin and saquinavir levels.

Route/Dosage

PO (Adults): *Pharyngitis/tonsillitis*—250 mg q 12 hr for 10 days; *Acute maxillary sinusitis*—500 mg q 12 hr for 14 days or 1000 mg once daily for 14 days as XL tablets; *Acute exacerbation of chronic bronchitis*—250–500 mg q 12 hr for 7–14 days or 1000 mg once daily for 7 days as XL tablets; *Community-Acquired pneumonia*—250 mg q 12 hr for 7–14 days or 1000 mg once daily for 7 days as XL tablets; *Skin/skin structure infections*—250 mg q 12 hr for 7–14 days; *H. pylori*—500 mg 2–3 times daily with a proton pump inhibitor (lansoprazole or omeprazole) or ranitidine with or without amoxicillin for 10–14 days; *Endocarditis prophylaxis*—500 mg 1 hr before procedure; *MAC prophylaxis/treatment*—500 mg twice daily, for active infection another antimycobacterial is required.

PO (Children): *Most infections*—15 mg/kg/day divided q 12 hr for 7–14 days (up to 500 mg/dose for

MAC). *Endocarditis prophylaxis*—15 mg/kg 1 hr before procedure.

Renal Impairment

PO (Adults): *CCr <30 mL/min*—250 mg 1–2 times daily, a 500-mg initial dose may be used.
PO (Children): *CCr <30 mL/min*—decrease dose by 50% or double dosing interval.

Availability (generic available)

Tablets: 250 mg, 500 mg. **Extended-release tablets:** 500 mg. **Oral suspension (fruit punch and vanilla flavors):** 125 mg/5 mL, 250 mg/5 mL. ***In combination with:*** amoxicillin and lansoprazole as part of a compliance package (Prevpac); See Appendix B.

NURSING IMPLICATIONS

Assessment

- Assess patient for infection (vital signs; appearance of wound, sputum, urine, and stool; WBC) at beginning of and during therapy.
- Obtain specimens for culture and sensitivity before initiating therapy. First dose may be given before receiving results.
- Monitor bowel function. Diarrhea, abdominal cramping, fever, and bloody stools should be reported to health care professional promptly as a sign of Clostridium difficile-associated diarrhea (CDAD). May begin up to several weeks following cessation of therapy.
- Assess patient for skin rash frequently during therapy. Discontinue clarithromycin at first sign of rash; may be life-threatening. Stevens-Johnson syndrome may develop. Treat symptomatically; may recur once treatment is stopped.
- **Ulcers:** Assess patient for epigastric or abdominal pain and frank or occult blood in the stool, emesis, or gastric aspirate.
- ***Lab Test Considerations:*** May rarely cause ↑ serum AST, ALT, total bilirubin, and alkaline phosphatase concentrations.
- May occasionally cause ↑ BUN.

Potential Nursing Diagnoses

Risk for infection (Indications, Side Effects)
Noncompliance (Patient/Family Teaching)

Implementation

- **PO:** Administer around the clock, without regard to meals; may be administered with milk. Food slows but does not decrease the extent of absorption.
- Administer XL tablets with food or milk; do not crush, break, or chew.
- Shake suspension well before administration. Store suspension at room temperature; do not refrigerate.
- Do not administer within 4 hr of zidovudine.

Patient/Family Teaching

- Instruct patient to take medication around the clock and to finish the drug completely as directed, even if feeling better. Take missed doses as soon as possible, unless almost time for next dose. Do not double doses. Advise patient that sharing of this medication may be dangerous.
- Advise patient to report the signs of superinfection (black, furry overgrowth on the tongue; vaginal itching or discharge; loose or foul-smelling stools).
- Instruct patient to notify health care professional if rash, or fever and diarrhea develop, especially if stool contains blood, pus, or mucus. Advise patient not to treat diarrhea without consulting health care professional.
- Caution patients taking zidovudine that clarithromycin and zidovudine must be taken at least 4 hr apart.
- Advise patient to notify health care professional immediately if pregnancy is planned or suspected or if breast feeding.
- Instruct the patient to notify health care professional if symptoms do not improve within a few days.

Evaluation/Desired Outcomes

- Resolution of the signs and symptoms of infection. Length of time for complete resolution depends on the organism and site of infection.
- Treatment of ulcers.
- Endocarditis prophylaxis.

clevidipine (kle-vi-di-peen)

Cleviprex

Classification
Therapeutic: antihypertensives
Pharmacologic: calcium channel blockers (dihydropyridine)

Indications

Reduction of BP when oral therapy is not feasible/desirable.

Action

Inhibits calcium transport into vascular smooth muscle, resulting in inhibition of excitation-contraction coupling and subsequent contraction. Decreases systemic vascular resistance; does not reduce cardiac filling pressure (pre-load). Has no effect on venous capacitance vessels. **Therapeutic Effects:** Decreases BP.

Pharmacokinetics

Absorption: IV administration results in complete bioavailibility.
Distribution: Unknown.
Protein Binding: >99.5%.
Metabolism and Excretion: Rapidly metabolized by esterases in plasma and tissue to inactive metabolites; metabolites are excreted in urine (63–74%) and feces (7–22%).
Half-life: *Initial phase*—1 min; *terminal phase*—15 min.

TIME/ACTION PROFILE

ROUTE	ONSET	PEAK	DURATION
IV	2–4 min	30 min*	end of infusion

*Time to target BP.

Contraindications/Precautions

Contraindicated in: Hypersensitivity; Allergy to soybeans or eggs/egg products; Defective lipid metabolism including pathologic hyperlipidemia, lipoid nephrosis or acute pancreatitis; Severe aortic stenosis.
Use Cautiously in: Geri: Titrate dose cautiously, initiate therapy at low end of dose range; consider age-related changes in hepatic, renal, or cardiac function, concomitant diseases, or other drug therapy; OB: Use only if maternal benefit outweighs potential risk to fetus; Lactation: Consider possible infant exposure; Pedi: Safety not established.

Adverse Reactions/Side Effects

CNS: headache. **CV:** HF, hypotension, rebound hypertension, reflex tachycardia. **Resp:** hypoxemia. **GI:** nausea, vomiting. **MS:** arthralgia.

Interactions

Drug-Drug: ↑ risk of excess hypotension with other **antihypertensives**. Does not protect against effects of abrupt **beta blocker** withdrawal.

Route/Dosage

IV (Adults): *Initial dose*— 1–2 mg/hr; *Dose titration*—Double dose every 90 sec initially; as BP approaches goal, ↑ dose by less than doubling and lengthen the time between dose adjustments to every 5–10 min. Usual dose required is 4–6 mg/hr. Severe hypertensive patients may require higher doses with a maximum of 16 mg/hr or less. Doses up to 32 mg/hr have been used, but generally should not exceed 21 mg/hr in a 24 hr period due to lipid load.

Availability

Emulsion for injection: 0.5 mg/mL.

NURSING IMPLICATIONS

Assessment

- Monitor BP and heart rate during infusion, and until vital signs stabilize. Hypotension and reflex tachycardia may occur with rapid upward titration. Monitor patients receiving prolonged clevidipine infusions and who have not been transitioned to other antihypertensive therapies for the possibility of rebound hypertension for at least 8 hr after infusion is stopped; additional adjustments may be needed.

Potential Nursing Diagnoses

Ineffective tissue perfusion (Indications)

Implementation

- Discontinue clevidipine or titrate downward during initiation of oral therapy; consider time to onset of the oral agent's effect. Continue BP monitoring until desired effect is achieved.

IV Administration

- **Intermittent Infusion:** ***Diluent:*** Do not dilute. Invert vial gently several times before use to ensure emulsion uniformity prior to administration. Solution is milky white; inspect for particulate matter and discoloration. Commercially available standard plastic cannulae may be used to administer the infusion. Administer via central line or peripheral line. Solution is in single-use vials; discard unused portion 4 hr after stopper puncture. Store in refrigerator; once emulsion reaches room temperature, stable for 2 mo, do not re-refrigerate. ***Rate:*** Initiate intravenous infusion at 1–2 mg/hr. Administer using an infusion device allowing calibrated infusion rates.
- **Y-Site Compatibility:** Water for Injection, USP, 0.9% NaCl, D5W, D5/0.9% NaCl, D5/LR, LR, 10% amino acid.
- **Y-Site Incompatibility:** Do not administer in the same line as other medications.

Patient/Family Teaching

- Inform patient of the rationale for use of clevidipine.
- Advise patients to contact a health care professional immediately if signs of a new hypertensive emergency (neurological symptoms, visual changes, evidence of HF) occur.
- Advise female patients to notify health care professional if pregnancy is planned or suspected or if breast feeding.
- Encourage patients with underlying hypertension to continue follow-up care and to continue taking their oral antihypertensive medication(s) as directed.

Evaluation/Desired Outcomes

- Decrease in BP.

clindamycin (klin-da-**mye**-sin)

Cleocin, Cleocin T, Clinda-Derm, ✱Clinda-T, Clindagel, Clindesse, Clindets, ✱Dalacin C, ✱Dalacin T, Evoclin

Classification
Therapeutic: anti-infectives

Pregnancy Category B

Indications

PO, IM, IV: Treatment of: Skin and skin structure infections, Respiratory tract infections, Septicemia, Intra-abdominal infections, Gynecologic infections, Osteomyelitis, Endocarditis prophylaxis. **Topical:** Severe acne. **Vag:** Bacterial vaginosis. **Unlabeled Use: PO, IM, IV:** Treatment of *Pneumocystis carinii* pneumonia, CNS toxoplasmosis, and babesiosis.

Action

Inhibits protein synthesis in susceptible bacteria at the level of the 50S ribosome. **Therapeutic Effects:** Bactericidal or bacteriostatic, depending on susceptibility and concentration. **Spectrum:** Active against most gram-positive aerobic cocci, including: Staphylococci, *Streptococcus pneumoniae*, other streptococci, but not enterococci. Has good activity against those anaerobic bacteria that cause bacterial vaginosis, including *Bacteroides fragilis*, *Gardnerella vaginalis*, *Mobiluncus* spp., *Mycoplasma hominis*, and *Corynebacterium*. Also active against *Pneumocystis jirovecii* and *Toxoplasma gondii*.

Pharmacokinetics

Absorption: Well absorbed following PO/IM administration. Minimal absorption following topical/vaginal use.

Distribution: Widely distributed. Does not significantly cross blood-brain barrier. Crosses the placenta; enters breast milk.

Protein Binding: 94%.

Metabolism and Excretion: Mostly metabolized by the liver.

Half-life: Neonates: 3.6–8.7 hr; Infants up to 1 yr: 3 hr; Children and adults: 2–3 hr.

TIME/ACTION PROFILE (blood levels)

ROUTE	ONSET	PEAK	DURATION
PO	rapid	60 min	6–8 hr
IM	rapid	1–3 hr	6–8 hr
IV	rapid	end of infusion	6–8 hr

Contraindications/Precautions

Contraindicated in: Hypersensitivity; Regional enteritis or ulcerative colitis (topical foam); Previous *Clostridium difficile*-associated diarrhea; Severe liver impairment; Diarrhea; Known alcohol intolerance (topical solution, suspension).

Use Cautiously in: OB: Safety not established for topical administration; systemic administration during 2nd and 3rd trimesters not associated with ↑ risk of congenital abnormalities; approved for vaginal use in 3rd trimester of pregnancy; injection contains benzyl alcohol which can cross placenta; Lactation: Has been used safely but appears in breast milk and exposes infant to drug and its side effects; Pedi: Injection contains benzyl alcohol which can cause gasping syndrome in infants and neonates.

Adverse Reactions/Side Effects

CNS: dizziness, headache, vertigo. **CV:** arrhythmias, hypotension. **GI:** ***CLOSTRIDIUM DIFFICILE*-ASSOCIATED DIARRHEA**, diarrhea, bitter taste (IV only), nausea, vomiting. **Derm:** DRUG REACTION WITH EOSINOPHILIA AND SYSTEMIC SYMPTOMS (DRESS), ERYTHEMA MULTIFORME, TOXIC EPIDERMAL NECROLYSIS, rash, urticaria. **Local:** local irritation (topical products), phlebitis at IV site.

Interactions

Drug-Drug: Kaolin/pectin may ↓ GI absorption. May enhance the neuromuscular blocking action of other **neuromuscular blocking agents**. **Topical:** Concurrent use with **irritants**, **abrasives**, or **desquamating agents** may result in additive irritation.

Route/Dosage

PO (Adults): *Most infections*—150–450 mg q 6 hr. P. carinii *pneumonia*—1200–1800 mg/day in divided doses with 15–30 mg Primaquine/day (unlabeled). *CNS toxoplasmosis*—1200–2400 mg/day in divided doses with pyrimethamine 50–100 mg/day (unlabeled); *Bacterial endocarditis prophylaxis*—600 mg 1 hr before procedure.

PO (Children >1 mo): 10–30 mg/kg/day divided q 6–8 hr; maximum dose 1.8 g/day. *Bacterial endocarditis prophylaxis*—20 mg/kg 1 hr before procedure.

IM, IV (Adults): *Most infections*—300–600 mg q 6–8 hr *or* 900 mg q 8 hr (up to 4.8 g/day IV has been used; single IM doses of >600 m g are not recommended). P. carinii *pneumonia*—2400–2700 mg/day in divided doses with Primaquine (unlabeled). *Toxoplasmosis*—1200–4800 mg/day in divided doses with pyrimethamine. *Bacterial endocarditis prophylaxis*—600 mg 30 min before procedure.

IM, IV (Children >1 mo): 25–40 mg/kg/day divided q 6–8 hr; maximum dose: 4.8 g/day. *Bacterial endocarditis prophylaxis*—20 mg/kg 30 min before procedure; maximum dose: 600 mg.

IM, IV (Infants <1 mo and <2 kg): 5 mg/kg q 8–12 hr; *≥2 kg*—20–30 mg/kg/day divided q 6–8 hr.

Vag (Adults and Adolescents): *Cleocin, Clindamax*—1 applicatorful (5 g) at bedtime for 3 or 7 days (7 days in pregnant patients); *Clindesse*—one applicatorful (5 g) single dose; *or* 1 suppository (100 mg) at bedtime for 3 nights.

Topical (Adults and Adolescents): *Solution*—1% solution/suspension applied twice daily (range 1–4 times daily). *Foam, gel*—1% foam or gel applied once daily.

Availability (generic available)

Capsules: 75 mg, 150 mg, 300 mg. **Oral suspension:** 75 mg/5 mL. **Injection:** 150 mg/mL. **Premixed infusion:** 300 mg/50 mL, 600 mg/50 mL, 900 mg/50 mL. **Topical:** 1% lotion, gel, foam, solution, suspension, single-use applicators. ***In combination with:*** benzoyl peroxide (Acanya, BenzaClin, Duac); (see Appendix B). **Vaginal cream:** 2%. **Vaginal suppositories (ovules):** 100 mg. ***In combination with:*** tretinoin (Ziana); (see Appendix B).

NURSING IMPLICATIONS

Assessment

- Assess for infection (vital signs; appearance of wound, sputum, urine, and stool; WBC) at beginning of and during therapy.

- Obtain specimens for culture and sensitivity prior to initiating therapy. First dose may be given before receiving results.
- Monitor bowel elimination. Diarrhea, abdominal cramping, fever, and bloody stools should be reported to health care professional promptly as a sign of Clostridium difficile-associated diarrhea (CDAD). May begin up to several weeks following the cessation of therapy.
- Assess patient for hypersensitivity (skin rash, urticaria).
- ***Lab Test Considerations:*** Monitor CBC; may cause transient ↓ in leukocytes, eosinophils, and platelets.
- May cause ↑ alkaline phosphatase, bilirubin, CPK, AST, and ALT concentrations.

Potential Nursing Diagnoses

Risk for infection (Indications, Side Effects)
Diarrhea (Side Effects)

Implementation

- Do not confuse Clindesse with Clindets.
- **PO:** Administer with a full glass of water. May be given with or without meals. Shake liquid preparations well. Do not refrigerate. Stable for 14 days at room temperature.
- **IM:** Inject undiluted. Do not administer >600 mg in a single IM injection.

IV Administration

- **Intermittent Infusion: *Diluent:*** Vials must be diluted before use. Dilute a dose of 300 mg or 600 mg in 50 mL and a dose of 900 mg or 1200 mg in 100 mL. Compatible diluents include D5W, 0.9% NaCl, D5/0.9% NaCl, D5/0.45% NaCl, or LR. Admixed solution stable for 16 days at room temperature. Premixed infusion is already diluted and ready to use. ***Concentration:*** Not to exceed 18 mg/mL. ***Rate:*** Infuse over 10–60 min. Not to exceed 30 mg/min. Hypotension and cardiopulmonary arrest have been reported following rapid IV administration.
- **Y-Site Compatibility:** acetaminophen, acyclovir, alemtuzumab, alfentanil, amifostine, amikacin, aminocaproic acid, aminophylline, amiodarone, amphotericin B lipid complex, amphotericin B liposome, anakinra, anidulafungin, argatroban, ascorbic acid, atropine, aztreonam, benztropine, bivalirudin, bleomycin, bumetanide, buprenorphine, butorphanol, calcium chloride, calcium gluconate, cangrelor, carboplatin, carmustine, cefazolin, cefotaxime, cefotetan, cefoxitin, ceftaroline, ceftazidime, cefuroxime, chloramphenicol, cisatracurium, cisplatin, cyanocobalamin, cyclophosphamide, cyclosporine, cytarabine, dacarbazine, dactinomycin, daptomycin, dexamethasone, dexmedetomidine, dexrazoxane, digoxin, diltiazem, dimehydrinate, diphenhydramine, dobutamine, docetaxel, dolasetron, dopamine, doxorubicin, doxorubicin liposomal, doxycycline, enalaprilat, ephedrine, epinephrine, epirubicin, epoetin alfa, eptifibatide, esmolol, etoposide, etoposide phosphate, famotidine, fenoldopam, fentanyl, fludarabine, fluorouracil, folic acid, foscarnet, fosphenytoin, furosemide, gemcitabine, gentamicin, glycopyrrolate, granisetron, heparin, hetastarch, hydrocortisone sodium succinate, hydromorphone, ifosfamide, imipenem/cilastatin, indomethacin, insulin, irinotecan, isoproterenol, ketamine, ketorolac, leucovorin, levofloxacin, lidocaine, linezolid, lorazepam, magnesium sulfate, mannitol, mechlorethamine, melphalan, meperidine, mesna, methotrexate, methylprednisolone, metoclopramide, metoprolol, metronidazole, milrinone, morphine, multivitamins, nafcillin, nalbuphine, naloxone, nesiritide, nitroglycerin, nitroprusside, norepinephrine, octreotide, ondansetron, oxacillin, oxaliplatin, oxytocin, paclitaxel, palonosetron, pamidronate, pancuronium, pemetrexed, penicillin G, pentazocine, perphenazine, phenobarbital, phenylephrine, phytonadione, piperacillin/tazobactam, potassium acetate, potassium chloride, procainamide, propofol, propranolol, protamine, pyridoxine, ranitidine, remifentanil, rituximab, rocuronium, sargramostim, sodium acetate, sodium bicarbonate, streptokinase, succinylcholine, sufentanil, tacrolimus, teniposide, theophylline, thiamine, thiotepa, tigecycline, tirofiban, tobramycin, vancomycin, vasopressin, vecuronium, verapamil, vinblastine, vincristine, vinorelbine, vitamin B complex with C, voriconazole, zidovudine, zoledronic acid.
- **Y-Site Incompatibility:** allopurinol, amphotericin B colloidal, azathioprine, caspofungin, ceftriaxone, chlorpromazine, dantrolene, daunorubicin hydrochloride, diazepam, filgrastim, ganciclovir, haloperidol, hydroxyzine, idarubicin, mitomycin, mitoxantrone, mycophenolate, papaverine, pentamidine, pentobarbital, phenytoin, prochlorperazine, promethazine, quinupristin/dalfopristin, topotecan, trastuzumab, trimethoprim/sulfamethoxazole.
- **Vag:** Applicators are supplied for vaginal administration. When treating bacterial vaginosis, concurrent treatment of male partner is not usually necessary.
- **Topical:** Contact with eyes, mucous membranes, and open cuts should be avoided during topical application. If accidental contact occurs, rinse with copious amounts of cool water.
- Wash affected areas with warm water and soap, rinse, and pat dry prior to application. Apply to entire affected area.

Patient/Family Teaching

- Instruct patient to take medication around the clock at evenly spaced times and to finish completely as directed, even if feeling better. Take missed doses as soon as possible unless almost time for next dose. Do not double doses. Advise patient that sharing of this medication may be dangerous.

- Instruct patient to notify health care professional immediately if diarrhea, abdominal cramping, fever, or bloody stools occur and not to treat with antidiarrheals without consulting health care professional.
- Advise patient to report signs of superinfection (furry overgrowth on the tongue, vaginal or anal itching or discharge).
- Notify health care professional if no improvement within a few days.
- Patients with a history of rheumatic heart disease or valve replacement need to be taught the importance of antimicrobial prophylaxis before invasive medical or dental procedures.
- **IV:** Inform patient that bitter taste occurring with IV administration is not clinically significant.
- **Vag:** Instruct patient on proper use of vaginal applicator. Insert high into vagina at bedtime. Instruct patient to remain recumbent for at least 30 min following insertion. Advise patient to use sanitary napkin to prevent staining of clothing or bedding. Continue therapy during menstrual period.
- Advise patient to refrain from vaginal sexual intercourse during treatment.
- Caution patient that mineral oil in clindamycin cream may weaken latex or rubber contraceptive devices. Such products should not be used within 72 hr of vaginal cream.
- **Topical:** Caution patient applying topical clindamycin that solution is flammable (vehicle is isopropyl alcohol). Avoid application while smoking or near heat or flame.
- Advise patient to notify health care professional if excessive drying of skin occurs.
- Advise patient to wait 30 min after washing or shaving area before applying.

Evaluation/Desired Outcomes

- Resolution of the signs and symptoms of infection. Length of time for complete resolution depends on the organism and site of infection.
- Endocarditis prophylaxis.
- Improvement in acne vulgaris lesions. Improvement should be seen in 6 wk but may take 8–12 wk for maximum benefit.

clobetasol, See CORTICOSTEROIDS (TOPICAL/LOCAL).

clocortolone, See CORTICOSTEROIDS (TOPICAL/LOCAL).

clonazePAM (kloe-na-ze-pam)

✽Clonapam, KlonoPIN, ✽Rivotril

Classification
Therapeutic: anticonvulsants
Pharmacologic: benzodiazepines

Schedule IV

Pregnancy Category D

Indications

Prophylaxis of: Petit mal, Lennox-Gastaut, Akinetic, Myoclonic seizures. Panic disorder with or without agoraphobia. **Unlabeled Use:** Uncontrolled leg movements during sleep. Neuralgias. Infantile spasms. Sedation. Adjunct management of acute mania, acute psychosis, or insomnia.

Action

Anticonvulsant effects may be due to presynaptic inhibition. Produces sedative effects in the CNS, probably by stimulating inhibitory GABA receptors. **Therapeutic Effects:** Prevention of seizures. Decreased manifestations of panic disorder.

Pharmacokinetics

Absorption: Well absorbed from the GI tract.
Distribution: Probably crosses the blood-brain barrier and the placenta.
Protein Binding: 85%.
Metabolism and Excretion: Mostly metabolized by the liver.
Half-life: 18–50 hr.

TIME/ACTION PROFILE (anticonvulsant activity)

ROUTE	ONSET	PEAK	DURATION
PO	20–60 min	1–2 hr	6–12 hr

Contraindications/Precautions

Contraindicated in: Hypersensitivity to clonazepam or other benzodiazepines; Severe hepatic impairment.
Use Cautiously in: All patients (may ↑ risk of suicidal thoughts/behaviors); Angle-closure glaucoma; Obstructive sleep apnea; Chronic respiratory disease; History of porphyria; Do not discontinue abruptly; OB: Safety not established; chronic use during pregnancy may result in withdrawal in the neonate; Lactation: May enter breast milk; discontinue drug or bottle feed; Geri: May experience excessive sedation at usual doses; ↓ dosage recommended.

Adverse Reactions/Side Effects

CNS: SUICIDAL THOUGHTS, behavioral changes, drowsiness, fatigue, slurred speech, ataxia, sedation, abnormal eye movements, diplopia, nystagmus. **Resp:** ↑ secretions. **CV:** palpitations. **Derm:** rash. **GI:**

constipation, diarrhea, hepatitis, weight gain. **GU:** dysuria, nocturia, urinary retention. **Hemat:** anemia, eosinophilia, leukopenia, thrombocytopenia. **Neuro:** ataxia, hypotonia. **Misc:** fever, physical dependence, psychological dependence, tolerance.

Interactions

Drug-Drug: **Alcohol**, **antidepressants**, **antihistamines**, other **benzodiazepines**, and **opioid analgesics**; concurrent use results in ↑ CNS depression. **Cimetidine**, **hormonal contraceptives**, **disulfiram**, **fluoxetine**, **isoniazid**, **ketoconazole**, **metoprolol**, **propranolol**, or **valproic acid** may ↓ metabolism and ↑ toxicity of clonazepam. May ↓ efficacy of **levodopa**. **Rifampin** or **barbiturates** may ↑ metabolism and ↓ effectiveness. Sedative effects may be ↓ by **theophylline**. May ↑ serum **phenytoin** levels. **Phenytoin** may ↓ levels.

Drug-Natural Products: Concomitant use of **kava-kava**, **valerian**, or **chamomile** can ↑ CNS depression.

Route/Dosage

PO (Adults): 0.5 mg 3 times daily; may ↑ by 0.5–1 mg q 3 days. Total daily maintenance dose not to exceed 20 mg. *Panic disorder*—0.125 mg twice daily; ↑ after 3 days toward target dose of 1 mg/day (some patients may require up to 4 mg/day).

PO (Children <10 yr or 30 kg): Initial daily dose 0.01–0.03 mg/kg/day (not to exceed 0.05 mg/kg/day) given in 2–3 equally divided doses; ↑ by no more than 0.25–0.5 mg q 3 days until therapeutic blood levels are reached (not to exceed 0.2 mg/kg/day).

Availability (generic available)

Tablets: 0.5 mg, 1 mg, 2 mg. **Cost:** *Generic*—0.5 mg $11.77/100, 1 mg $11.25/100, 2 mg $15.59/100. **Orally disintegrating tablets:** 0.125 mg, 0.25 mg, 0.5 mg, 1 mg, 2 mg. **Cost:** *Generic*—0.125 mg $77.93/60, 0.25 mg $77.93/60, 0.5 mg $77.80/60, 1 mg $88.91/60, 2 mg $123.19/60.

NURSING IMPLICATIONS

Assessment

- Observe and record intensity, duration, and location of seizure activity.
- Assess degree and manifestations of anxiety and mental status (orientation, mood, behavior) prior to and periodically during therapy.
- Assess need for continued treatment regularly.
- Assess patient for drowsiness, unsteadiness, and clumsiness. These symptoms are dose related and most severe during initial therapy; may decrease in severity or disappear with continued or long-term therapy.
- Monitor closely for notable changes in behavior that could indicate the emergence or worsening of suicidal thoughts or behavior or depression.
- ***Lab Test Considerations:*** Patients on prolonged therapy should have CBC and liver function test results evaluated periodically. May cause an ↑ in serum bilirubin, AST, and ALT.
- May cause ↓ thyroidal uptake of ^{123}I, and ^{131}I.
- ***Toxicity and Overdose:*** Therapeutic serum concentrations are 20–80 mg/mL. Flumazenil antagonizes clonazepam toxicity or overdose (may induce seizures in patients with history of seizure disorder or who are on tricyclic antidepressants).

Potential Nursing Diagnoses

Risk for injury (Indications, Side Effects)

Implementation

- Do not confuse clonazepam with clonidine, clozapine, clorazepate, or lorazepam. Do not confuse Klonopin with clonidine.
- Institute seizure precautions for patients on initial therapy or undergoing dose manipulations.
- **PO:** Administer with food to minimize gastric irritation. Tablets may be crushed if patient has difficulty swallowing. Administer largest dose at bedtime to avoid daytime sedation. Taper by 0.25 mg every 3 days to decrease signs and symptoms of withdrawal. Some patients may require longer taper period (months).
- Orally disintegrating tablets should be left in the package until use. Remove from the blister pouch. Do not push tablet through the blister; peel open the blister pack with dry hands and place tablet on tongue. Tablet will dissolve rapidly and be swallowed with saliva. No liquid is needed to take the orally disintegrating tablet.

Patient/Family Teaching

- Instruct patient to take medication exactly as directed. Take missed doses within 1 hr or omit; do not double doses. Abrupt withdrawal of clonazepam may cause status epilepticus, tremors, nausea, vomiting, and abdominal and muscle cramps. Instruct patient to read the *Medication Guide* before starting and with each Rx refill, changes may occur.
- Advise patient that clonazepam is usually prescribed for short-term use and does not cure underlying problems.
- Advise patient to not share medication with others.
- May cause drowsiness or dizziness. Advise patient to avoid driving or other activities requiring alertness until response to drug is known.
- Instruct patient to notify health care professional of all Rx or OTC medications, vitamins, or herbal products being taken and to consult health care professional before taking any other Rx, OTC, or herbal products. Caution patient to avoid taking alcohol or other CNS depressants concurrently with this medication.

- Advise patient to notify health care professional of medication regimen prior to treatment or surgery.
- Instruct patient and family to notify health care professional of unusual tiredness, bleeding, sore throat, fever, clay-colored stools, yellowing of skin, or behavioral changes. Advise patient and family to notify health care professional if thoughts about suicide or dying, attempts to commit suicide; new or worse depression; new or worse anxiety; feeling very agitated or restless; panic attacks; trouble sleeping; new or worse irritability; acting aggressive; being angry or violent; acting on dangerous impulses; an extreme increase in activity and talking; other unusual changes in behavior or mood occur.
- Advise female patients to notify health care professional if pregnancy is planned or suspected or if breast feeding. Encourage pregnant patients to enroll in North American Antiepileptic Drug (NAAED) Pregnancy Registry to collect information about safety of antiepileptic drugs during pregnancy. To enroll, patients can call 1-888-233-2334.
- Patient on anticonvulsant therapy should carry identification at all times describing disease process and medication regimen.
- Emphasize the importance of follow-up exams to determine effectiveness of the medication.

Evaluation/Desired Outcomes

- Decrease or cessation of seizure activity without undue sedation. Dose adjustments may be required after several months of therapy.
- Decrease in frequency and severity of panic attacks.
- Relief of leg movements during sleep.
- Decrease in pain from neuralgia.

cloNIDine (klon-i-deen)

Catapres, Catapres-TTS, ✦Dixarit, Duraclon, Kapvay

Classification

Therapeutic: antihypertensives

Pharmacologic: adrenergics (centrally acting)

Pregnancy Category C

Indications

PO, Transdermal: Mild to moderate hypertension. **PO:** Attention-deficit hyperactivity disorder (ADHD) (as monotherapy or as adjunctive to stimulants) (Kapvay only). **Epidural:** Management of cancer pain unresponsive to opioids alone. **Unlabeled Use:** Management of opioid withdrawal. Adjunctive treatment of neuropathic pain.

Action

Stimulates alpha-adrenergic receptors in the CNS, which results in decreased sympathetic outflow inhibiting cardioacceleration and vasoconstriction centers. Prevents pain signal transmission to the CNS by stimulating alpha-adrenergic receptors in the spinal cord. **Therapeutic Effects:** Decreased BP. Decreased pain. Improvement in ADHD symptoms.

Pharmacokinetics

Absorption: Well absorbed from the GI tract and skin. Enters systemic circulation following epidural use. Some absorption follows sublingual administration.

Distribution: Widely distributed; enters CNS. Crosses the placenta readily; enters breast milk in high concentrations.

Metabolism and Excretion: Mostly metabolized by the liver; 40–60% eliminated unchanged in urine.

Half-life: *Neonates*—44–72 hr; *Children*—8–12 hr; *Adults: Plasma*—12–16 hr (↑ in renal impairment); *CNS*—1.3 hr.

TIME/ACTION PROFILE (PO, TD = antihypertensive effect; epidural = analgesia)

ROUTE	ONSET	PEAK	DURATION
PO	30–60 min	1–3 hr	8–12 hr
Transdermal	2–3 days	unknown	7 days†
Epidural	unknown	unknown	unknown

†8 hr following removal of patch.

Contraindications/Precautions

Contraindicated in: Hypersensitivity; *Epidural*—injection site infection, anticoagulant therapy, or bleeding problems.

Use Cautiously in: Serious cardiac or cerebrovascular disease; Renal insufficiency; Pedi: Safety and efficacy not established for ADHD in children <6 yr; evaluation for cardiac disease should precede initiation of therapy for ADHD in children; Geri: Appear on Beers list due to ↑ risk of orthostatic hypotension and adverse CNS effects in geriatric patients (↓ dose recommended); OB, Lactation: Safety not established.

Adverse Reactions/Side Effects

CNS: drowsiness, depression, dizziness, hallucinations, nervousness, nightmares. **EENT:** dry eyes. **CV:** AV block, bradycardia, hypotension (↑ with epidural), palpitations. **GI:** dry mouth, constipation, nausea, vomiting. **GU:** erectile dysfunction. **Derm:** rash, sweating. **F and E:** sodium retention. **Metab:** weight gain. **Neuro:** paresthesia. **Misc:** withdrawal phenomenon.

Interactions

Drug-Drug: Additive sedation with **CNS depressants**, including **alcohol**, **antihistamines**, **opioid analgesics**, and **sedative/hypnotics**. Additive hypotension with other **antihypertensives** and **nitrates**. Additive bradycardia with **beta blockers**, **diltiazem**, **verapamil**, or **digoxin**. **MAO inhibitors**, **amphetamines**, or **tricyclic antidepressants** may ↓ antihypertensive effect. Withdrawal phenomenon may be ↑ by discontinuation of **beta blockers**. Epidural clonidine prolongs the effects of epidurally administered **local anesthetics**. May ↓ effectiveness of **levodopa**.

Route/Dosage

PO (Adults and Adolescents ≥12 yr): *Hypertension (immediate-release)*—100 mcg (0.1 mg) BID, ↑ by 100–200 mcg (0.1–0.2 mg)/day q 2–4 days; usual maintenance dose is 200–600 mcg (0.2–0.6 mg)/day in 2–3 divided doses (up to 2.4 mg/day). *Urgent treatment of hypertension (immediate-release)*—200 mcg (0.2 mg) loading dose, then 100 mcg (0.1 mg) q hr until BP is controlled or 800 mcg (0.8 mg) total has been administered; follow with maintenance dosing; *Opioid withdrawal (immediate-release)*—300 mcg (0.3 mg)–1.2 mg/day, may be ↓ by 50%/day for 3 days, then discontinued or ↓ by 100–200 mcg (0.1–0.2 mg)/day.

PO (Geriatric Patients): *Hypertension (immediate–release)*—100 mcg (0.1 mg) at bedtime initially, ↑ as needed.

PO (Children): *Hypertension (immediate-release)*—Initial 5–10 mcg/kg/day divided BID-TID, then ↑ gradually to 5–25 mcg/kg/day in divided doses q 6 hr; maximum dose: 0.9 mg/day. *ADHD (Kapvay-extended release) (children >6 yr)*—0.1 mg once daily at bedtime; after 1 wk, ↑ dose to 0.1 mg in AM and at bedtime; after 1 wk, ↑ dose to 0.1 mg in AM and 0.2 mg at bedtime; after 1 wk, ↑ dose to 0.2 mg in AM and at bedtime (max dose = 0.4 mg/day). *ADHD (Immediate release) (children >6 yr, <45 kg)*—0.05 mg once daily at bedtime; then ↑ q 3–7 days to 0.05 mg BID; then 0.05 mg TID; then 0.05 mg QID. *Neuropathic pain (immediate-release)*—2 mcg/kg/dose q 4–6 hr then ↑ gradually over days up to 4 mcg/kg/dose q 4–6 hr.

PO (Neonates): *Neonatal abstinence syndrome*—0.5–1 mcg/kg/dose q 4–6 hr. Once stabilized taper by 0.25 mcg/kg/dose q 6 hr.

Transdermal (Adults): *Hypertension*—Transdermal system delivering 100–300 mcg (0.1–0.3 mg)/24 hr applied every 7 days. Initiate with 100 mcg (0.1 mg)/24 hr system; dosage increments may be made q 1–2 wk when system is changed.

Transdermal (Children): Once stable oral dose is reached, children may be switched to a transdermal system equivalent closest to the total daily oral dose.

Epidural (Adults): 30 mcg/hr initially; titrated according to need.

Epidural (Children): 0.5 mcg/kg/hr initially; titrated according to need up to 2 mcg/kg/hr.

Availability (generic available)

Tablets: ✤25 mcg (0.025 mg), 100 mcg (0.1 mg), 200 mcg (0.2 mg), 300 mcg (0.3 mg). **Cost:** *Generic*—0.1 mg $6.80/100, 0.2 mg $6.99/100, 0.3 mg $6.99/100. **Extended-release tablets (Kapvay):** 0.1 mg, 0.2 mg. **Cost:** All strengths $366.60/60. **Transdermal systems:** Catapres-TTS 1, releases 0.1 mg/24 hr, Catapres-TTS 2, releases 0.2 mg/24 hr, Catapres-TTS 3, releases 0.3 mg/24 hr. **Cost:** *Generic*—0.1 mg/24 hr $132.49/4 patches, 0.2 mg/24 hr $223.06/4 patches, 0.3 mg/24 hr $309.44/4 patches. **Solution for epidural injection (Duraclon):** 100 mcg/mL, 500 mcg/mL. ***In combination with:*** chlorthalidone (Clorpres). See Appendix B.

NURSING IMPLICATIONS

Assessment

- **Hypertension:** Monitor intake and output ratios and daily weight, and assess for edema daily, especially at beginning of therapy.
- Monitor BP and pulse prior to starting, frequently during initial dose adjustment and dose increases and periodically throughout therapy. Titrate slowly in patients with cardiac conditions or those taking other sympatholytic drugs. Report significant changes.
- **Pain:** Assess location, character, and intensity of pain prior to, frequently during first few days, and routinely throughout administration.
- Monitor for fever as potential sign of catheter infection.
- **Opioid Withdrawal:** Monitor patient for signs and symptoms of opioid withdrawal (tachycardia, fever, runny nose, diarrhea, sweating, nausea, vomiting, irritability, stomach cramps, shivering, unusually large pupils, weakness, difficulty sleeping, gooseflesh).
- **ADHD:** Assess attention span, impulse control, and interactions with others.
- ***Lab Test Considerations:*** May cause transient ↑ in blood glucose levels.
- May cause ↓ urinary catecholamine and vanillylmandelic acid (VMA) concentrations; these may ↑ on abrupt withdrawal.
- May cause weakly positive Coombs' test result.

Potential Nursing Diagnoses

Chronic pain (Indications)
Impaired social interaction (Indications)
Risk for injury (Side Effects)

Implementation

- Do not confuse Catapres (clonidine) with Cataflam (diclofenac).
- Do not confuse clonidine with clonazepam (Klonopin).
- Do not confuse clonidine with clozapine.
- Do not substitute between clonidine products on a mg-per-mg basis, because of differing pharmacokinetic profiles.
- In the perioperative setting, continue clonidine up to 4 hr prior to surgery and resume as soon as possible thereafter. Do not interrupt *transdermal clonidine* during surgery. Monitor BP carefully.
- **PO:** Administer last dose of the day at bedtime. May be taken without regard for food.

- Swallow extended-release tablets whole; do not crush, break, or chew.
- **Transdermal:** Transdermal system should be applied once every 7 days. May be applied to any hairless site; avoid cuts or calluses. Absorption is greater when placed on chest or upper arm and decreased when placed on thigh. Rotate sites. Wash area with soap and water; dry thoroughly before application. Apply firm pressure over patch to ensure contact with skin, especially around edges. Remove old system and discard. System includes a protective adhesive overlay to be applied over medication patch to ensure adhesion, should medication patch loosen.
- **Epidural:** Dilute 500 mcg/mL with 0.9% NaCl for a concentration of 100 mcg/mL. Do not administer solutions that are discolored or contain a precipitate. Discard unused portion.

Patient/Family Teaching

- Instruct patient to take clonidine at the same time each day, even if feeling well. Take missed dosed as soon as remembered. If dose of extended-release product is missed, omit dose and take next dose as scheduled. Do not take more than the prescribed daily dose in any 24 hr. If more than 1 oral dose in a row is missed or if transdermal system is late in being changed by 3 or more days, consult health care professional. All routes of clonidine should be gradually discontinued over 2–4 days to prevent rebound hypertension.
- Advise patient to make sure enough medication is available for weekends, holidays, and vacations. A written prescription may be kept in wallet in case of emergency.
- May cause drowsiness, which usually diminishes with continued use. Advise patient to avoid driving or other activities requiring alertness until response to medication is known.
- Caution patient to avoid sudden changes in position to decrease orthostatic hypotension. Use of alcohol, standing for long periods, exercising, and hot weather may increase orthostatic hypotension.
- If dry mouth occurs, frequent mouth rinses, good oral hygiene, and sugarless gum or candy may decrease effect. If dry mouth continues for more than 2 wk, consult health care professional.
- Caution patients with contact lenses that clonidine may cause dryness of eyes.
- Caution patient to avoid concurrent use of alcohol or other CNS depressants with this medication.
- Instruct patient to notify health care professional of all Rx or OTC medications, vitamins, or herbal products being taken and to consult health care professional before taking any other Rx, OTC, or herbal products, especially cough, cold, or allergy remedies.
- Advise patient to notify health care professional of medication regimen prior to treatment or surgery.
- Advise patient to notify health care professional if itching or redness of skin (with transdermal patch), mental depression, swelling of feet and lower legs, paleness or cold feeling in fingertips or toes, or vivid dreams or nightmares occur. May require discontinuation of therapy, especially with depression.
- **Hypertension:** Encourage patient to comply with additional interventions for hypertension (weight reduction, low-sodium diet, discontinuation of smoking, moderation of alcohol consumption, regular exercise, and stress management). Medication helps control but does not cure hypertension.
- Instruct patient and family on proper technique for BP monitoring. Advise them to check BP at least weekly and report significant changes.
- **Transdermal:** Instruct patient on proper application of transdermal system. Do not cut or trim unit. Transdermal system can remain in place during bathing or swimming.
- Advise patient referred for MRI test to discuss patch with referring health care professional and MRI facility to determine if removal of patch is necessary prior to test and for directions for replacing patch.
- Pedi: Advise parents to notify school nurse of medication regimen.

Evaluation/Desired Outcomes

- Decrease in BP.
- Decrease in severity of pain.
- Decrease in the signs and symptoms of opioid withdrawal.
- Improved attention span and social interactions in ADHD.

clopidogrel (kloh-**pid**-oh-grel)

Plavix

Classification
Therapeutic: antiplatelet agents
Pharmacologic: platelet aggregation inhibitors

Pregnancy Category B

Indications

Reduction of atherosclerotic events (MI, stroke, vascular death) in patients at risk for such events including recent MI, acute coronary syndrome (unstable angina/non–Q-wave MI), stroke, or peripheral vascular disease.

Action

Inhibits platelet aggregation by irreversibly inhibiting the binding of ATP to platelet receptors. **Therapeutic Effects:** Decreased occurrence of atherosclerotic events in patients at risk.

Pharmacokinetics

Absorption: Well absorbed following oral administration; rapidly metabolized to an active antiplatelet compound. Parent drug has no antiplatelet activity.
Distribution: Unknown.

Protein Binding: *Clopidogrel*—98%; *active metabolite*—94%.
Metabolism and Excretion: Rapidly and extensively converted by the liver (CYP2C19) to its active metabolite, which is then eliminated 50% in urine and 45% in feces; 2% of Whites, 4% of Blacks, and 14% of Asians have CYP2C19 genotype that results in reduced metabolism of clopidogrel (poor metabolizers) into its active metabolite (may result in ↓ antiplatelet effects).
Half-life: 6 hr (active metabolite 30 min).

TIME/ACTION PROFILE (effects on platelet function)

ROUTE	ONSET	PEAK	DURATION
PO	within 24 hr	3–7 days	5 days†

†Following discontinuation.

Contraindications/Precautions

Contraindicated in: Hypersensitivity to clopidogrel or prasugrel; Pathologic bleeding (peptic ulcer, intracranial hemorrhage); Concurrent use of omeprazole or esomeprazole; Impaired CYP2C19 function due to genetic variation; Lactation: Lactation.
Use Cautiously in: Patients at risk for bleeding (trauma, surgery, or other pathologic conditions); History of GI bleeding/ulcer disease; Severe hepatic impairment; Hypersensitivity to another thienopyridine (prasugrel); OB: Use only if clearly indicated; Pedi: Safety and effectiveness not established.

Adverse Reactions/Side Effects

Incidence of adverse reactions similar to that of aspirin.
CNS: depression, dizziness, fatigue, headache. **EENT:** epistaxis. **Resp:** cough, dyspnea, eosinophilic pneumonia. **CV:** chest pain, edema, hypertension. **GI:** GI BLEEDING, abdominal pain, diarrhea, dyspepsia, gastritis. **Derm:** ACUTE GENERALIZED EXANTHEMATOUS PUSTULOSIS, DRUG RASH WITH EOSINOPHILIA AND SYSTEMIC SYMPTOMS, STEVENS-JOHNSON SYNDROME, TOXIC EPIDERMAL NECROLYSIS, pruritus, purpura, rash. **Hemat:** BLEEDING, NEUTROPENIA, THROMBOTIC THROMBOCYTOPENIC PURPURA. **Metab:** hypercholesterolemia. **MS:** arthralgia, back pain. **Misc:** fever, hypersensitivity reactions.

Interactions

Drug-Drug: Concurrent **abciximab**, **eptifibatide**, **tirofiban**, **aspirin**, **NSAIDs**, **heparin**, **LMWHs**, **thrombolytic agents**, **SSRIs**, **SNRIs**, **prasugrel**, or **warfarin** may ↑ risk of bleeding. May ↓ metabolism and ↑ effects of **phenytoin**, **tolbutamide**, **tamoxifen**, **torsemide**, **fluvastatin**, and many **NSAIDs**. Concurrent use with the CYP2C19 inhibitors, **omeprazole**, or **esomeprazole** may ↓ antiplatelet effects; avoid concurrent use; may consider using **H2 antagonist** or another **proton pump inhibitor** (e.g., **dexlansoprazole**, **lansoprazole**, or **pantoprazole**).
Drug-Natural Products: ↑ bleeding risk with **anise**, **arnica**, **chamomile**, **clove**, **fenugreek**, **feverfew**, **garlic**, **ginger**, **ginkgo**, **Panax ginseng**, and others.

Route/Dosage

Recent MI, Stroke, or Peripheral Vascular Disease

PO (Adults): 75 mg once daily.

Acute Coronary Syndrome

PO (Adults): 300 mg initially, then 75 mg once daily; aspirin 75–325 mg once daily should be given concurrently.

Availability (generic available)

Tablets: 75 mg, 300 mg. **Cost:** *Generic*—75 mg $23.46/90.

NURSING IMPLICATIONS

Assessment

- Assess patient for symptoms of stroke, peripheral vascular disease, or MI periodically during therapy.
- Monitor patient for signs of thrombotic thrombocytic purpura (thrombocytopenia, microangiopathic hemolytic anemia, neurologic findings, renal dysfunction, fever). May rarely occur, even after short exposure (<2 wk). Requires prompt treatment.
- ***Lab Test Considerations:*** Monitor bleeding time during therapy. Prolonged bleeding time, which is time- and dose-dependent, is expected.
- Monitor CBC with differential and platelet count periodically during therapy. Neutropenia and thrombocytopenia may rarely occur.
- May cause ↑ serum bilirubin, hepatic enzymes, total cholesterol, nonprotein nitrogen (NPN), and uric acid concentrations.

Potential Nursing Diagnoses

Risk for injury (Indications, Side Effects)

Implementation

- Do not confuse Plavix with Paxil.
- Discontinue clopidogrel 5–7 days before planned surgical procedures. If clopidogrel must be temporarily discontinued, restart as soon as possible. Premature discontinuation of therapy may increase risk of cardiovascular events.
- **PO:** Administer once daily without regard to food.

Patient/Family Teaching

- Instruct patient to take medication exactly as directed. Take missed doses as soon as possible unless almost time for next dose; do not double doses. Do not discontinue clopidogrel without consulting health care professional; may increase risk of cardiovascular events. Advise patient to read the *Medi-*

cation Guide before starting clopidogrel and with each Rx refill in case of changes.

- Advise patient to notify health care professional promptly if fever, weakness, chills, sore throat, rash, unusual bleeding or bruising, extreme skin paleness, purple skin patches, yellowing of skin or eyes, or neurological changes occur.
- Advise patient to notify health care professional of medication regimen prior to treatment or surgery.
- Instruct patient to notify health care professional of all Rx or OTC medications, vitamins, or herbal products being taken and to consult health care professional before taking any other Rx, OTC, or herbal products, especially those containing aspirin or NSAIDs or proton pump inhibitors.
- Advise female patient to notify health care professional if pregnancy is planned or suspected, or if breast feeding.

Evaluation/Desired Outcomes

- Prevention of stroke, MI, and vascular death in patients at risk.

clotrimazole, See ANTIFUNGALS (TOPICAL) and ANTIFUNGALS (VAGINAL).

REMS

cloZAPine (kloe-za-peen)

Clozaril, FazaClo, Versacloz

Classification

Therapeutic: antipsychotics

Pregnancy Category B

Indications

Schizophrenia unresponsive to or intolerant of standard therapy with other antipsychotics (treatment refractory). To reduce recurrent suicidal behavior in schizophrenic patients.

Action

Binds to dopamine receptors in the CNS. Also has anticholinergic and alpha-adrenergic blocking activity. Produces fewer extrapyramidal reactions and less tardive dyskinesia than standard antipsychotics but carries high risk of hematologic abnormalities. **Therapeutic Effects:** Diminished schizophrenic behavior. Diminished suicidal behavior.

Pharmacokinetics

Absorption: Well absorbed after oral administration.
Distribution: Rapid and extensive distribution; crosses blood-brain barrier and placenta.
Protein Binding: 95%.
Metabolism and Excretion: Mostly metabolized on first pass through the liver (by CYP1A2, CYP2D6, and CYP3A4 isoenzymes); (the CYP2D6 enzyme system exhibits genetic polymorphism; ~7% of population may be poor metabolizers and may have significantly ↑ clozapine concentrations and an ↑ risk of adverse effects).
Half-life: 8–12 hr.

TIME/ACTION PROFILE (antipsychotic effect)

ROUTE	ONSET	PEAK	DURATION
PO	unknown	wk	4–12 hr

Contraindications/Precautions

Contraindicated in: Hypersensitivity; Bone marrow depression; Severe CNS depression/coma; Uncontrolled epilepsy; Clozapine-induced agranulocytosis or severe granulocytopenia; Lactation: Discontinue drug or bottle-feed.

Use Cautiously in: Long QT syndrome; Risk factors for QT interval prolongation or ventricular arrhythmias (i.e., recent myocardial infarction, heart failure, arrhythmias); Concurrent use of CYP1A2, CYP2D6, or CYP3A4 inhibitors or QT-interval prolonging drugs; Hypokalemia or hypomagenesemia; Prostatic enlargement; Angle-closure glaucoma; Malnourished or dehydrated patients, patients with cardiovascular, cerebrovascular, hepatic, or renal disease, or patients on antihypertensives (use lower initial dose, titrate more slowly); Risk factors for stroke (↑ risk of stroke in patients with dementia); Diabetes; Seizure disorder; OB: Neonates at ↑ risk for extrapyramidal symptoms and withdrawal after delivery when exposed during the 3rd trimester; use only if benefit outweighs risk to fetus; Pedi: Children <16 yr (safety not established); Geri: ↑ risk of mortality in elderly patients treated for dementia-related psychosis.

Adverse Reactions/Side Effects

CNS: NEUROLEPTIC MALIGNANT SYNDROME, SEIZURES, dizziness, sedation. **EENT:** visual disturbances. **CV:** CARDIAC ARREST, DEEP VEIN THROMBOSIS, MYOCARDITIS, TORSADE DE POINTES, VENTRICULAR ARRHYTHMIAS, hypotension, tachycardia, bradycardia, ECG changes, hypertension, syncope, QT interval prolongation. **GI:** constipation, abdominal discomfort, dry mouth, ↑ salivation, nausea, vomiting, weight gain. **GU:** nocturnal enuresis. **Derm:** rash, sweating. **Endo:** hyperglycemia, hyperlipidemia, weight gain. **Hemat:** AGRANULOCYTOSIS, LEUKOPENIA. **Neuro:** extrapyramidal reactions. **Resp:** PULMONARY EMBOLISM. **Misc:** fever.

Interactions

Drug-Drug: ↑ anticholinergic effects with other **agents having anticholinergic properties**, including **antihistamines**, **quinidine**, **disopyramide**, and **antidepressants**. Concurrent use with strong **CYP1A2 inhibitors**, including **fluvoxamine** or **ciprofloxacin** may ↑ levels; ↓ clozapine dose to 1/3 of the original dose during concurrent use. Concurrent use with moderate or weak **CYP1A2 inhibitors**, including **oral contraceptives** or **caffeine** may ↑ levels; consider ↓

clozapine dose. Concurrent use with **CYP2D6 inhibitors** or **CYP3A4 inhibitors**, including **cimetidine**, **escitalopram**, **erythromycin**, **paroxetine**, **bupropion**, **fluoxetine**, **quinidine**, **duloxetine**, **terbinafine**, or **sertraline** may ↑ levels; consider ↓ clozapine dose. Concurrent use with **CYP1A2 inducers** or **CYP3A4 inducers**, including **nicotine**, **carbamazepine**, **phenytoin**, or **rifampin** may ↓ levels; concurrent use with strong CYP3A4 inducers not recommended. ↑ CNS depression with **alcohol**, **antidepressants**, **antihistamines**, **opioid analgesics**, or **sedative/hypnotics**. ↑ hypotension with **nitrates**, acute ingestion of **alcohol**, or **antihypertensives**. ↑ risk of bone marrow suppression with **antineoplastics** or **radiation therapy**. Use with **lithium** ↑ risk of adverse CNS reactions, including seizures. ↑ risk of QT interval prolongation with other **agents causing QT interval prolongation**.

Drug-Natural Products: Caffeine-containing herbs (**cola nut**, **tea**, **coffee**) may ↑ serum levels and side effects. **St. John's wort** may ↓ blood levels and efficacy.

Route/Dosage

PO (Adults): 12.5 mg 1–2 times daily initially; ↑ by 25–50 mg/day over a period of 2 wk up to target dose of 300–450 mg/day. May then be ↑ by up to 100 mg/day once or twice weekly (not to exceed 900 mg/day). Treatment should be continued for at least 2 yr in patients with suicidal behavior.

Availability (generic available)

Tablets: 25 mg, 100 mg. **Orally disintegrating tablets (mint):** 12.5 mg, 25 mg, 100 mg, 150 mg, 200 mg. **Oral suspension :** 50 mg/mL.

NURSING IMPLICATIONS

Assessment

- Monitor patient's mental status (orientation, mood, behavior) before and periodically during therapy. Titrate slowly and monitor closely; may cause orthostatic hypotension, bradycardia, syncope, and cardiac arrest.
- Monitor BP (sitting, standing, lying) and pulse rate before and frequently during initial dose titration.
- Assess weight and BMI initially and throughout therapy. Refer as appropriate for nutritional/weight management and medical management.
- Observe patient carefully when administering medication to ensure that medication is actually taken and not hoarded or cheeked.
- Monitor for signs of myocarditis (unexplained fatigue, dyspnea, tachypnea, fever, chest pain, palpitations, other signs and symptoms of heart failure, ECG changes, such as ST-T wave abnormalities, arrhythmias, or tachycardia during first month of therapy). If these occur, clozapine should be discontinued and not restarted.
- Monitor patient for onset of akathisia (restlessness or desire to keep moving) and extrapyramidal side effects (*parkinsonian*—difficulty speaking or swallowing, loss of balance control, pill-rolling motion of hands, mask-like face, shuffling gait, rigidity, tremors and dystonic muscle spasms, twisting motions, twitching, inability to move eyes, weakness of arms or legs) every 2 mo during therapy and 8–12 wk after therapy has been discontinued. Notify health care professional if these symptoms occur; reduction in dose or discontinuation of medication may be necessary. Trihexyphenidyl or benzotropine may be used to control these symptoms.
- Monitor for possible tardive dyskinesia (uncontrolled rhythmic movement of mouth, face, and extremities; lip smacking or puckering; puffing of cheeks; uncontrolled chewing; rapid or worm-like movements of tongue). Report these symptoms immediately; may be irreversible.
- Monitor frequency and consistency of bowel movements. Increasing bulk and fluids in the diet may help to minimize constipation.
- Clozapine lowers the seizure threshold. Institute seizure precautions for patients with history of seizure disorder.
- Transient fevers may occur, especially during first 3 wk of therapy. Fever is usually self-limiting but may require discontinuation of medication. Also, monitor for development of neuroleptic malignant syndrome (fever, respiratory distress, tachycardia, seizures, diaphoresis, hypertension or hypotension, pallor, tiredness). Notify health care professional immediately if these symptoms occur.
- Assess respiratory status during therapy. If deep-vein thrombosis, acute dyspnea, chest pain, or other respiratory signs and symptoms occur, consider pulmonary embolism.
- ***Lab Test Considerations:*** Monitor WBC, absolute neutrophil count (ANC), and differential count before initiation of therapy. ANC must be ≥2000/mm³ and WBC must be ≥3500/mm³ for patient to begin therapy. If ANC <1000/mm³ or WBC <2000/mm³, discontinue and do not rechallange. WBC and ANC must be monitored weekly for the first 6 mo, then biweekly for the second 6 mo, then, if maintained within acceptable parameters, every 4 wk during therapy and weekly for 4 wk after discontinuation of clozapine or until WBC ≥3500/mm³ and ANC ≥2000/mm³. If a substantial drop in ANC or WBC, single drop or cumulative drop within 3 wk of WBC ≤3,000/mm³ or ANC ≤1500/mm³, repeat WBC and ANC. If repeat values are: WBC 3000/mm³ to 3500/mm³ and/or ANC > 2000/mm³, then monitor twice weekly. If mild leukopenia or granulocyto-

penia occurs (WBC 3000/mm³ to 3500/mm³ and/or ANC 1500/mm³ to 2000/mm³), monitor twice weekly until WBC >3500/mm³ and ANC >2000/mm³, then return to previous monitoring frequency. If moderate leukopenia or granulocytopenia (WBC 2000/mm³ to 3000/mm³ and/or ANC 1000/mm³ to 1500/mm³), interrupt therapy. Monitor daily until WBC >3000/mm³ and ANC >1500/mm³, then twice weekly until WBC >3500/mm³ and ANC >2000/mm³, may rechallenge at this level. If rechallenged, monitor weekly for 1 yr before returning to usual monitoring schedule of every 2 wk for 6 mo and then every 4 weeks. Because of the risk of agranulocytosis, clozapine is available only through the **Clozaril National Registry, Fazaclo Patient Registry, or Versacloz Patient Registry,** which combines WBC testing, patient monitoring, and controlled distribution through participating pharmacies.

- Assess fasting blood glucose and cholesterol levels initially and throughout therapy.
- ***Toxicity and Overdose:*** Overdose is treated with activated charcoal and supportive therapy. Monitor patient for several days because of risk of delayed effects.
- Avoid use of epinephrine and its derivatives when treating hypotension, and avoid quinidine and procainamide when treating arrhythmias.

Potential Nursing Diagnoses

Risk for other-directed violence (Indications)
Disturbed thought process (Indications)
Risk for injury (Side Effects)

Implementation

- Do not confuse clozapine with clonazepam or clonidine. Do not confuse Clozaril with Colazal.
- **PO:** Administer capsules with food or milk to decrease gastric irritation.
- Leave oral disintegrating tablet in blister until time of use. Do not push tablet through foil. Just before use, peel foil and gently remove disintegrating tablet. Immediately place tablet in mouth and allow to disintegrate and swallow with saliva. If 1/2 tablet dose used, destroy other half of tablet.
- Oral solution may be taken without regard to food. Shake bottle for suspension for 10 sec prior to withdrawing. Use oral syringes and oral adaptor provided for accurate dosing. Do not store dose in syringe; wash between doses.

Patient/Family Teaching

- Instruct patient to take medication as directed. Patients on long-term therapy may need to discontinue gradually over 1–2 wk.
- Explain purpose and procedures for *Clozaril National Registry, Fazaclo Patient Registrry, Versacloz Patient Registry* to patient.
- Inform patient of possibility of extrapyramidal symptoms. Instruct patient to report these symptoms immediately.
- Inform patient that cigarette smoking can decrease clozapine levels. Risk for relapse increases if patient begins or increases smoking.
- Advise patient to change positions slowly to minimize orthostatic hypotension.
- May cause seizures and drowsiness. Caution patient to avoid driving or other activities requiring alertness while taking clozapine.
- Instruct patient to notify health care professional of all Rx or OTC medications, vitamins, or herbal products being taken and to consult health care professional before taking any other Rx, OTC, or herbal products. Caution patient to avoid concurrent use of alcohol and other CNS depressants.
- Instruct patient to use frequent mouth rinses, good oral hygiene, and sugarless gum or candy to minimize dry mouth.
- Advise patient to notify health care professional of medication regimen before treatment or surgery.
- Instruct patient to notify health care professional promptly if unexplained fatigue, dyspnea, tachypnea, chest pain, palpitations, sore throat, fever, lethargy, weakness, malaise, or flu-like symptoms occur.
- Advise female patients to notify health care professional if pregnancy is planned or suspected, or if breast feeding or planning to breast feed.
- Advise patient of need for continued medical follow-up for psychotherapy, eye exams, and laboratory tests.

Evaluation/Desired Outcomes

- Decreased positive symptoms (delusions, hallucinations) of schizophrenia.
- Decrease in negative symptoms (social withdrawal, flat, blunt affect) of schizophrenia.

HIGH ALERT

codeine (koe-deen)

Classification
Therapeutic: allergy, cold, and cough remedies, antitussives, opioid analgesics
Pharmacologic: opioid agonists

Schedule II, III, IV, V (depends on content)

Pregnancy Category C

Indications

Management of mild to moderate pain. Antitussive (in smaller doses). **Unlabeled Use:** Management of diarrhea.

Action

Binds to opiate receptors in the CNS. Alters the perception of and response to painful stimuli while producing generalized CNS depression. Decreases cough reflex. Decreases GI motility. **Therapeutic Effects:** Decreased severity of pain. Suppression of the cough reflex. Relief of diarrhea.

Pharmacokinetics

Absorption: 50% absorbed from the GI tract.
Distribution: Widely distributed. Crosses the placenta; enters breast milk.
Protein Binding: 7%.
Metabolism and Excretion: Mostly metabolized by the liver (primarily via CYP2D6); 10% converted to morphine; ⚕ the CYP2D6 enzyme system exhibits genetic polymorphism (some patients [1–10% Whites, 3% African Americans, 16–28% North Africans/Ethiopians/Arabs] may be ultra-rapid metabolizers and may have ↑ morphine concentrations and an ↑ risk of adverse effects); 5–15% excreted unchanged in urine.
Half-life: 2.5–4 hr.

TIME/ACTION PROFILE (analgesia)

ROUTE	ONSET	PEAK	DURATION
PO	30–45 min	60–120 min	4 hr

Contraindications/Precautions

Contraindicated in: Hypersensitivity.
Use Cautiously in: Head trauma; ↑ intracranial pressure; Severe renal, hepatic, or pulmonary disease; Hypothyroidism; Adrenal insufficiency; Alcoholism; Prostatic hyperplasia; Geri: Geriatric or debilitated patients (dose ↓ required; more susceptible to CNS depression, constipation); Undiagnosed abdominal pain; OB: Has been used during labor; respiratory depression may occur in the newborn; OB, Lactation: Avoid chronic use; Pedi: Children undergoing tonsillectomy or adenoidectomy for obstructive sleep apnea (↑ risk of respiratory depression and death).

Adverse Reactions/Side Effects

CNS: confusion, sedation, dysphoria, euphoria, floating feeling, hallucinations, headache, unusual dreams. **EENT:** blurred vision, diplopia, miosis. **Resp:** respiratory depression. **CV:** hypotension, bradycardia. **GI:** constipation, nausea, vomiting. **GU:** urinary retention. **Derm:** flushing, sweating. **Misc:** physical dependence, psychological dependence, tolerance.

Interactions

Drug-Drug: Use with extreme caution in patients receiving **MAO inhibitors** (↓ initial dose to 25% of usual dose). Additive CNS depression with **alcohol**, **antidepressants**, **antihistamines**, and **sedative/hypnotics**. Administration of **partial antagonists (buprenorphine**, **butorphanol**, **nalbuphine**, or **pentazocine)** may precipitate opioid withdrawal in physically dependent patients. **Nalbuphine** or **pentazocine** may ↓ analgesia.
Drug-Natural Products: Concomitant use of **kava-kava**, **valerian**, **skullcap**, **chamomile**, or **hops** can ↑ CNS depression.

Route/Dosage

PO (Adults): *Analgesic*— 15–60 mg q 3–6 hr as needed. *Antitussive*— 10–20 mg q 4–6 hr as needed (not to exceed 120 mg/day). *Antidiarrheal* —30 mg up to 4 times daily.
PO (Children 6–12 yr): *Analgesic*—0.5–1 mg/kg (up to 60 mg) q 4–6 hr (up to 4 times daily) as needed. *Antitussive*—5–10 mg q 4–6 hr as needed (not to exceed 60 mg/day). *Antidiarrheal*—0.5 mg/kg up to 4 times daily.
PO (Children 2–5 yr): *Analgesic*—0.5–1 mg/kg (up to 60 mg) q 4–6 hr (up to 4 times daily) as needed. *Antitussive*— 1–1.5 mg/kg divided q 4–6 hr as needed. *Antidiarrheal*—0.5 mg/kg up to 4 times daily.

Renal Impairment

(Adults and Children): *CCr 10–50 mL/min*—Administer 75% of the dose; *CCr <10 mL/min*—Administer 50% of the dose.

Availability (generic available)

Tablets: 15 mg, 30 mg, 60 mg. **Oral solution:** ✱10 mg/5 mL. ***In combination with:*** antihistamines, decongestants, antipyretics, caffeine, butalbital, and nonopioid analgesics. See Appendix B.

NURSING IMPLICATIONS

Assessment

- Assess BP, pulse, and respirations before and periodically during administration. If respiratory rate is <10/min, assess level of sedation. Physical stimulation may be sufficient to prevent significant hypoventilation. Dose may need to be decreased by 25–50%. Initial drowsiness will diminish with continued use.
- Assess bowel function routinely. Prevention of constipation should be instituted with increased intake of fluids, bulk, and laxatives to minimize constipating effects. Stimulant laxatives should be administered routinely if opioid use exceeds 2–3 days, unless contraindicated.
- **Pain:** Assess type, location, and intensity of pain before and 1 hr (peak) after administration. When titrating opioid doses, increases of 25–50% should be administered until there is either a 50% reduction in the patient's pain rating on a numerical or visual analogue scale or the patient reports satisfactory pain relief. A repeat dose can be safely administered at the time of the peak if previous dose is ineffective and side effects are minimal.
- An equianalgesic chart (see Appendix I) should be used when changing routes or when changing from one opioid to another.
- Prolonged use may lead to physical and psychological dependence and tolerance. This should not prevent patient from receiving adequate analgesia. Most

patients who receive codeine for pain do not develop psychological dependence. If progressively higher doses are required, consider conversion to a stronger opioid.

- **Cough:** Assess cough and lung sounds during antitussive use.
- ***Lab Test Considerations:*** May cause ↑ plasma amylase and lipase concentrations.
- ***Toxicity and Overdose:*** If an opioid antagonist is required to reverse respiratory depression or coma, naloxone (Narcan) is the antidote. Dilute the 0.4-mg ampule of naloxone in 10 mL of 0.9% NaCl and administer 0.5 mL (0.02 mg) by IV push every 2 min. For children and patients weighing <40 kg, dilute 0.1 mg of naloxone in 10 mL of 0.9% NaCl for a concentration of 10 mcg/mL and administer 0.5 mcg/kg every 2 min. Titrate dose to avoid withdrawal, seizures, and severe pain.

Potential Nursing Diagnoses

Acute pain (Indications)
Disturbed sensory perception (visual, auditory) (Side Effects)
Risk for injury (Side Effects)

Implementation

- ***High Alert:*** Accidental overdosage of opioid analgesics has resulted in fatalities. Before administering, clarify all ambiguous orders; have second practitioner independently check dose calculations and route of administration.
- ***High Alert:*** Do not confuse codeine with Lodine (etodolac).
- Explain therapeutic value of medication before administration to enhance the analgesic effect.
- Regularly administered doses may be more effective than prn administration. Analgesic is more effective if given before pain becomes severe.
- Coadministration with nonopioid analgesics may have additive analgesic effects and permit lower doses.
- Medications should be discontinued gradually after long-term use to prevent withdrawal symptoms.
- When combined with nonopioid analgesics (aspirin, acetaminophen) #2 = 15 mg, #3 = 30 mg, #4 = 60 mg codeine. Codeine as an individual drug is a Schedule II substance. In combination with other drugs, tablet form is Schedule III, and elixir or cough suppressant is Schedule V (see Appendix H).
- **PO:** Oral doses may be administered with food or milk to minimize GI irritation.

Patient/Family Teaching

- Instruct patient on how and when to ask for and take pain medication.
- May cause drowsiness or dizziness. Advise patient to call for assistance when ambulating or smoking. Caution ambulatory patient to avoid driving or other activities requiring alertness until response to medication is known.
- Advise patient to change positions slowly to minimize orthostatic hypotension.
- Caution patient to avoid concurrent use of alcohol or other CNS depressants with this medication.
- Encourage patient to turn, cough, and breathe deeply every 2 hr to prevent atelectasis.
- Advise patient that good oral hygiene, frequent mouth rinses, and sugarless gum or candy may decrease dry mouth.

Evaluation/Desired Outcomes

- Decrease in severity of pain without a significant alteration in level of consciousness or respiratory status.
- Suppression of cough.
- Control of diarrhea.

HIGH ALERT

colchicine (kol-chi-seen)

Colcrys, Mitigare

Classification
Therapeutic: antigout agents

Pregnancy Category C

Indications

Prophylaxis and treatment of acute attacks of gouty arthritis. Familial Mediterranean fever.

Action

Interferes with the functions of WBCs in initiating and perpetuating the inflammatory response to monosodium urate crystals. **Therapeutic Effects:** Decreased pain and inflammation in acute attacks of gout. Reduced number of attacks of gout and familial Mediterranean fever.

Pharmacokinetics

Absorption: 45% absorbed from the GI tract, then re-enters GI tract from biliary secretions, when more absorption may occur.
Distribution: Concentrates in WBCs.
Metabolism and Excretion: Partially metabolized by the liver by CYP3A4; also a substrate for P-glycoprotein. Secreted in bile back into GI tract; eliminated in the feces. 40–65% excreted in the urine as unchanged drug.
Half-life: 27–31 hr.

TIME/ACTION PROFILE (anti-inflammatory activity)

ROUTE	ONSET	PEAK	DURATION
PO	12 hr	24–72 hr	unknown

Contraindications/Precautions

Contraindicated in: Hypersensitivity; Use of P-glycoprotein inhibitors or strong CYP3A4 inhibitors in patients with renal or hepatic impairment; Renal and hepatic impairment.

Use Cautiously in: Geri: Elderly or debilitated patients (toxicity may be cumulative); Renal impairment (dose ↓ suggested if CCr <80 mL/min); OB, Lactation, Pedi: Safety not established for gout.

Adverse Reactions/Side Effects

GI: diarrhea, nausea, vomiting, abdominal pain. **Derm:** alopecia. **Hemat:** AGRANULOCYTOSIS, APLASTIC ANEMIA, leukopenia, thrombocytopenia. **Neuro:** peripheral neuritis.

Interactions

Drug-Drug: Concurrent use of strong **CYP3A4 inhibitors**, including **atazanavir**, **clarithromycin**, **darunavir/ritonavir**, **indinavir**, **itraconazole**, **ketoconazole**, **lopinavir/ritonavir**, **nefazodone**, **nelfinavir**, **ritonavir**, **saquinavir**, **telithromycin**, or **tipranavir/ritonavir**, may ↑ levels and risk of toxicity; ↓ colchicine dose in patients with normal renal or hepatic function; concurrent use in patients with renal or hepatic impairment is contraindicated. Concurrent use of **P-glycoprotein inhibitors**, including **cyclosporine** or **ranolazine** may ↑ levels and risk of toxicity; ↓ colchicine dose in patients with normal renal or hepatic function; concurrent use in patients with renal or hepatic impairment is contraindicated. Moderate **CYP3A4 inhibitors**, including **aprepitant**, **diltiazem**, **erythromycin**, **fluconazole**, **fosamprenavir**, or **verapamil** may ↑ levels and risk of toxicity; ↓ colchicine dose. Additive bone marrow depression may occur with **bone marrow depressants** or **radiation therapy**. ↑ risk of rhabdomyolysis with **HMG-CoA reductase inhibitors**, **gemfibrozil**, **fenofibrate**, or **digoxin**. Additive adverse GI effects with **NSAIDs**. May cause reversible malabsorption of **vitamin B_{12}**.
Drug-Food: **Grapefruit juice** may ↑ levels and risk of toxicity; ↓ colchicine dose.

Route/Dosage

Treatment of Acute Gout Attacks

PO (Adults): 1.2 mg initially, then 0.6 mg 1 hr later (maximum dose of 1.8 mg in 1 hr); *Concomitant use of strong CYP3A4 inhibitors in patients with normal renal and hepatic function (atazanavir, clarithromycin, darunavir/ritonavir, indinavir, itraconazole, ketoconazole, lopinavir/ritonavir, nefazodone, nelfinavir, ritonavir, saquinavir, telithromycin, tipranavir/ritonavir)*—0.6 mg × 1 dose, then 0.3 mg 1 hr later (do not repeat treatment course for ≥3 days); *Concomitant use of moderate CYP3A4 inhibitors (aprepitant, diltiazem, erythromycin, fluconazole, fosamprenavir, grapefruit juice, verapamil)*—1.2 mg × 1 dose (do not repeat for ≥3 days); *Concomitant use of P-glycoprotein inhibitors (cyclosporine, ranolazine) in patients with normal renal and hepatic function*—0.6 mg × 1 dose (do not repeat for ≥3 days).

Renal Impairment

PO (Adults): *CCr <30 mL/min*—1.2 mg initially, then 0.6 mg 1 hr later; do not repeat treatment course for ≥2 wk; *Dialysis*—0.6 mg × 1 dose; do not repeat treatment course for ≥2 wk.

Prevention of Acute Gout Attacks

PO (Adults): 0.6 mg once or twice daily; *Concomitant use of strong CYP3A4 inhibitors (atazanavir, clarithromycin, darunavir/ritonavir, indinavir, itraconazole, ketoconazole, lopinavir/ritonavir, nefazodone, nelfinavir, ritonavir, saquinavir, telithromycin, tipranavir/ritonavir) or P-glycoprotein inhibitors (cyclosporine, ranolazine) in patients with normal renal and hepatic function*—if original dose was 0.6 mg twice daily, ↓ to 0.3 mg once daily; if original dose was 0.6 mg once daily, ↓ to 0.3 mg every other day; *Concomitant use of moderate CYP3A4 inhibitors (aprepitant, diltiazem, erythromycin, fluconazole, fosamprenavir, grapefruit juice, verapamil)*—if original dose was 0.6 mg twice daily, ↓ to 0.3 mg twice daily or 0.6 mg once daily; if original dose was 0.6 mg once daily, ↓ to 0.3 mg once daily.

Renal Impairment

PO (Adults): *CCr <30 mL/min*—0.3 mg/day; *Dialysis*—0.3 mg twice weekly.

Familial Mediterranean Fever

PO (Adults and Children >12 yr): 1.2–2.4 mg daily (in 1–2 divided doses); may ↑ or ↓ dose in 0.3-mg/day increments based on safety and efficacy; *Concomitant use of strong CYP3A4 inhibitors (atazanavir, clarithromycin, darunavir/ritonavir, indinavir, itraconazole, ketoconazole, lopinavir/ritonavir, nefazodone, nelfinavir, ritonavir, saquinavir, telithromycin, tipranavir/ritonavir) or P-glycoprotein inhibitors (cyclosporine, ranolazine) in patients with normal renal and hepatic function*—Do not exceed 0.6 mg/day (may be given as 0.3 mg twice daily); *Concomitant use of moderate CYP3A4 inhibitors (aprepitant, diltiazem, erythromycin, fluconazole, fosamprenavir, grapefruit juice, verapamil)*—Do not exceed 1.2 mg/day (may be given as 0.6 mg twice daily).
PO (Children 6–12 yr): 0.9–1.8 mg daily (in 1–2 divided doses).
PO (Children 4–6 yr): 0.3–1.8 mg daily (in 1–2 divided doses).

Renal Impairment

PO (Adults): *CCr 30–50 mL/min*—dose ↓ may be necessary; *CCr <30 mL/min or dialysis*—0.3 mg/day.

Availability (generic available)

Tablets: 0.6 mg, 🍁1 mg. **Capsules:** 0.6 mg. ***In combination with:*** probenecid (Col-Probenecid). See Appendix B.

NURSING IMPLICATIONS

Assessment

- Monitor intake and output ratios. Fluids should be encouraged to promote a urinary output of at least 2000 mL/day.
- **Gout:** Assess involved joints for pain, mobility, and edema throughout therapy. During initiation of therapy, monitor for drug response every 1–2 hr.
- **Familial Mediterranean fever:** Assess for signs and symptoms of familial Mediterranean fever (abdominal pain, chest pain, fever, chills, recurrent joint pain, red and swollen skin lesions) periodically during therapy.
- ***Lab Test Considerations:*** In patients receiving prolonged therapy, monitor baseline and periodic CBC; report significant ↓ in values. May cause ↓ platelet count, leukopenia, aplastic anemia, and agranulocytosis.
- May cause ↑ in AST and alkaline phosphatase.
- May cause false-positive results for urine hemoglobin.
- May interfere with results of urinary 17-hydroxycorticosteroid concentrations.
- ***Toxicity and Overdose: High Alert:*** Assess patient for toxicity (muscle pain or weakness, tingling or numbness in fingers or toes; pale or gray color to lips, tongue, or palms of hands; severe diarrhea or vomiting; unusual bleeding, bruising, sore throat, fatigue, malaise, or weakness or tiredness). If these symptoms occur, discontinue colchicine and treat symptomatically. Opioids may be needed to treat diarrhea.

Potential Nursing Diagnoses

Acute pain (Indications)
Impaired walking (Indications)

Implementation

- Do not confuse colchicine with Cortrosyn.
- Intermittent therapy with 3 days between courses may be used to decrease risk of toxicity.
- **PO:** Administer without regard to meals.

Patient/Family Teaching

- Review medication administration schedule. Take missed doses as soon as remembered unless almost time for next dose. Do not double doses.
- Instruct patients taking prophylactic doses not to increase to therapeutic doses during an acute attack to prevent toxicity. An NSAID or corticosteroid, preferably via intrasynovial injection, should be used to treat acute attacks.
- Advise patient to avoid grapefruit and grapefruit juice during therapy; may increase risk of toxicity.
- Advise patient to follow recommendations of health care professional regarding weight loss, diet, and alcohol consumption.
- Instruct patient to report muscle pain or weakness, tingling or numbness in fingers or toes; pale or gray color to lips, tongue, or palms of hands; severe diarrhea or vomiting; unusual bleeding, bruising, sore throat, fatigue, malaise, or weakness or tiredness promptly. Medication should be withheld if symptoms of toxicity occur.
- Instruct patient to notify health care professional of all Rx or OTC medications, vitamins, or herbal products being taken and to notify health care professional before taking any other Rx, OTC, or herbal products.
- Surgery may precipitate an acute attack of gout. Advise patient to confer with health care professional regarding dose 3 days before surgical or dental procedures.
- Advise female patient to notify health care professional if pregnancy is planned or suspected or if breast feeding.

Evaluation/Desired Outcomes

- Decrease in pain and swelling in affected joints within 12 hr.
- Relief of symptoms within 24–48 hr.
- Prevention of acute gout attacks.
- Reduced number of attacks of familial Mediterranean fever.

colesevelam (koe-le-**sev**-e-lam)

✱Lodalis, Welchol

Classification
Therapeutic: lipid-lowering agents
Pharmacologic: bile acid sequestrants

Pregnancy Category B

Indications

Adjunctive therapy to diet and exercise for the reduction of LDL cholesterol in patients with primary hypercholesterolemia; may be used alone or in combination with statins. Adjunctive therapy to diet and exercise for the reduction of LDL cholesterol in children 10–17 yr with heterozygous familial hypercholesterolemia if diet therapy fails (LDL cholesterol remains ≥190 mg/dL or remains ≥160 mg/dL [with family history of premature cardiovascular disease or ≥2 risk factors for cardiovascular disease]); may be used alone or in combination with statin. Adjunctive therapy to diet and exercise to improve glycemic control in patients with type 2 diabetes.

Action

Binds bile acids in the GI tract. Result in increased clearance of cholesterol. Mechanism for lowering blood glucose unknown. **Therapeutic Effects:** Decreased cholesterol and blood glucose.

Pharmacokinetics

Absorption: Not absorbed; action is primarily local in the GI tract.
Distribution: Unknown.
Metabolism and Excretion: Unknown.

Half-life: Unknown.

TIME/ACTION PROFILE (cholesterol-lowering effect)

ROUTE	ONSET	PEAK	DURATION
PO	24–48 hr	2 wk	unknown

Contraindications/Precautions

Contraindicated in: Hypersensitivity; Bowel obstruction; Triglycerides >500 mg/dL; History of pancreatitis due to hypertriglyceridemia.

Use Cautiously in: Triglycerides >300 mg/dL; Dysphagia, swallowing disorders, severe GI motility disorders, or major GI tract surgery; OB, Lactation, Pedi: Pregnancy, lactation, or children <10 yr (safety not established).

Adverse Reactions/Side Effects

GI: constipation, dyspepsia.

Interactions

Drug-Drug: May ↓ absorption of **glyburide**, **glimepiride**, **glipizide**, **levothyroxine**, **olmesartan**, **phenytoin**, **cyclosporine**, **warfarin**, and **estrogen-containing oral contraceptives** (give ≥4 hr before colesevelam). May ↑ levels of **metformin extended-release**.

Route/Dosage

Hyperlipidemia

PO (Adults): 3 tablets twice daily or 6 tablets once daily.

PO (Adults and Children 10–17 yr): *Suspension*—one 3.75-g packet once daily or one 1.875-g packet twice daily.

Type 2 Diabetes

PO (Adults): 3 tablets twice daily or 6 tablets once daily; *Suspension*—one 3.75-g packet once daily or one 1.875-g packet twice daily.

Availability

Tablets: 625 mg. **Granules for oral suspension:** 1.875 g/packet (contains 13.5 mg phenylalanine), 3.75 g/packet (contains 27 mg phenylalanine).

NURSING IMPLICATIONS

Assessment

- **Hypercholesterolemia:** Obtain a diet history, especially in regard to fat consumption.
- **Type 2 Diabetes:** Observe patient for signs and symptoms of hypoglycemic reactions (sweating, hunger, weakness, dizziness, tremor, tachycardia, anxiety).
- ***Lab Test Considerations:*** Monitor serum total cholesterol, LDL, and triglyceride levels before initiating, 4–6 wk after starting, and periodically during therapy.
- Monitor serum glucose and glycosylated hemoglobin periodically during therapy in patients with diabetes.

C

Potential Nursing Diagnoses

Constipation (Side Effects)
Noncompliance (Patient/Family Teaching)

Implementation

- Patients stabilized on a diabetic regimen who are exposed to stress, fever, trauma, infection, or surgery may require administration of insulin.
- **PO:** Administer once or twice daily with meals. Colesevelam should be taken with a liquid. For oral suspension, empty the entire contents of one packet into a glass or cup. Add 1/2 to 1 cup (4 to 8 ounces) of water, fruit juice, or a diet soft drink; do not take in dry form to avoid espophgeal distress.

Patient/Family Teaching

- Instruct patient to take medication as directed; do not skip doses or double up on missed doses.
- Instruct patient to notify health care professional of all Rx or OTC medications, vitamins, or herbal products being taken and consult health care professional before taking other Rx, OTC, or herbal products. Advise patients taking oral vitamin supplementation or oral contraceptives to take their vitamins at least 4 hr prior to colesevelam.
- Instruct patient to consume a diet that promotes bowel regularity. Patients should be instructed to promptly discontinue colesevelam and notify health care professional if severe abdominal pain or severe constipation or symptoms of acute pancreatitis (severe abdominal pain with or without nausea and vomiting) occur.
- **Hypercholesterolemia:** Advise patient that this medication should be used in conjunction with diet restrictions (fat, cholesterol, carbohydrates, alcohol), exercise, and cessation of smoking.
- **Diabetes:** Explain to patient that this medication controls hyperglycemia but does not cure diabetes. Therapy is long term.
- Review signs of hypoglycemia and hyperglycemia with patient. If hypoglycemia occurs, advise patient to drink a glass of orange juice or ingest 2–3 tsp of sugar, honey, or corn syrup dissolved in water or an appropriate number of glucose tablets and notify health care professional.
- Encourage patient to follow prescribed diet, medication, and exercise regimen to prevent hypoglycemic or hyperglycemic episodes.
- Instruct patient in proper testing of serum glucose and ketones. These tests should be closely monitored during periods of stress or illness and health care professional notified if significant changes occur.

- Insulin is the recommended method of controlling blood sugar during pregnancy. Counsel female patients to use a form of contraception other than oral contraceptives and to notify health care professional promptly if pregnancy is planned or suspected.
- Advise patient to carry a form of sugar (sugar packets, candy) and identification describing disease process and medication regimen at all times.

Evaluation/Desired Outcomes

- Decrease in serum total choesterol, LDL cholesterol, apolipoprotein, and blood glucose levels.
- Control of blood glucose levels without the appearance of hypoglycemic or hyperglycemic episodes.

conivaptan (con-i-**vap**-tan)

Vaprisol

Classification
Therapeutic: electrolyte modifiers
Pharmacologic: vasopressin antagonists

Pregnancy Category C

Indications

To increase serum sodium in hospitalized patients with euvolemic or hypervolemic hyponatremia.

Action

Antagonizes vasopressin at V_2 receptor sites in renal collecting ducts, resulting in excretion of free water. **Therapeutic Effects:** Increased serum sodium concentrations. Improved fluid status.

Pharmacokinetics

Absorption: IV administration results in complete bioavailability.
Distribution: Unknown.
Protein Binding: 99% protein bound.
Metabolism and Excretion: Metabolized solely by the CYP3A4 enzyme system. 83% excreted in feces as metabolites, 12% in urine (as metabolites).
Half-life: 5 hr.

TIME/ACTION PROFILE

ROUTE	ONSET	PEAK	DURATION
IV	unknown	12 hr	end of infusion

Contraindications/Precautions

Contraindicated in: Hypersensitivity; Hypovolemic hyponatremia; Concurrent use of ketonconazole, itraconazole, clarithromycin, ritonavir, or indinavir.
Use Cautiously in: Moderate hepatic impairment (↓ dose recommended); Severe renal impairment (not recommended if CCr <30 mL/min); OB, Lactation: Safety not established; Pedi: Safety not established.

Adverse Reactions/Side Effects

CNS: headache, confusion, insomnia. **CV:** hypertension, hypotension. **GI:** diarrhea. **GU:** polyuria. **F and E:** dehydration, hypokalemia, hypomagnesemia, hyponatremia. **Local:** infusion reactions. **Misc:** fever, thirst.

Interactions

Drug-Drug: Blood levels and effects are ↑ by **ketoconazole**, **itraconazole**, **clarithromycin**, **ritonavir**, or **indinavir**; concurrent use is contraindicated. ↑ blood levels and may ↑ effects of **midazolam**, **simvastatin**, **lovastatin**, **amlodipine**, and **other drugs metabolized by CYP3A4**; careful monitoring recommended. May ↑ **digoxin** levels.

Route/Dosage

IV (Adults): 20 mg loading dose initially, followed by 20 mg/day as a continuous infusion for 2–4 days. May titrate conivaptan up to 40 mg/day as a continuous infusion if serum sodium is not rising at desired rate. Total duration of therapy should not exceed 4 days.

Hepatic Impairment

(Adults): *Moderate hepatic impairment*—10 mg loading dose initially, followed by 10 mg/day as a continuous infusion for 2–4 days; may titrate up to 20 mg/day as a continuous infusion if serum sodium is not rising at desired rate.

Availability

Premixed infusion: 20 mg/100 mL D5W.

NURSING IMPLICATIONS

Assessment

- Monitor injection site during administration. Frequently causes erythema, pain, swelling and phlebitis. May require discontinuation of therapy.
- Monitor vital signs frequently during therapy. Discontinue therapy if patient becomes hypovolemic and hypotensive. Therapy may be resumed at a reduced dose once patient is euvolemic and no longer hypotensive, if patient remains hyponatremic.
- Assess neurologic status during administration. Overly rapid rise in serum sodium may cause neurologic sequelae.
- ***Lab Test Considerations:*** Monitor serum sodium concentration frequently during therapy. If serum sodium rises at an undesirably rapid rate (>12 mEq/L/24 hr), discontinue administration of conivaptan. If serum sodium continues to rise, do not resume therapy. If hyponatremia persists or recurs (after discontinuation for rapid rise of serum sodium) and patient has no evidence of neurologic sequelae from rapid increase, conivaptan may be resumed at a reduced dose.
- May cause hyperglycemia, hypoglycemia, hypokalemia, hypomagnesemia, and hyponatremia.

Potential Nursing Diagnoses

Deficient knowledge, related to medication regimen (Patient/Family Teaching)

Implementation

IV Administration

- Administer IV through large veins and rotate infusion site every 24 hr to minimize risk if vascular irritation.

Loading Dose

- **Intermittent Infusion:** ***Diluent:*** Premixed containers require no further dilution. ***Concentration:*** 0.2 mg/mL. ***Rate:*** Administer over 30 min.

Continuous Infusion

- **Continuous Infusion:** ***Diluent:*** Premixed containers require no further dilution. ***Concentration:*** 0.2 mg/mL. ***Rate:*** Administer continuous infusion at a rate of 20 mg/24 hr. If patient requires 40 mg/24 hr continuous infusion, infuse 20 mg over 12 hr, followed by 20 mg over 12 hr.
- **Additive Incompatibility:** Do not admix with LR, furosemide, or combine with any other product in the same IV line or bag.

Patient/Family Teaching

- Explain purpose of medication to patient.
- Instruct patient to notify health care professional if pain or redness occurs at infusion site.

Evaluation/Desired Outcomes

- Restoration of normal fluid and electrolyte balance.

CONTRACEPTIVES, HORMONAL

MONOPHASIC ORAL CONTRACEPTIVES

ethinyl estradiol/desogestrel
(**eth**-in-il es-tra-**dye**-ole/dess-oh-**jess**-trel)
Apri-28, Desogen, Emoquette, Enskyce, Isibloom, Ortho-Cept, Reclipsen, Solia

ethinyl estradiol/drospirenone
(**eth**-in-il es-tra-**dye**-ole/droe-**spy**-re-nown)
Beyaz, Gianvi, Loryna, Nikki, Ocella, Safyral, Syeda, Vestura, Yaela, Yasmin, Yaz, Zarah

ethinyl estradiol/ethynodiol
(**eth**-in-il es-tra-**dye**-ole/e-thye-noe-**dye**-ole)
Kelnor, Zovia 1/35, Zovia 1/50

ethinyl estradiol/levonorgestrel
(**eth**-in-il es-tra-**dye**-ole/lee-voe-nor-**jess**-trel)
Altavera, Aubra, Aviane-28, Chateal, Falmina, Kurvelo, Lessina-28, Levora-28, Lutera, Marlissa, Orsythia, Portia-28, Sronyx, Vienva

ethinyl estradiol/norethindrone
(**eth**-in-il es-tra-**dye**-ole/nor-eth-**in**-drone)
Alyacen 1/35, Balziva-28, Brevicon-28, Briellyn, Cyclafem 1/35, Dasetta 1/35, Femcon Fe, Femhrt, Generess Fe, Gildagia, Gildess 1/20, Gildess Fe 1/20, Gildess 1.5/30, Gildess Fe 1.5/30, Jinteli, Junel 1/20, Junel 1.5/30, Junel Fe 1/20, Junel Fe 1.5/30, Larin 1/20, Larin 1.5/30, Larin Fe 1/20, Larin Fe 1.5/30, Loestrin 21 1/20, Loestrin 21 1.5/30, Loestrin Fe 1/20, Loestrin Fe 1.5/30, Microgestin 1/20, Microgestin 1.5/30, Microgestin Fe 1/20, Microgestin Fe 1.5/30, Minastrin 24 Fe, Modicon-28, Necon 0.5/35, Necon 1/35, Norinyl 1/35, Nortrel 0.5/35, Nortrel 1/35, Ortho-Novum 1/35, Philith, Pirmella 1/35, Vyfemla, Wera, Wymzya Fe, Zenchent, Zenchent Fe

ethinyl estradiol/norgestimate
(**eth**-in-il es-tra-**dye**-ole/nor-**jes**-ti-mate)
Estarylla, Mono-Linyah, Mononessa, Ortho-Cyclen-28, Previfem, Sprintec

ethinyl estradiol/norgestrel
(**eth**-in-il es-tra-**dye**-ole/nor-**jess**-trel)
Cryselle, Elinest, Lo/Ovral 28, Low-Ogestrel–28, Ogestrel–28

mestranol/norethindrone
(**mes**-tre-nole/nor-eth-**in**-drone)
Necon 1/50, Norinyl 1/50

BIPHASIC ORAL CONTRACEPTIVES

ethinyl estradiol/desogestrel
(**eth**-in-il es-tra-**dye**-ole/dess-oh-**jess**-trel)
Azurette, Bekyree, Kariva, Kimidess, Pimtrea, Viorele

ethinyl estradiol/norethindrone (**eth**-in-il es-tra-**dye**-ole/nor-eth-**in**-drone)
Lo Loestrin Fe, Lo Minastrin Fe, Necon 10/11

TRIPHASIC ORAL CONTRACEPTIVES

ethinyl estradiol/desogestrel (**eth**-in-il es-tra-**dye**-ole/dess-oh-**jess**-trel)
Caziant, Cyclessa, Velivet

ethinyl estradiol/levonorgestrel (**eth**-in-il ess-tra-**dye**-ole/lee-voe-nor-**jess**-trel)
Enpresse-28, Levonest, Myzilra, Trivora–28

ethinyl estradiol/norethindrone (**eth**-in-il es-tra-**dye**-ole/nor-eth-**in**-drone)
Alyacen 7/7/7, Aranelle, Cyclafem 7/7/7, Dasetta 7/7/7, Estrostep Fe, Leena, Necon 7/7/7, Nortrel 7/7/7, Ortho-Novum 7/7/7, Pirmella 7/7/7, Tilia Fe, Tri-Legest-21, Tri-Legest Fe, Tri-Norinyl

ethinyl estradiol/norgestimate (**eth**-in-il es-tra-**dye**-ole/nor-**jess**-ti-mate)
Ortho Tri-Cyclen, Ortho Tri-Cyclen Lo, Tri-Estarylla, Tri-Linyah, Tri-Lo-Estarylla, Tri-Previfem, Tri-Sprintec, Tri-Nessa

FOURPHASIC ORAL CONTRACEPTIVES

estradiol valerate/dienogest (es-tra-**dye**-ole **val**-er-ate/dye-**en**-oh-jest)
Natazia

EXTENDED-CYCLE ORAL CONTRACEPTIVE

ethinyl estradiol/levonorgestrel (**eth**-in-il ess-tra-**dye**-ole/lee-voe-nor-**jess**-trel)
Amethia, Amethia Lo, Amethyst, Ashlyna, Camrese, Camrese Lo, Daysee, Introvale, Jolessa, LoSeasonique, Quartette, Quasense, Seasonale, Seasonique, Setlakin

PROGESTIN-ONLY ORAL CONTRACEPTIVES

norethindrone (nor-eth-**in**-drone)
Camila, Errin, Jencycla, Jolivette, Micronor, Nor-Q D, Nora-BE, Ortho Micronor

CONTRACEPTIVE IMPLANT

etonogestrel (e-toe-no-**jess**-trel)
Implanon, Nexplanon

EMERGENCY CONTRACEPTIVE

levonorgestrel (**lee**-voe-nor-**jess**-trel)
Fallback Solo, Plan B

ulipristal (u-li-**priss**-tal)
Ella

INJECTABLE CONTRACEPTIVE

medroxyprogesterone (me-**drox**-ee-proe-**jess**-te-rone)
Depo-Provera, Depo-subQ Provera 104

INTRAUTERINE CONTRACEPTIVE

levonorgestrel (**lee**-voe-nor-**jess**-trel)
Mirena, Skyla

VAGINAL RING CONTRACEPTIVE

ethinyl estradiol/etonogestrel (**eth**-in-il ess-tra-**dye**-ole/e-toe-noe-**jess**-trel)
NuvaRing

TRANSDERMAL CONTRACEPTIVE

ethinyl estradiol/norelgestromin (**eth**-in-il ess-tra-**dye**-ole/nor-el-**jess**-troe-min)
Xulane

Classification
Therapeutic: contraceptive hormones

Pregnancy Category X

Indications

Prevention of pregnancy. Regulation of menstrual cycle. Emergency contraception (some products). Treatment of heavy menstrual bleeding in women who choose to use intrauterine contraception as their method of contraception (Mirena). Treatment of heavy menstrual bleeding in women who choose to use an oral contraceptive as their method of contraception (Natazia). Treatment of premenstrual dysphoric disorder (Beyaz, Yaz, Yasmin). Management of acne in women >14 yr who desire contraception, have no health problems, and have failed topical treatment. Increase folate levels in women who desire oral contraception to reduce the risk of neural tube defects in a pregnancy that occurs while taking or shortly after discontinuing the product.

Action

Monophasic Oral Contraceptives: Provide a fixed dosage of estrogen/progestin over a 21-day cycle. Ovulation is inhibited by suppression of follicle-stimulating hormone (FSH) and luteinizing hormone (LH). May alter cervical mucus and the endometrial environment, preventing penetration by sperm and implantation of the egg. **Biphasic Oral Contraceptives:** Ovulation is inhibited by suppression of FSH and LH. May alter cervical mucus and the endometrial environment, preventing penetration by sperm and implantation of the egg. In addition, smaller dose of progestin in phase 1 allows for proliferation of endometrium. Larger amount in phase 2 allows for adequate secretory development. **Triphasic Oral Contraceptives:** Ovulation is inhibited by suppression of FSH and LH. May alter cervical mucus and the endometrial environment, preventing penetration by sperm and implantation of the egg. Varying doses of estrogen/progestin may more closely mimic natural hormonal fluctuations. **Fourphasic Oral Contraceptives:** Ovulation is inhibited by suppression of FSH and LH. May alter cervical mucus and the endometrial environment, preventing penetration by sperm and implantation of the egg. Doses of estrogen decrease while doses of progestin increase over the 28-day cycle. **Extended-cycle:** Provides continuous estrogen/progestin for 84 days (365 days for Lybrel), then off for 7 days (low-dose estrogen-only tablet taken during these 7 days with LoSeasonique and Seasonique), resulting in 4 menstrual periods/year (no periods/year for Lybrel). **Progressive Estrogen:** Contains constant amount of progestin with 3 progressive doses of estrogen. **Progestin-Only Contraceptives/Contraceptive Implant/Intrauterine Levonorgestrel/ Medroxyprogesterone Injection:** Mechanism not clearly known. May alter cervical mucus and the endometrial environment, preventing penetration by sperm and implantation of the egg. Ovulation may also be suppressed. **Emergency Contraceptive Pills (ECPs):** Inhibit ovulation/fertilization; may also alter tubal transport of sperm/egg and prevent implantation. **Vaginal Ring, Transdermal Patch:** Inhibits ovulation, decreases sperm entry into uterus, decreases likelihood of implantation. **Anti-acne effect:** Combination of estrogen/progestin may increase sex hormone binding globulin (SHBG) resulting in decreased unbound testosterone, which may be a cause of acne. **Therapeutic Effects:** Prevention of pregnancy. Decreased severity of acne. Decrease in menstrual blood loss. Decrease in premenstrual disphoric disorder. Decrease in vasomotor symptoms or symptoms of vulvar and vaginal atrophy due to menopause. Increase in folate levels and prevention of neural tube defects.

Pharmacokinetics

Absorption: *Ethinyl estradiol*—rapidly absorbed; *Norethindrone*—65% absorbed; *Desogesrtrel and levonorgestrel*—100% absorbed; *Dienogest*—91% absorbed. Others are well absorbed after oral administration. Slowly absorbed from implant, subcutaneous or IM injection. Some absorption follows intrauterine implantation.

Distribution: Unknown.

Protein Binding: *Ethinyl estradiol*—97–98%; *Drospirenone*—97%; *Dienogest*—90%; *Ulipristal*—>94%.

Metabolism and Excretion: *Ethinyl estradiol and norethindrone*—undergo extensive first-pass hepatic metabolism. *Mestranol*—is rapidly converted to ethinyl estradol. *Desogestrel*—is rapidly metabolized to 3-keto-desogestgrel, the active metabolite. Most agents are metabolized by the liver.

Half-life: *Ethinyl estradiol*—6–20 hr; *Levonorgestrel*—45 hr; *Norethindrone*—5–14 hr; *Desogestrel (metabolite)*—38 ± 20 hr; *Drospirenone*—30 hr; *Norgestimate (metabolite)*—12–20 hr; *Dienogest*—11 hr; *others*—unknown; *Ulipristal*—32 hr.

TIME/ACTION PROFILE (prevention of pregnancy)

ROUTE	ONSET	PEAK	DURATION
PO	1 mo	1 mo	1 mo†
Implant	1 mo	1 mo	5 yr
Intrauterine system	1 mo	1 mo	5 yr
IM	1 mo	1 mo	3 mo
Subcut	unknown	1 wk	3 mo

†Only during month of taking contraceptive.

Contraindications/Precautions

Contraindicated in: Hypersensitivity; OB: Pregnancy; History of cigarette smoking or age >35 yr (↑ risk of cardiovascular or thromboembolic phenomenon); History of thromboembolic disease (e.g., DVT, PE, MI, stroke); Protein C, protein S, or antithrombin deficiency or other thrombophilic disorder; Valvular heart disease; Major surgery with extended periods of immobility; Diabetes with vascular involvement; Headache with focal neurological symptoms; Uncontrolled hypertension; History of breast, endometrial, or estrogen-dependent cancer; Abnormal genital bleeding;

Liver disease; Hypersensitivity to parabens (injectable only); *Drosperinone-containing products only*—Renal impairment, liver disease, or adrenal insufficiency (↑ risk of hyperkalemia); *Intrauterine levonorgestrel only*—Intrauterine anomaly, postpartum endometriosis, multiple sexual partners, pelvic inflammatory disease, liver disease, genital actinomycosis, immunosuppression, IV drug abuse, untreated genitourinary infection, history of ectopic pregnancy; Lactation: Avoid use.

Use Cautiously in: Presence of other cardiovascular risk factors (obesity, hyperglycemia, hypertension); History or family history of hypertriglyceridemia (↑ risk of pancreatitis); History of diabetes mellitus, bleeding disorders, concurrent anticoagulant therapy or headaches; History of hereditary angioedema; Pedi: Avoid use before menarche.

Adverse Reactions/Side Effects

CNS: depression, headache. **EENT:** contact lens intolerance, optic neuritis, retinal thrombosis. **CV:** THROMBOEMBOLISM (risk is greatest during first 6 mo of therapy or after restarting the same or different therapy), edema, hypertension, Raynaud's phenomenon, thrombophlebitis. **F and E:** *Drosperinone-containing products only*—hyperkalemia. **GI:** PANCREATITIS, abdominal cramps, bloating, cholestatic jaundice, gallbladder disease, liver tumors, nausea, vomiting. **GU:** amenorrhea, breakthrough bleeding, dysmenorrhea, spotting, *Intrauterine levonorgestrel only*—uterine imbedment/uterine rupture. **Derm:** melasma, rash. **Endo:** hyperglycemia. **MS:** *Injectable medroxyprogesterone only*—bone loss. **Misc:** weight change.

Interactions

Drug-Drug: Oral contraceptive efficacy may be ↓ by **penicillins, chloramphenicol, barbiturates,** chronic **alcohol** use, **carbamazepine, oxcarbazepine, bosentan, felbamate,** systemic **corticosteroids, phenytoin, topiramate, primidone, modafinil, rifampin, rifabutin, nelfinavir, ritonavir, darunavir/ritonavir, fosamprenavir/ritonavir, lopinavir/ritonavir, tipranavir/ritonavir, boceprevir, nevirapine, colesevelam,** or **tetracyclines. CYP3A4 inducers,** including **barbiturates, bosentan, carbamazepine, oxcarbazepine, phenytoin, topiramate, felbamate, rifampin** may ↓ effectiveness of ulipristal; avoid concomitant use. May ↑ effects/risk of toxicity of some **benzodiazepines, beta blockers, corticosteroids, cyclosporine, tizanidine, theophylline,** and **voriconazole.** ↑ risk of hepatic toxicity with **dantrolene** (estrogen only). **Indinavir, atazanavir/ritonavir, etravirine, itraconazole, ketoconazole, fluconazole, voriconazole, rosuvastatin,** and **atorvastatin** may ↑ effects/risk of toxicity. **Smoking** ↑ risk of thromboembolic phenomena (estrogen only). May ↓ levels of **acetaminophen, temazepam, lamotrigine, lorazepam, oxazepam,** or **morphine.** *Drosperinone-containing products only*—concurrent use with **NSAIDs, potassium-sparing diuretics, potassium supplements, ACE inhibitors, aldosterone receptor antagonists,** or **angiotensin II receptor antagonists** may result in hyperkalemia. *Drosperinone-containing products only*—concurrent use with strong **CYP3A4 inhibitors,** including **ketoconazole, itraconazole, voriconazole, protease inhibitors,** or **clarithromycin** may ↑ risk of hyperkalemia; consider monitoring K+ concentrations. Ulipristal may ↑ levels of **P-glycoprotein substrates,** including **dabigatran** and **digoxin.**

Drug-Natural Products: Concomitant use with **St. John's wort** may ↓ contraceptive efficacy and cause breakthrough bleeding and irregular menses.

Drug-Food: Grapefruit juice may ↑ effects/risk of toxicity.

Route/Dosage

Monophasic Oral Contraceptives

PO (Adults): On 21-day regimen, take first tablet on first Sunday after menses begins (take on Sunday if menses begins on Sunday) for 21 days, then skip 7 days and begin again. Regimen may also be started on first day of menses, continue for 21 days, then skip 7 days and begin again. Some regimens contain 7 placebo tablets, so that 1 tablet is taken every day for 28 days.

Biphasic Oral Contraceptives

PO (Adults): Given in 2 phases. First phase is 10 days of smaller amount of progestin. Second phase is larger amount of progestin. Amount of estrogen remains constant for same length of time (total of 21 days), then skip 7 days and begin again. Some regimens contain 7 placebo tablets for 28-day regimen.

Triphasic Oral Contraceptives

PO (Adults): Progestin amount varies throughout 21-day cycle. Estrogen component stays the same or may vary. Some regimens contain 7 placebo tablets for 28-day regimen.

Fourphasic Oral Contraceptives

PO (Adults): Given in 4 phases. First phase contains higher amount of estrogen and no progestin. Second and third phases contains lower amount of estrogen, and increasing amounts of progestin. Fourth phase contains low dose of estrogen only. Also contains 2 placebo tablets to complete 28-day regimen.

Extended-Cycle Contraceptive

PO (Adults): *Daysee, LoSeasonique, Quartette, Seasonale and Seasonique.* Start taking first active pill on first Sunday after menses begins (if first day is Sunday, begin then), continue for 84 days of active pill, followed by 7 days of placebo tablets (low-dose estrogen tablets for Daysee, LoSeasonique, Quartette, and Seasonique), then resume 84/7 cycle again. For *Lybrel,* begin taking the first pill during the first day of the menstrual cycle and start the next pack the day after the previous pack ends.

Progestin-Only Oral Contraceptives

PO (Adults): Start on first day of menses. Taken daily and continuously.

Progressive Estrogen Oral Contraceptives

PO (Adults): Estrogen amount increases q 7 days throughout 21-day cycle. Progestin component stays the same. Some regimens contain 7 placebo tablets for 28-day regimen.

Emergency Contraceptive

PO (Adults and Adolescents): *Plan B*—1 tablet within 72 hr of unprotected intercourse followed by 1 more tablet 12 hr later; *Lo/Ovral*—4 white tablets within 72 hr of unprotected intercourse followed by 4 more white tablets 12 hr later; *Levlen, Nordette*—4 light orange tablets within 72 hr of unprotected intercourse followed by 4 more light orange tablets 12 hr later; *Triphasil, Tri-Levlen*—4 yellow tablets within 72 hr of unprotected intercourse followed by 4 more yellow tablets 12 hr later; *Ulipristal*—1 tablet as soon as possible within 120 hr (5 days) after unprotected intercourse or known/suspected contraceptive failure.

Injectable Contraceptive

medroxyprogesterone (Depo-Provera)

IM (Adults): 150 mg within first 5 days of menses or within 5 days postpartum, if not breast feeding. If breast feeding, give 6 wk postpartum; repeat q 3 mo.

medroxyprogesterone (Depo-Sub Q Provera 104)

Subcut (Adults): 104 mg within first 5 days of menses or within 5 days postpartum, if not breast feeding. If breast feeding, give 6 wk postpartum; repeat q 12–14 wk.

Intrauterine Contraceptive

Intrauterine (Adults): Insert one device into uterine cavity within 7 days of menses or immediately after 1st trimester abortion. Mirena should be removed or replaced after 5 yr. Skyla should be removed or replaced after 3 yr.

Vaginal Ring Contraceptive

Vag (Adults): One ring inserted on or prior to day 5 of menstrual cycle. Ring is left in place for 3 wk, then removed for 1 wk, then a new ring is inserted.

Transdermal Patch

Transdermal (Adults): Patch is applied on day 1 of menstrual cycle (or convenient day in first week), changed weekly thereafter for 3 wk. Week 4 is patch-free. Cycle is then repeated.

Acne

PO (Adults): *Ortho Tri-Cyclen*—Take daily for 21 days, off for 7 days.

C

Availability

Combination Estrogen/Progestin Oral Contraceptives (generic available)

Oral contraceptive tablets: Usually in monthly packs with enough (21) active tablets to complete a 28-day cycle. Some contain 7 inert tablets to complete the cycle with or without supplemental iron, Beyaz and Safyral —contain 0.451 mg of levomefolate calcium/tablet.

Extended-Cycle Contraceptive

Tablets: *LoSeasonique*—active tablets containing 0.02 mg ethinyl estradiol, 0.1 mg levonorgestrel, and 7 tablets containing 0.01 mg ethinyl estradiol; *Quartette*—42 tablets containing 0.02 mg ethinyl estradiol and 0.15 mg levonorgestrel, 21 tablets containing 0.025 mg ethinyl estradiol and 0.15 mg levonorgestrel, 21 tablets containing 0.03 mg ethinyl estradiol and 0.15 mg levonorgestrel, and 7 tablets containing 0.01 mg ethinyl estradiol; *Seasonale*—84 active tablets containing 0.03 mg ethinyl estradiol and 0.15 mg levonorgestrel and 7 inactive tablets; *Daysee and Seasonique*—active tablets containing 0.03 mg ethinyl estradiol, 0.15 mg levonorgestrel, and 7 tablets containing 0.01 mg ethinyl estradiol; *Lybrel*—28 active tablets containing 0.09 mg levonorgestrel and 0.02 mg ethinyl estradiol.

Levonorgestrel (generic available)

Emergency contraceptives: 2 tablets containing 0.75 mg levonorgestrel (Plan B). **Implant:** Rod contains 68 mg etonogestrel. **Intrauterine system (Mirena):** contains 52 mg levonorgestrel (releases 20 mcg/day). **Intrauterine system (Skyla):** contains 13.5 mg levonorgestrel (releases 14 mcg/day).

Ulipristal

Tablets: 30 mg.

Medroxyprogesterone (generic available)

Injectable IM: 150 mg/mL. **Injectable Subcutaneous:** 104 mg/0.65 mL (in pre-filled syringes).

Vaginal Ring Contraceptive

Ring: delivers 0.015 mg ethinyl estradiol and 0.120 mg etonogestrel/day.

Transdermal Patch

Patch (Xulane): contains 0.53 mg ethinyl estradiol and 4.86 mg of norelgestromin; releases 35 mcg ethinyl estradiol/150 mcg norelgestromin per 24 hr.

NURSING IMPLICATIONS

Assessment

- Assess BP before and periodically during therapy.
- Exclude the possibility of pregnancy on the basis or history and/or physical exam or a pregnancy test before administering emergency contraceptives.
- **Acne:** Assess skin lesion before and periodically during therapy.
- **Menopausal Symptoms:** Assess vasomotor symptoms or symptoms of vulvar and vaginal atrophy due to menopause prior to and periodically during therapy.
- ***Lab Test Considerations:*** Monitor hepatic function periodically during therapy.
- *Estrogens only*—May cause ↑ serum glucose, sodium, triglyceride, VHDL, total cholesterol, prothrombin, and factors VII, VIII, IX, and X levels. May cause ↓ LDL and antithrombin III levels.
- May cause false interpretations of thyroid function tests.
- *Progestins only*—May cause ↑ LDL concentrations. May cause ↓ serum alkaline phosphatase and HDL concentrations.
- *Drosperidone-containing contraceptives* —monitor serum potassium during first treatment cycle in women on long-term treatment with strong CYP3A4 inhibitors; may ↑ serum potassium concentration.

Potential Nursing Diagnoses

Noncompliance (Patient/Family Teaching)

Implementation

- Do not confuse Ortho Tri-Cyclen with Ortho Tri-Cyclen Lo. Do not confuse Yasmin with Yaz.
- **PO:** Oral doses may be administered with or immediately after food to reduce nausea. Chewable tablets may be swallowed whole or chewed; if chewed follow with 8 ounces of liquid.
- For extended-cycle tablets, *Jolessa, Quasense, Seasonale, Seasonique,* or *LoSeasonique*—take active tablets for 84 days and followed by the placebo tablets for 7 days; for *Lybrel*—Take 1 pill each day for 28 days, then start the next set of pills daily for the next 28 days.
- For *Emergency Contraception:* Tablets are taken as soon as possible and within 72 hr after unprotected intercourse. Two doses are taken 12 hr apart. Emergency contraception products are available without a prescription to all women of child-bearing age.
- *Ulipristal:* Administer 1 tablet as soon as possible within 120 hr (5 days) after unprotected intercourse or a known or suspected contraceptive failure. May be taken without regard to food. If vomiting occurs within 3 hr of dose, may repeat. May be taken at any time during the menstrual cycle. Ulipristal may be less effective in women with a body mass index >30 kg/m^2.
- **Subcut:** Shake vigorously before use to form a uniform suspension. Inject slowly (over 5–7 sec) at a 45° angle into fatty area of anterior thigh or abdomen every 12 to 14 wk. If more than 14 wk elapse between injections, rule out pregnancy prior to administration. Do not rub area after injection.
- When switching from other hormonal contraceptives, administer within dosing period (7 days after taking last active pill, removing patch or ring, or within the dosing period for IM injection).
- **IM:** Shake vial vigorously just before use to ensure uniform suspension. Administer deep IM into gluteal or deltoid muscle. If period between injections is >14 wk, determine that patient is not pregnant before administering the drug.
- Injectable medroxyprogesterone may lead to bone loss, especially in women younger than 21 yr. Injectable medroxyprogesterone should be used for >2 yr only if other methods of contraception are inadequate. If used long term, women should use supplemental calcium and vitamin D, and monitor bone mineral density.
- **Intrauterine system:** Should be inserted by a trained health care provider. Health care providers are advised to become thoroughly familiar with the insertion instructions before attempting insertion. Following insertion counsel patient on what to expect following insertion. Give patient *Follow-up Reminder Card* provided with product. Discuss expected bleeding patterns during the first months of use. Prescribe analgesics, if indicated. Patients should be reexamined and evaluated 4 to 12 wk after insertion and once a year thereafter, or more frequently if clinically indicated.

Patient/Family Teaching

- Instruct patient to take oral medication as directed at the same time each day. Pills should be taken in proper sequence and kept in the original container. Advise patient not to skip pills even if not having sex very often. Advise patient to read *Patient Guide* before starting and with each Rx refill in case of changes.
- *If single daily dose is missed:* Take as soon as remembered; if not until next day, take 2 tablets and continue on regular dosing schedule. *If 2 days in a row are missed:* Take 2 tablets a day for the next 2 days and continue on regular dosing schedule, using a second method of birth control for the remaining cycle. *If 3 days in a row are missed:* Discontinue medication and use another form of birth control until period begins or pregnancy is ruled out; then begin a new cycle of tablets. *For 28-day dosing schedule:* If schedule is followed for first 21 days and 1 dose is missed of the last 7 tablets, it is important to take the 1st tablet of next month's cycle on the regularly scheduled day. Advise patient taking *Natazia* to follow *Patient Guide* for what to do if a pill is missed.
- Advise patient taking *Jolessa, Quasense, Seasonale, Sesonique,* or *LoSeasonique extended-cycle tab-*

lets that withdrawal bleeding should occur during the 7 days following discontinuation of the active tablets. If withdrawal bleeding does not occur, notify health care professional. Advise patient taking *Lybrel* that no withdrawal bleeding should occur.

- For initial use of *Jolessa, Quasense, Seasonale, Seasonique,* or *LoSeasonique extended cycle tablets*, caution patient to use a nonhormonal method of contraception until she has taken the first 7 days of active tablets. Each 91-day cycle should start on the same day of the week. If started later than the proper day or 2 or more days are missed, a second nonhormonal method of contraception should be used until she has taken the pink tablet for 7 days. Transient spotting or bleeding may occur. If bleeding is persistent or prolonged, notify health care professional.
- Advise patient taking extended cycle tablets that spotting or light bleeding may occur, especially during first 3 mo. Continue medication; notify health care professional if bleeding lasts >70 k days.
- Advise patient of the need to use another form of contraception for the first 3 wk when beginning to use *oral contraceptives*.
- Instruct patient to notify health care professional of all Rx or OTC medications, vitamins, or herbal products being taken and consult health care professional before taking any new medications.
- Advise patient that a second method of birth control should also be used during each cycle in which any of the following are used: *Oral contraceptives*—ampicillin, corticosteroids, antiretroviral protease inhibitors, barbiturates, carbamazepine, chloramphenicol, dihydroergotamine, corticosteroids (systemic), mineral oil, oral neomycin, oxcarbazapine, penicillin V, phenylbutazone, primidone, rifampin, sulfonamides, tetracyclines, topiramate, bosentan, or valproic acid.
- Explain dose schedule and maintenance routine. Discontinuing medication suddenly may cause withdrawal bleeding.
- If nausea becomes a problem, advise patient that eating solid food often provides relief. If nausea persists or vomiting or diarrhea occur, use a nonhormonal method of contraception and notify health care professional.
- Advise patient to report signs and symptoms of fluid retention (swelling of ankles and feet, weight gain), thromboembolic disorders (pain, swelling, tenderness in extremities, headache, chest pain, blurred vision), mental depression, hepatic dysfunction (yellowed skin or eyes, pruritus, dark urine, light-colored stools), or abnormal vaginal bleeding. Women with a strong family history of breast cancer, fibrocystic breast disease, abnormal mammograms, or cervical dysplasia should be monitored for breast cancer at least yearly.
- Instruct patient to stop taking medication and notify health care professional if pregnancy is suspected.
- Caution patient that cigarette smoking during estrogen therapy may increase risk of serious side effects, especially for women over age 35.
- Caution patients to use sunscreen and protective clothing to prevent increased pigmentation.
- Caution patient that hormonal contraceptives do not protect against HIV or other sexually transmitted diseases.
- Advise patient to notify health care professional of medication regimen before treatment or surgery.
- Emphasize the importance of routine follow-up physical exams including BP; breast, abdomen, and pelvic examinations; and Papanicolaou smears every 6–12 mo.
- **Emergency Contraception:** Instruct patient to take emergency contraceptive as directed. Advise patient that they should not take emergency contraceptives if they know or suspect they are pregnant; emergency contraceptives are not for use to end an existing pregnancy. Advise patient to contact health care professional if they vomit within 3 hr after taking ulipristal.
- Inform patient that *ulipristal* may reduce the effectiveness of hormonal contraceptives. Advise patient to use a non-hormonal contraceptive during that menstrual cycle. If a hormonal contraceptive is used, do not use less than 5 days after taking *ulipristal.*
- Advise patient to notify health care professional and consider the possibility of pregnancy of their period is delayed by more than 1 wk beyond the expected date after taking *ulipristal.*
- Inform patient that emergency contraceptives are not to be used as a routine form of contraception or to be used repeatedly within the same menstrual cycle.
- Advise patient to notify health care professional if severe lower abdominal pain occurs 3–5 wk after taking *ulipristal* to be evaluated for an ectopic pregnancy.
- Advise female patients to avoid breast feeding if taking *ulipristal.*
- **IM, Subcut:** Advise patient to maintain adequate amounts of dietary calcium and vitamin D to help prevent bone loss.
- **Transdermal:** Instruct patient on application of patch. First patch should be applied within 24 hr of menstrual period. If applied after Day 1 of menstrual period, a nonhormonal method of contraception should be used for the next 7 days. Day of application becomes *Patch Change Day*. Patches are worn for 1 wk and changed on the same day of each wk for 3 wk. Week 4 is patch-free. Withdrawal bleeding is expected during this time.

C

- Apply patch to clean, dry, intact, healthy skin on buttock, abdomen, upper outer arm, or upper torso in a place where it won't be rubbed by tight clothing. Do not place on skin that is red, irritated, or cut, and do not place on breasts. Do not apply make-up, creams, lotions, powders, or other topical products to area of patch application.
- To apply patch open foil pouch by tearing along edge using fingers. Peel pouch apart and open flat. Grasp a corner of the patch firmly and remove gently from foil pouch. Use fingernail to lift one corner of the patch and peel patch **and** the plastic liner off the foil liner. Do not remove clear liner as patch is removed. Peel away half of the clear liner without touching sticky surface. Apply the sticky surface and remove the rest of the liner. Press down firmly with palm of hand for 10 sec; make sure the edges stick well.
- On *Patch Change Day* remove patch and apply new one immediately. Used patch still contains some active hormones; fold in half so it sticks to itself and throw away. Apply new patches to a new spot to prevent skin irritation; may be applied in same anatomic area.
- Following patch-free week, apply a new patch on *Patch Change Day*, the day after Day 28, no matter when the menstrual cycle begins.
- If patch becomes partially or completely detached for less than 1 day, reapply patch or apply new patch. If patch is detached for more than 1 day, apply a new patch immediately and use a nonhormonal form of contraception for the next 7 days. Cycle will now start over with a new *Patch Change Day*. If patch is no longer sticky, apply a new patch; do not use tape or wraps to keep patch in place.
- If patch is not changed on *Patch Change Day* in the first week of the cycle, apply new patch immediately upon remembering and use a nonhormonal method of contraception for next 7 days. If patch change is missed in for 1 or 2 days during Week 2 or 3, apply new patch immediately and apply next patch on usual *Patch Change Day*. No backup contraception is needed. If patch change is missed for more than 2 days during Week 2 or 3, stop the cycle and start a new 4-wk contraceptive cycle by applying new patch immediately and using a nonhormonal method of contraception for the next 7 days. If patch is not removed on *Patch Change Day* in Week 4, remove as soon as remembered and start next cycle on usual *Patch Change Day*. No additional contraception is needed.
- Advise patient referred for MRI test to discuss patch with referring health care professional and MRI facility to determine if removal of patch is necessary prior to test and for directions for replacing patch.
- **NuvaRing:** *If a hormonal contraceptive was not used in the past month*, insert *NuvaRing* between Days 1 and 5 of the menstrual cycle (Day 1 = first day of menstrual period), even if bleeding has not finished. Use a nonhormonal method of birth control other than a diaphragm during the first 7 days of ring use. *If switching from a combination estrogen/progesterone oral contraceptive*, insert *NuvaRing* any time during first 7 days after last tablet and no later than the day a new pill cycle would have started. No extra birth control is needed. *If switching from a mini-pill*, start using *NuvaRing* on any day of the month; do not skip days between last pill and first day of *NuvaRing* use. *If switching from an implant*, start using *NuvaRing* on same day implant is removed. *If switching from an injectable contraceptive*, start using *NuvaRing* on the day when next injection is due. *If switching from a progestin-containing IUD*, start using *NuvaRing* on the same day as IUD is removed. A nonhormonal method of contraception, other than the diaphragm, should be used for the first 7 days of *NuvaRing* use when switching from the mini-pill, implant, injectable contraceptive, or IUD.
- *NuvaRing* comes in a reclosable foil pouch. Instruct patient to wash hands, then remove *NuvaRing* from pouch; keep pouch for ring disposal. Using a position of comfort (lying down, squatting, or standing with one leg up), hold *NuvaRing* between thumb and index finger and press opposite sides of the ring together. Gently push folded ring into vagina. Exact position is not important for function of *NuvaRing*. Most women do not feel *NuvaRing* once it is in place. If discomfort is felt, *NuvaRing* may not be inserted far enough into vagina; use finger to push further into vagina. *There is no danger of NuvaRing being pushed in too far or getting lost*. Once inserted, leave *NuvaRing* in place for 3 wk.
- Remove ring 3 wk after insertion on same day and time of insertion. Remove by hooking finger under forward rim or by holding ring between index and middle finger and pulling out. Place ring in foil pouch and dispose; do not throw in toilet. Menstrual period will usually start 2–3 days after ring is removed and may not have finished before next ring is inserted. To continue contraceptive protection, new ring must be inserted 1 wk after last one was removed, even if menstrual period has not stopped.
- If *NuvaRing* slips out of vagina and has been out less than 3 hr, contraceptive protection is still in place. *NuvaRing* can be rinsed in cool to tepid water and should be reinserted as soon as possible. If ring is lost, insert a new ring and continue same schedule as lost ring. If *NuvaRing* has been out of vagina for more than 3 hr, a nonhormonal method of contraception, other than a diaphragm, should be used for the next 7 days.
- *If NuvaRing has been left in for an extra wk or less (4 wk total or less)*, remove and insert a new ring after a 1-wk ring-free break. If *NuvaRing* has been left in place for more than 4 wk, woman should check to be sure she is not pregnant. A nonhor-

monal method of contraception, other than a diaphragm, must be used for the next 7 days.
- **Intrauterine system:** Advise patient to notify health care professional if pelvic pain or pain during sex, unusual vaginal discharge or genital sores, unexplained fever, exposure to sexually transmitted infections, very severe or migraine headaches, yellowing of skin or whites of the eyes, very severe vaginal bleeding or bleeding that lasts a long time occurs, if a menstrual period is missed, or if *Mirena's* threads cannot be felt.

Evaluation/Desired Outcomes
- Prevention of pregnancy.
- Regulation of the menstrual cycle.
- Decrease in menstrual blood loss.
- Decrease in acne.
- Decrease in symptoms of premenstrual dysphoric disorder.
- Decrease in vasomotor symptoms or symptoms of vulvar and vaginal atrophy due to menopause.

CORTICOSTEROIDS (INHALATION)

beclomethasone
(be-kloe-**meth**-a-sone)
QVAR

budesonide (byoo-**dess**-oh-nide)
Pulmicort Respules, Pulmicort Flexhaler

flunisolide (floo-**niss**-oh-lide)
Aerospan HFA

fluticasone (floo-**ti**-ka-sone)
Arnuity Ellipta, Flovent Diskus, Flovent HFA

mometasone (mo-**met**-a-sone)
Asmanex HFA, Asmanex Twisthaler

Classification
Therapeutic: antiasthmatics, anti-inflammatories (steroidal)
Pharmacologic: corticosteroids (inhalation)

Pregnancy Category B (budesonide), C (all others)

Indications
Maintenance treatment of asthma as prophylactic therapy. May decrease the need for or eliminate use of systemic corticosteroids in patients with asthma.

Action
Potent, locally acting anti-inflammatory and immune modifier. **Therapeutic Effects:** Decreased frequency and severity of asthma attacks. Improves asthma symptoms.

Pharmacokinetics
Absorption: *Beclomethasone*—20%; *budesonide*—6–13% (Flexhaler), 6% (Respules); *flunisolide*—40%; *fluticasone*—<7% (aerosol), 8–14% (powder); *mometasone*—<1%. Action is primarily local after inhalation.
Distribution: 10–25% is deposited in airways if a spacer device is not used. All cross the placenta and enter breast milk in small amounts.
Metabolism and Excretion: *Beclomethasone*—after inhalation, beclomethasone dipropionate is converted to beclomethasone monopropionate, an active metabolite that adds to its potency, primarily excreted in feces (<10% excreted in urine; *Budenoside, flunisolide, fluticasone, mometasone*—metabolized by the liver (primarily by CYP3A4) after absorption from lungs; *Budenoside*—60% excreted in urine, 40% in feces; *flunisolide*—50% excreted in urine, 50% in feces; *fluticasone*—primarily excreted in feces (<5% excreted in urine); *mometasone*—75% excreted in feces.
Half-life: *Beclomethasone*—2.8 hr; *budesonide*—2–3.6 hr; *flunisolide*—1.8 hr; *fluticasone*—7.8 hr (propionate); 24 hr (furoate); *mometasone*—5 hr.

TIME/ACTION PROFILE (improvement in symptoms)

ROUTE	ONSET	PEAK	DURATION
Inhalation	within 24 hr‡	1–4 wk†	unknown

†Improvement in pulmonary function; ↓ airway responsiveness may take longer.
‡2–8 days for budesonide respule.

Contraindications/Precautions
Contraindicated in: Some products contain alcohol or lactose and should be avoided in patients with known hypersensitivity or intolerance; Acute attack of asthma/status asthmaticus.
Use Cautiously in: Active untreated infections; Diabetes or glaucoma; Underlying immunosuppression (due to disease or concurrent therapy); Systemic corticosteroid therapy (should not be abruptly discontinued when inhalation therapy is started; additional corticosteroids needed in stress or trauma); Hepatic dysfunction (fluticasone); OB, Lactation: Safety not established; Pedi: Prolonged or high-dose therapy may lead to complications.

Adverse Reactions/Side Effects
CNS: headache, agitation, depression, dizziness, fatigue, insomnia, restlessness. **EENT:** dysphonia, hoarseness, cataracts, glaucoma, nasal congestion, pharyngitis, sinusitis. **Resp:** bronchospasm, cough,

wheezing. **GI:** diarrhea, dry mouth, dyspepsia, esophageal candidiasis, taste disturbances, nausea. **Endo:** adrenal suppression (↑ dose, long-term therapy only), ↓ growth (children), ↓ bone mineral density. **MS:** back pain. **Misc:** hypersensitivity reactions including ANAPHYLAXIS, LARYNGEAL EDEMA, URTICARIA, and BRONCHOSPASM, CHURG-STRAUSS SYNDROME.

Interactions

Drug-Drug: Strong **CYP3A4 inhibitors**, including **ritonavir**, **atazanavir**, **clarithromycin**, **conivaptan**, **indinavir**, **itraconazole**, **ketoconazole**, **lopinavir**, **nefazodone**, **nelfinavir**, **saquinavir**, **telithromycin**, and **voriconazole** ↓ metabolism and ↑ levels of budesonide, mometasone, and fluticasone; concurrent use with fluticasone not recommended.

Route/Dosage

Beclomethasone

Inhaln (Adults and Children ≥12 yr): *Previously on bronchodilators alone*—40–80 mcg twice daily (not to exceed 320 mcg twice daily); *Previously on inhaled corticosteroids*—40–160 mcg twice daily (not to exceed 320 mcg twice daily).
Inhaln (Children 5–11 yr): *Previously on bronchodilators alone*—40 mcg twice daily (not to exceed 80 mcg twice daily); *Previously on inhaled corticosteroids*—40 mcg twice daily (not to exceed 80 mcg twice daily).

Budesonide (Pulmicort Flexhaler)

Inhaln (Adults): 180–360 mcg twice daily (not to exceed 720 mcg twice daily).
Inhaln (Children ≥6 yr): 180–360 mcg twice daily (not to exceed 360 mcg twice daily).

Budesonide (Pulmicort Respules)

Inhaln (Children 1–8 yr): *Previously on bronchodilators alone*—0.5 mg once daily or 0.25 mg twice daily (not to exceed 0.5 mg/day); *Previously on other inhaled corticosteroids*—0.5 mg once daily or 0.25 mg twice daily (not to exceed 1 mg/day); *Previously on oral corticosteroids*—1 mg once daily or 0.5 mg twice daily (not to exceed 1 mg/day).

Flunisolide

Inhaln (Adults and Children ≥12 yr): 160 mcg (2 inhalations) twice daily (not to exceed 4 inhalations twice daily).
Inhaln (Children 6–11 yr): 80 mcg (1 inhalation) twice daily (not to exceed 2 inhalations twice daily).

Fluticasone (Aerosol Inhaler)

Inhaln (Adults and Children ≥12 yr): *Previously on bronchodilators alone*—88 mcg twice daily initially, may be ↑ up to 440 mcg twice daily; *Previously on other inhaled corticosteroids*—88–220 mcg twice daily initially, may be ↑ up to 440 mcg twice daily; *Previously on oral corticosteroids*—440 mcg twice daily initially, may be ↑ up to 880 mcg twice daily.
Inhaln (Children 4–11 yr): 88 mcg twice daily (not to exceed 88 mcg twice daily).

Fluticasone (Dry Powder Inhaler)

Inhaln (Adults and Children ≥12 yr): *Previously on bronchodilators alone*—Propionate: 100 mcg twice daily initially, may be ↑ up to 500 mcg twice daily; Furoate: 100 mcg once daily, may be ↑ up to 200 mcg once daily after 2 wk; *Previously on other inhaled corticosteroids*—Propionate: 100–250 mcg twice daily initially, may be ↑ up to 500 mcg twice daily; *Previously on oral corticosteroids*—Propionate: 500–1000 mcg twice daily.
Inhaln (Children 4–11 yr): *Previously on bronchodilators alone*—50 mcg twice daily initially, may be ↑ up to 100 mcg twice daily; *Previously on other inhaled corticosteroids*—50 mcg twice daily, may be ↑ up to 100 mcg twice daily.

Mometasone (Aerosol Inhaler)

Inhaln (Adults and Children ≥12 yr): *Previously on medium-dose inhaled corticosteroids*—Two 100–mcg inhalations twice daily; *Previously on high-dose inhaled corticosteroids or oral corticosteroids*—Two 200–mcg inhalations twice daily (not to exceed 800 mcg/day).

Mometasone (Dry Powder Inhaler)

Inhaln (Adults and Children ≥12 yr): *Previously on bronchodilators or other inhaled corticosteroids*—220 mcg once daily in evening, up to 440 mcg/day as a single dose or 2 divided doses; *Previously on oral corticosteroids*—440 mcg twice daily (not to exceed 880 mcg/day).
Inhaln (Children 4–11 yr): 110 mcg once daily in evening (not to exceed 110 mcg/day).

Availability

Beclomethasone

Inhalation aerosol: 40 mcg/metered inhalation in 8.7-g canister (delivers 120 metered inhalations), 80 mcg/metered inhalation in 8.7-g canister (delivers 120 metered inhalations). **Cost:** 40 mcg/metered inhalation $130.16/inhaler, 80 mcg/metered inhalation $173.67/inhaler.

Budesonide (generic available)

Inhalation powder (Flexhaler): 90 mcg/metered inhalation (delivers 60 metered inhalations), 180 mcg/metered inhalation (delivers 120 metered inhalations). **Cost:** 90 mcg/metered inhalation $143.87/inhaler, 180 mcg/metered inhalation $192.65/inhaler. **Inhalation suspension (Respules):** 0.25 mg/2 mL in single-dose ampules (5 ampules/envelope), 0.5 mg/2 mL in single-dose ampules (5 ampules/envelope), 1 mg/2 mL in single-dose ampules (5 ampules/envelope). ***In combination with:*** formoterol (Symbicort). See Appendix B.

C

Flunisolide

Inhalation aerosol: 80 mcg/metered inhalation in 5.1-g canisters (delivers 60 metered inhalations) or 8.9-g canisters (delivers 120 metered inhalations).

Fluticasone

Inhalation aerosol (propionate) (Flovent-HFA): 44 mcg/metered inhalation in 10.6-g canisters (delivers 120 metered inhalations), 110 mcg/metered inhalation in 12-g canisters (delivers 120 metered inhalations), 220 mcg/metered inhalation in 12-g canisters (delivers 120 metered inhalations). **Cost:** 44 mcg/inhalation $137.82/inhaler, 110 mcg/inhalation $181.43/inhaler, 220 mcg/inhalation $278.14/inhaler. **Powder for inhalation (propionate) (Flovent Diskus):** 50 mcg/blister, 100 mcg/blister, 250 mcg/blister. **Cost:** 50 mcg $144.47/60 blisters, 250 mcg $134.71/28 blisters. **Powder for inhalation (furoate) (Arnuity Ellipta):** 100 mcg/blister, 200 mcg/blister. ***In combination with:*** salmeterol (Advair), vilanterol (Breo Ellipta). See Appendix B.

Mometasone

Inhalation aerosol (Asmanex HFA): 100 mcg/metered inhalation in 13-g canisters (120 metered inhalations), 200 mcg/metered inhalation in 13-g canisters (120 metered inhalations). **Powder for inhalation (Asmanex Twisthaler):** 110 mcg (delivers 100 mcg/metered inhalation; in packages of 7 and 30 inhalation units), 220 mcg (delivers 200 mcg/metered inhalation; in packages of 14, 30, 60, and 120 inhalation units). **Cost:** 110 mcg $88.75/7 inhalation units, 110 mcg $157.90/30 inhalation units, 220 mcg $88.75/14 inhalation units, 220 mcg $170.47/30 inhalation units, 220 mcg $200.32/60 inhalation units, 220 mcg $287.09/120 inhalation units.

NURSING IMPLICATIONS

Assessment

- Monitor respiratory status and lung sounds. Assess pulmonary function tests periodically during and for several months after a transfer from systemic to inhalation corticosteroids.
- Assess patients changing from systemic corticosteroids to inhalation corticosteroids for signs of adrenal insufficiency (anorexia, nausea, weakness, fatigue, hypotension, hypoglycemia) during initial therapy and periods of stress. If these signs appear, notify health care professional immediately; condition may be life-threatening.
- Monitor for withdrawal symptoms (joint or muscular pain, lassitude, depression) during withdrawal from oral corticosteroids.
- Monitor growth rate in children receiving chronic therapy; use lowest possible dose.
- May cause decreased bone mineral density during prolonged therapy. Monitor patients with increased risk (prolonged immobilization, family history of osteoporosis, post-menopausal status, tobacco use, advanced age, poor nutrition, chronic use of drugs that can reduce bone mass [anticonvulsants, oral corticosteroids]) for fractures.
- Monitor for signs and symptoms of hypersensitivity reactions (rash, pruritis, swelling of face and neck, dyspnea) periodically during therapy.
- ***Lab Test Considerations:*** Periodic adrenal function tests may be ordered to assess degree of hypothalamic-pituitary-adrenal (HPA) axis suppression in chronic therapy. Children and patients using higher than recommended doses are at highest risk for HPA suppression.
- May cause ↑ serum and urine glucose concentrations if significant absorption occurs.

Potential Nursing Diagnoses

Ineffective airway clearance (Indications)
Risk for infection (Side Effects)
Deficient knowledge, related to medication regimen (Patient/Family Teaching)

Implementation

- Do not confuse Flovent with Flonase.
- After desired clinical effect has been obtained, attempts should be made to decrease dose to lowest amount required to control symptoms. Gradually decrease dose every 2–4 wk as long as desired effect is maintained. If symptoms return, dose may briefly return to starting dose.
- **Inhaln:** Allow at least 1 min between inhalations.

Patient/Family Teaching

- Advise patient to take medication as directed. Take missed doses as soon as remembered unless almost time for next dose. Instruct patient to read the *Patient Information and Instructions for Use* before using and with each Rx refill, in case of new information. Advise patient not to discontinue medication without consulting health care professional; gradual decrease is required.
- Advise patients using inhalation corticosteroids and bronchodilator to use bronchodilator first and to allow 5 min to elapse before administering the corticosteroid, unless otherwise directed by health care professional.
- Advise patient that inhalation corticosteroids should not be used to treat an acute asthma attack but should be continued even if other inhalation agents are used.
- Patients using inhalation corticosteroids to control asthma may require systemic corticosteroids for acute attacks. Advise patient to use regular peak flow monitoring to determine respiratory status.
- Caution patient to avoid smoking, known allergens, and other respiratory irritants.

- Advise patient to notify health care professional if sore throat or sore mouth occurs.
- Advise patient to stop using medication and notify health care professional immediately if signs and symptoms of hypersensitivity reactions occur.
- Advise female patients to notify health care professional if pregnancy is planned or suspected or if breast feeding.
- Instruct patient whose systemic corticosteroids have been recently reduced or withdrawn to carry a warning card indicating the need for supplemental systemic corticosteroids in the event of stress or severe asthma attack unresponsive to bronchodilators.
- **Metered-Dose Inhaler:** Instruct patient in proper use of metered-dose inhaler. Most inhalers require priming before first use. Shake inhaler well. Exhale completely, and then close lips firmly around mouthpiece. While breathing in deeply and slowly, press down on canister. Hold breath for as long as possible to ensure deep instillation of medication. Remove inhaler from mouth and breathe out gently. Allow 1–2 min between inhalations. Rinse mouth with water or mouthwash after each use to minimize fungal infections, dry mouth, and hoarseness. Clean mouthpiece weekly with clean, dry tissue or cloth. Do not place in water (see Appendix D).
- **Pulmicort Flexhaler:** Advise patient to follow instructions supplied. Before first-time use, prime unit by turning cover and lifting off; hold upright with mouthpiece up and twist brown grip fully to right, then fully to left until it clicks. To administer dose, hold upright, twist brown grip fully to right, then fully to left until it clicks. Turn head away from inhaler and exhale (do not blow into inhaler). Do not shake inhaler. Place mouthpiece between lips and inhale deeply and forcefully. Remove inhaler from mouth and exhale (do not exhale into mouthpiece). Repeat procedure if 2nd dose required. Replace cover; rinse mouth with water (do not swallow).
- **Pulmicort Respules:** Administer with a jet nebulizer connected to adequate air flow, equipped with a mouthpiece or face mask. Adjust face mask to avoid exposing eyes to nebulized medication. Wash face after use of face mask. Ultrasonic nebulizers are not adequate for administration and not recommended. Store respules upright, away from heat and protected from light. Do not refrigerate or freeze. Respules are stable for 2 wk at room temperature after opening aluminum foil envelope. Open respules must be used promptly. Unused respules should be returned to aluminum foil envelope.
- **Flovent Diskus/Arnuity Ellipta:** Do not use with a spacer. Exhale completely and then close lips firmly around mouthpiece. While breathing in deeply and slowly, press down on canister. Hold breath for as long as possible to ensure deep instillation of medication. Remove inhaler from mouth and breathe out gently. Allow 1–2 min between inhalations. After inhalation, rinse mouth with water and spit out (see Appendix D). Never wash the mouthpiece or any part of the Diskus inhaler. Discard Diskus inhaler device (Flovent Diskus) 6 wks (50-mcg strength) or 2 mo (100-mcg and 250-mcg strengths) or blister tray (Arnuity Ellipta) 6 wks after removal from protective foil overwrap pouch or after all blisters have been used (whichever comes first).
- **Asmanex Twisthaler:** Advise patient to remove cap while device is in upright position. To administer dose, exhale fully, then place mouthpiece between lips and inhale deeply and forcefully. Remove device from mouth and hold breath for 10 sec before exhaling (do not exhale into mouthpiece). Wipe the mouthpiece dry, if necessary, and replace the cap on the device. Rinse mouth with water. Advise patient to discard twisthaler 45 days from opening or when dose counter reads "00", whichever comes first.

Evaluation/Desired Outcomes

- Management of the symptoms of chronic asthma.
- Improvement in symptoms of asthma.

CORTICOSTEROIDS (NASAL)

beclomethasone
(be-kloe-**meth**-a-sone)
Beconase AQ, QNASL, 🍁Rivanase AQ

budesonide (byoo-**dess**-oh-nide)
Rhinocort Aqua

ciclesonide (sye-**kles**-oh-nide)
🍁Drymira, Omnaris, Zetonna

flunisolide (floo-**niss**-oh-lide)
~~Nasalide~~, 🍁Rhinalar

fluticasone (floo-**ti**-ka-sone)
🍁Avamys, Flonase, Veramyst

mometasone (moe-**met**-a-sone)
Nasonex

triamcinolone
(trye-am-**sin**-oh-lone)
Nasacort Allergy 24 HR

Classification
Therapeutic: anti-inflammatories (steroidal)
Pharmacologic: corticosteroids (nasal)

Pregnancy Category B (budesonide), C (all others)

Indications

Seasonal or perennial allergic rhinitis. Nonallergic rhinitis (fluticasone). Treatment of nasal polyps.

Action

Potent, locally acting anti-inflammatory and immune modifier. **Therapeutic Effects:** ↓ in symptoms of allergic or nonallergic rhinitis. ↓ in symptoms of nasal polyps.

Pharmacokinetics

Absorption: *Beclomethasone*—27–44% absorbed; *budesonide*—34% absorbed; *flunisolide*—50% absorbed; *ciclesonide, fluticasone, mometasone*—negligible absorption. Action of all agents is primarily local following nasal use.

Distribution: All agents cross the placenta and enter breast milk in small amounts.

Metabolism and Excretion: Following absorption from nasal mucosa, corticosteroids are rapidly and extensively metabolized by the liver.

Half-life: *Beclomethasone*—2.7 hr; *budesonide*—2–3 hr; *ciclesonide*—unknown; *flunisolide*—1–2 hr; *fluticasone*—7.8 hr; *mometasone*—5.8 hr; *triamcinolone*—3–5.4 hr.

TIME/ACTION PROFILE (improvement in symptoms)

ROUTE	ONSET	PEAK	DURATION
Beclomethasone	1–3 days	up to 2 wk	unknown
Budesonide	1–2 days	2 wk	unknown
Ciclesonide	1–2 days	2–5 wk	unknown
Flunisolide	few days	up to 3 wk	unknown
Fluticasone	few days	unknown	unknown
Mometasone	within 2 days	1–2 wk	unknown
Triamcinolone	few days	3–4 days	unknown

Contraindications/Precautions

Contraindicated in: Some products contain alcohol, propylene, or polyethylene glycol and should be avoided in patients with known hypersensitivity or intolerance.

Use Cautiously in: Active untreated infections; Diabetes or glaucoma; Underlying immunosuppression (due to disease or concurrent therapy); Systemic corticosteroid therapy (should not be abruptly discontinued when intranasal therapy is started); History of ↑ intraocular pressure, glaucoma, or cataracts; Recent nasal trauma, septal ulcers, or surgery (wound healing may be impaired by nasal corticosteroids); OB, Lactation, Pedi: Pregnancy, lactation, or children <12 yr (beclomethasone [QNASL]), <6 yr (beclomethasone [Beconase AQ], budesonide, ciclesonide, flunisolide) <4 yr (fluticasone [Flonase]) or <2 yr (fluticasone [Veramyst], mometasone, triamcinolone) (safety not established; prolonged or high-dose therapy may lead to complications).

Adverse Reactions/Side Effects

CNS: dizziness, headache. **EENT:** epistaxis, nasal burning, nasal congestion, nasal irritation, nasal perforation, nasal ulceration, pharyngitis, rhinorrhea, sneezing, tearing eyes. **GI:** dry mouth, esophageal candidiasis, nausea, vomiting. **Derm:** rash (fluticasone), urticaria (fluticasone). **Endo:** adrenal suppression (high-dose, long-term therapy only), growth suppression (children). **Resp:** bronchospasm, cough. **Misc:** ANAPHYLAXIS, ANGIOEDEMA.

C

Interactions

Drug-Drug: Ketoconazole ↑ effects of budesonide, ciclesonide, and fluticasone. **Ritonavir** ↑ effects of fluticasone (avoid concurrent use).

Route/Dosage

Beclomethasone

Intranasal (Adults and Children ≥12 yr): *Beconase AQ*—1–2 sprays in each nostril twice daily (not to exceed 2 metered sprays in each nostril twice daily); *QNASL*—2 sprays in each nostril once daily.
Intranasal (Children 6–12 yr): 1–2 sprays in each nostril twice daily; once adequate control achieved, ↓ dose to 1 spray in each nostril twice daily.

Budesonide

Intranasal (Adults and Children ≥12 yr): 1 spray in each nostril once daily (not to exceed 4 sprays in each nostril once daily).
Intranasal (Children 6–11 yr): 1 spray in each nostril once daily (not to exceed 2 sprays in each nostril once daily).

Ciclesonide

Intranasal (Adults and Children ≥12 yr): *Omnaris (for perennial allergic rhinitis only)*—2 sprays in each nostril once daily (not to exceed 2 sprays in each nostril/day); *Zetonna*—1 spray in each nostril once daily (not to exceed 1 spray in each nostril/day).
Intranasal (Adults and Children ≥6 yr): *Omnaris (for seasonal allergic rhinitis only)*—2 sprays in each nostril once daily (not to exceed 2 sprays in each nostril/day).

Flunisolide

Intranasal (Adults and Children >14 yr): 2 sprays in each nostril twice daily, may be ↑ to 2 sprays in each nostril 3 times daily if greater effect needed after 4–7 days (not to exceed 8 sprays in each nostril/day).
Intranasal (Children 6–14 yr): 1 spray in each nostril 3 times daily or 2 sprays in each nostril twice daily (not to exceed 4 sprays in each nostril/day).

Fluticasone

Intranasal (Adults and Children ≥12 yr): *Flonase*—2 sprays in each nostril once daily or 1 spray in each nostril twice daily; after several days, attempt to ↓ dose to 1 spray in each nostril once daily. Patients ≥12 yr with seasonal allergic rhinitis may also use 2 sprays

in each nostril once daily on an as-needed basis; *Veramyst*—2 sprays in each nostril once daily or 1 spray in each nostril twice daily; after several days, attempt to ↓ dose to 1 spray in each nostril once daily.
Intranasal (Children >4 yr): *Flonase*—1 spray in each nostril once daily (not to exceed 2 sprays in each nostril/day).
Intranasal (Children 2–11 yr): *Veramyst*—1 spray in each nostril daily; may ↑ to 2 sprays if no response. Once symptoms are controlled, attempt to ↓ dose to 1 spray/day.

Mometasone

Intranasal (Adults and Children >12 yr): *Treatment of seasonal and perennial allergic rhinitis*—2 sprays in each nostril once daily (not to exceed 2 sprays in each nostril once daily).
Intranasal (Adults): *Nasal polyps*—2 sprays in each nostril twice daily (not to exceed 2 sprays in each nostril twice daily).
Intranasal (Children 2–11 yr): *Treatment of seasonal and perennial allergic rhinitis*—1 spray in each nostril once daily.

Triamcinolone

Intranasal (Adults and Children ≥12 yr): 2 sprays in each nostril once daily.
Intranasal (Children 6–11 yr): 1 spray in each nostril once daily (not to exceed 2 sprays in each nostril/day).
Intranasal (Children 2–5 yr): 1 spray in each nostril once daily.

Availability

Beclomethasone

Nasal spray (Beconase AQ): 42 mcg/metered spray in 25-g bottles (delivers 180 metered sprays). **Cost:** $173.37/bottle. **Nasal spray (QNASL):** 80 mcg/metered spray in 8.7-g bottles (delivers 120 metered sprays). **Cost:** $139.94/bottle. **Nasal spray (Rivanase AQ):** ✱50 mcg/metered spray in 25-g bottles (delivers 200 metered sprays).

Budesonide (generic available)

Nasal spray: 32 mcg/metered spray in 8.6-g canister (delivers 120 metered sprays). **Cost:** $153.97/bottle.

Ciclesonide

Nasal spray (Omnaris): 50 mcg/metered spray in 12.5-g bottle (delivers 120 metered sprays). **Cost:** $152.07/bottle. **Nasal spray (Zetonna):** 37 mcg/actuation in 6.1-g bottle (delivers 60 metered sprays). **Cost:** $159.43/bottle.

Flunisolide (generic available)

Nasal solution: 25 mcg/metered spray in 25-mL bottle (delivers 200 metered sprays). **Cost:** *Generic*—$44.56/bottle.

Fluticasone (generic available)

Nasal spray (Flonase): 50 mcg/metered spray in 16-g bottle (delivers 120 metered sprays). **Cost:** *Generic*—$19.52/bottle. **Nasal spray (Veramyst):** 27.5 mcg/spray in a 10-g bottle (delivers 120 sprays). **Cost:** $122.29/bottle. ***In combination with:*** azelastine (Dymista); see Appendix B.

Mometasone

Nasal spray (scent-free): 50 mcg/metered spray in 17-g bottle (delivers 120 metered sprays). **Cost:** $162.27/bottle.

Triamcinolone (generic available)

Nasal spray: 55 mcg/metered spray in 16.5-g bottle (120 metered sprays)[OTC]. **Cost:** *Generic*—$86.05/bottle.

NURSING IMPLICATIONS

Assessment

- Monitor degree of nasal stuffiness, amount and color of nasal discharge, and frequency of sneezing.
- Patients on long-term therapy should have periodic otolaryngologic examinations to monitor nasal mucosa and passages for infection or ulceration.
- Monitor growth rate in children receiving chronic therapy; use lowest possible dose.
- ***Lab Test Considerations:*** Periodic adrenal function tests may be ordered to assess degree of hypothalamic-pituitary-adrenal (HPA) axis suppression in chronic therapy. Children and patients using higher than recommended doses are at highest risk for HPA suppression.

Potential Nursing Diagnoses

Ineffective airway clearance (Indications)
Risk for infection (Side Effects)
Deficient knowledge, related to medication regimen (Patient/Family Teaching)

Implementation

- Do not confuse Flonase with Flovent.
- After desired clinical effect has been obtained, attempt to decrease dose to lowest amount. Gradually decrease dose every 2–4 wk as long as desired effect is maintained. If symptoms return, dose may briefly return to starting dose.
- **Intranasal:** Patients also using a nasal decongestant should be given decongestant 5–15 min before corticosteroid nasal spray. If patient is unable to breathe freely through nasal passages, instruct patient to blow nose gently in advance of medication administration.

C

Patient/Family Teaching

- Advise patient to take medication as directed. Take missed doses as soon as remembered unless almost time for next dose.
- Caution patient not to exceed maximal daily dose of nasal spray.
- Instruct patient in correct technique for administering nasal spray (see Appendix D). Most nasal sprays include directions with pictures. Instruct patient to read patient information sheet prior to use. Most nasal sprays require priming prior to first use or use after 7 days. Shake well before use. Warn patient that temporary nasal stinging may occur.
- Instruct patient to gently blow nose to clear nostrils prior to administering dose.
- Instruct patient to stop medication and notify health care professional immediately if signs of anaphylaxis (rash, hives, difficulty breathing, swollen lips or throat) or if changes in vision occur.
- Instruct patient to notify health care professional of all Rx or OTC medications, vitamins, or herbal products being taken and consult health care professional before taking other Rx, OTC, or herbal products.
- Advise female patients to notify health care professional if pregnancy is planned or suspected or if breast feeding.
- Instruct patient to notify health care professional if symptoms do not improve within 1 mo, if symptoms worsen, or if sneezing or nasal irritation occurs.

Evaluation/Desired Outcomes

- Resolution of nasal stuffiness, discharge, and sneezing in seasonal or perennial allergic rhinitis or nonallergic rhinitis.
- Reduction in symptoms of nasal polyps.

CORTICOSTEROIDS (SYSTEMIC)

short-acting corticosteroids

cortisone (**kor**-ti-sone)

hydrocortisone
(hye-droe-**kor**-ti-sone)
A-Hydrocort, Cortef, Cortenema, ✱Hycort, Solu-CORTEF

intermediate-acting corticosteroids

methylPREDNISolone
(meth-ill-pred-**niss**-oh-lone)
A-Methapred, Depo-Medrol, Medrol, Solu-MEDROL

prednisoLONE
(pred-**niss**-oh-lone)
Orapred, Orapred ODT, Pediapred, Prelone

predniSONE (**pred**-ni-sone)
✱Winipred

triamcinolone
(trye-am-**sin**-oh-lone)
Aristospan, Kenalog

long-acting corticosteroids

betamethasone
(bay-ta-**meth**-a-sone)
✱Betaject, ~~Celestone~~

budesonide (byoo-**dess**-oh-nide)
Entocort EC, Uceris

dexamethasone
(dex-a-**meth**-a-sone)
~~Decadron~~, ✱Dexasone

Classification
Therapeutic: antiasthmatics, corticosteroids
Pharmacologic: corticosteroids (systemic)

Pregnancy Category B (prednisone), C (betamethasone, budesonide, dexamethasone, hydrocortisone, methylprednisolone, prednisolone, triamcinolone), D (cortisone)

Indications

Cortisone, hydrocortisone: Management of adrenocortical insufficiency. **Betamethasone, dexamethasone, hydrocortisone, prednisolone, prednisone, methylprednisolone, triamcinolone:** Used systemically and locally in a wide variety of chronic diseases including: Inflammatory, Allergic, Hematologic, Neoplastic, Autoimmune disorders. **Methylprednisolone, prednisone:** With other immunosuppressants in the prevention of organ rejection in transplantation surgery. Asthma. **Dexamethasone:** Management of cerebral edema: Diagnostic agent in adrenal disorders. **Budesonide (Entocort EC):** Treatment of mild to moderate Crohn's disease involving ileum and/or ascending colon. **Budesonide (Entocort EC):** Maintenance of clinical remission for up to 3 mo of mild to moderate Crohn's disease involving ileum and/or ascending colon. **Budesonide (Uceris):** Induction of remission of active, mild to moderate ulcerative colitis. **Unlabeled Use:** Short-term administration to high-risk mothers before delivery to prevent respiratory distress syndrome in the newborn (betamethasone, dexamethasone). Adjunctive therapy of hypercalcemia (prednisone, prednisolone, methylprednisolone). Management of acute spinal cord injury (methylprednisolone). Adjunctive management of nausea and vomiting from chemotherapy (dexamethasone, prednisone, prednisolone, methylprednisolone). Management of croup (dexamethasone). Treatment of airway edema prior to extubation (dexamethasone). Facilitation of ventilator weaning in neonates with bronchopulmonary dysplasia (dexamethasone).

Action

In pharmacologic doses, all agents suppress inflammation and the normal immune response. All agents have numerous intense metabolic effects (see Adverse Reactions/Side Effects). Suppress adrenal function at chronic doses of *betamethasone*—0.6 mg/day; *cortisone, hydrocortisone*—20 mg/day; *dexamethasone*—0.75 mg/day; *methylprednisolone, triamcinolone*—4 mg/day; *prednisone/prednisolone*—5 mg/day. **Cortisone, hydrocortisone:** Replace endogenous cortisol in deficiency states. **Cortisone, hydrocortisone:** Have potent mineralocorticoid (sodium-retaining) activity. **Prednisolone, prednisone:** Have minimal mineralocorticoid activity. **Betamethasone, dexamethasone, methylprednisolone, triamcinolone:** Have negligible mineralocorticoid activity. **Budesonide:** Local anti-inflammatory activity in the lumen of the GI tract. **Therapeutic Effects:** Suppression of inflammation and modification of the normal immune response. Replacement therapy in adrenal insufficiency. **Budesonide:** Improvement in symptoms/sequelae of Crohn's disease and induction of remission of ulcerative colitis.

Pharmacokinetics

Absorption: Well absorbed after oral administration (except budesonide). Sodium phosphate and sodium succinate salts are rapidly absorbed after IM administration. Acetate and acetonide salts are slowly but completely absorbed after IM administration. Absorption from local sites (intra-articular, intralesional) is slow but complete. Bioavailability of budesonide is 9–21%.
Distribution: All are widely distributed, cross the placenta, and probably enter breast milk.
Metabolism and Excretion: All are metabolized mostly by the liver to inactive metabolites. *Cortisone* is converted by the liver to hydrocortisone. *Prednisone* is converted by the liver to prednisolone, which is then metabolized by the liver.
Half-life: *Betamethasone*—3–5 hr (plasma), 36–54 hr (tissue). *Budesonide*—2.0–3.6 hr. *Cortisone*—0.5 hr (plasma), 8–12 hr (tissue). *Dexamethasone*—3–4.5 hr (plasma), 36–54 hr (tissue). *Hydrocortisone*—1.5–2 hr (plasma), 8–12 hr (tissue). *Methylprednisolone*—>3.5 hr (plasma), 18–36 hr (tissue). *Prednisolone*—2.1–3.5 hr (plasma), 18–36 hr (tissue). *Prednisone*—3.4–3.8 hr (plasma), 18–36 hr (tissue). *Triamcinolone*—2–5 hr (plasma), 18–36 hr (tissue).

TIME/ACTION PROFILE (anti-inflammatory activity)

ROUTE	ONSET	PEAK	DURATION
Betamethasone IM (acetate/sodium phosphate)	1–3 hr	unknown	1 wk
Budesonide PO	unknown	unknown	unknown
Cortisone PO	rapid	2 hr	1.25–1.5 days
Dexamethasone PO	unknown	1–3 hr	2.75 days
Dexamethasone IM, IV (sodium phosphate)	rapid	unknown	2.75 days
Hydrocortisone PO	unknown	1–2 hr	1.25–1.5 days
Hydrocortisone IM (sodium succinate)	rapid	1 hr	variable
Hydrocortisone IV (sodium succinate)	rapid	unknown	unknown
Methylprednisolone PO	unknown	1–2 hr	1.25–1.5 days
Methylprednisolone IM (acetate)	6–48 hr	4–8 days	1–4 wk
Methylprednisolone IM, IV (sodium succinate)	rapid	unknown	unknown
Prednisolone PO	unknown	1–2 hr	1.25–1.5 days
Prednisone PO	unknown	1–2 hr	1.25–1.5 days
Triamcinolone IM (acetonide)	24–48 hr	unknown	1–6 wk
Triamcinolone Intralesional (hexacetonide)	slow	unknown	4 days–4 wk

Contraindications/Precautions

Contraindicated in: Active untreated infections (may be used in patients being treated for some forms of meningitis); Lactation: Avoid chronic use; Known alcohol, bisulfite, or tartrazine hypersensitivity or intolerance (some products contain these and should be avoided in susceptible patients); Administration of live virus vaccines.

Use Cautiously in: Chronic treatment (will lead to adrenal suppression; use lowest possible dose for shortest period of time); Hypothyroidism; Immunosuppression; Cirrhosis; Pedi: Children (chronic use will result in ↓ growth; use lowest possible dose for shortest period of time); Stress (surgery, infections); supplemental doses may be needed; Potential infections may mask signs (fever, inflammation); Traumatic brain injury (high doses may be associated with ↑ mortality); OB: Safety not established; Pedi: Neonates (avoid use of benzyl alcohol containing injectable preparations; use preservative-free formulations).

Adverse Reactions/Side Effects

Adverse reactions/side effects are much more common with high-dose/long-term therapy.

CNS: depression, euphoria, headache, ↑ intracranial pressure (children only), personality changes, psychoses, restlessness. **EENT:** cataracts, ↑ intraocular pressure. **CV:** hypertension. **GI:** PEPTIC ULCERATION, anorexia, nausea, vomiting. **Derm:** acne, ↓ wound healing, ecchymoses, fragility, hirsutism, petechiae. **Endo:** adrenal suppression, hyperglycemia. **F and E:** fluid retention (long-term high doses), hypokalemia, hypokalemic alkalosis. **Hemat:** THROMBOEMBOLISM, thrombophlebitis. **Metab:** weight gain. **MS:** muscle wasting, osteoporosis, avascular necrosis of joints, muscle pain. **Misc:** cushingoid appearance (moon face, buffalo hump), ↑ susceptibility to infection.

Interactions

Drug-Drug: ↑ risk of hypokalemia with **thiazide** and **loop diuretics**, or **amphotericin B**. Hypokalemia may ↑ risk of **digoxin** toxicity. May increase requirement for **insulin** or **oral hypoglycemic agents**. **Phenytoin**, **phenobarbital**, and **rifampin** ↑ metabolism; may ↓ effectiveness. **Hormonal contraceptives** may ↓ metabolism. ↑ risk of adverse GI effects with **NSAIDs** (including aspirin). At chronic doses that suppress adrenal function, may ↓ antibody response to and ↑ risk of adverse reactions from **live-virus vaccines**. May ↑ serum concentrations of **cyclosporine** and **tacrolimus**. May ↑ risk of tendon rupture from **fluoroquinolones**. **Antacids** ↓ absorption of prednisone and dexamethasone. Known inhibitors of the CYP3A4 enzyme including **ketoconazole**, **itraconazole**, **ritonavir**, **indinavir**, **saquinavir**, and **erythromycin** may ↑ blood levels and effects of budesonide (↓ dose may be necessary). May ↓ **isoniazid** levels and effectiveness. May antagonize the effects of **anticholinergic agents** in myasthenia gravis.

Drug-Food: **Grapefruit juice** ↑ serum levels and effects of budesonide (avoid concurrent use).

Route/Dosage

Betamethasone

IM (Adults): 0.5–9 mg as betamethasone sodium phosphate/acetate suspension. *Prevention of respiratory distress syndrome in newborn*—12 mg daily for 2–3 days before delivery (unlabeled).

IM (Children): *Adrenocortical insufficiency*—17.5 mcg/kg/day (500 mcg/m²/day) in 3 divided doses every 3rd day or 5.8–8.75 mcg/kg (166–250 mcg/m²)/day as a single dose.

Budesonide

PO (Adults): *Active Crohn's disease (Entocort EC)*—9 mg once daily in the morning for ≤8 wk, may repeat 8-wk course for recurring episodes. *Maintenance of remission of Crohn's disease (Entocort EC)*—6 mg once daily for up to 3 mo; once symptoms are controlled, taper to complete cessation; *Induction of remission of ulcerative colitis (Uceris)*—9 mg once daily for up to 8 wk; once symptoms are controlled, taper to complete cessation.

Cortisone

PO (Adults): 25–300 mg/day in divided doses q 12–24 hr.

PO (Children): *Adrenocortical insufficiency*—0.7 mg/kg/day (20–25 mg/m²/day) in divided doses q 8 hr. *Other uses*—2.5–10 mg/kg/day (75–300 mg/m²/day) in divided doses q 6–8 hr.

Dexamethasone

PO, IM, IV (Adults): *Anti-inflammatory*—0.75–9 mg daily in divided doses q 6–12 hr. *Airway edema or extubation*—0.5–2 mg/kg/day divided q 6 hr; begin 24 hr prior to extubation and continue for 24 hr post-extubation. *Cerebral edema*—10 mg IV, then 4 mg IM or IV q 6 hr until maximal response achieved, then switch to PO regimen and taper over 5–7 days.

PO, IM, IV (Children): *Airway edema or extubation*—0.5–2 mg/kg/day divided q 6 hr; begin 24 hr prior to extubation and continue for 24 hr post-extubation. *Anti-inflammatory*—0.08–0.3 mg/kg/day or 2.5–10 mg/m²/day divided q 6–12 hr. *Physiologic replacement*—0.03–0.15 mg/kg/day or 0.6–0.75 mg/m²/day divided q 6–12 hr.

PO (Adults): *Suppression test*—1 mg at 11PM or 0.5 mg q 6 hr for 48 hr.

IV (Children): *Chemotherapy-induced emesis*—5–20 mg given 15–30 min before treatment; *Cerebral edema*—Loading dose 1–2 mg/kg followed by 1–1.5 mg/kg/day divided q 4–6 hr for 5 days (not to exceed 16 mg/day); then taper over 1–6 wk; *Bacterial meningitis*—0.6 mg/kg/day divided q 6 hr for 4 days (start at time of first antibiotic dose).

IV, PO (Adults): *Chemotherapy-induced emesis*—10–20 mg given 15–30 min before each treatment or

10 mg q 12 hr on each treatment day; *Delayed nausea/vomiting*—4–10 mg PO 1–2 times/day for 2–4 days *or* 8 mg PO q 12 hr for 2 days, then 4 mg PO q 12 hr for 2 days *or* 20 mg PO 1 hr before chemotherapy, then 10 mg PO q 12 hr after chemotherapy, then 8 mg PO q 12 hr for 2 days, then 4 mg PO q 12 hr for 2 days.
IS (Adults): 0.4–6 mg/day.

Hydrocortisone

PO (Adults): 20–240 mg/day in 1–4 divided doses.
PO (Children): *Adrenocortical insufficiency*—0.56 mg/kg/day (15–20 mg/m^2/day) as a single dose or in divided doses. *Other uses*—2–8 mg/kg/day (60–240 mg/m^2/day) as a single dose or in divided doses.
IM, IV (Adults): 100–500 mg q 2–6 hr (range 100–8000 mg/day).
IM, IV (Children): *Adrenocortical insufficiency*—0.186–0.28 mg/kg/day (10–12 mg/m^2/day) in 3 divided doses. *Other uses*—0.666–4 mg/kg (20–120 mg/m^2) q 12–24 hr.
Rect (Adults): *Retention enema*—100 mg nightly for 21 days or until remission occurs.

Methylprednisolone

PO (Adults): *Multiple sclerosis*—160 mg/day for 7 days, then 64 mg every other day for 1 mo. *Other uses*—2–60 mg/day as a single dose or in 2–4 divided doses. *Asthma exacerbations*—120–180 mg/day in divided doses 3–4 times/day for 48 hr, then 60–80 mg/day in 2 divided doses.
PO (Children): *Anti-inflammatory/Immunosuppressive*—0.5–1.7 mg/kg/day (5–25 mg/m^2/day) in divided doses q 6–12 hr. *Asthma exacerbations*—1 mg/kg q 6 hr for 48 hr, then 1–2 mg/kg/day (maximum: 60 mg/day) divided twice daily.
IM, IV (Adults): *Most uses: methylprednisolone sodium succinate*—40–250 mg q 4–6 hr. *High-dose "pulse" therapy: methylprednisolone sodium succinate*—30 mg/kg IV q 4–6 hr for up to 72 hr. *Status asthmaticus: methylprednisolone sodium succinate*—2 mg/kg IV, then 0.5–1 mg/kg IV q 6 hr for up to 5 days. *Multiple sclerosis: methylprednisolone sodium succinate*—160 mg/day for 7 days, then 64 mg every other day for 1 mo. *Adjunctive therapy of* Pneumocystis jirovecii *pneumonia in AIDS patients: methylprednisolone sodium succinate*—30 mg twice daily for 5 days, then 30 mg once daily for 5 days, then 15 mg once daily for 10 days. *Acute spinal cord injury: methylprednisolone sodium succinate*—30 mg/kg IV over 15 min initially, followed in 45 min with a continuous infusion of 5.4 mg/kg/hr for 23 hr (unlabeled).
IM, IV (Children): *Anti-inflammatory/Immunosuppressive*—0.5–1.7 mg/kg/day (5–25 mg/m^2/day) in divided doses q 6–12 hr. *Acute spinal cord injury: methylprednisolone sodium succinate*—30 mg/kg IV over 15 min initially, followed in 45 min with a continuous infusion of 5.4 mg/kg/hr for 23 hr (unlabeled). *Status asthmaticus*—2 mg/kg IV, then 0.5–1 mg/kg IV q 6 hr. *Lupus nephritis*—30 mg/kg IV every other day for 6 doses.
IM (Adults): *Methylprednisolone acetate*—40–120 mg daily, weekly, or every 2 wk.

Prednisolone

PO (Adults): *Most uses*—5–60 mg/day as a single dose or in divided doses. *Multiple sclerosis*—200 mg/day for 7 days, then 80 mg every other day for 1 mo. *Asthma exacerbations*—120–180 mg/day in divided doses 3–4 times/day for 48 hr, then 60–80 mg/day in 2 divided doses.
PO (Children): *Anti-inflammatory/Immunosuppressive*—0.1–2 mg/kg/day in 1–4 divided doses; *Nephrotic syndrome*—2 mg/kg/day (60 mg/m^2/day) in 1–3 divided doses daily (maximum dose: 80 mg/day) until urine is protein-free for 4–6 wk, followed by 2 mg/kg/dose (40 mg/m^2/dose) every other day in the morning; gradually taper off over 4–6 wk; *Asthma exacerbations*—1 mg/kg q 6 hr for 48 hr, then 1–2 mg/kg/day (maximum: 60 mg/day) divided twice daily.

Prednisone

PO (Adults): *Most uses*—5–60 mg/day as a single dose or in divided doses. *Multiple sclerosis*—200 mg/day for 1 wk, then 80 mg every other day for 1 mo. *Adjunctive therapy of* P. jirovecii *pneumonia in AIDS patients*—40 mg twice daily for 5 days, then 40 mg once daily for 5 days, then 20 mg once daily for 10 days.
PO (Children): *Nephrotic syndrome*—2 mg/kg/day initially given in 1–3 divided doses (maximum 80 mg/day) until urine is protein-free for 4–6 wk. Maintenance dose of 2 mg/kg/day every other day in the morning, gradually taper off after 4–6 wk. *Asthma exacerbation*—1 mg/kg q 6 hr for 48 hr, then 1–2 mg/kg/day (maximum 60 mg/day) in divided doses twice daily.

Triamcinolone

IM (Adults): *Triamcinolone acetonide*—40–80 mg q 4 wk.
Intra-articular (Adults): *Triamcinolone hexacetonide*—2–20 mg q 3–4 wk (dose depends on size of joint to be injected, amount of inflammation, and amount of fluid present).
IM (Children): *Triamcinolone acetonide*—40 mg q 4 wk or 30–200 mcg/kg (1–6.25 mg/m^2) q 1–7 days.

Availability

Betamethasone (generic available)

Suspension for injection (sodium phosphate and acetate): 6 mg (total)/mL.

Budesonide (generic available)

Capsules (Entocort EC): 3 mg. **Cost:** *Generic*—$397.88/30. **Extended-release tablets (Uceris):** 9 mg. **Cost:** $1,482.00/30.

Cortisone (generic available)

Tablets: 25 mg. **Cost:** *Generic*—$108.00/100.

Dexamethasone (generic available)

Tablets: 0.5 mg, 0.75 mg, 1 mg, 1.5 mg, 2 mg, 4 mg, 6 mg. **Cost:** *Generic*—0.5 mg $20.76/100, 0.75 mg $36.39/100, 1 mg $35.00/100, 1.5 mg $27.14/100, 2 mg $68.54/100, 4 mg $64.25/100, 6 mg $107.07/100. **Elixir (raspberry flavor):** 0.5 mg/5 mL. **Cost:** *Generic*—$63.68/237 mL. **Oral solution (cherry flavor):** 0.5 mg/5 mL, 1 mg/mL. **Cost:** *Generic*—0.5 mg/5 mL $63.69/240 mL, 1 mg/mL $23.74/30 mL. **Solution for injection (sodium phosphate):** 4 mg/mL, 10 mg/mL.

Hydrocortisone (generic available)

Tablets: 5 mg, 10 mg, 20 mg. **Cost:** *Generic*—5 mg $16.95/50, 10 mg $57.30/100, 20 mg $78.81/100. **Enema:** 100 mg/60 mL. **Cost:** *Generic*—$48.80/480 mL. **Powder for injection (sodium succinate):** 100 mg, 250 mg, 500 mg, 1 g.

Methylprednisolone (generic available)

Tablets: 4 mg, 8 mg, 16 mg, 32 mg. **Cost:** *Generic*—4 mg $142.93/100, 8 mg $50.26/25, 16 mg $155.29/50, 32 mg $115.62/25. **Powder for injection (sodium succinate):** 40 mg, 125 mg, 500 mg, 1 g, 2 g. **Suspension for injection (acetate):** 20 mg/mL, 40 mg/mL, 80 mg/mL.

Prednisolone (generic available)

Tablets: 5 mg. **Cost:** $256.35/30. **Orally disintegrating tablets (grape flavor):** 10 mg, 15 mg, 30 mg. **Cost:** 10 mg $394.84/48, 15 mg $593.71/48, 30 mg $846.02/48. **Oral solution:** 5 mg/5 mL, 10 mg/5 mL, 15 mg/5 mL, 20 mg/5 mL, 25 mg/5 mL. **Cost:** *Generic*—5 mg/5 mL $98.09/120 mL, 15 mg/5 mL $25.80/237 mL, 25 mg/5 mL $186.00/237 mL. **Oral suspension:** 15 mg/5 mL. **Cost:** $124.77/30 mL.

Prednisone (generic available)

Tablets: 1 mg, 2.5 mg, 5 mg, 10 mg, 20 mg, 50 mg. **Cost:** *Generic*—1 mg $11.04/30, 2.5 mg $7.41/30, 5 mg $8.32/30, 10 mg $10.84/30, 50 mg $13.77/30. **Oral solution:** 1 mg/mL, 5 mg/mL. **Cost:** *Generic*—1 mg/mL $24.45/120 mL, 5 mg/mL $42.32/30 mL.

Triamcinolone (generic available)

Suspension for injection (acetonide): 10 mg/mL, 40 mg/mL, 80 mg/mL. **Suspension for injection (hexacetonide):** 5 mg/mL, 20 mg/mL.

NURSING IMPLICATIONS

Assessment

- These drugs are indicated for many conditions. Assess involved systems before and periodically during therapy.
- Assess for signs of adrenal insufficiency (hypotension, weight loss, weakness, nausea, vomiting, anorexia, lethargy, confusion, restlessness) before and periodically during therapy.
- Monitor intake and output ratios and daily weights. Observe patient for peripheral edema, steady weight gain, rales/crackles, or dyspnea. Notify health care professional if these occur.
- Children should have periodic evaluations of growth.
- **Cerebral Edema:** Assess for changes in level of consciousness and headache during therapy.
- **Budesonide:** Assess signs of Crohn's disease and ulcerative colitis (diarrhea, crampy abdominal pain, fever, bleeding from rectum) during therapy. Monitor frequency and consistency of bowel movements periodically during therapy.
- **Rect:** Assess symptoms of ulcerative colitis (diarrhea, bleeding, weight loss, anorexia, fever, leukocytosis) periodically during therapy.
- ***Lab Test Considerations:*** Monitor serum electrolytes and glucose. May cause hyperglycemia, especially in persons with diabetes. May cause hypokalemia. Patients on prolonged therapy should routinely have CBC, serum electrolytes, and serum and urine glucose evaluated. May ↓ WBCs. May ↓ serum potassium and calcium and ↑ serum sodium concentrations.
- Guaiac-test stools. Promptly report presence of guaiac-positive stools.
- May ↑ serum cholesterol and lipid values. May ↓ uptake of thyroid ^{123}I or ^{131}I.
- Suppress reactions to allergy skin tests.
- Periodic adrenal function tests may be ordered to assess degree of hypothalamic-pituitary-adrenal axis suppression in systemic and chronic topical therapy.
- **Dexamethasone Suppression Test:** : To diagnose Cushing's syndrome: Obtain baseline cortisol level; administer dexamethasone at 11 PM and obtain cortisol levels at 8 AM the next day. Normal response is a ↓ cortisol level.
- Alternative method: Obtain baseline 24-hr urine for 17-hydroxycorticosteroid (OHCS) concentrations, then begin 48-hr administration of dexamethasone. Second 24-hr urine for 17-OHCS is obtained after 24 hr of dexamethasone.

Potential Nursing Diagnoses

Risk for infection (Side Effects)
Disturbed body image (Side Effects)

Implementation

- Do not confuse prednisone with prednisolone. Do not confuse Solu-Cortef with Solu-Medrol.
- If dose is ordered daily or every other day, administer in the morning to coincide with the body's normal secretion of cortisol.
- Periods of stress, such as surgery, may require supplemental systemic corticosteroids.
- Patients with mild to moderate Crohn's disease may be switched from oral prednisolone without adrenal

C

insufficiency by gradually decreasing prednisolone doses and adding budesonide.

- **PO:** Administer with meals to minimize GI irritation.
- Tablets may be crushed and administered with food or fluids for patients with difficulty swallowing. Capsules and extended-release tablets should be swallowed whole; do not open, crush, crush, break, or chew.
- Use calibrated measuring device to ensure accurate dose of liquid forms.
- For orally disintegrating tablets (ODT), remove tablet from blister just prior to dosing. Peel blister pack open, and place tablet on tongue; may be swallowed whole or allowed to dissolve in mouth, with or without water. Tablets are friable; do not cut, split, or break.
- Avoid consumption of grapefruit juice during therapy with budesonide or methylprednisolone.
- **IM, Subcut:** Shake suspension well before drawing up. IM doses should not be administered when rapid effect is desirable. Do not dilute with other solution or admix. Do not administer suspensions IV.

Dexamethasone

IV Administration

- **IV Push:** ***Diluent:*** May be given undiluted. ***Concentration:*** 4–10 mg/mL. ***Rate:*** Administer over 1–4 min if dose is <10 mg.
- **Intermittent Infusion:** ***Diluent:*** High-dose therapy should be added to D5W or 0.9% NaCl solution. Solution should be clear and colorless to light yellow; use diluted solution within 24 hr. ***Concentration:*** Up to 10 mg/mL. ***Rate:*** Administer infusions over 15–30 min.
- **Y-Site Compatibility:** acetaminpophen, acyclovir, alfentanil, allopurinol, amifostine, amikacin, aminophylline, amphotericin B cholesteryl, amphotericin B lipid complex, amphotericin B liposome, amsacrine, anidulafungin, argatroban, ascorbic acid, atracurium, atropine, azithromycin, aztreonam, benztropine, bivalirudin, bleomycin, bumetanide, buprenorphine, butorphanol, carboplatin, carmustine, cefazolin, cefepime, cefotaxime, cefotetan, cefoxitin, ceftaroline, ceftazidime, ceftriaxone, chloramphenicol, cisatracurium, cisplatin, cladribine, clindamycin, cyanocobalamin, cyclophosphamide, cyclosporine, cytarabine, dactinomycin, daptomycin, dexmedetomidine, digoxin, diltiazem, docetaxel, dopamine, doripenem, doxacurium, doxorubicin, doxorubicin liposome, enalaprilat, ephedrine, epinephrine, epoetin alfa, eptifibatide, ertapenem, etoposide, etoposide phosphate, famotidine, fentanyl, filgrastim, fluconazole, fludarabine, fluorouracil, folic acid, fosaprepitant, foscarnet, furosemide, ganciclovir, gemcitabine, glycopyrrolate, granisetron, heparin, hetastarch, hydrocortisone, hydromorphone, ifosfamide, imipenem/cilastatin, indomethacin, insulin, irinotecan, isoproterenol, ketorolac, leucovorin calcium, levofloxacin, lidocaine, linezolid, lorazepam, mannitol, mechlorethamine, melphalan, meropenem, metaraminol, methadone, methyldopate, methylprednisolone, metoclopramide, metoprolol, metronidazole, milrinone, morphine, moxifloxacin, multivitamin, nafcillin, nalbuphine, naloxone, nitroglycerin, nitroprusside, norepinephrine, octreotide, ondansetron, oxacillin, oxaliplatin, oxytocin, paclitaxel, palonosetron, pamidronate, pancuronium, pemetrexed, penicillin G, pentobarbital, phenobarbital, phenylephrine, phytonadione, piperacillin/tazobactam, potassium acetate, potassium chloride, procainamide, propofol, propranolol, pyridoxime, ranitidine, remifentanil, rituximab, sargramostim, sodium acetate, sodium bicarbonate, streptokinase, succinylcholine, sufentanil, tacrolimus, telavancin, teniposide, theophylline, thiamine, thiotepa, tigecycline, tirofiban, tolazoline, trastuzumab, vancomycin, vasopressin, vecuronium, verapamil, vinblastine, vincristine, vinorelbine, vitamin B complex with C, voriconazole, zidovudine, zoledronic acid.
- **Y-Site Incompatibility:** alemtuzumab, amphotericin B colloidal, calcium chloride, calcium gluconate, caspofungin, cefuroxime, chlorpromazine, ciprofloxacin, dantrolene, diazepam, diazoxide, diphenhydramine, dobutamine, doxycycline, epirubicin, erythromycin, esmolol, fenoldopam, gentamicin, haloperidol, hydroxyzine, idarubicin, labetalol, magnesium sulfate, midazolam, mitoxantrone, mycophenolate, nicardipine, pantoprazole, papaverine, pentamidine, pentazocine, phenytoin, prochlorperazine, promethazine, protamine, quinapristin/dalfopristin, tobramycin, topotecan, trimethoprim/sulfamethoxazole.

Hydrocortisone

IV Administration

- **IV Push:** ***Diluent:*** Reconstitute with provided solution (i.e., Act-O-Vials) or 2 mL of bacteriostatic water or saline for injection. ***Concentration:*** 50 mg/mL. ***Rate:*** Administer each 100 mg over at least 30 sec. Doses 500 mg and larger should be infused over at least 10 min.
- **Intermittent/Continuous Infusion:** ***Diluent:*** May be added to 50–1000 mL of D5W, 0.9% NaCl, or D5/0.9% NaCl. Diluted solutions should be used within 24 hr. ***Concentration:*** 1–5 mg/mL. Concentrations of up to 60 mg/mL have been used in fluid restricted adults. ***Rate:*** Administer over 20–30 min or at prescribed rate.
- **Hydrocortisone sodium succinateY-Site Compatibility:** acetaminophen, acyclovir, alemtuzumab, alfentanil, allopurinol, amifostine, amikacin, aminophylline, amphotericin B cholesteryl, amphotericin B lipid complex, amphotericin B liposome, amsacrine, anidulafungin, argatroban, ascorbic acid, atracurium, atropine, azithromycin, aztreonam,

benztropine, bivalirudin, bleomycin, bumetanide, buprenorphine, butorphanol, carboplatin, carmustine, caspofungin, cefazolin, cefepime, cefotaxime, cefotetan, cefoxitin, ceftaroline, ceftazidime, ceftriaxone, cefuroxime, chloramphenicol, chlorpromazine, cisatracurium, cisplatin, cladribine, clindamycin, cyanocobalamin, cyclophosphamide, cyclosporine, cytarabine, dactinomycin, daptomycin, dexamethasone, dexmedetomidine, dexrazoxane, digoxin, docetaxel, dopamine, doripenem, doxacurium, doxorubicin hydrochloride, doxorubicin liposome, droperidol, edrophonium, enalaprilat, ephedrine, epinephrine, epirubicin, epoetin alfa, eptifibatide, ertapenem, erythromycin, estrogens, conjugated, etoposide, famotidine, fenoldopam, fentanyl, filgrastim, fluconazole, fludarabine, fluorouracil, folic acid, foscarnet, furosemide, gemcitabine, glycopyrrolate, granisetron, heparin, hetastarch, hydromorphone, ifosfamide, imiepnem/cilastatin, indomethacin, insulin, irinotecan, isoproterenol, ketamine, ketorolac, leucovorin calcium, levofloxacin, lidocaine, linezolid, lorazepam, mannitol, mechlorethamine, melphalan, metaraminol, methotrexate, methoxamine, methyldopate, methylergonovine, metoclopramide, metoprolol, metronidazole, milrinone, mitoxantrone, morphine, moxifloxacin, multivitamins, nafcillin, naloxone, neostigmine, nesiritide, nitroglycerin, nitroprusside, norepinephrine, octreotide, ondansetron, oxacillin, oxaliplatin, oxytocin, paclitaxel, palonosetron, pamidronate, pancuronium, pantoprazole, pemetrexed, penicillin G, pentobarbital, phenobarbital, phenylephrine, phytonadione, piperacillin/tazobactam, potassium acetate, potassium chloride, procainamide, prochlorperazine, propofol, propranolol, pyridostigmine, ranitidine, remifentanil, rituximab, scopolamine, sodium acetate, sodium bicarbonate, streptokinase, succinylcholine, sufentanil, tacrolimus, telavancin, teniposide, theophylline, thiotepa, tigecycline, tirofiban, trastuzumab, trimetaphan, vasopressin, vecuronium, verapamil, vinblastine, vincristine, vinorelbine, voriconazole, zoledronic acid.

- **Y-Site Incompatibility:** amphotericin B colloidal, ampicillin/sulbactam, azathioprine, calcium chloride, ciprofloxacin, dacarbazine, dantrolene, diazepam, diazoxide, dobutamine, doxycycline, ganciclovir, haloperidol, idarubicin, labetalol, mycophenolate, nalbuphine, pentamidine, phenytoin, protamine, pyridoxime, quinupristin/dalfopristin, rocuronium, sargramostim, thiamine, trimethoprim/sulfamethoxazole.

Methylprednisolone sodium succinate

IV Administration

- **IV Push:** ***Diluent:*** Reconstitute with provided solution (Act-O-Vials, Univials) or 2 mL of bacteriostatic water (with benzyl alcohol) for injection. Use preservative-free diluent for use in neonates. Acetate injection is not for IV use. ***Concentration:*** Maximum concentration 125 mg/mL. ***Rate:*** Low dose (<1.8 mg/kg or <125 mg/dose): May be administered IV push over 1 to several minutes. Moderate dose (2 mg/kg or 250 mg/dose): give over 15–30 min. High dose (15 mg/kg or 500 mg/dose): give over 30 min. Doses 15 mg/kg or 1 g give over 1 hr.
- **Intermittent/Continuous Infusion:** ***Diluent:*** May be diluted further in D5W, 0.9% NaCl, or D5/0.9% NaCl and administered as intermittent or continuous infusion at the prescribed rate. ***Concentration:*** Maximum 2.5 mg/mL. Solution may form a haze upon dilution.
- **Y-Site Compatibility:** acetaminophen, acyclovir, alfentanil, alprostadil, amifostine, amikacin, aminophylline, amiodarone, amphotericin B cholesteryl, amphotericin B lipid complex, amphotericin B liposome, anidulafungin, argatroban, ascorbic acid, atracurium, atropine, azithromycin, aztreonam, benztropine, bivalirudin, bleomycin, bumetanide, buprenorphine, butorphanol, carboplatin, carmustine, cefazolin, cefepime, cefotetan, ceftaroline, ceftazidime, ceftriaxone, cefuroxime, chloramphenicol, chlorpromazine, cisplatin, cladribine, clindamycin, cyanocobalamin, cyclophosphamide, cyclosporine, cytarabine, dactinomycin, daptomycin, dexamethasone, dexmedetomidine, digoxin, dobutamine, dopamine, doripenem, doxacurium, doxorubicin liposome, enalaprilat, ephedrine, epinephrine, epoetin alfa, eptifibatide, ertapenem, erythromycin, etoposide, famotidine, fentanyl, fludarabine, fluorouracil, folic acid, fosaprepitant, furosemide, gentamicin, glycopyrrolate, granisetron, hetastarch, hydromorphone, ifosfamide, imipenem/cilastatin, insulin, isoproterenol, ketorolac, labetalol, levofloxacin, linezolid, lorazepam, mannitol, mechlorethamine, melphalan, metaraminol, methotrexate, methoxamine, methyldopate, metoclopramide, metoprolol, metronidazole, milrinone, morphine, moxifloxacin, multivitamin, nafcillin, naloxone, nesiritide, nitroglycerin, nitroprusside, norepinephrine, octreotide, oxaliplatin, oxytocin, pamidronate, pancuronium, pemetrexed, penicillin G, pentobarbital, phenobarbital, phenylephrine, piperacillin/tazobactam, potassium acetate, procainamide, prochlorperazine, propranolol, ranitidine, remifentanil, rituximab, sodium acetate, sodium bicarbonate, streptokinase, succinylcholine, sufentanil, tacrolimus, teniposide, theophylline, thiotepa, tirofiban, tobramycin, tolazoline, topotecan, trastuzumab, vasopressin, verapamil, vincristine, voriconazole, zoledronic acid.
- **Y-Site Incompatibility:** alemtuzumab, allopurinol, amphotericin B colloidal, ampicillin/sulbactam, amsacrine, calcium chloride, calcium gluconate, cas-

pofungin, cefotaxime, cefoxitin, ciprofloxacin, dantrolene, dexrazoxane, diazepam, diazoxide, diphenhydramine, docetaxel, doxycycline, epirubicin, etoposide phosphate, fenoldopam, filgrastim, foscarnet, ganciclovir, gemcitabine, haloperidol, hydralazine, idarubicin, irinotecan, magnesium sulfate, mitoxantrone, mycophenolate, nalbuphine, paclitaxel, palonosetron, pantoprazole, papaverine, pentamidine, pentazocine, phentolamine, phenytoin, promethazine, propofol, protamine, pyridoxime, quinupristin/dalfopristin, rocuronium, sargramostim, thiamine, trimethoprim/sulfamethoxazole, vancomycin, vecuronium, vinorelbine.

Patient/Family Teaching

- Instruct patient on correct technique of medication administration. Advise patient to take medication as directed. Take missed doses as soon as remembered unless almost time for next dose. Do not double doses. Stopping the medication suddenly may result in adrenal insufficiency (anorexia, nausea, weakness, fatigue, dyspnea, hypotension, hypoglycemia). If these signs appear, notify health care professional immediately. This can be life threatening.
- Advise patient to avoid consumption of grapefruit juice during therapy with *budesonide* or *methylprednisolone*.
- Corticosteroids cause immunosuppression and may mask symptoms of infection. Instruct patient to avoid people with known contagious illnesses and to report possible infections immediately.
- *Prelone* syrup should not be refrigerated, *Pediapred* solution may be refrigerated, *Orapred* solution should be refrigerated.
- Caution patient to avoid vaccinations without first consulting health care professional.
- Review side effects with patient. Instruct patient to inform health care professional promptly if severe abdominal pain or tarry stools occur. Patient should also report unusual swelling, weight gain, tiredness, bone pain, bruising, nonhealing sores, visual disturbances, or behavior changes.
- Instruct patient to notify health care professional of all Rx or OTC medications, vitamins, or herbal products being taken and to consult health care professional before taking any Rx, OTC, or herbal products.
- Instruct patient to notify health care professional immediately if exposed to chicken pox or measles.
- Advise patient to notify health care professional of medication regimen before treatment or surgery.
- Discuss possible effects on body image. Explore coping mechanisms.
- Instruct patient to inform health care professional if symptoms of underlying disease return or worsen.
- Advise patient to carry identification describing disease process and medication regimen in the event of emergency in which patient cannot relate medical history.
- Explain need for continued medical follow-up to assess effectiveness and possible side effects of medication. Periodic lab tests and eye exams may be needed.
- **Long-term Therapy:** Encourage patient to eat a diet high in protein, calcium, and potassium, and low in sodium and carbohydrates (see Appendix J). Alcohol should be avoided during therapy; may ↑ risk of GI irritation.
- If rectal dose used 21 days, decrease to every other night for 2–3 wk to decrease gradually.

Evaluation/Desired Outcomes

- Decrease in presenting symptoms with minimal systemic side effects.
- Suppression of the inflammatory and immune responses in autoimmune disorders, allergic reactions, and neoplasms.
- Management of symptoms in adrenal insufficiency.
- Improvement of symptoms/sequelae of Crohn's disease and ulcerative colitis (decreased frequency of liquid stools, decreased abdominal complaints, improved sense of well being).
- Improvement in symptoms of ulcerative colitis. Clinical symptoms usually improve in 3–5 days. Mucosal appearance may require 2–3 mo to improve.

CORTICOSTEROIDS (TOPICAL/LOCAL)

alclometasone
(al-kloe-**met**-a-sone)
Aclovate

amcinonide (am-**sin**-oh-nide)
✱Cyclocort

betamethasone
(bay-ta-**meth**-a-sone)
✱Betaderm, Beta-Val, ✱Celestoderm, Dermabet, Diprolene, Diprolene AF, ✱Diprosone, Luxiq, ✱Prevex, ✱Rivasone, ✱Rolene, ✱Rosone, ✱Valisone, Valnac

clobetasol (kloe-**bay**-ta-sol)
Clobex, Cormax, ✱Dermovate, Embeline, Embeline E, Olux, Olux-E, Temovate, Temovate E

clocortolone (kloe-**kore**-toe-lone)
Cloderm

desonide (**des**-oh-nide)
✱Desocort, Desonate, DesOwen, ✱Tridesilon, Verdeso

desoximetasone
(dess-ox-i-**met**-a-sone)
✱Desoxi, Topicort

diflorasone (dye-**flor**-a-sone)

fluocinolone (floo-oh-**sin**-oh-lone)
Capex, Derma-Smoothe/FS, ✤Fluoderm, Synalar

fluocinonide (floo-oh-**sin**-oh-nide)
✤Lidemol, ~~Lidex~~, ✤Lyderm, ✤Tiamol, ✤Topactin, Vanos

flurandrenolide (flure-an-**dren**-oh-lide)
Cordran, Cordran SP

fluticasone (floo-**ti**-ka-sone)
Cutivate

halcinonide (hal-**sin**-oh-nide)
Halog

halobetasol (hal-oh-**bay**-ta-sol)
Ultravate

hydrocortisone (hye-droe-**kor**-ti-sone)
Ala-Cort, Ala-Scalp, Anusol HC, ✤Barriere-HC, CaldeCORT Anti-Itch, Carmol HC, Cortaid, ✤Cortate, Corticaine, Cortifoam, Cortizone, ✤Cortoderm, ✤Emo-Cort, ✤Hyderm, ✤Hydroval, Lanacort 9-1-1, Locoid, Nutracort, Pandel, ✤Prevex HC, ✤Sarna HC, Synacort, Texacort, ✤Topiderm HC, ✤Uremol HC

mometasone (moe-**met**-a-sone)
✤Elocom, Elocon

prednicarbate (pred-ni-**kar**-bate)
Dermatop

triamcinolone (trye-am-**sin**-oh-lone)
✤Aristocort C, ✤Aristocort R, ✤Triaderm, Triderm

Classification
Therapeutic: anti-inflammatories (steroidal)
Pharmacologic: corticosteroids (topical)

Pregnancy Category C

Indications
Management of inflammation and pruritis associated with various allergic/immunologic skin problems. **Desoximetasone topical spray:** Plaque psoriasis.

Action
Suppress normal immune response and inflammation. **Therapeutic Effects:** Suppression of dermatologic inflammation and immune processes. Clearing of plaques.

Pharmacokinetics
Absorption: Minimal. Prolonged use on large surface areas, application of large amounts, or use of occlusive dressings may ↑ systemic absorption.
Distribution: Remain primarily at site of action.
Metabolism and Excretion: Usually metabolized in skin; some have been modified to resist local metabolism and have a prolonged local effect.
Half-life: *Betamethasone*—3–5 hr (plasma), 36–54 hr (tissue). *Dexamethasone*—3–4.5 hr (plasma), 36–54 hr (tissue). *Hydrocortisone*—1.5–2 hr (plasma), 8–12 hr (tissue). *Triamcinolone*—2–>5 hr (plasma), 18–36 hr (tissue).

TIME/ACTION PROFILE (response depends on condition being treated)

ROUTE	ONSET	PEAK	DURATION
Topical	min–hr	hr–days	hr–days

Contraindications/Precautions
Contraindicated in: Hypersensitivity or known intolerance to corticosteroids or components of vehicles (ointment or cream base, preservative, alcohol); Untreated bacterial or viral infections.
Use Cautiously in: Hepatic dysfunction; Diabetes mellitus, cataracts, glaucoma, or tuberculosis (use of large amounts of high-potency agents may worsen condition); Patients with pre-existing skin atrophy; OB, Lactation: Chronic use at high dosages may result in adrenal suppression in mother and growth suppression in children; Pedi: Children may be more susceptible to adrenal and growth suppression. Clobetasol not recommended for children <12 yr; desoximetasone not recommended for children <10 yr (cream, ointment, gel) or <18 yr (spray).

Adverse Reactions/Side Effects
Derm: allergic contact dermatitis, atrophy, burning, dryness, edema, folliculitis, hypersensitivity reactions, hypertrichosis, hypopigmentation, irritation, maceration, miliaria, perioral dermatitis, secondary infection, striae. **Misc:** adrenal suppression (↑ dose, long-term therapy).

Interactions
Drug-Drug: None significant.

Route/Dosage
Topical (Adults and Children): 1–4 times daily (depends on product, preparation, and condition being treated).

Rect (Adults): hydrocortisone *Aerosol foam*—90 mg 1–2 times/day for 2–3 wk; then adjusted.

Availability

Alclometasone (generic available)

Cream: 0.05%. **Cost:** *Generic*—$97.51/45 g. **Ointment:** 0.05%. **Cost:** *Generic*—$50.47/15 g.

Amcinonide (generic available)

Cream: 0.1%. **Cost:** *Generic*—$38.88/30 g. **Lotion:** 0.1%. **Cost:** *Generic*—$325.73/60 mL. **Ointment:** 0.1%. **Cost:** *Generic*—$388.80/60 g.

Betamethasone (generic available)

Cream: 0.05%, 0.1%. **Cost:** *Generic*—0.05% $39.51/15 g, 0.1% $24.17/15 g. **Gel:** 0.05%. **Cost:** *Generic*—$61.48/15 g. **Lotion:** 0.05%, 0.1%. **Cost:** *Generic*—0.05% $66.87/60 mL, 0.1% $78.09/60 mL. **Ointment:** 0.05%, 0.1%. **Cost:** *Generic*—0.05% $43.22/15 g, 0.1% $20.34/15 g. **Aerosol Foam:** 0.12%. **Cost:** *Generic*—$236.90/50 g. ***In combination with:*** clotrimazole (Lotrisone), calcipotriene (Taclonex); see Appendix B.

Clobetasol (generic available)

Cream: 0.05%. **Cost:** *Generic*—$24.94/30 g. **Emollient cream:** 0.05%. **Foam:** 0.05%. **Cost:** *Generic*—$551.63/100 g. **Gel:** 0.05%. **Cost:** *Generic*—$47.87/30 g. **Lotion:** 0.05%. **Cost:** *Generic*—$288.96/59 mL. **Ointment:** 0.05%. **Cost:** *Generic*—$22.96/30 g. **Scalp solution:** 0.05%. **Cost:** *Generic*—$21.31/25 mL. **Shampoo:** 0.05%. **Cost:** *Generic*—$385.29/118 mL. **Spray:** 0.05%. **Cost:** $335.22/59 mL.

Clocortolone

Cream: 0.1%. **Cost:** $183.74/30 g.

Desonide (generic available)

Cream: 0.05%. **Cost:** *Generic*—$88.27/15 g. **Foam:** 0.05%. **Cost:** $630.00/100 g. **Gel:** 0.05%. **Cost:** $449.16/60 g. **Ointment:** 0.05%. **Cost:** *Generic*—$70.30/15 g. **Lotion:** 0.05%. **Cost:** *Generic*—$274.42/59 mL.

Desoximetasone (generic available)

Cream: 0.05%, 0.25%. **Cost:** *Generic*—0.05% $195.09/100 g, 0.25% $197.03/60 g. **Gel:** 0.05%. **Cost:** *Generic*—$87.57/15 g. **Ointment:** 0.25%. **Cost:** *Generic*—$279.97/60 g. **Spray:** 0.25%. **Cost:** $502.50/100 mL.

Diflorasone (generic available)

Cream: 0.05%. **Cost:** *Generic*—$169.23/30 g. **Ointment:** 0.05%. **Cost:** *Generic*—$179.53/30 g.

Fluocinolone (generic available)

Cream: 0.01%, 0.025%. **Cost:** *Generic*—0.01% $44.57/15 g, 0.025% $33.93/15 g. **Ointment:** 0.025%. **Cost:** *Generic*—$33.93/15 g. **Solution:** 0.01%. **Cost:** *Generic*—$178.80/60 mL. **Shampoo:** 0.01%. **Cost:** $416.76/120 mL. **Oil:** 0.01%. **Cost:** *Generic*—$197.90/20 mL. ***In combination with:*** hydroquinone and tretinoin (Tri-Luma). See Appendix B.

Fluocinonide (generic available)

Cream: 0.05%, 0.1%. **Cost:** *Generic*—0.05% $22.32/30 g; *Vanos (0.1%)*—$965.89/60 g. **Gel:** 0.05%. **Cost:** *Generic*—$67.10/60 g. **Ointment:** 0.05%. **Cost:** *Generic*—$55.76/60 g. **Solution:** 0.05%. **Cost:** *Generic*—$100.99/60 mL.

Flurandrenolide

Cream: 0.025%, 0.05%. **Cost:** 0.05% $204.60/30 g. **Lotion:** 0.05%. **Cost:** $394.68/60 mL. **Tape:** 4 mcg/cm^2. **Cost:** $214.96/1 unit.

Fluticasone (generic available)

Cream: 0.05%. **Cost:** *Generic*—$34.37/30 g. **Lotion:** 0.05%. **Cost:** *Generic*—$389.95/60 mL. **Ointment:** 0.005%. **Cost:** *Generic*—$34.30/30 g.

Halcinonide

Cream: 0.1%. **Cost:** $226.55/60 g. **Ointment:** 0.1%. **Cost:** $133.22/30 g.

Halobetasol (generic available)

Cream: 0.05%. **Cost:** *Generic*—$193.26/50 g. **Ointment:** 0.05%. **Cost:** *Generic*—$88.67/15 g.

Hydrocortisone (generic available)

Cream: 0.1%, 0.2%, 0.5%$^{Rx, OTC}$, 1%$^{Rx, OTC}$, 2.5%. **Gel:** 1%$^{Rx, OTC}$. **Ointment:** 0.1%, 0.2%, 0.5%$^{Rx, OTC}$, 1%$^{Rx, OTC}$, 2.5%. **Lotion:** 1%$^{Rx, OTC}$, 2.5%. **Solution:** 1%, 2.5%. **Spray:** 0.5%$^{Rx, OTC}$, 1%$^{Rx, OTC}$. **Rectal cream:** 1%. **Rectal aerosol:** 10%. ***In combination with:*** acetic acid, antifungals, anti-infectives, antihistamines, urea, and benzoyl peroxide in various otic and topical preparations. See Appendix B.

Mometasone (generic available)

Cream: 0.1%. **Cost:** *Generic*—$15.59/15 g. **Ointment:** 0.1%. **Cost:** *Generic*—$28.10/15 g. **Lotion:** 0.1%. **Cost:** $58.20/30 mL.

Prednicarbate (generic available)

Cream: 0.1%. **Cost:** *Generic*—$23.08/15 g. **Ointment:** 0.1%. **Cost:** *Generic*—$30.00/15 g.

Triamcinolone (generic available)

Cream: 0.025%, 0.1%, 0.5%. **Cost:** *Generic*—0.025% $4.45/15 g, 0.1% $5.57/15 g, 0.5% $10.11/15 g. **Ointment:** 0.025%, 0.1%, 0.5%. **Cost:** *Generic*—0.025% $10.11/80 g, 0.1% $5.58/15 g, 0.5% $10.10/15 g. **Lotion:** 0.025%, 0.1%. **Cost:** *Generic*—0.025% $37.79/60 mL, 0.1% $90.00/60 mL. ***In combination with:*** acetic acid, antifungals, anti-infectives, antihistamines, urea, and benzoyl peroxide in various otic and topical preparations. See Appendix B.

NURSING IMPLICATIONS

Assessment

- Assess affected skin before and daily during therapy. Note degree of inflammation, pruritus, and/or plaques. Notify health care professional if symptoms of infection (increased pain, erythema, purulent exudate) develop.

- ***Lab Test Considerations:*** Adrenal function tests may be ordered to assess degree of hypothalamic-pituitary-adrenal (HPA) axis suppression in long-term topical therapy. Children and patients with dose applied to a large area, using an occlusive dressing, or using high-potency products are at highest risk for HPA suppression.
- May cause ↑ serum and urine glucose concentrations if significant absorption occurs.

Potential Nursing Diagnoses

Risk for impaired skin integrity (Indications)
Risk for infection (Side Effects)

Implementation

- Choice of vehicle depends on site and type of lesion. Ointments are more occlusive and preferred for dry, scaly lesions. Creams should be used on oozing or intertriginous areas, where the occlusive action of ointments might cause folliculitis or maceration. Creams may be preferred for esthetic reasons even though they may dry skin more than ointments. Gels, aerosols, lotions, and solutions are useful in hairy areas.
- **Topical:** Apply *ointments, creams,* or *gels* sparingly as a thin film to clean, slightly moist skin. Wear gloves. Apply occlusive dressing only if specified by health care professional.
- Apply *lotion, solution,* or *gel* to hair by parting hair and applying a small amount to affected area. Rub in gently. Protect area from washing, clothing, or rubbing until medication has dried. Hair may be washed as usual but not right after applying medication.
- Use *aerosols* by shaking well and spraying on affected area, holding container 3–6 in. away. Spray for about 2 sec to cover an area the size of a hand. Do not inhale. If spraying near face, cover eyes.

Patient/Family Teaching

- Instruct patient on correct technique of medication administration. Emphasize importance of avoiding the eyes. Apply missed doses as soon as remembered unless almost time for the next dose.
- Caution patient to use only as directed. Avoid using cosmetics, bandages, dressings, or other skin products over the treated area unless directed by health care professional.
- Advise parents of pediatric patients not to apply tight-fitting diapers or plastic pants on a child treated in the diaper area; these garments work as an occlusive dressing and may cause more of the drug to be absorbed.
- Advise patient to consult health care professional before using medicine for condition other than indicated.
- Caution women that medication should not be used extensively, in large amounts, or for protracted periods if they are pregnant or planning to become pregnant.
- Instruct patient to inform health care professional if symptoms of underlying disease return or worsen or if symptoms of infection develop.
- **Fluticasone:** Advise patient to avoid excessive natural or artificial exposure (tanning booth, sun lamp) to areas where lotion is applied.

Evaluation/Desired Outcomes

- Resolution of skin inflammation, pruritus, or other dermatologic conditions.
- Clearing of plaques in plaque psoriasis.

cortisone, See CORTICOSTEROIDS (SYSTEMIC).

⧖ crizotinib (kriz-oh-ti-nib)

Xalkori

Classification
Therapeutic: antineoplastics
Pharmacologic: kinase inhibitors

Pregnancy Category D

Indications

⧖ Metastatic non-small cell lung cancer (NSCLC) that is positive for anaplastic lymphoma kinase (ALK).

Action

Inhibits receptor tyrosine kinases including anaplastic lymphoma kinase (ALK), Hepatocyte Growth Factor Receptor (HGFR, c-Met), and Recepteur d'Origine Nantais (RON). **Therapeutic Effects:** Decreased spread of lung cancer.

Pharmacokinetics

Absorption: 43% absorbed following oral administration.
Distribution: Extensively distributed to tissues.
Metabolism and Excretion: Mostly metabolized by the liver (CYP3A4/5 enzyme system) also acts as a inhibitor of CYP3A. 53% excreted in feces unchanged, 2.3% eliminated unchanged in urine.
Half-life: 42 hr.

TIME/ACTION PROFILE (blood levels)

ROUTE	ONSET	PEAK	DURATION
PO	unknown	4–6 hr	unknown

Contraindications/Precautions

Contraindicated in: Concurrent use of strong inhibitors/inducers of the CYP3A enzyme system; Congenital long QT syndrome; OB: May cause fetal harm; Lactation: Breast feeding should be avoided.

Use Cautiously in: Heart failure, bradyarrhythmias, electrolyte abnormalities, concurrent medications that prolong QT interval (↑ risk of arrhythmias); Asian patients (↑ blood levels); Hepatic impairment; Severe renal impairment; Patients with childbearing potential; Pedi: Safety and effectiveness not established.

Adverse Reactions/Side Effects

CNS: fatigue, headache, insomnia. **EENT:** visual disturbances. **Resp:** PNEUMONITIS. **CV:** QT INTERVAL PROLONGATION, bradycardia, edema, chest pain. **GI:** HEPATOTOXICITY, constipation, diarrhea, nausea, vomiting, abdominal pain, dysgeusia, ↓ appetite, stomatitis. **Derm:** rash. **Neuro:** neuropathy. **Misc:** fever.

Interactions

Drug-Drug: **Strong CYP3A inhibitors** including **atazanavir**, **clarithromycin**, **indinavir**, **itraconazole**, **ketoconazole**, **nefazodone**, **nelfinavir**, **ritonavir**, **saquinavir**, **telithromycin**, **troleandomycin**, and **voriconazole** may ↑ levels; concurrent use should be avoided. **Strong CYP3A inducers** including **carbamazepine**, **phenobarbital**, **phenytoin**, **rifabutin**, and **rifampin** may ↓ levels and effectiveness; concurrent use should be avoided. May ↑ levels of **alfentanil**, **cyclosporine**, **dihydroergotamine**, **ergotamine**, **fentanyl**, **pimozide**, **quinidine**, **sirolimus**, and **tacrolimus**; avoid concurrent use. **Beta-blockers**, **verapamil**, **diltiazem**, **digoxin**, and **clonidine** may ↑ risk of bradycardia; avoid concurrent use, if possible.
Drug-Natural Products: Concurrent use of **St. John's wort** may ↓ levels and effectiveness and should be avoided.
Drug-Food: **Grapefruit** or **grapefruit juice** may ↑ levels and should be avoided.

Route/Dosage

PO (Adults): 250 mg twice daily; dose adjusted according to tolerance, toxicity or adverse effects.

Renal Impairment

PO (Adults): *CCr <30 mL/min (not on dialysis)*— 250 mg once daily.

Availability

Capsules: 200 mg, 250 mg.

NURSING IMPLICATIONS

Assessment

- Assess respiratory function (lung sounds, dyspnea, oxygen saturation) periodically during therapy.
- Monitor for signs and symptoms of pneumonitis (difficulty breathing, shortness or breath, cough with or without mucus, fever) periodically during therapy. *If any Grade of pneumonitis occurs,* permanently discontinue.
- Assess for signs and symptoms of neuropathy (burning, dysesthesia, hyperesthesia, hypoesthesia, neuralgia, paresthesia, peripheral neuropathy sensory and motor) periodically during therapy. Usually Grade 1.
- Monitor ECG periodically during therapy in patients with HF, bradyarrhythmias, electrolyte imbalances, or taking medications than may prolong QT interval. *If QTc >500 ms on at least 2 separate ECGs,* withhold until recovery to baseline or to a QTc <481 ms, then resume at reduced dose. *If QTc >500 ms or ≥60 ms change from baseline with Torsade de pointes or polymorphic ventricular tachycardia or signs/symptoms of serious arrhythmia,* permanently discontinue. *If symptomatic bradycardia occurs,* withhold dose until heart rate return to ≥60 bpm. Evaluate concomitant medications, if contributing medication is identified and dose reduced or discontinued, return to previous dose of crizotinib once heart rate is ≥60 bpm and/or bradycardia is asymptomatic. If no contributing medication is identified or dose modifications are not made, resume crizotinib at a reduced dose once heart rate ≥60 bpm and/or bradycardia is asymptomatic. *If bradycardia is life-threatening and no contributing medication identified,* discontinue crizotinib. If contributing medication is identified and dose is reduced or discontinued, reduce crizotinib dose to 250 mg once daily with frequent monitoring once heart rate ≥60 bpm and/or bradycardia is asymptomatic.
- Monitor vision during therapy. If visual loss (Grade 4 Ocular Disorder) occurs, discontinue crizotinib during evaluation of severe vision loss. Perform an ophthalmological evaluation consisting of best corrected visual acuity, retinal photographs, visual fields, optical coherence tomography (OCT) and other evaluations as appropriate for new onset of severe visual loss.
- ***Lab Test Considerations:*** Monitor CBC with differential monthly and as clinically indicated; more frequently if Grade 3 or 4 toxicities occur. *If Grade 3 hematologic toxicity occurs,* withhold dose until recovery to Grade ≤2, then resume same dose schedule. *If Grade 4 hematologic toxicity occurs,* withhold until recovery to Grade ≤2, then resume at 200 mg twice daily. May also cause Grade 3 or 4 neutropenia, thrombocytopenia, and lymphopenia.
- Monitor liver function tests monthly and as clinically indicated; more frequently if Grade 2, 3, 4 abnormalities occur. *If ALT or AST ↑ >5 x upper limit of normal (ULN) with total bilirubin ≤ 1.5 times ULN,* withhold crizotinib until recovery to baseline or ≤ 3 x ULN, then resume at reduced dose. *If ALT or AST ↑ >3 x ULN with concurrent total bilirubin ↑ >1.5 x ULN (in the absence of cholestasis or hemolysis),* permanently discontinue crizotinib. *If Grade 3 or 4 AST or ALT ↑ with Grade ≤1 total bilirubin occurs,* withhold until recovery to Grade ≤1 or baseline, then resume at 200 mg twice daily. *If Grade 2, 3, or 4 AST or ALT ↑ with concurrent Grade 2, 3, or 4 total bilirubin ↑ (with no cholestasis or hemolysis),* permanently discontinue.

Potential Nursing Diagnoses
Impaired gas exchange (Indications)

Implementation
- **PO:** Administer twice daily without regard to food. Swallow capsules whole, do not crush, dissolve, or open.

Patient/Family Teaching
- Instruct patient to take crizotinib as directed; do not change dose or stop taking without consulting health care professional. If vomiting occurs, do not take extra dose, just take next dose at regular scheduled time. Take missed doses as soon as remembered unless <6 hr until next dose. If <6 hr to next dose, skip dose and return to regular schedule; do not double doses. Advise patient to read the *Patient Information leaflet* before starting and with each Rx refill in case of changes.
- Advise patient to avoid eating grapefruit or drinking grapefruit juice during therapy.
- Caution patient that dizziness and visual disorders may occur. Advise patient to avoid driving or other activities requiring alertness until response to medication is known. Visual disturbances generally start within 2 wk of therapy. Instruct patient to notify health care professional if flashes of light, blurry vision, light sensitivity, or new or worse vitreous floaters occur; ophthalmological evaluation should be considered.
- Advise patient to notify health care professional immediately if symptoms of weakness, fatigue, anorexia, nausea, vomiting, abdominal pain (especially RUQ abdominal pain), jaundice, dark urine, generalized pruritus, and bleeding occur, especially in combination with fever and rash.
- Inform patient that nausea, diarrhea, vomiting, and constipation are common side effects and usually occur during first few days of therapy. Standard antiemetic, antidiarrheal, and laxative medications are usually effective.
- Instruct patient to notify health care professional of all Rx or OTC medications, vitamins, or herbal products being taken and consult health care professional before taking any new medications, especially St. John's Wort.
- Rep: Instruct women of childbearing age to use effective contraception during and for at least 45 days following discontinuation of therapy and to avoid breast feeding during therapy. Because of potential for genotoxicty, advise males with females partners of reproductive potential to use condoms during treatment and for at least 90 days after final dose. May cause reduced fertility in females and males of reproductive potential; may be irreversible.

Evaluation/Desired Outcomes
- Decrease spread of lung cancer.

crofelemer (kro-**fel**-e-mer)
Fulyzaq

Classification
Therapeutic: antidiarrheals
Pharmacologic: catechins

Pregnancy Category C

Indications
Symptomatic relief of non-infectious diarrhea in HIV-infected patients currently receiving antiretroviral therapy.

Action
A natural product derived from *Croton lechleri*, a species of flowering plant. Inhibits cyclic adenosine monophosphate (cAMP)-stimulated cystic fibrosis transmembrane conductance regulator (CTFR) chloride ion channels and the calcium-activated chloride channels on luminal membranes of enterocytes. Blocks chloride secretion and water loss by inhibiting chloride channels on the membranes of enterocytes. **Therapeutic Effects:** Decreased incidence and severity of diarrhea.

Pharmacokinetics
Absorption: Minimal absorption following oral administration.
Distribution: Unknown.
Metabolism and Excretion: Unknown.
Half-life: Unknown.

TIME/ACTION PROFILE

ROUTE	ONSET	PEAK	DURATION
PO	unknown	unknown	unknown

Contraindications/Precautions
Contraindicated in: None noted.
Use Cautiously in: Infectious causes of diarrhea (evaluate and treat prior to use); OB: Use during pregnancy only if clearly needed; Lactation: Breast feeding should be avoided by HIV-infected patients; Pedi: Safe and effective use in children <18 yr has not been established.

Adverse Reactions/Side Effects
CNS: anxiety. **EENT:** nasopharyngitis. **Resp:** bronchitis, cough, upper respiratory tract infection. **GI:** abdominal distention, flatulence, hemorrhoids, nausea, ↑ liver function tests. **GU:** urinary tract infection. **MS:** arthralgia, back pain, muscuoloskeletal pain.

Interactions
Drug-Drug: Due to minimal systemic absorption, interactions are unlikely.

Route/Dosage
PO (Adults): 125 mg twice daily.

Availability

Delayed-release tablets: 125 mg.

NURSING IMPLICATIONS

Assessment

- Assess for abdominal distention, presence of bowel sounds, and usual pattern of bowel function.
- Assess color, consistency, and amount of stool produced.

Potential Nursing Diagnoses

Diarrhea (Indications)

Implementation

- **PO:** Administer tablets twice daily with or without food. Swallow tablets whole; do not crush, break, or chew.

Patient/Family Teaching

- Instruct patient to take crofelemer as directed.
- Advise female patients to notify health care professional if pregnancy is planned or suspected or if breast feeding.

Evaluation/Desired Outcomes

- Decreased incidence and severity of diarrhea.

---

cyanocobalamin, See VITAMIN B_{12} PREPARATIONS.

---

cyclobenzaprine

(sye-kloe-**ben**-za-preen)

Amrix, ~~Flexeril~~

Classification

Therapeutic: skeletal muscle relaxants (centrally acting)

Pregnancy Category B

Indications

Management of acute painful musculoskeletal conditions associated with muscle spasm. **Unlabeled Use:** Management of fibromyalgia.

Action

Reduces tonic somatic muscle activity at the level of the brainstem. Structurally similar to tricyclic antidepressants. **Therapeutic Effects:** Reduction in muscle spasm and hyperactivity without loss of function.

Pharmacokinetics

Absorption: Well absorbed from the GI tract.
Distribution: Unknown.
Protein Binding: 93%.
Metabolism and Excretion: Mostly metabolized by the liver.
Half-life: 1–3 days.

TIME/ACTION PROFILE (skeletal muscle relaxation)

ROUTE	ONSET	PEAK†	DURATION
PO	within 1 hr	3–8 hr	12–24 hr
Extended release	unknown	unknown	24 hr

†Full effects may not occur for 1–2 wk.

Contraindications/Precautions

Contraindicated in: Hypersensitivity; Should not be used within 14 days of MAO inhibitor therapy; Immediate period after MI; Severe or symptomatic cardiovascular disease; Cardiac conduction disturbances; Hyperthyroidism.
Use Cautiously in: Cardiovascular disease; Geri: Appears on Beers list. Poorly tolerated due to anticholinergic effects; OB, Lactation, Pedi: Pregnancy, lactation, and children <15 yr (safety not established).

Adverse Reactions/Side Effects

CNS: dizziness, drowsiness, confusion, fatigue, headache, nervousness. **EENT:** dry mouth, blurred vision. **CV:** arrhythmias. **GI:** constipation, dyspepsia, nausea, unpleasant taste. **GU:** urinary retention.

Interactions

Drug-Drug: Additive CNS depression with other **CNS depressants**, including **alcohol**, **antihistamines**, **opioid analgesics**, and **sedative/hypnotics**. Additive anticholinergic effects with **drugs possessing anticholinergic properties**, including **antihistamines**, **antidepressants**, **atropine**, **disopyramide**, **haloperidol**, and **phenothiazines**. Avoid use within 14 days of **MAO inhibitors** (hyperpyretic crisis, seizures, and death may occur). Drugs that affect serotonergic neurotransmitter systems, including **tricyclic antidepressants**, **SSRIs**, **SNRIs**, **fentanyl**, **buspirone**, **tramadol**, and **triptans** ↑ risk of serotonin syndrome.
Drug-Natural Products: Concomitant use of **kava-kava**, **valerian**, **chamomile**, or **hops** can ↑ CNS depression.

Route/Dosage

PO (Adults): *Acute painful musculoskeletal conditions*—Immediate-release: 10 mg 3 times daily (range 20–40 mg/day in 2–4 divided doses; not to exceed 60 mg/day); Extended-release: 15–30 mg once daily. *Fibromyalgia*—5–40 mg at bedtime (unlabeled).

Availability (generic available)

Tablets: 5 mg, 10 mg. **Cost:** *Generic*—5 mg $9.43/100, 10 mg $8.32/100. **Extended-release capsules (Amrix):** 15 mg, 30 mg. **Cost:** All strengths $1,437.60/60.

NURSING IMPLICATIONS

Assessment

- Assess patient for pain, muscle stiffness, and range of motion before and periodically throughout therapy.

- Geri: Assess geriatric patients for anticholinergic effects (sedation and weakness).
- Assess for serotonin syndrome (mental changes [agitation, hallucinations, coma], autonomic instability [tachycardia, labile BP, hyperthermia], neuromuscular aberrations [hyperreflexia, incoordination], and/or GI symptoms [nausea, vomiting, diarrhea]), especially in patients taking other serotonergic drugs (SSRIs, SNRIs, triptans).

Potential Nursing Diagnoses

Acute pain (Indications)
Impaired physical mobility (Indications)
Risk for injury (Side Effects)

Implementation

- **PO:** May be administered with meals to minimize gastric irritation.
- Swallow extended-release capsules whole; do not open, crush, or chew.

Patient/Family Teaching

- Instruct patient to take medication as directed; do not take more than the prescribed amount. Take missed doses within 1 hr of time ordered; otherwise, return to normal dose schedule. Do not double doses.
- Medication may cause drowsiness, dizziness, and blurred vision. Caution patient to avoid driving or other activities requiring alertness until response to drug is known.
- Advise patient to avoid concurrent use of alcohol or other CNS depressants with this medication.
- If constipation becomes a problem, advise patient that increasing fluid intake and bulk in diet and stool softeners may alleviate this condition.
- Advise patient to notify health care professional if symptoms of urinary retention (distended abdomen, feeling of fullness, overflow incontinence, voiding small amounts) occur.
- Instruct patient to notify health care professional immediately if signs and symptoms of serotonin syndrome occur.
- Inform patient that good oral hygiene, frequent mouth rinses, and sugarless gum or candy may help relieve dry mouth.

Evaluation/Desired Outcomes

- Relief of muscular spasm in acute skeletal muscle conditions. Maximum effects may not be evident for 1–2 wk. Use is usually limited to 2–3 wk; however, has been effective for at least 12 wk in the management of fibromyalgia.

HIGH ALERT

cyclophosphamide

(sye-kloe-**fos**-fa-mide)
Cytoxan, ✱Procytox

Classification
Therapeutic: antineoplastics, immunosuppressants
Pharmacologic: alkylating agents

Pregnancy Category D

Indications

Alone or with other modalities in the management of: Hodgkin's disease, Malignant lymphomas, Multiple myeloma, Leukemias, Mycosis fungoides, Neuroblastoma, Ovarian carcinoma, Breast carcinoma, and a variety of other tumors. Minimal change nephrotic syndrome in children. **Unlabeled Use:** Severe active rheumatoid arthritis or granulomatosis with polyangiitis.

Action

Interferes with DNA replication and RNA transcription, ultimately disrupting protein synthesis (cell-cycle phase–nonspecific). **Therapeutic Effects:** Death of rapidly replicating cells, particularly malignant ones. Also has immunosuppressant action in smaller doses.

Pharmacokinetics

Absorption: Inactive parent drug is well absorbed from the GI tract. Converted to active drug by the liver.
Distribution: Widely distributed. Limited penetration of the blood-brain barrier. Crosses the placenta; enters breast milk.
Metabolism and Excretion: Converted to active drug by the liver; 30% eliminated unchanged by the kidneys.
Half-life: 4–6.5 hr.

TIME/ACTION PROFILE (effects on blood counts)

ROUTE	ONSET	PEAK	DURATION
PO, IV	7 days	7–15 days	21 days

Contraindications/Precautions

Contraindicated in: Hypersensitivity; OB, Lactation: Pregnancy or lactation.
Use Cautiously in: Active infections; Bone marrow depression; Other chronic debilitating illnesses; OB: Patients with childbearing potential.

Adverse Reactions/Side Effects

Resp: PULMONARY FIBROSIS. **CV:** MYOCARDIAL FIBROSIS, hypotension. **GI:** anorexia, nausea, vomiting. **GU:** HEMORRHAGIC CYSTITIS, hematuria. **Derm:** alopecia. **Endo:** gonadal suppression, syndrome of inappropriate antidiuretic hormone (SIADH). **Hemat:** LEUKOPENIA, thrombocytopenia, anemia. **Metab:** hyperuricemia. **Misc:** secondary neoplasms.

Interactions

Drug-Drug: Phenobarbital or **rifampin** may ↑ toxicity of cyclophosphamide. Concurrent **allopurinol** or **thiazide diuretics** may exaggerate bone marrow depression. May prolong neuromuscular blockade from **succinylcholine**. Cardiotoxicity may be additive with other **cardiotoxic agents** (e.g., **cytarabine, daunorubicin, doxorubicin**). May ↓ serum **digoxin** levels. Additive bone marrow depression with other **antineoplastics** or **radiation therapy**. May potentiate the effects of **warfarin**. May ↓ antibody response to **live-virus vaccines** and ↑ risk of adverse reactions. Prolongs the effects of **cocaine**.

Route/Dosage

Many regimens are used.

PO (Adults): 1–5 mg/kg/day.

PO (Children): *Induction*—2–8 mg/kg/day (60–250 mg/m²/day) in divided doses for 6 days or longer. *Maintenance*—2–5 mg/kg (50–150 mg/m²/day) twice weekly.

IV (Adults): 40–50 mg/kg in divided doses over 2–5 days *or* 10–15 mg/kg q 7–10 days *or* 3–5 mg/kg twice weekly *or* 1.5–3 mg/kg/day. Other regimens may use larger doses.

IV (Children): *Induction*—2–8 mg/kg/day (60–250 mg/m²/day) in divided doses for 6 days or longer. Total dose for 7 days may be given as a single weekly dose. *Maintenance*—10–15 mg/kg every 7–10 days or 30 mg/kg q 3–4 wk.

Availability (generic available)

Capsules: 25 mg, 50 mg. **Lyophilized powder for injection:** 500 mg/vial, 1 g/vial, 2 g/vial.

NURSING IMPLICATIONS

Assessment

- Monitor BP, pulse, respiratory rate, and temperature frequently during administration. Report significant changes.
- Monitor urinary output frequently during therapy. To reduce the risk of hemorrhagic cystitis and to promote excretion of uric acid, fluid intake should be at least 3000 mL/day for adults and 1000–2000 mL/day for children. May be administered with mesna. Alkalinization of the urine may be used to help prevent uric acid nephropathy.
- Monitor for bone marrow depression. Assess for bleeding (bleeding gums, bruising, petechiae, guaiac stools, urine, and emesis) and avoid IM injections and taking rectal temperatures if platelet count is low. Apply pressure to venipuncture sites for 10 min. Assess for signs of infection during neutropenia. Anemia may occur. Monitor for increased fatigue, dyspnea, and orthostatic hypotension.
- Assess nausea, vomiting, and appetite. Weigh weekly. Antiemetics may be given 30 min before administration of medication to minimize GI effects. Anorexia and weight loss can be minimized by feeding frequent light meals.
- Assess cardiac and respiratory status for dyspnea, rales/crackles, cough, weight gain, edema. Pulmonary toxicity may occur after prolonged therapy. Cardiotoxicity may occur early in therapy and is characterized by symptoms of HF.
- ***Lab Test Considerations:*** Monitor CBC with differential and platelet count before and periodically during therapy. The nadir of leukopenia occurs in 7–12 days (recovery in 17–21 days). Leukocytes should be maintained at 2500–4000/mm³. May also cause thrombocytopenia (nadir 10–15 days), and rarely causes anemia.
- Monitor BUN, creatinine, and uric acid before and frequently during therapy to detect nephrotoxicity.
- Monitor ALT, AST, LDH, and serum bilirubin before and frequently during therapy to detect hepatotoxicity.
- Urinalysis should be evaluated before initiating therapy and frequently during therapy to detect hematuria or change in specific gravity indicative of SIADH.
- May suppress positive reactions to skin tests for *Candida*, mumps, *Trichophyton*, and tuberculin purified-protein derivative (PPD). May also produce false-positive results in Papanicolaou smears.

Potential Nursing Diagnoses

Risk for infection (Side Effects)
Disturbed body image (Side Effects)

Implementation

- ***High Alert:*** Fatalities have occurred with chemotherapeutic agents. Before administering, clarify all ambiguous orders; double-check single, daily, and course-of-therapy dose limits; have second practitioner independently double-check original order, calculations, and infusion pump settings.
- **PO:** Administer in the morning. Swallow tablets whole; do not crush, break, or chew.
- **IV:** Solution should be prepared in a biologic cabinet. Wear gloves, gown, and mask while handling medication. If powder or solution comes in contact with skin or mucosa, wash thoroughly with soap and water. Discard equipment in specially designated containers.

IV Administration

- **IV Push:** Reconstitute each 100 mg with 5 mL of 0.9% NaCl. Swirl gently to dissolve. Do not reconstitute with sterile water for injection; results in a hypotonic solution not suitable for IV push. ***Concentration:*** 20 mg/mL. Administer reconstituted solution undiluted. ***Rate:*** Inject very slowly.
- **Intermittent Infusion:** Reconstitute each 100 mg with 5 mL of 0.9% NaCl or Sterile Water for injection. Swirl gently to dissolve. Use solution reconsti-

tuted with Sterile Water for injection immediately; solution reconstituted with 0.9% NaCl may be stored at room temperature for 24 hr or if refrigerated for 6 days. Do not administer solutions that contain clear or yellow viscous liquid. ***Diluent:*** May be further diluted in up to 250 mL of D5W, D5/0.9% NaCl, or 0.45% NaCl. ***Concentration:*** minimum 2 mg/mL. ***Rate:*** Infuse very slowly. May reduce rate-dependent adverse reactions (facial swelling, headache, nasal congestion, scalp burning).

- **Y-Site Compatibility:** acyclovir, alemtuzumab, alfentanil, allopurinol, amifostine, amikacin, aminocaproic acid, aminophylline, amiodarone, amphotericin B lipid complex, amphotericin B liposome, ampicillin/sulbactam, anidulafungin, argatroban, arsenic trioxide, azithromycin, aztreonam, bivalirudin, bleomycin, bumetanide, buprenorphine, butorphanol, calcium chloride, calcium gluconate, carboplatin, carmustine, caspofungin, cefazolin, cefepime, cefotaxime, cefotetan, cefoxitin, ceftazidime, ceftriaxone, cefuroxime, chloramphenicol, chlorpromazine, ciprofloxacin, cisatracurium, cisplatin, cladribine, clindamycin, cyclosporine, cytarabine, dacarbazine, dactinomycin, dapotomycin, daunorubicin hydrochloride, dexamethasone, dexmedetomidine, dexrazoxane, digoxin, diltiazem, diphenhydramine, dobutamine, docetaxel, dolasetron, dopamine, doripenem, doxorubicin, doxorubicin liposome, doxycycline, droperidol, enalaprilat, ephedrine, epinephrine, epirubicin, ertapenem, erythromycin, esmolol, etoposide, etoposide phosphate, famotidine, fenoldopam, fentanyl, filgrastim, fluconazole, fludarabine, fluorouracil, foscarnet, fosphenytoin, furosemide, ganciclovir, gemcitabine, gentamicin, granisetron, haloperidol, heparin, hetastarch, hydralazine, hydrocortisone, hydromorphone, idarubicin, imipenem/cilastatin, insulin, irinotecan, isoproterenol, ketorolac, labetalol, leucovorin calcium, levofloxacin, levorphanol, lidocaine, linezolid, lorazepam, magnesium sulfate, mannitol, mechlorethamine, melphalan, meperidine, meropenem, mesna, methotrexate, methylprednisolone, metoclopramide, metoprolol, metronidazole, midazolam, milrinone, mitomycin, mitoxantrone, morphine, moxifloxacin, nafcillin, nalbuphine, naloxone, nesiritide, nicardipine, nitroglycerin, nitroprusside, norepinephrine, octreotide, ondansetron, oxacillin, oxaliplatin, oxytocin, paclitaxel, palonosetron, pamidronate, pancuronium, pantoprazole, pemetrexed, penicillin G , pentamidine, pentobarbital, phenobarbital, phenylephrine, piperacillin/tazobactam, potassium acetate, potassium chloride, potassium phosphates, procainamide, prochlorperazine, promethazine, propofol, propranolol, quinupristin/dalfopristin, ranitidine, remifentanil, rituximab, rocuronium, sargramostim, sodium acetate, sodium bicarbonate, sodium phosphates, succinylcholine, sufentanil, tacrolimus, teniposide, theophylline, thiopental, thiotepa, tigecycline, tirofiban, tobramycin, topotecan, trastuzumab, trimethoprim/sulfamethoxazole, vancomycin, vasopressin, vecuronium, verapamil, vinblastine, vincristine, vinorelbine, voriconazole, zidovudine, zoledronic acid.
- **Y-Site Incompatibility:** amphotericin B colloidal, diazepam, phenytoin.

C

Patient/Family Teaching

- Instruct patient to take dose in early morning. Emphasize need for adequate fluid intake for 72 hr after therapy. Patient should void frequently to decrease bladder irritation from metabolites excreted by the kidneys. Report hematuria immediately. If a dose is missed, contact health care professional. Advise caregivers to use gloves when handling capsules. If capsule opens, wash hands thoroughly.
- Instruct patient to notify health care professional promptly if fever; sore throat; signs of infection; lower back or side pain; difficult or painful urination; sores in the mouth or on the lips; yellow discoloration of skin or eyes; bleeding gums; bruising; petechiae; blood in urine, stool, or emesis; unusual swelling of ankles or legs; joint pain; shortness of breath; cough, palpitations, weight gain of more than 5 lb in 24 hr, dizziness, loss of consciousness or confusion occurs. Caution patient to avoid crowds and persons with known infections. Instruct patient to use soft toothbrush and electric razor and to avoid falls. Patient should also be cautioned not to drink alcoholic beverages or to take products containing aspirin or NSAIDs; may precipitate GI hemorrhage.
- Discuss with patient the possibility of hair loss. Explore methods of coping. May also cause darkening of skin and fingernails.
- Instruct patient not to receive any vaccinations without advice of health care professional.
- Rep: Advise patient that this medication may cause sterility and menstrual irregularities or cessation of menses. This drug is also teratogenic; females should use highly effective contraceptive measures for up to 1 yr after completion and men should continue to wear condoms for at least 4 mo after completion of therapy.

Evaluation/Desired Outcomes

- Decrease in size or spread of malignant tumors.
- Improvement of hematologic status in patients with leukemia. Maintenance therapy is instituted if leukocyte count remains between 2500 and 4000/mm^3 and if patient does not demonstrate serious side effects.
- Management of minimal change nephrotic syndrome in children.

cycloSPORINE†
(sye-kloe-spor-een)
Gengraf, Neoral, SandIMMUNE

Classification
Therapeutic: immunosuppressants, antirheumatics (DMARD)
Pharmacologic: polypeptides (cyclic)

Pregnancy Category C

†See Appendix C for ophthalmic use

Indications
PO, IV: Prevention and treatment of rejection in renal, cardiac, and hepatic transplantation (with corticosteroids). **PO:** Treatment of severe active rheumatoid arthritis (Neoral only). Treatment of severe recalcitrant psoriasis in adult nonimmunocompromised patients (Neoral only). **Unlabeled Use:** Management of recalcitrant ulcerative colitis. Treatment of steroid-resistant nephrotic syndrome. Treatment of severe steroid-resistant autoimmune disease. Prevention and treatment of graft vs. host disease in bone marrow transplant patients.

Action
Inhibits normal immune responses (cellular and humoral) by inhibiting interleukin-2, a factor necessary for initiation of T-cell activity. **Therapeutic Effects:** Prevention of rejection reactions. Slowed progression of rheumatoid arthritis or psoriasis.

Pharmacokinetics
Absorption: Erratically absorbed (range 10–60%) after oral administration, with significant first-pass metabolism by the liver. Microemulsion (Neoral) has better bioavailability.
Distribution: Widely distributed, mainly into extracellular fluid and blood cells. Crosses the placenta; enters breast milk.
Protein Binding: 90–98%.
Metabolism and Excretion: Extensively metabolized by the liver by CYP3A4 (first pass); excreted in bile, small amounts excreted unchanged in urine.
Half-life: Children—7 hr; adults—19 hr.

TIME/ACTION PROFILE (blood levels)

ROUTE	ONSET	PEAK	DURATION
PO	unknown†	2–6 hr	unknown
IV	unknown	end of infusion	unknown

†Onset of action in rheumatoid arthritis is 4–8 wk and may last 4 wk after discontinuation; for psoriasis, onset is 2–6 wk and lasts 6 wk following discontinuation.

Contraindications/Precautions
Contraindicated in: Hypersensitivity to cyclosporine or polyoxyethylated castor oil (vehicle for IV form); OB, Lactation: Should not be given unless benefits outweigh risks; Disulfiram therapy or known alcohol intolerance (IV and oral liquid dose forms contain alcohol); Psoriasis patients receiving immunosuppressants or radiation; Renal impairment (in patients with rheumatoid arthritis or psoriasis); Uncontrolled hypertension.
Use Cautiously in: Severe hepatic impairment (dose ↓ recommended); Renal impairment (frequent dose changes may be necessary); Active infection; Pedi: Larger or more frequent doses may be required.

Adverse Reactions/Side Effects
CNS: POSTERIOR REVERSIBLE ENCEPHALOPATHY SYNDROME, PROGRESSIVE MULTIFOCAL LEUKOENCEPHALOPATHY, SEIZURES, tremor, confusion, flushing, headache, psychiatric problems. **CV:** hypertension. **GI:** HEPATOTOXICITY, diarrhea, nausea, vomiting, abdominal discomfort, anorexia, pancreatitis. **GU:** nephrotoxicity. **Derm:** hirsutism, acne, psoriasis. **F and E:** hyperkalemia, hypomagnesemia. **Hemat:** anemia, leukopenia, thrombocytopenia. **Metab:** hyperlipidemia, hyperuricemia. **Neuro:** hyperesthesia, paresthesia. **MS:** lower extremity pain. **Misc:** gingival hyperplasia, hypersensitivity reactions, infections (including activation of latent viral infections such as BK virus-associated nephropathy), malignancy.

Interactions
Drug-Drug: **Azithromycin**, **clarithromycin**, **allopurinol**, **amiodarone**, **bromocriptine**, **colchicine**, **danazol**, **digoxin**, **diltiazem**, **erythromycin**, **fluconazole**, **fluoroquinolones**, **imatinib**, **itraconazole**, **ketoconazole**, **voriconazole**, **metoclopramide**, **methylprednisolone**, **nefazodone**, **nicardipine**, **protease inhibitors**, **quinupristin/dalfopristin**, **verapamil**, **boceprevir**, or **hormonal contraceptives** may ↑ serum levels and risk of toxicity. ↑ immunosuppression with other **immunosuppressants** (cyclophosphamide, azathioprine, corticosteroids). **Carbamazepine**, **nafcillin**, **octreotide**, **orlistat**, **oxcarbazepine**, **phenobarbital**, **phenytoin**, **rifampin**, **rifabutin**, or **terbinafine** may ↓ levels and effect. **Bosentan** may significantly ↓ levels; avoid concurrent use. ↑ risk of hyperkalemia with **potassium-sparing diuretics**, **potassium supplements**, or **ACE inhibitors**. May ↑ levels and risk of toxicity of **aliskiren**, **bosentan**, **colchicine**, **digoxin**, **etoposide**, **HMG-CoA reductase inhibitors**, **methotrexate**, **nifedipine**, **repaglinide**, and **sirolimus**. May ↑ levels and risk of toxicity of **ambrisentan**; do not titrate dose of ambrisentan up to maximum daily dose. May ↑ levels of and risk of bleeding with **dabigatran**; avoid concurrent use. May ↓ antibody response to **live-virus vaccines** and ↑ risk of adverse reactions; avoid concurrent use. Concurrent use with **tacrolimus** should be avoided. ↑ risk of renal dysfunction with **ciprofloxacin**, **aminoglycosides**, **vancomycin**, **trimethoprim/sulfamethoxazole**, **melphalan**, **amphotericin B**, **ketoconazole**, **colchicine**, **NSAIDS**, **cimetidine**, **ranitidine**, or **fibric acid derivatives**.

Drug-Natural Products: Concomitant use with **echinacea** and **melatonin** may interfere with immunosuppression. Use with **St. John's wort** may cause ↓ serum levels and organ rejection for transplant patients.

Drug-Food: Concurrent ingestion of **grapefruit or grapefruit juice** may ↑serum levels and should be avoided. **Food** ↓ absorption of microemulsion products (Neoral).

Route/Dosage

Doses are adjusted on the basis of serum level monitoring.

Prevention of Transplant Rejection (Sandimmune)

PO (Adults and Children): 14–18 mg/kg/dose 4–12 hr before transplant then 5–15 mg/kg/day divided q 12–24 hr postoperatively, taper by 5% weekly to maintenance dose of 3–10 mg/kg/day.
IV (Adults and Children): 5–6 mg/kg/dose 4–12 hr before transplant, then 2–10 mg/kg/day in divided doses q 8–24 hr; change to PO as soon as possible.

Prevention of Transplant Rejection (Neoral)

PO (Adults and Children): 4–12 mg/kg/day divided q 12 hr (dose varies depending on organ transplanted).

Rheumatoid Arthritis (Neoral only)

PO (Adults and Children): 2.5 mg/kg/day given in 2 divided doses; may ↑ by 0.5–0.75 mg/kg/day after 8 and 12 wk, up to 4 mg/kg/day. ↓ dose by 25–50% if adverse reactions occur.

Severe Psoriasis (Neoral only)

PO (Adults): 2.5 mg/kg/day given in 2 divided doses, for at least 4 wk; then may ↑ by 0.5 mg/kg/day q 2 wk, up to 4 mg/kg/day. ↓ dose by 25–50% if adverse reactions occur.

Autoimmune Diseases (Neoral only)

PO (Adults and Children): 1–3 mg/kg/day.

Availability (generic available)

Microemulsion soft gelatin capsules (Gengraf, Neoral): 25 mg, 50 mg, 100 mg. **Microemulsion oral solution (Gengraf, Neoral):** 100 mg/mL. **Soft gelatin capsules (Sandimmune):** 25 mg, 100 mg. **Oral solution (Neoral, Sandimmune):** 100 mg/mL. **Injection (Sandimmune):** 50 mg/mL.

NURSING IMPLICATIONS

Assessment

- Monitor serum creatinine level, intake and output ratios, daily weight, and BP during therapy. Report significant changes.
- Assess for any new signs or symptoms that may be suggestive of progressive multifocal leukoencephalopathy (PML), an opportunistic infection of the brain caused by the Jakob Cruzfeldt (JC) virus, that may be fatal; withhold dose and notify health care professional promptly. PML symptoms may begin gradually (hemiparesis, apathy, confusion, cognitive deficiencies, and ataxia) and may include deteriorating renal function and renal graft loss.
- Monitor for signs and symptoms of posterior reversible encephalopathy syndrome (PRES) (impaired consciousness, convulsions, visual disturbances including blindness, loss of motor function, movement disorders and psychiatric disturbances, papilloedema, visual impairment). Usually reversible with discontinuation of cyclosporine. Occurs more often in patients with liver transplant than kidney transplant.
- **Prevention of Transplant Rejection:** Assess for symptoms of organ rejection throughout therapy.
- **IV:** Monitor patient for signs and symptoms of hypersensitivity (wheezing, dyspnea, flushing of face or neck) continuously during at least the first 30 min of each treatment and frequently thereafter. Oxygen, epinephrine, and equipment for treatment of anaphylaxis should be available with each IV dose.
- **Arthritis:** Assess pain and limitation of movement prior to and during administration.
- Prior to initiating therapy, perform a physical exam including BP on 2 occasions to determine baseline. Monitor BP every 2 wk during initial 3 mo, then monthly if stable. If hypertension occurs, dose should be reduced.
- **Psoriasis:** Assess skin lesions prior to and during therapy.
- ***Lab Test Considerations:*** Measure serum creatinine, BUN, CBC, magnesium, potassium, uric acid, and lipids at baseline, every 2 wk during initial therapy, and then monthly if stable. Nephrotoxicity may occur; report significant increases.
- May cause hepatotoxicity; monitor for ↑ AST, ALT, alkaline phosphatase, amylase, and bilirubin.
- May cause ↑ serum potassium and uric acid levels and ↓ serum magnesium levels.
- Serum lipid levels may be ↑.
- ***Toxicity and Overdose:*** Evaluate serum cyclosporine levels periodically during therapy. Dose may be adjusted daily, in response to levels, during initiation of therapy. Guidelines for desired serum levels will vary among institutions.

Potential Nursing Diagnoses

Chronic pain (Indications)
Risk for infection (Side Effects)

Implementation

- Do not confuse cycloSPORINE with cyclophosphamide or cycloSERINE. Do not confuse Sandimmune with Sandostatin.
- Given with other immunosuppressive agents. Protect transplant patients from staff and visitors who may carry infection. Maintain protective isolation as indicated.
- Microemulsion products (Neoral) and other products (Sandimmune) are not interchangeable.
- **PO:** Draw up oral solution in the pipette provided with the medication. Mix oral solution with milk, chocolate milk, apple juice, or orange juice, preferably at room temperature. Stir well and drink at once. Use a glass container and rinse with more diluent to ensure that total dose is taken. Administer oral doses with meals. Wipe pipette dry; do not wash after use.

IV Administration

- **Intermittent Infusion:** ***Diluent:*** Dilute each 1 mL (50 mg) of IV concentrate immediately before use with 20–100 mL of D5W or 0.9% NaCl for injection. Solution is stable for 24 hr in D5W. In 0.9% NaCl, it is stable for 6 hr in a polyvinylchloride container and 12 hr in a glass container at room temperature. ***Concentration:*** 2.5 mg/mL. ***Rate:*** Infuse slowly over 2–6 hr via infusion pump.
- **Continuous Infusion:** May be administered over 24 hr.
- **Y-Site Compatibility:** alemtuzumab, alfentanil, amikacin, aminocaproic acid, aminophylline, amphotericin B lipid complex, anidulafungin, argatroban, ascorbic acid, atropine, azithromycin, aztreonam, benztropine, bivalirudin, bleomycin, bumetanide, buprenorphine, butorphanol, calcium chloride, calcium gluconate, carboplatin, carmustine, caspofungin, cefazolin, cefotaxime, cefotetan, cefoxitin, ceftaroline, ceftazidime, ceftriaxone, cefuroxime, chloramphenicol, chlorpromazine, cisplatin, clindamycin, cyclophosphamide, cytarabine, dacarbazine, dactinomycin, daptomycin, daunorubicin hydrochloride, dexamethasone, dexmedetomidine, dexrazoxane, digoxin, diltiazem, diphenhydramine, dobutamine, docetaxel, dolasetron, dopamine, doripenem, doxorubicin hydrochloride, doxorubicin liposomal, doxycycline, enalaprilat, ephedrine, epinephrine, epirubicin, epoetin alfa, ertapenem, erythromycin, esmolol, etoposide, etoposide phosphate, famotidine, fenoldopam, fentanyl, fluconazole, fludarabine, fluorouracil, folic acid, foscarnet, fosphenytoin, furosemide, ganciclovir, gemcitabine, gentamicin, glycopyrrolate, granisetron, heparin, hetastarch, hydrocortisone, hydromorphone, ifosfamide, imipenem/cilastatin, indomethacin, irinotecan, isoproterenol, ketorolac, labetalol, leucovorin calcium, levofloxacin, lidocaine, linezolid, lorazepam, mannitol, mechlorethamine, meperidine, meropenem, methotrexate, methylprednisolone, metoclopramide, metoprolol, metronidazole, micafungin, midazolam, milrinone, mitoxantrone, morphine, moxifloxacin, multivitamins, nafcillin, nesiritide, nicardipine, nitroglycerin, nitroprusside, norepinephrine, octreotide, ondansetron, oxacillin, oxaliplatin, oxytocin, paclitaxel, palonosetron, pamidronate, pancuronium, papaverine, pemetrexed, penicillin G, pentamidine, pentazocine, phenylephrine, phytonadione, piperacillin/tazobactam, potassium acetate, potassium chloride, procainamide, prochlorperazine, promethazine, propofol, propranolol, protamine, pyridoxine, quinupristin/dalfopristin, ranitidine, sargramostim, sodium acetate, sodium bicarbonate, streptokinase, succinylcholine, sufentanil, tacrolimus, teniposide, theophylline, thiamine, thiotepa, tigecycline, tirofiban, tobramycin, vancomycin, vasopressin, vecuronium, verapamil, vinblastine, vincristine, vinorelbine, zoledronic acid.
- **Y-Site Incompatibility:** amphotericin B liposome, cyanocobalamin, dantrolene, diazepam, idarubicin, nalbuphine, pentobarbital, phenobarbital, phenytoin, rituximab, trastuzumab, trimethoprim/sulfamethoxazole, voriconazole.

Patient/Family Teaching

- Instruct patient to take medication at the same time each day with meals, as directed. Take missed doses as soon as remembered within 12 hr. Do not skip doses or double up on missed doses. Do not discontinue medication without advice of health care professional.
- Reinforce the need for lifelong therapy to prevent transplant rejection. Review symptoms of rejection for transplanted organ, and stress need to notify health care professional immediately if they occur.
- Instruct patients and/or parents to notify health care professional if diarrhea develops; decreases absorption of cyclosporine and can result in rejection.
- Instruct patient to avoid grapefruit and grapefruit juice to prevent interaction with cyclosporine.
- Advise patient of common side effects (nephrotoxicity, ↑ BP, hand tremors, increased facial and body hair, gingival hyperplasia). Advise patients that if hair growth is excessive, depilatories or waxing can be used.
- Teach patient the correct method for monitoring BP. Instruct patient to notify health care professional of significant changes in BP or if hematuria, increased frequency, cloudy urine, decreased urine output, fever, sore throat, tiredness, or unusual bruising occurs.
- Instruct patient on proper oral hygiene. Meticulous oral hygiene and dental examinations for teeth cleaning and plaque control every 3 mo will help decrease gingival inflammation and hyperplasia.
- Instruct patient to notify health care professional of all Rx or OTC medications, vitamins, or herbal products being taken and consult health care professional before taking other Rx, OTC, or herbal prod-

ucts or receiving any vaccinations while taking this medication.

- Advise patient to notify health care professional if pregnancy is planned or suspected, or if breast feeding.
- Emphasize the importance of follow-up exams and lab tests.

Evaluation/Desired Outcomes

- Prevention of rejection of transplanted tissues.
- Decrease in severity of pain in patients with rheumatoid arthritis.
- Increased ease of joint movement in patients with rheumatoid arthritis.
- Decrease in progression of psoriasis.

HIGH ALERT

cytarabine (sye-**tare**-a-been)

cytosine arabinoside, ✱Cytosar, Cytosar-U, DepoCyt

Classification
Therapeutic: antineoplastics
Pharmacologic: antimetabolites

Pregnancy Category D

Indications

IV: Used mainly in combination chemotherapeutic regimens for the treatment of leukemias and non-Hodgkin's lymphomas. **IT:** Treatment of lymphomatous meningitis.

Action

Inhibits DNA synthesis by inhibiting DNA polymerase (cell-cycle S-phase–specific). **Therapeutic Effects:** Death of rapidly replicating cells, particularly malignant ones.

Pharmacokinetics

Absorption: Absorption occurs from subcut sites, but blood levels are lower than with IV administration; IT administration results in negligible systemic exposure.

Distribution: Widely distributed; IV- and subcut-administered cytarabine crosses the blood-brain barrier but not in sufficient quantities. Crosses the placenta.

Metabolism and Excretion: Metabolized mostly by the liver; <10% excreted unchanged by the kidneys. Metabolism to inactive drug in the CSF is negligible because the enzyme that metabolizes it is present in very low concentrations in the CSF.

Half-life: *IV, subcut*—1–3 hr; *IT*—100–236 hr.

TIME/ACTION PROFILE (IV, subcut—effects on WBCs; IT—levels in CSF)

ROUTE	ONSET	PEAK	DURATION
Subcut, IV (1st phase)	24 hr	7–9 days	12 days
Subcut, IV (2nd phase)	15–24 days	15–24 days	25–34 days
IT	rapid	5 hr	14–28 days

Contraindications/Precautions

Contraindicated in: Hypersensitivity; OB, Lactation: Pregnancy or lactation; Active meningeal infection (IT only).

Use Cautiously in: Active infections; ↓ bone marrow reserve; Renal/hepatic impairment; Other chronic debilitating illnesses; OB: Patients with childbearing potential.

Adverse Reactions/Side Effects

CNS: CNS dysfunction (high dose), confusion, drowsiness, headache. **EENT:** corneal toxicity (high dose), hemorrhagic conjunctivitis (high dose), visual disturbances (including blindness). **Resp:** PULMONARY EDEMA (high dose). **CV:** edema. **GI:** nausea, vomiting, hepatotoxicity, severe GI ulceration (high dose), stomatitis. **GU:** urinary incontinence. **Derm:** alopecia, rash. **Endo:** sterility. **Hemat:** *(less with IT use)*—anemia, leukopenia, thrombocytopenia. **Metab:** hyperuricemia. **Neuro:** *Intrathecal only*—CHEMICAL ARACHNOIDITIS, abnormal gait. **Misc:** cytarabine syndrome, fever.

Interactions

Drug-Drug: ↑ bone marrow depression with other **antineoplastics** or **radiation therapy**. ↑ risk of cardiomyopathy when used in high-dose regimens with **cyclophosphamide**. May ↓ antibody response to **live-virus vaccines** and ↑ risk of adverse reactions. May ↓ absorption of **digoxin** tablets. May ↓ the efficacy of **gentamicin** when used to treat *Klebsiella pneumoniae* infections. Recent treatment with **asparaginase** may ↑ risk of pancreatitis. ↑ neurotoxicity with concurrently administered **IT antineoplastics** (IT only).

Route/Dosage

Dose regimens vary widely.

IV (Adults): *Induction dose*—200 mg/m²/day for 5 days q 2 wk as a single agent *or* 2–6 mg/kg/day (100–200 mg/m²/day) as a single daily dose *or* in 2–3 divided doses for 5–10 days or until remission occurs as part of combination chemotherapy. *Maintenance*—70–200 mg/m²/day for 2–5 days monthly. *Refractory leukemias/lymphomas*—3 g/m² q 12 hr for up to 12 doses.

Subcut (Adults): *Maintenance*—1–1.5 mg/kg q 1–4 wk.

IT (Adults): *Depo Cyt Induction*—50 mg (intraventricular or lumbar puncture) q 14 days for 2 doses (weeks 1 and 3); *consolidation*—50 mg (intraventricular or lumbar puncture) q 14 days for 3 doses (weeks 5, 7, and 9), followed by 1 additional dose at week 13; *maintenance*—50 mg (intraventricular or lumbar puncture) q 28 days for 4 doses (weeks 17, 21, 25, and 29). If drug-related neurotoxicity occurs, dose should be reduced to 25 mg or discontinued (dexamethasone 4 mg PO/IV twice daily for 5 days should be started concurrently with IT cytarabine).

Availability (generic available)

Powder for injection: 100 mg, 500 mg, 1 g, 2 g. **Solution for injection:** 20 mg/mL, 100 mg/mL. **Sustained-release liposome injection for IT use:** 10 mg/mL.

NURSING IMPLICATIONS

Assessment

- Monitor for bone marrow depression. Assess for bleeding (bleeding gums, bruising, petechiae, guaiac stools, urine, and emesis) and avoid IM injections and taking rectal temperatures if platelet count is low. Apply pressure to venipuncture sites for 10 min. Assess for signs of infection during neutropenia. Anemia may occur. Monitor for increased fatigue, dyspnea, and orthostatic hypotension.
- Monitor intake and output ratios and daily weights. Report significant changes in totals.
- Monitor for symptoms of gout (increased uric acid, joint pain, edema). Encourage patient to drink at least 2 L of fluid each day. Allopurinol may decrease uric acid levels. Alkalinization of urine may increase excretion of uric acid.
- Assess nutritional status. Nausea and vomiting may occur within 1 hr of administration, especially if IV dose is administered rapidly, less severe if medication is infused slowly. Administering an antiemetic prior to and periodically throughout therapy and adjusting diet as tolerated may help maintain fluid and electrolyte balance and nutritional status.
- Monitor patient for development of *cytarabine* or *ara-C syndrome* (fever, myalgia, bone pain, chest pain, maculopapular rash, conjunctivitis, malaise), which usually occurs 6–12 hr following administration. Corticosteroids may be used for treatment or prevention. If patient responds to corticosteroids, continue cytarabine and corticosteroids.
- Assess patient for respiratory distress and pulmonary edema. Occurs with high doses rarely; may be fatal.
- Monitor patient for signs of anaphylaxis (rash, dyspnea, swelling). Epinephrine, corticosteroids, and resuscitation equipment should be readily available.
- **IT:** CSF flow should be evaluated prior to IT therapy. Allow *DepoCyt* to warm to room temperature. Gently agitate or invert to re-suspend particles; do not shake. Administer directly into CSF via an intraventricular reservoir or by direct injection into the lumbar sac slowly over 1–5 min. Following administration by lumbar puncture, patient should lie flat for 1 hr. Chemical arachnoiditis (nausea, vomiting, headache, fever, back pain, CSF pleocytosis and neck rigidity, neck pain, or meningism) is an expected side effect of IT cytarabine. Incidence and severity of symptoms may be decreased with coadministration of dexamethasone. 4 mg bid, PO or IV, for 5 days beginning on day of injection.
- Monitor patients receiving IT therapy continuously for the development of neurotoxicity (myelopathy, personality changes, dysarthria, ataxia, confusion, somnolence, coma). If neurotoxicity develops, decrease amount of subsequent doses and discontinue if neurotoxicity persists. Risk may be increased if cytarabine is administered intrathecally and IV within a few days.
- ***Lab Test Considerations:*** Monitor CBC with differential and platelet count prior to and frequently during therapy. Leukocyte counts begin to drop within 24 hr of administration. The initial nadir occurs in 7–9 days. After a small ↑ in the count, the second, deeper nadir occurs 15–24 days after administration. Platelet counts begin to ↓ 5 days after a dose, with a nadir at 12–15 days. Leukocyte and thrombocyte counts usually begin to ↑ 10 days after the nadirs. Therapy is usually withdrawn if leukocyte count is $<1000/mm^3$ or platelet count is $<50,000/mm^3$. Bone marrow aspirations are recommended every 2 wk until remission occurs.
- Monitor renal (BUN and creatinine) and hepatic function (AST, ALT, bilirubin, alkaline phosphatase, and LDH) prior to and routinely during therapy.
- May cause ↑ uric acid concentrations.

Potential Nursing Diagnoses

Risk for infection (Adverse Reactions)
Risk for injury (Side Effects)

Implementation

- ***High Alert:*** Fatalities have occurred with chemotherapeutic agents. Before administering, clarify all ambiguous orders; double-check single, daily, and course-of-therapy dose limits; have second practitioner independently double-check original order, calculations, and infusion pump settings.
- ***High Alert:*** Do not confuse high-dose and regular therapy. Fatalities have occurred with high-dose therapy.
- Solution should be prepared in a biologic cabinet. Wear gloves, gown, and mask while handling IV medication. Discard IV equipment in specially designated containers.
- May be given subcut, direct IV, intermittent IV, continuous IV, or IT.

- **IV, Subcut:** Reconstitute 100-mg vials with 5 mL of bacteriostatic water for injection with benzyl alcohol 0.9% for a concentration of 20 mg/mL. Reconstitute 500-mg vials with 10 mL for a concentration of 50 mg/mL, 1-g vials with 10 mL, and 2-g vials with 20 mL for a concentration of 100 mg/mL. Reconstituted solution is stable for 48 hr. Do not administer a cloudy or hazy solution.

IV Administration

- **IV Push:** ***Diluent:*** Administer undiluted. ***Concentration:*** 100 mg/mL. ***Rate:*** Administer each 100 mg over 1–3 min.
- **Intermittent Infusion:** ***Diluent:*** May be further diluted in 0.9% NaCl, D5W, D10W, D5/0.9% NaCl, Ringer's solution, LR, or D5/LR. ***Concentration:*** Dilute doses in 100 mL of diluent. ***Rate:*** Infuse over 15–30 min.
- **Continuous Infusion:** Rate and concentration for IV infusion are ordered individually.
- **Y-Site Compatibility:** acyclovir, alemtuzumab, alfentanil, amifostine, amakacin, aminocaproic acid, aminophylline, amphotericin B cholesteryl, amphotericin B lipid complex, amphotericin B liposome, ampicillin, ampicillin/sulbactam, amsacrine, anidulafungin, argatroban, atracurium, azithromycin, aztreonam, bivalirudin, bleomycin, bumetanide, buprenorphine, butorphanol, calcium chloride, calcium gluconate, carboplatin, carmustine, cefazolin, cefepime, cefotaxime, cefotetan, cefoxitin, ceftazidime, ceftriaxone, cefuroxime, chlorpromazine, ciprofloxacin, cisatracurium, cisplatin, cladribine, clindamycin, cyclophosphamide, cyclosporine, daunorubicin hydrochloride, dexamethasone phosphate, dexmedetomidine, dexrazoxane, digoxin, diltiazem, diphenhydramine, dobutamine, docetaxel, dolasetron, dopamine, doxacurium, doxorubicin hydrochloride, doxorubicin liposome, doxycycline, droperidol, enalaprilat, ephedrine, epinephrine, ertapenem, erythromycin, esmolol, etoposide, etoposide phosphate, famotidine, fenoldopam, fentanyl, filgrastim, fluconazole, fludarabine, foscarnet, fosphenytoin, furosemide, gemcitabine, gentamicin, granisetron, haloperidol, heparin, hydrocortisone, hydromorphone, idarubicin, ifosfamide, imipenem/cilastatin, insulin, irinotecan, isoproterenol, ketorolac, labetalol, leucovorin, levofloxacin, levorphanol, lidocaine, linezolid, lorazepam, magnesium sulfate, mannitol, melphalan, meperidine, meropenem, mesna, methohexital, methotrexate, methylprednisolone, metoclopramide, metoprolol, metronidazole, midazolam, milrinone, mitoxantrone, morphine, nalbuphine, naloxone, nesiritide, nicardipine, nitroglycerin, nitroprusside, norepinephrine, octreotide, ondansetron, oxaliplatin, paclitaxel, palonosetron, pamidronate, pancuronium, pantoprazole, pemetrexed, pentamidine, pentobarbital, phenobarbital, phenylephrine, piperacillin/tazobactam, potassium acetate, potassium chloride, potassium phosphates, procainamide, prochlorperazine, promethazine, propofol, propranolol, quinupristin/dalfopristin, ranitidine, remifentanil, rituximab, rocuronium, sargramostim, sodium acetate, sodium bicarbonate, sodium phosphates, succinylcholine, sufentanil, tacrolimus, teniposide, theophylline, thiopental, thiotepa, tigecycline, tirofiban, tobramycin, trastuzumab, trimethoprim/sulfamethoxazole, vancomycin, vasopressin, vecuronium, verapamil, vincristine, vinorelbine, voriconazole, zidovudine, zoledronic acid.
- **Y-Site Incompatibility:** allopurinol, amiodarone, amphotericin B colloidal, daptomycin, diazepam, ganciclovir, phenytoin.
- **IT:** Patients receiving *liposomal cytarabine* should be started on dexamethasone 4 mg twice daily PO or IV for 5 days beginning on the day of liposomal cytarabine injection.
- Allow vial to warm to room temperature. Gently agitate or invert vial to resuspend particles immediately before withdrawal from vial. No further reconstitution or dilution is required with *liposomal cytarabine*. Reconstitute *conventional cytarabine* with preservative-free 0.9% NaCl or autologous spinal fluid. Use immediately to prevent bacterial contamination.
- Liposomal cytarabine must be used within 4 hr of withdrawal from the vial. Discard unused portions. Inject directly into CSF via intraventricular reservoir or by direct injection into lumbar sac. Do not use in-line filters.
- Instruct patient to lie flat for 1 hr following IT injection. Monitor for immediate toxic reactions.

Patient/Family Teaching

- Caution patient to avoid crowds and persons with known infections. Report symptoms of infection (fever, chills, cough, hoarseness, sore throat, lower back or side pain, painful or difficult urination) immediately.
- Instruct patient to report unusual bleeding. Advise patient of thrombocytopenia precautions (use soft toothbrush and electric razor, avoid falls, do not drink alcoholic beverages or take medication containing aspirin or NSAIDs; may precipitate gastric bleeding).
- Instruct patient to inspect oral mucosa for redness and ulceration. If mouth sores occur, advise patient to use sponge brush and rinse mouth with water after eating and drinking. Stomatitis may require treatment with opioid analgesics.
- Instruct patient not to receive any vaccinations without advice of health care professional.

- Advise patient that this medication may have teratogenic effects. Contraception should be used during therapy and for at least 4 mo after therapy is concluded.
- Emphasize the need for periodic lab tests to monitor for side effects.
- **IT:** Inform patient about the expected side effects (headache, nausea, vomiting, fever) and about early signs of neurotoxicity. Instruct patient to notify health care professional if these signs occur.
- Emphasize the importance of taking dexamethasone with lyposomal cytarabine.

Evaluation/Desired Outcomes

- Improvement of hematopoietic values in leukemias.
- Decrease in size and spread of the tumor in non-Hodgkin's lymphomas. Therapy is continued every 2 wk until patient is in complete remission or thrombocyte count or leukocyte count falls below acceptable levels.
- Treatment of lymphomatous meningitis.

dabigatran (da-bye-**gat**-ran)
Pradaxa

Classification
Therapeutic: anticoagulants
Pharmacologic: thrombin inhibitors

Pregnancy Category C

Indications
To reduce the risk of stroke/systemic embolization associated with nonvalvular atrial fibrillation. Treatment of deep vein thrombosis or pulmonary embolism in patients who have been treated with parenteral anticoagulant for 5–10 days. To reduce the risk of recurrence of deep vein thrombosis or pulmonary embolism in patients who have been previously treated.

Action
Acts as a direct inhibitor of thrombin. **Therapeutic Effects:** Lowered risk of thrombotic sequelae (stroke and systemic embolization) of nonvalvular atrial fibrillation.

Pharmacokinetics
Absorption: 3–7% absorbed following oral administration.
Distribution: Unknown.
Metabolism and Excretion: Of the amount absorbed, mostly excreted by kidneys (80%); 86% of ingested dose is eliminated in feces due to poor bioavailability.
Half-life: 12–17 hr.

TIME/ACTION PROFILE (effects on coagulation)

ROUTE	ONSET	PEAK	DURATION
PO	within hours	unknown	2 days†

†Following discontinuation, 3–5 days in renal impairment.

Contraindications/Precautions
Contraindicated in: Hypersensitivity; Active pathological bleeding; Concurrent use of P-glycoprotein (P-gp) inducers; Prosthetic heart valves (mechanical or bioprosthetic).
Use Cautiously in: Neuroaxial spinal anesthesia or spinal puncture, especially if concurrent with an indwelling epidural catheter, drugs affecting hemostasis, history of traumatic/repeated spinal puncture or spinal deformity (↑ risk of spinal hematoma); Concurrent medications/pre-existing conditions that ↑ bleeding-risk (other anticoagulants, antiplatelet agents, antifibrinolytics, heparins, chronic NSAID use, labor and delivery); Renal impairment; Surgical procedures (discontinue 1–2 days prior if CCr ≥50 mL/min or 3–4 days prior if CCr <50 mL/min; Geri: ↑ risk of bleeding; Lactation: Use cautiously during breast feeding; Pedi: Safety and effectiveness not established.

Adverse Reactions/Side Effects
GI: abdominal pain, diarrhea, dyspepsia, gastritis, esophageal ulceration, nausea. **Hemat:** BLEEDING, thrombocytopenia. **Misc:** ANGIOEDEMA, hypersensitivity reactions including ANAPHYLAXIS.

Interactions
Drug-Drug: Concurrent use of other **anticoagulants**, **antiplatelet agents**, **antifibrinolytics**, **heparins**, **prasugrel**, **clopidogrel**, or chronic use of **NSAIDs** ↑ risk of bleeding. Concurrent use of **P-gp inducers** including **rifampin** ↓ levels and effectiveness; avoid concurrent use. **P-gp inhibitors**, including **dronedarone**, **ketoconazole (systemic)**, **verapamil**, **quinidine**, and **ticagrelor** may ↑ levels and the risk of bleeding; concomitant use should be avoided in patients with CCr 15–30 mL/min.

Route/Dosage

Reduction in Risk of Stroke/Systemic Embolism in Nonvalvular Atrial Fibrillation
PO (Adults): 150 mg twice daily.

Renal Impairment
PO (Adults): *CCr 30–50 mL/min and taking dronedarone or systemic ketoconazole*—75 mg twice daily; *CCr <30 mL/min and taking P-gp inhibitor*—Avoid concomitant use; *CCr 15–30 mL/min*—75 mg twice daily; *CCr <15 mL/min or on dialysis*—Not recommended.

Treatment of and Reduction in Risk of Recurrence of Deep Vein Thrombosis or Pulmonary Embolism
PO (Adults): 150 mg twice daily.

Renal Impairment
PO (Adults): *CCr <50 mL/min and taking P-gp inhibitor*—Avoid concomitant use; *CCr <30 mL/min or on dialysis*—Not recommended.

Availability
Capsules: 75 mg, ✤ 110 mg, 150 mg.

NURSING IMPLICATIONS

Assessment
- Assess for symptoms of stroke or peripheral vascular disease periodically during therapy.
- Assess for symptoms of bleeding and blood loss; may be fatal.
- ***Lab Test Considerations:*** Use aPTT or ECT, not INR, to assess anticoagulant activity, if needed.
- Monitor renal function prior to and periodically during therapy. Patients with renal impairment may require dose reduction or discontinuation.

Potential Nursing Diagnoses

Activity intolerance

Implementation

- When *converting from warfarin*, discontinue warfarin and start dabigatran when INR is <2.0.
- When *converting from dabigatran to warfarin*, adjust starting time based on creatinine clearance. For *CCr >50 mL/min*, start warfarin 3 days before discontinuing dabigatran. For *CCr 31–50 mL/min*, start warfarin 2 days before discontinuing dabigatran. For *CCr 15–30 mL/min*, start warfarin 1 day before discontinuing dabigatran. For *CCr <15 mL/min*, no recommendations can be made. INR will better reflect warfarin's effect after dabigatran has been stopped for at least 2 days.
- When *converting from parenteral anticoagulants*, start dabigatran up to 2 hr before next dose of parenteral drug is due or at time of discontinuation of parenteral therapy.
- When *converting to dabigatran from parenteral anticoagulants*, wait 12 hrs (CCr ≥30 mL/min) or 24 hr (CCr <30 mL/min) after last dose of dabigatran before initiating parenteral anticoagulant therapy.
- *For surgery*, discontinue dabigatran 1–2 days (CrCL ≥50 mL/min) or 3–5 days (CCr <50 mL/min) before invasive or surgical procedures; consider longer times for major surgery, spinal puncture, or placement of a spinal or epidural catheter. If surgery cannot be delayed, bleeding risk is ↑. Assess bleeding risk with ecarin clotting time (ECT) or a PTT if ECT is not available.
- **PO:** Administer twice daily with a full glass of water without regard to food. Swallow capsule whole; do not open, crush, or chew; may result in increased exposure.
- If dabigatran is discontinued, consider starting another anticoagulant; discontinuation of dabigatran increases risk of thromboembolic events.

Patient/Family Teaching

- Instruct patient to take dabigatran as directed. Take missed doses as soon as remembered within 6 hr. If <6 hr until next dose, skip dose and take next dose when scheduled; do not double doses. Do not discontinue without consulting health care professional. If temporarily discontinued, restart as soon as possible. Store dabigatran at room temperature. After opening bottle, use within 4 mo; discard unused dabigatran after 4 mo.
- Inform patient that they may bleed more easily or longer than usual. Advise patient to notify health care professional immediately if signs of bleeding (unusual bruising; pink or brown urine; red or black, tarry stools; coughing up blood; vomiting blood; pain or swelling in a joint; headache; dizziness; weakness; recurring nose bleeds; unusual bleeding from gums; heavier than normal menstrual bleeding; dyspepsia; abdominal pain; epigastric pain) occur.
- Advise patient to notify health care professional of medication regimen prior to treatment or surgery.
- Instruct patient to notify health care professional of all Rx or OTC medications, vitamins, or herbal products being taken and consult health care professional before taking any new medications.
- Advise female patient to notify health care professional if pregnancy is planned or suspected or if breast feeding.

Evaluation/Desired Outcomes

- Reduction in the risk of stroke and systemic embolism.

⚞ **dabrafenib** (da-**braf**-e-nib)

Tafinlar

Classification

Therapeutic: antineoplastics

Pharmacologic: kinase inhibitors

Pregnancy Category D

Indications

⚞ Treatment of metastatic/unresectable melanoma in patients with the BRAF V600E mutation. ⚞ Treatment of metastatic/unresectable melanoma in patients with the BRAF V600E or V600K mutation (in combination with trametinib).

Action

Inhibits kinase, an enzyme that promotes cell proliferation. **Therapeutic Effects:** Decreased spread/progression of melanoma.

Pharmacokinetics

Absorption: Well absorbed (95%) following oral administration.

Distribution: Unknown.

Protein Binding: 99.7%.

Metabolism and Excretion: Mostly metabolized by CYP 2C8 and CYP3A4 enzyme systems, Two metabolites (hydroxy-dabrafenib and desmethyl-1–dabrafenib) have antineoplastic activity. Excreted as metabolites in feces (72%) and urine (23%).

Half-life: *Dabrafenib*—8 hr; *hydroxy-dabrafenib*—10 hr, *desmethyl-1–dabrafenib*—21–22 hr.

TIME/ACTION PROFILE (progression-free survival)

ROUTE	ONSET	PEAK	DURATION
PO	within 1 mo	1–2 mo	8 mo

Contraindications/Precautions

Contraindicated in: OB: Pregnancy (may cause fetal harm); Lactation: Breast feeding should be avoided; Concurrent use of CYP 3A4/CYP2C8 inhibitors or inducers (may significantly alter levels and effects).

Use Cautiously in: BRAF Wild-type melanoma (may ↑ proliferation); History of glucose-6–phosphate dehydrogenase deficiency (may cause hemolytic anemia); Moderate to severe hepatic impairment (blood levels may be ↑); Moderate to severe renal impairment; OB: Patients with reproductive potential (hormonal contraceptives may be less effective, additional methods required); Pedi: Safety and effectiveness not established.

Adverse Reactions/Side Effects

CNS: headache, fatigue. **CV:** HF, THROMBOEMBOLISM. **EENT:** iritis, retinal detachment, uveitis. **Endo:** hyperglycemia. **Resp:** cough, nasopharyngitis. **GI:** constipation, pancreatitis. **Derm:** alopecia, hyperkeratosis, palmar-plantar erythrodysesthesia, papilloma, cutaneous squamous cell carcinoma. **F and E:** hypophosphatemia, hyponatremia. **Hemat:** BLEEDING. **MS:** arthralgia, back pain, myalgia. **Misc:** MALIGNANCY, fever including serious febrile reactions, ↑ alkaline phosphatase, chills, tumor promotion.

Interactions

Drug-Drug: Concurrent use of strong inhibitors of CYP3A4 or CYP2C8, including **ketoconazole**, **nefazodone**, **clarithromycin** and **gemfibrozil** ↑ blood levels and the risk of toxicity and should be avoided. Careful monitoring for toxicity is required. Concurrent use of **strong inducers of CYP3A4 or CYP2C8** including **carbamazepine**, **phenobarbital**, **phenytoin**, and **rifampin** ↓ blood levels and may ↓ effectiveness. Careful monitoring for decreased results is required. **Drugs that ↑ gastric pH** including **antacids**, **H_2–receptor antagonists** and **proton pump inhibitors** may ↓ blood levels and effectiveness. May ↓ effectiveness of other **CYP3A4 substrates** and **CYP2C9 substrates**, including **midazolam**, **warfarin**, **dexamethasone**, and **hormonal contraceptives**.

Drug-Natural Products: **St. John's wort** ↓ blood levels and may ↓ effectiveness; concurrent use should be avoided.

Route/Dosage

PO (Adults): 150 mg twice daily, continued until disease progression or unacceptable toxicity. Dose modifications recommended for various levels of related toxicities.

Availability

Capsules: 50 mg, 75 mg.

NURSING IMPLICATIONS

Assessment

- Perform skin examinations prior to starting therapy and every 2 months during and for 6 months after completion of therapy. *If intolerable Grade 2 skin toxicity, Grade 3 or Grade 4 occurs,* withhold dabrafenib for up to 3 wks; if used with trametinib, withhold trametinib for up to 3 wks. If improved, resume at a lower dose. If not improved, permanently discontinue.
- Monitor temperature. *If fever is 101.3°F to 104°F,* withhold dabrafenib until fever resolves, then resume at same dose. *If fever is >104°F or complicated by rigors, hypotension, dehydration, or renal failure,* withhold until fever resolves, then resume at a reduced dose. *For first reduction,* decrease dose to 100 mg twice daily. *For second dose reduction,* decrease dose to 75 mg twice daily. *For third dose reduction,* decrease dose to 50 mg twice daily. *If unable to tolerate 50 mg twice daily,* discontinue dabrafenib.
- Monitor for signs and symptoms of ocular toxicities (blurred vision, loss of vision, other vision changes, see color dots, halo around objects), swelling, redness, photophobia, eye pain). May require steroid and mydriatic ophthalmic drops. *If Grade 2-3 retinal pigment epithelial detachments (RPED) occur,* do not modify dabrafenib dose. Withhold trametinib for up to 3 weeks. If improved to Grade 0-1, resume at lower dose. If not improved, permanently discontinue. *If retinal vein occlusion occurs,* do not modify dabrafenib dose. Discontinue trametinib permanently. *If uveitis and iritis occur,* withhold dabrafenib for up to 6 weeks. If improved to Grade 0-1, resume at same dose. If not improved, permanently discontinue dabrafenib. Do not modify trametinib dose.
- Monitor cardiac function during therapy. *If asymptomatic, absolute decrease in LVEF ≥10% from baseline occurs and is below institutional lower limits of normal (LLN) from pretreatment value,* do not modify dose if only taking dabrafenib. If also taking trametinib, withhold trametinib for up to 4 wks. If improved to normal LVEF, resume at lower dose. If not improved to normal LVEF value, permanently discontinue trametinib. *If symptomatic congestive heart failure occurs with absolute decrease in LVEF >20% from baseline that is below LLN,* withhold dabrafenib, if improved, resume at same dose. Permanently discontinue trametinib.
- Monitor for signs and symptoms of venous thromboembolism (shortness of breath, chest pain, arm or leg swelling, cool or pale arm or leg) during therapy. *If uncomplicated deep vein thrombosis (DVT) or pulmonary embolus (PE) occur,* do not modify dabrafenib dose. Withhold trametinib for up to 3 weeks. If improved to Grade 0-1, resume at lower dose. If not improved, permanently discontinue. *If life-threatening PE occurs,* permanently discontinue dabrafenib and trametinib.
- Monitor for signs and symptoms of interstitial lung disease or pneumonitis (cough, dyspnea, hypoxia, pleural effusion, infiltrates) during therapy. If signs

and symptoms occur, do not modify dabrafenib dose; permanently discontinue trametinib.

- Assess for bleeding (headaches, dizziness, feeling weak, coughing up blood or blood clots, vomiting blood or vomit looks like "coffee grounds", red or black stools that look like tar) during therapy. *If Grade 3 hemorrhagic event occurs,* withhold dabrafenib and trametinib for up to 3 wks, if improved resume at lower level. *If Grade 4 hemorrhagic event occurs,* permanently discontinue dabrafenib and trametinib.
- ***Lab Test Considerations:*** May cause hyperglycemia requiring increase in dose of or initiation of insulin or oral hypoglycemic agents. Monitor serum glucose levels in patients with pre-existing diabetes or hyperglycemia.
- May cause hypophosphatemia, ↑ alkaline phosphatase, and hyponatremia.
- Monitor for hemolytic anemia in patients with glucose-6-phosphate dehydrogenase (G6PD) deficiency.

Potential Nursing Diagnoses

Impaired skin integrity (Indications)

Implementation

- Evidence of BRAF V600E or V600K mutation status must be confirmed prior to starting therapy with dabrafenib.
- **PO:** Administer twice daily about 12 hrs apart. Administer on an empty stomach at least 1 hr before or 2 hrs after a meal. Swallow capsules whole; do not open, crush, break, or chew.
- When administered with trametinib, administer once-daily dose of trametinib at same time each day with either morning or evening dose of dabrafenib.

Patient/Family Teaching

- Instruct patient to take dabrafenib as directed at least 1 hr before or 2 hrs after meals. Take missed doses as soon as remembered unless within 6 hrs of next dose, then skip missed dose and take regularly scheduled dose.
- Inform patient that dabrafenib increases risk of developing new cutaneous malignancies. Notify health care professional immediately if new lesions (wart, skin sore or reddish bump that bleeds or does not heal) or changes in size or color of existing moles or lesions occur.
- Advise patient to notify health care professional of all Rx or OTC medications, vitamins, or herbal products being taken and to consult with health care professional before taking other medications, especially St. John's Wort.
- Inform patient of potential side effects. Advise patient to notify health care professional if fever, signs and symptoms of hyperglycemia (increased thirst, urinating more often than normal, breath smells like fruit), or eye problems, bleeding, thromboembolism, heart failure (heart pounding or racing, shortness of breath, swelling of ankles and feet, feeling lightheaded) occur.
- Rep: Advise female patient to use a highly effective form of contraception during and for at least 2 wks after dabrafenib alone or 4 months after treatment with dabrafenib and trametinib. Use a non-hormonal form of contraception; dabrafenib may decrease effectiveness of hormonal contraceptives. Advise patient to notify health care professional if pregnancy is suspected and to avoid breast feeding. Advise patients to seek counseling on fertility and family planning prior to beginning therapy; may impair fertility in females and may cause spermatogenesis in males.

Evaluation/Desired Outcomes

- Decrease in progression of malignant melanoma.

HIGH ALERT

dacarbazine (da-**kar**-ba-zeen)

DTIC, DTIC-Dome

Classification

Therapeutic: antineoplastics

Pharmacologic: alkylating agents

Pregnancy Category C

Indications

Treatment of metastatic malignant melanoma (single agent). Treatment of Hodgkin's disease as second-line therapy (with other agents).

Action

Disrupts DNA and RNA synthesis (cell-cycle phase–nonspecific). **Therapeutic Effects:** Death of rapidly growing tissue cells, especially malignant ones.

Pharmacokinetics

Absorption: IV administration results in complete bioavailability.

Distribution: Large volume of distribution; probably concentrates in liver; some CNS penetration.

Metabolism and Excretion: 50% metabolized by the liver, 50% excreted unchanged by the kidneys.

Half-life: 5 hr (↑ in renal and hepatic dysfunction).

TIME/ACTION PROFILE (effects on blood counts)

ROUTE	ONSET	PEAK	DURATION
IV (WBCs)	16–20 days	21–25 days	3–5 days
IV (platelets)	unknown	16 days	3–5 days

Contraindications/Precautions

Contraindicated in: Hypersensitivity; OB, Lactation: Pregnancy or lactation.

Use Cautiously in: Active infections; Bone marrow depression; Pedi: Children (safety not established); Renal dysfunction; Hepatic dysfunction.

Adverse Reactions/Side Effects

GI: HEPATIC NECROSIS, anorexia, nausea, vomiting, diarrhea, hepatic vein thrombosis. **Derm:** alopecia, facial flushing, photosensitivity, rash. **Endo:** gonadal suppression. **Hemat:** anemia, leukopenia, thrombocytopenia. **Local:** pain at IV site, phlebitis at IV site, tissue necrosis. **MS:** myalgia. **Neuro:** facial paresthesia. **Misc:** ANAPHYLAXIS, fever, flu-like syndrome, malaise.

Interactions

Drug-Drug: Additive bone marrow depression with other **antineoplastics**. **Carbamazepine**, **phenobarbital**, and **rifampin** may ↑ metabolism and decrease effectiveness. Blood levels may be ↑ with **amiodarone**, **ciprofloxacin**, **fluvoxamine**, **ketoconazole**, **ofloxacin**, **isoniazid**, or **miconazole**. May ↓ antibody response to **live-virus vaccines** and ↑ risk of adverse reactions.

Route/Dosage

Other regimens are used.

IV (Adults): *Malignant melanoma*—2–4.5 mg/kg/day for 10 days administered every 4 wk *or* 250 mg/m²/day for 5 days administered every 3 wk. *Hodgkin's disease*—150 mg/m²/day for 5 days (in combination with other agents) administered every 4 wk *or* 375 mg/m² (in combination with other agents) administered every 15 days.

Availability

Powder for injection: 200 mg.

NURSING IMPLICATIONS

Assessment

- Monitor vital signs prior to and frequently during therapy.
- Monitor for bone marrow depression. Assess for bleeding (bleeding gums, bruising, petechiae, guaiac stools, urine, and emesis) and avoid IM injections and rectal temperatures if platelet count is low. Apply pressure to venipuncture sites for 10 min. Assess for signs of infection during neutropenia. Anemia may occur. Monitor for increased fatigue, dyspnea, and orthostatic hypotension.
- Monitor IV site closely. Dacarbazine is an irritant. Instruct patient to notify health care professional immediately if discomfort at IV site occurs. Discontinue IV immediately if infiltration occurs. Applications of hot packs may relieve pain, burning sensation, and irritation at injection site.
- Monitor intake and output, appetite, and nutritional intake. Assess for nausea and vomiting, which may be severe and last 1–12 hr. Administration of an antiemetic prior to and periodically during therapy, restricting oral intake for 4–6 hr prior to administration, and adjusting diet as tolerated may help maintain fluid and electrolyte balance and nutritional status. Nausea usually decreases on subsequent doses.
- ***Lab Test Considerations:*** Monitor CBC and differential prior to and periodically throughout therapy. The nadir of thrombocytopenia occurs in 16 days. The nadir of leukopenia occurs in 3–4 wk. Recovery begins in 5 days. Withhold dose and notify physician if platelet count is <100,000/mm³ or leukocyte count is <4000/mm³.
- Monitor for increased AST, ALT, BUN, and serum creatinine. May cause hepatic necrosis.

Potential Nursing Diagnoses

Risk for infection (Side Effects)
Risk for injury (Side Effects)

Implementation

- ***High Alert:*** Fatalities have occurred with chemotherapeutic agents. Before administering, clarify all ambiguous orders; double-check single, daily, and course-of-therapy dose limits; have second practitioner independently double-check original order, calculations, and infusion pump settings.

IV Administration

- Prepare solution in a biologic cabinet. Wear gloves, gown, and mask while handling medication. Discard equipment in designated containers.
- Reconstitute each 200-mg vial with 19.7 mL of sterile water for injection. Solution is colorless or clear yellow. Do not use solution that has turned pink. ***Concentration:*** 10 mg/mL. Solution is stable for 8 hr at room temperature and for 72 hr if refrigerated.
- **Intermittent Infusion:** ***Diluent:*** Further dilute with up to 250 mL of D5W or 0.9% NaCl. Stable for 24 hr if refrigerated or 8 hr at room temperature. ***Rate:*** Administer over 30–60 min.
- **Y-Site Compatibility:** amifostine, aztreonam, bivalirudin, caspofungin, daptomycin, dexmedetomidine, docetaxel, doxorubicin liposome, ertapenem, etoposide phosphate, fenoldopam, filgrastim, fludarabine, granisetron, hetastarch, levofloxacin, mechlorethamine, melphalan, nesiritide, octreotide, ondansetron, oxaliplatin, paclitaxel, palonosetron, quinupristin/dalfopristin, sargramostim, teniposide, thiotepa, tigecycline, tirofiban, vinorelbine, voriconazole.
- **Y-Site Incompatibility:** allopurinol, amphotericin B liposome, cefepime, pantoprazole, pemetrexed, piperacillin/tazobactam.

Patient/Family Teaching

- Instruct patient to notify health care professional if fever; chills; sore throat; signs of infection; bleeding gums; bruising; petechiae; abdominal pain; yellowing of eyes; or blood in urine, stool, or emesis occurs. Caution patient to avoid crowds and persons with known infections. Instruct patient to use soft toothbrush and electric razor. Patients should be cautioned not to drink alcoholic beverages or take products containing aspirin or NSAIDs; may increase GI irritation.

- May cause photosensitivity. Instruct patient to avoid sunlight or wear protective clothing and use sunscreen for 2 days after therapy.
- Instruct patient to inform health care professional if flu-like syndrome occurs. Symptoms include fever, myalgia, and general malaise. May occur after several courses of therapy. Usually occurs 1 wk after administration. May persist for 1–3 wk. Acetaminophen may be used for relief of symptoms.
- Discuss with patient the possibility of hair loss. Explore coping strategies.
- Advise patient of the need for a nonhormonal method of contraception.
- Instruct patient not to receive any vaccinations without advice of health care professional.

Evaluation/Desired Outcomes

- Decrease in size and spread of malignant melanoma or Hodgkin's lymphoma.

daclatasvir (da-kla-**tass**-veer)

Daklinza

Classification

Therapeutic: antivirals

Pharmacologic: NS5A inhibitors

Indications

Treatment of chronic hepatitis C virus (HCV) genotype 3 infection in combination with sofosbuvir.

Action

Acts as a direct acting antiviral. Inhibits NS5A, a HCV-encoded protein, resulting in inhibited viral RNA replication and virion assembly. **Therapeutic Effects:** Decreased presence of HCV with decreased sequelae of HCV infection.

Pharmacokinetics

Absorption: Well absorbed (67%) following oral administration.

Distribution: Unknown.

Protein Binding: 99%.

Metabolism and Excretion: Metabolized mostly by the the CYP3A enzyme system. 88% excreted in feces (53% as unchanged drug); 6.6% excreted unchanged in urine.

Half-life: 12–15 hr.

TIME/ACTION PROFILE (blood levels)

ROUTE	ONSET	PEAK	DURATION
PO	unknown	2 hr	24 hr

Contraindications/Precautions

Contraindicated in: Strong CYP3A inhibitors.

Use Cautiously in: Cirrhosis (sustained virologic response is decreased); Decompensated cirrhosis/post liver transplant (safe and effective use has not been established); Concurrent use with dabigatran; OB: Consider benefits and risks carefully; Lactation: Beneficial effects of breast feeding should be weighed against potential adverse drug effects; Pedi: Safe and effective use in children <18 yr has not been established.

Exercise Extreme Caution in: Concurrent use of amiodarone (with sofosbuvir).

Adverse Reactions/Side Effects

CNS: fatigue, headache. **GI:** diarrhea, nausea.

Interactions

Drug-Drug: Strong inducers of CYP3A including **carbamazepine**, **phenytoin** and **rifampin** ↓ levels and effectiveness (concurrent use is contraindicated). **Moderate inducers of CYP3A** including **bosentan**, **dexamethasone**, **efavirenz**, **modafinil**, **nfacillin** and **rifapentine** ↓ levels and effectiveness (↑ dose required). Concurrent use with **amiodarone** and sofosbuvir ↑ risk of serious bradycardia and should be avoided, especially if **beta blockers** are being used/concurrent cardiovascular/liver disease is present. *Concurrent strong inhibitors of CYP3A*—including **atazanavir/ritonavir**, **clarithromycin**, **indinavir**, **itraconaole**, **ketoconazole**, **nefazodone**, **nelfinavir**, **posaconazole**, **saquinavir**, **telithromycine** and **voriconazole** ↑ blood levels and risk of adverse effects (↓ dose required). Concurrent use of moderate inhibitors of CYP3A including **atazanavir**, **ciprofloxacin**, **darunavir/ritonavir**, **diltiazem**, **erythromycin**, **fluconazole**, **fosamprenavir** and **verapamil** ↑ blood levels and may ↑ risk of adverse reactions (clinical monitoring recommeneded). ↑ levels and risk of toxicity with **digoxin** (↓ initial dose of digoxin/↓ dose of chronic digoxin may be necessary, careful clinical monitoring recommended). ↑ levels and risk of adverse effects including myopathy with **HMG-CoA reductase inhibitors (statins)** (monitor effects and ↓ dose if necessary).

Drug-Natural Products: Concurrent use of **St. John's wort** ↓ levels and effectiveness (concurrent use is contraindicated).

Route/Dosage

Must be taken concurrently with sofosbuvir

PO (Adults): 60 mg once daily for 12 wk; *Concurrent strong inhibitors of CYP3A*—30 mg once daily; *Concurrent moderate inducers of CYP3A*—90 mg once daily.

Availability

Tablets: 30 mg, 60 mg.

NURSING IMPLICATIONS

Assessment

- Monitor for signs and symptoms of chronic hepatitis C.

Potential Nursing Diagnoses

Risk for infection (Indications)

Implementation

- Must be administered in conjunction with sofosbuvir. If sofosbuvir is permanently discontinued, daclatasvir must also be discontinued.
- **PO:** Administer once daily without regard to food for 12 wk.

Patient/Family Teaching

- Instruct patient to take daclatasvir with sofosbuvir as directed. Take missed dose as soon as remembered in same day. If not until next day, skip dose and take next dose as scheduled; do not double doses. Advise patient to read *Patient Information* before starting therapy and with each Rx refill in case of changes.
- Advise patient receiving beta-blockers or having underlying significant cardiovascular/hepatic disease to notify health care professional if signs and symptoms of bradycardia (near-fainting or fainting, dizziness or lightheadedness, malaise, weakness, excessive tiredness, shortness of breath, chest pain, confusion, memory problems) occur.
- Instruct patient to notify health care professional of all Rx or OTC medications, vitamins, or herbal products being taken and consult health care professional before taking any new medications, especially St. John's Wort.
- Advise female patient to notify health care professional if pregnancy is planned or suspected or if breast feeding.

Evaluation/Desired Outcomes

- Decreased presence of HCV with decreased sequelae of HCV infection.

dalbavancin (dal-ba-**van**-sin)

Dalvance

Classification

Therapeutic: anti-infectives

Pharmacologic: lipoglycopeptides

Pregnancy Category C

Indications

Treatment of skin/skin structure infections due to susceptible bacteria.

Action

Binds to bacterial cell wall resulting in cell death. **Therapeutic Effects:** Bactericidal action against susceptible bacteria with resolution of infection. **Spectrum:** Active against *Staphylococcus aureus* (including methicillin-susceptible and resistant strains), *Streptococcus agalactiae*, *Streptococcus anginosus* (including *S. anginosus*, *S. intermidius* and *S. constellatus*) and *Streptococcus pyogenes*.

Pharmacokinetics

Absorption: IV administration results in complete bioavailability.

Distribution: Penetrates tissues and fluids.

Metabolism and Excretion: 33% eliminated unchanged in urine, 12% eliminated as inactive metabolite, 20% excreted in feces.

Half-life: 346 hr.

TIME/ACTION PROFILE (blood levels)

ROUTE	ONSET	PEAK	DURATION
IV	unknown	end of infusion	1 wk

Contraindications/Precautions

Contraindicated in: Hypersensitivity.

Use Cautiously in: Renal impairment (dose adjustment required for CCr <30 mL/min; Moderate to severe hepatic impairment; Geri: Consider age-related decrease in renal function; OB: Use during pregnancy only if potential benefit justifies potential risk to the fetus; Lactation: Use cautiously if breast feeding; Pedi: Safe and effective use in children has not been established.

Adverse Reactions/Side Effects

CNS: headache. **GI:** DIARRHEA INCLUDING CLOSTRIDIUM DIFFICILE, nausea, ↑ ALT. **Derm:** pruritus, rash. **Misc:** hypersensitivity reactions including ANAPHYLAXIS, infusion reactions including "Red-Man Syndrome".

Interactions

Drug-Drug: None noted.

Route/Dosage

IV (Adults): 1000 mg followed one wk later by 500 mg.

Renal Impairment

IV (Adults): *CCr <30 mL/min*—750 mg followed one wk later by 375 mg.

Availability

Lyophylized powder for intravenous injection (requires reconstitution and further dilution): 500 mg single-use vial.

NURSING IMPLICATIONS

Assessment

- Assess for infection (vital signs; appearance of wound, sputum, urine, and stool; WBC) at beginning of and during therapy.

- Obtain specimens for culture and sensitivity prior to therapy. First dose may be given before receiving results.
- Monitor bowel function. Diarrhea, abdominal cramping, fever, and bloody stools should be reported to health care professional promptly as a sign of Clostridium difficile-associated diarrhea (CDAD). May begin up to 2 mo following cessation of therapy.
- Monitor for infusion reactions (Red-man syndrome —flushing of upper body, urticaria, pruritus, rash). May resolve with stopping or slowing infusion.
- ***Lab Test Considerations:*** Monitor hepatic function tests. May cause ↑ ALT, AST, and bilirubin.

Potential Nursing Diagnoses

Risk for infection (Indications)
Diarrhea (Adverse Reactions)

Implementation

IV Administration

- **Intermittent Infusion:** Reconstitute with 25 mL of Sterile water in each 500 mg vial. Alternate gentle swirling and inverting to avoid foaming, until completely dissolved. Do not shake. Reconstituted vial contains a clear colorless to yellow solution. Do not administer solutions that are discolored or contain particulate matter. Transfer reconstituted solution into D5W. ***Concentration:*** 1 mg/mL to 5 mg/mL. Discard unused solution. May be refrigerated or kept at room temperature; do not freeze. Infuse within 48 hr of reconstitution. Do not administer solutions containing particulate matter. ***Rate:*** Infuse over 30 min.
- **Y-Site Incompatibility:** Do not infuse with other medications or electrolytes. Saline solutions may cause precipitation. Flush line before and after infusion with D5W.

Patient/Family Teaching

- Instruct patient to notify health care professional if signs and symptoms of hypersensitivity reactions (rash, hives, dyspnea, facial swelling) occur.
- Instruct patient to notify health care professional immediately if diarrhea, abdominal cramping, fever, or bloody stools occur and not to treat with antidiarrheals without consulting health care professionals.
- Advise patient to notify health care professional of all Rx or OTC medications, vitamins, or herbal products being taken and to consult with health care professional before taking other medications.
- Advise female patients to use effective contraception during therapy and to notify health care professional if pregnancy is suspected or if breast feeding.
- Instruct the patient to notify health care professional if symptoms do not improve.

Evaluation/Desired Outcomes

- Resolution of the signs and symptoms of infection. Length of time for complete resolution depends on the organism and site of infection.

dalfampridine

(dal-**fam**-pri-deen)
Ampyra, ✱Fampyra

Classification
Therapeutic: anti-multiple sclerosis agents
Pharmacologic: potassium channel blockers

Pregnancy Category C

Indications

Treatment of mutiple sclerosis, to improve walking speed.

Action

Acts as a potassium channel blocker, which may increase conduction of action potentials. **Therapeutic Effects:** Increased walking speed in patients with multiple sclerosis.

Pharmacokinetics

Absorption: Rapidly and completely absorbed (96%).
Distribution: Unknown.
Metabolism and Excretion: 96% eliminated in urine, 0.5% in feces.
Half-life: 5.2–6.5 hr.

TIME/ACTION PROFILE (improvement in walking speed)

ROUTE	ONSET	PEAK	DURATION
PO	unk	3–4 hr	24 hr

Contraindications/Precautions

Contraindicated in: Hypersensitivity; History of seizures; Moderate/severe renal impairment (CCr ≤50 mL/min) (↑ risk of seizures); Lactation: Avoid use.
Use Cautiously in: Mild renal impairment (CCr 51–80 mL/min) (↑ risk of seizures); Geri: Consider age-related ↓ in renal function; OB: Use only if potential benefit justifies potential risk to fetus; Pedi: Safety and effectiveness not established.

Adverse Reactions/Side Effects

CNS: SEIZURES, dizziness, headache, insomnia, weakness. **EENT:** nasopharyngitis, pharyngolaryngeal pain. **GI:** constipation, dyspepsia, nausea. **GU:** urinary tract infection. **MS:** back pain. **Neuro:** balance disorder, multiple sclerosis relapse, paresthesia. **Misc:** ANAPHYLAXIS.

Interactions

Drug-Drug: None noted.

Route/Dosage

PO (Adults): 10 mg twice daily.

Availability

Extended-release tablets: 10 mg.

NURSING IMPLICATIONS

Assessment

- Assess walking speed in patients with multiple sclerosis prior to and periodically during therapy.
- Monitor for seizures during therapy, risk increases with increased dose. If seizure occurs, discontinue therapy.
- Monitor for signs and symptoms of anaphylaxis (dyspnea, wheezing, urticaria, angioedema of the throat or tongue) during therapy.
- ***Lab Test Considerations:*** Monitor creatinine clearance prior to and at least yearly during therapy; renal impairment may require dose reduction or discontinuation.

Potential Nursing Diagnoses

Impaired walking (Indications)

Implementation

- Administer tablets twice daily approximately 12 hr apart without regard to food. Administer tablets whole; do not break, crush, chew, or dissolve.

Patient/Family Teaching

- Instruct patient to take dalfampridine as directed, with approximately 12 hrs between tablets. If a dose is missed, omit and take next scheduled dose on time; do not double doses. May increase risk of seizures. Advise patient to read *Medication Guide* prior to beginning therapy and with each Rx refill; new information may be available.
- Instruct patient to notify health care professional of all Rx or OTC medications, vitamins, or herbal products being taken and consult health care professional before taking any new medications.
- If a seizure or signs or symptoms of anaphylaxis occur, advise patient to notify health care professional immediately, to discontinue dalfampridine, and to report the event to Acorda (manufacturer) at 1-800-367-5109.
- Advise female patient to notify health care professional if pregnancy is planned or suspected or if breast feeding.

Evaluation/Desired Outcomes

- Improved walking and increased walking speed in patients with multiple sclerosis.

dalteparin, See HEPARINS (LOW MOLECULAR WEIGHT).

dantrolene (dan-troe-leen)

Dantrium, Ryanodex

Classification

Therapeutic: skeletal muscle relaxants (direct acting)

Pregnancy Category C

D

Indications

PO: Treatment of spasticity associated with: Spinal cord injury, stroke, cerebral palsy, multiple sclerosis. Prophylaxis of malignant hyperthermia. **IV:** Emergency treatment of malignant hyperthermia. Prevention of malignant hyperthermia in patients at high risk. **Unlabeled Use:** Management of neuroleptic malignant syndrome.

Action

Acts directly on skeletal muscle, causing relaxation by decreasing calcium release from sarcoplasmic reticulum in muscle cells. Prevents intense catabolic process associated with malignant hyperthermia. **Therapeutic Effects:** Reduction of muscle spasticity. Treatment and prevention of malignant hyperthermia.

Pharmacokinetics

Absorption: 35% absorbed after oral administration. IV administration results in complete bioavailability.

Distribution: Unknown.

Metabolism and Excretion: Almost entirely metabolized by the liver.

Half-life: 8.7–11.4 hr.

TIME/ACTION PROFILE (effects on spasticity)

ROUTE	ONSET	PEAK	DURATION
PO	1 wk	unknown	6–12 hr
IV	rapid	rapid	unknown

Contraindications/Precautions

Contraindicated in: No contraindications to IV form in treatment of malignant hyperthermia; Lactation: Lactation; Situations in which spasticity is used to maintain posture or balance.

Use Cautiously in: Cardiac, pulmonary, or previous liver disease; Women and patients >35 yr (↑ risk of hepatotoxicity); Geri: Use lowest possible dose (may have ↑ risk of hepatotoxicity); OB: Use only if benefit outweighs potential risk to fetus.

Adverse Reactions/Side Effects

CNS: drowsiness, muscle weakness, confusion, dizziness, headache, insomnia, malaise, nervousness.

EENT: excessive lacrimation, visual disturbances.

Resp: dyspnea, pleural effusions, respiratory depression. **CV:** changes in BP, heart failure, tachycardia. **GI:** HEPATOTOXICITY, diarrhea, anorexia, cramps, dysphagia, GI bleeding, nausea, vomiting. **GU:** crystalluria, dysuria, frequency, erectile dysfunction, incontinence, nocturia. **Derm:** flushing, pruritus, sweating, urticaria. **Hemat:** anemia, aplastic anemia, eosinophilia, leukopenia, thrombocytopenia. **Local:** irritation at IV site, phlebitis. **MS:** myalgia. **Misc:** ANAPHYLAXIS, chills, drooling, fever.

Interactions

Drug-Drug: Calcium channel blockers may ↑ risk of cardiovsacular collapse; avoid concomitant use. Additive CNS depression with **CNS depressants**, including **alcohol, antihistamines, opioid analgesics, sedative/hypnotics**, and parenteral **magnesium sulfate**. ↑ risk of hepatotoxicity with other **hepatotoxic agents** or **estrogens**. ↑ risk of arrhythmias with **verapamil**. ↑ neuromuscular blocking effects of **vecuronium**.

Drug-Natural Products: Concomitant use of **kava-kava, valerian, chamomile,** or **hops** can ↑ CNS depression.

Route/Dosage

PO (Adults): *Spasticity*—25 mg once daily for 7 days, then 25 mg 2 times daily for 7 days, then 50 mg 3 times daily for 7 days, then 100 mg 3 times daily; may ↑ to 100 mg 4 times daily, if needed. *Prevention of malignant hyperthermia*—4–8 mg/kg/day in 3–4 divided doses for 1–2 days before procedure, last dose 3–4 hr preop. *Posthyperthermic crisis follow-up*—4–8 mg/kg/day in 3–4 divided doses for 1–3 days after IV treatment.

PO (Children >5 yr): *Spasticity*—0.5 mg/kg once daily for 7 days, then 0.5 mg/kg 3 times daily for 7 days, then 1 mg/kg 3 times daily for 7 days, then 2 mg/kg 3 times daily (not to exceed 400 mg/day). *Prevention of malignant hyperthermia*—4–8 mg/kg/day in 3–4 divided doses for 1–2 days before procedure, last dose 3–4 hr preop. *Posthyperthermic crisis follow-up*—4–8 mg/kg/day in 3–4 divided doses for 1–3 days after IV treatment.

IV (Adults and Children): *Treatment of malignant hyperthermia*—at least 1 mg/kg, continued until symptoms ↓ or a cumulative dose of 10 mg/kg has been given. If symptoms reappear, dose may be repeated. *Prevention of malignant hyperthermia*—2.5 mg/kg given 75 min before surgery.

Availability (generic available)

Capsules: 25 mg, 50 mg, 100 mg. **Powder for injection:** 20 mg/vial, 250 mg/vial.

NURSING IMPLICATIONS

Assessment

- Assess bowel function periodically. Persistent diarrhea may warrant discontinuation of therapy.
- **Muscle Spasticity:** Assess neuromuscular status and muscle spasticity before initiating and periodically during therapy to determine response.
- **Malignant Hyperthermia:** Assess previous anesthesia history of all surgical patients. Also assess for family history of reactions to anesthesia (malignant hyperthermia or perioperative death).
- Monitor ECG, vital signs, electrolytes, and urine output continuously when administering IV for malignant hyperthermia.
- Monitor patient for difficulty swallowing and choking during meals on the day of administration.
- ***Lab Test Considerations:*** Monitor liver function frequently during therapy. Liver function abnormalities (↑ AST, ALT, alkaline phosphatase, bilirubin, GGTP) may require discontinuation of therapy.
- Evaluate renal function and CBC before and periodically during therapy in patients receiving prolonged therapy.

Potential Nursing Diagnoses

Impaired physical mobility (Indications)
Acute pain (Indications)
Risk for injury (Side Effects)

Implementation

- **PO:** If gastric irritation becomes a problem, may be administered with food. Oral suspensions may be made by opening capsules and adding them to fruit juices or other liquids. Drink immediately after mixing.
- Oral dose for spasticity should be divided into 4 doses/day.
- Oral dose is not indicated for neuroleptic malignant syndrome.

IV Administration

- Reconstitute each 20 mg of **Dantrium** with 60 mL of sterile water for injection (without a bacteriostatic agent). Shake until solution is clear. Solution must be used within 6 hr. Protect diluted solution from direct light.
- Reconstitute **Ryanodex** by adding 5 mL of Sterile Water for Injection; do not reconstitute with other solutions. Shake vial to ensure uniform orange suspension. Do not administer solutions that are discolored or contain particulate matter. Solution is stable for 6 hrs at room temperature.

Treatment of Malignant Hyperthermia

- **IV Push:** Administer reconstituted solution without further dilution. ***Rate:*** Administer each single dose by rapid continuous IV push through Y-tubing. Follow immediately with subsequent doses as indicated. Medication is very irritating to tissues; observe infusion site frequently to avoid extravasation.

Prevention of Malignant Hyperthermia

- **IV Push:** Rates of products for prevention differ. ***Rate:*** Inject **Ryanodex**over at least 1 min starting 75 min before surgery into catheter with free flowing

0.9% NaCl or D5W or into a patent indwelling catheter, flush before and after injection.

- **Intermittent Infusion:** Reconstitute required number of **Dantrium** vials as above and transfer to a larger volume sterile plastic bag (do not use glass bottles). ***Rate:*** Administer over 1 hr beginning 75 min before anesthesia.
- **Y-Site Compatibility:** acyclovir, paclitaxel, palonosetron.
- **Y-Site Incompatibility:** alemtuzumab, alfentanil, amikacin, aminophylline, amphotericin B colloidal, amphotericin B lipid complex, ampicillin, ampicillin/sulbactam, anidulafungin, argatroban, arsenic trioxide, ascorbic acid, asparaginase, atropine, azathioprine, aztreonam, benztropine, bivalirudin, bleomycin, bumetanide, buprenorphine, butorphanol, caclium chloride, calcium gluconate, carmustine, caspofungin, cefotaxime, cefotetan, cefoxitin, ceftazidime, ceftriaxone, cefuroxime, chloramphenicol, chlorpromazine, cisplatin, clindamycin, cyanocobalamin, cyclosporine, dactinomycin, daptomycin, dexamethasone, diazepam, diazoxide, digoxin, diltiazem, diphenhydramine, dobutamine, docetaxel, dopamine, doxorubicin liposome, doxycycline, enalaprilat, ephedrine, epinephrine, epoetin alfa, ertapenem, erythromycin, esmolol, etoposide, etoposide phosphate, famotidine, fenoldopam, fentanyl, fluconazole, fludarabine, folic acid, foscarnet, fosphenytoin, furosemide, ganciclovir, gemcitabine, gentamicin, glycopyrrolate, granisetron, haloperidol, heparin, hetastarch, hydralazine, hydrocortisone, hydromorphone, hydroxyzine, idarubicin, imipenem/cilastatin, indomethacin, insulin, irinotecan, isoproterenol, ketorolac, labetalol, leucovorin, lidocaine, linezolid, lorazepam, magnesium sulfate, mannitol, mechlorethamine, meperidine, mesna, metaraminol, methyldopate, methylprednisolone, metoclopramide, metoprolol, metronidazole, midazolam, milrinone, mitoxantrone, morphine, moxifloxacin, multivitamins, mycophenolate, nafcillin, nalbuphine, naloxone, nesiritide, nitroglycerin, nitroprusside, norepinephrine, octreotide, ondansetron, oxacillin, oxaliplatin, oxytocin, pamidronate, pancuronium, pantoprazole, papaverine, pemetrexed, penicillin G, pentamidine, pentazocine, pentobarbital, phenobarbital, phenylephrine, phenytoin, phytonadione, piperacillin/tazobactam, potassium acetate, potassium chloride, procainamide, prochlorperazine, promethazine, propranolol, protamine, pyridoxime, ranitidine, sodium acetate, sodium bicarbonate, streptokinase, succinylcholine, sufentanil, tacrolimus, teniposide, theophylline, thiamine, thiotepa, tigecycline, tirofiban, tobramycin, tolazoline, topotecan, trimethoprim/sulfamethoxazole, vancomycin, vasopressin, vecuronium, verapamil, vinblastine, vinorelbine, voriconazole, zoledronic acid.

Patient/Family Teaching

- Advise patient not to take more medication than the amount prescribed, to minimize risk of hepatotoxicity and other side effects. If a dose is missed, do not take unless remembered within 1 hr. Do not double doses.
- May cause dizziness, drowsiness, visual disturbances, and muscle weakness. Advise patient to avoid driving and other activities requiring alertness until response to drug is known. After IV dose for surgery, patients may experience decreased grip strength, leg weakness, light-headedness, and difficulty swallowing for up to 48 hr. Caution patients to avoid activities requiring alertness and to use caution when walking down stairs and eating during this period.
- Advise patient to avoid taking alcohol or other CNS depressants concurrently with this medication.
- Instruct patient to notify health care professional if rash; itching; yellow eyes or skin; dark urine; or clay-colored, bloody, or black, tarry stools occur or if nausea, weakness, malaise, fatigue, or diarrhea persists. May require discontinuation of therapy.
- Advise patient to wear sunscreen and protective clothing to prevent photosensitivity reactions.
- Emphasize the importance of follow-up exams to check progress in long-term therapy and blood tests to monitor for side effects.
- **Malignant Hyperthermia:** Patients with malignant hyperthemia should carry identification describing disease process at all times.

Evaluation/Desired Outcomes

- Relief of muscle spasm in musculoskeletal conditions. One wk or more may be required to see improvement; if there is no observed improvement in 45 days, the medication is usually discontinued.
- Prevention of or decrease in temperature and skeletal rigidity in malignant hyperthermia.

DAPTOmycin (dap-to-**mye**-sin)

Cubicin

Classification

Therapeutic: anti-infectives

Pharmacologic: cyclic lipopeptide antibacterial agents

Pregnancy Category B

Indications

Complicated skin and skin structure infections caused by aerobic Gram-positive bacteria.

D

Action

Causes rapid depolarization of membrane potential following binding to bacterial membrane; this results in inhibition of protein, DNA, and RNA synthesis. **Therapeutic Effects:** Death of bacteria with resolution of infection. **Spectrum:** Active against *Staphylococcus aureus* (including methicillin-resistant strains), *Streptococcus pyogenes*, *S. pyogenes agalactiae*, some *S. dysgalactiae*, and *Enterococcus faecalis* (vancomycin-susceptible strains).

Pharmacokinetics

Absorption: IV administration results in complete bioavailability.

Distribution: Unknown.

Protein Binding: 92%.

Metabolism and Excretion: Metabolism not known; mostly excreted by kidneys.

Half-life: 8.1 hr.

TIME/ACTION PROFILE

ROUTE	ONSET	PEAK	DURATION
IV	rapid	end of infusion	24 hr

Contraindications/Precautions

Contraindicated in: Hypersensitivity.

Use Cautiously in: CCr <30 mL/min (dose ↓ required); Moderate-to-severe renal impairment (may have ↓ clinical response); Geri: May have ↓ clinical response with ↑ risk of adverse reactions; OB: Use only if clearly needed; Lactation: Lactation; Pedi: Safety and effectiveness not established (↑ risk of muscular, neuromuscular, and CNS effects in children <1 yr; avoid use).

Adverse Reactions/Side Effects

CNS: dizziness. **Resp:** EOSINOPHILIC PNEUMONIA, dyspnea. **CV:** hypertension, hypotension. **GI:** CLOSTRIDIUM DIFFICILE-ASSOCIATED DIARRHEA (CDAD), constipation, diarrhea, nausea, vomiting, ↑ liver enzymes. **GU:** renal failure. **Derm:** DRUG RASH WITH EOSINOPHILIA AND SYSTEMIC SYMPTOMS (DRESS), pruritus, rash. **Hemat:** anemia. **Local:** injection site reactions. **MS:** ↑ CPK. **Misc:** ANGIOEDEMA, fever.

Interactions

Drug-Drug: Tobramycin ↑ blood levels. Concurrent **HMG-CoA reductase inhibitors** may ↑ the risk of myopathy.

Route/Dosage

IV (Adults): 4 mg/kg every 24 hr.

Renal Impairment

IV (Adults): *CCr <30 mL/min*—4 mg/kg every 48 hr.

Availability (generic available)

Powder for injection: 500 mg/vial.

NURSING IMPLICATIONS

Assessment

- Assess for infection (vital signs; appearance of wound, sputum, urine, and stool; WBC) at beginning of and throughout therapy.
- Monitor bowel function. Diarrhea, abdominal cramping, fever, and bloody stools should be reported to health care professional promptly as a sign of Clostridium difficile-associated diarrhea (CDAD). May begin up to several weeks following cessation of therapy.
- Monitor for signs and symptoms of eosinophilic pneumonia (new onset or worsening fever, dyspnea, difficulty breathing, new infiltrates on chest imaging studies). Discontinue daptomycin if symptoms occur.
- Monitor for development of muscle pain or weakness, particularly of distal extremities. Discontinue daptomycin in patients with unexplained signs and symptoms of myopathy in conjunction with CPK elevation >1000 U/L, or in patients without reported symptoms who have marked elevations in CPK >2000 U/L. Consider temporarily suspending agents associated with rhabdomyolysis (HMG-CoA reductase inhibitors) in patients receiving daptomycin.
- ***Lab Test Considerations:*** Monitor CPK weekly, more frequently in patients with unexplained ↑. Discontinue daptomycin if CPK >1000 units/L and signs and symptoms of myopathy occur. In patients with renal insufficiency, monitor both renal function and CPK more frequently.
- May cause false prolongation of PT and ↑ INR.

Potential Nursing Diagnoses

Risk for infection (Indications, Side Effects)

Implementation

- Do not confuse daptomycin with dactinomycin.

IV Administration

- **IV Push:** Reconstitute 500-mg vial with 10 mL of 0.9% NaCl inserted toward wall of vial. Rotate vial gently to wet powder. Allow to stand for 10 min undisturbed. Swirl vial gently to completely reconstitute solution. Reconstituted vials are stable for 12 hr at room temperature or 48 hr if refrigerated. ***Concentration:*** 50 mg/mL. ***Rate:*** Administer over 2 min.
- **Intermittent Infusion:** ***Diluent:*** Dilute further in 50 mL of 0.9% NaCl. Solution is stable for 12 hr at room temperature or 48 hr if refrigerated. Do not administer solutions that are cloudy or contain a precipitate. ***Rate:*** Infuse over 30 min. Do not infuse daptomycin with ReadyMED elastomeric infusion pumps due to incompatibility.
- **Y-Site Compatibility:** alfentanil, amifostine, amikacin, aminocaproic acid, aminophylline, amiodarone, amphotericin B liposome, ampicillin, ampicillin/sulbactam, argatroban, arsenic trioxide,

azithromycin, aztreonam, bivalirudin, bleomycin, bumetanide, buprenorphine, busulfan, butorphanol, calcium chloride, calcium gluconate, cangrelor, carboplatin, carmustine, caspofungin, cefazolin, cefepime, cefotaxime, cefotetan, cefoxitin, ceftazidime, ceftriaxone, cefuroxime, chloramphenicol, chlorpromazine, ciprofloxacin, cisatracurium, cisplatin, clindamycin, cyclophosphamide, cyclosporine, dacarbazine, dactinomycin, daunorubicin hydrochloride, dexamethasone sodium phosphate, dexmedetomidine, dexrazoxane, digoxin, diltiazem, diphenhydramine, dobutamine, docetaxel, dolasetron, dopamine, doripenem, doxorubicin hydrochloride, doxorubicin liposome, doxycycline, droperidol, enalaprilat, ephedrine, epinephrine, epirubicin, eptifibatide, ertapenem, erythromycin, esmolol, etoposide, etoposide phosphate, famotidine, fenoldopam, fentanyl, fluconazole, fludarabine, fluorouracil, foscarnet, fosphenytoin, furosemide, ganciclovir, gentamicin, glycopyrrolate, granisetron, haloperidol, heparin, hydralazine, hydrocortisone sodium succinate, hydromorphone, idarubicin, ifosfamide, insulin, irinotecan, isoproterenol, ketorolac, labetalol, leucovorin, levofloxacin, lidocaine, linezolid, lorazepam, magnesium sulfate, mannitol, mechlorethamine, melphalan, meperidine, meropenem, mesna, methylprednisolone sodium succinate, metoclopramide, metoprolol, midazolam, milrinone, mitoxantrone, morphine, moxifloxacin, mycophenolate, nafcillin, nalbuphine, naloxone, nicardipine, nitroprusside, norepinephrine, octreotide, ondansetron, oxaliplatin, oxytocin, paclitaxel, palonosetron, pamidronate, pancuronium, pemetrexed, pentamidine, phenobarbital, phenylephrine, piperacillin/tazobactam, potassium acetate, potassium chloride, potassium phosphates, procainamide, prochlorperazine, promethazine, propranolol, quinupristin/dalfopristin, ranitidine, rocuronium, sodium acetate, sodium bicarbonate, sodium citrate, sodium phosphates, succinylcholine, tacrolimus, teniposide, theophylline, thiotepa, tigecycline, tirofiban, tobramycin, topotecan, trimethoprim/sulfamethoxazole, vasopressin, vecuronium, verapamil, vinblastine, vincristine, vinorelbine, voriconazole, zidovudine, zoledronic acid.

- **Y-Site Incompatibility:** acyclovir, alemtuzumab, allopurinol, amphotericin B colloidal, amphotericin B lipid complex, cytarabine, dantrolene, gemcitabine, imipenem/cilastatin, methotrexate, metronidazole, mitomycin, nesiritide, nitroglycerin, pantoprazole, pentazocine, pentobarbital, phenytoin, remifentanil, streptozocin, sufentanil, thiopental, vancomycin.
- **Solution Incompatibility:** D5W.

Patient/Family Teaching

- Inform patient of purpose of daptomycin.
- Instruct patient to notify health care professional if fever and diarrhea develop, especially if stool contains blood, pus, or mucus. Advise patient not to treat diarrhea without consulting health care professional.
- May cause dizziness. Caution patient to avoid driving or other activities requiring alertness until response to medication is known.
- Advise patient to notify health care professional immediately if signs and symptoms of eosinophilic pneumonia occur.

Evaluation/Desired Outcomes

- Resolution of the signs and symptoms of infection. Length of time for complete resolution depends on the organism and site of infection.

REMS

darbepoetin (dar-be-**poh**-e-tin)

Aranesp

Classification

Therapeutic: antianemics

Pharmacologic: hormones (rDNA), erythropoiesis stimulating agents (ESA)

Pregnancy Category C

Indications

Anemia associated with chronic kidney disease (CKD). Chemotherapy-induced anemia in patients with nonmyeloid malignancies.

Action

Stimulates erythropoiesis (production of red blood cells). **Therapeutic Effects:** Maintains and may elevate red blood cell counts, decreasing the need for transfusions.

Pharmacokinetics

Absorption: 30–50% following subcut administration; IV administration results in complete bioavailability.

Distribution: Confined to the intravascular space.

Metabolism and Excretion: Unknown.

Half-life: *Subcut*—49 hr; *IV*—21 hr.

TIME/ACTION PROFILE (↑ in RBCs)

ROUTE	ONSET	PEAK	DURATION
IV, Subcut	2–6 wk	unknown	unknown

Contraindications/Precautions

Contraindicated in: Hypersensitivity; Uncontrolled hypertension; Patients receiving chemotherapy when anticipated outcome is cure.

Use Cautiously in: Cardiovascular disease or stroke; Underlying hematologic diseases, including hemolytic anemia, sickle-cell anemia, thalassemia and porphyria (safety not established); OB, Lactation: Safety not established.

Adverse Reactions/Side Effects

CNS: SEIZURES, dizziness, fatigue, headache, weakness. **Resp:** cough, dyspnea, bronchitis. **CV:** HF, MI, STROKE, THROMBOEMBOLIC EVENTS (especially with hemoglobin >11 g/dL), edema, hypertension, hypotension, chest pain. **GI:** abdominal pain, nausea, diarrhea, vomiting, constipation. **Derm:** pruritus. **Hemat:** pure red cell aplasia. **MS:** myalgia, arthralgia, back pain, limb pain. **Misc:** fever, allergic reactions, flu-like syndrome, sepsis, ↑ mortality and ↑ tumor growth (with hemoglobin ≥12 g/dL).

Interactions

Drug-Drug: None reported.

Route/Dosage

Anemia due to Chronic Kidney Disease

(Do not initiate if hemoglobin ≥10 g/dL; should only consider initiating therapy in patients not on dialysis if rate of hemoglobin decline indicates likelihood of requiring a red blood cell transfusion and a goal is to reduce the risk of alloimmunization and/or red blood cell transfusion risks).

IV, Subcut (Adults): *Starting treatment with darbepoetin (no previous epoetin)*—0.45 mcg/kg once weekly or 0.75 mcg/kg q 2 wk (for patients on dialysis); 0.45 mcg/kg q 4 wk (for patients not on dialysis); use lowest dose sufficient to ↓ the need for red blood cell transfusions (do not exceed hemoglobin of 10 g/dL [patients not on dialysis] or 11 g/dL [patients on dialysis]); if Hgb ↑ by >1.0 g/dL in 2 wk, ↓ dose by 25%; if Hgb ↑ by <1.0 g/dL after 4 wk of therapy (with adequate iron stores), ↑ dose by 25%; do not ↑ dose more frequently than q 4 wk. *Conversion from epoetin to darbepoetin*—weekly epoetin dose <2500 units = 6.25 mcg/week darbepoetin, weekly epoetin dose 2500–4999 units = 12.5 mcg/week darbepoetin, weekly epoetin dose 5000–10,999 units = 25 mcg/week darbepoetin, weekly epoetin dose 11,000–17,999 units = 40 mcg/week darbepoetin, weekly epoetin dose 18,000–33,999 units = 60 mcg/week darbepoetin, weekly epoetin dose 34,000–89,999 units = 100 mcg/week darbepoetin, weekly epoetin dose >90,000 units = 200 mcg/week darbepoetin.

IV, Subcut (Children): *Starting treatment with darbepoetin (no previous epoetin)*—0.45 mcg/kg once weekly (may also start with 0.75 mcg/kg q 2 wk in patients not on dialysis); use lowest dose sufficient to ↓ the need for red blood cell transfusions (do not exceed hemoglobin of 12 g/dL; if Hgb ↑ by >1.0 g/dL in 2 wk, ↓ dose by 25%; if Hgb ↑ by <1.0 g/dL after 4 wk of therapy (with adequate iron stores), ↑ dose by 25%; do not ↑ dose more frequently than q 4 wk.

Anemia due to Chemotherapy

(Use only for chemotherapy-related anemia and discontinue when chemotherapy course is completed; do not initiate if hemoglobin ≥10 g/dL.).

Subcut (Adults): 2.25 mcg/kg weekly or 500 mcg q 3 wk; target Hgb should not exceed 12 g/dL. If Hgb ↑ by >1.0 g/dL in 2 wk or or reaches a level needed to avoid red blood cell transfusions, ↓ dose by 40%; if Hgb ↑ by <1.0 g/dL after 6 wk of therapy, ↑ dose to 4.5 mcg/kg weekly.

Availability

Albumin solution for injection: 25 mcg/1 mL, 40 mcg/1 mL, 60 mcg/1 mL, 100 mcg/1 mL, 150 mcg/0.75-mL, 200 mcg/1 mL, 300 mcg/1 mL, 500 mcg/1 mL. **Pre-filled syringes:** 10 mcg/0.4 mL, 25 mcg/0.42 mL, 40 mcg/0.4 mL, 60 mcg/0.3 mL, 100 mcg/0.5 mL, 150 mcg/0.3 mL, 200 mcg/0.4 mL, 300 mcg/0.6 mL, 500 mcg/1 mL.

NURSING IMPLICATIONS

Assessment

- Monitor BP before and during therapy. Inform health care professional if severe hypertension is present or if BP begins to increase. Additional antihypertensive therapy may be required during initiation of therapy.
- Monitor response for symptoms of anemia (fatigue, dyspnea, pallor).
- Monitor dialysis shunts (thrill and bruit) and status of artificial kidney during hemodialysis. May need to increase heparin dose to prevent clotting. Monitor patients with underlying vascular disease for impaired circulation.
- Monitor for allergic reactions (rash, utricaria). Discontinue darbepoetin if signs of anaphylaxis (dyspnea, laryngeal swelling) occur.
- **Lab Test Considerations:** May cause ↑ in WBCs and platelets. May ↓ bleeding times.
- Monitor serum ferritin, transferrin, and iron levels prior to and during therapy to assess need for concurrent iron therapy. Administer supplemental iron therapy if transferrin saturation <20% or serum ferritin is <100 mcg/mL.
- Monitor hemoglobin before and weekly during initial therapy, for 4 wk after a change in dose, and regularly after target range has been reached and maintenance dose is determined. Monitor other hematopoietic parameters (CBC with differential and platelet count) before and periodically during therapy. *If hemoglobin ↑ of more than 1.0 g/dL in any 2-wk period or hemoglobin reaches a level needed to avoid RBC transfusion,* ↓ dose by 40%. *If hemoglobin exceeds a level needed to avoid RBC transfusion,* withhold dose until hemoglobin approaches level where RBC transfusions may be required and reinitiate at a dose 40% below the previous dose. *If hemoglobin ↑ by less than 1 g/dL and remains below 10 g/dL after 6 wk of therapy,* ↑ dose to 4.5

mcg/kg/wk (if on weekly therapy) or do not adjust dose (if on every 3 wk schedule). *If there is no response as measured by hemoglobin levels or if RBC transfusions are still required after 8 wks of therapy,* following completion of a chemotherapy course, discontinue darbepoetin. Hemoglobin >11 g/dL increases the likelihood of life-threatening cardiovascular complications, cardiac arrest, neurologic events (seizures, stroke), hypertensive reactions, HF, vascular thrombosis/ischemia/infarction, acute MI, and fluid overload/edema.

- Only prescribers and hospitals enrolled in the *ESA APPRISE Oncology Program* can provide darbepoetin for patients with cancer. Visit www.esa-apprise.com or call 1-866-284-8089.
- If ↑ in hemoglobin is less than 1 g/dL over 4 wk and iron stores are adequate, dose may be ↑ by 25% of previous dose. Use the lowest dose possible to avoid transfusions.
- Monitor renal function studies and electrolytes closely; resulting increased sense of well-being may lead to decreased compliance with other therapies for renal failure.

Potential Nursing Diagnoses

Activity intolerance (Indications)

Implementation

- Transfusions are still required for severe symptomatic anemia. Supplemental iron should be initiated with darbepoetin and continued during therapy. Correct deficiencies of folic acid or vitamin B_{12} prior to therapy.
- Institute seizure precautions in patients who experience greater than a 1.0 g/dL increase in hemoglobin in a 2-wk period or exhibit any change in neurologic status.
- *For conversion from epoetin alfa to darbepoetin,* if epoetin was administered 2–3 times/wk administer darbepoetin once a week. If patient was receiving epoetin once/wk, darbepoetin may be administered once every 2 wk. Route of administration should remain consistent.
- Dose adjustments should not be more frequent than once/month.
- Do not shake vial; inactivation of medication may occur. Do not administer vials containing solution that is discolored or contains particulate matter. Discard vial immediately after withdrawing dose. Do not pool unused portions.
- **Subcut:** This route is often used for patients not requiring dialysis.

IV Administration

- **IV Push:** Administer undiluted. ***Rate:*** May be administered as direct injection or bolus over 1–3 min into IV tubing or via venous line at end of dialysis session.
- **Y-Site Incompatibility:** Do not administer in conjunction with other drugs or solutions.

Patient/Family Teaching

- Explain *ESA APPRISE Oncology Program* and rationale for concurrent iron therapy (increased red blood cell production requires iron). Instruct patient to read the *Medication Guide* prior to beginning therapy. Inform patients of risks and benefits of darbepoetin. Inform patients with cancer that they must sign the patient-health care provider acknowledgment form before the start of each treatment course.
- Discuss ways of preventing self-injury in patients at risk for seizures. Driving and activities requiring continuous alertness should be avoided.
- Inform patient that use of darbepoetin may result in shortened overall survival and/or ↓ time to tumor progression. May also cause MI or stroke. Advise patient to notify health care professional immediately if chest pain; trouble breathing or shortness of breath; pain in legs, with or without swelling; a cool or pale arm or leg; sudden confusion, trouble speaking, or trouble understanding others' speech; sudden numbness or weakness in face, arm, or leg, especially on one side of body; sudden trouble seeing; sudden trouble walking, dizziness, loss of balance or coordination; loss of consciousness (fainting); or hemodialysis vascular access stops working.
- **Anemia of Chronic Kidney Disease**Stress importance of compliance with dietary restrictions, medications, and dialysis. Foods high in iron and low in potassium include liver, pork, veal, beef, mustard and turnip greens, peas, eggs, broccoli, kale, blackberries, strawberries, apple juice, watermelon, oatmeal, and enriched bread. Darbepoetin will result in increased sense of well-being, but it does not cure underlying disease.
- **Home Care Issues:** Home dialysis patients determined to be able to safely and effectively administer darbepoetin should be taught proper dose, administration technique with syringe, auto-injector or IV use, and disposal of equipment. *Information for Patients and Caregivers* should be provided to patient along with medication.

Evaluation/Desired Outcomes

- Increase in hemoglobin not to exceed 11 g/dL with improvement in symptoms of anemia in patients with chronic renal failure or with chemotherapy-induced anemia.

darifenacin (dar-i-fen-a-sin)

Enablex

Classification

Therapeutic: urinary tract antispasmodics

Pharmacologic: anticholinergics

Pregnancy Category C

Indications

Overactive bladder with symptoms (urge incontinence, urgency, frequency).

Action

Acts as a muscarinic (cholinergic) receptor antagonist; antagonizes bladder smooth muscle contraction.

Therapeutic Effects: Decreased symptoms of overactive bladder.

Pharmacokinetics

Absorption: 15–19% absorbed.

Distribution: Unknown.

Protein Binding: 98%.

Metabolism and Excretion: Extensively metabolized by the CYP2D6 enzyme system in most individuals; poor metabolizers (7% of Caucasians, 2% of African Americans) have less CYP2D6 activity with less metabolism occurring. Some metabolism via CYP3A4 enzyme system. 60% excreted renally as metabolites, 40% in feces as metabolites.

Half-life: 13–19 hr.

TIME/ACTION PROFILE

ROUTE	ONSET	PEAK	DURATION
PO	unknown	7 hr	24 hr

Contraindications/Precautions

Contraindicated in: Hypersensitivity; Urinary retention; Gastric retention; Uncontrolled angle-closure glaucoma; Severe hepatic impairment.

Use Cautiously in: Concurrent use of CYP3A4 inhibitors (use lower dose/clinical monitoring may be necessary); Moderate hepatic impairment (lower dose recommended); Bladder outflow obstruction; GI obstructive disorders, ↓ GI motility, severe constipation or ulcerative colitis; Myasthenia gravis; Angle-closure glaucoma; Lactation, Pedi: Safety not established; OB: Use only if maternal benefit outweighs fetal risk.

Adverse Reactions/Side Effects

CNS: confusion, dizziness, drowsiness, hallucinations, headache. **EENT:** blurred vision. **GI:** constipation, dry mouth, dyspepsia, nausea. **Metab:** heat intolerance. **Misc:** ANGIOEDEMA.

Interactions

Drug-Drug: Blood levels and risk of toxicity are ↑ by concurrent use of strong CYP3A4 inhibitors including **ketoconazole**, **itraconazole**, **ritonavir**, **nelfinavir**, **clarithromycin**, and **nefazodone**; daily dose should not exceed 7.5 mg. Concurrent use of moderate inhibitors of CYP3A4, especially those with narrow therapeutic indices, including **flecainide**, **thioridazine**, and **tricyclic antidepressants**, should be undertaken with caution.

Route/Dosage

PO (Adults): 7.5 mg once daily, may be ↑ after 2 wk to 15 mg once daily.

Availability

Extended-release tablets: 7.5 mg, 15 mg. **Cost:** All strengths $599.48/90.

NURSING IMPLICATIONS

Assessment

- Monitor voiding pattern and assess symptoms of overactive bladder (urinary urgency, urinary incontinence, urinary frequency) to and periodically during therapy.

Potential Nursing Diagnoses

Impaired urinary elimination (Indications)

Implementation

- Do not confuse Enablex with Effexor XR.
- **PO:** Administer once daily without regard to food. Extended-release tablets must be swallowed whole; do not break, crush, or chew.

Patient/Family Teaching

- Instruct patient to take darifenacin as directed. If a dose is missed, skip dose and take next day; do not take 2 doses in same day. Advise patient to read the *Patient Information* before starting therapy and with each Rx refill in case of changes.
- Do not share darifenacin with others; may be dangerous.
- Inform patient of potential anticholinergic side effects (constipation, urinary retention, blurred vision, heat prostration in a hot environment).
- May cause dizziness, drowsiness, confusion, and blurred vision. Caution patient to avoid driving and other activities that require alertness until response to medication is known.
- Instruct patient to notify health care professional of all Rx or OTC medications, vitamins, or herbal products being taken and consult health care professional before taking any new medications.
- Advise female patient to notify health care professional if pregnancy is planned or suspected or if breast feeding.

Evaluation/Desired Outcomes

- Decrease in symptoms of overactive bladder (urge urinary incontinence, urgency, frequency).

darunavir (da-ru-na-veer)

Prezista

Classification

Therapeutic: antiretrovirals

Pharmacologic: protease inhibitors

Pregnancy Category C

Indications

HIV infection (must be used with ritonavir and with other antiretrovirals).

Action

Inhibits HIV-1 protease, selectively inhibiting the cleavage of HIV-encoded specific polyproteins in infected cells. This prevents the formation of mature virus particles. **Therapeutic Effects:** Increased CD4 cell counts and decreased viral load with subsequent slowed progression of HIV infection and its sequelae.

Pharmacokinetics

Absorption: *Without ritonavir*—37% absorbed following oral administration; *with ritonavir*—82%. Food ↑ absorption by 30%.

Distribution: Unknown.

Protein Binding: 95% bound to plasma proteins.

Metabolism and Excretion: Extensively metabolized by CYP3A enzyme system. 41% eliminated unchanged in feces, 8% in urine.

Half-life: 15 hr.

TIME/ACTION PROFILE

ROUTE	ONSET	PEAK	DURATION
PO	unknown	2.5–4 hr	12 hr

Contraindications/Precautions

Contraindicated in: Concurrent alfuzosin, dronedarone, colchicine (in renal/hepatic impairment), ranolazine, sildenafil (Revatio), ergot derivatives, midazolam (PO), pimozide, triazolam, lovastatin, simvastatin, rifampin, or St. John's wort; Lactation: HIV may be transmitted in human milk; Pedi: Children <3 yr.

Use Cautiously in: Hepatic impairment; Sulfa allergy; Geri: Consider age-related impairment in hepatic function, concurrent chronic disease states and drug therapy; OB: Use only if maternal benefit outweighs fetal risk.

Adverse Reactions/Side Effects

Based on concurrent use with ritonavir.

GI: HEPATOTOXICITY, constipation, diarrhea, nausea, vomiting. **Endo:** hyperglycemia. **Metab:** body fat redistribution. **Derm:** DRUG RASH WITH EOSINOPHILIA AND SYSTEMIC SYMPTOMS, STEVENS-JOHNSON SYNDROME, TOXIC EPIDERMAL NECROLYSIS, rash, acute generalized exanthematous pustulosis. **Misc:** immune reconstitution syndrome.

Interactions

Drug-Drug: Darunavir and ritonavir are both inhibitors of CYP3A, CYP2D6, and P-gp and are metabolized by CYP3A. Multiple drug-drug interactions can be expected with drugs that share, inhibit, or induce these pathways. Consult product information for more specific details. ↑ blood levels and risk of toxicity from **ergot derivatives (dihydroergotamine, ergotamine, methylergonovine)**, **sildenafil (Revatio)**, **alfuzosin**, **dronedarone**, **ranolazine**, **pimozide**, **lovastatin**, **simvastatin**, **midazolam (oral)**, and **triazolam**; concurrent use is contraindicated. May ↑ **colchicine** levels and cause serious/life-threatening reactions; ↓ dose of colchicine; concurrent use contraindicated in patients with renal or hepatic impairment. **Rifampin** ↑ metabolism and may ↓ antiretroviral effectiveness, concurrent use is contraindicated. Concurrent use with **indinavir** may ↑ darunavir and indinavir levels. ↑ levels and risk of myopathy from **atorvastatin**, **rosuvastatin**, or **pravastatin**; use lowest dose of these agents; do not exceed atorvastatin dose of 20 mg/day. Concurrent use with **efavirenz** results in ↓ darunavir levels and ↑ efavirenz levels; use combination cautiously. **Lopinavir/ritonavir** may ↓ levels; concurrent use not recommended. **Saquinavir** may ↓ levels; concurrent use not recommended. May ↑ **maraviroc** levels; ↓ maraviroc dose to 150 mg twice daily. May ↑ levels of **lidocaine**, **quinidine**, **disopyramide**, **mexiletine**, **propafenone**, **flecainide**, and **amiodarone**; use cautiously and with available blood level monitoring. ↑ **digoxin** levels; blood level monitoring recommended. May ↑ **carbamazepine** levels; blood level monitoring recommended. May ↓ **phenytoin** or **phenobarbital** levels; blood level monitoring recommended. May ↓ levels of **warfarin**; monitor INR. May ↑ levels of **trazodone**, **amitriptyline**, **desipramine**, **imipramine**, and **nortriptyline**; use cautiously and ↓ dose if necessary. May ↑ levels of **clarithromycin**; ↓ dose of clarithromycin if CCr ≤60 mL/min. May ↑ levels of **ketoconazole** and **itraconazole**; do not exceed itraconazole or ketoconazole dose >200 m g/day. **Ketoconazole** and **itraconazole** may ↑ levels. May ↓ levels of **voriconazole**; concurrent use not recommended. Concurrent use with **rifabutin** ↑ rifabutin levels and ↑ darunavir levels; (may be due to ritonavir); ↓ rifabutin dose to 150 mg every other day. **Rifapentin** may ↓ levels; concurrent use not recommended. May ↑ levels of **beta-blockers**; may need to ↓ dose. May ↑ levels of **amlodipine**, **diltiazem**, **felodipine**, **nifedipine**, **nicardipine**, or **verapamil**; monitor clinical response carefully. **Dexamethasone** may ↓ levels and effectiveness. May ↑ levels and the risk of Cushing's syndrome and adrenal suppression with systemic **bu-**

desonide and **prednisone**; consider alternative therapy. May ↑ levels of inhaled/nasal **fluticasone** and **budesonide**; choose alternative inhaled/nasal corticosteroid. May ↑ levels of **cyclosporine**, **tacrolimus**, or **sirolimus**; blood level monitoring recommended. May ↑ levels of **everolimus**; concurrent use not recommended. May ↓ levels of **methadone**. May ↑ **risperidone** and **thioridazine** levels; may need to ↓ dose. May ↑ levels of **sildenafil**, **vardenafil**, **tadalafil**, or **avanafil**; single dose should not exceed the following(sildenafil 25 mg in 48 hr; vardenafil 2.5 mg in 72 hr; tadalafil 10 mg in 72 hr); concurrent use with avanafil not recommended. May ↓ levels of **sertraline** and **paroxetine**; adjust dose by clinical response. May ↓ levels and contraceptive efficacy of some estrogen-based **hormonal contraceptives** (alternative methods of nonhormonal contraception recommended). May ↑ levels of **salmeterol**; concurrent use not recommended. May ↑ **bosentan** levels; initiate bosentan at 62.5 mg once daily or every other day once patient receiving darunavir for ≥10 days; if patient already receiving bosentan, discontinue bosentan ≥36 hr before initiation of darunavir and then restart bosentan ≥10 days later at 62.5 mg once daily or every other day. May ↑ **tadalafil (Adcirca)** levels; initiate tadalafil (Adcirca) at 20 mg once daily once patient receiving darunavir for ≥1 wk; if patient already receiving tadalfil (Adcirca), discontinue tadalafil (Adcirca) ≥24 hr before initiation of darunavir and then restart tadalafil (Adcirca) ≥7 days later at 20 mg once daily. Concurrent use with **boceprevir** results in ↓ darunavir and boceprevir levels; concurrent use not recommended. Concurrent use with **simeprevir** results in ↑ darunavir levels and ↑ simeprevir levels; concurrent use not recommended. May ↑ **lumefantrine** levels and risk of QT interval prolongation. May ↑ **quetiapine** levels; ↓ quetiapine dose to 1/6 of current dose. May ↑ levels of and risk of bleeding with **apixaban**, **dabigatran**, and **rivaroxaban**; concurrent use not recommended. May ↑ **dasatinib** and **nilotinib** levels; may need to ↓ dose or ↑ dosing interval of dasatinib and nilotinib. May ↑ **vinblastine** and **vincristine** levels; may need to temporarily hold darunavir-ritonavir or initiate another antiretroviral regimen. May ↑ levels of **buspirone**, **diazepam**, **estazolam**, **midazolam (IV)**, and **zolpidem**; ↓ dose of sedative.

Drug-Natural Products: St. John's wort ↑ metabolism and may ↓ antiretroviral effectiveness; concurrent use contraindicated.

Route/Dosage

🧬 Genotypic testing of the baseline virus is recommended prior to initiating treatment in therapy-experienced patients. This testing is performed to screen for darunavir resistance associated substitutions, which may be helpful in determining whether the HIV virus will be susceptible to darunavir.

🧬 **PO (Adults):** *Therapy-naive*—800 mg once daily with ritonavir 100 mg once daily; *Therapy-experienced (with no darunavir resistance associated substitution)*—800 mg once daily with ritonavir 100 mg once daily; *Therapy-experienced (with ≥1 darunavir resistance associated substitution or if genotypic testing not performed)*—600 mg twice daily with ritonavir 100 mg twice daily.

PO (Oral suspension or tablets) (Children 3–17 yr and ≥40 kg): *Therapy-naive*—800 mg once daily with ritonavir 100 mg once daily; *Therapy-experienced (with no darunavir resistance associated substitution)*—800 mg once daily with ritonavir 100 mg once daily; *Therapy-experienced (with ≥1 darunavir resistance associated substitution or if genotypic testing not performed)*—600 mg twice daily with ritonavir 100 mg twice daily.

PO (Oral suspension or tablets) (Children 3–17 yr and 30–39.9 kg): *Therapy-naive*—675 mg once daily with ritonavir 100 mg once daily; *Therapy-experienced (with no darunavir resistance associated substitution)*—675 mg once daily with ritonavir 100 mg once daily; *Therapy-experienced (with ≥1 darunavir resistance associated substitution or if genotypic testing not performed)*—450 mg twice daily with ritonavir 60 mg twice daily.

PO (Oral suspension or tablets) (Children 3–17 yr and 15–29.9 kg): *Therapy-naive*—600 mg once daily with ritonavir 100 mg once daily; *Therapy-experienced (with no darunavir resistance associated substitution)*—600 mg once daily with ritonavir 100 mg once daily; *Therapy-experienced (with ≥1 darunavir resistance associated substitution or if genotypic testing not performed)*—375 mg twice daily with ritonavir 48 mg twice daily.

PO (Oral suspension only) (Children 3–17 yr and 14–14.9 kg): *Therapy-naive*—490 mg once daily with ritonavir 96 mg once daily; *Therapy-experienced (with no darunavir resistance associated substitution)*—490 mg once daily with ritonavir 96 mg once daily; *Therapy-experienced (with ≥1 darunavir resistance associated substitution or if genotypic testing not performed)*—280 mg twice daily with ritonavir 48 mg twice daily.

PO (Oral suspension only) (Children 3–17 yr and 13–13.9 kg): *Therapy-naive*—455 mg once daily with ritonavir 80 mg once daily; *Therapy-experienced (with no darunavir resistance associated substitution)*—455 mg once daily with ritonavir 80 mg once daily; *Therapy-experienced (with ≥1 darunavir resistance associated substitution or if genotypic testing not performed)*—260 mg twice daily with ritonavir 40 mg twice daily.

PO (Oral suspension only) (Children 3–17 yr and 12–12.9 kg): *Therapy-naive*—420 mg once daily with ritonavir 80 mg once daily; *Therapy-experienced (with no darunavir resistance associated substitution)*—420 mg once daily with ritonavir 80 mg once daily; *Therapy-experienced (with ≥1 darunavir resistance associated substitution or if genotypic* *testing not performed)*—240 mg twice daily with ritonavir 40 mg twice daily.

PO (Oral suspension only) (Children 3–17 yr and 11–11.9 kg): *Therapy-naive*—385 mg once daily with ritonavir 64 mg once daily; *Therapy-experienced (with no darunavir resistance associated substitution)*—385 mg once daily with ritonavir 64 mg once daily; *Therapy-experienced (with ≥1 darunavir resistance associated substitution or if genotypic testing not performed)*—220 mg twice daily with ritonavir 32 mg twice daily.

PO (Oral suspension only) (Children 3–17 yr and 10–10.9 kg): *Therapy-naive*—350 mg once daily with ritonavir 64 mg once daily; *Therapy-experienced (with no darunavir resistance associated substitution)*—350 mg once daily with ritonavir 64 mg once daily; *Therapy-experienced (with ≥1 darunavir resistance associated substitution or if genotypic testing not performed)*—200 mg twice daily with ritonavir 32 mg twice daily.

Availability

Tablets: 75 mg, 150 mg, 600 mg, 800 mg. **Oral suspension:** 100 mg/mL. ***In combination with:*** cobicistat (Prezcobix). See Appendix B.

NURSING IMPLICATIONS

Assessment

- Assess patient for change in severity of HIV symptoms and for symptoms of opportunistic infections during therapy.
- Assess for allergy to sulfonamides.
- Monitor patient for development of rash; usually maculopapular and self-limited. May cause Stevens-Johnson syndrome or toxic epidermal necrolysis. Discontinue therapy if severe or if accompanied with fever, general malaise, fatigue, muscle or joint aches, blisters, oral lesions, conjunctivitis, hepatitis, and/or eosinophilia.
- ***Lab Test Considerations:*** Monitor viral load and CD4 counts regularly during therapy.
- May cause ↑ serum AST, ALT, GGT, total bilirubin, alkaline phosphatase, pancreatic amylase, pancreatic lipase, triglycerides, total cholesterol, and uric acid concentrations. Monitor hepatic function prior to and periodically during therapy. Hepatotoxicity may require interruption or discontinuation of therapy.

Potential Nursing Diagnoses

Risk for infection (Indications)
Noncompliance (Patient/Family Teaching)

Implementation

- **PO:** Must be administered with a meal or light snack along with ritonavir 100 mg to be effective. The type of food is not important. Tablets should be swallowed whole with water or milk; do not chew.
- Administer oral suspension 8 mL dose and two 4-mL doses using syringe provided along with ritonavir and food.

Patient/Family Teaching

- Emphasize the importance of taking darunavir with ritonavir exactly as directed, at evenly spaced times throughout day. Do not take more than prescribed amount and do not stop taking without consulting health care professional. If a dose of darunavir or ritonavir is missed by more than 6 hr, wait and take next dose at regularly scheduled time. If missed by less than 6 hr, take darunavir and ritonavir immediately and then take next dose at regularly scheduled time. If a dose is skipped, do not double doses. Advise patient to read the *Patient Information* sheet before starting therapy and with each Rx renewal in case changes have been made.
- Instruct patient that darunavir should not be shared with others.
- Instruct patient to notify health care professional of all Rx or OTC medications, vitamins, or herbal products being taken and consult health care professional before taking any new medications.
- Inform patient that darunavir does not cure AIDS or prevent associated or opportunistic infections. Darunavir does not reduce the risk of transmission of HIV to others through sexual contact or blood contamination. Caution patient to use a condom during sexual contact and to avoid sharing needles or donating blood to prevent spreading the AIDS virus to others. Advise patient that the long-term effects of darunavir are unknown at this time.
- Inform patient that darunavir may cause hyperglycemia, hepatotoxicity, and severe skin reactions. Advise patient to notify health care professional promptly if signs of hyperglycemia (increased thirst or hunger; unexplained weight loss; increased urination; fatigue; or dry, itchy skin), hepatotoxicity (unexplained fatigue, anorexia, nausea, jaundice, abdominal pain, or dark urine), or rash occur.
- Inform patient that redistribution and accumulation of body fat may occur, causing central obesity, dorsocervical fat enlargement (buffalo hump), peripheral wasting, breast enlargement, and cushingoid appearance. The cause and long-term effects are not known.
- Rep: Instruct females using hormonal contraceptives to use an alternative nonhormonal method of contraception. Advise patient to notify health care professional if pregnancy is planned or suspected and to avoid breast feeding. If pregnant patient is exposed to darunavir, register patient in *Antiretroviral Pregnancy Registry* by calling 1-800-258-4263.
- Emphasize the importance of regular follow-up exams and blood counts to determine progress and monitor for side effects.

Evaluation/Desired Outcomes

- Delayed progression of AIDS and decreased opportunistic infections in patients with HIV.
- Decrease in viral load and improvement in CD4 cell counts.

HIGH ALERT

DAUNOrubicin hydrochloride

(daw-noe-**roo**-bi-sin **hye**-dro-**klor**-ide)

Cerubidine

Classification

Therapeutic: antineoplastics

Pharmacologic: anthracyclines

Pregnancy Category D

Indications

In combination with other antineoplastics in the treatment of leukemias.

Action

Forms a complex with DNA, which subsequently inhibits DNA and RNA synthesis (cell-cycle phase-nonspecific). **Therapeutic Effects:** Death of rapidly replicating cells, particularly malignant ones. Also has immunosuppressive properties.

Pharmacokinetics

Absorption: Administered IV only, resulting in complete bioavailability.

Distribution: Widely distributed. Crosses the placenta.

Metabolism and Excretion: Extensively metabolized by the liver. Converted partially to a compound that also has antineoplastic activity (daunorubicinol); 40% eliminated by biliary excretion.

Half-life: *Daunorubicin* —18.5 hr. *Daunorubicinol*—26.7 hr.

TIME/ACTION PROFILE (effects on blood counts)

ROUTE	ONSET	PEAK	DURATION
IV	7–10 days	10–14 days	21 days

Contraindications/Precautions

Contraindicated in: Hypersensitivity to daunorubucin or any other components in the formulation; Symptomatic HF/arrhythmias; Pregnant or lactating women.

Use Cautiously in: Active infections or decreased bone marrow reserve; Geriatric patients or patients with other chronic debilitating illnesses (dosage reduction recommended for patients ≥60 yr); May reactivate skin lesions produced by previous radiation therapy; Hepatic or renal impairment (dosage reduction recommended if serum creatinine >3 m g/dL or serum bilirubin >1.2 m g/dL); Patients who have received previous anthracycline therapy or who have underlying cardiovascular disease (increased risk of cardiotoxicity); Patients with child-bearing potential.

Adverse Reactions/Side Effects

EENT: rhinitis, abnormal vision, sinusitis. **CV:** CARDIOTOXICITY, arrhythmias. **GI:** nausea, vomiting, esophagitis, hepatoxicity, stomatitis. **GU:** red urine, gonadal suppression. **Derm:** alopecia. **Hemat:** anemia, leukopenia, thrombocytopenia. **Local:** phlebitis at IV site. **Metab:** hyperuricemia. **Misc:** chills, fever.

Interactions

Drug-Drug: Additive myelosuppression with other **antineoplastics**. May decrease antibody response to **live-virus vaccines** and increase risk of adverse reactions. **Cyclophosphamide** increases the risk of cardiotoxicity. Increased risk of hepatic toxicity with other **hepatotoxic agents**.

Route/Dosage

Other dose regimens are used. In adults, cumulative dose should not exceed 550 mg/m^2 (450 mg/m^2 if previous chest radiation).

IV (Adults <60 yr): 45 mg/m^2/day for 3 days in first course, then for 2 days of second course (as part of combination regimen).

IV (Adults ≥60 yr): 30 mg/m^2/day for 3 days in first course, then for 2 days of second course (as part of combination regimen).

IV (Children >2 yr): 25 mg/m^2 once weekly (as part of combination regimen). In children <2 yr or BSA <0.5 m^2, dosage should be determined on a mg/kg basis.

Availability (generic available)

Powder for injection: 20 mg/vial. **Solution for injection:** 5 mg/mL in 4-mL vials (20 mg).

NURSING IMPLICATIONS

Assessment

- Monitor vital signs before and frequently during therapy.
- Monitor for bone marrow depression. Assess for bleeding (bleeding gums; bruising; petechiae; guaiac stools, urine, and emesis) and avoid IM injections and taking rectal temperatures if platelet count is low. Apply pressure to venipuncture sites for 10 min. Assess for signs of infection during neutropenia. Anemia may occur. Monitor for increased fatigue, dyspnea, and orthostatic hypotension.
- Assess IV site frequently for inflammation or infiltration. Instruct patient to notify nurse immediately if pain or irritation at injection site occurs. If extravasation occurs, infusion must be stopped and restarted in another vein to avoid damage to subcut tissue. Notify physician immediately. Daunorubicin is a vesicant. Standard treatments include local injections of steroids and application of ice compresses.

- Monitor intake and output, appetite, and nutritional intake. Assess for nausea and vomiting, which, although mild, may persist for 24–48 hr. Administration of an antiemetic before and periodically during therapy and adjusting diet as tolerated may help maintain fluid and electrolyte balance and nutritional status. Encourage fluid intake of 2000–3000 mL/day. Allopurinol and alkalinization of the urine may be used to help prevent urate stone formation.
- Assess patient for evidence of cardiotoxicity, which manifests as HF (peripheral edema, dyspnea, rales/crackles, weight gain, jugular venous distention) and usually occurs 1–6 mo after initiation of therapy. Chest x ray, echocardiography, ECGs, and radionuclide angiography determination of ejection fraction may be ordered before and periodically throughout therapy. A 30% decrease in QRS voltage and decrease in systolic ejection fraction are early signs of cardiotoxicity. Patients who receive total cumulative doses >550/mm^2, who have a history of cardiac disease, or who have received mediastinal radiation are at greater risk of developing cardiotoxicity. May be irreversible and fatal, but usually responds to early treatment.
- ***Lab Test Considerations:*** Monitor uric acid levels.
- *Daunorubicin hydrochloride*: Monitor CBC and differential before and periodically throughout therapy. The leukocyte count nadir occurs 10–14 days after administration. Recovery usually occurs within 21 days after administration of daunorubicin.
- Monitor AST, ALT, LDH, and serum bilirubin. May cause transiently ↑ serum alkaline phosphatase, bilirubin, and AST concentrations.

Potential Nursing Diagnoses

Risk for infection (Adverse Reactions)
Decreased cardiac output (Side Effects)

Implementation

- ***High Alert:*** Fatalities have occurred with chemotherapeutic agents. Before administering, clarify all ambiguous orders; double-check single, daily, and course-of-therapy dose limits; have second practitioner independently double-check original order, calculations, and infusion pump settings. Do not confuse daunorubicin hydrochloride (Cerubidine) or with doxorubicin (Adriamycin, Rubex) or doxorubicin hydrochloride liposome (Doxil). To prevent confusion, orders should include generic and brand name.
- Solution should be prepared in a biologic cabinet. Wear gloves, gown, and mask while handling IV medication. Discard IV equipment in specially designated containers.
- **IV:** Reconstitute each 20 mg with 4 mL of sterile water for injection for a concentration of 5 mg/mL. Shake gently to dissolve. Reconstituted medication is stable for 24 hr at room temperature, 48 hr if refrigerated. Protect from sunlight.
- Do not use aluminum needles when reconstituting or injecting daunorubicin, as aluminum darkens the solution.

D

IV Administration

- **IV Push:** ***Diluent:*** Dilute further in 10–15 mL of 0.9% NaCl. Administer IV push through Y-site into free-flowing infusion of 0.9% NaCl or D5W. ***Rate:*** Administer over at least 2–3 min. Rapid administration rate may cause facial flushing or erythema along the vein.
- **Intermittent Infusion:** ***Diluent:*** May also be diluted in 50–100 mL of 0.9% NaCl. ***Rate:*** Administer 50 mL over 10–15 min or 100 mL over 30–45 min.
- **Y-Site Compatibility:** amifostine, etoposide, filgrastim, gemcitabine, granisetron, melphalan, methotrexate, ondansetron, sodium bicarbonate, teniposide, thiotepa, vinorelbine.
- **Y-Site Incompatibility:** allopurinol, aztreonam, cefepime, fludarabine, lansoprazole, piperacillin/tazobactam.
- **Additive Incompatibility:** Manufacturer does not recommend admixing daunorubicin hydrochloride.

Patient/Family Teaching

- Instruct patient to notify health care professional if fever; chills; sore throat; signs of infection; bleeding gums; bruising; petechiae; or blood in urine, stool, or emesis occurs. Caution patient to avoid crowds and persons with known infections. Instruct patient to use soft toothbrush and electric razor. Patient should be cautioned not to drink alcoholic beverages or take products containing aspirin or NSAIDs.
- Instruct patient to inspect oral mucosa for erythema and ulceration. If ulceration occurs, advise patient to use sponge brush and rinse mouth with water after eating and drinking. Stomatitis pain may require management with opioid analgesics. Period of highest risk is 3–7 days after administration of dose.
- Instruct patient to notify health care professional immediately if irregular heartbeat, shortness of breath, or swelling of lower extremities occurs.
- Discuss with patient possibility of hair loss. Explore methods of coping. Regrowth of hair usually begins within 5 wk after discontinuing therapy.
- Inform patient that medication may turn urine reddish color for 1–2 days after administration.
- Inform patient that this medication may cause irreversible gonadal suppression. Advise patient that this medication may have teratogenic effects. Contraception should be used during therapy and for at least 4 mo after therapy is concluded.
- Instruct patient not to receive any vaccinations without advice of health care professional.

- Emphasize the need for periodic lab tests to monitor for side effects.

Evaluation/Desired Outcomes

- Improvement of hematologic status in patients with leukemia.

deferoxamine

(de-fer-**ox**-a-meen)

Desferal

Classification

Therapeutic: antidotes

Pharmacologic: heavy metal antagonists

Pregnancy Category C

Indications

Acute toxic iron ingestion. Secondary iron overload syndromes associated with multiple transfusion therapy.

Action

Chelates unbound iron, forming a water-soluble complex (ferrioxamine) in plasma that is easily excreted by the kidneys. **Therapeutic Effects:** Removal of excess iron. Also chelates aluminum.

Pharmacokinetics

Absorption: Poorly absorbed after oral administration. Well absorbed after IM administration and subcut administration.

Distribution: Appears to be widely distributed.

Metabolism and Excretion: Metabolized by tissues and plasma enzymes. Unchanged drug and chelated form excreted by the kidneys; 33% of iron removed is eliminated in the feces via biliary excretion.

Half-life: 1 hr.

TIME/ACTION PROFILE (effects on hematologic parameters)

ROUTE	ONSET	PEAK	DURATION
IV	rapid	unknown	unknown
IM	unknown	unknown	unknown
Subcut	unknown	unknown	unknown

Contraindications/Precautions

Contraindicated in: Severe renal disease; Anuria; OB: Rep: Early pregnancy or childbearing potential (however, may be used safely in pregnant patients with moderate-to-severe acute iron intoxication).

Use Cautiously in: Pedi: Children <3 yr (safety not established).

Adverse Reactions/Side Effects

EENT: blurred vision, cataracts, ototoxicity. **CV:** hypotension, tachycardia. **GI:** abdominal pain, diarrhea. **GU:** red urine. **Derm:** erythema, flushing, urticaria. **Local:** induration at injection site, pain at injection site. **MS:** leg cramps. **Misc:** allergic reactions, fever, shock after rapid IV administration.

Interactions

Drug-Drug: Ascorbic acid may ↑ effectiveness of deferoxamine but may also ↑ cardiac iron toxicity.

Route/Dosage

Acute Iron Ingestion

IM, IV (Adults and Children ≥3 yr): 1 g, then 500 mg q 4 hr for 2 doses. Additional doses of 500 mg q 4–12 hr may be needed (not to exceed 6 g/24 hr).

Chronic Iron Overload

IM, IV (Adults and Children ≥3 yr): 500 mg–1 g daily IM; additional doses of 2 g should be given IV for each unit of blood transfused (not to exceed 1 g/day in absence of transfusions; 6 g/day if patient receives transfusions).

Subcut (Adults and Children ≥3 yr): 1–2 g/day (20–40 mg/kg/day) infused over 8–24 hr.

Availability (generic available)

Powder for injection: 500 mg/vial, 2 g/vial.

NURSING IMPLICATIONS

Assessment

- In acute poisoning, assess time, amount, and type of iron preparation ingested.
- Monitor signs of iron toxicity: early acute (abdominal pain, bloody diarrhea, emesis), late acute (decreased level of consciousness, shock, metabolic acidosis).
- Monitor vital signs closely, especially during IV administration. Report hypotension, erythema, urticaria, or signs of allergic reaction. Keep epinephrine, an antihistamine, and resuscitation equipment close by in the event of an anaphylactic reaction.
- May cause oculotoxicity or ototoxicity. Report decreased visual acuity or hearing loss. Audiovisual exams should be performed every 3 mo in patients with chronic iron overload.
- Monitor intake and output and urine color. Inform health care professional if patient is anuric. Chelated iron is excreted primarily by the kidneys; urine may turn red.
- ***Lab Test Considerations:*** Monitor serum iron, total iron binding capacity (TIBC), ferritin levels, and urinary iron excretion before and periodically during therapy.
- Monitor liver function studies to assess damage from iron poisoning.

Potential Nursing Diagnoses

Risk for injury poisoning (Indications)

Implementation

- IM route is preferred in acute iron intoxication unless patient is in shock.
- Reconstitute 500-mg vial with 2 mL and 2-g vial with 8 mL of sterile water for injection for a concentration of 213 mg/mL. Dissolve powder completely before administration. Solution is yellow and is stable

for 1 wk after reconstitution if protected from light. Discard unused portion.

- Used in conjunction with induction of emesis or gastric aspiration and lavage with sodium bicarbonate, and supportive measures for shock and metabolic acidosis in acute poisoning.
- **IM:** Administer deep IM and massage well. Rotate sites. IM administration may cause transient severe pain.
- **Subcut:** Reconstitute 500-mg vial with 5 mL and 2-g vial with 20 mL of sterile water for injection. ***Concentration:*** 95 mg/mL. Subcut route used to treat chronically elevated iron therapy is administered into abdominal subcut tissue via infusion pump for 8–24 hr per treatment.

IV Administration

- **IV:** Reconstitute 500-mg vial with 5 mL and 2-g vial with 20 mL of sterile water for injection. ***Concentration:*** 95 mg/mL. ***Diluent:*** D5W, 0.9% NaCl, 0.45% NaCl, or LR. Dissolve powder completely before administration. Solution is clear and colorless to slightly yellow. Administer within 3 hr of reconstitution; 24 hr if prepared under laminar flow hood. Discard unused portion. ***Rate:*** Maximum infusion rate is 15 mg/kg/hr for first 1000 mg. May be followed by 500 mg infused over 4 hr at a slower rate not to exceed 125 mg/hr. Rapid infusion rate may cause hypotension, erythema, urticaria, wheezing, convulsions, tachycardia, or shock.
- May be administered at the same time as blood transfusion in persons with chronically elevated serum iron levels. Use separate site for administration.

Patient/Family Teaching

- Reinforce need to keep iron preparations, all medications, and hazardous substances out of the reach of children.
- Reassure patient that red coloration of urine is expected and reflects excretion of excess iron.
- May cause dizziness or impairment of vision or hearing. Caution patient to avoid driving or other activities requiring alertness until response from medication is known.
- Advise patient not to take vitamin C preparations without consulting health care professional, because tissue toxicity may increase.
- Encourage patients requiring chronic therapy to keep follow-up appointments for lab tests. Eye and hearing exams may be monitored every 3 mo.

Evaluation/Desired Outcomes

- Return of serum iron concentrations to a normal level (50–150 mcg/100 mL).

degarelix (deg-a-rel-ix)

Firmagon

Classification

Therapeutic: antineoplastics

Pharmacologic: GnRH antagonist

Pregnancy Category X

Indications

Management of advanced prostate cancer.

Action

Reversibly brings to GnRH receptors in the pituitary gland, causing a decrease in the release of gonadotropins and testosterone. **Therapeutic Effects:** Decreased spread of prostate cancer.

Pharmacokinetics

Absorption: Well absorbed from depot following water.

Metabolism and Excretion: 70–80% undergoes hepatic metabolism and biliary excretion, most metabolites excreted in feces; 20–30% excreted unchanged in urine.

Half-life: 53 days.

TIME/ACTION PROFILE (decrease in testosterone levels)

ROUTE	ONSET	PEAK	DURATION
SC	within 1 wk	2 wk	1 mo

Contraindications/Precautions

Contraindicated in: Previous hypersensitivity; OB: Pregnancy (may cause fetal harm) or child-bearing women; Lactation: Not recommended for use in women.

Use Cautiously in: Severe hepatic/renal impairment; Previous history of cardiovascular disease including congenital long QT syndrome, electrolyte abnormalities, HF, concurrent use of class IA or class III antiarrhythmics (may ↑ the risk of QT prolongation); Geri: May be more sensitive to drug effects; Pedi: Safety and effectiveness not established.

Adverse Reactions/Side Effects

CNS: dizziness, headache, insomnia, weakness. **CV:** QT INTERVAL PROLONGATION. **GI:** ↑ liver enzymes, diarrhea, nausea. **GU:** erectile dysfunction, testicular atrophy. **Endo:** gynecomastia, pituitary gonadal suppression. **Local:** injection site reactions. **Metab:** hot flashes, weight gain, ↓ bone density. **Misc:** hypersensitivity reactions including ANAPHYLAXIS, ANGIOEDEMA, AND URTICARIA, fever, sweating.

Interactions

Drug-Drug: Concurrent use with **class IA antiarrhythmics**, including **procainamide** and **quinidine** or **class III antiarrhythmics** including **amiodarone** or **sotalol** may ↑ risk of QT prolongation and serious arrhythmias.

Route/Dosage

Subcut (Adults): 240 mg initially (given as two injections of 120 mg each), followed by maintenance dose of 80 mg every 28 days.

Availability

Powder for subcutaneous injection (requires reconstitution): 80 mg/vial, 120 mg/vial.

NURSING IMPLICATIONS

Assessment

- Assess patient for hot flashes and other side effects.
- Monitor for signs and symptoms of hypersensitivity reactions (rash, wheezing, shortness of breath). Treat symptomatically and discontinue degarelix if symptoms occur.
- Monitor ECG periodically during therapy, especially in patients with congenital long QT syndrome, HF, frequent electrolyte abnormalities, and in patients taking drugs known to prolong QT interval.
- ***Lab Test Considerations:*** Measure serum prostate-specific antigen (PSA) periodically to determine effect. If PSA ↑, measure serum testosterone concentrations.
- May effect pituitary gonadotropic or gonadal functions.
- Monitor electrolyte levels periodically during therapy; correct abnormalities.

Potential Nursing Diagnoses

Sexual dysfunction (Side Effects)

Implementation

- **Subcut:** Reconstitute each 120-mg vial with 3 mL and each 80-mg vial with 4.2 mL sterile water using 21 gauge, 2-inch reconstitution needle. Keep vial upright and swirl very gently until liquid is clear, without undissolved powder or particles. If powder adheres to vial over the liquid surface, vial can be tilted slightly to dissolve powder. Avoid shaking to prevent foam; ring of small air bubbles on surface of liquid is acceptable. Tilt vial slightly, keeping needle in lowest part of vial and withdraw 3 mL for 120-mg dose or 4 mL for 80-mg dose. Exchange reconstitution needle for 27 gauge, 1 1/4-inch administration needle. Remove air bubbles. Grasp abdominal skin and insert needle deeply at angle not <45°. Inject in an area free of pressure from belts, waistbands, or other types of clothing. Administer immediately after reconstitution. If administering 240-mg loading dose, repeat 120-mg injection for the second dose.

Patient/Family Teaching

- Explain purpose of medication to patient. Instruct patient to notify health care professional if an injection is missed. Advise patient to read *Patient Labeling* before starting and with each Rx refill in case of changes.
- Inform patient of possible side effects (hot flashes, flushing, increased weight, decreased sex drive, erectile dysfunction). Advise patient that redness, swelling, and itching at injection site is usually mild, self-limiting, and decreases within 3 days.
- Instruct patient to notify health care professional of all Rx or OTC medications, vitamins, or herbal products being taken and consult health care professional before taking any new medications.
- Advise female patient that women who are pregnant or who plan to become pregnant or breast feed should not take degarelix.

Evaluation/Desired Outcomes

- Decrease in the spread of prostate cancer.

REMS

denosumab (de-no-su-mab)

Prolia, Xgeva

Classification

Therapeutic: bone resorption inhibitors

Pharmacologic: monoclonal antibodies

Pregnancy Category X

Indications

Prolia. Treatment of osteoporosis in postmenopausal women who are at high risk for fracture or those who have failed/are intolerant of conventional osteoporosis therapy. To increase bone mass in men with osteoporosis who are at high risk for fracture or those who have failed/are intolerant of conventional osteoporosis therapy. To increase bone mass in men receiving androgen deprivation therapy for nonmetastatic prostate cancer who are at high risk for fracture. To increase bone mass in women receiving adjuvant aromatase inhibitor therapy for breast cancer who are at high risk for fracture.

Xgeva. Prevention of skeletal-related events in patients with bone metastases from solid tumors. Giant cell tumor of bone that is unresectable or where surgical resection is likely to result in severe morbidity. Treatment of hypercalcemia of malignancy that is refractory to bisphosphonate therapy.

Action

A monoclonal antibody that binds specifically to the human receptor activator of nuclear factor kappa-B-ligand (RANKL), which is required for formation, function, and survival of osteoclasts. Binding inhibits osteoclast formation, function, and survival. **Therapeutic Effects:** ↓ bone resorption with ↓ occurrence of fractures (vertebral, nonvertebral, hip) or other skeletal-related events (e.g., radiation therapy to bone, surgery to bone, spinal cord compression). ↑ bone mass.

Pharmacokinetics

Absorption: Well absorbed following subcutaneous administration.

Distribution: Unknown.

Metabolism and Excretion: Unknown.

Half-life: 25.4 days.

TIME/ACTION PROFILE (effects on bone resorption)

ROUTE	ONSET	PEAK	DURATION
Subcut	1 mo	unknown†	12 mo‡

†Maximum ↓ in serum calcium occurs at 10 days.
‡Following discontinuation.

Contraindications/Precautions

Contraindicated in: Hypersensitivity; Hypocalcemia (correct before administering); adequate supplemental calcium and vitamin D required; OB: May cause fetal harm; Lactation: Avoid use; ↓ mammary gland development and lactation.

Use Cautiously in: Conditions associated with hypocalcemia including hypoparathyroidism, previous thyroid/parathyroid surgery, malabsorption syndromes, history of small intestinal excision, inadequate/no calcium supplementation, renal impairment/hemodialysis (CCr <30 mL/min and/or on dialysis); monitoring of calcium levels and calcium and vitamin D intake recommended; Invasive dental procedures, cancer, receiving chemotherapy, corticosteroids, or angiogenesis inhibitors, poor oral hygiene, diabetes. gingival infections, periodontal disease, dental disease, anemia, coagulopathy, infection, or poorly-fitting dentures (may ↑ risk of jaw osteonecrosis).; Concurrent use of immunosuppressants or diseases resulting in immunosuppression (↑ risk of infection); Geri: May be more sensitive to drug effects; Pedi: Safety and effectiveness not established.

Adverse Reactions/Side Effects

CNS: headache. **GI:** PANCREATITIS, diarrhea, nausea. **GU:** cystitis. **Derm:** dermatitis, eczema, rashes. **F and E:** hypocalcemia, hypophosphatemia. **Metab:** hypercholesterolemia. **MS:** back pain, extremity pain, musculoskeletal pain, atypical femoral fracture, osteonecrosis of the jaw, suppression of bone turnover. **Resp:** dyspnea, cough. **Misc:** hypersensitivity reactions including ANAPHYLAXIS, infection.

Interactions

Drug-Drug: Concurrent use of **immunosuppressants** ↑ risk of infection.

Route/Dosage

Prolia

Subcut (Adults): 60 mg every 6 mo.

Xgeva

Subcut (Adults): *Bone metastasis from solid tumors*—120 mg every 4 weeks; *Giant cell tumor of bone*—120 mg every 4 weeks, with additional doses of 120 mg given on Days 8 and 15 of first month of therapy; *Hypercalcemia of malignancy*—120 mg every 4 weeks, with additional doses of 120 mg given on Days 8 and 15 of first month of therapy.

Availability

Injection (Prolia): 60 mg/mL. **Injection (Xgeva):** 120 mg/1.7 mL.

NURSING IMPLICATIONS

Assessment

- Assess patients via bone density study for low bone mass before and periodically during therapy.
- Perform a routine oral exam prior to initiation of therapy. Dental exam with appropriate preventative dentistry should be considered prior to therapy. Patients with history of tooth extraction, poor oral hygiene, gingival infections, diabetes, or use of a dental appliance or those taking immunosuppressive therapy, angiogenesis inhibitors, or systemic corticosteroids are at greater risk for osteonecrosis of the jaw.
- Monitor for signs and symptoms of hypersensitivity reactions (hypotension, dyspnea, upper airway edema, lip swelling, rash, pruritis, urticaria). Treat symptomatically and discontinue medication if symptoms occur.
- ***Lab Test Considerations:*** Assess serum calcium, phosphorous, and magnesium levels before and periodically during therapy, especially during first wks of therapy. Hypocalcemia and vitamin D deficiency should be treated before initiating therapy. May cause mild, transient ↑ of calcium and phosphate. Administer calcium, magnesium, and vitamin D as needed.
- May cause anemia.
- May cause hypercholesterolemia.

Potential Nursing Diagnoses

Risk for injury (Indications)

Implementation

- Grey needle cap on single-use prefilled *Prolia* syringe should not be handled by people sensitive to latex.
- **Subcut:** Remove from refrigerator and bring to room temperature by standing in original container for 15–30 min prior to administration; do not warm in any other way. Do not shake. Administer using a 27–gauge needle in the upper arm, upper thigh, or abdomen. Solution is clear and colorless to pale yellow, and may contain trace amounts of translucent to white proteinaceous particles. Do not use if solution is discolored or contains many particles. Manu-

ally activate the green safety guard *after* the injection is given, not before.

- Patients should receive calcium 1000 mg and 400 IU vitamin D daily.

Patient/Family Teaching

- Explain the purpose of denosumab to patient. If a dose is missed, administer injection as soon as possible.
- Advise patient to eat a balanced diet and consult health care professional about the need for supplemental calcium and vitamin D (see Appendix J).
- Advise patient to notify health care professional immediately if signs of hypersensitivity, hypocalcemia (spasms, twitches, or cramps in muscles; numbness or tingling in fingers, toes, or around mouth), infection (fever, chills, skin that is red, swollen, hot, or tender to touch; severe abdominal pain, frequent or urgent need to urinate or burning during urination), or skin reactions (redness, itching, rash, dry or leathery feeling, blisters that ooze or become crusty, peeling), or osteonecrosis of the jaw (pain, numbness, swelling of or drainage from the jaw, mouth, or teeth) occur.
- Encourage patient to participate in regular exercise and to modify behaviors that ↑ the risk of osteoporosis (stop smoking, reduce alcohol consumption).
- Advise patient to take good care of teeth and gums (brush and floss regularly) and to inform health care professional of therapy prior to dental surgery.
- Rep: Advise female patients to notify health care professional if pregnancy is planned or suspected or if breast feeding. Instruct female patient to use highly effective contraception during and for at least 5 mo after therapy is completed. Encourage women who become pregnant during Xgeva treatment to enroll in Amgen's Pregnancy Surveillance Program. Patients or their health care professional should call 1-800-77-AMGEN (1-800-772-6436) to enroll.

Evaluation/Desired Outcomes

- Reversal of the progression of osteoporosis with ↓ fractures and other sequelae.
- ↑ bone mass.
- Decreased growth of giant cell tumors.
- Reduction in hypercalcemia of malignancy that is refractory to bisphosphonate therapy.

desipramine

(dess-**ip**-ra-meen)

Norpramin

Classification

Therapeutic: antidepressants

Pharmacologic: tricyclic antidepressants

Pregnancy Category C

Indications

Depression. **Unlabeled Use:** Chronic pain syndromes. Anxiety. Insomnia.

Action

Potentiates the effect of serotonin and norepinephrine in the CNS. Has significant anticholinergic properties. **Therapeutic Effects:** Antidepressant action (may develop only over several weeks).

Pharmacokinetics

Absorption: Well absorbed from the GI tract.

Distribution: Widely distributed.

Protein Binding: 90–92%.

Metabolism and Excretion: Mostly metabolized by the liver (CYP2D6 isoenzyme); one metabolite is pharmacologically active (2-hydroxydesipramine); the CYP2D6 enzyme system exhibits genetic polymorphism; ~7% of population may be poor metabolizers (PMs) and may have significantly ↑desipramine concentrations and an ↑ risk of adverse effects. Small amounts enter breast milk.

Half-life: 12–27 hr.

TIME/ACTION PROFILE (antidepressant effect)

ROUTE	ONSET	PEAK	DURATION
PO	2–3 wk	2–6 wk	days–wk

Contraindications/Precautions

Contraindicated in: Angle-closure glaucoma; Recent MI, heart failure, known history of QTc prolongation.

Use Cautiously in: Patients with pre-existing cardiovascular disease; Family history of sudden death, cardiac arrhythmias, or conduction disturbances; Prostatic hyperplasia (↑ susceptibility to urinary retention); History of seizures (threshold may be ↓ seizures may precede the development of cardiac arrhythmias or death); May ↑ risk of suicide attempt/ideation especially during early treatment or dose adjustment; risk may be greater in children or adolescents; OB: Use during pregnancy only if potential maternal benefit outweighs risks to fetus; use during lactation may result in neonatal sedation; Pedi: Children <12 yr (safety not established); Geri: ↑ sensitivity to effects.

Adverse Reactions/Side Effects

CNS: drowsiness, fatigue. **EENT:** blurred vision, dry eyes, dry mouth. **CV:** ARRHYTHMIAS, hypotension, ECG changes. **GI:** constipation, drug-induced hepatitis, paralytic ileus, ↑ appetite, weight gain. **GU:** urinary retention, ↓ libido. **Derm:** photosensitivity. **Endo:** changes in blood glucose, gynecomastia. **Hemat:** blood dyscrasias.

Interactions

Drug-Drug: Desipramine is metabolized in the liver by the cytochrome P450 2D6 enzyme and its action may be affected by drugs which compete for metabolism by or alter the activity of this enzyme including other **anti-**

depressants, **phenothiazines**, **carbamazepine**, **class 1C antiarrthythmics** (**propafenone** or **flecainide**); when used concurrently dose ↓ of one or the other or both may be necessary. Concurrent use of other drugs that inhibit the activity of the enzyme, including **cimetidine**, **quinidine**, **amiodarone**, and **ritonavir**, may result in ↑ effects. May cause hypotension, tachycardia, and potentially fatal reactions when used with **MAO inhibitors** (avoid concurrent use—discontinue 2 wk prior to). Concurrent use with **SSRI antidepressants** may result in ↑ toxicity and should be avoided (fluoxetine should be stopped 5 wk before). Concurrent use with **clonidine** may result in hypertensive crisis and should be avoided. **Phenytoin** may ↓ levels and effectiveness; ↑ doses of desipramine may be required to treat depression. Concurrent use with **levodopa** may result in delayed/↓ absorption of levodopa or hypertension. Blood levels and effects may be ↓ by **rifampin**, **carbamazepine**, and **barbiturates**. Concurrent use with **moxifloxacin** ↑ risk of adverse cardiovascular reactions. ↑ CNS depression with other **CNS depressants** including **alcohol**, **antihistamines**, **clonidine**, **opioid analgesics**, and **sedative/hypnotics**. **Barbiturates** may alter blood levels and effects. **Adrenergic** and **anticholinergic** side effects may be ↑ with other **agents having these properties**. **Hormonal contraceptives** ↑ levels and may cause toxicity. **Cigarette smoking** may ↑ metabolism and alter effects.

Drug-Natural Products: Concomitant use of **kava-kava**, **valerian**, or **chamomile** can ↑ CNS depression. ↑ anticholinergic effects with **jimson weed** and **scopolia**.

Route/Dosage

PO (Adults): 100–200 mg/day as a single dose or in divided doses (up to 300 mg/day).

PO (Geriatric Patients): 25–50 mg/day in divided doses (up to 150 mg/day).

PO (Children >12 yr): 25–50 mg/day in divided doses, may ↑ as needed up to 100 mg/day.

PO (Children 6–12 yr): 10–30 mg/day (1–5 mg/kg/day) in divided doses.

Availability (generic available)

Tablets: 10 mg, 25 mg, 50 mg, 75 mg, 100 mg, 150 mg.

NURSING IMPLICATIONS

Assessment

- Obtain weight and BMI initially and periodically throughout therapy.
- Assess FBS and cholesterol levels for overweight/obese individuals.
- Refer as appropriate for nutrition/weight management and medical management.
- Monitor BP and pulse prior to and during initial therapy. Notify physician or other health care professional of decreases in BP (10–20 mm Hg) or sudden increase in pulse rate. Patients taking high doses or with a history of cardiovascular disease should have ECG monitored prior to and periodically during therapy.
- **Depression:** Monitor mental status (orientation, mood, behavior) frequently. Assess for suicidal tendencies, especially during early therapy. Restrict amount of drug available to patient.
- Assess mental status and mood changes, especially during initial few months of therapy and during dose changes. Risk may be increased in children, adolescents, and adults ≤24 yrs. Inform health care professional if patient demonstrates significant increase in signs of depression (depressed mood, loss of interest in usual activities, significant change in weight and/or appetite, insomnia or hypersomnia, psychomotor agitation or retardation, increased fatigue, feelings of guilt or worthlessness, slowed thinking or impaired concentration, suicide attempt or suicidal ideation). Restrict amount of drug available to patient.
- **Pain:** Assess intensity, quality, and location of pain periodically throughout therapy. Use pain scale to monitor effectiveness of medication.
- ***Lab Test Considerations:*** Assess leukocyte and differential blood counts, liver function, and serum glucose periodically. May cause an ↑ serum bilirubin and alkaline phosphatase. May cause bone marrow depression. Serum glucose may be ↑ or ↓.
- ***Lab Test Considerations:*** Serum levels may be monitored in patients who fail to respond to usual therapeutic dose.

Potential Nursing Diagnoses

Ineffective coping (Indications)
Risk for injury (Side Effects)
Chronic pain (Indications)

Implementation

- Do not confuse despiramine with disopyramide.
- Dose increases should be made at bedtime because of sedation. Dose titration is a slow process; may take wk to mo. May give entire dose at bedtime.
- Taper to avoid withdrawal effects. Reduce dose by half for 3 days then reduce again by half for 3 days, then discontinue.
- **PO:** Administer medication with or immediately after a meal to minimize gastric upset. Tablet may be crushed and given with food or fluids.

Patient/Family Teaching

- Instruct patient to take medication as directed. Take missed doses as soon as possible unless almost time for next dose; if regimen is a single dose at bedtime, do not take in the morning because of side effects. Advise patient that drug effects may not be noticed for at least 2 wk. Abrupt discontinuation may cause nausea; vomiting; diarrhea; headache; trouble sleeping, with vivid dreams; and irritability. Instruct patient to read the *Medication Guide* prior to starting and with each Rx refill in case of changes.

- May cause drowsiness and blurred vision. Caution patient to avoid driving and other activities requiring alertness until response to drug is known.
- Orthostatic hypotension, sedation, and confusion are common during early therapy, especially in the elderly. Protect patient from falls. Institute fall precautions. Advise patient to make position changes slowly.
- Advise patient to avoid alcohol or other CNS depressant drugs during and for 3–7 days after therapy has been discontinued.
- Advise patient, family, and caregivers to look for suicidality, especially during early therapy or dose changes. Notify health care professional immediately if thoughts about suicide or dying, attempts to commit suicide, new or worse depression or anxiety, agitation or restlessness, panic attacks, insomnia, new or worse irritability, aggressiveness, acting on dangerous impulses, mania, or other changes in mood or behavior occur.
- Instruct patient to notify health care professional if urinary retention, dry mouth, or constipation persists. Sugarless candy or gum may diminish dry mouth, and an increase in fluids or bulk may prevent constipation. If symptoms persist, dose reduction or discontinuation may be necessary. Consult health care professional if dry mouth persists for more than 2 wk.
- Caution patient to use sunscreen and protective clothing to prevent photosensitivity reactions.
- Inform patient of need to monitor dietary intake. Increase in appetite may lead to undesired weight gain.
- Alert patient that medication may turn urine blue-green in color.
- Advise patient to notify health care professional of medication regimen prior to treatment or surgery.
- Advise female patients to notify health care professional if pregnancy is planned or suspected.
- Therapy for depression is usually prolonged. Emphasize the importance of follow-up exams to monitor effectiveness and side effects and to improve coping skills.

Evaluation/Desired Outcomes

- Increased sense of well-being.
- Renewed interest in surroundings.
- Increased appetite.
- Improved energy level.
- Improved sleep.
- Decrease in chronic pain symptoms.
- Full therapeutic effects may be seen 2–6 wk after initiating therapy.

desmopressin
(des-moe-**press**-in)

DDAVP, DDAVP Rhinal Tube, DDAVP Rhinyle Drops, Stimate

Classification

Therapeutic: hormones

Pharmacologic: antidiuretic hormones

Pregnancy Category B

Indications

PO, Subcut, IV, Intranasal: Treatment of central diabetes insipidus caused by a deficiency of vasopressin. **IV, Intranasal:** Controls bleeding in certain types of hemophilia and von Willebrand's disease. **PO:** Primary nocturnal enuresis.

Action

An analogue of naturally occurring vasopressin (antidiuretic hormone). Primary action is enhanced reabsorption of water in the kidneys. **Therapeutic Effects:** Prevention of nocturnal enuresis. Maintenance of appropriate body water content in diabetes insipidus. Control of bleeding in certain types of hemophilia or von Willebrand's disease.

Pharmacokinetics

Absorption: < 1% absorbed following oral administration; nasal solution 10–20% absorbed; nasal spray 3–4% absorbed.

Distribution: Distribution not fully known. Enters breast milk.

Metabolism and Excretion: Unknown.

Half-life: *PO*–1.5–2.5 hr; *IV*—75 min (↑ in renal impairment); *Intranasal*—3.3–3.5 hr.

TIME/ACTION PROFILE (PO, intranasal = antidiuretic effect; IV = effect on factor VIII activity)

ROUTE	ONSET	PEAK	DURATION
PO	1 hr	4–7 hr	unknown
Intranasal	1 hr	1–5 hr	8–20 hr
IV	within min	15–30 min	3 hr†

†4–24 hr in mild hemophilia A.

Contraindications/Precautions

Contraindicated in: Hypersensitivity; Hypersensitivity to chlorobutanol; Patients with severe type I, type IIB, or platelet-type (pseudo) von Willebrand's disease, hemophilia A with factor VIII levels <5% or hemophilia B; Renal impairment (CCr < 50 mL/min); Hyponatremia.

Use Cautiously in: Angina pectoris; Hypertension; Patients at risk for hyponatremia; OB, Lactation: Safety not established.

Adverse Reactions/Side Effects

CNS: SEIZURES, drowsiness, headache, listlessness.

EENT: *intranasal*—nasal congestion, rhinitis.

Resp: dyspnea. **CV:** hypertension, hypotension, tachycardia (large IV doses only). **GI:** mild abdominal cramps, nausea. **GU:** vulval pain. **Derm:** flushing. **F and E:** water intoxication/hyponatremia. **Local:** phlebitis at IV site.

Interactions

Drug-Drug: Chlorpropamide, **clofibrate**, **chlorpromazine**, **lamotrigine**, **SSRIs**, or **carbamazepine** may enhance the antidiuretic response to desmopressin. **Demeclocycline**, **lithium**, or **norepinephrine** may diminish the antidiuretic response to desmopressin. Large doses may enhance the effects of **vasopressors**.

Route/Dosage

Primary Nocturnal Enuresis

PO (Adults and Children ≥6 yr): 0.2 mg at bedtime; may be titrated up to 0.6 mg at bedtime to achieve desired response.

Diabetes Insipidus

PO (Adults and Children): 0.05 mg twice daily; adjusted as needed (usual range: 0.1–1.2 mg/day for adults or 0.1–0.8 mg/day for children in 2–3 divided doses).

Intranasal (Adults and Children ≥ 12 yr): *DDAVP*—5–40 mcg (0.0.05–0.4 mL)in 1–3 divided doses.

Intranasal (Children 3 mo–12 yr): *DDAVP*—5–30 mcg (0.05–0.3 mL) in 1–2 divided doses.

Subcut, IV (Adults and Children≥12 yr): 2–4 mcg/day in 2 divided doses.

Subcut, IV (Children < 12 yr): 0.1–1 mcg/day in 1–2 divided doses.

Hemophilia A/von Willebrand's disease

Intranasal (Adults and Children >50 kg): *Stimate*—1 spray (150 mcg) in each nostril.

Intranasal (Adults and Children ≤50 kg): *Stimate*—1 spray (150 mcg) in one nostril.

IV (Adults and Children >3 mo): 0.3 mcg/kg, repeated as needed.

Availability (generic available)

Tablets: 0.1 mg, 0.2 mg. **Nasal spray (DDAVP):** 10 mcg/spray—5-mL bottle (0.1 mg/mL) contains 50 doses). **Nasal spray (Stimate):** 150 mcg/spray. **Rhinal tube delivery system-nasal solution:** 2.5-mL vials with applicator tubes (0.1 mg/mL). **Injection:** 4 mcg/mL.

NURSING IMPLICATIONS

Assessment

- Chronic intranasal use may cause tolerance or if administered more frequently than every 24–48 hr IV tachyphylaxis (short-term tolerance) may develop.
- **Nocturnal Enuresis:** Monitor frequency of enuresis throughout therapy. Use cautiously in patients at risk for water intoxication with hyponatremia.
- Do not use intranasal form for nocturnal enuresis.
- **Diabetes Insipidus:** Monitor urine and plasma osmolality and urine volume frequently. Assess patient for symptoms of dehydration (excessive thirst, dry skin and mucous membranes, tachycardia, poor skin turgor). Weigh patient daily and assess for edema.
- **Hemophilia:** Monitor plasma factor VIII coagulant, factor VIII antigen, and ristocetin cofactor. May also assess activated partial thromboplastin time (aPTT) for hemophilia A and skin bleeding time for von Willebrand's disease. Assess patient for signs of bleeding.
- Monitor BP and pulse during IV infusion.
- Monitor intake and output and adjust fluid intake (especially in children and elderly) to avoid overhydration in patients receiving desmopressin for hemophilia.
- ***Toxicity and Overdose:*** Signs and symptoms of water intoxication include confusion, drowsiness, headache, weight gain, difficulty urinating, seizures, and coma.
- Treatment of overdose includes decreasing dose and, if symptoms are severe, administration of furosemide.

Potential Nursing Diagnoses

Deficient fluid volume (Indications)
Excess fluid volume (Adverse Reactions)

Implementation

- IV desmopressin has 10 times the antidiuretic effect of intranasal desmopressin.
- **PO:** Begin oral doses 12 hr after last intranasal dose. Monitor response closely.
- **Diabetes Insipidus:** Parenteral dose for antidiuretic effect is administered IV push or subcut.
- **Hemophilia:** Parenteral dose for control of bleeding is administered via IV infusion. If used preoperatively, administer 30 min prior to procedure.

IV Administration

- **IV Push:** (for diabetes insipidus) ***Diluent:*** Administer undiluted. ***Concentration:*** 4 mcg/mL. ***Rate:*** Administer over 1 min.
- **Intermittent Infusion (for hemophilia and von Willebrand's disease):** ***Diluent:*** Dilute each dose in 50 mL of 0.9% NaCl for adults and children >10 kg and in 10 mL in children weighing <10 kg. ***Concentration:*** maximum 0.5 mcg/mL. ***Rate:*** Infuse slowly over 15–30 min.
- **Y-Site Compatibility:** No information available.
- **Intranasal:** If intranasal dose is used preoperatively, administer 2 hr before procedure.

Patient/Family Teaching

- Advise patient to notify health care professional if bleeding is not controlled or if headache, dyspnea, heartburn, nausea, abdominal cramps, vulval pain, or severe nasal congestion or irritation occurs.
- Caution patient to avoid concurrent use of alcohol with this medication.
- **Diabetes Insipidus:** Instruct patient on intranasal administration. Medication is supplied with a flexible calibrated catheter (rhinyle). Draw solution into rhinyle. Insert one end of tube into nostril, blow on the other end to deposit solution deep into nasal cavity. An air-filled syringe may be attached to the plastic catheter for children, infants, or obtunded patients. Tube should be rinsed under water after each use.
- If nasal spray is used, prime pump prior to first use by pressing down 4 times. Caution patient that nasal spray should not be used beyond the labeled number of sprays; subsequent sprays may not deliver accurate dose. Do not attempt to transfer remaining solution to another bottle.
- Instruct patient to take missed doses as soon as remembered but not if it is almost time for the next dose. Do not double doses.
- Advise patient that rhinitis or upper respiratory infection may decrease effectiveness of this therapy. If increased urine output occurs, patient should contact health care professional for dosage adjustment.
- Patients with diabetes insipidus should carry identification at all times describing disease process and medication regimen.

Evaluation/Desired Outcomes

- Decreased frequency of nocturnal enuresis.
- Decrease in urine volume.
- Relief of polydipsia.
- Increased urine osmolality.
- Control of bleeding in hemophilia.

desonide, See CORTICOSTEROIDS (TOPICAL/LOCAL).

desoximetasone, See CORTICOSTEROIDS (TOPICAL/LOCAL).

desvenlafaxine

(**des**-ven-la-**fax**-een)

Khedezla, Pristiq

Classification

Therapeutic: antidepressants

Pharmacologic: selective serotonin/norepinephrine reuptake inhibitors

Pregnancy Category C

Indications

Major depressive disorder.

Action

Inhibits serotonin and norepinephrine reuptake in the CNS. **Therapeutic Effects:** Decrease in depressive symptomatology, with fewer relapses/recurrences.

Pharmacokinetics

Absorption: 80% absorbed following oral administration.

Distribution: Enters breast milk.

Metabolism and Excretion: 55% metabolized by the liver, 45% excreted unchanged in urine.

Half-life: 10 hr.

TIME/ACTION PROFILE (blood levels)

ROUTE	ONSET	PEAK	DURATION
PO	unknown	7.5 hr	24 hr

Contraindications/Precautions

Contraindicated in: Hypersensitivity to venlafaxine or desvenlafaxine; Concurrent use of MAO inhibitors or MAO-like drugs (linezolid or methylene blue); Should not be used concurrently with venlafaxine.

Use Cautiously in: Untreated cerebrovascular or cardiovascular disease, including untreated hypertension (control BP before initiating therapy); Bipolar disorder (may activate mania/hypomania); Renal impairment (consider modifications, dose should not exceed 50 mg/day, especially in moderate to severe renal impairment); History of seizures or neurologic impairment; Hepatic impairment (dose should not exceed 100 mg/day); Angle-closure glaucoma; Geri: Consider age-related ↓ in renal function, ↓ body mass, concurrent disease states, and medications; OB, Lactation: Use only if maternal benefit outweighs fetal/infant risk; Pedi: ↑ risk of suicidal thinking and behavior (suicidality) in children and adolescents with major depressive disorder and other psychiatric disorders. Observe closely for suicidality and behavior changes.

Adverse Reactions/Side Effects

CNS: NEUROLEPTIC MALIGNANT SYNDROME, SEIZURES, SUICIDAL THOUGHTS, anxiety, dizziness, drowsiness, insomnia, headache, teeth grinding, vertigo. **EENT:** ↑ intraocular pressure, mydriasis. **Resp:** eosinophilic pneumonia, interstitial lung disease. **CV:** hypertension. **GI:** ↓ appetite, constipation, nausea. **GU:** male sexual dysfunction. **Derm:** ERYTHEMA MULTIFORME, STEVENS-JOHNSON SYNDROME, TOXIC EPIDERMAL NECROLYSIS, sweating. **F and E:** hyponatremia. **Hemat:** ↑ risk of bleeding. **Metab:** hypercholesterolemia, hyperlipidemia. **Misc:** SEROTONIN SYNDROME.

Interactions

Drug-Drug: Concurrent use with **MAO inhibitors** may result in serious, potentially fatal reactions (wait at least 2 wk after stopping MAO inhibitor before initiating desvenlafaxine; wait at least 1 wk after stopping desvenlafaxine before starting an MAO inhibitor). Concurrent use with **MAO-inhibitor like drugs**, such as **linezolid** or **methylene blue** may ↑ risk of serotonin syndrome; concurrent use contraindicated; do not start therapy in patients receiving **linezolid** or **methylene blue**; if **linezolid** or **methylene blue** need to be started in a patient receiving desvenlafaxine, immediately discontinue desvenlafaxine and monitor for signs/symptoms of serotonin syndrome for 2 wk or until 24 hr after last dose of linezolid or methylene blue, whichever comes first (may resume desvenlafaxine therapy 24 hr after last dose of linezolid or methylene blue). ↑ risk of bleeding with other **drugs that ↑ bleeding risk** including **anticoagulants**, **antithrombotics**, **platelet aggregation inhibitors**, and **NSAIDs**. Use cautiously with other **CNS-active drugs**, including **alcohol** or **sedative/hypnotics**; effects of combination are unknown. Drugs that affect serotonergic neurotransmitter systems, including **tricyclic antidepressants**, **SNRIs**, **fentanyl**, **buspirone**, **tramadol**, and **triptans** ↑ risk of serotonin syndrome. **Ketoconazole** may ↑ the effects of desvenlafaxine. May ↑ levels of CYP2D6 substrates, including **desipramine**, **atomoxetine**, **dextromethorphan**, **metoprolol**, **nebivolol**, **perphenazine**, and **tolterodine**; if using desvenlafaxine at dose of 400 mg/day, ↓ dose of CYP2D6 substrate by 50%.

Route/Dosage

PO (Adults): 50 mg once daily (range = 50–400 mg/day).

Renal Impairment

PO (Adults): *CCr 30–50 mL/min*—50 mg once daily; *CCr <30 mL/min*—50 mg every other day or 25 mg once daily.

Hepatic Impairment

PO (Adults): *Moderate-to-severe hepatic impairment*—50 mg once daily (not to exceed 100 mg/day).

Availability (generic available)

Extended-release tablets: 25 mg, 50 mg, 100 mg. **Cost:** *Generic*—All strengths $174.14/30.

NURSING IMPLICATIONS

Assessment

- Assess mental status and mood changes, especially during initial few months of therapy and during dose changes. Inform health care professional if patient demonstrates significant increase in signs of depression (depressed mood, loss of interest in usual activities, significant change in weight and/or appetite, insomnia or hypersomnia, psychomotor agitation or retardation, increased fatigue, feelings or guilt or worthlessness, slowed thinking or impaired concentration, suicide attempt or suicidal ideation).
- Assess suicidal tendencies, especially in early therapy. Restrict amount of drug available to patient. Risk may be increased in children, adolescents, and adults ≤24 yr.
- Monitor BP before and periodically during therapy. Sustained hypertension may be dose related; decrease dose or discontinue therapy if this occurs.
- Monitor appetite and nutritional intake; weigh weekly. Report continued weight loss. Adjust diet as tolerated to support nutritional status.
- Assess for serotonin syndrome (mental changes [agitation, hallucinations, coma], autonomic instability [tachycardia, labile BP, hyperthermia], neuromuscular aberations [hyperreflexia, incoordination], and/or GI symptoms [nausea, vomiting, diarrhea]), especially in patients taking other serotonergic drugs (SSRIs, SNRIs, triptans).
- Assess patient for skin rash frequently during therapy. Discontinue at first sign of rash; may be life-threatening. Stevens-Johnson syndrome may develop. Treat symptomatically; may recur once treatment is stopped.
- ***Lab Test Considerations:*** May cause ↑ fasting serum total cholesterol, LDL, cholesterol, and triglycerides.
- May cause transient proteinuria, not usually associated with ↑ BUN or creatinine.
- May cause hyponatremia.
- May cause false-positive immunoassay screening tests for phencyclidine (PCP) and amphetamine.

Potential Nursing Diagnoses

Ineffective coping (Indications)
Risk for injury (Side Effects)

Implementation

- Do not confuse Pristiq with Prilosec.
- **PO:** Administer at the same time each day, with or without food. Swallow tablets whole; do not crush, break, chew, or dissolve.

Patient/Family Teaching

- Instruct patient to take medication exactly as directed at the same time each day. Take missed doses as soon as possible unless almost time for next dose. Do not double doses or discontinue abruptly; gradually decrease before discontinuation to prevent dizziness, nausea, headache, irritability, insomnia, diarrhea, anxiety, fatigue, abnormal dreams, and hyperhidrosis.
- Advise patient, family, and caregivers to look for suicidality, especially during early therapy or dose changes. Notify health care professional immediately if thoughts about suicide or dying, attempts to commit suicide, new or worse depression or anxiety, agitation or restlessness, panic attacks, insomnia, new or worse irritability, aggressiveness, acting on dan-

gerous impulses, mania, or other changes in mood or behavior or if symptoms of serotonin syndrome occur.

- May cause drowsiness or dizziness. Caution patient to avoid driving or other activities requiring alertness until response to the drug is known.
- Caution patient to avoid taking alcohol or other CNS-depressant drugs during therapy and of increased risk of bleeding with concomitant use of NSAIDs, aspirin, or other drugs that affect coagulation or bleeding. Instruct patient to notify health care professional of all Rx or OTC medications, vitamins, or herbal products being taken and to consult health care professional before taking other Rx, OTC, or herbal products.
- Instruct patient to notify health care professional if signs of allergy (rash, hives, swelling, difficulty breathing) occur.
- Inform patient that remains of tablet may pass into stool, but medication has already been absorbed.
- Instruct female patients to inform health care professional if pregnancy is planned or suspected or if breast feeding.
- Emphasize the importance of follow-up exams to monitor progress.

Evaluation/Desired Outcomes

- Increased sense of well-being.
- Renewed interest in surroundings. Need for therapy should be periodically reassessed. Therapy is usually continued for several mo.

dexamethasone, See CORTICOSTEROIDS (SYSTEMIC).

dexlansoprazole

(dex-lan-**soe**-pra-zole)

Dexilant

Classification

Therapeutic: antiulcer agents

Pharmacologic: proton-pump inhibitors

Pregnancy Category B

Indications

Healing of erosive esophagitis (EE). Maintenance of healed EE and relief of heartburn. Treatment of heartburn from nonerosive gastroesopahageal reflux disease (GERD).

Action

Binds to an enzyme in the presence of acidic gastric pH, preventing the final transport of hydrogen ions into the gastric lumen. **Therapeutic Effects:** Diminished accumulation of acid in the gastric lumen, with lessened acid reflux.

Pharmacokinetics

Absorption: Well absorbed following oral administration.

Distribution: Unknown.

Protein Binding: 96–99%.

Metabolism and Excretion: Extensively metabolized by the liver (CYP2C19 and CYP3A4 enzyme systems are involved); the CYP2C19 enzyme system exhibits genetic polymorphism; 15–20% of Asian patients and 3–5% of Caucasian and Black patients may be poor metabolizers and may have significantly ↑ dexlansoprazole concentrations and an ↑ risk of adverse effects); no active metabolites. No renal elimination.

Half-life: 1–2 hr.

TIME/ACTION PROFILE (blood levels)

ROUTE	ONSET	PEAK*	DURATION
PO	unknown	1–2 hr (1st); 4–5 hr (2nd)	24 hr

*Reflects effects of delayed release capsule.

Contraindications/Precautions

Contraindicated in: Hypersensitivity; Severe hepatic impairment; Lactation: Lactation.

Use Cautiously in: Moderate hepatic impairment (daily dose should not exceed 30 mg); Patients using high doses for >1 year (↑ risk of hip, wrist, or spine fractures); Patients using therapy for >3 yr (↑ risk of vitamin B_{12} deficiency; Pedi: Safety not established.

Adverse Reactions/Side Effects

GI: CLOSTRIDIUM DIFFICILE-ASSOCIATED DIARRHEA (CDAD), abdominal pain, diarrhea, flatulence, nausea, vomiting. **F and E:** hypomagnesemia (especially if treatment duration ≥3 mo). **GU:** acute interstitial nephritis. **Hemat:** vitamin B_{12} deficiency. **MS:** bone fracture.

Interactions

Drug-Drug: May ↓ absorption of drugs requiring acid pH, including **ketoconazole**, **itraconazole**, **atazanavir ampicillin esters**, **iron salts**, **erlotinib**, and **mycophenolate mofetil**; avoid concurrent use with **atazanavir**. May ↑ levels of **digoxin** and **methotrexate**. May ↑ effect of **warfarin**. May ↑ **tacrolimus** and **methotrexate** levels. Hypomagnesemia ↑ risk of **digoxin** toxicity.

Route/Dosage

PO (Adults): *Healing of EE*—60 mg once daily for up to 8 wk; *Maintenance of healed EE*—30 mg once daily for up to 6 mo; *GERD*—30 mg once daily for 4 wk.

Hepatic Impairment

PO (Adults): *Moderate hepatic impairment*—daily dose should not exceed 30 mg.

Availability

Delayed release capsules: 30 mg, 60 mg.

NURSING IMPLICATIONS

Assessment

- Assess patient routinely for epigastric or abdominal pain and for frank or occult blood in stool, emesis, or gastric aspirate.
- Monitor bowel elimination. Diarrhea, abdominal cramping, fever, and bloody stools should be reported to health care professional promptly as a sign of Clostridium difficile-associated diarrhea (CDAD).
- ***Lab Test Considerations:*** May cause abnormal liver function tests, including ↑AST, ALT, and ↑ or ↓ serum bilirubin.
- May cause ↑ serum creatinine and BUN, ↑ blood glucose, and ↑ serum potassium, and ↓ serum magnesium levels.
- May cause ↓ platelet levels.
- May also cause ↑ gastrin and total protein levels.
- Monitor INR and prothrombin time in patients taking warfarin.

Potential Nursing Diagnoses

Acute pain (Indications)

Implementation

- **PO:** May be administered without regard to food. Swallow capsules whole or may be opened and sprinkled on 1 tbsp of applesauce and swallowed immediately, without crushing or chewing, for patients with difficulty swallowing.
- Capsules may be opened and granules emptied into 20 mL water. Withdraw entire mixture into syringe; swirl gently to mix. Administer mixture into mouth or NG tube immediately; do not save for later. Rinse syringe with 10 mL or water twice to ensure all medication administered.

Patient/Family Teaching

- Instruct patient to take medication as directed for the full course of therapy, even if feeling better. Take missed doses as soon as remembered. Brand name was formerly Kapidex.
- Advise patient to avoid alcohol, products containing aspirin or NSAIDs, and foods that may cause an increase in GI irritation.
- Advise patient to report onset of black, tarry stools; diarrhea; or abdominal pain to health care professional promptly, especially if accompanied by fever or bloody stools. Do not treat with antidiarrheals without consulting health care professional.
- Advise patient to notify health care professional if signs and symptoms of hypomagnesemia (seizures, dizziness, abnormal or fast heartbeat, jitteriness, jerking movements or shaking [tremors], muscle weakness, spasms of the hands and feet, cramps or muscle aches, spasm of the voice box) occur.
- Instruct patient to notify health care professional of all Rx or OTC medications, vitamins, or herbal products being taken and to consult with health care professional before taking other medications.
- Advise female patients to notify health care professional if pregnancy is planned or suspected or if breast feeding.

Evaluation/Desired Outcomes

- Decrease in abdominal pain, heartburn, gastric irritation, and bleeding in patients with GERD; may require up to 4 wk of therapy.
- Healing in patients with erosive esophagitis; may require up to 8 wk of therapy for healing and 6 mo of therapy for maintenance.

D

dexmedetomidine

(dex-me-de-**to**-mi-deen)

Precedex

Classification

Therapeutic: sedative/hypnotics

Pregnancy Category C

Indications

Sedation of initially intubated and mechanically ventilated patients during treatment in an intensive care setting; should not be used for >24 hr. Sedation of non-intubated patients before and/or during surgical and other procedures.

Action

Acts as a relatively selective alpha-adrenergic agonist with sedative properties. **Therapeutic Effects:** Sedation.

Pharmacokinetics

Absorption: IV administration results in complete bioavailability.

Distribution: Unknown.

Protein Binding: 94%.

Metabolism and Excretion: Mostly metabolized by the liver, some metabolism by P450 enzyme system. Metabolites are mostly excreted in urine.

Half-life: 2 hr.

TIME/ACTION PROFILE (sedation)

ROUTE	ONSET	PEAK	DURATION
IV	rapid	unknown	unknown

Contraindications/Precautions

Contraindicated in: Hypersensitivity.

Use Cautiously in: Hepatic impairment (lower doses may be required); Advanced heart block; Severe left ventricular dysfunction; Geri: ↑ risk of bradycardia and hypotension (consider dose ↓); OB, Lactation, Pedi: Safety not established.

Adverse Reactions/Side Effects

Resp: hypoxia. **CV:** BRADYCARDIA, SINUS ARREST, hypotension, transient hypertension. **GI:** dry mouth, nausea, vomiting. **Hemat:** anemia. **Misc:** fever.

Interactions

Drug-Drug: Sedation is enhanced by **anesthetics**, other **sedative/hypnotics**, and **opioid analgesics**.
Drug-Natural Products: Concomitant use of **kava-kava, valerian, skullcap, chamomile**, or **hops** can ↑ CNS depression.

Route/Dosage

ICU Sedation

IV (Adults): *Loading infusion*—1 mcg/kg over 10 min followed by *maintenance infusion* of 0.2–0.7 mcg/kg/hr for maximum of 24 hr; rate is adjusted to achieve desired level of sedation.
IV (Children): *Loading infusion*—0.5–1 mcg/kg followed by *maintenance infusion* of 0.2–1 mcg/kg/hr. Children <1 yr may require higher end of infusion rate.

Procedural Sedation

IV (Adults): *Loading infusion*—1 mcg/kg (0.5 mcg/kg for ophthalmic surgery or patients >65 yr) over 10 min followed by *maintenance infusion* of 0.6 mcg/kg/hr; rate is adjusted to achieve desired level of sedation (usual range 0.2–1 mcg/kg/hr) (maintenance infusion of 0.7 mcg/kg/hr recommended for fiberoptic intubation until endotracheal tube secured).

Availability (generic available)

Solution for injection (requires further dilution): 100 mcg/mL. **Premixed infusion (in 0.9% NaCl):** 4 mcg/mL.

NURSING IMPLICATIONS

Assessment

- Assess level of sedation throughout therapy. Dose is adjusted based on level of sedation.
- Monitor ECG and BP continuously throughout therapy. May cause hypotension, bradycardia, and sinus arrest.
- ***Toxicity and Overdose:*** Atropine IV may be used to modify the vagal tone.

Potential Nursing Diagnoses

Anxiety (Indications)

Implementation

- Dexmedetomidine should be administered only in intensive care settings with continuous monitoring.
- A loading dose may not be required when converting patient from another sedative.

IV Administration

- **Continuous Infusion:** ***Diluent:*** To prepare infusion, withdraw 2 mL of dexmedetomidine and add to 48 mL of 0.9 NaCl for a total of 50 mL. ***Concentration:*** 4 mcg/mL. Shake gently. Solution should be clear; do not administer solutions that are discolored or contain particulate matter. Ampules and vials are for single use only. ***Rate:*** Administer *loading infusion* over 10 minutes, followed by *maintenance infusion* of 0.2–0.7 mcg/kg/hr for ICU sedation and 0.2–1.0 mcg/kg/hr for procedural sedation. Adjust dose to achieve desired level of sedation. Administer via infusion pump to ensure accurate rate.
- **Y-Site Compatibility:** 20% mannitol, acyclovir, alemtuzumab, alfentanil, allopurinol, amifostine, amikacin, aminophylline, amiodarone, amphotericin B liposome, ampicillin, ampicillin/sulbactam, anidulafungin, argatroban, asparaginase, atropine, azithromycin, aztreonam, bivalirudin, bleomycin, bumetanide, buprenorphine, busulfan, butorphanol, calcium chloride, calcium gluconate, carboplatin, carmustine, caspofungin, cefazolin, cefepime, cefotaxime, cefotetan, cefoxitin, ceftazidime, ceftriaxone, cefuroxime, chlorpromazine, ciprofloxacin, cisatracurium, cisplatin, clindamycin, cyclophosphamide, cyclosporine, cytarabine, dacarbazine, dactinomycin, daptomycin, daunorubicin hydrochloride, dexamethasone, dexrazoxane, digoxin, diltiazem, diphenhydramine, dobutamine, docetaxel, dolasetron, dopamine, doxacurium, doxorubicin hydrochloride, doxycycline, droperidol, enalaprilat, ephedrine, epinephrine, ertapenem, erythromycin, esmolol, etomidate, etoposide, etoposide phosphate, famotidine, fenoldopam, fentanyl, fluconazole, fludarabine, fluorouracil, foscarnet, fosphenytoin, furosemide, ganciclovir, gemcitabine, gentamicin, glycopyrrolate, granisetron, haloperidol, heparin, hydrocortisone, hydromorphone, idarubicin, ifosfamide, imipenem/cilastatin, insulin, isoproterenol, ketorolac, labetalol, leucovorin, levofloxacin, levorphanol, lidocaine, linezolid, lorazepam, magnesium sulfate, mannitol, mechlorethamine, meperidine, meropenem, mesna, methohexital, methotrexate, methylprednisolone, metoclopramide, metoprolol, metronidazole, midazolam, milrinone, mitomycin, mitoxantrone, morphine, moxifloxacin, mycophenolate, nalbuphine, naloxone, nesiritide, nicardipine, nitroglycerin, nitroprusside, norepinephrine, octreotide, ondansetron, oxaliplatin, oxytocin, paclitaxel, palonosetron, pamidronate, pancuronium, pemetrexed, pentamidine, pentobarbital, phenobarbital, phenylephrine, piperacillin/tazobactam, plasma substitute, potassium acetate, potassium chloride, potassium phosphate, prochlorperazine, promethazine, propofol, propranolol, quinupristin/dalfopristin, ranitidine, remifentanil, rocuronium, sodium acetate, sodium bicarbonate, sodium phosphates, succinylcholine, sufentanil, tacrolimus, teniposide, theophylline, thiopental, thiotepa, tigecycline, tirofiban, tobramycin, topotecan, trimethoprin/sulfamethoxazole, vancomycin, vasopressin, vecuronium, verapamil, vinblastine, vincristine, vinorelbine, voriconazole, zidovudine, zoledronic acid.

- **Y-Site Incompatibility:** amphotericin B colloidal, amphotericin B lipid complex, blood, diazepam, irinotecan, pantoprazole, plasma, phenytoin.

Patient/Family Teaching

- Explain to patient and family the purpose of the medication.

Evaluation/Desired Outcomes

- Sedation for up to 24 hr.

dexrazoxane (dex-ra-**zox**-ane)

Totect, Zinecard

Classification

Therapeutic: cardioprotective agents

Pregnancy Category D

Indications

Reducing incidence and severity of cardiomyopathy from doxorubicin in women with metastatic breast cancer who have already received a cumulative dose of doxorubicin >300 m g/m². Treatment of extravasation resulting from IV anthracycline chemotherapy.

Action

Acts as an intracellular chelating agent. **Therapeutic Effects:** Diminishes the cardiotoxic effects of doxorubicin. Decreased damage from extravasation of anthracyclines.

Pharmacokinetics

Absorption: IV administration results in complete bioavailability.

Distribution: Unknown.

Metabolism and Excretion: Some metabolism occurs; 42% eliminated in urine.

Half-life: 2.1–2.5 hr.

TIME/ACTION PROFILE (cardioprotective effect)

ROUTE	ONSET	PEAK	DURATION
IV	rapid	unknown	unknown

Contraindications/Precautions

Contraindicated in: Any other type of chemotherapy except other anthracyclines (doxorubicin-like agents); May cause fetal harm.

Use Cautiously in: CCr <40 mL/min (dose ↓ required); Lactation: Lactation; Pedi: Safety and effectiveness not established.

Adverse Reactions/Side Effects

Hemat: myelosuppression. **Local:** pain at injection site. **Misc:** MALIGNANCY.

Interactions

Drug-Drug: Myelosuppression may be ↑ by **antineoplastics** or **radiation therapy**. Antitumor effects of concurrent combination chemotherapy with **fluorouracil** and **cyclophosphamide** may be ↓ by dexrazoxane.

Route/Dosage

Cardioprotective

IV (Adults): 10 mg of dexrazoxane/1 mg doxorubicin.

Renal Impairment

IV (Adults): ↓ dose by 50%.

Extravasation Protection

IV (Adults): 1000 mg/m² (maximum 2000 mg) given on days 1 and 2, and followed by a dose of 500 mg/m² (maximum 1000 mg) on day 3.

Renal Impairment

IV (Adults CCr <40 mL/min): ↓ dose by 50%.

Availability (generic available)

Injection (Zinecard): 250 mg/vial, 500 mg/vial. **Injection (Totect):** 500 mg/vial.

NURSING IMPLICATIONS

Assessment

- **Cardioprotective:** Assess extent of cardiomyopathy (cardiomegaly on x ray, basilar rales, S gallop, dyspnea, decline in left ventricular ejection fraction) prior to and periodically during therapy.
- **Extravasation protection:** Assess site of extravasation for pain, burning, swelling, and redness.
- ***Lab Test Considerations:*** Monitor CBC and platelet count frequently during therapy. Thrombocytopenia, leukopenia, neutropenia, and granulocytopenia from chemotherapy may be more severe at nadir with dexrazoxane therapy.
- Monitor liver function tests periodically during therapy. May cause reversible ↑ of liver enzymes.

Potential Nursing Diagnoses

Decreased cardiac output (Indications)
Risk for impaired skin integrity (Indications)

Implementation

- Solution should be prepared in a biologic cabinet. Wear gloves, gown, and mask while handling IV medication. Discard IV equipment in specially designated containers.
- Do not administer solutions that are discolored or contain particulate matter. Reconstituted solution and diluted solution are stable in an IV bag for 6 hr at room temperature or if refrigerated. Discard unused solutions.

IV Administration

- **Cardioprotective:** Doxorubicin should be administered within 30 min following dexrazoxane administration.
- **IV Push:** ***Diluent:*** Reconstitute dexrazoxane with 0.167 molar (M/6) sodium lactate injection. ***Concentration:*** 10 mg/mL. ***Rate:*** Administer via slow IV push.
- **Intermittent Infusion:** ***Diluent:*** Reconstituted solution may also be diluted with 0.9% NaCl or D5W. Solution is stable for 6 hr at room temperature or refrigerated. ***Concentration:*** 1.3–5 mg/mL. ***Rate:*** May also be administered via rapid IV infusion over 15–30 min.
- **Additive Incompatibility:** Do not mix with other medications.
- **Extravasation Protection:** Administer as soon as possible within 6 hr of extravasation. Remove cooling procedures, such as ice packs, at least 15 min before administration to allow sufficient blood flow to area of extravasation.
- **Intermittent Infusion:** ***Diluent:*** Dilute each vial in 50 mL of diluent provided by manufacturer. Add contents of all vials into 1000 mL of 0.9% NaCl for further dilution. Solution is slightly yellow. Use diluted solutions within 2 hr of dilution. Store at room temperature. ***Rate:*** Administer over 1–2 hr.
- **Y-Site Compatibility:** alemtuzumab, alfentanil, amifostine, amikacin, amiodarone, ampicillin, ampicillin/sulbactam, anidulafungin, argatroban, arsenic trioxide, atracurium, azithromycin, aztreonam, bivalirudin, bleomycin, bumetanide, buprenorphine, busulfan, buprenorphine, calcium chloride, calcium gluconate, carboplatin, carmustine, caspofungin, cefazolin, cefotaxime, cefotetan, cefoxitin, ceftazidime, ceftriaxone, cefuroxime, chloramphenicol, chlorpromazine, ciprofloxacin, cisatracurium, cisplatin, clindamycin, cyclophosphamide, cyclosporine, cytarabine, dactinomycin, daptomycin, dexmedetomidine, digoxin, diltiazem, diphenhydramine, docetaxel, dolasetron, dopamine, doxacurium, doxorubicin, doxorubicin liposomal, doxycycline, droperidol, enalaprilat, ephedrine, epinephrine, epirubicin, eptifibatide, srtapenem, erythromycin, esmolol, stoposide, famotidine, fenoldopam, fentanyl, fluconazole, fludarabine, fluorouracil, foscarnet, fosphenytoin, gentamycin, glycopyrrolate, granisetron, haloperidol, heparin, hetastarch, hydralazine, hydrocortisone sodium succinate, hydromorphone, idarubicin, ifosfamide, imipenem/cilastatin, insulin, irinotecan, isoproterenol, ketorolac, leucovorin, levofloxacin, lidocaine, linezolid, lorazepam, magnesium sulfate, mannitol, mechlorethamine, melphalan, meperidine, meropenem, metaraminol, methyldopate, metoclopramide, metoprolol, metronidazole, midazolam, milrinone, minocycline, mitoxantrone, morphine, mycophenolate, nalbuphine, naloxone, nesiritide, nicardipine, nitroglycerin, nitroprusside, norepinephrine, octreotide, ondansetron, oxaliplatin, paclitaxel, palonosetron, pamidronate, pancuronium, pemetrexed, pentamidine, pentazocine, phenobarbital, phentolamine, phenylephrine, piperacillin/tazobactam, polumyxin B, potassium acetate, potassium chloride, potassium phosphates, procainamide, prochlorperazine, promethazine, propranolol, quinupristin/dalfopristin, ranitidine, remifentanil, rituximab, rocuronium, sodium acetate, sodium bicarbonate, streptozocin, succinylcholine, sufentanil, tacrolimus, teniposide, theophylline, thiotepa, tigecycline, tirofiban, tobramycin, vancomycin, vasopressin, vecuronium, verapamil, vinblastine, vincristine, vinorelbine, voriconazole, zoledronic acid.
- **Additive Incompatibility:** acyclovir, allopurinol, aminophylline, amphotericin B colloidal, amphotericin B lipid complex, amphotericin B liposome, cefepime, dantrolene, diazepam, dobutamine, furosemide, ganciclovir, methotrexate, methylprednisolone, nafcillin, pantoprazole, pentobarbital, phenytoin, sodium phosphates, thiopental, trimethoprim/sulfamethoxazole, zidovudine.

Patient/Family Teaching

- Explain the purpose of the medication to the patient.
- Emphasize the need for continued monitoring of cardiac function.
- Advise patient to notify health care professional if pregnancy is suspected or planned or if breast feeding. Dexrazoxane may be teratogenic. Breast feeding should be avoided during therapy.

Evaluation/Desired Outcomes

- Reduction of incidence and severity of cardiomyopathy associated with doxorubicin administration in women with metastatic breast cancer.
- Decrease in late sequalae (site pain, fibrosis, atrophy, and local sensory disturbance) following extravasation of anthracycline chemotherapeutic agents.

dextromethorphan

(dex-troe-meth-**or**-fan)

✱Balminil DM, ✱Benylin DM, ✱Bronchophan Forte DM, ✱Buckley's DM, ✱Cough Syrup DM, Creo-Terpin, Creomulsion Adult Formula, Creomulsion for Children, Delsym, ✱Delsym DM, ✱DM Children's Cough Syrup, ✱DM Cough Syrup, ✱Dry Cough Syrup, Father John's, Hold DM, ✱Koffex DM, ✱Neocitran Thin Strips Cough, Pediacare Children's Long-Acting Cough, Robafin Cough, Robitussin Children's

Cough Long-Acting, Robitussin Cough Long-Acting, Robitussin CoughGels Long-Acting, Robitussin Lingering Cold Long-Acting CoughGels, Scot-Tussin Diabetes, ✤Sedatuss DM, ✤Sucrets Cough Control, ✤Sucrets DM, ✤Triaminic DM, ✤Triaminic Long-Acting Cough, Triaminic Thin Strips Children's Long-Acting Cough, Triaminic Children's Cough Long-Acting, Vicks 44 Cough Relief, ✤Vicks Custom Care Dry Cough, Vicks DayQuil Cough, Vicks Nature Fusion Cough

Classification
Therapeutic: allergy, cold, and cough remedies, antitussives

Pregnancy Category C

Indications

Symptomatic relief of coughs caused by minor viral upper respiratory tract infections or inhaled irritants. Most effective for chronic nonproductive cough. A common ingredient in nonprescription cough and cold preparations.

Action

Suppresses the cough reflex by a direct effect on the cough center in the medulla. Related to opioids structurally but has no analgesic properties. **Therapeutic Effects:** Relief of irritating nonproductive cough.

Pharmacokinetics

Absorption: Rapidly absorbed from the GI tract. Extended-release product is slowly absorbed.
Distribution: Unknown. Probably crosses the placenta and enters breast milk.
Metabolism and Excretion: Metabolized to dextrorphan, an active metabolite. Dextromethorphan and dextrorphan are renally excreted.
Half-life: Unknown.

TIME/ACTION PROFILE (cough suppression)

ROUTE	ONSET	PEAK	DURATION
PO	15–30 min	unknown	3–6 hr†
PO-ER	unknown	unknown	9–12 hr

†Up to 8 hr for gelcaps.

Contraindications/Precautions

Contraindicated in: Hypersensitivity; Patients taking MAO inhibitors or SSRIs; Should not be used for chronic productive coughs; Some products contain alcohol and should be avoided in patients with known intolerance.

Use Cautiously in: Cough that lasts more than 1 wk or is accompanied by fever, rash, or headache—health care professional should be consulted; History of drug abuse or drug-seeking behavior (capsules have been abused resulting in deaths); Diabetes (some products contain sucrose); OB: Pregnancy (has been used safely); Lactation: Lactation; Pedi: Children <4 yr (OTC cough and cold products containing this medication should be avoided).

D

Adverse Reactions/Side Effects

CNS: *high dose*—dizziness, sedation. **GI:** nausea.

Interactions

Drug-Drug: Use with **MAO inhibitors** may result in serotonin syndrome (nausea, confusion, changes in BP); concurrent use should be avoided. ↑ CNS depression with **antihistamines**, **alcohol**, **antidepressants**, **sedative/hypnotics**, or **opioids**. **Amiodarone**, **fluoxetine**, or **quinidine** may ↑ blood levels and adverse reactions from dextromethorphan.

Route/Dosage

PO (Adults and Children >12 yr): 10–20 mg q 4 hr *or* 30 mg q 6–8 hr *or* 60 mg of extended-release preparation bid (not to exceed 120 mg/day).
PO (Children 6–12 yr): 5–10 mg q 4 hr *or* 15 mg q 6–8 hr *or* 30 mg of extended-release preparation q 12 hr (not to exceed 60 mg/day).
PO (Children 4–6 yr): 2.5–5 mg q 4 hr *or* 7.5 mg q 6–8 hr *or* 15 mg of extended-release preparation q 12 hr (not to exceed 30 mg/day).

Availability (generic available)

Gelcaps: 30 mg^{OTC}. **Lozenges (cherry):** 2.5 mg^{OTC}, 5 mg^{OTC}. **Liquid (cherry, grape):** 3.5 mg/5 mL^{OTC}, 5 mg/5 mL, 7.5 mg/5 mL^{OTC}, 15 mg/5 mL^{OTC}, 30 mg/5 mL^{OTC}. **Syrup (cherry, cherry bubblegum):** 7.5 mg/5 mL^{OTC}, 15 mg/15 mL^{OTC}, 10 mg/5 mL^{OTC}. **Extended-release suspension (orange):** 30 mg/5 mL^{OTC}. **Drops (Grape):** 7.5 mg/0.8 mL^{OTC}, 7.5 mg/1 mL^{OTC}. **Orally-disintegrating strips (cherry, grape):** 7.5 mg^{OTC}, 15 mg^{OTC}. ***In combination with:*** antihistamines, decongestants, and expectorants in cough and cold preparations^{OTC}, quinidine sulfate (Nuedextra). See Appendix B.

NURSING IMPLICATIONS

Assessment

- Assess frequency and nature of cough, lung sounds, and amount and type of sputum produced. Unless contraindicated, maintain fluid intake of 1500–2000 mL to decrease viscosity of bronchial secretions.

Potential Nursing Diagnoses

Ineffective airway clearance (Indications)

Implementation

- Dextromethorphan 15–30 mg is equivalent in cough suppression to codeine 8–15 mg.
- **PO:** Do not give fluids immediately after administering to prevent dilution of vehicle. Shake oral suspension well before administration.

Patient/Family Teaching

- Instruct patient to cough effectively: Sit upright and take several deep breaths before attempting to cough.
- Advise patient to minimize cough by avoiding irritants, such as cigarette smoke, fumes, and dust. Humidification of environmental air, frequent sips of water, and sugarless hard candy may also decrease the frequency of dry, irritating cough.
- Caution patient to avoid taking more than the recommended dose or taking alcohol or other CNS depressants concurrently with this medication; fatalities have occurred. Caution parents to avoid OTC cough and cold products while breast feeding or to children <4 yrs.
- May occasionally cause dizziness. Caution patient to avoid driving or other activities requiring alertness until response to the medication is known.
- Advise patient that any cough lasting over 1 wk or accompanied by fever, chest pain, persistent headache, or skin rash warrants medical attention.

Evaluation/Desired Outcomes

- Decrease in frequency and intensity of cough without eliminating patient's cough reflex.

⧖ diazepam (dye-az-e-pam)

Diastat, ✱Diazemuls, Valium

Classification

Therapeutic: antianxiety agents, anticonvulsants, sedative/hypnotics, skeletal muscle relaxants (centrally acting)
Pharmacologic: benzodiazepines

Schedule IV

Pregnancy Category D

Indications

Adjunct in the management of: Anxiety Disorder, Athetosis, Anxiety relief prior to cardioversion (injection), Stiffman Syndrome, Preoperative sedation, Conscious sedation (provides light anesthesia and anterograde amnesia). Treatment of status epilepticus/uncontrolled seizures (injection). Skeletal muscle relaxant. Management of the symptoms of alcohol withdrawal. **Unlabeled Use:** Anxiety associated with acute myocardial infarction, insomnia.

Action

Depresses the CNS, probably by potentiating GABA, an inhibitory neurotransmitter. Produces skeletal muscle relaxation by inhibiting spinal polysynaptic afferent pathways. Has anticonvulsant properties due to enhanced presynaptic inhibition. **Therapeutic Effects:** Relief of anxiety. Sedation. Amnesia. Skeletal muscle relaxation. Decreased seizure activity.

Pharmacokinetics

Absorption: Rapidly absorbed from the GI tract. Absorption from IM sites may be slow and unpredictable. Well absorbed (90%) from rectal mucosa.
Distribution: Widely distributed. Crosses the blood-brain barrier. Crosses the placenta; enters breast milk.
Metabolism and Excretion: Highly metabolized by the hepatic P450 enzymes (CYP2C19 and CYP3A4); the CYP2C19 enzyme system exhibits genetic polymorphism; ⧖ 15–20% of Asian patients and 3–5% of Caucasian and Black patients may be poor metabolizers and may have significantly ↑ diazepam concentrations and an ↑ risk of adverse effects. Some products of metabolism are active as CNS depressants.
Half-life: Neonates: 50–95 hr; Infants 1 mo–2 yr: 40–50 hr; Children 2–12 yr: 15–21 hr; Children 12–16 yr: 18–20 hr; Adults: 20–50 hr (up to 100 hr for metabolites).

TIME/ACTION PROFILE (sedation)

ROUTE	ONSET	PEAK	DURATION
PO	30–60 min	1–2 hr	up to 24 hr
IM	within 20 min	0.5–1.5 hr	unknown
IV	1–5 min	15–30 min	15–60 min†
Rectal	2–10 min	1–2 hr	4–12 hr

†In status epilepticus, anticonvulsant duration is 15–20 min.

Contraindications/Precautions

Contraindicated in: Hypersensitivity; Cross-sensitivity with other benzodiazepines may occur; Comatose patients; Myasthenia gravis; Severe pulmonary impairment; Sleep apnea; Severe hepatic dysfunction; Pre-existing CNS depression; Uncontrolled severe pain; Angle-closure glaucoma; Some products contain alcohol, propylene glycol, or tartrazine and should be avoided in patients with known hypersensitivity or intolerance; OB: ↑ risk of congenital malformations; Pedi: Children <6 mo (for oral; safety not established); Lactation: Recommend to discontinue drug or bottle-feed.
Use Cautiously in: Severe renal impairment; History of suicide attempt or drug dependence; Debilitated patients (dose ↓ required); Patients with low albumin; Pedi: Metabolites can accumulate in neonates. Injection contains benzyl alcohol which can cause potentially fatal gasping syndrome in neonates; Geri: Long-acting benzodiazepines cause prolonged sedation in the elderly. Appears on *Beers list* and is associated with ↑ risk of falls (↓ dose required or consider short-acting benzodiazepine).

Adverse Reactions/Side Effects

CNS: dizziness, drowsiness, lethargy, depression, hangover, ataxia, slurred speech, headache, paradoxical excitation. **EENT:** blurred vision. **Resp:** RESPIRATORY DEPRESSION. **CV:** hypotension (IV only). **GI:** constipation, diarrhea (may be caused by propylene glycol content in oral solution), nausea, vomiting, weight gain. **Derm:** rashes. **Local:** pain (IM), phlebitis (IV), venous thrombosis. **Misc:** physical dependence, psychological dependence, tolerance.

Interactions

Drug-Drug: Alcohol, antidepressants, antihistamines, and **opioid analgesics**—concurrent use results in additive CNS depression. **Cimetidine, hormonal contraceptives, disulfiram, fluoxetine, isoniazid, ketoconazole, metoprolol, propranolol,** or **valproic acid** may ↓ the metabolism of diazepam, enhancing its actions. May ↓ the efficacy of **levodopa. Rifampin** or **barbiturates** may ↑ the metabolism and ↓ effectiveness of diazepam. Sedative effects may be ↓ by **theophylline**. Concurrent use of **ritonavir** is not recommended.
Drug-Natural Products: Concomitant use of **kava-kava, valerian,** or **chamomile** can ↑ CNS depression.

Route/Dosage

Antianxiety

PO (Adults): 2–10 mg 2–4 times daily.
IM, IV (Adults): 2–10 mg, may repeat in 3–4 hr as needed.
PO (Children >6 mo): 1–2.5 mg 3–4 times daily.
IM, IV (Children >1 mo): 0.04–0.3 mg/kg/dose q 2–4 hr to a maximum of 0.6 mg/kg within an 8 hr period if necessary.

Precardioversion

IV (Adults): 5–15 mg 5–10 min precardioversion.

Pre-endoscopy

IV (Adults): 2.5–20 mg.
IM (Adults): 5–10 mg 30 min pre-endoscopy.

Pediatric Conscious Sedation for Procedures

PO (Children >6 mo): 0.2–0.3 mg/kg (not to exceed 10 mg/dose) 45–60 min prior to procedure.

Status Epilepticus/Acute Seizure Activity

IV (Adults): 5–10 mg, may repeat q 10–15 min to a total of 30 mg, may repeat regimen again in 2–4 hr (IM route may be used if IV route unavailable); larger doses may be required.
IM, IV (Children ≥5 yr): 0.05–0.3 mg/kg/dose given over 3–5 min q 15–30 min to a total dose of 10 mg, repeat q 2–4 hr.
IM, IV (Children 1 mo–5 yr): 0.05–0.3 mg/kg/dose given over 3–5 min q 15–30 min to maximum dose of 5 mg, repeat in 2–4 hr if needed.
IV (Neonates): 0.1–0.3 mg/kg/dose given over 3–5 min q 15–30 min to maximum dose of 2 mg.
Rect (Adults and Children >12 yr): 0.2 mg/kg; may repeat 4–12 hr later.
Rect (Children 6–11 yr): 0.3 mg/kg; may repeat 4–12 hr later.
Rect (Children 2–5 yr): 0.5 mg/kg; may repeat 4–12 hr later.

Febrile Seizure Prophylaxis

PO (Children >1 mo): 1 mg/kg/day divided q 8 hr at first sign of fever and continue for 24 hr after fever is gone.

Skeletal Muscle Relaxation

PO (Adults): 2–10 mg 3–4 times daily.
PO (Geriatric Patients or Debilitated Patients): 2–2.5 mg 1–2 times daily initially.
PO (Children >6 mo): 1–2.5 mg 3–4 times daily.
IM, IV (Adults): 5–10 mg; may repeat in 2–4 hr (larger doses may be required for tetanus).
IM, IV (Geriatric Patients or Debilitated Patients): 2–5 mg; may repeat in 2–4 hr (larger doses may be required for tetanus).
IM, IV (Children ≥5 yr): *Tetanus*—5–10 mg q 3–4 hr.
IM, IV (Children >1 mo): *Tetanus*—1–2 mg q 3–4 hr.

Alcohol Withdrawal

PO (Adults): 10 mg 3–4 times in first 24 hr, ↓ to 5 mg 3–4 times daily.
IM, IV (Adults): 10 mg initially, then 5–10 mg in 3–4 hr as needed; larger or more frequent doses have been used.

Psychoneurotic Reactions

IM, IV (Adults): 2–10 mg, may be repeated in 3–4 hr.

Availability (generic available)

Tablets: 2 mg, 5 mg, 10 mg. **Cost:** *Generic*—2 mg $7.51/100, 5 mg $10.74/100, 10 mg $10.84/100. **Oral solution:** 1 mg/mL, 5 mg/mL (Intensol). **Cost:** *Generic*—1 mg/mL $2.44/5 mL, 5 mg/mL $33.98/30 mL. **Injection:** 5 mg/mL (contains 10% alcohol and 40% propylene glycol). **Rectal gel delivery system:** 2.5 mg, 10 mg, 20 mg.

NURSING IMPLICATIONS

Assessment

- Monitor BP, pulse, and respiratory rate prior to and periodically throughout therapy and frequently during IV therapy.
- Assess IV site frequently during administration; diazepam may cause phlebitis and venous thrombosis.
- Prolonged high-dose therapy may lead to psychological or physical dependence. Restrict amount of

drug available to patient. Observe depressed patients closely for suicidal tendencies.

- Conduct regular assessment of continued need for treatment.
- Geri: Assess risk of falls and institute fall prevention strategies.
- **Anxiety:** Assess mental status (orientation, mood, behavior) and degree of anxiety.
- Assess level of sedation (ataxia, dizziness, slurred speech) prior to and periodically throughout therapy.
- **Seizures:** Observe and record intensity, duration, and location of seizure activity. The initial dose of diazepam offers seizure control for 15–20 min after administration. Institute seizure precautions.
- **Muscle Spasms:** Assess muscle spasm, associated pain, and limitation of movement prior to and during therapy.
- **Alcohol Withdrawal:** Assess patient experiencing alcohol withdrawal for tremors, agitation, delirium, and hallucinations. Protect patient from injury.
- ***Lab Test Considerations:*** Evaluate hepatic and renal function and CBC periodically during prolonged therapy. May cause ↑ tranaminases and alkaline phosphatase.
- ***Toxicity and Overdose:*** Flumazenil is an adjunct in the management of toxicity or overdose. (Flumazenil may induce seizures in patients with a history of seizures disorder or who are on tricyclic antidepressants.).

Potential Nursing Diagnoses

Anxiety (Indications)
Impaired physical mobility (Indications)
Risk for injury (Side Effects)

Implementation

- Patient should be kept on bedrest and observed for at least 3 hr following parenteral administration.
- If opioid analgesics are used concurrently with parenteral diazepam, decrease opioid dose by 1/3 and titrate dose to effect.
- Use lowest effective dose. Taper by 2 mg every 3 days to decrease withdrawal symptoms. Some patients may require longer taper periods (mo).
- **PO:** Tablets may be crushed and taken with food or water if patient has difficulty swallowing.
- Mix Intensol preparation with liquid or semisolid food such as water, juices, soda, applesauce, or pudding. Administer entire amount immediately. Do not store.
- **IM:** IM injections are painful and erratically absorbed. If IM route is used, inject deeply into deltoid muscle for maximum absorption.

IV Administration

- **IV:** Resuscitation equipment should be available when diazepam is administered IV.
- **IV Push:** ***Diluent:*** For IV administration do not dilute or mix with any other drug. If IV push is not feasible, administer IV push into tubing as close to insertion site as possible. Continuous infusion is not recommended due to precipitation in IV fluids and absorption of diazepam into infusion bags and tubing. Injection may cause burning and venous irritation; avoid small veins. ***Concentration:*** 5 mg/mL. ***Rate:*** Administer slowly at a rate of 5 mg/min in adults. Infants and children should receive 1–2 mg/min. Rapid injection may cause apnea, hypotension, bradycardia, or cardiac arrest.
- **Y-Site Compatibility:** docetaxel, methadone, piperacillin/tazobactam, teniposide.
- **Y-Site Incompatibility:** acetaminophen, acyclovir, alemtuzumab, alfentanil, amikacin, aminocaproic acid, aminophylline, amphotericin B cholesteryl, amphotericin B colloidal, amphotericin B lipid complex, amphotericin B liposome, ampicillin, ampicillin/sulbactam, anidulafungin, argatroban, ascorbic acid, atracurium, atropine, azathioprine, aztreonam, azithromycin, benztropine, bivalirudin, bleomycin, bumetanide, buprenorphine, butorphanol, calcium chloride, calcium gluconate, carboplatin, carmustine, caspofungin, cefazolin, cefepime, cefotaxime, cefotetan, cefoxitin, ceftaroline, ceftazidime, ceftriaxone, cefuroxime, chloramphenicol, chlorpromazine, cisplatin, clindamycin, cyanocobalamin, cyclophosphamide, cyclosporine, cytarabine, dactinomycin, dantrolene, dexamethasone, dexmedetomidine, dexrazoxane, diazoxide, digoxin, diltiazem, diphenhydramine, dopamine, doripenem, doxacurium, doxorubicin, doxorubicin liposomal, doxycycline, enalaprilat, ephedrine, epinephrine, epirubicin, epoetin alfa, eptifibatide, ertapenem, erythromycin, esmolol, etoposide, etoposide phosphate, famotidine, fenoldopam, fluconazole, fludarabine, fluorouracil, folic acid, foscarnet, furosemide, ganciclovir, gemcitabine, gentamicin, glycopyrrolate, granisetron, haloperidol, heparin, hetastarch, hydralazine, hydrocortisone, hydroxycobalamin, hydroxyzine, idarubicin, ifosfamide, imipenem/cilastatin, indomethacin, insulin, irinotecan, isoproterenol, ketorolac, labetalol, leucovorin calcium, levofloxacin, lidocaine, linezolid, magnesium chloride, mannitol, mechlorethamine, meperidine, meropenem, metaraminol, methotrexate, methoxamine, methyldopate, methylprednisolone, metoclopramide, metoprolol, metronidazole, midazolam, milrinone, mitoxantrone, multivitamin, mycophenolate, nalbuphine, naloxone, nesiritide, nitroglycerin, nitroprusside, norepinephrine, octreotide, oxacillin, oxaliplatin, oxytocin, paclitaxel, palonosetron, pancuronium, pantoprazole, papaverine, pemetrexed, penicillin G, pentamidine, pentazocine, pentobarbital, phenobarbital, phentolamine, phenylephrine, phenytoin, phytonadione, potassium acetate, potassium chloride, procainamide, prochlorperazine, promethazine, propofol, propranolol, protamine, pyridoxime, quinupristin/dalfopristin, ranitidine, rocuronium, sodium acetate, sodium bicarbonate,

streptokinase, succinylcholine, tacrolimus, theophylline, thiamine, thiotepa, tigecycline, tirofiban, tobramycin, tolazoline, trimethoprim/sulfamethoxazole, vancomycin, vasopressin, vecuronium, verapamil, vinblastine, vincristine, vinorelbine, vitamin B complex with C, voriconazole, zoledronic acid.

- **Rect:** Do not repeat *Diastat* rectal dose more than 5 times/mo or 1 episode every 5 days. Round dose up to next available dose unit.
- Diazepam injection has been used for rectal administration. Instill via catheter or cannula fitted to the syringe or directly from a 1-mL syringe inserted 4–5 cm into the rectum. A dilution of diazepam injection with propylene glycol containing 1 mg/mL has also been used.
- Do not dilute with other solutions, IV fluids, or medications.

Patient/Family Teaching

- Instruct patient to take medication as directed and not to take more than prescribed or increase dose if less effective after a few weeks without checking with health care professional. Review package insert for Diastat rectal gel with patient/caregiver prior to administration. Abrupt withdrawal of diazepam may cause insomnia, unusual irritability or nervousness, and seizures. Advise patient that sharing of this medication may be dangerous.
- Medication may cause drowsiness, clumsiness, or unsteadiness. Advise patient to avoid driving or other activities requiring alertness until response to medication is known. Geri: Advise geriatric patients of increased risk for CNS effects and potential for falls.
- Caution patient to avoid taking alcohol or other CNS depressants concurrently with this medication.
- Advise patient to notify health care professional if pregnancy is planned or suspected or if breast feeding.
- Emphasize the importance of follow-up examinations to determine effectiveness of the medication.
- **Seizures:** Patients on anticonvulsant therapy should carry identification describing disease process and medication regimen at all times.

Evaluation/Desired Outcomes

- Decrease in anxiety level. Full therapeutic antianxiety effects occur after 1–2 wk of therapy.
- Decreased recall of surgical or diagnostic procedures.
- Control of seizures.
- Decrease in muscle spasms.
- Decreased tremulousness and more rational ideation when used for alcohol withdrawal.

DICLOFENAC† (dye-kloe-fen-ak)

diclofenac (oral)
Zorvolex

diclofenac potassium (oral)
Cambia, Cataflam, Zipsor

diclofenac sodium (injection)
Dyloject

diclofenac sodium (oral)
~~Voltaren~~, Voltaren XR

diclofenac sodium (topical gel)
Solaraze, Voltaren Gel

diclofenac sodium (topical solution)
Pennsaid

diclofenac epolamine (transdermal patch)
Flector

Classification
Therapeutic: nonopioid analgesics, nonsteroidal anti-inflammatory agents

Pregnancy Category B (3% gel), C (injection, oral, and topical solution [<30 wk gestation], 1% gel, patch), D (injection, oral, and topical solution [≥30 wk gestation)

†For ophthalmic use see Appendix C

Indications

PO: Management of inflammatory disorders including: Rheumatoid arthritis, Osteoarthritis, Ankylosing spondylitis. Primary dysmenorrhea. Relief of mild to moderate pain. Acute treatment of migraines (powder for oral solution). **Topical:** Management of: Actinic keratoses (Solaraze), Osteoarthritis (Voltaren Gel, Pennsaid [for knees]). **Transdermal:** Acute pain due to minor strains, sprains, and contusions. **IV:** Management of moderate to severe pain (alone or with opioids).

Action

Inhibits prostaglandin synthesis. **Therapeutic Effects:** Suppression of pain and inflammation. Relief of acute migraine attacks. **Topical (Solaraze):** Clearance of actinic keratosis lesions.

Pharmacokinetics

Absorption: Undergoes first-pass metabolism by liver which results in 50% bioavailability. Oral diclofenac sodium is a delayed-release dose form. Diclofenac potassium is an immediate-release dose form. 6–

10% of topical gel is systemically absorbed. IV administration results in complete bioavailability.
Distribution: Crosses the placenta.
Protein Binding: >99%.
Metabolism and Excretion: Metabolized by the liver (primarily by CYP2C9) to several metabolites; 65% excreted in urine, 35% in bile.
Half-life: 2 hr.

TIME/ACTION PROFILE

ROUTE	ONSET	PEAK	DURATION
IV	unknown	unknown	unknown
PO (inflammation)	few days–1 wk	≥2 wk	unknown
PO (pain)	30 min	unknown	up to 8 hr
Top (gel and patch)	unknown	10–20 hr	unknown
Top (solution)	unknown	unknown	unknown

Contraindications/Precautions

Contraindicated in: Hypersensitivity to diclofenac or other components of formulation; Cross-sensitivity may occur with other NSAIDs including aspirin; Active GI bleeding/ulcer disease; Peri-operative pain from coronary artery bypass graft (CABG) surgery; Exudative dermatitis, eczema, infectious lesions, burns, or wounds; Moderate-to-severe renal impairment in the perioperative period and at risk for volume depletion (IV only).
Use Cautiously in: Severe renal/hepatic disease; Cardiovascular disease or risk factors for cardiovascular disease (may ↑ risk of serious cardiovascular thrombotic events, myocardial infarction, and stroke, especially with prolonged use or use of higher doses); Heart failure or edema; History of porphyria; History of peptic ulcer disease and/or GI bleeding; Geri: Dose ↓ recommended; more susceptible to adverse effects, including GI bleeding; Bleeding tendency or concurrent anticoagulant therapy; OB, Lactation: Not recommended for use during second half of pregnancy; Pedi: Safety not established.

Adverse Reactions/Side Effects

CNS: dizziness, headache. **CV:** HF, MYOCARDIAL INFARCTION, STROKE, hypertension. **EENT:** tinnitus. **GI:** GI BLEEDING, HEPATOTOXICITY, abdominal pain, constipation, diarrhea, dyspepsia, flatulence, heartburn, ↑ liver enzymes, nausea, vomiting. **GU:** acute renal failure, hematuria. **Derm:** EXFOLIATIVE DERMATITIS, STEVENS-JOHNSON SYNDROME, TOXIC EPIDERMAL NECROLYSIS, pruritis, rashes, eczema, photosensitivity. **F and E:** edema. **Hemat:** anemia, prolonged bleeding time. **Local:** *Topical only*—contact dermatitis, dry skin, exfoliation. **Misc:** allergic reactions including ANAPHYLAXIS.

Interactions

Primarily noted for oral administration.

Drug-Drug: ↑ adverse GI effects with **aspirin**, other **NSAIDs**, or **corticosteroids**. May ↓ effectiveness of **diuretics** or **antihypertensives**. May ↑ levels/risk of toxicity from **cyclosporine**, **lithium**, or **methotrexate**. ↑ risk of bleeding with some **cephalosporins**, **thrombolytic agents**, **antiplatelet agents**, or **warfarin**. **CYP2C9 inhibitors**, including **voriconazole** may ↑ levels/risk of toxicity. **CYP2C9 inducers**, including **rifampin** may ↓ levels/effectivness. Concurrent use of oral **NSAIDs** during topical diclofenac therapy should be minimized.
Drug-Natural Products: ↑ bleeding risk with **arnica**, **chamomile**, **clove**, **dong quai**, **feverfew**, **garlic**, **ginger**, **ginkgo**, ***Panax ginseng***, and others.

Route/Dosage

Different formulations of oral diclofenac (diclofenac capsules, diclofenac sodium enteric-coated tablets, diclofenac sodium extended-release tablets, and diclofenac potassium immediate-release tablets) are not bioequivalent and should not be substituted on a mg-to-mg basis.

Diclofenac

PO (Adults): *Acute pain*—18–35 mg 3 times daily; *Osteoarthritis*—35 mg 3 times daily.

Hepatic Impairment

PO (Adults): Do not exceed dose of 18 mg 3 times daily.

Diclofenac Potassium

PO (Adults): *Analgesic/antidysmenorrheal (Cataflam)*—100 mg initially, then 50 mg 3 times daily as needed; *Analgesic (Zipsor)*—25 mg 4 times daily; *Rheumatoid arthritis (Cataflam)*—50 mg 3–4 times daily; *Osteoarthritis (Cataflam)*—50 mg 2–3 times daily; *Osteoarthritis (Cambia)*—one packet (50 mg) given as a single dose.

Diclofenac Sodium

PO (Adults): *Rheumatoid arthritis (delayed-release [enteric-coated] tablets)*—50 mg 3–4 times daily *or* 75 mg twice daily (usual maintenance dose 25 mg 3 times daily). *Rheumatoid arthritis (extended-release tablets)*—100 mg once daily; if unsatisfactory response, dose may be ↑ to 100 mg twice daily. *Osteoarthritis (delayed-release [enteric-coated] tablets)*—50 mg 2–3 times daily *or* 75 mg twice daily. *Osteoarthritis (extended-release tablets)*—100 mg once daily. *Ankylosing spondylitis (delayed-release [enteric-coated] tablets)*—25 mg 4 times daily, with an additional 25 mg given at bedtime, if necessary.
Topical (Adults): *Solaraze*—Apply to lesions twice daily for 60–90 days; *Voltaren gel*—Lower extremities (knees, ankles, feet): Apply 4 g to affected area 4 times daily (maximum of 16 g per joint/day); Upper extremities (elbows, wrists, hands): Apply 2 g to affected area 4 times daily (maximum of 8 g per joint/day); Maximum total body dose should not exceed 32 g/day; *Pennsaid*—Apply 40 drops to affected knee(s) 4 times daily.

IV (Adults): 37.5 mg every 6 hr as needed (maximum of 150 mg/day).

Diclofenac Epolamine

Topical (Adults): *Flector*—Apply 1 patch to most painful area twice daily.

Availability (generic available)

Diclofenac capsules (Zorvolex): 18 mg, 35 mg. **Diclofenac potassium immediate-release tablets (Cataflam):** 50 mg. **Cost:** *Generic*—$156.55/100. **Diclofenac potassium liquid-filled capsules (Zipsor):** 25 mg. **Cost:** $478.80/100. **Diclofenac potassium powder for oral solution (Cambia):** 50 mg/packet. **Cost:** $29.04/1 pkt. **Diclofenac sodium delayed-release (enteric-coated) tablets (Voltaren):** 25 mg, 50 mg, 75 mg. **Cost:** *Generic*—25 mg $142.18/100, 50 mg $147.23/100, 75 mg $177.39/100. **Diclofenac sodium extended-release tablets (Voltaren XR):** ✤75 mg, 100 mg. **Cost:** *Generic*—100 mg $281.42/100. **Diclofenac sodium gel:** 1% (Voltaren gel), 3% (Solaraze). **Cost:** 1% $46.48/100 g, 3% $931.92/100 g. **Diclofenac sodium solution for injection (Dyloject):** 37.5 mg/mL. **Diclofenac sodium topical solution:** 1.5%. **Cost:** $289.67/150 mL. **Diclofenac epolamine transdermal patch:** 180 mg/patch. **Cost:** $239.70/30. ***In combination with:*** misoprostol (Arthrotec). See Appendix B.

NURSING IMPLICATIONS

Assessment

- Patients who have asthma, aspirin-induced allergy, and nasal polyps are at ↑ risk for developing hypersensitivity reactions.
- Monitor BP closely during initiation of treatment and periodically during therapy in patients with hypertension.
- Assess patient for skin rash frequently during therapy. Discontinue at first sign of rash; may be life-threatening. Stevens-Johnson syndrome may develop. Treat symptomatically; may recur once treatment is stopped.
- **Pain:** Assess pain and limitation of movement; note type, location, and intensity before and 30–60 min after administration.
- **Arthritis:** Assess arthritic pain (note type, location, intensity) and limitation of movement before and periodically during therapy.
- **Actinic Keratosis:** Assess lesions prior to and periodically during therapy.
- ***Lab Test Considerations:*** Diclofenac has minimal effect on bleeding time and platelet aggregation.
- May cause ↓ in hemoglobin and hematocrit.
- Monitor CBC and liver function tests within 4–8 wk of initiating diclofenac and periodically during therapy. May cause ↑ serum alkaline phosphatase, LDH, AST, and ALT concentrations.
- Monitor BUN and serum creatinine periodically during therapy. May cause ↑ BUN and serum creatinine.

Potential Nursing Diagnoses

Acute pain (Indications)
Impaired physical mobility (Indications)

Implementation

- Administration in higher than recommended doses does not provide increased effectiveness but may cause increased side effects. Use lowest effective dose for shortest period of time.
- **PO:** Take with food or milk to minimize gastric irritation. May take first 1–2 doses on an empty stomach for more rapid onset. Do not crush or chew enteric-coated or extended-release tablets.
- **Dysmenorrhea:** Administer as soon as possible after the onset of menses. Prophylactic treatment has not been shown to be effective.
- **IV Push:** Patient must be well hydrated prior to administration to prevent renal adverse effects. Administer undiluted. Solution is clear and colorless; do not administer solution that are discolored or contain particulate matter. ***Rate:*** Inject over 15 seconds.
- **Topical: Gel** should be applied to intact skin; do not use on open wounds. An adequate amount of gel should be applied to cover the entire lesion.
- **Topical:** Dispense **solution** 10 drops at a time either directly onto knee or first into the hand and then onto knee. Spread solution evenly around front, back, and sides of the knee. Repeat until 40 drops have been applied and knee is completely covered with solution.
- **Transdermal:** Apply patch to the most painful area twice a day. Do not apply to nonintact or damaged skin resulting from any etiology (exudative dermatitis, eczema, infected lesion, burns, wounds). Avoid contact with eyes; wash hands after applying, handling, or removing patch.

Patient/Family Teaching

- Caution patient to avoid concurrent use of alcohol, aspirin, acetaminophen, other NSAIDs, or other OTC medications without consulting health care professional.
- Instruct patient to notify health care professional of medication regimen before treatment or surgery.
- May cause serious side effects: CV (MI or stroke), GI (ulcers, bleeding), skin (exfoliative dermatitis, Stevens-Johnson Syndrome, toxic epidermal necrolysis), and hypersensitivity (anaphylaxis). May occur without warning symptoms. Advise patient to stop medication and notify health care professional immediately if symptoms of CV side effects (chest pain, shortness of breath, weakness, slurring of speech), GI side effects (epigastric pain, dyspepsia, melana,

hematemesis), skin side effects (skin rash, blisters, fever, itching), or hypersensitivity reactions (difficulty breathing or swelling of face or throat) occur. Inform patient that risk for heart attack or stroke that can lead to death increases with longer use of NSAID medications and in people who have heart disease and that risk of ulcer increases with concurrent use of corticosteroids and anticoagulants, longer use, smoking, drinking alcohol, older age, and having poor health.

- Advise patient to notify health care professional promptly if unexplained weight gain, swelling of arms and legs or hands and feet, nausea, fatigue, lethargy, rash, pruritis, yellowing of skin or eyes, itching, stomach pain, vomiting blood, bloody or tarry stools, or flu-like symptoms occur.
- Instruct patient to notify health care professional of all Rx or OTC medications, vitamins, or herbal products being taken and to consult with health care professional before taking other medications.
- Instruct female patients to inform health care professional if they plan or suspect pregnancy. Caution female patient to avoid use of diclofenac in last trimester of pregnancy and to notify health care professional if breast feeding.
- **PO:** Instruct patient to take diclofenac with a full glass of water and to remain in an upright position for 15–30 min after administration. Take missed doses as soon as possible within 1–2 hr if taking once or twice a day or unless almost time for next dose if taking more than twice a day. Do not double doses.
- May cause drowsiness or dizziness. Caution patient to avoid driving or other activities requiring alertness until response to medication is known.
- Caution patient to wear sunscreen and protective clothing to prevent photosensitivity reactions.
- **Topical:** Advise patient to minimize use of concurrent NSAIDs during topical therapy. Instruct patient to read *Medication Guide* before starting therapy and with each Rx refill in case changes have been made.
- *Pennsaid:* Instruct patient to avoid touching treated knee and allowing another person to touch knee until completely dry. Cover knee with clothing until completely dry. Avoid covering lesion with occlusive dressing or tight clothing, and avoid applying sunscreen, insect repellent, lotion, moisturizer, cosmetics to the affected area. Do not use heating pads, sunlamps, and tanning beds. Protect treated knee from sunlight; wear protective clothes when in sunlight. Avoid showers or baths for at least 30 minutes after application.
- *Solarze:* Advise patient that it may take up to 1 mo for complete healing of the lesion to occur.
- **Transdermal:** Instruct patient on correct application procedure for patch. Apply patch to most painful area. Change patch every 12 hr. Remove patch if irritation occurs. Fold used patches so adhesive sticks to itself and discard where children and pets cannot get them. Encourage patient to read the *NSAID Medication Guide* that accompanies the prescription.
- Instruct patients if patch begins to peel off to tape the edges. Do not wear patch during bathing or showering. Bathing should take place between scheduled patch removal and application.
- Advise patient referred for MRI test to discuss patch with referring health care professional and MRI facility to determine if removal of patch is necessary prior to test and for directions for replacing patch.

Evaluation/Desired Outcomes

- Decrease in severity of mild-to-moderate pain.
- Increased ease of joint movement. Patients who do not respond to one NSAID may respond to another. May require 2 wk or more for maximum effects.
- Decrease in or healing of lesions in actinic keratosis. Optimal effect may not be seen until 30 days after discontinuation of therapy. Lesions that do not heal should be re-evaluated.

dicloxacillin, See PENICILLINS, PENICILLINASE RESISTANT.

dicyclomine

(dye-**sye**-kloe-meen)

Bentyl, ✱Bentylol, ✱Formulex, ✱Protylol

Classification

Therapeutic: antispasmodics

Pharmacologic: anticholinergics

Pregnancy Category B

Indications

Management of irritable bowel syndrome in patients who do not respond to usual interventions (sedation/ change in diet).

Action

May have a direct and local effect on GI smooth muscle, reducing motility and tone. **Therapeutic Effects:** Decreased GI motility.

Pharmacokinetics

Absorption: Well absorbed after oral and IM administration.

Distribution: Unknown.

Metabolism and Excretion: 80% eliminated in urine, 10% in feces.

Half-life: 1.8 hr (initial phase), 9–10 hr (terminal phase).

TIME/ACTION PROFILE (antispasmodic effect)

ROUTE	ONSET	PEAK	DURATION
PO, IM	unknown	unknown	unknown

Contraindications/Precautions

Contraindicated in: Hypersensitivity; Obstruction of the GI or GU tract; Reflux esophagitis; Severe ulcerative colitis (risk of paralytic ileus); Unstable cardiovascular status; Glaucoma; Myasthenia gravis; Pedi: Infants <6 mo; Lactation: Lactation.

Use Cautiously in: High environmental temperatures (risk of heat prostration); Hepatic/renal impairment; Autonomic neuropathy; Cardiovascular disease; Prostatic hyperplasia; Geri: Appears on Beers list. Geriatric patients have ↑ sensitivity to anticholinergics; OB: Safety not established.

Adverse Reactions/Side Effects

CNS: confusion, delirium, drowsiness, light-headedness (IM only), psychosis. **EENT:** blurred vision, ↑ intraocular pressure. **CV:** palpitations, tachycardia. **GI:** PARALYTIC ILEUS, <u>constipation</u>, <u>heartburn</u>, ↓ salivation, dry mouth, nausea, vomiting. **GU:** erectile dysfunction, urinary hesitancy, urinary retention. **Derm:** ↓ sweating. **Endo:** ↓ lactation. **Local:** pain/redness at IM site. **Misc:** allergic reactions including ANAPHYLAXIS.

Interactions

Drug-Drug: Additive anticholinergic effects with other **anticholinergics**, including **antihistamines**, **quinidine**, and **disopyramide**. May alter the absorption of **other orally administered drugs** by slowing motility of the GI tract. **Antacids** or **adsorbent antidiarrheals** ↓ the absorption of anticholinergics. May ↑ GI mucosal lesions in patients taking oral **potassium chloride** tablets.

Route/Dosage

PO (Adults): 10–20 mg 3–4 times daily (up to 160 mg/day).

PO (Children ≥2 yr): 10 mg 3–4 times daily, adjusted as tolerated.

PO (Children 6 mo–2 yr): 5–10 mg 3–4 times daily, adjusted as tolerated.

IM (Adults): 20 mg q 4–6 hr, adjusted as tolerated.

Availability (generic available)

Tablets: ✤10 mg, 20 mg. **Cost:** *Generic*—20 mg $7.18/100. **Capsules:** 10 mg. **Cost:** *Generic*—$6.99/100. **Solution for injection:** 10 mg/mL.

NURSING IMPLICATIONS

Assessment

- Assess for symptoms of irritable bowel syndrome (abdominal cramping, alternating constipation and diarrhea, mucus in stools) before and periodically during therapy.
- Assess patient routinely for abdominal distention and auscultate for bowel sounds. If constipation becomes a problem, increasing fluids and adding bulk to the diet may help alleviate the constipating effects of the drug.
- Monitor intake and output ratios; may cause urinary retention.
- ***Lab Test Considerations:*** Antagonizes effects of pentagastrin and histamine during the gastric acid secretion test. Avoid administration for 24 hr preceding the test.
- ***Toxicity and Overdose:*** Severe anticholinergic symptoms may be reversed with physostigmine or neostigmine.

Potential Nursing Diagnoses

Acute pain (Indications)
Diarrhea (Indications)

Implementation

- **PO:** Administer dicyclomine 30 min–1 hr before meals.
- **IM:** Monitor patient after administration; may cause light-headedness and irritation at injection site. Do not administer IV; may cause thrombosis and thrombophlebitis.

Patient/Family Teaching

- Instruct patient to take dicyclomine exactly as directed and not to take more than the prescribed amount. Missed doses should be taken as soon as remembered if not just before next dose.
- Medication may cause drowsiness and blurred vision. Caution patient to avoid driving or other activities requiring alertness until response to the medication is known.
- Advise patient to stay in temperature-controlled rooms. Fever and extremes of heat may cause confusional state, disorientation, amnesia, hallucinations, dysarthria, ataxia, coma, euphoria, fatigue, insomnia, agitation and mannerisms, inappropriate affect, psychosis and delirium. Usually resolves 12–24 hr after discontinuation of dicyclomine.
- Inform patient that frequent oral rinses, sugarless gum or candy, and good oral hygiene may help relieve dry mouth. Consult health care professional regarding use of saliva substitute if dry mouth persists for more than 2 wk.
- Advise patient receiving dicyclomine to make position changes slowly to minimize the effects of drug-induced orthostatic hypotension.
- Caution patient to avoid extremes of temperature. This medication decreases the ability to sweat and may increase the risk of heat stroke.
- Instruct patient to notify health care professional of all Rx or OTC medications, vitamins, or herbal products being taken and to consult health care profes-

sional before taking other Rx, OTC, or herbal products.

- Advise patient to notify health care professional immediately if eye pain or increased sensitivity to light occurs. Emphasize the importance of routine eye exams throughout therapy.

Evaluation/Desired Outcomes

- A decrease in the symptoms of irritable bowel syndrome.

diflorasone, See CORTICOSTEROIDS (TOPICAL/LOCAL).

HIGH ALERT

digoxin (di-jox-in)

Lanoxin, ✱Toloxin

Classification

Therapeutic: antiarrhythmics, inotropics

Pharmacologic: digitalis glycosides

Pregnancy Category C

Indications

Heart failure. Atrial fibrillation and atrial flutter (slows ventricular rate). Paroxysmal atrial tachycardia.

Action

Increases the force of myocardial contraction. Prolongs refractory period of the AV node. Decreases conduction through the SA and AV nodes. **Therapeutic Effects:** Increased cardiac output (positive inotropic effect) and slowing of the heart rate (negative chronotropic effect).

Pharmacokinetics

Absorption: 60–80% absorbed after oral administration of tablets; 70–85% absorbed after administration of elixir; 80% absorbed from IM sites (IM route not recommended due to pain/irritation).

Distribution: Widely distributed; crosses placenta and enters breast milk.

Metabolism and Excretion: Excreted almost entirely unchanged by the kidneys.

Half-life: 36–48 hr (↑ in renal impairment).

TIME/ACTION PROFILE (antiarrhythmic or inotropic effects, provided that a loading dose has been given)

ROUTE	ONSET	PEAK	DURATION
Digoxin–PO	30–120 min	2–8 hr	2–4 days†
Digoxin–IM	30 min	4–6 hr	2–4 days†
Digoxin–IV	5–30 min	1–4 hr	2–4 days†

†Duration listed is that for normal renal function; in impaired renal function, duration will be longer.

Contraindications/Precautions

Contraindicated in: Hypersensitivity; Uncontrolled ventricular arrhythmias; AV block (in absence of pacemaker); Idiopathic hypertrophic subaortic stenosis; Constrictive pericarditis; Known alcohol intolerance (elixir only).

Use Cautiously in: Hypokalemia (↑ risk of digoxin toxicity); Hypercalcemia (↑ risk of toxicity, especially with mild hypokalemia); Hypomagnesemia (↑ risk of digoxin toxicity); Diuretic use (may cause electrolyte abnormalities including hypokalemia and hypomagnesemia); Hypothyroidism; Myocardial infarction; Renal impairment (dose ↓ required); Obesity (base dose on ideal body weight); Geri: Very sensitive to toxic effects; dose adjustments required for age-related ↓ in renal function and body weight; OB: Although safety has not been established, has been used without adverse effects on the fetus; Lactation: Similar concentrations in serum and breast milk result in subtherapeutic levels in infant, use with caution.

Adverse Reactions/Side Effects

CNS: <u>fatigue</u>, headache, weakness. **EENT:** blurred vision, yellow or green vision. **CV:** ARRHYTHMIAS, <u>bradycardia</u>, ECG changes, AV block, SA block. **GI:** <u>anorexia</u>, <u>nausea</u>, <u>vomiting</u>, diarrhea. **Hemat:** thrombocytopenia. **Metab:** electrolyte imbalances with acute digoxin toxicity.

Interactions

Drug-Drug: **Thiazide** and **loop diuretics**, **piperacillin**, **ticarcillin**, **amphotericin B**, **corticosteroids**, and excessive use of **laxatives** may cause hypokalemia which may ↑ risk of toxicity. **Quinidine** and **ritonavir** may ↑ levels and lead to toxicity; ↓ digoxin dose by 30–50%. **Amiodarone** may ↑ levels and lead to toxicity; ↓ digoxin dose by 50%. , **Cyclosporine**, **itraconazole**, **propafenone**, **quinine**, **spironolactone**, and **verapamil** may ↑ levels and lead to toxicity; serum level monitoring/dose ↓ may be required. Levels may be ↓ by some **antineoplastics (bleomycin, carmustine, cyclophosphamide, cytarabine, doxorubicin, methotrexate, procarbazine, vincristine)**, **activated charcoal**, **cholestyramine**, **colestipol**, **kaolin/pectin**, **metoclopramide**, **penicillamine**, **rifampin**, or **sulfasalazine**. In a small percentage (10%) of patients gut bacteria metabolize digoxin to inactive compounds; **macrolide anti-infectives (erythromycin, azithromycin, clarithromycin)** and **tetracyclines**, by killing these bacteria, will cause ↑ levels and toxicity; dose may need to be ↓ for up to 9 wk. Additive bradycardia may occur with **beta—blockers**, **diltiazem**, **verapamil**, **clonidine**, and other **antiarrhythmics (quinidine, disopyramide)**. Concurrent use of **sympathomimetics** may ↑ risk of arrhythmias. **Thyroid hormones** may ↓ therapeutic effects.

Drug-Natural Products: **Licorice** and stimulant natural products (**aloe**) may ↑ risk of potassium depletion. **St. John's wort** may ↓ levels and effect.

Drug-Food: Concurrent ingestion of a **high-fiber meal** may ↓ absorption. Administer digoxin 1 hour before or 2 hours after such a meal.

Route/Dosage

For rapid effect, a larger initial loading/digitalizing dose should be given in several divided doses over 12–24 hr. Maintenance doses are determined for digoxin by renal function. All dosing must be evaluated by individual response. In general, doses required for atrial arrhythmias are higher than those for inotropic effect.

IV, IM (Adults): *Digitalizing dose*—0.5–1 mg given as 50% of the dose initially and one quarter of the initial dose in each of 2 subsequent doses at 6–12 hr intervals.

IV, IM (Children >10 yr): *Digitalizing dose*—8–12 mcg/kg given as 50% of the dose initially and one quarter of the initial dose in each of 2 subsequent doses at 6–12 hr intervals.

IV, IM (Children 5–10 yr): *Digitalizing dose*—15–30 mcg/kg given as 50% of the dose initially and one quarter of the initial dose in each of 2 subsequent doses at 6–12 hr intervals.

IV, IM (Children 2–5 yr): *Digitalizing dose*—25–35 mcg/kg given as 50% of the dose initially and one quarter of the initial dose in each of 2 subsequent doses at 6–12 hr intervals.

IV, IM (Children 1–24 mo): *Digitalizing dose*—30–50 mcg/kg given as 50% of the dose initially and one quarter of the initial dose in each of 2 subsequent doses at 6–12 hr intervals.

IV, IM (Infants –full term): 20–30 mcg/kg given as 50% of the dose initially and one quarter of the initial dose in each of 2 subsequent doses at 6–12 hr intervals.

IV, IM (Infants –premature): *Digitalizing dose*—15–25 mcg/kg given as 50% of the dose initially and one quarter of the initial dose in each of 2 subsequent doses at 6–12 hr intervals.

PO (Adults): *Digitalizing dose*—0.75–1.5 mg given as 50% of the dose initially and one quarter of the initial dose in each of 2 subsequent doses at 6–12 hr intervals. *Maintenance dose*—0.125–0.5 mg/day depending on patient's lean body weight, renal function, and serum level.

PO (Geriatric Patients): Initial daily dosage should not exceed 0.125 mg.

PO (Children >10 yr): *Digitalizing dose*—10–15 mcg/kg given as 50% of the dose initially and one quarter of the initial dose in each of 2 subsequent doses at 6–12 hr intervals. *Maintenance dose*—2.5–5 mcg/kg given daily as a single dose.

PO (Children 5–10 yr): *Digitalizing dose*—20–35 mcg/kg given as 50% of the dose initially and one quarter of the initial dose in each of 2 subsequent doses at 6–12 hr intervals. *Maintenance dose*—5–10 mcg/kg given daily in 2 divided doses.

PO (Children 2–5 yr): *Digitalizing dose*—30–40 mcg/kg given as 50% of the dose initially and one quarter of the initial dose in each of 2 subsequent doses at 6–12 hr intervals. *Maintenance dose*—7.5–10 mcg/kg given daily in 2 divided doses.

PO (Children 1–24 mo): *Digitalizing dose*—35–60 mcg/kg given as 50% of the dose initially and one quarter of the initial dose in each of 2 subsequent doses at 6–12 hr intervals. *Maintenance dose*—10–15 mcg/kg given daily in 2 divided doses.

PO (Infants –full term): *Digitalizing dose*—25–35 mcg/kg given as 50% of the dose initially and one quarter of the initial dose in each of 2 subsequent doses at 6–12 hr intervals. *Maintenance dose*—6–10 mcg/kg given daily in 2 divided doses.

PO (Infants –premature): *Digitalizing dose*—20–30 mcg/kg given as 50% of the dose initially and one quarter of the initial dose in each of 2 subsequent doses at 6–12 hr intervals. *Maintenance dose*—5–7.5 mcg/kg given daily in 2 divided doses.

Availability (generic available)

Tablets: 0.0625 mg, 0.125 mg, 0.1875 mg, 0.25 mg. **Cost:** *Generic*—All strengths $27.75/10. **Elixir (lime flavor):** 0.05 mg/mL. **Cost:** *Generic*—$42.10/60 mL. **Injection:** 0.25 mg/mL. **Pediatric injection:** 0.1 mg/mL.

NURSING IMPLICATIONS

Assessment

- Monitor apical pulse for 1 full min before administering. Withhold dose and notify health care professional if pulse rate is <60 bpm in an adult, <70 bpm in a child, or <90 bpm in an infant. Also notify health care professional promptly of any significant changes in rate, rhythm, or quality of pulse.
- Pedi: Heart rate varies in children depending on age, ask health care professional to specify at what heart rates digoxin should be withheld.
- Monitor BP periodically in patients receiving IV digoxin.
- Monitor ECG throughout IV administration and 6 hr after each dose. Notify health care professional if bradycardia or new arrhythmias occur.
- Observe IV site for redness or infiltration; extravasation can lead to tissue irritation and sloughing.
- Monitor intake and output ratios and daily weights. Assess for peripheral edema, and auscultate lungs for rales/crackles throughout therapy.
- Before administering initial loading dose, determine whether patient has taken any digoxin in the preceding 2–3 wk.
- ***Lab Test Considerations:*** Evaluate serum electrolyte levels (especially potassium, magnesium, and calcium) and renal and hepatic functions periodically during therapy. Notify health care professional before giving dose if patient is hypokalemic. Hypokalemia, hypomagnesemia, or hypercalcemia may make the patient more susceptible to digitalis toxic-

ity. Pedi: Neonates may have falsely elevated serum digoxin concentrations due to a naturally occurring substance chemically similar to digoxin.

- ***Toxicity and Overdose:*** Therapeutic serum digoxin levels range from 0.5–2 ng/mL. Serum levels may be drawn 6–8 hr after a dose is administered, although they are usually drawn immediately before the next dose. Geri: Older adults are at increased risk for toxic effects of digoxin (appears on Beers list) due to age-related decreased renal clearance, which can exist even when serum creatinine levels are normal. Digoxin requirements in the older adult may change and a formerly therapeutic dose can become toxic.
- Observe for signs and symptoms of toxicity. *In adults and older children,* the first signs of toxicity usually include abdominal pain, anorexia, nausea, vomiting, visual disturbances, bradycardia, and other arrhythmias. *In infants and small children,* the first symptoms of overdose are usually cardiac arrhythmias. If these appear, withhold drug and notify health care professional immediately.
- If signs of toxicity occur and are not severe, discontinuation of digoxin may be all that is required.
- Correct electrolyte abnormalities, thyroid dysfunction, and concomitant medications. Administer potassium so that serum potassium is maintained between 4.0 and 5.5 mmol/L. Monitor ECG for evidence of potassium toxicity (peaking of T waves).
- Treatment of life-threatening arrhythmias may include administration of digoxin immune Fab *(Digibind)*, which binds to the digitalis glycoside molecule in the blood and is excreted by the kidneys.

Potential Nursing Diagnoses

Decreased cardiac output (Indications)
Deficient knowledge, related to medication regimen (Patient/Family Teaching)

Implementation

- Do not confuse Lanoxin with levothyroxine or naloxone.
- ***High Alert:*** Digoxin has a narrow therapeutic range. Medication errors associated with digoxin include miscalculation of pediatric doses and insufficient monitoring of digoxin levels. Have second practitioner independently check original order and dose calculations.
- For rapid digitalization, initial dose is higher than maintenance dose; 50% of total digitalizing dose is given initially. Remainder of dose will be administered in 25% increments at 4–8 hr intervals.
- When changing from parenteral to oral dose forms, dose adjustments may be necessary because of pharmacokinetic variations in percentage of digoxin absorbed: 100 mcg (0.1 mg) digoxin injection = 125 mcg (0.125 mg) tablet or 125 mcg (0.125 mg) of elixir.
- **PO:** Administer oral preparations consistently with regard to meals. Tablets can be crushed and administered with food or fluids if patient has difficulty swallowing. Use calibrated measuring device for elixir; calibrated dropper is not accurate for doses of less than 0.2 mL or 10 mcg.
- **IM:** Administer deep into gluteal muscle and massage well to reduce painful local reactions. Do not administer more than 2 mL of digoxin in each IM site. IM administration is not generally recommended.

IV Administration

- **IV Push:** ***Diluent:*** May be administered undiluted. May also dilute 1 mL of digoxin in 4 mL of sterile water for injection, D5W, or 0.9% NaCl. Less diluent will cause precipitation. Use diluted solution immediately. ***Rate:*** Administer over at least 5 min.
- **Y-Site Compatibility:** acyclovir, alemtuzumab, alfentanil, amikacin, aminocaproic acid, aminophylline, amphotericin B lipid complex, anidulafungin, argatroban, ascorbic acid, atropine, azithromycin, aztreonam, benztropine, bivalirudin, bleomycin, bumetanide, buprenorphine, butorphanol, calcium chloride, calcium gluconate, cangrelor, carboplatin, carmustine, cefazolin, cefotaxime, cefotetan, cefoxitin, ceftaroline, ceftazidime, ceftriaxone, cefuroxime, chloramphenicol, chlorpromazine, ciprofloxacin, cisatracurium, cisplatin, clindamycin, cyanocobalamin, cyclophosphamide, cyclosporine, cytarabine, dacarbazine, dactinomycin, daptomycin, daunorubicin hydrochloride, dexamethasone, dexmedetomidine, dexrazoxane, diltiazem, dimenhydrinate, diphenhydramine, dobutamine, docetaxel, dopamine, doripenem, doxorubicin liposome, doxycycline, enalaprilat, ephedrine, epinephrine, epirubicin, epoetin alfa, eptifibatide, ertapenem, erythromycin, esmolol, etoposide, etoposide phosphate, famotidine, fenoldopam, fentanyl, fludarabine, fluorouracil, folic acid, furosemide, ganciclovir, gemcitabine, gentamicin, glycopyrrolate, granisetron, heparin, hetastarch, hydrocortisone sodium succinate, hydromorphone, ifosfamide, imipenem/cilastatin, indomethacin, irinotecan, isoproterenol, ketamine, ketorolac, labetalol, leucovorin calcium, levofloxacin, lidocaine, linezolid, lorazepam, magnesium sulfate, mannitol, mechlorethamine, meperidine, meropenem, mesna, methohexital, methotrexate, methyldopate, methylprednisolone sodium succinate, metoclopramide, metoprolol, metronidazole, midazolam, milrinone, morphine, moxifloxacin, multivitamins, mycophenolate, nafcillin, nalbuphine, naloxone, nesiritide, nicardipine, nitroglycerin, nitroprusside, norepinephrine, octreotide, ondansetron, oxacillin, oxaliplatin, oxytocin, palonosetron, pamidronate, pancuronium, pantoprazole, papaverine, pemetrexed, penicillin G, pentazocine, pentobarbital, phenobarbital, phenylephrine, phytonadione, piperacillin/tazobactam, potassium acetate, potassium chloride, procainamide, prochlorperazine, promethazine, propranolol, protamine, pyridoxine, ranitidine, remifentanil, rituxi-

mab, rocuronium, sodium acetate, sodium bicarbonate, streptokinase, succinylcholine, sufentanil, tacrolimus, teniposide, theophylline, thiamine, thiotepa, tigecycline, tirofiban, tobramycin, trastuzumab, vancomycin, vasopressin, vecuronium, verapamil, vinblastine, vincristine, vinorelbine, vitamin B complex with C, voriconazole, zoledronic acid.

- **Y-Site Incompatibility:** amiodarone, amphotericin B colloidal, amphotericin B liposome, caspofungin, dantrolene, diazepam, diazoxide, doxorubicin, foscarnet, idarubicin, mitoxantrone, paclitaxel, pentamidine, phenytoin, propofol, quinupristin/dalfopristin, telavancin, topotecan, trimethoprim/sulfamethoxazole.

Patient/Family Teaching

- Instruct patient to take medication as directed, at same time each day. Teach parents or caregivers of infants and children how to accurately measure medication. Take missed doses within 12 hr of scheduled dose or omit. Do not double doses. Consult health care professional if doses for 2 or more days are missed. Do not discontinue medication without consulting health care professional.
- Teach patient to take pulse and to contact health care professional before taking medication if pulse rate is <60 or >100.
- Pedi: Teach parents or caregivers that changes in heart rate, especially bradycardia, are among the first signs of digoxin toxicity in infants and children. Instruct parents or caregivers in apical heart rate assessment and ask them to notify health care professional if heart rate is outside of range set by health care professional before administering the next scheduled dose.
- Review signs and symptoms of digitalis toxicity with patient and family. Advise patient to notify health care professional immediately if these or symptoms of HF occur. Inform patient that these symptoms may be mistaken for those of colds or flu.
- Instruct patient to keep digoxin tablets in their original container and not to mix in pill boxes with other medications; they may look similar to and may be mistaken for other medications.
- Advise patient that sharing of this medication can be dangerous.
- Instruct patient to notify health care professional of all Rx or OTC medications, vitamins, or herbal products being taken and to consult health care professional before taking other Rx, OTC, or herbal products. Advise patient to avoid taking antacids or antidiarrheals within 2 hr of digoxin.
- Advise patient to notify health care professional of this medication regimen before treatment.
- Patients taking digoxin should carry identification describing disease process and medication regimen at all times.
- Geri: Review fall prevention strategies with older adults and their families.
- Advise female patient to notify health care professional if pregnancy is planned or suspected.
- Emphasize the importance of routine follow-up exams to determine effectiveness and to monitor for toxicity.

Evaluation/Desired Outcomes

- Decrease in severity of HF.
- Increase in cardiac output.
- Decrease in ventricular response in atrial tachyarrhythmias.
- Termination of paroxysmal atrial tachycardia.

D

diltiazem (dil-**tye**-a-zem)

Cardizem, Cardizem CD, Cardizem LA, Cartia XT, Taztia XT, Tiazac, ✤Tiazac XC

Classification

Therapeutic: antianginals, antiarrhythmics (class IV), antihypertensives

Pharmacologic: calcium channel blockers

Pregnancy Category C

Indications

Hypertension. Angina pectoris and vasospastic (Prinzmetal's) angina. Supraventricular tachyarrhythmias and rapid ventricular rates in atrial flutter or fibrillation.

Action

Inhibits transport of calcium into myocardial and vascular smooth muscle cells, resulting in inhibition of excitation-contraction coupling and subsequent contraction. **Therapeutic Effects:** Systemic vasodilation resulting in decreased BP. Coronary vasodilation resulting in decreased frequency and severity of attacks of angina. Reduction of ventricular rate in atrial fibrillation or flutter.

Pharmacokinetics

Absorption: Well absorbed, but rapidly metabolized after oral administration.

Distribution: Unknown.

Protein Binding: 70–80%.

Metabolism and Excretion: Mostly metabolized by the liver (CYP3A4 enzyme system).

Half-life: 3.5–9 hr.

TIME/ACTION PROFILE

ROUTE	ONSET	PEAK	DURATION
PO	30 min	2–3 hr	6–8 hr
PO–SR	unknown	unknown	12 hr
PO–CD, LA, XT	unknown	14 days†	up to 24 hr
IV	2–5 min	2–4 hr	unknown

†Maximum antihypertensive effect with chronic therapy.

Contraindications/Precautions

Contraindicated in: Hypersensitivity; Sick sinus syndrome; 2nd- or 3rd-degree AV block (unless an artificial pacemaker is in place); Systolic BP <90 mm Hg; Recent MI or pulmonary congestion; Concurrent use of rifampin.

Use Cautiously in: Severe hepatic impairment (↓ dose recommended); Geri: ↓ dose; slower IV infusion rate recommended; ↑ risk of hypotension; consider age-related decrease in body mass, ↓ hepatic/renal/cardiac function, concurrent drug therapy and other disease states); Severe renal impairment; Serious ventricular arrhythmias or HF; OB, Lactation, Pedi: Safety not established.

Adverse Reactions/Side Effects

CNS: abnormal dreams, anxiety, confusion, dizziness, drowsiness, headache, nervousness, psychiatric disturbances, weakness. **EENT:** blurred vision, disturbed equilibrium, epistaxis, tinnitus. **Resp:** cough, dyspnea. **CV:** ARRHYTHMIAS, HF, peripheral edema, bradycardia, chest pain, hypotension, palpitations, syncope, tachycardia. **GI:** ↑ liver enzymes, anorexia, constipation, diarrhea, dry mouth, dysgeusia, dyspepsia, nausea, vomiting. **GU:** dysuria, nocturia, polyuria, sexual dysfunction, urinary frequency. **Derm:** STEVENS-JOHNSON SYNDROME, dermatitis, erythema multiforme, flushing, sweating, photosensitivity, pruritus/urticaria, rash. **Endo:** gynecomastia, hyperglycemia. **Hemat:** anemia, leukopenia, thrombocytopenia. **Metab:** weight gain. **MS:** joint stiffness, muscle cramps. **Neuro:** paresthesia, tremor. **Misc:** gingival hyperplasia.

Interactions

Drug-Drug: ↑ hypotension may occur when used with **fentanyl**, other **antihypertensives**, **nitrates**, acute ingestion of **alcohol**, or **quinidine**. Antihypertensive effects may be ↓ by **NSAIDs**. May ↑ **digoxin** levels. May ↑ levels of and risk of myopathy from **simvastatin** and **lovastatin**. Concurrent use with **beta blockers**, **clonidine**, **digoxin**, **disopyramide**, or **phenytoin** may result in bradycardia, conduction defects, or HF. **Phenobarbital** and **phenytoin** may ↑ metabolism and ↓ effectiveness. May ↓ metabolism of and ↑ risk of toxicity from **cyclosporine**, **quinidine**, or **carbamazepine**. **Cimetidine** and **ranitidine** ↑ levels and effects. May ↑ or ↓ the effects of **lithium** or **theophylline**.

Drug-Food: **Grapefruit juice** ↑ levels and effect.

Route/Dosage

PO (Adults): 30–120 mg 3–4 times daily or 60–120 mg twice daily as SR capsules or 180–240 mg once daily as CD or XR capsules or LA tablets (up to 360 mg/day); *Concurrent simvastatin therapy*—Diltiazem dose should not exceed 240 mg/day and simvastatin dose should not exceed 10 mg/day.

IV (Adults): 0.25 mg/kg; may repeat in 15 min with a dose of 0.35 mg/kg. May follow with continuous infusion at 10 mg/hr (range 5–15 mg/hr) for up to 24 hr.

Availability (generic available)

Tablets: 30 mg, 60 mg, 90 mg, 120 mg. **Cost:** *Generic*—30 mg $10.44/100, 60 mg $22.25/100, 90 mg $26.89/100. **Sustained-release capsules:** 60 mg, 90 mg, 120 mg. **Cost:** *Generic*—60 mg $83.05/100, 90 mg $94.95/100, 120 mg $123.75/100. **Extended-release capsules (Cardizem CD, Tiazac, Cartia XT, Taztia XT):** 120 mg, 180 mg, 240 mg, 300 mg, 360 mg, 420 mg. **Cost:** *Generic*—180 mg $58.19/100, 240 mg $63.54/100, 420 mg $171.49/100. **Extended-release tablets (Cardizem LA):** 120 mg, 180 mg, 240 mg, 300 mg, 360 mg, 420 mg. **Injection:** 5 mg/mL.

NURSING IMPLICATIONS

Assessment

- Monitor BP and pulse prior to therapy, during dose titration, and periodically during therapy. Monitor ECG periodically during prolonged therapy. May cause prolonged PR interval.
- Monitor intake and output ratios and daily weight. Assess for signs of HF (peripheral edema, rales/crackles, dyspnea, weight gain, jugular venous distention).
- Monitor frequency of prescription refills to determine adherence.
- Patients receiving digoxin concurrently with calcium channel blockers should have routine serum digoxin levels checked and be monitored for signs and symptoms of digoxin toxicity.
- Assess for rash periodically during therapy. May cause Stevens-Johnson syndrome. Discontinue therapy if severe or if accompanied with fever, general malaise, fatigue, muscle or joint aches, blisters, oral lesions, conjunctivitis, hepatitis and/or eosinophilia.
- **Angina:** Assess location, duration, intensity, and precipitating factors of patient's anginal pain.
- **Arrhythmias:** Monitor ECG continuously during administration. Report bradycardia or prolonged hypotension promptly. Emergency equipment and medication should be available. Monitor BP and pulse before and frequently during administration.
- ***Lab Test Considerations:*** Total serum calcium concentrations are not affected by calcium channel blockers.
- Monitor serum potassium periodically. Hypokalemia ↑ the risk of arrhythmias and should be corrected.

- Monitor renal and hepatic functions periodically during long-term therapy. May cause ↑ in hepatic enzymes after several days of therapy, which return to normal on discontinuation of therapy.

Potential Nursing Diagnoses

Acute pain (Indications)
Decreased cardiac output (Adverse Reactions)

Implementation

- Do not confuse Cardizem (diltiazem) with Cardene (nicardipine). Do not confuse Tiazac (diltiazem) with Ziac (bisprolol/hydrochlorothiazide).
- **PO:** May be administered without regard to meals. May be administered with meals if GI irritation becomes a problem.
- Do not open, crush, break, or chew sustained-release capsules or extended-release tablets. Empty tablets that appear in stool are not significant.

IV Administration

- **IV Push:** ***Diluent:*** Administer bolus dose undiluted. ***Concentration:*** 5 mg/mL. ***Rate:*** Administer over 2 min.
- **Continuous Infusion:** ***Diluent:*** Dilute 125 mg in 100 mL, 250 mg in 250 mL, or 250 mg in 500 mL of 0.9% NaCl, D5W, or D5/0.45% NaCl. Infusion is stable for 24 hr at room temperature or if refrigerated. ***Concentration:*** 125 mg/125 mL (1 mg/mL), 250 mg/300 mL (0.83 mg/mL), 250 mg/550 mL (0.45 mg/mL). ***Rate:*** See Route/Dosage section. Titrate to patient's heart rate and BP response.
- **Y-Site Compatibility:** albumin, alemtuzumab, alfentanil, amifostine, amikacin, aminocaproic acid, amiodarone, amphotericin B colloidal, anidulafungin, argatroban, azithromycin, aztreonam, bivalirudin, bleomycin, bumetanide, buprenorphine, busulfan, butorphanol, calcium chloride, calcium gluconate, cangrelor, carboplatin, carmustine, caspofungin, cefazolin, cefotaxime, cefotetan, cefoxitin, ceftaroline, ceftazidime, ceftriaxone, cefuroxime, chlorpromazine, ciprofloxacin, cisatracurium, cisplatin, clindamycin, cyclophosphamide, cyclosporine, cytarabine, dactinomycin, daptomycin, daunorubicin, dexamethasone, dexmedetomidine, dexrazoxane, digoxin, diphenhydramine, dobutamine, docetaxel, dolasetron, dopamine, doripenem, doxorubicin, doxycycline, droperidol, enalaprilat, ephedrine, epinephrine, epirubicin, eptifibatide, ertapenem, erythromycin, esmolol, etoposide, etoposide phosphate, famotidine, fenoldopam, fentanyl, fluconazole, fludarabine, foscarnet, fosphenytoin, gemcitabine, gentamicin, glycopyrrolate, granisetron, haloperidol, hetastarch, hydralazine, hydromorphone, idarubicin, ifosfamide, imipenem/cilastatin, irinotecan, isoproterenol, labetalol, leucovorin calcium, levofloxacin, lidocaine, linezolid, lorazepam, magnesium sulfate, mannitol, mechlorethamine, melphalan, meperidine, meropenem, metoclopramide, metoprolol, metronidazole, midazolam, milrinone, mitoxantrone, morphine, moxifloxacin, multivitamins, mycophenolate, nalbuphine, naloxone, nesiritide, nicardipine, nitroglycerin, nitroprusside, norepinephrine, octreotide, ondansetron, oxacillin, oxaliplatin, oxytocin, paclitaxel, palonosetron, pamidronate, pancuronium, pemetrexed, penicillin G potassium, pentamidine, phenylephrine, potassium acetate, potassium chloride, potassium phosphates, prochlorperazine, promethazine, propranolol, quinupristin/dalfopristin, ranitidine, remifentanil, rocuronium, sodium acetate, streptozocin, succinylcholine, sufentanil, tacrolimus, telavancin, teniposide, theophylline, thiotepa, tigecycline, tirofiban, tobramycin, topotecan, trimethoprim/sulfamethoxazole, vancomycin, vasopressin, vecuronium, verapamil, vinblastine, vincristine, vinorelbine, voriconazole, zidovudine, zoledronic acid.
- **Y-Site Incompatibility:** allopurinol, amphotericin B lipid complex, amphotericin B liposome, cefepime, chloramphenicol, dantrolene, diazepam, doxorubicin liposomal, fluorouracil, furosemide, ganciclovir, ketorolac, methotrexate, micafungin, pantoprazole, pentobarbital, phenobarbital, phenytoin, piperacillin/tazobactam, rifampin, thiopental.

Patient/Family Teaching

- Advise patient to take medication as directed at the same time each day, even if feeling well. Take missed doses as soon as possible unless almost time for next dose; do not double doses. May need to be discontinued gradually.
- Advise patient to avoid large amounts (6–8 glasses of grapefruit juice/day) during therapy.
- Instruct patient on correct technique for monitoring pulse. Instruct patient to contact health care professional if heart rate is <50 bpm.
- Caution patient to change positions slowly to minimize orthostatic hypotension.
- May cause drowsiness or dizziness. Advise patient to avoid driving or other activities requiring alertness until response to the medication is known.
- Instruct patient on importance of maintaining good dental hygiene and seeing dentist frequently for teeth cleaning to prevent tenderness, bleeding, and gingival hyperplasia (gum enlargement).
- Instruct patient to notify health care professional of all Rx or OTC medications, vitamins, or herbal products being taken and to avoid concurrent use of alcohol or OTC medications and herbal products, especially NSAIDs and cold preparations, without consulting health care professional.
- Advise patient to notify health care professional if rash, irregular heartbeats, dyspnea, swelling of

hands and feet, pronounced dizziness, nausea, constipation, or hypotension occurs or if headache is severe or persistent.

- Caution patient to wear protective clothing and use sunscreen to prevent photosensitivity reactions.
- Advise female patient to notify health care professional if pregnancy is planned or suspected or if breast feeding.
- **Angina:** Instruct patient on concurrent nitrate or beta-blocker therapy to continue taking both medications as directed and to use SL nitroglycerin as needed for anginal attacks.
- Advise patient to contact health care professional if chest pain does not improve, worsens after therapy, or occurs with diaphoresis; if shortness of breath occurs; or if severe, persistent headache occurs.
- Caution patient to discuss exercise restrictions with health care professional before exertion.
- **Hypertension:** Encourage patient to comply with other interventions for hypertension (weight reduction, low-sodium diet, smoking cessation, moderation of alcohol consumption, regular exercise, and stress management). Medication controls but does not cure hypertension.
- Instruct patient and family in proper technique for monitoring BP. Advise patient to take BP weekly and to report significant changes to health care professional.

Evaluation/Desired Outcomes

- Decrease in BP.
- Decrease in frequency and severity of anginal attacks.
- Decrease in need for nitrate therapy.
- Increase in activity tolerance and sense of well-being.
- Suppression and prevention of tachyarrhythmias.

dimenhyDRINATE

(dye-men-**hye**-dri-nate)
✤Anti-Nauseant, Calm X, Dimetabs, ✤Dinate, Dramamine, Dramanate, ✤Gravol, Hydrate, ✤Nauseatol, ✤Traveltabs, Triptone Caplets

Classification
Therapeutic: antiemetics, antihistamines

Pregnancy Category B

Indications

Nausea, vomiting, dizziness, and vertigo accompanying motion sickness.

Action

Inhibits vestibular stimulation. Has significant CNS depressant, anticholinergic, antihistaminic, and antiemetic properties. **Therapeutic Effects:** Decreased vestibular stimulation, which may prevent motion sickness.

Pharmacokinetics

Absorption: Well absorbed after oral or IM administration.
Distribution: Probably crosses the placenta and enters breast milk.
Metabolism and Excretion: Metabolized by the liver.
Half-life: Unknown.

TIME/ACTION PROFILE (antimotion sickness, antiemetic activity)

ROUTE	ONSET	PEAK	DURATION
PO	15–60 min	1–2 hr	3–6 hr
Rect	30–45 min	unknown	6–12 hr
IM	20–30 min	1–2 hr	3–6 hr
IV	rapid	unknown	3–6 hr

Contraindications/Precautions

Contraindicated in: Hypersensitivity; Some products contain alcohol or tartrazine; in patients with known intolerance.
Use Cautiously in: Angle-closure glaucoma; Seizure disorders; Prostatic hyperplasia.

Adverse Reactions/Side Effects

CNS: drowsiness, dizziness, headache, paradoxical excitation (children). **EENT:** blurred vision, tinnitus. **CV:** hypotension, palpitations. **GI:** anorexia, constipation, diarrhea, dry mouth. **GU:** dysuria, frequency. **Derm:** photosensitivity. **Local:** pain at IM site.

Interactions

Drug-Drug: ↑ CNS depression with other **antihistamines**, **alcohol**, **opioid analgesics**, and **sedative/hypnotics**. May mask signs or symptoms of ototoxicity in patients receiving **ototoxic drugs (aminoglycosides, ethacrynic acid)**. ↑ anticholinergic properties with **tricyclic antidepressants**, **quinidine**, or **disopyramide**. **MAO inhibitors** intensify and prolong the anticholinergic effects of antihistamines.

Route/Dosage

PO (Adults): 50–100 mg q 4 hr (not to exceed 400 mg/day).
PO (Children 6–12 yr): 25–50 mg q 6–8 hr (not to exceed 300 mg/day).
Rect (Adults): 50–100 mg q 6–8 hr.
Rect (Children 8–12 yr): 25–50 mg q 8–12 hr.
Rect (Children 6–8 yr): 12.5–25 mg q 8–12 hr.
IM, IV (Adults): 50 mg q 4 hr as needed.
IM, IV (Children): 1.25 mg/kg (37.5 mg/m^2) q 6 hr as needed (not to exceed 300 mg/day).

Availability (generic available)

Tablets: ✤15 mg^{OTC}, 50 mg^{OTC}. **Chewable tablets (orange flavor):** ✤15 mg^{OTC}, 50 mg^{OTC}. **Capsules:** ✤50 mg^{OTC}. **Elixir (cherry flavor):** 12.5 mg/5 mL^{OTC}, ✤15 mg/5 mL^{OTC}. **Liquid:** 12.5 mg/4 mL^{OTC}. **Suppositories:** ✤100 mg^{OTC}. **Injection:** 50 mg/mL.

NURSING IMPLICATIONS

Assessment

- Assess nausea, vomiting, bowel sounds, and abdominal pain before and after administration of this drug. Dimenhydrinate may mask the signs of an acute abdomen.
- Monitor intake and output, including emesis. Assess for signs of dehydration (excessive thirst, dry skin and mucous membranes, tachycardia, increased urine specific gravity, poor skin turgor).
- ***Lab Test Considerations:*** Will cause false-negative allergy skin test results; discontinue 72 hr before testing.

Potential Nursing Diagnoses

Risk for deficient fluid volume (Indications)
Imbalanced nutrition: less than body requirements (Indications)
Risk for injury (Side Effects)

Implementation

- When used for prophylaxis of motion sickness, administer at least 30 min and preferably 1–2 hr before exposure to conditions that may precipitate motion sickness.
- **PO:** Use calibrated measuring device when administering liquid dose.
- **IM:** Administer into well-developed muscle; massage well.

IV Administration

- **IV Push:** ***Diluent:*** Dilute 50 mg in 0.9% NaCl for injection. ***Concentration:*** 5 mg/mL. ***Rate:*** Inject over 2 min.
- **Y-Site Compatibility:** acyclovir, ciprofloxacin, fluconazole, ketamine, metronidazole.
- **Solution Compatibility:** D5W, 0.45% NaCl, 0.9% NaCl, Ringer's solution, lactated Ringer's solution, dextrose/saline combinations, or dextrose/Ringer's combinations.

Patient/Family Teaching

- Instruct patient to take dimenhydrinate as directed.
- May cause drowsiness. Caution patient to avoid driving or other activities requiring alertness until response to the drug is known.
- Inform patient that this medication may cause dry mouth. Frequent oral rinses, good oral hygiene, and sugarless gum or candy may minimize this effect.
- Caution patient to avoid alcohol and other CNS depressants concurrently with this medication.
- Advise patient to use sunscreen and protective clothing to prevent photosensitivity reactions.

Evaluation/Desired Outcomes

- Prevention or decreased severity of nausea and vomiting, vertigo, or motion sickness.

D

dimethyl fumarate

(dye-**meth**-il **fue**-ma-rate)
Tecfidera

Classification
Therapeutic: anti-multiple sclerosis agents

Pregnancy Category C

Indications

Treatment of relapsing forms of multiple sclerosis.

Action

Activates nuclear factor (Nrf2) pathway involved in cellular response to oxidative stress. **Therapeutic Effects:** Decreased incidence/severity of relapse with decreased progression of lesions and disability.

Pharmacokinetics

Absorption: Following oral administration rapidly converted to active metabolite monomethyl fumarate (MMF) by enzymes in GI tract, blood, and tissue.
Distribution: Unknown.
Metabolism and Excretion: MMF is metabolized by the tricarboxylic acid (TCA) cycle. 60% eliminated via exhalation of CO_2. Minor amounts eliminated by renal (16%) and fecal (1%) routes, trace amounts in urine.
Half-life: *MMF*—1 hr.

TIME/ACTION PROFILE (effects on disability)

ROUTE	ONSET	PEAK	DURATION
PO	24 wk	60 wk	Unk

Contraindications/Precautions

Contraindicated in: Hypersensitivity.
Use Cautiously in: Serious infections (treatment may be withheld); OB: Use during pregnancy only if potential benefit justifies potential risk to fetus; Lactation: Use cautiously if breast feeding; Pedi: Safety and effectiveness not established.

Adverse Reactions/Side Effects

CNS: PROGRESSIVE MULTIFOCAL LEUKOENCEPHALOPATHY. **GI:** abdominal pain, diarrhea, nausea, dyspepsia, ↑ liver enzymes, vomiting. **Derm:** flushing, erythema, pruritus, rash. **Hemat:** lymphopenia. **Misc:** hypersensitivity reactions including ANAPHYLAXIS and ANGIOEDEMA.

Interactions

Drug-Drug: None noted.

Route/Dosage

PO (Adults): 120 mg twice daily for one week, then 240 mg twice daily.

Availability

Extended-release capsules: 120 mg, 240 mg.

NURSING IMPLICATIONS

Assessment

- Monitor for signs and symptoms of infections (fever, sore throat). Consider withholding medication until serious infections are resolved.
- ***Lab Test Considerations:*** Monitor CBC with lymphocyte count before initiating therapy, after 6 months, and every 6 to 12 months thereafter.
- May casue ↓ lymphocyte counts.
- May cause ↑ hepatic transaminases, mostly during first 6 mo of therapy.
- May cause transient ↑ mean eosinophil count during first 2 mo of therapy.

Potential Nursing Diagnoses

Deficient knowledge, related to disease process and medication regimen (Patient/Family Teaching)

Implementation

- **PO:** Administer 120 mg twice daily for 7 days then increase to maintenance dose of 240 mg twice daily without regard to food. For patients with difficulty tolerating maintenance dose, may temporarily decrease to 120 mg twice daily; resume maintenance dose within 4 wks. Swallow capsules whole; do not open, crush, chew, or sprinkle on food. Discard any unused capsules 90 days after opening.

Patient/Family Teaching

- Instruct patient to take dimethyl fumarate as directed. Advise patient to read *Patient Information* before starting therapy and with each Rx refill in case of changes.
- Caution patient not to share medication with others, even if they have the same symptoms; may be dangerous.
- May cause flushing (warmth, redness, itching, and/or burning sensation). Usually begins after starting and resolves over time. Administration of dimethyl fumarate with food or administration of non-enteric coated aspirin (up to a dose of 325 mg) 30 minutes prior to dimethyl fumarate dosing may decrease incidence or severity of flushing.
- Advise patient to notify health care professional promptly if signs and symptoms of PML (new or worsening weakness; trouble using their arms or legs; or changes to thinking, eyesight, strength or balance) or hypersensitivity reactions (difficulty breathing, urticaria, swelling of throat and tongue) occur.
- Advise patient to notify health care professional of all Rx or OTC medications, vitamins, or herbal products being taken and to consult with health care professional before taking other medications.
- Rep: Advise female patient to notify health care professional if pregnancy is planned or suspected, or if breast feeding. Patients who become pregnant should be encouraged to join the pregnancy registry by calling 1-866-810-1462 or visiting www.tecfiderapregnancyregistry.com.

Evaluation/Desired Outcomes

- Decreased incidence/severity of relapse of multiple sclerosis.

dinoprostone

(dye-noe-**prost**-one)

Cervidil Vaginal Insert, Prepidil Endocervical Gel, Prostin E Vaginal Suppository

Classification

Therapeutic: cervical ripening agent

Pharmacologic: oxytocics, prostaglandins

Pregnancy Category C

Indications

Endocervical Gel, Vaginal Insert: Used to "ripen" the cervix in pregnancy at or near term when induction of labor is indicated. Vaginal Suppository: Induction of midtrimester abortion, Management of missed abortion up to 28 wk, Management of nonmetastatic gestational trophoblastic disease (benign hydatidiform mole).

Action

Produces contractions similar to those occurring during labor at term by stimulating the myometrium (oxytocic effect). Initiates softening, effacement, and dilation of the cervix ("ripening"). Also stimulates GI smooth muscle. **Therapeutic Effects:** Initiation of labor. Expulsion of fetus.

Pharmacokinetics

Absorption: Rapidly absorbed.

Distribution: Unknown. Action is mostly local.

Metabolism and Excretion: Metabolized by enzymes in lung, kidneys, spleen, and liver tissue.

Half-life: Unknown.

TIME/ACTION PROFILE

ROUTE	ONSET	PEAK	DURATION
Cervical ripening (gel)	rapid	30–45 min	unknown
Cervical ripening (insert)	rapid	unknown	12 hr
Abortion time (suppository)	10 min	12–24 hr	2–3 hr

Contraindications/Precautions

Contraindicated in: Hypersensitivity to prostaglandins or additives in the gel or suppository; The gel/insert should be avoided in situations in which prolonged uterine contractions should be avoided, including: Previous cesarean section or uterine surgery; Cephalopelvic disproportion; Traumatic delivery or difficult labor; Multiparity (≥6 term pregnancies); Hyperactive or hypertonic uterus; Fetal distress (if delivery is not imminent); Unexplained vaginal bleeding; Placenta previa; Vasa previa; Active herpes genitalis; Obstetric emergency requiring surgical intervention; Situations in which vaginal delivery is contraindicated; Presence of acute pelvic inflammatory disease or ruptured membranes; Concurrent oxytocic therapy (wait for 30 min after removing insert before using oxytocin).

Use Cautiously in: Uterine scarring; Asthma; Hypotension; Cardiac disease; Adrenal disorders; Anemia; Jaundice; Diabetes mellitus; Epilepsy; Glaucoma; Pulmonary, renal, or hepatic disease; Multiparity (up to 5 previous term pregnancies); Women >30 yr, those with complications during pregnancy, and those with a gestational age >40 wk (↑ risk of disseminated intravascular coagulation).

Adverse Reactions/Side Effects

Endocervical Gel, Vaginal Insert.

GU: uterine contractile abnormalities, warm feeling in vagina. **MS:** back pain. **Misc:** AMNIOTIC FLUID EMBOLISM, fever.

Suppository

CNS: headache, drowsiness, syncope. **Resp:** coughing, dyspnea, wheezing. **CV:** hypotension, hypertension. **GI:** diarrhea, nausea, vomiting. **GU:** UTERINE RUPTURE, urinary tract infection, uterine hyperstimulation, vaginal/uterine pain. **Misc:** allergic reactions including ANAPHYLAXIS, chills, fever.

Interactions

Drug-Drug: Augments the effects of other **oxytocics**.

Route/Dosage

Cervical Ripening

Vag (Adults, Cervical): *Endocervical gel*—0.5 mg; if response is unfavorable, may repeat in 6 hr (not to exceed 1.5 mg/24 hr). *Vaginal insert*—one 10-mg insert.

Abortifacient

Vag (Adults): One 20-mg suppository, repeat q 3–5 hr (not to exceed 240 mg total or longer than 48 hr).

Availability

Endocervical gel (Prepidil): 0.5 mg dinoprostone in 3 g of gel vehicle in a prefilled syringe with catheters. **Vaginal insert (Cervidil):** 10 mg. **Vaginal suppository (Prostin E Vaginal):** 20 mg.

NURSING IMPLICATIONS

Assessment

- **Abortifacient:** Monitor frequency, duration, and force of contractions and uterine resting tone. Opioid analgesics may be administered for uterine pain.
- Monitor temperature, pulse, and BP periodically throughout therapy. Dinoprostone-induced fever (elevation >1.1°C or 2°F) usually occurs within 15–45 min after insertion of suppository. This returns to normal 2–6 hr after discontinuation or removal of suppository from vagina.
- Auscultate breath sounds. Wheezing and sensation of chest tightness may indicate hypersensitivity reaction.
- Assess for nausea, vomiting, and diarrhea in patients receiving suppository. Vomiting and diarrhea occur frequently. Patient should be premedicated with antiemetic and antidiarrheal.
- Monitor amount and type of vaginal discharge. Notify health care professional immediately if symptoms of hemorrhage (increased bleeding, hypotension, pallor, tachycardia) occur.
- **Cervical Ripening:** Monitor uterine activity, fetal status, and dilation and effacement of cervix continuously throughout therapy. Assess for hypertonus, sustained uterine contractility, and fetal distress. Insert should be removed at the onset of active labor.

Potential Nursing Diagnoses

Deficient knowledge, related to medication regimen (Patient/Family Teaching)

Implementation

- **Abortifacient:** Warm the suppository to room temperature just before use.
- Wear gloves when handling unwrapped suppository to prevent absorption through skin.
- Patient should remain supine for 10 min after insertion of suppository; then she may be ambulatory.
- **Vaginal Insert:** Place vaginal insert transversely in the posterior vaginal fornix immediately after removing from foil package. Warming of insert and sterile conditions are not required. Use vaginal insert only with a retrieval system. Use minimal amount of water-soluble lubricant during insertion; avoid excess because it may hamper release of dinoprostone from insert. Patient should remain supine for 2 hr after insertion, then may ambulate.
- Vaginal insert delivers dinoprostone 0.3 mg/hr over 12 hr. Remove insert at the onset of active labor, before amniotomy, or after 12 hr.
- Oxytocin should not be used during or less than 30 min after removal of insert.
- **Endocervical Gel:** Determine degree of effacement before insertion of the endocervical catheter. Do not administer above the level of the internal os. Use a 20-mm endocervical catheter if no effacement is present and a 10-mm catheter if the cervix is 50% effaced.

- Use caution to prevent contact of dinoprostone gel with skin. Wash hands thoroughly with soap and water after administration.
- Bring gel to room temperature just before administration. Do not force warming with external sources (water bath, microwave). Remove peel-off seal from end of syringe; then remove the protective end cap and insert end cap into plunger stopper assembly in barrel of syringe. Aseptically remove catheter from package. Firmly attach catheter hub to syringe tip; click is evidence of attachment. Fill catheter with sterile gel by pushing plunger to expel air from catheter before administration to patient. Gel is stable for 24 mo if refrigerated.
- Patient should be in dorsal position with cervix visualized using a speculum. Introduce gel with catheter into cervical canal using sterile technique. Administer gel by gentle expulsion from syringe and then remove catheter. Do not attempt to administer small amount of gel remaining in syringe. Use syringe for only 1 patient; discard syringe, catheter, and unused package contents after using.
- Patient should remain supine for 15–30 min after administration to minimize leakage from cervical canal.
- Oxytocin may be administered 6–12 hr after desired response from dinoprostone gel. If no cervical/uterine response to initial dose of dinoprostone is obtained, repeat dose may be administered in 6 hr.

Patient/Family Teaching

- Explain purpose of medication and vaginal exams.
- **Abortifacient:** Instruct patient to notify health care professional immediately if fever and chills, foul-smelling vaginal discharge, lower abdominal pain, or increased bleeding occurs.
- Provide emotional support throughout therapy.
- **Cervical Ripening:** Inform patient that she may experience a warm feeling in her vagina during administration.
- Advise patient to notify health care professional if contractions become prolonged.

Evaluation/Desired Outcomes

- Complete abortion. Continuous administration for more than 2 days is not usually recommended.
- Cervical ripening and induction of labor.

dinutuximab (di-noo-**tux**-i-mab)

Unituxin

Classification

Therapeutic: antineoplastics

Pharmacologic: monoclonal antibodies

Indications

Treatment (with granulocyte-macrophage colony-stimulating factor [GM-CSF], interleukin-2 [IL-2], and 13-cis-retinoic acid [RA]) of pediatric patients with high-risk neuroblastoma who have had at least a partial response to previous first-line multiagent, multimodality therapy.

Action

Acts as a glycolipid disialoganglioside (GD2)-binding monoclonal antibody that binds to specific cells in the CNS and peripheral nerves, inducing cell lysis through antibody-dependent cell-mediated cytotoxicity (ADCC) and complement-dependent cytotoxicity (CDC). **Therapeutic Effects:** Decreased progression of neuroblastoma.

Pharmacokinetics

Absorption: IV administration results in complete bioavailability.

Distribution: Unknown.

Metabolism and Excretion: Unknown.

Half-life: 10 days.

TIME/ACTION PROFILE (event-free survival probability)

ROUTE	ONSET	PEAK	DURATION
IV	6 mo	2 yr	unknown

Contraindications/Precautions

Contraindicated in: Previous anaphylactic reaction to dinutuximab; OB: May cause fetal harm; Lactation: Discontinue breast feeding.

Use Cautiously in: Female patients with reproductive potential (effective contraception is required); Geri: Safe and effective use in geriatric patients has not been established; Safe and effective use in renal or hepatic impairment has not been established; Pedi: Has been used in children.

Adverse Reactions/Side Effects

EENT: neurologic disorders of the eye. **Resp:** hypoxia. **CV:** HYPOTENSION, tachycardia. **GI:** ↓ appetite, diarrhea, ↑ liver enzymes, vomiting. **GU:** proteinuria. **Derm:** urticaria. **F and E:** HYPOKALEMIA, hypocalcemia, hyponatremia. **Hemat:** anemia, lymphopenia, neutropenia, thrombocytopenia. **Metab:** hyperglycemia, hypertriglyceridemia, hypoalbuminemia, ↑ weight. **Neuro:** neuropathic pain, peripheral neuropathy. **Misc:** CAPILLARY LEAK SYNDROME, FEBRILE NEUTROPENIA, INFUSION-RELATED REACTIONS, pain, ATYPICAL HEMOLYTIC UREMIC SYNDROME.

Interactions

Drug-Drug: ↑ risk of myelosuppression with other **myelosuppressants**, **antineoplastics** and **radiation therapy**.

Route/Dosage

Pretreatment with opioid analgesics, antihistamines and antipyretics is required.

IV (Adults): 17.5 mg/m^2/day for 4 consecutive days for up to 5 cycles. Infusion-related reactions may require slowed infusion rate, dose reduction or discontinuation.

Availability

Solution for IV administration (requires further dilution): 17.5 mg/5 mL (3.5 mg/mL) single-use vial.

NURSING IMPLICATIONS

Assessment

- Assess hematologic, respiratory, hepatic, and renal function prior to each course of dinutuximab to determine adequate function.
- Monitor for signs and symptoms of infusion reactions during and for at least 4 hrs following completion of infusion. Infusion reactions usually occur during or within 24 hours of completing infusion. *For mild to moderate infusion reactions* (transient rash, fever, rigors, localized urticaria) that respond promptly to antihistamines or antipyretics, decrease infusion rate to 50% previous rate and monitor closely. After resolution, gradually increase infusion rate up to maximum rate of 1.75 mg/m^2/hour. *For serious infusion reactions* (facial and upper airway edema, dyspnea, bronchospasm, stridor, urticaria, hypotension) immediately interrupt dinutuximab infusion and institute supportive therapy. If symptoms resolve rapidly, decrease infusion rate to 50% previous rate and monitor closely. For first recurrence of symptoms, discontinue dinutuximab until next day. If symptoms resolve and continued treatment is warranted, premedicate with hydrocortisone 1 mg/kg (maximum dose 50 mg) IV administer dinutuximab at rate of 0.875 mg/m^2/hour in an intensive care unit. Discontinue dintuximab permanently for life-threatening reactions.
- Assess pain (abdominal pain, generalized pain, extremity pain, back pain, neuralgia, musculoskeletal chest pain, arthralgia) frequently during and following therapy. See Implementation for analgesic guidelines.
- Assess for signs and symptoms of peripheral neuropathy (lower extremity weakness and inability to ambulate, neurogenic bladder) frequently during therapy. May occur more frequently in adult patients. Permanently discontinue dinutuximab in patients with Grade 2 peripheral motor neuropathy, Grade 3 sensory neuropathy that interferes with daily activities for more than 2 weeks, or Grade 4 sensory neuropathy.
- Monitor for signs and symptoms of capillary leak syndrome (severe hypotension, hypoalbuminemia, hemoconcentration). *At onset of moderate to severe, but not life threatening symptoms,* interrupt dinutuximab infusion; resume infusion at 50% previous rate when symptoms resolve. Then gradually increase infusion rate up to a maximum rate of 1.75 mg/m^2/hour. *For life-threatening symptoms,* discontinue current cycle of dinutuximab. Administer subsequent cycles at 50% of previous rate. Permanently discontinue dinutuximab if symptoms recur.
- Monitor BP closely during therapy. Administer required hydration prior to dinutuximab infusion. Interrupt therapy and institute supportive measures if symptomatic hypotension occurs. Resume at 50% infusion rate. If BP remains stable for at least 2 hours, increase infusion rate as tolerated up to a maximum rate of 1.75 mg/m^2/hour.
- Monitor for signs and symptoms of infection during therapy. If severe systemic infection or sepsis occur, discontinue dinutuximab until resolution of infection, then continue subsequent cycles.
- Monitor for neurological disorders of the eye (blurred vision, photophobia, mydriasis, fixed or unequal pupils, optic nerve disorder, eyelid ptosis, papilledema) during therapy. Interrupt therapy in patients with dilated pupil with sluggish light reflex or other visual disturbances not causing visual loss. Upon resolution and if continued treatment is warranted, decrease dinutuximab dose by 50%. Permanently discontinue dinutuximab in patients with recurrent signs or symptoms of eye disorder following dose reduction and in patients with loss of vision.
- Monitor for signs and symptoms of hemolytic uremic syndrome (fatigue, dizziness, fainting, pallor, edema, decreased urine output, hematuria) during therapy. Permanently discontinue dinutuximab and provide supportive therapy if signs occur.
- ***Lab Test Considerations:*** Monitor peripheral blood counts.
- Monitor serum electrolytes daily during therapy. May cause hypokalemia, hyponatremia, and hypocalcemia. Discontinue therapy if Grade 4 hyponatremia occurs despite appropriate fluid management.

Potential Nursing Diagnoses

Risk for infection (Adverse Reactions)
Acute pain (Adverse Reactions)

Implementation

- **Pretreatment:** Administer 10 mL/kg 0.9% NaCl as an infusion 1 hr prior to dinutuximab infusion.
- Administer 50 mcg/kg morphine immediately before dinutuximab infusion, then continue as morphine drip at infusion rate of 20 to 50 mcg/kg/hour during and for two hours following completion of dinutuximab. Give additional 25 mcg/kg to 50 mcg/kg IV morphine as needed for pain up to once every 2 hours followed by an increase in morphine infusion rate in clinically stable patient.
- Consider fentanyl or hydromorphone if morphine not tolerated.
- If pain is inadequately managed with opioids, consider gabapentin or lidocaine in conjunction with IV morphine.
- For severe pain, decrease dinutuximab infusion rate to 0.875 mg/m^2/hour. Discontinue dinutuximab per-

manently if Grade 3 pain unresponsive to maximum supportive measures occurs.

- Administer an antihistamine such as diphenhydramine (0.5 to 1 mg/kg; maximum dose 50 mg) IV over 10 to 15 minutes starting 20 min before initiation of dinutuximab and as tolerated every 4 to 6 hours during infusion.
- Administer acetaminophen (10 to 15 mg/kg; maximum dose 650 mg) 20 minutes before each dinutuximab infusion and every 4 to 6 hours as needed for fever or pain. Administer ibuprofen (5 to 10 mg/kg) every 6 hours as needed for control of persistent fever or pain.
- **Continuous Infusion:** Store vials in refrigerator protected from light. ***Diluent:*** Withdraw solution from vial and inject into 100 mL of 0.9% NaCl. Mix by gentle inversion; do not shake. Do not administer solutions that are discolored, cloudy, or contain particulate matter. Store diluted solution in refrigerator; administer within 4 hrs and discard after 24 hrs. ***Rate:*** Infuse over 10–20 hrs for 4 consecutive days for a maximum of 5 cycles. Begin with infusion rate of 0.875 mg/m²/hr for 30 min. Gradually increase for a maximum of 1.75 mg/m²/hr as tolerated.

Patient/Family Teaching

- Explain purpose of dinutuximab to patient and caregivers.
- Advise patient ton notify health care professional if signs and symptoms of infusion reaction (facial or lip swelling, urticaria, difficulty breathing, lightheadedness or dizziness occurring during or within 24 hours after infusion), capillary leak syndrome, hypotension, infection, or hemolytic uremic syndrome occur.
- Inform patient and caregiver of risk of pain and peripheral neuropathy. Advise patient to notify health care professional if pain, numbness, tingling, burning, or weakness occur.
- Advise patient to notify health care professional if signs and symptoms of neurological eye disorder (blurred vision, photophobia, ptosis, diplopia, unequal pupil size) occur.
- Caution female patients to use effective contraception during and for at least 2 months following therapy. Advise patient to avoid breast feeding during therapy.

Evaluation/Desired Outcomes

- Decreased progression of neuroblastoma.

diphenhydrAMINE (oral, parenteral)

(dye-fen-**hye**-dra-meen)

✤Aller-Aide, ✤Allerdryl, ✤Allergy Formula, AllerMax, ✤Allernix, Banophen, Benadryl Dye-Free Alergy, Benadryl Allergy, Benadryl, ✤Benylin, ✤Calmex, Compoz, Compoz Nighttime Sleep Aid, ✤Dimetane Allergy, Diphen AF, Diphen Cough, ✤Diphenhist, ✤Dormex, ✤Dormiphen, Genahist, 40 Winks, Hyrexin-50, ✤Insomnal, Maximum Strength Nytol, Maximum Strength Sleepinal, Midol PM, Miles Nervine, ✤Nadryl, Nighttime Sleep Aid, Nytol, Scot-Tussin Allergy DM, Siladril, Silphen, Sleep-Eze 3, Sleepwell 2-night, Sominex, Snooze Fast, Sominex, Tusstat, Twilite, Unisom Nighttime Sleep-Aid

Classification

Therapeutic: allergy, cold, and cough remedies, antihistamines, antitussives

Pregnancy Category B

Indications

Relief of allergic symptoms caused by histamine release including: Anaphylaxis, Seasonal and perennial allergic rhinitis, Allergic dermatoses. Parkinson's disease and dystonic reactions from medications. Mild nighttime sedation. Prevention of motion sickness. Antitussive (syrup only).

Action

Antagonizes the effects of histamine at H_1-receptor sites; does not bind to or inactivate histamine. Significant CNS depressant and anticholinergic properties. **Therapeutic Effects:** Decreased symptoms of histamine excess (sneezing, rhinorrhea, nasal and ocular pruritus, ocular tearing and redness, urticaria). Relief of acute dystonic reactions. Prevention of motion sickness. Suppression of cough.

Pharmacokinetics

Absorption: Well absorbed after oral or IM administration but 40–60% of an oral dose reaches systemic circulation due to first-pass metabolism.

Distribution: Widely distributed. Crosses the placenta; enters breast milk.

Metabolism and Excretion: 95% metabolized by the liver.

Half-life: 2.4–7 hr.

TIME/ACTION PROFILE (antihistaminic effects)

ROUTE	ONSET	PEAK	DURATION
PO	15–60 min	2–4 hr	4–8 hr
IM	20–30 min	2–4 hr	4–8 hr
IV	rapid	unknown	4–8 hr

Contraindications/Precautions

Contraindicated in: Hypersensitivity; Acute attacks of asthma; Lactation: Lactation; Known alcohol intolerance (some liquid products).

Use Cautiously in: Severe liver disease; Angle-closure glaucoma; Seizure disorders; Prostatic hyperplasia; Peptic ulcer; May cause paradoxical excitation in young children; Hyperthyroidism; OB: Safety not established; Geri: Appears on *Beers list*. Geriatric patients are more susceptible to adverse drug reactions and anticholinergic effects (delirium, acute confusion, dizziness, dry mouth, blurred vision, urinary retention, constipation, tachycardia); dose ↓ or nonanticholinergic antihistamine recommended.

Adverse Reactions/Side Effects

CNS: drowsiness, dizziness, headache, paradoxical excitation (increased in children). **EENT:** blurred vision, tinnitus. **CV:** hypotension, palpitations. **GI:** anorexia, dry mouth, constipation, nausea. **GU:** dysuria, frequency, urinary retention. **Derm:** photosensitivity. **Resp:** chest tightness, thickened bronchial secretions, wheezing. **Local:** pain at IM site.

Interactions

Drug-Drug: ↑ risk of CNS depression with other **antihistamines**, **alcohol**, **opioid analgesics**, and **sedative/hypnotics**. ↑ anticholinergic effects with **tricyclic antidepressants**, **quinidine**, or **disopyramide**. **MAO inhibitors** intensify and prolong the anticholinergic effects of antihistamines.

Drug-Natural Products: Concomitant use of **kava-kava**, **valerian**, or **chamomile** can ↑ CNS depression.

Route/Dosage

PO (Adults and Children >12 yr): *Antihistaminic/antiemetic/antivertiginic*—25–50 mg q 4–6 hr, not to exceed 300 mg/day. *Antitussive*—25 mg q 4 hr as needed, not to exceed 150 mg/day. *Antidyskinetic*—25–50 mg q 4 hr (not to exceed 400 mg/day). *Sedative/hypnotic*—50 mg 20–30 min before bedtime.

PO (Children 6–12 yr): *Antihistaminic/antiemetic/antivertiginic*—12.5–25 mg q 4–6 hr (not to exceed 150 mg/day). *Antidyskinetic*—1–1.5 mg/kg q 6–8 hr as needed (not to exceed 300 mg/day). *Antitussive*—12.5 mg q 4 hr (not to exceed 75 mg/day). *Sedative/hypnotic*—1 mg/kg/dose 20–30 min before bedtime (not to exceed 50 mg).

PO (Children 2–6 yr): *Antihistaminic/antiemetic/antivertiginic*—6.25–12.5 mg q 4–6 hr (not to exceed 37.5 mg/day). *Antidyskinetic*—1–1.5 mg/kg q 4–6 hr as needed (not to exceed 300 mg/day). *Antitussive*—6.25 mg q 4 hr (not to exceed 37.5 mg/24 hr). *Sedative/hypnotic*—1 mg/kg/dose 20–30 min before bedtime (not to exceed 50 mg).

IM, IV (Adults): 25–50 mg q 4 hr as needed (may need up to 100-mg dose, not to exceed 400 mg/day).

IM, IV (Children): 1.25 mg/kg (37.5 mg/m^2) 4 times daily (not to exceed 300 mg/day).

Topical (Adults and Children ≥2 yr): Apply to affected area up to 3–4 times daily.

Availability (generic available)

Capsules: 25 mg$^{Rx, OTC}$, 50 mg$^{Rx, OTC}$. **Tablets:** ✤ 12.5 mg$^{Rx, OTC}$, 25 mg$^{Rx, OTC}$, 50 mg$^{Rx, OTC}$. **Chewable tablets (grape flavor):** 25 mg$^{Rx, OTC}$. **Orally disintegrating strips (cherry and grape flavor):** 12.5 mg$^{Rx, OTC}$, 25 mg^{OTC}. **Orally disintegrating tablets:** 12.5 mg^{OTC}, 25 mg^{OTC}, 50 mg$^{Rx, OTC}$. **Elixir (cherry and other flavors):** 12.5 mg/5 mL$^{Rx, OTC}$. **Syrup (cherry and raspberry flavor):** ✤ 6.25 mg/5 mL$^{Rx, OTC}$, 12.5 mg/5 mL$^{Rx, OTC}$. **Cream:** 1%$^{Rx, OTC}$, 2%$^{Rx, OTC}$. **Topical gel:** 2%^{OTC}. **Topical spray:** 2%^{OTC}. **Topical stick:** 2%^{OTC}. **Injection:** 50 mg/mL. ***In combination with:*** analgesics, decongestants, and expectorants, in OTC pain, sleep, cough, and cold preparations. See Appendix B.

NURSING IMPLICATIONS

Assessment

- Diphenhydramine has multiple uses. Determine why the medication was ordered and assess symptoms that apply to the individual patient. Geri: Appears in the *Beers list.* May cause sedation and confusion due to increased sensitivity to anticholinergic effects. Monitor carefully, assess for confusion, delirium, other anticholinergic side effects and fall risk. Institute measures to prevent falls.
- **Prevention and Treatment of Anaphylaxis:** Assess for urticaria and for patency of airway.
- **Allergic Rhinitis:** Assess degree of nasal stuffiness, rhinorrhea, and sneezing.
- **Parkinsonism and Extrapyramidal Reactions:** Assess movement disorder before and after administration.
- **Insomnia:** Assess sleep patterns.
- **Motion Sickness:** Assess nausea, vomiting, bowel sounds, and abdominal pain.
- **Cough Suppressant:** Assess frequency and nature of cough, lung sounds, and amount and type of sputum produced. Unless contraindicated, maintain fluid intake of 1500–2000 mL daily to decrease viscosity of bronchial secretions.
- **Pruritus:** Assess degree of itching, skin rash, and inflammation.
- ***Lab Test Considerations:*** May ↓ skin response to allergy tests. Discontinue 4 days before skin testing.

Potential Nursing Diagnoses

Insomnia (Indications)
Risk for deficient fluid volume (Indications)
Risk for injury (Side Effects)

Implementation

- Do not confuse Benadryl with benazepril.
- When used for insomnia, administer 20 min before bedtime and schedule activities to minimize interruption of sleep.
- When used for prophylaxis of motion sickness, administer at least 30 min and preferably 1–2 hr before exposure to conditions that may precipitate motion sickness.
- **PO:** Administer with meals or milk to minimize GI irritation. Capsule may be emptied and contents taken with water or food.
- Orally disintegrating tablets and strips should be left in the package until use. Remove from the blister pouch. Do not push tablet through the blister; peel open the blister pack with dry hands and place tablet on tongue. Tablet will dissolve rapidly and be swallowed with saliva. No liquid is needed to take the orally disintegrating tablet.
- **IM:** Administer 50 mg/mL into well-developed muscle. Avoid subcut injections.

IV Administration

- **IV Push:** ***Diluent:*** May be further diluted in 0.9% NaCl, 0.45% NaCl, D5W, D10W, dextrose/saline combinations, Ringer's solution, LR, and dextrose/Ringer's combinations. ***Concentration:*** 25 mg/mL. ***Rate:*** Infuse at a rate not to exceed 25 mg/min.
- **Y-Site Compatibility:** acetaminophen, aldesleukin, alemtuzumab, alfentanil, amifostine, amikacin, aminocaproic acid, amphotericin B lipid complex, amphotericin B liposome, amsacrine, anidulafungin, argatroban, ascorbic acid, atropine, azithromycin, benztropine, bivalirudin, bleomycin, bumetanide, buprenorphine, butorphanol, calcium chloride, calcium gluconate, carboplatin, carmustine, caspofungin, ceftaroline, chlorpromazine, ciprofloxacin, cisatracurium, cisplatin, cladribine, clindamycin, cyanocobalamin, cyclophosphamide, cyclosporine, cytarabine, dactinomycin, daptomycin, dexmedetomidine, dexrazoxane, digoxin, diltiazem, dobutamine, docetaxel, dolasetron, dopamine, doripenem, doxorubicin, doxorubicin liposome, doxycycline, enalaprilat, ephedrine, epinephrine, epirubicin, epoetin alfa, eptifibatide, ertapenem, erythromycin, esmolol, etoposide, etoposide phosphate, famotidine, fenoldopam, fentanyl, filgrastim, fluconazole, fludarabine, folic acid, gemcitabine, gentamicin, glycopyrrolate, granisetron, hydromorphone, idarubicin, ifosfamide, imipenem/cilastatin, irinotecan, isoproterenol, ketamine, labetalol, leucovorin calcium, levofloxacin, lidocaine, linezolid, lorazepam, magnesium sulfate, mannitol, mechlorethamine, melphalan, meperidine, meropenem, metaraminol, methadone, methotrexate, methyldopate, metoclopramide, metoprolol, metronidazole, midazolam, mitomycin, mitoxantrone, morphine, moxifloxacin, multiple vitamins, mycophenolate, nalbuphine, naloxone, nesiritide, nicardipine, nitroglycerin, norepinephrine, octreotide, ondansetron, oxaliplatin, oxytocin, paclitaxel, palonosetron, pamidronate, papaverine, pemetrexed, penicillin G, pentamidine, pentazocine, phentolamine, phenylephrine, phytonadione, piperacillin/tazobactam, potassium acetate, potassium chloride, procainamide, prochlorperazine, promethazine, propofol, propranolol, protamine, pyridoxime, quinipristin/dalfopristin, ranitidine, remifentanil, rituximab, rocuronium, sargramostim, sodium acetate, streptokinase, succinylcholine, sufentanil, tacrolimus, teniposide, theophylline, thiamine, thiotepa, tigecycline, tirofiban, tobramycin, tolazoline, trastuzumab, vancomycin, vasopressin, vecuronium, verapamil, vinblastine, vincristine, vinorelbine, vitamin B complex with C, voriconazole, zoledronic acid.
- **Y-Site Incompatibility:** allopurinol, aminophylline, amphotericin B cholesteryl, amphotericin B colloidal, ampicillin, azathioprine, cefazolin, cefepime, cefotaxime, cefotetan, cefoxitin, ceftazidime, ceftriaxone, cefuroxime, chloramphenicol, dantrolene, dexamethasone, diazepam, diazoxide, fluorouracil, foscarnet, furosemide, ganciclovir, indomethacin, insulin, ketorolac, methylprednisolone, milrinone, nitroprusside, oxacillin, pantoprazole, pentobarbital, phenobarbital, phenytoin, sodium bicarbonate, trimethoprim/sulfamethoxazole.
- **Topical:** Apply a thin coat and rub gently until absorbed. Only for topical use; avoid ingestion.

Patient/Family Teaching

- Instruct patient to take medication as directed; do not exceed recommended amount. Caution patient not to use oral OTC diphenhydramine products with any other product containing diphenhydramine, including products used topically.
- May cause drowsiness. Caution patient to avoid driving or other activities requiring alertness until response to drug is known.
- May cause dry mouth. Inform patient that frequent oral rinses, good oral hygiene, and sugarless gum or candy may minimize this effect. Notify health care professional if dry mouth persists for more than 2 wk.
- Teach sleep hygiene techniques (dark room, quiet, bedtime ritual, limit daytime napping, avoidance of nicotine and caffeine) to patients taking diphenhydramine to aid sleep.
- Advise patient to use sunscreen and protective clothing to prevent photosensitivity reactions.
- Caution patient to avoid use of alcohol and other CNS depressants concurrently with this medication.
- Pedi: Can cause excitation in children. Caution parents or caregivers about proper dose calculation; overdose, especially in infants and children, can cause hallucinations, seizures, or death. Caution parents to avoid OTC cough and cold products while breast feeding or to children <4 yr.
- Geri: Instruct older adults to avoid OTC products that contain diphenhydramine due to increased sen-

sitivity to anticholinergic effects and potential for adverse reactions related to these effects.
- Advise patients taking diphenhydramine in OTC preparations to notify health care professional if symptoms worsen or persist for more than 7 days.

Evaluation/Desired Outcomes
- Prevention of, or decreased urticaria in, anaphylaxis or other allergic reactions.
- Decreased dyskinesia in parkinsonism and extrapyramidal reactions.
- Sedation when used as a sedative/hypnotic.
- Prevention of or decrease in nausea and vomiting caused by motion sickness.
- Decrease in frequency and intensity of cough without eliminating cough reflex.

DIURETICS (POTASSIUM-SPARING)

aMILoride (a-**mill**-oh-ride)
✱Midamor

spironolactone
(speer-oh-no-**lak**-tone)
Aldactone

triamterene (trye-**am**-ter-een)
Dyrenium

Classification
Therapeutic: diuretics
Pharmacologic: potassium-sparing diuretics

Pregnancy Category B (amiloride), C (spironolactone, triamterene)

Indications
Counteract potassium loss caused by other diuretics. Used with other agents (thiazides) to treat edema or hypertension. Primary hyperaldosteronism (spironolactone only). **Unlabeled Use: Spironolactone:** Management of HF (low doses).

Action
Inhibition of sodium reabsorption in the kidney while saving potassium and hydrogen ions (spironolactone achieves this effect by antagonizing aldosterone receptors). **Therapeutic Effects:** Weak diuretic and antihypertensive response when compared with other diuretics. Conservation of potassium.

Pharmacokinetics
Absorption: *Amiloride*— 30–90% absorbed; *spironolactone*— >90% absorbed; *triamterene*— 30–70% absorbed.
Distribution: *Amiloride* and *triamterene*— widely distributed; all cross the placenta and enter breast milk.
Protein Binding: *Spironolactone* >90%.
Metabolism and Excretion: *Amiloride*— 50% eliminated unchanged in urine, 40% excreted in the feces; *spironolactone*— converted by the liver to its active diuretic compound (canrenone); *triamterene*— 80% metabolized by the liver, some excretion of unchanged drug.
Half-life: *Amiloride*— 6–9 hr; *spironolactone*— 78–84 min (spironolactone); 13–24 hr (canrenone); *triamterene*— 1.7–2.5 hr.

TIME/ACTION PROFILE (diuretic effect)

ROUTE	ONSET	PEAK	DURATION
Amiloride	2 hr†	6–10 hr†	24 hr†
Spironolactone	unknown	2–3 days‡	2–3 days‡
Triamterene	2–4 hr†	1–several days‡	7–9 hr†

†Single dose.
‡Multiple doses.

Contraindications/Precautions
Contraindicated in: Hypersensitivity; Hyperkalemia; Anuria; Acute renal insufficiency; Significant renal dysfunction (CCr ≤30 mL/min or SCr >2.5 m g/dL).
Use Cautiously in: Hepatic dysfunction; Geri: Presence of age-related renal dysfunction may lead to ↑ risk of hyperkalemia; Diabetes (↑ risk of hyperkalemia); History of gout or kidney stones (triamterene only); Concurrent use of potassium supplements or potassium-containing salt substitutes; OB, Lactation, Pedi: Safety not established.

Adverse Reactions/Side Effects
CNS: dizziness; *spironolactone only*, clumsiness, headache. **CV:** arrhythmias. **GI:** *amiloride*— constipation, nausea, vomiting. **GU:** *spironolactone*— erectile dysfunction; *triamterene*—nephrolithiasis. **Derm:** STEVENS-JOHNSON SYNDROME, TOXIC EPIDERMAL NECROLYSIS; *triamterene*—photosensitivity. **Endo:** *spironolactone*— breast tenderness, gynecomastia, irregular menses, voice deepening. **F and E:** hyperkalemia, hyponatremia. **Hemat:** *spironolactone*—agranulocytosis; *triamterene*—hemolytic anemia, thrombocytopenia. **MS:** muscle cramps. **Misc:** allergic reactions.

Interactions
Drug-Drug: ↑ hypotension with acute ingestion of **alcohol**, other **antihypertensives**, or **nitrates**. Use with **ACE inhibitors**, **angiotensin II receptor antagonists**, **NSAIDS**, **potassium supplements**, **cyclosporine**, or **tacrolimus** ↑ risk of hyperkalemia. May ↑ levels/risk of toxicity from **lithium**. Effectiveness may be ↓ by **NSAIDs**. Spironolactone may ↑ effects of **digoxin**.

Route/Dosage

Amiloride

PO (Adults): *HTN*—5–10 mg/day (up to 20 mg).
PO (Children 1–17 yr): 0.4–0.625 mg/kg/day (maximum = 20 mg/day) (unlabeled use).

Spironolactone

PO (Adults): *Edema*—25–200 mg/day in 1–2 divided doses. *HTN*—50–100 mg/day in 1–2 divided doses. *Diuretic-induced hypokalemia*—25–100 mg/day in 1–2 divided doses. *Diagnosis of primary hyperaldosteronism*—100–400 mg/day in 1–2 divided doses. *HF*—12.5–25 mg/day (unlabeled use).
PO (Children 1–17 yr): *Diuretic, HTN*—1 mg/kg/day in 1–2 divided doses (should not exceed 3.3 mg/kg/day or 100 mg/day) (unlabeled use). *Diagnosis of primary hyperaldosteronism*—125–375 mg/m²/day in 1–2 divided doses (unlabeled use).
PO (Neonates): 1–3 mg/kg/day in 1–2 divided doses.

Triamterene

PO (Adults): *HTN*—100 mg twice daily (not to exceed 300 mg/day; lower doses in combination products).
PO (Children): *HTN*—1–2 mg/kg/day in 2 divided doses; should not exceed 4 mg/kg/day or 300 mg/day.

Availability

Amiloride (generic available)

Tablets: 5 mg. **Cost:** *Generic*—$59.00/100.

Spironolactone (generic available)

Tablets: 25 mg, 50 mg, 100 mg. **Cost:** *Generic*—25 mg $10.83/100, 50 mg $23.97/100, 100 mg $24.87/100. ***In combination with:*** hydrochlorothiazide (Aldactazide). See Appendix B.

Triamterene

Capsules: 50 mg, 100 mg. **Cost:** 50 mg $404.14/100, 100 mg $372.44/100. ***In combination with:*** hydrochlorothiazide (Dyazide, Maxzide). See Appendix B.

NURSING IMPLICATIONS

Assessment

- Monitor intake and output ratios and daily weight during therapy.
- If medication is given as an adjunct to antihypertensive therapy, monitor BP before administering.
- Assess patient frequently for development of hyperkalemia (fatigue, muscle weakness, paresthesia, confusion, dyspnea, ECG changes, cardiac arrhythmias). Patients who have diabetes mellitus or kidney disease and geriatric patients are at increased risk of developing these symptoms.
- Periodic ECGs are recommended in patients receiving prolonged therapy.
- Assess patient for skin rash frequently during therapy. Discontinue diuretic at first sign of rash; may be life-threatening. Stevens-Johnson syndrome or toxic epidermal necrolysis may develop. Treat symptomatically; may recur once treatment is stopped.
- ***Lab Test Considerations:*** Serum potassium levels should be evaluated before and routinely during therapy. Withhold drug and notify health care professional if patient becomes hyperkalemic.
- Monitor BUN, serum creatinine, and electrolytes before and periodically during therapy. May cause ↑ serum magnesium, BUN, creatinine, potassium, and urinary calcium excretion levels. May also cause ↓ sodium levels.
- Discontinue potassium-sparing diuretics 3 days before a glucose tolerance test because of risk of severe hyperkalemia.
- *Spironolactone* may cause false ↑ of plasma cortisol concentrations. Spironolactone should be withdrawn 4–7 days before test.
- Monitor platelet count and total and differential leukocyte count periodically during therapy in patients taking *triamterene*.

Potential Nursing Diagnoses

Excess fluid volume (Indications)

Implementation

- Do not confuse amiloride with amlodipine.
- **PO:** Administer in AM to avoid interrupting sleep pattern.
- Administer with food or milk to minimize gastric irritation and to increase bioavailability.
- *Triamterene* capsules may be opened and contents mixed with food or fluids for patients with difficulty swallowing.

Patient/Family Teaching

- Emphasize the importance of continuing to take this medication, even if feeling well. Instruct patient to take medication at the same time each day. Take missed doses as soon as remembered unless almost time for next dose. Do not double doses.
- Caution patient to avoid salt substitutes and foods that contain high levels of potassium or sodium unless prescribed by health care professional.
- May cause dizziness. Caution patient to avoid driving or other activities requiring alertness until response to medication is known.
- Instruct patient to notify health care professional of all Rx or OTC medications, vitamins, or herbal products being taken and to consult health care professional before taking any OTC medications concurrently with this therapy, especially OTC decongestants, cough or cold preparations, or appetite suppressants due to potential for increased BP.
- Advise patients taking *triamterene* to use sunscreen and protective clothing to prevent photosensitivity reactions.
- Instruct patient to notify health care professional of medication regimen before treatment or surgery.

- Advise patient to notify health care professional if rash, muscle weakness or cramps; fatigue; or severe nausea, vomiting, or diarrhea occurs.
- Emphasize the need for follow-up exams to monitor progress.
- **Hypertension:** Reinforce need to continue additional therapies for hypertension (weight loss, restricted sodium intake, stress reduction, moderation of alcohol intake, regular exercise, and cessation of smoking). Medication helps control but does not cure hypertension.
- Teach patient and family the correct technique for checking BP weekly.

Evaluation/Desired Outcomes

- Increase in diuresis and decrease in edema while maintaining serum potassium level in an acceptable range.
- Decrease in BP.
- Prevention of hypokalemia in patients taking diuretics.
- Treatment of hyperaldosteronism.

DIURETICS (THIAZIDE)

chlorothiazide
(klor-oh-**thye**-a-zide)
Diuril

chlorthalidone (thiazide–like)
(klor-**thal**-i-doan)
~~Thalitone~~

hydrochlorothiazide
(hye-droe-klor-oh-**thye**-a-zide)
Microzide, Oretic, ✤Urozide

Classification
Therapeutic: antihypertensives, diuretics
Pharmacologic: thiazide diuretics

Pregnancy Category B (chlorthalidone, hydrochlorothiazide), C (chlorothiazide)

Indications

Management of mild to moderate hypertension. Treatment of edema associated with: HF, Renal dysfunction, Cirrhosis, Glucocorticoid therapy, Estrogen therapy.

Action

Increases excretion of sodium and water by inhibiting sodium reabsorption in the distal tubule. Promotes excretion of chloride, potassium, magnesium, and bicarbonate. May produce arteriolar dilation. **Therapeutic Effects:** Lowering of BP in hypertensive patients and diuresis with mobilization of edema.

Pharmacokinetics

Absorption: All are rapidly absorbed after oral administration.
Distribution: All cross the placenta and enter breast milk.
Metabolism and Excretion: All are excreted mainly unchanged by the kidneys.
Half-life: *Chlorothiazide*—1–2 hr; *chlorthalidone*—35–50 hr; *hydrochlorothiazide*—6–15 hr.

TIME/ACTION PROFILE (diuretic effect)

ROUTE	ONSET	PEAK	DURATION
Chlorothiazide PO	2 hr	4 hr	6–12 hr
Chlorothiazide IV	15 min	30 min	2 hr
Chlorthalidone	2 hr	2 hr	48–72 hr
Hydrochlorothiazide†	2 hr	3–6 hr	6–12 hr

†Onset of antihypertensive effect is 3–4 days and does not become maximal for 7–14 days of dosing.

Contraindications/Precautions

Contraindicated in: Hypersensitivity (cross-sensitivity with other thiazides or sulfonamides may exist); Some products contain tartrazine and should be avoided in patients with known intolerance; Anuria; Lactation: Lactation.
Use Cautiously in: Renal or hepatic impairment; OB: Pregnancy (jaundice or thrombocytopenia may be seen in the newborn).

Adverse Reactions/Side Effects

CNS: dizziness, drowsiness, lethargy, weakness. **CV:** hypotension. **EENT:** acute angle-closure glaucoma (hydrochlorothiazide), acute myopia (hydrochlorothiazide). **GI:** anorexia, cramping, hepatitis, nausea, pancreatitis, vomiting. **Derm:** STEVENS-JOHNSON SYNDROME, photosensitivity, rash. **Endo:** hyperglycemia. **F and E:** hypokalemia, dehydration, hypercalcemia, hypochloremic alkalosis, hypomagnesemia, hyponatremia, hypophosphatemia, hypovolemia. **Hemat:** thrombocytopenia. **Metab:** hypercholesterolemia, hyperuricemia. **MS:** muscle cramps.

Interactions

Drug-Drug: Additive hypotension with other **antihypertensives**, acute ingestion of **alcohol**, or **nitrates**. Additive hypokalemia with **corticosteroids**, **amphotericin B**, or **piperacillin/tazobactam**. ↓ excretion of **lithium**. **Cholestyramine** or **colestipol** ↓ absorption. Hypokalemia ↑ risk of **digoxin** toxicity. **NSAIDs** may ↓ effectiveness.

Route/Dosage

When used as a diuretic in adults, generally given daily, but may be given every other day or 2–3 days/week.

Chlorothiazide

PO (Adults): 125 mg–2 g/day in 1–2 divided doses.
PO (Children >6 mos): 20 mg/kg/day in 1–2 divided doses (maximum dose = 1 g/day).
PO (Neonates ≤6 mo): 10–20 mg/kg q 12 hr (maximum dose = 375 mg/day).
IV (Adults): 500 mg–1 g/day in 1–2 divided doses.
IV (Children >6 mos): 4 mg/kg/day in 1–2 divided doses (maximum dose = 20 mg/kg/day) (unlabeled use).
IV (Neonates ≤6 mo): 1–4 mg/kg q 12 hr (maximum dose = 20 mg/kg/day) (unlabeled use).

Chlorthalidone

PO (Adults): 12.5–100 mg once daily (daily doses above 25 mg are associated with greater likelihood of electrolyte abnormalities).

Hydrochlorothiazide

PO (Adults): 12.5–100 mg/day in 1–2 divided doses (up to 200 mg/day); not to exceed 50 mg/day for hypertension; daily doses above 25 mg are associated with greater likelihood of electrolyte abnormalities.
PO (Children >6 mo): 1–3 mg/kg/day in 2 divided doses (not to exceed 37.5 mg/day).
PO (Children <6 mo): 1–3 mg/kg/day in 2 divided doses.

Availability

Chlorothiazide (generic available)

Tablets: 250 mg, 500 mg. **Cost:** *Generic*—250 mg $13.08/100, 500 mg $25.25/100. **Oral suspension:** 250 mg/5 mL. **Cost:** *Generic*—$63.36/237 mL. **Powder for injection:** 500 mg/vial.

Chlorthalidone (generic available)

Tablets: 25 mg, 50 mg. **Cost:** *Generic*—25 mg $55.17/100, 50 mg $68.04/100, 100 mg $101.25/100. ***In combination with:*** atenolol (Tenoretic), clonidine (Clorpres). See Appendix B.

Hydrochlorothiazide (generic available)

Tablets: 12.5 mg, 25 mg, 50 mg. **Cost:** *Generic*—12.5 mg $82.43/100, 25 mg $8.48/100, 50 mg $16.45/100. **Capsules:** 12.5 mg. ***In combination with:*** numerous antihypertensive agents. See Appendix B.

NURSING IMPLICATIONS

Assessment

- Monitor BP, intake, output, and daily weight and assess feet, legs, and sacral area for edema daily.
- Assess patient, especially if taking digoxin, for anorexia, nausea, vomiting, muscle cramps, paresthesia, and confusion. Notify health care professional if these signs of electrolyte imbalance occur. Patients taking digoxin are at risk of digoxin toxicity because of the potassium-depleting effect of the diuretic.
- If hypokalemia occurs, consideration may be given to potassium supplements or ↓ dose of diuretic.
- Assess patient for allergy to sulfonamides. Assess patient for skin rash frequently during therapy. Discontinue diuretic at first sign of rash; may be life-threatening. Stevens-Johnson syndrome may develop. Treat symptomatically; may recur once treatment is stopped.
- **Hypertension:** Monitor BP before and periodically during therapy.
- Monitor frequency of prescription refills to determine compliance.
- ***Lab Test Considerations:*** Monitor electrolytes (especially potassium), blood glucose, BUN, serum creatinine, and uric acid levels before and periodically throughout therapy.
- May cause ↑ in serum and urine glucose in diabetic patients.
- May cause ↑ in serum bilirubin, calcium, creatinine, and uric acid, and ↓ in serum magnesium, potassium, sodium, and urinary calcium concentrations.
- May cause ↑ serum cholesterol, low-density lipoprotein, and triglyceride concentrations.

Potential Nursing Diagnoses

Excess fluid volume (Indications)
Risk for deficient fluid volume (Side Effects)
Deficient knowledge, related to medication regimen (Patient/Family Teaching)

Implementation

- Administer in the morning to prevent disruption of sleep cycle.
- Intermittent dose schedule may be used for continued control of edema.
- **PO:** May give with food or milk to minimize GI irritation. Tablets may be crushed and mixed with fluid to facilitate swallowing.

IV Administration

- **Intermittent Infusion:** Reconstitute chlorothiazide with at least 18 mL of sterile water for injection. Shake to dissolve. Stable for 24 hr at room temperature. ***Diluent:*** May be given undiluted or may be diluted further with D5W or 0.9% NaCl. ***Concentration:*** Up to 28 mg/mL. ***Rate:*** If administered undiluted may give by IV push over 3–5 min. If diluted, may run over 30 min.
- **Y-Site Compatibility:** alprostadil, aminophylline, atropine, calcium chloride, calcium gluconate, chloramphenicol, cyclophosphamide, dexamethasone, digoxin, epinephrine, erythromycin, furosemide, gentamicin, heparin, hydrocortisone sodium succinate, isoproterenol, lidocaine, mechlorethamine, methohexital, methyodopate, norepinephrine, oxytocin, penicillin G, phenobarbital, potassium chloride, procainamide, propranolol, succinylcholine.
- **Y-Site Incompatibility:** chlorpromazine, hydralazine, prochlorperazine, promethazine.

Patient/Family Teaching

- Instruct patient to take this medication at the same time each day. Take missed dose as soon as remembered but not just before next dose is due. Do not double doses.
- Instruct patient to monitor weight biweekly and notify health care professional of significant changes.
- Caution patient to change positions slowly to minimize orthostatic hypotension. This may be potentiated by alcohol.
- Advise patient to use sunscreen and protective clothing to prevent photosensitivity reactions.
- Instruct patient to discuss dietary potassium requirements with health care professional (see Appendix J).
- Instruct patient to notify health care professional of medication regimen before treatment or surgery.
- Advise patient to report rash, muscle weakness, cramps, nausea, vomiting, diarrhea, or dizziness to health care professional.
- Emphasize the importance of routine follow-up exams.
- **Hypertension:** Advise patients to continue taking the medication even if feeling better. Medication controls but does not cure hypertension.
- Encourage patient to comply with additional interventions for hypertension (weight reduction, low-sodium diet, regular exercise, smoking cessation, moderation of alcohol consumption, and stress management).
- Instruct patient and family in correct technique for monitoring weekly BP.
- Instruct patient to notify health care professional of all Rx or OTC medications, vitamins, or herbal products being taken and to consult health care professional before taking other Rx, OTC, or herbal products, especially cough or cold preparations.

Evaluation/Desired Outcomes

- Decrease in BP.
- Increase in urine output.
- Decrease in edema.

divalproex sodium, See VALPROATES.

HIGH ALERT

DOBUTamine

(doe-**byoo**-ta-meen)
Dobutrex

Classification
Therapeutic: inotropics
Pharmacologic: adrenergics

Pregnancy Category B

Indications

Short-term (<48 hr) management of heart failure caused by depressed contractility from organic heart disease or surgical procedures.

Action

Stimulates $beta_1$ (myocardial)-adrenergic receptors with relatively minor effect on heart rate or peripheral blood vessels. **Therapeutic Effects:** Increased cardiac output without significantly increased heart rate.

Pharmacokinetics

Absorption: Administered by IV infusion only, resulting in complete bioavailability.
Distribution: Unknown.
Metabolism and Excretion: Metabolized by the liver and other tissues.
Half-life: 2 min.

TIME/ACTION PROFILE (inotropic effects)

ROUTE	ONSET	PEAK	DURATION
IV	1–2 min	10 min	brief (min)

Contraindications/Precautions

Contraindicated in: Hypersensitivity to dobutamine or bisulfites; Idiopathic hypertrophic subaortic stenosis.
Use Cautiously in: History of hypertension (increased risk of exaggerated pressor response); MI; Atrial fibrillation (pretreatment with digitalis glycosides recommended); History of ventricular atopic activity (may be exacerbated); Hypovolemia (correct before administration); Pregnancy or lactation (safety not established).

Adverse Reactions/Side Effects

CNS: headache. **Resp:** shortness of breath. **CV:** hypertension, increased heart rate, premature ventricular contractions, angina pectoris, arrhythmias, hypotension, palpitations. **GI:** nausea, vomiting. **Local:** phlebitis. **Misc:** hypersensitivity reactions including skin rash, fever, bronchospasm or eosinophilia, nonanginal chest pain.

Interactions

Drug-Drug: Use with **nitroprusside**; may have a synergistic effect on ↑ cardiac output. **Beta blockers** may negate the effect of dobutamine. ↑ risk of arrhythmias or hypertension with some **anesthetics** (**cyclopropane, halothane**), **MAO inhibitors**, **oxytocics**, or **tricyclic antidepressants**.

Route/Dosage

IV (Adults and Children): 2.5–15 mcg/kg/min titrate to response (up to 40 mcg/kg/min).
IV (Neonates): 2–15 mcg/kg/min.

Availability

Injection: 12.5 mg/mL in 20-, 40-, and 100-mL vials. **Premixed infusion:** 250 mg/250 mL, 500 mg/500 mL, 500 mg/250 mL, 1000 mg/250 mL.

NURSING IMPLICATIONS

Assessment

- Monitor BP, heart rate, ECG, pulmonary capillary wedge pressure (PCWP), cardiac output, CVP, and urinary output continuously during the administration. Report significant changes in vital signs or arrhythmias. Consult physician for parameters for pulse, BP, or ECG changes for adjusting dose or discontinuing medication.
- Palpate peripheral pulses and assess appearance of extremities routinely throughout dobutamine administration. Notify physician if quality of pulse deteriorates or if extremities become cold or mottled.
- ***Lab Test Considerations:*** Monitor potassium concentrations during therapy; may cause hypokalemia.
- Monitor electrolytes, BUN, creatinine, and prothrombin time weekly during prolonged therapy.
- ***Toxicity and Overdose:*** If overdose occurs, reduction or discontinuation of therapy is the only treatment necessary because of the short duration of dobutamine.

Potential Nursing Diagnoses

Decreased cardiac output (Indications)
Ineffective tissue perfusion (Indications)

Implementation

- ***High Alert:*** IV vasoactive medications are potentially dangerous. Have second practitioner independently check original order, dosage calculations, and infusion pump settings. Do not confuse dobutamine with dopamine. If available as floor stock, store in separate areas.
- Correct hypovolemia with volume expanders before initiating dobutamine therapy.
- Administer into a large vein and assess administration site frequently. Extravasation may cause pain and inflammation.

IV Administration

- **Continuous Infusion:** ***Diluent:*** Vials must be diluted before use. Dilute 250–1000 mg in 250–500 mL of D5W, 0.9% NaCl, 0.45% NaCl, D5/0.45% NaCl, D5/0.9% NaCl, or LR. Admixed infusions stable for 48 hr at room temperature and 7 days if refrigerated. Premixed infusions are already diluted and ready to use. ***Concentration:*** 0.25–5 mg/mL. ***Rate:*** Based on patient's weight (see Route/Dosage section). Administer via infusion pump to ensure precise amount delivered. Titrate to patient response (heart rate, presence of ectopic activity, BP, urine output, CVP, PCWP, cardiac index). Dose should be titrated so heart rate does not increase by >10% of baseline.
- **Y-Site Compatibility:** amifostine, amikacin, amiodarone, anidulafungin, argatroban, atracurium, atropine, aztreonam, bivalirudin, bumetanide, calcium chloride, calcium gluconate, caspofungin, cimetidine, ciprofloxacin, cisatracurium, cyclosporine, cladribine, dexmedetomidine, diazepam, digoxin, diltiazem, diphenhydramine, docetaxel, dopamine, doxorubicin liposome, doxycycline, enalaprilat, epinephrine, eptifibatide, erythromycin, esmolol, etoposide phosphate, famotidine, fenoldopam, fentanyl, fluconazole, gemcitabine, gentamicin, granisetron, haloperidol, hydromorphone, insulin, isoproterenol, labetalol, levofloxacin, lidocaine, linezolid, lorazepam, magnesium sulfate, meperidine, methylprednisolone sodium succinate, metoclopramide, metoprolol, milrinone, morphine, nafcillin, nicardipine, nitroglycerin, norepinephrine, ondansetron, oxaliplatin, palonosetron, pancuronium, phenylephrine, potassium chloride, procainamide, prochlorperazine, promethazine, propofol, propranolol, protamine, ranitidine, remifentanil, streptokinase, tacrolimus, theophylline, thiotepa, tigecycline, tirofiban, tobramycin, tolazoline, vancomycin, vasopressin, vecuronium, verapamil, voriconazole, zidovudine.
- **Y-Site Incompatibility:** acyclovir, alteplase, aminophylline, amphotericin B cholesteryl sulfate, ampicillin, ampicillin/sulbactam, amphotericin B, cefazolin, cefoxitin, ceftriaxone, cefuroxime, chloramphenicol, ertapenem, foscarnet, ganciclovir, hydrocortisone sodium succinate, indomethacin, ketorolac, lansoprazole, micafungin, pantoprazole, pemetrexed, penicillin G potassium, phenytoin, phytonadione, piperacillin/tazobactam, sodium bicarbonate, thiopental, trimethoprim/sulfamethoxazole, warfarin.

Patient/Family Teaching

- Explain to patient the rationale for instituting this medication and the need for frequent monitoring.
- Advise patient to inform nurse immediately if chest pain; dyspnea; or numbness, tingling, or burning of extremities occurs.
- Instruct patient to notify nurse immediately of pain or discomfort at the site of administration.
- **Home Care Issues:** Instruct caregiver on proper care of IV equipment.
- Instruct caregiver to report signs of worsening HF (shortness of breath, orthopnea, decreased exercise tolerance), abdominal pain, and nausea or vomiting to health care professional promptly.

Evaluation/Desired Outcomes

- Increase in cardiac output.
- Improved hemodynamic parameters.
- Increased urine output.

HIGH ALERT

DOCEtaxel (doe-se-**tax**-el)
Docefrez, Taxotere

Classification
Therapeutic: antineoplastics
Pharmacologic: taxoids

Pregnancy Category D

Indications

Breast cancer (locally advanced/metastatic breast cancer or with doxorubicin and cyclophosphamide as adjuvant treatment of node-positive disease). Non–small-cell lung cancer (locally advanced/metastatic) after failure on platinum regimen or with platinum as initial therapy). Advanced metastatic hormone-refractory prostate cancer (with prednisone). Squamous cell carcinoma of the head and neck (locally advanced) with cisplatin and fluorouracil. Gastric adenocarcinoma (locally advanced) with cisplatin and fluorouracil.

Action

Interferes with normal cellular microtubule function required for interphase and mitosis. **Therapeutic Effects:** Death of rapidly replicating cells, particularly malignant ones.

Pharmacokinetics

Absorption: IV administration results in complete bioavailability.

Distribution: Unknown.

Metabolism and Excretion: Extensively metabolized by the liver; metabolites undergo fecal elimination.

Half-life: 11.1 hr.

TIME/ACTION PROFILE (effect on blood counts)

ROUTE	ONSET	PEAK	DURATION
IV	rapid	5–9 days	7 days

Contraindications/Precautions

Contraindicated in: Hypersensitivity; Hypersensitivity to polysorbate 80; Known alcohol intolerance; Neutrophil count <1500/mm³; Liver impairment (serum bilirubin > upper limit of normal, ALT and/or AST >1.5 times upper limit of normal, with alkaline phosphatase >2.5 times upper limit of normal); OB, Lactation: Pregnancy or lactation.

Use Cautiously in: OB: Patients with child-bearing potential; Pedi: Efficacy not established.

Adverse Reactions/Side Effects

CNS: fatigue, weakness, alcohol intoxication. **EENT:** cystoid macular edema. **Resp:** ACUTE RESPIRATORY DISTRESS SYNDROME, INTERSTITIAL LUNG DISEASE, PULMONARY FIBROSIS, bronchospasm, dyspnea. **CV:** ASCITES, CARDIAC TAMPONADE, PERICARDIAL EFFUSION, PULMONARY EDEMA, peripheral edema. **GI:** diarrhea, nausea, stomatitis, vomiting. **Derm:** alopecia, edema, rash, dermatitis, desquamation, erythema, nail disorders. **Hemat:** anemia, leukopenia, thrombocytopenia, leukemia. **Local:** injection site reactions. **MS:** myalgia, arthralgia. **Neuro:** neurosensory deficits, peripheral neuropathy. **Misc:** hypersensitivity reactions, including ANAPHYLAXIS.

Interactions

Drug-Drug: ↑ bone marrow depression may occur with other **antineoplastics** or **radiation therapy**. Strong inhibitors of CYP3A4, including **atazanavir**, **clarithromycin**, **indinavir**, **itraconazole**, **ketoconazole**, **nefazodone**, **nelfinavir**, **ritonavir**, **saquinavir**, **telithromycin**, or **voriconazole** ↑ levels and the risk of toxicity; avoid concomitant use (if need to use, ↓ docetaxel dose by 50%).

Route/Dosage

IV (Adults): *Breast cancer*—60–100 mg/m² every 3 wk; *Breast cancer adjuvant therapy*—75 mg/m² every 3 wk for 6 cycles (with doxorubicin and cyclophosphamide); *Non–small-cell lung cancer*—75 mg/m² every 3 wk (alone or with platinum); *Prostate cancer*—75 mg/m² every 3 wk (with oral prednisone); *Squamous cell head and neck cancer*—75 mg/m² every 3 wk for 3–4 cycles (with cisplatin and fluorouracil); *Gastric adenocarcinoma*—75 mg/m² every 3 wk (with cisplatin and fluorouracil).

Availability (generic available)

Injection concentrate: 10 mg/mL (dose of 100 mg/m² contains 0.15 g/m² of ethanol), 20 mg/mL (dose of 100 mg/m² contains 1.975 g/m² of ethanol), 40 mg/mL (dose of 100 mg/m² contains 0.15 g/m² of ethanol). **Lyophilized powder for injection:** 20 mg/vial, 80 mg/vial.

NURSING IMPLICATIONS

Assessment

- Monitor vital signs before and after administration.
- Assess infusion site for patency. Docetaxel is not a vesicant. If extravasation occurs, discontinue docetaxel immediately and aspirate the IV needle. Apply cold compresses to the site for 24 hr.
- Monitor for hypersensitivity reactions continuously during infusion. These are most common after first and second doses of docetaxel. Reactions may consist of bronchospasm, hypotension, and/or erythema. Mild to moderate reactions may be treated symptomatically and infusion slowed or stopped until reaction subsides. Severe reactions require discontinuation of therapy and symptomatic treatment.

Do not readminister docetaxel to patients with previous severe reactions. Severe edema may also occur. Weigh patients before each treatment. Fluid accumulation may result in edema, ascites, and pleural or pericardial effusions. Pretreatment with corticosteroids (such as dexamethasone 8 mg PO twice daily for 3 days, starting 1 day before docetaxel) is recommended to minimize edema and hypersensitivity reactions. PO furosemide may be used to treat edema. For hormone-refractory metastatic prostate cancer (given with prednisone), recommended premedication regimen is dexamethasone 8 mg PO, at 12 hr, 3 hr and 1 hr before docetaxel infusion.

- Monitor for bone marrow depression. Assess for bleeding (bleeding gums, bruising, petechiae; guaiac stools, urine, and emesis) and avoid IM injections and taking rectal temperatures if platelet count is low. Apply pressure to venipuncture sites for 10 min. Assess for signs of infection during neutropenia. Anemia may occur. Monitor for increased fatigue, dyspnea, and orthostatic hypotension.
- Assess for rash. May occur on feet or hands but may also occur on arms, face, or thorax, usually with pruritus. Rash usually occurs within 1 wk after infusion and resolves before next infusion.
- Assess for development of neurosensory deficit (paresthesia, dysesthesia, pain, burning). May also cause weakness. Pyridoxine may be used to minimize symptoms. Severe symptoms may require dose reduction or discontinuation.
- Assess for arthralgia and myalgia, which are usually relieved by nonopioid analgesics but may be severe enough to require treatment with opioid analgesics.
- Assess for diarrhea and stomatitis. If Grade 3 or 4, reduce dose.
- ***Lab Test Considerations:*** Monitor CBC and differential before each treatment. Frequently causes neutropenia (<2000 neutrophils/mm^3); may require dose adjustment. If neutrophil count <1500/mm^3, hold dose. Neutropenia is reversible and not cumulative. The nadir is 8 days, with a duration of 7 days. May also cause thrombocytopenia and anemia.
- Monitor liver function studies (AST, ALT, alkaline phosphatase, bilirubin) before each cycle. If AST/ALT >2.5 to ≤5 x upper limit of normal and AP ≤2.5 x upper limit of normal, or AST/ALT >1.5 to ≤5 x upper limit of normal and AP >2.5 to ≤5 x ULN, reduce dose by 20%. If AST/ALT >5 x upper limit of normal and/or AP >5 x upper limit of normal discontinue therapy.

Potential Nursing Diagnoses

Risk for infection (Adverse Reactions)
Risk for injury (Adverse Reactions)

Implementation

- ***High Alert:*** Fatalities have occurred with chemotherapeutic agents. Before administering, clarify all ambiguous orders; double-check single, daily, and course-of-therapy dose limits; have second practitioner independently double-check original order, calculations, and infusion pump settings.
- ***High Alert:*** Do not confuse Taxotere (docetaxel) with Taxol (paclitaxel).
- Premedicate with dexamethasone 8 mg twice daily for 3 days starting 1 day before docetaxel infusion to reduce incidence and severity of fluid retention and hypersensitivity reactions. Premedicate patients with hormone-refractory metastatic prostate cancer with PO dexamethasone 8 mg, at 12 hr, 3 hr and 1 hr before docetaxel infusion.
- Solution should be prepared in a biologic cabinet. Wear gloves, gown, and mask while handling medication. If powder or solution comes in contact with skin or mucosa, wash thoroughly with soap and water. Discard equipment in specially designated containers.

IV Administration

- **Intermittent Infusion:** *For injection concentrate:* Before dilution, allow vials to stand at room temperature for 5 min. Solution is pale yellow to brownish yellow. *For powder for injection:* Allow number of vials required for dose to stand at room temperature for 5 min. Reconstitute with diluent provided, 1 mL for 20-mg vial or 4 mL for 80-mg vial. Shake vial to dissolve. Solution should be clear; do not administer solutions that are discolored or contain a precipitate. Allow solution to stand for a few minutes for air bubbles to dissipate. May be refrigerated for up to 8 hrs. ***Concentration:*** 20 mg/0.8 mL for 20-mg vial; 24 mg/mL for 80-mg vial. ***Diluent:*** Withdraw required amount and inject into 250-mL bag of 0.9% NaCl or D5W. If a dose greater than 200 mg is required, use a larger volume diluent so that concentration of 0.74 mg/mL is not exceeded. Rotate gently to mix. Do not administer solutions that are cloudy or contain a precipitate. Diluted solution must be infused within 4 hrs. ***Concentration:*** 0.3 mg/mL to 0.74 mg/mL. ***Rate:*** Administer over 1 hr.
- **Y-Site Compatibility:** acyclovir, alfentanil, allopurinol, amifostine, amikacin, aminocaproic acid, aminophylline, amiodarone, amphotericin B lipid complex, ampicillin, ampicillin/sulbactam, anidulafungin, argatroban, azithromycin, aztreonam, bivalirudin, bleomycin, bumetanide, buprenorphine, busulfan, butorphanol, calcium chloride, calcium gluconate, carboplatin, carmustine, caspofungin, cefazolin, cefepime, cefotaxime, cefotetan, cefoxitin, ceftazidime, ceftriaxone, cefuroxime, chlorpromazine, ciprofloxacin, cisatracurium, cisplatin, clindamycin, cyclophosphamide, cyclosporine, cytarabine, dacarbazine, dactinomycin, daptomycin, dexamethasone, dexmedetomidine, dexrazoxane, diazepam, digoxin, diltiazem, diphenhydramine, dobutamine, dolasetron, dopamine, doripenem, doxycycline, droperidol, enalaprilat, ephedrine, epinephrine, epirubicin, ertapenem, erythromycin, esmolol, etoposide, etoposide phosphate, famotidine, fenoldo-

pam, fentanyl, fluconazole, fludarabine, fluorouracil, foscarnet, fosphenytoin, furosemide, ganciclovir, gemcitabine, gentamicin, glycopyrrolate, granisetron, haloperidol, heparin, hydralazine, hydrocortisone, hydromorphone, ifosfamide, imipenem/cilastatin, insulin, irinotecan, isoproterenol, ketorolac, labetalol, leucovorin, levofloxacin, levorphanol, lidocaine, linezolid, lorazepam, magnesium sulfate, mannitol, meperidine, meropenem, mesna, methotrexate, methyldopate, metoclopramide, metoprolol, metronidazole, midazolam, milrinone, mitoxantrone, morphine, moxifloxacin, nafcillin, naloxone, nesiritide, nicardipine, nitroglycerin, nitroprusside, norepinephrine, octreotide, ondansetron, oxaliplatin, palonosetron, pamidronate, pancuronium, pantoprazole, pemetrexed, pentamidine, pentazocine, pentobarbital, phenobarbital, phenylephrine, piperacillin/tazobactam, potassium acetate, potassium chloride, potassium phosphates, procainamide, prochlorperazine, promethazine, propranolol, quinupristin/dalfopristin, ranitidine, remifentanil, rituximab, rocuronium, sodium acetate, sodium bicarbonate, sodium phosphates, succinylcholine, sufentanil, tacrolimus, teniposide, theophylline, thiotepa, tigecycline, tirofiban, tobramycin, trastuzumab, trimethoprim/sulfamethoxazole, vancomycin, vasopressin, vecuronium, verapamil, vinblastine, vincristine, vinorelbine, voriconazole, zidovudine, zoledronic acid.

- **Y-Site Incompatibility:** amphotericin B colloidal, amphotericin B liposome, dantrolene, doxorubicin liposome, idarubicin, methylprednisolone, nalbuphine, phenytoin.

Patient/Family Teaching

- Instruct patient to report symptoms of hypersensitivity reactions (trouble breathing; sudden swelling of face, lips, tongue, throat; trouble swallowing; hives; rash; redness all over body) to health care professional immediately.
- Advise patient to notify health care professional if fever >101°F; chills; sore throat; signs of infection; bleeding gums; bruising; petechiae; or blood in urine, stool, or emesis occur. Caution patient to avoid crowds and persons with known infections. Instruct patient to use soft toothbrush and electric razor.
- Patient should be cautioned not to drink alcoholic beverages or take products containing aspirin or NSAIDs.
- Fatigue is a frequent side effect of docetaxel. Advise patient that frequent rest periods and pacing of activities may minimize fatigue.
- Instruct patient to notify health care professional if signs of fluid retention (peripheral edema in the lower extremities, weight gain, dyspnea), abdominal pain, yellow skin, weakness, paresthesia, gait disturbances, swelling of the feet, or joint or muscle aches occur.
- Alcohol content of docetaxel may impair CNS. Caution patient to avoid driving or other activities requiring alertness until response to medication is known. Advise patient to avoid alcohol during therapy.
- Instruct patient to inspect oral mucosa for redness and ulceration. If mouth sores occur, advise patient to use sponge brush and rinse mouth with water after eating and drinking.
- Instruct patient to notify health care professional of all Rx or OTC medications, vitamins, or herbal products being taken and consult health care professional before taking any new medications.
- Advise patient to notify health care professional if changes in vision occur. Obtain a prompt and comprehensive ophthalmologic examination. May require discontinuation of docetaxel and a non-taxane cancer therapy used.
- Discuss with patient the possibility of hair loss. Complete hair loss usually begins after 1 or 2 treatments and is reversible after discontinuation of therapy. Explore coping strategies.
- Instruct patient not to receive any vaccinations without advice of health care professional.
- Advise female patients to use effective contraception during therapy and to notify health care professional if pregnancy is planned or suspected or if breast feeding.
- Emphasize the need for periodic lab tests to monitor for side effects.

Evaluation/Desired Outcomes

- Decrease in size or spread of malignancy in women with advanced breast cancer.
- Decrease in size or spread of malignancy in locally advanced or metastatic non–small-cell lung cancer, squamous cell carcinoma of the head and neck, and gastric adenocarcinoma.
- Decreased size or spread of advanced metastatic hormone-refractory prostate cancer.

DOCUSATE (dok-yoo-sate)

docusate calcium
Kao-Tin, Kaopectate Stool Softener

docusate sodium
Colace, Correctol, Diocto, Docu-Soft, Docusoft S, DOK, ✤Dosolax, DSS, Dulcolax, Dulcolax Stool Softener, Enemeez, Fleet Pedialax, Fleet Sof-Lax, Phillips Liquid-Gels, ✤Selax, Silace, ✤Soflax

Classification
Therapeutic: laxatives
Pharmacologic: stool softeners

Pregnancy Category C

Indications

PO: Prevention of constipation (in patients who should avoid straining, such as after MI or rectal surgery). **Rect:** Used as enema to soften fecal impaction.

Action

Promotes incorporation of water into stool, resulting in softer fecal mass. May also promote electrolyte and water secretion into the colon. **Therapeutic Effects:** Softening and passage of stool.

Pharmacokinetics

Absorption: Small amounts may be absorbed from the small intestine after oral administration. Absorption from the rectum is not known.
Distribution: Unknown.
Metabolism and Excretion: Amounts absorbed after oral administration are eliminated in bile.
Half-life: Unknown.

TIME/ACTION PROFILE (softening of stool)

ROUTE	ONSET	PEAK	DURATION
PO	12–72 hr	unknown	unknown
Rectal	2–15 min	unknown	unknown

Contraindications/Precautions

Contraindicated in: Hypersensitivity; Abdominal pain, nausea, or vomiting, especially when associated with fever or other signs of an acute abdomen.
Use Cautiously in: Excessive or prolonged use may lead to dependence; Should not be used if prompt results are desired; OB, Lactation: Has been used safely.

Adverse Reactions/Side Effects

EENT: throat irritation. **GI:** mild cramps, diarrhea. **Derm:** rashes.

Interactions

Drug-Drug: None significant.

Route/Dosage

Docusate Calcium

PO (Adults): 240 mg once daily.

Docusate Sodium

PO (Adults and Children >12 yr): 50–400 mg in 1–4 divided doses.
PO (Children 6–12 yr): 40–150 mg in 1–4 divided doses.
PO (Children 3–6 yr): 20–60 mg in 1–4 divided doses.
PO (Children <3 yr): 10–40 mg in 1–4 divided doses.
PO (Infants): 5 mg/kg/day in 1–4 divided doses.
Rect (Adults): 50–100 mg or 1 unit containing 283 mg docusate sodium, soft soap, and glycerin.

Availability (generic available)

Docusate Calcium

Capsules: 240 mg[OTC].

Docusate Sodium (generic available)

Tablets: 100 mg[OTC]. **Capsules:** 50 mg[OTC], 100 mg[OTC], 250 mg[OTC]. **Syrup:** 20 mg/5 mL[OTC]. **Liquid:** 50 mg/5 mL[OTC]. **Enema:** 283 mg/5 mL[OTC]. ***In combination with:*** stimulant laxatives[OTC]. See Appendix B.

NURSING IMPLICATIONS

Assessment

- Assess for abdominal distention, presence of bowel sounds, and usual pattern of bowel function.
- Assess color, consistency, and amount of stool produced.

Potential Nursing Diagnoses

Constipation (Indications)

Implementation

- Do not confuse Colace with Cozaar. Do not confuse Dulcolax (docusate sodium) with Dulcolax (bisacodyl). Do not confuse Kaopectate Stool Softener (docusate calcium) with Kaopectate (bismuth subsalicylate).
- This medication does not stimulate intestinal peristalsis; stimulant laxative may be required for constipation.
- **PO:** Administer with a full glass of water or juice. May be administered on an empty stomach for more rapid results.
- Oral solution may be diluted in milk, infant formula, or fruit juice to decrease bitter taste.
- Do not administer within 2 hr of other laxatives, especially mineral oil. May cause increased absorption.
- **Rect:** Administer as a retention or flushing enema.

Patient/Family Teaching

- Advise patients that laxatives should be used only for short-term therapy. Long-term therapy may cause electrolyte imbalance and dependence.
- Encourage patients to use other forms of bowel regulation, such as increasing bulk in the diet, increasing fluid intake (6–8 full glasses/day), and increasing mobility. Normal bowel habits are variable and may vary from 3 times/day to 3 times/wk.
- Instruct patients with cardiac disease to avoid straining during bowel movements (Valsalva maneuver).
- Advise patient not to use laxatives when abdominal pain, nausea, vomiting, or fever is present.
- Advise patient not to take docusate within 2 hr of other laxatives.

Evaluation/Desired Outcomes

- A soft, formed bowel movement, usually within 24–48 hr. Therapy may take 3–5 days for results. Rectal dose forms produce results within 2–15 min.

REMS

dofetilide (doe-fet-il-ide)

Tikosyn

Classification

Therapeutic: antiarrhythmics (class III)

Pregnancy Category C

Indications

Maintenance of normal sinus rhythm (delay in time to recurrence of atrial fibrillation/atrial flutter [AF/AFl]) in patients with AF/AFl lasting more than one week, and who have been converted to normal sinus rhythm. Conversion of AF and AFl to normal sinus rhythm.

Action

Blocks cardiac ion channels responsible for transport of potassium. Increases monophasic action potential duration. Increases effective refractory period. **Therapeutic Effects:** Prevention of recurrent AF/AFl. Conversion of AF/AFl to normal sinus rhythm.

Pharmacokinetics

Absorption: Well absorbed (>90%) following oral administration.

Distribution: Unknown.

Metabolism and Excretion: 80% excreted by kidneys via cationic renal secretion, mostly as unchanged drug; 20% excreted as inactive metabolites; some metabolism in the liver via cytochrome P450 system (CYP3A4 isoenzyme).

Half-life: 10 hr.

TIME/ACTION PROFILE (blood levels)

ROUTE	ONSET	PEAK	DURATION
PO	within hrs	2–3 hr†	12–24 hr

†Steady state levels are achieved after 2–3 days.

Contraindications/Precautions

Contraindicated in: Hypersensitivity; Congenital or acquired prolonged QT syndromes; Baseline QT interval or QTc of >440 msec (500 msec in patients with ventricular conduction abnormalities); Creatinine clearance <20 mL/min; Concurrent use of verapamil, cimetidine, dolutegravir, ketoconazole, itraconazole, trimethoprim, megestrol, prochlorperazine, hydrochlorothiazide, or other QT-interval prolonging drugs; Lactation: Avoid use.

Use Cautiously in: Underlying electrolyte abnormalities (↑ risk of serious arrhythmias; correct prior to administration); Creatinine clearance 20–60 mL/min (dose ↓ recommended); Severe hepatic impairment; OB: Use only when potential benefit to patient outweighs potential risk to fetus; Pedi: Safety not established.

Adverse Reactions/Side Effects

CNS: <u>dizziness</u>, <u>headache</u>. **CV:** VENTRICULAR ARRHYTHMIAS (including torsade de pointes), <u>chest pain</u>, QT interval prolongation.

Interactions

Drug-Drug: Hydrochlorothiazide, **verapamil**, **cimetidine**, **ketoconazole**, **itraconazole**, **trimethoprim**, **megestrol**, **dolutegravir**, and **prochlorperazine** ↑ dofetilide levels and the risk of QT interval prolongation with arrhythmias; concurrent use is contraindicated. **QT interval prolonging drugs** may ↑ the risk of QT interval prolongation with arrhythmias; concurrent use contraindicated. **Amiloride**, **metformin**, and **triamterene** may also ↑ dofetilide levels; use with caution. Inhibitors of the cytochrome P450 system (CY P450 3A4 isoenzyme) including **macrolide anti-infectives**, **azole antifungals**, **protease inhibitor antiretrovirals**, **SSRI antidepressants**, **amiodarone**, **diltiazem**, **nefazodone**, **quinine**, and **zafirlukast** may also ↑ blood levels and the risk of arrhythmias and concurrent use should be undertaken with caution. Should not be used concurrently with other **class I or III antiarrhythmics** due to ↑ risk of arrhythmias. Hypokalemia or hypomagnesemia from **potassium-depleting diuretics** ↑ the risk of arrhythmias; correct abnormalities prior to administration. Concurrent use of **digoxin** may ↑ the risk of arrhythmias.

Drug-Food: Grapefruit juice may ↑ levels; avoid concurrent use.

Route/Dosage

Dosing should be adjusted according to renal function and assessment of QT interval.

PO (Adults): *Starting dose*—500 mcg twice daily; *maintenance dose*—250 mcg twice daily (not to exceed 500 mcg twice daily).

Renal Impairment

PO (Adults): *CCr 40–60 mL/min Starting dose*—250 mcg twice daily; *maintenance dose*—125 mcg twice daily; *CCr 20– 40 mL/min Starting dose*—125 mcg twice daily; *maintenance dose*—125 mcg once daily.

Availability

Capsules: 125 mcg, 250 mcg, 500 mcg.

NURSING IMPLICATIONS

Assessment

- Monitor ECG, pulse, and BP continuously during initiation of therapy and for at least 3 days or a minimum of 12 hrs after electrical or pharmacological conversion to normal sinus rhythm, whichever is greater, then periodically during therapy. Evaluate QTc prior to initiation of therapy and every 3 mo

D

during therapy. If QTc exceeds 440 msec (500 msec in patients with ventricular conduction abnormalities), discontinue dofetilide and monitor patient until QTc returns to baseline.

- Assess the patient's medication history including OTC, Rx, and natural/herbal products, with emphasis on those that interact with dofetilide (see Interactions).
- ***Lab Test Considerations:*** Creatinine clearance must be calculated for all patients prior to administration and every 3 mo during therapy.
- Maintain serum potassium in normal range before and during dofetilide therapy.

Potential Nursing Diagnoses

Decreased cardiac output (Indications)

Implementation

- Dolfetilide must be initiated or reinitiated in a setting that provides continuous ECG monitoring and has personnel trained in the management of serious ventricular arrhythmias and pharmacists trained to dispense dofetilide. Due to the potential for life-threatening ventricular arrhythmias, dofetilide is usually used for patients with highly symptomatic AF/AFl.
- Patients with AF should be anticoagulated according to usual protocol prior to electrical or pharmacological cardioversion.
- Make sure patient has an adequate supply of dofetilide prior to discharge to prevent interruption of therapy.
- Patients should not be discharged from the hospital within 12 hr of electrical or pharmacological conversion to normal sinus rhythm.
- **PO:** Administer at the same time each day without regard to food.

Patient/Family Teaching

- Instruct patient to take medication as directed, even if feeling well. If a dose is missed, skip dose; do not double next dose. Take next dose at usual time.
- Advise patient to read *Medication Guide* prior to initiation of therapy and reread with each Rx refill in case of changes. Emphasize need for compliance with therapy, potential for drug interactions, and need for periodic monitoring to minimize the risk of serious arrhythmias.
- Instruct patient or family member on how to take pulse. Advise patient to report changes in pulse rate or rhythm to health care professional.
- May cause dizziness. Caution patient to avoid driving or other activities requiring alertness until response to medication is known.
- Advise patient to inform health care professional of medication regimen prior to treatment or surgery.
- Instruct patient to notify health care professional of all Rx or OTC medications, vitamins, or herbal products being taken and to consult health care professional before taking other Rx, OTC, or herbal products.
- Advise patient to consult health care professional immediately if they faint, become dizzy, or have fast heartbeats. If health care professional is unavailable, instruct patient to go to nearest hospital emergency department, take remaining dofetilide capsules, and show them to health care professional. If symptoms associated with altered electrolyte balance such as excessive or prolonged diarrhea, sweating, or vomiting or loss of appetite or thirst occur, health care professional should also be notified immediately.
- Advise female patient to notify health care professional if pregnancy is planned or suspected or if breast feeding.
- Emphasize the importance of routine follow-up exams to monitor progress.

Evaluation/Desired Outcomes

- Prevention of recurrent AF/AFl.
- Conversion of AF/AFl to normal sinus rhythm.
- If patients do not convert to normal sinus rhythm within 24 hr of initiation of therapy, electrical conversion should be considered.

dolasetron (dol-a-se-tron)

Anzemet

Classification

Therapeutic: antiemetics

Pharmacologic: 5-HT_3 antagonists

Pregnancy Category B

Indications

PO: Prevention of nausea and vomiting associated with emetogenic chemotherapy. **IV:** Prevention and treatment of postoperative nausea/vomiting.

Action

Blocks the effects of serotonin at receptor sites (selective antagonist) located in vagal nerve terminals and in the chemoreceptor trigger zone in the CNS. **Therapeutic Effects:** Decreased incidence and severity of nausea/vomiting associated with emetogenic chemotherapy or surgery.

Pharmacokinetics

Absorption: Well absorbed but rapidly metabolized to hydrodolasetron, the active metabolite.

Distribution: Unknown.

Metabolism and Excretion: 61% of hydrodolasetron is excreted unchanged by the kidneys.

Half-life: *Hydrodolasetron*—8.1 hr (shorter in children).

TIME/ACTION PROFILE (antiemetic effect)

ROUTE	ONSET	PEAK	DURATION
PO	unknown	1–2 hr	up to 24 hr
IV	unknown	15–30 min	up to 24 hr

Contraindications/Precautions

Contraindicated in: Hypersensitivity; Prevention of nausea and vomiting associated with emetogenic chemotherapy (for IV only) (may ↑ risk of QT interval prolongation); Congenital long QT syndrome; Complete heart block (unless pacemaker present).

Use Cautiously in: Patients with risk factors for cardiac conduction abnormalities (underlying structural heart disease, sick sinus syndrome, atrial fibrillation and slow ventricular rate, myocardial ischemia, concurrent beta-blocker, verapamil, diltiazem, or antiarrhythmic therapy); Hypokalemia, hypomagenesemia, concurrent therapy with diuretics, or history of cumulative high-dose anthracycline therapy; Geri: ↑ risk for cardiac conduction abnormalities; OB, Lactation: Safety not established.

Adverse Reactions/Side Effects

CNS: headache (increased in cancer patients), dizziness, fatigue, syncope. **CV:** CARDIAC ARREST, TORSADE DE POINTES, VENTRICULAR ARRHYTHMIAS, bradycardia, heart block, hypertension, hypotension, PR interval prolongation, QRS interval prolongation, QT interval prolongation, tachycardia. **GI:** diarrhea, dyspepsia. **GU:** oliguria. **Derm:** pruritus. **Misc:** SEROTONIN SYNDROME, chills, fever, pain.

Interactions

Drug-Drug: Concurrent **diuretic** or **antiarrhythmic** therapy or cumulative **high-dose anthracycline therapy** may ↑ risk of conduction abnormalities. Blood levels and effects of hydrodolasteron are ↑ by **atenolol** and **cimetidine**. Blood levels and effects of hydrodolasetron are ↓ by **rifampin**. ↑ risk of QT interval prolongation with other **agents causing QT interval prolongation**. Drugs that affect serotonergic neurotransmitter systems, including **SSRIs**, **SNRIs**, **tricyclic antidepressants**, **MAOIs**, **fentanyl**, **lithium**, **buspirone**, **tramadol**, **methylene blue**, and **triptans** ↑ risk of serotonin syndrome.

Route/Dosage

Prevention of Chemotherapy-Induced Nausea/Vomiting

PO (Adults): 100 mg given within 1 hr before chemotherapy.

PO (Children 2–16 yr): 1.8 mg/kg given within 1 hr before chemotherapy (not to exceed 100 mg).

Prevention/Treatment of Postoperative Nausea/Vomiting

IV (Adults): *Prevention or treatment*—12.5 mg given 15 min before cessation of anesthesia (prevention) or as soon as nausea or vomiting begins (treatment).

IV (Children 2–16 yr): *Prevention or treatment*—0.35 mg/kg (up to 12.5 mg) given 15 min before cessation of anesthesia (prevention) or as soon as nausea or vomiting begins (treatment).

Availability

Tablets: 50 mg, 100 mg. **Injection:** 20 mg/mL.

D

NURSING IMPLICATIONS

Assessment

- Assess patient for nausea, vomiting, abdominal distention, and bowel sounds before and after administration.
- Monitor vital signs after administration. IV administration may be followed by severe hypotension, bradycardia, and syncope.
- Monitor ECG in patients with HF, bradycardia, underlying heart disease, renal impairment, and elderly patients.
- ***Lab Test Considerations:*** Monitor serum potassium and magnesium prior to and periodically during therapy.

Potential Nursing Diagnoses

Imbalanced nutrition: less than body requirements (Indications)

Implementation

- Do not confuse Anzemet with Avandamet.
- **PO:** Administer within 1 hr before chemotherapy.
- Injectable dolasetron may be mixed in apple or apple-grape juice for oral dosing for pediatric patients. Recommended oral dose in patients 2 to 16 yr of age is 1.2 mg/kg (maximum 100 mg) given within 2 hr before surgery. Diluted product may be kept up to 2 hr at room temperature before use. May be stored at room temperature for 2 hr before use.

IV Administration

- Correct hypokalemia and hypomagnesemia before administering.
- **IV:** Administer 15 min before cessation of anesthesia, or postoperatively if nausea and vomiting occur shortly after surgery.
- **IV Push:** ***Diluent:*** May be administered undiluted. ***Concentration:*** 20 mg/mL. ***Rate:*** Administer 100 mg over at least 30 sec.
- **Intermittent Infusion:** ***Diluent:*** May be diluted in 50 mL of 0.9% NaCl, D5W, dextrose/saline combinations, D5/LR, LR, or 10% mannitol solution. Solution is clear and colorless. Stable for 24 hr at room temperature or 48 hr if refrigerated after dilution. ***Rate:*** Administer each dose as an IV infusion over up to 15 min.
- **Y-Site Compatibility:** acetaminophen, alfentanil, amifostine, amikacin, amiodarone, anidulafungin, argatroban, aztreonam, bivalirudin, bleomycin, bumetanide, buprenorphine, busulfan, butorphanol, calcium chloride, calcium gluconate, carboplatin, carmustine, caspofungin, ceftazidime, chlorproma-

zine, ciprofloxacin, cisplatin, clindamycin, cyclophosphamide, cyclosporine, cytarabine, daptomycin, dacarbazine, dactinomycin, daptomycin, daunorubicin, dexmedetomidine, dexrazoxane, digoxin, diltiazem, diphenhydramine, dobutamine, docetaxel, dopamine, doxorubicin hydrochloride, doxycycline, droperidol, enalaprilat, ephedrine, epinephrine, epirubicin, eptifibatide, ertapenem, erythromycin, esmolol, etoposide, etoposide phosphate, famotidine, fenoldopam, fentanyl, fluconazole, fludarabine, gemcitabine, gentamicin, haloperidol, hetastarch, hydromorphone, idarubicin, ifosfamide, imipenem/cilastatin, irinotecan, isoproterenol, labetalol, calcium, levofloxacin, levorphanol, lidocaine, linezolid, lorazepam, magnesium sulfate, mannitol, mechlorethamine, meperidine, mesna, methotrexate, metoclopramide, metronidazole, midazolam, milrinone, mitomycin, mitoxantrone, morphine, moxifloxacin, mycophenolate, nalbuphine, naloxone, nesiritide, nicardipine, nitroglycerin, nitroprusside, octreotide, oxaliplatin, oxytocin, paclitaxel, pamidronate, pancuronium, pemetrexed, pentamidine, phenylephrine, potassium acetate, potassium chloride, procainamide, prochlorperazine, promethazine, propranolol, quinupristin/dalfopristin, ranitidine, rocuronium, sodium acetate, streptozocin, sufentanil, tacrolimus, teniposide, theophylline, thiopental , thiotepa, tigecycline, tirofiban, tobramycin, vancomycin, vecuronium, verapamil, vinblastine, vincristine, vinorelbine, voriconazole, zidovudine, zoledronic acid.

- **Y-Site Incompatibility:** Manufacturer recommends not admixing with other medications, acyclovir, alemtuzumab, aminocaproic acid, aminophylline, amphotericin B colloidal, amphotericin B lipid complex, amphotericin B liposome, ampicillin, ampicillin/sulbactam, cefazolin, cefepime, cefotaxime, cefotetan, cefoxitin, ceftazidime, ceftriaxone, cefuroxime, diazepam, doxorubicin liposomal, fluorouracil, foscarnet, fosphenytoin, furosemide, ganciclovir, heparin, hydrocortisone, ketorolac, meropenem, methylprednisolone, pantoprazole, pentobarbital, phenobarbital, phenytoin, piperacillin/tazobactam, potassium phosphates, sodium bicarbonate, sodium phosphates, trimethoprim/sulfamethoxazole.

Patient/Family Teaching

- Explain purpose of dolasetron to patient.
- Advise patient to notify health care professional if nausea or vomiting occurs.
- Advise patient to notify health care professional symptoms of abnormal heart rate or rhythm (racing heart beat, shortness of breath, dizziness, fainting) occur.

Evaluation/Desired Outcomes

- Prevention of nausea and vomiting associated with emetogenic cancer chemotherapy.
- Prevention and treatment of postoperative nausea and vomiting.

dolutegravir

(doe-loo-**teg**-ra-vir)

Tivicay

Classification

Therapeutic: antiretrovirals

Pharmacologic: integrase strand transfer inhibitors (INSTI)

Pregnancy Category B

Indications

Treatment of HIV-1 infection, in combination with other antiretrovirals.

Action

Inhibits HIV-1 integrase, which is required for viral replication. **Therapeutic Effects:** Evidence of decreased viral replication and reduced viral load with slowed progression of HIV and its sequelae.

Pharmacokinetics

Absorption: Absorption follows oral administration; bioavailability is unknown.

Distribution: Enters CSF.

Protein Binding: >98.9%.

Metabolism and Excretion: Metabobolized primarily by the UGT1A1 enzyme system with some metabolism by CYP3A4. 53% excreted unchanged in feces. Metabolites are renally excreted, minimal renal elimination of unchanged drug. Poor metabolizers of dolutegravir have ↑ levels and ↓ clearance.

Half-life: 14 hr.

TIME/ACTION PROFILE (blood levels)

ROUTE	ONSET	PEAK	DURATION
PO	unk	2–3 hr	12–24 hr†

†Depends on concurrent use of metabolic inducers.

Contraindications/Precautions

Contraindicated in: Concurrent use of dofetilide; Severe hepatic impairment; Lactation: Breast feeding not recommended in HIV-infected patients.

Use Cautiously in: Underlying hepatic disease, including hepatitis B or C (↑ risk fo hepatotoxicity); Severe renal impairment; Geri: Consider age-related ↓ in cardiac, renal and hepatic function, chronic disease states and concurrent medications; OB: Use during pregnancy only if clearly needed; Pedi: Patients <12 yr, <40 kg or INSTI-experienced with resistance documented to other INSTIs (raltegravir or elvitegravir) (safety and effectiveness not established).

Adverse Reactions/Side Effects

CNS: <u>headache</u>, <u>insomnia</u>, fatigue. **GI:** HEPATOTOXICITY (↑ WITH HEPATITIS B OR C). **GU:** renal impairment.

Derm: pruritus. **Metab:** fat accumulation/redistribution. **MS:** myositis. **Misc:** HYPERSENSITIVITY REACTIONS (including rash, constitutional symptoms, and liver injury), immune reconstitution syndrome.

Interactions

Drug-Drug: May ↑ blood levels and toxicity from **dofetilide**; concurrent use contraindicated. Blood levels and effectiveness are ↓ by **etravirine** (should not be used concurrently without atazanavir/ritonavir, darunavir/ritonavir or lopinavir/ritonavir). Blood levels and effectiveness are ↓ by **efavirenz**, **fosamprenavir/ritonavir**, **tipranavir/ritonavir**, **carbamazepine**, and **rifampin**; ↑ dose of dolutegravir recommended. Blood levels and effectiveness may be ↓ by **nevirapine**; avoid concurrent use. May ↑ blood levels and toxicity from **metformin**; do not exceed metformin dose of 1000 mg/day. Blood levels and effectiveness may be ↓ by **oxcarbazepine**, **phenobarbital**, **phenytoin**; avoid concurrent use. Absorption and effectiveness may be ↓ by cation-containing **antacids**, **buffered medications**, **calcium supplements** (oral), **iron supplements** (oral), **laxatives**, or **sucralfate**; dolutegravir should be taken 2 hr before or 6 hr after; may also take dolutegravir and calcium or iron supplements with food.

Drug-Natural Products: Blood levels and effectiveness may be ↓ **St. John's wort**; avoid concurrent use.

Route/Dosage

PO (Adults): *Treatment-naïve or treatment-experienced INSTI-naïve patients*—50 mg once daily; *Treatment-naïve or treatment-experienced INSTI-naïve patients currently receiving efavirenz, fosamprenavir/ritonavir, tipranvir/ritonavir, carbamazepine, or rifampin*—50 mg twice daily; *INSTI-experienced with certain INSTI-associated resistance substitutions or clinically suspected INSTI resistance (consider other combinations that do not include metabolic inducers)*—50 mg twice daily.

PO (Children ≥ 12 yr and ≥40 kg): *Treatment-naïve or treatment-experienced INSTI-naïve patients*—50 mg once daily; *Treatment-naïve or treatment-experienced INSTI-naïve patients currently receiving efavirenz, fosamprenavir/ritonavir, tipranvir/ritonavir, carbamazepine, or rifampin*—50 mg twice daily.

Availability

Tablets: 50 mg. ***In combination with:*** abacavir and lamivudine (Triumeq). See Appendix B.

NURSING IMPLICATIONS

Assessment

- Assess patient for change in severity of HIV symptoms and for symptoms of opportunistic infections during therapy.
- Monitor for signs and symptoms of hypersensitivity reactions (rash, fever, malaise, fatigue, muscle or joint aches, blisters or peeling of skin, oral blisters or lesions, conjunctivitis, facial edema, hepatitis, eosinophilia, angioedema, difficulty breathing). Discontinue therapy and do not restart.
- ***Lab Test Considerations:*** Monitor viral load and CD4 counts regularly during therapy.
- May cause ↓ ANC, hemoglobin, total neutrophils, and platelet counts.
- May cause ↑ serum glucose, lipase, AST, ALT, total bilirubin, creatine kinase concentrations.

Potential Nursing Diagnoses

Risk for infection (Indications)
Noncompliance (Patient/Family Teaching)

Implementation

- **PO:** May be administered without regard to food.

Patient/Family Teaching

- Emphasize the importance of taking dolutegravir as directed. Do not take more than prescribed amount and do not stop taking without consulting health care professional. Take missed doses as soon as remembered unless within 4 hr of next dose; then skip dose. Do not double doses. Advise patient to read *Patient Information* before starting therapy and with each Rx renewal in case of changes.
- Instruct patient that dolutegravir should not be shared with others.
- Instruct patient to notify health care professional of all Rx or OTC medications, vitamins, or herbal products being taken and consult health care professional before taking any new medications.
- Inform patient that dolutegravir does not cure AIDS or prevent associated or opportunistic infections. Dolutegravir does not reduce the risk of transmission of HIV to others through sexual contact or blood contamination. Caution patient to use a condom during sexual contact and to avoid sharing needles or donating blood to prevent spreading the AIDS virus to others. Advise patient that the long-term effects of dolutegravir are unknown at this time.
- Advise patient to notify health care professional if signs and symptoms of hypersensitivity or infection occur.
- Inform patient that redistribution and accumulation of body fat may occur, causing central obesity, dorsocervical fat enlargement (buffalo hump), peripheral wasting, breast enlargement, and cushingoid appearance. The cause and long-term effects are not known.
- Rep: Advise patients to notify health care professional if pregnancy is planned or suspected. Breast feeding should be avoided during therapy. Pregnant

patients should be encouraged to enroll in the Antiretroviral Pregnancy Registry by calling 1-800-258-4263.

- Emphasize the importance of regular follow-up exams and blood counts to determine progress and monitor for side effects.

Evaluation/Desired Outcomes

- Delayed progression of AIDS and decreased opportunistic infections in patients with HIV.
- Decrease in viral load and improvement in CD4 cell counts.

donepezil (doe-**nep**-i-zill)

Aricept, ~~Aricept ODT~~

Classification

Therapeutic: anti-Alzheimer's agents

Pharmacologic: cholinergics (cholinesterase inhibitors)

Pregnancy Category C

Indications

Mild, moderate, or severe dementia/neurocognitive disorder associated with Alzheimer's disease.

Action

Inhibits acetylcholinesterase thus improving cholinergic function by making more acetylcholine available. **Therapeutic Effects:** May temporarily lessen some of the dementia associated with Alzheimer's disease. Enhances cognition. Does not cure the disease.

Pharmacokinetics

Absorption: Well absorbed after oral administration.

Distribution: Unknown.

Protein Binding: 96%.

Metabolism and Excretion: Partially metabolized by the liver (CYP2D6 and CYP3A4 enyzmes) and partially excreted by kidneys (17% unchanged). Two metabolites are pharmacologically active.

Half-life: 70 hr.

TIME/ACTION PROFILE (improvement in symptoms)

ROUTE	ONSET	PEAK	DURATION
PO	unknown	several wk	6 wk†

†Return to baseline after discontinuation.

Contraindications/Precautions

Contraindicated in: Hypersensitivity to donepezil or piperidine derivatives.

Use Cautiously in: Underlying cardiac disease, especially sick sinus syndrome or supraventricular conduction defects; History of ulcer disease or currently taking NSAIDs; History of seizures; History of asthma or obstructive pulmonary disease; OB, Lactation, Pedi: Safety not established; assumed to be secreted in breast milk. Discontinue drug or bottle-feed.

Adverse Reactions/Side Effects

CNS: headache, abnormal dreams, depression, dizziness, drowsiness, fatigue, insomnia, syncope, sedation (unusual). **CV:** atrial fibrillation, hypertension, hypotension, vasodilation. **GI:** diarrhea, nausea, anorexia, vomiting, weight gain (unusual). **GU:** frequent urination. **Derm:** ecchymoses. **Metab:** hot flashes, weight loss. **MS:** arthritis, muscle cramps.

Interactions

Drug-Drug: Exaggerates muscle relaxation from **succinylcholine**. Interferes with the action of **anticholinergics**. ↑ cholinergic effects of **bethanechol**. May ↑ risk of GI bleeding from **NSAIDs**. **Quinidine** and **ketoconazole** ↓ metabolism of donepezil. **Rifampin**, **carbamazepine**, **dexamethasone**, **phenobarbital**, and **phenytoin** induce the enzymes that metabolize donepezil and may ↓ its effects.

Drug-Natural Products: Jimson weed and **scopolia** may antagonize cholinergic effects.

Route/Dosage

Mild to Moderate Alzheimer's Disease

PO (Adults): 5 mg once daily; after 4–6 wk may ↑ to 10 mg once daily (dose should not exceed 5 mg/day in frail, elderly females).

Severe Alzheimer's Disease

PO (Adults): 5 mg once daily; may ↑ to 10 mg once daily after 4–6 wk; after 3 mo, may then ↑ to 23 mg once daily.

Availability (generic available)

Tablets: 5 mg, 10 mg, 23 mg. **Cost:** *Aricept*—23 mg $1,059.91/90; *Generic*—All strengths $23.97/90. **Orally disintegrating tablets:** 5 mg, 10 mg. **Cost:** *Generic*—All strengths $233.62/30. ***In combination with:*** memantine (Namzaric). See Appendix B.

NURSING IMPLICATIONS

Assessment

- Assess cognitive function (memory, attention, reasoning, language, ability to perform simple tasks) periodically during therapy.
- Monitor heart rate periodically during therapy. May cause bradycardia.

Potential Nursing Diagnoses

Disturbed thought process (Indications)

Impaired environmental interpretation syndrome (Indications)

Risk for injury (Indications)

Implementation

- Do not confuse Aricept with Aciphex or Azilect.
- **PO:** Administer in the evening just before going to bed. May be taken without regard to food.
- *Oral disintegrating tablets* should be allowed to dissolve on tongue; follow with water.
- Swallow *23 mg tablet* whole. Do not split, crush, or chew; may increase rate of absorption.

D

Patient/Family Teaching

- Emphasize the importance of taking donepezil daily, as directed. Missed doses should be skipped and regular schedule returned to the following day. Do not take more than prescribed; higher doses do not increase effects but may increase side effects.
- Inform patient/family that it may take weeks before improvement in baseline behavior is observed.
- Caution patient and caregiver that donepezil may cause dizziness.
- Advise patient and caregiver to notify health care professional if nausea, vomiting, diarrhea, or changes in color of stool occur or if new symptoms occur or previously noted symptoms increase in severity.
- Instruct patient to notify health care professional of all Rx or OTC medications, vitamins, or herbal products being taken and to consult health care professional before taking other Rx, OTC, or herbal products.
- Advise patient and caregiver to notify health care professional of medication regimen before treatment or surgery.
- Emphasize the importance of follow-up exams to monitor progress.

Evaluation/Desired Outcomes

- Improvement in cognitive function (memory, attention, reasoning, language, ability to perform simple tasks) in patients with Alzheimer's disease.

HIGH ALERT

DOPamine (dope-a-meen)

Intropin, ✱Revimine

Classification

Therapeutic: inotropics, vasopressors
Pharmacologic: adrenergics

Pregnancy Category C

Indications

Adjunct to standard measures to improve: BP, Cardiac output, Urine output in treatment of shock unresponsive to fluid replacement. Increase renal perfusion (low doses).

Action

Small doses (0.5–3 mcg/kg/min) stimulate dopaminergic receptors, producing renal vasodilation. Larger doses (2–10 mcg/kg/min) stimulate dopaminergic and beta$_1$-adrenergic receptors, producing cardiac stimulation and renal vasodilation. Doses greater than 10 mcg/kg/min stimulate alpha-adrenergic receptors and may cause renal vasoconstriction. **Therapeutic Effects:** Increased cardiac output, increased BP, and improved renal blood flow.

Pharmacokinetics

Absorption: Administered IV only, resulting in complete bioavailability.
Distribution: Widely distributed but does not cross the blood-brain barrier.
Metabolism and Excretion: Metabolized in liver, kidneys, and plasma.
Half-life: 2 min.

TIME/ACTION PROFILE (hemodynamic effects)

ROUTE	ONSET	PEAK	DURATION
IV	1–2 min	up to 10 min	<10 min

Contraindications/Precautions

Contraindicated in: Tachyarrhythmias; Pheochromocytoma; Hypersensitivity to bisulfites (some products).
Use Cautiously in: Hypovolemia; Myocardial infarction; Occlusive vascular diseases; Geri: Older patients may be more susceptible to adverse effects; OB: Pregnancy and lactation (safety not established).

Adverse Reactions/Side Effects

CNS: headache. **EENT:** mydriasis (high dose). **Resp:** dyspnea. **CV:** arrhythmias, hypotension, angina, ECG change, palpitations, vasoconstriction. **GI:** nausea, vomiting. **Derm:** piloerection. **Local:** irritation at IV site.

Interactions

Drug-Drug: Use with **MAO inhibitors**, **ergot alkaloids (ergotamine)**, **doxapram**, or some **antidepressants** results in severe hypertension. Use with IV **phenytoin** may cause hypotension and bradycardia. Use with **general anesthetics** may result in arrhythmias. **Beta blockers** may antagonize cardiac effects.

Route/Dosage

IV (Adults): *Dopaminergic (renal vasodilation) effects*—1–5 mcg/kg/min. *Beta-adrenergic (cardiac stimulation) effects*—5–15 mcg/kg/min. *Alpha-adrenergic (increased peripheral vascular resistance) effects*—>15 mcg/kg/min; infusion rate may be increased as needed.
IV (Children and Infants): 1–20 mcg/kg/min, depending on desired response (1–5 mcg/kg/min has been used to improve renal blood flow).
IV (Neonates): 1–20 mcg/kg/min.

Availability (generic available)

Injection for dilution: 40 mg/mL, 80 mg/mL, 160 mg/mL. **Premixed injection:** 200 mg/250 mL, 400 mg/250 mL, 800 mg/250 mL, 800 mg/500 mL.

NURSING IMPLICATIONS

Assessment

- Monitor BP, heart rate, pulse pressure, ECG, pulmonary capillary wedge pressure (PCWP), cardiac output, CVP, and urinary output continuously during administration. Report significant changes in vital signs or arrhythmias. Consult physician for parameters for pulse, BP, or ECG changes for adjusting dose or discontinuing medication.
- Monitor urine output frequently throughout administration. Report decreases in urine output promptly.
- Palpate peripheral pulses and assess appearance of extremities routinely during dopamine administration. Notify physician if quality of pulse deteriorates or if extremities become cold or mottled.
- If hypotension occurs, administration rate should be increased. If hypotension continues, more potent vasoconstrictors (norepinephrine) may be administered.
- ***Toxicity and Overdose:*** If excessive hypertension occurs, rate of infusion should be decreased or temporarily discontinued until BP is decreased.

Potential Nursing Diagnoses

Decreased cardiac output (Indications)
Ineffective tissue perfusion (Indications)

Implementation

- ***High Alert:*** IV vasoactive medications are potentially dangerous. Have second practitioner independently check original order, dose calculations, and infusion pump settings. Do not confuse dopamine with dobutamine. If both are available as floor stock, store in separate areas.
- Correct hypovolemia with volume expanders before initiating dopamine therapy.
- Extravasation may cause severe irritation, necrosis, and sloughing of tissue. Administer into a large vein and assess administration site frequently. If extravasation occurs, affected area should be infiltrated liberally with 10–15 mL of 0.9% NaCl containing 5–10 mg of phentolamine. For pediatric patients, use 1 mL of phentolamine dilution to infiltrate (do not exceed 5 mg total). Infiltration within 12 hr of extravasation produces immediate hyperemic changes.

IV Administration

- **Continuous Infusion: *Diluent:*** Dopamine vials must be diluted before use. Dilute 200–800 mg of dopamine in 250–500 mL of 0.9% NaCl, D5W, D5/LR, D5/0.45% NaCl, D5/0.9% NaCl, or LR. Admixed solution is stable for 24 hr. Discard solutions that are cloudy, discolored, or contain a precipitate. Premixed infusions are already diluted and ready to use. ***Concentration:*** 0.8–3.2 mg/mL. ***Rate:*** Based on patient's weight (see Route/Dosage section). Infusion must be administered via infusion pump to ensure precise amount delivered. Titrate to response (BP, heart rate, urine output, peripheral perfusion, presence of ectopic activity, cardiac index). Decrease rate gradually when discontinuing to prevent marked decreases in BP.
- **Y-Site Compatibility:** amifostine, amikacin, aminophylline, amiodarone, anidulafungin, argatroban, atracurium, atropine, aztreonam, bivalirudin, bumetanide, calcium chloride, calcium gluconate, caspofungin, cefotaxime, cefoxitin, ceftazidime, ceftriaxone, cefuroxime, cimetidine, ciprofloxacin, cisatracurium, cladribine, clindamycin, cyclosporine, daptomycin, dexamethasone sodium phosphate, dexmedetomidine, digoxin, diltiazem, diphenhydramine, dobutamine, docetaxel, doxorubicin liposome, doxycycline, droperidol, enalaprilat, epinephrine, ertapenem, erythromycin, esmolol, etoposide phosphate, famotidine, fenoldopam, fentanyl, fluconazole, foscarnet, gemcitabine, gentamicin, granisetron, haloperidol, heparin, hydrocortisone sodium succinate, hydromorphone, imipenem/cilastatin, isoproterenol, ketorolac, labetalol, levofloxacin, lidocaine, linezolid, lorazepam, magnesium sulfate, meperidine, methylprednisolone sodium succinate, metoclopramide, metoprolol, metronidazole, micafungin, midazolam, milrinone, morphine, nafcillin, nicardipine, nitroglycerin, nitroprusside, norepinephrine, ondansetron, oxaliplatin, palonosetron, pancuronium, pantoprazole, pemetrexed, penicillin G potassium, phenylephrine, phytonadione, piperacillin/tazobactam, potassium chloride, procainamide, prochlorperazine, promethazine, propofol, propranolol, protamine, ranitidine, remifentanil, sargramostim, streptokinase, tacrolimus, theophylline, thiotepa, tigecycline, tirofiban, tobramycin, tolazoline, vancomycin, vasopressin, vecuronium, verapamil, vitamin B complex with C, voriconazole, warfarin, zidovudine.
- **Y-Site Incompatibility:** acyclovir, alteplase, amphotericin B cholesteryl sulfate, ampicillin, cefazolin, chloramphenicol, diazepam, ganciclovir, indomethacin, insulin, lansoprazole, phenytoin, thiopental, trimethoprim/sulfamethoxazole.

Patient/Family Teaching

- Explain to patient the rationale for instituting this medication and the need for frequent monitoring.
- Advise patient to inform nurse immediately if chest pain; dyspnea; numbness, tingling, or burning of extremities occurs.
- Instruct patient to inform nurse immediately of pain or discomfort at the site of administration.

Evaluation/Desired Outcomes

- Increase in BP.
- Increase in peripheral circulation.
- Increase in urine output.

doripenem (do-ri-pen-em)

Doribax

Classification

Therapeutic: anti-infectives

Pharmacologic: carbapenems

Pregnancy Category B

Indications

Infections caused by susceptible organisms including: complicated intra-abdominal infections, complicated urinary tract infections, including pyelonephritis.

Action

Inhibits bacterial cell wall formation. **Therapeutic Effects:** Bactericidal action against susceptible bacteria. **Spectrum:** Active against the following gram-negative organisms: *Acinetobacter baumanii*, *Escherichia coli*, *Klebsiella pneumoniae*, *Proteus mirabilis*, and *Pseudomonas aeruginosa*. Also active against the following gram-positive organisms: *Streptococcus constellatus* and *S. intermedius*. Anaerobic spectrum includes *Bacteroides caccae*, *B. fragilis*, *B. thetaiotaomicron*, *B.uniformis*, *B. vulgatus*, and *Peptostreptococcus micros*.

Pharmacokinetics

Absorption: IV administration results in complete bioavailability.

Distribution: Penetrates renal and peritoneal and retroperitoneal tissues and fluids.

Metabolism and Excretion: 71% excreted unchanged in urine; minimal metabolism.

Half-life: 1 hr.

TIME/ACTION PROFILE (blood levels)

ROUTE	ONSET	PEAK	DURATION
IV	unknown	end of infusion	8 hr*

*Normal renal function.

Contraindications/Precautions

Contraindicated in: Hypersensitivity to doripenem, other carbapenems, or beta-lactams; Ventilator-associated pneumonia (↑ mortality).

Use Cautiously in: Renal impairment (↑ risk of seizures; dose ↓ recommended if CCr <50 mL/min); Geri: Consider age-related ↓ in renal function when choosing dose; Lactation: Use cautiously during lactation; Pedi: Safety not established.

Adverse Reactions/Side Effects

CNS: SEIZURES, headache. **GI:** CLOSTRIDIUM DIFFICILE-ASSOCIATED DIARRHEA (CDAD), nausea, diarrhea, ↑ liver enzymes. **Hemat:** anemia, thrombocytopenia. **Derm:** STEVENS-JOHNSON SYNDROME, TOXIC EPIDERMAL NECROLYSIS, pruritis, rash. **Local:** phlebitis. **Misc:** allergic reactions including ANAPHYLAXIS, infection with resistant organisms, superinfection.

Interactions

Drug-Drug: May ↓ serum **valproate** levels (↑ risk of seizures).

Drug-Natural Products: May ↓ blood levels of **valproic acid**; this may result in loss of seizure control. **Probenecid** ↓ renal clearance and ↑ blood levels.

Route/Dosage

IV (Adults): 500 mg every 8 hr.

Renal Impairment

IV (Adults): *CCr 30–50 mL/min*—250 mg every 8 hr; *CCr >10–<30 mL/min*—250 mg every 12 hr.

Availability

Powder for injection (requires reconstitution): 250 mg/vial, 500 mg/vial.

NURSING IMPLICATIONS

Assessment

- Assess patient for infection (vital signs; appearance of wound, sputum, urine, and stool; WBC) at beginning of and during therapy.
- Obtain a history before initiating therapy to determine previous use of and reactions to penicillins, cephalosporins, or carbapenems. Persons with a negative history of penicillin sensitivity may still have an allergic response.
- Obtain specimens for culture and sensitivity before initiating therapy. First dose may be given before receiving results.
- Observe patient for signs and symptoms of anaphylaxis (rash, pruritus, laryngeal edema, wheezing). Discontinue doripenem and notify health care professional immediately if these occur. Have epinephrine, an antihistamine, and resuscitative equipment close by in the event of an anaphylactic reaction.
- Monitor bowel function. Diarrhea, abdominal cramping, fever, and bloody stools should be reported to health care professional promptly as a sign of Clostridium difficile-associated diarrhea (CDAD). May begin up to several weeks following cessation of therapy.
- Assess patient for skin rash frequently during therapy. Discontinue at first sign of rash; may be life-threatening. Stevens-Johnson syndrome may develop. Treat symptomatically; may recur once treatment is stopped.
- ***Lab Test Considerations:*** May cause ↑ AST, ALT, serum alkaline phosphatase levels.
- May cause anemia.

Potential Nursing Diagnoses

Risk for infection (Indications, Side Effects)

Implementation

- Do not confuse Doribax with Zovirax.
- May switch to appropriate oral therapy after at least 3 days of parenteral therapy, once clinical improvement has been demonstrated.

IV Administration

- **Intermittent Infusion:** Reconstitute 500-mg vial with 10 mL of sterile injection or 0.9% NaCl and shake gently to form a suspension of 50 mg/mL. ***Diluent:*** Withdraw the resulting solution using a 21-gauge needle and add it to 100 mL of 0.9% NaCl or D5W; gently shake until clear. *For moderate or severe renal impairment, withdraw 55 mL of this solution from the bag and discard.* Solution should be clear and colorless to slightly yellow. ***Concentration:*** Final concentration is 4.5 mg/mL. Suspension is stable for 1 hr prior to dilution in infusion bag. Administer within 8 hr of reconstitution with 0.9% NaCl or 4 hr of reconstitution with D5W at room temperature or 24 hr if refrigerated; do not freeze. ***Rate:*** Administer over 1 hr. Do not administer IV push.
- **Y-Site Compatibility:** acyclovir, amikacin, aminophylline, amiodarone, anidulafungin, atropine, azithromycin, bumetanide, calcium gluconate, carboplatin, caspofungin, ceftaroline, ciprofloxacin, cisplatin, cyclophosphamide, cyclosporine, daptomycin, dexamethasone, digoxin, diltiazem, diphenhydramine, dobutamine, docetaxel, dopamine, doxorubicin, enalaprilat, esmolol, esomeprazole, etoposide phosphate, famotidine, fentanyl, fluconazole, fluorouracil, foscarnet, fucosemide, gemcitabine, gentamicin, granisetron, heparin, hydrocortisone sodium succinate, hydromorphone, ifosfamide, insulin, labetalol, levofloxacin, linezolid, lorazepam, magnesium sulfate, mannitol, meperidine, methotrexate, methylprednisolone, metoclopramide, metronidazole, micafungin, midazolam, milrinone, morphine, moxifloxacin, norepinephrine, ondansetron, paclitaxel, pantoprazole, phenobarbital, phenylephrine, potassium chloride, ranitidine, sodium bicarbonate, sodium phosphates, tacrolimus, telavancin, tigecycline, tobramycin, vancomycin, voriconazole, zidovudine.
- **Y-Site Incompatibility:** Do not mix with or physically add to solutions containing other medications, diazepam, potassium phosphates, propofol.

Patient/Family Teaching

- Advise patient to report the signs of superinfection (black, furry overgrowth on the tongue; vaginal itching or discharge; loose or foul-smelling stools) and allergy. Consult health care professional before treating with antidiarrheals.
- Caution patient to notify health care professional if rash or fever and diarrhea occur, especially if stool contains blood, pus, or mucus. Advise patient not to treat diarrhea without consulting health care professional. May occur up to several weeks after discontinuation of medication.

Evaluation/Desired Outcomes

- Resolution of the signs and symptoms of infection. Length of time for complete resolution depends on the organism and site of infection. Duration may be extended up to 14 days for patients with concurrent bacteremia.

doxazosin (dox-ay-zoe-sin)

Cardura, Cardura XL

Classification

Therapeutic: antihypertensives
Pharmacologic: peripherally acting antiadrenergics

Pregnancy Category C

Indications

Hypertension (alone or with other agents) (immediate-release only). Symptomatic benign prostatic hyperplasia (BPH).

Action

Dilates both arteries and veins by blocking postsynaptic alpha$_1$-adrenergic receptors. **Therapeutic Effects:** Lowering of BP. Increased urine flow and decreased symptoms of BPH.

Pharmacokinetics

Absorption: Well absorbed following oral administration.
Distribution: Probably enters breast milk; rest of distribution unknown.
Protein Binding: 98–99%.
Metabolism and Excretion: Extensively metabolized by the liver.
Half-life: 22 hr.

TIME/ACTION PROFILE

ROUTE	ONSET	PEAK	DURATION
PO†	1–2 hr	2–6 hr	24 hr
PO-XL‡	5 wk	unknown	unknown

† Antihypertensive effect.
‡ Improved urinary flow and BPH symptoms.

Contraindications/Precautions

Contraindicated in: Hypersensitivity.
Use Cautiously in: Hepatic dysfunction; Gastrointestinal narrowing (XL only); Geri: Appears on Beers list. Geriatric patients are at ↑ risk for hypotension; OB, Lactation, Pedi: Safety not established; Patients undergoing cataract surgery (↑ risk of intraoperative floppy iris syndrome).

Adverse Reactions/Side Effects

CNS: dizziness, headache, depression, drowsiness, fatigue, nervousness, weakness. **EENT:** abnormal vision, blurred vision, conjunctivitis, epistaxis, intraoperative floppy iris syndrome. **Resp:** dyspnea. **CV:** first-dose orthostatic hypotension, arrhythmias, chest pain, edema, palpitations. **GI:** abdominal discomfort, constipation, diarrhea, dry mouth, flatulence, nausea, vomiting. **GU:** ↓ libido, priapism, sexual dysfunction. **Derm:** flushing, rash, urticaria. **MS:** arthralgia, arthritis, gout, myalgia.

Interactions

Drug-Drug: ↑ risk of hypotension with **sildenafil**, **tadalafil**, **vardenafil**, other **antihypertensives**, **nitrates**, or acute ingestion of **alcohol**. **NSAIDs**, **sympathomimetics**, or **estrogens** may ↓ effects of antihypertensive therapy.

Route/Dosage

Hypertension

PO (Adults): —1 mg once daily, may be gradually ↑ at 2-wk intervals to 2–16 mg/day; incidence of postural hypotension greatly ↑ at doses >4 mg/day. *BPH*—1 mg once daily, may be gradually increased to 8 mg/day.

Benign Prostatic Hyperplasia

PO (Adults): *Immediate release*—1 mg once daily, may be ↑ every 1–2 wk up to 8 mg/day; *Extended release*—4 mg once daily (with breakfast), may be ↑ in 3–4 wk to 8 mg/day.

Availability (generic available)

Tablets: 1 mg, 2 mg, 4 mg, 8 mg. **Cost:** *Generic*—1 mg $60.00/100, 2 mg $79.89/100, 4 mg $85.34/100, 8 mg $60.41/100. **Extended-release tablets:** 4 mg, 8 mg. **Cost:** 4 mg $84.62/30, 8 mg $88.90/30.

NURSING IMPLICATIONS

Assessment

- Monitor BP and pulse 2–6 hr after first dose, with each increase in dose, and periodically during therapy. Report significant changes.
- Assess for first-dose orthostatic hypotension and syncope. Incidence may be dose related. Observe patient closely during this period and take precautions to prevent injury.
- Monitor intake and output ratios and daily weight, and assess for edema daily, especially at beginning of therapy. Report weight gain or edema.
- **BPH:** Assess patient for symptoms of prostatic hyperplasia (urinary hesitancy, feeling of incomplete bladder emptying, interruption of urinary stream, impairment of size and force of urinary stream, terminal urinary dribbling, straining to start flow, dysuria, urgency) prior to and periodically during therapy.

Potential Nursing Diagnoses

Impaired urinary elimination (Indications)
Risk for injury (Side Effects)

Implementation

- Do not confuse Cardura with Coumadin.
- **PO:** Administer daily dose at bedtime.
- XL tablets should be swallowed whole; do not break, crush, or chew.
- **Hypertension:** May be administered concurrently with a diuretic or other antihypertensive.

Patient/Family Teaching

- Emphasize the importance of continuing to take this medication, even if feeling well. Instruct patient to take medication at the same time each day. Take missed doses as soon as remembered unless almost time for next dose. Do not double doses.
- May cause drowsiness or dizziness. Advise patient to avoid driving or other activities requiring alertness until response to medication is known.
- Caution patient to change positions slowly to decrease orthostatic hypotension. May cause syncopal episodes, especially within first 24 hr of therapy, with dose increase, and with resumption of therapy after interruption.
- Instruct patient to notify health care professional of all Rx or OTC medications, vitamins, or herbal products being taken and to avoid concurrent use of alcohol or OTC medications and herbal products, especially cold preparations, without consulting health care professional, especially cough, cold, or allergy remedies.
- Advise male patient to notify health care professional if priapism or erection of longer than 4 hr occurs; may lead to permanent impotence if not treated.
- Advise female patient to notify health care professional if pregnancy is planned or suspected or if breast feeding.
- Emphasize the importance of follow-up visits to determine effectiveness of therapy.
- **Hypertension:** Instruct patient and family on proper technique for BP monitoring. Advise them to check BP at least weekly and report significant changes.
- Encourage patient to comply with additional interventions for hypertension (weight reduction, low-sodium diet, smoking cessation, moderation of alcohol consumption, regular exercise, and stress management).

Evaluation/Desired Outcomes

- Decrease in BP without appearance of side effects.
- Decrease in urinary symptoms of BPH.

doxepin (dox-e-pin)
Silenor, SINEquan, Zonalon

Classification
Therapeutic: antianxiety agents, antidepressants, antihistamines (topical), sedative/hypnotics
Pharmacologic: tricyclic antidepressants

Pregnancy Category C

Indications
PO: Management of: Depression, Insomnia. **Topical:** Short-term control of pruritus associated with: Eczematous dermatitis, Lichen simplex chronicus. **Unlabeled Use: PO:** Management of: Chronic pain syndromes, Pruritus, Dermatitis, Anxiety.

Action
PO: Prevents the reuptake of norepinephrine and serotonin by presynaptic neurons; resultant accumulation of neurotransmitters potentiates their activity. Also possesses significant anticholinergic properties. **Topical:** Antipruritic action due to antihistaminic properties.
Therapeutic Effects: PO: Relief of depression. Decreased anxiety. Sedation and improved sleep maintenance. **Topical:** Decreased pruritus.

Pharmacokinetics
Absorption: Well absorbed from the GI tract, although much is metabolized on first pass through the liver. Some systemic absorption follows topical application.
Distribution: Widely distributed. Enters breast milk; probably crosses the placenta.
Metabolism and Excretion: Metabolized by the liver by the CYP2C19 and CYP2D6 isoenzymes; the CYP2C19 enzyme system exhibits genetic polymorphism; 15–20% of Asian patients and 3–5% of Caucasian and Black patients may be poor metabolizers of CYP2C19 and may have significantly ↑ doxepin concentrations and an ↑ risk of adverse effects; the CYP2D6 enzyme system also exhibits genetic polymorphism; ~7% of population may be poor metabolizers of CYP2D6 and may have significantly ↑ doxepin concentrations and an ↑ risk of adverse effects. Some conversion to active antidepressant compound. May re-enter gastric juice via secretion from enterohepatic circulation, where more absorption may occur.
Half-life: 8–25 hr.

TIME/ACTION PROFILE (antidepressant activity)

ROUTE	ONSET	PEAK	DURATION
PO	2–3 wk	up to 6 wk	days–weeks

Contraindications/Precautions
Contraindicated in: Hypersensitivity; Concurrent use of MAO inhibitors; Some products contain bisulfites and should be avoided in patients with known intolerance; Untreated angle-closure glaucoma; Severe urinary retention; Period immediately after myocardial infarction; History of QTc prolongation, heart failure, cardiac arrhythmia.
Use Cautiously in: Geri: Pre-existing cardiovascular disease (↑ risk of adverse reactions); Prostatic enlargement (more susceptible to urinary retention); Seizures; OB: Use only if potential maternal benefit outweighs risks to fetus; Lactation: Use during lactation may result in neonatal sedation. Recommend discontinue drug or bottle-feed; Pedi: May ↑ risk of suicide attempt/ideation especially during dose early treatment or dose adjustment; risk may be greater in children or adolescents; safety not established; Geri: Appears on *Beers list* and is associated with ↑ falls risk secondary to anticholinergic and sedative effects. Geriatric patients should have initial dosage ↓.

Adverse Reactions/Side Effects
CNS: fatigue, sedation, agitation, confusion, hallucinations. **EENT:** blurred vision, ↑ intraocular pressure. **CV:** hypotension, arrhythmias, ECG abnormalities. **GI:** constipation, dry mouth, ↑ appetite, hepatitis, nausea, paralytic ileus, weight gain. **GU:** ↓ libido, urinary retention. **Derm:** photosensitivity, rash. **Hemat:** blood dyscrasias. **Misc:** hypersensitivity reactions.

Interactions
Apply to both topical and oral use.
Drug-Drug: Doxepin is metabolized in the liver by the cytochrome P450 2D6 enzyme and its action may be affected by drugs that compete for metabolism by this enzyme including other **antidepressants**, **phenothiazines**, **carbamazepine**, **propafenone**, **flecainide**; when used concurrently, dosage ↓ of one or the other or both may be necessary. Concurrent use of other drugs that inhibit the activity of the enzyme, including **cimetidine**, **quinidine**, **amiodarone**, and **ritonavir**, may result in ↑ effects of doxepin. May cause hypotension, tachycardia, and potentially fatal reactions when used with **MAO inhibitors** (avoid concurrent use—discontinue 2 wk prior to doxepin). Concurrent use with **SSRI antidepressants** may result in ↑ serotonin syndrome and should be avoided (fluoxetine should be stopped 5 wk before). Concurrent use with **clonidine** may result in hypertensive crisis and should be avoided. Concurrent use with **levodopa** may result in delayed/↓ absorption of levodopa or hypertension. Blood levels and effects may be ↓ by **rifamycins**. ↑ CNS depression with other **CNS depressants** including **alcohol**, **antihistamines**, **clonidine**, **opioid analgesics**, and **sedative/hypnotics**. **Barbiturates** may alter blood levels and effects. **Adrenergic** and **anticholinergic** side effects may be ↑ with other **agents having these properties**. **Phenothiazines** or **hormonal contraceptives** ↑ levels and may cause toxicity. **Smoking** may ↑ metabolism and alter effects.

Drug-Natural Products: Concomitant use of **kava-kava**, **valerian**, or **chamomile** can ↑ CNS depression. ↑ anticholinergic effects with **jimson weed** and **scopolia**.

Route/Dosage

PO (Adults): *Antidepressant/antianxiety*—25 mg 3 times daily, may be ↑ as needed (up to 150 mg/day in outpatients or 300 mg/day in inpatients; some patients may require only 25–50 mg/day). Once stabilized, entire daily dose may be given at bedtime. *Antipruritic*—10 mg at bedtime initially, may be ↑ up to 25 mg. *Insomnia*—6 mg at bedtime (should not exceed 3 mg/day if concurrently taking cimetidine).
PO (Geriatric Patients): *Antidepressant*—25–50 mg/day initially, may be ↑ as needed. *Insomnia*—3 mg at bedtime, may be ↑ as needed to 6 mg at bedtime (should not exceed 3 mg/day if concurrently taking cimetidine).
Topical (Adults): Apply 4 times daily (wait 3–4 hr between applications) for up to 8 days.

Availability (generic available)

Capsules: 10 mg, 25 mg, 50 mg, 75 mg, 100 mg, 150 mg. **Cost:** *Generic*—10 mg $32.45/100, 25 mg $42.85/100, 50 mg $56.86/100, 75 mg $124.29/100, 100 mg $102.79/100, 150 mg $299.49/90. **Tablets (Silenor):** 3 mg, 6 mg. **Cost:** All strengths $198.17/30. **Oral concentrate:** 10 mg/mL. **Cost:** *Generic*—$23.70/120 mL. **Topical cream:** 5%. **Cost:** $240.28/30 g.

NURSING IMPLICATIONS

Assessment

- Monitor BP and pulse rate prior to and during initial therapy. Patients taking high doses or with a history of cardiovascular disease should have ECG monitored prior to and periodically during therapy.
- Assess for sexual dysfunction (decreased libido; erectile dysfunction).
- Assess weight and BMI initially and throughout treatment. Obtain FBS and cholesterol levels in overweight/obese individuals.
- Geri: Assess falls risk and institute fall prevention strategies. Assess for anticholinergic effects.
- **Depression:** Assess mental status and mood changes (orientation, mood, behavior) frequently, especially during initial few months of therapy and during dose changes. Confusion, agitation, and hallucinations may occur during initiation of therapy and may require dose reduction. Assess for suicidal tendencies, especially during early therapy. Restrict amount of drug available to patient. Risk may be increased in children, adolescents, and adults ≤24 yr. Inform health care professional if patient demonstrates significant increase in signs of depression (depressed mood, loss of interest in usual activities, significant change in weight and/or appetite, insomnia or hypersomnia, psychomotor agitation or retardation, increased fatigue, feelings of guilt or worthlessness, slowed thinking or impaired concentration, suicide attempt or suicidal ideation). Restrict amount of drug available to patient.
- Assess for serotonin syndrome (mental changes [agitation, hallucinations, coma], autonomic instability [tachycardia, labile BP, hyperthermia], neuromuscular aberrations [hyperreflexia, incoordination], and/or GI symptoms [nausea, vomiting, diarrhea]), especially in patients taking other serotonergic drugs (SSRIs, SNRIs, triptans).
- **Anxiety:** Assess degree and manifestations of anxiety prior to and during therapy.
- **Pain:** Assess the type, location, and severity of pain prior to and periodically during therapy. Use pain scale to assess effectiveness of therapy.
- **Topical:** Assess pruritic area prior to and periodically during therapy.
- ***Lab Test Considerations:*** Monitor WBC and differential blood counts, hepatic function, and serum glucose periodically. May cause ↑ serum bilirubin and alkaline phosphatase levels. May cause bone marrow depression. Serum glucose may be ↑ or ↓.

Potential Nursing Diagnoses

Ineffective coping (Indications)
Risk for injury (Side Effects)
Sexual dysfunction (Side Effects)

Implementation

- Do not confuse Sinequan with Seroquel, saquinavir, Singulair, or Zonegran.
- May be given as a single dose 30 min before bedtime to minimize sedation during the day. Dose increases should be made at bedtime because of sedation. Dose titration is a slow process; may take weeks to months.
- To avoid withdrawal, taper by 50% for 3 days, then 50% again for 3 days, then discontinue.
- **PO:** Administer medication with or immediately following a meal to minimize gastric irritation. Capsules may be opened and mixed with foods or fluids if patient has difficulty swallowing.
- Oral concentrate must be diluted in at least 120 mL of water, milk, or fruit juice. Do not mix with carbonated beverages or grape juice. Use calibrated measuring device to ensure accurate amount.
- **Topical:** Apply thin film of doxepin cream only to affected areas, and rub in gently. Apply only to affected skin; not for ophthalmic, oral, or intravaginal use.

Patient/Family Teaching

- Inform patient that systemic side effects may occur with oral or topical use.

- May cause drowsiness and blurred vision. Caution patient to avoid driving and other activities requiring alertness until response to the medication is known.
- Orthostatic hypotension, sedation, and confusion are common during early therapy, especially in geriatric patients. Protect patient from falls. Institute fall precautions. Advise patient to change positions slowly.
- Advise patient to avoid alcohol or other CNS depressant drugs during and for at least 3–7 days after therapy has been discontinued.
- Inform patient that doxepin may cause getting up out of bed while not being fully awake and doing an activity that patient does not know he is doing. The next morning, he may not remember that he did anything during the night. May occur more frequently with alcohol or other sedatives. Advise patient to notify health care professional if this occurs.
- Instruct patient to notify health care professional if urinary retention occurs or if dry mouth or constipation persists. Sugarless candy or gum may diminish dry mouth, and an increase in fluid intake or bulk may prevent constipation. If symptoms persist, dose reduction or discontinuation may be necessary. Consult health care professional if dry mouth persists for more than 2 wk.
- Advise patient to notify health care professional of medication regimen prior to treatment or surgery.
- **PO:** Instruct patient to take medication as directed. Take missed doses as soon as possible unless almost time for next dose; if regimen is a single dose at bedtime, do not take in the morning because of side effects. Advise patient that drug effects may not be noticed for at least 2 wk. Abrupt discontinuation may cause nausea, vomiting, diarrhea, headache, trouble sleeping with vivid dreams, and irritability. Advise patient, family, and caregivers to look for suicidality, especially during early therapy or dose changes. Notify health care professional immediately if thoughts about suicide or dying, attempts to commit suicide, new or worse depression or anxiety, agitation or restlessness, panic attacks, insomnia, new or worse irritability, aggressiveness, acting on dangerous impulses, mania, or other changes in mood or behavior or if symptoms of serotonin syndrome occur.
- Caution patient to use sunscreen and protective clothing to prevent photosensitivity reactions.
- Inform patient that urine may turn blue-green in color.
- Inform patient of need to monitor dietary intake. Increase in appetite is possible and may lead to undesired weight gain.
- Therapy for depression is usually prolonged. Emphasize the importance of follow-up exams to monitor effectiveness and side effects.
- **Topical:** Instruct patient to apply a thin film of medication exactly as directed; do not use more medication than directed, apply to a larger area than directed, use more often than directed, or use longer than 8 days.
- Inform patient that topical preparation may cause burning, stinging, swelling, increased itching, or worsening of eczema. Notify health care professional if these symptoms become bothersome.
- Caution patient not to use occlusive dressings; may increase systemic absorption.
- Advise patient to notify health care professional if excessive drowsiness occurs with topical application. Number of applications per day, amount of cream applied, or area of application may be reduced. May require discontinuation of therapy.

Evaluation/Desired Outcomes

- Increased sense of well-being.
- Renewed interest in surroundings.
- Increased appetite.
- Improved energy level.
- Improved sleep.
- Decrease in anxiety.
- Decrease in chronic pain. Patients may require 2–6 wk of oral therapy before full therapeutic effects of medication are evident.
- Decrease in pruritus associated with eczema.

---

doxercalciferol, See VITAMIN D COMPOUNDS.

HIGH ALERT

DOXOrubicin

(dox-oh-**roo**-bi-sin)

✽Adriamycin, ✽Caelyx, ✽Myocet

Classification

Therapeutic: antineoplastics

Pharmacologic: anthracyclines

Pregnancy Category D

Indications

Alone or with other modalities in the treatment of various solid tumors including: Breast, Ovarian, Bladder, Bronchogenic carcinoma, Malignant lymphomas and leukemias.

Action

Inhibits DNA and RNA synthesis by forming a complex with DNA; action is cell-cycle S-phase–specific. Also has immunosuppressive properties. **Therapeutic Effects:** Death of rapidly replicating cells, particularly malignant ones.

Pharmacokinetics

Absorption: Administered IV only, resulting in complete bioavailability.

Distribution: Widely distributed; does not cross the blood-brain barrier; extensively bound to tissues.

Metabolism and Excretion: Mostly metabolized by the liver (primarily by CYP2D6 and CYP3A4). Con-

verted by liver to an active compound. Excreted predominantly in the bile, 50% as unchanged drug. Less than 5% eliminated unchanged in the urine.
Half-life: 16.7 hr.

TIME/ACTION PROFILE (effect on blood counts)

ROUTE	ONSET	PEAK	DURATION
IV	10 days	14 days	21–24 days

Contraindications/Precautions

Contraindicated in: Hypersensitivity; OB, Lactation: Pregnancy or lactation.
Use Cautiously in: History of cardiac disease or high cumulative doses of anthracyclines; Depressed bone marrow reserve; Liver impairment (reduce dose if serum bilirubin >1.2 m g/dL); Pedi, Geri: Children, geriatric patients, mediastinal radiation, concurrent cyclophosphamide (↑ risk of cardiotoxicity); Rep: Patients with childbearing potential.

Adverse Reactions/Side Effects

Resp: recall pneumonitis. **CV:** CARDIOMYOPATHY, ECG changes. **GI:** diarrhea, esophagitis, nausea, stomatitis, vomiting. **GU:** red urine. **Derm:** alopecia, photosensitivity. **Endo:** sterility, prepubertal growth failure with temporary gonadal impairment (children only). **Hemat:** anemia, leukopenia, thrombocytopenia. **Local:** phlebitis at IV site, tissue necrosis. **Metab:** hyperuricemia. **Misc:** hypersensitivity reactions.

Interactions

Drug-Drug: CYP2D6 inhibitors, **CYP3A4 inhibitors**, and **P-glycoprotein inhibitors** may ↑ risk of toxicity; avoid concurrent use. **CYP2D6 inducers**, **CYP3A4 inducers**, and **P-glycoprotein inducers** may ↓ effect and ↑ risk of therapeutic failure; avoid concurrent use. ↑ bone marrow depression with other **antineoplastics** or **radiation therapy**. Pediatric patients who have received concurrent doxorubicin and **dactinomycin** have an ↑ risk of recall pneumonitis at variable times following local radiation therapy. May ↑ skin reactions at previous **radiation therapy** sites. If **paclitaxel** is administered first, clearance of doxorubicin is ↓ and the incidence and severity of neutropenia and stomatitis are ↑ (problem is diminished if doxorubicin is administered first). Hematologic toxicity is ↑ and prolonged by concurrent use of **cyclosporine**; risk of coma and seizures is also ↑. Incidence and severity of neutropenia and thrombocytopenia are ↑ by concurrent **progesterone**. **Phenobarbital** may ↑ clearance and decrease effects of doxorubicin. Doxorubicin may ↓ metabolism and ↑ effects of **phenytoin**. **Streptozocin** may ↑ the half-life of doxorubicin (dosage ↓ of doxorubicin recommended). May ↑ risk of hemorrhagic cystitis from **cyclophosphamide**. May ↑ risk of hepatotoxicity from **mercaptopurine**. Cardiac toxicity may be ↑ by **radiation therapy** or **cyclophosphamide**. ↑ risk of cardiac toxicity with **trastuzumab**; avoid concurrent use. If **dexrazoxane** is administered at initiation of doxorubicin-containing regimens, may ↑ risk of therapeutic failure and tumor progression. May ↓ antibody response to **live-virus vaccines** and ↑ risk of adverse reactions.

D

Route/Dosage

Other regimens are used.
IV (Adults): 60–75 mg/m² daily, repeat q 21 days; or 25–30 mg/m² daily for 2–3 days, repeat q 3–4 wk or 20 mg/m²/wk. Total cumulative dose should not exceed 550 mg/m² without monitoring of cardiac function or 400 mg/m² in patients with previous chest radiation or other cardiotoxic chemotherapy.
IV (Children): 30 mg/m²/day for 3 days every 4 wk.

Hepatic Impairment

IV (Adults): Serum bilirubin 1.2–3mg/dL—50% of usual dose; serum bilirubin 3.1–5 mg/dL—25% of usual dose.

Availability (generic available)

Powder for injection: 10 mg/vial, 20 mg/vial, 50 mg/vial, ✤150 mg/vial. **Solution for injection:** 2 mg/mL.

NURSING IMPLICATIONS

Assessment

- Monitor BP, pulse, respiratory rate, and temperature frequently during administration. Report significant changes.
- Monitor for bone marrow depression. Assess for bleeding (bleeding gums, bruising, petechiae, guaiac stools, urine, and emesis) and avoid IM injections and taking rectal temperatures if platelet count is low. Apply pressure to venipuncture sites for 10 min. Assess for signs of infection during neutropenia. Anemia may occur. Monitor for increased fatigue, dyspnea, and orthostatic hypotension.
- Monitor intake and output ratios, and report occurrence of significant discrepancies. Encourage fluid intake of 2000–3000 mL/day. Allopurinol and alkalinization of the urine may be used to decrease serum uric acid levels and to help prevent urate stone formation.
- Severe and protracted nausea and vomiting may occur as early as 1 hr after therapy and may last 24 hr. Administer parenteral antiemetics 30–45 min prior to therapy and routinely around the clock for the next 24 hr as indicated. Monitor amount of emesis and notify physician or other health care professional if emesis exceeds guidelines to prevent dehydration.
- Monitor for development of signs of cardiac toxicity, which may be either acute and transient (ST segment

depression, flattened T wave, sinus tachycardia, and extrasystoles) or late onset (usually occurs 1–6 mo after initiation of therapy) and characterized by intractable HF (peripheral edema, dyspnea, rales/crackles, weight gain). Chest x ray, echocardiography, ECGs, and radionuclide angiography may be ordered prior to and periodically during therapy. Cardiotoxicity is more prevalent in children younger than 2 yr and geriatric patients. Dexrazoxane may be used to prevent cardiotoxicity in patients receiving cumulative doses of >300 m g/m^2.

- Assess injection site frequently for redness, irritation, or inflammation during and for up to 2 hr after completion of infusion. Doxorubicin is a vesicant but may infiltrate painlessly even if blood returns on aspiration of infusion needle. Severe tissue damage may occur if doxorubicin extravasates. If extravasation occurs, stop infusion immediately, restart, and complete dose in another vein. Local infiltration of antidote is not recommended. If extravasation is suspected, intermittent application of ice to site for 15 min. 4 times daily for 3 days may be useful. Because of the progressive nature of extravasation reactions, close observation and plastic surgery consultation are recommended. Blistering, ulceration and/or persistent pain are indications for wide excision surgery, followed by split- thickness skin grafting. May use dexrazoxane to treat extravasation. Administer first infusion of dexrazoxane as soon as possible within 6 hr of extravasation. Remove ice packs for at least 15 min prior to and during dexrazoxane administration. Recommended dose of dexrazoxane for day 1 is 1000 mg/m^2 (up to 2000 mg); the dose for day 2 is 1000 mg/m^2 (up to 2000 mg); the dose for day 3 is 500 mg/m^2 (up to 1000 mg). Dexrazoxane is admnistered as an IV infusion over 1–2 hr. If swelling, redness, and/or pain persists beyond 48 hr, immediate consultation for possible debridement is indicated.
- Assess oral mucosa frequently for development of stomatitis. Increased dosing interval and/or decreased dosing is recommended if lesions are painful or interfere with nutrition.
- ***Lab Test Considerations:*** Monitor CBC and differential prior to and periodically during therapy. WBC nadir occurs 10–14 days after administration, and recovery usually occurs by the 21st day. Thrombocytopenia and anemia may also occur. Increased dosing interval and/or decreased dose is recommended if ANC is <1000 cells/mm^3 and/or platelet count is <50,000 cells/mm^3.
- Monitor renal (BUN and creatinine) and hepatic (AST, ALT, LDH, and serum bilirubin) function prior to and periodically during therapy. Dose reduction is required for bilirubin >1.2 m g/dL or serum creatinine >3 m g/dL.
- May cause ↑ serum and urine uric acid concentrations.

Potential Nursing Diagnoses

Risk for infection (Adverse Reactions)
Decreased cardiac output (Adverse Reactions)

Implementation

- ***High Alert:*** Fatalities have occurred with incorrect administration of chemotherapeutic agents. Before administering, clarify all ambiguous orders; double-check single, daily, and course-of-therapy dose limits; have second practitioner independently double-check original order, calculations, and infusion pump settings.
- ***High Alert:*** Do not confuse doxorubicin hydrochloride with doxorubicin hydrochloride liposome (Doxil) or with daunorubicin hydrochloride (Cerubidine) or with idarubicin. Clarify orders that do not include generic and brand names.
- Solution should be prepared in a biologic cabinet. Wear gloves, gown, and mask while handling medication. Discard IV equipment in specially designated containers.
- Aluminum needles may be used to administer doxorubicin but should not be used during storage, because prolonged contact results in discoloration of solution and formation of a dark precipitate. Solution is red.

IV Administration

- **IV Push: *Diluent:*** Dilute each 10 mg with 5 mL of 0.9% NaCl (nonbacteriostatic) for injection. Shake to dissolve completely. Do not add to IV solution. Reconstituted medication is stable for 24 hr at room temperature and 48 hr if refrigerated. Protect from sunlight. ***Concentration:*** 2 mg/mL. ***Rate:*** Administer each dose over 3–5 min through Y-site of a free-flowing infusion of 0.9% NaCl or D5W. Facial flushing and erythema along involved vein frequently occur when administration is too rapid.
- **Intermittent Infusion:** Has also been mixed in 100–250 mL of 0.9% NaCl. ***Rate:*** Infuse over 30–60 min.
- **Y-Site Compatibility:** alemtuzumab, alfentanil, amifostine, amikacin, anidulafungin, argatroban, aztreonam, bivalirudin, bleomycin, bumetanide, buprenorphine, butorphanol, calcium chloride, calcium gluconate, carboplatin, carmustine, caspofungin, chlorpromazine, ciprofloxacin, cisplatin, cladribine, clindamycin, cyclophosphamide, cyclosporine, cytarabine, dacarbazine, dactinomycin, daptomycin, dexamethasone, dexmedetomidine, dexrazoxane, diltiazem, diphenhydramine, dobutamine, docetaxel, dolasetron, dopamine, doripenem, doxycycline, droperidol, enalaprilat, ephedrine, epinephrine, erythromycin, esmolol, etoposide, etoposide phosphate, famotidine, fenoldopam, fentanyl, filgrastim, fluconazole, fludarabine, gemcitabine, gentamicin, granisetron, haloperidol, hydrocortisone, hydromorphone, ifosfamide, imipenem/cilastatin, irinotecan, isoproterenol, ketorolac, labetalol,

leucovorin calcium, levorphanol, lidocaine, linezolid, lorazepam, mannitol, mechlorethamine, melphalan, meperidine, mesna, methotrexate, metoclopramide, metoprolol, metronidazole, midazolam, milrinone, mitomycin, morphine, moxifloxacin, nalbuphine, naloxone, nesiritide, nicardipine, nitroglycerin, nitroprusside, octreotide, ondansetron, oxaliplatin, paclitaxel, palonosetron, pamidronate, pancuronium, phenylephrine, potassium acetate, potassium chloride, procainamide, prochlorperazine, promethazine, propranolol, quinupristin/dalfopristin, ranitidine, sargramostim, sodium acetate, sufentanil, tacrolimus, teniposide, theophylline, thiotepa, tigecycline, tirofiban, tobramycin, topotecan, trastuzumab, vancomycin, vasopressin, vecuronium, verapamil, vinblastine, vincristine, vinorelbine, zidovudine, zoledronic acid.

- **Y-Site Incompatibility:** acyclovir, allopurinol, aminophylline, amiodarone, amphotericin B colloidal, amphotericin B lipid complex, amphotericin B liposome, ampicillin, ampicillin/sulbactam, azithromycin, cefazolin, cefepime, cefotaxime, cefotetan, cefoxitin, ceftazidime, ceftriaxone, cefuroxime, diazepam, digoxin, ertapenem, foscarnet, fosphenytoin, ganciclovir, magnesium sulfate, meropenem, methohexital, pantoprazole, pemetrexed, pentamidine, pentobarbital, phenobarbital, phenytoin, piperacillin/tazobactam, potassium phosphates, propofol, rituximab, sodium phosphates, thiopental, trimethoprim/sufamethoxazole, voriconazole.

Patient/Family Teaching

- Instruct patient to notify health care professional promptly if fever; sore throat; signs of infection; bleeding gums; bruising; petechiae; blood in stools, urine, or emesis; increased fatigue; dyspnea; or orthostatic hypotension occurs. Caution patient to avoid crowds and persons with known infections. Instruct patient to use soft toothbrush and electric razor and to avoid falls. Caution patient not to drink alcoholic beverages or take medication containing aspirin or NSAIDs, because these may precipitate gastric bleeding.
- Instruct patient to report pain at injection site immediately.
- Instruct patient to inspect oral mucosa for erythema and ulceration. If ulceration occurs, advise patient to use sponge brush, rinse mouth with water after eating and drinking, and confer with health care professional if mouth pain interferes with eating. Pain may require treatment with opioid analgesics. The risk of developing stomatitis is greatest 5–10 days after a dose; the usual duration is 3–7 days.
- Instruct patient to notify health care professional immediately if irregular heartbeat, shortness of breath, swelling of lower extremities, or skin irritation (swelling, pain, or redness of feet or hands) occurs.
- Discuss the possibility of hair loss with patient. Explore methods of coping. Regrowth usually occurs 2–3 mo after discontinuation of therapy.
- Instruct patient not to receive any vaccinations without advice of health care professional.
- Inform patient that medication may cause urine to appear red for 1–2 days.
- Instruct patient to notify health care professional if skin irritation occurs at site of previous radiation therapy.
- Advise family and/or caregivers to take precautions (i.e., latex gloves) in handling body fluids for at least 5 days post-treatment.
- Instruct patient to notify health care professional of all Rx or OTC medications, vitamins, or herbal products being taken and to consult health care professional before taking other Rx, OTC, or herbal products.
- Inform patient that doxorubicin may increase risk of developing secondary cancers.
- Rep: Advise patient that this medication may have teratogenic effects. Contraception should be used during and for at least 4 mo after therapy is concluded. Inform patient before initiating therapy that this medication may cause irreversible gonadal suppression.
- Emphasize the need for periodic lab tests to monitor for side effects.

Evaluation/Desired Outcomes

- Decrease in size or spread of malignancies in solid tumors.
- Improvement of hematologic status in leukemias.

HIGH ALERT

DOXOrubicin, liposomal

(dox-oh-**roo**-bi-sin **lye**-poe-sohm-al)

Doxil

Classification

Therapeutic: antineoplastics

Pharmacologic: anthracyclines

Pregnancy Category D

Indications

AIDS-related Kaposi's sarcoma (KS) in patients who cannot tolerate or fail conventional therapy. Ovarian cancer that has progressed or recurred after platinum-based chemotherapy. Multiple myeloma with bortezomib in patients who have not previously received bortezomib and have received at least one prior therapy.

Action

Inhibits DNA and RNA synthesis by forming a complex with DNA; action is cell-cycle S-phase–specific. Also has immunosuppressive properties. Encapsulation in a liposome increases uptake by tumors, prolongs action, and may decrease some toxicity. **Therapeutic Effects:** Death of rapidly replicating cells, particularly malignant ones.

Pharmacokinetics

Absorption: Administered IV only, resulting in complete bioavailability.

Distribution: Widely distributed; does not cross the blood-brain barrier; extensively bound to tissues (↑ concentrations delivered to KS lesions due to liposomal carrier).

Metabolism and Excretion: Mostly metabolized by the liver with conversion to an active compound. Excreted mostly in bile, 50% as unchanged drug. <5% eliminated unchanged in the urine.

Half-life: 55 hr.

TIME/ACTION PROFILE (effect on blood counts)

ROUTE	ONSET	PEAK	DURATION
IV	10 days	14 days	21–24 days

Contraindications/Precautions

Contraindicated in: Hypersensitivity; OB, Lactation: Fetal harm may occur.

Use Cautiously in: Pre-existing cardiac disease or ↑ cumulative doses of anthracyclines; Depressed bone marrow reserve; Liver impairment (dose ↓ required if serum bilirubin >1.2 m g/dL); Geri, Pedi: Children, geriatric patients, prior mediastinal radiation, concurrent cyclophosphamide (↑ risk of cardiotoxicity); OB: Patients with child-bearing potential.

Adverse Reactions/Side Effects

CNS: weakness. **CV:** CARDIOMYOPATHY. **GI:** nausea, diarrhea, ↑ alkaline phosphatase, moniliasis, ORAL MALIGNANCY, stomatitis, vomiting. **Derm:** hand-foot syndrome, alopecia. **Hemat:** anemia, leukopenia, thrombocytopenia. **Local:** injection site reactions. **Misc:** ANAPHYLACTOID ALLERGIC REACTIONS, acute infusion-related reactions, fever.

Interactions

Drug-Drug: ↑ bone marrow depression with other **antineoplastics** or **radiation therapy**. Pediatric patients who have received concurrent doxorubicin and **dactinomycin** have ↑ risk of recall pneumonitis following local radiation therapy. May ↑ skin reactions at previous **radiation therapy** sites. If **paclitaxel** is administered first, clearance of doxorubicin is ↓ and incidence and severity of neutropenia and stomatitis are ↑ (problem is less if doxorubicin is administered first). Hematologic toxicity is ↑ by concurrent use of **cyclosporine**; risk of coma and seizures is also ↑. Incidence and severity of neutropenia and thrombocytopenia are ↑ by concurrent **progesterone**. **Phenobarbital** may ↑ clearance and ↓ effects of doxorubicin. Doxorubicin may ↓ metabolism and ↑ effects of **phenytoin**. **Streptozocin** may ↑ the half-life of doxorubicin (dose reduction of doxorubicin recommended). May ↑ risk of hemorrhagic cystitis from **cyclophosphamide** or hepatitis from **mercaptopurine**. Cardiac toxicity may be ↑ by **radiation therapy** or **cyclophosphamide**. May ↓ antibody response to **live-virus vaccines** and ↑ risk of adverse reactions.

Route/Dosage

AIDS-Related KS

IV (Adults): 20 mg/m^2 every 3 wk until disease progression or unacceptable toxicity.

Ovarian Cancer

IV (Adults): 50 mg/m^2 every 4 wk until disease progression or unacceptable toxicity.

Multiple Myeloma

IV (Adults): 30 mg/m^2 on day 4 (after bortezomib) of each 21–day cycle for 8 cycles or until disease progression or unacceptable toxicity.

Availability (generic available)

Liposomal dispersion for injection: 2 mg/mL.

NURSING IMPLICATIONS

Assessment

- Monitor BP, pulse, respiratory rate, and temperature frequently during administration. Report significant changes.
- Monitor for acute infusion-related reactions consisting of flushing, shortness of breath, facial swelling, headache, chills, chest pain, back pain, chest or throat tightness, fever, tachycardia, pruritus, rash, cyanosis, syncope, bronchospasm, asthma, apnea, and hypotension. Reactions usually resolve over 1 day and are usually limited to first dose. Slowing infusion rate may minimize this reaction. Reaction is thought to be due to liposome.
- Observe for signs and symptoms of anaphylaxis (rash, pruritus, laryngeal edema, wheezing). Discontinue doxorubicin liposome and notify health care professional immediately if these problems occur. Keep epinephrine, an antihistamine, and resuscitation equipment close by in case of an anaphylactic reaction.
- Monitor for bone marrow depression. Assess for bleeding (bleeding gums, bruising, petechiae, guaiac stools, urine, and emesis) and avoid IM injections and taking rectal temperatures if platelet count is low. Apply pressure to venipuncture sites for 10 min. Assess for signs of infection during neutropenia. Anemia may occur. Monitor for increased fatigue, dyspnea, and orthostatic hypotension.
- Monitor intake and output ratios, and report occurrence of significant discrepancies. Encourage fluid intake of 2000–3000 mL/day. Allopurinol and alkalinization of the urine may be used to decrease se-

rum uric acid levels and to help prevent urate stone formation.

- Severe and protracted nausea and vomiting may occur as early as 1 hr after therapy and may last 24 hr. Administer parenteral antiemetics 30–45 min prior to therapy and routinely around the clock for the next 24 hr as indicated. Monitor amount of emesis and notify health care professional if emesis exceeds guidelines to prevent dehydration.
- Assess left ventricular cardiac function (MUGA or echocardiogram) prior to initiation of therapy, during treatment to detect acute changes, and after treatment to detect delayed cardiotoxicity. Monitor for development of signs of cardiac toxicity, which may be either acute and transient (ST segment depression, flattened T wave, sinus tachycardia, and extrasystoles) or late onset (usually occurs 1–6 mo after initiation of therapy) and characterized by intractable HF (peripheral edema, dyspnea, rales/crackles, weight gain); occurs more frequently in patients receiving a cumulative dose of ≥550 mg/m^2. Cardiotoxicity is more prevalent in children younger than 2 yr and geriatric patients. Dexrazoxane may be used to prevent cardiotoxicity in patients receiving cumulative doses of >300 m g/m^2.
- Assess injection site frequently for redness, irritation, or inflammation. Doxorubicin liposome is an irritant but may infiltrate painlessly even if blood returns on aspiration of infusion needle. Severe tissue damage may occur if doxorubicin liposome extravasates. If extravasation occurs, stop infusion immediately, restart, and complete dose in another vein. If possible, withdraw 3–5 mL of blood to remove doxorubicin liposome. Apply ice to site for 15 min. 4 times daily for 3 days. Local infiltration of antidote is not recommended. Delineate the infiltrated area on patient's skin with a felt-tip marker. Elevate for 48 hr above heart level using a sling or stockinette dressing with an observation window cut in the dressing. Avoid pressure or friction. Do not rub the area. Observe for signs of increased erythema, pain, or skin necrosis. If increased symptoms occur, consult a plastic surgeon. After 48 hr, encourage patient to use extremity normally to promote full range of motion.
- Assess oral mucosa frequently for development of stomatitis. Increased dosing interval and/or decreased dose is recommended if lesions are painful or interfere with nutrition.
- Continue to assess oral mucosa regularly during and for at least 6 yr for ulceration or any discomfort; may indicate secondary oral cancer. *For Grade 1: Painless ulcers, erythema, or mild soreness,* If no previous Grade 3 or 4 toxicity: no dose adjustment. If previous Grade 3 or 4 toxicity: delay up to 2 wks then ↓ dose by 25%. *For Grade 2: Painful erythema, edema, or ulcers, but can eat,* Delay dosing up to 2 wks or until resolved to Grade 0-1. Discontinue therapy if no resolution after 2 wks. If resolved to Grade 0-1 within 2 weeks: if no previous Grade 3 or 4 stomatitis: resume therapy at previous dose. If previous Grade 3 or 4 toxicity: ↓ dose by 25%. *For Grade 3: Painful erythema, edema, or ulcers, and cannot eat,* Delay dosing up to 2 wks or until resolved to Grade 0-1. ↓ dose by 25% and return to original dose interval. If no resolution after 2 wks, discontinue therapy. *For Grade 4: Requires parenteral or enteral support,* Delay dosing up to 2 wks or until resolved to Grade 0-1. ↓ dose by 25% and return to original dose interval. If no resolution after 2 wks, discontinue therapy.
- Monitor for skin toxicity with prolonged use; hand-foot syndrome (HFS) usually occurs after 6 wk of treatment and consists of swelling, pain, and erythema of the hands and feet. This may progress to desquamation but usually regresses after 2 wk. In severe cases, modification and delay of future doses of doxorubicin liposome may be necessary. *For Grade 1: Mild erythema, swelling, or desquamation not interfering with daily activities,* if no previous Grade 3 or 4 HFS: no dose adjustment. If previous Grade 3 or 4 HFS: delay dose up to 2 wks, then ↓ dose by 25%. *For Grade 2: Erythema, desquamation, or swelling interfering with, but not precluding normal physical activities; small blisters or ulcerations less than 2 cm in diameter,* delay dosing up to 2 wks or until resolved to Grade 0-1. Discontinue therapy if no resolution after 2 wks. If resolved to Grade 0-1 within 2 wks: if no previous Grade 3 or 4 HFS: continue treatment at previous dose. If previous Grade 3 or 4 toxicity: ↓ dose by 25%. *For Grade 3: Blistering, ulceration, or swelling interfering with walking or normal daily activities; cannot wear regular clothing,* Delay dosing up to 2 wks or until resolved to Grade 0-1, then ↓ dose by 25%. Discontinue therapy if no resolution after 2 wks. *For Grade 4: Diffuse or local process causing infectious complications, or a bed ridden state or hospitalization,* Delay dosing up to 2 wks or until resolved to Grade 0-1, then ↓ dose by 25%. Discontinue therapy if no resolution after 2 wks.
- ***Lab Test Considerations:*** Monitor CBC and differential prior to and periodically during therapy. The WBC nadir occurs 10–14 days after administration, and recovery usually occurs by the 21st day. Thrombocytopenia and anemia may also occur. ↑ dosing interval and/or ↓ dose is recommended if ANC is <1000 cells/mm^3 and/or platelet count is <50,000 cells/mm^3. *If ANC 1500 – 1900 cells/mm^3 and platelets 75,000–150,000 cells/mm^3 (Grade 1)*, resume treatment with no dose reduction. *If ANC 1000 – <1500 cells/mm^3 and platelets 50,000 –*

<75,000 cells/mm³ (Grade 2), wait until ANC >1500 and platelets >75,000; then redose with no dose reduction. *If ANC 500 – 999 cells/mm³ and platelets 25,000 – <50,000 cells/mm³ (Grade 3),* wait until ANC >1500 and platelets >75,000; then redose with no dose reduction. *If ANC <500 and platelets <25,000 cells/mm³ (Grade 4),* wait until ANC >1500 and platelets >75,000, then redose at 25% dose reduction or continue full dose with prophylactic granulocyte growth factor.

- **Recommended modifications of doxorubicin liposomal when administered with bortezomib.** *If fever ≥38°C and ANC <1,000/mm³,* withhold dose for this cycle if before Day 4; ↓ dose by 25%, if after Day 4 of previous cycle. *If on any day of drug administration after Day 1 of each cycle: Platelet count <25,000/mm³ or Hemoglobin <8 g/dL or ANC <500/mm³,* withhold dose for this cycle if before Day 4; ↓ dose by 25%, if after Day 4 of previous cycle AND if bortezomib is reduced for hematologic toxicity. *If Grade 3 or 4 non-hematologic drug related toxicity,* do not dose until recovered to Grade <2, then ↓ dose by 25%.
- Monitor renal (BUN and creatinine) and hepatic (AST, ALT, LDH, and serum bilirubin) function prior to and periodically during therapy. Dose reduction is required for bilirubin >1.2 m g/dL or serum creatinine >3 m g/dL.
- May cause ↑ serum and urine uric acid concentrations.

Potential Nursing Diagnoses

Risk for infection (Adverse Reactions)
Decreased cardiac output (Adverse Reactions)

Implementation

- ***High Alert:*** Fatalities have occurred with incorrect administration of chemotherapeutic agents. Before administering, clarify all ambiguous orders; double-check single, daily, and course-of-therapy dose limits; have second practitioner independently double-check original order, calculations, and infusion pump settings.
- ***High Alert:*** Do not confuse doxorubicin hydrochloride liposome (Doxil) with doxorubicin hydrochloride or with daunorubicin hydrochloride (Cerubidine). Do not confuse Doxil with Paxil. Clarify orders that do not include generic and brand names.
- Prepare solution in a biologic cabinet. Wear gloves, gown, and mask while handling medication. Discard IV equipment in specially designated containers.
- Aluminum needles may be used to administer doxorubicin but should not be used during storage, because prolonged contact results in discoloration of solution and formation of a dark precipitate. Solution is red.
- Do not increase dose if reduction is made due to toxicity.

IV Administration

- **Intermittent Infusion:** ***Diluent:*** Dilute dose, up to 90 mg, in 250 mL and doses >90 m g in 500 mL of D5W. Do not dilute with other diluents or diluents containing a bacteriostatic agent. Solution is not clear, but a translucent red liposomal dispersion. Do not use in-line filters. Refrigerate diluted solutions and administer within 24 hr of dilution. ***Rate:*** Initial rate of infusion should be 1 mg/min to minimize risk of infusion reactions. If no reactions occur, increase rate to complete administration within 1 hr. Do not administer as a bolus or undiluted solution. Rapid infusion may increase infusion-related reactions.
- **Y-Site Compatibility:** acyclovir, alfentanil, allopurinol, amifostine, amikacin, aminocaproic acid, aminophylline, amphotericin B lipid complex, amphotericin B liposomal, ampicillin, ampicillin/sulbactam, anidulafungin, argatroban, azithromycin, aztreonam, bivalirudin, bleomycin, bumetanide, butorphanol, calcium gluconate, carboplatin, caspofungin, cefazolin, cefepime, cefotaxime, cefotetan, cefoxitin, ceftriaxone, cefuroxime, chloramphenicol, chlorpromazine, ciprofloxacin, cisatracurium, cisplatin, clindamycin, cyclophosphamide, cyclosporine, cytarabine, dacarbazine, daptomycin, dexamethasone sodium phosphate, dexmedetomidine, dexrazoxane, digoxin, diphenhydramine, dobutamine, dopamine, droperidol, enalaprilat, ephedrine, epinephrine, eptifibatide, ertapenem, erythromycin, esmolol, etoposide, etoposide phosphate, famotidine, fenoldopam, fentanyl, fluconazole, fluorouracil, foscarnet, fosphenytoin, furosemide, ganciclovir, gentamicin, glycopyrrolate, granisetron, haloperidol, heparin, hydrocortisone sodium succinate, hydromorphone, ifosfamide, imipenem/cilastatin, insulin, irinotecan, isoproterenol, ketorolac, labetalol, leucovorin, levofloxacin, lidocaine, linezolid, lorazepam, magnesium sulfate, meropenem, mesna, methotrexate, methyldopate, methylprednisolone , metoprolol, metronidazole, midazolam, milrinone, moxifloxacin, mycophenolate, nafcillin, nalbuphine, naloxone, nesiritide, nicardipine, nitroglycerin, nitroprusside, norepinephrine, octreotide, ondansetron, oxaliplatin, palonosetron, pamidronate, pancuronium, pantoprazole, pemetrexed, pentamidine, pentazocine, pentobarbital, phenobarbital, phenylephrine, potassium acetate, potassium chloride, potassium phosphates, procainamide, prochlorperazine, propranolol, quinupristin/dalfopristin, ranitidine, remifentanil, rituximab, rocuronium, sodium acetate, sodium phosphates, succinylcholine, sufentanil, tacrolimus, thiopental, tigecycline, tirofiban, tobramycin, topotecan, trastuzumab, trimethoprim/sulfamethoxazole, vancomycin, vasopressin, vecuronium, verapamil, vinblastine, vincristine, vinorelbine, voriconazole, zidovudine, zoledronic acid.
- **Y-Site Incompatibility:** amiodarone, amphotericin B colloidal, buprenorphine, calcium chloride,

ceftazidime, dantrolene, diazepam, diltiazem, docetaxel, dolasetron, gemcitabine, hydralazine, hydroxyzine, mannitol, metoclopramide, mitoxantrone, morphine, paclitaxel, phenytoin, piperacillin/tazobactam, promethazine, sodium bicarbonate, theophylline.

Patient/Family Teaching

- Instruct patient to notify health care professional promptly if fever; sore throat; signs of infection; bleeding gums; bruising; petechiae; blood in stools, urine, or emesis; increased fatigue; dyspnea; or orthostatic hypotension occurs. Caution patient to avoid crowds and persons with known infections. Instruct patient to use soft toothbrush and electric razor and to avoid falls. Caution patient not to drink alcoholic beverages or take medication containing aspirin or NSAIDs; may precipitate gastric bleeding.
- Instruct patient to report pain at injection site immediately.
- Instruct patient to inspect oral mucosa for erythema and ulceration. If ulceration occurs, advise patient to use sponge brush, rinse mouth with water after eating and drinking, and confer with health care professional if mouth pain interferes with eating. Pain may require treatment with opioid analgesics. The risk of developing stomatitis is greatest 5–10 days after a dose; the usual duration is 3–7 days.
- Instruct patient to notify health care professional immediately if irregular heartbeat, shortness of breath, swelling of lower extremities, or skin irritation (swelling, pain, or redness of feet or hands) occurs.
- Discuss the possibility of hair loss with patient. Explore methods of coping. Regrowth usually occurs 2–3 mo after discontinuation of therapy.
- Instruct patient not to receive any vaccinations without advice of health care professional.
- Inform patient that medication may cause urine to appear red for 1–2 days.
- Instruct patient to notify health care professional if skin irritation occurs at site of previous radiation therapy.
- Advise family and/or caregivers to take precautions (i.e., latex gloves) in handling body fluids for at least 5 days post-treatment.
- Rep: Advise patient that this medication may have teratogenic effects. Contraception should be used during and for at least 6 mo after therapy is concluded. Inform patient before initiating therapy that this medication may cause irreversible gonadal suppression. In females, may cause infertility, amenorrhea, and premature menopause. In men, may result in oligospermia, azoospermia, and permanent loss of fertility. Some sperm counts have returned to normal several years after therapy ended. Advise female patient to avoid breast feeding during therapy.
- Emphasize the need for periodic lab tests to monitor for side effects.

Evaluation/Desired Outcomes

- Decrease in size or spread of malignancies.
- Arrested progression of KS in patients with HIV infection.

doxycycline, See TETRACYCLINES.

doxylamine/pyridoxine

(dox-**il**-a-meen peer-ih-**dox**-een)

Diclegis, ✱Diclectin

Classification

Therapeutic: antiemetics

Pharmacologic: antihistamines, vitamin B6 analogues

Pregnancy Category A

Indications

Treatment of nausea and vomiting during pregnancy that has not responded to conservative management.

Action

Combination of an antihistamine and a vitamin B_6 analog. Mechanism not known. **Therapeutic Effects:** Decreased nausea and vomiting associated with pregnancy.

Pharmacokinetics

Absorption: Well absorbed following oral administration. Food delays/decreases absorption.

Distribution: Doxylamine probably enters breast milk.

Metabolism and Excretion: Doxylamine is mostly metabolized by the liver, inactive metabolites are renally excreted. Pyridoxine is a pro-drug, converted to its active metabolite by the liver.

Half-life: *Doxylamine*—12.5 hr; *pyridoxine*—0.4–0.5 hr.

TIME/ACTION PROFILE (anti-emetic effect)

ROUTE	ONSET	PEAK	DURATION
PO	unk	unk	8–24 hr

Contraindications/Precautions

Contraindicated in: Hypersensitivity to doxylamine or pyridoxine; Concurrent use of MAOIs; Lactation: Doxylamine probably enters breast milk and may cause irritability, excitement, or sedation in infants; breast feeding should be avoided.

Use Cautiously in: Asthma; Increased intraocular pressure or narrow angle glaucoma; Stenosing peptic ulcer or pyloroduodenal obstruction; Urinary bladder-neck obstruction; Pedi: Safe and effective use in children <18 yr has not been established.

Adverse Reactions/Side Effects

CNS: drowsiness.

Interactions

Drug-Drug: ↑ risk of CNS depression with other **CNS depressants** including **alcohol**, other **antihistamines**, **opioid analgesics**, and **sedative/hypnotics**. Concurrent use of **MAOIs** ↑ intensity/duration of adverse CNS (anticholinergic) reactions.

Route/Dosage

PO (Adults): *Day 1*—Two tablets (doxylamine 10 mg/pyridoxine 10 mg) at bedtime, if symptoms are controlled continue this regimen; *Day 2, if symptoms persist into afternoon on day 2*—two tablets at bedtime on day 2 and then one tablet in the morning on day 3 and two tablets in the evening, if symptoms are controlled, continue this regimen; *Day 4, if symptoms persist*—one tablet in the morning, one tablet mid-afternoon and two tablets at bedtime (not to exceed four tablets daily).

Availability

Delayed-release tablets: doxylamine 10 mg/pyridoxine 10 mg.

NURSING IMPLICATIONS

Assessment

- Assess for frequency and amount of emesis daily during therapy. Reassess need for medication as pregnancy progresses.

Potential Nursing Diagnoses

Nausea (Indications)
Risk for injury (Adverse Reactions)

Implementation

- **PO:** Administer on an empty stomach with a full glass of water; food delays onset of medication. Swallow tablets whole; do not crush, break, or chew.

Patient/Family Teaching

- Instruct patient to take as directed.
- May cause drowsiness. Caution patient to avoid driving and other activities requiring alertness until response to medication is known.
- Advise patient to avoid alcohol and CNS depressants, including sedatives, tranquilizers, antihistamines, opioids, and some cough and cold medications with doxylamine pyridoxine.
- Instruct patient to notify health care professional of all Rx or OTC medications, vitamins, or herbal products being taken and consult health care professional before taking any new medications.
- Advise female patient to avoid breast feeding during therapy.

Evaluation/Desired Outcomes

- Decrease in frequency of nausea and vomiting during pregnancy.

REMS

dronedarone (droe-**ned**-a-rone)

Multaq

Classification
Therapeutic: antiarrhythmics
Pharmacologic: benzofurans

Pregnancy Category X

Indications

Reduces the risk of hospitalization for atrial fibrillation (AF) in patients in sinus rhythm with a history of paroxysmal or persistent AF.

Action

Has several antiarrhythmic properties; prolongs PR and QTc intervals. **Therapeutic Effects:** Suppression of AF/AFL.

Pharmacokinetics

Absorption: Poor bioavailability (4%) due to extensive first-pass hepatic metabolism (4%); food ↑ bioavailability (15%).
Distribution: Unknown.
Protein Binding: >98%.
Metabolism and Excretion: Undergoes extensive first-pass hepatic metabolism; mostly by the CYP3A enzyme system. 6% excreted in urine as metabolites, 84% was excreted in feces as metabolites. Minimal elimination as unchanged drug.
Half-life: 13–19 hr.

TIME/ACTION PROFILE (antiarrhythmic effect)

ROUTE	ONSET	PEAK	DURATION
PO	unknown†	3–6 hr‡	12 hr

† Steady state blood levels are attained at 4–8 days.
‡ Peak levels after individual doses.

Contraindications/Precautions

Contraindicated in: Class IV heart failure or Class II–III heart failure with recent decompensation requiring hospitalization; Permanent AF; Second- or third-degree atrioventricular (AV) block or sick sinus syndrome (unless a pacemaker is present); Heart rate <50 bpm; Concurrent use of strong CYP3A inhibitors or drugs/herbal products that prolong the QT interval; liver or lung toxicity related to previous amiodarone use; QTc interval ≥500 msec; PR interval >280 msec; Concurrent use of Class I or III antiarrhythmics including amiodarone, flecainide, propafenone, quinidine, disopyramide, dofetilide, and sotalol; must be discontinued prior to treatment; Severe hepatic impairment; OB: May cause fetal harm; Lactation: Avoid use.
Use Cautiously in: New/worsening heart failure; Hypokalemia or hypomagnesemia (may ↑ risk of ar-

rhythmias); Mild or moderate hepatic impairment; OB: Women with child-bearing potential; contraception should be used; Pedi: Safety and effectiveness not established.

Adverse Reactions/Side Effects

CNS: weakness. **CV:** HF, QTc prolongation. **GI:** HEPATOTOXICITY, abdominal pain, diarrhea, nausea, taste abnormality, vomiting. **Resp:** PNEUMONITIS, PULMONARY FIBROSIS. **GU:** ACUTE RENAL FAILURE, renal impairment. **Derm:** photosensitivity. **Misc:** ANGIOEDEMA.

Interactions

Drug-Drug: Dronedarone is metabolized by CYP3A and is a moderate inhibitor of CYP3A and CYP2D6 enzyme systems; interactions may occur with other drugs that are substrates for or are metabolized by these systems. Dronedarone also inhibits P-gp, which can result in ↑ absorption of certain drugs. Concurrent use of **strong CYP3A inhibitors** including **ketoconazole**, **itraconazole**, **voriconazole**, **cyclosporine**, **telithromycin**, **clarithromycin**, **nefazodone**, and **ritonavir** or **drugs that prolong the QT interval** including **phenothiazine antipsychotics**, **tricyclic antidepressants**, some oral **macrolide antibiotics**, and other **Class I and III antiarrhythmics** ↑ risk of serious adverse cardiovascular reactions; concurrent use contraindicated. Concurrent use of CYP3A4 inducers including **rifampin**, **phenobarbital**, **carbamazepine**, or **phenytoin** ↓ blood levels and effectiveness and should be avoided. ↑ **digoxin** levels and the risk of toxicity (discontinue or ↓ dose of digoxin by 50% before treatment and monitor carefully). May ↑ **dabigatran** and **warfarin** levels and the risk of bleeding. Avoid concurrent use of other **antiarrhythmics**, including **amiodarone**, **flecainide**, **propafenone**, **quinidine**, **disopyramide**, **dofetilide**, and **sotalol** due to ↑ risk of adverse cardiovascular reactions; discontinue prior to dronedarone therapy (concurrent use is contraindicated). Concurrent use of **diltiazem**, **verapamil**, **digoxin**, or **beta-blockers** ↑ risk of bradycardia (initiate at lower dose and ↑ only after ECG evaluation). May also ↑ levels and effects of**tricyclic antidepressants**, and **selective serotonin reuptake inhibitors (SSRIs)**. May ↑ levels and risk of toxicity of some **HMG-CoA reductase inhibitors (statins)**; do not exceed simvastatin dose of 10 mg/day. Concurrent use with **CYP 3A substrates** including **sirolimus** and **tacrolimus** may ↑ risk of serious adverse reactions; monitor and adjust dosage carefully.

Drug-Natural Products: St. John's wort ↓ blood levels and may ↓ effectiveness; avoid concurrent use.

Drug-Food: Grapefruit juice may ↑ levels and the risk of toxicity; avoid concurrent ingestion.

Route/Dosage

PO (Adults): 400 mg twice daily.

Availability

Tablets: 400 mg.

NURSING IMPLICATIONS

Assessment

- Assess for signs and symptoms of atrial fibrillation or atrial flutter (palpitations, abnormal ECG) periodically during therapy. If atrial fibrillation occurs, cardiovert or discontinue dronaderone; increases risk of stroke, hospitalization for HF, and death.
- Monitor ECG periodically and at least every 3 mo during therapy. If QTc ≥500 ms or PR interval >280 ms, discontinue therapy.
- Assess for signs and symptoms of hepatic injury (anorexia, nausea, vomiting, fever, malaise, fatigue, right upper quadrant pain, jaundice, dark urine, or itching) during therapy. If hepatic injury is suspected, discontinue therapy and test serum enzymes (AST, ALT), alkaline phosphatase, and serum bilirubin to determine liver injury. If liver injury occurs, begin treatment. Do not restart therapy without another explanation for liver injury.
- Assess for signs of pulmonary toxicity (dyspnea, nonproductive cough) periodically during therapy. If pulmonary toxicity occurs, discontinue therapy.
- ***Lab Test Considerations:*** Monitor serum hepatic enzymes periodically, especially during first 6 mo of therapy.
- Monitor serum potassium and magnesium levels during therapy and maintain within normal range. May cause hypokalemia and hypomagnesemia.
- Monitor serum creatinine levels periodically during therapy. Serum creatinine levels ↑ by about 0.1 mg/dL following initiation of therapy with a rapid onset and plateau after 7 days; reversible with discontinuation. If ↑ and plateau occurs, use increased value as new baseline.

Potential Nursing Diagnoses

Decreased cardiac output (Indications)

Implementation

- Patient should be on concurrent antithrombotic therapy.
- **PO:** Administer twice daily with morning and evening meals; avoid grapefruit juice.

Patient/Family Teaching

- Instruct patient to take dronedarone as directed. Do not stop taking dronedarone, even if feeling better, without consulting health care professional. If a dose is missed, omit and take next dose at regularly scheduled time; do not double dose. Advise patient to read *Medication Guide* before starting therapy and with each Rx refill in case of changes.
- Advise patient to avoid grapefruit juice during therapy.

- Advise patient to notify health care professional if signs and symptoms of heart failure (weight gain, dependent edema, increasing shortness of breath), hepatic injury, or pulmonary toxicity occur.
- Instruct patient to notify health care professional of all Rx or OTC medications, vitamins, or herbal products being taken and to consult with health care professional before taking other medications, especially St. John's wort.
- May be teratogenic. Caution female patients of childbearing age to use effective contraception during therapy and to notify health care professional if pregnancy is planned or suspected or if breast feeding.

Evaluation/Desired Outcomes

- Reduction in hospitalization of patients with paroxysmal or persistent atrial fibrillation or atrial flutter.

REMS

dulaglutide (doo-la-**gloo**-tide)

Trulicity

Classification

Therapeutic: antidiabetics

Pharmacologic: glucagon-like peptide-1 (GLP-1) receptor agonists

Pregnancy Category C

Indications

Adjunct treatment to diet and exercise in the management of adults with type 2 diabetes mellitus; not recommended as first line therapy, as a substitute for insulin, in patients with type 1 diabetes, or for ketoacidosis.

Action

Acts as an acylated human Glucagon-Like Peptide-1 (GLP-1, an incretin) receptor agonist; increases intracellular cyclic AMP (cAMP) leading to insulin release when glucose is elevated, which then subsides as blood glucose decreases toward euglycemia. Also decreases glucagon secretion and delays gastric emptying. **Therapeutic Effects:** Improved glycemic control.

Pharmacokinetics

Absorption: *0.75 mg dose*—65% absorbed following subcutaneous administration; *1.5 mg dose*—47% absorbed following subcutaneous administration.
Distribution: Unknown.
Metabolism and Excretion: Degraded by protein catabolic processes.
Half-life: 5 days.

TIME/ACTION PROFILE (↓ in HbA_{1c})

ROUTE	ONSET	PEAK	DURATION
subcut	within 4 wk	13 wk	unknown

Contraindications/Precautions

Contraindicated in: Hypersensitivity; Personal or family history of medullary thyroid carcinoma; Multiple Endocrine Neoplasia syndrome type 2; Type 1 diabetes; Diabetic ketoacidosis; Severe gastrointestinal disease (including severe gastroparesis); Lactation: Avoid use; Pedi: Not recommended.
Use Cautiously in: History of pancreatitis; History of angioedema to another GLP-1 receptor agonist; Hepatic/renal impairment; OB: Use only if potential benefit justifies potential risk to fetus.

Adverse Reactions/Side Effects

CNS: fatigue. **Derm:** pruritis, rash. **Endo:** THYROID C-CELL TUMORS. **GI:** PANCREATITIS, abdominal pain, nausea, vomiting, constipation, ↓ appetite, diarrhea, dyspepsia. **GU:** acute renal failure. **Local:** hypersensitivity reactions including ANAPHYLAXIS AND ANGIOEDEMA, injection site reactions.

Interactions

Drug-Drug: Concurrent use with **insulin** or **agents that increase insulin secretion** including **sulfonylureas** may ↑ the risk of serious hypoglycemia, use cautiously and consider dose ↓ of insulin or agents increasing insulin secretion. May alter absorption of concomitantly administered **oral medications** due to delayed gastric emptying.

Route/Dosage

Subcut (Adults): 0.75 mg once weekly; may ↑ to 1.5 mg once weekly to obtain glycemic control.

Availability

Solution for subcutaneous injection: 0.75 mg/0.5 mL single-dose pen, 0.75 mg/0.5 mL single-dose prefilled syringe, 1.5 mg/0.5 mL single-use pen, 1.5 mg/0.5 mL single-dose prefilled syringe.

NURSING IMPLICATIONS

Assessment

- Observe patient taking concurrent insulin for signs and symptoms of hypoglycemic reactions (sweating, hunger, weakness, dizziness, tremor, tachycardia, anxiety, headache, blurred vision, slurred speech, irritability).
- If thyroid nodules or elevated serum calcitonin are noted, patient should be referred to an endocrinologist.
- Monitor for pancreatitis (persistent severe abdominal pain, sometimes radiating to the back, with or without vomiting). If pancreatitis is suspected, discontinue dulaglutide; if confirmed, do not restart dulaglutide.
- ***Lab Test Considerations:*** Monitor serum HbA_{1c} periodically during therapy to evaluate effectiveness.
- May ↑ lipase and pancreatic amylase.

Potential Nursing Diagnoses

Imbalanced nutrition: more than body requirements (Indications)
Noncompliance (Patient/Family Teaching)

Implementation

- Patients stabilized on a diabetic regimen who are exposed to stress, fever, trauma, infection, or surgery may require administration of insulin.
- **Subcut:** Administer once weekly at any time of the day, without regard to food. Day of week may be changed as long as at least 72 hr before next dose. Inject into abdomen, thigh, or upper arm. Solution should be clear and colorless; do not administer solutions that are discolored or contain particulate matter.

Patient/Family Teaching

- Instruct patient on use of pen and to take dulaglutide as directed. Follow manufacturer's instructions for pen use. Pen should never be shared between patients, even if needle is changed. Store pen in refrigerator; do not freeze. After initial use, pen may be stored at room temperature up to 14 days. Advise patient to read the *Patient Medication Guide* before starting dulaglutide and with each Rx refill in case of changes.
- Take missed dose as soon as remembered as long as 3 days (72 hr) until next scheduled dose. If less than 3 days until next scheduled dose, skip and take next scheduled dose.
- Inform patient that nausea is the most common side effect, but usually decreases over time.
- Advise patient taking insulin and dulaglutide to never mix insulin and dulaglutide together. Give as 2 separate injections. Both injections may be given in the same body area, but should not be given right next to each other.
- Explain to patient that this medication controls hyperglycemia but does not cure diabetes. Therapy is long-term.
- Review signs of hypoglycemia and hyperglycemia with patient. If hypoglycemia occurs, advise patient to take a glass of orange juice or 2–3 tsp of sugar, honey, or corn syrup dissolved in water and notify health care professional.
- Encourage patient to follow prescribed diet, medication, and exercise regimen to prevent hypoglycemic or hyperglycemic episodes.
- Instruct patient in proper testing of serum glucose and ketones. These tests should be closely monitored during periods of stress or illness, and health care professional should be notified if significant changes occur.
- Advise patient to notify health care professional of all Rx or OTC medications, vitamins, or herbal products being taken and consult health care professional before taking any new medications.
- Advise patient to notify discontinue dulaglutide and health care professional immediately if signs of pancreatitis (nausea, vomiting, abdominal pain) occur.
- Inform patient of risk of benign and malignant thyroid C-cell tumors. Advise patient to notify health care professional if symptoms of thyroid tumors (lump in neck, hoarseness, trouble swallowing, shortness of breath) or if signs of allergic reaction (swelling of face, lips, tongue, or throat; fainting or feeling dizzy; very rapid heartbeat; problems breathing or swallowing; severe rash or itching) occur.
- Advise patient to inform health care professional of medication regimen before treatment or surgery.
- Advise patient to carry a form of sugar (sugar packets, candy) and identification describing disease process and medication regimen at all times.
- Insulin is the preferred method of controlling blood glucose during pregnancy. Counsel female patients to notify health care professional if pregnancy is planned or suspected or if breast feeding.
- Emphasize the importance of routine follow-up exams.

Evaluation/Desired Outcomes

- Improved glycemic control.

D

DULoxetine (do-**lox**-e-teen)

Cymbalta

Classification

Therapeutic: antidepressants

Pharmacologic: selective serotonin/norepinephrine reuptake inhibitors

Pregnancy Category C

Indications

Major depressive disorder. Diabetic peripheral neuropathic pain. Generalized anxiety disorder. Fibromyalgia. Chronic musculoskeletal pain (including chronic lower back pain and chronic pain from osteoarthritis). **Unlabeled Use:** Stress urinary incontinence.

Action

Inhibits serotonin and norepinephrine reuptake in the CNS. Both antidepressant and pain inhibition are centrally mediated. **Therapeutic Effects:** Decreased depressive symptomatology. Decreased neuropathic pain. Decreased symptoms of anxiety. Decreased pain.

Pharmacokinetics

Absorption: Well absorbed following oral administration.

Distribution: Unknown.

Protein Binding: Highly (> 90%) protein-bound.

Metabolism and Excretion: Mostly metabolized, primarily by the CYP2D6 and CYP1A2 enzyme pathways.

Half-life: 12 hr.

TIME/ACTION PROFILE (blood levels)

ROUTE	ONSET	PEAK	DURATION
PO	unknown	6 hr	12 hr

Contraindications/Precautions

Contraindicated in: Hypersensitivity; Concurrent use of MAO inhibitors or MAO-like drugs (linezolid or methylene blue); Severe renal impairment (CCr <30 mL/min); Chronic hepatic impairment or substantial alcohol use (↑ risk of hepatitis); Lactation: May enter breast milk; discontinue or bottle-feed.

Use Cautiously in: History of suicide attempt or ideation; History of mania (may activate mania/hypomania); Concurrent use of other centrally acting drugs (↑ risk of adverse reactions); History of seizure disorder; Diabetes (may worsen glycemic control); Angle-closure glaucoma; OB: Use during 3rd trimester may result in neonatal serotonin syndrome requiring prolonged hospitalization, respiratory and nutritional support; Pedi: May ↑ risk of suicide attempt/ideation especially during dose early treatment or dose adjustment; risk may be greater in children or adolescents.; Geri: ↑ risk of orthostatic hypotension and falls

Adverse Reactions/Side Effects

CNS: NEUROLEPTIC MALIGNANT SYNDROME, SEIZURES, SUICIDAL THOUGHTS, fatigue, drowsiness, insomnia, activation of mania, dizziness, fainting, falls, nightmares. **EENT:** blurred vision, ↑ intraocular pressure. **CV:** ↑ BP, orthostatic hypotension. **GI:** HEPATOTOXICITY, ↓ appetite, constipation, dry mouth, nausea, diarrhea, ↑ liver enzymes, gastritis, vomiting. **F and E:** hyponatremia. **GU:** dysuria, abnormal orgasm, erectile dysfunction, ↓ libido, urinary retention. **Derm:** ERYTHEMA MULTIFORME, STEVENS-JOHNSON SYNDROME, ↑ sweating, pruritus, rash. **Neuro:** tremor. **Misc:** SEROTONIN SYNDROME.

Interactions

Drug-Drug: Concurrent use with **MAO inhibitors** may result in serious potentially fatal reactions (Do not use within 14 days of discontinuing MAOI. Wait at least 5 days after stopping duloxetine to start MAOI). Concurrent use with **MAO-inhibitor-like drugs**, such as **linezolid** or **methylene blue** may ↑ risk of serotonin syndrome; concurrent use contraindicated; do not start therapy in patients receiving **linezolid** or **methylene blue**; if **linezolid** or **methylene blue** need to be started in a patient receiving duloxetine, immediately discontinue duloxetine and monitor for signs/symptoms of serotonin syndrome for 5 days or until 24 hr after last dose of linezolid or methylene blue, whichever comes first (may resume duloxetine therapy 24 hr after last dose of linezolid or methylene blue). ↑ risk of hepatotoxicity with alcohol use disorder/**alcohol** abuse. Drugs that affect serotonergic neurotransmitter systems, including **tricyclic antidepressants**, **SSRIs**, **fentanyl**, **buspirone**, **tramadol**, and **triptans** ↑ risk of serotonin syndrome. **Drugs that inhibit CYP1A2**, including **fluvoxamine** and some **fluoroquinolones**, ↑ levels of duloxetine and should be avoided. **Drugs that inhibit CYP2D6**, including **paroxetine**, **fluoxetine**, and **quinidine**↑ levels of duloxetine and may increase the risk of adverse reactions. Duloxetine also inhibits CYP2D6 and may ↑ levels of drugs metabolized by CYP2D6, including **tricyclic antidepressants**, **phenothiazines**, and **class Ic antiarrhythmics** (**propafenone** and **flecainide**); concurrent use should be undertaken with caution. ↑ risk of serious arrhythmias with **thioridazine**; avoid concurrent use. ↑ risk of bleeding with **aspirin**, **NSAIDs**, or **warfarin**.

Drug-Natural Products: Use with **St. John's wort** ↑ serotonin syndrome.

Route/Dosage

Major Depressive Disorder

PO (Adults): 40–60 mg/day (as 20 mg or 30 mg twice daily or as 60 mg once daily) as initial therapy, then 60 mg once daily as maintenance therapy.

Generalized Anxiety Disorder

PO (Adults ≥65 yr): 30 mg once daily for 2 wk; may then consider ↑ to 60 mg once daily, then may ↑ by 30 mg once daily to maintenance dose of 60–120 mg once daily.

PO (Adults <65 yr): 30–60 mg once daily as initial therapy (if initiated on 30 mg once daily, should titrate to 60 mg once daily after 1 wk), then may ↑ by 30 mg once daily to maintenance dose of 60–120 mg once daily.

PO (Children 7–17 yr): 30 mg once daily for 2 wk; may then consider ↑ to 60 mg once daily; recommended maintenance dose = 30–60 mg once daily (not to exceed 120 mg once daily).

Diabetic Peripheral Neuropathic Pain

PO (Adults): 60 mg once daily.

Fibromyalgia

PO (Adults): 30 mg once daily for 1 wk, then ↑ to 60 mg once daily.

Chronic Musculoskeletal Pain

PO (Adults): 60 mg once daily (may also be started on 30 mg once daily and ↑ to 60 mg once daily after 1 wk.

Availability (generic available)

Capsules: 20 mg, 30 mg, 40 mg, 60 mg. **Cost:** 20 mg $437.15/60, 30 mg $473.58/60, 60 mg $478.64/60.

NURSING IMPLICATIONS

Assessment

- Assess for sexual dysfunction (erectile dysfunction; decreased libido).
- Monitor BP before and periodically during therapy. Sustained hypertension may be dose related; decrease dose or discontinue therapy if this occurs.
- Monitor appetite and nutritional intake. Weigh weekly. Report continued weight loss. Adjust diet as tolerated to support nutritional status.

- Monitor closely for notable changes in behavior that could indicate the emergence or worsening of suicidal thoughts or behavior or depression, especially in early therapy or during dose changes. Risk may be increased in children, adolescents, and adults ≤24 yr. Restrict amount of drug available to patient.
- Assess for serotonin syndrome (mental changes [agitation, hallucinations, coma], autonomic instability [tachycardia, labile BP, hyperthermia], neuromuscular aberrations [hyperreflexia, incoordination], and/or GI symptoms [nausea, vomiting, diarrhea]), especially in patients taking other serotonergic drugs (SSRIs, SNRIs, triptans).
- Assess for rash periodically during therapy. May cause Stevens-Johnson syndrome. Discontinue therapy if severe or if accompanied with fever, general malaise, fatigue, muscle or joint aches, blisters, oral lesions, conjunctivitis, hepatitis and/or eosinophilia.
- **Depression:** Assess mental status (orientation, mood, and behavior). Inform health care professional if patient demonstrates significant increase in anxiety, nervousness, or insomnia.
- **Pain and Fibromyalgia:** Assess intensity, quality, and location of pain periodically during therapy. May require several weeks for effects to be seen.
- ***Lab Test Considerations:*** May cause ↑ ALT, AST, bilirubin, CPK, and alkaline phosphatase.
- May cause hyponatremia.
- Monitor blood sugar and hemoglobin A1c. May cause slight ↑ in blood glucose.

Potential Nursing Diagnoses

Ineffective coping (Indications)
Risk for suicide (Adverse Reactions)
Chronic pain (Indications)

Implementation

- Do not confuse duloxetine with fluoxetine or paroxetine. Do not confuse Cymbalta with Symbyax.
- **PO:** May be administered without regard to meals. Capsules should be swallowed whole. Do not crush, chew, or open and sprinkle contents on food or liquids; may affect enteric coating .

Patient/Family Teaching

- Instruct patient to take duloxetine as directed at the same time each day. Take missed doses as soon as possible unless time for next dose. Do not stop abruptly; may cause dizziness, headache, nausea, diarrhea, paresthesia, irritability, vomiting, insomnia, anxiety, hyperhidrosis, and fatigue; must be decreased gradually.
- Encourage patient and family to be alert for emergence of anxiety, agitation, panic attacks, insomnia, irritability, hostility, impulsivity, akathisia, hypomania, mania, worsening of depression and suicidal ideation, especially during early antidepressant therapy. If these symptoms occur, notify health care professional.
- May cause drowsiness. Caution patient to avoid driving or other activities requiring alertness until response to medication is known.
- Advise patient to make position changes slowly to minimize orthostatic hypotension and falls, especially in elderly patients and those taking antihypertensive medications.
- Instruct patient to notify health care professional of all Rx or OTC medications, vitamins, or herbal products being taken and to consult with health care professional before taking other medications.
- Instruct patient to notify health care professional if signs of serotonin syndrome (mental status changes: agitation, hallucinations, coma; autonomic instability: tachycardia, labile BP, hyperthermia; neuromuscular aberrations: hyperreflexia, incoordination; and/or gastrointestinal symptoms: nausea, vomiting, diarrhea), liver damage (pruritus, dark urine, jaundice, right upper quadrant tenderness, unexplained "flu-like" symptoms) or rash occur.
- Advise patient to avoid taking alcohol during duloxetine therapy.
- Instruct patient to notify health care professional if pregnancy is planned or suspected or if breast feeding. Encourage any patient exposed to duloxetine during pregnancy to register with the Cymbalta Pregnancy Registry at 1-866-814-6975 or www.cymbaltapregnancyregistry.com.

Evaluation/Desired Outcomes

- Increased sense of well-being.
- Renewed interest in surroundings. Need for therapy should be periodically reassessed. Patients may notice improvement within 1–4 wk, but should be advised to continue therapy as directed. Therapy is usually continued for several months.
- Decrease in neuropathic pain associated with diabetic peripheral neuropathy.
- Decrease in chronic musculoskeletal pain and pain and soreness associated with fibromyalgia.
- Decrease in anxiety.

dutasteride (doo-**tas**-te-ride)

Avodart

Classification

Therapeutic: benign prostatic hyperplasia (BPH) agents
Pharmacologic: androgen inhibitors

Pregnancy Category X

Indications

Management of the symptoms of benign prostatic hyperplasia (BPH) in men with an enlarged prostate gland (alone or with tamsulosin).

Action

Inhibits the enzyme 5-alpha-reductase, which is responsible for converting testosterone to its potent metabolite 5-alpha-dihydrotestosterone in the prostate gland and other tissues. 5-Alpha-dihydrotestosterone is partly responsible for prostatic hyperplasia. **Therapeutic Effects:** Reduced prostate size with associated decrease in urinary symptoms.

Pharmacokinetics

Absorption: Well absorbed (60%) following oral administration; also absorbed through skin.
Distribution: 11.5% of serum concentration partitions into semen.
Protein Binding: 99% bound to albumin; 96.6% bound to alpha-1 glycoprotein.
Metabolism and Excretion: Mostly metabolized by the liver via the CYP3A4 metabolic pathway; metabolites are excreted in feces.
Half-life: 5 wk.

TIME/ACTION PROFILE (reduction in dihydrotestosterone levels†)

ROUTE	ONSET	PEAK	DURATION
PO	unknown	1–2 wk	unknown

†Symptoms may only improve over 3–12 mo.

Contraindications/Precautions

Contraindicated in: Hypersensitivity; Cross-sensitivity with other 5-alpha-reductase inhibitors may occur; Women; Pedi: Children.
Use Cautiously in: Hepatic impairment.

Adverse Reactions/Side Effects

CNS: depressed mood. **GU:** PROSTATE CANCER (high-grade), ↓ libido, ejaculation disorders, erectile dysfunction, testicular pain, testicular swelling. **Endo:** gynecomastia. **Derm:** rash, urticaria. **Misc:** ALLERGIC REACTIONS, ANGIOEDEMA.

Interactions

Drug-Drug: Blood levels and effects may be ↑ by **ritonavir**, **ketoconazole**, **verapamil**, **diltiazem**, **cimetidine**, **ciprofloxacin**, or other **CYP3A4 enzyme inhibitors**.

Route/Dosage

PO (Adults): 0.5 mg once daily (with or without tamsulosin).

Availability (generic available)

Soft gelatin capsules: 0.5 mg. ***In combination with:*** tamsulosin (Jalyn); see Appendix B.

NURSING IMPLICATIONS

Assessment

- Assess patient for symptoms of prostatic hyperplasia (urinary hesitancy, feeling of incomplete bladder emptying, interruption of urinary stream, impairment of size and force of urinary stream, terminal urinary dribbling, straining to start flow, dysuria, urgency) before and periodically during therapy.
- Digital rectal examinations should be performed before and periodically during therapy for BPH.
- ***Lab Test Considerations:*** Serum prostate-specific antigen (PSA) concentrations, used to screen for prostate cancer, decrease by about 20% within the 1st mo of therapy and stabilize at about 50% of the pretreatment level within 6 mo. New baseline PSA concentrations should be established at 3 and 6 mo of therapy and evaluated periodically during therapy. Any increase in PSA during dutaseride therapy may be a sign of prostate cancer and should be evaluated, even those within normal limits. Isolated PSA values from men taking dutaseride for 3 mo or more should be doubled for comparison in untreated men.

Potential Nursing Diagnoses

Impaired urinary elimination (Indications)

Implementation

- **PO:** Administer once daily with or without meals. Do not break, crush, or chew capsule.

Patient/Family Teaching

- Instruct patient to take dutasteride at the same time each day as directed, even if symptoms improve or are unchanged. Take missed doses as soon as remembered later in the day or omit dose. Do not make up by taking double doses the next day.
- Caution patient that sharing of dutasteride may be dangerous.
- Inform patient that the volume of ejaculate may be decreased during therapy but that this will not interfere with normal sexual function.
- Advise patient to avoid donating blood for at least 6 mo after last dose of dutasteride to prevent a pregnant female from receiving dutasteride through a blood transfusion.
- Inform patient of potential increase risk in high-grade prostate cancer.
- Caution patient that dutasteride poses a potential risk to a male fetus. Women who are pregnant or may become pregnant should avoid exposure to semen of a partner taking dutasteride and should not handle dutasteride because of the potential for absorption.
- Emphasize the importance of periodic follow-up exams to determine whether a clinical response has occurred.

Evaluation/Desired Outcomes

- Decrease in urinary symptoms of BPH.

econazole, See ANTIFUNGALS (TOPICAL).

edoxaban (e-dox-a-ban)

Savaysa

Classification

Therapeutic: anticoagulants

Pharmacologic: factor Xa inhibitors

Pregnancy Category C

Indications

Reduction of stroke/systemic embolization (SE) risk associated with nonvalvular atrial fibrillation (NVAF).

Action

Selective inhibitor of factor Xa. Does not inhibit platelet aggregation directly, but does inhibit thrombin-induced platelet aggregation. Decreases thrombin generation and thrombus development. **Therapeutic Effects:** Decreased thrombotic events associated with atrial fibrillation including stroke and systemic embolization. Treatment of deep vein thrombosis (DVT) and plumonary embolism (PE) after 5–10 days of parenteral anticoagulant.

Pharmacokinetics

Absorption: 62% absorbed following oral administration.

Distribution: Unknown.

Metabolism and Excretion: Minimal metabolism, one metabolite is pharmacologically active. Excreted mostly unchanged in urine.

Half-life: 10–14 hr.

TIME/ACTION PROFILE (anticoagulant effect)

ROUTE	ONSET	PEAK	DURATION
PO	unknown	1–2 hr	24 hr

Contraindications/Precautions

Contraindicated in: Active bleeding; CCr >95 mL/min (↓ effectiveness); Concurrent use of other anticoagulants or rifampin; Presence of mechanical heart valves or severe mitral stenosis; Moderate to severe hepatic impairment; Lactation: Discontinue edoxaban or discontinue breast feeding.

Use Cautiously in: Elective/planned invasive/surgical procudures (discontinue at least 24 hr prior to ↓ risk of bleeding); Premature discontinuation (↑ risk of ischemic events); Neuroaxial anesthesia/spinal puncture (↑ risk of spinal/epidural hematoma and potential paralysis); Renal impairment (dose reduction required for CCr 15–50 mL/min); Deteriorating or improving renal function (may require dose change); Body weight ≤60 kg (requires lower dose); OB: Use during pregnancy only if potential benefit outweighs potential risk to fetus; Pedi: Safe and effective use in children has not been established.

Adverse Reactions/Side Effects

GI: abnormal liver function tests. **Hemat:** BLEEDING, anemia.

Interactions

Drug-Drug: Concurrent use of other **anticoagulants, antifibrotics, antiplatelet agents, aspirin, fibrinolytics, NSAIDs** or **SSRIs** may ↑ risk of bleeding. Rifampin may ↓ blood levels and effectiveness and is contraindicated. Concurrent use of **P-gp inhibitors** including **azithromycin, clarithromcyin, erythromycin, itraconazole** (oral), **ketoconazole** oral), **quinidine**, or **verapamil** ↑ blood levels and the risk of bleeding (lower dose required).

Route/Dosage

Treatment of NVAF

PO (Adults): 60 mg once daily.

Renal Impairment

PO (Adults): *CCr 15–50 mL/min*—30 mg once daily.

Treatment of DVT/PE

PO (Adults >60 kg): 60 mg once daily.

PO (Adults ≤60 kg or certain concurrent P-gp inhibitors): 30 mg once daily.

Renal Impairment

PO (Adults CCr 15–50 ml/min): 30 mg once daily.

Availability

Tablets: 15 mg, 30 mg, 60 mg.

NURSING IMPLICATIONS

Assessment

- Monitor for bleeding. Discontinue edoxaban if active pathological bleeding occurs. Concomitant drugs (aspirin, other antiplatelet agents, other antithrombotic agents, fibrinolytic therapy, chronic use of NSAIDs) may increase risk of bleeding. Anticoagulant effects of edoxaban persist for about 24 hr after last dose; there is no established way to reverse anticoagulant effects. Anticoagulant effects cannot be reliably monitored with standard laboratory tests. No reversal agent is available; protamine sulfate, vitamin K, and tranexamic acid do not reverse anticoagulant activity. Hemodialysis does not significantly contribute to edoxaban clearance.
- Monitor frequently for signs and symptoms of neurological impairment (numbness or weakness of legs, bowel, or bladder dysfunction, back pain, tingling, muscle weakness); if noted, urgent treatment

is required. Intrathecal or epidural catheters should not be removed earlier than 12 hr after last dose of edoxaban. Next dose of edoxaban should not be given less than 2 hr after removal of catheter.

- ***Lab Test Considerations:*** Assess creatinine clearance (CrCl) using Cockcroft-Gault equation (Cockcroft-Gault CrCl = (140-age) x (weight in kg) x (0.85 if female)/(72 x creatinine in mg/dL) before starting therapy.

Potential Nursing Diagnoses

Risk for injury (Adverse Reactions)

Implementation

- Discontinue edoxaban at least 24 hr prior to invasive or surgical procedures; may increase risk of bleeding. Edoxaban may be restarted as soon as adequate hemostasis is established; time to onset of pharmacodynamic effect is 1–2 hr.
- **PO: Nonvalvular Atrial Fibrillation:** Administer 60 mg once daily without regard to food. Do not use in patients with CrCl >95 mL/min. If CrCl 15 to 50 mL/min, decrease dose to 30 mg once daily.
- **Deep Vein Thrombosis and Pulmonary Embolism:** Administer 60 mg once daily without regard to food following 5 to 10 days of parenteral anticoagulant therapy. If CrCl 15 to 50 mL/min, patient weighs ≤60 kg, or patient taking concurrent verapamil, quinidine, azithromycin, clarithromycin, erythromycin, oral itraconazole or oral ketoconazole, decrease dose to 30 mg once daily.
- *If transitioning from warafarin or other vitamin K antagonists to edoxaban,* discontinue warfarin and start edoxaban when INR ≤2.5. *If transitioning from oral anticoagulants other than warfarin or other Vitamin K antagonists to edoxaban,* discontinue current oral anticoagulant and start edoxaban at time of next scheduled dose of other oral anticoagulant. *If transitioning from low molecular weight heparin (LMWH) to edoxaban,* discontinue LMWH and start edoxaban at time of next scheduled administration of LMWH. *If transitioning from unfractionated heparin to edoxaban,* discontinue infusion and start edoxaban 4 hr later.
- *If transitioning from edoxaban to warfarin,* Oral Option: For patients taking 60 mg of edoxaban, reduce dose to 30 mg and begin warfarin concomitantly. For patients taking 30 mg edoxaban, reduce dose to 15 mg and begin warfarin concomitantly. Measure INR at least weekly and just prior to daily dose of edoxaban to minimize influence of edoxaban on INR measurements. Once stable INR ≥2.0 achieved, discontinue edoxaban and continue warfarin. Parenteral Option: Discontinue edoxaban and administer a parenteral anticoagulant and warfarin at time of next scheduled edoxaban dose. Once stable INR ≥2.0 achieved, discontinue parenteral anticoagulant and continue warfarin. *If transitioning from edoxaban to non-Vitamin-K Dependant Oral anticoagulant,* discontinue edoxaban and start other oral anticoagulant at time of next dose of edoxaban. *If transitioning from edoxaban to parenteral anticoagulant,* discontinue edoxaban and start parenteral anticoagulant at time of next dose of edoxaban.

Patient/Family Teaching

- Instruct patient to take edoxaban as directed. Take missed doses as soon as remembered on same day. Return to regular schedule next day. Do not double doses in one day. Do not discontinue without consulting health care professional; stopping may increase risk of stroke.
- Caution patient that they may bleed more easily, longer, or bruise more easily during therapy. Advise patient to notify health care professional immediately if bleeding or a fall, especially with head injury, occurs.
- Advise patient to notify health care professional of all Rx or OTC medications, vitamins, or herbal products being taken and to consult with health care professional before taking other medications, especially other aspirin or NSAIDs.
- Advise patient to notify health care professional of therapy before surgery, medical, or dental procedures are scheduled.
- Advise female patient to notify health care professional if pregnancy is planned or suspected. Avoid breast feeding during therapy.

Evaluation/Desired Outcomes

- Decreased thrombotic events (stroke and systemic embolization) associated with atrial fibrillation.
- Treatment of deep vein thrombosis (DVT) and pulmonary embolism (PE).

efavirenz (e-fa-veer-enz)

Sustiva

Classification

Therapeutic: antiretrovirals

Pharmacologic: non-nucleoside reverse transcriptase inhibitors

Pregnancy Category D

Indications

HIV infection (in combination with one or more other antiretroviral agents).

Action

Inhibits HIV reverse transcriptase, which results in disruption of DNA synthesis. **Therapeutic Effects:** Slowed progression of HIV infection and decreased occurrence of sequelae. Increases CD4 cell counts and decreases viral load.

Pharmacokinetics

Absorption: 50% absorbed when ingested following a high-fat meal.

Distribution: 99.5–99.75% bound to plasma proteins; enters CSF.
Metabolism and Excretion: Mostly metabolized by the liver.
Half-life: *Following single dose*—52–76 hr. *Following multiple doses*—40–55 hr.

TIME/ACTION PROFILE (blood levels)

ROUTE	ONSET	PEAK	DURATION
PO	rapid	3–5 hr	24 hr

Contraindications/Precautions

Contraindicated in: Hypersensitivity; Moderate to severe hepatic impairment.
Use Cautiously in: History of mental illness or substance abuse (↑ risk of psychiatric symptomatology); Mild hepatic impairment; History of seizure disorders (↑ risk of seizures); OB: Use in pregnancy only if other options have been exhausted; birth defects have been reported; Lactation: Breast feeding not recommended for HIV-infected mothers; efavirenz passes into breast milk; Pedi: Children <3 mo (safety not established); ↑ incidence of rash; Geri: Cautious initial dosing due to ↑ incidence of renal or cardiac dysfunction.

Adverse Reactions/Side Effects

CNS: abnormal dreams, depression, dizziness, drowsiness, fatigue, headache, impaired concentration, insomnia, nervousness, psychiatric symptomatology. **GI:** HEPATOTOXICITY, nausea, abdominal pain, anorexia, diarrhea, dyspepsia, flatulence. **GU:** hematuria, renal calculi. **Derm:** rash, sweating, pruritus. **Endo:** hypercholesterolemia, hypertriglyceridemia. **Neuro:** hypoesthesia. **Misc:** fat redistribution, immune reconstitution syndrome.

Interactions

Drug-Drug: Induces (stimulates) the hepatic cytochrome P450 3A4 enzyme system and would be expected to influence the effects of other drugs that are metabolized by this system; efavirenz itself is also metabolized by this system. ↑ risk of CNS depression with other **CNS depressants**, including **alcohol**, **antidepressants**, **antihistamines**, and **opioid analgesics**. May ↓ the effectiveness of **progestin-containing hormonal contraceptives** (e.g., etonogestrel, norelgestromin, levonorgestrel). Use with **voriconazole** significantly ↓ voriconazole levels and ↑ efavirenz levels; avoid concurrent use with standard doses of voriconazole; if used together, ↑ dose of voriconazole to 400 mg q 12 hr and ↓ dose of efavirenz to 300 mg daily. May ↓ **posaconazole** levels; avoid concurrent use. May ↓ **itraconazole** levels; use alternative antifungal agent. May ↓ **ketoconazole** levels. May ↓ **indinavir** levels; ↑ dose of indinavir dose. May ↓ **fosamprenavir** levels; ↑ dose of ritonavir when given with fosamprenavir/ritonavir once daily. May ↓ **atazanavir** levels; dosage adjustments may be needed in treatment-naïve patients; avoid concurrent use in treatment-experienced patients. May ↓ **lopinavir** levels; ↑ dose of lopinavir/ritonavir; avoid concurrent use of lopinavir/ritonavir once daily. May ↑ **ritonavir** levels; monitor liver function tests. May ↓ **saquinavir** and **raltegravir** levels. ↓ **maraviroc** levels; ↑ maraviroc dose. May alter the effects of **warfarin**. May ↓ levels of **cyclosporine**, **tacrolimus**, and **sirolimus**. May ↓ levels of **bupropion** and **sertraline**. **Rifampin** may ↓ levels; ↑ dose of efavirenz. Concurrent use with other **NNRTIs** including **etravirine**, **nevirapine**, **rilpivirine**, and **delavirdine** may lead to ↓ effectiveness and should be avoided. May ↓ levels of **raltegravir**. May ↓ levels of **boceprevir** and **simeprevir**; avoid concurrent use. Concurrent use with **carbamazepine** may ↓ levels of carbamazepine and efavirenz; use alternative anticonvulsant agent. Concurrent use with **phenytoin** or **phenobarbital** may ↓ levels of phenytoin, carbamazepine, and efavirenz. May ↓ levels of **clarithromycin**; consider using azithromycin. May ↓ levels of **rifabutin**; ↑ daily dose of rifabutin by 50%. May ↓ levels of **calcium channel blockers**, **atorvastatin**, **pravastatin**, **simvastatin**, **methadone** and **artemether/lumefantrine**. May ↓ levels of **progestin-containing contraceptives** and **etonogestrel**; use reliable method of barrier contraception in addition to hormonal contraceptive agent.
Drug-Food: Ingestion following a **high-fat meal** ↑ absorption by 50%.

Route/Dosage

PO (Adults and Children ≥40 kg): 600 mg once daily; *Concurrent rifampin therapy (in patients >50 kg)*—800 mg once daily.
PO (Children ≥3 mo and 32.5–39.9 kg): 400 mg once daily.
PO (Children ≥3 mo and 25–32.4 kg): 350 mg once daily.
PO (Children ≥3 mo and 20–24.9 kg): 300 mg once daily.
PO (Children ≥3 mo and 15–19.9 kg): 250 mg once daily.
PO (Children ≥3 mo and 7.5–14.9 kg): 200 mg once daily.
PO (Children ≥3 mo and 5–7.4 kg): 150 mg once daily.
PO (Children ≥3 mo and 3.5–4.9 kg): 100 mg once daily.

Availability

Capsules: 50 mg, 200 mg. **Tablets:** 600 mg. ***In combination with:*** emtricitabine and tenofovir (Atripla) (See Appendix B).

NURSING IMPLICATIONS

Assessment

- Assess for change in severity of HIV symptoms and for symptoms of opportunistic infections during therapy.
- Assess for rash, especially during 1st mo of therapy. Onset is usually within 2 wk and resolves with continued therapy within 1 mo. May range from mild maculopapular with erythema and pruritus to exfoliative dermatitis and Stevens-Johnson syndrome. Occurs more often and may be more severe in children. If rash is severe or accompanied by blistering, desquamation, mucosal involvement, or fever, therapy must be discontinued immediately. Efavirenz may be reinstated concurrently with antihistamines or corticosteroids in patients discontinuing due to rash.
- Assess patient for CNS and psychiatric symptoms (dizziness, impaired concentration, somnolence, abnormal dreams, insomnia) during therapy. Symptoms usually begin during 1st or 2nd day of therapy and resolve after 2–4 wk. Administration at bedtime may minimize symptoms. Concurrent use with alcohol or psychoactive agents may cause additive CNS symptoms.
- ***Lab Test Considerations:*** Monitor viral load and CD4 cell count regularly during therapy.
- Monitor liver function tests in patients with a history of hepatitis B or C or underlying liver disease. May cause ↑ serum AST, ALT, and GGT concentrations. If moderate to severe liver function test abnormalities occur, efavirenz doses should be held until levels return to normal. Discontinue if liver function abnormalities recur when therapy is resumed.
- May cause ↑ in total cholesterol and serum triglyceride levels.
- Obtain a pregnancy test prior to starting therapy. May cause fetal harm if administered during first trimester of pregnancy.
- May cause false-positive urine cannabinoid results.

Potential Nursing Diagnoses

Risk for infection (Indications)
Noncompliance (Patient/Family Teaching)

Implementation

- **PO:** Administer on an empty stomach, preferably at bedtime to minimize nervous system side effects. Avoid taking with a high-fat meal. Do not break tablets.
- Capsule may be opened and contents sprinkled on a small amount (1 to 2 tsp) of food for children at least 3 mo old and weighing at least 3.5 kg and adults who cannot swallow capsules or tablets. Open capsule carefully; avoid spillage or dispersion of contents into the air. ***For infants receiving capsule sprinkle-infant formula mixture***, gently mix entire capsule contents into 2 tsp (10 mL) of reconstituted room temperature infant formula in a medicine cup, then draw up mixture into a 10 mL oral dosing syringe for administration. Use of infant formula for mixing should only be considered for those young infants who cannot consume solid foods. *For patients able to tolerate solid foods*, mix entire capsule contents gently with soft food (applesauce, grape jelly, yogurt). After administration of mixture, add a small amount (2 tsp) of food or formula to empty mixing container, stir to disperse any remaining efavirenz residue, and administer to patient. Administer mixture within 30 minutes of mixing. Avoid food for 2 hr after administration.

Patient/Family Teaching

- Emphasize the importance of taking efavirenz as directed. It must always be used in combination with other antiretroviral drugs. Do not take more than prescribed amount, and do not stop taking without consulting health care professional. Take missed doses as soon as remembered; do not double doses. Advise patient to read *Patient Information* before starting therapy and with each Rx refill in case of changes.
- Instruct patient that efavirenz should not be shared with others.
- May cause dizziness, impaired concentration, or drowsiness. Caution patient to avoid driving or other activities requiring alertness until response to medication is known.
- Instruct patient to notify health care professional immediately if rash occurs.
- Inform patient that efavirenz does not cure AIDS or prevent associated or opportunistic infections. Efavirenz does not reduce the risk of transmission of HIV to others through sexual contact or blood contamination. Caution patient to use a condom and to avoid sharing needles or donating blood to prevent spreading the AIDS virus to others. Advise patient that the long-term effects of efavirenz are unknown at this time.
- Inform patient that redistribution and accumulation of body fat may occur, causing central obesity, dorsocervical fat enlargement (buffalo hump), peripheral wasting, breast enlargement, and cushingoid appearance. The cause and long-term effects are not known.
- Instruct patient to notify health care professional of all Rx or OTC medications, vitamins, or herbal products being taken and to consult with health care professional before taking other medications.
- Rep: Advise patients taking oral contraceptives to use a nonhormonal method of birth control during efavirenz therapy and for at least 12 wk following discontinuation and to notify health care professional if they become pregnant while taking efavirenz. Encourage patients who become pregnant during therapy to join the registry by calling 1-800-258-4263.
- Emphasize the importance of regular follow-up exams and blood counts to determine progress and monitor for side effects.

Evaluation/Desired Outcomes

- Delayed progression of AIDS and decreased opportunistic infections in patients with HIV.
- Decrease in viral load and increase in CD4 cell counts.

elvitegravir (el-vi-teg-ra-vir)

Vitekta

Classification

Therapeutic: antiretrovirals

Pharmacologic: integrase strand transfer inhibitors (INSTI)

Pregnancy Category B

Indications

Treatment of HIV-1 infection, in combination with a protease inhibitor plus ritonavir and other antiretrovirals in treatment-experienced adults.

Action

Acts as an integrase strand transfer inhibitor; inhibits an enzyme necessary for viral replication. **Therapeutic Effects:** Slowed progression of HIV infection and decreased occurrence of sequelae.

Pharmacokinetics

Absorption: Absorption follows oral administration.

Distribution: Unknown.

Protein Binding: 98–99%.

Metabolism and Excretion: Metabolized by CYP3A, 94.5% eliminated in feces, 6.7% in urine.

Half-life: *Elvitegravir*—12.9 hr, *with ritonavir*—8.7 hr.

TIME/ACTION PROFILE (blood levels)

ROUTE	ONSET	PEAK	DURATION
PO	unknown	4 hr	24 hr

Contraindications/Precautions

Contraindicated in: Should not be used concurrently with cobicistat, efavirenz, nevirapine, rifampin, rifapentine, boceprevir, other elvitegravir-containing agents, norgestimate/ethinyl estradiol or St. John's wort; Severe hepatic impairment; Lactation: HIV-infected women should not breast feed due to risk of viral transmission.

Use Cautiously in: Concurrent use of drugs that induce the CYP3A enzyme system; Geri: May be more sensitive to drug effects (consider age-related ↓ in renal, hepatic and cardiac function, concurrent medications and medical conditions); OB: Use only if potential benefit justifies potential fetal risk; Pedi: Safety and effectiveness not established.

Adverse Reactions/Side Effects

GI: diarrhea. **Misc:** immune reconstitution syndrome.

Interactions

Drug-Drug: Strong **CYP3A inducers** including **carbamazepine**, **oxcarbazepine**, **phenobarbital**, and **phenytoin** can ↓ blood levels/effectiveness and ↑ risk of viral resistance (consider other anticonvulsants); similar effects may occur with **rifampin** and **rifapentine** (concurrent use not recommended); **dexamethasone** (consider alternative corticosteroid); **cobicistat**, **efavirenz**, and **nevirapine** (concurrent use should be avoided); and **bosentan** (discontinue bosentan at least 36 hr prior to starting elvitegravir, wait 10 days before restarting at ↓ dose of 62.5 mg once daily or ever other day with careful titration). **Antacids** may ↓ blood levels/effectiveness and ↑ risk of viral resistance by forming complexes in the GI (separate doses by 2 hr). Blood levels and the risk of toxicity are ↑ by **atazanavir/ritonavir** and **lopinavir/ritonavir** (↓ elvitegravir dose). May ↑ blood levels and risk of toxicity from **ketoconazole** (daily ketoconazole dose should not exceed 200 mg), **rifabutin** (↓ rifabutin dose to 150 mg every other day or 3 times weekly), **bosentan** (initiate bosentan at 62.5 mg once daily or every other day and titrate carefully), and **buprenorphine**. May ↓ blood levels and effectiveness of **boceprevir** (concurrent use not recommended). May ↓ levels of **ethinyl estradiol** in **hormonal contraceptives** leading to ↓ contraceptive efficacy (alternative non-hormonal contraceptive recommended). May ↓ **naloxone** and **methadone** levels (may need to ↑ methadone dose).

Drug-Natural Products: St. John's wort can ↓ blood levels/effectiveness and ↑ risk of viral resistance (concurrent use should be avoided).

Drug-Food: Didanosine (needs to be given on an empty stomach) should be given 1 hr before or 2 hr after elvitegravir (needs to be given with food).

Route/Dosage

An additional antiretroviral must be coadministered in addition to elvitegravir, a protease inhibitor, and ritonavir.

PO (Adults): *If used with ataznavir 300 mg once daily with 100 mg ritonavir once daily or lopinavir 400 mg once daily with ritonavir 100 mg twice daily*—85 mg once daily; *If used with darunavir 600 mg once daily with 100 mg ritonavir twice daily or fosamprenavir 700 mg twice daily with ritonavir 100 mg twice daily or tipranavir 500 mg twice daily with ritonavir 200 mg twice daily*—150 mg once daily.

Availability

Tablets: 85 mg, 150 mg.

NURSING IMPLICATIONS

Assessment

- Assess patient for change in severity of HIV symptoms and for symptoms of opportunistic infections during therapy.

Potential Nursing Diagnoses

Risk for infection (Indications)
Deficient knowledge, related to medication regimen (Patient/Family Teaching)

Implementation

- **PO:** Administer once daily with food with a protease inhibitor and with ritonavir.
- Administer antacids at least 2 hr before or after elvitegravir.

Patient/Family Teaching

- Explain purpose of elvitegravir to patient; elvitegravir does not treat HIV and must be taken with antiretroviral medications. Instruct patient to take elvitegravir as directed with food and with a protease inhibitor (atazanavir, darunavir, fosamprenavir, lopinavir/ritonavir, or tipranavir) and ritonavir on a regular dosing schedule. Do not stop taking elvitegravir without consulting health care professional. Advise patient to read *Patient Information* prior to starting therapy and with each Rx refill in case of change.
- Inform patient that elvitegravir does not cure AIDS or prevent associated or opportunistic infections. Elvitegravir does not reduce the risk of transmission of HIV to others through sexual contact or blood contamination. Caution patient to use a condom during sexual contact and to avoid sharing needles or donating blood to prevent spreading the AIDS virus to others.
- Advise patient to notify health care professional of all Rx or OTC medications, vitamins, or herbal products being taken and consult health care professional before taking any new medications, especially St. John's Wort. Elvitegravir interacts with many other drugs. Follow instructions for specific timing of or avoiding other medications.
- Advise patient to notify health care professional if signs and symptoms of immune reconstitution syndrome (signs and symptoms of infection or inflammation) occur.
- Rep: Advise female patient to notify health care professional if pregnancy is planned or suspected or if breast feeding. May decrease plasma concentrations of hormonal contraceptives. Use nonhormonal methods of contraception during therapy. Encourage pregnant patient to enroll in Antiretroviral Pregnancy Registry by calling 1-800-258-4263. Advise patient to avoid breast feeding.

Evaluation/Desired Outcomes

- Slowed progression of HIV infection and decreased occurrence of sequelae.

elvitegravir/cobicistat/emtricitabine/tenofovir

(el-vi-**teg**-ra vir/koe-**bis**-i-stat/em-tri-**si**-ti-been/te-**noe**-fo-veer)
Stribild

Classification
Therapeutic: antiretrovirals
Pharmacologic: integrase strand transfer inhibitors (INSTI), enzyme inhibitors, nucleoside reverse transcriptase inhibitors

Pregnancy Category B

Indications

Management of HIV infection, a complete regimen for treatment-naïve adults or in adults who are virologically suppressed (HIV—1 RNA <50 copies/mL) on a stable regimen for ≥6 mo with no history of treatment failure and no known substitutions associated with resistance to the individual components of this medication.

Action

Elvitegravir—An integrase strand transfer inhibitor that inhibits an enzyme necessary for viral replication. *Cobicistat*—A pharmacokinetic enhancer (inhibits CYP3A and CYP2D6) enhancing systemic exposure to elvitegravir. *Emtricitabine*—Phosphorylated intracellularly where it inhibits HIV reverse transcriptase, resulting in viral DNA chain termination. *Tenofovir*—Phosphorylated intracellularly where it inhibits HIV reverse transcriptase resulting in disruption of DNA synthesis. **Therapeutic Effects:** Slowed progression of HIV infection and decreased occurrence of sequelae.

Pharmacokinetics

elvitegravir

Absorption: Absorption follows oral administration.
Distribution: Unkown.
Protein Binding: 98–99%.
Metabolism and Excretion: Metabolized by CYP3A, 94.5% eliminated in feces, 6.7% in urine.
Half-life: 12.9 hr.

cobicistat

Absorption: Absorption follows oral administration.
Distribution: Unknown.
Protein Binding: 97–98%.
Metabolism and Excretion: Metabolized by CYP3A and to a small extent by CYP2D6, 86.2 eliminated in feces, 8.2% in urine.
Half-life: 3.5 hr.

emtricitabine

Absorption: Rapidly and extensively absorbed; 93% bioavailable.
Distribution: Unknown.
Metabolism and Excretion: Some metabolism, 86% renally excreted, 14% fecal excretion.
Half-life: 10 hr.

tenofovir

Absorption: Tenofovir disoproxil fumarate is a prodrug, which is split into tenofovir, the active component.

Distribution: Absorption is enhanced by food.

Metabolism and Excretion: 70–80% excreted unchanged in urine by glomerular filtration and active tubular secretion.

Half-life: Unknown.

TIME/ACTION PROFILE

ROUTE	ONSET	PEAK	DURATION
elivtegravir PO	unknown	4 hr	24 hr
cobicistat PO	unknown	3 hr	24 hr
emtricitabine PO	rapid	1–2 hr	24 hr
tenofovir PO	unknown	2 hr	24 hr

Contraindications/Precautions

Contraindicated in: Severe hepatic impairment; Concurrent administration of other drugs that depend mainly on CYP3A for metabolism and whose blood levels, when ↑, are associated with serious/life-threatening adverse reactions; Concurrent administration of other drugs that induce the CYP3A enzyme system which may ↓ blood levels/effectiveness and promote development of viral resistance; Should not be used concurrently with other antiretrovirals that contain cobicistat, elvitegravir, emtricitabine, tenofovir, lamivudine, adefovir, or ritonavir; Renal impairment (do not initiate if CCr < 70 mL/min, discontinue if CCr < 50 mL/min); Lactation: HIV-infected women should not breast feed due to risk of viral transmission.

Use Cautiously in: Female patients or obese patients (may be at ↑ risk for lactic acidosis/hepatic steatosis); Geri: Elderly may be more sensitive to drug effects; consider age-related ↓ in renal, hepatic, and cardiovascular function; concurrent disease states and medications; OB: Use during pregnancy only if potential benefits justify fetal risks; Pedi: Safety and effectiveness not established.

Exercise Extreme Caution in: Hepatitis B (may cause severe acute exacerbation).

Adverse Reactions/Side Effects

CNS: abnormal dreams, dizziness, headache, insomnia, drowsiness. **GU:** ACUTE RENAL FAILURE/FANCONI SYNDROME, proteinuria. **GI:** LACTIC ACIDOSIS/HEPATIC STEATOSIS, POST-TREATMENT ACUTE EXACERBATION OF HEPATITIS B, diarrhea, nausea. **Derm:** rash, hyperpigmentation. **F and E:** hypophosphatemia. **Metab:** ↑ lipids, redistribution of body fat. **MS:** bone pain, ↓ bone mineral density, muscle pain, osteomalacia. **Misc:** immune reconstitution syndrome.

Interactions

Drug-Drug: May alter blood levels and effects of other drugs metabolized by the CYP3A or CYP2D6 enzyme systems. Other drugs that induce the CYP3A system can alter blood levels and effects. Concurrent administration of other drugs that depend mainly on CYP3A for metabolism and whose blood levels, when ↑, are associated with serious/life-threatening adverse reactions including **alfuzosin**, **dihyroergotamine**, **ergotamine**, **lovastatin**, oral **midazolam**, **methylergonovine**, **pimozide**, **sildenafil** (when used for pulmonary hypertension), **simvastatin**, and **triazolam**; concurrent use contraindicated. **Carbamazepine**, **phenobarbital**, **phenytoin**, or **rifampin** may significantly ↓ levels/effectiveness of cobicistat and elvitegravir and ↑ risk of resistance; concurrent use contraindicated. Nephrotoxic agents, including **NSAIDs** ↑ risk of nephrotoxicity; avoid concurrent use. Drugs that induce CYP3A will ↓ levels/effectiveness of elvitegravir and cobicistat. Drugs that inhibit CYP3A will also ↑ levels/effectiveness of cobicistat. **Acyclovir**, **cidofovir**, **ganciclovir**, **valacyclovir**, and **valganciclovir** may ↓ renal elimination of emtricitabine and tenofovir, ↑ levels and effects. **Antacids**, including **aluminum and magnesium hydroxide**, may ↓ levels and effectiveness of elvitegravir (separate adminstration by at least 2 hr). ↑ blood levels and risk of toxicity from **amiodarone**, **digoxin**, **disopyramide**, **flecainide**, systemic **lidocaine**, **mexiletine**, **propafenone** or **quinidine**; careful monitoring recommended. May alter effects of **warfarin**. Concurrent use with **clarithromycin** or **telithromycin** can result in altered levels of clarithromycin and/or cobicistat (for patients with CCr 50–60 mL/min ↓ dose of clarithromycin by 50%), levels of telithromycin and/or cobicistat may be ↑. **Oxcarbamazepine**, may ↓ levels/effectiveness of cobicistat and elvitegravir; consider using alternative anticonvulsant. May ↑ levels of **clonazepam** and **ethosuximide** (clinical monitoring recommended). ↑ levels and risk of adverse effects with **SSRIs**, **tricyclic antidepressants**, and **trazodone** (careful titration and monitoring recommended). ↑ levels of **itraconazole**, **ketoconazole**, and **voriconazole** (maximum daily dose of ketoconazole or itraconazole should not exceed 300 mg, voriconazole with extreme caution). These **azole antifungals** may also ↑ levels of cobicistat and elvitegravir. ↑ levels and risk of toxicity from colchicine (concurrent use is contraindicated in patients with renal or hepatic impairment), *gout flares*—0.6 mg followed by 0.3 mg 1 hr later, do not repeat for at least three days; *prophylaxis of gout flares*—0.3 mg once daily if original regimen was 0.6 mg twice daily, 0.3 mg every other day if original regimen was 0.6 mg daily; *treatment of familial Mediterranean fever*—not to exceed 0.6 mg daily, may be given as 0.3 mg twice daily. Concurrent use with **rifabutin** or **rifapentine** may significantly ↓

levels/effectiveness of cobicistat and elvitegravir and may foster resistance, concurrent use is not recommended. May ↑ levels and effects of **beta blockers** including **metoprolol** and **timolol;** careful monitoring is recommended, ↓ dose of beta blocker if necessary. May ↑ levels and effects of **calcium channel blockers** including **amlodipine**, **diltiazem**, **felodipine**, **nicardipine**, **nifedipine**, and **verapamil;** careful monitoring is recommended. ↓ blood levels/effectiveness and ↑ risk of resistance with concurrent systemic **dexamethasone**, consider other corticosteroids. ↑ systemic levels from long term use of nasal or inhaled **fluticasone**, consider other corticosteroids. ↑ levels and effects of **bosentan** (initiate bosentan at 62.5 mg daily or every other day if already receiving elvitegravir/cobicistat/emtricitabine/tenofovir for at least 10 days, if already receiving bosentan discontinue at least 36 hr prior to starting elvitegravir/cobicistat/emtricitabine/tenofovir; after 10 days, bosentan may be restarted at 62.5 mg daily or every other day). ↑ levels and risk of adverse effect with **atorvastatin** (initiate atorvastatin at lowest dose and titrate cautiously). ↑ levels of **norgestimate** and ↓ levels of **ethinyl estradiol** (due to unpredictable effects, non-hormonal contraception should be considered). ↑ levels and effects of **immunosuppressants** including **cyclosporine**, **sirolimus**, and **tacrolimus**, careful monitoring recommended. ↑ levels and risk of adverse cardiovascular reactions with **salmeterol**, concurrent use is not recommended. ↑ blood levels and effects of **neuroleptics** including **perphenazine**, **risperidone**, and **thioridazine**, neuroleptic dose may need to ↓. ↑ levels and risk of serious cardiovascular adverse effects from **PDE5 inhibitors** including **sildenafil**, **tadalafil**, and **vardenafil** (*for pulmonary hypertension*—sildenafil is contraindicated; in patients who have received elvitegravir/cobicistat/emtricitabine/tenofovir for at least 7 days, tadalafil may be started at 20 mg/day and carefully titrated if necessary to 40 mg/day; in patients already receiving tadalafil, discontinue for at least 24 hr before initiating elvitegravir/cobicistat/emtricitabine/tenofovir; after 7 days, resume at 20 mg/day and titirate as necessary to 40 mg/day; *for erectile dysfunction*—sildenafil dose should not exceed 25 mg in 48 hr, vardenafil dose should not exceed 2.5 mg in 72 hr, and tadalafil dose should not exceed 10 mg in 72 hr). ↑ levels and risk of sedation with **sedative/hypnotics** including **midazolam**, **clorazepate**, **diazepam**, **estazolam**, **flurazepam**, **buspirone**, and **zolpidem**; concurrent use with oral midazolam is contraindicated, dose reduction of parenteral midazolam should be considered, clinical monitoring and dose reduction if necessary is recommended for others.

Drug-Natural Products: St. John's wort may significantly ↓ levels/effectiveness of cobicistat and elvitegravir and ↑ risk of resistance; concurrent use contraindicated.

Route/Dosage

PO (Adults): One tablet once daily.

Availability

Tablets: elvitegravir 150 mg/cobicistat 150 mg/emtricitabine 200 mg/tenofovir 300 mg.

NURSING IMPLICATIONS

Assessment

- Assess for change in severity of HIV symptoms and for symptoms of opportunistic infections during therapy.
- Monitor bone mineral density in patients who have a history of pathologic bone fracture or are at risk for osteoporosis or bone loss.
- ***Lab Test Considerations:*** Monitor viral load and CD4 cell count regularly during therapy.
- Assess for hepatitis B virus (HBV). *Stribild* is not approved for administration in patients with HIV and HBV.
- Monitor liver function tests before and periodically during therapy, especially in patients with underlying liver disease or marked ↑ transaminase. May cause ↑ serum creatinine, AST, ALT, total bilirubin, total cholesterol, LDL, amylase, and triglycerides. Lactic acidosis may occur with hepatic toxicity causing hepatic steatosis; may be fatal, especially in women.
- Calculate creatinine clearance (CCr), urine glucose, and urine protein prior to therapy. CCr should be >70 mL/min before starting therapy. Monitor CCr, urine glucose, and urine protein in all patients periodically during therapy and serum phosphorous in patients at risk for renal impairment. Assess patients with persistent or worsening bone pain, pain in extremities, fractures and/or muscular pain or weakness for proximal renal tubulopathy; evaluate renal function promptly.

Potential Nursing Diagnoses

Risk for infection (Indications)
Noncompliance (Patient/Family Teaching)

Implementation

- **PO:** Administer once daily with food.

Patient/Family Teaching

- Emphasize the importance of taking *Stribild* as directed, at the same time each day. Do not take more than prescribed amount and do not stop taking without consulting health care professional. Take missed doses with a meal if remembered unless almost time for next dose; do not double doses. Advise patient to read *Patient Information* prior to starting therapy and with each Rx refill in case of changes.
- Advise patient to take antacids 2 hr before or 4 hr after and H_2 antagonists 12 hr before or 4 hr after *Stribild*.
- Instruct patient that *Stribild* should not be shared with others.
- Inform patient that *Stribild* does not cure AIDS or prevent associated or opportunistic infections. Rilpivirine does not reduce the risk of transmission of HIV to others through sexual contact or blood con-

tamination. Caution patient to use a condom and to avoid sharing needles or donating blood to prevent spreading the AIDS virus to others. Advise patient that the long-term effects of *Stribild* are unknown at this time.

- Advise patient to notify health care professional immediately if symptoms of lactic acidosis (nausea, vomiting, unusual or unexpected stomach discomfort, and weakness) occur.
- Immune reconstitution syndrome may trigger opportunistic infections or autoimmune disorders. Notify health care professional if symptoms occur.
- May cause dizziness. Caution patient to avoid driving or other activities requiring alertness until response to medication is known.
- Advise patient to notify health care professional of all Rx or OTC medications, vitamins, or herbal products being taken and to consult with health care professional before taking other medications, especially St. John's wort.
- Inform patient that changes in body fat (increased fat in upper back and neck, breast, and around back, chest, and stomach area, loss of fats from legs, arms, and face) may occur.
- Rep: Advise patients to notify health care professional if pregnancy is planned or suspected. Advise patient to avoid breast feeding during *Stribild* therapy. Encourage women who become pregnant during *Stribild* therapy to enroll in Antiviral Pregnancy Registry by calling 1-800-258-4263.
- Emphasize the importance of regular follow-up exams and blood counts to determine progress and monitor for side effects.

Evaluation/Desired Outcomes

- Delayed progression of AIDS and decreased opportunistic infections in patients with HIV.
- Decrease in viral load and increase in CD4 cell counts.

empagliflozin

(em-pag-gli-**floe**-zin)

Jardiance

Classification

Therapeutic: antidiabetics

Pharmacologic: sodium-glucose co-transporter 2 (SGLT2) inhibitors

Pregnancy Category C

Indications

Adjunct to diet and exercise in the management of type 2 diabetes mellitus. May be used with other antidiabetic agents.

Action

Inhibits proximal renal tubular sodium-glucose co-transporter 2 (SGLT2) which determines reabsorption of glucose from the tubular lumen. Inhibits reabsorption of glucose, lowers renal threshold for glucose and increases excretion of glucose in urine. **Therapeutic Effects:** Improved glycemic control.

Pharmacokinetics

Absorption: Well absorbed following oral administration.

Distribution: Enters red blood cells, remainder of distribution unknown.

Metabolism and Excretion: Minimally metabolized; excreted in feces (41.2% mostly as unchanged drug) and urine (54.4% half as unchanged drug, half as metabolites).

Half-life: 12.4 hr.

TIME/ACTION PROFILE (↓ in A1c)

ROUTE	ONSET	PEAK	DURATION
PO	within 6 wk	12 wk	unknown

Contraindications/Precautions

Contraindicated in: Hypersensitivity; Renal impairment (eGFR< 45 mL/min/1.73 m^2/end-stage renal disease/dialysis); Type 1 diabetes; Diabetic ketoacidosis; Lactation: Avoid use, discontinue breast feeding or discontinue empagliflozin.

Use Cautiously in: Moderate renal impairment (↑ risk of adverse reactions related to ↓ intravascular volume); Hypotension (correct prior to treatment, especially in renal impairment, age >65 yr, or concurrent use of loop diuretics, ACE inhibitors, or ARBs; History of bladder cancer; OB: Use only if potential maternal benefit justifies potential fetal risk; Pedi: Safety and effectiveness not established; Geri: ↑ risk of adverse reactions related to ↓ intravascular volume.

Adverse Reactions/Side Effects

CV: hypotension, volume depletion. **GU:** genital mycotic infections, ↑ urination, urinary tract infections, renal impairment. **Endo:** hypoglycemia (↑ with other medications). **F and E:** hyperphosphatemia. **Metab:** hyperlipidemia.

Interactions

Drug-Drug: ↑ risk of hypotension with **antihypertensives** or **diuretics**. ↑ risk of hypoglycemia with other **antidiabetics** (dose adjustments maybe required).

Route/Dosage

PO (Adults): 10 mg once daily, may be ↑ to 25 mg once daily.

Availability

Tablets: 10 mg, 25 mg. ***In combination with:*** linagliptin (Glyxambi). See Appendix B.

NURSING IMPLICATIONS

Assessment

- Observe patient for signs and symptoms of hypoglycemic reactions (sweating, hunger, weakness, dizziness, confusion, headache, tremor, tachycardia, irritability, drowsiness).
- Monitor for signs and symptoms of volume depletion (dizziness, feeling faint, weakness, orthostatic hypotension) after initiating therapy, especially in elderly patients and patients with renal impairment, low systolic BP, or on diuretics.
- ***Lab Test Considerations:*** Monitor hemoglobin A1C prior to and periodically during therapy.
- May ↑ serum creatinine and ↓ eGFR. Monitor renal function prior to starting and periodically during therapy. Do not begin therapy if eGFR <45 mL/min/1.73 m^2. Discontinue therapy if eGFR is persistently <45 mL/min/1.73 m^2.
- May cause ↑ serum phosphate levels. Monitor electrolytes periodically during therapy.
- May cause ↑ LDL-C. Monitor serum lipid levels periodically during therapy.
- May cause ↑ hematocrit.

Potential Nursing Diagnoses

Imbalanced nutrition: more than body requirements (Indications)
Noncompliance (Patient/Family Teaching)

Implementation

- Patients stabilized on a diabetic regimen who are exposed to stress, fever, trauma, infection, or surgery may require administration of insulin.
- Correct volume depletion prior to beginning therapy with empagliflozin.
- **PO:** Administer once daily in the morning with or without food.

Patient/Family Teaching

- Instruct patient to take empagliflozin as directed. Take missed doses as soon as remembered, unless it is almost time for next dose; do not double doses. Advise patient to read the *Medication Guide* before starting and with each Rx refill in case of changes.
- Explain to patient that empagliflozin helps control hyperglycemia but does not cure diabetes. Therapy is usually long term.
- Instruct patient not to share this medication with others, even if they have the same symptoms; it may harm them.
- Encourage patient to follow prescribed diet, medication, and exercise regimen to prevent hyperglycemic or hypoglycemic episodes.
- Review signs of hypoglycemia and hyperglycemia with patient. If hypoglycemia occurs, advise patient to take a glass of orange juice or 2–3 tsp of sugar, honey, or corn syrup dissolved in water, and notify health care professional.
- Instruct patient in proper testing of blood glucose and urine ketones. Inform patient that empagliflozin will cause a positive test result when testing for urine glucose. Monitor closely during periods of stress or illness and health care professional notified if significant changes occur.
- Advise patient to notify health care professional if signs and symptoms of hypotension occur and to maintain adequate hydration as dehydration may increase risk of hypotension.
- Inform patient that empagliflozin may cause mycotic (yeast) infections. Women may have signs and symptoms of a vaginal yeast infection (vaginal odor, white or yellow vaginal discharge [may be lumpy or look like cottage cheese], vaginal itching). Men may have signs and symptoms of a yeast infection of the penis (redness, itching or swelling of penis; rash on penis; foul smelling discharge from penis; pain in skin around penis). Advise patient to notify health care professional if yeast infection occurs.
- Advise patient to notify health care professional if signs and symptoms of urinary tract infection (burning feeling when passing urine, cloudy urine, pain in pelvis or back) occur.
- Advise patient to notify health care professional of all Rx or OTC medications, vitamins, or herbal products being taken and to consult with health care professional before taking other medications, especially other oral hypoglycemic medications.
- Advise patient to notify health care professional if pregnancy is planned or suspected and to avoid breast feeding during therapy.
- Encourage patient to follow up with routine lab tests for blood glucose and renal function.

Evaluation/Desired Outcomes

- Improved hemoglobin A1C and glycemic control in adults with Type II diabetes.

emtricitabine

(em-tri-**si**-ti-been)
Emtriva

Classification
Therapeutic: antiretrovirals
Pharmacologic: nucleoside reverse transcriptase inhibitors

Pregnancy Category B

Indications

HIV infection (with other antiretrovirals).

Action

Phosphorylated intracellularly where it inhibits HIV reverse transcriptase, resulting in viral DNA chain termination. **Therapeutic Effects:** Slowed progression of

HIV infection and decreased occurrence of sequelae. Increases CD4 cell counts and decreases viral load.

Pharmacokinetics

Absorption: Rapidly and extensively absorbed; 93% bioavailable.
Distribution: Unknown.
Metabolism and Excretion: Some metabolism, 86% renally excreted, 14% fecal excretion.
Half-life: 10 hr.

TIME/ACTION PROFILE (blood levels†)

ROUTE	ONSET	PEAK	DURATION
PO	rapid	1–2 hr	24 hr

†Normal renal function.

Contraindications/Precautions

Contraindicated in: Hypersensitivity; Concurrent use of antiretroviral combination products containing emtricitabine or lamivudine-containing products; Lactation: Breast feeding not recommended in HIV-infected patients.
Use Cautiously in: Hepatitis B infection (may exacerbate following discontinuation); Renal impairment; OB: Use only if clearly needed; Geri: May be at ↑ risk for adverse effects.

Adverse Reactions/Side Effects

CNS: dizziness, headache, insomnia, weakness, depression, nightmares. **GI:** abdominal pain, diarrhea, nausea, SEVERE HEPATOMEGALY WITH STEATOSIS, dyspepsia, vomiting. **Derm:** rash, skin discoloration. **F and E:** LACTIC ACIDOSIS. **MS:** arthralgia, myalgia. **Neuro:** neuropathy, paresthesia. **Resp:** cough, rhinitis. **Misc:** fat redistribution, immune reconstitution syndrome.

Interactions

Drug-Drug: None noted.

Route/Dosage

PO (Adults ≥18 yr): 200 mg once daily.

Renal Impairment

PO (Adults ≥18 yr): *CCr 30–49 mL/min*—200 mg every 48 hr; *CCr 15–29 mL/min*—200 mg every 72 hr; *CCr <15 mL/min*—200 mg every 96 hr.

Availability

Capsules: 200 mg. **Oral solution (cotton candy flavor):** 10 mg/mL. ***In combination with:*** efavirenz and tenofovir (Atripla); tenofovir (Truvada); rilpivirine and tenofovir (Complera); elvitegravir, cobicistat, and tenofovir (Stribild). See Appendix B.

NURSING IMPLICATIONS

Assessment

- Assess patient for change in severity of HIV symptoms and for symptoms of opportunistic infections during therapy.
- May cause lactic acidosis and severe hepatomegaly with steatosis. These events are more likely to occur if patients are female, obese, or receiving nucleoside analogue medications for extended periods of time. Monitor patient for signs (increased serum lactate levels, elevated liver enzymes, liver enlargement on palpation). Therapy should be suspended if clinical or laboratory signs occur.
- Test patients for chronic hepatitis B virus (HBV) before initiating therapy. Emtricitabine is not indicated for treatment of HBV. Exacerbations of HBV have occurred upon discontinuation of emtricitabine.
- ***Lab Test Considerations:*** Monitor viral load and CD4 cell count regularly during therapy.
- May cause ↑ AST, ALT, bilirubin, creatine kinase, serum amylase, serum lipase, and triglycerides.May cause ↑ or ↓ serum glucose. May cause ↓ neutrophil count.

Potential Nursing Diagnoses

Risk for infection (Indications)
Noncompliance (Patient/Family Teaching)

Implementation

- **PO:** May be administered with or without food.

Patient/Family Teaching

- Emphasize the importance of taking emtricitabine as directed. It must always be used in combination with other antiretroviral drugs. Do not take more than prescribed amount and do not stop taking without consulting health care professional. Take missed doses as soon as remembered, but not if almost time for next dose; do not double doses.
- Instruct patient that emtricitabine should not be shared with others.
- Inform patient that emtricitabine does not cure AIDS or prevent associated or opportunistic infections. Emtricitabine does not reduce the risk of transmission of HIV to others through sexual contact or blood contamination. Caution patient to use a condom and to avoid sharing needles or donating blood to prevent spreading the AIDS virus to others. Advise patient that the long-term effects of emtricitabine are unknown at this time.
- Instruct patient to notify health care professional immediately if symptoms of lactic acidosis (tiredness or weakness, unusual muscle pain, trouble breathing, stomach pain with nausea and vomiting, cold especially in arms or legs, dizziness, fast or irregular heartbeat) or if signs of hepatotoxicity (yellow skin or whites of eyes, dark urine, light colored stools, lack of appetite for several days or longer, nausea, abdominal pain) occur. These symptoms may occur more frequently in patients that are female, obese, or have been taking medications like emtricitabine for a long time.

- Advise patient to notify health care professional if signs and symptoms of Immune Reconstitution Syndrome (signs and symptoms of an infection) occur.
- Inform patient that redistribution of body fat (central obesity, dorsocervical fat enlargement or buffalo hump, peripheral and facial wasting, breast enlargement, cushingoid appearance) and skin discoloration (hyperpigmentation on palms and soles) may occur.
- Advise patient to notify health care professional if she plans or suspects pregnancy or is breast feeding.
- Emphasize the importance of regular follow-up exams and blood counts to determine progress and monitor for side effects.

Evaluation/Desired Outcomes

- Delayed progression of AIDS and decreased opportunistic infections in patients with HIV.
- Decrease in viral load and increase in CD4 cell counts.

emtricitabine/rilpivirine/tenofovir

(em-tri-**si**-ti-been/**ril**–pi-vir-een/te-**noe**-fo-veer)

Complera

Classification

Therapeutic: antiretrovirals

Pharmacologic: nucleoside reverse transcriptase inhibitors, non-nucleoside reverse transcriptase inhibitors

Pregnancy Category B

Indications

Management of HIV infection in treatment-naïve adults with HIV-1 RNA <100,000 copies/mL at the start of therapy (for use as a complete regiment). Management of HIV infection in patients on a stable antiretroviral regimen with HIV-1 RNA <50 copies/mL (to replace their current antiretroviral regimen).

Action

Emtricitabine—Phosphorylated intracellularly where it inhibits HIV reverse transcriptase, resulting in viral DNA chain termination. *Rilpivirine*—Inhibits HIV-replication by noncompetitively inhibiting HIV reverse transcriptase. *Tenofovir*—Phosphorylated intracellularly where it inhibits HIV reverse transcriptase resulting in disruption of DNA synthesis. **Therapeutic Effects:** Slowed progression of HIV infection and decreased occurrence of sequelae.

Pharmacokinetics

emtricitabine

Absorption: Rapidly and extensively absorbed; 93% bioavailable.

Distribution: Unknown.

Metabolism and Excretion: Some metabolism, 86% renally excreted, 14% fecal excretion.

Half-life: 10 hr.

rilpivirine

Absorption: Well absorbed following oral administration.

Distribution: Unknown.

Protein Binding: 99.7%.

Metabolism and Excretion: Mostly metabolized by the liver (CYP3A enzyme system); 25% excreted in feces unchanged, <1% excreted unchanged in urine.

Half-life: 50 hr.

tenofovir

Absorption: Tenofovir disoproxil fumarate is a prodrug, which is split into tenofovir, the active component.

Distribution: Absorption is enhanced by food.

Metabolism and Excretion: 70–80% excreted unchanged in urine by glomerular filtration and active tubular secretion.

Half-life: Unknown.

TIME/ACTION PROFILE (blood levels)

ROUTE	ONSET	PEAK	DURATION
emtricitabine PO	rapid	1–2 hr	24 hr
rilpivirine PO	unknown	4–5 hr	24 hr
tenofovir PO	unknown	2 hr*	24 hr

* When taken with food.

Contraindications/Precautions

Contraindicated in: Drugs that may significantly ↓ rilpivirine levels (may ↓ virologic response, ↑ risk of resistance and cross-resistance); Concurrent use of other antiretrovirals; Concurrent use of carbamazepine, oxcarbazepine, phenobarbital, phenytoin, rifampin, rifapentine, proton pump inhibitors, dexamethasone (>1 dose), or St. John's wort; Concurrent use of other products containing emtricitabine, rilpivirine (unless dose adjustment needed with rifabutin), tenofovir, lamivudine, or adefovir; CCr <50 mL/min; Lactation: HIV-infected patients should not breast feed.

Use Cautiously in: History of suicidal ideation or depression; History of pathologic fractures/osteoporosis/bone loss; OB: Use during pregnancy only if potential benefit justifies potential fetal risk; Pedi: Safety and effectiveness not established.

Adverse Reactions/Side Effects

Combination.

GI: HEPATOTOXICITY. **GU:** renal impairment. **MS:** ↓ bone density. **Derm:** DRUG REACTION WITH EOSINOPHILIA AND SYSTEMIC SYMPTOMS (DRESS). **Misc:** POST-TREATMENT ACUTE EXACERBATION OF HEPATITIS B, fat redistribution, immune reconstitution syndrome.

rilpivirine

CNS: SUICIDAL THOUGHTS, depression, insomnia, headache.

emtricitabine/tenofovir

CNS: abnormal dreams, depression, dizziness, fatigue, headache, insomnia. **F and E:** hypophosphatemia. **GI:** diarrhea, nausea. **Derm:** rash. **GU:** ACUTE RENAL FAILURE/FANCONI SYNDROME. **MS:** bone pain, ↓ bone mineral density, muscle pain, osteomalacia.

Interactions

Drug-Drug: May ↑ risk of nephrotoxicity with other nephrotoxic drugs; avoid if possible. **Strong CYP3A4 inducers**, including **carbamazepine**, **oxcarbazepine**, **phenobarbital**, **phenytoin**, **dexamethasone** (more than a single dose), **rifabutin**, **rifampin**, and **rifapentine** may ↓ levels and effectiveness; concurrent use contraindicated; . **Proton pump inhibitors** including **esomeprazole**, **lansoprazole**, **omeprazole**, **pantoprazole**, and **rabeprazole** ↑ gastric pH and may ↓ blood levels and effectiveness; concurrent use contraindicated. **Antacids** including **aluminum hydroxide**, **magnesium hydroxide**, and **calcium carbonate** ↑ gastric pH and may ↓ blood levels; administer at least 2 hr before or 4 hr after. Blood levels and effectiveness may be ↓ by H_2-receptor antagonists including **cimetidine**, **famotidine**, **nizatidine**, and **ranitidine**; administer 12 hr after or 4 hr before. Nephrotoxic agents, including **NSAIDs** ↑ risk of nephrotoxicity; avoid concurrent use. Concurrent use of other **drugs that ↑ risk of torsade de pointes** may ↑ risk of serious arrhythmias. May alter requirements for **methadone** maintenance. Blood levels and risk of adverse effects may be ↑ by **clarithromycin**, **erythromycin**, and **troleandomycin**; consider azithromycin as an alternative.

Drug-Natural Products: St. John's wort may ↓ blood levels and effectiveness; concurrent use contraindicated.

Route/Dosage

PO (Adults): One tablet once daily. *Concurrent rifabutin therapy*—Give an additional 25 mg of rilpivirine once daily.

Availability

Tablets: emtricitabine 200 mg/rilpivirine 25 mg/ tenofovir 300 mg.

NURSING IMPLICATIONS

Assessment

- Assess for change in severity of HIV symptoms and for symptoms of opportunistic infections during therapy.
- Monitor closely for notable changes in behavior that could indicate the emergence or worsening of suicidal thoughts or behavior or depression.
- Monitor bone mineral density in patients who have a history of pathologic bone fracture or are at risk for osteoporosis or bone loss.
- Monitor for signs or symptoms of severe skin or hypersensitivity reactions (severe rash or rash accompanied by fever, blisters, mucosal involvement, conjunctivitis, facial edema, angioedema, hepatitis or eosinophilia). Discontinue *Complera* immediately if signs develop.
- Monitor bone mineral density in patients who have a history of pathologic bone fracture or are at risk for osteoporosis or bone loss.
- ***Lab Test Considerations:*** Monitor viral load and CD4 cell count regularly during therapy.
- Assess for hepatitis B virus (HBV). *Complera* is not approved for administration in patients with HIV and HBV.
- Monitor liver function tests before and periodically during therapy, especially in patients with underlying liver disease or marked ↑ transaminase. May cause ↑ serum creatinine, AST, ALT, total bilirubin, total cholesterol, LDL, and triglycerides. Lactic acidosis may occur with hepatic toxicity causing hepatic steatosis; may be fatal, especially in women.
- Calculate creatinine clearance (CCr), urine glucose, and urine protein prior to therapy. CCr should be >70 mL/min before starting therapy. Monitor CCr, urine glucose, and urine protein in all patients periodically during therapy and serum phosphorous in patients at risk for renal impairment. Assess patients with persistent or worsening bone pain, pain in extremities, fractures and/or muscular pain or weakness for proximal renal tubulopathy; evaluate renal function promptly.

Potential Nursing Diagnoses

Risk for infection (Indications)
Noncompliance (Patient/Family Teaching)

Implementation

- **PO:** Administer once daily with food.

Patient/Family Teaching

- Emphasize the importance of taking *Complera* as directed, at the same time each day. Do not take more than prescribed amount and do not stop taking without consulting health care professional. Take missed doses with a meal if remembered <12 hr from the time it is usually taken, then return to regular schedule. If more than 12 hr from time dose is usually taken, omit dose and resume dosing schedule; do not double doses. Advise patient to read *Patient Information* prior to starting therapy and with each Rx refill in case of changes.
- Advise patient to take antacids 2 hr before or 4 hr after and H_2-antagonists 12 hr before or 4 hr after *Complera*.
- Instruct patient that *Complera* should not be shared with others.
- Inform patient that *Complera* does not cure AIDS or prevent associated or opportunistic infections. Rilpi-

virine does not reduce the risk of transmission of HIV to others through sexual contact or blood contamination. Caution patient to use a condom and to avoid sharing needles or donating blood to prevent spreading the AIDS virus to others. Advise patient that the long-term effects of *Complera* are unknown at this time.

- Advise patient to notify health care professional immediately if symptoms of lactic acidosis (nausea, vomiting, unusual or unexpected stomach discomfort, and weakness) occur.
- Inform patients and families of risk of suicidal thoughts and behavior and advise that behavioral changes, emergency or worsening signs and symptoms of depression, unusual changes in mood, or emergence of suicidal thoughts, behavior, or thoughts of self-harm should be reported to health care professional immediately.
- Immune reconstitution syndrome may trigger opportunistic infections or autoimmune disorders. Notify health care professional if symptoms occur.
- May cause dizziness. Caution patient to avoid driving or other activities requiring alertness until response to medication is known.
- Advise patient to notify health care professional of all Rx or OTC medications, vitamins, or herbal products being taken and to consult with health care professional before taking other medications, especially St. John's wort.
- Inform patient that changes in body fat (increased fat in upper back and neck, breast, and around back, chest, and stomach area, loss of fats from legs, arms, and face) may occur.
- Rep: Advise patients to notify health care professional if pregnancy is planned or suspected. Advise patient to avoid breast feeding during *Complera* therapy. Encourage women who become pregnant during *Complera* therapy to enroll in Antiviral Pregnancy Registry by calling 1-800-258-4263.
- Emphasize the importance of regular follow-up exams and blood counts to determine progress and monitor for side effects.

Evaluation/Desired Outcomes

- Delayed progression of AIDS and decreased opportunistic infections in patients with HIV.
- Decrease in viral load and increase in CD4 cell counts.

---

enalapril/enalaprilat, See ANGIOTENSIN-CONVERTING ENZYME (ACE) INHIBITORS.

---

enoxaparin, See HEPARINS (LOW MOLECULAR WEIGHT).

---

entacapone (en-tak-a-pone)

Comtan

Classification
Therapeutic: antiparkinson agents
Pharmacologic: catechol-*O*-methyltransferase inhibitors

Pregnancy Category C

Indications

With levodopa/carbidopa to treat idiopathic Parkinson's disease when signs and symptoms of end-of-dose "wearing-off" (so-called fluctuating patients) occur.

Action

Acts as a selective and reversible inhibitor of the enzyme catechol *O*-methyltransferase (COMT). Inhibition of this enzyme prevents the breakdown of levodopa, increasing availability to the CNS. **Therapeutic Effects:** Prolongs duration of response to levodopa with end-of-dose motor fluctuations. Decreased signs and symptoms of Parkinson's disease.

Pharmacokinetics

Absorption: 35% absorbed following oral administration; absorption is rapid.
Distribution: Unknown.
Protein Binding: 98%.
Metabolism and Excretion: Minimal amounts excreted unchanged; highly metabolized followed by biliary excretion.
Half-life: *Initial phase*—0.4–0.7 hr; *second phase*—2.4 hr.

TIME/ACTION PROFILE (inhibition of COMT)

ROUTE	ONSET	PEAK	DURATION
PO	unknown	unknown	up to 8 hr

Contraindications/Precautions

Contraindicated in: Hypersensitivity; Concurrent nonselective MAO inhibitor therapy; Psychotic disorder.
Use Cautiously in: Hepatic impairment; Concurrent use of drugs that are metabolized by COMT; OB, Lactation: Safety not established; Pedi: No identified use in children.

Adverse Reactions/Side Effects

CNS: NEUROLEPTIC MALIGNANT SYNDROME, agitation, aggressive behavior, confusion, delirium, disorientation, dizziness, hallucinations, paranoid ideation, syncope, urges (gambling, sexual). **Resp:** pulmonary infiltrates, pleural effusion, pleural thickening. **CV:** hypotension. **Derm:** melanoma. **GI:** abdominal pain, colitis, diarrhea, nausea (during initiation), retroperitoneal fibrosis. **GU:** brownish-orange discoloration of urine. **MS:** RHABDOMYOLYSIS, dyskinesia. **Neuro:** dyskinesia.

Interactions

Drug-Drug: Concurrent use with selective **MAO inhibitors** is not recommended; both agents inhibit the metabolic pathways of catecholamines. Concurrent use of drugs that are metabolized by COMT such as **isoproterenol**, **epinephrine**, **norepinephrine**, **dopamine**, **dobutamine**, and **methyldopa** may ↑ risk of tachycardia, ↑ BP, and arrhythmias. **Probenecid**, **cholestyramine**, **erythromycin**, **rifampin**, **ampicillin**, and **chloramphenicol** may interfere with biliary elimination of entacapone; use concurrently with caution.

Route/Dosage

PO (Adults): 200 mg with each dose of levodopa/carbidopa up to a maximum of 8 times daily.

Availability (generic available)

Tablets: 200 mg. ***In combination with:*** levodopa/carbidopa (Stalevo), see Appendix B.

NURSING IMPLICATIONS

Assessment

- Assess parkinsonian and extrapyramidal symptoms (restlessness or desire to keep moving, rigidity, tremors, pill rolling, mask-like face, shuffling gait, muscle spasms, twisting motions, difficulty speaking or swallowing, loss of balance control) prior to and during therapy. Dyskinesia may increase with therapy.
- Monitor patient for development of diarrhea. Usually occurs within 4 to 12 wk of start of therapy, but may occur as early as the first week and as late as months after initiation of therapy.
- Monitor patient for signs and symptoms of neuroleptic malignant syndrome (elevated temperature, muscular rigidity, altered consciousness, elevated CPK). Symptoms have been associated with rapid dose reduction or withdrawal of other dopaminergic drugs. Withdrawal should be gradual.

Potential Nursing Diagnoses

Impaired physical mobility (Indications)
Risk for injury (Indications)

Implementation

- **PO:** Always administer entacapone with levodopa/carbidopa. Entacapone has no antiparkinsonism effects of its own.

Patient/Family Teaching

- Encourage patient to take entacapone as directed. Take missed doses as soon as possible, up to 2 hr before the next dose. Taper gradually when discontinuing or a withdrawal reaction may occur.
- May cause dizziness or hallucinations. Advise patient to avoid driving or other activities that require alertness until response to the drug is known.
- Inform patient that nausea may occur, especially at initiation of therapy and diarrhea. Advise patient with diarrhea to drink fluids to maintain adequate hydration and monitor for weight loss. If diarrhea is prolonged, may resolve with discontinuation. Therapy may cause change in urine color to brownish orange.
- Caution patient to change positions slowly to minimize orthostatic hypotension.
- Advise patient to notify health care professional if suspicious or unusual skin changes, agitation, aggression, delirium, hallucinations, or new or increased gambling, sexual, or other intense urges occur.
- Instruct patient to notify health care professional if pregnancy is planned or suspected, or if breast feeding.
- Emphasize the importance of routine follow-up exams.

Evaluation/Desired Outcomes

- Decreased signs and symptoms of Parkinson's disease.

E

entecavir (en-**tek**-aveer)

Baraclude

Classification
Therapeutic: antivirals
Pharmacologic: nucleoside analogues

Pregnancy Category C

Indications

Chronic hepatitis B infection with evidence of active viral replication and either persistent elevations in AST or ALT or histologically active disease.

Action

Phosphorylated intracellularly to active form which acts as an analogue of guanosine, interfering with viral DNA synthesis. **Therapeutic Effects:** Decreased hepatic damage due to chronic hepatitis B infection.

Pharmacokinetics

Absorption: Well absorbed following oral administration.
Distribution: Extensive tissue distribution.
Metabolism and Excretion: 62–73% excreted unchanged by kidneys.
Half-life: Plasma—128–149 hr; intracellular—15 hr.

TIME/ACTION PROFILE (blood levels)

ROUTE	ONSET	PEAK	DURATION
PO	rapid	0.5–1 hr	24 hr

Contraindications/Precautions

Contraindicated in: Hypersensitivity; Lactation: Potential for serious adverse effects in infant.

Use Cautiously in: Renal impairment (dose ↓ recommended if CCr <50 mL/min; Liver transplant recipients (careful monitoring of renal function recommended); Patients coinfected with HIV (unless receiving highly active antiretroviral therapy; at ↑ risk for resistance); OB: Use only if clearly needed, considering benefits and risks; Pedi: Children <2 yr (safety not established); Geri: ↑ risk of toxicity due to age-related ↓ in renal function.

Adverse Reactions/Side Effects

CNS: dizziness, fatigue, headache. **GI:** HEPATOMEGALY (WITH STEATOSIS), dyspepsia, nausea. **F and E:** LACTIC ACIDOSIS. **Derm:** alopecia, rash.

Interactions

Drug-Drug: Concurrent use of drugs which may impair renal function may ↑ blood levels and risk of toxicity.

Route/Dosage

PO (Adults and Children >16 yr): *Compensated liver disease*—0.5 mg once daily (1 mg once daily if history of lamivudine or telbivudine resistance); *Decompensated liver disease*—1 mg once daily.

Renal Impairment

PO (Adults and Children >16 yr): *CCr 30–<50 mL/min*—0.25 mg once daily or 0.5 mg q 48 hr (0.5 mg once daily or 1 mg q 48 hr if history of lamivudine resistance) *CCr 10– <30 mL/min*—0.15 mg once daily or 0.5 mg q 72 hr (0.3 mg once daily or 1 mg q 72 hr if history of lamivudine resistance); *CCr <10 mL/min*—0.05 mg once daily or 0.5 mg q 7 days (0.1 mg once daily or 1 mg q 7 days if history of lamivudine resistance).

PO (Children 2–<16 yr and 10–11 kg): 0.15 mg once daily (0.3 mg once daily if history of lamivudine resistance).

PO (Children 2–<16 yr and >11–14 kg): 0.2 mg once daily (0.4 mg once daily if history of lamivudine resistance).

PO (Children 2–<16 yr and >14–17 kg): 0.25 mg once daily (0.5 mg once daily if history of lamivudine resistance).

PO (Children 2–<16 yr and >17–20 kg): 0.3 mg once daily (0.6 mg once daily if history of lamivudine resistance).

PO (Children 2–<16 yr and >20–23 kg): 0.35 mg once daily (0.7 mg once daily if history of lamivudine resistance).

PO (Children 2–<16 yr and >23–26 kg): 0.4 mg once daily (0.8 mg once daily if history of lamivudine resistance).

PO (Children 2–<16 yr and >26–30 kg): 0.45 mg once daily (0.9 mg once daily if history of lamivudine resistance).

PO (Children 2–<16 yr and >30 kg): 0.5 mg once daily (1 mg once daily if history of lamivudine resistance).

Availability (generic available)

Tablets: 0.5 mg, 1 mg. **Oral solution (orange flavor):** 0.05 mg/mL.

NURSING IMPLICATIONS

Assessment

- Monitor signs of hepatitis (jaundice, fatigue, anorexia, pruritus) during and for several months following discontinuation of therapy. Exacerbations may occur when therapy is discontinued.
- May cause lactic acidosis and severe hepatomegaly with steatosis. Monitor patient for signs (↑ serum lactate levels, elevated liver enzymes, liver enlargement on palpation). Suspend therapy if clinical or laboratory signs occur.
- ***Lab Test Considerations:*** Monitor liver function closely during and for several months following discontinuation of therapy. May cause ↑ AST, ALT, bilirubin, amylase, lipase, creatinine, and serum glucose. May cause ↓ serum albumin.

Potential Nursing Diagnoses

Risk for infection (Indications)
Noncompliance (Patient/Family Teaching)

Implementation

- **PO:** Administer on an empty stomach at least 2 hr before or after a meal. Use oral solution for dose <0.5 mg and children up to 30 kg. Children >30 kg can use oral solution or tablet. Oral solution is ready to use and should not be diluted or mixed with water or any other liquid. Hold spoon in a vertical position and fill gradually to mark corresponding to the prescribed dose. Rinse dosing spoon with water after each daily dose. Store in outer carton at room temperature. After opening, solution can be used until expiration date on bottle.

Patient/Family Teaching

- Instruct patient to read the *Patient Information* with each refill and to take entecavir as directed. Take missed doses as soon as possible unless almost time for next dose. Do not run out of entecavir; get more when supply runs low. Do not double doses. Emphasize the importance of compliance with full course of therapy, not taking more than the prescribed amount, and not discontinuing without consulting health care professional. Inform patient that hepatitis exacerbation may occur upon discontinuation of therapy. Caution patient not to share medication with others.
- Inform patient that entecavir does not cure HBV disease, but may lower the amount of HBV in the body, lower the ability of HBV to multiply and infect new liver cells, and may improve the condition of the liver. Entecavir does not reduce the risk of transmission of HBV to others through sexual contact or blood contamination. Caution patient to use a condom during sexual contact and avoid sharing nee-

dles or donating blood to prevent spreading HBV to others.

- Advise patient to notify health care professional promptly if signs of lactic acidosis (weakness or tiredness; unusual muscle pain; trouble breathing; stomach pain with nausea and vomiting; feeling cold, especially in arms or legs; dizziness, fast or irregular heartbeat) or hepatotoxicity (jaundice, dark urine, light-colored bowel movements, anorexia, nausea, lower stomach pain) occur.
- May cause dizziness. Caution patient to avoid driving or other activities requiring alertness until response to medication is known.
- Instruct patient to notify health care professional of all Rx or OTC medications, vitamins, or herbal products being taken and to consult with health care professional before taking other medications.
- Discuss the possibility of hair loss with patient. Explore methods of coping.
- Advise patient to notify health care professional if pregnancy is planned or suspected or if breast feeding.
- Emphasize the importance of regular follow-up exams and blood tests to determine progress and monitor for side effects.

Evaluation/Desired Outcomes

- Decreased hepatic damage due to chronic hepatitis B infection.

enzalutamide

(en-za-**loo**-ta-mide)

Xtandi

Classification

Therapeutic: antineoplastics

Pharmacologic: androgen receptor inhibitors

Pregnancy Category X

Indications

Management of metastatic castration-resistant prostate cancer.

Action

Acts as an androgen receptor inhibitor, preventing the binding of androgen; also inhibits androgen nuclear translocation and DNA interaction. Decreases proliferation and induces cell death of prostate cancer cells.

Therapeutic Effects: Decreased growth and spread of prostate cancer.

Pharmacokinetics

Absorption: Well absorbed following oral administration.

Distribution: Unknown.

Protein Binding: *Enalutamide*—97–98%; *N-desmethylenzalutamide*—95%.

Metabolism and Excretion: Extensively metabolized by the liver (CYP2C8 and CYP3A4 enzyme systems); one metabolite (N-desmethylenzalutamide) has antineoplastic activity. Metabolites are primarily renally excreted, only minimal amounts as unchanged drug.

Half-life: *Enalutamide*—5.8 days; *N-desmethylenzalutamide*—7.8–8.6 days.

TIME/ACTION PROFILE (improved survival)

ROUTE	ONSET	PEAK	DURATION
PO	3 mo	unknown	unknown

Contraindications/Precautions

Contraindicated in: OB: Pregnancy (may cause fetal harm) or women with child-bearing potential.

Use Cautiously in: History of seizures, underlying brain pathology, cerebrovascular accident, transient ischemic attack (within 12 mo), brain metastases or brain arteriovenous malformation (may ↑ risk of seizures); Geri: May be more sensitive to drug effects; Pedi: Safety and effectiveness not established.

Adverse Reactions/Side Effects

CNS: POSTERIOR REVERSIBLE ENCEPHALOPATHY SYNDROME (PRES), SEIZURES, SPINAL CORD COMPRESSION/CAUDA EQUINA SYNDROME, headache, weakness, anxiety, dizziness, hallucinations, insomnia, mental impairment disorders. **EENT:** epistaxis. **CV:** peripheral edema, hypertension. **GI:** diarrhea. **GU:** hematuria, urinary frequency. **Derm:** hot flush, dry skin, pruritus. **MS:** arthralgia, musculoskeletal pain, muscular stiffness, musular weakness. **Neuro:** hypoesthesia, paresthesia.

Interactions

Drug-Drug: Strong inhibitors of the CYP2C8 enzyme system (including **gemfibrozil**) may ↑ blood levels and the risk of adverse reactions/toxicity and should be avoided; if concurrent administration is necessary, dose of enzalutamide should be ↓. **Strong/moderate inducers of the CYP3A4 or CYP2C8 enzyme systems** (including **rifampin**) may alter levels and response and should be avoided. **Substrates of the CYP3A4, CYP2C9 (including warfarin) and CYP2C19 systems that have narrow therapeutic indexes** should be avoided as their levels and activity may be ↓ careful monitoring is recommended. **Concurrent use of drugs that ↓ seizure threshold** may ↑ risk of seizures.

Route/Dosage

PO (Adults): 160 mg (four 40-mg capsules) once daily; if ≥Grade 3 toxicity or intolerable adverse reactions occur, discontinue for 1 wk and resume at the same or lower dose (80 or 120 mg). *Concurrent use of strong CYP2C8 inhibitors*—80 mg once daily.

Availability
Capsules: 40 mg.

NURSING IMPLICATIONS

Assessment
- Monitor for seizures. Implement seizure precautions. If a seizure occurs during therapy, permanently discontinue enzalutamine therapy.
- Monitor for signs and symptoms of PRES (seizure, headache, lethargy, confusion, blindness, other visual and neurological disturbances, hypertension) during therapy. Diagnosis is made with MRI. Discontinue enzalutamide in patients who develop PRES.
- ***Lab Test Considerations:*** May cause hematuria.

Potential Nursing Diagnoses
Activity intolerance

Implementation
- **PO:** Administer 4 capsules once daily without regard to food. Swallow capsules whole; do not open, dissolve, or chew.
- If ≥Grade 3 toxicity or intolerable side effects occur, withhold dose for 1 wk or until symptoms improve to <Grade 2, then resume at same or reduced dose (120 mg or 80 mg).

Patient/Family Teaching
- Instruct patient to take enzalutamide as directed at the same time each day. Take missed doses as soon as remembered within the same day. If a whole day is missed, omit dose and take next day's scheduled dose; do not double doses. Advise patient not to interrupt, modify dose, or stop taking enzalutamide without consulting health care professional. Advise patient to read *Patient Information* before starting therapy and with each Rx refill in case of changes.
- May cause seizures, dizziness, mental impairment, paresthesia, hypoesthesia, falls, and hallucinations. Caution patient to avoid driving and other activities requiring alertness until response to medication is known. Notify health care professional immediately if loss of consciousness, seizure, or signs and symptoms of PRES occur.
- Inform patient of common side effects associated with enzalutamide: asthenia/fatigue, back pain, diarrhea, arthralgia, hot flush, peripheral edema, musculoskeletal pain, headache, upper and lower respiratory infection, muscular weakness, dizziness, insomnia, spinal cord compression, cauda equina syndrome, hematuria, paresthesia, anxiety, and hypertension. Notify health care professional if falls or problems thinking clearly, or if side effects are bothersome.
- Instruct patient to notify health care professional of all Rx or OTC medications, vitamins, or herbal products being taken and to consult health care professional before taking other Rx, OTC, or herbal products.
- Rep: Caution patients that enzalutamide is teratogenic. Advise patient to avoid pregnancy and breast feeding during and for 3 mo following completion of therapy. Male patients should use a condom if having sex with a pregnant woman, and a condom and another effective method of birth control should be used if having sex with a woman of child-bearing potential.

Evaluation/Desired Outcomes
- Decreased growth and spread of prostate cancer.

EPIDURAL LOCAL ANESTHETICS

bupivacaine (byoo-**pi**-vi-kane)
Marcaine, Sensorcaine

ropivacaine (**roe**-pi-vi-kane)
Naropin

Classification
Therapeutic: epidural local anesthetics, anesthetics (topical/local)

Pregnancy Category B (ropivacaine), C (bupivacaine)

Indications
Local or regional anesthesia or analgesia for surgical, obstetric, or diagnostic procedures.

Action
Local anesthetics inhibit initiation and conduction of sensory nerve impulses by altering the influx of sodium and efflux of potassium in neurons, slowing or stopping pain transmission. Epidural administration allows action to take place at the level of the spinal nerve roots immediately adjacent to the site of administration. The catheter is placed as close as possible to the dermatomes (skin surface areas innervated by a single spinal nerve or group of spinal nerves) that, when blocked, will produce the most effective spread of analgesia for the site of injury. **Therapeutic Effects:** Decreased pain or induction of anesthesia; low doses have minimal effect on sensory or motor function; higher doses may produce complete motor blockade.

Pharmacokinetics
Absorption: Systemic absorption follows epidural administration, but amount absorbed depends on dose.
Distribution: Agents are lipid soluble, which selectively keeps them in the epidural space and limits systemic absorption. If systemic absorption occurs, these agents are widely distributed and cross the placenta.
Metabolism and Excretion: Small amounts that may reach systemic circulation are mostly metabolized by the liver. Very little excreted unchanged in the urine.
Half-life: *Bupivacaine*—1.5–5 hr (after epidural use); *ropivacaine*—4.2 hr (after epidural use).

TIME/ACTION PROFILE (analgesia)

ROUTE	ONSET	PEAK	DURATION
Epidural	10–30 min	unknown	2–8 hr†

†Duration of anesthetic block.

Contraindications/Precautions

Contraindicated in: Hypersensitivity; cross-sensitivity with other amide local anesthetics may occur (lidocaine, mepivacaine, prilocaine); Bupivacaine contains bisulfites and should be avoided in patients with known intolerance; OB: Bupivacaine only—Do not use 0.75% concentration. Only 0.5% and 0.25% concentrations should be used for obstetrical anesthesia due to reports of cardiac arrest and difficult resuscitation with the 0.75% concentration; Lactation: Discontinue nursing.
Use Cautiously in: Concurrent use of other local anesthetics; Liver disease; Concurrent use of anticoagulants (including low-dose heparin and low-molecular-weight heparins/heparinoids) ↑ the risk of spinal/epidural hematomas; OB: Bupivacaine and ropivacaine—both agents rapidly cross the placenta with obstetrical paracervical block anesthesia and can result in maternal, fetal, or neonatal toxicity with cardiac, central nervous system, or vascular tone abnormalities. May cause maternal hypotension; Pedi: Bupivacaine—safety not established in children <12 yr. Ropivacaine—safety not established in chlidren <18 yr; Geri: May require lower doses due to ↑ risk of hypotension and/or ↑ risk of toxicity due to age-related decline in renal function.

Adverse Reactions/Side Effects

CNS: SEIZURES, anxiety, dizziness, headache, irritability. **EENT:** blurred vision, tinnitus. **CV:** CARDIOVASCULAR COLLAPSE, arrhythmias, bradycardia, hypotension, tachycardia. **GI:** nausea, vomiting. **GU:** urinary retention. **Derm:** pruritus. **F and E:** metabolic acidosis. **Neuro:** circumoral tingling/numbness, tremor. **MS:** chondrolysis. **Misc:** allergic reactions, fever.

Interactions

Drug-Drug: Additive toxicity may occur with concurrent use of other **amide local anesthetics** (including **lidocaine**, **mepivacaine**, and **prilocaine**). Use of bupivacaine solution containing epinephrine with **MAO inhibitors** may cause hypertension. **Fluvoxamine**, **amiodarone**, **ciprofloxacin**, and **propofol** may ↑ effects of ropivacaine.

Route/Dosage

Solutions containing preservatives should not be used for caudal or epidural blocks.

Bupivacaine

Epidural (Adults and Children > 12 yr): 10–20 mL of 0.25% (partial to moderate block), 0.5% (moderate to complete block), or 0.75% (complete block) solution. Administer in increments of 3–5 mL allowing sufficient time to detect toxic signs/symptoms of inadvertent IV or IT administration. A test dose of 2–3 mL of 0.5% with epinephrine solution is recommended prior to epidural blocks.

Ropivacaine

Surgical Anesthesia

Epidural (Adults): *Lumbar epidural*—15–30 mL of 0.5% solution or 15–25 mL of 0.75% solution or 15–20 mL of 1% solution; *Lumbar epidural for cesarean section*—20–30 mL of 0.5% solution or 15–20 mL of 0.75% solution; *Thoracic epidural*—5–15 mL of 0.5–0.75% solution.

Labor Pain

Epidural (Adults): *Lumbar epidural*—10–20 mL of 0.2% solution initially, then continuous infusion of 6–14 mL/hr of 0.2% solution with incremental injection of 10–15 mL/hr of 0.2% solution.

Postoperative Pain

Epidural (Adults): *Lumbar or thoracic epidural*—Continuous infusion of 6–14 mL/hr of 0.2% solution.

Availability (generic available)

Bupivacaine

Solution for injection (preservative-free): 0.25%, 0.5%, 0.75%. ***In combination with:*** epinephrine 1:200,000.

Ropivacaine

Solution for injection (preservative-free): 0.2%, 0.5%, 0.75%, 1%.

NURSING IMPLICATIONS

Assessment

- Monitor for sensation during procedure and return of sensation after procedure.
- **Systemic Toxicity:** Assess for systemic toxicity (circumoral tingling and numbness, ringing in ears, metallic taste, dizziness, blurred vision, tremors, slow speech, irritability, twitching, seizures, cardiac dysrhythmias) each shift. Report to health care professional.
- **Orthostatic Hypotension:** Monitor BP, heart rate, and respiratory rate continuously while patient is receiving this medication. Mild hypotension is common because of the effect of local anesthetic block of nerve fibers on the sympathetic nervous system, causing vasodilation. Significant hypotension and bradycardia may occur, especially when rising from a prone position or following large dose increases or boluses. Treatment of unresolved hypotension may include hydration, decreasing the epidural infusion rate, and/or removal of local anesthetic from analgesic solution.
- **Unwanted Motor and Sensory Deficit:** The goal of adding low-dose local anesthetics to epidural opioids

for pain management is to provide analgesia, not to produce anesthesia. Patients should be able to ambulate if their condition allows, and epidural analgesic should not hamper this important recovery activity. However, many factors, including location of the epidural catheter, local anesthetic dose, and variability in patient response, can result in patients experiencing unwanted motor and sensory deficits. Pain is the first sensation lost, followed by temperature, touch, proprioception, and skeletal muscle tone.

- Assess for sensory deficit every shift. Ask patient to point to numb and tingling skin areas (numbness and tingling at the incision site is common and usually normal). Notify physician or other health care professional of unwanted motor and sensory deficits.
- Unwanted motor and sensory deficits often can be corrected with simple treatment. For example, a change in position may relieve temporary sensory loss in an extremity. Minor extremity muscle weakness is often treated by decreasing the epidural infusion rate and keeping the patient in bed until the weakness resolves. Sometimes removing the local anesthetic from the analgesic solution is necessary, such as when signs of local anesthetic toxicity are detected or when simple treatment of motor and sensory deficits has been unsuccessful.

Potential Nursing Diagnoses

Acute pain (Indications)
Impaired physical mobility (Side Effects)

Implementation

- See Route and Dosage section.

Patient/Family Teaching

- Instruct patient to notify nurse if signs or symptoms of systemic toxicity occur.
- Advise patient to request assistance during ambulation until orthostatic hypotension and motor deficits are ruled out.

Evaluation/Desired Outcomes

- Decrease in postoperative pain without unwanted sensory or motor deficits.

HIGH ALERT

EPINEPHrine (ep-i-nef-rin)

Adrenaclick, Adrenalin, ♣Allerject, ♣Anapen, ♣Anapen Junior, ~~AsthmaNefrin~~, Auvi-Q, EpiPen, ♣S-2 (racepinephrine), Twin-Ject

Classification
Therapeutic: antiasthmatics, bronchodilators, vasopressors
Pharmacologic: adrenergics

Pregnancy Category C
See Appendix C for ophthalmic use

Indications

Subcut, IV, Inhaln: Management of reversible airway disease due to asthma or COPD. **Subcut, IM, IV:** Management of severe allergic reactions. **IV, Intracardiac, Intratracheal, Intraosseous (part of advanced cardiac life support [ACLS] and pediatric advanced life support [PALS] guidelines):** Management of cardiac arrest (unlabeled). **Inhaln:** Management of upper airway obstruction and croup (racemic epinephrine). **Local/Spinal:** Adjunct in the localization/prolongation of anesthesia.

Action

Results in the accumulation of cyclic adenosine monophosphate (cAMP) at beta-adrenergic receptors. Affects both $beta_1$ (cardiac)-adrenergic receptors and $beta_2$ (pulmonary)-adrenergic receptor sites. Produces bronchodilation. Also has alpha-adrenergic agonist properties, which result in vasoconstriction. Inhibits the release of mediators of immediate hypersensitivity reactions from mast cells. **Therapeutic Effects:** Bronchodilation. Maintenance of heart rate and BP. Localization/prolongation of local/spinal anesthetic.

Pharmacokinetics

Absorption: Well absorbed following subcut administration; some absorption may occur following repeated inhalation of large doses.
Distribution: Does not cross the blood-brain barrier; crosses the placenta and enters breast milk.
Metabolism and Excretion: Action is rapidly terminated by metabolism and uptake by nerve endings.
Half-life: Unknown.

TIME/ACTION PROFILE (bronchodilation)

ROUTE	ONSET	PEAK	DURATION
Inhaln	1 min	unknown	1–3 hr
Subcut	5–10 min	20 min	<1–4 hr
IM	6–12 min	unknown	<1–4 hr
IV	rapid	20 min	20–30 min

Contraindications/Precautions

Contraindicated in: Hypersensitivity to adrenergic amines; Some products may contain bisulfites or fluorocarbons (in some inhalers) and should be avoided in patients with known hypersensitivity or intolerance.
Use Cautiously in: Cardiac disease (angina, tachycardia, MI); Hypertension; Hyperthyroidism; Diabetes; Cerebral arteriosclerosis; Glaucoma (except for ophthalmic use); Excessive use may lead to tolerance and paradoxical bronchospasm (inhaler); OB: Use only if potential maternal benefit outweighs potential risks to fetus; Lactation: High intravenous doses of epinephrine might ↓ milk production or letdown. Low-dose epidural, topical, inhaled, or ophthalmic epinephrine are unlikely to interfere with breast feeding (NIH); Geri: More susceptible to adverse reactions; may require ↓ dose.

Adverse Reactions/Side Effects

CNS: nervousness, restlessness, tremor, headache, insomnia. **Resp:** PARADOXICAL BRONCHOSPASM (EXCESSIVE

USE OF INHALERS). **CV:** angina, arrhythmias, hypertension, tachycardia. **GI:** nausea, vomiting. **Endo:** hyperglycemia.

Interactions

Drug-Drug: Concurrent use with other **adrenergic agents** will have additive adrenergic side effects. Use with **MAO inhibitors** may lead to hypertensive crisis. **Beta blockers** may negate therapeutic effect. **Tricyclic antidepressants** enhance pressor response to epinephrine.

Drug-Natural Products: Use with caffeine-containing herbs (**cola nut**, **guarana**, **mate**, **tea**, **coffee**) ↑ stimulant effect.

Route/Dosage

Subcut, IM (Adults): *Anaphylactic reactions/asthma*—0.1–0.5 mg (single dose not to exceed 1 mg); may repeat q 10–15 min for anaphylactic shock or q 20 min–4 hr for asthma.

Subcut (Children > 1 mo): *Anaphylactic reactions/asthma*—0.01 mg/kg (not to exceed 0.5 mg/dose) q 15 min for 2 doses, then q 4 hr.

IV (Adults): *Severe anaphylaxis*—0.1–0.25 mg q 5–15 min; may be followed by 1–4 mcg/min continuous infusion; *cardiopulmonary resuscitation (ACLS guidelines)*—1 mg q 3–5 min; *bradycardia (ACLS guidelines)*—2–10 mcg/min).

IV (Children): *Severe anaphylaxis*—0.1 mg (less in younger children); may be followed by 0.1 mcg/kg/min continuous infusion (may be ↑ up to 1.5 mcg/kg/min); *symptomatic bradycardia/pulseless arrest (PALS guidelines)*—0.01 mg/kg, may be repeated q 3–5 min, higher doses (up to 0.1–0.2 mg/kg) may be considered; may also be given by the intraosseous route. May also be given by the endotracheal route in doses of 0.1—0.2 mg/kg diluted to a volume of 3–5 mL with normal saline followed by several positive pressure ventilations.

Inhaln (Adults): *Inhalation solution*—1 inhalation of 1% solution; may be repeated after 1–2 min; additional doses may be given q 3 hr; *racepinephrine*—Via hand nebulizer, 2–3 inhalations of 2.25% solution; may repeat in 5 min with 2–3 more inhalations, up to 4–6 times daily.

Inhaln (Children > 1 mo): 0.25–0.5 mL of 2.25% racemic epinephrine solution diluted in 3 mL normal saline.

IV, Intratracheal (Neonates): 0.01–0.03 mg/kg q 3–5 min as needed.

IM (Children > 1 mo <30 kg): 0.15 mg (EpiPen Jr); > 30 kg: 0.3 mg (EpiPen).

Intracardiac (Adults): 0.3–0.5 mg.

Endotracheal (Adults): *Cardiopulmonary resuscitation (ACLS guidelines)*—2–2.5 mg.

Topical (Adults and Children ≥6 yr): *Nasal decongestant*—Apply 1% solution as drops, spray, or with a swab.

Intraspinal (Adults and Children): 0.2–0.4 mL of 1:1000 solution.

With Local Anesthetics (Adults and Children): Use 1:200,000 solution with local anesthetic.

Availability (generic available)

Inhalation solution (racepinephrine): ✤2.25%. **Intranasal solution:** 1 mg/mL (1:1000). **Solution for injection:** 0.1 mg/mL (1:10,000), 1 mg/mL (1:1000). **Autoinjector (Auvi-Q, EpiPen):** 0.15 mg/0.15 mL (1:1000), 0.15 mg/0.3 mL (1:2000), 0.3 mg/0.3 mL (1:1000).

NURSING IMPLICATIONS

Assessment

- **Bronchodilator:** Assess lung sounds, respiratory pattern, pulse, and BP before administration and during peak of medication. Note amount, color, and character of sputum produced, and notify health care professional of abnormal findings.
- Monitor pulmonary function tests before and periodically during therapy.
- Observe for paradoxical bronchospasm (wheezing). If condition occurs, withhold medication and notify health care professional immediately.
- Observe patient for drug tolerance and rebound bronchospasm. Patients requiring more than 3 inhalation treatments in 24 hr should be under close supervision. If minimal or no relief is seen after 3–5 inhalation treatments within 6–12 hr, further treatment with aerosol alone is not recommended.
- Assess for hypersensitivity reaction (rash; urticaria; swelling of the face, lips, or eyelids). If condition occurs, withhold medication and notify health care professional immediately.
- **Vasopressor:** Monitor BP, pulse, ECG, and respiratory rate frequently during IV administration. Continuous ECG, hemodynamic parameters, and urine output should be monitored continuously during IV administration.
- Monitor for chest pain, arrhythmias, heart rate >110 bpm, and hypertension. Consult physician for parameters of pulse, BP, and ECG changes for adjusting dose or discontinuing medication.
- **Shock:** Assess volume status. Correct hypovolemia prior to administering epinephrine IV.
- **Nasal Decongestant:** Assess patient for nasal and sinus congestion prior to and periodically during therapy.
- ***Lab Test Considerations:*** May cause transient ↓ in serum potassium concentrations with nebulization or at higher than recommended doses.
- May cause an ↑ in blood glucose and serum lactic acid concentrations.

- ***Toxicity and Overdose:*** Symptoms of overdose include persistent agitation, chest pain or discomfort, decreased BP, dizziness, hyperglycemia, hypokalemia, seizures, tachyarrhythmias, persistent trembling, and vomiting.
- Treatment includes discontinuing adrenergic bronchodilator and other beta-adrenergic agonists and symptomatic, supportive therapy. Cardioselective beta blockers are used cautiously because they may induce bronchospasm.

Potential Nursing Diagnoses

Ineffective airway clearance (Indications)
Ineffective tissue perfusion (Indications)

Implementation

- Do not confuse epinephrine with ephedrine.
- ***High Alert:*** Patient harm or fatalities have occurred from medication errors with epinephrine. Epinephrine is available in various concentrations, strengths, and percentages and used for different purposes. Packaging labels may be easily confused or products incorrectly diluted. Dilutions should be prepared by a pharmacist. IV doses should be expressed in milligrams not ampules, concentration, or volume. Prior to administration, have second practitioner independently check original order, dose calculations, concentration, route of administration, and infusion pump settings.
- Medication should be administered promptly at the onset of bronchospasm.
- Use a tuberculin syringe with a 26-gauge ½-in. needle for subcut injection to ensure that correct amount of medication is administered.
- Tolerance may develop with prolonged or excessive use. Effectiveness may be restored by discontinuing for a few days and then readministering.
- Do not use solutions that are pinkish or brownish or that contain a precipitate.
- For anaphylactic shock, volume replacement should be administered concurrently with epinephrine. Antihistamines and corticosteroids may be used in conjunction with epinephrine.
- **IM, Subcut:** Medication can cause irritation of tissue. Rotate injection sites to prevent tissue necrosis. Massage injection sites well after administration to enhance absorption and to decrease local vasoconstriction. Avoid IM administration in gluteal muscle.

IV Administration

- **IV Push:** ***Diluent:*** The 1:10,000 solution can be administered undiluted. Dilute 1 mg (1 mL) of a 1:1000 solution in 9 mL of 0.9% NaCl to prepare a 1:10,000 solution. ***Concentration:*** 0.1 mg/mL (1:10,000). ***Rate:*** Administer each 1 mg (10 mL) of a 1:10,000 solution over at least 1 min; more rapid administration may be used during cardiac resuscitation. Follow each dose with 20 mL IV saline flush.
- **Continuous Infusion:** ***Diluent:*** Dilute 1 mg (1 mL) of a 1:1000 solution in 250 mL of D5W or 0.9% NaCl. Protect from light. Infusion stable for 24 hr. ***Concentration:*** 4 mcg/mL. ***Rate:*** See Route/Dosage section. Titrate to response (BP, heart rate, respiratory rate).
- **Y-Site Compatibility:** alfentanil, amikacin, aminocaproic acid, amiodarone, amphotericin B lipid complex, amphotericin B liposome, anidulafungin, argatroban, ascorbic acid, atropine, azithromycin, aztreonam, benztropine, bivalirudin, bleomycin, bumetanide, buprenorphine, butorphanol, calcium chloride, calcium gluconate, cangrelor, carboplatin, caspofungin, cefazolin, cefotaxime, cefotetan, cefoxitin, ceftazidime, ceftriaxone, cefuroxime, chloramphenicol , chlorpromazine, cisatracurium, cisplatin, clindamycin, cyanocobalamin, cyclophosphamide, cyclosporine, cytarabine, dactinomycin, daptomycin, daunorubicin hydrochloride, dexamethasone, dexmedetomidine, dexrazoxane, digoxin, diltiazem, diphenhydramine, dobutamine, docetaxel, dolasetron, dopamine, doxorubicin hydrochloride, doxorubicin liposomal, doxycycline, enalaprilat, ephedrine, epirubicin, epoetin alfa, eptifibatide, ertapenem, erythromycin, esmolol, etoposide, etoposide phosphate, famotidine, fenoldopam, fentanyl, fluconazole, fludarabine, folic acid, foscarnet, fosphenytoin, furosemide, gemcitabine, gentamicin, glycopyrrolate, granisetron, heparin, hetastarch, hydrocortisone sodium succinate, hydromorphone, ibuprofen, idarubicin, ifosfamide, imipenem/cilastatin, irinotecan, isoproterenol, ketamine, ketorolac, labetalol, calcium, levofloxacin, lidocaine, linezolid, lorazepam, magnesium sulfate, mannitol, mechlorethamine, meperidine, mesna, methotrexate, methyldopate, methylprednisolone sodium succinate, metoclopramide, metoprolol, metronidazole, midazolam, milrinone, mitoxantrone, morphine, moxifloxacin, multiple vitamins, mycophenolate, nafcillin, nalbuphine, naloxone, nicardipine, nitroglycerin, nitroprusside, norepinephrine, octreotide, ondansetron, oxacillin, oxaliplatin, oxytocin, paclitaxel, palonosetron, pamidronate, pancuronium, pantoprazole, papaverine, pantoprazole, pemetrexed, penicillin G, pentamidine, pentazocine, phenylephrine, phytonadione, piperacillin/tazobactam, potassium acetate, potassium chloride, procainamide, prochlorperazine, promethazine, propranolol, protamine, pyridoxine, quinupristin/dalfopristin, ranitidine, remifentanil, rocuronium, sodium acetate, streptokinase, succinylcholine, sufentanil, tacrolimus, teniposide, theophylline, thiamine, thiotepa, tigecycline, tirofiban, tobramycin, vancomycin, vasopressin, vecuronium, verapamil, vinblastine, vincristine, vinorelbine, vitamin B complex with C, voriconazole, warfarin, zoledronic acid.
- **Y-Site Incompatibility:** acyclovir, alemtuzumab, aminophylline, amphotericin B colloidal, carmustine, dacarbazine, dantrolene, diazepam, fluorouracil, fosphenytoin, ganciclovir, indomethacin, micafungin, pentobarbital, phenobarbital, phenytoin,

sodium bicarbonate, thiopental, trimethoprim/sulfamethoxazole.

- **Inhaln:** When using epinephrine inhalation solution, 10 drops of 1% base solution should be placed in the reservoir of the nebulizer.
- The 2.25% inhalation solution of racepinephrine must be diluted for use in the combination nebulizer/respirator.
- Allow 1–2 min to elapse between inhalations of epinephrine inhalation solution to make certain the second inhalation is necessary.
- When epinephrine is used concurrently with corticosteroid or ipratropium inhalations, administer bronchodilator first and other medications 5 min apart to prevent toxicity from inhaled fluorocarbon propellants.
- **Endotracheal:** Epinephrine can be injected directly into the bronchial tree via the endotracheal tube if the patient has been intubated. Perform 5 rapid insufflations; forcefully administer 10 mL containing 2–2.5 mg epinephrine (1 mg/mL) directly into tube; follow with 5 quick insufflations.

Patient/Family Teaching

- Instruct patient to take medication exactly as directed. If on a scheduled dosing regimen, take a missed dose as soon as possible; space remaining doses at regular intervals. Do not double doses. Caution patient not to exceed recommended dose; may cause adverse effects, paradoxical bronchospasm, or loss of effectiveness of medication.
- Instruct patient to contact health care professional immediately if shortness of breath is not relieved by medication or is accompanied by diaphoresis, dizziness, palpitations, or chest pain.
- Advise patient to consult health care professional before taking any OTC medications or alcoholic beverages concurrently with this therapy. Caution patient also to avoid smoking and other respiratory irritants.
- **Inhaln:** Review correct administration technique (aerosolization, IPPB) with patient.
- Do not spray inhaler near eyes.
- Advise patients to use bronchodilator first if using other inhalation medications, and allow 5 min to elapse before administering other inhalant medications, unless otherwise directed.
- Advise patient to rinse mouth with water after each inhalation dose to minimize dry mouth.
- Advise patient to maintain adequate fluid intake (2000–3000 mL/day) to help liquefy tenacious secretions.
- Advise patient to consult health care professional if respiratory symptoms are not relieved or worsen after treatment or if chest pain, headache, severe dizziness, palpitations, nervousness, or weakness occurs.
- Advise patient to notify health care professional if pregnancy is planned or suspected or if breast feeding.
- **Autoinjector:** Instruct patients using auto-injector for anaphylactic reactions to remove gray safety cap, placing black tip on thigh at right angle to leg. Press hard into thigh until auto-injector functions, hold in place for 10 seconds, remove, and discard properly. Massage injected area for 10 sec. Pedi: Teach parents or caregivers signs and symptoms of anaphlyaxis, how to use auto-injector safely, and to get the child to a hospital as soon as possible. Instruct parents or caregivers to teach child how to manage his or her allergy, how to self-inject, and what to do in an emergency. For children too young to self-inject and who will be separated from parent, tell parents to always discuss allergy and use of auto-injector with responsible adult.

Evaluation/Desired Outcomes

- Prevention or relief of bronchospasm.
- Increase in ease of breathing.
- Prevention of bronchospasm or reduction of frequency of acute asthma attacks in patients with chronic asthma.
- Prevention of exercise-induced asthma.
- Reversal of signs and symptoms of anaphylaxis.
- Increase in cardiac rate and output, when used in cardiac resuscitation.
- Increase in BP, when used as a vasopressor.
- Localization of local anesthetic.
- Decrease in sinus and nasal congestion.

HIGH ALERT

epirubicin (ep-i-**roo**-bi-sin)

Ellence, ✤Pharmorubicin PFS

Classification

Therapeutic: antineoplastics

Pharmacologic: anthracyclines

Pregnancy Category D

Indications

A component of adjuvant therapy for evidence of axillary tumor involvement following resection of primary breast cancer.

Action

Inhibits DNA and RNA synthesis by forming a complex with DNA. **Therapeutic Effects:** Death of rapidly replicating cells, particularly malignant ones.

Pharmacokinetics

Absorption: IV administration results in complete bioavailability.

Distribution: Rapidly and widely distributed; concentrates in RBCs.

Metabolism and Excretion: Extensively and rapidly metabolized by the liver and other tissues.
Half-life: 35 hr.

TIME/ACTION PROFILE (effect on WBCs)

ROUTE	ONSET	PEAK	DURATION
IV	unknown	10–14 days	21 days

Contraindications/Precautions

Contraindicated in: Hypersensitivity to epirubicin, other anthracyclines, or related compounds; Baseline neutrophil count <1500 cells/mm^3; Heart failure; Recent MI; Severe arrhythmias; Previous treatment with anthracyclines up to the maximum cumulative dose; Severe hepatic dysfunction; Concurrent cimetidine therapy; OB, Lactation: Significant risk for fetal or infant harm.
Use Cautiously in: Cardiovascular disease, prior or concomitant radiation therapy to mediastinal or pericardial area, previous therapy with anthracyclines, or concomitant use of cardiotoxic drugs (↑ risk of cardiotoxicity); Severe renal impairment (serum creatinine >5 m g/dL); consider ↓ dose; Hepatic impairment (dose ↓ recommended for bilirubin >1.2 m g/dL or AST >2.2 m–4 times upper limit of normal); Depressed bone marrow reserve; Rep: Patients with child-bearing potential; Pedi: Safety not established; ↑ risk of acute cardiotoxicity and chronic HF; Geri: ↑ risk of toxicity in female patients ≥70 yr.

Adverse Reactions/Side Effects

CNS: lethargy. **CV:** CARDIOTOXICITY (dose-related), bradycardia, heart block, thromboembolism, ventricular tachycardia. **GI:** nausea, vomiting, anorexia, diarrhea, mucositis. **Derm:** alopecia, flushing, itching, photosensitivity, radiation-recall reaction, rash, skin/nail hyperpigmentation. **Endo:** gonadal suppression. **Hemat:** LEUKOPENIA, anemia, thrombocytopenia, treatment-related leukemia/myelodysplastic syndromes. **Local:** injection site reactions, phlebitis at IV site, tissue necrosis. **Metab:** hot flashes, hyperuricemia. **Misc:** ANAPHYLAXIS, INFECTION.

Interactions

Drug-Drug: Cimetidine ↑ blood levels and risk of serious toxicity; avoid concurrent use. Additive hematologic and gastrointestinal toxicity with other **antineoplastics** or **radiation therapy**. Use with other cardiotoxic drugs may ↑ risk of cardiotoxicity; avoid concurrent use. May ↓ antibody response to **live-virus vaccines** and ↑ risk of adverse reactions. **Trastuzumab** may ↑ risk of cardiotoxicity.

Route/Dosage

IV (Adults): 100–120 mg/m^2 repeated in 3–4 wk cycles (total dose may be given on day 1 or split and given in equally divided doses on day 1 and day 8 of each cycle (combination regimens may employ concurrent 5-fluorouracil and cyclophosphamide).

Hepatic Impairment

IV (Adults): *Bilirubin 1.2–3 mg/dL or AST 2–4 times upper limit of normal*—use 50% of recommended starting dose; *bilirubin >3 m g/dL or AST >4 times upper limit of normal*—use 25% of recommended starting dose.

Availability (generic available)

Powder for injection: ✱ 50 mg/vial. **Solution for injection (red):** 2 mg/mL.

NURSING IMPLICATIONS

Assessment

- Monitor for bone marrow depression. Assess for bleeding (bleeding gums, bruising, petechiae, guaiac stools, urine, and emesis) and avoid IM injections and taking rectal temperatures if platelet count is low. Apply pressure to venipuncture sites for 10 min. Assess for signs of infection during neutropenia. Anemia may occur. Monitor for increased fatigue, dyspnea, and orthostatic hypotension.
- Severe nausea and vomiting may occur. Administer parenteral antiemetic agents 30–45 min prior to therapy and routinely around the clock for next 24 hr as indicated. Monitor amount of emesis and notify health care professional if emesis exceeds guidelines to prevent dehydration.
- Measure cardiac function, using ECG and a multigated radionuclide angiography (MUGA) scan or an ECHO, prior to therapy. Perform repeated evaluations of left ventricular ejection fraction during therapy. Monitor for development of signs of cardiac toxicity, which may occur early (ST-T wave changes, sinus tachycardia, and extrasystoles) or late (may occur mo to yr after termination of therapy). Delayed cardiac toxicity is characterized by cardiomyopathy, tachycardia, peripheral edema, dyspnea, rales/crackles, weight gain, hepatomegaly, ascites, pleural effusion. Toxicity is usually dependent on cumulative dose.
- Assess injection site frequently for redness, irritation, or inflammation. Burning or stinging during infusion may indicate infiltration and infusion should be discontinued and restarted in another vein. Epirubicin is a vesicant but may infiltrate painlessly even if blood returns on aspiration of infusion needle. Severe tissue damage may occur if epirubicin extravasates. If extravasation occurs, stop infusion immediately, restart, and complete dose in another vein.
- Assess oral mucosa frequently for development of stomatitis (pain, burning, erythema, ulcerations, bleeding, infection). Increased dosing interval and/or decreased dosing is recommended if lesions are painful or interfere with nutrition.
- ***Lab Test Considerations:*** Monitor CBC and differential before and during each cycle of therapy. Epirubicin should not be administered to patients with a baseline neutrophil count <1500 cells/mm^3. The WBC nadir occurs 10–14 days after administra-

tion, and recovery usually occurs by the 21st day. Severe thrombocytopenia and anemia may also occur.
- Monitor renal (BUN and creatinine) and hepatic (AST, ALT, LDH, and serum bilirubin) function prior to and periodically during therapy. Dose reduction is required for bilirubin >1.2 m g/dL, AST 2–4 times the upper limit of normal, or serum creatinine >5 m g/dL.

Potential Nursing Diagnoses

Risk for infection (Adverse Reactions)
Decreased cardiac output (Adverse Reactions)

Implementation

- ***High Alert:*** Fatalities have occurred with incorrect administration of chemotherapeutic agents. Before administering, clarify ambiguous orders; double-check single, daily, and course-of-therapy dose limits; have second practitioner independently double-check original order, calculations and infusion pump settings. Epirubicin should be administered only under the supervision of a physician experienced in the use of cancer chemotherapeutic agents.
- ***High Alert:*** Do not confuse epirubicin with eribulin.
- Prepare solution in a biologic cabinet. Wear gloves, gown, and mask while handling medication. Discard IV equipment in specially designated containers.
- Administer prophylactic anti-infective therapy with trimethoprim/sulfamethoxazole or a fluoroquinolone and antiemetic therapy prior to administration of epirubicin.
- Do not administer subcut or IM.

IV Administration

- **Intermittent Infusion: *Diluent:*** Administer undiluted. Solution is clear red. Use epirubicin within 24 hr of penetration of rubber stopper. Discard unused solution. ***Concentration:*** 2 mg/mL. ***Rate:*** Administer initial dose of 100–120 mg/m^2 over 15–20 min through free-flowing infusion of 0.9% NaCl or D5W. Lower doses may be infused for shorter periods, but not less than over 3 min. Do not administer via IV push. Facial flushing and erythema along involved vein frequently occur when administration is too rapid. Venous sclerosis may result from injection into a small vein or repeated injections into the same vein. Avoid veins over joints or in extremities with compromised venous or lymphatic drainage.
- **Y-Site Compatibility:** alemtuzumab, alfentanil, amifostine, amikacin, aminocaproic acid, anidulafungin, argatroban, aztreonam, bivalirudin, bleomycin, bumetanide, buprenorphine, butorphanol, calcium chloride, calcium gluconate, carboplatin, caspofungin, cefazolin, cefotaxime, chlorpromazine, ciprofloxacin, cisatracurium, cisplatin, clindamycin, cyclophosphamide, cyclosporine, daptomycin, dexrazoxane, digoxin, diltiazem, diphenhydramine, dobutamine, docetaxel, dolasetron, dopamine, doxycycline, droperidol, enalaprilat, ephedrine, epinephrine, erythromycin, etoposide, etoposide phosphate, famotidine, fenoldopam, fentanyl, fluconazole, gemcitabine, gentamicin, granisetron, haloperidol, hydrocortisone sodium succinate, hydromorphone, ifosfamide, imipenem cilastatin, insulin, isoproterenol, labetalol, levofloxacin, levorphanol, lidocaine, linezolid, lorazepam, mannitol, meperidine, mesna, methotrexate, metoclopramide, metoprolol, metronidazole, midazolam, milrinone, mitomycin, morphine, moxifloxacin, nalbuphine, naloxone, nesiritide, nicardipine, nitroglycerin, nitroprusside, norepinephrine, octreotide, ondansetron, oxaliplatin, paclitaxel, palonosetron, pamidronate, pancuronium, pentamidine, pentazocine, phenylephrine, potassium acetate, potassium chloride, procainamide, prochlorperazine, promethazine, propranolol, quinapristin/dalfopristin, ranitidine, remifentanil, rocuronium, sodium acetate, succinylcholine, sufentanil, tacrolimus, teniposide, theophylline, thiotepa, tirofiban, tobramycin, vancomycin, vasopressin, vecuronium, verapamil, vinblastine, vincristine, vinorelbine, voriconazole, zidovudine, zoledronic acid.
- **Y-Site Incompatibility:** acyclovir, allopurinol, aminophylline, amphotericin B colloidal, amphotericin B lipid complex, amphotericin B liposome, ampicillin, ampicillin/sulbactam, azithromycin, cefepime, cefotetan, cefoxitin, ceftazidime, ceftriaxone, cefuroxime, dexamethasone sodium phosphate, diazepam, ertapenem, fluorouracil, foscarnet, fosphenytoin, furosemide, ganciclovir, heparin, hydrocortisone sodium phosphate, ketorolac, leucovorin, magnesium sulfate, meropenem, methylprednisolone, nafcillin, pantoprazole, pemetrexed, pentobarbital, phenobarbital, phenytoin, piperacillin/tazobactam, potassium phosphates, sodium bicarbonate, sodium phosphates, thiopental, tigecycline, trimethoprim/sulfamethoxazole.

Patient/Family Teaching

- Instruct patient to notify health care professional promptly if fever; sore throat; signs of infection; bleeding gums; bruising; petechiae; blood in stools, urine, or emesis; increased fatigue; dyspnea; or orthostatic hypotension occurs. Caution patient to avoid crowds and persons with known infections. Instruct patient to use soft toothbrush and electric razor and to avoid falls. Patient should be cautioned not to drink alcoholic beverages or take medication containing aspirin or NSAIDs, because these may precipitate gastric bleeding.
- Instruct patient to report pain at injection site immediately.

- Instruct patient to inspect oral mucosa for erythema and ulceration. If ulceration occurs, advise patient to use sponge brush, rinse mouth with water after eating and drinking, and confer with health care professional if mouth pain interferes with eating. Pain may require treatment with opioid analgesics. Patients usually recover by the third week of therapy.
- Instruct patient to notify health care professional of all Rx or OTC medications, vitamins, or herbal products being taken and to avoid concurrent use of alcohol or OTC medications and herbal products, especially cold preparations, without consulting health care professional, especially cimetidine.
- Instruct patient to notify health care professional immediately if vomiting, dehydration, fever, evidence of infection, symptoms of HF, or pain at injection site occurs. Patients should be informed of the risk of irreversible cardiac damage and treatment-related leukemia.
- Discuss the possibility of hair loss with patient. Explore methods of coping. Regrowth usually occurs 2–3 mo after discontinuation of therapy.
- Instruct patient not to receive any vaccinations without advice of health care professional.
- Inform patient that medication may cause urine to appear red for 1–2 days.
- Instruct patient to notify health care professional if skin irritation occurs at site of previous radiation therapy. May cause hyperpigmentation of the skin and nails. Advise patient to use sunscreen and protective clothing to prevent photosensitivity reactions.
- Rep: Advise patient that this medication may have teratogenic effects. Contraception should be used during and for at least 4 mo after therapy is concluded. Inform patient before initiating therapy that this medication may cause irreversible gonadal suppression.
- Emphasize the need for periodic lab tests to monitor for side effects.

Evaluation/Desired Outcomes

- Decrease in size or spread of malignancies in patients with axillary node tumor involvement following resection of primary breast cancer.

eplerenone (e-ple-re-none)

Inspra

Classification

Therapeutic: antihypertensives

Pharmacologic: aldosterone antagonists

Pregnancy Category B

Indications

Hypertension (alone, or with other agents). LV systolic dysfunction and evidence of HF post-MI.

Action

Blocks the effects of aldosterone by attaching to mineralocorticoid receptors. **Therapeutic Effects:** Lowering of BP. Improves survival in patients with evidence of HF post-MI.

Pharmacokinetics

Absorption: Well absorbed following oral administration.

Distribution: Unknown.

Metabolism and Excretion: Mostly metabolized by the liver (CYP3A4 enzyme system); <5% excreted unchanged by the kidneys.

Half-life: 4–6 hr.

TIME/ACTION PROFILE (antihypertensive effect)

ROUTE	ONSET	PEAK	DURATION
PO	unknown	4 wk	unknown

Contraindications/Precautions

Contraindicated in: Serum potassium >5.5 mEq/L; Type 2 diabetes with microalbuminuria (for patients with HTN; ↑ risk of hyperkalemia); Serum creatinine >2 mg/dL in males or > 1.8 mg/dL in females (for patients with HTN); CCr ≤30 mL/min (for all patients); CCr <50 mL/min (for patients with HTN); Concurrent use of potassium supplements or potassium-sparing diuretics (for patients with HTN); Concurrent use of strong inhibitors of the CYP3A4 enzyme system (ketoconazole, itraconazole, nefazodone, clarithromycin, ritonavir, or nelfinavir); Lactation: Lactation.

Use Cautiously in: Severe hepatic impairment; OB: Use only if clearly needed; Pedi: Safety not established.

Adverse Reactions/Side Effects

CNS: dizziness, fatigue. **GI:** abnormal liver function tests, abdominal pain, diarrhea. **GU:** albuminuria. **Endo:** abnormal vaginal bleeding, gynecomastia. **F and E:** HYPERKALEMIA. **Metab:** hypercholesterolemia, hypertriglyceridemia. **Misc:** flu-like symptoms.

Interactions

Drug-Drug: Concurrent use of strong inhibitors of the CYP3A4 enzyme system (**ketoconazole**, **itraconazole**, **nefazodone**, **clarithromycin**, **ritonavir**, or **nelfinavir**) significantly ↑ effects of eplerenone; concurrent use contraindicated. Concurrent use of weak inhibitors of the CYP3A4 enzyme system (**erythromycin**, **saquinavir**, **fluconazole**, **verapamil**) may ↑ effects of eplerenone; initial dose of eplerenone should be ↓ by 50%. **NSAIDs** may ↓ antihypertensive effects. Concurrent use of **ACE inhibitors** or **Angiotensin II receptor blockers** may ↑ risk of hyperkalemia.

Route/Dosage

Hypertension

PO (Adults): 50 mg daily initially; may be ↑ to 50 mg twice daily; *Patients receiving concurrent moderate*

CYP3A4 inhibitors (erythromycin, saquinavir, verapamil, fluconazole)—25 mg once daily initially.

HF Post-MI

PO (Adults): 25 mg daily initially; ↑ in 4 wk to 50 mg daily; subsequent dose adjustments may need to be made based on serum potassium concentrations.

Availability (generic available)

Tablets: 25 mg, 50 mg.

NURSING IMPLICATIONS

Assessment

- Monitor BP periodically during therapy.
- Monitor prescription refills to determine adherence.
- ***Lab Test Considerations:*** May cause hyperkalemia. Monitor serum potassium levels prior to starting therapy, within the first wk, at 1 mo following start of therapy or dose adjustment and periodically thereafter. Monitor serum potassium and serum creatinine in 3–7 days in patients who start taking a moderate CYP3A4 inhibitor.
- May cause ↓ serum sodium and ↑ serum triglyceride, cholesterol, ALT, GGT, creatinine, and uric acid levels.

Potential Nursing Diagnoses

Decreased cardiac output (Indications)
Noncompliance (Patient/Family Teaching)

Implementation

- Do not confuse Inspra with Spiriva.
- **PO:** Administer once daily. May be increased to twice daily if response is inadequate.

Patient/Family Teaching

- Instruct patient to take medication as directed at the same time each day, even if feeling well.
- Encourage patient to comply with additional interventions for hypertension (weight reduction, discontinuation of smoking, moderation of alcohol consumption, regular exercise, stress management). Medication controls, but does not cure, hypertension.
- Instruct patient and family on correct technique for monitoring BP. Advise them to monitor BP at least weekly, and notify health care professional of significant changes.
- Inform patient not to use potassium supplements, salt substitutes containing potassium, or other Rx, OTC, or herbal products without consulting health care professional.
- May cause dizziness. Caution patient to avoid driving or other activities requiring alertness until response to medication is known.
- Advise patient to notify health care professional if dizziness, diarrhea, vomiting, rapid or irregular heartbeat, lower extremity edema, or difficulty breathing occur.
- Advise patient to inform health care professional of treatment regimen prior to treatment or surgery.
- Advise patient to notify health care professional if pregnancy is planned or suspected. Advise patient to avoid breast feeding during therapy.
- Emphasize the importance of follow-up exams to check serum potassium.

Evaluation/Desired Outcomes

- Decrease in BP without appearance of side effects.
- Improvement in survival in patients with evidence of HF post-MI.

REMS

epoetin (e-poe-e-tin)

Epogen, ✱Eprex, Procrit

Classification
Therapeutic: antianemics
Pharmacologic: hormones, erythropoiesis stimulating agents (ESA)

Pregnancy Category C

Indications

Anemia associated with chronic kidney disease (CKD). Anemia secondary to zidovudine (AZT) therapy in HIV-infected patients. Anemia from chemotherapy in patients with nonmyeloid malignancies. Reduction of need for allogeneic red blood cell transfusions in patients undergoing elective, noncardiac, nonvascular surgery. **Unlabeled Use:** Anemia of prematurity in neonates.

Action

Stimulates erythropoiesis (production of red blood cells). **Therapeutic Effects:** Maintains and may elevate RBCs, decreasing the need for transfusions.

Pharmacokinetics

Absorption: Well absorbed after subcut administration.
Distribution: Unknown.
Metabolism and Excretion: Unknown.
Half-life: *Children and Adults*–4–13 hr; *Neonates*—11–17 hr.

TIME/ACTION PROFILE (increase in RBCs)

ROUTE	ONSET†	PEAK	DURATION
IV, Subcut	7–10 days	within 2 mo	2 wk‡

†Increase in reticulocytes.
‡After discontinuation.

Contraindications/Precautions

Contraindicated in: Hypersensitivity to albumin or mammalian cell-derived products; Uncontrolled hypertension; Patients with erythropoietin levels >200 m-Units/mL; Patients receiving chemotherapy when anticipated outcome is cure; Neutropenia in newborns.

Use Cautiously in: History of seizures or stroke; Cardiovascular disease; History of porphyria; OB: Evidence of fetal harm in animal studies—use only if potential benefit outweighs potential risk to fetus; OB, Lactation: Little published information, however, erythropoetin alfa is a normal constituent of breast milk; Pedi: Multidose vials contain benzyl alcohol, which can cause potentially fatal gasping syndrome in neonates.

Adverse Reactions/Side Effects

CNS: SEIZURES, headache. **CV:** HF, MI, STROKE, THROMBOEMBOLIC EVENTS (especially with hemoglobin >11 g/dL), hypertension. **Derm:** transient rashes. **Endo:** restored fertility, resumption of menses. **Misc:** ↑ mortality and ↑ tumor growth (with hemoglobin ≥12 g/dL).

Interactions

Drug-Drug: May ↑ requirement for **heparin** anticoagulation during hemodialysis.

Route/Dosage

Anemia of CKD

(Do not initiate if hemoglobin ≥10 g/dL).
Subcut, IV (Adults): 50–100 units/kg 3 times weekly initially; use lowest dose sufficient to ↓ the need for red blood cell transfusions (do not exceed hemoglobin of 11 g/dL [patients on dialysis] or 10 g/dL [patients not on dialysis]); if Hgb ↑ by >1.0 g/dL in 2 wk, ↓ dose by 25%; if Hgb ↑ by <1.0 g/dL after 4 wk of therapy (with adequate iron stores), ↑ dose by 25%; do not ↑ dose more frequently than q 4 wk.
Subcut, IV (Children 1 mo–16 yr): 50 units/kg 3 times weekly initially; use lowest dose sufficient to ↓ the need for red blood cell transfusions (do not exceed hemoglobin of 11 g/dL [patients on dialysis] or 10 g/dL [patients not on dialysis]); if Hgb ↑ by >1.0 g/dL in 2 wk, ↓ dose by 25%; if Hgb ↑ by <1.0 g/dL after 4 wk of therapy (with adequate iron stores), ↑ dose by 25%; do not ↑ dose more frequently than q 4 wk.

Anemia Secondary to AZT Therapy

Subcut, IV (Adults): 100 units/kg 3 times weekly for 8 wk; if inadequate response, may ↑ by 50–100 units/kg every 4–8 wk (max: 300 units/kg 3 times weekly).
Subcut, IV (Children 8 mo–17 yr): 50–400 units/kg 2–3 times weekly.

Anemia from Chemotherapy

(Use only for chemotherapy-related anemia and discontinue when chemotherapy course is completed; do not initiate if hemoglobin ≥10 g/dL).
Subcut (Adults): 150 units/kg 3 times weekly or 40,000 units weekly; adjust dose to maintain lowest hemoglobin level sufficient to avoid blood transfusions (do not exceed hemoglobin of 12 g/dL); if Hgb ↑ by >1.0 g/dL in 2 wk or reaches a level needed to avoid red blood cell transfusions, ↓ dose by 25%; if Hgb ↑ by <1.0 g/dL (and remains < 10 g/dL) after initial 4 wk of therapy (with adequate iron stores), ↑ dose to 300 units/kg 3 times weekly or 60,000 units weekly.
IV (Children 5–18 yr): 600 units/kg weekly; adjust dose to maintain lowest hemoglobin level sufficient to avoid blood transfusions (do not exceed hemoglobin of 12 g/dL); if Hgb ↑ by >1.0 g/dL in 2 wk or reaches a level needed to avoid red blood cell transfusions, ↓ dose by 25%; if Hgb ↑ by <1.0 g/dL (and remains < 10 g/dL) after initial 4 wk of therapy (with adequate iron stores), ↑ dose to 900 units/kg (maximum = 60,000 units) weekly.

Surgery

Subcut (Adults): 300 units/kg/day for 10 days before surgery, day of surgery, and 4 days after *or* 600 units/kg 21, 14, and 7 days before surgery and on day of surgery.

Anemia of Prematurity

IV, Subcut (Neonates): 500–1250 units/week divided into 2–5 doses for 10 doses. Supplement with oral iron therapy 3–8 mg/kg/day.

Availability

Injection: 2,000 units/mL, 3,000 units/mL, 4,000 units/mL, 10,000 units/mL, 20,000 units/mL, 40,000 units/mL.

NURSING IMPLICATIONS

Assessment

- Monitor BP before and during therapy. Inform health care professional if severe hypertension is present or if BP begins to increase. Additional antihypertensive therapy may be required during initiation of therapy.
- Monitor for symptoms of anemia (fatigue, dyspnea, pallor).
- Monitor dialysis shunts (thrill and bruit) and status of artificial kidney during hemodialysis. Heparin dose may need to be increased to prevent clotting. Monitor patients with underlying vascular disease for impaired circulation.
- **Lab Test Considerations:** May cause ↑ in WBCs and platelets. May ↓ bleeding times.
- Monitor serum ferritin, transferrin, and iron levels to assess need for concurrent iron therapy. Transferrin saturation should be at least 20% and ferritin should be at least 100 ng/mL.
- **Anemia of Chronic Kidney Disease:** Monitor hematocrit before and twice weekly during initial therapy, for 2–6 wk after a change in dose, and regularly after target range (30–36%) has been reached and maintenance dose is determined. Monitor other hematopoietic parameters (CBC with differential and platelet count) before and periodically during therapy. If hemoglobin ↑ and approached 11 g/dL or ↑ by more than 1 g/dL in a 2-wk period, ↓ dose by 25% and monitor hemoglobin twice weekly for 2–6 wk. If ↑ in hemoglobin continues and exceeds 11 g/dL, dose should be withheld until hemoglobin begins to ↓ epoetin is then reinitiated at a dose 25%

lower than previous dose. If hemoglobin ↑ by <1 g/dL over 4 wk (and iron stores are adequate), ↑ dose by 25%; monitor hemoglobin twice weekly for 2–6 wk; further dose ↑ may be made at 4-wk intervals until desired response attained. If no response after 12 wk of escalation, further dose ↑ is unlikely to improve response and may increase risks. Use lowest dose that will maintain Hgb level sufficient to reduce need for transfusions.

- Monitor renal function studies and electrolytes closely; resulting increased sense of well-being may lead to decreased compliance with other therapies for renal failure. Increases in BUN, creatinine, uric acid, phosphorus, and potassium may occur.
- **Anemia Secondary to Zidovudine Therapy:** Before initiating therapy, determine serum erythropoietin level before transfusion. Patients receiving zidovudine with endogenous serum erythropoietin levels >500 mUnits/mL may not respond to therapy. Monitor hemoglobin weekly during dose adjustment. If response does not reduce transfusion requirements or increase hemoglobin effectively after 8 wk of therapy, dose may be ↑ by 50–100 units/kg 3 times weekly. Evaluate response and adjust dose by 50–100 units/kg every 4–8 wk thereafter. If a satisfactory response is not obtained with a dose of 300 units/kg 3 times weekly, it is unlikely that a higher dose will produce a response. Once the desired response is attained, maintenance dose is titrated based on variations of zidovudine dose and concurrent infections. If hemoglobin exceeds 12 g/dL, discontinue dose until hemoglobin drops to <11 g/dL, then ↓ dose by 25%.
- **Anemia from Chemotherapy:** Monitor hemoglobin weekly until stable. Do not initiate if hemoglobin ≥10 g/dL. Patients with lower baseline serum erythropoietin levels may respond more rapidly; not recommended if levels >200 mUnits/mL. If hemoglobin exceeds 12 g/dL, withhold dose until hemoglobin approaches level where transfusions may be required and then reinitiate at a dose 25% lower than previous dose. If hemoglobin ↑ by >1.0 g/dL in any 2-wk period, ↓ dose by 25%. For 3 times weekly dosing regimens, if response is not adequate (no ↓ in transfusion requirements or no ↑ in hemoglobin) after 8 wk of therapy, dose may be ↑ up to 300 units/kg 3 times weekly. If no response is obtained to this dose, it is unlikely that higher doses will produce a response. For weekly dosing regimens, if response is not adequate (no ↑ in hemoglobin by ≥1 g/dL after 4 wk in absence of RBC transfusion), ↑ dose to 60,000 units weekly (adults) or 900 units/kg (max: 60,000 units) (children).
- **Surgery:** Determine that hemoglobin is >10 to ≤13 g/dL before therapy. Epoetin has been used for 10 days before surgery, on the day of surgery and for 4 days post surgery. Implement prophylaxis of deep venous thrombosis during surgical use.

Potential Nursing Diagnoses

Activity intolerance (Indications)
Noncompliance (Patient/Family Teaching)

Implementation

IV Administration

- Prescribers and hospitals must enroll in and comply with the *ESA APPRISE Oncology Program* to prescribe and/or dispense epoetin alfa to patients with cancer. Visit www.esa-apprise.com or call 1-866-284-8089.
- Transfusions are still required for severe symptomatic anemia. Supplemental iron should be initiated with epoetin and continued throughout therapy.
- Institute seizure precautions in patients who experience greater than a 4-point increase in hematocrit in a 2-wk period or exhibit any change in neurologic status. Risk of seizures is greatest during the first 90 days of therapy.
- Do not shake vial; inactivation of medication may occur. Solution is clear and colorless; do not administer solutions that are discolored, cloudy, or contain a precipitate. Discard vial immediately after withdrawing dose from single-use 1-mL vial. Refrigerate multidose 2-mL vial; stable for 21 days after initial entry.
- **Subcut:** This route is often used for patients not requiring dialysis.
- May be admixed in syringe immediately before administration with 0.9% NaCl with benzyl alcohol 0.9% in a 1:1 ratio to prevent injection site discomfort.
- **IV Push:** ***Diluent:*** Administer undiluted or dilute with an equal amount of 0.9% NaCl. ***Concentration:*** 1000–40,000 units/mL. ***Rate:*** May be administered as direct injection or bolus over 1–3 minutes into IV tubing or via venous line at end of dialysis session.
- **Y-Site Compatibility:** alfentanil, amikacin, aminophylline, ascorbic acid, atracurium, atropine, aztreonam, benztropine, bumetanide, buprenorphine, butorphanol, calcium chloride, calcium gluconate, cefazolin, cefotaxime, cefotetan, cefoxitin, ceftazidime, ceftriaxone, cefuroxime, chloramphenicol, clindamycin, cyanocobalamin, cyclosporine, dexamethasone, digoxin, diphenhydramine, dobutamine, dopamine, doxycycline, enalaprilat, ephedrine, epinephrine, erythromycin, esmolol, famotidine, fentanyl, fluconazole, folic acid, furosemide, ganciclovir, gentamicin, glycopyrrolate, heparin, hydrocortisone, imipenem-cilastatin, indomethacin, insulin, isoproterenol, ketorolac, labetalol, lidocaine, magnesium sulfate, mannitol, meperidine,

methyldopate, methylprednisolone, metoclopramide, metoprolol, morphine, multivitamins, nafcillin, nalbuphine, naloxone, nitroglycerin, nitroprusside, norepinephrine, ondansetron, oxacillin, oxytocin, penicillin G, pentazocine, pentobarbital, phenobarbital, phenylephrine, phytonadione, potassium chloride, procainamide, promethazine, propranolol, protamine, pyridoxine, ranitidine, sodium bicarbonate, streptokinase, succinylcholine, sufentanil, theophylline, tobramycin, vasopressin, verapamil.

- **Y-Site Incompatibility:** amphotericin B colloidal, chlorpromazine, dantrolene, diazepam, haloperidol, midazolam, pentamidine, phenytoin, prochlorperazine, trimethoprim/sulfamethoxazole, vancomycin.

Patient/Family Teaching

- Advise patient to read the *Medication Guide* prior to initiating therapy and with each Rx refill in case of changes. Patient must sign the patient-health care provider acknowledgment form before each course of therapy.
- Explain rationale for concurrent iron therapy (increased red blood cell production requires iron).
- Discuss ways of preventing self-injury in patients at risk for seizures. Driving and activities requiring continuous alertness should be avoided.
- Inform patient that use of epoetin may result in shortened overall survival and/or ↓ time to tumor progression.
- Advise patient to notify health care professional immediately if signs of blood clots (chest pain, trouble breathing or shortness of breath; pain in the legs, with or without swelling; a cool or pale arm or leg; sudden confusion; trouble speaking or trouble understanding others' speech; sudden numbness or weakness in the face, arm, or leg, especially on one side of the body; sudden trouble seeing; sudden trouble walking, dizziness, loss of balance or coordination; loss of consciousness or fainting; hemodialysis vascular access stops working) occur.
- Advise patient to inform health care professional of medication prior to treatment or surgery.
- Rep: Discuss possible return of menses and fertility in women of child-bearing age. Patient should discuss contraceptive options with health care professional.
- **Anemia of Chronic Renal Failure:** Stress importance of compliance with dietary restrictions, medications, and dialysis. Foods high in iron and low in potassium include liver, pork, veal, beef, mustard and turnip greens, peas, eggs, broccoli, kale, blackberries, strawberries, apple juice, watermelon, oatmeal, and enriched bread. Epoetin will result in increased sense of well-being, but it does not cure underlying disease.
- **Home Care Issues:** Home dialysis patients determined to be able to safely and effectively administer epoetin should be taught proper dosage, administration technique, and disposal of equipment. *Information for Home Dialysis Patients* should be provided to patient along with medication.

Evaluation/Desired Outcomes

- Increase in hematocrit to 30–36% with improvement in symptoms of anemia in patients with chronic renal failure.
- Increase in hematocrit in anemia secondary to zidovudine therapy.
- Increase in hematocrit in patients with anemia resulting from chemotherapy.
- Reduction of need for transfusions after surgery.

eprosartan, See ANGIOTENSIN II RECEPTOR ANTAGONISTS.

HIGH ALERT

eptifibatide (ep-ti-fib-a-tide)

Integrilin

Classification

Therapeutic: antiplatelet agents

Pharmacologic: glycoprotein IIb/IIIa inhibitors

Pregnancy Category B

Indications

Acute coronary syndrome (unstable angina/non-Q-wave MI), including patients who will be managed medically and those who will undergo percutaneous coronary intervention (PCI) that may consist of percutaneous transluminal angioplasty (PCTA) or atherectomy. Treatment of patients undergoing PCI. Usually used concurrently with aspirin and heparin.

Action

Decreases platelet aggregation by reversibly antagonizing the binding of fibrinogen to the glycoprotein IIb/IIIa binding site on platelet surfaces. **Therapeutic Effects:** Inhibition of platelet aggregation resulting in decreased incidence of new MI, death, or refractory ischemia, reducing the need for repeat urgent cardiac intervention.

Pharmacokinetics

Absorption: IV administration results in complete bioavailability.
Distribution: Unknown.
Metabolism and Excretion: 50% excreted by the kidneys.
Half-life: 2.5 hr.

TIME/ACTION PROFILE (effects on platelet function)

ROUTE	ONSET	PEAK	DURATION
IV	immediate	following bolus	brief†

†Inhibition is reversible following cessation of infusion.

Contraindications/Precautions

Contraindicated in: Hypersensitivity; Active internal bleeding or history of bleeding within previous 30 days; Severe uncontrolled hypertension (systolic BP >200 mm Hg and/or diastolic BP >110 mm Hg); Major surgical procedure within 6 wk; History of hemorrhagic stroke or other stroke within 30 days; Concurrent use of other glycoprotein IIb/IIIa receptor antagonists; Platelet count <100,000/mm^3; Severe renal insufficiency (serum creatinine ≥4 mg/dL) or dependency on renal dialysis.
Use Cautiously in: Geri: ↑ risk of bleeding ; Renal insufficiency (↓ infusion rate if CCr < 50 mL/min); OB, Pedi: Pregnancy, lactation, or children (safety not established; use in pregnancy only if clearly needed).

Adverse Reactions/Side Effects

Noted for patients receiving heparin and aspirin in addition to eptifibatide.
CV: hypotension. **Hemat:** BLEEDING (including GI and intracranial bleeding, hematuria, and hematomas), thrombocytopenia.

Interactions

Drug-Drug: ↑ risk of bleeding with other drugs that affect hemostasis (**heparins**, **warfarin**, **NSAIDs**, **thrombolytic agents**, **abciximab**, **dipyridamole**, **clopidogrel**, some **cephalosporins**, **valproates**).
Drug-Natural Products: ↑ bleeding risk with **arnica**, **chamomile**, **clove**, **dong quai**, **feverfew**, **garlic**, **ginger**, **ginkgo**, and ***Panax ginseng***.

Route/Dosage

Acute Coronary Syndrome

IV (Adults ≤121 kg): 180 mcg/kg as a bolus dose, followed by 2 mcg/kg/min until hospital discharge or surgical intervention (up to 72 hr).

Percutaneous Coronary Intervention

IV (Adults): 180 mcg/kg as a bolus dose, immediately before PCI, followed by 2 mcg/kg/min infusion; a second bolus of 180 mcg/kg is given 10 min after first bolus; infusion should continue for 18–24 or hospital discharge (minimum of 12 hr).

Renal Impairment

(Adults CCr <50 mL/min): 180 mcg/kg bolus followed by 1 mcg/kg/min infusion; second bolus of 180 mcg/kg is given 10 min after first bolus for patients undergoing PCI.

Availability

Solution for injection: 20 mg/10 mL, 75 mg/100 mL, 200 mg/100 mL.

E

NURSING IMPLICATIONS

Assessment

- Assess for bleeding. Most common sites are arterial access site for cardiac catheterization or GI or GU tract. Arterial and venous punctures, IM injections, and use of urinary catheters, nasotracheal intubation, and NG tubes should be minimized. Noncompressible sites for IV access should be avoided. If bleeding cannot be controlled with pressure, discontinue eptifibatide and heparin immediately.
- ***Lab Test Considerations:*** Prior to eptifibatide therapy, assess hemoglobin or hematocrit, platelet count, serum creatinine, and PT/aPTT. Activated clotting time (ACT) should also be measured in patients undergoing PCI.
- Maintain the aPTT between 50 and 70 sec unless PCI is to be performed. Maintain ACT between 300 and 350 sec during PCI.
- Arterial sheath should not be removed unless aPTT <45 sec.
- If platelet count decreases to <100,000 and is confirmed, eptifibatide and heparin should be discontinued and condition monitored and treated.

Potential Nursing Diagnoses

Ineffective tissue perfusion (Indications)

Implementation

- ***High Alert:*** Accidental overdose of antiplatelet medications has resulted in patient harm or death from internal hemorrhage or intracranial bleeding. Have second practitioner independently check original order, dose calculations, and infusion pump settings.
- Most patients receive heparin and aspirin concurrently with eptifibatide.
- After PCI, femoral artery sheath may be removed during eptifibatide treatment only after heparin has been discontinued and its effects mostly reversed.
- Do not administer solutions that are discolored or contain particulate matter. Discard unused portion.

IV Administration

- **IV Push:** ***High Alert: Diluent:*** Withdraw appropriate loading dose from bolus vial (20 mg/10-mL vial) into a syringe. Administer undiluted. ***Concentration:*** 2 mg/mL. ***Rate:*** Administer over 1–2 min.

- **Continuous Infusion:** ***Diluent:*** Administer undiluted directly from the 100-mL vial via an infusion pump. ***Concentration:*** 0.75 mg/mL or 2 mg/mL (depends on vial used). ***Rate:*** Based on patient's weight (see Route/Dosage section).
- **Y-Site Compatibility:** alemtuzumab, alfentanil, alteplase, amikacin, amiodarone, amphotericin B lipid complex, amphotericin B liposome, ampicillin, ampicillin/sulbactam, anidulafungin, argatroban, atracurium, atropine, azithromycin, aztreonam, bivalirudin, bumetanide, buprenorphine, butorphanol, calcium chloride, calcium gluconate, cefepime, cefotaxime, cefotetan, ceftazidime, ceftriaxone, cefuroxime, ciprofloxacin, cisatracurium, clindamycin, cyclosporine, daptomycin, dexamethasone, digoxin, diltiazem, diphenhydramine, dobutamine, dolasetron, dopamine, doxycycline, droperidol, enalaprilat, ephedrine, epinephrine, ertapenem, erythromycin, esmolol, famotidine, fentanil, fluconazole, fosphenytoin, ganciclovir, gentamicin, granisetron, haloperidol, heparin, hydrocortisone, hydromorphone, imipenem/cilastatin, isoproterenol, ketorolac, labetalol, leucovorin, levofloxacin, lidocaine, linezolid, lorazepam, magnesium sulfate, mannitol, meperidine, meropenem, methylprednisolone, metoclopramide, metoprolol, micafungin, midazolam, milrinone, morphine, nalbuphine, naloxone, nicardipine, nitroglycerin, nitroprusside, octreotide, ondansetron, oxytocin, palonosetron, pancuronium, pemetrexed, pentobarbital, phenobarbital, phenylephrine, piperacillin/tazobactam, potassium acetate, potassium chloride, potassium phosphates, procainamide, prochlorperazine, promethazine, propranolol, ranitidine, remifentanil, rocuronium, sodium bicarbonate, sodium phosphates, succinylcholine, sufentanil, teniposide, theophylline, tigecycline, tirofiban, tobramycin, vancomycin, vecuronium, verapamil, zidovudine, zoledronic acid.
- **Y-Site Incompatibility:** acyclovir, amphotericin B colloid, chlorpromazine, diazepam, furosemide, methohexital, mycophenolate, pentamidine, phenytoin, thiopental.

Patient/Family Teaching

- Inform patient of the purpose of eptifibatide.
- Instruct patient to notify health care professional immediately if any bleeding is noted.

Evaluation/Desired Outcomes

- Inhibition of platelet aggregation, resulting in decreased incidence of new MI, death, or refractory ischemia with the need for repeat urgent cardiac intervention.

ergocalciferol, See VITAMIN D COMPOUNDS.

eribulin (e-**rib**-yoo-lin)

Halaven

Classification

Therapeutic: antineoplastics

Pharmacologic: antimicrotubulars

Pregnancy Category D

Indications

Metastatic breast cancer that has progressed despite at least two previous regimens which included an anthracycline and a taxane in either regimen.

Action

Inhibits intracellular microtubule growth phase, causing G_2/M cell-cycle block resulting in apoptotic cell death. **Therapeutic Effects:** Death of rapidly replicating cells, particularly malignant ones. ↓ spread of breast cancer.

Pharmacokinetics

Absorption: IV administration results in complete bioavailability.

Distribution: Unknown.

Metabolism and Excretion: Minimal metabolism, mostly excreted unchanged in feces (82%) and less in urine (9%).

Half-life: 40 hr.

TIME/ACTION PROFILE (effects on blood counts)

ROUTE	ONSET	PEAK	DURATION
IV	within days	7–14 days	up to 2 wk

Contraindications/Precautions

Contraindicated in: Severe hepatic impairment; Severe renal impairment (CCr <15 mL/min); Congenital long QT syndrome; OB: Pregnancy; may cause fetal harm; Lactation: Avoid breast feeding.

Use Cautiously in: HF, bradyarrhythmias, concurrent use of drugs known to prolong the QT interval (including Class Ia and III antiarrhythmics), electrolyte abnormalities (↑ risk of arrhythmias); Moderate renal impairment; lower initial dose recommended for CCr 30–50 mL/min; Mild to moderate hepatic impairment; lower initial dose recommended; OB: Women with child-bearing potential; Pedi: Safety and effectiveness not established.

Adverse Reactions/Side Effects

CNS: fatigue, weakness, depression, dizziness, headache, insomnia. **EENT:** ↑ lacrimation. **CV:** QT INTERVAL PROLONGATION, peripheral edema. **Resp:** cough, dyspnea, upper respiratory tract infection. **GI:** PANCREATITIS, anorexia, constipation, nausea, abdominal pain, abnormal taste, dry mouth, dyspepsia, mucusitis, diarrhea, vomiting. **Derm:** alopecia, rash. **F and E:** hypokalemia. **Hemat:** ANEMIA, NEUTROPENIA. **MS:** arthralgia, myalgia. **Neuro:** peripheral neuropathy. **Misc:** fever, urinary tract infection.

Interactions

Drug-Drug: ↑ risk of bone marrow depression with other **antineoplastics** or **radiation therapy**. ↓ antibody response and ↑ risk of adverse reactions with **live virus vaccines**.

Route/Dosage

IV (Adults): 1.4 mg/m² on days 1 and 8 of a 21-day cycle; dose modifications required for neutropenia, thrombocytopenia, or peripheral neuropathy.

Renal Impairment

IV (Adults): *Moderate—to—severe renal impairment (CCr 15–49 mL/min)*—1.1 mg/m² on days 1 and 8 of a 21-day cycle.

Hepatic Impairment

IV (Adults): *Mild hepatic impairment (Child-Pugh A)*—1.1 mg/m² on days 1 and 8 of a 21-day cycle *Moderate hepatic impairment (Child-Pugh B)*—0.7 mg/m² on days 1 and 8 of a 21-day cycle.

Availability

Solution for IV administration: 0.5 mg/mL.

NURSING IMPLICATIONS

Assessment

- Assess for peripheral motor and sensory neuropathy (numbness, tingling, burning in hands or feet). Withhold eribulin in patients who experience Grade 3 or 4 peripheral neuropathy until resolution to Grade 2 or less.
- Monitor ECG periodically as indicated.
- ***Lab Test Considerations:*** Monitor CBC prior to each dose; ↑ frequency of monitoring in patients who develop Grade 3 or 4 cytopenias. Delay administration and reduce subsequent doses in patients who develop febrile neutropenia or Grade 4 neutropenia lasting longer than 7 days.
- Monitor electrolytes periodically during therapy.

Potential Nursing Diagnoses

Activity intolerance

Implementation

- Correct hypokalemia or hypomagnesemia prior to initiating therapy.

IV Administration

- *Do not administer on Day 1 or Day 8 if:* ANC <1000/mm³, platelets <75,000/mm³, or Grade 3 or 4 nonhematological toxicities occur.
- *Day 8 dose may be delayed for a maximum of 1 wk:* If toxicities do not resolve or improve to ≤Grade 2 severity by Day 15, omit dose.
- If toxicities resolve or improve to ≤Grade 2 by Day 15, administer eribulin at a reduced dose and initiate next cycle no sooner than 2 wk later.
- If a dose has been delayed for toxicity and toxicities have recovered to Grade 2 severity or less, resume eribulin at a reduced dose of 1.1 mg/m².
- *Permanently reduce 1.4 mg/m² eribulin dose to 1.1 mg/m² if:* ANC <500/mm³ for >7 days, ANC <1000/mm³ either fever or infection, platelets <25,000/mm³, platelets <50,000/mm³ requiring transfusion, nonhematologic Grade 3 or 4 toxicities, or omission or delay of Day 8 eribulin dose in previous cycle for toxicity.
- *Permanently reduce 1.4 mg/m² eribulin dose to 0.7 mg/m² if:* occurrence of any event requiring permanent dose reduction while receiving 1.1 mg/m² dose.
- *If occurrence of any event requiring permanent dose reduction while receiving 0.7 mg/m²:* discontinue eribulin.
- **IV Push:** ***Diluent:*** Administer undiluted or dilute in 100 mL of 0.9% NaCl. Store undiluted in syringe or diluted eribulin for up to 4 hr at room temperature or for up to 24 hr under refrigeration. Discard unused portion of vial. ***Rate:*** Infuse over 2–5 minutes on Days 1 and 8 of a 21-day cycle.
- **Y-Site Incompatibility:** Do not dilute in or administer through an IV line containing solutions with dextrose or other medications.

Patient/Family Teaching

- Advise patient to notify health care professional if fever of ≥100.5° F or other signs or symptoms of infection (chills, cough, burning or pain on urination) occur.
- Instruct patient to notify health care professional of all Rx or OTC medications, vitamins, or herbal products being taken and consult health care professional before taking any new medications.
- Advise patient not to receive vaccinations without consulting health care professional.
- Advise female patient to use effective contraception during therapy and to notify health care professional immediately if pregnancy is planned or suspected or if breast feeding.

Evaluation/Desired Outcomes

- ↓ spread of breast cancer.

erlotinib (er-lo-ti-nib)

Tarceva

Classification

Therapeutic: antineoplastics
Pharmacologic: enzyme inhibitors

Pregnancy Category D

Indications

First-line therapy of metastatic non–small-cell lung cancer that has epidermal growth factor exon 19 deletions or exon 21 substitution mutations. Maintenance treatment of locally advanced/metastatic non–small-cell lung cancer when disease has not progressed after four cycles of platinum-based first-line chemotherapy. Locally advanced/metastatic non–small-cell lung cancer that has not responded to ≥1 previous chemotherapy regimen. First-line therapy for locally advanced, surgically unresectable, or metastatic pancreatic cancer (with gemcitabine).

Action

Inhibits the enzyme tyrosine kinase, which is associated with human epidermal growth factor receptor (EGFR); blocks growth stimulation signals in cancer cells. **Therapeutic Effects:** Decreased spread of lung or pancreatic cancer with increased survival.

Pharmacokinetics

Absorption: 60% absorbed; bioavailability ↑ to 100% with food.

Distribution: Unknown.

Protein Binding: 93% protein bound.

Metabolism and Excretion: Mostly metabolized by the liver (CYP3A4 enzyme system).

Half-life: 36 hr.

TIME/ACTION PROFILE (blood levels)

ROUTE	ONSET	PEAK	DURATION
Oral	unknown	4 hr	24 hr

Contraindications/Precautions

Contraindicated in: OB, Lactation: Pregnancy or lactation.

Use Cautiously in: Hepatic impairment; Previous chemotherapy/radiation, pre-existing lung disease, metastatic lung disease (may ↑ risk of interstitial lung disease); Patients with child-bearing potential; Pedi: Safety not established.

Adverse Reactions/Side Effects

CNS: CEREBROVASCULAR ACCIDENT (pancreatic cancer patients), fatigue. **CV:** MYOCARDIAL INFARCTION/ISCHEMIA (pancreatic cancer patients). **EENT:** abnormal eyelash growth, conjunctivitis, corneal perforation, corneal ulceration, keratitis, ↓ tear production. **Resp:** INTERSTITIAL LUNG DISEASE, dyspnea, cough. **GI:** HEPATOTOXICITY, GI PERFORATION, diarrhea, abdominal pain, anorexia, nausea, stomatitis, vomiting, ↑ liver enzymes. **Derm:** BULLOUS AND EXFOLIATIVE SKIN DISORDERS, rash, dry skin, pruritus. **GU:** RENAL FAILURE. **Hemat:** microangiopathic hemolytic anemia with thrombocytopenia (pancreatic cancer patients).

Interactions

Drug-Drug: Strong inhibitors of CYP3A4, including **atazanavir**, **clarithromycin**, **indinavir**, **itraconazole**, **ketoconazole**, **nefazodone**, **nelfinavir**, **ritonavir**, **saquinavir**, **telithromycin**, or **voriconazole** ↑ levels and the risk of toxicity; consider dose reduction. Strong inducers of CYP3A4, including **rifampin**, **rifabutin**, **rifapentine**, **phenytoin**, **carbamazepine**, or **phenobarbital** ↓ levels and may ↓ response; alternative therapy or ↑ dose should be considered. **Ciprofloxacin** may ↑ levels and the risk of toxicity. **Smoking** may ↓ levels and may ↓ response; may consider ↑ dose if smoking continues. May ↓ **midazolam** levels. May ↑ risk of bleeding with **warfarin**. ↓ levels with **proton pump inhibitors** and **H_2 blockers**; avoid concurrent use.

Drug-Natural Products: St. John's wort may ↓ levels and may ↓ response; alternative therapy or ↑ dose should be considered.

Route/Dosage

PO (Adults): *Non–small-cell lung cancer*–150 mg daily taken at least 1 hr before or 2 hr after food; *Pancreatic cancer*—100 mg daily taken at least 1 hr before or 2 hr after food.

Availability (generic available)

Tablets: 25 mg, 100 mg, 150 mg.

NURSING IMPLICATIONS

Assessment

- Assess respiratory status prior to and periodically during therapy. If dyspnea, cough, or fever occur, discontinue erlotinib, assess for interstitial lung disease, and institute treatment as needed.
- Assess for diarrhea. Usually responds to loperamide but may require dose reduction or discontinuation of therapy if patient becomes dehydrated.
- Assess skin throughout therapy. If bullous, blistering, and exfoliative skin conditions, including Stevens-Johnson syndrome/toxic epidermal necrolysis, occur, interrupt or discontinue treatment. Skin rash may require treatment with corticosteroids or anti-infectives with anti-inflammatory properties; acne treatments may aggravate dry skin and erythema.
- Assess eyes periodically during therapy. If acute or worsening eye disorders or pain occur, interrupt or discontinue therapy.
- Assess for GI pain. Patients receiving concomitant antiangiogenic agents, corticosteroids, NSAIDs, and/or taxane-based chemotherapy, or who have prior history of peptic ulceration or diverticular disease, are at increased risk for GI perforation. Permanently discontinue erlotinib in patients who develop gastrointestinal perforation.
- ***Lab Test Considerations:*** Monitor liver function tests (AST, ALT, bilirubin, alkaline phosphatase) periodically during therapy. Dose reduction or discontinuation of therapy should be considered if severe changes in liver function (total bilirubin ≥3 times upper limit of normal and/or transaminases ≥5 times upper limit of normal) occur.

- Monitor renal function and electrolytes in patients at risk for dehydration. Withhold therapy if dehydration occurs.
- Monitor INR regularly in patients taking warfarin. May cause ↑ INR.

Potential Nursing Diagnoses
Ineffective breathing pattern (Side Effects)

Implementation
- **PO:** Administer at least 1 hr before or 2 hr after food.

Patient/Family Teaching
- Instruct patient to take erlotinib as directed.
- Advise patient to notify health care professional if severe or persistent diarrhea, nausea, anorexia, vomiting, onset or worsening of skin rash, unexplained dyspnea or cough, or eye irritation occur.
- Advise patient to wear sunscreen and protective clothing to decrease skin reactions.
- Instruct patient to discontinue smoking during therapy; smoking decreases blood levels of erlotinib.
- Rep: Caution patient to use highly effective contraceptive during and for at least 2 wk after completion of therapy. Advise female patients to notify health care professional if pregnancy is planned or suspected or if breast feeding.

Evaluation/Desired Outcomes
- Decrease in spread of non–small-cell lung or pancreatic cancer with increased survival.

ertapenem (er-ta-pen-em)
INVanz

Classification
Therapeutic: anti-infectives
Pharmacologic: carbapenems

Pregnancy Category B

Indications
Moderate to severe: complicated intra-abdominal infections, complicated skin and skin structure infections, community acquired pneumonia, complicated urinary tract infections (including pyelonephritis), acute pelvic infections including postpartum endomyometritis, septic abortion, and postsurgical gynecologic infections. Prophylaxis of surgical site infection following elective colorectal surgery.

Action
Binds to bacterial cell wall, resulting in cell death. Ertapenem resists the actions of many enzymes that degrade most other penicillins and penicillin-like anti-infectives. **Therapeutic Effects:** Bactericidal action against susceptible bacteria. **Spectrum:** Active against the following aerobic gram-positive organisms: *Staphylococcus aureus* (methicillin-susceptible strains only), *Staphylococcus epidermidis, Streptococcus agalactiae, S. pneumoniae* (penicillin-susceptible strains only), and *S. pyogenes*. Also active against the following gram-negative aerobic organisms: *Escherichia coli, Haemophilus influenzae* (beta-lactamase negative strains), *Klebsiella pneumonia, Moraxella catarrhalis*, and *Providencia rettgeri*. Addition anaerobic spectrum includes *Bacteroides fragilis, B. distasonis, B. ovatus, B. thetaiotamicron, B. uniformis, B. vulgatis, Clostridium clostrioforme, Eubacterium lentum, Peptostreptococcus, Porphyromonas asaccharolytica*, and *Prevotella bivia*.

Pharmacokinetics
Absorption: 90% after IM administration; IV administration results in complete bioavailability.
Distribution: Enters breast milk.
Metabolism and Excretion: Mostly excreted by the kidneys.
Half-life: 1.8 hr (↑ in renal impairment).

TIME/ACTION PROFILE (blood levels)

ROUTE	ONSET	PEAK	DURATION
IM	rapid	2 hr	24 hr
IV	rapid	end of infusion	24 hr

Contraindications/Precautions
Contraindicated in: Hypersensitivity; Cross-sensitivity may occur with penicillins, cephalosporins, and other carbapenems; Hypersensitivity to lidocaine (may be used as a diluent for IM administration).
Use Cautiously in: History of multiple hypersensitivity reactions; Seizure disorders; Renal impairment; OB: Use in pregnancy only if clearly needed; Lactation: Not expected to cause adverse effects in breast-fed infants (NIH); Pedi: Safety not established; Geri: ↑ sensitivity due to age-related ↓ in renal function.

Adverse Reactions/Side Effects
CNS: SEIZURES, headache. **GI:** CLOSTRIDIUM DIFFICILE-ASSOCIATED DIARRHEA (CDAD), diarrhea, nausea, vomiting. **GU:** vaginitis. **Local:** phlebitis at IV site, pain at IM site. **Misc:** hypersensitivity reaction including ANAPHYLAXIS.

Interactions
Drug-Drug: Probenecid ↓ excretion and ↑ blood levels. May ↓ serum **valproate** levels (↑ risk of seizures).

Route/Dosage
IV, IM (Adults and Children 13 yrs or older): 1 g once daily for up to 14 days (IV) or 7 days (IM).

IV, IM (Children 3 mo–12 yrs): 15 mg/kg twice daily (not to exceed 1 g/day) for up to 14 days (IV) or 7 days (IM).

Renal Impairment

IM, IV (Adults): *CCr ≤30 mL/min/1.73m²*—500 mg once daily.

Availability

Powder for injection: 1 g/vial.

NURSING IMPLICATIONS

Assessment

- Assess for infection (vital signs; appearance of wound, sputum, urine, and stool; WBC) at beginning of and during therapy.
- Obtain a history before initiating therapy to determine previous use of and reactions to penicillins, cephalosporins, or carbapenems. Persons with a negative history of penicillin sensitivity may still have an allergic response.
- Obtain specimens for culture and sensitivity before initiating therapy. First dose may be given before receiving results.
- Observe patient for signs and symptoms of anaphylaxis (rash, pruritus, laryngeal edema, wheezing). Discontinue the drug and notify the physician immediately if these occur. Have epinephrine, an antihistamine, and resuscitative equipment close by in the event of an anaphylactic reaction.
- Monitor bowel function. Diarrhea, abdominal cramping, fever, and bloody stools should be reported to health care professional promptly as a sign of Clostridium difficile-associated diarrhea (CDAD). May begin up to several weeks following cessation of therapy.
- ***Lab Test Considerations:*** May cause ↑ AST, ALT, serum alkaline phosphatase levels.
- May cause ↑ platelet and eosinophil counts.

Potential Nursing Diagnoses

Risk for infection (Indications, Side Effects)

Implementation

- Do not confuse Invanz with Avinza.
- **IM:** Reconstitute 1-g vial with 3.2 mL of 1% lidocaine without epinephrine. Shake well to form solution. Immediately withdraw contents and inject deep into large muscle mass. Use reconstituted solution within 1 hr.

IV Administration

- **Intermittent Infusion:** ***Diluent:*** Reconstitute 1-g vial with 10 mL of sterile water for injection or 0.9% NaCl and shake well. Further dilute in 50 mL of 0.9% NaCl. Administer within 6 hr of reconstitution. ***Rate:*** Infuse over 30 min.
- **Y-Site Compatibility:** acyclovir, alfentanil, amifostine, amikacin, aminocaproic acid, aminophylline, amphotericin B lipid complex, amphotericin B liposome, argatroban, arsenic trioxide, atracurium, azithromycin, aztreonam, bivalirudin, bleomycin, bumetanide, buprenorphine, busulfan, butorphanol, calcium chloride, calcium gluconate, carboplatin, carmustine, chloramphenicol, ciprofloxacin, cisatracurium, cyclophosphamide, cyclosporine, cytarabine, dacarbazine, daptomycin, dexamethasone sodium phosphate, dexmedetomidine, dexrazoxane, digoxin, diltiazem, diphenhydramine, docetaxel, dolasetron, dopamine, doxacurium, doxycycline, enalaprilat, ephedrine, epinephrine, eptifibatide, erythromycin, esmolol, etoposide phosphate, famotidine, fenoldopam, fluconazole, fludarabine, fluorouracil, foscarnet, fosphenytoin, furosemide, ganciclovir, gemcitabine, gentamicin, glycopyrrolate, granisetron, haloperidol, heparin, hydrocortisone, hydromorphone, ifosfamide, insulin, irinotecan, isoproterenol, ketorolac, labetalol, leucovorin, levofloxacin, lidocaine, linezolid, lorazepam, magnesium sulfate, mannitol, mechlorethamine, melphalan, meperidine, mesna, metaraminol, methotrexate, methyldopate, methylprednisolone sodium succinate, metoclopramide, metronidazole, milrinone, mitomycin, morphine, moxifloxacin, nalbuphine, naloxone, nesiritide, nitroglycerin, nitroprusside, norepinephrine, octreotide, oxaliplatin, oxytocin, paclitaxel, pamidronate, pancuronium, pantoprazole, pemetrexed, pentobarbital, phenobarbital, phentolamine, phenylephrine, potassium acetate, potassium chloride, potassium phosphates, procainamide, propranolol, ranitidine, remifentanil, rocuronium, sodium acetate, sodium bicarbonate, sodium phosphates, streptozocin, succinylcholine, sufentanil, tacrolimus, telavancin, teniposide, theophylline, thiotepa, tigecycline, tirofiban, tobramycin, trimethoprim/sulfamethoxazole, vancomycin, vasopressin, vecuronium, vinblastine, vincristine, vinorelbine, voriconazole, zidovudine, zoledronic acid.
- **Y-Site Incompatibility:** alemtuzumab, allopurinol, amiodarone, amphotericin B colloidal, anidulafungin, caspofungin, dantrolene, daunorubicin hydrochloride, diazepam, dobutamine, doxorubicin hydrochloride, droperidol, epirubicin, hydralazine, hydroxyzine, idarubicin, midazolam, mitoxantrone, nicardipine, ondansetron, pentamidine, phenytoin, prochlorperazine, promethazine, quinupristin/dalfopristin, thiopental, topotecan, verapamil.

Patient/Family Teaching

- Advise patient to report the signs of superinfection (black, furry overgrowth on the tongue; vaginal itching or discharge; loose or foul-smelling stools) and allergy.
- Caution patient to notify health care professional if fever and diarrhea occur, especially if stool contains blood, pus, or mucus. Advise patient not to treat diarrhea without consulting health care professional. May occur up to several weeks after discontinuation of medication. Consult health care professional before treating with antidiarrheals.

Evaluation/Desired Outcomes

- Resolution of the signs and symptoms of infection. Length of time for complete resolution depends on the organism and site of infection.

ERYTHROMYCIN†

(eh-rith-roe-**mye**-sin)

erythromycin base

~~E-Mycin~~, ✱Erybid, Eryc, Ery-Tab, PCE

erythromycin ethylsuccinate

E.E.S, EryPed, ✱Erythro-ES

erythromycin lactobionate

Erythrocin

erythromycin stearate

Erythrocin Stearate, ✱Erythro-S

erythromycin (topical)

Akne-Mycin, Erygel

Classification

Therapeutic: anti-infectives
Pharmacologic: macrolides

Pregnancy Category B

†See Appendix C for ophthalmic use

Indications

IV, PO: Infections caused by susceptible organisms including: Upper and lower respiratory tract infections, Otitis media (with sulfonamides), Skin and skin structure infections, Pertussis, Diphtheria, Erythrasma, Intestinal amebiasis, Pelvic inflammatory disease, Nongonococcal urethritis, Syphilis, Legionnaires' disease, Rheumatic fever. Useful when penicillin is the most appropriate drug but cannot be used because of hypersensitivity, including: Streptococcal infections, Treatment of syphilis or gonorrhea. **Topical:** Treatment of acne.

Action

Suppresses protein synthesis at the level of the 50S bacterial ribosome. **Therapeutic Effects:** Bacteriostatic action against susceptible bacteria. **Spectrum:** Active against many gram-positive cocci, including: Streptococci, Staphylococci. Gram-positive bacilli, including: *Clostridium*, *Corynebacterium*. Several gram-negative pathogens, notably: *Neisseria*, *Legionella pneumophila*. *Mycoplasma* and *Chlamydia* are also usually susceptible.

Pharmacokinetics

Absorption: Variable absorption from the duodenum after oral administration (dependent on salt form). Absorption of enteric-coated products is delayed. Minimal absorption may follow topical or ophthalmic use.

Distribution: Widely distributed. Minimal CNS penetration. Crosses placenta; enters breast milk.

Protein Binding: 70–80%.

Metabolism and Excretion: Partially metabolized by the liver, excreted mainly unchanged in the bile; small amounts excreted unchanged in the urine.

Half-life: Neonates: 2.1 hr; Adults: 1.4–2 hr.

TIME/ACTION PROFILE (blood levels)

ROUTE	ONSET	PEAK	DURATION
PO	1 hr	1–4 hr	6–12 hr
IV	rapid	end of infusion	6–12 hr

Contraindications/Precautions

Contraindicated in: Hypersensitivity; Concurrent use of pimozide, ergotamine, dihydroergotamine, procainamide, quinidine, dofetilide, amiodarone, or sotalol; Long QT syndrome; Hypokalemia; Hypomagnesemia; Heart rate <50 bpm; Known alcohol intolerance (most topicals); Tartrazine sensitivity (some products contain tartrazine—FDC yellow dye #5); Products containing benzyl alcohol should be avoided in neonates.

Use Cautiously in: Liver/renal disease; OB: May be used in pregnancy to treat chlamydial infections or syphilis; Myasthenia gravis (may worsen symptoms); Geri: ↑ risk of ototoxicity if parenteral dose >4 g/day, ↑ risk of QTc interval prolongation.

Adverse Reactions/Side Effects

CNS: seizures (rare). **EENT:** ototoxicity. **CV:** TORSADE DE POINTES, VENTRICULAR ARRHYTHMIAS, QT interval prolongation. **GI:** CLOSTRIDIUM DIFFICILE-ASSOCIATED DIARRHEA (CDAD), <u>nausea</u>, <u>vomiting</u>, abdominal pain, cramping, diarrhea, hepatitis, infantile hypertrophic pyloric stenosis, pancreatitis (rare). **GU:** interstitial nephritis. **Derm:** rash. **Local:** <u>phlebitis</u> at IV site. **Misc:** allergic reactions, superinfection.

Interactions

Drug-Drug: Concurrent use with **pimozide** may ↑ levels and the risk for serious arrhythmias (concurrent use contraindicated); similar effects may occur with **diltiazem**, **verapamil**, **ketoconazole**, **itraconazole**, **nefazodone**, and **protease inhibitors**; avoid concurrent use. May ↑ levels of **ergotamine** and **dihydroergotamine** and risk for acute ergot toxicity; concurrent use contraindicated. Concurrent use with **amiodarone**, **dofetilide**, or **sotalol** may ↑ risk of torsades de pointe; avoid concurrent use. May ↑ **verapamil** levels and the risk for hypotension, bradycardia, and lactic acidosis. ↑ blood levels and effects of **sildenafil**, **tadalafil**, and **vardenafil**; use lower doses. Concurrent **rifabutin** or **rifampin** may ↓ effect of erythromycin and ↑ risk of adverse GI reactions. ↑ levels and risk of toxicity from **alfentanil**, **alprazolam**, **bromocriptine**, **carbamazepine**, **cyclosporine**, **cilostazol**, **diazepam**, **disopyramide**, **ergot alkaloids**, **felodipine**, **methylprednisolone**, **midazolam**, **quinidine**, **rifabutin**, **tacrolimus**, **triazolam**, or **vinblastine**. May ↑ levels of **lovastatin** and **simvastatin** and ↑ the risk of myopathy/rhabdomyolysis. May ↑ serum **digoxin** levels. **Theophylline** may ↓ blood levels. May ↑ **colchicine** levels and the risk for toxicity; use lower starting and maximum dose of colchicine. May ↑ **theophylline** levels and the risk for toxicity; ↓ theophylline dose. May ↑ **warfarin** levels and the risk for bleeding.

Route/Dosage

250 mg of erythromycin base or stearate = 400 mg of erythromycin ethylsuccinate.

Most Infections

PO (Adults): *Base, stearate*—250 mg q 6 hr, *or* 333 mg q 8 hr, *or* 500 mg q 12 hr. *Ethylsuccinate*—400 mg q 6 hr *or* 800 mg q 12 hr.
PO (Children >1 mo): *Base and ethylsuccinate*—30–50 mg/kg/day divided q 6–8 hr (maximum 2 g/day as base or 3.2 g/day as ethylsuccinate). *Stearate*—30–50 mg/kg/day divided q 6 hr (maximum 2 g/day).
PO (Neonates): *Ethylsuccinate*—20–50 mg/kg/day divided q 6–12 hr.
IV (Adults): 250–500 mg (up to 1 g) q 6 hr.
IV (Children > 1 mo): 15–50 mg/kg/day divided q 6 hr, maximum 4 g/day.

Acne

Topical (Adults and Children >12 yr): 2% ointment, gel, solution, or pledgets twice daily.

Availability (generic available)

Erythromycin Base

Enteric-coated tablets: 250 mg, 333 mg, 500 mg. **Tablets with polymer-coated particles:** 333 mg, 500 mg. **Delayed-release capsules:** 250 mg.

Erythromycin Ethylsuccinate

Tablets: 400 mg, ✱600 mg. **Oral suspension (fruit flavor, cherry):** 200 mg/5 mL. **Oral suspension (orange, banana flavors):** 400 mg/5 mL.

Erythromycin Lactobionate

Powder for injection: 500 mg, 1 g.

Erythromycin Stearate

Film-coated tablets: 250 mg, ✱500 mg.

Topical Preparations

Ointment: 2%. **Gel:** 2%. **Solution:** 2%. **Pledgets:** 2%. ***In combination with:*** benzoyl peroxide (Benzamycin). See Appendix B.

NURSING IMPLICATIONS

Assessment

- Assess for infection (vital signs; appearance of wound, sputum, urine, and stool; WBC) at beginning of and during therapy.
- Obtain specimens for culture and sensitivity before initiating therapy. First dose may be given before receiving results.
- Monitor bowel function. Diarrhea, abdominal cramping, fever, and bloody stools should be reported to health care professional promptly as a sign of Clostridium difficile-associated diarrhea (CDAD). May begin up to several weeks following cessation of therapy.
- ***Lab Test Considerations:*** Monitor liver function tests periodically on patients receiving high-dose, long-term therapy.
- May cause ↑ serum bilirubin, AST, ALT, and alkaline phosphatase concentrations.
- May cause false ↑ of urinary catecholamines.

Potential Nursing Diagnoses

Risk for infection (Indications, Side Effects)
Noncompliance (Patient/Family Teaching)

Implementation

- **PO:** Administer around the clock. *Erythromycin film-coated tablets (base and stearate)* are absorbed better on an empty stomach, at least 1 hr before or 2 hr after meals; may be taken with food if GI irritation occurs. *Enteric-coated erythromycin (base)* may be taken without regard to meals. *Erythromycin ethylsuccinate* is best absorbed when taken with meals. Take each dose with a full glass of water.
- Use calibrated measuring device for liquid preparations. Shake well before using.
- Do not crush or chew delayed-release capsules or tablets; swallow whole. *Erythromycin base delayed-release capsules* may be opened and sprinkled on applesauce, jelly, or ice cream immediately before ingestion. Entire contents of the capsule should be taken.

IV Administration

- **IV:** Add 10 mL of sterile water for injection without preservatives to 250- or 500-mg vials and 20 mL to 1-g vial. Solution is stable for 7 days after reconstitution if refrigerated.
- **Intermittent Infusion:** ***Diluent:*** Dilute in 0.9% NaCl or D5W. ***Concentration:*** 1–5 mg/mL. ***Rate:*** Administer slowly over 20–60 min to avoid phlebitis. Assess for pain along vein; slow rate if pain occurs; apply ice and notify health care professional if unable to relieve pain.
- **Continuous Infusion:** May also be administered as an infusion over 4 hr. ***Diluent:*** 0.9% NaCl, D5W, or LR. ***Concentration:*** 1 g/L.

Erythromycin Lactobionate

- **Y-Site Compatibility:** acyclovir, alemtuzumab, alfentanil, amikacin, aminocaproic acid, aminophylline, amiodarone, anidulafungin, argatroban, atropine, azathioprine, benztropine, bivalirudin, bleomycin, bumetanide, buprenorphine, butorphanol, calcium chloride, calcium gluconate, cangrelor, carboplatin, carmustine, caspofungin, cefotaxime, ceftriaxone, cefuroxime, chlorpromazine, cisplatin, cyanocobalamin, cyclophosphamide, cyclosporine, cytarabine, dacarbazine, dactinomycin, daptomycin, daunorubicin hydrochloride, dexmedetomidine, dexrazoxane, digoxin, diltiazem, diphenhydramine, dobutamine, docetaxel, dolasetron, dopamine, doxorubicin, doxorubicin liposomal, enalaprilat, ephedrine, epinephrine, epirubicin, epoetin alfa, eptifibatide, ertapenem, esmolol, etoposide, etoposide phosphate, famotidine, fenoldopam, fentanyl, fluconazole, fludarabine, fluorouracil, folic acid, foscarnet, fosphenytoin, gemcitabine, gentamicin, glycopyrrolate, granisetron, hetastarch, hydrocortisone, hydromorphone, idarubicin, ifosfamide, imipenem/cilastatin, insulin, irinotecan, isoproterenol, labetalol, leucovorin, levofloxacin, lidocaine, lorazepam, mannitol, mechlorethamine, meperidine, mesna, methotrexate, methyldopate, methylprednisolone, metoclopramide, metoprolol, metronidazole, midazolam, milrinone, mitoxantrone, morphine, multivitamins, mycophenolate, nafcillin, nalbuphine, naloxone, nesiritide, nicardipine, nitroglycerin, norepinephrine, octreotide, ondansetron, oxacillin, oxaliplatin, oxytocin, paclitaxel, palonosetron, pamidronate, pancuronium, papaverine, pentamidine, pentazocine, perphenazine, phenylephrine, phytonadione, piperacillin/tazobactam, potassium acetate, potassium chloride, procainamide, prochlorperazine, promethazine, propranolol, protamine, pyridoxine, ranitidine, sodium acetate, sodium bicarbonate, streptokinase, succinylcholine, sufentanil, tacrolimus, teniposide, theophylline, thiamine, thiotepa, tigecycline, tirofiban, tobramycin, topotecan, vancomycin, vasopressin, vecuronium, verapamil, vinblastine, vincristine, vinorelbine, vitamin B complex with C, voriconazole, zidovudine, zoledronic acid.
- **Y-Site Incompatibility:** amphotericin B colloidal, amphotericin B lipid complex, amphotericin B liposome, ascorbic acid, aztreonam, cefazolin, cefepime, cefotetan, cefoxitin, dantrolene, diazepam, diazoxide, doxycycline, furosemide, ganciclovir, indomethacin, ketorolac, metaraminol, nitroprusside, pemetrexed, pentobarbital, phenytoin, trimethoprim/sulfamethoxazole.
- **Topical:** Cleanse area before application. Wear gloves during application.

Patient/Family Teaching

- Instruct patient to take medication around the clock and to finish the drug completely as directed, even if feeling better. Take missed doses as soon as remembered, with remaining doses evenly spaced throughout day. Advise patient that sharing of this medication may be dangerous.
- May cause nausea, vomiting, diarrhea, or stomach cramps; notify health care professional if these effects persist or if severe abdominal pain, yellow discoloration of the skin or eyes, darkened urine, pale stools, or unusual tiredness develops. May cause infantile hypertrophic pyloric stenosis in infants; notify health care professional if vomiting and irritability occur.
- Caution patient to notify health care professional if fever and diarrhea occur, especially if stool contains blood, pus, or mucus. Advise patient not to treat diarrhea without consulting health care professional. May occur up to several weeks after discontinuation of medication.
- Advise patient to report signs of superinfection (black, furry overgrowth on the tongue; vaginal itching or discharge; loose or foul-smelling stools).
- Instruct patient to notify health care professional if symptoms do not improve.

Evaluation/Desired Outcomes

- Resolution of the signs and symptoms of infection. Length of time for complete resolution depends on the organism and site of infection.
- Improvement of acne lesions.

escitalopram
(ess-sit-**al**-o-pram)
✱Cipralex, ✱Cipralex Meltz, Lexapro

Classification
Therapeutic: antidepressants
Pharmacologic: selective serotonin reuptake inhibitors (SSRIs)

Pregnancy Category C

Indications

Major depressive disorder. Generalized anxiety disorder (GAD). **Unlabeled Use:** Panic disorder. Obsessive-compulsive disorder (OCD). Post-traumatic stress disorder (PTSD). Social anxiety disorder (social phobia). Premenstrual dysphoric disorder (PMDD).

Action

Selectively inhibits the reuptake of serotonin in the CNS. **Therapeutic Effects:** Antidepressant action.

Pharmacokinetics

Absorption: 80% absorbed following oral administration.

Distribution: Enters breast milk.
Metabolism and Excretion: Mostly metabolized by the liver (primarily CYP3A4 and CYP2C19 isoenzymes); 7% excreted unchanged by kidneys.
Half-life: ↑ in elderly and patients with hepatic impairment.

TIME/ACTION PROFILE (antidepressant effect)

ROUTE	ONSET	PEAK	DURATION
PO	within 1–4 wk	unknown	unknown

Contraindications/Precautions

Contraindicated in: Hypersensitivity; Concurrent pimozide; Concurrent use of MAO inhibitors or MAO-like drugs (linezolid or methylene blue); Concurrent use of citalopram; Angle-closure glaucoma.
Use Cautiously in: History of mania (may activate mania/hypomania); History of seizures; Patients at risk for suicide; Hepatic impairment (dose ↓ recommended); Severe renal impairment; OB: Neonates exposed to SSRIs in the 3rd trimester may develop drug discontinuation syndrome manifested by respiratory distress, feeding difficulty, and irritability; Lactation: May cause adverse effects in infant; consider risk/benefit; Pedi: May ↑ risk of suicide attempt/ideation especially during early treatment or dose adjustment; safety not established in children <12 yr; Geri: ↓ doses recommended due to ↓ drug clearance in older patients.

Adverse Reactions/Side Effects

CNS: NEUROLEPTIC MALIGNANT SYNDROME, SUICIDAL THOUGHTS, insomnia, dizziness, drowsiness, fatigue. **GI:** diarrhea, nausea, abdominal pain, constipation, dry mouth, indigestion. **GU:** anorgasmia, ↓ libido, ejaculatory delay, erectile dysfunction. **Derm:** sweating. **Endo:** syndrome on inappropriate secretion of antidiuretic hormone (SIADH). **F and E:** hyponatremia. **Metab:** SEROTONIN SYNDROME, ↑ appetite.

Interactions

Drug-Drug: May cause serious, potentially fatal reactions when used with **MAO inhibitors**; allow at least 14 days between escitalopram and **MAO inhibitors**. Concurrent use with **MAO-inhibitor-like drugs**, such as **linezolid** or **methylene blue** may ↑ risk of serotonin syndrome; concurrent use contraindicated; do not start therapy in patients receiving **linezolid** or **methylene blue**; if **linezolid** or **methylene blue** need to be started in a patient receiving escitalopram, immediately discontinue escitalopram and monitor for signs/symptoms of serotonin syndrome for 2 wk or until 24 hr after last dose of linezolid or methylene blue, whichever comes first (may resume escitalopram therapy 24 hr after last dose of linezolid or methylene blue). Concurrent use with **pimozide** may result in prolongation of the QTc interval and is contraindicated. Use cautiously with other **centrally acting drugs** (including **alcohol**, **antihistamines**, **opioid analgesics**, and **sedative/hypnotics**; concurrent use with **alcohol** is not recommended). Drugs that affect serotonergic neurotransmitter systems, including **tricyclic antidepressants**, **SNRIs**, **fentanyl**, **buspirone**, **tramadol**, and **triptans** ↑ risk of serotonin syndrome. **Cimetidine** may ↑ levels. Serotonergic effects may be ↑ by **lithium** (concurrent use should be carefully monitored). **Carbamazepine** may ↓ levels. May ↑ levels of **metoprolol**. Use cautiously with **tricyclic antidepressants** due to unpredictable effects on serotonin and norepinephrine reuptake. ↑ risk of bleeding with **aspirin**, **NSAIDs**, **clopidogrel**, or **warfarin**.
Drug-Natural Products: ↑ risk of serotonin syndrome with **St. John's wort** and **SAMe**.

Route/Dosage

PO (Adults): *Depression and GAD*— 10 mg once daily, may be ↑ to 20 mg once daily after 1 wk.

Hepatic Impairment

PO (Adults): 10 mg once daily.
PO (Geriatric Patients): 10 mg once daily.
PO (Children ≥12 yr): *Depression*— 10 mg once daily, may be ↑ to 20 mg once daily after 3 wk.

Availability (generic available)

Tablets: 5 mg, 10 mg, 20 mg. **Cost:** *Generic*— 5 mg $13.16/100, 10 mg $13.87/100, 20 mg $18.01/100. **Orally disintegrating tablets:** 🍁 10 mg, 🍁 20 mg. **Oral solution (peppermint flavor):** 1 mg/mL. **Cost:** *Generic*— $190.20/240 mL.

NURSING IMPLICATIONS

Assessment

- Monitor mood changes and level of anxiety during therapy.
- Assess for suicidal tendencies, especially during early therapy. Restrict amount of drug available to patient. Risk may be increased in children, adolescents, and adults ≤24 yr. After starting therapy, children, adolescents, and young adults should be seen by health care professional at least weekly for 4 wk, every 3 wk for next 4 wk, and on advice of health care professional thereafter.
- Assess for sexual dysfunction (erectile dysfunction; decreased libido).
- Assess for serotonin syndrome (mental changes [agitation, hallucinations, coma], autonomic instability [tachycardia, labile BP, hyperthermia], neuromuscular aberrations [hyperreflexia, incoordination], and/or GI symptoms [nausea, vomiting, diarrhea]), especially in patients taking other serotonergic drugs (SSRIs, SNRIs, triptans).

Potential Nursing Diagnoses

Ineffective coping (Indications)
Risk for injury (Side Effects)
Sexual dysfunction (Side Effects)

Implementation

- Do not confuse Lexapro with Loxitane (loxapine).
- Do not administer escitalopram and citalopram concomitantly. Taper to avoid potential withdrawal reac-

tions. Reduce dose by 50% for 3 days, then again by 50% for 3 days, then discontinue.

- **PO:** Administer as a single dose in the morning or evening without regard to meals.

Patient/Family Teaching

- Instruct patient to take escitalopram as directed. Take missed doses on the same day as soon as remembered and consult health care professional. Resume regular dosing schedule next day. Do not double doses. Do not stop abruptly; should be discontinued gradually. Instruct patient to read *Medication Guide* before starting and with each Rx refill in case of changes.
- May cause dizziness. Caution patient to avoid driving or other activities requiring alertness until response to medication is known.
- Advise patient, family, and caregivers to look for suicidality, especially during early therapy or dose changes. Notify health care professional immediately if thoughts about suicide or dying, attempts to commit suicide, new or worse depression or anxiety, agitation or restlessness, panic attacks, insomnia, new or worse irritability, aggressiveness, acting on dangerous impulses, mania, or other changes in mood or behavior or if rash or symptoms of serotonin syndrome occur.
- Instruct patient to notify health care professional of all Rx or OTC medications, vitamins, or herbal products being taken and to consult health care professional before taking any other Rx, OTC, or herbal products, especially St. John's Wort, alcohol or other CNS depressants.
- Instruct female patients to notify health care professional if pregnancy is planned or suspected or if they plan to breast feed. If used during pregnancy, should be tapered during 3rd trimester to avoid neonatal serotonin syndrome.
- Emphasize importance of follow-up exams to monitor progress.

Evaluation/Desired Outcomes

- Increased sense of well-being.
- Renewed interest in surroundings. May require 1–4 wk of therapy to obtain antidepressant effects. Full antidepressant effects occur in 4–6 wk.
- Decrease in anxiety.

HIGH ALERT

esmolol (es-moe-lole)

Brevibloc

Classification

Therapeutic: antiarrhythmics (class II)

Pharmacologic: beta blockers

Pregnancy Category C

Indications

Management of sinus tachycardia and supraventricular arrhythmias.

Action

Blocks stimulation of $beta_1$ (myocardial)-adrenergic receptors. Does not usually affect $beta_2$ (pulmonary, vascular, or uterine)-receptor sites. **Therapeutic Effects:** Decreased heart rate. Decreased AV conduction.

Pharmacokinetics

Absorption: IV administration results in complete bioavailability.

Distribution: Rapidly and widely distributed.

Metabolism and Excretion: Metabolized by enzymes in RBCs and liver.

Half-life: 9 min.

TIME/ACTION PROFILE (antiarrhythmic effect)

ROUTE	ONSET	PEAK	DURATION
IV	within minutes	unknown	1–20 min

Contraindications/Precautions

Contraindicated in: Uncompensated HF; Pulmonary edema; Cardiogenic shock; Bradycardia or heart block; Known alcohol intolerance.

Use Cautiously in: Geri: ↑ sensitivity to the effects of beta blockers; Thyrotoxicosis (may mask symptoms); Diabetes mellitus (may mask symptoms of hypoglycemia); Patients with a history of severe allergic reactions (intensity of reactions may be increased); OB, Lactation, Pedi: Safety not established; neonatal bradycardia, hypotension, hypoglycemia, and respiratory depression may occur rarely.

Adverse Reactions/Side Effects

CNS: fatigue, agitation, confusion, dizziness, drowsiness, weakness. **CV:** hypotension, peripheral ischemia. **GI:** nausea, vomiting. **Derm:** sweating. **Local:** injection site reactions.

Interactions

Drug-Drug: General anesthesia, IV **phenytoin**, and **verapamil** may cause additive myocardial depression. Additive bradycardia may occur with **digoxin**. Additive hypotension may occur with other **antihypertensives**, acute ingestion of **alcohol**, or **nitrates**. Concurrent use with **amphetamine**, **cocaine**, **ephedrine**, **epinephrine**, **norepinephrine**, **phenylephrine**, or **pseudoephedrine** may result in unopposed alpha-adrenergic stimulation (excessive hypertension, bradycardia). Concurrent **thyroid hormone** administration may ↓ effectiveness. May alter the effectiveness of **insulins** or **oral hypoglycemic agents** (dose adjustments may be necessary). May ↓ effectiveness of **theophylline**. May ↓ beneficial beta cardiovascular effects of **dopamine** or **dobutamine**.

Use cautiously within 14 days of **MAO-inhibitor** therapy (may result in hypertension).

Route/Dosage

IV (Adults): *Antiarrhythmic*—500-mcg/kg loading dose over 1 min initially, followed by 50-mcg/kg/min infusion for 4 min; if no response within 5 min, give 2nd loading dose of 500 mcg/kg over 1 min, then ↑ infusion to 100 mcg/kg/min for 4 min. If no response, repeat loading dose of 500 mcg/kg over 1 min and ↑ infusion rate by 50-mcg/kg/min increments (not to exceed 200 mcg/kg/min for 48 hr). As therapeutic end point is achieved, eliminate loading doses and decrease dose increments to 25 mg/kg/min. *Intraoperative antihypertensive/antiarrhythmic*—250–500-mcg/kg loading dose over 1 min initially, followed by 50-mcg/kg/min infusion for 4 min; if no response within 5 min, give 2nd loading dose of 250–500 mcg/kg over 1 min, then ↑ infusion to 100 mcg/kg/min for 4 min. If no response, repeat loading dose of 250–500 mcg/kg over 1 min and ↑ infusion rate by 50-mcg/kg/min increments (not to exceed 200 mcg/kg/min for 48 hr).

IV (Children): *Antiarrhythmic*—50 mcg/kg/min, may be ↑ q 10 min up to 300 mcg/kg/min.

Availability

Solution for injection (prediluted for use as loading dose): 10 mg/mL, 20 mg/mL. **Premixed infusion:** 2000 mg/100 mL, 2500 mg/250 mL.

NURSING IMPLICATIONS

Assessment

- Monitor BP, ECG, and pulse frequently during dose adjustment period and periodically during therapy. The risk of hypotension is greatest within the first 30 min of initiating esmolol infusion.
- Monitor intake and output ratios and daily weights. Assess routinely for signs and symptoms of HF (dyspnea, rales/crackles, weight gain, peripheral edema, jugular venous distention).
- Assess infusion site frequently throughout therapy. Concentrations >10 m g/mL may cause redness, swelling, skin discoloration, and burning at the injection site. Do not use butterfly needles for administration. If venous irritation occurs, stop the infusion and resume at another site.
- ***Toxicity and Overdose:*** Monitor patients receiving esmolol for signs of overdose (bradycardia, severe dizziness or fainting, severe drowsiness, dyspnea, bluish fingernails or palms, seizures).
- IV glucagon and symptomatic care are used in the treatment of esmolol overdose. Because of the short action of esmolol, discontinuation of therapy may relieve acute toxicity.

Potential Nursing Diagnoses

Decreased cardiac output (Side Effects)

Implementation

- ***High Alert:*** IV vasoactive medications are inherently dangerous. Esmolol is available in different concentrations; fatalities have occurred when loading dose vial is confused with concentrated solution for injection, which contains 2500 mg in 10 mL (250 mg/mL) and must be diluted. Before administering, have second practitioner independently check original order, dose calculations, and infusion pump settings.
- ***High Alert:*** Do not confuse Brevibloc (esmolol) with Brevital (methohexital). If both are available as floor stock, store in separate areas.
- To convert to other antiarrhythmics following esmolol administration, administer the 1st dose of the antiarrhythmic agent and decrease the esmolol dose by 50% after 30 min. If an adequate response is maintained for 1 hr following the 2nd dose of the antiarrhythmic agent, discontinue esmolol.

IV Administration

- **IV Push:** ***Diluent:*** The 10-mg/mL and 20-mg/mL vials should be used for the loading dose. These vials are already diluted. No further dilution is needed. ***Concentration:*** Avoid concentrations >10 m g/mL. ***Rate:*** Administer over 1 min.
- **Continuous Infusion:** ***Diluent:*** Premixed infusions are already diluted and ready to use. Solution is clear, colorless to light yellow. ***Concentration:*** 10 mg/mL. ***Rate:*** Based on patient's weight (see Route/Dosage section). Titration of dose is based on desired heart rate or undesired decrease in BP. Esmolol infusions should not be abruptly discontinued; the infusion rate should be tapered.
- **Y-Site Compatibility:** alfentanil, amikacin, aminophylline, amiodarone, amphotericin B liposome, anidulafungin, ascorbic acid, atracurium, atropine, aztreonam, benztropine, bivalirudin, bleomycin, bumetanide, buprenorphine, butorphanol, calcium chloride, calcium gluconate, carboplatin, caspofungin, cefazolin, cefotaxime, cefoxitin, ceftazidime, ceftriaxone, cefuroxime, chlorpromazine, cimetidine, cisatracurium, cisplatin, clindamycin, cyanocobalamin, cyclophosphamide, cyclosporine, cytarabine, dactinomycin, daptomycin, dexmedetomidine, digoxin, diltiazem, diphenhydramine, dobutamine, docetaxel, dopamine, doripenem, doxorubicin, doxycycline, enalaprilat, ephedrine, epinephrine, epoetin alfa, eftifibatide, ertapenem, erythromycin, etoposide, etoposide phosphate, famotidine, fenoldopam, fentanyl, fluconazole, fludarabine, fluorouracil, folic acid, gemcitabine, gentamicin, glycopyrrolate, granisetron, hetastarch, hydromorphone, idarubicin, ifosfamide, imipenem/cilastatin, insulin, isoproterenol, labetalol, levofloxacin, lidocaine, linezolid, lorazepam, magnesium sulfate, mannitol, mechlorethamine, meperidine, metaraminol, methotrexate, methoxamine, methyldopate, metoclopramide, metoprolol, metronidazole, micafungin, midazolam, mitoxantrone, morphine, multivitamins, nalbuphine, naloxone, nesiritide, nicardipine, nitroglycerin, nitroprusside, norepinephrine, octreotide, ondanse-

tron, oxaliplatin, oxytocin, paclitaxel, palonosetron, pancuronium, papaverine, pemetrexed, penicillin G, pentamidine, pentazocine, phentolamine, phenylephrine, phytonadione, piperacillin/tazobactam, potassium chloride, potassium phosphates, procainamide, prochlorperazine, promethazine, propofol, propranolol, protamine, pyridoxime, quinupristin/dalfopristin, ranitidine, remifentanil, rocuronium, sodium acetate, sodium bicarbonate, streptokinase, succinylcholine, sufentanil, tacrolimus, teniposide, theophylline, thiamine, thiotepa, tigecycline, tirofiban, tobramycin, tolazoline, trimetaphan, vancomycin, vasopressin, vecuronium, verapamil, vincristine, voriconazole.
- **Y-Site Incompatibility:** acyclovir, amphotericin B cholesteryl, amphotericin B colloidal, azathioprine, cefotetan, dantrolene, dexamethasone, diazepam, diazoxide, furosemide, ganciclovir, indomethacin, ketorolac, milrinone, oxacillin, pantoprazole, phenobarbital, warfarin.

Patient/Family Teaching
- May cause drowsiness. Caution patients receiving esmolol to call for assistance during ambulation or transfer.
- Advise patients to change positions slowly to minimize orthostatic hypotension.
- Patients with diabetes should closely monitor blood glucose, especially if weakness, malaise, irritability, or fatigue occurs. Medication does not block dizziness or sweating as signs of hypoglycemia.

Evaluation/Desired Outcomes
- Control of arrhythmias without appearance of detrimental side effects.

esomeprazole
(es-o-**mep**-ra-zole)
NexIUM, NexIUM 24hr

Classification
Therapeutic: antiulcer agents
Pharmacologic: proton-pump inhibitors

Pregnancy Category C

Indications
PO, IV: GERD/erosive esophagitis (IV therapy should only be used if PO therapy is not possible/appropriate). **IV:** Reduction in risk of rebleeding following therapeutic endoscopy for acute bleeding gastric or duodenal ulcers. **PO:** Hypersecretory conditions, including Zollinger-Ellison syndrome. **PO:** With amoxicillin and clarithromycin to eradicate *Helicobacter pylori* in duodenal ulcer disease or history of duodenal ulcer disease. **PO:** Decrease risk of gastric ulcer during continuous NSAID therapy. **OTC:** Heartburn occurring ≥twice/wk.

Action
Binds to an enzyme on gastric parietal cells in the presence of acidic gastric pH, preventing the final transport of hydrogen ions into the gastric lumen. **Therapeutic Effects:** Diminished accumulation of acid in the gastric lumen with lessened gastroesophageal reflux. Healing of duodenal ulcers. Decreased incidence of gastric ulcer during continuous NSAID therapy.

Pharmacokinetics
Absorption: 90% absorbed following oral administration; food ↓ absorption.
Distribution: Unknown.
Protein Binding: 97%.
Metabolism and Excretion: Extensively metabolized by the liver (cytochrome P450 [CYP450] system, primarily CYP2C19 isoenzyme, but also the CYP3A4 isoenzyme) (the CYP2C19 enzyme system exhibits genetic polymorphism; 15–20% of Asian patients and 3–5% of Caucasian and Black patients may be poor metabolizers and may have significantly ↑ esomeprazole concentrations and an ↑ risk of adverse effects); <1% excreted unchanged in urine.
Half-life: *Children 1–11 yrs:* 0.42–0.88 hr; *Adults:* 1.0–1.5 hr.

TIME/ACTION PROFILE (blood levels*)

ROUTE	ONSET	PEAK	DURATION
PO	rapid	1.6 hr	24 hr
IV	rapid	end of infusion	24 hr

*Resolution of symptoms takes 5–8 days.

Contraindications/Precautions
Contraindicated in: Hypersensitivity to esomeprazole or related drugs (benzimidazoles); Hypersensitivity; Lactation: Not recommended.
Use Cautiously in: Severe hepatic impairment; Patients using high-doses for >1 year (↑ risk of hip, wrist, or spine fractures); Patients using therapy for >3 yr (↑ risk of vitamin B_{12} deficiency; OB: Use only if potential benefit outweighs potential risk.

Adverse Reactions/Side Effects
CNS: headache. **GI:** CLOSTRIDIUM DIFFICILE-ASSOCIATED DIARRHEA (CDAD), abdominal pain, constipation, diarrhea, dry mouth, flatulence, nausea. **F and E:** hypomagnesemia (especially if treatment duration ≥3 mo). **GU:** acute interstitial nephritis. **Hemat:** vitamin B_{12} deficiency. **MS:** bone fracture.

Interactions
Drug-Drug: May ↓ levels of **atazanavir** and **nelfinavir**; avoid concurrent use with either of these antiretrovirals. May ↑ levels and risk of toxicity of **saquinavir** (may need to ↓ dose of saquinavir). May ↓

absorption of drugs requiring acid pH, including **ketoconazole**, **itraconazole**, **ampicillin esters**, **iron salts**, **erlotinib**, and **mycophenolate mofetil**. May ↑ levels of **digoxin** and **methotrexate**. May ↑ risk of bleeding with **warfarin** (monitor INR and PT). **Voriconazole** may ↑ levels. May ↓ the antiplatelet effects of **clopidogrel**; avoid concurrent use. May ↑ levels of **cilostazol**; consider ↓ dose of cilostazol from 100 mg twice daily to 50 mg twice daily. **Rifampin** may ↓ levels and may ↓ response (avoid concurrent use). Hypomagnesemia ↑ risk of **digoxin** toxicity. May ↑ levels of **tacrolimus** and **methotrexate**.

Drug-Natural Products: St. John's wort may ↓ levels and may ↓ response (avoid concurrent use).

Route/Dosage

Gastroesophageal Reflux Disease

PO (Adults): *Healing of erosive esophagitis*—20 mg or 40 mg once daily for 4–8 wk; *Maintenance of healing of erosive esophagitis*—20 mg once daily; *Symptomatic GERD*—20 mg once daily for 4 wk (additional 4 wk may be considered for nonresponders); *Heartburn*—20 mg once daily for 2 wk.

PO (Children 12–17 yr): *Short-term treatment of GERD*—20–40 mg once daily for up to 8 wk.

PO (Children 1–11 yr): *Short-term treatment of GERD*—10 mg once daily for up to 8 wk; *Healing of erosive esophagitis*—<20 kg: 10 mg once daily for 8 wk; ≥20 kg: 10–20 mg once daily for 8 wk.

PO (Infants and Children 1 mo–<1 yr): *>7.5–12 kg*—10 mg once daily for up to 6 wk; *>5–7.5 kg*—5 mg once daily for up to 6 wk; *3–5 kg*—2.5 mg once daily for up to 6 wk.

IV (Adults): 20 or 40 mg once daily.

IV (Children 1–17 yr): *<55 kg*—10 mg once daily; *≥55 kg*—20 mg once daily.

IV (Children 1 mo-<1 yr): 0.5 mg/kg once daily.

Hepatic Impairment

PO, IV (Adults): *Severe hepatic impairment*—Dose should not exceed 20 mg/day.

Reduction of Risk of Rebleeding of Gastric or Duodenal Ulcers After Therapeutic Endoscopy

IV (Adults): 80 mg over 30 min, then 8 mg/hr continuous infusion for 71.5 hr.

Hepatic Impairment

IV (Adults): *Mild-to-moderate hepatic impairment*—Do not exceed continuous infusion rate of 6 mg/hr; *Severe hepatic impairment*—Do not exceed continuous infusion rate of 4 mg/hr.

H. pylori Eradication to Reduce the Risk of Duodenal Ulcer Recurrence (Triple Therapy)

PO (Adults): 40 mg once daily for 10 days with amoxicillin 1000 mg twice daily for 10 days and clarithromycin 500 mg twice daily for 10 days.

Hepatic Impairment

PO (Adults): *Severe hepatic impairment*—Dose should not exceed 20 mg/day.

Decrease Gastric Ulcer During Continuous NSAID Therapy

PO (Adults): 20 or 40 mg once daily for up to 6 mo.

Hepatic Impairment

PO (Adults): *Severe hepatic impairment*—Dose should not exceed 20 mg/day.

Pathological Hypersecretory Conditions Including Zollinger-Ellison Syndrome

PO (Adults): 40 mg twice daily.

Hepatic Impairment

PO (Adults): *Severe hepatic impairment*—Dose should not exceed 20 mg/day.

Availability (generic available)

Delayed-release capsules: 20 mg[Rx, OTC], 40 mg. **Cost:** 20 mg $713.55/90, 40 mg $731.22/90. **Delayed-release oral suspension packets:** 2.5 mg/pkt, 5 mg/pkt, 10 mg/pkt, 20 mg/pkt, 40 mg/pkt. **Cost:** All strengths $268.01/30 pkts. **Powder for injection (requires reconstitution):** 20 mg/vial, 40 mg/vial. ***In combination with:*** naproxen (Vimovo).

NURSING IMPLICATIONS

Assessment

- Assess routinely for epigastric or abdominal pain and frank or occult blood in the stool, emesis, or gastric aspirate.
- Monitor bowel function. Diarrhea, abdominal cramping, fever, and bloody stools should be reported to health care professional promptly as a sign of Clostridium difficile-associated diarrhea (CDAD).
- ***Lab Test Considerations:*** May cause ↑ serum creatinine, uric acid, total bilirubin, alkaline phosphatase, AST, and ALT.
- May alter hemoglobin, WBC, platelets, serum sodium, potassium, and thyroxine levels.
- May cause hypomagnesemia. Monitor serum magnesium prior to and periodically during therapy.
- May cause false positive results in diagnostic investigations for neuroendocrine tumors due to ↑ serum chromogranin A (CgA) levels secondary to drug-induced ↓ gastric acidity. Temporarily stop esomeprazole at least 14 days before assessing CgA levels and consider repeating test if initial CgA levels are high.

Potential Nursing Diagnoses

Acute pain (Indications)

Implementation

- ***High Alert:*** Do not confuse Nexium with Nexavar.
- Antacids may be used while taking esomeprazole.
- **PO:** Administer at least 1 hr before meals. Capsules should be swallowed whole.
- *Delayed-release capsules:* For patients with difficulty swallowing, place 1 tbsp of applesauce in an

empty bowl. Open capsule and carefully empty the pellets inside onto applesauce. Mix pellets with applesauce and swallow immediately. Applesauce should not be hot and should be soft enough to swallow without chewing. Do not store applesauce mixture for future use. Tap water, orange juice, apple juice, and yogurt have also been used. Do not crush or chew pellets.

- *For patients with an NG tube,* delayed-release capsules can be opened and intact granules emptied into a 60-mL syringe and mixed with 50 mL of water. Replace plunger and shake syringe vigorously for 15 sec. Hold syringe with tip up and check for granules in tip. Attach syringe to NG tube and administer solution. After administering, flush syringe with additional water. Do not administer if granules have dissolved or disintegrated. Administer immediately after mixing.
- For *Delayed-release oral suspension:* Mix contents of packet with 1 tbsp (15 mL) of water, leave 2–3 min to thicken, stir and drink within 30 min.
- *For Delayed-Release Oral Suspension Nasogastric or Gastric Tube:* Add 15 mL of water to a syringe and then add contents of packet. Shake the syringe, leave 2–3 min to thicken. Shake the syringe and inject through the nasogastric or gastric tube within 30 min.

IV Administration

- **IV Push:** Reconstitute each vial with 5 mL of 0.9% NaCl, LR, or D5W. Do not administer solutions that are discolored or contain a precipitate. Stable at room temperature for up to 12 hr. ***Rate:*** Administer over at least 3 min.
- **Intermittent Infusion: *Diluent:*** Dilute reconstituted solution to a volume of 50 mL with *D5W, 0.9% NaCl, or LR for adults* and *with 0.9% NaCl for pediatric patients.* ***Concentration:*** 0.8 mg/mL (40-mg vial) or 0.4 mg/mL (20-mg vial). Solutions diluted with 0.9% NaCl or LR are stable for 12 hr and those diluted with D5W are stable for 6 hr at room temperature. ***Rate:*** Administer over 10–30 min.
- **Continuous Infusion:** *For 80 mg Loading Dose,* reconstitute two 40 mg vials with 5 mL of 0.9% NaCl. ***Diluent:*** Further diluted in 100 mL 0.9% NaCl. ***Rate:*** Administer *loading dose* over 30 minutes. Follow with infusion at a rate of 8 mg/hr for 71.5 hrs.
- **Continuous Infusion:** *For 80 mg dose,* reconstitute two 40 mg vials with 5 mL of 0.9% NaCl. ***Diluent:*** Further diluted in 100 mL 0.9% NaCl. ***Rate:*** Follow loading dose with infusion at a rate of 8 mg/hr for 71.5 hrs.
- **Y-Site Compatibility:** ceftaroline, doripenem, fentanyl, furosemide, insulin, nitroglycerin.
- **Y-Site Incompatibility:** dobutamine, dopamine, midazolam, morphine, tacrolimus, telavancin, tigecycline. Do not administer with other medication or solutions. Flush line with 0.9% NaCl, LR, or D5W before and after administration.

Patient/Family Teaching

- Instruct patient to take medication as directed for the full course of therapy, even if feeling better. Take missed doses as soon as remembered but not if almost time for next dose. Do not double doses. Advise patient to read the *Patient Information* sheet prior to starting therapy and with each Rx refill in case of changes.
- Advise patient to avoid alcohol, products containing aspirin or NSAIDs, and foods that may cause an increase in GI irritation.
- Advise patient to report onset of black, tarry stools; diarrhea; abdominal pain; or persistent headache to health care professional promptly.
- Instruct patient to notify health care professional of all Rx or OTC medications, vitamins, or herbal products being taken and consult health care professional before taking any new medications, especially St. John's wort.
- Advise patient to notify health care professional if signs of hypomagnesemia (seizures, dizziness, abnormal or fast heartbeat, jitteriness, jerking movements or shaking, muscle weakness, spasms of the hands and feet, cramps or muscle aches, spasm of the voice box) occur.
- Caution patient to notify health care professional if fever and diarrhea occur, especially if stool contains blood, pus, or mucus. Advise patient not to treat diarrhea without consulting health care professional.
- Advise female patient to notify health care professional if pregnancy is planned or suspected or if breast feeding.

Evaluation/Desired Outcomes

- Decrease in abdominal pain or prevention of gastric irritation and bleeding. Healing of duodenal ulcers can be seen on x-ray examination or endoscopy.
- Decrease in symptoms of GERD and erosive esophagitis. Sustained resolution of symptoms usually occurs in 5–8 days. Therapy is continued for 4–8 wk after initial episode.
- Decreased incidence of gastric ulcer during continuous NSAID therapy.
- Eradication of *H. pylori* in duodenal ulcer disease.
- Decrease in symptoms of hypersecretory conditions, including Zollinger-Ellison.

E

ESTRADIOL (es-tra-**dye**-ole)
Estrace

estradiol acetate
Femtrace

estradiol cypionate
Depo-Estradiol

estradiol valerate
Delestrogen

estradiol topical emulsion
Estrasorb

estradiol topical gel
Divigel, Elestrin, EstroGel

estradiol transdermal spray
EvaMist

estradiol transdermal system
Alora, Climara, Estraderm, ✤Estradot, Menostar, Minivelle, ✤Oesclim, Vivelle-Dot

estradiol vaginal tablet
Vagifem

estradiol vaginal ring
Femring, Estring

Classification
Therapeutic: hormones
Pharmacologic: estrogens

Pregnancy Category X

Indications
PO, IM, Topical, Transdermal: Replacement of estrogen (HRT) to diminish moderate to severe vasomotor symptoms of menopause and of various estrogen deficiency states including: Female hypogonadism, Ovariectomy, Primary ovarian failure. Treatment and prevention of postmenopausal osteoporosis (not vaginal dose forms). **PO:** Inoperable metastatic postmenopausal breast or prostate carcinoma. **Vag:** Management of atrophic vaginitis that may occur with menopause (low dose), bothersome systemic symptoms of menopause (higher dose). Concurrent use of progestin is recommended during cyclical therapy to decrease the risk of endometrial carcinoma in patients with an intact uterus.

Action
Estrogens promote growth and development of female sex organs and the maintenance of secondary sex characteristics in women. Metabolic effects include reduced blood cholesterol, protein synthesis, and sodium and water retention. **Therapeutic Effects:** Restoration of hormonal balance in various deficiency states, including menopause. Treatment of hormone-sensitive tumors.

Pharmacokinetics
Absorption: Well absorbed after oral administration. Readily absorbed through skin and mucous membranes.
Distribution: Widely distributed. Crosses the placenta and enters breast milk.
Metabolism and Excretion: Mostly metabolized by the liver and other tissues. Enterohepatic recirculation occurs, and more absorption may occur from the GI tract.
Half-life: Gel: 36 hr.

TIME/ACTION PROFILE (estrogenic effects)

ROUTE	ONSET	PEAK	DURATION
PO	unknown	unknown	unknown
IM	unknown	unknown	unknown
TD	unknown	unknown	3–4 days (Estraderm), 7 days (Climara)
Topical	unknown	unknown	unknown
Vaginal ring	unknown	unknown	90 days
Vaginal tablet	unknown	unknown	3–4 days

Contraindications/Precautions
Contraindicated in: History of anaphylaxis or angioedema to estradiol; Thromboembolic disease (e.g., DVT, PE, MI, stroke); Protein C, protein S, or antithrombin deficiency or other thrombophilic disorder; History of breast cancer; History of estrogen-dependent cancer; Hepatic impairment; Undiagnosed vaginal bleeding; OB: Positive evidence of fetal risk.
Use Cautiously in: Underlying cardiovascular disease; Severe hepatic or renal disease; May ↑ the risk of endometrial carcinoma; History of porphyria; History of hereditary angioedema; Lactation: Usually compatible with breast feeding (AAP).

Adverse Reactions/Side Effects
CNS: headache, dizziness, lethargy. **EENT:** intolerance to contact lenses, worsening of myopia or astigmatism. **CV:** MI, THROMBOEMBOLISM, edema, hypertension. **GI:** nausea, weight changes, anorexia, ↑ appetite, jaundice, vomiting. **GU:** *women*—amenorrhea, dysmenorrhea, breakthrough bleeding, cervical erosions, loss of libido, vaginal candidiasis; *men*, erectile dysfunction, testicular atrophy. **Derm:** oily skin, acne, pigmentation, urticaria. **Endo:** gynecomastia (men), hyperglycemia. **F and E:** hypercalcemia, sodium and water retention. **MS:** leg cramps. **Misc:** breast tenderness.

Interactions
Drug-Drug: May alter requirement for **warfarin**, **oral hypoglycemic agents**, or **insulins**. **Barbiturates** or **rifampin** may ↓ effectiveness. **Smoking** ↑ risk of adverse CV reactions.

Route/Dosage

Estrogens should be used in the lowest doses for the shortest period of time consistent with desired therapeutic outcome.

Symptoms of Menopause, Atrophic Vaginitis, Female Hypogonadism, Ovarian Failure/Osteoporosis

PO (Adults): 0.45–2 mg daily or in a cycle.
IM (Adults): 1–5 mg monthly (estradiol cypionate) *or* 10–20 mg (estradiol valerate) monthly.
Topical Emulsion *(Estrasorb)* (Adults): Apply two 1.74-g pouches (4.35 mg estradiol) daily.
Gel (Adults): Apply contents of one packet *(Divigel)* or one actuation from pump *(EstroGel, Elestrin)* daily.
Spray *EvaMist* (Adults): 1 spray daily, may be ↑ to 2–3 sprays daily.
Transdermal (Adults): *Alora*—25–50–mcg/24-hr transdermal patch applied twice weekly. *Estraderm*—50–mcg/24-hr transdermal patch applied twice weekly. *Climara*—25-mcg/24-hr transdermal patch applied weekly. *Vivelle-Dot*—25–50–mcg/24-hr transdermal patch applied twice weekly. *Menostar*—14-mcg/24-hr transdermal patch applied q 7 days. Progestin may be administered for 10–14 days of each mo. *Minivelle*—37.5–mcg/24–hr transdermal patch applied twice weekly (for treatment of vasomotor symptoms); 25–mcg/24–hr transdermal patch applied twice weekly (for prevention of postmenopausal osteoporosis).
Vag (Adults): *Cream*—2–4 g (0.2–0.4 mg estradiol) daily for 1–2 wk, then ↓ to 1–2 g/day for 1–2 wk; then maintenance dose of 1 g 1–3 times weekly for 3 wk, then off for 1 wk; then repeat cycle once vaginal mucosa has been restored; *Vaginal ring (Estring)*—2-mg (releases 7.5 mcg estradiol/24 hr) q 3 mo; *Vaginal ring (Femring)*—12.4 mg (releases 50 mcg estradiol/24 hr) q 3 mo or 24.8 mg (releases 100 mcg estradiol/24 hr) q 3 mo (*Femring* requires concurrent progesterone); *Vaginal tablet*—1 tablet once daily for 2 wk, then twice weekly.

Postmenopausal Breast Carcinoma

PO (Adults): 10 mg 3 times daily.

Prostate Carcinoma

PO (Adults): 1–2 mg 3 times daily.
IM (Adults): 30 mg q 1–2 wk (estradiol valerate).

Availability (generic available)

Tablets: 0.45 mg, 0.5 mg, 0.9 mg, 1 mg, 1.8 mg, 2 mg. **Cost:** *Generic*—0.5 mg $10.83/100, 1 mg $10.83/100, 2 mg $10.83/100. **Injection (valerate in oil):** 10 mg/mL, 20 mg/mL, 40 mg/mL. **Injection (cypionate in oil):** 5 mg/mL. **Topical emulsion:** 4.35 mg/1.74-g pouch. **Cost:** $1.36/pouch. **Topical gel packet (Divigel):** 0.25 mg/packet, 0.5 mg/packet, 1 mg/packet. **Cost:** All strengths $3.45/pkt. **Topical gel pump (Elestrin):** 0.52 mg/actuation. **Cost:** *Elestrin (0.52 mg/actuation)*—$89.44/26 g. **Topical gel pump (Estrogel):** 0.75 mg/actuation. **Cost:** *EstroGel (0.75 mg/actuation)*—$103.80/50 g. **Transdermal spray:** 1.53 mg/spray. **Cost:** $108.76/9 mL. **Transdermal system:** 14 mcg/24-hr release rate, 25 mcg/24-hr release rate, 37.5 mcg/24-hr release rate, 50 mcg/24-hr release rate, 60 mcg/24-hr release rate, 75 mcg/24-hr release rate, 100 mcg/24-hr release rate. **Cost:** 14 mcg/24 hr $221.46/4, 25 mcg/24 hr $88.40/4, 37.5 mcg/24 hr $88.40/4, 50 mcg/24 hr $88.40/4, 60 mcg/24 hr $88.40/4, 75 mcg/24 hr $88.40/4, 100 mcg/24 hr $88.40/4. **Vaginal cream:** 0.01%. **Cost:** $165.70/43 g. **Vaginal ring (Estring):** 2 mg (releases 7.5 mcg/day over 90 days). **Cost:** $252.72/1 ring. **Vaginal ring (Femring):** 12.4 mg (releases 50 mcg/day over 90 days), 24.8 mg (releases 100 mcg/day over 90 days). **Cost:** 50 mcg/day $248.98/1 ring, 100 mcg/day $259.58/1 ring. **Vaginal tablet:** 10 mcg. **Cost:** $97.05/8. ***In combination with:*** norethindrone (Combipatch). See Appendix B.

E

NURSING IMPLICATIONS

Assessment

- Assess BP before and periodically during therapy.
- Monitor intake and output ratios and weekly weight. Report significant discrepancies or steady weight gain.
- **Menopause:** Assess frequency and severity of vasomotor symptoms.
- ***Lab Test Considerations:*** May cause ↑ HDL, phospholipids, and triglycerides and ↓ serum LDL and total cholesterol concentrations.
- May cause ↑ serum glucose, sodium, cortisol, prolactin, prothrombin, and factor VII, VIII, IX, and X levels. May ↓ serum folate, pyridoxine, antithrombin III, and urine pregnanediol concentrations.
- Monitor hepatic function before and periodically during therapy.
- May cause false interpretations of thyroid function tests, false ↑ in norepinephrine platelet-induced aggregability, and false ↓ in metyrapone tests.
- May cause hypercalcemia in patients with metastatic bone lesions.

Potential Nursing Diagnoses

Sexual dysfunction (Indications)

Implementation

- Do not confuse Alora with Aldara.
- **PO:** Administer with or immediately after food to reduce nausea.
- **Vag:** Manufacturer provides applicator with cream. Dose is marked on the applicator. Wash applicator with mild soap and warm water after each use.

- **Transdermal:** When switching from PO form, begin transdermal therapy 1 wk after the last dose or when symptoms reappear.
- **Topical:** In a comfortable position, apply *Estrasorb* to clean, dry skin of thighs each morning. Open each foil pouch individually. Cut or tear the first pouch at the notches near the top of the pouch. Apply the contents of pouch to top of left thigh; push entire contents from bottom through neck of pouch. Using one or both hands rub emulsion into thigh and calf for 3 min until completely absorbed. Rub any excess remaining on hands into buttocks. Repeat procedure with second pouch on right leg. Allow application sites to dry completely before covering with clothing to prevent transfer. Wash hands with soap and water to remove residual estradiol.
- Apply *Divigel* individual-use once-daily packets of quick drying gel to an area measuring 5 inches by 7 inches (size of 2 palm prints) on the thigh. Do not wash area for at least 1 hr after gel has dried.
- Spray *EvaMist* on inside of forearm at the same time each day. Do not massage or rub the spray into the skin. Allow to dry for 2 min before dressing and at least 1 hr before washing. Never spray *EvaMist* around breast or vagina. Do not use more than 56 doses, even if fluid remains in pump.
- **IM:** Injection has oil base. Roll syringe to ensure even dispersion. Administer deep IM. Avoid IV administration.

Patient/Family Teaching

- Instruct patient on correct method of administration. Instruct patient to take medication as directed. Take missed doses as soon as remembered as long as it is not just before next dose. If a dose of *EvaMist* is missed, apply if more than 12 hr before next dose; if less than 12 hr, omit dose and return to regular schedule. Do not double doses.
- Explain dose schedule and maintenance routine. Discontinuing medication suddenly may cause withdrawal bleeding.
- If nausea becomes a problem, advise patient that eating solid food often provides relief.
- Advise patient to report signs and symptoms of fluid retention (swelling of ankles and feet, weight gain), thromboembolic disorders (pain, swelling, tenderness in extremities, headache, chest pain, blurred vision), mental depression, or hepatic dysfunction (yellowed skin or eyes, pruritus, dark urine, light-colored stools) to health care professional.
- Advise patient to notify health care professional of medication regimen before treatment or surgery.
- Caution patient that cigarette smoking during estrogen therapy may cause increased risk of serious side effects, especially for women over age 35.
- Caution patient to use sunscreen and protective clothing to prevent increased pigmentation.
- Advise patient treated for osteoporosis that exercise has been found to arrest and reverse bone loss. Patient should discuss any exercise limitations with health care professional before beginning program.
- Inform patient that estrogens should not be used to decrease risk of cardiovascular disease. Estrogens may increase risk of cardiovascular disease and breast cancer.
- Instruct patient to stop taking medication and notify health care professional if pregnancy is planned or suspected.
- Emphasize the importance of routine follow-up physical exams, including BP; breast, abdomen, and pelvic examinations; Papanicolaou smears every 6–12 mo; and mammogram every 12 mo or as directed. Health care professional will evaluate possibility of discontinuing medication every 3–6 mo. If on continuous (not cyclical) therapy or without concurrent progestins, endometrial biopsy may be recommended, if uterus is intact.
- **Vag:** Instruct patient in the correct use of applicator. Patient should remain recumbent for at least 30 min after administration. May use sanitary napkin to protect clothing, but do not use tampon. If a dose is missed, do not use the missed dose, but return to regular dosing schedule.
- Instruct patient to use applicator provided with vaginal tablet. Insert as high up in the vagina as comfortable, without using force.
- **Vaginal Ring:** Instruct patient to press ring into an oval and insert into the upper third of the vaginal vault. Exact position is not critical. Once ring is inserted, patient should not feel anything. If discomfort is felt, ring is probably not in far enough; gently push farther into vagina. Leave in place continuously for 90 days. Ring does not interfere with sexual intercourse. If straining at defecation makes ring move to lower vagina, push up with finger. If expelled totally, rinse ring with lukewarm water and reinsert. To remove, hook a finger through the ring and pull it out.
- **Transdermal:** Instruct patient to wash and dry hands first. Apply disc to intact skin on hairless portion of abdomen (do not apply to breasts or waistline). Apply *Minivelle* patch to lower abdomen or buttocks. Press disc/patch for 10 sec to ensure contact with skin (especially around edges). Avoid areas where clothing may rub disc loose. Change site with each administration to prevent skin irritation. Do not reuse site for 1 wk; disc may be reapplied if it falls off.
- Advise patient referred for MRI test to discuss patch with referring health care professional and MRI facility to determine if removal of patch is necessary prior to test and for directions for replacing patch.
- *Evamist*: Caution patient to make sure children are not exposed to Evamist and do not come into contact with any skin area where the drug was applied. Women who cannot avoid contact with children should wear a garment with long sleeves to cover the application site.

Evaluation/Desired Outcomes

- Resolution of menopausal vasomotor symptoms.
- Decreased vaginal and vulvar itching, inflammation, or dryness associated with menopause.
- Normalization of estrogen levels in patients with ovariectomy or hypogonadism.
- Control of the spread of advanced metastatic breast or prostate cancer.
- Prevention of osteoporosis.

estradiol valerate/dienogest, See CONTRACEPTIVES, HORMONAL.

estrogens, conjugated (equine)

(**ess**-troe-jenz **con**-joo-gae-ted)

✱C.E.S, ✱Congest, Premarin

estrogens, conjugated (synthetic, A)

Cenestin

estrogens, conjugated (synthetic, B)

Enjuvia

Classification

Therapeutic: hormones

Pharmacologic: estrogens

Pregnancy Category X

Indications

PO: Treatment of moderate to severe vasomotor symptoms of menopause. Estrogen deficiency states, including: Female hypogonadism, Ovariectomy, Primary ovarian failure. Prevention of postmenopausal osteoporosis. Advanced inoperable metastatic breast and prostatic carcinoma. **IM, IV:** Uterine bleeding resulting from hormonal imbalance. **Vag:** Atrophic vaginitis. Moderate to severe dyspareunia due to menopause. Concurrent use of progestin is recommended during cyclical therapy to decrease the risk of endometrial carcinoma in patients with an intact uterus.

Action

Estrogens promote the growth and development of female sex organs and the maintenance of secondary sex characteristics in women. **Therapeutic Effects:** Restoration of hormonal balance in various deficiency states and treatment of hormone-sensitive tumors.

Pharmacokinetics

Absorption: Well absorbed after oral administration. Readily absorbed through skin and mucous membranes.

Distribution: Widely distributed. Crosses placenta and enters breast milk.

Metabolism and Excretion: Mostly metabolized by liver and other tissues. Enterohepatic recirculation occurs, with more absorption from GI tract.

Half-life: Unknown.

TIME/ACTION PROFILE (estrogenic effects†)

ROUTE	ONSET	PEAK	DURATION
PO	rapid	unknown	24 hr
IM	delayed	unknown	6–12 hr
IV	rapid	unknown	6–12 hr

†Tumor response may take several weeks.

Contraindications/Precautions

Contraindicated in: History of anaphylaxis or angioedema to estrogen; Thromboembolic disease (e.g., DVT, PE, MI, stroke); Undiagnosed vaginal bleeding; History of breast cancer; History of estrogen-dependent cancer; Hepatic impairment; Protein C, protein S, or antithrombin deficiency or other thrombophilic disorder; OB: May result in harm to the fetus; Lactation: Negatively affects quantity and quality of breast milk.

Use Cautiously in: Long-term use (more than 4–5 yr); may ↑ risk of myocardial infarction, stroke, invasive breast cancer, pulmonary emboli, deep vein thrombosis and dementia in postmenopausal women; Underlying cardiovascular disease; Hypertriglyceridemia; May ↑ risk of endometrial carcinoma.; History of hereditary angioedema

Adverse Reactions/Side Effects

(Systemic use) **CNS:** headache, dizziness, insomnia, lethargy, mental depression. **CV:** MI, THROMBOEMBOLISM, edema, hypertension. **GI:** nausea, weight changes, anorexia, ↑ appetite, jaundice, vomiting. **GU:** *women*—amenorrhea, breakthrough bleeding, dysmenorrhea, cervical erosion, loss of libido, vaginal candidiasis; *men*, erectile dysfunction, testicular atrophy. **Derm:** acne, oily skin, pigmentation, urticaria. **Endo:** gynecomastia (men), hyperglycemia. **F and E:** hypercalcemia, sodium and water retention. **MS:** leg cramps. **Misc:** ANAPHYLAXIS, ANGIOEDEMA, breast tenderness.

Interactions

Drug-Drug: May alter requirement for **warfarin**, **oral hypoglycemic agents**, or **insulins**. **Barbiturates**, **carbamazepine**, or **rifampin** may ↓ effectiveness. **Smoking** ↑ risk of adverse CV reactions. **Erythromycin**, **clarithromycin**, **itraconazole**, **ketoconazole**, and **ritonavir** may ↑ risk of adverse effects.

Drug-Food: Grapefruit juice may ↑ risk of adverse effects.

Route/Dosage

Estrogens should be used in the lowest doses for the shortest period of time consistent with desired therapeutic outcome.

Ovariectomy, Primary Ovarian Failure

PO (Adults): 1.25 mg daily administered cyclically (3 wk on, 1 wk off).

Osteoporosis/Menopausal Symptoms

PO (Adults): 0.3–1.25 mg daily or in a cycle.

Female Hypogonadism

PO (Adults): 0.3–0.625 mg daily administered cyclically (3 wk on, 1 wk off).

Inoperable Breast Carcinoma—Men and Postmenopausal Women

PO (Adults): 10 mg 3 times daily.

Inoperable Prostate Carcinoma

PO (Adults): 1.25–2.5 mg 3 times daily.

Uterine Bleeding

IM, IV (Adults): 25 mg, may repeat in 6–12 hr if necessary.

Atrophic Vaginitis

PO (Adults): 0.3–1.25 mg daily.
Vag (Adults): 0.5–2 g cream (0.3125 mg–1.25 g conjugated estrogens) daily for 3 wk, off for 1 wk, then repeat.

Moderate to Severe Dyspareunia

Vag (Adults): 0.5 g cream (0.3125 mg conjugated estrogens) twice weekly continuously or daily for 3 wk, off for 1 wk, then repeat.

Availability

Tablets: 0.3 mg, 0.45 mg, 0.625 mg, 0.9 mg, 1.25 mg. **Cost:** *Premarin*—0.3 mg $299.14/100, 0.45 mg $299.14/100, 0.625 mg $299.14/100, 0.9 mg $311.87/100, 1.25 mg $298.45/100. **Powder for injection:** 25 mg/vial. **Vaginal cream:** 0.625 mg/g. **Cost:** $208.20/30 g. ***In combination with:*** medroxyprogesterone (Prempro and Premphase [compliance package]); bazedoxifene (Duavee). See Appendix B.

NURSING IMPLICATIONS

Assessment

- Assess BP before and periodically during therapy.
- Monitor intake and output ratios and weekly weight. Report significant discrepancies or steady weight gain.
- **Menopause:** Assess frequency and severity of vasomotor symptoms.
- ***Lab Test Considerations:*** May cause ↑ HDL and triglycerides, and ↓ serum LDL and total cholesterol concentrations.
- May cause ↑ serum glucose, sodium, cortisol, prolactin, prothrombin, and factor VII, VIII, IX, and X levels. May ↓ serum folate, pyridoxine, antithrombin III, and urine pregnanediol concentrations.
- Monitor hepatic function before and periodically during therapy.
- May cause false interpretations of thyroid function tests.
- May cause hypercalcemia in patients with metastatic bone lesions.

Potential Nursing Diagnoses

Sexual dysfunction (Indications)

Implementation

- Do not confuse Enjuvia (conjugated estrogen) with Januvia (sitagliptin).
- Estrogens should be used in the lowest doses for the shortest period of time consistent with desired therapeutic outcome.
- **PO:** Administer with or immediately after food to reduce nausea.
- **Vag:** Manufacturer provides applicator with cream. Dose is marked on the applicator. Wash applicator with mild soap and warm water after each use.
- **IM:** To reconstitute, withdraw at least 5 mL of air from dry container and then slowly introduce the sterile diluent (bacteriostatic water for injection) against the container side. Gently agitate container to dissolve; do not shake vigorously. Solution is stable for 60 days if refrigerated. Do not use if precipitate is present or if solution is darkened.
- IV is preferred parenteral route because of rapid response.

IV Administration

- **IV Push:** ***Diluent:*** Reconstitute as for IM. Inject into distal port tubing of free-flowing IV of 0.9% NaCl, D5W, or lactated Ringer's solution. ***Concentration:*** 5 mg/mL. ***Rate:*** Administer slowly (no faster than 5 mg/min) to prevent flushing.
- **Y-Site Compatibility:** heparin, hydrocortisone sodium succinate, potassium chloride, vitamin B complex with C.

Patient/Family Teaching

- Instruct patient to take oral medication as directed. Advise patient to avoid drinking grapefruit juice during therapy. Take missed doses as soon as remembered, but not just before next dose. Do not double doses.
- Explain dose schedule and maintenance routine. Discontinuing medication suddenly may cause withdrawal bleeding. Bleeding is anticipated during the week when conjugated estrogens are withheld.
- If nausea becomes a problem, advise patient that eating solid food often provides relief.Inform patient that estrogens should not be used to decrease risk of cardiovascular disease. Estrogens may increase risk of cardiovascular disease and breast cancer.
- Advise patient to report signs and symptoms of fluid retention (swelling of ankles and feet, weight gain),

thromboembolic disorders (pain, swelling, tenderness in extremities; headache; chest pain; blurred vision), depression, hepatic dysfunction (yellowed skin or eyes, pruritus, dark urine, light-colored stools), or abnormal vaginal bleeding to health care professional.

- Caution patient that cigarette smoking during estrogen therapy may increase risk of serious side effects, especially for women over age 35.
- Inform patient that *Premarin* tablet may appear in stool; this is not harmful.
- Caution patient to use sunscreen and protective clothing to prevent increased pigmentation.
- Instruct patient to notify health care professional of all Rx or OTC medications, vitamins, or herbal products being taken and to consult with health care professional before taking other medications.
- Advise patient to notify health care professional of medication regimen before treatment or surgery.
- Advise patient treated for osteoporosis that exercise has been found to arrest and reverse bone loss. The patient should discuss any exercise limitations with health care professional before beginning program.
- Instruct patient to stop taking medication and notify health care professional if pregnancy is suspected.
- Emphasize the importance of routine follow-up physical exams, including BP; breast, abdomen, and pelvic examinations; Papanicolaou smears every 6–12 mo; and mammogram every 12 mo or as directed. Health care professional will evaluate possibility of discontinuing medication every 3–6 mo. If on continuous (not cyclical) therapy or without concurrent progestins, endometrial biopsy may be recommended if uterus is intact.
- **Vag:** Instruct patient in the correct use of applicator. Patient should remain recumbent for at least 30 min after administration. May use sanitary napkin to protect clothing, but do not use tampon. If a dose is missed, do not use the missed dose, but return to regular dosing schedule.

Evaluation/Desired Outcomes

- Resolution of menopausal vasomotor symptoms.
- Decreased vaginal and vulvar itching, inflammation, or dryness associated with menopause.
- Normalization of estrogen levels in patients with ovariectomy or hypogonadism.
- Control of the spread of advanced metastatic breast or prostate cancer.
- Prevention of osteoporosis.
- Relief of moderate to severe dyspareunia due to menopause.

eszopiclone (es-zop-i-klone)

Lunesta

Classification
Therapeutic: sedative/hypnotics
Pharmacologic: cyclopyrrolones

Schedule IV

Pregnancy Category C

E

Indications

Insomnia.

Action

Interacts with GABA-receptor complexes; not a benzodiazepine. **Therapeutic Effects:** Improved sleep with decreased latency and increased maintenance of sleep.

Pharmacokinetics

Absorption: Rapidly absorbed after oral administration.

Distribution: Unknown.

Metabolism and Excretion: Extensively metabolized by the liver (CYP3A4 and CYP2E1 enzyme systems); metabolites are renally excreted, <10% excreted unchanged in urine.

Half-life: 6 hr.

TIME/ACTION PROFILE (blood levels)

ROUTE	ONSET	PEAK	DURATION
PO	rapid	1 hr	6 hr

Contraindications/Precautions

Contraindicated in: Hypersensitivity.

Use Cautiously in: Debilitated patients may have ↓ metabolism or increased sensitivity; use lower initial dose; Conditions that may alter metabolic or hemodynamic function; Severe hepatic impairment (↓ dose recommended); OB, Pedi: Safety not established; Lactation: Occasional use while breast feeding an older infant should pose little risk; Geri: May impair motor and/or cognitive performance; see dosing guidelines.

Adverse Reactions/Side Effects

CNS: abnormal thinking, behavior changes, depression, hallucinations, headache, next day impairment, sleep-driving. **CV:** chest pain, peripheral edema. **GI:** dry mouth, unpleasant taste. **Derm:** rash.

Interactions

Drug-Drug: ↑ risk of CNS depression and next day impairment with other **CNS depressants** including **antihistamines**, **antidepressants**, **opioids**, **sedative/hypnotics**, and **antipsychotics**. ↑ levels and risk of CNS depression with **drugs that inhibit the**

CYP3A4 enzyme system, including **ketoconazole**, **itraconazole**, **clarithromycin**, **nefazodone**, **ritonavir**, and **nelfinavir**. Levels and effectiveness may be ↓ by **drugs that induce the CYP3A4 enzyme system**, including **rifampin**.

Route/Dosage

PO (Adults): 1 mg immediately before bedtime; may be ↑ to 2–3 mg if needed; *Geriatric patients*— 1 mg immediately before bedtime; may be ↑ to 2 mg if needed; *Concurrent use of CYP3A4 inhibitors*— 1 mg immediately before bedtime; may be ↑ to 2 mg if needed.

Hepatic Impairment

PO (Adults): *Severe hepatic impairment*— 1 mg immediately before bedtime; may be ↑ to 2 mg if needed.

Availability (generic available)

Tablets: 1 mg, 2 mg, 3 mg. **Cost:** 1 mg $338.76/30, 2 mg $300.85/30, 3 mg $300.85/30.

NURSING IMPLICATIONS

Assessment

- Assess sleep patterns prior to and during administration. Continued insomnia after 7–10 days of therapy may indicate primary psychiatric or mental illness.
- Assess mental status and potential for abuse prior to administration. Prolonged use of >7–10 days may lead to physical and psychological dependence. Limit amount of drug available to the patient.

Potential Nursing Diagnoses

Insomnia (Indications)

Implementation

- Do not confuse Lunesta with Neulasta.
- **PO:** Onset is rapid. Administer immediately before going to bed or after patient has gone to bed and has experienced difficulty falling asleep, only on nights when patient is able to get 8 or more hours of sleep before being active again.
- Swallow tablet whole; do not break, crush, or chew.
- Eszopiclone is more effective if not taken with or before a high-fat, heavy meal.

Patient/Family Teaching

- Instruct patient to take eszopiclone immediately before going to bed, as directed. May result in short-term memory impairment, hallucinations, impaired coordination, and dizziness. Do not increase dose or discontinue without notifying health care professional. Dose may need to be decreased gradually to minimize withdrawal symptoms. Rebound insomnia and/or anxiety may occur upon discontinuation and usually resolves within 1–2 nights.
- May cause daytime and next-day drowsiness. Caution patient to avoid driving or other activities requiring alertness until response to medication is known.
- Inform patient that after taking eszopiclone patient may get out of bed and perform activities (driving a car ("sleep-driving"), making and eating food, talking on the phone, having sex, sleep-walking) while unaware. Patient may not remember anything done during the night; increased risk with alcohol or other CNS depressants.
- Instruct patient to notify health care professional of all Rx or OTC medications, vitamins, or herbal products being taken and to consult health care professional before taking any other Rx, OTC, or herbal products.
- Caution patient to avoid concurrent use of alcohol or other CNS depressants.
- Advise patient to notify health care professional if pregnancy is planned or suspected.

Evaluation/Desired Outcomes

- Decreased sleep latency and improved sleep maintenance.

etanercept (e-tan-er-sept)

Enbrel

Classification

Therapeutic: antirheumatics (DMARDs)

Pharmacologic: anti-TNF agents

Pregnancy Category B

Indications

Moderately to severely active rheumatoid arthritis (may be used alone or with methotrexate). Moderate to severely active polyarticular juvenile idiopathic arthritis. Psoriatic arthritis (may be used alone or with methotrexate). Active ankylosing spondylitis. Moderate to severe chronic plaque psoriasis in patients who are candidates for systemic therapy or phototherapy.

Action

Binds to tumor necrosis factor (TNF), making it inactive. TNF is a mediator of inflammatory response.

Therapeutic Effects: Decreased pain and swelling with decreased rate of joint destruction in patients with rheumatoid arthritis, psoriatic arthritis, juvenile idiopathic arthritis, and ankylosing spondylitis. Reduced severity of plaques.

Pharmacokinetics

Absorption: 60% absorbed after subcut administration.

Distribution: Unknown.

Metabolism and Excretion: Unknown.

Half-life: 115 hr (range 98–300 hr).

TIME/ACTION PROFILE (symptom reduction)

ROUTE	ONSET	PEAK	DURATION
Subcut	2–4 wk	unknown	unknown

Contraindications/Precautions

Contraindicated in: Hypersensitivity; Active infection (including localized); Lactation: Lactation; Untreated infections; Granulomatosis with polyangiitis (receiving immunosuppressive agents); Concurrent cyclophosphamide or anakinra.

Use Cautiously in: History of chronic or recurrent infection or underlying illness/treatment predisposing to infection (including advanced or poorly controlled diabetes); History of exposure to tuberculosis; History of opportunistic infection; History of hepatitis B; Patients residing, or who have resided, where tuberculosis, histoplasmosis, coccidioidomycoses, or blastomycosis is endemic; Pre-existing or recent demyelinating disorders (multiple sclerosis, myelitis, optic neuritis); Latex allergy (needle cover of diluent syringe contains latex); Geri: May have ↑ risk of infection; Pedi: Children with significant exposure to varicella virus (temporarily discontinue etanercept; consider varicella zoster immune globulin); ↑ risk of lymphoma (including hepatosplenic T-cell lymphoma [HSTCL]), leukemia, and other malignancies; OB: Use only if needed.

Adverse Reactions/Side Effects

CNS: headache, dizziness, weakness. **EENT:** rhinitis, pharyngitis. **Resp:** upper respiratory tract infection, cough, respiratory disorder. **GI:** abdominal pain, dyspepsia. **Derm:** psoriasis, rash. **Hemat:** pancytopenia. **Local:** injection site reactions. **Misc:** INFECTIONS (including reactivation tuberculosis and other opportunistic infections due to bacterial, invasive fungal, viral, mycobacterial, and parasitic pathogens), MALIGNANCY (including lymphoma, HSTCL, leukemia, and skin cancer), SARCOIDOSIS.

Interactions

Drug-Drug: Concurrent use with **anakinra** ↑ risk of serious infections (not recommended). Concurrent use of **cyclophosphamide** may ↑ risk of malignancies. Concurrent use with **azathioprine** and/or **methotrexate** may ↑ risk of HSTCL. May ↓ antibody response to **live-virus vaccine** and ↑ risk of adverse reactions (do not administer concurrently).

Route/Dosage

Subcut (Adults): *Adult rheumatoid arthritis, ankylosing spondylitis, psoriatic arthritis*—50 mg once weekly; *adult plaque psoriasis*—50 mg twice weekly for 3 mo, then 50 mg once weekly, may also be given as 25–50 mg once weekly as an initial dose.

Subcut (Children 4–17 yr): *>63 kg*—0.8 mg/kg/wk (up to 50 mg) as a single injection; *31–62 kg*—0.8 mg/kg/wk either as two injections on the same day or divided and given on two separate days 3–4 days apart; *<31 kg*—0.8 mg/kg/wk as a single injection.

Availability

Pre-filled syringes: 50 mg/mL. **Powder for injection:** 25 mg/vial.

NURSING IMPLICATIONS

Assessment

- Assess range of motion, degree of swelling, and pain in affected joints before and periodically during therapy.
- Assess patient for injection site reaction (erythema, pain, itching, swelling). Reactions are usually mild to moderate and last 3–5 days after injection.
- Monitor patients who develop a new infection while taking etanercept closely. Discontinue therapy in patients who develop a serious infection or sepsis. Do not initiate therapy in patients with active infections.
- Assess for signs and symptoms of systemic fungal infections (fever, malaise, weight loss, sweats, cough, dypsnea, pulmonary infiltrates, serious systemic illness with or without concomitant shock). Ascertain if patient lives in or has traveled to areas of endemic mycoses. Consider empiric antifungal treatment for patients at risk of histoplasmosis and other invasive fungal infections until the pathogens are identified. Consult with an infectious diseases specialist. Consider stopping etanercept until the infection has been diagnosed and adequately treated.
- ***Lab Test Considerations:*** Monitor CBC with differential periodically during therapy. May cause leukopenia, neutropenia, thrombocytopenia, and pancytopenia. Discontinue etanercept if symptoms of blood dyscrasias (persistent fever) occur.

Potential Nursing Diagnoses

Impaired physical mobility (Indications)
Acute pain (Indications)

Implementation

- Do not confuse Enbrel with Levbid.
- Administer a tuberculin skin test prior to administration of etanercept. Patients with active latent TB should be treated for TB prior to therapy.
- Needle cover of the prefilled syringe contains latex and should not be handled by people with latex allergies.
- **Subcut:** Prepare injection with single dose pre-filled syringe or multidose vial for reconstitution.
- Solution in prefilled syringe may be allowed to reach room temperature (15–30 min); do not remove needle cap during this time.
- For multidose vial, reconstitute with 1 mL of the bacteriostatic sterile water supplied by manufacturer for a concentration of 25 mg/mL. If the vial is used for multiple doses, use a 25-gauge needle for reconstituting and withdrawing solution and apply "Mixing Date" sticker with date of reconstitution entered. Inject diluent slowly into vial to avoid foaming. Some foaming will occur. Swirl gently for dissolution; do not shake or vigorously agitate to prevent excess foaming. Solution should be clear and colorless; do

not administer solution that is discolored or contains particulate matter. Dissolution usually takes <10 min. Withdraw solution into syringe. Some foam may remain in vial. Amount in syringe should approximate 1 mL. Do not filter reconstituted solution during preparation or administration. Attach a 27-gauge needle to inject. Administer as soon as possible after reconstitution; stable up to 6 hr if refrigerated. Solution and pre-filled syringes are stable if refrigerated and used within 14 days.

- May be injected into abdomen, thigh, or upper arm. Rotate sites. Do not administer within 1 inch of an old site or into area that is tender, red, hard, or bruised.
- **Syringe Incompatibility:** Do not mix with other solutions or dilute with other diluents.

Patient/Family Teaching

- Instruct patient on self-administration technique, storage, and disposal of equipment. First injection should be administered under the supervision of health care professional. Provide patient with a puncture-proof container for used equipment.
- Advise patient not to receive live vaccines during therapy. Parents should be advised that children should complete immunizations to date before initiation of etanercept. Patients with significant exposure to varicella virus (chickenpox) should temporarily discontinue therapy and varicella immune globulin should be considered.
- Advise patient that methotrexate, analgesics, NSAIDs, corticosteroids, and salicylates may be continued during therapy.
- Instruct patient to notify health care professional if upper respiratory or other infections occur. Therapy may need to be discontinued if serious infection occurs.
- Advise patient of risk of malignancies such as hepatosplenic T-cell lymphoma. instruct patient to report signs and symptoms (splenomegaly, hepatomegaly, abdominal pain, persistent fever, night sweats, weight loss) to health care professional promptly.

Evaluation/Desired Outcomes

- Reduction in symptoms of rheumatoid arthritis. Symptoms may return within 1 mo of discontinuation of therapy.
- Reduced severity of plaques in chronic plaque psoriasis.

ethambutol (e-tham-byoo-tole)

✱Etibi, Myambutol

Classification
Therapeutic: antituberculars

Pregnancy Category C

Indications

Active tuberculosis or other mycobacterial diseases (with at least one other drug).

Action

Inhibits the growth of mycobacteria. **Therapeutic Effects:** Tuberculostatic effect against susceptible organisms.

Pharmacokinetics

Absorption: Rapidly and well absorbed (80%) from the GI tract.
Distribution: Widely distributed; crosses blood-brain barrier in small amounts; crosses placenta and enters breast milk.
Protein Binding: 20–30%.
Metabolism and Excretion: 50% metabolized by the liver, 50% eliminated unchanged by the kidneys.
Half-life: 3.3 hr (increased in renal or hepatic impairment).

TIME/ACTION PROFILE (blood levels)

ROUTE	ONSET	PEAK	DURATION
PO	rapid	2–4 hr	24 hr

Contraindications/Precautions

Contraindicated in: Hypersensitivity; Optic neuritis.
Use Cautiously in: Renal and severe hepatic impairment (dosage reduction required); OB: Although safety not established, ethambutol has been used with isoniazid in pregnant women without fetal adverse effects; Lactation: Usually compatible with breast feeding (AAP).

Adverse Reactions/Side Effects

CNS: confusion, dizziness, hallucinations, headache, malaise. **EENT:** optic neuritis. **GI:** HEPATITIS, abdominal pain, anorexia, nausea, vomiting. **Metab:** hyperuricemia. **MS:** joint pain. **Neuro:** peripheral neuritis. **Resp:** pulmonary infiltrates. **Misc:** anaphylactoid reactions, fever.

Interactions

Drug-Drug: Neurotoxicity may be ↑ with other **neurotoxic agents. Aluminum hydroxide** may decrease absorption (space doses 4 hr apart).

Route/Dosage

PO (Adults and Children >13 yr): 15–25 mg/kg/day (maximum 2.5 g/day) *or* 50 mg/kg (up to 2.5 g) twice weekly *or* 25–30 mg/kg (up to 2.5 g) 3 times weekly.
PO (Children 1 mo — 13 yr): *HIV negative*—15–20 mg/kg/day once daily (maximum: 1 g/day) or 50 mg/kg/dose twice weekly (maximum: 2.5 g/dose); *HIV-exposed/-infected*—15–25 mg/kg/day once daily (maximum: 2.5 g/day); *MAC, secondary prophylaxis, or treatment in HIV-exposed/-infected*—15–25 mg/kg/day once daily (maximum: 2.5 g/day) with clarithro-

mycin (or azithromycin) with or without rifabutin; *Nontuberculous mycobacterial infection*— 15–25 mg/kg/day once daily (maximum: 2.5 g/day).

Availability (generic available)

Tablets: 100 mg, 400 mg.

NURSING IMPLICATIONS

Assessment

- Mycobacterial studies and susceptibility tests should be performed before and periodically during therapy to detect possible resistance.
- Assess lung sounds and character and amount of sputum periodically during therapy.
- Assessments of visual function should be made frequently during therapy. Advise patient to report blurring of vision, constriction of visual fields, or changes in color perception immediately. Visual impairment, if not identified early, may lead to permanent sight impairment.
- ***Lab Test Considerations:*** Monitor renal and hepatic functions, CBC, and uric acid levels routinely. Frequently causes elevated uric acid concentrations, which may precipitate an attack of gout.

Potential Nursing Diagnoses

Risk for infection (Indications)
Disturbed sensory perception (Side Effects)

Implementation

- Ethambutol is given as a single daily dose and should be taken at the same time each day. Some regimens require dosing 2–3 times/week. Usually administered concurrently with other antitubercular medications to prevent development of bacterial resistance.
- **PO:** Administer with food or milk to minimize GI irritation.
- **PO:** Tablets may be crushed and mixed with apple juice or apple sauce.

Patient/Family Teaching

- Instruct patient to take medication as directed. Take missed doses as soon as possible unless almost time for next dose; do not double up on missed doses. A full course of therapy may take mo to yr. Do not discontinue without consulting health care professional, even though symptoms may disappear.
- Advise patient to notify health care professional if pregnancy is suspected.
- Instruct patient to notify health care professional if no improvement is seen in 2–3 wk. Health care professional should also be notified if unexpected weight gain or decreased urine output occurs.
- Emphasize the importance of routine exams to evaluate progress and ophthalmic examinations if signs of optic neuritis occur.

Evaluation/Desired Outcomes

- Resolution of clinical symptoms of tuberculosis.
- Decrease in acid-fast bacteria in sputum samples.
- Improvement seen in chest x rays. Therapy for tuberculosis is usually continued for at least 1–2 yr.

E

ethinyl estradiol/desogestrel, **See CONTRACEPTIVES, HORMONAL.**

ethinyl estradiol/drospirenone, **See CONTRACEPTIVES, HORMONAL.**

ethinyl estradiol/ethynodiol, **See CONTRACEPTIVES, HORMONAL.**

ethinyl estradiol/etonogestrel, **See CONTRACEPTIVES, HORMONAL.**

ethinyl estradiol/levonorgestrel, **See CONTRACEPTIVES, HORMONAL.**

ethinyl estradiol/norelgestromin, **See CONTRACEPTIVES, HORMONAL.**

ethinyl estradiol/norethindrone, **See CONTRACEPTIVES, HORMONAL.**

ethinyl estradiol/norgestimate, **See CONTRACEPTIVES, HORMONAL.**

ethinyl estradiol/norgestrel, **See CONTRACEPTIVES, HORMONAL.**

etodolac (ee-**toe**-doe-lak)
~~Lodine~~, ~~Lodine XL~~

Classification
Therapeutic: antirheumatics, nonopioid analgesics
Pharmacologic: pyranocarboxylic acid

Pregnancy Category C

Indications

Osteoarthritis. Rheumatoid arthritis. Mild to moderate pain (not XL tablets).

Action

Inhibits prostaglandin synthesis. Also has uricosuric action. **Therapeutic Effects:** Suppression of inflammation. Decreased severity of pain.

Pharmacokinetics

Absorption: Well absorbed after oral administration.
Distribution: Widely distributed.
Protein Binding: >99%.
Metabolism and Excretion: Mostly metabolized by the liver; <1% excreted unchanged in urine.
Half-life: 6–7 hr (single dose); 7.3 hr (chronic dosing).

TIME/ACTION PROFILE (analgesic effect)

ROUTE	ONSET	PEAK	DURATION
PO (analgesic)	0.5 hr	1–2 hr	4–12 hr
PO (anti-inflammatory)	days–wk	unknown	6–12 hr†

†Up to 24 hr as XL (extended-release) tablet.

Contraindications/Precautions

Contraindicated in: Hypersensitivity; Active GI bleeding or ulcer disease; Cross-sensitivity may exist with other NSAIDs, including aspirin; Peri-operative pain from coronary artery bypass graft (CABG) surgery; OB: Use during second half of pregnancy can result in premature closure of ductus arteriosis.
Use Cautiously in: Renal or hepatic disease; Cardiovascular disease or risk factors for cardiovascular disease (may ↑ risk of serious cardiovascular thrombotic events, myocardial infarction, and stroke, especially with prolonged use or use of higher doses); History of ulcer disease; Lactation: Limited information available; use other safer NSAID; Pedi: Safety not established; Geri: ↑ risk of GI bleeding.

Adverse Reactions/Side Effects

CNS: depression, dizziness, drowsiness, insomnia, malaise, nervousness, syncope, weakness. **EENT:** blurred vision, photophobia, tinnitus. **Resp:** asthma. **CV:** HF, MYOCARDIAL INFARCTION, STROKE, edema, hypertension, palpitations. **GI:** GI BLEEDING, dyspepsia, abdominal pain, constipation, diarrhea, drug-induced hepatitis, dry mouth, flatulence, gastritis, nausea, stomatitis, thirst, vomiting. **GU:** dysuria, renal failure, urinary frequency. **Derm:** EXFOLIATIVE DERMATITIS, STEVENS-JOHNSON SYNDROME, TOXIC EPIDERMAL NECROLYSIS, ecchymoses, flushing, hyperpigmentation, pruritus, rash, sweating. **Hemat:** anemia, prolonged bleeding time, thrombocytopenia. **Misc:** allergic reactions including ANAPHYLAXIS, ANGIOEDEMA, chills, fever.

Interactions

Drug-Drug: Concurrent use with **aspirin** may ↓ effectiveness. ↑ adverse GI effects with **aspirin**, other **NSAIDs, potassium supplements, corticosteroids, antiplatelet agents**, or **alcohol**. Chronic use with **acetaminophen** may ↑ risk of adverse renal reactions. May ↓ effectiveness of **diuretic** or **antihypertensive** therapy. May ↑ serum **lithium** levels and ↑ risk of toxicity. ↑ risk of toxicity from **methotrexate**. ↑ risk of bleeding with **cefotetan, valproic acid, thrombolytics, antiplatelet agents**, or **anticoagulants**. ↑ risk of adverse hematologic reactions with **antineoplastics** or **radiation therapy**. May ↑ the risk of nephrotoxicity from **cyclosporine**.
Drug-Natural Products: ↑ risk of bleeding with **arnica, chamomile, clove, dong quai, fever few, garlic, ginko**, and ***Panax ginseng***.

Route/Dosage

PO (Adults): *Analgesia*—200–400 mg q 6–8 hr (not to exceed 1200 mg/day). *Osteoarthritis/rheumatoid arthritis*—300 mg 2–3 times daily, 400 mg twice daily, or 500 mg twice daily; may also be given as 400–1200 mg once daily as XL tablets.

Availability (generic available)

Capsules: 200 mg, 300 mg. **Tablets:** 400 mg, 500 mg. **Extended-release tablets:** 400 mg, 500 mg, 600 mg.

NURSING IMPLICATIONS

Assessment

- Patients who have asthma, aspirin-induced allergy, and nasal polyps are at increased risk for developing hypersensitivity reactions. Monitor for rhinitis, asthma, and urticaria.
- Assess for rash periodically during therapy. May cause Stevens-Johnson syndrome. Discontinue therapy if severe or if accompanied with fever, general malaise, fatigue, muscle or joint aches, blisters, oral lesions, conjunctivitis, hepatitis, and/or eosinophilia.
- **Osteoarthritis/Rheumatoid Arthritis:** Assess pain and range of movement before and 1–2 hr after administration.
- **Pain:** Assess location, duration, and intensity of the pain before and 60 min after administration.
- ***Lab Test Considerations:*** May cause ↓ hemoglobin, hematocrit, leukocyte, and platelet counts.
- Monitor liver function tests within 8 wk of initiating etodolac therapy and periodically during therapy. May cause ↑ serum alkaline phosphatase, LDH, AST, and ALT concentrations.
- Monitor BUN, serum creatinine, and electrolytes periodically during therapy. May cause ↑ BUN, serum creatinine, and electrolyte concentrations and ↓ urine electrolyte concentrations.
- May cause ↓ serum and ↑ urine uric acid concentrations.

Potential Nursing Diagnoses

Acute pain (Indications)
Impaired physical mobility (Indications)

Implementation

Administration in higher-than-recommended doses does not provide increased effectiveness but may cause increased side effects.

- Use lowest effective dose for shortest period of time.
- **PO:** For rapid initial effect, administer 30 min before or 2 hr after meals. May be administered with food, milk, or antacids containing aluminum or magnesium to decrease GI irritation.
- Do not break, crush, or chew extended-release tablets.

Patient/Family Teaching

- Advise patients to take etodolac with a full glass of water and to remain in an upright position for 15–30 min after administration.
- Instruct patient to take medication as directed. Take missed doses as soon as possible within 1–2 hr if taking twice/day, or unless almost time for next dose if taking more than twice/day. Do not double doses.
- Etodolac may occasionally cause drowsiness or dizziness. Advise patient to avoid driving or other activities requiring alertness until response to the medication is known.
- Caution patient to avoid the concurrent use of alcohol, aspirin, acetaminophen, NSAIDs, or other OTC medications without consultation with health care professional.
- Advise patient to inform health care professional of medication regimen before treatment or surgery.
- Advise patient to consult health care professional if rash, itching, visual disturbances, tinnitus, weight gain, edema, black stools, persistent headache, or influenza-like syndrome (chills, fever, muscle aches, pain) occurs.
- Advise patient to notify health care professional if pregnancy is planned or suspected or if breast feeding.

Evaluation/Desired Outcomes

- Decreased severity of pain.
- Improved joint mobility. Patients who do not respond to one NSAID may respond to another. May require 2 wk or more for maximum anti-inflammatory effects.

etonogestrel, See CONTRACEPTIVES, HORMONAL.

⌘ everolimus (e-ve-ro-li-mus)

Afinitor, Afinitor Disperz, Zortress

Classification

Therapeutic: antineoplastics, immunosuppressants

Pharmacologic: kinase inhibitors

Pregnancy Category C (Zortress), D (Afinitor)

Indications

Afinitor. Advanced renal cell carcinoma that has failed treatment with sunitinib or sorafenib. Subependymal giant cell astrocytoma (SEGA) associated with tuberous sclerosis complex (TSC) in patients who are not candidates for curative surgical resection. Progressive neuroendocrine tumors of pancreatic origin (PNET) in patients with unresectable, locally advanced or metastatic disease. Renal angiomyolipoma with TSC in patients not requiring immediate surgery. ⌘ Treatment of postmenopausal women with advanced hormone receptor-positive, HER2-negative breast cancer in combination with exemestane, after failure of treatment with letrozole or anastrozole. **Zortress**. Prevention of organ rejection in patients who have received a kidney transplant and are at low-to-moderate immunologic risk. Prevention of organ rejection in patients who have received a liver transplant.

Action

Acts as a kinase inhibitor, decreasing cell proliferation. Inhibits activation and proliferation of T and B lymphocytes. **Therapeutic Effects:** Decreased spread of renal cell carcinoma. Improvement in progression-free survival in patients with PNET. Decreased volume of SEGA and angiomyolipoma lesions. Prevention of kidney transplant rejection.

Pharmacokinetics

Absorption: Well absorbed following oral administration.

Distribution: 20% confined to plasma.

Metabolism and Excretion: Mostly metabolized by liver and other systems (CYP3A4 and PgP; metabolites are mostly excreted in feces [80%] and urine [5%]).

Half-life: 30 hr.

TIME/ACTION PROFILE (blood levels))

ROUTE	ONSET	PEAK	DURATION
PO	unknown	1–2 hr	24 hr

Contraindications/Precautions

Contraindicated in: Hypersensitivity to everolimus or other rapamycins; Severe hepatic impairment (Child-Pugh class C); use only if benefit exceeds risk for renal cell carcinoma, PNET, breast cancer, and renal angiomyolipoma with TSC; Concurrent use with strong CYP3A4 inhibitors (i.e., ketoconazole, itraconazole, clarithromycin, atazanavir, nefazodone, saquinavir, telithromycin, ritonavir, indinavir, nelfinavir, voriconazole); Heart transplantation (Zortress) (↑ risk of mortality); Functional carcinoid tumors; OB: Avoid use during pregnancy (Afinitor); use only if benefit to

mother outweighs risk to fetus (Zortress); Lactation: Avoid breast feeding.
Use Cautiously in: Mild or moderate hepatic impairment (Child-Pugh class A or B); dose ↓ required; Concurrent use of moderate CYP3A4 and/or P-glycoprotein inhibitors; dose ↓ required; Exposure to sunlight/UV light (may ↑ risk of malignant skin changes); Geri: May be more sensitive to drug effects; consider age-related ↓ in hepatic function, concurrent disease states and drug therapy; Pedi: Safety not established for indications other than SEGA.

Adverse Reactions/Side Effects

CNS: fatigue, weakness, headache. **CV:** peripheral edema. **Resp:** PNEUMONITIS, cough, dyspnea, pulmonary embolism. **GI:** HEPATIC ARTERY THROMBOSIS, anorexia, constipation, diarrhea, mucositis, mouth ulcers, nausea, stomatitis, vomiting, dysgeusia. **GU:** acute renal failure, infertility, proteinuria. **Derm:** delayed wound healing, dry skin, pruritus, rash. **Hemat:** HEMOLYTIC UREMIC SYNDROME, THROMBOTIC MICROANGIOPATHY, THROMBOTIC THROMBOCYTOPENIC PURPURA, anemia, leukopenia, thrombocytopenia. **Metab:** hyperlipidemia, hyperglycemia, hypertriglyceridemia. **MS:** extremity pain. **Misc:** ANGIOEDEMA, fever, hypersensitivity reactions including ANAPHYLAXIS, infection (including activation of latent viral infections such as BK virus-associated nephropathy), kidney arterial/venous thrombosis (Zortress), ↑ risk of lymphoma/skin cancer (Zortress).

Interactions

Drug-Drug: Strong **CYP3A4 inhibitors**, including **atazanavir**, **clarithromycin**, **indinavir**, **itraconazole**, **ketoconazole**, **nefazodone**, **nelfinavir**, **ritonavir**, **saquinavir**, **telithromycin**, or **voriconazole** ↑ levels and the risk of toxicity; avoid concurrent use. Moderate inhibitors of CYP3A4, including **aprepitant**, **diltiazem**, **erythromycin**, **fluconazole**, **fosamprenavir**, and **verapamil** ↑ levels and the risk of toxicity; ↓ dose of everolimus (Afinitor). Avoid concurrent use with strong **CYP3A4 inducers** including **carbamazepine**, **dexamethasone**, **phenobarbital**, **phenytoin**, **rifabutin**, and **rifampin**; ↑ dose of everolimus may be required. **Cyclosporine**, **aprepitant**, **diltiazem**, **verapamil**, **fluconazole**, and **fosamprenavir** may ↑ levels. ↑ risk of nephrotoxicity with **aminoglycosides**, **amphotericin B**, **cisplatin**, or **cyclosporine**. **ACE inhibitors** may ↑ risk of angioedema. May ↓ antibody formation and ↑ risk of adverse reactions from **live-virus vaccines**; avoid use of live-virus vaccines during treatment.
Drug-Natural Products: **St. John's wort** may ↓ levels and efficacy; avoid concurrent use.
Drug-Food: ↑ blood levels and risk of toxicity with **grapefruit juice**; avoid concurrent use.

Route/Dosage

Advanced Renal Cell Carcinoma, Advanced PNET, Advanced Hormone Receptor-Positive, HER2-Negative Breast Cancer, and Renal Angiomyolipoma with TSC

PO (Adults): 10 mg once daily; *Concurrent use of moderate inhibitors of CYP3A4 and/or P-glycoprotein*—↓ dose to 2.5 mg daily; *Concurrent use of strong inducers of CYP3A4*—↑ dose in 5 mg increments up to 20 mg/daily.

Hepatic Impairment

PO (Adults): *Mild hepatic impairment (Child–Pugh Class A)*—7.5 mg once daily; may be ↓ to 5 mg once daily if not well tolerated; *Moderate hepatic impairment (Child–Pugh Class B)*—5 mg once daily; may be ↓ to 2.5 mg once daily if not well tolerated; *Severe hepatic impairment (Child–Pugh Class C)*—2.5 mg once daily.

SEGA with TSC

PO (Adults and Children ≥1 yr): 4.5 mg/m². Titrate, as needed, at 2-wk intervals to achieve recommended whole blood trough concentration *Concurrent use of moderate inhibitors of CYP3A4 and/or P-glycoprotein*—2.25 mg/m²; *Concurrent use of strong inducers of CYP3A4*—9 mg/m².

Hepatic Impairment

PO (Adults and Children ≥1 yr): *Severe hepatic impairment (Child–Pugh Class C)*—2.5 mg/m².

Kidney Transplantation

PO (Adults): 0.75 mg twice daily (with reduced-dose cyclosporine); titrate to achieve recommended whole blood trough concentration.

Hepatic Impairment

PO (Adults): *Mild hepatic impairment (Child–Pugh Class A)*—↓ daily dose by 33%; *Moderate or severe hepatic impairment (Child–Pugh Class B or C)*—↓ daily dose by 50%.

Liver Transplantation

PO (Adults): 1 mg twice daily (with reduced-dose tacrolimus) (start ≥30 days post-transplant); titrate to achieve recommended whole blood trough concentration.

Hepatic Impairment

PO (Adults): *Mild hepatic impairment (Child–Pugh Class A)*—↓ daily dose by 33%; *Moderate or severe hepatic impairment (Child–Pugh Class B or C)*—↓ daily dose by 50%.

Availability

Tablets (Afinitor): 2.5 mg, 5 mg, 7.5 mg, 10 mg. **Tablets for oral suspension (Afinitor Disperz):** 2 mg, 3 mg, 5 mg. **Tablets (Zortress):** 0.25 mg, 0.5 mg, 0.75 mg.

NURSING IMPLICATIONS

Assessment

- Assess for symptoms of noninfectious pneumonitis (hypoxia, pleural effusion, cough, dyspnea) during therapy. If symptoms are mild, therapy may continue. Therapy should be interrupted for moderate symptoms and corticosteroids may be used. Reinitiate everolimus at a 50% reduced dose when symptoms resolve. If symptoms are severe, discontinue therapy. Corticosteroids may be used until clinical symptoms resolve. Base reinitiation of therapy on individual clinical circumstances.
- Assess for mouth ulcers, stomatitis, or oral mucositis. Topical treatments may be used; avoid peroxide-containing mouthwashes and antifungals unless fungal infection has been diagnosed.
- Assess for signs and symptoms of systemic fungal infections (fever, malaise, weight loss, sweats, cough, dypsnea, pulmonary infiltrates, serious systemic illness with or without concomitant shock). Consider stopping therapy until infection has been diagnosed and adequately treated.
- ***Lab Test Considerations:*** Monitor renal function prior to and periodically during therapy. May cause ↑ BUN, serum creatinine, and proteinuria.
- Monitor fasting serum glucose and lipid profile prior to and periodically during therapy. May cause ↑ cholesterol, triglycerides, glucose. Attempt to achieve optimal glucose and lipid control prior to therapy.
- Monitor CBC prior to and periodically during therapy; may cause ↓ hemoglobin, lymphocytes, neutrophils, and platelets.
- May cause ↑ AST, ALT, phosphate, and bilirubin.
- **Affinitor:** Monitor *Affinitor* trough levels 2 wk after initiation of therapy, a change in dose, a change in co-administration of CYP3A4 and/or PgP inducers or inhibitors, change in hepatic function, or change in dose form between everolimus tablets and Disperz. Once at a stable dose, monitor trough concentrations every 3 to 6 mo in patients with changing body surface area or every 6 to 12 mo in patients with stable body surface area for duration of treatment. Therapeutic blood concentrations are 5–15 (*Affinitor*). If trough concentration is <5 ng/mL increase daily dose by 2.5 mg in patients taking tablets and 2 mg for Disperz. If trough concentration is >15 n g/mL decrease daily dose by 2.5 mg in patients taking tablets and 2 mg for Disperz. If dose reduction is required with lowest dose, administer every other day. Do not combine dose forms to achieve dose. **Zortress:** Therapeutic blood concentrations are 3–8 ng/mL via the LCMSMS assay (*Zortress*). Base dose adjustments of *Zortress* on trough concentrations obtained 4 or 5 days after a previous dosing change. Adjust dose if trough concentration is <3 ng/mL by doubling dose using available tablet strengths (0.25mg, 0.5mg or 0.75 mg). If trough concentration is >8 n g/mL on 2 consecutive measures; decrease dose of *Zortress* by 0.25 mg twice daily.

Potential Nursing Diagnoses

Risk for infection (Adverse Reactions)

Implementation

- **PO:** Administer at the same time each day consistently with or without food, followed by a whole glass of water. Swallow tablets whole; do not break, crush, or chew.
- Do not combine the 2 dose forms (Afinitor Tablets and Afinitor Disperz) to achieve the desired total dose. Use one dosage form or the other.
- Administer *Disperz*, dispersable tablet, as a suspension only. Wear gloves to avoid possible contact with everolimus when preparing suspensions for another person. Place dose in 10 mL syringe; do not exceed 10 mg/syringe. If higher dose required, use additional syringe. Do not break or crush tablets. Draw 5 mL water and 4 mL of air into syringe. Place filled syringe into container (tip up) for 3 min until tablets are in suspension. Invert syringe five times immediately prior to administration. Administer immediately after preparation; discard suspension if not administered within 60 minutes after preparation. After administration, draw 5 mL of water and 4 mL of air into same syringe, and swirl contents to suspend remaining particles. Administer entire contents of syringe. Can also be dispersed using same technique and 25 mL water in small glass.

Patient/Family Teaching

- Instruct patient to take everolimus at the same time each day as directed. Take missed doses as soon as remembered up to 6 hr after time of normal dose. If more than 6 hr after normal dose, omit dose for that day and take next dose next day; do not take two doses to make up missed dose. Do not eat grapefruit or drink grapefruit juice during therapy. Advise patient to read *Patient Information Leaflet* prior to beginning therapy and with each Rx refill in case of new information.
- Advise patient to report worsening respiratory symptoms or signs of infection (new or worsening cough, shortness of breath, chest pain, difficulty breathing or wheezing, fever, chills, skin rash, joint pain and inflammation, tiredness, loss of appetite, nausea, pale stool or dark urine, yellowing of the skin, pain in upper right side) to health care professional promptly.
- Inform patient that mouth sores may occur. Consult health care professional for treatment if pain, discomfort, or open sores in mouth occur. May require special mouthwash or gel.

- Instruct patient to avoid use of live vaccines and close contact with those who have received live vaccines.
- Instruct patient to notify health care professional of all Rx or OTC medications, vitamins, or herbal products being taken and to consult with health care professional before taking other medications.
- Rep: May have teratogenic effects and decrease male and female fertility. Advise female patients to use effective contraception during and for up to 8 wk following therapy and to notify health care professional if pregnancy is planned or suspected or if breast feeding.
- Emphasize the importance of routine blood tests to determine effectiveness and side effects.

Evaluation/Desired Outcomes

- Decreased spread of tumor. Continue treatment as long as clinical benefit is observed or until unacceptable toxicity occurs.
- Prevention of kidney transplant rejection.

evolocumab

(e-vo-**lo**-kyoo-mab)

Repatha

Classification

Therapeutic: lipid-lowering agents

Pharmacologic: proprotein convertase subtilisin kexin type 9 (PCSK9) inhibitor antibodies

Indications

Lowering of low density lipoprotein cholesterol (LDL-C) as an adjunct to diet and maximally tolerated statin (HMG CoA reductase inhibitor) therapy in patients with heterozygous familial hyercholesterolemia (HeFH) or cardiovascular disease who require supplemental agents. Additional lowering of low density lipoprotein cholesterol (LDL-C) as an adjunct to diet and maximally tolerated statin and other drug therapies in patients with homozygous familial hyercholesterolemia (HoFH).

Action

A human monoclonal immunoglobulin (IgG2) produced in genetically engineered Chinese hamster ovary cells that binds to PSCSK9 inhibiting its binding to the low density lipoprotein receptor (LDLR) resulting in ↑ number of LDLRs available to clear LDL from blood.
Therapeutic Effects: ↓ LDL-C.

Pharmacokinetics

Absorption: Well absorbed (72%) following subcut administration.
Distribution: Crosses the placenta.
Metabolism and Excretion: Eliminated by binding to PCSK9 and by proteolytic degradation.
Half-life: 11–17 days.

TIME/ACTION PROFILE (effect circulating unbound PCSK9)

ROUTE	ONSET	PEAK	DURATION
subcut	rapid	4 hr	2–4 wk

Contraindications/Precautions

Contraindicated in: History of serious hypersensitivity to evolocumab.
Use Cautiously in: Severe renal/hepatic impairment; Geri: Elderly patients may be more sensitive to drug effects; OB: Crosses the placenta, consider fetal risks; Lactation: Consider benefits of breast feeding against possible risk to infant.; Pedi: Safe and effective use in children <13 yr has not been established.

Adverse Reactions/Side Effects

Local: injection site reactions. **MS:** back pain. **Misc:** allergic reactions (including urticaria and rash), flu-like symptoms.

Interactions

Drug-Drug: None noted.

Route/Dosage

Subcut (Adults): *Primary hyperlipidemia with established CVD/HeFH*— 140 mg every two weeks or 420 mg monthly; *HoFH*—420 mg monthly.

Availability

Solution for subcutaneous injection (needle cover contains latex derivative): 140 mg/mL in prefilled syringe, 140 mg/mL in prefilled autoinjector.

NURSING IMPLICATIONS

Assessment

- Obtain a diet history, especially with regard to fat consumption.
- Monitor for signs and symptoms of hypersensitivity reactions (rash, urticaria) during therapy. If symptoms occur, discontinue therapy.
- Assess for latex allergy. Needle cover of the glass prefilled syringe and the autoinjector contain dry natural rubber (a derivative of latex); may cause allergic reactions.
- ***Lab Test Considerations:*** Assess LDL-C levels within 4 to 8 weeks of initiating; response to therapy depends on degree of LDL-receptor function.

Potential Nursing Diagnoses

Noncompliance, related to diet and medication regimen (Patient/Family Teaching)

Implementation

- **Subcut:** Administer 140 mg every 2 wks or 420 mg once monthly. To administer the 420 mg dose, give 3 injections, using 3 separate pens/syringes in 3 separate sites, consecutively within 30 minutes. When switching dose regimens, administer first dose of new regimen on next scheduled date of prior regimen. If stored in refrigerator allow solution to warm to room temperature for at least 30 min before injecting. May also be stored at room temperature, but only stable for 30 days. Solution is clear to opalescent and colorless to pale yellow; do not administer solutions that are cloudy or contain particulate matter. Do not shake. Inject into thigh, abdomen, or upper arm. Rotate sites with each injection. Do not inject into areas that are tender, bruised, red, or indurated. Do not re-use pre-filled pen or syringe. Do not administer other injectable drugs at same site.

Patient/Family Teaching

- Instruct patient in correct technique for self-injection, care and disposal of equipment. Administer missed doses within 7 days, then resume original schedule. If not administered within 7 days, wait until next dose on original schedule. Advise patient to read *Patient Information* before starting therapy and with each Rx refill in case of changes.
- Advise patient that this medication should be used in conjunction with diet restrictions (fat, cholesterol, carbohydrates, alcohol), exercise, and cessation of smoking.
- Instruct patient to notify health care professional of all Rx or OTC medications, vitamins, or herbal products being taken and to consult health care professional before taking any other Rx, OTC, or herbal products.
- Advise patient to notify health care professional of medication regimen prior to treatment or surgery.
- Advise patient to notify health care professional if pregnancy is planned or suspected or if breast feeding.

Evaluation/Desired Outcomes

- ↓ LDL-C levels.

exemestane (ex-e-mes-tane)

Aromasin

Classification

Therapeutic: antineoplastics

Pharmacologic: aromatase inhibitors

Pregnancy Category X

Indications

Adjuvant treatment of breast cancer in postmenopausal women who have estrogen-receptor positive early disease and who have already received 2–3 yr of tamoxifen and are then switched to exemestane to complete a total of 5 yr of adjuvant therapy. Treatment of advanced postmenopausal breast cancer that has progressed despite tamoxifen therapy.

Action

Inhibits aromatase, an enzyme responsible for the conversion of androgen to estrogen. In postmenopausal women, the primary source of estrogen is androgen. Decreases circulating estrogen. **Therapeutic Effects:** Decreased spread of estrogen-sensitive breast cancer.

Pharmacokinetics

Absorption: 42% absorbed following oral administration.

Distribution: Extensively distributed.

Metabolism and Excretion: Mostly metabolized by the liver (CYP3A4 enzyme system); metabolites are excreted in urine (40%) and feces (40%); <1% excreted unchanged in urine.

Half-life: 24 hr.

TIME/ACTION PROFILE (suppression of circulating estrogen)

ROUTE	ONSET	PEAK	DURATION
PO	unknown	2–3 days	4–5 days

Contraindications/Precautions

Contraindicated in: Hypersensitivity; Premenopausal status; OB: Pregnancy (may cause fetal harm); Lactation: Breast feeding should be avoided.

Use Cautiously in: Pedi: Safety and effectiveness not established.

Adverse Reactions/Side Effects

CNS: fatigue, depression, insomnia. **CV:** THROMBOEMBOLISM, hypertension. **GI:** diarrhea, nausea. **GU:** endometrial hyperplasia, uterine polyps. **Endo:** visual disturbances. **Derm:** alopecia, hot flashes, ↑ sweating, dermatitis. **MS:** arthralgia, musculoskeletal pain, carpal tunnel syndrome, muscle cramps, osteoporosis. **Neuro:** neuropathy, paresthesia.

Interactions

Drug-Drug: Strong **CYP3A4 inducers** including **rifampin** or **phenytoin** may ↓ levels and effectiveness; ↑ daily dose to 50 mg once daily. **Estrogens** can interfere with action.

Route/Dosage

PO (Adults): 25 mg once daily; *Concurrent use with strong CYP3A4 inducers*— 50 mg once daily.

Availability (generic available)

Tablets: 25 mg.

NURSING IMPLICATIONS

Assessment

- Assess patient for pain and other side effects periodically during therapy.
- ***Lab Test Considerations:*** May cause ↑ GTT, AST, ALT, alkaline phosphatase, bilirubin, and creatinine levels.
- Assess 25-hydroxy vitamin D levels prior to starting therapy. Supplement vitamin D deficiency with vita-

min D due to high prevalence of vitamin D deficiency in women with early breast cancer.

Potential Nursing Diagnoses

Acute pain (Side Effects)

Implementation

- Take 1 tablet daily after a meal.

Patient/Family Teaching

- Instruct patient to take exemestane as directed at the same time each day. Take missed doses as soon as remembered unless it is almost time for next dose. Do not double doses. Advise patient to read the *Patient Information* leaflet before starting and with each Rx refill in case of changes.
- Advise patient not to take other estrogen-containing agents; may interfere with action of exemestane.
- Inform patient that lower level of estrogen may lead to decreased bone mineral density over time and increased risk of osteoporosis and fracture. Women with osteoporosis or at risk of osteoporosis should have their bone mineral density formally assessed by bone densitometry at end of treatment. Monitor patients for bone mineral density loss and treat as appropriate.
- Advise patient to notify health care professional immediately if chest pain or signs of heart failure or stroke occur.
- Advise patient to notify health care professional of all Rx or OTC medications, vitamins, or herbal products being taken and to consult with health care professional before taking other medications.
- Exemestane is teratogenic; advise female patients to use effective contraception during therapy and to avoid breast feeding.
- Explain need for follow-up blood tests to check liver and kidney function.

Evaluation/Desired Outcomes

- Slowing of disease progression in women with breast cancer.

REMS

exenatide (ex-**en**-a-tide)

Bydureon, Byetta

Classification

Therapeutic: antidiabetics

Pharmacologic: incretin mimetic agents

Pregnancy Category C

Indications

Management of type 2 diabetes as an adjunct to diet and exercise (not recommended as first-line therapy).

Action

Mimics the action of incretin which promotes endogenous insulin secretion and promotes other mechanisms of glucose-lowering. **Therapeutic Effects:** Improved control of blood glucose.

Pharmacokinetics

Absorption: Well absorbed following subcutaneous administration.

Distribution: Unknown.

Metabolism and Excretion: Excreted mostly by glomerular filtration followed by degradation.

Half-life: *Immediate-release*—2.4 hr.

TIME/ACTION PROFILE (effects on postprandial blood glucose)

ROUTE	ONSET	PEAK	DURATION
Subcut (immediate-release)	within 30 min	2.1 hr	8 hr
Subcut (extended-release)	unknown	9 wk	unknown

Contraindications/Precautions

Contraindicated in: Hypersensitivity; Type 1 diabetes or diabetic ketoacidosis; Severe renal impairment or end-stage renal disease (CCr <30 mL/min); Severe gastrointestinal disease; Personal or family history of medullary thyroid carcinoma (extended-release only); Multiple Endocrine Neoplasia syndrome type 2 (extended-release only); OB: Has caused fetal physical defects and neonatal death in animal studies; Lactation: Excretion into breast milk unknown.

Use Cautiously in: History of pancreatitis; Moderate renal impairment (CCr 30–50 mL/min); Concurrent use of insulin (extended-release only); Pedi: Safety not established.

Adverse Reactions/Side Effects

CV: dizziness, headache, jitteriness, weakness. **GI:** PANCREATITIS, diarrhea, nausea, vomiting, dyspepsia, gastroinestinal reflux. **Endo:** THYROID C-CELL TUMORS (extended-release), hypoglycemia. **GU:** acute renal failure. **Derm:** hyperhydrosis. **Metab:** ↓ appetite, weight loss. **Misc:** injection site reactions.

Interactions

Drug-Drug: Concurrent use with **sulfonylureas** or **insulin** may ↑ risk of hypoglycemia (↓ dose of **sulfonylurea** or **insulin** if hypoglycemia occurs); concomitant use of **insulin** with extended-release exenatide not recommended. Concurrent use with **nateglinide** or **repaglinide** may ↑ risk of hypoglycemia. Due to slowed gastric emptying, may ↓ absorption of **orally administered medications**, especially those requiring rapid GI absorption or require a specific level for efficacy; take oral **anti-infectives** and **oral contraceptives** at least 1 hr before injecting exenatide).

Route/Dosage

Immediate Release (Byetta)

Subcut (Adults): 5 mcg within 60 min before morning and evening meal; after 1 mo, dose may be ↑ to 10 mcg depending on response.

Renal Impairment

Subcut (Adults): *CCr 30–50 mL/min*—Use caution when ↑ dose from 5 mcg to 10 mcg.

Extended Release (Bydureon)

Subcut (Adults): 2 mg every 7 days.

Availability

Solution for subcutaneous injection (Byetta): 250 mcg/mL in prefilled pen-injector that delivers either 5 mcg/dose (1.2-mL pen) or 10 mcg/dose (2.4-mL pen) for 60 doses (30 days of twice daily dosing). **Suspension for subcutaneous injection (Bydureon):** 2 mg/vial or pen.

NURSING IMPLICATIONS

Assessment

- Observe for signs and symptoms of hypoglycemic reactions (abdominal pain, sweating, hunger, weakness, dizziness, headache, drowsiness, tremor, tachycardia, anxiety, confusion, irritability, jitteriness), especially when combined with oral sulfonylureas.
- Assess for signs and symptoms of pancreatitis (persistent severe abdominal pain, sometimes radiating to the back, may or may not be accompanied by vomiting) at beginning of therapy and with dose increases. If suspected, promptly discontinue therapy and initiate appropriate management. If pancreatitis is confirmed, do not restart exenatide. Consider other antidiabetic therapies in patients with a history of pancreatitis.
- ***Lab Test Considerations:*** Monitor serum glucose and glycolysated hemoglobin periodically during therapy to evaluate effectiveness of therapy.
- Monitor renal function prior to and periodically during therapy. Renal dysfunction may be reversed with discontinuation of therapy.

Potential Nursing Diagnoses

Imbalanced nutrition: more than body requirements (Indications)
Noncompliance (Patient/Family Teaching)

Implementation

- Some medications may need to be taken 1 hr before exenatide.
- Patients stabilized on a diabetic regimen who are exposed to stress, fever, trauma, infection, or surgery may require administration of insulin.
- **Subcut:** *Immediate release:* Follow directions for *New Pen Setup* in *Information for Patient* prior to use of each new pen. Inject exenatide in thigh, abdomen, or upper arm at any time within the 60–min period **before** the morning and evening meals. Do not administer after a meal. Do not mix with insulin. Solution should be clear and colorless; do not administer solutions that are discolored or contain particulate matter. Refrigerate; discard pen 30 days after 1st use, even if some drug remains in pen. Do not freeze. Do not store pen with needle attached; medication may leak from pen or air bubbles may form in the cartridge.
- **Subcut:** *Extended release:* Dilute with diluent and needles included in tray. Suspension should be white or off-white and cloudy. Administer without regard to meals. Inject into upper arm, abdomen, or thigh; change site each week. Refrigerate; each tray can be kept at room temperature if not >77°F for up to 4 wks. Do not use beyond expiration date.

E

Patient/Family Teaching

- Instruct patient to take exenatide *immediate release* as directed within 60 min before a meal. Do not take after a meal. If a dose is missed, skip the dose and take the next dose at the prescribed time. Do not take an extra dose or increase the amount of the next dose to make up for missed dose. If a dose of exenatide *extended release* is missed, administer as soon as remembered as long as the next dose is due at least 3 days later; if 1 or 2 days later skip dose and administer next dose as scheduled. The day of weekly administration can be changed as long as the last dose was administered 3 or more days before.
- Instruct patient in proper technique for administration, timing of dose and concurrent oral medications, storage of medication, and disposal of used needles. Patients should read the *Information for Patient* insert prior to initiation of therapy and with each Rx refill. Advise patient that *New Pen Setup* should be done only with each new pen, not with each dose.
- Inform patient that pen needles are not included with pen and must be purchased separately. Advise patient which needle length and gauge should be used. Caution patient not to share pen and needles.
- Caution patient to never share pen with others, even if needle is changed. May cause transmission of blood-borne pathogens.
- Explain to patient that exenatide helps control hyperglycemia but does not cure diabetes. Therapy is usually long term.
- Encourage patient to follow prescribed diet, medication, and exercise regimen to prevent hyperglycemic or hypoglycemic episodes.
- Review signs of hypoglycemia and hyperglycemia with patient. If hypoglycemia occurs, advise patient to take a glass of orange juice or 2–3 tsp of sugar, honey, or corn syrup dissolved in water, and notify health care professional. Risk of hypoglycemia is increased if sulfonureas are taken concurrently with exenatide.
- Advise patient to notify health care professional immediately if symptoms of pancreatitis (unexplained,

persistent, severe abdominal pain which may or may not be accompanied by vomiting) occur.

- Inform patient that therapy may result in reduction of appetite, food intake, and/or body weight. Dose modification is not necessary. Nausea is more common at initiation of therapy and usually decreases over time.
- Instruct patient to notify health care professional of all Rx or OTC medications, vitamins, or herbal products being taken and to consult health care professional before taking any other Rx, OTC, or herbal products. Exenatide delays stomach emptying. Some medications (such as anti-infectives and oral contraceptives) may need to be taken 1 hr before exenatide injection.
- Instruct patient in proper testing of blood glucose and urine ketones. These tests should be monitored closely during periods of stress or illness and health care professional notified if significant changes occur.
- Advise patient to inform health care professional of medication regimen before treatment or surgery.
- Advise patient to notify health care professional if pregnancy is suspected or planned.
- Advise patient to carry a form of sugar (sugar packets, candy) and identification describing disease process and medication regimen at all times.
- Emphasize the importance of routine follow-up exams and regular testing of blood glucose and glycosylated hemoglobin.

Evaluation/Desired Outcomes

- Control of blood glucose levels without the appearance of hypoglycemic or hyperglycemic episodes.

ezetimibe (e-zet-i-mibe)

✱Ezetrol, Zetia

Classification

Therapeutic: lipid-lowering agents

Pharmacologic: cholesterol absorption inhibitors

Pregnancy Category C

Indications

Alone or with other agents (HMG-CoA reductase inhibitors) in the management of dyslipidemias including primary hypercholesterolemia, homozygous familial hypercholesterolemia, and homozygous sitosterolemia.

Action

Inhibits absorption of cholesterol in the small intestine.
Therapeutic Effects: Lowering of cholesterol, a known risk factor for atherosclerosis.

Pharmacokinetics

Absorption: Following absorption, rapidly converted to ezetimibe-glucaronide, which is active. Bioavailability is variable.
Distribution: Unknown.
Metabolism and Excretion: Undergoes enterhepatic recycling, mostly eliminated in feces, minimal renal excretion.
Half-life: 22 hr.

TIME/ACTION PROFILE

ROUTE	ONSET	PEAK	DURATION
PO	unknown	unknown	unknown

Contraindications/Precautions

Contraindicated in: Hypersensitivity; Acute liver disease or unexplained laboratory evidence of liver disease (when used with HMG-CoA reductase inhibitor); Moderate or severe hepatic impairment; Concurrent use of fibrates; OB: May cause fetal harm by interfering with cholesterol synthesis and, possibly, biologically active substances derived from cholesterol; Lactation: Potential for adverse effects in nursing infant.
Use Cautiously in: Pedi: Children <10 yr (safety not established).

Adverse Reactions/Side Effects

GI: cholecystitis, cholelithiasis, ↑ liver enzymes (with HMG-CoA reductase inhibitors), nausea, pancreatitis. **Derm:** rash. **Misc:** ANGIOEDEMA.

Interactions

Drug-Drug: Effects may be ↓ by **cholestyramine** or other **bile acid sequestrants**. Concurrent use of **fibrates** may ↑ levels and the risk of cholelithiasis. **Cyclosporine** may ↑ levels. May ↑ risk of rhabdomyolysis when used with **HMG CoA-reductase inhibitors**.

Route/Dosage

PO (Adults): 10 mg once daily.

Renal Impairment

PO (Adults): *CCr <60 mL/min and concurrent use with simvastatin*—Do not exceed simvastatin dose of 20 mg/day.

Availability (generic available)

Tablets: 10 mg. **Cost:** $517.89/90. ***In combination with:*** simvastatin (Vytorin); see Appendix B.

NURSING IMPLICATIONS

Assessment

- Obtain a diet history, especially with regard to fat consumption.
- ***Lab Test Considerations:*** Evaluate serum cholesterol and triglyceride levels before initiating, after 2–4 wk of therapy, and periodically thereafter.
- May cause ↑ liver transaminases when administered with HMG-CoA reductase inhibitors. Monitor liver enzymes prior to initiation and during therapy according to recommendations of HMG-CoA reductase inhibitor. Elevations are usually asymptomatic and return to baseline with continued therapy.

Potential Nursing Diagnoses

Noncompliance, related to diet and medication regimen (Patient/Family Teaching)

Implementation

- Do not confuse Zetia with Zebeta (bisoprolol) or Zestril (lisinopril).
- **PO:** Administer without regard to meals. May be taken at the same time as HMG-CoA reductase inhibitors.

Patient/Family Teaching

- Instruct patient to take ezetimibe as directed, at the same time each day, even if feeling well. Take missed doses as soon as remembered, but do not take more than 1 dose/day. Medication helps control but does not cure elevated serum cholesterol levels.
- Advise patient that this medication should be used in conjunction with diet restrictions (fat, cholesterol, carbohydrates, alcohol), exercise, and cessation of smoking. Ezetimibe does not assist with weight loss.
- Instruct patient to notify health care professional if unexplained muscle pain, tenderness, or weakness occur. Risk may increase when used with HMG-CoA reductase inhibitors.
- Instruct patient to notify health care professional of all Rx or OTC medications, vitamins, or herbal products being taken and to consult health care professional before taking any other Rx, OTC, or herbal products.
- Advise patient to notify health care professional of medication regimen prior to treatment or surgery.
- Instruct female patients to notify health care professional promptly if pregnancy is planned or suspected or if breast feeding. If regimen includes HMG-CoA reductase inhibitors, they are contraindicated in pregnancy.
- Emphasize the importance of follow-up exams to determine effectiveness and to monitor for side effects.

Evaluation/Desired Outcomes

- Decrease in serum LDL and total cholesterol levels.

E

famciclovir (fam-**sye**-kloe-veer)
Famvir

Classification
Therapeutic: antivirals

Pregnancy Category B

Indications

Acute herpes zoster infections (shingles). Treatment/suppression of recurrent herpes genitalis in immunocompetent patients. Treatment of recurrent herpes labialis (cold sores) in immunocompetent patients. Treatment of recurrent mucocutaneous herpes simplex virus (HSV) infection in HIV-infected patients.

Action

Inhibits viral DNA synthesis in herpes-infected cells only. **Therapeutic Effects:** Decreased duration of herpes zoster infection with decreased duration of viral shedding. Decreased time to healing for cold sores. Decreased lesion formation and improved healing in recurrent HSV infection.

Pharmacokinetics

Absorption: Following absorption, famciclovir is rapidly converted in the intestinal wall to penciclovir, the active compound.
Distribution: Unknown.
Metabolism and Excretion: Penciclovir is mostly excreted by the kidneys.
Half-life: *Penciclovir*—2.1–3 hr (↑ in renal impairment).

TIME/ACTION PROFILE (penciclovir blood levels)

ROUTE	ONSET	PEAK	DURATION
PO	rapid	0.9 hr	8–12 hr

Contraindications/Precautions

Contraindicated in: Hypersensitivity.
Use Cautiously in: Patients with impaired renal function (↑ dose interval/↓ dose recommended if CCr <40–60 mL/min); OB, Lactation: Limited information; use only if maternal benefit clearly outweighs potential risks to fetus or infant; Pedi: Safety not established in children <18 yr; Geri: Consider age-related ↓ in renal function when prescribing.

Adverse Reactions/Side Effects

CNS: headache, dizziness, fatigue. **CV:** leukocytoclastic vasculitis, palpitations. **GI:** diarrhea, nausea, vomiting.

Interactions

Drug-Drug: Probenecid ↑ plasma concentrations of penciclovir.

Route/Dosage

Herpes Zoster

PO (Adults): 500 mg q 8 hr for 7 days.

Renal Impairment

PO (Adults): *CCr 40–59 mL/min*—500 mg q 12 hr; *CCr 20–39mL/min*—500 mg q 24 hr; *CCr <20 mL/min*—250 mg q 24 hr; *Hemodialysis*—250 mg after each dialysis.

Recurrent Genital Herpes Simplex Infections

PO (Adults): 1000 mg twice daily for one day.

Renal Impairment

PO (Adults): *CCr 40–59 mL/min*—500 mg twice daily for 1 day; *CCr 20–39 mL/min*—500 mg as a single dose; *CCr <20 mL/min*—250 mg as a single dose; *Hemodialysis*—250 mg as a single dose after dialysis.

Suppression of Recurrent Herpes Simplex Infections

PO (Adults): 250 mg q 12 hr for up to 1 yr.

Renal Impairment

PO (Adults): *CCr 20–39 mL/min*—125 mg q 12 hr for 5 days; *CCr <20 mL/min*—125 mg q 24 hr for 5 days; *Hemodialysis*—125 mg after each dialysis.

Recurrent Herpes Labialis Infections (cold sores)

PO (Adults): 1500 mg as a single dose.

Renal Impairment

PO (Adults): *CCr 40–59 mL/min*—750 mg as a single dose; *CCr 20–39 mL/min*—500 mg as a single dose; *CCr <20 mL/min*—250 mg as a single dose; *Hemodialysis*—250 mg as a single dose after dialysis.

Herpes Simplex in HIV-Infected Patients

PO (Adults): 500 mg q 12 hr for 7 days.

Renal Impairment

PO (Adults): *CCr 20–39 mL/min*—500 mg q 24 hr for 7 days; *CCr <20 mL/min*—250 mg q 24 hr for 7 days; *Hemodialysis*—250 mg after each dialysis.

Availability (generic available)

Tablets: 125 mg, 250 mg, 500 mg.

NURSING IMPLICATIONS

Assessment

- Assess lesions prior to and daily during therapy.
- Assess patient for postherpetic neuralgia periodically during and following therapy.

F

Potential Nursing Diagnoses

Risk for impaired skin integrity (Indications)
Risk for infection (Indications, Patient/Family Teaching)

Implementation

- Famciclovir therapy should be started as soon as herpes zoster is diagnosed, at least within 72 hr, preferably within 48 hr.
- **PO:** Famciclovir may be administered without regard to meals.

Patient/Family Teaching

- Instruct patient to take famciclovir as directed for the full course of therapy. Take missed doses as soon as remembered, if not just before next dose.
- Inform patient that famciclovir does not prevent the spread of infection to others. Until all lesions have crusted, precautions should be taken around others who have not had chickenpox or varicella vaccine or people who are immunosuppressed.
- Advise patient that condoms should be used during sexual contact and that no sexual contact should be made while lesions are present.
- May cause dizziness. Caution patient to avoid driving and other activities requiring alertness until response to medication is known.
- Instruct women with genital herpes to have yearly Papanicolaou smears because these women may be more likely to develop cervical cancer.

Evaluation/Desired Outcomes

- Decrease in time to full crusting, loss of vesicles, loss of ulcers, and loss of crusts in patients with acute herpes zoster (shingles).
- Crusting over and healing of lesions in herpes labialis, genital herpes, and in recurrent mucocutaneous HSV infection in HIV-infected patients.
- Prevention of recurrence of herpes genitalis.
- Decreased time to healing for cold sores.

famotidine, See HISTAMINE H_2 ANTAGONISTS.

febuxostat (fe-bux-o-stat)

Uloric

Classification
Therapeutic: antigout agents
Pharmacologic: xanthine oxidase inhibitors

Pregnancy Category C

Indications

Chronic management of hyperuricemia in patients with a history of gout.

Action

Decreases production of uric acid by inhibiting xanthine oxidase. **Therapeutic Effects:** Lowering of serum uric acid levels with resultant decrease in gouty attacks.

Pharmacokinetics

Absorption: Well absorbed (49%) following oral administration.
Distribution: Unknown.
Protein Binding: 99.2%.
Metabolism and Excretion: Extensively metabolized by the liver; minimal renal excretion of unchanged drug, 45% eliminated in feces as unchanged drug, remainder is eliminated in urine and feces as inactive metabolites.
Half-life: 5–8 hr.

TIME/ACTION PROFILE (blood levels)

ROUTE	ONSET	PEAK	DURATION
PO	rapid	1–1.5 hr*	24 hr

*Maximum lowering of uric acid may take 2 wk.

Contraindications/Precautions

Contraindicated in: Concurrent azathioprine or mercaptopurine.
Use Cautiously in: Severe renal impairment (CCr <30 mL/min); Severe hepatic impairment; OB: Use only when potential maternal benefit outweighs potential fetal risk; Lactation: Unknown if excreted into breast milk; use caution when breast feeding; Pedi: Safety in children <18 yr not established.

Adverse Reactions/Side Effects

GI: ↑ liver function tests, nausea. **Derm:** rash. **MS:** gout flare, arthralgia.

Interactions

Drug-Drug: Significantly ↑ levels of and risk of serious toxicity from **azathioprine** and **mercaptopurine**; concurrent use is contraindicated. May ↑ levels of **theophylline**; use cautiously together.

Route/Dosage

PO (Adults): 40 mg once daily initially; if serum uric acid does not ↓ to <6 mg/dL, dose should be ↑ to 80 mg once daily.

Availability

Tablets: 40 mg, 80 mg.

NURSING IMPLICATIONS

Assessment

- Assess for joint pain and swelling, especially during early therapy. Changing serum uric acid levels from mobilization of urate from tissue deposits may cause gout flares. Use prophylactic NSAID or colchicine therapy for up to 6 mo. If a gout flare occurs, continue febuxostat therapy and treat flare concurrently.
- Monitor for signs and symptoms of MI and stroke.
- ***Lab Test Considerations:*** Monitor serum uric acid levels prior to, 2 wk after intiating, and periodically thereafter. If serum uric acid levels are ≥6 mg/

dL after 2 wk of daily 40 mg therapy, increase dose to 80 mg daily.
- Monitor liver function at 2 and 4 mo of therapy and periodically thereafter. May cause ↑ AST, ALT, CPK, LDH, alkaline phosphatase, and creatine.
- May cause prolonged aPTT and PT, and ↓ hematocrit, hemoglobin, RBC, platelet count, and lymphocyte, neutrohpil counts. May cause ↑ or ↓ WBC.
- May cause ↓ serum bicarbonate and ↑ serum sodium, glucose, potassium, and TSH levels.
- May cause ↑ serum cholesterol, triglycerides, amylase, and LDL levels.
- May cause ↑ BUN and serum creatinine and proteinuria.

Potential Nursing Diagnoses

Chronic pain (Indications)

Implementation

- **PO:** May be taken with or without food and with antacids.

Patient/Family Teaching

- Instruct patient to take febuxostat as directed. If a gout flare occurs, continue febuxostat and consult health care professional; medications to manage gout flare may be added.
- Advise patient to notify health care professional if rash, chest pain, shortness of breath, or stroke symptoms (weakness, headache, confusion, slurred speech) occur or if side effects are persistent or bothersome.
- Instruct patient to notify health care professional of all Rx or OTC medications, vitamins, or herbal products being taken and to consult health care professional before taking any other Rx, OTC, or herbal products.
- Advise female patient to notify health care professional if pregnancy is planned or suspected or if breast feeding.
- Emphasize the importance of follow-up lab tests to monitor therapy.

Evaluation/Desired Outcomes

- Reduction in serum uric acid levels and resultant gout attacks.

felodipine (fe-loe-di-peen)

Plendil, ✱Renedil

Classification

Therapeutic: antianginals, antihypertensives
Pharmacologic: calcium channel blockers

Pregnancy Category C

Indications

Management of hypertension, angina pectoris, and vasospastic (Prinzmetal's) angina.

Action

Inhibits the transport of calcium into myocardial and vascular smooth muscle cells, resulting in inhibition of excitation-contraction coupling and subsequent contraction. **Therapeutic Effects:** Systemic vasodilation resulting in decreased BP. Coronary vasodilation resulting in decreased frequency and severity of attacks of angina.

Pharmacokinetics

Absorption: Well absorbed after oral administration, but extensively metabolized, resulting in ↓ bioavailability.
Distribution: Unknown.
Protein Binding: >99%.
Metabolism and Excretion: Mostly metabolized; minimal amounts excreted unchanged by kidneys.
Half-life: 11–16 hr.

TIME/ACTION PROFILE (antihypertensive effect)

ROUTE	ONSET	PEAK	DURATION
PO	1 hr	2–4 hr	up to 24 hr

Contraindications/Precautions

Contraindicated in: Hypersensitivity (cross-sensitivity may occur); Sick sinus syndrome; 2nd- or 3rd-degree AV block (unless an artificial pacemaker is in place); Systolic BP <90 mm Hg.
Use Cautiously in: Severe hepatic impairment (dose ↓ recommended); Geri: Dose ↓ recommended; ↑ risk of hypotension; Severe renal impairment; History of serious ventricular arrhythmias or HF; OB, Lactation, Pedi: Safety not established.

Adverse Reactions/Side Effects

CNS: headache, abnormal dreams, anxiety, confusion, dizziness, drowsiness, nervousness, psychiatric disturbances, weakness. **EENT:** blurred vision, disturbed equilibrium, epistaxis, tinnitus. **Resp:** cough, dyspnea. **CV:** ARRHYTHMIAS, HF, peripheral edema, chest pain, hypotension, palpitations, syncope, tachycardia. **GI:** anorexia, constipation, diarrhea, dry mouth, dysgeusia, dyspepsia, ↑ liver enzymes, nausea, vomiting. **GU:** dysuria, nocturia, polyuria, sexual dysfunction, urinary frequency. **Derm:** dermatitis, erythema multiforme, flushing, ↑ sweating, photosensitivity, pruritus/urticaria, rash. **Endo:** gynecomastia, hyperglycemia. **Hemat:** anemia, leukopenia, thrombocytopenia. **Metab:** weight gain. **MS:** joint stiffness, muscle cramps. **Neuro:** paresthesia, tremor. **Misc:** STEVENS-JOHNSON SYNDROME, gingival hyperplasia.

Interactions

Drug-Drug: Additive hypotension may occur when used concurrently with **fentanyl**, other **anti-**

hypertensives, **nitrates**, acute ingestion of **alcohol**, or **quinidine**. Antihypertensive effects may be ↓ by concurrent use of **NSAIDs**. **Ketoconazole**, **itraconazole**, **propranolol**, and **erythromycin** ↓ metabolism and ↑ blood levels and the risk of toxicity (dose ↓ may be necessary).

Drug-Food: Grapefruit juice ↑ serum levels and effect.

Route/Dosage

PO (Adults): 5 mg/day (2.5 mg/day in geriatric patients); may ↑ q 2 wk (range 5–10 mg/day; not to exceed 10 mg/day).

Availability (generic available)

Extended-release tablets: 2.5 mg, 5 mg, 10 mg.

NURSING IMPLICATIONS

Assessment

- Monitor BP and pulse before therapy, during dosage titration, and periodically during therapy. Monitor ECG periodically during prolonged therapy.
- Monitor intake and output ratios and daily weight. Assess for signs of HF (peripheral edema, rales/crackles, dyspnea, weight gain, jugular venous distention).
- Assess for rash periodically during therapy. May cause Stevens-Johnson syndrome. Discontinue therapy if severe or if accompanied with fever, general malaise, fatigue, muscle or joint aches, blisters, oral lesions, conjunctivitis, hepatitis, and/or eosinophilia.
- **Angina:** Assess location, duration, intensity, and precipitating factors of patient's anginal pain.
- **Hypertension:** Check frequency of refills to monitor adherence.
- ***Lab Test Considerations:*** Total serum calcium concentrations are not affected by calcium channel blockers.
- Monitor serum potassium periodically. Hypokalemia ↑ risk of arrhythmias and should be corrected.
- Monitor renal and hepatic functions periodically during long-term therapy. May cause ↑ in hepatic enzymes after several days of therapy, which return to normal upon discontinuation of therapy.

Potential Nursing Diagnoses

Ineffective tissue perfusion (Indications)
Acute pain (Indications)

Implementation

- Do not confuse Plendil with Isordil.
- **PO:** May be administered without regard to meals. May be administered with meals if GI irritation becomes a problem.
- Swallow tablets whole; do not break, crush, or chew. Empty tablets that appear in stool are not significant.

Patient/Family Teaching

- Advise patient to take medication as directed, even if feeling well. If a dose is missed, take as soon as possible unless almost time for next dose; do not double doses. May need to be discontinued gradually.
- Instruct patient on correct technique for monitoring pulse. Instruct patient to contact health care professional if heart rate is <50 bpm.
- Advise patient to avoid grapefruit or grapefruit juice during therapy.
- Caution patient to change positions slowly to minimize orthostatic hypotension.
- May cause drowsiness or dizziness. Advise patient to avoid driving or other activities requiring alertness until response to the medication is known.
- Instruct patient on importance of maintaining good dental hygiene and seeing dentist frequently for teeth cleaning to prevent tenderness, bleeding, and gingival hyperplasia (gum enlargement).
- Instruct patient to notify health care professional of all Rx or OTC medications, vitamins, or herbal products being taken and to avoid concurrent use of alcohol or OTC medications and herbal products, especially cold preparations, without consulting health care professional.
- Advise patient to notify health care professional if rash, irregular heartbeat, dyspnea, swelling of hands and feet, pronounced dizziness, nausea, constipation, rash, or hypotension occurs or if headache is severe or persistent.
- Caution patient to wear protective clothing and to use sunscreen to prevent photosensitivity reactions.
- Advise patient to inform health care professional of medication regimen before treatment or surgery.
- **Angina:** Instruct patient on concurrent nitrate or beta-blocker therapy to continue taking both medications as directed and to use SL nitroglycerin as needed for anginal attacks.
- Advise patient to contact health care professional if chest pain does not improve or worsens after therapy; occurs with diaphoresis or shortness of breath; or if severe, persistent headache occurs.
- Caution patient to discuss exercise restrictions with health care professional before exertion.
- **Hypertension:** Encourage patient to comply with other interventions for hypertension (weight reduction, low-sodium diet, smoking cessation, moderation of alcohol consumption, regular exercise, and stress management). Medication controls but does not cure hypertension.
- Instruct patient and family in proper technique for monitoring BP. Advise patient to take BP weekly and to report significant changes.

Evaluation/Desired Outcomes

- Decrease in BP.
- Decrease in frequency and severity of anginal attacks.
- Decrease in need for nitrate therapy.
- Increase in activity tolerance and sense of well-being.

fenofibrate (fen-o-fi-brate)

Antara, Fenoglide, ✤Fenomax, ✤Lipidil EZ, ✤Lipidil Micro, ✤Lipidil Supra, Lipofen, Lofibra, Tricor, Triglide

Classification
Therapeutic: lipid-lowering agents
Pharmacologic: fibric acid derivatives

Pregnancy Category C

Indications

With dietary therapy to decrease LDL cholesterol, total cholesterol, triglycerides, and apolipoprotein B in adult patients with hypercholesterolemia or mixed dyslipidemia. With dietary management in the treatment of hypertriglyceridemia (types IV and V hyperlipidemia) in patients who are at risk for pancreatitis and do not respond to nondrug therapy.

Action

Fenofibric acid primarily inhibits triglyceride synthesis. **Therapeutic Effects:** Lowering of cholesterol and triglycerides with subsequent decreased risk of pancreatitis.

Pharmacokinetics

Absorption: Well absorbed (60%) after oral administration; absorption ↑ by food.
Distribution: Unknown.
Protein Binding: 99%.
Metabolism and Excretion: Rapidly converted to fenofibric acid, which is the active metabolite; fenofibric acid is metabolized by the liver. Fenofibric acid and its metabolites are primarily excreted in urine (60%).
Half-life: 20 hr.

TIME/ACTION PROFILE (lowering of triglycerides)

ROUTE	ONSET	PEAK	DURATION
PO	unknown	2 wk	unknown

Contraindications/Precautions

Contraindicated in: Hypersensitivity; Hepatic impairment (including primary biliary cirrhosis); Pre-existing gallbladder disease; Severe renal impairment; Concurrent use of HMG-CoA reductase inhibitors; Lactation: Potential for tumorigenicity noted in animal studies; discontinue breast feeding.
Use Cautiously in: Concurrent warfarin or HMG-CoA reductase inhibitor therapy; OB: Embryocidal and teratogenic in animal studies; use only if potential benefits outweigh risks to the fetus; Pedi: Safety not established; Geri: Age-related ↓ in renal function may make older patients more susceptible to adverse reactions.

Adverse Reactions/Side Effects

CNS: fatigue/weakness, headache. **CV:** PULMONARY EMBOLISM, arrhythmias, deep vein thrombosis. **GI:** cholelithiasis, pancreatitis. **Derm:** rash, urticaria. **Metab:** ↓ HDL levels. **MS:** rhabdomyolysis. **Misc:** hypersensitivity reactions.

Interactions

Drug-Drug: ↑ anticoagulant effects of **warfarin**. **HMG-CoA reductase inhibitors** ↑ risk of rhabdomyolysis (concurrent use should be avoided). Absorption is ↓ by **bile acid sequestrants** (fenofibrate should be given 1 hr before or 4–6 hr after). ↑ risk of nephrotoxicity with **cyclosporine**. Concurrent use with **colchicine** may ↑ risk of rhabdomyolysis.

Route/Dosage

Primary hypercholesterolemia/mixed dyslipidemia

PO (Adults): *Antara*—90 mg/day initially; *Fenoglide*—120 mg/day; *Lofibra*—200 mg/day initially; *Tricor*—145 mg/day initially; *Triglide*—160 mg/day initially; *Lipofen*—50 mg daily.

Hypertriglyceridemia

PO (Adults): *Antara*—30–90 mg/day; *Fenoglide*—40–120 mg/day; *Lofibra*—67–200 mg/day initially; *Tricor*—48–145 mg/day initially; *Triglide*—50–160 mg/day initially; *Lipofen*—50 mg daily.

Renal impairment/Geriatric patients

PO (Adults): *Antara*—30 mg/day; *Fenoglide*—start at 40 mg/day; *Lofibra*—67 mg/day; *Tricor*—48 mg/day.

Availability (generic available)

Tablets (Tricor): 48 mg, 145 mg. **Cost:** *Generic*—48 mg $171.86/90, 145 mg $515.58/90. **Tablets (Fenoglide):** 40 mg, 120 mg. **Cost:** 40 mg $289.44/90, 120 mg $869.40/90. **Tablets (Triglide):** 50 mg, 160 mg. **Cost:** *Generic*—160 mg $176.40/100. **Micronized tablets (Lofibra):** 54 mg, ✤100 mg, 160 mg. **Cost:** *Generic*—54 mg $71.29/90, 160 mg $213.88/90. **Micronized capsules (Antara):** 30 mg, 90 mg. **Capsules (Lipofen):** 50 mg, 150 mg. **Cost:** 50 mg $213.58/90, 150 mg $468.24/90. **Micronized capsules (Lofibra):** 67 mg, 134 mg, 200 mg. **Cost:** *Generic*—67 mg $74.95/100, 134 mg $199.62/100, 200 mg $266.45/100.

NURSING IMPLICATIONS

Assessment

- Obtain a diet history, especially with regard to fat consumption. Every attempt should be made to obtain normal serum triglyceride levels with diet, exercise, and weight loss in obese patients before fenofibrate therapy is instituted.

- Assess patient for cholelithiasis. If symptoms occur, gallbladder studies are indicated. Discontinue therapy if gallstones are found.
- ***Lab Test Considerations:*** Monitor serum lipids before therapy to determine consistent elevations, then monitor periodically during therapy.
- Monitor serum AST and ALT periodically during therapy. May cause ↑ levels. Therapy should be discontinued if levels rise >3 times the normal limit.
- If patient develops muscle tenderness during therapy, monitor CPK levels. If CPK levels are markedly ↑ or myopathy occurs, discontinue therapy.
- May cause mild to moderate ↓ in hemoglobin, hematocrit, and WBCs. Monitor periodically during first 12 mo of therapy. Levels usually stabilize during long-term therapy.
- Monitor prothrombin levels frequently until levels stabilize in patients taking anticoagulants concurrently.

Potential Nursing Diagnoses

Noncompliance (Patient/Family Teaching)

Implementation

- Do not confuse Tricor with Tracleer (bosentan).
- Place patients on a triglyceride-lowering diet before therapy and remain on this diet throughout therapy.
- Dose may be increased after repeated serum triglyceride levels every 4–8 wk.
- Brands are not interchangeable.
- **PO:** Administer *Antara, Fenoglide, Lipofen, Lipidil Micro, Lipidil Supra, Lofibra,* and *Tricor* products with meals. *Triglide* formulation may be taken without regard to meals.

Patient/Family Teaching

- Instruct patient to take medication as directed, not to skip doses or double up on missed doses. Medication helps control but does not cure elevated serum triglyceride levels.
- Advise patient that this medication should be used in conjunction with diet restrictions (fat, cholesterol, carbohydrates, alcohol), exercise, and cessation of smoking.
- Instruct patient to notify health care professional if unexplained muscle pain, tenderness, or weakness occurs, especially if accompanied by fever or malaise.
- Advise patient to notify health care professional of medication regimen before treatment or surgery.
- Instruct female patients to notify health care professional promptly if pregnancy is planned or suspected.
- Emphasize the importance of follow-up exams to determine effectiveness and to monitor for side effects.

Evaluation/Desired Outcomes

- Decrease in serum triglycerides and cholesterol to normal levels. Therapy should be discontinued in patients who do not have an adequate response in 2 mo of therapy.

fenofibric acid

(feen-oh**fye**-brik **as**-id)

Fibricor, TriLipix

Classification

Therapeutic: lipid-lowering agents

Pharmacologic: fibric acid derivatives

Indications

With a statin to reduce triglycerides (TG) and increase high density lipoprotein-C (HDL-C) in patients with mixed dyslipidemias and CHD or a CHD risk equivalent who are on statin therapy to achieve their low-density lipoprotein-C (LDL-C) goal (TriLipix only). As monotherapy to reduce TG in patients with severe hypertriglyceridemia. As monotherapy to reduce elevated LDL-C, total cholesterol (Total-C), TG and apolipoprotein B (Apo B), and increase HDL-C in patients with primary hyperlipidemia or mixed dyslipidemia. Part of a comprehensive program to decrease cardiovascular risk factors.

Action

Activates the peroxisome proliferator activated receptor α (PPARα), resulting in increased lipolysis and elimination of triglycerides from plasma. Activation of PPARα also increases production of HDL. **Therapeutic Effects:** Improvement in lipid profile with lowered triglycerides and LDL cholesterol, and increased HDL cholesterol.

Pharmacokinetics

Absorption: Well absorbed following oral administration.

Distribution: Unknown.

Protein Binding: 99%.

Metabolism and Excretion: Fenofibric acid is the active metabolite of fenofibrate. Fenofibric acid is mostly metabolized by glucuronidation and the metabolites are mostly excreted by the kidneys.

Half-life: 20 hr.

TIME/ACTION PROFILE (effects on blood lipids)

ROUTE	ONSET	PEAK	DURATION
PO	unknown	4–5 hr†	unknown

†Blood levels.

Contraindications/Precautions

Contraindicated in: Hypersensitivity to fenofibric acid, choline fenofibrate or fenofibrate; Severe renal impairment (CCr <30 mL/min); Active liver or gallbladder disease; Lactation: Avoid use during breast feeding.

Use Cautiously in: Mild/moderate renal impairment (dose ↓ required for CCr 30–80 mL/min); Concurrent use with statins in elderly patients, patients with diabetes, renal failure, or hypothyroidism (↑ risk of myopathy/rhabdomyolysis); Geri: Consider age-related ↓ in renal function, concurrent illnesses and drug therapy; OB: Use only if the potential benefit justifies the potential risk to the fetus; Pedi: Safety and effectiveness not established.

Adverse Reactions/Side Effects

CNS: headache. **GI:** diarrhea, nausea, cholelithiasis, ↑ liver enzymes, pancreatitis. **GU:** ↑ serum creatinine. **Metab:** ↓ HDL levels. **MS:** MYOPATHY/RHABDOMYOLYSIS, myalgia, back pain.

Interactions

Drug-Drug: ↑ effects and risk of bleeding with **warfarin**; monitor prothrombin time/INR. **Bile acid sequestrants** may ↓ absorption and effectiveness; administer at least 1 hr before or 4–6 hr after a bile acid sequestrant. Concurrent use with **nephrotoxic drugs** including **cyclosporine** may impair renal function and excretion, ↑ risk of adverse reactions. Concurrent use with **colchicine** may ↑ risk of rhabdomyolysis.

Route/Dosage

Mixed Dyslipidemia

PO (Adults): *TriLipix*—135 mg once daily; *Hypertriglyceridemia*—45–135 mg once daily.

Hypertriglyceridemia

PO (Adults): *Fibricor*—35–105 mg once daily; *TriLipix*—45–135 mg once daily.

Primary Hypercholesterolemia or Mixed Dyslipidemia

PO (Adults): *Fibricor*—105 mg once daily; *TriLipix*—135 mg once daily.

Renal Impairment

PO (Adults): *CCr 30–80 mL/min*—Fibricor: Initiate with 35 mg once daily; may titrate cautiously; TriLipix: Initiate with 45 mg once daily; may titrate cautiously; *CCr <30 mL/min*—Contraindicated.

Availability (generic available)

Delayed-release capsules (Fibricor): 35 mg, 105 mg. **Delayed-release capsules (TriLipix):** 45 mg, 135 mg.

NURSING IMPLICATIONS

Assessment

- Obtain a diet history, especially with regard to fat consumption. Every attempt should be made to obtain normal serum triglyceride levels with diet, exercise, and weight loss in obese patients before fenofibric acid therapy is instituted.
- Assess patient for cholelithiasis. If symptoms occur, gallbladder studies are indicated. Discontinue therapy if gallstones are found.
- ***Lab Test Considerations:*** Monitor serum lipids before therapy to determine consistent elevations, then monitor periodically during therapy.
- Monitor serum AST and ALT periodically during therapy. May cause ↑ levels. Discontinue therapy if levels rise >3 times the normal limit.
- If patient develops muscle tenderness during therapy, CPK levels should be monitored. If CPK levels are markedly ↑ or myopathy occurs, therapy should be discontinued.
- May cause reversible ↑ in serum creatinine. Monitor renal function in patients at risk for renal insufficiency (elderly, diabetics).
- May cause mild to moderate ↓ in hemoglobin, hematocrit, and WBCs. Monitor periodically during first 12 mo of therapy. Levels usually stabilize during long-term therapy.
- Monitor prothrombin time and INR monitored frequently until levels stabilize in patients taking anticoagulants concurrently.

Potential Nursing Diagnoses

Noncompliance (Patient/Family Teaching)

Implementation

- Patients should be placed on a triglyceride-lowering diet before therapy and remain on this diet throughout therapy.
- **PO:** Administer without regard to meals. Swallow capsules whole; do not open, crush, or chew. May be administered at same time as statin dose.

Patient/Family Teaching

- Instruct patient to take medication as directed. Take missed doses as soon as remembered; if time for next dose, skip dose and take next dose at regular time. Do not double doses. Medication helps control but does not cure elevated serum triglyceride levels. Advise patient to read *Medication Guide* before starting and with each Rx refill, as new information may be available.
- Advise patient that this medication should be used in conjunction with diet restrictions (fat, cholesterol, carbohydrates, alcohol), exercise, and cessation of smoking.
- Instruct patient to notify health care professional if unexplained muscle pain, tenderness, weakness, tiredness, fever, nausea, vomiting, or abdominal pain occurs, especially if accompanied by fever or malaise.
- Instruct female patients to notify health care professional promptly if pregnancy is planned or suspected.
- Advise patient to notify health care professional of all Rx or OTC medications, vitamins, or herbal products

being taken and to consult with health care professional before taking other medications.
- Advise patient to notify health care professional of medication regimen before treatment or surgery.
- Emphasize the importance of follow-up exams to determine effectiveness and to monitor for side effects.

Evaluation/Desired Outcomes
- Decrease in serum triglycerides and LDL cholesterol to normal levels with an increase in HDL levels.

HIGH ALERT

fentaNYL (parenteral)
(**fen**-ta-nil)
Sublimaze

Classification
Therapeutic: opioid analgesics
Pharmacologic: opioid agonists

Schedule II

Pregnancy Category C

Indications
Analgesic supplement to general anesthesia; usually with other agents (ultra–short-acting barbiturates, neuromuscular blocking agents, and inhalation anesthetics) to produce balanced anesthesia. Induction/maintenance of anesthesia (with oxygen or oxygen/nitrous oxide and a neuromuscular blocking agents). Neuroleptanalgesia/neuroleptanesthesia (with or without nitrous oxide). Supplement to regional/local anesthesia. Preoperative and postoperative analgesia. **Unlabeled Use:** Continuous IV infusion as part of PCA.

Action
Binds to opiate receptors in the CNS, altering the response to and perception of pain. Produces CNS depression. **Therapeutic Effects:** Supplement in anesthesia. Decreased pain.

Pharmacokinetics
Absorption: Well absorbed after IM administration.
Distribution: Unknown.
Metabolism and Excretion: Mostly metabolized by the liver, 10–25% excreted unchanged by the kidneys.
Half-life: Children: Bolus dose—2.4 hr, long-term continuous infusion—11–36 hr; Adults: 2–4 hr (↑ after cardiopulmonary bypass and in geriatric patients).

TIME/ACTION PROFILE (analgesia*)

ROUTE	ONSET	PEAK	DURATION
IM	7–15 min	20–30 min	1–2 hr
IV	1–2 min	3–5 min	0.5–1 hr

*Respiratory depression may last longer than analgesia.

Contraindications/Precautions
Contraindicated in: Hypersensitivity; cross-sensitivity among agents may occur; Known intolerance.
Use Cautiously in: Geri: Geriatric, debilitated, or critically ill patients; Diabetes; Severe renal, pulmonary, or hepatic disease; CNS tumors; ↑ intracranial pressure; Head trauma; Adrenal insufficiency; Undiagnosed abdominal pain; Hypothyroidism; Alcoholism; Cardiac disease (arrhythmias); OB, Lactation: Pregnancy and lactation.

Adverse Reactions/Side Effects
CNS: confusion, paradoxical excitation/delirium, postoperative depression, postoperative drowsiness.
EENT: blurred/double vision. **Resp:** APNEA, LARYNGOSPASM, allergic bronchospasm, respiratory depression.
CV: arrhythmias, bradycardia, circulatory depression, hypotension. **GI:** biliary spasm, nausea/vomiting.
Derm: facial itching. **MS:** skeletal and thoracic muscle rigidity (with rapid IV infusion).

Interactions
Drug-Drug: Avoid use in patients who have received **MAO inhibitors** within the previous 14 days (may produce unpredictable, potentially fatal reactions). Concomitant use of **CYP3A4 inhibitors** including **ritonavir**, **ketoconazole**, **itraconazole**, **clarithromycin**, **nelfinavir**, **nefazodone**, **diltiazem**, **aprepitant**, **fluconazole**, **fosamprenavir**, **verapamil**, and **erythromycin** may result in ↑ plasma levels and ↑ risk of CNS and respiratory depression. Additive CNS and respiratory depression with other **CNS depressants**, including **alcohol**, **antihistamines**, **antidepressants**, other **sedative/hypnotics**, and other **opioid analgesics**. ↑ risk of hypotension with **benzodiazepines**. **Nalbuphine**, **buprenorphine**, or **pentazocine** may ↓ analgesia.
Drug-Food: Grapefruit juice is a moderate inhibitor of the CYP3A4 enzyme system; concurrent use may ↑ blood levels and the risk of respiratory and CNS depression. Careful monitoring and dose adjustment is recommended.

Route/Dosage

Preoperative Use
IM, IV (Adults and Children >12 yr): 50–100 mcg 30–60 min before surgery.

Adjunct to General Anesthesia
IM, IV (Adults and Children >12 yr): *Low dose–minor surgery*—2 mcg/kg. *Moderate dose–major surgery*—2–20 mcg/kg. *High dose–major surgery*—20–50 mcg /kg.

Adjunct to Regional Anesthesia
IM, IV (Adults and Children >12 yr): 50–100 mcg.

Postoperative Use (Recovery Room)
IM, IV (Adults and Children >12 yr): 50–100 mcg; may repeat in 1–2 hr.

General Anesthesia

IV (Adults and Children >12 yr): 50–100 mcg/kg (up to 150 mcg/kg).
IV (Children 1–12 yr): 2–3 mcg/kg.

Sedation/Analgesia

IV (Adults and Children >12 yr): 0.5–1 mcg/kg/dose, may repeat after 30–60 min.
IV (Children 1–12 yr): *Bolus*—1–2 mcg/kg/dose, may repeat at 30–60 min intervals. *Continuous infusion*—1–5 mcg/kg/hr following bolus dose.
IV (Neonates): *Bolus*—0.5–3 mcg/kg/dose. *Continuous infusion*—0.5–2 mcg/kg/hr following bolus dose. *Continuous infusion during ECMO*—5–10 mcg/kg bolus followed by 1–5 mcg/kg/hr, may require up to 20 mcg/kg/hr after 5 days of therapy.

Availability (generic available)

Injection: 0.05 mg/mL.

NURSING IMPLICATIONS

Assessment

- Monitor respiratory rate and BP frequently throughout therapy. Report significant changes immediately. The respiratory depressant effects of fentanyl may last longer than the analgesic effects. Initial doses of other opioids should be reduced by 25–33% of the usually recommended dose. Monitor closely.
- Geri: Opioids have been associated with increased risk of falls in geriatric patients. Assess risk and implement fall prevention strategies.
- **IV, IM:** Assess type, location, and intensity of pain before and 30 min after IM administration or 3–5 min after IV administration when fentanyl is used to treat pain.
- ***Lab Test Considerations:*** May cause ↑ serum amylase and lipase concentrations.
- ***Toxicity and Overdose:*** Symptoms of toxicity include respiratory depression, hypotension, arrhythmias, bradycardia, and asystole. Atropine may be used to treat bradycardia. If respiratory depression persists after surgery, prolonged mechanical ventilation may be required. If an opioid antagonist is required to reverse respiratory depression or coma, naloxone (Narcan) is the antidote. Dilute the 0.4-mg ampule of naloxone in 10 mL of 0.9% NaCl and administer 0.5 mL (0.02 mg) by IV push every 2 min. Pedi: For children and patients weighing <40 kg, dilute 0.1 mg of naloxone in 10 mL of 0.9% NaCl for a concentration of 10 mcg/mL and administer 0.5 mcg/kg every 2 min. Titrate dose to avoid withdrawal, seizures, and severe pain. Administration of naloxone in these circumstances, especially in cardiac patients, has resulted in hypertension and tachycardia, occasionally causing left ventricular failure and pulmonary edema.

Potential Nursing Diagnoses

Acute pain (Indications)
Ineffective breathing pattern (Adverse Reactions)
Risk for injury (Side Effects)

Implementation

- ***High Alert:*** Accidental overdosage of opioid analgesics has resulted in fatalities. Before administering, clarify all ambiguous orders; have second practitioner independently check original order, dose calculations, route of administration, and infusion pump programming.
- Do not confuse fentanyl with sufentanil.
- Benzodiazepines may be administered before or after administration of fentanyl to reduce the induction dose requirements, decrease the time to loss of consciousness, and produce amnesia. This combination may also increase the risk of hypotension.

IV Administration

- **IV Push:** ***Diluent:*** Administer undiluted. ***Concentration:*** 50 mcg/mL. ***Rate:*** Injections should be administered slowly over 1–3 min. Administer doses >5 mcg/kg over 5–10 min. Slow IV administration may reduce the incidence and severity of muscle rigidity, bradycardia, or hypotension. Neuromuscular blocking agents may be administered concurrently to decrease chest wall muscle rigidity.
- **Intermittent Infusion:** ***Diluent:*** May be diluted in D5W or 0.9% NaCl. ***Concentration:*** Up to 50 mcg/mL. ***Rate:*** see IV Push.
- **Y-Site Compatibility:** acyclovir, alemtuzumab, alfentanil, alprostadil, amikacin, aminocaproic acid, aminophylline, amiodarone, amphotericin cholesteryl, amphotericin B lipid complex, amphotericin B liposome, anidulafungin, argatroban, ascorbic acid, atracurium, atropine, azathioprine, aztreonam, benztropine, bivalirudin, bumetanide, buprenorphine, butorphanol, calcium chloride, calcium gluconate, carboplatin, carmustine, caspofungin, cefazolin, cefotaxime, cefotetan, cefoxitin, ceftaroline, ceftazidime, ceftriaxone, cefuroxime, chloramphenicol, chlorpromazine, cisatracurium, cisplatin, clindamycin, cyanocobalamin, cyclophosphamide, cyclosporine, cytarabine, dactinomycin, daptomycin, dexamethasone, dexmedetomidine, digoxin, diltiazem, diphenhydramine, dobutamine, docetaxel, dopamine, doripenem, doxacurium, doxapram, doxorubicin, doxycycline, enalaprilat, ephedrine, epinephrine, epirubicin, epoetin alfa, eptifibatide, erythromycin, esmolol, etomidate, etoposide, etoposide phosphate, famotidine, fenoldopam, fluconazole, fludarabine, fluorouracil, folic acid, furosemide, ganciclovir, gemcitabine, gentamicin, glycopyrrolate, granisetron, heparin, hetastarch, hydrocortisone, hydromorphone, idarubicin, ifosfamide, imipenem/cilastatin, insulin, irinotecan, isopro-

terenol, ketorolac, labetalol, levofloxacin, lidocaine, linezolid, lorazepam, magnesium sulfate, mannitol, mechlorethamine, meperidine, metaraminol, methotrexate, methoxamine, methyldopate, methylprednisolone, metoclopramide, metoprolol, metronidazole, midazolam, milrinone, mitoxantrone, morphine, multivitamins, mycophenolate, nafcillin, nalbuphine, naloxone, nesiritide, nicardipine, nitroglycerin, nitroprusside, norepinephrine, octreotide, ondansetron, oxacillin, oxaliplatin, oxytocin, paclitaxel, palonosetron, pamidronate, pancuronium, papaverine, pemetrexed, penicillin G, pentamidine, pentobarbital, phenobarbital, phentolamine, phenylephrine, phytonadione, piperacillin/tazobactam, potassium acetate, potassium chloride, procainamide, prochlorperazine, promethazine, propofol, propranolol, protamine, pyridoxime, quinupristin/dalfopristin, ranitidine, remifentanil, rituximab, rocuronium, sargramostim, scopolamine, sodium acetate, sodium bicarbonate, streptokinase, succinylcholine, sufentanil, tacrolimus, teniposide, theophylline, thiamine, thiopental, thiotepa, tigecycline, tirofiban, tobramycin, tolazoline, trastuzumab, trimetaphan, vancomycin, vasopressin, vecuronium, verapamil, vincristine, vinorelbine, vitamin B complex with C, voriconazole, zoledronic acid.

- **Y-Site Incompatibility:** azithromycin, dantrolene, diazoxide, pantoprazole, phenytoin, trimethoprim/sulfamethoxazole.

Patient/Family Teaching

- Discuss the use of anesthetic agents and the sensations to expect with the patient before surgery.
- Explain pain assessment scale to patient.
- Caution patient to change positions slowly to minimize orthostatic hypotension. Geri: Geriatric patients may be at a greater risk for orthostatic hypotension and, consequently, falls. Teach patient to take precautions until drug effects have completely resolved.
- Medication causes dizziness and drowsiness. Advise patient to call for assistance during ambulation and transfer, and to avoid driving or other activities requiring alertness for 24 hr after administration during outpatient surgery.
- Instruct patient to avoid alcohol or other CNS depressants for 24 hr after administration for outpatient surgery.

Evaluation/Desired Outcomes

- General quiescence.
- Reduced motor activity.
- Pronounced analgesia.

REMS HIGH ALERT

fentaNYL (transdermal)

(**fen**-ta-nil)

Duragesic

Classification

Therapeutic: opioid analgesics, anesthetic adjuncts

Pharmacologic: opioid agonists

Schedule II

Pregnancy Category C

Indications

Moderate to severe chronic pain in opioid-tolerant patients requiring use of daily, around-the-clock long-term opioid treatment and for which alternative treatment options are inadequate (extended-release). Transdermal fentanyl is not recommended for the control of postoperative, mild, or intermittent pain, nor should it be used for short-term pain relief.

Action

Binds to opiate receptors in the CNS, altering the response to and perception of pain. **Therapeutic Effects:** Decrease in severity of chronic pain.

Pharmacokinetics

Absorption: Well absorbed (92% of dose) through skin surface under transdermal patch, creating a depot in the upper skin layers. Release from transdermal system into systemic circulation ↑ gradually to a constant rate, providing continuous delivery for 72 hr.

Distribution: Crosses the placenta; enters breast milk.

Metabolism and Excretion: Mostly metabolized by the liver (CYP3A4 enzyme system); 10–25% excreted unchanged by the kidneys.

Half-life: 17 hr after removal of a single application patch, ↑ to 21 hr after removal of multiple patches (because of continued release from deposition of drug in skin layers).

TIME/ACTION PROFILE (↓ pain)

ROUTE	ONSET	PEAK	DURATION
Transdermal	6 hr†	12–24 hr	72 hr‡

†Achievement of blood levels associated with analgesia. Maximal response and dose titration may take up to 6 days.
‡While patch is worn.

Contraindications/Precautions

Contraindicated in: Hypersensitivity to fentanyl or adhesives; Patients who are not opioid tolerant; Acute, mild, intermittent, or postoperative pain; Significant respiratory depression; Acute or severe bronchial asthma; Paralytic ileus; Severe hepatic or renal impairment; Alcohol intolerance (small amounts of alcohol released into skin); OB: Not recommended during labor and delivery; Lactation: May cause adverse affects in infant.

Use Cautiously in: Diabetes; Patients with severe pulmonary disease; Mild or moderate hepatic or renal impairment; CNS tumors; ↑ intracranial pressure; Head trauma; Adrenal insufficiency; Undiagnosed abdominal pain; Hypothyroidism; Alcoholism; Cardiac disease (particularly bradyarrhythmias); Fever or situations that ↑ body temperature (↑ release of fentanyl from delivery system); Titration period (additional analgesics may be required); Cachectic or debilitated patients (dose ↓ suggested because of altered drug disposition); OB: Avoid chronic use; prolonged use of transdermal fentanyl during pregnancy can result in neonatal opioid withdrawal syndrome; Pedi: Children <2 yr (safety not established); pediatric patients initiating therapy at 25 mcg/hr should be opioid tolerant and receiving at least 60 mg oral morphine equivalents per day; Geri: ↑ risk of respiratory depression; dose ↓ suggested.

Adverse Reactions/Side Effects

CNS: confusion, sedation, weakness, dizziness, restlessness. **Resp:** APNEA, bronchoconstriction, laryngospasm, RESPIRATORY DEPRESSION. **CV:** bradycardia, hypotension. **GI:** anorexia, constipation, dry mouth, nausea, vomiting. **Derm:** sweating, erythema. **Local:** application site reactions. **MS:** skeletal and thoracic muscle rigidity. **Misc:** physical dependence, psychological dependence.

Interactions

Drug-Drug: Avoid use in patients who have received **MAO inhibitors** within the previous 14 days (may produce unpredictable, potentially fatal reactions). Concomitant use of **CYP3A4 inhibitors** including **ritonavir, ketoconazole, itraconazole, clarithromycin, nelfinavir, nefazodone, amiodarone, diltiazem, aprepitant, fluconazole, fosamprenavir, verapamil**, and **erythromycin** may result in ↑ plasma levels and ↑ risk of CNS and respiratory depression. Levels and effectiveness may be ↓ by **CYP3A4 inducers** including **rifampin, carbamazepine**, and **phenytoin**. ↑ CNS and respiratory depression with other **CNS depressants**, including **alcohol, antihistamines, antidepressants, sedative/hypnotics**, and other **opioids**.

Drug-Natural Products: Concomitant use of **kava-kava, valerian**, or **chamomile** can ↑ CNS depression.

Drug-Food: Grapefruit juice is a moderate inhibitor of the CYP3A4 enzyme system; concurrent use may ↑ blood levels and the risk of respiratory and CNS depression. Careful monitoring and dose adjustment is recommended.

Route/Dosage

Transdermal (Adults): 25 mcg/hr is the initial dose; patients who have not been receiving opioids should receive not more than 25 mcg/hr. To calculate the dose of transdermal fentanyl required in patients who are already receiving opioid analgesics, assess the 24-hr requirement of currently used opioid. Using the equianalgesic table in Appendix I, convert this to an equivalent amount of morphine/24 hr. Conversion to fentanyl transdermal may be accomplished by using the fentanyl conversion table (Appendix I). During dose titration, additional short-acting opioids should be available for any breakthrough pain that may occur. Morphine 10 mg IM or 60 mg PO q 4 hr (60 mg/24 hr IM or 360 mg/24 hr PO) is considered to be approximately equivalent to transdermal fentanyl 100 mcg/hr. Transdermal patch lasts 72 hr in most patients. Some patients require a new patch every 48 hr.

Transdermal (Adults >60 yr, Debilitated, or Cachectic Patients): Initial dose should be 25 mcg/hr unless previous opioid use was >135 m g morphine PO/day (or other opioid equivalent).

Hepatic Impairment

Transdermal (Adults): *Mild-to-moderate hepatic impairment*—12 mcg/hr is the initial dose.

Renal Impairment

Transdermal (Adults): *Mild-to-moderate renal impairment*—12 mcg/hr is the initial dose.

Availability (generic available)

Transdermal systems: 12 mcg/hr, 25 mcg/hr, 50 mcg/hr, 75 mcg/hr, 100 mcg/hr. **Cost:** *Generic*—12 mcg/hr $101.51/5, 25 mcg/hr $72.17/5, 50 mcg/hr $131.92/5, 75 mcg/hr $201.23/5, 100 mcg/hr $267.07/5.

NURSING IMPLICATIONS

Assessment

- Assess type, location, and intensity of pain before and 24 hr after application and periodically during therapy. Monitor pain frequently during initiation of therapy and dose changes to assess need for supplementary analgesics for breakthrough pain.
- Assess BP, pulse, and respirations before and periodically during administration. If respiratory rate is <10/min, assess level of sedation. Physical stimulation may be sufficient to prevent significant hypoventilation. Dose may need to be decreased by 25–50%. Initial drowsiness will diminish with continued use.
- Prolonged use may lead to physical and psychological dependence and tolerance. This should not prevent patient from receiving adequate analgesia. Most patients who receive opioid analgesics for pain do not develop psychological dependence.
- Progressively higher doses may be required to relieve pain with long-term therapy. It may take up to 6 days after increasing doses to reach equilibrium, so

patients should wear higher dose through 2 applications before increasing dose again.

- Assess bowel function routinely. Prevent constipation with increased intake of fluids and bulk, and laxatives to minimize constipating effects. Administer stimulant laxatives routinely if opioid use exceeds 2–3 days, unless contraindicated.
- Assess risk for opioid addiction, abuse, or misuse prior to administration. Monitor for respiratory depression, especially during initiation or following dose increase; serious, life-threatening, or fatal respiratory depression may occur. Misuse or abuse of *transdermal fentanyl* by chewing, swallowing, snorting or injecting fentanyl extracted from transdermal system will result in the uncontrolled delivery of fentanyl and risk of overdose and death.
- ***Lab Test Considerations:*** May ↑ plasma amylase and lipase levels.
- ***Toxicity and Overdose:*** If an opioid antagonist is required to reverse respiratory depression or coma, naloxone is the antidote. Dilute the 0.4-mg ampule of naloxone in 10 mL of 0.9% NaCl and administer 0.5 mL (0.02 mg) by IV push every 2 min. For patients weighing <40 kg, dilute 0.1 mg of naloxone in 10 mL of 0.9% NaCl for a concentration of 10 mcg/mL and administer 0.5 mcg/kg every 2 min. Titrate dose to avoid withdrawal, seizures, and severe pain. Monitor patient closely; dose may need to be repeated or may need to be administered as an infusion because of long duration of action despite removal of patch.

Potential Nursing Diagnoses

Chronic pain (Indications)
Risk for injury (Side Effects)

Implementation

- Do not confuse fentanyl with sufentanil.
- ***High Alert:*** Accidental overdose of opioid analgesics has resulted in fatalities. Before administering, confirm patient is opioid tolerant and clarify ambiguous orders; have second practitioner independently check original order and dose calculations.
- 12-mcg patch delivers 12.5 mcg/hr of fentanyl. Use supplemental doses of short-acting opioid analgesics to manage pain until relief is obtained with the transdermal system. Patients may continue to require supplemental opioids for breakthrough pain. If >100 mcg/hr is required, use multiple transdermal systems.
- Titrate dose based on patient's report of pain until adequate analgesia (50% reduction in patient's pain rating on numerical or visual analogue scale or patient reports satisfactory relief) is attained. Determine dose by calculating the previous 24-hr analgesic requirement and converting to the equianalgesic morphine dose using Appendix I. The conversion ratio from morphine to transdermal fentanyl is conservative; 50% of patients may require a dose increase after initial application. Increase after 3 days based on required daily doses of supplemental analgesics. Increases should be based on ratio of 45 mg/24 hr of oral morphine to 12.5 mcg/hr increase in transdermal fentanyl dose.
- Coadministration with nonopioid analgesics may have additive analgesic effects and permit lower opioid doses.
- To convert to another opioid analgesic, remove transdermal fentanyl system and begin treatment with half the equianalgesic dose of the new analgesic in 12–18 hr.
- Medication should be discontinued gradually after long-term use to prevent withdrawal symptoms.
- **Transdermal:** Apply system to flat, nonirritated, and nonirradiated site such as chest, back, flank, or upper arm. If skin preparation is necessary, use clear water and clip, do not shave, hair. Allow skin to dry completely before application. Apply immediately after removing from package. Do not alter the system (i.e., cut) in any way before application. Remove liner from adhesive layer and press firmly in place with palm of hand for 30 sec, especially around the edges, to make sure contact is complete. Remove used system and fold so that adhesive edges are together. Flush system down toilet immediately on removal or follow the institutional policy. Apply new system to a different site.

Patient/Family Teaching

- Instruct patient in how and when to ask for and take pain medication.
- Instruct patient in correct method for application and disposal of transdermal system. Fatalities have occurred from children having access to improperly discarded patches. May be worn while bathing, showering, or swimming.
- Advise patient to avoid grapefruit juice during therapy.
- May cause drowsiness or dizziness. Caution patient to call for assistance when ambulating or smoking and to avoid driving or other activities requiring alertness until response to medication is known.
- Advise patient to change positions slowly to minimize dizziness.
- Caution patient to avoid concurrent use of alcohol or other CNS depressants with this medication.
- Advise patient that fever, electric blankets, heating pads, saunas, hot tubs, and heated water beds increase the release of fentanyl from the patch.
- Advise patient that good oral hygiene, frequent mouth rinses, and sugarless gum or candy may decrease dry mouth.
- Advise patient to notify health care professional of all Rx or OTC medications, vitamins, or herbal products being taken and to consult with health care professional before taking other medications.
- Instruct female patient to notify health care professional if pregnancy is planned or suspected or if breast feeding.

- Advise patient referred for MRI test to discuss patch with referring health care professional and MRI facility to determine if removal of patch is necessary prior to test and for directions for replacing patch.

Evaluation/Desired Outcomes

- Decrease in severity of pain without a significant alteration in level of consciousness, respiratory status, or BP.

REMS HIGH ALERT

FENTANYL (transmucosal)

(fen-ta-nil)

fentaNYL (buccal tablet)
Fentora

fentaNYL (nasal spray)
Lazanda

fentaNYL (oral transmucosal lozenge)
Actiq

fentaNYL (sublingual spray)
Subsys

fentaNYL (sublingual tablet)
Abstral

Classification
Therapeutic: opioid analgesics
Pharmacologic: opioid agonists

Schedule II

Pregnancy Category C

Indications

Management of breakthrough pain in cancer patients >18 yr old already receiving opioids and tolerant to around-the-clock opioids for persistent cancer pain (60 mg/day of oral morphine or equivalent).

Action

Binds to opioid receptors in the CNS, altering the response to and perception of pain. **Therapeutic Effects:** Decrease in severity of breakthrough pain.

Pharmacokinetics

Absorption: *Buccal tablet*—65% absorbed from buccal mucosa; 50% is absorbed transmucosally, remainder is swallowed and is absorbed slowly from the GI tract. Buccal absorption is enhanced by an effervescent reaction in the dose form; *Nasal spray*—Well absorbed from nasal mucosa (bioavailability higher than that of oral transmucosal lozenge); *Oral transmucosal lozenge*—Initial rapid absorption (25%) from buccal mucosa is followed by more prolonged absorption (25%) from GI tract (combined bioavailability 50%); *Sublingual spray*—76% absorbed through sublingual mucosa; *Sublingual tablets*—54% absorbed from oral mucosa following sublingual administration.
Distribution: Readily crosses the placenta and enters breast milk.
Metabolism and Excretion: Mostly metabolized in the liver and intestinal mucosa via the the CYP3A4 enzyme system; inactive metabolites are excreted in urine; <7% excreted unchanged in urine.
Half-life: *Buccal tablet*—2.6–11.7 hr (↑ with dose); *Nasal spray*—15–25 hr (↑ with dose); *Sublingual spray*—5–12 hr; *Sublingual tablet*—5–10 hr (↑ with dose); *Transmucosal lozenge*—7 hr.

TIME/ACTION PROFILE (↓ pain)

ROUTE	ONSET	PEAK	DURATION
Buccal tablet	15 min	40–60 min	60 min
Nasal spray	within 10 min	unknown	2–4 hr
Oral transmucosal lozenge	rapid	15–30 min	several hr
SL	within 30 min	30–60 min	2–4 hr

Contraindications/Precautions

Contraindicated in: Known intolerance or hypersensitivity; Acute/postoperative pain including headache/migraine, dental pain, or emergency room use; Opioid—naive (nontolerant) patients; Concurrent use of MAO inhibitors; OB: Labor and delivery; Lactation: Avoid use during breast feeding; may cause infant sedation and/or respiratory depression.
Use Cautiously in: Chronic obstructive pulmonary disease or pre-existing medical conditions predisposing to hypoventilation; Concurrent use of CNS active drugs; History of substance abuse; Severe renal/hepatic impairment (use lowest effective starting dose); Concurrent use of CYP3A4 inhibitors (use lowest effective dose); Bradyarrhythmias; OB: Use only if the potential benefit justifies the potential risk to the fetus. Chronic maternal treatment with opioids during pregnancy may result in neonatal abstinence syndrome; Geri: May be more sensitive to effects and may have an ↑ risk of adverse reactions; titrate dosage carefully; Pedi: Safety and effectiveness not established.
Exercise Extreme Caution in: Patients susceptible to intracranial effects of CO_2 retention including those with ↑ intracranial pressure, head injuries, or impaired consciousness.

Adverse Reactions/Side Effects

Opioid side effects ↑ with ↑ dosage.
CNS: dizziness, drowsiness, headache, confusion, depression, fatigue, hallucinations, headache, insomnia, weakness. **Resp:** RESPIRATORY DEPRESSION, dyspnea. **CV:** hypotension. **GI:** constipation, nausea, vomiting,

abdominal pain, anorexia, dry mouth. **Misc:** allergic reaction including ANAPHYLAXIS, physical dependence, psychological dependence.

Interactions

Drug-Drug: Should not be used within 14 days of **MAO inhibitors** because of possible severe and unpredictable reactions. Concurrent use of **CYP3A4 inhibitors** including **ritonavir**, **ketoconazole**, **itraconazole**, **fluconazole clarithromycin**, **erythromycin**, **nefazodone**, **diltiazem**, **verapamil**, **fosamprenavir**, **nelfinavir**, and **fosamprenavir** ↑ levels and risk of opioid toxicity; careful monitoring during initiation, dose changes, or discontinuation of the inhibitor is recommended. Concurrent use with **CYP3A4 inducers** including **barbiturates**, **carbamazepine**, **efavirenz**, **corticosteroids**, **modafinil**, **nevirapine**, **oxcarbazepine**, **phenobarbital**, **phenytoin**, **rifabutin**, or **rifampin** may ↓ fentanyl levels and analgesia; if inducers are discontinued or dosage ↓, patients should be monitored for signs of opioid toxicity and necessary dose adjustments made. **CNS depressants** including other **opioids**, **sedative/hypnotics**, **general anesthetics**, **phenothiazines**, **skeletal muscle relaxants**, sedating **antihistamines**, and **alcohol** may ↑ CNS depression, hypoventilation, and hypotension.
Drug-Natural Products: St. John's wort is an inducer of CYP3A4; concurrent use may ↓ levels and analgesia; if inducers are discontinued or dosage decreased, patients should be monitored for signs of opioid toxicity and necessary dosage adjustments made.
Drug-Food: Grapefuit juice is a moderate inhibitor of CYP3A4 enzyme system; concurrent use may ↑ levels and the risk of CNS and respiratory depression. Careful monitoring and dose adjustment may be necessary.

Route/Dosage

Transmucosal Products Are Not Equivalent on a mcg-to-mcg Basis

Buccal (Adults): *Tablets*–100 mcg, then titrate to dose that provides adequate analgesia without undue side effects.
Intranasal (Adults): One 100-mcg spray in one nostril initially, then titrate in a step-wise manner (↑ to one 100-mcg spray in each nostril [200 mcg total], then one 400-mcg spray in one nostril (or two 100–mcg sprays in each nostril [400 mcg total]), then one 400-mcg spray in each nostril [800 mcg total] to provide adequate analgesia without undue side effects (up to a maximum of one 400-mcg spray in each nostril).
Oral transmucosal (Adults): One 200-mcg unit dissolved in mouth (see Implementation section) over 15 min; additional unit may be used 15 min after first unit is completed. If more than 1 unit is required per episode (as evaluated over several episodes), dose may be ↑ as required to control pain. Optimal usage/titration should result in using no more than 4 units/day.
SL (Adults): *Tablets*—100 mcg initially, then titrate using 100-mcg increments to provide adequate analgesia without undue side effects (not to exceed 2 doses per episode; no more than 4 doses per day; separate by at least 2 hr); *Spray*—100 mcg initially; if pain not relieved within 30 min, repeat 100-mcg dose (do not take more than 2 doses per breakthrough pain episode); patients must wait ≥4 hr before treating another episode of breakthrough pain. Dose may be titrated during subsequent pain episodes to 200 mcg, then 400 mcg, then 600 mcg, then 800 mcg, then 1200 mcg, and then 1600 mcg to provide adequate analgesia and undue side effects.

Availability (generic available)

Buccal tablets: 100 mcg, 200 mcg, 300 mcg, 400 mcg, 600 mcg, 800 mcg. **Cost:** 200 mcg $1,006.04/28. **Nasal spray:** 100 mcg/spray, 400 mcg/spray. **Oral transmucosal lozenge on a stick (berry flavor-sugar free):** 200 mcg, 400 mcg, 600 mcg, 800 mcg, 1200 mcg, 1600 mcg. **Cost:** *Generic*—400 mcg $599.93/30, 1200 mcg $799.93/30, 1600 mcg $1,155.89/30. **Sublingual spray:** 100 mcg/spray, 200 mcg/spray, 400 mcg/spray, 600 mcg/spray, 800 mcg/spray. **Sublingual tablets:** 100 mcg, 200 mcg, 300 mcg, 400 mcg, 600 mcg, 800 mcg.

NURSING IMPLICATIONS

Assessment

- Monitor type, location, and intensity of pain before and 1 hr after administration of transmucosal fentanyl.
- Assess BP, pulse, and respirations before and periodically during administration. If respiratory rate is <10 min, assess level of sedation. Physical stimulation may be sufficient to prevent hypoventilation. Subsequent doses may need to be decreased. Patients tolerant to opioid analgesics are usually tolerant to the respiratory depressant effects also.
- Monitor for application site reactions (paresthesia, ulceration, bleeding, pain, ulcer, irritation). Reactions are usually self-limited and rarely require discontinuation.
- ***Lab Test Considerations:*** May cause anemia, neutropenia, thrombocytopenia, and leukopenia.
- May cause hypokalemia, hypoalbuminemia, hypercalcemia, hypomagnesemia, and hyponatremia.
- ***Toxicity and Overdose:*** If an opioid antagonist is required to reverse respiratory depression or coma, naloxone is the antidote. Dilute the 0.4-mg ampule of naloxone in 10 mL of 0.9% NaCl and administer 0.5 mL (0.02 mg) by IV push every 2 min. For patients weighing <40 kg, dilute 0.1 mg of naloxone in 10 mL of 0.9% NaCl for a concentration of 10 mcg/mL and administer 0.5 mcg every 2 min. Use extreme caution when titrating dose in patients physically dependent on opioid analgesics to avoid withdrawal, seizures, and severe pain. Duration of

respiratory depression may be longer than duration of opioid antagonist, requiring repeated doses.

Potential Nursing Diagnoses

Acute pain (Indications)
Risk for injury (Adverse Reactions)

Implementation

- ***High Alert:*** Accidental overdose of opioid analgesics has resulted in fatalities. Before administering, clarify all ambiguous orders; have second practitioner independently check original order and dose calculations.
- Do not confuse fentanyl with sufentanil.
- Patients considered opioid-tolerant are those who are taking ≥60 mg of oral morphine/day, at least 25 mcg transdermal fentanyl/hr, 30 mg of oxycodone/day, 8 mg of hydromorphone/day or an equianalgesic dose of another opioid for ≥1 wk.
- ***High Alert:*** Dose may be lethal to a child; keep out of reach of children.
- Do not substitute fentanyl products; doses are not equivalent.
- **REMS:** Health care professionals who prescribe transmucosal immediate-release fentanyl (TIRF) medicines for outpatient use are required to enroll in the TIRF REMS Access program. Health care professionals already enrolled in an individual Risk Evaluation and Mitigation Strategy (REMS) program for at least one TIRF medicine, will be automatically transitioned to the shared TIRF REMS Access program, and do not need to re-enroll. Enrollment renewal in TIRF REMS program is required every 2 yr from the date of enrollment. Information can be found at www.TIRFREMSaccess.com. A TIRF REMS Access Patient-Prescriber Agreement Form must be signed with each new patient before writing the patient's first TIRF prescription and health care professionals must also provide patients with a copy of the *Medication Guide* during counseling about the proper use of their TIRF medicine. Pharmacists who dispense TIRF medicines are also required to enroll in the TIRF REMS program and re-enroll every 2 yr. Patients are enrolled in the TIRF REMS Access program by the pharmacy at the time their first prescription is filled. Patients can locate a participating pharmacy by consulting their prescriber or calling the TIRF REMS Access program at 1-866-822-1483.
- **Buccal:** *Fentora*: Do not attempt to push tablet through blister, may cause damage to tablet. Open by tearing along perforations to separate from blister card. Then bend blister unit on line where indicated. Blister backing should then be peeled to expose tablets. Use immediately; do not store, may damage integrity of tablet. Tablets are not to be sucked, chewed, or swallowed whole; this will reduce medication effectiveness. Place between cheek and gum above a molar or under tongue and allow medication to dissolve, usually 14–25 min. May cause bubbling sensation between teeth and gum while tablet dissolves. Do not attempt to split tablet. After 30 min, if remnants of tablet remain, swallow with glass of water.
- For patients not previously using transmucosal fentanyl, initial dose should be 100 mcg. Titrate to provide adequate relief while minimizing side effects. For patients switching from oral transmucosal fentanyl to fentanyl buccal, if transmucosal dose is 200–400 mcg, switch to 100 mcg buccal; if transmucosal dose is 600–800 mcg, switch to 200 mcg buccal; if transmucosal dose is 1200–1600 mcg, switch to 400 mcg buccal fentanyl.
- Dose may be repeated once during a single episode of breakthrough pain if not adequately relieved. Redose may occur 30 min after start of administration of fentanyl buccal and the same dose should be used.
- If more than 1 dose is required per breakthrough pain episode for several consecutive episodes, dose of maintenance opioid and fentanyl buccal should be adjusted. To increase dose, use multiples of 100 mcg tablet, use two 100-mcg tablets (1 on each side of mouth in buccal cavity). If unsuccessful in controlling breakthrough pain episode, two 100-mcg tablets may be placed on each side of mouth in buccal cavity (four 100-mcg tablets). Titrate above 400 mcg by 200 mcg increments. To reduce risk of overdose, patients should have only one strength available at any one time.
- Once a successful dose has been established, if more than 4 breakthrough pain episodes/day occur, reevaluate opioid dose for persistent pain.
- Inform patient if medication is no longer needed they should contact Cephalon at 1-800-896-5855 or remove from blister pack and flush any remaining product down toilet.
- **Intranasal:** *Lazanda*: Prime the device before use by spraying into the pouch (4 sprays in total). Insert nozzle of the bottle a short distance (about 1/2 inch or 1 cm) into nose and point toward bridge of nose, tilting the bottle slightly. Press down firmly on finger grips until a "click" is heard and the number in the counting window advances by one. Advise patients that the fine-mist spray is not always felt on the nasal mucosal membrane and to rely on the audible click and advancement of dose counter to confirm a spray has been administered.
- All patients (including those switching from another fentanyl product) must start using one 100-mcg spray of fentanyl sublingual (1 spray in 1 nostril). If adequate analgesia is obtained within 30 min of administration of the 100-mcg single spray, treat subsequent episodes of breakthrough pain with this

dose. If adequate analgesia is not achieved with first 100-mcg dose, ↑ dose in a step-wise manner over consecutive episodes of breakthrough pain until adequate analgesia with tolerable side effects is achieved. Patients MUST wait at least 2 hr before treating another episode of breakthrough cancer pain with fentanyl intranasal. Confirm the dose of fentanyl intranasal that works for patient with a second episode of breakthrough pain and review their experience with their health care professional to determine if that dose is appropriate, or whether a further adjustment is warranted.

- During any episode of breakthrough cancer pain, if there is inadequate pain relief after 30 min following fentanyl intranasal dosing or if a separate episode of breakthrough cancer pain occurs before the next dose of fentanyl intranasal is permitted (i.e., within 2 hr), patients may use a rescue medication as directed by their health care professional.
- For patients no longer requiring opioid therapy, consider discontinuing fentanyl sublingual along with a gradual downward titration of other opioids to minimize possible withdrawal effects. In patients who continue to take chronic opioid therapy for persistent pain but no longer require treatment for breakthrough pain, fentanyl intranasal therapy can usually be discontinued immediately.
- **Transmucosal:** *Actiq*: Open the foil package immediately before use. Instruct patient to place unit in the mouth between the cheek and lower gum, moving it from one side to the other using the handle. Patient should suck, not chew, the lozenge. If it is chewed and swallowed, lower peak concentrations and lower bioavailability may occur. Instruct patient to consume lozenge over 15-min period; longer or shorter periods may be less efficacious. If signs of excessive opioid effects occur, remove from patient's mouth immediately and decrease future doses.
- Initial dose for breakthrough pain should be 200 mcg. Six 200-mcg units should be prescribed and should be used before increasing to a higher dose. If one unit is ineffective, a second unit may be started 15 min after the completion of the first unit. Do not use more than 2 units during a single episode of breakthrough pain during titration phase. With each new dose during titration, 6 units should be prescribed, allowing treatment of several episodes of breakthrough pain. Adequate dose is determined based on effective analgesia with acceptable side effects. Side effects during titration period are usually greater than after effective dose is determined.
- Once an effective dose is determined, instruct patient to limit dose to 4 units/day. If >4 units/day are required, consider increasing the dose of the long-acting opioid.
- Discontinue with a gradual decrease in dose to prevent signs and symptoms of abrupt withdrawal.
- To dispose of remaining unit, using wire-cutting pliers cut off the drug matrix end so that it falls into the toilet. Flush remaining drug matrix down toilet. Drug remaining on handle may be removed by placing under running warm water until dissolved. Dispose of drug-free handle according to institutional protocol. ***High Alert:*** Partially consumed units are no longer protected by child-resistant pouch; dose may still be fatal. A temporary child-resistant storage bottle is provided for partially consumed units that cannot be disposed of properly.
- **SL: Abstral**: Dose must start with 100 mcg initially, titrate to adequate pain relief; if initial dose is adequate, this will be the dose for subsequent breakthrough pain; if dose is inadequate within 30 min give supplemental 100-mcg dose and ↑ next breakthrough dose by 100 mcg; if inadequate continue to ↑ breakthrough dose to 300, then 400, then 600 mcg, then 800 mcg; limit treatment to 4 episodes/24 hr.
- If inadequate analgesia after first dose, a second dose may be used after 30 min. No more than 2 doses may be used to treat an episode of breakthrough pain. Episodes should be separated by at least 2 hr. Other rescue medications may be used as directed.
- Once a successful dose has been established, if more than 4 breakthrough pain episodes/day occur, reevaluate opioid dose for persistent pain.
- Place tablet on the floor of the mouth directly under the tongue and allow to dissolve completely; do not chew, suck, or swallow. Do not eat or drink anything until tablet is dissolved. In patients with dry mouth, water may be used to moisten oral mucosa *before* taking sublingual fentanyl. Advise patient to dispose of unused fentanyl sublingual tablets by removing from blister pack and flushing down toilet.
- **SL: Subsys**: Dose must start with 100 mcg initially, titrate to adequate pain relief; if initial dose is adequate, this will be the dose for subsequent breakthrough pain; if dose is inadequate within 30 min give supplemental 100-mcg dose and ↑ next breakthrough dose by 100 mcg; if inadequate continue to ↑ breakthrough dose to 400, then 600 mcg, then 800 mcg, then 1600 mcg.
- If inadequate analgesia after first dose, a second dose may be used after 30 min. No more than 2 doses may be used to treat an episode of breakthrough pain. Episodes should be separated by at least 4 hr. Other rescue medications may be used as directed.
- Spray contents under tongue. Follow instructions in *Medication Guide*.
- Before you throw away the *Subsys* spray units, empty all of medicine (up to 10 spray units) into charcoal-lined disposal pouch provided with each dose. Put nozzle of spray unit upside-down into opening of charcoal-lined disposal pouch. Squeeze fingers and thumb together to spray into the charcoal lined dis-

posal pouch. Place empty spray unit into pouch. To seal used charcoal-lined disposal pouch, remove backing from adhesive strip. Fold the flap down and press to seal charcoal-lined disposal pouch. Place sealed charcoal-lined disposal pouch into a disposal bag and seal. Discard sealed disposal bag in trash out of reach of children. This protects others, especially children from harm. Follow instructions for use of disposal pouch in *Medication Guide* and *Instructions for Use*.

Patient/Family Teaching

- Instruct patient to take fentanyl as directed. Do not take more often than prescribed, keep out of reach of children, protect it from being stolen, and do not share with others, even if they have the same symptoms. Open only when ready to administer. Advise patient to review *Medication Guide* before and with each Rx refill; new information may be available. Advise patient to notify health care professional if breakthrough pain is not alleviated, worsens, if >4 units/day are required to control pain, or if excessive opioid effects occur.
- Explain TIRF REMS program to patient and caregiver. Patients must sign the Patient-Prescriber Agreement Form to confirm they understand the risks, appropriate use, and storage of fentanyl transmucosal.
- Advise patient to avoid grapefruit juice during therapy.
- Caution patient to make position changes slowly to minimize orthostatic hypotension.
- Medication causes dizziness and drowsiness. Advise patient to call for assistance during ambulation and transfer, and to avoid driving or other activities requiring alertness until response to medication is known.
- Instruct patient to avoid concurrent use of alcohol or other CNS depressants, such as sleep aids.
- Advise patient to notify health care professional if sores on gums or inside cheek become a problem.
- Advise patient to notify health care professional of all Rx or OTC medications, vitamins, or herbal products being taken and to consult with health care professional before taking other medications.
- Advise patient to notify health care professional if pregnancy is planned or suspected or if breast feeding.
- *Actiq*: Inform patient that this drug may contain sugar and may cause dry mouth. Advise patient to maintain good oral hygiene regular dental exams.

Evaluation/Desired Outcomes

- Decrease in severity of pain during episodes of breakthrough pain in patients receiving long-acting opioids.

ferric citrate (fe-rik si-trate)

Auryxia

Classification
Therapeutic: electrolyte modifiers
Pharmacologic: phosphate binders

Pregnancy Category B

F

Indications

Control of serum phosphorous in chronic renal failure patients on dialysis.

Action

Binds phosphorous and precipitates it as ferric phosphate. **Therapeutic Effects:** Maintenance of normal phosphorous levels.

Pharmacokinetics

Absorption: Some absorption follows oral administration and may lead to iron overload.
Distribution: Unknown.
Metabolism and Excretion: Following binding, precipitated ferric phosphate is excreted in stool.
Half-life: Unknown.

TIME/ACTION PROFILE (lowering of serum phosphorous)

ROUTE	ONSET	PEAK	DURATION
PO	within 1 wk	unknown	unknown

Contraindications/Precautions

Contraindicated in: Iron overload syndromes including hemochromatosis.
Use Cautiously in: GI bleeding/inflammation; OB: Use cautiously during pregnancy (consider effects on vitamins/nutrient and potential iron overload); Lactation: Consider possible iron transport into milk; Pedi: Safety and effectiveness not established.

Adverse Reactions/Side Effects

GI: diarrhea, discolored feces, nausea, constipation, vomiting. **Misc:** iron overload.

Interactions

Drug-Drug: Binds and ↓ absorption of **doxycycline** (should be given ≥1 hr prior to ferric citrate). Binds and ↓ absorption of **ciprofloxacin** (should be given ≥2 hr prior to or after ferric citrate).

Route/Dosage

PO (Adults): 2 tablets (2 g ferric citrate) 3 times daily. Adjust by 1–2 tablets/day at weekly (or longer) intervals to attain target phosphorous levels.

Availability (generic available)

Tablets: 1 g (contains 210 mg ferric iron).

NURSING IMPLICATIONS

Assessment

- Monitor clinical responses or blood levels of concurrent medications; may decrease bioavailability of medications administered concurrently.
- ***Lab Test Considerations:*** Monitor serum phosphorous prior to starting and periodically during therapy to keep serum phosphorous at target levels.
- Assess iron parameters (serum ferritin and transferritin saturation TSAT) prior to starting and periodically during therapy. May cause ↑ serum ferritin and TSAT requiring reduced dose or discontinuation of IV iron therapy.

Potential Nursing Diagnoses

Deficient knowledge, related to medication regimen (Patient/Family Teaching)

Implementation

- **PO:** Administer 3 times daily with meals.

Patient/Family Teaching

- Instruct patient to take ferric citrate as directed and to continue with prescribed diet.
- Advise patient that ferric citrate may cause dark stools; this is normal for medications containing iron.
- Inform patient that ferric citrate may cause diarrhea, nausea, constipation, and vomiting. Notify health care professional if GI symptoms become severe or persistent.
- Advise patient to notify health care professional of all Rx or OTC medications, vitamins, or herbal products being taken and to consult with health care professional before taking other medications. Medications may need to be taken separately from ferric citrate.
- Advise female patient to notify health care professional if pregnancy is planned or suspected or if breast feeding.

Evaluation/Desired Outcomes

- Normal serum phosphorous levels.

ferrous fumarate, See IRON SUPPLEMENTS.

ferrous gluconate, See IRON SUPPLEMENTS.

ferrous sulfate, See IRON SUPPLEMENTS.

fesoterodine

(fee-soe-**ter**-o-deen)

Toviaz

Classification

Therapeutic: urinary tract antispasmodics

Pharmacologic: anticholinergics

Pregnancy Category C

Indications

Treatment of overactive bladder function that results in urinary frequency, urgency, or urge incontinence.

Action

Acts as a competitive muscarinic receptor antagonist resulting in inhibition of cholinergically mediated bladder contraction. **Therapeutic Effects:** Decreased urinary frequency, urgency, and urge incontinence.

Pharmacokinetics

Absorption: Rapidly absorbed following oral administration, but is rapidly converted to its active metabolite (bioavailability of metabolite 52%); further metabolism occurs in the liver via CYP2D6 and CYP3A4 enzyme systems. 16% of active metabolite is excreted in urine, most of the remainder of inactive metabolites are renally excreted. 7% excreted in feces.

Distribution: Unknown.

Metabolism and Excretion: Rapidly converted by esterases to active metabolite.

Half-life: 7 hr (following oral administration).

TIME/ACTION PROFILE (active metabolite)

ROUTE	ONSET	PEAK	DURATION
PO	rapid	5 hr	24 hr

Contraindications/Precautions

Contraindicated in: Hypersensitivity; Urinary retention; Gastric retention; Severe hepatic impairment; Uncontrolled narrow-angle glaucoma.

Use Cautiously in: Significant bladder outlet obstruction (↑ risk of retention); Severe renal insufficiency (dose adjustment required); ↓ GI motility including severe constipation; Treated narrow-angle glaucoma (use only if benefits outweigh risks); Myasthenia gravis; Severe renal impairment (dose should not exceed 4 mg/day); Geri: ↑ risk of anticholinergic side effects in patients >75 yr; OB, Lactation: Avoid using unless potential benefits outweighs potential risk to fetus/neonate; Pedi: Safety not established.

Adverse Reactions/Side Effects

CNS: dizziness, drowsiness, headache. **CV:** tachycardia (dose related). **GI:** dry mouth, constipation, nausea, upper abdominal pain. **GU:** dysuria, urinary retention. **MS:** back pain. **Misc:** ANGIOEDEMA.

Interactions

Drug-Drug: Concurrent use of **potent CYP3A4 enzyme inhibitors** including **ketoconazole, itraconazole**, and **clarithromycin** ↑ blood levels and risk of toxicity; daily dose should not exceed 4 mg. Use **less potent inhibitors of CYP3A4** (such as **erythromycin**) with caution; escalate dose carefully. Anticholinergic effects may alter the GI absorption of other drugs.

Route/Dosage

PO (Adults): 4 mg once daily initially may be ↑ to 8 mg/daily; *Concurrent potent CYP3A4 inhibitors or CCr <30 mL/min*—dose should not exceed 4 mg/day.

Availability

Extended-release tablets: 4 mg, 8 mg.

NURSING IMPLICATIONS

Assessment

- Assess for urinary urgency, frequency, and urge incontinence periodically throughout therapy.
- Monitor for signs and symptoms of angioedema (swelling of face, lips, tongue, and/or larynx). May occur with first or subsequent doses. Discontinue therapy and prove supportive therapy. Have epinephrine, corticosteroids, and resuscitation equipment available.
- ***Lab Test Considerations:*** May cause ↑ ALT and GGT.

Potential Nursing Diagnoses

Impaired urinary elimination (Indications)
Urinary retention (Indications)

Implementation

- **PO:** Administer without regard to food.
- Extended-release tablets should be swallowed whole; do not break, crush, or chew.

Patient/Family Teaching

- Instruct patient to take fesoterodine as directed. If a dose is missed, omit and begin taking again the next day; do not take 2 doses the same day. Advise patient to read the *Patient Information* sheet prior to initiation of therapy and with each Rx refill.
- May cause drowsiness, dizziness, and blurred vision. Caution patient to avoid driving or other activities requiring alertness until response to medication is known.
- Advise patient to avoid alcohol; may increase drowsiness.
- Advise patient to use caution in hot environments; may cause decreased sweating and severe heat illness.
- Instruct patient to notify health care professional of all Rx or OTC medications, vitamins, or herbal products being taken and to consult with health care professional before taking other medications.
- Advise patient to stop medication and notify health care professional if signs and symptoms of angioedema occur.
- Advise patient to notify health care professional if pregnancy is planned or suspected or if breast feeding.

Evaluation/Desired Outcomes

- Decreased urinary frequency, urgency, and urge incontinence.

F

fexofenadine

(fex-oh-**fen**-a-deen)
Allegra, Mucinex Allergy

Classification
Therapeutic: allergy, cold, and cough remedies, antihistamines

Pregnancy Category C

Indications

Relief of symptoms of seasonal allergic rhinitis. Management of chronic idiopathic urticaria.

Action

Antagonizes the effects of histamine at peripheral histamine–1 (H_1) receptors, including pruritus and urticaria. Also has a drying effect on the nasal mucosa. **Therapeutic Effects:** Decreased sneezing, rhinorrhea, itchy eyes, nose, and throat associated with seasonal allergies. Decreased urticaria.

Pharmacokinetics

Absorption: Rapidly absorbed after oral administration.
Distribution: Unknown.
Metabolism and Excretion: 80% excreted in urine, 11% excreted in feces.
Half-life: 14.4 hr (↑ in renal impairment).

TIME/ACTION PROFILE (antihistaminic effect)

ROUTE	ONSET	PEAK	DURATION
PO	within 1 hr	2–3 hr	12–24 hr

Contraindications/Precautions

Contraindicated in: Hypersensitivity.
Use Cautiously in: Impaired renal function (↑ dosing interval recommended); OB: use only if maternal benefit outweighs potential risk to fetus; Lactation: Usually compatible with breast feeding (AAP).

Adverse Reactions/Side Effects

CNS: drowsiness, fatigue. **GI:** dyspepsia. **Endo:** dysmenorrhea.

Interactions

Drug-Drug: Magnesium and aluminum-containing antacids ↓ absorption and may decrease effectiveness.

Drug-Food: Apple, orange, and **grapefruit juice** ↓ absorption and may decrease effectiveness.

Route/Dosage

PO (Adults and Children ≥12 yr): 60 mg twice daily, or 180 mg once daily.

PO (Children 2–11 yr): 30 mg twice daily.

PO (Children 6 mo–2 yr): 15 mg twice daily.

Renal Impairment

PO (Adults): 60 mg once daily as a starting dose.

PO (Children 6–11 yr): 30 mg once daily as a starting dose.

Availability (generic available)

Tablets: 30 mg[OTC], 60 mg[OTC], ✱ 120 mg[OTC], 180 mg[OTC]. **Orally disintegrating tablets:** 30 mg[OTC]. **Gelcaps:** 180 mg[OTC]. **Suspension (berry flavor):** 30 mg/5 mL[OTC]. ***In combination with:*** pseudoephedrine (Allegra-D). See Appendix B.

NURSING IMPLICATIONS

Assessment

- Assess allergy symptoms (rhinitis, conjunctivitis, hives) before and periodically during therapy.
- Assess lung sounds and character of bronchial secretions. Maintain fluid intake of 1500–2000 mL/day to decrease viscosity of secretions.
- ***Lab Test Considerations:*** Will cause false-negative reactions on allergy skin tests; discontinue 3 days before testing.

Potential Nursing Diagnoses

Ineffective airway clearance (Indications)
Risk for injury (Adverse Reactions)

Implementation

- Do not confuse Allegra with Viagra.
- **PO:** Administer with food or milk to decrease GI irritation. Capsules and tablets should be taken with water or milk, not juice.

Patient/Family Teaching

- Instruct patient to take medication as directed. Take missed doses as soon as remembered unless almost time for next dose.
- Inform patient that drug may cause drowsiness, although it is less likely to occur than with other antihistamines. Avoid driving or other activities requiring alertness until response to drug is known.
- Instruct patient to contact health care professional if symptoms persist.

Evaluation/Desired Outcomes

- Decrease in allergic symptoms.
- Decrease in urticaria.

fidaxomicin (fi-dax-oh-**mye**-sin)

Dificid

Classification
Therapeutic: anti-infectives
Pharmacologic: macrolides

Pregnancy Category B

Indications

Treatment of diarrhea associated with *Clostridium difficile*.

Action

Bactericial action mostly against clostridia; inhibits RNA synthesis. Acts locally in the GI tract to eliminate *Clostridium difficile*. **Therapeutic Effects:** Elimination of diarrhea caused by *Clostridium difficile*.

Pharmacokinetics

Absorption: Minimal systemic absorption.

Distribution: Stays primarily in the GI tract.

Metabolism and Excretion: Mostly transformed via hydrolysis in the GI tract to OP-1118, its active metabolite. Eliminated mostly (>92%) in feces: <1% excreted in urine.

Half-life: *Fidaxomicin*—11.7 hr; *OP-1118*—11.2 hr.

TIME/ACTION PROFILE

ROUTE	ONSET	PEAK	DURATION
PO	unknown	unknown	unknown

Contraindications/Precautions

Contraindicated in: Hypersensitivity.

Use Cautiously in: OB, Lactation: Use during pregnancy only if clearly needed, use cautiously during lactation; Pedi: Safe and effective use in children <18 yr has not been established.

Adverse Reactions/Side Effects

GI: GI HEMORRHAGE, nausea, abdominal pain. **Hemat:** anemia, neutropenia. **Misc:** HYPERSENSITIVITY REACTIONS.

Interactions

Drug-Drug: No significant interactions noted.

Route/Dosage

PO (Adults >18 yr): 200 mg twice daily for 10 days.

Availability

Tablets: 200 mg.

NURSING IMPLICATIONS

Assessment

- Monitor bowel function for diarrhea, abdominal cramping, fever, and bloody stools. May begin up to several weeks following cessation of antibiotic therapy.

- Monitor for signs and symptoms of hypersensitivity reactions (dyspnea, pruritus, rash, angioedema of mouth, throat, and face) periodically during therapy. Risk increases with a macrolide allergy.
- ***Lab Test Considerations:*** May cause ↑ serum alkaline phosphatase, and hepatic enzymes.
- May cause ↓ serum bicarbonate, ↓ platelet count, anemia, and neutropenia.
- May cause hyperglycemia and metabolic acidosis.

Potential Nursing Diagnoses

Risk for infection (Indications)
Diarrhea (Indications)

Implementation

- **PO:** Administer twice daily without regard to food.

Patient/Family Teaching

- Instruct patient to take fidamoxicin as directed for the full course of therapy, even if feeling better. Skipping doses or not completing full course of therapy may decrease effectiveness of therapy and increase risk that bacteria will develop resistance and not be treatable in the future.
- Advise female patients to notify health care professional if pregnancy is planned or suspected or if breast feeding.

Evaluation/Desired Outcomes

- Decrease in diarrhea caused by *Clostridium difficile.*

filgrastim (fil-gra-stim)

Neupogen, Zarxio

Classification

Therapeutic: colony-stimulating factors

Pregnancy Category C

Indications

Prevention of febrile neutropenia and associated infection in patients who have received bone marrow–depressing antineoplastics for the treatment of nonmyeloid malignancies. Reduction of time for neutrophil recovery and duration of fever in patients undergoing induction and consolidation chemotherapy for acute myelogenous leukemia. Reduction of time to neutrophil recovery and sequelae of neutropenia in patients with nonmyeloid malignancies undergoing myeloablative chemotherapy followed by bone marrow transplantation. Mobilization of hematopoietic progenitor cells into peripheral blood for collection by leukapheresis. Management of severe chronic neutropenia. Survival improvement in patients acutely exposed to myelosuppressive doses of radiation. **Unlabeled Use:** Neutropenia associated with HIV infection. Neonatal neutropenia.

Action

A glycoprotein, filgrastim binds to and stimulates immature neutrophils to divide and differentiate. Also activates mature neutrophils. **Therapeutic Effects:** Decreased incidence of infection in patients who are neutropenic from chemotherapy or other causes. Improved harvest of progenitor cells for bone marrow transplantation. Improved survival in patients exposed to myelosuppressive doses of radiation.

Pharmacokinetics

Absorption: Well absorbed after subcut administration.

Distribution: Unknown.

Metabolism and Excretion: Unknown.

Half-life: *Adults*—3.5 hr; *Neonates*—4.4 hr.

TIME/ACTION PROFILE

ROUTE	ONSET	PEAK	DURATION
IV, subcut	unknown	unknown	4 days†

†Return of neutrophil count to baseline.

Contraindications/Precautions

Contraindicated in: Hypersensitivity to filgrastim or *Escherichia coli*-derived proteins.

Use Cautiously in: Malignancy with myeloid characteristics; Pre-existing cardiac disease; OB: Use only if potential benefit justifies potential risk to fetus; Lactation: Unlikely to adversely affect breast-fed infant.

Adverse Reactions/Side Effects

CV: vasculitis. **GI:** SPLENIC RUPTURE, splenomegaly. **EENT:** hemoptysis. **GU:** glomerulonephritis. **Hemat:** excessive leukocytosis, sickle cell crises, thrombocytopenia. **Resp:** ACUTE RESPIRATORY DISTRESS SYNDROME, pulmonary infiltrates. **Local:** ALLERGIC REACTIONS, pain, redness at subcut site. **MS:** medullary bone pain.

Interactions

Drug-Drug: Simultaneous use with **antineoplastics** may have adverse effects on rapidly proliferating neutrophils—avoid use for 24 hr before and 24 hr after chemotherapy. **Lithium** may potentiate the release of neutrophils; concurrent use should be undertaken cautiously.

Route/Dosage

After Myelosuppressive Chemotherapy

IV, Subcut (Adults and Children): 5 mcg/kg/day as a single subcut injection, by short IV infusion, or via continuous IV infusion for up to 2 wk or until ANC reaches 10,000/mm^3. Initiate at least 24 hr after chemotherapy. Dose may be ↑ by 5 mcg/kg during each cycle of chemotherapy, depending on blood counts.

After Bone Marrow Transplantation

IV (Adults): 10 mcg/kg/day as a continuous IV infusion for up to 24 hr; initiate at least 24 hr after chemotherapy and at least 24 hr after bone marrow transplantation. Subsequent dose is adjusted according to blood counts.

Peripheral Blood Progenitor Cell Collection and Therapy

Subcut (Adults): 10 mcg/kg/day for at least 4 days before first leukapheresis and continued until last leukapheresis; Discontinue if WBC >100,000 cells/mm³.

Severe Chronic Neutropenia

Subcut (Adults): *Congenital neutropenia*—6 mcg/kg twice daily. *Idiopathic/cyclical neutropenia*—5 mcg/kg daily (↓ if ANC remains 7 gt;10,000/mm³).

After Myelosuppressive Radiation

Subcut (Adults): 10 mcg/kg once daily; initiate as soon as possible after exposure to radiation doses greater than 2 gray; continue until ANC remains >1000/mm³ for 3 consecutive blood counts (performed q 3 days) or is >10,000/mm³ after a radiation-induced nadir.

Neonatal Neutropenia

IV, Subcut (Neonates): 5–10 mcg/kg/day once daily for 3–5 days.

Availability

Injection: 300 mcg/1 mL, 480 mcg/1.6 mL. **Prefilled syringe:** 300 mcg/0.5 mL, 480 mcg/0.8 mL.

NURSING IMPLICATIONS

Assessment

- Monitor heart rate, BP, and respiratory status before and periodically during therapy.
- Assess bone pain throughout therapy. Pain is usually mild to moderate and controllable with nonopioid analgesics, but may require treatment with opioid analgesics, especially in patients receiving high-dose IV therapy. Loratadine 10 mg PO administered before filgrastim dose has been used to prevent bone pain.
- Monitor for signs and symptoms of allergic reactions (rash, urticaria, facial edema, wheezing, dyspnea, (hypotension, tachycardia). Usually occur within 30 min of administration. Treatment includes antihistamines, steroids, bronchodilators, and/or epinephrine; may recur with rechallenge.
- Assess for signs and symptoms of acute respiratory distress syndrome (fever, lung infiltrates, or respiratory distress). If symptoms occur, withhold filgrastim until symptoms resolve or discontinue.
- Monitor for signs and symptoms of splenic enlargement or rupture (left upper abdominal or shoulder pain).
- ***Lab Test Considerations:*** *After chemotherapy,* obtain a CBC with differential, including examination for the presence of blast cells, and platelet count before chemotherapy and twice weekly during therapy to avoid leukocytosis. Monitor ANC. A transient rise is seen 1–2 days after initiation of therapy, but therapy should not be discontinued until ANC >10,000/mm³.
- *After bone marrow transplant,* the daily dose is titrated by the neutrophil response. When the ANC is >1000/mm³ for 3 consecutive days, the dose should be reduced by 5 mcg/kg/day. If the ANC remains >1000/mm³ for 3 or more consecutive days, filgrastim is discontinued. If the ANC decreases to <1000/mm³, filgrastim should be resumed at 5 mcg/kg/day.
- *For chronic severe neutropenia,* monitor CBC with differential and platelet count twice weekly during initial 4 wk of therapy and during 2 wk after any dose adjustment.
- May cause ↓ platelet count and transient ↑ in uric acid, LDH, and alkaline phosphatase concentrations.

Potential Nursing Diagnoses

Risk for infection (Indications)
Acute pain (Side Effects)

Implementation

- Do not confuse Neupogen with Neumega (oprelvekin).
- Administer no earlier than 24 hr after cytotoxic chemotherapy, at least 24 hr after bone marrow infusion, and not during the 24 hr before administration of chemotherapy.
- Refrigerate; do not freeze. Do not shake. May warm to room temperature for up to 6 hr before injection. Discard if left at room temperature for >6 hr. Vial is for 1-time use only.
- **Subcut:** May be administered in outer area of upper arms, abdomen, thighs, or upper outer areas of buttock. If dose requires >1 mL of solution, may be divided into 2 injection sites.
- Cap of needle contains latex; avoid administration by persons with latex allergy.
- May also be administered as a continuous subcut infusion over 24 hr after bone marrow transplantation.

IV Administration

- **Continuous Infusion:** ***Diluent:*** Dilute in D5W; do not dilute with 0.9% NaCl, will precipitate. Refrigerate; do not freeze. Do not shake. May warm to room temperature for up to 6 hr before injection. Vial is for 1-time use only. ***Concentration:*** Dilute to a final concentration of at least 15 mcg/mL. If the final concentration is <15 mcg/mL, human albumin in a concentration of 2 mg/mL must be added to D5W before filgrastim to prevent adsorption of the components of the drug delivery system. ***Rate:*** *After chemotherapy* dose is administered via infusion over 15–60 min.
- *After chemotherapy* dose may also be administered as a continuous infusion.
- *After bone marrow transplant,* dose should be administered as an infusion over 4 or 24 hr.
- **Y-Site Compatibility:** acyclovir, allopurinol, amikacin, aminophylline, ampicillin, ampicillin/sulbactam, aztreonam, bleomycin, bumetanide, buprenorphine, butorphanol, calcium gluconate, carboplatin, carmustine, cefazolin, cefotetan, ceftazidime, chlor-

promazine, cisplatin, cyclophosphamide, cytarabine, dacarbazine, daunorubicin, dexamethasone, diphenhydramine, doxorubicin, doxycycline, droperidol, enalaprilat, famotidine, fluconazole, fludarabine, ganciclovir, granisetron, haloperidol, hydrocortisone, hydromorphone, idarubicin, ifosfamide, leucovorin calcium, levofloxacin, lorazepam, mechlorethamine, melphalan, meperidine, mesna, methotrexate, metoclopramide, mitoxantrone, morphine, nalbuphine, ondansetron, potassium chloride, promethazine, ranitidine, rituximab, sodium acetate, sodium bicarbonate, streptozocin, tobramycin, trastuzumab, trimethoprim/sulfamethoxazole, vancomycin, vinblastine, vincristine, vinorelbine, zidovudine.

- **Y-Site Incompatibility:** aminocaproic acid, amphotericin B colloidal, cefepime, cefotaxime, cefoxitin, ceftaroline, ceftriaxone, cefuroxime, clindamycin, dactinomycin, etoposide, fluorouracil, furosemide, heparin, mannitol, methylprednisolone sodium succinate, metronidazole, mitomycin, prochlorperazine, thiotepa.

Patient/Family Teaching

- Explain purpose of filgrastim to patient. Advise patient to notify health care professional regarding when to give next dose if a dose is missed. Instruct patient and caregiver to read *Instructions for Patients and Caregivers* before starting therapy and with each Rx refill in case of changes.
- Instruct patient to notify health care professional immediately if signs and symptoms of spleen enlargement or rupture, allergic reaction, ARDS, or vasculitis (skin redness, purple spots on skin) occur. Discuss risk of sickle cell crisis with patients with sickle cell disease before administering.
- Rep: Advise female patient to notify health care professional if pregnancy is planned or suspected or if breast feeding. Encourage patients that become pregnant during therapy to enroll in Amgen's Pregnancy Surveillance Program by calling 1-800-77AMGEN (1-800-772-6436). Encourage patients that breast feed during therapy to enroll in Amgen's Lactation Surveillance Program by calling 1-800-77AMGEN (1-800-772-6436).
- **Home Care Issues:** Instruct patient on correct technique and proper disposal for home administration. Caution patient not to reuse needle, vial, or syringe. Provide patient with a puncture-proof container for needle and syringe disposal.

Evaluation/Desired Outcomes

- Decreased incidence of infection in patients who receive bone marrow–depressing antineoplastics.
- Reduction of duration and sequelae of neutropenia after bone marrow transplantation.
- Reduction of the incidence and duration of sequelae of neutropenia in patients with severe chronic neutropenia.
- Improved harvest of progenitor cells for bone marrow transplantation.
- Improved survival in patients exposed to myelosuppressive doses of radiation.

finasteride (fi-nas-teer-ide)

Propecia, Proscar

Classification

Therapeutic: hair regrowth stimulants
Pharmacologic: androgen inhibitors

Pregnancy Category X

Indications

Benign prostatic hyperplasia (BPH); can be used with doxazosin. Androgenetic alopecia (male pattern baldness) in men only.

Action

Inhibits the enzyme 5-alpha-reductase, which is responsible for converting testosterone to its potent metabolite 5-alpha-dihydrotestosterone in prostate, liver, and skin; 5-alpha-dihydrotestosterone is partially responsible for prostatic hyperplasia and hair loss. **Therapeutic Effects:** Reduced prostate size with associated decrease in urinary symptoms. Decreases hair loss; promotes hair regrowth.

Pharmacokinetics

Absorption: Well absorbed after oral administration (63%).
Distribution: Enters prostatic tissue and crosses the blood-brain barrier. Remainder of distribution not known.
Protein Binding: 90%.
Metabolism and Excretion: Mostly metabolized; 39% excreted in urine as metabolites; 57% excreted in feces.
Half-life: 6 hr (range 6–15 hr; slightly ↑ in patients >70 yr).

TIME/ACTION PROFILE (↓ in dihydrotestosterone levels†)

ROUTE	ONSET	PEAK	DURATION
PO	rapid	8 hr	2 wk

†Clinical effects as noted by urinary tract symptoms and hair regrowth may not be evident for several months and remain for 4 mo after discontinuation.

Contraindications/Precautions

Contraindicated in: Hypersensitivity; Women.
Use Cautiously in: Patients with hepatic impairment or obstructive uropathy.

Adverse Reactions/Side Effects

Endo: gynecomastia. **GU:** PROSTATE CANCER (HIGH-GRADE), ↓ libido, ↓ volume of ejaculate, erectile dysfunction, infertility. **Misc:** ANGIOEDEMA, BREAST CANCER.

Interactions

Drug-Drug: None noted.

Route/Dosage

PO (Adults): *BPH*—5 mg once daily (Proscar); *Androgenetic alopecia*—1 mg once daily (Propecia).

Availability (generic available)

Tablets: 1 mg (Propecia), 5 mg (Proscar). **Cost:** *Generic*—1 mg $134.61/100, 5 mg $21.85/100.

NURSING IMPLICATIONS

Assessment

- Assess for symptoms of prostatic hyperplasia (urinary hesitancy, feeling of incomplete bladder emptying, interruption of urinary stream, impairment of size and force of urinary stream, terminal urinary dribbling, straining to start flow, dysuria, urgency) before and periodically during therapy.
- Digital rectal examinations should be performed before and periodically during therapy for BPH.
- ***Lab Test Considerations:*** Serum prostate-specific antigen (PSA) concentrations, which are used to screen for prostate cancer, may be evaluated before and periodically during therapy. Finasteride may cause a ↓ in serum PSA levels.

Potential Nursing Diagnoses

Impaired urinary elimination (Indications)

Implementation

- Do not confuse Proscar with Provera.
- **PO:** Administer once daily with or without meals.

Patient/Family Teaching

- Instruct patient to take finasteride as directed, even if symptoms improve or are unchanged. At least 6–12 mo of therapy may be necessary to determine whether or not an individual will respond to finasteride. Advise patient to read the *Patient Package Insert* prior to starting therapy and with each Rx refill in case of changes.
- Inform patient that the volume of ejaculate may be decreased and erectile dysfunction and decreased libido may occur during therapy and after therapy is completed.
- Advise patient to notify health care professional promptly if changes in breasts (lumps, pain, nipple discharge) occur.
- Inform patient that there is an increased risk of high grade prostate cancer in men taking this drug.
- Rep: Caution patient that finasteride poses a potential risk to a male fetus. Women who are pregnant or may become pregnant should avoid exposure to semen of a partner taking finasteride and should not handle crushed finasteride because of the potential for absorption.
- Emphasize the importance of periodic follow-up exams to determine whether a clinical response has occurred.

Evaluation/Desired Outcomes

- Decrease in urinary symptoms of benign prostatic hyperplasia.
- Hair regrowth in androgenetic alopecia. Evidence of hair growth usually requires 3 mo or longer. Continued use is recommended to sustain benefit. Withdrawal leads to reversal of effect within 12 mo.

REMS

fingolimod (fin-go-li-mod)

Gilenya

Classification

Therapeutic: anti-multiple sclerosis agents
Pharmacologic: receptor modulators

Pregnancy Category C

Indications

Treatment of relapsing forms of multiple sclerosis.

Action

Converted by sphingosine kinase to the active metabolite fingolimod-phosphate, which binds to sphingosine 1–phosphate receptors, resulting in ↓ migration of lymphocytes into peripheral blood. This may ↓ lymphocyte migration into the CNS. **Therapeutic Effects:** ↓ frequency of relapses/delayed accumulation of disability.

Pharmacokinetics

Absorption: Well absorbed (93%) following oral administration.

Distribution: Extensively distributed to body tissues; 86% of parent drug distributes into red blood cells; active metabolite uptake 17%.

Metabolism and Excretion: Converted to its active metabolite, then metabolized mostly by the CYP450 4F2 enzyme system, with further degradation by other enzyme systems. Most inactive metabolites excreted in urine (81%); <2.5% excreted as fingolimod and fingolimod-phosphate in feces.

Protein Binding: >99.7%.

Half-life: 6–9 hr.

TIME/ACTION PROFILE

ROUTE	ONSET	PEAK	DURATION
PO	unknown	1–2 mo*	2 mo†

*Time to steady state blood levels, peak blood levels after a single dose at 12–16 hr.

†Time for complete elimination.

Contraindications/Precautions

Contraindicated in: MI, unstable angina, stroke, TIA, or class III or IV HF within previous 6 mo; 2nd- or 3rd-degree heart block or sick sinus syndrome (in the absence of a pacemaker); QT interval ≥500 msec; Concurrent use of class Ia or III antiarrhythmics; Active acute/chronic untreated infections; Lactation: Breast feeding should be avoided.

Use Cautiously in: Concurrent use of beta blockers, diltiazem, verapamil, or digoxin (↑ risk of bradycardia/heart block); History of ischemic heart disease, MI, HF, cerebrovascular disease, uncontrolled hypertension, AV block, bradycardia, syncope, cardiac arrest, or severe sleep apnea (↑ risk of bradycardia/heart block); Severe hepatic impairment (↑ blood levels and risk of adverse reactions); Diabetes mellitus/history of uveitis (↑ risk of macular edema); Negative history for chickenpox or vaccination against varicella zoster virus vaccination; Geri: Risk of adverse reactions may be ↑ consider age-related ↓ in cardiac/renal/hepatic function, chronic illnesses, and concurrent drug therapy; Pedi: Safety and effectiveness not established; OB: Use only if potential benefit justifies potential risk to fetus.

Adverse Reactions/Side Effects

CNS: POSTERIOR REVERSIBLE ENCEPHALOPATHY SYNDROME (PRES), PROGRESSIVE MULTIFOCAL LEUKOENCEPHALOPATHY (PML), headache. **EENT:** blurred vision, eye pain, macular edema. **Resp:** cough, ↓ pulmonary function. **CV:** ASYSTOLE, BRADYCARDIA, HEART BLOCK, QT INTERVAL PROLONGATION, hypertension, syncope. **GI:** diarrhea, ↑ liver enzymes. **Hemat:** leukopenia, lymphopenia. **MS:** back pain. **Misc:** INFECTION (INCLUDING HERPES VIRAL INFECTIONS AND CRYPTOCOCCAL MENINGITIS).

Interactions

Drug-Drug: Concurrent use of **class Ia or class III antiarrhythmics** may ↑ risk of serious arrhythmias; careful monitoring recommended. Concurrent use of **beta blockers**, **diltiazem**, **verapamil**, or **digoxin** may ↑ risk of bradycardia; careful monitoring recommended. Concurrent use of **ketoconazole** may ↑ blood levels and of adverse reactions. ↑ risk of immunosuppression with **antineoplastics**, **immunosuppressants**, or **immune modulating therapies**. **Live-attenuated vaccines** ↑ risk of infection.

Route/Dosage

PO (Adults): 0.5 mg once daily.

Availability

Hard capsules: 0.5 mg.

NURSING IMPLICATIONS

Assessment

- Monitor pulse and BP hourly for bradycardia for at least 6 hr following first dose and periodically during therapy. Obtain baseline ECG before first dose and at end of observation period. If patient develops heart rate <45 bpm or new onset 2nd-degree or higher heart block, monitor until resolved. If bradycardia is symptomatic, patient has coexisting medical condition that affects heart rate, or if QTC prolongation occurs, monitor continuous ECG; if pharmacologic therapy is required, monitor in hospital overnight and repeat first-dose monitoring for 2nd dose. If fingolimod is stopped for 2 wk or more, first-dose monitoring must be followed when restarting. Have cardiologist perform cardiac evaluation on patients with a pre-existing CV condition prior to starting therapy. Monitor overnight with continuous ECG for 1st dose.
- Monitor for signs of infection (fever, sore throat) during and for 2 mo after discontinuation of therapy. Consider suspending therapy if serious infection develops.
- Perform an opthalmologic exam prior to starting fingolimod, at 3–4 mo after treatment initiation, and if visual disturbances occur. Monitor visual acuity at baseline and during routine exams. Patients with diabetes or history of uveitis are at ↑ risk and should have regular ophthalmologic exams.
- Monitor pulmonary function tests for decline periodically during therapy. Obtain spirometry and diffusion lung capacity for carbon monoxide when indicated clincally.
- Assess for any new signs or symptoms that may be suggestive of PML, an opportunistic infection of the brain caused by the Jakob Cruzfeldt (JC) virus, that may be fatal; withhold dose and notify health care professional promptly. PML symptoms may begin gradually (hemiparesis, apathy, confusion, cognitive deficiencies and ataxia) and may include deteriorating renal function.
- ***Lab Test Considerations:*** Obtain baseline liver function test before starting therapy. May cause ↑ liver transaminases. Monitor liver function tests if symptoms develop.
- Before initiating therapy, obtain a recent (within 6 mo) CBC. May cause ↓ lymphocyte counts.

Potential Nursing Diagnoses

Deficient knowledge, related to medication regimen (Patient/Family Teaching)

Implementation

- **PO:** Administer once daily without regard to food.

Patient/Family Teaching

- Instruct patient to take fingolimod as directed. Do not discontinue therapy without consulting health care professional. Advise patient to read the *Medication Guide* prior to starting therapy and with each Rx refill in case of changes.
- Advise patient to notify health care professional if signs and symptoms of liver dysfunction (unexplained nausea, vomiting, abdominal pain, fatigue, anorexia, jaundice, dark urine), infection, new onset of dyspnea, or changes in vision develop.

- Instruct patient not to receive live-attenuated vaccines during and for 2 mo after treatment due to risk of infection. Patients who have not had a healthcare professional confirmed history of chickenpox or documentation of a full course vaccination should be tested for antibodies to varicella zoster virus before starting therapy. Antibody-negative patients should receive vaccination prior to starting therapy, then postpone start of fingolimod for 1 mo to allow for full effect of vaccination.
- Rep: Advise female patients to use contraception during and for at least 2 mo after discontinuation of therapy and to notify health care professional immediately if pregnancy is planned or suspected or if breast feeding. Encourage pregnant patients to enroll in the pregnancy registry by calling 1-877-598-7237.

Evaluation/Desired Outcomes

- Reduction in frequency of clinical exacerbations and delay of accumulation of physical disability in patients with relapsing forms of multiple sclerosis.

REMS

flibanserin (flib- an-ser-in)

Addyi

Classification
Therapeutic: sexual dysfunction agents

Indications

Treatment of premenopausal women with hypoactive sexual desire disorder (HSDD) unrelated to concurrent medical/psychiatric diagnoses, relationship issues or substance abuse. Does not enhance sexual performance.

Action

May be explained by agonist activity at $5-HT_{1A}$ receptors and antagonist activity at $5-HT_{2A}$ receptors; also has moderate antagonist activity at $5-HT_{2B}$, $5-HT_{2C}$ and dopamine D_4 receptors. **Therapeutic Effects:** ↑ sexual desire with ↓ distress and interpersonal dysfunction.

Pharmacokinetics

Absorption: Moderately absorbed (33%) following oral administration.
Distribution: Unknown.
Protein Binding: 98%.
Metabolism and Excretion: Highly metabolized, mostly by the CYP3A4 enzyme system with lesser metabolized by CYP2C19. 44% excreted in urine, 51% in feces almost entirely as metabolites which do not appear to be pharmacologically active.
Half-life: 11 hr.

TIME/ACTION PROFILE (blood levels)

ROUTE	ONSET	PEAK	DURATION
PO	within 1 hr	1 hr	24 hr

Contraindications/Precautions

Contraindicated in: Alcohol ingeston (excess risk of hypotension/syncope); Concurrent use of strong/moderate CYP3A4 inhibitors; Concurrent use of CYP3A4 inducers; Hepatic impairment; Lactation: Breast feeding is not recommended.
Use Cautiously in: CYP2C19 Poor Metabolizers (↑ risk of adverse reactions including hypotension, syncope and drowsiness); Geri: Not indicated for use in the elderly; OB: Safe use during pregnancy has not been established; Pedi: Not indicated for use in children.

Adverse Reactions/Side Effects

CNS: dizziness, drowsiness, anxiety, fatigue, insomnia, vertigo. **CV:** HYPOTENSION/SYNCOPE. **GI:** nausea, constipation, dry mouth. **Derm:** rash.

Interactions

Drug-Drug: Concurrent use of **strong or moderate CYP3A4 inhibitors** including **atazanavir**, **boceprevir**, **ciprofloxacin**, **clarithromycin**, **conivaptan**, **diltiazem**, **erythromycin**, **fluconazole**, **fosamprenavir**, **indinavir**, **itraconazole**, **ketoconazole**, **indinavir**, **nelfinavir**, **posaconazole**, **ritonavir**, **saquinavir**, **telithromycin**, and **verapamil** ↑ blood levels, effects and risk of serious adverse reactions; concurrent use is contraindicated. Wait two weeks after discontinuing inhibitor before initiating fibanserin. If initiating inhibitor, wait two days after last dose of flibanserin. Concurrent use with **alcohol** ↑ risk of hypotension/syncope and excess sedation; concurrent use is contraindicated. Concurrent use of **oral hormonal contraceptives** and **weak CYP3A4 inhibitors** including **cimetidine**, **fluoxetine** and **ranitidine** may also ↑ blood levels, effects and the risk of adverse reactions; avoid use of multiple weak CYP3A4 inhibitors. **Strong CYP2C19 inhibitors** including **proton pump inhibitors**, **SSRIs**, **benzodiazepines** and **antifungals** ↑ blood levels, effects and the risk of adverse reactions including hypotension, syncope and CNS depression; concurrent use should be undertaken with caution. **CYP3A4 inducers** including **carbamazepine**, **phenobarbital**, **phenytoin**, **rifabutin**, **rifampin** and **rifapentine** ↓ blood levels and effectiveness; concurrent use in not recommended. ↑ **digoxin** and **sirolimus** levels and risk of toxicity; careful monitoring recommended. ↑ risk of CNS depression with other **CNS depressants** including **alcohol**, **antihistamines**, **opioids**, **sedative/hypnotics**, some **anti-anxiety agents**, **antidepressants**, and **antipsychotics**.
Natural-Natural: Concurrent use with **ginko** may also ↑ blood levels, effects and the risk of adverse reactions; avoid use with other weak CYP3A4 inhibitors. **St. John's wort** ↓ blood levels and effectiveness; concurrent use in not recommended.

Drug-Food: Concurrent ingestion of **grapefruit juice** ↑ blood levels, effects and risk of hypotension/syncope; concurrent ingestion is contraindicated.

Route/Dosage

PO (Adults): 100 mg once daily (at bedtime).

Availability

Tablets: 100 mg.

NURSING IMPLICATIONS

Assessment

- Assess sexual desire and related distress and interpersonal dysfunction before and periodically during therapy.
- Monitor for hypotension and syncope. Have patient lie supine if dizziness occurs.
- Assess likelihood of patient abstaining from alcohol, taking into account the patient's current and past drinking behavior, and other pertinent social and medical history. Counsel patients who are prescribed flibanserin about the importance of abstaining from alcohol use; interaction with alcohol increases risk of hypotension and syncope.

Potential Nursing Diagnoses

Sexual dysfunction (Indications)
Risk for injury (Adverse Reactions)

Implementation

- Administer once daily at bedtime; administration during waking hrs increases risks of hypotension, syncope, accidental injury, and central nervous system (CNS) depression.
- Only available through a restricted program, *Addyi REMS Program* due to increased risk of severe hypotension and syncope interaction with alcohol.

Patient/Family Teaching

- Instruct patient to take flibanserin as directed. If dose is missed, omit and take next dose at bedtime on next day. Advise patient to read *Patient Information* before starting therapy and with each Rx refill in case of changes.
- Advise patient to avoid grapefruit juice during therapy.
- Caution patient to alcohol during therapy; increases hypotensive effects. May cause dizziness and fainting.
- Advise patient if dizziness occurs, immediately lie supine and promptly seek medical help if symptoms do not resolve.
- May cause drowsiness. Caution patient to avoid driving and other activities requiring alertness until 6 hrs after each dose or until response to medication is known.
- Instruct patient to notify health care professional of all Rx or OTC medications, vitamins, or herbal products being taken and consult health care professional before taking any new medications, especially St. John's wort.
- Advise patient to notify health care professional if pregnancy is planned or suspected and to avoid breast feeding.

Evaluation/Desired Outcomes

- Increase in sexual desire. If no improvement in 8 wks, discontinue flibanserin.

F

fluconazole (floo-**kon**-a-zole)

✱Canesoral, Diflucan, ✱Diflucan One, ✱Monicure

Classification

Therapeutic: antifungals (systemic)

Pregnancy Category C (single-dose oral treatment of vaginal candidiasis), D (all other indications)

Indications

PO, IV: Fungal infections caused by susceptible organisms, including: Oropharyngeal or esophageal candidiasis, Serious systemic candidal infections, Urinary tract infections, Peritonitis, Cryptococcal meningitis. Prevention of candidiasis in patients who have undergone bone marrow transplantation. **PO:** Single-dose oral treatment of vaginal candidiasis. **Unlabeled Use:** Prevention of recurrent vaginal yeast infections.

Action

Inhibits synthesis of fungal sterols, a necessary component of the cell membrane. **Therapeutic Effects:** Fungistatic action against susceptible organisms. May be fungicidal in higher concentrations. **Spectrum:** *Cryptococcus neoformans. Candida* spp.

Pharmacokinetics

Absorption: Well absorbed after oral administration.
Distribution: Widely distributed, good penetration into CSF, saliva, sputum, vaginal fluid, skin, eye, and peritoneum. Excreted in breast milk.
Metabolism and Excretion: >80% excreted unchanged by the kidneys; <10% metabolized by the liver.
Half-life: Premature neonates: 46–74 hr; Children: 19–25 hr (PO) and 15–17 hr (IV); Adults: 30 hr (↑ in renal impairment).

TIME/ACTION PROFILE (blood levels)

ROUTE	ONSET	PEAK	DURATION
PO	unknown	2–4 hr	24 hr
IV	rapid	end of infusion	24 hr

Contraindications/Precautions

Contraindicated in: Hypersensitivity to fluconazole or other azole antifungals; Concurrent use with pimozide, erythromycin, or quinidine.

Use Cautiously in: Renal impairment (dose ↓ required if CCr <50 mL/min); Underlying liver disease; OB: Safety not established; congenital defects have occurred with use of high-dose fluconazole (400–800 mg/day); Lactation: Usually compatible with breast feeding; Geri: ↑ risk of adverse reactions (rash, vomiting, diarrhea, seizures); consider age-related ↓ in renal function in determining dose.

Adverse Reactions/Side Effects

Incidence of adverse reactions is increased in HIV patients.

CNS: headache, dizziness, seizures. **GI:** HEPATOTOXICITY, abdominal discomfort, diarrhea, nausea, vomiting. **Derm:** exfoliative skin disorders including STEVENS-JOHNSON SYNDROME. **Endo:** hypokalemia, hypertriglyceridemia. **Misc:** allergic reactions, including ANAPHYLAXIS.

Interactions

Drug-Drug: May ↑ levels of **pimozide**, **erythromycin**, and **quinidine** which can prolong the QT interval and ↑ the risk of torsade de pointes. May ↑ levels of and the risk of bleeding with **warfarin**. **Rifampin**, **rifabutin**, and **isoniazid** ↓ levels. Fluconazole at doses >200 mg/day may inhibit the CYP3A4 enzyme system and effect the activity of drugs metabolized by this system. ↑ hypoglycemic effects of **tolbutamide**, **glyburide**, or **glipizide**. ↑ levels and risk of toxicity from **cyclosporine**, **carbamazepine**, **celecoxib**, **rifabutin**, **tacrolimus**, **sirolimus**, **theophylline**, **zidovudine**, **alfentanil**, and **phenytoin**. ↑ levels and effects of **benzodiazepines**, **amlodipine**, **felodipine**, **isradipine**, **nifedipine**, **nisoldipine**, **verapamil**, **atorvastatin**, **fluvastatin**, **lovastatin**, **simvastatin**, **methadone**, **flurbiprofen**, **prednisone**, **saquinavir**, **tricyclic antidepressants**, and **losartan**. ↑ levels of **tofacitinib**; ↓ dose of tofacitinib to 5 mg once daily. May ↑ risk of bleeding with **warfarin**. May antagonize effects of **amphotericin B**. May ↑ **voriconazole** levels; avoid concurrent use.

Route/Dosage

Oropharyngeal Candidiasis

PO, IV (Adults): 200 mg initially, then 100 mg daily for at least 2 wk.

PO, IV (Children >14 days): 6 mg/kg initially, then 3 mg/kg/day for at least 2 wk.

PO, IV (Neonates <14 days, 30–36 weeks gestation): same dose as older children except frequency is q 48 hr; Premature neonates <29 wk gestation: 5–6 mg/kg/dose q 48–72 hr.

Esophageal Candidiasis

PO, IV (Adults): 200 mg initially, then 100 mg once daily for at least 3 wk (up to 400 mg/day).

PO, IV (Children >14 days): 6 mg/kg initially, then 3–12 mg/kg/day for at least 3 wk.

PO, IV (Neonates <14 days, 30–36 weeks gestation): same dose as older children except frequency is q 48 hr; Premature neonates <29 wk gestation: 5–6 mg/kg/dose q 48–72 hr.

Vaginal Candidiasis

PO (Adults): 150-mg single dose; prevention of recurrence (unlabeled)—150 mg daily for 3 days then weekly for 6 mo.

Systemic Candidiasis

PO, IV (Adults): 400 mg/day initially, then 200–800 mg/day for 28 days.

PO, IV (Children > 14 days): 6–12 mg/kg/day for 28 days.

PO, IV (Neonates <14 days, 30–36 weeks gestation): same dose as older children except frequency is q 48 hr; Premature neonates <29 wk gestation: 5–6 mg/kg/dose q 48–72 hr.

Cryptococcal Meningitis

PO, IV (Adults): *Treatment*—400 mg once daily until favorable clinical response, then 200–800 mg once daily for at least 10–12 wk after clearing of CSF; change to oral therapy as soon as possible. *Suppressive therapy*—200 mg once daily.

PO, IV (Children >14 days): 12 mg/kg/day initially, then 6–12 mg/kg/day for at least 10–12 wk after clearing of CSF; change to oral therapy as soon as possible. *Suppressive therapy*—6 mg/kg/day.

PO, IV (Neonates <14 days, 30–36 weeks gestation): same dose as older children except frequency is q 48 hr; Premature neonates <29 wk gestation: 5–6 mg/kg/dose q 48–72 hr.

Prevention of Candidiasis after Bone Marrow Transplant

PO, IV (Adults): 400 mg once daily; begin several days before procedure if severe neutropenia is expected, and continue for 7 days after ANC >1000 /mm^3.

PO, IV (Children >14 days): 10–12 mg/kg/day, not to exceed 600 mg/day.

Renal Impairment

PO, IV (Adults): *CCr ≤50 mL/min (no hemodialysis)*—Give 50% of the usual dose (not for single-dose therapy); *Hemodialysis*—Give 100% of the usual dose after each dialysis session; give reduced dose based on CCr on non-dialysis days (not for single-dose therapy).

Availability (generic available)

Tablets: 50 mg, 100 mg, 150 mg, 200 mg. **Cost:** *Generic*—100 mg $88.17/30, 150 mg $6.99/1. **Powder for oral suspension (orange flavor):** 10 mg/mL, 40 mg/mL. **Cost:** *Generic*—10 mg/mL $36.00/35 mL, 40 mg/mL $130.76/35 mL. **Premixed infusion:** 2 mg/mL.

NURSING IMPLICATIONS

Assessment

- Assess infected area and monitor CSF cultures before and periodically during therapy.
- Specimens for culture should be taken before instituting therapy. Therapy may be started before results are obtained.
- Assess patient for rash (mild to moderate rash usually occurs in the 2nd wk of therapy and resolves within 1–2 wk of continued therapy). If rash is severe (extensive erythematous or maculopapular rash with moist desquamation or angioedema), accompanied by systemic symptoms (serum sickness-like reaction, Stevens-Johnson syndrome, toxic epidermal necrolysis), or occurs during treatment for a superficial fungal infection, therapy must be discontinued immediately.
- ***Lab Test Considerations:*** Monitor BUN and serum creatinine before and periodically during therapy; patients with renal dysfunction will require dose adjustment.
- Monitor liver function tests before and periodically during therapy. May cause ↑ AST, ALT, serum alkaline phosphate, and bilirubin concentrations.

Potential Nursing Diagnoses

Risk for infection (Indications)

Implementation

- Do not confuse Diflucan (fluconazole) with Diprivan (propofol).
- **PO:** Shake oral suspension well before administration.

IV Administration

- **Intermittent Infusion: *Diluent:*** Premixed infusions are prediluted and ready to use. Do not unwrap until ready to use. Do not administer solution that is cloudy or has a precipitate. Check for leaks by squeezing inner bag. If leaks are found, discard container as unsterile. ***Concentration:*** 2 mg/mL. ***Rate:*** Infuse over 1–2 hr. Do not exceed a rate of 200 mg/hr. Pedi: For children receiving doses >6 mg/kg/day, give over 2 hr.
- **Y-Site Compatibility:** acyclovir, aldesleukin, alemtuzumab, alfentanil, allopurinol, amifostine, amikacin, aminocaproic acid, aminophylline, amiodarone, anidulafungin, argatroban, ascorbic acid, atropine, azathioprine, azithromycin, aztreonam, benztropine, bivalirudin, bleomycin, bumetanide, buprenorphine, butorphanol, calcium chloride, cangrelor, carboplatin, carmustine, caspofungin, cefazolin, cefepime, cefotetan, cefoxitin, ceftaroline, chlorpromazine, cisatracurium, cisplatin, cyanocobalamin, cyclophosphamide, cyclosporine, cytarabine, dactinomycin, daptomycin, dexamethasone sodium phosphate, dexmedetomidine, dexrazoxane, diltiazem, diphenhydramine, dobutamine, docetaxel, dolasetron, dopamine, doripenem, doxorubicin hydrochloride, doxorubicin liposome, doxycycline, droperidol, enalaprilat, ephedrine, epinephrine, epirubicin, epoetin alfa, eptifibatide, ertapenem, erythromycin, esmolol, etoposide, etoposide phosphate, famotidine, fenoldopam, fentanyl, filgrastim, fludarabine, fluorouracil, folic acid, foscarnet, fosphenytoin, ganciclovir, gemcitabine, gentamicin, glycopyrrolate, granisetron, heparin, hydrocortisone, hydromorphone, idarubicin, ifosfamide, indomethacin, insulin, irinotecan, isoproterenol, ketorolac, labetalol, leucovorin, levofloxacin, lidocaine, linezolid, lorazepam, magnesium sulfate, mannitol, mechlorethamine, melphalan, meperidine, meropenem, mesna, methotrexate, methyldopate, methylprednisolone sodium succinate, metoclopramide, metoprolol, metronidazole, midazolam, milrinone, mitoxantrone, morphine, multivitamins, mycophenolate, nafcillin, nalbuphine, naloxone, nesiritide, nicardipine, nitroglycerin, nitroprusside, norepinephrine, octreotide, ondansetron, oxacillin, oxaliplatin, oxytocin, paclitaxel, palonosetron, pamidronate, pancuronium, papaverine, pemetrexed, penicillin G, pentazocine, pentobarbital, phenobarbital, phenylephrine, phytonadione, piperacillin/tazobactam, potassium acetate, potassium chloride, procainamide, prochlorperazine, promethazine, propofol, propranolol, protamine, pyridoxine, quinupristin-dalfopristin, ranitidine, remifentanil, rituximab, rocuronium, sargramostim, sodium acetate, sodium bicarbonate, streptokinase, succinylcholine, sufentanil, tacrolimus, telavancin, teniposide, theophylline, thiotepa, tigecycline, tirofiban, tobramycin, topotecan, trastuzumab, vancomycin, vasopressin, vecuronium, verapamil, vinblastine, vincristine, vinorelbine, voriconazole, zidovudine, zoledronic acid.
- **Y-Site Incompatibility:** amphotericin B colloidal, amphotericin B lipid complex, ampicillin, dantrolene, diazepam, pantoprazole, trimethoprim/sulfamethoxazole.

Patient/Family Teaching

- Instruct patient to take medication as directed, even if feeling better. Doses should be taken at the same time each day. Take missed doses as soon as remembered, but not if almost time for next dose. Do not double doses.
- Instruct patient to notify health care professional if skin rash, abdominal pain, fever, or diarrhea becomes pronounced, if signs and symptoms of liver dysfunction (unusual fatigue, anorexia, nausea, vomiting, jaundice, dark urine, or pale stools) occur, if unusual bruising or bleeding occur, or if no improvement is seen within a few days of therapy.

F

- Advise patient to notify health care professional if pregnancy is planned or suspected or if breast feeding.

Evaluation/Desired Outcomes

- Resolution of clinical and laboratory indications of fungal infections. Full course of therapy may require weeks or months of treatment after resolution of symptoms.
- Prevention of candidiasis in patients who have undergone bone marrow transplantation.
- Decrease in skin irritation and vaginal discomfort in patients with vaginal candidiasis. Diagnosis should be reconfirmed with smears or cultures before a second course of therapy to rule out other pathogens associated with vulvovaginitis. Recurrent vaginal infections may be a sign of systemic illness.

fludrocortisone

(floo-droe-**kor**-ti-sone)

✱Florinef

Classification

Therapeutic: hormones

Pharmacologic: corticosteroids (mineralocorticoid)

Pregnancy Category C

Indications

Sodium loss and hypotension associated with adrenocortical insufficiency (given with hydrocortisone or cortisone). Management of sodium loss due to congenital adrenogenital syndrome (congenital adrenal hyperplasia). **Unlabeled Use:** Idiopathic orthostatic hypotension (with increased sodium intake). Type IV renal tubular acidosis.

Action

Causes sodium reabsorption, hydrogen and potassium excretion, and water retention by its effects on the distal renal tubule. **Therapeutic Effects:** Maintenance of sodium balance and BP in patients with adrenocortical insufficiency.

Pharmacokinetics

Absorption: Well absorbed following oral administration.

Distribution: Widely distributed; probably enters breast milk.

Protein Binding: High.

Metabolism and Excretion: Mostly metabolized by the liver.

Half-life: 3.5 hr.

TIME/ACTION PROFILE (mineralocorticoid activity)

ROUTE	ONSET	PEAK	DURATION
PO	unknown	unknown	1–2 days

Contraindications/Precautions

Contraindicated in: Hypersensitivity.

Use Cautiously in: HF; Addison's disease (patients may have exaggerated response); OB, Lactation, Pedi: Safety not established.

Adverse Reactions/Side Effects

CNS: dizziness, headache. **CV:** HF, arrhythmias, edema, hypertension. **GI:** anorexia, nausea. **Endo:** adrenal suppression, weight gain. **F and E:** hypokalemia, hypokalemic alkalosis. **MS:** arthralgia, muscular weakness, tendon contractures. **Neuro:** ascending paralysis. **Misc:** hypersensitivity reactions.

Interactions

Drug-Drug: Use with **thiazide or loop diuretics**, **piperacillin**, or **amphotericin B** may ↑ risk of hypokalemia. Hypokalemia may ↑ risk of **digoxin** toxicity. May produce prolonged neuromuscular blockade following the use of **nondepolarizing neuromuscular blocking agents**. **Phenobarbital** or **rifampin** may ↑ metabolism and ↓ effectiveness.

Drug-Food: Large amounts of **salt** or **sodium-containing foods** may cause excessive sodium retention and potassium loss.

Route/Dosage

PO (Adults): *Adrenocortical insufficiency*—100 mcg/day (range 100 mcg 3 times weekly—200 mcg daily). Doses as small as 50 mcg daily may be required by some patients. Use with 10–37.5 mg cortisone daily or 10–30 mg hydrocortisone daily. *Adrenogenital syndrome*—100–200 mcg/day. *Idiopathic hypotension*—50–200 mcg/day (unlabeled).

PO (Children): 50–100 mcg/day.

Availability (generic available)

Tablets: 100 mcg (0.1 mg).

NURSING IMPLICATIONS

Assessment

- Monitor BP periodically during therapy. Report significant changes. Hypotension may indicate insufficient dose.
- Monitor for fluid retention (weigh daily, assess for edema, and auscultate lungs for rales/crackles).
- Monitor patients with Addison's disease closely and stop treatment if a significant increase in weight or BP, edema, or cardiac enlargement occurs. Patients with Addison's disease are more sensitive to the action of fludrocortisone and may have an exaggerated response.
- ***Lab Test Considerations:*** Monitor serum electrolytes periodically during therapy. Fludrocortisone causes ↓ serum potassium levels.

Potential Nursing Diagnoses

Deficient fluid volume (Indications)

Excess fluid volume (Side Effects)

Implementation

- ***High Alert:*** Do not confuse Florinef with Floranex or Florastor.
- **PO:** Tablets are scored and may be broken if dose adjustment is necessary.

Patient/Family Teaching

- Instruct patient to take medication as directed. Take missed doses as soon as remembered but not just before next dose is due. Explain that lifelong therapy may be necessary and that abrupt discontinuation may lead to Addisonian Crisis. Patient should keep an adequate supply available at all times.
- Advise patient to follow dietary modification prescribed by health care professional. Instruct patient to follow a diet high in potassium (see Appendix J). Amount of sodium allowed in diet varies with pathophysiology.
- Instruct patient to inform health care professional if weight gain or edema, muscle weakness, cramps, nausea, anorexia, or dizziness occurs.
- Advise patient to carry identification at all times describing disease process and medication regimen.

Evaluation/Desired Outcomes

- Normalization of fluid and electrolyte balance without the development of hypokalemia or hypertension.

flumazenil (flu-maz-e-nil)

✱ Anexate, Romazicon

Classification
Therapeutic: antidotes

Pregnancy Category C

Indications

Complete/partial reversal of effects of benzodiazepines used as general anesthetics, or during diagnostic or therapeutic procedures. Management of intentional or accidental overdose of benzodiazepines.

Action

Flumazenil is a benzodiazepine derivative that antagonizes the CNS depressant effects of benzodiazepine compounds. It has no effect on CNS depression from other causes, including opioids, alcohol, barbiturates, or general anesthetics. **Therapeutic Effects:** Reversal of benzodiazepine effects.

Pharmacokinetics

Absorption: IV administration results in complete bioavailability.
Distribution: Unknown.
Protein Binding: 50% primarily to albumin.
Metabolism and Excretion: Metabolism of flumazenil occurs primarily in the liver.
Half-life: Children: 20–75 min; Adults: 41–79 min.

TIME/ACTION PROFILE (reversal of benzodiazepine effects)

ROUTE	ONSET	PEAK	DURATION
IV	1–2 min	6–10 min	1–2 hr†

†Depends on dose/concentration of benzodiazepine and dose of flumazenil.

Contraindications/Precautions

Contraindicated in: Hypersensitivity to flumazenil or benzodiazepines; Patients receiving benzodiazepines for life-threatening medical problems, including status epilepticus or ↑ intracranial pressure; Serious cyclic antidepressant overdosage.
Use Cautiously in: Mixed CNS depressant overdose (effects of other agents may emerge when benzodiazepine effect is removed); History of seizures (seizures are more likely to occur in patients who are experiencing sedative/hypnotic withdrawal, who have recently received repeated doses of benzodiazepines, or who have a previous history of seizure activity); Head injury (may ↑ intracranial pressure and risk of seizures); Severe hepatic impairment; OB, Lactation: Safety not established; Pedi: Children <1 yr (safety not established).

Adverse Reactions/Side Effects

CNS: SEIZURES, dizziness, agitation, confusion, drowsiness, emotional lability, fatigue, headache, sleep disorders. **EENT:** abnormal hearing, abnormal vision, blurred vision. **CV:** arrhythmias, chest pain, hypertension. **GI:** nausea, vomiting, hiccups. **Derm:** flushing, sweating. **Local:** pain/injection-site reactions, phlebitis. **Neuro:** paresthesia. **Misc:** rigors, shivering.

Interactions

Drug-Drug: None significant.

Route/Dosage

Reversal of Conscious Sedation or General Anesthesia

IV (Adults): 0.2 mg. Additional doses may be given at 1-min intervals until desired results are obtained, up to a total dose of 1 mg. If resedation occurs, regimen may be repeated at 20-min intervals, not to exceed 3 mg/hr.
IV (Children): 0.01 mg/kg (up to 0.2 mg); if the desired level of consciousness is not obtained after waiting an additional 45 sec, further injections of 0.01 mg/kg (up to 0.2 mg) can be administered and repeated at 60-sec intervals when necessary (up to a maximum of 4 additional times) to a maximum total dose of 0.05 mg/kg or 1 mg, whichever is lower. The dose should be individualized based on the patient's response.

Suspected Benzodiazepine Overdose

IV (Adults): 0.2 mg. Additional 0.3 mg may be given 30 sec later. Further doses of 0.5 mg may be given at 1-

min intervals, if necessary, to a total dose of 3 mg. Usual dose required is 1–3 mg. If resedation occurs, additional doses of 0.5 mg/min for 2 min may be given at 20-min intervals (given no more than 1 mg at a time, not to exceed 3 mg per hr).
IV (Children): *Unlabeled*—0.01 mg/kg (maximum dose 0.2 mg) with repeat doses every minute up to a cumulative dose of 1 mg. As an alternative to repeat doses, continuous infusions of 0.005–0.01 mg/kg/hr have been used.

Availability (generic available)

Injection: 0.1 mg/mL.

NURSING IMPLICATIONS

Assessment

- Assess level of consciousness and respiratory status before and during therapy. Observe patient for at least 2 hr after administration for the appearance of resedation. Hypoventilation may occur.
- **Overdose:** Attempt to determine time of ingestion and amount and type of benzodiazepine taken. Knowledge of agent ingested allows an estimate of duration of CNS depression.

Potential Nursing Diagnoses

Risk for injury (Indications)
Risk for poisoning (Indications)

Implementation

- Do not confuse flumazenil with influenza virus vaccine.
- Ensure that patient has a patent airway before administration of flumazenil.
- Observe IV site frequently for redness or irritation. Administer through a free-flowing IV infusion into a large vein to minimize pain at the injection site.
- Optimal emergence should be undertaken slowly to decrease undesirable effects including confusion, agitation, emotional lability, and perceptual distortion.
- Institute seizure precautions. Seizures are more likely to occur in patients who are experiencing sedative/hypnotic withdrawal, patients who have recently received repeated doses of benzodiazepines, or those who have a previous history of seizure activity. Seizures may be treated with benzodiazepines, barbiturates, or phenytoin. Larger than normal doses of benzodiazepines may be required.
- **Suspected Benzodiazepine Overdose:** If no effects are seen after administration of flumazenil, consider other causes of decreased level of consciousness (alcohol, barbiturates, opioid analgesics).

IV Administration

- **IV Push:** ***Diluent:*** May be administered undiluted or diluted in syringe with D5W, 0.9% NaCl, or LR. Diluted solution should be discarded after 24 hr. ***Concentration:*** Up to 0.1 mg/mL. ***Rate:*** Administer each dose over 15–30 sec into free-flowing IV in a large vein. Do not exceed 0.2 mg/min in children or 0.5 mg/min in adults.

Patient/Family Teaching

- Flumazenil does not consistently reverse the amnestic effects of benzodiazepines. Provide patient and family with written instructions for postprocedure care. Inform family that patient may appear alert at the time of discharge but the sedative effects of the benzodiazepine may recur. Instruct patient to avoid driving or other activities requiring alertness for at least 24 hr after discharge.
- Instruct patient not to take any alcohol or nonprescription drugs for at least 18–24 hr after discharge.
- Resumption of usual activities should occur only when no residual effects of the benzodiazepine remain.

Evaluation/Desired Outcomes

- Improved level of consciousness.
- Decrease in respiratory depression caused by benzodiazepines.

---

flunisolide, See CORTICOSTEROIDS (INHALATION) and CORTICOSTEROIDS (NASAL).

---

fluocinolone, See CORTICOSTEROIDS (TOPICAL/LOCAL).

---

fluocinonide, See CORTICOSTEROIDS (TOPICAL/LOCAL).

FLUOROQUINOLONES
(floor-oh-**kwin**-oh-lones)

ciprofloxacin†
(sip-roe-**flox**-a-sin)
Cipro, Cipro XR

gemifloxacin (gem-i-**flox**-a-sin)
Factive

levofloxacin (le-voe-**flox**-a-sin)
Levaquin

moxifloxacin† (mox-i-**flox**-a-sin)
Avelox

ofloxacin† (oh-**flox**-a-sin)
~~Floxin~~

Classification
Therapeutic: anti-infectives
Pharmacologic: fluoroquinolones

Pregnancy Category C

†See Appendix C for ophthalmic use

Indications

PO, IV: Treatment of the following bacterial infections: Urinary tract infections including cystitis and prostatitis (ciprofloxacin, levofloxacin, ofloxacin), Gonorrhea (may not be considered first-line agents due to increasing resistance), Gynecologic infections (ciprofloxacin, ofloxacin), Respiratory tract infections including acute sinusitis, acute exacerbations of chronic bronchitis, and pneumonia, Skin and skin structure infections (levofloxacin, moxifloxacin, ciprofloxacin, ofloxacin), Bone and joint infections (ciprofloxacin), Infectious diarrhea (ciprofloxacin), Intra-abdominal infections (ciprofloxacin, moxifloxacin). Febrile neutropenia (ciprofloxacin). Postexposure treatment of inhalational anthrax (ciprofloxacin, levofloxacin). Treatment and prophylaxis of plague (ciprofloxacin, levofloxacin, moxifloxacin).

Action

Inhibit bacterial DNA synthesis by inhibiting DNA gyrase. **Therapeutic Effects:** Death of susceptible bacteria. **Spectrum:** Broad activity includes many gram-positive pathogens: Staphylococci including methicillin-resistant *Staphylococcus aureus*, *Staphylococcus epidermidis*, *Staphylococcus saprophyticus*, *Streptococcus pneumoniae*, *Streptococcus pyogenes*, and *Bacillus anthracis*. Gram-negative spectrum notable for activity against: *Escherichia coli*, *Klebsiella*, *Enterobacter*, *Salmonella*, *Shigella*, *Proteus*, *Providencia*, *Morganella morganii*, *Pseudomonas aeruginosa*, *Serratia*, *Haemophilus*, *Acinetobacter*, *Neisseria gonorrhoeae*, *Moraxella catarrhalis*, *Campylobacter*, and *Yersinia pestis*. Additional spectrum includes: *Chlamydia pneumoniae*, *Legionella pneumoniae*, and *Mycoplasma pneumoniae*.

Pharmacokinetics

Absorption: Well absorbed after oral administration (*ciprofloxacin*—70%; *moxifloxacin*—90%; *gemifloxacin*—71%; *levofloxacin*—99%; *ofloxacin*—98%).

Distribution: Widely distributed. High tissue and urinary levels are achieved. All agents appear to cross the placenta. *Ciprofloxacin* and *ofloxacin* enter breast milk.

Metabolism and Excretion: *Ciprofloxacin*—15% metabolized by the liver, 40–50% excreted unchanged by the kidneys; *gemifloxacin*—Minimal metabolism, 61% excreted unchanged in feces, 36% excreted unchanged in urine; *levofloxacin*—87% excreted unchanged in urine, small amounts metabolized; *moxifloxacin*—mostly metabolized by the liver, 20% excreted unchanged in urine, 25% excreted unchanged in feces; *ofloxacin*—70–80% excreted unchanged by the kidneys.

Half-life: *Ciprofloxacin*—4 hr; *gemifloxacin*—7 hr; *levofloxacin*—8 hr; *moxifloxacin*—12 hr; *ofloxacin*—5–7 hr (all are ↑ in renal impairment).

F

TIME/ACTION PROFILE (blood levels)

ROUTE	ONSET	PEAK	DURATION
Ciprofloxacin—PO	rapid	1–2 hr	12 hr
Ciprofloxacin—PO-ER	rapid	1–4 hr	24 hr
Ciprofloxacin—IV	rapid	end of infusion	12 hr
Gemifloxacin—PO	rapid	0.5–2 hr	24 hr
Levofloxacin—PO	rapid	1–2 hr	24 hr
Levofloxacin—IV	rapid	end of infusion	24 hr
Moxifloxacin—PO	within 1 hr	1–3 hr	24 hr
Moxifloxacin—IV	rapid	end of infusion	24 hr
Ofloxacin—PO	rapid	1–2 hr	12 hr
Ofloxacin—IV	rapid	end of infusion	12 hr

Contraindications/Precautions

Contraindicated in: Hypersensitivity. Cross-sensitivity among agents within class may occur; History of myasthenia gravis (may worsen symptoms including muscle weakness and breathing problems); **Gemifloxacin and moxifloxacin**: Concurrent use of Class IA antiarrhythmics (disopyramide, quinidine, procainamide) or Class III antiarrhythmics (amiodarone, sotalol) (↑ risk of QTc interval prolongation and torsade de pointes); Known QT interval prolongation or concurrent use of agents causing prolongation; **Ciprofloxacin**: Concurrent use with tizanidine; OB: Do not use unless potential benefit outweighs potential fetal risk; Pedi: Use only for treatment of anthrax, plague, and complicated UTIs in children 1–17 yrs due to possible arthropathy.

Use Cautiously in: Known or suspected CNS disorder; Renal impairment (dose ↓ if CCr ≤50 mL/min for ciprofloxacin, levofloxacin, ofloxacin; <40 mL/min for gemifloxacin); Cirrhosis (levofloxacin, moxifloxacin); **Gemifloxacin and moxifloxacin**: Concurrent use of erythromycin, antipsychotics, and tricyclic antidepressants (↑ risk of QTc prolongation and torsades de pointes); **Gemifloxacin and moxifloxacin**: Bradycardia; **Gemifloxacin and moxifloxacin**: Acute myocardial ischemia; Concurrent use of corticosteroids (↑ risk of tendinitis/tendon rupture); Kidney, heart, or lung transplant patients (↑ risk of tendinitis/tendon rupture); Diabetes; Lactation: Safety not established except for treatment of anthrax; Geri: ↑ risk of adverse reactions.

Adverse Reactions/Side Effects

CNS: ELEVATED INTRACRANIAL PRESSURE (including pseudotumor cerebri), SEIZURES, dizziness, headache, insomnia, acute psychoses, agitation, confusion, depression, drowsiness, hallucinations, nightmares, paranoia, tremor. **CV:** *gemifloxacin, levofloxacin, moxifloxacin*—TORSADE DE POINTES, QT prolongation, vasodilation. **GI:** HEPATOTOXICITY (CIPROFLOXACIN), CLOSTRIDIUM DIFFICILE-ASSOCIATED DIARRHEA (CDAD), diarrhea, nausea, abdominal pain, ↑ liver enzymes (ciprofloxacin, moxifloxacin), vomiting. **GU:** vaginitis. **Derm:** photosensitivity, rash. **Endo:** hyperglycemia, hypoglycemia. **Local:** phlebitis at IV site. **MS:** tendinitis, tendon rupture. **Neuro:** peripheral neuropathy. **Misc:** hypersensitivity reactions including ANAPHYLAXIS, STEVENS-JOHNSON SYNDROME.

Interactions

Drug-Drug: Concurrent use of **amiodarone**, **disopyramide**, **erythromycin**, **procainamide**, **dofetilide**, **quinidine**, some **antipsychotics**, **sotalol**, or **tricyclic antidepressants** ↑ risk of torsade de pointes in susceptible individuals (avoid concurrent use). Ciprofloxacin ↑ serum **theophylline** levels and may lead to toxicity. Administration with **magnesium and aluminum-containing antacids**, **iron salts**, **bismuth subsalicylate**, **sucralfate**, **didanosine**, and **zinc salts** ↓ absorption of fluoroquinolones. May ↑ the effects of **warfarin**. Ciprofloxacin may ↓ levels and effectiveness of **phenytoin**. Levels of fluoroquinolones may be ↓ by **antineoplastics**. **Cimetidine** may interfere with elimination of fluoroquinolones. Beneficial effects of ciprofloxacin may be antagonized by **nitrofurantoin**. **Probenecid** ↓ renal elimination of fluoroquinolones. May ↑ risk of nephrotoxicity from **cyclosporine**. Concurrent use of ciprofloxacin with **foscarnet** may ↑ risk of seizures. Concurrent therapy with **corticosteroids** may ↑ the risk of tendon rupture. May ↑ risk of hypoglycemia when used with **antidiabetic agents**.

Drug-Natural Products: Fennel ↓ the absorption of ciprofloxacin.

Drug-Food: Absorption is impaired by **concurrent tube feeding** (because of metal cations). Absorption is ↓ if taken with **dairy products** or calcium-fortified juices.

Route/Dosage

Ciprofloxacin

PO (Adults): *Most infections*—500–750 mg q 12 hr. *Complicated urinary tract infections*—500 mg q 12 hr for 7–14 days (immediate-release); *or* 1000 mg q 24 hr for 7–14 days (extended-release). *Uncomplicated urinary tract infections*—250 mg every 12 hr for 3 days (immediate-release) *or* 500 mg every 24 hr for 3 days (extended-release). *Gonorrhea*—250-mg single dose. *Inhalational anthrax (postexposure) or cutaneous anthrax*—500 mg every 12 hr for 60 days; *Plague*—500–750 mg q 12 hr for 14 days.

PO (Children 1–17 yr): *Complicated urinary tract infections*—10–15 mg/kg q 12 hr (not to exceed 750 mg/dose) for 10–21 days. *Inhalational anthrax (postexposure) or cutaneous anthrax*—10–15 mg/kg q 12 hr (not to exceed 500 mg/dose) for 60 days; *Plague*—15 mg/kg q 8–12 hr (maximum: 500 mg/dose) for 10–21 days.

IV (Adults): *Most infections*—400 mg q 12 hr. *Complicated urinary tract infections*—400 mg q 12 hr for 7–14 days. *Uncomplicated urinary tract infections*—200 mg q 12 hr for 7–14 days. *Inhalational anthrax (post exposure)*—400 mg q 12 hr for 60 days; *Plague*—400 mg q 8–12 hr for 14 days.

IV (Children 1–17 yr): *Inhalational anthrax (post exposure)*—10 mg/kg q 12 hr (not to exceed 400 mg/dose) for 60 days; *Complicated urinary tract infections*—6–10 mg/kg q 8 hr (not to exceed 400 mg/dose) for 10–21 days; *Plague*—10 mg/kg q 8–12 hr (maximum: 400 mg/dose) for 10–21 days.

Renal Impairment

PO (Adults): *CCr 30–50 mL/min*—250–500 mg q 12 hr; *CCr 5–29 mL/min*—250–500 mg q 18 hr (immediate-release) *or* 500 mg q 24 hr (extended-release).

IV (Adults): *CCr 5–29 mL/min*—200–400 mg q 18–24 hr.

Gemifloxacin

PO (Adults): *Acute bacterial exacerbation of chronic bronchitis*—320 mg once daily for 5 days; *Community-acquired pneumonia (CAP) caused by* Klebsiella pneumoniae, Moraxella catarrhalis, *and multidrug resistant strains of* S. pneumonia—320 mg once daily for 7 days. *Community-acquired-pneumonia (CAP) caused by* S. pneumonia, Haemophilus influenzae, Mycoplasma pneumoniae, *or* Chlamydia pneumonia, *and multidrug resistant strains of* S. pneumonia—320 mg once daily for 5 days.

Renal Impairment

PO (Adults): *CCr ≤40 mL/min*—160 mg once daily for 5 days.

Levofloxacin

PO, IV (Adults): *Most infections*—250–750 mg q 24 hr; *inhalational anthrax (postexposure)*—500 mg once daily for 60 days.

PO, IV (Children >50 kg): *Inhalational anthrax (postexposure)*—500 mg daily for 60 days; *Plague*—500 mg daily for 10–14 days.

PO, IV (Children <50 kg and ≥6 mo): *Inhalational anthrax (postexposure)*–8 mg/kg (max: 250

mg/dose) every 12 hr for 60 days. *Plague*—8 mg/kg (max: 250 mg/dose) every 12 hr for 10–14 days; *Other infections*—10 mg/kg/dose every 24 hr (max: 500 mg/dose).

Renal Impairment

PO, IV (Adults): *Normal renal function dosing of 750 mg/day: CCr 20–49 mL/min*—750 mg q 48 hr; *CCr 10–19 mL/min*—750 mg initially, then 500 mg q 48 hr; *Normal renal function dosing of 500 mg/day: CCr 20–49 mL/min*—500 mg initially then 250 mg q 24 hr; *CCr 10–19 mL/min*—500 mg initially then 250 mg q 48 hr. *Normal renal function dosing of 250 mg/day: CCr 10–19 mL/min*—250 mg q 48 hr.

Moxifloxacin

PO, IV (Adults): *Bacterial sinusitis*—400 mg once daily for 10 days; *Community-acquired pneumonia*—400 mg once daily for 7–14 days. *Acute bacterial exacerbation of chronic bronchitis*—400 mg once daily for 5 days. *Complicated intra-abdominal infection*—400 mg once daily for 5–14 days. *Skin/skin structure infections*—400 mg/day for 7–21 days. *Treatment/prevention of plague*—400 mg once daily for 10–14 days.

Ofloxacin

PO (Adults): *Most infections*—400 mg q 12 hr. *Prostatitis*—300 mg q 12 hr for 6 wk. *Uncomplicated urinary tract infections*—200 mg q 12 hr for 3–7 days. *Complicated urinary tract infections*—200 mg q 12 hr for 10 days. *Gonorrhea*—400-mg single dose.

Renal Impairment

PO, IV (Adults): *CCr 20–50 mL/min*—100% of the usual dose q 24 hr; *CCr <20 mL/min*—50% of the usual dose q 24 hr.

Availability

Ciprofloxacin (generic available)

Tablets: 100 mg, 250 mg, 500 mg, 750 mg. **Cost:** *Generic*—100 mg $20.22/6, 250 mg $7.51/30, 500 mg $15.38/30, 750 mg $278.41/50. **Extended-release tablets:** 500 mg, 1000 mg. **Cost:** *Generic*—500 mg $489.94/50, 1000 mg $557.80/50. **Oral suspension (strawberry flavor):** 250 mg/5 mL, 500 mg/5 mL. **Cost:** *Generic*—250 mg/5 mL $123.24/100 mL, 500 mg/5 mL $144.28/100 mL. **Solution for injection:** 10 mg/mL. **Premixed infusion:** 200 mg/100 mL D5W, 400 mg/200 mL D5W. ***In combination with:*** hydrocortisone (Cipro HC) (see Appendix B).

Gemifloxacin (generic available)

Tablets: 320 mg. **Cost:** $239.20/5.

Levofloxacin (generic available)

Tablets: 250 mg, 500 mg, 750 mg. **Cost:** *Generic*—500 mg $13.77/50, 750 mg $24.22/20. **Oral solution:** 25 mg/mL. **Cost:** *Generic*—$579.42/480 mL. **Solution for injection:** 25 mg/mL. **Premixed infusion:** 250 mg/50 mL D5W, 500 mg/100 mL D5W, 750 mg/150 mL D5W.

Moxifloxacin (generic available)

Tablets: 400 mg. **Cost:** $769.58/30. **Premixed infusion:** 400 mg/250 mL 0.8% NaCl.

Ofloxacin (generic available)

Tablets: 200 mg, 300 mg, 400 mg. **Cost:** *Generic*—200 mg $239.20/50, 300 mg $284.66/50, 400 mg $600.36/100.

NURSING IMPLICATIONS

Assessment

- Assess for infection (vital signs; appearance of wound, sputum, urine, and stool; WBC; urinalysis; frequency and urgency of urination; cloudy or foul-smelling urine) prior to and during therapy.
- Obtain specimens for culture and sensitivity before initiating therapy. First dose may be given before receiving results.
- Observe for signs and symptoms of anaphylaxis (rash, pruritus, laryngeal edema, wheezing). Discontinue drug and notify health care professional immediately if these problems occur. Keep epinephrine, an antihistamine, and resuscitation equipment close by in case of an anaphylactic reaction. Patients taking gemifloxacin who are at greater risk for rash are those receiving gemifloxacin for >7 days, <40 yr of age, females, and postmenopausal females receiving hormone replacement therapy.
- Monitor bowel function. Diarrhea, abdominal cramping, fever, and bloody stools should be reported to health care professional promptly as a sign of Clostridium difficile-associated diarrhea (CDAD). May begin up to several weeks following cessation of therapy.
- Assess for rash periodically during therapy. May cause Stevens-Johnson syndrome. Discontinue therapy if severe or if accompanied with fever, general malaise, fatigue, muscle or joint aches, blisters, oral lesions, conjunctivitis, hepatitis and/or eosinophilia.
- Assess for signs and symptoms of peripheral neuropathy (pain, burning, tingling, numbness, and/or weakness or other alterations of sensation including light touch, pain, temperature, position sense, and vibratory sensation) periodically during therapy. Symptoms may be irreversible; discontinue fluoroquinolone if symptoms occur.
- ***Lab Test Considerations:*** May cause ↑ serum AST, ALT, LDH, bilirubin, and alkaline phosphatase.
- May also cause ↑ or ↓ serum glucose.
- Moxifloxacin may cause hyperglycemia, hyperlipidemia, and altered prothrombin time. It may also cause ↑ WBC; ↑ serum calcium, chloride, albumin,

and globulin; and ↓ hemoglobin, RBCs, neutrophils, eosinophils, and basophils.
- Monitor prothrombin time closely in patients receiving fluoroquinolones and warfarin; may enhance the anticoagulant effects of warfarin.

Potential Nursing Diagnoses

Risk for infection (Patient/Family Teaching)

Implementation

- Do not confuse levofloxacin with levetiracetam.
- **PO:** Administer *ofloxacin* on an empty stomach 1 hr before or 2 hr after meals, with a full glass of water. *Moxifloxacin, ciprofloxacin, levofloxacin,* and *gemifloxacin* may be administered without regard to meals. Should be taken at least 2 hr (3 hr for gemifloxacin, 4 hr for moxifloxacin) before or 2 hr (6 hr for *ciprofloxacin,* 8 hr for *moxifloxacin*) after antacids or other products containing calcium, iron, zinc, magnesium, or aluminum. Gemifloxacin should be taken at least 2 hr before sucralfate.
- If gastric irritation occurs, ciprofloxacin may be administered with meals.
- Ciprofloxacin 5% and 10% oral suspension should not be administered through a feeding tube (may ↓ absorption). Shake solution for 15 seconds prior to administration.
- *Gemifloxacin* and *ciprofloxacin extended-release tablets;* swallow whole; do not break, crush, or chew.

Ciprofloxacin

IV Administration

- **Intermittent Infusion:** ***Diluent:*** Dilute with 0.9% NaCl or D5W. Stable for 14 days at refrigerated or room temperature. ***Concentration:*** 1–2 mg/mL. ***Rate:*** Administer over 60 min into a large vein to minimize venous irritation.
- **Y-Site Compatibility:** alemtuzumab, amifostine, amiodarone, anakinra, anidulafungin, argatroban, aztreonam, bivalirudin, bleomycin, calcium gluconate, carboplatin, carmustine, caspofungin, ceftaroline, ceftazidime, cisatracurium, cisplatin, cyclophosphamide, cytarabine, dactinomycin, daptomycin, daunorubicin hydrochloride, dexmedetomidine, dexrazoxane, digoxin, diltiazem, diphenhydramine, dobutamine, docetaxel, dolasetron, dopamine, doxorubicin, doxorubicin liposome, epirubicin, eptifibatide, ertapenem, etoposide, etoposide phosphate, fenoldopam, fludarabine, gemcitabine, gentamicin, granisetron, hetastarch, hydromorphone, idarubicin, ifosfamide, irinotecan, leucovorin, lidocaine, linezolid, lorazepam, mechlorethamine, meperidine, mesna, methotrexate, metoclopramide, metronidazole, midazolam, milrinone, mitomycin, mitoxantrone, mycophentolate, naloxone, nesiritide, nicardipine, octreotide, ondansetron, oxaliplatin, oxytocin, paclitaxel, palonosetron, pamidronate, pancuronium, potassium acetate, potassium chloride, promethazine, quinupristin-dalfopristin, ranitidine, remifentanil, rocuronium, tacrolimus, telavancin, teniposide, thiotepa, tigecycline, tirofiban, tobramycin, topotecan, trastuzumab, vancomycin, vasopressin, vecuronium, verapamil, vinblastine, vincristine, vinorelbine, voriconazole, zoledronic acid.
- **Y-Site Incompatibility:** Manufacturer recommends temporarily discontinuing other solutions when administering ciprofloxacin, acyclovir, aminocaproic acid, aminophylline, amphotericin B lipid complex, amphotericin B liposome, ampicillin/sulbactam, cangrelor, cefepime, dexamethasone, fluorouracil, foscarnet, furosemide, heparin, hydrocortisone, magnesium sulfate, meropenem, methylprednisolone, pantoprazole, pemetrexed, phenytoin, piperacillin/tazobactam, potassium phosphates, propofol, rituxumab, sodium phosphates, warfarin.

Levofloxacin

IV Administration

- **Intermittent Infusion:** ***Diluent:*** Dilute with 0.9% NaCl, D5W, or dextrose/saline combinations. Also available in premixed bottles and flexible containers with D5W, which need no further dilution. ***Concentration:*** 5 mg/mL. Discard unused solution. Diluted solution is stable for 72 hr at room temperature and 14 days if refrigerated. ***Rate:*** Administer by infusion over at least 60 min for 250 mg or 500 mg doses and over 90 min for 750 mg dose. Avoid rapid bolus injection to prevent hypotension.
- **Y-Site Compatibility:** alemtuzumab, alfentanil, amifostine, amikacin, aminocaproic acid, aminophylline, ampicillin, ampicillin/sulbactam, anidulafungin, argatroban, aztreonam, bivalirudin, bleomycin, bumetanide, buprenorphine, busulfan, butorphanol, caffeine citrate, calcium gluconate, cangrelor, carboplatin, carmustine, caspofungin, cefepime, cefotetan, ceftaroline, ceftazidime, ceftriaxone, cefuroxime, chlorpromazine, cisatracurium, cisplatin, clindamycin, cyclophosphamide, cyclosporine, cytarabine, dacarbazine, dactomycin , daptomycin, dexamethasone, dexmedetomidine, dexrazoxane, digoxin, diltiazem, diphenhydramine, dobutamine, docetaxel, dolasetron, dopamine, doripenem, doxorubicin liposome, doxycycline, droperidol, enalaprilat, ephedrine, epinephrine, epirubicin, eptifibatide, ertapenem, erythromycin, esmolol, etoposide, etoposide phosphate, famotidine, fenoldopam, fentanyl, filgrastim, fluconazole, fludarabine, foscarnet, fosphenytoin, gemcitabine, gentamicin, granisetron, haloperidol, hydrocortisone, hydromorphone, idarubicin, ifosfamide, imipenem/cilastatin, irinotecan, isoproterenol, labetalol, leucovorin, levorphanol, lidocaine, linezolid, mannitol, mechlorethamine, meperidine, mesna, methylprednisolone, metoclopramide, metronidazole, midazo-

lam, milrinone, mitomycin, mitoxantrone, mycohpenolate, nalbuphine, naloxone, nesiritide, nicardipine, octreotide, ondansetron, oxacillin, oxaliplatin, oxytocin, paclitaxel, palonosetron, pamidronate, pancuronium, pemetrexed, penicillin G sodium, pentamidine, phenylephrine, potassium acetate, potassium chloride, promethazine, propranolol, quinapristin/dalfopristin, ranitidine, remifentanil, rocuronium, sargramostim, sodium bicarbonate, succinylcholine, sufentanil, tacrolimus, teniposide, theophylline, thiotepa, tigecycline, tirofiban, tobramycin, topotecan, trimethoprim/sulfamethoxazole, vancomycin, vasopressin, vecuronium, verapamil, vinblastine, vincristine, vinorelbine, voriconazole, zidovudine, zoledronic acid.

- **Y-Site Incompatibility:** acyclovir, alprostadil, amiodarone, amphotericin B colloidal, amphotericin B lipid complex, amphotericin B liposome, cefazolin, cefoxitin, daunorubicin hydrochloride, diazepam, fluorouracil, furosemide, ganciclovir, heparin, indomethacin, ketorolac, methotrexate, micafungin, nitroglycerin, nitroprusside, pantoprazole, pentobarbital, phenytoin, piperacillin/tazobactam, prochlorperazine, propofol, rituximab, streptozocin, telavancin, thiopental, trastuzumab.

Moxifloxacin

IV Administration

- **Intermittent Infusion:** ***Diluent:*** Premixed bags are diluted in sodium chloride 0.8% and should not be further diluted. Use transfer set whose piercing pin does not require excessive force; insert with a gentle twisting motion until pin is firmly seated. ***Concentration:*** 1.6 mg/mL. ***Rate:*** Administer over 60 min. Avoid rapid or bolus infusion.
- **Y-Site Compatibility:** alemtuzumab, amifostine, aminocaproic acid, anidulafungin, argatroban, atracurium, bivalirudin, bleomycin, bumetanide, busulfan, calcium acetate, caclium chloride, calcium gluconate, cangrelor, carboplatin, carmustine, caspofungin, ceftaroline, chlorpromazine, cisartacurium, cisplatin, cyclophosphamide, cyclosporine, cytarabine, dacarbacine, dactinomycin, daptomycin, daunorubicin hydrochloride, dexmedetonidine, dexrazoxane, digoxin, diltiazem, diphenhydramine, dobutamine, docetaxel, dolasetron, dopamine, doripenem, doxorubicin , doxorubicin liposome, droperidol, enalaprilat, epinephrine, epirubicin, ertapenem, esmolol, etoposide, etoposide phosphate, famotidine, fenoldopam, fludarabine, gemcitabine, glycopyrrolate, granisetron, haloperidol, heparin, hetastarch, hydralazine, hydrocortisone sodium succinate, idarubicin, ifosfamide, insulin, irinotecan, isoproterenol, ketorolac, labetolol, leucovorin, lidocaine, magnesium sulfate, mannitol, mechlorethamine, melphalan, mesna, methotrexate, methyldopate, methylprednisolone, metoclopramide, metoprolol, milrinone, mitomycin, mitoxantrone, mycophenolate, naloxone, nesiritide, nicardipine, nitroglycerin, norepinephrine, octreotide, ondansetron, oxaliplatin, oxytocin, paclitaxel, palonosetron, pamidronate, pancuronium, pemetrexed, phenylephrine, potassium acetate, potassium chloride, potassium phosphates, procainamide, prochlorperazine, promethazine, propranolol, ranitidine, rocuronium, sodium acetate, sodium bicarbonate, sodium phosphates, streptozocin, succinylcholine, tacrolimus, teniposide, theophylline, thiotepa, tigecycline, tirofiban, topotecan, vasopressin, vecuronium, verapamil, vinblastine, vincristine, vinorelbine, zoledronic acid.
- **Y-Site Incompatibility:** allopurinol, aminophylline, amphotericin B lipid complex, dantrolene, fluorouracil, fosphenytoin, furosemide, nitroprusside, pantoprazole, phenytoin, vancomycin, voriconazole.

Patient/Family Teaching

- Instruct patient to take medication as directed at evenly spaced times and to finish drug completely, even if feeling better. Take missed doses as soon as possible, unless almost time for next dose. Do not double doses. Advise patient that sharing of this medication may be dangerous.
- Advise patients to notify health care professional immediately if they are taking theophylline.
- Encourage patient to maintain a fluid intake of at least 1500–2000 mL/day to prevent crystalluria.
- Advise patient that antacids or medications containing iron or zinc will decrease absorption. *Ciprofloxacin, levofloxacin,* and *ofloxacin* should be taken at least 2 hr before (3 hr for *gemifloxacin*, 4 hr for *moxifloxacin*) or 2 hr after (6 hrs for *ciprofloxacin*, 8 hr for *moxifloxacin*) these products.
- May cause dizziness and drowsiness. Caution patient to avoid driving or other activities requiring alertness until response to medication is known.
- Advise patient to notify health care professional of any personal or family history of QTc prolongation or proarrhythmic conditions such as recent hypokalemia, significant bradycardia, or recent myocardial ischemia or if fainting spells or palpitations occur. Patients with this history should not receive gemifloxacin.
- Advise patient to stop taking fluoroquinolone and notify health care professional immediately if signs and symptoms of peripheral neuropathy occur.
- Caution patient to use sunscreen and protective clothing to prevent phototoxicity reactions during and for 5 days after therapy. Notify health care professional if a sunburn-like reaction or skin eruption occurs.
- Instruct patients being treated for gonorrhea that partners also must be treated.

- Advise patient to notify health care professional of all Rx or OTC medications, vitamins, or herbal products being taken and to consult with health care professional before taking other medications.
- Advise patient to report signs of superinfection (furry overgrowth on the tongue, vaginal itching or discharge, loose or foul-smelling stools).
- Instruct patient to notify health care professional if fever and diarrhea develop, especially if stool contains blood, pus, or mucus. Advise patient not to treat diarrhea without consulting health care professional.
- Instruct patient to notify health care professional immediately if rash, jaundice, signs of hypersensitivity, or tendon (shoulder, hand, Achilles, and other) pain, swelling, or inflammation occur. If tendon symptoms occur, avoid exercise and use of the affected area. Increased risk in >65 yrs old; kidney, heart and lung transplant recipients; and patients taking corticosteroids concurrently. Therapy should be discontinued.

Evaluation/Desired Outcomes

- Resolution of the signs and symptoms of infection. Time for complete resolution depends on organism and site of infection.
- Post exposure treatment of inhalational anthrax or cutaneous anthrax (ciprofloxacin and levofloxacin).
- Prevention and treatment of plague (ciprofloxacin, levofloxacin, and moxifloxacin).

HIGH ALERT

fluorouracil

(flure-oh-**yoor**-a-sill)

Carac, Efudex, Fluoroplex, 5-FU

Classification

Therapeutic: antineoplastics

Pharmacologic: antimetabolites

Pregnancy Category D

Indications

IV: Used alone and in combination with other modalities (surgery, radiation therapy, other antineoplastics) in the treatment of: Colon cancer, Breast cancer, Rectal cancer, Gastric cancer, Pancreatic carcinoma. **Topical:** Management of multiple actinic (solar) keratoses and superficial basal cell carcinomas.

Action

Inhibits DNA and RNA synthesis by preventing thymidine production (cell-cycle S-phase–specific). **Therapeutic Effects:** Death of rapidly replicating cells, particularly malignant ones.

Pharmacokinetics

Absorption: Minimal absorption (5–10%) after topical application.

Distribution: Widely distributed; concentrates and persists in tumors.

Metabolism and Excretion: Metabolized by dihydropyrimidine dehydrogenase to a less toxic compound; inactive metabolites are excreted primarily in urine.

Half-life: 20 hr.

TIME/ACTION PROFILE (IV = effects on blood counts, Top = dermatologic effects)

ROUTE	ONSET	PEAK	DURATION
IV	1–9 days	9–21 days (nadir)	30 days
Top	2–3 days	2–6 wk	1–2 mo

Contraindications/Precautions

Contraindicated in: Hypersensitivity; Dihydropyrimidine dehydrogenase deficiency (patients at ↑ risk of 5-FU toxicity); OB, Lactation: Pregnancy or lactation.

Use Cautiously in: Infections; Depressed bone marrow reserve; Other chronic debilitating illnesses; Obese patients, patients with edema or ascites (dose should be based on ideal body weight).

Adverse Reactions/Side Effects

More likely to occur with systemic use than with topical use.

CNS: acute cerebellar dysfunction. **GI:** diarrhea, nausea, stomatitis, vomiting. **Derm:** alopecia, maculopapular rash, local inflammatory reactions (topical only), melanosis of nails, nail loss, palmar-plantar erythrodysesthesia, phototoxicity. **Endo:** sterility. **Hemat:** anemia, leukopenia, thrombocytopenia. **Local:** thrombophlebitis. **Misc:** fever.

Interactions

Drug-Drug: Combination chemotherapy with **irinotecan** may produce unacceptable toxicity (dehydration, neutropenia, sepsis). Additive bone marrow depression with other **bone marrow depressants**, including other **antineoplastics** and **radiation therapy**. May ↓ antibody response to **live-virus vaccines** and ↑ risk of adverse reactions.

Route/Dosage

Doses may vary greatly, depending on tumor, patient condition, and protocol used.

Advanced Colorectal Cancer

IV (Adults): 370 mg/m² preceded by leucovorin *or* 425 mg/m² preceded by leucovorin daily for 5 days. May be repeated q 4–5 wk.

Other Tumors

IV (Adults): *Initial dose*— 12 mg/kg/day for 4 days, then 1 day of rest, then 6 mg/kg every other day for 4–5 doses *or* 7–12 mg/kg/day for 4 days followed by 3-day rest, then 7–10 mg/kg q 3–4 days for 3 doses. *Maintenance*— 7–12 mg/kg q 7–10 days *or* 300–500 mg/m²/day for 4–5 days, repeated monthly (no single daily dose should exceed 800 mg). **Poor-Risk Patients:** 3–6 mg/kg/day on days 1–3, 3 mg/kg/day on days 5, 7, 9 (not to exceed 400 mg/dose). Doses of 370–425 mg/m²/day for 5 days have been used in combination with leucovorin.

Actinic (Solar) Keratoses

Topical (Adults): *Carac*—Apply 0.5% cream to lesions once daily for up to 4 wk; *Efudex*—Apply 2% or 5% solution or cream to lesions twice daily for 2–4 wk; *Fluoroplex*—Apply 1% cream to lesions twice daily for 2–6 wk.

Superficial Basal Cell Carcinomas

Topical (Adults): *Efudex*—Apply 5% solution or cream to lesions twice daily for 3–6 wk (up to 12 wk).

Availability (generic available)

Injection: 50 mg/mL. **Cream:** 0.5%, 1%, 5%. **Solution:** 2%, 5%.

NURSING IMPLICATIONS

Assessment

- Monitor vital signs before and frequently during therapy.
- Assess mucous membranes, number and consistency of stools, and frequency of vomiting. Assess for signs of infection (fever, chills, sore throat, cough, hoarseness, pain in lower back or side, difficult or painful urination). Assess for bleeding (bleeding gums; bruising; petechiae; and guaiac test stools, urine, and emesis). Avoid IM injections and taking rectal temperatures. Apply pressure to venipuncture sites for 10 min. Notify health care professional if symptoms of toxicity (stomatitis or esophagopharyngitis, uncontrollable vomiting, diarrhea, GI bleeding, myocardial ischemia, leukocyte count <3500/mm³, platelet count <100,000/mm³, or hemorrhage from any site) occur; drug will need to be discontinued. May be reinitiated at a lower dose when side effects have subsided.
- Assess IV site frequently for inflammation or infiltration. Patient should notify nurse if pain or irritation at injection site occurs. May cause thrombophlebitis. If extravasation occurs, infusion must be stopped and restarted in another vein to avoid damage to subcut tissue. Report immediately. Standard treatment includes application of ice compresses.
- Assess skin for palmar-plantar erythrodysesthesia (tingling of hands and feet followed by pain, erythema, and swelling) throughout therapy.
- Monitor intake and output, appetite, and nutritional intake. GI effects usually occur on 4th day of therapy. Adjusting diet as tolerated may help maintain fluid and electrolyte balance and nutritional status.
- Monitor patient for cerebellar dysfunction (weakness, ataxia, dizziness). This may persist after discontinuation of therapy.
- **Topical:** Inspect involved skin before and throughout therapy.
- ***Lab Test Considerations:*** May cause ↓ in plasma albumin.
- Monitor hepatic (AST, ALT, LDH, and serum bilirubin), renal, and hematologic (hematocrit, hemoglobin, leukocyte, platelet count) functions before and periodically during therapy. Monitor CBC daily during IV therapy. Report WBC of <3500/mm³ or platelets <100,000/mm³ immediately; they are criteria for discontinuation. Nadir of leukopenia usually occurs in 9–14 days, with recovery by day 30. May also cause thrombocytopenia.
- May cause ↑ in urine excretion of 5-hydroxyindoleacetic acid (5-HIAA).

Potential Nursing Diagnoses

Risk for infection (Side Effects)
Imbalanced nutrition: less than body requirements (Side Effects)

Implementation

- ***High Alert:*** Fatalities have occurred with incorrect administration of chemotherapeutic agents. Before administering, clarify all ambiguous orders; double-check single, daily, and course-of-therapy dose limits; have second practitioner independently double-check original order, calculations, and infusion pump settings. The number 5 in 5-fluorouracil is part of the drug name and does not refer to the dose.
- Prepare solution in a biologic cabinet. Wear gloves, gown, and mask while handling IV medication. Discard IV equipment in specially designated containers.

IV Administration

- **IV Push:** ***Diluent:*** May be administered undiluted. ***Concentration:*** 50 mg/mL. ***Rate:*** Rapid IV push administration (over 1–2 min) is most effective, but there is a more rapid onset of toxicity.
- **Intermittent Infusion:** ***Diluent:*** May be diluted with D5W or 0.9% NaCl.
- Use plastic IV tubing and IV bags to maintain greater stability of medication. Solution is stable for 24 hr at room temperature; do not refrigerate. Solution is colorless to faint yellow. Discard highly discolored or cloudy solution. If crystals form, dissolve by warming solution to 140°F, shaking vigorously, and cooling to body temperature. ***Concentration:*** Up to 50 mg/mL. ***Rate:*** Onset of toxicity is greatly delayed by administering an infusion over 2–8 hr.
- **Y-Site Compatibility:** acyclovir, alfentanil, allopurinol, amifostine, amikacin, aminophylline, amphotericin B lipid complex, amphotericin B liposome, ampicillin, ampicillin/sulbactam, anidulafungin, argatroban, azithromycin, aztreonam, bivalirudin, bleomycin, bumetanide, butorphanol, calcium glu-

conate, carboplatin, carmustine, cefazolin, cefepime, cefotaxime, cefotetan, cefoxitin, ceftazidime, ceftriaxone, cefuroxime, cisatracurium, cisplatin, clindamycin, cyclophosphamide, cyclosporine, daptomycin, dexamethasone, dexmedetomidine, dexrazoxane, digoxin, docetaxel, dopamine, doripenem, doxorubicin liposome, enalaprilat, ephedrine, ertapenem, erythromycin, esmolol, etoposide phosphate, famotidine, fenoldopam, fentanyl, fluconazole, fludarabine, foscarnet, fosphenytoin, furosemide, ganciclovir, gemcitabine, gentamicin, granisetron, heparin, hetastarch, hydrocortisone, hydromorphone, ifosfamide, imipenem/cilastatin, isoproterenol, ketorolac, labetalol, leucovorin, levorphanol, lidocaine, linezolid, magnesium sulfate, mannitol, melphalan, meperidine, meropenem, mesna, methohexital, methotrexate, methylprednisolone, metoprolol, metronidazole, milrinone, mitomycin, mitoxantrone, morphine, nalbuphine, naloxone, nesiritide, nitroglycerin, nitroprusside, octreotide, paclitaxel, palonosetron, pamidronate, pancuronium, pantoprazole, pemetrexed, pentobarbital, phenobarbital, phenylephrine, piperacillin/tazobactam, potassium acetate, potassium chloride, potassium phosphates, procainamide, propofol, propranolol, ranitidine, remifentanil, rituximab, sargramostim, sodium acetate, sodium bicarbonate, sodium phosphates, succinylcholine, sufentanil, teniposide, theophylline, thiopental, thiotepa, tigecycline, tirofiban, tobramycin, trastuzumab, vasopressin, vecuronium, vinblastine, vincristine, vitamin B complex with C, voriconazole, zidovudine, zoledronic acid.

- **Y-Site Incompatibility:** aldesleukin, amiodarone, amphotericin B cholesteryl, amphotericin B colloidal, buprenorphine, calcium chloride, caspofungin, chlorpromazine, ciprofloxacin, diazepam, diltiazem, diphenhydramine, dobutamine, doxycycline, droperidol, epinephrine, epirubicin, filgrastim, haloperidol, hydroxyzine, idarubicin, irinotecan, levofloxacin, lorazepam, midazolam, nicardipine, pentamidine, phenytoin, prochlorperazine, promethazine, quinapristin/dalfopristin, topotecan, vancomycin, verapamil, vinorelbine.
- **Topical:** Consult health care professional before administering topical preparations to determine which skin preparation regimen should be followed. Tight occlusive dressings are not advised because of irritation to surrounding healthy tissue. A loose gauze dressing for cosmetic purposes is usually preferred. Wear gloves when applying medication. Do not use metallic applicator.

Patient/Family Teaching

- Instruct patient to notify health care professional if fever; chills; sore throat; signs of infection; yellowing of skin or eyes; abdominal pain; joint or flank pain; swelling of feet or legs; bleeding gums; bruising; petechiae; or blood in urine, stool, or emesis occurs. Caution patient to avoid crowds and persons with known infections. Instruct patient to use soft toothbrush and electric razor. Patients should be cautioned not to drink alcoholic beverages or take products containing aspirin or NSAIDs.
- Advise patient to rinse mouth with clear water after eating and drinking and to avoid flossing to minimize stomatitis. Viscous lidocaine may be used if mouth pain interferes with eating. Stomatitis pain may require treatment with opioid analgesics.
- Discuss with patient the possibility of hair loss. Explore methods of coping.
- Review with patient the need for contraception during therapy.
- Caution patient to use sunscreen and protective clothing to prevent phototoxicity reactions.
- Instruct patient not to receive any vaccinations without advice of health care professional.
- Emphasize the importance of routine follow-up lab tests to monitor progress and to check for side effects.
- **Topical:** Instruct patient in correct application of solution or cream. Emphasize importance of avoiding the eyes; caution should also be used when applying medication near mouth and nose. If patient uses clean finger to self-administer, emphasize importance of washing hands thoroughly after application. Explain that erythema, scaling, and blistering with pruritus and burning sensation are expected. Advise patient to avoid sunlight or ultraviolet light (tanning booths) as much as possible; may increase side effects. Therapy is discontinued when erosion, ulceration, and necrosis occur in 2–6 wk (10–12 wk for basal cell carcinomas). Skin heals 4–8 wk later.

Evaluation/Desired Outcomes

- Tumor regression.
- Removal of solar keratoses or superficial basal cell skin cancers.

FLUoxetine (floo-**ox**-uh-teen)

PROzac, PROzac Weekly, Sarafem, Selfemra

Classification

Therapeutic: antidepressants

Pharmacologic: selective serotonin reuptake inhibitors (SSRIs)

Pregnancy Category C

Indications

Major depressive disorder. Obsessive compulsive disorder (OCD). Bulimia nervosa. Panic disorder. Acute treatment of depressive episodes associated with bipolar I disorder (when used with olanzapine). Treatment-resistant depression (when used with olanzapine). **Sarafem and Selfemra:** Premenstrual dysphoric disorder

(PMDD). **Unlabeled Use:** Anorexia nervosa: ADHD, Diabetic neuropathy, Fibromyalgia, Obesity, Raynaud's phenomenon, Social anxiety disorder (social phobia), Posttraumatic stress disorder (PTSD).

Action

Selectively inhibits the reuptake of serotonin in the CNS. **Therapeutic Effects:** Antidepressant action. Decreased behaviors associated with: panic disorder, bulimia. Decreased mood alterations associated with PMDD.

Pharmacokinetics

Absorption: Well absorbed after oral administration.
Distribution: Crosses the blood-brain barrier.
Protein Binding: 94.5%.
Metabolism and Excretion: Converted by the liver to norfluoxetine (primarily by CYP2D6 isoenzyme), another antidepressant compound; ⧚ the CYP2D6 enzyme system exhibits genetic polymorphism (~7% of population may be poor metabolizers and may have significantly ↑ fluoxetine concentrations and an ↑ risk of adverse effects). Fluoxetine and norfluoxetine are mostly metabolized by the liver; 12% excreted by kidneys as unchanged fluoxetine, 7% as unchanged norfluoxetine.
Half-life: 1–3 days (norfluoxetine 5–7 days).

TIME/ACTION PROFILE (antidepressant effect)

ROUTE	ONSET	PEAK	DURATION
PO	1–4 wk	unknown	2 wk

Contraindications/Precautions

Contraindicated in: Hypersensitivity; Concurrent use of MAO inhibitors or MAO-like drugs (linezolid or methylene blue); Concurrent use of pimozide; Concurrent use of thioridazine (fluoxetine should be discontinued at least 5 wk before thioridazine therapy is initiated).
Use Cautiously in: History of seizures; Debilitated patients (↑ risk of seizures); Diabetes mellitus; Patients with concurrent chronic illness or multiple drug therapy (dose adjustments may be necessary); Hepatic impairment (↓ doses/↑ dosing interval may be necessary); May ↑ risk of suicide attempt/ideation especially during early treatment or dose adjustment; Congenital long QT syndrome, history of QT interval prolongation, family history of long QT syndrome or sudden cardiac death, concurrent use of QT interval prolonging drugs, hypokalemia, hypomagnesemia, recent MI, uncompensated HF, or bradycardia; Angle-closure glaucoma; OB: Use during first trimester may ↑ risk of cardiovascular malformations in infant. Use during third trimester may result in neonatal serotonin syndrome requiring prolonged hospitalization, respiratory and nutritional support. May cause sedation in infant. Use only if potential benefit justifies potential risk to fetus; Lactation: May cause sedation in infant; discontinue drug or bottle-feed; Pedi: Risk of suicide ideation or attempt may be greater in children or adolescents (safe use in children <7 yr not established); Geri: Appears on Beers list. Geriatric patients are at ↑ risk for excessive CNS stimulation, sleep disturbances, and agitation.

Adverse Reactions/Side Effects

CNS: NEUROLEPTIC MALIGNANT SYNDROME, SEIZURES, SUICIDAL THOUGHTS, anxiety, drowsiness, headache, insomnia, nervousness, abnormal dreams, dizziness, fatigue, hypomania, mania, weakness. **EENT:** mydriasis, stuffy nose, visual disturbances. **Resp:** cough. **CV:** TORSADES DE POINTES, chest pain, palpitations, QT interval prolongation. **GI:** diarrhea, abdominal pain, abnormal taste, anorexia, constipation, dry mouth, dyspepsia, nausea, vomiting, weight loss. **GU:** sexual dysfunction, urinary frequency. **Derm:** ↑ sweating, pruritus, erythema nodusum, flushing, rashes. **Endo:** dysmenorrhea. **F and E:** hyponatremia. **MS:** arthralgia, back pain, myalgia. **Neuro:** tremor. **Misc:** SEROTONIN SYNDROME, allergic reactions, fever, flu-like syndrome, hot flashes, sensitivity reaction.

Interactions

Drug-Drug: Discontinue use of **MAO inhibitors** for 14 days before fluoxetine therapy; combined therapy may result in confusion, agitation, seizures, hypertension, and hyperpyrexia (serotonin syndrome). Fluoxetine should be discontinued for at least 5 wk before MAO inhibitor therapy is initiated. Concurrent use with **MAO-inhibitor-like drugs**, such as **linezolid** or **methylene blue** may ↑ risk of serotonin syndrome; concurrent use contraindicated; do not start therapy in patients receiving **linezolid** or **methylene blue**; if **linezolid** or **methylene blue** need to be started in a patient receiving fluoxetine, immediately discontinue fluoxetine and monitor for signs/symptoms of serotonin syndrome for 2 wk or until 24 hr after last dose of linezolid or methylene blue, whichever comes first (may resume fluoxetine therapy 24 hr after last dose of linezolid or methylene blue). Concurrent use with **pimozide** may ↑ risk of QT interval prolongation. ↑ levels of **thioridazine** may ↑ risk of QT interval prolongation (concurrent use contraindicated; fluoxetine should be discontinued for at least 5 wk before thioridazine is initiated). **QT interval prolonging drugs** may ↑ the risk of QT interval prolongation with arrhythmias; avoid concurrent use. Inhibits the activity of cytochrome P450 2D6 enzyme in the liver and ↑ effects of drugs metabolized by this enzyme system. **Medications that inhibit the P450 enzyme system** (including **ritonavir**, **saquinavir**, and **efavirenz**) may ↑ risk of developing the serotonin syndrome). For concurrent use with **ritonavir** ↓ fluoxetine dose by 70%; if initiating fluoxetine, start with 10 mg/day dose. ↓ metabolism and ↑ effects of **alprazolam** (decrease alprazolam dose by 50%). Drugs that affect serotonergic neurotransmitter systems, including **tricyclic antidepressants, SNRIs, fentanyl, buspirone, tramadol**, and **triptans** ↑ risk of serotonin syndrome. ↑ CNS depression with **alcohol, antihistamines**, other **antidepressants, opioid analgesics**, or **sedative/hypnotics**. ↑ risk of side effects and adverse reactions with other **antidepressants, risperidone**, or **phenothiazines**. May ↑ effectiveness/risk of toxicity from **carbamazepine, clozapine, digoxin, haloperidol, phenytoin, lithium**, or **warfarin**. May ↓ the effects of **buspirone**. **Cyproheptadine** may ↓ or reverse effects of fluoxetine. May ↑ sensitivity to **adrenergics** and increase the risk of serotonin syndrome. May alter the activity of other **drugs that are highly bound to plasma proteins**. ↑ risk of serotonin syndrome with **$5HT_1$ agonists**. ↑ risk of bleeding with **NSAIDS, aspirin, clopidogrel**, or **warfarin**.

Drug-Natural Products: ↑ risk of serotonin syndrome with **St. John's wort** and **SAMe**.

Route/Dosage

PO (Adults): *Depression, OCD*—20 mg/day in the morning. After several weeks, may ↑ by 20 mg/day at weekly intervals. Doses greater than 20 mg/day should be given in 2 divided doses, in the morning and at noon (not to exceed 80 mg/day). Patients who have been stabilized on the 20 mg/day dose may be switched over to delayed-release capsules (Prozac Weekly) at dose of 90 mg weekly, initiated 7 days after the last 20-mg dose. *Panic disorder*—10 mg/day initially, may ↑ after 1 week to 20 mg/day (usual dose is 20 mg, but may be ↑ as needed/tolerated up to 60 mg/day). *Bulimia nervosa*—60 mg/day (may need to titrate up to dosage over several days). *PMDD*—20 mg/day (not to exceed 80 mg/day) *or* 20 mg/day starting 14 days prior to expected onset on menses, continued through first full day of menstruation, repeated with each cycle. *Depressive episodes associated with bipolar I disorder*—20 mg/day with olanzapine 5 mg/day (both given in evening); may ↑ fluoxetine dose up to 50 mg/day and olanzapine dose up to 12.5 mg/day; *Treatment-resistant depression*—20 mg/day with olanzapine 5 mg/day (both given in evening); may ↑ fluoxetine dose up to 50 mg/day and olanzapine dose up to 20 mg/day.

PO (Geriatric Patients): *Depression*—10 mg/day in the morning initially, may be ↑ (not to exceed 60 mg/day).

PO (Children 7–17 yr): *Depression and OCD (adolescents and higher weight children)*—10 mg/day may be ↑ after 2 wk to 20 mg/day; additional increases may be made after several more weeks (range 20–60 mg/day); *Depression and OCD (lower-weight children)*—10 mg/day initially, may be ↑ after several more weeks (range 20–30 mg/day).

PO (Children 10–17 yr): *Depressive episodes associated with bipolar I disorder*—20 mg/day with olanzapine 2.5 mg/day (both given in evening); may ↑ fluoxetine dose up to 50 mg/day and olanzapine dose up to 12 mg/day.

Availability (generic available)

Tablets: 10 mg, 15 mg, 20 mg. **Cost:** *Generic*—20 mg $73.03/100. **Capsules:** 10 mg, 20 mg, 40 mg. **Cost:** *Generic*—10 mg $10.83/100, 20 mg $8.62/100, 40 mg $41.03/100. **Delayed-release capsules (Prozac Weekly):** 90 mg. **Cost:** *Generic*—$147.96/4. **Oral solution (mint flavor):** 20 mg/5 mL. **Cost:** *Generic*—$118.00/120 mL. ***In combination with:*** olanzapine (Symbyax; see Appendix B).

NURSING IMPLICATIONS

Assessment

- Monitor mood changes. Inform health care professional if patient demonstrates significant increase in anxiety, nervousness, or insomnia.
- Assess for suicidal tendencies, especially during early therapy. Restrict amount of drug available to patient. Risk may be increased in children, adolescents, and adults ≤24 yr. After starting therapy, children, adolescents, and young adults should be seen by health care professional at least weekly for 4 wk, every 3 wk for next 4 wk, and on advice of health care professional thereafter.
- Monitor appetite and nutritional intake. Weigh weekly. Notify health care professional of continued weight loss. Adjust diet as tolerated to support nutritional status.
- Assess for sensitivity reaction (urticaria, fever, arthralgia, edema, carpal tunnel syndrome, rash, hives, lymphadenopathy, respiratory distress) and notify health care professional if present; symptoms usually resolve by stopping fluoxetine but may require administration of antihistamines or corticosteroids.
- Assess for sexual side effects (erectile dysfunction; decreased libido).
- Monitor for development of neuroleptic malignant syndrome (fever, respiratory distress, tachycardia, seizures, diaphoresis, arrhythmias, hypertension or hypotension, pallor, tiredness, severe muscle stiffness, loss of bladder control). Report immediately.
- Assess for serotonin syndrome (mental changes [agitation, hallucinations, coma], autonomic instability [tachycardia, labile BP, hyperthermia], neuromuscular aberrations [hyperreflexia, incoordination], and/or GI symptoms [nausea, vomiting, diarrhea]), especially in patients taking other serotonergic drugs (SSRIs, SNRIs, triptans).
- **OCD:** Assess for frequency of obsessive-compulsive behaviors. Note degree to which these thoughts and behaviors interfere with daily functioning.
- **Bulimia Nervosa:** Assess frequency of binge eating and vomiting during therapy.
- **PMDD:** Monitor mood prior to and periodically during therapy.

- ***Lab Test Considerations:*** Monitor CBC and differential periodically during therapy. Notify health care professional if leukopenia, anemia, thrombocytopenia, or increased bleeding time occurs.
- Proteinuria and mild ↑ in AST may occur during sensitivity reactions.
- May cause ↑ in serum alkaline phosphatase, ALT, BUN, creatine phosphokinase, hypouricemia, hypocalcemia, hypoglycemia or hyperglycemia, and hyponatremia.
- May cause hypoglycemia in patient with diabetes.

Potential Nursing Diagnoses

Ineffective coping (Indications)
Risk for injury (Side Effects)
Sexual dysfunction (Side Effects)

Implementation

- Do not confuse fluoxetine with duloxetine, paroxetine, or Loxitane (loxapine). Do not confuse Prozac with Prilosec (omeprazole), Prograf (tacrolimus), or Provera (medroxyprogesterone). Do not confuse Sarafem (fluoxetine) with Serophene (clomiphene).
- **PO:** Administer as a single dose in the morning. Some patients may require increased amounts, in divided doses, with a 2nd dose at noon.
- May be administered with food to minimize GI irritation. Do not open, dissolve, chew, or crush delayed-release capsules.

Patient/Family Teaching

- Instruct patient to take fluoxetine as directed. Take missed doses as soon as remembered unless almost time for next dose, then omit and return to regular schedule. Do not double doses or discontinue without consulting health care professional; discontinuation may cause anxiety, insomnia, nervousness.
- May cause drowsiness, dizziness, impaired judgment, and blurred vision. Caution patient to avoid driving and other activities requiring alertness until response to the drug is known.
- Advise patient, family, and caregivers to look for suicidality, especially during early therapy or dose changes. Notify health care professional immediately if thoughts about suicide or dying, attempts to commit suicide, new or worse depression or anxiety, agitation or restlessness, panic attacks, insomnia, new or worse irritability, aggressiveness, acting on dangerous impulses, mania, or other changes in mood or behavior or if symptoms of serotonin syndrome occur.
- Instruct patient to notify health care professional of all Rx or OTC medications, vitamins, or herbal products being taken and consult health care professional before taking any new medications. Advise patient to avoid taking other CNS depressants or alcohol.
- Caution patient to change positions slowly to minimize dizziness.
- Inform patient that frequent mouth rinses, good oral hygiene, and sugarless gum or candy may minimize dry mouth. If dry mouth persists for more than 2 wk, consult health care professional regarding use of saliva substitute.
- Caution patient to wear protective clothing and use sunscreen to prevent photosensitivity reactions.
- Inform patient that medication may cause decreased libido.
- Advise patient to notify health care professional if symptoms of sensitivity reaction occur or if headache, nausea, anorexia, anxiety, or insomnia persists.
- Instruct female patients to inform health care professional if pregnancy is planned or suspected, or if breast feeding.
- Emphasize the importance of follow-up exams to monitor progress.

Evaluation/Desired Outcomes

- Increased sense of well-being.
- Renewed interest in surroundings. May require 1–4 wk of therapy to obtain antidepressant effects.
- Decrease in obsessive-compulsive behaviors.
- Decrease in binge eating and vomiting in patients with bulimia nervosa.
- Decreased incidence frequency of panic attacks.
- Decreased mood alterations associated with PMDD.

flurandrenolide, See CORTICOSTEROIDS (TOPICAL/LOCAL).

fluticasone, See CORTICOSTEROIDS (INHALATION), CORTICOSTEROIDS (NASAL), and CORTICOSTEROIDS (TOPICAL/LOCAL).

fluvastatin, See HMG-CoA REDUCTASE INHIBITORS (statins).

fluvoxaMINE

(floo-**voks**-a-meen)

Luvox, Luvox CR

Classification

Therapeutic: antidepressants, antiobsessive agents

Pharmacologic: selective serotonin reuptake inhibitors (SSRIs)

Pregnancy Category C

Indications

Obsessive-compulsive disorder (OCD). **Unlabeled Use:** Depression. Generalized anxiety disorder (GAD). Social anxiety disorder (SAD). Post-traumatic stress disorder (PTSD).

Action

Inhibits the reuptake of serotonin in the CNS. **Therapeutic Effects:** Decrease in obsessive-compulsive behaviors.

Pharmacokinetics

Absorption: 53% absorbed after oral administration.

Distribution: Excreted in breast milk; enters the CNS. Remainder of distribution not known.

Metabolism and Excretion: Mostly metabolized by the liver (CYP2D6 isoenzyme); the CYP2D6 enzyme system exhibits genetic polymorphism; ~7% of population may be poor metabolizers (PMs) and may have significantly ↑ fluvoxamine concentrations and an ↑ risk of adverse effects.

Half-life: 13.6–15.6 hr.

TIME/ACTION PROFILE (improvement on obsessive-compulsive behaviors)

ROUTE	ONSET	PEAK	DURATION
PO	within 2–3 wk	several mo	unknown

Contraindications/Precautions

Contraindicated in: Hypersensitivity to fluvoxamine or other SSRIs; Concurrent use of MAOIs (or within 14 days of discontinuing fluvoxamine), MAOI-like drugs (linezolid or methylene blue), alosetron, pimozide, thioridazine, or tizanidine.

Use Cautiously in: Impaired hepatic function; Risk of suicide (may ↑ risk of suicide attempt/ideation especially during early treatment or dose adjustment); Angle-closure glaucoma; OB: Neonates exposed to SSRI in third trimester may develop drug discontinuation syndrome including respiratory distress, feeding difficulty, and irritability; Lactation: Discontinue drug or bottle-feed; Pedi: May ↑ risk of suicide attempt/ideation especially during early treatment or dose adjustment; may be greater in children and adolescents (safety not established in children <18 yr [controlled-release] and <8 yr [immediate-release]); Pedi: Safety not established in children <8 yr (for immediate-release); Geri: May have ↑ sensitivity; recommend lower initial dose and slower dosage titration.

Adverse Reactions/Side Effects

CNS: NEUROLEPTIC MALIGNANT SYNDROME, SUICIDAL THOUGHTS, sedation, dizziness, drowsiness, headache, insomnia, nervousness, weakness, agitation, anxiety, apathy, emotional lability, manic reactions, mental depression, psychotic reactions, syncope. **EENT:** sinusitis. **Resp:** cough, dyspnea. **CV:** edema, hypertension, palpitations, postural hypotension, tachycardia, vasodilation. **GI:** constipation, diarrhea, dry mouth, dyspepsia, nausea, anorexia, dysphagia, ↑ liver enzymes, flatulence, vomiting. **GU:** ↓ libido/sexual dysfunction. **Derm:** ↑ sweating. **Metab:** weight gain, weight loss. **MS:** hypertonia, myoclonus/twitching. **Neuro:** hypokinesia/hyperkinesia, tremor. **Misc:** SEROTONIN SYNDROME, allergic reactions, chills, flu-like symptoms, tooth disorder/caries, yawning.

Interactions

Drug-Drug: Concurrent use with **MAO inhibitors** may result in serious potentially fatal reactions (MAO inhibitors should be stopped at least 14 days before fluvoxamine therapy. Fluvoxamine should be stopped at least 14 days before MAO inhibitor therapy). Concurrent use with **MAO-inhibitor-like drugs**, such as **linezolid** or **methylene blue** may ↑ risk of serotonin syndrome; concurrent use contraindicated; do not start therapy in patients receiving **linezolid** or **methylene blue**; if **linezolid** or **methylene blue** need to be started in a patient receiving fluvoxamine, immediately discontinue fluvoxamine and monitor for signs/symptoms of serotonin syndrome for 2 wk or until 24 hr after last dose of linezolid or methylene blue, whichever comes first (may resume fluvoxamine therapy 24 hr after last dose of linezolid or methylene blue). **Smoking** may ↓ effectiveness of fluvoxamine. Concurrent use with **tricyclic antidepressants** may ↑ plasma levels of fluvoxamine. Drugs that affect serotonergic neurotransmitter systems, including **SSRIs**, **SNRIs**, **fentanyl**, **buspirone**, **tramadol**, and **triptans** ↑ risk of serotonin syndrome; ↓ metabolism and may ↑ effects of some **beta blockers** (**propranolol**), **alosetron** (avoid concurrent use), some **benzodiazepines** (avoid concurrent **diazepam**), **carbamazepine**, **methadone**, **lithium**, **theophylline** (↓ dose to 33% of usual dose), **ramelteon** (avoid concurrent use), **warfarin**, and **L-tryptophan**. ↑ risk of bleeding with **NSAIDS**, **aspirin**, **clopidogrel**, or **warfarin**. ↑ blood levels and risk of toxicity from **clozapine** (dosage adjustments may be necessary).

Drug-Natural Products: Use with **St. John's wort** ↑ of serotonin syndrome.

Route/Dosage

PO (Adults): *Immediate release*–50 mg daily at bedtime; ↑ by 50 mg q 4–7 days until desired effect is achieved. If daily dose >100 mg, give in 2 equally divided doses or give a larger dose at bedtime (not to ex-

ceed 300 mg/day); *Controlled release*– 100 mg at bedtime; ↑ by 50 mg q 7 days until desired effect is achieved, not to exceed 300 mg/day.
PO (Children 8–17 yr): *Immediate release*—25 mg at bedtime, may ↑ by 25 mg/day q 4–7 days (not to exceed 200 mg/day; daily doses >50 mg should be given in divided doses with a larger dose at bedtime).

Hepatic Impairment

PO (Adults): *Immediate release*—25 mg daily at bedtime initially, slower titration, and longer dosing intervals should be used.

Availability (generic available)

Tablets: 25 mg, 50 mg, 100 mg. **Controlled-release capsules:** 100 mg, 150 mg.

NURSING IMPLICATIONS

Assessment

- Monitor mood changes. Assess patient for frequency of obsessive-compulsive behaviors. Note degree to which these thoughts and behaviors interfere with daily functioning. Inform health care professional if patient demonstrates significant increase in anxiety, nervousness, or insomnia.
- Assess for suicidal tendencies, especially during early therapy. Restrict amount of drug available to patient. Risk may be increased in children, adolescents, and adults ≤24 yrs. After starting therapy, children, adolescents, and young adults should be seen by health care professional at least weekly for 4 wk, every 3 wk for next 4 wk, and on advice of health care professional thereafter.
- Monitor appetite and nutritional intake. Weigh weekly. Report significant changes in weight. Adjust diet as tolerated to support nutritional status.
- Assess for serotonin syndrome (mental changes [agitation, hallucinations, coma], autonomic instability [tachycardia, labile BP, hyperthermia], neuromuscular aberations [hyperreflexia, incoordination], and/or GI symptoms [nausea, vomiting, diarrhea]), especially in patients taking other serotonergic drugs (SSRIs, SNRIs, triptans).
- ***Toxicity and Overdose:*** Common symptoms of toxicity include drowsiness, vomiting, diarrhea, and dizziness. Coma, tachycardia, bradycardia, hypotension, ECG abnormalities, liver function abnormalities, and convulsions may also occur. Treatment is symptomatic and supportive.

Potential Nursing Diagnoses

Ineffective coping (Indications)
Risk for injury (Side Effects)

Implementation

- Do not confuse fluvoxamine with fluphenazine or flavoxate. Do not confuse Luvox with Lasix (furosemide).
- Taper to avoid withdrawal effects. Reduce dose by 50% for 3 days, then reduce by 50% for 3 days, then discontinue.
- **PO:** Initial therapy is administered as a single bedtime dose. May be increased every 4–7 days as tolerated.
- Fluvoxamine may be given without regard to meals. Do not open, break, crush, or chew controlled-release capsules.

Patient/Family Teaching

- Instruct patient to take fluvoxamine as directed. Do not skip or double up on missed doses. Improvement in symptoms may be noticed in 2–3 wk, but medication should be continued as directed.
- May cause drowsiness and dizziness. Caution patient to avoid driving and other activities requiring alertness until response to medication is known.
- Advise patient, family, and caregivers to look for suicidality, especially during early therapy or dose changes. Notify health care professional immediately if thoughts about suicide or dying, attempts to commit suicide, new or worse depression or anxiety, agitation or restlessness, panic attacks, insomnia, new or worse irritability, aggressiveness, acting on dangerous impulses, mania, or other changes in mood or behavior or if symptoms of serotonin syndrome occur.
- Advise patient to notify health care professional if rash or hives occur or if headache, nausea, anorexia, anxiety, or insomnia persists.
- Instruct patient to notify health care professional of all Rx or OTC medications, vitamins, or herbal products being taken and consult health care professional before taking any new medications, especially St. John's wort. Advise patient to avoid taking other CNS depressants or alcohol.
- Advise patient to avoid use of caffeine (chocolate, tea, cola).
- Instruct female patients to notify health care professional if breast feeding or if pregnancy is planned or suspected.
- Emphasize the importance of follow-up exams to monitor progress.

Evaluation/Desired Outcomes

- Decrease in symptoms of obsessive-compulsive disorder.

folic acid (foe-lik a -sid)

✤Apo-Folic, folate, Folvite,
✤Novofolacid, vitamin B

Classification
Therapeutic: antianemics, vitamins
Pharmacologic: water soluble vitamins

Pregnancy Category A

Indications
Prevention and treatment of megaloblastic and macrocytic anemias. Given during pregnancy to promote normal fetal development.

Action
Required for protein synthesis and red blood cell function. Stimulates the production of red blood cells, white blood cells, and platelets. Necessary for normal fetal development. **Therapeutic Effects:** Restoration and maintenance of normal hematopoiesis.

Pharmacokinetics
Absorption: Well absorbed from the GI tract and IM and subcut sites.
Distribution: Half of all stores are in the liver. Enters breast milk. Crosses the placenta.
Protein Binding: Extensive.
Metabolism and Excretion: Converted by the liver to its active metabolite, dihydrofolate reductase. Excess amounts are excreted unchanged by the kidneys.
Half-life: Unknown.

TIME/ACTION PROFILE (↑ in reticulocyte count)

ROUTE	ONSET	PEAK	DURATION
PO, IM, subcut, IV	30–60 min	1 hr	unknown

Contraindications/Precautions
Contraindicated in: Uncorrected pernicious, aplastic, or normocytic anemias (neurologic damage will progress despite correction of hematologic abnormalities); Pedi: Preparations containing benzyl alcohol should not be used in newborns.
Use Cautiously in: Undiagnosed anemias.

Adverse Reactions/Side Effects
Derm: rash. **CNS:** irritability, difficulty sleeping, malaise, confusion. **Misc:** fever.

Interactions
Drug-Drug: Pyrimethamine, **methotrexate**, **trimethoprim**, and **triamterene** prevent the activation of folic acid (leucovorin should be used instead to treat overdoses of these drugs). Absorption of folic acid is ↓ by **sulfonamides** (including **sulfasalazine**), **antacids**, and **cholestyramine**. Folic acid requirements are ↑ by **estrogens**, **phenytoin**, **phenobarbital**, **primidone**, **carbamazepine**, or **corticosteroids**. May ↓ **phenytoin** levels.

Route/Dosage

Therapeutic Dose (Folic acid deficiency)
PO, IM, IV, Subcut (Adults and Children >11 yr): 1 mg/day initial dose then 0.5 mg/day maintenance dose.
PO, IM, IV, Subcut (Children >1 yr): 1 mg/day initial dose then 0.1–0.4 mg/day maintenance dose.
PO, IM, IV, Subcut (Infants): 15 mcg/kg/dose daily or 50 mcg/day.

Recommended Daily Allowance
PO (Adults and Children >15 yr): 0.2 mg/day.
PO (Adults): *Females of child-bearing potential*—0.4–0.8 mg/day.
PO (Children 11–14 yr): 0.15 mg/day.
PO (Children 7–10 yr): 0.1 mg/day.
PO (Children 4–6 yr): 0.075 mg/day.
PO (Infants 6 mo–3 yr): 0.05 mg/day.

Availability (generic available)
Tablets: 0.4 mg, 0.8 mg, 1 mg, ✱5 mg. **Injection:** 5 mg/mL. ***In combination with:*** other vitamins and minerals as multiple vitamins[Rx, OTC].

NURSING IMPLICATIONS

Assessment
- Assess patient for signs of megaloblastic anemia (fatigue, weakness, dyspnea) before and periodically throughout therapy.
- ***Lab Test Considerations:*** Monitor plasma folic acid levels, hemoglobin, hematocrit, and reticulocyte count before and periodically during therapy.
- May cause ↓ serum concentrations of other B complex vitamins when given in high continuous doses.

Potential Nursing Diagnoses
Imbalanced nutrition: less than body requirements (Indications)
Activity intolerance (Indications)

Implementation
- Do not confuse folic acid with folinic acid (leucovorin calcium).
- Because of infrequency of solitary vitamin deficiencies, combinations are commonly administered (see Appendix B).
- May be given subcut, deep IM, or IV when PO route is not feasible.
- **PO:** Antacids should be given at least 2 hr after folic acid; folic acid should be given 2 hr before or 4–6 hr after cholestyramine. A 50-mcg/mL oral solution may be extemporaneously prepared by pharmacy for use in neonates and infants.
- **IV:** Solution ranges from yellow to orange-yellow in color.

IV Administration

- **IV Push:** ***Diluent:*** Dilute with dextrose or 0.9%NaCl. ***Concentration:*** 0.1 mg/mL. ***Rate:*** 5 mg/min.
- **Continuous Infusion:** May be added to hyperalimentation solution.
- **Y-Site Compatibility:** alfentanil, aminophylline, ascorbic acid, atracurium, atropine, azathioprine, aztreonam, benztropine, bumetanide, calcium gluconate, cefazolin, cefonocid, cefotaxime, cefotetan, cefoxitin, ceftazidime, ceftriaxone, cefuroxime, chloramphenicol, cimetidine, clindamycin, cyanoco-

balamin, cyclosporine, dexamethasone, digoxin, diphenhydramine, dopamine, enalaprilat, ephedrine, epinephrine, epoetin alfa, erythromycin, esmolol, famotidine, fentanyl, fluconazole, furosemide, ganciclovir, glycopyrrolate, heparin, hydrocortisone, imipenem/cilastatin, indomethacin, insulin, ketorolac, labetalol, lidocaine, magnesium sulfate, mannitol, meperidine, methylprednisolone, metoclopramide, metoprolol, midazolam, multivitamins, naloxone, nitroglycerin, nitroprusside, ondansetron, oxacillin, penicillin G, pentobarbital, phenobarbital, phentolamine, phenylephrine, phytonadione, potassium chloride, procainamide, propranolol, ranitidine, sodium bicarbonate, streptokinase, succinylcholine, sufentanil, theophylline, trimetaphan, vancomycin, vasopressin.

- **Y-Site Incompatibility:** amikacin, calcium chloride, chlorpromazine, dantrolene, diazepam, diazoxide, dobutamine, doxycycline, gentamicin, haloperidol, hydralazine, metaraminol, methoxamine, methyldopate, morphine, nafcillin, nalbuphine, norepinephrine, pentamidine, pentazocine, phenytoin, prochlorperazine, promethazine, protamine, pyridoxime, tacrolimus, thiamine, tobramycin, tolazoline, trimethoprim/sulfamethoxazole, verapamil.

Patient/Family Teaching

- Encourage patient to comply with diet recommendations of health care professional. Explain that the best source of vitamins is a well-balanced diet with foods from the 4 basic food groups. A diet low in vitamin B and folate will be used to diagnose folic acid deficiency without concealing pernicious anemia.
- Folic acid in early pregnancy is necessary to prevent neural tube defects.
- Foods high in folic acid include vegetables, fruits, and organ meats; heat destroys folic acid in foods.
- Patients self-medicating with vitamin supplements should be cautioned not to exceed RDA. The effectiveness of megadoses for treatment of various medical conditions is unproven and may cause side effects.
- Explain that folic acid may make urine more intensely yellow.
- Instruct patient to notify health care professional if rash occurs, which may indicate hypersensitivity.
- Emphasize the importance of follow-up exams to evaluate progress.

Evaluation/Desired Outcomes

- Reticulocytosis 2–5 days after beginning therapy.
- Resolution of symptoms of megaloblastic anemia.
- Prevention of neural tube defects.

HIGH ALERT

fondaparinux
(fon-da-**par**-i-nux)
Arixtra

Classification
Therapeutic: anticoagulants
Pharmacologic: active factor X inhibitors

Pregnancy Category B

Indications

Prevention and treatment of deep vein thrombosis and pulmonary embolism. **Unlabeled Use:** Systemic anticoagulation for other diagnoses.

Action

Binds selectively to antithrombin III (AT III). This binding potentiates the neutralization (inactivation) of active factor X (Xa). **Therapeutic Effects:** Interruption of the coagulation cascade resulting in inhibition of thrombus formation. Prevention of thrombus formation decreases the risk of pulmonary emboli.

Pharmacokinetics

Absorption: 100% absorbed following subcutaneous administration.
Distribution: Distributes mainly throughout the intravascular space.
Metabolism and Excretion: Eliminated mainly unchanged in urine.
Half-life: 17–21 hr.

TIME/ACTION PROFILE (anticoagulant effect)

ROUTE	ONSET	PEAK	DURATION
Subcut	rapid	3 hr	24 hr

Contraindications/Precautions

Contraindicated in: Hypersensitivity; Severe renal impairment (CCr <30 mL/min; ↑ risk of bleeding); Body weight <50 kg (for prophylaxis) (markedly ↑ risk of bleeding); Active major bleeding; Bacterial endocarditis; Thrombocytopenia due to fondaparinux antibodies.
Use Cautiously in: Mild-to-moderate renal impairment (CCr 30–50 mL/min); Untreated hypertension; Recent history of ulcer disease; Body weight <50 kg (for treatment of DVT or PE) (may ↑ risk of bleeding); Geri: Patients >65 yr (↑ risk of bleeding); Malignancy; History of heparin-induced thrombocytopenia; OB: Use during pregnancy only if clearly needed; Lactation, Pedi: Safety not established.
Exercise Extreme Caution in: History of congenital or acquired bleeding disorder; Severe uncontrolled hypertension; Hemorrhagic stroke; Recent CNS or ophthalmologic surgery; Active GI bleeding/ulceration; Ret-

inopathy (hypertensive or diabetic); Neuroaxial spinal anesthesia or spinal puncture, especially if concurrent with an indwelling epidural catheter, drugs affecting hemostasis, history of traumatic/repeated spinal puncture or spinal deformity (↑ risk of spinal/epidural hematoma that may lead to long-term or permanent paralysis).

Adverse Reactions/Side Effects

CNS: confusion, dizziness, headache, insomnia. **CV:** edema, hypotension. **GI:** constipation, diarrhea, dyspepsia, ↑ liver enzymes, nausea, vomiting. **GU:** urinary retention. **Derm:** bullous eruption, hematoma, purpura, rash. **Hemat:** bleeding, thrombocytopenia. **F and E:** hypokalemia. **Misc:** hypersensitivity reactions including ANGIOEDEMA, fever, ↑ wound drainage.

Interactions

Drug-Drug: Risk of bleeding may be ↑ by concurrent use of **warfarin** or **drugs that affect platelet function**, including **aspirin**, **NSAIDs**, **dipyridamole**, some **cephalosporins**, **valproates**, **clopidogrel**, **abciximab**, **eptifibatide**, **tirofiban**, and **dextran**.
Drug-Natural Products: ↑ risk of bleeding with **arnica**, **chamomile**, **clove**, **dong quai**, **feverfew**, **garlic**, **ginger**, **gingko**, ***Panax ginseng***, and others.

Route/Dosage

Treatment of DVT/PE

Subcut (Adults): *<50 kg*—5 mg once daily for at least 5 days until therapeutic anticoagulation with warfarin is achieved (INR >2 for 2 consecutive days); warfarin may be started within 72 hr of fondaparinux (has been used for up to 26 days); *50–100 kg*—7.5 mg once daily for at least 5 days until therapeutic anticoagulation with warfarin is achieved (INR >2 for 2 consecutive days); *>100 kg*—10 mg once daily for at least 5 days until therapeutic anticoagulation with warfarin is achieved (INR >2 for 2 consecutive days); warfarin may be started within 72 hr of fondaparinux.

Prevention of DVT/PE

Subcut (Adults): 2.5 mg once daily, starting 6–8 hr after surgery, continuing for 5–9 days (up to 11 days) following abdominal surgery or knee/hip replacement or continuing for 24 days following hip fracture surgery (up to 32 days).

Availability (generic available)

Solution for subcut injection (prefilled syringes): 2.5 mg/0.5 mL, 5 mg/0.4 mL, 7.5 mg/0.6 mL, 10 mg/0.8 mL.

NURSING IMPLICATIONS

Assessment

- Assess for signs of bleeding and hemorrhage (bleeding gums; nosebleed; unusual bruising; black, tarry stools; hematuria; fall in hematocrit; sudden drop in BP; guaiac positive stools); bleeding from surgical site. Notify health care professional if these occur.
- Assess for evidence of additional or increased thrombosis. Symptoms will depend on area of involvement. Monitor neurological status frequently for signs of impairment, especially in patients with indwelling epidural catheters for administration of analgesia or with concomitant use of drugs affecting hemostasis (NSAIDs, platelet inhibitors, other anticoagulants). Risk is increased by traumatic or repeated epidural or spinal puncture. May require urgent treatment.
- ***Lab Test Considerations:*** Monitor platelet count closely; may cause thrombocytopenia. If platelet count is <100,000/mm^3, discontinue fondaparinux.
- Fondaparinux is not accurately measured by prothrombin time (PT), activated thromboplastin time (aPTT), or international standards of heparin or low-molecular-weight heparins. If unexpected changes in coagulation parameters or major bleeding occurs, discontinue fondaparinux.
- Monitor CBC, serum creatinine levels, and stool occult blood tests routinely during therapy.
- May cause asymptomatic ↑ in AST and ALT. Elevations are fully reversible and not associated with ↑ in bilirubin.
- May cause ↑ aPTT temporally associated with bleeding with or without concomitant administration of other anticoagulants and thrombocytopenia with thrombosis similar to heparin-induced thrombocytopenia, with or without exposure to heparin or low-molecular-weight heparins.

Potential Nursing Diagnoses

Ineffective tissue perfusion (Indications)
Risk for injury (Side Effects)

Implementation

- ***High Alert:*** Do not confuse Arixtra with Arista AH (absorbable hemostatic agent).
- Fondaparinux cannot be used interchangeably with heparin, low-molecular-weight heparins, or heparinoids as they differ in manufacturing process, anti-Xa and anti-IIa activity, units, and dose. Each of these medications has its own instructions for use.
- Initial dose should be administered 6–8 hr after surgery. Administration before 6 hr after surgery has been associated with risk of major bleeding.
- **Subcut:** Administer subcut only into fatty tissue, alternating sites between right and left anterolateral or posterolateral abdominal wall. Inject entire length of needle at a 45° or 90° angle into a skin fold held between thumb and forefinger; hold skin fold throughout injection. Do not aspirate or massage. Rotate sites frequently. Do not administer IM because of danger of hematoma formation. Solution should be clear; do not inject solution containing particulate matter. Do not mix with other injections.
- Fondaparinux is provided in a single-dose prefilled syringe with an automatic needle protection system. Do not expel air bubble from prefilled syringe before injection to prevent loss of drug.

Patient/Family Teaching

- Advise patient to report any symptoms of unusual bleeding or bruising, dizziness, itching, rash, fever, swelling, or difficulty breathing to health care professional immediately.
- Instruct patient not to take aspirin or NSAIDs without consulting health care professional during therapy.

Evaluation/Desired Outcomes

- Prevention and treatment of deep vein thrombosis and pulmonary embolism.

formoterol (for-mo-te-role)

✤Oxeze Turbuhaler, Perforomist

Classification
Therapeutic: bronchodilators
Pharmacologic: adrenergics

Pregnancy Category C

Indications

Maintenance treatment to prevent bronchospasm in chronic obstructive pulmonary disease (COPD) including chronic bronchitis and emphysema.

Action

Produces accumulation of cyclic adenosine monophosphate (cAMP) at beta-adrenergic receptors, resulting in relaxation of airway smooth muscle. Relatively specific for $beta_2$ (pulmonary) receptors. **Therapeutic Effects:** Bronchodilation.

Pharmacokinetics

Absorption: Following inhalation, majority of inhaled drug is swallowed and absorbed.

Distribution: Unknown.

Metabolism and Excretion: Mostly metabolized by the liver; 10–18% excreted unchanged in urine.

Half-life: 10 hr.

TIME/ACTION PROFILE (bronchodilation)

ROUTE	ONSET	PEAK	DURATION
Inhaln	15 min	1–3 hr	12 hr

Contraindications/Precautions

Contraindicated in: Hypersensitivity; Acute attack of asthma (onset of action is delayed); Patients not receiving a long-term asthma-control medication (e.g. inhaled corticosteroid).

Use Cautiously in: Cardiovascular disease (including angina, hypertension, and arrhythmias); Diabetes; Seizure disorders; Glaucoma; Hyperthyroidism; Pheochromocytoma; Excessive use (may lead to tolerance and paradoxical bronchospasm); OB, Lactation, Pedi: Pregnancy, lactation, or children <5 yr (may inhibit contractions during labor; use only if potential benefits outweigh risks; in children, a fixed-dose combination product containing formoterol and an inhaled corticosteroid should be strongly considered to ensure adherence).

Adverse Reactions/Side Effects

CNS: dizziness, fatigue, headache, insomnia, malaise, nervousness. **Resp:** ASTHMA-RELATED DEATH, PARADOXICAL BRONCHOSPASM. **CV:** angina, arrhythmias, hypertension, hypotension, palpitations, tachycardia. **GI:** dry mouth, nausea. **F and E:** hypokalemia. **Metab:** hyperglycemia, metabolic acidosis. **MS:** muscle cramps. **Neuro:** tremor. **Derm:** rash. **Misc:** allergic reactions including ANAPHYLAXIS.

Interactions

Drug-Drug: Concurrent use with **MAO inhibitors, tricyclic antidepressants,** or other **agents that may prolong the QTc interval** may result in serious arrhythmias and should be undertaken with extreme caution. ↑ risk of hypokalemia with **theophylline, corticosteroids, potassium-losing diuretics. Beta blockers** may ↓ therapeutic effects. ↑ adrenergic effects may occur with concurrent use of **adrenergics.**

Route/Dosage

Inhaln (Adults): 20 mcg/2 mL-unit-dose vial twice daily via jet nebulizer.

Availability

Inhalation solution for nebulization (Perforomist): 20 mcg/2 mL. **Powder for oral inhalation (Oxeze Turbuhaler):** ✤6 mcg/inhalation (60 metered doses), ✤12 mcg/inhalation (60 metered doses). ***In combination with:*** budesonide (Symbicort) and mometasone (Dulera); see Appendix B).

NURSING IMPLICATIONS

Assessment

- Assess lung sounds, pulse, and BP before administration and during peak of medication. Note amount, color, and character of sputum produced. Closely monitor patients on higher dose for adverse effects.
- Monitor pulmonary function tests before initiating and periodically during therapy to determine effectiveness.
- Observe for paradoxical bronchospasm (wheezing, dyspnea, tightness in chest) and hypersensitivity reaction (rash; urticaria; swelling of the face, lips, or eyelids). If condition occurs, withhold medication and notify physician or other health care professional immediately.
- Monitor ECG periodically during therapy. May cause prolonged QTc interval.
- Monitor patient for signs of anaphylaxis (dyspnea, rash, laryngeal edema) throughout therapy.
- ***Lab Test Considerations:*** May cause ↑ serum glucose and decreased serum potassium.

F

Potential Nursing Diagnoses

Ineffective airway clearance (Indications)

Implementation

- Formoterol should be used along with an inhaled corticosteroid, not as monotherapy.
- **Inhaln:** *For use with nebulizer:* Administer via standard jet nebulizer via mouthpiece or face mask. Remove vial from foil immediately prior to use and discard via after use. May be stored in refrigerator for up to 3 mo.

Patient/Family Teaching

- Instruct patient to take fomoterol as directed. Do not discontinue therapy without discussing with health care professional, even if feeling better. If a dose is missed skip dose and take next dose at regularly scheduled time. Do not double doses. Use a rapid-acting bronchodilator if symptoms occur before next dose is due. Caution patient not to use more than 2 times a day or less than 12 hr apart; may cause adverse effects, paradoxical bronchospasm, or loss of effectiveness of medication. Instruct patient to review medication guide with each Rx refill in case of changes.
- Instruct patient to contact health care professional immediately if shortness of breath is not relieved by medication or nausea, vomiting, shakiness, headache, fast or irregular heartbeat, or sleeplessness occur.
- Advise patient to consult health care professional before taking any Rx, OTC, or herbal products or alcohol concurrently with this therapy. Caution patient also to avoid smoking and other respiratory irritants.
- Advise patient to notify health care professional if pregnancy is planned or suspected, or if nursing.

Evaluation/Desired Outcomes

- Bronchodilation.

foscarnet (foss-kar-net)

~~Foscavir~~

Classification

Therapeutic: antivirals

Pregnancy Category C

Indications

Treatment of cytomegalovirus (CMV) retinitis in HIV-infected patients (alone or with ganciclovir). Treatment of acyclovir-resistant mucocutaneous herpes simplex virus (HSV) infections in immunocompromised patients.

Action

Prevents viral replication by inhibiting viral DNA-polymerase and reverse transcriptase. **Therapeutic Effects:** Virustatic action against susceptible viruses including CMV.

Pharmacokinetics

Absorption: IV administration results in complete bioavailability.

Distribution: Variable penetration into CSF. May concentrate in and be slowly released from bone.

Metabolism and Excretion: 80–90% excreted unchanged in urine.

Half-life: 3 hr (in patients with normal renal function); longer half-life of 90 hr may reflect release of drug from bone.

TIME/ACTION PROFILE

ROUTE	ONSET	PEAK	DURATION
IV	rapid	end of infusion	8–24 hr

Contraindications/Precautions

Contraindicated in: Hypersensitivity; HF (due to sodium content); Patients on sodium-restricted diets; Hemodialysis; Lactation: Avoid breast feeding.

Use Cautiously in: Renal impairment (dose ↓ required if CCr ≤1.4–1.6 mL/min/kg; see product information); History of seizures; OB, Pedi: Safety not established.

Adverse Reactions/Side Effects

CNS: SEIZURES, headache, anxiety, confusion, dizziness, fatigue, malaise, mental depression, weakness. **EENT:** conjunctivitis, eye pain, vision abnormalities. **Resp:** coughing, dyspnea. **CV:** chest pain, ECG abnormalities, edema, palpitations. **GI:** diarrhea, nausea, vomiting, abdominal pain, abnormal taste sensation, anorexia, constipation, dyspepsia. **GU:** renal failure, albuminuria, dysuria, nocturia, polyuria, urinary retention. **Derm:** ↑ sweating, pruritus, rash, skin ulceration. **F and E:** hypocalcemia, hypokalemia, hypomagnesemia, hyperphosphatemia, hypophosphatemia. **Hemat:** anemia, granulocytopenia, leukopenia, neutropenia. **Local:** pain/inflammation at injection site. **MS:** arthralgia, myalgia, back pain, involuntary muscle contraction. **Neuro:** ataxia, hypoesthesia, neuropathy, paresthesia, tremor. **Misc:** fever, chills, flu-like syndrome, lymphoma, sarcoma.

Interactions

Drug-Drug: Concurrent use with parenteral **pentamidine** may result in severe, life-threatening hypocalcemia. Risk of nephrotoxicity may be ↑ by concurrent use of other **nephrotoxic agents** (**amphotericin B**, **aminoglycosides**, **cyclosporine**, **acyclovir**, **methotrexate**, **tacrolimus**, **pentamidine (IV)**).

Route/Dosage

IV (Adults): *CMV retinitis*—60 mg/kg q 8 hr or 90 mg/kg q 12 hr for 2–3 wk, then 90–120 mg/kg/day as a single dose. Dose ↓ required for any degree of renal impairment; *HSV*—40 mg/kg q 8–12 hr for 2–3 wk or until healing occurs.

Availability (generic available)

Solution for injection: 24 mg/mL.

NURSING IMPLICATIONS

Assessment

- **CMV Retinitis:** Diagnosis of CMV retinitis should be determined by ophthalmoscopy before treatment with foscarnet. Ophthalmologic examinations should also be performed at the conclusion of induction and every 4 wk during maintenance therapy.
- Culture for CMV (urine, blood, throat) may be taken before administration. However, a negative CMV culture does not rule out CMV retinitis.
- **HSV Infections:** Assess lesions before and daily during therapy.
- ***Lab Test Considerations:*** Monitor serum creatinine before and 2–3 times weekly during induction therapy and at least once every 1–2 wk during maintenance therapy. Monitor 24-hr CCr before and periodically throughout therapy. If CCr drops below 0.4 mL/min/kg, discontinue foscarnet.
- Monitor serum calcium, magnesium, potassium, and phosphorus before and 2–3 times weekly during induction therapy and at least weekly during maintenance therapy. May cause ↓ concentrations.
- May cause anemia, granulocytopenia, leukopenia, and thrombocytopenia. May cause ↑ AST and ALT levels and abnormal A-G ratios.

Potential Nursing Diagnoses

Risk for infection (Indications)

Implementation

- Adequately hydrate patient with 750–1000 mL of 0.9% NaCl or D5W before first infusion to establish diuresis, then administer 750–1000 mL with 120 mg/kg of foscarnet or 500 mL with 40–60 mg/kg of foscarnet with each dose to prevent renal toxicity.

IV Administration

- **Intermittent Infusion: *Diluent:*** May be administered via central line undiluted. If administered via peripheral line, ***must*** be diluted with D5W or 0.9% NaCl to prevent vein irritation. Do not administer solution that is discolored or contains particulate matter. Do not refrigerate or freeze; stable for 24 hrs at room temperature. Use diluted solution within 24 hr. ***Concentration:*** Undiluted: 24 mg/mL; Diluted: 12 mg/mL.
- Dose is based on patient weight; excess solution may be discarded from bottle before administration to prevent overdosage.
- Patients who experience progression of CMV retinitis during maintenance therapy may be retreated with induction therapy followed by maintenance therapy. ***Rate:*** Administer at a rate not to exceed 1 mg/kg/min.
- Infuse solution via infusion pump to ensure accurate infusion rate.
- **Y-Site Compatibility:** aldesleukin, alemtuzumab, alfentanil, amifostine, amikacin, aminophylline, amphotericin B liposome, ampicillin, ampicillin/sulbactam, anidulafungin, argatroban, asparaginase, azithromycin, aztreonam, bivalirudin, bleomycin, bumetanide, buprenorphine, busulfan, butorphanol, carboplatin, carmustine, cefazolin, cefotaxime, cefotetan, cefoxitin, ceftazidime, ceftriaxone, cefuroxime, chloramphenicol, cisatracurium, cisplatin, clindamycin, cyclophosphamide, cyclosporine, cytarabine, dacarbazine, dactinomycin, daptomycin, dexamethasone sodium phosphate, dexmedetomidine, dexrazoxane, diltiazem, docetaxel, dopamine, doripenem, doxacurium, enalaprilat, ephedrine, epinephrine, eptifibatide, ertapenem, erythromycin lactobionate, esmolol, etoposide, etoposide phosphate, famotidine, fenoldopam, fentanyl, fluconazole, flucytosine, fludarabine, fluorouracil, fosphenytoin, furosemide, gemcitabine, gentamicin, glycopyrrolate, granisetron, heparin, hetastarch, hydrocortisone, hydromorphone, ifosfamide, imipenem-cilastatin, insulin, irinotecan, isoproterenol, ketorolac, levofloxacin, lidocaine, linezolid, magnesium sulfate, mannitol, mechlorethamine, melphalan, meperidine, meropenem, mesna, methotrexate, metoclopramide, metoprolol, metronidazole, milrinone, mitomycin, morphine, nafcillin, nalbuphine, naloxone, nesiritide, nitroglycerin, nitroprusside, octreotide, oxacillin, oxaliplatin, oxytocin, paclitaxel, palonosetron, pamidronate, pancuronium, pantoprazole, pemetrexed, penicillin G potassium, pentobarbital, phenylephrine, piperacillin/tazobactam, potassium acetate, potassium chloride, potassium phosphates, procainamide, propranolol, ranitidine, remifentanil, rocuronium, sodium acetate, sodium bicarbonate, sodium phosphates, streptozocin, succinylcholine, sufentanil, tacrolimus, teniposide, theophylline, thiotepa, tigecycline, tirofiban, tobramycin, vancomycin, vecuronium, vinblastine, vincristine, voriconazole, zidovudine, zoledronic acid.
- **Y-Site Incompatibility:** Manufacturer recommends that foscarnet not be administered concurrently with other drugs or solutions in the same IV catheter except D5W or 0.9% NaCl, acyclovir, allopurinol, amphotericin B colloidal, amphotericin B lipid complex, calcium chloride, calcium gluconate, caspofungin, chlorpromazine, ciprofloxacin, dantrolene, daunorubicin, diazepam, digoxin, diphenhydramine, dobutamine, dolasetron, doxorubicin, droperidol, epirubicin, ganciclovir, haloperidol, idarubicin, labetalol, leucovorin, methylprednisolone, midazolam, mitoxantrone, mycophenolate, nicardipine, norepinephrine, ondansetron, pentami-

F

dine, pentazocine, prochlorperazine, promethazine, quinupristin/dalfopristin, thiopental, topotecan, verapamil, vinorelbine.

Patient/Family Teaching

- Inform patient that foscarnet is not a cure for CMV retinitis. Progression of retinitis may continue in immunocompromised patients during and after therapy. Advise patients to have regular ophthalmologic exams.
- May cause dizziness and seizures. Caution patient to avoid driving or other activities requiring alertness until response to medication is known.
- Advise patient to notify health care professional immediately if perioral tingling or numbness in the extremities or paresthesia occurs during or after infusion. If these signs of electrolyte imbalance occur during administration, infusion should be stopped and lab samples for serum electrolyte concentrations obtained immediately.
- Emphasize the importance of frequent follow-up exams to monitor renal function and electrolytes.

Evaluation/Desired Outcomes

- Management of the symptoms of CMV retinitis in patients with AIDS.
- Crusting over and healing of skin lesions in HSV infections.

fosinopril, See ANGIOTENSIN-CONVERTING ENZYME (ACE) INHIBITORS.

fosphenytoin

(foss-**fen**-i-toyn)

Cerebyx

Classification

Therapeutic: anticonvulsants

Pregnancy Category D

Indications

Short-term (<5 day) parenteral management of generalized, convulsive status epilepticus when use of phenytoin is not feasible. Treatment and prevention of seizures during neurosurgery when use of phenytoin is not feasible.

Action

Limits seizure propagation by altering ion transport. May also decrease synaptic transmission. Fosphenytoin is rapidly converted to phenytoin, which is responsible for its pharmacologic effects. **Therapeutic Effects:** Diminished seizure activity.

Pharmacokinetics

Absorption: Rapidly converted to phenytoin after IV administration and completely absorbed after IM administration.

Distribution: Distributes into CSF and other body tissues and fluids. Enters breast milk; crosses the placenta, achieving similar maternal/fetal levels. Preferentially distributes into fatty tissue.

Protein Binding: *Fosphenytoin*—95–99%; *phenytoin*—90–95%.

Metabolism and Excretion: Mostly metabolized by the liver; minimal amounts excreted in the urine.

Half-life: *Fosphenytoin*—15 min; *phenytoin*—22 hr (range 7–42 hr).

TIME/ACTION PROFILE (anticonvulsant effect)

ROUTE	ONSET	PEAK	DURATION
IM	unknown	30 min	up to 24 hr
IV	15–45 min	15–60 min	up to 24 hr

Contraindications/Precautions

Contraindicated in: Hypersensitivity; Sinus bradycardia, sinoatrial block, 2nd- or 3rd-degree AV heart block or Adams-Stokes syndrome; Concurrent use of delavirdine.

Use Cautiously in: Hepatic or renal disease (↑ risk of adverse reactions; dose reduction recommended for hepatic impairment); OB: Safety not established; may result in fetal hydantoin syndrome if used chronically or hemorrhage in the newborn if used at term; Lactation: Safety not established.

Exercise Extreme Caution in: Patients positive for HLA-B*1502 allele (unless exceptional circumstances exist where benefits clearly outweigh the risks).

Adverse Reactions/Side Effects

CNS: dizziness, drowsiness, nystagmus, agitation, brain edema, headache, stupor, vertigo. **EENT:** amblyopia, deafness, diplopia, tinnitus. **CV:** hypotension (with rapid IV administration), tachycardia. **GI:** dry mouth, nausea, taste perversion, tongue disorder, vomiting. **Derm:** pruritus, purple glove syndrome, rash, STEVENS-JOHNSON SYNDROME, TOXIC EPIDERMAL NECROLYSIS. **MS:** back pain. **Neuro:** ataxia, dysarthria, extrapyramidal syndrome, hypesthesia, incoordination, paresthesia, tremor. **Misc:** DRUG REACTION WITH EOSINOPHILIA AND SYSTEMIC SYMPTOMS (DRESS), pelvic pain.

Interactions

Drug-Drug: May ↓ the effects of **delavirdine**, resulting in loss of virologic response and potential resistant (concurrent use contraindicated). **Disulfiram**, acute ingestion of **alcohol**, **amiodarone**, **capecitabine**, **chloramphenicol**, **chlordiazepoxide**, **cimetidine**, **diazepam**, **estrogens**, **ethosuximide**, **felbamate**, **fluconazole**, **fluorouracil**, **fluoxetine**, **fluvastatin**, **fluvoxamine**, **halothane**, **isoniazid**, **itraconazole**, **ketoconazole**, **methylphenidate**, **miconazole**, **omeprazole**, **oxcarbazepine**, **phenothiazines**, **salicylates**, **sertraline**, **succinamides**, **sulfonamides**, **topiramate**, **trazodone**, **voriconazole**, and**warfarin** may ↑ phenytoin blood levels. **Barbiturates**, **bleomycin**, **carbamazepine**, **carbopla-**

tin, cisplatin, diazoxide, doxorubicin, folic acid, fosamprenavir, methotrexate, nelfinavir, reserpine, rifampin, ritonavir, theophylline, vigabatrin, and chronic ingestion of **alcohol** may ↓ phenytoin blood levels. Phenytoin may ↓ the effects of **albendazole, amiodarone, atorvastatin, benzodiazepines, carbamazepine, chloramphenicol, chlorpropamide, clozapine, corticosteroids, cyclosporine, digoxin, disopyramide, doxycycline, efavirenz, estrogens, felbamate, fluconazole, fluvastatin, folic acid, furosemide, indinavir, irinotecan, itraconazole, ketoconazole, lamotrigine, lopinavir/ritonavir, methadone, mexiletine, nelfinavir, nifedipine, nimodpine, nisoldipine, oral contraceptives, oxcarbazepine, paclitaxel, paroxetine, posaconazole, propafenone, quetiapine, quinidine, rifampin, ritonavir, saquinavir, sertraline, simvastatin, tacrolimus, teniposide, theophylline, topiramate, tricyclic antidepressants, verapamil vitamin D, voriconazole, warfarin**, and **zonisamide**.

Drug-Natural Products: St. John's wort may ↓ levels.

Route/Dosage

Note: Doses of fosphenytoin are expressed as phenytoin sodium equivalents [PE].

Status Epilepticus

IV (Adults): 15–20 mg PE/kg.

Nonemergent and Maintenance Dosing

IV, IM (Adults and Children > 16 yr): *Loading dose*— 10–20 mg PE/kg. *Maintenance dose*—4–6 mg PE/kg/day.
IV, IM (Children 10–16 yr): 6–7 mg PE/kg/day.
IV, IM (Children 7–9 yr): 7–8 mg PE/kg/day.
IV, IM (Children 4–6 yr): 7.5–9 mg PE/kg/day.
IV, IM (Children 0.5–3 yr): 8–10 mg PE kg/day.
IV, IM (Infants): 5 mg PE kg/day.
IV, IM (Neonates): 5–8 mg PE/kg/day.

Availability (generic available)

Injection: 50 mg PE/mL.

NURSING IMPLICATIONS

Assessment

- Assess location, duration, frequency, and characteristics of seizure activity. EEG may be monitored periodically during therapy.
- Monitor BP, ECG, and respiratory function continuously during administration of fosphenytoin and during period when peak serum phenytoin levels occur (15–30 min after administration).
- Observe patient for development of rash. Discontinue fosphenytoin at the first sign of skin reactions. Serious adverse reactions such as exfoliative, purpuric, or bullous rashes or the development of lupus erythematosus, Stevens-Johnson syndrome, or toxic epidermal necrolysis preclude further use of phenytoin or fosphenytoin. Stevens-Johnson syndrome and toxic epidermal necrolysis are significantly more common in patients with a particular human leukocyte antigen (HLA) allele, HLA-B*1502 (occurs almost exclusively in patients with Asian ancestry, including including Han Chinese, Filipinos, Malaysians, South Asian Indians, and Thais). Avoid using phenytoin or fosphenytoin as alternatives to carbamazepine for patients who test positive. If less serious skin eruptions (measles-like or scarlatiniform) occur, fosphenytoin may be resumed after complete clearing of the rash. If rash reappears, further use of fosphenytoin or phenytoin should be avoided.
- Assess mental status (orientation, mood, behavior) before and periodically during therapy. Monitor closely for notable changes in behavior that could indicate the emergence or worsening of suicidal thoughts or behavior or depression.
- Monitor injection site frequently during therapy for edema, discoloration, and pain distal to the site of injection (described as "purple glove syndrome"). May or may not be associated with extravasation. The syndrome may not develop for several days after injection of phenytoin or fosphenytoin.
- ***Lab Test Considerations:*** Fosphenytoin contains 0.0037 mmol phosphate per mg PE. Monitor serum phosphate concentrations in patients with renal insufficiency; may cause ↑ phosphate concentrations.
- May cause ↑ serum alkaline phosphatase, GTT, and glucose levels.
- Fosphenytoin therapy may be monitored using phenytoin levels. Optimal total plasma phenytoin concentrations are typically 10–20 mcg/mL (unbound plasma phenytoin concentrations of 1–2 mcg/mL).
- ***Toxicity and Overdose:*** Serum phenytoin levels should not be monitored until complete conversion from fosphenytoin to phenytoin has occurred (2 hr after IV or 4 hr after IM administration).
- Initial signs and symptoms of phenytoin toxicity include nystagmus, ataxia, confusion, nausea, slurred speech, and dizziness.

Potential Nursing Diagnoses

Risk for injury (Indications)

Implementation

- Do not confuse concentration of fosphenytoin with total amount of drug in vial.
- Implement seizure precautions.
- When substituting *fosphenytoin* for oral *phenytoin* therapy, the same total daily dose may be given as a single dose. Unlike parenteral phenytoin, fosphenytoin may be given safely by the IM route.

F

- The anticonvulsant effect of fosphenytoin is not immediate. Additional measures (including parenteral benzodiazepines) are usually required in the immediate management of status epilepticus. Loading dose of *fosphenytoin* should be followed with the institution of maintenance anticonvulsant therapy.

IV Administration

- **IV Push:** ***Diluent:*** D5W or 0.9% NaCl. ***Concentration:*** 1.5–25 mg PE/mL. May be refrigerated for up to 48 hr. ***Rate:*** Administer at a rate of <150 mg PE/min in adults and <3 mg/kg/min in children to minimize risk of hypotension.
- **Y-Site Compatibility:** acyclovir, alemtuzumab, alfentanil, allopurinol, amifostine, amikacin, aminocaproic acid, aminophylline, amphotericin B lipid complex, amphotericin B liposome, ampicillin, ampicillin/sulbactam, anidulafungin, argatroban, azithromycin, aztreonam, bivalirudin, bleomycin, bumetanide, buprenorphine, busulfan, butorphanol, carboplatin, carmustine, cefazolin, cefepime, cefotaxime, cefotetan, cefoxitin, ceftazidime, ceftriaxone, cefuroxime, chloramphenicol, ciprofloxacin, cisatracurium, cisplatin, clindamycin, cyclophosphamide, cyclosporine, cytarabine, dacarbazine, dactinomycin, daptomycin, dexamethasone, dexmedetomidine, dexrazoxane, digoxin, diltiazem, diphenhydramine, docetaxel, doxacurium, doxorubicin liposomal, enalaprilat, ephedrine, epinephrine, eptifibatide, ertapenem, erythromycin, esmolol, etoposide, etoposide phosphate, famotidine, fentanyl, fluconazole, fludarabine, fluorouracil, foscarnet, furosemide, foscarnet, gemcitabine, gentamicin, glycopyrrolate, granisetron, heparin, hetastarch, hydrocortisone, hydromorphone, ifosfamide, imipenem, insulin, isoproterenol, ketotolac, labetalol, leucovorin, levofloxacin, lidocaine, linezolid, lorazepam, magnesium sulfate, mannitol, mechlorethamine, mephalan, meperidine, meropenem, mesna, methotrexate, methyldopate, methylprednisolone, metoprolol, metronidazole, milrinone, mitomycin, morphine, nalbuphine, naloxone, nesiritide, nitroglycerin, nitroprusside, norepinephrine, octreotide, ondansetron, oxaliplatin, oxytocin, paclitaxel, palonosetron, pamidronate, pancuronium, pantoprazole, pemetrexed, pentobarbital, phenobarbital, phenylephrine, piperacillin/tazobactam, potassium acetate, potassium chloride, potassium phosphates, procainamide, propranolol, ranitidine, remifentanil, rocuronium, sodium acetate, sodium bicarbonate, sodium phosphates, succinylcholine, sufentanil, tacrolimus, teniposide, theophylline, thiotepa, tigecycline, tirofiban, tobramycin, trimethoprim/sulfamethoxazole, vancomycin, vasopressin, vecuronium, vinblastine, vincristine, vinorelbine, voriconazole, zidovudine, zoledronic acid.
- **Y-Site Incompatibility:** amiodarone, amphotericin B colloidal, calcium chloride, calcium gluconate, caspofungin, chlorpromazine, dantrolene, daunorubicin hydrochloride, diazepam, dobutamine, dolasetron, doxorubicin hydrochloride, droperidol, epirubicin, fenoldopam, haloperidol, hydralazine, idarubicin, irinotecan, midazolam, mitoxantrone, moxifloxacin, mycophenolate, nicardipine, pentamidine, pentazocine, phenytoin, prochlorperazine, quinupristin/dalfopristin, thiopental, topotecan, verapamil.

Patient/Family Teaching

- May cause drowsiness or dizziness. Caution patient to avoid driving or other activities requiring alertness until response to medication is known. Do not resume driving until physician gives clearance based on control of seizure disorder.
- Instruct patients that behavioral changes, skin rash, fever, sore throat, mouth ulcers, easy bruising, petechiae, unusual bleeding, abdominal pain, chills, pale stools, dark urine, jaundice, severe nausea or vomiting, drowsiness, slurred speech, unsteady gait, swollen glands,or persistent headache should be reported to health care professional immediately. Advise patient and family to notify health care professional if thoughts about suicide or dying, attempts to commit suicide; new or worse depression; new or worse anxiety; feeling very agitated or restless; panic attacks; trouble sleeping; new or worse irritability; acting aggressive; being angry or violent; acting on dangerous impulses; an extreme increase in activity and talking, other unusual changes in behavior or mood occur.
- Rep: Advise female patients to use an additional nonhormonal method of contraception during therapy and until next menstrual period. Instruct patient to notify health care professional if pregnancy is planned or suspected. Encourage patients who become pregnant to enroll in the North American Antiepileptic Drug (NAAED) Pregnancy Registry by calling 1-888-233-2334 or on the web at www.aedpregnancyregistry.org. Enrollment must be done by patients themselves.
- Advise patient to carry identification describing disease process and medication regimen at all times.
- Emphasize the importance of routine exams to monitor progress. Patient should have routine physical exams, especially monitoring skin and lymph nodes, and EEG testing.

Evaluation/Desired Outcomes

- Decrease or cessation of seizures without excessive sedation.

frovatriptan (froe-va-**trip**-tan)

Frova

Classification

Therapeutic: vascular headache suppressants

Pharmacologic: 5-HT_1 agonists

Pregnancy Category C

Indications

Acute treatment of migraine headache.

Action

Acts as an agonist at specific 5-HT receptor sites in intracranial blood vessels and sensory trigeminal nerves. **Therapeutic Effects:** Cranial vessel vasoconstriction with associated decrease in release of neuropeptides and resultant decrease in migraine headache.

Pharmacokinetics

Absorption: 20–30% following oral administration.
Distribution: Unknown.
Metabolism and Excretion: Mostly metabolized by the liver (P450 1A2 enzyme system); some metabolites eliminated in urine, <10% excreted unchanged.
Half-life: 26 hr.

TIME/ACTION PROFILE (blood levels)

ROUTE	ONSET	PEAK	DURATION
PO	unknown	2–4 hr	unknown

Contraindications/Precautions

Contraindicated in: Hypersensitivity; History, symptoms or findings consistent with; Cerebrovascular syndromes including; Uncontrolled hypertension; Hemiplegic or basilar migraine; Peripheral vascular disease, including ischemic bowel disease; Should not be used within 24 hr of any other 5-HT agonist or ergot-type compounds (e.g. dihydroergotamine, ergotamine); Pedi: Children <18 yr.
Use Cautiously in: Concurrent use of SSRIs or SNRIs (↑ risk of serotonin syndrome); Geri: May be more susceptible to adverse cardiovascular effects; OB, Lactation: Safety not established.
Exercise Extreme Caution in: Cardiovascular risk factors (hypertension, hypercholesterolemia, cigarette smoking, obesity, diabetes, strong family history, menopausal women or men >40 yr); use only if cardiovascular status has been evaluated and determined to be safe and first dose is administered under supervision.

Adverse Reactions/Side Effects

CNS: dizziness, drowsiness, fatigue. **CV:** CORONARY ARTERY VASOSPASM, MI, VENTRICULAR FIBRILLATION, VENTRICULAR TACHYCARDIA, chest pain, myocardial ischemia. **GI:** dry mouth, dyspepsia, nausea. **Derm:** flushing. **MS:** skeletal pain. **Neuro:** paresthesia. **Misc:** pain.

Interactions

Drug-Drug: Hormonal contraceptives or **propranolol** may ↑ levels. ↑ risk of serious vasospastic reactions with **dihydroergotamine** or **ergotamine** (concurrent use contraindicated). ↑ risk of serotonin syndrome when used with **fluoxetine**, **paroxetine**, **sertraline**, **fluvoxamine**, **citalopram**, **escitalopram**, **venlafaxine**, or **duloxetine**.

Route/Dosage

PO (Adults): 2.5 mg; if there has been initial relief, a second tablet may be taken after at least 2 hr (daily dose should not exceed 3 tablets and should not be used to treat more than 4 attacks/30 day period).

Availability (generic available)

Tablets: 2.5 mg.

NURSING IMPLICATIONS

Assessment

- Assess pain location, intensity, duration, and associated symptoms (photophobia, phonophobia, nausea, vomiting) during migraine attack.

Potential Nursing Diagnoses

Acute pain (Indications)

Implementation

- **PO:** Tablets may be administered at any time after the headache starts.

Patient/Family Teaching

- Inform patient that frovatriptan should be used only during a migraine attack. It is meant to be used to relieve migraine attack but not to prevent or reduce the number of attacks.
- Instruct patient to administer frovatriptan as soon as symptoms appear, but it may be administered any time during an attack. If migraine symptoms return, a second dose may be used. Allow at least 2 hr between doses, and do not use more than 3 tablets in any 24-hr period.
- If dose does not relieve headache, additional frovatriptan doses are not likely to be effective; notify health care professional.
- Caution patient not to take frovatriptan within 24 hr of another vascular headache suppressant.
- Advise patient that lying down in a darkened room following frovatriptan administration may further help relieve headache.
- May cause dizziness or drowsiness. Caution patient to avoid driving or other activities requiring alertness until response to medication is known.
- Advise patient that overuse (use more than 10 days/month) may lead to exacerbation of headache (mi-

graine-like daily headaches, or as a marked increase in frequency of migraine attacks). May require gradual withdrawal of frovatriptan and treatment of symptoms (transient worsening of headache).

- Advise patient to notify health care professional prior to next dose of frovatriptan if pain or tightness in the chest occurs during use. If pain is severe or does not subside, notify health care professional immediately. If wheezing; heart throbbing; swelling of eyelids, face, or lips; skin rash; skin lumps; or hives occur, notify health care professional immediately and do not take more frovatriptan without approval of health care professional. If feelings of tingling, heat, flushing, heaviness, pressure, drowsiness, dizziness, tiredness, or sickness develop, discuss with health care professional at next visit.
- Advise patient to avoid alcohol, which aggravates headaches, during frovatriptan use.
- Advise patient to notify health care professional of all Rx or OTC medications, vitamins, or herbal products being taken and to consult with health care professional before taking other medications.
- Advise patient to notify health care professional immediately if signs or symptoms of serotonin syndrome occur.
- Caution patient not to use frovatriptan if pregnancy is planned or suspected, or if breast feeding. Adequate contraception should be used during therapy.

Evaluation/Desired Outcomes

- Relief of migraine attack.

furosemide (fur-oh-se-mide)

Lasix

Classification

Therapeutic: diuretics

Pharmacologic: loop diuretics

Pregnancy Category C

Indications

Edema due to heart failure, hepatic impairment or renal disease. Hypertension.

Action

Inhibits the reabsorption of sodium and chloride from the loop of Henle and distal renal tubule. Increases renal excretion of water, sodium, chloride, magnesium, potassium, and calcium. Effectiveness persists in impaired renal function. **Therapeutic Effects:** Diuresis and subsequent mobilization of excess fluid (edema, pleural effusions). Decreased BP.

Pharmacokinetics

Absorption: 60–67% absorbed after oral administration (↓ in acute HF and in renal failure); also absorbed from IM sites.

Distribution: Crosses placenta, enters breast milk.

Protein Binding: 91–99%.

Metabolism and Excretion: Minimally metabolized by liver, some nonhepatic metabolism, some renal excretion as unchanged drug.

Half-life: 30–60 min (↑ in renal impairment).

TIME/ACTION PROFILE (diuretic effect)

ROUTE	ONSET	PEAK	DURATION
PO	30–60 min	1–2 hr	6–8 hr
IM	10–30 min	unknown	4–8 hr
IV	5 min	30 min	2 hr

Contraindications/Precautions

Contraindicated in: Hypersensitivity; Cross-sensitivity with thiazides and sulfonamides may occur; Hepatic coma or anuria; Some liquid products may contain alcohol, avoid in patients with alcohol intolerance.

Use Cautiously in: Severe liver disease (may precipitate hepatic coma; concurrent use with potassium-sparing diuretics may be necessary); Electrolyte depletion; Diabetes mellitus; Hypoproteinemia (↑ risk of ototoxicity); Severe renal impairment (↑ risk of ototoxicity); OB, Lactation: Safety not established; Pedi: ↑ risk for renal calculi and patent ductus arteriosis in premature neonates; Geri: May have ↑ risk of side effects, especially hypotension and electrolyte imbalance, at usual doses.

Adverse Reactions/Side Effects

CNS: blurred vision, dizziness, headache, vertigo. **EENT:** hearing loss, tinnitus. **CV:** hypotension. **GI:** anorexia, constipation, diarrhea, dry mouth, dyspepsia, ↑ liver enzymes, nausea, pancreatitis, vomiting. **GU:** ↑ BUN, excessive urination, nephrocalcinosis. **Derm:** ERYTHEMA MULTIFORME, STEVENS-JOHNSON SYNDROME, TOXIC EPIDERMAL NECROLYSIS, photosensitivity, pruritis, rash, urticaria. **Endo:** hypercholesterolemia, hyperglycemia, hypertriglyceridemia, hyperuricemia. **F and E:** dehydration, hypocalcemia, hypochloremia, hypokalemia, hypomagnesemia, hyponatremia, hypovolemia, metabolic alkalosis. **Hemat:** APLASTIC ANEMIA, AGRANULOCYTOSIS, hemolytic anemia, leukopenia, thrombocytopenia. **MS:** muscle cramps. **Neuro:** paresthesia. **Misc:** fever.

Interactions

Drug-Drug: ↑ risk of hypotension with **antihypertensives**, **nitrates**, or acute ingestion of **alcohol**. ↑ risk of hypokalemia with other **diuretics**, **amphotericin B**, **stimulant laxatives**, and **corticosteroids**. Hypokalemia may ↑ risk of **digoxin** toxicity and ↑ risk of arrhythmia in patients taking drugs that prolong the QT interval. ↓ **lithium** excretion, may cause **lithium** toxicity. ↑ risk of ototoxicity with **aminoglycosides** or **cisplatin**. ↑ risk of nephrotoxicity with **cisplatin**. **NSAIDS**↓ effects of furosemide. May ↑ risk of **methotrexate** toxicity. ↓ effects of furosemide when given at same time as **sucralfate**, **cholestyramine**,or **colestipol**. ↑ risk of **salicylate** toxicity (with use of high-dose **salicylate** therapy).

Concurrent use with **cyclosporine** may ↑ risk of gouty arthritis.

Route/Dosage

Edema

PO (Adults): 20–80 mg/day as a single dose initially, may repeat in 6–8 hr; may ↑ dose by 20–40 mg q 6–8 hr until desired response. Maintenance doses may be given once or twice daily (doses up to 2.5 g/day have been used in patients with HF or renal disease). *Hypertension*—40 twice daily initially (when added to regimen, ↓ dose of other antihypertensives by 50%); adjust further dosing based on response; *Hypercalcemia*—120 mg/day in 1–3 doses.
PO (Children > 1 mo): 2 mg/kg as a single dose; may be ↑ by 1–2 mg/kg q 6–8 hr (maximum dose = 6 mg/kg).
PO (Neonates): 1–4 mg/kg/dose 1–2 times/day.
IM, IV (Adults): 20–40 mg, may repeat in 1–2 hr and ↑ by 20 mg every 1–2 hr until response is obtained, maintenance dose may be given q 6–12 hr; *Continuous infusion*—Bolus 0.1 mg/kg followed by 0.1 mg/kg/hr, double q 2 hr to a maximum of 0.4 mg/kg/hr.
IM, IV (Children): 1–2 mg/kg/dose q 6–12 hr *Continuous infusion*—0.05 mg/kg/hr, titrate to clinical effect.
IM, IV (Neonates): 1–2 mg/kg/dose q 12–24 hr.

Hypertension

PO (Adults): 40 twice daily initially (when added to regimen, ↓ dose of other antihypertensives by 50%); adjust further dosing based on response.

Availability (generic available)

Tablets: 20 mg, 40 mg, 80 mg, ✤500 mg. **Cost:** *Generic*—20 mg $6.50/100, 40 mg $7.11/100, 80 mg $10.83/100. **Oral solution (10 mg/mL—orange flavor, 8 mg/mL—pineapple—peach flavor):** 8 mg/mL, 10 mg/mL. **Cost:** *Generic*—10 mg/mL $10.40/60 mL. **Solution for injection:** 10 mg/mL.

NURSING IMPLICATIONS

Assessment

- Assess fluid status. Monitor daily weight, intake and output ratios, amount and location of edema, lung sounds, skin turgor, and mucous membranes. Notify health care professional if thirst, dry mouth, lethargy, weakness, hypotension, or oliguria occurs.
- Monitor BP and pulse before and during administration. Monitor frequency of prescription refills to determine compliance in patients treated for hypertension.
- Geri: Diuretic use is associated with increased risk for falls in older adults. Assess falls risk and implement fall prevention strategies.
- Assess patients receiving digoxin for anorexia, nausea, vomiting, muscle cramps, paresthesia, and confusion. Patients taking digoxin are at increased risk of digoxin toxicity because of the potassium-depleting effect of the diuretic. Potassium supplements or potassium-sparing diuretics may be used concurrently to prevent hypokalemia.
- Assess patient for tinnitus and hearing loss. Audiometry is recommended for patients receiving prolonged high-dose IV therapy. Hearing loss is most common after rapid or high-dose IV administration in patients with decreased renal function or those taking other ototoxic drugs.
- Assess for allergy to sulfonamides.
- Assess patient for skin rash frequently during therapy. Discontinue furosemide at first sign of rash; may be life-threatening. Stevens-Johnson syndrome, toxic epidermal necrolysis, or erythema multiforme may develop. Treat symptomatically; may recur once treatment is stopped.
- ***Lab Test Considerations:*** Monitor electrolytes, renal and hepatic function, serum glucose, and uric acid levels before and periodically throughout therapy. Commonly ↓ serum potassium. May cause ↓ serum sodium, calcium, and magnesium concentrations. May also cause ↑ BUN, serum glucose, creatinine, and uric acid levels.

Potential Nursing Diagnoses

Excess fluid volume (Indications)
Deficient fluid volume (Side Effects)

Implementation

- Do not confuse Lasix with Luvox.
- If administering twice daily, give last dose no later than 5 PM to minimize disruption of sleep cycle.
- IV route is preferred over IM route for parenteral administration.
- **PO:** May be taken with food or milk to minimize gastric irritation. Tablets may be crushed if patient has difficulty swallowing.
- Do not administer discolored solution or tablets.

IV Administration

- **IV Push: *Diluent:*** Administer undiluted (larger doses may be diluted and administered as intermittent infusion [see below]). ***Concentration:*** 10 mg/mL. ***Rate:*** Administer at a rate of 20 mg/min. Pedi: Administer at a maximum rate of 0.5–1 mg/kg/min (for doses <120 mg) with infusion not exceeding 10 min.
- **Intermittent Infusion: *Diluent:*** Dilute larger doses in 50 mL of D5W, D10W, D20W, D5/0.9% NaCl, D5/LR, 0.9% NaCl, 3% NaCl, or LR. Infusion stable for 24 hr at room temperature. Do not refrigerate. Protect from light. ***Concentration:*** 1 mg/mL. ***Rate:*** Administer at a rate not to exceed 4 mg/

min (for doses > 120 mg) in adults to prevent ototoxicity. Pedi: not to exceed 1 mg/kg/min with infusion not exceeding 10 min. Use an infusion pump to ensure accurate dose.

- **Y-Site Compatibility:** acyclovir, alfentanil, allopurinol, alprostadil, amifostine, amikacin, aminocaproic acid, aminophylline, amphotericin B cholesteryl, amphotericin B lipid complex, amphotericin B liposome, anidulafungin, argatroban, ascorbic acid, atropine, azathioprine, aztreonam, bivalirudin, bleomycin, bumetanide, calcium chloride, calcium gluconate, carboplatin, carmustine, cefazolin, cefepime, cefotaxime, cefotetan, cefoxitin, ceftaroline, ceftazidime, ceftriaxone, cefuroxime, chloramphenicol, cisplatin, cladribine, clindamycin, cyanocobalamin, cyclophosphamide, cyclosporine, cytarabine, dactinomycin, daptomycin, dexamethasone, dexmedetomidine, digoxin, docetaxel, doripenem, doxacurium, doxorubicin liposome, enalaprilat, ephedrine, epinephrine, epoetin alfa, ertapenem, esomeprazole, etoposide, etoposide phosphate, fentanyl, fludarabine, fluorouracil, folic acid, foscarnet, ganciclovir, granisetron, hydrocortisone sodium succinate, hydromorphone, ibuprofen, ifosfamide, imipenem/cilastatin, indomethacin, ketorolac, leucovorin calcium, lidocaine, linezolid, lorazepam, mannitol, mechlorethamine, melphalan, meropenem, methotrexate, methylprednisolone, metoprolol, metronidazole, micafungin, mitomycin, multivitamins, nafcillin, naloxone, nitroprusside, octreotide, oxacillin, oxaliplatin, oxytocin, paclitaxel, palonosetron, pamidronate, pemetrexed, penicillin G, pentobarbital, phenobarbital, phytonadione, piperacillin/tazobactam, potassium acetate, potassium chloride, procainamide, propofol, propranolol, ranitidine, remifentanil, sargramostim, sodium acetate, sodium bicarbonate, streptokinase, succinylcholine, sufentanil, teniposide, theophylline, thiotepa, tigecycline, tirofiban, tobramycin, vitamin B complex with C, voriconazole, zoledronic acid.
- **Y-Site Incompatibility:** alemtuzumab, amsacrine, atracurium, benztropine, butorphanol, caspofungin, chlorpromazine, ciprofloxacin, dantrolene, dexrazoxane, diazepam, diazoxide, diltiazem, diphenhydramine, dolasetron, doxycycline, droperidol, epirubicin, eptifibitide, erythromycin, esmolol, fenoldopam, filgrastim, gemcitabine, gentamicin, glycopyrrolate, haloperidol, hydroxyzine, idarubicin, irinotecan, ketamine, levofloxacin, metaraminol, methyldopate, midazolam, milrinone, mitoxantrone, moxifloxacin, mycophenolate, nalbuphine, nesiritide, nicardipine, ondansetron, pancuronium, papaverine, pentamidine, pentazocine, phentolamine, phenylephrine, phenytoin, prochlorperazine, promethazine, protamine, pyridoxime, quinupristin/dalfopristin, rituximab, rocuronium, telavancin, thiamine, trastuzumab, trimethoprim/sulfamethoxazole, vancomycin, vecuronium, verapamil, vinblastine, vinorelbine.

Patient/Family Teaching

- Instruct patient to take furosemide as directed. Take missed doses as soon as possible; do not double doses.
- Caution patient to change positions slowly to minimize orthostatic hypotension. Caution patient that the use of alcohol, exercise during hot weather, or standing for long periods during therapy may enhance orthostatic hypotension.
- Instruct patient to consult health care professional regarding a diet high in potassium (see Appendix J).
- Advise patient to contact health care professional of weight gain more than 3 lbs in 1 day.
- Instruct patient to notify health care professional of all Rx or OTC medications, vitamins, or herbal products being taken and to consult health care professional before taking any OTC medications concurrently with this therapy.
- Instruct patient to notify health care professional of medication regimen before treatment or surgery.
- Caution patient to use sunscreen and protective clothing to prevent photosensitivity reactions.
- Advise patient to contact health care professional immediately if rash, muscle weakness, cramps, nausea, dizziness, numbness, or tingling of extremities occurs.
- Advise diabetic patients to monitor blood glucose closely; may cause increased blood glucose levels.
- Emphasize the importance of routine follow-up examinations.
- Geri: Caution older patients or their caregivers about increased risk for falls. Suggest strategies for fall prevention.
- **Hypertension:** Advise patients on antihypertensive regimen to continue taking medication even if feeling better. Furosemide controls but does not cure hypertension.
- Reinforce the need to continue additional therapies for hypertension (weight loss, exercise, restricted sodium intake, stress reduction, regular exercise, moderation of alcohol consumption, cessation of smoking).

Evaluation/Desired Outcomes

- Decrease in edema.
- Decrease in abdominal girth and weight.
- Increase in urinary output.
- Decrease in BP.

gabapentin (ga-ba-**pen**-tin)

Gralise, Horizant, Neurontin

Classification

Therapeutic: analgesic adjuncts, therapeutic, anticonvulsants, mood stabilizers

Pregnancy Category C

Indications

Partial seizures (adjunct treatment) (immediate-release only). Postherpetic neuralgia. Restless legs syndrome (Horizant only). **Unlabeled Use:** Neuropathic pain. Prevention of migraine headache. Bipolar disorder. Anxiety. Diabetic peripheral neuropathy.

Action

Mechanism of action is not known. May affect transport of amino acids across and stabilize neuronal membranes. **Therapeutic Effects:** Decreased incidence of seizures. Decreased postherpetic pain. Decreased leg restlessness.

Pharmacokinetics

Absorption: Well absorbed after oral administration by active transport. At larger doses, transport becomes saturated and absorption ↓ (bioavailability ranges from 60% for a 300-mg dose to 35% for a 1600-mg dose).
Distribution: Crosses blood-brain barrier; enters breast milk.
Metabolism and Excretion: Eliminated mostly by renal excretion of unchanged drug.
Half-life: *Adults*—5–7 hr (normal renal function); up to 132 hr in anuria; *Children*—4.7 hr.

TIME/ACTION PROFILE (blood levels)

ROUTE	ONSET	PEAK	DURATION
PO-IR	rapid	2–4 hr	8 hr
PO-SR	unknown	5–8 hr	24 hr

Contraindications/Precautions

Contraindicated in: Hypersensitivity.
Use Cautiously in: All patients (may ↑ risk of suicidal thoughts/behaviors); Renal insufficiency (↓ dose and/or ↑ dosing interval if CCr ≤60 mL/min); OB: Pregnancy; Pedi: Children <18 yr (sustained-/extended-release) or <3 yr (immediate-release) (safety not established); Lactation: Discontinue drug or bottle-feed; Geri: May be more susceptible to toxicity due to age-related ↓ in renal function.

Adverse Reactions/Side Effects

CNS: SUICIDAL THOUGHTS, confusion, depression, dizziness, drowsiness, sedation, anxiety, concentration difficulties (children), emotional lability (children), hostility, hyperkinesia (children), malaise, vertigo, weakness. **EENT:** abnormal vision, nystagmus. **CV:** hypertension. **GI:** weight gain, anorexia, flatulence, gingivitis. **MS:** RHABDOMYOLYSIS, arthralgia, ↑ creatine kinase. **Neuro:** ataxia, altered reflexes, hyperkinesia, paresthesia. **Misc:** MULTIORGAN HYPERSENSITIVITY REACTIONS, facial edema.

Interactions

Drug-Drug: Antacids may ↓ absorption of gabapentin. ↑ risk of CNS depression with other **CNS depressants**, including **alcohol**, **antihistamines**, **opioids**, and **sedative/hypnotics**. **Morphine** ↑ gabapentin levels and may ↑ risk of toxicity, dosage adjustments may be required.
Drug-Natural Products: Kava-kava, **valerian**, or **chamomile** can ↑ CNS depression.

Route/Dosage

The sustained/extended-release formulations should not be interchanged with the immediate-release products.

Epilepsy

PO (Adults and Children >12 yr): 300 mg 3 times daily initially. Titration may be continued until desired (range is 900–1800 mg/day in 3 divided doses; doses should not be more than 12 hr apart). Doses up to 2400–3600 mg/day have been well tolerated.
PO (Children ≥5–12 yr): 10–15 mg/kg/day in 3 divided doses initially titrated upward over 3 days to 25–35 mg/kg/day in 3 divided doses; dosage interval should not exceed 12 hr (doses up to 50 mg/kg/day have been used).
PO (Children 3–4 yrs): 10–15 mg/kg/day in 3 divided doses initially titrated upward over 3 days to 40 mg/kg/day in 3 divided doses; dosage interval should not exceed 12 hr (doses up to 50 mg/kg/day have been used).

Renal Impairment

PO (Adults and Children >12 yr): *CCr 30–59 mL/min*—200–700 mg twice daily; *CCr 15–29 mL/min*—200–700 mg once daily; *CCr 15 mL/min*—100–300 mg once daily; *CCr <15 mL/min*—Reduce daily dose in proportion to CCr.

Postherpetic Neuralgia

PO (Adults): *Immediate-release*—300 mg once daily on first day, then 300 mg 2 times daily on second day, then 300 mg 3 times/day on day 3, may then be titrated upward as needed up to 600 mg 3 times/day; *Sustained-release (Gralise)*—300 mg once daily on first day, then 600 mg once daily on second day, then 900 mg once daily on days 3–6, then 1200 mg once daily on days 7–10, then 1500 mg once daily on days 11–14, then 1800 mg once daily thereafter; *Extended-release (Horizant)*—600 mg once daily in the morning on days 1–3, then 600 mg twice daily thereafter.

Renal Impairment

PO (Adults): *CCr 30–59 mL/min*—200–700 mg twice daily (immediate-release); 600–1800 mg once daily (sustained-release [Gralise]); 300 mg once daily in the morning on days 1–3, then 300 mg twice daily thereafter (may ↑ to 600 mg twice daily, as needed) (extended-release [Horizant]); *CCr 15–29 mL/min*—200–700 mg once daily (immediate-release); sustained release [Gralise] not recommended; 300 mg in the morning on days 1 and 3, then 300 mg once daily in the morning thereafter (may ↑ to 300 mg twice daily, as needed) (extended-release [Horizant]); *CCr 15 mL/min*—100–300 mg once daily (immediate-release); sustained release [Gralise] not recommended; *CCr <15 mL/min*—↓ daily dose in proportion to CCr (immediate release); sustained release [Gralise] not recommended; 300 mg every other day in the morning (may ↑ to 300 mg once daily in the morning, as needed) (extended-release [Horizant]); *CCr <15 mL/min (on hemodialysis)*—300 mg after each dialysis session (may ↑ to 600 mg after each dialysis sessions, as needed) (extended-release [Horizant]).

Restless Legs Syndrome

PO (Adults): *Extended-release (Horizant)*—600 mg once daily at 5 PM.

Renal Impairment

(Adults): *CCr 30–59 mL/min*—300 mg once daily at 5 PM; may ↑ to 600 mg once daily at 5 PM as needed; *CCr 15–29 mL/min*—300 mg once daily at 5 PM; *CCr <15 mL/min*—300 mg every other day; *CCr <15 mL/min (on hemodialysis)*—Not recommended.

Neuropathic Pain (unlabeled use)

PO (Adults): 100 mg 3 times daily initially. Titrate weekly by 300 mg/day up to 900–2400 mg/day (maximum: 3600 mg/day).

PO (Children): 5 mg/kg/dose at bedtime initially then ↑ to 5 mg/kg BID on day 2 and 5 mg/kg TID on day 3. Titrate to effect up to 8–35 mg/kg/day in 3 divided doses.

Availability (generic available)

Capsules: 100 mg, 300 mg, 400 mg. **Cost:** *Generic*—100 mg $11.45/100, 300 mg $15.18/100, 400 mg $12.36/100. **Tablets:** 600 mg, 800 mg. **Cost:** *Generic*—600 mg $33.96/100, 800 mg $49.20/100. **Extended-release tablets (Horizant):** 600 mg. **Sustained-release tablets (Gralise):** 300 mg, 600 mg. **Cost:** 300 mg $99.00/30, 600 mg $329.40/90. **Oral solution (cool strawberry anise flavor):** 250 mg/5 mL. **Cost:** *Generic*—$148.91/470 mL.

NURSING IMPLICATIONS

Assessment

- Monitor closely for notable changes in behavior that could indicate the emergence or worsening of suicidal thoughts or behavior or depression.
- **Seizures:** Assess location, duration, and characteristics of seizure activity.
- **Postherpetic Neuralgia & Neuropathic Pain:** Assess location, characteristics, and intensity of pain periodically during therapy.
- **Migraine Prophylaxis:** Monitor frequency and intensity of pain on pain scale.
- **Restless Leg Syndrome**Assess frequency and intensity of restless leg syndrome prior to and periodically during therapy.
- ***Lab Test Considerations:*** May cause false-positive readings when testing for urinary protein with *Ames N-Multistix SG* dipstick test; use sulfosalicylic acid precipitation procedure.
- May cause leukopenia.

Potential Nursing Diagnoses

Risk for injury (Side Effects)
Chronic pain (Indications)
Ineffective coping (Indications)

Implementation

- Doses of *Gralise* and *Horizant* are not interchangeable with other dose forms of gabapentin.
- **PO:** May be administered without regard to meals.
- 600-mg and 800-mg tablets are scored and can be broken to administer a half-tablet. If half-tablet is used, administer other half at the next dose. Discard half-tablets not used within several days.
- Administer *Gralise* with evening meal. Swallow tablet whole; do not crush, break, or chew.
- Administer *Horizant for Restless Leg Syndrome* with evening meal at 5 PM. *Horizant for Postherpetic Neuralgia* is administered twice daily. Swallow tablet whole; do not crush, break, or chew.
- Gabapentin should be discontinued gradually over at least 1 wk. If dose is 600 mg/day, may discontinue without tapering. If >600 m g/day, titrate daily to 600 mg for 1 week, then discontinue. If patient is taking 600 mg twice daily, taper to once daily before discontinuing. Abrupt discontinuation may cause increase in seizure frequency.

Patient/Family Teaching

- Instruct patient to take medication exactly as directed. Patients on tid dosing should not exceed 12 hr between doses. Take missed doses as soon as possible; if less than 2 hr until next dose, take dose immediately and take next dose 1–2 hr later, then resume regular dosing schedule. Do not double dose. Do not discontinue abruptly; may cause increase in frequency of seizures. Instruct patient to read the *Medication Guide* before starting and with each Rx refill, as changes may occur.
- Advise patient not to take gabapentin within 2 hr of an antacid.
- Gabapentin may cause dizziness and drowsiness. Caution patient to avoid driving or activities requiring alertness until response to medication is known. Seizure patients should not resume driving until phy-

sician gives clearance based on control of seizure disorder.
- Advise patient and family to notify health care professional if thoughts about suicide or dying, attempts to commit suicide; new or worse depression; new or worse anxiety; feeling very agitated or restless; panic attacks; trouble sleeping; new or worse irritability; acting aggressive; being angry or violent; acting on dangerous impulses; an extreme increase in activity and talking; or other unusual changes in behavior or mood occur.
- Instruct patient to notify health care professional of medication regimen before treatment or surgery.
- Advise female patient to notify health care professional if pregnancy is planned or suspected or if breast feeding.
- Advise patient to carry identification describing disease process and medication regimen at all times.

Evaluation/Desired Outcomes
- Decreased frequency of or cessation of seizures.
- Decreased postherpetic neuralgia pain.
- Decreased intensity of neuropathic pain.
- Decreased frequency of migraine headaches.
- Increased mood stability.
- Decrease effects of restless leg syndrome.

galantamine
(ga-**lant**-a-meen)
Razadyne, Razadyne ER, Reminyl ER

Classification
Therapeutic: anti-Alzheimer's agents
Pharmacologic: cholinergics (cholinesterase inhibitors)

Pregnancy Category B

Indications
Mild to moderate dementia/neurocognitive disorder of the Alzheimer's type.

Action
Enhances cholinergic function by reversible inhibition of cholinesterase. **Therapeutic Effects:** Decreased dementia/cognitive decline (temporary) associated with Alzheimer's disease. Cognitive enhancer.

Pharmacokinetics
Absorption: Well absorbed (90%) following oral administration.
Distribution: Unknown.
Metabolism and Excretion: Mostly metabolized by the liver (primarily by CYP2D6 and CYP3A4 isoenzymes); the CYP2D6 enzyme system exhibits genetic polymorphism; ~7% of population may be poor metabolizers (PMs) and may have significantly ↑ galantamine concentrations and an ↑ risk of adverse effects. 20% excreted unchanged in urine.
Half-life: 7 hr.

TIME/ACTION PROFILE (antihcholinesterase activity)

ROUTE	ONSET	PEAK	DURATION
PO	unknown	1 hr	12 hr
PO-ER	unknown	1 hr	24 hr

Contraindications/Precautions
Contraindicated in: Hypersensitivity; Severe hepatic or renal impairment; Pedi, Lactation: Children or lactation.
Use Cautiously in: Patients with supraventricular cardiac conduction defects or concurrent use of drugs that may slow heart rate (↑ risk of bradycardia); History of ulcer disease/GI bleeding/concurrent NSAID use; Severe asthma or obstructive pulmonary disease; Mild to moderate renal impairment (avoid use if CCr <9 mL/min); Mild to moderate hepatic impairment (cautious dose titration recommended); May ↑ risk of cardiovascular mortality; OB: Use only if potential benefit outweighs potential risk to fetus.

Adverse Reactions/Side Effects
CNS: fatigue, dizziness, headache, syncope. **CV:** bradycardia, chest pain. **GI:** anorexia, diarrhea, dyspepsia, flatulence, nausea, vomiting. **GU:** bladder outflow obstruction, incontinence. **Neuro:** tremor. **Derm:** STEVENS-JOHNSON SYNDROME, ACUTE GENERALIZED EXANTHEMATOUS PUSTULOSIS. **Misc:** weight loss.

Interactions
Drug-Drug: Will ↑ neuromuscular blockade from **succinylcholine-type neuromuscular blocking agents**. May ↑ effects of other **cholinesterase inhibitors** or other **cholinergic agonists**, including **bethanechol**. May ↓ effectiveness of **anticholinergic medications**. Blood levels and effects may be ↑ by **ketoconazole**, **paroxetine**, **amitriptyline**, **fluvoxamine**, or **quinidine**.

Route/Dosage
PO (Adults): *Immediate-release tablets*—4 mg twice daily initially, dose increments of 4 mg should be made at 4 wk intervals, up to 12 mg twice daily. Doses up to 16 mg twice daily have been used (range 16–32 mg/day; *Extended-release capsules*—8 mg/day as a single dose in the morning, may be ↑ to 16 mg/day after 4 wk, then up to 24 mg/day after 4 wk; increments based on benefit/tolerability.

Renal Impairment
PO (Adults): *Moderate renal impairment*—Daily dose should not exceed 16 mg.

Hepatic Impairment

PO (Adults): *Moderate hepatic impairment*—Daily dose should not exceed 16 mg.

Availability (generic available)

Immediate-release tablets: 4 mg, 8 mg, 12 mg. **Extended-release capsules:** 8 mg, 16 mg, 24 mg. **Oral solution:** 4 mg/mL.

NURSING IMPLICATIONS

Assessment

- Assess cognitive function (memory, attention, reasoning, language, ability to perform simple tasks) periodically during therapy.
- Monitor heart rate periodically during therapy. May cause bradycardia.

Potential Nursing Diagnoses

Disturbed thought process (Indications)
Risk for injury (Indications)
Impaired environmental interpretation syndrome (Indications)

Implementation

- Do not confuse Razadyne with Rozerem (ramelteon).
- Patient should be maintained on a stable dose for a minimum of 4 wk prior to increasing dose.
- If dose has been interrupted for several days or longer, restart at the lowest dose and escalate to the current dose.
- **PO:** Administer twice daily, preferably with morning and evening meal. Administration with food, the use of antiemetic medications, and ensuring adequate fluid intake may decrease nausea and vomiting.
- Administer extended-release capsules in the morning, preferably with food. Swallow whole; do not open, crush, or chew.
- Use pipette provided with oral solution to administer accurate amount.

Patient/Family Teaching

- Emphasize the importance of taking galantamine daily, as directed. Instruct patient and/or caregiver in correct use of pipette if using oral solution. Skip missed doses and return to regular schedule the following day; do not double doses. Do not discontinue abruptly; although no increase in frequency of adverse events may occur, beneficial affects of galantamine are lost when the drug is discontinued.
- Caution patient and caregiver that galantamine may cause dizziness. Monitor and assist with ambulation and caution patient to avoid driving and other activities requiring alertness until response to medication is known.
- Instruct patient to maintain adequate fluid intake during therapy.
- Advise patient and caregiver to stop taking galantamine and notify health care professional immediately if rash occurs.
- Advise patient and caregiver to notify health care professional if nausea or vomiting persists beyond 7 days or if new symptoms occur or previously noted symptoms increase in severity.
- Advise patient and caregiver to notify health care professional of medication regimen prior to treatment or surgery.
- Emphasize the importance of follow-up exams to monitor progress.
- Teach patient and caregivers that improvements in cognitive functioning may take weeks to months to stabilize.
- Caution that disease is not cured and degenerative process is not reversed.

Evaluation/Desired Outcomes

- Improvement in cognitive function (memory, attention, reasoning, language, ability to perform simple tasks) in patients with Alzheimer's disease.

ganciclovir (gan-**sye**-kloe-vir)

Cytovene

Classification
Therapeutic: antivirals

Pregnancy Category C

Indications

IV: Treatment of cytomegalovirus (CMV) retinitis in immunocompromised patients, including HIV-infected patients (may be used with foscarnet). Prevention of CMV infection in transplant patients at risk. Congenital CMV infection in neonates.

Action

CMV converts ganciclovir to its active form (ganciclovir phosphate) inside the host cell, where it inhibits viral DNA polymerase. **Therapeutic Effects:** Antiviral effect directed preferentially against CMV-infected cells.

Pharmacokinetics

Absorption: IV administration results in complete bioavailability.
Distribution: Widely distributed; enters CSF.
Protein Binding: 1–2%.
Metabolism and Excretion: 90% excreted unchanged by the kidneys.
Half-life: *Adults:* 2.9 hr; *Children 9 mo–12 yr:* 2.4 ± 0.7 hr; *Neonates:* 2.4 hr (↑ in renal impairment).

TIME/ACTION PROFILE (antiviral levels)

ROUTE	ONSET	PEAK	DURATION
IV	rapid	end of infusion	12–24 hr

Contraindications/Precautions

Contraindicated in: Hypersensitivity to ganciclovir or acyclovir; Bone marrow depression or immunosuppression or thrombocytopenia (do not administer if ANC <500/mm³ or platelet count <25,000/mm³).

Use Cautiously in: Renal impairment (dose ↓ required if CCr <80 mL/min); Geri: Dose ↓ recommended.

Adverse Reactions/Side Effects

CNS: SEIZURES, abnormal dreams, coma, confusion, dizziness, drowsiness, headache, malaise, nervousness. **Resp:** dyspnea. **CV:** arrhythmias, edema, hypertension, hypotension. **GI:** GI BLEEDING, abdominal pain, ↑ liver enzymes, nausea, vomiting. **GU:** gonadal suppression, hematuria, renal toxicity. **Derm:** alopecia, photosensitivity, pruritus, rash, urticaria. **Endo:** hypoglycemia. **Hemat:** neutropenia, thrombocytopenia, anemia, eosinophilia. **Local:** pain/phlebitis at IV site. **Neuro:** ataxia, tremor. **Misc:** fever.

Interactions

Drug-Drug: ↑ risk of bone marrow depression with **antineoplastics**, **radiation therapy**, or **zidovudine**. Toxicity may be ↑ by **probenecid**. ↑ risk of seizures with **imipenem/cilastatin**. Concurrent use of other **nephrotoxic drugs**, **cyclosporine**, or **amphotericin B** ↑ risk of nephrotoxicity.

Route/Dosage

IV (Adults and Children >3 mo): *Induction*—5 mg/kg q 12 hr for 14–21 days. *Maintenance regimen*—5 mg/kg/day or 6 mg/kg for 5 days of each week. If progression occurs, ↑ to q 12 hr regimen. *Prevention*—5 mg/kg q 12 hr for 7–14 days, then 5 mg/kg/day or 6 mg/kg for 5 days of each week.

IV (Neonates): *Congenital CMV infection*—12 mg/kg/day divided q 12 hr x 6 weeks.

Renal Impairment

IV (Adults and Children): *Induction*—CCr 50–69 mL/min: 2.5 mg/kg/dose q 12 hr; CCr 25–49 mL/min: 2.5 mg/kg/dose q 24 hr; CCr 10–24 mL/min: 1.25 mg/kg/dose q 24 hr; CCr <10 mL/min: 1.25 mg/kg 3 times/week after hemodialysis; *Maintenance*—CCr 50–69 mL/min: 2.5 mg/kg/dose q 24 hr; CCr 25–49 mL/min: 1.25 mg/kg/dose q 24 hr; CCr 10–24 mL/min: 0.625 mg/kg/dose q 24 hr; CCr <10 mL/min: 0.625 mg/kg 3 times/week after hemodialysis.

Availability (generic available)

Powder for injection: 500 mg/vial.

NURSING IMPLICATIONS

Assessment

- Diagnosis of CMV retinitis should be determined by ophthalmoscopy before treatment with ganciclovir.
- Culture for CMV (urine, blood, throat) may be taken before administration. However, a negative CMV culture does not rule out CMV retinitis. If symptoms do not respond after several weeks, resistance to ganciclovir may have occurred. Ophthalmologic exams should be performed weekly during induction and every 2 wk during maintenance or more frequently if the macula or optic nerve is threatened. Progression of CMV retinitis may occur during or after ganciclovir treatment.
- Assess for signs of infection (fever, chills, cough, hoarseness, lower back or side pain, sore throat, difficult or painful urination). Notify health care professional if these symptoms occur.
- Assess for bleeding (bleeding gums, bruising, petechiae; guaiac stools, urine, and emesis). Avoid IM injections and taking rectal temperatures. Apply pressure to venipuncture sites for 10 min.
- ***Lab Test Considerations:*** Monitor neutrophil and platelet count at least every 2 days during bid therapy and weekly thereafter. Granulocytopenia usually occurs during the first 2 wk of treatment but may occur anytime during therapy. Do not administer if neutrophil count <500/mm³ or platelet count <25,000/mm³. Recovery begins within 3–7 days of discontinuation of therapy.
- Monitor BUN and serum creatinine at least once every 2 wk throughout therapy.
- Monitor liver function tests (AST, ALT, serum bilirubin, alkaline phosphatase) periodically during therapy. May cause ↑ levels.
- May cause ↓ blood glucose.

Potential Nursing Diagnoses

Risk for infection (Indications, Patient/Family Teaching)

Implementation

- Do not confuse Cytovene (ganciclovir) with Cytosar (cytarabine).
- Prepare solution in a biologic cabinet. Wear gloves, gown, and mask while handling medication. Discard IV equipment in specially designated containers.
- Do not administer subcut or IM; severe tissue irritation may result.
- **IV:** Observe infusion site for phlebitis. Rotate infusion site to prevent phlebitis.
- Maintain adequate hydration throughout therapy.

IV Administration

- **Intermittent Infusion:** Reconstitute 500 mg with 10 mL of sterile water for injection for a concentration of 50 mg/mL. Do not reconstitute with bacteriostatic water with parabens; precipitation will occur. Shake well to dissolve completely. Discard vial if particulate matter or discoloration occurs. Reconstituted solution is stable for 12 hr at room temperature; do not refrigerate.
- ***Diluent:*** Dilute in 100 mL of D5W, 0.9% NaCl, Ringer's or LR. Once diluted for infusion, solution should be used within 24 hr. Refrigerate but do not

freeze. ***Concentration:*** 10 mg/mL. ***Rate:*** Administer slowly, via infusion pump, over 1 hr using an in-line filter. Rapid administration may increase toxicity.

- **Y-Site Compatibility:** alemtuzumab, alfentanyl, allopurinol, amphotericin B cholesteryl, amphotericin B lipid complex, anidulafungin, argatroban, atropine, azithromycin, bivalirudin, bleomycin, calcium chloride, calcium gluconate, carboplatin, carmustine, caspofungin, cisplatin, cyanocobalamin, cyclophosphamide, cyclosporine, dactinomycin, daptomycin, dexamethasone, dexmedetomidine, digoxin, docetaxel, doxacurium, doxorubicin liposome, enalaprilat, epoetin alfa, eptifibatide, ertapenem, etoposide, etoposide phosphate, fentanyl, filgrastim, fluconazole, fluorouracil, folic acid, furosemide, glycopyrrolate, granisetron, heparin, hetastarch, hydromorphone, ifosfamide, indomethacin, insulin, labetalol, leucovorin calcium, linezolid, lorazepam, mannitol, mechlorethamine, melphalan, methotrexate, metoprolol, milrinone, mitoxantrone, nafcillin, naloxone, nesiritide, nitroglycerin, nitroprusside, octreotide, oxytocin, paclitaxel, pancuronium, pantoprazole, pemetrexed, pentobarbital, phenobarbital, phytonadione, potassium chloride, propofol, propranolol, protamine, ranitidine, remifentanil, rituximab, rocuronium, sodium acetate, sufentanil, teniposide, thiotepa, tigecycline, tirofiban, trastuzumab, vasopressin, vinblastine, vincristine, voriconazole, zoledronic acid.
- **Y-Site Incompatibility:** aldesleukin, amifostine, amikacin, aminophylline, amphotericin B colloidal, ampicillin, ampicillin/sulbactam, amsacrine, ascorbic acid, atracurium, azathioprine, aztreonam, benztropine, bumetanide, butorphanol, cefazolin, cefepime, cefotaxime, cefotetan, cefoxitin, ceftazidime, ceftriaxone, cefuroxime, chloramphenicol, chlorpromazine, clindamycin, cytarabine, dantrolene, dexrazoxane, diazepam, diazoxide, diltiazem, diphenhydramine, dobutamine, dolasetron, dopamine, doxorubicin, doxycycline, ephedrine, epinephrine, epirubicin, erythromycin, esmolol, famotidine, fenoldopam, fludarabine, foscarnet, gemcitabine, gentamicin, haloperidol, hydralazine, hydrocortisone, hydroxyzine, idarubicin, imipenem/cilastatin, irinotecan, isoproterenol, ketorolac, levofloxacin, lidocaine, magnesium sulfate, meperidine, metaraminol, methyldopa, methylprednisolone, metoclopramide, metronidazole, midazolam, morphine, multivitamins, mycophenolate, nalbuphine, nicardipine, norepinephrine, ondansetron, oxacillin, palonosetron, papaverine, penicillin G, pentamidine, pentazocine, phentolamine, phenylephrine, phenytoin, piperacillin/tazobactam, potassium acetate, procainamide, prochlorperazine, promethazine, pyridoxime, quinupristin/dalfopristin, sargramostim, sodium bicarbonate, streptokinase, succinylcholine, tacrolimus, theophylline, thiamine, tobramycin, tolazoline, trimethoprim/sulfamethoxazole, vancomycin, vecuronium, verapamil, vinorelbine.

Patient/Family Teaching

- Inform patient that ganciclovir is not a cure for CMV retinitis. Progression of retinitis may continue in immunocompromised patients during and after therapy. Advise patients to have regular ophthalmic exams at least every 6 wk. Duration of therapy for CMV prevention is based on the duration and degree of immunosuppression.
- Advise patient to notify health care professional if fever; chills; sore throat; other signs of infection; bleeding gums; bruising; petechiae; or blood in urine, stool, or emesis occurs. Caution patient to avoid crowds and persons with known infections. Instruct patient to use soft toothbrush and electric razor. Patient should be cautioned not to drink alcoholic beverages or take products containing aspirin or NSAIDs.
- Advise patient that ganciclovir may have teratogenic effects. A nonhormonal method of contraception should be used during and for at least 90 days after therapy.
- Caution patient to use sunscreen and protective clothing to prevent photosensitivity reactions.
- Emphasize the importance of frequent follow-up exams to monitor blood counts.

Evaluation/Desired Outcomes

- Treatment of the symptoms of CMV retinitis in immunocompromised patients.
- Prevention of CMV retinitis in transplant patients at risk.

gefitinib (je-fit-in-ib)

Iressa

Classification

Therapeutic: antineoplastics

Pharmacologic: enzyme inhibitors

Pregnancy Category D

Indications

First-line treatment of patients with metastatic non–small-cell lung cancer (NSCLC) whose tumors have epidermal growth factor receptor (EGFR) exon 19 deletions or exon 21 (L858R) substitution mutations.

Action

Inhibits activation of kinases found in transmembrane cell surface receptors, including EGFR. **Therapeutic Effects:** Prolonged progression-free survival.

Pharmacokinetics

Absorption: 60% absorbed following oral administration.

Distribution: Extensively distributed.

Metabolism and Excretion: Mostly metabolized by the liver (CYP3A4 enzyme system); excreted in feces, <4% excreted in urine.
Half-life: 48 hr.

TIME/ACTION PROFILE (plasma levels)

ROUTE	ONSET	PEAK	DURATION
PO	unknown	3–7 hr	unknown

Contraindications/Precautions

Contraindicated in: Hypersensitivity; OB: May cause fetal harm; Lactation: Safety not established; Pedi: Safety and effectiveness not established.
Use Cautiously in: Idiopathic pulmonary fibrosis (↑ risk of pulmonary toxicity); Concurrent use of strong inhibitors of the CYP3A4 enzyme system (may ↑ risk of toxicity); OB: Women with childbearing potential.

Adverse Reactions/Side Effects

EENT: aberrant eyelash growth, blepharitis, conjunctivitis, corneal erosion/ulcer, dry eye, nose bleeding. **Resp:** INTERSTITIAL LUNG DISEASE, dyspnea. **GI:** GI PERFORATION, HEPATOTOXICITY, anorexia, diarrhea, nausea, vomiting, dry mouth, mouth ulceration. **GU:** ↓ fertility (females), hematuria, ↑ serum creatinine. **Derm:** ERYTHEMA MULTIFORME, STEVENS-JOHNSON SYNDROME, TOXIC EPIDERMAL NECROLYSIS, rash, alopecia, pruritus. **F and E:** dehydration. **Metab:** weight loss. **Misc:** allergic reactions including ANGIOEDEMA, fever.

Interactions

Drug-Drug: Strong inducers of the CYP3A4 enzyme system, including **rifampin** and **phenytoin**, ↓ blood levels and effects (↑ dose of gefitinib to 500 mg/day). Strong inhibitors of the CYP3A4 enzyme system, including **ketoconazole** and **itraconazole**, ↑ blood levels and effects. Absorption and efficacy may be ↓ by **drugs that ↑ gastric pH** including **H_2 receptor antagonist**, **proton pump inhibitors**, and **antacids**; take geftinib 12 hr after last dose or 12 hr before the next dose of proton pump inhibitor; take geftinib 6 hr after last dose or 6 hr before next dose H_2 receptor antagonist or antacid. May ↑ the risk of bleeding with **warfarin**.

Route/Dosage

PO (Adults): 250 mg once daily; *Concurrent use of rifampin or phenytoin*—500 mg once daily (resume 250 mg once daily dose 7 days after discontinuing strong CYP3A4 inducer).

Availability

Tablets: 250 mg.

NURSING IMPLICATIONS

Assessment

- Assess for signs of pulmonary toxicity (dyspnea, cough, fever). Withhold gefitinib during diagnosis. If interstitial lung disease is confirmed, discontinue gefitinib and treat appropriately.
- Assess patient for eye symptoms such as pain during therapy. May require interruption of therapy and removal of aberrant eyelash. After symptoms and eye changes have resolved, may reinstate therapy.
- Monitor for rash. Interrupt or discontinue therapy if severe bullous, blistering or exfoliating conditions develop.
- ***Lab Test Considerations:*** Monitor liver function tests periodically. May cause ↑ transaminases, bilirubin, and alkaline phosphatase. Withhold gefitinib in patients with worsening liver function tests; discontinue gefitinib if elevations are severe.
- Monitor for changes in prothrombin time and INR in patients taking warfarin. May cause ↑ levels.

Potential Nursing Diagnoses

Diarrhea (Adverse Reactions)
Impaired skin integrity (Side Effects)
Ineffective breathing pattern (Adverse Reactions)

Implementation

- Available only through the *Iressa Access Program*. Patients must be currently on the medication or in an approved study and must sign the Patient Consent Form. Physicians and prescribers must enroll in program.
- 🧬 FDA-approved test must be used to detect of EGFR mutations in NSCLC. Patients must have EGFR exon 19 deletions or exon 21 substitutions use gefitinib.
- **PO:** Administer one tablet daily without regard to food. Tablets can also be dispersed in half a glass of drinking water (noncarbonated). No other liquids should be used. Drop the tablet in the water, without crushing it, stir until the tablet is dispersed (approximately 10 min), and drink the liquid immediately. Rinse the glass with half a glass of water and drink. The liquid can also be administered through a nasogastric tube.
- May interrupt therapy briefly (14 days) for patients with poorly tolerated diarrhea with dehydration or skin adverse reactions. Follow by restarting 250 mg dose.

Patient/Family Teaching

- Instruct patient to take gefitinib as directed. Take missed doses up to 12 hrs of next dose. Advise patient to read the *Instruction Sheet* with each Rx refill; new information may be available.
- Advise patient to notify health care professional promptly if severe persistent diarrhea, nausea, vomiting, or anorexia occur; if shortness of breath or cough occur or worsen; or if eye irritation or other new symptoms develop.
- Rep: Instruct female patient to use effective contraception during and for 2 wks after last dose and no-

tify health care professional if pregnancy is suspected or if breast feeding.

Evaluation/Desired Outcomes

- Decrease in size and spread of tumors in non-small-cell lung cancer.

HIGH ALERT

gemcitabine (jem-**site**-a-been)

Gemzar

Classification

Therapeutic: antineoplastics

Pharmacologic: antimetabolites, nucleoside analogues

Pregnancy Category D

Indications

Pancreatic cancer (locally advanced or metastatic). Inoperable locally advanced/metastatic non–small-cell lung cancer (with cisplatin). Metastatic breast cancer (with paclitaxel). Advanced ovarian cancer that has relapsed 6 mo after completion of platinum-based therapy (with carboplatin).

Action

Interferes with DNA synthesis (cell-cycle phase–specific). **Therapeutic Effects:** Death of rapidly replicating cells, particularly malignant ones.

Pharmacokinetics

Absorption: IV administration results in complete bioavailability.

Distribution: Unknown.

Metabolism and Excretion: Converted in cells to active diphosphate and triphosphate metabolites; these are excreted primarily by the kidneys.

Half-life: 32–94 min.

TIME/ACTION PROFILE (effect on blood counts)

ROUTE	ONSET	PEAK	DURATION
IV	unknown	unknown	unknown

Contraindications/Precautions

Contraindicated in: Hypersensitivity; OB: Can cause fetal malformation; Lactation: Can expose infant to serious adverse effects. Bottle-feed if gemcitabine therapy is necessary.

Use Cautiously in: History of cardiovascular disease; Impaired hepatic or renal function (↑ risk of toxicity); Other chronic debilitating illness; Rep: Patients with childbearing potential.

Adverse Reactions/Side Effects

CNS: POSTERIOR REVERSIBLE ENCEPHALOPATHY SYNDROME (PRES). **Resp:** PULMONARY TOXICITY, dyspnea, bronchospasm. **CV:** ARRHYTHMIAS, CAPILLARY LEAK SYNDROME, CEREBROVASCULAR ACCIDENT, MI, edema, hypertension. **GI:** HEPATOTOXICITY, diarrhea, ↑ liver enzymes, nausea, stomatitis, vomiting. **GU:** HEMOLYTIC UREMIC SYNDROME, hematuria, proteinuria. **Derm:** alopecia, rash. **Hemat:** anemia, leukopenia, thrombocytopenia. **Local:** injection site reactions. **Neuro:** paresthesias. **Misc:** flu-like symptoms, fever, anaphylactoid reactions.

Interactions

Drug-Drug: ↑ bone marrow depression with other **antineoplastics** or **radiation therapy**. May ↓ antibody response to **live virus vaccines** and ↑ risk of adverse reactions.

Route/Dosage

Other regimens are used.

Pancreatic Cancer

IV (Adults): 1000 mg/m^2 once weekly for 7 wk, followed by a week of rest. May be followed by cycles of once-weekly administration for 3 wk followed by a week of rest.

Non–Small-Cell Lung Cancer (with Cisplatin)

IV (Adults): 1000 mg/m^2 on days 1, 8, and 15 of each 28-day cycle (cisplatin is also given on day 1) *or* 1250 mg/m^2 on days 1 and 8 of each 21-day cycle (cisplatin is also given on day 1).

Breast Cancer

IV (Adults): 1250 mg/m^2 on days 1 and 8 of each 21-day cycle (paclitaxel is also given on day 1).

Ovarian Cancer

IV (Adults): 1000 mg/m^2 on days 1 and 8 of each 21-day cycle.

Availability (generic available)

Powder for injection: 200 mg/vial, 1 g/vial, ✱ 2 g/vial.

NURSING IMPLICATIONS

Assessment

- Monitor vital signs before and frequently during therapy.
- Assess injection site during administration. Although gemcitabine is not considered a vesicant, local reactions may occur.
- Monitor for bone marrow depression. Assess for bleeding (bleeding gums, bruising, petechiae; guaiac stools, urine, and emesis) and avoid IM injections and taking rectal temperatures if platelet count is low. Apply pressure to venipuncture sites for 10 min. Assess for signs of infection during neutropenia. Anemia may occur. Monitor for increased fatigue, dyspnea, and orthostatic hypotension.
- Monitor intake and output, appetite, and nutritional intake. Mild to moderate nausea and vomiting occur frequently. Antiemetics may be used prophylactically.

- Assess for signs and symptoms of capillary leak syndrome (severe hypotension, hypoalbuminemia, hemoconcentration). Discontinue therapy if symptoms occur.
- Monitor respiratory status during therapy. Discontinue gemcitabine if unexplained dyspnea or other evidence of severe pulmonary toxicity occurs. May occur up to 2 wks after last dose.
- Monitor for signs and symptoms of posterior reversible encephalopathy syndrome (PRES) (headache, seizure, lethargy, hypertension, confusion, blindness, and other visual and neurologic disturbances) during therapy. Confirm diagnosis of PRES with magnetic resonance imaging (MRI). Discontinue gemcitabine if PRES develops during therapy.
- ***Lab Test Considerations:*** Monitor CBC, including differential and platelet count, before each dose. Dose guidelines are based on CBC. **For single-agent use:** *If absolute granulocyte count is >1000 and platelet count is >100,000,* full dose may be administered. *If absolute granulocyte count is 500–999 or platelet count is 50,000–99,000,* 75% of dose may be given. *If absolute granulocyte count is <500 or platelet count is <50,000,* withhold further doses. **For gemcitabine with paclitaxel (breast cancer):** *If absolute granulocyte count is >1200 and platelet count is >75,000,* full dose may be administered. *If absolute granulocyte count is 1000–1199 or platelet count is 50,000–75,000,* 75% of dose may be given. *If absolute granulocyte count is 700–999 or platelet count is ≥50,000,* 50% of dose may be given. *If absolute granulocyte count is <700 or platelet count is <50,000,* withhold further doses. **For gemcitabine with carboplatin (ovarian cancer):** *If absolute granulocyte count is >1500 and platelet count is >100,000,* full dose may be administered. *If the absolute granulocyte count is 1000–1499 or platelet count is 75,000–99,000,* 75% of dose may be given. *If the absolute granulocyte count is <1000 or the platelet count is <75,000,* withhold further doses.
- Monitor serum creatinine, potassium, calcium, and magnesium in patients taking cisplatin with gemcitabine.
- Monitor hepatic and renal function before and periodically during therapy. May cause transient ↑ in serum AST, ALT, alkaline phosphatase, and bilirubin concentrations. Discontinue gemcitabine for severe hepatic toxicity or hemolytic-uremic syndrome.
- May also cause ↑ BUN and serum creatinine concentrations, proteinuria, and hematuria.

Potential Nursing Diagnoses

Risk for infection (Adverse Reactions)

Implementation

- ***High Alert:*** Fatalities have occurred with incorrect administration of chemotherapeutic agents. Before administering, clarify all ambiguous orders; double-check single, daily, and course-of-therapy dose limits; have second practitioner independently double-check original order, calculations, and infusion pump settings.
- Solution should be prepared in a biologic cabinet. Wear gloves, gown, and mask while handling IV medication. Discard IV equipment in specially designated containers.

IV Administration

- **Intermittent Infusion:** To reconstitute, add 5 mL of 0.9% NaCl without preservatives to 200-mg vial or 25 mL of 0.9% NaCl to the 1-g vial of gemcitabine for a concentration of 40 mg/mL. Incomplete dissolution may result in concentrations greater than 40 mg/mL. ***Diluent:*** May be further diluted with 0.9% NaCl. Solution is colorless to light straw color. Do not administer solutions that are discolored or contain particulate matter. Solution is stable for 24 hr at room temperature. Discard unused portions. Do not refrigerate; crystallization may occur. ***Concentration:*** 0.1–38 mg/mL. ***Rate:*** Administer dose over 30 min. Infusions longer than 60 min have a greater incidence of toxicity.
- **Y-Site Compatibility:** alemtuzumab, alfentanil, allopurinol, amifostine, amikacin, aminocaproic acid, aminophylline, amiodarone, ampicillin, ampicillin/sulbactam, anidulafungin, argatroban, azithromycin, aztreonam, bivalirudin, bleomycin, bumetanide, buprenorphine, butorphanol, calcium acetate, calcium chloride, calcium gluconate, carboplatin, carmustine, caspofungin, cefazolin, cefotetan, cefoxitin, ceftazidime, ceftriaxone, cefuroxime, chlorpromazine, ciprofloxacin, cisatracurium, cisplatin, clindamycin, cyclophosphamide, cyclosporine, cytarabine, dacarbazine, dactinomycin, daunorubicin, dexamethasone, dexmedetomidine, dexrazoxane, digoxin, diltiazem, diphenhydramine, dobutamine, docetaxel, dolasetron, dopamine, doripenem, doxacurium, doxorubicin, doxycycline, droperidol, enalaprilat, ephedrine, epinephrine, epirubicin, ertapenem, erythromycin, esmolol, etoposide, etoposide phosphate, famotidine, fenoldopam, fentanyl, floxuridine, fluconazole, fludarabine, fluorouracil, foscarnet, fosphenytoin, gentamicin, glycopyrrolate, granisetron, haloperidol, heparin, hydralazine, hydrocortisone, hydromorphone, idarubicin, ifosfamide, insulin, isoproterenol, labetalol, leucovorin, levofloxacin, lidocaine, linezolid, lorazepam, magnesium sulfate, mannitol, meperidine, meropenem, mesna, metaraminol, methyldopate, metoclopramide, metoprolol, metronidazole, midazolam, milri-

none, mitoxantrone, morphine, moxifloxacin, nalbuphine, naloxone, nesiritide, nicardipine, nitroglycerin, nitroprusside, norepinephrine, octreotide, ondansetron, oxaliplatin, paclitaxel, palonosetron, pamidronate, pancuronium, pentamidine, pentazocine, pentobarbital, phenobarbital, potassium acetate, potassium chloride, potassium phosphates, procainamide, promethazine, propranolol, quinupristin/dalfopristin, ranitidine, remifentanil, rituxumab, rocuronium, sodium acetate, sodium bicarbonate, sodium phosphates, streptozocin, succinylcholine, sufentanil, tacrolimus, teniposide, theophylline, thiotepa, tigecycline, tirofiban, tobramycin, tolazoline, topotecan, trastuzumab, trimethoprim/sulfamethoxazole, vancomycin, vasopressin, vecuronium, verapamil, vinblastine, vincristine, vinorelbine, voriconazole, zidovudine, zoledronic acid.

- **Y-Site Incompatibility:** acyclovir, amphotericin B colloidal, amphotericin B lipid complex, amphotericin B liposome, cefepime, cefotaxime, chloramphenicol, dantrolene, daptomycin, diazepam, doxorubicin liposomal, furosemide, ganciclovir, imipenem-cilastatin, irinotecan, ketorolac, methotrexate, methoprednisolone, mitomycin, nafcillin, pantoprazole, pemetrexed, phenytoin, piperacillin/tazobactam, prochlorperazine, thiopental.

Patient/Family Teaching

- Instruct patient to notify health care professional if fever; chills; sore throat; signs of infection; bleeding gums; bruising; petechiae; or blood in urine, stool, or emesis occurs. Caution patient to avoid crowds and persons with known infections. Instruct patient to use soft toothbrush and electric razor. Patient should be cautioned not to drink alcoholic beverages or take products containing aspirin or NSAIDs.
- Instruct patient to inspect oral mucosa for erythema and ulceration. If ulceration occurs, advise patient to use sponge brush and rinse mouth with water after eating and drinking. Stomatitis pain may require management with opioid analgesics.
- Instruct patient to notify health care professional if flu-like symptoms (fever, anorexia, headache, cough, chills, myalgia), swelling of feet or legs, signs and symptoms of pulmonary toxicity (shortness of breath, wheezing, cough), hemolytic-uremic syndrome (changes in color or volume of urine output, increased bruising or bleeding), or hepatic toxicity (jaundice, pain/tenderness in right upper abdominal quadrant) occur.
- Discuss with patient the possibility of hair loss. Explore methods of coping.
- Instruct patient not to receive any vaccinations without advice of health care professional.
- Rep: Advise patient that medication may have teratogenic effects. Contraception should be used during therapy.
- Emphasize the need for periodic lab tests to monitor for side effects.

Evaluation/Desired Outcomes

- Palliative, symptomatic improvement in patients with pancreatic cancer.
- Decrease in size and spread of malignancy in lung, ovarian, and breast cancer.

gemfibrozil (gem-**fye**-broe-zil)

Lopid

Classification
Therapeutic: lipid-lowering agents
Pharmacologic: fibric acid derivatives

Pregnancy Category C

Indications

Management of type II-b hyperlipidemia (decreased HDL, increased LDL, increased triglycerides) in patients who do not yet have clinical coronary artery disease and have failed therapy with diet, exercise, weight loss, or other agents (niacin, bile acid sequestrants).

Action

Inhibits peripheral lipolysis. Decreases triglyceride production by the liver. Decreases production of the triglyceride carrier protein. Increases HDL. **Therapeutic Effects:** Decreased plasma triglycerides and increased HDL.

Pharmacokinetics

Absorption: Well absorbed after oral administration.
Distribution: Unknown.
Metabolism and Excretion: Some metabolism by the liver, 70% excreted by the kidneys (mostly unchanged), 6% excreted in feces.
Half-life: 1.3–1.5 hr.

TIME/ACTION PROFILE (triglyceride-VLDL–lowering effect)

ROUTE	ONSET	PEAK	DURATION
PO	2–5 days	4 wk	several mo

Contraindications/Precautions

Contraindicated in: Hypersensitivity; Primary biliary cirrhosis; Concurrent use of HMG-CoA reductase inhibitors or repaglinide.
Use Cautiously in: Gallbladder disease; Liver disease; Severe renal impairment; OB, Lactation, Pedi: Safety not established.

Adverse Reactions/Side Effects

CNS: dizziness, headache. **EENT:** blurred vision. **GI:** abdominal pain, diarrhea, epigastric pain, flatulence, gallstones, heartburn, nausea, vomiting. **Derm:** alopecia, rash, urticaria. **Hemat:** anemia, leukopenia. **MS:** myositis.

Interactions

Drug-Drug: Repaglinide may ↑ the risk of severe hypoglycemia; concurrent use contraindicated. May ↑

the effects of **warfarin** or **sulfonylurea oral hypoglycemic agents**. Concurrent use with **HMG-CoA reductase inhibitors** may ↑ risk of rhabdomyolysis (avoid concurrent use). Concurrent use with **colchicine** may ↑ risk of rhabdomyolysis, especially in patients with renal dysfunction or elderly. May ↓ the effect of **cyclosporine**. **Cholestyramine** and **colestipol** may ↓ absorption; separate administration by ≥2 hr.

Route/Dosage

PO (Adults): 600 mg twice daily 30 min before breakfast and dinner.

Availability (generic available)

Tablets: 600 mg. **Cost:** *Generic*—$24.07/100. **Capsules:** ✱ 300 mg.

NURSING IMPLICATIONS

Assessment

- Obtain patient's diet history, especially regarding fat and alcohol consumption.
- ***Lab Test Considerations:*** Monitor serum triglyceride and cholesterol levels before and periodically during therapy. Assess LDL and VLDL levels before and periodically during therapy. Discontinue gemfibrozil if paradoxical ↑ in lipid levels occurs.
- Assess liver function tests before and periodically during therapy. May cause ↑ serum bilirubin, alkaline phosphatase, CK, LDH, AST, and ALT. If hepatic function tests rise significantly, discontinue therapy and do not resume.
- Evaluate CBC and electrolytes every 3–6 mo and then yearly during therapy. May cause mild ↓ in hemoglobin, hematocrit, and leukocyte counts. May cause ↓ serum potassium concentrations.
- May cause slight ↑ in serum glucose.

Potential Nursing Diagnoses

Noncompliance (Patient/Family Teaching)

Implementation

- **PO:** Administer 30 min before breakfast or dinner.

Patient/Family Teaching

- Instruct patient to take medication as directed, not to skip doses or double up on missed doses. Take missed doses as soon as remembered unless almost time for next dose.
- Advise patient that gemfibrozil should be used in conjunction with dietary restrictions (fat, cholesterol, carbohydrates, alcohol), exercise, and cessation of smoking.
- Instruct patient to notify health care professional promptly if any of the following symptoms occur: severe stomach pains with nausea and vomiting, fever, chills, sore throat, rash, diarrhea, muscle cramping, general abdominal discomfort, or persistent flatulence.
- Advise female patient to notify health care professional if pregnancy is planned or suspected or if breast feeding.

Evaluation/Desired Outcomes

- Decrease in serum triglyceride and cholesterol levels and improved HDL to total cholesterol ratios. If response is not seen within 3 mo, medication is usually discontinued.

gentamicin, See AMINOGLYCOSIDES.

glimepiride, See SULFONYLUREAS.

glipiZIDE, See SULFONYLUREAS.

glucagon (gloo-ka-gon)

GlucaGen

Classification

Therapeutic: hormones

Pharmacologic: pancreatics

Pregnancy Category B

Indications

Acute management of severe hypoglycemia when administration of glucose is not feasible. Facilitation of radiographic examination of the GI tract. **Unlabeled Use:** Antidote to: Beta blockers, Calcium channel blockers.

Action

Stimulates hepatic production of glucose from glycogen stores (glycogenolysis). Relaxes the musculature of the GI tract (stomach, duodenum, small bowel, and colon), temporarily inhibiting movement. Has positive inotropic and chronotropic effects. **Therapeutic Effects:** Increase in blood glucose. Relaxation of GI musculature, facilitating radiographic examination.

Pharmacokinetics

Absorption: Well absorbed following IM and subcut administration.

Distribution: Unknown.

Metabolism and Excretion: Extensively metabolized by the liver, plasma, and kidneys.

Half-life: 8–18 min.

TIME/ACTION PROFILE

ROUTE	ONSET	PEAK	DURATION
IM (hyperglycemic action)	within 10 min	30 min	12–27 min
IV (hyperglycemic action)	1 min	5 min	9–17 min
Subcut (hyperglycemic action)	within 10 min	30–45 min	60–90 min
IV (effect on GI musculature)	45 sec (for 0.25–2-mg dose)	unknown	9–17 min (0.25–0.5-mg dose); 22–25 min (2-mg dose)
IM (effect on GI musculature)	8–10 min (1-mg dose); 4–7 min (2-mg dose)	unknown	9–27 min (1-mg dose); 21–32 min (2-mg dose)

Contraindications/Precautions

Contraindicated in: Hypersensitivity; Pheochromocytoma; Some products contain glycerin and phenol—avoid use in patients with hypersensitivities to these ingredients.

Use Cautiously in: History suggestive of insulinoma or pheochromocytoma; Prolonged fasting, starvation, adrenal insufficiency or chronic hypoglycemia (low levels of releasable glucose); When used to inhibit GI motility, use cautiously in geriatric patient with cardiac disease or diabetics; OB: Should be used during pregnancy only if clearly needed; Lactation: Safety not established.

Adverse Reactions/Side Effects

CV: hypotension. **GI:** nausea, vomiting. **Misc:** hypersensitivity reactions including ANAPHYLAXIS.

Interactions

Drug-Drug: Large doses may enhance the effect of **warfarin**. Negates the response to **insulin** or **oral hypoglycemic agents**. **Phenytoin** inhibits the stimulant effect of glucagon on insulin release. Hyperglycemic effect is intensified and prolonged by **epinephrine**. Patients on concurrent **beta blocker** therapy may have a greater increase in heart rate and BP.

Route/Dosage

Hypoglycemia

IV, IM, Subcut (Adults and Children ≥20 kg): 1 mg; may be repeated in 15 min if necessary.

IV, IM, Subcut (Children <20 kg): 0.5 mg or 0.02–0.03 mg/kg; may be repeated in 15 min if necessary.

Radiographic Examination of the GI Tract

IM, IV (Adults): 0.25–2 mg; depending on location and duration of examination (0.5 mg IV or 2 mg IM for relaxation of stomach; for examination of the colon 2 mg IM 10 min before procedure).

Antidote (unlabeled)

IV (Adults): *To beta blockers*—50–150 mcg (0.05–0.15 mg)/kg, followed by 1–5 mg/hr infusion. *To calcium channel blockers*—2 mg; additional doses determined by response.

Availability

Powder for injection: 1-mg (equivalent to 1 unit) vials as an emergency kit for low blood glucose and a diagnostic kit.

NURSING IMPLICATIONS

Assessment

- Assess for signs of hypoglycemia (sweating, hunger, weakness, headache, dizziness, tremor, irritability, tachycardia, anxiety) prior to and periodically during therapy.
- Assess neurologic status throughout therapy. Institute safety precautions to protect patient from injury caused by seizures, falling, or aspiration. For insulin shock therapy, 0.5–1 mg is administered after 1 hr of coma; patient usually awakens in 10–25 min. If no response occurs, repeat the dose. Feed patient supplemental carbohydrates orally to replenish liver glycogen and prevent secondary hypoglycemia as soon as possible after awakening, especially pediatric patients.
- Assess nutritional status. Patients who lack liver glycogen stores (starvation, chronic hypoglycemia, adrenal insufficiency) will require glucose instead of glucagon.
- Assess for nausea and vomiting after administration of dose. Protect patients with depressed level of consciousness from aspiration by positioning on side; ensure that a suction unit is available. Notify health care professional if vomiting occurs; patient will require parenteral glucose to prevent recurrent hypoglycemia.
- ***Lab Test Considerations:*** Monitor serum glucose levels throughout episode, during treatment, and for 3–4 hr after patient regains consciousness. Use of bedside fingerstick blood glucose determination methods is recommended for rapid results. Follow-up lab results may be ordered to validate fingerstick values, but do not delay treatment while awaiting lab results, as this could result in neurologic injury or death.
- Large doses of glucagon may cause a ↓ in serum potassium concentrations.

Potential Nursing Diagnoses

Risk for injury (Indications)
Noncompliance (Patient/Family Teaching)

Implementation

- May be given subcut, IM, or IV. Reconstitute with diluent supplied in kit by manufacturer. Inspect solution prior to use; use only clear, water-like solution. Solution is stable for 48 hr if refrigerated, 24 hr at room temperature. Unmixed medication should be stored at room temperature.

- Administer supplemental carbohydrates IV or orally to facilitate increase of serum glucose levels.

IV Administration

- **IV Push:** ***Diluent:*** Reconstitute each vial with 1 mL of an appropriate diluent. For doses ≤2 mg, use diluent provided by manufacturer. For doses >2 mg, use sterile water for injection instead of diluent supplied by manufacturer to minimize risk of thrombophlebitis, CNS toxicity, and myocardial depression from phenol preservative in diluent supplied by manufacturer. Reconstituted vials should be used immediately. ***Concentration:*** Not exceed 1 mg/mL. ***Rate:*** Administer at a rate not exceeding 1 mg/min. May be administered through IV line containing D5W.
- **Continuous Infusion:** ***Diluent:*** Reconstitute vials as per directions above (use sterile water for injection). Further dilute 10 mg of glucagon in 100 mL of D5W. ***Concentration:*** 0.1 mg/mL. ***Rate:*** See Route/Dosage section.
- **Y-Site Compatibility:** No information available.

Patient/Family Teaching

- Teach patient and family signs and symptoms of hypoglycemia. Instruct patient to take oral glucose as soon as symptoms of hypoglycemia occur—glucagon is reserved for episodes when patient is unable to swallow because of decreased level of consciousness.
- **Home Care Issues:** Instruct family on correct technique to prepare, draw up, and administer injection. Health care professional must be contacted immediately after each dose for orders regarding further therapy or adjustment of insulin dose or diet.
- Advise family that patient should receive oral glucose when alertness returns.
- Instruct family to position patient on side until fully alert. Explain that glucagon may cause nausea and vomiting. Aspiration may occur if patient vomits while lying on back.
- Instruct patient to check expiration date monthly and to replace outdated medication immediately.
- Review hypoglycemic medication regimen, diet, and exercise programs.
- Patients with diabetes mellitus should carry a source of sugar (such as a packet of sugar or candy) and identification describing disease process and treatment regimen at all times.

Evaluation/Desired Outcomes

- Increase of serum glucose to normal levels with improved level of consciousness.
- Smooth muscle relaxation of the stomach, duodenum, and small and large intestine in patients undergoing radiologic examination of the GI tract.

glyBURIDE, See SULFONYLUREAS.

glycopyrrolate

(glye-koe-**pye**-roe-late)

Cuvposa, Robinul, Robinul-Forte

Classification

Therapeutic: antispasmodics

Pharmacologic: anticholinergics

Pregnancy Category B (oral, parenteral), C (oral solution)

Indications

Inhibits salivation and excessive respiratory secretions when given preoperatively. Reverses some of the secretory and vagal actions of cholinesterase inhibitors used to treat nondepolarizing neuromuscular blockade (cholinergic adjunct). Adjunctive management of peptic ulcer disease. **Oral solution:** Reduce chronic severe drooling in children with neurologic conditions associated with drooling.

Action

Inhibits the action of acetylcholine at postganglionic sites located in smooth muscle, secretory glands, and the CNS (antimuscarinic activity). Low doses decrease sweating, salivation, and respiratory secretions. Intermediate doses result in increased heart rate. Larger doses decrease GI and GU tract motility. **Therapeutic Effects:** Decreased GI and respiratory secretions.

Pharmacokinetics

Absorption: Incompletely absorbed (<10%) after oral administration. Well absorbed after IM administration.

Distribution: Distribution not fully known. Does not significantly cross the blood-brain barrier or eye. Crosses the placenta.

Metabolism and Excretion: Eliminated primarily unchanged in the urine and bile.

Half-life: 1.7 hr (0.6–4.6 hr).

TIME/ACTION PROFILE (anticholinergic effects)

ROUTE	ONSET	PEAK	DURATION
PO	1 hr	unknown	8–12 hr
IM	15–30 min	30–45 min	2–7 hr*
IV	1–10 min	unknown	2–7 hr*

*Antisecretory effect lasts up to 7 hr; vagal blockade lasts 2–3 hr.

Contraindications/Precautions

Contraindicated in: Hypersensitivity; Angle-closure glaucoma; Acute hemorrhage; Tachycardia secondary to cardiac insufficiency or thyrotoxicosis; Severe ulcerative colitis; Toxic megacolon; Myasthenia gravis; Obstructive uropathy; Paralytic ileus; Concurrent use of oral potassium chloride dosage forms (oral solution only); Pedi: Injection contains benzyl alcohol and should not be given to neonates.

Use Cautiously in: Patients who may have intra-abdominal infections; Prostatic hyperplasia; Chronic renal, hepatic, pulmonary, or cardiac disease; Hyperthyroidism; Down syndrome and children with spastic paralysis or brain damage (may be hypersensitive to antimuscarinic effects); OB, Lactation: Safety not established; Pedi: ↑ sensitivity to anticholinergic effects and adverse reactions; Geri: ↑ sensitivity to anticholinergic effects and adverse reactions.

Adverse Reactions/Side Effects

CNS: headache, confusion, drowsiness. **EENT:** nasal congestion, blurred vision, cycloplegia, dry eyes, mydriasis. **CV:** tachycardia, orthostatic hypotension, palpitations. **GI:** dry mouth, vomiting, constipation. **GU:** urinary hesitancy, urinary retention. **Derm:** flushing.

Interactions

Drug-Drug: May ↑ GI mucosal lesions in patients taking oral **potassium chloride** tablets; concurrent use with oral glycopyrrolate solution contraindicated. Additive anticholinergic effects with other **anticholinergics**, including **antihistamines**, **phenothiazines**, **meperidine**, **amantadine**, **tricyclic antidepressants**, **quinidine**, and **disopyramide**. May alter the absorption of other **orally administered drugs** by slowing motility of the GI tract. May ↑ GI transit time of oral **digoxin** and ↑ digoxin levels. **Antacids** or **adsorbent antidiarrheal agents** ↓ absorption of anticholinergics. May ↑ GI mucosal lesions in patients taking oral **potassium chloride** tablets. May ↑ **atenolol** and **metformin** levels. May ↓ levels of **haloperidol** and **levodopa**. Concurrent use may ↓ absorption of **ketoconazole** (administer 2 hr after ketoconazole).

Route/Dosage

Control of Secretions during Surgery

IM (Adults): 4.4 mcg/kg 30–60 min preop (not to exceed 0.1 mg).
IM (Children >2 yr): 4.4 mcg/kg 30–60 min preop.
IM (Children <2 yr): 4.4–8.8 mcg/kg 30–60 min preop.

Control of Secretions (chronic)

IM, IV (Children): 4–10 mcg/kg/dose q 3–4 hr.
PO (Children): 40–100 mcg/kg/dose 3–4 times/day.

Cholinergic Adjunct

IV (Adults and Children): 200 mcg for each 1 mg of neostigmine or 5 mg of pyridostigmine given at the same time.

Antiarrhythmic

IV (Adults): 100 mcg, may be repeated q 2–3 min.
IV (Children): 4.4 mcg/kg (up to 100 mcg); may be repeated q 2–3 min.

Peptic Ulcer

PO (Adults): 1–2 mg 2–3 times daily. An additional 2 mg may be given at bedtime; may be ↓ to 1 mg twice daily (not to exceed 8 mg/day).
IM, IV (Adults): 100–200 mcg q 4 hr up to 4 times daily.

Chronic Severe Drooling

PO (Children 3–16 yr): *Oral solution*—0.02 mg/kg 3 times daily; may ↑ by 0.02 mg/kg 3 times daily every 5–7 days (not to exceed 0.1 mg/kg 3 times daily or 1.5–3 mg/dose).

Availability (generic available)

Tablets: 1 mg, 2 mg. **Injection:** 200 mcg (0.2 mg)/mL. **Oral solution (cherry-flavor):** 1 mg/5 mL.

NURSING IMPLICATIONS

Assessment

- Assess heart rate, BP, and respiratory rate before and periodically during parenteral therapy.
- Monitor intake and output ratios in geriatric or surgical patients; glycopyrrolate may cause urinary retention. Instruct patient to void before parenteral administration.
- Assess patient routinely for abdominal distention and auscultate for bowel sounds. If constipation becomes a problem, increasing fluids and adding bulk to the diet may help alleviate the constipating effects of the drug.
- Periodic intraocular pressure determinations should be made for patients receiving long-term therapy.
- Pedi: Monitor amount and frequency of drooling periodically during therapy.
- Assess for hyperexcitability, a paradoxical response that may occur in children.
- ***Lab Test Considerations:*** Antagonizes effects of pentagastrin and histamine during the gastric acid secretion test. Avoid administration for 24 hr preceding the test.
- May cause ↓ uric acid levels in patients with gout or hyperuricemia.
- ***Toxicity and Overdose:*** If overdose occurs, neostigmine is the antidote.

Potential Nursing Diagnoses

Impaired oral mucous membrane (Side Effects)
Constipation (Side Effects)

Implementation

- Do not administer cloudy or discolored solution.
- **PO:** Administer 30–60 min before meals to maximize absorption.
- For drooling: Administer at least 1 hr before or 2 hr after meals.

- Do not administer within 1 hr of antacids or antidiarrheal medications.
- Oral dose is 10 times the parenteral dose.
- **IM:** May be administered undiluted (200 mcg/mL).

IV Administration

- **IV Push:** ***Diluent:*** May be given undiluted through Y-site. ***Concentration:*** 200 mcg/mL. ***Rate:*** Administer at a maximum rate of 20 mcg over 1 min.
- **Y-Site Compatibility:** acyclovir, alfentanil, amikacin, aminophylline, anidulafungin, argatroban, ascorbic acid, atracurium, atropine, azithromycin, aztreonam, benztropine, bivalirudin, bleomycin, bumetanide, buprenorphine, butorphanol, calcium chloride, calcium gluconate, carmustine, caspofungin, cefazolin, cefotaxime, cefotetan, cefoxitin, ceftazidime, ceftriaxone, cefuroxime, chloramphenicol, chlorpromazine, cisplatin, clindamycin, cyanocobalamin, cyclosporine, dactinomycin, daptomycin, dexamethasone, dexmedetomidine, digoxin, diltiazem, diphenhydramine, dobutamine, docetaxel, dopamine, doxycycline, enalaprilat, ephedrine, epinephrine, epoetin alfa, ertapenem, erythromycin, esmolol, etoposide, etoposide phosphate, famotidine, fenoldopam, fentanyl, fluconazole, fludarabine, folic acid, ganciclovir, gemcitabine, gentamicin, granisetron, heparin, hydrocortisone, hydromorphone, idarubicin, imipenem/cilastatin, isoproterenol, ketorolac, labetalol, lidocaine, linezolid, lorazepam, magnesium sulfate, mannitol, mechlorethamine, meperidine, metaraminol, methoxamine, methyldopate, methylprednisolone, metoclopramide, metoprolol, metronidazole, midazolam, milrinone, mitoxantrone, morphine, multivitamins, mycophenolate, nafcillin, nalbuphine, naloxone, nesiritide, nitroglycerin, nitroprusside, norepinephrine, octreotide, ondansetron, oxacillin, oxaliplatin, oxytocin, paclitaxel, palonosetron, pamidronate, pancuronium, papaverine, pemetrexed, penicillin G, pentamidine, pentazocine, pentobarbital, phenobarbital, phentolamine, phenylephrine, phytonadione, potassium acetate, potassium chloride, procainamide, promethazine, propofol, propranolol, protamine, pyridoxime, ranitidine, sodium bicarbonate, streptokinase, succinylcholine, sufentanil, tacrolimus, teniposide, theophylline, thiamine, thiotepa, tigecycline, tirofiban, tobramycin, tolazoline, trimetaphan, vancomycin, vasopressin, vecuronium, verapamil, vinorelbine, voriconazole, zoledronic acid.
- **Y-Site Incompatibility:** amphotericin B colloidal, amphotericin B lipid complex, dantrolene, diazepam, diazoxide, indomethacin, irinotecan, pantoprazole, phenytoin, piperacillin/tazobactam, trimethoprim/sulfamethoxazole.
- **Solution Compatibility:** D5/0.45% NaCl, D5W, 0.9% NaCl, Ringer's solution. Administer immediately after admixing.
- **Additive Incompatibility:** methylprednisolone sodium succinate.

Patient/Family Teaching

- Instruct patient to take glycopyrrolate as directed and not to take more than the prescribed amount. Take missed doses as soon as remembered if not just before next dose.
- Medication may cause drowsiness and blurred vision. Caution patient to avoid driving or other activities requiring alertness until response to the medication is known.
- Inform patient that frequent oral rinses, sugarless gum or candy, and good oral hygiene may help relieve dry mouth. Consult health care professional regarding use of saliva substitute if dry mouth persists for more than 2 wk.
- Advise patient to change positions slowly to minimize the effects of drug-induced orthostatic hypotension.
- Caution patient to avoid extremes of temperature. This medication decreases the ability to sweat and may increase the risk of heat stroke.
- Advise patient to notify health care professional immediately if eye pain or increased sensitivity to light occurs. Emphasize the importance of routine eye exams throughout therapy.
- Advise patient to consult health care professional before taking any OTC medications concurrently with this therapy.
- Geri: Advise geriatric patients about increased susceptibility to side effects and to call health care professional immediately if they occur.
- Pedi: Instruct parents to use a calibrated measuring device with solution for accurate dosing.
- Advise parents to stop glycopyrrolate and notify health care professional if constipation; signs of urinary retention (inability to urinate, dry diapers or undergarments, irritability or crying); or rash, hives, or an allergic reaction occurs.
- Glycopyrrolate reduces sweating. Advise parents to avoid exposure of the patient to hot or very warm environmental temperatures to avoid overheating and heat exhaustion or heat stroke.

Evaluation/Desired Outcomes

- Mouth dryness preoperatively.
- Reversal of cholinergic medications.
- Decrease in GI motility and pain in patients with peptic ulcer disease.
- Reduce chronic severe drooling in children with neurologic conditions associated with drooling.

golimumab (go-li-mu-mab)

Simponi, Simponi Aria

Classification
Therapeutic: antirheumatics
Pharmacologic: DMARDs, monoclonal antibodies, anti-TNF agents

Pregnancy Category B

Indications

Simponi and Simponi Aria: Treatment of moderately to severely active rheumatoid arthritis (with methotrexate). **Simponi:** Treatment of active psoriatic arthritis (alone or with methotrexate). **Simponi:** Treatment of active ankylosing spondylitis. **Simponi:** Moderately to severely active ulcerative colitis in patients who have demonstrated corticosteroid dependence or have responded inadequately to immunosuppressants such as aminosalicylates, corticosteroids, azathioprine, or 6–mercaptopurine.

Action

Inhibits binding of TNFα to receptors inhibiting activity and resulting in anti-inflammatory and antiproliferative activity. **Therapeutic Effects:** Decreased pain and swelling with decreased joint destruction in patients with rheumatoid arthritis, psoriatic arthritis, and ankylosing spondylitis. Induction and maintenance of clinical remission of ulcerative colitis.

Pharmacokinetics

Absorption: Well absorbed following subcutaneous administration. IV administration results in complete bioavailability.
Distribution: Distributed primarily in the circulatory system with limited extravascular distribution.
Metabolism and Excretion: Unknown.
Half-life: 2 wk.

TIME/ACTION PROFILE (improvement)

ROUTE	ONSET	PEAK	DURATION
Subcut	within 3 mo	2–7 days†	unknown
IV	within 3 mo	unknown	unknown

† Blood levels.

Contraindications/Precautions

Contraindicated in: Active infection (including localized); Concurrent use of abatacept or anakinra (↑ risk of infections); Lactation: Avoid during breast feeding.
Use Cautiously in: History of chronic or recurrent infection or underlying illness/treatment predisposing to infection; History of exposure to tuberculosis; History of opportunistic infection; Patients residing, or who have resided, where tuberculosis, histoplasmosis, coccidioidomycoses, or blastomycosis is endemic; History of HF (may worsen); Pre-existing or recent-onset CNS demyelinating disorders; History of cytopenias (may worsen); History of psoriasis (may exacerbate); Hepatitis B virus carriers (risk of reactivation); Geri: Use cautiously in elderly patients due to ↑ risk of infection; OB: Use during pregnancy only if clearly needed; Pedi: Safety not established; ↑ risk of lymphoma (including hepatosplenic T-cell lymphoma [HSTCL]), leukemia, and other malignancies.

Adverse Reactions/Side Effects

CNS: CENTRAL NERVOUS SYSTEM DEMYELINATING DISORDERS, Guillain-Barre syndrome, multiple sclerosis. **EENT:** nasopharyngitis, optic neuritis. **Resp:** upper respiratory tract infection. **CV:** HF, hypertension. **GI:** ↑ liver enzymes. **Derm:** psoriasis. **Hemat:** aplastic anemia, leukopenia, neutropenia, pancytopenia, thrombocytopenia. **Local:** injection site reactions. **Neuro:** paresthesia. **Misc:** ANAPHYLAXIS, HYPERSENSITIVITY REACTIONS, INFECTIONS (including reactivation tuberculosis and other opportunistic infections due to bacterial, invasive fungal, viral, mycobacterial, and parasitic pathogens), MALIGNANCY (including lymphoma, HSTCL, leukemia, and skin cancer), fever.

Interactions

Drug-Drug: Abatacept, **anakinra**, **corticosteroids**, or **methotrexate** ↑ risk of serious infections; concurrent use with anakinra or abatacept is not recommended. Use of **live virus vaccines** or therapeutic infectious agents may ↑ risk of infection; avoid concurrent use. Concurrent use with **azathioprine** and/or **6–mercaptopurine** may ↑ risk of HSTCL. May normalize previously suppressed levels of CYP450 enzymes, following initiation or discontinuation of golimumab, effects of substrates of this system may be altered and should be monitored, including **warfarin**, **theophylline**, and **cyclosporine**.

Route/Dosage

Rheumatoid Arthritis

Subcut (Adults): 50 mg once monthly.
IV (Adults): 2 mg/kg initially and 4 wk later, then 2 mg/kg every 8 wk.

Psoriatic Arthritis and Ankylosing Spondylitis

Subcut (Adults): 50 mg once monthly.

Ulcerative Colitis

Subcut (Adults): 200 mg initially, then 100 mg 2 wk later, then 100 mg every 4 wk.

Availability

Solution for subcutaneous injection: 50 mg/0.5 mL in single-dose prefilled syringes and Smartject autoinjectors, 100 mg/mL in single-dose prefilled syringes and Smartject autoinjectors. **Solution for intravenous injection (Simponi Aria):** 12.5 mg/mL.

NURSING IMPLICATIONS

Assessment

- Assess for signs and symptoms of infection (fever, dyspnea, flu-like symptoms, frequent or painful urination, redness or swelling at the site of a wound) prior to, during, and after therapy. Discontinue therapy if serious or opportunistic infection or sepsis occurs. If new infection develops during therapy, assess patient and institute antimicrobial therapy. Patients who tested negative for latent tuberculosis (TB) prior to therapy may develop TB during therapy. Initiate treatment for latent TB prior to initiating therapy.
- Test for HBV prior to therapy and monitor carriers of HBV for signs of reactivation during and for several months after therapy. If reactivation occurs, discontinue golimumab and institute antiviral therapy.
- Monitor patients with HF for new or worsening symptoms. Discontinue therapy if symptoms occur.
- Assess for exacerbations and new onset psoriasis. Discontinue therapy of these occur.
- Assess patient for latex allergy. Needle cover of syringe contains latex and should not be handled by persons sensitive to latex.
- Assess for signs and symptoms of systemic fungal infections (fever, malaise, weight loss, sweats, cough, dypsnea, pulmonary infiltrates, serious systemic illness with or without concomitant shock). Ascertain if patient lives in or has traveled to areas of endemic mycoses. Consider empiric antifungal treatment for patients at risk of histoplasmosis and other invasive fungal infections until the pathogens are identified. Consult with an infectious diseases specialist. Consider stopping golimumab until the infection has been diagnosed and adequately treated.
- Observe for signs and symptoms of anaphylaxis (rash, pruritus, laryngeal edema, wheezing). Discontinue drug and notify physician or other health care professional immediately if these problems occur. Keep epinephrine, an antihistamine, and resuscitation equipment close by in case of an anaphylactic reaction.
- **Rheumatoid Arthritis:** Assess pain and range of motion prior to and periodically during therapy.
- **Ulcerative Colitis:** Assess for signs and symptoms before, during, and after therapy.
- ***Lab Test Considerations:*** Monitor liver function tests periodically during therapy. May cause ↑ serum AST and ALT.
- Monitor CBC with differential periodically during therapy. May cause leukopenia, neutropenia, thrombocytopenia, and pancytopenia. Discontinue golimumab if symptoms of blood dyscrasias (persistent fever) occur.
- Monitor for HBV blood tests before starting during, and for several months after therapy is completed.

Potential Nursing Diagnoses

Chronic pain (Indications)
Risk for infection (Adverse Reactions)

Implementation

- Administer a tuberculin skin test prior to administration of golimumab. Assess if treatment for latent tuberculosis is needed; an induration of 5 mm or greater is a positive tuberculin skin test, even for patients previously vaccinated with Bacille Calmette-Guerin (BCG). Consider antituberculosis therapy prior to therapy in patients with a history of latent or active tuberculosis if an adequate course of treatment cannot be confirmed, and for patients with risk factors for tuberculosis infection.
- Initial injection should be supervised by health care professional.
- Refrigerate solution; do not freeze. Allow prefilled syringe or autoinjector to sit at room temperature for 30 min prior to injection; do not warm in any other way. Do not shake. Solution is clear to slightly opalescent and colorless to light yellow. Do not administer solutions that are discolored, cloudy, or contain particulate matter. Discard unused solution.
- **Subcut:** Remove the needle cover or autoinjector cap just prior to injection. Inject into front of middle thigh, lower part of abdomen 2 inches from navel, or caregiver may administer into outer area of upper arm. Do not inject in areas where skin is tender, bruised, red, scaly, or hard; avoid scars or stretch marks. Press a cotton ball or gauze over injection site for 10 sec; do not rub.
- *Autoinjector:* Press open end of autoinjector against skin at 90° angle. Use free hand to pinch and hold skin at injection site. Press button with fingers or thumb; button will stay pressed and does not need to be held. Injection will begin following a loud click. Keep holding the autoinjector against skin until a second loud click is heard (usually 3–6 sec, but may take up to 15 sec). Lift autoinjector from skin following second click. Yellow indicator in viewing window indicates autoinjector worked correctly. If yellow does not appear in viewing window call 1-800-457-6399 for help.
- *Prefilled syringe:* Hold body of syringe between thumb and index finger. Do not pull back on plunger at any time. Pinch skin. Using a dart-like motion, insert needle into pinched skin at 45° angle. Inject all medication by pushing plunger until plunger head is between needle guard wings. Take needle out of skin and let go of skin. Slowly take thumb off plunger to allow empty syringe to move up until entire needle is covered by needle guard.

Patient/Family Teaching

- Instruct patient on correct technique for administration. Review patient information sheet, preparation of dose, administration sites and technique, and disposal of equipment into a puncture-resistant container. Advise patient of risks and benefits of golimumab therapy. Inject missed doses as soon as remembered, then return to regular schedule. Instruct patient to read *Medication Guide* before starting therapy and with each Rx refill; new information may be available.

- Caution patient not to share this medication with others, even with the same symptoms; may be harmful.
- Inform patient of increased risk of infections, malignancies, cardiac and nervous system disorders during therapy.
- Caution patient to notify health care professional promptly if any signs of infection, including TB, invasive fungal infections (fever, malaise, weight loss, sweats, cough, dypsnea, pulmonary infiltrates, serious systemic illness with or without concomitant shock), reactivation of HBV (muscle aches, clay-colored bowel movements, feeling very tired, fever, dark urine, chills, skin or eyes look yellow, stomach discomfort, little or no appetite, skin rash, vomiting), hypersensitivity reactions, or nervous system problems (vision changes, weakness in arms or legs, numbness or tingling in any part of the body) develop.
- Advise patient to examine skin periodically during therapy and notify health care professional of any changes in appearance of skin or growths on skin.
- Advise patient to notify health care professional of all Rx or OTC medications, vitamins, or herbal products being taken and to consult with health care professional before taking other medications.
- Inform patient to avoid receiving live vaccinations; other vaccinations may be given.
- Inform patient of increased risk of cancer. Advise patient of need for screening for dysplasia (colonoscopy, skin cancer examinations, biopsy) periodically during therapy.
- Advise patient to notify health care professional of pregnancy is planned or suspected or if breast feeding.

Evaluation/Desired Outcomes

- Decreased pain and swelling with decreased rate of joint destruction in patients with rheumatoid arthritis.
- Decreased signs and symptoms, slowed progression of joint destruction, and improved physical function in patients with psoriatic arthritis.
- Reduced signs and symptoms of ankylosing spondylitis.
- Decreased symptoms, maintaining remission and mucosal healing with decreased corticosteroid use in ulcerative colitis.

goserelin (goe-se-rel-lin)
Zoladex

Classification
Therapeutic: antineoplastics, hormones
Pharmacologic: gonadotropin-releasing hormones

Pregnancy Category D (breast cancer), X (endometriosis)

Indications
Prostate cancer in patients who cannot tolerate orchiectomy or estrogen therapy (palliative). With flutamide and radiation therapy in the treatment of locally confined stage T2b–T4 (stage B2–C) prostate cancer. Advanced breast cancer in peri- and postmenopausal women (palliative). Endometriosis. Produces thinning of the endometrium before endometrial ablation for dysfunctional uterine bleeding.

Action
Acts as a synthetic form of luteinizing hormone–releasing hormone (LHRH, GnRH). Inhibits the production of gonadotropins by the pituitary gland. Initially, levels of luteinizing hormone (LH), follicle-stimulating hormone (FSH), and testosterone increase. Continued administration leads to decreased production of testosterone and estradiol. **Therapeutic Effects:** Decreased spread of cancer of the prostate or breast. Regression of endometriosis with decreased pain. Thinning of the endometrium.

Pharmacokinetics
Absorption: Well absorbed from subcut implant. Absorption is slower in first 8 days, then is faster and continuous for remainder of 28-day dosing cycle.
Distribution: Unknown.
Metabolism and Excretion: Some metabolism by the liver (<10%), some excretion by kidneys (>90%, only 20% as unchanged drug).
Half-life: 4.2 hr.

TIME/ACTION PROFILE (↓ in serum testosterone levels)

ROUTE	ONSET	PEAK	DURATION
Subcut	unknown	2–4 wk	length of therapy

Contraindications/Precautions
Contraindicated in: Hypersensitivity; Undiagnosed vaginal bleeding; OB, Lactation: Pregnancy or lactation.
Use Cautiously in: Congenital long QT syndrome, HF, hypokalemia, or hypomagnesemia; Concurrent use of other drugs known to prolong the QTc interval; Low BMI (↑ risk of bleeding complications); Concurrent use of anticoagulant therapy (↑ risk of bleeding complications); Pedi: Safety not established.

Adverse Reactions/Side Effects

CNS: STROKE, headache, anxiety, depression, dizziness, fatigue, insomnia, mood swings, seizures, weakness. **Resp:** dyspnea. **CV:** MYOCARDIAL INFARCTION, QT INTERVAL PROLONGATION, vasodilation, chest pain, hypertension, palpitations. **GI:** anorexia, constipation, diarrhea, nausea, ulcer, vomiting. **GU:** renal insufficiency, urinary obstruction. **Derm:** sweating, acne, rash. **Endo:** ↓ libido, erectile dysfunction, breast swelling, breast tenderness, infertility, ovarian cysts, ovarian hyperstimulation syndrome (with gonadotropins). **F and E:** peripheral edema. **Hemat:** anemia. **Metab:** gout, hyperglycemia, ↑ lipids. **MS:** ↑ bone pain, arthralgia, ↓ bone density. **Misc:** hot flashes, chills, fever, injection site/vascular injury, weight gain.

Interactions

Drug-Drug: None significant.

Route/Dosage

Subcut (Adults): 3.6 mg every 4 wk or 10.8 mg q 12 wk. *Endometrial thinning*— 1 or 2 depots given 4 wk apart; if 1 depot used, surgery is performed at 4 wk; if 2 depots used, surgery is performed 2–4 wk after 2nd depot.

Availability

Implant: 3.6 mg, 10.8 mg.

NURSING IMPLICATIONS

Assessment

- Monitor for signs and symptoms of injection site injury/abdominal hemorrhage (abdominal pain, abdominal distension, dyspnea, dizziness, hypotension and/or any altered levels of consciousness) following administration. Advise patient to report symptoms immediately to health care professional.
- **Cancer:** Monitor patients with vertebral metastases for increased back pain and decreased sensory/motor function.
- Monitor intake and output ratios and assess for bladder distention in patients with urinary tract obstruction during initiation of therapy.
- **Endometriosis:** Assess patient for signs and symptoms of endometriosis before and periodically during therapy. Amenorrhea usually occurs within 8 wk of initial administration and menses usually resume 8 wk after completion.
- ***Lab Test Considerations:*** Initially ↑, then ↓ LH and FSH. This leads to castration levels of testosterone in men 2–4 wk after initial increase in concentrations.
- Monitor serum acid phosphatase and prostate-specific antigen concentrations periodically during therapy. May cause transient ↑ in serum acid phosphatase concentrations, which usually return to baseline by the 4th wk of therapy and may ↓ to below baseline or return to baseline if elevated before therapy.
- May cause hypercalcemia in patients with breast or prostate cancer with bony metastases.
- May cause an ↑ in serum HDL, LDL, and triglycerides.
- May cause hyperglycemia. Monitor blood glucose and HbA1c periodically during therapy.

Potential Nursing Diagnoses

Sexual dysfunction (Side Effects)

Implementation

- **Subcut:** Implant is inserted in upper subcut tissue of upper abdominal wall every 28 days. Local anesthesia may be used before injection.
- If the implant needs to be removed for any reason, it can be located by ultrasound.

Patient/Family Teaching

- Explain purpose of goserelin to patient. Emphasize importance of adhering to the schedule of monthly or every-3-mo administration.
- Advise patient that bone pain may increase at initiation of therapy. This will resolve with time. Patient should discuss use of analgesics to control pain with health care professional.
- Advise female patients to notify health care professional if regular menstruation persists.
- Inform diabetic patients of potential for hyperglycemia. Encourage close monitoring of serum glucose.
- Advise patient that medication may cause hot flashes. Notify health care professional if these become bothersome. Hormone replacement therapy may be added to decrease vasomotor symptoms and vaginal dryness without compromising beneficial effect.
- Instruct patient to notify health care professional promptly if difficulty urinating or if symptoms of myocardial infarction or stroke (chest pain, difficulty breathing, weakness, loss of consciousness) occur.
- Rep: Advise premenopausal women to notify health care professional if pregnancy is planned or suspected or if breast feeding. Effective contraception should be used during and for 12 wk after treatment ends.

Evaluation/Desired Outcomes

- Decrease in the spread of prostate cancer.
- Reduction of symptoms of advanced breast cancer in peri- and postmenopausal women.
- Decrease in the signs and symptoms of endometriosis. Symptoms are usually reduced within 4 wk of implantation.
- Thinning of the endometrium before endometrial ablation for dysfunctional uterine bleeding.

G

granisetron (oral and IV)

(gra-**nees**-e-tron)

~~Kytril~~, ✤Kytril

granisetron (transdermal)

Sancuso

Classification

Therapeutic: antiemetics

Pharmacologic: 5-HT_3 antagonists

Pregnancy Category B

Indications

PO: Prevention of nausea and vomiting due to emetogenic chemotherapy or radiation therapy. Prevention and treatment of postoperative nausea and vomiting. **Transdermal:** Prevention of nausea and vomiting due to moderately/highly emetogenic chemotherapy.

Action

Blocks the effects of serotonin at receptor sites (selective antagonist) located in vagal nerve terminals and in the chemoreceptor trigger zone in the CNS. **Therapeutic Effects:** Decreased incidence and severity of nausea and vomiting following emetogenic chemotherapy, radiation therapy, or surgery.

Pharmacokinetics

Absorption: 50% absorbed following oral administration; transdermal enters systemic circulation via passive diffusion through intact skin.

Distribution: Distributes into erythrocytes; remainder of distribution is unknown.

Protein Binding: 65%.

Metabolism and Excretion: Mostly metabolized by the liver; 12% excreted unchanged in urine.

Half-life: *Patients with cancer*—10–12 hr (range 0.9–31.1 hr); *healthy volunteers* —3–4 hr (range 0.9–15.2 hr); *geriatric patients*—7.7 hr (range 2.6–17.7 hr).

TIME/ACTION PROFILE

ROUTE	ONSET	PEAK	DURATION
PO	rapid	60 min	24 hr
IV	1–3 min	30 min	up to 24 hr
TD*	unknown	48 hr	unknown

* Blood levels.

Contraindications/Precautions

Contraindicated in: Hypersensitivity; Some products contain benzyl alcohol; avoid use in neonates.

Use Cautiously in: History of arrhythmias or conduction disorders; OB, Lactation: Safety not established; Pedi: Safe use of IV route not established in children <2 yr; safe use of PO or transdermal route not established in children <18 yr.

Adverse Reactions/Side Effects

CNS: <u>headache</u>, agitation, anxiety, CNS stimulation, drowsiness, weakness. **CV:** hypertension, QT interval prolongation. **GI:** constipation, diarrhea, e↑ liver enzymes, taste disorder. **Derm:** *Topical*—application site reactions, photosensitivity. **Misc:** SEROTONIN SYNDROME, anaphylactoid reactions, fever.

Interactions

Drug-Drug: ↑ risk of extrapyramidal reactions with other **agents causing extrapyramidal reactions.** ↑ risk of QT interval prolongation with other **agents causing QT interval prolongation**. Drugs that affect serotonergic neurotransmitter systems, including **SSRIs**, **SNRIs**, **tricyclic antidepressants**, **MAOIs**, **fentanyl**, **lithium**, **buspirone**, **tramadol**, **methylene blue**, and **triptans** ↑ risk of serotonin syndrome.

Route/Dosage

Prevention of Nausea and Vomiting Due to Emetogenic Chemotherapy

PO (Adults): 1 mg twice daily; 1st dose given at least 60 min prior to chemotherapy and 2nd dose 12 hr later only on days when chemotherapy is administered; may also be given as 2 mg once daily at least 60 min prior to chemotherapy.

IV (Adults and Children 2–16 yr): 10 mcg/kg within 30 min prior to chemotherapy or 20–40 mcg/kg/day divided once or twice daily (maximum: 3 mg/dose or 9 mg/day).

Transdermal (Adults): One 34.3-mg patch (delivers 3.1 mg/24 hr) applied up to 48 hr prior to chemotherapy, leave in place for at least 24 hr following chemotherapy, may be left in place for a total of 7 days.

Prevention of Nausea and Vomiting Associated with Radiation Therapy

PO (Adults): 2 mg taken once daily within 1 hr of radiation therapy.

Prevention and Treatment of Postoperative Nausea and Vomiting

IV (Adults): *Prevention*—1 mg prior to induction of anesthesia or just prior to reversal of anesthesia; *Treatment*—1 mg.

IV (Children ≥4 yr): 20–40 mcg/kg as a single dose (maximum: 1 mg).

Availability (generic available)

Tablets: 1 mg. **Solution for injection:** 0.1 mg/mL, 1 mg/mL. **Transdermal patch:** 3.1 mg/24 hr.

NURSING IMPLICATIONS

Assessment

- Assess patient for nausea, vomiting, abdominal distention, and bowel sounds prior to and following administration.
- Assess for extrapyramidal symptoms (involuntary movements, facial grimacing, rigidity, shuffling walk,

trembling of hands) during therapy. This occurs rarely and is usually associated with concurrent use of other drugs known to cause this effect.

- Monitor ECG in patients with HF, bradycardia, underlying heart disease, renal impairment and elderly patients.
- Monitor for signs and symptoms of serotonin syndrome (mental status changes [agitation, hallucinations, delirium, and coma], autonomic instability [tachycardia, labile BP, dizziness, diaphoresis, flushing, hyperthermia], neuromuscular symptoms [tremor, rigidity, myoclonus, hyperreflexia, incoordination], seizures, with or without gastrointestinal symptoms [nausea, vomiting, diarrhea]). If symptoms occur discontinue granisetron and treat symptomatically.
- **Transdermal:** Monitor application site. If allergic, erythematous, macular, or papular rash or pruritus occurs, remove patch.
- ***Lab Test Considerations:*** May cause ↑ AST and ALT levels.

Potential Nursing Diagnoses

Imbalanced nutrition: less than body requirements (Indications)

Implementation

- Correct hypokalemia and hypomagnesemia before administering.
- For chemotherapy or radiation, granisetron is administered only on the day(s) chemotherapy or radiation is given. Continued treatment when not on chemotherapy or radiation therapy has not been found to be useful.
- **PO:** Administer 1st dose up to 1 hr before chemotherapy or radiation therapy and 2nd dose 12 hr after the first.

IV Administration

- **IV Push: *Diluent:*** May be administered undiluted or diluted in 20–50 mL of 0.9% NaCl or D5W. Solution should be prepared at time of administration but is stable for 24 hr at room temperature. ***Concentration:*** Up to 1 mg/mL. ***Rate:*** Administer undiluted granisetron over 30 sec or as a diluted solution over 5 min.
- **Y-Site Compatibility:** acetaminophen, alemtuzumab, alfentanil, allopurinol, amifostine, amikacin, aminocaproic acid, aminophylline, amiodarone, amphotericin B lipid complex, amphotericin B liposome, ampicillin, ampicillin/sulbactam, anidulafungin, argatroban, azithromycin, aztreonam, bivalirudin, bleomycin, bumetanide, buprenorphine, busulfan, butorphanol, calcium acetate, calcium chloride, calcium gluconate, carboplatin, carmustine, caspofungin, cefazolin, cefepime, cefotaxime, cefotetan, cefoxitin, ceftaroline, ceftazidime, ceftriaxone, cefuroxime, chloramphenicol, chlorpromazine, ciprofloxacin, cisatracurium, cisplatin, cladribine, clindamycin, cyclophosphamide, cyclosporine, cytarabine, dacarbazine, dactinomycin, daptomycin, daunorubicin hydrochloride, dexamethasone, dexmedetomidine, dexrazoxane, digoxin, diltiazem, diphenhydramine, dobutamine, docetaxel, dopamine, doripenem, doxorubicin hydrochloride, doxorubicin liposome, doxycycline, droperidol, enalaprilat, ephedrine, epinephrine, epirubicin, eptifibatide, ertapenem, erythromycin, esmolol, etoposide, etoposide phosphate, famotidine, fenoldopam, fentanyl, filgrastim, floxuridine, fluconazole, fludarabine, fluorouracil, fosaprepitant, foscarnet, fosphenytoin, furosemide, ganciclovir, gemcitabine, gentamicin, glycopyrrolate, haloperidol, heparin, hetastarch, hydralazine, hydrocortisone, hydromorphone, idarubicin, ifosfamide, imipenem/cilastatin, insulin, irinotecan, isoproterenol, ketorolac, labetalol, leucovorin, levofloxacin, lidocaine, linezolid, lorazepam, magnesium sulfate, mannitol, mechlorethamine, melphalan, meperidine, meropenem, mesna, methotrexate, methyldopate, methylprednisolone, metoclopramide, metoprolol, metronidazole, midazolam, milrinone, mitomycin, mitoxantrone, morphine, moxifloxacin, mycophenolate, nafcillin, nalbuphine, naloxone, nesiritide, nicardipine, nitroglycerin, nitroprusside, norepinephrine, octreotide, oxaliplatin, oxytocin, paclitaxel, pamidronate, pancuronium, pantoprazole, pemetrexed, pentamidine, pentazocine, pentobarbital, phenobarbital, phenylephrine, piperacillin/tazobactam, potassium acetate, potassium chloride, potassium phosphates, procainamide, prochlorperazine, promethazine, propofol, propranolol, quinupristin/dalfopristin, ranitidine, remifentanil, rituximab, rocuronium, sargramostim, sodium acetate, sodium bicarbonate, sodium phosphates, streptozocin, succinylcholine, sufentanil, tacrolimus, teniposide, theophylline, thiopental, thiotepa, tigecycline, tirofiban, tobramycin, topotecan, trastuzumab, trimethoprim/sulfamethoxazole, vancomycin, vasopressin, vecuronium, verapamil, vinblastine, vincristine, vinorelbine, voriconazole, zidovudine, zoledronic acid.
- **Y-Site Incompatibility:** amphotericin B colloidal, dantrolene, diazepam, phenytoin.
- **Additive Incompatibility:** Granisetron should not be admixed with other medications.
- **Transdermal:** Apply system to clear, dry, intact healthy skin on upper outer arm 24–48 hr before chemotherapy. Do not use creams, lotions, or oils that may keep patch from sticking. Do not apply to skin that is red, irritated, or damaged. Apply immediately after removing from package. Do not cut patch into pieces. Remove liner from adhesive layer and press firmly in place with palm of hand for 30

sec, especially around the edges, to make sure contact is complete. Patch should be worn throughout chemotherapy. If patch does not stick, bandages or medical adhesive tape may be applied on edges of patch; do not cover patch with tape or bandages or wrap completely around arm. Patient may shower and wash normally while wearing patch; avoid swimming, strenuous exercise, sauna, or whirlpool during patch use. Remove patch gently at least 24 hr after completion of chemotherapy; may be worn for up to 7 days. Fold so that adhesive edges are together. Throw away in garbage out of reach of children and pets on removal. Do not reuse patch. Use soap and water to remove remaining adhesive; do not use alcohol or acetone.

Patient/Family Teaching

- Instruct patient to take granisetron as directed.
- Advise patient to notify health care professional immediately if involuntary movement of eyes, face, or limbs occurs.
- May cause dizziness and drowsiness. Caution patient to avoid driving and other activities requiring alertness until response to medication is known.
- Advise patient to notify health care professional symptoms of abnormal heart rate or rhythm (racing heartbeat, shortness of breath, dizziness, fainting) or serotonin syndrome occur.
- Advise patient to notify health care professional of all Rx or OTC medications, vitamins, or herbal products being taken and to consult with health care professional before taking other medications.
- Advise female patient to notify health care professional if pregnancy is planned or suspected or if breast feeding.
- **Transdermal:** Instruct patient on correct application, removal, and disposal of patch. Advise patient to read *Patient Information* sheet prior to using and with each Rx refill in case of new information. Inform patient that additional granisetron should not be taken during patch application unless directed by health care professional.
- Advise patient referred for MRI test to discuss patch with referring health care professional and MRI facility to determine if removal of patch is necessary prior to test and for directions for replacing patch.
- Advise patient to cover patch application site with clothing to avoid exposure to sunlight, sunlamp, or tanning beds during and for 10 days following removal of patch.
- Instruct patient to notify health care professional if pain or swelling in the abdomen occurs or if redness at patch removal site remains for more than 3 days.

Evaluation/Desired Outcomes

- Prevention of nausea and vomiting associated with emetogenic cancer chemotherapy or radiation therapy.
- Prevention and treatment of postoperative nausea and vomiting.

guaiFENesin (gwye-**fen**-e-sin)

Alfen Jr, Altarussin, ✤Balminil Expectorant, ✤Benylin Chest Congestion Extra Strength, Breonesin, ✤Bronchophan Expectorant, ✤Chest Congestion, ✤Cough Syrup Expectorant, Diabetic Tussin, ✤Expectorant Syrup, Ganidin NR, Guiatuss, Hytuss, Hytuss-2X, ✤Jack & Jill Expectorant, Mucinex, Naldecon Senior EX, Organidin NR, Robitussin, Scot-tussin Expectorant, Siltussin SA, Siltussin DAS, ✤Vicks Chest Congestion Relief, ✤Vicks Dayquil Mucus Control

Classification

Therapeutic: allergy, cold, and cough remedies, expectorant

Pregnancy Category C

Indications

Coughs associated with viral upper respiratory tract infections.

Action

Reduces viscosity of tenacious secretions by increasing respiratory tract fluid. **Therapeutic Effects:** Mobilization and subsequent expectoration of mucus.

Pharmacokinetics

Absorption: Well absorbed after oral administration.
Distribution: Unknown.
Metabolism and Excretion: Renally excreted as metabolites.
Half-life: Unknown.

TIME/ACTION PROFILE (expectorant action)

ROUTE	ONSET	PEAK	DURATION
PO	30 min	unknown	4–6 hr
PO-ER	unknown	unknown	12 hr

Contraindications/Precautions

Contraindicated in: Hypersensitivity; Some products contain alcohol; Avoid in patients with known intolerance; Some products contain aspartame and should be avoided in patients with phenylketonuria.
Use Cautiously in: Cough lasting >1 wk or accompanied by fever, rash, or headache; Patients receiving disulfiram (liquid products may contain alcohol); Diabetic patients (some products may contain sugar); OB: Although safety has not been established, guaifenesin has been used without adverse effects; Pedi: OTC cough and cold products containing this medication should be avoided in children <4 yr.

Adverse Reactions/Side Effects

CNS: dizziness, headache. **GI:** nausea, diarrhea, stomach pain, vomiting. **Derm:** rash, urticaria.

Interactions

Drug-Drug: None significant.

Route/Dosage

PO (Adults): 200–400 mg q 4 hr or 600–1200 mg q 12 hr as extended-release product (not to exceed 2400 mg/day).
PO (Children 6–12 yr): 100–200 mg q 4 hr or 600 mg q 12 hr as extended-release product (not to exceed 1200 mg/day).
PO (Children 4–6 yr): 50–100 mg q 4 hr (not to exceed 600 mg/day).

Availability (generic available)

Syrup: 100 mg/5 mL[OTC]. **Oral solution:** 100 mg/5 mL[Rx, OTC], 200 mg/5 mL[OTC]. **Capsules:** 200 mg[OTC]. **Tablets:** 100 mg[OTC], 200 mg[Rx, OTC], 1200 mg. **Extended-release tablets (Mucinex):** 600 mg, 1200 mg. ***In combination with:*** analgesics/antipyretics, antihistamines, decongestants, and cough suppressants[Rx, OTC].

NURSING IMPLICATIONS

Assessment

- Assess lung sounds, frequency and type of cough, and character of bronchial secretions periodically during therapy. Maintain fluid intake of 1500–2000 mL/day to decrease viscosity of secretions.

Potential Nursing Diagnoses

Ineffective airway clearance (Indications)

Implementation

- ***High Alert:*** Do not confuse guaifenesin with guanfacine. Do not confuse Mucinex with Mucomyst. Do not confuse Mucinex with Mucinex Allergy.
- **PO:** Administer each dose of guaifenesin followed by a full glass of water to decrease viscosity of secretions.
- Extended-release tablets should be swallowed whole; do not open, break, crush, or chew.

Patient/Family Teaching

- Instruct patient to cough effectively. Patient should sit upright and take several deep breaths before attempting to cough.
- Caution parents to avoid OTC cough and cold products while breast feeding or administering to children <4 yrs.
- Inform patient that drug may occasionally cause dizziness. Avoid driving or other activities requiring alertness until response to drug is known.
- Advise patient to limit talking, stop smoking, maintain moisture in environmental air, and take some sugarless gum or hard candy to help alleviate the discomfort caused by a chronic nonproductive cough.
- Instruct patient to contact health care professional if cough persists longer than 1 wk or is accompanied by fever, rash, or persistent headache or sore throat.

Evaluation/Desired Outcomes

- Easier mobilization and expectoration of mucus from cough associated with upper respiratory infection.

guanFACINE (gwahn-fa-seen)

Intuniv, ✱Intuniv XR, Tenex

Classification
Therapeutic: antihypertensives
Pharmacologic: centrally acting antiadrenergics

Pregnancy Category B

Indications

Hypertension (with thiazide-type diuretics) (immediate-release). Treatment of attention-deficit hyperactivity disorder (ADHD) as monotherapy or as adjunctive therapy to stimulants (extended-release).

Action

Stimulates CNS $alpha_2$-adrenergic receptors, producing a decrease in sympathetic outflow to heart, kidneys, and blood vessels. Result is decreased BP and peripheral resistance, a slight decrease in heart rate, and no change in cardiac output. Mechanism of action in ADHD is unknown. **Therapeutic Effects:** Lowering of BP in hypertension. Increased attention span in ADHD.

Pharmacokinetics

Absorption: Immediate-release is well absorbed (80%); extended-release has lower rate and extent of absorption (↑ absorption with high-fat meals).
Distribution: Appears to be widely distributed.
Metabolism and Excretion: 50% metabolized by the liver, 50% excreted unchanged by the kidneys.
Half-life: 17 hr.

TIME/ACTION PROFILE (antihypertensive effect)

ROUTE	ONSET	PEAK	DURATION
PO (single dose)	unknown	8–12 hr	24 hr
PO (multiple doses)	within 1 wk	1–3 mo	unknown

Contraindications/Precautions

Contraindicated in: Hypersensitivity.
Use Cautiously in: Severe coronary artery disease or recent myocardial infarction; Geri: May have ↑ sensi-

tivity, especially those with hepatic, cardiac, or renal dysfunction; Cerebrovascular disease; Severe renal or liver disease; History of hypotension, heart block, bradycardia, or cardiovascular disease; OB, Lactation, Pedi: Pregnancy, lactation, or children <6 yr (safety not established).

Adverse Reactions/Side Effects

CNS: drowsiness, headache, weakness, depression, dizziness, fatigue, insomnia, irritability. **EENT:** tinnitus. **Resp:** dyspnea. **CV:** bradycardia, chest pain, hypotension, palpitations, rebound hypertension, syncope. **GI:** constipation, dry mouth, abdominal pain, nausea. **GU:** erectile dysfunction.

Interactions

Drug-Drug: ↑ hypotension with other **antihypertensives**, **nitrates**, and acute ingestion of **alcohol**. ↑ CNS depression may occur with other **CNS depressants**, including **alcohol**, **antihistamines**, **opioid analgesics**, **tricyclic antidepressants**, and **sedative/hypnotics**. **NSAIDs** may ↓ effectiveness. **Adrenergics** may ↓ effectiveness. ↑ risk of hypotension and bradycardia with strong **CYP3A4 inhibitors**, including **ketoconazole**. Strong **CYP3A4 inducers**, including **rifampin** may ↓ effects (an ↑ in dose of guanfacine may be needed). May ↑ levels of **valproic acid**.

Route/Dosage

Immediate-release and extended-release tablets should not be interchanged.

Hypertension

PO (Adults): 1 mg daily given at bedtime, may be ↑ if necessary at 3–4 wk intervals up to 2 mg/day; may also be given in 2 divided doses.

ADHD

PO (Adults and Children ≥6 yr): 1 mg once daily in morning or evening; may be ↑ by 1 mg/day at weekly intervals to achieve dose of 1–4 mg/day (6–12 yr) or 1–7 mg-day (13–17 yr) when used as monotherapy or 1–4 mg/day when used as adjunctive therapy.

Availability (generic available)

Immediate-release tablets (Tenex): 1 mg, 2 mg. **Cost:** *Generic*—1 mg $10.34/100, 2 mg $25.67/100. **Extended-release tablets (Intuniv):** 1 mg, 2 mg, 3 mg, 4 mg. **Cost:** All strengths $884.11/100.

NURSING IMPLICATIONS

Assessment

- **Hypertension:** Monitor BP (lying and standing) and pulse frequently during initial dose adjustment and periodically during therapy. Report significant changes.
- Monitor frequency of prescription refills to determine adherence.
- **ADHD:** Assess attention span, impulse control, and interactions with others.
- Monitor BP and heart rate prior to starting therapy, following dose increases, and periodically during therapy. May cause hypotension, orthostatic hypotension, and bradycardia.
- ***Lab Test Considerations:*** May cause temporary, clinically insignificant ↑ in plasma growth hormone levels.
- May cause ↓ in urinary catecholamines and vanillylmandelic acid levels.

Potential Nursing Diagnoses

Risk for injury (Side Effects)
Noncompliance (Patient/Family Teaching)

Implementation

- Do not confuse guanfacine with guaifenesin.
- Do not substitute extended-release tablets for immediate-release tablets on a mg-mg basis. Doses are not the same.
- **PO:** *For hypertension:* Administer daily dose at bedtime to minimize daytime sedation.
- *For ADHD:* Administer once daily. Swallow extended-release tablets whole; do not crush, break, or chew. Do not administer with high fat meals, due to increased exposure.

Patient/Family Teaching

- Advise patient to notify health care professional of all Rx or OTC medications, vitamins, or herbal products being taken and to consult with health care professional before taking other medications, especially cough, cold, or allergy remedies.
- Caution patient to avoid alcohol and other CNS depressants while taking guanfacine.
- Advise patient to notify health care professional if dry mouth or constipation persists. Frequent mouth rinses, good oral hygiene, and sugarless gum or candy may minimize dry mouth. Increase in fluid and fiber intake and exercise may decrease constipation.
- Instruct patient to notify health care professional of medication regimen prior to treatment or surgery.
- Advise patient to notify health care professional if dizziness, prolonged drowsiness, fatigue, weakness, depression, headache, sexual dysfunction, mental depression, or sleep pattern disturbance occurs. Discontinuation may be required if drug-related mental depression occurs.
- Advise female patients to notify health care professional if pregnancy is planned or suspected or if breast feeding.
- Emphasize the importance of follow-up exams to evaluate effectiveness of medication.
- **Hypertension:** Emphasize the importance of continuing to take medication as directed, even if feeling well. Medication controls but does not cure hypertension. Instruct patient to take medication at the same time each day. Take missed doses as soon as remembered; do not double doses. If 2 or more doses are missed, consult health care professional.

Do not discontinue abruptly; may cause sympathetic overstimulation (nervousness, anxiety, rebound hypertension, chest pain, tachycardia, increased salivation, nausea, trembling, stomach cramps, sweating, difficulty sleeping). These effects may occur 2–7 days after discontinuation, although rebound hypertension is rare and more likely to occur with high doses.

- Advise patient to make sure enough medication is available for weekends, holidays, and vacations. A written prescription may be kept in wallet in case of emergency.
- Encourage patient to comply with additional interventions for hypertension (weight reduction, low-sodium diet, smoking cessation, moderation of alcohol consumption, regular exercise, and stress management).
- Instruct patient and family on proper technique for BP monitoring. Advise them to check BP at least weekly and to report significant changes.
- May cause drowsiness or dizziness. Advise patient to avoid driving or other activities requiring alertness until response to the medication is known.
- **ADHD:** Instruct patient to take medication as directed at the same time each day. Take missed doses as soon as possible, but should not take more than the total daily amount in any 24-hr period. Do not stop taking abruptly; discontinue gradually at no more than 1 mg/3–7 days. Advise patient and parents to read the *Medication Guide* prior to starting therapy and with each Rx refill.
- Inform patient that sharing this medication may be dangerous.
- Pedi: Advise parents to notify school nurse of medication regimen.

Evaluation/Desired Outcomes

- Decrease in BP without excessive side effects.
- Improved attention span and social interactions in ADHD. Re-evaluate use if used for >9 wk.

G

halcinonide, See CORTICOSTEROIDS (TOPICAL/LOCAL).

halobetasol, See CORTICOSTEROIDS (TOPICAL/LOCAL).

haloperidol (ha-loe-per-i-dole)

Haldol, Haldol Decanoate

Classification
Therapeutic: antipsychotics
Pharmacologic: butyrophenones

Pregnancy Category C

Indications

Acute and chronic psychotic disorders including: schizophrenia, manic states, drug-induced psychoses. Patients with schizophrenia who require long-term parenteral (IM) antipsychotic therapy. Also useful in managing aggressive or agitated patients. Tourette's syndrome. Severe behavioral problems in children which may be accompanied by: unprovoked, combative, explosive hyperexcitability, hyperactivity accompanied by conduct disorders (short-term use when other modalities have failed). Considered second-line treatment after failure with atypical antipsychotic. **Unlabeled Use:** Nausea and vomiting from surgery or chemotherapy.

Action

Alters the effects of dopamine in the CNS. Also has anticholinergic and alpha-adrenergic blocking activity. **Therapeutic Effects:** Diminished signs and symptoms of psychoses. Improved behavior in children with Tourette's syndrome or other behavioral problems.

Pharmacokinetics

Absorption: Well absorbed following PO/IM administration. Decanoate salt is slowly absorbed and has a long duration of action.
Distribution: Concentrates in liver. Crosses placenta; enters breast milk.
Protein Binding: 92%.
Metabolism and Excretion: Mostly metabolized by the liver.
Half-life: 21–24 hr.

TIME/ACTION PROFILE (antipsychotic activity)

ROUTE	ONSET	PEAK	DURATION
PO	2 hr	2–6 hr	8–12 hr
IM	20–30 min	30–45 min	4–8 hr†
IM (decanoate)	3–9 days	unknown	1 mo

†Effect may persist for several days.

Contraindications/Precautions

Contraindicated in: Hypersensitivity; Angle-closure glaucoma; Bone marrow depression; CNS depression; Parkinsonism; Severe liver or cardiovascular disease (QT interval prolonging conditions); Some products contain tartrazine, sesame oil, or benzyl alcohol and should be avoided in patients with known intolerance or hypersensitivity.
Use Cautiously in: Debilitated patients (dose ↓ required); Cardiac disease (risk of QT prolongation with high doses); Diabetes; Respiratory insufficiency; Prostatic hyperplasia; CNS tumors; Intestinal obstruction; Seizures; OB: Neonates at ↑ risk for extrapyramidal symptoms and withdrawal after delivery when exposed during the 3rd trimester; use only if benefit outweighs risk to fetus; Lactation: Discontinue drug or bottle-feed; Geri: Dose ↓ required due to ↑ sensitivity; ↑ risk of mortality in elderly patients treated for dementia-related psychosis.

Adverse Reactions/Side Effects

CNS: SEIZURES, extrapyramidal reactions, confusion, drowsiness, restlessness, tardive dyskinesia. **EENT:** blurred vision, dry eyes. **Resp:** respiratory depression. **CV:** hypotension, tachycardia, ECG changes (QT prolongation, torsade de pointes), ventricular arrhythmias. **GI:** constipation, dry mouth, anorexia, drug-induced hepatitis, ileus, weight gain. **GU:** impotence, urinary retention. **Derm:** diaphoresis, photosensitivity, rashes. **Endo:** amenorrhea, galactorrhea, gynecomastia. **Hemat:** AGRANULOCYTOSIS, anemia, leukopenia, neutropenia. **Metab:** hyperpyrexia. **Misc:** NEUROLEPTIC MALIGNANT SYNDROME, hypersensitivity reactions.

Interactions

Drug-Drug: May enhance the QTc-prolonging effect of **QTc-prolonging agents**. ↑ hypotension with **antihypertensives**, **nitrates**, or acute ingestion of **alcohol**. ↑ anticholinergic effects with **drugs having anticholinergic properties**, including **antihistamines**, **antidepressants**, **atropine**, **phenothiazines**, **quinidine**, and **disopyramide**. ↑ CNS depression with other **CNS depressants**, including **alcohol**, **antihistamines**, **opioid analgesics**, and **sedative/hypnotics**. Concurrent use with **epinephrine** may result in severe hypotension and tachycardia. May ↓ therapeutic effects of **levodopa**. Acute encephalopathic syndrome may occur when used with **lithium**. Dementia may occur with **methyldopa**.
Drug-Natural Products: Kava-kava, **valerian**, or **chamomile** can ↑ CNS depression.

Route/Dosage

Haloperidol

PO (Adults): 0.5–5 mg 2–3 times daily. Patients with severe symptoms may require up to 100 mg/day.

H

PO (Geriatric Patients or Debilitated Patients): 0.5–2 mg twice daily initially; may be gradually ↑ as needed.
PO (Children 3–12 yr or 15–40 kg): 0.25–0.5 mg/day given in 2–3 divided doses; increase by 0.25–0.5 mg every 5–7 days; maximum dose: 0.15 mg/kg/day (up to 0.75 mg/kg/day for Tourette's syndrome or 0.15 mg/kg/day for psychoses).
IM (Adults): 2–5 mg q 1–8 hr (not to exceed 100 mg/day).
IM (Children 6–12 yr): 1–3 mg/dose every 4–8 hours to a maximum of 0.15 mg/kg/day.
IV (Adults): 0.5–5 mg, may be repeated q 30 min (unlabeled).

Haloperidol Decanoate

IM (Adults): 10–15 times the previous daily PO dose but not to exceed 100 mg initially, given monthly (not to exceed 300 mg/mo).

Availability (generic available)

Tablets: 0.5 mg, 1 mg, 2 mg, 5 mg, 10 mg, 20 mg. **Oral concentrate:** 2 mg/mL. **Haloperidol lactate injection:** 5 mg/mL. **Haloperidol decanoate injection:** 50 mg/mL, 100 mg/mL.

NURSING IMPLICATIONS

Assessment

- Assess mental status (orientation, mood, behavior) prior to and periodically during therapy.
- Assess positive (hallucination, delusions) and negative (social isolation) symptoms of schizophrenia.
- Monitor BP (sitting, standing, lying) and pulse prior to and frequently during the period of dose adjustment. May cause QT interval changes on ECG.
- Observe patient carefully when administering medication, to ensure that medication is actually taken and not hoarded.
- Monitor intake and output ratios and daily weight. Assess patient for signs and symptoms of dehydration (decreased thirst, lethargy, hemoconcentration), especially in geriatric patients.
- Assess fluid intake and bowel function. Increased bulk and fluids in the diet help minimize constipating effects.
- Monitor patient for onset of akathisia (restlessness or desire to keep moving), which may appear within 6 hr of 1st dose and may be difficult to distinguish from psychotic agitation. Benztropine may be used to differentiate agitation from akathisia. Observe closely for extrapyramidal side effects (*parkinsonian*—difficulty speaking or swallowing, loss of balance control, pill rolling of hands, mask-like face, shuffling gait, rigidity, tremors; and *dystonic*—muscle spasms, twisting motions, twitching, inability to move eyes, weakness of arms or legs). Trihexyphenidyl or benzotropine may be used to control these symptoms. Benzodiazepines may alleviate akathisia.
- Monitor for tardive dyskinesia (uncontrolled rhythmic movement of mouth, face, and extremities; lip smacking or puckering; puffing of cheeks; uncontrolled chewing; rapid or worm-like movements of tongue, excessive eye blinking). Report immediately; may be irreversible.
- Monitor for symptoms related to hyperprolactinemia (menstrual abnormalities, galactorrhea, sexual dysfunction).
- Monitor for development of neuroleptic malignant syndrome (fever, respiratory distress, tachycardia, seizures, diaphoresis, hypertension or hypotension, pallor, tiredness, severe muscle stiffness, loss of bladder control). Report symptoms immediately. May also cause leukocytosis, elevated liver function tests, elevated CPK.
- ***Lab Test Considerations:*** Monitor CBC with differential and liver function tests periodically during therapy.
- Monitor serum prolactin prior to and periodically during therapy. May cause ↑ serum prolactin levels.

Potential Nursing Diagnoses

Disturbed thought process (Indications)
Disturbed sensory perception (specify: visual, auditory, kinesthetic, gustatory, tactile, olfactory) (Indications)

Implementation

- Avoid skin contact with oral solution; may cause contact dermatitis.
- **PO:** Administer with food or full glass of water or milk to minimize GI irritation.
- Use calibrated measuring device for accurate dosage. Do not dilute concentrate with coffee or tea; may cause precipitation. May be given undiluted or mixed with water or juice.
- **IM:** Inject slowly, using 2-in., 21-gauge needle into well-developed muscle via Z-track technique. Do not exceed 3 mL per injection site. Slight yellow color does not indicate altered potency. Keep patient recumbent for at least 30 min following injection to minimize hypotensive effects.

IV Administration

- **IV:** Haloperidol decanoate should not be administered IV.
- **IV Push:** ***Diluent:*** May be administered undiluted for rapid control of acute psychosis or delirium. ***Concentration:*** 5 mg/mL. ***Rate:*** Administer at a rate of 5 mg/min.
- **Intermittent Infusion:** ***Diluent:*** May be diluted in 30–50 mL of D5W. ***Rate:*** Infuse over 30 min.
- **Y-Site Compatibility:** alemtuzumab, amifostine, aminocaproic acid, amiodarone, amphotericin B liposome, amsacrine, anidulafungin, argatroban, azithromycin, bleomycin, carboplatin, carmustine, caspofungin, ceftaroline, cisatracurium, cisplatin, cladribine, clonidine, cyclophosphamide, cytarabine, dactinomycin, daptomycin, dexmedetomidine, dexrazoxane, diltiazem, docetaxel, doxacurium,

doxorubicin hydrochloride, doxorubicin liposome, epirubicin, eptifibatide, ertapenem, etoposide, etoposide phosphate, fenoldopam, filgrastim, fludarabine, gemcitabine, granisetron, hetastarch, hydromorphone, idarubicin, ifosfamide, irinotecan, ketamine, leucovorin calcium, levofloxacin, linezolid, lorazepam, mechlorethamine, melphalan, methadone, metronidazole, milrinone, mitoxantrone, morphine, moxifloxacin, mycophenolate, nesiritide, nicardipine, octreotide, oxaliplatin, paclitaxel, palonosetron, pamidronate, pancuronium, pemetrexed, potassium acetate, propofol, quinupristin/dalfopristin, remifentanil, rituximab, rocuronium, sodium acetate, tacrolimus, teniposide, thiotepa, tigecycline, tirofiban, trastuzumab, vecuronium, vinblastine, vincristine, vinorelbine, voriconazole, zoledronic acid.

- **Y-Site Incompatibility:** acyclovir, allopurinol, aminophylline, amphotericin B cholesteryl, amphotericin B colloidal, amphotericin B lipid complex, ampicillin, ampicillin/sulbactam, azathioprine, bumetanide, calcium chloride, cefazolin, cefepime, cefonocid, cefotaxime, cefotetan, cefoxitin, ceftazidime, ceftriaxone, cefuroxime, chloramphenicol, clindamycin, dantrolene, dexamethasone sodium phosphate, diazepam, diazoxide, epoetin alfa, fluorouracil, folic acid, foscarnet, furosemide, ganciclovir, heparin, hydralazine, hydrocortisone, imipenem/cilastatin, indomethacin, ketorolac, magnesium sulfate, methylprednisolone sodium succinate, nafcillin, oxacillin, pantoprazole, penicillin G, pentobarbital, phenobarbital, phenytoin, piperacillin/tazobactam, potassium chloride, sargramostim, sodium bicarbonate, trimethoprim/sulfamethoxazole.

Patient/Family Teaching

- Advise patient to take medication as directed. Take missed doses as soon as remembered, with remaining doses evenly spaced throughout the day. May require several weeks to obtain desired effects. Do not increase dose or discontinue medication without consulting health care professional. Abrupt withdrawal may cause dizziness; nausea; vomiting; GI upset; trembling; or uncontrolled movements of mouth, tongue, or jaw.
- Inform patient of possibility of extrapyramidal symptoms, tardive dyskinesia, and neuroleptic malignant syndrome. Caution patient to report symptoms immediately.
- Advise patient to change positions slowly to minimize orthostatic hypotension.
- May cause drowsiness. Caution patient to avoid driving or other activities requiring alertness until response to medication is known.
- Caution patient to avoid taking alcohol or other CNS depressants concurrently with this medication.
- Advise patient to use sunscreen and protective clothing when exposed to the sun to prevent photosensitivity reactions. Extremes of temperature should also be avoided; drug impairs body temperature regulation.
- Instruct patient to use frequent mouth rinses, good oral hygiene, and sugarless gum or candy to minimize dry mouth.
- Advise patient to notify health care professional of medication regimen prior to treatment or surgery.
- Instruct patient to notify health care professional promptly if weakness, tremors, visual disturbances, dark-colored urine or clay-colored stools, sore throat, fever, menstrual abnormalities, galactorrhea or sexual dysfunction occur.
- Emphasize the importance of routine follow-up exams to monitor response to medication and detect side effects.

Evaluation/Desired Outcomes

- Decrease in hallucinations, insomnia, agitation, hostility, and delusions.
- Decreased tics and vocalization in Tourette's syndrome.
- Improved behavior in children with severe behavioral problems. If no therapeutic effects are seen in 2–4 wk, dosage may be increased.

HIGH ALERT

heparin (hep-a-rin)

✱Hepalean, Hep-Lock, Hep-Lock U/P

Classification

Therapeutic: anticoagulants
Pharmacologic: antithrombotics

Pregnancy Category C

Indications

Prophylaxis and treatment of various thromboembolic disorders including: Venous thromboembolism, Pulmonary emboli, Atrial fibrillation with embolization, Acute and chronic consumptive coagulopathies, Peripheral arterial thromboembolism. Used in very low doses (10–100 units) to maintain patency of IV catheters (heparin flush).

Action

Potentiates the inhibitory effect of antithrombin on factor Xa and thrombin. In low doses, prevents the conversion of prothrombin to thrombin by its effects on factor Xa. Higher doses neutralize thrombin, preventing the conversion of fibrinogen to fibrin. **Therapeutic Effects:** Prevention of thrombus formation. Prevention of extension of existing thrombi (full dose).

Pharmacokinetics

Absorption: Erratically absorbed following subcut or IM administration.

Distribution: Does not cross the placenta or enter breast milk.

Protein Binding: Very high (to low-density lipoproteins, globulins, and fibrinogen).

Metabolism and Excretion: Probably removed by the reticuloendothelial system (lymph nodes, spleen).

Half-life: 1–2 hr (↑ with increasing dose); affected by obesity, renal and hepatic function, malignancy, presence of pulmonary embolism, and infections.

TIME/ACTION PROFILE (anticoagulant effect)

ROUTE	ONSET	PEAK	DURATION
Heparin subcut	20–60 min	2 hr	8–12 hr
Heparin IV	immediate	5–10 min	2–6 hr

Contraindications/Precautions

Contraindicated in: Hypersensitivity; Uncontrolled bleeding; Severe thrombocytopenia; Open wounds (full dose); Avoid use of products containing benzyl alcohol in premature infants.

Use Cautiously in: Severe liver or kidney disease; Retinopathy (hypertensive or diabetic); Untreated hypertension; Ulcer disease; Spinal cord or brain injury; History of congenital or acquired bleeding disorder; Malignancy; OB: May be used during pregnancy, but use with caution during the last trimester and in the immediate postpartum period; Geri: Women >60 yr have ↑ risk of bleeding.

Exercise Extreme Caution in: Severe uncontrolled hypertension; Bacterial endocarditis, bleeding disorders; GI bleeding/ulceration/pathology; Hemorrhagic stroke; Recent CNS or ophthalmologic surgery; Active GI bleeding/ulceration; History of thrombocytopenia related to heparin.

Adverse Reactions/Side Effects

GI: drug-induced hepatitis. **Derm:** alopecia (long-term use), rashes, urticaria. **Hemat:** BLEEDING, HEPARIN-INDUCED THROMBOCYTOPENIA (HIT) (WITH OR WITHOUT THROMBOSIS), anemia. **Local:** pain at injection site. **MS:** osteoporosis (long-term use). **Misc:** fever, hypersensitivity.

Interactions

Heparin is frequently used concurrently or sequentially with other agents affecting coagulation. The risk of potentially serious interactions is greatest with full anticoagulation.

Drug-Drug: Risk of bleeding may be ↑ by concurrent use of **drugs that affect platelet function**, including **aspirin**, **NSAIDs**, **clopidogrel**, **dipyridamole**, some **penicillins**, **abciximab**, **eptifibitide**, **tirofiban**, and **dextran**. Risk of bleeding may be ↑ by concurrent use of **drugs that cause hypoprothrombinemia**, including **quinidine**, **cefotetan**, and **valproic acid**. Concurrent use of **thrombolytics** ↑ risk of bleeding. Heparins affect the prothrombin time used in assessing the response to **warfarin**. **Digoxin**, **tetracyclines**, **nicotine**, and **antihistamines** may ↓ anticoagulant effect of heparin. **Streptokinase** may be followed by relative resistance to heparin.

Drug-Natural Products: ↑ risk of bleeding with **arnica**, **anise**, **chamomile**, **clove**, **dong quai**, **fever few**, **garlic**, **ginger**, and **Panax ginseng**.

Route/Dosage

Therapeutic Anticoagulation

IV (Adults): *Intermittent bolus*—10,000 units, followed by 5000–10,000 units q 4–6 hr. *Continuous infusion*—5000 units (35–70 units/kg), followed by 20,000–40,000 units infused over 24 hr (approx. 1000 units/hr or 15–18 units/kg/hr).

IV (Children > 1 yr): *Intermittent bolus*—50–100 units/kg, followed by 50–100 units/kg q 4 hr. *Continuous infusion*—Loading dose 75 units/kg, followed by 20 units/kg/hr, adjust to maintain aPTT of 60–85 sec.

IV (Neonates and Infants <1 yr): *Continuous infusion*—Loading dose 75 units/kg, followed by 28 units/kg/hr, adjust to maintain aPTT of 60–85 sec.

Subcut (Adults): 5000 units IV, followed by initial subcut dose of 10,000–20,000 units, then 8000–10,000 units q 8 hr or 15,000–20,000 units q 12 hr.

Prophylaxis of Thromboembolism

Subcut (Adults): 5000 units q 8–12 hr (may be started 2 hr prior to surgery).

Cardiovascular Surgery

IV (Adults): At least 150 units/kg (300 units/kg if procedure <60 min; 400 units/kg if >60 min).

Intra-arterial (Neonates, Infants, and Children): 100–150 units/kg via an artery prior to cardiac catheterization.

Line Flushing

IV (Adults and Children): 10–100 units/mL (10 units/mL for infants <10 kg, 100 units/mL for all others) solution to fill heparin lock set to needle hub; replace after each use.

Total Parenteral Nutrition

IV (Adults and Children): 0.5–1 units/mL (final solution concentration) to maintain line patency.

Arterial Line Patency

Intra-arterial (Neonates): 0.5–2 units/mL.

Availability (generic available)

Heparin Sodium

Solution for injection: 10 units/mL, 100 units/mL, 1000 units/mL, 5000 units/mL, 7500 units/mL, 10,000 units/mL, 20,000 units/mL, 40,000 units/mL. **Pre-**

mixed solution: 1000 units/500 mL, 2000 units/1000 mL, 12,500 units/250 mL, 25,000 units in 250 and 500 mL.

NURSING IMPLICATIONS

Assessment

- Assess for signs of bleeding and hemorrhage (bleeding gums; nosebleed; unusual bruising; black, tarry stools; hematuria; fall in hematocrit or BP; guaiac-positive stools). Notify health care professional if these occur.
- Assess patient for evidence of additional or increased thrombosis. Symptoms will depend on area of involvement.
- Monitor patient for hypersensitivity reactions (chills, fever, urticaria).
- **Subcut:** Observe injection sites for hematomas, ecchymosis, or inflammation.
- ***Lab Test Considerations:*** Monitor activated partial thromboplastin time (aPTT) and hematocrit prior to and periodically during therapy. When *intermittent IV* therapy is used, draw aPTT levels 30 min before each dose during initial therapy and then periodically. During *continuous* administration, monitor aPTT levels every 4 hr during early therapy. For *Subcut* therapy, draw blood 4–6 hr after injection.
- Monitor platelet count every 2–3 days throughout therapy. May cause mild thrombocytopenia, which appears on 4th day and resolves despite continued heparin therapy. Heparin-induced thrombocytopenia (HIT), a more severe form which necessitates discontinuing medication, may develop on 8th day of therapy; may reduce platelet count to as low as 5000/mm^3 and lead to increased resistance to heparin therapy. HIT may progress to development of venous and arterial thrombosis (HITT) and may occur up to several wk after discontinuation. Patients who have received a previous course of heparin may be at higher risk for severe thrombocytopenia for several months after the initial course.
- May cause hyperkalemia and ↑ AST and ALT levels.
- ***Toxicity and Overdose:*** Protamine sulfate is the antidote. Due to short half-life, overdose can often be treated by withdrawing the drug.

Potential Nursing Diagnoses

Ineffective tissue perfusion (Indications)
Risk for injury (Side Effects)

Implementation

- ***High Alert:*** Fatal hemorrhages have occurred in pediatric patients due to errors in which heparin sodium injection vials were confused with heparin flush vials. Carefully examine all heparin sodium injection vials to confirm the correct vial choice prior to administration. Have second practitioner independently check original order, dose calculation, and infusion pump settings. Unintended concomitant use of two heparin products (unfractionated heparin and LMW heparins) has resulted in serious harm or death. Review patients' recent (emergency department, operating room) and current medication administration records before administering any heparin or LMW heparin product. Do not confuse heparin with Hespan (hetastarch in sodium chloride). Do not confuse vials of heparin with vials of insulin.
- Inform all personnel caring for patient of anticoagulant therapy. Venipunctures and injection sites require application of pressure to prevent bleeding or hematoma formation. Avoid IM injections of other medications; hematomas may develop.
- In patients requiring long-term anticoagulation, oral anticoagulant therapy should be instituted 4–5 days prior to discontinuing heparin therapy.
- Solution is colorless to slightly yellow.

IV Administration

- **Subcut:** Administer deep into subcut tissue. Alternate injection sites between arm and the left and right abdominal wall above the iliac crest. Inject entire length of needle at a 45°- or 90°-angle into a skin fold held between thumb and forefinger; hold skin fold throughout injection. Do not aspirate or massage. Rotate sites frequently. Do not administer IM because of danger of hematoma formation. Solution should be clear; do not inject solution containing particulate matter.
- **IV Push:** ***Diluent:*** Administer loading dose undiluted. ***Concentration:*** Varies depending upon vial used. ***Rate:*** Administer over at least 1 min. Loading dose given before continuous infusion.
- **Continuous Infusion:** ***Diluent:*** Dilute 25,000 units of heparin in 250–500 mL of 0.9% NaCl or D5W. Premixed infusions are already diluted and ready to use. Admixed solutions stable for 24 hr at room temperature or if refrigerated. Premixed infusion stable for 30 days once overwrap removed. ***Concentration:*** 50–100 units/mL. ***Rate:*** See Route/Dosage section. Adjust to maintain therapeutic aPTT. Use an infusion pump to ensure accuracy.
- **Flush:** To prevent clot formation in intermittent infusion (heparin lock) sets, inject dilute heparin solution of 10–100 units/0.5–1 mL after each medication injection or every 8–12 hr. To prevent incompatibility of heparin with medication, flush lock set with sterile water or 0.9% NaCl for injection before and after medication is administered.
- **Y-Site Compatibility:** acyclovir, alemtuzumab, alfentanil, allopurinol, amifostine, aminocaproic acid, aminophylline, amphotericin B lipid complex, amphotericin B liposome, anidulafungin, argatroban,

ascorbic acid, atropine, azathioprine, aztreonam, benztropine, bivalirudin, bleomycin, bumetanide, buprenorphine, butorphanol, calcium chloride, calcium gluconate, carboplatin, carmustine, cefazolin, cefotaxime, cefotetan, cefoxitin, ceftaroline, ceftazidime, ceftriaxone, cefuroxime, chloramphenicol, cisplatin, cladribine, clindamycin, cyanocobalamin, cyclosporine, cytarabine, dactinomycin, daptomycin, dexamethasone, dexmedetomidine, digoxin, docetaxel, dopamine, doripenem, doxacurium, doxapram, doxorubicin liposome, edrophonium, enalaprilat, ephedrine, epinephrine, epoetin alfa, eptifibatide, ertapenem, estrogens, conjugated, etoposide, etoposide phosphate, famotidine, fenoldopam, fentanyl, fluconazole, fludarabine, flumazenil, fluorouracil, folic acid, foscarnet, ganciclovir, gemcitabine, glycopyrrolate, granisetron, hydrocortisone, hydromorphone, ifosfamide, imipenem/cilastatin, indomethacin, irinotecan, isoproterenol, ketorolac, leucovorin, lidocaine, linezolid, lorazepam, magnesium sulfate, mannitol, mechlorethamine, melphalan, meropenem, metaraminol, methotrexate, methoxamine, methyldopate, methylergonovine, metoclopramide, metoprolol, metronidazole, micafungin, midazolam, milrinone, mitomycin, morphine, multiple vitamins, nafcillin, nalbuphine, naloxone, neostigmine, nitroglycerin, nitroprusside, norepinephrine, octreotide, ondansetron, oxacillin, oxaliplatin, oxytocin, paclitaxel, palonosetron, pamidronate, pancuronium, pemetrexed, penicillin G, pentobarbital, phenobarbital, phentolamine, phenylephrine, phytonadione, piperacillin/tazobactam, potassium acetate, potassium chloride, procainamide, propofol, propranolol, pyridostigmine, pyridoxime, ranitidine, remifentanil, rituximab, rocuronium, sargramostim, scopolamine, sodium acetate, sodium bicarbonate, streptokinase, succinylcholine, sufentanil, tacrolimus, theophylline, thiamine, thiopental, thiotepa, tigecycline, tirofiban, tolazoline, tranexamic acid, trastuzumab, trimetaphan, vasopressin, vecuronium, verapamil, vinblastine, vincristine, voriconazole, warfarin, zidovudine, zoledronic acid.

- **Y-Site Incompatibility:** alteplase, amikacin, amiodarone, amphotericin B cholesteryl, amsacrine, caspofungin, ciprofloxacin, dantrolene, diazepam, diazoxide, doxycycline, epirubicin, filgrastim, gentamicin, haloperidol, hydroxyzine, idarubicin, ketamine, levofloxacin, mitoxantrone, mycophenolate, palifermin, papaverine, pentamidine, phenytoin, protamine, quinupristin/dalfopristin, reteplase, tobramycin, trimethoprim/sulfamethoxazole, vancomycin.
- **Additive Compatibility:** It is recommended that heparin not be mixed in solution with other medications when given for anticoagulation, even those that are compatible, because changes in rate of heparin infusion may be required that would also affect admixtures.

Patient/Family Teaching

- Advise patient to report any symptoms of unusual bleeding or bruising to health care professional immediately.
- Instruct patient not to take medications containing aspirin or NSAIDs while on heparin therapy.
- Caution patient to avoid IM injections and activities leading to injury and to use a soft toothbrush and electric razor during heparin therapy.
- Advise patient to inform health care professional of medication regimen prior to treatment or surgery.
- Patients on anticoagulant therapy should carry an identification card with this information at all times.

Evaluation/Desired Outcomes

- Prolonged partial thromboplastin time (PTT) of 1.5–2.5 times the control, without signs of hemorrhage.
- Prevention of deep vein thrombosis and pulmonary emboli.
- Patency of IV catheters.

HIGH ALERT

HEPARINS (LOW MOLECULAR WEIGHT)

dalteparin (dal-**te**-pa-rin)
Fragmin

enoxaparin (e-nox-a-**pa**-rin)
Lovenox

Classification
Therapeutic: anticoagulants
Pharmacologic: antithrombotics

Pregnancy Category B

Indications

Enoxaparin and dalteparin: Prevention of venous thromboembolism (VTE) (deep vein thrombosis (DVT) and/or pulmonary embolism (PE)) in surgical or medical patients. **Dalteparin only:** Extended treatment of symptomatic DVT and/or PE in patients with cancer. **Enoxaparin only:** Treatment of DVT with or without PE (with warfarin). **Enoxaparin and dalteparin:** Prevention of ischemic complications (with aspirin) from unstable angina and non-ST-segment-elevation MI. **Enoxaparin only:** Treatment of acute ST-segment-elevation MI (with thrombolytics or percutaneous coronary intervention).

Action

Potentiate the inhibitory effect of antithrombin on factor Xa and thrombin. **Therapeutic Effects:** Prevention of thrombus formation.

Pharmacokinetics

Absorption: Well absorbed after subcut administration (87% for dalteparin, 92% for enoxaparin).
Distribution: Unknown.

Metabolism and Excretion: *Dalteparin*—unknown; *enoxaparin*—primarily eliminated renally.
Half-life: *Dalteparin*—2.1–2.3 hr; *enoxaparin*—3–6 hr (all are ↑ in renal insufficiency).

TIME/ACTION PROFILE (anticoagulant effect)

ROUTE	ONSET	PEAK	DURATION
Dalteparin subcut	rapid	4 hr	up to 24 hr
Enoxaparin subcut	unknown	3–5 hr	12 hr

Contraindications/Precautions

Contraindicated in: Hypersensitivity to specific agents or pork products; cross-sensitivity may occur; Some products contain sulfites or benzyl alcohol and should be avoided in patients with known hypersensitivity or intolerance; Active major bleeding; History of heparin-induced thrombocytopenia; *Dalteparin*—regional anesthesia during treatment for unstable angina/non–Q-wave MI.
Use Cautiously in: Severe hepatic or renal disease (adjust dose of enoxaparin if CCr <30 mL/min); Women <45 kg or men <57 kg; Retinopathy (hypertensive or diabetic); Untreated hypertension; Geri: May have ↑ risk of bleeding due to age-related ↓ in renal function; *Dalteparin*— Geri: ↑ mortality in patients >70 yrs with renal insufficiency; Recent history of ulcer disease; History of congenital or acquired bleeding disorder; OB, Lactation, Pedi: Safety not established; should not be used in pregnant patients with prosthetic heart valves without careful monitoring.
Exercise Extreme Caution in: Spinal/epidural anesthesia (↑ risk of spinal/epidural hematomas, especially with concurrent NSAIDs, repeated or traumatic epidural puncture, or indwelling epidural catheter); Severe uncontrolled hypertension; Bacterial endocarditis; Bleeding disorders.

Adverse Reactions/Side Effects

CNS: dizziness, headache, insomnia. **CV:** edema. **GI:** constipation, ↑ liver enzymes, nausea, vomiting. **GU:** urinary retention. **Derm:** alopecia, ecchymoses, pruritus, rash, urticaria. **Hemat:** BLEEDING, anemia, eosinophilia, thrombocytopenia. **Local:** erythema at injection site, hematoma, irritation, pain. **MS:** osteoporosis. **Misc:** fever.

Interactions

Drug-Drug: Risk of bleeding may be ↑ by concurrent use of **drugs that affect platelet function and coagulation**, including **warfarin**, **aspirin**, **NSAIDs**, **dipyridamole**, **clopidogrel**, **abciximab**, **eptifibatide**, **tirofiban**, and **thrombolytics**.
Drug-Natural Products: ↑ bleeding risk with, **arnica**, **chamomile**, **clove**, **feverfew**, **garlic**, **ginger**, **ginkgo**, **Panax ginseng**, and others.

Route/Dosage

Dalteparin

Subcut (Adults): *Prophylaxis of DVT following abdominal surgery*—2500 units 1–2 hr before surgery, then once daily for 5–10 days; *Prophylaxis of VTE in high-risk patients undergoing abdominal surgery*—5000 units evening before surgery, then once daily for 5–10 days *or* in patients with malignancy, 2500 units 1–2 hr before surgery, another 2500 units 12 hr later, then 5000 units once daily for 5–10 days; *Prophylaxis of VTE in patients undergoing hip replacement surgery*—2500 units within 2 hr before surgery, then 2500 units 4–8 hr after surgery, then 5000 units once daily (start at least 6 hr after postsurgical dose) for 5–10 days *or* 5000 units evening before surgery (10–14 hr before surgery), then 5000 units 4–8 hr after surgery, then 5000 units once daily for 5–10 days *or* 2500 units 4–8 hr after surgery, then 5000 units once daily (start at least 6 hr after postsurgical dose); *Prophylaxis of VTE in medical patients with severely restricted mobility during acute illness:* 5000 units once daily for 12 to 14 days. *Unstable angina/non–ST-segment-elevation MI*—120 units/kg (not to exceed 10,000 units) q 12 hr for 5–8 days with concurrent aspirin; *Extended treatment of symptomatic VTE in cancer patients*—200 units/kg (not to exceed 18,000 units) once daily for first 30 days, followed by 150 units/kg (not to exceed 18,000 units) once daily for months 2–6.

Renal Impairment

Subcut (Adults): *Cancer patients receiving extended treatment of symptomatic VTE with CCr <30 mL/min*—Monitor anti-Xa levels (target 0.5–1.5 IU/mL).

Enoxaparin

Subcut (Adults): *VTE prophylaxis in patients undergoing knee replacement surgery*—30 mg q 12 hr starting 12–24 hr postop for 7–10 days; *VTE prophylaxis in patients undergoing hip replacement surgery*—30 mg q 12 hr starting 12–24 hr postop *or* 40 mg once daily starting 12 hr before surgery (either dose may be continued for 7–14 days; continued prophylaxis with 40 mg once daily may be continued for up to 3 wk); *VTE prophylaxis following abdominal surgery*—40 mg once daily starting 2 hr before surgery and then continued for 7–12 days or until ambulatory (up to 14 days); *VTE prophylaxis in medical patients with acute illness*—40 mg once daily for 6–14 days; *Treatment of DVT/PE (outpatient)*—1 mg/kg q 12 hr. Warfarin should be started within 72 hr; enoxaparin may be continued for a minimum of 5 days and until therapeutic anticoagulation with warfarin is achieved (INR >2 for 2 consecutive days); *Treatment of DVT/PE (inpatient)*—1 mg/kg q 12 hr *or* 1.5 mg/kg once

H

daily. Warfarin should be started within 72 hr; enoxaparin may be continued for a minimum of 5 days and until therapeutic anticoagulation with warfarin is achieved (INR >2 for two consecutive days); *Unstable angina/non—ST-segment-elevation MI*—1 mg/kg q 12 hr for 2–8 days (with aspirin).

IV, Subcut (Adults <75 yr): *Acute ST–segment-elevation MI*—Administer single IV bolus of 30 mg plus 1 mg/kg subcut dose (maximum of 100 mg for first 2 doses only), followed by 1 mg/kg subcut q 12 hr. The usual duration of treatment is 2–8 days. In patients undergoing percutaneous coronary intervention, if last subcut dose was <8 hr before balloon inflation, no additional dosing needed; if last subcut dose was ≥8 hr before balloon inflation, administer single IV bolus of 0.3 mg/kg.

Subcut (Adults ≥75 yr): *Acute ST-segment-elevation MI*—0.75 mg/kg every 12 hr (no IV bolus needed) (maximum of 75 mg for first 2 doses only; no initial bolus). The usual duration of treatment is 2–8 days.

Renal Impairment

Subcut (Adults CCr <30 mL/min): *VTE prophylaxis for abdominal or knee/hip replacement surgery*—30 mg once daily. *Treatment of DVT/PE*—1 mg/kg once daily. *Unstable angina/non-ST-segment-elevation MI*—1 mg/kg once daily. *Acute ST-segment-elevation MI (patients <75 yr)*—Single IV bolus of 30 mg plus 1 mg/kg subcut dose, followed by 1 mg/kg subcut once daily. *Acute ST-segment-elevation MI (patients ≥75 yr)*—1 mg/kg once daily (no initial bolus).

Availability

Dalteparin

Solution for injection (prefilled syringes): 2500 units/0.2 mL, 5000 units/0.2 mL, 7500 units/0.3 mL, 10,000 units/1 mL, 12,500 units/0.5 mL, 15,000 units/0.6 mL, 18,000 units/0.72 mL. **Solution for injection (multidose vials):** 25,000 IU/mL.

Enoxaparin (generic available)

Solution for injection (prefilled syringes): 30 mg/0.3 mL, 40 mg/0.4 mL, 60 mg/0.6 mL, 80 mg/0.8 mL, 100 mg/1 mL, 120 mg/0.8 mL, 150 mg/mL. **Solution for injection (multidose vials):** 300 mg/3 mL.

NURSING IMPLICATIONS

Assessment

- Assess for signs of bleeding and hemorrhage (bleeding gums; nosebleed; unusual bruising; black, tarry stools; hematuria; fall in hematocrit or BP; guaiac-positive stools); bleeding from surgical site. Notify health care professional if these occur.
- Assess patient for evidence of additional or increased thrombosis. Symptoms depend on area of involvement.
- Assess for evidence of additional or increased thrombosis. Symptoms depend on area of involvement. Monitor neurological status frequently for signs of neurological impairment. May require urgent treatment.
- Monitor for hypersensitivity reactions (chills, fever, urticaria). Report signs to health care professional.
- Monitor patients with epidural catheters frequently for signs and symptoms of neurologic impairment. Delay placement or removal of catheter for at least 12 hours after administration of lower doses (30 mg once or twice daily or 40 mg once daily) and at least 24 hours after administration of higher doses (0.75 mg/kg twice daily, 1 mg/kg twice daily, or 1.5 mg/kg once daily) of enoxaparin. Do not give 2nd enoxaparin dose in twice daily regimen to patients receiving 0.75 mg/kg twice daily dose or 1 mg/kg twice daily dose to allow a longer delay before catheter placement or removal, then delay next dose for at least 4 hrs. For patients with creatinine clearance <30 mL/minute, double timing of removal of catheter, at least 24 hrs for lower dose (30 mg once daily) and at least 48 hrs for higher dose (1 mg/kg/day). Monitor for signs and symptoms of neurological impairment (midline back pain, sensory and motor deficits [numbness or weakness in lower limbs], bowel and/or bladder dysfunction) frequently if epidural or spinal anesthesia or lumbar puncture is done during therapy.
- **Subcut:** Observe injection sites for hematomas, ecchymosis, or inflammation.
- ***Lab Test Considerations:*** Monitor CBC, platelet count, and stools for occult blood periodically during therapy. If thrombocytopenia occurs (platelet count <100,000/mm³), discontinue therapy. If hematocrit ↓ unexpectedly, assess patient for potential bleeding sites. For *dalteparin* use for extended treatment of symptomatic VTE in cancer patients, if platelets ↓ to 50,000–100,000/mm³, reduce dose to 2500 units once daily until recovery to ≥100,000/mm³; if platelets <50,000/mm³, discontinue until count returns to ≥50,000/mm³.
- Special monitoring of aPTT is not necessary. Monitoring of anti-Xa levels may be considered in patients who are obese or have renal dysfunction (for *enoxaparin*, obtain 4 hr after injection).
- Monitoring of antifactor Xa levels may be necessary to titrate doses in pediatric patients (therapeutic range 0.5–1 unit/mL).
- May cause ↑ in AST and ALT levels.
- ***Toxicity and Overdose:*** For *enoxaparin* overdose, protamine sulfate 1 mg for each mg of *enoxaparin* should be administered by slow IV injection. For *dalteparin* overdose, protamine sulfate 1 mg for each 100 anti-factor Xa IU of *dalteparin* should be administered by slow IV injection. If the aPTT measured 2–4 hr after protamine administration remains prolonged, a 2nd infusion of protamine 0.5 mg/100 anti-factor Xa IU of *dalteparin* may be administered.

Potential Nursing Diagnoses

Ineffective tissue perfusion (Indications)
Risk for injury (Side Effects)

Implementation

- ***High Alert:*** Unintended concomitant use of two heparin products (unfractionated heparin and low molecular weight heparins) has resulted in serious harm and death. Review patients' recent and current medication administration records before administering any heparin or low-molecular-weight heparin product.
- Do not confuse Lovenox with Levemir.
- Cannot be used interchangeably (unit for unit) with unfractionated heparin or other low-molecular-weight heparins.
- **Subcut:** Administer deep into subcut tissue. Alternate injection sites daily between the left and right anterolateral and left and right posterolateral abdominal wall, the upper thigh, or buttocks. Inject entire length of needle at a 45° or 90° angle into a skin fold held between thumb and forefinger; hold skin fold throughout injection. Do not aspirate or massage. Rotate sites frequently. Do not administer IM because of danger of hematoma formation. Solution should be clear and colorless to slightly yellow; do not inject solution containing particulate matter.
- If excessive bruising occurs, ice cube massage of site before injection may lessen bruising.
- **Enoxaparin:** To avoid the loss of drug, do not expel the air bubble from the syringe before the injection.
- **Subcut:** Per manufacturer's recommendations, to enhance absorption, inject enoxaparin into left or right anterolateral or posterolateral abdominal wall only.
- To minimize risk of bleeding after vascular instrumentation for unstable angina, recommended intervals between doses should be followed closely. Leave vascular access sheath in place for 6–8 hr after enoxaparin dose. Give next enoxaparin dose ≥6–8 hr after sheath removal. Observe site for bleeding or hematoma formation.

IV Administration

- **IV Push:** (for treatment of STEMI only) Use multiple-dose vial. Inject via IV line. Flush with 0.9% NaCl or D5W prior to and following administration to avoid mixture with other drugs and clear the port of the drug. May be administered with 0.9% NaCl or D5W. ***Rate:*** Inject as a bolus.
- **Y-Site Incompatibility:** Do not mix or co-administer with other medications.

Patient/Family Teaching

- Instruct patient in correct technique for self injection, care and disposal of equipment.
- Advise patient to report any symptoms of unusual bleeding or bruising, dizziness, itching, rash, fever, swelling, or difficulty breathing to health care professional immediately.
- Instruct patient not to take aspirin or NSAIDs without consulting health care professional while on therapy.

Evaluation/Desired Outcomes

- Prevention of DVT and pulmonary emboli (enoxaparin and dalteparin).
- Resolution of DVT and pulmonary embolism (enoxaparin only).
- Prevention of ischemic complications (with aspirin) in patients with unstable angina or non–ST—segment—elevation MI (enoxaparin and dalteparin).
- Treatment of acute ST-segment elevation myocardial infarction (enoxaparin only).

HISTAMINE H_2 ANTAGONISTS

cimetidine (sye-**me**-ti-deen)
Tagamet, Tagamet HB

famotidine (fa-**moe**-ti-deen)
✱Acid Control, Pepcid, Pepcid AC, ✱Peptic Guard, ✱Ulcidine

nizatidine (ni-**za**-ti-deen)
Axid, Axid AR

ranitidine (ra-**ni**-ti-deen)
✱Acid Reducer, Zantac, Zantac EFFERdose, Zantac 75, Zantac 150

Classification
Therapeutic: antiulcer agents
Pharmacologic: histamine H_2 antagonists

Pregnancy Category B

Indications

Short-term treatment of active duodenal ulcers and benign gastric ulcers. Maintenance therapy for duodenal and gastric ulcers after healing of active ulcers. Management of GERD. Treatment of heartburn, acid indigestion, and sour stomach (OTC use). **Cimetidine, famotidine, ranitidine:** Management of gastric hypersecretory states (Zollinger-Ellison syndrome). **Famotidine, ranitidine IV:** Prevention and treatment of stress-induced upper GI bleeding in critically ill patients. **Ranitidine:** Treatment of and maintenance therapy for erosive esophagitis. **Unlabeled Use:** Management of GI symptoms associated with the use of NSAIDs. Prevention of acid inactivation of supplemental pancreatic enzymes in patients with pancreatic insufficiency. Management of urticaria.

Action

Inhibits the action of histamine at the H_2-receptor site located primarily in gastric parietal cells, resulting in inhibition of gastric acid secretion. **Therapeutic Effects:** Healing and prevention of ulcers. Decreased symptoms of gastroesophageal reflux. Decreased secretion of gastric acid.

Pharmacokinetics

Absorption: *Cimetidine*—well absorbed after oral administration. *Famotidine*—40–45% absorbed after oral administration. *Nizatidine*—70–95% absorbed after oral administration. *Ranitidine*—50% absorbed after PO and IM administration.

Distribution: All agents enter breast milk and cerebrospinal fluid.

Metabolism and Excretion: *Cimetidine*—30% metabolized by the liver; remainder is eliminated unchanged by the kidneys. *Famotidine*—up to 70% excreted unchanged by the kidneys, 30–35% metabolized by the liver. *Nizatidine*—60% excreted unchanged by the kidneys; some hepatic metabolism; at least 1 metabolite has histamine-blocking activity. *Ranitidine*—metabolized by the liver, mostly on first pass; 30% excreted unchanged by the kidneys after PO administration, 70% after parenteral administration.

Half-life: *Cimetidine*—2 hr; *famotidine*—2.5–3.5 hr; *nizatidine*—1.6 hr; *ranitidine*—2–2.5 hr (all are ↑ in renal impairment).

TIME/ACTION PROFILE

ROUTE	ONSET	PEAK	DURATION
Cimetidine PO	30 min	45–90 min	4–5 hr
Famotidine PO	within 60 min	1–4 hr	6–12 hr
Famotidine IV	within 60 min	0.5–3 hr	8–15 hr
Nizatidine PO	unknown	unknown	8–12 hr
Ranitidine PO	unknown	1–3 hr	8–12 hr
Ranitidine IM	unknown	15 min	8–12 hr
Ranitidine IV	unknown	15 min	8–12 hr

Contraindications/Precautions

Contraindicated in: Hypersensitivity; Some products contain alcohol and should be avoided in patients with known intolerance; Some products contain aspartame and should be avoided in patients with phenylketonuria.

Use Cautiously in: Renal impairment (more susceptible to adverse CNS reactions; ↑ dose interval recommended for *cimetidine* and *nizatidine* if CCr ≤50 mL/min, and for *famotidine* and *ranitidine* if CCr <50 mL/min; Hepatic impairment (for *ranitidine*); Acute porphyria (for *ranitidine*); Geri: More susceptible to adverse CNS reactions; dose ↓ recommended; OB, Lactation: Pregnancy or lactation.

Adverse Reactions/Side Effects

CNS: confusion, dizziness, drowsiness, hallucinations, headache. **CV:** ARRHYTHMIAS. **GI:** constipation, diarrhea, drug-induced hepatitis (nizatidine, cimetidine), nausea. **GU:** ↓ sperm count, erectile dysfunction (cimetidine). **Endo:** gynecomastia. **Hemat:** AGRANULOCYTOSIS, APLASTIC ANEMIA, anemia, neutropenia, thrombocytopenia. **Local:** pain at IM site. **Misc:** hypersensivity reactions, vasculitis.

Interactions

Drug-Drug: Cimetidine is a moderate inhibitor of the CYP1A2, CYP2C9, CYP2D6, and CYP3A4 isoenzymes in the liver; may lead to ↑ levels and toxicity with **benzodiazepines** (especially **chlordiazepoxide, diazepam**, and **midazolam**), some **beta blockers (labetalol, metoprolol, propranolol)**, **caffeine, calcium channel blockers, carbamazepine, cyclosporine, dofetilide, lidocaine, metronidazole, mexiletine, nefazodone, pentoxifylline, phenytoin, procainamide, propafenone, quinidine, metformin, risperidone, ritonavir, ropinirole, selective serotonin reuptake inhibitors, sildenafil, sulfonylureas, tacrolimus, theophylline, tricyclic antidepressants, venlafaxine**, and **warfarin**. Famotidine, nizatidine, and ranitidine have a much smaller and less significant effect on the metabolism of other drugs. Cimetidine may ↑ myelosuppressive effects of **carmustine** (avoid concurrent use). All may ↓ absorption of **ketoconazole, itraconazole, atazanavir, delavirdine**, and **gefitinib**. Ranitidine may ↑ absorption of **triazolam, midazolam**, and **glipizide**. Ranitidine may ↑ **procainamide** levels. Ranitidine may ↑ the effects of **warfarin**.

Route/Dosage

Cimetidine

PO (Adults): *Short-term treatment of active ulcers*—300 mg 4 times daily *or* 800 mg at bedtime *or* 400–600 mg twice daily (not to exceed 2.4 g/day) for up to 8 wk. *Duodenal ulcer prophylaxis*—300 mg twice daily *or* 400 mg at bedtime. *GERD*—400 mg q 6 hr *or* 800 mg twice daily for 12 wk. *Gastric hypersecretory conditions*—300–600 mg q 6 hr (up to 2400 mg/day). *OTC use*—up to 200 mg may be taken twice daily (for not more than 2 wk).

PO (Children): *Short-term treatment of active ulcers*—5–10 mg/kg q 6 hr.

Renal Impairment

PO (Adults): *CCr 10–50 mL/min*—Administer 50% of normal dose; *CCr <10 mL/min*—Administer 25% of normal dose.

Renal Impairment

PO (Children): 10–15 mg/kg/day.

Famotidine

PO (Adults): *Short-term treatment of active duodenal ulcers*—40 mg/day at bedtime or 20 mg twice daily for up to 8 wk. *Treatment of benign gastric ulcers*—40 mg/day at bedtime. *Maintenance treatment of duodenal ulcers*—20 mg once daily at bedtime. *GERD*—20 mg twice daily for up to 6 wk; up to 40 mg twice daily for up to 12 wk for esophagitis with erosions, ulcerations, and continuing symptoms. *Gastric hypersecretory conditions*—20 mg q 6 hr initially, up

to 160 mg q 6 hr. *OTC use*—10 mg for relief of symptoms; for prevention—10 mg 60 min before eating or take 10 mg as chewable tablet 15 minutes before heartburn-inducing foods or beverages (not to exceed 20 mg/24 hr for up to 2 wk).
PO, IV (Children 1–16 yr): *Peptic ulcer*—0.5 mg/kg/day as a single bedtime dose or in 2 divided doses (up to 40 mg daily); *GERD*—1 mg/kg/day in 2 divided doses(up to 80 mg twice daily).
PO (Infants >3 mo–1 yr): *GERD*—0.5 mg/kg/dose twice daily.
PO (Infants and neonates <3 mo): *GERD*—0.5 mg/kg/dose once daily.
IV (Adults): 20 mg q 12 hr.

Renal Impairment

PO (Adults): *CCr <50 mL/min*—administer normal dose q 36–48 hr *or* 50% of normal dose at normal dosing interval. *CCr <10 mL/min*—dosing interval may need to be ↑ to q 36–48 hr.

Nizatidine

PO (Adults): *Short-term treatment of active duodenal or benign gastric ulcers*—300 mg once daily at bedtime. *Maintenance treatment of duodenal ulcers*—150 mg once daily at bedtime. *GERD*—150 mg twice daily. *OTC use*—75 mg twice daily given 30–60 min before foods or beverages expected to cause symptoms.

Renal Impairment

PO (Adults): *Short-term treatment of active ulcers—CCr 20–50 mL/min*—150 mg once daily; *CCr <20 mL/min*—150 mg every other day. *Maintenance treatment of duodenal ulcers—CCr 20–50 mL/min*—150 mg every other day; *CCr <20 mL/min*—150 mg every 3 days.

Ranitidine

PO (Adults): *Short-term treatment of active duodenal of benign gastric ulcers*—150 mg twice daily *or* 300 mg once daily at bedtime. *Maintenance treatment of duodenal or gastric ulcers*—150 mg once daily at bedtime. *GERD*—150 mg twice daily. *Erosive esophagitis*—150 mg 4 times daily initially, then 150 mg twice daily as maintenance. *Gastric hypersecretory conditions*—150 mg twice daily initially; up to 6 g/day have been used. *OTC use*—75 mg 30–60 min before foods or beverages expected to cause symptoms (up to twice daily) (not to be used for more than 2 wk).
PO (Children 1 mo–16 yr): *Treatment of gastric/duodenal ulcers*—2–4 mg/kg/day in 2 divided doses (up to 300 mg/day); *Maintenance treatment of ulcers*—2–4 mg/kg once daily (up to 150 mg/day); *GERD/erosive esophagitis*—5–10 mg/kg/day in 2 divided doses (up to 300 mg/day for GERD or 600 mg/day for erosive esophagitis).
PO (Neonates): 2 mg/kg/day in 2 divided doses.
IV, IM (Adults): 50 mg q 6–8 hr. *Continuous IV infusion*—6.25 mg/hr. *Gastric hypersecretory conditions*—1 mg/kg/hr; may be ↑ by 0.5 mg/kg/hr (not to exceed 2.5 mg/kg/hr).
IV, IM (Children 1 mo–16 yr): *Treatment of gastric/duodenal ulcers*—2–4 mg/kg/day divided q 6–8 hr (up to 200 mg/day). *Continuous infusion*—1 mg/kg/dose followed by 0.08–0.17 mg/kg/hr.
IV (Neonates): 1.5 mg/kg/dose load, then in 12 hr start maintenance of 1.5–2 mg/kg/day divided q 12 hr. *Continuous IV infusion*—1.5 mg/kg/dose load followed by 0.04–0.08 mg/kg/hr infusion.

Renal Impairment

PO (Adults): *CCr <50 mL/min*—150 mg q 24 hr.

Renal Impairment

IV (Adults): *CCr <50 mL/min*—50 mg q 24 hr.

Availability

Cimetidine (generic available)

Tablets: 200 mg[Rx, OTC], 300 mg, 400 mg, ✤ 600 mg, 800 mg. **Cost:** *Generic*—200 mg $82.15/100, 300 mg $90.45/100, 400 mg $146.85/100, 800 mg $220.00/100. **Oral liquid (mint-peach flavor):** 200 mg/5 mL[OTC], 300 mg/5 mL. **Cost:** *Generic*—300 mg/5 mL $89.00/237 mL.

Famotidine (generic available)

Tablets: 10 mg[OTC], 20 mg[Rx, OTC], 40 mg. **Cost:** *Generic*—20 mg $173.50/100, 40 mg $335.00/100. **Gelcaps:** 10 mg[OTC]. **Oral suspension (cherry-banana-mint flavor):** 40 mg/5 mL. **Cost:** *Generic*—$176.95/50 mL. **Premixed infusion:** 20 mg/50 mL 0.9% NaCl. **Solution for injection:** 10 mg/mL. ***In combination with:*** ibuprofen (Duexis), calcium carbonate and magnesium hydroxide[OTC] (Pepcid Complete, see Appendix B).

Nizatidine (generic available)

Tablets: 75 mg[OTC]. **Capsules:** 150 mg, 300 mg. **Cost:** *Generic*—150 mg $143.28/60, 300 mg $142.98/30. **Oral solution (bubble gum flavor):** 15 mg/mL. **Cost:** *Generic*—$347.65/473 mL.

Ranitidine (generic available)

Tablets: 75 mg[OTC], 150 mg, 300 mg. **Cost:** *Generic*—150 mg $156.20/100, 300 mg $87.85/30. **Capsules:** 150 mg, 300 mg. **Cost:** *Generic*—150 mg $91.27/60, 300 mg $82.30/30. **Effervescent tablets (EFFERdose):** 25 mg. **Syrup (peppermint flavor):** 15 mg/mL. **Cost:** *Generic*—$350.49/473 mL. **Premixed infusion:** 50 mg/50 mL 0.45% NaCl. **Solution for injection:** 25 mg/mL.

NURSING IMPLICATIONS

Assessment

- Assess for epigastric or abdominal pain and frank or occult blood in the stool, emesis, or gastric aspirate.
- Geri: Assess geriatric and debilitated patients routinely for confusion. Report promptly.
- ***Lab Test Considerations:*** Monitor CBC with differential periodically during therapy.
- Antagonize effects of pentagastrin and histamine during gastric acid secretion testing. Avoid administration for 24 hr before the test.
- May cause false-negative results in skin tests using allergenic extracts. Histamine H_2 antagonists should be discontinued 24 hr before the test.
- May cause ↑ in serum transaminases and serum creatinine.
- Serum prolactin concentration may be ↑ after IV bolus of *cimetidine*. May also cause ↓ parathyroid concentrations.
- *Nizatidine* may cause ↑ alkaline phosphatase concentrations.
- *Ranitidine* and *famotidine* may cause false-positive results for urine protein; test with sulfosalicylic acid.

Potential Nursing Diagnoses

Acute pain (Indications)

Implementation

- Do not confuse Zantac (ranitidine) with Xanax (alprazolam) or Zyrtec (cetirizine).
- **PO:** Administer with meals or immediately afterward and at bedtime to prolong effect.
- If antacids or sucralfate are used concurrently for relief of pain, avoid administration of antacids within 30 min–1 hr of the H_2 antagonist and take sucralfate 2 hr after H_2 antagonist; may ↓ absorption of H_2 antagonist.
- Doses administered once daily should be administered at bedtime to prolong effect.
- Shake oral suspension before administration. Discard unused suspension after 30 days.
- Remove foil from *ranitidine effervescent tablets* and dissolve in 6–8 oz water before drinking.

Famotidine

IV Administration

- **IV Push:** ***Diluent:*** 0.9% NaCl, D5W, D10W, or LR. ***Concentration:*** 4 mg/mL. ***Rate:*** Administer at a rate of 10 mg/min. Rapid administration may cause hypotension.
- **Intermittent Infusion:** ***Diluent:*** Dilute each 20 mg in 100 mL of 0.9% NaCl, D5W, D10W, or LR. Diluted solution is stable for 48 hr at room temperature. Do not use solution that is discolored or contains a precipitate. ***Concentration:*** 0.2 mg/mL. ***Rate:*** Administer over 15–30 min.
- **Y-Site Compatibility:** acyclovir, alemtuzumab, alfentanil, allopurinol, amifostine, amikacin, aminocaproic acid, aminophylline, amiodarone, amphotericin B lipid complex, amphotericin B liposome, amsacrine, anakinra, anidulafungin, argatroban, ascorbic acid, atracurium, atropine, aztreonam, benztropine, bleomycin, bumetanide, buprenorphine, butorphanol, calcium chloride, calcium gluconate, carboplatin, carmustine, caspofungin, cefotaxime, ceftaroline, ceftazidime, cefuroxime, chlorpromazine, cisatracurium, cisplatin, cladribine, clindamycin, cyanocobalamin, cyclophosphamide, cyclosporine, cytarabine, dactinomycin, daptomycin, dexamethasone, dexmedetomidine, dexrazoxane, digoxin, diltiazem, diphenhydramine, dobutamine, docetaxel, dolasetron, dopamine, doripenem, doxacurium, doxorubicin, doxorubicin liposome, doxycycline, droperidol, enalaprilat, ephedrine, epinephrine, epirubicin, epoetin alfa, eptifibitide, ertapenem, erythromycin lactobionate, esmolol, etoposide, etoposide phosphate, fenoldopam, fentanyl, filgrastim, fluconazole, fludarabine, fluorouracil, folic acid, foscarnet, gemcitabine, gentamicin, glycopyrrolate, granisetron, heparin, hydrocortisone, hydromorphone, idarubicin, ifosfamide, imipenem/cilastatin, irinotecan, isoproterenol, ketorolac, labetalol, calcium, levofloxacin, lidocaine, linezolid, lorazepam, magnesium sulfate, mannitol, mechlorethamine, melphalan, meperidine, metaraminol, methotrexate, methyldopate, methylprednisolone, metoclopramide, metoprolol, metronidazole, midazolam, milrinone, mitoxantrone, morphine, moxifloxacin, multivitamins, mycophenolate, nafcillin, nalbuphine, naloxone, nesiritide, nicardipine, nitroglycerin, nitroprusside, norepinephrine, octreotide, ondansetron, oxacillin, oxaliplatin, oxytocin, paclitaxel, palonosetron, pamidronate, pancuronium, papaverine, pemetrexed, penicillin G, pentamidine, pentazocine, pentobarbital, perphenazine, phenobarbital, phentolamine, phenylephrine, phytonadione, potassium acetate, potassium chloride, potassium phosphates, procainamide, prochlorperazine, promethazine, propofol, propranolol, protamine, pyridoxime, ranitidine, remifentanil, rituximab, sargramostim, sodium acetate, sodium bicarbonate, streptokinase, succinylcholine, sufentanil, tacrolimus, telavancin, teniposide, theophylline, thiamine, thiotepa, tigecycline, tirofiban, tobramycin, tolazoline, trastuzumab, vancomycin, vasopressin, vecuronium, verapamil, vinblastine, vincristine, vinorelbine, voriconazole, zoledronic acid.
- **Y-Site Incompatibility:** amphotericin B cholesteryl, amphotericin B colloidal, azathioprine, cefepime, chloramphenicol, dantrolene, diazepam, diazoxide, ganciclovir, indomethacin, pantoprazole, piperacillin/tazobactam, trimethoprim/sulfamethoxazole.

Ranitidine

IV Administration

- **IV Push:** ***Diluent:*** 0.9% NaCl or D5W for injection. ***Concentration:*** 2.5 mg/mL. ***Rate:*** Administer over at least 5 min not to exceed 10 mg/min. Rapid administration may cause hypotension and arrhythmias.

- **Intermittent Infusion:** ***Diluent:*** Dilute each 50 mg in 100 mL of 0.9% NaCl or D5W. Diluted solution is stable for 48 hr at room temperature. Do not use solution that is discolored or that contains precipitate. ***Concentration:*** 0.5 mg/mL. ***Rate:*** Administer over 15–30 min.
- **Continuous Infusion:** ***Diluent:*** D5W. ***Concentration:*** 150 mg/250 mL (no greater than 2.5 mg/mL for Zollinger-Ellison patients). ***Rate:*** Administer at a rate of 6.25 mg/hr. In patients with Zollinger-Ellison syndrome, start infusion at 1 mg/kg/hr. If gastric acid output is >10 mEq/hr or patient becomes symptomatic after 4 hr, adjust dose by 0.5 mg/kg/hr increments and remeasure gastric output.
- **Y-Site Compatibility:** acyclovir, aldesleukin, alemtuzumab, alfentanil, allopurinol, amifostine, amikacin, aminocaproic acid, aminophylline, amphotericin B lipid complex, amphotericin B liposome, amsacrine, anikinra, anidulafungin, argatroban, ascorbic acid, atracurium, atropine, azithromycin, aztreonam, benztropine, bivalirudin, bleomycin, bumetanide, buprenorphine, butorphanol, calcium chloride, calcium gluconate, carboplatin, carmustine, cefazolin, cefepime, cefotaxime, cefotetan, cefoxitin, ceftaroline, ceftazidime, ceftriaxone, cefuroxime, chloramphenicol, chlorpromazine, ciprofloxacin, cisatracurium, cisplatin, cladribine, clindamycin, cyanocobalamin, cyclophosphamide, cyclosporine, cytarabine, dactinomycin, daptomycin, dexamethasone, dexmedetomidine, dexrazoxane, digoxin, diltiazem, diphenhydramine, dobutamine, docetaxel, dolasetron, dopamine, doripenem, doxacurium, doxapram, doxorubicin hydrochloride, doxorubicin liposome, doxycycline, enalaprilat, ephedrine, epinephrine, epirubicin, epoetin alfa, eptifibatide, ertapenem, erythromycin, esmolol, etoposide, etoposide phosphate, famotidine, fenoldopam, fentanyl, filgrastim, fluconazole, fludarabine, fluorouacil, folic acid, foscarnet, furosemide, ganciclovir, gemcitabine, gentamicin, glycopyrrolate, granisetron, heparin, hydrocortisone, hydromorphone, idarubicin, ifosfamide, imipenem/cilastatin, indomethacin, irinotecan, isoproterenol, ketamine, ketorolac, labetalol, leucovorin calcium, levofloxacin, lidocaine, linezolid, lorazepam, magnesium sulfate, mannitol, mechlorethamine, melphalan, meperidine, metaraminol, methotrexate, methyldopate, methylprednisolone, metoclopramide, metoprolol, metronidazole, midazolam, milrinone, mitoxantrone, morphine, moxifloxacin, multivitamins, mycophenolate, nafcillin, nalbuphine, naloxone, nesiritide, nitroglycerin, nitroprusside, norepinephrine, octreotide, ondansetron, oxacillin, oxaliplatin, oxytocin, paclitaxel, palonosetron, pamidronate, pancuronium, papaverine, pemetrexed, penicillin G, pentamidine, pentazocine, pentobarbital, phenobarbital, phentolamine, phenylephrine, phytonadione, piperacillin/tazobactam, potassium acetate, potassium chloride, procainamide, prochlorperazine, promethazine, propofol, propranolol, protamine, pyridoxime, remifentanil, rituximab, rocuronium, sargramostim, sodium acetate, sodium bicarbonate, strepotkinase, succinylcholine, sufentanil, tacrolimus, telavancin, teniposide, theophylline, thiamine, thiopental, thiotepa, tigecycline, tirofiban, tobramycin, tolazoline, trastuzumab, vancomycin, vasopressin, vecuronium, verapamil, vinblastine, vincristine, vinorelbine, warfarin, zidovudine, zoledronic acid.
- **Y-Site Incompatibility:** amphotericin B cholesteryl, caspofungin, dantrolene, diazepam, diazoxide, pantoprazole, phenytoin, quinupristin/dalfopristin, trimethoprim/sulfamethoxazole.

H

Patient/Family Teaching

- Instruct patient to take medication as directed for the full course of therapy, even if feeling better. Take missed doses as soon as remembered but not if almost time for next dose. Do not double doses.
- Advise patients taking OTC preparations not to take the maximum dose continuously for more than 2 wk without consulting health care professional. Notify health care professional if difficulty swallowing occurs or abdominal pain persists.
- Inform patient that smoking interferes with the action of histamine antagonists. Encourage patient to quit smoking or at least not to smoke after last dose of the day.
- May cause drowsiness or dizziness. Caution patient to avoid driving or other activities requiring alertness until response to the drug is known.
- Advise patient to avoid alcohol, products containing aspirin or NSAIDs, and foods that may cause an increase in GI irritation.
- Inform patient that increased fluid and fiber intake and exercise may minimize constipation.
- Advise patient to report onset of black, tarry stools; fever; sore throat; diarrhea; dizziness; rash; confusion; or hallucinations to health care professional promptly.

Evaluation/Desired Outcomes

- Decrease in abdominal pain.
- Treatment and prevention of gastric or duodenal irritation and bleeding. Healing of duodenal ulcers can be seen by x-rays or endoscopy. Therapy is continued for at least 6 wk in treatment of ulcers but not usually longer than 8 wk.
- Decreased symptoms of esophageal reflux.
- Treatment of heartburn, acid indigestion, and sour stomach (OTC use).

HMG-CoA REDUCTASE INHIBITORS (statins)

atorvastatin (a-**tore**-va-stat-in)
Lipitor

fluvastatin (**floo**-va-sta-tin)
Lescol, Lescol XL

lovastatin (**loe**-va-sta-tin)
Altoprev, ~~Mevacor~~

pitavastatin (pi-**tava**-sta-tin)
Livalo

pravastatin (**pra**-va-sta-tin)
Pravachol

rosuvastatin (roe-**soo**-va-sta-tin)
Crestor

simvastatin (**sim**-va-sta-tin)
Zocor

Classification
Therapeutic: lipid-lowering agents
Pharmacologic: HMG-CoA reductase inhibitors

Pregnancy Category X

Indications

Adjunctive management of primary hypercholesterolemia and mixed dyslipidemias. **Atorvastatin:** Primary prevention of cardiovascular disease (↓ risk of MI or stroke) in patients with multiple risk factors for coronary heart disease CHD or type 2 diabetes mellitus (also ↓ risk of angina or revascularization procedures in patients with multiple risk factors for CHD). **Atorvastatin and pravastatin:** Secondary prevention of cardiovascular disease (↓ risk of MI, stroke, revascularization procedures, angina, and hospitalizations for HF) in patients with clinically evident CHD. **Fluvastatin:** Secondary prevention of coronary revascularizations procedures in patients with clinically evident CHD. **Fluvastatin and lovastatin:** Slow progression of coronary atherosclerosis in patients with CHD. **Lovastatin:** Primary prevention of CHD (↓ risk of MI, unstable angina, and coronary revascularization) in patients without symptomatic cardiovascular disease with ↑ total and low-density lipoprotein (LDL) cholesterol and ↓ high-density lipoprotein (HDL) cholesterol. **Pravastatin:** Primary prevention of CHD (↓ risk of MI, coronary revascularization, and cardiovascular mortality) in patients without clinically evident CHD. **Simvastatin:** Secondary prevention of cardiovascular events (↓ risk of MI, coronary revascularization, stroke, and cardiovascular mortality) in patients with clinically evident CHD or those at high-risk for CHD (history of diabetes, peripheral arterial disease, or stroke). **Rosuvastatin:** Slow progression of coronary atherosclerosis. **Rosuvastatin:** Primary prevention of cardiovascular disease (reduces risk of stroke, myocardial infarction, and revascularization) in patients without clinically evident coronary heart disease but with an increased risk of cardiovascular disease because of age (≥50 yr for men; ≥60 yr for women), hsCRP ≥2 mg/L, and the presence of ≥1 risk factor for cardiovascular disease (hypertension, low HDL-C, smoking, or premature family history of coronary heart disease).

Action

Inhibit an enzyme, 3-hydroxy-3-methylglutaryl-coenzyme A (HMG-CoA) reductase, which is responsible for catalyzing an early step in the synthesis of cholesterol. **Therapeutic Effects:** Lowers total and LDL cholesterol and triglycerides. Slightly increase HDL. Slows of the progression of coronary atherosclerosis with resultant decrease in CHD-related events (all agents except rosuvastatin have indication for ↓ events).

Pharmacokinetics

Absorption: *Atorvastatin*—rapidly absorbed but undergoes extensive GI and hepatic metabolism, resulting in 14% bioavailability; *fluvastatin*—98% absorbed after oral administration, but undergoes extensive first-pass metabolism resulting in 24% bioavailability; *lovastatin, pravastatin*—poorly and variably absorbed after oral administration; *pitavastatin*-well absorbed (51%) after oral administration; *rosuvastatin*—20% absorbed following oral administration; *simvastatin*—85% absorbed but rapidly metabolized.
Distribution: *Atorvastatin*—probably enters breast milk. *Fluvastatin*—enters breast milk. *Lovastatin*—crosses the blood-brain barrier and placenta. *Pravastatin*—small amounts enter breast milk. *Pitavastatin, rosuvastatin, and simvastatin*—unknown.
Protein Binding: *Atorvastatin, fluvastatin, pitavastatin, and simvastatin*—>98%.
Metabolism and Excretion: All agents are extensively metabolized by the liver; amount excreted unchanged in urine: *atorvastatin*—<2%, *lovastatin*—10%, *fluvastatin*—5%, *pitavastatin*—15%, *pravastatin*—20%, and *simvastatin*—13%.
Half-life: *Atorvastatin*—14 hr; *fluvastatin*—1.2 hr; *lovastatin*—3 hr; *pitavastatin*—12 hr; *pravastatin*—1.3–2.7 hr; *rosuvastatin*—19 hr; *simvastatin*—unknown.

TIME/ACTION PROFILE (cholesterol-lowering effect)

ROUTE	ONSET	PEAK	DURATION*
Atorvastatin	unknown	unknown	20–30 hr
Fluvastatin	1–2 wk	4–6 wk	unknown
Lovastatin	2 wk	4–6 wk	6 wk
Pitavastatin	within 4 wk	4 wk	unknown
Pravastatin	several days	2–4 wk	unknown
Rosuvastatin	unknown	2–4 wk	unknown
Simvastatin	several days	2–4 wk	unknown

*After discontinuation.

Contraindications/Precautions

Contraindicated in: Hypersensitivity; Active liver disease or unexplained persistent ↑ in AST or ALT; *Simvastatin and lovastatin*—Concurrent use of strong CYP3A4 inhibitors (↑ risk of myopathy/rhabdomyolysis); *Pitavastatin*—Concurrent use of cyclosporine; *Pitavastatin*—severe renal impairment (CCr <30 mL/min); *Simvastatin*—Concurrent use of cyclosporine, gemfibrozil, or danazol (↑ risk of myopathy/rhabdomyolysis); OB: Potential for fetal anomalies; Lactation: May disrupt infant lipid metabolism.

Use Cautiously in: History of liver disease; Alcoholism; ⧖ *Rosuvastatin*—patients with Asian ancestry (may have ↑ blood levels and ↑ risk of rhabdomyolysis); *Atorvastatin*—Concurrent use of gemfibrozil, azole antifungals, erythromycin, clarithromycin, protease inhibitors, niacin, or cyclosporine (higher risk of myopathy/rhabdomyolysis); *Lovastatin*—Concurrent use of gemfibrozil, niacin, cyclosporine, amiodarone, danazol, diltiazem, verapamil, colchicine, or ranolazine (higher risk of myopathy/rhabdomyolysis); *Pitavastatin*—Hypothyroidism, concurrent use of fibrates or lipid-lowering doses of niacin (higher risk of myopathy/rhabdomyolysis); *Rosuvastatin*—Concurrent use of gemfibrozil, azole antifungals, protease inhibitors, niacin, cyclosporine, amiodarone, or verapamil (higher risk of myopathy/rhabdomyolysis); *Simvastatin*—Concurrent use of amiodarone, amlodipine, diltiazem, dronedarone, verapamil, lomitapide, or ranolazine (↑ risk of myopathy/rhabdomyolysis); ⧖ *Simvastatin*—Chinese patients receiving ≥1 g/day of niacin (↑ risk of myopathy; do not use simvastatin 80 mg/day in these patients); Renal impairment; Geri: *Pitavastatin*—↑ risk of myopathy (age >65 yr); OB: Women of childbearing age; Pedi: Safety not established in children <8 yr (some products approved for use in older children only.

Adverse Reactions/Side Effects

CNS: amnesia, confusion, dizziness, headache, insomnia, memory loss, weakness. **CV:** chest pain, peripheral edema. **EENT:** rhinitis; *lovastatin*, blurred vision. **Resp:** bronchitis. **GI:** abdominal cramps, constipation, diarrhea, flatus, heartburn, altered taste, drug-induced hepatitis, dyspepsia, elevated liver enzymes, nausea, pancreatitis. **GU:** erectile dysfunction. **Derm:** rashes, pruritus. **Endo:** hyperglycemia. **MS:** RHABDOMYOLYSIS, arthralgia, arthritis, immune-mediated necrotizing myopathy, myalgia, myopathy (↑ with simvastatin 80 mg/day dose). **Misc:** hypersensitivity reactions.

Interactions

Atorvastatin, lovastatin, simvastatin, and rosuvastatin are metabolized by the CYP3A4 metabolic pathway. Fluvastatin is metabolized by CYP 2C9. Pravastatin is not metabolized by the CYP P450 system.

Drug-Drug: Atorvastatin, lovastatin, and simvastatin may interact with **CYP3A4 inhibitors**. Risk of myopathy with lovastatin is ↑ by concurrent use of **strong CYP3A4 inhibitors**, including **ketoconazole**, **itraconazole**, **posaconazole**, **voriconazole protease inhibitors**, **boceprevir**, **clarithromycin**, **erythromycin**, **telithromycin**, **nefazodone**, and **cobicistat-containing products**; concurrent use contraindicated. Risk of myopathy with simvastatin is ↑ by concurrent use of **cyclosporine**, **gemfibrozil**, **danazol**, **erythromycin**, **clarithromycin**, **telithromycin**, **protease inhibitors**, **nefazodone**, **boceprevir**, **ketoconazole**, **itraconazole**, **voriconazole posaconazole** and **cobicistat-containing products**; concurrent use contraindicated. Risk of myopathy with pitavastatin is ↑ by concurrent use of **cyclosporine**; concurrent use contraindicated. Bioavailability and effectiveness may be ↓ by **cholestyramine** and **colestipol**. Risk of myopathy with atorvastatin is ↑ by concurrent use of **cyclosporine**, **gemfibrozil**, **itraconazole**, **colchicine**, **erythromycin**, **clarithromycin**, **nelfinavir**, **ritonavir/saquinavir**, **lopinavir/ritonavir**, **tipranavir/ritonavir**, **saquinavir/ritonavir**, **darunavir/ritonavir**, **fosamprenavir**, **fosamprenavir/ritonavir**, and large doses of **niacin**; concurrent use with gemfibrozil, cyclosporine, or tipranavir/ritonavir should be avoided; use lowest dose with lopinavir/ritonavir; use ↓ doses with nelfinavir, clarithromycin, itraconazole, saquinavir/ritonavir, darunavir/ritonavir, fosamprenavir, or fosamprenavir/ritonavir. Risk of myopathy with fluvastatin is ↑ by concurrent use of **gemfibrozil**, **erythromycin**, **colchicine**, **cyclosporine**, **azole antifungal agents**, or large doses of **niacin** may ↑ risk of myopathy; concurrent use with gemfibrozil should be avoided; use ↓ doses with cyclosporine, and fluconazole. Risk of myopathy with lovastatin is ↑ by concurrent use of **amiodarone cyclosporine**, **gemfibrozil**, **diltiazem**, **verapamil**, **danazol**, and large doses of **niacin**; concurrent use with gemfibrozil or cyclosporine should be avoided; use ↓ doses with danazol, amiodarone, diltiazem, or verapamil. Risk of myopathy with pitavastatin is ↑ by concurrent use of **erythromycin**, **rifampin**, **colchicine**, **fibrates**, or large doses of **niacin**; use ↓ doses with erythromycin, rifampin, and niacin; concurrent use with gemfibrozil should be avoided. Risk of myopathy with pravastatin is ↑ by concurrent use of **cyclosporine**, **fibrates**, **colchicine**, **erythromycin**, **clarithromycin**, or large doses of **niacin**; concurrent use with gemfibrozil should be avoided; consider lower dose with niacin. Risk of myopathy with rosuvastatin is ↑ by concurrent use of **cyclosporine**, **lopinavir/ritonavir**, **atazanavir/ritonavir**, **simeprevir**, **colchicine**, **fibrates** or large doses of **niacin**; concurrent use of gemfibrozil should be avoided, if possible; use ↓ doses with cyclosporine, lopinavir/ritonavir, and ataza-

H

navir/ritonavir. Risk of myopathy with simvastatin is ↑ by concurrent use of **amiodarone**, **amlodipine**, **diltiazem**, **dronedarone**, **verapamil**, **lomitapide**, **ranolazine**, or **niacin**. Atorvastatin, fluvastatin, and simvastatin may slightly ↑ serum **digoxin** levels. Atorvastatin and rosuvastatin may ↑ levels of **hormonal contraceptives**. Atorvastatin, fluvastatin, lovastatin, rosuvastatin, and simvastatin may ↑ risk of bleeding with **warfarin**. **Alcohol**, **cimetidine**, **ranitidine**, and **omeprazole** may ↑ fluvastatin levels. **Rifampin** may ↓ fluvastatin levels. **Antacids** ↓ absorption of rosuvastatin (administer 2 hr after rosuvastatin. **Lopinavir/ritonavir** may ↑ rosuvastatin levels. Fluvastatin ↑ levels of **glyburide**.

Drug-Natural Products: St. John's wort may ↓ levels and effectiveness (lovastatin and simvastatin).

Drug-Food: Large quantities of **grapefruit juice** may ↑ blood levels and ↑ risk of rhabdomyolysis (atorvastatin, lovastatin, and simvastatin); concurrent use contraindicated. **Food** ↑ blood levels of lovastatin.

Route/Dosage

Atorvastatin

PO (Adults): 10–20 mg once daily initially; (may start with 40 mg/day if LDL-C needs to be ↓ by >45%); may be ↑ every 2–4 wk up to 80 mg/day; *Concurrent nelfinavir therapy*—Dose should not exceed 40 mg/day; *Concurrent clarithromycin, itraconazole, saquinavir/ritonavir, darunavir/ritonavir, fosamprenavir, or fosamprenavir/ritonavir therapy*—Dose should not exceed 20 mg/day.

PO (Children 10–17 yr): 10 mg/day initially, may be ↑ every 4 wk up to 20 mg/day; *Concurrent nelfinavir therapy*—Dose should not exceed 40 mg/day; *Concurrent clarithromycin, itraconazole, saquinavir/ritonavir, darunavir/ritonavir, fosamprenavir, or fosamprenavir/ritonavir therapy*—Dose should not exceed 20 mg/day.

Fluvastatin

PO (Adults): 20–40 mg (immediate-release) once daily at bedtime. May be ↑ to 40 mg twice daily (immediate-release) or 80 mg once daily (extended-release); *Concurrent fluconazole or cyclosporine therapy*—Dose should not exceed 20 mg twice daily.

Lovastatin

PO (Adults): 20 mg once daily with evening meal. May be ↑ at 4-wk intervals to a maximum of 80 mg/day (immediate-release) or 60 mg/day (extended-release); *Concurrent danazol, verapamil, or diltiazem therapy*—Initiate at 10 mg/day; do not exceed 20 mg/day; *Concurrent amiodarone therapy*—Dose should not exceed 40 mg/day.

Renal Impairment

PO (Adults): *CCr <30 mL/min*—dosage should not exceed 20 mg/day unless carefully titrated.

PO (Children /Adolescents 10–17 yr): *Familial heterozygous hypercholesterolemia*—10–40 mg/day adjusted at 4-wk intervals.

Pitavastatin

PO (Adults): 2 mg once daily initially, may be ↑ up to 4 mg depending on response. *Concurrent erythromycin therapy*—Dose should not exceed 1 mg/day; *Concurrent rifampin therapy*—Dose should not exceed 2 mg/day.

Renal Impairment

PO (Adults): *CCr 30–<60 mL/min*—1 mg once daily initially, may be ↑ up to 2 mg daily.

Pravastatin

PO (Adults): 10–20 mg once daily at bedtime, may be adjusted at 4-wk intervals as needed (usual range 10–40 mg/day); *Concurrent cyclosporine therapy*—Dose should not exceed 20 mg/day; *Concurrent clarithromycin therapy*—Dose should not exceed 40 mg/day.

PO (Children 14–18 yrs): 40 mg once daily.

PO (Children 8–13 yrs): 20 mg once daily.

Hepatic/Renal Impairment

PO (Adults): 10–20 mg once daily at bedtime; ↑ at 4-wk intervals as needed (usual range = 10–20 mg/day).

Rosuvastatin

PO (Adults): 10 mg once daily initially (range 5–20 mg initially) (20 mg initial dose may be considered for patients with LDL-C >190 m g/dL or homozygous familial hypercholesterolemia); dose may be adjusted at 2–4 wk intervals, some patients may require up to 40 mg/day, however this dose is associated with ↑ risk of rhabdomyolysis; *Patients with Asian ancestry*—initial dose should be 5 mg; *Concurrent cyclosporine therapy*—Dose should not exceed 5 mg/day; *Concurrent lopinavir/ritonavir, atazanavir/ritonavir, or simeprevir therapy*—Dose should not exceed 10 mg/day; *Concurrent gemfibrozil therapy*—Dose should not exceed 10 mg/day (avoid if possible).

PO (Children 10–17 yr): 5–20 mg once daily.

Renal Impairment

PO (Adults): *CCr <30 mL/min*—5 mg once daily initially; dose may be ↑ but should not exceed 10 mg/day.

Simvastatin

The 80 mg dose should be restricted to patients who have been taking this dose for ≥12 mo without evidence of muscle toxicity.

PO (Adults): 5–40 mg once daily in the evening; if LDL goal cannot be achieved with 40 mg/day dose, add another lipid-lowering therapy (do not ↑ simvastatin dose to 80 mg/day). *Concurrent verapamil, diltiazem, or dronedarone therapy*—Dose should not exceed 10 mg/day. *Concurrent amiodarone, amlodipine or ranolazine therapy*—Dose should not exceed 20 mg/day; *Concurrent lomitapide therapy*—↓ dose by 50% (dose should not exceed 20 mg/day or 40 mg/day for patients who previously received 80 mg/day chronically [for ≥12 mo] without evidence of myopathy).

PO (Children 10–17 yr): 10 mg once daily initially, may be ↑ at 4–wk intervals up to 40 mg/day. *Concurrent verapamil or diltiazem therapy*—Dose should not exceed 10 mg/day. *Concurrent amiodarone, amlodipine or ranolazine therapy*—Dose should not exceed 20 mg/day.

Renal Impairment

PO (Adults): *CCr <10 mL/min*—5 mg/day initially, titrate carefully.

Availability

Atorvastatin (generic available)

Tablets: 10 mg, 20 mg, 40 mg, 80 mg. **Cost:** *Generic*—10 mg $33.25/100, 20 mg $48.75/100, 40 mg $40.42/100, 80 mg $49.20/100. ***In combination with:*** amlodipine (Caduet); see Appendix B.

Fluvastatin (generic available)

Capsules: 20 mg, 40 mg. **Cost:** *Generic*—All strengths $113.40/30. **Extended-release tablets:** 80 mg. **Cost:** $194.69/30.

Lovastatin (generic available)

Immediate-release tablets : 10 mg, 20 mg, 40 mg. **Cost:** *Generic*—10 mg $10.83/100, 20 mg $10.83/100, 40 mg $16.50/100. **Extended-release tablets:** 20 mg, 40 mg, 60 mg. **Cost:** All strengths $555.98/30. ***In combination with:*** Niacin (Advicor). See Appendix B.

Pitavastatin

Tablets: 1 mg, 2 mg, 4 mg. **Cost:** All strengths $492.48/90.

Pravastatin (generic available)

Tablets: 10 mg, 20 mg, 40 mg, 80 mg. **Cost:** *Generic*—20 mg $10.83/100, 40 mg $29.82/100, 80 mg $142.06/100.

Rosuvastatin

Tablets: 5 mg, 10 mg, 20 mg, 40 mg. **Cost:** 5 mg $609.27/100, 10 mg $600.47/100, 20 mg $609.27/100, 40 mg $541.62/100.

Simvastatin (generic available)

Tablets: 5 mg, 10 mg, 20 mg, 40 mg, 80 mg. **Cost:** *Generic*—5 mg $7.11/100, 10 mg $10.83/100, 20 mg $10.83/100, 40 mg $10.83/100, 80 mg $9.83/100. ***In combination with:*** ezetimibe (Vytorin). See Appendix B.

NURSING IMPLICATIONS

Assessment

- Obtain a dietary history, especially with regard to fat consumption.
- ***Lab Test Considerations:*** Evaluate serum cholesterol and triglyceride levels before initiating, after 4–6 wk of therapy, and periodically thereafter.
- Monitor liver function tests, including AST and ALT, before initiating therapy and if signs of liver injury (fatigue, anorexia, right upper abdominal discomfort, dark urine or jaundice) occur. May also cause ↑ alkaline phosphatase and bilirubin levels.
- If patient develops muscle tenderness during therapy, monitor CK levels. If CK levels are >10 times the upper limit of normal or myopathy occurs, therapy should be discontinued. Monitor for signs and symptoms of immune-mediated necrotizing myopathy (IMNM) (proximal muscle weakness and ↑ serum creatine kinase), persisting despite discontinuation of statin therapy. Perform muscle biopsy to diagnose; shows necrotizing myopathy without significant inflammation. Treat with immunosuppressive agents.

Potential Nursing Diagnoses

Noncompliance (Patient/Family Teaching)

Implementation

- Do not confuse Lipitor with Loniten or Zyrtec. Do not confuse Mevacor with Benicar.
- **PO:** Administer *lovastatin* with food. Administration on an empty stomach decreases absorption by approximately 30%. Initial once-daily dose is administered with the evening meal.
- Administer extended-release tablets at bedtime. Extended-release tablets should be swallowed whole, do not break, crush, chew or open capsules.
- Administer *fluvastatin, pravastatin,* and *simvastatin* once daily in the evening. Do not take two 40 mg fluvastatin tablets at one time. *Atorvastatin, pitavastatin,* and *rosuvastatin* can be taken any time of day. May be administered without regard to food.
- Avoid large amounts of grapefruit juice during therapy; may ↑ risk of toxicity.
- If *fluvastatin* or *pravastatin* is administered in conjunction with bile acid sequestrants (cholestyramine, colestipol), administer at least 4 hr after bile acid sequestrant.
- If *rosuvastatin* is administered in conjunction with magnesium or aluminum-containing antacids, administer antacid at least 2 hr after *rosuvastatin*.

Patient/Family Teaching

- Instruct patient to take medication as directed and not to skip doses or double up on missed doses. Advise patient to avoid drinking more that 200 mL/day of grapefruit juice during therapy. Medication helps control but does not cure elevated serum cholesterol levels.

- Advise patient that this medication should be used in conjunction with diet restrictions (fat, cholesterol, carbohydrates, alcohol), exercise, and cessation of smoking.
- Instruct patient to notify health care professional if signs of liver injury or if unexplained muscle pain, tenderness, or weakness occurs, especially if accompanied by fever or malaise.
- Advise patient to notify health care professional of all Rx or OTC medications, vitamins, or herbal products being taken and to consult with health care professional before taking other medications.
- Advise patient to notify health care professional of medication regimen before treatment or surgery.
- Instruct female patients to notify health care professional promptly if pregnancy is planned or suspected. Advise women of childbearing age to use effective contraception during therapy and discuss plans to discontinue statins if trying to conceive. Advise patients to avoid breast feeding during therapy.
- Emphasize the importance of follow-up exams to determine effectiveness and to monitor for side effects.

Evaluation/Desired Outcomes

- Decrease in LDL and total cholesterol levels.
- Increase in HDL cholesterol levels.
- Decrease in triglyceride levels.
- Slowing of the progression of coronary artery disease.
- Prevention of cardiovascular disease.

HUMAN PAPILLOMAVIRUS VACCINE

(hyoo-man pa-pil-lo-ma)

human papillomavirus quadrivalent (types 6, 11, 16, and 18) vaccine, recombinant
Gardasil

human papillomavirus bivalent (types 16 and 18) vaccine, recombinant
Cervarix

human papillomavirus 9-valent (types 6, 11, 16, 18, 31, 33, 45, 52, and 58) vaccine, recombinant
Gardasil 9

Classification
Therapeutic: vaccines/immunizing agents

Indications

Gardasil and Gardasil 9: Prevention of cervical, vulvar, vaginal, and anal cancers and genital warts (in females) and anal cancer and genital warts (in males). **Cervarix:** Prevention of cervical cancer.

Action

Vaccination results in antibodies to HPV viruses that are causative agents for cervical, vulvar, vaginal, and anal cancers and genital warts. **Therapeutic Effects:** Prevention of cervical, vulvar, vaginal, and anal cancers and genital warts.

Pharmacokinetics

Absorption: Well absorbed following IM administration.
Distribution: Unknown.
Metabolism and Excretion: Unknown.
Half-life: Unknown.

TIME/ACTION PROFILE (antibody response)

ROUTE	ONSET	PEAK	DURATION
IM	unknown	6 mo*	unknown

*After third vaccination.

Contraindications/Precautions

Contraindicated in: Hypersensitivity; Thrombocytopenia/bleeding disorder; OB: Limited data available; use only if potential benefit justifies potential risk to fetus.
Use Cautiously in: Current/recent febrile illness; Immunosuppression may ↓ antibody response; Lactation: Excretion into breast milk unknown; Pedi: Children <9 yr (safety not established).

Adverse Reactions/Side Effects

Neuro: fainting. **Local:** injection site reactions.
Misc: ANAPHYLAXIS (RARE).

Interactions

Drug-Drug: Immunosuppressants or **antineoplastics** may ↓ antibody response.

Route/Dosage

IM (Adults and Children —males and females 9–26 yr): *Gardasil and Gardasil 9*—Three 0.5 mL doses at 0, 2, and 6 mo.
IM (Adults and Children —females 9–25 yr): *Cervarix*—Three 0.5 mL doses at 0, 2, and 6 mo.

Availability

Sterile preparation for intramuscular administration (Gardasil): 20 mcg of HPV 6 L1 protein, 40 mcg of HPV 11 L1 protein, 40 mcg of HPV 16 L1 protein, and 20 mcg of HPV 18 L1 protein/0.5-mL dose. **Sterile preparation for intramuscular administration (Gardasil 9):** 30 mcg of HPV 6 L1 protein, 40 mcg of HPV 11 L1 protein, 60 mcg of HPV 16 L1 protein, 40 mcg of HPV 18 L1 protein, 20 mcg of HPV 31 L1 protein, 20 mcg of HPV 33 L1 protein, 20 mcg of HPV 45 L1 protein, 20 mcg of HPV 52 L1 protein, and 20 mcg of HPV 58 L1 protein/0.5-mL dose. **Sterile preparation for intramuscular administration (Cervarix):** 20 mcg of HPV type 16 L1 protein and 20 mcg of HPV type 18 L1 protein.

NURSING IMPLICATIONS

Assessment

- Assess vital signs prior to administration. Do not administer to patient with a current or recent febrile illness; low grade fever (<100°F) and mild upper respiratory infection are usually not contraindicated.
- Monitor patient for 15 min following injection for fainting. Patient should remain lying down or seated to prevent falls or injury.

Potential Nursing Diagnoses

Risk for infection (Indications)

Implementation

- Vaccine is not intended for treatment of active genital warts or cervical cancer and will not protect from diseases not caused by HPV.
- **IM:** *Gardasil and Gardisil 9:* Prefilled syringe is for single use; do not use for more than one person. Administer as supplied; do not dilute; administer full dose. Shake well prior to administration to maintain suspension of vaccine. Solution is cloudy and white; do not administer solution that is discolored or contains particulate matter. If using single-dose vial, withdraw 0.5 mL dose and administer entire contents of syringe. Administer intramuscularly in the deltoid or in the high anterolateral area of the thigh.
- **IM:** *Cervarix:* Prefilled syringe is for single use; do not use for more than one person. Administer as supplied; do not dilute; administer full dose. Shake vial or syringe well before use. Solution is a turbid, white suspension; do not administer if it is discolored or contains particulate matter. The tip cap and rubber plunger of needleless prefilled syringes contain dry natural latex rubber; may cause allergic reactions in latex sensitive individuals. Vial stopper does not contain latex.

Patient/Family Teaching

- Provide information about vaccine and the importance of completing immunization series, unless contraindicated, to patient and guardian.
- Inform patient that vaccine does not replace routine cervical cancer screening or prevent other sexually transmitted diseases; such screening should be continued as usual.
- Advise patient to notify health care professional of all Rx or OTC medications, vitamins, or herbal products being taken and to consult with health care professional before taking other medications.
- Rep: Advise patient to notify health care professional if pregnancy is planned or suspected. Women exposed to *Gardasil or Gardisil 9* vaccine during pregnancy are encouraged to call manufacturer pregnancy registry at 800-986-8999. Women exposed to *Cervarix* vaccine during pregnancy are encouraged to call manufacturer pregnancy registry at 800-452-9622.
- Instruct patient to report any adverse reactions to health care professional.

Evaluation/Desired Outcomes

- Prevention of cervical cancer, genital warts, cervical adenocarcinoma in situ, cervical, vulvar, anal, and vaginal intraepithelial neoplasia caused by HPV.

H

hydrALAZINE

(hye-**dral**-a-zeen)

~~Apresoline~~, Apresoline

Classification
Therapeutic: antihypertensives
Pharmacologic: vasodilators

Pregnancy Category C

Indications

Moderate to severe hypertension (with a diuretic). **Unlabeled Use:** HF unresponsive to conventional therapy with digoxin and diuretics.

Action

Direct-acting peripheral arteriolar vasodilator. **Therapeutic Effects:** Lowering of BP in hypertensive patients and decreased afterload in patients with HF.

Pharmacokinetics

Absorption: Rapidly absorbed following oral administration; well absorbed from IM sites.
Distribution: Widely distributed. Crosses the placenta; enters breast milk in minimal concentrations.
Metabolism and Excretion: Mostly metabolized by the GI mucosa and liver by N-acetyltransferase (rate of acetylation is genetically determined [slow acetylators have ↑ hydralazine levels and ↑ risk of toxicity; fast acetylators have ↓ hydralazine levels and ↓ response]).
Half-life: 2–8 hr.

TIME/ACTION PROFILE (antihypertensive effect)

ROUTE	ONSET	PEAK	DURATION
PO	45 min	2 hr	2–4 hr
IM	10–30 min	1 hr	3–8 hr
IV	5–20 min	15–30 min	2–6 hr

Contraindications/Precautions

Contraindicated in: Hypersensitivity; Some products contain tartrazine and should be avoided in patients with known intolerance.
Use Cautiously in: Cardiovascular or cerebrovascular disease; Severe renal and hepatic disease (dose

modification may be necessary); OB, Lactation: Has been used safely during pregnancy.

Adverse Reactions/Side Effects

CNS: dizziness, drowsiness, headache. **CV:** tachycardia, angina, arrhythmias, edema, orthostatic hypotension. **GI:** diarrhea, nausea, vomiting. **Derm:** rash. **F and E:** sodium retention. **MS:** arthralgias, arthritis. **Neuro:** peripheral neuropathy. **Misc:** drug-induced lupus syndrome.

Interactions

Drug-Drug: ↑ hypotension with acute ingestion of **alcohol**, other **antihypertensives**, or **nitrates**. **MAO inhibitors** may exaggerate hypotension. May ↓ pressor response to **epinephrine**. **NSAIDs** may ↓ antihypertensive response. **Beta blockers** ↓ tachycardia from hydralazine (therapy may be combined for this reason). **Metoprolol** and **propranolol** ↑ hydralazine levels. ↑ blood levels of **metoprolol** and **propranolol**.

Route/Dosage

PO (Adults): *Hypertension*—10 mg 4 times daily initially. After 2–4 days may ↑ to 25 mg 4 times daily for the rest of the 1st week; may then ↑ to 50 mg 4 times daily (up to 300 mg/day). Once maintenance dose is established, twice-daily dosing may be used. *HF*—25–37.5 mg 4 times daily; may be ↑ up to 300 mg/day in 3–4 divided doses.

PO (Children > 1 mo): Initial—0.75–1 mg/kg/day in 2–4 divided doses, not to exceed 25 mg/dose; may ↑ gradually to 5 mg/kg/day in infants and 7.5 mg/kg/day in children (not to exceed 200 mg/day) in 2–4 divided doses.

IM, IV (Adults): *Hypertension*—5–40 mg repeated as needed. *Eclampsia*—5 mg q 15–20 min; if no response after a total of 20 mg, consider an alternative agent.

IM, IV (Children > 1 mo): Initial—0.1–0.2 mg/kg/dose (not to exceed 20 mg) q 4–6 hr as needed, up 1.7–3.5 mg/kg/day in 4–6 divided doses.

Availability (generic available)

Tablets: 10 mg, 25 mg, 50 mg, 100 mg. **Injection:** 20 mg/mL. ***In combination with:*** isosorbide dinitrate (BiDil). See Appendix B.

NURSING IMPLICATIONS

Assessment

- Monitor BP and pulse frequently during initial dose adjustment and periodically during therapy. About 50–65% of Caucasians, Black, South Indians, and Mexicans are slow acetylators at risk for toxicity, while 80–90% of Eskimos, Japanese, and Chinese are rapid acetylators at risk for decreased levels and treatment failure.
- Monitor frequency of prescription refills to determine adherence.
- ***Lab Test Considerations:*** Monitor CBC, electrolytes, LE cell prep, and ANA titer prior to and periodically during prolonged therapy.
- May cause a positive direct Coombs' test result.

Potential Nursing Diagnoses

Ineffective tissue perfusion (Indications)
Noncompliance (Patient/Family Teaching)

Implementation

- Do not confuse hydralazine with hydroxyzine.
- IM or IV route should be used only when drug cannot be given orally.
- May be administered concurrently with diuretics or beta blockers to permit lower doses and minimize side effects.
- **PO:** Administer with meals consistently to enhance absorption.
- Pharmacist may prepare oral solution from hydralazine injection for patients with difficulty swallowing.

IV Administration

- **IV Push: *Diluent:*** Administer undiluted. Use solution as quickly as possible after drawing through needle into syringe. ***Concentration:*** 20 mg/mL. ***Rate:*** Administer over at least 1 min. Pedi: Administer at a rate of 0.2 mg/kg/min in children. Monitor BP and pulse in all patients frequently after injection.
- **Y-Site Compatibility:** alemtuzumab, amiodarone, anidulafungin, argatroban, bivalirudin, bleomycin, carmustine, cyclophosphamide, dactinomycin, daptomycin, daunorubicin hydrochloride, dexrazoxane, diltiazem, docetaxel, etoposide, etoposide phosphate, fenoldopam, fludarabine, gemcitabine, granisetron, hetastarch, hydromorphone, idarubicin, irinotecan, leucovorin, linezolid, mechlorethamine, mesna, metronidazole, milrinone, mitomycin, mitoxantrone, moxifloxacin, mycophenolate, octreotide, oxaliplatin, paclitaxel, palonosetron, pamidronate, pancuronium, prochlorperazine, tacrolimus, teniposide, thiotepa, tirofiban, topotecan, vecuronium, vinblastine, vincristine, vinorelbine, vitamin B complex with C, voriconazole, zoledronic acid.
- **Y-Site Incompatibility:** acyclovir, amphotericin B colloidal, amphotericin B lipid complex, ampicillin/sulbactam, ascorbic acid, cefazolin, cefotaxime, cefoxitin, ceftazidime, ceftriaxone, cefuroxime, dantrolene, diazepam, doxorubicin liposomal, ertapenem, folic acid, foscarnet, fosphenytoin, ganciclovir, haloperidol, indomethacin, lorazepam, methylprednisolone, multivitamins, nafcillin, nitroprusside, oxacillin, pantoprazole, pemetrexed, pentobarbital, phenytoin, piperacillin/tazobactam, potassium acetate, sodium acetate, tigecycline, trimethoprim/sulfamethoxazole.

Patient/Family Teaching

- Emphasize the importance of continuing to take this medication, even if feeling well. Instruct patient to take medication at the same time each day; last dose of the day should be taken at bedtime. Take missed doses as soon as remembered; do not double doses. If more than 2 doses in a row are missed, consult health care professional. Must be discontinued gradually to avoid sudden increase in BP. Hydralazine controls but does not cure hypertension.

- Encourage patient to comply with additional interventions for hypertension (weight reduction, low-sodium diet, smoking cessation, moderation of alcohol intake, regular exercise, and stress management). Instruct patient and family on proper technique for BP monitoring. Advise them to check BP at least weekly and report significant changes.
- Patients should weigh themselves twice weekly and assess feet and ankles for fluid retention.
- May occasionally cause drowsiness. Advise patient to avoid driving or other activities requiring alertness until response to medication is known.
- Caution patient to avoid sudden changes in position to minimize orthostatic hypotension.
- Advise patient to notify health care professional of all Rx or OTC medications, vitamins, or herbal products being taken and to consult with health care professional before taking other medications, especially cough, cold, or allergy remedies.
- Instruct patient to notify health care professional of medication prior to treatment or surgery.
- Advise patient to notify health care professional immediately if general tiredness; fever; muscle or joint aching; chest pain; skin rash; sore throat; or numbness, tingling, pain, or weakness of hands and feet occurs. Vitamin B_6 (pyridoxine) may be used to treat peripheral neuritis.
- Emphasize the importance of follow-up exams to evaluate effectiveness of medication.

Evaluation/Desired Outcomes

- Decrease in BP without appearance of side effects.
- Decreased afterload in patients with HF.

hydralazine/isosorbide dinitrate

(hye-**dral**-a-zeen eye-so-**sor**-bide di-**ni**-trate)

BiDil

Classification

Therapeutic: vasodilators

Pharmacologic: vasodilators, nitrates

Pregnancy Category C

Indications

Management of heart failure in black patients.

Action

BiDil is a fixed-dose combination of **isosorbide dinitrate**, a vasodilator with effects on both arteries and veins, and **hydralazine**, a predominantly arterial vasodilator. **Therapeutic Effects:** Improved survival, increased time to hospitalization and decreased symptoms of heart failure in black patients.

Pharmacokinetics

See pharmacokinetic sections in hydralazine and isosorbide dinitrate monographs of Davis's Drug Guide for Nurses for more information.

Absorption: *Hydralazine*—10–26% absorbed in HF patients, absorption can be saturated leading to large ↑ in absorption with higher doses; *isosorbide dinitrate*—variable absorbed (10–90%) reflecting first-pass hepatic metabolism.

Distribution: *Hydralazine*—widely distributed, crosses the placenta, minimal amounts in breast milk; *isosorbide dinitrate*—accumulates in muscle and venous wall.

Metabolism and Excretion: *Hydralazine*—mostly metabolized by GI mucosa and liver; *isosorbide dinitrate*—undergoes extensive first-pass metabolism in the liver mostly metabolized by the liver, some metabolites are vasodilators.

Half-life: *Hydralazine*—4 hr; *isosorbide dinitrate*—2 hr.

TIME/ACTION PROFILE (effect on BP)

ROUTE	ONSET	PEAK	DURATION
hydralazine	45 min	2 hr	2–4 hr
isosorbide	15–40 min	unknown	4 hr

Contraindications/Precautions

Contraindicated in: Hypersensitivity to either component; Concurrent use of PDE-5 inhibitor (avanafil, sildenafil, tadalafil, vardenafil) or riociguat.

Use Cautiously in: Severe renal/hepatic disease (dose modification may be necessary); Head trauma or cerebral hemorrhage; Geri: Start with lower doses; OB: May compromise maternal/fetal circulation; Lactation: Safety not established; Pedi: Safety not established.

Adverse Reactions/Side Effects

Hydralazine **CNS:** dizziness, drowsiness, headache. **CV:** tachycardia, angina, arrhythmias, edema, orthostatic hypotension. **GI:** diarrhea, nausea, vomiting. **Derm:** rash. **F and E:** sodium retention. **MS:** arthralgias, arthritis. **Neuro:** peripheral neuritis. **Misc:** drug-induced lupus syndrome.

Isosorbide Dinitrate

CNS: dizziness, headache, apprehension, weakness. **CV:** hypotension, tachycardia, paradoxic bradycardia, syncope. **GI:** abdominal pain, nausea, vomiting. **Misc:** cross-tolerance, flushing, tolerance.

Interactions

Drug-Drug: Concurrent use of **avanafil**, **sildenafil**, **tadalafil**, or **vardenafil** may result in severe hypotension; concurrent use contraindicated. Concurrent use of **riociguat** may result in severe hypotension; concurrent use contraindicated. ↑ risk of hypotension with other **antihypertensives**, acute ingestion of **alcohol**, and **phenothiazines**. **MAO inhibitors** may exaggerate hypotension. May ↓ the pressor response to **epinephrine**. **Beta blockers** ↓ tachycardia from hydralazine (therapy may be combined for this reason). **Metoprolol** and **propranolol** may ↑ hydralazine levels. Hydralazine ↑ levels of **metoprolol** and **propranolol**.

Route/Dosage

PO (Adults): 1 tablet 3 times daily, may be ↑ to 2 tablets 3 times daily.

Availability

Tablets: hydralazine 37.5 mg/isosorbide dinitrate 20 mg.

NURSING IMPLICATIONS

Assessment

- Monitor BP and pulse routinely during period of dose adjustment. Symptomatic hypotension may occur even with small doses. Use caution with patients who are volume depleted or hypotensive.
- Assess for signs and symptoms of peripheral neuritis (paresthesia, numbness, tingling) periodically during therapy. Adding pyridoxine may cause symptoms to decrease.
- ***Lab Test Considerations:*** If symptoms of systemic lupus erythematosus (SLE) occur obtain a CBC and ANA titer. If positive for SLE, carefully weigh risks/benefits of continued therapy.

Potential Nursing Diagnoses

Ineffective tissue perfusion (Indications)
Activity intolerance (Indications)

Implementation

- Dose may be titrated rapidly over 3–5 days, but may need to decrease if side effects occur. May decrease to one-half tablet 3 times daily if intolerable side effects occur. Titrate up as soon as side effects subside.

Patient/Family Teaching

- Instruct patient to take medication as directed on a regular schedule.
- Caution patient to make position changes slowly to minimize orthostatic hypotension.
- May cause dizziness. Caution patient to avoid driving or other activities requiring alertness until response to medication is known.
- Advise patient to avoid concurrent use of alcohol or medications for erectile dysfunction with this medication. Patient should also consult health care professional before taking Rx, OTC, or herbal products while taking this medication.
- Caution patient that inadequate fluid intake or excessive fluid loss from perspiration, diarrhea or vomiting may lead to a fall in BP, dizziness or syncope. If syncope occurs, discontinue medication and notify health care professional promptly.
- Inform patient that headache is a common side effect that should decrease with continuing therapy. Aspirin or acetaminophen may be ordered to treat headache. Notify health care professional if headache is persistent or severe. Do not alter dose to avoid headache.
- Advise patient to notify health care professional if symptoms of systemic lupus erythematosus occur (arthralgia, fever, chest pain, prolonged malaise or other unexplained symptoms).
- Advise female patient to notify health care professional if pregnancy is planned or suspected or if breast feeding.

Evaluation/Desired Outcomes

- Improved survival, increased time to hospitalization and decreased symptoms of heart failure in black patients.

---

hydrochlorothiazide, See DIURETICS (THIAZIDE).

REMS HIGH ALERT

HYDROcodone

(hye-droe-**koe**-done)
✱Hycodan, Hysingla ER, Zohydro ER

HYDROcodone/acetaminophen

Anexsia, Norco

HYDROcodone/ibuprofen

Reprexain, Vicoprofen

Classification
Therapeutic: allergy, cold, and cough remedies (antitussive), opioid analgesics
Pharmacologic: opioid agonists/nonopioid analgesic combinations

Schedule II

Pregnancy Category C

For information on the acetaminophen and ibuprofen components of these formulations, see the acetaminophen and ibuprofen monographs

Indications

Extended-release product: Management of pain that is severe enough to warrant daily, around-the-clock, long-term opioid treatment where alternative treatment options are inadequate. **Combination products**: Management of moderate to severe pain. Antitussive (usually in combination products with decongestants).

Action

Bind to opiate receptors in the CNS. Alter the perception of and response to painful stimuli while producing generalized CNS depression: Suppress the cough reflex via a direct central action. **Therapeutic Effects:** Decrease in severity of moderate pain. Suppression of the cough reflex.

Pharmacokinetics

Absorption: Well absorbed following oral administration.

Distribution: Unknown.

Metabolism and Excretion: Mostly metabolized by the liver; eliminated in the urine (50–60% as metabolites, 10% as unchanged drug).

Half-life: 2.2 hr; *Extended-release*—8 hr.

TIME/ACTION PROFILE (analgesic effect)

ROUTE	ONSET	PEAK	DURATION
PO	10–30 min	30–60 min	4–6 hr
PO-ER	unknown	unknown	unknown

Contraindications/Precautions

Contraindicated in: Hypersensitivity to hydrocodone (cross-sensitivity may exist to other opioids); Significant respiratory depression; Paralytic ileus; Acute or severe bronchial asthma or hypercarbia; Congenital long QT syndrome (Hysingla only); Hypersensitivity to acetaminophen/ibuprofen (for combination products); Ibuprofen-containing products should be avoided in patients with bleeding disorders or thrombocytopenia; Acetaminophen-containing products should be avoided in patients with severe hepatic or renal disease; Ibuprofen-containing products should be avoided in patients undergoing coronary artery bypass graft surgery; OB, Lactation: Avoid chronic use;; Products containing alcohol, aspartame, saccharin, sugar, or tartrazine (FDC yellow dye #5) should be avoided in patients who have hypersensitivity or intolerance to these compounds.

Use Cautiously in: Head trauma; ↑ intracranial pressure; Severe renal, hepatic, or pulmonary disease; Cardiovascular disease (ibuprofen-containing products only); History of peptic ulcer disease (ibuprofen-containing products only); Alcoholism; Difficulty swallowing; Patients with undiagnosed abdominal pain; Prostatic hyperplasia; Geri: Geriatric or debilitated patients (initial dose ↓ required; more prone to CNS depression, constipation).

Adverse Reactions/Side Effects

Noted for hydrocodone only; see acetaminophen/ibuprofen monographs for specific information on individual components.

CNS: confusion, dizziness, sedation, euphoria, hallucinations, headache, unusual dreams. **EENT:** blurred vision, diplopia, miosis. **Resp:** respiratory depression. **CV:** hypotension, bradycardia, QT interval prolongation (Hysingla only). **GI:** constipation, dyspepsia, nausea, choking, dysphagia, esophageal obstruction, vomiting. **GU:** urinary retention. **Derm:** sweating. **Misc:** physical dependence, psychological dependence, tolerance.

Interactions

Drug-Drug: Use with extreme caution in patients receiving **MAO inhibitors**; may produce severe, unpredictable reactions—do not use within 14 days of each other. **CYP3A4 inhibitors**, including **erythromycin**, **ketoconazole**, **itraconazole**, and **protease inhibitors** may ↑ levels and effects. **CYP3A4 inducers** may ↓ levels and effects. Additive CNS depression with **alcohol**, **antihistamines**, and **sedative/hypnotics**. Administration of partial antagonist opioids (**buprenorphine**, **butorphanol**, **nalbuphine**, or **pentazocine**) may ↓ analgesia or precipitate opioid withdrawal in physically dependent patients. **Anticholinergic drugs** may ↑ risk of urinary retention and constipation.

Drug-Natural Products: Concomitant use of **kava-kava**, **valerian**, **skullcap**, **chamomile**, or **hops** can ↑ CNS depression.

Route/Dosage

PO (Adults): *Analgesic*—2.5–10 mg q 3–6 hr as needed; if using combination products, acetaminophen dosage should not exceed 4 g/day and should not exceed 5 tablets/day of ibuprofen-containing products; *Antitussive*—5 mg q 4–6 hr as needed; *Extended-release (Zohydro ER)*—10 mg q 12 hr; may ↑ as needed in increments of 10 mg q 12 hr q 3–7 days; *Extended-release (Hysingla)*—20 mg once daily; may ↑ as needed in increments of 10–20 mg/day q 3–5 days.

PO (Children): *Analgesic (1–13 yr)*—0.1–0.2 mg/kg q 3–4 hr. *Antitussive* —0.6 mg/kg/day divided q 6–8 hr; (maximum doses <2 yr: 1.25 mg/dose; 2–12 yr: 5 mg/dose; >12 yr: 10 mg/dose).

Renal Impairment

PO (Adults): *CCr <45 mL/min*—Extended-release (Hysingla): ↓ initial dose by 50%.

Hepatic Impairment

PO (Adults): *Extended-release (Hysingla)*—↓ initial dose by 50%.

Availability

Hydrocodone

Extended-release capsules (Zohydro ER): 10 mg, 15 mg, 20 mg, 30 mg, 40 mg, 50 mg. **Extended-release tablets (Hysingla ER):** 20 mg, 30 mg, 40 mg, 60 mg, 80 mg, 100 mg, 120 mg. **Syrup:** ✤1 mg/mL). ***In combination with:*** chlorpheniramine (Tussionex); chlorpheniramine and pseudoephedrine (Zutripro); chlorpheniramine (Vituz); guaifenesin (Obredon). See Appendix B.

Hydrocodone/Acetaminophen (generic available)

Tablets: 2.5 mg hydrocodone/325 mg acetaminophen, 5 mg hydrocodone/325 mg acetaminophen (Anexsia 5/325, Norco), 7.5 mg hydrocodone/325 mg acetaminophen (Anexsia 7.5/325, Norco), 10 mg hydrocodone/325 mg acetaminophen (Norco). **Cost:** *Generic*—5 mg/325 mg $15.08/100, 7.5 mg/325 mg $30.93/100, 10 mg/325 mg $41.59/100. **Elixir/oral solution:** 7.5 mg hydrocodone plus 325 mg acetaminophen/15 mL, 10 mg hydrocodone plus 325 mg acetaminophen/15 mL. **Cost:** *Generic*—$58.12/473 mL.

Hydrocodone/Ibuprofen (generic available)

Tablets: 2.5 mg hydrocodone/200 mg ibuprofen (Reprexain), 5 mg hydrocodone/200 mg ibuprofen (Reprexain), 7.5 mg hydrocodone/200 mg ibuprofen (Vicoprofen), 10 mg hydrocodone/200 mg ibuprofen (Reprexain). **Cost:** *Generic*—7.5 mg/200 mg $48.40/100.

NURSING IMPLICATIONS

Assessment

- Assess BP, pulse, and respirations before and periodically during administration. If respiratory rate is <10/min, assess level of sedation. Physical stimulation may be sufficient to prevent significant hypoventilation. Dose may need to be decreased by 25–50%. Initial drowsiness will diminish with continued use.
- Assess bowel function routinely. Prevention of constipation should be instituted with increased intake of fluids and bulk, and laxatives to minimize constipating effects. Stimulant laxatives should be administered routinely if opioid use exceeds 2–3 days, unless contraindicated.
- **Pain:** Assess type, location, and intensity of pain prior to and 1 hr (peak) following administration. When titrating opioid doses, increases of 25–50% should be administered until there is either a 50% reduction in the patient's pain rating on a numerical or visual analogue scale or the patient reports satisfactory pain relief. A repeat dose can be safely administered at the time of the peak if previous dose is ineffective and side effects are minimal.
- Patients taking extended-release hydrocodone may require additional short-acting or rapid-onset opioid doses for breakthrough pain. Doses of short-acting opioids should be equivalent to 10–20% of 24 hr total and given every 2 hr as needed.
- An equianalgesic chart (see Appendix I) should be used when changing routes or when changing from one opioid to another.
- Prolonged use may lead to physical and psychological dependence and tolerance. This should not prevent patient from receiving adequate analgesia. Most patients who receive opioids for pain do not develop psychological dependence. If progressively higher doses are required, consider conversion to a stronger opioid.
- Assess risk for opioid addiction, abuse, or misuse prior to administration. Abuse or misuse of extended-release preparations by crushing, chewing, snorting, or injecting dissolved product will result in uncontrolled delivery of hydrocodone and can result in overdose and death.
- **Cough:** Assess cough and lung sounds during antitussive use.
- ***Lab Test Considerations:*** May cause ↑ plasma amylase and lipase concentrations.
- ***Toxicity and Overdose:*** If an opioid antagonist is required to reverse respiratory depression or coma, naloxone is the antidote. Dilute the 0.4-mg ampule of naloxone in 10 mL of 0.9% NaCl and administer 0.5 mL (0.02 mg) by IV push every 2 min. For children and patients weighing <40 kg, dilute 0.1 mg of naloxone in 10 mL of 0.9% NaCl for a concentration of 10 mcg/mL and administer 0.5 mcg/kg every 2 min. Titrate dose to avoid withdrawal, seizures, and severe pain.

Potential Nursing Diagnoses

Acute pain (Indications)
Chronic pain (Indications)
Risk for injury (Side Effects)

Implementation

- ***High Alert:*** Do not confuse hydrocodone with oxycodone. Do not confuse Reprexain with Zyprexa.
- Explain therapeutic value of medication prior to administration to enhance the analgesic effect.
- Regularly administered doses may be more effective than prn administration. Analgesic is more effective if given before pain becomes severe.
- Combination with nonopioid analgesics may have additive analgesic effects and permit lower doses. Maximum doses of nonopioid agents limit the titration of hydrocodone doses.
- Medication should be discontinued gradually after long-term use to prevent withdrawal symptoms.
- **PO:** May be administered with food or milk to minimize GI irritation.
- Swallow extended-release capsules whole; do not open, crush, dissolve, or chew.

Patient/Family Teaching

- Advise patient to take medication as directed and not to take more than the recommended amount. Severe and permanent liver damage may result from prolonged use or high doses of acetaminophen. Renal damage may occur with prolonged use of acetaminophen or ibuprofen. Doses of nonopioid agents should not exceed the maximum recommended daily dose. Do not stop taking without discussing with health care professional; my cause withdrawal symptoms if discontinued abruptly after prolonged use.

- Instruct patient on how and when to ask for and take pain medication.
- Advise patient that hydrocodone is a drug with known abuse potential. Protect it from theft, and never give to anyone other than the individual for whom it was prescribed.
- May cause drowsiness or dizziness. Advise patient to call for assistance when ambulating or smoking. Caution patient to avoid driving or other activities requiring alertness until response to the medication is known.
- Advise patient to notify health care professional if pain control is not adequate or if severe or persistent side effects occur.
- Advise patient to change positions slowly to minimize orthostatic hypotension.
- Caution patient to avoid concurrent use of alcohol or other CNS depressants with this medication.
- Instruct patient to notify health care professional of all Rx or OTC medications, vitamins, or herbal products being taken and consult health care professional before taking any new medications.
- Emphasize the importance of aggressive prevention of constipation with the use of hydrocodone.
- Encourage patient to turn, cough, and breathe deeply every 2 hr to prevent atelectasis.
- Advise patient that good oral hygiene, frequent mouth rinses, and sugarless gum or candy may decrease dry mouth.
- Advise patient to notify health care professional if pregnancy is planned or suspected, or if breast feeding.

Evaluation/Desired Outcomes

- Decrease in severity of pain without a significant alteration in level of consciousness or respiratory status.
- Suppression of nonproductive cough.

hydrocortisone, See CORTICOSTEROIDS (SYSTEMIC) and CORTICOSTEROIDS (TOPICAL/LOCAL).

REMS HIGH ALERT

HYDROmorphone

(hye-droe-**mor**-fone)

Dilaudid, Dilaudid-HP, Exalgo, ✱Hydromorph Contin, ✱Jurnista

Classification

Therapeutic: allergy, cold, and cough remedies (antitussives), opioid analgesics

Pharmacologic: opioid agonists

Schedule II

Pregnancy Category C

H

Indications

Moderate to severe pain (alone and in combination with nonopioid analgesics). Moderate to severe chronic pain in opioid-tolerant patients requiring use of daily, around-the-clock long-term opioid treatment and for which alternative treatment options are inadequate (extended-release). Antitussive (lower doses).

Action

Binds to opiate receptors in the CNS. Alters the perception of and response to painful stimuli while producing generalized CNS depression. Suppresses the cough reflex via a direct central action. **Therapeutic Effects:** Decrease in moderate to severe pain. Suppression of cough.

Pharmacokinetics

Absorption: Well absorbed following oral, rectal, subcut, and IM administration. Extended-release product results in an initial release of drug, followed by a second sustained phase of absorption.

Distribution: Widely distributed. Crosses the placenta; enters breast milk.

Metabolism and Excretion: Mostly metabolized by the liver.

Half-life: *Oral (immediate-release), or injection*—2–4 hr; *Oral (extended-release)*—8–15 hr.

TIME/ACTION PROFILE (analgesic effect)

ROUTE	ONSET	PEAK	DURATION
PO-IR	30 min	30–90 min	4–5 hr
PO-ER	unknown	unknown	unknown
Subcut	15 min	30–90 min	4–5 hr
IM	15 min	30–60 min	4–5 hr
IV	10–15 min	15–30 min	2–3 hr
Rect	15–30 min	30–90 min	4–5 hr

Contraindications/Precautions

Contraindicated in: Hypersensitivity; Some products contain bisulfites and should be avoided in patients with known hypersensitivity; Severe respiratory depression (in absence of resuscitative equipment) (extended-release only); Acute or severe bronchial asthma (extended-release only); Paralytic ileus (extended-release only); Acute, mild, intermittent, or postoperative pain (extended-release only); Prior GI surgery or narrowing of GI tract (extended-release only); Opioid nontolerant patients (extended-release only); Severe hepatic impairment (extended-release only).

Use Cautiously in: Head trauma; ↑ intracranial pressure; Severe pulmonary disease; Moderate or severe renal disease (extended-release only) (dose ↓ recommended); Moderate hepatic impairment (extended-release only) (dose ↓ recommended); Hypothyroidism; Seizure disorder; Adrenal insufficiency; Alcoholism; Undiagnosed abdominal pain; Prostatic hypertrophy; Biliary tract disease (including pancreatitis); OB, Lactation: Avoid chronic use; prolonged use of extended-release hydromorphone during pregnancy can result in neonatal opioid withdrawal syndrome; Geri: Geriatric or debilitated patients (↑ risk of respiratory depression; dose ↓ suggested).

Adverse Reactions/Side Effects

CNS: confusion, sedation, dizziness, dysphoria, euphoria, floating feeling, hallucinations, headache, unusual dreams. **EENT:** blurred vision, diplopia, miosis. **Resp:** RESPIRATORY DEPRESSION. **CV:** hypotension, bradycardia. **GI:** constipation, dry mouth, nausea, vomiting. **GU:** urinary retention. **Derm:** flushing, sweating. **Misc:** physical dependence, psychological dependence, tolerance.

Interactions

Drug-Drug: Exercise extreme caution with **MAO inhibitors** (may produce severe, unpredictable reactions—reduce initial dose of hydromorphone to 25% of usual dose, discontinue MAO inhibitors 2 wk prior to hydromorphone). ↑ risk of CNS depression with **alcohol**, **antidepressants**, **antihistamines**, and **sedative/hypnotics** including **benzodiazepines** and **phenothiazines**. Administration of partial antagonists (**buprenorphine**, **butorphanol**, **nalbuphine**, or **pentazocine**) may precipitate opioid withdrawal in physically dependent patients. **Nalbuphine** or **pentazocine** may ↓ analgesia.

Drug-Natural Products: Concomitant use of **kava-kava**, **valerian**, **chamomile**, or **hops** can ↑ CNS depression.

Route/Dosage

Doses depend on level of pain and tolerance. Larger doses may be required during chronic therapy.

Analgesic

PO (Adults ≥50 kg): *Immediate-release*—4–8 mg q 3–4 hr initially (some patients may respond to doses as small as 2 mg initially); *or* once 24-hr opioid requirement is determined, convert to *extended-release* by administering total daily oral dose once daily.

PO (Adults and Children <50 kg): 0.06 mg/kg q 3–4 hr initially, younger children may require smaller initial doses of 0.03 mg/kg. Maximum dose 5 mg.

IV, IM, Subcut (Adults ≥50 kg): 1.5 mg q 3–4 hr as needed initially; may be ↑.

IV, IM, Subcut (Adults and Children <50 kg): 0.015 mg/kg mg q 3–4 hr as needed initially; may be ↑.

IV (Adults): *Continuous infusion (unlabeled)*—0.2–30 mg/hr depending on previous opioid use. An initial bolus of twice the hourly rate in mg may be given with subsequent breakthrough boluses of 50–100% of the hourly rate in mg.

Rect (Adults): 3 mg q 6–8 hr initially as needed.

Hepatic Impairment

PO (Adults): *Moderate hepatic impairment (extended–release)*—↓ initial dose by 75%.

Renal Impairment

PO (Adults): *Moderate renal impairment (extended–release)*—↓ initial dose by 50%; *Severe renal impairment (extended–release)*—↓ initial dose by 75%.

Antitussive

PO (Adults and Children >12 yr): 1 mg q 3–4 hr.

PO (Children 6–12 yr): 0.5 mg q 3–4 hr.

Availability (generic available)

Immediate-release tablets: 2 mg, 4 mg, 8 mg. **Extended-release tablets:** ✱ 4 mg, 8 mg, 12 mg, 16 mg, 32 mg. **Controlled-release capsules:** ✱ 3 mg, ✱ 4.5 mg, ✱ 6 mg, ✱ 9 mg, ✱ 12 mg, ✱ 18 mg, ✱ 24 mg, ✱ 30 mg. **Oral solution:** 1 mg/mL. **Injection:** 1 mg/mL, 2 mg/mL, 4 mg/mL, 10 mg/mL. **Suppositories:** 3 mg.

NURSING IMPLICATIONS

Assessment

- Assess BP, pulse, and respirations before and periodically during administration. If respiratory rate is <10/min, assess level of sedation. Dose may need to be decreased by 25–50%. Initial drowsiness will diminish with continued use.Geri, Pedi: Assess geriatric and pediatric patients frequently; more sensitive to the effects of opioid analgesics and may experience side effects and respiratory complications more frequently.

- Assess bowel function routinely. Institute prevention of constipation with increased intake of fluids and bulk, and laxatives to minimize constipating effects. Administer stimulant laxatives routinely if opioid use exceeds 2–3 days, unless contraindicated.
- **Pain:** Assess type, location, and intensity of pain prior to and 1 hr following IM or PO and 5 min (peak) following IV administration. When titrating opioid doses, increases of 25–50% should be administered until there is either a 50% reduction in the patient's pain rating on a numerical or visual analogue scale or the patient reports satisfactory pain relief. When titrating doses of short-acting hydromorphone, a repeat dose can be safely administered at the time of the peak if previous dose is ineffective and side effects are minimal.
- Patients on a continuous infusion should have additional bolus doses provided every 15–30 min, as needed, for breakthrough pain. The bolus dose is usually set to the amount of drug infused each hour by continuous infusion.
- Patients taking extended-release hydromorphone may require additional short-acting or rapid-onset opioid doses for breakthrough pain. Doses of short-acting opioids should be equivalent to 10–20% of 24 hr total and given every 2 hr as needed.
- An equianalgesic chart (see Appendix I) should be used when changing routes or when changing from one opioid to another.
- Prolonged use may lead to physical and psychological dependence and tolerance. This should not prevent patient from receiving adequate analgesia. Most patients who receive hydromorphone for pain do not develop psychological dependence. Progressively higher doses may be required to relieve pain with long-term therapy.
- Assess risk for opioid addiction, abuse, or misuse prior to administration. Abuse or misuse of extended-release preparations by crushing, chewing, snorting, or injecting dissolved product will result in uncontrolled delivery of hydromorphone and can result in overdose and death.
- **Cough:** Assess cough and lung sounds during antitussive use.
- ***Lab Test Considerations:*** May ↑ plasma amylase and lipase concentrations.
- ***Toxicity and Overdose:*** If an opioid antagonist is required to reverse respiratory depression or coma, naloxone (Narcan) is the antidote. Dilute the 0.4-mg ampule of naloxone in 10 mL of 0.9% NaCl and administer 0.5 mL (0.02 mg) by IV push every 2 min. For children and patients weighing <40 kg, dilute 0.1 mg of naloxone in 10 mL of 0.9% NaCl for a concentration of 10 mcg/mL and administer 0.5 mcg every 2 min. Titrate dose to avoid withdrawal, seizures, and severe pain.

Potential Nursing Diagnoses

Acute pain (Indications)
Chronic pain (Indications)
Risk for injury (Side Effects)

Implementation

- ***High Alert:*** Accidental overdose of opioid analgesics has resulted in fatalities. Before administering, check infusion pump settings. Pedi: Medication errors with opioid analgesics are common in pediatric patients; calculate doses carefully. Use appropriate measuring devices.
- ***High Alert:*** Do not confuse with morphine; fatalities have occurred. Do not confuse high-potency (HP) dose forms with regular dose forms.
- Explain therapeutic value of medication prior to administration to enhance the analgesic effect.
- Regularly administered doses may be more effective than prn administration. Analgesic is more effective if given before pain becomes severe.
- Coadministration with nonopioid analgesics may have additive analgesic effects and permit lower opioid doses.
- Medication should be discontinued gradually after long-term use to prevent withdrawal symptoms.
- When converting from immediate-release to extended-release hydromorphone administer total daily oral hydromorphone dose once daily; dose of extended-release product can be titrated q 3–4 days. To convert from another opioid to extended-release hydromorphone, convert to total daily dose of hydromorphone and then administer 50% of this dose as extended-release hydromorphone once daily; can then titrate dose q 3–4 days. When converting from transdermal fentanyl, initiate extended-release hydromorphone 18 hr after removing transdermal fentanyl patch; for each 25 mcg/hr fentanyl transdermal dose, the equianalgesic dose of extended-release hydromorphone is 12 mg once daily (should initiate at 50% of this calculated total daily dose given once daily).
- **PO:** May be administered with food or milk to minimize GI irritation.
- Swallow extended-release tablets whole; do not break, crush, dissolve, or chew.

IV Administration

- **IV Push:** ***Diluent:*** Dilute with at least 5 mL of sterile water or 0.9% NaCl for injection. Inspect solution for particulate matter. Slight yellow color does not alter potency. Store at room temperature. ***Rate:*** Administer slowly, at a rate not to exceed 2 mg over 3–5 min. ***High Alert:*** Rapid administration may lead to increased respiratory depression, hypotension, and circulatory collapse.

- **Y-Site Compatibility:** acetaminophen, acyclovir, alemtuzumab, allopurinol, amifostine, amikacin, aminocaproic acid, aminophylline, amphotericin B colloidal, amphotericin B lipid complex, amphotericin B liposome, ampicillin/sulbactam, anidulafungin, argatroban, atropine, azithromycin, aztreonam, bivalirudin, bleomycin, bumetanide, busulfan, calcium chloride, calcium gluconate, cangrelor, carboplatin, carmustine, caspofungin, cefepime, cefotaxime, cefoxitin, ceftaroline, ceftazidime, ceftriaxone, cefuroxime, chloramphenicol, chlorpromazine, ciprofloxacin, cisatracurium, cisplatin, cladribine, clindamycin, cyclophosphamide, cyclosporine, cytarabine, dacarbazine, dactinomycin, daptomycin, daunorubicin hydrochloride, dexamethasone, dexmedetomidine, dexrazoxane, digoxin, diltiazem, diphenhydramine, dobutamine, docetaxel, dolasetron, dopamine, doripenem, doxorubicin, doxorubicin liposome, doxycycline, droperidol, enalaprilat, ephedrine, epinephrine, epirubicin, eptifibatide, ertapenem, erythromycin, esmolol, etoposide, etoposide phosphate, famotidine, fenoldopam, fentanyl, filgrastim, fluconazole, fludarabine, fluorouracil, foscarnet, fosphenytoin, furosemide, ganciclovir, gemcitabine, gentamicin, glycopyrrolate, granisetron, haloperidol, heparin, hydralazine, hydrocortisone, idarubicin, ifosfamide, imipenem/cilastatin, insulin, irinotecan, isoproterenol, ketorolac, labetalol, leucovorin, levofloxacin, lidocaine, linezolid, lorazepam, magnesium sulfate, mannitol, mechlorethamine, melphalan, meropenem, mesna, methotrexate, methyldopate, methylprednisolone, metoclopramide, metoprolol, metronidazole, micafungin, midazolam, milrinone, mitoxantrone, mitomycin, morphine, mycophenolate, nafcillin, naloxone, nesiritide, nicardipine, nitroglycerin, nitroprusside, norepinephrine, octreotide, ondansetron, oxacillin, oxaliplatin, oxytocin, paclitaxel, palonosetron, pamidronate, pancuronium, pemetrexed, penicillin G potassium, pentamidine, pentobarbital, phenylephrine, piperacillin/tazobactam, potassium acetate, potassium chloride, potassium phosphates, procainamide, prochlorperazine, promethazine, propofol, propranolol, quinupristin/dalfopristin, ranitidine, remifentanil, rituximab, rocuronium, scopolamine, sodium acetate, sodium phosphates, streptozocin, succinylcholine, tacrolimus, teniposide, theophylline, thiotepa, tigecycline, tirofiban, tobramycin, topotecan, trastuzumab, trimethoprim/sulfamethoxazole, vancomycin, vasopressin, vecuronium, verapamil, vinblastine, vincristine, vinorelbine, zidovudine, zoledronic acid.
- **Y-Site Incompatibility:** dantrolene, dimenhydrate, phenytoin, sargramostim, thiopental.

Patient/Family Teaching

- Instruct patient on how and when to ask for pain medication. Do not stop taking without discussing with health care professional; my cause withdrawal symptoms if discontinued abruptly after prolonged use.
- Advise patient that hydromorphone is a drug with known abuse potential. Protect it from theft, and never give to anyone other than the individual for whom it was prescribed.
- May cause drowsiness or dizziness. Advise patient to call for assistance when ambulating or smoking. Caution patient to avoid driving or other activities requiring alertness until response to medication is known.
- Advise patient to notify health care professional if pain control is not adequate or if side effects occur.
- Advise patient to change positions slowly to minimize orthostatic hypotension.
- Instruct patient to avoid concurrent use of alcohol or other CNS depressants.
- Instruct patient to notify health care professional of all Rx or OTC medications, vitamins, or herbal products being taken and consult health care professional before taking any new medications.
- Encourage patient to turn, cough, and breathe deeply every 2 hr to prevent atelectasis.
- Advise patient to notify health care professional if pregnancy is planned or suspected, or if breast feeding.
- **Home Care Issues:** Explain to patient and family how and when to administer hydromorphone, discuss safe storage of medication, and how to care for infusion equipment properly. Pedi: Teach parents or caregivers how to accurately measure liquid medication and to use only measuring device dispensed with medication.
- Emphasize the importance of aggressive prevention of constipation with the use of hydromorphone.

Evaluation/Desired Outcomes

- Decrease in severity of pain without a significant alteration in level of consciousness or respiratory status.
- Suppression of cough.

hydroxocobalamin, See VITAMIN B_{12} PREPARATIONS.

hydroxychloroquine
(hye-drox-ee-**klor**-oh-kwin)
Plaquenil

Classification
Therapeutic: antimalarials, antirheumatics (DMARDs)

Pregnancy Category C

Indications
Suppression/chemoprophylaxis of malaria. Treatment of severe rheumatoid arthritis/systemic lupus erythematosus.

Action
Inhibits protein synthesis in susceptible organisms by inhibiting DNA and RNA polymerase. **Therapeutic Effects:** Death of plasmodia responsible for causing malaria. Also has anti-inflammatory properties.

Pharmacokinetics
Absorption: Highly variable (31–100%) following oral administation.
Distribution: Widely distributed; high concentrations in RBCs; crosses the placenta; excreted into breast milk.
Metabolism and Excretion: Partially metabolized by the liver to active metabolites; partially excreted unchanged by the kidneys.
Half-life: 72–120 hr.

TIME/ACTION PROFILE (blood levels)

ROUTE	ONSET	PEAK	DURATION
PO	rapid†	1–2 hr	days–weeks

†Onset of antirheumatic action may take 6 wk.

Contraindications/Precautions
Contraindicated in: Hypersensitivity to hydroxychloroquine or chloroquine; Previous visual damage from hydroxychloroquine or chloroquine.
Use Cautiously in: Concurrent use of hepatotoxic drugs; History of liver disease, alcoholism or renal impairment; Severe neurological disorders; Severe blood disorders; Retinal or visual field changes; G6PD deficiency; Psoriasis; Bone marrow depression; Obesity (determine dose by ideal body weight); OB, Lactation: Avoid use unless treating/preventing malaria or treating amebic abscess; Pedi: Long-term use may ↑ sensitivity to effects.

Adverse Reactions/Side Effects
CNS: SEIZURES, aggressiveness, anxiety, apathy, confusion, fatigue, headache, irritability, personality changes, psychoses. **EENT:** keratopathy, ototoxicity, retinopathy, tinnitus, visual disturbances. **CV:** ECG changes, hypotension. **GI:** abdominal cramps, anorexia, diarrhea, epigastric discomfort, nausea, vomiting, hepatic failure. **Derm:** bleaching of hair, alopecia, hyperpigmentation, photosensitivity, Stevens-Johnson syndrome. **Hemat:** AGRANULOCYTOSIS, APLASTIC ANEMIA, leukopenia, thrombocytopenia. **Neuro:** neuromyopathy, peripheral neuritis.

Interactions
Drug-Drug: May ↑ the risk of hepatotoxicity when administered with **hepatotoxic drugs**. May ↑ the risk of hematologic toxicity when administered with **penicillamine**. May ↑ risk of dermatitis when administered with other **agents having dermatologic toxicity**. May ↓ serum titers of rabies antibody when given concurrently with **human diploid cell rabies vaccine**. **Urinary acidifiers** may ↑ renal excretion. May ↑ levels of **digoxin**.

Route/Dosage
Antimalarial doses expressed as mg of base; antirheumatic and lupus doses expressed as mg of hydroxychloroquine sulfate (200 mg hydroxychloroquine sulfate = 155 mg of hydroxychloroquine base).

Malaria
PO (Adults): *Suppression or chemoprophylaxis*—310 mg once weekly; start 1–2 wk prior to entering malarious area; continue for 4 wk after leaving area. *Treatment*—620 mg, then 310 mg at 6 hr, 24 hr, and 48 hr after initial dose.
PO (Children): *Suppression or chemoprophylaxis*—5 mg/kg once weekly; start 1–2 wk prior to entering malarious area; continue for 4 wk after leaving area. *Treatment*—10 mg/kg initially, then 5 mg/kg at 6–8 hr, 24 hr, and 48 hr after initial dose.

Rheumatoid Arthritis
PO (Adults): 400–600 mg once daily initially, maintenance 200–400 mg/day divided 1–2 times/day.
PO (Children): 3–5 mg/kg/day divided 1–2 times/day to a maximum of 400 mg/day; not to exceed 7 mg/kg/day.

Systemic Lupus Erythematosus
PO (Adults): 400 mg once or twice daily, maintenance 200–400 mg/day.
PO (Children): 3–5 mg/kg/day divided 1–2 times/day to a maximum of 400 mg/day; not to exceed 7 mg/kg/day.

Availability (generic available)
Tablets: 200 mg (155-mg base). **Cost:** *Generic*—$14.88/100.

NURSING IMPLICATIONS

Assessment

- Assess deep tendon reflexes periodically to determine muscle weakness. Therapy may be discontinued should this occur.
- Patients on prolonged high-dose therapy should have eye exams prior to and every 3–6 mo during therapy to detect retinal damage.
- **Malaria or Lupus Erythematosus:** Assess patient for improvement in signs and symptoms of condition daily throughout course of therapy.
- **Rheumatoid Arthritis:** Assess patient monthly for pain, swelling, and range of motion.
- ***Lab Test Considerations:*** Monitor CBC and platelet count periodically throughout therapy. May cause decreased RBC, WBC, and platelet counts. If severe decreases occur that are not related to the disease process, hydroxychloroquine should be discontinued.

Potential Nursing Diagnoses

Risk for infection (Indications)
Chronic pain (Indications)

Implementation

- **PO:** Administer with milk or meals to minimize GI distress.
- Tablets may be crushed and placed inside empty capsules for patients with difficulty swallowing. Contents of capsules may also be mixed with a teaspoonful of jam, jelly, or Jell-O prior to administration.
- **Malaria Prophylaxis:** Hydroxychloroquine therapy should be started 2 wk prior to potential exposure and continued for 4–6 wk after leaving the malarious area.

Patient/Family Teaching

- Instruct patient to take medication exactly as directed and continue full course of therapy even if feeling better. Missed doses should be taken as soon as remembered unless it is almost time for next dose. Do not double doses.
- Advise patients to avoid use of alcohol while taking hydroxychloroquine.
- Caution patient to keep hydroxychloroquine out of reach of children; fatalities have occurred with ingestion of 3 or 4 tablets.
- Explain need for periodic ophthalmic exams for patients on prolonged high-dose therapy. Advise patient that the risk of ocular damage may be decreased by the use of dark glasses in bright light. Protective clothing and sunscreen should also be used to reduce risk of dermatoses.
- Advise patient to notify health care professional promptly if sore throat, fever, unusual bleeding or bruising, blurred vision, visual changes, ringing in the ears, difficulty hearing, or muscle weakness occurs.
- Advise female patient to notify health care professional if pregnancy is planned or suspected or if breast feeding.
- **Malaria Prophylaxis:** Review methods of minimizing exposure to mosquitoes with patients receiving hydroxychloroquine prophylactically (use repellent, wear long-sleeved shirt and long trousers, use screen or netting).
- Advise patient to notify health care professional if fever develops while traveling or within 2 mo of leaving an endemic area.
- **Rheumatoid Arthritis:** Instruct patient to contact health care professional if no improvement is noticed within a few days. Treatment for rheumatoid arthritis may require up to 6 mo for full benefit.

Evaluation/Desired Outcomes

- Prevention or resolution of malaria.
- Improvement in signs and symptoms of rheumatoid arthritis.
- Improvement in symptoms of lupus erythematosus.

hydroxyprogesterone caproate

(hye-drox-ee-pro-**jess**-te-rone **kap**-roe-ate)
Makena

Classification
Therapeutic: hormones
Pharmacologic: progestins

Pregnancy Category B

Indications

To ↓ the risk of preterm birth in women with a singleton pregnancy who have a history of previous singleton preterm birth.

Action

A synthetic analog of progesterone. Produces secretory changes in the endometrium. ↑s basal temperature. Produces changes in the vaginal epithelium. Relaxes uterine smooth muscle. Stimulates mammary alveolar growth. Inhibits pituitary function. Action in reducing risk of recurrent preterm birth is unknown. **Therapeutic Effects:** ↓ risk of preterm birth in women at risk.

Pharmacokinetics

Absorption: Slowly absorbed following IM administration.
Distribution: Unknown.
Protein Binding: Extensively bound to plasma proteins.
Metabolism and Excretion: Extensively metabolized by the liver.
Half-life: 7.8 days.

TIME/ACTION PROFILE (blood levels)

ROUTE	ONSET	PEAK	DURATION
IM	unknown	4.6 days	7 days

Contraindications/Precautions

Contraindicated in: Hypersensitivity to hydroxyprogesterone or castor oil; History of or known thrombosis/thromboembolic disorder; History of or known/suspected breast cancer or other hormone-sensitive cancer; Unexplained abnormal vaginal bleeding unrelated to pregnancy; Cholestatic jaundice of pregnancy; Benign/malignant liver tumors or active liver disease; Uncontrolled hypertension.

Use Cautiously in: Risk factors for thromboembolic disorders (may ↑ risk); Diabetes mellitus or risk factors for diabetes mellitus (may impair glucose tolerance); History of preeclampsia, epilepsy, cardiac or renal impairment (may be adversely affected by fluid retention); History of depression (may worsen); Safe and effective use in children <16 yr has not been established.

Adverse Reactions/Side Effects

CNS: depression. **CV:** hypertension. **GI:** diarrhea, jaundice, nausea. **Derm:** urticaria, pruritus. **F and E:** fluid retention. **Hemat:** THROMBOEMBOLISM. **Local:** injections site reactions. **Misc:** allergic reactions including ANGIOEDEMA.

Interactions

Drug-Drug: May ↑ metabolism and ↓ blood levels and effectiveness of **drugs metabolized by the CYP1A2, CYP2A6 and CYP2B6 enzyme systems**.

Route/Dosage

IM (Adults): 250 mg once weekly starting between 16 wks, 0 days and 20 wks, 6 days continuing until wk 37 of gestation or delivery, whichever occurs first.

Availability

Solution for IM injection (contains castor oil): 1250 mg/5 mL vial (250 mg/mL).

NURSING IMPLICATIONS

Assessment

- Monitor for signs and symptoms of thromboembolic disorders throughout therapy.
- Monitor vital signs during therapy. If hypertension occurs, consider discontinuation of therapy.
- Assess for signs and symptoms of allergic reactions (urticaria, pruritus, angioedema) during therapy. Consider discontinuation if allergic reactions occur.
- Monitor for fluid retention during therapy, especially in patients at ↑ risk for complications (preeclampsia, epilepsy, migraine, asthma, cardiac or renal dysfunction).
- Assess mental status and mood changes, especially in women with a history of depression. Discontinue hydroxyprogesterone if depression recurs or worsens.
- ***Lab Test Considerations:*** May ↓ glucose tolerance. Monitor serum glucose in prediabetic and diabetic women during therapy.

Potential Nursing Diagnoses

Deficient knowledge, related to disease process and medication regimen (Patient/Family Teaching)

Implementation

- **IM:** Draw up 1 mL of solution into a 3 mL syringe with an 18 gauge needle. Solution is clear, yellow, viscous and oily. Do not administer solutions that are cloudy or contain particles. Change needle to 21 gauge 1 1/2 inch needle. Inject into upper outer quadrant of gluteus maximus slowly, over 1 min or longer. Apply pressure to injection site to minimize bruising and swelling. Store hydroxyprogesterone in original box, at room temperature, protected from light. Discard unused product after 5 wks from first use.

Patient/Family Teaching

- Instruct patient to continue to receive injection weekly from health care professional. If a dose is missed, consult health care professional for instructions regarding returning to schedule.
- Advise patient to notify health care professional if signs and symptoms of blood clots (leg swelling, redness in your leg, a spot on your leg that is warm to touch, leg pain that worsens when you bend your foot), allergic reactions (hives, itching, swelling of the face), depression, or yellowing of skin and whites of the eyes occur.
- Inform patient that injection site reactions (pain, swelling, itching, bruising, nodule formation) may occur. If ↑ pain over time, oozing of blood or fluid, or swelling occur, notify health care professional.

Evaluation/Desired Outcomes

- ↓ risk of preterm birth in women at risk.

hydrOXYzine (hye-drox-i-zeen)

✱Atarax, Vistaril

Classification
Therapeutic: antianxiety agents, antihistamines, sedative/hypnotics

Pregnancy Category C

Indications

Treatment of anxiety. Preoperative sedation. Antiemetic. Antipruritic. May be combined with opioid analgesics.

H

Action

Acts as a CNS depressant at the subcortical level of the CNS. Has anticholinergic, antihistaminic, and antiemetic properties. Blocks histamine 1 receptors. **Therapeutic Effects:** Sedation. Relief of anxiety. Decreased nausea and vomiting. Decreased allergic symptoms associated with release of histamine, including pruritus.

Pharmacokinetics

Absorption: Well absorbed following PO/IM administration.

Distribution: Unknown.

Metabolism and Excretion: Completely metabolized by the liver; eliminated in the feces via biliary excretion.

Half-life: 3 hr.

TIME/ACTION PROFILE (sedative, antiemetic, antipruritic effects)

ROUTE	ONSET	PEAK	DURATION
PO	15–30 min	2–4 hr	4–6 hr
IM	15–30 min	2–4 hr	4–6 hr

Contraindications/Precautions

Contraindicated in: Hypersensitivity; OB: Potential for congenital defects (oral clefts and hypoplasia of cerebral hemisphere; Lactation: Safety not established.

Use Cautiously in: Severe hepatic dysfunction; OB: Has been used safely during labor; Pedi: Injection contains benzyl alcohol, which can cause potentially fatal gasping syndrome in neonates; Geri: Appears on *Beers list*. Geriatric patients are more susceptible to adverse reactions due to anticholinergic effects; dose ↓ recommended.

Adverse Reactions/Side Effects

CNS: drowsiness, agitation, ataxia, dizziness, headache, weakness. **Resp:** wheezing. **GI:** dry mouth, bitter taste, constipation, nausea. **GU:** urinary retention. **Derm:** flushing, rash. **Local:** pain at IM site, abscesses at IM sites. **Misc:** chest tightness.

Interactions

Drug-Drug: Additive CNS depression with other **CNS depressants**, including **alcohol**, **antidepressants**, **antihistamines**, **opioid analgesics**, and **sedative/hypnotics**. Additive anticholinergic effects with other **drugs possessing anticholinergic properties**, including **antihistamines**, **antidepressants**, **atropine**, **haloperidol**, **phenothiazines**, **quinidine**, and **disopyramide**. Can antagonize the vasopressor effects of **epinephrine**.

Drug-Natural Products: Concomitant use of **kava-kava**, **valerian**, or **chamomile** can ↑ CNS depression. ↑ anticholinergic effects with **angel's trumpet**, **jimson weed**, and **scopolia**.

Route/Dosage

PO (Adults): *Antianxiety*—25–100 mg 4 times/day, not to exceed 600 mg/day. *Preoperative sedation*—50–100 mg single dose. *Antipruritic*—25 mg 3–4 times daily.

PO (Children): —2 mg/kg/day divided q 6–8 hr.

IM (Adults): *Preoperative sedation*—25–100 mg single dose. *Antiemetic, adjunct to opioid analgesics*—25–100 mg q 4–6 hr as needed.

IM (Children): —0.5–1 mg/kg/dose q 4–6 hr as needed.

Availability (generic available)

Tablets: 10 mg, 25 mg, 50 mg. **Cost:** *Generic*—10 mg $10.03/100, 25 mg $13.87/100, 50 mg $17.50/100. **Capsules:** 🍁 10 mg, 25 mg, 50 mg, 100 mg. **Cost:** *Generic*—25 mg $29.94/100, 50 mg $32.19/100, 100 mg $62.69/100. **Syrup:** 10 mg/5 mL. **Cost:** *Generic*—$19.94/473 mL. **Injection:** 25 mg/mL, 50 mg/mL.

NURSING IMPLICATIONS

Assessment

- Assess patient for profound sedation and provide safety precautions as indicated (side rails up, bed in low position, call bell within reach, supervision of ambulation and transfer). Geri: Older adults are more sensitive to CNS and anticholinergic effects (delirium, acute confusion, dizziness, dry mouth, blurred vision, urinary retention, constipation, tachycardia). Monitor for drowsiness, agitation, over sedation, and other systemic side effects. Assess falls risk and implement prevention strategies.
- **Anxiety:** Assess mental status (orientation, mood, and behavior).
- **Nausea and Vomiting:** Assess degree of nausea and frequency and amount of emesis.
- **Pruritus:** Assess degree of itching and character of involved skin.
- ***Lab Test Considerations:*** May cause false-negative skin test results using allergen extracts. Discontinue hydroxyzine at least 72 hr before test.

Potential Nursing Diagnoses

Anxiety (Indications)
Impaired skin integrity (Indications)
Risk for injury (Side Effects)

Implementation

- Do not confuse hydroxyzine with hydralazine or Atarax (hydroxyzine) with Ativan (lorazepam).
- **PO:** Tablets may be crushed and capsules opened and administered with food or fluids for patients having difficulty swallowing.
- **IM:** Administer *only* IM deep into well-developed muscle, preferably with Z-track technique. Injection is extremely painful. Do not use deltoid site. If must be administered to children, midlateral muscles of the thigh are preferred. Significant tissue damage, necrosis, and sloughing may result from subcut or intra-arterial injections. Hemolysis may result from IV injections. Rotate injection sites frequently.
- **Syringe Compatibility:** atropine, buprenorphine, butorphanol, chlorpromazine, diphenhydramine,

doxapram, droperidol, fentanyl, fluphenazine, glycopyrrolate, hydromorphone, lidocaine, meperidine, metoclopramide, midazolam, morphine, nalbuphine, oxymorphone, pentazocine, perphenazine, prochlorperazine, promethazine, scopolamine, sufentanil.

- **Syringe Incompatibility:** dimenhydrinate, haloperidol, heparin, ketorolac, penicillin G potassium, pentobarbital, phenobarbital, phenytoin.

Patient/Family Teaching

- Instruct patient to take medication exactly as directed. Missed doses should be taken as soon as remembered unless it is almost time for next dose; do not double doses.
- May cause drowsiness or dizziness. Caution patient to avoid driving and other activities requiring alertness until response to medication is known. Geri: Warn patients or caregivers that older adults are at increased risk for CNS effects and falls.
- Advise patient to avoid concurrent use of alcohol or other CNS depressants with this medication.
- Inform patient that frequent mouth rinses, good oral hygiene, and sugarless gum or candy may help decrease dry mouth. If dry mouth persists for more than 2 wk, consult dentist about saliva substitute.
- Advise female patient to notify health care professional if pregnancy is planned or suspected or if breast feeding.

Evaluation/Desired Outcomes

- Decrease in anxiety.
- Relief of nausea and vomiting.
- Relief of pruritus.
- Sedation when used as a sedative/hypnotic.

H

ibandronate (i-ban-dro-nate)
Boniva

Classification
Therapeutic: bone resorption inhibitors
Pharmacologic: biphosphonates

Pregnancy Category C

Indications
Treatment/prevention of postmenopausal osteoporosis.

Action
Inhibits resorption of bone by inhibiting osteoclast activity. **Therapeutic Effects:** Reversal/prevention of progression of osteoporosis with decreased fractures.

Pharmacokinetics
Absorption: 0.6% absorbed following oral administration (significantly ↓ by food).
Distribution: Rapidly binds to bone.
Protein Binding: 90.9–99.5%.
Metabolism and Excretion: 50–60% excreted in urine; unabsorbed drug is eliminated in feces.
Half-life: *PO*—10–60 hr; *IV*—4.6–25.5 hr.

TIME/ACTION PROFILE

ROUTE	ONSET	PEAK	DURATION
PO	unknown	0.5–2 hr	up to 1 mo
IV	unknown	3 hr	up to 3 mo

Contraindications/Precautions
Contraindicated in: Hypersensitivity; Abnormalities of the esophagus which delay esophageal emptying (i.e. strictures, achalasia); Uncorrected hypocalcemia; Inability to stand/sit upright for at least 60 min; CCr <30 mL/min.
Use Cautiously in: History of upper GI disorders; Concurrent use of NSAIDs or aspirin; Invasive dental procedures, cancer, receiving chemotherapy, corticosteroids, or angiogenesis inhibitors, poor oral hygiene, periodontal disease, dental disease, anemia, coagulopathy, infection, or poorly-fitting dentures (may ↑ risk of jaw osteonecrosis); OB: Use only if potential benefit outweighs risks to mother and fetus; Lactation: Lactation; Pedi: Children <18 yr (safety not established); Geri: Consider age related ↓ in body mass, renal and hepatic function, concurrent disease states and drug therapy.

Adverse Reactions/Side Effects
GI: diarrhea, dyspepsia, dysphagia, esophageal cancer, esophagitis, esophageal/gastric ulcer. **MS:** musculoskeletal pain, pain in arms/legs, femur fractures, osteonecrosis (primarily of jaw). **Derm:** ERYTHEMA MULTIFORME, STEVENS-JOHNSON SYNDROME. **Resp:** asthma exacerbation. **Misc:** ANAPHYLAXIS, injection site reactions.

Interactions
Drug-Drug: Calcium-, aluminum-, magnesium-, and **iron-**containing products, including **antacids** ↓ absorption (ibandronate should be taken 60 min before). Concurrent use of **NSAIDs** including **aspirin,** may ↑ risk of gastric irritation.
Drug-Food: Milk and other foods ↓ absorption.

Route/Dosage
PO (Adults): 150 mg once monthly.
IV (Adults): 3 mg every 3 mo.

Availability (generic available)
Tablets: 150 mg. **Injection:** 3 mg/3 mL in prefilled single-use syringe.

NURSING IMPLICATIONS
Assessment
- **Osteoporosis:** Assess patients for low bone mass before and periodically during therapy.
- **IV:** Monitor for signs and symptoms of anaphylactic reactions (swelling of face, lips, mouth or tongue; trouble breathing; wheezing; severe itching; skin rash, redness or swelling; dizziness or fainting; fast heartbeat or pounding in chest; sweating) during therapy. Discontinue injection immediately and begin supportive treatment if symptoms occur.
- Perform a routine oral exam prior to initiation of therapy. Dental exam with appropriate preventative dentistry should be considered prior to therapy. Patients with history of tooth extraction, poor oral hygiene, gingival infections, diabetes, or use of a dental appliance or those taking immunosuppressive therapy, angiogenesis inhibitors, or systemic corticosteroids are at greater risk for osteonecrosis of the jaw.
- ***Lab Test Considerations:*** Assess serum calcium before and periodically during therapy. Hypocalcemia and vitamin D deficiency should be treated before initiating ibandronate therapy.
- May cause ↓ total alkaline phosphatase levels.
- May cause hypercholesterolemia.

Potential Nursing Diagnoses
Risk for injury (Indications)

Implementation
- **PO:** Administer first thing in the morning with 6–8 oz plain water 30 min before other medications, beverages, or food. Tablet should be swallowed whole; do not break, crush, or chew.
- *Once-monthly tablet* should be administered on the same date each month.

IV Administration

- **IV:** Administer using prefilled syringe. Do not administer solution that is discolored or contains particulate matter. Administer IV only; other routes may cause tissue damage.

- ***Rate:*** Administer as a 15–30 second bolus.
- **Y-Site Incompatibility:** Do not administer with calcium-containing solutions or other IV drugs.

Patient/Family Teaching

- Advise patient to eat a balanced diet and consult health care professional about the need for supplemental calcium and vitamin D. Wait at least 60 min after administration before taking supplemental calcium and vitamin D.
- Encourage patient to participate in regular exercise and to modify behaviors that increase the risk of osteoporosis (stop smoking, reduce alcohol consumption).
- Inform patient that severe musculoskeletal pain may occur within days, months, or yr after starting ibandronate. Symptoms may resolve completely after discontinuation or slow or incomplete resolution may occur. Notify health care professional if severe pain occurs.
- Advise patient to notify health care professional if rash or signs and symptoms of osteonecrosis of the jaw (pain, numbness, swelling of or drainage from the jaw, mouth, or teeth) occur.
- Instruct patient to notify health care professional if swallowing difficulties, chest pain, new or worsening heartburn, or trouble or pain when swallowing occurs; may be signs of problems of the esophagus.
- Advise patient to inform health care professional of ibandronate therapy prior to dental surgery.
- Advise female patient to notify health care professional if pregnancy is planned or suspected or if breast feeding.
- **PO:** Instruct patient on the importance of taking as directed, first thing in the morning, 60 min before other medications, beverages, or food. Ibandronate should be taken with 6–8 oz plain water (mineral water, orange juice, coffee, and other beverages decrease absorption). Do not chew or suck on tablet. If a dose is missed, skip dose and resume the next morning; do not double doses or take later in the day. If a once-monthly dose is missed and the next scheduled dose is >7 days away, take in the morning following the date it is remembered. Resume original schedule the following month. If the next dose is <7 days away, omit dose and take next scheduled dose. Do not discontinue without consulting health care professional.
- Caution patient to remain upright for 60 min following dose to facilitate passage to stomach and minimize risk of esophageal irritation. Advise patient to stop taking ibandronate and contact health care professional if symptoms of esophageal irritation (new or worsening dysphagia, pain on swallowing, retrosternal pain, or heartburn) occur.
- **IV:** Advise patient that IV doses should not be administered sooner that every 3 mo. If a dose is missed, have health care professional administer as soon as possible; next injection should be scheduled 3 mo from last injection.

Evaluation/Desired Outcomes

- Prevention of or decrease in the progression of osteoporosis in postmenopausal women. Discontinuation after 3–5 years should be considered for women with low risk for fractures.

ibuprofen (eye-byoo-**proe**-fen)

Advil, Advil Migraine Liqui-Gels, Children's Advil, Children's Motrin, Excedrin IB, Junior Strength Advil, Medipren, Midol Maximum Strength Cramp Formula, Motrin, Motrin Drops, Motrin IB, Motrin Junior Strength, Motrin Migraine Pain, Nuprin, PediaCare Children's Fever

ibuprofen (injection)

Caldolor, NeoProfen (ibuprofen lysine)

Classification

Therapeutic: antipyretics, antirheumatics, nonopioid analgesics, nonsteroidal anti-inflammatory agents

Pharmacologic: nonopioid analgesics

Pregnancy Category C (up to 30 wk gestation), D (starting at 30 wk gestation)

Indications

PO, IV: Treatment of: Mild to moderate pain, Fever. **PO:** Treatment of: Inflammatory disorders including rheumatoid arthritis (including juvenile) and osteoarthritis, Dysmenorrhea. **IV:** Moderate to severe pain with opioid analgesics. Closure of a clinically significant PDA in neonates weighing 500–1500 g and ≤32 weeks gestational age (ibuprofen lysine only)

Action

Inhibits prostaglandin synthesis. **Therapeutic Effects:** Decreased pain and inflammation. Reduction of fever.

Pharmacokinetics

Absorption: Oral formulation is well absorbed (80%) from the GI tract; IV administration results in complete bioavailability.

Distribution: Does not enter breast milk in significant amounts.

Protein Binding: 99%.

Metabolism and Excretion: Mostly metabolized by the liver; small amounts (1%) excreted unchanged by the kidneys.

Half-life: Neonates: 26–43 hr; Children: 1–2 hr; Adults: 2–4 hr.

TIME/ACTION PROFILE

ROUTE	ONSET	PEAK	DURATION
PO (antipyretic)	0.5–2.5 hr	2–4 hr	6–8 hr
PO (analgesic)	30 min	1–2 hr	4–6 hr
PO (anti-inflammatory)	≤7 days	1–2 wk	unknown
IV (analgesic)	unknown	unknown	6 hr
IV (antipyretic)	within 2 hr	10–12 hr†	4–6 hr

† With repeated dosing.

Contraindications/Precautions

Contraindicated in: Hypersensitivity (cross-sensitivity may exist with other NSAIDs, including aspirin); Active GI bleeding or ulcer disease; Chewable tablets contain aspartame and should not be used in patients with phenylketonuria; Peri-operative pain from coronary artery bypass graft (CABG) surgery; OB: Avoid after 30 wk gestation (may cause premature closure of fetal ductus arteriosus); Pedi: Ibuprofen lysine: Preterm neonates with untreated infection, congenital heart disease where patency of PDA is necessary for pulmonary or systemic blood flow, bleeding, thrombocytopenia, coagulation defects, necrotizing enterocolitis, significant renal dysfunction.

Use Cautiously in: Cardiovascular disease or risk factors for cardiovascular disease (may ↑ risk of serious cardiovascular thrombotic events, myocardial infarction, and stroke, especially with prolonged use or use of higher doses); Renal or hepatic disease, dehydration, or patients on nephrotoxic drugs (may ↑ risk of renal toxicity); Aspirin triad patients (asthma, nasal polyps, and aspirin intolerance); can cause fatal anaphylactoid reactions; Chronic alcohol use/abuse; Geri: ↑ risk of adverse reactions secondary to age-related ↓ in renal and hepatic function, concurrent illnesses, and medications; Coagulation disorders; OB: Use cautiously up to 30 wk gestation; avoid after that; Lactation: Use cautiously; Pedi: Safety not established for infants <6 mo (oral) and children <17 yr (IV Caldolor); Ibuprofen lysine: Hyperbilirubinemia in neonates (may displace bilirubin from albumin-binding sites).

Exercise Extreme Caution in: History of GI bleeding or GI ulcer disease.

Adverse Reactions/Side Effects

CNS: headache, dizziness, drowsiness, intraventricular hemorrhage (ibuprofen lysine), psychic disturbances. **EENT:** amblyopia, blurred vision, tinnitus. **CV:** HF, MYOCARDIAL INFARCTION, STROKE, arrhythmias, edema, hypertension. **GI:** GI BLEEDING, HEPATITIS, constipation, dyspepsia, nausea, necrotizing enterocolitis (ibuprofen lysine), vomiting, abdominal discomfort. **GU:** cystitis, hematuria, renal failure. **Derm:** EXFOLIATIVE DERMATITIS, STEVENS-JOHNSON SYNDROME, TOXIC EPIDERMAL NECROLYSIS, rash, injection site reaction. **Hemat:** anemia, blood dyscrasias, prolonged bleeding time. **Misc:** allergic reactions including ANAPHYLAXIS.

Interactions

Drug-Drug: May limit the cardioprotective effects of low-dose **aspirin**. Concurrent use with **aspirin** may ↓ effectiveness of ibuprofen. Additive adverse GI side effects with **aspirin**, **oral potassium**, other **NSAIDs**, **corticosteroids**, or **alcohol**. Chronic use with **acetaminophen** may ↑ risk of adverse renal reactions. May ↓ effectiveness of **diuretics**, **ACE inhibitors**, or other **antihypertensives**. May ↑ hypoglycemic effects of **insulin** or **oral hypoglycemic agents**. May ↑ serum **lithium** levels and risk of toxicity. ↑ risk of toxicity from **methotrexate**. **Probenecid** ↑ risk of toxicity from ibuprofen. ↑ risk of bleeding with **cefotetan**, **corticosteroids**, **valproic acid**, **thrombolytics**, **warfarin**, and **drugs affecting platelet function** including **clopidogrel**, **abciximab**, **eptifibatide**, or **tirofiban**. ↑ risk of adverse hematologic reactions with **antineoplastics** or **radiation therapy**. ↑ risk of nephrotoxicity with **cyclosporine**.

Drug-Natural Products: ↑ bleeding risk with, **arnica**, **chamomile**, **feverfew**, **garlic**, **ginger**, **ginkgo**, **Panax ginseng**, and others.

Route/Dosage

Analgesia

PO (Adults): *Anti-inflammatory*—400–800 mg 3–4 times daily (not to exceed 3200 mg/day). *Analgesic/antidysmenorrheal/antipyretic*—200–400 mg q 4–6 hr (not to exceed 1200 mg/day).

PO (Children 6 mo–12 yr): *Anti-inflammatory*—30–50 mg/kg/day in 3–4 divided doses (maximum dose: 2.4 g/day). *Antipyretic*—5 mg/kg for temperature <102.5°F (39.17°C) or 10 mg/kg for higher temperatures (not to exceed 40 mg/kg/day); may be repeated q 4–6 hr. *Cystic fibrosis (unlabeled)*—20–30 mg/kg/day divided twice daily.

PO (Infants and Children): *Analgesic*—4–10 mg/kg/dose q 6–8 hr.

IV (Adults): *Analgesic*—400–800 mg q 6 hr as needed (not to exceed 3200 mg/day); *Antipyretic*—400 mg initially, then 400 mg q 4–6 hr or 100–200 mg q 4 hr as needed (not to exceed 3200 mg/day).

Pediatric OTC Dosing

PO (Children 11 yr/72–95 lb): 300 mg q 6–8 hr.
PO (Children 9–10 yr/60–71 lb): 250 mg q 6–8 hr.
PO (Children 6–8 yr/48–59 lb): 200 mg q 6–8 hr.
PO (Children 4–5 yr/36–47 lb): 150 mg q 6–8 hr.
PO (Children 2–3 yr/24–35 lb): 100 mg q 6–8 hr.

PO (Children 12–23 mo/18–23 lb): 75 mg q 6–8 hr.
PO (Infants 6–11 mo/12–17 lb): 50 mg q 6–8 hr.

PDA Closure

IV (Neonates Gestational age ≤32 weeks, 500–1500 g): 10 mg/kg followed by two doses of 5 mg/kg at 24 and 48 hr after initial dose.

Availability (generic available)

Tablets: 100 mg^OTC^, 200 mg^OTC^, 300 mg, 400 mg, 600 mg, 800 mg. **Capsules (liqui-gels):** 200 mg^OTC^. **Chewable tablets (fruit, grape, orange, and citrus flavor):** 50 mg^OTC^, 100 mg^OTC^. **Liquid (berry flavor):** 100 mg/5 mL^OTC^. **Oral suspension (fruit, berry, grape flavor):** 100 mg/5 mL^OTC^, 100 mg/2.5 mL^OTC^. **Pediatric drops (berry flavor):** 50 mg/1.25 mL^OTC^. **Solution for injection:** 100 mg/mL (Caldolor), 17.1 mg/mL as lysine, 10 mg/mL as ibuprofen base (Neoprofen). ***In combination with:*** decongestants, ^OTC^, hydrocodone (Vicoprofen), famotidine (Duexis). See Appendix B.

NURSING IMPLICATIONS

Assessment

- Patients who have asthma, aspirin-induced allergy, and nasal polyps are at increased risk for developing hypersensitivity reactions. Assess for rhinitis, asthma, and urticaria.
- Assess for signs and symptoms of GI bleeding (tarry stools, lightheadedness, hypotension), renal dysfunction (elevated BUN and creatinine levels, decreased urine output), and hepatic impairment (elevated liver enzymes, jaundice). Geri: Higher risk for poor outcomes or death from GI bleeding. Age-related renal impairment increases risk of hepatic and renal toxicity.
- Assess patient for skin rash frequently during therapy. Discontinue ibuprofen at first sign of rash; may be life-threatening. Stevens-Johnson syndrome or toxic epidermal necrolysis may develop. Treat symptomatically; may recur once treatment is stopped.
- **Pain:** Assess pain (note type, location, and intensity) prior to and 1–2 hr following administration.
- **Arthritis:** Assess pain and range of motion prior to and 1–2 hr following administration.
- **Fever:** Monitor temperature; note signs associated with fever (diaphoresis, tachycardia, malaise).
- **PDA Closure:** Monitor preterm neonates for signs of bleeding, infection and decreased urine output. Monitor IV site for signs of extravasation. If ductus arteriosus closes or size significantly decreases, 2nd and 3rd doses are unnecessary.
- ***Lab Test Considerations:*** BUN, serum creatinine, CBC, and liver function tests should be evaluated periodically in patients receiving prolonged therapy.
- Serum potassium, BUN, serum creatinine, alkaline phosphatase, LDH, AST, and ALT may show ↑ levels. Blood glucose, hemoglobin, and hematocrit concentrations, leukocyte and platelet counts, and CCr may be ↓.
- May cause prolonged bleeding time; may persist for <1 day following discontinuation.
- **PDA Closure:** If urinary output <0.6 mL/kg/hr at time of 2nd or 3rd dose, hold dose until renal function has returned to normal.

Potential Nursing Diagnoses

Acute pain (Indications)
Impaired physical mobility (Indications)
Ineffective thermoregulation (Indications)

Implementation

- Do not confuse Motrin (ibuprofen) with Neurontin (gabapentin).
- Administration of higher than recommended doses does not provide increased pain relief but may increase incidence of side effects.
- Patient should be well hydrated before administration to prevent renal adverse reactions. Do not give to neonates with urine output < 0.6 mL/kg/hour.
- Use lowest effective dose for shortest period of time, especially in the elderly.
- Coadministration with opioid analgesics may have additive analgesic effects and may permit lower opioid doses.
- **PO:** For rapid initial effect, administer 30 min before or 2 hr after meals. May be administered with food, milk, or antacids to decrease GI irritation. Tablets may be crushed and mixed with fluids or food; 800-mg tablet can be dissolved in water.
- **Dysmenorrhea:** Administer as soon as possible after the onset of menses. Prophylactic treatment has not been shown to be effective.

IV Administration

- **Intermittent Infusion:** ***Diluent:*** 0.9% NaCl, D5W, or LR. ***Concentration:*** *Ibuprofen injection:* Dilute the 800 mg dose in at least 200 mL and the 400 mg dose in at least 100 mL for a concentration of 4 mg/mL. *Ibuprofen lysine:* Dilute in appropriate volume of D5W or 0.9% NaCl and infuse over 15 minutes. Do not administer solutions that are discolored or contain particulate matter. Stable for up to 24 hr at room temperature. Discard remaining solution; does not contain preservatives. ***Rate:*** Infuse over at least 30 min.

Patient/Family Teaching

- Advise patients to take ibuprofen with a full glass of water and to remain in an upright position for 15–30 min after administration.
- Instruct patient to take medication as directed. Take missed doses as soon as remembered but not if almost time for next dose. Do not double doses. Pedi: Teach parents and caregivers to calculate and measure doses accurately and to use measuring device supplied with product.

- May cause drowsiness or dizziness. Advise patient to avoid driving or other activities requiring alertness until response to medication is known.
- Caution patient to avoid the concurrent use of alcohol, aspirin, acetaminophen, and other OTC or herbal products without consulting health care professional.
- Advise patient to inform health care professional of medication regimen prior to treatment or surgery.
- Instruct patients not to take OTC ibuprofen preparations for more than 10 days for pain or more than 3 days for fever, and to consult health care professional if symptoms persist or worsen. Many OTC products contain ibuprofen; avoid duplication.
- Caution patient that use of ibuprofen with 3 or more glasses of alcohol per day may increase the risk of GI bleeding.
- Advise patient to consult health care professional if rash, itching, visual disturbances, tinnitus, weight gain, edema, epigastric pain, dyspepsia, black stools, hematemasis, persistent headache, or influenza-like syndrome (chills, fever, muscle aches, pain) occurs.
- Pedi: Advise parents or caregivers not to administer ibuprofen to children who may be dehydrated (can occur with vomiting, diarrhea, or poor fluid intake); dehydration increases risk of renal dysfunction.
- Advise female patients to notify health care professional if pregnancy is planned or suspected.

Evaluation/Desired Outcomes

- Decrease in severity of pain.
- Improved joint mobility. Partial arthritic relief is usually seen within 7 days, but maximum effectiveness may require 1–2 wk of continuous therapy. Patients who do not respond to one NSAID may respond to another.
- Reduction in fever.
- Closure of PDA.

ibutilide (eye-**byoo**-ti-lide)

Corvert

Classification

Therapeutic: antiarrhythmics (class III)

Pregnancy Category C

Indications

Rapid conversion of recent-onset atrial flutter or fibrillation to normal sinus rhythm, including management of atrial flutter or fibrillation occurring within 1 wk of coronary artery bypass or cardiac valve surgery.

Action

Activates slow inward current of sodium in cardiac tissue, resulting in delayed repolarization, prolonged action potential duration, and increased refractoriness. Mildly slows sinus rate and AV conduction. **Therapeutic Effects:** Conversion to normal sinus rhythm.

Pharmacokinetics

Absorption: IV administration results in complete bioavailability.

Distribution: Unknown.

Metabolism and Excretion: Highly metabolized by the liver, one metabolite is active; metabolites excreted by kidneys.

Half-life: 6 hr (2–12 hr).

TIME/ACTION PROFILE (antiarrhythmic effect)

ROUTE	ONSET	PEAK	DURATION
IV	within 30–90 min	unknown	up to 24 hr

Contraindications/Precautions

Contraindicated in: Hypersensitivity.

Use Cautiously in: HF or left ventricular dysfunction (↑ risk of more serious arrhythmias during infusion); OB, Lactation, Pedi: Pregnancy, lactation, or children <18 yr (safety not established).

Adverse Reactions/Side Effects

CNS: headache. **CV:** arrhythmias. **GI:** nausea.

Interactions

Drug-Drug: Amiodarone, **disopyramide**, **procainamide**, **quinidine**, and **sotalol** should not be given concurrently or within 4 hr because of additive effects on refractoriness. Proarrhythmic effects may be ↑ by **phenothiazines**, **tricyclic** and **tetracyclic antidepressants**, some **antihistamines**, and **histamine H_2-receptor blocking agents**; concurrent use should be avoided.

Route/Dosage

Atrial Fibrillation/Flutter

IV (Adults ≥60 kg): 1 mg infusion; may be repeated 10 min after end of first infusion.

IV (Adults <60 kg): 0.01 mg/kg infusion; may be repeated 10 min after end of first infusion.

Atrial Fibrillation/Flutter After Cardiac Surgery

IV (Adults ≥60 kg): 0.5 mg infusion, may be repeated once.

IV (Adults <60 kg): 0.005 mg/kg infusion, may be repeated once.

Availability (generic available)

Solution for injection: 0.1 mg/mL.

NURSING IMPLICATIONS

Assessment

- Monitor ECG continuously throughout and for 4 hr after infusion or until QT interval normalizes. Discontinue if arrhythmia terminates or if sustained ventricular tachycardia, prolonged QT, or QT develops. Ibutilide may have proarrhythmic effects. These arrhythmias may be serious and potentially life threatening. Clinicians trained to treat ventricular arrhythmias, medications, and equipment (defibrillator/cardioverter) should be available during therapy and monitoring of patient.

Potential Nursing Diagnoses

Decreased cardiac output (Indications)

Implementation

- Oral antiarrhythmic therapy may be instituted 4 hr after ibutilide infusion.

IV Administration

- **Intermittent Infusion:** ***Diluent:*** May be administered undiluted or diluted in 50 mL of 0.9% NaCl or D5W. Diluted solution is stable for 24 hr at room temperature or 48 hr if refrigerated. ***Concentration:*** Undiluted: 0.1 mg/mL; Diluted: 0.017 mg/mL. ***Rate:*** Administer over 10 min.
- **Additive Incompatibility:** Information unavailable; do not admix with other solutions or medications.

Patient/Family Teaching

- Inform patient of the purpose of ibutilide.

Evaluation/Desired Outcomes

- Conversion of recent-onset atrial flutter or fibrillation to normal sinus rhythm.

idarucizumab

(eye-da-roo-**siz**-ue-mab)
Praxbind

Classification
Therapeutic: antidotes
Pharmacologic: monoclonal antibodies

Indications

To counteract the anticoagulant effect of dabigatran for emergency surgery/urgent procedures or life-threatening uncontrolled bleeding.

Action

Human monoclonal antibody fragment (Fab) that selectively binds to dabigatran and its metabolites, preventing its binding to thrombin and negating its anticoagulant effects. Does not reverse any other anticoagulants. **Therapeutic Effects:** Reversal of the anticoagulant effect of dabigatran.

Pharmacokinetics

Absorption: IV administration results in complete bioavailability.
Distribution: Unknown.
Metabolism and Excretion: Biodegraded to smaller molecules. 60% excreted in urine, remainder via protein catabolism primarily in the kidneys.
Half-life: 10.3 hr.

TIME/ACTION PROFILE

ROUTE	ONSET	PEAK	DURATION
IV	immediate	unknown	24 hr

Contraindications/Precautions

Contraindicated in: None noted.
Use Cautiously in: Geri: Elderly patients may be more sensitive to drug effects; OB: Safe use not established. Consider maternal benefits and fetal risks; Lactation: Safe use not established, consider beneficial effects of breast feeding and possible adverse effects in infant; Pedi: Safe and effective use in children has not been established.
Exercise Extreme Caution in: Hereditary fructose intolerance (risk of serious adverse reactions due to sorbitol excipient); History of serious hypersensivity (including anaphylactoid reactions) to idarucizumab.

Adverse Reactions/Side Effects

CNS: delerium. **CV:** THROMBOEMBOLISM. **GI:** constipation. **F and E:** hypokalemia. **Misc:** hypersensitivity reactions, fever.

Interactions

Drug-Drug: None noted.

Route/Dosage

IV (Adults): 5 g.

Availability

Solution for IV injection (contains sorbitol): 2.5 g/50 mL single use vial.

NURSING IMPLICATIONS

Assessment

- Reversal of dabigatran exposes patient to thrombotic risk of their underlying disease; may cause thromboembolism. Resume anticoagulant therapy as soon as medically appropriate. Dabigatran therapy can be reinstituted 24 hr after idarucizumab infusion.
- Monitor for signs and symptoms of hypersensitivity reactions (rash, urticaria, fever, pruritus, dyspnea, orofacial swelling). Contains sorbitol; reactions in patients with hereditary fructose intolerance have included hypoglycemia, hypophosphatemia, metabolic acidosis, increase in uric acid, acute liver failure. If symptoms occur discontinue therapy and treat symptomatically.
- ***Lab Test Considerations:*** Monitor coagulation parameters (activated partial thromboplastin time [aPTT], ecarin clotting time [ECT]) 12–24 hrs after infusion.
- May cause hypokalemia.

Potential Nursing Diagnoses

Ineffective tissue perfusion (Adverse Reactions)

Implementation

- **Intermittent Infusion:** Flush IV line with 0.9% NaCl prior to and following infusion. Solution is clear to opalescent, colorless to slightly yellow; do not administer solutions that are discolored or contain precipitates. Administer as 2 consecutive infusion or inject both vials consecutively via syringe. Must be administered within 1 hr when removed from vial. Store in refrigerator; stable for 48 hrs at room temperature and 6 hrs if exposed to light.

Patient/Family Teaching

- Explain purpose of idarucizumab to patient.
- Instruct patient to notify health care professional immediately if bleeding occurs.
- Advise patient to notify health care professional if pregnancy is planned or suspected or if breast feeding.

Evaluation/Desired Outcomes

- Reversal of the anticoagulant effect of dabigatran.

ifosfamide (eye-foss-fam-ide)

Ifex

Classification
Therapeutic: antineoplastics
Pharmacologic: alkylating agents

Pregnancy Category D

Indications

Germ cell testicular carcinoma (with other agents). Used with mesna, which prevents ifosfamide-induced hemorrhagic cystitis.

Action

Following conversion to active compounds, interferes with DNA replication and RNA transcription, ultimately disrupting protein synthesis (cell-cycle phase–nonspecific). **Therapeutic Effects:** Death of rapidly replicating cells, particularly malignant ones.

Pharmacokinetics

Absorption: Administered IV only; inactive prior to conversion to metabolites.
Distribution: Excreted in breast milk.
Metabolism and Excretion: Metabolized by the liver to active antineoplastic compounds.
Half-life: 15 hr.

TIME/ACTION PROFILE (effects on blood counts)

ROUTE	ONSET	PEAK	DURATION
IV	unknown	7–14 days	21 days

Contraindications/Precautions

Contraindicated in: Hypersensitivity; OB, Lactation: Pregnancy or lactation.
Use Cautiously in: Patients with childbearing potential; Active infections; ↓ bone marrow reserve; Geri: Geriatric patients; Other chronic debilitating illness; Renal impairment; Pedi: Children.

Adverse Reactions/Side Effects

CNS: CNS toxicity (somnolence, confusion, hallucinations, coma), cranial nerve dysfunction, disorientation, dizziness. **CV:** cardiotoxicity. **GI:** nausea, vomiting, anorexia, constipation, diarrhea, hepatotoxicity. **GU:** hemorrhagic cystitis, dysuria, sterility, renal toxicity. **Derm:** alopecia. **Hemat:** ANEMIA, LEUKOPENIA, THROMBOCYTOPENIA. **Local:** phlebitis. **Misc:** allergic reactions.

Interactions

Drug-Drug: CYP3A4 inhibitors, including **ketoconazole**, **fluconazole**, **itraconazole**, **sorafenib**, and **aprepitant** may ↓ its effectiveness. **CYP3A4 inducers**, including **carbamazepine**, **phenytoin**, **phenytoin**, **phenobarbital**, and **rifampin** may ↑ the formation of a toxic metabolite and may ↑ risk of toxicity. ↑ myelosuppression with other **antineoplastics** or **radiation therapy**. Toxicity may be ↑ by **allopurinol** or **phenobarbital**. May ↓ antibody response to and ↑ risk of adverse reactions from **live-virus vaccines**.
Drug-Food: Grapefruit juice may ↑ levels; avoid concurrent use.

Route/Dosage

Other Regimens are Used

IV (Adults): 1.2 g/m²/day for 5 days; coadminister with mesna. May repeat cycle q 3 wk.

Availability (generic available)

Powder for injection (requires reconstitution): 1 g/vial, 3 g/vial. **Solution for injection:** 50 mg/mL.

NURSING IMPLICATIONS

Assessment

- Monitor BP, pulse, respiratory rate, and temperature frequently during administration. Report significant changes.
- Monitor urinary output frequently during therapy. Notify health care professional if hematuria occurs. To reduce the risk of hemorrhagic cystitis, fluid intake should be at least 3000 mL/day for adults and 1000–2000 mL/day for children. Mesna is given concurrently to prevent hemorrhagic cystitis.

- Monitor neurologic status. Ifosfamide should be discontinued if severe CNS symptoms (agitation, confusion, hallucinations, unusual tiredness) occur. Symptoms usually abate within 3 days of discontinuation of ifosfamide but may persist for longer; fatalities have been reported.
- Assess nausea, vomiting, and appetite. Weigh weekly. Premedication with an antiemetic may be used to minimize GI effects. Adjust diet as tolerated.
- Monitor for bone marrow depression. Assess for bleeding (bleeding gums, bruising, petechiae, guaiac stools, urine, and emesis) and avoid IM injections and taking rectal temperatures if platelet count is low. Apply pressure to venipuncture sites for 10 min. Assess for signs of infection during neutropenia. Anemia may occur. Monitor for increased fatigue, dyspnea, and orthostatic hypotension.
- ***Lab Test Considerations:*** Monitor CBC, differential, and platelet count prior to and periodically during therapy. Withhold dose if WBC <2000/mm^3 or platelet count is <50,000/mm^3. Nadir of leukopenia and thrombocytopenia occurs within 7–14 days and usually recovers within 21 days of therapy.
- Urinalysis should be evaluated before each dose. Withhold dose until recovery if urinalysis shows >10 RBCs per high-power field.
- May cause ↑ in liver enzymes and serum bilirubin.
- Monitor AST, ALT, serum alkaline phosphatase, bilirubin, and LDH prior to and periodically during therapy. May cause ↑ in liver enzymes and serum bilirubin.
- Monitor BUN, serum creatinine, phosphate, and potassium periodically during therapy. May cause hypokalemia.

Potential Nursing Diagnoses

Risk for infection (Side Effects)
Disturbed body image (Side Effects)

Implementation

- Prepare solution in a biologic cabinet. Wear gloves, gown, and mask while handling IV medication. Discard IV equipment in specially designated containers.

IV Administration

- **IV:** Prepare solution by diluting each 1-g vial with 20 mL of sterile water or bacteriostatic water for injection containing parabens. Use solution prepared without bacteriostatic water within 6 hr. Solution prepared with bacteriostatic water is stable for 1 wk at 30°C or 6 wk at 5°C.
- **Intermittent Infusion:** ***Diluent:*** May be further diluted in D5W, 0.9% NaCl, LR, or sterile water for injection. ***Concentration:*** 0.6 to 20 mg/mL (maximum 40 mg/mL). Dilute solution is stable for 7 days at room temperature or 6 wk if refrigerated. ***Rate:*** Administer over at least 30 min.
- **Continuous Infusion:** Has also been administered as a continuous infusion over 72 hr.
- **Y-Site Compatibility:** acyclovir, alemtuzumab, alfentanil, allopurinol, amifostine, amikacin, aminocaproic acid, aminophylline, amiodarone, amphotericin B cholesteryl, amphotericin B colloidal, amphotericin B lipid complex, amphotericin B liposome, ampicillin, ampicillin/sulbactam, anidulafungin, argatroban, azithromycin, aztreonam, bivalirudin, bleomycin, bumetanide, buprenorphine, butorphanol, calcium chloride, calcium gluconate, carboplatin, caspofungin, cefazolin, cefotaxime, cefotetan, cefoxitin, ceftazidime, ceftriaxone, cefuroxime, chlorpromazine, ciprofloxacin, cisatracurium, cisplatin, clindamycin, cyclosporine, cytarabine, dacarbazine, dactinomycin, daptomycin, dexamethasone, dexmedetomidine, dexrazoxane, digoxin, diltiazem, diphenhydramine, dobutamine, docetaxel, dolasetron, dopamine, doripenem, doxorubicin hydrochloride, doxorubicin liposome, doxycycline, droperidol, enalaprilat, ephedrine, epinephrine, epirubicin, ertapenem, erythromycin, esmolol, etoposide, etoposide phosphate, famotidine, fenoldopam, fentanyl, filgrastim, fluconazole, fludarabine, fluorouracil, foscarnet, fosphenytoin, furosemide, ganciclovir, gemcitabine, gentamicin, granisetron, haloperidol, heparin, hetastarch, hydrocortisone, hydromorphone, idarubicin, imipenem/cilastatin, insulin, isoproterenol, ketorolac, labetalol, leucovorin calcium, levofloxacin, levorphanol, lidocaine, linezolid, lorazepam, magnesium sulfate, mannitol, melphalan, meperidine, meropenem, mesna, methylprednisolone, metoclopramide, metoprolol, metronidazole, midazolam, milrinone, minocycline, mitomycin, mitoxantrone, morphine, moxifloxacin, nalbuphine, naloxone, nesiritide, nicardipine, nitroglycerin, nitroprusside, norepinephrine, octreotide, ondansetron, oxaliplatin, paclitaxel, palonosetron, pamidronate, pancuronium, pemetrexed, pentamidine, pentobarbital, phenobarbital, phenylephrine, piperacillin/tazobactam, potassium acetate, potassium chloride, procainamide, prochlorperazine, promethazine, propofol, propranolol, quinupristin/dalfopristin, ranitidine, remifentanil, rituximab, rocuronium, sargramostim, sodium acetate, sodium bicarbonate, sodium phosphates, succinylcholine, sufentanil, tacrolimus, teniposide, theophylline, thiopental, thiotepa, tigecycline, tirofiban, tobramycin, topotecan, trastuzumab, trimethoprim/sulfamethoxazole, vancomycin, vasopressin, vecuronium, verapamil, vinblastine, vincristine, vinorelbine, voriconazole, zidovudine, zoledronic acid.
- **Y-Site Incompatibility:** cefepime, diazepam, methotrexate, pantoprazole, phenytoin, potassium phosphates.

Patient/Family Teaching

- Emphasize need for adequate fluid intake throughout therapy. Patient should void frequently to decrease bladder irritation from metabolites excreted by the kidneys. Notify health care professional immediately if hematuria is noted.

- Instruct patient to drink at least 8 glasses of water/day during and for 3 days after completion of therapy.
- Advise patient to avoid grapefruit and grapefruit juice during therapy.
- Instruct patient to notify health care professional promptly if fever; chills; cough; hoarseness; sore throat; signs of infection; lower back or side pain; painful or difficult urination; bleeding gums; bruising; petechiae; blood in urine, stool, or emesis; or confusion occurs.
- Caution patient to avoid crowds and persons with known infections. Instruct patient to use soft toothbrush and electric razor and to avoid falls. Patients should also be cautioned not to drink alcoholic beverages or to take products containing aspirin or NSAIDs, as these may precipitate GI hemorrhage.
- Discuss with patient the possibility of hair loss. Explore methods of coping.
- Instruct patient to notify health care professional of all Rx or OTC medications, vitamins, or herbal products being taken and to consult with health care professional before taking other medications.
- Instruct patient not to receive any vaccinations without advice of health care professional; ifosfamide may decrease antibody response to and increase risk of adverse reactions from live-virus vaccines.
- Review with patient the need for contraception during therapy and for at least 6 months after therapy. Women should avoid pregnancy and breast feeding and men should avoid fathering a child during and for at least 6 months after end of therapy.
- Rep: Caution patient about the potential for amenorrhea, premature menopause, and sterility from this medication.

Evaluation/Desired Outcomes

- Decrease in size or spread of malignant germ cell testicular carcinoma.

⧖ iloperidone

(eye-loe-**per**-i-done)

Fanapt

Classification

Therapeutic: antipsychotics

Pharmacologic: benzisoxazoles

Pregnancy Category C

Indications

Schizophrenia.

Action

May act by antagonizing dopamine and serotonin in the CNS. **Therapeutic Effects:** Decreased symptoms of schizophrenia.

Pharmacokinetics

Absorption: Well absorbed (96%) following oral administration.

Distribution: Unknown.

Metabolism and Excretion: Extensively metabolized by the liver. ⧖ Metabolism is genetically determined; primarily by CYP3A4 and CYP2D6 enzyme systems, with individual variability in metabolism via CYP2D6 (extensive metabolizers [EM] and poor metabolizers [PM] and some in-between; 7–10% of Caucasians and 3–8% of Black/African Americans are considered PM). Two major metabolites (P88 and P95) may be partially responsible for pharmacologic activity. 58% excreted in urine as metabolites in EM and 45% in PM; 20% eliminated in feces in EM and 22.1% in PM.

Half-life: *EMs*—iloperidone–18 hr, P88–26 hr, P95–23 hr; *PMs*—iloperidone–33 hr, P88–37 hr, P95–31 hr.

TIME/ACTION PROFILE (antipsychotic effect)

ROUTE	ONSET	PEAK	DURATION
PO	2–4 wk	2–4 hr†	unknown

† Blood level.

Contraindications/Precautions

Contraindicated in: Hypersensitivity; Concurrent use of drugs known to prolong QTc interval; Bradycardia, recent MI or uncompensated heart failure (↑ risk of serious arrhythmias); Congenital long QT syndrome, QTc interval >500 msec or history of cardiac arrhythmias; Severe hepatic impairment; Geri: Elderly patients with dementia-related psychoses (↑ risk of death, CVA or TIA); Lactation: Breast feeding should be avoided.

Use Cautiously in: Known cardiovascular disease including heart failure, history of MI/ischemia, conduction abnormalities, cerebrovascular disease, or other conditions known to predispose to hypotension including dehydration, hypovolemia, concurrent antihypertensive therapy (↑ risk of orthostatic hypotension); Electrolyte abnormalities, especially hypomagnesemia or hypokalemia (correct prior to therapy); Concurrent use of CYP3A4 or CYP2D6 inhibitors; Known ↓ WBC or history of drug-induced leukopenia/neutropenia; Circumstances that may result in ↑ body temperature, including strenuous exercise, exposure to extreme heat, concurrent anticholinergic activity, or dehydration (may impair thermoregulation); Patients at risk for aspiration; Moderate hepatic impairment; Geri: May have ↑ sensitivity and risk of adverse reactions; OB: Neonates at ↑ risk for extrapyramidal symptoms and withdrawal after delivery when exposed during the 3rd trimester; use only if potential maternal benefit justifies potential fetal risk; Pedi: Safety and effectiveness not established.

Adverse Reactions/Side Effects

CNS: NEUROLEPTIC MALIGNANT SYNDROME, SUICIDAL THOUGHTS, dizziness, drowsiness, fatigue, agitation, delusion, restlessness, extrapyramidal disorders. **EENT:** nasal congestion. **CV:** orthostatic hypotension, tachycardia, palpitations, QTc interval prolongation. **GI:** dry mouth, nausea, abdominal discomfort, diarrhea. **GU:** priapism, urinary incontinence. **Endo:** dyslipidemia, hyperglycemia, hyperprolactinemia. **Neuro:** tardive dyskinesia. **Metab:** weight gain, weight loss. **MS:** ↓ bone density, musculoskeletal stiffness.

Interactions

Drug-Drug: Avoid use of drugs known to prolong QTc including the **antiarrhythmics quinidine**, **procainamide**, **amiodarone**, and **sotalol**; **antipsychotics** including **chlorpromazine** and **thioridazine**, the **antibiotic moxifloxacin**, or any other **medications known to prolong the QTc interval** including **pentamidine**, **levomethadyl**, and **methadone**; concurrent use may result in serious, life-threatening arrhythmias. Concurrent use of strong **CYP2D6 inhibitors** including **fluoxetine** and **paroxetine** ↑ levels and the risk of toxicity; dose ↓ is required. Concurrent use of strong **CYP3A4 inhibitors** including **ketoconazole** and **clarithromycin** ↑ levels and the risk of toxicity; dosage ↓ is required. Concurrent use of **antihypertensives** including **diuretics** may ↑ risk of orthostatic hypotension. Concurrent **anticholinergics** may ↑ risk of impaired thermoregulation.

Route/Dosage

PO (Adults): Initiate treatment with 1 mg twice daily on the first day, then 2 mg twice daily the second day, then ↑ by 2 mg/day every day until a target dose of 12–24 mg/day given in two divided doses is reached; *Concurrent strong CYP2D6 or CYP3A4 inhibitors*—↓ dose by 50%, if inhibitor is withdrawn ↑ dose to previous amount. Re-titration is required if iloperidone is discontinued >300 days; *Poor metabolizers of CYP2D6*—↓ dose by 50%.

Availability

Tablets: 1 mg, 2 mg, 4 mg, 6 mg, 8 mg, 10 mg, 12 mg.

NURSING IMPLICATIONS

Assessment

- Monitor patient's mental status (delusions, hallucinations, and behavior) before and periodically during therapy.
- Monitor mood changes. Assess for suicidal tendencies, especially during early therapy. Restrict amount of drug available to patient.
- Monitor BP (sitting, standing, lying down) and pulse before and periodically during therapy. May cause prolonged QT interval, tachycardia, and orthostatic hypotension.
- Assess weight and BMI initially and throughout therapy.
- Observe patient when administering medication to ensure that medication is actually swallowed and not hoarded.
- Monitor patient for onset of extrapyramidal side effects (*akathisia*—restlessness; *dystonia*—muscle spasms and twisting motions; or *pseudoparkinsonism*—mask-like face, rigidity, tremors, drooling, shuffling gait, dysphagia). Report these symptoms; reduction of dose or discontinuation of medication may be necessary.
- Monitor for tardive dyskinesia (involuntary rhythmic movement of mouth, face, and extremities). Report immediately and discontinue therapy; may be irreversible.
- Monitor for development of neuroleptic malignant syndrome (fever, respiratory distress, tachycardia, seizures, diaphoresis, hypertension or hypotension, pallor, tiredness). Discontinue iloperidone and notify health care professional immediately if these symptoms occur.
- Monitor for symptoms related to hyperprolactinemia (menstrual abnormalities, galactorrhea, sexual dysfunction).
- ***Lab Test Considerations:*** Monitor fasting blood glucose before and periodically during therapy in diabetic patients.
- Monitor CBC frequently during initial months of therapy in patients with pre-existing or history of low WBC. May cause leukopenia, neutropenia, or agranulocytosis. Discontinue therapy if this occurs.
- Monitor serum potassium and magnesium levels in patients at risk for electrolyte disturbances.
- Monitor serum prolactin prior to and periodically during therapy. May cause ↑ serum prolactin levels.

Potential Nursing Diagnoses

Risk for self-directed violence (Indications)
Disturbed thought process (Indications)
Risk for injury (Side Effects)

Implementation

- Do not confuse Fanapt (iloperidone) with Xanax (alprazolam).
- **PO:** Administer twice daily without regard to food.

Patient/Family Teaching

- Instruct patient to take medication exactly as directed. Advise patient that appearance of tablets in stool is normal and not of concern.
- Inform patient of the possibility of extrapyramidal symptoms. Instruct patient to report these symptoms immediately to health care professional.
- Advise patient to change positions slowly to minimize orthostatic hypotension.
- May cause drowsiness. Caution patient to avoid driving or other activities requiring alertness until response to medication is known.
- Extremes in temperature should also be avoided; this drug impairs body temperature regulation.
- Instruct patient to notify health care professional promptly if sore throat, fever, unusual bleeding or

bruising, rash, tremors, palpitations, fainting, menstrual abnormalities, galactorrhea or sexual dysfunction occur.
- Advise patient and family to notify health care professional if thoughts about suicide or dying, attempts to commit suicide; new or worse depression; new or worse anxiety; feeling very agitated or restless; panic attacks; trouble sleeping; new or worse irritability; acting aggressive; being angry or violent; acting on dangerous impulses; an extreme increase in activity and talking; other unusual changes in behavior or mood occur.
- Caution patient to avoid concurrent use of alcohol and other CNS depressants.
- Advise patient to notify health care professional of all Rx or OTC medications, vitamins, or herbal products being taken and to consult with health care professional before taking other medications.
- Advise patient to notify health care professional of medication regimen before treatment or surgery.
- Advise female patients to notify health care professional if pregnancy is planned or suspected or if breast feeding.
- Emphasize the need for continued follow-up for psychotherapy and monitoring for side effects.

Evaluation/Desired Outcomes
- Decrease in excited, paranoid, or withdrawn behavior.

HIGH ALERT

imatinib (i-mat-i-nib)
Gleevec

Classification
Therapeutic: antineoplastics
Pharmacologic: enzyme inhibitors

Pregnancy Category D

Indications
Newly diagnosed Philadelphia positive (Ph+) chronic myeloid leukemia (CML). CML in blast crisis, accelerated phase, or in chronic phase after failure of interferon-alpha treatment. Kit (CD117) positive metastatic/unresectable malignant gastrointestinal stomal tumors (GIST). Adjuvant treatment following resection of Kit (CD117) positive GIST. Pediatric patients with Ph+ CML after failure of bone marrow transplant or resistance to interferon-alpha. Adult patients with relapsed or refractory Ph+ acute lymphoblastic leukemia (ALL). Newly diagnosed Ph+ ALL (in combination with chemotherapy). Myelodysplastic/myeloproliferative disease (MDS/MPD) associated with platelet-derived growth factor receptor (PDGFR) gene re-arrangements. Aggressive systemic mastocytosis (ASM) without the D816V c-Kit mutation or with c-Kit mutational status unknown. Hypereosinophilic syndrome and/or chronic eosinophilic leukemia (HES/CEL). Unresectable, recurrent, or metastatic dermatofibrosarcoma protuberans (DFSP).

Action
Inhibits kinases which may be produced by malignant cell lines. **Therapeutic Effects:** Inhibits production of malignant cell lines with decreased proliferation of leukemic cells in CML, HES/CEL, and ALL and malignant cells in GIST, MDS/MPD, ASM, and DFSP.

Pharmacokinetics
Absorption: Well absorbed (98%) following oral administration.
Distribution: Unknown.
Protein Binding: 95%.
Metabolism and Excretion: Mostly metabolized by the CYP3A4 enzyme system to N-demethyl imatinib, which is as active as imatinib. Excreted mostly in feces as metabolites. 5% excreted unchanged in urine.
Half-life: *Imatinib*—18 hr; *N-desmethyl imatinib*—40 hr.

TIME/ACTION PROFILE (blood levels of imatinib)

ROUTE	ONSET	PEAK	DURATION
PO	unknown	2–4 hr	24 hr

Contraindications/Precautions
Contraindicated in: Hypersensitivity; OB: Potential for fetal harm; Lactation: Potential for serious adverse reactions in nursing infants; breast feeding should be avoided.
Use Cautiously in: Hepatic impairment (dose ↓ recommended if bilirubin >3 times normal or liver transaminases >5 times normal); Cardiac disease (severe HF and left ventricular dysfunction may occur); Pedi: Children <1 yr (safety not established); Geri: ↑ risk of edema.

Adverse Reactions/Side Effects
CNS: fatigue, headache, weakness, dizziness, somnolence. **CV:** HF. **EENT:** epistaxis, nasopharyngitis, blurred vision. **Resp:** cough, dyspnea, pneumonia. **GI:** HEPATOTOXICITY, abdominal pain, anorexia, constipation, diarrhea, dyspepsia, nausea, vomiting. **Derm:** DRUG RASH WITH EOSINOPHILIA AND SYSTEMIC SYMPTOMS (DRESS), petechiae, pruritus, skin rash. **F and E:** edema (including pleural effusion, pericardial infusion, pulmonary edema, and superficial edema), hypokalemia. **Endo:** ↓ growth (in children), hypothyroidism. **Hemat:** BLEEDING, NEUTROPENIA, THROMBOCYTOPENIA. **Metab:** weight gain. **MS:** arthralgia, muscle cramps, musculoskeletal pain, myalgia. **Misc:** TUMOR LYSIS SYNDROME, fever, night sweats.

Interactions

Drug-Drug: Blood levels and effects are ↑ by concurrent use of potent CYP3A4 inhibitors (e.g. **ketoconazole**, **itraconazole**, **clarithromycin**, **atazanavir**, **indinavir**, **nefazodone**, **nelfinavir**, **ritonavir**, **saquinavor**, **telithromycin**, or **voriconazole**). Blood levels and effects may be ↓ by potent CYP3A4 inducers (e.g., **dexamethasone**, **phenytoin**, **carbamazepine**, **rifampin**, **rifabutin**, and **phenobarbital**; if used concurrently, ↑ dose of imatinib by 50%. ↑ blood levels of **simvastatin**. Imatinib inhibits the following enzyme systems: CYP2C9, CYP2D6, CYP3A4/5 and may be expected to alter the effects of other drugs metabolized by these systems.

Drug-Food: Blood levels and effects are ↑ by **grapefruit juice**; concurrent use should be avoided.

Route/Dosage

Chronic Myeloid Leukemia

PO (Adults): *Chronic phase*—400 mg once daily, may be ↑ to 600 mg once daily; *accelerated phase or blast crisis*—600 mg once daily; may be ↑ to 800 mg/day given as 400 mg twice daily based on response and circumstances.

PO (Children): *Newly diagnosed Ph+ CML*—340 mg/m²/day (not to exceed 600 mg); *CML recurrent after failure of bone marrow transplant or resistance to interferon-alpha*—260 mg/m²/day.

Gastrointestinal Stromal Tumors

PO (Adults): *Metastatic or unresectable*—400 mg/day; may be ↑ to 400 mg twice daily if well tolerated and response insufficient; *Adjuvant treatment after resection*—400 mg/day.

Ph+ Acute Lymphoblastic Leukemia

PO (Adults): 600 mg/day.

PO (Children): 340 mg/m²/day (not to exceed 600 mg).

Myelodysplastic/Myeloproliferative Diseases

PO (Adults): 400 mg/day.

Aggressive Systemic Mastocytosis

PO (Adults): 400 mg/day. *For patients with eosinophilia*—100 mg/day; ↑ to 400 mg/day if well tolerated and response insufficient.

Hypereosinophilic Syndrome and/or Chronic Eosinophilic Leukemia

PO (Adults): 400 mg/day. *For patients with FIP1L1–PDGFRa fusion kinase* 100 mg/day; increase to 400 mg/day if well tolerated and response insufficient.

Dermatofibrosarcoma Protuberans

PO (Adults): 800 mg/day.

Hepatic Impairment

PO (Adults): ↓ dose by 25% in severe hepatic impairment.

Renal Impairment

PO (Adults): *CCr 40–59 mL/min*—Do not exceed dose of 600 mg/day; *CCr 20–39 mL/min*—↓ initial dose by 50%; ↑ as tolerated.

Availability

Tablets: 100 mg, 400 mg.

NURSING IMPLICATIONS

Assessment

- Monitor for fluid retention. Weigh regularly, and assess for signs of pleural effusion, pericardial effusion, pulmonary edema, ascites (dyspnea, periorbital edema, swelling in feet and ankles, weight gain). Evaluate unexpected weight gain. Edema is usually managed with diuretics. General fluid retention is usually dose related, more common in accelerated phase or blast crisis, and is more common in the elderly. Treatment usually involves diuretics, supportive therapy, and interruption of imatinib.
- Monitor growth rate in children and adolescents; may cause decrease in growth.
- Monitor vital signs; may cause fever.
- Monitor for tumor lysis syndrome (malignant disease progression, high WBC counts, hyperuricemia, hyperkalemia, hyperphosphatemia, hypocalcamia, and/or dehydration). Prevent by maintain adequate hydration and correcting uric acid levels prior to starting imatinib.
- ***Lab Test Considerations:*** Monitor liver function before and monthly during treatment or when clinically indicated. May cause ↑ transamininases and bilirubin which usually lasts 1 wk and may require dose reduction or interruption. If bilirubin is >3 times the upper limit of normal or transaminases are >5 times the upper limit of normal withhold dose until bilirubin levels return to <1.5 times the upper limit of normal and transaminase levels to <2.5 times the upper limit of normal. Treatment may then be continued at reduced levels (patients on 400 mg/day should receive 300 mg/day and patients receiving 600 mg/day should receive 400 mg/day).
- Monitor CBC weekly for the first month, biweekly for the second month, and periodically during therapy. May cause neutropenia and thrombocytopenia, usually lasting 2–3 wk or 3–4 wk, respectively, and anemia. Usually requires dose reduction, but may require discontinuation (see Implementation).
- Patients receiving *chronic phase, myelodysplastic/myeloproliferative disease, aggressive systemic mastocytosis, and hypereosinophilic syndrome and/or chronic eosinophilic leukemia* treatment who develop an ANC <1.0 × 10⁹/L and/or platelets <50 × 10⁹L should stop imatinib until ANC ≥1.5 × 10⁹/L and platelets are ≥75 × 10⁹/L. Then resume imatinib treatment at 400 mg or 600 mg/day.
- ***Patients receiving accelerated phase and blast crisis treatment or Ph+ acute lymphoblastic leukemia*** who develop an ANC <0.5 × 10⁹/L and/or

platelets <10 × 10⁹/L should determine if cytopenia is related to leukemia via marrow aspirate or biopsy. If cytopenia is unrelated to leukemia, reduce dose to 400 mg/day. If cytopenia persists for 2 wk, reduce dose to 300 mg/day. If cytopenia persists for 4 wk and is still unrelated to leukemia, stop imatinib until ANC ≥1 × 10^9/L and platelets are ≥20 × 10^9/L. Then resume imatinib treatment at 300 mg/day.

- *Patients receiving aggressive systemic mastocytosis with eosinophilia or hypereosinohpilic syndrome and/or chronic eosinophilic leukemia with FIP1L1–PDGFRa fusion kinase*—who develop ANC <1.0 × 10^9/L and platelets <50 × 10^9/L should stop imatinib until ANC ≥1.5 × 10^9/L and platelets ≥75 × 10^9/L. Resume treatment at previous dose.
- May cause hypokalemia.

Potential Nursing Diagnoses

Risk for injury (Adverse Reactions)

Implementation

- ***High Alert:*** Fatalities have occurred with incorrect administration of chemotherapeutic agents. Before administering, clarify all ambiguous orders; double check single, daily, and course-of-therapy dose limits; have second practitioner independently double check original order and dose calculations. Therapy should be initiated by physician experienced in the treatment of patients with chronic myeloid leukemia.
- Patients requiring anticoagulation should receive low-molecular-weight or standard heparin, not warfarin.
- Treatment should be continued as long as patient continues to benefit.
- **PO:** Administer with food and a full glass of water to minimize GI irritation.
- Tablets may be dispersed in water or apple juice (50 mL for the 100 mg and 100 mL for the 400 mg tablet) and stirred with a spoon for patients unable to swallow pills. Administer immediately after suspension.
- Doses for children may be given once daily or divided into two doses, one in morning and one in evening.
- Administer doses >800 m g/day as 400 mg twice daily to decrease exposure to iron.

Patient/Family Teaching

- Explain purpose of imatinib to patient.
- Advise patient to avoid grapefruit and grapefruit juice during therapy.
- May cause drowsiness or dizziness. Caution patient to avoid driving or other activities requiring alertness until response to medication is known.
- Advise female patient to notify health care professional if pregnancy is planned or suspected; avoid breast feeding.

Evaluation/Desired Outcomes

- Decrease in production of leukemic cells in patients with CML, HES/CEL, and ALL and malignant cells in GIST, MDS/MPD, ASM, and DFSP.

imipenem/cilastatin

(i-me-**pen**-em/sye-la-**stat**-in)
Primaxin

Classification
Therapeutic: anti-infectives
Pharmacologic: carbapenems

Pregnancy Category C

Indications

Treatment of: Lower respiratory tract infections, Urinary tract infections, Abdominal infections, Gynecologic infections, Skin and skin structure infections, Bone and joint infections, Bacteremia, Endocarditis, Polymicrobic infections.

Action

Imipenem binds to the bacterial cell wall, resulting in cell death. Combination with cilastatin prevents renal inactivation of imipenem, resulting in high urinary concentrations. Imipenem resists the actions of many enzymes that degrade most other penicillins and penicillin-like anti-infectives. **Therapeutic Effects:** Bactericidal action against susceptible bacteria. **Spectrum:** Spectrum is broad. Active against most gram-positive aerobic cocci: *Streptococcus pneumoniae*, Group A beta-hemolytic streptococci, *Enterococcus*, *Staphylococcus aureus*. Active against many gram-negative bacillary organisms: *Escherichia coli*, *Klebsiella*, *Acinetobacter*, *Proteus*, *Serratia*, *Pseudomonas aeruginosa*. Also displays activity against: *Salmonella*, *Shigella*, *Neisseria gonorrhoeae*, Numerous anaerobes.

Pharmacokinetics

Absorption: Well absorbed after IM administration (imipenem 95%, cilastatin 75%). IV administration results in complete bioavailability.
Distribution: Widely distributed. Crosses the placenta; enters breast milk.
Metabolism and Excretion: *Imipenem and cilastatin* —70% excreted unchanged by the kidneys.
Half-life: *Imipenem and cilastatin*—1 hr (↑ in renal impairment).

TIME/ACTION PROFILE (blood levels)

ROUTE	ONSET	PEAK	DURATION
IM	rapid	1–2 hr	12 hr
IV	rapid	end of infusion	6–8 hr

Contraindications/Precautions

Contraindicated in: Hypersensitivity; Cross-sensitivity may occur with penicillins and cephalosporins.

Use Cautiously in: Previous history of multiple hypersensitivity reactions; Seizure disorders; Renal impairment (dose ↓ required if CCr ≤70 mL/min/1.73 m^2); OB, Lactation, Pedi: Safety not established; Geri: May be at ↑ risk for toxic reactions due to age-related ↑ in renal function.

Adverse Reactions/Side Effects

CNS: SEIZURES, dizziness, somnolence. **CV:** hypotension. **GI:** CLOSTRIDIUM DIFFICILE-ASSOCIATED DIARRHEA (CDAD), diarrhea, nausea, vomiting. **Derm:** rash, pruritus, sweating, urticaria. **Hemat:** eosinophilia. **Local:** phlebitis at IV site. **Misc:** allergic reaction including ANAPHYLAXIS, fever, superinfection.

Interactions

Drug-Drug: Do not admix with **aminoglycosides** (inactivation may occur). **Probenecid** ↓ renal excretion and ↑ blood levels. ↑ risk of seizures with **ganciclovir** or **cyclosporine** (avoid concurrent use of ganciclovir). May ↓ serum **valproate** levels (↑ risk of seizures).

Route/Dosage

IV (Adults): *Mild infections*—250–500 mg q 6 hr. *Moderate infections*—500 mg q 6–8 hr *or* 1 g q 8 hr. *Serious infections*—500 mg q 6 hr to 1 g q 6–8 hr.

IV (Children ≥3 mo [non-CNS infections]): 15–25 mg/kg q 6 hr; higher doses have been used in older children with cystic fibrosis.

IV (Children 4 wk–3 mo): 25 mg/kg q 6 hr.

IV (Children 1–4 wk): 25 mg/kg q 8 hr.

IV (Children <1 wk): 25 mg/kg q 12 hr.

IM (Adults): 500–750 mg q 12 hr.

IM (Children): 10–15 mg/kg q 6 hr.

Renal Impairment

IV (Adults): If dose for normal renal function is 1 g/day *CCr 41–70 mL/min*—125–250 mg q 6–8 hr, *CCr 21–40 mL/min*—125–250 mg q 8–12 hr, *CCr 6–20 mL/min*—125–250 mg q 12 hr; **if dose for normal renal function is 1.5 g/day** *CCr 41–70 mL/min*—125–250 mg q 6–8 hr, *CCr 21–40 mL/min*—125–250 mg q 8–12 hr, *CCr 6–20 mL/min*—125–250 mg q 12 hr; **if dose for normal renal function is 2 g/day** *CCr 41–70 mL/min*—125–500 mg q 6–8 hr, *CCr 21–40 mL/min*—125–250 mg q 8–12 hr, *CCr 6–20 mL/min*—125–250 mg q 12 hr; **if dose for normal renal function is 3 g/day** *CCr 41–70 mL/min*—250–500 mg q 6–8 hr, *CCr 21–40 mL/min*—250–500 mg q 6–8 hr, *CCr 6–20 mL/min*—250–500 mg q 12 hr; **if dose for normal renal function is 4 g/day** *CCr 41–70 mL/min*—250–750 mg q 6–8 hr, *CCr 21–40 mL/min*—250–500 mg q 6–8 hr, *CCr 6–20 mL/min*—250–250 mg q 12 hr.

Availability (generic available)

Powder for IV injection: 250 mg imipenem/250 mg cilastatin, 500 mg imipenem/500 mg cilastatin. **Powder for IM injection:** 500 mg imipenem/500 mg cilastatin, 750 mg imipenem/750 mg cilastatin.

NURSING IMPLICATIONS

Assessment

- Assess patient for infection (vital signs; appearance of wound, sputum, urine, and stool; WBC) at beginning of and throughout therapy.
- Obtain a history before initiating therapy to determine previous use of and reactions to penicillins. Persons with a negative history of penicillin sensitivity may still have an allergic response.
- Obtain specimens for culture and sensitivity before initiating therapy. First dose may be given before receiving results.
- Observe patient for signs and symptoms of anaphylaxis (rash, pruritus, laryngeal edema, wheezing). Discontinue the drug and notify the physician immediately if these occur. Have epinephrine, an antihistamine, and resuscitative equipment close by in the event of an anaphylactic reaction.
- ***Lab Test Considerations:*** BUN, AST, ALT, LDH, serum alkaline phosphatase, bilirubin, and creatinine may be transiently ↑.
- Hemoglobin and hematocrit concentrations may be ↓.
- May cause positive direct Coombs' test.

Potential Nursing Diagnoses

Risk for infection (Indications, Side Effects)

Implementation

- **IM: Only the IM formulation can be used for IM administration.** Reconstitute 500-mg vial with 2 mL and 750-mg vial with 3 mL of lidocaine without epinephrine. Shake well to form a suspension. Withdraw and inject entire contents of vial IM.

IV Administration

- **Intermittent Infusion: Only the IV formulation can be used for IV administration.** ***Diluent:*** Reconstitute each 250- or 500-mg vial with 10 mL of D5W or 0.9% NaCl and shake well. Further dilute in 100 mL of D5W or 0.9% NaCl. Solution may range from clear to yellow in color. Infusion is stable for 4 hr at room temperature and 24 hr if refrigerated. ***Concentration:*** 2.5 mg/mL (with 250–mg vial); 5 mg/mL (with 500-mg vial). ***Rate:*** Infuse doses ≤500 mg over 20–30 min. Infuse doses ≥750 mg over 40–60 min. Pedi: Infuse doses ≤500 mg over 15–30 min. Infuse doses >500 m g over 40–60 min.
- Rapid infusion may cause nausea and vomiting. If these symptoms develop, slow infusion.
- **Y-Site Compatibility:** acyclovir, alfentanil, amifostine, amikacin, aminocaproic acid, anidulafungin, argatroban, ascorbic acid, atracurium, atropine,

benztropine, bivalirudin, bleomycin, bumetanide, buprenorphine, butorphanol, carboplatin, carmustine, caspofungin, cefazolin, cefepime, cefotaxime, cefoxitin, ceftazidime, cefuroxime, chloramphenicol, cisatracurium, clindamycin, cyanocobalamin, cyclophosphamide, cyclosporine, cytarabine, dactinomycin, dexamethasone sodium phosphate, dexmedetomidine, dexrazoxane, digoxin, diltiazem, diphenhydramine, docetaxel, dolasetron, dopamine, doxacurium, doxorubicin, doxorubicin liposomal, doxycycline, enalaprilat, ephedrine, epinephrine, epirubicin, epoetin, eptifibatide, erythromycin, esmolol, etoposide, famotidine, fenoldopam, fentanyl, fludarabine, fluorouracil, folic acid, foscarnet, furosemide, gentamicin, glycopyrrolate, granisetron, heparin, hydrocortisone sodium succinate, hydromorphone, idarubicin, ifosfamide, indomethacin, insulin, irinotecan, isoproterenol, ketorolac, labetalol, leucovorin, levofloxacin, lidocaine, linezolid, magnesium sulfate, melphalan, methotrexate, methylprednisolone sodium succinate, metoclopramide, metoprolol, metronidazole, mitoxantrone, morphine, multivitamins, nafcillin, naloxone, nesiritide, nitroglycerin, norepinephrine, octreotide, ondansetron, oxacillin, oxaliplatin, oxytocin, paclitaxel, pamidronate, pancuronium, pantoprazole, pemetrexed, penicillin G , pentobarbital, phentolamine, phenylephrine, phytonadione, potassium acetate, potassium chloride, propranolol, propofol, propranolol, protamine, ranitidine, remifentanil, rituximab, rocuronium, sodium acetate, streptokinase, succinylcholine, sufentanil, tacrolimus, teniposide, theophylline, thiotepa, tigecycline, tirofiban, tobramycin, tolazoline, trastuzumab, vasopressin, verapamil, vinblastine, vincristine, vinorelbine, voriconazole, zidovudine.

- **Y-Site Incompatibility:** alemtuzumab, alopurinol, amiodarone, amphotericin B cholesteryl sulfate, amphotericin B lipid complex, amphotericin B liposome, azathioprine, ceftriaxone, chlorpromazine, dantrolene, daptomycin, diazepam, diazoxide, etoposide phosphate, gallium nitrate, ganciclovir, gemcitabine, haloperidol, lorazepam, mannitol, mechlorethamine, metaraminol, methyldopate, milrinone, mycophenolate, nalbuphine, nicardipine, palonosetron, phenytoin, prochlorperazine, pyridoxime, quinupristin/dalfopristin, sargramostim, sodium bicarbonate, thiamine, trimethoprim/sulfamethoxazole, vecuronium.
- **Additive Incompatibility:** May be inactivated if administered concurrently with aminoglycosides. If administered concurrently, administer in separate sites, if possible, at least 1 hr apart. If second site is unavailable, flush lines between medications.

Patient/Family Teaching

- Advise patient to report the signs of superinfection (black, furry overgrowth on the tongue; vaginal itching or discharge; loose or foul-smelling stools) and allergy. Consult health care professional before treating with antidiarrheals.
- Caution patient to notify health care professional if fever and diarrhea occur, especially if stool contains blood, pus, or mucus. Advise patient not to treat diarrhea without consulting health care professional. May occur up to several weeks after discontinuation of medication.

Evaluation/Desired Outcomes

- Resolution of the signs and symptoms of infection. Length of time for complete resolution depends on the organism and site of infection.

I

⌘ imipramine (im-**ip**-ra-meen)

✱Impril, Tofranil, Tofranil PM

Classification

Therapeutic: antidepressants

Pharmacologic: tricyclic antidepressants

Pregnancy Category C

Indications

Various forms of depression. Enuresis in children. **Unlabeled Use:** Adjunct in the management of chronic pain, incontinence (in adults), vascular headache prophylaxis, cluster headache, insomnia.

Action

Potentiates the effect of serotonin and norepinephrine. Has significant anticholinergic properties. **Therapeutic Effects:** Antidepressant action that develops slowly over several weeks.

Pharmacokinetics

Absorption: Well absorbed from the GI tract.

Distribution: Widely distributed. Probably crosses the placenta and enters breast milk.

Protein Binding: 89–95%.

Metabolism and Excretion: Mostly metabolized by the liver (CYP2D6 isoenzyme) to desipramine; ⌘ the CYP2D6 enzyme system exhibits genetic polymorphism; ~7% of population may be poor metabolizers (PMs) and may have significantly ↑ imipramine concentrations and an ↑ risk of adverse effects.

Half-life: 8–16 hr.

TIME/ACTION PROFILE (antidepressant effect)

ROUTE	ONSET	PEAK	DURATION
PO	hours	2–6 wk	weeks

Contraindications/Precautions

Contraindicated in: Hypersensitivity; Cross-sensitivity with other antidepressants may occur; Angle-closure glaucoma; Hypersensitivity to tartrazine or sulfites (in some preparations); Recent MI, known history of QTc interval prolongation, heart failure; Concurrent use of MAO inhibitors or MAO-like drugs (linezolid or methylene blue).

Use Cautiously in: Pre-existing cardiovascular disease; Seizures or history of seizure disorder; May ↑ risk of suicide attempt/ideation especially during early treatment or dose adjustment; Lactation: Drug is present in breast milk; discontinue imipramine or bottle feed; Pedi: Suicide risk may be greater in children or adolescents. Safety not established in children <6 yr; Geri: More susceptible to adverse reactions. Geriatric males with prostatic hyperplasia are more susceptible to urinary retention.

Adverse Reactions/Side Effects

CNS: SUICIDAL THOUGHTS, drowsiness, fatigue, agitation, confusion, hallucinations, insomnia. **EENT:** blurred vision, dry eyes. **CV:** ARRHYTHMIAS, hypotension, ECG changes. **GI:** constipation, dry mouth, nausea, paralytic ileus, weight gain. **GU:** urinary retention, ↓ libido. **Derm:** photosensitivity. **Endo:** gynecomastia. **Hemat:** blood dyscrasias.

Interactions

Drug-Drug: Concurrent use with **MAO inhibitors** may result in serious potentially fatal reactions (MAO inhibitors should be stopped at least 14 days before imipramine therapy. Imipramine should be stopped at least 14 days before MAO inhibitor therapy). Concurrent use with **MAO-inhibitor like drugs**, such as **linezolid** or **methylene blue** may ↑ risk of serotonin syndrome; concurrent use contraindicated; do not start therapy in patients receiving **linezolid** or **methylene blue**; if **linezolid** or **methylene blue** need to be started in a patient receiving imipramine, immediately discontinue imipramine and monitor for signs/symptoms of serotonin syndrome for 2 wk or until 24 hr after last dose of linezolid or methylene blue, whichever comes first (may resume imipramine therapy 24 hr after last dose of linezolid or methylene blue). Concurrent use with **SSRI antidepressants** may result in ↑ toxicity and should be avoided (**fluoxetine** should be stopped 5 wk before). Hypertensive crisis may occur with **clonidine**. Imipramine is metabolized in the liver by the **cytochrome P450 2D6 enzyme** and its action may be affected by drugs that compete for metabolism by this enzyme including **other antidepressants**, **phenothiazines**, **carbamazepine**, **class 1C antiarrhythmics (propafenone, flecainide)**; when used concurrently, dose reduction of one or the other or both may be necessary. Concurrent use of other drugs that inhibit the activity of the enzyme, including **cimetidine**, **quinidine**, **amiodarone**, and **ritonavir**, may result in ↑ effects of imipramine. Concurrent use with **levodopa** may result in delayed/↓ absorption of levodopa or hypertension. Blood levels and effects may be ↓ by **rifamycins**. ↑ CNS depression with other CNS **depressants** including **alcohol**, **antihistamines**, **clonidine**, **opioids**, and **sedative/hypnotics**. **Barbiturates** may alter blood levels and effects. **Adrenergic** and **anticholinergic** side effects may be ↑ with other **agents having these properties**. **Phenothiazines** or **hormonal contraceptives** ↑ levels and may cause toxicity. **Cigarette smoking (nicotine)** may ↑ metabolism and alter effects. Drugs that affect serotonergic neurotransmitter systems, including **SSRIs**, **SNRIs**, **fentanyl**, **buspirone**, **tramadol** and **triptans** ↑ risk of serotonin syndrome.

Drug-Natural Products: Use with **St. John's wort** ↑ of serotonin syndrome. Concomitant use of **kava-kava**, **valerian**, or **chamomile** can ↑ CNS depression. ↑ anticholinergic effects with **jimson weed** and **scopolia**.

Route/Dosage

PO (Adults): 25–50 mg 3–4 times daily (not to exceed 300 mg/day); total daily dose may be given at bedtime.

PO (Geriatric Patients): 25 mg at bedtime initially, up to 100 mg/day in divided doses.

PO (Children >12 yr): *Antidepressant*—25–50 mg/day in divided doses (not to exceed 100 mg/day).

PO (Children 6–12 yr): *Antidepressant*—10–30 mg/day in 2 divided doses.

PO (Children ≥6 yr): *Enuresis*—25 mg once daily 1 hr before bedtime; ↑ if necessary by 25 mg at weekly intervals to 50 mg in children <12 yr, up to 75 mg in children >12 yr.

Availability (generic available)

Tablets: 10 mg, 25 mg, 50 mg, 🍁 75 mg. **Capsules:** 75 mg, 100 mg, 125 mg, 150 mg.

NURSING IMPLICATIONS

Assessment

- Monitor BP and pulse rate prior to and during initial therapy.
- Monitor plasma levels in treatment-resistant patients.
- Monitor weight and BMI initially and periodically throughout therapy.
- For overweight/obese individuals, obtain FBS and cholesterol levels. Refer as appropriate for nutrition/weight management and medical management.
- Obtain weight and BMI initially and regularly throughout therapy.
- Assess for sexual dysfunction (decreased libido; erectile dysfunction).
- Assess for suicidal tendencies, especially during early therapy. Restrict amount of drug available to patient. Risk may be increased in children, adolescents, and adults ≤24 yrs. After starting therapy, children, adolescents, and young adults should be seen by health care professional at least weekly for 4

wk, every 3 wk for next 4 wk, and on advice of health care professional thereafter.

- Pedi, Geri: Monitor baseline and periodic ECGs in elderly patients or patients with heart disease and before increasing dose with children treated for enuresis. May cause prolonged PR and QT intervals and may flatten T waves.
- **Depression:** Assess mental status (orientation, mood, behavior) frequently. Confusion, agitation, and hallucinations may occur during initiation of therapy and may require dosage reduction. Assess for suicidal tendencies, especially during early therapy. Restrict amount of drug available to patient.
- **Enuresis:** Assess frequency of bedwetting during therapy. Ask patient or caretaker to maintain diary.
- **Pain:** Assess location, duration, and severity of pain periodically during therapy. Use pain scale to monitor effectiveness of therapy.
- ***Lab Test Considerations:*** Assess leukocyte and differential blood counts and renal and hepatic functions prior to and periodically during prolonged or high-dose therapy.
- Serum levels may be monitored in patients who fail to respond to usual therapeutic dose. Therapeutic plasma concentration range for depression is 150–300 ng/mL.
- May cause alterations in blood glucose levels.
- ***Toxicity and Overdose:*** Symptoms of acute overdose include disturbed concentration, confusion, restlessness, agitation, seizures, drowsiness, mydriasis, arrhythmias, fever, hallucinations, vomiting, and dyspnea.
- Treatment of overdose includes gastric lavage, activated charcoal, and a stimulant cathartic. Maintain respiratory and cardiac function (monitor ECG for at least 5 days) and temperature. Medications may include digoxin for HF, antiarrhythmics, and anticonvulsants.

Potential Nursing Diagnoses

Ineffective coping (Indications)
Impaired urinary elimination (Indications, Side Effects)
Sexual dysfunction (Side Effects)

Implementation

- Dose increases should be made at bedtime because of sedation. Dose titration is a slow process; may take weeks to months. May be given as a single dose at bedtime to minimize sedation during the day.
- Taper to avoid withdrawal effects. Reduce by 50% for 3 days, then reduce by 50% for 3 days, then discontinue.
- **PO:** Administer medication with or immediately following a meal to minimize gastric irritation.
- **IM:** May be slightly yellow or red in color. Crystals may develop if solution is cool; place ampule under warm running water for 1 min to dissolve.

Patient/Family Teaching

- Instruct patient to take medication as directed. Take missed doses as soon as possible unless almost time for next dose; if regimen is a single dose at bedtime, do not take in the morning because of side effects. Advise patient that drug effects may not be noticed for at least 2 wk. Abrupt discontinuation may cause nausea, vomiting, diarrhea, headache, trouble sleeping with vivid dreams, and irritability.
- May cause drowsiness and blurred vision. Caution patient to avoid driving and other activities requiring alertness until response to drug is known.
- Instruct patient to notify health care professional if visual changes occur. Inform patient that periodic glaucoma testing may be needed during long-term therapy.
- Caution patient to change positions slowly to minimize orthostatic hypotension. Advise patient, family, and caregivers to look for suicidality, especially during early therapy or dose changes. Notify health care professional immediately if thoughts about suicide or dying, attempts to commit suicide, new or worse depression or anxiety, agitation or restlessness, panic attacks, insomnia, new or worse irritability, aggressiveness, acting on dangerous impulses, mania, or other changes in mood or behavior or if symptoms of serotonin syndrome occur.
- Advise patient to avoid alcohol or other CNS depressant drugs during therapy and for at least 3–7 days after therapy has been discontinued.
- Instruct patient to notify health care professional if urinary retention, dry mouth, or constipation persists. Sugarless candy or gum may diminish dry mouth and an increase in fluid intake or bulk may prevent constipation. If symptoms persist, dose reduction or discontinuation may be necessary. Consult health care professional if dry mouth persists for more than 2 wk.
- Caution patient to use sunscreen and protective clothing to prevent photosensitivity reactions.
- Alert patient that urine may turn blue-green in color.
- Inform patient of need to monitor dietary intake, as possible increase in appetite may lead to undesired weight gain. Inform patient that increased amounts of riboflavin in the diet may be required; consult health care professional.
- Advise patient to notify health care professional of medication regimen prior to treatment or surgery.
- Therapy for depression is usually prolonged. Emphasize the importance of follow-up exams to evaluate progress and improve coping skills.
- Instruct female patients to notify health care professional if pregnancy is planned or suspected, or if breast feeding.
- Pedi: Inform parents that the side effects most likely to occur include nervousness, insomnia, unusual

tiredness, and mild nausea and vomiting. Notify health care professional if these symptoms become pronounced.
- Advise parents to keep medication out of reach of children to prevent inadvertent overdose.

Evaluation/Desired Outcomes
- Increased sense of well-being.
- Renewed interest in surroundings.
- Increased appetite.
- Improved energy level.
- Pain relief.
- Diminished incidence of enuresis.
- Improved sleep in patients treated for depression. Patient may require 2–6 wk of therapy before full therapeutic effects of medication are noticeable.
- Control of bedwetting in children >6 yr.
- Decrease in chronic neurogenic pain.

indacaterol (in-da-**kat**-e-role)
Arcapta Neohaler, ✤Onbrez Breezhaler

Classification
Therapeutic: bronchodilators, COPD agents
Pharmacologic: adrenergics

Pregnancy Category C

Indications
Long-term maintenance treatment of airflow obstruction associated with chronic obstructive pulmonary disease (COPD).

Action
Produces accumulation of cyclic adenosine monophosphate (cAMP) at $beta_2$-adrenergic receptors. Relatively specific for pulmonary receptors. Acts as a long-acting beta-agonist (LABA). **Therapeutic Effects:** Bronchodilation, with improvement in symptoms of COPD.

Pharmacokinetics
Absorption: Some systemic absorption from lungs and GI tract (43–45%).
Distribution: Extensively distributed.
Metabolism and Excretion: 54% excreted unchanged in feces; absorbed drug is mostly metabolized; 23% excreted in feces as metabolites.
Half-life: 45.5–126 hr.

TIME/ACTION PROFILE (blood levels)

ROUTE	ONSET	PEAK	DURATION
Inhaln	unknown	15 min	24 hr†

† Bronchodilation.

Contraindications/Precautions
Contraindicated in: Hypersensitivity; Acutely deteriorating COPD or acute respiratory symptoms; Asthma.
Use Cautiously in: OB: Use during pregnancy only if potential benefit justifies potential fetal risks; may interfere with uterine contractility during labor; Pedi: Safety and effectiveness not established.
Exercise Extreme Caution in: Concurrent use of MAO inhibitors, tricyclic antidepressants or drugs that prolong the QTc interval (↑ risk of adverse cardiovascular reactions).

Adverse Reactions/Side Effects
CNS: headache. **EENT:** nasopharyngitis, oropharyngeal pain. **Resp:** PARADOXICAL BRONCHOSPASM, cough. **GI:** nausea. **Misc:** ALLERGIC REACTIONS.

Interactions
Drug-Drug: ↑ risk of serious adverse cardiovascular effects with **MAO inhibitors**, **tricyclic antidepressants**, **drugs that prolong the QTc interval**; use with extreme caution. Effectiveness may be ↓ by beta-blockers; use cautiously and only when necessary. Concurrent use with other **adrenergics** may ↑ adrenergic adverse reactions (↑ heart rate, BP, jitteriness). ↑ risk of hypokalemia or ECG changes with **xanthine derivatives**, **corticosteroids**, **diuretics**, or **non-potassium sparing diuretics**.
Drug-Natural Products: Use with **caffeine-containing herbs (cola nut, guarana, mate, tea, coffee)** ↑ stimulant effect.

Route/Dosage
Inhaln (Adults): 75 mcg once daily.

Availability
Capsules for inhalation: 75 mcg.

NURSING IMPLICATIONS
Assessment
- Assess respiratory status (rate, breath sounds, degree of dyspnea, pulse) before administration and at peak of medication. Consult health care professional about alternative medication if severe bronchospasm is present; onset of action is too slow for patients in acute distress. If paradoxical bronchospasm (wheezing) occurs, withhold medication and notify health care professional immediately.
- Monitor for signs and symptoms of allergic reactions (difficulties in breathing or swallowing, swelling of tongue, lips and face, urticaria, skin rash). Discontinue therapy if symptoms occur.
- ***Lab Test Considerations:*** May cause transient hypokalemia and hyperglycemia.

Potential Nursing Diagnoses
Ineffective airway clearance (Indications)
Risk for activity intolerance (Indications)

Implementation
- **Inhaln:** Pull cap off *Neohaler*. Open inhaler by holding the base and tilting the mouthpiece. Tear perforation to separate one blister from blister card; peal away protective back to expose foil. With dry hands, push capsule through foil to remove. Insert capsule into capsule chamber; do not swallow cap-

sule or place directly into mouthpiece. Close inhaler until it clicks. Press both buttons fully 1 time; click is heard as capsule is pierced; do not press piercing buttons more than 1 time. Release buttons fully. Breathe out; do not blow into mouthpiece. Close lips around mouthpiece; hold inhaler with buttons left and right (not up and down). Breathe in rapidly and steadily, as deep as possible, a whirring noise is heard. Continue to hold breath as long as possible while removing inhaler from mouth. Open inhaler, if powder remains in capsule, close inhaler and inhale again. Usually requires 1–2 breaths. Remove capsule.

Patient/Family Teaching

- Instruct patient in the correct use of capsules and *Neohaler*. Advise patient not to discontinue without consulting health care professional; symptoms may recur.
- Inform patient that indacaterol is not a bronchodilator and should not be used for treating sudden breathing problems.
- Advise patient to notify health care professional if signs and symptoms of allergic reaction, worsening symptoms; decreasing effectiveness of inhaled, short-acting $beta_2$-agonists; need for more inhalations than usual of inhaled, short-acting $beta_2$-agonists; or significant decrease in lung function occur.
- Instruct patient to notify health care professional of all Rx or OTC medications, vitamins, or herbal products being taken and to avoid concurrent use of Rx, OTC, and herbal products without consulting health care professional.
- Advise female patient to notify health care professional if pregnancy is planned or suspected or if breast feeding.

Evaluation/Desired Outcomes

- Decrease in the number of flare-ups or the worsening of COPD symptoms (exacerbations).

indomethacin

(in-doe-**meth**-a-sin)

Indocin, Tivorbex

Classification

Therapeutic: antirheumatics, ductus arteriosus patency adjuncts (IV only), nonsteroidal anti-inflammatory agents

Pregnancy Category C (<30 wk gestation), D (≥30 wk gestation)

Indications

PO: Inflammatory disorders including: Rheumatoid arthritis, Gouty arthritis, Osteoarthritis, Ankylosing spondylitis. Mild-to-moderate acute pain. **IV:** Alternative to surgery in the management of patent ductus arteriosus (PDA) in premature neonates.

Action

Inhibits prostaglandin synthesis. In the treatment of PDA, decreased prostaglandin production allows the ductus to close. **Therapeutic Effects: PO:** Suppression of pain and inflammation. **IV:** Closure of PDA.

Pharmacokinetics

Absorption: Well absorbed after oral administration in adults, incomplete oral absorption in neonates.

Distribution: Crosses the blood-brain barrier and the placenta. Enters breast milk.

Protein Binding: 99%.

Metabolism and Excretion: Mostly metabolized by the liver.

Half-life: Neonates <2 weeks: 20 hr; >2 weeks: 11 hr; Adults: 2.6–11 hr.

TIME/ACTION PROFILE

ROUTE	ONSET	PEAK	DURATION
PO (analgesic)	30 min	0.5–2 hr	4–6 hr
PO-ER (analgesic)	30 min	unknown	4–6 hr
PO (anti-inflammatory)	up to 7 days	1–2 wk	4–6 hr
PO-ER (anti-inflammatory)	up to 7 days	1–2 wk	4–6 hr
IV (closure of PDA)	up to 48 hr	unknown	unknown

Contraindications/Precautions

Contraindicated in: Hypersensitivity; Known alcohol intolerance (suspension); Cross-sensitivity may exist with other NSAIDs, including aspirin; Active GI bleeding; Ulcer disease; Proctitis or recent history of rectal bleeding; Intraventricular hemorrhage; Thrombocytopenia; Perioperative pain from coronary artery bypass graft (CABG) surgery; Pedi: ↑ risk of necrotizing enterocolitis and bowel perforation in premature infants with PDA.

Use Cautiously in: Severe renal or hepatic disease; Cardiovascular disease or risk factors for cardiovascular disease (may ↑ risk of serious cardiovascular thrombotic events, myocardial infarction, and stroke, especially with prolonged use or use of higher doses); History of ulcer disease; Seizure disorders; Hypertension; OB: Not recommended starting at 30 wk gestation (potential for causing premature closure of ductus arteriosus); Lactation: Usually compatible with breast feeding (AAP); Geri: ↑ risk of adverse reactions.

Adverse Reactions/Side Effects

CNS: dizziness, drowsiness, headache, psychic disturbances. **EENT:** blurred vision, tinnitus. **CV:** HF, MYOCARDIAL INFARCTION, STROKE, edema, hypertension. **GI:** *PO*—DRUG-INDUCED HEPATITIS, GI BLEEDING, constipation, dyspepsia, nausea, vomiting, discomfort, necrotizing enterocolitis. **GU:** cystitis, hematuria, renal failure. **Derm:** rash. **F and E:** hyperkalemia; *IV*, dilutional hyponatremia; *IV*, hypoglycemia. **Hemat:** thrombocytopenia, blood dyscrasias, prolonged bleeding time. **Local:** phlebitis at IV site. **Misc:** allergic reactions including ANAPHYLAXIS.

Interactions

Drug-Drug: Concurrent use with **aspirin** may ↓ effectiveness. Additive adverse GI effects with **aspirin**, other **NSAIDs**, **corticosteroids**, or **alcohol**. Chronic use of **acetaminophen** ↑ risk of adverse renal reactions. May ↓ effectiveness of **diuretics** or **antihypertensives**. May ↑ hypoglycemia from **insulins** or **oral hypoglycemic agents**. May ↑ risk of toxicity from **lithium** or **zidovudine** (avoid concurrent use with zidovudine). ↑ risk of toxicity from **methotrexate**. **Probenecid** ↑ risk of toxicity from indomethacin. ↑ risk of bleeding with **cefotetan**, **valproic acid**, **thrombolytics**, **warfarin**, and **drugs affecting platelet function** including **clopidogrel**, **abciximab**, **eptifibatide**, or **tirofiban**. ↑ risk of adverse hematologic reactions with **antineoplastics** or **radiation therapy**. ↑ risk of nephrotoxicity with **cyclosporine**. Concurrent use with **potassium-sparing diuretics** may result in hyperkalemia. May ↑ levels of **digitalis glycosides**, **methotrexate**, **lithium**, and **aminoglycosides** when used IV in neonates.

Drug-Natural Products: ↑ bleeding risk with **anise**, **arnica**, **chamomile**, **clove**, **dong quai**, **feverfew**, **garlic**, **ginger**, **ginkgo**, **Panax ginseng**.

Route/Dosage

Anti-inflammatory

PO (Adults): *Antiarthritic*—25–50 mg 2–4 times daily *or* 75-mg extended-release capsule once or twice daily (not to exceed 200 mg or 150 mg of SR/day). A single bedtime dose of 100 mg may be used. *Antigout*—100 mg initially, followed by 50 mg 3 times daily for relief of pain, then ↓ further. *Mild-to-moderate acute pain (Tivorbex)*—20 mg 3 times daily or 40 mg 2–3 times daily.

PO (Children >2 yr): 1–2 mg/kg/day in 2–4 divided doses (not to exceed 4 mg/kg/day or 150–200 mg/day).

PDA Closure

IV (Neonates): *Treatment*—0.2 mg/kg initially, then 2 subsequent doses at 12–24 hr intervals of 0.1 mg/kg if age <48 hr at time of initial dose; 0.2 mg/kg if 2–7 days at initial dose; 0.25 mg/kg if age >7 days at initial dose *Prophylaxis*—0.1–0.2 mg/kg initially, then 0.1 mg/kg q 12–24 hr for 2 doses.

Availability (generic available)

Capsules: 25 mg, 50 mg. **Capsules (Tivorbex):** 20 mg, 40 mg. **Sustained-release capsules:** 75 mg. **Oral suspension (fruit mint, pineapple coconut mint flavors):** 5 mg/mL. **Rectal suppository:** 50 mg. **Powder for injection:** 1 mg/vial.

NURSING IMPLICATIONS

Assessment

- Patients who have asthma, aspirin-induced allergy, and nasal polyps are at increased risk for developing hypersensitivity reactions. Monitor for rhinitis, asthma, and urticaria.
- Assess patient for skin rash frequently during therapy. Discontinue ibuprofen at first sign of rash; may be life-threatening. Stevens-Johnson syndrome or toxic epidermal necrolysis may develop. Treat symptomatically; may recur once treatment is stopped.
- **Arthritis:** Assess limitation of movement and pain—note type, location, and intensity before and 1–2 hr after administration.
- **PDA:** Monitor respiratory status, heart rate, BP, echocardiogram, and heart sounds routinely throughout therapy.
- Monitor intake and output. Fluid restriction is usually instituted throughout therapy.
- **Acute pain:** Assess type, location, and intensity of pain prior to and 2 hrs (peak) following administration.
- ***Lab Test Considerations:*** Evaluate BUN, serum creatinine, CBC, serum potassium levels, and liver function tests periodically in patients receiving prolonged therapy.
- Serum potassium, BUN, serum creatinine, AST, and ALT tests may show ↑ levels. Blood glucose concentrations may be altered. Hemoglobin and hematocrit concentrations, leukocyte and platelet counts, and CCr may be ↓.
- Urine glucose and urine protein concentrations may be ↑.
- Leukocyte and platelet count may be ↓. Bleeding time may be prolonged for several days after discontinuation.

Potential Nursing Diagnoses

Acute pain (Indications)
Impaired physical mobility (Indications)

Implementation

- If prolonged therapy is used, dose should be reduced to the lowest level that controls symptoms.
- **PO:** Administer after meals, with food, or with antacids to decrease GI irritation. Do not break, crush, or chew sustained-release capsules.
- Shake suspension before administration. Do not mix with antacid or any other liquid.

IV Administration

- **IV Push:** ***Diluent:*** Preservative-free 0.9% NaCl or preservative-free sterile water. Reconstitute with 1 or

2 mL of diluent. ***Concentration:*** 0.5–1 mg/mL. Reconstitute immediately before use and discard any unused solution. Do not dilute further or admix. Do not administer via umbilical catheter into vessels near the superior mesenteric artery, as these can cause vasoconstriction and compromise blood flow to the intestines. Do not administer intra-arterially. ***Rate:*** Administer over 20–30 min. Avoid extravasation, as solution is irritating to tissues.

- **Y-Site Compatibility:** aminophylline, ascorbic acid, atropine, bumetanide, cefazolin, cefotaxime, cefoxitin, ceftazidime, ceftriaxone, cefuroxime, chloramphenicol, cisplatin, clindamycin, cyanocobalamin, cyclosporine, dexamethasone, digoxin, enalaprilat, ephedrine, epoetin alfa, fentanyl, fluconazole, folic acid, furosemide, ganciclovir, heparin, hydrocortisone, imipenem/cilastatin, insulin, ketorolac, lidocaine, mannitol, metoclopramide, metoprolol, multivitamins, nafcillin, nitroglycerin, nitroprusside, penicillin G, pentobarbital, phenobarbital, phytonadione, potassium chloride, procainamide, ranitidine, sodium bicarbonate, streptokinase, theophylline.
- **Y-Site Incompatibility:** amikacin, amino acid injection, aztreonam, benztropine, buprenorphine, butorphanol, calcium chloride, calcium gluconate, cefotetan, chlorpromazine, dactinomycin, dantrolene, daunorubicin hydrochloride, diazepam, diphenhydramine, dobutamine, dopamine, doxycycline, epinephrine, erythromycin, esmolol, etoposide, famotidine, gentamicin, glycopyrrolate, haloperidol, isoproterenol, labetalol, levofloxacin, magnesium sulfate, meperidine, methyldopate, midazolam, morphine, nalbuphine, norepinephrine, ondansetron, oxytocin, paclitaxel, pantoprazole, papaverine, pentamidine, pentazocine, phenylephrine, phenytoin, prochlorperazine, promethazine, propranolol, protamine, pyridoxine, succinylcholine, sufentanil, thiamine, tobramycin, trimethoprim/sulfamethoxazole, vancomycin, vasopressin, verapamil.

Patient/Family Teaching

- Advise patient to take this medication with a full glass of water and to remain in an upright position for 15–30 min after administration.
- Instruct patient to take medication as directed. Take missed doses as soon as remembered if not almost time for next dose. Do not double doses.
- May cause drowsiness or dizziness. Advise patient to avoid driving or other activities requiring alertness until response to medication is known.
- Caution patient to avoid the concurrent use of alcohol, aspirin, other NSAIDs, acetaminophen, or other OTC medications without consulting health care professional.
- Caution patient to wear sunscreen and protective clothing to prevent photosensitivity reactions.
- Advise patient to inform health care professional of medication regimen before treatment or surgery.
- Instruct patient to notify health care professional if rash, itching, chills, fever, muscle aches, visual disturbances, weight gain, edema, abdominal pain, black stools, or persistent headache occurs.
- **PDA:** Explain to parents the purpose of medication and the need for frequent monitoring.

Evaluation/Desired Outcomes

- Decrease in severity of mild to moderate pain.
- Improved joint mobility. Partial arthritic relief is usually seen within 2 wk, but maximum effectiveness may require up to 1 mo of continuous therapy. Patients who do not respond to one NSAID may respond to another.
- Successful PDA closure.

I

inFLIXimab (in-flix-i-mab)

♣ Inflectra, Remicade, ♣ Remsima

Classification

Therapeutic: antirheumatics (DMARDs), gastrointestinal anti-inflammatories
Pharmacologic: monoclonal antibodies

Pregnancy Category C

Indications

Active rheumatoid arthritis (moderate to severe, with methotrexate). Active Crohn's disease (moderate to severe). Active psoriatic arthritis. Active ankylosing spondylitis. Active ulcerative colitis (moderate to severe) with inadequate response to conventional therapy: reducing signs and symptoms, and inducing and maintaining clinical remission and mucosal healing, and eliminating corticosteroid use. Plaque psoriasis (chronic severe).

Action

Neutralizes and prevents the activity of tumor necrosis factor-alpha (TNF-alpha), resulting in anti-inflammatory and antiproliferative activity. **Therapeutic Effects:** Decreased pain and swelling, decreased rate of joint destruction and improved physical function in ankylosing spondylitis, rheumatoid or psoriatic arthritis. Reduction and maintenance of closure of fistulae in Crohn's disease. Decreased symptoms, maintaining remission and mucosal healing with decreased corticosteroid use in ulcerative colitis. Decrease in induration, scaling and erythema of psoriatic lesions.

Pharmacokinetics

Absorption: IV administration results in complete bioavailability.

Distribution: Predominantly distributed within the vascular compartment.

Metabolism and Excretion: Unknown.
Half-life: 9.5 days.

TIME/ACTION PROFILE (symptoms of Crohn's disease)

ROUTE	ONSET	PEAK	DURATION
IV	1–2 wk	unknown	12–48 wk†

†After infusion.

Contraindications/Precautions

Contraindicated in: Hypersensitivity to infliximab, murine (mouse) proteins, or other components in the formulation; HF; Concurrent anakinra or abatacept; Lactation: Lactation.

Use Cautiously in: History of chronic or recurrent infection or underlying illness/treatment predisposing to infection; Patients being retreated after 2 yr without treatment (↑ risk of adverse reactions); History of tuberculosis or exposure (latent tuberculosis should be treated prior to infliximab therapy); History of opportunistic infection; Patients residing, or who have resided, where tuberculosis, histoplasmosis, coccidioidomycoses, or blastomycosis is endemic; Chronic obstructive pulmonary disease (↑ risk of malignancy); Geri: Geriatric patients; OB: Use only if clearly needed; Pedi: Children <6 yr (safety not established); ↑ risk of lymphoma (including hepatosplenic T-cell lymphoma [HSTCL] in patients with Crohn's disease or ulcerative colitis), leukemia, and other malignancies.

Adverse Reactions/Side Effects

CNS: fatigue, headache, anxiety, depression, dizziness, insomnia. **EENT:** conjunctivitis. **Resp:** upper respiratory tract infection, bronchitis, cough, dyspnea, laryngitis, pharyngitis, respiratory tract allergic reaction, rhinitis, sinusitis. **CV:** chest pain, hypertension, hypotension, pericardial effusion, tachycardia, HF. **GI:** abdominal pain, nausea, vomiting, constipation, diarrhea, dyspepsia, flatulence, hepatotoxicity, intestinal obstruction, oral pain, tooth pain, ulcerative stomatitis. **GU:** dysuria, urinary frequency, urinary tract infection. **Derm:** acne, alopecia, dry skin, ecchymosis, eczema, erythema, flushing, hematoma, hot flashes, pruritus, psoriasis, rash, sweating, urticaria. **Hemat:** neutropenia. **MS:** arthralgia, arthritis, back pain, involuntary muscle contractions, myalgia. **Neuro:** paresthesia. **Misc:** INFECTIONS (including reactivation tuberculosis and other opportunistic infections due to bacterial, invasive fungal, viral, mycobacterial, and parasitic pathogens), MALIGNANCY (including lymphoma, HSTCL, leukemia, and skin cancer), fever, SARCOIDOSIS, infusion reactions, chills, flu-like syndrome, herpes simplex, herpes zoster, hypersensitivity reactions, lupus-like syndrome, moniliasis, pain, peripheral edema, vasculitis.

Interactions

Drug-Drug: Concurrent use with **anakinra** or **abatacept** ↑ risk of serious infections (not recommended). Concurrent use with **azathioprine** and/or **methotrexate** may ↑ risk of HSTCL. Use of **live virus vaccines** or therapeutic infectious agents may ↑ risk of infection; avoid concurrent use.

Route/Dosage

Rheumatoid Arthritis

IV (Adults): 3 mg/kg initially, then repeat at 2 and 6 wk after initial infusion, then repeat qy 8 wk; dose may be adjusted in partial responders up to 10 mg/kg or treatment as often as q 4 wk (to be used with methotrexate).

Crohn's Disease

IV (Adults): 5 mg/kg initially, then repeat at 2 and 6 wk after initial infusion, then maintenance dose of 5 mg/kg q 8 wk; dose may be adjusted up to 10 mg/kg in patients who initially respond and then lose their response.

IV (Children): 5 mg/kg initially, then repeat at 2 and 6 wk after initial infusion, then maintenance dose of 5 mg/kg q 8 wk.

Ankylosing Spondylitis

IV (Adults): 5 mg/kg initially, then repeat at 2 and 6 wk after initial infusion, then maintenance dose of 5 mg/kg q 6 wk.

Psoriatic Arthritis

IV (Adults): 5 mg/kg initially, then repeat at 2 and 6 wk after initial infusion, then maintenance dose of 5 mg/kg q 8 wk (to be used with or without methotrexate).

Ulcerative Colitis

IV (Adults and Children ≥6 yr): 5 mg/kg initially, then repeat at 2 and 6 wk after initial infusion, then maintenance dose of 5 mg/kg q 8 wk.

Plaque Psoriasis

IV (Adults): 5 mg/kg initially, then repeat at 2 and 6 wk after initial infusion, then maintenance dose of 5 mg/kg q 8 wk.

Availability

Powder for injection: 100 mg/vial.

NURSING IMPLICATIONS

Assessment

- Assess for infusion-related reactions (fever, chills, urticaria, pruritus) during and for 2 hr after infusion. Symptoms usually resolve when infusion is discontinued. Reactions are more common after 1st or 2nd infusion. Frequency of reactions may be reduced with immunosuppressant agents.
- Monitor patients who develop a new infection while taking infliximab closely. Discontinue therapy in patients who develop a serious infection or sepsis. Do not initiate therapy in patients with active infections.
- Assess for signs and symptoms of systemic infections (fever, malaise, weight loss, sweats, cough, dyspnea,

pulmonary infiltrates, serious systemic illness with or without concomitant shock). Ascertain if patient lives in or has traveled to areas of endemic mycoses. Consider empiric antifungal treatment for patients at risk of histoplasmosis and other invasive fungal infections until the pathogens are identified. Consult with an infectious diseases specialist. Consider stopping infliximab until the infection has been diagnosed and adequately treated.

- Assess for latent tuberculosis with a tuberculin skin test prior to initiation of therapy. Treatment of latent tuberculosis should be initiated prior to therapy with infliximab.
- Observe patient for hypersensitivity reactions (urticaria, dyspnea, hypotension) during infusion. Discontinue infliximab if severe reaction occurs. Have medications (antihistamines, acetaminophen, corticosteroids, epinephrine) and equipment readily available in the event of a severe reaction.
- **Rheumatoid Arthritis:** Assess pain and range of motion prior to and periodically during therapy.
- **Crohn's Disease and Ulcerative Colitis:** Assess for signs and symptoms before, during, and after therapy.
- **Psoriasis:** Assess lesions periodically during therapy.
- ***Lab Test Considerations:*** May cause ↑ in positive ANA. Frequency may be decreased with baseline immunosuppressant therapy.
- Monitor liver function tests periodically during therapy. May cause mild to moderate AST and ALT ↑ without progressing to liver dysfunction. If patient develops jaundice or liver enzyme elevations ≥5 times the upper limits of normal, discontinue infliximab.
- Monitor CBC with differential periodically during therapy. May cause leukopenia, neutropenia, thrombocytopenia, and pancytopenia. Discontinue infliximab if symptoms of blood dyscrasias (persistent fever) occur.

Potential Nursing Diagnoses

Chronic pain (Indications)
Diarrhea (Indications)

Implementation

- Do not confuse infliximab with rituximab.

IV Administration

- **Intermittent Infusion:** Calculate the total number of vials needed. Reconstitute each vial with 10 mL of sterile water for injection using a syringe with a 21-gauge needle or smaller. Direct stream to sides of vial. Do not use if vacuum is not present in vial. Gently swirl solution by rotating vial to dilute; do not shake. May foam on reconstitution; allow to stand for 5 min. Solution is colorless to light yellow and opalescent; a few translucent particles may develop because infliximab is a protein. Do not use if opaque particles, discoloration, or other particles occur. ***Diluent:*** Withdraw volume of total infliximab dose from infusion container containing 250 mL with 0.9% NaCl. Slowly add total dose of infliximab. Do not dilute with other solutions. ***Concentration:*** 0.4 to 4 mg/mL. Mix gently. Infusion should begin within 3 hr of preparation. Solution is incompatible with polyvinyl chloride equipment. Prepare in glass infusion bottle or polypropylene or polyolefin bags. Do not reuse or store any portion of infusion solution. ***Rate:*** Administer over at least 2 hr through polyethylene-lined administration set with an in-line, sterile, nonpyrogenic, low protein-building filter with ≤1.2-micron pore size.
- **Y-Site Incompatibility:** Do not administer concurrently in the same line with any other agents.

Patient/Family Teaching

- Advise patient that adverse reactions (myalgia, rash, fever, polyarthralgia, pruritus) may occur 3–12 days after delayed (>2 yr) retreatment with infliximab. Symptoms usually decrease or resolve within 1–3 days. Instruct patient to notify health care professional if symptoms occur.
- May cause dizziness. Caution patient to avoid driving or other activities requiring alertness until response to medication is known.
- Advise patient to notify health care professional promptly if symptoms of fungal infection occur.
- Advise patient of risk of malignancies such as hepatosplenic T-cell lymphoma. Instruct patient to report signs and symptoms (splenomegaly, hepatomegaly, abdominal pain, persistent fever, night sweats, weight loss) to health care professional promptly.
- Advise patient to examine skin periodically during therapy and notify health care professional of any changes in appearance of skin or growths on skin.
- Instruct patient not to receive live vaccines during therapy.
- Rep: Advise female patient to notify health care professional if pregnancy is planned or suspected or if breast feeding. Infants exposed to inflixmab in utero should wait at least 6 months before receiving any live vaccine; may be at increased risk of infection.

Evaluation/Desired Outcomes

- Decreased pain and swelling with decreased rate of joint destruction and improved physical function in patients with ankylosing spondylitis, psoriatic, or rheumatoid arthritis.
- Decrease in the signs and symptoms of Crohn's disease and a decrease in the number of draining enterocutaneous fistulas. Decreased symptoms, maintaining remission and mucosal healing with decreased corticosteroid use in ulcerative colitis.

- Decrease in induration, scaling and erythema of psoriatic lesions.

insulin degludec
(**in**-soo-lin **deg**-lu-dek)
Tresiba

Classification
Therapeutic: antidiabetics, hormones
Pharmacologic: pancreatics

See Appendix K for more information concerning insulins

Indications
Improvement of glycemic control in adults with diabetes mellitus. Considered to be an ultra-long acting basal insulin analog.

Action
Lowers blood glucose by: stimulating glucose uptake in skeletal muscle and fat, inhibiting hepatic glucose production. Other actions: inhibition of lipolysis and proteolysis, enhanced protein synthesis. **Therapeutic Effects:** Control of hyperglycemia in diabetic patients.

Pharmacokinetics
Absorption: Absorption is slow and delayed.
Distribution: Widely distributed.
Protein Binding: >99%.
Metabolism and Excretion: Metabolized by liver, spleen, kidney, and muscle.
Half-life: 25 hr (as a result of rate of absorption).

TIME/ACTION PROFILE (effect on blood sugar)

ROUTE	ONSET	PEAK	DURATION
subcut	within 2 hr	12 hr	up to 42 hr†

†following discontinuation after chronic use.

Contraindications/Precautions
Contraindicated in: Hypersensitivity to insulin degludec; Hypoglycemia.
Use Cautiously in: Stress and infection (may temporarily ↑ insulin requirements); Renal/hepatic impairment (may ↓ insulin requirements); Concomitant use with pioglitazone or rosiglitazone (↑ risk of fluid retention and worsening HF); Effects may be ↓ in obese patients; Geri: Elderly may be ↑ sensitive to drug effects; OB: Pregnancy may temporarily ↑ insulin requirements; Lactation: Consider possible effects on infant (lactating females may require adjustments in insulin dose and/or meal plan); Pedi: Safe and effective use in children or adolescents <18 yr has not been established.

Adverse Reactions/Side Effects
Endo: HYPOGLYCEMIA. **Local:** lipodystrophy, pruritus, erythema, swelling. **F and E:** hypokalemia. **Misc:** allergic reactions including ANAPHYLAXIS.

Interactions
Drug-Drug: Beta blockers, clonidine, and **reserpine** may mask some of the signs and symptoms of hypoglycemia. **Corticosteroids, thyroid supplements, estrogens, isoniazid, niacin, phenothiazines,** and **rifampin** may ↑ insulin requirements. **Alcohol, ACE inhibitors, MAO inhibitors, octreotide, oral hypoglycemic agents,** and **salicylates,** may ↓ insulin requirements. Concurrent use with **pioglitazone** or **rosiglitazone** may ↑ risk of fluid retention and worsening HF.
Drug-Natural Products: Glucosamine may worsen blood glucose control. **Fenugreek, chromium,** and **coenzyme Q-10** may produce additive hypoglycemic effects.

Route/Dosage
Subcut (Adults): Dose individualized based on type of diabetes mellitus, metabolic needs, results of blood glucose monitoring and goals of glycemic control.

Availability
Solution for subcutaneous injection: 100 units/mL (U-100) in 3 mL FlexTouch system, 200 units/mL (U-200) in 3 mL FlexTouch system. ***In combination with:*** insulin aspart (Rysodeg 70/30) See Appendix B.

NURSING IMPLICATIONS

Assessment
- Assess patient for signs and symptoms of hypoglycemia (anxiety; restlessness; tingling in hands, feet, lips, or tongue; chills; cold sweats; confusion; cool, pale skin; difficulty in concentration; drowsiness; nightmares or trouble sleeping; excessive hunger; headache; irritability; nausea; nervousness; tachycardia; tremor; weakness; unsteady gait) and hyperglycemia (confusion, drowsiness; flushed, dry skin; fruit-like breath odor; rapid, deep breathing, polyuria; loss of appetite; nausea; vomiting; unusual thirst) periodically during therapy.
- Monitor body weight periodically. Changes in weight may necessitate changes in insulin dose.
- Monitor for signs and symptoms of hypersensitivity reactions (swelling of tongue and lips, diarrhea, nausea, tiredness, itching, urticaria). Discontinue insulin degludec and treat symptomatically.
- ***Lab Test Considerations:*** Monitor blood glucose during therapy, more frequently in ketoacidosis and times of stress. Hemoglobin A_{1C} may be monitored every 3–6 mo to determine effectiveness.
- Monitor serum potassium periodically during therapy, especially in patients at risk (patients using potassium-lowering medications, patients taking medications sensitive to serum potassium concentrations). May cause hypokalemia.
- ***Toxicity and Overdose:*** Overdose is manifested by symptoms of hypoglycemia. Mild hypoglycemia may be treated by ingestion of oral glucose. Severe hypoglycemia is a life-threatening emergency; treat-

ment consists of IV glucose, glucagon, or epinephrine.

Potential Nursing Diagnoses

Deficient knowledge, related to diet and medication regimen (Patient/Family Teaching)

Implementation

- ***High Alert:*** Insulin-related medication errors have resulted in patient harm and death. Clarify ambiguous orders; do not accept orders using the abbreviation "u" for units, (can be misread as a zero or the numeral 4; has resulted in tenfold overdoses). Insulins are available in different types, strengths. Check type, dose, and expiration date. Do not interchange insulins without consulting health care professional.
- **Subcut:** Inject once daily at any time of the day. Administer into thigh, upper arm, or abdomen. Press and hold down the dose button until dose counter shows 0 and then keep needle in the skin and count slowly to 6. When dose counter returns to 0, prescribed dose is not completely delivered until 6 seconds later. If the needle is removed earlier, a stream of insulin may be seen coming from the needle tip. If so, full dose will not be delivered; frequently check blood glucose levels, may need additional insulin. Use a new needle for each dose; do not reuse needles. Rotate injection sites to reduce risk of lipodystrophy. Do not administer IV, IM, or in an insulin infusion pump. Store unopened prefilled pens in refrigerator; do not freeze. Do not store opened (in-use) prefilled pens in refrigerator; stable at controlled room temperature, protected from light for 56 days (8 wks).
- Do not mix with other insulins or solutions.
- Do not transfer from pen into a syringe for administration.
- Dose increases should be made every 3–4 days as needed.
- Do not perform dose conversion when using the *Tresiba* U-100 or U-200 *FlexTouch* pens. Dose window for both the *Tresiba* U-100 and U-200 *FlexTouch* pens shows number of insulin units to be delivered and no conversion is needed.
- **Starting Dose in Insulin Naïve Patients :** *Type 1 Diabetes Mellitus:* Starting dose is one-third to one-half total daily insulin dose. Administer remainder of total daily insulin dose as short-acting insulin divided between daily meals. Generally, 0.2 to 0.4 units of insulin/kg can be used to calculate initial total daily insulin dose in insulin naïve patients with type 1 diabetes. *Type 2 Diabetes Mellitus:* 10 units once daily.
- **Starting Dose in Patients Already on Insulin Therapy :** *Type 1 and Type 2 Diabetes Mellitus:* Start insulin degludec at same unit dose as total daily long or intermediate-acting insulin unit dose.

Patient/Family Teaching

- Instruct patient on proper technique for administration. Include type of insulin, equipment (syringe, cartridge pens, alcohol swabs), storage, and place to discard syringes. If a dose is missed, inject daily dose during waking hrs upon discovering missed dose. Ensure that at least 8 hours have elapsed between consecutive injections. Discuss importance of not changing brands of insulin or syringes, selection and rotation of injection sites, and compliance with therapeutic regimen. Advise patient to read *Patient Information* before starting therapy and with each Rx refill in case of changes.
- Caution patient not to share pen device with another person, even if needle is changed; may risk transmission of blood-borne pathogens.
- Explain to patient that this medication controls hyperglycemia but does not cure diabetes. Therapy is long term.
- Instruct patient in proper testing of serum glucose and ketones. These tests should be closely monitored during periods of stress or illness and health care professional notified of significant changes.
- Emphasize the importance of compliance with nutritional guidelines and regular exercise as directed by health care professional.
- Instruct patient to notify health care professional of all Rx or OTC medications, vitamins, or herbal products being taken and to consult health care professional before taking other Rx, OTC, herbal products, or alcohol.
- Advise patient to notify health care professional of medication regimen prior to treatment or surgery.
- Advise patient to notify health care professional if nausea, vomiting, or fever develops, if unable to eat regular diet, or if blood glucose levels are not controlled.
- Instruct patient and caregiver on signs and symptoms of hypoglycemia and hyperglycemia and what to do if they occur.
- Patients with diabetes mellitus should carry a source of sugar (candy, glucose gel) and identification describing their disease and treatment regimen at all times.
- Advise patient to notify health care professional if pregnancy is planned or suspected or if breast feeding.
- Emphasize the importance of regular follow-up, especially during first few weeks of therapy.

Evaluation/Desired Outcomes

- Control of blood glucose levels in diabetic patients without the appearance of hypoglycemic or hyperglycemic episodes.

REMS

insulin, human inhalation
(in-soo-lin)
Afrezza

Classification
Therapeutic: antidiabetics
Pharmacologic: hormones

Pregnancy Category C

Indications
Control of hyperglycemia in patients with diabetes mellitus.

Action
Lowers blood glucose by: stimulating glucose uptake in skeletal muscle and fat, inhibiting hepatic glucose production. Other actions: inhibition of lypolysis and proteolysis, enhanced protein synthesis. **Therapeutic Effects:** Control of hyperglycemia in diabetic patients.

Pharmacokinetics
Absorption: Rapidly absorbed from lungs.
Distribution: Widely distributed.
Metabolism and Excretion: Metabolized by liver, spleen, kidney, and muscle.
Half-life: 28–39 min.

TIME/ACTION PROFILE (effect on blood glucose)

ROUTE	ONSET	PEAK	DURATION
Inhaln	within 30 min	30–60 min	160 min

Contraindications/Precautions
Contraindicated in: Hypersensitivity to regular insulin or any other components of the formulation; Hypoglycemia; Smokers or those who have recently stopped smoking; Lung disease, including asthma, COPD and active lung cancer; Lactation: Discontinue breast feeding.
Use Cautiously in: Stress and infection (may temporarily ↑ insulin requirements); Renal/hepatic dysfunction (may ↓ insulin requirements); Concomitant use with thiazolidinediones including pioglitazone or rosiglitazone (↑ risk of fluid retention and worsening HF); OB: Pregnancy may temporarily ↑ insulin requirements, should not be used during pregnancy unless potential benefit justifies potential risk to the fetus; Pedi: Safety not established in children <18 yr.

Adverse Reactions/Side Effects
CNS: fatigue. **Resp:** BRONCHOSPASM, cough, ↓ lung function, throat pain/irritation. **GI:** diarrhea, nausea. **Endo:** HYPOGLYCEMIA. **F and E:** hypokalemia. **Metab:** weight gain. **Misc:** allergic reactions including ANAPHYLAXIS.

Interactions
Drug-Drug: Concurrent use of **other antidiabetics, ACE inhibitors, ARBs, disopyrimide, fibrates, fluoxetine, MAOIs, pentoxifyllin, pramlintide, salicylates, somastatin analogs** including **octreotide**, and **sulfonamide anti-infectives**↑ risk of hypoglycemia, dose modifications may be necessary. Glucose lowering effects may be ↓ by **atypical antipsychotics** including **clozapine**, and **olanzapine**, **corticosteroids**, **danazol**, **diuretics**, **estrogens**, **glucagon**, **isonazid**, **niacin**, **oral (hormonal contraceptives)**, **phenothiazines**, **progestogens** (in hormonal contraceptives), **protease inhibitors**, **somatropin**, **sympathomimetic agents** including **albuterol**, **epinephrine** and **terbutabline** and **thyroid hormones**. Concurrent use of **anti-adrenergics** including **beta-blockers**, **clonidine**, or **reserpine** may ↓ signs any symptoms of hypoglycemia. Concomitant use with **thiazolidinediones** including **pioglitazone** or **rosiglitazone** (↑ risk of fluid retention and worsening HF). Concurrent use of **inhaled albuterol** may ↑ absorpion.
Drug-Natural Products: Glucosamine may worsen blood glucose control. **Fenugreek**, **chromium**, and **coenzyme Q-10** may produce additive hypoglycemic effects.

Route/Dosage
Inhaln (Adults): 4 or 8 units inhaled at the beginning of a meal; dose depends on a variety of patient factors.

Availability
Single-use cartridge for inhalation using Afrezza-specific inhaler: 4 units, 8 units, 12 units.

NURSING IMPLICATIONS
Assessment
- Before starting therapy perform a detailed medical history, physical examination, and spirometry (FEV_1) to determine potential lung disease. Assess pulmonary function via spirometry at baseline, after 6 mo and annually thereafter; more frequently if patient has pulmonary symptoms such as wheezing, bronchospasm, breathing difficulties, or persistent, recurring cough. May require discontinuation of inhalation therapy.
- Assess patient periodically for symptoms of hypoglycemia (anxiety; restlessness; tingling in hands, feet, lips, or tongue; chills; cold sweats; confusion; cool, pale skin; difficulty in concentration; drowsiness; nightmares or trouble sleeping; excessive hunger; headache; irritability; nausea; nervousness; tachycardia; tremor; weakness; unsteady gait) and hyperglycemia (confusion, drowsiness; flushed, dry skin; fruit-like breath odor; rapid, deep breathing, polyuria; loss of appetite; unusual thirst) during therapy.
- Monitor for bronchospasm. Occurs rarely, but if bronchospasm occurs, discontinue therapy and notify health care professional immediately. Re-admin-

istration should be attempted during close monitoring.

- Assess for respiratory illness. Monitor blood glucose concentrations closely; may require dose adjustments.
- Monitor body weight periodically. May cause weight gain. Changes in weight may necessitate changes in insulin dose.
- ***Lab Test Considerations:*** Monitor blood glucose every 6 hr during therapy, more frequently in ketoacidosis and times of stress. A1C may be monitored every 3–6 mo to determine effectiveness.
- Monitor serum potassium in patients at risk for hypokalemia (those using potassium-lowering agents, those receiving IV insulin) periodically during therapy.
- ***Toxicity and Overdose:*** Overdose is manifested by symptoms of hypoglycemia. Mild hypoglycemia may be treated by ingestion of oral glucose. Severe hypoglycemia is a life-threatening emergency; treatment consists of IV glucose, glucagon, or epinephrine.

Potential Nursing Diagnoses

Noncompliance (Patient/Family Teaching)

Implementation

- Inhalation insulin must be used in combination with long-acting subcutaneous insulin.
- *Afrezza* should only be used with *Afrezza inhaler*.
- **Inhaln:** Administer at beginning of meal. Keep inhaler level; white mouthpiece on top and purple base on the bottom after inserting cartridge. Loss of drug effect occurs if inhaler is upside down, held with mouthpiece pointing down, shaken, or dropped after cartridge is inserted but before dose given. If these occur, replace cartridge before use.
- Dosing: *Insulin naive patients:* Start with 4 units before each meal. *Patients using subcut mealtime (Prandial) Insulin:* Determine appropriate dose for each meal by converting from injected dose using dose conversion. *Patients using subcut pre-mixed insulin:* Estimate mealtime injected dose by dividing half total daily injected pre-mixed insulin dose equally among three meals. Convert each estimated injected mealtime dose to appropriate inhalation dose using dose conversion. Administer half of total daily injected pre-mixed dose as an injected basal insulin dose.
- Dose conversion: *If injected mealtime insulin dose is up to 4 units:* Administer one 4-unit inhalation dose. *If injected mealtime insulin dose is 5–8 units:* Administer one 8-unit inhalation dose. *If injected mealtime insulin dose is 9–12 units:* Administer one 12-unit inhalation dose. *If injected mealtime insulin dose is 13–16 units:* Administer one 4–unit inhalation dose and one 12-unit inhalation dose (16 units). *If injected mealtime insulin dose is 17–20 units:* Administer one 8–unit inhalation dose and one 12–unit inhalation doses (20 units). *If injected mealtime insulin dose is 21–24 units:* Administer two 12–unit inhalation doses (24 units).
- Adjust dose based on metabolic needs, blood glucose monitoring results, and glycemic control goal. Dose may need to be adjusted with changes in physical activity, meal patterns, renal and hepatic function, or during acute illness.
- Monitor blood glucose carefully in patients receiving high doses of inhalation insulin. If blood glucose control is not achieved with increased inhalation doses, consider use of subcut mealtime insulin.

Patient/Family Teaching

- Instruct patient on proper technique for administration. Advise patient to read Medication Guide before starting therapy and with each Rx refill in case of changes.
- Advise patient to notify health care professional immediately of signs and symptoms of allergic reaction (rash, trouble breathing, fast heartbeat, sweating) occur.
- Explain to patient that this medication controls hyperglycemia but does not cure diabetes. Therapy is long term.
- Instruct patient in proper testing of serum glucose and ketones. These tests should be closely monitored during periods of stress or illness and health care professional notified of significant changes.
- May cause dizziness. Caution patient to avoid driving or other activities requiring alertness until response to medication is known.
- Caution patient to avoid smoking while taking inhaled insulin.
- Emphasize the importance of compliance with nutritional guidelines and regular exercise as directed by health care professional.
- Instruct patient to notify health care professional of all Rx or OTC medications, vitamins, or herbal products being taken and to consult health care professional before taking other Rx, OTC, or herbal products, especially inhaled medications.
- Advise patient to notify health care professional of medication regimen prior to treatment or surgery.
- Advise patient to notify health care professional if nausea, vomiting, or fever develops, if unable to eat regular diet, or if blood glucose levels are not controlled.
- Instruct patient on signs and symptoms of hypoglycemia and hyperglycemia and what to do if they occur.
- Advise patient to notify health care professional if pregnancy is planned or suspected or if breast feeding or planning to breast feed.

- Patients with diabetes mellitus should carry a source of sugar (candy, glucose gel) and identification describing their disease and treatment regimen at all times.
- Emphasize the importance of regular follow-up, especially during first few weeks of therapy.

Evaluation/Desired Outcomes

- Control of blood glucose levels in diabetic patients without the appearance of hypoglycemic or hyperglycemic episodes.

HIGH ALERT

INSULIN (mixtures) (in-su-lin)

insulin lispro protamine suspension/insulin lispro injection mixtures, rDNA origin
HumaLOG Mix 75/25, HumaLOG Mix 50/50

insulin aspart protamine suspension/insulin aspart injection mixtures, rDNA origin
NovoLOG Mix 70/30

NPH/regular insulin mixtures
HumuLIN 70/30, NovoLIN 70/30

Classification
Therapeutic: antidiabetics, hormones
Pharmacologic: pancreatics

Pregnancy Category B (insulin lispro protamine suspension/insulin lispro injection mixtures), C (insulin aspart protamine suspension/insulin aspart injection mixtures, NPH/regular insulin mixtures)

See Appendix K for more information concerning insulins

Indications

Control of hyperglycemia in patients with type 1 or type 2 diabetes mellitus.

Action

Lower blood glucose by: stimulating glucose uptake in skeletal muscle and fat, inhibiting hepatic glucose production. Other actions: inhibition of lipolysis and proteolysis, enhanced protein synthesis. **Therapeutic Effects:** Control of hyperglycemia in diabetic patients.

Pharmacokinetics

Absorption: Well absorbed from subcutaneous administration sites. Absorption rate is determined by type of insulin, injection site, volume of injectate, and other factors.
Distribution: Widely distributed.
Metabolism and Excretion: Metabolized by liver, spleen, kidney, and muscle.
Half-life: 5–6 min (prolonged in patients with diabetes; biologic half-life is 1–1.5 hr).

TIME/ACTION PROFILE (hypoglycemic effect)

ROUTE	ONSET	PEAK	DURATION
insulin lispro protamine suspension/ insulin lispro injection mixture subcut	15–30 min	2.8 hr	24 hr
insulin aspart protamine suspension/ insulin aspart injection mixture subcut	15 min	1–4 hr	18–24 hr
NPH/Regular Insulin mixture subcutaneous	30 min	2–12 hr	24 hr

Contraindications/Precautions

Contraindicated in: Hypoglycemia; Allergy or hypersensitivity to a particular type of insulin, preservatives, or other additives.
Use Cautiously in: Stress and infection (may temporarily ↑ insulin requirements); Renal/hepatic impairment (may ↓ insulin requirements); Concomitant use with pioglitazone or rosiglitazone (↑ risk of fluid retention and worsening HF); OB: Pregnancy may temporarily ↑ insulin requirements; Pedi: Safety of Humalog not established.

Adverse Reactions/Side Effects

Endo: HYPOGLYCEMIA. **F and E:** hypokalemia. **Local:** erythema, lipodystrophy, pruritis, swelling. **Misc:** allergic reactions including ANAPHYLAXIS.

Interactions

Drug-Drug: Beta blockers, clonidine, and **reserpine** may mask some of the signs and symptoms of hypoglycemia. **Corticosteroids, thyroid supplements, estrogens, isoniazid, niacin, phenothiazines**, and **rifampin** may ↑ insulin requirements. **Alcohol, ACE inhibitors, MAO inhibitors, octreotide, oral hypoglycemic agents**, and **salicylates**, may ↓ insulin requirements. Concurrent use with **pioglitazone** or **rosiglitazone** may ↑ risk of fluid retention and worsening HF.
Drug-Natural Products: Glucosamine may worsen blood glucose control. **Fenugreek, chromium**, and **coenzyme Q-10** may produce additive hypoglycemic effects.

Route/Dosage

Dose depends on blood glucose, response, and many other factors.

Subcut (Adults and Children): 0.5–1 unit/kg/day. *Adolescents during rapid growth*—0.8–1.2 units/kg/day.

Availability

NPH insulin/regular insulin suspension mixture: 70 units NPH/30 units regular insulin/mL—Novolin 70/30, Humulin 70/30 (100 units/mL total) in 10-mL vials and 3-mL prefilled pens[OTC]. **Insulin lispro protamine suspension/insulin lispro injection mixture:** 75% insulin lispro protamine suspension and 25% insulin lispro injection—Humalog Mix 75/25 100 units/mL in 10-mL vials and 3-mL prefilled pens, 50% insulin lispro protamine suspension and 50% insulin lispro injection—Humalog Mix 50/50 100 units/mL in 10-mL vials and 3-mL prefilled pens. **Insulin aspart protamine suspension/insulin aspart injection mixture:** 70% insulin aspart protamine suspension and 30% insulin aspart inection—NovoLog Mix 70/30 100 units/mL in 10-mL vials and 3-mL prefilled pens.

NURSING IMPLICATIONS

Assessment

- Assess for symptoms of hypoglycemia (anxiety; restlessness; tingling in hands, feet, lips, or tongue; chills; cold sweats; confusion; cool, pale skin; difficulty in concentration; drowsiness; excessive hunger; headache; irritability; nightmares or trouble sleeping; nausea; nervousness; tachycardia; tremor; weakness; unsteady gait) and hyperglycemia (confusion, drowsiness; flushed, dry skin; fruit-like breath odor; rapid, deep breathing, polyuria; loss of appetite; nausea; vomiting; unusual thirst) periodically during therapy.
- Monitor body weight periodically. Changes in weight may necessitate changes in insulin dose.
- ***Lab Test Considerations:*** Monitor blood glucose every 6 hr during therapy, more frequently in ketoacidosis and times of stress. Hemoglobin A_{1C} may also be monitored every 3–6 mo to determine effectiveness.
- Monitor serum potassium in patients at risk for hypokalemia (those using potassium-lowering agents, those receiving IV insulin) periodically during therapy.
- ***Toxicity and Overdose:*** Overdose is manifested by symptoms of hypoglycemia. Mild hypoglycemia may be treated by ingestion of oral glucose. Severe hypoglycemia is a life-threatening emergency; treatment consists of IV glucose, glucagon, or epinephrine.

Potential Nursing Diagnoses

Noncompliance (Patient/Family Teaching)

Implementation

- ***High Alert:*** Insulin-related medication errors have resulted in patient harm and death. Clarify ambiguous orders; do not accept orders using the abbreviation "u" for units, (can be misread as a zero or the numeral 4; has resulted in tenfold overdoses).
- Insulins are available in different types and strengths. Check type, dose, and expiration date with another licensed nurse. Do not interchange insulins without consulting health care professional.
- Do not confuse Humalog with Humulin. Do not confuse Novolin with Novolog.
- Use *only* insulin syringes to draw up dose. The unit markings on the insulin syringe must match the insulin's units/mL.
- Store insulin in refrigerator. May also be kept at room temperature for up to 28 days. Do not use if cloudy, discolored, or unusually viscous. Store Humalog KwikPens at room temperature and discard after 10 days.
- NPH insulins should not be used in the management of ketoacidosis.
- **Subcut:** Rotate injection sites.
- Administer into abdominal wall, thigh, or upper arm subcutaneously.

Patient/Family Teaching

- Instruct patient on proper technique for administration. Include type of insulin, equipment (syringe, cartridge pens, alcohol swabs), storage, and place to discard syringes. Discuss the importance of not changing brands of insulin or syringes, selection and rotation of injection sites, and compliance with therapeutic regimen. Caution patient that insulin pens should not be shared with others, even if clean needles are used.
- Caution patient not to share pen device with another person, even if needle is changed; may risk transmission of blood-borne pathogens.
- Explain to patient that this medication controls hyperglycemia but does not cure diabetes. Therapy is long term.
- Instruct patient in proper testing of serum glucose and ketones. These tests should be closely monitored during periods of stress or illness and health care professional notified of significant changes.
- Emphasize the importance of compliance with nutritional guidelines and regular exercise as directed by health care professional.
- Advise patient to notify health care professional of all Rx or OTC medications, vitamins, or herbal products being taken and to consult with health care professional before taking other medications or alcohol.
- Advise patient to notify health care professional of medication regimen prior to treatment or surgery.
- Advise patient to notify health care professional if nausea, vomiting, or fever develops, if unable to eat

regular diet, or if blood glucose levels are not controlled.
- Instruct patient on signs and symptoms of hypoglycemia and hyperglycemia and what to do if they occur.
- Advise patient to notify health care professional if pregnancy is planned or suspected or if breast feeding or planning to breast feed.
- Patients with diabetes mellitus should carry a source of sugar (candy, glucose gel) and identification describing their disease and treatment regimen at all times.
- Emphasize the importance of regular follow-up, especially during first few weeks of therapy.

Evaluation/Desired Outcomes
- Control of blood glucose levels in diabetic patients without the appearance of hypoglycemic or hyperglycemic episodes.

HIGH ALERT

NPH insulin (isophane insulin suspension)
HumuLIN N, Novolin ge NPH, NovoLIN N

Classification
Therapeutic: antidiabetics, hormones
Pharmacologic: pancreatics

Pregnancy Category B

See Appendix K for more information concerning insulins

Indications
Control of hyperglycemia in patients with diabetes mellitus.

Action
Lowers blood glucose by: stimulating glucose uptake in skeletal muscle and fat, inhibiting hepatic glucose production. Other actions of insulin: inhibition of lipolysis and proteolysis, enhanced protein synthesis. **Therapeutic Effects:** Control of hyperglycemia in diabetic patients.

Pharmacokinetics
Absorption: Rapidly absorbed from subcutaneous administration sites. Presence of protamine delays peak effect and prolongs action.
Distribution: Identical to endogenous insulin.
Metabolism and Excretion: Metabolized by liver, spleen, kidney, and muscle.
Half-life: Unknown.

TIME/ACTION PROFILE (hypoglycemic effect)

ROUTE	ONSET	PEAK	DURATION
NPH subcutaneous	2–4 hr	4–10 hr	10–16 hr
70% NPH/30% Regular Insulin mixture	30 min	2–12 hr	24 hr

Contraindications/Precautions
Contraindicated in: Hypoglycemia; Allergy or hypersensitivity to a particular type of insulin, preservatives, or other additives.
Use Cautiously in: Stress or infection (may temporarily ↑ insulin requirements); Renal/hepatic impairment (may ↓ insulin requirements); Concomitant use with pioglitazone or rosiglitazone (↑ risk of fluid retention and worsening HF); OB: Pregnancy may temporarily ↑ insulin requirements.

Adverse Reactions/Side Effects
Endo: HYPOGLYCEMIA. **F and E:** hypokalemia. **Local:** lipodystrophy, pruritus, erythema, swelling. **Misc:** allergic reactions including ANAPHYLAXIS.

Interactions
Drug-Drug: **Beta blockers**, **clonidine**, and **reserpine** may mask some of the signs and symptoms of hypoglycemia. **Corticosteroids**, **thyroid supplements**, **estrogens**, **isoniazid**, **niacin**, **phenothiazines**, and **rifampin** may ↑ insulin requirements. **Alcohol**, **ACE inhibitors**, **MAO inhibitors**, **octreotide**, **oral hypoglycemic agents**, and **salicylates**, may ↓ insulin requirements. Concurrent use with **pioglitazone** or **rosiglitazone** may ↑ risk of fluid retention and worsening HF.
Drug-Natural Products: **Glucosamine** may worsen blood glucose control. **Fenugreek**, **chromium**, and **coenzyme Q-10** may produce additive hypoglycemic effects.

Route/Dosage
Dose depends on blood glucose, response, and many other factors.
Subcut (Adults and Children): 0.5–1 unit total insulin/kg/day. *Adolescents during rapid growth*—0.8–1.2 units total insulin/kg/day.

Availability
Isophane insulin suspension (NPH insulin): 100 units/mL in 10–mL vials and 3–mL prefilled pens.

NURSING IMPLICATIONS
Assessment
- Assess patient periodically for symptoms of hypoglycemia (anxiety; restlessness; tingling in hands, feet, lips, or tongue; chills; cold sweats; confusion; cool, pale skin; difficulty in concentration; drowsiness; nightmares or trouble sleeping; excessive hunger; headache; irritability; nausea; nervousness; tachy-

cardia; tremor; weakness; unsteady gait) and hyperglycemia (confusion, drowsiness; flushed, dry skin; fruit-like breath odor; rapid, deep breathing, polyuria; loss of appetite; unusual thirst) during therapy.

- Monitor body weight periodically. Changes in weight may necessitate changes in insulin dose.
- ***Lab Test Considerations:*** Monitor blood glucose every 6 hr during therapy, more frequently in ketoacidosis and times of stress. A1C may be monitored every 3–6 mo to determine effectiveness.
- Monitor serum potassium in patients at risk for hypokalemia (those using potassium-lowering agents, those receiving IV insulin) periodically during therapy.
- ***Toxicity and Overdose:*** Overdose is manifested by symptoms of hypoglycemia. Mild hypoglycemia may be treated by ingestion of oral glucose. Severe hypoglycemia is a life-threatening emergency; treatment consists of IV glucose, glucagon, or epinephrine.

Potential Nursing Diagnoses

Noncompliance (Patient/Family Teaching)

Implementation

- ***High Alert:*** Medication errors involving insulins have resulted in serious patient harm and death. Clarify all ambiguous orders and do not accept orders using the abbreviation "u" for units, which can be misread as a zero or the numeral 4 and has resulted in tenfold overdoses. Insulins are available in different types and strengths. Check type, dose, and expiration date with another licensed nurse. Do not interchange insulins without consulting physician or other health care professional.
- Do not confuse Humulin with Humalog. Do not confuse Novolin with Novolog.
- Use *only* insulin syringes to draw up dose. The unit markings on the insulin syringe must match the insulin's units/mL. Special syringes for doses <50 units are available. Prior to withdrawing dose, rotate vial between palms to ensure uniform solution; do not shake.
- When mixing insulins, draw regular insulin or insulin lispro into syringe first to avoid contamination of regular insulin vial.
- Insulin should be stored in a cool place but does not need to be refrigerated.
- When transferring from once-daily NPH human insulin to *insulin glargine*, the dose usually remains unchanged. When transferring from twice-daily NPH human insulin to insulin glargine, the initial dose of insulin glargine is usually reduced by 20%.
- NPH insulin should not be used in the management of ketoacidosis.
- **Subcut:** Administer NPH insulin within 30–60 min before a meal.

Patient/Family Teaching

- Instruct patient on proper technique for administration. Include type of insulin, equipment (syringe, cartridge pens, alcohol swabs), storage, and place to discard syringes. Discuss the importance of not changing brands of insulin or syringes, selection and rotation of injection sites, and compliance with therapeutic regimen. Caution patient that insulin pens should not be shared with others, even if clean needles are used.
- Demonstrate technique for mixing insulins by drawing up regular insulin or insulin lispro first and rolling intermediate-acting insulin vial between palms to mix, rather than shaking (may cause inaccurate dose).
- Caution patient not to share pen device with another person, even if needle is changed; may risk transmission of blood-borne pathogens.
- Explain to patient that this medication controls hyperglycemia but does not cure diabetes. Therapy is long term.
- Instruct patient in proper testing of serum glucose and ketones. These tests should be closely monitored during periods of stress or illness and health care professional notified of significant changes.
- Emphasize the importance of compliance with nutritional guidelines and regular exercise as directed by health care professional.
- Advise patient to notify health care professional of all Rx or OTC medications, vitamins, or herbal products being taken and to consult with health care professional before taking other medications or alcohol.
- Advise patient to notify health care professional of medication regimen prior to treatment or surgery.
- Advise patient to notify health care professional if nausea, vomiting, or fever develops, if unable to eat regular diet, or if blood glucose levels are not controlled.
- Instruct patient on signs and symptoms of hypoglycemia and hyperglycemia and what to do if they occur.
- Advise patient to notify health care professional if pregnancy is planned or suspected or if breast feeding or planning to breast feed.
- Patients with diabetes mellitus should carry a source of sugar (candy, glucose gel) and identification describing their disease and treatment regimen at all times.
- Emphasize the importance of regular follow-up, especially during first few weeks of therapy.

Evaluation/Desired Outcomes

- Control of blood glucose levels in diabetic patients without the appearance of hypoglycemic or hyperglycemic episodes.

HIGH ALERT

insulin, regular (injection, concentrated) (in-su-lin)

HumuLIN R, ✤ Novolin geToronto, NovoLIN R, HumuLIN R U-500 (Concentrated)

Classification

Therapeutic: antidiabetics, hormones
Pharmacologic: pancreatics

Pregnancy Category B

See Appendix K for more information concerning insulins

Indications

Control of hyperglycemia in patients with diabetes mellitus. **Concentrated regular insulin U-500:** Only for use in patients with insulin requirements >200 units/day. **Unlabeled Use:** Treatment of hyperkalemia.

Action

Lowers blood glucose by: stimulating glucose uptake in skeletal muscle and fat, inhibiting hepatic glucose production. Other actions of insulin: inhibition of lipolysis and proteolysis, enhanced protein synthesis. **Therapeutic Effects:** Control of hyperglycemia in diabetic patients.

Pharmacokinetics

Absorption: Rapidly absorbed from subcutaneous administration sites. U-100 regular insulin is absorbed slightly more quickly than U-500.
Distribution: Identical to endogenous insulin.
Metabolism and Excretion: Metabolized by liver, spleen, kidney, and muscle.
Half-life: 30–60 min.

TIME/ACTION PROFILE (hypoglycemic effect)

ROUTE	ONSET	PEAK	DURATION
Regular insulin IV	10–30 min	15–30 min	30–60 min
Regular insulin subcutaneous	30–60 min	2–4 hr	5–7 hr

Contraindications/Precautions

Contraindicated in: Hypoglycemia; Allergy or hypersensitivity to a particular type of insulin, preservatives, or other additives.
Use Cautiously in: Stress or infection—may temporarily ↑ insulin requirements; Renal/hepatic impairment—may ↓ insulin requirements; Concomitant use with pioglitazone or rosiglitazone (↑ risk of fluid retention and worsening HF); OB: Pregnancy may temporarily ↑ insulin requirements.

Adverse Reactions/Side Effects

Endo: HYPOGLYCEMIA. **F and E:** hypokalemia. **Local:** lipodystrophy, pruritus, erythema, swelling. **Misc:** allergic reactions including ANAPHYLAXIS.

Interactions

Drug-Drug: Beta blockers, clonidine, and **reserpine** may mask some of the signs and symptoms of hypoglycemia. **Corticosteroids, thyroid supplements, estrogens, isoniazid, niacin, phenothiazines,** and **rifampin** may ↑ insulin requirements. **Alcohol, ACE inhibitors, MAO inhibitors, octreotide, oral hypoglycemic agents,** and **salicylates,** may ↓ insulin requirements. Concurrent use with **pioglitazone** or **rosiglitazone** may ↑ risk of fluid retention and worsening HF.
Drug-Natural Products: Glucosamine may worsen blood glucose control. **Fenugreek, chromium,** and **coenzyme Q-10** may produce additive hypoglycemic effects.

Route/Dosage

Dose depends on blood glucose, response, and many other factors.

Ketoacidosis—Regular (100 units/mL) Insulin Only

IV (Adults): 0.1 unit/kg/hr as a continuous infusion.
IV (Children): Loading dose—0.1 unit/kg, then maintenance continuous infusion 0.05–0.2 unit/kg/hr, titrate to optimal rate of decrease of serum glucose of 80–100 mg/dL/hr.

Maintenance Therapy

Subcut (Adults and Children): 0.5–1 unit/kg/day in divided doses. *Adolescents during rapid growth*—0.8–1.2 unit/kg/day in divided doses.

Treatment of Hyperkalemia

Subcut, IV (Adults and Children): dextrose 0.5–1 g/kg combined with insulin 1 unit for every 4–5 g dextrose given.

Availability

Insulin injection (regular insulin): 100 units/mL in 10–mL vials and 3–mL prefilled pens[OTC]. **Regular (concentrated) insulin injection:** 500 units/mL in 20–mL vials. ***In combination with:*** NPH insulins (Humulin 70/30, Novolin 70/30).

NURSING IMPLICATIONS

Assessment

- Assess patient periodically for symptoms of hypoglycemia (anxiety; restlessness; tingling in hands, feet, lips, or tongue; chills; cold sweats; confusion; cool, pale skin; difficulty in concentration; drowsiness; nightmares or trouble sleeping; excessive hunger; headache; irritability; nausea; nervousness; tachycardia; tremor; weakness; unsteady gait) and hyperglycemia (confusion, drowsiness; flushed, dry skin;

fruit-like breath odor; rapid, deep breathing, polyuria; loss of appetite; unusual thirst) during therapy.

- Monitor body weight periodically. Changes in weight may necessitate changes in insulin dose.
- ***Lab Test Considerations:*** Monitor blood glucose every 6 hr during therapy, more frequently in ketoacidosis and times of stress. A1C may be monitered every 3–6 mo to determine effectiveness.
- Monitor serum potassium in patients at risk for hypokalemia (those using potassium-lowering agents, those receiving IV insulin) periodically during therapy.
- ***Toxicity and Overdose:*** Overdose is manifested by symptoms of hypoglycemia. Mild hypoglycemia may be treated by ingestion of oral glucose. Severe hypoglycemia is a life-threatening emergency; treatment consists of IV glucose, glucagon, or epinephrine.

Potential Nursing Diagnoses

Noncompliance (Patient/Family Teaching)

Implementation

- ***High Alert:*** Medication errors involving insulins have resulted in serious patient harm and death. Clarify all ambiguous orders and do not accept orders using the abbreviation "u" for units, which can be misread as a zero or the numeral 4 and has resulted in tenfold overdoses. Insulins are available in different types and strengths. Check type, dose, and expiration date with another licensed nurse. Do not interchange insulins without consulting health care professional. Do not confuse regular **concentrated (U-500)** insulin with regular insulin.To prevent errors between regular U-100 insulin and concentrated U-500 insulin, concentrated U-500 insulin is marked with a band of diagonal brown strips and "U-500" is highlighted in red on the label and a conversion chart should always be available.
- Do not confuse Humulin with Humalog. Do not confuse Novolin with Novolog.
- Use ***only*** insulin syringes to draw up dose. The unit markings on the insulin syringe must match the insulin's units/mL. Special syringes for doses <50 units are available. Prior to withdrawing dose, rotate vial between palms to ensure uniform solution; do not shake.
- When mixing insulins, draw regular insulin into syringe first to avoid contamination of regular insulin vial.
- Insulin should be stored in a cool place but does not need to be refrigerated.
- **Subcut:** Administer regular insulin within 15–30 min before a meal.

IV Administration

- **IV:** Do not use if cloudy, discolored, or unusually viscous. ***High Alert:*** Do not administer regular (concentrated) insulin U-500 IV.
- **IV Push:** ***Diluent:*** May be administered IV undiluted directly into vein or through Y-site. ***Rate:*** Administer up to 50 units over 1 min.
- **Continuous Infusion:** ***Diluent:*** May be diluted in 0.9% NaCl using polyvinyl chloride infusion bags. ***Concentration:*** 0.1 unit/mL to 1 unit/mL in infusion systems with the infusion fluids. ***Rate:*** Rate should be ordered by health care professional, and infusion placed on an IV pump for accurate administration.
- Rate of administration should be decreased when serum glucose level reaches 250 mg/dL.
- **Y-Site Compatibility:** acyclovir, alfentanil, aminophylline, amphotericin B lipid complex, anidulafungin , argatroban, ascorbic acid, atropine, aztreonam, benztropine, bivalirudin, bleomycin, bumetanide, buprenorphine, calcium chloride, calcium gluconate, carboplatin, carmustine, caspofungin, cefazolin, cefepime, ceftaroline, ceftazidime, ceftriaxone, cefuroxime, chloramphenicol, clindamycin, cyanocobalamin, cyclophosphamide, cytarabine, dacarbazine, dactinomycin, daptomycin, daunorubicin hydrochloride, dexamethasone, dexmedetomidine, dexrazoxane, docetaxel, doripenem, doxorubicin liposomal, doxycycline, enalapril, ephedrine, epirubicin, epoetin alfa, ertapenem, erythromycin, esmolol, esomeprazole, etoposide, etoposide phosphate, fenoldopam, fentanyl, fluconazole, fludarabine, folic acid, foscarnet, fosphenytoin, ganciclovir, gemcitabine, granisetron, hetastarch, hydrocortisone, hydromorphone, ibuprofen, idarubicin, ifosfamide, imipenem/cilastatin, indomethacin, irinotecan, ketorolac, leucovorin calcium, lidocaine, linezolid, lorazepam, magnesium sulfate, mannitol, mechlorethamine, meperidine, meropenem, mesna, methotrexate, methyldopate, methylprednisolone, metoclopramide, metoprolol, metronidazole, milrinone, mitoxantrone, moxifloxacin, mycophenolate, nalbuphine, naloxone, nitroglycerin, nitroprusside, octreotide, oxacillin, oxaliplatin, paclitaxel, palonosetron, pamidronate, pancuronium, papaverine, pemetrexed, penicillin G, pentazocine, pentobarbital, phenobarbital, phytonadione, potassium acetate, potassium chloride, procainamide, promethazine, propofol, pyridoxine, remifentanil, sodium bicarbonate, streptokinase, sufentanil, tacrolimus, teniposide, terbutaline, theophylline, thiamine, thiotepa, tigecycline, tirofiban, topotecan, vancomycin, vecuronium, verapamil, vinblastine, vincristine, vinorelbine, vitamin B complex with C, voriconazole, zoledronic acid.

I

- **Y-Site Incompatibility:** alemtuzumab, butorphanol, cefoxitin, chlorpromazine, cisplatin, dantrolene, diazepam, diphenhydramine, glycopyrrolate, hydroxyzine, isoproterenol, ketamine, labetalol, micafungin, mitomycin, nesiritide, pentamidine, phenylephrine, phenytoin, piperacillin/tazobactam, prochlorperazine, propranolol, protamine, quinupristin/dalfopristin, rocuronium, trimethoprim/sulfamethoxazole.
- **Additive Compatibility:** May be added to total parenteral nutrition (TPN) solutions.

Patient/Family Teaching

- Instruct patient on proper technique for administration. Include type of insulin, equipment (syringe, cartridge pens, alcohol swabs), storage, and place to discard syringes. Discuss the importance of not changing brands of insulin or syringes, selection and rotation of injection sites, and compliance with therapeutic regimen. Opened, unused insulin vials should be discarded 1 mo after opening.
- Demonstrate technique for mixing insulins by drawing up regular insulin first and rolling intermediate-acting insulin vial between palms to mix, rather than shaking (may cause inaccurate dose).
- Caution patient not to share pen device with another person, even if needle is changed; may risk transmission of blood-borne pathogens.
- Explain to patient that this medication controls hyperglycemia but does not cure diabetes. Therapy is long term.
- Instruct patient in proper testing of serum glucose and ketones. These tests should be closely monitored during periods of stress or illness and health care professional notified of significant changes.
- Emphasize the importance of compliance with nutritional guidelines and regular exercise as directed by health care professional.
- Instruct patient to notify health care professional of all Rx or OTC medications, vitamins, or herbal products being taken and to consult health care professional before taking other Rx, OTC, herbal products, or alcohol.
- Advise patient to notify health care professional of medication regimen prior to treatment or surgery.
- Advise patient to notify health care professional if nausea, vomiting, or fever develops, if unable to eat regular diet, or if blood glucose levels are not controlled.
- Instruct patient on signs and symptoms of hypoglycemia and hyperglycemia and what to do if they occur.
- Advise patient to notify health care professional if pregnancy is planned or suspected or if breast feeding or planning to breast feed.
- Patients with diabetes mellitus should carry a source of sugar (candy, glucose gel) and identification describing their disease and treatment regimen at all times.
- Emphasize the importance of regular follow-up, especially during first few weeks of therapy.

Evaluation/Desired Outcomes

- Control of blood glucose levels in diabetic patients without the appearance of hypoglycemic or hyperglycemic episodes.

HIGH ALERT

INSULINS (long-acting)

(in-su-lin)

insulin detemir

Levemir

insulin glargine

Lantus, Toujeo

Classification

Therapeutic: antidiabetics, hormones

Pharmacologic: pancreatics

Pregnancy Category B (Levemir), C (Lantus, Toujeo)

See Appendix K for more information concerning insulins

Indications

Control of hyperglycemia in patients with type 1 or type 2 diabetes mellitus.

Action

Lower blood glucose by: stimulating glucose uptake in skeletal muscle and fat, inhibiting hepatic glucose production. Other actions: inhibition of lipolysis and proteolysis, enhanced protein synthesis. **Therapeutic Effects:** Control of hyperglycemia in diabetic patients.

Pharmacokinetics

Absorption: Physiochemical characteristics of long-acting insulins result in delayed and prolonged absorption.

Distribution: Widely distributed.

Metabolism and Excretion: Metabolized by liver, spleen, kidney, and muscle.

Half-life: 5–6 min (prolonged in patients with diabetes); biologic half-life is 1–1.5 hr; *insulin detemir* 5–7 hr (dose-dependent).

TIME/ACTION PROFILE (hypoglycemic effect)

ROUTE	ONSET	PEAK	DURATION
Insulin detemir	3–4 hr	3–14 hr†	6–24 hr‡
Insulin glargine	3–4 hr	none†	24 hr

†Small amounts of insulin glargine and insulin detemir are slowly released resulting in a relatively constant effect over time.

‡Duration is dose dependent; duration increases as dose increases.

Contraindications/Precautions

Contraindicated in: Hypoglycemia; Allergy or hypersensitivity to a particular type of insulin, preservatives, or other additives.

Use Cautiously in: Stress and infection (may temporarily ↑ insulin requirements); Renal/hepatic impairment (may ↓ insulin requirements); Concomitant use with pioglitazone or rosiglitazone (↑ risk of fluid retention and worsening HF); OB: Pregnancy may temporarily ↑ insulin requirements; Pedi: Children <18 yr (Toujeo), <6 yr (Lantus), or <2 yr (detemir) (safety not established).

Adverse Reactions/Side Effects

Endo: HYPOGLYCEMIA. **F and E:** hypokalemia. **Local:** lipodystrophy, pruritis, erythema, swelling. **Misc:** allergic reactions including ANAPHYLAXIS.

Interactions

Drug-Drug: Beta blockers, **clonidine**, and **reserpine** may mask some of the signs and symptoms of hypoglycemia. **Corticosteroids**, **thyroid supplements**, **estrogens**, **isoniazid**, **niacin**, **phenothiazines**, and **rifampin** may ↑ insulin requirements. **Alcohol**, **ACE inhibitors**, **MAO inhibitors**, **octreotide**, **oral hypoglycemic agents**, and **salicylates**, may ↓ insulin requirements. Concurrent use with **pioglitazone** or **rosiglitazone** may ↑ risk of fluid retention and worsening HF.

Drug-Natural Products: Glucosamine may worsen blood glucose control. **Fenugreek**, **chromium**, and **coenzyme Q-10** may produce additive hypoglycemic effects.

Route/Dosage

Toujeo has a lower glucose lowering effect than Lantus on a unit-to-unit basis

Subcut (Adults and Children):.

Insulin Detemir

Subcut (Adults and Children ≥6 yr): *Type 2 diabetes patients who are insulin-naive*—0.1–0.2 units/kg once daily in the evening (or divided into a twice daily regimen) *or* 10 units once daily in the evening (or divided into a twice daily regimen). *Patients with type 1 or 2 diabetes receiving basal insulin or basal bolus therapy*—May substitute on an equivalent unit-per-unit basis.

Insulin Glargine (Lantus)

Subcut (Adults and Children ≥6 yr): *Type 1 diabetes (insulin naïve)*—1/3 of the total daily insulin dose given once daily, then adjust on the basis of patient's needs (remainder of insulin dose should be given as a short-acting insulin) (usual starting total daily insulin dose = 0.2–0.4 units/kg); *Type 2 diabetes (insulin naïve)*—0.2 units/kg or up to 10 units once daily; then adjust on the basis of patient's needs; *Type 1 or 2 diabetes (and converting from Toujeo)*—Give 80% of Toujeo dose as Lantus once daily, then adjust on the basis of patient's needs; *Type 1 or 2 diabetes (and converting from once daily NPH)*—Give the same dose once daily, then adjust on the basis of patient's needs; *Type 1 or 2 diabetes (and converting from twice daily NPH)*—Give 80% of the total daily NPH dose once daily, then adjust on the basis of patient's needs.

Insulin Glargine (Toujeo)

Subcut (Adults): *Type 1 diabetes (insulin naïve)*—1/3 to 1/2 of the total daily insulin dose given once daily, then adjust on the basis of patient's needs (range = 1–80 units/day), (remainder of insulin dose should be given as a short-acting insulin) (usual starting total daily insulin dose = 0.2–0.4 units/kg); *Type 2 diabetes (insulin naïve)*—0.2 units/kg once daily, then adjust on the basis of patient's needs; *Type 1 or 2 diabetes (and converting from intermediate or long-acting insulin)*—Use same total daily dose and give once daily, then adjust on the basis of patient's needs; *Type 1 or 2 diabetes (and converting from NPH insulin)*—Use 80% of the total daily NPH and give once daily, then adjust on the basis of patient's needs.

Availability

Insulin detemir: 100 units/mL in 10-mL vials and 3-mL prefilled pens. **Cost:** $177.61/10-ml vial *Levemir Flexpen (3 mL)*—$290.07/5 pens. **Insulin glargine (Lantus):** 100 units/mL in 10-mL vials and 3-mL prefilled pens. **Cost:** $180.34/10-mL vial *Lantus Solostar (3 mL)*—$306.22/5 pens. **Insulin glargine (Toujeo):** 300 units/mL in 1.5-mL prefilled pens.

NURSING IMPLICATIONS

Assessment

- Assess patient for signs and symptoms of hypoglycemia (anxiety; restlessness; mood changes; tingling in hands, feet, lips, or tongue; chills; cold sweats; confusion; cool, pale skin; difficulty in concentration; drowsiness; nightmares or trouble sleeping; excessive hunger; headache; irritability; nausea; nervousness; tachycardia; tremor; weakness; unsteady gait) and hyperglycemia (confusion, drowsiness; flushed, dry skin; fruit-like breath odor; rapid, deep breathing, polyuria; loss of appetite; nausea; vomiting; tiredness; unusual thirst) periodically during therapy.
- Monitor body weight periodically. Changes in weight may necessitate changes in insulin dose.
- ***Lab Test Considerations:*** Monitor blood glucose every 6 hr during therapy, more frequently in ketoacidosis and times of stress. Hemoglobin A_{1C} may

also be monitored every 3–6 mo to determine effectiveness.

- Monitor serum potassium in patients at risk for hypokalemia (those using potassium-lowering agents, those receiving IV insulin) periodically during therapy.
- ***Toxicity and Overdose:*** Overdose is manifested by symptoms of hypoglycemia. Mild hypoglycemia may be treated by ingestion of oral glucose. Severe hypoglycemia is a life-threatening emergency; treatment consists of IV glucose, glucagon, or epinephrine. Recovery from hypoglycemia may be delayed due to the prolonged effect of long-acting insulins.

Potential Nursing Diagnoses

Noncompliance (Patient/Family Teaching)

Implementation

- ***High Alert:*** Insulin-related medication errors have resulted in patient harm and death. Clarify ambiguous orders; do not accept orders using the abbreviation "u" for units, (can be misread as a zero or the numeral 4; has resulted in tenfold overdoses).
- Insulins are available in different types and strengths. Check type, dose, and expiration date with another licensed nurse. Do not interchange insulins without consulting health care professional.
- Do not confuse Levemir (insulin detemir) with Lovenox (enoxaparin).
- Use *only* insulin syringes to draw up dose. The unit markings on the insulin syringe must match the insulin's units/mL. Special syringes for doses <50 units are available. Prior to withdrawing dose, rotate vial between palms to ensure uniform solution; do not shake.
- ***High Alert:*** Do not mix ***insulin glargine or insulin detemir*** with any other insulin or solution, or use syringes containing any other medicinal product or residue. If giving with a short-acting insulin, use separate syringes and different injection sites. Solution should be clear and colorless with no particulate matter.
- Do not use if cloudy, discolored, or unusually viscous. Store unopened vials and cartridges of ***insulin glargine and insulin detemir*** in the refrigerator; do not freeze. If unable to refrigerate, the 10-mL vial of ***insulin glargine*** can be kept in a cool place unrefrigerated for up to 28 days. Once the cartridge is placed in a pen, do not refrigerate. After initial use, ***insulin detemir*** vials, cartridges, or a prefilled syringe may be stored in a cool place for 42 days. Do not store in-use cartridges and pre-filled syringes in refrigerator or with needle in place. Keep away from direct heat and sunlight.
- When transferring from once-daily NPH human insulin to ***insulin glargine***, the dose usually remains unchanged. When transferring from twice-daily NPH human insulin to insulin glargine, the initial dose of insulin glargine is usually reduced by 20%.
- **Subcut:** Rotate injection sites.
- Administer ***insulin glargine*** once daily at the same time each day.
- Administer ***daily insulin detemir*** with evening meal or at bedtime. With ***twice daily insulin detemir***, administer evening dose with evening meal, at bedtime, or 12 hr after morning dose.
- Do not administer ***insulin detemir*** or ***insulin glargine*** IV or in insulin pumps.

Patient/Family Teaching

- Instruct patient on proper technique for administration. Include type of insulin, equipment (syringe, cartridge pens, alcohol swabs), storage, and place to discard syringes. Discuss the importance of not changing brands of insulin or syringes, selection and rotation of injection sites, and compliance with therapeutic regimen. Patients taking insulin detemir should be given the *Patient Information* circular for this product.
- Caution patient not to share pen device with another person, even if needle is changed; may risk transmission of blood-borne pathogens.
- Explain to patient that this medication controls hyperglycemia but does not cure diabetes. Therapy is long term.
- Instruct patient in proper testing of serum glucose and ketones. These tests should be closely monitored during periods of stress or illness and health care professional notified of significant changes.
- Emphasize the importance of compliance with nutritional guidelines and regular exercise as directed by health care professional.
- Instruct patient to notify health care professional of all Rx or OTC medications, vitamins, or herbal products being taken and to consult health care professional before taking other Rx, OTC, herbal products, or alcohol.
- Advise patient to notify health care professional of medication regimen prior to treatment or surgery.
- Advise patient to notify health care professional if nausea, vomiting, or fever develops, if unable to eat regular diet, or if blood glucose levels are not controlled.
- Instruct patient on signs and symptoms of hypoglycemia and hyperglycemia and what to do if they occur.
- Patients with diabetes mellitus should carry a source of sugar (candy, glucose gel) and identification describing their disease and treatment regimen at all times.
- Advise patient to notify health care professional if pregnancy is planned or suspected or if breast feeding or planning to breast feed.
- Emphasize the importance of regular follow-up, especially during first few weeks of therapy.

Evaluation/Desired Outcomes

- Control of blood glucose levels in diabetic patients without the appearance of hypoglycemic or hyperglycemic episodes.

HIGH ALERT

INSULINS (rapid acting)
(in-su-lin)

insulin aspart, rDNA origin
NovoLOG, ✱NovoRapid

insulin glulisine
Apidra

insulin lispro, rDNA origin
HumaLOG

Classification
Therapeutic: antidiabetics, hormones
Pharmacologic: pancreatics

Pregnancy Category B (insulin aspart, insulin lispro), C (insulin glulisine)

See Appendix K for more information concerning insulins

Indications
Control of hyperglycemia in patients with type 1 or type 2 diabetes mellitus.

Action
Lower blood glucose by: stimulating glucose uptake in skeletal muscle and fat, inhibiting hepatic glucose production. Other actions: inhibition of lypolysis and proteolysis, enhanced protein synthesis. These are rapid-acting insulins with a more rapid onset and shorter duration than regular insulin; should be used with an intermediate- or long-acting insulin. **Therapeutic Effects:** Control of hyperglycemia in diabetic patients.

Pharmacokinetics
Absorption: Very rapidly absorbed from subcut administration sites.

Distribution: Widely distributed.

Metabolism and Excretion: Metabolized by liver, spleen, kidney, and muscle.

Half-life: *Insulin aspart*—1–1.5 hr; *Insulin lispro*—1 hr; *insulin glulisine*—42 min.

TIME/ACTION PROFILE (hypoglycemic effect)

ROUTE	ONSET	PEAK	DURATION
Insulin aspart	within 15 min	1–2 hr	3–4 hr
Insulin glulisine	within 15 min	1–2 hr	3–4 hr
Insulin lispro	within 15 min	1–2 hr	3–4 hr

Contraindications/Precautions
Contraindicated in: Hypoglycemia; Allergy or hypersensitivity to a particular type of insulin, preservatives, or other additives.

Use Cautiously in: Stress and infection (may temporarily ↑ insulin requirements); Renal/hepatic dysfunction (may ↓ insulin requirements); Concomitant use with pioglitazone or rosiglitazone (↑ risk of fluid retention and worsening HF); OB: Pregnancy may temporarily ↑ insulin requirements; Pedi: Safety not established in children <3 yr (for insulin lispro),<4 yr (insulin glulisine), <6 yr (for insulin aspart).

Adverse Reactions/Side Effects
Endo: HYPOGLYCEMIA. **F and E:** hypokalemia. **Local:** erythema, lipodystrophy, pruritis, swelling. **Misc:** allergic reactions including ANAPHYLAXIS.

Interactions
Drug-Drug: Beta blockers, **clonidine**, and **reserpine** may mask some of the signs and symptoms of hypoglycemia. **Corticosteroids**, **thyroid supplements**, **estrogens**, **isoniazid**, **niacin**, **phenothiazines**, and **rifampin** may ↑ insulin requirements. **Alcohol**, **ACE inhibitors**, **MAO inhibitors**, **octreotide**, **oral hypoglycemic agents**, and **salicylates**, may ↓ insulin requirements. Concurrent use with **pioglitazone** or **rosiglitazone** may ↑ risk of fluid retention and worsening HF.

Drug-Natural Products: Glucosamine may worsen blood glucose control. **Fenugreek**, **chromium**, and **coenzyme Q-10** may produce additive hypoglycemic effects.

Route/Dosage
Dose depends on blood glucose, response, and many other factors. Only insulin aspart and insulin glulisine can be administered IV.

Subcut (Adults and Children): Total insulin dose determined by needs of patient; generally 0.5–1 unit/kg/day; 50–70% of this dose may be given as meal-related boluses of rapid-acting insulin, and the remainder as an intermediate or long-acting insulin. *Subcutaneous infusion pump*—~50% of total dose can be given as meal-related boluses and ~50% of total dose can be given as basal infusion.

Availability
Insulin aspart: 100 units/mL in 10–mL vials and 3–mL prefilled cartridges or pens. **Cost:** $163.68/10–mL vial *NovoLog Flexpen (3 mL)*—$310.56/5 pens; *NovoLog Pen Fill (3 mL)*—$298.95/5 cartridges. **Insulin aspart 70/30 mix (Novolog Mix 70/30):** 70% insulin aspart protamine suspension and 30% insulin aspart solution mix 100 units/mL in 10-mL vials and 3-mL prefilled pens. **Cost:** $169.64/10–mL vial *NovoLog Mox 70/30 Flexpen (3 mL)*—$310.56/5 pens. **Insulin glulisine:** 100 units/mL in 10-mL vials and 3-mL prefilled pens. **Cost:** $158.53/10–mL vial *Apidra Solostar (3 mL)*—, $294.61/5 pens. **Insulin lispro:** 100 units/mL in 10-mL vials and 3-mL prefilled cartridges and pens, 200 units/mL in 3–mL prefilled cartridges and pens. **Cost:** $163.56/10-mL vial *Humalog Kwikpen (3 mL)*—$309.53/5 pens. **Insulin lispro**

75/25 mix (Humalog Mix 75/25): 75% lispro insulin protamine suspension and 25% insulin lispro mix 100 units/mL in 10-mL vials and 3-mL prefilled pens. **Cost:** $165.07/10-mL vial. **Insulin lispro 50/50 mix (Humalog Mix 50/50):** 50% lispro insulin protamine suspension and 50% insulin lispro mix 100 units/mL in 10-mL vials and 3-mL prefilled pens. **Cost:** *Humalog Mix 50/50 Kwikpen (3 mL)*—$303.58/5 pens.

NURSING IMPLICATIONS

Assessment

- Assess for symptoms of hypoglycemia (anxiety; restlessness; tingling in hands, feet, lips, or tongue; chills; cold sweats; confusion; cool, pale skin; difficulty in concentration; drowsiness; nightmares or trouble sleeping; excessive hunger; headache; irritability; nausea; nervousness; tachycardia; tremor; weakness; unsteady gait) and hyperglycemia (confusion, drowsiness; flushed, dry skin; fruit-like breath odor; rapid, deep breathing, polyuria; loss of appetite; nausea; vomiting; unusual thirst) periodically during therapy.
- Monitor body weight periodically. Changes in weight may necessitate changes in insulin dose.
- Assess patient for signs of allergic reactions (rash, shortness of breath, wheezing, rapid pulse, sweating, low BP) during therapy.
- ***Lab Test Considerations:*** Monitor blood glucose every 6 hr during therapy, more frequently in ketoacidosis and times of stress. HbA_{1C} may also be monitored every 3–6 mo to determine effectiveness.
- Monitor serum potassium in patients at risk for hypokalemia (those using potassium-lowering agents, those receiving IV insulin) periodically during therapy.
- ***Toxicity and Overdose:*** Overdose is manifested by symptoms of hypoglycemia. Mild hypoglycemia may be treated by ingestion of oral glucose. Severe hypoglycemia is a life-threatening emergency; treatment consists of IV glucose, glucagon, or epinephrine. Early signs of hypoglycemia may be less pronounced by long duration of diabetes, diabetic nerve disease, and use of beta blockers; may result in loss of consciousness prior to patient's awareness of hypoglycemia.

Potential Nursing Diagnoses

Noncompliance (Patient/Family Teaching)

Implementation

- ***High Alert:*** Insulin-related medication errors have resulted in patient harm and death. Clarify ambiguous orders; do not accept orders using the abbreviation "u" for units, (can be misread as a zero or the numeral 4; has resulted in tenfold overdoses).
- Insulins are available in different types and strengths. Check type, dose, and expiration date with another licensed nurse. Do not interchange insulins without consulting health care professional.
- Do not confuse Humalog with Humulin. Do not confuse Novolog with Novolin.
- Use *only* insulin syringes to draw up dose. The unit markings on the insulin syringe must match the insulin's units/mL. Special syringes for doses <50 units are available. Do not draw up dose into a syringe from the Kwik Pens; syringe markings do not match-up and could lead to a medication error. Use *only* U-100 insulin syringes to draw up *insulin lispro* dose. Prior to withdrawing dose, rotate vial between palms to ensure uniform solution; do not shake.
- *Insulin aspart, insulin glulisine,* and *insulin lispro* may be mixed with NPH insulin. When mixing insulins, draw insulin aspart, insulin glulisine, or insulin lispro into syringe first to avoid contamination of rapid-acting insulin vial. Mixed insulins should never be used in a pump or for IV infusion.
- Store vials in refrigerator. Vials may also be kept at room temperature for up to 28 days. Do not use if cloudy, discolored, or unusually viscous. Cartridges and pens should be stored at room temperature and used within 28 days. Never use the PenFill cartridge after the expiration date on the PenFill cartridge or on the box.
- Because of their short duration, *insulin lispro, insulin glulisine,* and *insulin aspart,* must be used with a longer-acting insulin or insulin infusion pump. In patients with type 2 diabetes, *insulin lispro* may be used without a longer-acting insulin when used in combination with an oral sulfonylurea agent.
- Humalog U-200 should not be mixed with other insulins, administered IV, or used in insulin pumps.
- **Subcut:** Administer into abdominal wall, thigh, or upper arm subcut. Rotate injection sites.
- Administer *insulin aspart* within 5–10 min before a meal.
- When used as meal time insulin, administer *insulin glulisine* 15 min before or within 20 min after starting a meal.
- Administer *insulin lispro* within 15 min before or immediately after a meal.
- May also be administered subcut via external insulin pump. Do not mix with other insulins or solution when used with a pump. Change the solution in the reservoir at least every 6 days, change the infusion set, and the infusion set insertion site at least every 3 days. Do not mix with other insulins or with a diluent when used in the pump.
- **IV:** *Insulin aspart* and *insulin glulisine* may be administered IV in selected situations under appropriate medical supervision. ***Diluent:*** Dilute *insulin aspart* with 0.9% NaCl or D5W in infusion systems using polypropylene infusion bags. Dilute *insulin glulisine* with 0.9% NaCl, using polyvinyl chloride (PVC) Viaflex infusion bags and Polyvinyl chloride (PVC) tubing (Clearlink System Continu-Flo solution

set) with a dedicated infusion line. ***Concentration:*** 0.05–1 unit/mL. *Insulin lispro Humalog U-100* can be administered IV under medical supervision ONLY with close monitoring of blood glucose and potassium levels to avoid hypoglycemia and hypokalemia. ***Concentration:*** 0.1 unit/mL to 1 unit/mL. ***Diluent:*** 0.9% NaCl. Solutions of insulin lispro and 0.9% NaCl can be stored for 48 hrs in refrigerator, then used at room temperature for another 48 hr.

Patient/Family Teaching

- Instruct patient on proper technique for administration. Include type of insulin, equipment (syringe, cartridge pens, external pump, alcohol swabs), storage, and place to discard syringes. Discuss the importance of not changing brands of insulin or syringes, selection and rotation of injection sites, and compliance with therapeutic regimen. Caution patient that insulin pens should not be shared with others, even if clean needles are used.
- Demonstrate technique for mixing insulins by drawing up insulin aspart, insulin glulisine, or insulin lispro first. Roll intermediate-acting insulin vial between palms to mix, rather than shaking (may cause inaccurate dose).
- Caution patient not to share pen device with another person, even if needle is changed; may risk transmission of blood-borne pathogens.
- Explain to patient that this medication controls hyperglycemia but does not cure diabetes. Therapy is long term.
- Instruct patient in proper testing of serum glucose and ketones. These tests should be closely monitored during periods of stress or illness and health care professional notified of significant changes.
- Emphasize the importance of compliance with nutritional guidelines and regular exercise as directed by health care professional.
- Advise patient to notify health care professional of all Rx or OTC medications, vitamins, or herbal products being taken and to consult with health care professional before taking other medications or alcohol.
- Advise patient to notify health care professional of medication regimen prior to treatment or surgery.
- Advise patient to notify health care professional if nausea, vomiting, or fever develops, if unable to eat regular diet, or if blood glucose levels are not controlled.
- Instruct patient on signs and symptoms of hypoglycemia and hyperglycemia and what to do if they occur.
- Advise patient to notify health care professional if pregnancy is planned or suspected or if breast feeding or planning to breast feed.
- Patients with diabetes mellitus should carry a source of sugar (candy, glucose gel) and identification describing their disease and treatment regimen at all times.
- Emphasize the importance of regular follow-up, especially during first few weeks of therapy.

Evaluation/Desired Outcomes

- Control of blood glucose levels without the appearance of hypoglycemic or hyperglycemic episodes.

INTERFERONS, ALPHA

(in-ter-**feer**-onz)

peginterferon alpha-2a
Pegasys

interferon alpha-2b
Intron A

peginterferon alpha-2b
Sylatron

interferon alpha-n3
Alferon N

Classification
Therapeutic: immune modifiers
Pharmacologic: interferons

Pregnancy Category C

Indications

Peginterferon alpha-2a: Treatment of: Chronic hepatitis C (alone or with ribavirin) (should only be used as monotherapy if patients have contraindication to or do not tolerate other antiviral drugs), Chronic hepatitis B. **Interferon alpha-2b:** Treatment of: Hairy cell leukemia, Malignant melanoma, AIDS-related Kaposi's sarcoma, Condylomata acuminata (intralesional), Chronic hepatitis B, Chronic hepatitis C (with oral ribavirin) which has relapsed following previous treatment with interferon alone, Follicular non-Hodgkin's lymphoma. **Peginterferon alpha–2b:** Adjuvant treatment of melanoma with microscopic or gross nodal involvement within 84 days of definitive surgical resection including complete lymphadenectomy. **Interferon alpha-n3:** Treatment of condylomata acuminata (intralesional).

Action

Interferons are proteins capable of modifying the immune response and have antiproliferative action against tumor cells. Interferon alpha-2b is produced by recombinant DNA techniques, peginterferon is a "pegylated" formulation of interferon alpha-2b formulated to have a longer duration of action; interferon alpha-n3 is from pooled human leukocytes. Interferons also have antiviral activity. Unknown mechanism for melanoma. **Therapeutic Effects:** Antineoplastic, antiviral, and antiproliferative activity. Decreased progression of hepatic damage (for patients with hepatitis). Improved relapse-free survival (for melanoma).

Pharmacokinetics

Absorption: Not absorbed orally. Well absorbed (>80%) following IM and subcut administration. Minimal systemic absorption follows intralesional administration.

Distribution: Unknown.

Metabolism and Excretion: Filtered by the kidneys and subsequently degraded in the renal tubule; *peginterferon alpha-2b*—30% renally excreted.

Half-life: *Peginterferon alpha-2a*—50–160 hr; *interferon alpha-2b*—2–3 hr; *peginterferon alpha-2b*—40 hr.

TIME/ACTION PROFILE (clinical effects)

ROUTE	ONSET	PEAK	DURATION
Interferon alpha-2b IM, subcut	1–3 mo	unknown	unknown (CR)
Interferon alpha-2b IM, subcut	unknown	3–5 days	3–5 days (BC)
Interferon alpha-2b IM, subcut	2 wk	unknown	unknown (LFT)
Interferon alpha-2b and n3	unknown	4–8 wk	unknown (IL)
Peginterferon alpha-2b subcut	unknown	6 mos or more	unknown

BC = effects on platelet counts; CR = clinical response; IL= regression of lesions; LFT = effects on liver function in patients with hepatitis.

Contraindications/Precautions

Contraindicated in: Hypersensitivity to alpha interferons or human serum albumin; Autoimmune hepatitis; Hepatic decompensation (Child-Pugh class B and C) before or during therapy; Pedi: Products containing benzyl alcohol should not be used in neonates.

Use Cautiously in: Severe cardiovascular, pulmonary, renal, or hepatic disease; CCr <50 mL/min (dose of peginterferon alfa-2b ↓ may be necessary; do not use combination therapy); Active infections; Underlying CNS pathology or psychiatric history; ↓ bone marrow reserve or underlying immunosuppression; Current history of chickenpox, herpes zoster, or herpes labialis (may reactivate or disseminate disease); Previous or concurrent radiation therapy; Autoimmune disorders (may ↑ risk of exacerbation); OB: ↑ risk of spontaneous abortion in animal studies; use only if potential fetal risks are outweighed by potential maternal benefit; women with childbearing potential should be advised of potential risk to fetus; ribavirin is contraindicated in pregnancy and lactation and in men whose female partners are pregnant; Lactation: Usually compatible with breast feeding (AAP); Pedi: Children <3 yr (<18 yr for Sylatron) (safety not established); Geri: ↑ risk of adverse reactions.

Exercise Extreme Caution in: History of depression/suicide attempt.

Adverse Reactions/Side Effects

All are more prominent with subcut, IV, or IM administration.

CNS: HOMICIDAL IDEATION, SUICIDAL IDEATION/ATTEMPTS, confusion, depression, dizziness, fatigue, headache, insomnia, irritability, aggression, anxiety. **EENT:** blurred vision, nose bleeds, rhinitis. **CV:** ISCHEMIC DISORDERS, edema, arrhythmias, chest pain, heart block. **GI:** COLITIS, HEPATOTOXICITY, PANCREATITIS, anorexia, abdominal pain, diarrhea, dry mouth, ↑ liver enzymes, nausea, taste disorder, vomiting, weight loss, flatulence. **Derm:** alopecia, dry skin, pruritus, rash, sweating. **Endo:** ↓ growth (children), thyroid disorders. **Hemat:** LEUKOPENIA, THROMBOCYTOPENIA, anemia, hemolytic anemia (with ribavirin). **MS:** arthralgia, myalgia, leg cramps. **Neuro:** paresthesia. **Resp:** cough, dyspnea. **Local:** injection site reactions. **Misc:** AUTOIMMUNE DISORDERS, INFECTIOUS DISORDERS, allergic reactions including ANAPHYLAXIS, chills, fever, flu-like syndrome.

Interactions

Drug-Drug: Additive myelosuppression with other **antineoplastic agents** or **radiation therapy**. ↑ CNS depression may occur with **CNS depressants**, including **alcohol**, **antihistamines**, **sedative/hypnotics**, and **opioids**. May ↓ metabolism and ↑ blood levels and toxicity of **theophylline** and **methadone**. ↑ risk of adverse reactions with **zidovudine**. **Ribavirin** ↑ risk of hemolytic anemia, especially if CCr <50 mL/min (avoid if possible). May ↓ effects of **immunosuppressant agents**. Peginterferon alfa-2b may ↑ levels and effects of **CYP1A2 substrates** and **CYP2D6 substrates**.

Route/Dosage

Peginterferon Alpha-2a

Subcut (Adults): *Chronic hepatitis C*—180 mcg once weekly for 48 wk for Genotypes 1,4 (24 wk for Genotypes 2,3). ***Patients with chronic hepatitis C co-infected with HIV***—180 mcg once weekly for 48 wk. *Chronic hepatitis B*—180 mcg once weekly for 48 wk.

Subcut (Children 5–17 yr): *Chronic hepatitis C (Genotype 1 or 4)*—180 mcg/1.73 m^2 X BSA once weekly (not to exceed 180 mcg) (with PO ribavirin) for 48 wk (should be used in combination with hepatitis C virus NS3/4A protease inhibitor in patients with genotype 1 infection); *Chronic hepatitis C (Genotype 2 or 3)*—180 mcg/1.73 m^2 X BSA once weekly (not to exceed 180 mcg) (with PO ribavirin) for 24 wk.

Renal Impairment

Subcut (Adults): *CCr 30–50 mL/min*—180 mcg once weekly (with PO ribavirin 200 mg alternating with

400 mg every other day) *CCr <30 mL/min (including hemodialysis)*—135 mcg once weekly (with PO ribavirin 200 mg once daily).

Interferon Alpha-2b

IV (Adults): *Malignant melanoma (induction)*—20 million units/m² for 5 days of each week for 4 wk initially, followed by subcut maintenance dosing.
IM, Subcut (Adults): *Hairy cell leukemia*—2 million units/m² IM or subcut 3 times weekly for up to 6 mo. *Malignant melanoma (maintenance)*—10 million units/m² subcut 3 times weekly for 48 wk, following initial IV dosing. *AIDS-related Kaposi's sarcoma*—30 million units/m² IM or subcut 3 times weekly until disease progression or maximum response has been achieved after 16 wk. *Chronic hepatitis C*—3 million units IM or subcut 3 times weekly. If normalization of ALT occurs after 16 wk of therapy, continue treatment for total of 18–24 mo. If normalization of ALT does not occur after 16 wk of therapy, may consider discontinuing treatment. *Chronic hepatitis B*—5 million units/day IM or subcut *or* 10 million units IM or subcut 3 times weekly for 16 wk. *Follicular non-Hodgkin's lymphoma*—5 million units subcut 3 times weekly for up to 18 mo (to be used following completion of anthracycline-containing chemotherapy).
Subcut (Children >3 yr): *Chronic hepatitis B*—3 million units/m² 3 times weekly for the first week of therapy then increase to 6 million units/m² 3 times weekly (not to exceed 10 million units/dose) for 16 to 24 weeks.
IL (Adults): *Condylomata acuminata*—1 million units/lesion 3 times weekly for 3 wk; treat only 5 lesions per course. An additional course of treatment may be initiated at 12–16 wk.

Peginterferon Alpha-2b

Subcut (Adults): 6 mcg/kg/wk for 8 doses, then 3 mcg/kg/wk for up to 5 yr.

Renal Impairment

Subcut (Adults): *CCr 30–50 mL/min*—4.5 mcg/kg/wk for 8 doses, then 2.25 mcg/kg/wk for up to 5 yr; *CCr <30 mL/min or on hemodialysis*—3 mcg/kg/wk for 8 doses, then 1.5 mcg/kg/wk for up to 5 yr.

Interferon Alpha-n3

IL (Adults): 250,000 units/lesion twice weekly for up to 8 wk; for large lesions, divide dose and inject at several sites.

Availability

Peginterferon Alpha-2a

Solution for injection: 180 mcg/mL in single use vials, 180 mcg/0.5 mL in prefilled syringes and pens, 135 mcg/0.5 mL in prefilled pens.

Interferon Alpha-2b

Powder for injection: 10 million units/vial, 18 million units/vial, 50 million units/vial. **Solution for injection:** 6 million units/mL, 10 million units/mL.

Peginterferon Alpha-2b

Powder for injection (Sylatron): 200 mcg/vial, 300 mcg/vial, 600 mcg/vial.

Interferon Alpha-n3

Solution for injection: 5 million units/mL.

NURSING IMPLICATIONS

Assessment

- Assess for signs of neuropsychiatric disorders (irritability, anxiety, depression, suicidal ideation, aggressive behavior). For patients taking interferon alfa 2a, *if depression is mild*, visit weekly by phone or in person. *If depression is moderate*, decrease interferon alfa 2a dose to 135 mcg or to 90 mcg if needed; see in office at least every other week. Consider psychiatric counseling. If symptoms improve and are stable for 4 wks, may return to regular visit schedule and may increase dose. *If depression is severe*, obtain psychiatric consultation and discontinue interferon alfa 2a or peginterferon alpha 2b permanently.
- Monitor for signs of infection (vital signs, WBC) during therapy. Discontinue drug therapy in cases of severe infection, and antibiotic therapy instituted.
- Assess for cardiovascular disorders (pulse, BP, chest pain). An ECG should be performed before and periodically during the course of therapy in patients with a history of cardiovascular disease.
- Assess for signs of colitis (abdominal pain, bloody diarrhea, fever) and pancreatitis (nausea, vomiting, abdominal pain) during therapy. Discontinue therapy if these occur; may be fatal. Colitis usually resolves within 1–3 wk of discontinuation.
- Assess for development of flu-like syndrome (fever, chills, myalgia, headache). Symptoms often appear suddenly 3–6 hr after therapy. Symptoms tend to decrease, even with continued therapy. Acetaminophen may be used for control of these symptoms.
- Monitor for bone marrow depression. Assess for bleeding (bleeding gums; bruising; petechiae; guaiac stools, urine, and emesis) and avoid IM injections and rectal temperatures if platelet count is low. Apply pressure to venipuncture sites for 10 min. Assess for signs of infection during neutropenia. Anemia may occur. Monitor for increased fatigue, dyspnea, and orthostatic hypotension.
- May cause nausea and vomiting. Antiemetics may be used prophylactically. Monitor intake and output, daily weight, and appetite. Adjust diet as tolerated for anorexia. Encourage fluid intake of at least 2 L/day.

- Assess pulmonary status (lung sounds, respirations) periodically during therapy.
- Perform a baseline eye exam in all patients prior to initiation of therapy. Eye exams should be performed periodically during therapy in patients with pre-existing diabetic or hypertensive retinopathy. Discontinue therapy if patients develop new or worsening eye disorders.
- Assess for signs of thyroid dysfunction, as hypothyroidism or hyperthyroidism may occur. Discontinue therapy if the patient's thyroid function cannot be controlled with medications (e.g., thyroid hormone supplementation, antithyroid medications).
- **Kaposi's Sarcoma:** Monitor number, size, and character of lesions prior to and throughout therapy.
- ***Lab Test Considerations:*** **Systemic:** Monitor for CBC and differential and electrolytes prior to and periodically during therapy. May cause leukopenia, neutropenia, thrombocytopenia, ↓ hemoglobin and hematocrit, and hemolytic anemia. The nadirs of leukopenia and thrombocytopenia occur in 3–5 days, with recovery 3–5 days after withdrawal of *interferon alpha-2b*. For malignant melanoma, if granulocyte count >250/mm³ but <500/mm³, discontinue *interferon alpha-2b* until platelet or granulocyte counts return to normal or baseline levels, then reinstitute at 50% of dose. If granulocyte count <250/mm³ with *interferon alpha-2b*, discontinue permanently. For follicular non-Hodgkin's lymphoma, if granulocyte count <1000/mm³ or platelet count <50,000/mm³, discontinue *interferon alpha-2b*. *Peginterferon alpha-2b* should be discontinued if granulocyte count <1000/mm³ or platelet count <50,000/mm³. *Peginterferon alpha-2a* should be discontinued if ANC <500/mm³ or platelet count <25,000/mm³ and then may be restarted at a lower dose if the ANC >1000/mm³.
- Platelet count should be ≥90,000 cells/mm³ and ANC ≥1500 cells/mm³ prior to initiation of peginterferon therapy. Commonly causes ↓ hemoglobin, hematocrit, WBC, ANC, lymphocytes and platelet counts within first 2 wk of therapy.
- *For interferon alpha 2b:* Monitor hepatic function with serum bilirubin, ALT, AST, alkaline phosphatase, and LDH at 2, 8 and 12 wks following initiation of therapy, then every 6 months while receiving therapy. Permanently discontinue interferon alpha 2b for severe hepatic injury.
- *For Peginterferon alpha-2a:* Monitor liver function tests (AST, ALT, LDH, bilirubin, alkaline phosphatase), triglycerides, and renal function tests (BUN, creatinine, uric acid, urinalysis) prior to and periodically during therapy. CCr should be >50 mL/min prior to initiation of peginterferon therapy. *Peginterferon alpha-2a* should be discontinued if liver function diminishes.
- Monitor TSH at baseline and if patients develop symptoms consistent with hypothyroidism or hyperthyroidism. TSH must be within normal limits at start of therapy. Monitor at 3 and 6 months.
- **Chronic Hepatitis C:** *For interferon alpha 2b:* Monitor CBC and platelet counts prior to initiation of therapy to establish baselines for monitoring toxicity. Repeat tests at at Wks 1 and 2 following initiation of therapy, and monthly thereafter. Evaluate serum ALT at 3-month intervals to assess response to treatment. **Chronic Hepatitis B:** *For interferon alpha 2b:* Monitor CBC and platelet counts prior to initiation of therapy to establish baselines for monitoring toxicity. Repeat tests at treatment Weeks 1, 2, 4, 8, 12, and 16. Monitor liver function tests (serum ALT, albumin, bilirubin) at treatment Weeks 1, 2, 4, 8, 12, and 16. Evaluate HBeAg, HBsAg, and ALT at the end of therapy, 3- and 6-months posttherapy; patients may become virologic responders during 6-month period following end of therapy. If ALT ↑ continue therapy unless signs and symptoms of liver failure occur. During ↑ monitor clinical symptoms and liver function tests (ALT, prothrombin time, alkaline phosphatase, albumin, bilirubin) at 2-wk intervals. Discontinue therapy if signs and symptoms of liver failure occur. **Hairy Cell Leukemia:** Monitor number of peripheral blood hairy cells and bone marrow hairy cells prior to and during therapy.

Potential Nursing Diagnoses

Risk for injury (Side Effects)
Risk for infection (Side Effects)

Implementation

- Solution should be prepared in a biologic cabinet. Wear gloves, gown, and mask while handling medication. Discard equipment in specially designated containers.

Interferon Alpha-2b

- **IM, Subcut:** Subcut route is preferred for patients with a platelet count <50,000/mm³.
- Reconstitute 10-, 18-, and 50-million-unit vials with 1 mL of diluent provided by manufacturer (sterile water for injection). Agitate gently. Solution may be colorless to light yellow. Solution should be used immediately; stable for up to 24 hr if refrigerated.
- The solution for injection vials do not require reconstitution prior to use and may be used for IM, subcut, or intralesional administration.
- The solution for injection in multidose pens are for subcut use only. Only the needles provided in the package should be used with the pen. A new needle should be used with each dose. Follow instructions in *Medication Guide* for use of multidose pens.
- **IL:** Reconstitute 10-million-unit vial with 1 mL of diluent provided by manufacturer (sterile water for injection). Use a TB syringe with 25–30-gauge needle to administer. Each 0.1-mL dose is injected into the center of the base of the wart using the intradermal injection approach. As many as 5 lesions can be treated at one time.

IV Administration

- **Intermittent Infusion:** (For Malignant Melanoma). ***Diluent:*** Add 1 mL of diluent provided by manufacturer (sterile water for injection) to vial. Further dilute appropriate dose in 100 mL of 0.9% NaCl. Solution should be used immediately; stable for 24 hr if refrigerated. The solution for injection vials are not recommended for IV administration. ***Concentration:*** Final concentration of infusion should not be less than 10 million units/100 mL. ***Rate:*** Infuse over 20 min.

Peginterferon Alpha-2a

- Vials and pre-filled syringes should be stored in refrigerator. Do not administer solution that is cloudy or contains a precipitate.
- Follow instructions in *Medication Guide* for use of pre-filled syringes.

Peginterferon Alpha-2b

- Reconstitute vial with 0.7 mL of diluent provided by manufacturer (sterile water for injection). Administer immediately; stable for 24 hr if refrigerated. Solution should be clear and colorless. Discard unused solution.

Interferon Alpha-n3

- Vials should be refrigerated.

Patient/Family Teaching

- Advise patient to take medication as directed. If a dose is missed, omit dose and return to the regular schedule. Notify health care professional if more than 1 dose is missed.
- **Home Care Issues:** Instruct patient and family on preparation and correct technique for administration of injection and care and disposal of equipment. Advise patient to read *Medication Guide* prior to administration and with each prescription refill to check for changes. Explain to patient that brands should not be switched without consulting health care professional; may result in a change of dose.
- Discuss possibility of flu-like reaction 3–6 hr after dose. Acetaminophen may be taken prior to injection and every 3–4 hr afterward as needed to control symptoms.
- Review side effects with patient. Interferon may be temporarily discontinued or dose decreased by 50% if serious side effects occur.
- Instruct patient to notify health care professional promptly if fever; chills; cough; hoarseness; sore throat; signs of infection; lower back or side pain; painful or difficult urination; bleeding gums; bruising; petechiae; blood in stools, urine, or emesis; increased fatigue; dyspnea; or orthostatic hypotension occurs. Caution patient to avoid crowds and persons with known infections. Instruct patient to use soft toothbrush and electric razor and to avoid falls. Caution patient not to drink alcoholic beverages or take medication containing aspirin or NSAIDs; may precipitate gastric bleeding.
- Advise patient and family to notify health care professional if thoughts about suicide or dying, attempts to commit suicide; new or worse depression; new or worse anxiety; feeling very agitated or restless; panic attacks; trouble sleeping; new or worse irritability; acting aggressive; being angry or violent; acting on dangerous impulses; an extreme increase in activity and talking, other unusual changes in behavior or mood occur.
- Discuss with patient the possibility of hair loss. Explore coping strategies.
- Explain to patient that fertility may be impaired and that contraception is needed during treatment to prevent potential harm to the fetus.
- Instruct patient not to receive any vaccinations without advice of health care professional.
- Emphasize need for periodic lab tests to monitor for side effects.
- Inform patient that peginterferon alpha-2a may not reduce the risk of transmission of HCV to others or prevent cirrhosis, liver failure, or liver cancer.

Evaluation/Desired Outcomes

- Normalized blood parameters (hemoglobin, neutrophils, platelets, monocytes, and bone marrow and peripheral hairy cells) in hairy cell leukemia. Response may not be seen for 6 mo with *interferon alpha-2b*.
- Decrease in the size and number of lesions in Kaposi's sarcoma. Therapy may be required for 6 mo before full response is seen. Therapy is continued until disease progresses or a maximum response has been achieved after 4 mo of therapy.
- Increase in time to relapse and overall survival in patients with malignant melanoma.
- Disappearance of or decrease in size and number of genital warts. Condylomata acuminata usually respond in 4–8 wk. A second course of therapy may be required if genital warts persist and laboratory values remain in acceptable limits.
- Decrease in symptoms and improvement in liver function tests and ↓ progression of hepatic damage in patients with hepatitis B or hepatitis C infection. Discontinue *Peginterferon alpha-2a* therapy if patient fails to demonstrate at least a 2 log10 reduction from baseline in HCV RNA titer by 12 weeks of therapy or undetectable HCV RNA after 24 weeks of therapy.

INTERFERONS, BETA
(in-ter-**feer**-on)

inteferon beta-1a
Avonex, Rebif

interferon beta-1b
Betaseron, Extavia

Classification
Therapeutic: anti-multiple sclerosis agents, immune modifiers
Pharmacologic: interferons

Pregnancy Category C

Indications
Relapsing forms of multiple sclerosis.

Action
Antiviral and immunoregulatory properties produced by interacting with specific receptor sites on cell surfaces may explain beneficial effects. Produced by recombinant DNA technology. **Therapeutic Effects:** Reduce incidence of relapse (neurologic dysfunction) and slow physical disability.

Pharmacokinetics
Absorption: *Interferon beta-1b*—50% absorbed following subcut administration.
Distribution: Unknown.
Metabolism and Excretion: Unknown.
Half-life: *Interferon beta-1a*—69 hr (subcut), 10 hr (IM); *interferon beta-1b*—8 min–4.3 hr.

TIME/ACTION PROFILE (serum concentrations)

ROUTE	ONSET	PEAK	DURATION
Interferon beta-1a IM, subcut	unknown	3–15 h	unknown
Interferon beta-1b subcut	rapid	16 h	unknown

Contraindications/Precautions
Contraindicated in: Hypersensitivity to natural or recombinant interferon beta or human albumin.
Use Cautiously in: History of suicide attempt or depression; History of seizures (interferon beta-1a); Cardiovascular disease; Congestive HF (may worsen HF); Liver disease (interferon beta-1a); History of alcohol abuse (interferon beta-1a); Patients with childbearing potential; OB: May ↑ risk of spontaneous abortion; use only if potential maternal benefit outweighs potential fetal risk; Lactation: Safety not established; Pedi: Safety not established.

Adverse Reactions/Side Effects
CNS: SEIZURES (↑ WITH INTERFERON BETA-1A), depression, dizziness, fatigue, headache, insomnia, drowsiness, incoordination, rigors, suicidal ideation. **EENT:** sinusitis, vision abnormalities. **Resp:** dyspnea, upper respiratory tract infection. **CV:** chest pain, edema, hypertension. **GI:** constipation, nausea, vomiting, abdominal pain, autoimmune hepatitis, dry mouth, ↑ liver enzymes. **GU:** cystitis, erectile dysfunction, polyuria, urinary incontinence. **Derm:** ERYTHEMA MULTIFORME, STEVENS-JOHNSON SYNDROME, rash, alopecia, ↑ sweating. **Endo:** menstrual disorders, hyperthyroidism, hypothyroidism, menorrhagia, spontaneous abortion. **Hemat:** neutropenia, anemia, eosinophilia, thrombocytopenia. **Local:** injection-site reactions, injection site necrosis. **MS:** myalgia, arthralgia, muscle spasm. **Misc:** allergic reactions including ANAPHYLAXIS, chills, fever, flu-like symptoms, pain.

Interactions
(All interactions below are for Interferon beta-1b).
Drug-Drug: ↑ myelosuppression may occur with other myelosuppressives including **antineoplastics**. Concurrent use of **hepatotoxic agents** may ↑ the risk of hepatotoxicity (↑ liver enzymes).
Drug-Natural Products: Avoid concommitant use with immmunomodulating natural products such as **astragalus**, **echinacea**, and **melatonin**.

Route/Dosage

Interferon Beta-1a
IM (Adults): *Avonex*—30 mcg once weekly.
Subcut (Adults): *Rebif (target dose of 22 mcg 3 times/wk)*—Start with 4.4 mcg 3 times/wk for 2 wk, then ↑ to 11 mcg 3 times/wk for 2 wk, then ↑ to maintenance dose of 22 mcg 3 times/wk. *Rebif (target dose of 44 mcg 3 times/wk)*—Start with 8.8 mcg 3 times/wk for 2 wk, then ↑ to 22 mcg 3 times/wk for 2 wk, then ↑ to maintenance dose of 44 mcg 3 times/wk.

Interferon Beta-1b
Subcut (Adults): Initiate with 0.0625 mg (2 million units) every other day and then ↑ dose by 0.0625 mg q 2 wk over a 6-wk period up to target dose of 0.25 mg (8 million units) every other day.

Availability

Interferon Beta-1a
Powder for injection (Avonex): 30 mcg/vial. **Prefilled syringes (Avonex):** 30 mcg/0.5 mL. **Prefilled pens (Avonex):** 30 mcg/0.5 mL. **Pre-illed syringes (Rebif):** 22 mcg/0.5 mL, 44 mcg/0.5 mL, titration pack of 6 syringes prefilled with 8.8 mcg/0.2 mL and 6 syringes prefilled with 22 mcg/0.5 mL.

Interferon Beta-1b
Powder for injection: 0.3 mg/vial.

NURSING IMPLICATIONS

Assessment
- Assess frequency of exacerbations of symptoms of multiple sclerosis periodically during therapy.

- Monitor patient for signs of depression during therapy. If depression occurs, notify health care professional immediately; discontinuation of therapy should be considered.
- ***Lab Test Considerations:*** Monitor hemoglobin, WBC, platelets, and blood chemistries including liver function tests prior to and 1, 3, and 6 mo after initiation of therapy and periodically thereafter. Therapy may be temporarily discontinued if the absolute neutrophil count is <750/mm^3, if AST or ALT exceeds 10 times the upper limit of normal, or if serum bilirubin exceeds 5 times the upper limit of normal. Once the absolute neutrophil count is >750/mm^3 or the hepatic enzymes have returned to normal, therapy can be restarted at 50% of the original dose.
- Thyroid function tests should be monitored every 6 mo, especially in patients with a history of thyroid abnormalities.

Potential Nursing Diagnoses

Deficient knowledge, related to medication regimen (Patient/Family Teaching)

Implementation

- Do not confuse products. Interferon beta-1a and interferon beta-1b are not interchangeable.
- **Interferon Beta-1a:** *Avonex:* Reconstitute with 1.1 mL of diluent and swirl gently to dissolve. Do not shake the vial. Inject into the thigh or upper arm. Keep reconstituted solution in refrigerator; inject within 6 hr of reconstitution.
- *Rebif:* Administer subcut via pre-filled, single-use syringe at the same time (afternoon or evening) on the same days (Monday, Wednesday, Friday) at least 48 hr apart each wk. Rotate sites with each injection to minimize risk of injection site reactions (pain, erythema, edema, cellulitis, abcess, necrosis). Avoid areas that are inflamed, edematous, erythematous, ecchymotic, or has signs of infection. Discard unused portions. Store in refrigerator.
- **Interferon Beta-1b:** To reconstitute, inject 1.2 mL of diluent supplied into interferon beta-1b vial for a concentration of 0.25 mg/mL. Swirl gently to dissolve completely; do not shake. Do not use solutions that are discolored or contain particulate matter. Keep reconstituted solution refrigerated; inject within 3 hr of reconstitution.
- Following reconstitution, withdraw 1 mL into a syringe with a 27-gauge needle and inject subcut into arm, abdomen, hip, or thigh. Pinch skin during injection and inject at a 90° angle. Gently massage injection site. Rotate sites with each injection to minimize risk of injection site reactions. Discard unused portion; vials are for single dose only.

Patient/Family Teaching

- **Home Care Issues:** Instruct patient in correct technique for injection and care and disposal of equipment. Caution patient not to reuse needles or syringes and provide patient with a puncture-resistant container for disposal.
- Instruct patient to take medication as directed; do not change dose or schedule without consulting health care professional. Patients should receive a medication guide with each product.
- Advise patient and family to notify health care professional if thoughts about suicide or dying, attempts to commit suicide; new or worse depression; new or worse anxiety; feeling very agitated or restless; panic attacks; trouble sleeping; new or worse irritability; acting aggressive; being angry or violent; acting on dangerous impulses; an extreme increase in activity and talking, other unusual changes in behavior or mood occur.
- Inform patient that flu-like symptoms (fever, chills, myalgia, sweating, malaise) may occur during therapy. Acetaminophen may be used for relief of fever and myalgias.
- Advise patient to notify health care professional if pregnancy is planned or suspected or if breast feeding.

Evaluation/Desired Outcomes

- Decrease in the frequency of relapse (neurologic dysfunction) in patients with relapsing-remitting multiple sclerosis.

IODINE, IODIDE

potassium iodide†
Pima, SSKI, ThyroSafe, ThyroShield

strong iodine solution
Lugol's solution

Classification
Therapeutic: antithyroid agents
Pharmacologic: iodine containing agents

Pregnancy Category D

†For more information on potassium iodide as a radiation protectant see *Potassium Iodide as a Thyroid Blocking Agent in Radiation Emergencies* at www.fda.gov

Indications

Adjunct with other antithyroid drugs in preparation for thyroidectomy. Treatment of thyrotoxic crisis. Radiation protectant following radiation emergencies or administration of radioactive iodine.

Action

Rapidly inhibits the release and synthesis of thyroid hormones. Decreases the vascularity of the thyroid gland. Decreases thyroidal uptake of radioactive iodine following radiation emergencies or administration of radioactive isotopes of iodine. Iodine is a necessary component of thyroid hormone. **Therapeutic Effects:** Control of hyperthyroidism. Decreased bleeding during thyroid surgery. Decreased incidence of thyroid cancer following radiation emergencies.

Pharmacokinetics

Absorption: Converted in the GI tract and enters the circulation as iodine; also absorbed through skin and lungs; may also be obtained via recycling of iodothyronines.

Distribution: Concentrates in the thyroid gland and muscle; also found in skin, skeleton, breasts, and hair. Readily crosses the placenta; enters breast milk.

Metabolism and Excretion: Taken up by the thyroid gland, then eliminated via kidneys, liver, skin, lungs, and intestines.

Half-life: Unknown.

TIME/ACTION PROFILE (effects on thyroid)

ROUTE	ONSET	PEAK	DURATION
PO	24 hr	10–15 days	variable†

†Radiation protection lasts 24 hr.

Contraindications/Precautions

Contraindicated in: Hypersensitivity; Hyperkalemia; Pulmonary edema; Impaired renal function.

Use Cautiously in: Tuberculosis; Bronchitis; Cardiovascular disease; OB, Pedi: Pregnancy or lactation (although iodine is required during pregnancy, excess amounts may cause thyroid abnormalities/goiter in the newborn; excess use during lactation may cause skin rash or thyroid suppression in the infant).

Adverse Reactions/Side Effects

CNS: confusion, weakness. **GI:** GI BLEEDING, diarrhea, nausea, vomiting. **Derm:** acneiform eruptions. **Endo:** hypothyroidism, goiter, hyperthyroidism. **F and E:** hyperkalemia. **Neuro:** tingling. **MS:** joint pain. **Misc:** hypersensitivity, iodism.

Interactions

Drug-Drug: Use with **lithium** may cause ↑ hypothyroidism. ↑ antithyroid effect of **methimazole** and **propylthiouracil**. ↑ hyperkalemia may result from combined use with **potassium-sparing diuretics**, **ACE inhibitors**, **angiotensin II receptor antagonists** or **potassium supplements**.

Route/Dosage

Preparation for Thyroidectomy

PO (Adults and Children): *Strong iodine solution*—3–5 drops (0.1–0.3 mL) 3 times daily for 10 days prior to surgery. *Potassium iodide saturated solution* (SSKI)—1–5 drops (50–250 mg) 3 times daily for 10 days prior to surgery.

Hyperthyroidism

PO (Adults and Children): *Strong iodine solution*—1 mL in water 3 times daily. *Potassium iodide saturated solution (SSKI)*—6–10 drops (300–500 mg) 3 times daily.

PO (Infants <1 yr): 3–5 drops (150–250 mg) 3 times daily.

Radiation Protectant to Radioactive Isotopes of Iodine

PO (Adults): *Pima*—195 mg once daily for 10 days (start 24 hr prior to exposure (continue until risk of exposure has passed or other measures have been implemented).

PO (Children >1 yr): 130 mg once daily for 10 days (start 24 hr prior to exposure).

PO (Infants <1 yr): 65 mg once daily for 10 days (start 24 hr prior to exposure).

Reduction of Thyroid Cancer after Nuclear Accident

PO (Adults and Children >68 kg, including pregnant/lactating women): *Iosat, ThyroSafe, ThyroShield*—130 mg once daily (continue until risk of exposure has passed or other measures have been implemented).

PO (Children 3–18 yr): 65 mg once daily.

PO (Children 1 mo–3 yr): 32.5 mg once daily.

PO (Infants <1 mo): 16.25 mg once daily.

Availability

Potassium Iodide (generic available)

Oral solution: 65 mg/mL (ThyroShield), 1 g potassium iodide/mL (SSKI). **Syrup (Pima) (black-raspberry flavor):** 325 mg potassium iodide/5 mL. **Tablets:** 65 mg^{OTC}, 130 mg^{OTC}(available only through state and federal agencies).

Strong Iodine Solution (generic available)

Oral solution: Iodine 50 mg/mL plus potassium iodide 100 mg/mL.

NURSING IMPLICATIONS

Assessment

- Assess for signs and symptoms of iodism (metallic taste, stomatitis, skin lesions, cold symptoms, severe GI upset). Report these symptoms promptly.
- Monitor response symptoms of hyperthyroidism (tachycardia, palpitations, nervousness, insomnia, diaphoresis, heat intolerance, tremors, weight loss).
- Monitor for hypersensitivity reaction (rash, pruritus, laryngeal edema, wheezing). Discontinue drug and notify physician immediately if these problems occur.
- ***Lab Test Considerations:*** Monitor thyroid function before and periodically during therapy. May alter results of radionuclide thyroid imaging and may ↓ thyroidal uptake of ^{131}I, ^{123}I, and sodium pertechnetate ^{99m}Tc in thyroid uptake tests.

- Monitor serum potassium levels periodically during therapy.
- ***Lab Test Considerations:*** Monitor thyroid stimulating hormone (TSH) and free T_4 in neonates (within the first month of life) treated with potassium iodide for development of hypothyroidism. Thyroid hormone therapy should be instituted if hypothyroidism develops.

Potential Nursing Diagnoses

Deficient knowledge, related to medication regimen (Patient/Family Teaching)

Implementation

- Do not confuse iodine with Lodine (etodolac).
- For protection against inhaled radioiodines, administer potassium iodide prior to or immediately coincident with passage of the radioactive cloud, though a substantial protective effect lasts 3–4 hr after exposure.
- **PO:** Mix solutions in a full glass of fruit juice, water, broth, formula, or milk. Administer after meals to minimize GI irritation.
- Solution is normally clear and colorless. Darkening upon standing does not affect potency of drug. Solutions that are brownish yellow should be discarded.
- Crystals may form, especially if refrigerated, but redissolve upon warming and shaking.

Patient/Family Teaching

- Instruct patient to take medication as directed. Take missed doses as soon as possible but not just before next dose; do not double doses.
- Instruct patient to report suspected pregnancy to health care professional before therapy is initiated.
- Advise patient to consult health care professional about avoiding foods high in iodine (seafood, iodized salt, cabbage, kale, turnips) or potassium (see Appendix J).
- Advise patient to consult health care professional before using OTC or herbal cold remedies. Some cold remedies use iodide as an expectorant.
- **Hyperthyroidism:** Instruct patient to take medication as ordered. Missing a dose may precipitate hyperthyroidism.

Evaluation/Desired Outcomes

- Resolution of the symptoms of thyroid crisis.
- Decrease in size and vascularity of the gland before thyroid surgery. Use of iodides in the treatment of hyperthyroidism is usually limited to 2 wk.
- Protection of the thyroid gland from the effects of radioactive iodine.

REMS

ipilimumab (i-pil-li-moo-mab)

Yervoy

Classification
Therapeutic: antineoplastics
Pharmacologic: monoclonal antibodies

Pregnancy Category C

Indications

Treatment of unresectable/metastatic melanoma. Adjuvant treatment of cutaneous melanoma with pathologic involvement of regional lymph nodes >1 mm in patients who have undergone complete resection, including total lymphadenectomy.

Action

Binds to cytotoxic T-lymphocyte-associated antigen 4 (CTLA-4) and prevents it from binding to CD80/CD86 ligands. CTLA-4 is a negative regulator of T-cell activation; binding results in augmented T-cell activation and proliferation as well as enhanced T-cell responsiveness. **Therapeutic Effects:** ↓ spread or recurrence of melanoma.

Pharmacokinetics

Absorption: IV administration results in complete bioavailability.
Distribution: Crosses the placenta.
Metabolism and Excretion: Unknown.
Half-life: 14.7 days.

TIME/ACTION PROFILE

ROUTE	ONSET	PEAK	DURATION
IV	unknown	unknown	unknown

Contraindications/Precautions

Contraindicated in: Lactation: Avoid breast feeding.
Use Cautiously in: OB: Use only if potential maternal benefit justifies potential risk to the fetus; may cause fetal harm; Pedi: Safety and effectiveness not established.

Adverse Reactions/Side Effects

CNS: ENCEPHALITIS, fatigue. **EENT:** hearing loss, immune-mediated ocular disease. **GI:** IMMUNE-MEDIATED COLITIS, IMMUNE-MEDIATED HEPATITIS, colitis, diarrhea. **Derm:** immune-mediated dermatitis including TOXIC EPIDERMAL NECROLYSIS, pruritus, rash. **Endo:** IMMUNE-MEDIATED ENDROCRINOPATHIES including HYPOPITUITARISM, HYPOTHYROIDISM, HYPERTHYROIDISM, ADRENAL INSUFFICIENCY, CUSHING'S SYNDROME, AND HYPOGONADISM. **MS:** myositis. **Neuro:** IMMUNE-MEDIATED NEUROPATHY. **Misc:** SARCOIDOSIS.

Interactions

Drug-Drug: Concurrent use with **vemurafenib** may ↑ risk of hepatic dysfunction.

Route/Dosage

Unresectable/Metastatic Melanoma

IV (Adults): 3 mg/kg every 3 wk for a total of 4 doses.

Adjuvant Treatment of Melanoma

IV (Adults): 10 mg/kg every 3 wk for 4 doses, then 10 mg/kg every 12 wk for up to 3 yr.

Availability

Solution for IV infusion (requires further dilution): 5 mg/mL.

NURSING IMPLICATIONS

Assessment

- Monitor for signs and symptoms of entercolitis (diarrhea, abdominal pain, mucus or blood in stool, with or without fever) and bowel perforation (peritoneal signs, ileus). Rule out infection and consider endoscopic evaluation. If severe enterocolitis occurs, discontinue ilipimumab and start systemic corticosteroids at doses of 1–2 mg/kg/day of prednisone or equivalents. At improvement to Grade 1 or less, taper corticosteroid over at least 1 mo. Consider adding anti-TNF therapy or other immunosuppressive therapy if signs and symptoms of enterocolitis persist despite systemic corticosteroid therapy within 3–5 days or if they recur after symptomatic improvement. Withhold dose for moderate enterocolitis; administer anti-diarrheal treatment and if persists for >1 wk, start corticosteroids at a dose of 0.5 mg/kg/day of prednisone or equivalent.
- Assess for signs and symptoms of hepatotoxicity (yellowing of skin or whites of eyes, unusual darkening of urine, unusual tiredness, pain in right upper stomach) before each dose. If hepatotoxicity occurs, rule out infectious or malignant causes. Permanently discontinue ipilimumab if Grade 3–5 hepatotoxicity occurs and start systemic corticosteroids at a dose of 1–2 mg/kg/day of prednisone or equivalent. When liver function tests show sustained improvement or return to baseline, start corticosteroid taper over 1 mo. May administer mycophenolate in patients with persistent severe hepatitis despite high-dose corticosteroids. Withhold ipilimumab in patients with Grade 2 hepatotoxicity.
- Monitor for signs and symptoms of dermatitis (rash, pruritus). Unless other causes are identified, assume immune-mediated dermatitis. Permanently discontinue ipilimumab in patients with Stevens-Johnson syndrome, toxic epidermal necrolysis, or rash complicated by full thickness dermal ulceration, or necrotic, bullous, or hemorrhagic manifestations. Administer corticosteroids at a dose of 1–2 mg/kg/day of prednisone or equivalent. When dermatitis is controlled, taper corticosteroids over at least 1 mo. Withhold ipilimumab in patients with moderate to severe signs and symptoms. Treat mild to moderate dermatitis symptomatically. Administer topical or systemic corticosteroids if there is no improvement of symptoms within 1 wk.
- Monitor for symptoms of motor or sensory neuropathy (unilateral or bilateral weakness, sensory alterations, paresthesia). Permanently discontinue ipilimumab in patients with severe neuropathy (interfering with daily activities). Institute treatment as needed. Consider systemic corticosteroids of 1–2 mg/kg/day of prednisone or equivalent for severe neuropathy. Withhold dose of ipilimumab in patients with moderate neuropathy (not interfering with daily activities).
- Monitor for clinical signs and symptoms of hypophysitis, adrenal insufficiency (including adrenal crisis), and hyper or hypothyroidism (fatigue, headache, mental status changes, abdominal pain, unusual bowel habits, hypotension). Unless other causes are determined, consider signs and symptoms as immune-mediated endocrinopathies. Withhold ipilimumab in symptomatic patients and initiate corticosteroids at 1–2 mg/kg/day of prednisone or equivalents. Initiate hormone replacement therapy as needed.
- Assess eyes for signs and symptoms of uveitis, iritis, or episcleritis. Administer corticosteroid eyedrops if these occur. Permanently discontinue ipilimumab for immune-mediated occular disease unresponsive to local immunosuppressive therapy.
- ***Lab Test Considerations:*** Monitor liver function tests (AST, ALT, bilirubin) prior to each dose of ipilimumab; ↑ frequency of monitoring if levels ↑. Withhold ipilimumab in patients with Grade 2 hepatotoxicity. With complete or partial resolution (Grade 0–1), and patient receiving <7.5 mg prednisone, resume at a dose of 3 mg/kg every 3 weeks until administration of all 4 planned doses or 16 weeks from first dose, whichever occurs earlier. Discontinue ipilimumab permanently with Grade 3–5 hepatotoxicity and administer systemic corticosteroids at a dose of 1 to 2 mg/kg/day of prednisone or equivalent. Initiate corticosteroid taper when liver function tests show sustained improvement or return to baseline; continue to taper over 1 mo.
- Monitor thyroid function tests and serum chemistries at start of therapy, before each dose, and as clinically indicated.

Potential Nursing Diagnoses

Impaired skin integrity (Indications)

Implementation

- For unresectable/metastatic melanoma, doses may be delayed in the event of toxicity, but must be administered with 16 wks from 1st dose. For adjuvant treatment of melanoma, doses can be omitted, but not delayed in the event of toxicity.

- Withhold dose for any moderate immune-mediated adverse reactions or for symptomatic endocrinopathy. For patients with complete or partial resolution of adverse reactions (Grade 0–1), who are receiving equivalents of <7.5 mg prednisone/day, resume ipilimumab therapy.
- Permanently discontinue if persistent moderate adverse reactions or inability to reduce corticosteroid dose to equivalent of prednisone 7.5 mg/day, failure to complete full treatment course within 16 wks from infusion of 1st dose, or severe or life threatening adverse reactions occur including: Colitis with abdominal pain, fever, or peritoneal signs; ↑ in stool frequency of 7 or more over baseline, stool incontinence. Need for IV hydration for >24 hrs, GI hemorrhage and GI perforation; AST or ALT >5 times the upper limits of normal or total bilirubin >3 times the upper limit of normal; Stevens-Johnson syndome, toxic epidermal necrolysis, or rash complicated by full-thickness dermal ulceration, or necrotic, bullous, or hemorrhagic manifestations; Severe motor or sensory neuropathy, Guillian-Barre syndrome, or myasthenia gravis; Severe immune-mediated reactions involving any organ system (nephritis, pneumonitis, pancreatitis, non-infectious myocarditis); and Immune-mediated ocular disease that is unresponsive to topical immunosuppressive therapy.
- Allow vial to stand at room temperature for 5 min prior to preparation of infusion. Withdraw amount of ipilimumab required and transfer to IV bag. ***Diluent:*** Dilute with 0.9% NaCL or D5W. ***Concentration:*** 1 mg/mL to 2 mg/mL. Mix slowly by gentle inversion; do not shake. Solution is clear, pale yellow, and may contain translucent-to-white amorphous particles; do not administer if cloudy, discolored, or contains particulate matter. Store for up to 24 hr at room temperature or refrigerated; do not freeze, protect from light. Discard partially used vials. ***Rate:*** Infuse over 90 min through a sterile, non-pyrogenic, low-protein-binding in-line filter. Flush the IV line with 0.9% NaCl or D5W after each dose.
- **Y-Site Incompatibility:** Do not mix with or infuse with other solutions or products.

Patient/Family Teaching

- Inform patient of the risk of immune-mediated reactions due to T-cell activation and proliferation. Advise patients these may be severe and fatal. Instruct patient to notify health care professional immediately if signs and symptoms occur.
- Instruct patient to read the *Medication Guide* before starting therapy and before each dose of ipilimumab.
- Advise female patients to notify health care professional if pregnancy is planned or suspected or if breast feeding. Contraception should be used throughout therapy. Women must choose to discontinue breast feeding or ipilimumab.

Evaluation/Desired Outcomes

- ↓ spread or recurrence of melanoma.

ipratropium (i-pra-**troe**-pee-um)

Atrovent, Atrovent HFA

Classification

Therapeutic: allergy, cold, and cough remedies, bronchodilators

Pharmacologic: anticholinergics

Pregnancy Category B

Indications

Inhaln: Maintenance therapy of reversible airway obstruction due to COPD, including chronic bronchitis and emphysema. **Intranasal:** Rhinorrhea associated with allergic and nonallergic perennial rhinitis (0.03% solution) or the common cold (0.06% solution). **Unlabeled Use: Inhaln:** Adjunctive management of bronchospasm caused by asthma.

Action

Inhaln: Inhibits cholinergic receptors in bronchial smooth muscle, resulting in decreased concentrations of cyclic guanosine monophosphate (cGMP). Decreased levels of cGMP produce local bronchodilation. **Intranasal:** Local application inhibits secretions from glands lining the nasal mucosa. **Therapeutic Effects: Inhaln:** Bronchodilation without systemic anticholinergic effects. **Intranasal:** Decreased rhinorrhea.

Pharmacokinetics

Absorption: Minimal systemic absorption (2% for inhalation solution; 20% for inhalation aerosol; <20% following nasal use).

Distribution: 15% of dose reaches lower airways after inhalation.

Metabolism and Excretion: Small amounts absorbed are metabolized by the liver.

Half-life: 2 hr.

TIME/ACTION PROFILE (bronchodilation)

ROUTE	ONSET	PEAK	DURATION
Inhalation	1–3 min	1–2 hr	4–6 hr
Intranasal	15 min	unknown	6–12 hr

Contraindications/Precautions

Contraindicated in: Hypersensitivity to ipratropium, atropine, belladonna alkaloids, or bromide; Avoid use during acute bronchospasm; **Note: Atrovent HFA has replaced the discontinued Atrovent CFC (chlorofluorocarbon). Soy and CFC-allergic pa-**

tients can now safely use the Atrovent HFA formulation. However, Combivent (ipratropium/albuterol combination) MDI does contain soya lecithin and is contraindicated in patients with a history of hypersensitivity to soy and peanuts.
Use Cautiously in: Patients with bladder neck obstruction, prostatic hyperplasia, glaucoma, or urinary retention; Geri: May be more sensitive to effects.

Adverse Reactions/Side Effects

CNS: dizziness, headache, nervousness. **EENT:** blurred vision, sore throat; *nasal only*, epistaxis, nasal dryness/irritation. **Resp:** bronchospasm, cough. **CV:** hypotension, palpitations. **GI:** GI irritation, nausea. **Derm:** rash. **Misc:** allergic reactions.

Interactions

Drug-Drug: ↑ anticholinergic effects with other **drugs having anticholinergic properties (antihistamines, phenothiazines, disopyramide)**.

Route/Dosage

Inhaln (Adults and Children >12 yr): *Metered-dose inhaler (nonacute)*—2 inhalations 4 times daily (not to exceed 12 inhalations/24 hr or more frequently than q 4 hr). *Acute exacerbations*—4–8 puffs using a spacer device as needed. *Via nebulization (nonacute)*—500 mcg 3–4 times daily. *Via nebulization (acute exacerbations)*—500 mcg q 30 min for 3 doses then q 2–4 hr as needed.
Inhaln (Children 5–12 yr): *Metered-dose inhaler (nonacute)*—1–2 inhalations q 6 hr as needed (not to exceed 12 inhalations/24 hr). *Acute exacerbations*—4–8 puffs as needed *Via nebulization (nonacute)*—250–500 mcg 4 times daily given q 6 hr. *Acute exacerbations*—250 mcg q 20 min for 3 doses then q 2–4 hr as needed.
Inhaln (Infants): *Nebulization*—125–250 mcg 3 times a day.
Inhaln (Neonates): *Nebulization*—25 mcg/kg/dose 3 times a day.
Intranasal (Adults and Children >6 yr): *0.03% solution*—2 sprays in each nostril 2–3 times daily (21 mcg/spray).
Inhaln (Adults and Children >5 yr): *0.06% solution*—2 sprays in each nostril 3–4 times daily (42 mcg/spray).

Availability (generic available)

Aerosol inhaler (HFA) (chlorofluorocarbon-free): 17 mcg/spray in 12.9-g canister (200 inhalations). **Inhalation solution:** 🍁0.0125%, 0.02% in single-dose vials containing 500 mcg, 🍁0.025%. **Nasal spray:** 0.03% solution—21 mcg/spray in 30-mL bottle (345 sprays/bottle), 0.06% solution—42 mcg/spray in 15-mL bottle (165 sprays). ***In combination with:*** albuterol (Combivent, Duoneb). See Appendix B.

NURSING IMPLICATIONS

Assessment

- Assess for allergy to atropine and belladonna alkaloids; patients with these allergies may also be sensitive to ipratropium. Atrovent HFA MDI does not contain CFC or soy and may be used safely in soy or CFC-allergic patients. However, Combivent MDI should be avoided in soy or peanut-allergic patients.
- **Inhaln:** Assess respiratory status (rate, breath sounds, degree of dyspnea, pulse) before administration and at peak of medication. Consult health care professional about alternative medication if severe bronchospasm is present; onset of action is too slow for patients in acute distress. If paradoxical bronchospasm (wheezing) occurs, withhold medication and notify health care professional immediately.
- **Nasal Spray:** Assess patient for rhinorrhea.

Potential Nursing Diagnoses

Ineffective airway clearance (Indications)
Activity intolerance (Indications)

Implementation

- **Inhaln:** See Appendix D for administration of inhalation medications.
- When ipratropium is administered concurrently with other inhalation medications, administer adrenergic bronchodilators first, followed by ipratropium, then corticosteroids. Wait 5 min between medications.
- Solution for *nebulization* can be diluted with preservative-free 0.9% NaCl. Diluted solution should be used within 24 hr at room temperature or 48 hr if refrigerated. Solution can be mixed with preservative-free albuterol, cromolyn, or metaproterenol if used within 1 hr of mixing.

Patient/Family Teaching

- Instruct patient in proper use of inhaler, nebulizer, or nasal spray and to take medication as directed. Take missed doses as soon as remembered unless almost time for the next dose; space remaining doses evenly during day. Do not double doses.
- Advise patient that rinsing mouth after using inhaler, good oral hygiene, and sugarless gum or candy may minimize dry mouth. Health care professional should be notified if stomatitis occurs or if dry mouth persists for more than 2 wk.
- **Inhalation:** Caution patient not to exceed 12 doses within 24 hr. Patient should notify health care professional if symptoms do not improve within 30 min after administration of medication or if condition worsens.
- Explain need for pulmonary function tests prior to and periodically during therapy to determine effectiveness of medication.
- Caution patient to avoid spraying medication in eyes; may cause blurring of vision or irritation.

- Advise patient to inform health care professional if cough, nervousness, headache, dizziness, nausea, or GI distress occurs.
- **Nasal Spray:** Instruct patient in proper use of nasal spray. Clear nasal passages gently before administration. Do not inhale during administration, so medication remains in nasal passages. Prime pump initially with 7 actuations. If used regularly, no further priming is needed. If not used in 24 hr, prime with 2 actuations. If not used for >7 days, prime with 7 actuations.
- Advise patient to contact health care professional if symptoms do not improve within 1–2 wk or if condition worsens.

Evaluation/Desired Outcomes

- Decreased dyspnea.
- Improved breath sounds.
- Decrease in rhinorrhea from perennial rhinitis or the common cold.

irbesartan, See ANGIOTENSIN II RECEPTOR ANTAGONISTS.

irinotecan

(eye-ri-noe-**tee**-kan)

Camptosar

Classification

Therapeutic: antineoplastics

Pharmacologic: enzyme inhibitors

Pregnancy Category D

Indications

Metastatic colorectal cancer (with 5-fluorouracil and leucovorin).

Action

Interferes with DNA synthesis by inhibiting the enzyme topoisomerase. **Therapeutic Effects:** Death of rapidly replicating cells, particularly malignant ones.

Pharmacokinetics

Absorption: IV administration results in complete bioavailability.

Distribution: Unknown.

Protein Binding: *Irinotecan*—30–68%; *SN–38 (active metabolite)*—95%.

Metabolism and Excretion: Converted by the liver to SN–38, its active metabolite, which is metabolized by the liver by UDP-glucuronosyl 111 transferase 1A1 (UGT1A1) and CYP3A4. Small amounts excreted by kidneys.

Half-life: 6 hr.

TIME/ACTION PROFILE (hematologic effects)

ROUTE	ONSET	PEAK	DURATION
IV	unknown	21–29 days	27–34 days

Contraindications/Precautions

Contraindicated in: Hypersensitivity; Hereditary fructose intolerance (contains sorbitol); Concurrent use of ketoconazole and St. John's wort; OB, Lactation: Pregnancy or lactation.

Use Cautiously in: Previous pelvic or abdominal irradiation or age ≥65 yr (↑ risk of myelosuppression); Presence of infection, underlying bone marrow depression, or concurrent chronic illness; History of prior pelvic/abdominal irradiation and serum bilirubin >1–2 mg/dL (initial dose reduction recommended); Geri: ↑ sensitivity to adverse effects (myelosuppression); initiate at lower dose; Hepatic impairment; Previous severe myelosuppression or diarrhea (reinstitute at lower dose following resolution); Patients with genetically reduced UGT1A1 activity (↑ risk of neutropenia); Rep: Patients with childbearing potential;; Pedi: Safety not established.

Adverse Reactions/Side Effects

CNS: dizziness, headache, insomnia, weakness. **EENT:** rhinitis. **Resp:** INTERSTITAL LUNG DISEASE, coughing, dyspnea. **CV:** edema, vasodilation. **GI:** DIARRHEA, ↑ LIVER ENZYMES, abdominal pain/cramping, anorexia, constipation, dyspepsia, flatulence, nausea, stomatitis, vomiting, abdominal enlargement, colonic ulceration. **Derm:** alopecia, rash, sweating. **F and E:** dehydration. **Hemat:** anemia, leukopenia, neutropenia, thrombocytopenia. **Local:** injection site reactions. **Metab:** weight loss. **MS:** back pain. **Misc:** chills, fever.

Interactions

Drug-Drug: Combination with **fluorouracil** may result in serious toxicity (dehydration, neutropenia, sepsis). ↑ bone marrow depression may occur with other **antineoplastics** or **radiation therapy**. Strong **CYP3A4 inhibitors (ketoconazole, clarithromycin, indinavir, itraconazole, lopinavir, nefazodone, nelfinavir, ritonavir, saquinavir, teleprevir,** and **voriconazole**) and strong**UGT1A1 inhibitors** (**atazanavir, gemfibrozil,** and **indinavir**) may ↑ levels of irinotecan and its active metabolite; should be discontinued ≥1 wk before initiating irinotecan. **Phenobarbital, phenytoin, carbamazepine, rifampin,** or **rifabutin** may ↓ levels of irinotecan and its active metabolite; consider using an alternative anticonvulsant at least 2 wk before initiating irinotecan. **Laxatives** should be avoided (diarrhea may be ↑). **Diuretics** ↑ risk of dehydration (may discontinue during therapy). **Dexamethasone** may ↑ risk of hyperglycemia and lymphocytopenia. **Prochlorperazine** given on the same day as irinotecan ↑ risk of akathisia. May ↓ antibody response to and ↑ risk of adverse reactions from **live virus vaccines**.

Drug-Natural Products: St. John's wort ↓ levels of the active metabolite; concurrent use is contraindicated; should be discontinued at least 2 wk before initiating irinotecan.

Route/Dosage

Other regimens are used; careful modification required for all levels of toxicity/tolerance.

Single Agent

IV (Adults): *Weekly dosage schedule*—125 mg/m² once weekly for 4 wk, followed by a 2-wk rest period. Cycle may be repeated using doses which depend on patient tolerance and degree of toxicity encountered. *Once-every-3-wk schedule*—350 mg/m² once every 3 wk. Cycle may be repeated using doses which depend on patient tolerance and degree of toxicity encountered.

IV (Geriatric Patients >70 yr): *Weekly dosage schedule*—125 mg/m² once weekly for 4 wk, followed by a 2-wk rest period. Cycle may be repeated using doses which depend on patient tolerance and degree of toxicity encountered. *Once-every-3-wk schedule*—300 mg/m² once every 3 wk. Cycle may be repeated using doses which depend on patient tolerance and degree of toxicity encountered.

IV (Adults Patients with Reduced UGT1A1 Activity): *Weekly dosage schedule*—100 mg/m² once weekly for 4 wk, followed by a 2-wk rest period. Cycle may be repeated using doses which depend on patient tolerance and degree of toxicity encountered. *Once-every-3-wk schedule*—300 mg/m² once every 3 wk. Cycle may be repeated using doses which depend on patient tolerance and degree of toxicity encountered.

Hepatic Impairment

IV (Adults): *Bilirubin 1–2 mg/dL and history of prior pelvic/abdominal irradiation— Weekly dosage schedule*—Initiate therapy at lower dose (100 mg/m²); once weekly for 4 wk, followed by a 2-wk rest period. Cycle may be repeated with dose adjusted as tolerated. *Once-every-3-wk schedule*—300 mg/m² once every 3 wk. Cycle may be repeated with dose adjusted as tolerated.

As Part of Combination Therapy with Leucovorin and 5-Fluorouracil

IV (Adults): *Regimen 1 (Bolus regimen)*—125 mg/m² once weekly for 4 wk, followed by a 2-wk rest period. Cycle may be repeated using doses that depend on patient tolerance and degree of toxicity encountered; *Regimen 2 (Infusional regimen)*—180 mg/m² every 2 wk for 3 doses, followed by a 3-wk rest period. Cycle may be repeated using doses that depend on patient tolerance and degree of toxicity encountered.

IV (Adults Patients with Reduced UGT1A1 Activity): *Regimen 1 (Bolus regimen)*—100 mg/m² once weekly for 4 wk, followed by a 2-wk rest period. Cycle may be repeated using doses that depend on patient tolerance and degree of toxicity encountered; *Regimen 2 (Infusional regimen)*—150 mg/m² every 2 wk for 3 doses, followed by a 3-wk rest period. Cycle may be repeated using doses that depend on patient tolerance and degree of toxicity encountered.

Availability (generic available)

Solution for injection: 20 mg/mL.

NURSING IMPLICATIONS

Assessment

- Monitor vital signs frequently during administration.
- Monitor for bone marrow depression. Assess for bleeding (bleeding gums, bruising, petechiae, guaiac stools, urine, and emesis) and avoid IM injections and taking rectal temperatures if platelet count is low. Apply pressure to venipuncture sites for 10 min. Assess for signs of infection during neutropenia. Anemia may occur. Monitor for increased fatigue, dyspnea, and orthostatic hypotension.
- Monitor closely for the development of diarrhea. Two types may occur. The early type occurs within 24 hr of administration and may be preceded by cramps and sweating. Atropine 0.25–1 mg IV may be given to decrease symptoms. Potentially life-threatening diarrhea may occur more than 24 hr after a dose and may be accompanied by severe dehydration and electrolyte imbalance. Loperamide 4 mg initially, followed by 2 mg every 2 hr until diarrhea ceases for at least 12 hr (or 4 mg every 4 hr if given during sleeping hours) should be administered promptly to treat late-occurring diarrhea. Do not administer loperamide at these doses for >48 hr. Careful fluid and electrolyte replacement should be instituted to prevent complications. Subsequent doses should be delayed in patients with active diarrhea until diarrhea is resolved for 24 hr. If diarrhea is grade 2, 3, or 4, decrease subsequent doses of irinotecan.
- Nausea and vomiting are common. Pretreatment with dexamethasone 10 mg along with agents such as ondansetron or granisetron should be started on the same day as irinotecan at least 30 min before administration. Prochlorperazine may be used on subsequent days but may increase risk of akathisia if given on the same day as irinotecan.
- Assess IV site frequently for inflammation. Avoid extravasation. If extravasation occurs, infusion must be stopped and restarted in another vein to avoid damage to subcut tissue. Flushing site with sterile water and application of ice over the extravasated site are recommended.
- If signs of pulmonary toxicity (dyspnea, cough, fever) occur, interrupt therapy. If interstitial pulmonary disease is determined, discontinue irinotecan.
- Assess for cholinergic symptoms (rhinitis, increased salivation, miosis, lacrimation, diaphoresis, flushing,

abdominal cramping, diarrhea) during therapy. Atropine 0.25–1 mg subcut or IV may be used to prevent or treat symptoms.

- ***Lab Test Considerations:*** Monitor CBC with differential and platelet count prior to each dose. Temporarily discontinue irinotecan if absolute neutrophil count is <500 cells/mm^3 or if neutropenic fever occurs. Administration of a colony-stimulating factor may be considered if clinically significant decreases in WBC (<2000/mm^3), neutrophil count (<1000/mm^3), hemoglobin (<9 g/dL), or platelet count (<100,000 cells/mm^3) occur.
- May cause ↑ serum alkaline phosphatase and AST concentrations.

Potential Nursing Diagnoses

Risk for infection (Adverse Reactions)

Implementation

- Prepare solution in a biologic cabinet. Wear gloves, gown, and mask while handling IV medication. Discard IV equipment in specially designated containers.

IV Administration

- **Intermittent Infusion:** ***Diluent:*** Dilute before infusion with D5W or 0.9% NaCl. Usual diluent is 500 mL of D5W. ***Concentration:*** 0.12–2.8 mg/mL. Solution is pale yellow. Do not administer solutions that are cloudy or contain particulate matter. Solution is stable for 24 hr at room temperature or 48 hr if refrigerated. To prevent microbial contamination, solutions should be used within 24 hr of dilution if refrigerated or 6 hr at room temperature. Do not refrigerate solutions diluted with 0.9% NaCl. ***Rate:*** Administer dose over 90 min.
- **Y-Site Compatibility:** alemtuzumab, alfentanil, amifostine, amikacin, aminophylline, amiodarone, ampicillin, ampicillin/sulbactam, anidulafungin, argatroban, azithromycin, aztreonam, bivalirudin, bleomycin, bumetanide, buprenorphine, butorphanol, calcium chloride, calcium gluconate, carboplatin, caspofungin, cefazolin, cefotetan, cefoxitin, ceftazidime, cefuroxime, ciprofloxacin, cisatracurium, cisplatin, clindamycin, cyclophosphamide, cyclosporine, cytarabine, dacarbazine, daptomycin, daunorubicin, dexamethasone, dexrazoxane, digoxin, diltiazem, diphenhydramine, dobutamine, docetaxel, dolasetron, dopamine, doxacurium, doxorubicin, doxycycline, enalaprilat, ephedrine, epinephrine, ertapenem, erythromycin, esmolol, etoposide , etoposide phosphate, famotidine, fenoldopam, fentanyl, fluconazole, foscarnet, gentamicin, granisetron, haloperidol, heparin, hetastarch, hydralazine, hydrocortisone, hydromorphone, idarubicin, imipenem/cilastatin, insulin, isoproterenol, ketorolac, labetalol, leucovorin, levofloxacin, levoleucovorin, levorphanol, lidocaine, linezolid, lorazepam, magnesium sulfate, mannitol, meperidine, meropenem, mesna, metaraminol, methyldopate, metoclopramide, metoprolol, metronidazole, midazolam, milrinone, mitoxantrone, morphine, moxifloxacin, nalbuphine, naloxone, nesiritide, nicardipine, nitroglycerin, norepinephrine, octreotide, ondansetron, oxaliplatin, paclitaxel, palonosetron, pancuronium, pantoprazole, pentamidine, pentazocine, pentobarbital, phenobarbital, phenylephrine, potassium acetate, potassium chloride, potassium phosphates, procainamide, prochlorperazine, promethazine, propranolol, quinupristin/dalfopristin, ranitidine, remifentanyl, rituximab, rocuronium, sodium acetate, sodium bicarbonate, sodium phosphates, succinylcholine, sufentanil, tacrolimus, teniposide, theophylline, thiotepa, tigecycline, tirofiban, tobramycin, tolazoline, trimethoprim/sulfamethoxazole, vancomycin, vasopressin, vecuronium, verapamil, vinblastine, vinorelbine, voriconazole, zidovudine, zoledronic acid.
- **Y-Site Incompatibility:** acyclovir, allopurinol, amphotericin B colloidal, amphotericin B lipid complex, amphotericin B liposome, cefepime, cefotaxime, ceftriaxone, chloramphenicol, chlorpromazine, dantrolene, dexmedetomidine, diazepam, droperidol, fluorouracil, fosphenytoin, furosemide, ganciclovir, gemcitabine, glycopyrrolate, methohexital, methylprednisolone, mitomycin, nafcillin, nitroprusside, pemetrexed, phenytoin, piperacillin/tazobactam, thiopental, trastuzumab.
- **Additive Incompatibility:** Information unavailable. Do not admix with other solutions or medications.

Patient/Family Teaching

- Instruct patient to report occurrence of diarrhea to health care professional immediately, especially if it occurs more than 24 hr after dose. Diarrhea may be accompanied by severe dehydration and electrolyte imbalance. It may be life-threatening and should be treated promptly. Patient should have loperamide for treatment.
- Instruct patient to notify health care professional promptly if fever; chills; sore throat; signs of infection; bleeding gums; bruising; petechiae; blood in urine, stool, or emesis occurs. Caution patient to avoid crowds and persons with known infections. Instruct patient to use soft toothbrush and electric razor. Caution patient not to drink alcoholic beverages or take products containing aspirin or other NSAIDs.
- Instruct patient to notify nurse of pain at injection site immediately.
- Instruct patient to notify health care professional if vomiting, fainting, or dizziness occurs.

- Discuss with patient possibility of hair loss. Explore methods of coping.
- Instruct patient not to receive any vaccinations without consulting health care professional.
- Rep: Advise patient that this medication may have teratogenic effects. Contraception should be used during therapy.
- Emphasize the need for periodic lab tests to monitor for side effects.

Evaluation/Desired Outcomes

- Decrease in size and spread of malignancy.

IRON SUPPLEMENTS

carbonyl iron (100%)
(**kar**-bo-nil **eye**-ern)
Feosol, Icar

ferrous fumarate (33% elemental iron) (**fer**-us **fyoo**-ma-rate)
Femiron, Feostat, Fumasorb, Fumerin, Hemocyte, Neo-Fer, Span-FF

ferrous gluconate (12% elemental iron) (**fer**-us **gloo**-koe-nate)
Fergon, Ferralet, Simron

ferrous sulfate (30% elemental iron) (**fer**-us **sul**-fate)
ED-IN-SOL, Fe50, Feosol, Feratab, Fergen-sol, Fer-In-Sol, Fer-Iron, Slow FE

iron dextran (**eye**-ern **dex**-tran)
DexFerrum, ✤Dexiron, InFeD, ✤Infufer

iron polysaccharide
(**eye**-ern poll-ee-**sak**-a-ride)
Hytinic, Niferex, Nu-Iron

iron sucrose (**eye**-ern **su**-krose)
Venofer

sodium ferric gluconate complex
(**so**-dee-yum **ferr**-ic **gloo**-ko-nate)
Ferrlecit

Classification
Therapeutic: antianemics
Pharmacologic: iron supplements

Pregnancy Category A (ferrous gluconate, ferrous sulfate, iron polysaccharide), B (sodium ferric gluconate, iron sucrose), C (iron dextran)

Indications

PO: Prevention/treatment of iron-deficiency anemia. **IM, IV:** *Iron dextran*—Treatment of iron-deficiency anemia in patients who cannot tolerate or receive oral iron. *Sodium ferric gluconate complex*—Treatment of iron deficiency in patients undergoing chronic hemodialysis or peritoneal dialysis who are concurrently receiving erythropoietin. Treatment of iron-deficiency anemia in patients with chronic kidney disease including patients who are not on dialysis (with or without erythropoietin) and patients dependent on dialysis (with erythropoietin).

Action

An essential mineral found in hemoglobin, myoglobin, and many enzymes. Enters the bloodstream and is transported to the organs of the reticuloendothelial system (liver, spleen, bone marrow), where it is separated out and becomes part of iron stores. **Therapeutic Effects:** Prevention/treatment of iron deficiency.

Pharmacokinetics

Absorption: 5–10% of dietary iron is absorbed (up to 30% in deficiency states). Therapeutically administered PO iron may be 60% absorbed via an active and passive transport process. Well absorbed following IM administration.
Distribution: Remains in the body for many months. Crosses the placenta; enters breast milk.
Protein Binding: ≥90%.
Metabolism and Excretion: Mostly recycled; small daily losses occurring via desquamation, sweat, urine, and bile.
Half-life: *Iron dextran, iron sucrose*—6 hr.

TIME/ACTION PROFILE (effects on erythropoiesis)

ROUTE	ONSET	PEAK	DURATION
PO	4 days	7–10 days	2–4 mo
IM, IV	4 days	1–2 wk	wk–mos

Contraindications/Precautions

Contraindicated in: Hemochromatosis, hemosiderosis, or other evidence of iron overload; Anemias not due to iron deficiency; Some products contain alcohol, tartrazine, or sulfites and should be avoided in patients with known intolerance or hypersensitivity.
Use Cautiously in: Peptic ulcer; Ulcerative colitis or regional enteritis (condition may be aggravated); Alcoholism; Severe hepatic impairment; Severe renal impairment (oral products); Pre-existing cardiovascular disease (iron dextran) (may be exacerbated by adverse reactions to this drug); Significant allergies or asthma (iron dextran); History of drug allergy or multiple drug allergies (iron dextran) (may be at ↑ risk for anaphylactic reaction); Rheumatoid arthritis (iron dextran) (may have exacerbation of joint swelling); OB, Lactation: Pregnancy or lactation (safety of some parenteral products not established); Pedi: Safety not established for infants <4 mo (iron dextran) or children <6 yr (sodium ferric gluconate complex); safety may not be established for other products in the pediatric population.

Adverse Reactions/Side Effects

CNS: *IM, IV*—SEIZURES, dizziness, headache, syncope. **CV:** *IM, IV*—hypotension, hypertension, tachycardia. **GI:** nausea; *PO*, constipation, dark stools, diarrhea, epigastric pain, GI bleeding; *IM, IV*, taste disorder, vomiting. **Derm:** *IM, IV*—flushing, urticaria. **Resp:** *IV*—cough, dyspnea. **Local:** pain at IM site (iron dextran), phlebitis at IV site, skin staining at IM site (iron dextran). **MS:** *IM, IV*—arthralgia, myalgia. **Misc:** *PO*—staining of teeth (liquid preparations); *IM, IV*, allergic reactions including ANAPHYLAXIS, fever, lymphadenopathy, sweating.

Interactions

Drug-Drug: Oral iron supplements ↓ absorption of **tetracyclines**, **bisphosphonates**, **fluoroquinolones**, **levothyroxine**, **mycophenolate mofetil**, and **penicillamine** (simultaneous administration should be avoided). ↓ absorption of and may ↓ effects of **levodopa** and **methyldopa**. Concurrent administration of **H_2 antagonists**, **proton pump inhibitors**, and **cholestyramine** may ↓ absorption of iron. Doses of **ascorbic acid** ≥200 mg may ↑ absorption of iron up to ≥30%. **Chloramphenicol** and **vitamin E** may ↓ hematologic response to iron therapy. **ACE inhibitors** may ↑ risk of anaphylactic reaction with iron dextran.
Drug-Food: Iron absorption is ↓ 33–50% by concurrent administration of food.

Route/Dosage

Oral Iron Dosage for Iron Deficiency (expressed as mg elemental iron, note individual salt forms, multiple ones exist—see approximate equivalent doses below for dose conversions).

Approximate Equivalent Doses (mg of iron salt): *Ferrous fumarate*—197; *Ferrous gluconate*—560; *Ferrous sulfate*—324; *Ferrous sulfate, exsiccated*—217.

PO (Adults): *Deficiency*— 120—240 mg/day (2–3 mg/kg/day) in 2–4 divided doses. *Prophylaxis*—60–100 mg/day.
PO (Infants and Children): *Severe deficiency*—4–6 mg/kg/day in 3 divided doses. *Mild to moderate deficiency*—3 mg/kg/day in 1–2 divided doses. *Prophylaxis*—1–2 mg/kg/day in 1–2 divided dose (maximum: 15 mg/day).
PO (Neonates, premature): 2–4 mg/kg/day in 1–2 divided doses, maximum: 15 mg/day.

Iron Dextran

IM, IV (Adults and Children): Test dose of 0.5 mL (25 mg) is given 1 hr prior to therapy.
IM, IV (Infants): Test dose of 0.25 mL (12.5 mg) is given 1 hr prior to therapy.
IM, IV (Adults and Children >15 kg): *Iron deficiency*—Total dose (mL) = 0.0442 × (desired Hgb− actual Hgb) × lean body weight (kg) + [0.26 × lean body weight (kg)]. Divided up and given in small daily doses until total is reached; not to exceed 100 mg/day. *Total dose IV infusion*—Total dose may be diluted and infused over 4–5 hr following a test dose of 10 drops (unlabeled).
IM, IV (Adults): *Blood loss*—Dose (mL) = (Blood loss [mL] × hematocrit) × 0.02.
IM, IV (Children 5–15 kg): *Iron deficiency*—Total dose (mL) = 0.042 (desired Hgb− actual Hgb) × weight (kg) + [0.26 × weight (kg)]. Divided up and given in small daily doses until total is reached; not to exceed 25 mg/day in children <5 kg; 50 mg/day in children 5–10 kg; or 100 mg/day in children > 10 kg.

Iron Polysaccharide Complex

PO (Adults): 50–100 mg twice daily of tablets/elixir or 150–300 mg/day of the capsules.
PO (Children >6yr): 50–100 mg/day (may be given in divided doses).
PO (Infants): 1–2 mg/kg/day.
PO (Adults—Pregnant Women): 30–60 mg/day.

Iron Sucrose

IV (Adults): *Hemodialysis dependent patients*—100 mg (5 mL) during each dialysis session for 10 doses (total of 1000 mg) additional smaller doses may be necessary; *Peritoneal dialysis dependent patients*—300 mg (15 mL) infusion, followed by another 300 mg (15 mL) infusion 14 days later, followed by 400 mg (20 mL) infusion 14 days later; *Non-dialysis dependent patients*—200 mg (10 mL) on 5 different days within a 14 day period to a total of 1000 mg, may also be given as infusion of 500 mg on day 1 and day 14.

Sodium Ferric Gluconate Complex

IV (Adults): 10 mL (125 mg elemental iron) repeated during 8 sequential dialysis treatments to a total cumulative dose of 1 g.
IV (Children >6 yr): 0.12 mL/kg (not to exceed 125 mg/dose) repeated during 8 sequential dialysis treatments.

Availability

Carbonyl Iron (100% Iron)

Tablets: 50 mg^OTC. **Oral suspension:** 15 mg/1.25 mL^OTC.

Ferrous Fumarate (33% Elemental Iron) (generic available)

Tablets: 63 mg^OTC, 195 mg^OTC, 200 mg^OTC, 324 mg^OTC, 325 mg^OTC. **Chewable tablets:** 100 mg^OTC. **Controlled-release capsules:** 325 mg^OTC. **Suspension (butterscotch flavor):** 100 mg/5 mL^OTC, ✱300 mg/5 mL^OTC. **Drops:** 45 mg/0.6 mL^OTC, ✱60 mg/1 mL^OTC.

Ferrous Gluconate (11.6% Elemental Iron) (generic available)
Tablets: 300 mg[OTC], 320 mg[OTC], 325 mg[OTC]. **Sustained-release tablets:** 320 mg[OTC]. **Soft gelatin capsules:** 86 mg[OTC]. **Elixir:** 300 mg/5 mL[OTC]. **Syrup:** ✱300 mg/5 mL[OTC].

Ferrous Sulfate (20–30% Elemental Iron)
Tablets: 195 mg[OTC], 300 mg[OTC], 325 mg[OTC]. **Capsules:** 150 mg[OTC], 250 mg[OTC]. **Timed-release tablets:** 525 mg[OTC]. **Syrup:** 90 mg/5 mL[OTC]. **Elixir:** 220 mg/5 mL[OTC]. **Drops:** 75 mg/0.6 mL[OTC], 125 mg/1 mL[OTC].

Iron Dextran
Injection: 50 mg/mL, ✱100 mg/mL.

Iron Polysaccharide (mg Iron)
Capsules: 150 mg[OTC]. **Tablets:** 50 mg[OTC].

Iron Sucrose
Aqueous complex for injection: 20 mg/mL.

Sodium Ferric Gluconate Complex (generic available)
Injection: 62.5 mg/5 mL.

NURSING IMPLICATIONS

Assessment
- Assess nutritional status and dietary history to determine possible cause of anemia and need for patient teaching.
- Assess bowel function for constipation or diarrhea. Notify health care professional and use appropriate nursing measures should these occur.
- **Iron Dextran, Iron Sucrose, and Sodium Ferric Gluconate Complex:** Monitor BP and heart rate frequently following IV administration until stable. Rapid infusion rate may cause hypotension and flushing.
- Assess patient for signs and symptoms of anaphylaxis (rash, pruritus, laryngeal edema, wheezing) for at least 30 min following injection. Notify health care professional immediately if these occur. Keep epinephrine and resuscitation equipment close by in the event of an anaphylactic reaction.
- ***Lab Test Considerations:*** Monitor hemoglobin, hematocrit, and reticulocyte values prior to and every 3 wk during the first 2 mo of therapy and periodically thereafter. Serum ferritin and iron levels may also be monitored to assess effectiveness of therapy.
- Occult blood in stools may be obscured by black coloration of iron in stool. Guaiac test results may occasionally be false-positive.
- **Iron Dextran:** Monitor hemoglobin, hematocrit, reticulocyte values, transferrin, ferritin, total iron-binding capacity, and plasma iron concentrations periodically during therapy. Serum ferritin levels peak in 7–9 days and return to normal in 3 wk. Serum iron determinations may be inaccurate for 1–2 wk after therapy with large doses; therefore, hemoglobin and hematocrit are used to gauge initial response.
- May impart a brownish hue to blood drawn within 4 hr of administration. May cause false ↑ in serum bilirubin and false decrease in serum calcium values.
- Prolonged PTT may be calculated when blood sample is anticoagulated with citrate dextrose solution; use sodium citrate instead.
- **Iron Sucrose:** Monitor hemoglobin, hematocrit, serum ferritin, and transferritin saturation prior to and periodically during therapy. Transferrin saturation values increase rapidly after IV administration; therefore, serum iron values may be reliably obtained 48 hr after IV administration. Withhold iron therapy if evidence of iron overload occurs.
- May cause ↑ liver enzymes.
- ***Toxicity and Overdose:*** Early symptoms of overdose include stomach pain, fever, nausea, vomiting (may contain blood), and diarrhea. Late symptoms include bluish lips, fingernails, and palms; drowsiness; weakness; tachycardia; seizures; metabolic acidosis; hepatic injury; and cardiovascular collapse. Patient may appear to recover prior to the onset of late symptoms. Hospitalization continues for 24 hr after patient becomes asymptomatic to monitor for delayed onset of shock or GI bleeding. Late complications of overdose include intestinal obstruction, pyloric stenosis, and gastric scarring.
- If patient is comatose or seizing, gastric lavage with sodium bicarbonate is performed. Deferoxamine is the antidote. Additional supportive treatments to maintain fluid and electrolyte balance and correction of metabolic acidosis are also indicated.
- If signs of overdose occur during IV administration of iron sucrose, treatment includes IV fluids, corticosteroids, and/or antihistamines. Administering at a slower rate usually relieves symptoms.

Potential Nursing Diagnoses
Activity intolerance (Indications)

Implementation
- Discontinue oral iron preparations prior to parenteral administration.
- Sodium ferric gluconate and iron sucrose are for IV use only.
- **PO:** Oral preparations are most effectively absorbed if administered 1 hr before or 2 hr after meals. If gastric irritation occurs, administer with meals. Take tablets and capsules with a full glass of water or juice. Do not crush or chew enteric-coated tablets and do not open capsules.
- Liquid preparations may stain teeth. Dilute in water or fruit juice, full glass (240 mL) for adults and 1/2 glass (120 mL) for children, and administer with a straw or place drops at back of throat.
- Avoid using antacids, coffee, tea, dairy products, eggs, or whole-grain breads with or within 1 hr after administration of ferrous salts. Iron absorption is decreased by 33% if iron and calcium are given with

meals. If calcium supplementation is needed, calcium carbonate does not decrease absorption of iron salts if supplements are administered between meals.

- **Iron Dextran:** The 2-mL ampule may be used for IM or IV administration.
- Prior to initial IM or IV dose, a test dose of 25 mg should be given by the same route as the dose will be given, to determine reaction. The IV test dose should be administered over 5 min. The IM dose should be administered in the same injection site and by same technique as the therapeutic dose. The remaining portion may be administered after 1 hr, if no adverse symptoms have occurred.
- **IM:** Inject deeply via Z-track technique into upper outer quadrant of buttock, never into arm or other exposed areas. Use a 2–3 in., 19- or 20-gauge needle. Change needles between withdrawal from container and injection to minimize staining of subcut tissues. Stains are usually permanent.

IV Administration

- **IV: Iron Dextran**: Following IV administration, patient should remain recumbent for at least 30 min to prevent orthostatic hypotension.
- **IV Push:** ***Diluent:*** May administer undiluted or dilute in 0.9% NaCl or D5W. ***Concentration:*** 50 mg/mL. ***Rate:*** Administer slowly at a rate of 50 mg (1 mL) over at least 1 min.
- **Intermittent Infusion:** May be diluted in 200–1000 mL of 0.9% NaCl or D5W; 0.9% NaCl is the preferred diluent; dilution in D5W increases incidence of pain and phlebitis. ***Rate:*** Administer over 1–6 hr following a test dose of 10 drops/min for 10 min. Flush line with 10 mL of 0.9% NaCl at completion of infusion.
- **Y-Site Incompatibility:** Discontinue other IV solutions during infusion.
- **Additive Incompatibility:** Manufacturers recommend that iron dextran not be mixed with other solutions; however, iron dextran has been added to total parenteral nutrition solutions.
- **Sodium Ferric Gluconate Complex:** ***Diluent:*** Dilute test dose in 50 mL of 0.9% NaCl and administer IV over 60 min. ***Concentration:*** 12.5 mg/mL.
- To administer therapeutic dose of 10 mL (125 mg of elemental iron) dilute in 100 mL of 0.9% NaCl. Dialysis patients frequently require a cumulative dose of 1 g of elemental iron, administered over 8 sessions of sequential dialysis. ***Rate:*** Administer at a maximum rate of 12.5 mg/min.
- **Iron Sucrose:** Each 5-mL vial contains 100 mg of elemental iron.
- *Hemodialysis*—Most patients require a minimum cumulative dose of 1000 mg of elemental iron, administered over 10 sequential dialysis sessions, to achieve a favorable hemoglobin or hematocrit response.
- Solution is brown. Inspect for particulate matter or discoloration. Do not administer solutions that contain particulate matter or are discolored.
- **IV Push:** May be administered undiluted by slow injection into dialysis line. ***Rate:*** Administer at a rate of 1 mL undiluted solution per minute, not to exceed one vial per injection. Discard any unused portion.
- **Intermittent Infusion:** May also be administered via infusion, into dialysis line for hemodialysis patients. May reduce risk of hypotensive episodes. ***Diluent:*** Each vial must be diluted in a maximum of 100 mL of 0.9% NaCl immediately prior to infusion. Unused diluted solution should be discarded. ***Concentration:*** 1–2 mg/mL. ***Rate:*** Infuse at a rate of 100 mg of iron over at least 15 min, large doses (500 mg) should be given over 3.5–4 hr.
- **Intermittent Infusion:** *For Peritoneal Dialysis Patients*—***Diluent:*** Dilute each dose in a maximum of 250 mL of 0.9% NaCl. ***Rate:*** Administer doses of 300 mg over 1.5 hr and doses of 400 mg over 2.5 hr.
- **IV Push:** *For Non-dialysis dependent patients*—May be administered as a slow injection of 200 mg undiluted. ***Rate:*** Administer over 2–5 min.
- **Intermittent Infusion:** Dilute 500 mg in 250 mL 0.9% NaCl. ***Rate:*** Infuse over 3.5–4 hr on days 1 and 14. May cause hypotension; monitor closely.
- **Additive Incompatibility:** Do not mix iron sucrose with other medications or add to parenteral nutrition solutions for IV infusion.

Patient/Family Teaching

- Explain purpose of iron therapy to patient.
- Encourage patient to comply with medication regimen. Take missed doses as soon as remembered within 12 hr; otherwise, return to regular dosing schedule. Do not double doses.
- Advise patient that stools may become dark green or black and that this change is harmless.
- Instruct patient to follow a diet high in iron (see Appendix J).
- Discuss with parents the risk of children's overdosing on iron. Medication should be stored in the original childproof container and kept out of reach of children. Do not refer to vitamins as candy. In the event of a suspected overdose, parents or guardians should contact the poison control center (1-800-222-1222) or emergency medical services (911) immediately.
- **Iron Dextran:** Delayed reaction may occur 1–2 days after administration and last 3–4 days if IV route used, 3–7 days with IM route. Instruct patient to contact physician if fever, chills, malaise, muscle and joint aches, nausea, vomiting, dizziness, and backache occur.

- **Iron sucrose and sodium ferric gluconate complex:** Instruct patient to immediately report symptoms of hypersensitivity reaction to health care professional.

Evaluation/Desired Outcomes

- Increase in hemoglobin, which may reach normal parameters after 1–2 mo of therapy. May require 3–6 mo for normalization of body iron stores.
- Improvement in iron deficiency anemia or anemia of chronic renal failure.

isavuconazonium

(eye-sa-vue-kon-a-**zoe**-nee-um)
Cresemba

Classification
Therapeutic: antifungals
Pharmacologic: azoles

Pregnancy Category C

Indications

Treatment of invasive aspergillosis and mucormycosis.

Action

A prodrug that is converted (rapidly hydrolyzed) to isavuconazole. Inhibits the synthesis of ergosterol, a key component of fungal cell walls. **Therapeutic Effects:** Resolution of invasive fungal infections. **Spectrum:** Active against *Aspergillus flavus*, *Aspergillus fumigatus*, *Aspergillus niger* and Mucormycetes species including *Rhizopus oryzae*.

Pharmacokinetics

Absorption: Prodrug is rapidly converted to isavuconazole, the active component. 98% absorbed following oral administration. Similar conversion follows intravenous administration, resulting in complete bioavailability.
Distribution: Extensively distributed.
Protein Binding: >99%.
Metabolism and Excretion: Extensively metabolized (mostly by CYP3A4 and CYPA5); inactive metabolites are mostly renally eliminated, <1% excreted unchanged in urine.
Half-life: 130 hr.

TIME/ACTION PROFILE (blood levels)

ROUTE	ONSET	PEAK	DURATION
PO	unk	2 hr	unk
IV	unk	end of infusion	unk

Contraindications/Precautions

Contraindicated in: Known hypersensitivity; Strong CYP3A4 inhibitors; Familial short QT syndrome; Strong CYP3A4 inducers; Lactation: Discontinue breast feeding.

Use Cautiously in: Severe hepatic impairment (use only if benefits outweigh risks, monitor carefully for adverse reactions); OB: Use during pregnancy only if maternal benefits outweigh risks to the fetus; Pedi: Safe and effective use in children <18 yr has not been established.

Adverse Reactions/Side Effects

CNS: fatigue, insomnia, headache, anxiety, delerium. **Resp:** cough, dyspnea, respiratory failure. **CV:** peripheral edema, chest pain, hypotension. **GI:** constipation, diarrhea, ↑ liver enzymes, nausea, vomiting, ↓ appetite, dyspepsia. **GU:** renal failure. **Derm:** pruritus, rash. **F and E:** hypokalemia, hypomagnesemia. **Local:** injection site reactions. **MS:** back pain. **Misc:** infusion-related reactions.

Interactions

Drug-Drug: ↑ levels and risk of toxicity with **strong inhibitors of CYP3A4**, including **ketoconazole** or high-dose **ritonavir**; concurrent use is contraindicated. **Lopinavir/ritonavir** significantly ↑ levels and risk of toxicity; concurrent use should be undertaken with caution. Isavuconazonium ↓ levels and effectiveness of **lopinavir/ritonavir**. Isavuconzonium ↑ levels and risk of toxicity with **atorvastatin**, **cyclosporine**, **digoxin**, **midazolam**, **mycophenolate**, **sirolimus**, **tacrolimus**; undertake concurrent use with caution, monitoring drug effects and making adjustments if necessary. **Strong inducers of CYP3A4** including long-acting **barbiturates**, **carbamazepine** or **rifampin** ↓ levels and effectiveness; concurrent use is contraindicated. ↓ levels and effectiveness of **bupropion**; bupropion dose may need to be ↑ but should not exceed maximum recommended dose.
Drug-Natural Products: St. John's wort ↓ blood levels and effectiveness; concurrent use in contraindicated.

Route/Dosage

186 mg isavuconazonium = 100 mg isavuconazole; doses expressed as isavuconazole.

PO, IV (Adults ≥18 yr): *Loading dose*—200 mg every 8 hr for six doses; *maintenance dose*—200 mg once daily starting 12–24 hr after last loading dose.

Availability

186 mg isavuconazonium = 100 mg isavuconazole; strength expressed as isavuconazole

Capsules: 100 mg. **Lyophilized powder for intravenous injection (requires reconstitution):** 200 mg.

NURSING IMPLICATIONS

Assessment

- Obtain specimens for culture and sensitivity prior to therapy. First dose may be given before receiving results.
- Monitor for signs and symptoms of infusion-related reactions (hypotension, dyspnea, chills, dizziness, paresthesia, hypoesthesia) periodically during therapy. Discontinue infusion if symptoms occur.
- Monitor skin for hypersensitivity reactions during therapy.
- ***Lab Test Considerations:*** Monitor liver function tests prior to and periodically during therapy. Discontinue therapy if clinical signs of liver disease occur.
- May cause hypokalemia and hypomagnesemia.

Potential Nursing Diagnoses

Risk for infection (Indications)

Implementation

- Oral and IV formulations are bioequivalent; may be used interchangeably. Loading dose is not needed when switching.
- **PO:** Administer without regard to food. Swallow capsule whole; do not open, dissolve, crush or chew.

IV Administration

- Reconstitute by adding 5 mL sterile water to vial. Shake gently to dissolve powder completely. Solution should be clear and colorless; do not administer solutions that are discolored or contain particulate matter. Solution is stable for 1 hr at room temperature.
- **Intermittent Infusion: *Diluent:*** Remove 5 mL of reconstituted solution from vial and add to 250 mL 0.9% NaCl or D5W. ***Concentration:*** 1.5 mg isavuconazonium/mL. Diluted solution may show visible translucent to white particulates; removed with in-line filter. Roll bag to mix gently; avoid shaking. Solution is stable if infused at room temperature within 6 hrs; may refrigerate for up to 24 hrs.; do not freeze. Flush line with 0.9% NaCl or D5W prior to and following infusion. ***Rate:*** Infuse over at least 1 hr to minimize infusion—related reactions. Infuse through a 0.2–1.2 micron in-line filter. Do not administer as a bolus injection.
- **Y-Site Incompatibility:** Do not infuse with other medication.

Patient/Family Teaching

- Instruct patient to take isavuconazonium as directed. Do not stop taking isavuconazonium without consulting heath care professional. Advise patient to read *Patient Information* before starting and with each Rx refill in case of changes.
- Advise patient to notify health care professional promptly of signs and symptoms of liver disease (itchy skin, nausea, vomiting, yellowing of eyes, feeling very tired, flu-like symptoms), infusion-related reactions, or rash occur.
- Instruct patient to notify health care professional of all Rx or OTC medications, vitamins, or herbal products being taken and consult health care professional before taking any new medications.
- Advise female patient to notify health care professional if pregnancy is planned or suspected or if breast feeding.
- Emphasize the importance of lab tests to monitor for side effects during therapy.

Evaluation/Desired Outcomes

- Resolution of signs and symptoms of invasive fungal infection.

isocarboxazid, See MONOAMINE OXIDASE (MAO) INHIBITORS.

isoniazid (eye-soe-**nye**-a-zid)

INH, Isotamine

Classification

Therapeutic: antituberculars

Pregnancy Category C

Indications

First-line therapy of active tuberculosis, in combination with other agents. Prevention of tuberculosis in patients exposed to active disease (alone).

Action

Inhibits mycobacterial cell wall synthesis and interferes with metabolism. **Therapeutic Effects:** Bacteriostatic or bactericidal action against susceptible mycobacteria.

Pharmacokinetics

Absorption: Well absorbed following PO/IM administration.

Distribution: Widely distributed; readily crosses the blood-brain barrier. Crosses the placenta; enters breast milk in concentrations equal to plasma.

Protein Binding: 10–15%.

Metabolism and Excretion: 50% metabolized by the liver by N-acetyltransferase (rate of acetylation is genetically determined [slow acetylators have ↑ isoniazid levels and ↑ risk of toxicity; fast acetylators have ↓ isoniazid levels and ↑ risk for treatment failure]); 50% excreted unchanged by the kidneys.

Half-life: 1–4 hr in patients with normal renal and hepatic function; 0.5–1.6 hr in fast acetylators; 2–5 hr in slow acetylators.

TIME/ACTION PROFILE (blood levels)

ROUTE	ONSET	PEAK	DURATION
PO	rapid	1–2 hr	up to 24 hr
IM	rapid	1–2 hr	up to 24 hr

Contraindications/Precautions

Contraindicated in: Hypersensitivity; Acute liver disease; History of hepatitis from previous use.

Use Cautiously in: History of liver damage or chronic alcohol ingestion; Black and Hispanic women, women in the postpartum period, or patients >50 yr (↑ risk of drug-induced hepatitis); Severe renal impairment (dose ↓ may be necessary); Malnourished patients, patients with diabetes, or chronic alcoholics (↑ risk of neuropathy); OB, Lactation: Although safety is not established, isoniazid has been used with ethambutol to treat tuberculosis in pregnant women without harm to the fetus.

Adverse Reactions/Side Effects

CNS: psychosis, seizures. **EENT:** visual disturbances. **GI:** DRUG-INDUCED HEPATITIS, nausea, vomiting. **Derm:** rashes. **Endo:** gynecomastia. **Hemat:** blood dyscrasias. **Neuro:** peripheral neuropathy. **Misc:** fever.

Interactions

Drug-Drug: Additive CNS toxicity with other **antituberculars**. **BCG vaccine** may not be effective during isoniazid therapy. Isoniazid ↓ metabolism of and may ↑ levels of **phenytoin**. **Aluminum-containing antacids** may ↓ absorption. Psychotic reactions and coordination difficulties may result with **disulfiram**. Concurrent administration of **pyridoxine** may prevent neuropathy. ↑ risk of hepatotoxicity with other **hepatotoxic agents** including **alcohol**, **acetaminophen** and **rifampin**. Isoniazid may ↓ blood levels and effectiveness of **ketoconazole**. May ↑ **carbamazepine** levels and risk of hepatotoxicity. May ↓ effectiveness of **clopidogrel** (avoid concurrent use).

Drug-Food: Severe reactions may occur with ingestion of foods containing high concentrations of **tyramine** (see Appendix J).

Route/Dosage

PO, IM (Adults): 300 mg/day (5 mg/kg) *or* 15 mg/kg (up to 900 mg) 2–3 times weekly.

PO, IM (Children <40 kg): *Latent TB infection*—10–20 mg/kg/day (up to 300 mg/day) *or* 20–40 mg/kg (up to 900 mg) 2 times weekly; *Active TB infection*—10–15 mg/kg/day (up to 300 mg/day) *or* 20–40 mg/kg (up to 900 mg) 2 times weekly.

Availability (generic available)

Tablets: 100 mg, 300 mg. **Oral solution (orange, raspberry flavor):** 50 mg/5 mL. **Injection:** 100 mg/mL. ***In combination with:*** rifampin (Rifamate); rifampin and pyrazinamide (Rifater). See Appendix B.

NURSING IMPLICATIONS

Assessment

- Mycobacterial studies and susceptibility tests should be performed prior to and periodically throughout therapy to detect possible resistance. About 50% to 65% of Caucasians, Black, South Indians and Mexicans are slow acetylators at risk for toxicity, while 80 to 90% of Eskimos, Japanese, and Chinese are rapid acetylators at risk for decreased levels and treatment failure.
- ***Lab Test Considerations:*** Hepatic function should be evaluated prior to and monthly throughout therapy. Increased AST, ALT, and serum bilirubin may indicate drug-induced hepatitis. Black and Hispanic women, postpartal women, and patients >50 yr are at highest risk. Risk is lower in children; therefore, liver function tests are usually ordered less frequently for children.
- ***Toxicity and Overdose:*** If isoniazid overdosage occurs, treatment with pyridoxine (vitamin B) is instituted.

Potential Nursing Diagnoses

Risk for infection (Indications)
Noncompliance (Patient/Family Teaching)

Implementation

- **PO:** May be administered with food or antacids if GI irritation occurs, although antacids containing aluminum should not be taken within 1 hr of administration.
- **IM:** Medication may cause discomfort at injection site. Massage site after administration and rotate injection sites.
- Solution may form crystals at low temperatures; crystals will redissolve upon warming to room temperature.

Patient/Family Teaching

- Advise patient to take medication as directed. Take missed doses as soon as possible unless almost time for next dose; do not double up on missed doses. Emphasize the importance of continuing therapy even after symptoms have subsided. Therapy may be continued for 6 mo–2 yr.
- Advise patient to notify health care professional promptly if signs and symptoms of hepatitis (yellow eyes and skin, nausea, vomiting, anorexia, dark urine, unusual tiredness, or weakness) or peripheral neuritis (numbness, tingling, paresthesia) occur. Pyridoxine may be used concurrently to prevent neuropathy. Any changes in visual acuity, eye pain, or blurred vision should also be reported immediately.
- Caution patient to avoid the use of alcohol during this therapy, as this may increase the risk of hepatotoxicity. Ingestion of Swiss or Cheshire cheeses, fish (tuna, skipjack, and sardinella), and possibly tyramine-containing foods (see Appendix J) should also be avoided, as they may result in redness or itching

of the skin; hot feeling; rapid or pounding heartbeat; sweating; chills; cold, clammy feeling; headache; or light-headedness.

- Emphasize the importance of regular follow-up physical and ophthalmologic exams to monitor progress and to check for side effects.

Evaluation/Desired Outcomes

- Resolution of signs and symptoms of tuberculosis.
- Negative sputum cultures.
- Prevention of activation of tuberculosis in persons known to have been exposed.

ISOSORBIDE

isosorbide dinitrate
(eye-soe-**sor**-bide dye-**nye**-trate)
Dilatrate-SR, Isordil

isosorbide mononitrate
(eye-soe-**sor**-bide mo-noe-**nye**-trate)
~~Imdur~~, ✱Imdur, ~~Ismo~~, Monoket

Classification
Therapeutic: antianginals
Pharmacologic: nitrates

Pregnancy Category C

Indications

Prophylactic management of angina pectoris. **Unlabeled Use:** Treatment of chronic heart failure (unlabeled).

Action

Produce vasodilation (venous greater than arterial). Decrease left ventricular end-diastolic pressure and left ventricular end-diastolic volume (preload). Net effect is reduced myocardial oxygen consumption. Increase coronary blood flow by dilating coronary arteries and improving collateral flow to ischemic regions. **Therapeutic Effects:** Prevention of anginal attacks.

Pharmacokinetics

Absorption: Isosorbide dinitrate undergoes extensive first-pass metabolism by the liver, resulting in 25% bioavailability; isosorbide mononitrate has 100% bioavailability (does not undergo first-pass metabolism).
Distribution: Unknown.
Metabolism and Excretion: Isosorbide dinitrate is metabolized by the liver to 2 active metabolites (5–mononitrate and 2–mononitrate). Isosorbide mononitrate is primarily meteabolized by the liver to inactive metabolites; primarily excreted in urine as metabolites.
Half-life: *Isosorbide dinitrate*—1 hr; *isosorbide mononitrate*—5 hr.

TIME/ACTION PROFILE (cardiovascular effects)

ROUTE	ONSET	PEAK	DURATION
ISDN-PO	45–60 min	unknown	4 hr
ISDN-PO-ER	30 min	unknown	up to 12 hr
ISMN-PO	30–60 min	unknown	7 hr
ISMN-ER	unknown	unknown	12 hr

Contraindications/Precautions

Contraindicated in: Hypersensitivity; Concurrent use of PDE-5 inhibitor (sildenafil, tadalafil, vardenafil) or riociguat.
Use Cautiously in: Volume depleted patients; Right ventricular infarction; Hypertrophic cardiomyopathy; OB: May compromise maternal/fetal circulation; Lactation: No data available; Pedi: Safety not established; Geri: Initial dose ↓ required due to ↑ potential for hypotension.

Adverse Reactions/Side Effects

CNS: <u>dizziness</u>, <u>headache</u>. **CV:** <u>hypotension</u>, <u>tachycardia</u>, paradoxic bradycardia, syncope. **GI:** nausea, vomiting. **Misc:** flushing, tolerance.

Interactions

Drug-Drug: Concurrent use of **sildenafil**, **tadalafil**, or **vardenafil** may result in severe hypotension (do not use within 24 hr of isosorbide dinitrate or mononitrate); concurrent use contraindicated. Concurrent use of **riociguat** may result in severe hypotension; concurrent use contraindicated. Additive hypotension with **antihypertensives**, acute ingestion of **alcohol**, **beta blockers**, **calcium channel blockers**, and **phenothiazines**.

Route/Dosage

Isosorbide Dinitrate

PO (Adults): *Prophylaxis of angina pectoris*—5–20 mg 2–3 times daily; usual maintenance dose is 10–40 mg q 6 hr (immediate-release) or 40–80 mg q 8–12 hr (sustained-release).

Isosorbide Mononitrate

PO (Adults): *ISMO, Monoket*—5–20 mg twice daily with the 2 doses given 7 hr apart. *Imdur*—30–60 mg once daily; may ↑ to 120 mg once daily (maximum dose = 240 mg/day).

Availability

Isosorbide Dinitrate (generic available)

Tablets: 5 mg, 10 mg, 20 mg, 30 mg, 40 mg. **Cost:** *Isordil*—40 mg $191.65/100; *Generic*—5 mg $15.54/100, 10 mg $32.96/100, 20 mg $18.85/100, 30 mg $23.32/100. **Extended-release tablets:** 40 mg. **Sustained-release capsules:** 40 mg. ***In combination with:*** hydralazine (BiDil). See Appendix B.

Isosorbide Mononitrate (generic available)

Tablets (Monoket): 10 mg, 20 mg. **Cost:** *Generic*—10 mg $55.97/180, 20 mg $48.99/180. **Extended-release tablets:** 30 mg, 60 mg, 120 mg. **Cost:** *Generic*—30 mg $10.00/90, 60 mg $10.00/90, 120 mg $61.18/90.

NURSING IMPLICATIONS

Assessment

- Assess location, duration, intensity, and precipitating factors of anginal pain.
- Monitor BP and pulse routinely during period of dose adjustment.
- ***Lab Test Considerations:*** Excessive doses may ↑ methemoglobin concentrations.

Potential Nursing Diagnoses

Ineffective tissue perfusion (Indications)
Activity intolerance (Indications)

Implementation

Isosorbide Dinitrate

- Do not confuse Isordil (isosorbide dinitrate) with Plendil (felodipine).
- **PO:** Swallow extended-release capsules whole; do not break, crush, or chew .

Isosorbide Mononitrate

- **PO:** Extended-release tablets should be swallowed whole. Do not break, crush, or chew.

Patient/Family Teaching

- Instruct patient to take medication as directed, even if feeling better. Take missed doses as soon as remembered; doses of isosorbide dinitrate should be taken at least 2 hr apart (6 hr with extended-release preparations); daily doses of isosorbide mononitrate should be taken 7 hr apart. Do not double doses. Do not discontinue abruptly.
- Caution patient to make position changes slowly to minimize orthostatic hypotension.
- May cause dizziness. Caution patient to avoid driving or other activities requiring alertness until response to medication is known.
- Instruct patient to take last dose of day (when taking 2–4 doses/day) no later than 7 pm to prevent the development of tolerance.
- Advise patient to avoid concurrent use of alcohol with this medication. Instruct patient to notify health care professional of all Rx or OTC medications, vitamins, or herbal products being taken and to consult health care professional before taking other Rx, OTC, or herbal products.
- Inform patient that headache is a common side effect that should decrease with continuing therapy. Aspirin or acetaminophen may be ordered to treat headache. Notify health care professional if headache is persistent or severe. Do not alter dose to avoid headache.
- Advise patient to notify health care professional if dry mouth or blurred vision occurs.

Evaluation/Desired Outcomes

- Decrease in frequency and severity of anginal attacks.
- Increase in activity tolerance.

REMS

ISOtretinoin

(eye-soe-**tret**-i-noyn)
Absorica, ~~Accutane~~, ✱Accutane, Amnesteem, Claravis, ✱Clarus, ✱Epuris, Myorisan, Sotret, Zenatane

Classification
Therapeutic: antiacne agents
Pharmacologic: retinoids

Pregnancy Category X

Indications

Management of severe nodular acne resistant to more conventional therapy, including topical therapy and systemic antibiotics. Not to be used under any circumstances in pregnant patients.

Action

A metabolite of vitamin A (retinol); reduces sebaceous gland size and differentiation. **Therapeutic Effects:** Diminution and resolution of severe acne. May also prevent abnormal keratinization.

Pharmacokinetics

Absorption: Rapidly absorbed following (23–25%) oral administration; absorption ↑ when taken with a high-fat meal.
Distribution: Appears to be widely distributed; crosses the placenta.
Protein Binding: 99.9%.
Metabolism and Excretion: Metabolized by the liver and excreted in the urine and feces.
Half-life: 10–20 hr.

TIME/ACTION PROFILE (diminution of acne)

ROUTE	ONSET	PEAK	DURATION
PO	unknown	up to 8 wk	unknown

Contraindications/Precautions

Contraindicated in: Hypersensitivity to retinoids, glycerin, soybean oil, or parabens; OB, Lactation: Pregnancy and lactation; Rep: Women of childbearing age who may become or who intend to become pregnant; Patients planning to donate blood.
Use Cautiously in: Pre-existing hypertriglyceridemia; Diabetes mellitus; History of alcohol abuse, psychosis, depression, or suicide attempt; Obese patients;

Inflammatory bowel disease.; Pedi: Children <12 yr (safety not established)

Adverse Reactions/Side Effects

CNS: SUICIDE ATTEMPT, behavior changes, depression, PSEUDOTUMOR CEREBRI, psychosis, suicidal ideation. **EENT:** conjunctivitis, epistaxis, blurred vision, contact lens intolerance, corneal opacities, ↓ night vision, dry eyes. **CV:** edema. **GI:** cheilitis, dry mouth, nausea, vomiting, abdominal pain, anorexia, hepatitis, pancreatitis, ↑ appetite. **Derm:** STEVENS-JOHNSON SYNDROME, TOXIC EPIDERMAL NECROLYSIS, pruritus, palmar desquamation, photosensitivity, skin infections, thinning of hair. **Hemat:** anemia. **Metab:** ↓ high-density lipoprotein cholesterol, hypercholesterolemia, hypertriglyceridemia, hyperglycemia, hyperuricemia. **MS:** arthralgia, back pain, muscle/bone pain (↑ in adolescents), hyperostosis. **Misc:** SEVERE BIRTH DEFECTS, ↑ thirst.

Interactions

Drug-Drug: Additive toxicity with **vitamin A** and **drugs having anticholinergic properties**. ↑ risk of pseudotumor cerebri with **tetracycline** or **minocycline**. Concurrent use with **alcohol** ↑ risk of hypertriglyceridemia. Drying effects ↑ by concurrent use of **benzoyl peroxide**, **sulfur**, **tretinoin**, and **other topical agents**.

Drug-Food: Excessive ingestion of **foods high in vitamin A** may result in additive toxicity.

Route/Dosage

PO (Adults and Children ≥12 yr): 0.5–1 mg/kg/day (up to 2 mg/kg/day) in 2 divided doses for 15–20 wk. Once discontinued, if relapse occurs, therapy may be reinstituted after an 8-wk rest period.

Availability (generic available)

Capsules: 10 mg, 20 mg, 25 mg, 30 mg, 35 mg, 40 mg.

NURSING IMPLICATIONS

Assessment

- Verify that patient receiving isotretinoin is registered with the *iPLEDGE program* and is completing all required interactions with their health care provider.
- Assess skin prior to and periodically during therapy. Transient worsening of acne may occur at initiation of therapy. Note number and severity of cysts, degree of skin dryness, erythema, and itching.
- Assess for allergy to parabens; capsules contain parabens as a preservative.
- Monitor patient for behavioral changes throughout therapy. May cause depression, psychosis, and suicide ideation. If behavioral changes occur, they usually resolve with discontinuation of therapy.
- Assess for rash periodically during therapy. May cause Stevens-Johnson syndrome or toxic epidermal necrolysis. Discontinue therapy if severe or if accompanied with fever, general malaise, fatigue, muscle or joint aches, blisters, oral lesions, conjunctivitis, hepatitis and/or eosinophilia.
- ***Lab Test Considerations:*** Obtain 2 negative sequential serum or urine pregnancy tests with a sensitivity ≥25 mIU/mL before receiving initial prescription and monthly before each new Rx.
- Monitor liver function (AST, ALT, and LDH) prior to therapy, after 1 mo of therapy, and periodically thereafter. Inform health care professional if these values become ↑ therapy may need to be discontinued.
- Monitor blood lipids (cholesterol, HDL, triglycerides) under fasting conditions prior to beginning therapy, at 1–2 wk intervals until lipid response to isotretinoin is established (usually within 1 mo), and periodically thereafter. Report ↑ cholesterol and triglyceride levels or ↓ HDL.
- Obtain baseline and periodic CBC, urinalysis, and SMA-12. May cause ↑ blood glucose, CPK, platelet counts, and sedimentation rate. May ↓ RBC and WBC parameters. May cause proteinuria, red and white blood cells in urine, and ↑ uric acid.

Potential Nursing Diagnoses

Risk for impaired skin integrity (Indications, Side Effects)

Disturbed body image (Indications)

Implementation

- Do not confuse isotretinoin with tretinoin.
- Isotretinoin is approved for marketing only under the *iPLEDGE program*, a special restricted distribution program approved by the FDA.
- Only patients who meet all requirements of the *iPLEDGE program* may receive isotretinoin.
- Isotretinoin may only be prescribed by health care providers registered and activated with the *iPLEDGE program*.
- Isotretinoin may only be dispensed by pharmacies registered with the *iPLEDGE program*.
- **PO:** Administer with meals. Do not crush or open capsules.

Patient/Family Teaching

- Explain the *iPLEDGE program* and its requirements to patient and parent.
- Instruct patient to take isotretinoin as directed. Do not take more than the amount prescribed. Take missed doses as soon as remembered if not almost time for next dose. Do not double doses. Patients must read *Medication Guide* and sign consent form prior to initiation of therapy.
- Explain to patient that a temporary worsening of acne may occur at beginning of therapy.
- Rep: Instruct female patients to use 2 forms of contraception 1 mo before therapy, throughout therapy,

I

and for at least 1 mo after discontinuation of drug. This drug is contraindicated during pregnancy and may cause birth defects. Patient must have 2 negative serum or urine pregnancy tests with a sensitivity ≥25 mIU/mL before receiving initial prescription. First test is obtained by prescriber when decision is made to prescribe isotretinoin. Second pregnancy test should be done during first 5 days of menstrual period immediately preceding beginning of therapy. For patients with amenorrhea, second test should be done 11 days after last act of unprotected sexual intercourse. Each month of therapy patient must have a negative result from a urine or serum pregnancy test. Pregnancy test must be repeated every month prior to female patient receiving prescription. Manufacturer will make available pregnancy test kits to female patients. Patient should discontinue medication and inform health care professional immediately if pregnancy is suspected. Recommended consent form prepared by manufacturer stresses fetal risk. Parents of minors should also read and sign form. Yellow self-adhesive qualification stickers completed by prescriber must accompany prescription.

- Advise patient and family to notify health care professional if rash or thoughts about suicide or dying, attempts to commit suicide; new or worse depression; new or worse anxiety; feeling very agitated or restless; panic attacks; trouble sleeping; new or worse irritability; acting aggressive; being angry or violent; acting on dangerous impulses; an extreme increase in activity and talking; other unusual changes in behavior or mood occur.
- May cause sudden decrease in night vision. Caution patient to avoid driving at night until response to the medication is known.
- Advise patient to consult with health care professional before using other acne preparations while taking isotretinoin. Soaps, cosmetics, and shaving lotion may also worsen dry skin.
- Advise patient to notify health care professional of all Rx or OTC medications, vitamins, or herbal products being taken and to consult with health care professional before taking other medications.
- Inform patient that dry skin and chapped lips will occur. Lubricant to lips may help cheilitis.
- Instruct patient that oral rinses, good oral hygiene, and sugarless gum or candy may help minimize dry mouth. Notify health care professional if dry mouth persists for more than 2 wk.
- Discuss possibility of excessively dry eyes with patients who wear contact lenses. Patient should contact health care professional about eye lubricant. Patient may need to switch to glasses during course of therapy and for up to 2 wk following discontinuation.
- Advise patient to avoid alcoholic beverages while taking isotretinoin, as this may further increase triglyceride levels.
- Caution patient to use sunscreen and protective clothing to prevent photosensitivity reactions. Health care professional should be consulted about sunscreen, as some sunscreens may worsen acne.
- Instruct patient not to take vitamin A supplements and to avoid excessive ingestion of foods high in vitamin A (liver; fish liver oils; egg yolks; yellow-orange fruits and vegetables; dark green, leafy vegetables; whole milk; vitamin A–fortified skim milk; butter; margarine) while taking isotretinoin; this may result in hypervitaminosis.
- Advise patient not to donate blood while receiving this medication. After discontinuing isotretinoin, wait at least 1 mo before donating blood to prevent the possibility of a pregnant patient receiving the blood.
- Inform diabetic patients that difficulty controlling blood glucose may occur.
- Instruct patient to report burning of eyes, visual changes, rash, abdominal pain, diarrhea, headache, nausea, and vomiting to health care professional.
- Inform patient of need for medical follow-up. Periodic lab tests may be required.

Evaluation/Desired Outcomes

- Decrease in the number and severity of cysts in severe acne. Therapy may take 4–5 mo before full effects are seen. Therapy is discontinued when the number of cysts is reduced by 70% or after 5 mo. Improvement may occur after discontinuation of therapy; therefore, a delay of at least 8 wk is recommended before a second course of therapy is considered.

ivabradine (eye-**vab**-ra-deen)

Corlanor

Classification
Therapeutic: heart failure agents
Pharmacologic: hyperpolarization-activated cyclic nucleotide-gated channel blockers

Indications

To decrease the need for hospitalization due to worsening HF in patients with stable, but symptomatic chronic HF (ejection fraction <35%, sinus rhythm ≥70 bpm, receiving highest tolerated doses of beta-blockers or are unable to tolerate beta-blockers).

Action

Inhibits the cardiac pacemaker I_f-current by acting as a hyperpolarization-activated cyclic nucleoside-gated channel blocker, resulting in ↓ spontaneous pacemaker activity of sinus node. Decreases heart rate without effecting contractility or ventricular repolarization. **Therapeutic Effects:** Lowering of heart rate with reduced need for hospitalization in HF patients.

Pharmacokinetics

Absorption: 40% absorbed following oral administration (undergoes first pass metabolism); food delays absorption and ↑ blood levels.

Distribution: Unknown.

Metabolism and Excretion: Extensively metabolized, primarily by the CYP3A4 enzyme system. The major metabolite is pharmacologically active and has the same potency as ivabradine. Metabolites excreted equally in urine and feces; 4% excreted unchanged in urine.

Half-life: 6 hr.

TIME/ACTION PROFILE (blood levels)

ROUTE	ONSET	PEAK	DURATION
PO	unknown	1 hr	12 hr

Contraindications/Precautions

Contraindicated in: Acute decompensated heart failure; BP <90/50 mmHg; Sick sinus syndrome, sinoatrial block or 3rd degree heart block (unless a functioning demand pacemaker is in place, ↑ risk of bradycardia); Resting heart rate <60 bpm (before treatment); Severe hepatic impairment; Concurrent use of demand pacemaker set at ≥60 bpm; Pacemaker dependence; Concurrent use of strong CYP3A4 inhibitors; Second degree AV block; OB: Pregnancy (may cause fetal harm); Lactation: Discontinue ivabradine or discontinue breast feeding.

Use Cautiously in: Female patients with reproductive potential (effective contraception required); Pedi: Safe and effective use in children has not been established.

Adverse Reactions/Side Effects

EENT: phosphenes (luminous phenomena). **CV:** atrial fibrillation, bradycardia, heart block, hypertension, sinus arrest.

Interactions

Drug-Drug: Blood levels and risk of adverse effects ↑ by concurrent use of **CYP3A4 inhibitors**; concurrent use of **strong inhibitors** including **azole antifungals**, **macolide anti-infectives**, **HIV protease inhibitors** and **nefazodone** is contraindicated. Use of **moderate inhibitors** including **diltiazem** and **verapamil** should be avoided. Blood levels and effectiveness may be ↓ by concurrent use of **CYP3A4 inducers** including **barbiturates**, **phenytoin** and **rifampicin**; concurrent use should be avoided. ↑ risk of bradycardia with concurrent use of **negative chronotropes** including **amiodarone**, **beta-blockers**, and **digoxin**; monitoring of heart rate is recommended.

Drug-Natural Products: Concurrent use of **St. John's wort** may ↓ blood levels and effectiveness and should be avoided.

Drug-Food: Concurrent ingestion of **grapefruit juice** may ↑ blood levels and the risk of adverse effects and should be avoided.

Route/Dosage

PO (Adults): 5 mg twice daily for two weeks, dose may then be adjusted based on heart rate, not to exceed 7.5 mg twice daily; *patients with conduction defects or bradycardia*—2.5 mg twice daily initially.

Availability

Tablets: 5 mg, 7.5 mg.

NURSING IMPLICATIONS

Assessment

- Assess heart rate prior to, after 2 wks, and periodically during therapy. Adjust dose for a resting heart rate 50–60 bpm. *If heart rate >60 bpm,* increase dose by 2.5 mg given twice daily up to 7.5 mg twice daily. *If heart rate 50–60 bpm,* maintain dose. *If heart rate <50 bpm or signs and symptoms of bradycardia (dizziness, fatigue, hypotension) occur,* decrease dose by 2.5 mg given twice daily; if current dose is 2.5 mg given twice daily, discontinue ivabradine.
- Monitor ECG periodically during therapy. May cause atrial fibrillation. Discontinue ivabradine of atrial fibrillation occurs.

Potential Nursing Diagnoses

Decreased cardiac output (Indications)

Implementation

- **PO:** Administer twice daily with meals.

Patient/Family Teaching

- Instruct patient to take ivabradine as directed.
- Advise patient to avoid taking grapefruit juice during therapy; may increase risk of side effects.
- Inform patient that ivabradine may cause phosphenes or luminous phenomena, a transiently enhanced brightness in a limited area of the visual field, halos, image decomposition, colored bright lights, or multiple images. Phosphenes are usually triggered by sudden variations in light intensity. Usually begin within first 2 months of therapy, may occur repeatedly of mild to moderate intensity, and resolve after therapy is discontinued.
- Instruct patient to notify health care professional of all Rx or OTC medications, vitamins, or herbal products being taken and to consult health care professional before taking any other Rx, OTC, or herbal products, especially St. John's wort.
- May be teratogenic. Advise female patient to use effective contraception during therapy and to notify health care professional if pregnancy is planned or suspected or if breast feeding.

Evaluation/Desired Outcomes

- Lowering of heart rate to prevent hospitalization in patients with HF.

ixabepilone (icks-a-**bep**-i-lone)

Ixempra

Classification

Therapeutic: antineoplastics

Pharmacologic: epothilone B analogues

Pregnancy Category D

Indications

Combination use with capecitabine for the treatment of metastatic or locally advanced breast cancer currently resistant to a taxane and anthracycline or resistant to a taxane and cannot tolerate further anthracycline. May also be used as monotherapy for breast cancers that are not responding to anthracyclines, taxane, or capecitabine.

Action

Binds to β-tubulin subunits on microtubules; this action blocks cells in mitosis, leading to cell death. Also has antiangiogenic activity. **Therapeutic Effects:** Decreased spread of breast cancer.

Pharmacokinetics

Absorption: IV administration results in complete bioavailablity.

Distribution: Unknown.

Metabolism and Excretion: Extensively metabolized by the liver, primarily by the CYP3A4 enzyme system. Metabolites are not active and are excreted mainly by the kidneys.

Half-life: 52 hr.

TIME/ACTION PROFILE (blood levels)

ROUTE	ONSET	PEAK	DURATION
IV	unknown	end of infusion	unknown

Contraindications/Precautions

Contraindicated in: Previous hypersensitivity to any medications containing Cremophor EL or similar derivatives (polyoxyethylated castor oil); Neutrophils <1500 cells/m^3 or platelets <100,000 cells/m^3; Severe hepatic impairment; Use with capecitabine is contraindicated for hepatic impairment (AST or ALT >2.5 × upper limits of normal or bilirubin >1 × upper limit of normal) due to ↑ risk of toxicity and death associated with neutropenia; OB, Lactation: Pregnancy or lactation.

Use Cautiously in: Toxicity; dose adjustments may be required for neuropathy/arthralgia/myalgia/fatigue, neutropenia, thrombocytopenia, moderate hepatic impairment or palmar-plantar erythrodysesthesia; Diluent contains dehydrated alcohol; consider possible CNS effects; Diabetes or history of neuropathy (↑ risk of severe neuropathy); History of cardiac disease (may ↑ risk of myocardial ischemia or ventricular dysfunction; OB: Patients with childbearing potential; Pedi: Effectiveness not established.

Adverse Reactions/Side Effects

CNS: fatigue, weakness, dizziness, headache, insomnia. **EENT:** ↑ lacrimation. **CV:** chest pain, edema, left ventricular dysfunction, myocardial ischemia. **Resp:** dyspnea. **GI:** abdominal pain, anorexia, constipation, diarrhea, mucositis, nausea, stomatitis, vomiting, altered taste. **Derm:** alopecia, hyperpigmentation, nail disorder, palmar-plantar erythrodysesthesia (combination therapy with capecitabine), exfoliation, pruritus, rash, hot flushes. **Hemat:** MYELOSUPPRESSION. **MS:** arthralgia, musculoskeletal pain, myalgia. **Neuro:** peripheral neuropathy. **Misc:** hypersensitivity reactions.

Interactions

Drug-Drug: Strong CYP3A4 inhibitors including **ketoconazole**, **itraconazole**, **voriconazole**, **clarithromycin**, **telithromycin**, **atazanavir**, **delavirdine**, **ritonavir**, **saquinavir**, **nefazodone** ↑ blood levels and the risk of serious toxicities, concurrent use should be avoided if possible. If concurrent use is required, dose reduction of ixabepilone is recommended. Inducers of the **CYP3A4 enzyme system** including **dexamathasone**, **phenytoin**, **carbamazepine**, **phenobarbital**, **rifampin**, **rifampicin**, or **rifabutin** may ↓ levels and effectiveness, avoid if possible.

Drug-Natural Products: St. John's wort may ↓ blood levels and should be avoided.

Drug-Food: Grapefruit juice may ↑ blood levels and toxicity; avoid concurrent use.

Route/Dosage

IV (Adults): 40 mg/m^2 every 3 wk; not to exceed dose greater than that calculated for 2.2 m^2 (88 mg/dose).

Hepatic Impairment

IV (Adults): *Moderate Impairment*—20 mg/m^2 every 3 wk; not to exceed 30 mg/m^2.

Availability

Powder for injection (requires specific diluent for initial reconstitution): 15-mg vial (contains 16 mg ixabepilone to allow for withdrawal losses) with 8 mL of diluent in a separate vial as a kit, 45-mg vial (contains 47 mg ixabepilone to allow for withdrawal losses) with 23.5 mL of diluent in a separate vial.

NURSING IMPLICATIONS

Assessment

- Monitor for hypersensitivity reaction (flushing, rash, dyspnea, bronchospasm). If severe reactions occur stop infusion and provide aggressive supportive treatment with epinephrine and corticosteroids. In subsequent cycles, add corticosteroids to the premedication regimen.

- Monitor for myelosuppression frequently during therapy. Assess for signs of infection during neutropenia. Assess for bleeding (bleeding gums, bruising, petechiae, blood in stools, urine, and emesis) and avoid IM injections and taking rectal temperatures if platelet count is low. Apply pressure to venipuncture sites for 10 min.
- Assess patient for signs of peripheral neuropathy (burning sensation, hyperesthesia, hypoesthesia, paresthesia, discomfort, neuropathic pain); may occur early during treatment within the first 3 cycles. Patients experiencing new or worsening symptoms may require a reduction or delay in dose of ixabepilone. If neuropathy is Grade 2 (moderate) lasting for ≥7 days or Grade 3 (severe) lasting for <7 days decrease dose by 20%. If neuropathy is Grade 3 lasting ≥7 days or is disabling discontinue treatment.
- ***Lab Test Considerations:*** Monitor CBC and platelets frequently during therapy. If neutrophil count is <500 cells/mm^3 for ≥7 days or patient has febrile neutropenia or if platelet count is <25,000/mm^3 or platelets are <50,000/mm^3 with bleeding decrease the dose by 20%. Begin new treatment cycle only if neutrophil count is at least 1500 cells/mm^3 and nonhematologic toxicities have improved to Grade 1 (mild) or resolved. May also cause leukopenia and anemia.
- Monitor hepatic function prior to therapy. Patients with decreased hepatic function require a decreased dose. If AST and ALT ≤2.5 × the upper limits of normal (ULN) and bilirubin ≤1 × ULN administer ixabepilone at 40 mg/m^2. If AST and ALT ≤10 × the upper limits of normal (ULN) and bilirubin ≤1 X ULN administer ixabepilone at 32mg/m^2. If AST and ALT ≤10 × the upper limits of normal (ULN) and bilirubin >1.5 × ULN—≤3 × ULN administer ixabepilone at 20–30 mg/m^2.

Potential Nursing Diagnoses

Risk for injury (Adverse Reactions)

Implementation

- Premedicate patient with an H_1 and an H_2 antagonist approximately 1 hr before ixabepilone infusion. Patients who experienced a hypersensitivity reaction in a previous ixabepilone cycle should also be premedicated with corticosteroids and extension of the infusion time should be considered.
- To minimize risk of dermal exposure, wear impervious gloves when handling ixabepilone vials regardless of setting (unpacking and inspection, transport within a facility, dose preparation and administration).

IV Administration

- **Intermittent Infusion:** Remove *Ixempra kit* (containing ixabepilone vial and diluent vial) from refrigerator and allow to stand at room temperature for 30 min prior to diluting. *Ixempra kit* must be stored in refrigerator. When vials are first removed from refrigerator, a white precipitate may be observed in the diluent vial; precipitate will dissolve to form a clear solution once diluent warms to room temperature. Use only diluent supplied in kit for reconstitution. Reconstitute 15-mg vial with 8 mL and 45-mg vial with 23.5 mL of diluent. Gently swirl and invert vial until powder is completely dissolved. ***Diluent:*** Prior to administration, dilute constituted solution further with only LR supplied in DEHP-free bags. Dilute as soon as possible after constitution, but may be stored at room temperature and room light for up to 1 hr. For most doses use 250 mL bag of LR, 0.9% NaCl (pH adjusted 6.0–9.0 with sodium bicarbonate), or Plasma-lyte A injection (pH 7.4). ***Concentration:*** If final concentration is not between 0.2 mg/mL and 0.6 mg/mL add to appropriate size bag of LR. Thoroughly mix infusion bag by manual rotation. Diluted solution is stable for up to 6 hr at room temperature and room light; must complete infusion during 6-hr period. Administer through an in-line filter with a microporous membrane of 0.2–1.2 microns. DEHP-free infusion containers and administration sets must be used. Discard remaining solution. ***Rate:*** Infuse over 3 hr.

Patient/Family Teaching

- Advise patient to avoid grapefruit juice during therapy; may lead to increased levels and side effects.
- Solution contains alcohol and may cause drowsiness or dizziness. Caution patient to avoid driving and other activities requiring alertness until response to medication is known.
- Instruct patient to notify health care professional promptly if fever >100.5°F; chills; cough; hoarseness; sore throat; signs of infection; lower back or side pain; burning, painful or difficulty urination; bleeding gums; bruising; petechiae; blood in stools, urine, or emesis; increased fatigue; dyspnea; or orthostatic hypotension occurs. Caution patient to avoid crowds and persons with known infections. Instruct patients to use a soft toothbrush and electric razor and to avoid falls. Caution patient not to drink alcoholic beverages or take medication containing aspirin or NSAIDs; may precipitate bleeding.
- Instruct patient to notify health care professional promptly if signs and symptoms of hypersensitivity (hives, urticaria, pruritus, rash, flushing, swelling, dyspnea, chest tightness), peripheral neuropathy (numbness and tingling in hands and feet), or car-

diac adverse reactions (chest pain, difficulty breathing, palpitations, unusual weight gain) occur.
- Advise patient to notify health care professional of all Rx or OTC medications, vitamins, or herbal products being taken and to consult health care professional before taking other Rx, OTC, or herbal products, especially St. John's wort.
- Instruct patient not to receive any vaccinations without advice of health care professional.
- Discuss the possibility of hair loss with patient. Explore methods of coping. Regrowth usually occurs 2–3 mo after discontinuation of therapy.
- Advise women of childbearing potential to use effective contraception during therapy and to avoid breast feeding during therapy.

Evaluation/Desired Outcomes

- Decreased progression of breast cancer.

ketoconazole, See ANTIFUNGALS (TOPICAL).

ketoprofen (kee-toe-proe-fen)

Classification
Therapeutic: antipyretics, antirheumatics, nonopioid analgesics, nonsteroidal anti-inflammatory agents
Pharmacologic: nonopioid analgesics

Pregnancy Category C

Indications
Inflammatory disorders, including: Rheumatoid arthritis, Osteoarthritis. Mild to moderate pain, including dysmenorrhea and fever.

Action
Inhibits prostaglandin synthesis. **Therapeutic Effects:** Suppression of pain and inflammation. Reduction of fever.

Pharmacokinetics
Absorption: Well absorbed from the GI tract.
Distribution: Unknown.
Protein Binding: 99%.
Metabolism and Excretion: Mostly (60%) metabolized by the liver; some renal excretion.
Half-life: 2–4 hr.

TIME/ACTION PROFILE

ROUTE	ONSET	PEAK	DURATION
PO (analgesic)	within 60 min	1 hr	4–6 hr
PO (anti-inflammatory)	few days–1 wk	unknown	up to 24 hr (SR products)

Contraindications/Precautions
Contraindicated in: Hypersensitivity; Cross-sensitivity may exist with other NSAIDs, including aspirin; Active GI bleeding; Ulcer disease; Some products contain tartrazine and should be avoided in patients with known intolerance; Peri-operative pain from coronary artery bypass graft (CABG) surgery; OB: Should not be used in late pregnancy (may cause premature closure of the ductus arteriosus).
Use Cautiously in: Cardiovascular disease or risk factors for cardiovascular disease (may ↑ risk of serious cardiovascular thrombotic events, myocardial infarction, and stroke, especially with prolonged use or use of higher doses); Severe renal or hepatic disease; History of ulcer disease; Renal impairment (dosage ↓ suggested); Geri: Extended-release product should not be used in geriatric patients, patients of small stature, or patients with renal impairment; ↑ risk of bleeding; Chronic alcohol use/abuse; Lactation, Pedi: Safety not established.

Adverse Reactions/Side Effects
CNS: drowsiness, headache, dizziness. **EENT:** blurred vision, tinnitus. **CV:** HF, MYOCARDIAL INFARCTION, STROKE, edema, hypertension. **GI:** DRUG-INDUCED HEPATITIS, GI BLEEDING, constipation, diarrhea, dyspepsia, nausea, vomiting, anorexia, discomfort, flatulence. **GU:** cystitis, hematuria, renal failure. **Derm:** EXFOLIATIVE DERMATITIS, STEVENS-JOHNSON SYNDROME, TOXIC EPIDERMAL NECROLYSIS, photosensitivity, rashes. **Endo:** gynecomastia. **Hemat:** blood dyscrasias, prolonged bleeding time. **MS:** myalgia. **Misc:** allergic reactions including ANAPHYLAXIS, fever.

Interactions
Drug-Drug: Aspirin alters distribution, metabolism, and excretion of ketoprofen (concurrent use not recommended). ↑ adverse GI effects with other **NSAIDs**, **corticosteroids**, or **alcohol**. Chronic use with **acetaminophen** may ↑ risk of adverse renal reactions. May ↓ effectiveness of **diuretics** or **antihypertensives**. May ↑ hypoglycemic effects of **insulin** or sulfonylurea **oral hypoglycemic agents**. May ↑ serum **lithium** levels and risk of toxicity. ↑ risk of toxicity from **methotrexate**. **Probenecid** ↑ risk of toxicity from ketoprofen (concurrent use not recommended). ↑ risk of bleeding with **cefotetan**, **valproic acid**, **thrombolytic agents**, **clopidogrel**, **eptifibatide**, **tirofiban**, or **anticoagulants**. ↑ risk of adverse hematologic reactions with **antineoplastics** or **radiation therapy**. ↑ risk of nephrotoxicity with **cyclosporine**.
Drug-Natural Products: ↑ bleeding risk with **arnica**, **chamomile**, **clove**, **dong quai**, **feverfew**, **garlic**, **ginger**, **ginkgo**, and **Panax ginseng**.

Route/Dosage
PO (Adults): *Anti-inflammatory*—150–300 mg/day in 3–4 divided doses or 150–200 mg once daily as extended-release product; *Analgesic*—25–50 mg q 6–8 hr.

Availability (generic available)
Capsules: 25 mg, 50 mg, 75 mg. **Extended-release capsules:** 100 mg, 150 mg, 200 mg.

NURSING IMPLICATIONS

Assessment
- Patients who have asthma, aspirin-induced allergy, and nasal polyps are at increased risk for developing hypersensitivity reactions. Assess for rhinitis, wheezing, and urticaria.
- Assess for rash periodically during therapy. May cause Stevens-Johnson syndrome or toxic epidermal

K

necrolysis. Discontinue therapy if severe or if accompanied with fever, general malaise, fatigue, muscle or joint aches, blisters, oral lesions, conjunctivitis, hepatitis and/or eosinophilia.

- **Arthritis:** Assess pain and range of motion prior to and 1 hr following administration.
- **Pain:** Assess pain (note type, location, and intensity) prior to and 1 hr following administration.
- **Fever:** Monitor temperature; note signs associated with fever (diaphoresis, tachycardia, malaise).
- ***Lab Test Considerations:*** Evaluate BUN, serum creatinine, CBC, and liver function tests periodically in patients receiving prolonged therapy.
- Serum potassium, BUN, serum creatinine, alkaline phosphatase, LDH, AST, and ALT tests may show ↑ levels. Blood glucose, hemoglobin and hematocrit concentrations, leukocyte and platelet counts, and CCr may be ↓.
- May prolong bleeding time by 3–4 min.
- May alter results of urine albumin, bilirubin, 17-ketosteroid, and 17-hydroxycorticosteroid determinations.

Potential Nursing Diagnoses

Acute pain (Indications)
Impaired physical mobility (Indications)

Implementation

- Administration in higher-than-recommended doses does not provide increased effectiveness but may cause increased side effects. Use lowest effective dose for shortest period of time.
- Coadministration with opioid analgesics may have additive analgesic effects and may permit lower opioid doses.
- Analgesic is more effective if given before pain becomes severe.
- **PO:** For rapid initial effect, administer 30 min before or 2 hr after meals. Capsules may be administered with food, milk, or antacids containing aluminum hydroxide and magnesium hydroxide to decrease GI irritation.
- Extended-release capsules should be swallowed whole; do not open or chew.
- **Dysmenorrhea:** Administer as soon as possible after the onset of menses.

Patient/Family Teaching

- Advise patient to take this medication with a full glass of water and to remain in an upright position for 15–30 min after administration.
- Instruct patient to take medication exactly as directed. Take missed doses as soon as remembered but not if almost time for the next dose. Do not double doses.
- May cause drowsiness or dizziness. Advise patient to avoid driving or other activities requiring alertness until response to medication is known.
- Caution patient to avoid the concurrent use of alcohol, aspirin, acetaminophen, or other OTC medications without consulting health care professional.
- Advise patient to inform health care professional of medication regimen prior to treatment or surgery.
- Caution patient to wear sunscreen and protective clothing to prevent photosensitivity reactions.
- Instruct patients not to take OTC ketoprofen preparations for more than 10 days for pain or more than 3 days for fever and to consult health care professional if symptoms persist or worsen.
- Caution patient that use of ketoprofen with 3 or more glasses of alcohol may increase risk of GI bleeding.
- Advise patient to consult health care professional if rash, itching, visual disturbances, tinnitus, weight gain, edema, black stools, persistent headache, or influenza-like syndrome (chills, fever, muscle aches, pain) occurs.
- Advise patient to notify health care professional if pregnancy is planned or suspected or if breast feeding.

Evaluation/Desired Outcomes

- Improved joint mobility.
- Decrease in severity of pain. Improvement in arthritis may be seen in a few days to 1 wk; 1–2 wk may be required for maximum effectiveness. Patients who do not respond to one NSAID may respond to another.
- Reduction of fever.

ketorolac† (kee-**toe**-role-ak)

Sprix, ~~Toradol~~, ✱Toradol

Classification
Therapeutic: nonsteroidal anti-inflammatory agents, nonopioid analgesics
Pharmacologic: pyrroziline carboxylic acid

Pregnancy Category C (oral, nasal spray [<30 wk gestation]), D (nasal spray [≥30 wk gestation)

†See Appendix C for ophthalmic use

Indications

Short-term management of pain (not to exceed 5 days total for all routes combined).

Action

Inhibits prostaglandin synthesis, producing peripherally mediated analgesia. Also has antipyretic and anti-inflammatory properties. **Therapeutic Effects:** Decreased pain.

Pharmacokinetics

Absorption: Rapidly and completely absorbed following all routes of administration.
Distribution: Enters breast milk in low concentrations.
Protein Binding: 99%.
Metabolism and Excretion: Primarily metabolized by the liver. Ketorolac and its metabolites are ex-

creted primarily by the kidneys (92%); 6% excreted in feces.

Half-life: 4.5 hr (range 3.8–6.3 hr; ↑ in geriatric patients and patients with impaired renal function).

TIME/ACTION PROFILE (analgesic effects)

ROUTE	ONSET	PEAK	DURATION
PO	unknown	2–3 hr	4–6 hr or longer
IM, IV	10 min	1–2 hr	6 hr or longer
IN	unknown	unknown	6–8 hr or longer

Contraindications/Precautions

Contraindicated in: Hypersensitivity; Cross-sensitivity with other NSAIDs may exist; Preoperative use; Active or history of peptic ulcer disease or GI bleeding; Known alcohol intolerance (injection only); Perioperative pain from coronary artery bypass graft (CABG) surgery; Cerebrovascular bleeding; Advanced renal impairment or at risk for renal failure due to volume depletion; Concurrent use of pentoxifylline or probenecid; OB: Chronic use in 3rd trimester may cause constriction of ductus arteriosus. May inhibit labor and ↑ maternal bleeding at delivery.

Use Cautiously in: Cardiovascular disease or risk factors for cardiovascular disease (may ↑ risk of serious cardiovascular thrombotic events, myocardial infarction, and stroke, especially with prolonged use or use of higher doses); Heart failure; Coagulation disorders; Mild-to-moderate renal impairment (↓ dose may be required); Hepatic impairment; Pedi: Safety not established in neonates; Geri: Appears on Beers list; ↑ risk of GI bleeding.; Lactation: Lactation.

Adverse Reactions/Side Effects

CNS: drowsiness, abnormal thinking, dizziness, euphoria, headache. **EENT:** ↑ lacrimation (spray), nasal discomfort (spray), throat irritation (spray). **Resp:** asthma, dyspnea. **CV:** HF, MYOCARDIAL INFARCTION, STROKE, edema, pallor, vasodilation. **GI:** GI BLEEDING, abnormal taste, diarrhea, dry mouth, dyspepsia, GI pain, ↑ liver enzymes, nausea. **GU:** oliguria, renal toxicity, urinary frequency. **Derm:** EXFOLIATIVE DERMATITIS, STEVENS-JOHNSON SYNDROME, TOXIC EPIDERMAL NECROLYSIS, pruritus, purpura, sweating, urticaria. **Hemat:** prolonged bleeding time. **Local:** injection site pain. **Neuro:** paresthesia. **Misc:** allergic reactions including, anaphylaxis.

Interactions

Drug-Drug: Probenecid ↑ levels and the risk of adverse reactions; concurrent use is contraindicated. ↑ risk of bleeding when used with **pentoxifylline**; concurrent use is contraindicated. Concurrent use with **aspirin** may ↓ effectiveness. ↑ adverse GI effects with **aspirin**, other **NSAIDs**, **potassium supplements**, **corticosteroids**, or **alcohol**. May ↓ effectiveness of **diuretics** or **antihypertensives**. May ↑ serum **lithium** levels and ↑ risk of toxicity. ↑ risk of toxicity from **methotrexate**. ↑ risk of bleeding with **cefotetan**, **valproic acid**, **clopidogrel**, **tirofiban**, **eptifibatide**, **thrombolytic agents**, or **anticoagulants**. ↑ risk of adverse hematologic reactions with **antineoplastics** or **radiation therapy**. May ↑ risk of nephrotoxicity from **cyclosporine**.

Drug-Natural Products: ↑ bleeding risk with **arnica**, **chamomile**, **clove**, **dong quai**, **feverfew**, **garlic**, **ginger**, **ginkgo**, **Panax ginseng**.

Route/Dosage

Oral therapy is indicated only as a continuation of parenteral therapy. Total duration of therapy by all routes should not exceed 5 days.

PO (Adults <65 yr): 20 mg initially, followed by 10 mg q 4–6 hr (not to exceed 40 mg/day).

PO (Adults ≥65 yr, <50 kg, or with renal impairment): 10 mg q 4–6 hr (not to exceed 40 mg/day).

PO (Children 2–16 yr, <50 kg): 1 mg/kg as a single dose. No data available for multiple doses.

IM (Adults <65 yr): *Single dose*—60 mg. *Multiple dosing*—30 mg q 6 hr (not to exceed 120 mg/day).

IM (Adults ≥65 yr, <50 kg, or with renal impairment): *Single dose*—30 mg. *Multiple dosing*—15 mg q 6 hr (not to exceed 60 mg/day).

IM (Children 2–16 yr, <50 kg): *Single dose*—0.4–1 mg/kg (maximum: 30 mg/dose). *Multiple dosing*—0.5 mg/kg q 6 hr.

IV (Adults <65 yr): *Single dose*—30 mg. *Multiple dosing*—30 mg q 6 hr (not to exceed 120 mg/day).

IV (Adults ≥65 yr, <50 kg, or with renal impairment): *Single dose*—15 mg. *Multiple dosing*—15 mg q 6 hr (not to exceed 60 mg/day).

IV (Children 2–16 yr, <50 kg): *Single dose*—0.4–1 mg/kg (maximum: 15 mg/dose). *Multiple dosing*—0.5 mg/kg q 6 hr.

Intranasal (Adults <65 yr): 1 spray in each nostril q 6–8 hr (not to exceed 4 sprays in each nostril/day).

Intranasal (Adults ≥65 yr, <50 kg, or with renal impairment): 1 spray in only one nostril q 6–8 hr (not to exceed 4 sprays in one nostril/day).

Availability (generic available)

Tablets: 10 mg. **Injection:** 15 mg/mL, 30 mg/mL. **Nasal spray (Sprix):** 15.75 mg/spray in 1.7–g bottle (delivers 8 sprays).

NURSING IMPLICATIONS

Assessment

- Patients who have asthma, aspirin-induced allergy, and nasal polyps are at increased risk for developing hypersensitivity reactions. Assess for rhinitis, asthma, and urticaria.

- Assess for rash periodically during therapy. May cause Stevens-Johnson syndrome or toxic epidermal necrolysis. Discontinue therapy if severe or if accompanied with fever, general malaise, fatigue, muscle or joint aches, blisters, oral lesions, conjunctivitis, hepatitis and/or eosinophilia.
- **Pain:** Assess pain (note type, location, and intensity) prior to and 1–2 hr following administration.
- ***Lab Test Considerations:*** Evaluate liver function tests, especially AST and ALT, periodically in patients receiving prolonged therapy. May cause ↑ levels.
- May cause prolonged bleeding time that may persist for 24–48 hr following discontinuation of therapy.
- May cause ↑ BUN, serum creatinine, or potassium concentrations.

Potential Nursing Diagnoses

Acute pain (Indications)

Implementation

- Do not confuse Toradol (ketorolac) with tramadol (Ultram).
- Administration in higher-than-recommended doses does not provide increased effectiveness but may cause increased side effects. Duration of ketorolac therapy, by all routes combined, should not exceed 5 days. Use lowest effective dose for shortest period of time.
- Coadministration with opioid analgesics may have additive analgesic effects and may permit lower opioid doses.
- **PO:** Ketorolac therapy should always be given initially by the IM or IV route. Use oral therapy *only* as a continuation of parenteral therapy.

IV Administration

- **IV Push:** Administer undiluted. ***Concentration:*** 15–30 mg/mL. ***Rate:*** Administer over at least 15 sec.
- **Y-Site Compatibility:** acetaminophen, alfentanil, amikacin, aminocaproic acid, aminophylline, amphotericin B lipid complex, amphotericin B liposome, anidulafungin, argatroban, ascorbic acid, atropine, aztreonam, benztropine, bivalirudin, bleomycin, bumetanide, buprenorphine, butorphanol, carboplatin, carmustine, cefazolin, cefotaxime, cefotetan, cefoxitin, ceftazidime, ceftriaxone, cefuroxime, chloramphenicol, cisatracurium, cisplatin, clindamycin, cyanocobalamin, cyclophosphamide, cyclosporine, cytarabine, dactinomycin, daptomycin, daunorubicin hydrochloride, dexamethasone, dexmedetomidine, dexrazoxane, digoxin, docetaxel, dopamine, doxorubicin hydrochloride, doxorubicin liposomal, enalaprilat, ephedrine, epinephrine, epoetin alfa, eptifibatide, ertapenem, etoposide, etoposide phosphate, famotidine, fentanyl, fluconazole, fludarabine, fluorouracil, folic acid, foscarnet, fosphenytoin, furosemide, gentamicin, glycopyrrolate, granisetron, heparin, hydrocortisone, hydromorphone, ifosfamide, imipenem/cilastatin, indomethacin, insulin, irinotecan, isoproterenol, leucovorin calcium, lidocaine, linezolid, lorazepam, magnesium sulfate, mannitol, mechlorethamine, meperidine, mesna, methotrexate, methylprednisolone, metoclopramide, metoprolol, metronidazole, milrinone, mitoxantrone, morphine, moxifloxacin, multivitamins, nafcillin, naloxone, nesiritide, nitroglycerin, nitroprusside, norepinephrine, octreotide, ondansetron, oxacillin, oxaliplatin, oxytocin, paclitaxel, palonosetron, pamidronate, pancuronium, pemetrexed, penicillin G, phenobarbital, phenylephrine, phytonadione, piperacillin/tazobactam, potassium acetate, potassium chloride, procainamide, propranolol, ranitidine, remifentanil, sodium acetate, sodium bicarbonate, streptokinase, succinylcholine, sufentanil, tacrolimus, teniposide, theophylline, thiotepa, tigecycline, tirofiban, tobramycin, vasopressin, verapamil, vinblastine, vincristine, voriconazole, zoledronic acid.
- **Y-Site Incompatibility:** acyclovir, alemtuzumab, amiodarone, amphotericin B colloidal, azithromycin, calcium chloride, caspofungin, chlorpromazine, dacarbazine, dantrolene, daunorubicin hydrochloride, diazepam, diltiazem, diphenhydramine, dobutamine, dolasetron, doxycycline, epirubicin, erythromycin, esmolol, fenoldopam, ganciclovir, gemcitabine, haloperidol, hydroxyzine, idarubicin, labetalol, levofloxacin, midazolam, mycophenolate, nalbuphine, nicardipine, pantoprazole, papaverine, pentamidine, pentazocine, phenytoin, prochlorperazine, promethazine, protamine, pyridoxine, quinupristin/dalfopristin, rocuronium, topotecan, trimethoprim/sulfamethoxazole, vancomycin, vecuronium, vinorelbine.
- **Intranasal:** Activate pump before first use by holding bottle arm's length away with index finger and middle finger resting on top of finger flange and thumb supporting base. Press down evenly and release pump 5 times to activate. Prior to each use, blow nose gently to clear nostrils. Sit up straight or stand. Tilt head slightly forward. Insert tip of container into nostril. Point container away from center of nose. Push down to spray. Bottles are for 24 hr use; discard bottle no more than 24 hours after taking first dose, even if the bottle still contains some liquid.

Patient/Family Teaching

- Instruct patient on how and when to ask for and take pain medication.
- Instruct patient to take medication exactly as directed. Take missed doses as soon as remembered if not almost time for next dose. Do not double doses. Do not take more than prescribed or for longer than 5 days.
- May cause drowsiness or dizziness. Advise patient to avoid driving or other activities requiring alertness until response to the medication is known.

- Caution patient to avoid the concurrent use of alcohol, aspirin, NSAIDs, acetaminophen, or other OTC medications without consulting health care professional.
- Advise patient to inform health care professional of medication regimen prior to treatment or surgery.
- Advise patient to consult health care professional if rash, itching, visual disturbances, tinnitus, weight gain, edema, black stools, persistent headache, or influenza-like syndrome (chills, fever, muscle aches, pain) occurs.
- Advise female patient to notify health care professional if pregnancy is planned or suspected or if breast feeding.
- **Intranasal:** Instruct patient on correct technique for administration, need to open a new bottle every 24 hr, and the 5 day limit for use.

Evaluation/Desired Outcomes

- Decrease in severity of pain. Patients who do not respond to one NSAID may respond to another.

HIGH ALERT

labetalol (la-**bet**-a-lole)
✱Trandate

Classification
Therapeutic: antianginals, antihypertensives
Pharmacologic: beta blockers

Pregnancy Category C

Indications

Management of hypertension.

Action

Blocks stimulation of $beta_1$ (myocardial)- and $beta_2$ (pulmonary, vascular, and uterine)-adrenergic receptor sites. Also has $alpha_1$-adrenergic blocking activity, which may result in more orthostatic hypotension.
Therapeutic Effects: Decreased BP.

Pharmacokinetics

Absorption: Well absorbed but rapidly undergoes extensive first-pass hepatic metabolism, resulting in 25% bioavailability.
Distribution: Some CNS penetration; crosses the placenta.
Protein Binding: 50%.
Metabolism and Excretion: Undergoes extensive hepatic metabolism.
Half-life: 3–8 hr.

TIME/ACTION PROFILE (cardiovascular effects)

ROUTE	ONSET	PEAK	DURATION
PO	20 min–2 hr	1–4 hr	8–12 hr
IV	2–5 min	5 min	16–18 hr

Contraindications/Precautions

Contraindicated in: Uncompensated HF; Pulmonary edema; Cardiogenic shock; Bradycardia or heart block.
Use Cautiously in: Renal impairment; Hepatic impairment; Pulmonary disease (including asthma); Diabetes mellitus (may mask signs of hypoglycemia); Thyrotoxicosis (may mask symptoms); Patients with a history of severe allergic reactions (intensity of reactions may be ↑); OB: May cause fetal/neonatal bradycardia, hypotension, hypoglycemia, or respiratory depression; Lactation: Usually compatible with breast feeding (AAP); Pedi: Limited data available; Geri: ↑ sensitivity to beta blockers (↑ risk of orthostatic hypotension); initial dosage ↓ recommended.

Adverse Reactions/Side Effects

CNS: fatigue, weakness, anxiety, depression, dizziness, drowsiness, insomnia, memory loss, mental status changes, nightmares. **EENT:** blurred vision, dry eyes, intraoperative floppy iris syndrome, nasal stuffiness. **Resp:** bronchospasm, wheezing. **CV:** ARRHYTHMIAS, BRADYCARDIA, CHF, PULMONARY EDEMA, orthostatic hypotension. **GI:** constipation, diarrhea, nausea. **GU:** erectile dysfunction, ↓ libido. **Derm:** itching, rashes. **Endo:** hyperglycemia, hypoglycemia. **MS:** arthralgia, back pain, muscle cramps. **Neuro:** paresthesia.

Interactions

Drug-Drug: General anesthesia and **verapamil** may cause additive myocardial depression. Additive bradycardia may occur with **digoxin**, **verapamil**, or **diltiazem**. Additive hypotension may occur with other **antihypertensives**, acute ingestion of **alcohol**, or **nitrates**. Concurrent **thyroid** administration may ↓ effectiveness. May alter the effectiveness of **insulin** or **oral hypoglycemic agents** (dose adjustments may be necessary). May ↓ the effectiveness of **adrenergic bronchodilators** and **theophylline**. May ↓ beneficial beta cardiovascular effects of **dopamine** or **dobutamine**. Use cautiously within 14 days of **MAO inhibitor** therapy (may result in hypertension). Effects may be ↑ by **propranolol** or **cimetidine**. Concurrent **NSAIDs** may ↓ antihypertensive action.

Route/Dosage

PO (Adults): 100 mg twice daily initially, may be ↑ by 100 mg twice daily q 2–3 days as needed (usual range 400–800 mg/day in 2–3 divided doses; doses up to 1.2–2.4 g/day have been used).
PO (Infants and Children): 1–3 mg/kg/day divided BID (maximum dose: 10–12 mg/kg/day, up to 1200 mg/day).
IV (Adults): 20 mg (0.25 mg/kg) initially, additional doses of 40–80 mg may be given q 10 min as needed (not to exceed 300 mg total dose) *or* 2 mg/min infusion (range 50–300 mg total dose required).
IV (Infants and Children): 0.2–1 mg/kg/dose (maximum: 40 mg/dose).

Availability (generic available)

Tablets: 100 mg, 200 mg, 300 mg. **Injection:** 5 mg/mL.

NURSING IMPLICATIONS

Assessment

- Monitor BP and pulse frequently during dose adjustment and periodically during therapy. Assess for orthostatic hypotension when assisting patient up from supine position.
- Check frequency of refills to determine compliance.
- Patients receiving *labetalol IV* must be supine during and for 3 hr after administration. Vital signs should be monitored every 5–15 min during and for several hours after administration.
- Monitor intake and output ratios and daily weight. Assess patient routinely for evidence of fluid over-

L

load (peripheral edema, dyspnea, rales/crackles, fatigue, weight gain, jugular venous distention).

- ***Lab Test Considerations:*** May cause ↑ BUN, serum lipoprotein, potassium, triglyceride, and uric acid levels.
- May cause ↑ ANA titers.
- May cause ↑ in blood glucose levels.
- May cause ↑ serum alkaline phosphatase, LDH, AST, and ALT levels. Discontinue if jaundice or laboratory signs of hepatic function impairment occur.
- ***Toxicity and Overdose:*** Monitor patients receiving beta blockers for signs of overdose (bradycardia, severe dizziness or fainting, severe drowsiness, dyspnea, bluish fingernails or palms, seizures). Notify health care professional immediately if these signs occur.
- Glucagon has been used to treat bradycardia and hypotension.

Potential Nursing Diagnoses

Decreased cardiac output (Side Effects)
Noncompliance (Patient/Family Teaching)

Implementation

- ***High Alert:*** IV vasoactive medications are inherently dangerous. Before administering intravenously, have second practitioner independently check original order, dosage calculations, and infusion pump settings.
- Do not confuse labetalol with Lamictal.
- Discontinuation of concurrent clonidine should take place gradually, with beta blocker discontinued first. Then, after several days, discontinue clonidine.
- **PO:** Take apical pulse prior to administering. If <50 bpm or if arrhythmia occurs, withhold medication and notify health care professional.
- Administer with meals or directly after eating to enhance absorption.

IV Administration

- **IV Push:** ***Diluent:*** Administer undiluted. ***Concentration:*** 5 mg/mL. ***Rate:*** Administer slowly over 2 min.
- **Continuous Infusion:** ***Diluent:*** Add 200 mg of labetalol to 160 mL of diluent. May also be administered as undiluted drug. Compatible diluents include D5W, 0.9% NaCl, D5/0.9% NaCl, and LR. ***Concentration:*** Diluted: 1 mg/mL; Undiluted: 5 mg/mL. ***Rate:*** Administer at a rate of 2 mg/min. Titrate for desired response. Infuse via infusion pump to ensure accurate dose.
- **Y-Site Compatibility:** alemtuzumab, alfentanil, amikacin, aminocaproic acid, aminophylline, amiodarone, anidulafungin, argatroban, ascorbic acid, atracurium, atropine, aztreonam, bivalirudin, bleomycin, bumetanide, buprenorphine, butorphanol, calcium chloride, calcium gluconate, carboplatin, carmustine, caspofungin, cefazolin, ceftazidime, chlorpromazine, cisplatin, clonidine, cyanocobalamin, cyclophosphamide, cyclosporine, dactinomycin, daptomycin, dexmedetomidine, digoxin, diltiazem, diphenhydramine, dobutamine, docetaxel, dopamine, doripenem, doxorubicin hydrochloride, doxycycline, enalaprilat, ephedrine, epinephrine, epirubicin, epoetin alfa, eptifibatide, ertapenem, erythromycin lactobionate, esmolol, etoposide, etoposide phosphate, famotidine, fenoldopam, fentanyl, fluconazole, fludarabine, fluorouracil, folic acid, ganciclovir, gemcitabine, gentamicin, glycopyrrolate, granisetron, hydromorphone, idarubicin, ifosfamide, imipenem/cilastatin, irinotecan, isoproterenol, levofloxacin, lidocaine, linezolid, lorazepam, magnesium sulfate, mannitol, mechlorethamine, meperidine, methoxamine, methyldopate, methylprednisolone sodium succinate, metoclopramide, metoprolol, metronidazole, midazolam, milrinone, mitoxantrone, morphine, multivitamins, mycophenolate, nalbuphine, naloxone, nicardipine, nitroglycerin, nitroprusside, norepinephrine, octreotide, ondansetron, oxacillin, oxaliplatin, oxytocin, palonosetron, pamidronate, pancuronium, papaverine, pemetrexed, pentamidine, pentazocine, pentobarbital, phenobarbital, phentolamine, phenylephrine, phytonadione, potassium acetate, potassium chloride, potassium phosphates, procainamide, prochlorperazine, promethazine, propofol, propranolol, protamine, pyridoxime, quinupristin/dalfopristin, ranitidine, rocuronium, sodium acetate, sodium bicarbonate, streptokinase, succinylcholine, sufentanil, tacrolimus, telavancin, teniposide, theophylline, thiamine, thiotepa, tigecycline, tirofiban, tobramycin, tolazoline, trimetaphan, vancomycin, vasopressin, vecuronium, verapamil, vincristine, vinorelbine, voriconazole, zoledronic acid.
- **Y-Site Incompatibility:** acyclovir, amphotericin B cholesteryl, amphotericin B colloidal, amphotericin B lipid complex, amphotericin B liposome, azathioprine, cefotaxime, cefotetan, cefoxitin, ceftaroline, ceftriaxone, cefuroxime, dantrolene, dexamethasone sodium phosphate, diazepam, diazoxide, hydrocortisone sodium succinate, indomethacin, insulin, ketorolac, micafungin, nesiritide, paclitaxel, pantoprazole, penicillin G, phenytoin, piperacillin/tazobactam, thiopental, warfarin.

Patient/Family Teaching

- Instruct patient to take medication as directed, at the same time each day, even if feeling well; do not skip or double up on missed doses. Take missed doses as soon as possible up to 8 hr before next dose. **Abrupt withdrawal may precipitate life-threatening arrhythmias, hypertension, or myocardial ischemia.**
- Advise patient to make sure enough medication is available for weekends, holidays, and vacations. A written prescription may be kept in wallet in case of emergency.
- Teach patient and family how to check pulse and BP. Instruct them to check pulse daily and BP biweekly. Advise patient to hold dose and contact health care

professional if pulse is <50 bpm or BP changes significantly.

- May cause drowsiness or dizziness. Caution patients to avoid driving or other activities that require alertness until response to the drug is known. Caution patients receiving labetalol IV to call for assistance during ambulation or transfer.
- Advise patients to make position changes slowly to minimize orthostatic hypotension, especially during initiation of therapy or when dose is increased. Patients taking oral labetalol should be especially cautious when drinking alcohol, standing for long periods, or exercising, and during hot weather, because orthostatic hypotension is enhanced.
- Caution patient that this medication may increase sensitivity to cold.
- Instruct patient to notify health care professional of all Rx or OTC medications, vitamins, or herbal products being taken and to consult health care professional before taking any Rx, OTC, or herbal products, especially cold preparations, concurrently with this medication. Patients on antihypertensive therapy should also avoid excessive amounts of coffee, tea, and cola.
- Patients with diabetes should closely monitor blood glucose, especially if weakness, malaise, irritability, or fatigue occurs. Medication may mask tachycardia and increased BP as signs of hypoglycemia, but dizziness and sweating may still occur.
- Advise patient to notify health care professional if slow pulse, difficulty breathing, wheezing, cold hands and feet, dizziness, light-headedness, confusion, depression, rash, fever, sore throat, unusual bleeding, or bruising occurs.
- Instruct patient to inform health care professional of medication regimen prior to treatment or surgery.
- Advise patient to carry identification describing disease process and medication regimen at all times.
- **Hypertension:** Reinforce the need to continue additional therapies for hypertension (weight loss, sodium restriction, stress reduction, regular exercise, moderation of alcohol consumption, and smoking cessation). Medication controls but does not cure hypertension.

Evaluation/Desired Outcomes

- Decrease in BP.

lacosamide (la-**kose**-a-mide)

Vimpat

Classification

Therapeutic: anticonvulsants

Schedule V

Pregnancy Category C

Indications

Treatment of partial-onset seizures as either monotherapy or adjunctive therapy.

Action

Mechanism is not known, but may involve enhancement of slow inactivation of sodium channels with resultant membrane stabilization. **Therapeutic Effects:** Decreased incidence and severity of partial-onset seizures.

Pharmacokinetics

Absorption: 100% absorbed following oral administration; IV administration results in complete bioavailability.

Distribution: Unknown.

Protein Binding: <15%.

Metabolism and Excretion: Partially metabolized by the liver; 40% excreted in urine as unchanged drug, 30% as a metabolite.

Half-life: 13 hr.

TIME/ACTION PROFILE (blood levels)

ROUTE	ONSET	PEAK	DURATION
PO	unknown	1–4 hr	12 hr
IV	unknown	end of infusion	12 hr

Contraindications/Precautions

Contraindicated in: Hypersensitivity; Severe hepatic impairment; Lactation: Lactation.

Use Cautiously in: CCr <30 mL/min (use lower daily dose); All patients (may ↑ risk of suicidal thoughts/behaviors); Hepatic or renal impairment and taking strong inhibitor of CYP3A4 or CYP2C9 (dose ↓ may be needed); Mild to moderate hepatic impairment; titrate dose carefully, use lower daily dose; Known cardiac conduction problems or severe cardiac disease (heart block or sick sinus syndrome without a pacemaker, Brugada syndrome, taking medications that prolong PR interval, MI or HF); Diabetic neuropathy or cardiac disease (↑ risk for atrial fibrillation/flutter); OB: Use only if potential benefit justifies risk to the fetus; Pedi: Children <17 yr (safety and effectiveness not established); Geri: Titrate dose carefully.

Adverse Reactions/Side Effects

CNS: SUICIDAL THOUGHTS, dizziness, headache, hallucinations, syncope, vertigo. **EENT:** diplopia. **CV:** atrial fibrillation/flutter, bradycardia, heart block, syncope. **Derm:** DRUG REACTION WITH EOSINOPHILIA AND SYSTEMIC SYMPTOMS, STEVENS-JOHNSON SYNDROME, TOXIC EPIDERMAL NECROLYSIS, rash. **GI:** nausea, vomiting. **Hemat:** AGRANULOCYTOSIS. **Neuro:** ataxia. **Misc:** physical dependence, psychological dependence, multiorgan hypersensitivity reactions (Drug Reaction with Eosinophilia and Systemic Symptoms—DRESS).

Interactions

Drug-Drug: Use cautiously with other **drugs that affect cardiac conduction**.

Route/Dosage

PO, IV (Adults): *Monotherapy*—100 mg twice daily; may be ↑ weekly by 100 mg/day in two divided doses up to a maintenance dose of 300–400 mg/day given in two divided doses; may also initiate therapy with 200 mg single loading dose followed 12 hr later by 100 mg twice daily; may be ↑ weekly by 100 mg/day in two divided doses up to a maintenance dose of 300–400 mg/day given in two divided doses; *Adjunctive therapy*—50 mg twice daily; may be ↑ weekly by 100 mg/day in two divided doses up to a maintenance dose of 200–400 mg/day given in two divided doses; may also initiate therapy with 200 mg single loading dose followed 12 hr later by 100 mg twice daily for 1 wk; may be ↑ weekly by 100 mg/day in two divided doses up to a maintenance dose of 400 mg/day given in two divided doses;.

Hepatic/Renal Impairment

PO, IV (Adults): *CCr ≤30 mL/min or mild to moderate hepatic impairment*—Do not exceed 300 mg/day.

Availability

Tablets: 50 mg, 100 mg, 150 mg, 200 mg. **Solution for injection:** 10 mg/mL. **Oral solution:** 10 mg/mL.

NURSING IMPLICATIONS

Assessment

- Assess location, duration, and characteristics of seizure activity. Institute seizure precautions.
- Monitor closely for notable changes in behavior that could indicate the emergence or worsening of suicidal thoughts or behavior or depression.
- Assess patient for skin rash frequently during therapy. Discontinue at first sign of rash; may be life-threatening. Stevens-Johnson syndrome may develop. Treat symptomatically; may recur once treatment is stopped.
- **IV:** Assess ECG prior to therapy in patients with pre-existing cardiac disease. Monitor patients with cardiac conduction problems, on medications that prolong PR interval, or with severe cardiac disease (myocardial ischemia, heart failure) closely, as IV lacosamide may cause bradycardia or AV block.
- ***Lab Test Considerations:*** May cause ↑ALT, which may return to normal without treatment.
- Monitor CBC and platelets periodically during therapy.

Potential Nursing Diagnoses

Risk for injury (Indications)

Implementation

- IV administration is indicated for short term replacement (up to 5 days) when PO administration is not feasible. When switching from PO to IV, initial total daily dose should be equivalent to total daily dose and frequency of PO therapy. At end of IV period, may switch to PO at equivalent daily dose and frequency of IV therapy.
- When switching from another antiepileptic drug to lacosamide, administer 150 mg-200 mg twice daily for at least 3 days before beginning withdrawal of other antiepileptic drug. Gradually decrease other antiepileptic drug over 6 wks.
- When administering loading dose, monitor for CNS adverse reactions (dizziness, headache, nausea, somnolence, fatigue). May occur more frequently.
- When discontinuing lacosamide, gradually decrease dose over 1 wk.
- **PO:** May be administered with or without food.
- Use a calibrated measuring device for accurate dosing of oral solution; household measures are not accurate.

IV Administration

- **Intermittent Infusion:** ***Diluent:*** May be administered undiluted or diluted with 0.9% NaCl, D5W, or LR. ***Concentration:*** 10 mg/mL. Solution is clear and colorless; do not administer solutions that are discolored or contain a precipitate. Solution is stable for 4 hr at room temperature. Discard unused portion. ***Rate:*** Infuse over 15–60 min, preferably 30–60 min.

Patient/Family Teaching

- Instruct patient to take lacosamide around the clock, as directed. Medication should be gradually discontinued over at least 1 wk to prevent seizures. Advise patient to read the *Medication Guide* before starting therapy and with each Rx refill.
- May cause dizziness, ataxia, and syncope. Caution patient to avoid driving or other activities requiring alertness until response to medication is known. Tell patient not to resume driving until physician gives clearance based on control of seizure disorder. If syncope occurs, advise patient to lay down with legs raised until recovered and notify health care professional.
- Inform patients and families of risk of suicidal thoughts and behavior and advise that behavioral changes, emergency or worsening signs and symptoms of depression, unusual changes in mood, or emergence of suicidal thoughts, behavior, or thoughts of self-harm should be reported to health care professional immediately.
- Instruct patient to notify health care professional if signs of multiorgan hypersensitivity reactions (fever, rash, fatigue, jaundice, dark urine) occur.
- Advise patient to consult health care professional before taking other Rx, OTC, or herbal preparation and to avoid taking alcohol or other CNS depressants concurrently with lacosamide.
- Rep: Advise female patients to notify health care professional if pregnancy is planned or suspected or if breast feeding. Encourage pregnant patients to en-

roll in the pregnancy registry by calling 1-888-233-2334, call must be made by patient. Information on registry can be found at the website http://www.aedpregnancyregistry.org/.

Evaluation/Desired Outcomes

- Decreased seizure activity.

lactulose (lak-tyoo-lose)

Cholac, Constilac, Constulose, Enulose, Generlac, Kristalose

Classification
Therapeutic: laxatives
Pharmacologic: osmotics

Pregnancy Category B

Indications

Treatment of chronic constipation. Adjunct in the management of portal-systemic (hepatic) encephalopathy (PSE).

Action

Increases water content and softens the stool. Lowers the pH of the colon, which inhibits the diffusion of ammonia from the colon into the blood, thereby reducing blood ammonia levels. **Therapeutic Effects:** Relief of constipation. Decreased blood ammonia levels with improved mental status in PSE.

Pharmacokinetics

Absorption: Less than 3% absorbed after oral administration.
Distribution: Unknown.
Metabolism and Excretion: Absorbed lactulose is excreted unchanged in the urine. Unabsorbed lactulose is metabolized by colonic bacteria to lactic, acetic, and formic acids.
Half-life: Unknown.

TIME/ACTION PROFILE (relief of constipation)

ROUTE	ONSET	PEAK	DURATION
PO	24–48 hr	unknown	unknown

Contraindications/Precautions

Contraindicated in: Patients on low-galactose diets.
Use Cautiously in: Diabetes mellitus; Excessive or prolonged use (may lead to dependence); OB, Lactation: Safety not established.

Adverse Reactions/Side Effects

GI: belching, cramps, distention, flatulence, diarrhea. **Endo:** hyperglycemia (diabetic patients).

Interactions

Drug-Drug: Should not be used with other **laxatives** in the treatment of hepatic encephalopathy (leads to inability to determine optimal dose of lactulose). **Anti-infectives** may ↓ effectiveness in treatment of hepatic encephalopathy.

Route/Dosage

Constipation

PO (Adults): 15–30 mL/day up to 60 mL/day as liquid or 10–20 g as powder for oral solution (up to 40 g/day has been used).
PO (Children): 7.5 mL daily after breakfast (unlabeled).

PSE

PO (Adults): 30–45 mL 3–4 times/day; may be given q 1–2 hr initially to induce laxation.
PO (Infants): 2.5–10 mL daily in 3–4 divided doses (unlabeled).
PO (Children and Adolescents): 40–90 mL daily in 3–4 divided doses (unlabeled).
Rect (Adults): 300 mL diluted and administered as a retention enema q 4–6 hr.

Availability (generic available)

Oral solution: 10 g lactulose/15 mL. **Rectal solution:** 10 g lactulose/15 mL. **Single-use packets (Kristalose):** 10 g (equal to 15 mL liquid lactulose), 20 g (equal to 30 mL liquid lactulose).

NURSING IMPLICATIONS

Assessment

- Assess patient for abdominal distention, presence of bowel sounds, and normal pattern of bowel function.
- Assess color, consistency, and amount of stool produced.
- **PSE:** Assess mental status (orientation, level of consciousness) before and periodically throughout course of therapy.
- ***Lab Test Considerations:*** ↓ blood ammonia concentrations by 25–50%.
- May cause ↑ blood glucose levels in diabetic patients.
- Monitor serum electrolytes periodically when used chronically. May cause diarrhea with resulting hypokalemia and hypernatremia.

Potential Nursing Diagnoses

Constipation (Indications)

Implementation

- When used in hepatic encephalopathy, adjust dose until patient averages 2–3 soft bowel movements per day. During initial therapy, 30–45 mL may be given hourly to induce rapid laxation.

L

- Darkening of solution does not alter potency.
- **PO:** Mix with fruit juice, water, milk, or carbonated citrus beverage to improve flavor. Administer with a full glass (240 mL) of water or juice. May be administered on an empty stomach for more rapid results.
- Dissolve single dose packets (Kristalose) in 4 oz of water. Solution should be colorless to slightly pale yellow.
- **Rect:** To administer enema, use rectal balloon catheter. Mix 300 mL of lactulose with 700 mL of water or 0.9% NaCl. Enema should be retained for 30–60 min. If inadvertently evacuated, may repeat administration.

Patient/Family Teaching

- Encourage patients to use other forms of bowel regulation, such as increasing bulk in the diet, increasing fluid intake, and increasing mobility. Normal bowel habits are individualized and may vary from 3 times/day to 3 times/wk.
- Caution patients that this medication may cause belching, flatulence, or abdominal cramping. Health care professional should be notified if this becomes bothersome or if diarrhea occurs.

Evaluation/Desired Outcomes

- Passage of a soft, formed bowel movement, usually within 24–48 hr.
- Clearing of confusion, apathy, and irritation and improved mental status in PSE. Improvement may occur within 2 hr after enema and 24–48 hr after oral administration.

lamiVUDine (la-mi-vyoo-deen)

✤3TC, Epivir, Epivir-HBV, ✤Heptovir

Classification

Therapeutic: antiretrovirals, antivirals

Pharmacologic: nucleoside reverse transcriptase inhibitors

Pregnancy Category C

Indications

HIV infection (with other antiretrovirals). Chronic hepatitis B infection. **Unlabeled Use:** Part of HIV-post-exposure prophylaxis with zidovudine and indinavir.

Action

After intracellular conversion to its active form (lamivudine-5-triphosphate), inhibits viral DNA synthesis by inhibiting the enzyme reverse transcriptase. **Therapeutic Effects:** Slows the progression of HIV infection and decreases the occurrence of its sequelae. Increases CD4 cell counts and decreases viral load. Protection from liver damage caused by chronic hepatitis B infection; decreases viral load.

Pharmacokinetics

Absorption: Well absorbed after oral administration (86% in adults, 66% in infants and children).

Distribution: Distributes into the extravascular space. Some penetration into CSF; remainder of distribution unknown.

Metabolism and Excretion: Mostly excreted unchanged in urine; <5% metabolized by the liver.

Half-life: *Adults*—3.7 hr; *children*—2 hr.

TIME/ACTION PROFILE (blood levels)

ROUTE	ONSET	PEAK	DURATION
PO	unknown	0.9 hr†	12 hr

†On an empty stomach; peak levels occur at 3.2 hr if lamivudine is taken with food. Food does not affect total amount of drug absorbed.

Contraindications/Precautions

Contraindicated in: Hypersensitivity; Concurrent use of antiretroviral combination products containing lamivudine or emtricitabine; Lactation: Breast feeding not recommended for HIV positive mothers.

Use Cautiously in: Impaired renal function (↑ dosing interval/↓ dose if CCr <50 mL/min); Women, prolonged exposure, obesity, history of liver disease (↑ risk of lactic acidosis and severe hepatomegaly with steatosis); Coinfection with hepatitis B (hepatitis may recur after discontinuation of lamivudine); OB, Pedi: Pregnancy or children <3 mo (safety not established); Geri: ↓ dose may be necessary due to age-related ↓ in renal function.

Exercise Extreme Caution in: Pedi: Pediatric patients with a history of or significant risk factors for pancreatitis (use only if no alternative).

Adverse Reactions/Side Effects

Noted for combination of lamivudine plus zidovudine.

CNS: SEIZURES, fatigue, headache, insomnia, malaise, depression, dizziness. **Resp:** cough. **GI:** HEPATOMEGALY WITH STEATOSIS, PANCREATITIS (↑ in pediatric patients), anorexia, diarrhea, nausea, vomiting, abdominal discomfort, ↑ liver enzymes, dyspepsia. **Derm:** alopecia, erythema multiforme, rash, urticaria. **Endo:** fat redistribution, hyperglycemia. **F and E:** lactic acidosis. **Hemat:** anemia, neutropenia, pure red cell aplasia. **MS:** musculoskeletal pain, arthralgia, muscle weakness, myalgia, rhabdomyolysis. **Neuro:** neuropathy. **Misc:** hypersensitivity reactions including ANAPHYLAXIS, immune reconstitution syndrome.

Interactions

Drug-Drug: Trimethoprim/sulfamethoxazole ↑ levels (dose alteration may be necessary in renal impairment). ↑ risk of pancreatitis with concurrent use of other **drugs causing pancreatitis.** ↑ risk of neuropathy with concurrent use of other **drugs causing neuropathy**. Combination therapy with **tenofovir** and **abacavir** may lead to virologic nonresponse and should not be used.

Route/Dosage

HIV infection

PO (Adults and Children >16 yr and ≥50 kg): 150 mg twice daily or 300 mg once daily.
PO (Adults <50 kg): 2 mg/kg twice daily.
PO (Children 3 mo–16 yr): *Oral solution*—4 mg/kg twice daily or 8 mg/kg once daily (up to 300 mg/day); *Tablets*—14–19 kg: 75 mg twice daily or 150 mg once daily; 20–24 kg: 75 mg in AM, 150 mg in PM or 225 mg once daily; ≥25 kg: 150 mg twice daily or 300 mg once daily.

Renal Impairment

PO (Adults): *CCr 30–49 mL/min*—150 mg once daily; *CCr 15–29 mL/min*—150 mg first dose, then 100 mg once daily; *CCr 5–14 mL/min*—150 mg first dose, then 50 mg once daily; *CCr <5 mL/min*—50 mg first dose, then 25 mg once daily.

Chronic Hepatitis B

PO (Adults): 100 mg once daily.

Renal Impairment

PO (Adults): *CCr 30–49 mL/min*—100 mg first dose, then 50 mg once daily; *CCr 15–29 mL/min*—100 mg first dose, then 25 mg once daily; *CCr 5–14 mL/min*—35 mg first dose, then 15 mg once daily; *CCr <5 mL/min*—35 mg first dose, then 10 mg once daily.
PO (Children 2–17 yr): 3 mg/kg once daily (up to 100 mg/day).

Availability (generic available)

Epivir

Tablets: 150 mg, 300 mg. **Oral solution (strawberry-banana flavor):** 10 mg/mL. ***In combination with:*** abacavir (Epzicom); zidovudine (Combivir); zidovudine and abacavir (Trizivir); abacavir and dolutegravir (Triumeq). See Appendix B.

Epivir-HBV

Tablets: 100 mg. **Oral solution (strawberry-banana flavor):** 5 mg/mL.

NURSING IMPLICATIONS

Assessment

- Assess patient, especially pediatric patients, for signs of pancreatitis (nausea, vomiting, abdominal pain) periodically during therapy. May require discontinuation of therapy.
- **HIV:** Assess patient for change in severity of symptoms of HIV infection and for symptoms of opportunistic infection during therapy.
- Monitor patient for signs and symptoms of peripheral neuropathy (tingling, burning, numbness, or pain in hands or feet); may be difficult to differentiate from peripheral neuropathy of severe HIV disease. May require discontinuation of therapy.
- **Chronic Hepatitis B Infection:** Monitor signs of hepatitis (jaundice, fatigue, anorexia, pruritus) during therapy.
- ***Lab Test Considerations:*** Monitor viral load and CD4 levels before and periodically during therapy.
- Monitor serum amylase, lipase, and triglycerides periodically during therapy. Elevated serum levels may indicate pancreatitis and require discontinuation.
- Monitor liver function. May cause ↑ levels of AST, ALT, CPK, bilirubin, and alkaline phosphatase, which usually resolve after interruption of therapy. Lactic acidosis may occur with hepatic toxicity causing hepatic steatosis; may be fatal, especially in women.
- May rarely cause neutropenia and anemia.

Potential Nursing Diagnoses

Risk for infection (Indications)

Implementation

- Do not confuse lamivudine with lamotrigine. Do not confuse Epivir tablets and oral solution with Epivir-HBV tablets and oral solutions. Epivir Tablets and Oral Solution contain a higher dose of the same active ingredient (lamivudine) than in Epivir-HBV Tablets and Oral Solution. Epivir-HBV was developed for patients with hepatitis B and should not be used for patients dually infected with HIV and hepatitis B; use may lead to lamivudine-resistant HIV due to subtherapeutic dose.
- **PO:** May be administered without regard to food.

Patient/Family Teaching

- Instruct patient to take lamivudine as directed, every 12 hr. Explain the difference between Epivir and Epivir-HBV to patients. Emphasize the importance of compliance with full course of therapy, not taking more than the prescribed amount, and not discontinuing without consulting health care professional. Take missed doses as soon as possible unless almost time for next dose. Do not double doses. Caution patient not to share medication with others.
- Inform patient that lamivudine does not cure HIV disease or prevent associated or opportunistic infections. Lamivudine does not reduce the risk of transmission of HIV to others through sexual contact or blood contamination. Caution patient to use a condom during sexual contact and avoid sharing needles or donating blood to prevent spreading HIV to others. Advise patient that the long-term effects of lamivudine are unknown at this time.
- Instruct patient to notify health care professional promptly if signs of peripheral neuropathy, pancreatitis, or Immune Reconstitution Syndrome (signs and symptoms of an infection, Mycobacterium avium infection, cytomegalovirus, Pneumocystis jirovecii pneumonia, tuberculosis) occur.

- Inform patient that redistribution and accumulation of body fat may occur, causing central obesity, dorsocervical fat enlargement (buffalo hump), peripheral wasting, breast enlargement, and cushingoid appearance. The cause and long-term effects are not known.
- Instruct patient to notify health care professional of all Rx or OTC medications, vitamins, or herbal products being taken and to consult health care professional before taking other Rx, OTC, or herbal products.
- Rep: Instruct females using hormonal contraceptives to use an alternative nonhormonal method of contraception. Advise patient to notify health care professional if pregnancy is planned or suspected and to avoid breast feeding. If pregnant patient is exposed to lamivudine, register patient in *Antiretroviral Pregnancy Registry* by calling 1-800-258-4263.
- Emphasize the importance of regular follow-up exams and blood tests to determine progress and monitor for side effects.

Evaluation/Desired Outcomes

- Slowing of the progression of HIV infection and its sequelae.
- Decrease in viral load and improvement in CD4 levels in patients with advanced HIV infection.
- Protection from liver damage caused by chronic hepatitis B infection; decreases viral load.

lamoTRIgine (la-moe-tri-jeen)

LaMICtal, LaMICtal CD, LaMICtal ODT, LaMICtal XR

Classification
Therapeutic: anticonvulsants

Pregnancy Category C

Indications

Adjunct treatment of partial seizures in adults and children with epilepsy (immediate-release, extended-release, chewable, and orally disintegrating tablets). Lennox-Gastaut syndrome (immediate-release, chewable, and orally disintegrating tablets only). Adjunct treatment of primary generalized tonic-clonic seizures in adults and children (immediate-release, extended-release, chewable, and orally disintegrating tablets). Conversion to monotherapy in adults with partial seizures receiving carbamazepine, phenytoin, phenobarbital, primidone, or valproate as the single antiepileptic drug (immediate-release, extended-release, chewable, and orally disintegrating tablets only). Maintenance treatment of bipolar disorder (immediate-release, chewable, and orally disintegrating tablets only).

Action

Stabilizes neuronal membranes by inhibiting sodium transport. **Therapeutic Effects:** Decreased incidence of seizures. Delayed time to recurrence of mood episodes in bipolar disorder.

Pharmacokinetics

Absorption: 98% absorbed following oral administration.

Distribution: Enters breast milk. Highly bound to melanin-containing tissues (eyes, pigmented skin).

Metabolism and Excretion: Mostly metabolized by the liver via glucuronidation to inactive metabolites; 10% excreted unchanged by the kidneys.

Half-life: Children taking enzyme–inducing antiepileptic drugs (AEDs): 7–10 hr; Children taking enzyme inducers and valproic acid: 15–27 hr; Children taking valproic acid: 44–94 hr; Adults: 25.4 hr (during chronic therapy of lamotrigine alone).

TIME/ACTION PROFILE (blood levels)

ROUTE	ONSET	PEAK	DURATION
PO	unknown	1.4–4.8 hr; 4–10 hr (XR)	unknown

Contraindications/Precautions

Contraindicated in: Hypersensitivity; Acute manic or mixed episodes.

Use Cautiously in: All patients (may ↑ risk of suicidal thoughts/behaviors); Patients with renal dysfunction, impaired cardiac function, and hepatic dysfunction (lower maintenance doses may be required); Prior history of rash to lamotrigine; OB: Exposure during first trimester may ↑ risk of cleft lip/palate; Lactation: Enters breast milk; use cautiously during lactation; Pedi: Immediate-release, chewable, and orally disintegrating tablets not safe for children <2 yr; extended-release tablets not approved for use in children <13 yr.

Adverse Reactions/Side Effects

CNS: ASEPTIC MENINGITIS, SUICIDAL THOUGHTS, ataxia, dizziness, headache, behavior changes, depression, drowsiness, insomnia, tremor. **EENT:** blurred vision, double vision, rhinitis. **GI:** HEPATIC FAILURE, nausea, vomiting. **GU:** vaginitis. **Derm:** photosensitivity, rash (higher incidence in children, patients taking valproic acid, high initial doses, or rapid dose increases). **MS:** arthralgia. **Misc:** MULTI-ORGAN HYPERSENSITIVITY REACTIONS, STEVENS-JOHNSON SYNDROME.

Interactions

Drug-Drug: Concurrent use with **carbamazepine** may ↑ levels of an active metabolite of carbamazepine. Concurrent use with drugs that induce glucuronidation, including **phenobarbital**, **phenytoin**, **primidone**, **carbamazepine**, **estrogen-containing oral contraceptives rifampin**, **lopinavir/ritonavir**, or **atazanavir/ritonavir** may ↓ levels; lamotrigine dose adjustments may be necessary when starting and stopping oral contraceptive or atazanavir/ritonavir therapy. Concurrent use with drugs that inhibit glucuronidation, including **valproic acid**, may ↑ levels and ↑ incidence of rash; may also ↓ valproic acid levels (↓ lamotrigine dose by at least 50%).

Route/Dosage

Epilepsy

In Combination with Other Antiepileptic Agents

PO (Adults and Children >12 yr; Immediate-release, chewable, or orally disintegrating tablets): *Patients taking anti-epileptic drugs other than carbamazepine, phenobarbital, phenytoin, primidone, or valproate*—25 mg daily for first 2 wk, then 50 mg daily for next 2 wk; then ↑ by 50 mg/day every 1–2 wk to maintenance dose of 225–375 mg/day (in 2 divided doses); *Patients taking carbamazepine, phenobarbital, phenytoin, or primidone (and not valproate)*—50 mg daily for first 2 wk, then 50 mg twice daily for next 2 wk; then ↑ by 100 mg/day every 1–2 wk to maintenance dose of 300–500 mg/day (in 2 divided doses); *Patients taking regimen containing valproate*—25 mg every other day for first 2 wk, then 25 mg daily for next 2 wk; then ↑ by 25–50 mg/day every 1–2 wk to maintenance dose of 100–400 mg/day (in 1–2 divided doses) (maintenance dose of 100–200 mg/day if receiving valproate alone).

PO (Adults and Children ≥13 yr; Extended-release tablets): *Patients taking anti-epileptic drugs other than carbamazepine, phenobarbital, phenytoin, primidone, or valproate*—25 mg daily for first 2 wk, then 50 mg daily for next 2 wk; then 100 mg daily for 1 wk, then 150 mg daily for 1 wk, then 200 mg daily for 1 wk, then ↑ by 100 mg/day every week to maintenance dose of 300–400 mg daily; *Patients taking carbamazepine, phenobarbital, phenytoin, or primidone (and not valproate)*—50 mg daily for first 2 wk, then 100 mg daily for next 2 wk, then 200 mg daily for 1 wk, then 300 mg daily for 1 wk, then 400 mg daily for 1 wk, then ↑ by 100 mg/day every week to maintenance dose of 400–600 mg daily; *Patients taking regimen containing valproate*—25 mg every other day for first 2 wk, then 25 mg daily for next 2 wk, then 50 mg daily for 1 wk, then 100 mg daily for 1 wk, then 150 mg daily for 1 wk, then maintenance dose of 200–250 mg daily.

PO (Children 2–12 yr; Immediate-release, chewable, or orally disintegrating tablets): *Patients taking anti-epileptic drugs other than carbamazepine, phenobarbital, phenytoin, primidone, or valproate* —0.3 mg/kg/day in 1–2 divided doses (rounded down to nearest whole tablet) for first 2 wk, then 0.6 mg/kg/day in 2 divided doses (rounded down to nearest whole tablet) for next 2 wk; then ↑ by 0.6 mg/kg/day (rounded down to nearest whole tablet) every 1–2 wk to maintenance dose of 4.5–7.5 mg/kg/day (not to exceed 300 mg/day in 2 divided doses); *Patients taking carbamazepine, phenobarbital, phenytoin, or primidone (and not valproate)*—0.6 mg/kg/day in 2 divided doses (rounded down to nearest whole tablet) for first 2 wk, then 1.2 mg/kg/day in 2 divided doses (rounded down to nearest whole tablet) for next 2 wk; then ↑ by 1.2 mg/kg/day (rounded down to nearest whole tablet) every 1–2 wk to maintenance dose of 5–15 mg/kg/day (not to exceed 400 mg/day in 2 divided doses). *Patients taking regimen containing valproate*—0.15 mg/kg/day in 1–2 divided doses (rounded down to nearest whole tablet) for first 2 wk, then 0.3 mg/kg in 1–2 divided doses (rounded down to nearest whole tablet) for next 2 wk; then ↑ by 0.3 mg/kg/day (rounded down to nearest whole tablet) every 1–2 wk to maintenance dose of 1–5 mg/kg/day (not to exceed 200 mg/day in 1–2 divided doses) (maintenance dose of 1–3 mg/kg/day if receiving valproate alone).

Conversion to Monotherapy

PO (Adults and Children ≥16 yr; Immediate-release, chewable, or orally disintegrating tablets): *Patients taking carbamazepine, phenobarbital, phenytoin, or primidone (and not valproate)*—After achieving a dose of 500 mg/day (as per dosing guidelines above), ↓ dose of other antiepileptic by 20% weekly over 4 wk; *Patients taking regimen containing valproate*—After achieving a dose of 200 mg/day (as per dosing guidelines above), ↓ valproate dose by 500 mg/day on a weekly basis until a dose of 500 mg/day is achieved. Maintain the valproate dose of 500 mg/day and the lamotrigine dose of 500 mg/day for 1 wk. Then ↑ lamotrigine dose to 300 mg/day and ↓ valproate dose to 250 mg/day, and maintain these doses for 1 wk. Then discontinue valproate and ↑ lamotrigine dose by 100 mg/day every wk until maintenance dose of 500 mg/day is achieved.

PO (Adults and Children ≥13 yr; Extended-release tablets): *Patients taking carbamazepine, phenobarbital, phenytoin, or primidone (and not valproate)*—After achieving a dose of 500 mg/day (as per dosing guidelines above), ↓ dose of other antiepileptic by 20% weekly over 4 wk. Two wk later, ↓ dose of lamotrigine by 100 mg/day every wk to achieve maintenance dose of 250–300 mg/day; *Patients taking regimen containing valproate*—After achieving a dose of 150 mg/day (as per dosing guidelines above), ↓ valproate dose by 500 mg/day on a weekly basis until a dose of 500 mg/day is achieved. Maintain the valproate dose of 500 mg/day and the lamotrigine dose of 150 mg/day for 1 wk. Then ↑ lamotrigine dose to 200 mg/day and ↓ valproate dose to 250 mg/day, and maintain these doses for 1 wk. Then discontinue valproate and ↑ lamotrigine dose to 250–300 mg/day; *Patients taking anti-epileptic drugs other than carbamazepine, phenobarbital, phenytoin, primidone, or val-*

proate —After achieving a dose of 250–300 mg/day (as per dosing guidelines above), ↓ dose of other antiepileptic by 20% weekly over 4 wk.

Bipolar Disorder

Escalation Regimen

PO (Adults): *Patients not taking cabamazepine, phenobarbital, phenytoin, primidone, rifampin, or valproate*—25 mg daily for first 2 wk, then 50 mg daily for next 2 wk, then 100 mg daily for 1 wk, then 200 mg daily; *Patients taking valproate*—25 mg every other day for first 2 wk, then 25 mg daily for next 2 wk, then 50 mg daily for 1 wk, then 100 mg daily; *Patients taking carbamazepine, phenobarbital, phenytoin, primidone, or rifampin (and not valproate)* 50 mg daily for first 2 wk, then 100 mg/day (in divided doses) for next 2 wk, then 200 mg/day (in divided doses) for one wk, then 300 mg/day (in divided doses) for 1 wk, then up to 400 mg/day (in divided doses).

Dosage Adjustment Following Discontinuation of Other Psychotropics

PO (Adults): *Following discontinuation of valproate (if current dose 100 mg/day)*—↑ to 150 mg/day for 1 wk, then 200 mg/day; *Following discontinuation of carbamazepine, phenobarbital, phenytoin, primidone, or rifampin (if current dose 400 mg/day)*—400 mg/day for 1 wk, then 300 mg/day for 1 wk, then 200 mg/day; *Following discontinuation of other psychotropics*—maintain previous dose.

Availability (generic available)

Immediate-release tablets: 25 mg, 100 mg, 150 mg, 200 mg. **Cost:** *Generic*—25 mg $415.96/100, 100 mg $475.12/100, 150 mg $312.44/100, 200 mg $340.15/100. **Chewable dispersible tablets:** 2 mg, 5 mg, 25 mg. **Cost:** *Generic*—5 mg $305.33/100, 25 mg $319.80/100. **Orally disintegrating tablets:** 25 mg, 50 mg, 100 mg, 200 mg. **Cost:** 25 mg $218.27/30, 50 mg $233.78/30, 100 mg $249.29/30, 200 mg $297.47/30. **Extended-release tablets:** 25 mg, 50 mg, 100 mg, 200 mg, 250 mg, 300 mg. **Cost:** *Generic*—25 mg $196.43/30, 50 mg $392.81/30, 100 mg $420.77/30, 200 mg $448.70/30, 250 mg $611.88/30, 300 mg $673.07/30.

NURSING IMPLICATIONS

Assessment

- Monitor closely for notable changes in behavior that could indicate the emergence or worsening of suicidal thoughts or behavior or depression.
- Assess patient for skin rash frequently during therapy. Discontinue lamotrigine at first sign of rash; may be life-threatening. Stevens-Johnson syndrome or toxic epidermal necrolysis may develop. Rash usually occurs during the initial 2–8 wk of therapy and is more frequent in patients taking multiple antiepileptic agents, especially valproic acid, and much more frequent in patients <16 yr.
- Monitor for signs and symptoms of multiorgan hypersensitivity reactions—DRESS (rash, fever, lymphadenopathy). May be associated with other organ involvement (hepatitis, hepatic failure, blood dyscrasias, acute multiorgan failure). If cause cannot be determined, discontinue lamotrigine immediately.
- **Seizures:** Assess location, duration, and characteristics of seizure activity.
- **Bipolar disorders:** Assess mood, ideation, and behaviors frequently. Initiate suicide precautions if indicated.
- ***Lab Test Considerations:*** Lamotrigine plasma concentrations may be monitored periodically during therapy, especially in patients concurrently taking other anticonvulsants. Therapeutic plasma concentration range has not been established, proposed therapeutic range: 1–5 mcg/mL.
- May cause false-positive results for phencyclidine (PCP) in some rapid urine drug screens. Use a more specific analytical method to confirm results.

Potential Nursing Diagnoses

Risk for impaired skin integrity (Adverse Reactions)
Risk for injury (Side Effects)

Implementation

- Do not confuse lamotrigine (Lamictal) with lamivudine (Epivir) or levothyroxine.
- When converting from immediate-release to XR form, initial dose of XR should match the total daily dose of immediate-release lamotrigine; monitor closely and adjust and needed.
- **PO:** May be administered without regard to meals. Swallow XR tablets whole; do not break, crush, or chew.
- Lamotrigine should be discontinued gradually over at least 2 wk, unless safety concerns require a more rapid withdrawal. Abrupt discontinuation may cause increase in seizure frequency.
- **Orally Disintegrating Tablets:** Place on the tongue and move around the mouth. Tablet will rapidly disintegrate, can be swallowed with or without water, and can be taken with or without food.
- **Chewable/Dispersible Tablets:** May be swallowed whole, chewed, or dispersed in water or dispersed in fruit juice. If chewed, follow with water or fruit juice to aid in swallowing. Only use whole tablets, do not attempt to administer partial quantities of dispersible tablets.

Patient/Family Teaching

- Instruct patient to take medication exactly as directed. Take missed doses as soon as possible unless almost time for next dose. Do not double doses. Do not discontinue abruptly; may cause increase in frequency of seizures. Instruct patient to read the *Medication Guide* before starting and with each Rx refill, changes may occur.
- Advise patient to notify health care professional immediately if skin rash, fever, or swollen lymph glands occur or if frequency of seizures increases.

- May cause dizziness, drowsiness, and blurred vision. Caution patient to avoid driving or activities requiring alertness until response to medication is known. Do not resume driving until physician gives clearance based on control of seizure disorder.
- Caution patient to wear sunscreen and protective clothing to prevent photosensitivity reactions.
- Advise patient and family to notify health care professional if thoughts about suicide or dying, attempts to commit suicide; new or worse depression; new or worse anxiety; feeling very agitated or restless; panic attacks; trouble sleeping; new or worse irritability; acting aggressive; being angry or violent; acting on dangerous impulses; an extreme increase in activity and talking; other unusual changes in behavior or mood or if symptoms of aseptic meningitis (headache, fever, nausea, vomiting, and nuchal rigidity, rash, photophobia, myalgia, chills, altered consciousness, somnolence) occur.
- Advise patient to notify health care professional if pregnancy is planned or suspected or if breast feeding.
- Instruct patient to notify health care professional of medication regimen prior to treatment or surgery.
- Rep: Advise female patients to use a nonhormonal form of contraception while taking lamotrigine, to avoid breast feeding, and to notify health care professional if pregnancy is planned or suspected or if breast feeding. Encourage patients who become pregnant to enroll in the North American Antiepileptic Drug Pregnancy Registry. Must be done by patients themselves by calling 1-888-233-2334 or on the website http://www.aedpregnancyregistry.org.
- Advise patient to carry identification at all times describing disease process and medication regimen.

Evaluation/Desired Outcomes

- Decrease in the frequency of or cessation of seizures.
- Delay in time to occurrence of mood episodes (depression, mania, hypomania, mixed episodes) in patients with Bipolar I disorder.

lansoprazole (lan-**soe**-pra-zole)

Prevacid, Prevacid 24 Hr

Classification

Therapeutic: antiulcer agents

Pharmacologic: proton-pump inhibitors

Pregnancy Category B

Indications

Erosive esophagitis. Duodenal ulcers (with or without anti-infectives for *Helicobacter pylori*). Active benign gastric ulcer. Short-term treatment of symptomatic GERD. Healing and risk reduction of NSAID-associated gastric ulcer. Pathologic hypersecretory conditions, including Zollinger-Ellison syndrome. **OTC:** Heartburn occurring ≥twice/wk.

Action

Binds to an enzyme in the presence of acidic gastric pH, preventing the final transport of hydrogen ions into the gastric lumen. **Therapeutic Effects:** Diminished accumulation of acid in the gastric lumen, with lessened acid reflux. Healing of duodenal ulcers and esophagitis.

Pharmacokinetics

Absorption: 80% absorbed after oral administration.

Distribution: Unknown.

Protein Binding: 97%.

Metabolism and Excretion: Extensively metabolized by the liver to inactive compounds. Converted intracellularly to at least two other antisecretory compounds.

Half-life: Children: 1.2–1.5 hr; Adults: 1.3–1.7 hr (↑ in geriatric patients and patients with impaired hepatic function).

TIME/ACTION PROFILE (acid suppression)

ROUTE	ONSET	PEAK	DURATION
PO	rapid	1.7 hr	more than 24 hr

Contraindications/Precautions

Contraindicated in: Hypersensitivity.

Use Cautiously in: Solutabs contain aspartame; use caution when used in phenylketonurics; Severe hepatic impairment (not to exceed 30 mg/day in these patients); Patients using high-doses for >1 year (↑ risk of hip, wrist, or spine fractures); Patients using therapy for >3 yr (↑ risk of vitamin B_{12} deficiency; OB, Lactation: Safety not established; Pedi: Children <1 yr (safety not established); Geri: Maintenance dose not to exceed 30 mg/day unless additional acid suppression is required.

Adverse Reactions/Side Effects

CNS: dizziness, headache. **GI:** CLOSTRIDIUM DIFFICILE-ASSOCIATED DIARRHEA (CDAD), diarrhea, abdominal pain, nausea. **Derm:** rash. **F and E:** hypomagnesemia (especially if treatment duration ≥3 mo). **GU:** acute interstitial nephritis. **Hemat:** vitamin B_{12} deficiency. **MS:** bone fracture.

Interactions

Drug-Drug: Sucralfate ↓ absorption of lansoprazole (take 30 min before sucralfate). May ↓ absorption of drugs requiring acid pH, including **ketoconazole**, **itraconazole**, **atazanavir ampicillin esters**, **iron**

salts, **erlotinib**, and **mycophenolate mofetil**; concomitant use with **atazanavir** not recommended. May ↑ levels of **digoxin tacrolimus**, and **methotrexate**. May ↑ risk of bleeding with **warfarin** (monitor INR/PT). Hypomagnesemia ↑ risk of **digoxin** toxicity.

Route/Dosage

PO (Adults and children ≥12 yr): *Short-term treatment of duodenal ulcer*—15 mg once daily for 4 wk; *H. pylori eradication to reduce the risk of duodenal ulcer recurrence*—30 mg twice daily with clarithromycin 500 mg twice daily and amoxicillin 1000 mg twice daily for 10–14 days (triple therapy) or 30 mg 3 times daily with 1000 mg amoxicillin 3 times daily for 14 days (dual therapy); *Maintenance of healed duodenal ulcers*—15 mg once daily; *Short-term treatment of gastric ulcers/healing of NSAID-associated gastric ulcer*—30 mg once daily for up to 8 wk; *Risk reduction of NSAID-associated gastric ulcer*—15 mg once daily for up to 12 wk; *Short-term treatment of symptomatic GERD*—15 mg once daily for up to 8 wk; *Short-term treatment of erosive esophagitis*—30 mg once daily for up to 8 wk (8 additional weeks may be necessary); *Maintenance of healing of erosive esophagitis*—15 mg once daily; *Pathologic hypersecretory conditions*—60 mg once daily intially, up to 90 mg twice daily (daily dose >120 mg should be given in divided doses).

PO (Adults): *OTC*—15 mg once daily for up to 14 days (14 day course may be repeated every 4 mo).

PO (Children 1–11 yr and >30 k g): *GERD*—30 mg once to twice daily.

PO (Children 1–11 yr and 10–30 kg): *GERD*—15 mg once or twice daily.

PO (Children 1–11 yr and <10 kg): *GERD*—7.5 mg once daily.

Availability (generic available)

Delayed-release capsules: 15 mg[Rx, OTC], 30 mg. **Delayed-release orally disintegrated tablets (SoluTabs):** 15 mg, 30 mg. ***In combination with:*** amoxicillin and clarithromycin as part of a compliance package (Prevpac). See Appendix B.

NURSING IMPLICATIONS

Assessment

- Assess patient routinely for epigastric or abdominal pain and for frank or occult blood in stool, emesis, or gastric aspirate.
- Monitor bowel function. Diarrhea, abdominal cramping, fever, and bloody stools should be reported to health care professional promptly as a sign of Clostridium difficile-associated diarrhea (CDAD). May begin up to several weeks following cessation of therapy.
- ***Lab Test Considerations:*** May cause abnormal liver function tests, including ↑ AST, ALT, alkaline phosphatase, LDH, and bilirubin.
- May cause ↑ serum creatinine and ↑ or ↓ electrolyte levels.
- May alter RBC, WBC, and platelet levels.
- May also cause ↑ gastrin levels, abnormal A/G ratio, hyperlipidemia, and ↑ or ↓ cholesterol.
- Monitor INR and prothrombin time in patients taking warfarin.
- May cause hypomagnesemia. Monitor serum magnesium prior to and periodically during therapy.
- May cause vitamin B_{12} deficiency with long term use (>3 yrs).

Potential Nursing Diagnoses

Acute pain (Indications)

Implementation

- **PO:** *Delayed-release capsules:* Administer before meals. Swallow whole; do not crush or chew capsule contents. Capsules may be opened and sprinkled on 1 tbsp of applesauce, *Ensure* pudding, cottage cheese, yogurt or strained pears and swallowed immediately for patients with difficulty swallowing.
- For patients with an NG tube, capsules may be opened and intact granules may be mixed in 40 mL of apple juice and injected through the NG tube into stomach. Flush NG tube with additional apple juice to clear tube.
- *Orally disintegrating tablets* may be placed on tongue, allowed to disintegrate and swallowed with or without water. Do not cut or break tablet. For administration via oral syringe or nasogastric tube, *Prevacid SoluTab* can be administered by placing a 15-mg tablet in oral syringe and drawing up 4 mL of water, or a 30-mg tablet in oral syringe and drawing up 10 mL of water. Shake gently to allow for a quick dispersal. After tablet has dispersed, administer the contents within 15 minutes. Refill syringe with 2 mL (5 mL for the 30-mg tablet) of water, shake gently, and administer any remaining contents and flush nasogastric tube.
- Antacids may be used concurrently.

Patient/Family Teaching

- Instruct patient to take medication as directed for the full course of therapy, even if feeling better. Take missed doses as soon as remembered unless almost time for next dose; do not double doses.
- May occasionally cause dizziness. Caution patient to avoid driving and other activities that require alertness until response to medication is known.
- Advise patient to avoid alcohol, products containing aspirin or NSAIDs, and foods that may cause an increase in GI irritation.
- Advise patient to report onset of black, tarry stools; diarrhea; or abdominal pain to health care professional promptly. Instruct patient to notify health care professional immediately if rash, diarrhea, abdominal cramping, fever, or bloody stools occur and not to treat with antidiarrheals without consulting health care professional.
- Instruct patient to notify health care professional of all Rx or OTC medications, vitamins, or herbal prod-

ucts being taken and consult health care professional before taking any new medications.
- Advise female patient to notify health care professional if pregnancy is planned or suspected or if breast feeding.

Evaluation/Desired Outcomes
- Decrease in abdominal pain or prevention of gastric irritation and bleeding. Healing of duodenal ulcers can be seen on x-ray examination or endoscopy. Therapy is continued for at least 2–4 wk. Therapy for pathologic hypersecretory conditions may be long term.
- Healing in patients with erosive esophagitis. Therapy is continued for up to 8 wk, and an additional 8-wk course may be used for patients who do not heal in 8 wk or whose ulcer recurs.

lanthanum carbonate
(**lan**-than-um)
Fosrenol

Classification
Therapeutic: hypophosphatemics
Pharmacologic: phosphate binders

Pregnancy Category C

Indications
Reduction of serum phosphate levels associated with end-stage renal disease.

Action
Dissociates in the upper GI tract forming lanthanate ions, which form an insoluble complex with phosphate. **Therapeutic Effects:** Decreased serum phosphate levels.

Pharmacokinetics
Absorption: Negligible absorption.
Distribution: Stays within the GI tract.
Metabolism and Excretion: Eliminated almost entirely in feces.
Half-life: 53 hr (in plasma).

TIME/ACTION PROFILE (effect on phosphate levels)

ROUTE	ONSET	PEAK	DURATION
PO	unknown	2–3 wk	unknown

Contraindications/Precautions
Contraindicated in: Bowel obstruction; Ileus; Fecal impaction; OB: Congenital abnormalities noted in animal studies; Pedi: Potential negative effect on developing bone.
Use Cautiously in: Patients with risk factors for bowel obstruction, including history of GI surgery, colon cancer, constipation, ileus, diabetes, or taking medications that cause constipation; Lactation: Safety not established.

Adverse Reactions/Side Effects
GI: nausea, vomiting, diarrhea, fecal impaction, GI obstruction, ileus. **F and E:** hypocalcemia.

Interactions
Drug-Drug: May ↓ absorption of **fluoroquinolones**, **tetracyclines**, and **levothyroxine**; administer at least 1 hr before or 3 hr after lanthanum carbonate.

Route/Dosage
PO (Adults): 1500 mg/day in divided doses; may be titrated upward every 2–3 wk in increments of 750 mg/day up to 4500 mg/day (usual range 1500–3000 mg/day).

Availability (generic available)
Chewable tablets: ✦ 250 mg, 500 mg, 750 mg, 1000 mg. **Oral powder:** 750 mg/pkt, 1000 mg/pkt.

NURSING IMPLICATIONS
Assessment
- Assess patient for nausea and vomiting during therapy.
- ***Lab Test Considerations:*** Monitor serum phosphate levels prior to and periodically during therapy.

Potential Nursing Diagnoses
Nausea (Side Effects)

Implementation
- Do not confuse lanthanum carbonate with lithium carbonate.
- Divide total daily dose and administer with meals.
- **PO:** Administer with or immediately after meals. Tablets should be crushed or chewed completely before swallowing; intact tablets should not be swallowed.
- Sprinkle powder on small quantity of applesauce or other similar food; consume immediately. Consider powder formulation for patients with poor dentition.

Patient/Family Teaching
- Instruct patient to take lanthanum as directed.

Evaluation/Desired Outcomes
- Decrease in serum phosphate to below than 6.0 mg/dL in patients with end stage renal disease.

lapatinib (la-pat-i-nib)

Tykerb

Classification

Therapeutic: antineoplastics

Pharmacologic: enzyme inhibitors, kinase inhibitors

Pregnancy Category D

Indications

Advanced or metastatic breast cancer with tumor overexpression of the Human Epidermal Receptor Type 2 (HER2) and past therapy with an anthracycline, a taxane and trastuzumab (used in combination with capecitabine). Postmenopausal women with hormone-receptor positive metastatic breast cancer that overexpresses HER2 for whom hormonal therapy is indicated (used in combination with letrozole).

Action

Acts as an inhibitor of intracellular tyrosine kinase affecting Epidermal Growth Factor (EGFR, ErbB1) and HER2 (ErbB2). Inhibits the growth of ErbB-driven tumors. Effect is additive with capecitabine. **Therapeutic Effects:** Decreased/slowed spread of metastatic breast cancer.

Pharmacokinetics

Absorption: Incompletely and variably absorbed following oral administration; blood levels ↑ by food.

Distribution: Unknown.

Protein Binding: >99%.

Metabolism and Excretion: Extensively metabolized by, mostly by CYP3A4 and CYP3A5 enzyme systems; <2% excreted by kidneys.

Half-life: 24 hr.

TIME/ACTION PROFILE (blood levels)

ROUTE	ONSET	PEAK	DURATION
PO	unknown	4 hr	24 hr

Contraindications/Precautions

Contraindicated in: Hypersensitivity; ↓ left ventricular ejection fraction (Grade 2 or greater); OB, Lactation: Pregnancy or lactation.

Use Cautiously in: Concurrent use of CYP3A4 inhibitors including ketoconazole, itraconazole, clarithromycin, atazanavir, indinavir, nefazodone, nelfinavir, ritoanvir, saquinavir, telithromycin, and voriconazole should be avoided (if necessary, ↓ lapatinib dose); Concurrent use of CYP3A4 inducers including dexamathasone, phenytoin, carbamazepine, rifampin, rifabutin, rifapentin, phenobarbital, and St. John's wort should be avoided (if necassary, ↑ lapatinib dose; Severe hepatic impairment (dose ↓ recommended for Child-Pugh Class C); Known QTc interval prolongation or co-existing risk factors for QTc interval prolongation including hypokalemia, hypomagnesemia, concurrent antiarrhythmics or medications that are known to prolong the QTc interval; Geri: May be more sensitive to effects; Pedi: Safety not established.

Adverse Reactions/Side Effects

CNS: fatigue, insomnia. **Resp:** dyspnea, interstitial lung disease, pneumonitis. **CV:** ↓ left ventricular ejection fraction, QT interval prolongation. **GI:** DIARRHEA, HEPATOTOXICITY, nausea, vomiting, dyspepsia, ↑ liver enzymes, stomatitis. **Derm:** ERYTHEMA MULTIFORM, STEVENS-JOHNSON SYNDROME, TOXIC EPIDERMAL NECROLYSIS, palmar-plantar erythrodysesthesia, rash, dry skin, nail disorders. **Hemat:** neutropenia. **MS:** back pain, extremity pain.

Interactions

Drug-Drug: Lapatinib inhibits CYP3A4, CYP28 and P-glycoprotein; concurrent use of drugs, which are substrates for these enzymes should be undertaken with caution. May ↑ effects of **midazolam**, **paclitaxel**, and **digoxin**. Concurrent use of **strong CYP3A4 inhibitors** including **ketoconazole**, **itraconazole**, **clarithromycin**, **atazanavir**, **indinavir**, **nefazodone**, **nelfinavir**, **ritonavir**, **saquinavir**, **telithromycin**, and **voriconazole** may ↑ blood levels and the risk of toxicity. Concurrent use should be avoided, but if necessary, dose of lapatinib should be ↓. Concurrent use of **strong CYP3A4 inducers** including **dexamethasone**, **phenytoin**, **carbamazepine**, **rifampin**, **rifabutin**, **rifapentin**, and **phenobarbital** may ↓ blood levels and effectiveness. Concurrent use should be avoided, but if necessary, dose of lapatinib should be ↑.

Drug-Natural Products: Concurrent use of **St. John's wort** may ↓ blood levels and effectiveness. Concurrent use should be avoided, but if necessary dose of lapatinib should be ↑.

Drug-Food: Concurrent **grapefruit juice** may ↑ blood levels and the risk of toxicity and should be avoided.

Route/Dosage

PO (Adults): *HER2 positive metastatic breast cancer*—1250 mg once daily for 21 days; *Hormone receptor positive, HER2 positive metastatic breast cancer*—1500 mg once daily; *Concurrent use of strong CYP3A4 inhibitor*—↓ dose to 500 mg once daily; *Concurrent use of strong CYP3A4 inducer*—HER2 positive metastatic breast cancer: Gradually titrate dose from 1250 mg once daily up to 4500 mg once daily as tolerated; Hormone receptor positive, HER2 positive metastatic breast cancer: Gradually titrate dose from 1500 mg once daily up to 5500 mg once daily as tolerated.

Hepatic Impairment

PO (Adults): *Severe hepatic impairment*—HER2 positive metastatic breast cancer: 750 mg/day; Hormone receptor positive, HER2 positive metastatic breast cancer: 1000 mg/day.

Availability

Tablets: 250 mg.

NURSING IMPLICATIONS

Assessment

- Evaluate left ventricular ejection fraction (LVEF) prior to therapy to determine if within institution's normal limits. Continue to monitor periodically during therapy to ensure it does not fall below limits. If LVEF decreases to Grade 2 or greater discontinue therapy. If returns to normal and patient is asymptomatic after 2 wk, may restart therapy at a reduced dose of 1000 mg/day (with cabcitabine) or 1250 mg/day (with letrazole).
- Monitor for diarrhea; usually occurs within first 6 days of therapy and lasts 4–5 days. Treat with antidiarrheals (loperamide) after first loose stool. If diarrhea is severe, treat with oral or intravenous fluids, antibiotics (fluoroquinolones) especially if diarrhea persists >24 hrs or accompanied by fever; may require interruption or discontinuation of therapy. If accompanied by moderate to severe abdominal cramping, nausea or vomiting, decreased performance status, fever, sepsis, neutropenia, frank bleeding, or dehydration, interrupt therapy and reintroduce at lower dose (from 1,250 mg/day to 1,000 mg/day or from 1,500 mg/day to 1,250 mg/day) when diarrhea <Grade 1. If Grade 4 diarrhea occurs, discontinue therapy.
- Monitor ECG prior to and periodically during therapy to monitor QT.
- Monitor for respiratory status for symptoms of interstitial lung disease and pneumonitis (dyspnea, cough); may require discontinuation of therapy.
- Monitor for signs and symptoms of skin reactions (progressive skin rash often with blisters or mucosal lesions). Discontinue lapatinib if erythema multiforme, Stevens-Johnson syndrome, or toxic epidermal necrolysis are suspected.
- ***Lab Test Considerations:*** Monitor liver function tests prior to initiation and every 4–6 wk during therapy and as clinically indicated. Discontinue and do not restart lapatinib if patients experience severe changes in liver function tests.
- Monitor serum potassium and magnesium prior to and periodically during therapy.

Potential Nursing Diagnoses

Diarrhea (Adverse Reactions)

Implementation

- Correct hypokalemia and hypomagnesemia prior to therapy.
- **PO:** Administer tablets once daily at least 1 hr before or 1 hr after a meal for 21 days. Do not divide daily dose.

Patient/Family Teaching

- Instruct patient to take lapatinib as directed and to review the *Patient Information Sheet* prior to therapy and with each refill for new information. If a dose is missed take as soon remembered that day. If a day is missed, skip the dose; do not double doses. Caution patient not to share this medication with others, even with same condition; may be harmful.
- Advise patient to avoid drinking grapefruit juice or eating grapefruit during therapy.
- Advise patient to report signs or decreased LVEF (shortness of breath, palpitations, fatigue) and skin rash to health care professional promptly.
- Instruct patient to notify health care professional of all Rx or OTC medications, vitamins, or herbal products being taken and consult health care professional before taking any new medications, especially St. John's wort.
- Advise patient that lapatinib may cause diarrhea, which may become severe. Instruct patient in how to prevent and manage diarrhea and to notify health care professional if severe.
- Advise female patients to notify health care professional if pregnancy is planned or suspected; therapy may be teratogenic.

Evaluation/Desired Outcomes

- Decreased/slowed spread of metastatic breast cancer.

L

ledipasvir/sofosbuvir

(led-i-**pas**-vir/soe-**fos**-bue-vir)

Harvoni

Classification

Therapeutic: antivirals

Pharmacologic: NS5A inhibitors, polymerase inhibitors

Pregnancy Category B

Indications

Treatment of adults with chronic hepatitis C (CHC) genotype 1 infection.

Action

Ledipasvir—inhibits NS5A, a protein required for viral replication. *Sofosbuvir*—inhibits RNA-dependent RNA polymerase, resulting in inhibition of viral replication.

Therapeutic Effects: Decreased HCV RNA levels with decreased severity and sequelae of CHC.

Pharmacokinetics

Ledipasvir

Absorption: Well absorbed following oral administration.

Distribution: Unknown.

Protein Binding: >99.8%.

Metabolism and Excretion: Minimal metabolism, undergoes biliary excretion. Mostly excreted unchanged in feces (86%), 1% eliminated in urine.

Half-life: 47 hr.

Sofosbuvir

Absorption: Rapidly metabolized following absorption (extensive first-pass effect).

Distribution: Unknown.

Protein Binding: 61–65%.

Metabolism and Excretion: Extensively metabolized with much conversion to GS-461203, an active antiviral moiety, then converted GS-331007, which does not have antiviral activity. 80% excreted in urine mostly as GS-331007 (3.5% as unchanged drug), 14% excreted in feces, 2.5% excreted in expired air.

Half-life: *Sofosbuvir*—0.4 hr; *GS-331007*—27 hr.

TIME/ACTION PROFILE (blood levels)

ROUTE	ONSET	PEAK	DURATION
ledipasvir	unknown	4–5 hr	24 hr
sofosbuvir	unknown	0.8–1 hr†	24 hr

† Sofosbuvir (2–4 hr for GS-331007).

Contraindications/Precautions

Contraindicated in: Should not be used with other drugs/regimens that already containing sofosbuvir; Concurrent use of P-gp inducers, some anticonvulsants, some antivirals and rosuvastatin; Severe renal impairment (eGFR <30 mL/min/1.73 m^2) or end stage renal disease (no dose recommendation).

Use Cautiously in: Decompensated cirrhosis (safety and effectiveness not established); Geri: May be more sensitive to drug effects; Lactation: Weigh benefits of breast feeding against possible adverse effects; OB: Use only if potential benefit justifies fetal risk; Pedi: Safety and effectiveness not established.

Adverse Reactions/Side Effects

CNS: fatigue, headache, insomnia. **GI:** diarrhea, nausea.

Interactions

Drug-Drug: Concurrent use of **P-gp inducers** including **rifampin** ↓ levels and effectiveness of both ledipasvir and sofosbuvir; concurrent use contraindicated. Ledipasvir inhibits P-gp and may ↑ levels of **substrates of P-gp**. **Amiodarone** may ↑ risk of symptomatic bradycardia; concurrent use not recommended; if amiodarone necessary, monitor patients in inpatient setting for first 48 hr of concomitant use and then monitor heart rate on outpatient basis for at least the first 2 wk of treatment (follow same monitoring procedure if discontinuing amiodarone immediately before initiation of ledipasvir/sofosbuvir therapy). **Acid-reducing agents** may ↓ levels of ledipasvir; separate **antacids** including **magnesium and aluminum hydroxide** by 4 hr, administer **H_2-receptor antagonists** including **famotidine** simultaneously or 12 hr apart (dose of antagonist should not exceed famotidine 40 mg twice daily or equivalent), **proton-pump inhibitors** including **omeprazole** 20 mg daily or equivalent may be given simultaneously. May ↑ levels/effects/risk of toxicity with **digoxin** (therapeutic monitoring recommended). Level and effectiveness ↓ by **carbamazepine**, **phenytoin**, **phenobarbital** and **oxcarbazepine** concurrent use in not recommended. Levels and effectiveness may be ↓ by concurrent use of **rifabutin** and **rifapentine**; concurrent use not recommended. ↑ levels and risk of adverse reactions from **tenofovir** and **tenofovir-containing combinations** (dosage adjustments may be necessary, consider alternative regimens). Levels and effectiveness are ↓ by **tipranavir/ritonavir**; concurrent use not recommended. Concurrent use with **simeprevir** may ↑ levels of simeprevir and ledipasvir; concurrent use not recommended. ↑ levels and risk of myopathy/rhabdomyolysis with **rosuvastatin**; concurrent use not recommended.

Drug-Natural Products: Concurrent use with **St. John's wort** ↓ blood levels and effectiveness; concurrent use contraindicated.

Route/Dosage

PO (Adults): Ledipasvir 90 mg/sofosbuvir 400 mg (one tablet) once daily for 12 wk in patients who are treatment naïve with/without cirrhosis or who are treatment-experienced without cirrhosis and for 24 wk in patients who are treatment-experienced with cirrhosis.

Availability

Tablets: ledipasvir 90 mg/sofosbuvir 400 mg.

NURSING IMPLICATIONS

Assessment

- Monitor symptoms of hepatitis during therapy.
- ***Lab Test Considerations:*** May cause ↑ serum bilirubin and lipase levels.

Potential Nursing Diagnoses

Risk for infection (Indications)

Implementation

- **PO:** Administer once daily with or without food.

Patient/Family Teaching

- Instruct patient to take ledipasvir/sofosbuvir at the same time each day for the full course of therapy. Take missed doses as soon as remembered on same day; do not take more than 1 tablet in a day. Do not stop taking ledipasvir/sofosbuvir without consulting health care professional. Advise patient to read *Patient Information* prior to starting therapy and with each Rx refill in case of changes.
- Inform patient that ledipasvir/sofosbuvir may not reduce the risk of transmission of CHC to others; use appropriate precautions to prevent transmission.
- Instruct patient that ledipasvir/sofosbuvir should not be shared with others; may be harmful.
- Advise patient to notify health care professional of all Rx or OTC medications, vitamins, or herbal products being taken and consult health care professional before taking any new medications, especially St. John's Wort.

- Instruct patient to take antacids containing aluminum or magnesium 4 hrs before or 4 hrs after ledipasvir/sofosbuvir.
- Advise female patient to notify health care professional if pregnancy is planned or suspected or if breast feeding.

Evaluation/Desired Outcomes

- Decreased HCV RNA levels with decreased severity and sequelae of CHC.

leflunomide (le-flu-noe-mide)

Arava

Classification

Therapeutic: antirheumatics (DMARDs)
Pharmacologic: immune response modifiers, pyrimidine synthesis inhibitors

Pregnancy Category X

Indications

Rheumatoid arthritis (disease-modifying agent).

Action

Inhibits an enzyme required for pyrimidine synthesis; has antiproliferative and anti-inflammatory effects. **Therapeutic Effects:** Decreased pain and inflammation, slowed structural progression and improved physical function.

Pharmacokinetics

Absorption: Tablets are 80% absorbed following oral administration; rapidly converted to the M1 metabolite, which is responsible for pharmacologic activity.
Distribution: Crosses the placenta.
Protein Binding: 99%.
Metabolism and Excretion: Extensively metabolized with metabolites excreted in urine (43%) and feces (48%). Also undergoes biliary recycling.
Half-life: 14–18 days.

TIME/ACTION PROFILE (antirheumatic effect)

ROUTE	ONSET	PEAK	DURATION
PO	1 mo	3–6 mo	wk–mos†

†Due to persistence of active metabolite.

Contraindications/Precautions

Contraindicated in: Hypersensitivity to leflunomide or teriflunomide; Compromised immune function, including bone marrow dysplasia or severe uncontrolled infection; Concurrent vaccination with live vaccines; Hepatic impairment; OB: May cause fetal abnormalities or death. Contact Pregnancy Registry if accidental exposure occurs; Lactation: Lactation.
Use Cautiously in: Renal insufficiency; History of interstitial lung disease; Patients >60 yr, with diabetes, or taking neurotoxic medications (↑ risk of peripheral neuropathy); Pedi: Safety and effectiveness not established; OB: Women with childbearing potential must use two forms of birth control. Should not be used in men attempting to father a child.
Exercise Extreme Caution in: Concurrent use of other hepatotoxic agents (↑ risk of hepatotoxicity).

Adverse Reactions/Side Effects

CNS: headache, dizziness, weakness. **Resp:** INTERSTITIAL LUNG DISEASE, bronchitis, cough, pharyngitis, pneumonia, respiratory infection, rhinitis, sinusitis. **CV:** chest pain, hypertension. **GI:** HEPATOTOXICITY, diarrhea, nausea, abdominal pain, anorexia, dyspepsia, gastroenteritis, ↑ liver enzymes, mouth ulcers, vomiting. **GU:** urinary tract infection. **Derm:** STEVENS-JOHNSON SYNDROME, TOXIC EPIDERMAL NECROLYSIS, alopecia, rash, dry skin, eczema, pruritus. **F and E:** hypokalemia. **Metab:** weight loss. **MS:** arthralgia, back pain, joint disorder, leg cramps, synovitis, tenosynovitis. **Neuro:** paresthesia, peripheral neuropathy. **Misc:** DRUG REACTION WITH EOSINOPHILIA AND SYSTEMIC SYMPTOMS (DRESS), allergic reactions, flu syndrome, infections including sepsis and tuberculosis reactivation, pain.

Interactions

Drug-Drug: Cholestyramine and **activated charcoal** cause a rapid and significant ↓ in blood levels of active metabolite. Concurrent use of **methotrexate** and other **hepatotoxic drugs** ↑ risk of hepatotoxicity. Concurrent administration of **rifampin** ↑ blood levels of the active metabolite. May ↑ risk of bleeding with **warfarin**.

Route/Dosage

PO (Adults): *Loading dose*—100 mg daily for 3 days; *maintenance dosing*—20 mg/day (if intolerance occurs, dose may be ↓ to 10 mg/day).

Availability (generic available)

Tablets: 10 mg, 20 mg, 100 mg.

NURSING IMPLICATIONS

Assessment

- Assess range of motion and degree of swelling and pain in affected joints before and periodically during therapy.
- Monitor for signs and symptoms of interstitial lung disease (new onset or worsening cough or dyspnea, associated with fever). May require discontinuation of therapy; consider drug elimination procedure if needed.
- Assess for rash periodically during therapy. May cause Stevens-Johnson syndrome or toxic epidermal necrolysis. Discontinue therapy if severe or if accompanied with fever, general malaise, fatigue, mus-

cle or joint aches, blisters, oral lesions, conjunctivitis, hepatitis and/or eosinophilia.

- ***Lab Test Considerations:*** Monitor liver function throughout therapy. Assess ALT at baseline, then monthly during initial 6 mo of therapy, then every 6–8 wk. If given concurrently with methotrexate, monitor ALT, AST, and serum albumin monthly. May cause ↑ ALT and AST, which are usually reversible with reduction in dose or discontinuation, but may be fatal. If ALT is 2–3 times the upper limit of normal, reduce dose to 10 mg/day and continue therapy. Monitor closely after dose reduction; plasma levels may not ↓ for several weeks due to long half-life. If ALT ↑ of 2–3 times the upper limit of normal persists despite dose reduction or if ALT >3 times the upper limit of normal occurs, discontinue leflunomide and administer cholestyramine (see Toxicity and Overdose). Monitor closely and readminister cholestyramine as indicated.
- Monitor CBC with platelets monthly for 6 mo following initiation of therapy and every 6–8 wk thereafter. If used with methotrexate or other immunosuppressive therapy continue monitoring monthly. If bone marrow depression occurs, discontinue leflunomide and begin decreasing levels with cholestyramine (see Implementation).
- May rarely cause ↑ of alkaline phosphatase and bilirubin.
- ***Toxicity and Overdose:*** If overdose or significant toxicity occurs, cholestyramine 8 g 3 times a day for 24 hr, or activated charcoal orally or via nasogastric tube, 50 g every 6 hr for 24 hr, is recommended to accelerate elimination.

Potential Nursing Diagnoses

Impaired physical mobility (Indications)
Acute pain (Indications)

Implementation

- Administer a tuberculin skin test prior to administration of leflunomide. Patients with active latent TB should be treated for TB prior to therapy.
- **PO:** Initiate therapy with loading dose of 100 mg/day for 3 days, followed by 20 mg/day dose. May decrease to 10 mg/day if not well tolerated.
- **Drug Elimination Procedure:** Recommended to achieve nondetectable plasma levels <0.02 mg/L after stopping treatment with leflunomide. Administer cholestyramine 8 g 3 times daily for 11 days. (Days do not need to be consecutive unless rapid lowering of levels is desired.) Verify plasma levels <0.02 mg/L by 2 separate tests at least 14 days apart. If plasma levels >00.02 mg/L, consider additional cholestyramine treatment. Plasma levels may take up to 2 yr to reach nondetectable levels without drug elimination procedure.

Patient/Family Teaching

- Instruct patient to take leflunomide as directed.
- May cause dizziness. Caution patient to avoid driving or other activities requiring alertness until response to medication is known.
- Advise patient to consult health care professional prior to taking other Rx, OTC, or herbal products concurrently with leflunomide. Aspirin, NSAIDs, or low-dose corticosteroids may be continued during therapy, but other agents for treatment of rheumatoid arthritis may require discontinuation.
- Discuss the possibility of hair loss with patient. Explore methods of coping.
- Advise patient to notify health care professional if rash, mucous membrane lesions, unusual tiredness, abdominal pain, jaundice, or symptoms of interstitial lung disease occur.
- Instruct patient to avoid vaccinations with live vaccines during and following therapy without consulting health care professional.
- Rep: Caution patients of childbearing age that leflunomide has teratogenic effects. Women wishing to become pregnant must undergo the drug elimination procedure (see Implementation) and verify that the M1 metabolite plasma levels are <0.02 mg/L. Men wishing to father a child should also take cholestyramine 8 g 3 times daily for 11 days to minimize any possible risk.
- Emphasize the importance of routine lab tests to monitor for side effects.

Evaluation/Desired Outcomes

- Decrease in signs and symptoms of rheumatoid arthritis and slowing of structural damage as evidenced by x-ray erosions and joint narrowings.
- Improved physical function.

lenvatinib (len-**va**-ti-nib)

Lenvima

Classification
Therapeutic: antineoplastics
Pharmacologic: kinase inhibitors

Indications

Treatment of locally recurrent or metastatic/progressive, radioactive-iodine-refractory differentiated thyroid cancer.

Action

Acts as a receptor tyrosine kinase inhibitor; inhibits kinase activities of various vascular endoethelial growth factor receptors (VEGFRs), resulting in decreased pathogenic angiogenesis, tumor growth and spread. **Therapeutic Effects:** Decreased progression of differentiated thyroid cancer.

Pharmacokinetics

Absorption: Well absorbed following oral administration.

Distribution: Unknown.
Protein Binding: 98–99%.
Metabolism and Excretion: Metabolized by CYP3A and aldehyde oxidase; 64% eliminated in feces, 25% in urine.
Half-life: 28 hr.

TIME/ACTION PROFILE (improvement in progression-free survival)

ROUTE	ONSET	PEAK	DURATION
PO	within 2 mo	8 mo	throughout treatment

Contraindications/Precautions

Contraindicated in: Lactation: Discontinue lenvatinib or discontinue breast feeding; OB: Pregnancy (may cause fetal harm, effective contraception required, may result in reduced fertility).

Use Cautiously in: Hypertension (control BP before initiating treatment, may need to withhold/discontinue for life-threatening elevation); History of heart failure (may need to withhold/discontinue for worsening HF); History of congenital long QTc syndrome, HF, bradyarrhythmias, concurrent use of drugs that prolong QTc, including Class Ia and III antiarrhythmics (↑ risk of further QTc prolongation and serious arrthythmias, may require interruption/discontinuation of lenvatinib); Severe hepatic or renal impairment (lower dose required); Dehydration/volume depletion (↑ risk of renal impairment, may need to withhold/discontinue for worsening renal function); Hypocalcemia (replace calcium, if persistent may require dose adjustment/interruption); History of reversible posterior leukencephalopathy syndrome (may require dose adjustment/interruption); May damage male reproductive tissue resulting in decreased fertility; Pedi: Safe and effective use in children has not been established.

Adverse Reactions/Side Effects

CNS: fatigue, insomnia, headache. **Resp:** cough. **CV:** ARTERIAL THROMBOEMBOLIC EVENTS, HEART FAILURE, HYPERTENSION, QTC PROLONGATION, hypotension. **EENT:** dysphonia, epistaxis. **GI:** GASTROINTESTINAL PERFORATION/FISTULA FORMATION, HEPATOTOXICITY, abdominal pain, ↓ appetite, diarrhea, dry mouth, dysgeusia, nausea, stomatitis, vomiting, ↑ liver enzymes. **GU:** NEPHROTIC SYNDROME, proteinuria, renal impairment. **Derm:** alopecia, palmar-plantar erythrodysesthesia syndrome, rash, hyperkeratosis. **Endo:** impaired thyroid stimulating hormone suppression. **F and E:** dehydration, hypocalcemia, hypokalemia. **Hemat:** hemorrhagic events, thrombocytopenia. **Metab:** ↓ weight. **MS:** arthralgia/myalgia. **Neuro:** reversible posterior leukoencephalopathy syndrome (RPLS).

Interactions

Drug-Drug: Concurrent use of drugs that prolong QTc, including Class Ia and III antiarrhythmics may ↑ risk of further QTc prolongation and serious arrhythmias (may require interruption/discontinuation of lenvatinib).

Route/Dosage

PO (Adults): 24 mg once daily.

Renal Impairment

PO (Adults): *CCr <30 mL/min*—14 mg once daily.

Hepatic Impairment

PO (Adults): *Child–Pugh C or worse*—14 mg once daily.

Availability

Capsules: 4 mg, 10 mg.

L

NURSING IMPLICATIONS

Assessment

- Assess BP prior to and after 1 wk, then every 2 wks for first 2 mo, and then at least monthy thereafter during therapy. Initiate or adjust medication management to control BP. Withhold lenvatinib for Grade 3 hypertension that persists despite antihypertensive therapy. Resume at a reduced dose (*1st occurrence* – 20 mg/day; *2nd occurrence* —14 mg/day; *3rd occurrence* —10 mg/day) when hypertension is controlled or ≤Grade 2. Discontinue lenvatinib for life-threatening hypertension.
- Monitor for clinical signs and symptoms of cardiac decompensation (shortness of breath, swollen ankles) during therapy. Withhold lenvatinib for Grade 3 cardiac dysfunction until improved to Grade 0 or 1 or baseline. Resume at reduced dose (*1st occurrence* – 20 mg/day; *2nd occurrence* —14 mg/day; *3rd occurrence* —10 mg/day) or discontinue depending of severity and persistence of cardiac dysfunction.
- Monitor for signs and symptoms of arterial thromboembolic events (chest pain, acute neurologic symptoms of MI or stroke) during therapy. Discontinue lenvatinib if event occurs.
- Assess for signs and symptoms of gastrointestinal perforation or fistula formation (severe abdominal pain) during therapy. Discontine lenvatinib if gastrointestinal perforation or fistula occurs.
- Monitor ECG for patients with congential long QT syndrome, congestive heart failure, bradyarrhythmias, or those taking drugs known to prolong QT interval. Withhold lenvatinib for development of ≥Grade 3 QT interval prolongation. Resume at reduced dose (*1st occurrence* – 20 mg/day; *2nd occurrence* —14 mg/day; *3rd occurrence* —10 mg/day) when QT prolongation resolves to Grade 0 or 1.

- Monitor for signs and symptoms of reversible posterior leukoencephalopathy syndrome (RPLS) (severe headache, seizures, weakness, confusion, blindness or change in vision) during therapy. If symptoms occur, confirm diagnosis with MRI. Withhold lenvatinib for RPLS until fully resolved. Resume at reduced dose (*1st occurrence* – 20 mg/day; *2nd occurrence* —14 mg/day; *3rd occurrence* —10 mg/day) or discontinue depending on severity and persistence of neurologic symptoms.
- Monitor for bleeding (severe and persistent nose bleeds, vomiting blood, red or black stools, coughing up blood or blood clots, heavy or new onset vaginal bleeding) during therapy. Withhold lenvatinib for Grade 3 hemorrhage until resolved to Grade 0 or 1. Resume at reduced dose (*1st occurrence* – 20 mg/day; *2nd occurrence* —14 mg/day; *3rd occurrence* —10 mg/day) or discontinue depending on severity and persistence of hemorrhage. Discontinue lenvatinib if Grade 4 hemorrhage occurs.
- ***Lab Test Considerations:*** Monitor serum ALT and AST levels for hepatotoxicity prior to and every 2 wks for first 2 mo, and at least monthy thereafter during therapy. Withhold lenvatinib for Grade 3 cardiac dysfunction until improved to Grade 0 or 1 or baseline. Resume at reduced dose (*1st occurrence*—20 mg/day; *2nd occurrence*—14 mg/day; *3rd occurrence*—10 mg/day) or discontinue depending of severity and persistence of hepatotoxicity. May cause hypoalbuminemia, ↑ alkaline phosphatase, and hyperbilirubinemia.
- Monitor for proteinuria prior to and periodically during therapy. If urine dipstick proteinuria ≥2+ is detected, obtain 24 hr urine protein. Withhold lenvatinib for ≥2 g proteinuria/24 hrs and resume at reduced dose (*1st occurrence*—20 mg/day; *2nd occurrence*—14 mg/day; *3rd occurrence*—10 mg/day) when proteinuria <2 g/24 hrs. Discontinue lenvatinib for nephrotic syndrome.
- Monitor BUN and creatinine prior to and periodically during therapy. Withhold lenvatinib for Grade 3 or 4 renal failure/impairment until resolved to Grade 0 or 1 or baseline. Resume at reduced dose (*1st occurrence*—20 mg/day; *2nd occurrence*—14 mg/day; *3rd occurrence*—10 mg/day) or discontinue depending of severity and persistence of renal impairment.
- Monitor and correct electrolyte abnormalities. Monitor serum calcium levels at least monthy and replace calcium as needed during therapy. Interrupt and adjust lenvatinib dose based on severity, presence of ECG changes, and persistence of hypocalcemia. May cause hypokalemia, hypomegnesemia, hypoglycemia, hypercalcemia, and hyperkalemia.
- Monitor TSH levels monthy and adjust thyroid replacement medication as needed in patients with ↓ thyroid levels.
- May cause ↑ serum lipase and amylase, hypercholesterolemia, and ↓ platelet count.

Potential Nursing Diagnoses

Deficient knowledge, related to medication regimen (Adverse Reactions)

Implementation

- **PO:** Administer two 10–mg capsules and one 4–mg capsule to make 24 mg at the same time each day without regard to food.

Patient/Family Teaching

- Instruct patient to take lenvatinib as directed at the same time each day. Take missed dose within 12 hrs or omit and take next dose at usual time; do not double doses. Advise patient to read *Patient Information* before starting therapy and with each Rx refill in case of changes.
- Advise patient to notify health care professional promptly if signs and symptoms of high BP, heart problems, blood clots (severe chest pain or pressure; pain in arms, back, or jaw; shortness of breath; numbness or weakness on 1 side of body; trouble talking; sudden severe headache; sudden vision changes), liver problems (yellow skin or whites of eyes, dark tea colored urine, light-colored bowel movements), severe stomach pain, RPLS, or bleeding occur.
- Advise patient to notify health care professional of all Rx or OTC medications, vitamins, or herbal products being taken and to consult with health care professional before taking other medications.
- May be teratogenic. May cause fertility problems in males and females. Advise female patient to use effective contraception during and for at least 2 wks following completion of therapy and to notify health care professional if pregnancy is planned or suspected. Advise patient to avoid breast feeding during therapy.
- Emphasize importance of lab tests to monitor for adverse reactions.

Evaluation/Desired Outcomes

- Decreased progression of thyroid cancer.

letrozole (let-roe-zole)

Femara

Classification

Therapeutic: antineoplastics

Pharmacologic: aromatase inhibitors

Pregnancy Category X

Indications

First-line or second-line treatment of postmenopausal women with hormone receptor positive or hormone receptor unknown advanced breast cancer. Adjuvant treatment of postmenopausal women with hormone receptor positive early breast cancer. Extended adjuvant treatment of postmenopausal early breast cancer already treated with 5 yr of tamoxifen.

Action

Inhibits the enzyme aromatase, which is partially responsible for conversion of precursors to estrogen. **Therapeutic Effects:** Lowers levels of circulating estrogen, which may halt progression of estrogen-sensitive breast cancer. Decreased risk of recurrence/metastatic disease.

Pharmacokinetics

Absorption: Rapidly and completely absorbed.
Distribution: Unknown.
Metabolism and Excretion: Mostly metabolized by the liver.
Half-life: 2 days.

TIME/ACTION PROFILE (effect on lowering of serum estradiol levels)

ROUTE	ONSET	PEAK	DURATION
PO	unknown	2–3 days	unknown

Contraindications/Precautions

Contraindicated in: Hypersensitivity; Premenopausal women; OB: Potential for fetal harm.
Use Cautiously in: Severe hepatic impairment; Lactation, Pedi: Safety not established.

Adverse Reactions/Side Effects

CNS: anxiety, depression, dizziness, drowsiness, fatigue, headache, vertigo, weakness. **Resp:** coughing, dyspnea, pleural effusion. **CV:** chest pain, edema, hypertension, cerebrovascular events, thromboembolic events. **GI:** nausea, abdominal pain, anorexia, constipation, diarrhea, dyspepsia, vomiting. **Derm:** alopecia, hot flashes, ↑ sweating, pruritus, rash. **F and E:** hypercalcemia. **Metab:** hypercholesterolemia, weight gain. **MS:** musculoskeletal pain, arthralgia, ↓ bone density, fractures.

Interactions

Drug-Drug: None significant.

Route/Dosage

PO (Adults): 2.5 mg daily.

Hepatic Impairment

PO (Adults): *Severe hepatic impairment*—2.5 mg every other day.

Availability (generic available)

Tablets: 2.5 mg.

NURSING IMPLICATIONS

Assessment

- Assess patient for pain and other side effects periodically throughout therapy.
- ***Lab Test Considerations:*** May cause elevated AST, ALT, alkaline phosphatase, bilirubin, GGT and cholesterol levels.

Potential Nursing Diagnoses

Acute pain (Side Effects)

Implementation

- Do not confuse Femara (letrozole) with Femhrt (ethinyl estradiol/norethindrone).
- **PO:** May be taken without regard to food.

Patient/Family Teaching

- Instruct patient to take medication as directed.
- May cause dizziness and fatigue. Caution patient to avoid driving and other activities requiring awareness until response to medication is known.
- Inform patient of potential for adverse reactions and advise her to notify health care professional if side effects are problematic.
- Caution women who are perimenopausal or who recently became menopausal to use adequate contraception during therapy; letrozole may cause fetal harm.

Evaluation/Desired Outcomes

- Slowing of disease progression in women with advanced breast cancer.
- Decreased risk of recurrence/metastatic disease.

leucovorin calcium

(loo-koe-**vor**-in)

Classification
Therapeutic: antidotes (for methotrexate), vitamins
Pharmacologic: folic acid analogues

Pregnancy Category C

Indications

Minimizes hematologic effects of high-dose methotrexate therapy (leucovorin rescue). Advanced colorectal carcinoma (with 5-fluorouracil). Management of overdoses/prevention of toxicity from folic acid antagonists (pyrimethamine, trimethoprim). Folic acid deficiency (megaloblastic anemia) unresponsive to oral replacement.

Action

The reduced form of folic acid that serves as a cofactor in the synthesis of DNA and RNA. **Therapeutic Effects:** Reversal of toxic effects of folic acid antagonists. Reversal of folic acid deficiency.

Pharmacokinetics

Absorption: Well absorbed (38%) following PO administration. ↓ bioavailability with larger doses. Oral absorption is saturated at doses >25 mg.
Distribution: Widely distributed. Concentrates in the CNS and liver.

Metabolism and Excretion: Extensively converted to tetrahydrofolic derivatives, including 5-methyltetrahydrofolate, a major storage form.
Half-life: 3.5 hr.

TIME/ACTION PROFILE (serum folate levels)

ROUTE	ONSET	PEAK	DURATION
PO	20–30 min	unknown	3–6 hr
IM	10–20 min	unknown	3–6 hr
IV	<5 min	unknown	3–6 hr

Contraindications/Precautions

Contraindicated in: Hypersensitivity; Pedi: Preparations containing benzyl alcohol should not be used in neonates.

Use Cautiously in: Undiagnosed anemia (may mask the progression of pernicious anemia); OB, Lactation: Safety not established but has been used safely to treat megaloblastic anemia in pregnancy; Coadministration with high-dose methotrexate requires crucial timing of dosing and knowledge of methotrexate levels; Ascites; Renal failure; Dehydration; Pleural effusions; Urine pH <7.

Adverse Reactions/Side Effects

Hemat: thrombocytosis. **Misc:** allergic reactions (rash, urticaria, wheezing).

Interactions

Drug-Drug: May ↓ anticonvulsant effect of **barbiturates, phenytoin**, or **primidone**. High doses of the liquid contain significant **alcohol** and may cause ↑ CNS depression when used with **CNS depressants**. Concurrent use with **trimethoprim/sulfamethoxazole** may result in ↓ anti-infective efficacy and poor therapeutic outcome when used to treat *Pneumocystis jirovecii* pneumonia in HIV patients. May ↑ therapeutic effects and toxicity of **fluorouracil**; therapy may be combined for this purpose.

Route/Dosage

High-Dose Methotrexate—Leucovorin Rescue. Must start within 24 hr of methotrexate.

PO, IM, IV (Adults and Children): *Normal methotrexate elimination*—10 mg/m^2 q 6 hr (1st dose IV/IM, then change to PO) until methotrexate level is $<5 \times 10^{-8}$ M (0.05 micromolar). Larger doses/longer duration may be required in patients with aciduria, ascites, dehydration, renal impairment, GI obstruction, pleural/peritoneal effusions. Dose of leucovorin should be determined on the basis of plasma methotrexate levels.

Advanced Colorectal Cancer

IV (Adults): 200 mg/m^2 followed by 5-fluorouracil 370 mg/m^2 or leucovorin 20 mg/m^2 is followed by 5-fluorouracil 425 mg/m^2. Regimen is given daily for 5 days q 4–5 wk.

Prevention of Hematologic Toxicity from Pyrimethamine

PO, IV (Adults and Children): 5–15 mg/day.

Inadvertent Overdose of Folic Acid Antagonists

IM, IV (Adults and Children): *Methotrexate–large doses*—75 mg IV followed by 12 mg IM q 6 hr for 4 doses; *methotrexate–average doses*—6–12 mg IM q 6 hr for 4 doses; *other folic acid antagonists*—amount equal in mg to folic acid antagonist.

Megaloblastic Anemia

PO, IM, IV (Adults and Children): Up to 1 mg/day (up to 6 mg/day for dihydrofolate reductase deficiency).

Availability (generic available)

Tablets: 5 mg, 10 mg, 15 mg, 25 mg. **Solution for injection (preservative-free):** 10 mg/mL. **Powder for injection:** 50 mg/vial, 100 mg/vial, 200 mg/vial, 350 mg/vial, 500 mg/vial.

NURSING IMPLICATIONS

Assessment

- Assess patient for nausea and vomiting secondary to methotrexate therapy or folic acid antagonists (pyrimethamine and trimethoprim) overdose. Parenteral route may be necessary to ensure that patient receives dose.
- Monitor for development of allergic reactions (rash, urticaria, wheezing). Notify health care professional if these occur.
- **Megaloblastic Anemia:** Assess degree of weakness and fatigue.
- ***Lab Test Considerations:*** **Leucovorin rescue:** Monitor serum methotrexate levels to determine dose and effectiveness of therapy. Leucovorin calcium levels should be equal to or greater than methotrexate level. Rescue continues until serum methotrexate level is $<5 \times 10$M.
- Monitor CCr and serum creatinine prior to and every 24 hr during therapy to detect methotrexate toxicity. An increase >50% over the pretreatment concentration at 24 hr is associated with severe renal toxicity.
- Monitor urine pH every 6 hr during therapy; pH should be maintained >7 to decrease nephrotoxic effects of high-dose methotrexate. Sodium bicarbonate or acetazolamide may be ordered to alkalinize urine.
- *Megaloblastic anemia*—Monitor plasma folic acid levels, hemoglobin, hematocrit, and reticulocyte count prior to and periodically during therapy.

Potential Nursing Diagnoses

Risk for injury (Indications)
Imbalanced nutrition: less than body requirements (Indications)

Implementation

- Do not confuse folinic acid (leucovorin calcium) with folic acid. Do not confuse leucovorin calcium with levoleucovorin (Fusilev). Do not confuse leucovorin with Leukeran (chlorambucil).

- Make sure leucovorin calcium is available before administering high-dose methotrexate. Administration must be initiated within 24 hr of methotrexate therapy.
- Administer as soon as possible after toxic dose of folic acid antagonists (pyrimethamine and trimethoprim). Effectiveness of therapy begins to decrease 1 hr after overdose.
- **PO:** Parenteral therapy should be used in patients with GI toxicity, with nausea and vomiting, or with doses >25 m g.
- **IM:** IM route is preferred for treatment of megaloblastic anemia. Ampules of leucovorin calcium injection for IM use do not require reconstitution.

IV Administration

- **IV Push:** Bacteriostatic water or sterile water. Do not use product containing benzyl alcohol. Use immediately if reconstituted with sterile water for injection. Stable for 7 days when reconstituted with bacteriostatic water. ***Concentration:*** reconstitute 50-mg, 100-mg, and 200-mg vials to a concentration of 10 mg/mL; reconstitute 350-mg vial to a concentration of 20 mg/mL. ***Rate:*** Administer by slow injection over a minimum of 3 min; not to exceed 160 mg/min.
- **Intermittent Infusion: *Diluent:*** May be diluted in 100–500 mL of D5W, D10W, 0.9% NaCl, Ringer's, or LR. Stable for 24 hr.
- **Y-Site Compatibility:** acyclovir, alemtuzumab, alfentanil, allopurinol, amifostine, amikacin, aminocaproic acid, aminophylline, ampicillin, ampicillin/sulbactam, anidulafungin, argatroban, azithromycin, aztreonam, bivalirudin, bleomycin, bumetamide, buprenorphine, busulfan, butorphanol, calcium acetate, calcium chloride, calcium gluconate, carmustine, caspofungin, cefepime, cefotaxime, cefotetan, cefoxitin, ceftazidime, cefuroxime, chloramphenicol, ciprofloxacin, cisatracurium, cisplatin, cladribine, clindamycin, cyclophosphamide, cyclosporine, cytarabine, dacarbazine, dactinomycin, daptomycin, daunorubicin hydrochloride, dexamethasone, dexamedetomidine, dexrazoxane, digoxin, diltiazem, diphenhydramine, dobutamine, docetaxel, dolasetron, dopamine, doxorubicin hydrochloride, doxorubicin liposomal, doxycycline, enalaprilat, ephedrine, epinephrine, eptifibatide, ertapenem, erythromycin, esmolol, etoposide, etoposide phosphate, famotidine, fenoldopam, fentanyl, filgrastim, fluconazole, fludarabine, fluorouracil, fosphenytoin, furosemide, ganciclovir, gemcitabine, gentamicin, glycopyrrolate, granisetron, haloperidol, heparin, hetastarch, hydralazine, hydrocortisone, hydromorphone, idarubicin, ifosfamide, imipenem/cilastatin, insulin, irinotecan, isoproterenol, ketorolac, labetalol, levofloxacin, lidocaine, linezolid, lorazepam, magnesium sulfate, mannitol, mechlorethamine, melphalan, meperidine, meropenem, mesna, methotrexate, methyldopate, metoclopramide, metoprolol, metronidazole, midazolam, milrinone, mitomycin, mitoxantrone, morphine, moxifloxacin, mycophenolate, nafcillin, nalbuphine, nesiritide, nicardipine, nitroglycerin, nitroprusside, norepinephrine, octreotide, ondansetron, oxaliplatin, oxytocin, paclitaxel, palonosetron, pancuronium, pemetrexed, pentazocine, pentobarbital, phenobarbital, phenylephrine, piperacillin/tazobactam , potassium acetate, potassium chloride, procainamide, prochlorperazine, promethazine, propranolol, ranitidine, remifentanil, rituximab, rocuronium , sodium acetate, sodium phosphates, streptozocin, succinylcholine, sufentanil, tacrolimus, teniposide, theophylline, thiotepa, tigecycline, tirofiban, tobramycin, topotecan, trastuzumab, trimethopeim/sulfamethoxazole, vasopressin, vecuronium, verapamil, vinblastine, vincristine, vinorelbine, voriconazole, zidovudine.
- **Y-Site Incompatibility:** amiodarone, amphotericin B colloidal, amphotericin B lipid complex, amphotericin B liposome, carboplatin, ceftriaxone, chlorpromazine, dantrolene, diazepam, droperidol, epirubicin, foscarnet, methylprednisolone, naloxone, pamidronate, pantoprazole, pentamidine, phenytoin, potassium phosphates, quinupristin/dalfopristin, sodium bicarbonate, thiopental, vancomycin.

Patient/Family Teaching

- Explain purpose of medication to patient. Emphasize need to take exactly as ordered. Advise patient to contact health care professional if a dose is missed.
- **Leucovorin Rescue:** Instruct patient to drink at least 3 liters of fluid each day during leucovorin rescue.
- **Folic Acid Deficiency:** Encourage patient to eat a diet high in folic acid (meat proteins; bran; dried beans; and green, leafy vegetables).

Evaluation/Desired Outcomes

- Reversal of bone marrow and GI toxicity in patients receiving methotrexate or in overdose of folic acid antagonists.
- Increased sense of well-being and increased production of normoblasts in patients with megaloblastic anemia.

L

leuprolide (loo-**proe**-lide)
Eligard, ~~Lupron~~, ✱Lupron, Lupron Depot, Lupron Depot-Ped

Classification
Therapeutic: antineoplastics
Pharmacologic: hormones, gonadotropin-releasing hormones

Pregnancy Category X

Indications
Advanced prostate cancer in patients who are unable to tolerate orchiectomy or estrogen therapy (may be used in combination with flutamide or bicalutamide). Central precocious puberty (CPP). Endometriosis. Uterine fibroids (with iron therapy).

Action
A synthetic analogue of luteinizing hormone–releasing hormone (LHRH). Initially causes a transient increase in testosterone; however, with continuous administration, testosterone levels are decreased. Reduces gonadotropins, testosterone, and estradiol. **Therapeutic Effects:** Decreased testosterone levels and resultant decrease in spread of prostate cancer. Reduction of pain/lesions in endometriosis. Decreased growth of fibroids. Delayed puberty.

Pharmacokinetics
Absorption: Rapidly and almost completely absorbed following subcut administration. More slowly absorbed following IM administration of depot form.
Distribution: Unknown.
Metabolism and Excretion: Unknown.
Half-life: 3 hr.

TIME/ACTION PROFILE (effect on hormone levels)

ROUTE	ONSET†	PEAK‡	DURATION§
Subcut	within 1st wk	2–4 wk	4–12 wk
IM	within 1st wk	2–4 wk	4–12 wk
IM-depot	within 1st wk	2–4 wk	4–12 wk

†Initial transient ↑ in testosterone and estradiol levels.
‡Maximum decline in testosterone and estradiol levels.
§Restoration of normal pituitary–gonadal function; in amenorrheic patients, normal menses usually returns 60–90 days after treatment is discontinued.

Contraindications/Precautions
Contraindicated in: Intolerance to synthetic analogues of LHRH (GnRH); OB: Potential for fetal harm or spontaneous abortion; Lactation: Potentially serious adverse effects.
Use Cautiously in: Hypersensitivity to benzyl alcohol (results in induration and erythema at subcut site); Congenital long QT syndrome, HF, hypokalemia, or hypomagnesemia; Concurrent use of other drugs known to prolong the QTc interval.

Adverse Reactions/Side Effects
CNS: STROKE, dizziness, headache, seizures, syncope; *Depot*, depression, drowsiness, personality disorder; ***Subcut***, anxiety, blurred vision, lethargy, memory disorder, mood swings. **EENT:** blurred vision; ***Subcut***, hearing disorder. **Resp:** hemoptysis; *Depot*, epistaxis, throat nodules; ***Subcut***, cough, pleural rub, pulmonary fibrosis, pulmonary infiltrate. **CV:** MYOCARDIAL INFARCTION, PULMONARY EMBOLI, angina, arrhythmias; *Depot*, QT INTERVAL PROLONGATION, vasodilation. **GI:** anorexia, diarrhea, dysphagia, nausea, vomiting; *Depot*, HEPATOTOXICITY, gingivitis; ***Subcut***, GI BLEEDING, hepatic dysfunction, peptic ulcer, rectal polyps, taste disorders. **GU:** ↓ testicular size, dysuria, incontinence, testicular pain; *Depot*, cervix disorder; ***Subcut***, bladder spasm, penile swelling, prostate pain, urinary obstruction. **Derm:** *Depot*—hair growth, rash; ***Subcut***, dry skin, hair loss, pigmentation, skin cancer, skin lesions. **Endo:** breast swelling, breast tenderness, hyperglycemia. **F and E:** hypercalcemia, lower extremity edema. **Local:** burning, itching, swelling at injection site. **Metab:** *Depot*—hyperuricemia, ↓ bone density. **MS:** fibromyalgia, transient ↑ in bone pain (prostate cancer only); ***Subcut***, ankylosing spondylitis, joint pain, pelvic fibrosis, temporal bone pain. **Neuro:** *Subcut*—peripheral neuropathy. **Misc:** hot flashes, chills, ↓ libido, fever; *Depot*, body odor, epistaxis.

Interactions
Drug-Drug: ↑ antineoplastic effects with **antiandrogens**, (**megestrol**, **flutamide**).

Route/Dosage
Prostate Cancer
Subcut (Adults): *Leuprolide acetate*—1 mg/day *or Eligard*—7.5 mg once monthly, 22.5 mg every 3 mo, 30 mg q 4 mo, or 45 mg q 6 mo.
IM (Adults): *Lupron Depot*—7.5 mg once monthly *or* 22.5 mg q 3 mo *or* 30 mg q 4 mo *or* 45 mg q 6 mo.

Endometriosis
IM (Adults): *Lupron Depot*—3.75 mg once monthly for up to 6 mo *or* 11.25 mg q 3 mo for up to 2 doses.

Uterine Fibroids (with iron therapy)
IM (Adults): *Lupron Depot*—3.75 mg once monthly for up to 3 mo *or* 11.25 mg single injection.

Central Precocious Puberty (CPP)
Subcut (Children): *Leuprolide acetate*—50 mcg/kg/day, may ↑ by 10 mcg/kg/day as required.
IM (Children >37.5 kg): *Lupron Depot-Ped*—15 mg q 4 wk; may ↑ by 3.75 mg q 4 wk as required.
IM (Children 26–37.5 kg): *Lupron Depot-Ped*—11.25 mg q 4 wk; may ↑ by 3.75 mg q 4 wk as required.
IM (Children ≤25 kg): *Lupron Depot-Ped*—7.5 mg q 4 wk; may ↑ by 3.75 mg q 4 wk as required.
IM (Children): *Lupron Depot-Ped*—11.25 or 30 mg q 3 mo.

Availability (generic available)

Solution for subcut injection (leuprolide acetate): 5 mg/mL. **Lyophilized microspheres for depot injection (Lupron Depot):** 3.75 mg, 7.5 mg, 11.25 mg, 22.5 mg, 30 mg, 45 mg. **Lyophilized microspheres for pediatric depot injection (Lupron Depot-Ped):** 7.5 mg, 11.25 mg, 15 mg, 30 mg. **Polymeric matrix injectable formulation for subcut injection (Eligard):** 7.5 mg, 22.5 mg, 30 mg, 45 mg.

NURSING IMPLICATIONS

Assessment

- **Prostate Cancer:** Assess for an increase in bone pain, especially during the first few weeks of therapy. Monitor patients with vertebral metastases for increased back pain and decreased sensory/motor function.
- Monitor intake and output ratios; assess for bladder distention in patients with urinary tract obstruction during initiation of therapy.
- **Fibroids:** Assess for severity of symptoms (bloating, pelvic pain, pressure, excessive vaginal bleeding) periodically during therapy.
- **Endometriosis:** Assess for endometrial pain prior to and periodically during therapy.
- **CPP:** Prior to therapy, diagnosis of CPP should be confirmed by onset of secondary sex characteristics in girls <8 yr or boys <9 yr; a complete physical and endocrinologic examination, including height, weight, hand and wrist x-ray; total sex steroid level (estradiol or testosterone); adrenal steroid level; beta human chorionic gonadotropin level; GnRH stimulation test; and computerized tomography of the head must be performed. These parameters are monitored after 1–2 mo and every 6–12 mo during therapy.
- Assess for signs of precocious puberty (menses, breast development, testicular growth) periodically during therapy. Dose is increased until no progression of the disease is noted either clinically or by lab test parameters, then usually maintained throughout therapy. Discontinuation of therapy should be considered before age 11 in girls and age 12 in boys.
- ***Lab Test Considerations:*** Initially ↑, then ↓ luteinizing hormone (LH) and follicle-stimulating hormone (FSH). This leads to castration levels of testosterone in boys 2–4 wk after initial increase in concentrations.
- Monitor testosterone, prostatic acid phosphate, and prostate-specific antigen (PSA) levels to evaluate response to therapy. Transient ↑ in levels may occur during the 1st month of therapy for prostate cancer.
- May cause ↑ BUN, serum calcium, uric acid, hypoproteinemia, LDH, alkaline phosphatase, AST, hyperglycemia, hyperlipidemia, hyperphosphatemia, WBC, PT, or PTT. May also cause ↓ platelets and serum potassium.
- Monitor blood sugar and glycosylated hemoglobin periodically during therapy.

Potential Nursing Diagnoses

Sexual dysfunction (Side Effects)

Implementation

- Do not confuse Lupron Depot with Lupron Depot-Ped.
- Norethindrone acetate 5 mg daily may be used to prevent bone density loss from leuprolide.
- **Subcut** *Eligard subcut formulation:* **Bring to room temperature before mixing. Assemble the Eligard kit and reconstitute solution using syringes provided, as directed by manufacturer. Wearing gloves, mix in syringes as directed by manufacturer, do not shake. Solution must reach room temperature before administration and must be administered within 30 min of mixing, or be discarded. Solution is light tan to tan in color. Inject into abdomen, upper buttocks, or anywhere that has adequate amounts of subcut tissue without excessive pigment, nodules, lesions, or hair. Vary site with each injection.**
- **IM:** Use syringe supplied by manufacturer. Rotate sites.
- Leuprolide depot is *only* for IM injection.
- *Lupron Depot formulation:* To prepare for injection screw white plunger into end stopper until stopper begins to turn. Hold syringe upright; release diluent by slowly pushing, over 6–8 seconds, until the first stopper is at the blue line in the middle of the barrel. Keep syringe upright. Mix microspheres by shaking syringe until power forms a unified suspension. Tap syringe if caking or clumping occurs. Suspension will appear milky. Do not use if powder does not go into suspension. Keep syringe upright, remove cap and expel air. Inject at 90° angle in gluteal area, anterior thigh, or deltoid; rotate injection sites. Suspension settles very quickly; mix and administer immediately.
- Store at room temperature; stable for 24 hr following reconstitution.

Patient/Family Teaching

- Advise patient that medication may cause hot flashes. Notify health care professional if these become bothersome.
- Leuprolide depot usually causes a temporary discontinuation of menstruation. Advise patient to notify health care professional if menstruation persists or if intermittent bleeding occurs.
- Inform patient of the possibility of the development or worsening of depression and occurrence of memory disorders.

- **Prostate Cancer:** Instruct patient and family on subcut injection technique. Review patient insert provided with leuprolide patient-administration kit.
- Instruct patient to take medication exactly as directed. Take missed doses as soon as remembered unless not remembered until next day.
- Advise patient that bone pain may increase at initiation of therapy, but will resolve with time. Patient should discuss with health care professional use of analgesics to control pain.
- Instruct patient to notify health care professional promptly if difficulty urinating, weakness, or numbness occurs.
- **Endometriosis:** Advise patient to use a form of contraception other than oral contraceptives during therapy. Inform patient that amenorrhea is expected but does not guarantee contraception. Advise patient breast feeding should be avoided during therapy.
- **Central Precocious Puberty:** Instruct patient and family on the proper technique for subcut injection. Emphasize the importance of administering the medication at the same time each day. Rotate injection sites periodically.
- Inform patient and parents that if injections are not given daily, pubertal process may be reactivated.
- Advise patient and parents that during the first 2 mo of therapy patient may experience a light menstrual flow or spotting. Health care professional should be notified if this continues beyond 2nd mo.
- Instruct patient and parents to notify health care professional immediately if irritation at the injection site or unusual signs or symptoms occur.

Evaluation/Desired Outcomes

- Decrease in the spread of prostate cancer.
- Decrease in lesions and pain in endometriosis.
- Resolution of the signs of CPP.
- Improvement in preoperative hematologic parameters in patients with anemia from uterine fibroids.

levalbuterol

(leev-al-**byoo**-ter-ole)

Xopenex, Xopenex HFA

Classification

Therapeutic: bronchodilators

Pharmacologic: adrenergics

Pregnancy Category C

Indications

Bronchospasm due to reversible airway disease (short-term control agent).

Action

R-enantiomer of racemic albuterol. Binds to beta-2 adrenergic receptors in airway smooth muscle leading to activation of adenylcyclase and increased levels of cyclic-3', 5'-adenosine monophosphate (cAMP). Increases in cAMP activate kinases, which inhibit the phosphorylation of myosin and decrease intracellular calcium. Decreased intracellular calcium relaxes bronchial smooth muscle. **Therapeutic Effects:** Relaxation of airway smooth muscle with subsequent bronchodilation. Relatively selective for beta-2 (pulmonary) receptors.

Pharmacokinetics

Absorption: Some absorption occurs following inhalation.

Distribution: Unknown.

Metabolism and Excretion: Metabolized in the liver to an inactive sulfate and 3–6% excreted unchanged in the urine.

Half-life: 3.3–4 hr.

TIME/ACTION PROFILE (bronchodilation)

ROUTE	ONSET	PEAK	DURATION
Inhaln	10–17 min	90 min	5–6 hr

Contraindications/Precautions

Contraindicated in: Hypersensitivity to levalbuterol or albuterol.

Use Cautiously in: Cardiovascular disorders (including coronary insufficiency, hypertension, and arrhythmias); History of seizures; Hypokalemia; Hyperthyroidism; Diabetes mellitus; Unusual sensitivity to adrenergic amines; OB, Lactation, Pedi: Pregnancy, lactation, or children <6 yr (for nebulized solution) or <4 yr (for metered-dose inhaler) (safety not established).

Exercise Extreme Caution in: Concurrent use or use within 2 weeks of **tricyclic antidepressants** or **MAO inhibitors** (may ↑ risk of adverse cardiovascular reactions).

Adverse Reactions/Side Effects

CNS: anxiety, dizziness, headache, nervousness. **Resp:** PARADOXICAL BRONCHOSPASM (excessive use of inhalers), increased cough, turbinate edema. **CV:** tachycardia. **GI:** dyspepsia, vomiting. **Endo:** hyperglycemia. **F and E:** hypokalemia. **Neuro:** tremor.

Interactions

Drug-Drug: Concurrent use or use within 2 weeks of **tricyclic antidepressants** or **MAO inhibitors** may ↑ risk of adverse cardiovascular reactions (use with extreme caution). **Beta blockers** block the beneficial pulmonary effects of adrenergic bronchodilators (choose cardioselective beta blockers if necessary and with caution). May ↑ risk of hypokalemia from **potassium-losing diuretics**. May ↓ serum **digoxin** levels. May ↑ risk of arrhythmias with **hydrocarbon inhalation anesthetics** or **cocaine**.

Drug-Natural Products: Use with caffeine-containing herbs (**guarana, tea, coffee**) ↑ stimulant effect.

Route/Dosage

Inhaln (Adults and Children ≥4 yr): 2 inhalations q 4–6 hr; some patients may respond to 1 inhalation q 4 hr.

Inhaln (Adults and Children >12 yr): 0.63 mg via nebulization 3 times daily (every 6–8 hr); may be ↑ to 1.25 mg 3 times daily (every 6–8 hr).
Inhaln (Children 6–11 yr): 0.31 mg via nebulization 3 times daily (not to exceed 0.63 mg 3 times daily).

Availability (generic available)

Metered-dose inhaler: 45 mcg/actuation in 15-g (200 metered actuations) canisters. **Cost:** $54.23/15 g. **Inhalation solution:** 0.31 mg/3 mL in green foil pouch containing 12 vials, 0.63 mg/3 mL in yellow foil pouch containing 12 vials, 1.25 mg/3 mL in red foil pouch containing 12 vials, 1.25 mg/0.5 mL in unit-dose vials. **Cost:** *Generic*—All strengths $6.71/3 mL.

NURSING IMPLICATIONS

Assessment

- Assess lung sounds, pulse, and BP before administration and during peak of medication. Note amount, color, and character of sputum produced. Closely monitor patients on higher dose for adverse effects.
- Monitor pulmonary function tests before initiating therapy and periodically during course to determine effectiveness of medication.
- Observe for paradoxical bronchospasm (wheezing, dyspnea, tightness in chest). If condition occurs, withhold medication and notify health care provider immediately.
- ***Lab Test Considerations:*** May cause ↑ serum glucose and ↓ serum potassium.

Potential Nursing Diagnoses

Ineffective airway clearance (Indications)

Implementation

- **Inhaln:** Allow at least 1 min between inhalations of aerosol medication.
- For nebulization, levalbuterol solution does not require dilution prior to administration. Once the foil pouch is opened, vials must be used within 2 weeks; open vials may be stored for 1 week. Discard vial if solution is not clear or colorless.

Patient/Family Teaching

- Instruct patient in the proper use of metered-dose inhaler and nebulizer (see Appendix D) and to take levalbuterol as directed. Caution patient not to exceed recommended dose; may cause adverse effects, paradoxical bronchospasm, or loss of effectiveness of medication.
- Instruct patient to notify health care professional of all Rx or OTC medications, vitamins, or herbal products being taken and to consult health care professional before taking any OTC medications or alcoholic beverages concurrently with this therapy. Caution patient also to avoid smoking and other respiratory irritants.
- Instruct patient to contact health care professional immediately if shortness of breath is not relieved by medication or is accompanied by diaphoresis, dizziness, palpitations, or chest pain.
- Advise patients to use levalbuterol first if using other inhalation medications, and allow 5 min to elapse before administering other inhalant medications unless otherwise directed.
- Advise patient to rinse mouth with water after each inhalation dose to minimize dry mouth.
- Instruct patient to notify health care professional if no response to the usual dose of levalbuterol.

Evaluation/Desired Outcomes

- Prevention or relief of bronchospasm.

levetiracetam

(le-ve-teer-**a**-se-tam)
Keppra, Keppra XR

Classification
Therapeutic: anticonvulsants
Pharmacologic: pyrrolidines

Pregnancy Category C

Indications

Partial onset seizures (adjunct). Primary generalized tonic-clonic seizures (adjunct) (immediate-release and injection only). Myoclonic seizures in patients with juvenile myoclonic epilepsy (adjunct) (immediate-release and injection only).

Action

Appears to inhibit burst firing without affecting normal neuronal excitability and may selectively prevent hypersynchronization of epileptiform burst firing and propagation of seizure activity. **Therapeutic Effects:** Decreased incidence and severity of seizures.

Pharmacokinetics

Absorption: Rapidly and completely absorbed following oral administration.
Distribution: Unknown.
Protein Binding: <10%.
Metabolism and Excretion: 66% excreted unchanged by the kidneys; some metabolism by the liver (metabolites inactive).
Half-life: 7.1 hr (↑ in renal impairment).

TIME/ACTION PROFILE (blood levels)

ROUTE	ONSET	PEAK	DURATION
PO	rapid	1–1.5 hr†‡	12 hr

†1 hr in the fasting state, 1.5 hr when taken with food.
‡ 4 hr with extended-release.

L

Contraindications/Precautions

Contraindicated in: Hypersensitivity; Lactation: Lactation.

Use Cautiously in: All patients (may ↑ risk of suicidal thoughts/behaviors); Renal impairment (dose ↓ recommended if CCr ≤80 mL/min); Pedi: Safety and effectivness not established in children <16 yr (injection) <12 yr (extended-release); OB: Use only if potential benefit justifies potential risk to fetus; blood levels may be ↓ during pregnancy (especially during 3rd trimester); Geri: ↓ renal elimination (dose ↓ may be necessary).

Adverse Reactions/Side Effects

CNS: SUICIDAL THOUGHTS, aggression, agitation, anger, anxiety, apathy, depersonalization, depression, dizziness, drowsiness, fatigue, hostility, irritability, personality disorder, psychosis, weakness, drowsiness, fatigue, hyperkinesia. **CV:** hypertension. **Neuro:** coordination difficulties (adults only). **Derm:** STEVENS-JOHNSON SYNDROME, TOXIC EPIDERMAL NECROLYSIS. **Hemat:** AGRANULOCYTOSIS, anemia, eosinophilia, neutropenia. **Misc:** DRUG REACTION WITH EOSINOPHILIA AND SYSTEMIC SYMPTOMS (DRESS).

Interactions

Drug-Drug: None noted.

Route/Dosage

Only the oral solution should be used in patients ≤20 kg.

Partial Onset Seizures

PO, IV (Adults and Children ≥16 yr): 500 mg 2 times daily initially; may ↑ by 1000 mg/day at 2-wk intervals up to 3000 mg/day.

PO (Adults and Children ≥12 yr): *Extended-release*—1000 mg daily; may ↑ by 1000 mg/day at 2-wk intervals up to 3000 mg/day.

PO, IV (Children 4–15 yr): 10 mg/kg twice daily; ↑ by 20 mg/kg/day at 2-wk intervals to recommended dose of 30 mg/kg twice daily (maximum dose: 3000 mg/day).

PO, IV (Children 6 mo–3 yr): 10 mg/kg twice daily; ↑ by 20 mg/kg/day at 2-wk intervals to recommended dose of 25 mg/kg twice daily.

PO, IV (Children 1–5 mo): 7 mg/kg twice daily; ↑ by 14 mg/kg/day at 2-wk intervals to recommended dose of 21 mg/kg twice daily.

Primary Generalized Tonic-Clonic Seizures

PO, IV (Adults and Children ≥16 yr): 500 mg twice daily initially; ↑ by 1000 mg/day at 2-wk intervals to recommended dose of 3000 mg/day.

PO, IV (Children 6–15 yr): 10 mg/kg twice daily; ↑ by 20 mg/kg/day at 2-wk intervals to recommended dose of 30 mg/kg twice daily.

Myoclonic Seizures

PO, IV (Adults and Children ≥12 yr): 500 mg twice daily initially; ↑ by 1000 mg/day at 2-wk intervals to recommended dose of 3000 mg/day.

Status Epilepticus

IV (Infants and Children <16yr): 50 mg/kg/dose followed by maintenance dose of 30–55 mg/kg/day IV/PO divided BID.

IV (Neonates): 20–30 mg/kg/dose loading followed by neonatal seizure dosing.

Neonatal Seizures

IV (Neonates): 10 mg/kg/day divided BID; ↑ by 10 mg/kg at 3 day intervals to 30 mg/kg/day. May ↑ to 45–60 mg/kg/day with persistent seizure activity.

PO (Neonates): 10 mg/kg/day in 1–2 divided doses initially; ↑ daily by 10 mg/kg up to 30 mg/kg/day (maximum reported dose: 60 mg/kg/day).

Renal Impairment

PO, IV (Adults): *CCr 50–80 mL/min*—500–1000 mg q 12 hr (1000–2000 mg q 24 hr for extended-release); *CCr 30–50 mL/min*—250–750 mg q 12 hr (500–1500 mg q 24 hr for extended-release); *CCr <30 mL/min*—250–500 mg q 12 hr (500–1000 mg q 24 hr for extended-release); *Dialysis (immediate-release and injection)*—500–1000 mg q 24 hr with a 250–500-mg supplemental dose after dialysis.

Availability (generic available)

Tablets: 250 mg, 500 mg, 750 mg, 100 mg. **Cost:** *Generic*—250 mg $29.94/100, 500 mg $43.36/100, 750 mg $55.11/100, 1000 mg $148.42/180. **Extended-release tablets:** 500 mg, 750 mg. **Cost:** *Generic*—500 mg $266.82/60, 750 mg $400.64/60. **Oral solution (grape-flavored):** 100 mg/mL. **Cost:** *Generic*—$307.74/473 mL. **Solution for injection:** 100 mg/mL. **Premixed infusion:** 500 mg/100 mL 0.82% NaCl, 1000 mg/100 mL 0.75% NaCl, 1500 mg/100 mL 0.54% NaCl.

NURSING IMPLICATIONS

Assessment

- Assess location, duration, and characteristics of seizure activity.
- Assess patient for CNS adverse effects throughout therapy. These adverse effects are categorized as somnolence and fatigue (asthenia), coordination difficulties (ataxia, abnormal gait, or incoordination), and behavioral abnormalities (agitation, hostility, anxiety, apathy, emotional lability, depersonalization, depression) and usually occur during the first 4 wk of therapy.
- Monitor mood changes. Assess for suicidal tendencies, especially during early therapy. Restrict amount of drug available to patient.
- Assess for rash periodically during therapy. May cause Stevens-Johnson syndrome. Discontinue therapy if severe or if accompanied with fever, general

malaise, fatigue, muscle or joint aches, blisters, oral lesions, conjunctivitis, hepatitis and/or eosinophilia.
- Pedi: Monitor patients 1 month to <4 years of age for increases in diastolic BP.
- ***Lab Test Considerations:*** May cause ↓ RBC and WBC and abnormal liver function tests.

Potential Nursing Diagnoses

Risk for injury (Side Effects)

Implementation

- Do not confuse Keppra (levetiracetam) with Kaletra (lopinavir/ritonavir).
- IV doses should be used temporarily when oral route is not feasible. To convert IV to PO, equivalent dose and frequency may be used.
- **PO:** May be administered without regard to meals.
- Administer tablets whole; do not administer partial tablets. Do not break, crush, or chew XR tablets.
- Pedi: Patients <20 kg should receive oral solution. Administer with calibrated measuring device for accurate dose.
- Discontinue gradually to minimize the risk of increase in seizure frequency.

IV Administration

- **Intermittent Infusion: *Diluent:*** Dilute dose in 100 mL of 0.9% NaCl, D5W, or LR. If a smaller volume is required (e.g. pediatric patients), concentration should not exceed 15 mg/mL. Do not administer solutions that are cloudy or contain particulate matter. ***Rate:*** Infuse over 15 min.
- **Y-Site Compatibility:** diazepam, lorazepam, valproate.

Patient/Family Teaching

- Instruct patient to take medication as directed. Pedi: Explain to parents the importance of using calibrated measuring device for accurate dosing. Take missed doses as soon as possible unless almost time for next dose. Do not double doses. Do not discontinue abruptly; may cause increase in frequency of seizures. Advise patient to read the *Medication Guide* prior to starting therapy and with each Rx refill in case of changes.
- May cause dizziness and somnolence. Caution patient to avoid driving or activities requiring alertness until response to medication is known. Do not resume driving until physician gives clearance based on control of seizure disorder.
- Advise patient and family to notify health care professional if thoughts about suicide or dying, attempts to commit suicide; new or worse depression; new or worse anxiety; feeling very agitated or restless; panic attacks; trouble sleeping; new or worse irritability; acting aggressive; being angry or violent; acting on dangerous impulses; an extreme increase in activity and talking; other unusual changes in behavior or mood or if skin rash occur.
- Advise patient to notify health care professional of all Rx or OTC medications, vitamins, or herbal products being taken and to consult with health care professional before taking other medications.
- Instruct patient to notify health care professional of medication regimen prior to treatment or surgery.
- Rep: Advise female patients to notify health care professional if pregnancy is planned or suspected or if breast feeding. Encourage pregnant patients to enroll in the North American Antiepileptic Drug (NAAED) Pregnancy Registry by calling 1-888-233-2334; information is available at www.aedpregnancyregistry.org.
- Advise patient to carry identification describing disease process and medication regimen at all times.

Evaluation/Desired Outcomes

- Decrease in the frequency of or cessation of seizures.

levomilnacipran

(lee-voe-mil-**na**-si-pran)

Fetzima

Classification

Therapeutic: antidepressants

Pharmacologic: selective serotonin/norepinephrine reuptake inhibitors

Pregnancy Category C

Indications

Treatment of major depressive disorder.

Action

Inhibits neuronal reuptake of norepinephrine and serotonin in the CNS (SNRI). **Therapeutic Effects:** Decrease in depressive symptomatology, with fewer relapses/recurrences.

Pharmacokinetics

Absorption: Well absorbed (92%) following oral administration.

Distribution: Widely distributed.

Metabolism and Excretion: 58% eliminated unchanged in urine; 42% metabolized, primarily by the CYP3A4 enzyme system; metabolites are renally eliminated.

Half-life: 12 hr.

TIME/ACTION PROFILE

ROUTE	ONSET	PEAK	DURATION
PO	Unk	6–8 hr (blood level)	Unk

Contraindications/Precautions

Contraindicated in: Hypersensitivity to levomilnacipran or milnacipran; Uncontrolled narrow-angle glaucoma; Concurrent use of or in close temporal proximity to MAO inhibitors, linezolid or methylene blue (risk of serotonin syndrome); Concurrent use of alcohol.

Use Cautiously in: History of hypertension, cardiovascular or cerebrovascular disease (BP should be controlled prior to treatment); History of bipolar disorder (may activate mania/hypomania); Renal impairment (dose ↓ required for CCr< 60 mL/min); Geri: Consider age-related ↓ in renal function, chronic disease state and concurrent drug therapy; may have ↑ risk of hyponatremia; OB: Use only if clearly required during pregnancy weighing benefit to mother versus potential harm to fetus; Lactation: Potential for serious adverse reactions in infant; discontinue drug or discontinue breast feeding; Pedi: ↑ risk of suicidal thinking and behavior (suicidality) in adolescents and young adults up to 24 yrs with MDD.

Exercise Extreme Caution in: Concurrent use with other serotonergic drugs (↑ risk of serotonin syndrome especially during initiation and dose adjustment).

Adverse Reactions/Side Effects

CNS: activation of mania/hypomania. **EENT:** mydrasis. **CV:** hypertension, hypotension, palpitations, tachycardia. **GI:** nausea, ↓ appetite, constipation, vomiting. **GU:** ejaculation disorder, erectile dysfunction, testicular pain, urinary hesitation/retention. **Derm:** hot flush, hyperhydrosis, rash. **F and E:** hyponatremia (in association with syndrome of inappropriate antidiuretic hormone [SIADH]). **Hemat:** bleeding. **Misc:** SEROTONIN SYNDROME.

Interactions

Drug-Drug: Concurrent use with **MAO inhibitors used for psychiatric disorders** may result in serious, potentially fatal reactions; wait at least 14 days following discontinuation of MAO inhibitor before initiation of levomilnacipran. Wait at least 7 days after discontinuing levomilnacipran before initiation of MAO inhibitor. Concurrent use of **serotonergic drugs** (including **triptans**, **lithium**, **buspirone**, **fentanyl**, **tricyclics** and **tramadol**) may ↑ the risk of serotonin syndrome, especially during initiation and dose adjustment; also ↑ risk of coronary vasoconstriction and hypertension. Concurrent use with **methylene blue** or **linezolid** is contraindicated due to risk of serotonin syndrome. Concurrent use of **NSAIDs**, **aspirin**, **warfarin** or other**drugs that affect coagulation** may ↑ the risk of bleeding. Blood levels and risk of toxicity ↑ by concurrent use of **CYP3A4 inhitors** including **ketoconazole**, **clarithromycin**, **ritonavir**; daily dose should not exceed 80 mg. Concurrent use of other **medications that may ↑ BP** may ↑ risk of hypertension. Concurrent use with **alcohol** may cause a rapid release of drug and should be avoided. Concurrent use with other **CNS-active medications**, especially other **NSRIs**.

Drug-Natural Products: Concurrent use with **St. John's wort** or **tryptophan** may ↑ the risk of serotinin syndrome; also ↑ risk of coronary vasoconstriction and hypertension.

Route/Dosage

PO (Adults): 20 mg once daily for two days, then increase to 40 mg once daily, may then be ↑ by 40 mg every two or more days; may be ↑ up to 120 mg/day; *Concurrent use of CYP3A4 inhibitors (including ketoconazole, clarithromycin, ritonavir)*—not to exceed 80 mg/day.

Renal Impairment

PO (Adults): *CCr 30–59 mL/min*—not to exceed 80 mg/day; *CCr 15–29 mL/min*—not to exceed 40 mg/day.

Availability

Extended-release capsules: 20 mg, 40 mg, 80 mg, 120 mg.

NURSING IMPLICATIONS

Assessment

- Monitor BP and heart rate before and periodically during therapy. Treat per-existing hypertension and cardiac disease prior to therapy. Sustained hypertension may require discontinuation of therapy.
- Monitor closely for notable changes in behavior that could indicate the emergence or worsening of suicidal thoughts or behavior or depression.
- ***Lab Test Considerations:*** May cause hyponatremia.

Potential Nursing Diagnoses

Ineffective coping (Indications)
Risk for suicide (Adverse Reactions)

Implementation

- ***High Alert:*** Do not confuse Fetzima with Farxiga.
- **PO:** Administer daily without regard to food. Swallow capsule whole; do not open, crush, or chew.

Patient/Family Teaching

- Instruct patient to take levomilnacipran as directed at the same time each day. Take missed doses as soon as possible unless time for next dose; do not double dose. Do not stop abruptly; must be decreased gradually. Abrupt discontinuation may cause dysphoric mood, irritability, agitation, dizziness, paresthesia, electric shock sensation, anxiety, confusion, headache, lethargy, emotional lability, insomnia, hypomania, tinnitus and seizures. Advise patient to read *Medication Guide* prior to therapy and with each Rx refill in case of changes.
- May cause drowsiness and may affect ability to make decisions or react quickly. Caution patient to avoid driving or other activities requiring alertness until response to medication is known.

- Advise patient, family, and caregivers to look for activation of mania/hypomania and suicidality, especially during early therapy or dose changes. Notify health care professional immediately if thoughts about suicide or dying, attempts to commit suicide; new or worse depression or anxiety; agitation or restlessness; panic attacks; insomnia; new or worse irritability; aggressiveness; acting on dangerous impulses, mania, or other changes in mood or behavior or if symptoms of serotonin syndrome occur.
- Caution patient of the risk or serotonin syndrome (agitation, hallucinations, changes in mental status, muscle twitching, fast heartbeat, high or low BP, sweating or fever, nausea or vomiting, diarrhea, muscle stiffness or tightness), especially when taking triptans, tramadol, tryptophan supplements and other serotonergic or antipsychotic agents.
- Instruct patient to notify health care professional of all Rx or OTC medications, vitamins, or herbal products being taken and to avoid concurrent use of Rx, OTC, and herbal products, especially NSAIDs, aspirin, and warfarin, without consulting health care professional; may increase bleeding.
- Instruct patient to notify health care professional if signs of hyponatremia (headache, difficulty concentrating, memory impairment, confusion, weakness, unsteadiness) occur.
- Advise patient to avoid taking alcohol during levomilnacipran therapy.
- Instruct patient to notify health care professional if pregnancy is planned or suspected or if breast feeding.
- Encourage patient to maintain routine follow-up visits with health care provider to determine effectiveness.

Evaluation/Desired Outcomes

- Increased sense of well-being.
- Renewed interest in surroundings. Need for therapy should be periodically reassessed.

levonorgestrel, See CONTRACEPTIVES, HORMONAL.

levothyroxine

(lee-voe-thye-**rox**-een)

✱ Eltroxin, ✱ Euthyrox, Levo-T, Levoxyl, Synthroid, T_4, Tirosint, Unithroid

Classification

Therapeutic: hormones

Pharmacologic: thyroid preparations

Pregnancy Category A

Indications

Thyroid supplementation in hypothyroidism. Treatment or suppression of euthyroid goiters. Adjunctive treatment for thyrotropin-dependent thyroid cancer.

Action

Replacement of or supplementation to endogenous thyroid hormones. Principal effect is increasing metabolic rate of body tissues: Promote gluconeogenesis, Increase utilization and mobilization of glycogen stores, Stimulate protein synthesis, Promote cell growth and differentiation, Aid in the development of the brain and CNS. **Therapeutic Effects:** Replacement in hypothyroidism to restore normal hormonal balance. Suppression of thyroid cancer.

Pharmacokinetics

Absorption: Levothyroxine is variably (40–80%) absorbed from the GI tract.

Distribution: Distributed into most body tissues. Thyroid hormones do not readily cross the placenta; minimal amounts enter breast milk.

Protein Binding: >99%.

Metabolism and Excretion: Metabolized by the liver and other tissues to active T3. Thyroid hormone undergoes enterohepatic recirculation and is excreted in the feces via the bile.

Half-life: 6–7 days.

TIME/ACTION PROFILE

ROUTE	ONSET	PEAK	DURATION
Levothyroxine PO	unknown	1–3 wk	1–3 wk
Levothyroxine IV	6–8 hr	24 hr	unknown

Contraindications/Precautions

Contraindicated in: Hypersensitivity; Recent MI; Hyperthyroidism.

Use Cautiously in: Cardiovascular disease (initiate therapy with lower doses); Severe renal insufficiency; Uncorrected adrenocortical disorders; Pedi: Monitor neonates and infants for cardiac overload, arrhythmias, and aspiration during first 2 wk of therapy; Geri: Extremely sensitive to thyroid hormones; initial dose should be ↓.

Adverse Reactions/Side Effects

Usually only seen when excessive doses cause iatrogenic hyperthyroidism.

CNS: headache, insomnia, irritability. **CV:** angina pectoris, arrhythmias, tachycardia. **GI:** abdominal cramps, diarrhea, vomiting. **Derm:** sweating. **Endo:** hyperthyroidism, menstrual irregularities. **Metab:** heat intolerance, weight loss. **MS:** accelerated bone maturation in children.

Interactions

Drug-Drug: Bile acid sequestrants and **orlistat** ↓ absorption of orally administered thyroid preparations. May ↑ the effects of **warfarin.** May ↑ requirement for **insulin** or **oral hypoglycemic agents** in diabetics. Concurrent **estrogen** therapy may ↑ thyroid replacement requirements. ↑ cardiovascular effects with **adrenergics** (sympathomimetics).
Drug-Food: Foods or supplements containing calcium, iron, magnesium, or zinc may bind levothyroxine and prevent complete absorption.

Route/Dosage

PO (Adults): *Hypothyroidism*—50 mcg as a single dose initially; may be ↑ q 2–3 wk by 25 mcg/day; usual maintenance dose is 75–125 mcg/day (1.5 mcg/kg/day).
PO (Geriatric Patients and Patients with Increased Sensitivity to Thyroid Hormones): 12.5–25 mcg as a single dose initially; may be ↑ q 6–8 wk; usual maintenance dose is 75 mcg/day.
PO (Children >12 yr): 2–3 mcg/kg/day (≥150 mcg/day).
PO (Children 6–12 yr): 4–5 mcg/kg/day (100–125 mcg/day).
PO (Children 1–5 yr): 5–6 mcg/kg/day (75–100 mcg/day).
PO (Children 6–12 mo): 6–8 mcg/kg/day (50–75 mcg/day).
PO (Infants 3–6 mo): 8–10 mcg/kg/day (25–50 mcg/day).
PO (Infants 0–3 mo or Infants at Risk for Cardiac Failure): 10–15 mcg/kg/day or 25 mcg/day; may be ↑ after 4–6 wk to 50 mcg.
IM, IV (Adults): *Hypothyroidism*—50–100 mcg/day as a single dose. *Myxedema coma/stupor*—300–500 mcg IV; additional 100–300 mcg may be given on 2nd day, followed by daily administration of smaller doses.
IM, IV (Children): *Hypothyroidism*—50–80% of the oral dose.

Availability (generic available)

Capsules (Tirosint): 13 mcg, 25 mcg, 50 mcg, 75 mcg, 88 mcg, 100 mcg, 112 mcg, 125 mcg, 137 mcg, 150 mcg. **Tablets:** 25 mcg, 50 mcg, 75 mcg, 88 mcg, 100 mcg, 112 mcg, 125 mcg, 137 mcg, 150 mcg, 175 mcg, 200 mcg, 300 mcg. **Powder for injection:** 100 mcg/vial, 200 mcg/vial, 500 mcg/vial.

NURSING IMPLICATIONS

Assessment

- Assess apical pulse and BP prior to and periodically during therapy. Assess for tachyarrhythmias and chest pain.
- **Children:** Monitor height, weight, and psychomotor development.
- ***Lab Test Considerations:*** Monitor thyroid function studies prior to and during therapy. Monitor thyroid-stimulating hormone serum levels in adults 8–12 wks after changing from one brand to another.
- Monitor blood and urine glucose in diabetic patients. Insulin or oral hypoglycemic dose may need to be increased.
- ***Toxicity and Overdose:*** Overdose is manifested as hyperthyroidism (tachycardia, chest pain, nervousness, insomnia, diaphoresis, tremors, weight loss). Usual treatment is to withhold dose for 2–6 days then resume at a lower dose. Acute overdose is treated by induction of emesis or gastric lavage, followed by activated charcoal. Sympathetic overstimulation may be controlled by antiadrenergic drugs (beta blockers), such as propranolol. Oxygen and supportive measures to control symptoms are also used.

Potential Nursing Diagnoses

Deficient knowledge, related to medication regimen (Patient/Family Teaching)

Implementation

- ***High Alert:*** Do not confuse levothyroxine with lamotrigine or Lanoxin (digoxin). Do not confuse levothyroxine with liothyronine.
- **PO:** Administer with a full glass of water, on an empty stomach, 30–60 min before breakfast, to prevent insomnia.
- Initial dose is low, especially in geriatric and cardiac patients. Dose is increased gradually, based on thyroid function tests.
- For patients with difficulty swallowing, tablets can be crushed and placed in 5–10 mL of water and administered immediately via dropper or spoon; do not store suspension.

IV Administration

- **IV Push:** Reconstitute the 200-mcg and 500-mcg vials with 2 or 5 mL, respectively, of 0.9% NaCl without preservatives (diluent usually provided). ***Concentration:*** 100 mcg/mL. Shake well to dissolve completely. Administer solution immediately after preparation; discard unused portion. ***Rate:*** Administer at a rate of 100 mcg over 1 min. Do not add to IV infusions; may be administered through Y-tubing.
- **Y-Site Incompatibility:** Do not admix with other IV solutions.

Patient/Family Teaching

- Instruct patient to take medication as directed at the same time each day. Take missed doses as soon as remembered unless almost time for next dose. If more than 2–3 doses are missed, notify health care professional. Do not discontinue without consulting health care professional.
- Explain to patient that medication does not cure hypothyroidism; it provides a thyroid hormone supplement. Therapy is lifelong.
- Advise patient to notify health care professional if headache, nervousness, diarrhea, excessive sweat-

ing, heat intolerance, chest pain, increased pulse rate, palpitations, weight loss >2 lb/wk, or any unusual symptoms occur.

- Caution patient to avoid taking other medications concurrently with thyroid preparations unless instructed by health care professional. Advise patient to take 4 hrs apart from antacids, iron, and calcium supplements.
- Instruct patient to inform health care professionals of thyroid therapy.
- Emphasize importance of follow-up exams to monitor effectiveness of therapy. Thyroid function tests are performed at least yearly.
- Pedi: Discuss with parents the need for routine follow-up studies to ensure correct development. Inform patient that partial hair loss may be experienced by children on thyroid therapy. This is usually temporary.

Evaluation/Desired Outcomes

- Resolution of symptoms of hypothyroidism and normalization of hormone levels.

HIGH ALERT

LIDOCAINE

lidocaine (parenteral)
(**lye**-doe-kane)
Xylocaine, ✤Xylocard

lidocaine (local anesthetic)
Xylocaine

lidocaine (mucosal)
✤Jampocaine Viscous, Xylocaine Viscous

lidocaine (transdermal)
Lidoderm

lidocaine (topical)
✤Betacaine, ✤Cathejell, Glydo, ✤Lidodan, L-M-X 4, L-M-X 5, ✤Lyracaine, ✤Maxilene, ✤Stallion, ✤Topicaine, Xylocaine

Classification
Therapeutic: anesthetics (topical/local), antiarrhythmics (class IB)

Pregnancy Category B

Indications

IV: Ventricular arrhythmias. **IM:** Self-injected or when IV unavailable (during transport to hospital facilities). **Local:** Infiltration/mucosal/topical anesthetic. **Transdermal:** Pain due to post-herpetic neuralgia.

Action

IV, IM: Suppresses automaticity and spontaneous depolarization of the ventricles during diastole by altering the flux of sodium ions across cell membranes with little or no effect on heart rate. **Local:** Produces local anesthesia by inhibiting transport of ions across neuronal membranes, thereby preventing initiation and conduction of normal nerve impulses. **Therapeutic Effects:** Control of ventricular arrhythmias. Local anesthesia.

Pharmacokinetics

Absorption: Well absorbed after administration into the deltoid muscle; some absorption follows local use.
Distribution: Widely distributed. Concentrates in adipose tissue. Crosses the blood-brain barrier and placenta; enters breast milk.
Metabolism and Excretion: Mostly metabolized by the liver; <10% excreted in urine as unchanged drug.
Half-life: Biphasic—initial phase, 7–30 min; terminal phase, 90–120 min; ↑ in HF and liver impairment.

TIME/ACTION PROFILE (IV, IM = antiarrhythmic effects; local = anesthetic effects)

ROUTE	ONSET	PEAK	DURATION
IV	immediate	immediate	10–20 min (up to several hours after continuous infusion)
IM	5–15 min	20–30 min	60–90 min
Local	rapid	unknown	1–3 hr

Contraindications/Precautions

Applies mainly to systemic use

Contraindicated in: Hypersensitivity; cross-sensitivity may occur; Third-degree heart block; Pedi: Children <3 yr (↑ risk of seizures, cardiac arrest and death with viscous lidocaine); viscous lidocaine should not be used for teething pain; should only be used for other indications when safer alternatives are not available or have failed.
Use Cautiously in: Liver disease, HF, patients weighing <50 kg, and geriatric patients (↓ bolus and/or maintenance dose); Respiratory depression; Shock; Heart block; OB, Lactation: Safety not established; Pedi: Safety not established for transdermal patch.

Adverse Reactions/Side Effects

Applies mainly to systemic use.
CNS: SEIZURES, <u>confusion</u>, <u>drowsiness</u>, blurred vision, dizziness, nervousness, slurred speech, tremor. **EENT:** *mucosal use*—↓ or absent gag reflex. **CV:** CARDIAC

ARREST, arrhythmias, bradycardia, heart block, hypotension. **GI:** nausea, vomiting. **Resp:** bronchospasm. **Hemat:** methemoglobinemia. **Local:** stinging, burning, contact dermatitis, erythema. **MS:** chondrolysis. **Misc:** allergic reactions, including ANAPHYLAXIS.

Interactions

Applies mainly to systemic use.

Drug-Drug: ↑ cardiac depression and toxicity with **phenytoin, amiodarone, quinidine, procainamide**, or **propranolol. Cimetidine, azole antifungals, clarithromycin, erythromycin, fluoxetine, nefazodone, paroxetine, protease inhibitors, ritonavir, verapamil**, and **beta blockers** may ↓ metabolism and ↑ risk of toxicity. Lidocaine may ↑ levels of **calcium channel blockers**, certain **benzodiazepines, cyclosporine, fluoxetine, lovastatin, simvastatin, mirtazapine, paroxetine, ritonavir, tacrolimus, theophylline, tricyclic antidepressants**, and **venlafaxine**. Effects of lidocaine may be ↓ by **carbamazepine, phenobarbital, phenytoin**, and **rifampin**.

Route/Dosage

Ventricular Tachycardia (with a Pulse) or Pulseless Ventricular Tachycardia/Ventricular Fibrillation

IV (Adults): 1–1.5 mg/kg bolus; may repeat doses of 0.5–0.75 mg/kg q 5–10 min up to a total dose of 3 mg/kg; may then start continuous infusion of 1–4 mg/min.
Endotracheal (Adults): Give 2–2.5 times the IV loading dose down the endotracheal tube, followed by a 10 mL saline flush.
IV (Children): 1 mg/kg bolus (not to exceed 100 mg), followed by 20–50 mcg/kg/min continuous infusion (range 20–50 mcg/kg/min); may administer second bolus of 0.5–1 mg/kg if delay between bolus and continuous infusion.
Endotracheal (Children): Give 2–3 mg/kg down the endotracheal tube followed by a 5 mL saline flush.
IM (Adults and Children ≥50 kg): 300 mg (4.5 mg/kg); may be repeated in 60–90 min.

Local

Infiltration (Adults and Children): Infiltrate affected area as needed (increased amount and frequency of use increases likelihood of systemic absorption and adverse reactions).
Topical (Adults): Apply to affected area 2–3 times daily.
Mucosal (Adults): *For anesthetizing oral surfaces*—20 mg as 2 sprays/quadrant (not to exceed 30 mg/quadrant) may be used. 15 mL of the viscous solution may be used q 3 hr for oral or pharyngeal pain. *For anesthetizing the female urethra*—3–5 mL of the jelly or 20 mg as 2% solution may be used. *For anesthetizing the male urethra*—5–10 mL of the jelly or 5–15 mL of 2% solution may be used before catheterization or 30 mL of jelly before cystoscopy or similar procedures. Topical solutions may be used to anesthetize mucous membranes of the larynx, trachea, or esophagus.
Mucosal (Children ≥3 yr): Do not exceed 4.5 mg/kg/dose (or 300 mg/dose) of viscous solution; swish in the mouth and spit out no more frequently than q 3 hr (maximum: 4 doses per 12-hour period).
Mucosal (Children <3 yr): ≤1.2 mL applied to area with a cotton-tipped applicator no more frequently than q 3 hr (maximum: 4 doses per 12-hour period); use only if the underlying condition requires treatment with product volume of ≤1.2 mL.
Patch (Adults): Up to 3 patches may be applied once for up to 12 hr in any 24-hr period; consider smaller areas of application in geriatric or debilitated patients.

Availability (generic available)

Autoinjector for IM injection: 300 mg/3 mL. **IV push injection:** 5 mg/mL (0.5%), 10 mg/mL (1%), 15 mg/mL (1.5%), 20 mg/mL (2%). **For IV admixture:** 100 mg/mL (10%). **Premixed solution for IV infusion:** 200 mg/100 mL D5W (0.2%), 400 mg/100 mL D5W (0.4%), 1000 mg/250 mL D5W (0.4%), 2000 mg/500 mL D5W (0.4%), 800 mg/100 mL D5W (0.8%), 2000 mg/250 mL D5W (0.8%). **Injection for local infiltration/nerve block:** 0.5%, 1%, 2%, 4%. ***In combination with:*** epinephrine for local infiltration. **Cream:** 4% OTC. **Gel:** 0.5%OTC, 2.5%OTC, ✱ 5%OTC. **Jelly:** 2%. **Liquid:** 5%. **Ointment:** 5%. **Transdermal system:** 5% patch. **Cost:** $309.45/30. **Solution:** 4%. **Spray:** 10%. **Viscous solution:** 2%. ***In combination with:*** prilocaine (as EMLA cream, Oraquix); with tetracaine (Synera); with bupivacaine (Duocaine); with epinephrine (LidoSite).

NURSING IMPLICATIONS

Assessment

- **Antiarrhythmic:** Monitor ECG continuously and BP and respiratory status frequently during administration.
- **Anesthetic:** Assess degree of numbness of affected part.
- **Transdermal:** Monitor for pain intensity in affected area periodically during therapy.
- ***Lab Test Considerations:*** Serum electrolyte levels should be monitored periodically during prolonged therapy.
- IM administration may cause ↑ CPK levels.
- ***Toxicity and Overdose:*** Monitor serum lidocaine levels periodically during prolonged or high-dose IV therapy. Therapeutic serum lidocaine levels range from 1.5 to 5 mcg/mL.
- Signs and symptoms of toxicity include confusion, excitation, blurred or double vision, nausea, vomiting, ringing in ears, tremors, twitching, seizures, difficulty breathing, severe dizziness or fainting, and unusually slow heart rate.

- If symptoms of overdose occur, stop infusion and monitor patient closely.

Potential Nursing Diagnoses

Decreased cardiac output (Indications)
Acute pain (Indications)

Implementation

- ***High Alert:*** Lidocaine is readily absorbed through mucous membranes. Inadvertent overdose of lidocaine jelly and spray has resulted in patient harm or death from neurologic and/or cardiac toxicity. Do not exceed recommended doses.
- **Throat Spray:** Ensure that gag reflex is intact before allowing patient to drink or eat.
- **IM:** IM injections are recommended only when ECG monitoring is not available and benefits outweigh risks. Administer IM injections only into deltoid muscle while frequently aspirating to prevent IV injection.

IV Administration

- **IV Push:** Only 1% and 2% solutions are used for IV push injection. ***Diluent:*** Administer undiluted. ***Rate:*** Administer loading dose over 2–3 min. Follow by IV continuous infusion.
- **Continuous Infusion: *Diluent:*** Lidocaine vials need to be further diluted. Dilute 2 g of lidocaine in 250 mL or 500 mL of D5W or 0.9% NaCl. Admixed infusion stable for 24 hr at room temperature. Premixed infusions are already diluted and ready to use. ***Concentration:*** 4–8 mg/mL. ***Rate:*** See Route/Dosage section. Administer via infusion pump for accurate dose.
- **Y-Site Compatibility:** acetaminophen, alemtuzumab, alfentanil, alteplase, amikacin, aminocaproic acid, aminophylline, amiodarone, amphotericin B lipid complex, amphotericin B liposome, anidulafungin, argatroban, ascorbic acid, atropine, azithromycin, aztreonam, benztropine, bivalirudin, bleomycin, bumetanide, buprenorphine, butorphanol, calcium chloride, calcium gluconate, cangrelor, carboplatin, carmustine, cefazolin, cefotaxime, cefoxitin, ceftaroline, ceftazidime, ceftriaxone, cefuroxime, chloramphenicol, chlorpromazine, ciprofloxacin, cisatracurium, cisplatin, clindamycin, cyanocobalamin, cyclophosphamide, cyclosporine, cytarabine, dacarbazine, dactinomycin, daptomycin, dexamethasone, dexmedetomidine, dexrazoxane, digoxin, diltiazem, diphenhydramine, dobutamine, docetaxel, dolasetron, dopamine, doxorubicin hydrochloride, doxorubicin liposomal, doxycycline, enalaprilat, ephedrine, epinephrine, epirubicin, epoetin alfa, eptifibatide, ertapenem, erythromycin, esmolol, etomidate, etoposide, etoposide phosphate, famotidine, fenoldopam, fentanyl, fluconazole, fludarabine, fluorouracil, folic acid, foscarnet, fosphenytoin, furosemide, gemcitabine, gentamicin, glycopyrrolate, granisetron, heparin, hetastarch, hydrocortisone, hydromorphone, idarubicin, ifosfamide, imipenem/cilastatin, indomethacin, insulin, irinotecan, isoproterenol, ketorolac, labetalol, levofloxacin, linezolid, lorazepam, magnesium sulfate, mannitol, mechlorethamine, meperidine, mesna, methotrexate, methyldopate, methylprednisolone, metoclopramide, metronidazole, micafungin, midazolam, mitoxantrone, morphine, moxifloxacin, multivitamins, mycophenolate, nafcillin, nalbuphine, naloxone, nicardipine, nitroglycerin, nitroprusside, norepinephrine, octreotide, ondansetron, oxacillin, oxaliplatin, oxytocin, paclitaxel, palonosetron, pamidronate, pancuronium, papaverine, pemetrexed, penicillin G, pentamidine, pentazocine, phenylephrine, phytonadione, piperacillin/tazobactam, potassium acetate, potassium chloride, procainamide, prochlorperazine, promethazine, propranolol, protamine, pyridoxine, quinupristin/dalfopristin, ranitidine, remifentanil, rocuronium, sodium acetate, sodium bicarbonate, streptokinase, succinylcholine, sufentanil, tacrolimus, teniposide, theophylline, thiamine, thiotepa, tigecycline, tirofiban, tobramycin, trimetaphan, vancomycin, vasopressin, vecuronium, verapamil, vinblastine, vincristine, vinorelbine, vitamin B complex with C , voriconazole, warfarin, zoledronic acid.
- **Y-Site Incompatibility:** acyclovir, amphotericin B cholesteryl, amphotericin B colloidal, caspofungin, dantrolene, diazepam, ganciclovir, milrinone, pantoprazole, pentobarbital, phenobarbital, phenytoin, thiopental, trimethoprim/sulfamethoxazole.
- **Infiltration:** Lidocaine with epinephrine may be used to minimize systemic absorption and prolong local anesthesia.
- **Transdermal:** When used concomitantly with other products containing local anesthetic agents, consider amount absorbed from all formulations.

Patient/Family Teaching

- May cause drowsiness and dizziness. Advise patient to call for assistance during ambulation and transfer.
- **IM:** Available in LidoPen Auto-Injector for use outside the hospital setting. Advise patient to telephone health care professional immediately if symptoms of a heart attack occur. Do not administer unless instructed by health care professional. To administer, remove safety cap and place back end on thickest part of thigh or deltoid muscle. Press hard until needle prick is felt. Hold in place for 10 sec, then massage area for 10 sec. Do not drive after administration unless absolutely necessary.
- **Topical:** Apply *Lidoderm Patch* to intact skin to cover the most painful area. Patch may be cut to smaller sizes with scissors before removing release liner. Clothing may be worn over patch. Avoid con-

L

tact with water (bathing, swimming, showering), may not stick if it gets wet. If irritation or burning sensation occurs during application, remove patch until irritation subsides. Wash hands after application; avoid contact with eyes. Dispose of used patch to avoid access by children or pets.

- Caution women to consult health care professional before using a topical anesthetic for a mammogram or other procedures. If recommended, use lowest drug concentration, and apply sparingly. Do not apply to broken or irritated skin, do not wrap skin, and do not apply heat to area (heating pad/electric blanket), to decrease chance that drug may be absorbed into the body. May result in seizures, cardiac arrhythmias, respiratory failure, coma, and death.
- Advise patient referred for MRI test to discuss patch with referring health care professional and MRI facility to determine if removal of patch is necessary prior to test and for directions for replacing patch.
- **Mucosal:** Caution parent to administer as directed, not to use more or more often than directed, and to use measuring device for accurate dose in children younger than 3 yrs. Advise parent that if signs and symptoms of toxicity (lethargy, shallow breathing, seizure activity) occur to seek emergency attention and not to administer more lidocaine.
- Caution parents that oral lidocaine causes numbness and may impair swallowing; do not administer food and/or chewing gum for at least 60 min after administration.

Evaluation/Desired Outcomes

- Decrease in ventricular arrhythmias.
- Local anesthesia.

lidocaine/prilocaine

(**lye**-doe-kane/**pri**-loe-kane)

EMLA, Oraqix

Classification

Therapeutic: anesthetics (topical/local)

Pregnancy Category B

Indications

Produces local anesthesia prior to minor painful procedures including: Insertion of cannulae or needles, Arterial/venous/lumbar puncture, Intramuscular injections, Subcutaneous injections, Dermal procedures, Laser treatments, Circumcision. When applied to genital mucous membranes in preparation for superficial minor surgery or as preparation for infiltration anesthesia. Produces localized anesthesia in periodontal pockets during scaling and/or root planing (Oraqix only).

Action

Produces local anesthesia by inhibiting transport of ions across neuronal membranes, thereby preventing initiation and conduction of normal nerve impulses. Combination of two anesthetics is applied as a system consisting of a cream under an occlusive dressing. Active drug is released into the dermal and epidermal skin layers, resulting in accumulation of local anesthetic in the regions of dermal pain receptors and nerve endings. **Therapeutic Effects:** Anesthetic action localized to the area of the application.

Pharmacokinetics

Absorption: Small amounts are systemically absorbed.

Distribution: Small amounts absorbed are widely distributed and cross the placenta and blood-brain barrier.

Metabolism and Excretion: *Lidocaine*—mostly metabolized by the liver. *Prilocaine*—metabolized by the liver and kidneys.

Half-life: *Lidocaine*—90–120 min (EMLA); 2–6 hr (Oraqix): *Prilocaine*—10–50 min (EMLA); 2–6 hr (Oraqix).

TIME/ACTION PROFILE (local anesthesia)

ROUTE	ONSET	PEAK	DURATION
Top	1 hr(EMLA); 30 sec (Oraqix)	3 hr (EMLA)	1–2 hr (EMLA)† 20 min (Oraqix)

†Following removal of occlusive dressing.

Contraindications/Precautions

Contraindicated in: Hypersensitivity to lidocaine, prilocaine, or any other amide-type local anesthetic; Hypersensitivity to any other product in the formulation; Should not be applied to middle ear, mucous membranes, or broken/inflamed skin; Pedi: Congenital or idiopathic methemoglobinemia; Infants <1 mo if gestational age is <37 weeks; Infants <12 mo receiving methemoglobin-inducing agents.

Use Cautiously in: Repeated use or use on large areas of skin (more likely to result in systemic absorption); Acutely ill, or debilitated patients (↑ risk of absorption and systemic effects); Severe liver disease; Any conditions associated with methemoglobinemia (including glucose-6-phosphate dehydrogenase deficiency); OB: Use only if clearly needed; Lactation: Usually compatible with breast feeding (AAP); Pedi: Area/duration of treatment should be limited in neonates and children <20 kg or 37 weeks gestation (↑ susceptibility to methemoglobinemia); Geri: May have ↑ absorption and risk of systemic effects.

Adverse Reactions/Side Effects

Local: blanching, redness, alteration in temperature sensation, edema, itching, rash, hyperpigmentation.

Misc: allergic reactions including ANAPHYLAXIS.

Interactions

Drug-Drug: Concurrent use with class I antiarrhythmics including **mexiletine** may result in adverse cardiovascular effects. Concurrent use with other **local**

anesthetics may result in ↑ toxicity. Concurrent use with **sulfonamides, acetaminophen, chloroquine, nitroglycerin, nitroprusside, phenobarbital, phenytoin,** or **quinine** in children ↑ the risk of methemoglobinemia (avoid concurrent use in children <12 mo).

Route/Dosage

EMLA

Topical (Adults and Children): *Minor dermal procedures including venipuncture and IV cannulation*—2.5 g (½ of the 5-g tube) applied to 20–25 cm^2 (2 in. by 2 in.) area of skin, covered with an occlusive dressing applied for at least 1 hr. *Major dermal procedures including split-thickness skin graft harvesting*—2 g/10 cm^2 area of skin, covered with an occlusive dressing for at least 2 hr. *Adult male genital skin*—as an adjunct prior to local anesthetic infiltration, apply a thick layer (1 g/10 cm^2) to skin surface for 15 min; local infiltration anesthesia should be performed immediately after removal of cream. *Adult female genital mucous membranes*—apply a thick layer (5–log) for 5–10 min.

Topical (Children 7–12 yr and >20 kg): Dose should not exceed 20 g over more than 200 cm^2 for more than 4 hr.

Topical (Children 1–6 yr and >10 kg): Dose should not exceed 10 g over more than 100 cm^2 for more than 4 hr.

Topical (Children 3 mo–12 mo and >5 kg): Dose should not exceed 2 g over more than 20 cm^2 for more than 4 hr.

Topical (Children 0–3 mo or <5 kg): Dose should not exceed 1 g over more than 10 cm^2 for more than 1 hr.

Oraqix

Topical (Adults): Apply on gingival margin around the selected teeth using the blunt-tipped applicator included in package; wait 30 seconds, then fill the periodontal pockets with gel using the blunt-tipped applicator until the gel becomes visible at the gingival margin; wait another 30 seconds before starting treatment; maximum recommended dose at one treatment session is 5 cartridges (8.5 g).

Availability (generic available)

Cream: 2.5% lidocaine with 2.5% prilocaine. **Periodontal gel:** 2.5% lidocaine with 2.5% prilocaine; 1.7 g/dental cartridge.

NURSING IMPLICATIONS

Assessment

- Assess application site for open wounds. Apply only to intact skin.
- Assess application site for anesthesia following removal of system and prior to procedure.

Potential Nursing Diagnoses

Acute pain (Indications)

Implementation

- **Topical:** *EMLA:* When used for minor dermal procedures (venipuncture, IV cannulation, arterial puncture, lumbar puncture), apply the 2.5-g tube of cream (½ of the 5-g tube) to each 2 in. by 2 in. area of skin in a ***thick*** layer at the site of the impending procedure. Remove the center cutout piece from an occlusive dressing (supplied with the 5-g tube) and peel the paper liner from the paper-framed dressing. Cover the lidocaine/prilocaine cream so that there is a ***thick*** layer of cream underneath the occlusive dressing. Do not spread out or rub in the cream. Smooth the dressing edges carefully and ensure it is secure to avoid leakage. Remove the paper frame and mark the time of application on the occlusive dressing. Lidocaine/prilocaine cream must be applied *at least 1 hr* before the start of a minor dermal procedure (venipuncture, IV cannulation). Anesthesia may be more profound with 90 min–2 hr application. Remove the occlusive dressing and wipe off the lidocaine/prilocaine cream. Clean the entire area with antiseptic solution and prepare the patient for the procedure.
- For major dermal procedures (skin graft harvesting), follow the same procedure using larger amounts of lidocaine/prilocaine cream and the appropriate-size occlusive dressing. Lidocaine/prilocaine cream must be applied *at least 2 hr* before major dermal procedures.

Patient/Family Teaching

- Explain the purpose of cream and occlusive dressing to patient and parents. Inform the patient that lidocaine/prilocaine cream may block all sensations in the treated skin. Caution patient to avoid trauma to the area from scratching, rubbing, or exposure to extreme heat or cold temperatures until all sensation has returned.
- **Home Care Issues:** Instruct patient or parent in proper application. Provide a diagram of location for application.

Evaluation/Desired Outcomes

- Anesthesia in the area of application.

---

linagliptin (lin-a-**glip**-tin)
Tradjenta, ✤Trajenta

Classification
Therapeutic: antidiabetics
Pharmacologic: dipeptidyl peptidase-4 (DDP-4) inhibitors, enzyme inhibitors

Pregnancy Category B

Indications

Adjunct to diet and exercise in the management of type 2 diabetes mellitus.

Action

Inhibits the enzyme dipeptidyl peptidase-4 (DPP-4), which slows the inactivation of incretin hormones, resulting in increased levels of active incretin hormones. These hormones are released by the intestine throughout the day, and are involved in regulation of glucose. Increased/prolonged incretin levels increase insulin release and decrease glucagon levels. **Therapeutic Effects:** Improved control of blood glucose.

Pharmacokinetics

Absorption: 30% absorbed following oral administration.
Distribution: Extensively distributed to tissues.
Metabolism and Excretion: Approximately 90% excreted unchanged in urine; mininally metabolized.
Half-life: >100 hr (due to saturable binding to DPP-4).

TIME/ACTION PROFILE

ROUTE	ONSET	PEAK	DURATION
PO	unknown	1.5 hr†	24 hr

† Blood level.

Contraindications/Precautions

Contraindicated in: Hypersensitivity. Cross-sensitivity may exist with sitagliptin, alogliptin, or saxagliptin; Type 1 diabetes mellitus; Diabetic ketoacidosis.
Use Cautiously in: History of pancreatitis; Geri: Elderly may have greater sensitivity to drug effects; OB: Use during pregnancy only if clearly needed; Lactation: Excretion in breast milk unknown, use cautiously; Pedi: Safety and effectiveness not established.

Adverse Reactions/Side Effects

Resp: bronchial hyperreactivity. **GI:** PANCREATITIS. **Derm:** localized exfoliation, urticaria. **Metab:** hypoglycemia, hypertriglyceridemia. **MS:** arthralgia. **Misc:** hypersensitivity reactions including ANGIOEDEMA. ANAPHYLAXIS, EXFOLIATIVE SKIN CONDITIONS, URTICARIA, OR BRONCHOSPASM.

Interactions

Drug-Drug: ↑ risk of hypoglycemia with **sulfonylureas** or **insulin**; dose ↓ of sulfonylurea or insulin may be necessary. Concurrent use of P-glycoprotein or CYP3A4 inducers, including **rifampin** may ↓ blood levels and effectiveness and should be avoided.

Route/Dosage

PO (Adults): 5 mg once daily.

Availability

Tablets: 5 mg. ***In combination with:*** metformin (Jentadueto); empagliflozin (Glyxambi). See Appendix B.

NURSING IMPLICATIONS

Assessment

- Observe patient for signs and symptoms of hypoglycemic reactions (abdominal pain, sweating, hunger, weakness, dizziness, headache, tremor, tachycardia, anxiety).
- Monitor for signs of pancreatitis (nausea, vomiting, anorexia, persistent severe abdominal pain, sometimes radiating to the back) during therapy. If pancreatitis occurs, discontinue linagliptin and monitor serum and urine amylase, amylase/creatinine clearance ratio, electrolytes, serum calcium, glucose, and lipase.
- Monitor for arthralgia. Severe joint pain usually disappears with discontinuation of linagliptin.
- ***Lab Test Considerations:*** Monitor hemoglobin A1C prior to and periodically during therapy.
- May cause ↑ uric acid levels.

Potential Nursing Diagnoses

Imbalanced nutrition: more than body requirements (Indications)
Noncompliance (Patient/Family Teaching)

Implementation

- Patients stabilized on a diabetic regimen who are exposed to stress, fever, trauma, infection, or surgery may require administration of insulin.
- **PO:** May be administered without regard to food.

Patient/Family Teaching

- Instruct patient to take linagliptin as directed. Take missed doses as soon as remembered, unless it is almost time for next dose; do not double doses. Advise patient to read the *Patient Package Insert* before starting and with each Rx refill in case of changes.
- Explain to patient that linagliptin helps control hyperglycemia but does not cure diabetes. Therapy is usually long term.
- Instruct patient not to share this medication with others, even if they have the same symptoms; it may harm them.
- Encourage patient to follow prescribed diet, medication, and exercise regimen to prevent hyperglycemic or hypoglycemic episodes.
- Review signs of hypoglycemia and hyperglycemia with patient. If hypoglycemia occurs, advise patient to take a glass of orange juice or 2–3 tsp of sugar, honey, or corn syrup dissolved in water, and notify health care professional.
- Instruct patient in proper testing of blood glucose and urine ketones. These tests should be monitored closely during periods of stress or illness and health care professional notified if significant changes occur.
- Advise patient to notify health care professional promptly if signs and symptoms of pancreatitis or if rash; hives; or swelling of face, lips, or throat occur.
- Advise patient to notify health care professional of all Rx or OTC medications, vitamins, or herbal products

being taken and to consult with health care professional before taking other medications, especially other oral hypoglycemic medications.

- Advise patient to notify health care professional if pregnancy is planned or suspected or if breast feeding.

Evaluation/Desired Outcomes

- Improved hemoglobin A1C, fasting plasma glucose and 2–hr post-prandial glucose levels.

lindane (lin-dane)

gamma benzene hexachloride, ✱GBH, ✱Hexit, ✱PMS Lindane

Classification

Therapeutic: pediculocides, scabicides

Pregnancy Category B

Indications

Second-line treatment of parasitic arthropod infestation (scabies and head, body, and crab lice) for use only in patients who are intolerant to or do not respond to less toxic agents.

Action

Causes seizures and death in parasitic arthropods. **Therapeutic Effects:** Cure of infestation by parasitic arthropods.

Pharmacokinetics

Absorption: Significant systemic absorption (9–13%) greater with topical application to damaged skin.

Distribution: Stored in fat.

Metabolism and Excretion: Metabolized by the liver.

Half-life: 17–22 hr (infants and children).

TIME/ACTION PROFILE (antiparasitic action)

ROUTE	ONSET	PEAK	DURATION
Top	rapid	6 hr	190 min

Contraindications/Precautions

Contraindicated in: Hypersensitivity; Areas of skin rash, abrasion, or inflammation (absorption is increased); History of seizures; Lactation: Potentially toxic to infants; may ↓ milk supply; Pedi: Premature neonates (↑ risk of CNS toxicity).

Use Cautiously in: Patients with skin conditions (↑ risk of systemic absorption); OB: Do not exceed recommended dose; do not use >2 courses of therapy; Pedi: Geri: Children ≤2 yr and geriatric patients (↑ risk of systemic absorption and CNS side effects).

Adverse Reactions/Side Effects

All adverse reactions except dermatologic are signs of systemic absorption and toxicity.

CNS: SEIZURES, headache. **CV:** tachycardia. **GI:** nausea, vomiting. **Derm:** contact dermatitis (repeated application), local irritation.

Interactions

Drug-Drug: Concurrent use of **medications that lower seizure threshold** (may ↑ risk of seizures). Simultaneous topical use of **skin, scalp,** or **hair** products may ↑ systemic absorption.

Route/Dosage

Scabies

Topical (Adults and Children >1 mo): 1% lotion applied to all skin surfaces from neck to toes; wash off 6 hr after application in infants, after 6–8 hr in children or after 8–12 hr in adults; may require a 2nd treatment 1 wk later.

Head Lice or Crab Lice

Topical (Adults and Children): 15–30 mL of shampoo applied and lathered for 4 min; may require a 2nd treatment 1 wk later.

Availability (generic available)

Lotion: 1%. **Shampoo:** 1%.

NURSING IMPLICATIONS

Assessment

- Assess skin and hair for signs of infestation before and after treatment.
- Examine family members and close contacts for infestation. When used in treatment of pediculosis pubis or scabies, sexual partners should receive concurrent prophylactic therapy.

Potential Nursing Diagnoses

Risk for impaired skin integrity (Indications)

Implementation

- Due to serious side effects, no more than 2 oz may be dispensed at a time and no refills are allowed.
- **Topical:** When applying medication to another person, wear gloves to prevent systemic absorption.
- Do not apply to open wounds (scratches, cuts, sores on skin or scalp) to minimize systemic absorption. Avoid contact with the eyes. If eye contact occurs, flush thoroughly with water and notify physician or other health care professional.
- Institute appropriate isolation techniques.
- **Lotion:** Instruct patient to bathe with soap and water. Dry skin well and allow to cool before application. Apply lotion in amount sufficient to cover entire body surface with a thin film from neck down (60 mL for an adult). Leave medication on for an age appropriate time frame (see dosing), then remove by washing. If rash, burning, or itching develops, wash off medication and notify physician or other health care professional.

- **Shampoo:** Use a sufficient amount of shampoo to wet hair and scalp (30 mL for short hair, 45 mL for medium hair, 60 mL for long hair). Rub thoroughly into hair and scalp and leave in place for 4 min. Then use enough water to work up a good lather; follow with thorough rinsing and drying. If applied in shower or bath, do not let shampoo run down on other parts of body or into water in which patient is sitting. When hair is dry, use fine-toothed comb to remove remaining nits or nit shells. Shampoo may also be used on combs and brushes to prevent spread of infestation.

Patient/Family Teaching

- Instruct patient on application technique and provide with a medication guide. Patient should repeat therapy only at the recommendation of health care professional. Discuss hygienic measures to prevent and to control infestation. Discuss potential for infectious contacts with patient. Explain why household members should be examined and sexual partners treated simultaneously.
- Instruct patient to wash all recently worn clothing and used bed linens and towels in very hot water or to dry clean to prevent reinfestation or spreading.
- Instruct patient not to apply other oils or creams during therapy; these increase the absorption of lindane and may lead to toxicity.
- Explain to patient that itching may persist after treatment; consult health care professional about use of topical hydrocortisone or systemic antihistamines.
- Advise patient that eyelashes can be treated by applying petroleum jelly 3 times/day for 1 wk.
- **Instruct patient not to reapply sooner than 1 week if live mites appear.**
- **Shampoo:** Advise patient that shampoo should not be used as a regular shampoo in the absence of infestation. Emphasize need to avoid contact with eyes.
- Pedi: Advise parents to monitor young children closely for evidence of CNS toxicity (seizures, dizziness, clumsiness, fast heartbeat, muscle cramps, nervousness, restlessness, irritability, nausea, vomiting) during and immediately after treatment.
- Pedi: Cover hands of young children to prevent accidental ingestion from thumbsucking.

Evaluation/Desired Outcomes

- Resolution of signs of infestation with scabies or lice.

linezolid (li-nez-o-lid)

Zyvox, ✱Zyvoxam

Classification

Therapeutic: anti-infectives

Pharmacologic: oxazolidinones

Pregnancy Category C

Indications

Treatment of: Infections caused by vancomycin-resistant *Enterococcus faecium*, Nosocomial pneumonia caused by *Staphylococcus aureus* (methicillin-susceptible and -resistant strains), Complicated skin/skin structure infections caused by *Staphylococcus aureus* (methicillin-susceptible and -resistant strains), *Streptococcus pyogenes* or *Streptococcus agalactiae* (including diabetic foot infections), Uncomplicated skin/skin structure infections caused by *Staphylococcus aureus* (methicillin-susceptible and -resistant strains), *Streptococcus pyogenes*, Community-acquired pneumonia caused by *Streptococcus pneumoniae* (including multi-drug resistant strains) or *Staphylococcus aureus* (methicillin-susceptible strains only).

Action

Inhibits bacterial protein synthesis at the level of the 23S ribosome of the 50S subunit. **Therapeutic Effects:** Bactericidal action against streptococci; bacteriostatic action against enterococci and staphylococci.

Pharmacokinetics

Absorption: Rapidly and extensively (100%) absorbed following oral administration.

Distribution: Readily distributes to well-perfused tissues.

Metabolism and Excretion: 65% metabolized, mostly by the liver; 30% excreted unchanged by the kidneys.

Half-life: 6.4 hr.

TIME/ACTION PROFILE

ROUTE	ONSET	PEAK	DURATION
PO	rapid	1–2 hr	12 hr
IV	rapid	end of infusion	12 hr

Contraindications/Precautions

Contraindicated in: Hypersensitivity; Phenylketonuria (suspension contains aspartame); Uncontrolled HTN, pheochromocytoma, thyrotoxicosis, or concurrent use of sympathomimetic agents, vasopressors, or dopaminergic agents (↑ risk of hypertensive response); Concurrent or recent (<2 wk) use of monoamine oxidase (MAO) inhibitors (↑ risk of hypertensive response); Carcinoid syndrome or concurrent use of SSRIs, TCAs, triptans, meperidine, or buspirone (↑ risk of serotonin syndrome).

Use Cautiously in: Thrombocytopenia, concurrent use of antiplatelet agents or bleeding diathesis (platelet counts should be monitored more frequently); Diabetes (↑ risk of hypoglycemia); OB: Safety not established; use only if maternal benefit outweighs potential risk to fetus; Lactation: Lactation.

Adverse Reactions/Side Effects

CV: headache, insomnia. **EENT:** teeth discoloration, tongue discoloration. **GI:** CLOSTRIDIUM DIFFICILE-ASSOCIATED DIARRHEA (CDAD), diarrhea, ↑ liver enzymes, nausea, taste alteration, vomiting. **Endo:** hypoglycemia. **F and E:** lactic acidosis. **Hemat:** thrombocytopenia. **Neuro:** optic neuropathy, peripheral neuropathy. **Misc:** SEROTONIN SYNDROME.

Interactions

Drug-Drug: ↑ risk of hypertensive response with **MAO inhibitors**, **sympathomimetics** (e.g., **pseudoephedrine**), **vasopressors** (e.g., **epinephrine**, **norepinephrine**), and **dopaminergic agents** (e.g., **dopamine**, **dobutamine**); concurrent or recent use should be avoided. ↑ risk of serotonin syndrome with **SSRIs**, **TCAs**, **triptans**, **meperidine**, **bupropion**, or **buspirone**; avoid concurrent use. **Rifampin**, **carbamazepine**, **phenytoin**, and **phenobarbital** may ↓ levels. Concurrent use with **oral hypoglycemics** or **insulin** may ↑ risk of hypoglycemia.
Drug-Food: Because of monoamine oxidase inhibitory properties, consumption of large amounts of foods or beverages containing tyramine should be avoided (↑ risk of pressor response. See Appendix J).

Route/Dosage

Vancomycin-Resistant *Enterococcus faecium* Infections

PO, IV (Adults): 600 mg every 12 hr for 14–28 days.
PO, IV (Children birth-11 yr): (in the first week of life, pre-term neonates may initially receive 10 mg/kg every 12 hr).

Pneumonia, Complicated Skin/Skin Structure Infections

PO, IV (Adults): 600 mg every 12 hr for 10–14 days.
PO, IV (Children birth-11 yr): 10 mg/kg every 8 hr for 10–14 days (in the first week of life, pre-term neonates may initially receive 10 mg/kg every 12 hr).

Uncomplicated Skin/Skin Structure Infections

PO (Adults): 400 mg q 12 hr for 10–14 days.
PO, IV (Children 5–11 yr): 10 mg/kg every 12 hr for 10–14 days.
PO, IV (Children <5 yr): 10 mg/kg every 8 hr for 10–14 days (in the first week of life, pre-term neonates may initially receive 10 mg/kg every 12 hr).

Availability (generic available)

Oral suspension: (orange-flavored): 20 mg/mL. **Tablets:** 600 mg. **Premixed infusion:** 200 mg/100 mL, 400 mg/200 mL, 600 mg/300 mL.

NURSING IMPLICATIONS

Assessment

- Assess for infection (vital signs; appearance of wound, sputum, urine, and stool; WBC) at beginning of and during therapy.
- Obtain specimens for culture and sensitivity prior to initiating therapy. First dose may be given before receiving.
- May cause lactic acidosis. Notify health care professional if recurrent nausea and vomiting, unexplained acidosis or low bicarbonate levels occur.
- Monitor visual function in patients receiving linezolid for ≥3 mo or who report visual symptoms (changes in acuity or color vision, blurred vision, visual field defect) regardless of length of therapy. If optic neuropathy occurs therapy should be reconsidered.
- Monitor bowel function. Diarrhea, abdominal cramping, fever, and bloody stools should be reported to health care professional promptly as a sign of Clostridium difficile-associated diarrhea (CDAD). May begin up to several weeks following cessation of therapy.
- Monitor patient taking serotonergic drugs for signs of serotonin syndrome (hyperthermia, rigidity, myoclonus, autonomic instability, mental status changes (extreme agitation progressing to delirium and coma) for two weeks (five weeks if fluoxetine was taken) or until 24 hours after the last dose of linezolid, whichever comes first.
- ***Lab Test Considerations:*** May cause bone marrow suppression, anemia, leukopenia, pancytopenia. Monitor CBC and platelet count weekly, especially in patients at risk for increased bleeding, having pre-existing bone marrow suppression, receiving concurrent medications that may cause myelosuppression, or requiring >2 weeks of therapy. Discontinue therapy if bone marrow suppression occurs or worsens.
- May cause ↑ AST, ALT, LDH, alkaline phosphatase and BUN.
- May cause hypoglycemia requiring decrease in dose of antidiabetic agent or discontinuation of linezolid.

Potential Nursing Diagnoses

Risk for infection (Indications)
Diarrhea (Adverse Reactions)

Implementation

- ***High Alert:*** Do not confuse Zyvox with Vioxx or Zovirax.
- Dose adjustment is not necessary when switching from IV to oral dose.
- **PO:** May be administered with or without food.
- Before using oral solution gently invert 3–5 times to mix; do not shake. Store at room temperature.

IV Administration

- **Intermittent Infusion: *Diluent:*** Premixed infusions are already diluted and ready to use. Solution is yellowish in color which may intensify over time without affecting its potency. ***Concentration:*** 2

mg/mL. ***Rate:*** Infuse over 30–120 minutes. Flush line before and after infusion.

- **Y-Site Compatibility:** acyclovir, alemtuzumab, alfentanil, allopurinol, amifostine, amikacin, aminocaproic acid, aminophylline, amiodarone, amphotericin B lipid complex, amphotericin B liposome, ampicillin, ampicillin/sulbactam, anidulafungin, argatroban, azithromycin, aztreonam, bivalirudin, bleomycin, bumetanide, buprenorphine, busulfan, butorphanol, calcium acetate, calcium chloride, calcium gluconate, cangrelor, carboplatin, carmustine, caspofungin, cefazolin, cefepime, cefotaxime, cefotetan, cefoxitin, ceftazidime, ceftriaxone, cefuroxime, chloramphenicol, ciprofloxacin, cisatracurium, cisplatin, clindamycin, cyclophosphamide, cyclosporine, cytarabine, dacarbazine, dactinomycin, daptomycin, daunorubicin hydrochloride, dexamethasone, dexmedetomidine, dexrazoxane, digoxin, diltiazem, diphenhydramine, dobutamine, docetaxel, dolasetron, dopamine, doripenem, doxorubicin hydrochloride, doxorubicin liposomal, doxycycline, droperidol, enalaprilat, ephedrine, epinephrine, epirubicin, eptifibatide, ertapenem, esmolol, etoposide, etoposide phosphate, famotidine, fenoldopam, fentanyl, fluconazole, fludarabine, fluorouracil, foscarnet, fosphenytoin, furosemide, ganciclovir, gemcitabine, gentamicin, glycopyrrolate, granisetron, haloperidol, heparin, hydralazine, hydrocortisone, hydromorphone, idarubicin, ifosfamide, imipenem/cilastatin, insulin, irinotecan, isoproterenol, ketorolac, labetalol, leucovorin, levofloxacin, lidocaine, lorazepam, magnesium sulfate, mannitol, mechlorethamine, melphalan, meperidine, meropenem, mesna, methotrexate, methyldopate, methylprednisolone, metoclopramide, metoprolol, metronidazole, midazolam, milrinone, mitomycin, mitoxantrone, morphine, mycophenolate, nafcillin, nalbuphine, naloxone, nesiritide, nicardipine, nitroglycerin, nitroprusside, norepinephrine, octreotide, ondansetron, oxaliplatin, oxytocin, paclitaxel, palonosetron, pamidronate, pancuronium, pemetrexed, pentazocine, pentobarbital, phenobarbital, phenylephrine, piperacillin/tazobactam, potassium acetate, potassium chloride, potassium phosphates, procainamide, prochlorperazine, promethazine, propranolol, quinupristin/dalfopristin, ranitidine, remifentanil, rocuronium, sodium acetate, sodium bicarbonate, sodium phosphates, streptozocin, succinylcholine, sufentanil, tacrolimus, teniposide, theophylline, thiotepa, tigecycline, tirofiban, tobramycin, topotecan, trimethoprim/sulfamethoxazole, vancomycin, vasopressin, vecuronium, verapamil, vinblastine, vincristine, vinorelbine, voriconazole, zidovudine, zoledronic acid.
- **Y-Site Incompatibility:** amphotericin B colloidal, chlorpromazine, dantrolene, diazepam, pantoprazole, pentamidine, phenytoin, thiopental.

Patient/Family Teaching

- Advise patients taking oral linezolid to take as directed, for full course of therapy, even if feeling better. Take missed doses as soon as remembered unless almost time for next dose; do not double dose.
- Instruct patient to avoid large quantities of foods or beverages containing tyramine (See Appendix J). May cause hypertensive response.
- Instruct patient to notify health care professional if patient has a history of hypertension or seizures.
- Advise patient to notify health care professional of all Rx or OTC medications, vitamins, or herbal products being taken and to consult with health care professional before taking other medications, especially cold remedies, decongestants, or antidepressants.
- Instruct patient to notify health care professional if changes in vision occur or immediately if diarrhea, abdominal cramping, fever, or bloody stools occur and not to treat with antidiarrheals without consulting health care professionals.
- Advise female patient to notify health care professional if pregnancy is planned or suspected or if breast feeding.
- Advise patient to notify health care professional if no improvement is seen in a few days.

Evaluation/Desired Outcomes

- Resolution of signs and symptoms of infection. Length of time for complete resolution depends on organism and site of infection.

REMS

liraglutide (lir-a-gloo-tide)

Saxenda, Victoza

Classification

Therapeutic: antidiabetics

Pharmacologic: glucagon-like peptide-1 (GLP-1) receptor agonists

Pregnancy Category C (Victoza), X (Saxenda)

Indications

Victoza: Adjunct treatment to diet and exercise in the management of adults with type 2 diabetes mellitus; not recommended as first line therapy, as a substitute for insulin, in patients with type 1 diabetes, or for ketoacidosis. **Saxenda**: Chronic weight management in patients in patients who are obese (body mass index [BMI] $\geq$30 kg/m^2) or are overweight (BMI $\geq$27 kg/m^2) with $\geq$1 weight-related comorbid condition (e.g. hypertension, dyslipidemia, type 2 diabetes).

Action

Acts as an acylated human glucagon-like peptide-1 (GLP-1, an incretin) receptor agonist; increases intracellular cyclic AMP (cAMP) leading to insulin release when glucose is elevated, which then subsides as blood glucose decreases toward euglycemia. Also decreases glucagon secretion and delays gastric emptying. Also helps to suppress appetite, leading to decreased caloric intake. **Therapeutic Effects:** Improved glycemic control. Reduction in body weight.

Pharmacokinetics

Absorption: 55% absorbed following subcutaneous injection.
Distribution: Unknown.
Protein Binding: >98%.
Metabolism and Excretion: Endogenously metabolized.
Half-life: 13 hr.

TIME/ACTION PROFILE

ROUTE	ONSET	PEAK	DURATION
Subcut	within 4 wk† within 2 wk‡	8 wk† 40 wk‡	unk†‡

† ↓ in HbA1c.
‡ ↓ in body weight.

Contraindications/Precautions

Contraindicated in: Hypersensitivity; Personal or family history of medullary thyroid carcinoma; Multiple Endocrine Neoplasia syndrome type 2; Type 1 diabetes (Victoza only); Diabetic ketoacidosis (Victoza only); History of suicidal attempts or suicidal thoughts (Saxenda only); OB: Weight loss not recommended during pregnancy (Saxenda only); Lactation: Avoid use; Pedi: Not recommended.
Use Cautiously in: History of pancreatitis; History of angioedema to another GLP-1 receptor agonist; Hepatic/renal impairment; OB: Use only if potential benefit justifies potential risk to fetus (Victoza only).

Adverse Reactions/Side Effects

CNS: SUICIDAL THOUGHTS (Saxenda only), headache. **CV:** tachycardia. **Derm:** pruritis, rash. **Endo:** THYROID C-CELL TUMORS. **GI:** PANCREATITIS, diarrhea, nausea, vomiting, cholelithiasis (Saxenda only), constipation. **GU:** acute renal failure. **Local:** HYPERSENSITIVITY REACTIONS INCLUDING ANAPHYLAXIS AND ANGIOEDEMA, injection site reactions.

Interactions

Drug-Drug: Concurrent use with **agents that increase insulin secretion** including **sulfonylureas** may ↑ the risk of serious hypoglycemia, use cautiously and consider dose ↓ of agent increasing insulin secretion. May alter absorption of concomitantly administered **oral medications** due to delayed gastric emptying.

Route/Dosage

Victoza

Subcut (Adults): 0.6 mg once daily initially for 1 wk, then 1.2 mg once daily for 1 wk; may then ↑ dose, if needed up to 1.8 mg once daily.

Saxenda

Subcut (Adults): 0.6 mg once daily for 1 wk (Wk 1), then 1.2 mg once daily for 1 wk (Wk 2), then 1.8 mg once daily for 1 wk (Wk 3), then 2.4 mg once daily for 1 wk (Wk 4), then 3 mg once daily.

Availability

Solution for subcutaneous injection (Victoza): Pre-filled, multi-dose pen that delivers doses of 0.6 mg, 1.2 mg, or 1.8 mg. **Solution for subcutaneous injection (Saxenda):** Pre-filled, multi-dose pen that delivers doses of 0.6 mg, 1.2 mg, 1.8 mg, 2.4 mg, or 3 mg.

L

NURSING IMPLICATIONS

Assessment

- If thyroid nodules or elevated serum calcitonin are noted, patient should be referred to an endocrinologist.
- Monitor for pancreatitis (persistent severe abdominal pain, sometimes radiating to the back, with or without vomiting). If pancreatitis is suspected, discontinue liraglutide; if confirmed, do not restart liraglutide.
- **Victoza:** Observe patient taking concurrent insulin for signs and symptoms of hypoglycemic reactions (sweating, hunger, weakness, dizziness, tremor, tachycardia, anxiety).
- **Saxenda:** Monitor patients for weight loss and adjust concurrent medications (antihypertensives, antidiabetics, lipid-lowering agents) as needed.
- ***Lab Test Considerations:*** Monitor serum HbA1c periodically during therapy to evaluate effectiveness.

Potential Nursing Diagnoses

Imbalanced nutrition: more than body requirements (Indications)
Noncompliance (Patient/Family Teaching)

Implementation

- Patients stabilized on a diabetic regimen who are exposed to stress, fever, trauma, infection, or surgery may require administration of insulin.
- **Subcut:** Administer once daily at any time of the day, without regard to food. Inject into abdomen, thigh, or upper arm. Solution should be clear and colorless; do not administer solutions that are discolored or contain particulate matter.
- Initial dose of 0.6 mg/day is increased after 1 wk to 1.2 mg/day. If glycemic control is not acceptable, in-

crease to 1.8 mg/day. Available in a prefilled pen without needle; patient may require Rx for needles.

- *First Time Use for Each New Pen*—Follow manufacturer's instructions only once with each new pen or if pen is dropped.

Patient/Family Teaching

- Instruct patient on use of pen injector and to take liraglutide as directed. If a dose is missed, omit and take next dose as scheduled; do not double doses. If >3 days dosing missed, reinitiate with 0.6 mg dose; titrate at direction of health care professional. Pen should never be shared between patients, even if needle is changed. Store pen in refrigerator; do not freeze. After initial use, pen may be stored at room temperature or refrigerated up to 30 days. Keep pen cap on when not in use. Protect from excessive heat and sunlight. Remove and safely discard needle after each injection and store pen without needle attached. Advise patient to read the *Patient Medication Guide* before starting liraglutide and with each Rx refill.
- If a dose is missed do not make up, skip and take next scheduled dose the next day. If more than 3 days are missed, reinitiate at 0.6 mg to minimize GI effects. Notify health care professional and increase dose as directed.
- Inform patient that nausea is the most common side effect, but usually decreases over time.
- Advise patient taking insulin and liraglutide to never mix insulin and liraglutide together. Give as 2 separate injections. Both injections may be given in the same body area, but should not be given right next to each other.
- Explain to patient that this medication controls hyperglycemia but does not cure diabetes. Therapy is long-term.
- Review signs of hypoglycemia and hyperglycemia with patient. If hypoglycemia occurs, advise patient to take a glass of orange juice or 2–3 tsp of sugar, honey, or corn syrup dissolved in water and notify health care professional.
- Encourage patient to follow prescribed diet, medication, and exercise regimen to prevent hypoglycemic or hyperglycemic episodes.
- Instruct patient in proper testing of serum glucose and ketones. These tests should be closely monitored during periods of stress or illness, and health care professional should be notified if significant changes occur.
- Advise patient to tell health care professional what medications they are taking and to avoid taking new Rx, OTC, vitamins, or herbal products without consulting health care professional.
- Advise patient to notify discontinue liraglutide and health care professional immediately if signs of pancreatitis (nausea, vomiting, abdominal pain) occur.
- Advise patient to inform health care professional of medication regimen before treatment or surgery.
- Inform patient of risk of benign and malignant thyroid C-cell tumors. Advise patient to notify health care professional if symptoms of thyroid tumors (lump in neck, hoarseness, trouble swallowing, shortness of breath) or if signs of allergic reaction (swelling of face, lips, tongue, or throat; fainting or feeling dizzy; very rapid heartbeat; problems breathing or swallowing; severe rash or itching) occur.
- Insulin is the preferred method of controlling blood glucose during pregnancy. Counsel female patients to notify health care professional if pregnancy is planned or suspected or if breast feeding.
- Advise patient to carry a form of sugar (sugar packets, candy) and identification describing disease process and medication regimen at all times.
- Emphasize the importance of routine follow-up exams.

Evaluation/Desired Outcomes

- Improved glycemic control.
- Reduction in body weight. If patient has not lost at least 4% of body weight after 16 wks of therapy, it is unlikely that patient will achieve and sustain clinically meaningful weight loss with continued treatment.

lisinopril, See ANGIOTENSIN-CONVERTING ENZYME (ACE) INHIBITORS.

lithium (lith-ee-um)

✱Carbolith, ✱Lithane, ✱Lithmax, Lithobid

Classification
Therapeutic: mood stabilizers

Pregnancy Category D

Indications

Manic episodes of bipolar I disorder (treatment, maintenance, prophylaxis).

Action

Alters cation transport in nerve and muscle. May also influence reuptake of neurotransmitters. **Therapeutic Effects:** Prevents/decreases incidence of acute manic episodes.

Pharmacokinetics

Absorption: Completely absorbed after oral administration.

Distribution: Widely distributed into many tissues and fluids; CSF levels are 50% of plasma levels. Crosses the placenta; enters breast milk.

Metabolism and Excretion: Excreted almost entirely unchanged by the kidneys.

Half-life: 20–27 hr.

TIME/ACTION PROFILE (antimanic effects)

ROUTE	ONSET	PEAK	DURATION
PO, PO–ER	5–7 days	10–21 days	days

Contraindications/Precautions

Contraindicated in: Hypersensitivity; Severe cardiovascular or renal disease; Dehydrated or debilitated patients; Brugada syndrome; Should be used only where therapy, including blood levels, may be closely monitored; Some products contain alcohol or tartrazine and should be avoided in patients with known hypersensitivity or intolerance; Lactation: Lactation.

Use Cautiously in: Any degree of cardiac, renal, or thyroid disease; Diabetes mellitus; OB: Fetal cardiac anomalies are associated with lithium use; however, potential maternal benefit may warrant use in some pregnant women; Geri: Initial dosage ↓ recommended.

Adverse Reactions/Side Effects

CNS: SEIZURES, fatigue, headache, impaired memory, ataxia, sedation, confusion, dizziness, drowsiness, psychomotor retardation, restlessness, stupor. **EENT:** aphasia, blurred vision, dysarthria, tinnitus. **CV:** ECG changes, arrhythmias, edema, hypotension, unmasking of Brugada syndrome. **GI:** abdominal pain, anorexia, bloating, diarrhea, nausea, dry mouth, metallic taste. **GU:** polyuria, glycosuria, nephrogenic diabetes insipidus, renal toxicity. **Derm:** acneiform eruption, folliculitis, alopecia, diminished sensation, pruritus. **Endo:** hypothyroidism, goiter, hyperglycemia, hyperthyroidism. **F and E:** hyponatremia. **Hemat:** leukocytosis. **Metab:** weight gain. **MS:** muscle weakness, hyperirritability, rigidity. **Neuro:** tremors.

Interactions

Drug-Drug: May prolong the action of **neuromuscular blocking agents**. ↑ risk of neurologic toxicity with **haloperidol**. **Diuretics**, **methyldopa**, **probenecid**, **fluoxetine**, and **NSAIDs** may ↑ risk of toxicity. Blood levels may be ↑ by **ACE inhibitors**. Lithium may ↓ effects of **chlorpromazine**. **Chlorpromazine** may mask early signs of lithium toxicity. Hypothyroid effects may be additive with **potassium iodide** or **antithyroid agents**. **Aminophylline**, **phenothiazines**, and **drugs containing large amounts of sodium** ↑ renal elimination and ↓ effectiveness. **Psyllium** can ↓ **lithium** levels.

Drug-Natural Products: Caffeine-containing herbs (**cola nut**, **guarana**, **mate**, **tea**, **coffee**) may ↓ **lithium** serum levels and efficacy.

Drug-Food: Large changes in **sodium** intake may alter the renal elimination of lithium. ↑ sodium intake will ↑ renal excretion.

Route/Dosage

Precise dosing is based on serum lithium levels. 300 mg lithium carbonate contains 8–12 mEq lithium.

PO (Adults and children ≥12 yr): *Tablets/capsules*—300–600 mg 3 times daily initially; usual maintenance dose is 300 mg 3–4 times daily. *Extended-release tablets*—450–900 mg twice daily *or* 300–600 mg 3 times daily initially; usual maintenance dose is 450 mg twice daily *or* 300 mg 3 times daily.

PO (Children <12 yr): 15–20 mg (0.4–0.5 mEq)/kg/day in 2–3 divided doses; dosage may be adjusted weekly.

Availability (generic available)

Capsules: 150 mg, 300 mg, 600 mg. **Cost:** *Generic*—150 mg $13.97/100, 300 mg $17.91/100, 600 mg $39.11/100. **Tablets:** 300 mg. **Cost:** *Generic*—$21.52/100. **Extended-release tablets:** 300 mg, 450 mg. **Cost:** *Generic*—300 mg $46.52/100, 450 mg $50.05/100. **Oral solution:** 300 mg (8 mEq lithium)/5 mL.

L

NURSING IMPLICATIONS

Assessment

- Assess mental status (orientation, mood, behavior) initially and periodically. Initiate suicide precautions if indicated.
- Monitor intake and output ratios. Report significant changes in totals. Unless contraindicated, fluid intake of at least 2000–3000 mL/day should be maintained. Weight should also be monitored at least every 3 mo.
- ***Lab Test Considerations:*** Evaluate renal and thyroid function, WBC with differential, serum electrolytes, and glucose periodically during therapy.
- ***Toxicity and Overdose:*** Monitor serum lithium levels twice weekly during initiation of therapy and every 2 mo during chronic therapy. Draw blood samples in the morning immediately before next dose. Therapeutic levels range from 0.5 to 1.5 mEq/L for acute mania and 0.6–1.2 mEq/L for long term control. Serum concentrations should not exceed 2.0 mEq/L.
- Assess patient for signs and symptoms of lithium toxicity (vomiting, diarrhea, slurred speech, decreased coordination, drowsiness, muscle weakness, or twitching). If these occur, report before administering next dose.

Potential Nursing Diagnoses

Disturbed thought process (Indications)
Ineffective coping (Indications)
Imbalanced nutrition: risk for more than body requirements (Side Effects)

Implementation

- Do not confuse lithium carbonate with lanthanum carbonate. Do not confuse lithium with Ultram (tramadol).
- **PO:** Administer with food or milk to minimize GI irritation. Extended-release preparations should be swallowed whole; do not break, crush, or chew.

Patient/Family Teaching

- Instruct patient to take medication as directed, even if feeling well. Take missed doses as soon as remembered unless within 2 hr of next dose (6 hr if extended release).
- Lithium may cause dizziness or drowsiness. Caution patient to avoid driving or other activities requiring alertness until response to medication is known.
- Low sodium levels may predispose patient to toxicity. Advise patient to drink 2000–3000 mL fluid each day and eat a diet with consistent and moderate sodium intake. Excessive amounts of coffee, tea, and cola should be avoided because of diuretic effect. Avoid activities that cause excess sodium loss (heavy exertion, exercise in hot weather, saunas). Notify health care professional of fever, vomiting, and diarrhea, which also cause sodium loss.
- Advise patient that weight gain may occur. Review principles of a low-calorie diet.
- Advise patient to notify health care professional of all Rx or OTC medications, vitamins, or herbal products being taken and to consult with health care professional before taking other medications, especially NSAIDs.
- Review side effects and symptoms of toxicity with patient. Instruct patient to stop medication and report signs of toxicity to health care professional promptly.
- Advise patient to notify health care professional if fainting, irregular pulse, or difficulty breathing occurs.
- Advise patient to use contraception and to consult health care professional if pregnancy is planned or suspected or if breast feeding. Lithium may be teratogenic.
- Emphasize the importance of periodic lab tests to monitor for lithium toxicity.

Evaluation/Desired Outcomes

- Resolution of the symptoms of mania (hyperactivity, pressured speech, poor judgment, need for little sleep).
- Decreased incidence of mood swings in bipolar disorders.
- Improved affect in unipolar disorders. Improvement in condition may require 1–3 wk.
- Decreased incidence of acute manic episodes.

loperamide (loe-**per**-a-mide)

Imodium, Imodium A-D, Neo-Diaral

Classification
Therapeutic: antidiarrheals

Pregnancy Category B

Indications

Adjunctive therapy of acute diarrhea. Chronic diarrhea associated with inflammatory bowel disease. Decreases the volume of ileostomy drainage.

Action

Inhibits peristalsis and prolongs transit time by a direct effect on nerves in the intestinal muscle wall. Reduces fecal volume, increases fecal viscosity and bulk while diminishing loss of fluid and electrolytes. **Therapeutic Effects:** Relief of diarrhea.

Pharmacokinetics

Absorption: Not well absorbed following oral administration.

Distribution: Unknown. Does not cross the blood-brain barrier.

Protein Binding: 97%.

Metabolism and Excretion: Metabolized partially by the liver, undergoes enterohepatic recirculation; 30% eliminated in the feces. Minimal excretion in the urine.

Half-life: 10.8 hr.

TIME/ACTION PROFILE (relief of diarrhea)

ROUTE	ONSET	PEAK	DURATION
PO	1 hr	2.5–5 hr	10 hr

Contraindications/Precautions

Contraindicated in: Hypersensitivity; Patients in whom constipation must be avoided; Abdominal pain of unknown cause, especially if associated with fever; Alcohol intolerance (liquid only).

Use Cautiously in: Hepatic dysfunction; Lactation: Usually compatible with breast feeding; OB: Safety not established; Pedi: Children <2 yr (safety not established); Geri: ↑ sensitivity to effects.

Adverse Reactions/Side Effects

CNS: drowsiness, dizziness. **GI:** constipation, abdominal pain/distention/discomfort, dry mouth, nausea, vomiting. **Misc:** allergic reactions.

Interactions

Drug-Drug: ↑ CNS depression with other **CNS depressants**, including **alcohol**, **antihistamines**, **opioid analgesics**, and **sedative/hypnotics**. ↑ anticholinergic properties with other **drugs having anticholinergic properties**, including **antidepressants** and **antihistamines**.

Drug-Natural Products: Kava-kava, valerian, skullcap, chamomile, or **hops** can ↑ CNS depression.

Route/Dosage

Acute and Chronic Diarrhea

PO (Adults and Children >12 yr): 4 mg initially, then 2 mg after each loose stool. Maintenance dose usually 4–8 mg/day in divided doses (not to exceed 8 mg/day for OTC use or 16 mg/day for Rx use).

Acute Diarrhea

PO (Children 9–11 yr or 30–47 kg): 2 mg initially; then 1 mg after each loose stool (not to exceed 6 mg/24 hr; OTC use should not exceed 2 days).
PO (Children 6–8 yr or 24–30 kg): 1 mg initially, then 1 mg after each loose stool (not to exceed 4 mg/24 hr; OTC use should not exceed 2 days).
PO (Children 2–5 yr or 13–20 kg): 1 mg initially, then 0.1 mg/kg after each loose stool (not to exceed 3 mg/24 hr; OTC use should not exceed 2 days).

Chronic Diarrhea

PO (Children): 0.08–0.24 mg/kg/day divided 2–3 times/day (not to exceed 2 mg/dose).

Availability (generic available)

Tablets: 2 mg^OTC^. **Capsules:** 2 mg. **Liquid (mint):** 1 mg/7.5 mL^OTC^. ***In combination with:*** simethicone (Imodium Multi-Symptom Relief^OTC^, see Appendix B).

NURSING IMPLICATIONS

Assessment

- Assess frequency and consistency of stools and bowel sounds prior to and during therapy.
- Assess fluid and electrolyte balance and skin turgor for dehydration.

Potential Nursing Diagnoses

Diarrhea (Indications)
Risk for injury (Side Effects)

Implementation

- **PO:** Administer with clear fluids to help prevent dehydration, which may accompany diarrhea.

Patient/Family Teaching

- Instruct patient to take medication as directed. Do not take missed doses, and do not double doses. In acute diarrhea, medication may be ordered after each unformed stool. Advise patient not to exceed the maximum number of doses.
- May cause drowsiness. Advise patient to avoid driving or other activities requiring alertness until response to drug is known.
- Advise patient that frequent mouth rinses, good oral hygiene, and sugarless gum or candy may relieve dry mouth.
- Caution patient to avoid using alcohol and other CNS depressants concurrently with this medication.
- Instruct patient to notify health care professional if diarrhea persists or if fever, abdominal pain, or distention occurs.

Evaluation/Desired Outcomes

- Decrease in diarrhea.
- In acute diarrhea, treatment should be discontinued if no improvement is seen in 48 hr.
- In chronic diarrhea, if no improvement has occurred after at least 10 days of treatment with maximum dose, loperamide is unlikely to be effective.

lopinavir/ritonavir

(loe-**pin**-a-veer/ri-**toe**-na-veer)
Kaletra

Classification
Therapeutic: antiretrovirals
Pharmacologic: protease inhibitors, metabolic inhibitors

Pregnancy Category C

Indications

HIV infection (with other antiretrovirals).

Action

Lopinavir: Inhibits HIV viral protease. **Ritonavir:** Although ritonavir has antiretroviral activity of its own (inhibits the action of HIV protease and prevents the cleavage of viral polyproteins), it is combined with lopinavir to inhibit the metabolism of lopinavir thus increasing its plasma levels. **Therapeutic Effects:** Increased CD4 cell counts and decreased viral load with subsequent slowed progression of HIV infection and its sequelae.

Pharmacokinetics

Absorption: Well absorbed following oral administration; food enhances absorption.
Distribution: *Ritonavir*—poor CNS penetration.
Protein Binding: *Lopinavir*—98–99% bound to plasma proteins.
Metabolism and Excretion: *Lopinavir*—completely metabolized in the liver by cytochrome P450 3A (CYP450 3A); ritonavir is a potent inhibitor of this enzyme. *Ritonavir*—highly metabolized by the liver (by CYP450 3A and CYP2D6 enzymes); one metabolite has antiretroviral activity; 3.5% excreted unchanged in urine.
Half-life: *Lopinavir*—5–6 hr *Ritonavir*—3–5 hr.

TIME/ACTION PROFILE (blood levels)

ROUTE	ONSET	PEAK	DURATION
Lopinavir PO	rapid	4 hr	12 hr
Ritonavir PO	rapid	4 hr*	12 hr

*Non-fasting.

Contraindications/Precautions

Contraindicated in: Hypersensitivity (including toxic epidermal necrolysis, Stevens-Johnson syndrome, or erythema multiforme); Concurrent use of dihydroergotamine, ergotamine, lovastatin, methylergonovine, midazolam (PO), pimozide, sildenafil (Revatio), alfuzosin, simvastatin, and triazolam (may result in serious and/or life-threatening events); Concurrent use with St. John's wort or rifampin (may lead to ↓ virologic response and possible resistance); Hypersensitivity or intolerance to alcohol or castor oil (present in liquid); Congenital long QT syndrome, concurrent use of QT-interval prolonging drugs, or hypokalemia (↑ risk of QT interval prolongation); OB: Not recommended in pregnancy if ≥1 lopinavir resistance-associated substitution present; Lactation: Breast feeding not recommended in HIV-infected patients; Pedi: Preterm infants (should be avoided until 14 days after their due date) or full-term infants <14 days old (↑ risk of toxicity from alcohol and propylene glycol in oral solution).

Use Cautiously in: Known alcohol intolerance (oral solution contains alcohol); Impaired hepatic function, history of hepatitis (for ritonavir content); Pre-existing conduction system disease (marked first-degree AV block or second- or third-degree AV block), ischemic heart disease, or concurrent use of other drugs that increase the PR interval (especially those metabolized by CYP3A4 including verapamil or diltiazem); OB: Once daily regimen should not be used in pregnancy; Pedi: Children ≤6 mo (↑ risk of toxicity from alcohol and propylene glycol in oral solution); should not be used once daily in children.

Adverse Reactions/Side Effects

CNS: headache, insomnia, weakness. **CV:** TORSADES DE POINTES, ↑ PR interval, heart block, QT interval prolongation. **GI:** HEPATOTOXICITY, PANCREATITIS, diarrhea (↑ in children), abdominal pain, nausea, taste aversion (in children), vomiting (↑ in children). **Derm:** ERYTHEMA MULTIFORME, STEVENS JOHNSON SYNDROME, TOXIC EPIDERMAL NECROLYSIS, rash. **Misc:** immune reconstitution syndrome.

Interactions

Drug-Drug: ↑ blood levels and risk of toxicity from **ergot derivatives (dihydroergotamine, ergotamine, methylergonovine)**, **pimozide**, **sildenafil (Revatio)**, **alfuzosin**, **simvastatin**, **lovastatin**, **midazolam (oral)**, and **triazolam**; avoid concomitant use. Concurrent use of **rifampin** ↓ effectiveness of lopinavir/ritonavir (contraindicated). ↑ risk of myopathy with **atorvastatin** or **rosuvastatin**; use lowest possible dose of statin; do not exceed rosuvastatin dose of 10 mg/day. Concurrent use with **efavirenz** or **nevirapine** ↓ lopinavir/ritonavir levels and effectiveness; dose ↑ recommended; once daily lopinavir/ritonavir regimen not recommended when these drugs are used. **Delavirdine** ↑ lopinavir levels. May ↑ **tenofovir** and **rilpivirine** levels. May ↓ **abacavir**, **etravirine**, and **zidovudine** levels. Concurrent use with **fosamprenavir** ↓ lopinavir and **fosamprenavir** levels. Concurrent use with **nelfinavir** ↓ lopinavir levels and ↑ **nelfinavir** levels; ↑ dose of lopinavir/ritonavir; once daily lopinavir/ritonavir regimen not recommended when these drugs are used. ↑ **indinavir** levels; indinavir dose should be ↓. ↑ **saquinavir** levels. **Tipranavir** ↓ lopinavir levels. ↑ **maraviroc** levels; maraviroc dose should be ↓ to 150 mg twice daily. ↑ levels of **amiodarone**, **lidocaine**, and **quinidine** (blood level monitoring recommended, if possible). Concurrent use of **carbamazepine**, **phenobarbital**, or **phenytoin** may ↓ effectiveness of lopinavir (blood level monitoring recommended; once daily lopinavir/ritonavir regimen not recommended when these drugs are used); lopinavir may also ↓ **phenytoin** levels. May ↓ **bupropion** levels/effects. ↑ levels/effects of **trazodone**. ↑ levels of dihydropyridine calcium channel blockers including **felodipine**, **nifedipine**, **amlodipine**, and **nicardipine**. May alter levels and effectiveness of **warfarin**. ↑ levels of **clarithromycin** (dose ↓ recommended for patients with CCr ≤60 mL/min. ↑ blood levels of **itraconazole** and **ketoconazole** (high antifungal doses not recommended). ↓ levels of **voriconazole**; concurrent use not recommended. ↑ levels of **rifabutin** (dose ↓ recommended). ↓ levels of **atovaquone** (may require dose ↑). **Dexamethasone** ↓ levels/effectiveness of lopinavir. Oral solution contains alcohol may produce intolerance when administered with **disulfiram** or **metronidazole**. May ↑ levels and risk of toxicity with immunosuppressants including **cyclosporine**, **tacrolimus**, or **sirolimus** (blood level monitoring recommended). May ↓ levels and effects of **methadone** (dose of **methadone** may need to be ↑). May ↑ levels and effects of **fentanyl**; monitor for respiratory depression. May ↓ levels and contraceptive efficacy of some estrogen-based **hormonal contraceptives** including **ethinyl estradiol** (alternative or additional methods of contraception recommended). ↑ levels of **fluticasone** and **budesonide**; avoid concurrent use. May ↑ **vincristine** and **vinblastine** levels; consider holding or switching to another antiretroviral regimen that does not contain a CYP3A or P-glycoprotein inhibitor. May ↑ **dasatinib** and **nilotinib** levels; may need to ↓ doses of dasatinib and nilotinib. Concurrent use of other **drugs known to ↑ PR interval** may ↑ risk of heart block. Concurrent use of other **drugs known to ↑ QT interval** should be avoided. May ↑ risk of adverse effects with **salmeterol**; concurrent use not recommended. May ↑ **bosentan** levels; initiate bosentan at 62.5 mg once daily or every other day; if patient already receiving bosentan, discontinue bosentan at least 36 hr before initiation of tipranavir and then restart bosentan at least 10 days later at 62.5 mg once daily or every other day. May ↑ levels of **sildenafil** (Viagra), **vardenafil**, **tadalafil** (Cialis) or **avanafil**; may result in hypotension, syncope, visual changes, and prolonged erection (↓ dose of sildenafil to 25 mg q 48 hr, vardenafil to 2.5 mg q 72 hr, and tadalafil to 10 mg q 72 hr recommended; do not use with avanafil). May ↑ **tadalafil (Adcirca)** levels; initiate tadalafil (Adcirca) at 20 mg once daily; if patient already receiving tadalfil (Adcirca), discontinue tadalafil (Adcirca) at least 24 hr before initiation of tipranavir and then restart tadalafil (Adcirca) at least 7 days later at 20 mg once daily. May ↑ **colchicine** levels; ↓ dose of colchicine; do not administer colchicine if patients have renal or hepatic impairment. Concurrent use with **boceprevir** may ↓ levels of boceprevir, lopinavir, and ritonavir; avoid concurrent use. May ↑ levels of **simeprevir**; avoid concurrent use. May ↓ levels of **valproate** and **lamotrigine**; may need to ↑ dose of valproate or lamotrigine. May ↑ levels of **rivaroxaban**; avoid concurrent use. May ↑ **quetiapine** levels; ↓ quetiapine dose to 1/6 of current dose.

Drug-Natural Products: Concurrent use with **St. John's wort** may ↓ levels and beneficial effect of lopinavir/ritonavir (contraindicated).

Route/Dosage

PO (Adults): *Patients with <3 lopinavir resistance-associated substitutions*—400/100 mg (two 200/50-mg tablets or 5 mL oral solution) twice daily *or* 800/200 mg (four 200/50–mg tablets or 10 mL oral solution) once daily; *Patients with ≥3 lopinavir resistance-associated substitutions*—400/100 mg (two 200/50-mg tablets or 5 mL oral solution) twice daily; *Pregnant women with no lopinavir resistance-associated substitutions*—400/100 mg (two 200/50-mg tablets) twice daily; *Pregnant women with ≥1 lopinavir resistance-associated substitution*—Not recommended.

PO (Children ≥6 mo and 15–40 kg): *Oral solution*—10/2.5 mg/kg lopinavir/ritonavir twice daily.

PO (Children ≥6 mo and <15 kg): *Oral solution*—12/3 mg/kg lopinavir/ritonavir twice daily.

PO (Children ≥6 mo): *Tablets*—15–25 kg: 200/50 mg (two 100/25-mg tablets) twice daily; 26–35 kg: 300/75 mg (three 100/25-mg tablets) twice daily; >35 kg: 400/100 mg (four 100/25-mg tablets or two 200/50-mg tablets) twice daily.

PO (Children 14 days–6 mo): *Oral solution*—16/4 mg/kg lopinavir/ritonavir content twice daily.

With Concurrent Efavirenz, Nevirapine, or Nelfinavir

PO (Adults): *Therapy-naive or therapy-experienced*—500/125 mg (two 200/50-mg tablets and one 100/25-mg tablet or 6.5 mL oral solution) twice daily.

PO (Children ≥6 mo and 15–45 kg): *Oral solution*—11/2.75 mg/kg lopinavir/ritonavir twice daily.

PO (Children ≥6 mo and <15 kg): *Oral solution*—13/3.25 mg/kg lopinavir/ritonavir twice daily.

PO (Children ≥6 mo): *Tablets*—15–20 kg: 200/50 mg (two 100/25-mg tablets) twice daily; 21–30 kg: 300/75 mg (three 100/25-mg tablets) twice daily; 31–45 kg: 400/100 mg (four 100/25-mg tablets or two 200/50-mg tablets) twice daily.

PO (Children 14 days–6 mo): Not recommended for concomitant administration with these drugs.

Availability

Tablets: 100 mg lopinavir/25 mg ritonavir, 200 mg lopinavir/50 mg ritonavir. **Oral solution:** 80 mg lopinavir/20 mg ritonavir per mL (contains 42.4% alcohol).

NURSING IMPLICATIONS

Assessment

- Assess for change in severity of HIV symptoms and for symptoms of opportunistic infections during therapy.
- Assess patient for signs of pancreatitis (nausea, vomiting, abdominal pain, increased serum lipase or amylase) periodically during therapy. May require discontinuation of therapy.
- Assess patient for rash (mild to moderate rash usually occurs in the 2nd wk of therapy and resolves within 1–2 wk of continued therapy). If rash is severe (extensive erythematous or maculopapular rash with moist desquamation or angioedema) or accompanied by systemic symptoms (serum sickness-like reaction, Stevens-Johnson syndrome, toxic epidermal necrolysis), therapy must be discontinued immediately.
- ***Lab Test Considerations:*** Monitor viral load and CD4 counts regularly during therapy.
- Monitor triglyceride and cholesterol levels prior to initiating therapy and periodically during therapy.
- May cause hyperglycemia.
- Monitor liver function before and during therapy, especially in patients with underlying hepatic disease, including hepatitis B and hepatitis C, or marked transaminase elevations. May cause ↑ serum AST, ALT, GGT, and total bilirubin concentrations.
- Monitor serum lipase and amylase levels during therapy.

Potential Nursing Diagnoses

Risk for infection (Indications)
Noncompliance (Patient/Family Teaching)

Implementation

- Do not confuse Kaletra (lopinavir/ritonavir) with Keppra (levetiracetam).
- Patients taking didanosine with Kaletra solution should take didanosine 1 hr before or 2 hr after taking lopinavir/ritonavir.

L

- **PO:** Tablets may be administered with or without food. Swallow whole, do not break, crush, or chew.
- Oral solution must be taken with food. Oral solution is light yellow to orange. Solution is stable if refrigerated until expiration date on label or 2 mo at room temperature. Oral solution should be avoided in premature babies until 14 days after their due date, or in full-term babies younger than 14 days of age unless a health care professional believes that the benefit of using *Kaletra* oral solution to treat HIV infection immediately after birth outweighs the potential risks. If oral solution is used in babies younger than 14 days, monitor for increases in serum osmolality, serum creatinine, and other signs of toxicity.

Patient/Family Teaching

- Emphasize the importance of taking lopinavir/ritonavir as directed, at evenly spaced times throughout day. Do not take more than prescribed amount, and do not stop taking this or other antiretrovirals without consulting health care professional. Take missed doses as soon as remembered; do not double doses. Advise patient to read the *Patient Information* prior to taking this medication and with each Rx refill in case of changes.
- Instruct parent/patient to measure oral solution carefully.
- Instruct patient that lopinavir/ritonavir should not be shared with others.
- Advise patient to notify health care professional of all Rx or OTC medications, vitamins, or herbal products being taken and to consult with health care professional before taking other medications, especially St. John's wort.
- Inform patient that lopinavir/ritonavir does not cure AIDS or prevent associated or opportunistic infections. Lopinavir/ritonavir does not reduce the risk of transmission of HIV to others through sexual contact or blood contamination. Caution patient to use a condom during sexual contact and to avoid sharing needles or donating blood to prevent spreading the AIDS virus to others. Advise patient that the long-term effects of lopinavir/ritonavir are unknown at this time.
- Instruct patient to notify health care professional immediately if rash, symptoms of lactic acidosis (tiredness or weakness, unusual muscle pain, trouble breathing, stomach pain with nausea and vomiting, cold especially in arms or legs, dizziness, fast or irregular heartbeat) or if signs of hepatotoxicity (yellow skin or whites of eyes, dark urine, light-colored stools, lack of appetite for several days or longer, nausea, abdominal pain) occur.
- Inform patient that lopinavir/ritonavir may cause hyperglycemia. Advise patient to notify health care professional if increased thirst or hunger; unexplained weight loss; or increased urination occurs.
- Caution patients taking sildenafil, vardenafil, or tadalafil of increased risk of associated side effects (hypotension, visual changes, sustained erection). Notify health care professional promptly if these occur.
- Inform patient that redistribution and accumulation of body fat may occur causing central obesity, dorsocervical fat enlargement (buffalo hump), peripheral wasting, breast enlargement, and cushingoid appearance. The cause and long-term effects are not known.
- Rep: Advise patients taking oral contraceptives to use a nonhormonal method of birth control during lopinavir/ritonavir therapy. Instruct patient to notify health care professional if pregnancy is planned or suspected and to avoid breast feeding. Encourage pregnant women exposed to lopinavir/ritonavir to enroll in the Antiviral Pregnancy Registry by calling 1–800–258–4263 to monitor maternal/fetal outcomes.
- Emphasize the importance of regular follow-up exams and blood counts to determine progress and monitor for side effects.

Evaluation/Desired Outcomes

- Delayed progression of AIDS and decreased opportunistic infections in patients with HIV.
- Decrease in viral load and improvement in CD4 cell counts.

loratadine (lor-a-ta-deen)

Alavert Allergy 24 Hour, Alavert Children's Allergy, ✤Claritin, Claritin 24-Hour Allergy, Claritin Children's Allergy, Claritin Liqui–Gels 24-Hour Allergy, Claritin Reditabs 24 Hour Allergy, Loradamed, Tavist ND Allergy

Classification
Therapeutic: antihistamines

Pregnancy Category B

Indications

Relief of symptoms of seasonal allergies. Management of chronic idiopathic urticaria. Management of hives.

Action

Blocks peripheral effects of histamine released during allergic reactions. **Therapeutic Effects:** Decreased symptoms of allergic reactions (nasal stuffiness; red, swollen eyes, itching).

Pharmacokinetics

Absorption: Rapidly absorbed after oral administration (80%).
Distribution: Unknown.
Protein Binding: *Loratadine*—97%; *descarboethoxyloratadine*—73–77%.
Metabolism and Excretion: Rapidly and extensively metabolized during first pass through the liver. Much is converted to descarboethoxyloratadine, an active metabolite.

Half-life: *Loratadine*—8.4 hr; *descarboethoxyloratadine*—28 hr.

TIME/ACTION PROFILE (antihistaminic effects)

ROUTE	ONSET	PEAK	DURATION
PO	1–3 hr	8–12 hr	>24 hr

Contraindications/Precautions

Contraindicated in: Hypersensitivity.

Use Cautiously in: Hepatic impairment or CCr <30 mL/min (↓ dose to 10 mg every other day); Lactation: Usually compatible with breast feeding (AAP); OB, Pedi: Pregnancy or children <2 yr (safety not established). Syrup contains sodium benzoate, avoid use in neonates; Geri: ↑ risk of adverse reactions.

Adverse Reactions/Side Effects

CNS: confusion, drowsiness (rare), paradoxical excitation. **EENT:** blurred vision. **GI:** dry mouth, GI upset. **Derm:** photosensitivity, rash. **Metab:** weight gain.

Interactions

Drug-Drug: The following interactions may occur, but are less likely to occur with loratidine than with more sedating antihistamines. **MAO inhibitors** may intensify and prolong effects of antihistamines. ↑ CNS depression may occur with other **CNS depressants**, including **alcohol**, **antidepressants**, **opioid analgesics**, and **sedative/hypnotics**. **Amiodarone** may ↑ loratadine levels and ↑ risk of QTc interval prolongation.

Drug-Natural Products: **Kava-kava**, **valerian**, or **chamomile** can ↑ CNS depression.

Route/Dosage

PO (Adults and Children ≥6 yr): 10 mg once daily.
PO (Children ≥2–5 yr): 5 mg once daily.

Renal Impairment

PO (Adults): *CCr <30 mL/min*—10 mg every other day.

Hepatic Impairment

PO (Adults): 10 mg every other day.

Availability (generic available)

Rapidly disintegrating tablets (mint): 10 mg[OTC]. **Tablets:** 10 mg[OTC]. **Capsules:** 10 mg[OTC]. **Chewable tablets:** 5 mg[OTC] (grape flavored). **Syrup (grape, fruit):** 5 mg/5 mL[OTC]. ***In combination with:*** pseudoephedrine (Claritin-D)[OTC]. See Appendix B.

NURSING IMPLICATIONS

Assessment

- Assess allergy symptoms (rhinitis, conjunctivitis, hives) before and periodically during therapy.
- Assess lung sounds and character of bronchial secretions. Maintain fluid intake of 1500–2000 mL/day to decrease viscosity of secretions.
- ***Lab Test Considerations:*** May cause false-negative result on allergy skin testing.

Potential Nursing Diagnoses

Ineffective airway clearance (Indications)
Risk for injury (Adverse Reactions)

Implementation

- Do not confuse Claritin (loratadine) with Claritin Eye (ketotifen fumarate).
- **PO:** Administer once daily.
- *For rapidly disintegrating tablets (Alavert, Claritin Reditabs)*—place on tongue. Tablet disintegrates rapidly. May be taken with or without water.

Patient/Family Teaching

- Instruct patient to take medication as directed.
- May cause dizziness or drowsiness. Caution patient to avoid driving or other activities requiring alertness until response to medication is known.
- Caution patient to use sunscreen and protective clothing to prevent photosensitivity reactions.
- Advise patient to avoid taking alcohol or other CNS depressants concurrently with this drug.
- Advise patient that good oral hygiene, frequent rinsing of mouth with water, and sugarless gum or candy may minimize dry mouth. Patient should notify dentist if dry mouth persists >2 wk.
- Instruct patient to contact health care professional immediately if dizziness, fainting, or fast or irregular heartbeat occurs or if symptoms persist.

Evaluation/Desired Outcomes

- Decrease in allergic symptoms.
- Management of chronic idiopathic urticaria.
- Management of hives.

LORazepam (lor-az-e-pam)

Ativan

Classification
Therapeutic: anesthetic adjuncts, antianxiety agents, sedative/hypnotics
Pharmacologic: benzodiazepines

Schedule IV

Pregnancy Category D

Indications

Anxiety disorder (oral). Preoperative sedation (injection). Decreases preoperative anxiety and provides amnesia. **Unlabeled Use: IV:** Antiemetic prior to chemotherapy. Insomnia, panic disorder, as an adjunct with acute mania or acute psychosis.

Action

Depresses the CNS, probably by potentiating GABA, an inhibitory neurotransmitter. **Therapeutic Effects:** Sedation. Decreased anxiety. Decreased seizures.

Pharmacokinetics

Absorption: Well absorbed following oral administration. Rapidly and completely absorbed following IM administration. Sublingual absorption is more rapid than oral and is similar to IM.

Distribution: Widely distributed. Crosses the blood-brain barrier. Crosses the placenta; enters breast milk.

Metabolism and Excretion: Highly metabolized by the liver.

Half-life: Full-term neonates: 18–73 hr; Older children: 6–17 hr; Adults: 10–16 hr.

TIME/ACTION PROFILE (sedation)

ROUTE	ONSET	PEAK	DURATION
PO	15–60 min	1–6 hr	8–12 hr
IM	30–60 min	1–2 hr†	8–12 hr
IV	15–30 min	15–20 min	8–12 hr

†Amnestic response.

Contraindications/Precautions

Contraindicated in: Hypersensitivity; Cross-sensitivity with other benzodiazepines may exist; Comatose patients or those with pre-existing CNS depression; Uncontrolled severe pain; Angle-closure glaucoma; Severe hypotension; Sleep apnea; OB, Lactation: Use in pregnancy and lactation may cause CNS depression, flaccidity, feeding difficulties, hypothermia, seizures, and respiratory problems in the neonate; discontinue drug or bottle-feed.

Use Cautiously in: Severe hepatic/renal/pulmonary impairment; Myasthenia gravis; Depression; Psychosis; History of suicide attempt or drug abuse/substance use disorder; COPD; Sleep apnea; Pedi: Use cautiously in children under 12 yr. In ↑ doses, benzyl alcohol in injection may cause potentially fatal "gasping syndrome" in neonates; Geri: Lower doses recommended for geriatric or debilitated patients; Hypnotic use should be short-term.

Adverse Reactions/Side Effects

CNS: dizziness, drowsiness, lethargy, hangover, headache, ataxia, slurred speech, forgetfulness, confusion, mental depression, rhythmic myoclonic jerking in preterm infants, paradoxical excitation. **EENT:** blurred vision. **Resp:** respiratory depression. **CV:** *rapid IV use only*—APNEA, CARDIAC ARREST, bradycardia, hypotension. **GI:** constipation, diarrhea, nausea, vomiting, weight gain (unusual). **Derm:** rashes. **Misc:** physical dependence, psychological dependence, tolerance.

Interactions

Drug-Drug: Additive CNS depression with other **CNS depressants** including **alcohol**, **antihistamines**, **antidepressants**, **opioid analgesics**, **clozapine**, and other **sedative/hypnotics** including other benzodiazepines. May ↓ the efficacy of **levodopa**. **Smoking** may ↑ metabolism and ↓ effectiveness. **Valproate** and can ↑ levels (↓ dose by 50%). **Oral contraceptives** may ↓ levels.

Drug-Natural Products: Concomitant use of **kava-kava**, **valerian**, or **chamomile** can ↑ CNS depression.

Route/Dosage

PO (Adults): *Anxiety*—1–3 mg 2–3 times daily (up to 10 mg/day). *Insomnia*—2–4 mg at bedtime.

PO (Geriatric Patients or Debilitated Patients): *Anxiety*—0.5–2 mg/day in divided doses initially. *Insomnia*—0.25–1 mg initially, ↑ as needed.

PO (Children): *Anxiety/sedation*—0.02–0.1 mg/kg/dose (not to exceed 2 mg) q 4–8 hr. *Preoperative sedation*—0.02–0.09 mg/kg/dose.

PO (Infants): *Anxiety/sedation*—0.02–0.1 mg/kg/dose (not to exceed 2 mg) q 4–8 hr. *Preoperative sedation*—0.02–0.09 mg/kg/dose.

SL (Adults and adolescents >18 yr): *Anxiety*—2–3 mg/day in divided doses, not to exceed 6 mg/day; *preoperative sedation*—0.05 mg/kg, up to 4 mg total given 1–2 hr before surgery.

SL (Geriatric Patients and debilitated patients): 0.5 mg/day, dose may be adjusted as necessary.

IM (Adults): *Preoperative sedation*—50 mcg (0.05 mg)/kg 2 hr before surgery (not to exceed 4 mg).

IM (Children): *Preoperative sedation*—0.02–0.09 mg/kg/dose.

IM (Infants): *Preoperative sedation*—0.02–0.09 mg/kg/dose.

IV (Adults): *Preoperative sedation*—44 mcg (0.044 mg)/kg (not to exceed 2 mg) 15–20 min before surgery. *Operative amnestic effect*—up to 50 mcg/kg (not to exceed 4 mg). *Antiemetic*—2 mg 30 min prior to chemotherapy; may be repeated q 4 hr as needed (unlabeled). *Anticonvulsant*—50 mcg (0.05 mg)/kg, up to 4 mg; may be repeated after 10–15 min (not to exceed 8 mg/12 hr; unlabeled).

IV (Children): *Preoperative sedation*—0.02–0.09 mg/kg/dose; may use smaller doses (0.01–0.03 mg/kg) and repeat q 20 min. *Antiemetic*—Single dose: 0.04–0.08 mg/kg/dose prior to chemotherapy (not to exceed 4 mg). Multiple doses: 0.02–0.05 mg/kg/dose q 6 hr prn (not to exceed 2 mg). *Anxiety/sedation*—0.02–0.1 mg/kg (not to exceed 2 mg) q 4–8 hr. *Status epilepticus*—0.1 mg/kg over 2–5 min (not to exceed 4 mg); may repeat with 0.05 mg/kg if needed.

IV (Infants): *Preoperative sedation*—0.02–0.09 mg/kg/dose; may use smaller doses (0.01–0.03 mg/kg) and repeat q 20 min. *Anxiety/sedation*—0.02–0.1 mg/kg/dose (not to exceed 2 mg) q 4–8 hr. *Status epilepticus*—0.1 mg/kg over 2–5 min (not to exceed 4 mg); may repeat with 0.05 mg/kg if needed.

IV (Neonates): *Status epilepticus*—0.05 mg/kg over 2–5 min; may repeat in 10–15 min.

Availability (generic available)

Tablets: 0.5 mg, 1 mg, 2 mg. **Cost:** *Generic*—0.5 mg $6.99/100, 1 mg $9.73/100, 2 mg $10.34/100. **Concentrated oral solution:** 2 mg/mL. **Cost:** *Generic*—$39.80/30 mL. **Sublingual tablets :** ✱0.5 mg, ✱1 mg, ✱2 mg. **Injection:** 2 mg/mL, 4 mg/mL.

NURSING IMPLICATIONS

Assessment

- Conduct regular assessment of continued need for treatment.
- Pedi: Assess neonates for prolonged CNS depression related to inability to metabolize lorazepam.
- Geri: Assess geriatric patients carefully for CNS reactions as they are more sensitive to these effects. Assess falls risk.
- **Anxiety:** Assess degree and manifestations of anxiety and mental status (orientation, mood, behavior) prior to and periodically throughout therapy.
- Prolonged high-dose therapy may lead to psychological or physical dependence. Restrict amount of drug available to patient.
- **Status Epilepticus:** Assess location, duration, characteristics, and frequency of seizures. Institute seizure precautions.
- ***Lab Test Considerations:*** Patients on high-dose therapy should receive routine evaluation of renal, hepatic, and hematologic function.
- ***Toxicity and Overdose:*** If overdose occurs, flumazenil (Romazicon) is the antidote. Do not use with patients with seizure disorder. May induce seizures.

Potential Nursing Diagnoses

Anxiety (Indications)
Risk for injury (Indications, Side Effects)

Implementation

- Do not confuse Ativan (lorazepam) with Atarax (hydroxyzine). Do not confuse lorazepam with alprazolam or clonazepam.
- Following parenteral administration, keep patient supine for at least 8 hr and observe closely.
- **PO:** Tablet may also be given sublingually (unlabeled) for more rapid onset.
- Take concentrated liquid solution with water, soda, pudding, or applesauce.
- **IM:** Administer IM doses deep into muscle mass at least 2 hr before surgery for optimum effect.

IV Administration

- **IV Push:** ***Diluent:*** Dilute immediately before use with an equal amount of sterile water for injection, D5W, or 0.9% NaCl for injection. Pedi: To decrease the amount of benzyl alcohol delivered to neonates, dilute the 4 mg/mL injection with preservative-free sterile water for injection to make a 0.4 mg/mL dilution for IV use. Do not use if solution is colored or contains a precipitate. ***Rate:*** Administer at a rate not to exceed 2 mg/min or 0.05 mg/kg over 2–5 min. Rapid IV administration may result in apnea, hypotension, bradycardia, or cardiac arrest.
- **Y-Site Compatibility:** acyclovir, albumin, alemtuzumab, alfentanil, allopurinol, amifostine, amikacin, aminocaproic acid, aminophylline, amiodarone, amphotericin B cholesteryl, amphotericin B colloidal, amphotericin B lipiod complex, amsacrine, anakinra, anidulafungin, argatroban, atracurium, bivalirudin, bleomycin, bumetanide, buprenorphine, bulsulfan, butorphanol, calcium chloride, calcium gluconate, carboplatin, carmustine, cefazolin, cefepime, cefotaxime, cefotetan, cefoxitin, ceftaroline, ceftazidime, ceftriaxone, cefuroxime, chloramphenicol, ciprofloxacin, cisatracurium, cisplatin, cladribine, clindamycin, cyclophosphamide, cyclosporine, cytarabine, dactinomycin, daptomycin, dexamethasone sodium phosphate, dexmedetomidine, digoxin, diltiazem, diphenhydramine, dobutamine, docetaxel, dopamine, doxorubicin, doxorubicin liposome, doxycycline, droperidol, enalaprilat, ephedrine, epinephrine, epirubicin, eptifibatide, ertapenem, erythromycin lactobionate, esmolol, etomidate, etoposide phosphate, famotidine, fenoldopam, fentanyl, filgrastim, fluconazole, fludarabine, fosphenytoin, furosemide, gemcitabine, gentamicin, glycopyrrolate, granisetron, haloperidol, heparin, hydrocortisone sodium succinate, hydromorphone, ifosfamide, insulin, irinotecan, isoproterenol, ketorolac, labetalol, lidocaine, linezolid, magnesium sulfate, mannitol, mechlorethamine, melphalan, meropenem, metaraminol, methadone, methotrexate, methyldopate, methylprednisolone sodium succinate, metoclopramide, metoprolol, metronidazole, micafungin, midazolam, milrinone, mitoxantrone, morphine, mycophenolate, nafcillin, nalbuphine, naloxone, nesiritide, nicardipine, nitroglycerin, nitroprusside, norepinephrine, octreotide, oxaliplatin, oxytocin, paclitaxel, palonosetron, pamidronate, pancuronium, pemetrexed, pentamidine, pentobarbital, phenobarbital, phenylephrine, piperacillin/tazobactam, potassium acetate, potassium chloride, procainamide, prochlorperazine, promethazine, propofol, propranolol, quinupristin/dalfopristin, ranitidine, remifentanil, rituximab, sodium acetate, sodium bicarbonate, sodium phosphates, streptozocin, succinylcholine, tacrolimus, teniposide, theophylline, thiotepa, tigecycline, tirofiban, tobramycin, trastuzumab, trimethoprim/sulfamethoxazole, vancomycin, vasopressin, vecuronium, verapamil, vincristine, vinorelbine, voriconazole, zidovudine, zoledronic acid.
- **Y-Site Incompatibility:** aldesleukin, ampicillin, ampicillin/sulbactam, aztreonam, dantrolene, doxa-

curium, fluorouracil, hydralazine, idarubicin, imipenem/cilastatin, meperidine, omeprazole, ondansetron, pantoprazole, phenytoin, potassium phosphates, rocuronium, sargramostim, sufentanil.

Patient/Family Teaching

- Instruct patient to take medication exactly as directed and not to skip or double up on missed doses. If medication is less effective after a few weeks, check with health care professional; do not increase dose.
- Advise patient that lorazepam is usually prescribed for short-term use and does not cure underlying problem.
- Advise patient to decrease lorazepam dose gradually to minimize withdrawal symptoms; abrupt withdrawal may cause tremors, nausea, vomiting, and abdominal and muscle cramps.
- Teach other methods to decrease anxiety, such as increased exercise, support groups, relaxation techniques. Emphasize that psychotherapy is beneficial in addressing source of anxiety and improving coping skills.
- May cause drowsiness or dizziness. Advise patient to avoid driving or other activities requiring alertness until response to medication is known.
- Caution patient to avoid taking alcohol or other CNS depressants concurrently with this medication.
- Instruct patient to contact health care professional immediately if pregnancy is planned or suspected.
- Emphasize the importance of follow-up exams to determine effectiveness of the medication.

Evaluation/Desired Outcomes

- Increase in sense of well-being.
- Decrease in subjective feelings of anxiety without excessive sedation.
- Reduction of preoperative anxiety.
- Postoperative amnesia.
- Improvement in sleep patterns.

lorcaserin (lor-ca-**ser**-in)

Belviq

Classification

Therapeutic: weight control agents

Pharmacologic: serotonin 2C receptor agonists

Schedule IV

Pregnancy Category X

Indications

In conjunction with a reduced-calorie diet and increased physical activity for chronic weight management in patients with a body mass index (BMI) of ≥30 kg/m^2 or 27 kg/m^2 with a weight-related comorbidity (hypertension, type 2 diabetes, dyslipidemia).

Action

Acts as a serotonin 2C receptor agonist; increases satiety by activating 5−HT$_{2C}$ receptors located on anorexigenic neurons in the hypothalmus. **Therapeutic Effects:** Decreased appetite with subsequent weight loss and health benefits.

Pharmacokinetics

Absorption: Well absorbed following oral administration.

Distribution: Enters cerebrospinal fluid and central nervous system.

Metabolism and Excretion: Extensively metabolized by the liver; metabolites are mostly excreted in urine (92.3%), minimal amounts in feces (2.2%).

Half-life: 11 hr.

TIME/ACTION PROFILE (weight loss)

ROUTE	ONSET	PEAK	DURATION
PO	within 1 mo	6–9 mo	unknown

Contraindications/Precautions

Contraindicated in: Severe renal impairment/end stage renal disease; OB: Pregnancy (weight loss may result in fetal harm); Lactation: Breast feeding not recommended; Pedi: Not recommended (safety and effectiveness not established).

Use Cautiously in: History of priapism or risk of priapism (including sickle-cell anemia, multiple myeloma, leukemia or penile deformity); History of heart failure, bradycardia or 2nd/3rd-degree heart block; History of suicidal thoughts/behavior; History of type 2 diabetes (weight loss may ↑ risk of hypoglycemia); Concurrent use of CYP2D6 substrates; Moderate renal impairment; Severe hepatic impairment; Geri: May have ↑ risk of adverse reactions due to age-related ↓ in renal function.

Exercise Extreme Caution in: Concurrent use of serotoninergic or antidopaminergic agents.

Adverse Reactions/Side Effects

CNS: NEUROLEPTIC MALIGNANT SYNDROME, SEROTONIN SYNDROME, cognitive impairment, depression, dizziness, fatigue, psychiatric disorders, suicidality. **CV:** VALVULOPATHY, bradycardia, hypertension, peripheral edema. **GI:** constipation, dry mouth, nausea. **GU:** priapism. **Endo:** hypoglycemia, ↑ prolactin. **Hemat:** ↓ RBC count.

Interactions

Drug-Drug: Concurrent use with **serotonergic** or **antidopaminergic** medications, including **antipsychotics** may ↑ risk of serotonin syndrome or neuroleptic malignant syndrome; use extreme caution. Concurrent use with serotonergic/dopaminergic agents that are potent 5−HT$_{2B}$ agonists may ↑ risk of cardiac valvulopathy. May ↑ blood levels and effects of other **drugs metabolized by the CYP 2D6 system**, including **dextromethorphan**; locaserin is an inhibitor of the CYP 2D6 system.

Route/Dosage

PO (Adults): 10 mg twice daily; discontinue if 5% weight loss has not been observed at 12 wk.

Availability

Tablets: 10 mg.

NURSING IMPLICATIONS

Assessment

- Monitor patients for weight loss and adjust concurrent medications (antihypertensives, antidiabetics, lipid-lowering agents) as needed.
- Assess for serotonin syndrome (mental changes [agitation, hallucinations, coma], autonomic instability [tachycardia, labile BP, hyperthermia], neuromuscular aberrations [hyper-reflexia, incoordination], and/or GI symptoms [nausea, vomiting, diarrhea]), especially in patients taking other serotonergic drugs (SSRIs, SNRIs, triptans).
- Monitor for signs and symptoms of neuroleptic malignant syndrome (hyperthermia, muscle rigidity, autonomic instability with possible rapid fluctuation of vital signs, mental status changes) during therapy.
- Assess for signs and symptoms of valvular heart disease (dyspnea, dependent edema, CHF, new cardiac murmur) during therapy. If these develop, consider discontinuing lorcaserin.
- Monitor closely for notable changes in behavior that could indicate the emergence or worsening of suicidal thoughts or behavior or depression. Discontinue lorcaserin if these occur.
- Monitor for symptoms related to hyperprolactinemia (menstrual abnormalities, galactorrhea, gynecomastia).
- ***Lab Test Considerations:*** Monitor CBC periodically during therapy. May cause leukopenia, lymphopenia, neutropenia, anemia, and ↓ WBC, hemoglobin, and hematocrit.
- May cause ↑ prolactin levels.
- Monitor blood sugar closely in patients with diabetes.

Potential Nursing Diagnoses

Disturbed body image (Indications)
Imbalanced nutrition: more than body requirements (Indications)
Deficient knowledge, related to medication regimen (Patient/Family Teaching)

Implementation

- **PO:** May be administered with or without food.

Patient/Family Teaching

- Instruct patient to take lorcaserin as directed and not to increase dose.
- May impair cognitive function. Caution patient to avoid driving or other activities that require alertness until response to medication is known.
- Advise patient and family to notify health care professional if thoughts about suicide or dying, attempts to commit suicide; new or worse depression; new or worse anxiety; feeling very agitated or restless; panic attacks; trouble sleeping; new or worse irritability; acting aggressive; being angry or violent; acting on dangerous impulses; an extreme increase in activity and talking; other unusual changes in behavior or mood or if symptoms of serotonin syndrome, neuroleptic malignant syndrome, or valvular heart disease occur.
- Instruct patient to notify health care professional of all Rx or OTC medications, vitamins, or herbal products being taken and to consult with health care professional before taking other medications, especially St. John's Wort.
- Advise patients with diabetes to monitor blood sugar closely during therapy.
- Inform male patient that priapism may occur. If an erection lasts longer than 4 hrs, whether painful or not, immediately discontinue lorcaserin and seek emergency attention.
- Advise patient to notify health care professional if pregnancy is planned or suspected or if breast feeding.

Evaluation/Desired Outcomes

- Decrease in weight and BMI. If 5% of baseline body weight is not lost by Week 12, discontinue lorcaserin, as it is unlikely patient will achieve and sustain clinically meaningful weight loss with continued treatment.

losartan, See ANGIOTENSIN II RECEPTOR ANTAGONISTS.

lovastatin, See HMG-CoA REDUCTASE INHIBITORS (statins).

lurasidone (loo-ras-i-done)

Latuda

Classification
Therapeutic: antipsychotics
Pharmacologic: benzoisothiazole

Pregnancy Category B

Indications

Treatment of schizophrenia. Depressive episodes associated with bipolar I disorder (as monotherapy or with lithium or valproate).

Action

Effect may mediated via effects on central dopamine Type 2 (D_2) and serotonin Type 2 ($5HT_{2A}$) receptor antagonism. **Therapeutic Effects:** ↓ schizophrenic behavior.

Pharmacokinetics

Absorption: 9–19% absorbed following oral administration.

Distribution: Unknown.

Protein Binding: >99%.

Metabolism and Excretion: Mostly metabolized by the CYP3A4 enzyme system. Two metabolites are pharmacologically active; 80% eliminated in feces, 8% in urine primarily as metabolites.

Half-life: 18 hr.

TIME/ACTION PROFILE

ROUTE	ONSET	PEAK	DURATION
PO	unknown	1–3 hr*	24 hr

*Blood level.

Contraindications/Precautions

Contraindicated in: Hypersensitivity; Concurrent use of strong CYP3A4 inhibitors or inducers.

Use Cautiously in: Renal/hepatic impairment (dose adjustment recommended for CCr of 10 mL/min–<50 mL/min or Child-Pugh Class B and C); History of suicide attempt; Diabetes mellitus; Overheating/dehydration (may ↑ risk of serious adverse reactions); History of leukopenia or previous drug-induced leukopenia/neutropenia; Geri: ↑ risk of seizures; elderly patients with dementia-related psychoses (↑ risk of cerebrovascular adverse reactions); use cautiously in elderly females (↑ risk of tardive dyskinesia); OB: Use in pregnancy only if potential benefit justifies potential risk to fetus; Lactation: Breast feeding should only be considered if potential benefit justifies risk to child; Pedi: May ↑ risk of suicide attempt/ideation especially during dose early treatment or dose adjustment; risk may be greater in children, adolescents, and young adults taking antidepressants (safe use in children/adolescents not established).

Adverse Reactions/Side Effects

CNS: NEUROLEPTIC MALIGNANT SYNDROME, SEIZURES, SUICIDAL THOUGHTS, akathisia, drowsiness, parkinsonism, agitation, anxiety, cognitive/motor impairment, dizziness, dystonia, tardive dyskinesia. **EENT:** blurred vision. **CV:** bradycardia, orthostatic hypotension, syncope, tachycardia. **GI:** nausea, esophageal dysmotility. **Derm:** pruritus, rash. **Endo:** hyperglycemia, hyperprolactinemia. **Hemat:** AGRANULOCYTOSIS, anemia, leukopenia. **Metab:** dyslipidemia, weight gain.

Interactions

Drug-Drug: **Strong CYP3A4 inhibitors**, including **ketoconazole, clarithromycin, ritonavir**, and **voriconazole** ↑ blood levels and risk of adverse reactions; concurrent use contraindicated. **Strong CYP3A4 inducers**, including **rifampin**, **phenytoin**, and **carbamazepine** ↓ blood levels and effectiveness; concurrent use contraindicated. **Moderate inhibitors of the CYP3A4 enzyme system**, including **diltiazem**, **atazanavir**, **erythromycin**, **fluconazole**, and **verapamil** ↑ blood levels; if used concurrently, dose of lurasidone should not exceed 40 mg/day. ↑ sedation may occur with other **CNS depressants**, including **alcohol**, **sedative/hypnotics**, **opioids**, some **antidepressants** and **antihistamines**.

Drug-Natural Products: **St. John's wort** ↓ blood levels and effectiveness; concurrent use contraindicated.

Drug-Food: **Grapefruit juice** ↑ blood levels and risk of adverse reactions; concurrent use contraindicated.

Route/Dosage

Schizophrenia

PO (Adults): 40 mg once daily (not to exceed 160 mg once daily); *Addition of moderate CYP3A4 inhibitor to existing lurasidone therapy*— ↓ lurasidone dose by 50%; *Addition of lurasidone to existing moderate CYP3A4 inhibitor therapy*— 20 mg once daily (not to exceed 80 mg once daily).

Renal Impairment

PO (Adults): *CCr <50 mL/min*— 20 mg once daily (not to exceed 80 mg once daily).

Hepatic Impairment

PO (Adults): *Child-Pugh Class B*— 20 mg once daily (not to exceed 80 mg once daily); *Child-Pugh Class C*— 20 mg once daily (not to exceed 40 mg once daily).

Depressive Episodes Associated with Bipolar I Disorder

PO (Adults): 20 mg once daily (not to exceed 120 mg once daily); *Addition of moderate CYP3A4 inhibitor to existing lurasidone therapy*— ↓ lurasidone dose by 50%; *Addition of lurasidone to existing moderate CYP3A4 inhibitor therapy*— 20 mg once daily (not to exceed 80 mg once daily).

Renal Impairment

PO (Adults): *CCr <50 mL/min*— 20 mg once daily (not to exceed 80 mg once daily).

Hepatic Impairment

PO (Adults): *Child-Pugh Class B*— 20 mg once daily (not to exceed 80 mg once daily); *Child-Pugh Class C*— 20 mg once daily (not to exceed 40 mg once daily).

Availability

Tablets: 20 mg, 40 mg, 60 mg, 80 mg, 120 mg.

NURSING IMPLICATIONS

Assessment

- Monitor patient's mental status (orientation, mood, behavior) before and periodically during therapy.
- Assess weight and BMI initially and throughout therapy.
- Monitor mood changes. Assess for suicidal tendencies, especially during early therapy. Restrict amount of drug available to patient.
- Monitor BP (sitting, standing, lying down) and pulse before and frequently during initial dose titration. May cause tachycardia and orthostatic hypotension. If hypotension occurs, dose may need to be ↓.
- Observe patient when administering medication to ensure medication is swallowed and not hoarded or cheeked.
- Monitor patient for onset of extrapyramidal side effects (*akathisia*—restlessness; *dystonia*—muscle spasms and twisting motions; or *pseudoparkinsonism*—mask-like face, rigidity, tremors, drooling, shuffling gait, dysphagia). Report these symptoms; reduction of dose or discontinuation may be necessary. Trihexyphenidyl or benztropine may be used to control symptoms.
- Monitor for tardive dyskinesia (involuntary rhythmic movement of mouth, face, and extremities). Report immediately; may be irreversible.
- Monitor for development of neuroleptic malignant syndrome (fever, respiratory distress, tachycardia, seizures, diaphoresis, hypertension or hypotension, pallor, tiredness). Notify health care professional immediately if these symptoms occur.
- Monitor for symptoms of hyperglycemia (polydipsia, polyuria, polyphagia, weakness) periodically during therapy.
- ***Lab Test Considerations:*** May cause ↑ serum prolactin levels.
- May cause ↑ CPK.
- Obtain fasting blood glucose and cholesterol levels initially and periodically during therapy.
- Monitor CBC frequently during initial mo of therapy in patients with pre-existing or history of low WBC. May cause leukopenia, neutropenia, or agranulocytosis. Discontinue therapy if this occurs.

Potential Nursing Diagnoses

Risk for self-directed violence (Indications)
Disturbed thought process (Indications)
Risk for injury (Side Effects)

Implementation

- ***High Alert:*** Do not confuse Latuda with Lantus.
- **PO:** Administer once daily with food of at least 350 calories.

Patient/Family Teaching

- Instruct patient to take medication as directed. Emphasize the caloric food needs for taking medication.
- Inform patient of the possibility of extrapyramidal symptoms. Instruct patient to report these symptoms immediately to health care professional.
- Advise patient to change positions slowly to minimize orthostatic hypotension.
- May cause drowsiness and cognitive and motor impairment. Caution patient to avoid driving or other activities requiring alertness until response to medication is known.
- Advise patient and family to notify health care professional if thoughts about suicide or dying, attempts to commit suicide; new or worse depression; new or worse anxiety; feeling very agitated or restless; panic attacks; trouble sleeping; new or worse irritability; acting aggressive; being angry or violent; acting on dangerous impulses; an extreme ↑ in activity and talking, other unusual changes in behavior or mood occur.
- Advise patient to avoid extremes in temperature; this drug impairs body temperature regulation.
- Advise patient to tell health care professional what medications they are taking and to avoid taking new Rx, OTC, vitamins, or herbal products without consulting health care professional, especially alcohol and other CNS depressants.
- Advise patient to notify health care professional of medication regimen before treatment or surgery.
- Instruct patient to notify health care professional promptly if sore throat, fever, unusual bleeding or bruising, rash, or tremors occur.
- Advise female patients to notify health care professional if pregnancy is planned or suspected, or if breast feeding.
- Emphasize the importance of routine follow up exams to monitor side effects.

Evaluation/Desired Outcomes

- ↓ in symptoms of schizophrenia (delusions, hallucinations, social withdrawal, flat, blunted affects).

L

magaldrate, See MAGNESIUM AND ALUMINUM SALTS.

MAGNESIUM AND ALUMINUM SALTS

magaldrate (with simethicone)
(**mag**-al-drate)
Riopan Plus

magnesium hydroxide/aluminum hydroxide
(mag-**nee**-zhum hye-**drox**-ide/ a-**loo**-mi-num hye-**drox**-ide)
Alamag, ✱Diovol Plus, Maalox, Rulox

Classification
Therapeutic: antiulcer agents
Pharmacologic: antacids

Pregnancy Category C

Indications
Useful in a variety of GI complaints, including: Hyperacidity, Indigestion, GERD, Heartburn.

Action
Neutralize gastric acid following dissolution in gastric contents. Inactivate pepsin if pH is raised to ≥4. **Therapeutic Effects:** Neutralization of gastric acid with healing of ulcers and decrease in associated pain.

Pharmacokinetics
Absorption: During routine use, antacids are nonabsorbable. With chronic use, 15–30% of magnesium and smaller amounts of aluminum may be absorbed.
Distribution: Small amounts absorbed are widely distributed, cross the placenta, and appear in breast milk. Aluminum concentrates in the CNS.
Metabolism and Excretion: Excreted by the kidneys.
Half-life: Unknown.

TIME/ACTION PROFILE (effect on gastric pH)

ROUTE	ONSET	PEAK	DURATION
Aluminum PO	slightly delayed	30 min	30 min–1 hr (empty stomach); 3 hr (after meals)
Magnesium PO	slightly delayed	30 min	30 min–1 hr (empty stomach); 3 hr (after meals)

Contraindications/Precautions
Contraindicated in: Severe abdominal pain of unknown cause, especially if accompanied by fever; Renal failure (CrCl <30 mL/min); Products containing tartrazine or sugar in patients with known intolerance.
Use Cautiously in: Antacids containing magnesium in patients with any degree of renal insufficiency; ↓ bowel motility; Dehydration; Upper GI hemorrhage; Pedi: Children <12 yr (safety not established).

Adverse Reactions/Side Effects
GI: *aluminum salts*—constipation; *magnesium salts*, diarrhea. **F and E:** *magnesium salts*—hypermagnesemia; *aluminum salts*, hypophosphatemia.

Interactions
Drug-Drug: Absorption of **tetracyclines**, **phenothiazines**, **ketoconazole**, **itraconazole**, **iron salts**, **fluoroquinolones**, and **isoniazid** may be ↓ (separate by at least 2 hr).

M

Route/Dosage
Magaldrate/Simethicone
PO (Adults): 5–10 mL (540–1080 mg) between meals and at bedtime.

Magnesium Hydroxide/Aluminum Hydroxide
PO (Adults and Children ≥12 yr): 5–30 mL or 1–2 tablets 1–3 hr after meals and at bedtime.

Availability
Magaldrate/Simethicone (generic available)
Suspension: 540 mg magaldrate/20 mg simethicone/5 mL[OTC], 1080 mg magaldrate/40 mg simethicone/5 mL[OTC].

Magnesium Hydroxide/Aluminum Hydroxide (generic available)
Chewable Tablets: 300 mg aluminum hydroxide/150 mg magnesium hydroxide[OTC]. **Suspension:** 225 mg aluminum hydroxide/200 mg magnesium hydroxide/5 mL[OTC], 500 mg aluminum hydroxide/500 mg magnesium hydroxide/5 mL[OTC]. ***In combination with:*** simethicone[OTC]. See Appendix B.

NURSING IMPLICATIONS
Assessment
- **Antacid:** Assess for heartburn and indigestion as well as location, duration, character, and precipitating factors of gastric pain.
- ***Lab Test Considerations:*** Monitor serum phosphate, potassium, and calcium levels periodically during chronic use. May cause ↑ serum calcium and ↓ serum phosphate concentrations.

Potential Nursing Diagnoses

Acute pain (Indications)

Implementation

- Magnesium and aluminum are combined as antacids to balance the constipating effects of aluminum with the laxative effects of magnesium.
- **PO:** To prevent tablets from entering small intestine in undissolved form, they must be chewed thoroughly before swallowing. Follow with at least ½ glass of water.
- Shake suspensions well before administration.
- For an antacid effect, administer 1–3 hr after meals and at bedtime.

Patient/Family Teaching

- Caution patient to consult health care professional before taking antacids for more than 2 wk if problem is recurring, if relief is not obtained, or if symptoms of gastric bleeding (black, tarry stools; coffee-ground emesis) occur.
- Advise patient not to take this medication within 2 hr of taking other medications.
- Pedi: Aluminum- or magnesium-containing medicines can cause serious side effects in children, especially when given to children with renal disease or dehydration. Advise parents or caregivers not to administer OTC antacids to children without consulting health care professional.

Evaluation/Desired Outcomes

- Relief of gastric pain and irritation.

magnesium salicylate, See SALICYLATES.

MAGNESIUM SALTS (ORAL)

magnesium chloride (12% Mg; 9.8 mEq Mg/g)
(mag-**nee**-zhum **klor**-ide)
Chloromag, Slo-Mag

magnesium citrate (16.2% Mg; 4.4 mEq Mg/g)
(mag-**nee**-zhum **si**-trate)
Citrate of Magnesia, Citroma,
✱Citromag

magnesium gluconate (5.4% Mg; 4.4 mEq/g)
(mag-**nee**-zhum **gloo**-con-ate)
Magtrate, Magonate

magnesium hydroxide (41.7% Mg; 34.3 mEq Mg/g)
(mag-**nee**-zhum hye-**drox**-ide)
Dulcolax Magnesia Tablets, Phillips Magnesia Tablets, Phillips Milk of Magnesia, MOM

magnesium oxide (60.3% Mg; 49.6 mEq Mg/g)
(mag-**nee**-zhum **ox**-ide)
Mag-Ox 400, Uro-Mag

Classification
Therapeutic: mineral and electrolyte replacements/supplements, laxatives
Pharmacologic: salines

Pregnancy Category UK

Indications

Treatment/prevention of hypomagnesemia. As a: Laxative, Bowel evacuant in preparation for surgical/radiographic procedures. Milk of Magnesia has also been used as an antacid.

Action

Essential for the activity of many enzymes. Play an important role in neurotransmission and muscular excitability. Are osmotically active in GI tract, drawing water into the lumen and causing peristalsis. **Therapeutic Effects:** Replacement in deficiency states. Evacuation of the colon.

Pharmacokinetics

Absorption: Up to 30% may be absorbed orally.
Distribution: Widely distributed. Cross the placenta and are present in breast milk.
Metabolism and Excretion: Excreted primarily by the kidneys.
Half-life: Unknown.

TIME/ACTION PROFILE (laxative effect)

ROUTE	ONSET	PEAK	DURATION
PO	3–6 hr	unknown	unknown

Contraindications/Precautions

Contraindicated in: Hypermagnesemia; Hypocalcemia; Anuria; Heart block; OB: Unless used for preterm labor, use during active labor or within 2 hr of delivery may ↑ potential for magnesium toxicity in newborn.
Use Cautiously in: Any degree of renal insufficiency.

Adverse Reactions/Side Effects

GI: <u>diarrhea</u>. **Derm:** flushing, sweating.

Interactions

Drug-Drug: Potentiates **neuromuscular blocking agents**. May ↓ absorption of **fluoroquinolones, nitrofurantoin**, and **tetracyclines** and **penicillamine**.

Route/Dosage

Prevention of Deficiency (in mg of Magnesium)

PO (Adults and Children >10 yr): *Adolescent and adult men*—270–400 mg/day; *adolescent and adult women*—280–300 mg/day; *pregnant women*—320 mg/day; *breast-feeding women*—340–355 mg/day.
PO (Children 7–10 yr): 170 mg/day.
PO (Children 4–6 yr): 120 mg/day.
PO (Children birth–3 yr): 40–80 mg/day.

Treatment of Deficiency (Expressed as mg of Magnesium)

PO (Adults): 200–400 mg/day in 3–4 divided doses.
PO (Children 6–11 yr): 3–6 mg/kg/day in 3–4 divided doses.

Laxative

PO (Adults): *Magnesium citrate*—240 mL; *magnesium hydroxide (Milk of Magnesia)*—30–60 mL single or divided dose or 10–20 mL as concentrate.
PO (Children 6–12 yr): *Magnesium citrate*—100 mL; *magnesium hydroxide (Milk of Magnesia)*—15–30 mL single or divided dose.
PO (Children 2–5 yr): *magnesium hydroxide (Milk of Magnesia)*—5–15 mL single or divided dose.

Availability

Magnesium Chloride (generic available)

Sustained-release tablets: 535 mg (64 mg magnesium)^{OTC}. **Enteric-coated tablets:** 833 mg (100 mg magnesium)^{OTC}.

Magnesium Citrate (generic available)

Oral solution: 240-, 296-, and 300-mL bottles (77 mEq magnesium/100 mL)^{OTC}.

Magnesium Gluconate (generic available)

Tablets: 500 mg^{OTC}. **Liquid:** 54 mg/5 mL^{OTC}.

Magnesium Hydroxide (generic available)

Liquid: 400 mg/5 mL (164 mg magnesium/5 mL)^{OTC}. **Concentrated liquid:** 800 mg/5 mL (328 mg magnesium/5 mL)^{OTC}. **Chewable tablets:** 300 mg (130 mg magnesium)^{OTC}, 600 mg (260 mg magnesium)^{OTC}.

Magnesium Oxide (generic available)

Tablets: 400 mg (241.3 mg magnesium)^{OTC}. **Capsules:** 140 mg (84.5 mg magnesium)^{OTC}.

NURSING IMPLICATIONS

Assessment

- **Laxative:** Assess patient for abdominal distention, presence of bowel sounds, and usual pattern of bowel function.
- Assess color, consistency, and amount of stool produced.
- **Antacid:** Assess for heartburn and indigestion as well as location, duration, character, and precipitating factors of gastric pain.

Potential Nursing Diagnoses

Constipation (Indications)

Implementation

- **PO:** To prevent tablets entering small intestine in undissolved form, they must be chewed thoroughly before swallowing. Follow with ½ glass of water.
- *Magnesium citrate:* Refrigerate solutions to ensure they retain potency and palatability. May be served over ice. Magnesium citrate in an open container will lose carbonation upon standing; this will not affect potency but may reduce palatability.
- *Magnesium hydroxide:* Shake solution well before administration.
- **Antacid:** Administer 1–3 hr after meals and at bedtime.
- Powder and liquid forms are considered more effective than tablets.
- **Laxative:** Administer on empty stomach for more rapid results. Follow all oral laxative doses with a full glass of liquid to prevent dehydration and for faster effect. Do not administer at bedtime or late in the day.

Patient/Family Teaching

- Advise patient not to take this medication within 2 hr of taking other medications, especially fluoroquinolones, nitrofurantoin, and tetracyclines.
- **Antacids:** Caution patient to consult health care professional before taking antacids for more than 2 wk if problem is recurring, if relief is not obtained, or if symptoms of gastric bleeding (black, tarry stools; coffee-ground emesis) occur.
- **Laxatives:** Advise patient that laxatives should be used only for short-term therapy. Long-term therapy may cause electrolyte imbalance and dependence.
- Encourage patient to use other forms of bowel regulation, such as increasing bulk in the diet, fluid intake, and mobility. Normal bowel habits are individualized; frequency of bowel movement may vary from 3 times/day to 3 times/wk.
- Advise patient to notify health care professional if unrelieved constipation, rectal bleeding, or symptoms of electrolyte imbalance (muscle cramps or pain, weakness, dizziness) occur.

Evaluation/Desired Outcomes

- Relief of gastric pain and irritation.
- Passage of a soft, formed bowel movement, usually within 3–6 hr.
- Prevention and treatment of magnesium deficiency.

M

HIGH ALERT

magnesium sulfate (IV, parenteral) (9.9% Mg; 8.1 mEq Mg/g)

(mag-**nee**-zhum **sul**-fate)

Classification

Therapeutic: mineral and electrolyte replacements/supplements

Pharmacologic: minerals/electrolytes

Pregnancy Category D

Indications

Treatment/prevention of hypomagnesemia. Treatment of hypertension. Prevention of seizures associated with severe eclampsia, pre-eclampsia, or acute nephritis. **Unlabeled Use:** Preterm labor. Treatment of torsade de pointes. Adjunctive treatment for bronchodilation in moderate to severe acute asthma.

Action

Essential for the activity of many enzymes. Plays an important role in neurotransmission and muscular excitability. **Therapeutic Effects:** Replacement in deficiency states. Resolution of eclampsia.

Pharmacokinetics

Absorption: IV administration results in complete bioavailability; well absorbed from IM sites.
Distribution: Widely distributed. Crosses the placenta and is present in breast milk.
Metabolism and Excretion: Excreted primarily by the kidneys.
Half-life: Unknown.

TIME/ACTION PROFILE (anticonvulsant effect)

ROUTE	ONSET	PEAK	DURATION
IM	60 min	unknown	3–4 hr
IV	immediate	unknown	30 min

Contraindications/Precautions

Contraindicated in: Hypermagnesemia; Hypocalcemia; Anuria; Heart block; OB: Avoid using for more than 5–7 days for preterm labor (may ↑ risk of hypocalcemia and bone changes in newborn); avoid continuous use during active labor or within 2 hr of delivery due to potential for magnesium toxicity in newborn.
Use Cautiously in: Any degree of renal insufficiency; Geri: May require ↓ dosage due to age-related ↓ in renal function.

Adverse Reactions/Side Effects

CNS: drowsiness. **Resp:** ↓ respiratory rate. **CV:** arrhythmias, bradycardia, hypotension. **GI:** diarrhea. **MS:** muscle weakness. **Derm:** flushing, sweating. **Metab:** hypothermia.

Interactions

Drug-Drug: May potentiate **calcium channel blockers** and **neuromuscular blocking agents.**

Route/Dosage

Treatment of Deficiency (Expressed as mg of Magnesium)

IM, IV (Adults): *Severe deficiency*—8–12 g/day in divided doses; *mild deficiency*—1 g q 6 hr for 4 doses or 250 mg/kg over 4 hr.
IM, IV (Children >1 mo): 25–50 mg/kg/dose q 4–6 hr for 3–4 doses, maximum single dose: 2 g.
IV (Neonates): 25–50 mg/kg/dose q 8–12 hr for 2–3 doses.

Seizures/Hypertension

IM, IV (Adults): 1 g q 6 hr for 4 doses as needed.
IM, IV (Children): 20–100 mg/kg/dose q 4–6 hr as needed, may use up to 200 mg/kg/dose in severe cases.

Torsade de Pointes

IV (Infants and Children): 25–50 mg/kg/dose, maximum dose: 2 g.

Bronchodilation

IV (Adults): 2 g single dose.
IV (Children): 25 mg/kg/dose, maximum dose: 2 g.

Eclampsia/Pre-Eclampsia

IV, IM (Adults): 4–5 g by IV infusion, concurrently with up to 5 g IM in each buttock; then 4–5 g IM q 4 hr *or* 4 g by IV infusion followed by 1–2 g/hr continuous infusion (not to exceed 40 g/day or 20 g/48 hr in the presence of severe renal insufficiency).

Part of Parenteral Nutrition

IV (Adults): 4–24 mEq/day.
IV (Children): 0.25–0.5 mEq/kg/day.

Availability (generic available)

Injection: 500 mg/mL (50%). **Premixed infusion:** 1 g/100 mL, 2 g/100 mL, 4 g/50 mL, 4 g/100 mL, 20 g/500 mL, 40 g/1000 mL.

NURSING IMPLICATIONS

Assessment

- **Hypomagnesemia/Anticonvulsant:** Monitor pulse, BP, respirations, and ECG frequently throughout administration of parenteral magnesium sulfate. Respirations should be at least 16/min before each dose.
- Monitor neurologic status before and throughout therapy. Institute seizure precautions. Patellar reflex (knee jerk) should be tested before each parenteral dose of magnesium sulfate. If response is absent, no additional doses should be administered until positive response is obtained.
- Monitor newborn for hypotension, hyporeflexia, and respiratory depression if mother has received magnesium sulfate.

- Monitor intake and output ratios. Urine output should be maintained at a level of at least 100 mL/4 hr.
- ***Lab Test Considerations:*** Monitor serum magnesium levels and renal function periodically throughout administration of parenteral magnesium sulfate.

Potential Nursing Diagnoses

Risk for injury (Indications, Side Effects)

Implementation

- ***High Alert:*** Accidental overdosage of IV magnesium has resulted in serious patient harm and death. Have second practitioner independently double-check original order, dose calculations, and infusion pump settings. Do not confuse milligram (mg), gram (g), or millequivalent (mEq) dosages.
- **IM:** Administer deep IM into gluteal sites. Administer subsequent injections in alternate sides. Dilute to a concentration of 200 mg/mL prior to injection.

IV Administration

- **IV Push:** ***Diluent:*** 50% solution must be diluted in 0.9% NaCl or D5W to a concentration of ≤20% prior to administration. ***Concentration:*** ≤20%. ***Rate:*** Administer at a rate not to exceed 150 mg/min.
- **Continuous Infusion:** ***Diluent:*** Dilute in D5W, 0.9% NaCl, or LR. ***Concentration:*** 0.5 mEq/mL (60 mg/mL) (may use maximum concentration of 1.6 mEq/mL) (200 mg/mL) in fluid-restricted patients). ***Rate:*** Infuse over 2–4 hr. Do not exceed a rate of 1 mEq/kg/hr (125 mg/kg/hr). When rapid infusions are needed (severe asthma or torsade de pointes) may infuse over 10–20 min.
- **Y-Site Compatibility:** acyclovir, aldesleukin, alemtuzumab, alfentanil, amifostine, amikacin, argatroban, ascorbic acid, atropine, azithromycin, aztreonam, benztropine, bivalirudin, bleomycin, bumetanide, buprenorphine, butorphanol, calcium gluconate, carboplatin, carmustine, caspofungin, cefotaxime, cefoxitin, ceftazidime, chloramphenicol, chlorpromazine, cisatracurium, cisplatin, clindamycin, clonidine, cyanocobalamin, cyclophosphamide, cytarabine, dactinomycin, daptomycin, dexmedetomidine, dexrazoxane, digoxin, diltiazem, diphenhydramine, dobutamine, docetaxel, dolasetron, dopamine, doripenem, doxacurium, doxorubicin liposome, doxycycline, enalaprilat, ephedrine, epinephrine, epoetin alfa, eptifibatide, ertapenem, esmolol, etoposide, etoposide phosphate, famotidine, fenoldopam, fentanyl, fluconazole, fludarabine, fluorouracil, folic acid, foscarnet, gemcitabine, gentamicin, glycopyrrolate, granisetron, heparin, hetastarch, hydromorphone, idarubicin, ifosfamide, imipenem/cilastatin, insulin, irinotecan, isoproterenol, ketamine, ketorolac, labetalol, calcium, lidocaine, linezolid, lorazepam, mannitol, mechlorethamine, methotrexate, methyldopate, metoclopramide, metoprolol, metronidazole, micafungin, midazolam, milrinone, mitoxantrone, morphine, moxifloxacin, multivitamins, mycophenolate, nafcillin, nalbuphine, nesiritide, nicardipine, nitroglycerin, nitroprusside, norepinephrine, octreotide, ondansetron, oxaliplatin, oxytocin, paclitaxel, palonosetron, pamidronate, pancuronium, pantoprazole, papaverine, pemetrexed, penicillin G, pentazocine, pentobarbital, phenobarbital, phentolamine, phenylephrine, piperacillin/tazobactam, potassium acetate, potassium chloride, procainamide, prochlorperazine, promethazine, propranolol, propofol, propranolol, pyridoxime, quinupristin/dalfopristin, ranitidine, remifentanil, rituximab, rocuronium, sargramostim, sodium acetate, sodium bicarbonate, streptokinase, succinylcholine, sufentanil, tacrolimus, telavancin, teniposide, theophylline, thiamine, thiotepa, tigecycline, tirofiban, tobramycin, tolazoline, trastuzumab, trimetaphan, vancomycin, vasopressin, vecuronium, verapamil, vinblastine, vincristine, vinorelbine, vitamin B complex with C, voriconazole, zoledronic acid.
- **Y-Site Incompatibility:** aminophylline, amphotericin B cholesteryl sulfate, amphotericin B lipid complex, amphotericin B liposome, anidulafungin, azathioprine, calcium chloride, cefepime, ceftriaxone, cefuroxime, ciprofloxacin, dantrolene, dexamethasone sodium phosphate, diazepam, diazoxide, doxorubicin hydrochloride, epirubicin, ganciclovir, haloperidol, indomethacin, methylprednisolone sodium succinate, pentamidine, phenytoin, phytonadione.

Patient/Family Teaching

- Explain purpose of medication to patient and family.

Evaluation/Desired Outcomes

- Normal serum magnesium concentrations.
- Control of seizures associated with toxemias of pregnancy.

mannitol (man-i-tol)
Osmitrol, Resectisol

Classification
Therapeutic: diuretics
Pharmacologic: osmotic diuretics

Pregnancy Category C

Indications

IV: Adjunct in the treatment of: Acute oliguric renal failure, Edema, Increased intracranial or intraocular pressure, Toxic overdose. **GU irrigant:** During transurethral procedures (2.5–5% solution only).

Action

Increases the osmotic pressure of the glomerular filtrate, thereby inhibiting reabsorption of water and electrolytes. Causes excretion of: Water, Sodium, Potassium, Chloride, Calcium, Phosphorus, Magnesium, Urea, Uric acid. **Therapeutic Effects:** Mobilization of excess fluid in oliguric renal failure or edema. Reduction of intraocular or intracranial pressure. Increased urinary excretion of toxic materials. Decreased hemolysis when used as an irrigant after transurethral prostatic resection.

Pharmacokinetics

Absorption: IV administration produces complete bioavailability. Some absorption may follow use as a GU irrigant.
Distribution: Confined to the extracellular space; does not usually cross the blood-brain barrier or eye.
Metabolism and Excretion: Excreted by the kidneys; minimal liver metabolism.
Half-life: 100 min.

TIME/ACTION PROFILE (diuretic effect)

ROUTE	ONSET	PEAK	DURATION
IV	30–60 min	1 hr	6–8 hr

Contraindications/Precautions

Contraindicated in: Hypersensitivity; Anuria; Dehydration; Active intracranial bleeding; Severe pulmonary edema or congestion.
Use Cautiously in: OB, Lactation: Safety not established.

Adverse Reactions/Side Effects

CNS: confusion, headache. **EENT:** blurred vision, rhinitis. **CV:** transient volume expansion, chest pain, HF, pulmonary edema, tachycardia. **GI:** nausea, thirst, vomiting. **GU:** renal failure, urinary retention. **F and E:** dehydration, hyperkalemia, hypernatremia, hypokalemia, hyponatremia. **Local:** phlebitis at IV site.

Interactions

Drug-Drug: Hypokalemia ↑ the risk of **digoxin** toxicity.

Route/Dosage

IV (Adults): *Edema, oliguric renal failure*—50–100 g as a 5–25% solution; may precede with a test dose of 0.2 g/kg over 3–5 min. *Reduction of intracranial/intraocular pressure*—0.25–2 g/kg as 15–25% solution over 30–60 min (500 mg/kg may be sufficient in small or debilitated patients). *Diuresis in drug intoxications*—50–200 g as a 5–25% solution titrated to maintain urine flow of 100–500 mL/hr.
IV (Children): *Initial*—0.5–1 g/kg as a 15–20% solution; may precede with a test dose of 0.2 g/kg over 3–5 min. *Maintenance*—0.25–0.5 g/kg q 4–6 hrs. *Reduction of intracranial/intraocular pressure*—1–2 g/kg (30–60 g/m²) as a 15–20% solution over 30–60 min (500 mg/kg may be sufficient in small or debilitated patients). *Diuresis in drug intoxications*—up to 2 g/kg (60 g/m²) as a 5–10% solution.
IV (Neonates): *Acute renal failure*—0.5–1 g/kg/dose.

Availability (generic available)

IV injection: 5%, 10%, 15%, 20%, 25%. **GU irrigant:** 5%.

NURSING IMPLICATIONS

Assessment

- Monitor vital signs, urine output, CVP, and pulmonary artery pressures (PAP) before and hourly throughout administration. Assess patient for signs and symptoms of dehydration (decreased skin turgor, fever, dry skin and mucous membranes, thirst) or signs of fluid overload (increased CVP, dyspnea, rales/crackles, edema).
- Assess patient for anorexia, muscle weakness, numbness, tingling, paresthesia, confusion, and excessive thirst. Report signs of electrolyte imbalance.
- **Increased Intracranial Pressure:** Monitor neurologic status and intracranial pressure readings in patients receiving this medication to decrease cerebral edema.
- **Increased Intraocular Pressure:** Monitor for persistent or increased eye pain or decreased visual acuity.
- ***Lab Test Considerations:*** Renal function and serum electrolytes should be monitored routinely throughout therapy.

Potential Nursing Diagnoses

Excess fluid volume (Indications)
Risk for deficient fluid volume (Side Effects)

Implementation

- Observe infusion site frequently for infiltration. Extravasation may cause tissue irritation and necrosis.
- Do not administer electrolyte-free mannitol solution with blood. If blood must be administered simultaneously with mannitol, add at least 20 mEq NaCl to each liter of mannitol.
- Confer with health care professional regarding placement of an indwelling Foley catheter (except when used to decrease intraocular pressure).
- **IV:** Administer by IV infusion undiluted. If solution contains crystals, warm bottle in hot water and shake vigorously. Do not administer solution in which crystals remain undissolved. Cool to body temperature. Use an in-line filter for 15%, 20%, and 25% infusions.
- **Test Dose:** Administer over 3–5 min to produce a urine output of 30–50 mL/hr. If urine flow does not increase, administer 2nd test dose. If urine output is not at least 30–50 mL/hr for 2–3 hr after 2nd test dose, patient should be re-evaluated.
- **Oliguria:** Administration rate should be titrated to produce a urine output of 30–50 mL/hr. Administer child's dose over 2–6 hr.

- **Increased Intracranial Pressure:** Infuse dose over 30–60 min in adults and children.
- **Intraocular Pressure:** Administer dose over 30 min. When used preoperatively, administer 60–90 min before surgery.
- **Y-Site Compatibility:** acetaminophen, acyclovir, alemtuzumab, alfentanil, allopurinol, amifostine, amikacin, aminocaproic acid, aminophylline, amiodarone, amphotericin B lipid complex, ampicillin, anidulafungan, argatroban, ascorbic acid, atropine, azithromycin, aztreonam, benztropine, bivalirudin, bleomycin, bumetanide, buprenorphine, butorphanol, calcium chloride, calcium gluconate, cangrelor, carboplatin, carmustine, caspofungin, cefazolin, cefotaxime, cefotetan, cefoxitin, ceftaroline, ceftazidime, ceftriaxone, cefuroxime, chloramphenicol, chlorpromazine, cisatracurium, cisplatin, cladribine, clindamycin, cyanocobalamin, cyclophosphamide, cyclosporine, cytarabine, dacarbazine, dactinomycin, daptomycin, daunorubicin hydrochloride, dexamethasone, dexmedetomidine, dexrazoxane, digoxin, diltiazem, diphenhydramine, dobutamine, docetaxel, dolasetron, dopamine, doripenem, doxorubicin hydrochloride, doxycycline, enalaprilat, ephedrine, epinephrine, epirubicin, epoetin alfa, eptifibatide, ertapenem, erythromycin, esmolol, etoposide, etoposide phosphate, famotidine, fenoldopam, fentanyl, fluconazole, fludarabine, fluorouracil, folic acid, foscarnet, fosphenytoin, furosemide, ganciclovir, gemcitabine, gentamicin, glycopyrrolate, granisetron, heparin, hetastarch, hydrocortisone, hydromorphone, idarubicin, ifosfamide, indomethacin, insulin, irinotecan, isoproterenol, ketorolac, labetalol, leucovorin, levofloxacin, lidocaine, linezolid, lorazepam, magnesium sulfate, melphalan, meperidine, mesna, methotrexate, methyldopate, methylprednisolone, metoclopramide, metoprolol, metronidazole, midazolam, milrinone, mitomycin, mitoxantrone, morphine, moxifloxacin, multivitamins, mycophenolate, nafcillin, nalbuphine, naloxone, nesiritide, nicardipine, nitroglycerin, nitroprusside, norepinephrine, octreotide, ondansetron, oxacillin, oxaliplatin, oxytocin, paclitaxel, palonosetron, pamidronate, pancuronium, papaverine, pemetrexed, penicillin G, pentamidine, pentazocine, pentobarbital, phenobarbital, phenylephrine, phytonadione, piperacillin/tazobactam, potassium acetate, potassium chloride, procainamide, prochlorperazine, promethazine, propofol, propranolol, protamine, pyridoxine, quinupristin/dalfopristin, ranitidine, remifentanil, rituximab, rocuronium, sargramostim, sodium acetate, sodium bicarbonate, streptokinase, succinylcholine, sufentanil, tacrolimus, telavancin, teniposide, theophylline, thiamine, thiotepa , tigecycline, tirofiban, tobramycin, topotecan, trastuzumab, vancomycin, vasopressin, vecuronium, verapamil, vinblastine, vincristine, vinorelbine, voriconazole, zoledronic acid.
- **Y-Site Incompatibility:** amphotericin B liposome, cefepime, dantrolene, diazepam, doxorubicin liposomal, filgrastim, imipenem/cilastatin, phenytoin, trimethoprim/sulfamethoxazole.
- **Irrigation:** Add contents of two 50-mL vials of 25% mannitol to 900 mL of sterile water for injection for a 2.5% solution for irrigation. Use only clear solutions.

Patient/Family Teaching

- Explain purpose of therapy to patient.

Evaluation/Desired Outcomes

- Urine output of at least 30–50 mL/hr or an increase in urine output in accordance with parameters set by health care professional.
- Reduction in intracranial pressure.
- Reduction of intraocular pressure.
- Excretion of certain toxic substances.
- Irrigation during transurethral prostate resection.

M

meclizine (mek-li-zeen)

Antivert, Bonine, Dramamine Less Drowsy Formula

Classification

Therapeutic: antiemetics, antihistamines

Pregnancy Category B

Indications

Management/prevention of: Motion sickness, Vertigo.

Action

Has central anticholinergic, CNS depressant, and antihistaminic properties. Decreases excitability of the middle ear labyrinth and depresses conduction in middle ear vestibular-cerebellar pathways. **Therapeutic Effects:** Decreased motion sickness. Decreased vertigo from vestibular pathology.

Pharmacokinetics

Absorption: Absorbed after oral administration.
Distribution: Unknown.
Metabolism and Excretion: Unknown.
Half-life: 6 hr.

TIME/ACTION PROFILE (antihistaminic effects)

ROUTE	ONSET	PEAK	DURATION
PO	1 hr	unknown	8–24 hr

Contraindications/Precautions

Contraindicated in: Hypersensitivity; OB: Has caused congenital malformations (cleft palate) in animal studies.

Use Cautiously in: Prostatic hyperplasia; Angle-closure glaucoma; Lactation: Occasional use may be acceptable; prolonged use may expose infant to drug effects or may interfere with milk supply; Pedi: Children <12 yr (safety not established); Geri: ↑ sensitivity and risk of adverse reactions.

Adverse Reactions/Side Effects

CNS: drowsiness, fatigue. **EENT:** blurred vision. **GI:** dry mouth.

Interactions

Drug-Drug: Additive CNS depression with other **CNS depressants**, including **alcohol**, other **antihistamines**, **opioid analgesics**, and **sedative/hypnotics**. Additive anticholinergic effects with other **drugs possessing anticholinergic properties**, including some **antihistamines**, **antidepressants**, **atropine**, **haloperidol**, **phenothiazines**, **quinidine**, and **disopyramide**. **CYP2D6 inhibitors** may ↑ levels.

Route/Dosage

PO (Adults and Children ≥12 yr): *Motion sickness*—25–50 mg 1 hr before exposure; may repeat in 24 hr; *vertigo*—25–100 mg/day in divided doses.

Availability (generic available)

Tablets: 12.5 mg, 25 mg$^{Rx, OTC}$, 50 mg.

NURSING IMPLICATIONS

Assessment

- Assess patient for level of sedation after administration.
- **Motion Sickness:** Assess patient for nausea and vomiting before and 60 min after administration.
- **Vertigo:** Assess degree of vertigo periodically in patients receiving meclizine for labyrinthitis.
- ***Lab Test Considerations:*** May cause false-negative results in skin tests using allergen extracts. Discontinue meclizine 72 hr before testing.

Potential Nursing Diagnoses

Risk for injury (Side Effects)

Implementation

- Do not confuse Antivert (meclizine) with Axert (almotriptan).
- **PO:** Administer oral doses with food, water, or milk to minimize GI irritation.

Patient/Family Teaching

- Instruct patient to take meclizine exactly as directed. If a dose is missed, take as soon as possible unless almost time for next dose. Do not double doses.
- May cause drowsiness. Caution patient to avoid driving or other activities requiring alertness until response to the medication is known.
- Advise patient that frequent mouth rinses, good oral hygiene, and sugarless gum or candy may decrease dryness of mouth.
- Caution patient to avoid concurrent use of alcohol and other CNS depressants with this medication.
- **Motion Sickness:** When used as prophylaxis for motion sickness, advise patient to take medication at least 1 hr before exposure to conditions that may cause motion sickness.

Evaluation/Desired Outcomes

- Prevention and relief of symptoms in motion sickness.
- Prevention and treatment of vertigo due to vestibular pathology.

medroxyPROGESTERone†

(me-**drox**-ee-proe-**jess**-te-rone)

Depo-Provera, Depo-Sub Q Provera 104, ✤Medroxy, Provera

Classification

Therapeutic: antineoplastics, contraceptive hormones

Pharmacologic: hormones, progestins

Pregnancy Category X

†For contraceptive use see Contraceptives, Hormonal monograph

Indications

To decrease endometrial hyperplasia in postmenopausal women receiving concurrent estrogen (0.625 mg/day conjugated estrogens). Treatment of secondary amenorrhea and abnormal uterine bleeding caused by hormonal imbalance. **IM:** Treatment of advanced unresponsive endometrial or renal carcinoma. †Prevention of pregnancy. Management of endometriosis-associated pain (Depo-Sub Q Provera 104 only). **Unlabeled Use:** Obesity-hypoventilation (pickwickian) syndrome. Sleep apnea. Hypersomnolence.

Action

A synthetic form of progesterone—actions include secretory changes in the endometrium, increases in basal body temperature, histologic changes in vaginal epithelium, relaxation of uterine smooth muscle, mammary alveolar tissue growth, pituitary inhibition, and withdrawal bleeding in the presence of estrogen. **Therapeutic Effects:** Decreased endometrial hyperplasia in postmenopausal women receiving concurrent estrogen (combination with estrogen decreases vasomotor symptoms and prevents osteoporosis). Restoration of hormonal balance with control of uterine bleeding. Management of endometrial or renal cancer. Prevention of pregnancy.

Pharmacokinetics

Absorption: 0.6–10% absorbed after oral administration.

Distribution: Enters breast milk.
Metabolism and Excretion: Metabolized by the liver.
Half-life: *1st phase*—52 min; *2nd phase*—230 min; *biological*—14.5 hr.

TIME/ACTION PROFILE (IM = antineoplastic effects)

ROUTE	ONSET	PEAK	DURATION
PO	unknown	unknown	unknown
IM	wk–mos	mo	unknown†
SC	unknown	1 wk	3 mo

†Contraceptive effect lasts 3 mo.

Contraindications/Precautions

Contraindicated in: Hypersensitivity; Hypersensitivity to parabens (IM suspension only); Missed abortion; Thromboembolic disease; Cerebrovascular disease; Severe liver disease; Breast or genital cancer; Porphyria; OB: May ↑ risk of fetal genitourinary malformation.
Use Cautiously in: History of liver disease; Renal disease; Cardiovascular disease; Seizure disorders; Mental depression; Lactation: If used as a contraceptive, wait 6 wk after delivery if breast feeding.

Adverse Reactions/Side Effects

CNS: depression. **EENT:** retinal thrombosis. **CV:** PULMONARY EMBOLISM, thromboembolism, thrombophlebitis. **GI:** drug-induced hepatitis, gingival bleeding. **GU:** cervical erosions. **Derm:** chloasma, melasma, rashes. **Endo:** amenorrhea, breakthrough bleeding, breast tenderness, changes in menstrual flow, galactorrhea, hyperglycemia, spotting. **F and E:** edema. **Metab:** bone loss. **Misc:** allergic reactions including ANAPHYLAXIS and ANGIOEDEMA, BREAST CANCER, weight gain, weight loss.

Interactions

Drug-Drug: Strong **CYP3A4 inhibitors**, including **ketoconazole**, **itraconazole**, **clarithromycin**, **atazanavir**, **indinavir**, **nefazodone**, **nelfinavir**, **ritonavir**, **saquinavir**, and **voriconazole** may ↑ levels; avoid concurrent use. Strong **CYP3A4 inducers**, including **phenytoin**, **carbamazepine**, **rifampin**, **rifabutin**, **rifapentin**, and **phenobarbital** may ↓ levels; avoid concurrent use. May ↓ effectiveness of **bromocriptine** when used concurrently for galactorrhea/amenorrhea. Contraceptive effectiveness may be ↓ by **carbamazepine**, **phenobarbital**, **phenytoin**, **rifampin**, or **rifabutin**.
Drug-Natural Products: St. John's wort may ↓ levels; avoid concurrent use.

Route/Dosage

Postmenopausal Women Receiving Concurrent Estrogen

PO (Adults): 2.5–5 mg daily concurrently with 0.625 mg conjugated estrogens (monophasic regimen) *or* 5 mg daily on days 15–28 of the cycle with 0.625 mg conjugated estrogens taken daily throughout cycle (biphasic regimen).

Secondary Amenorrhea

PO (Adults): 5–10 mg/day for 5–10 days; start at any time in cycle.

Dysfunctional Uterine Bleeding/Induction of Menses

PO (Adults): 5–10 mg/day for 5–10 days, starting on day 16 or day 21 of menstrual cycle.

Renal or Endometrial Carcinoma

IM (Adults): 400–1000 mg, may be repeated weekly; if improvement occurs, attempt to decrease dose to 400 mg monthly.

Endometriosis-Associated Pain

Subcut (Adults): 104 mg every 12–14 wk (3 mo), beginning on day 5 of normal menses (not recommended for more than 2 yr).

Availability (generic available)

Tablets: 2.5 mg, 5 mg, 10 mg, 🍁100 mg. **Suspension for depot injection:** 🍁50 mg/mL, 150 mg/mL, 400 mg/mL. **Suspension for subcutaneous injection (Depo-Sub Q Provera 104):** 104 mg/0.65 mL. ***In combination with:*** conjugated estrogens as Prempro (single combination tablet of 0.626 mg conjugated estrogens plus 2.5 or 5 mg medroxyprogesterone) or Premphase (0.625 mg conjugated estrogens tablet for 14 days followed by combination tablet of 0.625 mg conjugated estrogens plus 5 mg medroxyprogesterone for days 15–28) in convenience packages. See Appendix B.

NURSING IMPLICATIONS

Assessment

- Monitor BP periodically during therapy.
- Assess patient's usual menstrual history. Administration of drug may begin on any day of cycle in patients with amenorrhea and on day 16 or 21 of cycle in patients with dysfunctional bleeding.
- Monitor intake and output ratios and weekly weight. Report significant discrepancies or steady weight gain.
- ***Lab Test Considerations:*** Monitor hepatic function before and periodically during therapy.
- May cause ↑ alkaline phosphatase levels. May ↓ pregnanediol excretion concentrations.

M

- May cause ↑ serum LDL concentrations or ↓ HDL concentrations.
- May alter thyroid hormone assays.

Potential Nursing Diagnoses

Sexual dysfunction (Indications)
Ineffective tissue perfusion (Side Effects)

Implementation

- Do not confuse Depo-Provera with Depo-subQ Provera 104. Do not confuse Provera (medroxyprogesterone) with Proscar (finasteride) or Prozac (fluoxetine).
- Only the 150 mg/mL vial should be used for contraception.
- Injectable medroxyprogesterone may lead to bone loss, especially in women younger than 21 yr. Injectable medroxyprogesterone should be used for >2 yr only if other methods of contraception are inadequate. If used long term, women should use supplemental calcium and vitamin D, and monitor bone mineral density.
- **Subcut:** Shake vigorously before use to form a uniform suspension. Inject slowly (over 5–7 seconds) at a 45° angle into fatty area of anterior thigh or abdomen every 12 to 14 wk. If more than 14 wk elapse between injections, rule out pregnancy prior to administration. **Do not rub area after injection**.
- When switching from other hormonal contraceptives, administer within dosing period (7 days after taking last active pill, removing patch or ring, or within the dosing period for IM injection).
- **IM:** Shake vial vigorously before preparing IM dose. Administer deep IM into gluteal or deltoid muscle. If period between injections is >14 wk, determine that patient is not pregnant before administering the drug.
- In patients with cancer, IM dose may initially be required weekly. Once stabilized, IM dose may be required only monthly.

Patient/Family Teaching

- Explain the dose schedule. Instruct patient to take medication at the same time each day. Take missed doses as soon as remembered, but do not double doses.
- Advise patients receiving medroxyprogesterone for menstrual dysfunction to anticipate withdrawal bleeding 3–7 days after discontinuing medication.
- Review patient package insert (PPI) with patient. Emphasize the importance of notifying health care professional if the following side effects occur: visual changes, sudden weakness, incoordination, difficulty with speech, headache, leg or calf pain, shortness of breath, chest pain, changes in vaginal bleeding pattern, yellow skin, swelling of extremities, depression, or rash. Patients receiving medroxyprogesterone for cancer may not receive PPI.
- Advise patient to keep a 1-mo supply of medroxyprogesterone available at all times.
- Instruct patient in correct method of monthly breast self-examination. Increased breast tenderness may occur.
- Advise patient that gingival bleeding may occur. Instruct patient to use good oral hygiene and to receive regular dental care and examinations.
- Medroxyprogesterone may cause melasma (brown patches of discoloration) on face when patient is exposed to sunlight. Advise patient to avoid sun exposure and to wear sunscreen or protective clothing when outdoors.
- Rep: Instruct patient to notify health care professional if menstrual period is missed or if pregnancy is suspected. Patient should not attempt conception for 3 mo after discontinuing medication in order to decrease risk to fetus.
- Emphasize the importance of routine follow-up physical exams, including BP; breast, abdomen, and pelvic exams; and Papanicolaou smears every 6–12 mo.
- **IM, Subcut:** Advise patient to maintain adequate amounts of dietary calcium and vitamin D to help prevent bone loss.

Evaluation/Desired Outcomes

- Regular menstrual periods.
- Decrease in endometrial hyperplasia in postmenopausal women receiving concurrent estrogen.
- Control of the spread of endometrial or renal cancer.
- Prevention of pregnancy.

medroxyprogesterone, See CONTRACEPTIVES, HORMONAL.

megestrol (me-jess-trole)

Megace, Megace ES, ✦Megace OS

Classification
Therapeutic: antineoplastics, hormones
Pharmacologic: progestins

Pregnancy Category D (tablets), X (suspension)

Indications

Palliative treatment of endometrial and breast carcinoma, either alone or with surgery or radiation (tablets only). Treatment of anorexia, weight loss, and cachexia associated with AIDS (oral suspension only).

Action

Antineoplastic effect may result from inhibition of pituitary function. **Therapeutic Effects:** Regression of tumor. Increased appetite and weight gain in patients with AIDS.

Pharmacokinetics

Absorption: Well absorbed from the GI tract.
Distribution: Unknown.
Protein Binding: ≥90%.
Metabolism and Excretion: Completely metabolized by the liver.
Half-life: 38 hr (range 13–104 hr).

TIME/ACTION PROFILE (antineoplastic activity)

ROUTE	ONSET	PEAK	DURATION
PO	wk–mos	2 mo	unknown

Contraindications/Precautions

Contraindicated in: Hypersensitivity; Undiagnosed vaginal bleeding; Severe liver disease; Suspension contains alcohol and should be avoided in patients with known intolerance; OB, Lactation: Pregnancy or lactation.
Use Cautiously in: Diabetes; Mental depression; Renal disease; History of thrombophlebitis; Cardiovascular disease; Seizure disorders.

Adverse Reactions/Side Effects

CV: THROMBOEMBOLISM, edema. **GI:** GI irritation. **Derm:** alopecia. **Endo:** asymptomatic adrenal suppression (chronic therapy). **GU:** vaginal bleeding. **Hemat:** thrombophlebitis. **MS:** carpal tunnel syndrome.

Interactions

Drug-Drug: None significant.

Route/Dosage

PO (Adults): *Breast carcinoma*— 160 mg/day single dose or divided doses; *Endometrial/ovarian carcinoma*— 40–320 mg/day in divided doses; *Anorexia associated with AIDS*—Megace: 800 mg once daily; may ↓ to 400 mg/day after 1 mo (range 400–800 mg/day); Megace ES: 625 mg once daily.

Availability (generic available)

Tablets: 20 mg, 40 mg, ✱160 mg. **Oral suspension (lemon-lime flavor):** 40 mg/mL, 125 mg/mL (Megace ES).

NURSING IMPLICATIONS

Assessment

- Assess for swelling, pain, or tenderness in legs. Report these signs of deep vein thrombophlebitis.
- **Anorexia:** Monitor weight, appetite, and nutritional intake in patients with AIDS.

Potential Nursing Diagnoses

Imbalanced nutrition: less than body requirements (Indications)

Implementation

- Because of high dose, suspension is most convenient form for patients with AIDS.
- Do not confuse *Megace* 40 mg/mL with *Megace ES* 125 mg/mL.
- **PO:** May be administered with meals if GI irritation becomes a problem.
- Shake suspension well before administering.

Patient/Family Teaching

- Instruct patient to take megestrol as directed; do not skip or double up on missed doses. Missed doses may be taken as long as not right before next dose. Gradually decrease dose prior to discontinuation.
- Advise patient to report to health care professional any unusual vaginal bleeding or signs of deep vein thrombophlebitis.
- Discuss with patient the possibility of hair loss. Explore methods of coping.
- Advise patient that this medication may have teratogenic effects. Contraception should be used during and for at least 4 mo after therapy is completed. Advise patient to notify health care professional immediately if pregnancy is planned or suspected or if breast feeding.

Evaluation/Desired Outcomes

- Slowing or arresting the spread of endometrial or breast malignancy. Therapeutic effects usually occur within 2 mo of initiating therapy.
- Increased appetite and weight gain in patients with AIDS.

M

meloxicam (me-lox-i-kam)

Mobic, ✱Mobicox

Classification
Therapeutic: nonsteroidal anti-inflammatory agents
Pharmacologic: nonopioid analgesics

Pregnancy Category C

Indications

Relief of signs and symptoms of osteoarthritis and rheumatoid arthritis (including juvenile rheumatoid arthritis).

Action

Inhibits prostaglandin synthesis, probably by inhibiting the enzyme cyclooxygenase. **Therapeutic Effects:** Decreased pain and inflammation associated with osteoarthritis. Also decreases fever.

Pharmacokinetics

Absorption: Well absorbed following oral administration.
Distribution: Unknown.
Protein Binding: 99.4%.

Metabolism and Excretion: Mostly metabolized to inactive metabolites by the liver via the P450 enzyme system; metabolites are excreted in urine and feces.
Half-life: 20.1 hr.

TIME/ACTION PROFILE

ROUTE	ONSET	PEAK†	DURATION
PO	unknown	5–6 hr	24 hr

†Blood levels.

Contraindications/Precautions

Contraindicated in: Hypersensitivity; Cross-sensitivity may occur with other NSAIDs, including aspirin; Severe renal impairment (CCr ≤15 mL/min); Concurrent use of aspirin (↑ risk of adverse reactions); Perioperative pain from coronary artery bypass graft (CABG) surgery; OB: Can cause premature closure of ductus arteriosus if used during third trimester.
Use Cautiously in: Cardiovascular disease or risk factors for cardiovascular disease (may ↑ risk of serious cardiovascular thrombotic events, myocardial infarction, and stroke, especially with prolonged use or use of higher doses); Dehydration (correct deficits before initiating therapy); Impaired renal function, heart failure, liver dysfunction, concurrent ACE inhibitor or diuretic therapy (↑ risk of renal dysfunction); Coagulation disorders or concurrent anticoagulant therapy (may ↑ risk of bleeding); Lactation: Safety not established; Pedi: Children <2 yr (safety not established); Geri: ↑ risk of GI bleeding and renal dysfuntion.

Adverse Reactions/Side Effects

CV: HF, MYOCARDIAL INFARCTION, STROKE, edema, hypertension. **GI:** GI BLEEDING, ↑ liver enzymes, diarrhea, dyspepsia, nausea. **Derm:** EXFOLIATIVE DERMATITIS, STEVENS-JOHNSON SYNDROME, TOXIC EPIDERMAL NECROLYSIS, pruritus. **GU:** delayed ovulation. **Hemat:** anemia, leukopenia, thrombocytopenia.

Interactions

Drug-Drug: May ↓ antihypertensive effects of **ACE inhibitors**. May ↓ diuretic effects of **furosemide** or **thiazide diuretics**. Concurrent use with **aspirin** ↑ meloxicam blood levels and may ↑ risk of adverse reactions. Concurrent use with **cholestyramine** ↓ blood levels. ↑ plasma **lithium** levels (close monitoring recommended when meloxicam is introduced or withdrawn). May ↑ risk of bleeding with **anticoagulants**, including **warfarin**. Concurrent use with **sodium polystyrene sulfonate** may ↑ risk of colonic necrosis; concurrent use should be avoided.

Route/Dosage

PO (Adults): 7.5 mg once daily; some patients may require 15 mg/day.
PO (Children 2–17 yr and >12 kg): 0.125 mg/kg once daily up to 7.5 mg/day.

Availability (generic available)

Tablets: 7.5 mg, 15 mg. **Cost:** *Generic*—7.5 mg $9.02/100, 15 mg $7.41/100.

NURSING IMPLICATIONS

Assessment

- Patients who have asthma, aspirin-induced allergy, and nasal polyps are at increased risk for developing hypersensitivity reactions. Assess for rhinitis, asthma, and urticaria.
- Assess pain and range of motion prior to and 1–2 hr following administration.
- Assess for rash periodically during therapy. May cause Stevens-Johnson syndrome or toxic epidermal necrolysis. Discontinue therapy if severe or if accompanied with fever, general malaise, fatigue, muscle or joint aches, blisters, oral lesions, conjunctivitis, hepatitis and/or eosinophilia.
- ***Lab Test Considerations:*** Evaluate BUN, serum creatinine, CBC, and liver function periodically in patients receiving prolonged therapy. May cause anemia, thrombocytopenia, leukopenia, and abnormal liver or renal function tests.
- Bleeding time may be prolonged.

Potential Nursing Diagnoses

Acute pain (Indications)
Impaired physical mobility (Indications)

Implementation

- Administration in higher than recommended doses does not provide increased effectiveness but may cause increased side effects. Use lowest effective dose for shortest period of time.
- **PO:** May be administered without regard to food.

Patient/Family Teaching

- Advise patient to take this medication with a full glass of water and to remain in an upright position for 15–30 min after administration.
- Instruct patient to take medication as directed. Take missed doses as soon as remembered but not if almost time for the next dose. Do not double doses. Instruct parent/caregiver to read the *Medication Guide* prior to use and with each Rx refill in case of changes.
- Caution patient to avoid the concurrent use of alcohol, aspirin, acetaminophen, or other OTC medications without consulting health care professional.
- Inform patient that meloxicam may increase the risk for heart attack and stroke; risk increases with longer use or in patients with heart disease.
- Advise patient to inform health care professional of medication regimen prior to treatment or surgery, especially right before or after coronary artery bypass graft (CABG).
- Advise patient to consult health care professional if rash, itching, visual disturbances, weight gain, edema, black stools, or signs of hepatotoxicity (nausea, fatigue, lethargy, jaundice, upper right quadrant tenderness, flu-like symptoms) occur.
- Advise female patient to notify health care professional if pregnancy is planned or suspected or if

breast feeding. Avoid especially after 30 wks of pregnancy.

Evaluation/Desired Outcomes

- Relief of pain.
- Improved joint mobility. Patients who do not respond to one NSAID may respond to another.

melphalan (mel-fa-lan)

Alkeran

Classification

Therapeutic: antineoplastics

Pharmacologic: alkylating agents

Pregnancy Category D

Indications

Alone or with other therapies for: Multiple myeloma, Ovarian cancer. **Unlabeled Use:** Breast cancer. Prostate cancer. Testicular carcinoma. Chronic myelogenous leukemia. Osteogenic sarcoma.

Action

Inhibits DNA and RNA synthesis by alkylation (cell-cycle phase–nonspecific). **Therapeutic Effects:** Death of rapidly replicating cells, particularly malignant ones. Also has immunosuppressive properties.

Pharmacokinetics

Absorption: Incompletely and variably absorbed following oral administration.

Distribution: Rapidly distributed throughout total body water.

Protein Binding: ≤30%.

Metabolism and Excretion: Rapidly metabolized in the bloodstream. Small amounts (10%) excreted unchanged by the kidneys.

Half-life: 1.5 hr.

TIME/ACTION PROFILE (effects on blood counts)

ROUTE	ONSET	PEAK	DURATION
PO	5 days	2–3 wk	5–6 wk

Contraindications/Precautions

Contraindicated in: Hypersensitivity to melphalan or chlorambucil; OB, Lactation: Pregnancy or lactation.

Use Cautiously in: Active infections; ↓ bone marrow reserve; Impaired renal function (dose ↓ recommended if BUN ≥30 mg/dL); OB: Women with child-bearing potential (should be counseled to avoid pregnancy during treatment); Pedi: Safety not established; Geri: Begin at lower end of dosing range due to potential for age-related ↓ in renal, hepatic, or cardiac function.

Adverse Reactions/Side Effects

Resp: bronchopulmonary dysplasia, pulmonary fibrosis. **GI:** diarrhea, hepatitis, nausea, stomatitis, vomiting. **GU:** infertility. **Derm:** alopecia, pruritus, rashes. **Endo:** menstrual irregularities. **Hemat:** leukopenia, thrombocytopenia, anemia. **Metab:** hyperuricemia. **Misc:** allergic reactions, including ANAPHYLAXIS (more common after IV use).

Interactions

Drug-Drug: ↑ bone marrow depression with other **antineoplastics** or **radiation therapy**. May ↓ antibody response to **live-virus vaccines** and ↑ risk of adverse reactions. May ↑ the risk of pulmonary toxicity with **carmustine**. Concurrent IV use with **cyclosporine** may ↑ risk of renal failure. Risk of enterocolitis may be ↑ with concurrent **nalidixic acid**.

Route/Dosage

Multiple Myeloma

PO (Adults): 150 mcg (0.15 mg)/kg/day for 7 days, followed by 3-wk rest, then 50 mcg (0.05 mg)/kg/day maintenance dose *or* 100–150 mcg/kg/day or 250 mg (0.25 mg)/kg/day for 4 days followed by 2–4-wk rest, then 2–4 mg/day maintenance dose *or* 7 mg/m^2 *or* 250 mcg (0.25 mg)/kg daily for 5 days q 5–6 wk.

IV (Adults): 16 mg/m^2 q 2 wk for 4 doses, then q 4 wk.

Ovarian Carcinoma

PO (Adults): 200 mcg (0.2 mg)/kg/day for 5 days q 4–5 wk.

Availability (generic available)

Tablets: 2 mg. **Powder for injection:** 50 mg/vial.

NURSING IMPLICATIONS

Assessment

- Assess for signs of infection (fever, chills, sore throat, cough, hoarseness, lower back or side pain, difficult or painful urination). Notify health care professional if these symptoms occur.
- Assess for bleeding (bleeding gums, bruising, petechiae, guaiac stools, urine, and emesis). Avoid IM injections and taking rectal temperatures. Apply pressure to venipuncture sites for 10 min.
- May cause nausea and vomiting. Monitor intake and output, appetite, and nutritional intake. Prophylactic antiemetics may be used. Adjust diet as tolerated.
- Monitor for symptoms of gout (increased uric acid, joint pain, edema). Encourage patient to drink at least 2 L of fluid per day. Allopurinol may be given to decrease uric acid levels.
- Anemia may occur. Monitor for increased fatigue and dyspnea.
- Assess patient for allergy to chlorambucil. Patients may have cross-sensitivity.

- ***Lab Test Considerations:*** Monitor CBC and differential weekly during therapy. The nadir of leukopenia occurs in 2–3 wk. Notify physician if leukocyte count is <3000/mm³. The nadir of thrombocytopenia occurs in 2–3 wk. Notify physician if platelet count is <100,000/mm³. Recovery of leukopenia and thrombocytopenia occurs in 5–6 wk.
- Monitor liver function studies (AST, ALT, LDH, bilirubin) and renal function studies (BUN, creatinine) prior to and periodically during therapy to detect hepatotoxicity and nephrotoxicity.
- May cause ↑ uric acid. Monitor periodically during therapy.
- May cause ↑ 5-hydroxyindoleacetic acid (5-HIAA) concentrations as a result of tumor breakdown.

Potential Nursing Diagnoses

Risk for injury (Side Effects)
Risk for infection (Side Effects)

Implementation

- Do not confuse Alkeran (melphalan) with Leukeran (chlorambucil) or Myleran (busulfan).
- Solution should be prepared in a biologic cabinet. Wear gloves, gown, and mask while handling medication. Discard IV equipment in specially designated container.
- If solution contacts skin or mucosa, immediately wash skin or mucosa with soap and water.
- **PO:** May be ordered in divided doses or as a single daily dose.

IV Administration

- **Intermittent Infusion:** Reconstitute with 10 mL of diluent supplied for a concentration of 5 mg/mL and shake vigorously until solution is clear. ***Diluent:*** Dilute dose immediately with 0.9% NaCl. ***Concentration:*** Not to exceed 2 mg/mL for central line or 0.45 mg/mL for a peripheral line. Administer within 60 min of reconstitution. ***Rate:*** Administer over at least 15 min (not to exceed 10 mg/min).
- **Y-Site Compatibility:** acyclovir, alemtuzumab, amikacin, aminophylline, amphotericin B lipid complex, ampicillin, anidulafungin, argatroban, aztreonam, bivalirudin, bleomycin, bumetanide, buprenorphine, butorphanol, calcium gluconate, carboplatin, carmustine, caspofungin, cefazolin, cefepime, cefotaxime, ceftazidime, ceftriaxone, cefuroxime, cisplatin, clindamycin, cyclophosphamide, cytarabine, dacarbazine, dactinomycin, daunorubicin, dexamethasone, diltiazem, diphenhydramine, doxorubicin, doxycycline, droperidol, enalaprilat, ertapenem, etoposide, famotidine, filgrastim, floxuridine, fluconazole, fludarabine, fluorouracil, furosemide, ganciclovir, gentamicin, granisetron, haloperidol, heparin, hetastarch, hydrocortisone, hydromorphone, idarubicin, ifosfamide, imipenem/cilastatin, linezolid, lorazepam, mannitol, mechlorethamine, meperidine, mesna, methotrexate, methylprednisolone, metoclopramide, metronidazole, milrinone, mitomycin, mitoxantrone, morphine, nalbuphine, nesiritide, octreotide, ondansetron, palonosetron, pamidronate, pancuronium, pentostatin, piperacillin/tazobactam, potassium acetate, potassium chloride, prochlorperazine, promethazine, ranitidine, sodium bicarbonate, streptozocin, teniposide, thiotepa, tigecycline, tirofiban, tobramycin, trimethoprim/sulfamethoxazole, vancomycin, vasopressin, vecuronium, vinblastine, vincristine, vinorelbine, voriconazole, zidovudine, zoledronic acid.
- **Y-Site Incompatibility:** amphotericin B colloidal, chlorpromazine, pantoprazole.

Patient/Family Teaching

- Instruct patient to take melphalan as directed, even if nausea and vomiting occur. If vomiting occurs shortly after dose is taken, consult health care professional. If a dose is missed, do not take at all.
- Advise patient to notify health care professional if fever; chills; dyspnea; persistent cough; sore throat; signs of infection; bleeding gums; bruising; petechiae; or blood in urine, stool, or emesis occurs. Caution patient to avoid crowds and persons with known infections. Instruct patient to use soft toothbrush and electric razor. Caution patient not to drink alcoholic beverages or take products containing aspirin or other NSAIDs.
- Instruct patient to notify health care professional if skin rash, vasculitis, bleeding, fever, persistent cough, nausea, vomiting, amenorrhea, weight loss, or unusual lumps/masses occur.
- Instruct patient to inspect oral mucosa for redness and ulceration. If ulceration occurs, advise patient to use sponge brush and to rinse mouth with water after eating and drinking. Consult health care professional if pain interferes with eating. Stomatitis pain may require treatment with opioid analgesics.
- Instruct patient not to receive any vaccinations without advice of health care professional.
- Advise patient that although fertility may be decreased, contraception should be used during melphalan therapy because of potential teratogenic effects on the fetus.
- Emphasize need for periodic lab tests to monitor for side effects.

Evaluation/Desired Outcomes

- Decrease in size and spread of malignant tissue.

memantine (me-man-teen)

✱Ebixa, Namenda, Namenda XR

Classification

Therapeutic: anti-Alzheimer's agents
Pharmacologic: N-methyl-D-aspartate antagonist

Pregnancy Category B

Indications

Moderate to severe dementia/neurocognitive disorder associated with Alzheimer's disease.

Action

Binds to CNS N-methyl-D-aspartate (NMDA) receptor sites, preventing binding of glutamate, an excitatory neurotransmitter. **Therapeutic Effects:** Decreased symptoms of dementia/cognitive decline. Does not slow progression. Cognitive enhancement. Does not cure disease.

Pharmacokinetics

Absorption: Well absorbed after oral administration.
Distribution: Unknown.
Metabolism and Excretion: 57–82% excreted unchanged in urine by active tubular secretion moderated by pH dependent tubular reabsorption. Remainder metabolized; metabolites are not pharmacologically active.
Half-life: 60–80 hr.

TIME/ACTION PROFILE (blood levels)

ROUTE	ONSET	PEAK	DURATION
PO	unknown	3–7 hr	12 hr
PO-ER	unknown	9–12 hr	24 hr

Contraindications/Precautions

Contraindicated in: Hypersensitivity.
Use Cautiously in: Severe renal impairment (↓ dose); Severe hepatic impairment; Concurrent use of other NMDA antagonists (amantadine, rimantadine, ketamine, dextromethorphan); Concurrent use of drugs or diets that cause alkaline urine; Conditions that ↑ urine pH including severe urinary tract infections or renal tubular acidosis (lead to ↓ excretion and ↑ levels); OB, Lactation: Safety not established; Pedi: Safety and effectiveness not established.

Adverse Reactions/Side Effects

CNS: dizziness, fatigue, headache, sedation. **CV:** hypertension. **Derm:** rash. **GI:** diarrhea, weight gain. **GU:** urinary frequency. **Hemat:** anemia.

Interactions

Drug-Drug: Medications that ↑ urine pH (e.g. **carbonic anhydrase inhibitors, sodium bicarbonate**) may↓ excretion and ↑ blood levels.

Route/Dosage

PO (Adults): *Immediate-release*— 5 mg once daily initially, ↑ at weekly intervals to 10 mg/day (5 mg twice daily), then 15 mg/day (5 mg once daily, 10 mg once daily as separate doses), then to target dose of 20 mg/day (10 mg twice daily); *Extended-release*— 7 mg once daily, ↑ at weekly intervals by 7 mg/day to target dose of 28 mg once daily.

Renal Impairment

(Adults): *CCr 5–29 mL/min*—Immediate-release (solution): Target dose is 10 mg/day (5 mg twice daily); Extended-release: Target dose is 14 mg once daily.

Availability (generic available)

Immediate-release tablets: 5 mg, 10 mg, titration package containing twenty-eight 5–mg tablets and twenty-one 10–mg tablets. **Cost:** 5 mg $887.69/180. **Extended-release capsules:** 7 mg, 14 mg, 21 mg, 28 mg. **Cost:** 7 mg $302.62/30, 14 mg $907.85/90, 21 mg $302.62/30, 28 mg $907.85/90. **Oral solution, sugar-free, alcohol-free (peppermint):** 2 mg/mL. **Cost:** $668.50/360 mL. ***In combination with:*** donepezil (Namzaric). See Appendix B.

NURSING IMPLICATIONS

Assessment

- Assess cognitive function (memory, attention, reasoning, language, ability to perform simple tasks) periodically during therapy.
- ***Lab Test Considerations:*** May cause anemia.

Potential Nursing Diagnoses

Disturbed thought process (Indications)
Risk for injury (Side Effects)
Impaired environmental interpretation syndrome

Implementation

- Dose increases should occur no more frequently than weekly.
- To switch from *Namenda* to Namenda XR, patients taking 10 mg twice daily of *Namenda* tablets may be switched to *Namenda XR* 28 mg once daily capsules the day following the last dose of a 10 mg *Namenda* tablet. Patients with renal impairment may use the same procedure to switch from *Namenda* 5 mg twice daily to *Namenda XR* 14 mg once daily.
- **PO:** May be administered without regard to food.
- Administer oral solution using syringe provided. Do not dilute or mix with other fluids.
- Swallow extended release capsules whole; do not crush, chew, or divide. Capsules may be opened, sprinkled on applesauce, and swallowed. Entire contents of each capsule should be consumed; do not divide dose.

Patient/Family Teaching

- Instruct patient and caregiver on how and when to administer memantine and how to titrate dose. Take missed doses as soon as remembered but not just before next dose; do not double doses. If several days doses are missed, may need to resume at a lower dose and re-titrate up to previous dose; consult health care professional. Advise patient and caregiver to read *Patient Instructions* before starting and with each Rx refill in case of changes.

M

- Caution patient and caregiver that memantine may cause dizziness. Monitor and assist with ambulation and caution patient to avoid driving and other activities requiring alertness until response to medication is known.
- Advise patient and caregiver to notify health care professional of all Rx or OTC medications, vitamins, or herbal products being taken and to consult with health care professional before taking other medications.
- Teach patient and caregivers that improvement in cognitive functioning may take months; degenerative process is not reversed.

Evaluation/Desired Outcomes

- Improvement in neurocognitive decline (memory, attention, reasoning, language, ability to perform simple tasks) in patients with Alzheimer's disease.

HIGH ALERT

meperidine (me-per-i-deen)

Demerol

Classification

Therapeutic: opioid analgesics

Pharmacologic: opioid agonists

Schedule II

Pregnancy Category C

Indications

Moderate or severe pain (alone or with nonopioid agents). Anesthesia adjunct. Analgesic during labor. Preoperative sedation. **Unlabeled Use:** Rigors.

Action

Binds to opiate receptors in the CNS. Alters the perception of and response to painful stimuli, while producing generalized CNS depression. **Therapeutic Effects:** Decrease in severity of pain.

Pharmacokinetics

Absorption: 50% from the GI tract; well absorbed from IM sites. Oral doses are about half as effective as parenteral doses.

Distribution: Widely distributed. Crosses the placenta; enters breast milk.

Protein Binding: Neonates: 52%; Infants 3–18 mo: 85%; Adults: 60–80%.

Metabolism and Excretion: Mostly metabolized by the liver; some converted to normeperidine, which may accumulate and cause seizures. 5% excreted unchanged by the kidneys.

Half-life: Neonates: 12–39 hr; Infants 3–18 mo: 2.3 hr; Children 5–8 yr: 3 hr; Adults: 2.5–4 hr (↑ in impaired renal or hepatic function [7–11 hr]).

TIME/ACTION PROFILE (analgesia)

ROUTE	ONSET	PEAK	DURATION
PO	15 min	60 min	2–4 hr
IM	10–15 min	30–50 min	2–4 hr
Subcut	10–15 min	40–60 min	2–4 hr
IV	immediate	5–7 min	2–3 hr

Contraindications/Precautions

Contraindicated in: Hypersensitivity; Hypersensitivity to bisulfites (some injectable products); Recent (within 14 days) MAO inhibitor therapy; Severe respiratory insufficiency; OB: Chronic use may pose risk to the fetus including possible addiction; Lactation: Excreted in breast milk and can cause respiratory depression in the infant.

Use Cautiously in: Head trauma; ↑ intracranial pressure; Severe renal or hepatic impairment; Acute asthma attack, COPD, hypoxia, or hypercapnea; Hypothyroidism; Adrenal insufficiency; Alcoholism; Debilitated patients (dose ↓ suggested); Undiagnosed abdominal pain or prostatic hyperplasia; Patients with renal impairment, or extensive burns; High-dose or prolonged therapy (>600 mg/day or >2 days; ↑ risk of CNS stimulation and seizures due to accumulation of normeperidine); Sickle cell anemia (may require ↓ initial doses); OB: Use during labor and delivery can cause respiratory depression in the newborn; Pedi: Syrup contains benzyl alcohol, which can cause "gasping syndrome" in neonates. Children have ↑ risk of seizures due to accumulation of normeperidine; Geri: Appears on Beers list; morphine recommended.

Adverse Reactions/Side Effects

CNS: SEIZURES, confusion, sedation, dysphoria, euphoria, floating feeling, hallucinations, headache, unusual dreams. **EENT:** blurred vision, diplopia, miosis. **Resp:** respiratory depression. **CV:** hypotension, bradycardia. **GI:** constipation, nausea, vomiting. **GU:** urinary retention. **Derm:** flushing, sweating. **Misc:** allergic reactions including ANAPHYLAXIS, physical dependence, psychological dependence, tolerance.

Interactions

Drug-Drug: Do not use in patients receiving **MAO inhibitors** or **procarbazine** (may cause fatal reaction—contraindicated within 14 days of MAO inhibitor therapy). ↑ CNS depression with **alcohol**, **antihistamines**, and **sedative/hypnotics**. Administration of **agonist/antagonist opioid analgesics** may precipitate opioid withdrawal in physically dependent patients. **Nalbuphine** or **pentazocine** may ↓ analgesia. **Protease inhibitors** may ↑ effects and adverse reactions (concurrent use should be avoided). **Phenytoin** ↑ metabolism and may ↓ effects. **Chlorpromazine** and **thioridazine** may ↑ the risk of adverse reactions (concurrent use should be avoided). May aggravate side effects of **isoniazid**. **Acyclovir** may ↑ plasma concentrations of meperidine and normeperidine.

Drug-Natural Products: Concomitant use of **kava-kava, valerian,** or **chamomile** can ↓ CNS depression. **St. John's wort** may ↑ serious side effects, concurrent use is not recommended.

Route/Dosage

PO, IM, Subcut (Adults): *Analgesia*—50 mg q 3–4 hr; may be ↑ as needed (not to exceed 600 mg/24 hr). *Analgesia during labor*—50–100 mg IM or subcut when contractions become regular; may repeat q 1–3 hr. *Preoperative sedation*—50–100 mg IM or subcut 30–90 min before anesthesia.

PO, IM, Subcut (Children): *Analgesia*—1–1.5 mg/kg q 3–4 hr (should not exceed 100 mg/dose). *Preoperative sedation*—1–2 mg/kg 30–90 min before anesthesia (not to exceed adult dose).

IV (Adults): 15–35 mg/hr as a continuous infusion; *PCA*—10 mg initially; with a range of 1–5 mg/incremental dose, recommended lockout interval is 6–10 min (minimum 5 min).

IV (Children): *Continuous infusion*—0.5–1 mg/kg loading dose followed by 0.3 mg/kg/hr, titrate to effect up to 0.5–0.7 mg/kg/hr.

Availability (generic available)

Tablets: 50 mg, 100 mg. **Syrup (banana flavor):** 50 mg/5 mL. **Injection:** 10 mg/mL, 25 mg/0.5 mL, 25 mg/mL, 50 mg/mL, 75 mg/mL, 100 mg/mL.

NURSING IMPLICATIONS

Assessment

- Assess type, location, and intensity of pain prior to and 1 hr following PO, subcut, and IM doses and 5 min (peak) following IV administration. When titrating opioid doses, increases of 25–50% should be administered until there is either a 50% reduction in the patient's pain rating on a numerical or visual analogue scale or the patient reports satisfactory pain relief. A repeat dose can be safely administered at the time of the peak if previous dose is ineffective and side effects are minimal.
- An equianalgesic chart (see Appendix I) should be used when changing routes or when changing from one opioid to another.
- Assess BP, pulse, and respirations before and periodically during administration. If respiratory rate is <10/min, assess level of sedation. Dose may need to be decreased by 25–50%. Initial drowsiness will diminish with continued use.
- Assess bowel function routinely. Prevention of constipation should be instituted with increased intake of fluids and bulk and with laxatives to minimize constipating effects. Stimulant laxatives should be administered routinely if opioid use exceeds 2–3 days, unless contraindicated.
- Prolonged use may lead to physical and psychological dependence and tolerance. This should not prevent patient from receiving adequate analgesia. Most patients who receive meperidine for pain do not develop psychological dependence. Progressively higher doses may be required to relieve pain with long-term therapy.
- Monitor patients on chronic or high-dose therapy for CNS stimulation (restlessness, irritability, seizures) due to accumulation of normeperidine metabolite. Risk of toxicity increases with doses >600 m g/24 hr, chronic administration (>2 days), and renal impairment.
- Geri: Meperidine has been reported to cause delirium in the elderly; older adults are at increased risk for normeperidine toxicity. Monitor frequently.
- Pedi: Assess pediatric patient frequently; neonates, infants, and children are more sensitive to the effects of opioid analgesics and may experience respiratory complications, excitability, and restlessness more frequently.
- ***Lab Test Considerations:*** May ↑ plasma amylase and lipase concentrations.
- ***Toxicity and Overdose:*** If an opioid antagonist is required to reverse respiratory depression or coma, naloxone (Narcan) is the antidote. Dilute the 0.4-mg ampule of naloxone in 10 mL of 0.9% NaCl and administer 0.5 mL (0.02 mg) by IV push every 2 min. For children and patients weighing <40 kg, dilute 0.1 mg of naloxone in 10 mL of 0.9% NaCl for a concentration of 10 mcg/mL and administer 0.5 mcg/kg every 2 min. Titrate dose to avoid withdrawal, seizures, and severe pain. In patients receiving meperidine chronically, naloxone may precipitate seizures by eliminating the CNS depressant effects of meperidine, allowing the convulsant activity of normeperidine to predominate. Monitor patient closely.

Potential Nursing Diagnoses

Acute pain (Indications)
Disturbed sensory perception (visual, auditory) (Side Effects)
Risk for injury (Side Effects)

Implementation

- ***High Alert:*** Accidental overdose of opioid analgesics has resulted in fatalities. Before administering, clarify all ambiguous orders; have second practitioner independently check original order, dose calculations, and infusion pump settings. Pedi: Medication errors with opioid analgesics are common in the pediatric population and include misinterpretation or miscalculation of doses and use of inappropriate measuring devices.
- Explain therapeutic value of medication prior to administration to enhance the analgesic effect.
- Regularly administered doses may be more effective than prn administration. Analgesic is more effective if given before pain becomes severe.

- Coadministration with nonopioid analgesics may have additive analgesic effects and permit lower doses.
- Oral dose is <50% as effective as parenteral. When changing to oral administration, dose may need to be increased (see Appendix I).
- Medication should be discontinued gradually after long-term use to prevent withdrawal symptoms.
- May be administered via PCA pump.
- **PO:** Doses may be administered with food or milk to minimize GI irritation. Syrup should be diluted in half-full glass of water.
- **IM:** Administration of repeated subcut doses may cause local irritation.

IV Administration

- **IV Push:** ***Diluent:*** Dilute with sterile water or 0.9% NaCl for injection. ***Concentration:*** ≤10 mg/mL. ***Rate: High Alert:*** Administer slowly over at least 5 min. Rapid administration may lead to increased respiratory depression, hypotension, and circulatory collapse.
- **Intermittent Infusion:** ***Diluent:*** Dilute with D5W, D10W, dextrose/saline combinations, dextrose/Ringer's or lactated Ringer's injection combinations, 0.45% NaCl, 0.9% NaCl, or Ringer's or LR. Administer via infusion pump. ***Concentration:*** 1 mg/mL. ***Rate:*** Administer over 15–30 min.
- **Y-Site Compatibility:** alemtuzumab, alfentanil, amifostine, amikacin, aminocaproic acid, aminophylline, amiodarone, anidulafungin, argatroban, ascorbic acid, atracurium, atropine, azithromycin, aztreonam, benztropine, bivalirudin, bleomycin, bumetanide, busulfan, calcium chloride, calcium gluconate, carboplatin, carmustine, caspofungin, cefazolin, cefotaxime, cefoxitin, ceftaroline, ceftazidime, ceftriaxone, cefuroxime, chlorpromazine, ciprofloxacin, cisatracurium, cisplatin, cladribine, clindamycin, cyanocobalamin, cyclophosphamide, cyclosporine, cytarabine, dactinomycin, daptomycin, daunorubicin, daunorubicin liposome, dexmedetomidine, dexrazoxane, digoxin, diltiazem, diphenhydramine, dobutamine, docetaxel, dolasetron, dopamine, doripenem, doxacurium, doxorubicin hydrochloride, doxycycline, droperidol, enalaprilat, ephedrine, epinephrine, epirubicin, epoetin alfa, eptifibatide, ertapenem, erythromycin, esmolol, etoposide, etoposide phosphate, famotidine, fenoldopam, fentanyl, filgrastim, floxuridine, fluconazole, fludarabine, fluorouracil, folic acid, fosphenytoin, gemcitabine, gentamicin, glycopyrrolate, granisetron, hetastarch, hydrocortisone sodium phosphate, ifosfamide, insulin, irinotecan, isoproterenol, ketamine, ketorolac, labetalol, leucovorin calcium, levofloxacin, lidocaine, linezolid, mannitol, mechlorethamine, melphalan, mesna, metaraminol, methotrexate, methyldopate, metoclopramide, metoprolol, metronidazole, midazolam, milrinone, mitomycin, mitoxantrone, morphine, multivitamins, mycophenolate, naloxone, nitroglycerin, nitroprusside, norepinephrine, octreotide, ondansetron, oxacillin, oxaliplatin, oxytocin, paclitaxel, palonosetron, pamidronate, pancuronium, papaverine, pemetrexed, penicillin G, pentamidine, phentolamine, phenylephrine, phytonadione, piperacillin/tazobactam, potassium acetate, potassium chloride, procainamide, prochlorperazine, promethazine, propofol, propranolol, protamine, pyridoxime, quinupristin/dalfopristin, ranitidine, remifentanil, rituximab, rocuronium, sargramostim, sodium acetate, streptokinase, streoptzocin, succinylcholine, sufentanil, tacrolimus, teniposide, theophylline, thiamine, thiotepa, tigecycline, tirofiban, tobramycin, tolazoline, topotecan, trastuzumab, trimetaphan, vancomycin, vasopressin, vecuronium, verapamil, vinblastine, vincristine, vinorelbine, voriconazole, zidovudine, zoledronic acid.
- **Y-Site Incompatibility:** allopurinol, amphotericin B cholesteryl, amphotericin B colloidal, amphotericin B liposome, azathioprine, cefepime, dantrolene, diazepam, diazoxide, ganciclovir, idarubicin, indomethacin, lorazepam, micafungin, nafcillin, pantoprazole, pentobarbital, phenobarbital, phenytoin, sodium bicarbonate, thiopental.

Patient/Family Teaching

- Instruct patient on how and when to ask for and take pain medication.
- Instruct patient to take meperidine as directed. If dose is less effective after a few weeks, do not increase dose without consulting health care professional. Pedi: Teach parents or caregivers how to accurately measure liquid medication and to use only the measuring device dispensed with the medication.
- May cause drowsiness or dizziness. Advise patient to call for assistance when ambulating or smoking. Caution patient to avoid driving or other activities requiring alertness until response to medication is known.
- Advise patient to change positions slowly to minimize orthostatic hypotension.
- Instruct patient to avoid concurrent use of alcohol or other CNS depressants.
- Advise ambulatory patients that nausea and vomiting may be decreased by lying down.
- Encourage patient to turn, cough, and breathe deeply every 2 hr to prevent atelectasis.

Evaluation/Desired Outcomes

- Decrease in severity of pain without a significant alteration in level of consciousness or respiratory status.

meropenem (mer-oh-**pen**-nem)
Merrem

Classification
Therapeutic: anti-infectives
Pharmacologic: carbapenems

Pregnancy Category B

Indications
Treatment of: Intra-abdominal infections, Bacterial meningitis. Skin and skin structure infections. **Unlabeled Use:** Febrile neutropenia. Hospital-acquired pneumonia and sepsis.

Action
Binds to bacterial cell wall, resulting in cell death. Meropenem resists the actions of many enzymes that degrade most other penicillins and penicillin-like anti-infectives. **Therapeutic Effects:** Bactericidal action against susceptible bacteria. **Spectrum:** Active against the following gram-positive organisms: *Staphylococcus aureus*, *Streptococcus pneumoniae*, Viridans group streptococci, *Enterococcus faecalis*. Also active against the following gram-negative pathogens: *Escherichia coli*, *Haemophilus influenzae*, *Klebsiella pneumoniae*, *Neisseria meningitidis*, *Pseudomonas aeruginosa*, *Proteus mirabilis*. Active against the following anaerobes: *Bacteroides fragilis*, *Bacteroides fragilis* group, *Peptostreptococcus* species.

Pharmacokinetics
Absorption: IV administration results in complete bioavailability.
Distribution: Widely distributed into body tissues and fluids; enters CSF when meninges are inflamed.
Metabolism and Excretion: 50–75% excreted unchanged by the kidneys.
Half-life: Premature neonates: 3 hr; Term neonates: 2 hr; Infants 3 mo–2 yr: 1.4 hr; Children >2 yr and Adults: 1 hr (↑ in renal impairment).

TIME/ACTION PROFILE (blood levels)

ROUTE	ONSET	PEAK	DURATION
IV	rapid	end of infusion	8 hr

Contraindications/Precautions
Contraindicated in: Hypersensitivity to meropenem or imipenem; Serious hypersensitivity to other beta-lactams (penicillins or cephalosporins; cross-sensitivity may occur).
Use Cautiously in: Renal impairment (↑ risk of thrombocytopenia and seizures; dose reduction recommended if CCr <50 mL/min); History of seizures, brain lesions, or meningitis; OB, Lactation: Safety not established; Pedi: Children <3 mo (safety not established for skin/skin structure infections and meningitis).

Adverse Reactions/Side Effects
CNS: SEIZURES, dizziness, headache. **Resp:** APNEA. **GI:** CLOSTRIDIUM DIFFICILE-ASSOCIATED DIARRHEA (CDAD), constipation, diarrhea, glossitis (↑ in children), nausea, thrush (↑ in children), vomiting. **Derm:** moniliasis (children only), pruritus, rash. **Local:** inflammation at injection site, phlebitis. **Neuro:** paresthesias. **Misc:** allergic reactions including ANAPHYLAXIS.

Interactions
Drug-Drug: Probenecid ↓ renal excretion and increases blood levels (coadministration not recommended). May ↓ serum **valproate** levels (↑ risk of seizures).

Route/Dosage
Skin/Skin Structure Infections
IV (Adults): 500 mg q 8 hr or 1 g q 8 hr (if caused by *Pseudomonas aeruginosa*).
IV (Children ≥3 mo–12 yr): 10 mg/kg (max of 500 mg) q 8 hr or 20 mg/kg (max of 1 g) q 8 hr (if caused by *Pseudomonas aeruginosa*).

Intra-abdominal Infections
IV (Adults): 1 g q 8 hr.
IV (Children ≥3 mo–12 yr): 20 mg/kg (max of 1 g) q 8 hr.
IV (Children <3 mo): *<32 wk gestational age (GA) and postnatal age (PNA) <2 wk*—20 mg/kg q 12 hr; *<32 wk GA and PNA ≥2 wk*—20 mg/kg q 8 hr; *≥32 wk GA and PNA <2 wk*—20 mg/kg q 8 hr; *≥32 wk GA and PNA ≥2 wk*—30 mg/kg q 8 hr.

Meningitis
IV (Adults): 2 g q 8 hr.
IV (Children ≥3 mo–12 yr): 40 mg/kg (max of 2 g) q 8 hr.

Renal Impairment
IV (Adults): *CCr 26–50 mL/min*—1 g q 12 hr; *CCr 10–25 mL/min*—500 mg q 12 hr; *CCr <10 mL/min*—500 mg q 24 hr.

Availability (generic available)
Powder for injection: 500 mg, 1 g.

NURSING IMPLICATIONS
Assessment
- Assess for infection (vital signs; appearance of wound, sputum, urine, and stool; WBC) at beginning of and throughout therapy.
- Obtain a history before initiating therapy to determine previous use of and reactions to penicillins.

M

Persons with a negative history of penicillin sensitivity may still have an allergic response.

- Obtain specimens for culture and sensitivity prior to initiating therapy. First dose may be given before receiving results.
- Observe for signs and symptoms of anaphylaxis (rash, pruritus, laryngeal edema, wheezing). Discontinue the drug and notify physician immediately if these symptoms occur. Have epinephrine, an antihistamine, and resuscitative equipment close by in the event of an anaphylactic reaction.
- Assess injection site for phlebitis, pain, and swelling periodically during administration.
- ***Lab Test Considerations:*** Monitor hematologic, hepatic, and renal functions periodically during therapy.
- BUN, AST, ALT, LDH, serum alkaline phosphatase, bilirubin, and creatinine may be transiently ↑.
- Hemoglobin and hematocrit concentrations may be ↓.
- May cause positive direct or indirect Coombs' test.

Potential Nursing Diagnoses

Risk for infection (Indications, Side Effects)
Deficient knowledge, related to medication regimen (Patient/Family Teaching)

Implementation

IV Administration

- **IV Push:** Reconstitute 500-mg and 1-g vials with 10 mL and 20 mL, respectively, of sterile water for injection. ***Concentration:*** 50 mg/mL. ***Rate:*** Administer over 3–5 min.
- **Intermittent Infusion:** Reconstitute 500-mg and 1-g vials with 10 mL and 20 mL, respectively, of sterile water for injection, 0.9% NaCl, or D5W. Vials reconstituted with sterile water for injection are stable for 3 hr at room temperature and 13 hr if refrigerated; if reconstituted with 0.9% NaCl, stable for 1 hr at room temperature and 15 hr if refrigerated; if reconstituted with D5W, should be used immediately. ***Diluent:*** Further dilute in 0.9% NaCl or D5W to achieve concentration below. Infusions further diluted in 0.9% NaCl are stable for 4 hr at room temperature and 24 hr if refrigerated. Infusions further diluted in D5W are stable for 1 hr at room temperature and 4 hr if refrigerated. ***Concentration:*** 1–20 mg/mL. ***Rate:*** Infuse over 15–30 min.
- **Y-Site Compatibility:** alemtuzumab, aminophylline, anidulafungin, argatroban, atropine, azithromycin, bivalirudin, bleomycin, cangrelor, carboplatin, carmustine, caspofungin, cisplatin, cyclophosphamide, cyclosporine, cytarabine, dactinomycin, daptomycin, daunorubicin hydrochloride, dexamethasone, dexmedetomidine, dexrazoxane, digoxin, diltiazem, diphenhydramine, docetaxel, doxorubicin liposomal, enalaprilat, eptifibatide, etoposide, etoposide phosphate, fluconazole, fludarabine, fluorouracil, foscarnet, fosphenytoin, furosemide, gemcitabine, gentamicin, granisetron, heparin, hetastarch, hydromorphone, ifosfamide, insulin, irinotecan, leucovorin calcium, linezolid, lorazepam, mechlorethamine, mesna, methotrexate, metoclopramide, metronidazole, milrinone, mitomycin, mitoxantrone, morphine, naloxone, nesiritide, norepinephrine, octreotide, oxaliplatin, oxytocin, paclitaxel, palonosetron, pamidronate, pancuronium, pemetrexed, phenobarbital, potassium acetate, potassium chloride, rocuronium, tacrolimus, telavancin, teniposide, thiotepa, tigecycline, tirofiban, vancomycin, vasopressin, vecuronium, vinblastine, vincristine, vinorelbine, voriconazole, zoledronic acid.
- **Y-Site Incompatibility:** amiodarone, amphotericin B colloidal, amphotericin B lipid complex, amphotericin B liposome, ciprofloxacin, dacarbazine, diazepam, dolasetron, doxorubicin hydrochloride, epirubicin, fenoldopam, idarubicin, ketamine, mycophenolate, nicardipine, pantoprazole, quinupristin/dalfopristin, topotecan.

Patient/Family Teaching

- Advise patient to report the signs of superinfection (black, furry overgrowth on the tongue; vaginal itching or discharge; loose or foul-smelling stools) and allergy.
- May cause dizziness. Caution patient to avoid driving or other activities requiring alertness until response to drug is known.
- Caution patient to notify health care professional if fever and diarrhea occur, especially if stool contains blood, pus, or mucus. Advise patient not to treat diarrhea without consulting health care professional. May occur up to several weeks after discontinuation of medication.
- Advise patient to notify health care professional of all Rx or OTC medications, vitamins, or herbal products being taken and to consult with health care professional before taking other medications.
- Advise female patient to notify health care professional if pregnancy is planned or suspected or if breast feeding.

Evaluation/Desired Outcomes

- Resolution of the signs and symptoms of infection. Length of time for complete resolution depends on the organism and site of infection.

mesalamine (me-sal-a-meen)

Apriso, ~~Asacol~~, ✱Asacol, ✱Asacol 800, Asacol HD, Canasa, Delzicol, Lialda, ✱Mesasal, ✱Mezavant, Pentasa, Rowasa, ✱Salofalk, ✱Teva 5-ASA

Classification

Therapeutic: gastrointestinal anti-inflammatories

Pregnancy Category B

Indications

Delzicol, Lialda, and Pentasa—Treatment and maintenance of remission of mildly-to-moderately-active ulcerative colitis. *Apriso*—Maintenance of remission of ulcerative colitis. *Asacol HD*—Treatment of moderately-active ulcerative colitis. *Canasa*—Treatment of active ulcerative proctitis. *Rowasa*—Treatment of active mild-to-moderate distal ulcerative colitis, proctosigmoiditis, or proctitis.

Action

Locally acting anti-inflammatory action in the colon, where activity is probably due to inhibition of prostaglandin synthesis. **Therapeutic Effects:** Reduction in the symptoms of ulcerative colitis, proctosigmoiditis, and proctitis.

Pharmacokinetics

Absorption: 28% absorbed following oral administration; 10–30% absorbed from the colon, depending on retention time, following rectal administration.
Distribution: Unknown.
Metabolism and Excretion: Some metabolism occurs, site unknown; mostly eliminated unchanged in the feces.
Half-life: *Oral*—12 hr (range 2–15 hr); *Rectal*—0.5–1.5 hr.

TIME/ACTION PROFILE (clinical improvement)

ROUTE	ONSET	PEAK	DURATION
PO	unknown	unknown	6–8 hr
ER	2 hr	9–12 hr	24 hr
Rectal	3–21 days	unknown	24 hr

Contraindications/Precautions

Contraindicated in: Hypersensitivity reactions to sulfonamides, salicylates, mesalamine, or sulfasalazine; Cross-sensitivity with furosemide, sulfonylurea hypoglycemic agents, or carbonic anhydrase inhibitors may exist; G6PD deficiency; Hypersensitivity to bisulfites (mesalamine enema only); Urinary tract or intestinal obstruction; Porphyria.

Use Cautiously in: Severe hepatic or renal impairment; OB: Safety not established; use tablets only if potential benefits outweigh risk to fetus (enteric coating contains dibutyl phthalate, which has been shown to cause congenital malformations in animals); Lactation: Has caused side effects in some infants; careful observation required.

Adverse Reactions/Side Effects

CNS: <u>headache</u>, dizziness, malaise, weakness. **EENT:** pharyngitis, rhinitis. **CV:** pericarditis. **GI:** diarrhea, eructation (PO), flatulence, nausea, vomiting. **GU:** interstitial nephritis, pancreatitis, renal failure. **Derm:** STEVENS-JOHNSON SYNDROME, hair loss, rash. **Local:** anal irritation (enema, suppository). **MS:** back pain, myalgia. **Misc:** ANAPHYLAXIS, ANGIOEDEMA, DRUG REACTION WITH EOSINOPHILIA AND SYSTEMATIC SYMPTOMS (DRESS), acute intolerance syndrome, fever.

Interactions

Drug-Drug: May ↓ metabolism and ↑ effects/toxicity of **mercaptopurine** or **thioguanine**.

Route/Dosage

One Asacol HD 800-mg tablet is NOT bioequivalent to two Delzicol 400-mg capsules.

Treatment of Ulcerative Colitis

PO (Adults): *Delzicol*—800 mg (two 400-mg capsules) 3 times daily for 6 wk; *Asacol HD*—1.6 g (two 800-mg tablets) 3 times daily for 6 wk; *Lialda*—2.4–4.8 g (two to four 1.2-g tablets) once daily for up to 8 wk; *Pentasa*—1 g (four 250-mg capsules or two 500-mg capsules) 4 times daily for up to 8 wk.
Rect (Adults): *Rowasa*—4-g enema (60 mL) at bedtime, retained for 8 hr for 3–6 wk.
PO (Children ≥12 yr and 54–90 kg): *Delzicol*—27–44 mg/kg/day in 2 divided doses (max dose = 2.4 g/day) for 6 wk.
PO (Children ≥12 yr and 33–53 kg): *Delzicol*—37–61 mg/kg/day in 2 divided doses (max dose = 2 g/day) for 6 wk.
PO (Children ≥12 yr and 17–32 kg): *Delzicol*—36–71 mg/kg/day in 2 divided doses (max dose = 1.2 g/day) for 6 wk.

Maintenance of Remission of Ulcerative Colitis

PO (Adults): *Apriso*—1.5 g (four 375-mg capsules) once daily in the morning; *Delzicol*—800 mg (two 400-mg capsules) 2 times daily; *Lialda*—2.4 g (two 1.2-g tablets) once daily; *Pentasa*—1 g (four 250-mg capsules or two 500-mg capsules) 4 times daily.

Treatment of Ulcerative Proctosigmoiditis

Rect (Adults): *Rowasa*—4-g enema (60 mL) at bedtime, retained for 8 hr (treatment duration = 3–6 wk).

Treatment of Ulcerative Proctitis

Rect (Adults): *Rowasa*—4-g enema (60 mL) at bedtime, retained for 8 hr (treatment duration = 3–6 wk); *Canasa*—Insert a 1–g suppository at bedtime, retain for at least 1–3 hr (treatment duration = 3–6 wk).

Availability (generic available)

Delayed-release tablets: ✤400 mg, ✤500 mg, 800 mg (Asacol HD), ✤1 g, 1.2 g (Lialda). **Controlled-release capsules (Pentasa):** 250 mg, 500 mg. **Delayed-release capsules (Delzicol):** 400 mg. **Extended-release capsules (Apriso):** 375 mg. **Rectal suppository (Canasa):** ✤500 mg, 1 g. **Rectal suspension (Rowasa):** ✤1 g/100 mL, ✤2 g/60 mL, 4 g/60 mL, ✤4 g/100 mL.

NURSING IMPLICATIONS

Assessment

- Assess abdominal pain and frequency, quantity, and consistency of stools at the beginning of and during therapy.
- Assess for allergy to sulfonamides and salicylates. Patients allergic to sulfasalazine may take mesalamine or olsalazine without difficulty, but therapy should be discontinued if rash or fever occurs.
- Monitor intake and output ratios. Fluid intake should be sufficient to maintain a urine output of at least 1200–1500 mL daily to prevent crystalluria and stone formation.
- ***Lab Test Considerations:*** Monitor urinalysis, BUN, and serum creatinine prior to and periodically during therapy. Mesalamine may cause renal toxicity.
- Mesalamine may cause ↑ AST and ALT levels, serum alkaline phosphatase, GGTP, LDH, amylase, and lipase.

Potential Nursing Diagnoses

Acute pain (Indications)
Diarrhea (Indications)

Implementation

- Do not confuse Asacol (mesalamine) with Os-Cal (calcium carbonate).
- **PO:** Administer with a full glass of water. Tablets should be swallowed whole; do not break the outer coating, which is designed to remain intact. Take *Lialda* tablets with a meal. Take *Apriso* capsules in the morning without regard to meals. Do not co-administer with antacids; may effect dissolution of the coating of the granules in *Apriso* capsules. Intact or partially intact tablets may occasionally be found in the stool. If this occurs repeatedly, advise patient to notify health care professional. Swallow *Delzicol* capsules whole; do not break, crush, or chew. Administer without regard to meals. Intact or partially intact tablets may occasionally be found in the stool. If this occurs repeatedly, advise patient to notify health care professional. Two *Delzicol* 400 mg capsules are not equal to one *Asacol HD* (mesalamine) delayed-release 800 mg tablet. *Pentasa* capsules may be swallowed whole or opened and sprinkled onto applesauce or yogurt. Consume entire contents immediately. Avoid crushing or chewing capsules and capsule contents.
- **Rect:** Patient should empty bowel prior to administration of rectal dose forms.
- Avoid excessive handling of *suppository*. Remove foil wrapper and insert pointed end first into rectum with gentle pressure. Suppository should be retained for 1–3 hr or more for maximum benefit.
- Administer 60-mL retention enema once daily at bedtime. Solution should be retained for approximately 8 hr. Prior to administration of *rectal suspension*, shake bottle well and remove the protective cap. Have patient lie on left side with the lower leg extended and the upper leg flexed for support or place the patient in knee-chest position. Gently insert the applicator tip into the rectum, pointing toward the umbilicus. Squeeze the bottle steadily to discharge most of the preparation.

Patient/Family Teaching

- Instruct patient on the correct method of administration. Advise patient to take medication as directed, even if feeling better. Take missed doses as soon as remembered unless almost time for next dose.
- Advise patient not to change brands of mesalamine without consulting health care professional.
- May cause dizziness. Caution patient to avoid driving or other activities that require alertness until response to medication is known.
- Advise patient to notify health care professional if skin rash, sore throat, fever, mouth sores, unusual bleeding or bruising, wheezing, fever, or hives occur.
- Instruct patient to notify health care professional if symptoms do not improve after 1–2 mo of therapy.
- Instruct patient to notify health care professional if symptoms worsen or do not improve. If symptoms of acute intolerance (cramping, acute abdominal pain, bloody diarrhea, fever, headache, rash) occur, discontinue therapy and notify health care professional immediately.
- Advise female patient to notify health care professional if pregnancy is planned or suspected or if breast feeding.
- Inform patient that proctoscopy and sigmoidoscopy may be required periodically during treatment to determine response.
- **Rect:** Instruct patient to use *rectal suspension* at bedtime and retain suspension all night for best results.

Evaluation/Desired Outcomes

- Decrease in diarrhea and abdominal pain.
- Return to normal bowel pattern in patients with inflammatory bowel disease. Effects may be seen

within 3–21 days. The usual course of therapy is 3–6 wk.

- Maintenance of remission in patients with inflammatory bowel disease.

mesna (mes-na)

Mesnex, ♣Uromitexan

Classification

Therapeutic: antidotes

Pharmacologic: ifosfamide detoxifying agents

Pregnancy Category B

Indications

Prevention of ifosfamide-induced hemorrhagic cystitis (see Ifosfamide monograph). **Unlabeled Use:** May also prevent hemorrhagic cystitis from cyclophosphamide.

Action

Binds to the toxic metabolites of ifosfamide in the kidneys. **Therapeutic Effects:** Prevents hemorrhagic cystitis from ifosfamide.

Pharmacokinetics

Absorption: IV administration results in complete bioavailability; 45–79% absorbed after oral administration. Following IV with PO dosing ↑ systemic exposure.

Distribution: Unknown.

Metabolism and Excretion: Rapidly converted to mesna disulfide, then back to mesna in the kidneys, where it binds to toxic metabolites of ifosfamide (18–26% excreted as free mesna in urine after IV and PO dosing).

Half-life: *Mesna*—0.36 hr (IV); 1.2—8.3 hr (IV followed by PO); *mesna disulfide*—1.17 hr.

TIME/ACTION PROFILE (detoxifying action)

ROUTE	ONSET	PEAK	DURATION
PO, IV	rapid	unknown	4 hr

Contraindications/Precautions

Contraindicated in: Hypersensitivity to mesna or other thiol (rubber) compounds.

Use Cautiously in: OB, Lactation: Safety not established.

Adverse Reactions/Side Effects

CNS: dizziness, drowsiness, headache. **GI:** anorexia, diarrhea, nausea, unpleasant taste, vomiting. **Derm:** flushing. **Local:** injection site reactions. **Misc:** flu-like symptoms.

Interactions

Drug-Drug: None significant.

Route/Dosage

IV (Adults): Give a dose of mesna equal to 20% of the ifosfamide dose at the same time as ifosfamide and 4 and 8 hr after.

PO, IV (Adults): Give a dose of IV mesna equal to 20% of the ifosfamide dose at the same time as ifosfamide; then give PO mesna equal to 40% of the ifosfamide dose 2 and 6 hr after ifosfamide (total mesna dose is 100% of ifosfamide dose).

Availability (generic available)

Tablets: 400 mg. **Injection:** 100 mg/mL.

NURSING IMPLICATIONS

Assessment

- Monitor for development of hemorrhagic cystitis in patients receiving ifosfamide.
- ***Lab Test Considerations:*** Causes a false-positive result when testing urinary ketones.

M

Potential Nursing Diagnoses

Deficient knowledge, related to medication regimen (Patient/Family Teaching)

Implementation

- Initial IV bolus is to be given at time of ifosfamide administration.
- **PO:** If second and third doses are given orally, administer 2 and 6 hr after IV dose.
- If PO mesna is vomited within 2 hr of administration, repeat dose or use IV mesna.

IV Administration

- **Intermittent Infusion:** 2nd IV dose is given 4 hr later, 3rd dose is given 8 hr after initial dose. This schedule must be repeated with each subsequent dose of ifosfamide. ***Diluent:*** Dilute 2-, 4-, and 10-mL ampules, containing a concentration of 100 mg/mL in 8 mL, 16 mL, or 50 mL, respectively, of D5W, 0.9% NaCl, D5/0.9% NaCl, D5/0.2% NaCl, D5/0.33% NaCl, or LR. ***Concentration:*** 20 mg/mL. Refrigerate to store. Use within 6 hr. Discard unused solution. ***Rate:*** Administer over 15–30 min or as a continuous infusion.
- **Syringe Compatibility:** ifosfamide.
- **Y-Site Compatibility:** alemtuzumab, alfentanil, allopurinol, amifostine, amikacin, aminocaproic acid, aminophylline, amiodarone, amphotericin B liposome, ampicillin, ampicillin/sulbactam, anidulafungin, argatroban, azithromycin, aztreonam, bivalirudin, bleomycin, bumetanide, buprenorphine, butorphanol, calcium acetate, calcium chloride, calcium gluconate, carmustine, caspofungin, cefazolin, cefepime, cefotaxime, cefotetan, cefoxitin, ceftriaxone, cefuroxime, chloramphenicol, chlorpromazine, ciprofloxacin, cisatracurium, cladribine, clindamycin, cyclophosphamide, cytarabine, dactinomycin,

dexamethasone, dexmedetomidine, dexrazoxane, digoxin, diltiazem, diphenhydramine, dobutamine, docetaxel, dolasetron, dopamine, doxorubicin hydrochloride, doxorubicin liposomal, doxycycline, droperidol, enalaprilat, ephedrine, epinephrine, epirubicin, ertapenem, erythromycin, esmolol, etoposide, etoposide phosphate, famotidine, fentanyl, filgrastim, fluconazole, fludarabine, fluorouracil, foscarnet, fosphenytoin, furosemide, gemcitabine, gentamicin, glycopyrrolate, granisetron, haloperidol, heparin, hetastarch, hydralazine, hydrocortisone, hydromorphone, idarubicin, ifosfamide, imipenem/cilastatin, insulin, irinotecan, isoproterenol, ketorolac, labetalol, leucovorin, levofloxacin, lidocaine, linezolid, lorazepam, magnesium sulfate, mannitol, mechlorethamine, melphalan, meperidine, meropenem, methotrexate, methyldopate, methylprednisolone, metoclopramide, metoprolol, metronidazole, micafungin, midazolam, milrinone, mitomycin, mitoxantrone, morphine, moxifloxacin, mycophenolate, nafcillin, nalbuphine, naloxone, nesiritide, nitroglycerin, norepinephrine, octreotide, ondansetron, oxaliplatin, paclitaxel, palonosetron, pamidronate, pancuronium, pantoprazole, pemetrexed, pentamidine, pentazocine, pentobarbital, phenobarbital, phenylephrine, piperacillin/tazobactam, potassium acetate, potassium chloride, potassium phosphates, procainamide, prochlorperazine, promethazine, propranolol, ranitidine, remifentanil, rituximab, rocuronium, sargramostim, sodium acetate, sodium bicarbonate, sodium phosphates, streptozocin, succinylcholine, sufentanil, tacrolimus, teniposide, theophylline, thiotepa, tigecycline, tirofiban, tobramycin, topotecan, trastuzumab, vancomycin, vasopressin, vecuronium, verapamil, vinblastine, vincristine, vinorelbine, voriconazole, zidovudine, zoledronic acid.

- **Y-Site Incompatibility:** acyclovir, amphotericin B colloidal, amphotericin B lipid complex, dacarbazine, dantrolene, diazepam, fenoldopam, ganciclovir, nicardipine, nitroprusside, phenytoin, quinupristin/dalfopristin, thiopental.

Patient/Family Teaching

- Inform patient that unpleasant taste may occur during administration.
- Advise patient to notify health care professional if nausea, vomiting, or diarrhea persists or is severe.
- Advise female patient to notify health care professional if pregnancy is planned or suspected and to avoid breast feeding.

Evaluation/Desired Outcomes

- Prevention of hemorrhagic cystitis associated with ifosfamide therapy.

mestranol/norethindrone, See CONTRACEPTIVES, HORMONAL.

metaxalone (me-tax-a-lone)

Skelaxin

Classification

Therapeutic: skeletal muscle relaxants (centrally acting)

Pregnancy Category UK

Indications

Muscle spasm associated with acute painful musculoskeletal conditions (with rest and physical therapy).

Action

Skeletal muscle relaxation, probably as a result of CNS depression. **Therapeutic Effects:** Skeletal muscle relaxation.

Pharmacokinetics

Absorption: Well absorbed following oral administration.

Distribution: Unknown.

Metabolism and Excretion: Mostly metabolized by the liver; metabolites excreted in urine.

Half-life: 2–3 hr.

TIME/ACTION PROFILE

ROUTE	ONSET	PEAK	DURATION
PO	1 hr	2 hr	4–6 hr

Contraindications/Precautions

Contraindicated in: Hypersensitivity; Significant hepatic/renal impairment; History of drug-induced hemolytic anemia or other anemia.

Use Cautiously in: Hepatic impairment; History of seizures; OB, Lactation, Pedi: Pregnancy, lactation or children ≤12 yr (safety not established); Geri: Appears on Beers list. Poorly tolerated due to anticholinergic effects.

Adverse Reactions/Side Effects

CNS: drowsiness, dizziness, confusion, headache, irritability, nervousness. **GI:** nausea, anorexia, dry mouth, GI upset, vomiting. **GU:** urinary retention.

Interactions

Drug-Drug: ↑ CNS depression with other **CNS depressants** including **alcohol**, **antihistamines**, **opioid analgesics**, and **sedative/hypnotics**.

Drug-Natural Products: Concomitant use of **kava-kava**, **valerian**, or **chamomile** can ↑ CNS depression.

Route/Dosage

PO (Adults): 800 mg 3–4 times daily.

Availability (generic available)

Tablets: 800 mg. **Cost:** *Generic*—$409.39/100.

NURSING IMPLICATIONS

Assessment

- Assess for pain, muscle stiffness, and range of motion before and periodically during therapy.
- Geri: Assess geriatric patients for anticholinergic effects (sedation and weakness).
- ***Lab Test Considerations:*** Monitor hepatic function tests closely in patients with pre-existing liver damage.
- May cause false-positive Benedict's tests.

Potential Nursing Diagnoses

Acute pain (Indications)
Impaired bed mobility (Indications)
Risk for injury (Side Effects)

Implementation

- Provide safety measures as indicated. Supervise ambulation and transfer.
- **PO:** Administer 3–4 times daily.

Patient/Family Teaching

- Instruct patient to take medication as directed. Take missed doses within 1 hr; if not, return to regular dosing schedule. Do not double doses.
- Encourage patient to comply with additional therapies prescribed for muscle spasm (rest, physical therapy, heat).
- Medication may cause dizziness, drowsiness, and blurred vision. Advise patient to avoid driving and other activities requiring alertness until response to drug is known.
- Instruct patient to make position changes slowly to minimize orthostatic hypotension.
- Advise patient to avoid concurrent use of alcohol and other CNS depressants while taking this medication.
- Instruct patient to notify health care professional if skin rash or yellowish discoloration of the skin or eyes occurs.
- Emphasize the importance of routine follow-up exams to monitor progress.

Evaluation/Desired Outcomes

- Decreased musculoskeletal pain and muscle spasticity.
- Increased range of motion.

metFORMIN (met-for-min)

Fortamet, Glucophage, Glucophage XR, Glumetza, ✤Glycon, Riomet

Classification
Therapeutic: antidiabetics
Pharmacologic: biguanides

Pregnancy Category B

Indications

Management of type 2 diabetes mellitus; may be used with diet, insulin, or sulfonylurea oral hypoglycemics.

Action

Decreases hepatic glucose production. Decreases intestinal glucose absorption. Increases sensitivity to insulin.
Therapeutic Effects: Maintenance of blood glucose.

Pharmacokinetics

Absorption: 50–60% absorbed after oral administration.
Distribution: Enters breast milk in concentrations similar to plasma.
Metabolism and Excretion: Eliminated almost entirely unchanged by the kidneys.
Half-life: 17.6 hr.

TIME/ACTION PROFILE (blood levels)

ROUTE	ONSET	PEAK	DURATION
PO	unknown	unknown	12 hr
XR	unknown	4–8 hr	24 hr

Contraindications/Precautions

Contraindicated in: Hypersensitivity; Metabolic acidosis; Dehydration, sepsis, hypoxemia, hepatic impairment, excessive alcohol use (acute or chronic); Renal dysfunction (SCr >1.5 mg/dL in men or >1.4 mg/dL in women); Radiographic studies requiring IV iodinated contrast media (withhold metformin); HF.
Use Cautiously in: Concurrent renal disease; Geri: Geriatric/debilitated patients (↓ doses may be required; avoid in patients >80 yr unless renal function is normal); Chronic alcohol use/abuse; Serious medical conditions (MI, stroke); Patients undergoing stress (infection, surgical procedures); Hypoxia; Pituitary deficiency or hyperthyroidism; OB, Lactation, Pedi: Pregnancy, lactation, or children <10 yr (safety not established; extended release for use in patients >17 yr only).

Adverse Reactions/Side Effects

GI: abdominal bloating, diarrhea, nausea, vomiting, unpleasant metallic taste. **F and E:** LACTIC ACIDOSIS.
Misc: decreased vitamin B_{12} levels.

Interactions

Drug-Drug: Acute or chronic **alcohol** ingestion or **iodinated contrast media** ↑ risk of lactic acidosis. **Amiloride**, **digoxin**, **morphine**, **procainamide**, **quinidine**, **ranitidine**, **triamterene**, **trimethoprim**, **calcium channel blockers**, and **vancomycin** may compete for elimination pathways with metformin. Altered responses may occur. **Cimetidine** and **furosemide** may ↑ effects of metformin. **Nifedipine** ↑ absorption and effects.

Drug-Natural Products: Glucosamine may worsen blood glucose control. **Chromium**, and **coenzyme Q-10** may produce ↑ hypoglycemic effects.

Route/Dosage

PO (Adults and children >17 yr): 500 mg twice daily; may ↑ by 500 mg at weekly intervals up to 2000 mg/day. If doses >2000 mg/day are required, give in 3 divided doses (not to exceed 2500 mg/day) or 850 mg once daily; may ↑ by 850 mg at 2-wk intervals (in divided doses) up to 2550 mg/day in divided doses (up to 850 mg 3 times daily); *Extended-release tablets*—500–1000 mg once daily with evening meal, may ↑ by 500 mg at weekly intervals up to 2500 mg once daily. If 2000 mg once daily is inadequate, 1000 mg twice daily may be used.

PO (Children >10 yr): 500 mg twice daily, may be ↑ by 500 mg/day at 1-wk intervals, up to 2000 mg/day in 2 divided doses.

Availability (generic available)

Tablets: 500 mg, 850 mg, 1000 mg. **Cost:** *Generic*—500 mg $6.99/100, 850 mg $7.18/100, 1000 mg $7.01/100. **Extended-release tablets (Fortamet, Glucophage XR, Glumetza):** 500 mg, 750 mg, 1000 mg. **Cost:** *Generic*—500 mg $74.50/100, 750 mg $119.70/100. **Oral solution (Riomet) (cherry flavor):** 100 mg/mL. **Cost:** $59.30/118 mL. ***In combination with:*** glyburide (Glucovance) glipizide (Metaglip), pioglitazone (Actoplus Met, Actoplus Met XR), repaglinide (PrandiMet), rosiglitazone (Avandamet), alogliptin (Kazano), sitagliptin (Janumet, Janumet XR), saxagliptin (Kombiglyze XR), linagliptin (Jentadueto), canagliflozin (Invokamet), and dapagliflozin (Xigduo XR). See Appendix B.

NURSING IMPLICATIONS

Assessment

- When combined with oral sulfonylureas, observe for signs and symptoms of hypoglycemic reactions (abdominal pain, sweating, hunger, weakness, dizziness, headache, tremor, tachycardia, anxiety).
- Patients who have been well controlled on metformin who develop illness or laboratory abnormalities should be assessed for ketoacidosis or lactic acidosis. Assess serum electrolytes, ketones, glucose, and, if indicated, blood pH, lactate, pyruvate, and metformin levels. If either form of acidosis is present, discontinue metformin immediately and treat acidosis.
- ***Lab Test Considerations:*** Monitor serum glucose and glycosylated hemoglobin periodically during therapy to evaluate effectiveness of therapy. May cause false-positive results for urine ketones.
- Assess renal function before initiating and at least annually during therapy. Discontinue metformin if renal impairment occurs.
- Monitor serum folic acid and vitamin B_{12} every 1–2 yr in long-term therapy. Metformin may interfere with absorption.

Potential Nursing Diagnoses

Imbalanced nutrition: more than body requirements (Indications)
Noncompliance (Patient/Family Teaching)

Implementation

- Do not confuse metformin with metronidazole.
- Patients stabilized on a diabetic regimen who are exposed to stress, fever, trauma, infection, or surgery may require administration of insulin. Withhold metformin and reinstitute after resolution of acute episode.
- Metformin should be temporarily discontinued in patients requiring surgery involving restricted intake of food and fluids. Resume metformin when oral intake has resumed and renal function is normal.
- Withhold metformin before or at the time of studies requiring IV administration of iodinated contrast media and for 48 hr after study.
- **PO:** Administer metformin with meals to minimize GI effects.
- XR tablets must be swallowed whole; do not crush, dissolve, or chew.

Patient/Family Teaching

- Instruct patient to take metformin at the same time each day, as directed. Take missed doses as soon as possible unless almost time for next dose. Do not double doses. Instruct parent/caregiver to read the *Medication Guide* prior to use and with each Rx refill; new information may be available.
- Explain to patient that metformin helps control hyperglycemia but does not cure diabetes. Therapy is usually long term.
- Encourage patient to follow prescribed diet, medication, and exercise regimen to prevent hyperglycemic or hypoglycemic episodes.
- Review signs of hypoglycemia and hyperglycemia with patient. If hypoglycemia occurs, advise patient to take a glass of orange juice or 2–3 tsp of sugar, honey, or corn syrup dissolved in water, and notify health care professional.
- Instruct patient in proper testing of blood glucose and urine ketones. These tests should be monitored closely during periods of stress or illness and health care professional notified if significant changes occur.
- Explain to patient the risk of lactic acidosis and the potential need for discontinuation of metformin therapy if a severe infection, dehydration, or severe or continuing diarrhea occurs or if medical tests or surgery is required. Symptoms of lactic acidosis (chills, diarrhea, dizziness, low BP, muscle pain, sleepiness, slow heartbeat or pulse, dyspnea, or weakness) should be reported to health care professional immediately.
- Advise patient to notify health care professional of all Rx or OTC medications, vitamins, or herbal products being taken and to consult with health care professional before taking other medications or alcohol.

- Inform patient that metformin may cause an unpleasant or metallic taste that usually resolves spontaneously.
- Inform patients taking XR tablets that inactive ingredients resembling XR tablet may appear in stools.
- Advise patient to inform health care professional of medication regimen before treatment or surgery.
- Advise patient to report the occurrence of diarrhea, nausea, vomiting, and stomach pain or fullness to health care professional.
- Insulin is the recommended method of controlling blood glucose during pregnancy. Counsel female patients to use a form of contraception other than oral contraceptives and to notify health care professional promptly if pregnancy is planned or suspected, or if breast feeding.
- Advise patient to carry a form of sugar (sugar packets, candy) and identification describing disease process and medication regimen at all times.
- Emphasize the importance of routine follow-up exams and regular testing of blood glucose, glycosylated hemoglobin, renal function, and hematologic parameters.

Evaluation/Desired Outcomes

- Control of blood glucose levels without the appearance of hypoglycemic or hyperglycemic episodes. Control may be achieved within a few days, but full effect of therapy may be delayed for up to 2 wk. If patient has not responded to metformin after 4 wk of maximum dose therapy, an oral sulfonylurea may be added. If satisfactory results are not obtained with 1–3 mo of concurrent therapy, oral agents may be discontinued and insulin therapy instituted.

REMS HIGH ALERT

methadone (meth-a-done)

Dolophine, ✱Metadol, ✱Metadol-D, Methadose

Classification

Therapeutic: opioid analgesics
Pharmacologic: opioid agonists

Schedule II

Pregnancy Category C

Indications

Moderate to severe chronic pain in opioid-tolerant patients requiring use of daily, around-the-clock long-term opioid treatment and for which alternative treatment options are inadequate (extended-release). Detoxification and maintenance therapy for opioid use disorder. **Unlabeled Use:** Neonatal abstinence syndrome.

Action

Binds to opiate receptors in the CNS. Alters the perception of and response to painful stimuli, while producing generalized CNS depression. **Therapeutic Effects:** Decrease in severity of pain. Suppression of withdrawal symptoms during detoxification and maintenance from heroin and other opioids.

Pharmacokinetics

Absorption: Well absorbed from all sites (50% absorbed following oral administration).

Distribution: Widely distributed. Crosses the placenta; enters breast milk.

Protein Binding: High.

Metabolism and Excretion: Mostly metabolized by the liver; some metabolites are active and may accumulate with chronic administration.

Half-life: 15–25 hr; ↑ with chronic use.

TIME/ACTION PROFILE (analgesic effect)

ROUTE	ONSET	PEAK	DURATION
PO	30–60 min	90–120 min	4–12 hr
IM, subcut	10–20 min	60–120 min	4–6 hr

Contraindications/Precautions

Contraindicated in: Hypersensitivity; Significant respiratory depression; Acute or severe bronchial asthma; Paralytic ileus; Known alcohol intolerance (some oral solutions); Concurrent MAO inhibitor therapy.

Use Cautiously in: Structural heart disease, concomitant diuretic use, hypokalemia, hypomagnesemia, history of arrhythmia/syncope, or other risk factors for arrhythmias; Concurrent use of drugs that prolong the QTc interval or are CYP3A4 inhibitors; Head trauma; Seizure disorders; ↑ intracranial pressure; Severe renal, hepatic, or pulmonary disease; Hypothyroidism; Adrenal insufficiency; Alcoholism; Undiagnosed abdominal pain; Prostatic hyperplasia or ureteral stricture; OB: Use with addiction control: weigh risk against potential for illicit drug use. Counsel mother about potential harm to fetus. Prolonged use of methadone during pregnancy can result in neonatal opioid withdrawal syndrome; Lactation: Appears in breast milk. Weigh risks against potential for illicit drug use. Counsel mother about potential harm to infant and to wean breast feeding slowly to prevent abstinence syndrome; Geri: ↑ risk of respiratory depression (dose ↓ suggested).

Adverse Reactions/Side Effects

CNS: <u>confusion</u>, <u>sedation</u>, dizziness, dysphoria, euphoria, floating feeling, hallucinations, headache, unusual dreams. **EENT:** blurred vision, diplopia, miosis. **Resp:** RESPIRATORY DEPRESSION. **CV:** TORSADES DE

M

POINTES, hypotension, bradycardia, QT interval prolongation. **GI:** constipation, nausea, vomiting. **GU:** urinary retention. **Derm:** flushing, sweating. **Misc:** physical dependence, psychological dependence, tolerance.

Interactions

Drug-Drug: Use with extreme caution in patients receiving **MAO inhibitors** (may result in severe, unpredictable reactions—↓ initial dose of methadone to 25% of usual dose). Use with extreme caution with any drug known to potentially prolong QT interval, including **class I and III antiarrhythmics**, some **neuroleptics** and **tricyclic antidepressants**, and **calcium channel blockers**. Use with extreme caution with CYP3A4 inhibitors, including **ketoconazole, itraconazole, erythromycin, clarithromycin, calcium channel blockers**, or **voriconazole**. Concurrent use with **laxatives, diuretics**, or **mineralocorticoids** may ↑ risk of hypomagnesemia or hypokalemia and ↑ risk of arrhythmias. ↑ CNS depression with **alcohol, antihistamines**, and **sedative/hypnotics**. Administration of **agonist/antagonist opioids** may precipitate opioid withdrawal in physically dependent patients. **Nalbuphine** or **pentazocine** may ↓ analgesia. **Interferons (alpha)** may ↓ metabolism and ↑ effects. **Abacavir, darunavir/ritonavir, nelfinavir, nevirapine, efavirenz, ritonavir, ritonavir/lopinavir, saquinavir/ritonavir, tipranavir/ritonavir, phenobarbital, carbamazepine phenytoin**, and **rifampin** may ↑ metabolism and ↓ analgesia; withdrawal may occur. **Fluvoxamine** may ↑ CNS depression; with **fluvoxamine**, opioid withdrawal may occur. May ↑ blood levels and effects of **zidovudine** and **desipramine**. May ↓ level and effects of **didanosine** and **stavudine**. Concurrent abuse of methadone with **benzodiazepines** has resulted in death.

Drug-Natural Products: St. John's wort ↑ metabolism and ↓ blood levels, concurrent use may result in withdrawal. **Kava-kava, valerian**, or **chamomile**, can ↑ CNS depression.

Route/Dosage

Larger doses may be required for analgesia during chronic therapy; interval may be ↓/dose ↑ if pain recurs.

PO (Adults and Children ≥50 kg): *Usual starting dose for moderate to severe pain in opioid-naive patients*—2.5 mg q 8–12 hr; *Opioid detoxification*—15–40 mg once daily or amount needed to prevent withdrawal. Dose may be ↓ q 1–2 days; maintenance dose is determined on an individual basis.

PO (Adults and Children <50 kg): *Analgesic*—0.1 mg/kg/dose q 4 hr for 2–3 doses then q 6–8 hr prn; maximum: 10 mg/dose. *Iatrogenic narcotic dependency*—0.05–0.1 mg/kg/dose q 6 hr; ↑ by 0.05 mg/kg/dose until withdrawal symptoms controlled; after 1–2 days lengthen dosing interval to q 12–24 hr; taper by ↓ dose by 0.05 mg/kg/day.

PO, IV (Neonates): Initial 0.05–0.2 mg/kg/dose q 12–24 hr or 0.5 mg/kg/day divided q 8 hr; taper dose by 10–20% per week over 1–1 1/2 mo.

IV, IM, Subcut (Adults and Children ≥50 kg): *Analgesic*—10 mg q 6–8 hr. *Opioid detoxification*—15–40 mg once daily or amount needed to prevent withdrawal. Dose may be ↓ q 1–2 days; maintenance dose is determined on an individual basis.

IV, IM, Subcut (Adults and Children <50 kg): *Analgesic*—0.1 mg/kg q 6–8 hr; maximum: 10 mg/dose.

Availability (generic available)

Tablets: 🍁1 mg, 5 mg, 10 mg, 🍁25 mg. **Dispersible tablets (diskettes):** 40 mg (available only to licensed detoxification/maintenance programs). **Injection:** 10 mg/mL. **Oral solution (contains alcohol) (citrus):** 5 mg/5 mL, 10 mg/5 mL. **Oral concentrate (cherry and unflavored):** 10 mg/mL.

NURSING IMPLICATIONS

Assessment

- **Pain:** Assess type, location, and intensity of pain prior to and 1–2 hr (peak) following administration. When titrating opioid doses, increases of 25–50% should be administered until there is either a 50% reduction in the patient's pain rating on a numeric or visual analogue scale or the patient reports satisfactory pain relief. Dose increases should be made no more frequently than every 3–5 days because of variability in half-life between patients. Cumulative effects of this medication may require periodic dose adjustments.
- Doses of methadone for patients on methadone maintenance only prevent withdrawal symptoms; *no analgesia is provided*. Additional opioid doses are required for treatment of pain.
- An equianalgesic chart (see Appendix I) should be used when changing routes or when changing from one opioid to another.
- Assess BP, pulse, and respirations before and periodically during administration. If respiratory rate is <10/min, assess level of sedation. Dose may need to be decreased by 25–50%. Initial drowsiness will diminish with continued use.
- Assess bowel function routinely. Prevention of constipation should be instituted with increased intake of fluids and bulk and with laxatives to minimize constipating effects. Stimulant laxatives should be administered routinely if opioid use exceeds 2–3 days, unless contraindicated.
- Prolonged use may lead to physical and psychological dependence and tolerance. This should not prevent patient from receiving adequate analgesia. Most patients who receive methadone for pain do not develop psychological dependence. Progressively higher doses may be required to relieve pain with long-term therapy.
- Assess for history of structural heart disease, arrhythmia, and syncope. Obtain a pretreatment ECG

to measure QTc interval and follow-up ECG within 30 days and annually. Additional ECGs recommended if dose >100 m g/day or if patients have unexplained syncope or seizures. If QTc interval is >450 ms but <500 ms, discuss potential risks and benefits with patients and monitor more frequently. If the QTc interval >500 ms, consider discontinuing or reducing dose; eliminating contributing factors (drugs that promote hypokalemia) or using an alternative therapy.

- Assess risk for opioid addiction, abuse, or misuse prior to administration. Abuse or misuse of extended-release preparations by crushing, chewing, snorting, or injecting dissolved product will result in uncontrolled delivery of methadone and can result in overdose and death.
- **Opioid Detoxification:** Assess patient for signs of opioid withdrawal (irritability, runny nose and eyes, abdominal cramps, body aches, sweating, loss of appetite, shivering, unusually large pupils, trouble sleeping, weakness, yawning). Methadone maintenance is undertaken only by federally approved treatment centers. This does not preclude maintenance for addicts hospitalized for other conditions and who require temporary maintenance during their care.
- ***Lab Test Considerations:*** May ↑ plasma amylase and lipase levels.
- ***Toxicity and Overdose:*** If an opioid antagonist is required to reverse respiratory depression or coma, naloxone is the antidote. Dilute the 0.4-mg ampule of naloxone in 10 mL of 0.9% NaCl and administer 0.5 mL (0.02 mg) by IV push every 2 min. For children and patients weighing <40 kg, dilute 0.1 mg of naloxone in 10 mL of 0.9% NaCl for a concentration of 10 mcg/mL and administer 0.5 mcg/kg every 2 min. Titrate dose to avoid withdrawal, seizures, and severe pain.

Potential Nursing Diagnoses

Acute pain (Indications)
Disturbed sensory perception (visual, auditory) (Side Effects)
Risk for injury (Side Effects)

Implementation

- ***High Alert:*** Do not confuse methadone with dexmethylphenidate, ketorolac, Mephyton (phytonadione), Metadate ER/CD (methylphenidate), or methylphenidate.
- Explain therapeutic value of medication prior to administration to enhance the analgesic effect.
- Regularly administered doses may be more effective than prn administration. Analgesic is more effective if administered before pain becomes severe. For patients in chronic severe pain, the oral solution containing 5 or 10 mg/5 mL is recommended on a fixed dose schedule.
- Coadministration with nonopioid analgesics may have additive analgesic effects and may permit lower doses.
- Medication should be discontinued gradually after long-term use to prevent withdrawal symptoms.
- **PO:** Doses may be administered with food or milk to minimize GI irritation.
- Dilute each dose of 10 mg/mL oral concentrate with at least 30 mL of water or other liquid prior to administration.
- Diskettes (dispersible tablets) are to be dissolved and used for detoxification and maintenance treatment only. Available only to licensed detoxification/maintenance programs.
- **Subcut, IM:** IM is the preferred parenteral route for repeated doses. Subcut administration may cause tissue irritation.

M

Patient/Family Teaching

- Instruct patient on how and when to ask for and take pain medication.
- Instruct patient to take methadone exactly as directed. If dose is less effective after a few weeks, do not increase dose without consulting health care professional.
- May cause drowsiness or dizziness. Advise patient to call for assistance when ambulating or smoking and to avoid driving or other activities requiring alertness until response to medication is known.
- Inform patient of the potential for arrhythmias and emphasize the importance of regular ECGs.
- Caution patient to notify health care professional if signs of overdose (difficult or shallow breathing, extreme tiredness or sleepiness, blurred vision, inability to think, talk, or walk normally, and feelings of faintness, dizziness, or confusion) occur. Methadone has a prolonged action causing increased risk of overdose.
- Advise patient to change positions slowly to minimize orthostatic hypotension.
- Advise patient to tell health care professional what medications they are taking and to avoid taking new Rx, OTC, vitamins, or herbal products without consulting health care professional. Caution patient to avoid concurrent use of alcohol or other CNS depressants with this medication.
- Encourage patient to turn, cough, and breathe deeply every 2 hr to prevent atelectasis.

Evaluation/Desired Outcomes

- Decrease in severity of pain without a significant alteration in level of consciousness or respiratory status.
- Prevention of withdrawal symptoms in detoxification from heroin and other opioid analgesics.

methimazole (meth-im-a-zole)

Tapazole

Classification

Therapeutic: antithyroid agents

Pregnancy Category D

Indications

Palliative treatment of hyperthyroidism. Used as an adjunct to control hyperthyroidism in preparation for thyroidectomy or radioactive iodine therapy.

Action

Inhibits the synthesis of thyroid hormones. **Therapeutic Effects:** Decreased signs and symptoms of hyperthyroidism.

Pharmacokinetics

Absorption: Rapidly absorbed following oral administration.

Distribution: Crosses the placenta and enters breast milk in high concentrations.

Metabolism and Excretion: Mostly metabolized by the liver; <10% eliminated unchanged by the kidneys.

Half-life: 3–5 hr.

TIME/ACTION PROFILE (effect on thyroid function)

ROUTE	ONSET	PEAK	DURATION
PO	1 wk	4–10 wk	wk

Contraindications/Precautions

Contraindicated in: Hypersensitivity; Lactation: Lactation.

Use Cautiously in: Patients with ↓ bone marrow reserve; Patients >40 yr (↑ risk of agranulocytosis); OB: May be used cautiously; however, thyroid problems may occur in the fetus.

Adverse Reactions/Side Effects

CNS: drowsiness, headache, vertigo. **GI:** diarrhea, hepatotoxicity, loss of taste, nausea, parotitis, vomiting. **Derm:** rash, skin discoloration, urticaria. **Hemat:** AGRANULOCYTOSIS, anemia, leukopenia, thrombocytopenia. **MS:** arthralgia. **Misc:** fever, lymphadenopathy.

Interactions

Drug-Drug: Additive bone marrow depression with **antineoplastics** or **radiation therapy**. Antithyroid effect may be ↓ by **potassium iodide** or **amiodarone**. ↑ risk of agranulocytosis with **phenothiazines**. May alter response to **warfarin** and **digoxin**.

Route/Dosage

PO (Adults): *Thyrotoxic crisis*—15–20 mg q 4 hr during the first 24 hr (with other interventions). *Hyperthyroidism*—15–60 mg/day as a single dose or divided doses for 6–8 wk. *Maintenance*—5–30 mg/kg as a single dose or 2 divided doses.

PO (Children): *Initial*—400 mcg (0.4 mg)/kg/day in single dose or 2 divided doses. *Maintenance*—200 mcg/kg/day in single dose or 2 divided doses.

Availability (generic available)

Tablets: 5 mg, 10 mg.

NURSING IMPLICATIONS

Assessment

- Monitor response for symptoms of hyperthyroidism or thyrotoxicosis (tachycardia, palpitations, nervousness, insomnia, fever, diaphoresis, heat intolerance, tremors, weight loss, diarrhea).
- Assess for development of hypothyroidism (intolerance to cold, constipation, dry skin, headache, listlessness, tiredness, or weakness). Dose adjustment may be required.
- Assess for skin rash or swelling of cervical lymph nodes. Treatment may be discontinued if this occurs.
- ***Lab Test Considerations:*** Monitor thyroid function studies prior to therapy, monthly during initial therapy, and every 2–3 mo during therapy.
- Monitor WBC and differential counts periodically during therapy. Agranulocytosis may develop rapidly; usually occurs during the first 2 mo and is more common in patients over 40 yr and those receiving >40 mg/day. This necessitates discontinuation of therapy.
- May cause ↑ AST, ALT, LDH, alkaline phosphatase, serum bilirubin, and prothrombin time.

Potential Nursing Diagnoses

Noncompliance (Patient/Family Teaching)

Implementation

- Do not confuse methimazole with metolazone.
- **PO:** Administer at same time in relation to meals every day. Food may either increase or decrease absorption.

Patient/Family Teaching

- Instruct patient to take medication as directed, around the clock. Take missed doses as soon as remembered; take both doses together if almost time for next dose; check with health care professional if more than 1 dose is missed. Consult health care professional prior to discontinuing medication.
- Instruct patient to monitor weight 2–3 times weekly. Notify health care professional of significant changes.
- May cause drowsiness. Caution patient to avoid driving or other activities requiring alertness until response to medication is known.
- Advise patient to consult health care professional regarding dietary sources of iodine (iodized salt, shellfish).
- Advise patient to report sore throat, fever, chills, headache, malaise, weakness, yellowing of eyes or

skin, unusual bleeding or bruising, rash, or symptoms of hyperthyroidism or hypothyroidism promptly.
- Instruct patient to notify health care professional of all Rx or OTC medications, vitamins, or herbal products being taken and to consult with health care professional before taking other medications.
- Advise patient to carry identification describing medication regimen at all times.
- Advise patient to notify health care professional of medication regimen prior to treatment or surgery.
- Emphasize the importance of routine exams to monitor progress and to check for side effects.

Evaluation/Desired Outcomes
- Decrease in severity of symptoms of hyperthyroidism (lowered pulse rate and weight gain).
- Return of thyroid function studies to normal.
- May be used as short-term adjunctive therapy to prepare patient for thyroidectomy or radiation therapy or may be used in treatment of hyperthyroidism. Treatment from 6 mo to several yr may be necessary, usually averaging 1 yr.

methocarbamol
(meth-oh-**kar**-ba-mole)
✱Robaximol, Robaxin

Classification
Therapeutic: skeletal muscle relaxants (centrally acting)

Pregnancy Category C

Indications
Adjunctive treatment of muscle spasm associated with acute painful musculoskeletal conditions (with rest and physical therapy).

Action
Skeletal muscle relaxation, probably as a result of CNS depression. **Therapeutic Effects:** Skeletal muscle relaxation.

Pharmacokinetics
Absorption: Rapidly absorbed from the GI tract.
Distribution: Widely distributed. Crosses the placenta; enters breast milk in small amounts.
Metabolism and Excretion: Metabolized by the liver.
Half-life: 1–2 hr.

TIME/ACTION PROFILE (skeletal muscle relaxation)

ROUTE	ONSET	PEAK	DURATION
PO	30 min	2 hr	unknown
IM	rapid	unknown	unknown
IV	immediate	end of infusion	unknown

Contraindications/Precautions
Contraindicated in: Hypersensitivity; Hypersensitivity to polyethylene glycol (parenteral form); Renal impairment (parenteral form).
Use Cautiously in: Seizure disorders (parenteral form); OB, Pedi, Lactation: Safety not established; Geri: Appears on Beers list. Poorly tolerated due to anticholinergic effects.

Adverse Reactions/Side Effects
CNS: SEIZURES (IV, IM only), dizziness, drowsiness, light-headedness. **EENT:** blurred vision, nasal congestion. **CV:** *IV*—bradycardia, hypotension. **GI:** anorexia, GI upset, nausea. **GU:** brown, black, or green urine. **Derm:** flushing (IV only), pruritus, rashes, urticaria. **Local:** pain at IM site, phlebitis at IV site. **Misc:** allergic reactions including ANAPHYLAXIS (IM, IV use only), fever.

Interactions
Drug-Drug: Additive CNS depression with other **CNS depressants**, including **alcohol**, **antihistamines**, **opioid analgesics**, and **sedative/hypnotics**.
Drug-Natural Products: Concomitant use of **kava-kava**, **valerian**, **chamomile**, or **hops** can ↑ CNS depression.

Route/Dosage
PO (Adults): 1.5 g 4 times daily initially (up to 8 g/day) for 2–3 days, then 4–4.5 g/day in 3–6 divided doses; may be followed by maintenance dosing of 750 mg q 4 hr or 1 g 4 times daily or 1.5 g 3 times daily.
IM, IV (Adults): 1–3 g/day for not more than 3 days; course may be repeated after a 48-hr rest.

Availability (generic available)
Tablets: 500 mg, 750 mg. **Cost:** *Generic*—500 mg $41.79/100, 750 mg $60.28/100. **Injection:** 100 mg/mL.

NURSING IMPLICATIONS
Assessment
- Assess patient for pain, muscle stiffness, and range of motion before and periodically throughout therapy.
- Monitor pulse and BP every 15 min during parenteral administration.
- Geri: Assess geriatric patients for anticholinergic effects (sedation and weakness).

M

- Assess patient for allergic reactions (skin rash, asthma, hives, wheezing, hypotension) after parenteral administration. Keep epinephrine and oxygen on hand in the event of a reaction.
- Monitor IV site. Injection is hypertonic and may cause thrombophlebitis. Avoid extravasation.
- ***Lab Test Considerations:*** Monitor renal function periodically during prolonged parenteral therapy (>3 days), because polyethylene glycol 300 vehicle is nephrotoxic.
- May cause falsely increased urinary 5-hydroxyindoleacetic acid (5-HIAA) and vanillylmandelic acid (VMA) determinations.

Potential Nursing Diagnoses

Acute pain (Indications)
Impaired physical mobility (Indications)
Risk for injury (Side Effects)

Implementation

- Provide safety measures as indicated. Supervise ambulation and transfer of patients.
- **PO:** May be administered with food to minimize GI irritation. Tablets may be crushed and mixed with food or liquids to facilitate swallowing. For administration via NG tube, crush tablet and suspend in water or saline.
- **IM:** Do not administer subcut. IM injections should contain no more than 5 mL (500 mg) at a time in the gluteal region.

IV Administration

- **IV Push:** ***Diluent:*** Administer undiluted. ***Concentration:*** 100 mg/mL. ***Rate:*** Administer at a maximum rate of 180 mg/m^2/min but not >3 mL (300 mg)/min.
- **Intermittent Infusion:** ***Diluent:*** Dilute each dose in no more than 250 mL of 0.9% NaCl or D5W for injection. ***Concentration:*** 4 mg/mL for slower infusions. Do not refrigerate after dilution.
- Have patient remain recumbent during and for at least 10–15 min after infusion to avoid orthostatic hypotension.

Patient/Family Teaching

- Advise patient to take medication as directed. Take missed doses within 1 hr; if not, return to regular dosing schedule. Do not double doses.
- Encourage patient to comply with additional therapies prescribed for muscle spasm (rest, physical therapy, heat).
- May cause dizziness, drowsiness, and blurred vision. Advise patient to avoid driving and other activities requiring alertness until response to drug is known.
- Instruct patient to change positions slowly to minimize orthostatic hypotension.
- Advise patient to avoid concurrent use of alcohol and other CNS depressants.
- Inform patient that urine may turn black, brown, or green, especially if left standing.
- Instruct patient to notify health care professional if skin rash, itching, fever, or nasal congestion occurs.
- Emphasize the importance of routine follow-up exams to monitor progress.

Evaluation/Desired Outcomes

- Decreased musculoskeletal pain and muscle spasticity.
- Increased range of motion.

HIGH ALERT

methotrexate (meth-o-**trex**-ate)

Metoject, Otrexup, Rasuvo, Rheumatrex, Trexall

Classification
Therapeutic: antineoplastics, antirheumatics (DMARDs), immunosuppressants
Pharmacologic: antimetabolites

Pregnancy Category X

Indications

Alone or with other treatment modalities in the treatment of: Trophoblastic neoplasms (choriocarcinoma, chorioadenoma destruens, hydatidiform mole), Leukemias, Breast carcinoma, Head carcinoma, Neck carcinoma, Lung carcinoma. Severe psoriasis, rheumatoid arthritis, and polyarticular juvenile idiopathic arthritis unresponsive to conventional therapy. Treatment of mycosis fungoides (cutaneous T-cell lymphoma).

Action

Interferes with folic acid metabolism. Result is inhibition of DNA synthesis and cell reproduction (cell-cycle S-phase–specific). Also has immunosuppressive activity. **Therapeutic Effects:** Death of rapidly replicating cells, particularly malignant ones, and immunosuppression.

Pharmacokinetics

Absorption: Small doses are well absorbed from the GI tract. Larger doses incompletely absorbed.
Distribution: Actively transported across cell membranes, widely distributed. Does not reach therapeutic concentrations in the CSF. Crosses placenta; enters breast milk in low concentrations. Absorption in children is variable (23–95%) and dose-dependent.
Metabolism and Excretion: Excreted mostly unchanged by the kidneys.
Half-life: *Low dose*—3–10 hr; *high dose*—8–15 hr (↑ in renal impairment).

TIME/ACTION PROFILE (effects on blood counts)

ROUTE	ONSET	PEAK	DURATION
PO, IM, IV	4–7 days	7–14 days	21 days
Subcut	unknown	unknown	unknown

Contraindications/Precautions

Contraindicated in: Hypersensitivity; Alcoholism or hepatic impairment; Immunosuppresion; ↓ bone marrow reserve; OB, Lactation: Pregnancy or lactation; Pedi: Products containing benzyl alcohol should not be used in neonates.

Use Cautiously in: Renal impairment (CCr must be ≥60 mL/min prior to therapy); Patients with childbearing potential; Active infections; Geri: May be more sensitive to toxicity and adverse events.

Adverse Reactions/Side Effects

CNS: arachnoiditis (IT use only), dizziness, drowsiness, headache, malaise, seizures. **EENT:** blurred vision, dysarthriatransient blindness. **Resp:** PULMONARY FIBROSIS, interstitial pneumonitis. **GI:** HEPATOTOXICITY, anorexia, diarrhea, nausea, stomatitis, vomiting. **GU:** acute renal failure, infertility. **Derm:** ERYTHEMA MULTIFORME, STEVENS-JOHNSON SYNDROME, TOXIC EPIDERMAL NECROLYSIS, alopecia, painful plaque erosions (during psoriasis treatment), photosensitivity, pruritus, rashes, skin ulceration, urticaria. **Hemat:** APLASTIC ANEMIA, anemia, leukopenia, thrombocytopenia. **Metab:** hyperuricemia. **MS:** osteonecrosis, stress fracture.
Misc: nephropathy, chills, fever, soft tissue necrosis.

Interactions

Drug-Drug: The following drugs may ↑ hematologic toxicity of methotrexate: high-dose **salicylates**, **NSAIDs**, **oral hypoglycemic agents (sulfonylureas)**, **phenytoin**, **tetracyclines**, **probenecid**, **trimethoprim/sulfamethoxazole**, **pyrimethamine**, **proton pump inhibitors** and **chloramphenicol**. ↑ hepatotoxicity with other **hepatotoxic drugs** including **azathioprine**, **sulfasalazine**, and **retinoids**. ↑ nephrotoxicity with other **nephrotoxic drugs**. ↑ bone marrow depression with other **antineoplastics** or **radiation therapy**. **Radiation therapy** ↑ risk of soft tissue necrosis and osteonecrosis. May ↓ antibody response to **live-virus vaccines** and ↑ risk of adverse reactions. ↑ risk of neurologic reactions with **acyclovir** (IT methotrexate only). **Asparaginase** may ↓ effects of methotrexate.

Drug-Natural Products: Concomitant use with **echinacea** and **melatonin** may interfere with immunosuppression. **Caffeine** may ↓ efficacy of methotrexate, similar effect may occur with **guarana**.

Route/Dosage

Trophoblastic Neoplasms

PO, IM (Adults): 15–30 mg/day for 5 days; repeat after 1 or more weeks for 3–5 courses.

Breast Cancer

IV (Adults): 40 mg/m² on days 1 and 8 (with other agents; many regimens are used).

Leukemia

PO (Adults): *Induction*—3.3 mg/m²/day, usually with prednisone.
PO, IM (Adults): *Maintenance*—20–30 mg/m² twice weekly.
IV (Adults): 2.5 mg/kg q 2 wk.
IT (Adults): 12 mg/m² or 15 mg.
IT (Children ≥3 yr): 12 mg.
IT (Children 2 yr): 10 mg.
IT (Children 1 yr): 8 mg.
IT (Children <1 yr): 6 mg.

Osteosarcoma

IV (Adults): 12 g/m² as a 4-hr infusion followed by leucovorin rescue, usually as part of a combination chemotherapeutic regimen (or increase dose until peak serum methotrexate level is 1 × 10^{-3} M/L but not to exceed 15 g/m²; 12 courses are given starting 4 wk after surgery and repeated at scheduled intervals.

M

Psoriasis

Therapy may be preceded by a 5–10-mg test dose.
PO, IM, Subcut, IV (Adults): 10–25 mg/weekly (not to exceed 30 mg/wk); Otrexup may be used when dose is 10–25 mg/wk.

Rheumatoid Arthritis

PO, Subcut (Adults): 7.5 mg weekly (not to exceed 20 mg/wk); when response is obtained, dose should be ↓ Otrexup may be used when dose is 10–20 mg/wk.

Polyarticular Juvenile Idiopathic Arthritis

PO (Children): 10 mg/m² once weekly initially, may be ↑ up to 20–30 mg/m², however response may be better if doses >20 mg/m² are given IM or subcut; Otrexup may be used when dose is 10–25 mg/wk.

Mycosis Fungoides

PO, IM, Subcut (Adults): 5–50 mg once weekly, if response is poor, dose may be changed to 15–37.5 mg twice weekly.
IM (Adults): 50 mg once weekly or 25 mg twice weekly.

Availability (generic available)

Tablets: 2.5 mg, 5 mg, 7.5 mg, 10 mg, 15 mg. **Cost:** 2.5 mg $96.36/30, 5 mg $352.75/30, 7.5 mg $529.13/30, 10 mg $705.50/30, 15 mg $1,058.27/30. **Injection:** 25 mg/mL. **Cost:** *Generic*—$115.02/30 mL. **Powder for injection:** 1 g/vial. **Preservative-free injection:** 25 mg/mL. **Solution for subcutaneous injection (Otrexup):** 7.5 mg/0.4 mL, 10 mg/0.4 mL, 15 mg/0.4 mL, 20 mg/0.4 mL, 25 mg/0.4 mL. **Solution for subcutaneous injection (Rasuvo):** 7.5 mg/0.15 mL, 10 mg/0.2 mL, 12.5 mg/0.25 mL, 15 mg/0.3 mL, 17.5 mg/0.35 mL, 20 mg/0.4 mL, 22.5 mg/0.45 mL, 25 mg/0.5 mL, 27.5 mg/0.55 mL, 30 mg/0.6 mL.

NURSING IMPLICATIONS

Assessment

- Monitor vital signs periodically during administration. Report significant changes.
- Monitor for abdominal pain, diarrhea, or stomatitis; therapy may need to be discontinued.
- Monitor for bone marrow depression. Assess for bleeding (bleeding gums, bruising, petechiae, guaiac stools, urine, and emesis) and avoid IM injections and taking rectal temperatures if platelet count is low. Apply pressure to venipuncture sites for 10 min. Assess for signs of infection during neutropenia. Anemia may occur. Monitor for increased fatigue, dyspnea, and orthostatic hypotension.
- Monitor intake and output ratios and daily weights. Report significant changes in totals.
- Monitor for symptoms of pulmonary toxicity, which may manifest early as a dry, nonproductive cough.
- Monitor for symptoms of gout (increased uric acid, joint pain, edema). Encourage patient to drink at least 2 L of fluid each day. Allopurinol and alkalinization of urine may be used to decrease uric acid levels.
- Assess nutritional status. Administering an antiemetic prior to and periodically during therapy and adjusting diet as tolerated may help maintain fluid and electrolyte balance and nutritional status.
- Assess for rash periodically during therapy. May cause Stevens-Johnson syndrome. Discontinue therapy if severe or if accompanied with fever, general malaise, fatigue, muscle or joint aches, blisters, oral lesions, conjunctivitis, hepatitis and/or eosinophilia.
- **IT:** Assess for development of nuchal rigidity, headache, fever, confusion, drowsiness, dizziness, weakness, or seizures.
- **Rheumatoid Arthritis:** Assess patient for pain and range of motion prior to and periodically during therapy.
- **Psoriasis:** Assess skin lesions prior to and periodically during therapy.
- ***Lab Test Considerations:*** Monitor CBC and differential prior to and frequently during therapy. The nadir of leukopenia and thrombocytopenia occurs in 7–14 days. Leukocyte and thrombocyte counts usually recover 7 days after the nadirs. Notify health care professional of any sudden drop in values.
- Monitor renal (BUN and creatinine) and hepatic function (AST, ALT, bilirubin, and LDH) prior to and every 1–2 months during therapy. Urine pH should be monitored prior to high-dose methotrexate therapy and every 6 hr during leucovorin rescue. Urine pH should be kept above 7.0 to prevent renal damage.
- May cause ↑ serum uric acid concentrations, especially during initial treatment of leukemia and lymphoma.
- ***Toxicity and Overdose:*** Monitor serum methotrexate levels every 12–24 hr during high-dose therapy until levels are $<5 \times 10$ M. This monitoring is essential to plan correct leucovorin dose and determine duration of rescue therapy.
- With high-dose therapy, patient must receive leucovorin rescue within 24–48 hr to prevent fatal toxicity. In cases of massive overdose, hydration and urinary alkalization with sodium bicarbonate are required to prevent renal tubule damage. Monitor fluid and electrolyte status; patients must be well hydrated. Intermittent hemodialysis using a high-flux dialyzer may be used for clearance until levels are <0.05 micromolar. Methotrexate should be delayed until recovery if WBC <1500/microliter, neutrophil count <200/microliter, platelet count <75,000/microliter, serum bilirubin level >1.2m g/dL, AST level >450 U, mucositis is present, until evidence of healing, persistent pleural effusion is present, should be drained dry prior to infusion. Adequate renal function is required. Serum creatinine must be normal, creatinine clearance must be >60 mL/min, before initiation of therapy. Serum creatinine must be measured before each course of therapy. If ↑ by ≥50% of a prior value, creatinine clearance must be >60 mL/min, even if serum creatinine is within normal range.

Potential Nursing Diagnoses

Risk for infection (Adverse Reactions)

Imbalanced nutrition: less than body requirements (Adverse Reactions)

Implementation

- ***High Alert:*** Fatalities have occurred with chemotherapeutic agents. Before administering, clarify all ambiguous orders; double-check single, daily, and course-of-therapy dose limits; have second practitioner independently double-check original order, calculations and infusion pump settings. Methotrexate for non-oncologic use is given at a much lower dose and frequency—often just once a week. Do not confuse non-oncologic dosing regimens with dosing regimens for cancer patients.
- Solutions for injection should be prepared in a biologic cabinet. Wear gloves, gown, and mask while handling medication. Discard equipment in specially designated containers.
- *Otrexup* and *Rasuvo* are not indicated for treatment of neoplastic diseases. Not for patients requiring oral, IM, IV, intra-arterial, or IT dosing, doses <10 mg/week, doses >25 mg/week, high-dose regimens, or dose adjustments of less than 5 mg increments.
- **Subcut:** *Otrexup* and *Rasuvo* are single-dose auto-injectors. Inject once weekly in abdomen or upper thigh. Avoid areas where skin is tender, bruised, red, scaly, hard, or has scars or stretch marks. Solution is clear and yellow; do not inject solutions that are discolored or contain particulate matter.

IV Administration

- **IV Push:** ***Diluent:*** Reconstitute each vial with 25 mL of 0.9% NaCl. Use sterile preservative-free diluents for high-dose regimens to prevent complications from large amounts of benzyl alcohol. Do not use preparations that are discolored or that contain a precipitate. Reconstitute immediately before use. Discard unused portion. ***Concentration:*** <25 mg/mL for IV push and intermittent/continuous infusions. ***Rate:*** Administer at a rate of 10 mg/min into Y-site of a free-flowing IV.

- **Intermittent/Continuous Infusion:** ***Diluent:*** Doses >100–300 mg/m^2 may also be diluted in D5W, D5/0.9% NaCl, or 0.9% NaCl and infused as intermittent or continuous infusion. ***Rate:*** Administration rates of 4–20 mg/hr have been used.
- **Y-Site Compatibility:** acyclovir, alemtuzumab, alfentanil, allopurinol, amifostine, amikacin, aminophylline, amphotericin B lipid complex, amphotericin B liposome, ampicillin, ampicillin/sulbactam, anidulafungin, argatroban, azithromycin, aztreonam, bivalirudin, bleomycin, bumetanide, buprenorphine, butorphanol, calcium chloride, calcium gluconate, carboplatin, carmustine, cefazolin, cefepime, cefotaxime, cefotetan, cefoxitin, ceftazidime, ceftriaxone, cefuroxime, ciprofloxacin, cisatracurium, cisplatin, clindamycin, cyclophosphamide, cyclosporine, cytarabine, dactinomycin, daunorubicin hydrochloride, dexmedetomidine, digoxin, diphenhydramine, docetaxel, dolasetron, doripenem, doxorubicin hydrochloride, doxorubicin liposomal, enalaprilat, ephedrine, epinephrine, epirubicin, ertapenem, erythromycin, esmolol, etoposide, etoposide phosphate, famotidine, fenoldopam, fentanyl, filgrastim, fluconazole, fludarabine, fluorouracil, foscarnet, fosphenytoin, furosemide, ganciclovir, granisetron, heparin, hydrocortisone, hydromorphone, imipenem/cilastatin, insulin, isoproterenol, ketorolac, leucovorin, levorphanol, lidocaine, linezolid, lorazepam, magnesium sulfate, mannitol, melphalan, meperidine, meropenem, mesna, methylprednisolone, metoclopramide, metoprolol, metronidazole, milrinone, mitomycin, mitoxantrone, morphine, moxifloxacin, naloxone, nesiritide, nitroglycerin, norepinephrine, octreotide, ondansetron, oxacillin, paclitaxel, palonosetron, pamidronate, pancuronium, pentobarbital, phenobarbital, phenylephrine, piperacillin/tazobactam, potassium acetate, potassium chloride, potassium phosphate, procainamide, prochlorperazine, propranolol, ranitidine, remifentanil, rituximab, rocuronium, sargramostim, sodium acetate, sodium bicarbonate, sodium phosphate, succinylchloride, sufentanil, tacrolimus, teniposide, theophylline, thiopental, thiotepa, tigecycline, tirofiban, tobramycin, trastuzumab, trimethoprim/sulfamethoxazole, vasopressin, vecuronium, verapamil, vinblastine, vincristine, vinorelbine, voriconazole, zidovudine, zoledronic acid.
- **Y-Site Incompatibility:** amiodarone, amphotericin B colloidal, caspofungin, chlorpromazine, daptomycin, dexrazoxane, diazepam, diltiazem, dobutamine, dopamine, doxycycline, gemcitabine, gentamicin, idarubicin, ifosfamide, levofloxacin, midazolam, mycophenolate, nalbuphine, nicardipine, pantoprazole, pentamidine, phenytoin, propofol, quinupristin/dalfopristin.
- **IT:** Reconstitute preservative-free methotrexate with preservative-free 0.9% NaCl, Elliot's B solution, or patient's CSF to a concentration not greater than 2 mg/mL. May be administered via lumbar puncture or Ommaya reservoir. To prevent bacterial contamination, use immediately.

Patient/Family Teaching

- Instruct patient to take medication as directed. If a dose is missed, it should be omitted. Consult health care professional if vomiting occurs shortly after a dose is taken.
- Instruct patient to notify health care professional promptly if rash, fever; chills; cough; hoarseness; sore throat; signs of infection; lower back or side pain; painful or difficult urination; bleeding gums; bruising; petechiae; blood in stools, urine, or emesis; increased fatigue; dyspnea; or orthostatic hypotension occurs. Caution patient to avoid crowds and persons with known infections. Instruct patient to use soft toothbrush and electric razor and to avoid falls. Caution patient not to drink alcoholic beverages or take medication containing aspirin or other NSAIDs; may precipitate gastric bleeding.
- Instruct patient to inspect oral mucosa for erythema and ulceration. If ulceration occurs, advise patient to use sponge brush and to rinse mouth with water after eating and drinking. Topical therapy may be used if mouth pain interferes with eating. Stomatitis pain may require treatment with opioid analgesics.
- Advise patient to tell health care professional what medications they are taking and to avoid taking new Rx, OTC, vitamins, or herbal products without consulting health care professional.
- Discuss the possibility of hair loss with patient. Explore methods of coping.
- Instruct patient not to receive any vaccinations without advice of health care professional.
- Caution patient to use sunscreen and protective clothing to prevent photosensitivity reactions.
- Rep: Advise patient that this medication may have teratogenic effects. Contraception should be used during therapy and for at least 3 mo for men and 1 ovulatory cycle for women after completion of therapy.
- Emphasize the need for periodic lab tests to monitor for side effects.
- **Subcut:** Instruct patient on correct technique for injection and care and disposal of equipment.

M

Evaluation/Desired Outcomes

- Improvement of hematopoietic values in leukemia.
- Decrease in symptoms of meningeal involvement in leukemia.
- Decrease in size and spread of non-Hodgkin's lymphomas and other solid cancers.
- Resolution of skin lesions in severe psoriasis.
- Decreased joint pain and swelling.
- Improved mobility in patients with rheumatoid arthritis.
- Regression of lesions in mycosis fungoides.

methyldopa (meth-ill-**doe**-pa)

~~Aldomet~~

Classification

Therapeutic: antihypertensives

Pharmacologic: centrally acting antiadrenergics

Pregnancy Category B

Indications

Management of moderate to severe hypertension (with other agents).

Action

Stimulates CNS alpha-adrenergic receptors, producing a decrease in sympathetic outflow to heart, kidneys, and blood vessels. Result is decreased BP and peripheral resistance, a slight decrease in heart rate, and no change in cardiac output. **Therapeutic Effects:** Lowering of BP.

Pharmacokinetics

Absorption: 50% absorbed from the GI tract. Parenteral form, methyldopate hydrochloride, is slowly converted to methyldopa.

Distribution: Crosses the blood-brain barrier. Crosses the placenta; small amounts enter breast milk.

Metabolism and Excretion: Partially metabolized by the liver, partially excreted unchanged by the kidneys.

Half-life: 1.7 hr.

TIME/ACTION PROFILE (antihypertensive effect)

ROUTE	ONSET	PEAK	DURATION
PO	4–6 hr	12–24 hr	24–48 hr
IV	4–6 hr	unknown	10–16 hr

Contraindications/Precautions

Contraindicated in: Hypersensitivity; Active liver disease.

Use Cautiously in: Previous history of liver disease; OB: Has been used safely (may be used for treatment of hypertension in pregnancy); Lactation: Usually compatible with breast feeding; Geri: ↑ risk of adverse reactions; consider age-related impairment of hepatic, renal and cardiovascular function as well as other chronic illnesses. Appears on Beers list. May cause bradycardia and exacerbate depression.

Adverse Reactions/Side Effects

CNS: sedation, ↓ mental acuity, depression. **EENT:** nasal stuffiness. **CV:** MYOCARDITIS, bradycardia, edema, orthostatic hypotension. **GI:** DRUG-INDUCED HEPATITIS, diarrhea, dry mouth. **GU:** erectile dysfunction. **Hemat:** eosinophilia, hemolytic anemia. **Misc:** fever.

Interactions

Drug-Drug: Additive hypotension with other **antihypertensives**, acute ingestion of **alcohol**, **anesthesia**, and **nitrates**. **Amphetamines**, **barbiturates**, **tricyclic antidepressants**, **NSAIDs**, and **phenothiazines** may ↓ antihypertensive effect of methyldopa. ↑ effects and risk of psychoses with **haloperidol**. Excess sympathetic stimulation may occur with concurrent use of **MAO inhibitors** or other **adrenergics**. May ↑ **lithium** toxicity. Additive hypotension and CNS toxicity with **levodopa**. Additive CNS depression may occur with **alcohol**, **antihistamines**, **sedative/hypnotics**, some **antidepressants**, and **opioid analgesics**. Concurrent use with **nonselective beta blockers** may rarely cause paradoxical hypertension.

Route/Dosage

PO (Adults): 250–500 mg 2–3 times daily (not to exceed 500 mg/day if used with other agents); may be ↑ every 2 days as needed; usual maintenance dose is 500 mg–2 g/day (not to exceed 3 g/day).

PO (Children): 10 mg/kg/day (300 mg/m^2/day); may be ↑ every 2 days up to 65 mg/kg/day in divided doses (not to exceed 3 g/day).

IV (Adults): 250–500 mg q 6 hr (up to 1 g q 6 hr).

IV (Children): 5–10 mg/kg q 6 hr; up to 65 mg/kg/day in divided doses (not to exceed 3 g/day).

Availability (generic available)

Tablets: 250 mg, 500 mg. **Injection:** 50 mg/mL. ***In combination with:*** hydrochlorothiazide. See Appendix B.

NURSING IMPLICATIONS

Assessment

- Monitor BP and pulse frequently during initial dose adjustment and periodically during therapy. Report significant changes.
- Monitor frequency of prescription refills to determine compliance.
- Monitor intake and output ratios and weight and assess for edema daily, especially at beginning of therapy. Report weight gain or edema; sodium and water retention may be treated with diuretics.
- Assess patient for depression or other alterations in mental status. Notify health care professional promptly if these symptoms develop.

- Monitor temperature during therapy. Drug fever may occur shortly after initiation of therapy and may be accompanied by eosinophilia and hepatic function changes. Monitor hepatic function test if unexplained fever occurs.
- ***Lab Test Considerations:*** Monitor renal and hepatic function and CBC before and periodically during therapy.
- Monitor direct Coombs' test before and after 6 and 12 mo of therapy. May cause a positive direct Coombs' test, rarely associated with hemolytic anemia.
- May cause ↑ BUN, serum creatinine, potassium, sodium, prolactin, uric acid, AST, ALT, alkaline phosphatase, and bilirubin concentrations.
- May cause prolonged prothrombin times.
- May interfere with serum creatinine and AST measurements.

Potential Nursing Diagnoses

Risk for injury (Side Effects)
Noncompliance (Patient/Family Teaching)

Implementation

- Fluid retention and expanded volume may cause tolerance to develop within 2–3 mo after initiation of therapy. Diuretics may be added to regimen at this time to maintain control.
- Dose increases should be made with the evening dose to minimize drowsiness.
- When changing from IV to oral forms, dose should remain consistent.
- **PO:** Shake suspension before administration.

IV Administration

- **Intermittent Infusion: *Diluent:*** Dilute in 100 mL of D5W, 0.9% NaCl, D5/0.9% NaCl, 5% sodium bicarbonate, or Ringer's solution. ***Concentration:*** ≤10 mg/mL. ***Rate:*** Infuse slowly over 30–60 min.
- **Y-Site Compatibility:** alemtuzumab, alfentanil, amikacin, aminophylline, anidulafungin, argatroban, ascorbic acid, atracurium, atropine, aztreonam, benztropine, bivalirudin, bleomycin, bumetanide, buprenorphine, butorphanol, calcium chloride, calcium gluconate, carmustine, caspofungin, cefazolin, cefotaxime, cefotetan, cefoxitin, ceftazidime, ceftriaxone, cefuroxime, chlorpromazine, clindamycin, cyanocobalamin, cyclosporine, dactinomycin, daptomycin, dexamethasone, digoxin, diltiazem, diphenhydramine, dobutamine, docetaxel, dopamine, doxycycline, enalaprilat, ephedrine, epinephrine, epoetin alfa, ertapenem, erythromycin, esmolol, etoposide, etoposide phosphate, famotidine, fenoldopam, fentanyl, fluconazole, fludarabine, gemcitabine, gentamicin, glycopyrrolate, granisetron, heparin, hetastarch, hydrocortisone, hydromorphone, idarubicin, insulin, irinotecan, isoproterenol, labetalol, lidocaine, linezolid, lorazepam, magnesium sulfate, mannitol, mechlorethamine, meperidine, metaraminol, methoxamine, methylprednisolone, metoclopramide, metoprolol, metronidazole, midazolam, milrinone, mitoxantrone, morphine, multivitamins, nafcillin, nalbuphine, naloxone, nitroglycerin, nitroprusside, norepinephrine, octreotide, ondansetron, oxacillin, oxaliplatin, oxytocin, paclitaxel, palonosetron, pamidronate, pancuronium, pantoprazole, papaverine, pemetrexed, penicillin G, pentazocine, phentolamine, phenylephrine, phytonadione, potassium acetate, potassium chloride, procainamide, prochlorperazine, promethazine, propranolol, protamine, pyridoxime, ranitidine, sodium bicarbonate, streptokinase, succinylcholine, sufentanil, tacrolimus, teniposide, theophylline, thiamine, thiotepa, tigecycline, tirofiban, tobramycin, tolazoline, trimetaphan, vancomycin, vasopressin, vecuronium, verapamil, vinorelbine, voriconazole, zoledronic acid.
- **Y-Site Incompatibility:** acyclovir, amphotericin B colloidal, amphotericin B lipid complex, azathioprine, chloramphenicol, dantrolene, diazepam, diazoxide, folic acid, furosemide, ganciclovir, imipenem/cilastatin, indomethacin, pentamidine, pentobarbital, phenobarbital, phenytoin, piperacillin/tazobactam, trimethoprim/sulfamethoxazole.

Patient/Family Teaching

- Emphasize the importance of continuing to take this medication, even if feeling well. Instruct patient to take medication at the same time each day; last dose of the day should be taken at bedtime. Take missed doses as soon as remembered but not if almost time for next dose. Do not double doses.
- Encourage patient to comply with additional interventions for hypertension (weight reduction, low-sodium diet, smoking cessation, moderation of alcohol consumption, regular exercise, and stress management). Methyldopa controls but does not cure hypertension.
- Instruct patient and family on proper technique for monitoring BP. Advise them to check BP at least weekly and to report significant changes.
- Instruct patient to notify health care professional if fever, muscle aches, or flu-like syndrome occurs.
- Inform patient that urine may darken or turn red-black when left standing.
- May cause drowsiness. Advise patient to avoid driving or other activities requiring alertness until response to medication is known. Drowsiness usually subsides after 7–10 days of continuous use.
- Caution patient to avoid sudden changes in position to decrease orthostatic hypotension.
- Advise patient that frequent mouth rinses, good oral hygiene, and sugarless gum or candy may minimize

M

dry mouth. Notify health care professional if dry mouth continues for >2 wk.

- Caution patient to avoid concurrent use of alcohol or other CNS depressants.
- Advise patient to notify health care professional of all Rx or OTC medications, vitamins, or herbal products being taken and to consult with health care professional before taking other medications, especially cough, cold, or allergy remedies.
- Advise patient to notify health care professional of medication regimen before treatment or surgery.

Evaluation/Desired Outcomes

- Decrease in BP without appearance of side effects.

methylergonovine

(meth-ill-er-goe-**noe**-veen)

Methergine

Classification

Therapeutic: oxytocic

Pharmacologic: ergot alkaloids

Pregnancy Category C

Indications

Prevention and treatment of postpartum or postabortion hemorrhage caused by uterine atony or subinvolution.

Action

Directly stimulates uterine and vascular smooth muscle. **Therapeutic Effects:** Uterine contraction.

Pharmacokinetics

Absorption: Well absorbed following oral or IM administration.

Distribution: Unknown. Enters breast milk in small quantities.

Metabolism and Excretion: Probably metabolized by the liver.

Half-life: 30–120 min.

TIME/ACTION PROFILE (effects on uterine contractions)

ROUTE	ONSET	PEAK	DURATION
PO	5–15 min	unknown	3 hr
IM	2–5 min	unknown	3 hr
IV	immediate	unknown	45 min–3 hr

Contraindications/Precautions

Contraindicated in: Hypersensitivity; OB: Should not be used to induce labor; Lactation: Do not breast feed during treatment and for 12 hours after the last dose; Concurrent use of potent CYP3A4 inhibitors.

Use Cautiously in: Hypertensive or eclamptic patients (more susceptible to hypertensive and arrhythmogenic side effects); History of or risk factors for coronary artery disease; Severe hepatic or renal disease; Sepsis.; Concurrent use of moderate CYP3A4 inhibitors

Exercise Extreme Caution in: OB: Third stage of labor.

Adverse Reactions/Side Effects

CNS: STROKE, dizziness, headache. **EENT:** tinnitus. **Resp:** dyspnea. **CV:** HYPERTENSION, arrhythmias, AV block, chest pain, palpitations. **GI:** nausea, vomiting. **GU:** cramps. **Derm:** diaphoresis. **Neuro:** paresthesia. **Misc:** allergic reactions.

Interactions

Drug-Drug: Excessive vasoconstriction may result when used with heavy cigarette smoking (**nicotine**), other **vasopressors**, such as **dopamine**, or **beta-blockers**. Potent **CYP3A4 inhibitors**, including **erythromycin**, **clarithromycin**, **troleandomycin**, **ritonavir**, **indinavir**, **nelfinavir**, **delavirdine**, **ketoconazole**, **itraconazole**, or **voriconazole** may ↑ levels and ↑ risk of ischemia; concurrent use contraindicated. Moderate **CYP3A4 inhibitors** including **saquinavir**, **nefazodone**, **fluconazole**, **fluoxetine**, **fluvoxamine**, **zileuton**, or **clotrimazole** may ↑ levels; use with caution. **CYP3A4 inducers** including **nevirapine** and **rifampin** may ↓ levels. **Anesthetics** may ↓ its oxytocic properties. May ↓ the antianginal effects of **nitrates**.

Drug-Food: **Grapefruit juice** may ↑ levels; use with caution.

Route/Dosage

PO (Adults): 200–400 mcg (0.2–0.4 mg) q 6–12 hr for 2–7 days.

IM, IV (Adults): 200 mcg (0.2 mg) q 2–4 hr for up to 5 doses.

Availability (generic available)

Tablets: 200 mcg (0.2 mg). **Injection:** 200 mcg (0.2 mg)/mL.

NURSING IMPLICATIONS

Assessment

- Monitor BP, heart rate, and uterine response frequently during medication administration. Notify health care professional promptly if uterine relaxation becomes prolonged or if character of vaginal bleeding changes.
- Assess for signs of ergotism (cold, numb fingers and toes, chest pain, nausea, vomiting, headache, muscle pain, weakness).
- ***Lab Test Considerations:*** If no response to methylergonovine, calcium levels may need to be assessed. Effectiveness of medication is ↓ with hypocalcemia.
- May cause ↓ serum prolactin levels.

Potential Nursing Diagnoses

Acute pain (Side Effects)

Implementation

IV Administration

- **IV:** IV administration is used for emergencies only. Oral and IM routes are preferred.
- **IV Push:** ***Diluent:*** May be given undiluted or diluted in 5 mL of 0.9% NaCl and administered through Y site. Do not add to IV solutions. Do not mix in syringe with any other drug. Refrigerate; stable for storage at room temperature for 60 days; deteriorates with age. Use only solution that is clear and colorless and that contains no precipitate. ***Concentration:*** 0.2 mg/mL. ***Rate:*** Administer at a rate of 0.2 mg over at least 1 min.
- **Y-Site Compatibility:** heparin, hydrocortisone sodium succinate, potassium chloride, vitamin B complex with C.

Patient/Family Teaching

- Instruct patient to take medication as directed; do not skip or double up on missed doses. If a dose is missed, omit it and return to regular dose schedule.
- Advise patient that medication may cause menstrual-like cramps.
- Caution patient to avoid smoking, because nicotine constricts blood vessels.
- Instruct patient to notify health care professional if infection develops, as this may cause increased sensitivity to the medication.
- Advise patient to notify health care professional of all Rx or OTC medications, vitamins, or herbal products being taken and to consult with health care professional before taking other medications.

Evaluation/Desired Outcomes

- Contractions that maintain uterine tone and prevent postpartum hemorrhage.

methylnaltrexone
(me-thil-nal-**trex**-one)
Relistor

Classification
Therapeutic: laxatives
Pharmacologic: opioid antagonists

Pregnancy Category B

Indications

Treatment of constipation caused by opioid use in patients being treated palliatively, when laxative therapy has failed. Treatment of constipation caused by opioid use in patients with chronic, non-cancer pain.

Action

Acts peripherally as mu-opioid receptor antagonist, blocking opioid effects on the GI tract. **Therapeutic Effects:** Blocks constipating effects of opioids on the GI tract without loss of analgesia.

Pharmacokinetics

Absorption: Rapidly absorbed after subcutaneous administration.
Distribution: Moderate tissue distribution, does not cross the blood-brain barrier.
Metabolism and Excretion: Some metabolism; 85% excreted unchanged in urine.
Half-life: 8 hr.

TIME/ACTION PROFILE

ROUTE	ONSET	PEAK	DURATION
Subcut	rapid	0.5 hr	24–48 hr

Contraindications/Precautions

Contraindicated in: Known/suspected mechanical GI obstruction.
Use Cautiously in: Known/suspected lesions of GI tract (↑ risk for GI perforation); OB, Lactation: Use in pregnancy only if clearly needed; use cautiously during lactation; Pedi: Safety and effectiveness not established.

Adverse Reactions/Side Effects

CNS: dizziness. **GI:** GI PERFORATION, abdominal pain, flatulence, nausea, diarrhea. **Derm:** hyperhidrosis. **Misc:** opioid withdrawal.

Interactions

Drug-Drug: None noted.

Route/Dosage

Opioid-Induced Constipation in Patients with Advanced Illness

Subcut (Adults): *38–<62 kg*—8 mg every other day, not to exceed every 24 hr; *62–114 kg*—12 mg every other day, not to exceed every 24 hr; *other weights*—0.15 mg/kg every other day, not to exceed every 24 hr.

Renal Impairment

(Adults): *CCr <30 mL/min*—use 50% of recommended dose based on weight.

Opioid-Induced Constipation in Patients with Non-Cancer Pain

Subcut (Adults): 12 mg once daily.

Availability

Solution for subcutaneous injection (single-use vial): 12 mg/0.6 mL. **Cost:** $500.22/7 vials. **Solution for subcutaneous injection (prefilled syringes):** 8 mg/0.4 mL, 12 mg/0.6 mL. **Cost:** All strengths $71.46/syringe.

NURSING IMPLICATIONS

Assessment

- Assess bowel sounds and frequency, quantity, and consistency of stools periodically during therapy.
- Monitor pain intensity during therapy. Methylnaltrexone does not affect pain or effects of opioid analgesics on pain control.

Potential Nursing Diagnoses

Constipation (Indications)
Diarrhea (Adverse Reactions)

Implementation

- Maintenance laxative must be stopped prior to administration of methylnaltrexone. If response is not sufficient after 3 days, laxatives may be restarted.
- **Subcut:** Pinch skin and administer in upper arm, abdomen, or thigh at a 45° angle using a 1-mL syringe with a 27-gauge needle inserted the full length of the needle. Do not rub the injection site. Solution is clear and colorless to pale yellow. Do not administer solutions that are discolored or contain a precipitate. Solution is stable for 24 hr at room temperature. Protect vials from light. Do not freeze. Do not use single-use vials for more than 1 dose.

Patient/Family Teaching

- Instruct patient on administration of methylnaltrexone and disposal of supplies. Usual schedule is one dose every other day, as needed, but no more than one dose in a 24-hr period. Advise patient to read the *Patient Information* prior to starting therapy and with each Rx refill.
- Advise patient that laxation may occur within 30 min, so toilet facilities should be available following administration.
- Advise patient to continue taking other medications for constipation unless told not to by health care professional.
- May cause dizziness. Caution patient to avoid driving and other activities requiring alertness until response to medication is known.
- Advise patient to notify health care professional and discontinue therapy if severe or persistent diarrhea occurs or if abdominal pain, nausea, or vomiting persists or worsens.
- Instruct patient to stop taking methylnaltrexone if they stop taking opioid medications.
- Advise patient to consult health care professional prior to taking other Rx, OTC, or herbal products.
- Advise female patients to notify health care professional if pregnancy is planned or suspected or if breast feeding.

Evaluation/Desired Outcomes

- Laxation and relief of opioid-induced constipation.

methylphenidate (oral)

(meth-ill-**fen**-i-date)
Aptensio XR, ✱Biphentin, Concerta, Metadate CD, Metadate ER, Methylin, Methylin ER, Quillivant XR, Ritalin, Ritalin LA, Ritalin SR

methylphenidate (transdermal)

Daytrana

Classification
Therapeutic: central nervous system stimulants

Schedule II

Pregnancy Category C

Indications

Treatment of ADHD (adjunct). **Oral**: Symptomatic treatment of narcolepsy. **Unlabeled Use:** Management of some forms of refractory depression.

Action

Produces CNS and respiratory stimulation with weak sympathomimetic activity. **Therapeutic Effects:** Increased attention span in ADHD. Increased motor activity, mental alertness, and diminished fatigue in narcoleptic patients.

Pharmacokinetics

Absorption: Slow and incomplete after oral administration; absorption of sustained or extended-release tablet (SR) is delayed and provides continuous release; well absorbed from skin. *Aptensio XR, Metadate CD, Concerta, Ritalin LA*—provides initial rapid release followed by a second continuous release (biphasic release).
Distribution: Unknown.
Metabolism and Excretion: Mostly metabolized (80%) by the liver.
Half-life: 2–4 hr.

TIME/ACTION PROFILE (CNS stimulation)

ROUTE	ONSET	PEAK	DURATION
PO	unknown	1–3 hr	4–6 hr
PO-ER	unknown	4–7 hr	3–12 hr†
Transdermal	unknown	unknown	12 hr

†Depends on formulation.

Contraindications/Precautions

Contraindicated in: Hypersensitivity; Hyperexcitable states; Hyperthyroidism; Patients with psychotic personalities or suicidal or homicidal tendencies; Personal or family history of Tourette's syndrome; Glaucoma; Motor tics; Concurrent use or use within 14 days of MAO inhibitors; Fructose intolerance, glucose-galactose malabsorption, or sucrose-isomaltase insufficiency; Surgery.

Use Cautiously in: History of cardiovascular disease (sudden death has occurred in children with structural cardiac abnormalities or other serious heart problems); Hypertension; Diabetes mellitus; History of contact sensitization with transdermal product (may be at ↑ risk for systemic sensitization reactions with oral products); History or family history of vitiligo (may be at ↑ risk for loss of skin pigmentation with transdermal product); Geri: Geriatric or debilitated patients; Continual use (may result in psychological or physical dependence); Seizure disorders (may lower seizure threshold); Concerta product should be used cautiously in patients with esophageal motility disorders or severe GI narrowing (may ↑ the risk of obstruction); OB, Lactation: Safety not established; Pedi: Growth suppression may occur in children with long-term use; children <6 yr (transdermal only).

Adverse Reactions/Side Effects

CNS: hyperactivity, insomnia, restlessness, tremor, behavioral disturbances, dizziness, hallucinations, headache, irritability, mania, thought disorder. **EENT:** blurred vision, teeth grinding. **CV:** SUDDEN DEATH, hypertension, palpitations, tachycardia, hypotension, peripheral vasculopathy. **GI:** anorexia, constipation, cramps, diarrhea, dry mouth, metallic taste, nausea, vomiting. **Derm:** contact sensitization (erythema, edema, papules, vesicles) (transdermal), erythema, loss of skin pigmentation (transdermal), rash. **Metab:** growth suppression, weight loss (may occur with prolonged use). **Neuro:** akathisia, dyskinesia, tics. **GU:** priapism. **MS:** RHABDOMYOLYSIS. **Misc:** ANAPHYLAXIS, ANGIOEDEMA, fever, physical dependence, psychological dependence, tolerance.

Interactions

Drug-Drug: ↑ sympathomimetic effects with other **adrenergics**, including **vasoconstrictors**, **decongestants**, and **halogenated anesthetics**. Use with **MAO inhibitors** or **vasopressors** may result in hypertensive crisis (concurrent use or use within 14 days of MAO inhibitors is contraindicated). Metabolism of **warfarin**, **phenytoin**, **phenobarbital**, **primidone**, **phenylbutazone**, **selective serotonin reuptake inhibitors**, and **tricyclic antidepressants** may be ↓ and effects ↑. Avoid concurrent use with **pimozide** (may mask cause of tics). May ↓ the effectiveness of **antihypertensives**. **Alcohol** may ↑ rate of release of drug from some methylphenidate formulations (Metadate CD, Ritalin LA).

Drug-Natural Products: Use with caffeine-containing herbs (**guarana**, **tea**, **coffee**) ↑ stimulant effect. **St. John's wort** may ↑ serious side effects (concurrent use is NOT recommended).

Drug-Food: Excessive use of **caffeine**-containing foods or beverages (**coffee**, **cola**, **tea**) may cause ↑ CNS stimulation.

Route/Dosage

PO (Adults): *ADHD*—5–20 mg 2–3 times daily as prompt-release tablets. When maintenance dose is determined, may change to extended-release formulation. *Narcolepsy*—10 mg 2–3 times/day; maximum dose 60 mg/day.

PO (Children >6 yr): *Prompt release tablets*—0.3 mg/kg/dose or 2.5–5 mg before breakfast and lunch; ↑ by 0.1 mg/kg/dose or by 5–10 mg/day at weekly intervals (not to exceed 60 mg/day or 2 mg/kg/day). When maintenance dose is determined, may change to extended-release formulation. *Ritalin SR, Metadate ER*—may be used in place of the prompt-release tablets when the 8-hour dose corresponds to the titrated 8-hour dosage of the prompt-release tablets; *Ritalin LA*—can be used in place of twice daily regimen given once daily at same total dose, or in place of SR product at same dose; *Concerta (patients who have not taken methylphenidate previously)*—18 mg once daily in the morning initially, may be titrated as needed up to 54 mg/day. *Concerta (patients are currently taking other forms of methylphenidate)*—18 mg once daily in the morning if previous dose was 5 mg 2–3 times daily or 20 mg daily as SR product, 36 mg once daily in the morning if previous dose was 10 mg 2–3 times daily or 40 mg daily as SR product, 54 mg once daily in the morning if previous dose was 15 mg 2–3 times daily or 60 mg once daily as SR product. *Aptensio XR*—10 mg once daily. Dose may be adjusted in weekly 10-mg increments to a maximum of 60 mg/day taken once daily in the morning. *Metadate CD*—20 mg once daily. Dose may be adjusted in weekly 20-mg increments to a maximum of 60 mg/day taken once daily in the morning. *Quillivant XR*—20 mg once daily. Dose may be adjusted in weekly 10–20-mg increments to a maximum of 60 mg/day taken once daily in the morning.

Transdermal (Children 6–17 yr): Apply one 10-mg patch initially (should be applied 2 hr before desired effect and removed 9 hr after application); may be titrated based on response and tolerability; may ↑ to 15-mg patch after 1 wk, and then to 20-mg patch after another week, and then to 30-mg patch after another week.

Availability (generic available)

Immediate-release tablets (Ritalin): 5 mg, 10 mg, 20 mg. **Cost:** *Generic*—5 mg $73.08/100, 10 mg $104.19/100, 20 mg $149.81/100. **Extended-release tablets (Metadate ER):** 20 mg. **Extended-release tablets (Methylin ER):** 10 mg, 20 mg. **Cost:** *Generic*—10 mg $171.91/100, 20 mg $247.21/100. **Ex-**

M

tended-release tablets (Concerta): 18 mg, 27 mg, 36 mg, 54 mg. **Cost:** *Generic*—18 mg $622.18/100, 27 mg $637.78/100, 36 mg $657.86/100, 54 mg $715.83/100. **Sustained-release tablets (Ritalin SR):** 20 mg. **Cost:** $266.65/100. **Extended-release capsules (Aptensio XR):** 10 mg, 15 mg, 20 mg, 30 mg, 40 mg, 50 mg, 60 mg. **Extended-release capsules (Metadate CD):** 10 mg, 20 mg, 30 mg, 40 mg, 50 mg, 60 mg. **Cost:** *Generic*—10 mg $560.21/100, 20 mg $560.21/100, 30 mg $560.21/100, 40 mg $711.52/100, 50 mg $944.19/100, 60 mg $944.19/100. **Extended-release capsules (Ritalin LA):** 10 mg, 20 mg, 30 mg, 40 mg, 60 mg. **Cost:** *Generic*—10 mg $630.47/100, 20 mg $630.47/100, 30 mg $644.82/100, 40 mg $66.274/100. **Extended-release oral suspension (Quillivant XR):** 5 mg/mL. **Chewable tablets (Methylin) (grape flavor):** 2.5 mg, 5 mg, 10 mg. **Cost:** 2.5 mg $351.16/100, 5 mg $501.16/100, 10 mg $715.09/100. **Oral solution (Methylin) (grape flavor):** 5 mg/5 mL, 10 mg/5 mL. **Cost:** *Generic*—5 mg/5 mL $451.61/500 mL, 10 mg/5 mL $643.82/500 mL. **Transdermal patch:** 10 mg/9 hr, 15 mg/9 hr, 20 mg/9 hr, 30 mg/9 hr. **Cost:** All strengths $249.35/30.

NURSING IMPLICATIONS

Assessment

- Monitor BP, pulse, and respiration before administering and periodically during therapy. Obtain a history (including assessment of family history of sudden death or ventricular arrhythmia), physical exam to assess for cardiac disease, and further evaluation (ECG and echocardiogram), if indicated. If exertional chest pain, unexplained syncope, or other cardiac symptoms occur, evaluate promptly.
- Monitor closely for behavior change.
- Monitor for signs and symptoms of peripheral vasculopathy (numbness and burning in fingers, digital changes). May require reduction in dose or discontinuation.
- Pedi: Monitor growth, both height and weight, in children on long-term therapy.
- May produce a false sense of euphoria and well-being. Provide frequent rest periods and observe patient for rebound depression after the effects of the medication have worn off.
- Methylphenidate has a high abuse potential; may lead to tolerance and psychological dependence.
- **ADHD:** Assess children for attention span, impulse control, and interactions with others. Therapy may be interrupted at intervals to determine whether symptoms are sufficient to continue therapy.
- **Narcolepsy:** Observe and document frequency of episodes.
- **Transdermal:** Assess skin for signs of contact sensitization (erythema with edema, papules, or vesicles that does not improve within 48 hr or spreads beyond patch site) during therapy. May lead to systemic sensitization to other forms of methylphenidate (flare-up of previous dermatitis or prior positive patch-test sites, generalized skin eruptions, headache, fever, malaise, arthralgia, diarrhea, vomiting). If contact sensitization develops and oral methylphenidate is instituted, monitor closely.
- Monitor for signs of skin depigmentation. May cause persistent loss of skin pigmentation at and around the application site and at other sites distant from application site. Discontinue transdermal if depigmentation occurs.
- ***Lab Test Considerations:*** Monitor CBC, differential, and platelet count periodically in patients receiving prolonged therapy.

Potential Nursing Diagnoses

Disturbed thought process (Side Effects)

Implementation

- Do not confuse Metadate ER/CD (methylphenidate), or methylphenidate with methadone. Do not confuse Metadate CD with Metadate ER. Do not confuse Ritalin LA with Ritalin SR.
- **PO:** Administer immediate and sustained-release tablets on an empty stomach (30–45 min before a meal). Sustained-release tablets should be swallowed whole; do not break, crush, or chew. Aptensio XL, Metadate CD and Ritalin LA capsules may be opened and sprinkled on cool applesauce; entire mixture should be ingested immediately and followed by a drink of water. Do not store for future use. Concerta may be administered without regard to food, but must be taken with water, milk, or juice.
- Shake extended-release oral suspension for 10 seconds before administering. May be given with or without food.
- **Transdermal:** Apply patch to a clean, dry site on the hip which is not oily, damaged, or irritated; do not apply to waistline where tight clothing may rub it. Press firmly in place with palm of hand for 30 seconds to make sure of good contact with skin, especially around edges. Alternate site daily. Apply patch 2 hr before desired effect and remove 9 hr after applied; effects last several more hours. Do not apply or reapply with dressings, tape, or other adhesives. Do not cut patches.
- If difficulty in separating patch from release liner, tearing, or other damage occurs during removal from liner, discard patch and apply a new patch. Inspect release liner to ensure no adhesive containing medication has transferred to liner; if transfer has occurred, discard patch. Avoid touching adhesive during application; wash hands immediately after application.
- If patch does not fully adhere or partially detaches, remove and replace with another patch. Wear patched for a total of 9 hr, regardless of number used. Exposure to water during bathing, swimming, or showering may affect patch adherence.

- Patches may be removed earlier before decreasing dose if an unacceptable loss of appetite or insomnia occurs.
- Store patches at room temperature in a safe place to prevent abuse and misuse; do not refrigerate or freeze.
- To remove patch, peel off slowly. An oil-based product (petroleum jelly, olive oil, mineral oil) may be applied gently to facilitate removal. Upon removal, fold so that adhesive side of patch adheres to itself and flush down toilet or dispose of in an appropriate lidded container.

Patient/Family Teaching

- Instruct patient to take medication as directed. If an oral dose is missed, take the remaining doses for that day at regularly spaced intervals; do not double doses. Take the last dose before 6 PM to minimize the risk of insomnia. Instruct patient not to alter dose without consulting health care professional. Abrupt cessation of high doses may cause extreme fatigue and mental depression. Instruct parent/caregiver to read the *Medication Guide* prior to use and with each Rx refill; new information may be available.
- Advise patient to check weight 2–3 times weekly and report weight loss to health care professional.
- May cause dizziness or blurred vision. Caution patient to avoid driving or activities requiring alertness until response to medication is known.
- Inform patient and/or parents that shell of *Concerta* tablet may appear in the stool. This is no cause for concern.
- Advise patient to avoid using caffeine-containing beverages concurrently with this therapy.
- Advise patient to notify health care professional if nervousness, insomnia, palpitations, vomiting, skin rash, or fever occurs.
- Advise patient and/or parents to notify health care professional of behavioral changes.
- Advise patient to notify health care professional of all Rx or OTC medications, vitamins, or herbal products being taken and to consult with health care professional before taking other medications.
- Inform patient that health care professional may order periodic holidays from the drug to assess progress and to decrease dependence.
- Emphasize the importance of routine follow-up exams to monitor progress.
- **Transdermal:** Encourage parent or caregiver to use the administration chart included in package to monitor application and removal time and disposal method.
- Caution patient to avoid exposing patch to direct external heat sources (hair dryers, heating pads, electric blankets, heated water beds, etc.). May increase rate and extent of absorption.
- Inform parent/caregiver that skin redness, itching and small bumps on the skin are common. If swelling or blistering occurs, the patch should not be worn and health care professional notified. Caution parent/caregiver not to apply hydrocortisone or other solutions, creams, ointments, or emollients prior to application.
- Advise patient referred for MRI test to discuss patch with referring health care professional and MRI facility to determine if removal of patch is necessary prior to test and for directions for replacing patch.
- **Home Care Issues:** Pedi: Advise parents to notify school nurse of medication regimen.

Evaluation/Desired Outcomes

- Improved attention span and social interactions in ADHD.
- Decreased frequency of narcoleptic symptoms.

M

methylPREDNISolone, See CORTICOSTEROIDS (SYSTEMIC).

metoclopramide

(met-oh-**kloe**-pra-mide)

✱Metonia, Metozolv ODT, Reglan

Classification
Therapeutic: antiemetics

Pregnancy Category B

Indications

Prevention of chemotherapy-induced emesis. Treatment of postsurgical and diabetic gastric stasis. Facilitation of small bowel intubation in radiographic procedures. Management of gastroesophageal reflux. Treatment and prevention of postoperative nausea and vomiting when nasogastric suctioning is undesirable. **Unlabeled Use:** Treatment of hiccups. Adjunct management of migraine headaches.

Action

Blocks dopamine receptors in chemoreceptor trigger zone of the CNS. Stimulates motility of the upper GI tract and accelerates gastric emptying. **Therapeutic Effects:** Decreased nausea and vomiting. Decreased symptoms of gastric stasis. Easier passage of nasogastric tube into small bowel.

Pharmacokinetics

Absorption: Well absorbed from the GI tract, from rectal mucosa, and from IM sites.
Distribution: Widely distributed into body tissues and fluids. Crosses blood-brain barrier and placenta.

Enters breast milk in concentrations greater than plasma.
Metabolism and Excretion: Partially metabolized by the liver; 25% eliminated unchanged in the urine.
Half-life: 2.5–6 hr.

TIME/ACTION PROFILE (effects on peristalsis)

ROUTE	ONSET	PEAK	DURATION
PO	30–60 min	unknown	1–2 hr
IM	10–15 min	unknown	1–2 hr
IV	1–3 min	immediate	1–2 hr

Contraindications/Precautions

Contraindicated in: Hypersensitivity; Possible GI obstruction or hemorrhage; History of seizure disorders; Pheochromocytoma; Parkinson's disease.
Use Cautiously in: History of depression; Diabetes (may alter response to insulin); Renal impairment (↓ dose in CCr <50 mL/min); Chronic use >3 mo (↑ risk for tardive dyskinesia); OB, Lactation: Safety not established; Pedi: Prolonged clearance in neonates can result in high serum concentrations and ↑ the risk for methemoglobinemia. Side effects are more common in children, especially extrapyramidal reactions; Geri: More susceptible to oversedation, extrapyramidal reactions, and tardive dyskinesia.

Adverse Reactions/Side Effects

CNS: drowsiness, extrapyramidal reactions, restlessness, NEUROLEPTIC MALIGNANT SYNDROME, anxiety, depression, irritability, tardive dyskinesia. **CV:** arrhythmias (supraventricular tachycardia, bradycardia), hypertension, hypotension. **GI:** constipation, diarrhea, dry mouth, nausea. **Endo:** gynecomastia. **Hemat:** methemoglobinemia, neutropenia, leukopenia, agranulocytosis.

Interactions

Drug-Drug: Additive CNS depression with other **CNS depressants**, including **alcohol**, **antidepressants**, **antihistamines**, **opioid analgesics**, and **sedative/hypnotics**. May ↑ absorption and risk of toxicity from **cyclosporine**. May affect the GI absorption of other **orally administered drugs** as a result of effect on GI motility. May exaggerate hypotension during **general anesthesia**. ↑ risk of extrapyramidal reactions with agents such as **haloperidol** or **phenothiazines**. **Opioids** and **anticholinergics** may antagonize the GI effects of metoclopramide. Use cautiously with **MAO inhibitors** (causes release of catecholamines). May ↑ neuromuscular blockade from **succinylcholine**. May ↓ effectiveness of **levodopa**. May ↑ **tacrolimus** serum levels.

Route/Dosage

Prevention of Chemotherapy-Induced Vomiting

PO, IV (Adults and Children): 1–2 mg/kg 30 min before chemotherapy. Additional doses of 1–2 mg/kg may be given q 2–4 hr, pretreatment with diphenhydramine will ↓ the risk of extrapyramidal reactions to this dose.

Facilitation of Small Bowel Intubation

IV (Adults and Children >14 yr): 10 mg over 1–2 min.
IV (Children 6–14 yr): 2.5–5 mg (dose should not exceed 0.5 mg/kg) over 1–2 min.
IV (Children <6 yr): 0.1 mg/kg over 1–2 min.

Diabetic Gastroparesis

PO, IV (Adults): 10 mg 30 min before meals and at bedtime for 2–8 weeks.

Gastroesophageal Reflux

PO, IM, IV (Adults): 10–15 mg 30 min before meals and at bedtime (not to exceed 0.5 mg/kg/day). A single dose of 20 mg may be given preventively. Some patients may respond to doses as small as 5 mg.
PO, IM, IV (Neonates, Infants, and Children): 0.4–0.8 mg/kg/day in 4 divided doses.

Postoperative Nausea/Vomiting

IM, IV (Adults and Children >14 yr): 10 mg at the end of surgical procedure, repeat in 6–8 hr if needed.
IM, IV (Children <14 yr): 0.1–0.2 mg/kg/dose, repeat in 6–8 hr if needed.

Treatment of Hiccups

PO, IM (Adults): 10–20 mg 4 times daily PO; may be preceded by a single 10-mg dose IM (unlabeled).

Availability (generic available)

Tablets: 5 mg, 10 mg. **Cost:** *Generic*—5 mg $11.04/100, 10 mg $7.18/100. **Orally disintegrating tablets:** 5 mg, 10 mg. **Cost:** $26.40/10. **Oral solution (apricot-peach flavor):** 5 mg/5 mL. **Solution for injection:** 5 mg/mL.

NURSING IMPLICATIONS

Assessment

- Assess for nausea, vomiting, abdominal distention, and bowel sounds before and after administration.
- Assess for extrapyramidal side effects (*parkinsonian*—difficulty speaking or swallowing, loss of balance control, pill rolling, mask-like face, shuffling gait, rigidity, tremors; and *dystonic*—muscle spasms, twisting motions, twitching, inability to move eyes, weakness of arms or legs) periodically throughout course of therapy. May occur weeks to months after initiation of therapy and are reversible on discontinuation. Dystonic reactions may occur within minutes of IV infusion and stop within 24 hr

of discontinuation of metoclopramide. May be treated with 50 mg of IM diphenhydramine or diphenhydramine 1 mg/kg IV may be administered prophylactically 15 min before metoclopramide IV infusion.

- Monitor for tardive dyskinesia (uncontrolled rhythmic movement of mouth, face, and extremities; lip smacking or puckering; puffing of cheeks; uncontrolled chewing; rapid or worm-like movements of tongue). Usually occurs after a year or more of continued therapy; risk of tardive dyskinesia increases with total cumulative dose. Report immediately and discontinue metoclopramide; may be irreversible.
- Monitor for neuroleptic malignant syndrome (hyperthermia, muscle rigidity, altered consciousness, irregular pulse or BP, tachycardia, and diaphoresis).
- Assess for signs of depression periodically throughout therapy.
- ***Lab Test Considerations:*** May alter hepatic function test results.
- May cause ↑ serum prolactin and aldosterone concentrations.

Potential Nursing Diagnoses

Imbalanced nutrition: less than body requirements (Indications)
Risk for injury (Side Effects)

Implementation

- **PO:** Administer doses 30 min before meals and at bedtime.
- Do not to remove *orally disintegrating tablets* from the bottle until just prior to dosing. Remove tablet from bottle with dry hands and immediately place on tongue to disintegrate and swallow with saliva. Tablet typically disintegrates in 1–1.5 minutes. Administration with liquid is not necessary.
- **IM:** For prevention of postoperative nausea and vomiting, inject IM near the end of surgery.

IV Administration

- **IV Push:** Administer IV dose 30 min before administration of chemotherapeutic agent. ***Rate:*** Doses may be given slowly over 1–2 min. Rapid administration causes a transient but intense feeling of anxiety and restlessness followed by drowsiness.
- **Intermittent Infusion:** ***Diluent:*** May be diluted for IV infusion in 50 mL of D5W, 0.9% NaCl, D5/0.45% NaCl, Ringer's solution, or LR. Diluted solution is stable for 48 hr if protected from light or 24 hr under normal light. ***Concentration:*** May dilute to 0.2 mg/mL or give undiluted at 5 mg/mL. ***Rate:*** Infuse slowly (maximum rate 5 mg/min) over at least 15–30 min.
- **Y-Site Compatibility:** aldesleukin, alemtuzumab, alfentanil, amifostine, amikacin, aminophylline, amphotericin B lipid complex, anidulafungin, argatroban, ascorbic acid, atropine, aztreonam, benztropine, bivalirudin, bleomycin, bumetanide, buprenorphine, butorphanol, calcium chloride, calcium gluconate, carboplatin, caspofungin, cefazolin, cefotaxime, cefotetan, cefoxitin, ceftaroline, ceftazidime, ceftriaxone, cefuroxime, chloramphenicol, chlorpromazine, ciprofloxacin, cisatracurium, cisplatin, cladribine, clindamycin, cyanocobalamin, cyclophosphamide, cyclosporine, cytarabine, dactinomycin, daptomycin, dexamethasone, dexmedetomidine, digoxin, diltiazem, diphenhydramine, dobutamine, docetaxel, dopamine, doripenem, doxorubicin hydrochloride, doxycycline, droperidol, enalaprilat, ephedrine, epinephrine, epirubicin, epoetin alfa, eptifibatide, ertapenem, erythromycin, esmolol, etoposide, etoposide phosphate, famotidine, fenoldopam, fentanyl, filgrastim, fluconazole, fludarabine, folic acid, foscarnet, gemcitabine, gentamicin, glycopyrrolate, granisetron, heparin, hetastarch, hydrocortisone, hydromorphone, idarubicin, ifosfamide, imipenem/cilastatin, indomethacin, insulin, irinotecan, isoproterenol, ketamine, ketorolac, labetalol, leucovorin, levofloxacin, lidocaine, linezolid, lorazepam, magnesium sulfate, mannitol, mechlorethamine, melphalan, meperidine, meropenem, methadone, methotrexate, methyldopate, methylprednisolone, metoprolol, metronidazole, midazolam, milrinone, mitomycin, mitoxantrone, morphine, multiple vitamins, mycophenolate, nafcillin, nalbuphine, naloxone, nesiritide, nitroglycerin, nitroprusside, norepinephrine, octreotide, ondansetron, oxacillin, oxaliplatin, oxytocin, paclitaxel, palonosetron, pamidronate, pancuronium, pantoprazole, papaverine, pemetrexed, penicillin G, pentamidine, pentazocine, pentobarbital, phenobarbital, phenylephrine, phytonadione, piperacillin/tazobactam, potassium acetate, potassium chloride, procainamide, prochlorperazine, promethazine, propranolol, protamine, pyridoxine, quinupristin/dalfopristin, ranitidine, remifentanil, rituximab, rocuronium, sargramostim, sodium acetate, sodium bicarbonate, streptokinase, succinylcholine, sufentanil, tacrolimus, telavancin, teniposide, theophylline, thiamine, thiotepa, tigecycline, tirofiban, tobramycin, topotecan, trastuzumab, vancomycin, vasopressin, vecuronium, verapamil, vinblastine, vincristine, vinorelbine, voriconazole, zidovudine, zoledronic acid.
- **Y-Site Incompatibility:** amphotericin B cholesteryl, amphotericin B colloidal, amphotericin B liposome, carmustine, cefepime, dantrolene, diazepam, doxorubicin liposome, ganciclovir, phenytoin, propofol, trimethoprim/sulfamethoxazole.

M

Patient/Family Teaching

- Instruct patient to take metoclopramide as directed. Take missed doses as soon as remembered if not almost time for next dose. Advise patient to read the *Medication Guide* before starting therapy and with each Rx refill in case of changes.
- Pedi: Unintentional overdose has been reported in infants and children with the use of metoclopramide oral solution. Teach parents how to accurately read labels and administer medication.
- May cause drowsiness. Caution patient to avoid driving or other activities requiring alertness until response to medication is known.
- Advise patient to avoid concurrent use of alcohol and other CNS depressants while taking this medication.
- Inform patient of risk of extrapyramidal symptoms, tardive dyskinesia, and neuroleptic malignant syndrome. Advise patient to notify health care professional immediately if involuntary or repetitive movements of eyes, face, or limbs occur.
- Advise female patient to notify health care professional if pregnancy is planned or suspected or if breast feeding.

Evaluation/Desired Outcomes

- Prevention or relief of nausea and vomiting.
- Decreased symptoms of gastric stasis.
- Facilitation of small bowel intubation.
- Decreased symptoms of esophageal reflux.
- Metoclopramide should not be used for more than 12 wk due to risk of tardive dyskinesia.

metolazone (me-tole-a-zone)

Zaroxolyn

Classification

Therapeutic: antihypertensives, diuretics

Pharmacologic: thiazide-like diuretics

Pregnancy Category B

Indications

Mild to moderate hypertension. Edema associated with HF or the nephrotic syndrome.

Action

Increases excretion of sodium and water by inhibiting sodium reabsorption in the distal tubule. Promotes excretion of chloride, potassium, magnesium, and bicarbonate. May produce arteriolar dilation. **Therapeutic Effects:** Lowering of BP in hypertensive patients. Diuresis with subsequent mobilization of edema. Effect may continue in renal impairment.

Pharmacokinetics

Absorption: Absorption is variable.

Distribution: Unknown.

Protein Binding: 95%.

Metabolism and Excretion: Excreted mainly unchanged by the kidneys.

Half-life: 6–20 hr.

TIME/ACTION PROFILE (diuretic effect†)

ROUTE	ONSET	PEAK	DURATION
PO	1 hr	2 hr	12–24 hr

†Full antihypertensive effect may take days–weeks.

Contraindications/Precautions

Contraindicated in: Hypersensitivity; Cross-sensitivity with other sulfonamides may exist; Anuria; Lactation: Avoid breastfeeding.

Use Cautiously in: Severe hepatic impairment; OB: Safety not established; Geri: ↑ sensitivity to drug effects.

Adverse Reactions/Side Effects

CNS: drowsiness, lethargy. **CV:** chest pain, hypotension, palpitations. **GI:** anorexia, bloating, cramping, drug-induced hepatitis, nausea, pancreatitis, vomiting. **Derm:** photosensitivity, rashes. **Endo:** hyperglycemia. **F and E:** hypokalemia, dehydration, hypercalcemia, hypochloremic alkalosis, hypomagnesemia, hyponatremia, hypophosphatemia, hypovolemia. **Hemat:** blood dyscrasias. **Metab:** hyperuricemia. **MS:** muscle cramps.

Interactions

Drug-Drug: ↑ risk of hypotension with **nitrates**, acute ingestion of **alcohol**, or other **antihypertensives**. ↑ risk of hypokalemia with **corticosteroids**, **amphotericin B**, or **piperacillin/tazobactam**. May ↑ the risk of **digoxin** toxicity. ↓ the excretion of **lithium**; may cause toxicity. May ↓ the effectiveness of **methenamine**. **Stimulant laxatives** (including **aloe**, **senna**) may ↑ risk of potassium depletion.

Drug-Food: Food may ↑ extent of absorption.

Route/Dosage

PO (Adults): *Hypertension*—2.5–5 mg/day; *edema*—5–20 mg/day.

PO (Children): 0.2–0.4 mg/kg/day divided q 12–24 hr.

Availability (generic available)

Tablets: 2.5 mg, 5 mg, 10 mg.

NURSING IMPLICATIONS

Assessment

- Monitor BP, intake and output, and daily weight, and assess feet, legs, and sacral area for edema daily.
- Assess patient, especially if taking digoxin, for anorexia, nausea, vomiting, muscle cramps, paresthesia, and confusion. Notify health care professional if these signs of electrolyte imbalance occur. Patients taking digoxin are at risk of digoxin toxicity because of the potassium-depleting effect of the diuretic.
- Assess patient for allergy to sulfonamides.

- **Hypertension:** Monitor BP before and periodically during therapy.
- Monitor frequency of prescription refills to determine compliance.
- ***Lab Test Considerations:*** Monitor electrolytes (especially potassium), blood glucose, BUN, and serum creatinine and uric acid levels before and periodically during therapy.
- May cause ↑ in serum and urine glucose in diabetic patients.
- May cause an ↑ in serum bilirubin, calcium, creatinine, and uric acid, and a ↓ in serum magnesium, potassium, and sodium and urinary calcium concentrations.
- May cause ↓ serum protein-bound iodine (PBI) concentrations.
- May cause ↑ serum cholesterol, low-density lipoprotein, and triglyceride concentrations.

Potential Nursing Diagnoses

Excess fluid volume (Indications)
Risk for deficient fluid volume (Side Effects)

Implementation

- Do not confuse metolazone with methimazole. Do not confuse metolazone with methadone.
- Administer in the morning to prevent disruption of sleep cycle.
- Intermittent dose schedule may be used for continued control of edema.
- **PO:** May give with food or milk to minimize GI irritation.

Patient/Family Teaching

- Instruct patient to take metolazone at the same time each day. Take missed doses as soon as remembered but not just before next dose is due. Do not double doses.
- Instruct patient to monitor weight biweekly and notify health care professional of significant changes.
- Caution patient to change positions slowly to minimize orthostatic hypotension; may be potentiated by alcohol.
- Advise patient to use sunscreen and protective clothing in the sun to prevent photosensitivity reactions.
- Instruct patient to discuss dietary potassium requirements with health care professional (see Appendix J).
- Instruct patient to notify health care professional of medication regimen before treatment or surgery.
- Advise patient to report muscle weakness, cramps, nausea, vomiting, diarrhea, or dizziness to health care professional.
- Emphasize the importance of routine follow-up exams.
- **Hypertension:** Advise patient to continue taking the medication even if feeling better. Medication controls but does not cure hypertension.
- Encourage patient to comply with additional interventions for hypertension (weight reduction, low-sodium diet, regular exercise, smoking cessation, moderation of alcohol consumption, and stress management).
- Instruct patient and family in correct technique for monitoring weekly BP.
- Advise patient to notify health care professional of all Rx or OTC medications, vitamins, or herbal products being taken and to consult with health care professional before taking other medications, especially cough or cold preparations, concurrently with this therapy.

Evaluation/Desired Outcomes

- Decrease in BP.
- Increase in urine output.
- Decrease in edema.

M

HIGH ALERT

⌘ metoprolol (me-toe-proe-lole)

♣Betaloc, ♣Lopresor, ♣Lopresor SR, Lopressor, Toprol-XL

Classification
Therapeutic: antianginals, antihypertensives
Pharmacologic: beta blockers

Pregnancy Category C

Indications

Hypertension. Angina pectoris. Prevention of MI and decreased mortality in patients with recent MI. Management of stable, symptomatic (class II or III) heart failure due to ischemic, hypertensive or cardiomyopathc origin (may be used with ACE inhibitors, diuretics and/or digoxin; Toprol XL only). **Unlabeled Use:** Ventricular arrhythmias/tachycardia. Migraine prophylaxis. Tremors. Aggressive behavior. Drug-induced akathisia. Anxiety.

Action

Blocks stimulation of $beta_1$ (myocardial)-adrenergic receptors. Does not usually affect $beta_2$ (pulmonary, vascular, uterine)-adrenergic receptor sites. **Therapeutic Effects:** Decreased BP and heart rate. Decreased frequency of attacks of angina pectoris. Decreased rate of cardiovascular mortality and hospitalization in patients with heart failure.

Pharmacokinetics

Absorption: Well absorbed after oral administration.
Distribution: Crosses the blood-brain barrier, crosses the placenta; small amounts enter breast milk.
Metabolism and Excretion: Mostly metabolized by the liver (primarily by CYP2D6; the CYP2D6 enzyme

system exhibits genetic polymorphism); 🧬 ~7% of population may be poor metabolizers and may have significantly ↑ metoprolol concentrations and an ↑ risk of adverse effects.

Half-life: 3–7 hr.

TIME/ACTION PROFILE (cardiovascular effects)

ROUTE	ONSET	PEAK	DURATION
PO†	15 min	unknown	6–12 hr
PO–ER	unknown	6–12 hr	24 hr
IV	immediate	20 min	5–8 hr

†Maximal effects on BP (chronic therapy) may not occur for 1 wk. Hypotensive effects may persist for up to 4 wk after discontinuation.

Contraindications/Precautions

Contraindicated in: Uncompensated HF; Pulmonary edema; Cardiogenic shock; Bradycardia, heart block, or sick sinus syndrome (in absence of a pacemaker).

Use Cautiously in: Renal impairment; Hepatic impairment; Geri: ↑ sensitivity to beta blockers; initial dose reduction recommended; Pulmonary disease (including asthma; $beta_1$ selectivity may be lost at higher doses); Diabetes mellitus (may mask signs of hypoglycemia); Thyrotoxicosis (may mask symptoms); Patients with a history of severe allergic reactions (intensity of reactions may be increased); Untreated pheochromocytoma (initiate only after alpha blocker therapy started); OB, Lactation, Pedi: Safety not established; all agents cross the placenta and may cause fetal/neonatal bradycardia, hypotension, hypoglycemia, or respiratory depression.

Adverse Reactions/Side Effects

CNS: fatigue, weakness, anxiety, depression, dizziness, drowsiness, insomnia, memory loss, mental status changes, nervousness, nightmares. **EENT:** blurred vision, stuffy nose. **Resp:** bronchospasm, wheezing. **CV:** BRADYCARDIA, HF, PULMONARY EDEMA, hypotension, peripheral vasoconstriction. **GI:** constipation, diarrhea, drug-induced hepatitis, dry mouth, flatulence, gastric pain, heartburn, ↑ liver enzymes, nausea, vomiting. **GU:** erectile dysfunction, ↓ libido, urinary frequency. **Derm:** rash. **Endo:** hyperglycemia, hypoglycemia. **MS:** arthralgia, back pain, joint pain. **Misc:** drug-induced lupus syndrome.

Interactions

Drug-Drug: General anesthesia, IV phenytoin, and **verapamil** may cause ↑ myocardial depression. ↑ risk of bradycardia when used with **digoxin, verapamil, diltiazem,** or **clonidine**. ↑ hypotension may occur with other **antihypertensives**, acute ingestion of **alcohol**, or **nitrates**. Concurrent use with **amphetamines, cocaine, ephedrine, epinephrine, norepinephrine, phenylephrine,** or **pseudoephedrine** may result in unopposed alpha-adrenergic stimulation (excessive hypertension, bradycardia). Concurrent administration of **thyroid** administration may ↓ effectiveness. May alter the effectiveness of **insulins** or **oral hypoglycemic agents** (dose adjustments may be necessary). May ↓ the effectiveness of **theophylline**. May ↓ the beneficial $beta_1$-cardiovascular effects of **dopamine** or **dobutamine**. Use cautiously within 14 days of **MAO inhibitor** therapy (may result in hypertension).

Route/Dosage

When switching from immediate-release to extended-release product, the same total daily dose can be used

PO (Adults): *Antihypertensive/antianginal*—25–100 mg/day as a single dose initially or 2 divided doses; may be ↑ q 7 days as needed up to 450 mg/day (immediate-release) or 400 mg/day (extended-release) (for angina, give in divided doses). Extended-release products are given once daily. *MI*—25–50 mg (starting 15 min after last IV dose) q 6 hr for 48 hr, then 100 mg twice daily. *Heart failure*—12.5–25 mg once daily (of extended-release), can be doubled every 2 wk up to 200 mg/day. *Migraine prevention*—50–100 mg 2–4 times daily (unlabeled).

IV (Adults): *MI*—5 mg q 2 min for 3 doses, followed by oral dosing.

Availability (generic available)

Tablets (tartrate): 25 mg, 50 mg, 100 mg. **Cost:** *Generic*—All strengths $7.18/100. **Extended-release tablets (succinate; Toprol XL):** 25 mg, 50 mg, 100 mg, 200 mg. **Cost:** *Generic*—25 mg $35.68/100, 50 mg $41.93/100, 100 mg $53.95/100, 200 mg $84.54/100. **Solution for injection:** 1 mg/mL. ***In combination with:*** hydrochlorothiazide (Dutoprol, Lopressor HCT). See Appendix B.

NURSING IMPLICATIONS

Assessment

- Monitor BP, ECG, and pulse frequently during dose adjustment and periodically during therapy.
- Monitor frequency of prescription refills to determine compliance.
- Monitor vital signs and ECG every 5–15 min during and for several hours after parenteral administration. If heart rate <40 bpm, especially if cardiac output is also decreased, administer atropine 0.25–0.5 mg IV.
- Monitor intake and output ratios and daily weights. Assess routinely for signs and symptoms of HF (dyspnea, rales/crackles, weight gain, peripheral edema, jugular venous distention).
- **Angina:** Assess frequency and characteristics of anginal attacks periodically during therapy.
- ***Lab Test Considerations:*** May cause ↑ BUN, serum lipoprotein, potassium, triglyceride, and uric acid levels.

- May cause ↑ ANA titers.
- May cause ↑ in blood glucose levels.
- May cause ↑ serum alkaline phosphatase, LDH, AST, and ALT levels.

Potential Nursing Diagnoses

Decreased cardiac output (Side Effects)
Noncompliance (Patient/Family Teaching)

Implementation

- ***High Alert:*** IV vasoactive medications are inherently dangerous. Before administering intravenously, have second practitioner independently check original order and dose calculations.
- ***High Alert:*** Do not confuse Toprol-XL (metoprolol) with Topamax (topiramate). Do not confuse Lopressor with Lyrica. Do not confuse metoprolol tartrate with metoprolol succinate.
- **PO:** Take apical pulse before administering. If <50 bpm or if arrhythmia occurs, withhold medication and notify health care professional.
- Administer metoprolol with meals or directly after eating.
- Extended-release tablets should be swallowed whole; do not break, crush, or chew.

IV Administration

- **IV Push:** ***Diluent:*** Administer undiluted. ***Concentration:*** 1 mg/mL. ***Rate:*** Administer over 1 min.
- **Y-Site Compatibility:** acyclovir, alemtuzumab, alfentanil, alteplase, amikacin, aminocaproic acid, aminophylline, amiodarone, amphotericin B liposome, anidulafungin, argatroban, ascorbic acid, atropine, aztreonam, benztropine, bivalirudin, bleomycin, bumetanide, buprenorphine, butorphanol, calcium chloride, calcium gluconate, cangrelor, carboplatin, carmustine, caspofungin, cefazolin, cefonocid, cefotaxime, cefotetan, cefoxitin, ceftaroline, ceftazidime, ceftriaxone, cefuroxime, chloramphenicol, chlorpromazine, cisplatin, clindamycin, cyanocobalamin, cyclophosphamide, cyclosporine, cytarabine, dactinomycin, daptomycin, dexamethasone, dexmedetomidine, digoxin, diltiazem, diphenhydramine, dobutamine, docetaxel, dopamine, doxorubicin hydrochloride, doxycycline, enalaprilat, ephedrine, epinephrine, epirubicin, epoetin alfa, eptifibatide, esmolol, etoposide, etoposide phosphate, famotidine, fenoldopam, fentanyl, fluconazole, fludarabine, fluorouracil, folic acid, foscarnet, fosphenytoin, furosemide, ganciclovir, gemcitabine, gentamicin, glycopyrrolate, granisetron, heparin, hetastarch, hydrocortisone, hydromorphone, idarubicin, ifosfamide, imipenem/cilastatin, indomethacin, insulin, irinotecan, isoproterenol, ketorolac, labetalol, leucovorin, linezolid, lorazepam, magnesium sulfate, mannitol, mechlorethamine, meperidine, methotrexate, methyldopate, methylprednisolone, metoclopramide, metronidazole, midazolam, milrinone, mitoxantrone, morphine, multivitamins, mycophenolate, nafcillin, nalbuphine, naloxone, nitroprusside, norepinephrine, octreotide, ondansetron, oxacillin, oxaliplatin, oxytocin, paclitaxel, palonosetron, pamidronate, pancuronium, papaverine, pemetrexed, penicillin G, pentamidine, pentazocine, pentobarbital, phenobarbital, phenylephrine, phytonadione, piperacillin/tazobactam, potassium acetate, potassium chloride, procainamide, prochlorperazine, promethazine, propranolol, protamine, pyridoxine, quinupristin/dalfopristin, ranitidine, rocuronium, sodium bicarbonate, streptokinase, succinylcholine, sufentanil, tacrolimus, teniposide, theophylline, thiamine, thiotepa, tigecycline, tirofiban, tobramycin, vancomycin, vasopressin, vecuronium, verapamil, vincristine, vinorelbine, voriconazole, zoledronic acid.
- **Y-Site Incompatibility:** allopurinol, amphotericin B colloidal, amphotericin B lipid complex, dantrolene, diazepam, pantoprazole, phenytoin, trimethoprim/sulfamethoxazole.

Patient/Family Teaching

- Instruct patient to take medication as directed, at the same time each day, even if feeling well; do not skip or double up on missed doses. Take missed doses as soon as possible up to 8 hr before next dose. Abrupt withdrawal may precipitate life-threatening arrhythmias, hypertension, or myocardial ischemia.
- Teach patient and family how to check pulse daily and BP biweekly and to report significant changes to health care professional.
- May cause drowsiness. Caution patient to avoid driving or other activities that require alertness until response to the drug is known.
- Advise patient to change positions slowly to minimize orthostatic hypotension.
- Caution patient that this medication may increase sensitivity to cold.
- Instruct patient to notify health care professional of all Rx or OTC medications, vitamins, or herbal products being taken and to consult health care professional before taking any Rx, OTC, or herbal products, especially cold preparations, concurrently with this medication. Patients on antihypertensive therapy should also avoid excessive amounts of coffee, tea, and cola.
- Diabetics should closely monitor blood glucose, especially if weakness, malaise, irritability, or fatigue occurs. Medication does not block sweating as a sign of hypoglycemia.
- Advise patient to notify health care professional if slow pulse, difficulty breathing, wheezing, cold hands and feet, dizziness, light-headedness, confu-

M

sion, depression, rash, fever, sore throat, unusual bleeding, or bruising occurs.
- Instruct patient to inform health care professional of medication regimen before treatment or surgery.
- Advise patient to carry identification describing disease process and medication regimen at all times.
- **Hypertension:** Reinforce the need to continue additional therapies for hypertension (weight loss, sodium restriction, stress reduction, regular exercise, moderation of alcohol consumption, and smoking cessation). Medication controls but does not cure hypertension.

Evaluation/Desired Outcomes
- Decrease in BP.
- Reduction in frequency of anginal attacks.
- Increase in activity tolerance.
- Prevention of MI.

metroNIDAZOLE
(me-troe-**ni**-da-zole)
Flagyl, Flagyl ER, MetroCream, MetroGel, MetroGel-Vaginal, MetroLotion, Metro IV, ✱Nidagel, Noritate, ✱Novo-Nidazol, Nuvessa, Vandazole

Classification
Therapeutic: anti-infectives, antiprotozoals, antiulcer agents

Pregnancy Category B

Indications
PO, IV: Treatment of the following anaerobic infections: Intra-abdominal infections (may be used with a cephalosporin), Gynecologic infections, Skin and skin structure infections, Lower respiratory tract infections, Bone and joint infections, CNS infections, Septicemia, Endocarditis. **IV:** Perioperative prophylactic agent in colorectal surgery. **PO:** Amebicide in the management of amebic dysentery, amebic liver abscess, and trichomoniasis: Treatment of peptic ulcer disease caused by *Helicobacter pylori*. **Topical:** Treatment of acne rosacea. **Vag:** Management of bacterial vaginosis. **Unlabeled Use:** Treatment of giardiasis. Treatment of anti-infective associated Clostridium difficile-associated diarrhea (CDAD).

Action
Disrupts DNA and protein synthesis in susceptible organisms. **Therapeutic Effects:** Bactericidal, trichomonacidal, or amebicidal action. **Spectrum:** Most notable for activity against anaerobic bacteria, including: *Bacteroides*, *Clostridium*. In addition, is active against: *Trichomonas vaginalis*, *Entamoeba histolytica*, *Giardia lamblia*, *H. pylori*, *Clostridium difficile*.

Pharmacokinetics
Absorption: 80% absorbed after oral administration. Minimal absorption after topical or vaginal application.
Distribution: Widely distributed into most tissues and fluids, including CSF. Crosses the placenta and enters fetal circulation rapidly; enters breast milk in concentrations equal to plasma levels.
Metabolism and Excretion: Partially metabolized by the liver (30–60%), partially excreted unchanged in the urine, 6–15% eliminated in the feces.
Half-life: Neonates: 25–75 hr; Children and adults: 6–12 hr.

TIME/ACTION PROFILE (PO, IV = blood levels; topical = improvement in rosacea)

ROUTE	ONSET	PEAK	DURATION
PO	rapid	1–3 hr	8 hr
PO-ER	rapid	unknown	up to 24 hr
IV	rapid	end of infusion	6–8 hr
Topical	3 wk	9 wk	12 hr
Vaginal	unknown	6–12 hr	12 hr

Contraindications/Precautions
Contraindicated in: Hypersensitivity; Hypersensitivity to parabens (topical only); OB: First trimester of pregnancy.
Use Cautiously in: History of blood dyscrasias; History of seizures or neurologic problems; Severe hepatic impairment (dose ↓ suggested); OB: Although safety not established, has been used to treat trichomoniasis in 2nd- and 3rd-trimester pregnancy—but not as single-dose regimen; Lactation: If needed, use single dose and interrupt nursing for 24 hr thereafter; Patients receiving corticosteroids or predisposed to edema (injection contains 28 mEq sodium/g metronidazole).

Adverse Reactions/Side Effects
CNS: SEIZURES, <u>dizziness</u>, <u>headache</u>, <u>aseptic meningitis (IV)</u>, <u>encephalopathy (IV)</u>. **EENT:** optic neuropathy, tearing (topical only). **GI:** <u>abdominal pain</u>, <u>anorexia</u>, <u>nausea</u>, diarrhea, dry mouth, furry tongue, glossitis, unpleasant taste, vomiting. **Derm:** STEVENS-JOHNSON SYNDROME, rash, urticaria; *topical only*, burning, mild dryness, skin irritation, transient redness. **Hemat:** leukopenia. **Local:** phlebitis at IV site. **Neuro:** peripheral neuropathy. **Misc:** superinfection.

Interactions
Drug-Drug: Cimetidine may ↓ metabolism. **Phenobarbital** and **rifampin** ↑ metabolism and may ↓ effectiveness. Metronidazole ↑ the effects of **phenytoin**, **lithium**, and **warfarin**. Disulfiram-like reaction may occur with **alcohol** ingestion. May cause acute psychosis and confusion with **disulfiram**. ↑ risk of leukopenia with **fluorouracil** or **azathioprine**.

Route/Dosage
PO (Adults): *Anaerobic infections*—7.5 mg/kg q 6 hr (not to exceed 4 g/day). *Trichomoniasis*—250 mg

q 8 hr for 7 days *or* single 2-g dose *or* 1 g twice daily for 1 day. *Amebiasis*—500–750 mg q 8 hr for 5–10 days. *H. pylori*—250 mg 4 times daily *or* 500 mg twice daily for 1–2 wk (with other agents). *Bacterial vaginoses*—750 mg once daily as ER tablets for 7 days. *Antibiotic associated Clostridium difficile-associated diarrhea (CDAD)*—250–500 mg 3–4 times/day for 10–14 days.

PO (Infants and Children): *Anaerobic infections*—30 mg/kg/day divided q 6 hr, maximum dose: 4 g/day *Trichomoniasis*—15–30 mg/kg/day divided q 8 hr for 7–10 days. *Amebiasis*—35–50 mg/kg/day divided q 8 hr for 5–10 days (not to exceed 750 mg/dose). *Antibiotic associated Clostridium difficile-associated diarrhea (CDAD)*—30 mg/kg/day divided q 6 hr for 7–10 days. *H. pylori*—15–20 mg/kg/day divided twice daily for 4 wk.

IV, PO (Neonates 0–4 weeks, <1200 g): 7.5 mg/kg q 48 hr. *Postnatal age <7 days, 1200–2000 g*—7.5 mg/kg/day q 24 hr. *Postnatal age <7 days, >2000 g*—15 mg/kg/day divided q 12 hr. *Postnatal age >7 days, 1200–2000 g*—15 mg/kg/day divided q 12 hr. *Postnatal age >7 days, >2000 g*—30 mg/kg/day divided q 12 hr.

IV (Adults): *Anaerobic infections*—Initial dose 15 mg/kg, then 7.5 mg/kg q 6–8 hr *or* 500 mg q 6–8 hr (not to exceed 4 g/day). *Perioperative prophylaxis*—Initial dose 15 mg/kg 1 hr before surgery, then 7.5 mg/kg 6 and 12 hr later. *Amebiasis*—500–750 mg q 8 hr for 5–10 days.

IV (Children): *Anaerobic infections*—30 mg/kg/day divided q 6 hr, maximum dose: 4 g/day.

Topical (Adults): *Acne rosacea*—Apply thin film to affected area bid.

Vag (Adults): *Bacterial vaginosis*—*MetroGel Vaginal*—One applicatorful (37.5 mg) of 0.75% gel 1–2 times daily for 5 days; *Nuvessa*—One applicatorful (65 mg) of 1.3% gel as a single dose at bedtime; *Vandazole*—One applicatorful (37.5 mg) of 0.75% gel once daily for 5 days.

Availability (generic available)

Tablets: 250 mg, 500 mg. **Extended-release tablets:** 750 mg. **Capsules:** 375 mg, ✱500 mg. **Premixed injection:** 500 mg/100 mL. **Topical gel:** 0.75%, 1%. **Topical cream:** 0.75%, 1%. **Topical lotion:** 0.75%. **Vaginal gel:** 0.75% (37.5 mg/5 g applicatorful), 1.3% (65 mg/5 g applicatorful). ***In combination with:*** bismuth subcitrate potassium and tetracycline (Pylera). See Appendix B.

NURSING IMPLICATIONS

Assessment

- Assess for infection (vital signs; appearance of wound, sputum, urine, and stool; WBC) at beginning of and throughout therapy.
- Obtain specimens for culture and sensitivity before initiating therapy. First dose may be given before receiving results.
- Monitor neurologic status during and after IV infusions. Inform health care professional if numbness, paresthesia, weakness, ataxia, or seizures occur.
- Monitor intake and output and daily weight, especially for patients on sodium restriction. Each 500 mg of premixed injection for dilution contains 14 mEq of sodium.
- Assess for rash periodically during therapy. May cause Stevens-Johnson syndrome. Discontinue therapy if severe or if accompanied with fever, general malaise, fatigue, muscle or joint aches, blisters, oral lesions, conjunctivitis, hepatitis and/or eosinophilia.
- **Giardiasis:** Monitor three stool samples taken several days apart, beginning 3–4 wk after treatment.
- ***Lab Test Considerations:*** May alter results of serum AST, ALT, and LDH tests.

M

Potential Nursing Diagnoses

Risk for infection (Indications)
Diarrhea (Indications)

Implementation

- Do not confuse metronidzole with metformin.
- **PO:** Administer on an empty stomach, or may administer with food or milk to minimize GI irritation. Tablets may be crushed for patients with difficulty swallowing. Swallow extended-release tablets whole; do not break, crush, or chew.

IV Administration

- **Intermittent Infusion:** ***Diluent:*** Administer premixed injection (500 mg/100 mL) undiluted. Do not refrigerate. Once taken out of overwrap, premixed infusion stable for 30 days at room temperature. ***Concentration:*** 5 mg/mL. ***Rate:*** Infuse over 30–60 min.
- **Y-Site Compatibility:** acyclovir, alemtuzumab, alfentanil, allopurinol, amifostine, amikacin, aminocaproic acid, aminophylline, amiodarone, ampicillin, ampicillin/sulbactam, anidulafungin, argatroban, bivalirudin, bleomycin, bumetanide, buprenorphine, busulfan, butorphanol, calcium acetate, calcium chloride, calcium gluconate, carboplatin, carmustine, cefazolin, cefepime, cefotaxime, cefotetan, cefoxitin, ceftaroline, ceftazidime, ceftriaxone, cefuroxime, chloramphenicol, chlorpromazine, ciprofloxacin, cisatracurium, cisplatin, clindamycin, cyclophosphamide, cyclosporine, cytarabine, dactinomycin, dexamethasone, dexmedetomidine, dexrazoxane, digoxin, diltiazem, dimenhydrinate, diphenhydramine, dobutamine, docetaxel, dopamine, doripenem, doxorubicin hydrochloride, doxorubicin liposomal, doxycycline, droperidol, enalaprilat,

ephedrine, epinephrine, epirubicin, eptifibatide, ertapenem, erythromycin, esmolol, etoposide, etoposide phosphate, famotidine, fenoldopam, fentanyl, fluconazole, fludarabine, fluorouracil, foscarnet, fosphenytoin, furosemide, gemcitabine, gentamicin, glycopyrrolate, granisetron, haloperidol, heparin, hetastarch, hydralazine, hydrocortisone, hydromorphone, idarubicin, ifosfamide, imipenem/cilastatin, insulin, irinotecan, isoproterenol, ketamine, ketorolac, labetalol, leucovorin, levofloxacin, lidocaine, linezolid, lorazepam, magnesium sulfate, mannitol, mechlorethamine, melphalan, meperidine, meropenem, mesna, methotrexate, methyldopate, methylprednisolone, metoclopramide, metoprolol, midazolam, milrinone, mitoxantrone, morphine, mycophenolate, nafcillin, nalbuphine, naloxone, nesiritide, nicardipine, nitroglycerin, nitroprusside, norepinephrine, octreotide, ondansetron, oxaliplatin, oxytocin, paclitaxel, palonosetron, pamidronate, pancuronium, pentamidine, pentazocine, pentobarbital, pentobarbital, phenylephrine, piperacillin/tazobactam, potassium acetate, potassium chloride, potassium phosphates, prochlorperazine, promethazine, propranolol, ranitidine, remifentanil, rituximab, rocuronium, sargramostim, sodium acetate, sodium bicarbonate, sodium phosphates, streptozocin, succinylcholine, sufentanil, tacrolimus, teniposide, theophylline, thiopental, thiotepa, tigecycline, tirofiban, tobramycin, trastuzumab, trimethoprim/sulfamethoxazole, vancomycin, vasopressin, vecuronium, verapamil, vincristine, vinorelbine, voriconazole, zidovudine, zoledronic acid.

- **Y-Site Incompatibility:** amphotericin B colloidal, amphotericin B lipid complex, amphotericin B liposome, aztreonam, dantrolene, daptomycin, diazepam, filgrastim, ganciclovir, pantoprazole, pemetrexed, phenytoin, procainamide, quinupristin/dalfopristin.
- **Topical:** Cleanse affected area before application. Apply and rub in a thin film twice daily, morning and evening. Avoid contact with eyes.
- **Vag:** Administer once daily dosing at bedtime.

Patient/Family Teaching

- Instruct patient to take medication as directed with evenly spaced times between doses, even if feeling better. Do not skip doses or double up on missed doses. Take missed doses as soon as remembered if not almost time for next dose.
- Advise patients treated for trichomoniasis that sexual partners may be asymptomatic sources of reinfection and should be treated concurrently. Patient should also refrain from intercourse or use a condom to prevent reinfection.
- Caution patient to avoid intake of alcoholic beverages or preparations containing alcohol during and for at least 3 days after treatment with metronidazole, including vaginal gel. May cause a disulfiram-like reaction (flushing, nausea, vomiting, headache, abdominal cramps).
- May cause dizziness or light-headedness. Caution patient to avoid driving or other activities requiring alertness until response to medication is known.
- Instruct patient to notify health care professional promptly if rash occurs.
- Inform patient that medication may cause an unpleasant metallic taste.
- Advise patient to notify health care professional of all Rx or OTC medications, vitamins, or herbal products being taken and to consult with health care professional before taking other medications.
- Advise patient that frequent mouth rinses, good oral hygiene, and sugarless gum or candy may minimize dry mouth. Notify health care professional if dry mouth persists for more than 2 wk.
- Inform patient that medication may cause urine to turn dark.
- Advise patient to consult health care professional if no improvement in a few days or if signs and symptoms of superinfection (black, furry overgrowth on tongue; vaginal itching or discharge; loose or foul-smelling stools) develop.
- Advise patient to inform health care professional if pregnancy is planned or suspected or if breast feeding.
- **Vag:** Instruct patient in correct technique for intravaginal instillation. Advise patient to avoid intercourse during treatment with vaginal gel.
- **Topical:** Instruct patient on correct technique for application of topical gel. Cosmetics may be used after application of gel.

Evaluation/Desired Outcomes

- Resolution of the signs and symptoms of infection. Length of time for complete resolution depends on organism and site of infection.
- Significant results should be seen within 3 wk of application of topical gel. Application may be continued for 9 wk.

micafungin (my-ka-**fun**-gin)

Mycamine

Classification
Therapeutic: antifungals
Pharmacologic: echinocandins

Pregnancy Category C

Indications

Esophageal candidiasis. Candidemia/acute disseminated candidiasis/Candidal peritonitis and abscesses. Prophylaxis of *Candida* infections during hematopoetic stem cell transplantation.

Action

Inhibits synthesis of glucan required for the formation of fungal cell wall. **Therapeutic Effects:** Death of susceptible fungi. **Spectrum:** Active against the following *Candida* spp.: *C. albicans*, *C. glabrata*, *C. krusei*, *C. parapsilosis*, *C. tropicalis*.

Pharmacokinetics

Absorption: IV administration results in complete bioavailability.

Distribution: Unknown.

Protein Binding: >99 %.

Metabolism and Excretion: Mostly metabolized; 71% fecal elimination.

Half-life: 15 hr.

TIME/ACTION PROFILE

ROUTE	ONSET	PEAK	DURATION
IV	rapid	end of infusion	24 hr

Contraindications/Precautions

Contraindicated in: Hypersensitivity.

Use Cautiously in: Severe hepatic impairment; OB: Use only if clearly needed; Lactation, Pedi: Children <4 mo (safety not established).

Adverse Reactions/Side Effects

GI: worsening hepatic function/hepatitis. **GU:** renal impairment. **Hemat:** hemolysis/hemolytic anemia. **Local:** injection site reactions. **Misc:** allergic reactions including ANAPHYLAXIS (rare).

Interactions

Drug-Drug: ↑ blood levels and risk of toxicity with **sirolimus** and **nifedipine** (dose adjustments may be necessary).

Route/Dosage

IV (Adults): *Esophageal candidiasis*—150 mg daily for 15 days (range 10–30 days); *Candidemia/acute disseminated candidiasis/Candida peritonitis and abscesses*—100 mg daily for 15 days (range 10–47 days); *Prevention of Candida infections in stem cell transplantation*—50 mg daily (duration range 6–51 days).

IV (Children ≥4 mo and >30 kg): *Esophageal candidiasis*—2.5 mg/kg daily (maximum daily dose = 150 mg); *Candidemia/acute disseminated candidiasis/Candida peritonitis and abscesses*—2 mg/kg daily (maximum daily dose = 100 mg); *Prevention of Candida infections in stem cell transplantation*—1 mg/kg daily (maximum daily dose = 50 mg).

IV (Children ≥4 mo and ≤30 kg): *Esophageal candidiasis*—3 mg/kg daily; *Candidemia/acute disseminated candidiasis/Candida peritonitis and abscesses*—2 mg/kg daily; *Prevention of Candida infections in stem cell transplantation*—1 mg/kg daily.

IV (Neonates): 7–10 mg/kg daily. Higher dose should be used in neonates <27 weeks gestation and those with meningitis.

Availability

Lyophilized powder for injection: 50 mg/vial, 100 mg/vial.

NURSING IMPLICATIONS

Assessment

- Assess symptoms of esophageal candidiasis (dysphagia, odynophagia, retrosternal pain) prior to and during therapy.
- Monitor for signs of anaphylaxis (rash, pruritus, wheezing, laryngeal edema, abdominal pain). Discontinue micafungin and notify health care professional immediately if these occur.
- Assess for injection site reactions (phlebitis, thrombophlebitis) during therapy. These occur more frequently in patients receiving micafungin via peripheral IV infusion.
- ***Lab Test Considerations:*** May cause ↑ serum alkaline phosphatase, bilirubin, ALT, AST, and LDH levels. If elevations occur, monitor for worsening liver function; may require discontinuation of therapy.
- May cause ↑ BUN and serum creatinine.
- May cause leukopenia, neutropenia, thrombocytopenia, and anemia. Monitor for worsening levels; may require discontinuation of therapy.
- May cause hypokalemia, hypocalcemia, and hypomagnesemia.

Potential Nursing Diagnoses

Risk for infection (Indications)

Implementation

IV Administration

- **Intermittent Infusion:** ***Diluent:*** *For Adults:* Reconstitute each 50-mg vial with 5 mL of 0.9% NaCl or D5W to achieve concentration of 10 mg/mL. Reconstitute each 100-mg vial with 5 mL of 0.9% NaCl or D5W to achieve concentration of 20 mg/mL. Dissolve by gently swirling vial; do not shake vigorously. Directions for further dilution based on indication for use. For prophylaxis of *Candida* infections, add 50 mg of micafungin to 100 mL of 0.9% NaCl or D5W. For treatment of esophageal candidiasis, add 150 mg of micafungin to 100 mL of 0.9% NaCl or D5W. Reconstituted vials and infusion are stable for 24 hr at room temperature. Protect diluted solution from light. ***Concentration:*** 0.5–1.5 mg/mL.
- *For Children:* Determine dose and divide by final concentration (10 or 20 mg/mL). Add withdrawn volume to 0.9% NaCl or D5W in IV bag or syringe. ***Concentration:*** 0.5 mg/mL–4 mg/mL. Concentrations >1.5 m g/mL should be administered via central venous catheter to minimize infusion reactions. Discard unused vials. ***Rate:*** Flush line with 0.9%

M

NaCl prior to administration. Infuse over 1 hr. More rapid infusions may result in more frequent histamine mediated reactions.

- **Y-Site Compatibility:** aminophylline, bumetanide, calcium chloride, calcium gluconate, carboplatin, cyclosporine, dopamine, doripenem, eptifibatide, esmolol, rtoposide, fenoldopam, furosemide, heparin, hydromorphone, lidocaine, lorazepam, magnesium sulfate, mesna, milrinone, nitroglycerin, nitroprusside, norepinephrine, phenylephrine, potassium chloride, potassium phosphates, sodium phosphates, tacrolimus, theophylline, vasopressin.
- **Y-Site Incompatibility:** amiodarone, cisatracurium, diltiazem, dobutamine, epinephrine, insulin, labetalol, levofloxacin, meperidine, midazolam, morphine, mycophenolate mofetil, nesiritide, nicardipine, octreotide, ondansetron, phenytoin, rocuronium, telavancin, vecuronium.

Patient/Family Teaching

- Inform patient of the purpose of micafungin.
- Advise patient to notify health care professional immediately if signs of anaphylaxis occur.

Evaluation/Desired Outcomes

- Resolution of signs and symptoms of esophageal candidiasis, candidemia, acute disseminated candidiasis, candidal peritonitis, and abscesses.
- Prevention of *Candida* infections during hematopoetic stem cell transplantation.

miconazole, See ANTIFUNGALS (TOPICAL) and ANTIFUNGALS (VAGINAL).

HIGH ALERT

midazolam (mid-ay-zoe-lam)

~~Versed~~

Classification

Therapeutic: antianxiety agents, sedative/hypnotics

Pharmacologic: benzodiazepines

Schedule IV

Pregnancy Category D

Indications

PO: Preprocedural sedation and anxiolysis in pediatric patients. **IM, IV:** Preoperative sedation/anxiolysis/amnesia. **IV:** Provides sedation/anxiolysis/amnesia during therapeutic, diagnostic, or radiographic procedures (conscious sedation): Aids in the induction of anesthesia and as part of balanced anesthesia. As a continuous infusion, provides sedation of mechanically ventilated patients during anesthesia or in a critical care setting, Status epilepticus.

Action

Acts at many levels of the CNS to produce generalized CNS depression. Effects may be mediated by GABA, an inhibitory neurotransmitter. **Therapeutic Effects:** Short-term sedation. Postoperative amnesia.

Pharmacokinetics

Absorption: Rapidly absorbed following oral and nasal administration; undergoes substantial intestinal and first-pass hepatic metabolism. Well absorbed following IM administration; IV administration results in complete bioavailability.

Distribution: Crosses the blood-brain barrier and placenta; excreted in breast milk.

Protein Binding: 97%.

Metabolism and Excretion: Almost exclusively metabolized by the liver, resulting in conversion to hydroxymidazolam, an active metabolite, and 2 other inactive metabolites (metabolized by cytochrome P450 3A4 enzyme system); metabolites are excreted in urine.

Half-life: Preterm neonates: 2.6–17.7 hr; Neonates: 4–12 hr; Children: 3–7 hr; Adults: 2–6 hr (increased in renal impairment, HF, or cirrhosis).

TIME/ACTION PROFILE (sedation)

ROUTE	ONSET	PEAK	DURATION
IN	5 min	10 min	30–60 min
IM	15 min	30–60 min	2–6 hr
IV	1.5–5 min	rapid	2–6 hr

Contraindications/Precautions

Contraindicated in: Hypersensitivity; Cross-sensitivity with other benzodiazepines may occur; Shock; Comatose patients or those with pre-existing CNS depression; Uncontrolled severe pain; Acute angle-closure glaucoma; OB: Benzodiazepine drugs may ↑ risk of congenital malformations; use in the last weeks of pregnancy has caused CNS depression in the neonate; Lactation: Lactation; Pedi: Products containing benzyl alcohol should not be used in neonates.

Use Cautiously in: Pulmonary disease; HF; Renal impairment; Severe hepatic impairment; Obese pediatric patients (calculate dose on the basis of ideal body weight); Pedi: Rapid injection in neonates has caused severe hypotension and seizures, especially when used with fentanyl; Geri: Older patients (especially >70 yr) are more susceptible to cardiorespiratory depressant effects; dosage ↓ required.

Adverse Reactions/Side Effects

CNS: agitation, drowsiness, excess sedation, headache. **EENT:** blurred vision. **Resp:** APNEA, LARYNGOSPASM, RESPIRATORY DEPRESSION, bronchospasm, coughing. **CV:** CARDIAC ARREST, arrhythmias. **GI:** hiccups, nausea, vomiting. **Derm:** rashes. **Local:** phlebitis at IV site, pain at IM site.

Interactions

Drug-Drug: ↑ CNS depression with **alcohol**, **antihistamines**, **opioid analgesics**, and other **sedative/**

hypnotics (↓ midazolam dose by 30–50% if used concurrently). ↑ risk of hypotension with **antihypertensives**, **opioid analgesics**, acute ingestion of **alcohol**, or **nitrates**. Midazolam is metabolized by the cytochrome P450 3A4 enzyme system; drugs that induce or inhibit this system may be expected to alter the effects of midazolam. **Carbamazepine**, **phenytoin**, **rifampin**, **rifabutin**, and **phenobarbital** ↓ levels. **Erythromycin**, **cimetidine**, **ranitidine**, **diltiazem**, **verapamil**, **fluconazole**, **itraconazole**, and **ketoconazole** ↓ metabolism and may ↑ risk of toxicity.
Drug-Natural Products: Concomitant use of **kava-kava**, **valerian**, or **chamomile** can ↑ CNS depression. Long-term use of **St. John's wort** may significantly ↓ levels.
Drug-Food: Grapefruit juice ↓ metabolism and may ↑ risk of toxicity.

Route/Dosage

Dose must be individualized, taking caution to reduce dose in geriatric patients and in those who are already sedated.

Preoperative Sedation/Anxiolysis/Amnesia

PO (Children 6 mo–16 yr): 0.25–0.5 mg/kg, may require up to 1 mg/kg (dose should not exceed 20 mg); *patients with cardiac/respiratory compromise or concurrent CNS depressants*—0.25 mg/kg.
IM (Adults Otherwise Healthy and <60 yr): 0.07–0.08 mg/kg 1 hr before surgery (usual dose 5 mg).
IM (Adults ≥60 yr, Debilitated or Chronically Ill): 0.02–0.03 mg/kg 1 hr before surgery (usual dose 1–3 mg).
IM (Children): 0.1–0.15 mg/kg up to 0.5 mg/kg 30–60 min prior to procedure; not to exceed 10 mg/dose.

Conscious Sedation for Short Procedures

IV (Adults and Children Otherwise Healthy >12 yr and <60 yr): 1–2.5 mg initially; dosage may be ↑ further as needed. Total doses >5 mg are rarely needed (↓ dose by 50% if other CNS depressants are used). Maintenance doses of 25% of the dose required for initial sedation may be given as necessary.
IV (Children 6–12 yr): 0.025–0.05 mg/kg initially, then titrate dose carefully, may need up to 0.4 mg/kg total, maximum dose 10 mg.
IV (Children 6 mo–5 yr): 0.05 mg/kg initially, then titrate dose carefully, may need up to 0.6 mg/kg total, maximum dose 6 mg.
IV (Geriatric Patients ≥60 yr, Debilitated or Chronically Ill): 1–1.5 mg initially; dose may be ↑ further as needed. Total doses >3.5 mg are rarely needed (↓ dose by 30% if other CNS depressants are used). Maintenance doses of 25% of the dose required for initial sedation may be given as necessary.
Intranasal (Children): 0.2–0.3 mg/kg, may repeat in 5–15 min.

Status Epilepticus

IV (Children >2 mo): 0.15 mg/kg load followed by a continuous infusion of 1 mcg/kg/min. Titrate dose upward q 5 min until seizure controlled, range: 1–18 mcg/kg/min.

Induction of Anesthesia (Adjunct)

May give additional dose of 25% of initial dose if needed.
IV (Adults Otherwise Healthy and <55 yr): 300–350 mcg/kg initially (up to 600 mcg/kg total). If patient is premedicated, initial dose should be further ↓.
IV (Geriatric Patients >55 yr): 150–300 mcg/kg as initial dose. If patient is premedicated, initial dose should be further ↓.
IV (Adults —Debilitated): 150–250 mcg/kg initial dose. If patient is premedicated, initial dose should be further ↓.

Sedation in Critical Care Settings

IV (Adults): 0.01–0.05 mg/kg (0.5–4 mg in most adults) initially if a loading dose is required; may repeat q 10–15 min until desired effect is obtained; may be followed by infusion at 0.02–0.1 mg/kg/hr (1–7 mg/hr in most adults).
IV (Children): *Intubated patients only*—0.05–0.2 mg/kg initially as a loading dose; follow with infusion at 0.06–0.12 mg/kg/hr (1–2 mcg/kg/min), titrate to effect, range: 0.4–6 mcg/kg/min.
IV (Neonates >32 wk): *Intubated patients only*—0.06 mg/kg/hr (1 mcg/kg/min).
IV (Neonates <32 wk): *Intubated patients only*—0.03 mg/kg/hr (0.5 mcg/kg/min).

Availability (generic available)

Injection: 1 mg/mL, 5 mg/mL. **Syrup (cherry flavor):** 2 mg/mL.

NURSING IMPLICATIONS

Assessment

- Assess level of sedation and level of consciousness throughout and for 2–6 hr following administration.
- Monitor BP, pulse, and respiration continuously during IV administration. Oxygen and resuscitative equipment should be immediately available.
- ***Toxicity and Overdose:*** If overdose occurs, monitor pulse, respiration, and BP continuously. Maintain patent airway and assist ventilation as needed. If hypotension occurs, treatment includes IV fluids, repositioning, and vasopressors.
- The effects of midazolam can be reversed with flumazenil (Romazicon).

Potential Nursing Diagnoses

Ineffective breathing pattern (Adverse Reactions)
Risk for injury (Side Effects)

Implementation

- ***High Alert:*** Accidental overdose of oral midazolam syrup in children has resulted in serious harm or death. Do not accept orders prescribed by volume (5 mL or 1 tsp); instead, request dose be expressed in milligrams. Have second practitioner independently check original order and dose calculations. Midazolam syrup should only be administered by health care professionals authorized to administer conscious sedation.
- **PO:** To use the *Press-in Bottle Adaptor (PIBA)*, remove the cap and push bottle adaptor into neck of bottle. Close bottle tightly with cap. Solution is a clear red to purplish-red cherry-flavored syrup. Then remove cap and insert tip of oral dispenser in bottle adaptor. Push the plunger completely down toward tip of oral dispenser and insert firmly into bottle adaptor. Turn entire unit (bottle and oral dispenser) upside down. Pull plunger out slowly until desired amount of medication is withdrawn into oral dispenser. Turn entire unit right side up and slowly remove oral dispenser from the bottle. Tip of dispenser may be covered with tip of cap until time of use. Close bottle with cap after each use.
- Dispense directly into mouth. Do not mix with any liquid prior to dispensing.
- **Intranasal:** Administer using a 1 mL needleless syringe into the nares over 15 sec. Using the 5 mg/mL injection, administer half dose into each nare.
- **IM:** Administer IM doses deep into muscle mass, maximum concentration 1 mg/mL.

IV Administration

- **IV Push: *Diluent:*** Administer undiluted or diluted with D5W or 0.9% NaCl. ***Concentration:*** Undiluted: 1 mg/mL or 5 mg/mL. Diluted: 0.03–3 mg/mL. ***Rate:*** Administer slowly over at least 2–5 min. Titrate dose to patient response. Rapid injection, especially in neonates, has caused severe hypotension.
- **Continuous Infusion: *Diluent:*** Dilute with 0.9% NaCl or D5W. ***Concentration:*** 0.5–1 mg/mL. ***Rate:*** Based on patient's weight (see Route/Dosage section). Titrate to desired level of sedation. Assess sedation at regular intervals and adjust rate up or down by 25–50% as needed. Dose should also be decreased by 10–25% every few hours to find minimum effective infusion rate, which prevents accumulation of midazolam and provides more rapid recovery upon termination.
- **Y-Site Compatibility:** alemtuzumab, alfentanil, amikacin, amiodarone, anidulafungin, argatroban, atracurium, atropine, aztreonam, benztropine, bivalirudin, bleomycin, buprenorphine, calcium chloride, calcium gluconate, carboplatin, carmustine, caspofungin, cefazolin, cefotaxime, cefoxitin, ceftaroline, ceftriaxone, ciprofloxacin, cisatracurium, cisplatin, cyanocobalamin, cyclophosphamide, cyclosporine, cytarabine, dactinomycin, daptomycin, dexmedetomidine, digoxin, diltiazem, diphenhydramine, docetaxel, dopamine, doripenem, doxacurium, doxarubicin hydrochloride, doxycycline, enalaprilat, epinephrine, epirubicin, eptifibatide, erythromycin lactobionate, esmolol, etomidate, etoposide, etoposide phosphate, famotidine, fenoldopam, fentanyl, fluconazole, fludarabine, folic acid, gemcitabine, gentamicin, glycopyrrolate, granisetron, heparin, hydromorphone, idarubicin, ifosfamide, irinotecan, isoproterenol, labetalol, levofloxacin, lidocaine, linezolid, lorazepam, magnesium sulfate, mannitol, mechlorethamine, meperidine, metaraminol, methadone, methoxamine, methyldopate, metoclopramide, metoprolol, metronidazole, milrinone, mitoxantrone, morphine, multivitamins, mycophenolate, nalbuphine, naloxone, nesiritide, nicardipine, nitroglycerin, nitroprusside, norepinephrine, octreotide, ondansetron, oxacillin, oxaliplatin, oxytocin, paclitaxel, palonosetron, pamidronate, pancuronium, papaverine, pemetrexed, penicillin G potassium, pentamidine, pentazocine, phentolamine, phenylephrine, phytonadione, potassium chloride, procainamide, promethazine, propranolol, protamine, pyridoxime, quinupristin/dalfopristin, ranitidine, remifentanil, rifampin, rocuronium, streptokinase, succinylcholine, sufentanil, tacrolimus, teniposide, theophylline, thiotepa, tigecycline, tirofiban, tobramycin, tolazoline, trimetaphan, vancomycin, vasopressin, vecuronium, verapamil, vincristine, vinorelbine, voriconazole, zoledronic acid.
- **Y-Site Incompatibility:** acyclovir, aminocaproic acid, aminophylline, amphotericin B cholesteryl, amphotericin B colloidal, amphotericin B lipid complex, amphotericin B liposome, ampicillin, ampicillin/sulbactam, ascorbic acid, azathioprine, cefepime, ceftazidime, cefuroxime, chloramphenicol, dantrolene, dexamethasone sodium phosphate, diazepam, diazoxide, epoetin alfa, ertapenem, fluorouracil, foscarnet, fosphenytoin, furosemide, ganciclovir, indomethacin, ketorolac, methotrexate, micafungin, omeprazole, pantoprazole, pentobarbital, phenobarbital, phenytoin, piperacillin/tazobactam, potassium acetate, prochlorperazine, sodium bicarbonate, thiopental, trimethoprim/sulfamethoxazole.

Patient/Family Teaching

- Inform patient that this medication will decrease mental recall of the procedure.
- May cause drowsiness or dizziness. Advise patient to request assistance prior to ambulation and transfer and to avoid driving or other activities requiring alertness for 24 hr following administration.
- Instruct patient to inform health care professional prior to administration if pregnancy is suspected.

- Advise patient to avoid alcohol or other CNS depressants for 24 hr following administration of midazolam.

Evaluation/Desired Outcomes

- Sedation during and amnesia following surgical, diagnostic, and radiologic procedures.
- Sedation and amnesia for mechanically ventilated patients in a critical care setting.

REMS

mifepristone (mi-fe-priss-tone)

Korlym, Mifeprex

Classification

Therapeutic: abortifacients, antidiabetics
Pharmacologic: antiprogestational agents

Pregnancy Category UK (Mifeprex), X (Korlym)

Indications

Mifeprex: Medical termination of intrauterine pregnancy up to day 49 of pregnancy. **Korlym**: Hyperglycemia secondary to hypercortisolism in patients with endogenous Cushing's syndrome who have type 2 diabetes or glucose intolerance and have failed or are not candidates for surgery.

Action

Antagonizes endometrial and myometrial effects of progesterone. Sensitizes the myometrium to contraction-inducing activity of prostaglandins. Antagonizes the glucocorticoid receptor. **Therapeutic Effects:** Termination of pregnancy. Improved control of blood glucose.

Pharmacokinetics

Absorption: Rapidly absorbed following oral administration (69% bioavailability); absorption enhanced with food.

Distribution: Unknown.

Protein Binding: 98%.

Metabolism and Excretion: Mostly metabolized by the liver (CYP3A4 enzyme system); primarily excreted in the feces.

Half-life: 18 hr.

TIME/ACTION PROFILE (termination of pregnancy)

ROUTE	ONSET	PEAK	DURATION
PO	unknown	within 2 days	unknown

Contraindications/Precautions

Contraindicated in: Hypersensitivity; Presence of an intrauterine device (IUD) (Mifeprex); OB: Confirmed or suspected ectopic pregnancy (Mifeprex); Undiagnosed adnexal mass (Mifeprex); Chronic adrenal failure (Mifeprex); Concurrent long-term corticosteroid therapy; Bleeding disorders or concurrent anticoagulant therapy (Mifeprex); Inherited porphyrias (Mifeprex); Severe hepatic impairment (Korlym); OB: Pregnancy (Korlym); Concurrent use with simvastatin, lovastatin, cyclosporine, dihydroergotamine, ergotamine, fentanyl, pimozide, quinidine, sirolimus, or tacrolimus (Korlym); Vaginal bleeding; Endometrial hyperplasia with atypia or endometrial carcinoma (Korlym).

Use Cautiously in: Chronic medical conditions such as cardiovascular, hypertensive, hepatic, renal, or respiratory disease (safety and efficacy not established) (Mifeprex); Women >35 yrs old or who smoke ≥10 cigarettes/day (Mifeprex); Concurrent use with moderate CYP3A4 inhibitors; Bleeding disorders or concurrent anticoagulant therapy (Korlym).

Exercise Extreme Caution in: Concurrent use with strong CYP3A4 inhibitors (Korlym).

M

Adverse Reactions/Side Effects

CNS: anxiety (Korlym), headache, dizziness, fainting (Mifeprex), fatigue (Korlym), weakness (Mifeprex). **CV:** peripheral edema (Korlym), hypertension (Korlym), QT interval prolongation (Korlym). **GI:** abdominal pain (Mifeprex), anorexia (Korlym), constipation (Korlym), diarrhea, dry mouth (Korlym), nausea, vomiting. **Resp:** dyspnea (Korlym), *Pneumocystis jiroveci* pneumonia. **Endo:** hypothyroidism (Korlym), adrenal insufficiency (Korlym), ↓ HDL cholesterol (Korlym). **F and E:** hypokalemia (Korlym). **MS:** arthralgia (Korlym), myalgia (Korlym). **Derm:** rash (Korlym). **GU:** uterine bleeding, uterine cramping (Mifeprex), ruptured ectopic pregnancy (Mifeprex), pelvic pain (Mifeprex).

Interactions

Drug-Drug: Mifeprisone is a substrate and inhibitor of the **CYP3A4** enzyme system. ↑ blood levels and risk of toxicity from **dihydroergotamine**, **ergotamine**, **lovastatin**, **simvastatin**, **cyclosporine**, **fentanyl**, **pimozide**, **quinidine**, **sirolimus**, or **tacrolimus**; concurrent use with Korlym is contraindicated. **Strong CYP3A4 inhibitors**, including **ketoconazole**, **itraconazole**, **nefazodone**, **ritonavir**, **nelfinavir**, **indinavir**, **atazanavir**, **fosamprenavir**, **boceprevir**, **clarithromycin**, **conivaptan**, **lopinavir**, **posaconazole**, **saquinavir**, **telithromycin**, or **voriconazole** may ↑ levels; extreme caution with concurrent use of Korlym. **Moderate CYP3A4 inhibitors**, including **aprepitant**, **diltiazem**, **fluconazole**, **imatinib**, or **verapamil** may ↑ levels; caution with concurrent use of Korlym. Blood levels and effects may be ↓ by **rifampin**, **rifabutin dexamethasone**, **phenytoin**,

phenobarbital, and **carbamazepine**; avoid concurrent use with Korlym.

Drug-Natural Products: Blood levels and effects may be ↓ by **St. John's wort**; avoid concurrent use with Korlym.

Drug-Food: Blood levels and effects may be ↑ by **grapefruit juice**; caution with concurrent use of Korlym.

Route/Dosage

Mifeprex

PO (Adults): *Day 1*—600 mg (given as three 200 mg tablets) as a single dose, followed on *day 3* by 400 mcg misoprostol (Cytotec), unless abortion has occurred and has been confirmed by clinical or ultrasonographic examination (see misoprostol monograph).

Korlym

PO (Adults): 300 mg once daily; may ↑ by 300 mg/day every 2–4 wk (maximum dose = 1200 mg/day or 20 mg/kg/day); *Concurrent strong CYP3A4 inhibitor therapy*—300 mg once daily (maximum dose = 300 mg/day).

Renal Impairment

PO (Adults): 300 mg once daily; may ↑ by 300 mg/day every 2–4 wk (maximum dose = 600 mg/day).

Hepatic Impairment

PO (Adults): 300 mg once daily; may ↑ by 300 mg/day every 2–4 wk (maximum dose = 600 mg/day).

Availability

Tablets (Mifeprex): 200 mg. **Tablets (Korlym):** 300 mg.

NURSING IMPLICATIONS

Assessment

- **Mifeprex**: Determine duration of pregnancy. Pregnancy is dated from the first day of the last menstrual period in a presumed 28-day cycle with ovulation occurring at mid-cycle and can be determined by menstrual history and clinical examination; use ultrasound if duration is uncertain or if ectopic pregnancy is suspected.
- Assess amount of bleeding and cramping during treatment. Determine if termination is complete on day 14.
- **Korlym:** Monitor for changes in cushingoid appearance (acne, hirsutism, striae, body weight) during therapy.
- Monitor for signs and symptoms of adrenal insufficiency (weakness, nausea, increased fatigue, hypotension, hypoglycemia) during therapy. If adrenal insufficiency is suspected, discontinue Korlym and administer glucortocoids immediately.
- ***Lab Test Considerations:*** **Mifeprex:** ↓ hemoglobin, hematocrit, and RBCs may occur in women who bleed heavily.
- Changes in quantitative human chorionic gonadotropin (hCG) levels are not accurate until at least 10 days after mifepristone administration; complete termination of pregnancy must be confirmed by clinical examination.
- **Korlym:** Correct hypokalemia prior to initiating therapy. Assess serum potassium 1–2 wk after starting or increasing dose of Korlym and periodically thereafter.
- Obtain a negative pregnancy test in women prior to starting therapy or before restarting therapy if stopped for more than 14 days.
- Monitor Hemoglobin A_{1c} periodically during therapy.

Potential Nursing Diagnoses

Acute pain (Side Effects)
Deficient knowledge, related to medication regimen (Patient/Family Teaching)

Implementation

- Do not confuse mifepristone with misoprostol.
- **Mifeprex:** Mifepristone should be administered only by health care professionals who have read and understood the prescribing information, are able to assess gestational age of an embryo and diagnose ectopic pregnancies, and who are able to provide surgical intervention in cases of incomplete abortion or severe bleeding.
- Any IUD should be removed prior to mifepristone administration.
- Measures to prevent rhesus immunization, similar to those of surgical abortion, should be taken.
- **PO:** On *day 1*, after the patient has read the *Medication Guide* and signed the Patient Agreement, administer three 200 mg tablets of mifepristone as a single dose. On *day 3*, unless abortion has occurred and been confirmed by clinical examination or ultrasound, administer two 200-mcg tablets of misoprostol. On *day 14*, confirm that termination of pregnancy has occurred by clinical examination or ultrasound.
- **Korlym:** Administer with a meal. Swallow tablet whole; do not crush, break, or chew.
- If Korlym therapy is interrupted, reinitiate at lowest dose (300 mg).

Patient/Family Teaching

- **Mifeprex:** Advise patient of the treatment and its effects. Patients must be given a copy of the *Medication Guide and Patient Agreement.* Patient must understand the necessity of completing the treatment schedule of three office visits (day 1, day 3, and day 14).
- Inform patient that vaginal bleeding and uterine cramping will probably occur and that prolonged or heavy vaginal bleeding is not proof of complete expulsion. Bleeding or spotting occurs for an average of 9–16 days; but may continue for more than 30

days. Advise patient that if the treatment fails, there is a risk of fetal malformation; medical abortion failures are managed by surgical termination.

- Caution patient to notify health care professional immediately if she develops weakness, nausea, vomiting, diarrhea, with or without abdominal pain or fever more than 24 hr after taking mifepristone; may indicate life-threatening sepsis.
- Instruct patient in the steps to take in an emergency situation, including precise instructions and a telephone number to call if she has problems or concerns.
- May cause dizziness or fainting. Caution patient to avoid driving or other activities requiring alertness until response to medication is known.
- Caution patient that pregnancy can occur following termination of pregnancy and before resumption of normal menses. Contraception can be initiated as soon as pregnancy termination is confirmed, or before sexual intercourse is resumed.
- Advise patient to notify health care professional if she smokes at least 10 cigarettes a day.
- **Korlym:** Instruct patient to take Korlym as directed. Advise patient to read *Medication Guide* prior to starting therapy and with each refill in case of changes.
- Caution patient to avoid drinking grapefruit juice during therapy; may increase risk of side effects.
- Instruct patient to notify health care professional if signs and symptoms of adrenal insufficiency, abnormal vaginal bleeding, or low potassium (muscle weakness, aches, cramps, palpitations) occur.
- Advise patient to notify health care professional of all Rx or OTC medications, vitamins, or herbal products being taken and to consult with health care professional before taking other medications.
- Advise female patient to use a nonhormonal form of contraception during and for at least 1 month after therapy. Notify health care professional immediately if pregnancy is suspected; Korlym is teratogenic. Advise female patient to avoid breast feeding during therapy.

Evaluation/Desired Outcomes

- **Mifeprex:** Termination of an intrauterine pregnancy of less than 49 days' duration.
- **Korlym:** Improved control of blood glucose.

milnacipran (mil-na-**sip**-ran)

Savella

Classification

Therapeutic: antifibromyalgia agents

Pharmacologic: selective norepinephrine reuptake inhibitors

Pregnancy Category C

Indications

Management of fibromyalgia.

Action

Inhibits neuronal reuptake of norepinephrine and serotonin. **Therapeutic Effects:** Decreased pain associated with fibromyalgia.

Pharmacokinetics

Absorption: 85–90% absorbed following oral administration.

Distribution: Unknown.

Metabolism and Excretion: Mostly excreted urine as unchanged drug (55%) and inactive metabolites.

Half-life: *D*—isomer 8–10 hr; *L*—isomer 4–6 hr.

TIME/ACTION PROFILE (↓ in pain)

ROUTE	ONSET	PEAK	DURATION
PO	1 wk	unknown	unknown

M

Contraindications/Precautions

Contraindicated in: Concurrent use of MAO inhibitors or MAO-like drugs (linezolid or methylene blue); End-stage renal disease; Significant history of alcohol use/abuse; Chronic liver disease.

Use Cautiously in: History of suicide risk or attempt; History of seizures; Moderate-to-severe renal impairment (↓ dose if CCr <30 mL/min); Hypertension; Severe hepatic impairment; Obstructive uropathy (↑ risk of adverse genitourinary effects); Angle-closure glaucoma; Geri: Consider age-related ↓ in renal function, chronic disease state and concurrent drug therapy; OB: Use only if clearly required during pregnancy weighing benefit to mother versus potential harm to fetus; Lactation: Potential for serious adverse reactions in infant; discontinue drug or discontinue breast feeding; Pedi: ↑ risk of suicidal thinking and behavior (suicidality) in adolescents and young adults up to 24 yr with Major Depressive Disorder (MDD) and other psychiatric disorders.

Adverse Reactions/Side Effects

CNS: NEUROLEPTIC MALIGNANT SYNDROME, SUICIDAL THOUGHTS, dizziness, headache, insomnia. **CV:** hypertension, tachycardia. **F and E:** hyponatremia. **GI:** constipation, dry mouth, ↑ liver enzymes, nausea, vomiting. **Derm:** hot flushes, hyperhidrosis. **Misc:** SEROTONIN SYNDROME.

Interactions

Drug-Drug: Concurrent use with **MAO inhibitors** may result in serious, potentially fatal reactions; wait at least 14 days following discontinuation of MAO inhibitor before initiation of milnacipran. Wait at least 5 days after discontinuing milnacipran before initiation of

MAO inhibitor. Concurrent use with **MAO-inhibitor-like drugs**, such as **linezolid** or **methylene blue** may ↑ risk of serotonin syndrome; concurrent use contraindicated; do not start therapy in patients receiving **linezolid** or **methylene blue**; if **linezolid** or **methylene blue** need to be started in a patient receiving milnacipran, immediately discontinue milnacipran and monitor for signs/symptoms of serotonin syndrome for 5 days or until 24 hr after last dose of linezolid or methylene blue, whichever comes first (may resume milnacipran therapy 24 hr after last dose of linezolid or methylene blue). Drugs that affect serotonergic neurotransmitter systems, including **tricyclic antidepressants**, **SSRIs**, **fentanyl**, **buspirone**, **tramadol**, and **triptans** ↑ risk of serotonin syndrome. Concurrent use of **NSAIDs**, **aspirin**, or other **drugs that affect coagulation** may ↑ the risk of bleeding. May ↓ antihypertensive effectiveness of **clonidine**. ↑ risk of hypertension and arrhythmias with **epinephrine** or **norepinephrine**. ↑ risk of euphoria and hypotension when switching from **clomipramine**. Concurrent use with **digoxin** may result in adverse hemodynamics, including hypotension and tachycardia; avoid concurrent use with IV digoxin.

Drug-Natural Products: Use with **St. John's wort** ↑ serotonin syndrome.

Route/Dosage

PO (Adults): *Day 1*— 12.5 mg; *Day 2–3*— 12.5 mg twice daily; *Day 4–7*— 25 mg twice daily; *After Day 7*— 50 mg twice daily. Some patients may require up to 100 mg twice daily depending on response.

Renal Impairment

PO (Adults): *CCr 5–29 mL/min*— maintenance dose is 25 mg twice daily; some patients may require up to 50 mg twice daily depending on response.

Availability

Tablets (contain tartrazine): 12.5 mg, 25 mg, 50 mg, 100 mg.

NURSING IMPLICATIONS

Assessment

- Assess intensity, quality, and location of pain periodically during therapy. May require several weeks for effects to be seen.
- Monitor BP and heart rate before and periodically during therapy. Treat pre-existing hypertension and cardiac disease prior to therapy. Sustained hypertension may be dose related; decrease dose or discontinue therapy if this occurs.
- Monitor closely for changes in behavior that could indicate the emergence or worsening of suicidal thoughts or behavior or depression.
- Monitor for development of neuroleptic malignant syndrome (fever, respiratory distress, tachycardia, convulsions, diaphoresis, hypertension or hypotension, pallor, tiredness, severe muscle stiffness, loss of bladder control). Report symptoms immediately.
- ***Lab Test Considerations:*** May cause ↑ ALT, AST, and bilirubin.
- May cause hyponatremia.

Potential Nursing Diagnoses

Chronic pain (Indications)
Risk for suicide (Adverse Reactions)

Implementation

- **PO:** May be administered without regard to meals; may be more tolerable if taken with food.

Patient/Family Teaching

- Instruct patient to take milnacipran as directed at the same time each day. Take missed doses as soon as possible unless time for next dose. Do not stop abruptly; must be decreased gradually. Advise patient to read the *Medication Guide* prior to therapy and with each Rx refill.
- Encourage patient and family to be alert for emergence of anxiety, agitation, panic attacks, insomnia, irritability, hostility, impulsivity, akathisia, hypomania, mania, worsening of depression and suicidal ideation, especially during early antidepressant therapy. Assess symptoms on a day-to-day basis as changes may be abrupt. If these symptoms occur, notify health care professional.
- May cause dizziness. Caution patient to avoid driving or other activities requiring alertness until response to medication is known.
- Advise patient to notify health care professional of all Rx or OTC medications, vitamins, or herbal products being taken and to consult with health care professional before taking other medications, especially St. John's wort. Avoid use of aspirin, NSAIDs, and warfarin due to increased risk for bleeding.
- Instruct patient to notify health care professional if signs of liver damage (pruritus, dark urine, jaundice, right upper quadrant tenderness, unexplained "flu-like" symptoms) or hyponatremia (headache, difficulty concentrating, memory impairment, confusion, weakness, unsteadiness), hyponatremia (headache, difficulty concentrating, memory impairment, confusion, weakness, unsteadiness, falls), rash, or serotonin syndrome (mental status changes: agitation, hallucinations, coma; autonomic instability: tachycardia, labile BP, hyperthermia; neuromuscular aberrations: hyperreflexia, incoordination; and/or gastrointestinal symptoms: nausea, vomiting, diarrhea) occur.
- Advise patient to avoid taking alcohol during milnacipran therapy.
- Rep: Instruct patient to notify health care professional if pregnancy is planned or suspected or if breast feeding. Encourage patients who become pregnant while taking milnacipran to enroll in the pregnancy registry by calling 1-800-643-3010 or at www.savellapregnancyregistry.com.
- Encourage patient to maintain routine follow-up visits with health care provider to determine effectiveness.

Evaluation/Desired Outcomes

- Reduction in pain and soreness associated with fibromyalgia.

HIGH ALERT

milrinone (mill-ri-none)

~~Primacor~~

Classification

Therapeutic: inotropics

Pregnancy Category C

Indications

Short-term treatment of HF unresponsive to conventional therapy with digoxin, diuretics, and vasodilators.

Action

Increases myocardial contractility. Decreases preload and afterload by a direct dilating effect on vascular smooth muscle. **Therapeutic Effects:** Increased cardiac output (inotropic effect).

Pharmacokinetics

Absorption: IV administration results in complete bioavailability.

Distribution: Unknown.

Metabolism and Excretion: 80–90% excreted unchanged by the kidneys.

Half-life: 2.3 hr (↑ in renal impairment).

TIME/ACTION PROFILE (hemodynamic effects)

ROUTE	ONSET	PEAK	DURATION
IV	5–15 min	unknown	3–6 hr

Contraindications/Precautions

Contraindicated in: Hypersensitivity; Severe aortic or pulmonic valvular heart disease; Hypertrophic subaortic stenosis (may ↑ outflow tract obstruction).

Use Cautiously in: History of arrhythmias, electrolyte abnormalities, abnormal digoxin levels, or insertion of vascular catheters (↑ risk of ventricular arrhythmias); Renal impairment (↓ infusion rate if CCr is <50 mL/min); OB, Lactation: Pregnancy or lactation.

Adverse Reactions/Side Effects

CNS: headache, tremor. **CV:** VENTRICULAR ARRHYTHMIAS, angina pectoris, chest pain, hypotension, supraventricular arrhythmias. **CV:** skin rash. **GI:** ↑ liver enzymes. **F and E:** hypokalemia. **Hemat:** thrombocytopenia.

Interactions

Drug-Drug: None significant.

Route/Dosage

IV (Adults): *Loading dose*—50 mcg/kg followed by *continuous infusion* at 0.5 mcg/kg/min (range 0.375–0.75 mcg/kg/min).

IV (Infants and Children): *Loading dose*—50 mcg/kg over 10 min followed by *continuous infusion* at 0.5 mcg/kg/min (range 0.25–0.75 mcg/kg/min).

Availability (generic available)

Injection: 1 mg/mL. **Premixed infusion:** 20 mg/100 mL, 40 mg/200 mL.

NURSING IMPLICATIONS

Assessment

- Monitor heart rate and BP continuously during administration. Slow or discontinue if BP drops excessively.
- Monitor intake and output and daily weight. Assess patient for resolution of signs and symptoms of HF (peripheral edema, dyspnea, rales/crackles, weight gain) and improvement in hemodynamic parameters (increase in cardiac output and cardiac index, decrease in pulmonary capillary wedge pressure). Correct effects of previous aggressive diuretic therapy to allow for optimal filling pressure.
- Monitor ECG continuously during infusion. Arrhythmias are common and may be life threatening. The risk of ventricular arrhythmias is increased in patients with a history of arrhythmias, electrolyte abnormalities, abnormal digoxin levels, or insertion of vascular catheters.
- ***Lab Test Considerations:*** Monitor electrolytes and renal function frequently during administration. Correct hypokalemia prior to administration to decrease the risk of arrhythmias.
- Monitor platelet count during therapy.
- ***Toxicity and Overdose: High Alert:*** Overdose manifests as hypotension. Dose should be decreased or discontinued. Supportive measures may be necessary.

Potential Nursing Diagnoses

Decreased cardiac output (Indications)

Implementation

- ***High Alert:*** Accidental overdose of milrinone can cause patient harm or death. Have second practitioner independently check original order, dose calculations, and infusion pump settings.

IV Administration

- **IV Push:** ***Diluent:*** Loading dose may be administered undiluted. May also be diluted in 0.9% NaCl, 0.45% NaCl, or D5W for ease of administration. ***Concentration:*** 1 mg/mL. ***Rate:*** Administer the loading dose over 10 min.
- **Continuous Infusion:** ***Diluent:*** Milrinone drawn from vials must be diluted. Dilute 10 mg (10 mL) of

M

milrinone in 40 mL of diluent or 20 mg (20 mL) of milrinone in 80 mL of diluent. Compatible diluents include 0.45% NaCl, 0.9% NaCl, and D5W. Premixed infusions are already diluted and ready to use. Admixed solutions are stable for 72 hr at room temperature. Stability of premixed infusions based on manufacturer's expiration date. Do not use solutions that are discolored or contain particulate matter. ***Concentration:*** 200 mcg/mL. ***Rate:*** Based on patient's weight (see Route/Dosage section). Titrate according to hemodynamic and clinical response.

- **Y-Site Compatibility:** acyclovir, alfentanil, allopurinol, amifostine, amikacin, aminophylline, amiodarone, amphotericin B liposome, ampicillin, anidulafungin, argatroban, atracurium, aztreonam, bivalirudin, bleomycin, bumetanide, buprenorphine, busulfan, butorphanol, calcium chloride, calcium gluconate, carboplatin, carmustine, caspofungin, cefazolin, cefepime, cefotaxime, cefotetan, cefoxitin, ceftaroline, ceftazidime, ceftriaxone, cefuroxime, chloramphenicol, chlorpromazine, ciprofloxacin, cisatracurium, cisplatin, clindamycin, cyclophosphamide, cyclosporine, cytarabine, dactinomycin, daptomycin, dexamethasone sodium phosphate, dexmedetomidine, digoxin, diltiazem, dobutamine, docetaxel, dopamine, doripenem, doxacurium, doxorubicin, doxycycline, droperidol, enalaprilat, ephedrine, epinephrine, epirubicin, eptifibatide, ertapenem, erythromycin, etoposide, etoposide phosphate, fenoldopam, fentanyl, fluconazole, fludarabine, fluorouracil, ganciclovir, gemcitabine, gentamicin, glycopyrrolate, granisetron, haloperidol, heparin, hetastarch, hydralazine, hydrocortisone, hydromorphone, idarubicin, ifosfamide, insulin, irinotecan, isoproterenol, ketamine, ketorolac, labetalol, levofloxacin, linezolid, lorazepam, magnesium sulfate, mannitol, mechlorethamine, melphalan, meperidine, meropenem, methohexital, methotrexate, methyldopate, methylprednisolone sodium succinate, metoclopramide, metoprolol, metronidazole, micafungin, midazolam, mitoxantrone, morphine, mycophenolate, nafcillin, nalbuphine, naloxone, nesiritide, nicardipine, nitroglycerin, nitroprusside, norepinephrine, octreotide, oxacillin, oxaliplatin, oxytocin, paclitaxel, palonosetron, pamidronate, pancuronium, pemetrexed, pentobarbital, phenobarbital, phenylephrine, piperacillin/tazobactam, potassium acetate, potassium chloride, potassium phosphates, prochlorperazine, promethazine, propofol, propranolol, quinupristin/dalfopristin, ranitidine, remifentanil, rocuronium, sodium acetate, sodium bicarbonate, sodium phosphates, streptozocin, succinylcholine, sufentanil, tacrolimus, telavancin, teniposide, theophylline, thiopental, thiotepa, tigecycline, tirofiban, tobramycin, torsemide, vancomycin, vasopressin, vecuronium, verapamil, vincristine, vinorelbine, voriconazole, zidovudine, zoledronic acid.
- **Y-Site Incompatibility:** amphotericin B colloidal, amphotericin B lipid complex, dantrolene, diazepam, diphenhydramine, esmolol, furosemide, hydroxyzine, imipenem/cilastatin, lidocaine, ondansetron, pantoprazole, phenytoin, procainamide.

Patient/Family Teaching

- Inform patient and family of reasons for administration. Milrinone is not a cure but is a temporary measure to control the symptoms of HF.

Evaluation/Desired Outcomes

- Decrease in the signs and symptoms of HF.
- Improvement in hemodynamic parameters.

---

minocycline, See TETRACYCLINES.

---

mirabegron (mye-ra-**beg**-ron)

Myrbetriq

Classification

Therapeutic: urinary tract antispasmodics
Pharmacologic: beta-adrenergic agonists

Pregnancy Category C

Indications

Treatment of symptoms of overactive bladder (OAB) including urge urinary incontinence, urgency, and frequency.

Action

Acts as a selective beta-3 adrenergic agonist. Increases bladder capacity by relaxing detusor smooth muscle during storage phase of bladder fill-void cycle. **Therapeutic Effects:** Decreased symptoms of OAB.

Pharmacokinetics

Absorption: 29–35% absorbed following oral administration.

Distribution: Widely distributed.

Metabolism and Excretion: Extensively metabolized, 6% excreted unchanged in urine (25 mg dose), remainder excreted in urine and feces as metabolites.

Half-life: 50 hr.

TIME/ACTION PROFILE (effects on bladder)

ROUTE	ONSET	PEAK	DURATION
PO	unknown	3.5 hr†	24 hr

†Blood level.

Contraindications/Precautions

Contraindicated in: Hypersensitivity; Severe uncontrolled hypertension; End-stage renal disease or severe hepatic impairment (Child-Pugh Class C); Lactation: Probably enters breast milk and may cause adverse reactions in infant.

Use Cautiously in: Hypertension; Bladder outlet obstruction/concurrent antimuscarics (↑ risk of urinary retention); Concurrent use of antimuscarinics used to treat OAB; OB: Use only if potential maternal benefit outweighs risk to etus; Pedi: Safety and effectiveness not established.

Adverse Reactions/Side Effects

CNS: dizziness, headache. **EENT:** nasopharyngitis. **CV:** ↑ BP, tachycardia. **GI:** constipation, diarrhea, nausea. **GU:** urinary tract infection. **Misc:** ANGIOEDEMA.

Interactions

Drug-Drug: Acts as a moderate inhibitor of the CYP2D6 enzyme system. May ↑ levels and risk of adverse reactions of **drugs metabolized by the the CYP2D6 enzyme system** including **desipramine**, **flecainide**, **metoprolol**, **propafenone**, and **thioridazine**. May ↑ levels and risk of toxicity with **digoxin**; use lowest effective level of digoxin/monitor serum levels).

Route/Dosage

PO (Adults): 25 mg once daily; may be ↑ to 50 mg once daily based on need/tolerance after 8 wk.

Renal Impairment

PO (Adults): *CCr 15–20 mL/min*—Dose should not exceed 25 mg/day.

Hepatic Impairment

PO (Adults): *Moderate hepatic impairment (Child-Pugh Class B)*—Dose should not exceed 25 mg/day.

Availability

Extended-release tablets: 25 mg, 50 mg.

NURSING IMPLICATIONS

Assessment

- Assess patient for urinary urgency, frequency, and urge incontinence periodically during therapy.
- Monitor BP prior to starting and periodically during therapy; may cause ↑ BP.
- Monitor for signs and symptoms of angioedema (swelling of face, lips, tongue and/or larynx). Discontinue mirabegron and treat symptomatically.

Potential Nursing Diagnoses

Impaired urinary elimination (Indications)
Urinary retention (Indications)

Implementation

- **PO:** Administer without regard to food.
- Swallow tablets whole with water; do not break, crush, or chew.

Patient/Family Teaching

- Instruct patient to take mirabegron as directed. If a dose is missed, omit dose and begin taking next day; do not take 2 doses on the same day. Advise patient to read *Patient Information* sheet prior to starting and with each Rx refill in case of changes.
- Inform patient that mirabegron may cause an increase in BP. Advise patient to have BP checked periodically during therapy.
- May cause dizziness. Caution patient to avoid driving or other activities requiring alertness until response to medication is known.
- Advise patient to notify health care professional if difficulty emptying bladder occurs.
- Advise patient to notify health care professional of all Rx or OTC medications, vitamins, or herbal products being taken and to consult with health care professional before taking other medications.
- Advise female patients to notify health care professional if pregnancy is planned or suspected or if breast feeding.

Evaluation/Desired Outcomes

- Decreased urinary frequency, urgency, and urge incontinence.

mirtazapine (meer-taz-a-peen)

Remeron, ✱Remeron RD, Remeron SolTab

Classification
Therapeutic: antidepressants
Pharmacologic: tetracyclic antidepressants

Pregnancy Category C

Indications

Major depressive disorder. **Unlabeled Use:** Panic disorder. Generalized anxiety disorder (GAD). Post-traumatic stress disorder (PTSD).

Action

Potentiates the effects of norepinephrine and serotonin. **Therapeutic Effects:** Antidepressant action, which may develop only after several weeks.

Pharmacokinetics

Absorption: Well absorbed but rapidly metabolized, resulting in 50% bioavailability.
Distribution: Unknown.
Protein Binding: 85%.
Metabolism and Excretion: Extensively metabolized by the liver (P450 2D6, 1A2 and 3A enzymes involved); metabolites excreted in urine (75%) and feces (15%).
Half-life: 20–40 hr.

TIME/ACTION PROFILE (antidepressant effect)

ROUTE	ONSET	PEAK	DURATION
PO	1–2 wk	6 wk or more	unknown

Contraindications/Precautions

Contraindicated in: Hypersensitivity; Concurrent use of MAO inhibitors or MAO-like drugs (linezolid or methylene blue).

Use Cautiously in: History of seizures; History of suicide attempt; May ↑ risk of suicide attempt/ideation especially during early treatment or dose adjustment; History of mania/hypomania; Patients with hepatic or renal impairment; Angle-closure glaucoma; OB: Safety not established; Lactation: Discontinue drug or bottle-feed; Pedi: Safety not established. Suicide risk may be greater in children or adolescents; Geri: ↑ sensitivity to CNS effects and oversedation. Begin at lower doses and titrate carefully.

Adverse Reactions/Side Effects

CNS: NEUROLEPTIC MALIGNANT SYNDROME, SUICIDAL THOUGHTS, drowsiness, abnormal dreams, abnormal thinking, agitation, akathisia, anxiety, apathy, confusion, dizziness, malaise, weakness. **EENT:** sinusitis. **Resp:** dyspnea, cough. **CV:** edema, hypotension, vasodilation. **GI:** constipation, dry mouth, ↑ appetite, abdominal pain, anorexia, ↑ liver enzymes, nausea, vomiting. **GU:** urinary frequency. **Derm:** pruritus, rash. **F and E:** ↑ thirst. **Hemat:** AGRANULOCYTOSIS. **Metab:** weight gain, hypercholesterolemia, hyponatremia, ↑ triglycerides. **MS:** arthralgia, back pain, myalgia. **Neuro:** hyperkinesia, hypesthesia, twitching. **Misc:** SEROTONIN SYNDROME, flu-like syndrome.

Interactions

Drug-Drug: May cause hypertension, seizures, and death when used with **MAO inhibitors**; do not use within 14 days of MAO inhibitor therapy. Concurrent use with **MAO-inhibitor like drugs**, such as **linezolid** or **methylene blue** may ↑ risk of serotonin syndrome; concurrent use contraindicated; do not start therapy in patients receiving **linezolid** or **methylene blue**; if **linezolid** or **methylene blue** need to be started in a patient receiving mirtazapine, immediately discontinue mirtazapine and monitor for signs/symptoms of serotonin syndrome for 2 wk or until 24 hr after last dose of linezolid or methylene blue, whichever comes first (may resume mirtazapine therapy 24 hr after last dose of linezolid or methylene blue). Drugs that affect serotonergic neurotransmitter systems, including **tricyclic antidepressants**, **SNRIs**, **fentanyl**, **buspirone**, **tramadol**, and **triptans** ↑ risk of serotonin syndrome. ↑ CNS depression with other **CNS depressants**, including **alcohol** and **benzodiazepines**. **Ketoconazole**, **cimetidine**, **clarithromycin**, **erythromycin**, **indinavir**, **itraconazole**, **ketoconazole**, **nefazodone**, **nelfinavir**, **ritonavir**, or **saquinavir** may ↑ levels. **Phenobarbital**, **phenytoin**, **carbamazepine**, **rifampin**, or **rifabutin** may ↓ levels; may need to ↑ mirtazapine dose. May ↑ the effects and risk of bleeding from **warfarin**.

Drug-Natural Products: Concomitant use of **kava-kava**, **valerian**, **skullcap**, **chamomile**, or **hops** can ↑ CNS depression. ↑ risk of serotonin syndrome with **St. John's wort** and **SAMe**.

Route/Dosage

PO (Adults): 15 mg/day as a single bedtime dose initially; may be ↑ q 1–2 wk up to 45 mg/day.

Availability (generic available)

Tablets: 7.5 mg, 15 mg, 30 mg, 45 mg. **Cost:** *Generic*—7.5 mg $158.00/60, 15 mg $81.40/30, 30 mg $83.00/30, 45 mg $85.50/30. **Orally disintegrating tablets (orange flavor):** 15 mg, 30 mg, 45 mg. **Cost:** *Generic*—15 mg $77.90/30, 30 mg $80.27/30, 45 mg $85.53/30.

NURSING IMPLICATIONS

Assessment

- Assess mental status (orientation, mood, behavior) frequently. Assess for suicidal tendencies, especially during early therapy. Restrict amount of drug available to patient.
- Monitor closely for changes in behavior that could indicate the emergence or worsening of suicidal thoughts or behavior or depression.
- Assess weight and BMI initially and throughout therapy. For overweight/obese individuals, obtain fasting blood glucose and cholesterol levels. Refer as appropriate for nutritional/weight management and medical management.
- Monitor BP and pulse rate periodically during initial therapy. Report significant changes.
- Monitor for seizure activity in patients with a history of seizures or alcohol abuse. Institute seizure precautions.
- Assess for serotonin syndrome (mental changes [agitation, hallucinations, coma], autonomic instability [tachycardia, labile BP, hyperthermia], neuromuscular aberations [hyper reflexia, incoordination], and/or GI symptoms [nausea, vomiting, diarrhea]), especially in patients taking other serotonergic drugs (SSRIs, SNRIs, triptans).
- Monitor for development of neuroleptic malignant syndrome (fever, respiratory distress, tachycardia, seizures, diaphoresis, hypertension or hypotension, pallor, tiredness). Discontinue mirtazapine and notify health care professional immediately if these symptoms occur.
- ***Lab Test Considerations:*** Assess CBC and hepatic function before and periodically during therapy.

Potential Nursing Diagnoses

Ineffective coping (Indications)
Anxiety (Indications)

Imbalanced nutrition: risk for more than body requirements (Side Effects)

Implementation

- May be given as a single dose at bedtime to minimize excessive drowsiness or dizziness.
- May be taken without regard to food.
- For *orally disintegrating tablets*, do not attempt to push through foil backing; with dry hands, peal back backing and remove tablet. Immediately place tablet on tongue; tablet will dissolve in seconds, then swallow with saliva. Administration with liquid is not necessary.

Patient/Family Teaching

- Instruct patient to take mirtazapine as directed. Take missed doses as soon as remembered; if almost time for next dose, skip missed dose and return to regular schedule. If single bedtime dose regimen is used, do not take missed dose in morning, but consult health care professional. Do not discontinue abruptly; gradual dose reduction may be required.
- May cause drowsiness and dizziness. Caution patient to avoid driving and other activities requiring alertness until response to drug is known.
- Encourage patient and family to be alert for emergence of anxiety, agitation, panic attacks, insomnia, irritability, hostility, impulsivity, akathisia, hypomania, mania, worsening of depression and suicidal ideation, especially during early antidepressant therapy. Assess symptoms on a day-to-day basis as changes may be abrupt. If these symptoms occur, notify health care professional.
- Caution patient to change positions slowly to minimize orthostatic hypotension.
- Advise patient to avoid alcohol or other CNS depressant drugs during and for at least 3–7 days after therapy has been discontinued.
- Instruct patient to notify health care professional of signs and symptoms of serotonin syndrome (mental status changes: agitation, hallucinations, coma; autonomic instability: tachycardia, labile BP, hyperthermia; neuromuscular aberrations: hyperreflexia, incoordination; and/or gastrointestinal symptoms: nausea, vomiting, diarrhea) occur.
- Advise patient to notify health care professional if dry mouth, urinary retention, or constipation occurs. Frequent rinses, good oral hygiene, and sugarless candy or gum may diminish dry mouth. An increase in fluid intake, fiber, and exercise may prevent constipation.
- Inform patient of need to monitor dietary intake. Increase in appetite may lead to undesired weight gain.
- Advise patient to notify health care professional of all Rx or OTC medications, vitamins, or herbal products being taken and to consult with health care professional before taking other medications, especially St. John's wort.
- Advise patient to notify health care professional of medication regimen before treatment or surgery.
- Advise female patient to notify health care professional if pregnancy is planned or suspected or if breast feeding.
- Therapy for depression may be prolonged. Emphasize the importance of follow-up exam to monitor effectiveness and side effects.

Evaluation/Desired Outcomes

- Resolution of the symptoms of depression.
- Increased sense of well-being.
- Renewed interest in surroundings.
- Increased appetite.
- Improved energy level.
- Improved sleep.
- Therapeutic effects may be seen within 1 wk, although several wk are usually necessary before improvement is observed.

M

misoprostol

(mye-soe-**prost**-ole)

Cytotec

Classification

Therapeutic: antiulcer agents, cytoprotective agents

Pharmacologic: prostaglandins

Pregnancy Category X

Indications

Prevention of gastric mucosal injury from NSAIDs, including aspirin, in high-risk patients (geriatric patients, debilitated patients, or those with a history of ulcers). With mifepristone for termination of pregnancy. **Unlabeled Use:** Treatment of duodenal ulcers. Cervical ripening and labor induction.

Action

Acts as a prostaglandin analogue, decreasing gastric acid secretion (antisecretory effect) and increasing the production of protective mucus (cytoprotective effect). Causes uterine contractions. **Therapeutic Effects:** Prevention of gastric ulceration from NSAIDs. With mifepristone terminates pregnancy of less than 49 days.

Pharmacokinetics

Absorption: Well absorbed following oral administration and rapidly converted to its active form (misoprostol acid).

Distribution: Unknown.

Protein Binding: 85%.

Metabolism and Excretion: Undergoes some metabolism and is then excreted by the kidneys.

Half-life: 20–40 min.

TIME/ACTION PROFILE (effect on gastric acid secretion)

ROUTE	ONSET	PEAK	DURATION
PO	30 min	unknown	3–6 hr

Contraindications/Precautions

Contraindicated in: Hypersensitivity to prostaglandins; OB: Should not be used to prevent NSAID-induced gastric injury due to potential for fetal harm or death; Lactation: May cause severe diarrhea in the nursing infant.

Use Cautiously in: OB: Patients with childbearing potential should be counseled to avoid pregnancy during misoprostol therapy for prevention of NSAID-induced gastric injury. Pregnancy status should be determined before initiating therapy; Pedi: Safety not established.

Exercise Extreme Caution in: When used for cervical ripening (unlabeled use) may cause uterine rupture (risk factors are late trimester pregnancy, previous caesarian section or uterine surgery or ≥5 previous pregnancies).

Adverse Reactions/Side Effects

CNS: headache. **GI:** abdominal pain, diarrhea, constipation, dyspepsia, flatulence, nausea, vomiting. **GU:** miscarriage, menstrual disorders.

Interactions

Drug-Drug: ↑ risk of diarrhea with **magnesium-containing antacids**.

Route/Dosage

PO (Adults): *Antiulcer*—200 mcg 4 times daily with or after meals and at bedtime, *or* 400 mcg twice daily, with the last dose at bedtime. If intolerance occurs, dose may be ↓ to 100 mcg 4 times daily. *Termination of pregnancy*—400 mcg single dose 2 days after mifepristone if abortion has not occurred.

Intravaginally (Adults): 25 mcg (1/4 of 100–mcg tablet); may repeat q 3–6 hr, if needed.

Availability (generic available)

Tablets: 100 mcg (0.1 mg), 200 mcg (0.2 mg). ***In combination with:*** diclofenac (Arthrotec). See Appendix B.

NURSING IMPLICATIONS

Assessment

- Assess patient routinely for epigastric or abdominal pain and for frank or occult blood in the stool, emesis, or gastric aspirate.
- Assess women of childbearing age for pregnancy. Misoprostol is usually begun on 2nd or 3rd day of menstrual period following a negative pregnancy test result.
- **Termination of pregnancy:** Monitor uterine cramping and bleeding during therapy.
- **Cervical Ripening:** Assess dilation of cervix periodically during therapy.

Potential Nursing Diagnoses

Acute pain (Indications)

Implementation

- Do not confuse Cytotec (misoprostol) with Mifeprex (mifepristone).
- Misoprostol therapy should be started at the onset of treatment with NSAIDs.
- **PO:** Administer medication with meals and at bedtime to reduce severity of diarrhea.
- Antacids may be administered before or after misoprostol for relief of pain. Avoid those containing magnesium, because of increased diarrhea with misoprostol.

Patient/Family Teaching

- Instruct patient to take medication as directed for the full course of therapy, even if feeling better. Take missed doses as soon as possible unless next dose is due within 2 hr; do not double doses. Emphasize that sharing of this medication may be dangerous.
- Advise patient not to share misoprostol with others, even if they have similar symptoms; may be dangerous.
- Inform patient that misoprostol will cause spontaneous abortion. Women of childbearing age must be informed of this effect through verbal and written information and must use contraception throughout therapy. If pregnancy is suspected, the woman should stop taking misoprostol and immediately notify her health care professional.
- Inform patient that diarrhea may occur. Health care professional should be notified if diarrhea persists for more than 1 wk. Also advise patient to report onset of black, tarry stools or severe abdominal pain.
- Advise patient to avoid alcohol and foods that may cause an increase in GI irritation.

Evaluation/Desired Outcomes

- The prevention of gastric ulcers in patients receiving chronic NSAID therapy.
- Termination of pregnancy.
- Cervical ripening and induction of labor.

mitoMYcin (mye-toe-**mye**-sin)

~~Mutamycin~~

Classification

Therapeutic: antineoplastics

Pharmacologic: antitumor antibiotics

Pregnancy Category D

Indications

Used with other agents in the management of disseminated adenocarcinoma of the stomach or pancreas.

Unlabeled Use: Palliative treatment of: Carcinoma

of the colon or breast, Head and neck tumors, Advanced biliary, lung, and cervical squamous cell carcinomas.

Action

Primarily inhibits DNA synthesis by causing cross-linking; also inhibits RNA and protein synthesis (cell-cycle phase–nonspecific but is most active in S and G phases). **Therapeutic Effects:** Death of rapidly replicating cells, particularly malignant ones.

Pharmacokinetics

Absorption: IV administration results in complete bioavailability.
Distribution: Widely distributed, concentrates in tumor tissue. Does not enter CSF.
Metabolism and Excretion: Mostly metabolized by the liver. Small amounts (<10%) excreted unchanged by the kidneys and in bile.
Half-life: 50 min.

TIME/ACTION PROFILE (effects on blood counts)

ROUTE	ONSET	PEAK	DURATION
IV	3–8 wk	4–8 wk	up to 3 mo

Contraindications/Precautions

Contraindicated in: Hypersensitivity; Pregnancy or lactation.
Use Cautiously in: Active infections; ↓ bone marrow reserve; Hepatic dysfunction; History of pulmonary problems; OB: Patients with childbearing potential should be counseled to avoid pregnancy during treatment; Geri: May have ↑ sensitivity to drug effects.

Adverse Reactions/Side Effects

Resp: PULMONARY TOXICITY. **CV:** edema. **GI:** nausea, vomiting, anorexia, stomatitis. **GU:** infertility, renal failure. **Derm:** alopecia, desquamation. **Hemat:** leukopenia, thrombocytopenia, anemia. **Local:** phlebitis at IV site. **Misc:** HEMOLYTIC UREMIC SYNDROME, fever, prolonged malaise.

Interactions

Drug-Drug: Additive bone marrow depression with other **antineoplastics** or **radiation therapy**. May ↓ antibody response to **live-virus vaccines** and ↑ risk of adverse reactions. Concurrent or sequential use with **vinca alkaloids** may result in respiratory toxicity.

Route/Dosage

IV (Adults): 20 mg/m² every 6–8 wk.

Availability (generic available)

Powder for injection (requires reconstitution): 5 mg/vial, 20 mg/vial, 40 mg/vial.

NURSING IMPLICATIONS

Assessment

- Monitor vital signs periodically during administration.
- Monitor for bone marrow depression. Assess for bleeding (bleeding gums, bruising, petechiae, guaiac stools, urine, and emesis) and avoid IM injections and taking rectal temperatures if platelet count is low. Apply pressure to venipuncture sites for 10 min. Assess for signs of infection during neutropenia. Anemia may occur. Monitor for increased fatigue, dyspnea, and orthostatic hypotension.
- Monitor intake and output, appetite, and nutritional intake. Nausea and vomiting usually occur within 1–2 hr. Vomiting may stop within 3–4 hr; nausea may persist for 2–3 days. Antiemetics may be administered prophylactically. Adjust diet as tolerated to help maintain fluid and electrolyte balance and nutritional status.
- Assess respiratory status and chest x-ray examination prior to and periodically throughout course of therapy. Cough, bronchospasm, hemoptysis, or dyspnea usually occurs after several doses and may be indicative of pulmonary toxicity, which may be life threatening.
- Monitor for potentially fatal hemolytic uremic syndrome in patients receiving long-term therapy. Symptoms include microangiopathic hemolytic anemia, thrombocytopenia, renal failure, and hypertension.
- ***Lab Test Considerations:*** Monitor CBC with differential, platelet count, and observation for fragmented RBCs on peripheral blood smears prior to and periodically throughout therapy and for several months following therapy.
- The nadirs of leukopenia and thrombocytopenia occur in 4–8 wk. Notify health care professional if leukocyte count is <4000/mm³ or if platelet count is <150,000/mm³ or is progressively declining. Recovery from leukopenia and thrombocytopenia occurs within 10 wk after cessation of therapy. Myelosuppression is cumulative and may be irreversible. Repeat courses of therapy are held until leukocyte count is >4000/mm³ and platelet count is >100,000/mm³.
- Monitor liver function studies (AST, ALT, LDH, bilirubin) and renal function studies (BUN, creatinine) prior to and periodically throughout therapy to detect hepatotoxicity and nephrotoxicity. Notify health care professional if creatinine is >1.7 m g/dL.

Potential Nursing Diagnoses

Risk for injury (Side Effects)
Risk for infection (Side Effects)
Disturbed body image (Side Effects)

Implementation

- Do not confuse mitomycin with mitoxantrone.
- Solution should be prepared in a biologic cabinet. Wear gloves, gown, and mask while handling medication. Discard equipment in designated containers.
- Ensure patency of IV. Extravasation may cause severe tissue necrosis. If patient complains of discomfort at IV site, discontinue immediately and restart infusion at another site. Promptly notify physician of extravasation.

IV Administration

- **IV Push:** Reconstitute 5-mg vial with 10 mL and 10-mg vial with 40 mL of sterile water for injection. Shake the vial; may need to stand at room temperature for additional time to dissolve. Final solution is blue-gray. Reconstituted solution is stable for 7 days at room temperature, 14 days if refrigerated. ***Diluent:*** 0.9% NaCl. ***Concentration:*** 20–40 mcg/mL for administration. ***Rate:*** May be administered IV push over 5–10 min through free-flowing IV of 0.9% NaCl or D5W.
- **Y-Site Compatibility:** alfentanil, amifostine, amphotericin B lipid complex, amphotericin B liposome, ampicillin, ampicillin/sulbactam, anidulafungin, argatroban, bivalirudin, bleomycin, bumetamide, buprenorphine, butorphanol, calcium chloride, calicum gluconate, carboplatin, caspofungin, cefoxitin, ceftazidime, ceftriaxone, chloramphenicol, chlorpromazine, ciprofloxacin, cisplatin, cyclophosphamide, cyclophosphamide, cyclosporine, dactinomycin, dexamethasone, dexmedetomidine, doxorubicin hydrochloride, droperidol, epirubicin , ertapenem, fentanyl, fluconazole, fludarabine, fluorouracil, foscarnet, fosphenytoin, furosemide, granisetron, heparin, hydrocortisone, hydromorphone, ifosfamide, imipenem/cilastatin, ketorolac, leucovorin calcium, levofloxacin, linezolid, magnesium sulfate, mannitol, melphalan, meperidine, methotrexate, methylprednisolone, metoclopramide, metronidazole, moxifloxacin, nesiritide, nitroglycerin, octreotide, ondansetron, ondansetron, oxaliplatin, paclitaxel, palonosetron, pemetrexed, potassium chloride, procainamide, quinupristin/dalfopristin, ranitidine, rituximab, sodium bicarbonate, tacrolimus, teniposide, thiotepa, tigecycline, tirofiban, tobramycin, trastuzumab, vasopressin, verapamil, vinblastine, vincristine, voriconazole, zidovudine, zoledronic acid.
- **Y-Site Incompatibility:** acyclovir, allopurinol, amikacin, aminophylline, amiodarone, amphotericin B colloidal, aztreonam, cefepime, cefotaxime, cefotetan, cefuroxime, clindamycin, dacarbazine, daptomycin, dexrazoxane, diazepam, dobutamine, docetaxel, dopamine, doxycycline, esmolol, etoposide, etoposide phosphate, famotidine, fenoldopam, filgrastim, gemcitabine, gentamicin, glycopyrrolate, haloperidol, idarubicin, insulin, irinotecan, isoproterenol, labetalol, lorazepam, midazolam, milrinone, morphine, naloxone, pantoprazole, phenytoin, piperacillin/tazobactam, promethazine, propranolol, sargramostim, succinylcholine, topotecan, vancomycin, vecuronium, vinorelbine.

Patient/Family Teaching

- Instruct patient to notify health care professional promptly if fever; chills; cough; hoarseness; sore throat; signs of infection; lower back or side pain; painful or difficult urination; bleeding gums; bruising; petechiae; blood in stools, urine, or emesis; increased fatigue; dyspnea; or orthostatic hypotension occurs. Caution patient to avoid crowds and persons with known infections. Instruct patient to use soft toothbrush and electric razor and to avoid falls. Caution patient not to drink alcoholic beverages or take medication containing aspirin or NSAIDs; may precipitate gastric bleeding.
- Instruct patient to notify health care professional if decreased urine output, edema in lower extremities, shortness of breath, skin ulceration, or persistent nausea occurs.
- Instruct patient to inspect oral mucosa for redness and ulceration. If ulceration occurs, advise patient to use sponge brush and rinse mouth with water after eating and drinking. Topical agents may be used if pain interferes with eating. Stomatitis pain may require treatment with opioid analgesics.
- Discuss with patient the possibility of hair loss. Explore coping strategies.
- Instruct patient not to receive any vaccinations without advice of health care professional.
- Rep: Advise patient that, although mitomycin may cause infertility, contraception during therapy is necessary because of teratogenic effects.
- Emphasize need for periodic lab tests to monitor for side effects.

Evaluation/Desired Outcomes

- Decrease in size and spread of malignant tissue.

mitoXANtrone

(mye-toe-**zan**-trone)
Novantrone

Classification
Therapeutic: antineoplastics, immune modifiers
Pharmacologic: antitumor antibiotics

Pregnancy Category D

Indications

Acute nonlymphocytic leukemia (ANLL) in adults (with other antineoplastics). Initial chemotherapy for patients with pain associated with advanced hormone-refractory prostate cancer. Secondary (chronic) progressive, progressive relapsing, or worsening relapsing-remitting multiple sclerosis (MS). **Unlabeled Use:** Breast cancer, liver cancer, and non-Hodgkin's lymphoma.

Action

Inhibits DNA synthesis (cell-cycle phase–nonspecific). **Therapeutic Effects:** Death of rapidly replicating cells, particularly malignant ones. Decreased pain in patients with advanced prostate cancer. Decreased disability and slowed progression of MS.

Pharmacokinetics

Absorption: IV administration results in complete bioavailability.
Distribution: Widely distributed; limited penetration of CSF.
Metabolism and Excretion: Mostly eliminated by hepatobiliary clearance; <10% excreted unchanged by the kidneys.
Half-life: 5.8 days.

TIME/ACTION PROFILE (effects on blood counts)

ROUTE	ONSET	PEAK	DURATION
IV	unknown	10 days	21 days

Contraindications/Precautions

Contraindicated in: Hypersensitivity; OB, Lactation: Pregnancy or lactation.
Use Cautiously in: Presence or history of cardiovascular disease (↑ risk of heart failure); OB: Patients with childbearing potential; Active infection; ↓ bone marrow reserve; Previous mediastinal radiation or use of anthracyclines (↑ risk of heart failure); Impaired hepatobiliary function; Pedi: Safety not established; Geri: May have ↑ sensitivity to drug effects.

Adverse Reactions/Side Effects

CNS: SEIZURES, headache. **EENT:** blue-green sclera, conjunctivitis. **Resp:** cough, dyspnea. **CV:** CARDIOTOXICITY, arrhythmias, ECG changes. **GI:** abdominal pain, diarrhea, hepatic toxicity, nausea, stomatitis, vomiting. **GU:** blue-green urine, gonadal suppression, renal failure. **Derm:** alopecia, rashes. **Hemat:** anemia, leukopenia, secondary leukemia, thrombocytopenia. **Metab:** hyperuricemia. **Misc:** fever, hypersensitivity reactions.

Interactions

Drug-Drug: ↑ bone marrow depression with other **antineoplastics** or **radiation therapy**. Risk of cardiomyopathy ↑ by previous **anthracycline antineoplastics (daunorubicin, doxorubicin, idarubicin)** or **mediastinal radiation**. May ↓ antibody response to **live-virus vaccines** and ↑ risk of adverse reactions.

Route/Dosage

Acute Nonlymphatic Leukemia

IV (Adults): *Induction*— 12 mg/m²/day for 3 days (usually given with cytosine arabinoside 100 mg/m²/day for 7 days); if incomplete remission occurs, a 2nd induction may be given. *Consolidation*— 12 mg/m²/day for 2 days (usually given with cytosine arabinoside 100 mg/m²/day for 5 days), given 6 wk after induction with another course 4 wk later.

Advanced Prostate Cancer

IV (Adults): 12–14 mg/m² single dose as a short infusion (with corticosteroids).

Multiple Sclerosis

IV (Adults): 12 mg/m² q 3 mo.

Availability (generic available)

Solution for injection: 2 mg/mL.

M

NURSING IMPLICATIONS

Assessment

- Monitor for hypersensitivity reaction (rash, urticaria, bronchospasm, tachycardia, hypotension). If these occur, stop infusion and notify physician. Keep epinephrine, an antihistamine, and resuscitation equipment close by in the event of an anaphylactic reaction.
- Monitor for bone marrow depression. Assess for bleeding (bleeding gums, bruising, petechiae, guaiac stools, urine, and emesis) and avoid IM injections and taking rectal temperatures if platelet count is low. Apply pressure to venipuncture sites for 10 min. Assess for signs of infection during neutropenia. Anemia may occur. Monitor for increased fatigue, dyspnea, and orthostatic hypotension.
- Monitor intake and output, appetite, and nutritional intake. Assess patient for nausea and vomiting. Antiemetics may be administered prophylactically. Adjust diet as tolerated to help maintain fluid and electrolyte balance and nutritional status.
- Monitor chest x-ray, ECG, echocardiography or MUGA, and radionuclide angiography to determine ejection fraction prior to and periodically during therapy. Multiple sclerosis patients with baseline left ventricular ejection fraction (LVEF) <50% should not receive mitoxantrone. May cause cardiotoxicity, especially in patients who have received daunorubicin or doxorubicin. Assess for rales/crackles, dyspnea, edema, jugular vein distention, ECG changes, arrhythmias, and chest pain. Monitor LVEF with echocardiogram or MUGA if signs of HF occur, prior to each dose, and yearly after stopping therapy in patients with multiple sclerosis. Potentially fatal HF may occur during or for months or years after therapy.

Risk is greater in patients receiving a cumulative dose >140m g/m^2.

- Monitor for symptoms of gout (↑ uric acid levels and joint pain and swelling). Encourage patient to drink at least 2 L of fluid per day. Allopurinol may be given to decrease serum uric acid levels.
- **Multiple sclerosis:** Asses frequency of exacerbations of symptoms of multiple sclerosis periodically during therapy.
- ***Lab Test Considerations:*** Monitor CBC with differential and platelet count prior to and periodically during therapy. The nadir of leukopenia usually occurs within 10 days, and recovery usually occurs within 21 days.
- Monitor liver function studies (AST, ALT, LDH, bilirubin) and renal function studies (BUN, creatinine) prior to and periodically during therapy to detect hepatotoxicity and nephrotoxicity.
- May cause ↑ uric acid concentrations. Monitor periodically during therapy.

Potential Nursing Diagnoses

Risk for injury (Side Effects)
Risk for infection (Side Effects)
Disturbed body image (Side Effects)

Implementation

- Do not confuse mitoxantrone with mitomycin.
- Solution should be prepared in a biologic cabinet. Wear gloves, gown, and mask while handling medication. Discard equipment in designated containers.
- Avoid contact with skin. Use Luer-Lok tubing to prevent accidental leakage. If contact with skin occurs, immediately wash skin with soap and water.
- Clean all spills with an aqueous solution of calcium hypochlorite. Mix solution by adding 5.5 parts (per weight) of calcium hypochlorite to 13 parts water.

IV Administration

- **IV:** Monitor IV site. If extravasation occurs, discontinue IV and restart at another site. Elevate extremity with extravasation and place ice packs over area. Monitor closely and obtain surgical consultation if local reaction occurs. Mitoxantrone is not a vesicant.
- **IV Push:** ***Diluent:*** Dilute dark blue mitoxantrone solution in at least 50 mL of 0.9% NaCl or D5W. Discard unused solution appropriately. ***Rate:*** Administer slowly over at least 3 min into the tubing of a free-flowing IV of 0.9% NaCl or D5W.
- **Intermittent Infusion:** May be further diluted in D5W, 0.9% NaCl, or D5/0.9% NaCl and used immediately. ***Concentration:*** 0.02–0.5 mg/mL. ***Rate:*** Administer over 15–30 min.
- **Continuous Infusion:** May also be administered over 24 hr.
- **Y-Site Compatibility:** acyclovir, alfentanil, allopurinol, amikacin, aminophylline, amindarone, anidulafungin, argatroban, atracurium, bivalirudin, bleomycin, bumetanide, buprenorphine, butorphanol, calcium chloride, calcium gluconate, carboplatin, carmustin, caspofungin, chloramphenicol, chrlopromazine, ciprofloxacin, cisatracurium, cisplatin, cladribine, cyclophosphamide, cyclosporine, cytarabine, dactinomycin, daptomycin, dexmedetomidine, dexrazoxane, diltiazem, diphenhydramine, dobutamine, doxacurium, doxycycline, droperidol, enalaprilat, ephedrine, epinephrine, erythromycin, esmolol, etoposide, etoposide phosphate, famotidine, fenoldopam, fentanyl, filgrastim, fluconazole, fludarabine, fluorouracil, ganciclovir, gemcitabine, gentamicin, glycopyrrolate, granisetron, haloperidol, hydralazine, hydrocortisone, hydromorphone, ifosfamide, imipenem/cilastatin, insulin, irinotecan, isoproterenol, ketorolac, labetalol, leucovorin, levofloxacin, levorphanol, lidocaine, linezolid, lorazepam, magnesium sulfate, mannitol, melphalan, meperidine, meropenem, mesna, metaraminol, methohexital, methotrexate, methyldopate, metoclopramide, metoprolol, metronidazole, midazolam, milrinone, morphine, nalbuphine, naloxone, nesiritide, nicardipine, nitroglycerin, norepinephrine, octreotide, ondansetron, oxaliplatin, palonosetron, pamidronate, pancuronium, pantamidine, pentazocine, pentobarbital, phenobarbital, phentolamine, phenylephrine, potassium acetate, potassium chloride, procainamide, prochlorperazine, promethazine, propranolol, quinupristin/dalfopristin, ranitidine, remifentanil, rituximab, rocuronium, sargramostim, sodium acetate, sodium bicarbonate, succinylcholine, sufentanil, tacrolimus, teniposide, theophylline, thiopental, thiotepa, tigecycline, tirofiban, tobramycin, tolazoline, trastuzumab, trimethiprom/sulfamethoxazole, vancomycin, vasopressin, vecuronium, verapamil, vincristine, vinorelbine, zidovudine, zoledronic acid.
- **Y-Site Incompatibility:** amphotericin B cholesteryl, amphotericin B colloidal, amphotericin B lipid complex, amphotericin B liposome, ampicillin, ampicillin/sulbactam, azithromycin, aztreonam, cefazolin, cefepime, cefotaxime, cefoxitin, ceftazidime, ceftriaxone, cefuroxime, clindamycin, dantrolene, dexamethasone, diazepam, digoxin, doxorubicin liposome, ertapenem, foscarnet, fosphenytoin, furosemide, heparin, idarubicin, methylprednisolone, nafcillin, nitroprusside, paclitaxel, pantoprazole, pemetrexed, phenytoin, piperacillin/tazobactam, potassium phosphates, propofol, sodium phosphates, voriconazole.

Patient/Family Teaching

- Advise patient to read the *Patient Package Insert* before starting therapy and before each dose in case of changes.
- Instruct patient to notify health care professional promptly if fever; chills; cough; hoarseness; sore throat; signs of infection; lower back or side pain; painful or difficult urination; bleeding gums; bruising; petechiae; blood in stools, urine, or emesis; in-

creased fatigue; dyspnea; or orthostatic hypotension occurs. Caution patient to avoid crowds and persons with known infections. Instruct patient to use soft toothbrush and electric razor and to avoid falls. Caution patient not to drink alcoholic beverages or take medication containing aspirin or NSAIDS; may precipitate gastric bleeding.

- Instruct patient to notify health care professional if abdominal pain, yellow skin, cough, diarrhea, or decreased urine output occurs.
- Inform patient that medication may cause the urine and sclera to turn blue-green.
- Instruct patient to inspect oral mucosa for redness and ulceration. If mouth sores occur, advise patient to use sponge brush and rinse mouth with water after eating and drinking. Topical agents may be used if pain interferes with eating. Stomatitis pain may require treatment with opioid analgesics.
- Discuss with patient the possibility of hair loss. Explore coping strategies.
- Instruct patient not to receive any vaccinations without advice of health care professional.
- Advise patient that, although mitoxantrone may cause infertility, contraception during therapy is necessary because of possible teratogenic effects.
- Emphasize need for periodic lab tests to monitor for side effects.

Evaluation/Desired Outcomes

- Decrease in the production and spread of leukemic cells.
- Decreased pain in patients with prostate cancer.
- Decrease in the frequency of relapse (neurologic dysfunction) in patients with relapsing-remitting multiple sclerosis.

modafinil (mo-daf-i-nil)

✤Alertec, Provigil

Classification

Therapeutic: central nervous system stimulants

Pregnancy Category C

Indications

To improve wakefulness in patients with excessive daytime drowsiness due to narcolepsy, obstructive sleep apnea, or shift work sleep disorder.

Action

Produces CNS stimulation. **Therapeutic Effects:** Decreased daytime drowsiness in patients with narcolepsy and obstructive sleep apnea. Decreased drowsiness during work in patients with shift work sleep disorder.

Pharmacokinetics

Absorption: Rapidly absorbed; bioavailability unknown.

Distribution: Well distributed; moderately (60%) bound to plasma proteins.

Metabolism and Excretion: Highly (90%) metabolized by the liver; <10% eliminated unchanged.

Half-life: 15 hr.

TIME/ACTION PROFILE (blood levels)

ROUTE	ONSET	PEAK	DURATION
PO	rapid	2–4 hr	24 hr

Contraindications/Precautions

Contraindicated in: Hypersensitivity; History of left ventricular hypertrophy or ischemic ECG changes, chest pain, arrhythmia, or other significant manifestations of mitral valve prolapse in association with CNS stimulant use.

Use Cautiously in: History of MI or unstable angina; Severe hepatic impairment with or without cirrhosis (dosage ↓ recommended); Concurrent use of MAO inhibitors; OB, Lactation, Pedi: Safety not established; Geri: Lower doses may be necessary due to ↑ sensitivity to drug effects.

Adverse Reactions/Side Effects

CNS: SUICIDAL IDEATION, headache, aggression, amnesia, anxiety, cataplexy, confusion, delusions, depression, dizziness, hallucinations, insomnia, mania, nervousness, seizures. **EENT:** rhinitis, abnormal vision, amblyopia, epistaxis, pharyngitis. **Resp:** dyspnea, lung disorder. **CV:** arrhythmias, chest pain, hypertension, hypotension, syncope, vasodilation. **GI:** ↑ liver enzymes, nausea, anorexia, diarrhea, gingivitis, mouth ulcers, thirst, vomiting. **GU:** abnormal ejaculation, albuminuria, urinary retention. **Derm:** STEVENS-JOHNSON SYNDROME, dry skin, herpes simplex, rash. **Endo:** hyperglycemia. **Hemat:** eosinophilia. **MS:** joint disorder, neck pain. **Neuro:** ataxia, dyskinesia, hypertonia, paresthesia, tremor. **Misc:** infection.

Interactions

Drug-Drug: May ↓ the metabolism and ↑ the effects of **diazepam**, **phenytoin**, **propranolol**, or **tricyclic antidepressants** (dosage adjustments may be necessary). May ↑ the metabolism and ↓ the effects of **hormonal contraceptives**, **cyclosporine**, and **theophylline** (dosage adjustments or additional methods of contraception may be necessary).

Drug-Natural Products: Use with caffeine-containing herbs (**cola nut**, **guarana**, **mate**, **tea**, **coffee**) may ↑ stimulant effect.

Route/Dosage

PO (Adults): 200 mg/day as a single dose.

M

Hepatic Impairment

PO (Adults): *Severe hepatic impairment*—100 mg/day as a single dose.

Availability (generic available)

Tablets: 100 mg, 200 mg.

NURSING IMPLICATIONS

Assessment

- Observe and document frequency of narcoleptic episodes.
- Monitor closely for changes in behavior that could indicate the emergence or worsening of suicidal thoughts or behavior or depression.
- Assess for rash periodically during therapy. May cause Stevens-Johnson syndrome. Discontinue therapy if severe or if accompanied with fever, general malaise, fatigue, muscle or joint aches, blisters, oral lesions, conjunctivitis, hepatitis and/or eosinophilia.
- Monitor for signs and symptoms of angioedema or anaphylaxis (rash, swelling of face, eyes, lips, tongue or larynx; difficulty in swallowing or breathing; hoarseness).
- ***Lab Test Considerations:*** May cause elevated liver enzymes.

Potential Nursing Diagnoses

Disturbed thought process (Side Effects)
Deficient knowledge, related to medication regimen (Patient/Family Teaching)

Implementation

- **PO:** Administer as a single dose in the morning for patients with narcolepsy or obstructive sleep apnea. Administer 1 hr before the start of work shift for patients with shift work sleep disorder.

Patient/Family Teaching

- Instruct patient to take medication as directed. Advise patient to read the *Medication Guide* prior to starting therapy and with each Rx refill, in case of changes.
- Medication may impair judgment. Advise patient to use caution when driving or during other activities requiring alertness.
- Encourage patient and family to be alert for emergence of anxiety, agitation, panic attacks, insomnia, irritability, hostility, impulsivity, akathisia, hypomania, mania, worsening of depression and suicidal ideation, especially during early antidepressant therapy. Assess symptoms on a day-to-day basis as changes may be abrupt. If these symptoms occur, notify health care professional.
- Advise patient to notify health care professional immediately if rash or symptoms of anaphylaxis occur.
- Advise patient to notify health care professional of all Rx or OTC medications, vitamins, or herbal products being taken and to consult with health care professional before taking other medications. If alcohol is used during therapy, intake should be limited to moderate amounts.
- Nonhormonal methods of contraception should be used during and for 1 mo following discontinuation of therapy. Instruct patient to notify health care professional promptly if pregnancy is planned or suspected or if breast feeding.

Evaluation/Desired Outcomes

- Decrease in narcoleptic symptoms and an enhanced ability to stay awake.

---

moexipril, See ANGIOTENSIN-CONVERTING ENZYME (ACE) INHIBITORS.

---

mometasone, See CORTICOSTEROIDS (INHALATION), CORTICOSTEROIDS (NASAL), and CORTICOSTEROIDS (TOPICAL/LOCAL).

---

montelukast (mon-te-loo-kast)

Singulair

Classification

Therapeutic: allergy, cold, and cough remedies, bronchodilators
Pharmacologic: leukotriene antagonists

Pregnancy Category B

Indications

Prevention and chronic treatment of asthma. Management of seasonal allergic rhinitis. Prevention of exercise-induced bronchoconstriction in patients 6 yr and older.

Action

Antagonizes the effects of leukotrienes, which mediate the following: Airway edema, Smooth muscle constriction, Altered cellular activity. Result is decreased inflammatory process, which is part of asthma and allergic rhinitis. **Therapeutic Effects:** Decreased frequency and severity of acute asthma attacks. Decreased severity of allergic rhinitis. Decreased attacks of exercise-induced bronchoconstriction.

Pharmacokinetics

Absorption: Rapidly absorbed (63–73%) following oral administration.
Distribution: Unknown.
Protein Binding: 99%.
Metabolism and Excretion: Mostly metabolized by the liver (by P450 3A4 and 2C9 enzyme systems); metabolites eliminated in feces via bile; negligible renal excretion.
Half-life: 2.7–5.5 hr.

TIME/ACTION PROFILE (improved symptoms of asthma)

ROUTE	ONSET	PEAK†	DURATION
PO (swallow)	within 24 hr	3–4 hr	24 hr
PO (chew)	within 24 hr	2–2.5 hr	24 hr

†Blood levels.

Contraindications/Precautions

Contraindicated in: Hypersensitivity.

Use Cautiously in: Acute attacks of asthma; Phenylketonuria (chewable tablets contain aspartame); Hepatic impairment (may need ↓ doses); Reduction of corticosteroid therapy (may ↑ the risk of eosinophilic conditions); OB, Lactation, Pedi: Pregnancy, lactation, or children <1 yr (safety not established).

Adverse Reactions/Side Effects

CNS: SUICIDAL THOUGHTS, agitation, aggression, anxiety, depression, disorientation, dream abnormalities, fatigue, hallucinations, headache, insomnia, irritability, restlessness, tremor, weakness. **EENT:** nosebleed, otitis (children), sinusitis (children). **Resp:** cough, rhinorrhea. **GI:** abdominal pain, diarrhea (children), dyspepsia, nausea (children), ↑ liver enzymes. **Neuro:** tremor. **Derm:** STEVENS-JOHNSON SYNDROME, TOXIC EPIDERMAL NECROLYSIS, rash. **Misc:** eosinophilic conditions (including CHURG-STRAUSS SYNDROME), fever.

Interactions

Drug-Drug: Drugs which induce the CYP450 enzyme system (**phenobarbital** and **rifampin**) may ↓ the effects of montelukast.

Route/Dosage

Asthma and Allergic Rhinitis

PO (Adults and Children ≥14 yr): 10 mg once daily.

PO (Children 6–14 yr): 5 mg once daily (as chewable tablet).

PO (Children 2–5 yr): 4 mg once daily (as chewable tablet or granules).

PO (Children 6–23 months): 4 mg once daily (as oral granules).

Exercise-Induced Bronchoconstriction (EIB)

PO (Adults and Children ≥6 yrs): 10 mg at least 2 hr before exercise. Do not take within 24 hr of another dose; if taking daily doses, do not take dose for EIB.

Availability (generic available)

Tablets: 10 mg. **Cost:** *Generic*—$169.72/30. **Chewable tablets (cherry flavor):** 4 mg, 5 mg. **Cost:** *Generic*—All strengths $169.72/30. **Oral granules:** 4 mg/packet. **Cost:** *Generic*—$169.72/30 pkts.

NURSING IMPLICATIONS

Assessment

- Assess lung sounds and respiratory function prior to and periodically during therapy.
- Assess allergy symptoms (rhinitis, conjunctivitis, hives) before and periodically during therapy.
- Monitor closely for changes in behavior that could indicate the emergence or worsening of depression or suicidal thoughts.
- Assess for rash periodically during therapy. May cause Stevens-Johnson syndrome. Discontinue therapy if severe or if accompanied with fever, general malaise, fatigue, muscle or joint aches, blisters, oral lesions, conjunctivitis, hepatitis and/or eosinophilia.
- ***Lab Test Considerations:*** May cause ↑ AST and ALT concentrations.

Potential Nursing Diagnoses

Ineffective airway clearance (Indications)

Implementation

- Do not confuse Singulair with Sinequan.
- Doses of inhaled corticosteroids may be gradually decreased with supervision of health care professional; do not discontinue abruptly.
- **PO:** For asthma, administer once daily in the evening. For allergic rhinitis, may be administered at any time of day.
- Administer granules directly into mouth or mixed in a spoonful of cold or room temperature foods (use only applesauce, mashed carrots, rice, or ice cream). Do not open packet until ready to use. After opening packet, administer full dose within 15 min. Do not store mixture. Discard unused portion. Do not dissolve granules in fluid, but fluid may be taken following administration. Granules may be administered without regard to meals.
- For Exercise Induced Bronchoconstriction: Administer one tablet at least 2 hrs before exercise; do not take within 24 hr of another dose.

Patient/Family Teaching

- Instruct patient to take medication daily in the evening or at least 2 hr before exercise, even if not experiencing symptoms of asthma. Do not double doses. Do not discontinue therapy without consulting health care professional.
- Instruct patient not to discontinue or reduce other asthma medications without consulting health care professional.
- Advise patient that montelukast is not used to treat acute asthma attacks, but may be continued during an acute exacerbation. Patient should carry rapid-acting therapy for bronchospasm at all times. Advise patient to notify health care professional if more than the maximum number of short-acting bron-

M

chodilator treatments prescribed for a 24-hr period are needed.

- Encourage patient and family to be alert for emergence of anxiety, agitation, panic attacks, insomnia, irritability, hostility, impulsivity, akathisia, hypomania, mania, worsening of depression and suicidal ideation, especially during early antidepressant therapy. Assess symptoms on a day-to-day basis as changes may be abrupt. If these symptoms or rash occurs, notify health care professional.

Evaluation/Desired Outcomes

- Prevention of and reduction in symptoms of asthma.
- Decrease in severity of allergic rhinitis.
- Prevention of exercise-induced bronchoconstriction.

REMS HIGH ALERT

morphine (mor-feen)

Astramorph, ~~AVINza~~, ✤ Doloral, Duramorph, Embeda, Infumorph, Kadian, ✤ M-Eslon, ✤ Morphine EPD, ✤ Morphine Extra Forte, ✤ Morphine Forte, ✤ Morphine HP, ✤ Morphine LP Epidural, ✤ M.O.S, ✤ M.O.S.-S.R, MS Contin, ✤ MS Contin SRT, ~~Roxanol~~, ✤ Statex

Classification

Therapeutic: opioid analgesics

Pharmacologic: opioid agonists

Schedule II

Pregnancy Category C

Indications

Severe pain (the 20 mg/mL oral solution concentration should only be used in opioid-tolerant patients). Moderate to severe chronic pain in opioid-tolerant patients requiring use of daily, around-the-clock long-term opioid treatment and for which alternative treatment options are inadequate (extended-release). Pulmonary edema. Pain associated with MI.

Action

Binds to opiate receptors in the CNS. Alters the perception of and response to painful stimuli while producing generalized CNS depression. **Therapeutic Effects:** Decrease in severity of pain. Addition of naltrexone in *Embeda* product is designed to prevent abuse or misuse by altering the formulation. Naltrexone has no effect unless the capsule is crushed or chewed.

Pharmacokinetics

Absorption: Variably absorbed (about 30%) following oral administration. More reliably absorbed from rectal, subcut, and IM sites. Following epidural administration, systemic absorption and absorption into the intrathecal space via the meninges occurs.

Distribution: Widely distributed. Crosses the placenta; enters breast milk in small amounts.

Protein Binding: Premature infants: <20%; Adults: 35%.

Metabolism and Excretion: Mostly metabolized by the liver. Active metabolites excreted renally.

Half-life: Premature neonates: 10–20 hr; Neonates: 7.6 hr; Infants 1–3 mo: 6.2 hr; Children 6 mo–2.5 yr: 2.9 hr; Children 3–6 yr: 1–2 hr; Children 6–19 yr with sickle cell disease: 1.3 hr; Adults: 2–4 hr.

TIME/ACTION PROFILE (analgesia)

ROUTE	ONSET	PEAK	DURATION
PO	unknown	60 min	4–5 hr
PO-ER	unknown	3–4 hr	8–24 hr
IM	10–30 min	30–60 min	4–5 hr
Subcut	20 min	50–90 min	4–5 hr
Rect	unknown	20–60 min	3–7 hr
IV	rapid	20 min	4–5 hr
Epidural	6–30 min	1 hr	up to 24 hr
IT	rapid (min)	unknown	up to 24 hr

Contraindications/Precautions

Contraindicated in: Hypersensitivity; Some products contain tartrazine, bisulfites, or alcohol and should be avoided in patients with known hypersensitivity; Acute, mild, intermittent, or postoperative pain (extended/sustained-release); Significant respiratory depression (extended-release); Acute or severe bronchial asthma (extended-release); Paralytic ileus (extended-release).

Use Cautiously in: Head trauma; ↑ intracranial pressure; Severe renal, hepatic, or pulmonary disease; Hypothyroidism; Seizure disorder; Adrenal insufficiency; History of substance abuse; Undiagnosed abdominal pain; Prostatic hyperplasia; Patients undergoing procedures that rapidly ↓ pain (cordotomy, radiation); long-acting agents should be discontinued 24 hr before and replaced with short-acting agents; Geri: Geriatric or debilitated patients (↑ risk of respiratory depression; dose ↓ suggested); OB, Lactation: Avoid chronic use; has been used during labor but may cause respiratory depression in the newborn; prolonged use of extended-release morphine during pregnancy can result in neonatal opioid withdrawal syndrome; Pedi: Neonates and infants <3 mo (more susceptible to respiratory depression); Pedi: Neonates (oral solution contains sodium benzoate which can cause potentially fatal gasping syndrome).

Adverse Reactions/Side Effects

CNS: confusion, sedation, dizziness, dysphoria, euphoria, floating feeling, hallucinations, headache, unusual dreams. **EENT:** blurred vision, diplopia, miosis. **Resp:** RESPIRATORY DEPRESSION. **CV:** hypotension, bradycardia. **GI:** constipation, nausea, vomiting. **GU:** urinary retention. **Derm:** flushing, itching, sweating. **Misc:** physical dependence, psychological dependence, tolerance.

Interactions

Drug-Drug: Use with **extreme caution** in patients receiving **MAO inhibitors** within 14 days prior (may result in unpredictable, severe reactions—↓ initial dose of morphine to 25% of usual dose). ↑ CNS depression with **alcohol**, **sedative/hypnotics**, **clomipramine**, **barbiturates**, **tricyclic antidepressants**, and **antihistamines**. **Alcohol** may ↑ levels and ↑ the risk of toxicity. Administration of **partial-antagonist opioid analgesics** may precipitate opioid withdrawal in physically dependent patients. **Buprenorphine**, **nalbuphine**, **butorphanol**, or **pentazocine** may ↓ analgesia. May ↑ the anticoagulant effect of **warfarin**. **Cimetidine** ↓ metabolism and may ↑ effects.
Drug-Natural Products: Concomitant use of **kava-kava**, **valerian**, or **chamomile** can ↑ CNS depression.

Route/Dosage

Larger doses may be required during chronic therapy.
PO, Rect (Adults ≥50 kg): *Usual starting dose for moderate to severe pain in opioid-naive patients*—30 mg q 3–4 hr initially *or* once 24-hr opioid requirement is determined, convert to extended-release morphine by administering total daily oral morphine dose every 24 hr (as *Kadian* or other ER capsules), 50% of the total daily oral morphine dose every 12 hr (as *Kadian, MS Contin*), or 33% of the total daily oral morphine dose every 8 hr (as *MS Contin*). See equianalgesic chart, Appendix I. Dose of ER capsules (not *Kadian*) should not exceed 1600 mg/day because of fumaric acid in formulation.
PO, Rect (Adults and Children <50 kg): *Usual starting dose for moderate to severe pain in opioid-naive patients*—0.3 mg/kg q 3–4 hr initially.
PO (Children >1 mo): *Prompt-release tablets and solution*—0.2–0.5 mg/kg/dose q 4–6 hr as needed. *Controlled-release tablet*—0.3–0.6 mg/kg/dose q 12 hr.
IM, IV, Subcut (Adults ≥50 kg): *Usual starting dose for moderate to severe pain in opioid-naive patients*—4–10 mg q 3–4 hr. *MI*—8–15 mg, for very severe pain additional smaller doses may be given every 3–4 hr.
IM, IV, Subcut (Adults and Children <50 kg): *Usual starting dose for moderate to severe pain in opioid-naive patients*—0.05–0.2 mg/kg q 3–4 hr, maximum: 15 mg/dose.
IM, IV, Subcut (Neonates): 0.05 mg/kg q 4–8 hr, maximum dose: 0.1 mg/kg. Use preservative-free formulation.
IV, Subcut (Adults): *Continuous infusion*—0.8–10 mg/hr; may be preceded by a bolus of 15 mg (infusion rates vary greatly; up to 80 mg/hr have been used).
IV, Subcut (Children >1 mo): *Continuous infusion, postoperative pain*—0.01–0.04 mg/kg/hr. *Continuous infusion, sickle cell or cancer pain*—0.02–2.6 mg/kg/hr.
IV (Neonates): *Continuous infusion*—0.01–0.03 mg/kg/hr.
Epidural (Adults): *Intermittent injection*—5 mg/day (initially); if relief is not obtained at 60 min, 1–2 mg increments may be made (total dose not to exceed 10 mg/day. *Continuous infusion*—2–4 mg/24 hr; may ↑ by 1–2 mg/day (up to 30 mg/day).
Epidural (Children >1 mo): 0.03–0.05 mg/kg, maximum dose: 0.1 mg/kg or 5 mg/24 hr. Use preservative-free formulation.
IT (Adults): 0.2–1 mg. Use preservative-free formulation.

Availability (generic available)

Immediate-release tablets: 15 mg, 30 mg. **Cost:** *Generic*—15 mg $22.17/100, 30 mg $37.77/100. **Extended-release tablets (MS Contin):** 15 mg, 30 mg, 60 mg, 100 mg, 200 mg. **Cost:** *Generic*—15 mg $167.57/100, 30 mg $317.19/100, 60 mg $532.39/100, 100 mg $763.63/100, 200 mg $1,838.19/100. **Extended-release capsules (Kadian):** 10 mg, 20 mg, 30 mg, 40 mg, 50 mg, 60 mg, 70 mg, 80 mg, 100 mg, 130 mg, 150 mg, 200 mg. **Cost:** 10 mg $609.60/100, 20 mg $673.20/100, 30 mg $732.00/100, 40 mg $976.80/100, 50 mg $1,224.00/100, 60 mg $1,465.20/100, 70 mg $1,708.80/100, 80 mg $1,951.20/100, 100 mg $2,407.20/100, 130 mg $3,182.40/100, 150 mg $3,672.00/100, 200 mg $4,946.40/100. **Extended-release capsules:** 30 mg, 45 mg, 60 mg, 75 mg, 90 mg, 120 mg. **Cost:** 30 mg $606.31/100, 45 mg $898.99/100, 60 mg $1,177.88/100, 75 mg $1,498.31/100, 90 mg $1,770.29/100, 120 mg $2,088.66/100. **Oral solution:** ✱1 mg/mL, 2 mg/mL, 4 mg/mL, ✱5 mg/mL, 20 mg/mL (concentrated). **Cost:** *Generic*—4 mg/mL $17.51/100 mL, 20 mg/mL $25.20/30 mL. **Rectal suppositories:** 5 mg, 10 mg, 20 mg, 30 mg. **Cost:** *Generic*—5 mg $60.00/12, 10 mg $75.00/12, 20 mg $90.00/12, 30 mg $112.50/12. **Solution for IM, subcut, IV injection:** 1 mg/mL, 2 mg/mL, 4 mg/mL, 5 mg/mL, 8 mg/mL, 10 mg/mL, 15 mg/mL, 25 mg/mL, 50 mg/mL. **Solution for epidural, IV injection (preservative-free):** 0.5 mg/mL, 1 mg/mL. **Solution for epidural or IT use (continuous microinfusion device; preservative-free):** 10 mg/mL, 25 mg/mL. **Solution for IV injection (PCA device):** 1 mg/mL, 2 mg/mL, 3 mg/mL, 5 mg/mL.

NURSING IMPLICATIONS

Assessment

- Assess type, location, and intensity of pain prior to and 1 hr following PO, subcut, IM, and 20 min (peak) following IV administration. When titrating opioid doses, increases of 25–50% should be administered until there is either a 50% reduction in

M

the patient's pain rating on a numerical or visual analogue scale or the patient reports satisfactory pain relief. When titrating doses of short-acting morphine, a repeat dose can be safely administered at the time of the peak if previous dose is ineffective and side effects are minimal.

- Patients on a continuous infusion should have additional bolus doses provided every 15–30 min, as needed, for breakthrough pain. The bolus dose is usually set to the amount of drug infused each hour by continuous infusion.
- Patients taking extended-release morphine may require additional short-acting opioid doses for breakthrough pain. Doses of short-acting opioids should be equivalent to 10–20% of 24 hr total and given every 2 hr as needed.
- An equianalgesic chart (see Appendix I) should be used when changing routes or when changing from one opioid to another.
- ***High Alert:*** Assess level of consciousness, BP, pulse, and respirations before and periodically during administration. If respiratory rate is <10/min, assess level of sedation. Physical stimulation may be sufficient to prevent significant hypoventilation. Subsequent doses may need to be decreased by 25–50%. Initial drowsiness will diminish with continued use. Geri: Assess geriatric patients frequently; older adults are more sensitive to the effects of opioid analgesics and may experience side effects and respiratory complications more frequently. Pedi: Assess pediatric patient frequently; children are more sensitive to the effects of opioid analgesics and may experience respiratory complications, excitability and restlessness more frequently.
- Prolonged use may lead to physical and psychological dependence and tolerance. This should not prevent patient from receiving adequate analgesia. Most patients who receive morphine for pain do not develop psychological dependence. Progressively higher doses may be required to relieve pain with long-term therapy.
- Assess bowel function routinely. Institute prevention of constipation with increased intake of fluids and bulk and with laxatives to minimize constipating effects. Administer stimulant laxatives routinely if opioid use exceeds 2–3 days, unless contraindicated.
- Assess risk for opioid addiction, abuse, or misuse prior to administration. Abuse or misuse of extended-release preparations by crushing, chewing, snorting, or injecting dissolved product will result in uncontrolled delivery of morphine and can result in overdose and death.
- ***Lab Test Considerations:*** May ↑ plasma amylase and lipase levels.
- ***Toxicity and Overdose:*** If an opioid antagonist is required to reverse respiratory depression or coma, naloxone is the antidote. Dilute the 0.4-mg ampule of naloxone in 10 mL of 0.9% NaCl and administer 0.5 mL (0.02 mg) by IV push every 2 min. For children and adults weighing <40 kg, dilute 0.1 mg of naloxone in 10 mL of 0.9% NaCl for a concentration of 10 mcg/mL and administer 0.5 mcg/kg every 2 min. Titrate dose to avoid withdrawal, seizures, and severe pain.

Potential Nursing Diagnoses

Acute pain (Indications)
Chronic pain (Indications)
Risk for injury (Side Effects)

Implementation

- ***High Alert:*** Do not confuse MS Contin (morphine sulfate) with Oxycontin (oxycodone). Do not confuse morphine (non-concentrated oral liquid) with morphine (concentrated oral liquid).
- ***High Alert:*** Do not confuse morphine with hydromorphone—errors have resulted in death. Use only preservative-free formulations for neonates, and for epidural and intrathecal routes in all patients.
- Explain therapeutic value of medication prior to administration to enhance the analgesic effect.
- Regularly administered doses may be more effective than prn administration. Analgesic is more effective if given before pain becomes severe.
- Coadministration with nonopioid analgesics may have additive analgesic effects and may permit lower doses.
- When transferring from other opioids or other forms of morphine to extended-release tablets, administer a total daily dose of oral morphine equivalent to previous daily dose (see Appendix I) and divided every 8 hr (MS Contin), every 12 hr (Embeda, Kadian, MS Contin), every 24 hr (Kadian).
- Morphine should be discontinued gradually to prevent withdrawal symptoms after long-term use.
- **PO:** Doses may be administered with food or milk to minimize GI irritation.
- Administer oral solution with properly calibrated measuring device; may be diluted in a glass of fruit juice just prior to administration to improve taste. Verify correct dose (mg) and correct volume (mL) prior to administration. Use an oral syringe when using 20 mg/mL concentration of oral solution.
- Swallow extended-release tablets whole; do not break, crush, dissolve, or chew (could result in rapid release and absorption of a potentially toxic dose).
- *Embeda and Kadian* capsules may be opened and the pellets sprinkled onto applesauce immediately prior to administration. Patients should rinse mouth and swallow to assure ingestion of entire dose. Pellets should not be chewed, crushed, or dissolved. *Kadian* capsules may also be opened and sprinkled on approximately 10 mL of water and flushed while swirling through a pre-wetted 16 French gastrostomy tube fitted with a funnel at the port end. Addi-

tional water should be used to transfer and flush any remaining pellets. *Kadian* should not be administered via a nasogastric tube.

- **Rect:** *MS Contin* has been administered rectally.
- **IM, Subcut:** Use IM route for repeated doses, because morphine is irritating to subcut tissues.

IV Administration

- **IV:** Solution is colorless; do not administer discolored solution.
- **IV Push:** ***Diluent:*** Dilute with at least 5 mL of sterile water or 0.9% NaCl for injection. ***Concentration:*** 0.5–5 mg/mL. ***Rate: High Alert:*** Administer 2.5–15 mg over 5 min. Rapid administration may lead to increased respiratory depression, hypotension, and circulatory collapse.
- **Continuous Infusion:** ***Diluent:*** May be added to D5W, D10W, 0.9% NaCl, 0.45% NaCl, Ringer's or LR, dextrose/saline solution, or dextrose/Ringer's or LR. ***Concentration:*** 0.1–1 mg/mL or greater for continuous infusion. ***Rate:*** Administer via infusion pump to control the rate. Dose should be titrated to ensure adequate pain relief without excessive sedation, respiratory depression, or hypotension. May be administered via patient-controlled analgesia (PCA) pump.
- **Y-Site Compatibility:** acetaminophen, aldesleukin, alfentanil, allopurinol, amifostine, amikacin, aminocaproic acid, aminophylline, amiodarone, anakinra, anidulafungin, argatroban, ascorbic acid, atropine, aztreonam, benztropine, bivalirudin, bleomycin, bumetanide, buprenorphine, butorphanol, calcium chloride, calcium gluconate, cangrelor, carboplatin, carmustine, caspofungin, cefazolin, cefotaxime, cefotetan, cefoxitin, ceftaroline, ceftazidime, ceftriaxone, cefuroxime, chloramphenicol, chlorpromazine, cisatracurium, cladribine, clindamycin, cyanocobalamin, cyclophosphamide, cyclosporine, cytarabine, dactinomycin, daptomycin, dexamethasone, dexmedetomidine, dexrazoxane, digoxin, diltiazem, diphenhydramine, dobutamine, docetaxel, dolasetron, dopamine, doripenem, doxorubicin hydrochloride, doxycycline, droperidol, enalaprilat, ephedrine, epinephrine, epirubicin, epoetin alfa, eptifibatide, ertapenem, erythromycin, esmolol, etomidate, etoposide, etoposide phosphate, famotidine, fenoldopam, fentanyl, filgrastim, fluconazole, fludarabine, fluorouracil, foscarnet, fosphenytoin, gemcitabine, gentamicin, glycopyrrolate, granisetron, heparin, hydrocortisone, hydromorphone, idarubicin, ifosfamide, imipenem/cilastatin, irinotecan, isoproterenol, ketorolac, labetalol, leucovorin calcium, lidocaine, linezolid, lorazepam, magnesium sulfate, mannitol, mechlorethamine, melphalan, meperidine, meropenem, mesna, methotrexate, methyldopate, methylprednisolone, metoclopramide, metoprolol, metronidazole, midazolam, milrinone, mitoxantrone, multivitamins, mycophenolate, nafcillin, nalbuphine, naloxone, nicardipine, nitroglycerin, nitroprusside, norepinephrine, octreotide, ondansetron, oxacillin, oxaliplatin, oxytocin, paclitaxel, palonosetron, pamidronate, pancuronium, papaverine, pemetrexed, penicillin G, phenobarbital, phenylephrine, phytonadione, piperacillin/tazobactam, potassium acetate, potassium chloride, procainamide, prochlorperazine, promethazine, propranolol, protamine, pyridoxine, quinupristin/dalfopristin, ranitidine, remifentanil, rituximab, rocuronium, sodium acetate, sodium bicarbonate, streptokinase, succinylcholine, sufentanil, tacrolimus, teniposide, theophylline, thiamine, thiotepa, tigecycline, tirofiban, tobramycin, vancomycin, vasopressin, vecuronium, verapamil, vinblastine, vincristine, vinorelbine, vitamin B complex with C, voriconazole, warfarin, zidovudine, zoledronic acid.
- **Y-Site Incompatibility:** alemtuzumab, amphotericin B colloidal, amphotericin B lipid complex, amphotericin B liposome, dantrolene, doxorubicin liposomal, folic acid, ganciclovir, indomethacin, micafungin, pentamidine, pentobarbital, phenytoin, sargramostim, trastuzumab.
- **Epidural:** Administer undiluted. Do not use an in-line filter. Do not admix or administer other medications in epidural space for 48 hr after administration. Administer within 4 hr after removing from vial. Store in refrigerator; do not freeze.

Patient/Family Teaching

- Instruct patient how and when to ask for pain medication.
- May cause drowsiness or dizziness. Caution patient to call for assistance when ambulating or smoking and to avoid driving or other activities requiring alertness until response to medication is known.
- Advise patient to change positions slowly to minimize orthostatic hypotension.
- Caution patient to avoid concurrent use of alcohol or other CNS depressants with this medication.
- Encourage patients who are immobilized or on prolonged bedrest to turn, cough, and breathe deeply every 2 hr to prevent atelectasis.
- Advise patient to notify health care professional if pregnancy is planned or suspected, or if breast feeding.
- **Home Care Issues:** ***High Alert:*** Explain to patient and family how and when to administer morphine and how to care for infusion equipment properly. Pedi: Teach parents or caregivers how to accurately measure liquid medication and to use only the measuring device dispensed with the medication.
- Emphasize the importance of aggressive prevention of constipation with the use of morphine.

M

Evaluation/Desired Outcomes

- Decrease in severity of pain without a significant alteration in level of consciousness or respiratory status.
- Decrease in symptoms of pulmonary edema.

mupirocin (myoo-peer-oh-sin)

Bactroban, Bactroban Nasal, Centany

Classification
Therapeutic: anti-infectives

Pregnancy Category B

Indications

Topical: Treatment of: Impetigo, Secondarily infected traumatic skin lesions (up to 10 cm in length or 100 cm^2 area) caused by *Staphylococcus aureus* and *Streptococcus pyogenes*. **Intranasal:** Eradicates nasal colonization with methicillin-resistant *S. aureus*.

Action

Inhibits bacterial protein synthesis. **Therapeutic Effects:** Inhibition of bacterial growth and reproduction. **Spectrum:** Greatest activity against gram-positive organisms, including: *S. aureus*, Beta-hemolytic streptococci. Resolution of impetigo. Eradication of *S. aureus* carrier state.

Pharmacokinetics

Absorption: Minimal systemic absorption.
Distribution: Remains in the stratum corneum after topical use for prolonged periods of time (72 hr).
Metabolism and Excretion: Metabolized in the skin, removed by desquamation.
Half-life: 17–36 min.

TIME/ACTION PROFILE (anti-infective effect)

ROUTE	ONSET	PEAK	DURATION
Nasal	unknown	unknown	12 hr
Topical†	unknown	3–5 days	72 hr

†Resolution of lesions.

Contraindications/Precautions

Contraindicated in: Hypersensitivity to mupirocin or polyethylene glycol.
Use Cautiously in: Renal impairment; Burn patients; OB, Lactation: Safety not established.

Adverse Reactions/Side Effects

CNS: *nasal only*—headache. **EENT:** *nasal only*—cough, itching, pharyngitis, rhinitis, upper respiratory tract congestion. **GI:** nausea; *nasal only*, altered taste. **Derm:** *topical only*—burning, itching, pain, stinging.

Interactions

Drug-Drug: Nasal mupirocin should not be used concurrently with other **nasal products**.

Route/Dosage

Topical (Adults and Children ≥2 mo): Ointment: Apply 3–5 times daily for 5–14 days.
Topical (Adults and Children ≥3 mo): Cream: Apply small amount 3 times/day for 10 days.
Intranasal (Adults and Children ≥1 yr): Apply small amount nasal ointment to each nostril 2–4 times/day for 5–14 days.

Availability (generic available)

Ointment: 2%. **Cost:** *Generic*—$17.20/22 g. **Cream:** 2%. **Cost:** *Generic*—$69.25/15 g. **Nasal ointment:** 2%. **Cost:** $14.14/1 g.

NURSING IMPLICATIONS

Assessment

- Assess lesions before and daily during therapy.

Potential Nursing Diagnoses

Impaired skin integrity (Indications)
Risk for infection (Indications, Patient/Family Teaching)

Implementation

- **Topical:** Wash affected area with soap and water and dry thoroughly. Apply a small amount of mupirocin to the affected area 3 times daily and rub in gently. Treated area may be covered with gauze if desired.
- **Nasal:** Apply one half of the ointment from the single-use tube to each nostril twice daily (morning and evening) for 5 days. After application, close nostrils by pressing together and releasing sides of the nose repeatedly for 1 min.

Patient/Family Teaching

- Instruct patient on the correct application of mupirocin. Advise patient to apply medication exactly as directed for the full course of therapy. If a dose is missed, apply as soon as possible unless almost time for next dose. Avoid contact with eyes.
- **Topical:** Teach patient and family appropriate hygienic measures to prevent spread of impetigo.
- Instruct parents to notify school nurse for screening and prevention of transmission.
- Patient should consult health care professional if symptoms have not improved in 3–5 days.

Evaluation/Desired Outcomes

- Healing of skin lesions. If no clinical response is seen in 3–5 days, condition should be re-evaluated.
- Eradication of methicillin-resistant *S. aureus* carrier state in patients and health care workers during institutional outbreaks.

muromonab-CD3
(myoo-roe-**moe**-nab CD3)
Orthoclone OKT3

Classification
Therapeutic: immunosuppressants
Pharmacologic: monoclonal antibodies

Pregnancy Category C

Indications
Acute renal allograft rejection reactions in transplant patients that have occurred despite conventional antirejection therapy. Acute corticosteroid-resistant hepatic or cardiac allograft rejection reactions.

Action
A purified immunoglobulin antibody that acts as an immunosuppressant by interfering with normal T-cell function. **Therapeutic Effects:** Reversal of graft rejection in transplant patients.

Pharmacokinetics
Absorption: Administered IV only, resulting in complete bioavailability.
Distribution: Unknown.
Metabolism and Excretion: Eliminated by binding to T lymphocytes.
Half-life: 18 hr.

TIME/ACTION PROFILE (noted as levels of circulating CD3-positive T cells)

ROUTE	ONSET	PEAK	DURATION
IV	mins	2–7 days	1 wk

Contraindications/Precautions
Contraindicated in: Hypersensitivity to muromonab-CD3, murine (mouse) proteins, or polysorbate; Previous muromonab therapy; Fluid overload; Fever >37.8°C or 100°F; Chickenpox or recent exposure to chickenpox; Herpes zoster.
Use Cautiously in: Active infections; Depressed bone marrow reserve; Chronic debilitating illnesses; HF; OB, Lactation, Pedi: Pregnancy, lactation, or children <2 yr (safety not established).

Adverse Reactions/Side Effects
CNS: tremor, aseptic meningitis, dizziness. **Resp:** PULMONARY EDEMA, dyspnea, shortness of breath, wheezing. **CV:** chest pain. **GI:** diarrhea, nausea, vomiting. **Misc:** CYTOKINE RELEASE SYNDROME, INFECTIONS, chills, fever, hypersensitivity reactions, ↑ risk of lymphoma.

Interactions
Drug-Drug: Additive immunosuppression with other **immunosuppressives**. Concurrent **prednisone** and **azathioprine** dosages should be ↓ during muromonab therapy (↑ risk of infection and lymphoproliferative disorders). **Cyclosporine** should be ↓ or discontinued during muromonab-CD3 therapy (↑ risk of infection and lymphoproliferative disorders). ↑ risk of adverse CNS reactions with **indomethacin**. May ↓ antibody response to and ↑ risk of adverse reactions from **live-virus vaccines**.
Drug-Natural Products: Concomitant use with **astragalus**, **echinacea**, and **melatonin** may interfere with immunosuppression.

Route/Dosage
IV (Adults): 5 mg/day for 10–14 days (pretreatment with corticosteroids, acetaminophen, and/or antihistamines recommended).
IV (Children): 0.1 mg (100 mcg)/kg/day for 10–14 days.

Availability
Solution for injection: 1 mg/mL.

M

NURSING IMPLICATIONS
Assessment
- Assess for fluid overload (monitor weight and intake and output, assess for edema and rales/crackles). Notify health care professional if patient has experienced 3% or more weight gain in the previous week. Chest x-ray examination should be obtained within 24 hr before beginning therapy. Fluid-overloaded patients are at high risk of developing pulmonary edema. Monitor vital signs and breath sounds closely.
- Assess for cytokine release syndrome (CRS), usually manifested by high fever and chills, headache, tremor, nausea and vomiting, chest pain, muscle and joint pain, generalized weakness, shortness of breath, dizziness, abdominal pain, malaise, diarrhea, and trembling of hands, but may occasionally cause a severe, life-threatening, shock-like reaction. The severity of this reaction is greatest with initial dose. Reaction occurs within 30–48 hr and may persist for up to 6 hr. Acetaminophen and antihistamines may be used to treat early reactions. Patient temperature should be maintained below 37.8°C (100°F) at administration of each dose. Manifestations of CRS may be prevented or minimized by pretreatment with methylprednisolone sodium succinate 8 mg/kg IV given 1–4 hr before 1st dose of muromonab-CD3. Hydrocortisone 100 mg IV may also be given 30 min after the 1st and possibly 2nd dose to control respiratory side effects. Serious symptoms of CRS may require oxygen, IV fluids, corticosteroids, vasopressors, antihistamines, and intubation.

- Monitor for signs of anaphylactic or hypersensitivity reactions at each dose. Resuscitation equipment should be readily available.
- Monitor for infection (fever, chills, rash, sore throat, purulent discharge, dysuria). Notify physician immediately if these symptoms occur; may necessitate discontinuation of therapy.
- Monitor for development of aseptic meningitis. Onset is usually within 3 days of beginning therapy. Assess for fever, headache, nuchal rigidity, and photophobia.
- ***Lab Test Considerations:*** Monitor CBC with differential and platelet count before and periodically throughout therapy.
- Monitor assays of T cells (CD3, CD4, CD8); target CD3 is <25 cells/mm^3 or plasma levels as determined by ELISA daily; target levels should be ≥800 ng/mL.
- Monitor BUN, serum creatinine, and hepatic enzymes (AST, ALT, alkaline phosphatase, bilirubin), especially during the first 1–3 days of therapy. May cause transient ↑.

Potential Nursing Diagnoses

Risk for infection (Side Effects)
Excess fluid volume (Side Effects)

Implementation

- Physician will reduce dose of corticosteroids and azathioprine and discontinue cyclosporine during 10–14-day course of muromonab-CD3. Cyclosporine may be resumed 3 days before end of therapy.
- Initial dose is administered during hospitalization; patient should be monitored closely for 48 hr. Subsequent doses may be administered on outpatient basis.
- Keep medication refrigerated at 2–8°C. Do not shake vial. Solution may contain a few fine translucent particles that do not affect potency. Discard unused portion.

IV Administration

- **IV Push:** Draw solution into syringe via low-protein-binding 0.2- or 0.22-micrometer filter to ensure removal of translucent protein particles that may be present. Discard filter and attach 20-gauge needle for IV administration.
- ***Concentration:*** 1 mg/mL (undiluted). ***Rate:*** Administer IV push over <1 min. Do not administer as an infusion.
- **Y-Site Incompatibility:** Do not admix; do not administer in IV line containing other medications. If line must be used for other medications, flush with 0.9% NaCl before and after muromonab-CD3.

Patient/Family Teaching

- Explain purpose of medication to patient. Inform patient of possible initial-dose side effects, which are markedly reduced in subsequent doses. Explain that patient will need to resume lifelong therapy with other immunosuppressive drugs after completion of muromonab-CD3 course.
- Inform patient of potential for CRS. Describe reportable symptoms.
- Instruct patient to continue to avoid crowds and persons with known infections, as this drug also suppresses the immune system.
- Advise patient to notify health care professional at first sign of rash, urticaria, tachycardia, dyspnea, or difficulty swallowing.
- May cause dizziness. Caution patient to avoid driving or other activities requiring alertness until response is known.
- Instruct patient not to receive any vaccinations and to avoid contact with persons receiving oral polio vaccine without advice of health care professional.

Evaluation/Desired Outcomes

- Reversal of the symptoms of acute organ rejection.

REMS

mycophenolate mofetil

(mye-koe-**fee**-noe-late **moe**-fe-til)
CellCept

mycophenolic acid

(mye-koe-**fee**-noe-lik)
Myfortic

Classification
Therapeutic: immunosuppressants

Pregnancy Category D

Indications

Mycophenolate mofetil: Prevention of rejection in allogenic renal, hepatic, and cardiac transplantation (used concurrently with cyclosporine and corticosteroids). **Mycophenolic acid**: Prevention of rejection in allogenic renal transplantation (used concurrently with cyclosporine and corticosteroids). **Unlabeled Use:** Nephrotic syndrome.

Action

Inhibits the enzyme inosine monophosphate dehydrogenase, which is involved in purine synthesis. This inhibition results in suppression of T- and B-lymphocyte proliferation. **Therapeutic Effects:** Prevention of heart, kidney, or liver transplant rejection.

Pharmacokinetics

Absorption: Following oral and IV administration, mycophenolate mofetil is rapidly hydrolyzed to mycophenolic acid (MPA), the active metabolite. Absorption of enteric-coated mycophenolic acid (Myfortic) is delayed compared with mycophenolate mofetil (CellCept).

Distribution: Cross the placenta and enter breast milk.

Protein Binding: *MPA*—97%.
Metabolism and Excretion: MPA is extensively metabolized; <1% excreted unchanged in urine. Some enterohepatic recirculation of MPA occurs.
Half-life: *MPA*—8–18 hr.

TIME/ACTION PROFILE (blood levels of MPA)

ROUTE	ONSET	PEAK	DURATION
mycophenolate mofetil-PO	rapid	0.25–1.25 hr	N/A
mycophenolic acid	rapid	1.5–2.75 hr	N/A

Contraindications/Precautions

Contraindicated in: Hypersensitivity; Hypersensitivity to polysorbate 80 (for IV mycophenolate mofetil); OB, Lactation: ↑ risk of congenital anomalies or spontaneous abortion.
Use Cautiously in: Active serious pathology of the GI tract (including history of ulcer disease or GI bleeding); Phenylketonuria (oral suspension contains aspartame); Severe chronic renal impairment (dose not to exceed 1 g twice daily (CellCept) if CCr <25 mL/min/1.73 m²); careful monitoring recommended; Delayed graft function following transplantation (observe for ↑ toxicity); Geri: ↑ risk of adverse reactions related to immunosuppression; Rep: Women with childbearing potential; Pedi: Mycophenolate mofetil approved in children ≥3 mo for renal transplant; mycophenolic acid approved in children ≥5 yr for renal transplant; safety not established for other age groups.

Adverse Reactions/Side Effects

CNS: PROGRESSIVE MULTIFOCAL LEUKOENCEPHALOPATHY (PML), anxiety, dizziness, headache, insomnia, paresthesia, tremor. **CV:** edema, hypertension, hypotension, tachycardia. **Derm:** rashes. **Endo:** hypercholesterolemia, hyperglycemia, hyperkalemia, hypocalcemia, hypokalemia, hypomagnesemia. **GI:** GI BLEEDING, anorexia, constipation, diarrhea, nausea, vomiting, abdominal pain. **GU:** renal dysfunction. **Hemat:** leukocytosis, leukopenia, thrombocytopenia, anemia, pure red cell aplasia. **Resp:** cough, dyspnea. **Misc:** fever, infection (including activation of latent viral infections such as Polyomavirus-associated nephropathy or Hepatitis B/C), ↑ risk of malignancy.

Interactions

Drug-Drug: Combined use with **azathioprine** is not recommended (effects unknown). **Acyclovir** and **ganciclovir** compete with MPA for renal excretion and, in patients with renal dysfunction, may ↑ each other's toxicity. **Magnesium and aluminum hydroxide** antacids ↓ the absorption of MPA (avoid simultaneous administration). **Proton pump inhibitors**, including **dexlansoprazole**, **esomeprazole**, **lansoprazole**, **omeprazole**, **pantoprazole**, and **rabeprazole** may ↓ levels. **Cholestyramine** and **colestipol** ↓ the absorption of MPA (avoid concurrent use). May ↓ the effectiveness of **oral contraceptives** (additional contraceptive method should be used). May ↓ the antibody response to and ↑ risk of adverse reactions from **live-virus vaccines**, although influenza vaccine may be useful. **Amoxicillin/clavulanic acid** or **ciprofloxacin** may ↓ MPA trough levels. **Cyclosporine** may ↓ levels; use caution when discontinuing cyclosporine (may ↑ mycophenolate levels) or when switching from cyclosporine to another immunosupressant, such as tacrolimus or belatacept. **Telmisartan** may ↓ levels.
Drug-Food: When administered with food, peak blood levels of MPA are significantly ↓ (should be administered on an empty stomach).

Route/Dosage

Mycophenolate Mofetil

Renal Transplantation

PO, IV (Adults): 1 g twice daily; IV should be started ≤24 hr after transplantation and switched to PO as soon as possible (IV not recommended for ≥14 days).
PO (Children 3 mo–18 yr): 600 mg/m² twice daily (not to exceed 2 g/day).

Hepatic Transplantation

PO, IV (Adults): 1 g twice daily IV, or 1.5 g twice daily PO. IV should be started ≤24 hr after transplantation and switched to PO as soon as possible (IV not recommended for ≥14 days).

Cardiac Transplantation

PO, IV (Adults): 1.5 g twice daily; IV should be started ≤24 hr after transplantation and switched to PO as soon as possible (IV not recommended for ≥14 days).

Nephrotic syndrome

PO (Children): *Frequent relapses*—12.5–18 mg/kg/dose twice daily; maximum: 2 g/day. *Steroid-dependent*—12–18 mg/kg/dose or 600 mg/m² twice daily; maximum: 2 g/day.

Renal Impairment

PO, IV (Adults): *CCr <25 mL/min*—daily dose should not exceed 2 g.

Mycophenolic Acid

Mycophenolate mofetil and mycophenolic acid should not be used interchangeably without the advice of a health care professional.

Renal Transplantation

PO (Adults): 720 mg twice daily.
PO (Children 5–16 yr and ≥1.19 m²): 400–450 mg/m² twice daily (not to exceed 720 mg twice daily).

Availability (generic available)

Mycophenolate Mofetil

Capsules: 250 mg. **Tablets:** 500 mg. **Oral suspension (fruit flavor):** 200 mg/mL. **Powder for injection (requires reconstitution):** 500 mg/vial.

Mycophenolic Acid

Delayed-release tablets: 180 mg, 360 mg.

NURSING IMPLICATIONS

Assessment

- Assess for symptoms of organ rejection throughout therapy.
- Assess for signs of PML (hemiparesis, apathy, confusion, cognitive deficiencies, and ataxia) periodically during therapy.
- ***Lab Test Considerations:*** Obtain a urine pregnancy test with a specificity of 25 mIU/mL immediately prior to beginning therapy and again 8–10 days later. Repeat pregnancy tests should be preformed during routine follow-up visits.
- Monitor CBC with differential weekly during the 1st month, twice monthly for the 2nd and 3rd month of therapy, and then monthly during the 1st yr. Neutropenia occurs most frequently from 31–180 days post-transplant. If ANC is <1000/mm^3, dose should be reduced or discontinued.
- Monitor hepatic and renal status and electrolytes periodically during therapy. May cause ↑ serum alkaline phosphatase, AST, ALT, LDH, BUN, and creatinine. May also cause hyperkalemia, hypokalemia, hypocalcemia, hypomagnesemia, hyperglycemia, and hyperlipidemia.

Potential Nursing Diagnoses

Risk for infection (Adverse Reactions)

Implementation

- The initial dose of mycophenolate (usually IV) should be given within 24 hr of transplant.
- Women of childbearing yr should have a negative serum or urine pregnancy test within 1 wk prior to initiation of therapy.
- Mycophenolate mofetil (Cellcept) and mycophenolic acid (Myfortic) are not interchangeable; rate of absorption is different.
- **PO:** Administer on an empty stomach, 1 hr before or 2 hr after meals. Capsules and delayed-release tablets should be swallowed whole; do not open, crush, or chew. Mycophenolate may be teratogenic; contents of capsules should not be inhaled or come in contact with skin or mucous membranes.
- Do not administer mycophenolate concurrently with antacids containing magnesium or aluminum.

IV Administration

- **IV:** IV route should only be used for patients unable to take oral medication and should be switched to oral dose form as soon as patient can tolerate capsules or tablets.
- **Intermittent Infusion:** ***Diluent:*** Reconstitute each vial with 14 mL of D5W. Shake gently to dissolve. Solution is slightly yellow; discard if solution is discolored or contains particulate matter. Dilute contents of 2 vials (1-g dose) further with 140 mL of D5W or 3 vials (1.5-g dose) with 210 mL of D5W. ***Concentration:*** 6 mg/mL. Solution is stable for 4 hr. ***Rate:*** Administer via slow IV infusion over 2 hr. Do not administer as a bolus or via rapid infusion.
- **Y-Site Compatibility:** alemtuzumab, alfentanil, amikacin, amiodarone, anidulafungin, argatroban, bivalirudin, bumetanide, buprenorphine, butorphanol, calcium chloride, caspofungin, chlorpromazine, ciprofloxacin, cisatracurium, daptomycin, dexmedetomidine, dexrazoxane, digoxin, diltiazem, diphenhydramine, dobutamine, dolasetron, dopamine, doxorubicin liposomal, doxycycline, droperidol, enalaprilat, ephedrine, epinephrine, erythromycin, esmolol, famotidine, fenoldopam, fentanyl, fluconazole, gentamicin, glycopyrrolate, granisetron, haloperidol, hydralazine, hydromorphone, insulin, isoproterenol, labetalol, leucovorin, levofloxacin, lidocaine, linezolid, lorazepam, magnesium sulfate, mannitol, meperidine, mesna, methyldopate, metoclopramide, metoprolol, metronidazole, midazolam, milrinone, morphine, moxifloxacin, nalbuphine, naloxone, nesiritide, nicardipine, nitroglycerin, norepinephrine, octreotide, ondansetron, oxytocin, pamidronate, pancuronium, pentamidine, phenylephrine, potassium chloride, procainamide, prochlorperazine, promethazine, propranolol, quinupristin/dalfopristin, ranitidine, remifentanil, rocuronium, succinylcholine, sufentanil, tacrolimus, theophylline, tigecycline, tirofiban, tobramycin, vancomycin, vasopressin, vecuronium, verapamil, voriconazole, zidovudine, zoledronic acid.
- **Y-Site Incompatibility:** acyclovir, allopurinol, amifostine, aminophylline, amphotericin B colloidal, amphotericin B lipid complex, amphotericin B liposome, ampicillin, ampicillin/sulbactam, azithromycin, aztreonam, calcium gluconate, cangrelor, cefazolin, cefotaxime, cefotetan, cefoxitin, ceftazidime, ceftriaxone, cefuroxime, chloramphenicol, clindamycin, dantrolene, dexamethasone, diazepam, eptifibatide, foscarnet, fosphenytoin, furosemide, ganciclovir, heparin, hydrocortisone, imipenem/cilastatin, ketorolac, meropenem, methotrexate, methylprednisolone, micafungin, nafcillin, nitroprusside, pantoprazole, pentobarbital, phenobarbital, phenytoin, piperacillin/tazobactam, potassium acetate, potassoim phosphates, sodium acetate, sodium phosphates, trimethoprim/sulfamethoxazole.

Patient/Family Teaching

- Instruct patient to take medication as directed, at the same time each day. Take missed dose as soon as remembered, but not if almost time for next dose. Do not skip or double up on missed doses. Do not discontinue without consulting health care professional.

- Reinforce the need for lifelong therapy to prevent transplant rejection. Review symptoms of rejection for the transplanted organ, and stress need to notify health care professional immediately if signs of rejection or infection occur.
- Instruct patient to notify health care professional immediately if signs and symptoms of infection (temperature ≥100.5°F, cold symptoms [runny nose, sore throat], flu symptoms [upset stomach, stomach pain, vomiting, diarrhea], earache or headache, pain during urination, frequent urination, white patches in mouth or throat, unexpected bruising or bleeding, cuts, scrapes, or incisions that are red, warm, and oozing pus) or PML.
- Advise patient to avoid contact with persons with contagious diseases.
- Advise patient to avoid vaccinations with live attenuated virus during therapy.
- Inform patient of the increased risk of lymphoma and other malignancies. Advise patient to use sunscreen and wear protective clothing to decrease risk of skin cancer.
- Advise patient to notify health care professional of all Rx or OTC medications, vitamins, or herbal products being taken and to consult with health care professional before taking other medications.
- Rep: Inform female patients of the importance of simultaneously using two reliable forms of contraception, unless abstinence is the chosen method, prior to beginning, during, and for 6 wk following discontinuation of therapy and to avoid breast feeding. Discuss acceptable forms of contraception with health care professional. Encourage patients who become pregnant during or within 6 wk after therapy to enroll in the Pregnancy Registry by calling 1–800–617–8191 to help the Health Care Community better understand the effects of mycophenolate during pregnancy.
- Emphasize the importance of routine follow-up laboratory tests.

M

Evaluation/Desired Outcomes

- Prevention of rejection of transplanted organs.

nadolol (nay-doe-lole)

Corgard, ✱Syn-Nadolol

Classification

Therapeutic: antianginals, antihypertensives

Pharmacologic: beta blockers

Pregnancy Category C

Indications

Management of hypertension. Management of angina pectoris. **Unlabeled Use:** Arrhythmias. Migraine prophylaxis. Tremors (essential, lithium-induced, parkinsonian). Aggressive behavior. Antipsychotic-associated akathisia. Situational anxiety. Esophageal varices. Reduction of intraocular pressure.

Action

Blocks stimulation of $beta_1$ (myocardial) and $beta_2$ (pulmonary, vascular, and uterine) receptor sites. **Therapeutic Effects:** Decreased heart rate and BP.

Pharmacokinetics

Absorption: 30% absorbed after oral administration.

Distribution: Minimal penetration of the CNS. Crosses the placenta and enters breast milk.

Metabolism and Excretion: 70% excreted unchanged by the kidneys.

Half-life: 10–24 hr (↑ in renal impairment).

TIME/ACTION PROFILE (anithypertensive effects)

ROUTE	ONSET	PEAK	DURATION
PO†	up to 5 days	6–9 days	24 hr

†With chronic dosing.

Contraindications/Precautions

Contraindicated in: Uncompensated HF; Pulmonary edema; Cardiogenic shock; Bradycardia or heart block.

Use Cautiously in: Renal impairment (CCr <50 mL/min); Hepatic impairment; Pulmonary disease (including asthma); Diabetes mellitus (may mask signs of hypoglycemia); Thyrotoxicosis (may mask symptoms); Patients with a history of severe allergic reactions (intensity of reactions may be ↑); OB: Crosses the placenta and may cause fetal/neonatal bradycardia, hypotension, hypoglycemia, or respiratory depression; Lactation: Pedi: Safety not established; Geri: ↑ sensitivity to beta blockers; initial dose ↓ recommended.

Adverse Reactions/Side Effects

CNS: fatigue, weakness, anxiety, depression, dizziness, drowsiness, insomnia, memory loss, mental status changes, nightmares. **EENT:** blurred vision, dry eyes, nasal stuffiness. **Resp:** bronchospasm, wheezing. **CV:** ARRHYTHMIAS, BRADYCARDIA, HF, PULMONARY EDEMA, orthostatic hypotension, peripheral vasoconstriction. **GI:** constipation, diarrhea, nausea. **GU:** erectile dysfunction, ↓ libido. **Derm:** itching, rashes. **Endo:** hyperglycemia, hypoglycemia. **MS:** arthralgia, back pain, muscle cramps. **Neuro:** paresthesia. **Misc:** drug-induced lupus syndrome.

Interactions

Drug-Drug: General anesthesia, IV phenytoin, diltiazem, and **verapamil** may cause additive myocardial depression. Additive bradycardia may occur with **digoxin**. Additive hypotension may occur with other **antihypertensives**, acute ingestion of **alcohol**, or **nitrates**. Concurrent use with **amphetamines, cocaine, ephedrine, epinephrine, norepinephrine, phenylephrine**, or **pseudoephedrine** may result in unopposed alpha-adrenergic stimulation (excessive hypertension, bradycardia). Concurrent use with **clonidine** ↑ hypotension and bradycardia. Concurrent **thyroid** administration may ↓ effectiveness. May alter the effectiveness of **insulins** or **oral hypoglycemic agents** (dosage adjustments may be necessary). May ↓ the effectiveness of **theophylline**. May ↓ the effects of **dopamine** or **dobutamine**. Use cautiously within 14 days of **MAO inhibitor therapy** (may result in hypertension). Concurrent **NSAIDs** may ↓ antihypertensive action.

N

Route/Dosage

PO (Adults): *Antianginal*—40 mg once daily initially; may ↑ by 40–80 mg/day q 3–7 days as needed (up to 240 mg/day). *Antihypertensive*—40 mg once daily initially; may ↑ by 40–80 mg/day q 7 days as needed (up to 320 mg/day).

Renal Impairment

PO (Adults): *CCr 31–50 mL/min*—↑ dosing interval to 24–36 hr; *CCr 10–30 mL/min*—↑ dosing interval to 24–48 hr; *CCr <10 mL/min*—↑ dosing interval to 40–60 hr.

Availability (generic available)

Tablets: 20 mg, 40 mg, 80 mg. ***In combination with:*** bendroflumethiazide (Corzide). See Appendix B.

NURSING IMPLICATIONS

Assessment

- Monitor BP and pulse frequently during dose adjustment and periodically during therapy. Assess for orthostatic hypotension when assisting patient up from supine position.
- Monitor intake and output ratios and daily weight. Assess patient routinely for evidence of fluid overload (peripheral edema, dyspnea, rales/crackles, fatigue, weight gain, jugular venous distention).

- **Hypertension:** Check frequency of refills to determine compliance.
- **Angina:** Assess frequency and characteristics of angina periodically during therapy.
- ***Lab Test Considerations:*** May cause increased BUN, serum lipoprotein, potassium, triglyceride, and uric acid levels.
- May cause increased ANA titers.
- May cause increase in blood glucose levels.
- ***Toxicity and Overdose:*** Monitor patients receiving beta blockers for signs of overdose (bradycardia, severe dizziness or fainting, severe drowsiness, dyspnea, bluish fingernails or palms, seizures). Notify physician or other health care professional immediately if these signs occur.

Potential Nursing Diagnoses

Decreased cardiac output (Side Effects)
Noncompliance (Patient/Family Teaching)

Implementation

- Discontinuation of concurrent clonidine should be done gradually, with beta blocker discontinued first; then, after several days, discontinue clonidine.
- **PO:** Take apical pulse before administering. If <50 bpm or if arrhythmia occurs, withhold medication and notify physician or other health care professional.
- May be administered with food or on an empty stomach.
- Tablets may be crushed and mixed with food.

Patient/Family Teaching

- Instruct patient to take medication exactly as directed, at the same time each day, even if feeling well; do not skip or double up on missed doses. Take missed doses as soon as possible up to 8 hr before next dose. Abrupt withdrawal may precipitate life-threatening arrhythmias, hypertension, or myocardial ischemia.
- Advise patient to ensure that enough medication is available for weekends, holidays, and vacations. A written prescription may be kept in wallet for emergencies.
- Teach patient and family how to check pulse and BP. Instruct them to check pulse daily and BP biweekly. Advise patient to hold dose and contact health care professional if pulse is <50 bpm or if BP changes significantly.
- May cause drowsiness or dizziness. Caution patients to avoid driving or other activities that require alertness until response to the drug is known.
- Advise patients to make position changes slowly to minimize orthostatic hypotension, especially during initiation of therapy or when dose is increased.
- Caution patient that this medication may increase sensitivity to cold.
- Instruct patient to consult health care professional before taking any OTC medications, especially cold preparations, concurrently with this medication.
- Patients with diabetes should closely monitor blood glucose, especially if weakness, malaise, irritability, or fatigue occurs. Medication may mask some signs of hypoglycemia, but dizziness and sweating may still occur.
- Advise patient to notify health care professional if slow pulse, difficulty breathing, wheezing, cold hands and feet, dizziness, confusion, depression, rash, fever, sore throat, unusual bleeding, or bruising occurs.
- Instruct patient to inform health care professional of medication regimen before treatment or surgery.
- Advise patient to carry identification describing disease process and medication regimen at all times.
- **Hypertension:** Reinforce the need to continue additional therapies for hypertension (weight loss, sodium restriction, stress reduction, regular exercise, moderation of alcohol consumption, and smoking cessation). Medication controls but does not cure hypertension.
- **Angina:** Caution patient to avoid overexertion with decrease in chest pain.

Evaluation/Desired Outcomes

- Decrease in BP.
- Reduction in frequency of angina.
- Increase in activity tolerance. May require up to 5 days before therapeutic effects are seen.

nafarelin (na-**fare**-e-lin)

Synarel

Classification
Therapeutic: hormones
Pharmacologic: gonadotropin-releasing hormones

Pregnancy Category X

Indications

Endometriosis. Central precocious puberty (gonadotropin-dependent) in children.

Action

Acts as a synthetic analogue of gonadotropin-releasing hormone (GnRH). Initially increases pituitary production of luteinizing hormone (LH) and follicle-stimulating hormone (FSH), which cause ovarian steroid production. Chronic administration leads to decreased production of gonadotropins. Endometriotic lesions are sensitive to ovarian hormones. **Therapeutic Effects:** Reduction in lesions and associated pain in endometriosis. Arrest and regression of puberty in children with central precocious puberty.

Pharmacokinetics

Absorption: Well absorbed following intranasal administration.
Distribution: Unknown.
Metabolism and Excretion: 20–40% excreted in feces; 3% excreted unchanged by the kidneys.

Half-life: 3 hr.

TIME/ACTION PROFILE (↓ ovarian steroid production)

ROUTE	ONSET	PEAK	DURATION
Intranasal	within 4 wk	3–4 wk	3–6 mo†

†Relief of symptoms of endometriosis following discontinuation.

Contraindications/Precautions

Contraindicated in: Hypersensitivity to GnRH, its analogues, or sorbitol; OB, Lactation: Pregnancy or lactation.

Use Cautiously in: Rhinitis.

Adverse Reactions/Side Effects

CNS: STROKE, emotional instability, headaches, depression, insomnia. **EENT:** nasal irritation. **CV:** MYOCARDIAL INFARCTION, edema. **GU:** vaginal dryness. **Derm:** acne, hirsutism, seborrhea. **Endo:** cessation of menses, impaired fertility, ↓ breast size. **Metab:** hyperglycemia. **MS:** ↓ bone density, myalgia. **Misc:** ↓ libido, hot flashes, hypersensitivity reactions, weight gain.

Interactions

Drug-Drug: Concurrent **topical nasal decongestants** may ↓ absorption of nafarelin (administer decongestant at least 2 hr after nafarelin).

Route/Dosage

Intranasal (Adults): *Endometriosis*—1 spray (200 mcg) in 1 nostril in the morning and 1 spray in the other nostril in the evening (400 mcg/day). May ↑ to 1 spray in each nostril in the morning and evening (800 mcg/day).

Intranasal (Children): *Central precocious puberty*—2 sprays in each nostril in the morning and in the evening (1600 mcg/day); may ↑ up to 1800 mcg/day (3 sprays in alternating nostrils 3 times daily).

Availability

Nasal spray: 2 mg/mL (200 mcg/spray).

NURSING IMPLICATIONS

Assessment

- **Endometriosis:** Assess patient for endometriotic pain periodically during therapy.
- **Central Precocious Puberty:** Prior to therapy, a complete physical and endocrinologic examination including height, weight, hand and wrist x-ray, total sex steroid level (estradiol or testosterone), adrenal steroid level, beta human chorionic gonadotropin level, GnRH stimulation test, pelvic/adrenal/testicular ultrasound, and CT of the head must be performed. These parameters are monitored after 6–8 wk and every 3–6 mo during therapy.
- Assess patient for signs of precocious puberty (menses, breast development, testicular growth) periodically during therapy.
- Nafarelin is discontinued when the onset of normal puberty is desired. Monitor the onset of normal puberty and assess menstrual cycle, reproductive function, and final adult height.

Potential Nursing Diagnoses

Acute pain (Indications)
Sexual dysfunction (Indications, Side Effects)

Implementation

- **Endometriosis:** Treatment should be started between days 2 and 4 of the menstrual cycle and continued for up to 6 mo.

Patient/Family Teaching

- Instruct patient on the correct technique for nasal spray: The head should be tilted back slightly; wait 30 sec between sprays.
- Advise patient to consult health care professional if rhinitis occurs during therapy. If a topical decongestant is needed, do not use decongestant until 2 hr after nafarelin dosing. If possible, avoid sneezing during and immediately after nafarelin dose.
- **Endometriosis:** Inform patient that 1 spray should be administered into 1 nostril in the morning and 1 spray into the other nostril in the evening for the 400 mcg/day dose. If dose is increased to 800 mcg/day, administer 1 spray to each nostril (2 sprays) morning and evening; 1 bottle should provide a 30-day supply at the 400 mcg/day dose.
- Advise patient to use a form of contraception other than oral contraceptives during therapy. Inform patient that amenorrhea is expected. Instruct patient to notify health care professional if regular menstruation persists or if successive doses are missed.
- Advise patient that medication may cause hot flashes. Notify health care professional if these become bothersome.
- **Central Precocious Puberty:** Instruct patient on correct timing and number of sprays. The 1600 mcg/day dose is achieved by 2 sprays to each nostril in the morning (4 sprays) and 2 sprays to each nostril in the evening (4 sprays), for a total of 8 sprays. The 1800 mcg/day dose is achieved by 3 sprays into alternating nostrils 3 times per day, for a total of 9 sprays. Inform patient and parents that if doses are not taken as directed pubertal process may be reactivated. One bottle should provide a 7-day supply at the 1600 mcg/day dose.
- Advise patient and parents that during 1st mo of therapy some signs of puberty (vaginal bleeding, breast enlargement) may occur. These should resolve after the 1st mo of therapy. If these signs persist after the 2nd mo of therapy, notify health care professional.

Evaluation/Desired Outcomes

- Reduction in lesions and associated pain in endometriosis.
- Resolution of the signs of precocious puberty.

nafcillin, See PENICILLINS, PENICILLINASE RESISTANT.

naftifine, See ANTIFUNGALS (TOPICAL).

HIGH ALERT

nalbuphine (nal-byoo-feen)

~~Nubain~~, ✽Nubain

Classification

Therapeutic: opioid analgesics

Pharmacologic: opioid agonists/analgesics

Pregnancy Category C

Indications

Moderate to severe pain. Also provides: Analgesia during labor, Sedation before surgery, Supplement to balanced anesthesia. Prevention or treatment of opioid-induced pruritus.

Action

Binds to opiate receptors in the CNS. Alters the perception of and response to painful stimuli while producing generalized CNS depression. In addition, has partial antagonist properties, which may result in opioid withdrawal in physically dependent patients. **Therapeutic Effects:** Decreased pain.

Pharmacokinetics

Absorption: Well absorbed after IM and subcut administration.

Distribution: Probably crosses the placenta and enters breast milk.

Protein Binding: 50%.

Metabolism and Excretion: Mostly metabolized by the liver and eliminated in the feces via biliary excretion. Minimal amounts excreted unchanged by the kidneys.

Half-life: Children 1–8 yrs: 0.9 hr; Adults: 3.5–5 hr.

TIME/ACTION PROFILE (analgesia)

ROUTE	ONSET	PEAK	DURATION
IM	<15 min	60 min	3–6 hr
Subcut	<15 min	unknown	3–6 hr
IV	2–3 min	30 min	3–6 hr

Contraindications/Precautions

Contraindicated in: Hypersensitivity to nalbuphine or bisulfites; Patients physically dependent on opioids and who have not been detoxified (may precipitate withdrawal).

Use Cautiously in: Head trauma; ↑ intracranial pressure; Severe renal, hepatic, or pulmonary disease; Hypothyroidism; Adrenal insufficiency; Alcoholism; Undiagnosed abdominal pain; Prostatic hyperplasia; Patients who have recently received opioid agonists; OB: Has been used during labor but may cause respiratory depression in the newborn; Geri: Dose ↓ suggested.

Adverse Reactions/Side Effects

CNS: dizziness, headache, sedation, confusion, dysphoria, euphoria, floating feeling, hallucinations, unusual dreams. **EENT:** blurred vision, diplopia, miosis (high doses). **Resp:** respiratory depression. **CV:** hypertension, orthostatic hypotension, palpitations. **GI:** dry mouth, nausea, vomiting, constipation, ileus. **GU:** urinary urgency. **Derm:** clammy feeling, sweating. **Misc:** physical dependence, psychological dependence, tolerance.

Interactions

Drug-Drug: Use with extreme caution in patients receiving **MAO inhibitors** (may result in unpredictable, severe reactions—↓ initial dose of nalbuphine to 25% of usual dose). Additive CNS depression with **alcohol**, **antihistamines**, and **sedative/hypnotics**. May precipitate withdrawal in patients who are physically dependent on **opioid agonists**. Avoid concurrent use with other **opioid analgesic agonists** (may diminish analgesic effect).

Drug-Natural Products: Concomitant use of **kava-kava**, **valerian**, **skullcap**, **chamomile**, or **hops** can ↑ CNS depression.

Route/Dosage

Analgesia

IM, Subcut, IV (Adults): Usual dose is 10 mg q 3–6 hr (maximum: 20 mg/dose or 160 mg/day).

IM, Subcut, IV (Children): 0.1–0.15 mg/kg q 3–6 hr (maximum: 20 mg/dose or 160 mg/day).

Supplement to Balanced Anesthesia

IV (Adults): *Initial*—0.3–3 mg/kg over 10–15 min. *Maintenance*—0.25–0.5 mg/kg as needed.

Opioid-induced pruritus

IV (Adults): 2.5–5 mg; may repeat dose.

Availability (generic available)

Solution for injection: 10 mg/mL, 20 mg/mL.

NURSING IMPLICATIONS

Assessment

- Assess type, location, and intensity of pain before and 1 hr after IM or 30 min (peak) after IV administration. When titrating opioid doses, increases of 25–50% should be administered until there is either a 50% reduction in the patient's pain rating on a numeric or visual analogue scale or the patient reports satisfactory pain relief. A repeat dose can be safely administered at the time of the peak if previous dose is ineffective and side effects are minimal. Patients requiring doses higher than 20 mg should be converted to an opioid agonist. Nalbuphine is not recommended for prolonged use or as first-line therapy for acute or cancer pain.

- An equianalgesic chart (see Appendix I) should be used when changing routes or when changing from one opioid to another.
- Assess BP, pulse, and respirations before and periodically during administration. If respiratory rate is <10/min, assess level of sedation. Physical stimulation may be sufficient to prevent significant hypoventilation. Dose may need to be decreased by 25–50%. Nalbuphine produces respiratory depression, but this does not markedly increase with increased doses.
- Assess previous analgesic history. Antagonistic properties may induce withdrawal symptoms (vomiting, restlessness, abdominal cramps, and increased BP and temperature) in patients physically dependent on opioids.
- Although this drug has a low potential for dependence, prolonged use may lead to physical and psychological dependence and tolerance. This should not prevent patient from receiving adequate analgesia. Most patients who receive nalbuphine for pain do not develop psychological dependence. If tolerance develops, changing to an opioid agonist may be required to relieve pain.
- ***Lab Test Considerations:*** May cause ↑ serum amylase and lipase concentrations.
- ***Toxicity and Overdose:*** If an opioid antagonist is required to reverse respiratory depression or coma, naloxone (Narcan) is the antidote. Dilute the 0.4-mg ampule of naloxone in 10 mL of 0.9% NaCl and administer 0.5 mL (0.02 mg) by IV push every 2 min. For children and patients weighing <40 kg, dilute 0.1 mg of naloxone in 10 mL of 0.9% NaCl for a concentration of 10 mcg/mL and administer 0.5 mcg/kg every 2 min. Titrate dose to avoid withdrawal, seizures, and severe pain.

Potential Nursing Diagnoses

Acute pain (Indications)
Risk for injury (Side Effects)
Disturbed sensory perception (visual, auditory) (Side Effects)

Implementation

- ***High Alert:*** Do not confuse nalbuphine with naloxone.
- Explain therapeutic value of medication before administration to enhance the analgesic effect.
- Regularly administered doses may be more effective than prn administration. Analgesic is more effective if administered before pain becomes severe.
- Coadministration with nonopioid analgesics may have additive effects and permit lower opioid doses.
- **IM:** Administer deep into well-developed muscle. Rotate sites of injections.

IV Administration

- **IV Push:** May give IV undiluted.
- ***Concentration:*** 10–20 mg/mL. ***Rate:*** Administer slowly, each 10 mg over 3–5 min.
- **Y-Site Compatibility:** acetaminophen, alfentanil, amifostine, amikacin, aminocaproic acid, aminophylline, amiodarone, argatroban, atropine, azithromycin, aztreonam, benztropine, bivalirudin, cisatracurium, cladribine, bleomycin, bumetanide, buprenorphine, butorphanol, calcium chloride, calcium gluconate, cangrelor, carboplatin, carmustine, cefazolin, cefotaxime, cefoxitin, ceftazidime, ceftriaxone, cefuroxime, chlorpromazine, cisatracurium, cladribine, clindamycin, cyanocobalamin, cyclophosphamide, cytarabine, dacarbazine, dactinomycin, daptomycin, daunorubicin hydrochloride, dexamethasone, dexmedetomidine, dexrazoxane, digoxin, diltiazem, diphenhydramine, dobutamine, dolasetron, dopamine, doxorubicin hydrochloride, doxorubicin liposomal, enalaprilat, ephedrine, epinephrine, epirubicin, epoetin alfa, eptifibatide, ertapenem, erythromycin, esmolol, etoposide, etoposide phosphate, famotidine, fenoldopam, fentanyl, filgrastim, fluconazole, fludarabine, fluorouracil, foscarnet, fosphenytoin, gemcitabine, gentamicin, glycopyrrolate, granisetron, heparin, hetastarch, idarubicin, ifosfamide, insulin, irinotecan, isoproterenol, labetalol, leucovorin, levofloxacin, lidocaine, linezolid, lorazepam, magnesium sulfate, mannitol, mechlorethamine, melphalan, meperidine, mesna, methyldopate, metoclopramide, metoprolol, midazolam, milrinone, mitoxantrone, morphine, multivitamins, mycophenolate, naloxone, nesiritide, nicardipine, nitroglycerin, nitroprusside, norepinephrine, octreotide, ondansetron, oxaliplatin, oxytocin, paclitaxel, palosetron, pamidronate, pancuronium, papaverine, penicillin G, phenylephrine, phytonadione, potassium acetate, potassium chloride, procainamide, prochlorperazine, promethazine, propofol, propranolol, protamine, pyridoxine, ranitidine, remifentanil, rituximab, rocuronium, sodium acetate, succinylcholine, sufentanil, tacrolimus, teniposide, theophylline, thiamine, thiotepa, tigecycline, tirofiban, tobramycin, topotecan, vancomycin, vasopressin, vecuronium, verapamil, vinblastine, vincristine, vinorelbine, voriconazole, zoledronic acid.
- **Y-Site Incompatibility:** alemtuzumab, allopurinol, amphotericin B colloidal, amphotericin B lipid com-

N

plex, amphotericin B liposome, anidulafungin, cefepime, cholramphenicol, cyclosporine, dantrolene, diazepam, docetaxel, folic acid, furosemide, ganciclovir, hydrocortisone, imipenem/cilastatin, indomethacin, ketorolac, methotrexate, methylprednisolone, mitomycin, pantoprazole, pemetrexed, pentamidine, pentobarbital, phenobarbital, phenytoin, piperacillin/tazobactam, sargramostim, sodium bicarbonate, streptokinase, trastuzumab, trimethoprim/sulfamethoxazole.

Patient/Family Teaching

- Instruct patient on how and when to ask for pain medication.
- May cause drowsiness or dizziness. Advise patient to call for assistance when ambulating and to avoid driving or other activities requiring alertness until response to the medication is known.
- Caution patient to change positions slowly to minimize orthostatic hypotension.
- Advise patient that frequent mouth rinses, good oral hygiene, and sugarless gum or candy may decrease dry mouth.
- Encourage patient to turn, cough, and breathe deeply every 2 hr to prevent atelectasis.
- Advise patient to avoid concurrent use of alcohol or other CNS depressants with this medication.
- Advise patient to notify health care professional if pregnancy is planned or suspected, or if breast feeding.

Evaluation/Desired Outcomes

- Decrease in severity of pain without significant alteration in level of consciousness or respiratory status.

naloxegol (nal-ox-ee-gol)

Movantik

Classification
Therapeutic: laxatives
Pharmacologic: opioid antagonists

Schedule II

Pregnancy Category C

Indications

Treatment of opioid-caused constipation (OIC) in patients receiving chronic opioids for chronic non-cancer pain when traditional laxatives have failed.

Action

Acts peripherally as a mu receptor antagonist, blocking opioid receptors in the GI tract. **Therapeutic Effects:** Blocks constipating effects of opioids on the GI tract without loss of analgesia.

Pharmacokinetics

Absorption: Systemic absorption follows oral administration. A high-fat meal ↑ absorption.

Distribution: Does not cross the blood-brain barrier.

Metabolism and Excretion: Metabolized primarily by the CYP3A4 enzyme system; 68% excreted in feces, 16% in urine mostly as metabolites.

Half-life: 6–11 hr.

TIME/ACTION PROFILE (spontaneous bowel movement)

ROUTE	ONSET	PEAK	DURATION
PO	within 24 hr	unknown	unknown

Contraindications/Precautions

Contraindicated in: Hypersensitivity; Known/suspected/history of gastrointestinal obstruction; Severe hepatic impairment; Concurrent use of strong CYP3A4 inhibitors, strong CYP3A4 inducers, other opioid antagonists or grapefruit/grapefruit juice; Severe hepatic impairment; Lactation: May precipitate opioid withdrawal in infant.

Use Cautiously in: Patients with disruption of the blood-brain barrier (may precipitate opioid withdrawal); Geri: Blood levels are ↑ in elderly Japanese patients; OB: May precipitate fetal opioid withdrawal (use only if potential benefit justifies potential risk to fetus); Pedi: Safe and effective use in children has not been established.

Adverse Reactions/Side Effects

CNS: headache. **GI:** GASTROINTESTINAL PERFORATION, abdominal pain, diarrhea, flatulence, nausea, vomiting. **Derm:** sweating. **Misc:** opioid withdrawal.

Interactions

Drug-Drug: Concurrent use of **strong CYP3A4 inhibitors** including **clarithromycin** and **ketoconazole** ↑ risk of toxicity/adverse reactions and is contraindicated. Concurrent use of **moderate CYP3A4 inhibitors** including **diltiazem**, **erythromycin**, and **verapamil** may also↑ risk of toxicity/adverse reactions; dose reduction and careful monitoring recommended. Concurrent use of **strong CYP3A4 inducers** including **rifampin** may ↓ blood levels/effectiveness and is contraindicated. Concurrent use of other **opioid antagonists** may precipitate opioid withdrawal and is contraindicated. Concurrent use of **methadone** for pain ↑ risk of stomach pain and diarrhea.

Drug-Food: Grapefruit/grapefruit juice may ↑ blood levels and the risk of toxicity/adverse reactions and should be avoided.

Route/Dosage

PO (Adults): 25 mg once daily, if poorly tolerated decrease dose to 12.5 mg; *concurrent use of moderate CYP3A4 inhibitors*— 12.5 mg daily (careful monitoring recommended).

Renal Impairment

PO (Adults): *CCr <60 mL/min*— 12.5 mg daily initially, may be cautiously increased to 25 mg/day if necessary with careful monitoring.

Availability
Tablets: 12.5 mg, 25 mg.

NURSING IMPLICATIONS
Assessment
- Assess bowel sounds and frequency, quantity, and consistency of stools periodically during therapy.
- Monitor pain intensity during therapy. Naloxegol does not affect pain or effects of opioid analgesics on pain control. Discontinue naloxegol if opioid analgesic is discontinued.
- Monitor for signs and symptoms of gastrointestinal perforation (severe, persistent or worsening abdominal pain) periodically during therapy. Discontinue naloxegol if symptoms occur.

Potential Nursing Diagnoses
Constipation (Indications)
Diarrhea (Adverse Reactions)

Implementation
- Discontinue all maintenance laxative therapy before starting naloxegol. If a suboptimal response occurs with naloxegol, laxatives may be used after 3 days.
- **PO:** Administer on an empty stomach at least 1 hr before first meal in morning or 2 hrs after meal. Swallow tablet whole; do not break, crush, or chew.
- Avoid grapefruit and grapefruit juice during therapy.

Patient/Family Teaching
- Instruct patient to take naloxegol on an empty stomach as directed. Laxatives should be stopped before starting naloxegol, but may be restarted after 3 days if needed. Advise patient to read *Medication Guide* prior to starting therapy and with each refill in case of changes.
- Caution patient to avoid grapefruit and grapefruit juice during therapy.
- Advise patient to notify health care professional immediately if stomach pain that does not go away occurs.
- Advise patient to notify health care professional if signs and symptoms of opioid withdrawal (sweating, chills, diarrhea, stomach pain, anxiety, irritability, yawning) occur. Patients taking methadone for pain are at increased risk for stomach pain and diarrhea.
- Instruct patient to stop taking naloxegol if they stop taking opioid medications.
- Instruct patient to notify health care professional of all Rx or OTC medications, vitamins, or herbal products being taken and consult health care professional before taking any new medications.
- Advise female patients to notify health care professional if pregnancy is planned or suspected or if breast feeding.

Evaluation/Desired Outcomes
- Relief of opioid induced constipation, especially if opioid therapy has been for 4 wks or more.

naloxone (nal-ox-one)
Evzio, ~~Narcan~~

Classification
Therapeutic: antidotes (for opioids)
Pharmacologic: opioid antagonists

Pregnancy Category B

Indications
Reversal of CNS depression and respiratory depression because of suspected opioid overdose. **Unlabeled Use:** Opioid-induced pruritus (low-dose IV infusion). Management of refractory circulatory shock.

Action
Competitively blocks the effects of opioids, including CNS and respiratory depression, without producing any agonist (opioid-like) effects. **Therapeutic Effects:** Reversal of signs of opioid excess.

Pharmacokinetics
Absorption: Well absorbed after IM or subcut administration. Rapidly absorbed from nasal mucosa.
Distribution: Rapidly distributed to tissues. Crosses the placenta.
Metabolism and Excretion: Metabolized by the liver.
Half-life: 60–90 min (up to 3 hr in neonates).

TIME/ACTION PROFILE (reversal of opioid effects)

ROUTE	ONSET	PEAK	DURATION
IV	1–2 min	unknown	45 min
IM, Subcut	2–5 min	unknown	>45 min
Intranasal	8–13 min	unknown	unknown

Contraindications/Precautions
Contraindicated in: Hypersensitivity.
Use Cautiously in: Cardiovascular disease; Patients physically dependent on opioids (may precipitate severe withdrawal); OB: May cause acute withdrawal syndrome in mother and fetus if mother is opioid dependent; Lactation: Safety not established; Pedi: May cause acute withdrawal syndrome in neonates of opioid-dependent mothers.

Adverse Reactions/Side Effects
CV: VENTRICULAR ARRHYTHMIAS, hypertension, hypotension. **GI:** nausea, vomiting.

Interactions
Drug-Drug: Can precipitate withdrawal in patients physically dependent on **opioid analgesics**. Larger

doses may be required to reverse the effects of **buprenorphine**, **butorphanol**, **nalbuphine**, or **pentazocine**. Antagonizes postoperative **opioid analgesics**.

Route/Dosage

Postoperative Opioid-Induced Respiratory Depression

IV (Adults): 0.02–0.2 mg q 2–3 min until response obtained; repeat q 1–2 hr if needed.
IV (Children): 0.01 mg/kg; may repeat q 2–3 min until response obtained. Additional doses may be given q 1–2 hr if needed.
IM, IV, Subcut (Neonates): 0.01 mg/kg; may repeat q 2–3 min until response obtained. Additional doses may be given q 1–2 hr if needed.

Opioid-Induced Respiratory Depression During Chronic (>1 wk) Opioid Use

IV, IM, Subcut (Adults >40 kg): 20–40 mcg (0.02–0.04 mg) given as small, frequent (q min) boluses or as an infusion titrated to improve respiratory function without reversing analgesia.
IV, IM, Subcut (Adults and Children <40 kg): 0.005–0.02 mg/dose given as small, frequent (q min) boluses or as an infusion titrated to improve respiratory function without reversing analgesia.

Overdose of Opioids

IV, IM, Subcut (Adults): *Patients not suspected of being opioid dependent*—0.4 mg (10 mcg/kg); may repeat q 2–3 min (IV route is preferred). Some patients may require up to 2 mg. *Patients suspected to be opioid dependent*—Initial dose should be ↓ to 0.1–0.2 mg q 2–3 min. May also be given by IV infusion at rate adjusted to patient's response.
IM, Subcut (Adults and Children): *Evzio*—0.4 mg; may repeat q 2–3 min until emergency medical assistance arrives.
IV, IM, Subcut (Children >5 yr or >20 kg): 2 mg/dose, may repeat q 2–3 min.
IV, IM, Subcut (Infants up to 5 yr or 20 kg): 0.1 mg/kg, may repeat q 2–3 min.
Intranasal (Adults): 2 mg (1 mg in each nostril); may repeat in 5 min.

Opioid-Induced Pruritus

IV (Children): 2 mcg/kg/hr continuous infusion, may ↑ by 0.5 mcg/kg/hr every few hours if pruritus continues.

Availability (generic available)

Injection: 0.4 mg/0.4 mL prefilled syringe, 0.4 mg/mL, 1 mg/mL. ***In combination with:*** pentazocine; buprenorphine (Suboxone, Zubsolv). See Appendix B.

NURSING IMPLICATIONS

Assessment

- Monitor respiratory rate, rhythm, and depth; pulse, ECG, BP; and level of consciousness frequently for 3–4 hr after the expected peak of blood concentrations. After a moderate overdose of a short half-life opioid, physical stimulation may be enough to prevent significant hypoventilation. The effects of some opioids may last longer than the effects of naloxone, and repeat doses may be necessary.
- Patients who have been receiving opioids for >1 wk are extremely sensitive to the effects of naloxone. Dilute and administer carefully.
- Assess patient for level of pain after administration when used to treat postoperative respiratory depression. Naloxone decreases respiratory depression but also reverses analgesia.
- Assess patient for signs and symptoms of opioid withdrawal (vomiting, restlessness, abdominal cramps, increased BP, and temperature). Symptoms may occur within a few minutes to 2 hr. Severity depends on dose of naloxone, the opioid involved, and degree of physical dependence.
- Lack of significant improvement indicates that symptoms are caused by a disease process or other non-opioid CNS depressants not affected by naloxone.
- ***Toxicity and Overdose:*** Naloxone is a pure antagonist with no agonist properties and minimal toxicity.

Potential Nursing Diagnoses

Ineffective breathing pattern (Indications)
Ineffective coping (Indications)
Acute pain

Implementation

- Do not confuse naloxone with Lanoxin (digoxin). Do not confuse Narcan (naloxone) with Norcuron (vecuronium).
- Larger doses of naloxone may be necessary when used to antagonize the effects of buprenorphine, butorphanol, nalbuphine, and pentazocine.
- Resuscitation equipment, oxygen, vasopressors, and mechanical ventilation should be available to supplement naloxone therapy as needed.
- Doses should be titrated carefully in postoperative patients to avoid interference with control of postoperative pain.
- **Evzio:** A take-home naloxone auto-injector that patients, family members, and other caregivers can have close by in case an opioid overdose occurs. Has visual and voice instructions.
- Inject into upper outer thigh.
- **Intranasal:** Prefilled syringe is used with mucosal atomizer device (MAD) for intranasal administration.

IV Administration

- **IV Push:** ***Diluent:*** Administer undiluted for *suspected opioid overdose*. For *opioid-induced respiratory depression*, dilute with sterile water for injection. For children or adults weighing <40 kg, dilute 0.1 mg of naloxone in 10 mL of sterile water or 0.9% NaCl for injection. ***Concentration:*** 0.4 mg/mL, 1 mg/mL, or 10 mcg/mL (depending on preparation used). ***Rate:*** Administer over 30 seconds for patients with a *suspected opioid overdose*. For patients who develop *opioid-induced respiratory depression*, administer dilute solution of 0.4 mg/10 mL at a rate of 0.5 mL (0.02 mg) IV push every 2 min. Titrate to avoid withdrawal and severe pain. Excessive dose in postoperative patients may cause excitement, pain, hypotension, hypertention, pulmonary edema, ventricular tachycardia and fibrillation, and seizures. For children and adults weighing <40 kg, administer 10 mcg/mL solution at a rate of 0.5 mcg/kg every 1–2 min.

- **Continuous Infusion:** ***Diluent:*** Dilute 2 mg of naloxone in 500 mL of 0.9% NaCl or D5W. Infusion is stable for 24 hr. ***Concentration:*** 4 mcg/mL. ***Rate:*** Titrate dose according to patient response.
- **Y-Site Compatibility:** alfentanil, amikacin, aminocaproic acid, amiodarone, anidulafungin, argatroban, ascorbic acid, atropine, aztreonam, benztropine, bivalirudin, bleomycin, bumetanide, buprenorphine, butorphanol, calcium chloride, calcium gluconate, carboplatin, carmustine, caspofungin, cefazolin, cefotaxime, cefotetan, cefoxitin, ceftazidime, ceftriaxone, cefuroxime, chloramphenicol, chlorpromazine, cisplatin, clindamycin, cyanocobalamin, cyclophosphamide, cyclosporine, cytarabine, dactinomycin, daptomycin, dexamethasone sodium phosphate, dexmedetomidine, digoxin, diltiazem, dimenhydrinate, diphenhydramine, dobutamine, docetaxel, dolasetron, dopamine, doxorubicin hydrochloride, doxorubicin liposomal, doxycycline, enalaprilat, ephedrine, epinephrine, epirubicin, epoetin alfa, eptifibatide, ertapenem, erythromycin, esmolol, etoposide, etoposide phosphate, famotidine, fenoldopam, fentanyl, fluconazole, fludarabine, fluorouracil, folic acid, foscarnet, fosphenytoin, furosemide, ganciclovir, gemcitabine, gentamicin, glycopyrrolate, granisetron, heparin, hetastarch, hydrocortisone, hydromorphone, idarubicin, ifosfamide, imipenem/cilastatin, indomethacin, insulin, irinotecan, isoproterenol, ketamine, ketorolac, labetalol, levofloxacin, lidocaine, linezolid, lorazepam, mannitol, mechlorethamine, meperidine, meropenem, mesna, methotrexate, methyldopate, methylprednisolone, metoclopramide, metoprolol, metronidazole, midazolam, milrinone, mitoxantrone, morphine, moxifloxacin, multivitamins, mycophenolate, nafcillin, nalbuphine, nesiritide, nitroglycerin, nitroprusside, norepinephrine, octreotide, ondansetron, oxacillin, oxaliplatin, oxytocin, paclitaxel, palonosetron, pamidronate, pancuronium, papaverine, pemetrexed, penicillin G, pentamidine, pentazocine, pentobarbital, phenobarbital, phenylephrine, phytonadione, piperacillin/tazobactam, potassium acetate, potassium chloride, procainamide, prochlorperazine, promethazine, propofol, propranolol, protamine, pyridoxine, quinupristin/dalfopristin, ranitidine, rocuronium, sodium acetate, sodium bicarbonate, streptokinase, succinylcholine, sufentanil, tacrolimus, teniposide, theophylline, thiamine, tigecycline, tirofiban, tobramycin, vancomycin, vasopressin, vecuronium, verapamil, vincristine, vinorelbine, voriconazole, zoledronic acid.
- **Y-Site Incompatibility:** amphotericin B lipid complex, amphotericin B liposome, dantrolene, diazepam, leucovorin, mitomycin, pantoprazole, phenytoin, thiotepa.
- **Additive Incompatibility:** Incompatible with preparations containing bisulfite, sulfite, and solutions with an alkaline pH.

Patient/Family Teaching

- As medication becomes effective, explain purpose and effects of naloxone to patient.
- **Evzio:** Explain purpose and instructions for use to caregiver. Advise to continue monitoring patient after injection and notify emergency medical assistance. Repeated doses may be required due to duration of naloxone.

Evaluation/Desired Outcomes

- Adequate ventilation following opioid excess.
- Alertness without significant pain or withdrawal symptoms.

naproxen (na-**prox**-en)

Aleve, Anaprox, Anaprox DS, ✱Maxidol, EC-Naprosyn, Naprelan, Naprosyn

Classification

Therapeutic: nonopioid analgesics, nonsteroidal anti-inflammatory agents, antipyretics

Pregnancy Category C

Indications

Mild to moderate pain. Dysmenorrhea. Fever. Inflammatory disorders, including: Rheumatoid arthritis (adults and children), Osteoarthritis.

Action

Inhibits prostaglandin synthesis. **Therapeutic Effects:** Decreased pain. Reduction of fever. Suppression of inflammation.

Pharmacokinetics

Absorption: Completely absorbed from the GI tract. Sodium salt is more rapidly absorbed.

Distribution: Crosses the placenta; enters breast milk in low concentrations.

N

Protein Binding: >99%.
Metabolism and Excretion: Mostly metabolized by the liver.
Half-life: Children <8 yr: 8–17 hr; Children 8–14 yr: 8–10 hr; Adults: 10–20 hr.

TIME/ACTION PROFILE

ROUTE	ONSET	PEAK	DURATION
PO (analgesic)	1 hr	unknown	8–12 hr
PO (anti-inflammatory)	14 days	2–4 wk	unknown

Contraindications/Precautions

Contraindicated in: Hypersensitivity; Cross-sensitivity may occur with other NSAIDs, including aspirin; Active GI bleeding; Ulcer disease; Perioperative pain from coronary artery bypass graft (CABG) surgery; Lactation: Passes into breast milk and should not be used by nursing mothers.
Use Cautiously in: Severe renal or hepatic disease; Cardiovascular disease or risk factors for cardiovascular disease (may ↑ risk of serious cardiovascular thrombotic events, myocardial infarction, and stroke, especially with prolonged use or use of higher doses); History of ulcer disease or any other history of gastrointestinal bleeding (may ↑ risk of GI bleeding); Chronic alcohol use/abuse; Geri: ↑ risk of adverse reactions; OB: Avoid using during third trimester; may cause premature closure of the ductus arteriosus; Pedi: Children <2 yr (safety not established).

Adverse Reactions/Side Effects

CNS: dizziness, drowsiness, headache. **EENT:** tinnitus, visual disturbances. **Resp:** dyspnea. **CV:** HF, MYOCARDIAL INFARCTION, STROKE, edema, hypertension, palpitations, tachycardia. **GI:** DRUG-INDUCED HEPATITIS, GI BLEEDING, constipation, dyspepsia, nausea, anorexia, diarrhea, discomfort, flatulence, vomiting. **GU:** cystitis, hematuria, renal failure. **Derm:** photosensitivity, rashes, sweating, pseudoporphyria (12% incidence in children with juvenile rheumatoid arthritis—discontinue therapy if this occurs). **Hemat:** blood dyscrasias, prolonged bleeding time. **Misc:** allergic reactions including ANAPHYLAXIS and STEVENS-JOHNSON SYNDROME.

Interactions

Drug-Drug: Concurrent use with **aspirin** ↓ levels and may ↓ effectiveness. ↑ risk of bleeding with **anticoagulants**, **thrombolytic agents**, **eptifibatide**, **tirofiban**, **cefotetan**, **valproic acid**, **corticosteroids**, and **clopidogrel**. Additive adverse GI side effects with **aspirin**, **corticosteroids**, **alcohol**, and other **NSAIDs**. **Probenecid** ↑ blood levels and may ↑ toxicity. May ↑ risk of toxicity from **methotrexate**, **antineoplastics**, or **radiation therapy**. May ↑ serum levels and risk of toxicity from **lithium**. ↑ risk of adverse renal effects with **cyclosporine**, **ACE inhibitors**, **angiotensin II antagonists**, or chronic use of **acetaminophen**. May ↓ response to **antihypertensives** or **diuretics**. May ↑ risk of hypoglycemia with **insulin** or **oral hypoglycemic agents**. **Oral potassium supplements** may ↑ GI adverse effects.
Drug-Natural Products: ↑ anticoagulant effect and bleeding risk with **anise**, **arnica**, **chamomile**, **clove**, **dong quai**, **feverfew**, **garlic**, **ginger**, **ginkgo**, **Panax ginseng**, **licorice**, and others.

Route/Dosage

275 mg naproxen sodium is equivalent to 250 mg naproxen.

Anti-Inflammatory/Analgesic/Antidysmenorrheal

PO (Adults): *Naproxen*—250–500 mg twice daily (up to 1.5 g/day). *Delayed-release naproxen*—375–500 mg twice daily. *Naproxen sodium*—275–550 mg twice daily (up to 1.65 g/day).
PO (Children >2 yr): *Analgesia:* 5–7 mg/kg/dose q 8–12 hr. *Inflammatory disease:* 10–15 mg/kg/day divided q 12 hr, maximum: 1000 mg/day.

Antigout

PO (Adults): *Naproxen*—750 mg naproxen initially, then 250 mg q 8 hr. *Naproxen sodium*—825 mg initially, then 275 mg q 8 hr.

OTC Use (naproxen sodium)

PO (Adults): 200 mg q 8–12 hr or 400 mg followed by 200 mg q 12 hr (not to exceed 600 mg/24 hr).
PO (Geriatric Patients >65 yr): Not to exceed 200 mg q 12 hr.

Availability

Naproxen (generic available)

Tablets (Naprosyn): ❖125 mg, 250 mg, 375 mg, 500 mg. **Delayed-release tablets (EC-Naprosyn):** 375 mg, 500 mg. **Extended-release tablets:** ❖750 mg. **Oral suspension (Naprosyn):** 125 mg/5 mL. **Rectal suppositories :** ❖500 mg. ***In combination with:*** esomeprazole (Vimovo).

Naproxen Sodium (generic available)

Capsules (Maxidol): ❖220 mg[OTC]. **Tablets (Aleve, Anaprox, Anaprox DS):** 220 mg[OTC], 275 mg, 550 mg. **Extended-release tablets (Naprelan):** 375 mg, 500 mg, 750 mg. ***In combination with:*** pseudoephedrine (Aleve-D Sinus and Cold), sumatriptan (Treximet). See Appendix B.

NURSING IMPLICATIONS

Assessment

- Patients who have asthma, aspirin-induced allergy, and nasal polyps are at increased risk for developing hypersensitivity reactions. Assess for rhinitis, asthma, and urticaria.
- **Pain:** Assess pain (note type, location, and intensity) prior to and 1–2 hr following administration.

- **Arthritis:** Assess pain and range of motion prior to and 1–2 hr following administration.
- **Fever:** Monitor temperature; note signs associated with fever (diaphoresis, tachycardia, malaise).
- ***Lab Test Considerations:*** Evaluate BUN, serum creatinine, CBC, and liver function tests periodically in patients receiving prolonged therapy.
- May ↑ serum potassium, BUN, serum creatinine, alkaline phosphatase, LDH, AST, and ALT tests levels. May ↓ blood glucose, hemoglobin, and hematocrit concentrations, leukocyte and platelet counts, and CCr.
- Bleeding time may be prolonged up to 4 days following discontinuation of therapy.
- May alter test results for urine 5-HIAA and urine steroid determinations.

Potential Nursing Diagnoses

Acute pain (Indications)
Chronic pain (Indications)
Impaired physical mobility (Indications)

Implementation

- Administration in higher than recommended doses does not provide increased effectiveness but may cause increased side effects. Use lowest effective dose for the shortest duration possible to minimize cardiac risks.
- Coadministration with opioid analgesics may have additive analgesic effects and may permit lower opioid doses.
- Analgesic is more effective if given before pain becomes severe.
- **PO:** For rapid initial effect, administer 30 min before or 2 hr after meals. May be administered with food, milk, or antacids to decrease GI irritation. Food slows but does not reduce the extent of absorption. Do not mix suspension with antacid or other liquid prior to administration. Swallow extended-release, delayed-release, and controlled-release tablets whole; do not break, crush, or chew.
- **Dysmenorrhea:** Administer as soon as possible after the onset of menses. Prophylactic treatment has not been shown to be effective.

Patient/Family Teaching

- Advise patient to take this medication with a full glass of water and to remain in an upright position for 15–30 min after administration.
- Instruct patient to take medication as directed. Take missed doses as soon as remembered but not if almost time for the next dose. Do not double doses.
- May cause drowsiness or dizziness. Advise patient to avoid driving or other activities requiring alertness until response to the medication is known.
- Caution patient to avoid the concurrent use of alcohol, aspirin, acetaminophen, or other OTC medications without consulting health care professional. Use of naproxen with 3 or more glasses of alcohol per day may increase risk of GI bleeding.
- Advise patient to inform health care professional of medication regimen prior to treatment or surgery.
- Caution patient to wear sunscreen and protective clothing to prevent photosensitivity reactions (especially in children with JRA).
- Instruct patients not to take OTC naproxen preparations for more than 3 days for fever and to consult health care professional if symptoms persist or worsen.
- Advise patient to consult health care professional if rash, itching, visual disturbances, tinnitus, weight gain, edema, black stools, persistent headache, or influenza-like syndrome (chills, fever, muscle aches, pain) occurs.
- Advise patient to notify health care professional if pregnancy is planned or suspected or if breast feeding.

Evaluation/Desired Outcomes

- Relief of pain.
- Improved joint mobility. Partial arthritic relief is usually seen within 2 wk, but maximum effectiveness may require 2–4 wk of continuous therapy. Patients who do not respond to one NSAID may respond to another.
- Reduction of fever.

N

naratriptan (nar-a-**trip**-tan)

Amerge

Classification

Therapeutic: vascular headache suppressants

Pharmacologic: 5-HT_1 agonists

Pregnancy Category C

Indications

Acute treatment of migraine headache.

Action

Acts as an agonist at specific 5-HT_1 receptor sites in intracranial blood vessels and sensory trigeminal nerves. **Therapeutic Effects:** Cranial vessel vasoconstriction with resultant decrease in migraine headache.

Pharmacokinetics

Absorption: Well absorbed (70%) following oral administration.

Distribution: Unknown.

Metabolism and Excretion: 60% excreted unchanged in urine; 30% metabolized by the liver.

Half-life: 6 hr (↑ in renal impairment).

TIME/ACTION PROFILE (↓ migraine pain)

ROUTE	ONSET	PEAK	DURATION
PO	30–60 min	2–3 hr†	up to 24 hr

†3–4 hr during migraine attack.

Contraindications/Precautions

Contraindicated in: Hypersensitivity; Ischemic heart disease or Prinzmetal's angina; Uncontrolled hypertension; Wolff-Parkinson-White syndrome or other arrhythmias involving conduction pathways; Hemiplegic or basilar migraine; Stroke or transient ischemic attack; Peripheral vascular disease; Ischemic bowel disease; Severe renal impairment (CCr <15 mL/min); Severe hepatic impairment; Should not be used within 24 hr of other 5-HT_1 agonists or ergot-type compounds (dihydroergotamine); Geri: Age-related ↓ in renal function and ↑ likelihood of CAD greatly ↑ risk of fatal adverse events.

Use Cautiously in: Mild to moderate renal or hepatic impairment (dose should not exceed 2.5 mg/24 hr; initial dose should be ↓); OB, Lactation, Pedi: Safety not established.

Exercise Extreme Caution in: Cardiovascular risk factors (hypertension, hypercholesterolemia, cigarette smoking, obesity, diabetes, strong family history, menopausal women or men >40 yr); use only if cardiovascular status has been evaluated and determined to be safe and 1st dose is administered under supervision.

Adverse Reactions/Side Effects

CNS: dizziness, drowsiness, malaise/fatigue. **CV:** CORONARY ARTERY VASOSPASM, MI, VENTRICULAR FIBRILLATION, VENTRICULAR TACHYCARDIA, myocardial ischemia. **GI:** nausea. **Neuro:** paresthesia. **Misc:** pain/pressure sensation in throat/neck.

Interactions

Drug-Drug: ↑ risk of serotonin syndrome when used with **SSRI or SNRI antidepressants**. **Cigarette smoking** ↑ the metabolism of naratriptan. Blood levels and effects are ↑ by **hormonal contraceptives**. Avoid concurrent use (within 24 hr of each other) with **ergot-containing drugs (dihydroergotamine)** may result in prolonged vasospastic reactions. Avoid concurrent (within 2 wk) use with **MAO inhibitors**; produces ↑ systemic exposure and risk of adverse reactions to naratriptan.

Drug-Natural Products: ↑ risk of serotinergic side effects including serotonin syndrome with **St. John's wort** and **SAMe**.

Route/Dosage

PO (Adults): 1 or 2.5 mg; dose may be repeated in 4 hr if response is inadequate (not to exceed 5 mg/24 hr or treatment of more than 4 headaches/mo).

Availability (generic available)

Tablets: 1 mg, 2.5 mg.

NURSING IMPLICATIONS

Assessment

- Assess pain location, character, intensity, and duration and associated symptoms (photophobia, phonophobia, nausea, vomiting) during migraine attack.
- Monitor for serotonin syndrome in patients taking SSRIs or SNRIs concurrently with naratriptan.

Potential Nursing Diagnoses

Acute pain (Indications)

Implementation

- **PO:** Tablets may be administered at any time after the headache starts.

Patient/Family Teaching

- Inform patient that naratriptan should be used only during a migraine attack. It is meant to be used for relief of migraine attacks but not to prevent or reduce the number of attacks.
- Instruct patient to administer naratriptan as soon as symptoms of a migraine attack appear, but it may be administered any time during an attack. If migraine symptoms return, a 2nd dose may be used. Allow at least 4 hr between doses, and do not use more than 2 tablets in any 24-hr period. Do not use to treat more than 4 headaches per month.
- Advise patient that lying down in a darkened room following naratriptan administration may further help relieve headache.
- Advise patient that overuse (use more than 10 days/month) may lead to exacerbation of headache (migraine-like daily headaches, or as a marked increase in frequency of migraine attacks). May require gradual withdrawal of naratriptan and treatment of symptoms (transient worsening of headache).
- Advise patient to notify health care professional prior to next dose of naratriptan if pain or tightness in the chest occurs during use. If pain is severe or does not subside, notify health care professional immediately. If wheezing; heart throbbing; swelling of eyelids, face, or lips; skin rash; skin lumps; or hives occur, notify health care professional immediately and do not take more naratriptan without approval of health care professional. If feelings of tingling, heat, flushing, heaviness, pressure, drowsiness, dizziness, tiredness, or sickness develop, discuss with health care professional at next visit.
- Instruct patient not to take additional naratriptan if no response is seen with initial dose without consulting health care professional. There is no evidence that 5 mg provides greater relief than 2.5-mg dose. Additional naratriptan doses are not likely to be effective, and alternative medications, as previously discussed with health care professional, may be used.
- Naratriptan may cause dizziness or drowsiness. Caution patient to avoid driving or other activities requiring alertness until response to medication is known.

- Advise patient to avoid alcohol, which aggravates headaches, during naratriptan use.
- Advise patient to notify health care professional of all Rx or OTC medications, vitamins, or herbal products being taken and to consult with health care professional before taking other medications. Patients concurrently taking SSRI or SNRI antidepressants should notify health care professional promptly if signs of serotonin syndrome (mental status changes: agitation, hallucinations, coma; autonomic instability: tachycardia, labile BP, hyperthermia; neuromuscular aberrations: hyperreflexia, incoordination; and/or gastrointestinal symptoms: nausea, vomiting, diarrhea) occur.
- Caution patient not to use naratriptan if pregnancy is planned or suspected or if breast feeding. Adequate contraception should be used during therapy.

Evaluation/Desired Outcomes

- Relief of migraine attack.

nebivolol (ne-bi-vi-lole)

Bystolic

Classification

Therapeutic: antihypertensives

Pharmacologic: beta blockers (selective)

Pregnancy Category C

Indications

Hypertension (alone and with other antihypertensives).

Action

Blocks stimulation of beta adrenergic receptor sites; selective for beta$_1$ (myocardial) receptors in most patients. In some patients (poor metabolizers, higher blood levels may result in some beta$_2$ [pulmonary, vascular, uterine] adrenergic) blockade. **Therapeutic Effects:** Lowering of BP.

Pharmacokinetics

Absorption: Well absorbed following oral administration.

Distribution: Unknown.

Protein Binding: 98%.

Metabolism and Excretion: Mostly metabolized by the liver, including the CYP2D6 enzyme system; some have antihypertensive action; minimal excretion of unchanged drug.

Half-life: *Extensive metabolizers*— 12 hr; *poor metabolizers*— 19 hr.

TIME/ACTION PROFILE (blood levels)

ROUTE	ONSET	PEAK	DURATION
PO	unknown	1.5–4 hr	24 hr

Contraindications/Precautions

Contraindicated in: Hypersensitivity; Severe bradycardia, heart block greater than first degree cardiogenic shock, decompensated heart failure, or sick sinus syndrome (without pacemaker); Severe hepatic impairment (Child-Pugh >B); Bronchospastic disease; OB: Lactation.

Use Cautiously in: Coronary artery disease (rapid cessation should be avoided); Compensated HF; Major surgery (anesthesia may augment myocardial depression); Diabetes mellitus (may mask signs of hypoglycemia); Thyrotoxicosis (may mask symptoms); Moderate hepatic impairment (↓ metabolism); Severe renal impairment (↓ initial dose if CCr <30 mL/min); History of severe allergic reactions (↑ intensity of reactions); Pheochromocytoma (alpha blockers required prior to beta blockers); Geri: Consider increased sensitivity, concurrent chronic diseases, medications and presence of age-related decrease in clearance; OB: Use in pregnancy only if maternal benefit outweighs fetal risk; Pedi: Safe use in children <18 yr not established.

N

Adverse Reactions/Side Effects

CNS: dizziness, fatigue, headache.

Interactions

Drug-Drug: Drugs that affect the CYP2D6 enzyme system are expected to alter levels and possibly effects of nebivolol; dose alterations may be required. **Fluoxetine**, a known inhibitor of CYP2D6, ↑ levels and effects; similar effects may be expected from **quinidine**, **propafenone**, and **paroxetine**. Blood levels are also ↑ by **cimetine**. **Anesthetic agents** including **ether**, **trichloroethylene**, and **cyclopropane** as well as **other myocardial depressants** or **inhibitors of AV conduction**, such as **diltiazem** and **verapamil** may ↑ risk of myocardial depression and bradycardia. Avoid concurrent use with **beta blockers**. Concurrent use with **reserpine** may excessively reduce sympathetic activity. If used concurrently with **clonidine**, nebivolol should be tapered and discontinued several days prior to gradual withdrawal of clonidine.

Route/Dosage

PO (Adults): 5 mg once daily initially, may increase at 2 wk intervals up to 40 mg/day.

Hepatic/Renal Impairment

PO (Adults): 2.5 mg once daily initially; titrate upward cautiously.

Availability

Tablets: 2.5, 5 mg, 10 mg.

NURSING IMPLICATIONS

Assessment

- Monitor BP, ECG, and pulse prior to and periodically during therapy.

- Monitor intake and output ratios and daily weights. Assess routinely for signs and symptoms of HF (dyspnea, rales/crackles, weight gain, peripheral edema, jugular venous distention).
- ***Lab Test Considerations:*** May cause ↑ BUN, uric acid, triglycerides and ↓ HDL cholesterol and platelet court.

Potential Nursing Diagnoses

Decreased cardiac output (Side Effects)

Implementation

- **PO:** May be administered without regard to food.
- When discontinuation is planned, observe patient carefully and advise to minimize physical activity. Taper over 1–2 wk when possible. If angina worsens or acute coronary insufficiency develops, reinstitute nebivolol promptly, at least temporarily.

Patient/Family Teaching

- Instruct patient to take nebivolol as directed, at the same time each day, even if feeling well. If a dose is missed, skip missed dose and take next scheduled dose; do not double doses. Do not discontinue without consulting health care professional. Abrupt withdrawal may precipitate life-threatening arrhythmias, hypertension, or myocardial ischemia.
- Advise patient to ensure that enough medication is available for weekends, holidays, and vacations. A written prescription may be kept in the wallet for emergencies.
- Reinforce the need to continue additional therapies for hypertension (weight loss, sodium restriction, stress reduction, regular exercise, moderation of alcohol consumption, and smoking cessation). Medication controls but does not cure hypertension.
- Teach patient and family how to check pulse and BP. Instruct them to check pulse daily and BP biweekly and to report significant changes to health care professional.
- Instruct patient to consult health care professional before taking any Rx, OTC, or herbal products, especially cold preparations, concurrently with this medication. Patients on antihypertensive therapy should also avoid excessive amounts of coffee, tea, and cola.
- May mask some signs of hypoglycemia, especially tachycardia. Diabetics should closely monitor blood sugar, especially if weakness, malaise, irritability, or fatigue occurs. Medication does not block dizziness or sweating as signs of hypoglycemia.
- May cause dizziness. Caution patients to avoid driving or other activities requiring alertness until response to medication is known.
- Advise patient to notify health care professional if difficulty breathing or signs and symptoms of worsening HF (weight gain, increasing shortness or breath, excessive bradycardia) occur.
- Instruct patient to inform health care professional of medication regimen before treatment or surgery.
- Advise patient to carry identification describing disease process and medication regimen at all times.
- Advise female patients that breast feeding should be avoided during nebivolol therapy.

Evaluation/Desired Outcomes

- Decrease in BP.

neomycin, See AMINOGLYCOSIDES.

netupitant/palonosetron

(ne-**too**-pi-tant/pa-lone-**o**-se-tron)
Akynzeo

Classification
Therapeutic: antiemetics
Pharmacologic: neurokinin antagonists, 5-HT_3 antagonists

Pregnancy Category C

Indications

Treatment of acute and delayed nausea and vomiting associated with chemotherapy including highly emetogenic chemotherapy.

Action

Netupitant—Acts as a selective antagonist at substance P/neurokinin 1 (NK1) receptors in the CNS; prevents nausea and vomiting in the acute and delayed phases after chemotherapy. *Palonosetron*—Blocks the effects of serotonin at receptor sites (selective antagonist) located in vagal nerve terminals and in the chemoreceptor trigger zones in the CNS; prevents nausea and vomiting in the acute phase. **Therapeutic Effects:** Decreased incidence and severity of nausea and vomiting following emetogenic chemotherapy.

Pharmacokinetics

Netupitant

Absorption: Absorption follows oral administration.
Distribution: Unknown.
Protein Binding: >99.5%.
Metabolism and Excretion: Extensively metabolized, three metabolites have anti-emetic activity, <1% excreted unchanged in urine.
Half-life: 80 hr.

Palonosetron

Absorption: 97% absorbed following oral administration.
Distribution: Unknown.
Metabolism and Excretion: 50% metabolized (mostly by CYP2D6, and to a lesser extent by CYP3A4 and CYP1A2); 40% excreted unchanged in urine.
Half-life: 40 hr.

TIME/ACTION PROFILE

ROUTE	ONSET	PEAK	DURATION
netupitant PO	15 min-3 hr	5 hr	days
palonosetron PO	within 1 hr	5 hr	days

Contraindications/Precautions

Contraindicated in: Severe/end stage hepatic or renal impairment; Cross-sensitivity may occur with other 5–HT_3 antagonists; Lactation: Discontinue netupitant/palonosetron or discontinue breast feeding.

Use Cautiously in: Geri: Consider age-related ↓ in renal, hepatic and cardiac function, concurrent disease states and drug therapies; OB: Use only if potential benefit justifies potential fetal risk; Pedi: Safety and effectiveness not established.

Adverse Reactions/Side Effects

CNS: fatigue, headache, weakness. **GI:** constipation, dyspepsia. **Derm:** erythema. **Misc:** hypersensitivity reactions including ANAPHYLAXIS, SEROTONIN SYNDROME.

Interactions

Drug-Drug: Netupitant is a moderate inhibitor of CYP3A4 and can ↑ levels of drugs that are **CYP3A4 substrates** including **alprazolam**, **cyclophosphamide**, **dexamethasone**, **docetaxel**, **etoposide**, **ifosfamide**, **imatinib**, **irinotecan**, **midazolam**, **erythromycin**, **paclitaxel**, **triazolam**, **vinorelbine**, **vinblastine**, and **vincristine** for 4 days or more; concurrent use should be undertaken with caution and necessary dose adjustments made. **Inducers of CYP3A4** including **rifampin** may ↓ levels and effectiveness; avoid concurrent use. Concurrent use of **other serotonergic drugs** may ↑ risk of serotonin syndrome.

Route/Dosage

PO (Adults): *Highly emetogenic chemotherapy (included cisplatin-based)*—One capsule (netupitant 300 mg/palonosetron 0.5 mg) 1 hr before chemotherapy on day 1. *Anthracycline and cyclophosphamide=based chemotherapy and other chemotherapy not considered highly emetogenic*—One capsule (netupitant 300 mg/palonosetron 0.5 mg) 1 hr before chemotherapy.

Availability

Capsules: netupitant 300 mg/palonosetron 0.5 mg.

NURSING IMPLICATIONS

Assessment

- Assess patient for nausea, vomiting, abdominal distention, and bowel sounds prior to and following administration.
- Assess for serotonin syndrome (mental changes [agitation, hallucinations, delirium, coma], autonomic instability [tachycardia, labile BP, dizziness, diaphoresis, flushing, hyperthermia], neuromuscular aberrations [tremor, rigidity, myoclonus, hyperreflexia, incoordination], seizure, and/or GI symptoms [nausea, vomiting, diarrhea]), especially in patients taking other serotonergic drugs (SSRIs, SNRIs, triptans).
- ***Lab Test Considerations:*** May cause transient ↑ in serum bilirubin, AST, and ALT levels.

Potential Nursing Diagnoses

Imbalanced nutrition: less than body requirements (Indications)

Implementation

- *For highly emetogenic chemotherapy,* administer with dexamethasone PO 12 mg 30 min prior to chemotherapy on day 1 and 8 mg PO on days 2 and 4. *For chemotherapy not considered highly emetogenic,* administer dexamethasone 30 min prior to chemotherapy on Day 1 (day 2 and 4 not needed).
- **PO:** Administer netupitant/palonosetron 1 hr prior to start of chemotherapy without regard to food.

N

Patient/Family Teaching

- Instruct patient to take netupitant/palonosetron as directed. Advise patient to reach *Patient Information* prior to starting therapy and with each Rx refill in case of changes.
- Advise patient to notify health care professional promptly if signs and symptoms of anaphylaxis (shortness or breath, rash, hives, swelling of mouth, throat, and lips) or serotonin syndrome occur.
- Advise female patient to notify health care professional if pregnancy is planned or suspected or if breast feeding.

Evaluation/Desired Outcomes

- Decrease in frequency and severity of nausea and vomiting.

niacin (**nye**-a-sin)
Niacor, Niaspan, Nicobid, Nicolar, Nicotinex, nicotinic acid, Slo-Niacin, vitamin B_3

niacinamide (nye-a-**sin**-a-mide)
nicotinamide

Classification
Therapeutic: lipid-lowering agents, vitamins
Pharmacologic: water soluble vitamins

Pregnancy Category C

Indications

Treatment and prevention of niacin deficiency (pellagra). Adjunctive therapy in certain hyperlipidemias (niacin only).

Action

Required as coenzymes (for lipid metabolism, glycogenolysis, and tissue respiration). Large doses decrease lipoprotein and triglyceride synthesis by inhibiting the release of free fatty acids from adipose tissue and decreasing hepatic lipoprotein synthesis (niacin only). Cause peripheral vasodilation in large doses (niacin only). **Therapeutic Effects:** Decreased blood lipids (niacin only). Supplementation in deficiency states.

Pharmacokinetics

Absorption: Well absorbed following oral administration.

Distribution: Widely distributed following conversion to niacinamide. Enters breast milk.

Metabolism and Excretion: Amounts required for metabolic processes are converted to niacinamide. Large doses of niacin are excreted unchanged in the urine.

Half-life: 45 min.

TIME/ACTION PROFILE (effects on blood lipids)

ROUTE	ONSET	PEAK	DURATION
PO (cholesterol)	several days	unknown	unknown
PO (triglycerides)	several hr	unknown	unknown

Contraindications/Precautions

Contraindicated in: Hypersensitivity to niacin; Some products may contain tartrazine and should be avoided in patients with known hypersensitivity; Alcohol intolerance (Nicotinex only).

Use Cautiously in: Liver disease; Arterial bleeding; History of peptic ulcer disease; Gout; Glaucoma; Diabetes mellitus.

Adverse Reactions/Side Effects

Adverse reactions and side effects refer to doses used to treat hyperlipidemia.

CNS: dizziness, nervousness, panic. **EENT:** blurred vision, loss of central vision, proptosis, toxic amblyopia. **CV:** orthostatic hypotension. **GI:** HEPATOTOXICITY, GI upset, bloating, diarrhea, dry mouth, flatulence, heartburn, hunger pains, nausea, peptic ulceration. **Derm:** flushing of the face and neck, pruritus, burning, dry skin, hyperpigmentation, ↑ sebaceous gland activity, rashes, stinging or tingling of skin. **Metab:** glycosuria, hyperglycemia, hyperuricemia. **MS:** myalgia.

Interactions

Drug-Drug: ↑ risk of myopathy with concurrent use of **HMG-CoA reductase inhibitors**. Additive hypotension with **antihypertensive agents**. Large doses may ↓ uricosuric effects of **probenecid**.

Route/Dosage

PO (Adults and Children): *Dietary supplement*—10–20 mg/day. *Dietary deficiency*—Up to 500 mg/day in divided doses. *Hyperlipidemias–Niacin only*—Immediate-release: 250 mg once daily; ↑ dose every 4–7 days to desired response (usual dose = 1.5–2 g/day in 2–3 divided doses); after 2–3 mo, may ↑ at 2–4 wk intervals to 1 g 3 times daily; Extended-release: 500 mg at bedtime for 4 wk, then 1 g at bedtime for 4 wk; may then ↑ dose every 4 wk by 500 mg/day to maximum of 2 g/day.

PO (Children 7–10 yr): *Prevention of deficiency*—13 mg/day.

PO (Children 4–6 yr): *Prevention of deficiency*—12 mg/day.

PO (Children birth–3 yr): *Prevention of deficiency*—5–9 mg/day.

Availability

Niacin (generic available)

Tablets: 25 mg[OTC], 50 mg[OTC], 100 mg[OTC], 125 mg[OTC], 250 mg[OTC], 400 mg[OTC], 500 mg[Rx, OTC]. **Extended-release tablets:** 125 mg[Rx, OTC], 250 mg[Rx, OTC], 400 mg[OTC], 500 mg[Rx, OTC], 750 mg[Rx, OTC], 1000 mg[Rx, OTC]. **Cost:** 500 mg $399.90/100, 750 mg $562.53/100, 1000 mg $707.90/100. **Extended-release capsules:** 125 mg[Rx, OTC], 250 mg[Rx, OTC], 300 mg[Rx, OTC], 400 mg[Rx, OTC], 500 mg[Rx, OTC]. **Elixir:** 50 mg/5 mL in pints and gallons[OTC]. ***In combination with:*** lovastatin (Advicor); simvastatin (Simcor). See Appendix B.

Niacinamide (generic available)

Tablets: 50 mg[OTC], 100 mg[OTC], 125 mg[OTC], 250 mg[OTC], 500 mg[Rx, OTC].

NURSING IMPLICATIONS

Assessment

- **Vitamin Deficiency:** Assess patient for signs of niacin deficiency (*pellagra*—dermatitis, stomatitis, glossitis, anemia, nausea and vomiting, confusion, memory loss, and delirium) prior to and periodically during therapy.
- **Hyperlipidemia:** Obtain a diet history, especially with regard to fat consumption.
- ***Lab Test Considerations:*** Monitor serum glucose and uric acid levels and hepatic function tests periodically during prolonged high-dose therapy. Notify health care professional if AST, ALT, or LDH becomes elevated. May ↑ prothrombin times and ↓ serum albumin.
- High-dose therapy may cause ↑ serum glucose and uric acid levels.
- When niacin is used as a lipid-lowering agent, serum cholesterol and triglyceride levels should be monitored prior to and periodically during therapy.

Potential Nursing Diagnoses

Imbalanced nutrition: less than body requirements (Indications)

Noncompliance (Patient/Family Teaching)

Implementation

- Because of infrequency of single B-vitamin deficiencies, combinations are commonly administered.

- **PO:** Administer with meals or milk to minimize GI irritation.
- Extended-release tablets and capsules should be swallowed whole, without breaking, crushing, or chewing. Use calibrated measuring device to ensure accurate dose of solution.

Patient/Family Teaching

- Inform patient that cutaneous flushing and a sensation of warmth, especially in the face, neck, and ears; itching or tingling; and headache may occur within the first 2 hr after taking the drug. These effects are usually transient and subside with continued therapy. If flushing is distressing or persistent, aspirin 300 mg given 30 min before each dose or slow upward titration of dose may decrease flushing.
- Advise patient to change positions slowly to minimize orthostatic hypotension.
- Instruct patients taking long-term OTC extended-release niacin to report signs of hepatotoxicity (darkening of urine, light gray–colored stool, loss of appetite, severe stomach pain, yellow eyes or skin) to health care professional.
- Emphasize the importance of follow-up examinations to evaluate progress.
- **Vitamin Deficiency:** Encourage patient to comply with dietary recommendations of health care professional. Explain that the best source of vitamins is a well-balanced diet with foods from the four basic food groups.
- Foods high in niacin include meats, eggs, milk, and dairy products; little is lost during ordinary cooking.
- Patients self-medicating with vitamin supplements should be cautioned not to exceed RDA. The effectiveness of megadoses for treatment of various medical conditions is unproved and may cause side effects.
- **Hyperlipidemia:** Advise patient that this medication should be used in conjunction with dietary restrictions (fat, cholesterol, carbohydrates, alcohol), exercise, and cessation of smoking.

Evaluation/Desired Outcomes

- Prevention and treatment of niacin deficiency.
- Decrease in serum cholesterol and triglyceride levels.

niCARdipine (nye-kar-di-peen)

Cardene, Cardene IV

Classification

Therapeutic: antianginals, antihypertensives

Pharmacologic: calcium channel blockers

Pregnancy Category C

Indications

Management of: Hypertension, Angina pectoris, Vasospastic (Prinzmetal's) angina.

Action

Inhibits the transport of calcium into myocardial and vascular smooth muscle cells, resulting in inhibition of excitation-contraction coupling and subsequent contraction. **Therapeutic Effects:** Systemic vasodilation resulting in decreased BP. Coronary vasodilation resulting in decreased frequency and severity of attacks of angina.

Pharmacokinetics

Absorption: Well absorbed following oral administration but extensively metabolized, resulting in ↓ bioavailability.

Distribution: Unknown.

Metabolism and Excretion: Mostly metabolized by the liver; ≤10% excreted unchanged by kidneys.

Half-life: 2–4 hr.

TIME/ACTION PROFILE (cardiovascular effects)

ROUTE	ONSET	PEAK	DURATION
PO	20 min	0.5–2 hr	8 hr
IV	within min	45 min	50 hr†

†Following discontinuation.

Contraindications/Precautions

Contraindicated in: Hypersensitivity; Sick sinus syndrome; 2nd- or 3rd-degree AV block (unless an artificial pacemaker is in place); SBP <90 mm Hg; Advanced aortic stenosis.

Use Cautiously in: Severe hepatic impairment (dose ↓ recommended); Severe renal impairment (dose ↓ may be necessary); History of serious ventricular arrhythmias or HF; OB, Lactation, Pedi: Safety not established; Geri: Dose ↓/slower IV infusion rates recommended due to↑ risk of hypotension.

Adverse Reactions/Side Effects

CNS: abnormal dreams, anxiety, confusion, dizziness, drowsiness, headache, jitteriness, nervousness, psychiatric disturbances, weakness. **EENT:** blurred vision, disturbed equilibrium, epistaxis, tinnitus. **Resp:** cough, dyspnea, shortness of breath. **CV:** ARRHYTHMIAS, HF, peripheral edema, bradycardia, chest pain, hypotension, palpitations, syncope, tachycardia. **GI:** ↑ liver function tests, anorexia, constipation, diarrhea, dry mouth, dysgeusia, dyspepsia, nausea, vomiting. **GU:** dysuria, nocturia, polyuria, sexual dysfunction, urinary frequency. **Derm:** dermatitis, erythema multiforme, flushing, ↑ sweating, photosensitivity, pruritus/urticaria, rash. **Endo:** gynecomastia, hyperglycemia. **Hemat:** anemia, leukopenia, thrombocytopenia. **Metab:**

weight gain. **MS:** joint stiffness, muscle cramps. **Neuro:** paresthesia, tremor. **Misc:** STEVENS-JOHNSON SYNDROME, gingival hyperplasia.

Interactions

Drug-Drug: Additive hypotension may occur when used concurrently with **fentanyl**, other **antihypertensives**, **nitrates**, acute ingestion of **alcohol**, or **quinidine**. Antihypertensive effects may be ↓ by concurrent use of **NSAIDs**. Concurrent use with **beta blockers**, **digoxin**, **disopyramide**, or **phenytoin** may result in bradycardia, conduction defects, or HF. **Cimetidine** and **propranolol** may ↓ metabolism and ↑ risk of toxicity. May ↓ the metabolism of and ↑ risk of toxicity from **cyclosporine**, **prazosin**, **quinidine**, or **carbamazepine**.
Drug-Food: Grapefruit and Grapefruit juice ↑ serum levels and effect.

Route/Dosage

PO (Adults): 20 mg 3 times daily, may ↑ q 3 days (range 20–40 mg 3 times daily).
IV (Adults): *Substitute for PO nicardipine*—if PO dose is 20 mg q 8 hr, then infusion rate is 0.5 mg/hr; if PO dose is 30 mg q 8 hr, then infusion rate is 1.2 mg/hr; if PO dose is 40 mg q 8 hr, then infusion rate is 2.2 mg/hr. *Patients not receiving PO nicardipine*—initiate therapy at 5 mg/hr, may be increased by 2.5 mg q 5–15 min as needed (up to 15 mg/hr).

Availability (generic available)

Capsules: 20 mg, 30 mg. **Injection:** 2.5 mg/mL. **Premixed infusion:** 20 mg/200 mL D5W or 0.9% NaCl.

NURSING IMPLICATIONS

Assessment

- Monitor BP and pulse prior to therapy, during dose titration, and periodically throughout therapy. Monitor ECG periodically during prolonged therapy.
- Monitor intake and output ratios and daily weight. Assess for signs of HF (peripheral edema, rales/crackles, dyspnea, weight gain, jugular venous distention).
- Assess for rash periodically during therapy. May cause Stevens-Johnson syndrome. Discontinue therapy if severe or if accompanied with fever, general malaise, fatigue, muscle or joint aches, blisters, oral lesions, conjunctivitis, hepatitis, and/or eosinophilia.
- **Angina:** Assess location, duration, intensity, and precipitating factors of patient's anginal pain.
- ***Lab Test Considerations:*** Total serum calcium concentrations are not affected by calcium channel blockers.
- Monitor serum potassium periodically. Hypokalemia ↑ risk of arrhythmias; should be corrected.
- Monitor renal and hepatic functions periodically during long-term therapy. Several days of therapy may cause ↑ hepatic enzymes, which return to normal upon discontinuation of therapy.

Potential Nursing Diagnoses

Decreased cardiac output (Indications)
Acute pain (Indications)

Implementation

- Do not confuse Cardene with Cardizem. Do not confuse nicardipine with nifedipine or nimodipine.
- To transfer from IV nicardipine infusion to oral therapy with other antihypertensive, start oral therapy simultaneously with discontinuation of nicardipine infusion. If transferring to oral nicardipine therapy, administer first dose of a 3-times-a-day regimen 1 hr prior to discontinuation of infusion.
- Dose adjustments of nicardipine should be made no more frequently than every 3 days.
- **PO:** May be administered without regard to meals. May be administered with meals if GI irritation becomes a problem.

IV Administration

- **Continuous Infusion:** ***Diluent:*** Dilute each 25-mg ampule with 240 mL of D5W, D5/0.45% NaCl, D5/0.9% NaCl, 0.45% NaCl, or 0.9% NaCl. Infusion is stable for 24 hr at room temperature. ***Concentration:*** 0.1 mg/mL. ***Rate:*** Titrate rate according to BP response. Administer through large peripheral veins or central veins to reduce risk of venous thrombosis, phlebitis, local irritation, swelling, extravasation, and vascular impairment. Change infusion site every 12 hours to minimize risk of peripheral venous irritation.
- **Y-Site Compatibility:** alemtuzumab, alfentanil, amikacin, amiodarone, anidulafungin, argatroban, aztreonam, bivalirudin, bleomycin, bumetanide, buprenorphine, butorphanol, calcium gluconate, carboplatin, carmustine, caspofungin, cefazolin, cefotaxime, cefotetan, cefoxitin, ceftriaxone, chloramphenicol, chlorpromazine, ciprofloxacin, cisatracurium, cisplatin, cyclophosphamide, cyclosporine, cytarabine, dacarbazine, daptomycin, dexmedetomidine, dexrazoxane, digoxin, diltiazem, diphenhydramine, dobutamine, docetaxel, dolasetron, dopamine, doxorubicin, doxorubicin liposomal, doxycycline, droperidol, enalaprilat, ephedrine, epinephrine, epirubicin, eptifibatide, erythromycin, esmolol, etoposide, etoposide phosphate, famotidine, fenoldopam, fentanyl, fluconazole, gemcitabine, gentamicin, granisetron, haloperidol, hetastarch, hydromorphone, idarubicin, ifosfamide, irinotecan, isoproterenol, labetalol, leucovorin, levofloxacin, levorphanol, lidocaine, linezolid, magnesium sulfate, mannitol, mechlorethamine, meperidine, metoclopramide, metoprolol, metronidazole, midazolam, milrinone, mitoxantrone, morphine, moxifloxacin, mycophenolate, nafcillin, nalbuphine, naloxone, nesiritide, nitroglycerin, nitroprusside, norepinephrine, octreotide, ondansetron, oxaliplatin, oxytocin, paclitaxel, palonosetron, pamidronate, pancuronium, penicillin G potassium, pentamidine, phenyl-

ephrine, potassium chloride, procainamide, prochlorperazine, promethazine, propranolol, quinupristin/dalfopristin, remifentanil, rocuronium, sodium phosphates, succinylcholine, sufentanil, tacrolimus, teniposide, theophylline, tirofiban, tobramycin, vancomycin, vasopressin, vecuronium, vincristine, voriconazole, zidovudine, zoledronic acid.

- **Y-Site Incompatibility:** acyclovir, aminocaproic acid, amphotericin B colloidal, amphotericin B lipid complex, amphotericin B liposome, ampicillin, ampicillin/sulbactam, azithromycin, ceftazidime, cefuroxime, dexamethasone, diazepam, ertapenem, fludarabine, fluorouracil, foscarnet, fosphenytoin, furosemide, ganciclovir, hydrocortisone sodium phosphate, imipenem/cilastatin, ketorolac, meropenem, mesna, methotrexate, micafungin, pantoprazole, pemetrexed, pentobarbital, phenobarbital, phenytoin, piperacillin/tazobactam, potassium acetate, sodium bicarbonate, thiopental, thiotepa, tigecycline.

Patient/Family Teaching

- Advise patient to take medication exactly as directed, even if feeling well. Take missed doses as soon as possible unless almost time for next dose; do not double doses. May need to be discontinued gradually.
- Instruct patient on technique for monitoring pulse. Instruct patient to contact health care professional if heart rate is <50 bpm.
- Advise patient to avoid grapefruit or grapefruit juice during therapy.
- Caution patient to change positions slowly to minimize orthostatic hypotension.
- May cause drowsiness or dizziness. Advise patient to avoid driving or other activities requiring alertness until response to the medication is known.
- Instruct patient to notify health care professional of all Rx or OTC medications, vitamins, or herbal products being taken and to avoid concurrent use of alcohol or OTC medications and herbal products, especially NSAIDs and cold preparations, without consulting health care professional.
- Advise patient to notify health care professional if rash, irregular heartbeat, dyspnea, swelling of hands and feet, pronounced dizziness, nausea, constipation, or hypotension occurs or if headache is severe or persistent.
- Caution patient to wear protective clothing and to use sunscreen to prevent photosensitivity reactions.
- Advise female patient to notify health care professional if pregnancy is planned or suspected or if breast feeding.
- **Angina:** Instruct patient on concurrent nitrate or beta-blocker therapy to continue taking both medications as directed and to use SL nitroglycerin as needed for anginal attacks.
- Advise patient to contact health care professional if chest pain does not improve, worsens after therapy, or occurs with diaphoresis; if shortness of breath; or if persistent headache occurs.
- Caution patient to discuss exercise restrictions with health care professional prior to exertion.
- **Hypertension:** Encourage patient to comply with other interventions for hypertension (weight reduction, low-sodium diet, smoking cessation, moderation of alcohol consumption, regular exercise, and stress management). Medication controls but does not cure hypertension.
- Instruct patient and family in proper technique for monitoring BP. Advise patient to take BP weekly and to report significant changes to health care professional.

Evaluation/Desired Outcomes

- Decrease in BP.
- Decrease in frequency and severity of anginal attacks.
- Decrease in need for nitrate therapy.
- Increase in activity tolerance and sense of well-being.

N

NICOTINE (nik-o-teen)

nicotine chewing gum
Nicorette, Thrive

nicotine inhaler
Nicotrol Inhaler

nicotine lozenge
Commit, Nicorette

nicotine nasal spray
Nicotrol NS

nicotine transdermal
Nicoderm CQ

Classification
Therapeutic: smoking deterrents

Pregnancy Category D

Indications

Adjunct therapy (with behavior modification) in the management of nicotine withdrawal in patients desiring to give up cigarette smoking.

Action

Provides a source of nicotine during controlled withdrawal from cigarette smoking. **Therapeutic Effects:** Lessened sequelae of nicotine withdrawal (irritability, insomnia, somnolence, headache, and increased appetite).

Pharmacokinetics

Absorption: *Gum, lozenge*—Slowly absorbed from buccal mucosa during chewing/sucking. *Inhaler*—50% of dose is systemically absorbed; most of nicotine released from inhaler is deposited in the mouth; absorption from buccal mucosa is slow. *Nasal spray*—53% absorbed from nasal mucosa. *Transdermal*—70% of nicotine released from the system is absorbed through the skin.
Distribution: Enter breast milk.
Metabolism and Excretion: Mostly metabolized by the liver. Small amounts are metabolized by kidneys and lungs; 10–20% excreted unchanged by kidneys.
Half-life: 1–2 hr.

TIME/ACTION PROFILE (nicotine blood levels)

ROUTE	ONSET	PEAK	DURATION
gum	rapid	15–30 min	unknown
inhaler	slow	within 15 min	unknown
lozenge	unknown	unknown	unknown
nasal spray	rapid	4–15 min	unknown
transdermal	rapid	2–4 hr	unknown

Contraindications/Precautions

Contraindicated in: Hypersensitivity; Recent history of MI (inhaler or nasal spray); Arrhythmias (inhaler or nasal spray); Severe or worsening angina (inhaler or nasal spray); Severe cardiovascular disease; OB: Effects on fetus unknown; spontaneous abortion has been reported. Encourage behavioral approaches to smoking cessation. Lactation: Excreted in breast milk; weigh risks of nicotine product use against risk of continued smoking. Pedi: Safety not established.
Use Cautiously in: Cardiovascular disease (including hypertension); Recent history of MI (gum, lozenge, patch); Arrhythmias (gum, lozenge, patch); Severe or worsening angina (gum, lozenge, patch); Diabetes mellitus; Pheochromocytoma; Peripheral vascular diseases; Hyperthyroidism; Diabetes; Continued smoking; Peptic ulcer disease; Hepatic disease; Bronchospastic lung disease (inhaler or nasal spray); Geri: Begin at lower dosages.

Adverse Reactions/Side Effects

CNS: headache, insomnia, abnormal dreams, dizziness, drowsiness, impaired concentration, nervousness, weakness. **EENT:** sinusitis; *gum*, pharyngitis; *nasal spray*, nasopharyngeal irritation, sneezing, watering eyes, change in smell, earache, epistaxis, eye irritation, hoarseness; *inhaler*, local mouth/throat irritation. **Resp:** *Nasal spray, inhaler*—cough, dyspnea. **CV:** tachycardia, chest pain, hypertension. **GI:** abdominal pain, abnormal taste, constipation, diarrhea, dry mouth, dyspepsia, hiccups, nausea, vomiting; *gum*, belching, ↑ appetite, ↑ salivation, oral injury, sore mouth. **Derm:** *transdermal*—burning at patch site, erythema, pruritus, cutaneous hypersensitivity, rash, sweating. **Endo:** dysmenorrhea. **MS:** arthralgia, back pain, myalgia; *gum*, jaw muscle ache. **Neuro:** paresthesia. **Misc:** allergy.

Interactions

Drug-Drug: Effects of **acetaminophen**, **caffeine**, **imipramine**, **insulin**, **oxazepam**, **pentazocine**, **propranolol**, or other **beta blockers**, **adrenergic antagonists** (**prazosin**, **labetalol**), and **theophylline** may be ↑ upon smoking cessation; dose ↓ at cessation may be necessary. Effects of adrenergic agonists (e.g., **isoproterenol**, **phenylephrine**) may be ↓ upon smoking cessation; dose ↑ at cessation may be necessary. Concurrent treatment with **bupropion** may cause treatment-emergent hypertension.

Route/Dosage

Gum (Adults): If first cigarette is desired >30 min after awakening, start with 2 mg gum, if first cigarette is desired <30 min after awakening, start with 4 mg gum. Patients should chew one piece of gum every 1–2 hr for 6 wk, then one piece of gum every 2–4 hr for 3 wk, then one piece of gum every 4–8 hr for 3 wk, then discontinue. Should not exceed 24 pieces of gum/day.
Lozenge (Adults): If first cigarette is desired >30 min after awakening, start with 2 mg lozenge, if first cigarette is desired <30 min after awakening, start with 4 mg lozenge. Patients should use one lozenge every 1–2 hr for 6 wk, then one lozenge every 2–4 hr for 3 wk, then one lozenge every 4–8 hr for 3 wk, then discontinue. Should not exceed 20 lozenges/day or more than 5 lozenges in 6 hr.
Intranasal (Adults): One spray in each nostril 1–2 times/hr (up to 5 times/hr); may be ↑ up to maximum of 40 times/day (should not exceed 3 mo of therapy).
Inhaln (Adults): Patients are encouraged to use at least 6 cartridges/day for first 3–6 wk, with additional cartridges as necessary (up to 16/day) for 12 wk. Patients are self-titrated to level of nicotine they require (usual usage 6–16 cartridges/day) followed by gradual withdrawal over 6–12 wk (maximum duration of use = 6 mo).
Transdermal (Adults): *Patients smoking >10 cigarettes/day*—Begin with Step 1 (21 mg/day) for 6 wk, followed by Step 2 (14 mg/day) for 2 wk, and then Step 3 (7 mg/day) for 2 wk, then stop (total of 10 wk) (new patch should be applied every 24 hr); *Patients smoking ≤10 cigarettes/day*—Begin with Step 2 (14 mg/day) for 6 wk, followed by Step 3 (7 mg/day) for 2 wk, then stop (total of 8 wk) (new patch should be applied every 24 hr).

Availability (generic available)

Chewing gum (cinnamon, mint, orange, and fruit chill flavors): 2 mg^OTC^, 4 mg^OTC^. **Inhalation:** each system contains 168 cartridges, each containing 10 mg of nicotine (deliver 4 mg). **Lozenge (original, mint, cherry, and cappuccino flavors):** 2 mg^OTC^, 4 mg^OTC^. **Nasal spray:** 10 mg/mL (0.5 mg/spray) in 10-mL bottles (200 sprays). **Transdermal patch:** 7 mg/day^OTC^, 14 mg/day^OTC^, 21 mg/day^OTC^.

NURSING IMPLICATIONS

Assessment

- Prior to therapy, assess smoking history (number of cigarettes smoked daily, smoking patterns, nicotine content of preferred brand, degree to which patient inhales smoke).
- Assess patient for symptoms of smoking withdrawal (irritability, drowsiness, fatigue, headache, nicotine craving) periodically during nicotine replacement therapy (NRT).
- Evaluate progress in smoking cessation periodically during therapy.
- ***Toxicity and Overdose:*** Monitor for nausea, vomiting, diarrhea, increased salivation, abdominal pain, headache, dizziness, auditory and visual disturbances, weakness, dyspnea, hypotension, and irregular pulse.

Potential Nursing Diagnoses

Ineffective coping (Indications)

Implementation

- **Gum:** Protect gum from light; exposure to light causes gum to turn brown.
- **Lozenge:** Lozenge should be allowed to dissolve slowly in the mouth; it should not be chewed or swallowed.
- **Transdermal:** Patch can be worn for 16 or 24 hr; the patch can be removed before the patient goes to bed (especially if patient has vivid dreams or sleep disturbances) or can remain on while the patient sleeps (especially if patient craves cigarettes upon awakening).
- **Nasal Spray and Inhaler:** Regular use of the spray or inhaler during the first week of therapy may help patient adjust to irritant effects of the spray.

Patient/Family Teaching

- Encourage patient to participate in a smoking cessation program while using this product.
- Review the patient instruction sheet enclosed in the package.
- Instruct patient in proper method of disposal of unit. Emphasize need to keep out of the reach of children or pets.
- Nicotine in any form can be harmful to a pregnant woman and/or the fetus. Assist patient in determining risk/benefit of nicotine replacement therapy (NRT) and harm to the fetus versus the likelihood of stopping smoking without NRT.
- Emphasize the importance of regular visits to health care professional to monitor progress of smoking cessation.
- **Gum:** Explain purpose of nicotine gum to patient. Patient should chew 1 piece of gum whenever a craving for nicotine occurs or according to a fixed schedule (every 1–2 hr while awake) as directed. Chew gum slowly until a tingling sensation is felt (about 15 chews). Then, patient should stop chewing and store the gum between the cheek and gums until the tingling sensation disappears (about 1 min). Process of stopping, then resuming chewing should be repeated for approximately 30 min until most of the tingle has disappeared. Rapid, vigorous chewing may result in side effects similar to those of smoking too many cigarettes (headache, dizziness, nausea, increased salivation, heartburn, and hiccups). For best chances of quitting, chew at least 9 piece of gum/day during 1st 6 wk.
- Inform patient that the gum has a slight tobacco/pepper-like taste. Many patients initially find it unpleasant and slightly irritating to the mouth. This usually resolves after several days of therapy.
- Advise patient to carry gum at all times during therapy.
- Advise patient to avoid eating or drinking for 15 min before and during chewing of nicotine gum; these interfere with buccal absorption of nicotine.
- The gum usually can be chewed by denture wearers. Contact dentist if the gum adheres to bridgework.
- Inform patient that if they still feel need to use gum after completion of treatment period, advise them to contact a health care professional.
- Instruct patient not to swallow gum.
- Dispose of the gum by wrapping in wrapper to prevent ingestion by children and animals. Call the poison control center, emergency department, or health care professional immediately if a child ingests the gum.
- Emphasize the need to discontinue the gum and to inform health care professional if pregnancy occurs.
- **Transdermal:** Instruct patient in application and use of patch. Apply patch at the same time each day. Keep patch in sealed pouch until ready to apply. Apply to clean, dry skin of upper arm or torso free of oil, hair, scars, cuts, burns, or irritation. Press patch firmly in place with palm for 10 sec, making sure there is good contact, especially around the edges. Keep patch in place during showering, bathing, or swimming; replace patches that have fallen off. Wash hands with soap and water after handling patches. Do not trim or cut patch. No more than 1 patch should be worn at a time. Alternate application sites. Dispose of used patches by folding adhesive sides together and replacing in protective pouch or aluminum foil; keep out of reach of children.
- Advise patient that redness, itching, and burning at application site usually subside within 1 hr. Instruct patient to notify health care professional and not apply new patch if signs of allergic reaction (urticaria, generalized rash, hives) or persistent local skin reactions (severe erythema, pruritus, edema) occur.

N

- May cause drowsiness or dizziness. Caution patient to avoid driving or other activities requiring alertness until response to medication is known.
- Advise patient referred for MRI test to discuss patch with referring health care professional and MRI facility to determine if removal of patch is necessary prior to test and for directions for replacing patch.
- **Nasal Spray:** Instruct patient in proper use of spray. Tilt head back slightly. Do not sniff, swallow, or inhale through nose as spray is being administered. Patients who have successfully stopped smoking should continue to use the same dose for up to 8 wk, after which the spray should be discontinued over the next 4–6 wk.
- Discontinue nasal spray by using ½ dose (1 spray at a time), using the spray less frequently, skipping a dose by not using every hour, or setting a planned stop date for use of the spray.
- Treatment should be discontinued in patients who are unable to stop smoking by the 4th wk of therapy (patient is unlikely to quit on that attempt).
- Patients who fail to stop smoking should be given a therapy holiday before another attempt.
- Instruct patient to replace childproof cap after using and before disposal.
- **Inhalation:** Inhalation regimens should consist of frequent, continuous puffing for 20 minutes.
- Treatment should be discontinued in patients who are unable to stop smoking by the 4th wk of therapy (patient is unlikely to quit on that attempt).
- Patients who fail to stop smoking should be given a therapy holiday before another attempt.
- **Lozenge:** Instruct patient to place lozenge in mouth and allow it to slowly dissolve (20–30 min). Minimize swallowing; advise patient not to chew or swallow lozenge. May cause a warm tingling sensation in mouth. Advise patient to occasionally move lozenge from side to side of mouth until completely dissolved. Instruct patient not to eat or drink 15 min before or while lozenge is in mouth. For best chances of quitting, use at least 9 lozenges/day during 1st 6 wk. Do not use more than 1 lozenge at a time or use continuously one after the another. Lozenge should not be used after 12 wk without consulting health care professional.

Evaluation/Desired Outcomes

- Lessened sequelae of nicotine withdrawal (irritability, insomnia, somnolence, headache, and increased appetite) during smoking cessation.

NIFEdipine (nye-**fed**-i-peen)

Adalat CC, ✱Adalat XL, Afeditab CR, Procardia, Procardia XL

Classification

Therapeutic: antianginals, antihypertensives

Pharmacologic: calcium channel blockers

Pregnancy Category C

Indications

Management of: Hypertension (extended-release only), Angina pectoris, Vasospastic (Prinzmetal's) angina. **Unlabeled Use:** Prevention of migraine headache. Management of HF or cardiomyopathy.

Action

Inhibits calcium transport into myocardial and vascular smooth muscle cells, resulting in inhibition of excitation-contraction coupling and subsequent contraction. **Therapeutic Effects:** Systemic vasodilation, resulting in decreased BP. Coronary vasodilation, resulting in decreased frequency and severity of attacks of angina.

Pharmacokinetics

Absorption: Well absorbed after oral administration, but large amounts are rapidly metabolized (primarily by CYP3A4 enzyme system), resulting in ↓ bioavailability (45–70%); bioavailability is ↑ (80%) with long-acting (CC, PA, XL) forms.

Distribution: Unknown.

Protein Binding: 92–98%.

Metabolism and Excretion: Mostly metabolized by the liver.

Half-life: 2–5 hr.

TIME/ACTION PROFILE

ROUTE	ONSET	PEAK	DURATION
PO	20 min	unknown	6–8 hr
PO–PA	unknown	4 hr	12 hr
PO–CC, PA, XL	unknown	6 hr	24 hr

Contraindications/Precautions

Contraindicated in: Hypersensitivity; Sick sinus syndrome; 2nd- or 3rd-degree AV block (unless an artificial pacemaker is in place); Systolic BP <90 mm Hg; Coadministration with grapefruit juice, rifampin, rifabutin, phenobarbital, phenytoin, carbamazepine, or St. John's wort.

Use Cautiously in: Severe hepatic impairment (↓ dose recommended); History of porphyria; Severe renal impairment (↓ dose may be necessary); History of serious ventricular arrhythmias or HF; OB, Lactation: Use only if potential benefit justifies potential risks; Pedi: Safety not established; Geri: Short-acting forms appear on Beers list due to ↑ risk of hypotension and constipation (↓ dose recommended); also associated with ↑ incidence of falls.

Adverse Reactions/Side Effects

CNS: headache, abnormal dreams, anxiety, confusion, dizziness, drowsiness, jitteriness, nervousness, psychiatric disturbances, weakness. **EENT:** blurred vision, disturbed equilibrium, epistaxis, tinnitus. **Resp:** cough, dyspnea, shortness of breath. **CV:** ARRHYTHMIAS, HF, peripheral edema, bradycardia, chest pain, hypotension, palpitations, syncope, tachycardia. **GI:** ↑ liver enzymes, anorexia, constipation, diarrhea, dry mouth, dysgeusia, dyspepsia, GI obstruction, nausea, ulcer, vomiting. **GU:** dysuria, nocturia, polyuria, sexual dysfunction, urinary frequency. **Derm:** flushing, dermatitis, erythema multiforme, ↑ sweating, photosensitivity, pruritus/urticaria, rash. **Endo:** gynecomastia, hyperglycemia. **Hemat:** anemia, leukopenia, thrombocytopenia. **Metab:** weight gain. **MS:** joint stiffness, muscle cramps. **Neuro:** paresthesia, tremor. **Misc:** STEVENS-JOHNSON SYNDROME, gingival hyperplasia.

Interactions

Drug-Drug: Rifampin, **rifabutin**, **phenobarbital**, **phenytoin**, or **carbamazepine** may significantly ↓ levels and effects; concurrent use is contraindicated. **Ketoconazole**, **fluconazole**, **itraconazole**, **clarithromycin**, **erythromycin**, **nefazodone**, **saquinavir**, **indinavir**, **nelfinavir**, or **ritonavir** may ↑ levels and effects; consider initiating nifedipine at lowest dose. Additive hypotension may occur when used concurrently with **fentanyl**, other **antihypertensives**, **nitrates**, acute ingestion of **alcohol**, or **quinidine**. Antihypertensive effects may be ↓ by concurrent use of **NSAIDs**. May ↑ serum levels and risk of toxicity from **digoxin**. Concurrent use with **beta blockers**, **digoxin**, or **disopyramide** may result in bradycardia, conduction defects, or HF. **Cimetidine** and **propranolol** may ↓ metabolism and ↑ risk of toxicity. May ↓ metabolism of and ↑ risk of toxicity from **cyclosporine**, **tacrolimus**, **prazosin**, **quinidine**, or **carbamazepine**. ↑ risk of GI obstruction when used concurrently with **H_2 blockers**, **opioids**, **NSAIDS**, **laxatives**, **anticholinergic drugs**, **levothyroxine**, or **neuromuscular blockers**. **Strong CYP3A4 inducers**, including **carbamazepine**, **phenobarbital**, **phenytoin**, and **rifampin** may ↓ levels and effects; avoid concurrent use.

Drug-Natural Products: St. John's wort may significantly ↓ levels and effects; concurrent use is contraindicated.

Drug-Food: Grapefruit and **grapefruit juice** ↑ serum levels and effect; avoid concurrent use.

Route/Dosage

PO (Adults): 10–30 mg 3 times daily (not to exceed 180 mg/day), *or* 10–20 mg twice daily as immediate-release form, *or* 30–90 mg once daily as sustained-release (CC, XL) form (not to exceed 90–120 mg/day).

Availability (generic available)

Capsules: ✱5 mg, 10 mg, 20 mg. **Tablets:** ✱10 mg. **Extended-release tablets, (Adalat CC, Afeditab CR, Nifedical XL, Procardia XL):** ✱10 mg, ✱20 mg, 30 mg, 60 mg, 90 mg.

NURSING IMPLICATIONS

Assessment

- Monitor BP and pulse before therapy, during dose titration, and periodically during therapy. Monitor ECG periodically during prolonged therapy.
- Monitor intake and output ratios and daily weight. Assess for signs of HF (peripheral edema, rales/crackles, dyspnea, weight gain, jugular venous distention).
- Patients receiving digoxin concurrently with nifedipine should have routine tests of serum digoxin levels and be monitored for signs and symptoms of digoxin toxicity.
- Assess for rash periodically during therapy. May cause Stevens-Johnson syndrome. Discontinue therapy if severe or if accompanied with fever, general malaise, fatigue, muscle or joint aches, blisters, oral lesions, conjunctivitis, hepatitis and/or eosinophilia.
- **Angina:** Assess location, duration, intensity, and precipitating factors of patient's anginal pain.
- ***Lab Test Considerations:*** Total serum calcium concentrations are not affected by calcium channel blockers.
- Monitor serum potassium periodically. Hypokalemia increases risk of arrhythmias; should be corrected.
- Monitor renal and hepatic functions periodically during long-term therapy. Several days of therapy may cause ↑ hepatic enzymes, which return to normal upon discontinuation of therapy.
- Nifedipine may cause positive ANA and direct Coombs' test results.

Potential Nursing Diagnoses

Decreased cardiac output (Indications)
Acute pain (Indications)

Implementation

- Do not confuse with nicardipine or nimodipine.
- **PO:** May be administered without regard to meals. May be administered with meals if GI irritation becomes a problem.
- Do not open, break, crush, or chew extended-release tablets. Empty tablets that appear in stool are not significant.
- Avoid administration with grapefruit juice.
- Sublingual use is not recommended due to serious adverse drug reactions.

Patient/Family Teaching

- Advise patient to take medication as directed, even if feeling well. Take missed doses as soon as possible

N

unless almost time for next dose; do not double doses. May need to be discontinued gradually.

- Instruct patient on technique for monitoring pulse. Instruct patient to contact health care professional if heart rate is <50 bpm.
- Advise patient to avoid grapefruit or grapefruit juice during therapy.
- Caution patient to change positions slowly to minimize orthostatic hypotension.
- May cause drowsiness or dizziness. Advise patient to avoid driving or other activities requiring alertness until response to the medication is known.
- Geri: Teach patients and family about risk for falls and how to reduce risk in the home.
- Instruct patient on importance of maintaining good dental hygiene and seeing dentist frequently for teeth cleaning to prevent tenderness, bleeding, and gingival hyperplasia (gum enlargement).
- Instruct patient to notify health care professional of all Rx or OTC medications, vitamins, or herbal products being taken and to avoid concurrent use of alcohol or OTC medications and herbal products, especially cold preparations, without consulting health care professional.
- Advise patient to notify health care professional if rash, irregular heartbeat, dyspnea, swelling of hands and feet, pronounced dizziness, nausea, constipation, or hypotension occurs or if headache is severe or persistent.
- Caution patient to wear protective clothing and use sunscreen to prevent photosensitivity reactions.
- **Angina:** Instruct patient on concurrent nitrate or beta-blocker therapy to continue taking both medications as directed and use SL nitroglycerin as needed for anginal attacks.
- Inform patient that anginal attacks may occur 30 min after administration because of reflex tachycardia. This is usually temporary and is not an indication for discontinuation.
- Advise patient to contact health care professional if chest pain does not improve, worsens after therapy, or occurs with diaphoresis; if shortness of breath occurs; or if persistent headache occurs.
- Caution patient to discuss exercise restrictions with health care professional before exertion.
- **Hypertension:** Encourage patient to comply with other interventions for hypertension (weight reduction, low-sodium diet, smoking cessation, moderation of alcohol consumption, regular exercise, and stress management). Medication controls but does not cure hypertension.
- Instruct patient and family in proper technique for monitoring BP. Advise patient to take BP weekly and to report significant changes to health care professional.

Evaluation/Desired Outcomes

- Decrease in BP.
- Decrease in frequency and severity of anginal attacks.
- Decrease in need for nitrate therapy.
- Increase in activity tolerance and sense of well-being.

nilotinib (ni-lo-ti-nib)

Tasigna

Classification

Therapeutic: antineoplastics

Pharmacologic: enzyme inhibitors, kinase inhibitors

Pregnancy Category D

Indications

Newly diagnosed Philadelphia chromosome positive (Ph+) chronic myelogenous leukemia (CML) in chronic phase. Chronic or accelerated phase Ph+ CML that has not responded to other treatment, including imatinib.

Action

Inhibits kinases which may be produced by malignant cell lines. **Therapeutic Effects:** Inhibits production of malignant cells lines with decreased proliferation of leukemic cells.

Pharmacokinetics

Absorption: Well absorbed following oral administration. Blood levels are significantly ↑ by food.

Distribution: Unknown.

Metabolism and Excretion: Mostly metabolized by the liver; metabolites are not active.

Half-life: 17 hr.

TIME/ACTION PROFILE (blood levels)

ROUTE	ONSET	PEAK	DURATION
PO	unknown	3 hr	12 hr

Contraindications/Precautions

Contraindicated in: Hypokalemia or hypomagnesemia; Long QT syndrome; Concurrent use of medications known to prolong QT interval; Concurrent use of strong inhibitors of the CYP3A4 enzyme system (e.g. ketoconazole, itraconazole, clarithromycin, atazanavir, indinavir, nefazodone, nelfinavir, ritonavir, saquinavir, telithromycin, voriconazole, grapefruit juice); Concurrent use of strong inducers of the CYP3A4 enzyme system (e.g. dexamethasone, phenytoin, carbamazepine, rifampin, rifabutin, rifapentine, phenobarbital, St. John's wort); Galactose intolerance, severe lactase deficiency or glucose-galactose malabsorption (capsules contain lactose); OB, Lactation: Pregnancy or lactation.

Use Cautiously in: Concurrent use of other drugs that prolong QT interval; Concurrent use of proton pump inhibitors (may ↓ bioavailability of nilotinib); Electrolyte abnormalities; correct prior to administration to ↓ risk of arrhythmias; Hepatic impairment (↓ dose required for Grade 3 elevated bilirubin, transaminases or lipase); Total gastrectomy (may need to ↑ dose or use alterative therapy); History of pancreatitis; OB: Women with child-bearing potential (effective contraception required); Pedi: Safety not established.

Adverse Reactions/Side Effects

CNS: fatigue, headache, dizziness. **EENT:** vertigo. **CV:** MI, STROKE, TORSADES DE POINTES, hypertension, palpitations, pericardial effusion, peripheral arterial disease, QT interval prolongation. **GI:** HEPATOTOXICITY, ↑ lipase, constipation, diarrhea, nausea, vomiting, abdominal discomfort, anorexia, ascites, dyspepsia, flatulence. **Derm:** pruritus, rash, alopecia, flushing. **F and E:** hyperkalemia, hypocalcemia, hypokalemia, hyponatremia, hypophosphatemia. **Hemat:** BLEEDING, MYELOSUPRESSION. **Metab:** hyperglycemia. **MS:** musculoskeletal pain. **Neuro:** paresthesia. **Resp:** pleural effusion, pulmonary edema. **Misc:** fever, night sweats, tumor lysis syndrome.

Interactions

Drug-Drug: Strong **CYP3A4 inhibitors** including **ketoconazole**, **itraconaole**, **voriconazole**, **clarithromycin**, **telithromycin**, **atazanavir**, **indinavir**, **nelfinavir**, **ritonavir**, **saquinavir**, and **nefazodone** may result in ↑ blood levels and toxicity and should be avoided if possible; if concurrent use is necessary, ↓ nilotinib dose. Strong **CYP3A4 inducers** including **carbamazepine**, **dexamethasone**, **phenobarbital**, **phenytoin**, **rifabutin**, **rifampin**, and **rifapentin** may ↓ blood levels and effectiveness and should be avoided. May ↑ levels of **CYP3A4 substrates**, including **alfentanil**, **cyclosporine**, **dihydroergotamine**, **ergotamine**, **fentanyl**, **midazolam**, **sirolimus**, and **tacrolimus**. May ↑ levels of **CYP3A4 substrates**, including **alfentanil**, **atorvastatin**, **cyclosporine**, **dihydroergtamine**, **ergotamine**, **fentanyl**, **lovastatin**, **midazolam**, **simvastatin**, **sirolimus**, and **tacrolimus**. Concurrent use of other **drugs that prolong QT interval**; may ↑ risk of serious arrhythmias; avoid concomitant use. **Proton pump inhibitors**, **H_2 receptor antagonists**, and **antacids** may ↓ the bioavailability of nilotinib; avoid concurrent use of proton pump inhibitors; doses of H_2 receptor antagonists may be administered 10 hr before or 2 hr after nilotinib; doses of antacids may be administered 2 hr before or after nilotinib.

Drug-Natural Products: **St. John's wort** may ↓ levels and effectiveness; avoid concurrent use.

Drug-Food: **Grapefruit juice** may ↑ blood levels and toxicity and should be avoided.

Route/Dosage

Newly Diagnosed Ph+ CML Chronic Phase

PO (Adults): 300 mg twice daily; adjustment may be required for toxicity; *Concurrent use of strong CYP3A4 inhibitor (ketoconazole, itraconazole, clarithromycin, atazanavir, indinavir, nefazodone, nelfinavir, ritonavir, saquinavir, telithromycin, voriconazole)*—200 mg once daily.

Hepatic Impairment

PO (Adults): *Mild, moderate or severe hepatic impairment*—200 mg twice daily; may ↑ to 300 mg twice daily if tolerates.

Resistant or Intolerant Ph+ CML Chronic or Accelerated Phase

PO (Adults): 400 mg twice daily; adjustment may be required for toxicity; *Concurrent use of strong CYP3A4 inhibitor (ketoconazole, itraconazole, clarithromycin, atazanavir, indinavir, nefazodone, nelfinavir, ritonavir, saquinavir, telithromycin, voriconazole)*—300 mg once daily.

Hepatic Impairment

PO (Adults): *Mild or moderate hepatic impairment*—300 mg twice daily; may ↑ to 400 mg twice daily if tolerates; *Severe hepatic impairment*—200 mg twice daily; may ↑ to 300 mg twice daily, and eventually to 400 mg twice daily if tolerates.

Availability

Capsules: 150 mg, 200 mg.

NURSING IMPLICATIONS

Assessment

- Monitor ECG to assess the QTc interval at baseline, 7 days after initiation of therapy, after any dose adjustment, and periodically thereafter. For ECGs with QTc >480 msec, withhold nilotinib and check serum potassium and magnesium. If below lower limit of normal, correct to normal with supplements. Review concomitant medications for effects on electrolytes. If QTc returns to <450 msec and within 20 msec of baseline within 2 wk, return ot prior dose. If QTc is <480 msec and >450 msec after 2 wk, reduce nilotinib dose to 400 mg once daily. Following dose reduction to 400 mg once daily, if QTc return to >480 msec, discontinue nilotinib. Repeat ECG approximately 7 days after any dose adjustment.
- Monitor for myelosuppression. Assess for bleeding (bleeding gums, bruising, petechiae, blood in stools, urine, emesis) and avoid IM injections and taking rectal temperatures if platelet count is low. Apply pressure to venipuncture sites for at least 10 min. Assess for signs of infection during neutropenia. Anemia may occur. Monitor for fatigue, dyspnea, and othrostatic hypotension.
- Monitor for tumor lysis syndrome (malignant disease progression, high WBC counts, hyperuricemia, hyperkalemia, hyperphosphatemia, hypocalcamia, and/or dehydration). Prevent by maintain adequate

N

hydration and correcting uric acid levels prior to starting nilotinib.

- Monitor for signs of severe fluid retention (unexpected rapid weight gain or swelling) and for symptoms of respiratory or cardiac compromise (shortness of breath) periodically during therapy; evaluate cause and treat patients as needed.
- ***Lab Test Considerations:*** Monitor serum electrolytes prior to and periodically during therapy. May cause hypokalemia, hypomagnesemia, hypophosphatemia, hyperkalemia, hypocalcemia, hyperglycemia, and hyponatremia.
- Monitor CBC every 2 wk for first 2 mo and monthly thereafter or as indicated. May cause Grade 3/4 thrombocytopenia, neutropenia, and anemia. If ANC is $<1.0 \times 10^9$/L and/or platelet counts $<50 \times 10^9$/L, stop nilotinib and monitor blood counts. Resume within 2 wk at prior dose if ANC $>1.0 \times 10^9$/L and platelets $>50 \times 10^9$/L. If blood counts remain low for >2 wk, reduce dose to 400 mg once daily. Myelosuppression is generally reversible.
- May cause ↑ serum lipase or amylase. If ↑ to ≥Grade 3, withhold nilotinib and monitor serum levels. Resume treatment at 400 mg once daily if serum lipase or amylase return to ≤Grade 1.
- May cause ↑ serum bilirubin. If ↑ to ≥Grade 3, withhold nilotinib and monitor bilirubin. Resume treatment at 400 mg once daily if serum lipase or amylase return to ≤Grade 1.
- May cause ↑ serum hepatic tranaminases. If ↑ to ≥Grade 3, withhold nilotinib and monitor serum ALT, AST, and alkaline phosphatase. Resume treatment at 400 mg once daily if serum lipase or amylase return to ≤Grade 1.
- Monitor lipid panel and glucose prior to and periodically during first year of therapy, and then yearly during chronic therapy.

Potential Nursing Diagnoses

Deficient knowledge, related to medication regimen (Patient/Family Teaching)

Implementation

- Correct hypokalemia and hypomagnesemia prior to beginning therapy.
- **PO:** Administer twice daily at 12-hr intervals on an empty stomach, at least 1 hr before and 2 hr after food. Capsule should be swallowed whole with water; do not open capsule.
- Patients unable to swallow capsule may open capsule and sprinkle contents of each capsule in 1 teaspoon of applesauce. Swallow mixture within 15 minutes. Do not use more than 1 teaspoon of applesauce and use only applesauce.
- Avoid antacids less than 2 hr before or after and H_2 antagonists less than 10 hr before or less than 2 hr after administration.

Patient/Family Teaching

- Instruct patient to take nilotinib as directed, approximately 12 hr apart. If a dose is missed, skip dose and resume taking next prescribed dose. Nilotinib is a long-term treatment; do not stop medication or change dose without consulting health care professional. Advise patient to read the *Medication Guide* before starting and with each Rx refill, in case of changes.
- Advise patient to avoid grapefruit, grapefruit juice or products with grapefruit extract during therapy; may cause toxicity.
- May cause dizziness. Caution patient to avoid driving or other activities requiring alertness until response to medication is known.
- Advise patient to notify health care professional of all Rx or OTC medications, vitamins, or herbal products being taken and to consult with health care professional before taking other medications, especially St. John's wort, during therapy.
- Instruct patient to notify health care professional promptly if fever; chills; cough; hoarseness; sore throat; signs of infection; lower back or side pain; painful or difficulty urination; bleeding gums; bruising; petechiae; blood in stools, urine, or emesis; increased fatigue; dyspnea; signs of fluid retention, or orthostatic hypotension occurs. Caution patient to avoid crowds and persons with known infections. Instruct patients to use a soft toothbrush and electric razor and to avoid falls. Caution patient not to drink alcoholic beverages or take medication containing aspirin or NSAIDs; may precipitate bleeding.
- Instruct patient not to receive any vaccinations without advice of health care professional.
- Discuss the possibility of hair loss with patient. Explore methods of coping. Regrowth usually occurs 2–3 mo after discontinuation of therapy.
- Advise women of childbearing potential to use highly effective contraception during therapy and to avoid breast feeding.

Evaluation/Desired Outcomes

- Decrease in production of leukemic cells.

niMODipine (nye-moe-di-peen)

✱Nimotop, Nymalize

Classification

Therapeutic: subarachnoid hemorrhage therapy agents

Pharmacologic: calcium channel blockers

Pregnancy Category C

Indications

Management of subarachnoid hemorrhage.

Action

Inhibits the transport of calcium into vascular smooth muscle cells, resulting in inhibition of excitation-contraction coupling and subsequent contraction. Potent peripheral vasodilator. **Therapeutic Effects:** Prevention of vascular spasm after subarachnoid hemorrhage, resulting in decreased neurologic impairment.

Pharmacokinetics

Absorption: Well absorbed following oral administration but extensively metabolized, resulting in ↓ bioavailability.

Distribution: Crosses the blood-brain barrier; remainder of distribution unknown.

Protein Binding: >95%.

Metabolism and Excretion: Mostly metabolized by the liver; ≤10% excreted unchanged by kidneys.

Half-life: 1–2 hr.

TIME/ACTION PROFILE (vasodilation)

ROUTE	ONSET	PEAK	DURATION
PO	unknown	1 hr	4 hr

Contraindications/Precautions

Contraindicated in: Hypersensitivity; Systolic BP <90 mm Hg; Concurrent use of strong CYP3A4 inhibitors (↑ risk of hypotension); Concurrent use of strong CYP3A4 inducers (↓ efficacy).

Use Cautiously in: Severe hepatic impairment (dose ↓ recommended); Severe renal impairment; History of serious ventricular arrhythmias or HF; OB, Lactation, Pedi: Safety not established; Geri: Dose ↓ recommended due to↑ risk of hypotension.

Adverse Reactions/Side Effects

CNS: abnormal dreams, anxiety, confusion, dizziness, drowsiness, headache, nervousness, psychiatric disturbances, weakness. **EENT:** blurred vision, disturbed equilibrium, epistaxis, tinnitus. **Resp:** cough, dyspnea. **CV:** ARRHYTHMIAS, HF, chest pain, hypotension, palpitations, peripheral edema, syncope, tachycardia. **GI:** ↑ liver enzymes, anorexia, constipation, diarrhea, dry mouth, dysgeusia, dyspepsia, nausea, vomiting. **GU:** dysuria, nocturia, polyuria, sexual dysfunction, urinary frequency. **Derm:** dermatitis, erythema multiforme, flushing, ↑ sweating, photosensitivity, pruritus/urticaria, rash. **Endo:** gynecomastia, hyperglycemia. **Hemat:** anemia, leukopenia, thrombocytopenia. **Metab:** weight gain. **MS:** joint stiffness, muscle cramps. **Neuro:** paresthesia, tremor. **Misc:** STEVENS-JOHNSON SYNDROME, gingival hyperplasia.

Interactions

Drug-Drug: **Strong CYP3A4 inhibitors**, including **clarithromycin**, **telithromycin**, **indinavir**, **nelfinavir**, **ritonavir**, **saquinavir**, **boceprevir**, **ketoconazole**, **itraconazole**, **posaconazole**, **voriconazole**, **conivaptan**, and **nefazodone** may ↑ levels and the risk of hypotension; avoid concurrent use. **Strong CYP3A4 inducers**, including **carbamazepine**, **phenobarbital**, **phenytoin**, and **rifampin** may ↓ levels and effects; avoid concurrent use. Additive hypotension may occur when used concurrently with **fentanyl**, other **antihypertensives**, **nitrates**, acute ingestion of **alcohol**, or **quinidine**.

Drug-Natural Products: **St. John's wort** may ↓ levels and effect; avoid concurrent use.

Drug-Food: **Grapefruit** and **grapefruit juice** ↑ levels and effect; avoid concurrent use.

Route/Dosage

PO (Adults): 60 mg every 4 hr for 21 days; therapy should be started within 96 hr of subarachnoid hemorrhage.

Hepatic Impairment

PO (Adults): 30 mg every 4 hr for 21 days; therapy should be started within 96 hr of subarachnoid hemorrhage.

Availability (generic available)

Capsules: 30 mg. **Oral solution:** 3 mg/mL.

N

NURSING IMPLICATIONS

Assessment

- Assess patient's neurologic status (level of consciousness, movement) prior to and periodically following administration.
- Monitor BP and pulse prior to therapy and periodically during therapy.
- Monitor intake and output ratios and daily weight. Assess for signs of HF (peripheral edema, rales/crackles, dyspnea, weight gain, jugular venous distention).
- Assess for rash periodically during therapy. May cause Stevens-Johnson syndrome. Discontinue therapy if severe or if accompanied with fever, general malaise, fatigue, muscle or joint aches, blisters, oral lesions, conjunctivitis, hepatitis, and/or eosinophilia.
- ***Lab Test Considerations:*** Total serum calcium concentrations are not affected by calcium channel blockers.
- Monitor serum potassium periodically. Hypokalemia ↑ risk of arrhythmias; should be corrected.
- Monitor renal and hepatic functions periodically. Several days of therapy may cause ↑ hepatic enzymes, which return to normal upon discontinuation of therapy.
- May occasionally cause ↓ platelet count.

Potential Nursing Diagnoses

Ineffective tissue perfusion (Indications)

Implementation

- Do not confuse nimodipine with nicardipine or nifedipine.
- Begin administration within 96 hr of subarachnoid hemorrhage and continue every 4 hr for 21 consecutive days.

- Administer by PO route ONLY; when administered IV or parenterally, may cause serious adverse events, including death.
- **PO:** If patient is unable to swallow capsule, make a hole in both ends of the capsule with a sterile 18-gauge needle and extract the contents into a syringe. Empty contents into water or nasogastric tube and flush with 30 mL normal saline.
- Administer oral solution 1 hr before or 2 hr after meals. For administration via NG or gastric tube, administer via syringe included, then refill syringe with 20 mL of 0.9% saline water solution; flush remaining contents from NG or gastric tube into stomach.

Patient/Family Teaching

- Advise patient to take medication as directed, even if feeling well. Take missed doses as soon as possible unless almost time for next dose; do not double doses. May need to be discontinued gradually.
- Advise patient to avoid grapefruit or grapefruit juice during therapy.
- Caution patient to change positions slowly to minimize orthostatic hypotension.
- May cause drowsiness or dizziness. Advise patient to avoid driving or other activities requiring alertness until response to the medication is known.
- Instruct patient to notify health care professional of all Rx or OTC medications, vitamins, or herbal products being taken and to avoid concurrent use of alcohol or OTC medications and herbal products, especially cold preparations, without consulting health care professional.
- Advise patient to notify health care professional if rash, irregular heartbeats, dyspnea, swelling of hands and feet, pronounced dizziness, nausea, constipation, or hypotension occurs or if headache is severe or persistent.
- Caution patient to wear protective clothing and use sunscreen to prevent photosensitivity reactions.
- Advise female patient to notify health care professional if pregnancy is planned or suspected or if breast feeding.

Evaluation/Desired Outcomes

- Improvement in neurologic deficits due to vasospasm following subarachnoid hemorrhage.

nitrofurantoin

(nye-troe-fyoor-**an**-toyn)

Furadantin, Furantoin, Macrobid, Macrodantin

Classification

Therapeutic: anti-infectives

Pregnancy Category B

Indications

Prevention and treatment of urinary tract infections caused by susceptible organisms; not effective in systemic bacterial infections.

Action

Interferes with bacterial enzymes. **Therapeutic Effects:** Bactericidal or bacteriostatic action against susceptible organisms. **Spectrum:** Many gram-negative and some gram-positive organisms, specifically: *Citrobacter*, *Corynebacterium*, *Enterobacter*, *Escherichia coli*, *Klebsiella*, *Neisseria*, *Salmonella*, *Shigella*, *Staphylococcus aureus*, *Staphylococcus epidermidis*, *Enterococcus*.

Pharmacokinetics

Absorption: Readily absorbed after oral administration. Absorption is slower but more complete with macrocrystals (Macrodantin).

Distribution: Crosses placenta; enters breast milk.

Protein Binding: 40%.

Metabolism and Excretion: Partially metabolized by the liver; 30–50% excreted unchanged by the kidneys.

Half-life: 20 min (↑ in renal impairment).

TIME/ACTION PROFILE (urine levels)

ROUTE	ONSET	PEAK	DURATION
PO	unknown	30 min	6–12 hr

Contraindications/Precautions

Contraindicated in: Hypersensitivity; Hypersensitivity to parabens (suspension); Oliguria, anuria, or significant renal impairment (CCr <60 mL/min); History of cholestatic jaundice or hepatic impairment with previous use of nitrofurantoin; Pregnancy near term and infants <1 mo (↑ risk of hemolytic anemia).

Use Cautiously in: Glucose–6–phosphate dehydrogenase (G6PD) deficiency (↑ risk of hemolytic anemia, especially in Blacks and Mediterranean and Near-Eastern ethnic groups); Patients with diabetes or debilitated patients (neuropathy may be more common); OB: Safety not established but has been used safely in pregnant women. Lactation: May cause hemolysis in infants with G6PD deficiency who are breast fed; Geri: Appears on Beers list; ↑ risk for renal, hepatic, and pulmonary reactions.

Adverse Reactions/Side Effects

CNS: dizziness, drowsiness, headache. **EENT:** nystagmus. **Resp:** PNEUMONITIS, PULMONARY FIBROSIS. **CV:** chest pain. **GI:** HEPATOTOXICITY, CLOSTRIDIUM DIFFICILE-ASSOCIATED DIARRHEA (CDAD), anorexia, nausea, vomiting, abdominal pain, diarrhea. **GU:** rust/brown discoloration of urine. **Derm:** photosensitivity. **Hemat:** blood dyscrasias, hemolytic anemia. **Neuro:** peripheral neuropathy. **Misc:** hypersensitivity reactions.

Interactions

Drug-Drug: Probenecid prevents high urinary concentrations; may ↓ effectiveness. **Antacids** may ↓ absorption. ↑ risk of neurotoxicity with **neurotoxic drugs**. ↑ risk of hepatotoxicity with **hepatotoxic drugs**. ↑ risk of pneumonitis with **drugs having pulmonary toxicity**.

Route/Dosage

PO (Adults): *Treatment of active infection*—50–100 mg q 6–8 hr *or* 100 mg q 12 hr as extended-release product. *Chronic suppression*—50–100 mg single evening dose.

PO (Children >1 mo): *Treatment of active infection*—5–7 mg/kg/day divided q 6 hr; maximum dose: 400 mg/day. *Chronic suppression*—1–2 mg/kg/day as a single dose at bedtime; maximum dose: 100 mg/day (unlabeled).

Availability (generic available)

Oral suspension: 25 mg/5 mL. **Cost:** *Generic*—$608.68/230 mL. **Capsules:** 25 mg, 50 mg, 100 mg. **Cost:** *Generic*—50 mg $199.00/100, 100 mg $338.00/100. **Extended-release capsules:** 100 mg. **Cost:** *Generic*—$320.92/100.

NURSING IMPLICATIONS

Assessment

- Assess for signs and symptoms of urinary tract infection (frequency, urgency, pain, and burning on urination; fever; cloudy or foul-smelling urine) before and periodically during therapy.
- Obtain specimens for culture and sensitivity before and during drug administration.
- Monitor intake and output ratios. Report significant discrepancies in totals.
- Monitor bowel function. Diarrhea, abdominal cramping, fever, and bloody stools should be reported to health care professional promptly as a sign of Clostridium difficile-associated diarrhea (CDAD). May begin up to several weeks following cessation of therapy.
- Assess for signs and symptoms of pulmonary reactions periodically during therapy. Acute reactions (fever, chills, cough, chest pain, dyspnea, pulmonary infiltration with consolidation or pleural effusion on x-ray, eosinophilia) usually occur within first week of treatment and resolve when therapy is discontinued. Chronic reactions (malaise, dyspnea on exertion, cough, altered pulmonary function) may indicate pneumonitis or pulmonary fibrosis and are more common in patients taking nitrofurantoin for 6 mo or longer.
- ***Lab Test Considerations:*** Monitor CBC routinely with patients on prolonged therapy.
- Monitor liver function tests periodically during therapy. May cause ↑ serum glucose, bilirubin, alkaline phosphatase, BUN, and creatinine. If hepatotoxicity occurs, discontinue therapy.
- Monitor renal function periodically during therapy.

Potential Nursing Diagnoses

Risk for infection (Indications)

Implementation

- **PO:** Administer with food or milk to minimize GI irritation, to delay and increase absorption, to increase peak concentration, and to prolong duration of therapeutic concentration in the urine.
- Do not crush tablets or open capsules.
- Administer liquid preparations with calibrated measuring device. Shake well before administration. Oral suspension may be mixed with water, milk, fruit juices, or infant formula. Rinse mouth with water after administration of oral suspension to avoid staining teeth.

Patient/Family Teaching

- Instruct patient to take medication around the clock, as directed. Take missed doses as soon as remembered and space next dose 2–4 hr apart. Do not skip or double up on missed doses.
- May cause dizziness or drowsiness. Caution patient to avoid driving or other activities requiring alertness until response to medication is known.
- Inform patient that medication may cause a rust-yellow to brown discoloration of urine, which is not significant.
- Advise patient to notify health care professional if fever, chills, cough, chest pain, dyspnea, skin rash, numbness or tingling of the fingers or toes, or intolerable GI upset occurs. Signs of superinfection (milky, foul-smelling urine; perineal irritation; dysuria) should also be reported.
- Instruct patient to notify health care professional if fever and diarrhea develop, especially if stool contains blood, pus, or mucus. Advise patient not to treat diarrhea without consulting health care professional.
- Instruct patient to consult health care professional if no improvement is seen within a few days after initiation of therapy.

Evaluation/Desired Outcomes

- Resolution of the signs and symptoms of infection. Therapy should be continued for a minimum of 7 days and for at least 3 days after the urine has become sterile.
- Decrease in the frequency of infections in chronic suppressive therapy.

NITROGLYCERIN
(nye-tro-**gli**-ser-in)

nitroglycerin extended-release capsules

Nitro-Time, ✱Nitrogard SR

N

nitroglycerin intravenous
~~Nitro-Bid IV~~, ✽Nitroject, ~~Tridil~~

nitroglycerin sublingual tablets
Nitrostat

nitroglycerin transdermal ointment
Nitro-Bid, ✽Nitrol

nitroglycerin transdermal patch
Minitran, Nitro-Dur, ✽Trinipatch

nitroglycerin translingual spray
Nitrolingual, Nitromist, ✽Rho-Nitro

Classification
Therapeutic: antianginals
Pharmacologic: nitrates

Pregnancy Category B (tablets), C (capsules, IV, spray, ointment, patch)

Indications
Acute (**translingual, SL, ointment**) and long-term prophylatic (**oral, transdermal**) management of angina pectoris. **PO:** Adjunct treatment of HF. **IV:** Adjunct treatment of acute MI. Production of controlled hypotension during surgical procedures. Treatment of HF.

Action
Increases coronary blood flow by dilating coronary arteries and improving collateral flow to ischemic regions. Produces vasodilation (venous greater than arterial). Decreases left ventricular end-diastolic pressure and left ventricular end-diastolic volume (preload). Reduces myocardial oxygen consumption. **Therapeutic Effects:** Relief or prevention of anginal attacks. Increased cardiac output. Reduction of BP.

Pharmacokinetics
Absorption: Well absorbed after oral, buccal, and sublingual administration. Also absorbed through skin. Orally administered nitroglycerin is rapidly metabolized, leading to ↓ bioavailability.
Distribution: Unknown.
Metabolism and Excretion: Undergoes rapid and almost complete metabolism by the liver; also metabolized by enzymes in bloodstream.
Half-life: 1–4 min.

TIME/ACTION PROFILE (cardiovascular effects)

ROUTE	ONSET	PEAK	DURATION
SL/Translingual	1–3 min	unknown	30–60 min
PO-ER	40–60 min	unknown	8–12 hr
Oint	20–60 min	unknown	4–8 hr
Patch	40–60 min	unknown	8–24 hr
IV	immediate	unknown	several min

Contraindications/Precautions
Contraindicated in: Hypersensitivity; Severe anemia; Pericardial tamponade; Constrictive pericarditis; Alcohol intolerance (large IV doses only); Concurrent use of PDE-5 inhibitor (sildenafil, tadalafil, vardenafil) or riociguat.
Use Cautiously in: Head trauma or cerebral hemorrhage; Glaucoma; Hypertrophic cardiomyopathy; Severe liver impairment; Malabsorption or hypermotility (PO); Hypovolemia (IV); Normal or ↓ pulmonary capillary wedge pressure (IV); Cardioversion (remove transdermal patch before procedure); OB: May compromise maternal/fetal circulation; Lactation, Pedi: Safety not established.

Adverse Reactions/Side Effects
CNS: dizziness, headache, apprehension, restlessness, weakness. **EENT:** blurred vision. **CV:** hypotension, tachycardia, syncope. **GI:** abdominal pain, nausea, vomiting. **Derm:** contact dermatitis (transdermal). **Misc:** alcohol intoxication (large IV doses only), cross-tolerance, flushing, tolerance.

Interactions
Drug-Drug: Concurrent use of **sildenafil**, **tadalafil**, or **vardenafil** may result in severe hypotension (do not use within 24 hr of isosorbide dinitrate or mononitrate); concurrent use contraindicated. Concurrent use of **riociguat** may result in severe hypotension; concurrent use contraindicated. Additive hypotension with **antihypertensives**, acute ingestion of **alcohol**, **beta blockers**, **calcium channel blockers**, **haloperidol**, or **phenothiazines**. Agents having anticholinergic properties (**tricyclic antidepressants**, **antihistamines**, **phenothiazines**) may ↓ absorption of translingual or sublingual nitroglycerin.

Route/Dosage
SL (Adults): 0.3–0.6 mg; may repeat q 5 min for 2 additional doses for acute attack.
Translingual Spray (Adults): 1–2 sprays; may be repeated q 5 min for 2 additional doses for acute attack. Both may also be used prophylactically 5–10 min before activities that may precipitate an acute attack.
PO (Adults): 2.5–9 mg q 8–12 hr.
IV (Adults): 5 mcg/min; ↑ by 5 mcg/min q 3–5 min to 20 mcg/min; if no response, ↑ by 10–20 mcg/min q 3–5 min (dosing determined by hemodynamic parameters; max: 200 mcg/min).
Transdermal (Adults): *Ointment*—1–2 in. q 6–8 hr. *Transdermal patch*—0.2–0.4 mg/hr initially; may titrate up to 0.4–0.8 mg/hr. Patch should be worn 12–14 hr/day and then taken off for 10–12 hr/day.

Availability (generic available)
Extended-release capsules: 2.5 mg, 6.5 mg, 9 mg. **Sublingual tablets:** 0.3 mg, 0.4 mg, 0.6 mg. **Translingual spray:** 400 mcg/spray in 4.9–g bottle (60 doses) or 14.6-g bottle (200 doses) (Nitrolingual), 400 mcg/spray in 8.5–g bottle (230 doses) (Nitro-

mist). **Transdermal patch:** 0.1 mg/hr, 0.2 mg/hr, 0.3 mg/hr, 0.4 mg/hr, 0.6 mg/hr, 0.8 mg/hr. **Transdermal ointment:** 2%. **Solution for injection:** 5 mg/mL. **Premixed solution (in D5W):** 25 mg/250 mL, 50 mg/250 mL, 100 mg/250 mL.

NURSING IMPLICATIONS

Assessment

- Assess location, duration, intensity, and precipitating factors of patient's anginal pain.
- Monitor BP and pulse before and after administration. Patients receiving IV nitroglycerin require continuous ECG and BP monitoring. Additional hemodynamic parameters may be monitored.
- ***Lab Test Considerations:*** May cause ↑ urine catecholamine and urine vanillylmandelic acid concentrations.
- Excessive doses may cause ↑ methemoglobin concentrations.
- May cause falsely ↑ serum cholesterol levels.

Potential Nursing Diagnoses

Acute pain (Indications)
Ineffective tissue perfusion (Indications)

Implementation

- **PO:** Administer dose 1 hr before or 2 hr after meals with a full glass of water for faster absorption. Sustained-release preparations should be swallowed whole; do not break, crush, or chew.
- **SL:** Tablet should be held under tongue until dissolved. Avoid eating, drinking, or smoking until tablet is dissolved.
- **Translingual spray:** Spray *Nitrolingual* under tongue. Spray *Nitromist* on or under tongue.

IV Administration

- **IV:** Doses must be diluted and administered as an infusion. Standard infusion sets made of polyvinyl chloride (PVC) plastic may absorb up to 80% of the nitroglycerin in solution. Use glass bottles only and special tubing provided by manufacturer.
- **Continuous Infusion:** ***Diluent:*** Vials must be diluted in D5W or 0.9% NaCl. Premixed infusions already diluted in D5W and are ready to be administered (no further dilution needed). Admixed solutions stable for 48 hr at room temperature or 7 days if refrigerated. Stability of premixed solutions based on manufacturer's expiration date. ***Concentration:*** Should not exceed 400 mcg/mL. ***Rate:*** See Route/Dosage section. Administer via infusion pump to ensure accurate rate. Titrate rate according to patient response.
- **Y-Site Compatibility:** acyclovir, alemtuzumab, alfentanil, amikacin, aminocaproic acid, aminophylline, amiodarone, amphotericin B lipid complex, amphotericin B liposome, anidulafungin, argatroban, ascorbic acid, atropine, azithromycin, aztreonam, benztropine, bivalirudin, bleomycin, bumetanide, buprenorphine, butorphanol, calcium chloride, calcium gluconate, cangrelor, carboplatin, carmustine, caspofungin, cefazolin, cefotaxime, cefotetan, cefoxitin, ceftazidime, ceftriaxone, cefuroxime, chloramphenicol, chlorpromazine, cisatracurium, cisplatin, clindamycin, cyanocobalamin, cyclophosphamide, cyclosporine, cytarabine, dactinomycin, dexamethasone, dexmedetomidine, dexrazoxane, digoxin, diltiazem, diphenhydramine, dobutamine, docetaxel, dolasetron, dopamine, doxorubicin hydrochloride, doxorubicin liposomal, doxycycline, enalaprilat, ephedrine, epinephrine, epirubicin, epoetin alfa, eptifibatide, ertapenem, erythromycin, esmolol, etoposide, etoposide phosphate, famotidine, fenoldopam, fentanyl, fluconazole, fludarabine, fluorouracil, folic acid, foscarnet, fosphenytoin, ganciclovir, gemcitabine, gentamicin, glycopyrrolate, granisetron, heparin, hydrocortisone, hydromorphone, idarubicin, ifosfamide, imipenem-cilastatin, indomethacin, insulin, irinotecan, isoproterenol, ketorolac, labetalol, leucovorin, lidocaine, linezolid, lorazepam, magnesium sulfate, mannitol, mechlorethamine, meperidine, mesna, methotrexate, methyldopate, methylprednisolone, metoclopramide, metronidazole, metoprolol, metronidazole, micafungin, midazolam, milrinone, minocycline, mitoxantrone, morphine, moxifloxacin, multivitamins, mycophenolate, nafcillin, nalbuphine, naloxone, nesiritide, nicardipine, nitroprusside, norepinephrine, octreotide, ondansetron, oxacillin, oxaliplatin, oxytocin, paclitaxel, palonosetron, pamidronate, pancuronium, pantoprazole, papaverine, pemetrexed, penicillin G, pentamidine, pentazocine, pentobarbital, phenobarbital, phenylephrine, phytonadione, piperacillin/tazobactam, potassium acetate, potassium chloride, procainamide, prochlorperazine, promethazine, propofol, propranolol, protamine, pyridoxine, quinupristin-dalfopristin, ranitidine, remifentanil, rocuronium, sodium bicarbonate, streptokinase, succinylcholine, sufentanil, tacrolimus, teniposide, theophylline, thiamine, thiopental, thiotepa, tigecycline, tirofiban, tobramycin, topotecan, vancomycin, vasopressin, vecuronium, verapamil, vincristine, vinorelbine, voriconazole, warfarin, zoledronic acid.
- **Y-Site Incompatibility:** alteplase, dantrolene, daptomycin, diazepam, hydroxycobalamin, levofloxacin, phenytoin, trimethoprim/sulfamethoxazole.
- **Additive Incompatibility:** Manufacturer recommends that nitroglycerin not be admixed with other medications.
- **Topical:** Sites of topical application should be rotated to prevent skin irritation. Remove patch or ointment from previous site before application.

N

- Doses may be increased to the highest dose that does not cause symptomatic hypotension.
- Apply ointment by using dose-measuring application papers supplied with ointment. Squeeze ointment onto measuring scale printed on paper. Use paper to spread ointment onto nonhairy area of skin (chest, abdomen, thighs; avoid distal extremities) in a thin, even layer, covering a 2–3-in. area. Do not allow ointment to come in contact with hands. Do not massage or rub in ointment; this will increase absorption and interfere with sustained action. Apply occlusive dressing if ordered.
- Transdermal patches may be applied to any hairless site (avoid distal extremities or areas with cuts or calluses). Apply firm pressure over patch to ensure contact with skin, especially around edges. Apply a new dose unit if the first one becomes loose or falls off. Units are waterproof and not affected by showering or bathing. Do not cut or trim system to adjust dosage. Do not alternate between brands of transdermal products; dose may not be equivalent. Remove patches before MRI, cardioversion or defibrillation to prevent patient burns. Patch may be worn for 12–14 hr and removed for 10–12 hr at night to prevent development of tolerance.

Patient/Family Teaching

- Instruct patient to take medication as directed, even if feeling better. Take missed doses as soon as remembered unless next dose is scheduled within 2 hr (6 hr with extended-release preparations). Do not double doses. Do not discontinue abruptly; gradual dose reduction may be necessary to prevent rebound angina.
- Caution patient to change positions slowly to minimize orthostatic hypotension. First dose should be taken while in a sitting or reclining position, especially in geriatric patients.
- Advise patient to avoid concurrent use of alcohol with this medication. Patient should also consult health care professional before taking OTC medications while taking nitroglycerin.
- Inform patient that headache is a common side effect that should decrease with continuing therapy. Aspirin or acetaminophen may be ordered to treat headache. Notify health care professional if headache is persistent or severe.
- Advise patient to notify health care professional if dry mouth or blurred vision occurs.
- **Acute Anginal Attacks:** Advise patient to sit down and use medication at first sign of attack. Relief usually occurs within 5 min. Dose may be repeated if pain is not relieved in 5–10 min. Call health care professional or go to nearest emergency room if anginal pain is not relieved by 3 tablets in 15 min.
- **SL:** Inform patient that tablets should be kept in original glass container or in specially made metal containers, with cotton removed to prevent absorption. Tablets lose potency in containers made of plastic or cardboard or when mixed with other capsules or tablets. Exposure to air, heat, and moisture also causes loss of potency. Instruct patient not to open bottle frequently, handle tablets, or keep bottle of tablets next to body (i.e., shirt pocket) or in automobile glove compartment. Advise patient that tablets should be replaced 6 mo after opening to maintain potency.
- **Lingual Spray:** Instruct patient to lift tongue and spray dose under tongue (*Nitrolingual, NitroMist*) or on tongue (*NitroMist*).

Evaluation/Desired Outcomes

- Decrease in frequency and severity of anginal attacks.
- Increase in activity tolerance. During long-term therapy, tolerance may be minimized by intermittent administration in 12–14 hr or 10–12 hr off intervals.
- Controlled hypotension during surgical procedures.
- Treatment of HF associated with acute MI.

HIGH ALERT

nitroprusside

(nye-troe-**pruss**-ide)

Nitropress

Classification

Therapeutic: antihypertensives

Pharmacologic: vasodilators

Pregnancy Category C

Indications

Hypertensive crises. Controlled hypotension during anesthesia. Cardiac pump failure or cardiogenic shock (alone or with dopamine).

Action

Produces peripheral vasodilation by a direct action on venous and arteriolar smooth muscle. **Therapeutic Effects:** Rapid lowering of BP. Decreased cardiac preload and afterload.

Pharmacokinetics

Absorption: IV administration results in complete bioavailability.

Distribution: Unknown.

Metabolism and Excretion: Rapidly metabolized in RBCs and tissues to cyanide and subsequently by the liver to thiocyanate.

Half-life: 2 min.

TIME/ACTION PROFILE (hypotensive effect)

ROUTE	ONSET	PEAK	DURATION
IV	immediate	rapid	1–10 min

Contraindications/Precautions

Contraindicated in: Hypersensitivity; ↓ cerebral perfusion.

Use Cautiously in: Renal disease (↑ risk of thiocyanate accumulation); Hepatic disease (↑ risk of cyanide accumulation); Hypothyroidism; Hyponatremia; Vitamin B deficiency; OB, Lactation: Safety not established; Geri: May have ↑ sensitivity to drug effects.

Adverse Reactions/Side Effects

CNS: dizziness, headache, restlessness. **EENT:** blurred vision, tinnitus. **CV:** dyspnea, hypotension, palpitations. **GI:** abdominal pain, nausea, vomiting. **F and E:** acidosis. **Local:** phlebitis at IV site. **Misc:** CYANIDE TOXICITY, thiocyanate toxicity.

Interactions

Drug-Drug: ↑ hypotensive effect with **ganglionic blocking agents**, **general anesthetics**, and other **antihypertensives**. **Estrogens** and **sympathomimetics** may ↓ the response to nitroprusside.

Route/Dosage

IV (Adults and Children): 0.3 mcg/kg/min initially; may be ↑ as needed up to 10 mcg/kg/min (usual dose is 3 mcg/kg/min; not to exceed 10 min of therapy at 10 mcg/kg/min infusion rate).

Availability (generic available)

Injection: 25 mg/mL.

NURSING IMPLICATIONS

Assessment

- Monitor BP, heart rate, and ECG frequently throughout therapy; continuous monitoring is preferred. Consult physician for parameters. Monitor for rebound hypertension following discontinuation of nitroprusside.
- Pulmonary capillary wedge pressure (PCWP) may be monitored in patients with MI or HF.
- ***Lab Test Considerations:*** May cause ↓ bicarbonate concentrations, P_{CO_2}, and p H.
- May cause ↑ lactate concentrations.
- May cause ↑ serum cyanide and thiocyanate concentrations.
- Monitor serum methemoglobin concentrations in patients receiving >10 mg/kg and exhibiting signs of impaired oxygen delivery despite adequate cardiac output and arterial P_{CO_2} (blood is chocolate brown without change on exposure to air). Treatment of methemoglobinemia is 1–2 mg/kg of methylene blue IV administered over several minutes.
- ***Toxicity and Overdose:*** If severe hypotension occurs, drug effects are quickly reversed, within 1–10 min, by decreasing rate or temporarily discontinuing infusion. May place patient in Trendelenburg position to maximize venous return.
- Monitor plasma thiocyanate levels daily in patients receiving prolonged infusions at a rate >3 mcg/kg/min or 1 mcg/kg/min in patients with anuria. Thiocyanate levels should not exceed 1 millimole/L.
- Signs and symptoms of thiocyanate toxicity include tinnitus, toxic psychoses, hyperreflexia, confusion, weakness, seizures, and coma.
- Cyanide toxicity may manifest as lactic acidosis, hypoxemia, tachycardia, altered consciousness, seizures, and characteristic breath odor similar to almonds.
- Acute treatment of cyanide toxicity includes 4–6 mg/kg of *sodium nitrite* (as a 3% solution) over 2–4 min. This acts as a buffer for cyanide by converting 10% of hemoglobin to methemoglobin. If administration of sodium nitrite is delayed, inhalation of crushed ampule (vaporole, aspirole) of *amyl nitrite* for 15–30 sec of every minute should be started until sodium nitrite is running. Following completion of sodium nitrite infusion, administer *sodium thiosulfate* 150–200 mcg/kg (available as 25% and 50% solutions). This will convert cyanide to thiocyanate, which may then be eliminated. If required, entire regimen may be repeated in 2 hr at 50% of the initial doses.

N

Potential Nursing Diagnoses

Ineffective tissue perfusion (Indications)

Implementation

- If infusion of 10 mcg/kg/min for 10 min does not produce adequate reduction in BP, manufacturer recommends nitroprusside be discontinued.
- May be administered in left ventricular HF concurrently with an inotropic agent (dopamine, dobutamine) when effective doses of nitroprusside restore pump function and cause excessive hypotension.

IV Administration

- **Continuous Infusion:** ***Diluent:*** Dilute 50 mg of nitroprusside in 250–1000 mL of D5W. Wrap infusion in aluminum foil to protect from light; administration set tubing need not be covered. Amber plastic bags do not offer sufficient protection from light; wrap must be opaque. Freshly prepared solution has a slight brownish tint; discard if solution is dark brown, orange, blue, green, or dark red. Solution must be used within 24 hr of preparation. ***Concentration:*** 50–200 mcg/mL. ***Rate:*** Based on patient's weight (see Route/Dosage section). Administer via infusion pump to ensure accurate dosage rate.
- **Y-Site Compatibility:** amikacin, aminophylline, argatroban, atropine, aztreonam, bivalirudin, bumetanide, calcium chloride, calcium gluconate, cefazolin, cefotaxime, cefoxitin, ceftriaxone, cefuroxime, chloramphenicol, cimetidine, clindamycin, cyclosporine, daptomycin, dexamethasone sodium phosphate, digoxin, diltiazem, dopamine, doxycycline, enalaprilat, epinephrine, ertapenem, esmolol, famotidine, fenoldopam, fentanyl, fluconazole, furosem-

ide, ganciclovir, gentamicin, granisetron, heparin, hydrocortisone sodium succinate, hydromorphone, insulin, isoproterenol, ketorolac, labetalol, lidocaine, linezolid, lorazepam, magnesium sulfate, meperidine, methylprednisolone sodium succinate, metoclopramide, metoprolol, metronidazole, micafungin, midazolam, milrinone, morphine, nafcillin, nesiritide, nicardipine, nitroglycerin, norepinephrine, ondansetron, palonosetron, pancuronium, pantoprazole, penicillin G potassium, phenylephrine, phytonadione, piperacillin/tazobactam, potassium chloride, potassium phosphate, procainamide, propofol, propranolol, protamine, ranitidine, sodium bicarbonate, tacrolimus, tirofiban, tobramycin, vancomycin, vasopressin, verapamil.

- **Y-Site Incompatibility:** acyclovir, ampicillin, caspofungin, ceftazidime, diazepam, diphenhydramine, erythromycin, hydralazine, hydroxyzine, levofloxacin, phenytoin, prochlorperazine, promethazine, quinupristin/dalfopristin, trimethoprim/sulfamethoxazole, voriconazole.

Patient/Family Teaching

- Advise patient to report the onset of tinnitus, dyspnea, dizziness, headache, or blurred vision immediately.

Evaluation/Desired Outcomes

- Decrease in BP without the appearance of side effects.
- Treatment of cardiac pump failure or cardiogenic shock.

nivolumab (nye-**vol**-ue-mab)

Opdivo

Classification

Therapeutic: antineoplastics

Pharmacologic: antibodies

Pregnancy Category UK

Indications

Progressive unresectable/metastatic melanoma previously treated with ipilimumab and if BRAF V600 mutation positive, a BRAF inhibitor. Metastatic squamous non-small cell lung cancer (NSCLC) with progression on or after platinum-based chemotherapy.

Action

Acts as a human programmed death receptor-1 (PD-1) blocking antibody. Inhibits T-cell proliferation and cytokine production. **Therapeutic Effects:** Decreased spread of melanoma. Decreased progression of and improved survival with NSCLC.

Pharmacokinetics

Absorption: IV administration results in complete bioavailability.

Distribution: Unknown.

Metabolism and Excretion: Unknown.

Half-life: 26.7 days.

TIME/ACTION PROFILE

ROUTE	ONSET	PEAK	DURATION
IV	unknown	unknown	unknown

Contraindications/Precautions

Contraindicated in: OB: Pregnancy (may cause fetal harm); Lactation: Discontinue breast feeding.

Use Cautiously in: Pedi: Safety and effectiveness not established; Rep: Women with childbearing potential.

Adverse Reactions/Side Effects

Resp: IMMUNE-MEDIATED PNEUMONITIS, cough. **CV:** peripheral edema. **GI:** IMMUNE-MEDIATED COLITIS, immune-mediated hepatitis. **GU:** immune-mediated nephritis/renal dysfunction. **Derm:** rash. **Endo:** immune-mediated hyper/hypothyroidism. **F and E:** hyperkalemia.

Interactions

Drug-Drug: None noted.

Route/Dosage

IV (Adults): 3 mg/kg every 2 weeks; immune-mediated adverse reactions may require dose modification/ discontinuation.

Availability

Solution for intravenous use: 10 mg/mL.

NURSING IMPLICATIONS

Assessment

- Monitor for signs and symptoms of immune-mediated pneumonitis (shortness of breath, chest pain, new or worse cough) periodically during therapy. Treat with corticosteroids 1–2 mg/kg/day prednisone equivalents for ≥Grade 2 pneumonitis followed by corticosteroid taper. Withhold nivolumab and monitor symptoms for moderate (Grade 2) pneumonitis; resume therapy when recovery to Grade 0 to 1. Permanently discontinue for severe (Grade 3) or life-threatening (Grade 4) pneumonitis.
- Monitor for signs and symptoms of immune-mediated colitis (diarrhea, abdominal pain, mucus or blood in stool, with or without fever). Treat with corticosteroids at doses of 1–2 mg/kg/day of prednisone or equivalents followed by corticosteroid taper for severe (Grade 3) or life-threatening (Grade 4) colitis. Treat with corticosteroids at a dose of 0.5 mg/kg/day of prednisone or equivalent followed by corticosteroid taper for moderate (Grade 2) colitis or > 5 days; if worsening or no improvement despite corticosteroids increase dose to 1–2 mg/kg/day prednisone equivalents. Withhold nivolumab for Grade 2 or 3 colitis; permanently discontinue nivolumab for Grade 4 colitis or for recurrent colitis upon restarting nivolumab.
- ***Lab Test Considerations:*** Monitor for abnormal liver tests prior to and periodically during therapy.

Administer corticosteroids at dose of 1–2 mg/kg/day prednisone equivalents for ≥Grade 2 transaminase ↑, with or without ↑ in total bilirubin. Withhold for moderate (Grade 2) and permanently discontinue for severe (Grade 3) or life-threatening (Grade 4) immune-mediated hepatitis.

- Monitor for ↑ serum creatinine prior to and periodically during therapy. Administer corticosteroids at a dose of 1–2 mg/kg/day prednisone equivalents followed by corticosteroid taper for life-threatening (Grade 4) ↑ serum creatinine and permanently discontinue nivolumab. Withhold nivolumab for severe (Grade 3) or moderate (Grade 2) ↑ serum creatinine and administer corticosteroids at a dose of 0.5–1 mg/kg/day prednisone equivalents followed by corticosteroid taper. If worsening or no improvement occurs, increase dose of corticosteroids to 1–2 mg/kg/day prednisolone equivalents and permanently discontinue nivolumab.
- Monitor thyroid function prior to and periodically during therapy. Treat hypothyroidism with replacement therapy. Use medical management for hyperthyroidism. Immune-mediated thyroid dysfunction does not require dose modification of nivolumab.

Potential Nursing Diagnoses

Diarrhea (Adverse Reactions)
Deficient knowledge, related to medication regimen (Patient/Family Teaching)

Implementation

IV Administration

- **Intermittent Infusion:** ***Diluent:*** 0.9% NaCl or D5W. ***Concentration:*** 1 mg/mL to 10 mg/mL. Mix by gentle inversion; do not shake. Solution is clear to slightly opalescent, colorless to slightly yellow; do not administer solution if discolored or contains particulate matter other than translucent to white proteinaceous particles. Solution is stable at room temperature for up to 4 hr and 24 hr if refrigerated. ***Rate:*** Infuse through a sterile, non-pyrogenic, low-protein binding 0.2 micrometer to 1.2 micrometer in-line filter over 60 min. Flush line at end of infusion.
- **Y-Site Incompatibility:** Do not administer other drugs through same infusion line.

Patient/Family Teaching

- Explain purpose of nivolumab to patient.
- Advise patient to notify health care professional immediately if signs and symptoms of pneumonitis, colitis, hepatitis (jaundice, severe nausea or vomiting, pain on right side of abdomen, lethargy, easy bruising or bleeding), kidney problems (decreased urine output, blood in urine, swollen ankles, loss of appetite), hormone gland problems (rapid heart beat, weight loss, increased sweating, weight gain, hair loss, feeling cold, constipation, deepening of voice, muscle aches, dizziness or fainting, persistent or unusual headache) occur.
- Instruct patient to notify health care professional of all Rx or OTC medications, vitamins, or herbal products being taken and to consult with health care professional before taking other medications.
- Rep: Advise female patient of reproductive potential to use highly effective contraception during and for 5 mo after last dose; may cause fetal harm. Avoid breast feeding during therapy.
- Emphasize importance of keeping scheduled appointments for blood work or other laboratory tests.

Evaluation/Desired Outcomes

- ↓ spread of melanoma.
- ↓ spread of NSCLC.

nizatidine, See HISTAMINE H_2 ANTAGONISTS.

HIGH ALERT

norepinephrine

(**nor**-ep-i-nef-rin)
Levophed

Classification
Therapeutic: vasopressors

Pregnancy Category C

Indications

Produces vasoconstriction and myocardial stimulation, which may be required after adequate fluid replacement in the treatment of severe hypotension and shock.

Action

Stimulates alpha-adrenergic receptors located mainly in blood vessels, causing constriction of both capacitance and resistance vessels. Also has minor beta-adrenergic activity (myocardial stimulation). **Therapeutic Effects:** Increased BP. Increased cardiac output.

Pharmacokinetics

Absorption: IV administration results in complete bioavailability.
Distribution: Concentrates in sympathetic nervous tissue. Does not cross the blood-brain barrier but readily crosses the placenta.
Metabolism and Excretion: Taken up and metabolized rapidly by sympathetic nerve endings.
Half-life: Unknown.

TIME/ACTION PROFILE (effects on BP)

ROUTE	ONSET	PEAK	DURATION
IV	immediate	rapid	1–2 min

Contraindications/Precautions

Contraindicated in: Vascular, mesenteric, or peripheral thrombosis; OB: ↓ uterine blood flow; Hypoxia; Hypercarbia; Hypotension secondary to hypovolemia (without appropriate volume replacement); Hypersensitivity to bisulfites.
Use Cautiously in: Hypertension; Concurrent use of MAO inhibitors, tricyclic antidepressants, or cyclopropane or halothane anesthetics; Hyperthyroidism; Cardiovascular disease; Lactation: Safety not established.

Adverse Reactions/Side Effects

CNS: anxiety, dizziness, headache, insomnia, restlessness, tremor, weakness. **Resp:** dyspnea. **CV:** arrhythmias, bradycardia, chest pain, hypertension. **GU:** ↓ urine output, renal failure. **Endo:** hyperglycemia. **F and E:** metabolic acidosis. **Local:** phlebitis at IV site. **Misc:** fever.

Interactions

Drug-Drug: Use with **cyclopropane** or **halothane anesthesia**, **cardiac glycosides**, **doxapram**, or local use of **cocaine** may result in ↑ myocardial irritability. Use with **MAO inhibitors**, **methyldopa**, **doxapram**, or **tricyclic antidepressants** may result in severe hypertension. **Alpha-adrenergic blockers** can prevent pressor response. **Beta blockers** may exaggerate hypertension or block cardiac stimulation. Concurrent use with **ergot alkaloids (ergotamine, methylergonovine**, or **oxytocin** may result in enhanced vasoconstriction and hypertension.

Route/Dosage

IV (Adults): 0.5–1 mcg/min initially, followed by maintenance infusion of 2–12 mcg/min titrated by BP response (average rate 2–4 mcg/min, up to 30 mcg/min for refractory shock have been used).
IV (Children): 0.1 mcg/kg/min initially; may be followed by infusion titrated to BP response, up to 1 mcg/kg/min.

Availability (generic available)

Injection: 1 mg/mL.

NURSING IMPLICATIONS

Assessment

- Monitor BP every 2–3 min until stabilized and every 5 min thereafter. Systolic BP is usually maintained at 80–100 mm Hg or 30–40 mm Hg below the previously existing systolic pressure in previously hypertensive patients. Consult physician for parameters. Continue to monitor BP frequently for hypotension following discontinuation of norepinephrine.
- ECG should be monitored continuously. CVP, intra-arterial pressure, pulmonary artery diastolic pressure, pulmonary capillary wedge pressure (PCWP), and cardiac output may also be monitored.
- Monitor urine output and notify health care professional if it decreases to <30 mL/hr.
- Assess IV site frequently throughout infusion. A large vein should be used to minimize risk of extravasation, which may cause tissue necrosis. If prolonged therapy is required or if blanching along the course of the vein occurs, change injection sites to provide relief from vasoconstriction.
- ***Toxicity and Overdose:*** If overdose occurs, discontinue norepinephrine and administer fluid and electrolyte replacement therapy. An alpha-adrenergic blocking agent may be administered intravenously to treat hypertension.

Potential Nursing Diagnoses

Decreased cardiac output (Indications)
Ineffective tissue perfusion (Indications)

Implementation

- ***High Alert:*** Vasoactive medications are inherently dangerous. Have second practitioner independently check original order, dose calculations, and infusion pump programming. Establish maximum dose limits. Norepinephrine overdose can result in severe peripheral vasoconstriction with resultant ischemia and necrosis of peripheral tissue. Assess peripheral circulation frequently.
- Volume depletion should be corrected, if possible, prior to initiation of norepinephrine.
- Heparin may be added to each 500 mL of solution to prevent thrombosis in the infused vein, perivenous reactions, and necrosis in patients with severe hypotension following MI.
- Norepinephrine may deplete plasma volume and cause ischemia of vital organs, resulting in hypotension when discontinued, if used for prolonged periods. Prolonged or large doses may also decrease cardiac output.
- Infusion should be discontinued gradually, upon adequate tissue perfusion and maintenance of BP, to prevent hypotension. Do not resume therapy unless BP falls to 70–80 mm Hg.

IV Administration

- **Continuous Infusion: *Diluent:*** Dilute 4 mg in 1000 mL of D5W or D5/0.9% NaCl. Do not dilute in 0.9% NaCl without dextrose. ***Concentration:*** 4 mcg/mL. Do not use discolored solutions (pink, yellow, brown) or those containing a precipitate. ***Rate:*** Titrate infusion rate according to patient response, using slowest possible rate to correct hypotension. Administer via infusion pump to ensure accurate dosage.
- **Y-Site Compatibility:** alemtuzumab, alfentanil, amikacin, anidulafungin, argatroban, ascorbic acid, atracurium, atropine, aztreonam, benztropine, bivalirudin, bleomycin, bumetanide, buprenorphine, butorphanol, calcium chloride, calcium gluconate,

carboplatin, carmustine, caspofungin, cefazolin, cefotaxime, cefotetan, cefoxitin, ceftaroline, ceftazidime, ceftriaxone, cefuroxime, chloramphenicol, chrlopromazine, cisatracurium, cisplatin, clindamycin, cyanocobalamin, cyclophosphamide, cyclosporine, cytarabine, dactinomycin, daptomycin, dexamethasone, dexrazoxane, digoxin, diltiazem, diphenhydramine, dobutamine, docetaxel, dopamine, doripenem, doxycycline, doxorubicin liposomal, enalaprilat, ephedrine, epinephrine, epirubicin, epoetin alfa, ertapenem, erythromycin, esmolol, etoposide, etoposide phosphate, famotidine, fenoldopam, fentanyl, fluconazole, fludarabine, gemcitabine, gentamicin, glycopyrrolate, granisetron, heparin, hetastarch, hydrocortisone sodium succinate, hydromorphone, idarubicin, ifosfamide, imipenem/cilastatin, irinotecan, isoproterenol, ketorolac, labetalol, leucovorin calcium, lidocaine, linezolid, lorazepam, magnesium sulfate, mannitol, mechlorethamine, meperidine, meropenem, metaraminol, methotrexate, methoxamine, methyldopate, methylprednisolone, metoclopramide, metoprolol, metronidazole, micafungin, midazolam, milrinone, mitoxantrone, morphine, moxifloxacin, multivitamins, mycophenolate, nafcillin, nalbuphine, naloxone, nicardipine, nitroglycerin, nitroprusside, octreotide, ondansetron, oxacillin, oxaliplatin, oxytocin, paclitaxel, palonosetron, pamidronate, pancuronium, papaverine, pemetrexed, penicillin G, pentamidine, pentazocine, phenylephrine, phytonadione, piperacillin/tazobactam, potassium acetate, potassium chloride, procainamide, prochlorperazine, promethazine, propofol, propranolol, protamine, pyridoxime, ranitidine, remifentanil, streptokinase, succinylcholine, sufentanil, tacrolimus, telavancin, teniposide, theophylline, thiamine, thiotepa, tigecycline, tirofiban, tobramycin, tolazoline, vancomycin, vasopressin, vecuronium, verapamil, vinblastine, vincristine, vinorelbine, vitamin B complex with C, voriconazole, zoledronic acid.

- **Y-Site Incompatibility:** aminophylline, amphotericin B colloidal, amphotericin B lipid complex, azathioprine, dantrolene, diazepam, diazoxide, folic acid, foscarnet, ganciclovir, indomethacin, pentobarbital, phenobarbital, phenytoin, sodium bicarbonate, thiopental, trimethoprim/sulfamethoxazole.

Patient/Family Teaching

- Instruct patient to report headache, dizziness, dyspnea, chest pain, or pain at infusion site promptly.

Evaluation/Desired Outcomes

- Increase in BP to normal range.
- Increased tissue perfusion.

norethindrone, See CONTRACEPTIVES, HORMONAL.

⧖ nortriptyline (nor-**trip**-ti-leen)

✱Aventyl, ✱Norventyl, Pamelor

Classification
Therapeutic: antidepressants
Pharmacologic: tricyclic antidepressants

Pregnancy Category D

Indications

Various forms of depression. **Unlabeled Use:** Management of chronic neurogenic pain.

Action

Potentiates the effect of serotonin and norepinephrine. Has significant anticholinergic properties. **Therapeutic Effects:** Antidepressant action that develops slowly over several weeks.

Pharmacokinetics

Absorption: Well absorbed after oral administration.
Distribution: Widely distributed. Enters breast milk in small amounts; probably crosses the placenta.
Protein Binding: 92%.
Metabolism and Excretion: Mostly metabolized by the liver (CYP2D6 isoenzyme); ⧖ the CYP2D6 enzyme system exhibits genetic polymorphism; ~7% of population may be poor metabolizers (PMs) and may have significantly ↑ nortriptyline concentrations and an ↑ risk of adverse effects.
Half-life: 18–28 hr.

TIME/ACTION PROFILE (antidepressant effect)

ROUTE	ONSET	PEAK	DURATION
PO	2–3 wk	6 wk	unknown

Contraindications/Precautions

Contraindicated in: Hypersensitivity; Angle-closure glaucoma; Alcohol intolerance (solution only); Concurrent use of MAO inhibitors or MAO-like drugs (linezolid or methylene blue).

Use Cautiously in: Pre-existing cardiovascular disease; History of seizures; Asthma; May ↑ risk of suicide attempt/ideation especially during early treatment or dose adjustment; OB: Use only if clearly needed and maternal benefits outweigh risk to fetus; Lactation: May result in sedation in infant; discontinue drug or bottle-feed; Pedi: Suicide risk may be greater in children or adolescents. Safety not established in children; Geri: More susceptible to adverse reactions; dose ↓ recommended. Geriatric men with prostatic hyperplasia may be more susceptible to urinary retention.

N

Adverse Reactions/Side Effects

CNS: SUICIDAL THOUGHTS, drowsiness, fatigue, lethargy, agitation, confusion, extrapyramidal reactions, hallucinations, headache, insomnia. **EENT:** blurred vision, dry eyes, dry mouth. **CV:** ARRHYTHMIAS, hypotension, ECG changes. **GI:** constipation, nausea, paralytic ileus, unpleasant taste, weight gain. **GU:** urinary retention. **Derm:** photosensitivity. **Endo:** gynecomastia. **Hemat:** blood dyscrasias.

Interactions

Drug-Drug: Concurrent use with **MAO inhibitors** may result in serious potentially fatal reactions (MAO inhibitors should be stopped at least 14 days before nortriptyline therapy. Nortriptyline should be stopped at least 14 days before MAO inhibitor therapy). Concurrent use with **MAO-inhibitor like drugs**, such as **linezolid** or **methylene blue** may ↑ risk of serotonin syndrome; concurrent use contraindicated; do not start therapy in patients receiving **linezolid** or **methylene blue**; if **linezolid** or **methylene blue** need to be started in a patient receiving nortriptyline, immediately discontinue nortriptyline and monitor for signs/symptoms of serotonin syndrome for 2 wk or until 24 hr after last dose of linezolid or methylene blue, whichever comes first (may resume nortriptyline therapy 24 hr after last dose of linezolid or methylene blue). May prevent the therapeutic response to most **antihypertensives**. Hypertensive crisis may occur with **clonidine**. ↑ CNS depression with other **CNS depressants**, including **alcohol**, **antihistamines**, **opioids**, and **sedative/hypnotics**. Adrenergic effects may be ↑ with other **adrenergic agents**, including **vasoconstrictors** and **decongestants**. ↑ anticholinergic effects with other **drugs possessing anticholinergic properties**, including **antihistamines**, **antidepressants**, **atropine**, **haloperidol**, **phenothiazines**, **quinidine**, and **disopyramide**. **Cimetidine**, **fluoxetine**, or **hormonal contraceptives** ↑ blood levels and risk of toxicity. ↑ risk of agranulocytosis with **antithyroid agents**. Drugs that affect serotonergic neurotransmitter systems, including **SSRIs**, **SNRIs**, **fentanyl**, **buspirone**, **tramadol** and **triptans** ↑ risk of serotonin syndrome.

Drug-Natural Products: Concomitant use of **kava-kava**, **valerian**, or **chamomile** can ↑ CNS depression. Use with **St. John's wort** ↑ of serotonin syndrome. ↑ anticholinergic effects with **jimson weed** and **scopolia**.

Route/Dosage

PO (Adults): 25 mg 3–4 times daily, up to 150 mg/day.

PO (Geriatric Patients or Adolescents): 30–50 mg/day in divided doses or as a single dose.

Availability (generic available)

Capsules: 10 mg, 25 mg, 50 mg, 75 mg. **Cost:** *Generic*—10 mg $40.50/100, 25 mg $80.31/100, 50 mg $145.55/100, 75 mg $221.95/100. **Oral solution:** 10 mg/5 mL. **Cost:** *Generic*—$182.95/473 mL.

NURSING IMPLICATIONS

Assessment

- Monitor mental status (orientation, mood, behavior).
- Assess weight and BMI initially and throughout treatment. For overweight/obese individuals, monitor fasting blood glucose and cholesterol levels.
- Monitor BP and pulse rate before and during initial therapy. Report significant decreases in BP or a sudden increase in pulse rate.
- Monitor baseline and periodic ECGs in geriatric patients or patients with heart disease. May cause prolonged PR and QT intervals and may flatten T waves.
- Assess for suicidal tendencies, especially during early therapy. Restrict amount of drug available to patient. Risk may be increased in children, adolescents, and adults ≤24 yrs. After starting therapy, children, adolescents, and young adults should be seen by health care professional at least weekly for 4 wk, every 3 wk for next 4 wk, and on advice of health care professional thereafter.
- **Pain:** Assess type, location, and severity of pain before and periodically during therapy. Use pain scale to monitor effectiveness of medication.
- ***Lab Test Considerations:*** Assess leukocyte and differential blood counts, liver function, and serum glucose periodically. May cause ↑ serum bilirubin and alkaline phosphatase. May cause bone marrow depression. Serum glucose may be ↑ or ↓.
- Serum levels may be monitored in patients who fail to respond to usual therapeutic dose. Therapeutic plasma concentration range is 50–150 ng/mL.
- May cause alterations in blood glucose levels.
- ***Toxicity and Overdose:*** Symptoms of acute overdose include disturbed concentration, confusion, restlessness, agitation, seizures, drowsiness, mydriasis, arrhythmias, fever, hallucinations, vomiting, and dyspnea.
- Treatment of overdose includes gastric lavage, activated charcoal, and a stimulant cathartic. Maintain respiratory and cardiac function (monitor ECG for at least 5 days) and temperature. Medications may include digoxin for HF, antiarrhythmics, and anticonvulsants.

Potential Nursing Diagnoses

Ineffective coping (Indications)
Risk for injury (Side Effects)
Sexual dysfunction (Side Effects)

Implementation

- Do not confuse Pamelor (nortriptyline) with Tambocor (flecainide).
- Taper to avoid withdrawal effects. Reduce dose 50% for 3 days, then by 50% for 3 more days, then discontinue.

- **PO:** Administer medication with meals to minimize gastric irritation.
- May be given as a single dose at bedtime to minimize sedation during the day. Dose increases should be made at bedtime because of sedation.

Patient/Family Teaching

- Instruct patient to take medication as directed. Take missed doses as soon as possible unless almost time for next dose; if regimen is a single dose at bedtime, do not take in the morning because of side effects. Advise patient that drug effects may not be noticed for at least 2 wk. Abrupt discontinuation may cause nausea, vomiting, diarrhea, headache, trouble sleeping with vivid dreams, and irritability.
- May cause drowsiness and blurred vision. Caution patient to avoid driving and other activities requiring alertness until response to drug is known.
- Instruct patient to notify health care professional if visual changes occur. Inform patient that periodic glaucoma testing may be required during long-term therapy.
- Caution patient to make position changes slowly to minimize orthostatic hypotension. (This side effect is less pronounced with this medication than with other tricyclic antidepressants.).
- Advise patient, family, and caregivers to look for suicidality, especially during early therapy or dose changes. Notify health care professional immediately if thoughts about suicide or dying, attempts to commit suicide, new or worse depression or anxiety, agitation or restlessness, panic attacks, insomnia, new or worse irritability, aggressiveness, acting on dangerous impulses, mania, or other changes in mood or behavior or if symptoms of serotonin syndrome occur.
- Advise patient to avoid alcohol or other CNS depressant drugs during therapy and for at least 3–7 days after therapy has been discontinued.
- Instruct patient to notify health care professional if urinary retention occurs or if dry mouth or constipation persists. Sugarless candy or gum may diminish dry mouth, and an increase in fluid intake or bulk may prevent constipation. If symptoms persist, dose reduction or discontinuation may be necessary. Consult health care professional if dry mouth persists for more than 2 wk.
- Caution patient to use sunscreen and protective clothing to prevent photosensitivity reactions.
- Alert patient that urine may turn blue-green in color.
- Inform patient of need to monitor dietary intake. Increase in appetite may lead to undesired weight gain. Refer as appropriate for nutritional, weight, or medical management.
- May have teratogenic effects. Instruct patient to notify health care professional immediately if pregnancy is planned or suspected.
- Advise patient to notify health care professional of medication regimen before treatment or surgery.
- Therapy for depression is usually prolonged. Emphasize the importance of follow-up exams.

Evaluation/Desired Outcomes

- Increased sense of well-being.
- Renewed interest in surroundings.
- Increased appetite.
- Improved energy level.
- Improved sleep.
- Decrease in severity of chronic neurogenic pain. Patients may require 2–6 wk of therapy before full therapeutic effects of medication are seen.

NPH/regular insulin mixtures, See INSULIN (mixtures).

nystatin (nye-**stat**-in)

Mycostatin, ✱Nadostine, Nilstat, ✱PMS-Nystatin

Classification

Therapeutic: antifungals (topical/local)

Pregnancy Category B

For other nystatin dosage forms, see antifungals (topical) and antifungals (vaginal)

Indications

Lozenges, oral suspension: Local treatment of oropharyngeal candidiasis. Treatment of intestinal candidiasis.

Action

Binds to fungal cell membrane, allowing leakage of cellular contents. **Therapeutic Effects:** Fungistatic or fungicidal action. **Spectrum:** Active against most pathogenic *Candida* species, including *C. albicans*.

Pharmacokinetics

Absorption: Poorly absorbed; action is primarily local.

Distribution: Unknown.

Metabolism and Excretion: Excreted unchanged in the feces after oral administration.

Half-life: Unknown.

TIME/ACTION PROFILE (antifungal effects)

ROUTE	ONSET	PEAK	DURATION
Top	rapid	unknown	2 hr†

†Maintenance of saliva levels required to inhibit growth of Candida species after oral dissolution of 2 lozenges.

Contraindications/Precautions

Contraindicated in: Hypersensitivity; Some products may contain ethyl alcohol or benzyl alcohol—avoid use in patients who may be hypersensitive to or intolerant of these additives.
Use Cautiously in: Denture wearers (dentures require soaking in nystatin suspension); Pedi: Lozenges, pastilles, or troches may pose a choking risk for children <5 yr.

Adverse Reactions/Side Effects

GI: diarrhea, nausea, stomach pain (large doses), vomiting. **Derm:** contact dermatitis, Stevens-Johnson syndrome.

Interactions

Drug-Drug: None significant.

Route/Dosage

PO (Adults and Children): 400,000–600,000 units 4 times daily as oral suspension or 200,000–400,000 units 4–5 times daily as pastilles (lozenges).
PO (Infants): 200,000 units 4 times daily or 100,000 units to each side of the mouth 4 times daily.
PO (Neonates, Premature, and Low Birth Weight): 100,000 units 4 times daily or 50,000 units to each side of the mouth 4 times a day.

Availability (generic available)

Oral suspension: 100,000 units/mL. **Oral pastilles (lozenges, troches):** 200,000 units/troche. **Powder for oral suspension:** 1/8 tsp = 500,000 units. **Oral tablets:** 500,000 units.

NURSING IMPLICATIONS

Assessment

- Inspect oral mucous membranes before and frequently throughout therapy. Increased irritation of mucous membranes may indicate need to discontinue medication.

Potential Nursing Diagnoses

Risk for impaired skin integrity (Indications)
Risk for infection (Indications)

Implementation

- **PO:** Suspension should be administered by placing ½ of dose in each side of mouth. Patient should hold suspension in mouth or swish throughout mouth for several minutes before swallowing, then gargle and swallow. Use calibrated measuring device for liquid doses. Shake well before administration. Pedi: For neonates and infants, paint suspension into recesses of the mouth.
- To prepare oral solution from powder, add 1/8 tsp (approximately 500,000 units) to 120 mL of water and stir well. Prepare immediately before use; contains no preservatives.
- Lozenges (pastilles) should be allowed to dissolve slowly and completely in mouth; do not chew or swallow whole. Nystatin vaginal tablets can be administered orally for treatment of oral candidiasis.

Patient/Family Teaching

- Instruct patient to take medication as directed. If a dose is missed, take as soon as remembered but not if almost time for next dose. Do not double doses. Therapy should be continued for at least 2 days after symptoms subside.
- Pedi: Instruct parents or caregivers of infants and children on correct dose and administration. Remind them to use only the measuring devise dispensed with the product.
- Advise patient to report increased irritation of mucous membranes or lack of therapeutic response to health care professional.

Evaluation/Desired Outcomes

- Decrease in stomatitis.
- To prevent relapse after oral therapy, therapy should be continued for 48 hr after symptoms have disappeared and cultures are negative.
- Therapy for a period of 2 wk is usually sufficient, but more prolonged therapy may be necessary.

nystatin, See ANTIFUNGALS (TOPICAL).

octreotide (ok-**tree**-oh-tide)
SandoSTATIN, SandoSTATIN LAR

Classification
Therapeutic: antidiarrheals, hormones

Pregnancy Category B

Indications

Treatment of severe diarrhea and flushing episodes in patients with GI endocrine tumors, including metastatic carcinoid tumors and vasoactive intestinal peptide tumors (VIPomas). Treatment of acromegaly. **Unlabeled Use:** Management of diarrhea in AIDS patients, patients with fistulas, chemotherapy-induced diarrhea, and graft- vs. host–disease-induced diarrhea. Treatment of hyperinsulinemic hypoglycemia of infancy. Management of postoperative chylothorax.

Action

Suppresses secretion of serotonin and gastroenterohepatic peptides. Increases absorption of fluid and electrolytes from the GI tract and increases transit time. Decreases levels of serotonin metabolites. Also suppresses growth hormone, insulin, and glucagon. **Therapeutic Effects:** Control of severe flushing and diarrhea associated with GI endocrine tumors.

Pharmacokinetics

Absorption: Well absorbed following subcut administration and IM administration of depot form.
Distribution: Unknown.
Protein Binding: 65%.
Metabolism and Excretion: Extensive hepatic metabolism; 32% excreted unchanged in urine.
Half-life: 1.5 hr.

TIME/ACTION PROFILE (control of symptoms)

ROUTE	ONSET	PEAK	DURATION
Subcut, IV	unknown	unknown	up to 12 hr
IM (LAR)	unknown	2 wk	up to 4 wk

Contraindications/Precautions

Contraindicated in: Hypersensitivity.
Use Cautiously in: Gallbladder disease (↑ risk of stone formation); Renal impairment (dose ↓ may be necessary); Hyperglycemia or hypoglycemia (changes in blood glucose may occur); Fat malabsorption (may be aggravated); OB, Lactation: Safety not established.

Adverse Reactions/Side Effects

CNS: dizziness, drowsiness, fatigue, headache, weakness. **EENT:** visual disturbances. **CV:** bradycardia, edema, orthostatic hypotension, palpitations. **GI:** ILEUS, abdominal pain, cholelithiasis, diarrhea, fat malabsorption, nausea, vomiting. **Derm:** flushing. **Endo:** hyperglycemia, hypoglycemia, hypothyroidism. **Local:** injection-site pain.

Interactions

Drug-Drug: May alter requirements for **insulin** or **oral hypoglycemic agents**. May ↓ blood levels of **cyclosporine**. May ↑ levels of QTc-prolonging agents.

Route/Dosage

Carcinoid Tumors

Subcut, IV (Adults): *Sandostatin*—100–600 mcg/day in 2–4 divided doses during first 2 wk of therapy (range 50–1500 mcg/day).
IM (Adults): *Sandostatin LAR*—20 mg q 4 wk for 2 mo; dose may be further adjusted.

VIPomas

Subcut, IV (Adults): *Sandostatin*—200–300 mcg/day in 2–4 divided doses during first 2 wk of therapy (range 150–750 mcg/day).
IM (Adults): *Sandostatin LAR*—20 mg q 2 wk for 2 mo; dose may be further adjusted.

Suppression of Growth Hormone (Acromegaly)

Subcut, IV (Adults): *Sandostatin*—50–100 mcg 3 times daily; titrate to achieve growth hormone levels <5 ng/mL or IGF-I levels <1.9 units/mL (males) or <2.2 units/mL (females) (usual effective dose = 100–200 mcg 3 times daily.
IM (Adults): *Sandostatin LAR*—20 mg q 4 wk for 3 mo, then adjusted on the basis of growth hormone levels.

Antidiarrheal

Subcut, IV (Adults): *AIDS-related*—100–1800 mcg/day (unlabeled).
Subcut, IV (Children): 1–10 mcg/kg q 12 hr or 1 mcg/kg IV bolus followed by a continuous infusion of 1 mcg/kg/hr.

Persistent Hyperinsulinemic Hypoglycemia of Infancy

IV (Infants): Initially 2–10 mcg/kg/day divided q 12 hr up to 40 mcg/kg/day divided q 6–8 hr.

Chylothorax

Subcut (Adults): 50–100 mcg q 8 hr.
Subcut (Children): 40 mcg/kg/day.
IV (Children): 0.3–10 mcg/kg/hr continuous infusion.

Availability (generic available)

Injection: 50 mcg/mL, 100 mcg/mL, 200 mcg/mL, 500 mcg/mL, 1000 mcg/mL. **Depot injection:** 10 mg, 20 mg, 30 mg.

NURSING IMPLICATIONS

Assessment

- Assess frequency and consistency of stools and bowel sounds throughout therapy.
- Monitor pulse and BP prior to and periodically during therapy.
- Assess patient's fluid and electrolyte balance and skin turgor for dehydration.
- Monitor diabetic patients for signs of hypoglycemia. May require reduction in requirements for insulin and sulfonylureas and treatment with diazoxide.
- Assess for gallbladder disease; assess for pain and monitor ultrasound examinations of gallbladder and bile ducts prior to and periodically during prolonged therapy.
- ***Lab Test Considerations:*** Monitor 5-HIAA (urinary 5-hydroxyindoleacetic acid), plasma serotonin, and plasma substance P in patients with carcinoid; plasma vasoactive intestinal peptide (VIP) in patients with VIPoma; and free T_4 and serum glucose concentrations prior to and periodically during therapy in all patients taking octreotide.
- Monitor quantitative 72-hr fecal fat and serum carotene determinations periodically for possible drug-induced aggravations of fat malabsorption.
- May cause a slight ↑ in liver enzymes.
- May cause ↓ serum thyroxine (T_4) concentrations.

Potential Nursing Diagnoses

Diarrhea (Indications)

Implementation

- Do not confuse Sandostatin (octreotide) with Sandimmune (cyclosporine).
- Do not use solution that is discolored or contains particulate matter. Ampules should be refrigerated but may be stored at room temperature for the days they will be used. Discard unused solution.
- **Subcut:** Administer the smallest volume needed to achieve required dose to prevent pain at injection site. Rotate injection sites; avoid multiple injections in same site within short periods of time. Preferred injection sites are the hip, thigh, or abdomen.
- Administer injections between meals and at bedtime to avoid GI side effects.
- Allow medication to reach room temperature prior to injection to minimize local reactions at injection site.
- **IM:** Mix IM solution by adding diluent included in kit. Administer immediately after mixing into the gluteal muscle. Avoid using deltoid site due to pain of injection.
- Patients with carcinoid tumors and VIPomas should continue to receive subcut dose for 2 wk following switch to IM depot form to maintain therapeutic level.

IV Administration

- **IV Push: *Diluent:*** May be administered undiluted. ***Rate:*** Administer over 3 min.
- **Intermittent Infusion: *Diluent:*** Dilute in 50–200 mL of 0.9% NaCl or D5W. ***Concentration:*** 1.5–250 mcg/mL. ***Rate:*** Infuse over 15–30 min.
- **Y-Site Compatibility:** acyclovir, alfentanyl, allopurinol, amifostine, amikacin, aminocaproic acid, aminophylline, amiodarone, amphotericin B colloidal, amphotericin B lipid complex, amphotericin B liposome, ampicillin, ampicillin/sulbactam, anidulafungin, argatroban, atracurium, azithromycin, aztreonam, bivalirudin, bleomycin, bumetanide, buprenorphine, busulfan, butorphanol, calcium chloride, calcium gluconate, capreomycin, carboplatin, carmustine, caspofungin, cefazolin, cefepime, cefotaxime, cefotetan, cefoxitin, ceftazidime, ceftriaxone, cefuroxime, chloramphenicol, chlorpromazine, ciprofloxacin, cisatracurium, cisplatin, clindamycin, cyclosporine, cytarabine, dacarbazine, dactinomycin, daptomycin, daunorubicin hydrochloride, daunorubicin liposome, dexamethasone sodium phosphate, dexmedetomidine, dexrazoxane, digoxin, diltiazem, diphenhydramine, dobutamine, docetaxel, dolasetron, dopamine, doxorubicin hydrochloride, doxorubicin liposome, doxycycline, droperidol, enalaprilat, ephedrine, epinephrine, epirubicin, eptifibitide, ertapenem, erythromycin, esmolol, etoposide, etoposide phosphate, famotidine, fenoldopam, fentanyl, fluconazole, fludarabine, fluorouracil, foscarnet, fosphenytoin, furosemide, ganciclovir, gemcitabine, gentamicin, glycopyrrolate, granisetron, haloperidol, heparin, hydralazine, hydrocortisone, hydromorphone, idarubicin, ifosfamide, imipenem/cilastatin, insulin, irinotecan, isoproterenol, ketorolac, labetalol, leucovorin calcium, levofloxacin, lidocaine, linezolid, lorazepam, magnesium hydroxide, mannitol, mechlorethamine, melphalan, meperidine, meropenem, mesna, methohexital, methotrexate, methylprednisolone, methyldopate, metoclopramide, metoprolol, metronidazole, midazolam, milrinone, minocycline, mitomycin, mitoxantrone, morphine, mycophenolate, nafcillin, nalbuphine, naloxone, nesiritide, nicardipine, nitroglycerin, nitroprusside, norepinephrine, ondansetron, oxaliplatin, paclitaxel, palonosetron, pamidronate, pancuronium, pemetrexed, pentamidine, pentazocine, pentobarbital, phenobarbital, phentolamine, phenylephrine, piperacillin/tazobactam, potassium acetate, potassium chloride, potassium phosphates, procainamide, prochlorperazine, promethazine, propranolol, quinapristin/dalfopristin, ranitidine, remifentanyl, rocuronium, sodium acetate, sodium bicarbonate, sodium phosphates, streptozocin, succinylcholine, sufentanil, tacrolimus, teniposide, thiopental, thiotepa, tigecycline, tirofiban, tobramycin, topotecan, trimethoprim/sulfamethoxazole, vancomycin, vasopressin, vecuronium, verapamil, vinblastine, vincristine, vinorelbine, voriconazole, zidovudine, zoledronic acid.

- **Y-Site Incompatibility:** dantrolene, diazepam, micafungin, phenytoin.

Patient/Family Teaching

- May cause dizziness, drowsiness, or visual disturbances. Caution patient to avoid driving or other activities requiring alertness until response to medication is known.
- Advise patient to change positions slowly to minimize orthostatic hypotension.
- **Home Care Issues:** Instruct patients administering octreotide at home on correct technique for injection, storage, and disposal of equipment.
- Instruct patient to administer octreotide exactly as directed. If a dose is missed, administer as soon as possible, then return to regular schedule. Do not double doses.

Evaluation/Desired Outcomes

- Decrease in severity of diarrhea and improvement of electrolyte imbalances in patients with carcinoid or VIP-secreting tumors.
- Relief of symptoms and suppressed tumor growth in patients with pituitary tumors associated with acromegaly.
- Management of diarrhea in patients with AIDS.

OLANZapine (oh-**lan**-za-peen)

ZyPREXA, ✤ZyPREXA Intramuscular, ZyPREXA Relprevv, ZyPREXA Zydis

Classification

Therapeutic: antipsychotics, mood stabilizers

Pharmacologic: thienobenzodiazepines

Pregnancy Category C

Indications

Schizophrenia. Acute therapy of manic or mixed episodes associated with bipolar I disorder (as monotherapy [adults and adolescents] or with lithium or valproate [adults only]). Maintenance therapy of bipolar I disorder. Acute agitation due to schizophrenia or bipolar I mania (IM). Depressive episodes associated with bipolar I disorder (when used with fluoxetine). Treatment-resistant depression (when used with fluoxetine). **Unlabeled Use:** Management of anorexia nervosa. Treatment of nausea and vomiting related to highly emetogenic chemotherapy.

Action

Antagonizes dopamine and serotonin type 2 in the CNS. Also has anticholinergic, antihistaminic, and anti–alpha$_1$-adrenergic effects. **Therapeutic Effects:** Decreased manifestations of psychoses.

Pharmacokinetics

Absorption: Well absorbed but rapidly metabolized by first-pass effect, resulting in 60% bioavailability. Conventional tablets and orally disintegrating tablets (Zydis) are bioequivalent. IM administration results in significantly higher blood levels (5 times that of oral).
Distribution: Extensively distributed.
Protein Binding: 93%.
Metabolism and Excretion: Highly metabolized (mostly by the hepatic P450 CYP 1A2 system); 7% excreted unchanged in urine.
Half-life: 21–54 hr.

TIME/ACTION PROFILE (antipsychotic effects)

ROUTE	ONSET	PEAK*	DURATION
PO	unknown	6 hr	unknown
IM	rapid	15–45 min	2–4 hr

*Blood levels.

Contraindications/Precautions

Contraindicated in: Hypersensitivity; Lactation: Discontinue drug or bottle feed; Phenylketonuria (orally disintegrating tablets contain aspartame).
Use Cautiously in: Patients with hepatic impairment; Patients at risk for aspiration; Cardiovascular or cerebrovascular disease; History of seizures; History of attempted suicide; Diabetes or risk factors for diabetes (may worsen glucose control); Prostatic hyperplasia; Angle-closure glaucoma; History of paralytic ileus; Dysphagia and aspiration have been associated with antipsychotic drug use; use with caution in patients at risk for aspiration; OB: Neonates at ↑ risk for extrapyramidal symptoms and withdrawal after delivery when exposed during the 3rd trimester; use only if maternal benefit outweighs risk to fetus; Pedi: Children <13 yr (safety not established); adolescents at ↑ risk for weight gain and hyperlipidemia; Geri: May require ↓ doses; ↑ risk of mortality in elderly patients treated for dementia-related psychosis.

Adverse Reactions/Side Effects

CNS: NEUROLEPTIC MALIGNANT SYNDROME, SEIZURES, SUICIDAL THOUGHTS, agitation, delirium, dizziness, headache, restlessness, sedation, weakness, dystonia, insomnia, mood changes, personality disorder, speech impairment, tardive dyskinesia. **EENT:** amblyopia, rhinitis, ↑ salivation, pharyngitis. **Resp:** cough, dyspnea. **CV:** orthostatic hypotension, bradycardia, chest pain, tachycardia. **GI:** constipation, dry mouth, ↑ liver enzymes, weight loss or gain, abdominal pain, ↑ appetite, nausea, ↑ thirst. **GU:** impotence, ↓ libido, urinary incontinence. **Hemat:** AGRANULOCYTOSIS, leukopenia, neutropenia. **Derm:** photosensitivity. **Endo:** amenorrhea, galactorrhea, goiter, gynecomastia, hyperglycemia. **Metab:** dyslipidemia. **MS:** hypertonia, joint pain. **Neuro:** tremor. **Misc:** fever, flu-like syndrome.

O

Interactions

Drug-Drug: Effects may be ↓ by concurrent **carbamazepine**, **omeprazole**, or **rifampin**. ↑ hypotension may occur with **antihypertensives**. ↑ CNS depression may occur with concurrent use of **alcohol** or other **CNS depressants**; concurrent use of IM olanzapine and parenteral benzodiazepines should be avoided. May antagonize the effects of **levodopa** or other **dopamine agonists**. **Fluvoxamine** may ↑ levels. **Nicotine** can ↓ olanzapine levels.

Route/Dosage

Schizophrenia

PO (Adults —Most Patients): 5–10 mg/day initially; may ↑ at weekly intervals by 5 mg/day (target dose = 10 mg/day; not to exceed 20 mg/day).
PO (Adults —Debilitated or Nonsmoking Female Patients ≥65 yr): Initiate therapy at 5 mg/day.
PO (Children 13–17 yr): 2.5–5 mg/day initially; may ↑ at weekly intervals by 2.5–5 mg/day (target dose = 10 mg/day; not to exceed 20 mg/day).
IM (Adults): *Oral olanzapine dose = 10 mg/day*—210 mg every 2 wk or 410 mg every 4 wk for the first 8 wk, then 150 mg every 2 wk or 300 mg every 4 wk as maintenance therapy; *Oral olanzapine dose = 15 mg/day*—300 mg every 2 wk for the first 8 wk, then 210 mg every 2 wk or 405 mg every 4 wk as maintenance therapy; *Oral olanzapine dose = 20 mg/day*—300 mg every 2 wk for the first 8 wk, then 300 mg every 2 wk as maintenance therapy.
IM (Adults —Debilitated or Nonsmoking Female Patients ≥65 yr): Initiate therapy at 150 mg every 4 wk.

Acute Manic or Mixed Episodes Associated with Bipolar I Disorder

PO (Adults): 10–15 mg/day initially (use 10 mg/day when used with lithium or valproate); may ↑ every 24 hr by 5 mg/day (not to exceed 20 mg/day).
PO (Children 13–17 yr): 2.5–5 mg/day initially; may ↑ by 2.5–5 mg/day (target dose = 10 mg/day; not to exceed 20 mg/day).

Maintenance Treatment of Bipolar I Disorder

PO (Adults): Continue at the dose required to maintain symptom remission (usual dose: 5–20 mg/day).
PO (Children 13–17 yr): Continue at the lowest dose required to maintain symptom remission.

Acute Agitation due to Schizophrenia or Bipolar I Mania

IM (Adults): 10 mg, may repeat in 2 hr, then 4 hr later.
IM (Adults >65 yr): Initiate therapy with 5 mg.

Depressive Episodes Associated with Bipolar I Disorder

PO (Adults): 5 mg/day with fluoxetine 20 mg/day (both given in evening); may ↑ fluoxetine dose up to 50 mg/day and olanzapine dose up to 12.5 mg/day.
PO (Children 10–17 yr): 20 mg/day with olanzapine 2.5 mg/day (both given in evening); may ↑ fluoxetine dose up to 50 mg/day and olanzapine dose up to 12 mg/day.

Treatment-Resistant Depression

PO (Adults): 5 mg/day with fluoxetine 20 mg/day (both given in evening); may ↑ fluoxetine dose up to 50 mg/day and olanzapine dose up to 20 mg/day.

Availability (generic available)

Tablets: 2.5 mg, 5 mg, 7.5 mg, 10 mg, 15 mg, 20 mg. **Cost:** *Generic*—2.5 mg $31.23/90, 5 mg $24.47/90, 7.5 mg $30.83/90, 10 mg $37.19/90, 15 mg $53.38/90, 20 mg $71.55/90. **Orally disintegrating tablets (Zydis):** 5 mg, 10 mg, 15 mg, 20 mg. **Cost:** 5 mg $1,298.66/90, 15 mg $2,880.85/90. **Powder for intramuscular injection (requires reconstitution):** 10 mg/vial. **Extended-release powder for suspension for intramuscular injection (requires reconstitution) (Zyprexa Relprevv):** 210 mg/vial, 300 mg/vial, 405 mg/vial. ***In combination with:*** fluoxetine (Symbyax; see Appendix B).

NURSING IMPLICATIONS

Assessment

- Assess mental status (orientation, mood, behavior) before and periodically during therapy. Monitor closely for notable changes in behavior that could indicate the emergence or worsening of suicidal thoughts or behavior or depression.
- Monitor BP (sitting, standing, lying), ECG, pulse, and respiratory rate before and frequently during dose adjustment.
- Assess weight and BMI initially and throughout therapy.
- Observe patient carefully when administering medication to ensure that medication is taken and not hoarded or cheeked.
- Assess fluid intake and bowel function. Increased bulk and fluids in the diet may help minimize constipation.
- Monitor patient for onset of akathisia (restlessness or desire to keep moving) and extrapyramidal side effects (*parkinsonian*—difficulty speaking or swallowing, loss of balance control, pill rolling of hands, mask-like face, shuffling gait, rigidity, tremors; and *dystonic*—muscle spasms, twisting motions, twitching, inability to move eyes, weakness of arms or legs) every 2 mo during therapy and 8–12 wk after therapy has been discontinued. Report these symptoms if they occur, as reduction in dose or discontinuation of medication may be necessary. Tri-

hexyphenidyl or benztropine may be used to control symptoms.

- Monitor for tardive dyskinesia (uncontrolled rhythmic movement of mouth, face, and extremities; lip smacking or puckering; puffing of cheeks; uncontrolled chewing; rapid or worm-like movements of tongue, excessive blinking of eyes). Report immediately; may be irreversible.
- Monitor for development of neuroleptic malignant syndrome (fever, respiratory distress, tachycardia, seizures, diaphoresis, hypertension or hypotension, pallor, tiredness, severe muscle stiffness, loss of bladder control). Notify health care professional immediately if these symptoms occur.
- Monitor for symptoms related to hyperprolactinemia (menstrual abnormalities, galactorrhea, sexual dysfunction).
- *Zyprexa Relprevv*: Observe for signs and symptoms of Post-injection Delirium/Sedation Syndrome (dizziness, confusion, disorientation, slurred speech, altered gait, difficulty ambulating, weakness, agitation, extrapyramidal symptoms, hypertension, convulsion, reduced level of consciousness ranging from mild sedation to coma) for at least 3 hr after injection.
- ***Lab Test Considerations:*** Evaluate CBC, liver function tests, and ocular examinations periodically during therapy. May cause ↓ platelets. May cause ↑ bilirubin, AST, ALT, GGT, CPK, and alkaline phosphatase.
- Monitor blood glucose prior to and periodically during therapy.
- Monitor serum prolactin prior to and periodically during therapy. May cause ↑ serum prolactin levels.
- Monitor CBC frequently during initial months of therapy in patients with pre-existing or history of low WBC. May cause leukopenia, neutropenia, or agranulocytosis. Discontinue therapy if this occurs.
- May cause hyperlipidemia; monitor serum lipids prior to and periodically during therapy.

Potential Nursing Diagnoses

Disturbed thought process (Indications)
Impaired oral mucous membrane (Side Effects)
Sexual dysfunction (Side Effects)

Implementation

- Do not confuse Zyprexa (olanzapine) with Celexa (citalopram), quetiapine, Zyrtec (cetirizine), Reprexain (hydrocodone/ibuprofen), Zestril (lisinopril), or Zelapar (selegiline).
- *Zyprexa Relprevv* is only prescribed through the *Zyprexa Relprevv Patient Care Program*. Prescribers, pharmacies, and patients must be educated about the program and must comply with the program requirements.
- **PO:** May be administered without regard to meals.
- For orally disintegrating tablets, peel back foil on blister, do not push tablet through foil. Using dry hands, remove from foil and place entire tablet in mouth. Tablet will disintegrate with or without liquid.
- **IM:** Reconstitute with 2.1 mL of sterile water for injection for a concentration of 5 mg/mL. Solution should be clear and yellow; do not administer solutions that are discolored or contain particulate matter. Inject slowly, deep into muscle. Do not administer IV or subcutaneously. Administer within 1 hr of reconstitution. Discard unused solution.
- For *Zyprexa Relprevv*: Use gloves when preparing; solution may be irritating to skin. Use only diluent provided by manufacturer. Dilute 150 mg or 210 mg dose with 1.3 mL, 300 mg with 1.8 mL, and 405 mg with 2.3 mL of diluent. Loosen powder by tapping vial; inject diluent into powder. Remove needle from vial holding vial upright to prevent loss of solution. Engage needle safety device as explained by manufacturer. Pad a hard surface and tap vial repeatedly until no powder or yellow, dry clumps are visible. Shake vial vigorously until suspension appears smooth and consistent in color and texture. Solution will be yellow and opaque. Allow foam to dissipate. Suspension is stable for 24 hr at room temperature; if not used immediately, shake to resuspend. ***Concentration:*** 150 mg/mL. Replace needle with 19 gauge, 1.5 inch or 2 inch for obese patients. Slowly withdraw desired amount from vial; 150 mg = 1 mL, 210 mg = 1.4 mL, 300 mg = 2 mL, 405 mg = 2.7 mL. Administer immediately deep IM gluteal after withdrawing. Do not massage injection site. Patient must be observed for at least 3 hr after injection for Post-Injection Delirium/Sedation Syndrome.

Patient/Family Teaching

- Advise patient to take medication as directed and not to skip doses or double up on missed doses. May need to discontinue gradually. Advise patient to read the *Medication Guide* prior to starting therapy and with each Rx refill in case of changes. Explain the *Zyprexa Relprevv Patient Care Program* to patient and encourage patient to enroll in the *Zyprexa Relprevv Patient Care Program* registry.
- Inform patient of possibility of extrapyramidal symptoms and tardive dyskinesia. Instruct patient to report these symptoms immediately to health care professional.
- Advise patient to change positions slowly to minimize orthostatic hypotension.
- Medication may cause drowsiness. Caution patient to avoid driving or other activities requiring alertness until response to the medication is known. Patients receiving *Zyprexa Relprevv* should not drive for 24 hr following injection.

- Advise patient and family to notify health care professional if thoughts about suicide or dying, attempts to commit suicide; new or worse depression; new or worse anxiety; feeling very agitated or restless; panic attacks; trouble sleeping; new or worse irritability; acting aggressive; being angry or violent; acting on dangerous impulses; an extreme increase in activity and talking, other unusual changes in behavior or mood occur.
- Advise patient to notify health care professional of all Rx or OTC medications, vitamins, or herbal products being taken and to consult with health care professional before taking other medications and alcohol.
- Advise patient to use sunscreen and protective clothing when exposed to the sun. Extremes of temperature (exercise, hot weather, hot baths or showers) should also be avoided; this drug impairs body temperature regulation.
- Instruct patient to use saliva substitute, frequent mouth rinses, good oral hygiene, and sugarless gum or candy to minimize dry mouth. Consult dentist if dry mouth continues for >2 wk.
- Advise patient to notify health care professional of medication regimen before treatment or surgery.
- Instruct patient to notify health care professional promptly if sore throat, fever, unusual bleeding or bruising, rash, symptoms of Post-Injection Delirium/Sedation Syndrome, or weakness, tremors, visual disturbances, dark-colored urine, clay-colored stools, menstrual abnormalities, galactorrhea or sexual dysfunction occur.
- Advise patient to notify health care professional if pregnancy is planned or suspected, or if breast feeding.
- Emphasize the importance of routine follow-up exams and continued participation in psychotherapy.

Evaluation/Desired Outcomes
- Decrease in excitable, manic behavior.
- Decrease in positive symptoms (delusions, hallucinations) of schizophrenia.
- Decrease in negative symptoms (social withdrawal, flat, blunted affect) of schizophrenia.
- Increased sense of well-being.
- Decreased agitation.

olaparib (oh-lap-a-rib)
Lynparza

Classification
Therapeutic: antineoplastics
Pharmacologic: enzyme inhibitors

Pregnancy Category D

Indications
Treatment of deleterious/suspected deleterious documented germline BRCA mutated advanced ovarian cancer following three previous lines of chemotherapy.

Action
Acts as a poly (ADP-ribose) polymerase (PARP) inhibitor; disrupts DNA transcription, cell cycle regulation and DNA repair. **Therapeutic Effects:** Decreased growth and spread of ovarian cancer.

Pharmacokinetics
Absorption: Well absorbed following oral administration.
Distribution: Unknown.
Metabolism and Excretion: Extensively metabolized (mostly by CYP3A enzyme system); 15% excreted unchanged in urine, 6% in feces.
Half-life: 11.9 hr.

TIME/ACTION PROFILE (blood levels)

ROUTE	ONSET	PEAK	DURATION
PO	unknown	1–3 hr	12 hr†

† Median duration of tumor response 7.9 mo.

Contraindications/Precautions
Contraindicated in: OB: May cause fetal harm; Lactation: Discontinue olaparib or discontinue breast feeding.
Use Cautiously in: Concurrent use of strong/moderate CYP3A inhibitors (avoid if possible, if concurrent use is necessary ↓ olaparib dose); Concurrent use of strong/moderate CYP3A inducers (avoid if possible, if concurrent use is necessary effectiveness of olaparib may be ↓); Hepatic impairment; Renal impairment (CCr <50 mL/min); Pedi: Safe and effective use in children has not been established.

Adverse Reactions/Side Effects
CNS: fatigue, headache, weakness. **Resp:** PNEUMONITIS, cough. **GI:** abdominal pain, ↓ appetite, diarrhea, dyspepsia, nausea, vomiting, dysgeusia. **Derm:** dermatitis/rash. **Hemat:** MYELODYSPLASTIC SYNDROME/ACUTE MYELOID LEUKEMIA, anemia, lymphopenia, neutropenia, thrombocytopenia. **MS:** arthralgia, back pain, musculoskeletal pain, myalgia.

Interactions
Drug-Drug: ↑ risk of prolonged myelosuppression with other **antineoplastics**. Concurrent use with strong/moderate CYP3A inhibitors including **aprepitant**, **atazanavir**, **boceprevir**, **ciprofloxacin**, **clarithromycin**, **crizotinib**, **darunavir/ritonavir**, **diltiazem**, **erythromycin**, **fluconazole**, **fosamprenavir**, **imatinib**, **indinavir**, **itraconazole**, **ketoconazole**, **lopinavir/ritonavir**, **nefazodone**, **nelfinavir**, **posaconazole**, **ritonavir**, **saquinavir**, **telithromycin**, **verapamil**, and **voriconazole** ↑ blood levels and the risk of toxicity (avoid concurrent use if possible but if necessary olaparib dose should be ↓). Concurrent use with **strong CYP3A inducers** including **carbamazepine**, **phenytoin**, and **rifampicin** ↓ blood levels and effectiveness and should be avoided. Concurrent use with **moderate CYP3A inducers** in-

cluding **bosentan**, **efavirenz**, **etravirine**, **modafinil**, and **nafcillin**↓ blood levels and effectiveness; avoid if possible.
Drug-Natural Products: St. John's wort may ↓ blood levels and effectiveness and should be avoided.
Drug-Food: Concurrent ingestion of **grapefruit** and **Seville oranges** may ↑ blood levels and the risk of toxicity and should be avoided.

Route/Dosage

PO (Adults): 400 mg twice daily continued until disease progression or unacceptable toxicity; dose disruption/reduction may be required.

Availability

Capsules: 50 mg.

NURSING IMPLICATIONS

Assessment

- Monitor for signs and symptoms of pneumonitis (new or worsening respiratory symptoms, dyspnea, fever, cough, wheezing, radiological abnormality) during therapy. Interrupt therapy; if pneumonitis confirmed, discontinue therapy.
- ***Lab Test Considerations:*** Monitor CBC at baseline and moly during therapy. Do not start olaparib until patient has recovered from hematological toxicities from previous chemotherapy (≤CTCAE Grade 1). For prolonged hematological toxicities, interrupt olaparib and monitor CBC weekly until recovery. If levels have not recovered to Grade ≤1 after 4 wks, refer to hematologist. Discontinue olaparib if myelodysplastic syndrome or acute myeloid leukemia is confirmed.
- May cause ↓ hemoglobin, neutrophils, platelets, and lymphocytes. May cause ↑ mean corpuscular volume and creatinine.

Potential Nursing Diagnoses

Nausea (Side Effects)
Risk for infection (Adverse Reactions)

Implementation

- **PO:** Take eight 50 mg capsules twice daily (800 mg/day). Swallow capsules whole; do not open, chew, or dissolve capsule; do not take capsules that are deformed or leak.
- If dose reduction is needed, reduce dose to 200 mg (four 50 mg capsules) twice daily or 400 mg/day. If further final dose reduction is needed, reduce to 100 mg (two 50 mg capsules) twice daily or 200 mg.

Patient/Family Teaching

- Instruct patient to take olaparib as directed. If a dose is missed, do not take another to make up; omit dose and take next scheduled dose.
- Inform patient that mild to moderate nausea and/or vomiting is common when taking olaparib. Notify health care professional for antiemetic options if this is problematic.
- Advise patient to avoid grapefruit or Seville oranges during therapy.
- Advise patient to notify health care professional if signs and symptoms of pneumonitis or hematological toxicity (weakness, feeling tired, fever, weight loss, frequent infections, bruising, bleeding easily, shortness of breath, blood in urine or stool, low blood cell counts on laboratory findings, need for blood transfusions). May also be myelodysplastic syndrome (MDS) or acute myeloid leukemia (AML).
- Instruct patient to notify health care professional of all Rx or OTC medications, vitamins, or herbal products being taken and to consult with health care professional before taking other medications.
- Inform female patient that olaparib is teratogenic and to use effective contraception during and for at least 1 mo after last dose. Advise patient to notify health care professional if pregnancy is planned or suspected. Advise patient to avoid breast feeding during therapy.
- Emphasize importance of lab test to monitor for side effects.

Evaluation/Desired Outcomes

- Decreased growth and spread of ovarian cancer.

olmesartan, See ANGIOTENSIN II RECEPTOR ANTAGONISTS.

olodaterol (oh-loh-**dat**-er-ole)

Striverdi

Classification
Therapeutic: bronchodilators
Pharmacologic: beta-adrenergic agonists

Pregnancy Category C

Indications

Maintenance treatment of airflow obstruction in patients with COPD including chronic bronchitis and emphysema.

Action

A long-acting beta$_2$-adrenergic agonist (LABA) that stimulates adenyl cyclase, resulting in accumulation of cyclic adenosine monophosphate (cAMP) at beta$_2$-adrenergic receptors resulting in bronchodilation. **Therapeutic Effects:** Bronchodilation with decreased airflow obstruction.

Pharmacokinetics

Absorption: 30% absorbed following oral inhalation (from lung surface); swallowed drug is minimally absorbed.

Distribution: Extensive tissue distribution; probably enters breast milk.

Metabolism and Excretion: Extensively metabolized (some by CYP 3A4), only one metabolite binds to B_2adrenergic receptors. Following inhalation, 5–7% excreted unchanged in urine, remainder in feces as drug and metabolites (84%).

Half-life: 45 hr (following inhalation).

TIME/ACTION PROFILE (improvement in FEV_1)

ROUTE	ONSET	PEAK	DURATION
inhaln	within 1 hr	1–5 hr	24 hr

Contraindications/Precautions

Contraindicated in: Severe/acute/deteriorating symptoms of airflow obstruction.

Use Cautiously in: History of seizures; Thyrotoxicosis; History of cardiovascular disorders (coronary insufficiency, arrhythmias, hypertension); Sensitivity to sympathomimetics (adrenergics); Severe hepatic impairment; OB: Use during pregnancy only if potential benefit justifies potential risk to the fetus; Lactation: Use cautiously if breast feeding (probably enters breast milk); Pedi: Safe and effective use in children has not been established.

Exercise Extreme Caution in: Concurrent use with MAOIs, tricyclic antidepressants or drugs that prolong QTc (↑ risk of adverse cardiovascular reactions).

Adverse Reactions/Side Effects

CNS: dizziness. **EENT:** nasopharyngitis. **Resp:** PARADOXICAL BRONCHOSPASM, cough. **CV:** ↑ BP, ECG changes, tachycardia. **GI:** diarrhea. **Endo:** hyperglycemia. **F and E:** hypokalemia. **MS:** arthralgia, back pain. **Misc:** hypersensitivity reactions including ANGIOEDEMA.

Interactions

Drug-Drug: Concurrent use with **MAOIs**, **tricyclic antidepressants**, or **drugs that prolong QTc** ↑ risk of adverse cardiovascular reactions (use with extreme caution). Concurrent use of other **adrenergics** ↑ risk of adverse adrenergic adverse reactions (tachycardia, ↑ BP). Concurrent use with **corticosteroids**, **non-potassium sparing diuretics**, or **xanthine derivatives** (including **theophylline**) may ↑ risk of hypokalemia and adverse cardiovascular reactions (use cautiously). Concurrent use with **beta blockers** may ↓ effectiveness and cause severe bronchospasm (use cautiously). Should not be used concurrently with any other **long-acting beta2-adrenergic blockers** (LABAs). Blood levels may be ↑ by ketoconazole.

Route/Dosage

Inhaln (Adults): 2 inhalations once daily.

Availability

Inhalation spray: 2.7 mcg (delivers 2.5 mcg) per actuation in cartridges containing 14 doses/cartridge (one actuation lost in priming) for use with Respimat inhaler.

NURSING IMPLICATIONS

Assessment

- Assess respiratory status (rate, breath sounds, degree of dyspnea, pulse) before administration and at peak of medication. Consult health care professional about alternative medication if severe bronchospasm is present; onset of action is too slow for patients in acute distress. If paradoxical bronchospasm (wheezing) occurs, withhold medication and notify health care professional immediately.
- Monitor for signs and symptoms of allergic reactions (difficulties in breathing or swallowing, swelling of tongue, lips and face, urticaria, skin rash). Discontinue therapy if symptoms occur.
- ***Lab Test Considerations:*** May cause transient hypokalemia and hyperglycemia.

Potential Nursing Diagnoses

Ineffective airway clearance (Indications)
Risk for activity intolerance (Indications)

Implementation

- **Inhaln:** Prior to first use, prime the inhaler by actuating toward ground until aerosol cloud is visible, then repeat procedure 3 more times. If not used for 3 days, actuate inhaler once to prepare for use. *Striverdi Respimat* has a slow-moving mist to assist with inhalation. Use once (2 puffs), at the same time daily.
- A rescue inhaler of short-acting $beta_2$-agonists should always be available to treat sudden bronchospasm.

Patient/Family Teaching

- Instruct patient in the correct use of *Striverdi Respimat*. Take missed doses as soon as remembered. Do not take more than 1 dose (2 puffs) in 24 hr. Advise patient not to discontinue without consulting health care professional; symptoms may recur.
- Inform patient that olodaterol is not an rapid-actinga long-acting bronchodilator and should not be used for treating sudden breathing problems.
- Advise patient to notify health care professional if signs and symptoms of allergic reaction, worsening symptoms; decreasing effectiveness of inhaled, short-acting $beta_2$–agonists; need for more inhalations than usual of inhaled, short-acting $beta_2$-agonists; or significant decrease in lung function occur.
- Instruct patient to notify health care professional of all Rx or OTC medications, vitamins, or herbal products being taken and to avoid concurrent use of Rx, OTC, and herbal products without consulting health care professional.

- Advise female patient to notify health care professional if pregnancy is planned or suspected or if breast feeding.

Evaluation/Desired Outcomes

- Bronchodilation with decreased airflow obstruction.

olsalazine (ole-sal-a-zeen)

Dipentum

Classification

Therapeutic: gastrointestinal anti-inflammatories

Pregnancy Category C

Indications

Ulcerative colitis (when patients cannot tolerate sulfasalazine).

Action

Locally acting anti-inflammatory action in the colon, where activity is probably due to inhibition of prostaglandin synthesis. **Therapeutic Effects:** Reduction in the symptoms of inflammatory bowel disease.

Pharmacokinetics

Absorption: Acts locally in colon, where 98–99% is converted to mesalamine (5-aminosalicylic acid).

Distribution: Action is primarily local and remains in the colon.

Metabolism and Excretion: 2% absorbed into systemic circulation is rapidly metabolized; mostly eliminated as mesalamine in the feces.

Half-life: 0.9 hr.

TIME/ACTION PROFILE (levels)

ROUTE	ONSET	PEAK	DURATION
PO	unknown	1 hr; 4–8 hr	12 hr

Contraindications/Precautions

Contraindicated in: Hypersensitivity reactions to salicylates; Cross-sensitivity with furosemide, sulfonylurea hypoglycemic agents, or carbonic anhydrase inhibitors may exist; Glucose-6–phosphate dehydrogenase (G6PD) deficiency; Urinary tract or intestinal obstruction; Porphyria; Lactation: Lactation; Pedi: Children <2 yr (safety not established).

Use Cautiously in: Severe hepatic or renal impairment; Renal impairment (↑ risk of renal tubular damage); OB: Pregnancy; Geri: Consider ↓ body mass, hepatic/renal/cardiac function, intercurrent illness and drug therapies.

Adverse Reactions/Side Effects

CNS: ataxia, confusion, dizziness, drowsiness, headache, mental depression, psychosis, restlessness. **GI:** diarrhea, abdominal pain, anorexia, exacerbation of colitis, drug-induced hepatitis, nausea, vomiting. **Derm:** itching, rash. **Hemat:** blood dyscrasias.

Interactions

Drug-Drug: ↑ risk of bleeding after neuraxial anesthesia with **low molecular weight heparins** and **heparinoids**; discontinue olsalazine before initiation of therapy or monitor closely if discontinuation not possible. May ↓ metabolism, and ↑ effects/toxicity of **mercaptopurine** or **thioguanine** with and ↑ risk of myelosuppression (use lowest possible dose and monitor closely). ↑ risk of developing Reye's syndrome; avoid olsalazine during 6 wk after **varicella vaccine**.

Route/Dosage

PO (Adults): 500 mg twice daily.

Availability

Capsules: 250 mg.

NURSING IMPLICATIONS

Assessment

- Assess patient for allergy to sulfonamides and salicylates. Patients allergic to sulfasalazine may take mesalamine or olsalazine without difficulty, but therapy should be discontinued if rash or fever occur.
- Monitor intake and output ratios. Fluid intake should be sufficient to maintain a urine output of at least 1200–1500 mL daily to prevent crystalluria and stone formation.
- **Inflammatory Bowel Disease:** Assess abdominal pain and frequency, quantity, and consistency of stools at the beginning of and throughout therapy.
- ***Lab Test Considerations:*** Monitor urinalysis, BUN, and serum creatinine prior to and periodically during therapy.
- Olsalazine may cause ↑ AST and ALT levels.
- ***Lab Test Considerations:*** Monitor CBC prior to and every 3–6 mo during prolonged therapy. Discontinue olsalazine if blood dyscrasias occur.

Potential Nursing Diagnoses

Acute pain (Indications)
Diarrhea (Indications)

Implementation

- **PO:** Administer with food in evenly divided doses every 12 hr.

Patient/Family Teaching

- Instruct patient to take medication as directed, even if feeling better. Take missed doses as soon as remembered unless almost time for next dose.
- May cause dizziness. Caution patient to avoid driving or other activities that require alertness until response to medication is known.
- Advise patient to notify health care professional if skin rash, sore throat, fever, mouth sores, unusual

O

bleeding or bruising, wheezing, fever, or hives occurs.

- Instruct patient to notify health care professional if symptoms do not improve after 1–2 mo of therapy.
- Instruct patient to notify health care professional if symptoms worsen or do not improve. If symptoms of acute intolerance (cramping, acute abdominal pain, bloody diarrhea, fever, headache, rash) occur, discontinue therapy and notify health care professional immediately.
- Inform patient that proctoscopy and sigmoidoscopy may be required periodically during treatment to determine response.

Evaluation/Desired Outcomes

- Decrease in diarrhea and abdominal pain.
- Return to normal bowel pattern in patients with inflammatory bowel disease. Effects may be seen within 3–21 days. The usual course of therapy is 3–6 wk.
- Maintenance of remission in patients with inflammatory bowel disease.
- Decrease in pain and inflammation, and increase in mobility in patients with rheumatoid arthritis.

ombitasvir/paritaprevir/ritonavir

(om-**bit**-as-vir/par-i-**ta**-pre-vir/ri-**toe**-na-vir)

Technivie

Classification

Therapeutic: antivirals

Pharmacologic: NS5 inhibitors, protease inhibitors, enzyme inhibitors

Pregnancy Category B

Indications

Treatment of genotype 4 chronic hepatitis C infection (HVC) without cirrhosis (with ribavirin unless patient is treatment-naïve or cannot tolerate ribavirin).

Action

Ombitasvir—is an inhibitor of HCV NS5A which is necessary for RNA replication and virion assembly. *Paritaprevir*—is an inhibitor of NS3/4A protease an enzyme necessary for viral replication. *Ritonavir*is not active against HCV, but inhibits CYP3A resulting in ↑ blood levels and effectiveness of paritaprevir. **Therapeutic Effects:** Decreased levels of HCV with sustained virologic response and lessened sequelae of chronic HCV infection.

Pharmacokinetics

Absorption: Well absorbed following oral administration: *ombitasvir*—48%, *paritaprevir*—53%.

Distribution: *Ritonavir*—poor CNS penetration.

Protein Binding: *Ombitasvir*—99.9%, *paritaprevir*—97–98.6%, *ritonavir*—> 99%.

Metabolism and Excretion: *Ombitasvir*—metabolized by amide hydrolysis and then oxidative metabolism, excreted mainly in feces mostly as unchanged drug, minimal urinary excretion; *paritaprevir*—primarily metabolized by CYP3A, 88% excreted in feces mostly as metabolites; negligable urinary excretion; *ritonavir*—highly metabolized by CYP3A and CYP2D6, 86% excreted in feces (mostly as metabolites), 11.8% excreted in urine.

Half-life: *Ombitasvir*—21–25 hr, *paritaprevir*—5.5 hr, *ritonavir*—4 hr.

TIME/ACTION PROFILE (blood levels)

ROUTE	ONSET	PEAK	DURATION
ombitasvir PO	unk	4–5 hr	24 hr
paritaprevir PO	unk	4–5 hr	24 hr
ritonavir PO	rapid	4 hr	24 hr

Contraindications/Precautions

Contraindicated in: Hypersensitivity to any components including previous history of Stevens-Johnson syndrome or toxic epidermal necrolysis from ritonvir; Concurrent use of medications that are metabolized by CYP3A4 or strong/moderate inducers of CYP3A4; Hepatic impairment (contraindication in Child-Pugh Class C, not recommended in Child-Pugh Class B); OB: When used with ribavirin should not be used in pregnant patients or male patients whose partners are pregnant.

Use Cautiously in: Diabetes mellitus; Hemophilia (↑ risk of bleeding); Structural heart disease, conduction abnormalities, ischemic heart disease, or heart failure (↑ risk of heart block); Females with reproductive potential (ethinyl estradiol-containing medications including oral hormonal contraceptives are contraindicated due to ↑ risk of liver impairment; effective alternative contraception is recommended); Concurrent HIV infection (additional HIV-suppressive regimen required); OB: If used without ribavirin consider maternal benefits and possible adverse effects on the fetus; Lactation: Consider maternal benefits and possible adverse effects on infants; breast feeding not recommended in concurrently HIV-infected patients; Pedi: Safe and effective use in children < 18 yr has not been estabished.

Adverse Reactions/Side Effects

CNS: fatigue (↑ when used with ribavirin), insomnia (↑ when used with ribavirin), weakness(↑ when use with ribavirin). **GI:** nausea, HEPATOTOXICITY, ↑ bilirubin. **Hemat:** anemia. **Metab:** hypersensitivity reactions including ANGIOEDEMA..

Interactions

Drug-Drug: ↑ levels and risk of serious adverse reactions with **alfuzosin** (hypotension), **dihydroergotamine**, **ergotamine**, **methylergonovine** (ergot toxicity), **lovastatin** or **simvastatin** (myopathy/rhabdomyolysis), **pimozide** (arrhythmias), **efavirenz**

(↑ liver enzymes/↓ritonavir tolerance), **sildenafil** (when used for pulmonary hypertension ↑ risk of visual disturances/hypotension/priapism/syncope), oral **midazolam**; (↑ sedation/respiratory depression), **ethinyl estradiol** containing preparations including oral hormonal contraceptives; concurrent use is contraindicated. Levels and antiviral effectiveness are ↓ by **carbamazepine**, **phenobarbital**, **phenytoin**, and **rifampin**; concurrent use is contraindicated. ↑ levels and risk of **digoxin** toxicity; ↓ digoxin dose by 30–50%, monitor carefully. ↑ levels and risk of adverse cardiovascular reactions with **amiodarone**, **disopyramide**, **flecainide**, **lidocaine**, **mexiletine**, **propafenone**, and **quinidine**; careful monitoring recommended. ↑ levels and risk of adverse reactions with **ketoconazole**(daily dose of ketoconazole should not exceed 200 mg). ↓ levels and effectiveness of **voriconazole**; concurrrent use is not recommended. ↑ levels and risk of adverse reactions with **quetiapine**; ↓ quetiapine dose to 1/6th and monitor carefully, consider alternative anti-HCV treatments). ↑ levels and risk of hypotension with **amlodipine**; ↓ dose of amlodipine may be necessary. ↑ levels and effects of **furosemide**; monitor and adjust dose. Concurrent use with **atazanavir**, **atazanavir/ritonavir** or **lopinair/riotanivir**↑ levels of paritaprevir; concurrent use is not recommended. ↓ levels and may ↓ effectiveness of **darunavir**; darunavir (800 mg) without ritonavir should be taken at the same time as ombitasvir/peritaprevir/ritonavir. ↑ levels and risk of adverse cardiovascular reactions with **rilpivirine**; concurrent use is not recommended. ↑ levels and risk of adverse muscular reactions with **pravastatin**; pravastin dose should not exceed 40 mg/day. ↑ levels and risk of adverse reactions with **cyclosporine**; ↓ cyclosporine dose to 1/5th, monitor and readjust carefully. ↑ levels and effects of **tacrolimus**; omit tacrolimus on day of initiation ombitasvir/peritaprevir/ritonavir and ↓ dose (0.5 mg every 7 days) adjust by blood level monitoring. ↑ levels and risk of adverse cardiovascular reactions with **salmeterol**; Concurrent use is not recommended. ↑ levels of **buprenorphine**; monitor for sedation/congitive impairment. ↓ levels and effectiveness of **omeprazole**; ↑ dose of omeprazole if necesssary, but should not exced 40 mg/day. ↑ levels and effects of **alprazolam**; monitor for sedation/congitive impairment and adjust dose.

Drug-Natural Products: Levels and antiviral effectiveness are ↓ by **St. John's wort**; concurrent use is contraindicated.

Route/Dosage

PO (Adults): Two tablets (each tablet containing ombitasvir 12.5 mg/paritaprevir 75 mg/ritonavir 50 mg) once daily for 12 wk given concurrently with ribavirin 500 mg twice daily in patients < 75 kg or 600 mg twice daily in patients ≥ 75kg; may be used without ribavirin in treatment-naïve patients or patients who do not tolerate ribavarin.

Availability

Tablets: ombitasvir 12.5 mg/paritaprevir 75 mg/ritonavir 50 mg.

NURSING IMPLICATIONS

Assessment

- Monitor signs of hepatitis (jaundice, fatigue, anorexia, pruritus) during therapy.
- ***Lab Test Considerations:*** Monitor liver function tests during first 4 wks of therapy. If ALT is ↑, repeat test and monitor closely. Discontinue therapy if ALT levels are persistently ↑ >10 x upper limit of normal or if accompanied by signs of liver inflammation or ↑ direct bilirubin, alkaline phosphatase, or INR.
- May cause ↑ serum bilirubin; peaks by wk 1 of therapy and not associated with ↑ ALT.
- May cause ↓ hemoglobin requiring dose reduction.

Potential Nursing Diagnoses

Risk for injury (Indications)

Implementation

- **PO:** Administer 2 tablets once daily, in the morning, with a meal without regard to fat or calorie content. Usually given in combination with ribavirin.

Patient/Family Teaching

- Instruct patient to take *Technivie* as directed. Take missed dose within 12 hrs; if more than 12 hrs since missed dose, skip dose and take next dose at scheduled time; do not double doses. Advise patient to read *Medication Guide* before starting therapy and with each Rx refill in case of changes.
- Advise patient to notify health care professional promptly if signs and symptoms of liver dysfunction (fatigue, weakness, lack of appetite, nausea and vomiting, jaundice, discolored feces) occur.
- Instruct patient to notify health care professional of all Rx or OTC medications, vitamins, or herbal products being taken and to consult health care professional before taking other Rx, OTC, or herbal products, especially St. John's wort. Medications containing ethinyl estradiol must be stopped; if taking for birth control, another method must be used.
- Inform patient about teratogenic effects of *Technivie* and ribavirin. Instruct women with childbearing potential, and men, to use 2 forms of effective non-hormonal contraception during and for at least 6 mo following conclusion of therapy. Men must use a condom. Avoid breast feeding during use. Advise patient to notify health care professional if pregnancy occurs.

Evaluation/Desired Outcomes

- Protection from liver damage caused by chronic hepatitis C infection; decreases viral load.

O

ombitasvir/paritaprevir/ritonavir/dasabuvir

(om-**bit**-as-vir/par-i-**ta**-pre-vir/ri-**toe**-na-vir/da-**sa**-bue-vir)

Viekira Pak

Classification

Therapeutic: antivirals

Pharmacologic: NS5 inhibitors, protease inhibitors, enzyme inhibitors, non-nucleoside NS5B palm polymerase inhibitors

Pregnancy Category B

Indications

Treatment of (with or without ribavirin) genotype 1 chronic hepatitis C infection (HVC) including those with compensated cirrhosis.

Action

Ombitasvir—is an inhibitor of HCV NS5A which is necessary for RNA replication and virion assembly. *Paritaprevir*—is an inhibitor of NS3/4A protease an enzyme necessary for viral replication. *Ritonaviris* not active against HCV, but inhibits CYP3A resulting in ↑ blood levels and effectiveness of paritaprevir. *Dasabuvir*—inhibits RNA-dependent RNA polymerase necessary for viral genome replication. **Therapeutic Effects:** Decreased levels of HCV with sustained virologic response and lessened sequelae of chronic HCV infection.

Pharmacokinetics

Absorption: Well absorbed following oral administration: *ombitasvir*—48%, *paritaprevir*—53%, *dasabuvir*—70%.

Distribution: *Ritonavir*—poor CNS penetration.

Protein Binding: *Ombitasvir*—99.9%, *paritaprevir*—97–98.6%, *ritonavir*—> 99%, *dasabuvir*—>99.5%.

Metabolism and Excretion: *Ombitasvir*—metabolized by amide hydrolysis and then oxidative metabolism, excreted mainly in feces mostly as unchanged drug, minimal urinary excretion; *paritaprevir*—primarily metabolized by CYP3A, 88% excreted in feces mostly as metabolites; negligable urinary excretion; *ritonavir*—highly metabolized by CYP3A and CYP2D6, 86% excreted in feces (mostly as metabolites), 11.8% excreted in urine, *dasabuvir*—mostly metabolized by CYP2C8 and smaller amounts by CYP3A, 95% excreted in feces (26% as unchanged drug), minimal urinary excretion.

Half-life: *Ombitasvir*—21–25 hr, *paritaprevir*—5.5 hr, *ritonavir*—4 hr, *dasabuvir*—5.5–6 hr.

TIME/ACTION PROFILE (blood levels)

ROUTE	ONSET	PEAK	DURATION
ombitasvir PO	unknown	4–5 hr	24 hr
paritaprevir PO	unknown	4–5 hr	24 hr
ritonavir PO	rapid	4 hr	24 hr
dasabuvir	unknown	45 hr	12 hr

Contraindications/Precautions

Contraindicated in: Hypersensitivity to any components including previous history of Stevens-Johnson syndrome or toxic epidermal necrolysis from ritonvir; Concurrent use of medications that are metabolized by CYP3A4 or strong/moderate inducers of CYP3A4; Decompensated cirrhosis/severe hepatic impairment, not recommended in moderate hepatic impairment; OB: When used with ribavirin should not be used in pregnant patients or male patients whose partners are pregnant.

Use Cautiously in: Diabetes mellitus; Hemophilia (↑ risk of bleeding); Structural heart disease, conduction abnormalities, ischemic heart disease, or heart failure (↑ risk of heart block); Females with reproductive potential (ethinyl estradiol-containing medications including oral hormonal contraceptives are contraindicated due to ↑ risk of liver impairment; effective alternative contraception is recommended); Concurrent HIV infection (additional HIV-suppressive regimen required); OB: If used without ribavirin consider maternal benefits and possible adverse effects on the fetus; Lactation: Consider maternal benefits and possible adverse effects on infants; breast feeding not recommended in concurrently HIV-infected patients; Pedi: Safe and effective use in children < 18 yr has not been established.

Adverse Reactions/Side Effects

CNS: fatigue, insomnia (↑ with ribavirin), weakness (↑ with ribavirin). **GI:** HEPATOTOXICITY, nausea (↑ with ribavirin), ↑ liver enzymes. **Derm:** skin reactions including pruritus (↑ with ribavirin), rash, STEVENS-JOHNSON SYNDROME and TOXIC EPIDERMAL NECROLYSIS.

Interactions

Drug-Drug: ↑ levels and risk of serious adverse reactions with **alfuzosin** (hypotension), **dihydroergotamine**, **ergotamine**, **methylergonovine** (ergot toxicity), **lovastatin** or **simvastatin** (myopathy/rhabdomyolysis), **pimozide** (arrhythmias), **efavirenz** (↑ liver enzymes/↓ritonavir tolerance), **sildenafil** (when used for pulmonary hypertension ↑ risk of visual disturances/hypotension/priapism/syncope), oral **midazolam**; (↑ sedation/respiratory depression), **ethinyl estradiol** containing preparations including oral hormonal contraceptives; concurrent use is contraindicated. Levels and antiviral effectiveness are ↓ by **carbamazepine**, **phenobarbital**, **phenytoin**, and **rifampin**; concurrent use is contraindicated. Dasabuvir ↑ **gemfibrozil** levels and risk of cardiovascular toxicity; concurrent use in contraindicated. ↑ levels and risk of **digoxin** toxicity; ↓ digoxin dose by 30–50%, monitor carefully. ↑ levels and risk of adverse cardiovascular reactions with **amiodarone**, **disopyramide**, **flecainide**, **lidocaine**, **mexiletine**, **propafenone**, and **quinidine**; careful monitoring recommended. ↑ levels and risk of adverse reactions with **ketoconazole** (daily dose of ketoconazole should not exceed 200 mg). ↓ levels and effectiveness of **voriconazole**; concurrrent use is not recommended. ↑ levels and risk of adverse reactions with **quetiapine**; ↓ quetiapine dose to 1/6th and monitor carefully, consider alternative anti-HCV treatments). ↑ levels and risk of hypotension with **amlodipine**; ↓ dose of amlodipine may be necessary. ↑ levels and effects of **furosemide**; monitor and adjust dose. Concurrent use with **atazanavir**, **atazanavir/ritonavir**, or **lopinair/riotanivir**↑ levels of paritaprevir; concurrent use is not recommended. ↓ levels and may ↓ effectiveness of **darunavir**; darunavir (800 mg) without ritonavir should be taken at the same time as ombitasvir/peritaprevir/ritonavir. ↑ levels and risk of adverse cardiovascular reactions with **rilpivirine**; concurrent use is not recommended. ↑ levels and risk of adverse muscular reactions with **pravastatin**; pravastin dose should not exceed 40 mg/day. ↑ levels and risk of adverse reactions with **cyclosporine**; ↓ cyclosporine dose to 1/5th, monitor and readjust carefully. ↑ levels and effects of **tacrolimus**; omit tacrolimus on day of initiation ombitasvir/peritaprevir/ritonavir and ↓ dose (0.5 mg every 7 days) adjust by blood level monitoring. ↑ levels and risk of adverse cardiovascular reactions with **salmeterol**; Concurrent use is not recommended. ↑ levels of **buprenorphine**; monitor for sedation/congitive impairment. ↓ levels and effectiveness of **omeprazole**; ↑ dose of omeprazole if necessary, but should not exced 40 mg/day. ↑ levels and effects of **alprazolam**; monitor for sedation/cognitive impairment and adjust dose.

Drug-Natural Products: Levels and antiviral effectiveness are ↓ by **St. John's wort**; concurrent use is contraindicated.

Route/Dosage

PO (Adults): *Genotype 1a without cirrhosis*—Two tablets (each tablet containing ombitasvir 12.5 mg/paritaprevir 75 mg/ritonavir 50 mg) once daily with dasabuvir 250 mg twice daily with ribavirin for 12 wk; *Genotype 1a with cirrhosis or liver tranplant patients with normal hepatic function and mild fibrosis*—Two tablets (each tablet containing ombitasvir 12.5 mg/paritaprevir 75 mg/ritonavir 50 mg) once daily with dasabuvir 250 mg twice daily with ribavirin for 24 wk (some non-transplant patients may respond to 12 wk); *Genotype 1b without cirrhosis*—Two tablets (each tablet containing ombitasvir 12.5 mg/paritaprevir 75 mg/ritonavir 50 mg) once daily with dasabuvir 250 mg twice daily for 12 wk; *Genotype 1b with cirrhosis*—Two tablets (each tablet containing ombitasvir 12.5 mg/paritaprevir 75 mg/ritonavir 50 mg) once daily with dasabuvir 250 mg twice daily with ribavirin for 12 wk.

Availability

Tablets: ombitasvir 12.5 mg/paritaprevir 75 mg/ritonavir 50 mg copackaged with dasabuvir 250 mg in a 28–day convenience pak separated into weekly amounts.

NURSING IMPLICATIONS

Assessment

- Monitor signs of hepatitis (jaundice, fatigue, anorexia, pruritus) during therapy.
- Monitor for signs and symptoms of worsening liver disease (ascites, hepatic encephalopathy, variceal hemorrhage, increases in direct serum bilirubin).
- ***Lab Test Considerations:*** Monitor liver function tests prior to and during first 4 wks of therapy. If ALT is ↑, repeat test and monitor closely. Discontinue therapy if ALT levels are persistently ↑ >10 x upper limit of normal or if accompanied by signs of liver inflammation or ↑ direct bilirubin, alkaline phosphatase, or INR.
- May cause ↑ serum bilirubin; peaks by wk 1 of therapy and not associated with ↑ ALT.
- May cause ↓ hemoglobin requiring dose reduction.

Potential Nursing Diagnoses

Risk for injury (Indications)

Implementation

- **PO:** Administer 2 ombitasvir, paritaprevir, ritonavir 12.5/75/50 mg tablets once daily (in the morning) and 1 dasabuvir 250 mg tablet twice daily (morning and evening) with a meal without regard to fat or calorie content. Usually given in combination with ribavirin.

Patient/Family Teaching

- Instruct patient to take *Viekira Pak* as directed. Take missed doses of ombitasvir, paritaprevir, ritonavir within 12 hrs or of dasabuvir within 6 hrs; if more than 12 hrs or 6 hrs, respectively, since missed dose, skip dose and take next dose at scheduled time; do not double doses. Advise patient to read *Medication Guide* before starting therapy and with each Rx refill in case of changes.
- Advise patient to notify health care professional promptly if signs and symptoms of liver dysfunction (fatigue, weakness, lack of appetite, nausea and vomiting, jaundice, discolored feces) occur.
- Instruct patient to notify health care professional of all Rx or OTC medications, vitamins, or herbal prod-

O

ucts being taken and to consult health care professional before taking other Rx, OTC, or herbal products, especially St. John's wort. Medications containing ethinyl estradiol must be stopped; if taking for birth control, another method must be used.

- Inform patient about teratogenic effects of *Viekira Pak* and ribavirin. Instruct women with childbearing potential, and men, to use 2 forms of effective nonhormonal contraception during and for at least 2 mo following conclusion of therapy. Men must use a condom. Avoid breast feeding during use. Advise patient to notify health care professional if pregnancy occurs.

Evaluation/Desired Outcomes

- Protection from liver damage caused by chronic hepatitis C infection; decreases viral load.

omega-3-acid ethyl esters

(ohme-ga three as-id eth-il es-ters)

Lovaza, Omtryg

Classification

Therapeutic: lipid-lowering agents

Pharmacologic: fatty acids

Pregnancy Category C

Indications

Hypertriglyceridemia (triglycerides ≥500 mmg/dL) in adults; used with specific diet.

Action

Inhibits synthesis of triglycerides. **Therapeutic Effects:** Lowering of triglycerides.

Pharmacokinetics

Absorption: Well absorbed.

Distribution: Unknown.

Metabolism and Excretion: Incorporated into phospholipids.

Half-life: Unknown.

TIME/ACTION PROFILE (lowering of triglycerides)

ROUTE	ONSET	PEAK	DURATION
PO	unknown	2 mo	unknown

Contraindications/Precautions

Contraindicated in: Hypersensitivity.

Use Cautiously in: Allergy/hypersensitivity to fish; OB, Lactation: Pregnancy or lactation; Pedi: Safety not established.

Adverse Reactions/Side Effects

GI: altered taste, eructation, ↑ liver enzymes. **Derm:** rash.

Interactions

Drug-Drug: May ↑ risk of bleeding with **aspirin** or **warfarin**.

Route/Dosage

PO (Adults): *Lovaza*—4 g/day; may be given as a single dose or 2 g twice daily; *Omtryg*—4.8 g once daily or 2.4 g twice daily.

Availability (generic available)

Gelatin capsules (oil-filled) (Lovaza): 1 g. **Cost:** $196.69/100. **Gelatin capsules (oil-filled) (Omtryg):** 1.2 g.

NURSING IMPLICATIONS

Assessment

- Obtain a diet history, especially with regard to fat consumption.
- ***Lab Test Considerations:*** Monitor serum triglyceride levels prior to and periodically during therapy.
- Monitor serum ALT periodically during therapy. May cause ↑ serum ALT without concurrent ↑ in AST levels.
- Monitor serum LDL cholesterol levels periodically during therapy. May cause ↑ in serum LDL levels.

Potential Nursing Diagnoses

Noncompliance (Patient/Family Teaching)

Implementation

- Do not confuse Lovaza with lorazepam.
- An appropriate lipid-lowering diet should be followed before therapy and should continue during therapy.
- **PO:** May be taken as a single 4-g dose or as 2 g twice daily. May be administered with meals. Swallow capsules whole; do not break, dissolve, or chew.

Patient/Family Teaching

- Instruct patient to take medication as directed, not to skip doses or double up on missed doses. Take missed doses as soon as remembered, but if a day is missed, do not double doses the next day. Medication helps control but does not cure elevated serum triglyceride levels.
- Advise patient that this medication should be used in conjunction with diet restrictions (fat, cholesterol, carbohydrates, alcohol), exercise, weight loss in overweight patients, and control of medical problems (such as diabetes mellitus and hypothyroidism) that may contribute to hypertriglyceridemia.
- Emphasize the importance of follow-up exams to determine effectiveness.

Evaluation/Desired Outcomes

- Lowering of serum triglyceride levels. Patients who do not have an adequate response after 2 mo of treatment should be withdrawn from therapy.

omeprazole (o-mep-ra-zole)

Losec, Olex, PriLOSEC, PriLOSEC OTC

Classification
Therapeutic: antiulcer agents
Pharmacologic: proton-pump inhibitors

Pregnancy Category C

Indications

GERD/maintenance of healing in erosive esophagitis. Duodenal ulcers (with or without anti-infectives for *Helicobacter pylori*). Short-term treatment of active benign gastric ulcer. Pathologic hypersecretory conditions, including Zollinger-Ellison syndrome. Reduction of risk of GI bleeding in critically ill patients. **OTC:** Heartburn occurring ≥twice/wk.

Action

Binds to an enzyme on gastric parietal cells in the presence of acidic gastric pH, preventing the final transport of hydrogen ions into the gastric lumen. **Therapeutic Effects:** Diminished accumulation of acid in the gastric lumen with lessened gastroesophageal reflux. Healing of duodenal ulcers.

Pharmacokinetics

Absorption: Rapidly absorbed following oral administration; immediate release formulation contains bicarbonate to prevent acid degradation.
Distribution: Good distribution into gastric parietal cells.
Protein Binding: 95%.
Metabolism and Excretion: Mostly metabolized by the liver via the cytochrome P450 (CYP) system (primarily CYP2C19 isoenzyme, but also the CYP3A4 isoenzyme) (the CYP2C19 enzyme system exhibits genetic polymorphism; 15–20% of Asian patients and 3–5% of Caucasian and Black patients may be poor metabolizers and may have significantly ↑ omeprazole concentrations and an ↑ risk of adverse effects); inactive metabolites are excreted in urine (77%) and feces.
Half-life: 0.5–1 hr (↑ in liver disease to 3 hr).

TIME/ACTION PROFILE (antisecretory effects)

ROUTE	ONSET	PEAK	DURATION
PO-delayed release	within 1 hr	within 2 hr	72–96 hr

Contraindications/Precautions

Contraindicated in: Hypersensitivity to omeprazole or related drugs (benzimidazoles); Lactation: Discontinue omeprazole or discontinue breast feeding.
Use Cautiously in: Liver disease (dose ↓ may be necessary); Patients using high-doses for >1 year (↑ risk of hip, wrist, or spine fractures); Patients using therapy for >3 yr (↑ risk of vitamin B_{12} deficiency; OB, Lactation, Pedi: Safety not established in pregnant or breast-feeding women, or children <1 yr.

Adverse Reactions/Side Effects

CNS: dizziness, drowsiness, fatigue, headache, weakness. **CV:** chest pain. **GI:** CLOSTRIDIUM DIFFICILE-ASSOCIATED DIARRHEA (CDAD), abdominal pain, acid regurgitation, constipation, diarrhea, flatulence, nausea, vomiting. **F and E:** hypomagnesemia (especially if treatment duration ≥3 mo). **GU:** acute interstitial nephritis. **Derm:** itching, rash. **Hemat:** vitamin B_{12} deficiency. **MS:** bone fracture. **Misc:** allergic reactions.

Interactions

Drug-Drug: Omeprazole is metabolized by the CYP450 enzyme system and may compete with other agents metabolized by this system. ↓ metabolism and may ↑ effects of **antifungal agents**, **diazepam**, **digoxin**, **flurazepam**, **triazolam**, **cyclosporine**, **phenytoin**, **saquinavir**, **tacrolimus**, and **warfarin**. May ↓ absorption of drugs requiring acid pH, including **ketoconazole**, **itraconazole**, **ampicillin esters**, **iron salts**, **erlotinib**, and **mycophenolate mofetil**; concomitant use with **atazanavir** not recommended. Has been used safely with **antacids**. May significantly ↓ effects of **atazanavir** and **nelfinavir**; concurrent use not recommended. May ↑ risk of bleeding with **warfarin** (monitor INR/PT). May ↑ levels of **digoxin** and **methotrexate**. **Voriconazole** may ↑ levels. May ↓ the antiplatelet effects of **clopidogrel**; avoid concurrent use. May ↑ levels of **cilostazol**; consider ↓ dose of cilostazol from 100 mg twice daily to 50 mg twice daily. **Rifampin** may ↓ levels and may ↓ response; avoid concurrent use. Hypomagnesemia ↑ risk of **digoxin** toxicity. May ↑ levels of **tacrolimus** and **methotrexate**.
Drug-Natural Products: **St. John's wort** may ↓ levels and may ↓ response; avoid concurrent use.

Route/Dosage

PO (Adults): *GERD/erosive esophagitis and maintenance of healing of erosive esophagitis*—20 mg once daily. *Duodenal ulcers associated with H. pylori*—40 mg once daily in the morning with clarithromycin for 2 wk, then 20 mg once daily for 2 wk *or* 20 mg twice daily with clarithromycin 500 mg twice daily and amoxicillin 1000 mg twice daily for 10 days (if ulcer is present at beginning of therapy, continue omeprazole 20 mg daily for 18 more days); has also been used with clarithromycin and metronidazole. *Gastric ulcer*—40 mg once daily for 4–6 wk. *Reduction of the risk of GI bleeding in critically ill patients*—40 mg initially, then another 40 mg 6–8 hr later, followed by 40 mg once daily for up to 14 days. *Gastric hypersecretory conditions*—60 mg once daily initially; may

O

be increased up to 120 mg 3 times daily (doses >80 m g/day should be given in divided doses); *OTC*—20 mg once daily for up to 14 days.
PO (Children 1–16 yr and 5–9 kg): *GERD/erosive esophagitis*—5 mg once daily.
PO (Children 1–16 yr and 10–19 kg): *GERD/erosive esophagitis*—10 mg once daily.
PO (Children 1–16 yr and ≥20 kg): *GERD/erosive esophagitis*—20 mg once daily.

Availability (generic available)

Delayed-release capsules: 10 mg, 20 mg, 40 mg. **Delayed-release tablets:** 20 mg^{OTC}. **Delayed-release powder for oral suspension (peach-mint):** 2.5 mg/packet, 10 mg/packet. ***In combination with:*** metronidazole and clarithromycin in a compliance package (Losec 1-2-3 M); with amoxicillin and clarithromycin in a compliance package (Losec 1-2-3-A) (both in Canada only); with sodium bicarbonate (Zegerid [OTC] see Appendix B).

NURSING IMPLICATIONS

Assessment

- Assess patient routinely for epigastric or abdominal pain and frank or occult blood in the stool, emesis, or gastric aspirate.
- Monitor bowel function. Diarrhea, abdominal cramping, fever, and bloody stools should be reported to health care professional promptly as a sign of Clostridium difficile-associated diarrhea (CDAD). May begin up to several weeks following cessation of therapy.
- ***Lab Test Considerations:*** Monitor CBC with differential periodically during therapy.
- May cause ↑ AST, ALT, alkaline phosphatase, and bilirubin.
- May cause serum gastrin concentrations to ↑ during first 1–2 wk of therapy. Levels return to normal after discontinuation of omeprazole.
- Monitor INR and prothrombin time in patients taking warfarin.
- May cause hypomagnesemia. Monitor serum magnesium prior to and periodically during therapy.
- May cause false positive results in diagnostic investigations for neuroendocrine tumors due to ↑ serum chromogranin A (CgA) levels secondary to drug-induced ↓ gastric acidity. Temporarily stop esomeprazole at least 14 days before assessing CgA levels and consider repeating test if initial CgA levels are high.

Potential Nursing Diagnoses

Acute pain (Indications)

Implementation

- Do not confuse Prilosec (omeprazole) with Prozac (fluoxetine) or Pristiq (desvenlafaxine). Do not confuse omeprazole with fomepizole.
- **PO:** Administer doses before meals, preferably in the morning. Capsules and tablets should be swallowed whole; do not crush or chew. Capsules may be opened and sprinkled on cool applesauce, entire mixture should be ingested immediately and followed by a drink of water. Do not store for future use.
- *Powder for oral suspension:* Administer on empty stomach, as least 1 hr before a meal. Empty contents of 2.5 mg packet into 5 mL of water or contents of 10 mg packet into 15 mL of water. Stir. Leave 2 to 3 minutes to thicken. Stir and drink within 30 min. If material remains after drinking, add more water, stir and drink immediately. For patients with nasogastric or enteral feeding, suspend feeding for 3 hr before and 1 hr after administration. Empty packet contents into a small cup containing 5 mL of water for 2.5 mg dose or 15 mL water for 10 mg dose using a catheter tipped syringe. **Do not use other liquids or foods.** Immediately shake syringe and leave 2 to 3 minutes to thicken. Administer within 30 min. Refill the syringe with an equal amount of water. Shake and flush remaining contents from nasogastric or gastric tube into stomach.
- May be administered concurrently with antacids.

Patient/Family Teaching

- Instruct patient to take medication as directed for the full course of therapy, even if feeling better. Take missed doses as soon as remembered but not if almost time for next dose. Do not double doses.
- May cause occasional drowsiness or dizziness. Caution patient to avoid driving or other activities requiring alertness until response to medication is known.
- Instruct patient to notify health care professional of all Rx or OTC medications, vitamins, or herbal products being taken and consult health care professional before taking any new medications, especially St. John's wort.
- Advise patient to avoid alcohol, products containing aspirin or NSAIDs, and foods that may cause an increase in GI irritation.
- Advise patient to report onset of black, tarry stools; diarrhea; abdominal pain; or persistent headache to health care professional promptly.
- Instruct patient to notify health care professional of onset of black, tarry stools; diarrhea; abdominal pain; or persistent headache or if fever and diarrhea develop, especially if stool contains blood, pus, or mucus. Advise patient not to treat diarrhea without consulting health care professional.
- Advise female patient to notify health care professional if pregnancy is planned or suspected or if breast feeding.

Evaluation/Desired Outcomes

- Decrease in abdominal pain or prevention of gastric irritation and bleeding. Healing of duodenal ulcers can be seen on x-ray examination or endoscopy.

- Decrease in symptoms of GERD and erosive esophagitis. Therapy is continued for 4–8 wk after initial episode.

ondansetron (on-dan-se-tron)

✤Ondissolve ODF, Zofran, Zofran ODT, Zuplenz

Classification

Therapeutic: antiemetics

Pharmacologic: 5-HT_3 antagonists

Pregnancy Category B

Indications

Prevention of nausea and vomiting associated with highly or moderately emetogenic chemotherapy. **PO:** Prevention of nausea and vomiting associated with radiation therapy. Prevention and treatment of postoperative nausea and vomiting.

Action

Blocks the effects of serotonin at 5-HT_3–receptor sites (selective antagonist) located in vagal nerve terminals and the chemoreceptor trigger zone in the CNS. **Therapeutic Effects:** Decreased incidence and severity of nausea and vomiting following chemotherapy or surgery.

Pharmacokinetics

Absorption: IV administration results in complete bioavailability; 100% absorbed following oral administration.

Distribution: Unknown.

Metabolism and Excretion: Extensively metabolized by the liver (primarily by CYP3A4); 5% excreted unchanged by the kidneys.

Half-life: *Adults*—3.5–5.5 hr; *Children 5 mo–12 yr*—2.9 hr.

TIME/ACTION PROFILE (antiemetic effect)

ROUTE	ONSET	PEAK	DURATION
PO, IV	rapid	15–30 min	4–8 hr
IM	rapid	40 min	unknown

Contraindications/Precautions

Contraindicated in: Hypersensitivity; Orally disintegrating tablets contain aspartame and should not be used in patients with phenylketonuria; Congenital long QT syndrome; Concurrent use of apomorphine.

Use Cautiously in: Hepatic impairment (daily dose not to exceed 8 mg); Abdominal surgery (may mask ileus); OB, Lactation, Pedi: Pregnancy, lactation, or children ≤3 yr (PO) or <1 mo (parenteral) (safety not established).

Adverse Reactions/Side Effects

CNS: SEROTONIN SYNDROME, headache, dizziness, drowsiness, fatigue, weakness. **CV:** TORSADE DE POINTES, QT interval prolongation. **GI:** constipation, diarrhea, abdominal pain, dry mouth, ↑ liver enzymes. **Neuro:** extrapyramidal reactions. **Derm:** STEVENS-JOHNSON SYNDROME, TOXIC EPIDERMAL NECROLYSIS.

Interactions

Drug-Drug: Use with **apomorphine** ↑ risk of severe hypotension and loss of consciousness; concurrent use contraindicated. **Carbamazepine**, **phenytoin**, and **rifampin** may ↓ levels. Drugs that affect serotonergic neurotransmitter systems, including **SSRIs**, **SNRIs**, **tricyclic antidepressants**, **MAOIs**, **fentanyl**, **lithium**, **buspirone**, **tramadol**, **methylene blue**, and **triptans** ↑ risk of serotonin syndrome.

Route/Dosage

PO (Adults): *Prevention of nausea/vomiting associated with highly-emetogenic chemotherapy*—24 mg 30 min prior to chemotherapy.

PO (Adults and Children >11 yr): *Prevention of nausea/vomiting associated with moderately emetogenic chemotherapy*—8 mg 30 min prior to chemotherapy and repeated 8 hr later; 8 mg q 12 hr may be given for 1–2 days following chemotherapy. *Prevention of radiation-induced nausea/vomiting*—8 mg 1–2 hr prior to radiation; may be repeated q 8 hr, depending on type, location, and extent of radiation. *Prevention of postoperative nausea/vomiting*—16 mg 1 hr before induction of anesthesia.

PO (Children 4–11 yr): *Prevention of nausea/vomiting associated with moderately emetogenic chemotherapy*—4 mg 30 min prior to chemotherapy and repeated 4 and 8 hr later; 4 mg q 8 hr may be given for 1–2 days following chemotherapy.

IV (Adults): *Prevention of chemotherapy-induced nausea/vomiting*—0.15 mg/kg (max dose = 16 mg) 30 min prior to chemotherapy, repeated 4 and 8 hr later.

IM, IV (Adults): *Prevention of postoperative nausea/vomiting*—4 mg before induction of anesthesia or postoperatively.

IV (Children 6 mo–18 yr): *Prevention of chemotherapy-induced nausea/vomiting*—0.15 mg/kg (max dose = 16 mg) 30 min prior to chemotherapy, repeated 4 and 8 hr later.

IV (Children 1 mo–12 yr and >40 k g): *Prevention of postoperative nausea/vomiting*—4 mg.

IV (Children 1 mo–12 yr and ≤40 kg): *Prevention of postoperative nausea/vomiting*—0.1 mg/kg.

Hepatic Impairment

PO, IM, IV (Adults): *Severe hepatic impairment*—Not to exceed 8 mg/day.

O

Availability (generic available)

Orally disintegrating tablets (contain aspartame) (strawberry flavor): 4 mg, 8 mg. **Cost:** *Generic*—4 mg $668.78/30, 8 mg $1,113.95/30. **Oral soluble film (Zuplenz):** 4 mg, 8 mg. **Cost:** All strengths $16.50/1. **Tablets:** 4 mg, 8 mg, 24 mg. **Cost:** *Generic*—4 mg $735.05/30, 8 mg $1,217.42/30, 24 mg $105.50/1. **Oral solution (strawberry flavor):** 4 mg/5 mL. **Cost:** $269.74/50 mL. **Solution for injection:** 2 mg/mL.

NURSING IMPLICATIONS

Assessment

- Assess patient for nausea, vomiting, abdominal distention, and bowel sounds prior to and following administration.
- Assess patient for extrapyramidal effects (involuntary movements, facial grimacing, rigidity, shuffling walk, trembling of hands) periodically during therapy.
- Monitor ECG in patients with hypokalemia, hypomagnesemia, HF, bradyarrhythmias, or patients taking concomitant medications that prolong the QT interval.
- Monitor for signs and symptoms of serotonin syndrome (mental status changes [agitation, hallucinations, delirium, coma], autonomic instability [tachycardia, labile BP, dizziness, diaphoresis, flushing, hyperthermia], neuromuscular symptoms [tremor, rigidity, myoclonus, hyperreflexia, incoordination], seizures, gastrointestinal symptoms [nausea, vomiting, diarrhea]. If symptoms occur, discontinue therapy.
- ***Lab Test Considerations:*** May cause transient ↑ in serum bilirubin, AST, and ALT levels.

Potential Nursing Diagnoses

Imbalanced nutrition: less than body requirements (Indications)
Diarrhea (Side Effects)
Constipation (Side Effects)

Implementation

- First dose is administered prior to emetogenic event.
- **PO:** For orally disintegrating tablets, do not attempt to push through foil backing; with dry hands, peel back backing and remove tablet. Immediately place tablet on tongue; tablet will dissolve in seconds, then swallow with saliva. Administration of liquid is not necessary.

IV Administration

- **IV Push:** Administer undiluted (2 mg/mL) immediately before induction of anesthesia or postoperatively if nausea and vomiting occur shortly after surgery. ***Rate:*** Administer over at least 30 sec and preferably over 2–5 min.
- **Intermittent Infusion:** ***Diluent:*** Dilute doses for prevention of nausea and vomiting associated with chemotherapy in 50 mL of D5W, 0.9% NaCl, D5/0.9% NaCl, D5/0.45% NaCl. Solution is clear and colorless. Stable for 7 days at room temperature following dilution. ***Concentration:*** 1 mg/mL. ***Rate:*** Administer each dose over 15 min.
- **Y-Site Compatibility:** acetaminophen, aldesleukin, alemtuzumab, alfentanil, amifostine, amikacin, aminocaproic acid, anakinra, anidulafungin, argatroban, ascorbic acid, atropine, azithromycin, aztreonam, benztropine, bivalirudin, bleomycin, bumetanide, buprenorphine, busulfan, butorphanol, calcium chloride, calcium gluconate, carboplatin, carmustine, caspofungin, cefazolin, cefotaxime, cefoxitin, ceftaroline, ceftazidime, cefuroxime, chlorpromazine, ciprofloxacin, cisatracurium, cisplatin, cladribine, clindamycin, cyanocobalamin, cyclophosphamide, cyclosporine, cytarabine, dacarbazine, dactinomycin, daunorubicin hydrochloride, dexamethasone, dexmedetomidine, dexrazoxane, digoxin, diltiazem, diphenhydramine, dobutamine, docetaxel, dopamine, doripenem, doxorubicin hydrochloride, doxorubicin liposomal, doxycycline, droperidol, enalaprilat, ephedrine, epinephrine, epirubicin, epoetin alfa, eptifibatide, erythromycin, esmolol, etoposide, etoposide phosphate, famotidine, fenoldopam, fentanyl, filgrastim, floxuridine, fluconazole, fludarabine, folic acid, fosaprepritant, fosphenytoin, gemcitabine, gentamicin, glycopyrrolate, heparin, hetastarch, hydrocortisone, hydromorphone, idarubicin, ifosfamide, imipenem/cilastatin, irinotecan, isoproterenol, ketorolac, labetalol, levofloxacin, lidocaine, linezolid, magnesium sulfate, mannitol, mechlorethamine, melphalan, meperidine, mesna, methotrexate, methyldopate, metoclopramide, metoprolol, metronidazole, midazolam, mitomycin, mitoxantrone, morphine, moxifloxacin, multivitamins, mycophenolate, nafcillin, nalbuphine, naloxone, nesiritide, nitroglycerin, nitroprusside, norepinephrine, octreotide, oxacillin, oxaliplatin, oxytocin, paclitaxel, pamidronate, pancuronium, papaverine, penicillin G, pentamidine, pentazocine, pentostatin, phenylephrine, phytonadione, piperacillin/tazobactam, potassium acetate, potassium chloride, potassium phosphates, procainamide, prochlorperazine, promethazine, propranolol, protamine, pyridoxine, ranitidine, remifentanil, rocuronium, sodium acetate, sodium phosphates, streptokinase, streptozocin, succinylcholine, sufentanil, tacrolimus, telavancin, teniposide, theophylline, thiotepa, tigecycline, tirofiban, tobramycin, topotecan, vancomycin, vasopressin, vecuronium, verapamil, vinblastine, vincristine, vinorelbine, voriconazole, zidovudine, zoledronic acid.
- **Y-Site Incompatibility:** acyclovir, allopurinol, aminophylline, amphotericin B colloidal, amphotericin B lipid complex, amphotericin B liposome, ampicillin, ampicillin/sulbactam, cefepime, chloramphenicol, dantrolene, ertapenem, foscarnet, furosemide, ganciclovir, indomethacin, lorazepam,

micafungin, milrinone, pantoprazole, pemetrexed, pentobarbital, phenobarbital, phenytoin, rituximab, sargramostim, sodium bicarbonate, thiopental, trastuzumab, trimethoprin/sulfamethoxazole.

Patient/Family Teaching

- Instruct patient to take ondansetron as directed.
- Advise patient to notify health care professional immediately if symptoms of irregular heart beat, serotonin syndrome, or involuntary movement of eyes, face, or limbs occur.

Evaluation/Desired Outcomes

- Prevention of nausea and vomiting associated with emetogenic cancer chemotherapy.
- Prevention of postoperative nausea and vomiting.
- Prevention of nausea and vomiting due to radiation therapy.

oritavancin (oh-rit-a-van-sin)

Orbactiv

Classification
Therapeutic: anti-infectives
Pharmacologic: lipoglycopeptides

Pregnancy Category C

Indications

Treatment of acute bacterial skin and skin structure infections caused by or suspected to be caused by susceptible designated Gram-positive bacteria.

Action

Binds to bacterial cell wall resulting in cell death. **Therapeutic Effects:** Bactericidal action against susceptible bacteria with resolution of infection. **Spectrum:** Active against *Staphylococcus aureus* (including methicillin-susceptible and resistant strains), *Streptococcus pyogenes*, *Streptococcus agalactiae*, *Streptococcus dysgalactiae*, *Streptococcus anginosus* (including *S. anginosus*, *S. intermidius* and *S. constellatus*) and *Enterococcus faecalis* (vancomycin-susceptible strains only).

Pharmacokinetics

Absorption: IV administration results in complete bioavailability.
Distribution: Penetrates skin/skin structures.
Metabolism and Excretion: Slowly excreted unchanged in urine (5% in two weeks) and feces (1% in two weeks).
Half-life: 245 hr (terminal).

TIME/ACTION PROFILE (blood levels)

ROUTE	ONSET	PEAK	DURATION
IV	rapid	end of infusion	at least 2 wk

Contraindications/Precautions

Contraindicated in: Hypersensitivity (cross-sensitivity with other glycopeptides may occur); Heparin use within 48 hr following administration of oritavancin (causes false ↑ aPTT); Concurrent warfarin (↑ risk of bleeding, use only if benefit outweighs bleeding risk); Confirmed/suspected osteomyelitis (alternate treatment required).
Use Cautiously in: Concurrent use of drugs with narrow therapeutic indices that are metabolized by the CYP450 enzyme system (effects may be altered); Severe hepatic/renal impairment; Geri: Elderly patients may be ↑ sensitive to drug effects; OB: Use during pregnancy only if potential benefit justifies fetal risk; Lactation: Use cautiously if breast feeding; Pedi: Safe and effective use in patients <18 yr has not been established.

O

Adverse Reactions/Side Effects

CNS: headache. **CV:** tachycardia. **GI:** diarrhea including CLOSTRIDIUM DIFFICILE, ↑ liver enzymes, nausea, vomiting. **Local:** infusion site reactions. **Misc:** hypersensitivity reactions including ANAPHYLAXIS, infusion reactions including "Red-Man Syndrome", limb/subcutaneous abscess formation.

Interactions

Drug-Drug: ↑ risk of bleeding with **warfarin** (avoid if possible). Affects the activities of several CYP450 enzymes (careful monitoring of other **drugs metabolized by the CYP450 system** that have narrow therapeutic indices to assess for toxicity or ineffectiveness is recommended).

Route/Dosage

IV (Adults >18 yr): 1200 mg single dose.

Availability

Lyophylized powder for intravenous administration (requires reconstitution): 400 mg/vial.

NURSING IMPLICATIONS

Assessment

- Assess for infection (vital signs; appearance of wound, sputum, urine, and stool; WBC) at beginning of and during therapy.
- Obtain specimens for culture and sensitivity prior to therapy. First dose may be given before receiving results.
- Monitor bowel function. Diarrhea, abdominal cramping, fever, and bloody stools should be reported to health care professional promptly as a sign

of Clostridium difficile-associated diarrhea (CDAD). May begin up to 2 mo following cessation of therapy.

- Monitor for infusion reactions (Red-man syndrome—flushing of upper body, urticaria, pruritus, rash). May resolve with stopping or slowing infusion.
- ***Lab Test Considerations:*** Monitor hepatic function tests. May cause ↑ ALT, AST, and bilirubin.
- May cause hyperuricemia and hypoglycemia.
- Causes falsely ↑ aPTT for 48 hr after infusion. Avoid heparin administration during this time. Use a non-phospholipid dependent coagulation test such as Factor Xa assay if needed.
- Artificially prolongs PT and INR for up to 24 hr. May increase risk of bleeding with warfarin.

Potential Nursing Diagnoses

Risk for infection (Indications)
Diarrhea (Adverse Reactions)

Implementation

- Using three 400 mg vials, add 40 mL of Sterile Water for Injection to each vial for a 10 mg/mL solution/vial. Swirl gently to avoid foaming and ensure powder is completely reconstituted. Solution is clear and colorless to pale yellow; do not administer solutions that are discolored or contain particulate matter. ***Diluent:*** Withdraw and discard 120 mL from 1000 mL bag of D5W. Withdraw 40 mL from each vial and add to D5W bag. Do not use 0.9% NaCl; may cause precipitation. ***Concentration:*** 1.2 mg/mL. Use within 6 hr at room temperature or 12 hr if refrigerated, including 3 hr infusion. ***Rate:*** Infuse over 3 hr.
- **Y-Site Incompatibility:** Do not mix with other solutions or medications. Flush line before and after infusion.

Patient/Family Teaching

- Instruct patient to notify health care professional if signs and symptoms of hypersensitivity reactions (rash, hives, dyspnea, facial swelling) occur.
- Instruct patient to notify health care professional immediately if diarrhea, abdominal cramping, fever, or bloody stools occur and not to treat with antidiarrheals without consulting health care professionals.
- Advise patient to notify health care professional of all Rx or OTC medications, vitamins, or herbal products being taken and to consult with health care professional before taking other medications.
- Advise female patients to notify health care professional if pregnancy is planned or suspected or if breast feeding.
- Instruct the patient to notify health care professional if symptoms do not improve.

Evaluation/Desired Outcomes

- Resolution of the signs and symptoms of infection. Length of time for complete resolution depends on the organism and site of infection.

oseltamivir (o-sel-tam-i-vir)

Tamiflu

Classification
Therapeutic: antivirals
Pharmacologic: neuraminidase inhibitors

Pregnancy Category C

Indications

Treatment of uncomplicated acute illness due to influenza infection in adults and children ≥2 wk who have had symptoms for ≤2 days. Prevention of influenza in patients ≥1 yr.

Action

Inhibits the enzyme neuraminidase, which may alter virus particle aggregation and release. **Therapeutic Effects:** Reduced duration or prevention of flu-related symptoms.

Pharmacokinetics

Absorption: Rapidly absorbed from the GI tract and converted by the liver to the active form, oseltamivir carboxylate. 75% reaches systemic circulation as the active drug.
Distribution: Unknown.
Protein Binding: oseltamivir phosphate: 42%; oseltamivir carboxylate: 3%.
Metabolism and Excretion: Rapidly metabolized by the liver to oseltamivir carboxylate, the active drug. >99% excreted unchanged in urine.
Half-life: *Oseltamivir carboxylate*—6–10 hr.

TIME/ACTION PROFILE (blood levels)

ROUTE	ONSET	PEAK	DURATION
PO	unknown	unknown	12 hr

Contraindications/Precautions

Contraindicated in: Hypersensitivity; End stage renal disease and not receiving dialysis; Pedi: Children <1 yr.
Use Cautiously in: Renal impairment (↓ dose if CCr ≤60 mL/min); Pedi: Children <2 wk (safety and efficacy not established for treatment); children <1 yr (safety and efficacy not established for prevention). Oral suspension contains sodium benzoate, avoid use in neonates; OB, Lactation: Safety not established; use only if potential benefits outweigh possible risks.

Adverse Reactions/Side Effects

CNS: SEIZURES, abnormal behavior, agitation, confusion, delirium, hallucinations, insomnia, nightmares, vertigo. **Resp:** bronchitis. **GI:** nausea, vomiting.

Interactions

Drug-Drug: May ↓ the therapeutic effect of **influenza virus vaccine** avoid use 2 days prior to and 2 weeks after vaccine administration.

Route/Dosage

Treatment of Influenza

PO (Adults and Children ≥13 yr): 75 mg twice daily for 5 days.
PO (Children 1–12 yr and >40 kg): 75 mg twice daily for 5 days.
PO (Children 1–12 yr and 23.1–40 kg): 60 mg twice daily for 5 days.
PO (Children 1–12 yr and 15.1–23 kg): 45 mg twice daily for 5 days.
PO (Children 1–12 yr and ≤15 kg): 30 mg twice daily for 5 days.
PO (Infants 2 wk–<1 yr): 3 mg/kg/dose twice daily for 5 days.

Renal Impairment

PO (Adults): *CCr 30–60 mL/min*—30 mg twice daily for 5 days; *CCr 10–30 mL/min*—30 mg once daily for 5 days; *CCr ≥10 mL/min and on HD*—30 mg after each HD session (not to exceed 5 days); *CCr ≥10 mL/min and on PD*—30 mg single dose immediately after a dialysis exchange; *CCr <10 mL/min and not on dialysis*—Not recommended.

Influenza Prevention

PO (Adults and Children ≥13 yr): 75 mg once daily for at least 10 days.
PO (Children 1–12 yr and >40 k g): 75 mg once daily for 10 days.
PO (Children 1–12 yr and 23.1–40 kg): 60 mg once daily for 10 days.
PO (Children 1–12 yr and 15.1–23 kg): 45 mg once daily for 10 days.
PO (Children 1–12 yr and ≤15 kg): 30 mg once daily for 10 days.

Renal Impairment

PO (Adults): *CCr 30–60 mL/min*—30 mg once daily for at least 10 days; *CCr 10–30 mL/min*—30 mg every other day for at least 10 days; *CCr ≥10 mL/min and on HD*—30 mg after alternate HD sessions (treatment duration at least 10 days); *CCr ≥10 mL/min and on PD*—30 mg once weekly immediately after a dialysis exchange (treatment duration at least 10 days); *CCr <10 mL/min and not on dialysis*—Not recommended.

Availability

Capsules: 30 mg, 45 mg, 75 mg. **Oral suspension (tutti-frutti flavor):** 6 mg/mL.

NURSING IMPLICATIONS

Assessment

- Monitor influenza symptoms (sudden onset of fever, cough, headache, fatigue, muscular weakness, sore throat). Additional supportive treatment may be indicated to treat symptoms.

Potential Nursing Diagnoses

Risk for infection (Indications)

Implementation

- Treatment with oseltamivir should be started as soon as possible from the first sign of flu symptoms within 2 days of exposure.
- Consider available information on influenza drug susceptibility patterns and treatment effects before using oseltamivir for prophylaxis.
- **PO:** May be administered with food or milk to minimize GI irritation.
- Use correct oral dosing device for measuring oral solution. Dosing errors have occurred due to oseltamivir dosing in mg and solution in mL. Make sure units of measure on prescription instructions match dosing device provided with the drug.
- If oral suspension is not available, capsules can be opened and mixed with flavored foods (regular or sugar-free chocolate syrup, corn syrup, caramel topping, light brown sugar dissolved in water). If correct dose and oral suspension are not available, pharmacist may compound emergency supply of oral suspension from 75 mg capsules.

Patient/Family Teaching

- Instruct patient to take oseltamivir as soon as influenza symptoms appear and to continue to take it as directed, for the full course of therapy, even if feeling better. Take missed doses as soon as remembered unless within 2 hr of next dose. Do not double doses.
- Caution patient that oseltamivir should not be shared with anyone, even if they have the same symptoms.
- Advise patient that oseltamivir is not a substitute for a flu shot. Patients should receive annual flu shot according to immunization guidelines.
- Advise patients to report behavioral changes (hallucinations, delirium, and abnormal behavior) to health care professional immediately.
- Advise patient to consult health care professional before taking other medications concurrently with oseltamivir.

Evaluation/Desired Outcomes

- Reduced duration or prevention of flu-related symptoms.

ospemifene (os- pem-i-feen)

Osphena

Classification
Therapeutic: hormones
Pharmacologic: estrogen agonists/antagonists

Pregnancy Category X

Indications
Moderate to severe dyspareunia due to menopausal vulvar/vaginal atrophy.

Action
Has agonist (estrogen-like) effects on the endometrium of the uterus; effects are tissue-specific. **Therapeutic Effects:** Decreased dyspareunuia.

Pharmacokinetics
Absorption: Well absorbed following oral administration; food enhances absorption 2–3 fold.
Distribution: Unknown.
Protein Binding: >99%.
Metabolism and Excretion: Mostly metabolized by the liver (CYP3A4 and CYP2C9 enzyme systems); 75% excreted in feces, 7% in urine as metabolites; minimal amounts excreted unchanged in urine.
Half-life: 26 hr.

TIME/ACTION PROFILE (improvement in symptoms)

ROUTE	ONSET	PEAK	DURATION
PO	within 12 wk	unknown	unknown

Contraindications/Precautions
Contraindicated in: Hypersensitivity; Undiagnosed abnormal genital bleeding; History/ suspicion of estrogen-dependent cancer; History of/current thromboembolic disorder, including DVT, PE, MI, or stroke; Concurrent use of estrogens, estrogen agonists/antagonists, fluconazole, or rifampin; OB: Known/suspected pregnancy (may cause fetal harm); Lactation: Breast feeding should be avoided.
Use Cautiously in: Patients with risk factors for cardiovascular disease, arterial vascular disease or venous thromboembolism (including hypertension, obesity, family history, tobacco use, diabetes mellitus, history of DVT/PE or systemic lupus erythematosus); Known or suspected breast cancer; Severe hepatic impairment.

Adverse Reactions/Side Effects
CV: STROKE, DEEP VEIN THROMBOSIS/PE. **GU:** ENDOMETRIAL CANCER, genital/vaginal discharge. **Derm:** hot flush, hyperhydrosis. **MS:** muscle spasms. **Misc:** hypersensitivity reactions including ANGIOEDEMA.

Interactions
Drug-Drug: Blood levels, effects and risk of adverse reactions ↑ by **fluconazole**, avoid concurrent use. Blood levels and effects may be ↑ by **ketoconazole** or other **drugs that inhibit the CYP3A4 or CYP2C9 enzyme systems**. Blood levels and beneficial effects ↓ by **rifampin**, avoid concurrent use. Avoid concurrent use of other **estrogens** or **estrogen agonist/antagonists** due to ↑ estrogen effects. May displace or be displaced by other **drugs that are highly protein bound**.

Route/Dosage
PO (Adults): 60 mg once daily.

Availability
Tablets: 60 mg.

NURSING IMPLICATIONS

Assessment
- Assess amount of pain during intercourse prior to and periodically during therapy.
- Determine methods previously use to treat dyspareunia.
- Assess BP before and periodically during therapy.
- Monitor for hypersensitivity reactions (angioedema, urticaria, rash, pruritus). If symptoms occur discontinue ospemifene and treat symptomatically.

Potential Nursing Diagnoses
Sexual dysfunction (Indications)
Deficient knowledge, related to medication regimen (Patient/Family Teaching)

Implementation
- **PO:** Administer once daily with food.

Patient/Family Teaching
- Instruct patient to take ospemifene as directed. Advise patient to read *Patient Information* sheet before starting therapy and with each Rx refill in case of changes.
- Advise patient to report signs and symptoms of unusual vaginal bleeding, changes in vision or speech, sudden new severe headaches, severe pains in chest or legs with or without shortness of breath, weakness, or fatigue promptly to health care professional.
- Inform patient that ospemifene may cause hot flashes, vaginal discharge, muscle spasm, and increased sweating.
- Patients who still have a uterus should discuss addition of progestin with health care professional.
- Instruct patient to notify health care professional of all Rx or OTC medications, vitamins, or herbal products being taken and consult health care professional before taking any new medications.
- Advise patient to notify health care professional of medication regimen before treatment or surgery.
- Women should be monitored for breast and uterine cancer (pelvic exam, breast exam, mammogram) at least yearly.
- Caution patient that cigarette smoking, high BP, high cholesterol, diabetes, and being overweight during estrogen therapy may increase risk of heart disease.
- Ospemifene should not be taken during pregnancy. Instruct patient to notify health care professional immediately if pregnancy is planned or suspected or if breast feeding.
- Advise patient to discuss dose and need for ospemifene every 3–6 mo.

Evaluation/Desired Outcomes

- Decrease in pain during intercourse.

oxacillin, See PENICILLINS, PENICILLINASE RESISTANT.

oxaliplatin (ox-a-li-pla-tin)

Eloxatin

Classification
Therapeutic: antineoplastics
Pharmacologic: alkylating agents

Pregnancy Category D

Indications

Adjuvant treatment of stage III colon cancer in patients who have undergone complete resection of the primary tumor (in combination with 5–fluorouracil and leucovorin). Treatment of advanced colorectal cancer (in combination with 5–fluorouracil and leucovorin). **Unlabeled Use:** Treatment of ovarian cancer that has progressed despite treatment with other agents.

Action

Inhibits DNA replication and transcription by incorporating platinum into normal cross-linking (cell-cycle nonspecific). **Therapeutic Effects:** Death of rapidly replicating cells, particularly malignant ones.

Pharmacokinetics

Absorption: IV administration results in complete bioavailability.
Distribution: Extensive tissue distribution.
Protein Binding: >90% (platinum).
Metabolism and Excretion: Undergoes rapid and extensive nonenzymatic biotransformation; excreted mostly by the kidneys.
Half-life: 391 hours.

TIME/ACTION PROFILE

ROUTE	ONSET	PEAK	DURATION
IV	unknown	unknown	unknown

Contraindications/Precautions

Contraindicated in: Hypersensitivity; Hypersensitivity to other platinum compounds; OB, Lactation: Pregnancy or lactation.
Use Cautiously in: Renal impairment; Geri: ↑ risk of adverse reactions; Pedi: Safety not established.

Adverse Reactions/Side Effects

Adverse reactions are noted for the combination of oxaliplatin, 5–FU and leucovorin.

CNS: REVERSIBLE POSTERIOR LEUKOENCEPHALOPATHY SYNDROME, fatigue. **CV:** chest pain, edema, thromboembolism. **EENT:** visual abnormalities. **Resp:** PULMONARY FIBROSIS, coughing, dyspnea. **GI:** diarrhea, nausea, vomiting, abdominal pain, anorexia, gastroesophageal reflux, stomatitis. **F and E:** dehydration, hypokalemia. **Hemat:** leukopenia, NEUTROPENIA, THROMBOCYTOPENIA, anemia. **Local:** injection site reactions. **MS:** back pain. **Neuro:** neurotoxicity. **Misc:** ANAPHYLAXIS/ANAPHYLACTOID REACTIONS, fever.

Interactions

Drug-Drug: Concurrent use of **nephrotoxic agents** may ↑ toxicity.

Route/Dosage

IV (Adults): *Day 1*—85 mg/m² with leucovorin 200 mg/m² at the same time over 2 hr, followed by 5–fluorouracil 400 mg/m² bolus over 2–4 min, then 5–fluorouracil 600 mg/m² as a 22 hr infusion. *Day 2*—leucovorin 200 mg/m² over 2 hr, followed by 5–fluorouracil 400 mg/m² bolus over 2–4 min, then 5–fluorouracil 600 mg/m² as a 22 hr infusion. Cycle is repeated every 2 wk. Dosage reduction/alteration may be required for neurotoxicity or other serious adverse effects.

Renal Impairment

IV (Adults): *CCr <30 mL/min*—↓ dose on Day 1 to 65 mg/m².

Availability (generic available)

Solution for injection: 5 mg/mL.

NURSING IMPLICATIONS

Assessment

- Assess for peripheral sensory neuropathy. *Acute onset* occurs within hr to 1–2 days of dosing, resolves within 14 days, and frequently recurs with further dosing (transient paresthesia, dysesthesia and hypothesia of hands, feet, perioral area, or throat). Symptoms may be precipitated or exacerbated by exposure to cold or cold objects; avoid ice during symptoms. May also cause jaw spasm, abnormal tongue sensation, dysarthria, eye pain, and a feeling of chest pressure. *Persistent* (>14 days) causes paresthesias, dysethesias, and hypoesthesias, but may also include deficits in proprioception that may interfere with daily activities (walking, writing, swallowing). Persistent neuropathy may occur without prior acute neuropathy and may improve upon discontinuation of oxaliplatin.
- Assess for signs of pulmonary fibrosis (non-productive cough, dyspnea, crackles, radiological; infiltrates). May be fatal. Discontinue oxaliplatin if pulmonary fibrosis occurs.
- Monitor for signs of anaphylaxis (rash, hives, swelling or lips or tongue, sudden cough). Epinephrine,

O

corticosteroids, and antihistamines should be readily available.

- Monitor for signs and symptoms of reversible posterior leukoencephalopathy syndrome (headache, altered mental functioning, seizures, abnormal vision from blurriness to blindness, associated or not with hypertension).
- ***Lab Test Considerations:*** Monitor WBC with differential, hemoglobin, platelet count, and blood chemistries (ALT, AST, bilirubin, and creatinine) before each oxaliplatin cycle.

Potential Nursing Diagnoses

Nausea (Adverse Reactions)

Implementation

- Extravasation may result in local pain and inflammation that may be severe and lead to necrosis.
- Premedicate patient with antiemetics with or without dexamethasone. Prehydration is not required.

IV Administration

- **Intermittent Infusion:** Protect concentrated solution from light; do not freeze. ***Diluent:*** Must be further diluted with 250–500 mL of D5W. **Do not use 0.9% NaCl or any other chloride-containing solution for final solution.** Do not use aluminum needles or administration sets containing aluminum parts; aluminum may cause degradation of platinum compounds. May be stored in refrigerator for 24 hr or 6 hr at room temperature. Diluted solution is not light-sensitive. Do not administer solutions that are discolored or contain particulate matter. ***Concentration:*** 0.2–0.6 mg/mL. ***Rate:*** Administer oxaliplatin simultaneously with leucovorin in separate bags via Y-line over 120 min. Prolonging infusion time to 6 hr may decrease acute toxicities. Infusion times for fluorouracil and leucovorin do not need to change.
- **Y-Site Compatibility:** alemtuzumab, alfentanil, amifostine, amikacin, aminocaproic acid, amiodarone, amphotericin B colloid, amphotericin B lipid complex, amphotericin B liposome, ampicillin, ampicillin/sulbactam, anidulafungin, argatroban, atracurium, azithromycin, aztreonam, bivalirudin, bleomycin, bumetanide, buprenorphine, butorphanol, calcium chloride, calcium gluconate, carboplatin, caspofungin, cefotetan, cefoxitin, ceftazidime, ceftriaxone, cefuroxime, chloramphenicol, ciprofloxacin, cisatracurium, cisplatin, clindamycin, cyclophosphamide, cyclosporine, cytarabine, dacarbazine, dactinomycin, daptomycin, daunorubicin, dexamethasone sodium phosphate, dexmedetomidine, dexrazoxane, digoxin, diltiazem, diphenhydramine, dobutamine, docetaxel, dolasetron, dopamine, doxacurium, doxorubicin, doxorubicin liposomal, doxycycline, droperidol, enalaprilat, ephedrine, epinephrine, epirubicin, ertapenem, erythromycin, esmolol, etoposide, etoposide phosphate, famotidine, fenoldopam, fentanyl, fluconazole, fludarabine, foscarnet, fosphenytoin, furosemide, gemcitabine, gentamicin, glycopyrrolate, granisetron, haloperidol, heparin, hetastarch, hydralazine, hydrocortisone, hydromorphone, idarubicin, ifosfamide, imipenem/cilastatin, insulin, irinotecan, isoproterenol, ketorolac, labetalol, leucovorin calcium, levofloxacin, leucovorin calcium, levorphanol, lidocaine, linezolid, lorazepam, magnesium sulfate, mannitol, meperidine, meropenem, mesna, metaraminol, methyldopate, methylprednisolone sodium succinate, metoclopramide, metoprolol, metronidazole, midazolam, milrinone, mitoxantrone, morphine, moxifloxacin, nafcillin, nalbuphine, naloxone, nesiritide, nicardipine, nitroglycerin, nitroprusside, norepinephrine, octreotide, ondansetron, paclitaxel, palonosetron, pancuronium, pemetrexed, pentamidine, pentazocine, phentolamine, phenylephrine, potassium acetate, potassium chloride, potassium phosphates, procainamide, prochlorperazine, promethazine, propranolol, quinupristin/dalfopristin, ranitidine, rocuronium, sodium acetate, sodium phosphates, succinylcholine, sufentanil, tacrolimus, teniposide, theophylline, thiotepa, tigecycline, tirofiban, tobramycin, tolazoline, topotecan, trimethoprim/sulfamethoxazole, vancomycin, vasopressin, vecuronium, verapamil, vinblastine, vincristine, vinorelbine, voriconazole, zidovudine, zoledronic acid.
- **Y-Site Incompatibility:** cefepime, dantrolene, diazepam.Alkaline solutions, chloride-containing solutions. Infusion line should be flushed with D5W prior to administration of other solutions or medications.

Patient/Family Teaching

- Inform patients and caregivers of potential for peripheral neuropathy and potentiation by exposure to cold or cold objects. Advise patient to avoid cold drinks, use of ice in drinks or as ice packs, and to cover exposed skin prior to exposure to cold temperature or cold objects. Caution patients to cover themselves with a blanket during infusion, do not breathe deeply when exposed to cold air, wear warm clothing, and cover mouth and nose with a scarf or pull-down ski cap to warm the air that goes to their lungs, do not take things from the freezer or refrigerator without wearing gloves, drink fluids warm or at room temperature, always drink through a straw, do not use ice chips for nausea, be aware that most metals (car doors, mailbox) are cold; wear gloves to touch, do not run air conditioning at high levels in house or car, if hands get cold wash them with warm water. Advise health care professional of how you did since last treatment before next infusion.
- Instruct patient to notify health care professional immediately if signs of reversible posterior leukoencephalopathy syndrome, low blood cell counts (fever, persistent diarrhea, infection) or if persistent

vomiting, signs of dehydration, cough or breathing difficulty, thirst, dry mouth, dizziness, decreased urination, signs of infection (fever, temperature of ≥100.5° F, cough that brings up mucus, chills or shivering, burning or pain on urination, pain on swallowing, sore throat, redness or swelling at intravenous site) or signs of allergic reactions occur.
- Advise female patient to use effective contraception during therapy and to avoid breasfeeeding; oxaliplatin is teratogenic.

Evaluation/Desired Outcomes
- Decrease in size and spread of malignancies.

oxazepam (ox-az-e-pam)
♣Novoxapam, ♣Oxpam, Serax

Classification
Therapeutic: antianxiety agents, sedative/hypnotics
Pharmacologic: benzodiazepines

Schedule IV

Pregnancy Category D

Indications
Management of anxiety, anxiety associated with depression. Symptomatic treatment of alcohol withdrawal.

Action
Depresses the CNS, probably by potentiating GABA, an inhibitory neurotransmitter. **Therapeutic Effects:** Decreased anxiety. Diminished symptoms of alcohol withdrawal.

Pharmacokinetics
Absorption: Well absorbed following oral administration. Absorption is slower than with other benzodiazepines.
Distribution: Widely distributed. Crosses the blood-brain barrier. May cross the placenta and enter breast milk.
Metabolism and Excretion: Metabolized by the liver to inactive compounds.
Protein Binding: 97%.
Half-life: 5–15 hr.

TIME/ACTION PROFILE (sedation)

ROUTE	ONSET	PEAK	DURATION
PO	45–90 min	unknown	6–12 hr

Contraindications/Precautions
Contraindicated in: Hypersensitivity; Cross-sensitivity with other benzodiazepines may exist; Comatose patients or those with pre-existing CNS depression; Uncontrolled severe pain; Angle-closure glaucoma; Some products contain tartrazine and should be avoided in patients with known intolerance; OB, Lactation: Pregnancy or lactation.
Use Cautiously in: Hepatic dysfunction (may be preferred over some benzodiazepines due to short half-life); History of suicide attempt or substance use disorder; Debilitated patients (initial dosage ↓ recommended); Severe chronic obstructive pulmonary disease; Myasthenia gravis; Pedi: Children <6 yr (safety not established); Geri: Appears on Beers list (associated with ↑ risk of falls; ↓ dose required); ↑sensitivity to benzodiazepines.

Adverse Reactions/Side Effects
CNS: <u>dizziness</u>, <u>drowsiness</u>, confusion, hangover, headache, impaired memory, mental depression, paradoxical excitation, slurred speech. **EENT:** blurred vision. **Resp:** respiratory depression. **CV:** tachycardia. **GI:** constipation, diarrhea, drug-induced hepatitis, nausea, vomiting, weight gain (unusual). **GU:** urinary problems. **Derm:** rashes. **Hemat:** leukopenia. **Misc:** physical dependence, psychological dependence, tolerance.

O

Interactions
Drug-Drug: Additive CNS depression with other **CNS depressants**, including **alcohol**, **antihistamines**, **antidepressants**, **opioid analgesics**, and other **sedative/hypnotics** (including other **benzodiazepines**). May ↓ the therapeutic effectiveness of **levodopa**. **Hormonal contraceptives** or **phenytoin** may ↓ effectiveness. **Theophylline** may ↓ sedative effects.
Drug-Natural Products: Concomitant use of **kava-kava**, **valerian**, **skullcap**, **chamomile**, or **hops** can ↑ CNS depression.

Route/Dosage
PO (Adults): *Antianxiety agent*— 10–30 mg 3–4 times daily. *Sedative/hypnotic/management of alcohol withdrawal*— 15–30 mg 3–4 times daily.
PO (Geriatric Patients): 5 mg 1–2 times daily initially or 10 mg 3 times daily; may be ↑ as needed.

Availability (generic available)
Capsules: 10 mg, 15 mg, 30 mg. **Tablets:** ♣10 mg, 15 mg, ♣30 mg.

NURSING IMPLICATIONS
Assessment
- Assess patient for anxiety and orientation, mood and behavior.
- Assess level of sedation (ataxia, dizziness, slurred speech) periodically throughout therapy.
- Assess regularly for continued need for treatment.
- Prolonged high-dose therapy may lead to psychological or physical dependence. Restrict the amount of drug available to patient.

- Geri: Assess CNS effects and risk of falls. Institute falls prevention strategies.
- ***Lab Test Considerations:*** Monitor CBC and liver function tests periodically during prolonged therapy.
- May cause decreased thyroidal uptake of ^{123}I and ^{131}I.

Potential Nursing Diagnoses

Anxiety (Indications)
Ineffective coping (Indications)
Risk for injury (Side Effects)

Implementation

- Medication should be tapered at the completion of therapy (taper by 0.5 mg q 3 days). Sudden cessation of medication may lead to withdrawal (insomnia, irritability, nervousness, tremors).
- **PO:** Administer with food if GI irritation becomes a problem.

Patient/Family Teaching

- Instruct patient to take oxazepam exactly as directed. Missed doses should be taken within 1 hr; if remembered later, omit and return to regular dosing schedule. Do not double or increase doses. If dose is less effective after a few weeks, notify health care professional.
- Inform patient that oxazepam is usually prescribed for short-term use. Encourage patient to participate in psychotherapy to address source of anxiety and improve coping skills.
- Encourage patient to participate in psychotherapy to address source of anxiety and improve coping skills.
- Teach other methods to decrease anxiety, such as increased exercise, support group, relaxation techniques.
- May cause drowsiness or dizziness. Caution patient to avoid driving or other activities requiring alertness until response to medication is known.
- Advise patient to avoid the use of alcohol and to consult health care professional prior to the use of OTC preparations that contain antihistamines or alcohol.
- Advise patient to notify health care professional of medication regimen prior to treatment or surgery.
- Advise patient to inform health care professional if pregnancy is planned or suspected.
- Emphasize the importance of follow-up exams to monitor effectiveness of medication.
- Geri: Instruct patient and family how to reduce falls risk at home.

Evaluation/Desired Outcomes

- Decreased sense of anxiety.
- Increased ability to cope.
- Prevention or relief of acute agitation, tremor, and hallucinations during alcohol withdrawal.

OXcarbazepine

(ox-kar-**baz**-e-peen)
Oxtellar XR, Trileptal

Classification
Therapeutic: anticonvulsants
Pharmacologic: carbamazepine analogues

Pregnancy Category C

Indications

Monotherapy or adjunctive therapy of partial seizures in adults and children 4 yr and older with epilepsy (extended-release tablets only indicated for adjunctive therapy). Adjunctive therapy in patients 2–16 yr with epilepsy. **Unlabeled Use:** Management of trigeminal neuralgia.

Action

Blocks sodium channels in neural membranes, stabilizing hyperexcitable states, inhibiting repetitive neuronal firing, and decreasing propagation of synaptic impulses. **Therapeutic Effects:** Decreased incidence of seizures.

Pharmacokinetics

Absorption: Rapidly absorbed after oral administration and rapidly converted to the active 10-hydroxy metabolite (MHD).
Distribution: Enters breast milk in significant amounts.
Metabolism and Excretion: Extensively converted to MHD, which is then primarily excreted by the kidneys.
Half-life: *Oxcarbazepine*—2 hr; *MHD*—9 hr.

TIME/ACTION PROFILE (blood levels)

ROUTE	ONSET	PEAK	DURATION
PO 12 hr	PO	rapid	4.5 hr†

†Steady-state levels of MHD are reached after 2–3 days during twice-daily dosing.

Contraindications/Precautions

Contraindicated in: Hypersensitivity; cross-sensitivity with carbamazepine may occur; Lactation: Lactation.
Use Cautiously in: All patients (may ↑ risk of suicidal thoughts/behaviors); Renal impairment (dose ↓ recommended if CCr <30 mL/min); Severe hepatic impairment; OB: May be teratogenic; use only if potential benefit justifies potential risk to the fetus; Pedi: Children <4 yr (safety not established).
Exercise Extreme Caution in: Patients positive for HLA-B*1502 alleles (unless benefits clearly outweigh the risks) (↑ risk of serious skin reactions).

Adverse Reactions/Side Effects

CNS: SUICIDAL THOUGHTS, dizziness/vertigo, drowsiness/fatigue, headache, cognitive symptoms. **EENT:**

abnormal vision, diplopia, nystagmus. **GI:** abdominal pain, dyspepsia, nausea, vomiting, thirst. **Derm:** STEVENS-JOHNSON SYNDROME, TOXIC EPIDERMAL NECROLYSIS, acne, rash, urticaria. **Endo:** hypothyroidism. **F and E:** hyponatremia. **Neuro:** ataxia, gait disturbances, tremor. **Misc:** DRUG REACTION WITH EOSINOPHILIA AND SYSTEMIC SYMPTOMS (DRESS), allergic reactions, lymphadenopathy.

Interactions

Drug-Drug: May inhibit the CYP 2C19 enzyme system and would be expected to alter the effects of other drugs that are metabolized by this system. Oxcarbazepine and MHD induce the P450 3A4/5 enzyme systems and would be expected to alter the effects of other drugs that are metabolized by this system. This may result in ↓ levels and effectiveness of **hormonal contraceptives**, **felodipine**, **isradipine**, **nicardipine**, **nifedipine**, **nimodipine**, and **cyclosporine**. In addition, oxcarbazepine itself is metabolized by cytochrome P450 system and other **drugs that alter the activity of this system**. ↑ CNS depression may occur with other CNS depressants, including **alcohol**, **antihistamines**, **antidepressants**, **sedative/hypnotics**, and **opioids**. **Carbamazepine**, **phenobarbital**, **phenytoin**, **valproic acid**, and **verapamil** ↓ levels. May ↑ serum levels and effects of **phenytoin** (dose ↓ of phenytoin may be required).

Route/Dosage

(Immediate-release tablets and oral suspension can be interchanged at equal doses.)

PO (Adults): *Adjunctive therapy (immediate–release)*—300 mg twice daily, may be ↑ by up to 600 mg/day at weekly intervals up to 1200 mg/day (up to 2400 mg/day may be needed); *Adjunctive therapy (extended–release)*—600 mg once daily for 1 wk; may ↑ by 600 mg/day at weekly intervals up to 1200–2400 mg once daily; *Conversion to monotherapy*—300 mg twice daily; may be ↑ by 600 mg/day at weekly intervals, whereas other antiepileptic drugs are tapered over 3–6 wk; dose of oxcarbazepine should be ↑ up to 2400 mg/day over a period of 2–4 wk; *Initiation of monotherapy*—300 mg twice daily, ↑ by 300 mg/day every 3rd day, up to 1200 mg/day. Maximum maintenance dose should be achieved over 2–4 wk.

PO (Children 2–16 yr): *Adjunctive therapy (immediate release)*—4–5 mg/kg twice daily (up to 600 mg/day), ↑ over 2 wk to achieve 900 mg/day in patients 20–29 kg, 1200 mg/day in patients 29.1–39 kg and 1800 mg/day in patients >39 kg (range 6–51 mg/kg/day). In patients <20 kg, initial dose of 16–20 mg/kg/day may be used not to exceed 60 mg/kg/day. *Conversion to monotherapy (immediate release)*—8–10 mg/kg/day given twice daily; may be ↑ by 10 mg/kg/day at weekly intervals, whereas other antiepileptic drugs are tapered over 3–6 wk; dose of oxcarbazepine should be ↑ up to 600–900 mg/day in patients ≤20 kg, 900–1200 mg/day in patients 25–30 kg, 900–1500 mg/day in patients 35–40 kg. 1200–1500 mg/day in patients 45 kg, 1200–1800 mg/day in patients 50–55 kg, 1200–2100 mg/day in patients 60–65 kg, and 1500–2100 mg/day in patients 70 kg. Maximum maintenance dose should be achieved over 2–4 wk.

PO (Children 6–17 yr): *Adjunctive therapy (extended-release)*—8–10 mg/kg once daily (up to 600 mg/day) for 1 wk; may ↑ by 8–10 mg/kg/day at weekly intervals over 2–3 wk to achieve 900 mg/day in patients 20–29 kg, 1200 mg/day in patients 29.1–39 kg and 1800 mg/day in patients >39 kg.

Renal Impairment

PO (Adults): *CCr<30 mL/min (immediate and extended–release)*. Initiate therapy at 300 mg/day and ↑ slowly to achieve desired response.

Availability (generic available)

Immediate-release tablets: 150 mg, 300 mg, 600 mg. **Cost:** *Generic*—150 mg $145.36/100, 300 mg $264.46/100, 600 mg $487.92/100. **Extended-release tablets:** 150 mg, 300 mg, 600 mg. **Cost:** 150 mg $357.60/100, 300 mg $496.80/100, 600 mg $909.60/100. **Oral suspension (lemon-flavor):** 60 mg/mL. **Cost:** *Generic*—$206.80/250 ml.

O

NURSING IMPLICATIONS

Assessment

- Monitor closely for notable changes in behavior that could indicate the emergence or worsening of suicidal thoughts or behavior or depression.
- **Seizures:** Assess frequency, location, duration, and characteristics of seizure activity. Hyponatremia may increase frequency and severity of seizures.
- Monitor patient for CNS changes. May manifest as cognitive symptoms (psychomotor slowing, difficulty with concentration, speech or language problems), somnolence or fatigue, or coordination abnormalities (ataxia, gait disturbances).
- 🧬 Monitor for skin reactions (rash, erythema, urticaria, pruritus, fever, blistering). Patients with HLA-B*1502 alleles are at increased risk for Stevens Johnson syndrome and toxic epidermal necrolysis. Discontinue oxcarbazepine if symptoms occur.
- ***Lab Test Considerations:*** Monitor ECG and serum electrolytes before and periodically during therapy. May cause hyponatremia. Usually occurs during the first 3 mo of therapy. May require dose reduction, fluid restriction, or discontinuation of therapy. Sodium levels return to normal within a few days of discontinuation.

Potential Nursing Diagnoses

Risk for injury (Indications, Side Effects)

Implementation

- Do not confuse oxcarbazepine with carbamazepine.
- Implement seizure precautions as indicated.
- **PO:** Administer twice daily with or without food.
- Administer extended-release tablets on an empty stomach, at least 1 hr before or 2 hr after meals; giving with food increases risks of adverse effects. Swallow extended-release tablets whole, do not crush, break, or chew.
- Shake oral suspension well and prepare dose immediately after. Withdraw using oral dosing syringe supplied by manufacturer. May be mixed in a small glass of water just prior to administration or swallowed directly from syringe. Rinse syringe with warm water and allow to dry.

Patient/Family Teaching

- Instruct patient to take oxcarbazepine in equally spaced doses, as directed. Take missed doses as soon as possible but not just before next dose; do not double dose. Notify health care professional if more than 1 dose is missed. Medication should be gradually discontinued to prevent seizures. Instruct patient to read the *Medication Guide* before starting and with each Rx refill, changes may occur.
- May cause dizziness, drowsiness, or CNS changes. Advise patients to avoid driving or other activities requiring alertness until response to medication is known. Do not resume driving until physician gives clearance based on control of seizure disorder.
- Instruct patient to notify health care professional of all Rx or OTC medications, vitamins, or herbal products being taken and to consult with health care professional before taking other medications. Advise patient not to take alcohol or other CNS depressants concurrently with this medication.
- Advise patient and family to notify health care professional if thoughts about suicide or dying, attempts to commit suicide; new or worse depression; new or worse anxiety; feeling very agitated or restless; panic attacks; trouble sleeping; new or worse irritability; acting aggressive; being angry or violent; acting on dangerous impulses; an extreme increase in activity and talking, other unusual changes in behavior or mood occur.
- Instruct patient to notify health care professional of medication regimen before treatment or surgery. Rep: Advise female patients to use an additional nonhormonal method of contraception during therapy and until next menstrual period. Instruct patient to notify health care professional if pregnancy is planned or suspected. Encourage patients who become pregnant to enroll in the North American Antiepileptic Drug (NAAED) Pregnancy Registry by calling 1-888-233-2334 or on the web at www.aedpregnancyregistry.org. Enrollment must be done by patients themselves.
- Advise patients to carry identification describing disease and medication regimen at all times.

Evaluation/Desired Outcomes

- Absence or reduction of seizure activity.

oxiconazole, See ANTIFUNGALS (TOPICAL).

OXYBUTYNIN (ox-i-byoo-ti-nin)

oxybutynin (oral)
~~Ditropan~~, Ditropan XL

oxybutynin (gel)
Gelnique

oxybutynin (transdermal system)
Oxytrol, Oxytrol for Women

Classification
Therapeutic: urinary tract antispasmodics
Pharmacologic: anticholinergics

Pregnancy Category B

Indications

Urinary symptoms that may be associated with neurogenic bladder including: Frequent urination, Urgency, Nocturia, Urge incontinence. Overactive bladder with symptoms of urge incontinence, urgency, and frequency.

Action

Inhibits the action of acetylcholine at postganglionic receptors. Has direct spasmolytic action on smooth muscle, including smooth muscle lining the GU tract, without affecting vascular smooth muscle. **Therapeutic Effects:** Increased bladder capacity. Delayed desire to void. Decreased urge incontinence, urinary urgency, and frequency and decreased number of urinary accidents associated with overactive bladder.

Pharmacokinetics

Absorption: Rapidly absorbed following oral administration, but undergoes extensive first-pass metabolism; XL tablets provide extended release. Transdermal absorption occurs by passive diffusion through intact skin and bypasses the first-pass effect.

Distribution: Highly bound (>99%) to plasma proteins. Widely distributed.

Metabolism and Excretion: Extensively metabolized by the liver (CYP3A4 enzyme system); 1 metabolite is pharmacologically active; metabolites are renally excreted with negligible (<0.1%) excretion of unchanged drug.

Half-life: 7–8 hr (oral and patch); 30–64 hr (gel).

TIME/ACTION PROFILE (urinary spasmolytic effect)

ROUTE	ONSET	PEAK	DURATION
PO	30–60 min	3–6 hr	6–10 hr (up to 24 hr with XL tablet)
TD-patch	within 24 hr	36 hr	3–4 days
TD-gel	unknown	unknown	24 hr

Contraindications/Precautions

Contraindicated in: Hypersensitivity; Uncontrolled angle-closure glaucoma; Intestinal obstruction or atony; Urinary retention.

Use Cautiously in: Hepatic/renal impairment; Bladder outflow obstruction; Ulcerative colitis; Benign prostatic hyperplasia; Cardiovascular disease; Reflux esophagitis or gastrointestinal obstructive disorders; Patients with dementia receiving acetylcholinesterase inhibitors; Myasthenia gravis; Parkinson's disease (may worsen symptoms); Autonomic neuropathy (may worsen ↓ GI motility); OB, Lactation: Pregnancy or lactation; Pedi: Oral: Safety not established in children <5 yr; Patch and gel: Safety not established in children <18 yr; Geri: Appears on Beers list. Poorly tolerated due to anticholinergic effects. Initiate treatment at lower doses.

Adverse Reactions/Side Effects

CNS: dizziness, drowsiness, agitation, confusion, hallucinations, headache. **EENT:** blurred vision, hoarseness. **CV:** chest pain, edema, tachycardia. **GI:** constipation, dry mouth, nausea, abdominal pain, anorexia, diarrhea, dysphagia. **GU:** ↑ thirst, urinary retention. **Derm:** ↓ sweating, hot flushes, *transdermal only:* application site reactions, pruritus. **Metab:** hyperthermia. **Misc:** ANAPHYLAXIS, ANGIOEDEMA.

Interactions

Drug-Drug: ↑ anticholinergic effects with other **agents having anticholinergic properties**, including **amantadine**, **antidepressants**, **phenothiazines**, **disopyramide**, and **haloperidol**. Additive CNS depression with other **CNS depressants**, including **alcohol**, **antihistamines**, **antidepressants**, **opioids**, and **sedative/hypnotics**. **Ketoconazole**, **itraconazole**, **erythromycin**, and **clarithromycin** may ↑ effects. May ↓ the GI promotility effects of **metoclopramide**.

Route/Dosage

PO (Adults): *Immediate-release tablets*—5 mg 2–3 times daily (not to exceed 5 mg 4 times daily) (may start with 2.5 mg 2–3 times daily in elderly). *Extended-release tablets*—5–10 mg once daily; may ↑, as needed (in 5-mg increments) up to maximum dose of 30 mg/day.

PO (Children >5 yr): *Immediate-release tablets*—5 mg 2–3 times daily (not to exceed 15 mg/day). *Extended-release tablets (children ≥6 yr)*—5 mg once daily; may ↑, as needed, (in 5-mg increments) up to maximum dose of 20 mg/day.

PO (Children 1–5 yr): 0.2 mg/kg/dose 2–3 times daily.

Transdermal (Adults): *Patch*—Apply one 3.9 mg system twice weekly (every 3–4 days); *Gel*—Apply contents of one sachet once daily.

Availability (generic available)

Immediate-release tablets: 5 mg. **Cost:** *Generic*—$52.94/100. **Extended-release tablets:** 5 mg, 10 mg, 15 mg. **Cost:** *Generic*—5 mg $105.23/100, 10 mg $106.08/100, 15 mg $117.04/100. **Syrup:** 5 mg/5 mL. **Cost:** *Generic*—$38.95/473 mL. **Topical gel:** 10%. **Cost:** 3% $224.11/92 g, 10% $30.12/3 g. **Transdermal patch:** 3.9 mg/24 hr[OTC].

NURSING IMPLICATIONS

Assessment

- Monitor voiding pattern and intake and output ratios, and assess abdomen for bladder distention prior to and periodically during therapy. Catheterization may be used to assess postvoid residual. Cystometry is usually performed to diagnose type of bladder dysfunction prior to prescription of oxybutynin.
- Geri: Assess geriatric patients for anticholinergic effects (sedation and weakness).

Potential Nursing Diagnoses

Impaired urinary elimination (Indications)
Acute pain (Indications)

Implementation

- Do not confuse Ditropan XL (oxybutynin) with Diprivan (propofol).
- **PO:** Immediate release tabs should be administered on an empty stomach; XL tablets may be given with or without food. XL tablets should be swallowed whole; do not break, crush, or chew.
- **Transdermal patch:** Apply patch on same two days each week (Sunday/Wednesday, Monday/Thursday) to hip, abdomen, or buttock in an area that is clean, dry, and without irritation. Patch should be worn continuously.
- **Transdermal gel:** Apply clear, colorless gel once daily to intact skin on abdomen (avoid area around navel), upper arms/shoulders, or thighs until dry. Rotate sites; do not use same site on consecutive days.

Patient/Family Teaching

- Instruct patient to take oxybutinin as directed. Take missed doses as soon as remembered unless almost

O

time for next dose. Advise patient to read *Information for the Patient* prior to beginning therapy and with each Rx refill in case of new information.

- May cause drowsiness or blurred vision. Advise patient to avoid driving and other activities requiring alertness until response to medication is known.
- Advise patient to avoid concurrent use of alcohol and other CNS depressants while taking this medication.
- Instruct patient that frequent rinsing of mouth, good oral hygiene, and sugarless gum or candy may decrease dry mouth. Health care professional should be notified if mouth dryness persists >2 wk.
- Advise patient to stop taking oxybutinin and notify health care professional immediately if signs of angioedema and/or anaphylaxis (swelling of face, tongue, or throat; rash; dyspnea).
- Inform patient that oxybutynin decreases the body's ability to perspire. Avoid strenuous activity in a warm environment because overheating may occur.
- Advise patient to notify health care professional if urinary retention occurs or if constipation persists. Discuss methods of preventing constipation, such as increasing dietary bulk, increasing fluid intake, and increasing mobility.
- Advise patient to notify health care professional of all Rx or OTC medications, vitamins, or herbal products being taken and to consult with health care professional before taking other medications.
- Advise patient to notify health care professional if pregnancy is planned or suspected or if breast feeding.
- Discuss need for continued medical follow-up. Periodic cystometry may be used to evaluate effectiveness. Ophthalmic exams should be performed periodically to detect glaucoma, especially in patients over 40 yr of age.
- **Transdermal patch:** Instruct patient on correct application and disposal of patch. Open pouch by tearing along arrows; apply immediately. Apply 1/2 patch to skin by removing 1/2 protective cover and applying firmly to skin. Apply second half by bending in half and rolling patch onto skin while removing protective liner. Press patch firmly in place.
- Remove slowly; fold in half, sticky sides together, and discard. Wash site with mild soap and water or a small amount of baby oil.
- Advise patient referred for MRI to remove patch prior to test and give directions for replacing patch.
- **Transdermal gel:** Instruct patient on correct application of oxybutynin gel. Do not apply to recently shaved skin, skin with rashes, or areas treated with lotions, oils, or powders; may be used with sunscreen. Wash area with mild soap and water and dry completely before applying. Tear packet open just before use and squeeze entire contents into hand or directly onto application site of abdomen, arms/shoulders, or thighs. Amount of gel will be size of a nickel on the skin. Gently rub into skin until dry. Wash hands immediately following application. Avoid application near open fire or when smoking; medication is flammable. Do not shower, bathe, swim, exercise, or immerse the application site in water within 1 hr after application. Cover application site with clothing if close skin-to-skin contact at application site is anticipated.

Evaluation/Desired Outcomes

- Relief of bladder spasm and associated symptoms (frequency, urgency, nocturia, and incontinence) in patients with a neurogenic or overactive bladder.

REMS HIGH ALERT

oxyCODONE (ox-i-**koe**-done)

Oxaydo, OxyCONTIN, ✱Oxy IR, ✱OxyNEO, Roxicodone, ✱Supeudol

Classification

Therapeutic: opioid analgesics

Pharmacologic: opioid agonists, opioid agonists/nonopioid analgesic combinations

Schedule II

Pregnancy Category B

Indications

Moderate to severe pain. Moderate to severe chronic pain in opioid-tolerant patients requiring use of daily, around-the-clock long-term opioid treatment and for which alternative treatment options are inadequate (extended-release) (children ≥11 yr should be tolerating a minimum opioid dose of ≥20 mg of oxycodone or equivalent for ≥5 days before initiating extended-release oxycodone therapy.

Action

Binds to opiate receptors in the CNS. Alters the perception of and response to painful stimuli, while producing generalized CNS depression. **Therapeutic Effects:** Decreased pain.

Pharmacokinetics

Absorption: Well absorbed from the GI tract.
Distribution: Widely distributed. Crosses the placenta; enters breast milk.
Protein Binding: 38–45%.
Metabolism and Excretion: Mostly metabolized by the liver by the CYP3A4 isoenzyme.
Half-life: 2–3 hr.

TIME/ACTION PROFILE (analgesic effects)

ROUTE	ONSET	PEAK	DURATION
PO	10–15 min	60–90 min	3–6 hr
PO-ER†	10–15 min	3 hr	12 hr

†Extended-release.

Contraindications/Precautions

Contraindicated in: Hypersensitivity; Some products contain alcohol or bisulfites and should be avoided in patients with known intolerance or hypersensitivity; Significant respiratory depression; Paralytic ileus; Acute or severe bronchial asthma; Acute, mild, intermittent, or postoperative pain (extended-release).

Use Cautiously in: Head trauma; ↑ intracranial pressure; Severe renal or hepatic disease; Hypothyroidism; Adrenal insufficiency; Alcoholism; Seizure disorders; Undiagnosed abdominal pain; Prostatic hyperplasia; Difficulty swallowing or GI disorders that may predispose patient to obstruction (↑ risk for GI obstruction); OB, Lactation: Avoid chronic use; prolonged use of extended-release morphine during pregnancy can result in neonatal opioid withdrawal syndrome; Children <11 yr (safety and effectiveness of extended-release products not established); Geri: Elderly or debilitated patients (↑ risk of respiratory depression; initial dose ↓ recommended).

Adverse Reactions/Side Effects

CNS: confusion, sedation, dizziness, dysphoria, euphoria, floating feeling, hallucinations, headache, unusual dreams. **EENT:** blurred vision, diplopia, miosis. **Resp:** RESPIRATORY DEPRESSION. **CV:** orthostatic hypotension. **GI:** constipation, dry mouth, choking, GI obstruction, nausea, vomiting. **GU:** urinary retention. **Derm:** flushing, sweating. **Misc:** physical dependence, psychological dependence, tolerance.

Interactions

Drug-Drug: Use with caution in patients receiving **MAO inhibitors** (may result in unpredictable reactions—↓ initial dose of oxycodone to 25% of usual dose). Additive CNS depression with **alcohol**, **antihistamines**, and **sedative/hypnotics**. Administration of **partial-antagonist opioid analgesics** may precipitate withdrawal in physically dependent patients. **Nalbuphine**, **buprenorphine**, or **pentazocine** may ↓ analgesia. Potent **CYP3A4 inhibitors** including **erythromycin**, **ketoconazole**, **itraconazole**, **voriconazole**, or **ritonavir** may ↑ levels. Potent **CYP3A4 inducers** including **rifampin**, **carbamazepine**, and **phenytoin** may ↓ levels.

Route/Dosage

Larger doses may be required during chronic therapy.

PO (Adults ≥50 kg): *Opioid-naive patients*—5–10 mg q 3–4 hr initially, as needed. Once optimal analgesia is obtained, patients with chronic pain may be converted to an equivalent 24-hr dose given as extended-release tablets every 12 hr.

PO (Adults <50 kg): *Opioid-naive patients*—0.2 mg/kg q 3–4 hr initially, as needed. Once optimal analgesia is obtained, patients with chronic pain may be converted to an equivalent 24-hr dose given as extended-release tablets every 12 hr.

PO (Children ≥11 yr): 0.05–0.15 mg/kg q 4–6 hr as needed, as immediate-release product. Once optimal analgesia is obtained, patients with chronic pain may be converted to an equivalent 24-hr dose given as extended-release tablets every 12 hr.

Rect (Adults): 10–40 mg 3–4 times daily initially, as needed.

Hepatic Impairment

PO (Adults): ↓ initial dose by 50–66%.

Availability (generic available)

Immediate-release tablets (Roxicodone): 5 mg, 10 mg, 15 mg, 20 mg, 30 mg. **Cost:** *Generic*—5 mg $47.99/100, 10 mg $62.50/100, 15 mg $75.90/100, 20 mg $110.30/100, 30 mg $145.47/100. **Immediate-release tablets (abuse-deterrent) (Oxaydo):** 5 mg, 7.5 mg. **Capsules:** 5 mg. **Cost:** *Generic*—$79.59/100. **Extended-release tablets (abuse-deterrent) (Oxycontin):** 10 mg, 15 mg, 20 mg, 30 mg, 40 mg, 60 mg, 80 mg. **Cost:** 10 mg $52.54/20, 15 mg $78.60/20, 20 mg $100.42/20, 30 mg $142.16/20, 40 mg $178.10/20, 60 mg $259.32/20, 80 mg $335.08/20. **Oral solution:** 1 mg/mL. **Cost:** *Generic*—$142.50/500 mL. **Concentrated oral solution:** 20 mg/mL. **Cost:** *Generic*—$218.75/30 mL. **Suppositories:** ✱10 mg, ✱20 mg. ***In combination with:*** aspirin (Endodan, Percodan), acetaminophen (Endocet, Magnacet, Oxycet, Percocet, Roxicet, Xartemis XR); see Appendix B.

O

NURSING IMPLICATIONS

Assessment

- Assess type, location, and intensity of pain prior to and 1 hr (peak) after administration. When titrating opioid doses, increases of 25–50% should be administered until there is either a 50% reduction in the patient's pain rating on a numerical or visual analog scale or the patient reports satisfactory pain relief. A repeat dose can be safely administered at the time of the peak if previous dose is ineffective and side effects are minimal.
- Patients taking extended-release tablets may also be given supplemental short-acting opioid doses for breakthrough pain.
- An equianalgesic chart (see Appendix I) should be used when changing routes or when changing from one opioid to another.
- Assess BP, pulse, and respirations before and periodically during administration. If respiratory rate is <10/min, assess level of sedation. Physical stimulation may be sufficient to prevent significant hypoventilation. Dose may need to be decreased by 25–

50%. Initial drowsiness will diminish with continued use.

- Prolonged use may lead to physical and psychological dependence and tolerance. This should not prevent patient from receiving adequate analgesia. Most patients who receive oxycodone for pain do not develop psychological dependence. Progressively higher doses may be required to relieve pain with long-term therapy.
- Assess bowel function routinely. Prevention of constipation should be instituted with increased intake of fluids and bulk, and laxatives to minimize constipating effects. Stimulant laxatives should be administered routinely if opioid use exceeds 2–3 days, unless contraindicated.
- Assess risk for opioid addiction, abuse, or misuse prior to administration. Abuse or misuse of extended-release preparations by crushing, chewing, snorting, or injecting dissolved product will result in uncontrolled delivery of oxycodone and can result in overdose and death.
- ***Lab Test Considerations:*** May ↑ plasma amylase and lipase levels.
- ***Toxicity and Overdose:*** If an opioid antagonist is required to reverse respiratory depression or coma, naloxone is the antidote. Dilute the 0.4-mg ampule of naloxone in 10 mL of 0.9% NaCl and administer 0.5 mL (0.02 mg) by IV push every 2 min. For children and patients weighing <40 kg, dilute 0.1 mg of naloxone in 10 mL of 0.9% NaCl for a concentration of 10 mcg/mL and administer 0.5 mcg/kg every 2 min. Titrate dose to avoid withdrawal, seizures, and severe pain.

Potential Nursing Diagnoses

Acute pain (Indications)
Chronic pain (Indications)
Risk for injury (Side Effects)

Implementation

- ***High Alert:*** Accidental overdose of opioid analgesics has resulted in fatalities. Before administering, clarify all ambiguous orders; have second practitioner independently check original order and dose calculations.
- Do not confuse short-acting oxycodone with long-acting Oxycontin. Do not confuse oxycodone with hydrocodone. Do not confuse Oxycontin with MS Contin.
- Explain therapeutic value of medication prior to administration to enhance the analgesic effect.
- Regularly administered doses may be more effective than prn administration. Analgesic is more effective if given before pain becomes severe.
- Coadministration with nonopioid analgesics may have additive analgesic effects and may permit lower doses.
- Oxycodone should be discontinued gradually after long-term use to prevent withdrawal symptoms.
- **PO:** May be administered with food or milk to minimize GI irritation.
- Administer solution with properly calibrated measuring device.
- **Extended-Release:** Take 1 tablet at a time. Swallow extended-release tablet whole; do not crush, break, or chew. Taking broken, chewed, crushed or dissolved extended-release tablets may lead to rapid release and absorption of a potentially fatal dose of oxycodone. Advise patients not to pre-soak, lick, or wet controlled-release tablets prior to placing in the mouth. Take each tablet with enough water to ensure complete swallowing immediately after placing in mouth. Dose should be based on 24-hr opioid requirement determined with short-acting opioids then converted to extended-release form.
- Do not use *Oxaydo* for administration via nasogastric, gastric or other feeding tubes as it may cause obstruction of feeding tubes.

Patient/Family Teaching

- Instruct patient on how and when to ask for and take pain medication.
- Advise patient that oxycodone is a drug with known abuse potential. Protect it from theft, and never give to anyone other than the individual for whom it was prescribed.
- Medication may cause drowsiness or dizziness. Advise patient to call for assistance when ambulating or smoking. Caution patient to avoid driving and other activities requiring alertness until response to medication is known.
- Advise patients taking *Oxycontin* tablets that empty matrix tablets may appear in stool.
- Advise patient to make position changes slowly to minimize orthostatic hypotension.
- Advise patient to avoid concurrent use of alcohol or other CNS depressants with this medication.
- Instruct patient to notify health care professional of all Rx or OTC medications, vitamins, or herbal products being taken and consult health care professional before taking any new medications.
- Encourage patient to turn, cough, and breathe deeply every 2 hr to prevent atelectasis.
- Advise patient to notify health care professional if pregnancy is planned or suspected, or if breast feeding.

Evaluation/Desired Outcomes

- Decrease in severity of pain without a significant alteration in level of consciousness or respiratory status.

REMS HIGH ALERT

oxymorphone (ox-i-**mor**-fone)
Opana, Opana ER

Classification
Therapeutic: opioid analgesics
Pharmacologic: opioid agonists

Schedule II

Pregnancy Category C

Indications

Management of moderate to severe pain. Moderate to severe chronic pain in opioid-tolerant patients requiring use of daily, around-the-clock long-term opioid treatment and for which alternative treatment options are inadequate (extended/sustained-release). Supplement in balanced anesthesia.

Action

Binds to opiate receptors in the CNS. Alters the perception of and response to painful stimuli, while producing generalized CNS depression. **Therapeutic Effects:** Decrease in pain.

Pharmacokinetics

Absorption: 10% absorbed following oral administration. Food and alcohol significantly ↑absorption (38%). Well absorbed following IM or subcut administration.
Distribution: Widely distributed; crosses placenta, enters breast milk.
Metabolism and Excretion: Mostly metabolized by the liver; at least 2 metabolites are pharmacologically active, <1% excreted unchanged in urine.
Half-life: 2.6–4 hr.

TIME/ACTION PROFILE (analgesic effects)

ROUTE	ONSET	PEAK	DURATION
PO	unknown	unknown	4–6 hr
PO ER	unknown	unknown	12 hr
IM	10–15 min	30–90 min	3–6 hr
IV	5–10 min	15–30 min	3–6 hr
Subcut	10–20 min	unknown	3–4 hr

Contraindications/Precautions

Contraindicated in: Hypersensitivity; Concurrent alcohol; Moderate/severe hepatic impairment; Significant respiratory depression (unless monitoring and resuscitative equipment are readily available); Acute or severe bronchial asthma (extended-release); Acute, mild, intermittent, or postoperative pain (extended-release); Paralytic ileus.
Use Cautiously in: Acute alcoholism or delirium tremens or other toxic psychoses; Mild hepatic impairment; Head injury/↑ intracranial pressure (may obscure neurologic signs and further ↑ pressure); Volume depletion or drugs that may cause hypotension including diuretics and phenothiazines (↑ risk of severe hypotension); Circulatory shock (may ↑ risk of severe hypotension); Adrenocortical insufficiency; Seizure disorders; Hypothyroidism; Prostatic hypertrophy or ureteral stricture; Severe pulmonary or renal impairment; Biliary tract disease or pancreatitis; OB, Lactation: Avoid chronic use; prolonged use of extended-release oxymorphine during pregnancy can result in neonatal opioid withdrawal syndrome; Geri: Geriatric or debilitated patients (↑ risk of respiratory depression; dose ↓ suggested).
Exercise Extreme Caution in: Conditions association with hypoxia, hypercapnea, ↓ respiratory reserve (including asthma, COPD, cor pulmonale, morbid obesity, sleep apnea, myxedema, kyphoscoliosis, CNS depression and coma).

Adverse Reactions/Side Effects

CNS: confusion, sedation, dizziness, dysphoria, euphoria, floating feeling, hallucinations, headache, unusual dreams. **EENT:** blurred vision, diplopia, miosis. **Resp:** RESPIRATORY DEPRESSION. **CV:** orthostatic hypotension. **GI:** constipation, dry mouth, nausea, vomiting. **GU:** urinary retention. **Derm:** flushing, sweating. **Misc:** physical dependence, psychological dependence, tolerance.

O

Interactions

Drug-Drug: Use with caution in patients receiving **MAO inhibitors** (may result in unpredictable reactions—↓ initial dose of oxymorphone to 25% of usual dose). ↑ risk of CNS depression, hypotension and respiratory depression with **alcohol**, other **opioids** or **CNS depressants** including **sedatives**, **hypnotics**, **general anesthetics**, **phenothiazines**, **tranquilizers**, **skeletal muscle relaxants**, or **sedating antihistamines**; may initiate therapy with 1/3 to 1/2 usual starting dose. **Alcohol** may ↑ levels and ↑ the risk of toxicity. **Drugs that may cause volume depletion or hypotension** including **diuretics**, **phenothiazines** may ↑ risk of severe hypotension. Administration of **partial-antagonist opioid analgesics** may precipitate withdrawal in physically dependent patients. **Nalbuphine**, **buprenorphine**, or **pentazocine** ↓ analgesia.
Drug-Natural Products: Concomitant use of **kava-kava**, **valerian**, or **chamomile** can ↑ CNS depression.

Route/Dosage

Larger doses may be required during chronic therapy.
PO (Adults): *Opioid-naive patients*—10–20 mg every 4–6 hr, some patients may require initial dose of

5 mg, not to exceed 20 mg. Once optimal analgesia is obtained, chronic pain patients may be converted to an equivalent 24-hr dose given as extended release tablets every 12 hr.
Subcut, IM (Adults): 1–1.5 mg q 3–6 hr as needed. *Analgesia during labor*—0.5–1 mg.
IV (Adults): 0.5 mg q 3–6 hr as needed; ↑ as needed.

Hepatic Impairment

PO (Adults): *Mild hepatic impairment (extended-release)*—Initiate treatment with 5 mg q12h in opioid naïve patients; if on prior opioid therapy, ↓ dose by 50%.

Renal Impairment

PO (Adults): *CCr <50 mL/min (extended-release)*—Initiate treatment with 5 mg q12h in opioid naïve patients; if on prior opioid therapy, ↓ dose by 50%.

Availability (generic available)

Immediate-release tablets (Opana): 5 mg, 10 mg. **Extended-release tablets (abuse-deterrent) (Opana ER):** 5 mg, 7.5 mg, 10 mg, 15 mg, 20 mg, 30 mg, 40 mg. **Solution for injection:** 1 mg/mL.

NURSING IMPLICATIONS

Assessment

- Assess type, location, and intensity of pain prior to and 1 hr following IM and 15–30 min (peak) following IV administration. When titrating opioid doses, increases of 25–50% should be administered until there is either a 50% reduction in the patient's pain rating on a numerical or visual analogue scale or the patient reports satisfactory pain relief. A repeat dose can be safely administered at the time of the peak if previous dose is ineffective and side effects are minimal.
- Patients taking controlled-release tablets should also be given supplemental short-acting opioid doses for breakthrough pain.
- An equianalgesic chart (see Appendix I) should be used when changing routes or when changing from one opioid to another.
- Assess BP, pulse, and respirations before and periodically during administration. If respiratory rate is <10/min, assess level of sedation. Physical stimulation may be sufficient to prevent significant hypoventilation. Dose may need to be decreased by 25–50%. Initial drowsiness will diminish with continued use.
- Prolonged use may lead to physical and psychological dependence and tolerance. This should not prevent patient from receiving adequate analgesia. Most patients who receive oxymorphone for pain do not develop psychological dependence. Progressively higher doses may be required to relieve pain with long-term therapy.
- Assess bowel function routinely. Prevention of constipation should be instituted with increased intake of fluids and bulk, and laxatives. Stimulant laxatives should be administered routinely if opioid use exceeds 2–3 days, unless contraindicated.
- Assess risk for opioid addiction, abuse, or misuse prior to administration. Abuse or misuse of extended-release preparations by crushing, chewing, snorting, or injecting dissolved product will result in uncontrolled delivery of oxymorphone and can result in overdose and death.
- ***Lab Test Considerations:*** May ↑ plasma amylase and lipase levels.
- ***Toxicity and Overdose:*** If an opioid antagonist is required to reverse respiratory depression or coma, naloxone is the antidote. Dilute the 0.4-mg ampule of naloxone in 10 mL of 0.9% NaCl and administer 0.5 mL (0.02 mg) by IV push every 2 min. For children and patients weighing <40 kg, dilute 0.1 mg of naloxone in 10 mL of 0.9% NaCl for a concentration of 10 mcg/mL and administer 0.5 mcg/kg every 2 min. Titrate dose to avoid withdrawal, seizures, and severe pain.

Potential Nursing Diagnoses

Acute pain (Indications)
Chronic pain (Indications)
Risk for injury (Side Effects)

Implementation

- ***High Alert:*** Accidental overdose of opioid analgesics has resulted in fatalities. Before administering, clarify all ambiguous orders.
- Explain therapeutic value of medication prior to administration to enhance the analgesic effect.
- Regularly administered doses may be more effective than prn administration. Analgesic is more effective if given before pain becomes severe.
- Coadministration with nonopioid analgesics may have additive analgesic effects and may permit lower doses.
- Medication should be discontinued gradually after long-term use to prevent withdrawal symptoms.
- **PO:** Administer at least 1 hr prior to or 2 hr after eating.
- **Extended Release:** Swallow controlled-release tablets whole; do not break, crush, or chew. Titrate to mild to no pain with regular use of no more than 2 doses of supplemental analgesia (rescue) per 24 hr. Dose should be based on 24-hr opioid requirement determined with short-acting opioids then converted to controlled-release form. Taking broken, chewed, crushed or dissolved extended-release tablets may lead to rapid release and absorption of a potentially fatal dose of oxymorphone.
- If patient is opioid-naive, start with 5 mg every 12 hr, then titrate in increments of 5–10 mg every 12 hr every 3–7 days to a level that provides adequate analgesia with minimal side effects.
- If converting from *Opana* to *Opana ER*, administer half the patient's total daily dose of *Opana* as *Opana ER* every 12 hr.

- Do not use *Opana ER* for administration via nasogastric, gastric or other feeding tubes as it may cause obstruction of feeding tubes.
- If converting from parenteral oxymorphone, administer 10 times the patient's total daily parenteral oxymorphone dose as *Opana ER* in two equally divided doses every 12 hr.
- If converting from other opioids, 10 mg of oral oxymorphone is equianalgesic to hydrocodone 20 mg, oxycodone 20 mg, methadone 20 mg, and morphine 30 mg orally.

IV Administration

- **IV Push:** Administer undiluted. ***Concentration:*** 1 mg/mL. ***Rate:*** Give over 2–3 min.

Patient/Family Teaching

- Instruct patient on how and when to ask for pain medication.
- Instruct patient to take oxymorphone as directed and not to adjust dose without consulting health care professional. Take missed doses as soon as possible if on chronic therapy. If almost time for next dose, skip dose and return to regular schedule. Do not double doses unless advised by health care professional. Do not stop taking oxymorphone abruptly, may cause withdrawal symptoms. Discontinue gradually under supervision of health care professional. Caution patient to keep medication out of reach of children and pets.
- Advise patient that oxymorphone is a drug with known abuse potential. Protect it from theft, and never give to anyone other than the individual for whom it was prescribed.
- Caution patient not to share this medication; may cause harm or death and is against the law.
- Medication may cause drowsiness or dizziness. Advise patient to call for assistance when ambulating or smoking. Caution patient to avoid driving and other activities requiring alertness until response to medication is known.
- Advise patient to make position changes slowly to minimize orthostatic hypotension.
- Advise patient to avoid concurrent use of alcohol or other CNS depressants with this medication.
- Advise patient to notify health care professional of all Rx or OTC medications, vitamins, or herbal products being taken and to consult with health care professional before taking other medications.
- Encourage patient to turn, cough, and breathe deeply every 2 hr to prevent atelectasis.
- Inform patients taking *Opana ER* tablets that soft mass resembling tablets may appear in stool; active medication was already absorbed.
- Advise patient to notify health care professional if pregnancy is planned or suspected, or if breast feeding.

Evaluation/Desired Outcomes

- Decrease in severity of pain without a significant alteration in level of consciousness or respiratory status.

HIGH ALERT

oxytocin (ox-i-toe-sin)

Pitocin

Classification

Therapeutic: hormones

Pharmacologic: oxytocics

Pregnancy Category X

Indications

IV: Induction of labor at term. **IV:** Facilitation of threatened abortion. **IV, IM:** Postpartum control of bleeding after expulsion of the placenta.

Action

Stimulates uterine smooth muscle, producing uterine contractions similar to those in spontaneous labor. Has vasopressor and antidiuretic effects. **Therapeutic Effects:** Induction of labor. Control of postpartum bleeding.

Pharmacokinetics

Absorption: IV administration results in 100% bioavailability.

Distribution: Widely distributed in extracellular fluid. Small amounts reach fetal circulation.

Metabolism and Excretion: Rapidly metabolized by liver and kidneys.

Half-life: 3–9 min.

TIME/ACTION PROFILE (reduction in uterine contractions)

ROUTE	ONSET	PEAK	DURATION
IV	immediate	unknown	1 hr
IM	3–5 min	unknown	30–60 min

Contraindications/Precautions

Contraindicated in: Hypersensitivity; Anticipated nonvaginal delivery.

Use Cautiously in: OB: First and second stages of labor; slow infusion over 24 hr has caused water intoxication with seizure and coma or maternal death due to oxytocin's antidiuretic effect.

Adverse Reactions/Side Effects

Maternal adverse reactions are noted for IV use only.

CNS: *maternal*—COMA, SEIZURES; *fetal*, INTRACRANIAL HEMORRHAGE. **Resp:** *fetal*—ASPHYXIA, hypoxia. **CV:** *maternal*—hypotension; *fetal*, arrhythmias. **F and E:** *maternal*—hypochloremia, hyponatremia, water

0

intoxication. **Misc:** *maternal*—↑ uterine motility, painful contractions, abruptio placentae, ↓ uterine blood flow, hypersensitivity.

Interactions

Drug-Drug: Severe hypertension may occur if oxytocin follows administration of **vasopressors**.

Route/Dosage

Induction/Stimulation of Labor

IV (Adults): 0.5–1 milliunits/min; ↑ by 1–2 milliunits/min q 30–60 min until desired contraction pattern established; dose may be ↓ after desired frequency of contractions is reached and labor has progressed to 5–6 cm dilation.

Postpartum Hemorrhage

IV (Adults): 10 units infused at 20–40 milliunits/min.
IM (Adults): 10 units after delivery of placenta.

Incomplete/Inevitable Abortion

IV (Adults): 10 units at a rate of 20–40 milliunits/min.

Availability (generic available)

Solution for injection: 10 units/mL.

NURSING IMPLICATIONS

Assessment

- Fetal maturity, presentation, and pelvic adequacy should be assessed prior to administration of oxytocin for induction of labor.
- Assess character, frequency, and duration of uterine contractions; resting uterine tone; and fetal heart rate frequently throughout administration. If contractions occur <2 min apart and are >50–65 mm Hg on monitor, if they last 60–90 sec or longer, or if a significant change in fetal heart rate develops, stop infusion and turn patient on her left side to prevent fetal anoxia. Notify health care professional immediately.
- Monitor maternal BP and pulse frequently and fetal heart rate continuously throughout administration.
- This drug occasionally causes water intoxication. Monitor patient for signs and symptoms (drowsiness, listlessness, confusion, headache, anuria) and notify physician or other health care professional if they occur.
- ***Lab Test Considerations:*** Monitor maternal electrolytes. Water retention may result in hypochloremia or hyponatremia.

Potential Nursing Diagnoses

Deficient knowledge, related to medication regimen (Patient/Family Teaching)

Implementation

- Do not administer oxytocin simultaneously by more than one route.

IV Administration

- **Continuous Infusion:** Rotate infusion container to ensure thorough mixing. Store solution in refrigerator, but do not freeze.
- Infuse via infusion pump for accurate dose. Oxytocin should be connected via Y-site injection to an IV of 0.9% NaCl for use during adverse reactions.
- Magnesium sulfate should be available if needed for relaxation of myometrium.
- **Induction of Labor:** ***Diluent:*** Dilute 1 mL (10 units) in 1 L of compatible infusion fluid (0.9% NaCl, D5W, or LR). ***Concentration:*** 10 milliunits/mL. ***Rate:*** Begin infusion at 0.5–2 milliunits/min (0.05–0.2 mL); increase in increments of 1–2 milliunits/min at 15–30-min intervals until contractions simulate normal labor.
- **Postpartum Bleeding:** ***Diluent:*** For control of postpartum bleeding, dilute 1–4 mL (10–40 units) in 1 L of compatible infusion fluid. ***Concentration:*** 10–40 milliunits/mL. ***Rate:*** Begin infusion at a rate of 20–40 milliunits/min to control uterine atony. Adjust rate as indicated.
- **Incomplete or Inevitable Abortion:** ***Diluent:*** For incomplete or inevitable abortion, dilute 1 mL (10 units) in 500 mL of 0.9% NaCl or D5W. ***Concentration:*** 20 milliunits/mL. ***Rate:*** Infuse at a rate of 20–40 milliunits/min.
- **Y-Site Compatibility:** acyclovir, alfentanil, allopurinol, amikacin, aminocaproic acid, aminophylline, amphotericin B liposome, anidulafungin, argatroban, ascorbic acid, atropine, azathioprine, azithromycin, aztreonam, benztropine, bivalirudin, bumetanide, buprenorphine, butorphanol, calcium chloride, calcium gluconate, capreomycin, caspofungin, cefazolin, cefepime, cefotaxime, cefotetan, cefoxitin, ceftazidime, ceftriaxone, cefuroxime, chloramphenicol, ciprofloxacin, cisatracurium, clindamycin, cyanocobalamin, cyclosporine, daptomycin, dexamethasone, dexmedetomidine, digoxin, digoxin, diphenhydramine, dobutamine, dolasetron, dopamine, doxycycline, droperidol, enalaprilat, ephedrine, epinephrine, epoetin alfa, eptifibatide, ertapenem, erythromycin, esmolol, famotidine, fenoldopam, fentanyl, fluconazole, folic acid, foscarnet, fosphenytoin, furosemide, ganciclovir, gentamicin, glycopyrrolate, granisetron, heparin, hydrocortisone sodium succinate, hydromorphone, imipenem/cilastatin, isoproterenol, ketamine, ketorolac, labetalol, leucovorin calcium, levofloxacin, lidocaine, linezolid, lorazepam, magnesium sulfate, mannitol, meperidine, meropenem, metaraminol, methyldopate, methylprednisolone, metoclopramide, metoprolol, metronidazole, midazolam, milrinone, morphine, moxifloxacin, multivitamins, mycophenolate, nafcillin, nalbuphine, naloxone, nesiritide, nicardipine, nitroglycerin, nitroprusside, norepinephrine, ondansetron, oxacillin, palonosetron, pamidronate, papaverine, penicillin G, pentamidine, pentazocine,

pentobarbital, phenobarbital, phentolamine, phenylephrine, phytonadione, piperacillin/tazobactam, potassium acetate, potassium chloride, potassium phosphates, procainamide, prochlorperazine, promethazine, propranolol, protamine, pyridoxime, quinupristin/dalfopristin, ranitidine, sodium acetate, sodium bicarbonate, sodium phosphates, streptokinase, succinylcholine, sufentanil, tacrolimus, theophylline, thiamine, tigecycline, tirofiban, tobramycin, tolazoline, vancomycin, vasopressin, verapamil, vitamin B complex with C, voriconazole, warfarin, zidovudine, zoledronic acid.

- **Y-Site Incompatibility:** dantrolene, diazepam, diazoxide, indomethacin, methohexital, phenytoin, remifentanil, trimethoprim/sulfamethoxazole.
- **Solution Compatibility:** dextrose/Ringer's or lactated Ringer's combinations, dextrose/saline combinations, Ringer's or lactated Ringer's injection, D5W, D10W, 0.45% NaCl, 0.9% NaCl.

Patient/Family Teaching

- Advise patient to expect contractions similar to menstrual cramps after administration has started.

Evaluation/Desired Outcomes

- Onset of effective contractions.
- Increase in uterine tone.
- Reduction in postpartum bleeding.

O

PACLitaxel (pak-li-tax-el)

~~Taxol~~

PACLitaxel protein-bound particles (albumin-bound)

Abraxane

Classification

Therapeutic: antineoplastics

Pharmacologic: taxoids

Pregnancy Category D

Indications

Paclitaxel: Advanced ovarian cancer (with cisplatin). Non-small cell lung cancer (NSCLC) when potentially curative surgery and/or radiation therapy is not an option. Metastatic breast cancer unresponsive to other therapy. Node-positive breast cancer when administered sequentially to standard combination chemotherapy that includes doxorubicin. Treatment of AIDS-related Kaposi's sarcoma. **Paclitaxel (albumin-bound):** Metastatic breast cancer after treatment failure or relapse where therapy included an anthracycline. Locally advanced or metastatic NSCLC when potentially curative surgery or radiation therapy is not an option (with carboplatin). Metastatic pancreatic adenocarcinoma (with gemcitabine).

Action

Interferes with the normal cellular microtubule function that is required for interphase and mitosis. **Therapeutic Effects:** Death of rapidly replicating cells, particularly malignant ones.

Pharmacokinetics

Absorption: IV administration results in complete bioavailability.

Distribution: Cross the placenta.

Protein Binding: 89–98%.

Metabolism and Excretion: Highly metabolized by the liver (primarily by CYP2C8 and CYP3A4), <10% excreted unchanged in urine.

Half-life: *Paclitaxel*—13–52 hr; *Paclitaxel protein-bound particles (albumin-bound)*—27 hr.

TIME/ACTION PROFILE (effect on WBCs)

ROUTE	ONSET	PEAK	DURATION
IV	unknown	11 days	3 wk

Contraindications/Precautions

Contraindicated in: Hypersensitivity to paclitaxel or to castor oil (non-protein-bound vehicle contains polyoxyethylated castor oil); AST >10 x ULN or total bilirubin >5 x ULN (paclitaxel protein-bound particles); Moderate or severe hepatic impairment (pancreatic adenocarcinoma only for paclitaxel protein-bound particles); Known alcohol intolerance; OB, Lactation: Pregnancy or lactation; ANC ≤1500/mm³ in patients with ovarian, lung, or breast cancer; ANC ≤1000/mm³ in patients with AIDS-related Kaposi's sarcoma.

Use Cautiously in: Moderate or severe hepatic impairment (↓ dose); Geri: ↑ risk of adverse reactions; OB: Childbearing potential; Active infection; ↓ bone marrow reserve; Pedi: Safety and effectiveness not established.

Adverse Reactions/Side Effects

CNS: dizziness, headache, seizures. **CV:** <u>ECG changes</u>, <u>edema</u>, <u>hypotension</u>, bradycardia. **GI:** <u>diarrhea</u>, <u>↑ liver enzymes</u>, <u>mucositis</u>, <u>nausea</u>, <u>vomiting</u>, pancreatitis. **Derm:** <u>alopecia</u>. **Hemat:** <u>anemia</u>, <u>neutropenia</u>, <u>thrombocytopenia</u>. **MS:** <u>arthralgia</u>, <u>myalgia</u>. **GU:** renal failure. **Neuro:** <u>peripheral neuropathy</u>. **Resp:** PULMONARY EMBOLISM, PULMONARY FIBROSIS, cough, dyspnea, interstitial pneumonia. **Local:** injection site reactions. **Misc:** hypersensitivity reactions including ANAPHYLAXIS and STEVENS-JOHNSON SYNDROME, SEPSIS, TOXIC EPIDERMAL NECROLYSIS.

P

Interactions

Drug-Drug: CYP3A4 inhibitors including **atazanavir**, **clarithromycin**, **indinavir**, **itraconazole**, **ketoconazole**, **nefazodone**, **nelfinavir**, **ritonavir**, **saquinavir**, and **telithromycin** may ↑ levels and risk of toxicity; concurrent use should be undertaken with caution. **CYP3A4 inducers** including **carbamazepine**, **rifampin**, and **phenytoin** may ↓ levels and ↑ risk of treatment failure; concurrent use should be undertaken with caution. **Gemfibrozil** may ↑ levels and risk of toxicity; concurrent use should be undertaken with caution. ↑ risk of myelosuppression with other **antineoplastics** or **radiation therapy**. Myelosuppression ↑ when given after **cisplatin**. May ↑ levels and toxicity of **doxorubicin**. May ↓ antibody response to and ↑ risk of adverse reactions from **live-virus vaccines**.

Route/Dosage

Many other regimens are used.

Paclitaxel

Ovarian Cancer

IV (Adults): *Previously untreated patients*—175 mg/m² over 3 hr every 3 wk, or 135 mg/m² over 24 hr every 3 wk, followed by cisplatin; *Previously treated patients*—135 mg/m² or 175 mg/m² over 3 hr every 3 wk.

Breast Cancer

IV (Adults): *Adjuvant treatment of node-positive breast cancer*—175 mg/m² over 3 hr every 3 wk for 4 courses administered sequentially to doxorubicin-containing combination chemotherapy; *Failure of initial therapy for metastatic disease or relapse within 6 mo of adjuvant therapy*—175 mg/m² over 3 hr every 3 wk.

NSCLC

IV (Adults): 135 mg/m² over 24 hr every 3 wk, followed by cisplatin.

AIDS-Related Kaposi's Sarcoma

IV (Adults): 135 mg/m² over 3 hr every 3 wk or 100 mg/m² over 3 hr every 2 wk (dose ↓/adjustment may be necessary in patients with advanced HIV infection).

Paclitaxel Protein-Bound Particles (albumin-bound)

Breast Cancer

IV (Adults): 260 mg/m² over 30 min every 3 wk.

Hepatic Impairment

IV (Adults): *Moderate hepatic impairment (AST levels <10 × ULN and bilirubin levels 1.51–3 × ULN)*—200 mg/m² over 30 min every 3 wk; dose may be ↑ to 260 mg/m² for the 3rd course based on individual tolerance; *Severe hepatic impairment (AST levels <10 × ULN and bilirubin levels 3.01–5× ULN)*—200 mg/m² over 30 min every 3 wk; dose may be ↑ to 260 mg/m² for the 3rd course based on individual tolerance; *Severe hepatic impairment (AST levels >10× ULN or bilirubin levels >5 × ULN)*—Avoid use.

NSCLC

IV (Adults): 100 mg/m² over 30 min on Days 1, 8, and 15 of each 21-day cycle.

Hepatic Impairment

IV (Adults): *Moderate hepatic impairment (AST levels <10 × ULN and bilirubin levels 1.51–3 × ULN)*—80 mg/m² over 30 min on Days 1, 8, and 15 of each 21–day cycle; dose may be ↑ to 100 mg/m² for the 3rd course based on individual tolerance; *Severe hepatic impairment (AST levels <10 × ULN and bilirubin levels 3.01–5 × ULN)*—80 mg/m² over 30 min on Days 1, 8, and 15 of each 21–day cycle; dose may be ↑ to 100 mg/m² for the 3rd course based on individual tolerance; *Severe hepatic impairment (AST levels >10 × ULN or bilirubin levels >5 × ULN)*—Avoid use.

Pancreatic Adenocarcinoma

IV (Adults): 125 mg/m² over 30–40 min on Days 1, 8, and 15 of each 28–day cycle.

Hepatic Impairment

IV (Adults): *Moderate or severe hepatic impairment*—Avoid use.

Availability

Paclitaxel (generic available)

Solution for injection (requires dilution): 6 mg/mL.

Paclitaxel Protein-Bound Particles (albumin-bound)

Powder for injection (requires reconstitution): 100 mg/vial.

NURSING IMPLICATIONS

Assessment

- Monitor vital signs frequently, especially during first hour of the infusion.
- Monitor cardiovascular status especially during first 3 hr of infusion. Hypotension and bradycardia are common but usually do not require treatment. Continuous ECG monitoring is recommended only for patients with serious underlying conduction abnormalities or those concurrently taking doxorubicin.
- Monitor for bone marrow depression. Assess for bleeding (bleeding gums, bruising, petechiae, guaiac stools, urine, and emesis) and avoid IM injections and taking rectal temperatures if platelet count is low. Apply pressure to venipuncture sites for 10 min. Assess for signs of infection during neutropenia. Anemia may occur. Monitor for dyspnea and orthostatic hypotension. Granulocyte-colony stimulating factor (G-CSF) may be used if necessary.
- Assess for development of peripheral neuropathy. If severe symptoms occur, subsequent dose should be reduced by 20%.
- Monitor intake and output, appetite, and nutritional intake. Paclitaxel causes nausea and vomiting in 50% of patients. Prophylactic antiemetics may be used. Adjust diet as tolerated to help maintain fluid and electrolyte balance and nutritional status.
- Assess patient for arthralgia and myalgia, which usually begin 2–3 days after therapy and resolve within 5 days. Pain is usually relieved by nonopioid analgesics but may be severe enough to require treatment with opioid analgesics.
- Assess for rash periodically during therapy. May cause Stevens-Johnson syndrome and toxic epidermal necrolysis. Discontinue therapy if severe or if accompanied with fever, general malaise, fatigue, muscle or joint aches, blisters, oral lesions, conjunctivitis, hepatitis, and/or eosinophilia.
- **Paclitaxel:** Monitor for hypersensitivity reactions continuously during the first 30 min and frequently thereafter. These occur frequently (19%), usually during the first 10 min of paclitaxel infusion, after the first or second dose. Pretreatment is recommended for **all** patients and should include dexamethasone 20 mg PO (10 mg for patients with advanced HIV disease) 12 and 6 hr prior to paclitaxel, diphenhydramine 50 mg IV 30–60 min prior to paclitaxel, and ranitidine 50 mg IV 30–60 min prior to paclitaxel. Most common manifestations are dyspnea, flushing, tachycardia, rash, hypotension, and chest pain. If these occur, stop infusion and notify health care professional. Treatment may include

bronchodilators, epinephrine, antihistamines, and corticosteroids. Keep these agents and resuscitative equipment close by in the event of an anaphylactic reaction. Other manifestations of hypersensitivity reactions include flushing and rash.

- No premedication for hypersensitivity is required for *paclitaxel protein-bound (albumin-bound)*.
- ***Lab Test Considerations:*** **Paclitaxel:** Monitor CBC and differential prior to and periodically during therapy. The nadir of leukopenia occurs in 11 days, with recovery by days 15–21. Notify health care professional if the leukocyte count is <1500/mm^3 (1000/mm^3 in AIDS-related Kaposi's sarcoma) or if the platelet count is <100,000/mm^3. Subsequent doses are usually held until leukocyte count is >1500/mm^3 (1000/mm^3 in AIDS-related Kaposi's sarcoma) and platelet count is >100,000/mm^3.
- **Paclitaxel Protein-Bound Particles (albumin-bound)**Monitor CBC and differential prior to therapy and prior to dosing on Days 1, 8, and 15. Do not administer if neutrophil count is <1500/mm^3. If severe neutropenia (neutrophils <500 cells/mm3 for seven days or more), reduce dose in subsequent courses., Monitor liver function studies (AST, ALT, LDH, bilirubin) prior to and periodically during therapy to detect hepatotoxicity.

Potential Nursing Diagnoses

Risk for infection (Adverse Reactions)
Risk for injury (Adverse Reactions)

Implementation

- Do not confuse Taxol (paclitaxel) with Taxotere (docetaxel). Do not confuse Taxol (paclitaxel) with Paxil (paroxetine).

Paclitaxel

IV Administration

- **Continuous Infusion:** Paclitaxel must be diluted prior to injection. ***Diluent:*** Dilute contents of 5-mL (30-mg) vials with the following diluents: 0.9% NaCl, D5W, D5/0.9% NaCl, or dextrose in Ringer's solution. ***Concentration:*** 0.3–1.2 mg/mL. Although haziness in solution is normal, inspect for particulate matter or discoloration before use. Use an in-line filter of not >0.22-micron pore size. Solutions are stable for 27 hr at room temperature and lighting. Do not use PVC containers or administration sets. ***Rate:*** Dose for *breast cancer or AIDS-related Kaposi's sarcoma* is administered over 3 hr. Dose for *ovarian cancer* is administered as a 24-hr infusion.
- **Y-Site Compatibility:** acyclovir, alemtuzumab, alfentanil, allopurinol, amifostine, amikacin, aminophylline, amphotericin B lipid complex, ampicillin, ampicillin/sulbactam, anidulafungin, argatroban, azithromycin, aztreonam, bivalirudin, bleomycin, bumetanide, buprenorphine, busulfan, butorphanol, calcium chloride, calcium gluconate, carboplatin, carmustine, caspofungin, cefazolin, cefepime, cefotaxime, cefotetan, cefoxitin, ceftazidime, ceftriaxone, cefuroxime, chloramphenicol, ciprofloxacin, cisatracurium, cisplatin, cladribine, clindamycin, cyclophosphamide, cyclosporine, cytarabine, dacarbazine, dactinomycin, dantrolene, daptomycin, daunorubicin hydrochloride, dexamethasone, dexmedetomidine, dexrazoxane, diltiazem, diphenhydramine, dobutamine, dolasetron, dopamine, doripenem, doxorubicin hydrochloride, doxycycline, droperidol, enalaprilat, ephedrine, epinephrine, epirubicin, ertapenem, erythromycin , esmolol, etoposide, etoposide phosphate, famotidine, fenoldopam, fentanyl, floxuridine, fluconazole, fludarabine, fluorouracil, foscarnet, fosphenytoin, furosemide, ganciclovir, gemcitabine, gentamicin, glycopyrrolate, granisetron, haloperidol, heparin, hetastarch, hydralazine, hydrocortisone, hydromorphone, ifosfamide, imipenem/cilastatin, insulin, irinotecan, isoproterenol, ketorolac, leucovorin, levofloxacin, levorphanol, lidocaine, linezolid, lorazepam, magnesium sulfate, mannitol, meperidine, meropenem, mesna, methotrexate, methyldopate, metoclopramide, metoprolol, metronidazole, midazolam, milrinone, mitomycin, morphine, moxifloxacin, nafcillin, nalbuphine, naloxone, nesiritide, nicardipine, nitroglycerin, nitroprusside, norepinephrine, octreotide, ondansetron, oxaliplatin, palonosetron, pamidronate, pancuronium, pantoprazole, pemetrexed, pentamidine, pentazocine, pentobarbital, pentostatin, phenobarbital, phenylephrine, piperacillin/tazobactam, potassium acetate, potassium chloride, potassium phosphates, procainamide, prochlorperazine, promethazine, propofol, quinupristin/dalfopristin, ranitidine, remifentanil, rituximab, sodium acetate, sodium bicarbonate, sodium phosphates, streptozocin, succinylcholine, sufentanil, tacrolimus, teniposide, theophylline, thiopental, thiotepa, tigecycline, tirofiban, tobramycin, topotecan, trastuzumab, trimethoprim/sulfamethoxazole, vancomycin, vasopressin, vecuronium, verapamil, vinblastine, vincristine, vinorelbine, voriconazole, zidovudine, zoledronic acid.
- **Y-Site Incompatibility:** amiodarone, amphotericin B cholesteryl, amphotericin B colloidal, amphotericin B liposome, chlorpromazine, diazepam, digoxin, doxorubicin liposomal, hydroxyzine, idarubicin, indomethacin, labetalol, methyl-

P

prednisolone, mitoxantrone, phenytoin, propranolol.

Paclitaxel Protein-Bound Particles (albumin-bound)

IV Administration

- **Intermittent Infusion:** Reconstitute by slowly adding 20 mL to each vial over at least 1 min for a concentration of 5 mg/mL. Direct solution to inside wall of vial to prevent foaming. Allow vial to sit for at least 5 min to ensure proper wetting of cake/powder. Gently swirl or invert vial for at least 2 min until powder is completely dissolved; avoid foaming. If foaming or clumping occurs, allow vial to stand for 15 min until foaming dissolves. Solution should be milky and homogenous without visible particles. If particles or settling are visible, gently invert vial to resuspend. Inject appropriate amount into sterile PVC IV bag. Do not use an in-line filter during administration. Do not administer solutions that are discolored or contain particulate matter. Reconstituted solution should be administered immediately but is stable for 8 hr if refrigerated. Discard unused portion. ***Rate:*** Administer over 30–40 min. Monitor infusion site closely for infiltration.

Patient/Family Teaching

- Explain purpose of paclitaxel to patient.
- Advise patient to notify health care professional immediately of rash, difficulty breathing, or symptoms of hypersensitivity reaction occurs.
- Instruct patient to notify health care professional promptly if fever; chills; cough; hoarseness; sore throat; signs of infection; lower back or side pain; painful or difficult urination; bleeding gums; bruising; petechiae; blood in stools, urine, or emesis; dyspnea; or orthostatic hypotension occurs. Caution patient to avoid crowds and persons with known infections. Instruct patient to use soft toothbrush and electric razor and to avoid falls. Caution patient not to drink alcoholic beverages or to take medication containing aspirin or NSAIDs; may precipitate gastric bleeding.
- May cause dizziness. Caution patient to avoid driving or other activities requiring alertness until response to medication is known.
- Instruct patient to notify health care professional if abdominal pain, yellow skin, weakness, paresthesia, gait disturbances, or joint or muscle aches occur.
- Instruct patient to inspect oral mucosa for redness and ulceration. If mouth sores occur, advise patient to use sponge brush and rinse mouth with water after eating and drinking. Stomatitis usually resolves in 5–7 days.
- Discuss with patient the possibility of hair loss. Complete hair loss usually occurs between days 14 and 21 and is reversible after discontinuation of therapy. Explore coping strategies.
- Instruct patient not to receive any vaccinations without advice of health care professional.
- Rep: Advise patient to use a nonhormonal method of contraception and to avoid breast feeding during therapy. Advise male patients not to father a child while receiving paclitaxel.
- Emphasize the need for periodic lab tests to monitor for side effects.

Evaluation/Desired Outcomes

- Decrease in size or spread of malignancy.

palbociclib (pal-**bo**-si-klib)

Ibrance

Classification
Therapeutic: antineoplastics
Pharmacologic: kinase inhibitors

Indications

In combination with letrozole in the treatment of metastatic estrogen (ER)-positive human epidermal growth factor 2 (HER2)-negative advanced breast cancer in post-menopausal patients (part of initial endocrine-based therapy).

Action

Inhibits kinases (cyclin-dependent kinases 4 and 6) that are part of the signaling pathway for cell proliferation. **Therapeutic Effects:** Decreased spread of breast cancer.

Pharmacokinetics

Absorption: 46% absorbed following oral administration.
Distribution: Unknown.
Metabolism and Excretion: Mostly metabolized (by CYP3A and sulfontransferase [SULT]); also acts as an inhibitor of CYP3A; 6.9% excreted unchanged in urine, 2.3% in feces.
Half-life: 29 hr.

TIME/ACTION PROFILE (improvement in progression-free survival)

ROUTE	ONSET	PEAK	DURATION
PO	within 4 mos	unknown	maintained throughout treatment

Contraindications/Precautions

Contraindicated in: Stong/moderate inhibitors of CYP3A (if necessary ↓ dose of palbociclib); CYP3A inducers (may ↓ effectiveness); OB: Pregnancy (may cause fetal harm); Lactation: Discontinue palbociclib or discontinue breast feeding.
Use Cautiously in: Concurrent use of sensitive CYP3A substrates (narrow therapeutic indices), dose of substrate may need to be ↓; Severe renal impairment;

OB: Patients with child-bearing potential; Pedi: Safe and effective use in children has not been established.

Adverse Reactions/Side Effects

CNS: weakness. **CV:** PULMONARY EMBOLISM. **EENT:** epistaxis. **GI:** ↓appetite, diarrhea, nausea, stomatitis, vomiting. **Derm:** alopecia. **Hemat:** NEUTROPENIA, anemia, leukopenia, thrombocytopenia. **Neuro:** peripheral neuropathy. **Misc:** FEBRILE NEUTROPENIA.

Interactions

Drug-Drug: Concurrent use with **CYP3A inhibitors** including **clarithromycin**, **indinavir**, **itraconazole**, **ketoconazole**, **lopinavir/ritonavir**, **nefazodone**, **nelfinavir**, **posaconazole**, **ritonavir**, **saquinavir**, **telithromycin**, **verapamil** and **voraconazole** ↑ levels and the risk of toxicity; avoid if possible but if unavoidable ↓ dose of palbociclib (resume original dose after 3–5 half-lives of offending drug have passed following discontinuation). **Strong CYP3A inducers** including **carbamazepine**, **phenytoin**, **rifampin** can ↓ levels and effectiveness; concurrent use should be avoided. Moderate CYP inducers including **bosentan**, **efavirenz**, **etravirine**, **modafinil** and **nafcillin** may also ↓ levels and effectiveness; avoid concurrent use. ↑ levels and effects/toxicity of **alfentanil**, **cyclosporine**, **dihydroergotamine**, **ergotamine**, **everolimus**, **fentanyl**, **midazolam**, **pimozide**, **quinidine**, **sirolimus** and **tacrolimus**; if concurrent use is required dose ↓ may be necessary.

Drug-Natural Products: **St. John's wort** may ↓ levels and effectiveness; avoid concurrent use.

Drug-Food: **Grapefruit/grapefruit juice** ↑ levels and the risk of toxicity, avoid ingestion.

Route/Dosage

PO (Adults): 125 mg daily for 21 days, followed by 7 days off. Dose alteration may be required, depending on tolerance/toxicity. Letrozole 2.5 mg PO daily should be given concurrently.

Availability

Capsules: 75 mg, 100 mg, 125 mg.

NURSING IMPLICATIONS

Assessment

- Monitor for signs and symptoms of infection (fever, chills, dizziness, shortness of breath, weakness, increased bleeding or bruising) during therapy. Treat as medically appropriate. No dose adjustment is needed for Grade 1 or 2 non-hematologic toxicities. *For Grade ≥3 (if persisting despite medical treatment),* withhold palbociclib until symptoms resolve to: Grade ≤1; Grade ≤2 (if not considered a safety risk for patient). Resume at next lower dose.
- Monitor for signs and symptoms of pulmonary embolism (shortness or breath, chest pain, tachypnea, tachycardia) during therapy.
- ***Lab Test Considerations:*** Monitor CBC prior to and at beginning of each cycle, on Day 14 of first 2 cycles, and as clinically indicated. May cause ↓ neutrophil counts; median time to first episode is 15 days (13–117 days) and median duration of Grade ≥3 neutropenia was 7 days. May cause febrile neutropenia.
- No dose reduction is needed for Grade 1 or 2 hematologic toxicities. *For Grade 3,* no dose adjustment required. Consider repeating CBC monitoring in 1 wk. Withhold initiation of next cycle until recovery to Grade ≤2. *For Grade 3 ANC (<1000 to 500/mm³) plus Fever ≥38.5°C and/or infection,* withhold palbociclib and initiation of next cycle until recovery to Grade ≤2 (≥1000/mm³. Resume at next lower dose. *For Grade 4,* withhold palbociclib and initiation of next cycle until recovery to Grade ≤2. Resume at lower dose.
- May cause ↓ WBC, lymphocytes, hemoglobin, and platelets.

Potential Nursing Diagnoses

Risk for infection (Adverse Reactions)

Implementation

- **PO:** Administer once daily at the same time each day, for 21 consecutive days followed by 7 days off treatment, with food in combination with letrozole once daily given throughout 28 day cycle. Swallow capsules whole; do not open, crush, or chew; do not swallow capsules that are broken, cracked, or not intact.
- If dose reduction needed for adverse reactions starting dose is 125 mg/day. First dose reduction is to 100 mg/day, second dose reduction is to 75 mg/day; if further dose reduction needed, discontinue therapy.

Patient/Family Teaching

- Instruct patient to take palbociclib as directed. If a dose is vomited or missed, omit dose and take next dose at usual time; do not take an additional dose that day. Do not change dose or stop taking without consulting health care professional. Advise patient to read *Patient Information* before starting therapy and with each Rx refill in case of changes.
- Advise patient to avoid grapefruit or grapefruit products during therapy; may increase amount of palbociclib in blood.
- Advise patient to notify health care professional if signs and symptoms of infection or pulmonary embolism occur.
- Instruct patient to notify health care professional of all Rx or OTC medications, vitamins, or herbal products being taken and to consult with health care professional before taking other medications.

- Advise female patient to use effective contraception during and for at least 2 wks after last dose. Advise patient to notify health care professional if pregnancy is planned or suspected or if breast feeding. Inform male patient that palbociclib may compromise fertility.

Evaluation/Desired Outcomes

- Decrease in the spread of breast cancer.

palifermin (pa-liff-er-min)

Kepivance

Classification
Therapeutic: cytoprotective agents
Pharmacologic: keratinocyte growth factors (rDNA)

Pregnancy Category C

Indications

To decrease incidence/duration of severe oral mucositis (at least WHO grade 3) associated with myelotoxic therapy in patients requiring stem cell support for hematologic malignancies.

Action

Enhances proliferation of epithelial cells. **Therapeutic Effects:** Decreased incidence/duration of mucositis.

Pharmacokinetics

Absorption: IV administration results in complete bioavailability.
Distribution: Distributes into extravascular space.
Metabolism and Excretion: Unknown.
Half-life: 4.5 hr.

TIME/ACTION PROFILE (levels)

ROUTE	ONSET	PEAK	DURATION
IV	unknown	end of dose	unknown

Contraindications/Precautions

Contraindicated in: Hypersensitivity to palifermin or other *E. coli*-derived proteins.
Use Cautiously in: OB: Use only if maternal benefit outweighs fetal risk; Lactation, Pedi: Safety not established.

Adverse Reactions/Side Effects

Derm: skin toxicity. **GI:** oral toxicity. **Metab:** ↑ amylase, ↑ lipase. **MS:** arthralgia. **Neuro:** dysesthesia.

Interactions

Drug-Drug: Unfractionated heparin and **low-molecular weight heparin** ↑ levels (flush tubing with saline between use). Administration within 24 hr after **myelotoxic therapy (chemotherapy/radiation)** ↑ severity and duration of mucositis.

Route/Dosage

IV (Adults): 60 mcg/kg/day for 3 days before and 3 days after myelotoxic therapy.

Availability

Powder for injection (requires reconstitution): 6.25 mg/vial.

NURSING IMPLICATIONS

Assessment

- Assess level of oral mucositis prior to and periodically during therapy.
- ***Lab Test Considerations:*** May cause ↑ serum lipase and amylase; usually reversible.
- May cause proteinuria.

Potential Nursing Diagnoses

Acute pain (Indications)
Impaired oral mucous membrane (Indications)

Implementation

- Do not administer palifermin within 24 hr before, during infusion, or 24 hr after infusion of myelotoxic chemotherapy.
- Administer doses for 3 consecutive days before (third dose 24–48 hr prior to chemotherapy) and 3 consecutive days after myelotoxic chemotherapy (fourth dose on same day as hematopoietic stem cells infusion after infusion is completed and at least 4 days after most recent palifermin administration) for a total of 6 doses.

IV Administration

- **IV Push: *Diluent:*** Reconstitute palifermin powder by slowly injecting 1.2 mL of sterile water for injection aseptically. ***Concentration:*** 5 mg/mL. Swirl gently; do not shake or vigorously agitate. Solution should be clear and colorless; do not administer solution that is discolored or contains particulate matter. Dissolution usually takes less than 3 minutes. Administer immediately after reconstitution or refrigerate and administer within 24 hr. Do not freeze. Allow to reach room temperature for up to 1 hr. Protect from light. Discard palifermin after expiration date or if left at room temperature for more than 1 hr. ***Rate:*** Administer via bolus injection. Do not use a filter.
- **Y-Site Incompatibility:** heparin. If heparin solution is used to maintain IV line, flush with 0.9% NaCl prior to and after use of palifermin.

Patient/Family Teaching

- Explain the purpose of palifermin to patient.
- Inform patient of evidence of tumor growth and stimulation in cell culture and animal models.
- Advise patient to notify health care professional if rash, erythema, edema, pruritus, oral/perioral dysesthesia (tongue discoloration, tongue thickening, alteration of taste) occur.

Evaluation/Desired Outcomes

- Decrease in incidence and duration of oral mucositis in patients receiving myelotoxic therapy requiring hematopoietic stem cell support.

paliperidone (pa-li-per-i-done)

Invega, Invega Sustenna, Invega Trinza

Classification

Therapeutic: antipsychotics

Pharmacologic: benzisoxazoles

Pregnancy Category C

Indications

PO, IM: Acute and maintenance treatment of schizophrenia (Invega and Invega Sustenna). **IM:** Maintenance treatment of schizophrenia after patients have been adequately treated with Invega Sustenna for at least 4 mo (Invega Trinza). **PO, IM:** Acute treatment of schizoaffective disorder (as monotherapy or as adjunct to mood stabilizers and/or antidepressants) (Invega and Invega Sustenna).

Action

May act by antagonizing dopamine and serotonin in the CNS. Paliperidone is the active metabolite of risperidone. **Therapeutic Effects:** Decreased manifestations of schizophrenia. Decreased manifestations of schizoaffective disorder.

Pharmacokinetics

Absorption: 28% absorbed following oral administration, food ↑ absorption; slowly absorbed after IM administration (concentrations higher and more rapidly achieved with administration into deltoid muscle).

Distribution: Unknown.

Metabolism and Excretion: 59% excreted unchanged in urine; 32% excreted in urine as metabolites.

Half-life: 23 hr (PO); 25–49 days (IM —Sustenna); 84–139 days (IM —Trinza).

TIME/ACTION PROFILE (blood levels)

ROUTE	ONSET	PEAK	DURATION
PO	unknown	24 hr	24 hr
IM —Sustenna	unknown	13 days	1 mo
IM —Trinza	unknown	30–33 days	3 mo

Contraindications/Precautions

Contraindicated in: Hypersensitivity to paliperidone or risperidone; Concurrent use of drugs known to cause QTc prolongation (including quinidine, procainamide, sotalol, amiodarone, chlorpromazine, thioridazine, moxifloxacin); History of congenital QTc prolongation or other cardiac arrhythmias; Bradycardia, hypokalemia, hypomagnesemia (↑ risk of QTc prolongation); Pre-existing severe GI narrowing (due to nature of tablet formulation); CCr <50 mL/min (for IM); Lactation: Discontinue drug or bottle feed.

Use Cautiously in: Patients with Parkinson's disease or dementia with Lewy Bodies (↑ sensitivity to effects of antipsychotics); History of suicide attempt; History of HF, MI, conduction abnormalities, stroke, TIA (↑ risk of orthostatic hypotension and syncope); Patients at risk for aspiration pneumonia; History of seizures; Conditions which may ↑ body temperature (strenuous exercise, exposure to extreme heat, concurrent anticholinergics or risk of dehydration); ↓ GI transit time (may ↑ blood levels); May mask symptoms of some drug overdoses, intestinal obstruction, Reye's Syndrome or brain tumor (due to antiemetic effect); Diabetes mellitus; Severe hepatic impairment; Renal impairment (dose ↓ recommended if CCr <80 mL/min); OB: Neonates at ↑ risk for extrapyramidal symptoms and withdrawal after delivery when exposed during the 3rd trimester; use only if maternal benefit outweighs fetal risk; Pedi: Children <12 yr (safety not established); Geri: ↑ risk of mortality and stroke/TIA in elderly patients treated for dementia-related psychosis; consider age-related ↓ in renal function.

Adverse Reactions/Side Effects

CNS: NEUROLEPTIC MALIGNANT SYNDROME, SEIZURES, SUICIDAL THOUGHTS, drowsiness, extrapyramidal disorders (dose related), headache, insomnia, anxiety, confusion, dizziness, dysarthria, fatigue, syncope, tardive dyskinesia, weakness. **EENT:** blurred vision. **Resp:** dyspnea, cough. **CV:** QT INTERVAL PROLONGATION, palpitations, tachycardia (dose related), bradycardia, orthostatic hypotension. **GI:** abdominal pain, dry mouth, dyspepsia, nausea, swollen tongue. **GU:** impotence, priapism. **Endo:** amenorrhea, dyslipidemia, galactorrhea, gynecomastia, hyperglycemia, weight gain. **Hemat:** AGRANULOCYTOSIS, leukopenia, neutropenia. **MS:** back pain, dystonia (dose related). **Neuro:** akathisia, dyskinesia, tremor (dose related). **Misc:** fever.

Interactions

Drug-Drug: ↑ risk of CNS depression with other **CNS depressants** including **alcohol**, **antihistamines**, **sedative/hypnotics**, or **opioid analgesics**. May antagonize the effects of **levodopa** or other **dopamine agonists**. ↑ risk of orthostatic hypotension with **antihypertensives**, **nitrates**, or other **agents that lower BP**. **Carbamazepine** may ↓ levels/effects (may need to ↑ dose of paliperidone). **Valproic acid** may ↑ levels (may need to ↓ dose of paliperidone).

Route/Dosage

Schizophrenia

PO (Adults): 6 mg once daily; may titrate by 3 mg/day at intervals of at least 5 days (range 3–12 mg/day).
PO (Children 12–17 yr): 3 mg once daily; may titrate by 3 mg/day at intervals of at least 5 days (not to exceed 6 mg if <51 kg or 12 mg if ≥51 kg).
IM (Adults): *Invega Sustenna*—234 mg initially, then 156 mg one week later; continue with monthly maintenance dose of 117 mg (range of 39–234 mg based on efficacy and/or tolerability); *Invega Trinza*—Dose should be based on dose of previous 1–month injection dose of Invega Sustenna. If last dose of Invega Sustenna was 78 mg, administer 273 mg of Invega Trinza; if last dose of Invega Sustenna was 117 mg, administer 410 mg of Invega Trinza; if last dose of Invega Sustenna was 156 mg, administer 546 mg of Invega Trinza; if last dose of Invega Sustenna was 234 mg, administer 819 mg of Invega Trinza. Administer dose q 3 mo; may adjust dose based on efficacy and/or tolerability (range: 273–819 mg).

Renal Impairment

PO (Adults): *CCr 50–79 mL/min*—3 mg/day initially; dose may be ↑ to maximum of 6 mg/day; *CCr 10–<50 mL/min*—1.5 mg/day initially; dose may be ↑ to maximum of 3 mg/day.

Renal Impairment

IM (Adults): *CCr 50–79 mL/min*—Invega Sustenna: 156 mg initially, then 117 mg one week later; continue with monthly maintenance dose of 78 mg; Invega Trinza: once stabilized on Invega Sustenna, can then transition to appropriate dose of Invega Trinza (see above) *CCr <50 mL/min*—Contraindicated.

Schizoaffective Disorder

PO (Adults): 6 mg/day; may titrate by 3 mg/day at intervals of at least 4 days (range 3–12 mg/day).

Renal Impairment

PO (Adults): *CCr 50–79 mL/min*—3 mg/day initially; dose may be ↑ to maximum of 6 mg/day; *CCr 10–<50 mL/min*—1.5 mg/day initially; dose may be ↑ to maximum of 3 mg/day.

Availability

Extended-release tablets (Invega): 1.5 mg, 3 mg, 6 mg, 9 mg. **Extended-release intramuscular injection (Invega Sustenna):** 39 mg, 78 mg, 117 mg, 156 mg, 234 mg. **Extended-release intramuscular injection (Invega Trinza):** 273 mg, 410 mg, 546 mg, 819 mg.

NURSING IMPLICATIONS

Assessment

- Monitor patient's mental status (orientation, mood, behavior) before and periodically during therapy. Monitor closely for notable changes in behavior that could indicate the emergence or worsening of suicidal thoughts or behavior or depression, especially during early therapy. Restrict amount of drug available to patient.
- Assess weight and BMI initially and throughout therapy.
- Monitor BP (sitting, standing, lying down) and pulse before and periodically during therapy. May cause prolonged QT interval, tachycardia, and orthostatic hypotension.
- Observe patient when administering medication to ensure that medication is actually swallowed and not hoarded or cheeked.
- Monitor patient for onset of extrapyramidal side effects (*akathisia*—restlessness; *dystonia*—muscle spasms and twisting motions; or *pseudoparkinsonism*—mask-like face, rigidity, tremors, drooling, shuffling gait, dysphagia). Report these symptoms; reduction of dose or discontinuation of medication may be necessary.
- Monitor for tardive dyskinesia (involuntary rhythmic movement of mouth, face, and extremities). Report immediately; may be irreversible.
- Monitor for development of neuroleptic malignant syndrome (fever, respiratory distress, tachycardia, seizures, diaphoresis, hypertension or hypotension, pallor, tiredness). Discontinue paliperidone and notify health care professional immediately if these symptoms occur.
- Monitor for symptoms related to hyperprolactinemia (menstrual abnormalities, galactorrhea, sexual dysfunction).
- ***Lab Test Considerations:*** Monitor fasting blood glucose and cholesterol levels before and periodically during therapy.
- Monitor serum prolactin prior to and periodically during therapy. May cause ↑ serum prolactin levels.
- Monitor CBC frequently during initial months of therapy in patients with pre-existing or history of low WBC. May cause leukopenia, neutropenia, or agranulocytosis. Discontinue therapy if this occurs.

Potential Nursing Diagnoses

Risk for self-directed violence (Indications, Adverse Reactions)
Disturbed sensory perception (specify: visual, auditory, kinesthetic, gustatory, tactile, olfactory) (Indications)

Implementation

- ***High Alert:*** Do not confuse *Invega Sustenna* with *Invega Trinza*.
- **PO:** Administer once daily in the morning without regard to food. Tablets should be swallowed whole; do not crush, break or chew.
- **IM:** *Invega Sustenna:* Administer initial and second doses in deltoid using a 1 1/2-inch, 22 gauge needle for patients ≥90 kg (≥200 lb) or 1-inch 23 gauge needle for patients <90 kg (<200 lb). Monthly maintenance doses can be administered

in either deltoid or gluteal sites. For gluteal injection, use 1 1/2-inch, 22 gauge needle regardless of patient weight. To avoid missed dose, may give second dose 4 days before or after the 1-wk timepoint. Monthly doses may be given up to 7 days before or after the monthly timepoint. *After 1st month, if missed dose is within 4 wk of scheduled dose,* administer 2nd dose of 156 mg as soon as possible. Give 3rd dose of 117 mg in either deltoid or gluteal muscle 5 wk after first injection (regardless of timing of 2nd injection). Then return to normal monthly injections in either deltoid or gluteal muscle. *If >4 wk and <7 wk since 1st injection,* resume by administering 156 mg dose in deltoid as soon as possible, a second 156 mg dose in deltoid in 1 wk, followed by monthly doses in deltoid or gluteal sites. *If > 7 months since scheduled dose,* administer using initial dosing schedule. During regular monthly dose schedule, *if <6 wks since last injection*, administer previously stabilized dose as soon as possible, then monthly. *If >6 wks since last injection*, resume dose previously stabilized on, unless stabilized on 234 mg (then 1st two injections should be 156 mg). Administer 1 dose in deltoid as soon as possible, then another deltoid injection of same dose 1 wk later, then resume regular monthly schedule. *If >6 months since last injection*, administer using initial dosing schedule.

- **IM:** *Invega Trinza:* Use only after at least 4 months of monthly *Invega Sustenna* therapy. Prior to administration, shake the prefilled syringe vigorously for at least 15 seconds within 5 minutes prior to administration to ensure a homogeneous suspension. *Deltoid injection:* For patients weighing <90 kg, use the 1-inch 22 gauge thin wall needle. For patients weighing ≥90 kg, use the 1½-inch 22 gauge thin wall needle. *Gluteal injection:* Regardless of patient weight, use 1½-inch 22 gauge thin wall needle. Initiate *Invega Trinza* when next 1-month paliperidone dose is scheduled. *Avoid missed doses;* dose may be given 2 wks before or after 3 month scheduled dose. *If more than 3½ months (up to but <4 months) since last dose,* administer previously administered dose as soon as possible, then continue with 3-month injections. *If 4 months up to and including 9 months since last dose,* do NOT administer next dose. *If last dose was 273 mg,* administer 2 doses of 78 mg of *Invega Sustenna* one week apart into deltoid muscle, then one dose of *Invega Trinza*273 mg one month after second dose of *Invega Sustenna. If last dose was 410 mg,* administer 2 doses of 117 mg of *Invega Sustenna* one week apart into deltoid muscle, then one dose of *Invega Trinza*410 mg one month after second dose of *Invega Sustenna. If last dose was 819 mg,* administer 2 doses of 156 mg of *Invega Sustenna* one week apart into deltoid muscle, then one dose of *Invega Trinza*819 mg one month after second dose of *Invega Sustenna.* If >9 months have elapsed since last injection of *Invega Trinza*, re-initiate treatment with *Invega Sustenna*. Then resume *Invega Trinza* after at least 4 months of *Invega Sustenna*.

Patient/Family Teaching

- Instruct patient to take medication as directed. Advise patient that appearance of tablets in stool is normal and not of concern.
- Inform patient of the possibility of extrapyramidal symptoms. Instruct patient to report these symptoms immediately to health care professional.
- Advise patient to change positions slowly to minimize orthostatic hypotension.
- May cause drowsiness. Caution patient to avoid driving or other activities requiring alertness until response to medication is known.
- Advise patient and family to notify health care professional if thoughts about suicide or dying, attempts to commit suicide; new or worse depression; new or worse anxiety; feeling very agitated or restless; panic attacks; trouble sleeping; new or worse irritability; acting aggressive; being angry or violent; acting on dangerous impulses; an extreme increase in activity and talking, other unusual changes in behavior or mood occur.
- Advise patient that extremes in temperature should also be avoided; this drug impairs body temperature regulation.
- Advise patient to notify health care professional of all Rx or OTC medications, vitamins, or herbal products being taken and to consult with health care professional before taking other medications and alcohol.
- Advise patient to seek nutritional, weight, or medical management as needed for weight gain or cholesterol elevation.
- Instruct patient to notify health care professional promptly if sore throat, fever, unusual bleeding or bruising, rash, tremors, menstrual abnormalities, galactorrhea, or sexual dysfunction occur.
- Advise patient to notify health care professional of medication regimen before treatment or surgery.
- Advise female patients to notify health care professional if pregnancy is planned or suspected, or if breast feeding or planning to breast feed.
- Emphasize the importance of routine follow-up exams to monitor side effects and continued participation in psychotherapy to improve coping skills.

P

Evaluation/Desired Outcomes

- Decrease in excited, manic behavior.
- Decrease in positive symptoms (delusions, hallucinations) of schizophrenia.
- Decrease in negative symptoms (social withdrawal, flat, blunted affect) of schizophrenia.

palonosetron

(pa-lone-**o**-se-tron)

Aloxi

Classification

Therapeutic: antiemetics

Pharmacologic: 5-HT_3 antagonists

Pregnancy Category B

Indications

Prevention of acute and delayed nausea and vomiting caused by initial or repeat courses of moderately or highly emetogenic chemotherapy (moderately emetogenic chemotherapy for adults only). Prevention of postoperative nausea and vomiting (PONV) for up to 24 hr after surgery.

Action

Blocks the effects of serotonin at receptor sites (selective antagonist) located in vagal nerve terminals and in the chemoreceptor trigger zones in the CNS. **Therapeutic Effects:** Decreased incidence and severity of nausea and vomiting following emetogenic chemotherapy or surgery.

Pharmacokinetics

Absorption: IV administration results in complete bioavailability.

Distribution: Unknown.

Metabolism and Excretion: 50% metabolized; 40% excreted unchanged in urine.

Half-life: 40 hr.

TIME/ACTION PROFILE

ROUTE	ONSET	PEAK	DURATION
IV	within 30 min	unknown	7 days

Contraindications/Precautions

Contraindicated in: Hypersensitivity; cross sensitivity with other 5-HT_3 antagonists may occur; Lactation: Lactation.

Use Cautiously in: OB: Safety not established; Pedi: Neonates <1 mo (safety not established).

Adverse Reactions/Side Effects

CNS: dizziness, headache. **GI:** constipation, diarrhea. **Misc:** SEROTONIN SYNDROME.

Interactions

Drug-Drug: Drugs that affect serotonergic neurotransmitter systems, including **SSRIs**, **SNRIs**, **tricyclic antidepressants**, **MAOIs**, **fentanyl**, **lithium**, **buspirone**, **tramadol**, **methylene blue**, and **triptans** ↑ risk of serotonin syndrome.

Route/Dosage

Prevention of Chemotherapy-Induced Nausea/Vomiting

IV (Adults): 0.25 mg given 30 min before start of chemotherapy.

IV (Children 1 mo–<17 yr): 20 mcg/kg (max = 1.5 mg) given 30 min before start of chemotherapy.

Prevention of PONV

IV (Adults): 0.075 mg given immediately before induction of anesthesia.

Availability (generic available)

Solution for injection: 0.05 mg/mL.

NURSING IMPLICATIONS

Assessment

- Assess patient for nausea, vomiting, abdominal distention, and bowel sounds prior to and following administration.
- ***Lab Test Considerations:*** May cause transient ↑ in serum bilirubin, AST, and ALT levels.

Potential Nursing Diagnoses

Imbalanced nutrition: less than body requirements (Indications)

Diarrhea (Side Effects)

Constipation (Side Effects)

Implementation

- First dose is administered prior to emetogenic event.
- Repeated dose within a 7-day period is not recommended.

IV Administration

- **IV Push:** Administer dose undiluted 30 min prior to chemotherapy or immediately prior to the induction of anesthesia. Flush line prior to and after administration with 0.9% NaCl. Do not administer solutions that are discolored or contain particulate matter.
- ***Concentration:*** 0.05 mg/mL. ***Rate:*** Administer over 30 seconds in adults and 15 seconds in children 30 min before starting chemotherapy and over 10 seconds for postoperative nausea and vomiting.
- **Y-Site Compatibility:** alemtuzumab, alfentanil, amifostine, amikacin, aminocaproic acid, aminophylline, amiodarone, amphotericin B liposome, ampicillin, ampicillin/sulbactam, anidulafungin, argatroban, atropine, azithromycin, aztreonam, bivalirudin, bleomycin, bumetanide, buprenorphine, busulfan, butorphanol, calcium acetate, calcium chloride, calcium gluconate, carboplatin, carmustine, caspofungin, cefazolin, cefepime, cefotaxime, cefotetan, cefoxitin, ceftazidime, ceftriaxone, cefuroxime, chloramphenicol, chlorpromazine, ciprofloxacin, cisatracurium, cisplatin, clindamycin, cy-

clophosphamide, cyclosporine, cytarabine, dacarbazine, dactinomycin, dantrolene, daptomycin, daunorubicin hydrochloride, dexamethasone, dexmedetomidine, dexrazoxane, digoxin, diltiazem, diphenhydramine, dobutamine, docetaxel, dopamine, doxorubicin hydrochloride, droperidol, enalaprilat, ephedrine, epinephrine, epirubicin, eptifibitide, erythromycin, esmolol, etoposide, etoposide phosphate, famotidine, fenoldopam, fentanyl, fluconazole, fludarabine, fluorouracil, foscarnet, fosphenytoin, furosemide, gemcitabine, gentamicin, glycopyrrolate, haloperidol, heparin, hydralazine, hydrocortisone, hydromorphone, idarubicin, ifosfamide, insulin, irinotecan, isoproterenol, ketorolac, labetalol, leucovorin, levofloxacin, lidocaine, linezolid, lorazepam, magnesium sulfate, mannitol, melphalan, meperidine, meropenem, mesna, methotrexate, methyldopate, metoclopramide, metoprolol, metronidazole, midazolam, milrinone, mitomycin, mitoxantrone, morphine, moxifloxacin, nalbuphine, naloxone, neostigmine, nesiritide, nicardipine, nitroglycerin, nitroprusside, norepinephrine, octreotide, oxaliplatin, oxytocin, paclitaxel, pamidronate, pancuronium, pentazocine, phenobarbital, phenylephrine, piperacillin/tazobactam, potassium acetate, potassium chloride, potassium phosphates, procainamide, prochlorperazine, promethazine, propranolol, quinupristin/dalfopristin, ranitidine, remifentanil, rocuronium, sodium acetate, sodium bicarbonate, sodium phosphates, streptozocin, succinylcholine, sufentanil, tacrolimus, teniposide, theophylline, thiotepa, tigecycline, tirofiban, tobramycin, topotecan, trimethoprim/sulfamethoxazole, vancomycin, vasopressin, vecuronium, verapamil, vinblastine, vincristine, vinorelbine, zidovudine.

- **Y-Site Incompatibility:** acyclovir, allopurinol, amphotericin B colloidal, diazepam, doxycycline, ganciclovir, imipenem/cilastatin, methylprednisolone, minocycline, nafcillin, pantoprazole, pentamidine, pentobarbital, phenytoin, thiopental.

Patient/Family Teaching

- Inform patient of purpose of medication.
- Advise patient to notify health care professional if nausea or vomiting occur.

Evaluation/Desired Outcomes

- Prevention of nausea and vomiting associated with initial and repeat courses of emetogenic cancer chemotherapy or surgery.

pamidronate (pa-**mid**-roe-nate)

Aredia

Classification
Therapeutic: bone resorption inhibitors
Pharmacologic: biphosphonates, hypocalcemics

Pregnancy Category D

Indications

Moderate to severe hypercalcemia associated with malignancy. Osteolytic bone lesions associated with multiple myeloma or breast cancer. Moderate to severe Paget's disease.

Action

Inhibits resorption of bone. **Therapeutic Effects:** Decreased serum calcium. Decreased skeletal destruction in multiple myeloma or breast cancer. Decreased skeletal complications in Paget's disease.

Pharmacokinetics

Absorption: IV administration results in complete bioavailability.
Distribution: Rapidly absorbed by bone. Reaches high concentrations in bone, liver, spleen, teeth, and tracheal cartilage. Approximately 50% of a dose is retained by bone and then slowly released.
Metabolism and Excretion: 50% is excreted unchanged in the urine.
Half-life: Elimination half-life from plasma is biphasic— 1st phase 1.6 hr, 2nd phase 27.2 hr. Elimination half-life from bone is 300 days.

TIME/ACTION PROFILE (effect on serum calcium)

ROUTE	ONSET	PEAK	DURATION
IV	24 hr	7 days	unknown

Contraindications/Precautions

Contraindicated in: Hypersensitivity to pamidronate, other biphosphonates, or mannitol; OB, Lactation: Pregnancy or lactation.
Use Cautiously in: Underlying cardiovascular disease, especially HF (initiate saline hydration cautiously); Invasive dental procedures, cancer, receiving chemotherapy or corticosteroids, poor oral hygiene, periodontal disease, dental disease, anemia, coagulopathy, infection, or poorly-fitting dentures (may ↑ risk of jaw osteonecrosis); History of thyroid surgery (may be at ↑ risk for hypocalcemia); Renal impairment (dose ↓ recommended); Pedi: Safety not established.

Adverse Reactions/Side Effects

CNS: fatigue. **EENT:** conjunctivitis, blurred vision, eye pain/inflammation, rhinitis. **Resp:** rales. **CV:** arrhyth-

P

mias, hypertension, syncope, tachycardia. **GI:** nausea, abdominal pain, anorexia, constipation, vomiting. **F and E:** hypocalcemia, hypokalemia, hypomagnesemia, hypophosphatemia, fluid overload. **GU:** nephrotoxicity. **Hemat:** leukopenia, anemia. **Local:** phlebitis at injection site. **Metab:** hypothyroidism. **MS:** muscle stiffness, musculoskeletal pain, femur fractures, osteonecrosis (primarily of jaw). **Misc:** fever, generalized pain.

Interactions

Drug-Drug: Hypokalemia and hypomagnesemia may ↑ risk of **digoxin** toxicity. **Calcium** and **vitamin D** will antagonize the beneficial effects of pamidronate. Concurrent use of **thalidomide** may ↑ risk of renal dysfunction.

Route/Dosage

Single doses should not exceed 90 mg.

Hypercalcemia of Malignancy

IV (Adults): *Moderate hypercalcemia*—30–90 mg; may be repeated after 7 days.

Osteolytic Lesions from Multiple Myeloma

IV (Adults): 90 mg monthly.

Osteolytic Lesions from Metastatic Breast Cancer

IV (Adults): 90 mg q 3–4 wk.

Paget's Disease

IV (Adults): 90–180 mg/treatment; may be given as 30 mg daily for 3 days up to 30 mg/wk for 6 wk. Single doses of 60–90 mg may also be effective.

Availability (generic available)

Powder for injection: 30 mg/vial, 90 mg/vial.

NURSING IMPLICATIONS

Assessment

- Monitor intake/output ratios and BP frequently during therapy. Assess for signs of fluid overload (edema, rales/crackles).
- Monitor symptoms of hypercalcemia (nausea, vomiting, anorexia, weakness, constipation, thirst, and cardiac arrhythmias).
- Observe for evidence of hypocalcemia (paresthesia, muscle twitching, laryngospasm, and Chvostek's or Trousseau's sign). Protect symptomatic patients by elevating and padding side rails; keep bed in low position.
- Monitor IV site for phlebitis (pain, redness, swelling). Symptomatic treatment should be used if this occurs.
- Assess for bone pain. Treatment with nonopioid or opioid analgesics may be necessary.
- ***Lab Test Considerations:*** Assess serum creatinine prior to each treatment. Withhold dose if renal function has deteriorated in patients treated for bone metastases.
- Monitor serum electrolytes (including calcium, phosphate, potassium, and magnesium), hemoglobin, and creatinine closely. Monitor CBC and platelet count during the first 2 wk of therapy. May cause hyperkalemia or hypokalemia, hypernatremia, and hematuria.
- Monitor renal function periodically during therapy.

Potential Nursing Diagnoses

Acute pain (Indications, Side Effects)
Risk for injury (Indications)

Implementation

- Initiate a vigorous saline hydration, maintaining a urine output of 2000 mL/24 hr, concurrently with pamidronate therapy. Patients should be adequately hydrated, but avoid overhydration. Use caution in patients with underlying cardiovascular disease, especially HF. Do not use diuretics prior to treatment of hypovolemia.
- Patients with severe hypercalcemia should be started at the 90-mg dose.
- **IV:** Reconstitute by adding 10 mL of sterile water for injection to each vial. ***Concentration:*** 30 mg/10 mL or 90 mg/10 mL. Allow drug to dissolve before withdrawing. Solution is stable for 24 hr if refrigerated.
- **Hypercalcemia:** ***Diluent:*** Dilute further in 1000 mL of 0.45% NaCl, 0.9% NaCl, or D5W. Solution is stable for 24 hr at room temperature. ***Rate:*** Administer 60-mg infusion over at least 4 hr and 90-mg infusion over 24 hr.
- **Multiple Myeloma:** ***Diluent:*** Dilute reconstituted solution in 500 mL of 0.45% NaCl, 0.9% NaCl, or D5W. ***Rate:*** Administer over 4 hr.
- **Paget's Disease:** Dilute reconstituted solution in 500 mL of 0.45% NaCl, 0.9% NaCl, or D5W.
- ***Rate:*** Administer over 4 hr.
- **Y-Site Compatibility:** acyclovir, alemtuzumab, alfentanil, allopurinol, amifostine, amikacin, aminophylline, amphotericin B lipid complex, amphotericin B liposome, ampillicin, ampicillin/sulbactam, anidulafungin, argatroban, atracurium, azithromycin, aztreonam, bivalirudin, bleomycin, bumetanide, buprenorphine, butorphanol, carboplatin, carmustine, cefazolin, cefepime, cefotaxime, cefotetan, cefoxitin, ceftazidime, ceftriaxone, cefuroxime, chloramphenicol, chlorpromazine, ciprofloxacin, cisatracurium, cisplatin, clindamycin, cyclophosphamide, cyclosporine, cytarabine, dacarbazine, daptomycin, dexamethasone, dexmedetomidine, dexrazoxane, digoxin, diltiazem, diphenhydramine, dobutamine, docetaxel, dolasetron, dopamine, doxacurium, doxorubicin, doxorubicin liposomal, doxycycline, droperidol, enalaprilat, ephedrine, epinephrine, epirubicin, ertapenem, erythromycin, esmolol, etoposide, etoposide phosphate, famotidine,

fenoldopam, fentanyl, fluconazole, fludarabine, fluorouracil, foscarnet, fosphenytoin, furosemide, ganciclovir, gemcitabine, gentamicin, glycopyrrolate, granisetron, haloperidol, heparin, hydralazine, hydrocortisone, hydromorphone, ifosfamide, imipenem/cilastatin, insulin, isoproterenol, ketorolac, labetalol, levofloxacin, levorphanol, lidocaine, linezolid, lorazepam, magnesium sulfate, mannitol, mechlorethamine, melphalan, meperidine, meropenem, mesna, metaraminol, methotrexate, methyldopate, methylprednisolone, metoclopramide, metoprolol, metronidazole, midazolam, milrinone, mitoxantrone, morphine, moxifloxacin, mycophenolate, nafcillin, nalbuphine, naloxone, nesiritide, nicardipine, nitroglycerin, nitroprusside, norepinephrine, octreotide, ondansetron, oxytocin, paclitaxel, palonosetron, pancuronium, pemetrexed, pentamidine, pentazocine, pentobarbital, phenobarbital, phentolamine, phenylephrine, piperacillin/tazobactam, potassium acetate, potassium chloride, potassium phosphates, procainamide, prochlorperazine, promethazine, propranolol, quinupristin/dalfopristin, ranitidine, remifentanil, rocuronium, sodium acetate, sodium bicarbonate, sodium phosphates, succinylcholine, sufentanil, tacrolimus, teniposide, theophylline, thiopental, thiotepa, tigecycline, tirofiban, tobramycin, tolazoline, topotecan, trimethoprim/sulfamethoxazole, vancomycin, vasopressin, vecuronium, verapamil, vinblastine, vincristine, vinorelbine, voriconazole, zidovudine.

- **Y-Site Incompatibility:** amphotericin B colloidal, caspofungin, dantrolene, diazepam, leucovorin, phenytoin.
- **Additive Incompatibility:** Calcium-containing solutions, such as Ringer's solution.

Patient/Family Teaching

- Advise patient to report signs of hypercalcemic relapse (bone pain, anorexia, nausea, vomiting, thirst, lethargy) or eye problems (pain, inflammation, blurred vision, conjunctivitis) to health care professional promptly.
- Advise patient to notify nurse of pain at the infusion site.
- Encourage patient to comply with dietary recommendations. Diet should contain adequate amounts of calcium and vitamin D.
- Advise patient to notify health care professional if bone pain is severe or persistent.
- Advise patient to maintain good oral hygiene and have regular dental examinations. Instruct patient to inform health care professional of pamidronate therapy prior to dental surgery.
- Emphasize the need for keeping follow-up exams to monitor progress, even after medication is discontinued, to detect relapse.

Evaluation/Desired Outcomes

- Lowered serum calcium levels.
- Decreased pain from lytic lesions.

pancrelipase (pan-kre-li-pase)

✱Cotazym, Creon, ✱Pancrease MT, ✱Pancrease-V, Pancreaze, Pertyze, Ultresa, Viokace, Zenpep

Classification
Therapeutic: digestive agent
Pharmacologic: pancreatic enzymes

Pregnancy Category C

Indications

Pancreatic insufficiency associated with: Chronic pancreatitis, Pancreatectomy, Cystic fibrosis, GI bypass surgery, Ductal obstruction secondary to tumor.

Action

Contains lipolytic, amylolytic, and proteolytic activity. **Therapeutic Effects:** Increased digestion of fats, carbohydrates, and proteins in the GI tract.

Pharmacokinetics

Absorption: Unknown.
Distribution: Unknown.
Metabolism and Excretion: Unknown.
Half-life: Unknown.

TIME/ACTION PROFILE (digestant effects)

ROUTE	ONSET	PEAK	DURATION
PO	rapid	unknown	unknown

Contraindications/Precautions

Contraindicated in: Hypersensitivity to hog proteins.
Use Cautiously in: Gout, renal impairment, or hyperuricemia (may ↑ uric acid levels); OB, Lactation: Safety not established.

Adverse Reactions/Side Effects

EENT: nasal stuffiness. **Resp:** dyspnea, shortness of breath, wheezing. **GI:** FIBROSING COLONOPATHY (high doses only), abdominal pain (high doses only), diarrhea, nausea, stomach cramps, oral irritation. **GU:** hematuria. **Derm:** hives, rash. **Metab:** hyperuricemia. **Misc:** allergic reactions.

Interactions

Drug-Drug: Antacids (**calcium carbonate** or **magnesium hydroxide**) may ↓ effectiveness of pancrelipase. May ↓ the absorption of concurrently administered **iron supplements**.

P

Drug-Food: Alkaline foods destroy coating on enteric-coated products.

Route/Dosage

PO (Adults and Children ≥4 yr): Initiate with 500 lipase units/kg/meal; dose should be adjusted based on weight, clinical symptoms, and stool fat content; maximum dose = 2500 lipase units/kg/meal (or 10,000 lipase units/kg/day).
PO (Children >1 yr and <4 yr): Initiate with 1000 lipase units/kg/meal; dose should be adjusted based on weight, clinical symptoms, and stool fat content; maximum dose = 2500 lipase units/kg/meal (or 10,000 lipase units/kg/day).
PO (Children ≤1 yr): 2000–4000 lipase units per 120 mL of formula or breast milk.

Availability (generic available)

Delayed-release capsules: 2600 units lipase/6200 units protease/10,850 units amylase, 3000 units lipase/9500 units protease/15,000 units amylase, 3000 units lipase/10,000 units protease/16,000 units amylase, 4000 units lipase/8,000 units protease/8,000 units amylase, 4000 units lipase/12,000 units protease/12,000 units amylase, 4200 units lipase/10,000 units protease/17,500 units amylase, 5000 units lipase/17,000 units protease/27,000 units amylase, 6000 units lipase/19,000 units protease/30,000 units amylase, 8000 units lipase/28,750 units protease/30,250 units amylase, 🍁 8000 units lipase/30,000 units protease/30,000 units amylase, 10,000 units lipase/30,000 units protease/30,000 units amylase, 10,000 units lipase/34,000 units protease/55,000 units amylase, 10,500 units lipase/25,000 units protease/43,750 units amylase, 12,000 units lipase/38,000 units protease/60,000 units amylase, 13,800 units lipase/27,600 units protease/27,600 units amylase, 15,000 units lipase/51,000 units protease/82,000 units amylase, 16,000 units lipase/57,500 units protease/60,500 units amylase, 16,800 units lipase/40,000 units protease/70,000 units amylase, 20,000 units lipase/44,000 units protease/56,000 units amylase, 🍁 20,000 units lipase/55,000 units protease/55,000 units amylase, 20,000 units lipase/68,000 units protease/109,000 units amylase, 20,700 units lipase/41,400 units protease/41,400 units amylase, 21,000 units lipase/37,000 units protease/61,000 units amylase, 23,000 units lipase/46,000 units protease/46,000 units amylase, 24,000 units lipase/76,000 units protease/120,000 units amylase, 25,000 units lipase/85,000 units protease/136,000 units amylase, 36,000 units lipase/114,000 units protease/180,000 units amylase, 40,000 units lipase/136,000 units protease/218,000 units amylase. **Tablets:** 10,440 units lipase/39,150 units protease/39,150 units amylase, 20,880 units lipase/78,300 units protease/78,300 units amylase.

NURSING IMPLICATIONS

Assessment

- Assess patient's nutritional status (height, weight, skin-fold thickness, arm muscle circumference, and lab values) prior to and periodically throughout therapy.
- Monitor stools for high fat content (steatorrhea). Stools will be foul-smelling and frothy.
- Assess patient for allergy to pork; sensitivity to pancrelipase may exist.
- ***Lab Test Considerations:*** May cause ↑ serum and urine uric acid concentrations.

Potential Nursing Diagnoses

Imbalanced nutrition: less than body requirements (Indications)

Implementation

Pancreaze is not interchangerable with any other pancrelipase product.

- **PO:** Administer immediately before or with meals and snacks.
- Swallow tablets whole; do not crush, break, or chew.
- Swallow capsules whole. If unable to swallow, capsules may be opened and sprinkled on foods. Delayed-release capsules filled should not be chewed (sprinkle on soft, acidic foods that can be swallowed without chewing, such as applesauce or Jell-O) and followed immediately by water or juice to ensure complete ingestion. These medications should not be chewed or mixed with alkaline foods prior to ingestion or coating will be destroyed.
- Half of the prescribed *Pancreaze* dose for an individualized full meal should be given with each snack. The total daily dose should reflect approximately three meals plus two or three snacks per day.
- Do not mix contents of *Pancreaze* or *Creon* capsules directly into breast milk or formula. Capsule contents may be sprinkled on small amounts of acidic soft food with a pH of 4.5 or less (applesauce) and given to the infant within 15 minutes. Contents of the capsule may also be administered directly to the mouth. Follow administration with breast milk or formula.
- Do not mix *Zenpep* capsule contents directly into formula or breast milk prior to administration. Administer with applesauce, bananas, or pears (commercially prepared) and follow with breast milk or formula.
- Do not chew or retain *Ultressa* capsule in mouth.

Patient/Family Teaching

- Encourage patients to comply with diet recommendations of health care professional (generally high-calorie, high-protein, low-fat). Dose should be adjusted for fat content of diet. Usually 300 mg of pancrelipase is necessary to digest every 17 g of dietary fat. If a dose is missed, it should be omitted and next dose taken with next snack, as directed. Do not increase dose without consulting health care professional. Several days may be required to determine correct dose. Advise patient to read *Medication Guide* before starting therapy and with each Rx refill; information may be updated.

- Instruct patient not to chew tablets and to swallow them quickly with plenty of liquid to prevent mouth and throat irritation. Sit upright to enhance swallowing. Eating immediately after taking medication helps further ensure that the medication is swallowed and does not remain in contact with mouth and esophagus for a prolonged period. Patient should avoid sniffing powdered contents of capsules, as sensitization of nose and throat may occur (nasal stuffiness or respiratory distress).
- Advise patients and caregivers notify health care professional if symptoms of fibrosing colonopathy (abdominal pain, distention, vomiting, constipation) occur. Occur more frequently with doses exceeding 6000 lipase units/kg of body weight per meal (10,000 lipase units/kg of body weight/day) and have been associated with colonic strictures in children below the age of 12 years.
- Instruct patient to notify health care professional if joint pain, swelling of legs, gastric distress, or rash occurs.
- Advise female patients to notify health care professional if pregnancy is planned or suspected, or if breast feeding.

Evaluation/Desired Outcomes

- Improved nutritional status in patients with pancreatic insufficiency.
- Normalization of stools in patients with steatorrhea.

HIGH ALERT

pancuronium

(pan-cure-**oh**-nee-yum)

~~Pavulon~~

Classification

Therapeutic: neuromuscular blocking agents—nondepolarizing

Pregnancy Category C

Indications

Induction of skeletal muscle paralysis and facilitation of intubation after induction of anesthesia in surgical procedures. Facilitation of compliance during mechanical ventilation.

Action

Prevents neuromuscular transmission by blocking the effect of acetylcholine at the myoneural junction. Has no analgesic or anxiolytic properties. **Therapeutic Effects:** Skeletal muscle paralysis.

Pharmacokinetics

Absorption: Following IV administration, absorption is essentially complete.

Distribution: Rapidly distributes into extracellular fluid; small amounts cross the placenta.

Metabolism and Excretion: Excreted mostly unchanged by the kidneys; small amounts are eliminated in bile.

Half-life: 2 hr.

TIME/ACTION PROFILE (neuromuscular blockade)

ROUTE	ONSET	PEAK	DURATION
IV	30–45 sec	3–4.5 min	40–60 min

Contraindications/Precautions

Contraindicated in: Hypersensitivity; Hypersensitivity to bromides; Pedi: Products containing benzyl alcohol should be avoided in neonates.

Use Cautiously in: Underlying cardiovascular disease (↑ risk of arrhythmias); Dehydration or electrolyte abnormalities (should be corrected); Situations in which histamine release would be problematic; Fractures or muscle spasm; Renal impairment (↓ elimination); Hyperthermia (↑ duration/intensity of paralysis); Hepatic impairment (altered response); Shock; Extensive burns (may be more resistant to effects); Low plasma pseudocholinesterase levels (may be seen in association with anemia, dehydration, cholinesterase inhibitors/insecticides, severe liver disease, pregnancy, or hereditary predisposition); Obese patients; OB, Lactation: Safety not established; may be used during caesarian section; Pedi: Contains benzyl alcohol which can cause potentially fatal gasping syndrome in neonates; Geri: Age-related ↓ in renal function may result in prolonged effects.

Exercise Extreme Caution in: Patients with neuromuscular diseases such as myasthenia gravis (small test dose may be used to assess response).

Adverse Reactions/Side Effects

Resp: bronchospasm. **CV:** hypertension, tachycardia. **GI:** excessive salivation. **Derm:** rash. **Misc:** allergic reactions including ANAPHYLAXIS.

Interactions

Drug-Drug: Intensity and duration of paralysis may be prolonged by pretreatment with **succinylcholine**, **general anesthesia** (inhalation), **aminoglycosides**, **vancomycin**, **tetracyclines**, **polymyxin B**, **colistin**, **cyclosporine**, **calcium channel blockers**, **clindamycin**, **lidocaine**, and other **local anesthetics**, **lithium**, **quinidine**, **procainamide**, **beta blockers**, **potassium-losing diuretics**, or **magnesium**. **Inhalation anesthetics** including **enflurane**, **isoflurane**, **halothane**, **desflurane**, **sevoflurane** may enhance effects. Higher infusion rates may be required and duration of action may be shortened in patients receiving long-term **carbamazepine**, **steroids (chronic)**, **azathioprine** or **phenytoin**.

Route/Dosage

IV (Adults and Children >1 mo): *Initial intubating dose*—0.06–0.1 mg/kg initially; additional doses of 0.01 mg/kg may be given q 25–60 min to maintain paralysis. *Continuous infusion*—1–2 mcg/kg/min.

Availability (generic available)

Injection: 1 mg/mL.

NURSING IMPLICATIONS

Assessment

- Assess respiratory status continuously throughout therapy with neuromuscular blocking agents. These medications should be used only to facilitate intubation or in patients already intubated.
- Neuromuscular response should be monitored with a peripheral nerve stimulator intraoperatively. Paralysis is initially selective and usually occurs sequentially in the following muscles: levator muscles of eyelids, muscles of mastication, limb muscles, abdominal muscles, muscles of the glottis, intercostal muscles, and the diaphragm. Recovery of muscle function usually occurs in reverse order.
- Monitor ECG, heart rate, and BP throughout administration.
- Observe the patient for residual muscle weakness and respiratory distress during the recovery period.
- Monitor infusion site frequently. If signs of tissue irritation or extravasation occur, discontinue and restart in another vein.
- ***Toxicity and Overdose:*** If overdose occurs, use peripheral nerve stimulator to determine the degree of neuromuscular blockade. Maintain airway patency and ventilation until recovery of normal respirations occurs.
- Administration of anticholinesterase agents (neostigmine, pyridostigmine) may be used to antagonize the action of neuromuscular blocking agents once the patient has demonstrated some spontaneous recovery from neuromuscular block. Atropine is usually administered prior to or concurrently with anticholinesterase agents to counteract the muscarinic effects.
- Administration of fluids and vasopressors may be necessary to treat severe hypotension or shock.

Potential Nursing Diagnoses

Ineffective breathing pattern (Indications)
Impaired verbal communication (Side Effects)
Fear (Side Effects)

Implementation

- ***High Alert:*** Unintended administration of a neuromuscular blocking agent instead of administration of the intended medication or administration of a neuromuscular blocking agent in the absence of ventilatory support has resulted in serious harm or death. Confusing similarities in packaging and insufficiently controlled access to these medications are often implicated in these medication errors. Store these products in a separate, locked container.
- Dose is titrated to patient response.
- Neuromuscular blocking agents have *no* effect on consciousness or pain threshold. Adequate anesthesia/analgesia should *always* be used when neuromuscular blocking agents are used as an adjunct to surgical procedures or when painful procedures are performed. Benzodiazepines and/or analgesics should be administered concurrently when prolonged neuromuscular blocker therapy is used for ventilator patients, because patient is awake and able to feel all sensations.
- If eyes remain open throughout prolonged administration, protect corneas with artificial tears.
- Store pancuronium in refrigerator. To prevent absorption by plastic, pancuronium should not be stored in plastic syringes. May be administered in plastic syringes.
- Most neuromuscular blocking agents are incompatible with barbiturates and sodium bicarbonate. Do not admix.

IV Administration

- **IV Push: *Diluent:*** May be administered undiluted. ***Concentration:*** 1 mg/mL (10-mL vial); 2 mg/mL (2-mL or 5-mL vial). ***Rate:*** Administer over 1–2 min.
- **Intermittent Infusion: *Diluent:*** Add 100 mg of pancuroniuum to 250 mL of D5W, 0.9% NaCl, D5/0.9% NaCl, or LR. ***Concentration:*** 0.4 mg/mL. ***Rate:*** Based on patient's weight (see Route/Dosage section).
- **Y-Site Compatibility:** acyclovir, alemtuzumab, alfentanil, amifostine, amikacin, aminocaproic acid, aminophylline, amphotericin B liposome, ampicillin, ampicillin/sulbactam, anidulafungin, argatroban, azithromycin, aztreonam, bivalirudin, bleomycin, bumetanide, buprenorphine, busulfan, butorphanol, calcium chloride, calcium gluconate, carboplatin, carmustine, cefazolin, cefepime, cefotaxime, cefotetan, cefoxitin, ceftazidime, ceftriaxone, cefuroxime, chloramphenicol, chlorpromazine, ciprofloxacin, cisplatin, clindamycin, cyclophosphamide, cyclosporine, cytarabine, dactinomycin, daptomycin, dexamethasone, dexmedetomidine, dexrazoxane, diltiazem, diphenhydramine, dobutamine, docetaxel, dolasetron, dopamine, doxorubicin, doxorubicin liposomal, doxycycline, droperidol, enalaprilat, ephedrine, epinephrine, epirubicin, eptifibatide, ertapenem, erythromycin, esmolol, etomidate, etoposide, etoposide phosphate, famotidine, fenoldopam, fentanyl, fluconazole, fludarabine, fluorouracil, foscarnet, ganciclovir, gemcitabine, gentamicin, glycopyrrolate, granisetron, haloperidol, heparin, hydralazine, hydrocortisone sodium succinate,

hydromorphone, idarubicin, ifosfamide, imipenem-cilastatin, insulin, irinotecan, isoproterenol, ketamine, ketorolac, labetalol, leucovorin calcium, levofloxacin, lidocaine, linezolid, lorazepam, magnesium sulfate, mannitol, mechlorethamine, melphalan, meperidine, meropenem, methohexital, methotrexate, methyldopate, methylprednisolone, metoclopramide, metoprolol, metronidazole, midazolam, milrinone, mitoxantrone, morphine, moxifloxacin, mycophenolate, nafcillin, nalbuphine, naloxone, nesiritide, nitroglycerin, nitroprusside, norepinephrine, octreotide, ondansetron, oxaliplatin, paclitaxel, palonosetron, pamidronate, pemetrexed, pentamidine, pentazocine, pentobarbital, phenobarbital, phenylephrine, piperacillin/tazobactam, potassium acetate, potassium chloride, potassium phosphates, procainamide, prochlorperazine, promethazine, propranolol, quinupristin/dalfopristin, ranitidine, remifentanil, sodium acetate, sodium bicarbonate, sodium phosphates, streptozocin, sufentanil, tacrolimus, teniposide, theophylline, thiotepa, tigecycline, tirofiban, tobramycin, trimethoprim/sulfamethoxazole, vancomycin, verapamil, vinblastine, vincristine, vinorelbine, voriconazole, zidovudine, zoledronic acid.

- **Y-Site Incompatibility:** allopurinol, amphotericin B colloidal, amphotericin B lipid comples, caspofungin, dantrolene, diazepam, furosemide, pantoprazole, phenytoin, thiopental.

Patient/Family Teaching

- Explain all procedures to patient receiving neuromuscular blocker therapy without general anesthesia, because consciousness is not affected by neuromuscular blocking agents alone.
- Reassure patient that communication abilities will return as the medication wears off.

Evaluation/Desired Outcomes

- Adequate suppression of the twitch response when tested with peripheral nerve stimulation and subsequent muscle paralysis.
- Improved compliance during mechanical ventilation.

ⵗ panitumumab

(pan-i-**tu**-mu-mab)
Vectibix

Classification
Therapeutic: antineoplastics
Pharmacologic: monoclonal antibodies

Pregnancy Category C

Indications

ⵗ Treatment of wild-type *KRAS* (exon 2 in codons 12 or 13) metastatic colorectal cancer that has failed fluoropyrimidine-, oxaliplatin-, and irinotecan-containing chemotherapy (to be used as monotherapy). ⵗ Treatment of wild-type *KRAS* (exon 2 in codons 12 or 13) metastatic colorectal cancer (as first-line therapy with FOLFOX).

Action

ⵗ Binds to EGFR resulting in inactivation of kinases that regulate proliferation and transformation. **Therapeutic Effects:** Decreased progression of colorectal cancer.

Pharmacokinetics

Absorption: IV administration results in complete bioavailability.
Distribution: Monoclonal antibodies cross the placenta and enter breast milk.
Metabolism and Excretion: Unknown.
Half-life: 7.5 days.

TIME/ACTION PROFILE

ROUTE	ONSET	PEAK	DURATION
IV	unknown	end of infusion	unknown

Contraindications/Precautions

Contraindicated in: Concurrent leucovorin; ⵗ *RAS*—mutant metastatic colorectal cancer or unknown *RAS* mutation status (↑ mortality and tumor progression); OB, Lactation: Pregnancy or lactation.
Use Cautiously in: Pedi: Safety not established.

Adverse Reactions/Side Effects

CNS: fatigue. **EENT:** OCULAR TOXICITY, eyelash growth. **Resp:** INTERSTITIAL LUNG DISEASE, PULMONARY FIBROSIS, cough. **GI:** abdominal pain, constipation, diarrhea, nausea, vomiting, stomatitis. **Derm:** NECROTIZING FASCIITIS, acneiform dermatitis, dry skin, erythema, paronychia, pruritis, rash, skin exfoliation, skin fissures, abscesses, photosensitivity. **F and E:** edema, hypocalcemia, hypomagnesemia. **GU:** acute renal failure. **Misc:** INFUSION REACTIONS, SEPSIS.

Interactions

Drug-Drug: None noted.

Route/Dosage

IV (Adults): 6 mg/kg as a 60-min infusion every 14 days; ↓ infusion rates and dose modifications are recommended for infusion reactions and other serious toxicities.

Availability

Solution for IV administration (requires dilution): 20 mg/mL.

P

NURSING IMPLICATIONS

Assessment

- Assess for dermatologic toxicity (dermatitis acneiform, pruritus, erythema, rash, skin exfoliation, paronychia, dry skin, skin fissures). If severe, may lead to infection (sepsis, septic death, abscesses requiring incision and drainage). With severe reactions, withhold panitumumab and monitor for inflammatory or infectious sequelae.
- Monitor for severe infusion reactions (anaphylactic reaction, bronchospasm, fever, chills, hypotension). If severe reaction occurs, stop panitumumab; may require permanent discontinuation.
- Assess for pulmonary fibrosis (cough, wheezing, exertional dyspnea, interstitial lung disease, pneumonitis, lung infiltrates). Permanently discontinue panitumumab if these signs occur.
- Monitor for diarrhea and dehydration during therapy.
- Monitor for signs and symptoms of interstitial lung disease (persistent or recurrent coughing, wheezing, dyspnea) during therapy; discontinue panitumumab if symptoms occur.
- ***Lab Test Considerations:*** Monitor electrolyte levels periodically during and for 8 wk after completion of therapy. May cause hypomagnesemia, hypocalcemia, and hypokalemia. Replace electrolytes as needed.

Potential Nursing Diagnoses

Risk for impaired skin integrity (Adverse Reactions)
Impaired gas exchange (Adverse Reactions)

Implementation

- Prior to administration, assess RAS mutational status in colorectal tumors and confirm the absence of a RAS mutation.
- **Intermittent Infusion:** ***Diluent:*** Withdraw necessary amount of panitumumab. Dilute to a volume of 100 mL with 0.9% NaCl; dilute doses >1000 mg with 150 mL. ***Concentration:*** 10 mg/mL. Mix by inverting gently; do not shake. Administer via infusion pump using a low-protein binding 0.2 mcg or 0.22 mcg in-line filter. Solution is colorless and may contain a small amount of visible translucent to white, amorphous, proteinaceous particles. Do not administer solutions that are discolored or contain particulate matter. Store in refrigerator; do not freeze. Use diluted solution within 6 hr of preparation if stored at room temperature or within 24 hr if refrigerated. ***Rate:*** Administer over 60 min every 14 days. If first infusion is tolerated, subsequent infusions may be infused over 30–60 min. Administer doses >1000 mg over 90 min.
- If mild to moderate infusion reaction (Grade 1 or 2) occurs decrease infusion rate by 50%. If severe reaction (Grade 3 or 4) occurs, immediately and permanently discontinue panitumumab.
- If severe dermatologic toxicities (Grade 3 or higher) or those considered intolerable occur, withhold panitumumab. Upon 1st occurrence of a grade 3 dermatologic toxicity, withhold 1 to 2 doses; if skin improves to <Grade 3, reinitiate at original dose. For 2nd occurrence of a grade 3 dermatologic toxicity, withhold 1 to 2 doses; if skin improves to <Grade 3, reinitiate at 80% of original dose. For 3rd occurrence of a grade 3 dermatologic toxicity, withhold 1 to 2 doses; if skin improves to <Grade 3, reinitiate at 60% of original dose. For 4th occurrence of a grade 3 dermatologic toxicity, permanently discontinue panitumumab.
- **Y-Site Incompatibility:** Flush line before and after administration with 0.9% NaCl. Do not mix with other medications or solutions.

Patient/Family Teaching

- Explain purpose of panitumumab to patient.
- May cause photosensitivity. Caution patient to wear sunscreen and hats and to limit sun exposure.
- Advise patient to notify health care professional if signs and symptoms of dermatologic toxicity, infusion reactions, pulmonary fibrosis, or ocular changes occur.
- Advise patient that panitumumab may cause fertility impairment and may have teratogenic effects. Caution women of childbearing yr to use contraception during and for at least 6 mo after last dose and not to breast feed during and for at least 2 mo after the last dose of panitumumab. Encourage women who become pregnant to enroll in *Amgen's Pregnancy Surveillance Program* by calling 1-800-772-6436.
- Emphasize the need for periodic blood tests to monitor electrolyte levels.

Evaluation/Desired Outcomes

- Decreased progression of colorectal cancer.

pantoprazole

(pan-**toe**-pra-zole)

Panto IV, Pantoloc, Protonix, Protonix IV, Tecta

Classification

Therapeutic: antiulcer agents
Pharmacologic: proton-pump inhibitors

Pregnancy Category B

Indications

Erosive esophagitis associated with GERD. Maintenance of healing of erosive esophagitis. Pathologic gastric hypersecretory conditions. **Unlabeled Use:** Adjunctive treatment of duodenal ulcers associated with *Helicobacter pylori*.

Action

Binds to an enzyme in the presence of acidic gastric pH, preventing the final transport of hydrogen ions into the gastric lumen. **Therapeutic Effects:** Diminished accumulation of acid in the gastric lumen, with lessened acid reflux. Healing of duodenal ulcers and esophagitis. Decreased acid secretion in hypersecretory conditions.

Pharmacokinetics

Absorption: Tablet is enteric-coated; absorption occurs only after tablet leaves the stomach.
Distribution: Unknown.
Protein Binding: 98%.
Metabolism and Excretion: Mostly metabolized by the liver via the cytochrome P450 (CYP) system (primarily CYP2C19 isoenzyme, but also the CYP3A4 isoenzyme) (the CYP2C19 enzyme system exhibits genetic polymorphism; 15–20% of Asian patients and 3–5% of Caucasian and Black patients may be poor metabolizers and may have significantly ↑ pantoprazole concentrations and an ↑ risk of adverse effects); inactive metabolites are excreted in urine (71%) and feces (18%).
Half-life: 1 hr.

TIME/ACTION PROFILE (effect on acid secretion)

ROUTE	ONSET†	PEAK	DURATION†
PO	2.5 hr	unknown	1 wk
IV	15–30 min	2 hr	unknown

†Onset = 51% inhibition; duration = return to normal following discontinuation.

Contraindications/Precautions

Contraindicated in: Hypersensitivity to rabeprazole or related drugs (benzimidazoles); OB: Should be used during pregnancy only if clearly needed; Lactation: Discontinue breast feeding due to potential for serious adverse reactions in infants.
Use Cautiously in: Patients using high-doses for >1 year (↑ risk of hip, wrist, or spine fractures); Patients using therapy for >3 yr (↑ risk of vitamin B_{12} deficiency; Pedi: Safety not established.

Adverse Reactions/Side Effects

CNS: headache. **GI:** CLOSTRIDIUM DIFFICILE-ASSOCIATED DIARRHEA (CDAD), abdominal pain, diarrhea, eructation, flatulence. **Endo:** hyperglycemia. **F and E:** hypomagnesemia (especially if treatment duration ≥3 mo). **GU:** acute interstitial nephritis. **Hemat:** vitamin B_{12} deficiency. **MS:** bone fracture.

Interactions

Drug-Drug: May ↓ levels of **atazanavir** and **nelfinavir**; avoid concurrent use with either of these antiretrovirals. May ↓ absorption of drugs requiring acid pH, including **ketoconazole**, **itraconazole**, **ampicillin esters**, **iron salts**, **erlotinib**, and **mycophenolate mofetil**; concomitant use with **atazanavir** not recommended. May ↑ risk of bleeding with **warfarin** (monitor INR/PT). Hypomagnesemia ↑ risk of **digoxin** toxicity. May ↑ **methotrexate** levels.

Route/Dosage

GERD

PO (Adults): *Short-term treatment of erosive esophagitis associated with GERD*—40 mg once daily for up to 8 wk; *Maintenance of healing of erosive esophagitis*—40 mg once daily.
PO (Children ≥5 yr): *15–39 kg*–20 mg once daily for up to 8 wk; ≥*40 kg*–40 mg once daily for up to 8 wk.
IV (Adults): 40 mg once daily for 7–10 days.

Gastric Hypersecretory Conditions

PO (Adults): 40 mg twice daily, up to 120 mg twice daily.
IV (Adults): 80 mg q 12 hr (up to 240 mg/day).

Availability (generic available)

Delayed-release tablets: 20 mg, 40 mg. **Cost:** *Generic*—All strengths $368.22/90. **Powder for injection (requires reconstitution):** 40 mg/vial. **Delayed-release oral suspension:** 40 mg/packet. **Cost:** $7.60/1 pkt.

P

NURSING IMPLICATIONS

Assessment

- Assess patient routinely for epigastric or abdominal pain and for frank or occult blood in stool, emesis, or gastric aspirate.
- ***Lab Test Considerations:*** May cause abnormal liver function tests, including ↑ AST, ALT, alkaline phosphatase, and bilirubin.
- May cause hypomagnesemia. Monitor serum magnesium prior to and periodically during therapy.

Potential Nursing Diagnoses

Acute pain (Indications)

Implementation

- Do not confuse Protonix (pantoprazole) with Lotronex (alosetron) or protamine.
- Patients receiving pantoprazole IV should be converted to PO dosing as soon as possible.
- Monitor bowel function. Diarrhea, abdominal cramping, fever, and bloody stools should be reported to health care professional promptly as a sign of Clostridium difficile-associated diarrhea (CDAD). May begin up to several weeks following cessation of therapy.
- **PO:** May be administered with or without food. Do not break, crush, or chew tablets.
- Antacids may be used concurrently.

IV Administration

- **IV:** Reconstitute each vial with 10 mL of 0.9% NaCl. Reconstituted solution is stable for 6 hr at room temperature.
- **IV Push:** ***Diluent:*** Administer undiluted. ***Concentration:*** 4 mg/mL. ***Rate:*** Administer over at least 2 min.
- **Intermittent Infusion:** ***Diluent:*** Dilute further with D5W, 0.9% NaCl, or LR. ***Concentration:*** 0.4–0.8 mg/mL. Diluted solution is stable for 24 hr at room temperature. ***Rate:*** Administer over 15 min at a rate of <3 mg/min.
- **Y-Site Compatibility:** allopurinol, alprostadil, amifostine, aminocaproic acid, amikacin, aminophylline, amphotericin B lipid complex, amphotericin B liposome, ampicillin, ampicillin/sulbactam, anidulafungin, argatroban, azithromycin, bleomycin, bumetanide, cangrelor, carboplatin, carmustine, ceftaroline, ceftriaxone, cyclophosphamide, cytarabine, docetaxel, doripenem, doxorubicin liposomal, doxycycline, ertapenem, fluorouracil, foscarnet, fosphenytoin, ganciclovir, granisetron, imipenem/cilastatin, irinotecan, mesna, methyldopate, paclitaxel, penicillin G sodium, pentazocine, pentobarbital, phenobarbital, phenylephrine, potassium chloride, procainamide, rifampin, succinylcholine, sufentanil, telavancin, teniposide, theophylline, tigecycline, tirofiban, vasopressin, zidovudine, zoledronic acid.
- **Y-Site Incompatibility:** alemtuzumab, alfentanil, amphotericin B colloidal, atropine, aztreonam, buprenorphine, butorphanol, calcium acetate, calcium chloride, cefepime, cefotaxime, cefotetan, chloramphenicol, chlorpromazine, ciprofloxacin, cisatracurium, cisplatin, dacarbazine, dactinomycin, dantrolene, daptomycin, daunorubicin hydrochloride, dexamethasone, dexmedetomidine, dexrazoxane, diazepam, diltiazem, diphenhydramine, dobutamine, dolasetron, doxorubicin hydrochloride, droperidol, ephedrine, epirubicin, esmolol, etoposide, etoposide phosphate, famotidine, fenoldopam, fentanyl, fluconazole, fludarabine, furosemide, gemcitabine, glycopyrrolate, haloperidol, hydralazine, hydromorphone, hydroxyzine, idarubicin, ifosfamide, insulin, ketorolac, labetalol, leucovorin, levofloxacin, levorphanol, lidocaine, linezolid, lorazepam, mechlorethamine, melphalan, meperidine, meropenem, methotrexate, methylprednisolone, metoprolol, metronidazole, midazolam, milrinone, mitomycin, mitoxantrone, moxifloxacin, multivitamins, mycophenolate, nalbuphine, naloxone, nesiritide, nicardipine, norepinephrine, ondansetron, palonosetron, pancuronium, pemetrexed, pentamidine, phenytoin, potassium acetate, potassium phosphates, prochlorperazine, promethazine, propranolol, quinupristin/dalfopristin, ranitidine, remifentanil, rocuronium, sodium acetate, sodium phosphates, streptozocin, thiotepa, topotecan, vecuronium, verapamil, vinblastine, vincristine, vinorelbine, voriconazole, solutions containing zinc.

Patient/Family Teaching

- Instruct patient to take medication as directed for the full course of therapy, even if feeling better.
- Advise patient to avoid alcohol, products containing aspirin or NSAIDs, and foods that may cause an increase in GI irritation.
- Advise patient to report onset of black, tarry stools; diarrhea; or abdominal pain to health care professional promptly. Instruct patient to notify health care professional immediately if rash, diarrhea, abdominal cramping, fever, or bloody stools occur and not to treat with antidiarrheals without consulting health care professional.
- Instruct patient to notify health care professional of all Rx or OTC medications, vitamins, or herbal products being taken and consult health care professional before taking any new medications.
- Advise female patients to notify health care professional if pregnancy is planned or suspected or if breast feeding.

Evaluation/Desired Outcomes

- Decrease in abdominal pain heartburn, gastric irritation and bleeding in patients with GERD; may require up to 4 wk of therapy.
- Healing in patients with erosive esophagitis. Therapy is continued for up to 8 wk.

paricalcitol, See VITAMIN D COMPOUNDS.

PARoxetine hydrochloride

(par-**ox**-e-teen)

Paxil, Paxil CR

PARoxetine mesylate

Brisdelle, Pexeva

Classification

Therapeutic: antianxiety agents, antidepressants

Pharmacologic: selective serotonin reuptake inhibitors (SSRIs)

Pregnancy Category D

Indications

Paxil, Paxil CR, Pexeva: Major depressive disorder, panic disorder. **Paxil, Pexeva**: Obsessive compulsive disorder (OCD), generalized anxiety disorder (GAD). **Paxil, Paxil CR**: Social anxiety disorder. **Paxil**: Posttraumatic stress disorder (PTSD). **Paxil CR**: Premenstrual dysphoric disorder (PMDD). **Brisdelle**: Moderate to severe vasomotor symptoms associated with menopause.

Action

Inhibits neuronal reuptake of serotonin in the CNS, thus potentiating the activity of serotonin; has little effect on norepinephrine or dopamine; mechanism for benefit in treating vasomotor symptoms unknown. **Therapeutic Effects:** Antidepressant action. Decreased frequency of panic attacks, OCD, or anxiety. Improvement in manifestations of post-traumatic stress disorder. Decreased dysphoria prior to menses. Decreased vasomotor symptoms in postmenopausal women.

Pharmacokinetics

Absorption: Completely absorbed following oral administration. Controlled-release tablets are enteric-coated and control medication release over 4–5 hr.
Distribution: Widely distributed throughout body fluids and tissues, including the CNS; cross the placenta and enter breast milk.
Protein Binding: 95%.
Metabolism and Excretion: Highly metabolized by the liver (partly by P450 2D6 enzyme system); ⧖ the CYP2D6 enzyme system exhibits genetic polymorphism; ~7% of population may be poor metabolizers (PMs) and may have significantly ↑paroxetine concentrations and an ↑ risk of adverse effects. 2% excreted unchanged in urine.
Half-life: 21 hr.

TIME/ACTION PROFILE (antidepressant action)

ROUTE	ONSET	PEAK	DURATION
PO	1–4 wk	unknown	unknown

Contraindications/Precautions

Contraindicated in: Hypersensitivity; Concurrent use of MAO inhibitors or MAO-like drugs (linezolid or methylene blue); Concurrent use of thioridazine or pimozide.
Use Cautiously in: Risk of suicide (may ↑ risk of suicide attempt/ideation especially during early treatment or dose adjustment); History of seizures; History of bipolar disorder; Angle-closure glaucoma; OB: Use during the first trimester may be associated with an ↑ risk of cardiac malformations—consider fetal risk/maternal benefit; use during third trimester may result in neonatal serotonin syndrome requiring prolonged hospitalization, respiratory and nutritional support; Lactation: Safety not established; discontinue drug or bottle feed; Pedi: May ↑ risk of suicide attempt/ideation especially during early treatment or dose adjustment; may be greater in children and adolescents (safety in children/adolescents not established); Geri: Severe renal hepatic impairment; geriatric or debilitated patients (daily dose should not exceed 40 mg); history of mania/risk of suicide.

Adverse Reactions/Side Effects

CNS: NEUROLEPTIC MALIGNANT SYNDROME, SUICIDAL THOUGHTS, anxiety, dizziness, drowsiness, headache, insomnia, weakness, agitation, amnesia, confusion, emotional lability, hangover, impaired concentration, malaise, mental depression, syncope. **EENT:** blurred vision, rhinitis. **Resp:** cough, pharyngitis, respiratory disorders, yawning. **CV:** chest pain, edema, hypertension, palpitations, postural hypotension, tachycardia, vasodilation. **GI:** constipation, diarrhea, dry mouth, nausea, abdominal pain, ↓/↑ appetite, dyspepsia, flatulence, taste disturbances, vomiting. **GU:** ejaculatory disturbance, ↓ libido, genital disorders, infertility, urinary disorders, urinary frequency. **Derm:** STEVENS-JOHNSON SYNDROME, sweating, photosensitivity, pruritus, rash. **F and E:** hyponatremia. **Metab:** weight gain/loss. **MS:** back pain, bone fracture, myalgia, myopathy. **Neuro:** paresthesia, tremor. **Misc:** SEROTONIN SYNDROME, chills, fever.

Interactions

Drug-Drug: Concurrent use with **MAO inhibitors** may result in serious, potentially fatal reactions (wait at least 2 wk after stopping MAO inhibitor before initiating paroxetine; wait at least 2 wk after stopping paroxetine before starting MAO inhibitors). Concurrent use with **MAO-inhibitor like drugs**, such as **linezolid** or **methylene blue** may ↑ risk of serotonin syndrome; concurrent use contraindicated; do not start therapy in patients receiving **linezolid** or **methylene blue**; if **linezolid** or **methylene blue** need to be started in a patient receiving paroxetine, immediately discontinue paroxetine and monitor for signs/symptoms of serotonin syndrome for 2 wk or until 24 hr after last dose of linezolid or methylene blue, whichever comes first (may resume paroxetine therapy 24 hr after last dose of linezolid or methylene blue). Concurrent use with **pimozide** or **thioridazine** may ↑ risk of QT interval prolongation and torsades de pointes; concurrent use contraindicated. May ↓ metabolism and ↑ effects of certain **drugs that are metabolized by the liver**, including other **antidepressants**, **phenothiazines**, **class IC antiarrhythmics**, **risperidone**, **atomoxetine**, **theophylline**, and **quinidine**. Concurrent use should be undertaken with caution. **Cimetidine** ↑ blood levels. **Phenobarbital** and **phenytoin** may ↓ effectiveness. Concurrent use with **alcohol** is not recommended. May ↓ the effectiveness of **digoxin** and **tamoxifen**. May ↑ risk of bleeding with **warfarin**, **aspirin**, or **NSAIDS**. Drugs that affect serotonergic neurotransmitter systems, including **tricyclic antide-**

P

pressants, **SNRIs**, **fentanyl**, **buspirone**, **tramadol** and **triptans** ↑ risk of serotonin syndrome.
Drug-Natural Products: ↑ risk of serotonergic side effects including serotonin syndrome with **St. John's wort**, **SAMe**, and **tryptophan**.

Route/Dosage

Depression

PO (Adults): 20 mg as a single dose in the morning; may ↑ by 10 mg/day at weekly intervals (not to exceed 50 mg/day). *Controlled-release tablets*—25 mg once daily initially. May ↑ at weekly intervals by 12.5 mg (not to exceed 62.5 mg/day).
PO (Geriatric Patients or Debilitated Patients): 10 mg/day initially; may be slowly ↑ (not to exceed 40 mg/day). *Controlled-release tablets*—12.5 mg once daily initially; may be slowly ↑ (not to exceed 50 mg/day).

Obsessive-Compulsive Disorder

PO (Adults): 20 mg/day initially; ↑ by 10 mg/day at weekly intervals up to 40 mg (not to exceed 60 mg/day).

Panic Disorder

PO (Adults): 10 mg/day initially; ↑ by 10 mg/day at weekly intervals up to 40 mg (not to exceed 60 mg/day). *Controlled-release tablets*—12.5 mg/day initially; ↑ by 12.5 mg/day at weekly intervals (not to exceed 75 mg/day).

Social Anxiety Disorder

PO (Adults): 20 mg/day. *Controlled-release tablets*—12.5 mg/day initially; may ↑ by 12.5 mg/day weekly intervals (not to exceed 37.5 mg/day).

Generalized Anxiety Disorder

PO (Adults): 20 mg once daily initially; ↑ by 10 mg/day at weekly intervals (not to exceed 50 mg/day).

Post-Traumatic Stress Disorder

PO (Adults): 20 mg/day initially; may ↑ by 10 mg/day at weekly intervals (not to exceed 50 mg/day).

Premenstrual Dysphoric Disorder

PO (Adults): *Controlled-release tablets*—12.5 mg once daily throughout menstrual cycle or during luteal phase of menstrual cycle only; may ↑ to 25 mg/day after one week.

Menopausal Vasomotor Symptoms

PO (Adults): 7.5 mg once daily at bedtime.

Hepatic Impairment

PO (Adults): Paxil, Paxil CR, or Pexeva: *Severe hepatic impairment*—10 mg/day initially; may slowly ↑ (not to exceed 40 mg/day). *Controlled-release tablets*—12.5 mg once daily initially; may slowly ↑ (not to exceed 50 mg/day).

Renal Impairment

PO (Adults): Paxil, Paxil CR, or Pexeva: *Severe renal impairment*—10 mg/day initially; may slowly ↑ (not to exceed 40 mg/day). *Controlled-release tablets*—12.5 mg once daily initially; may slowly ↑ (not to exceed 50 mg/day).

Availability (generic available)

Paroxetine hydrochloride tablets: 10 mg, 20 mg, 30 mg, 40 mg. **Cost:** *Generic*—10 mg $9.93/90, 20 mg $9.93/90, 30 mg $18.82/90, 40 mg $14.88/90. **Paroxetine hydrochloride controlled-release tablets:** 12.5 mg, 25 mg, 37.5 mg. **Cost:** *Generic*—12.5 mg $263.62/90, 25 mg $254.13/90, 37.5 mg $270.06/90. **Paroxetine hydrochloride oral suspension (orange flavor):** 10 mg/5 mL. **Cost:** $268.35/250 mL. **Paroxetine mesylate tablets (Pexeva):** 10 mg, 20 mg, 30 mg, 40 mg. **Cost:** 10 mg $235.38/30, 20 mg $244.69/30, 30 mg $253.99/30, 40 mg $263.33/30. **Paroxetine mesylate capsules (Brisdelle):** 7.5 mg. **Cost:** $161.64/30.

NURSING IMPLICATIONS

Assessment

- Monitor appetite and nutritional intake. Weigh weekly. Notify health care professional of continued weight loss. Adjust diet as tolerated to support nutritional status.
- **Depression:** Monitor mental status (orientation, mood, behavior). Inform health care professional if patient demonstrates significant increase in anxiety, nervousness, or insomnia.
- Assess for suicidal tendencies, especially during early therapy. Restrict amount of drug available to patient. Risk may be increased in children, adolescents, and adults ≤24 yr.
- Assess for serotonin syndrome (mental changes [agitation, hallucinations, coma], autonomic instability [tachycardia, labile BP, hyperthermia], neuromuscular aberations [hyper reflexia, incoordination], and/or GI symptoms [nausea, vomiting, diarrhea]), especially in patients taking other serotonergic drugs (SSRIs, SNRIs, triptans).
- Monitor for development of neuroleptic malignant syndrome (fever, respiratory distress, tachycardia, seizures, diaphoresis, hypertension or hypotension, pallor, tiredness). Discontinue paroxetine and notify health care professional immediately if these symptoms occur.
- Assess for rash periodically during therapy. May cause Stevens-Johnson syndrome. Discontinue therapy if severe or if accompanied with fever, general malaise, fatigue, muscle or joint aches, blisters, oral lesions, conjunctivitis, hepatitis and/or eosinophilia.
- **OCD:** Assess patient for frequency of obsessive-compulsive behaviors. Note degree to which these thoughts and behaviors interfere with daily functioning.

- **Panic Attacks:** Assess frequency and severity of panic attacks.
- **Social Anxiety Disorder:** Assess frequency and severity of episodes of anxiety.
- **Post-traumatic Stress Disorder:** Assess manifestations of post-traumatic stress disorder periodically during therapy.
- **Premenstrual Dysphoria:** Assess symptoms of premenstrual distress prior to and during therapy.
- ***Lab Test Considerations:*** Monitor CBC and differential periodically during therapy. Report leukopenia or anemia.

Potential Nursing Diagnoses

Ineffective coping (Indications)
Risk for injury (Side Effects)

Implementation

- Do not confuse paroxetine with fluoxetine, duloxetine, or piroxicam. Do not confuse Paxil (paroxetine) with Doxil (doxorubicin liposomal), Taxol (paclitaxel), or Plavix (clopidogrel). Do not confuse Pexeva (paroxetine mesylate) with Lexiva (fosamprenavir).
- Paroxetine mesylate (Pexeva) cannot be substituted with paroxetine (Paxil or Paxil CR) or generic paroxetine.
- Periodically reassess dose and continued need for therapy.
- **PO:** Administer as a single dose in the morning. May administer with food to minimize GI irritation.
- Swallow tablets whole. Do not crush, break, or chew. Shake suspension before administering.
- Taper to avoid potential withdrawal reactions.

Patient/Family Teaching

- Instruct patient to take paroxetine as directed. Take missed doses as soon as possible and return to regular dosing schedule. Do not double doses. Caution patient to consult health care professional before discontinuing paroxetine. Daily doses should be decreased slowly. Abrupt withdrawal may cause dizziness, sensory disturbances, agitation, anxiety, nausea, and sweating. Advise patient to read *Medication Guide* before starting and with each Rx refill in case of changes.
- May cause drowsiness or dizziness. Caution patient to avoid driving and other activities requiring alertness until response to the drug is known.
- Advise patient, family and caregivers to look for suicidality, especially during early therapy or dose changes. Notify health care professional immediately if thoughts about suicide or dying, attempts to commit suicide, new or worse depression or anxiety, agitation or restlessness, panic attacks, insomnia, new or worse irritability, aggressiveness, acting on dangerous impulses, mania, or other changes in mood or behavior or if symptoms of serotonin syndrome or neuroleptic malignant syndrome occur.
- Instruct patient to notify health care professional of all Rx or OTC medications, vitamins, or herbal products being taken and consult health care professional before taking any new medications and to avoid alcohol or other CNS-depressant drugs during therapy.
- Inform patient that frequent mouth rinses, good oral hygiene, and sugarless gum or candy may minimize dry mouth. Saliva substitute may be used. Consult dentist if dry mouth persists for more than 2 wk.
- Advise patient to notify health care professional if headache, weakness, nausea, anorexia, anxiety, or insomnia persists.
- Instruct female patient to inform health care professional if pregnancy is planned or suspected or if breast feeding.
- Emphasize the importance of follow-up exams to monitor progress. Encourage patient participation in psychotherapy to improve coping skills.

Evaluation/Desired Outcomes

- Increased sense of well-being.
- Renewed interest in surroundings. May require 1–4 wk of therapy to obtain antidepressant effects.
- Decrease in obsessive-compulsive behaviors.
- Decrease in frequency and severity of panic attacks.
- Decrease in frequency and severity of episodes of anxiety.
- Improvement in manifestations of post-traumatic stress disorder.
- Decreased dysphoria prior to menses.

P

pazopanib (pah-zoe-puh-nib)

Votrient

Classification
Therapeutic: antineoplastics
Pharmacologic: kinase inhibitors

Pregnancy Category D

Indications

Advanced renal cell carcinoma. Advanced soft tissue sarcoma in patients who have previously received chemotherapy.

Action

Acts as a tyrosine kinase inhibitor of several vascular endothelial growth factor (VEGF) receptors, platelet-derived growth factor receptor, fibroblast growth factor receptor, cytokine receptor, interleukin-2 receptor inducible T-cell kinase, leukocyte-specific protein tyrosine kinase, and transmembrane glycoprotein receptor tyrosine kinase. Overall effect is decreased angiogenesis in tumors. **Therapeutic Effects:** Decreased growth and spread of renal cell carcinoma. Improvement in progression-free survival.

Pharmacokinetics

Absorption: Well absorbed following oral administration; crushing tablet and ingesting food ↑ absorption.
Distribution: unknown.
Protein Binding: >99%.
Metabolism and Excretion: Mostly metabolized by the liver (primarily by the CYP3A4 enzyme system, minor amounts by CYP1A2 and CYP2C8) followed by elimination in feces; <4% excreted by the kidneys.
Half-life: 30.9 hr.

TIME/ACTION PROFILE (blood levels)

ROUTE	ONSET	PEAK	DURATION
PO	PO	2–4 hr	24 hr

Contraindications/Precautions

Contraindicated in: Severe hepatic impairment; History of hemoptysis, cerebral or GI bleeding in preceding 6 mo; Risk/history of arterial thrombotic events, including MI, angina or ischemic stroke within preceding 6 mo; Concurrent use of strong CYP3A4 inhibitors (if concurrent use is necessary, ↓ dose of pazopanib); Concurrent use of strong CYP3A4 inducers (may ↓ effectiveness); Concurrent use of drugs that have narrow therapeutic windows and that are metabolized by CYP3A4, CYP2D6, or CYP2C8 enzyme systems; OB: May cause fetal harm, avoid use during pregnancy; Lactation: Avoid use during breast feeding.
Use Cautiously in: Congenital prolonged QTc interval or concurrent medications/diseases that prolong QTc (may ↑ risk of torsades de pointes); Electrolyte abnormalities (correct prior to use; may ↑ risk of potentially serious arrhythmia); Patients at risk for gastrointestinal perforation/fistula; Surgery; interruption of therapy recommended; Hypertension; control before therapy is initiated; Hypothyroidism (may worsen condition); Concurrent use of inducers of the CYP3A4 enzyme system; consider alternate concurrent medication with little or no enzyme induction potential or avoid pazopanib; Moderate hepatic impairment (dose ↓ recommended); Geri: May be more sensitive to drug effects, consider age-related ↓ in cardiac, renal, and hepatic function, concurrent disease states and drug therapy; ↑ risk of hepatotoxicity; Rep: Women with childbearing potential; Pedi: Safety and effectiveness not established.

Adverse Reactions/Side Effects

CNS: REVERSIBLE POSTERIOR LEUKOENCEPHALOPATHY SYNDROME, STROKE, fatigue, weakness. **CV:** HF, MYOCARDIAL INFARCTION, QT INTERVAL PROLONGATION, DEEP VEIN THROMBOSIS, bradycardia, hypertension, altered taste, chest pain, dyspepsia, heart failure. **GI:** GI PERFORATION/FISTULA, HEPATOTOXICITY, PANCREATITIS, abdominal pain, anorexia, diarrhea, nausea, vomiting. **GU:** HEMOLYTIC UREMIC SYNDROME, proteinuria. **Derm:** alopecia, facial edema, palmar-plantar erythrodysesthesia (hand-foot syndrome), rash, skin depigmentation. **Endo:** hypothyroidism. **Hemat:** BLEEDING, THROMBOEMBOLIC EVENTS, THROMBOTIC THROMBOCYTOPENIC PURPURA. **Metab:** ↑ lipase, weight loss. **MS:** arthralgia, muscle spasms. **Resp:** INTERSTITIAL LUNG DISEASE, PULMONARY EMBOLISM. **Misc:** hair color changes (depigmentation).

Interactions

Drug-Drug: Concurrent use of **strong CYP3A4 inhibitors**, including **ketoconazole**, **ritonavir** and **clarithromycin** may ↑ levels and should be avoided; if required, dose of pazopanib should be ↓ to 400 mg daily or more if necessary. Concurrent use of **strong CYP3A4 inducers**, including **rifampin**, may ↓ levels and effectiveness and should be avoided. Concurrent use with **drugs with narrow therapeutic windows that are metabolized by CYP3A4, CYP2D6, or CYP2C8** may ↑ levels of such drugs and the risk of toxicity/adverse reactions is not recommended. ↑ risk of hepatotoxicity with **simvastatin**. **Drugs that ↑ the pH**, including **proton pump inhibitors** and **H_2 receptor antagonists** may ↓ levels; avoid concurrent use; use short-acting antacid instead. **Antacids** may ↓ levels; separate doses by several hours.
Drug-Food: **Grapefruit juice** may ↑ levels; avoid concurrent use.

Route/Dosage

PO (Adults): 800 mg once daily; *Concurrent use of strong CYP3A4 inhibitors*—400 mg once daily, further reductions may be necessary.

Hepatic Impairment

PO (Adults): *Moderate hepatic impairment*—200 mg once daily.

Availability

Tablets: 200 mg.

NURSING IMPLICATIONS

Assessment

- Monitor BP during frequent therapy; may cause hypertension. BP should be well-controlled prior to initiating therapy. If persistent hypertension occurs despite antihypertensive therapy, reduce dose. If hypertension persists and is severe, discontinue therapy. Baseline and periodic evaluation of LVEF is recommended in patients at risk of cardiac dysfunction.
- Obtain baseline ECG and monitor periodically during therapy. Maintain serum calcium, magnesium, and potassium within normal range during therapy.
- Monitor for signs and symptoms of GI perforation and fistula (abdominal pain; swelling in stomach area; vomiting blood; black sticky stools; GI bleeding) during therapy.

- ***Lab Test Considerations:*** Monitor serum liver tests before initiation and wks 3, 5, 7, and 9, then at month 3 and month 4 if symptoms occur. Monitor periodically after month 4. *If isolated ALT ↑ between 3 and 8 times the upper limit of normal,* therapy may continue with weekly monitoring of liver function until ALT returns to Grade 1 or baseline. *If isolated ALT ↑ >8 times the upper limit of normal,* stop therapy until ALT returns to Grade 1 or baseline. If benefit outweighs risk, may reintroduce at reduced dose of 400 mg/day with weekly serum liver tests for 8 wk. Following reintroduction, if ALT ↑ >3 times the upper limit of normal recurs, permanently discontinue pazopanib. *If ALT ↑ occurs concurrently with ↑ serum bilirubin >2 times the upper limit of normal,* discontinue pazopanib permanently. Monitor liver function tests until return to baseline. *Patients with only mild indirect hyperbilirubinemia (Gilbert's syndrome) and ↑ ALT >3 times the upper limit of normal* should be managed as per recommendations for ↑ ALT.
- Monitor thyroid function periodically during therapy. May cause hypothyroidism.
- Obtain baseline urinalysis and monitor periodically. May cause proteinuria. Discontinue therapy if Grade 4 proteinuria develops.
- May cause leukopenia, neutropenia, thrombocytopenia, and lymphocytopenia.
- May cause ↑ AST and ↓ serum phosphorous, sodium, and magnesium. May cause ↑ or ↓ serum glucose.

Potential Nursing Diagnoses

Deficient knowledge, related to medication regimen (Patient/Family Teaching)

Implementation

- **PO:** Administer at least 1 hr before or 2 hr after a meal. Swallow tablets whole; do not crush tablets.

Patient/Family Teaching

- Instruct patient to take pazopanib on an empty stomach as directed. Take missed doses as soon as remembered; if less than 12 hr before next dose, omit dose. Advise patient to read the *Medication Guide* prior to taking pazopanib and with each Rx refill; new information may be available.
- Advise patient to avoid drinking grapefruit juice or eating grapefruit during therapy; may increase amounts of panopanib absorbed.
- Advise patient to notify health care professional immediately if signs and symptoms of liver problems (yellowing of skin or whites of eyes, unusual darkening of urine, unusual tiredness, pain in the right upper stomach area), heart failure (shortness of breath), heart attack or stroke (chest pain or pressure; pain in arms, back, neck or jaw; shortness of breath; numbness or weakness on one side of body; trouble talking; headache; dizziness), blood clots (new chest pain, trouble breathing or shortness of breath that starts suddenly; leg pain; swelling of arms and hands, or legs and feet; cool or pale arm or leg), bleeding problems (unusual bleeding, bruising, wounds that do not heal), GI perforation or fistula, reversible posterior leukoencephalopathy syndrome (headaches, seizures, lack of energy, confusion, high BP, loss of speech, blindness or changes in vision, and problems thinking), severe increase in BP (severe chest pain, severe head ache, blurred vision, confusion, nausea and vomiting, severe anxiety, shortness of breath, seizures, unconsciousness), interstitial lung disease (persistent cough, shortness of breath) or severe infections (fever; cold symptoms such as runny nose or sore throat that do not go away; flu symptoms such as cough, tiredness, and body aches; pain when urinating; cuts, scrapes or wounds that are red, warm, swollen or painful) occur.
- Inform patient that diarrhea frequently occurs. Instruct patient on ways to manage diarrhea and to notify health care professional if moderate to severe diarrhea occurs.
- Inform patient that loss of color (depigmentation) of skin or hair may occur during therapy. Explore methods of coping.
- Instruct patient to notify health care professional of all Rx or OTC medications, vitamins, or herbal products being taken and consult health care professional before taking any new medications.
- Advise patient to notify health care professional of any impending surgery. Panzopanib must be stopped for at least 7 days prior to surgery due to the affects on healing.
- Advise female patients to use effective contraception during therapy and to notify health care professional immediately if pregnancy is suspected.

Evaluation/Desired Outcomes

- Decreased growth and spread of renal cell carcinoma.
- Improvement in spread of sarcoma.

P

pegaspargase

(peg-ass-**par**-jase)

Oncaspar

Classification

Therapeutic: antineoplastics

Pharmacologic: enzymes

Pregnancy Category C

Indications

Treatment (usually with other agents) of acute lymphoblastic leukemia (ALL) in patients who have had a previous hypersensitivity reaction to native asparaginase.

Action

Consists of L-asparaginase bound to polyethylene glycol (PEG). This compound depletes asparagine, which leukemic cells cannot synthesize. Normal cells are able to produce their own asparagine and are less susceptible to the effects of asparaginase. Binding to PEG renders asparaginase less antigenic and therefore less likely to induce hypersensitivity reactions. **Therapeutic Effects:** Death of leukemic cells.

Pharmacokinetics

Absorption: IV administration results in complete bioavailability.

Distribution: Unknown.

Metabolism and Excretion: Metabolized by serum proteases and in the reticuloendothelial system.

Half-life: 5.7 days (less in patients with previous hypersensitivity to native L-asparaginase).

TIME/ACTION PROFILE (hematologic effects)

ROUTE	ONSET	PEAK	DURATION
IV	rapid	unknown	14 days

Contraindications/Precautions

Contraindicated in: Pancreatitis or history of pancreatitis; History of previous hemorrhagic reaction to asparaginase therapy; Previous hypersensitivity reactions to pegaspargase.

Use Cautiously in: History of previous hypersensitivity reactions to other drugs; Rep: Women with childbearing potential; OB, Lactation: Safety not established.

Adverse Reactions/Side Effects

CNS: SEIZURES, headache, malaise. **GI:** HEPATOTOXICITY, PANCREATITIS, abdominal pain, anorexia, diarrhea, lip edema, nausea, vomiting. **Derm:** jaundice. **Endo:** hypercholesterolemia, hyperglycemia, hypertriglyceridemia. **F and E:** peripheral edema. **Hemat:** ↓ fibrinogen, disseminated intravascular coagulation, hemolytic anemia, ↑ thromboplastin, leukopenia, pancytopenia, thrombocytopenia. **Local:** injection site hypersensitivity, injection site pain, thrombosis. **MS:** arthralgia, myalgia, pain in extremities. **Neuro:** paresthesia. **Misc:** chills, hypersensitivity reactions, night sweats.

Interactions

Drug-Drug: May alter response to **anticoagulants** or **antiplatelet agents**. May alter the response to other **drugs that are metabolized by the liver**.

Route/Dosage

IM, IV (Adults up to 21 yr, and Children with Body Surface Area ≥0.6 m^2): 2500 units/m^2 q 14 days (usually in combination with other agents).

IM, IV (Children with Body Surface Area <0.6 m^2): 82.5 units/kg q 14 days (usually in combination with other agents).

Availability

Injection: 750 units/mL.

NURSING IMPLICATIONS

Assessment

- Assess patient for previous hypersensitivity reactions to native L-asparaginase. Monitor for hypersensitivity reaction (urticaria, diaphoresis, facial swelling, joint pain, hypotension, bronchospasm) for at least 1 hr following administration. Epinephrine and resuscitation equipment should be readily available. Reaction may occur up to 2 hr after administration.
- Monitor for development of bone marrow depression. Assess for fever, sore throat, and signs of infection. Monitor platelet count throughout therapy. Assess for bleeding (bleeding gums, bruising, petechiae, guaiac test stools, urine, and emesis). Avoid giving IM injections and taking rectal temperatures. Apply pressure to venipuncture sites for 10 min. Anemia may occur. Monitor for increased fatigue, dyspnea, and orthostatic hypotension.
- Monitor patient frequently for signs of pancreatitis (nausea, vomiting, abdominal pain).
- Assess nausea, vomiting, and appetite. Weigh patient weekly. Prophylactic antiemetics may be used prior to administration.
- ***Lab Test Considerations:*** Monitor CBC prior to and periodically throughout therapy. May alter coagulation studies. Fibrinogen may be decreased; PT and partial thromboplastin time (PTT) may be ↑.
- Monitor serum amylase frequently to detect pancreatitis.
- Monitor blood glucose; may cause hyperglycemia.
- May cause elevated BUN and serum creatinine.
- Hepatotoxicity may be manifested by increased AST, ALT, alkaline phosphatase, or bilirubin. Liver function tests usually return to normal after therapy.
- May cause ↓ serum calcium.
- May cause elevated serum and urine uric acid and hyponatremia.
- May cause hypercholesterolemia and hypertriglyceridemia.

Potential Nursing Diagnoses

Risk for infection (Adverse Reactions)

Implementation

- IM is the preferred route because of a lower incidence of adverse reactions.
- Solutions should be prepared in a biologic cabinet. Wear gloves, gown, and mask while handling medication. Discard equipment in specially designated containers.
- **IM:** Limit single injection volume to 2 mL. If volume of injection is >2 mL, use multiple injection sites.

IV Administration

- **Intermittent Infusion:** ***Diluent:*** Dilute each dose in 100 mL of 0.9% NaCl or D5W. Do not shake or agitate. Do not use if solution is cloudy or has formed a precipitate.
- Use only 1 dose per vial; do not re-enter the vial. Discard unused portions.
- Keep refrigerated but do not freeze. Freezing destroys activity but does not change the appearance of pegaspargase. ***Rate:*** Administer over 1–2 hr via Y-site through an infusion that is already running.
- **Additive Incompatibility:** Information unavailable. Do not admix with other medications or solutions.

Patient/Family Teaching

- Inform patient of the possibility of hypersensitivity reactions, including anaphylaxis.
- Advise patient that concurrent use of other medications may increase the risk of bleeding and the toxicity of pegaspargase. Consult health care professional before taking any other medications, including OTC drugs.
- Instruct patient to notify health care professional if abdominal pain, severe nausea and vomiting, jaundice, fever, chills, sore throat, bleeding or bruising, excess thirst or urination, or mouth sores occur. Caution patient to avoid crowds and persons with known infections. Instruct patient to use soft toothbrush, electric razor, and to be especially careful to avoid falls. Patients should also be cautioned not to drink alcoholic beverages or take medications containing aspirin or NSAIDs because these may precipitate gastric bleeding.
- Instruct patient not to receive any vaccinations without advice of health care professional. Advise parents that this may alter child's immunization schedule.
- Advise female patient to notify health care professional if pregnancy is planned or suspected or if breast feeding.
- Emphasize the need for periodic lab tests to monitor for side effects.

Evaluation/Desired Outcomes

- Improvement of hematologic status in patients with leukemia.

pegfilgrastim (peg-fil-**gra**-stim)

Neulasta

Classification

Therapeutic: colony-stimulating factors

Pregnancy Category C

Indications

To decrease the incidence of infection (febrile neutropenia) in patients with nonmyeloid malignancies receiving myelosuppressive antineoplastics associated with a high risk of febrile neutropenia.

Action

Filgrastim is a glycoprotein that binds to and stimulates neutrophils to divide and differentiate. Also activates mature neutrophils. Binding to a polyethylene glycol molecule prolongs its effects. **Therapeutic Effects:** Decreased incidence of infection in patients who are neutropenic from chemotherapy.

Pharmacokinetics

Absorption: Well absorbed following subcut administration.

Distribution: Unknown.

Metabolism and Excretion: Unknown.

Half-life: 15–80 hr.

TIME/ACTION PROFILE

ROUTE	ONSET	PEAK	DURATION
Subcut	unknown	unknown	unknown

P

Contraindications/Precautions

Contraindicated in: Hypersensitivity to filgrastim or *Escherichia coli*-derived proteins.

Use Cautiously in: Patients with sickle cell disease (↑ risk of sickle cell crisis); Concurrent use of lithium; Malignancy with myeloid characteristics; **OB, Lactation:** Pregnancy or lactation; **Pedi:** 6 mg fixed dose should not be used in infants, children, and adolescents weighing <45 kg.

Adverse Reactions/Side Effects

Resp: ADULT RESPIRATORY DISTRESS SYNDROME (ARDS). **GI:** SPLENIC RUPTURE. **GU:** glomerulonephritis. **Hemat:** SICKLE CELL CRISIS, leukocytosis. **MS:** medullary bone pain. **Misc:** allergic reaction including ANAPHYLAXIS, CAPILLARY LEAK SYNDROME.

Interactions

Drug-Drug: Simultaneous use with **antineoplastics** may have adverse effects on rapidly proliferating neutrophils; avoid use for 24 hr before and 24 hr following chemotherapy. **Lithium** may potentiate the release of neutrophils; concurrent use should be undertaken cautiously.

Route/Dosage

Subcut (Adults and Children >45 kg): 6 mg per chemotherapy cycle.

Availability

Solution for injection: 6 mg/0.6 mL in prefilled syringes.

NURSING IMPLICATIONS

Assessment

- Assess patient for bone pain throughout therapy. Pain is usually mild to moderate and usually controllable with nonopioid analgesics, but may require opioid analgesics.
- Assess patient periodically for signs of ARDS (fever, lung infiltration, respiratory distress). If ARDS occurs, treat condition and discontinue pegfilgrastim and/or withold until symptoms resolve.
- Monitor for signs and symptoms of capillary leak syndrome (hypotension, hypoalbuminemia, edema, hemoconcentration). Treat symptomatically.
- ***Lab Test Considerations:*** Obtain CBC and platelet count before chemotherapy. Monitor hematocrit, WBC, and platelet count regularly.
- May cause elevated LDH, alkaline phosphatase, and uric acid.

Potential Nursing Diagnoses

Risk for infection (Indications)
Acute pain (Side Effects)

Implementation

- Do not confuse Neulasta (pegfilgrastim) with Lunesta (eszopiclone) or Neumega (oprelvekin).
- Pegfilgrastim should not be administered between 14 days before and 24 hrs after administration of cytotoxic chemotherapy.
- Keep patients with sickle cell disease receiving pegfilgrastim well hydrated and monitor for sickle cell crisis.
- **Subcut:** Administer subcut once per chemotherapy cycle. Do not administer solutions that are discolored or contain particulate matter. Do not shake. Store refrigerated; may be allowed to reach room temperature for a maximum of 48 hr, but protect from light.
- Supplied in prefilled syringes. Following administration, activate UltraSafe Needle Guard to prevent needle sticks by placing hands behind needle, grasping guard with one hand, and sliding guard forward until needle is completely covered and guard clicks into place. If audible click is not heard, guard may not be completely activated. Dispose of by placing entire prefilled syringe with guard activated into puncture-proof container.
- **On-body Injector**: Small, one-time use, lightweight, battery-powered, and waterproof up to 8 feet for 1 hr. Fill by health care professional with a prefilled syringe before application. The prefilled syringe with *Neulasta* and the *On-body Injector* are part of *Neulasta Onpro kit*. The *On-body Injector* is applied directly to skin using a self-adhesive backing. The *On-body Injector* uses sounds and lights to informs its status. The prefilled syringe gray needle cap contains dry natural rubber, a derived from latex; do not use if allergic to latex. Apply to intact, non-irritated skin on abdomen or back of arm. Back of arm may only be used if there is a caregiver available to monitor the status of the *On-body Injector*. Approximately 27 hours after the *On-body Injector* is applied, *Neulasta* will be delivered over approximately 45 minutes. Follow manufacturer's instructions for monitoring and removal.

Patient/Family Teaching

- Advise patient to notify health care professional immediately if signs of allergic reaction (shortness of breath, hives, rash, pruritus, laryngeal edema) or signs of splenic rupture (left upper abdominal or shoulder tip pain) occur.
- Emphasize the importance of compliance with therapy and regular monitoring of blood counts.
- **Home Care Issues:** Instruct patient on correct disposal technique for home administration. Caution patient not to reuse needle, syringe, or drug product. Provide patient with a puncture-proof container for disposal of prefilled syringe.

Evaluation/Desired Outcomes

- Decreased incidence of infection in patients who receive bone marrow–depressing antineoplastics.

peginterferon alpha-2a, See INTERFERONS, ALPHA.

peginterferon alpha-2b, See INTERFERONS, ALPHA.

peginterferon beta-1a

(peg-in-ter-**feer**-on **bay**-ta)

Plegridy

Classification

Therapeutic: immune modifiers

Pharmacologic: interferons

Pregnancy Category C

Indications

Treatment of relapsing forms of multiple sclerosis.

Action

Antiviral and immunoregulatory properties produced by interacting with specific receptor sites on cell surfaces may explain beneficial effects. Produced by recombinant DNA technology. Pegylation prolongs duration of action. **Therapeutic Effects:** Reduced incidence of relapse (neurologic dysfunction) and slowed physical disability.

Pharmacokinetics

Absorption: Absorption follows subcutaneous administration.

Distribution: Unknown.
Metabolism and Excretion: Undergoes catabolism; excretion is mainly renal.
Half-life: 78 hr.

TIME/ACTION PROFILE (reduction in relapse rate)

ROUTE	ONSET	PEAK	DURATION
subcutaneous	within one mo	24–36 wk	unknown

Contraindications/Precautions

Contraindicated in: Hypersensitivity to natural or recombinant interferon beta or peginterferon.
Use Cautiously in: History of depression or suicidal ideation; History of seizures; Renal impairment (risk of adverse reactions may be ↑); Geri: Safe and effective use in geriatric patients has not been established; OB: Use during pregnancy only if potential benefit justifies potential fetal risk; Lactation: Use cautiously if breast feeding; Pedi: Safe and effective use in children has not been established.

Adverse Reactions/Side Effects

CNS: SEIZURES, SUICIDAL IDEATION, headache, depression, weakness. **CV:** HF. **GI:** HEPATOTOXICITY, nausea, vomiting. **Derm:** pruritus. **Hemat:** ↓ peripheral blood counts. **Local:** injection site pain/pruritus/reactions. **MS:** arthralgia, myalgia. **Misc:** allergic reactions including ANAPHYLAXIS, AUTOIMMUNE DISORDERS, chills, fever, flu-like symptoms.

Interactions

Drug-Drug: ↑ myelosuppression may occur with other **myelosuppressives** including **antineoplastics**. Concurrent use of **hepatotoxic agents** may ↑ the risk of hepatotoxicity (↑ liver enzymes).
Drug-Natural Products: Avoid concommitant use with **immunomodulating natural products** such as **astragalus**, **echinacea**, and **melatonin**.

Route/Dosage

Subcut (Adults): 63 mcg initially, followed by 94 mcg on day 15, then 125 mcg every 14 days.

Availability

Solution for subcutaneous injection in prefilled pens and syringes: 63 mcg/0.5 mL, 94 mcg/0.5 ml, 125 mcg/0.5 mL.

NURSING IMPLICATIONS

Assessment

- Assess frequency of exacerbations of symptoms of multiple sclerosis periodically during therapy.
- Monitor patient for signs of depression during therapy. If depression occurs, notify health care professional immediately.
- Monitor for injection site reactions (erythema, pain, pruritus, edema, bruising, drainage, necrosis,) Avoid injecting near area of reaction.
- Monitor patient with significant cardiac disease for worsening symptoms during initiation and periodically during therapy.
- ***Lab Test Considerations:*** Monitor serum AST, ALT and bilirubin periodically during therapy.
- Monitor CBC with differential and platelet counts periodically during therapy. May cause anemia, ↓ lymphocyte, ↓ neutrophil, and ↓ platelet counts.

Potential Nursing Diagnoses

Deficient knowledge, related to medication regimen (Patient/Family Teaching)

Implementation

- Administer prophylactic analgesics and/or antipyretics to prevent or minimize flu-like symptoms.
- **Subcut:** Inject subcut in abdomen, back of upper arm, and thigh every 14 days; rotate sites. Prefilled pens are for single dose; discard after use.

Patient/Family Teaching

- Instruct patient in correct technique for injection and care and disposal of equipment. Avoid injecting into areas of skin irritation, redness, bruising, infection, or scarring. Check injection site 2 hr after injection for redness, swelling, and tenderness. Notify health care professional if skin reaction does not clear in a few days. Caution patient not to reuse needles or syringes and provide patient with a puncture-resistant container for disposal.
- Instruct patient to take medication as directed; do not change dose or schedule without consulting health care professional. Advise patient to read *Medication Guide* prior to starting therapy and with each Rx refill in case of changes.
- Inform patient that flu-like symptoms (headache, fever, chills, myalgia, sweating, malaise, tiredness) may occur during therapy. Acetaminophen may be used for relief of fever and myalgias. Flu-like symptoms are not contagious.
- Advise patient to notify health care professional immediately if signs and symptoms of liver disease (yellowing of skin or whites of eyes, nausea, loss of appetite, tiredness, bleeding easily, confusion, sleepiness, dark colored urine, pale stools), depression, suicidal thoughts, seizures, allergic reactions (itching; swelling of face, eyes, lips, tongue, throat; trouble breathing; feeling faint; anxiousness; rash; hives) or autoimmune diseases (easy bleeding or bruising, thyroid gland problems, autoimmune hepatitis) occur.
- Instruct patient to notify health care professional of all Rx or OTC medications, vitamins, or herbal prod-

P

ucts being taken and to consult with health care professional before taking other medications.

- Advise patient to notify health care professional if pregnancy is planned or suspected or if breast feeding.

Evaluation/Desired Outcomes

- Decrease in the frequency of relapse (neurologic dysfunction) in patients with relapsing-remitting multiple sclerosis.

REMS

pegloticase (peg-loe-ti-kase)

Krystexxa

Classification

Therapeutic: antigout agents
Pharmacologic: enzymes

Pregnancy Category C

Indications

Treatment of chronic gout in adults who have not responded to/cannot tolerate xanthine oxidase inhibitors, including allopurinol.

Action

Consists of recombinant uricase covalently bonded to monomethoxypoly(ethylene glycol) [mPEG] uricase catalyzes the oxidation of uric acid to allantoin, a water soluble byproduct that is readily excreted in urine.
Therapeutic Effects: ↓ serum uric acid levels with resultant ↓ in attacks of gout and its sequelae.

Pharmacokinetics

Absorption: IV administration results in complete bioavailability.
Distribution: Unknown.
Metabolism and Excretion: Unknown.
Half-life: Unknown.

TIME/ACTION PROFILE (effects on serum uric acid)

ROUTE	ONSET	PEAK	DURATION
IV	rapid	within 24 hr	>300 hr

Contraindications/Precautions

Contraindicated in: Glucose-6–phosphate dehydrogenase (G6–PD) deficiency (risk of hemolysis and methemoglobinemia); Lactation: Breast feeding is not recommended.
Use Cautiously in: HF (may ↑ risk of exacerbation); Retreatment after a drug-free interval (↑ risk of allergic reactions, monitor carefully); Geri: May be more sensitive to drug effects; OB: Use during pregnancy only if clearly needed; Pedi: Safety and effectiveness not established.

Adverse Reactions/Side Effects

CV: chest pain. **EENT:** nasopharyngitis. **GI:** nausea, constipation, vomiting. **Derm:** contusion/ecchymoses. **Metab:** gout flare. **Misc:** allergic reactions including ANAPHYLAXIS, INFUSION REACTIONS.

Interactions

Drug-Drug: May interfere with the action of other **PEG-containing therapies**.

Route/Dosage

IV (Adults): 8 mg every 2 wk.

Availability

Injection: 8 mg/mL.

NURSING IMPLICATIONS

Assessment

- Monitor for joint pain and swelling. Gout flares frequently occur upon initiation of therapy, but do not require discontinuation. Administer prophylactic doses of colchicine or an NSAID at least 1 wk before and concurrently during the first 6 mo of therapy.
- Monitor for signs and symptoms of anaphylaxis (wheezing, peri-oral or lingual edema, hemodynamic instability, rash, urticaria) during and following infusion. May occur with any infusion, including initial infusion; usually occurs with 2 hr of infusion. Delayed reactions have also been reported. Risk is higher in patients with uric acid level >6 m g/dL.
- Monitor for infusion reactions (rash, redness of skin, dyspnea, flushing, chest discomfort, chest pain) during and periodically after infusion. If infusion reaction occurs, slow or stop infusion; restart at slower rate. If severe reaction occurs, discontinue infusion and treat as needed. Risk is greater in patients who have lost therapeutic response. Monitor patient for at least 1 hr following infusion.
- ***Lab Test Considerations:*** Monitor serum uric acid levels prior to infusion. Consider discontinuing therapy if levels ↑ to >6 m g/dL, especially if 2 consecutive levels are >6 m g/dL.

Potential Nursing Diagnoses

Chronic pain (Indications)

Implementation

- Premedicate patient with antihistamines and corticosteroids prior to infusion to minimize risk of anaphylaxis and infusion reaction. Administer in a setting with professionals prepared to manage anaphylaxis and infusion reactions.
- Discontinue all oral urate-lowering medications prior to and during therapy.

IV Administration

- **Intermittent Infusion:** Withdraw 1 mL of pegloticase from vial and inject into 250 mL bag of NaCl; discard unused portion. Invert bag several times to mix; do not shake. Solution is clear and colorless;

do not administer solutions that are discolored or contain a precipitate. Solution is stable for 4 hr if refrigerated or at room temperature. Store in refrigerator and protect from light; do not freeze. Allow solution to reach room temperature before administering; do not use artificial heating. ***Rate:*** Infuse over 120 min. Do not administer via IV push or bolus.

- **Additive Incompatibility:** Do not mix with other medications.

Patient/Family Teaching

- Explain purpose of pegloticase to patient. Instruct patient to read *Medication Guide* before starting therapy before each infusion.
- Advise patient to notify health care professional immediately if signs of anaphylaxis or infusion reaction occur.
- 🧬 Advise patient not to take pegloticase if they have G6PD deficiency.
- Inform patient that gout flares may initially ↑ at the start of pegloticase. Advise patient to not to stop therapy but to take medication (colchicine, NSAID) to reduce flares regularly for the first few months of pegloticase therapy.
- Instruct patient to not to take oral urate-lowering medications before or during therapy.
- Advise female patient to notify health care professional if pregnancy is planned or suspected or if breast feeding.

Evaluation/Desired Outcomes

- ↓ in uric acid levels with resultant improvement in gout symptoms in patients with chronic gout.

pembrolizumab

(pem-broe-**li**-zoo-mab)

Keytruda

Classification

Therapeutic: antineoplastics

Pharmacologic: monoclonal antibodies

Pregnancy Category D

Indications

Treatment of unresectable or metastatic melanoma with disease progression despite ipilimumab and a BRAF inhibitor (if positive for the BRAF V600 mutation).

Action

Programmed death (PD) receptor-1–blocking antibody (an IgG4 kappa immunglobulin) that blocks the interaction between PD-1 and its ligands PD-L1 and PD-L2 resuling in inhibition of T-cell proliferation and decreased cytokine production. **Therapeutic Effects:** Decreased spread of melanoma.

Pharmacokinetics

Absorption: IV administration results in complete bioavailability.

Distribution: Unknown.

Metabolism and Excretion: Unknown.

Half-life: 26 days.

TIME/ACTION PROFILE (response)

ROUTE	ONSET	PEAK	DURATION
IV	within 3 mo	unk	may persist for > 8.8 mos

Contraindications/Precautions

Contraindicated in: OB: Pregnancy (may cause fetal harm); Lactation: Discontinue pembrolizumab or discontinue breast feeding.

Use Cautiously in: Moderate to severe hepatic impairment; Rep: Females with reproductive potential; Pedi: Safe and effective use in children has not been established.

Adverse Reactions/Side Effects

CNS: <u>dizziness</u>, <u>fatigue</u>, <u>headache</u>, <u>insomnia</u>. **EENT:** immune-mediated optic neuritis. **Resp:** IMMUNE-MEDIATED PNEUMONITIS. **GI:** IMMUNE-MEDIATED COLITIS, IMMUNE-MEDIATED HEPATITIS, <u>↓ appetite</u>, <u>constipation</u>, <u>diarrhea</u>, <u>nausea</u>. **GU:** IMMUNE-MEDIATED NEPHRITIS. **Derm:** <u>pruritus</u>, <u>rash</u>, immune-mediated dermatitis, vitiligo. **Endo:** IMMUNE-MEDIATED HYPOPHYSITIS, immune-mediated hyperthyroidism, immune-mediated hypothyroidism, immune-mediated type 1 diabetes. **MS:** IMMUNE-MEDIATED RHABDOMYOLYSIS, <u>arthralgia</u>, <u>back pain</u>, <u>extremity pain</u>, <u>mylagia</u>, immune-mediated myasthenic syndrome. **Hemat:** <u>anemia</u>. **Misc:** INFUSION-RELATED REACTIONS, SEPSIS.

Interactions

Drug-Drug: None noted.

Route/Dosage

IV (Adults): 2 mg/kg every 3 wk.

Availability

Lyophilized powder for injection (requires reconstitution): 50 mg/vial.

NURSING IMPLICATIONS

Assessment

- Monitor for signs and symptoms of immune-mediated pneumonitis (shortness of breath, chest pain, new or worse cough) periodically during therapy. Evaluate with x-ray. Treat with corticosteroids for ≥Grade 2 pneumonitis. Withhold pembrolizumab and monitor symptoms for moderate (Grade 2) pneumonitis; resume therapy when recovery to Grade 0 to 1. Permanently discontinue for severe

P

(Grade 3) or life-threatening (Grade 4) pneumonitis.

- Monitor for signs and symptoms of colitis (diarrhea, abdominal pain, mucus or blood in stool, with or without fever). Treat with corticosteroids for ≥Grade 2 colitis. Withhold pembrolizumab and monitor symptoms for moderate (Grade 2) or severe (Grade 3) colitis; resume therapy when recovery to Grade 0 to 1. Permanently discontinue for life-threatening (Grade 4) colitis.
- Assess for signs and symptoms of immune-mediated hepatitis (yellowing of skin or whites of eyes, unusual darkening of urine, unusual tiredness, pain in right upper stomach) before each dose. Treat with corticosteroids for ≥Grade 2. Withhold or discontinue pembrolizumab depending on severity of liver enzyme elevations. Resume therapy when recovery to Grade 0 to 1.
- Monitor for clinical signs and symptoms of hypophysitis (persistent or unusual headache, extreme weakness, dizziness or fainting, vision changes) during therapy. Treat with corticosteroids for ≥Grade 2 hypophysitis. Withhold pembrolizumab and monitor symptoms for moderate (Grade 2) hypophysitis; withhold or discontinue for severe (Grade 3), and resume therapy when recovery to Grade 0 to 1. Permanently discontinue for life-threatening (Grade 4) hypophysitis.
- ***Lab Test Considerations:*** Monitor for changes in renal function. Treat with corticosteroids for ≥Grade 2 nephritis. Withhold pembrolizumab and monitor symptoms for moderate (Grade 2) nephritis; resume therapy when recovery to Grade 0 to 1. Permanently discontinue for severe (Grade 3) or life-threatening (Grade 4) nephritis.
- Monitor for changes in thyroid function at start of and periodically during therapy, and as indicated based on clinical evaluation. Administer corticosteroids for ≥Grade 3 hyperthyroidism, withhold pembrolizumab for severe (Grade 3) hyperthyroidism and resume therapy when recovery to Grade 0 to 1. Permanently discontinue for life-threatening (Grade 4) hyperthyroidism. Manage hypothyroidism with thyroid replacement without interruption of therapy or corticosteroids.

Potential Nursing Diagnoses

Diarrhea (Adverse Reactions)
Deficient knowledge, related to medication regimen (Patient/Family Teaching)

Implementation

IV Administration

- **Intermittent Infusion:** Reconstitute by injecting 2.3 mL of sterile water for injection along vial walls; swirl slowly, do not shake. Allow up to 5 min for bubbles to clear. Solution is clear to slightly opalescent, colorless to slightly yellow; do not administer solution if discolored or contains particulate matter other than translucent to white proteinaceous particles. Solution is stable at room temperature for up to 4 hr and 24 hr if refrigerated. ***Diluent:*** 0.9% NaCl. Mix using gently inversion. ***Concentration:*** 1 mg/mL to 10 mg/mL. ***Rate:*** Infuse through a sterile, non-pyrogenic, low-protein binding 0.2 micron to 0.5 micron in-line or add-on filter over 30 min.
- **Y-Site Incompatibility:** Do not administer other drugs through same infusion line.

Patient/Family Teaching

- Explain purpose of pembrolizumab to patient.
- Advise patient to notify health care professional immediately if signs and symptoms of pneumonitis, colitis, hepatitis, kidney problems (change in amount or color of urine), hormone gland problems (rapid heart beat, weight loss, increased sweating, weight gain, hair loss, feeling cold, constipation, deepening of voice, muscle aches, dizziness or fainting, persistent or unusual headache) occur.
- Instruct patient to notify health care professional of all Rx or OTC medications, vitamins, or herbal products being taken and to consult with health care professional before taking other medications.
- Rep: Advise female patient of reproductive potential to use highly effective contraception during and for 4 mo after last dose; may cause fetal harm. Avoid breast feeding during therapy.
- Emphasize importance of keeping scheduled appointments for blood work or other laboratory tests.

Evaluation/Desired Outcomes

- ↓ spread of melanoma.

PEMEtrexed (pe-me-trex-ed)

Alimta

Classification

Therapeutic: antineoplastics
Pharmacologic: antimetabolites, folate antagonists

Pregnancy Category D

Indications

Malignant pleural mesothelioma (with cisplatin) when tumor is unresectable or patient is not a candidate for surgery. Local advanced or metastatic nonsquamous non–small cell lung cancer as initial therapy (with cisplatin), in previously treated patients (as monotherapy), or as maintenance treatment in patients whose disease has not progressed after 4 cycles of platinum-based chemotherapy.

Action

Disrupts folate dependent metabolic processes involved in thymidine and purine synthesis. Converted intracellularly to polyglutamate form which increases duration of action. **Therapeutic Effects:** Decreases growth and spread of mesothelioma. Improved survival in patients with nonsquamous non–small cell lung cancer.

Pharmacokinetics

Absorption: IV administration results in complete bioavailability.
Distribution: Unknown.
Metabolism and Excretion: Minimal metabolism; 70–90% excreted unchanged in urine.
Half-life: 3.5 hr (normal renal function).

TIME/ACTION PROFILE (hematologic effects)

ROUTE	ONSET	PEAK	DURATION
IV	unknown	8–15 days	21 days

Contraindications/Precautions

Contraindicated in: Hypersensitivity; CCr <45 mL/min; OB, Lactation: Pregnancy, lactation.
Use Cautiously in: Concurrent use of NSAIDs in patients with CCr 45–79 mL/min (avoid those with short half-lives); 3rd space fluid accumulation (ascites, pleural effusions); consider drainage prior to therapy; Hepatic impairment (dose alteration recommended); Pedi: Safety not established.

Adverse Reactions/Side Effects

Resp: pharyngitis. **CV:** chest pain. **GI:** constipation, nausea, stomatitis, vomiting, anorexia, diarrhea, esophagitis, mouth pain. **Derm:** desquamation, rash. **Hemat:** anemia, hemolytic anemia, leukopenia, thrombocytopenia. **Neuro:** neuropathy. **Misc:** fever, infection.

Interactions

Drug-Drug: NSAIDs, especially those with short half-lives, ↑ blood levels and risk of toxicity; avoid for 2 days before, day of, and 2 days after treatment. **Probenecid** ↑ blood levels. Concurrent use of **nephrotoxic agents** ↑ risk of nephrotoxicity.

Route/Dosage

IV (Adults): *Mesothelioma and non–small cell lung cancer (with cisplatin)* 500—mg/m² on day 1 of each 21-day cycle (with cisplatin); concurrent hydration, folic acid, and vitamin B_{12} therapy, and pretreatment with dexamethasone required. *Non–small cell lung cancer (as monotherapy)*—500 mg/m² on day 1 of each 21-day cycle (concurrent folic acid, and vitamin B_{12} therapy, and pretreatment with dexamethasone required).

Availability

Lyophilized powder for IV infusion: 100 mg/vial, 500 mg/vial.

NURSING IMPLICATIONS

Assessment

- Monitor for rash during therapy. Pretreatment with dexamethasone 4 mg orally twice daily the day before, the day of, and the day after administration reduces incidence and severity or reaction.
- Monitor for hematologic and GI (mucositis, diarrhea) toxicities. If any Grade 3 or 4 toxicities, except mucositis or diarrhea, requiring hospitalization occur, decrease doses of pemetrexed and cisplatin by 75%. If Grade 3 or 4 mucositis occurs decrease pemetrexed dose by 50% and cisplatin by 100% of previous dose.
- Monitor for bone marrow depression. Assess for bleeding (bleeding gums, bruising, petechiae, guaiac stools, urine, and emesis) and avoid IM injections and taking rectal temperatures if platelet count is low. Apply pressure to venipuncture sites for 10 min. Assess for signs of infection during neutropenia. Anemia may occur; monitor for increased fatigue, dyspnea, and orthostatic hypotension.
- Assess for neurotoxicity during therapy. If Grade 0–1 neurotoxicity occurs, decrease pemetrexed and cisplatin doses by 100% of previous dose. If Grade 2 neurotoxicity occurs, decrease pemetrexed dose by 100% and cisplatin dose by 50% of previous dose. If Grade 3 or 4 neurotoxicity occurs, discontinue therapy.
- ***Lab Test Considerations:*** Monitor CBC and platelet counts for nadir and recovery and renal function, before each dose and on days 8 and 15 of each cycle and chemistry for renal and liver functions periodically. May cause neutropenia, thrombocytopenia, leukopenia, and anemia. A new cycle should not be started unless the ANC is at least 1500 cells/mm³, platelet count is at least 100,000 cells/mm³, and creatinine clearance is at least 45 mL/min. If nadir of ANC is less than 500/mm³ and nadir of platelets are at least 50,000/mm³ decrease doses of pemetrexed and cisplatin by 75%. If nadir of platelets is less than 50,000/mm³ regardless of ANC nadir decrease pemetrexed and cisplatin doses by 50%.

Potential Nursing Diagnoses

Risk for injury (Adverse Reactions)

Implementation

- Do not confuse pemetrexed with pralatrexate.
- Pemetrexed should be administered under supervision of a physician experienced in the use of chemotherapeutic agents.

P

- Prepare solution in a biologic cabinet. Wear gloves, gown, and mask while handling medication. Discard equipment in designated containers.
- To reduce toxicity, 0.4–1 mg of folic acid must be taken daily for 7 days preceding first dose of pemetrexed and should continue during and for 21 days after last dose. Patients must also receive an injection of vitamin B_{12} 1 mg IM during the week preceding first dose of pemetrexed and every 3 cycles thereafter. Subsequent doses of vitamin B_{12} may be given on same day as pemetrexed. Also administer dexamethasone 4 mg twice daily the day before, the day of, and the day after pemetrexed administration.

IV Administration

- **Intermittent Infusion:** Calculate number of pemetrexed 500-mg vials needed; vials contain excess to facilitate delivery. Reconstitute 500 mg with 20 mL of preservative–free 0.9% NaCl. ***Concentration:*** 25 mg/mL. Swirl gently until powder is completely dissolved. Solution is clear and colorless to yellow or green-yellow. Do not administer if discolored or containing particulate matter ***Diluent:*** Dilute further to 100 mL with preservative–free 0.9% NaCl. Solution is stable at room temperature or if refrigerated for up to 24 hr. ***Rate:*** Administer over 10 min.
- **Y-Site Compatibility:** acyclovir, alfentanil, allopurinol, amifostine, amikacin, aminocaproic acid, aminophylline, amiodarone, amphotericin B lipid complex, amphotericin B liposome, ampicillin, ampicillin/sulbactam, atracurium, azithromycin, aztreonam, bivalirudin, bleomycin, bumetanide, buprenorphine, butorphanol, carboplatin, carmustine, ceftriaxone, cefuroxime, cisatracurium, cisplatin, clindamycin, cyclophosphamide, cyclosporine, cytarabine, dactinomycin, daptomycin, dexamethasone sodium phosphate, dexmedetomidine, dexrazoxane, digoxin, diltiazem, diphenhydramine, docetaxel, dolasetron, dopamine, doxacurium, doxorubicin liposome, enalaprilat, ephedrine, epinephrine, eptifibitide, ertapenem, esmolol, etoposide, etoposide phosphate, famotidine, fenoldopam, fentanyl, fluconazole, fludarabine, fluorouracil, foscarnet, fosphenytoin, furosemide, ganciclovir, glycopyrrolate, granisetron, haloperidol, heparin, hydrocortisone sodium succinate, hydromorphone, ifosfamide, imipenem/cilastatin, insulin, isoproterenol, ketorolac, labetalol, leucovorin, levofloxacin, lidocaine, linezolid, lorazepam, magnesium sulfate, mannitol, meperidine, meropenem, mesna, methyldopate, methylprednisolone sodium succinate, metoclopramide, metoprolol, midazolam, milrinone, mitomycin, morphine, moxifloxacin, nafcillin, naloxone, nesiritide, nitroglycerin, norepinephrine, octreotide, oxaliplatin, paclitaxel, pamidronate, pancuronium, pentobarbital, phenobarbital, phentolamine, piperacillin/tazobactam, potassium acetate, potassium chloride, potassium phosphates, procainamide, promethazine, propranolol, ranitidine, remifentanil, rocuronium, sodium acetate, sodium bicarbonate, sodium phosphates, succinylcholine, sufentanil, tacrolimus, theophylline, thiopental, thiotepa, tigecycline, tirofiban, trimethoprim/sulfamethoxazole, vancomycin, vecuronium, verapamil, vinblastine, vincristine, vinorelbine, zidovudine, zoledronic acid.
- **Y-Site Incompatibility:** amphotericin B colloidal, anidulafungin, calcium acetate, calcium chloride, calcium gluconate, caspofungin, cefazolin, cefepime, cefotaxime, cefotetan, cefoxitin, ceftazidime, chloramphenicol, chlorpromazine, ciprofloxacin, dacarbazine, dantrolene, daunorubicin hydrochloride, diazepam, dobutamine, doxorubicin, doxycycline, droperidol, epirubicin, erythromycin, gemcitabine, gentamicin, hydralazine, idarubicin, irinotecan, metronidazole, mitoxantrone, nalbuphine, nicardipine, nitroprusside, ondansetron, pantoprazole, pentamidine, pentazocine, phenytoin, prochlorperazine, quinupristin/dalfopristin, tobramycin, topotecan, vasopressin.
- **Additive Incompatibility:** Solutions containing calcium, including Lactated Ringer's and Ringer's solution.

Patient/Family Teaching

- Emphasize the importance of taking prophylactic folic acid and vitamin B_{12} to reduce treatment-related hematologic and GI toxicity.
- Advise patient to notify health care professional immediately if signs and symptoms of infection (fever, sore throat), anemia, or neurotoxicity occur.
- Instruct patients to notify health care professional if persistent vomiting, diarrhea, or signs of dehydration appear.
- Instruct patient to notify health care professional of all Rx or OTC medications, vitamins, or herbal products being taken and consult health care professional before taking any new medications, especially NSAIDs and to avoid alcohol during therapy.
- Advise patient to avoid becoming pregnant during therapy. If pregnancy is planned or suspected, notify health care professional promptly.

Evaluation/Desired Outcomes

- Decreased growth and spread of mesothelioma or non–small cell lung cancer.

PENICILLINS (pen-i-sill-ins)

penicillin G
✱Crystapen, ~~Pfizerpen~~

penicillin V
✱Pen-VK

procaine penicillin G
~~Wycillin~~

benzathine penicillin G
Bicillin L-A, Permapen

Classification
Therapeutic: anti-infectives
Pharmacologic: penicillins

Pregnancy Category B

Indications

Treatment of a wide variety of infections including: Pneumococcal pneumonia, Streptococcal pharyngitis, Syphilis, Gonorrhea strains. Treatment of enterococcal infections (requires the addition of an aminoglycoside). Prevention of rheumatic fever. Should not be used as a single agent to treat anthrax. **Unlabeled Use:** Treatment of Lyme disease. Prevention of recurrent *Streptococcal pneumoniae* septicemia in children with sickle-cell disease.

Action

Bind to bacterial cell wall, resulting in cell death. **Therapeutic Effects:** Bactericidal action against susceptible bacteria. **Spectrum:** Active against: Most gram-positive organisms, including many streptococci (*Streptococcus pneumoniae*, group A beta-hemolytic streptococci), staphylococci (non–penicillinase-producing strains) and *Bacillus anthracis*, Some gram-negative organisms, such as *Neisseria meningitidis* and *Neisseria gonorrhoeae* (only penicillin susceptible strains), Some anaerobic bacteria and spirochetes including *Borellia burgdorferi*.

Pharmacokinetics

Absorption: Variably absorbed from the GI tract. *Penicillin V*—resists acid degradation in the GI tract. *Procaine and benzathine penicillin*—IM absorption is delayed and prolonged and results in sustained therapeutic blood levels.
Distribution: Widely distributed, although CNS penetration is poor in the presence of uninflamed meninges. Cross the placenta and enter breast milk.
Metabolism and Excretion: Minimally metabolized by the liver, excreted mainly unchanged by the kidneys.
Half-life: 30–60 min.

TIME/ACTION PROFILE (blood levels)

ROUTE	ONSET	PEAK	DURATION
Penicillin V PO	rapid	0.5–1 hr	4–6 hr
Penicillin G IM	rapid	0.25–0.5 hr	4–6 hr
Penicillin G IV	rapid	end of infusion	4–6 hr
Benzathine penicillin IM	delayed	12–24 hr	3 wk
Procaine penicillin IM	delayed	1–4 hr	12 hr

Contraindications/Precautions

Contraindicated in: Previous hypersensitivity to penicillins (cross-sensitivity may exist with cephalosporins and other beta-lactams); Hypersensitivity to procaine or benzathine (procaine and benzathine preparations only); Some products may contain tartrazine and should be avoided in patients with known hypersensitivity.
Use Cautiously in: Severe renal insufficiency (dose ↓ recommended); OB: Although safety not established, has been used safely; Lactation: Safety not established; Geri: Consider ↓ body mass, age-related ↓ in renal, hepatic, and cardiac function, comorbidities, and concurrent drug therapy when prescribing and dosing.

Adverse Reactions/Side Effects

CNS: SEIZURES. **GI:** CLOSTRIDIUM DIFFICILE-ASSOCIATED DIARRHEA (CDAD), diarrhea, epigastric distress, nausea, vomiting. **GU:** interstitial nephritis. **Derm:** rash, urticaria. **Hemat:** eosinophilia, hemolytic anemia, leukopenia. **Local:** pain at IM site, phlebitis at IV site. **Misc:** allergic reactions including ANAPHYLAXIS and SERUM SICKNESS, superinfection.

Interactions

Drug-Drug: May ↓ effectiveness of oral contraceptive agents. **Probenecid** ↓ renal excretion and ↑ levels therapy may be combined for this purpose. **Neomycin** may ↓ absorption of penicillin V. ↓ elimination of **methotrexate** and ↑ risk of serious toxicity.

Route/Dosage

Penicillin G (aqueous)

IM, IV (Adults): *Most infections*—1–5 million units q 4–6 hr.
IM, IV (Children): 8333–16,667 units/kg q 4 hr; 12,550–25,000 units/kg q 6 hr; up to 250,000 units/kg/day in divided doses, some infections may require up to 300,000 units/kg/day.
IV (Infants >7 days): 25,000 units/kg q 8 hr; *meningitis*—50,000–75,000 units/kg q 6 hr.

✱ = Canadian drug name. ⧖ = Genetic implication. ~~Strikethrough~~ = Discontinued.
*CAPITALS indicates life-threatening; underlines indicate most frequent.

IV (Infants <7 days): 25,000 units/kg q 12 hr; *Streptococcus B meningitis*—100,000–150,000 units/kg/day in divided doses.

Penicillin V

PO (Adults and Children ≥12 yr): *Most infections*—125–500 mg q 6–8 hr. *Rheumatic fever prevention*—125–250 mg q 12 hr.
PO (Children <12 yr): *Lyme disease*—12.5 mg/kg q 6 hr (unlabeled); prevention of *Streptococcus pneumoniae* sepsis in children with sickle cell disease—125 mg twice daily.

Benzathine Penicillin G

IM (Adults): *Streptococcal infections/erysipeloid*—1.2 million units single dose. *Primary, secondary, and early latent syphilis*—2.4 million units single dose. *Tertiary and late latent syphilis (not neurosyphilis)*—2.4 million units once weekly for 3 wk. *Prevention of rheumatic fever*—1.2 million units q 3–4 wk.
IM (Children >27 kg): *Streptococcal infections/erysipeloid*—900,000–1.2 million units (single dose). *Primary, secondary, and early latent syphilis*—up to 2.4 million units single dose. *Late latent or latent syphilis of undetermined duration*—50,000 units/kg weekly for 3 wk. *Prevention of rheumatic fever*—1.2 million units q 2–3 wk.
IM (Children <27 kg): *Streptococcal infections/erysipeloid*—300,000–600,000 units single dose. *Primary, secondary, and early latent syphilis*—up to 2.4 million units single dose. *Late latent or latent syphilis of undetermined duration*—50,000 units/kg weekly for 3 wk. *Prevention of rheumatic fever*—1.2 million units q 2–3 wk.

Procaine Penicillin G

IM (Adults): *Moderate or severe infections*—600,000–1.2 million units/day as a single dose or in 2 divided doses. *Neurosyphilis*—2.4 million units/day with 500 mg probenecid PO 4 times daily for 10–14 days.
IM (Children): *Congenital syphilis*—50,000 units/kg/day for 10–14 days.

Availability

Penicillin G Potassium (generic available)

Powder for injection: 1 million units/vial, 5 million units/vial, 20 million units/vial. **Premixed (frozen) solution for injection:** 1 million units/50 mL, 2 million units/50 mL, 3 million units/50 mL.

Penicillin G Sodium (generic available)

Powder for injection: 5 million units/vial.

Penicillin V Potassium (generic available)

Tablets: 250 mg, 500 mg. **Cost:** *Generic*—250 mg $45.75/100, 500 mg $77.77/100. **Oral solution:** 125 mg/5 mL, 250 mg/5 mL. **Cost:** *Generic*—125 mg/5 mL $3.84/100 mL, 250 mg/5 mL $4.31/100 mL.

Procaine Penicillin G (generic available)

Suspension for IM injection: 300,000 units/mL, 600,000 units/mL.

Benzathine Penicillin G

Suspension for IM injection: 600,000 units/mL.

NURSING IMPLICATIONS

Assessment

- Assess for infection (vital signs; appearance of wound, sputum, urine, and stool; WBC) at beginning of and during therapy.
- Obtain a history to determine previous use of and reactions to penicillins, cephalosporins, or other beta-lactam antibiotics. Persons with a negative history of penicillin sensitivity may still have an allergic response.
- Obtain specimens for culture and sensitivity before initiating therapy. First dose may be given before receiving results.
- Observe patient for signs and symptoms of anaphylaxis (rash, pruritus, laryngeal edema, wheezing). Discontinue drug and notify health care professional immediately if these symptoms occur. Keep epinephrine, an antihistamine, and resuscitation equipment close by in case of an anaphylactic reaction.
- Monitor bowel function. Diarrhea, abdominal cramping, fever, and bloody stools should be reported to health care professional promptly as a sign of Clostridium difficile-associated diarrhea (CDAD). May begin up to several weeks following cessation of therapy.
- ***Lab Test Considerations:*** May cause positive direct Coombs' test results.
- Hyperkalemia may develop after large doses of penicillin G potassium.
- Monitor serum sodium concentrations in patient with hypertension or HF. Hypernatremia may develop after large doses of penicillin sodium.
- May cause ↑ AST, ALT, LDH, and serum alkaline phosphatase concentrations.
- May cause leukopenia and neutropenia, especially with prolonged therapy or hepatic impairment.

Potential Nursing Diagnoses

Risk for infection (Indications, Side Effects)
Noncompliance (Patient/Family Teaching)

Implementation

- Do not confuse penicillin with penicillamine. Do not confuse penicillin G aqueous (potassium or sodium salt) with penicillin G procaine.
- **PO:** Administer around the clock. Penicillin V may be administered without regard for meals.
- Use calibrated measuring device for liquid preparations. Solution is stable for 14 days if refrigerated.

- **IM:** Reconstitute according to manufacturer's directions with sterile water for injection, D5W, or 0.9% NaCl.
- **IM:** Shake medication well before injection. Inject penicillin deep into a well-developed muscle mass at a slow, consistent rate to prevent blockage of the needle. Massage well. Accidental injury near or into a nerve can result in severe pain and dysfunction.
- Penicillin G potassium or sodium may be diluted with lidocaine (without epinephrine) 1% or 2% to minimize pain from IM injection.
- Never give penicillin G benzathine or penicillin G procaine suspensions IV. May cause embolism or toxic reactions.

IV Administration

- **IV:** Change IV sites every 48 hr to prevent phlebitis.
- Administer slowly and observe patient closely for signs of hypersensitivity.
- **Intermittent Infusion:** ***Diluent:*** Doses of 3 million units or less should be diluted in at least 50 mL of D5W or 0.9% NaCl; doses of more than 3 million units should be diluted with 100 mL. ***Concentration:*** 100,000–500,000 units/mL (50,000 units/mL in neonates). ***Rate:*** Infuse over 1–2 hr in adults or 15–30 min in children.
- **Continuous Infusion:** Doses of 10 million units or more may be diluted in 1 or 2 L.
- ***Rate:*** Infuse over 24 hr.

Penicillin G Potassium

- **Y-Site Compatibility:** acyclovir, amiodarone, ascorbic acid, atropine, aztreonam, benztropine, bumetanide, buprenorphine, butorphanol, calcium chloride, calcium gluconate, cefazolin, cefotaxime, ceftazidime, ceftriaxone, cefuroxime, chloramphenicol, chlorpromazine, clindamycin, cyanocobalamin, cyclophosphamide, cyclosporine, dexamethasone, digoxin, diltiazem, diphenhydramine, dopamine, enalaprilat, ephedrine, epinephrine, epoetin alfa, esmolol, famotidine, fentanyl, fluconazole, folic acid, foscarnet, furosemide, glycopyrrolate, heparin, hydrocortisone, hydromorphone, imipenem/cilastatin, indomethacin, insulin, isoproterenol, ketamine, ketorolac, lidocaine, magnesium sulfate, mannitol, meperidine, methyldopate, methylprednisolone, metoclopramide, metoprolol, midazolam, morphine, nafcillin, nalbuphine, naloxone, nicardipine, nitroglycerin, nitroprusside, norepinephrine, ondansetron, oxacillin, oxytocin, penicillin G sodium, phenylephrine, phytonadione, potassium chloride, procainamide, prochlorperazine, propranolol, pyridoixine, ranitidine, sodium bicarbonate, streptokinase, succinylcholine, tacrolimus, theophylline, thiamine, tobramycin, vancomycin, vasopressin, verapamil, vitamin B complex with C.
- **Y-Site Incompatibility:** If aminoglycosides and penicillins must be administered concurrently, administer in separate sites at least 1 hr apart, aminophylline, amphotericin B colloidal, ampicilliin, dantrolene, diazepam, dobutamine, doxycycline, erythromycin, ganciclovir, haloperidol, papaverine, pentamidine, pentazocine, pentobarbital, phenobarbital, phentolamine, phenytoin, promethazine, protamine, tranexamic acid, trimethoprim/sulfamethoxazole.

Penicillin G Sodium

- **Y-Site Compatibility:** alfentanil, ascorbic acid, atropine, aztreonam, benztropine, bumetanide, buprenorphine, butorphanol, calcium chloride, calcium gluconate, chloramphenicol, clindamycin, cyanocobalamin, cyclosporine, dexamethasone, digoxin, diphenhydramine, dopamine, enalaprilat, ephedrine, epinephrine, epoetin alfa, esmolol, famotidine, fentanyl, fluconazole, folic acid, furosemide, glycopyrrolate, heparin, hydrocortisone, imipenem/cilastatin, indomethacin, insulin, isoproterenol, ketamine, ketorolac, levofloxacin, lidocaine, magnesium sulfate, mannitol, meperidine, methyldopate, methylprednisolone, metoclopramide, metoprolol, morphine, multivitamins, nafcillin, naloxone, nitroglycerin, nitroprusside, norepinephrine, ondansetron, oxacillin, oxytocin, penicillin G potassium, phenylephrine, phytonadione, potassium chloride, procainamide, prochlorperazine, propranolol, pyridoxine, ranitidine, sodium bicarbonate, streptokinase, sufentanil, theophylline, thiamine, vancomycin, vasopressin, verapamil.
- **Y-Site Incompatibility:** If aminoglycosides and penicillins must be administered concurrently, administer in separate sites at least 1 hr apart, aminophylline, amphotericin B colloidal, dantrolene, diazepam, dobutamine, doxycycline, erythromycin, ganciclovir, haloperidol, labetalol, papaverine, pentamidine, pentazocine, pentobarbital, phenobarbital, phenytoin, promethazine, protamine, succinylcholine, tranexamic acid, trimethoprim/sulfamethoxazole.
- **Additive Incompatibility:** Incompatible with aminoglycosides; do not admix.

Patient/Family Teaching

- Instruct patient to take medication around the clock and to finish drug completely as directed, even if feeling better. Advise patient that sharing this medication may be dangerous.
- Advise patient to report signs of superinfection (black, furry overgrowth on tongue; vaginal itching or discharge; loose or foul-smelling stools) and allergy.

P

- Instruct patient to notify health care professional if fever and diarrhea develop, especially if stool contains blood, pus, or mucus. Advise patient not to treat diarrhea without consulting health care professional.
- Instruct patient to notify health care professional if symptoms do not improve.
- Advise patient taking oral contraceptives to use an additional nonhormonal method of contraception during therapy with penicillin and until next menstrual period.
- Patient with an allergy to penicillin should be instructed to always carry an identification card with this information.

Evaluation/Desired Outcomes

- Resolution of signs and symptoms of infection. Length of time for complete resolution depends on the organism and site of infection.

PENICILLINS, PENICILLINASE RESISTANT

dicloxacillin (dye-klox-a-**sill**-in)
Nallpen

nafcillin (naf-**sill**-in)

oxacillin (ox-a-**sill**-in)
Bactocill

Classification
Therapeutic: anti-infectives
Pharmacologic: penicillinase resistant penicillins

Pregnancy Category B

Indications

Treatment of the following infections due to penicillinase-producing staphylococci: Respiratory tract infections, Sinusitis, Skin and skin structure infections. **Dicloxacillin:** Osteomyelitis. **Nafcillin, oxacillin:** Are also used to treat: Bone and joint infections, Urinary tract infections, Endocarditis, Septicemia, Meningitis.

Action

Bind to bacterial cell wall, leading to cell death. Not inactivated by penicillinase enzymes. **Therapeutic Effects:** Bactericidal action. **Spectrum:** Active against most gram-positive aerobic cocci but less so than penicillin. Spectrum is notable for activity against: Penicillinase-producing strains of *Staphylococcus aureus*, *Staphylococcus epidermidis*. Not active against methicillin-resistant staphylococci.

Pharmacokinetics

Absorption: *Dicloxacillin*—Rapidly but incompletely (35–76%) absorbed from the GI tract. *Nafcillin and oxacillin*—Completely absorbed following IV administration; well absorbed from IM sites.
Distribution: Widely distributed; penetration into CSF is minimal, but sufficient in the presence of inflamed meninges; cross the placenta and enter breast milk.
Metabolism and Excretion: *Dicloxacillin*—Some metabolism by the liver (6–10%) and some renal excretion of unchanged drug (60%); small amounts eliminated in the feces via the bile. *Nafcillin, oxacillin*—Partially metabolized by the liver (nafcillin 60%, oxacillin 49%), partially excreted unchanged by the kidneys.
Half-life: *Dicloxacillin*—0.5–1.1 hr (↑ in severe hepatic and renal dysfunction); *Nafcillin*—Neonates: 1–5 hr; Children 1 mo – 14 yr: 0.75–1.9 hr; Adults: 0.5–1.5 hr (↑ in renal impairment); *Oxacillin*—Neonates: 1.6 hr; Children up to 2 yr: 0.9–1.8 hr; Adults: 0.3–0.8 hr (↑ in severe hepatic impairment).

TIME/ACTION PROFILE (blood levels)

ROUTE	ONSET	PEAK	DURATION
Dicloxacillin	30 min	30–120 min	6 hr
Nafcillin IM	30 min	60–120 min	4–6 hr
Nafcillin IV	rapid	end of infusion	4–6 hr
Oxacillin IM	rapid	30 min	4–6 hr
Oxacillin IV	rapid	end of infusion	4–6 hr

Contraindications/Precautions

Contraindicated in: Hypersensitivity to penicillins (cross-sensitivity with cephalosporins may exist).
Use Cautiously in: Severe renal or hepatic impairment; OB, Lactation: Safety not established.

Adverse Reactions/Side Effects

CNS: SEIZURES (high doses). **GI:** CLOSTRIDIUM DIFFICILE-ASSOCIATED DIARRHEA (CDAD), diarrhea, nausea, vomiting, drug-induced hepatitis. **GU:** interstitial nephritis. **Derm:** rashes, urticaria. **Hemat:** eosinophilia, leukopenia. **Local:** pain at IM sites, phlebitis at IV sites. **Misc:** allergic reactions including ANAPHYLAXIS and SERUM SICKNESS, superinfection.

Interactions

Drug-Drug: Probenecid ↓ renal excretion and ↑ blood levels (treatment may be combined for this purpose). May ↓ effectiveness of **oral contraceptive agents**. May ↓ elimination of **methotrexate** and ↑ risk of serious toxicity.

Route/Dosage

Dicloxacillin

PO (Adults and Children ≥40 kg): 125–250 mg q 6 hr (up to 2 g/day).
PO (Children <40 kg): 6.25–12.5 mg/kg q 6 hr; (up to 12.25 mg/kg q 6 hr has been used for osteomyelitis), maximum: 2 g/day.

Nafcillin

IM (Adults): 500 mg q 4–6 hr.
IM, IV (Children and Infants): 50–200 mg/kg/day divided q 4–6 hr, maximum: 12 g/day.
IM, IV (Neonates 0–4 weeks, <1200 g): 25 mg/kg q 12 hr.
IM, IV (Neonates 1.2–2 kg): —25 mg/kg q 12 hr for the first 7 days of life, then 25 mg/kg q 8 hr.
IM, IV (Neonates >2 kg): —25 mg/kg q 8 hr for the first 7 days of life, then 25 mg/kg q 6 hr.
IV (Adults): 500–2000 mg q 4–6 hr.

Oxacillin

IM, IV (Adults and Children ≥40 kg): 250–2000 mg q 4–6 hr (up to 12 g/day).
IM, IV (Children <40 kg): 100–200 mg/kg/day divided q 4–6 hr, maximum: 12 g/day.
IM, IV (Neonates <1200 g): —25 mg/kg q 12 hr.
IM, IV (Neonates ≥2 kg): —25 mg/kg q 8 hr for the first 7 days of life, then 25 mg/kg q 6 hr.
IM, IV (Neonates 1.2–2 kg): —25 mg/kg q 12 hr for the first 7 days of life, then 25 mg/kg q 8 hr.

Availability

Dicloxacillin (generic available)

Capsules: 250 mg, 500 mg. **Oral suspension:** 62.5 mg/5 mL.

Nafcillin (generic available)

Powder for injection: 1 g/vial, 2 g/vial, 10 g/vial.

Oxacillin (generic available)

Powder for injection: 1 g/vial, 2 g/vial, 10 g/vial.

NURSING IMPLICATIONS

Assessment

- Assess patient for infection (vital signs; appearance of wound, sputum, urine, and stool; WBC) at beginning of and throughout therapy.
- Obtain a history before initiating therapy to determine previous use of and reactions to penicillins, cephalosporins, or other beta-lactam antibiotics. Persons with a negative history of penicillin sensitivity may still have an allergic response.
- Obtain specimens for culture and sensitivity prior to initiating therapy. First dose may be given before receiving results.
- Observe patient for signs and symptoms of anaphylaxis (rash, pruritus, laryngeal edema, wheezing, abdominal pain). Discontinue the drug and notify health care professional immediately if these occur. Keep epinephrine, an antihistamine, and resuscitation equipment close by in the event of an anaphylactic reaction.
- Assess vein for signs of irritation and phlebitis. Change IV site every 48 hr to prevent phlebitis.
- ***Lab Test Considerations:*** May cause leukopenia and neutropenia, especially with prolonged therapy or hepatic impairment.
- May cause positive direct Coombs' test result.
- May cause ↑ AST, ALT, LDH, and serum alkaline phosphatase concentrations.

Potential Nursing Diagnoses

Risk for infection (Indications, Side Effects)
Noncompliance (Patient/Family Teaching)

Implementation

- **PO:** Administer around the clock on an empty stomach at least 1 hr before or 2 hr after meals. Take with a full glass of water; acidic juices may decrease absorption of penicillins.
- Use calibrated measuring device for liquid preparations. Shake well. Solution is stable for 14 days if refrigerated.

Nafcillin

IV Administration

- **IV, IM:** To reconstitute, add 3.4 mL to each 1-g vial or 6.8 mL to each 2-g vial, for a concentration of 250 mg/mL. Stable for 2–7 days if refrigerated.
- **IV Push:** ***Diluent:*** Dilute reconstituted solution with 15–30 mL of sterile water, 0.45% NaCl, or 0.9% NaCl for injection. ***Concentration:*** 100 mg/mL. ***Rate:*** Administer over 5–10 min.
- **Intermittent Infusion:** ***Diluent:*** Dilute with sterile water for injection, 0.9% NaCl, D5W, D10W, D5/0.25% NaCl, D5/0.45% NaCl, D5/0.9% NaCl, D5/LR, Ringer's or LR. Stable for 24 hr at room temperature, 96 hr if refrigerated. ***Concentration:*** 2–40 mg/mL. ***Rate:*** Infuse over at least 30–60 min to avoid vein irritation.
- **Y-Site Compatibility:** acyclovir, alfentanil, aminophylline, amphotericin B lipid complex, anidulafungin, argatroban, ascorbic acid, atracurium, atropine, aztreonam, benztropine, bivalirudin, bleomycin, bumetanide, buprenorphine, butorphanol, calcium chloride, calcium gluconate, carboplatin, carmustine, chlorpromazine, cisplatin, clindamycin, cyanocobalamin, cyclophosphamide, dactinomycin, daptomycin, dexamethasone, digoxin, dobutamine, docetaxel, dopamine, enalaprilat, ephedrine, epinephrine, epoetin alfa, erythromycin, etoposide, etoposide phosphate, famotidine, fenoldopam, fentanyl, fluconazole, fludarabine, foscarnet, furosemide, ganciclovir, glycopyrrolate, granisetron, heparin, hetastarch, hydrocortisone, hydromorphone, imipenem/cilastatin, indomethacin, isoproterenol, ketorolac, lidocaine, linezolid, lorazepam, magnesium sulfate, mannitol, methoxamine, methyldopate, methylprednisolone, metoclopramide, metoprolol, metronidazole, milrinone, morphine, multivitamins,

P

naloxone, nicardipine, nitroglycerin, nitroprusside, norepinephrine, octreotide, ondansetron, oxacillin, oxytocin, paclitaxel, pamidronate, pnacuronium, pantoprazole, pemetrexed, penicillin G, pentobarbital, perphenazine, phenobarbital, phentolamine, phenylephrine, phytonadione, potassium acetate, potassium chloride, procainamide, prochlorperazine, propofol, propranolol, ranitidine, sodium bicarbonate, streptokinase, sufentanil, tacrolimus, teniposide, theophylline, thiamine, thiotepa, tigecycline, tirofiban, tolazoline, trimetaphan, vasopressin, voriconazole, zidovudine, zoledronic acid.

- **Y-Site Incompatibility:** alemtuzumab, amphotericin B colloidal, ampicillin, azathioprine, caspofungin, chloramphenicol, dantrolene, diazoxide, doxycycline, droperidol, epirubicin, folic acid, gemcitabine, haloperidol, hydralazine, hydroxyzine, idarubicin, irinotecan, meperidine, metaraminol, mitoxantrone, mycophenolate, nesiritide, palonosetron, pentamidine, pentazocine, phenytoin, promethazine, protamine, pyridoxime, succinylcholine, trimethoprim/sulfamethoxazole, vecuronium, vincristine, vinrelbine. If penicillins and aminoglycosides must be administered concurrently, administer at separate sites.

Oxacillin

IV Administration

- **IV, IM:** To reconstitute for IM or IV use, add 1.4 mL of sterile water for injection to each 250-mg vial, 2.7 mL to each 500-mg vial, 5.7 mL to each 1-g vial, 11.5 mL to each 2-g vial, and 23 mL to each 4-g vial, for a concentration of 250 mg/1.5 mL. Stable for 3 days at room temperature or 7 days if refrigerated.
- **IV Push:** ***Diluent:*** Further dilute each reconstituted 250-mg or 500-mg vial with 5 mL of sterile water or 0.9% NaCl for injection, 10 mL for each 1-g vial, 20 mL for each 2-g vial, and 40 mL for each 4-g vial. ***Concentration:*** 100 mg/mL. ***Rate:*** Administer slowly over 10 min.
- **Intermittent Infusion:** ***Diluent:*** Dilute with 0.9% NaCl, D5W, D5/0.9% NaCl, or LR. ***Concentration:*** 0.5–40 mg/mL. ***Rate:*** May be infused for up to 6 hr.
- **Y-Site Compatibility:** acyclovir, alfentanil, aminophylline, ascorbic acid, atracurium, atropine, aztreonam, benztropine, bumetanide, buprenorphine, butorphanol, chloramphenicol, chlorpromazine, clindamycin, cyanocobalamin, cyclophosphamide, cyclosporine, dexamethasone, digoxin, diltiazem, dopamine, doxapram, enalaprilat, ephedrine, epinephrine, epoetin alfa, erythromycin, famotidine, fentanil, fluconazole, folic acid, foscarnet, furosemide, glycopyrrolate, heparin, hydrocortisone sodium succinate, hydromorphone, imipenem/cilastatin, insulin, isoproterenol, ketorolac, labetalol, levofloxacin, lidocaine, mannitol, methotrexate, methoxamine, methyldopate, metoclopramide, metoprolol, midazolam, milrinone, morphine, multivitamins, nafcillin, naloxone, nitroglycerin, nitroprusside, norepinephrine, ondansetron, oxytocin, papaverine, penicillin G, pentobarbital, perphenazine, phenobarbital, phenylephrine, phytonadione, potassium chloride, procainamide, prochlorperazine, propranolol, ranitidine, streptokinase, sufentanil, tacrolimus, theophylline, thiamine, tolazoline, trimetaphan, vancomycin, vasopressin, vitamin B complex with C, zidovudine.
- **Y-Site Incompatibility:** amphotericin B colloidal, calcium chloride, calcium gluconate, dantrolene, diazepam, diazoxide, dobutamine, doxycycline, esmolol, haloperidol, hydralazine, metaraminol, pentamidine, pentazocine, phenytoin, promethazine, pyridoxime, succinylcholine, trimethoprim/sulfamethoazole. If penicillins and aminoglycosides must be administered concurrently, administer at separate sites.

Patient/Family Teaching

- Instruct patient to take medication around the clock and to finish the drug completely as directed, even if feeling better. Missed doses should be taken as soon as remembered. Advise patient that sharing of this medication may be dangerous.
- Advise patient to report signs of superinfection (black, furry overgrowth on the tongue; vaginal itching or discharge; loose or foul-smelling stools) and allergy.
- Instruct patient to notify health care professional if fever and diarrhea develop, especially if stool contains blood, pus, or mucus. Advise patient not to treat diarrhea without consulting health care professional.
- Instruct patient to notify health care professional if symptoms do not improve.

Evaluation/Desired Outcomes

- Resolution of the signs and symptoms of infection. Length of time for complete resolution depends on the organism and site of infection.

pentamidine (pen-**tam**-i-deen)

NebuPent, Pentam 300

Classification

Therapeutic: anti-infectives

Pregnancy Category C

Indications

IV, IM: Treatment of *Pneumocystis jirovecii* pneumonia (PJP). **Inhaln:** Prevention of PJP in AIDS or HIV-positive patients who have had PJP or who have a peripheral CD4 lymphocyte count of $\leq 200/mm^3$.
Unlabeled Use: Inhaln: Treatment of PJP.

Action

Appears to disrupt DNA or RNA synthesis. Also has a direct toxic effect on pancreatic islet cells. **Therapeutic Effects:** Death of susceptible organism.

Pharmacokinetics

Absorption: Well absorbed parenterally; Minimal systemic absorption occurs following inhalation.
Distribution: Widely and extensively distributed but does not cross the blood-brain barrier. Concentrates in liver, kidneys, lungs, and spleen, with prolonged storage in some tissues.
Metabolism and Excretion: 1–30% excreted unchanged by the kidneys. Remainder of metabolic fate unknown.
Half-life: 5–11 hr (↑ in renal impairment).

TIME/ACTION PROFILE (blood levels)

ROUTE	ONSET	PEAK	DURATION
IV	unknown	end of infusion	24 hr
Inhaln	unknown	unknown	unknown

Contraindications/Precautions

Contraindicated in: History of previous anaphylactic reaction to pentamidine.
Use Cautiously in: Hypotension; Hypertension; Hypoglycemia; Hyperglycemia; Hypocalcemia; Leukopenia; Thrombocytopenia; Anemia; Renal impairment (dose ↓ required); Diabetes mellitus; Liver impairment; Cardiovascular disease; Bone marrow depression, previous antineoplastic therapy, or radiation therapy; Asthma (aerosol can induce bronchospasm); OB, Lactation: Safety not established during pregnancy; breast feeding not recommended.

Adverse Reactions/Side Effects

For parenteral form, unless otherwise indicated.
CNS: anxiety, headache, confusion, dizziness, hallucinations. **EENT:** *inhalation*—burning in throat. **Resp:** *inhalation*—bronchospasm, cough. **CV:** ARRHYTHMIAS, HYPOTENSION, chest pain. **GI:** PANCREATITIS, abdominal pain, anorexia, drug-induced hepatitis, nausea, unpleasant metallic taste, vomiting. **GU:** nephrotoxicity. **Derm:** pallor, rash. **Endo:** HYPOGLYCEMIA, hyperglycemia. **F and E:** hyperkalemia, hypocalcemia. **Hemat:** anemia, leukopenia, thrombocytopenia. **Local:** *IV*—phlebitis, pruritus, urticaria at IV site; *IM*, sterile abscesses at IM sites. **Misc:** allergic reactions including ANAPHYLAXIS, STEVENS-JOHNSON SYNDROME, chills, fever.

Interactions

Interactions listed for parenteral administration.
Drug-Drug: Concurrent use with **erythromycin** IV may ↑ risk of potentially fatal arrhythmias. Additive nephrotoxicity with other **nephrotoxic agents**, including **aminoglycosides**, **amphotericin B**, and **vancomycin**. Additive bone marrow depression with **antineoplastics** or previous **radiation therapy**. ↑ risk of pancreatitis with **didanosine**. ↑ risk of nephrotoxicity, hypocalcemia, and hypomagnesemia with **foscarnet**.

Route/Dosage

IV, IM (Adults and Children >5 mo): 4 mg/kg once daily for 14–21 days (longer treatment may be required in AIDS patients; some patients may respond to 3 mg/kg/day).
Inhaln (Adults): *NebuPent*—300 mg q 4 wk, using a Respirgard II jet nebulizer (150 mg q 2 wk has also been used).
Inhaln (Children >5 yr): *NebuPent*—300 mg q 4 wk, using a Respirgard II jet nebulizer (for patients who cannot tolerate trimethoprim/sulfamethoxazole; unlabeled).

Renal Impairment

IV (Adults): CCr 10–30 mL/min- Administer normal dose q 24 hr; CCr <10 ml/min- Administer normal dose q 48 hr.

Availability (generic available)

Powder for injection: 300 mg/vial. **Solution for aerosol use (NebuPent):** 300 mg.

P

NURSING IMPLICATIONS

Assessment

- Assess patient for infection (vital signs, sputum, WBC) and monitor respiratory status (rate, character, lung sounds, dyspnea, sputum) at beginning of and throughout therapy.
- Obtain specimens for culture and sensitivity prior to initiating therapy. First dose may be given before receiving results.
- Assess for rash periodically during therapy. May cause Stevens-Johnson syndrome or toxic epidermal necrolysis. Discontinue therapy if severe or if accompanied with fever, general malaise, fatigue, muscle or joint aches, blisters, oral lesions, conjunctivitis, hepatitis and/or eosinophilia.
- **IV, IM:** Monitor BP frequently during and following IM or IV administration of pentamidine. Patient should be lying down during administration. Sudden, severe hypotension may occur following a single dose. Resuscitation equipment should be immediately available.
- Assess patient for signs of hypoglycemia (anxiety; chills; diaphoresis; cold, pale skin; headache; increased hunger; nausea; nervousness; shakiness) and hyperglycemia (drowsiness; flushed, dry skin; fruit-like breath odor; increased thirst; increased urination; loss of appetite), which may occur up to several months after therapy is discontinued.

- Pulse and ECG should be monitored prior to and periodically during therapy. Fatalities due to cardiac arrhythmias, tachycardia, and cardiotoxicity have been reported.
- Assess patient for signs of pancreatitis (nausea, vomiting, abdominal pain, increased serum lipase or amylase) periodically during therapy. May require discontinuation of therapy.
- **Inhaln:** A tuberculin skin test, chest x-ray, and sputum culture should be performed prior to administration to rule out tuberculosis.
- ***Lab Test Considerations:*** *IM, IV*—Monitor blood glucose concentrations prior to, daily during, and for several months following therapy. Severe hypoglycemia and permanent diabetes mellitus have occurred.
- Monitor BUN and serum creatinine prior to and daily during therapy to monitor for nephrotoxicity. Concentrations may be ↑.
- Monitor CBC and platelet count prior to and every 3 days during therapy. Pentamidine may cause leukopenia, anemia, and thrombocytopenia.
- May cause ↑ serum bilirubin, alkaline phosphatase, AST, and ALT concentrations. Monitor liver function tests prior to and every 3 days during therapy.
- Monitor serum calcium and magnesium concentrations prior to and every 3 days during therapy; may cause hypocalcemia and hypomagnesemia.
- May cause ↑ serum potassium concentrations.

Potential Nursing Diagnoses

Risk for infection (Indications, Side Effects)

Implementation

- Pentamidine must be given on a regular schedule for the full course of therapy. Administer missed doses as soon as remembered. If almost time for the next dose, skip the missed dose and return to the regular schedule. Do not double doses.
- **IM:** Dilute 300 mg of pentamidine with 3 mL of sterile water for injection for a concentration of 100 mg/mL. IM administration should be used only for patients with adequate muscle mass and given deep IM via Z-track technique. May cause sterile abscesses.

IV Administration

- **Intermittent Infusion:** ***Diluent:*** To reconstitute, add 3–5 mL of sterile water for injection or D5W to each 300-mg vial for a concentration of 100, 75, or 60 mg/mL, respectively. Withdraw dose and dilute further in 50–250 mL of D5W. Solution is stable for 48 hr at room temperature. Discard unused portions. ***Concentration:*** Not to exceed 6 mg/mL for administration. ***Rate:*** Administer slowly over 1–2 hr.
- **Y-Site Compatibility:** alemtuzumab, alfentanyl, aminocaproic acid, anidulafungin, argatroban, atracurium, atropine, benztropine, bleomycin, buprenorphine, calcium gluconate, carboplatin, caspofungin, chlorpromazine, cisplatin, cyanocobalamin, cyclophosphamide, cyclosporine, cytarabine, dactinomycin, daptomycin, dexmedetomidine, diltiazem, diphenhydramine, dobutamine, docetaxel, dopamine, doxacurium, doxycycline, enalaprilat, epinephrine, epirubicin, erythromycin, esmolol, etoposide, etoposide phosphate, famotidine, fenoldopam, fentanyl, fludarabine, gemcitabine, glycopyrrolate, granisetron, hetastarch, hydromorphone, idarubicin, ifosfamide, irinotecan, isoproterenol, labetalol, levofloxacin, lidocaine, lorazepam, mannitol, mechlorethamine, meperidine, metaraminol, methoxamine, metoclopramide, metoprolol, metronidazole, miconazole, midazolam, milrinone, mitoxantrone, multivitamins, naloxone, nesiritide, nitroglycerin, nitroprusside norepinephrine, octreotide, ondansetron, oxaliplatin, oxytocin, paclitaxel, pamidronate, pancuronium, papaverine, pentazocine, phentolamine, phytonadione, potassium acetate, procainamide, promethazine, propranolol, pyridoxime, quinupristin/dalfopristin, ranitidine, rituximab, rocuronium, sodium acetate, succinylcholine, sufentanil, tacrolimus, teniposide, theophylline, thiamine, thiotepa, tigecycline, tolazoline, trastuzumab, trimetaphan, vancomycin, vasopressin, verapamil, vincristine, vinorelbine, voriconazole, zidovudine, zoledronic acid.
- **Y-Site Incompatibility:** acyclovir, aldesleukin, amikacin, aminophylline, amphotericin B colloidal, amphotericin B lipid complex, amphotericin B liposome, ampicillin, ampicillin/sulbactam, ascorbic acid, azathioprine, aztreonam, bivalirudin, bumetanide, butorphanol, cefazolin, cefotaxime, cefotetan, cefoxitin, ceftazidime, ceftriaxone, cefuroxime, chloramphenicol, clindamycin, dantrolene, dexamethasone, diazepam, diazoxide, digoxin, doxorubicin, ephedrine, epoetin alfa, eptifibatide, ertapenem, fluorouracil, folic acid, foscarnet, furosemide, gentamicin, heparin, hydrocortisone, indomethacin, insulin, ketorolac, linezolid, magnesium sulfate, methotrexate, methyldopate, methylprednisolone, morphine, nafcillin, nalbuphine, oxacillin, palonosetron, pantoprazole, pemetrexed, penicillin G, pentobarbital, phenobarbital, phenylephrine, phenytoin, piperacillin/tazobactam, potassium chloride, prochlorperazine, protamine, sodium bicarbonate, streptokinase, tobramycin, trimethoprim/sulfamethoxazole, vecuronium.
- **Inhaln:** If using inhalation bronchodilator, administer bronchodilator 5–10 min prior to pentamidine administration.
- Administer in a well-ventilated area.
- Administration with patient in supine or recumbent position appears to provide a more uniform distribution of pentamidine.
- *NebuPent* Dilute 300 or 600 mg (for prophylaxis or treatment, respectively) in 6 mL of sterile water for injection. Place reconstituted solution into Respir-

gard II nebulizer. Do not dilute with 0.9% NaCl or admix with other medications, as solution will form a precipitate. Do not use Respirgard II nebulizer for other medications.

- Administer inhalation dose through nebulizer until chamber is empty, approximately 30–45 min.
- Administer with the flow rate of the nebulizer at the midflow mark (5–7 L/min) over approximately 15 min until the chamber is empty.

Patient/Family Teaching

- Inform patient of the importance of completing the full course of pentamidine therapy, even if feeling better.
- **IV:** Instruct patient to notify health care professional promptly if signs and symptoms of pancreatitis, rash, fever; sore throat; signs of infection; bleeding of gums; unusual bruising; petechiae; or blood in stool, urine, or emesis occurs. Caution patient to avoid crowds and persons with known infections. Instruct patient to use soft toothbrush and electric razor and to avoid falls. Patient should not be given IM injections or rectal thermometers. Caution patient not to drink alcoholic beverages or take medication containing aspirin or NSAIDs, as these may precipitate gastric bleeding.
- Caution patient to make position changes slowly to minimize orthostatic hypotension.
- **Inhaln:** Advise patient that an unpleasant metallic taste may occur with pentamidine administration but is not significant.
- Inform patients who continue to smoke that bronchospasm and coughing during therapy are more likely.

Evaluation/Desired Outcomes

- Prevention or resolution of the signs and symptoms of PJP in HIV-positive patients.

pentosan (pen-toe-san)

Elmiron

Classification

Therapeutic: interstitial cystitis agents
Pharmacologic: heparin-like compounds

Pregnancy Category B

Indications

Management symptoms (bladder pain/discomfort) of chronic interstitial cystitis (IC).

Action

Adheres to uroepithelium, providing a protective barrier against irritating solutes in urine. Has anticoagulant and fibrinolytic properties. **Therapeutic Effects:** ↓ pain and discomfort in chronic IC.

Pharmacokinetics

Absorption: 6% absorbed following oral administrations.

Distribution: Distributes into uroepithelium of the genitourinary tract with less found in liver, spleen, lung, skin, perisoteum, and bone marrow.

Metabolism and Excretion: Metabolized by saturable enzyme systems in liver, spleen and kidney. Majority (58–84%) excreted in feces as unchanged (unabsorbed drug). Metabolites of absorbed drug are renally excreted; minimal renal excretion of unchanged drug.

Half-life: 27 hr.

TIME/ACTION PROFILE (↓ symptoms)

ROUTE	ONSET	PEAK	DURATION
PO	within 4 wk-6 mos	unknown	unknown

Contraindications/Precautions

Contraindicated in: Hypersensitivity.

Use Cautiously in: Underlying coagulopathy, concurrent medications that ↑ bleeding risk, history of aneurysms. thrombocytopenia, hemophilia, GI ulceration/bleeding, polyps, diverticula; History of heparin-induced thrombocytopenia; risk of bleeding may be ↑ Hepatic insufficiency; OB: Use in pregnancy only if clearly needed; Lactation: Use cautiously in breast-feeding women; Pedi: Safe and effective use in children <16 yr has not been established.

Adverse Reactions/Side Effects

CNS: dizziness, headache. **EENT:** epistaxis. **GI:** abdominal pain, diarrhea, dyspepsia, gum bleeding, ↑ liver enzymes, nausea, rectal bleeding. **Derm:** alopecia, ecchymosis, rash. **Hemat:** bleeding, ↑ bleeding time.

Interactions

Drug-Drug: Concurrent use of **coumarin anticoagulants**, **heparins**, **t-PA**, **streptokinase**, high dose **aspirin**, or **NSAIDs** may ↑ risk of bleeding.

Route/Dosage

PO (Adults): 100 mg three times daily.

Availability

Capsules: 100 mg.

NURSING IMPLICATIONS

Assessment

- Assess pain intensity, frequency, and duration in patient with interstitial cystitis.
- ***Lab Test Considerations:*** Doses of <1200 mg/day are unlikely to affect PT or PTT.
- May cause liver function abnormalities.

- May rarely cause anemia, ↑ PT, ↑ PTT, leukopenia, and thrombocytopenia.

Potential Nursing Diagnoses

Chronic pain (Indications)

Implementation

- **PO:** Administer on an empty stomach 3 times daily, at least 1 hr before or 2 hr after meals.

Patient/Family Teaching

- Instruct patient to take pentosan as directed, taking no more or no more frequently than prescribed.
- Advise patient to notify health care professional if surgery, anticoagulant therapy (warfarin, heparin), or therapy with high doses of aspirin or NSAIDs is planned.
- Advise patient to notify health care professional if pregnancy is planned or suspected or if breast feeding.

Evaluation/Desired Outcomes

- ↓ in pain and discomfort of interstitial cystitis. Reassess after 3 mo of therapy. If no improvement but no limiting adverse events are present, may be continued for 3 more mo.

perampanel (per-am-pa-nel)

Fycompa

Classification

Therapeutic: anticonvulsants

Pharmacologic: glutamate receptor antagonists

Schedule III

Pregnancy Category C

Indications

Adjunctive treatment (with other anti-epileptic drugs [AEDs]) of partial-onset seizures with or without secondarily generalized seizures. Adjunctive treatment (with other AEDs) of primary generalized tonic-clonic seizures.

Action

Acts as a non-competitive α-amino-3–hydroxy-5–methyl-4–isoxazolepropionic acid (AMPA) antagonist on post-synaptic neuronal glutamate (excitatory) receptors. **Therapeutic Effects:** Decreased incidence and severity of partial-onset seizures and primary generalized tonic-clonic seizures.

Pharmacokinetics

Absorption: Rapidly and completely absorbed following oral administration.

Distribution: Unknown.

Protein Binding: 95–96%.

Metabolism and Excretion: Extensively metabolized by CYP3A4/5 enzyme systems; excreted in urine and feces primarily as metabolites.

Half-life: 105 hr.

TIME/ACTION PROFILE

ROUTE	ONSET	PEAK	DURATION†
PO	unknown	unknown	2 wk

†Duration of effects following cessation.

Contraindications/Precautions

Contraindicated in: Strong P450 inducers (other than AEDs); Severe hepatic impairment.

Use Cautiously in: History of homicidal/suicidal ideation or other psychiatric/behavioral issues; Geri: ↑ risk of adverse reactions; slower titration recommended; OB: Use in pregnancy only when potential benefits outweigh potential fetal risks; Lactation: Use cautiously; Pedi: Children <12 yr (safety and effectiveness not established).

Adverse Reactions/Side Effects

CNS: dizziness, drowsiness, headache, aggression, anger, fatigue, psychiatric/behavioral problems, hostility, irritability, suicidal ideation, vertigo. **Metab:** weight gain. **Neuro:** ataxia, balance disorder, gait disturbance. **Misc:** falls.

Interactions

Drug-Drug: Doses >12 m g/day may ↓ effectiveness of **levonorgestrel-containing hormonal contraceptives. CYPP450 inducers** including **carbamazepine, oxcarbazepine, phenobarbital, phenytoin, primidone**, and **topiramate** can ↓ levels and effectiveness; careful monitoring is required especially during initiation and withdrawal. Dosage adjustments may be required. ↑ risk of CNS depression with other **CNS depressants** including **alcohol**, sedating **antihistamines, barbiturates, benzodiazepines, opioids** and **sedative/hypnotics**.

Drug-Natural Products: Levels and effectiveness may be ↓ by **St. John's wort**; concurrent use should be avoided.

Route/Dosage

Partial-Onset Seizures

PO (Adults and Children ≥12 yr): 2 mg once daily at bedtime initially, may be ↑ by 2 mg/day weekly up to 4–12 mg once daily; *Concurrent enzyme-inducers*—4 mg once daily at bedtime initially may be ↑ by 2 mg/day weekly up to 12 mg once daily.

PO (Geriatric Patients): 2 mg once daily at bedtime initially, may be ↑ by 2 mg/day every 2 wk up to 4–12 mg once daily; *Concurrent enzyme-inducers*—4 mg once daily at bedtime initially may be ↑ by 2 mg/day every 2 wk up to 12 mg once daily.

Hepatic Impairment

PO (Adults and Children ≥12 yr): *Mild hepatic impairment*—2 mg once daily at bedtime initially, may be ↑ by 2 mg/day every 2 wk up to 6 mg once daily; *Moderate hepatic impairment*—2 mg once daily at bedtime initially, may be ↑ by 2 mg/day after 2 wk up to 4 mg once daily.

Primary Generalized Tonic-Clonic Seizures

PO (Adults and Children ≥12 yr): 2 mg once daily at bedtime initially, may be ↑ by 2 mg/day weekly up to 8–12 mg once daily; *Concurrent enzyme-inducers*—4 mg once daily at bedtime initially may be ↑ by 2 mg/day weekly up to 12 mg once daily.
PO (Geriatric Patients): 2 mg once daily at bedtime initially, may be ↑ by 2 mg/day every 2 wk up to 4–12 mg once daily; *Concurrent enzyme-inducers*—4 mg once daily at bedtime initially may be ↑ by 2 mg/day every 2 wk up to 12 mg once daily.

Hepatic Impairment

PO (Adults and Children ≥12 yr): *Mild hepatic impairment*—2 mg once daily at bedtime initially, may be ↑ by 2 mg/day every 2 wk up to 6 mg once daily; *Moderate hepatic impairment*—2 mg once daily at bedtime initially, may be ↑ by 2 mg/day after 2 wk up to 4 mg once daily.

Availability

Tablets: 2 mg, 4 mg, 6 mg, 8 mg, 10 mg, 12 mg.

NURSING IMPLICATIONS

Assessment

- Assess location, duration, and characteristics of seizure activity. Institute seizure precautions. Assess response to and continued need for perampanel periodically during therapy.
- Monitor closely for notable changes in behavior that could indicate the emergence or worsening of suicidal thoughts or behavior, new or worse aggressive behavior, or depression.

Potential Nursing Diagnoses

Risk for injury (Indications)

Implementation

- **PO:** Administer once daily at bedtime.

Patient/Family Teaching

- Instruct patient to take perampanel as directed. Missed doses should be omitted and dosing resumed the following day. Notify health care professional if more than 1 day of dosing is missed. Medication should be gradually discontinued, do not stop abruptly, to prevent seizures. Advise patient to read the *Medication Guide* prior to starting perampanel and with each Rx refill in case of changes.
- May cause dizziness, sleepiness, fatigue and gait disturbance, increasing risk of falls. Caution patient to avoid driving or other activities requiring alertness until response to medication is known.
- Inform patients and families of risk of suicidal thoughts and behavior (behavioral changes, emergency or worsening signs and symptoms of depression, unusual changes in mood, or emergence of suicidal thoughts, behavior, or thoughts of self-harm) and aggressive behavior (hostility, anger, anxiety, irritability, being suspicious or distrustful, believing things that are not true). Advise that these should be reported to health care professional immediately.
- Instruct patient to notify health care professional of all Rx or OTC medications, vitamins, or herbal products being taken and consult health care professional before taking any new medications, especially carbamazepine, phenytoin, oxcarbazepine, rifampin, and St. John's wort. Advise patient to avoid taking other CNS depressants or alcohol.
- Perampanel decreases efficacy of levonorgestrel; advise patients to use a non-hormonal form of birth control during therapy. Advise female patients to notify health care professional if pregnancy is planned or suspected or if breast feeding. Encourage pregnant patients to enroll in the North American Antiepileptic Drug (NAAED) Pregnancy Registry by calling 1-888-233-2334; information is available at www.aedpregnancyregistry.org.

Evaluation/Desired Outcomes

- Decreased seizure activity.

perindopril, See ANGIOTENSIN-CONVERTING ENZYME (ACE) INHIBITORS.

permethrin (per-meth-rin)

Elimite

Classification
Therapeutic: pediculocides

Pregnancy Category B

Indications

5% cream: Eradication of *Sarcoptes scabiei* (scabies).

Action

Causes repolarization and paralysis in scabies by disrupting sodium transport in normal nerve cells. **Therapeutic Effects:** Death of parasites.

Pharmacokinetics

Absorption: Small amounts (<2%) systemically absorbed.
Distribution: Unknown.

Metabolism and Excretion: Rapidly inactivated by enzymes.
Half-life: Unknown.

TIME/ACTION PROFILE (pediculocidal action)

ROUTE	ONSET	PEAK	DURATION
Topical	10 min	unknown	14 days

Contraindications/Precautions

Contraindicated in: Hypersensitivity to permethrin, pyrethrins (insecticides or veterinary pesticides), chrysanthemums, or isopropyl alcohol; Lactation: Lactation.
Use Cautiously in: OB: Use only if clearly needed; Pedi: Children <2 mo.

Adverse Reactions/Side Effects

Derm: burning, itching, rash, redness, stinging, swelling. **Neuro:** numbness, tingling.

Interactions

Drug-Drug: No significant interactions.

Route/Dosage

Topical (Adults and Children): Massage into all skin surfaces. Leave on for 8–14 hr, then wash off.
Topical (Infants >2 mo): Massage into hairline, scalp, neck, temple, and forehead. Leave on for 8–14 hr, then wash off.

Availability (generic available)

Cream: 5%.

NURSING IMPLICATIONS

Assessment

- **Scabies:** Assess skin for scabies prior to and following therapy.

Potential Nursing Diagnoses

Impaired home maintenance (Indications)
Bathing/hygiene self-care deficit (Indications)

Implementation

- **Topical:** For topical application only.

Patient/Family Teaching

- Instruct patient to notify health care professional if scalp itching, numbness, redness, or rash occurs.
- Instruct patient to avoid getting Elimite cream in eyes. If this occurs, eyes should be flushed thoroughly with water. Health care professional should be contacted if eye irritation persists.
- Instruct patient on methods of preventing reinfestation. All clothes, including outdoor apparel and household linens, should be machine-washed using very hot water and dried for at least 20 min in a hot dryer. Dry-clean nonwashable clothes. Brushes and combs should be soaked in hot (130°F), soapy water for 5–10 min. Remind patient that brushes and combs should not be shared. Wigs and hairpieces should be shampooed. Rugs and upholstered furniture should be vacuumed. Toys should be washed in hot, soapy water. Items that cannot be washed should be sealed in a plastic bag for 2 wk.
- If patient is a child, instruct parents to notify school nurse or day care center so that classmates and playmates can be checked.
- **Scabies:** Instruct patient to massage thoroughly into the skin from head to soles of feet. Treat infants on the hairline, neck, scalp, temple, and forehead. Remove the cream by washing after 8–14 hr. Usually 30 g (½ tube) is sufficient for adults. One application is curative.

Evaluation/Desired Outcomes

- Eradication of scabies following one application.
- If resistance to permethrin develops, malathion may be used.

pertuzumab

(per-**tue**-zue-mab)
Perjeta

Classification
Therapeutic: antineoplastics
Pharmacologic: HER2/neu receptor antagonists, monoclonal antibodies

Pregnancy Category D

Indications

Treatment of HER2-positive metastatic breast cancer in patients who have not yet been treated with anti-HER2 agents or chemotherapy; used in combination with docetaxel and trastuzumab. Neoadjuvant treatment of HER2-positive locally advanced, inflammatory, or early stage breast cancer (either >2 cm in diameter or node-positive); used in combination with docetaxel and trastuzumab.

Action

A monoclonal antibody that attaches to and blocks the human epidermal growth factor receptor 2 protein (HER2), resulting in cell growth arrest and apoptosis.
Therapeutic Effects: Decreased spread of metastatic breast cancer.

Pharmacokinetics

Absorption: IV administration results in complete bioavailability.
Distribution: Unknown.
Metabolism and Excretion: Unknown.
Half-life: 18 days.

TIME/ACTION PROFILE

ROUTE	ONSET	PEAK	DURATION
IV	unknown	unknown	20 mo†

† Median duration of response.

Contraindications/Precautions

Contraindicated in: Hypersensitivity; OB: Avoid use during pregnancy; Lactation: Discontinue drug or discontinue breast feeding.

Use Cautiously in: ⧖ HER2 testing is required prior to treatment; ⧖ Asian patients (↑ incidence of febrile neutropenia); Rep: Women with reproductive potential; Pedi: Safety and effectiveness not established.

Adverse Reactions/Side Effects

May reflect combination treatment with docetaxel and trastuzumab..

CNS: dizziness, fatigue, headache, insomnia, weakness. **EENT:** ↑ lacrimation. **Resp:** dyspnea. **CV:** ↓ left ventricular ejection fraction (LVEF), peripheral edema. **GI:** ↓ appetite, diarrhea, dysgeusia, nausea, vomiting. **Derm:** alopecia, rash, dry skin, itching, nail disorder. **Hemat:** ANEMIA, LEUKOPENIA, NEUTROPENIA. **MS:** arthralgia, myalgia. **Neuro:** peripheral neuropathy. **Misc:** allergic reactions including ANAPHYLAXIS, chills, infusion reactions, fever, hypersensitivity reactions.

Interactions

Drug-Drug: ↑ risk of bone marrow depression/immunosuppression with other **bone marrow depressants/immunosuppressabts** or **radiation therapy**.

Route/Dosage

Metastatic Breast Cancer

IV (Adults): 840 mg initially, then 420 mg every 3 wk. If less than 6 wk passes between infusions, continue with 420 mg dosing, if 6 wk or more passes between infusions, restart with initial 840 mg dose followed by 420 mg every 3 wk.

Neoadjuvant Treatment of Breast Cancer

IV (Adults): 840 mg initially, then 420 mg every 3 wk for 3–6 cycles given preoperatively. If less than 6 wk passes between infusions, continue with 420 mg dosing, if 6 wk or more passes between infusions, restart with initial 840 mg dose followed by 420 mg every 3 wk.

Availability

Solution for intravenous injection (requires dilution): 30 mg/mL.

NURSING IMPLICATIONS

Assessment

- Monitor left ventricular ejection fraction (LVEF) prior to and every 3 mo with metastatic disease and every 6 wk in neoadjuvant setting during therapy. If LVEF drops to <40% or LVEF of 45–49% with a ≥10% absolute decrease below pretreatment values withhold pertuzumab and trastuzumab and repeat LVEF within 3 wks. Pertuzumab may be resumed if LVEF >45% or to 40–45% associated with a <10% absolute decrease below pretreatment values. If after a repeat assessment LVEF has not improved or further declined, discontinue pertuzumab and trastuzumab, unless benefits outweigh risks. Patients who received anthracyclines are at increased risk for ↓ LVEF.
- If trastuzumab is withheld or discontinued, withhold or discontinue pertuzumab. If docetaxel is discontinued, pertuzumab and trastuzumab therapy may continue. Dose reductions are not recommended for pertuzumab.
- Assess patient closely for 60 min after initial infusion and 30 min after subsequent infusions for signs and symptoms of infusion-associated reactions (pyrexia, chills, fatigue, headache, asthenia, hypersensitivity, vomiting). If a significant infusion-associated reaction occurs, slow or interrupt infusion and administer appropriate medical therapies. Monitor until complete resolution of signs and symptoms. If severe infusion reactions occur, consider discontinuation of pertuzumab.
- ***Lab Test Considerations:*** ⧖ Determine HER protein overexpression prior to therapy.
- Verify pregnancy status prior to initiation of pertuzumab.
- Monitor CBC with differential periodically during therapy.

Potential Nursing Diagnoses

Decreased cardiac output (Adverse Reactions)

Implementation

IV Administration

- When administered with pertuzumab, initial dose of trastuzumab is 8 mg/kg infused over 90 min, followed every 3 wks by 6 mg/kg infused over 30–90 min.
- When administered with pertuzumab, initial dose of docetaxel is 75 mg/m² as an IV infusion. Dose of docetaxel may be ↑ to 100 mg/m² every 3 wks if initial dose is tolerated.
- Administer pertuzumab, trastuzumab, and docetaxel. Administer pertuzumab and trastuzumab in any order. Administer docetaxel after pertuzumab and trastuzumab. Observe patient for 30 to 60 min after pertuzumab infusion and before any subsequent infusion of trastuzumab or docetaxel.
- **Intermittent Infusion:** ***Diluent:*** 0.9% NaCl; do not use D5W. Withdraw appropriate volume of pertuzumab and dilute in 250 mL using a PVC or non-PVC polyolefin infusion bag. Gently invert to mix; do not shake. If not administered immediately, may be refrigerated for 24 hrs. ***Rate:*** Infuse initial 840 mg over 60 min, followed every 3 wks by 420 mg over 30–60 min.

P

- For delayed or missed doses, if time between 2 sequential infusions is <6 wk, administer 420 mg dose of pertuzumab; do not wait until next planned dose. If time between 2 sequential infusions ≥6 wk, re-administer initial 840 mg dose over 60 min, followed every 3 wk by 420 mg dose over 30–60 min.

Patient/Family Teaching

- Explain purpose of medication to patient.
- Advise patient to report signs and symptoms of infusion-associated reactions immediately.
- Instruct patient to notify health care professional promptly if fever; chills; cough; hoarseness; sore throat; signs of infection; lower back or side pain; painful or difficult urination; bleeding gums; bruising; petechiae; blood in stools, urine, or emesis; increased fatigue; dyspnea. Caution patient to avoid crowds and persons with known infections. Instruct patient to use soft toothbrush and electric razor and to avoid falls. Caution patient not to drink alcoholic beverages or take medication containing aspirin or NSAIDs; may precipitate gastric bleeding.
- Instruct patient to notify health care professional of all Rx or OTC medications, vitamins, or herbal products being taken and consult health care professional before taking any new medications.
- Rep: Advise female patient that pertuzumab is teratogenic and to notify health care professional immediately if pregnancy is planned or suspected or if breast feeding. Caution patient to use effective contraception during and for 7 mo following the last dose. Women who are breast feeding should be advised to discontinue nursing or discontinue pertuzumab. Encourage women who may be exposed during pregnancy to enroll in the MotHER Pregnancy Registry by contacting 1-800-690-6720 and report exposure to the Genentech Adverse Event Line at 1-888-835-2555. Monitor patients who become pregnant for oligohydramnios.

Evaluation/Desired Outcomes

- Decreased spread of metastatic breast cancer.

phenazopyridine

(fen-az-oh-**peer**-i-deen)

Baridium, ✱Phenazo, Pyridium, Pyridium Plus

Classification

Therapeutic: nonopioid analgesics
Pharmacologic: urinary tract analgesics

Pregnancy Category B

Indications

Provides relief from the following urinary tract symptoms, which may occur in association with infection or following urologic procedures: Pain, Itching, Burning, Urgency, Frequency.

Action

Acts locally on the urinary tract mucosa to produce analgesic or local anesthetic effects. Has no antimicrobial activity. **Therapeutic Effects:** Diminished urinary tract discomfort.

Pharmacokinetics

Absorption: Appears to be well absorbed following oral administration.
Distribution: Unknown. Small amounts cross the placenta.
Metabolism and Excretion: Rapidly excreted unchanged in the urine.
Half-life: Unknown.

TIME/ACTION PROFILE (urinary analgesia)

ROUTE	ONSET	PEAK	DURATION
PO	unknown	5–6 hr	6–8 hr

Contraindications/Precautions

Contraindicated in: Hypersensitivity; Glomerulonephritis; Severe hepatitis, uremia, or renal failure; Renal insufficiency; Glucose-6–phosphate dehydrogenase (G6PD) deficiency.
Use Cautiously in: Hepatitis; OB, Lactation: Safety not established.

Adverse Reactions/Side Effects

CNS: headache, vertigo. **GI:** hepatotoxicity, nausea. **GU:** bright-orange urine, renal failure. **Derm:** rash. **Hemat:** hemolytic anemia, methemoglobinemia.

Interactions

Drug-Drug: None significant.

Route/Dosage

PO (Adults): 200 mg 3 times daily for 2 days.
PO (Children): 4 mg/kg 3 times daily for 2 days.

Availability (generic available)

Tablets: 95 mg^{OTC}, 100 mg, ✱100 mg^{OTC}, ✱200 mg^{OTC}, 200 mg.

NURSING IMPLICATIONS

Assessment

- Assess patient for urgency, frequency, and pain on urination prior to and throughout therapy.
- ***Lab Test Considerations:*** Renal function should be monitored periodically during course of therapy.
- Interferes with urine tests based on color reactions (glucose, ketones, bilirubin, steroids, protein).

Potential Nursing Diagnoses

Acute pain (Indications)
Impaired urinary elimination (Indications)

Implementation

- ***High Alert:*** Do not confuse Pyridium (phenazopyridine) with pyridoxine.

- Medication should be discontinued after pain or discomfort is relieved (usually 2 days for treatment of urinary tract infection). Concurrent antibiotic therapy should continue for full prescribed duration.
- **PO:** Administer medication with or following meals to decrease GI irritation. Do not crush, break, or chew tablet.

Patient/Family Teaching

- Instruct patient to take medication exactly as directed. If a dose is missed, take as soon as remembered unless almost time for next dose.
- Advise patient that while phenazopyridine administration is stopped once pain or discomfort is relieved, concurrent antibiotic therapy must be continued for full duration of therapy. Do not save unused portion of phenazopyridine without consulting health care professional.
- Inform patient that drug causes reddish-orange discoloration of urine that may stain clothing or bedding. Sanitary napkin may be worn to avoid clothing stains. May also cause staining of soft contact lenses.
- Instruct patient to notify health care professional if rash, skin discoloration, or unusual tiredness occurs.

Evaluation/Desired Outcomes

- Decrease in pain and burning on urination.

phenelzine, See MONOAMINE OXIDASE (MAO) INHIBITORS.

PHENobarbital

(fee-noe-**bar**-bi-tal)

✱Ancalixir, ~~Luminal~~

Classification

Therapeutic: anticonvulsants, sedative/hypnotics

Pharmacologic: barbiturates

Schedule IV

Pregnancy Category D

Indications

Anticonvulsant in tonic-clonic (grand mal), partial, and febrile seizures in children. Preoperative sedative and in other situations in which sedation may be required. Hypnotic (short-term). **Unlabeled Use:** Prevention/treatment of hyperbilirubinemia in neonates.

Action

Produces all levels of CNS depression. Depresses the sensory cortex, decreases motor activity, and alters cerebellar function. Inhibits transmission in the nervous system and raises the seizure threshold. Capable of inducing (speeding up) enzymes in the liver that metabolize drugs, bilirubin, and other compounds. **Therapeutic Effects:** Anticonvulsant activity. Sedation.

Pharmacokinetics

Absorption: Absorption is slow but relatively complete (70–90%).

Distribution: Unknown.

Metabolism and Excretion: 75% metabolized by the liver, 25% excreted unchanged by the kidneys.

Half-life: Neonates: 1.8–8.3 days; Infants: 0.8–5.5 days; Children: 1.5–3 days; Adults: 2–6 days.

TIME/ACTION PROFILE (sedation†)

ROUTE	ONSET	PEAK	DURATION
PO	30–60 min	unknown	>6 hr
IM, subcut	10–30 min	unknown	4–6 hr
IV	5 min	30 min	4–6 hr

†Full anticonvulsant effects occur after 2–3 wk of chronic dosing unless a loading dose has been used.

Contraindications/Precautions

Contraindicated in: Hypersensitivity; Comatose patients or those with pre-existing CNS depression; Severe respiratory disease with dyspnea or obstruction; Uncontrolled severe pain; Known alcohol intolerance (elixir only); Lactation: Discontinue drug or bottle feed.

Use Cautiously in: Hepatic dysfunction; Severe renal impairment; History of suicide attempt or drug abuse; Hypnotic use should be short-term. Chronic use may lead to dependence; OB: Chronic use during pregnancy results in drug dependency in the infant; may result in coagulation defects and fetal malformation; acute use at term may result in respiratory depression in the newborn; Geri: Initial dose ↓ recommended.

Adverse Reactions/Side Effects

CNS: <u>hangover</u>, delirium, depression, drowsiness, excitation, lethargy, vertigo. **Resp:** respiratory depression; *IV*, LARYNGOSPASM, bronchospasm. **CV:** *IV*—hypotension. **GI:** constipation, diarrhea, nausea, vomiting. **Derm:** photosensitivity, rashes, urticaria. **Local:** phlebitis at IV site. **MS:** arthralgia, myalgia, neuralgia. **Misc:** hypersensitivity reactions including ANGIOEDEMA and SERUM SICKNESS, physical dependence, psychological dependence.

Interactions

Drug-Drug: Additive CNS depression with other **CNS depressants**, including **alcohol**, **antihistamines**, **opioid analgesics**, and other **sedative/hypnotics**. May induce hepatic enzymes that metabolize other drugs, ↓ their effectiveness, including **hormonal contraceptives**, **warfarin**, **chloramphenicol**, **cyclo-**

P

sporine, **dacarbazine**, **corticosteroids**, **tricyclic antidepressants**, **felodipine**, **clonazepam**, **carbamazepine**, **verapamil**, **theophylline**, **metronidazole**, and **quinidine**. May ↑ risk of hepatic toxicity of **acetaminophen**. **MAO inhibitors**, **valproic acid**, or **divalproex** may ↓ metabolism of phenobarbital, ↑ sedation. **Rifampin** may ↑ metabolism of and ↓ effects of phenobarbital. May ↑ risk of hematologic toxicity with **cyclophosphamide**.

Drug-Natural Products: Concomitant use of **kava-kava**, **valerian**, **chamomile**, or **hops** can ↑ CNS depression. **St. John's wort** may ↓ effects.

Route/Dosage

Status Epilepticus

IV (Adults and Children >1 mo): 15–18 mg/kg in a single or divided dose, maximum loading dose 20 mg/kg.

IV (Neonates): 15–20 mg/kg in a single or divided dose.

Maintenance Anticonvulsant

IV, PO (Adults and Children >12 yr): 1–3 mg/kg/day as a single dose or 2 divided doses.

IV, PO (Children 5–12 yr): 4–6 mg/kg/day in 1–2 divided doses.

IV, PO (Children 1–5 yr): 6–8 mg/kg/day in 1–2 divided doses.

IV, PO (Infants): 5–6 mg/kg/day in 1–2 divided doses.

IV, PO (Neonates): 3–4 mg/kg/day once daily, may need to increase up to 5 mg/kg/day by 2nd week of therapy.

Sedation

PO, IM (Adults): 30–120 mg/day in 2–3 divided doses. *Preoperative sedation*—100–200 mg IM 1–1.5 hours before the procedure.

PO (Children): 2 mg/kg 3 times daily. *Preoperative sedation*—1–3 mg/kg PO/IM/IV 1–1.5 hours before the procedure.

Hypnotic

PO, Subcut, IV, IM (Adults): 100–320 mg at bedtime.

IV, IM, Subcut (Children): 3–5 mg/kg at bedtime.

Hyperbilirubinemia

PO (Adults): 90–180 mg/day in 2–3 divided doses.

PO (Children <12 yr): 3–8 mg/kg/day in 2–3 divided doses, doses up to 12 mg/kg/day have been used.

Availability (generic available)

Tablets: 15 mg, 30 mg, 60 mg, 100 mg. **Elixir:** 20 mg/5 mL. **Injection:** 65 mg/mL, 130 mg/mL.

NURSING IMPLICATIONS

Assessment

- Monitor respiratory status, pulse, and BP and signs and symptoms of angioedema (swelling of lips, face, throat, dyspnea) frequently in patients receiving phenobarbital IV. Equipment for resuscitation and artificial ventilation should be readily available. Respiratory depression is dose-dependent.
- Prolonged therapy may lead to psychological or physical dependence. Restrict amount of drug available to patient, especially if depressed, suicidal, or with a history of addiction.
- Geri: Elderly patients may react to phenobarbital with marked excitement, depression, and confusion. Monitor for these adverse reactions.
- **Seizures:** Assess location, duration, and characteristics of seizure activity.
- **Sedation:** Assess level of consciousness and anxiety when used as a preoperative sedative.
- Assess postoperative patients for pain with a pain scale. Phenobarbital may increase sensitivity to painful stimuli.
- ***Lab Test Considerations:*** Patients on prolonged therapy should have hepatic and renal function and CBC evaluated periodically.
- Monitor serum folate concentrations periodically during therapy because of increased folate requirements of patients on long-term anticonvulsant therapy with phenobarbital.
- May cause ↓ serum bilirubin concentrations in neonates, in patients with congenital nonhemolytic unconjugated hyperbilirubinemia, and in epileptics.
- ***Toxicity and Overdose:*** Serum phenobarbital levels may be monitored when used as an anticonvulsant. Therapeutic blood levels are 10–40 mcg/mL. Symptoms of toxicity include confusion, drowsiness, dyspnea, slurred speech, and staggering.

Potential Nursing Diagnoses

Risk for injury (Indications, Side Effects)
Acute confusion (Side Effects)

Implementation

- Do not confuse phenobarbital with pentobarbital.
- Supervise ambulation and transfer of patients following administration. Two side rails should be raised and call bell within reach at all times. Keep bed in low position. Institute seizure and fall precautions.
- When changing from phenobarbital to another anticonvulsant, gradually decrease phenobarbital dose while concurrently increasing dose of replacement medication to maintain anticonvulsant effects.
- **PO:** Tablets may be crushed and mixed with food or fluids (do not administer dry) for patients with difficulty swallowing. Oral solution may be taken undiluted or mixed with water, milk, or fruit juice. Use calibrated measuring device for accurate measurement of liquid doses.
- **IM:** Injections should be given deep into the gluteal muscle to minimize tissue irritation. Do not inject >5 mL into any one site, because of tissue irritation.

IV Administration

- **IV:** Doses may require 15–30 min to reach peak concentrations in the brain. Administer minimal dose and wait for effectiveness before administering 2nd dose to prevent cumulative barbiturate-induced depression.

- **IV Push:** ***Diluent:*** Reconstitute sterile powder for IV dose with a minimum of 3 mL of sterile water for injection. Dilute further with 10 mL of sterile water. Do not use solution that is not absolutely clear within 5 min after reconstitution or that contains a precipitate. Discard powder or solution that has been exposed to air for longer than 30 min.
- Solution is highly alkaline; avoid extravasation, which may cause tissue damage and necrosis. If extravasation occurs, injection of 5% procaine solution into affected area and application of moist heat may be ordered.
- ***Concentration:*** 130 mg/mL (undiluted). ***Rate:*** Do not inject IV faster than 1 mg/kg/min with a maximum of 30 mg over 1 min in infants and children and 60 mg over 1 min in adults. Titrate slowly for desired response. Rapid administration may result in respiratory depression.
- **Y-Site Compatibility:** acyclovir, alfentanil, amikacin, aminocaproic acid, aminophylline, amphotericin B lipid complex, amphotericin B liposome, anidulafungin, argatroban, ascorbic acid, atropine, azathioprine, aztreonam, benztropine, bivalirudin, bleomycin, bumetanide, butorphanol, calcioum chloride, calcium gluconate, carboplatin, cefazolin, ceftazidime, ceftriaxone, chloramphenicol, cisplatin, clindamycin, cyanocobalamin, cyclophosphamide, cytarabine, dactinomycin, daptomycin, dexamethasone, dexmedetomidine, digoxin, docetaxel, dopamine, doripenem, doxacurium, doxapram, enalaprilat, ephedrine, epoetin alfa, eptifibatide, ertapenem, etoposide, etoposide phosphate, famotidine, fenoldopam, fentanyl, fluconazole, fludarabine, fluorouracil, folic acid, fosphenytoin, furosemide, ganciclovir, gemcitabine, gentamicin, glycopyrrolate, granisetron, heparin, hetastarch, hydrocortisone, ifosfamide, indomethacin, insulin, irinotecan, ketorolac, labetalol, linezolid, lorazepam, magnesium sulfate, mannitol, meropenem, metaraminol, methadone, methotrexate, methoxamine, methylprednisolone, metoclopramide, metoprolol, metronidazole, milrinone, mitoxantrone, morphine, multivitamins, nafcillin, naloxone, nesiritide, nitroglycerin, nitroprusside, octreotide, oxacillin, oxytocin, paclitaxel, palonosetron, pamidronate, pancuronium, pantoprazole, pemetrexed, pentobarbital, phenylephrine, phytonadione, piperacillin/tazobactam, potassium acetate, potassium chloride, procainamide, propofol, propranolol, ranitidine, rocuronium, sodium acetate, sodium bicarbonate, streptokinase, sufentanil, teniposide, theophylline, thiotepa, tigecycline, tirofiban, tobramycin, tolazoline, trimetaphan, vancomycin, vasopressin, vecuronium, vincristine, voriconazole, zoledronic acid.
- **Y-Site Incompatibility:** alemtuzumab, amphotericin B cholesteryl, ampicillin, atracurium, buprenorphine, carmustine, caspofungin, cefotaxime, cefotetan, cefoxitin, cefuroxime, chlorpromazine, cyclophosphamide, dantrolene, diazepam, diazoxide, diltiazem, diphenhydramine, dobutamine, doxorubicin, doxycycline, epinephrine, erythromycin, esmolol, haloperidol, hydroxyzine, idarubicin, isoproterenol, lidocaine, mechlorethamine, meperidine, methyldopate, midazolam, mycophenolate, nalbuphine, norepinephrine, ondansetron, papaverine, penicillin G, pentamidine, pentazocine, phenytoin, prochlorperazine, promethazine, protamine, pyridoxime, quinupristin/dalfopristin, succinylcholine, thiamine, trimethoprim/sulfamethoxazole, verapamil, vinorelbine.

Patient/Family Teaching

- Advise patient to take medication as directed. Take missed doses as soon as remembered if not almost time for next dose; do not double doses.
- Advise patients on prolonged therapy not to discontinue medication without consulting health care professional. Abrupt withdrawal may precipitate seizures or status epilepticus.
- Medication may cause daytime drowsiness. Caution patient to avoid driving and other activities requiring alertness until response to medication is known. Do not resume driving until physician gives clearance based on control of seizure disorder.
- Caution patient to avoid taking alcohol or other CNS depressants concurrently with this medication.
- Advise patient to notify health care professional if signs and symptoms of angioedema, fever, sore throat, mouth sores, unusual bleeding or bruising, nosebleeds, or petechiae occur.
- Teach sleep hygiene techniques (dark room, quiet, bedtime ritual, limit daytime napping, avoid nicotine and caffeine).
- Advise female patients using oral contraceptives to use an additional nonhormonal contraceptive during therapy and until next menstrual period. Instruct patient to contact health care professional immediately if pregnancy is planned or suspected.
- Pedi: Advise parents or caregivers that child may experience irritability, hyperactivity, and/or sleep disturbances, which may diminish in a few days to a few weeks or may persist until drug is stopped. An alternative medication can be considered. Instruct parents to monitor for skin rash occurring 7–20 days after treatment begins and to contact a health care provider if rash occurs. Teach family about symptoms of toxicity (staggering, drowsiness, slurred speech).

P

Evaluation/Desired Outcomes

- Decrease or cessation of seizure activity without excessive sedation. Several weeks may be required to achieve maximum anticonvulsant effects.
- Preoperative sedation.
- Improvement in sleep patterns.
- Decrease in serum bilirubin levels.

REMS

phentermine/topiramate

(**fen**-ter-meen/toe-**pyre**-a-mate)
Qsymia

Classification
Therapeutic: weight control agents
Pharmacologic: appetite suppressants

Schedule IV

Pregnancy Category X

Indications

Weight management as part of a program including caloric restriction and increased exercise in patients with an initial body mass index (BMI) of ≥30 kg/m^2 or a BMI of ≥27 kg/m^2 with at least one other risk factor (hypertension, type 2 diabetes mellitus or dyslipidemia).

Action

Phentermine—↓ appetite and food consumption;. *Topiramate*—↓ appetite and enhances satiety. **Therapeutic Effects:** Weight loss.

Pharmacokinetics

Absorption: *Phentermine*—Unknown; *Topiramate*—80% absorbed following oral administration.
Distribution: *Phentermine*—Unknown; *Topiramate*—Unknown.
Metabolism and Excretion: *Phentermine*—metabolized by the liver; *Topiramate*—70% excreted unchanged in urine.
Half-life: *Phentermine*—19–24 hr; *Topiramate*—21 hr.

TIME/ACTION PROFILE (phentermine—appetite suppression, topiramate—blood levels)

ROUTE	ONSET	PEAK	DURATION
PO (weight loss)	within 8 wk	16–32 wk	unknown

Contraindications/Precautions

Contraindicated in: Hypersensitivity/idiosyncracy to sympathomimetics; OB: Pregnancy (may cause fetal harm); Lactation: Breast feeding should be avoided; Glaucoma; Hyperthyroidism; During/within 14 days of MAO inhibitors; Severe renal impairment (CCr <30 mL/min); Severe hepatic impairment; History of suicidal thought/active suicidal ideation.
Use Cautiously in: Diabetes (weight loss may ↑ risk of hypoglycemia); Females with reproductive potential (negative pregnancy test and contraception required); History of substance abuse; Geri: ↑ risk of adverse effects, consider age-related decrease in cardiac, renal and hepatic function, concurrent chronic disease states and medications; Pedi: Safety and effectiveness not established.

Adverse Reactions/Side Effects

CNS: SEIZURES (FOLLOWING ABRUPT DISCONTINUATION), headache, insomnia, cognitive impairment, dizziness, mood disorders, suicidal ideation. **EENT:** acute myopia, blurred vision, eye pain, secondary angle closure glaucoma. **CV:** tachycardia, hypotension, palpitations. **GI:** HEPATOTOXICITY, altered taste, constipation, dry mouth. **GU:** ↑ creatinine, kidney stones. **Derm:** serious skin reactions including ERYTHEMA MULTIFORME, STEVENS-JOHNSON SYNDROME and TOXIC EPIDERMAL NECROLYSIS, alopecia, oligohydrosis (↓ sweating). **Endo:** hypoglycemia. **F and E:** metabolic acidosis, hypokalemia. **Neuro:** paraesthesia. **Misc:** hyperthermia.

Interactions

Drug-Drug: ↑ risk of hypokalemia with **non-potassium sparing diuretics**. ↑ risk of CNS depression with **other CNS depressants** including **alcohol**, some **antihistamines**, **sedative/hypnotics**, **antipsychotics**, and **opioid analgesics**; avoid concurrent use of alcohol. Altered exposure to **oral contraceptives** may ↑ risk of irregular bleeding. Blood levels of topiramate may be ↓ by **carbamazepine** or **phenytoin**. Concurrent use of topiramate with **valproic acid** may ↑ risk of hyperammonemia. Concurrent use of topiramate with **carbonic anhydrase inhibitors** may ↑ risk of metabolic acidosis and kidney stones. ↑ risk of hypotension with **antihypertensive** and **diuretics**.

Route/Dosage

PO (Adults): *Initial dose*—one phentermine 3.75 mg/topiramate 23 mg capsule daily for 14 days, then increase to one phentermine 7.5 mg/topiramate 46 mg capsule daily for 12 wk, then assess weight loss. If weight loss has not exeeded 3% of baseline, discontinue or escalate dose to one phentermine 11.25 mg/topiramate 69 mg capsule daily for 14 days, then one phentermine 15 mg/topiramate 92 mg capsule daily for 12 wk, if weight loss has not exceeded 5% of baseline, discontinue as success is unlikely. Discontinuation should proceed by taking the phentermine 15 mg/topiramate 92 mg capsule every other day for 1 wk.

Renal Impairment

PO (Adults): *CCr ≥30 mL/min–<50 mL/min*—daily dose should not exceed one phentermine 7.5 mg/topiramate 46 mg capsule daily.

Hepatic Impairment

PO (Adults): *Child-Pugh score 7–9*—daily dose should not exceed one phentermine 7.5 mg/topiramate 46 mg capsule daily.

Availability

Phentermine immediate-release/topiramate extended-release capsules: phentermine 3.75 mg/topiramate 23 mg (for titration only), phentermine 7.5 mg/topiramate 46 mg, phentermine 11.25 mg/topiramate 69 mg (for titration only), phentermine 15 mg/topiramate 92 mg. **Cost:** 3.75 mg/23 mg $163.24/30, 7.5 mg/46 mg $184.49/30, 11.25 mg/69 mg $221.38/30, 15 mg/92 mg $239.40/30.

NURSING IMPLICATIONS

Assessment

- Monitor patients for weight loss and adjust concurrent medications (antihypertensives, antidiabetics, lipid-lowering agents) as needed. Evaluate weight loss after each 12 wks of therapy.
- Monitor closely for notable changes in behavior that could indicate the emergence or worsening of suicidal thoughts or behavior or depression. Discontinue phentermine/topiramate if these occur.
- Monitor BP and heart rate periodically during therapy; may cause increase in resting heart rate. May cause hypotension in patients treated with antihypertensives.
- ***Lab Test Considerations:*** Obtain a pregnancy test prior to starting therapy and monthly during therapy.
- May cause hypoglycemia; monitor blood glucose closely in diabetic patients.
- May cause metabolic acidosis; monitor serum bicarbonate, prior to starting and periodically during therapy.
- May cause ↑ serum creatinine; peak increases observed after 4–8 wks of therapy. Monitor serum creatinine prior to and periodically during therapy; if persistent elevations occur, decrease dose or discontinue therapy.
- May cause hypokalemia; monitor serum potassium periodically during therapy.

Potential Nursing Diagnoses

Disturbed body image (Indications)
Imbalanced nutrition: more than body requirements (Indications)
Deficient knowledge, related to medication regimen (Patient/Family Teaching)

Implementation

- Qsymia is only available through certified pharmacies that are enrolled in the Qsymia certified pharmacy network. Information can be obtained at www.QsymiaREMS.com or by calling 1-888-998-4887.
- **PO:** Administer once daily in the morning without regard to food. Avoid dosing in the evening; may cause insomnia.

Patient/Family Teaching

- Instruct patient to take phentermine/topiramate as directed. Do not stop taking without consulting health care professional. Discontinue gradually taking 1 dose every other day for at least 1 wk to prevent seizures.
- Advise patient to notify health care professional if sustained periods of heart pounding or racing while at rest; severe and persistent eye pain or significant changes in vision; changes in attention, concentration, memory, and/or difficulty finding words; factors that can increase risk or acidosis (prolonged diarrhea, surgery, high protein/low carbohydrate diet, and/or concomitant medications).
- Inform patients and families of risk of suicidal thoughts and behavior (behavioral changes, emergency or worsening signs and symptoms of depression, unusual changes in mood, or emergence of suicidal thoughts, behavior, or thoughts of self-harm). Advise that these should be reported to health care professional immediately.
- May cause changes in mental performance, motor performance, and/or vision. Caution patients to avoid driving and other activities requiring alertness until response to medication is known.
- Instruct patient to increase fluid intake to increase urinary output and decrease risk of kidney stones.
- Advise patient to monitor for decreased sweating and increased body temperature during physical activity, especially in hot weather.
- Instruct patient to notify health care professional of all Rx or OTC medications, vitamins, or herbal products being taken and consult health care professional before taking any new medications. Advise patient to avoid taking other CNS depressants or alcohol.
- Phentermine/topiramate is teratogenic. Advise female patient to use effective contraception during therapy. Advise female patients to notify health care professional if pregnancy is planned or suspected or if breast feeding.

Evaluation/Desired Outcomes

- Decrease in weight and BMI. If 3% of baseline body weight is not lost by Week 12, increase dose or discontinue phentermine/topiramate. Evaluate after second 12 wk of therapy. If 5% of baseline body weight is not lost by second 12 wks of therapy, as it is unlikely patient will achieve and sustain clinically meaningful weight loss with continued treatment.

P

HIGH ALERT

phenylephrine (fen-il-eff-rin)

✱Neo-Synephrine, Vazculep

Classification

Therapeutic: vasopressors

Pharmacologic: adrenergics, alpha adrenergic agonists, vasopressors

Pregnancy Category B, C (Ophth, Parenteral)

For ophthalmic use see Appendix C

Indications

Management of hypotension associated with shock that may persist after adequate fluid replacement. Management of hypotension associated with anesthesia. **Anesthesia adjunct:** Prolongation of the duration of spinal anesthesia. Localization of the effect of regional anesthesia.

Action

Constricts blood vessels by stimulating alpha-adrenergic receptors. **Therapeutic Effects:** Increased BP.

Pharmacokinetics

Absorption: Well absorbed from IM sites. IV administration results in complete bioavailability.

Distribution: Highly distributed into organs and tissues.

Metabolism and Excretion: Metabolized by the liver into inactive metabolites.

Half-life: 2.5 hr.

TIME/ACTION PROFILE (vasopressor effects)

ROUTE	ONSET	PEAK	DURATION
IV	immediate	unknown	15–20 min
IM	10–15 min	unknown	0.5–2 hr
Subcut	10–15 min	unknown	50–60 min

Contraindications/Precautions

Contraindicated in: Hypersensitivity to bisulfites.

Use Cautiously in: HF, coronary artery disease, or peripheral arterial disease; OB, Lactation: Safety not established.

Adverse Reactions/Side Effects

CNS: blurred vision, headache, insomnia, nervousness, tremor. **Resp:** dyspnea. **CV:** ARRHYTHMIAS, bradycardia, chest pain, hypertension, ischemia, tachycardia. **Derm:** pruritis. **GI:** epigastric pain, nausea, vomiting. **Local:** phlebitis, sloughing at IV sites.

Interactions

Drug-Drug: Use with **general anesthetics** may result in myocardial irritability; use with extreme caution. Use with **MAO inhibitors, ergot alkaloids (methylergonovine), oxytocics, tricyclic antidepressants, atropine, corticosteroids,** or **atomoxetine** results in severe hypertension. **Alpha-adrenergic blockers, phosphodiesterase-5 inhibitors, calcium channel blockers, benzodiazepines, ACE inhibitors,** or **guanfacine** may antagonize vasopressor effects.

Route/Dosage

Hypotension

Subcut, IM (Adults): 2–5 mg.

Subcut, IM (Children): 0.1 mg/kg/dose q 1–2 hr as needed, maximum dose 5 mg.

IV (Adults): 0.2 mg (range 0.1–0.5 mg), may be repeated q 10–15 min *or* as an infusion at 100–180 mcg/min initially, 40–60 mcg/min maintenance.

IV (Children): 5–20 mcg/kg/dose q 10–15 min as needed or 0.1–0.5 mcg/kg/min infusion, titrate to effect.

Hypotension during Anesthesia

Subcut, IM (Adults): 2–3 mg has been used 3–4 min before spinal anesthesia to prevent hypotension.

IM, Subcut (Children): —0.5–1 mg/25 lb body weight.

IV (Adults): 40–100 mcg; may repeat q 1–2 min as needed (not to exceed total dose of 200 mcg); if BP remains low, initiate continuous infusion at 10–35 mcg/min (not to exceed 200 mcg/min).

Vasoconstrictor for Regional Anesthesia

Local (Adults): Add 1 mg to every 20 mL of local anesthetic (yields a 1:20,000 solution).

Prolongation of Spinal Anesthesia

Spinal (Adults): 2–5 mg added to anesthetic solution.

Availability (generic available)

Injection: 10 mg/mL.

NURSING IMPLICATIONS

Assessment

- Monitor BP every 2–3 min until stabilized and every 5 min thereafter during IV administration.
- Monitor ECG continuously for arrhythmias during IV administration.
- Assess IV site frequently throughout infusion. Antecubital or other large vein should be used to minimize risk of extravasation, which may cause tissue necrosis.

Potential Nursing Diagnoses

Decreased cardiac output (Indications)

Ineffective tissue perfusion (Indications)

Implementation

- ***High Alert:*** Patient harm and fatalities have occurred from medication errors with phenylephrine. Prior to administration, have second practitioner independently check original order, dose calculations, concentration, route of administration and infusion pump settings.

IV Administration

- **IV:** Blood volume depletion should be corrected, if possible, before initiation of IV phenylephrine.
- **IV Push:** ***Diluent:*** Dilute each 1 mg with 9 mL of sterile water for injection or D5W. ***Rate:*** Administer each single dose over 1 min.
- **Continuous Infusion:** ***Diluent:*** Dilute 10 mg in 250 or 500 mL of D5W or 0.9% NaCl. ***Concentration:*** 125,000 or 150,000 solution, respectively. ***Rate:*** Titrate rate according to patient response. Infuse via infusion pump to ensure accurate dose rate.
- **Y-Site Compatibility:** alemtuzumab, alfentanil, amikacin, aminophylline, amiodarone, amphotericin B liposome, anidulafungin, argatroban, ascorbic acid, asparaginase, atracurium, atropine, aztreonam, benztropine, bivalirudin, bleomycin, bumetanide, buprenorphine, butorphanol, calcium chloride, calcium gluconate, cangrelor, carboplatin, carmustine, caspofungin, cefazolin, cefotaxime, cefotetan, cefoxitin, ceftazidime, ceftriaxone, chloramphenicol, cisatracurium, cisplatin, clindamycin, cyanocobalamin, cyclophosphamide, cyclosporine, cytarabine, dactinomycin, daptomycin, daunorubicin, dexamethasone, dexmedetomidine, dexrazoxane, digoxin, diltiazem, diphenhydramine, dobutamine, docetaxel, dolasetron, dopamine, doripenem, doxacurium, doxorubicin hydrochloride, doxycycline, enalaprilat, ephedrine, epinephrine, epirubicin, epoetin alfa, eptifibatide, ertapenem, erythromycin, esmolol, etomidate, etoposide, etoposide phosphate, famotidine, fenoldopam, fentanyl, fluconazole, fludarabine, fluorouracil, folic acid, foscarnet, fosphenytoin, gentamicin, glycopyrrolate, granisetron, heparin, hetastarch, hydrocortisone, hydromorphone, idarubicin, ifosfamide, imipenem/cilastatin, irinotecan, isoproterenol, ketorolac, labetalol, leucovorin calcium, levofloxacin, lidocaine, linezolid, lorazepam, magnesium sulfate, mannitol, mechlorethamine, meperidine, mesna, metaraminol, methotrexate, methtylprednisolone, metoclopramide, metoprolol, metronidazole, micafungin, midazolam, milrinone, mitoxantrone, morphine, multivitamins, mycophenolate, nafcillin, nalbuphine, naloxone, nicardipine, nitroglycerin, nitroprusside, norepinephrine, octreotide, ondansetron, oxacillin, oxaliplatin, oxytocin, paclitaxel, palonosetron, pamidronate, pancuronium, pantoprazole, penicillin G , pentobarbital, phenobarbital, phytonadione, piperacillin/tazobactam, potassium acetate, potassium chloride, procainamide, prochlorperazine, promethazine, propranolol, protamine, pyridoxime, quinupristin/dalfopristin, ranitidine, remifentanil, rocuronium, sodium acetate, sodium bicarbonate, streptokinase, succinylcholine, sufentanil, tacrolimus, telavancin, teniposide, theophylline, thiamine, thiotepa, tigecycline, tirofiban, tobramycin, tolazoline, topotecan, vancomycin, vasopressin, vecuronium, verapamil, vinblastine, vincristine, vinorelbine, voriconazole, zidovudine, zoledronic acid.
- **Y-Site Incompatibility:** acyclovir, amphotericin B colloidal, amphotericin B lipid complex, azathioprine, dantrolene, diazepam, diazoxide, ganciclovir, indomethacin, insulin, mitomycin, pentamidine, phenytoin, trimethoprim/sulfamethoxazole, thiopental.
- **Anesthesia:** Phenylephrine 2–5 mg may be added to spinal anesthetic solution to prolong anesthesia.
- Phenylephrine 1 mg may be added to each 20 mL of local anesthetic to produce vasoconstriction.

Patient/Family Teaching

- **IV:** Instruct patient to report headache, dizziness, dyspnea, or pain at IV infusion site promptly.

Evaluation/Desired Outcomes

- Increase in BP to normal range.
- Prolonged duration of spinal anesthesia.
- Localization of regional anesthesia.

phenytoin (fen-i-toyn)

Dilantin, Phenytek, ✱Tremytoine

Classification

Therapeutic: antiarrhythmics (group IB), anticonvulsants

Pharmacologic: hydantoins

Pregnancy Category D

P

Indications

Treatment/prevention of tonic-clonic (grand mal) seizures and complex partial seizures. **Unlabeled Use:** As an antiarrhythmic, particularly for ventricular arrhythmias associated with digoxin toxicity, prolonged QT interval, and surgical repair of congenital heart diseases in children. Management of neuropathic pain, including trigeminal neuralgia.

Action

Limits seizure propagation by altering ion transport. May also decrease synaptic transmission. Antiarrhythmic properties as a result of shortening the action potential and decreasing automaticity. **Therapeutic Effects:** Diminished seizure activity. Termination of ventricular arrhythmias.

Pharmacokinetics

Absorption: Absorbed slowly from the GI tract. Bioavailability differs among products; the Dilantin and Phenytek preparations are considered to be "extended" products. Other products are considered to be prompt release.

Distribution: Distributes into CSF and other body tissues and fluids. Enters breast milk; crosses the placenta, achieving similar maternal/fetal levels. Preferentially distributes into fatty tissue.
Protein Binding: Adults 90–95%; ↓ protein binding in neonates (up to 20% free fraction available), infants (up to 15% free), and patients with hyperbilirubinemia, hypoalbuminemia, severe renal dysfunction or uremia.
Metabolism and Excretion: Mostly metabolized by the liver; minimal amounts excreted in the urine.
Half-life: 22 hr (range 7–42 hr).

TIME/ACTION PROFILE (anticonvulsant effect)

ROUTE	ONSET	PEAK	DURATION
PO	2–24 hr (1 wk)*	1.5–3 hr	6–12 hr
PO-ER	2–24 hr (1 wk)	4–12 hr	12–36 hr
IV	0.5–1 hr (1 wk)	rapid	12–24 hr

*() = time required for onset of action without a loading dose.

Contraindications/Precautions

Contraindicated in: Hypersensitivity; Hypersensitivity to propylene glycol (phenytoin injection only); Alcohol intolerance (phenytoin injection and liquid only); Sinus bradycardia, sinoatrial block, 2nd- or 3rd-degree heart block, or Stokes-Adams syndrome (phenytoin injection only); Concurrent use of delavirdine.
Use Cautiously in: All patients (may ↑ risk of suicidal thoughts/behaviors); Hepatic or renal disease (↑ risk of adverse reactions; dose reduction recommended for hepatic impairment); Patients with severe cardiac or respiratory disease (use of IV phenytoin may result in an ↑ risk of serious adverse reactions); OB: ↑ risk of congenital anomalies; ↑ risk of hemorrhage in newborn if used at term; use with extreme caution; Lactation: Safety not established; Pedi: Suspension contains sodium benzoate, a metabolite of benzyl alcohol that can cause potentially fatal gasping syndrome in neonates; Geri: Use of IV phenytoin may result in an ↑ risk of serious adverse reactions.
Exercise Extreme Caution in: Patients positive for HLA-B*1502 allele (unless exceptional circumstances exist where benefits clearly outweigh the risks).

Adverse Reactions/Side Effects

Most listed are for chronic use of phenytoin.
CNS: SUICIDAL THOUGHTS, ataxia, agitation, confusion, dizziness, drowsiness, dysarthria, dyskinesia, extrapyramidal syndrome, headache, insomnia, vertigo, weakness. **EENT:** diplopia, nystagmus. **CV:** hypotension (↑ with IV phenytoin), tachycardia. **GI:** ACUTE HEPATIC FAILURE, gingival hyperplasia, nausea, constipation, drug-induced hepatitis, vomiting. **Derm:** STEVENS-JOHNSON SYNDROME, TOXIC EPIDERMAL NECROLYSIS, hypertrichosis, rash, exfoliative dermatitis, pruritus, purple glove syndrome. **Hemat:** AGRANULOCYTOSIS, APLASTIC ANEMIA, leukopenia, megaloblastic anemia, thrombocytopenia. **MS:** osteomalacia, osteoporosis. **Misc:** DRUG REACTION WITH EOSINOPHILIA AND SYSTEMIC SYMPTOMS (DRESS), fever, lymphadenopathy.

Interactions

Drug-Drug: May ↓ the effects of **delavirdine**, resulting in loss of virologic response and potential resistant (concurrent use contraindicated). Acute ingestion of **alcohol**, **amiodarone**, **benzodiazepines**, **capecitabine**, **chloramphenicol**, **chlordiazepoxide**, **cimetidine**, **disulfiram estrogens**, **ethosuximide**, **felbamate**, **fluconazole**, **fluorouracil**, **fluoxetine**, **fluvastatin**, **fluvoxamine**, **halothane**, **isoniazid**, **itraconazole**, **ketoconazole**, **methylphenidate**, **miconazole**, **oxcarbazepine**, **omeprazole**, **phenothiazines**, **salicylates**, **sertraline**, **succinamides**, **sulfonamides**, **tolbutamide**, **trazodone**, **voriconazole** and **warfarin** may ↑ levels. Chronic ingestion of **alcohol**, **barbiturates**, **carbamazepine**, **diazepam**, **diazoxide**, **fosamprenavir**, **nelfinavir**, **reserpine**, **rifampin**, **ritonavir**, **sucralfate**, **theophylline**, and **vigabatrin** may ↓ levels. May ↓ the effects of **albendazole**, **amiodarone**, **atorvastatin**, **benzodiazepines**, **carbamazepine**, **chlorpropamide**, **clozapine**, **cyclosporine**, **digoxin**, **efavirenz**, **estrogens**, **felbamate fluvastatin**, **indinavir**, **lamotrigine**, **lopinavir/ritonavir**, **methadone**, **mexiletine**, **nelfinavir**, **nifedipine**, **nimodipine**, **nisoldipine**, **oxcarbazepine**, **oral contraceptives**, **quetiapine**, **quinidine**, **rifampin**, **ritonavir**, **saquinavir**, **simvastatin**, **tacrolimus**, **theophylline**, **topiramate**, **verapamil**, and **warfarin**. IV phenytoin and **dopamine** may cause additive hypotension. Additive CNS depression with other **CNS depressants**, including **alcohol**, **antihistamines**, **antidepressants**, **opioids**, and **sedative/hypnotics**. **Antacids** may ↓ absorption of orally administered phenytoin. ↑ systemic clearance of antileukemic drugs **teniposide** and **methotrexate** which has been associated with a worse event free survival, phenytoin use is not recommended in children undergoing chemotherapy for acute lymphocytic leukemia.
Drug-Natural Products: **St. John's wort** may ↓ levels.
Drug-Food: Phenytoin may ↓ absorption of **folic acid**. Concurrent administration of **enteral tube feedings** may ↓ phenytoin absorption. **Folic acid** may ↓ levels.

Route/Dosage

IM administration is not recommended due to erratic absorption and pain on injection. Oral route should be used whenever possible.

Anticonvulsant

PO (Adults): Loading dose of 15–20 mg/kg as extended capsules in 3 divided doses given every 2–4 hr;

maintenance dose 5–6 mg/kg/day given in 1–3 divided doses; usual dosing range = 200–1200 mg/day.
PO (Children 10–16 yr): 6–7 mg/kg/day in 2–3 divided doses.
PO (Children 7–9 yr): 7–8 mg/kg/day in 2–3 divided doses.
PO (Children 4–6 yr): 7.5–9 mg/kg/day in 2–3 divided doses.
PO (Children 0.5–3 yr): 8–10 mg/kg/day in 2–3 divided doses.
PO (Neonates up to 6 mo): 5–8 mg/kg/day in 2 divided doses, may require q 8 hr dosing.
IV (Adults): *Status epilepticus loading dose*—15–20 mg/kg. Rate not to exceed 25–50 mg/min. *Maintenance dose*—same as PO dosing above.
IV (Children): *Status epilepticus loading dose*—15–20 mg/kg at 1–3 mg/kg/min. *Maintenance dose*—same as PO dosing above.

Antiarrhythmic

IV (Adults): 50–100 mg q 10–15 min until arrhythmia is abolished, or a total of 15 mg/kg has been given, or toxicity occurs.
PO (Adults): Loading dose: 250 mg 4 times daily for 1 day, then 250 mg twice daily for 2 days, then maintenance at 300–400 mg/day in divided doses 1–4 times/day.
IV (Children): 1.25 mg/kg q 5 min, may repeat up to total loading dose of 15 mg/kg. *Maintenance dose*—5–10 mg/kg/day in 2–3 divided doses IV or PO.

Availability (generic available)

Chewable tablets: 50 mg. **Cost:** *Generic*—$52.63/100. **Oral suspension:** 125 mg/5 mL. **Cost:** $36.97/237 mL. **Extended-release capsules:** 30 mg, 100 mg, 200 mg, 300 mg. **Cost:** *Generic*—100 mg $33.90/100, 200 mg $24.00/30, 300 mg $34.94/30. **Injection:** 50 mg/mL.

NURSING IMPLICATIONS

Assessment

- Monitor closely for notable changes in behavior that could indicate the emergence or worsening of suicidal thoughts or behavior or depression.
- Assess oral hygiene. Vigorous cleaning beginning within 10 days of initiation of phenytoin therapy may help control gingival hyperplasia.
- Assess patient for phenytoin hypersensitivity syndrome (fever, skin rash, lymphadenopathy). Rash usually occurs within the first 2 wk of therapy. Hypersensitivity syndrome usually occurs at 3–8 wk but may occur up to 12 wk after initiation of therapy. May lead to renal failure, rhabdomyolysis, or hepatic necrosis; may be fatal.
- Observe patient for development of rash. Discontinue phenytoin at the first sign of skin reactions. Serious adverse reactions such as exfoliative, purpuric, or bullous rashes or the development of lupus erythematosus, Stevens-Johnson syndrome, or toxic epidermal necrolysis preclude further use of phenytoin or fosphenytoin. 🧬 Stevens-Johnson syndrome and toxic epidermal necrolysis are significantly more common in patients with a particular human leukocyte antigen (HLA) allele, HLA-B*1502 (occurs almost exclusively in patients with Asian ancestry, including including Han Chinese, Filipinos, Malaysians, South Asian Indians, and Thais). Avoid using phenytoin or fosphenytoin as alternatives to carbamazepine for patients who test positive. If less serious skin eruptions (measles-like or scarlatiniform) occur, phenytoin may be resumed after complete clearing of the rash. If rash reappears, further use of fosphenytoin or phenytoin should be avoided.
- Assess mental status (orientation, mood, behavior) before and periodically during therapy. Monitor closely for notable changes in behavior that could indicate the emergence or worsening of suicidal thoughts or behavior or depression.
- **Seizures:** Assess location, duration, frequency, and characteristics of seizure activity. EEG may be monitored periodically throughout therapy.
- Monitor BP, ECG, and respiratory function continuously during administration of IV phenytoin and throughout period when peak serum phenytoin levels occur (15–30 min after administration).
- **Arrhythmias:** Monitor ECG continuously during treatment of arrhythmias.
- ***Lab Test Considerations:*** Monitor CBC, serum calcium, albumin, and hepatic function tests prior to and monthly for the first several months, then periodically during therapy.
- May cause ↑ serum alkaline phosphatase, GGT, and glucose levels.
- Monitor serum folate concentrations periodically during prolonged therapy.
- ***Toxicity and Overdose:*** Monitor serum phenytoin levels routinely. Therapeutic blood levels are 10–20 mcg/mL (8–15 mcg/mL in neonates) in patients with normal serum albumin and renal function. In patients with altered protein binding (neonates, patients with renal failure, hypoalbuminemia, acute trauma), free phenytoin serum concentrations should be monitored. Therapeutic serum free phenytoin levels are 1–2 mcg/mL.
- Progressive signs and symptoms of phenytoin toxicity include nystagmus, ataxia, confusion, nausea, slurred speech, and dizziness.

Potential Nursing Diagnoses

Risk for injury (Indications)
Impaired oral mucous membrane (Side Effects)

P

Implementation

- Implement seizure precautions.
- When transferring from phenytoin to another anticonvulsant, dosage adjustments are made gradually over several weeks.
- When substituting *fosphenytoin* for oral *phenytoin* therapy, the same total daily dose may be given as a single dose. Unlike parenteral phenytoin, fosphenytoin may be given safely by the IM route.
- **PO:** Administer with or immediately after meals to minimize GI irritation. Shake liquid preparations well before pouring. Use a calibrated measuring device for accurate dose. Chewable tablets must be crushed or chewed well before swallowing. Capsules may be opened and mixed with food or fluids for patients with difficulty swallowing. To prevent direct contact of alkaline drug with mucosa, have patient swallow a liquid first, follow with mixture of medication, then follow with a full glass of water or milk or with food.
- If patient is receiving enteral tube feedings, 2 hr should elapse between feeding and phenytoin administration. If phenytoin is administered via nasogastric tube, flush tube with 2–4 oz water before and after administration.
- Do not interchange chewable phenytoin tablets with phenytoin sodium capsules, because they are not bioequivalent.
- Capsules labeled "extended" may be used for once-a-day dose; those labeled "prompt" may result in toxic serum levels if used for once-a-day dose.

IV Administration

- **IV:** Slight yellow color will not alter solution potency. If refrigerated, may form precipitate, which dissolves after warming to room temperature. Discard solution that is not clear.
- To prevent precipitation and minimize local venous irritation, follow infusion with 0.9% NaCl through the same needle or catheter. Avoid extravasation; phenytoin is caustic to tissues; may lead to purple glove syndrome. Monitor infusion site closely.
- **IV Push:** Administer undiluted. ***Rate:*** Administer at a rate not to exceed 50 mg over 1 min in adults or 1–3 mg/kg/min in neonates. Rapid administration may result in severe hypotension, cardiovascular collapse, or CNS depression.
- **Intermittent Infusion:** ***Diluent:*** Administer by mixing with no more than 50 mL of 0.9% NaCl. ***Concentration:*** 1–10 mg/mL. Administer immediately following admixture. Use tubing with a 0.45- to 0.22-micron in-line filter. ***Rate:*** Complete infusion within 1 hr at a rate not to exceed 50 mg/min. In patients who may develop hypotension, patients with cardiovascular disease, or geriatric patients maximum rate of 25 mg/min [may be as low as 5–10 mg/min]. Maximum rate in neonates is 1–3 mg/kg/min. Monitor cardiac function and BP throughout infusion.
- **Y-Site Compatibility:** cisplatin.
- **Y-Site Incompatibility:** acyclovir, alemtuzumab, alfentanil, amikacin, aminocaproic acid, aminophylline, amphotericin B colloidal, amphotericin B lipid complex, amphotericin B liposome, ampicillin, ampicillin/sulbactam, anidulafungin, argatroban, ascorbic acid, atropine, aztreonam, benztropine, bivalirudin, bumetanide, buprenorphine, butorphanol, calcium chloride, calcium gluconate, carboplatin, carmustine, caspofungin, cefazolin, cefepime, cefotaxime, cefotetan, cefoxitin, ceftazidime, ceftriaxone, cefuroxime, chloramphenicol, chlorpromazine, ciprofloxacin, clindamycin, cyanocobalamin, cyclophosphamide, cyclosporine, cytarabine, dactinomycin, dantrolene, daptomycin, dexamethasone, dexmedetomidine, dexrazoxane, diltiazem, digoxin, diltiazem, diphenhydramine, dobutamine, docetaxel, dolasetron, dopamine, doxorubicin hydrochloride, doxorubicin liposomal, doxycycline, enalaprilat, ephedrine, epinephrine, epirubicin, epoetin alfa, eptifibatide, ertapenem, erythromycin, etoposide, etoposide phosphate, fenoldopam, fentanyl, fludarabine, fluorouracil, folic acid, furosemide, ganciclovir, gemcitabine, gentamicin, glycopyrrolate, granisetron, haloperidol, heparin, hetastarch, hydralazine, hydrocortisone, hydromorphone, hydroxyzine, idarubicin, ifosfamide, imipenem/cilastatin, indomethacin, insulin, irinotecan, isoproterenol, ketamine, ketorolac, labetalol, levofloxacin, lidocaine, linezolid, lorazepam, magnesium sulfate, mannitol, mechlorethamine, meperidine, mesna, methadone, methotrexate, methyldopate, methylprednisolone, metoclopramide, micafungin, midazolam, milrinone, mitoxantrone, morphine, moxifloxacin, multivitamin infusion, mycophenolate, nafcillin, nalbuphine, naloxone, nesiritide, nicardipine, nitroglycerin, nitroprusside, norepinephrine, octreotide, ondansetron, oxacillin, oxytocin, paclitaxel, palonosetron, pamidronate, pantoprazole, papaverine, pemetrexed, penicillin G, pentamidine, pentazocine, pentobarbital, phenobarbital, phenylephrine, phytonadione, piperacillin/tazobactam, potassium acetate, potassium chloride, procainamide, prochlorperazine, promethazine, propofol, propranolol, protamine, pyridoxine, quinupristin/dalfopristin, ranitidine, rocuronium, sodium acetate, sodium bicarbonate, streptokinase, succinylcholine, sufentanil, tacrolimus, teniposide, theophylline, thiamine, thiotepa, tigecycline, tirofiban, tobramycin, trimethoprim/sulfamethoxazole, vancomycin, vasopressin, vecuronium, verapamil, vinblastine, vincristine, vinorelbine, vitamin B complex with C, voriconazole, zoledronic acid.
- **Additive Incompatibility:** Do not admix with other solutions or medications, especially dextrose, because precipitation will occur.

Patient/Family Teaching

- Instruct patient to take medication as directed, at the same time each day. If a dose is missed from a once-a-day schedule, take as soon as possible and return to regular dosing schedule. If taking several doses a day, take missed dose as soon as possible within 4 hr of next scheduled dose; do not double doses. Consult health care professional if doses are missed for 2 consecutive days. Abrupt withdrawal may lead to status epilepticus.

- May cause drowsiness or dizziness. Caution patient to avoid driving or other activities requiring alertness until response to medication is known. Do not resume driving until physician gives clearance based on control of seizure disorder.
- Caution patient to avoid alcohol and CNS depressants. Advise patient to notify health care professional of all Rx or OTC medications, vitamins, or herbal products being taken and to consult with health care professional before taking other medications and alcohol.
- Instruct patient on importance of maintaining good dental hygiene and seeing dentist frequently for teeth cleaning to prevent tenderness, bleeding, and gingival hyperplasia. Institution of oral hygiene program within 10 days of initiation of phenytoin therapy may minimize growth rate and severity of gingival enlargement. Patients under 23 yr of age and those taking doses >500 mg/day are at increased risk for gingival hyperplasia.
- Advise patient that brands of phenytoin may not be equivalent. Check with health care professional if brand or dose form is changed.
- Advise diabetic patients to monitor blood glucose carefully and to notify health care professional of significant changes.
- Instruct patient to notify health care professional of medication regimen prior to treatment or surgery.
- Advise patient not to take phenytoin within 2–3 hr of antacids.
- Advise patient to carry identification describing disease process and medication regimen at all times.
- Instruct patients that behavioral changes, skin rash, fever, sore throat, mouth ulcers, easy bruising, petechiae, unusual bleeding, abdominal pain, chills, pale stools, dark urine, jaundice, severe nausea or vomiting, drowsiness, slurred speech, unsteady gait. swollen glands,or persistent headache should be reported to health care professional immediately. Advise patient and family to notify health care professional if thoughts about suicide or dying, attempts to commit suicide; new or worse depression; new or worse anxiety; feeling very agitated or restless; panic attacks; trouble sleeping; new or worse irritability; acting aggressive; being angry or violent; acting on dangerous impulses; an extreme increase in activity and talking, other unusual changes in behavior or mood occur.
- Rep: Advise female patients to use an additional nonhormonal method of contraception during therapy and until next menstrual period. Instruct patient to notify health care professional if pregnancy is planned or suspected. Encourage patients who become pregnant to enroll in the North American Antiepileptic Drug (NAAED) Pregnancy Registry by calling 1-888-233-2334 or on the web at www.aedpregnancyregistry.org. Enrollment must be done by patients themselves.
- Emphasize the importance of routine exams to monitor progress. Patient should have routine physical exams, especially monitoring skin and lymph nodes, and EEG testing.

Evaluation/Desired Outcomes

- Decrease or cessation of seizures without excessive sedation.
- Suppression of arrhythmias.
- Relief of neuropathic pain.

phosphate/biphosphate

(**foss**-fate/bye-**foss** -fate)

Fleet Enema, OsmoPrep

Classification

Therapeutic: laxatives (saline)

Pregnancy Category C

Indications

Intermittent treatment of chronic constipation. **OsmoPrep:** Cleansing of the bowel as a preparation for colonoscopy.

Action

Osmotically active in the lumen of the GI tract. Produces laxative effect by causing water retention and stimulation of peristalsis. Stimulates motility and inhibits fluid and electrolyte absorption from the small intestine. **Therapeutic Effects:** Relief of constipation. Emptying of the bowel.

Pharmacokinetics

Absorption: 1–20% of rectally administered sodium and phosphate may be absorbed; some absorption follows oral administration.

Distribution: Unknown.

Metabolism and Excretion: Excreted by the kidneys.

Half-life: Unknown.

TIME/ACTION PROFILE (laxative effect)

ROUTE	ONSET	PEAK	DURATION
PO	0.5–3 hr	unknown	unknown
Rect	2–5 min	unknown	unknown

Contraindications/Precautions

Contraindicated in: Hypersensitivity; Abdominal pain, nausea, or vomiting, especially when associated with fever or other signs of an acute abdomen; Severe renal or cardiovascular disease; Intestinal obstruction; OB: Not recommended for use at term; *OsmoPrep*—HF, ascites, unstable angina, acute colitis, toxic megacolon, or hypomotility syndrome; Pedi: Children <2 yr.
Use Cautiously in: Excessive or chronic use (may lead to dependence); Renal or cardiovascular disease, dehydration or concurrent use of diuretics or other drugs known to alter electrolytes (correct abnormalities prior to administration); Dehydration, renal dysfunction, bowel obstruction, active colitis, or concurrent use of diuretics, ACE inhibitors, ARBs, or NSAIDs (↑ risk of acute phosphate nephropathy); OB: May cause sodium retention and edema; Geri: May be more sensitive to effects.

Adverse Reactions/Side Effects

CNS: *Visicol*—dizziness, headache. **CV:** ARRHYTHMIAS. **GI:** cramping, nausea, colonic aphtous ulcerations, ischemic colitis; *OsmoPrep*, abdominal bloating, abdominal pain, vomiting. **F and E:** hyperphosphatemia, hypocalcemia, hypokalemia, sodium retention. **GU:** renal dysfunction.

Interactions

Drug-Drug: *OsmoPrep*—Concurrently administered oral medications may not be absorbed due to rapid peristalsis and diarrhea.

Route/Dosage

Each Fleet Enema contains 4.4 g sodium/118 mL.

Bowel Cleansing

PO (Adults): *OsmoPrep*—evening before colonoscopy: 4 tablets every 15 min (with at least 8 oz of water) for a total of 20 tablets; on morning of colonoscopy starting 3–5 hr before procedure, 4 tablets every 15 min (with at least 8 oz of clear liquids), for a total of 12 tablets; should not be repeated in less than 7 days.

Constipation

PO (Adults): 15 mL as single dose.
PO (Children 5–9 yr): 7.5 mL as single dose.
Rect (Adults and Children >12 yr): 118 mL Fleet Enema.
Rect (Children >2 yr): ½ of the adult dose.

Availability (generic available)

Oral solution: 0.9 g dibasic sodium phosphate and 2.4 g monobasic sodium biphosphate/5 mL. **Enema:** 7 g dibasic sodium phosphate and 19 g monobasic sodium biphosphate/118 mL. **Tablets (OsmoPrep):** 1.5 g.

NURSING IMPLICATIONS

Assessment

- Assess patient for fever, abdominal distention, presence of bowel sounds, and usual pattern of bowel function.
- Assess color, consistency, and amount of stool produced.
- May rarely cause arrhythmias. Monitor patients with underlying cardiovascular disease, renal disease, bowel perforation, misuse or overdose.
- ***Lab Test Considerations:*** May cause ↑ serum sodium and phosphorus levels, ↓ serum calcium and potassium levels, and acidosis. Electrolyte changes are transient, self-limiting, do not require treatment and are not usually associated with adverse clinical events.

Potential Nursing Diagnoses

Constipation (Indications)

Implementation

- Do not administer at bedtime or late in the day.
- **PO:** Administer on an empty stomach for more rapid results. Mix dose in at least ½ glass cold water. May be followed by carbonated beverage or fruit juice to improve flavor.
- See Route and Dosage section for dosing of *OsmoPrep*.
- *Osmoprep:* Do not drink any red—or purple-colored liquids.
- **Rect:** Position patient on left side with knee slightly flexed. Insert prelubricated tip about 2 inches into rectum, aiming toward the umbilicus. Gently squeeze bottle until empty. Discontinue if resistance is met, because perforation may occur if contents are forced into rectum.

Patient/Family Teaching

- Advise patient that laxatives should be used only for short-term therapy. Avoid using more than 1 dose of OTC laxatives/day. Long-term therapy may cause electrolyte imbalance and dependence.
- Caution patient on sodium restriction that this product has a high sodium content.
- Advise patient not to take oral form of this medication within 2 hr of other medications.
- Encourage patient to use other forms of bowel regulation, such as increasing bulk in the diet, fluid intake, and mobility. Normal bowel habits may vary from 3 times/day to 3 times/wk.
- Advise patient to notify health care professional if unrelieved constipation, rectal bleeding, or symptoms of electrolyte imbalance (muscle cramps or pain, weakness, dizziness, and so forth) occur.

Evaluation/Desired Outcomes

- Soft, formed bowel movement.
- Evacuation of the bowel.

phytonadione
(fye-toe-na-**dye**-one)
Mephyton, vitamin K

Classification
Therapeutic: antidotes, vitamins
Pharmacologic: fat-soluble vitamins

Pregnancy Category C

Indications
Prevention and treatment of hypoprothrombinemia, which may be associated with: Excessive doses of oral anticoagulants, Salicylates, Certain anti-infective agents, Nutritional deficiencies, Prolonged total parenteral nutrition. Prevention of hemorrhagic disease of the newborn.

Action
Required for hepatic synthesis of blood coagulation factors II (prothrombin), VII, IX, and X. **Therapeutic Effects:** Prevention of bleeding due to hypoprothrombinemia.

Pharmacokinetics
Absorption: Well absorbed following oral or subcut administration. Oral absorption requires presence of bile salts. Some vitamin K is produced by bacteria in the GI tract.
Distribution: Crosses the placenta; does not enter breast milk.
Metabolism and Excretion: Rapidly metabolized by the liver.
Half-life: Unknown.

TIME/ACTION PROFILE

ROUTE	ONSET	PEAK†	DURATION‡
PO	6–12 hr	unknown	unknown
Subcut	1–2 hr	3–6 hr	12–14 hr
IV	1–2 hr	3–6 hr	12 hr

†Control of hemorrhage.
‡Normal PT achieved.

Contraindications/Precautions
Contraindicated in: Hypersensitivity; Hypersensitivity or intolerance to benzyl alcohol (injection only).
Use Cautiously in: Impaired liver function.
Exercise Extreme Caution in: Severe life-threatening reactions have occurred following IV administration, use other routes unless risk is justified.

Adverse Reactions/Side Effects
GI: gastric upset, unusual taste. **Derm:** flushing, rash, urticaria. **Hemat:** hemolytic anemia. **Local:** erythema, pain at injection site, swelling. **Misc:** allergic reactions, hyperbilirubinemia (large doses in very premature infants), kernicterus.

Interactions
Drug-Drug: Large doses will counteract the effect of **warfarin**. Large doses of **salicylates** or broad-spectrum **anti-infectives** may ↑ vitamin K requirements. **Bile acid sequestrants**, **mineral oil**, and **sucralfate** may ↓ vitamin K absorption from the GI tract.

Route/Dosage
IV use of phytonadione should be reserved for patients with serious or life-threatening bleeding and elevated INR. Oral route is preferred in patients with elevated INRs and no serious or life-threatening bleeding. IM route should generally be avoided because of risk of hematoma formation.

Treatment of Hypoprothrombinemia due to Vitamin K Deficiency (from factors other than warfarin)
Subcut, IV (Adults): 10 mg.
PO (Adults): 2.5–25 mg/day.
Subcut, IV (Children >1 mo): 1–2 mg single dose.
PO (Children >1 mo): 2.5–5 mg/day.

Vitamin K Deficiency (Supratherapeutic INR) Secondary to Warfarin
PO (Adults): *INR ≥5 and <9 (no significant bleeding)*—Hold warfarin and give 1–2.5 mg vitamin K; if more rapid reversal required, given ≤5 mg vitamin K; *INR >9 (no significant bleeding)*—Hold warfarin and give 2.5–5 mg vitamin K.
IV (Adults): *Elevated INR with serious or life-threatening bleeding*—10 mg slow infusion.

Prevention of Hypoprothrombinemia during Total Parenteral Nutrition
IV (Adults): 5–10 mg once weekly.
IV (Children): 2–5 mg once weekly.

Prevention of Hemorrhagic Disease of Newborn
IM (Neonates): 0.5–1 mg, within 1 hr of birth, may repeat in 6–8 hr if needed. May be repeated in 2–3 wk if mother received previous anticonvulsant/anticoagulant/anti-infective/antitubercular therapy. 1–5 mg may be given IM to mother 12–24 hr before delivery.

Treatment of Hemorrhagic Disease of Newborn
IM, Subcut (Neonates): 1–2 mg/day.

Availability (generic available)
Tablets: 5 mg. **Injection:** 1 mg/0.5 mL, 10 mg/mL.

P

NURSING IMPLICATIONS

Assessment

- Monitor for frank and occult bleeding (guaiac stools, Hematest urine, and emesis). Monitor pulse and BP frequently; notify health care professional immediately if symptoms of internal bleeding or hypovolemic shock develop. Inform all personnel of patient's bleeding tendency to prevent further trauma. Apply pressure to all venipuncture sites for at least 5 min; avoid unnecessary IM injections.
- Pedi: Monitor for side effects and adverse reactions. Children may be especially sensitive to the effects and side effects of vitamin K. Neonates, especially premature neonates, may be more sensitive than older children.
- ***Lab Test Considerations:*** Monitor prothrombin time (PT) prior to and throughout vitamin K therapy to determine response to and need for further therapy.

Potential Nursing Diagnoses

Imbalanced nutrition: less than body requirements (Indications)
Ineffective tissue perfusion (Indications)

Implementation

- Do not confuse Mephyton (phytonadione) with methadone.
- The parenteral route is preferred for phytonadione therapy but, because of severe, potentially fatal hypersensitivity reactions, IV vitamin K is not recommended.
- Administration of whole blood or plasma may also be required in severe bleeding because of the delayed onset of this medication.
- Phytonadione is an antidote for warfarin overdose but does not counteract the anticoagulant activity of heparin.

IV Administration

- **Intermittent Infusion: *Diluent:*** Dilute in 0.9% NaCl, D5W, or D5/0.9% NaCl. ***Rate:*** Administer over 30–60 min. Rate should not exceed 1 mg/min.
- **Y-Site Compatibility:** alfentanil, amikacin, aminophylline, ascorbic acid, atracurium, atropine, azathioprine, aztreonam, benztropine, bumetanide, buprenorphine, butorphanol, calcium chloride, calcium gluconate, cefazolin, cefotaxime, cefotetan, cefoxitin, ceftazidime, ceftriaxone, cefuroxime, chloramphenicol, chlorpromazine, clindamycin, cyanocobalamin, cyclosporine, dexamethasone sodium phosphate, digoxin, diphenhydramine, dopamine, doxycycline, enalaprilat, ephedrine, epinephrine, epoetin alfa, erythromycin, esmolol, famotidine, fentanyl, fluconazole, folic acid, furosemide, ganciclovir, gentamicin, glycopyrrolate, heparin, hydrocortisone sodium succinate, imipenem/cilastatin, indomethacin, insulin, isoproterenol, ketorolac, labetalol, lidocaine, mannitol, meperidine, metaraminol, methoxamine, methyldopate, metoclopramide, metoprolol, metronidazole, midazolam, morphine, multivitamins, nafcillin, nalbuphine, naloxone, nitroglycerin, nitroprusside, norepinephrine, ondansetron, oxacillin, oxytocin, papaverine, penicillin G, pentamidine, pentazocine, pentobarbital, phenobarbital, phentolamine, phenylephrine, potassium chloride, procainamide, prochlorperazine, propranolol, pyridoxime, ranitidine, sodium bicarbonate, streptokinase, succinylcholine, sufentanil, theophylline, thiamine, tobramycin, tolazoline, trimetaphan, vancomycin, vasopressin, verapamil, vitamin B complex with C.
- **Y-Site Incompatibility:** dantrolene, diazepam, diazoxide, magnesium sulfate, phenytoin, trimethoprim/sulfamethoxazole.

Patient/Family Teaching

- Instruct patient to take phytonadione as directed. Take missed doses as soon as remembered unless almost time for next dose. Notify health care professional of missed doses.
- Cooking does not destroy substantial amounts of vitamin K. Patient should not drastically alter diet while taking vitamin K. See Appendix J for foods high in vitamin K.
- Caution patient to avoid IM injections and activities leading to injury. Use a soft toothbrush, do not floss, and shave with an electric razor until coagulation defect is corrected.
- Advise patient to report any symptoms of unusual bleeding or bruising (bleeding gums; nosebleed; black, tarry stools; hematuria; excessive menstrual flow).
- Advise patient to notify health care professional of all Rx or OTC medications, vitamins, or herbal products being taken and to consult with health care professional before taking other medications and alcohol.
- Advise patient to inform health care professional of medication regimen prior to treatment or surgery.
- Advise patient to carry identification at all times describing disease process.
- Emphasize the importance of frequent lab tests to monitor coagulation factors.

Evaluation/Desired Outcomes

- Prevention of spontaneous bleeding or cessation of bleeding in patients with hypoprothrombinemia secondary to impaired intestinal absorption or oral anticoagulant, salicylate, or anti-infective therapy.
- Prevention of hemorrhagic disease in the newborn.

pilocarpine (oral)†
(pye-loe-**kar**-peen)
Salagen

Classification
Therapeutic: none assigned
Pharmacologic: cholinergics

Pregnancy Category C

†For ophthalmic use of pilocarpine, see Appendix C

Indications
Management of xerostomia, which may occur as a consequence of radiation therapy for cancer of the head and neck. Treatment of dry mouth in patients with Sjögren's syndrome.

Action
Stimulates cholinergic receptors, resulting in primarily muscarinic action, including stimulation of exocrine glands. Other effects include: Increased sweating, gastric secretions, Increased bronchial secretions, Increased tone and motility of the urinary tract, gallbladder, and biliary duct smooth muscle. **Therapeutic Effects:** Increased salivary gland secretion.

Pharmacokinetics
Absorption: Well absorbed after oral administration.
Distribution: Unknown.
Metabolism and Excretion: Inactivated at neuronal synapses and in plasma. Some unchanged pilocarpine and metabolites are excreted in urine.
Half-life: *After 5-mg dose for 2 days*—0.8 hr; *after 10-mg dose for 2 days*—1.3 hr.

TIME/ACTION PROFILE

ROUTE	ONSET	PEAK	DURATION
PO	20 min	1 hr	3–5 hr

Contraindications/Precautions
Contraindicated in: Hypersensitivity; Uncontrolled asthma; Angle-closure glaucoma; Iritis.
Use Cautiously in: History of pulmonary disease (asthma, bronchitis, or chronic obstructive pulmonary disease); Biliary tract disease or cholelithiasis; Cardiovascular disease; Retinal disease; Nephrolithiasis; History of psychiatric or cognitive disorders; OB, Lactation, Pedi: Safety not established.

Adverse Reactions/Side Effects
CNS: dizziness, headache, weakness. **EENT:** amblyopia, epistaxis, rhinitis. **CV:** edema, hypertension, tachycardia. **GI:** nausea, vomiting, dyspepsia, dysphagia. **GU:** urinary frequency. **Derm:** flushing, sweating. **Neuro:** tremors. **Misc:** chills, voice change.

Interactions
Drug-Drug: Concurrent use of **anticholinergics** will ↓ the effectiveness of pilocarpine. Concurrent use of **bethanechol** or **ophthalmic cholinergics** may result in ↑ cholinergic effects. Concurrent use with **beta blockers** may ↑ the risk of adverse cardiovascular reactions (conduction disturbances).

Route/Dosage

Head and Neck Cancer Patients
PO (Adults): 5 mg three times daily initially, then titrated to need/response, usual range 15–30 mg/day (no single should exceed 10 mg).

Patients with Sjögren's Syndrome
PO (Adults): 5 mg four times daily.

Availability
Tablets: 5 mg, 7.5 mg.

P

NURSING IMPLICATIONS

Assessment
- Assess oral mucosa for dryness and ulceration periodically during therapy.

Potential Nursing Diagnoses
Impaired oral mucous membrane (Indications)

Implementation
- Do not confuse Salagen (pilocarpine) with selegiline.
- **PO:** Use lowest dose that is tolerated and effective for maintenance.

Patient/Family Teaching
- Instruct patient to take medication as directed.
- Caution patient that pilocarpine may cause visual changes, especially at night; avoid driving or other activities requiring alertness until effects of medication are known.
- Advise patient to drink adequate daily fluids (1500–2000 mL/day), especially if sweating occurs. Less than adequate fluid intake may lead to dehydration.

Evaluation/Desired Outcomes
- Increased salivary gland secretion in patients with xerostomia.
- Decrease in dry mouth in patients with Sjögren's syndrome. Full effects in cancer patients may not be seen for up to 12 wk or 6 wk in patients with Sjögren's syndrome.

pimecrolimus
(pi-me-**cro**-li-mus)
Elidel

Classification
Therapeutic: immunosuppressants (topical)

Indications
Short-term and intermittent long-term management of mild to moderate atopic dermatitis unresponsive to or in patients intolerant of conventional treatment.

Action
Inhibits T-cell and mast cell activation by interfering with production of inflammatory cytokines. **Therapeutic Effects:** Decreased severity of atopic dermatatis.

Pharmacokinetics
Absorption: Minimally absorbed through intact skin.
Distribution: Local distribution after topical administration.
Metabolism and Excretion: Systemic metabolism and excretion is negligible with local application.
Half-life: Not applicable.

TIME/ACTION PROFILE (improvement in symptoms)

ROUTE	ONSET	PEAK	DURATION
topical	within 6 days	unknown	unknown

Contraindications/Precautions
Contraindicated in: Hypersensitivity; Should not be applied to areas of active cutaneous viral infections (↑ risk of dissemination); Concurrent use of occlusive dressings; Netherton's syndrome (↑ absorption of pimecrolimus); Lactation: Discontinue breast feeding.
Use Cautiously in: Possible risk of cancer. Do not use as first-line therapy; Clinical infection at treatment site (infection should be treated/cleared prior to use); Skin papillomas (warts); allow treatment/resolution prior to use; Natural/artificial sunlight (minimize exposure); OB: Use only if clearly needed; Pedi: Children <2 yr (safety not established); use only if other treatments have failed.

Adverse Reactions/Side Effects
Local: burning. **Misc:** ↑ risk of lymphoma/skin cancer.

Interactions
Drug-Drug: None significant as systemic absorption is negligible.

Route/Dosage
Topical (Adults and Children ≥2 yr): Apply thin film twice daily; rub in gently and completely.

Availability
Cream: 1%.

NURSING IMPLICATIONS

Assessment
- Assess skin lesions prior to and periodically during therapy. Discontinue therapy after signs and symptoms of atopic dermatitis have resolved. Resume treatment at the first signs and symptoms of recurrence.

Potential Nursing Diagnoses
Impaired skin integrity (Indications)

Implementation
- **Topical:** Apply a thin layer to affected area twice daily and rub in gently and completely. May be used on all skin areas including head, neck, and intertriginous areas. Do not use with occlusive dressings.

Patient/Family Teaching
- Instruct patient on correct technique for application. Apply only as directed to external areas. Wash hands following application, unless hands are areas of application. Advise patient to read *Medication Guide* before starting and with each Rx refill in case of changes.
- Caution patient to avoid exposure to natural or artificial sunlight, including tanning beds, while using cream.
- Advise patient that pimecrolimus may cause skin burning. This occurs most commonly during first few days of application, is of mild to moderate severity, and improves within 5 days or as atopic dermatitis resolves.
- Advise patient to notify health care provider if no improvement is seen following 6 wk of treatment or at any time if condition worsens.

Evaluation/Desired Outcomes
- Resolution of signs and symptoms of atopic dermatitis.

pioglitazone (pi-o-**glit**-a-zone)
Actos

Classification
Therapeutic: antidiabetics (oral)
Pharmacologic: thiazolidinediones

Pregnancy Category C

Indications
Type 2 diabetes mellitus (with diet and exercise); may be used with metformin, sulfonylureas, or insulin.

Action
Improves sensitivity to insulin by acting as an agonist at receptor sites involved in insulin responsiveness and subsequent glucose production and utilization. Re-

quires insulin for activity. **Therapeutic Effects:** Decreased insulin resistance, resulting in glycemic control without hypoglycemia.

Pharmacokinetics

Absorption: Well absorbed following oral administration.

Distribution: Unknown.

Protein Binding: >99% bound to plasma proteins. Active metabolites are also highly (>99%) bound.

Metabolism and Excretion: Extensively metabolized by the liver (primarily by CYP2C8); at least two metabolites have pharmacologic activity. Minimal renal excretion of unchanged drug.

Half-life: *Pioglitazone*—3–7 hr; *total pioglitazone (pioglitazone plus metabolites)*—16–24 hr.

TIME/ACTION PROFILE (effects on blood glucose)

ROUTE	ONSET	PEAK	DURATION
PO	30 min	2–4 hr	24 hr

Contraindications/Precautions

Contraindicated in: Hypersensitivity; Type 1 diabetes; Diabetic ketoacidosis; Clinical evidence of active liver disease or ↑ ALT (>2.5 times upper limit of normal); Active bladder cancer; OB, Lactation: Insulin should be used to control blood glucose levels; Pedi: Children.

Use Cautiously in: Edema; HF (avoid use in moderate to severe HF); Hepatic impairment; History of bladder cancer; Women (may ↑ distal upper and lower limb fractures); Women with childbearing potential (may restore ovulation and ↑ risk of pregnancy).

Adverse Reactions/Side Effects

CV: CHF, edema. **EENT:** macular edema. **GI:** LIVER FAILURE, ↑ liver enzymes. **GU:** BLADDER CANCER (especially after >1 yr). **Hemat:** anemia. **MS:** RHABDOMYOLYSIS. **Misc:** fractures (arm, hand, foot) in female patients.

Interactions

Drug-Drug: May ↓ efficacy of **hormonal contraceptives**. Strong **CYP2C8 inhibitors**, including **gemfibrozil** may ↑ levels. **Ketoconazole** may ↑ effects of pioglitazone. Concurrent use with **insulin** may ↑ risk of fluid retention and worsening HF.

Drug-Natural Products: **Glucosamine** may worsen blood glucose control. **Chromium**, and **coenzyme Q-10** may produce ↑ hypoglycemic effects.

Route/Dosage

PO (Adults): *No heart failure*—15–30 mg once daily, may be ↑ in increments of 15 mg/day to 45 mg/day if needed; *NYHA class I-II heart failure*—15 mg once daily; may be ↑ in increments of 15 mg/day to 45 mg/day if needed; *Concurrent use of gemfibrozil*—do not exceed 15 mg once daily.

Availability (generic available)

Tablets: 15 mg, 30 mg, 45 mg. **Cost:** *Generic*—15 mg $25.49/90, 30 mg $22.75/90, 45 mg $38.12/90. ***In combination with:*** metformin (Actoplus Met, Actoplus Met XR), glimepride (Duetact), alogliptin (Oseni); see Appendix B.

NURSING IMPLICATIONS

Assessment

- Observe patient taking concurrent insulin for signs and symptoms of hypoglycemic reactions (sweating, hunger, weakness, dizziness, tremor, tachycardia, anxiety).
- Assess for signs and symptoms of heart failure (edema, dyspnea, rapid weight gain, unusual tiredness) after initiation and with dose increases.
- ***Lab Test Considerations:*** Monitor serum glucose and Hb A_{1c} periodically during therapy to evaluate effectiveness.
- Monitor CBC with differential periodically during therapy. May cause ↓ in hemoglobin and hematocrit, usually during the first 4–12 wk of therapy; then levels stabilize.
- Monitor serum AST, ALT, alkaline phosphatase, and total bilirubin levels before starting therapy and periodically thereafter or if jaundice or symptoms of hepatic dysfunction occur. Pioglitazone should not be started in patients with active liver disease or ALT levels >2.5 times the upper limit of normal. Patients with mild ALT ↑ should have more frequent monitoring. If ALT ↑ to >3 times the upper limit of normal, recheck ALT promptly. Discontinue pioglitazone if ALT remains >3 times normal.
- May cause transient ↑ in CPK levels.

Potential Nursing Diagnoses

Imbalanced nutrition: more than body requirements (Indications)
Noncompliance (Patient/Family Teaching)

Implementation

- Do not confuse Actos (pioglitazone) with Actonel (risedronate).
- Patients stabilized on a diabetic regimen who are exposed to stress, fever, trauma, infection, or surgery may require administration of insulin.
- **PO:** May be administered with or without meals.

Patient/Family Teaching

- Instruct patient to take medication as directed. If dose for 1 day is missed, do not double dose the next day.

P

- Explain to patient that this medication controls hyperglycemia but does not cure diabetes. Therapy is long-term.
- Review signs of hypoglycemia and hyperglycemia with patient. If hypoglycemia occurs, advise patient to take a glass of orange juice or 2–3 tsp of sugar, honey, or corn syrup dissolved in water and notify health care professional.
- Encourage patient to follow prescribed diet, medication, and exercise regimen to prevent hypoglycemic or hyperglycemic episodes.
- Instruct patient in proper testing of serum glucose and ketones. These tests should be closely monitored during periods of stress or illness, and health care professional should be notified if significant changes occur.
- Advise patient to notify health care professional immediately if signs of hepatic dysfunction (nausea, vomiting, upper right abdominal pain, fatigue, anorexia, dark urine, jaundice), bladder cancer (hematuria, dysuria, urinary urgency), or HF (edema, shortness of breath, rapid weight gain, tiredness) occur.
- Advise patient to inform health care professional of medication regimen before treatment or surgery.
- Insulin is the preferred method of controlling blood glucose during pregnancy. Counsel female patients that higher doses of oral contraceptives or a form of contraception other than oral contraceptives may be required and to notify health care professional promptly if pregnancy is planned or suspected.
- Advise patient to carry a form of sugar (sugar packets, candy) and identification describing disease process and medication regimen at all times.
- Emphasize the importance of routine follow-up exams.

Evaluation/Desired Outcomes

- Control of blood glucose levels.

piperacillin/tazobactam

(pi-**per**-a-sill-in/tay-zoe-**bak**-tam)

✤Tazocin, Zosyn

Classification

Therapeutic: anti-infectives

Pharmacologic: extended spectrum penicillins

Pregnancy Category B

Indications

Appendicitis and peritonitis. Skin and skin structure infections. Gynecologic infections. Community-acquired and nosocomial pneumonia caused by piperacillin-resistant, beta-lactamase–producing bacteria.

Action

Piperacillin: Binds to bacterial cell wall membrane, causing cell death. Spectrum is extended compared with other penicillins. **Tazobactam:** Inhibits beta-lactamase, an enzyme that can destroy penicillins. **Therapeutic Effects:** Death of susceptible bacteria. **Spectrum:** Active against piperacillin-resistant, beta-lactamase–producing: *Bacteroides fragilis*, *E. coli*, *Acinetobacter baumanii*, *Klebsiella pneumoniae*, *Pseudomonas aeruginosa*, *Staphylococcus aureus*, *Haemophilus influenzae*.

Pharmacokinetics

Absorption: Piperacillin is well absorbed (80%) from IM sites.

Distribution: Widely distributed. Enter CSF well only when meninges are inflamed. Crosses the placenta and enters breast milk in low concentrations.

Metabolism and Excretion: Piperacillin (68%) and tazobactam (80%) are mostly excreted unchanged by the kidneys.

Half-life: Adults: 0.7–1.2 hr; Children 6 mo–12 yr: 0.7–0.9 hr; Infants 2–5 mo: 1.4 hr.

TIME/ACTION PROFILE (piperacillin blood levels)

ROUTE	ONSET	PEAK	DURATION
IV	rapid	end of infusion	4–6 hr

Contraindications/Precautions

Contraindicated in: Hypersensitivity to penicillins, beta-lactams, cephalosporins, or tazobactam (cross-sensitivity may occur).

Use Cautiously in: Renal impairment (dosage reduction or increased interval recommended if CCr <40 mL/min); Sodium restriction; OB, Lactation: Safety not established.

Adverse Reactions/Side Effects

CNS: SEIZURES (higher doses), confusion, dizziness, headache, insomnia, lethargy. **GI:** CLOSTRIDIUM DIFFICILE-ASSOCIATED DIARRHEA (CDAD), diarrhea, constipation, drug-induced hepatitis, nausea, vomiting. **GU:** interstitial nephritis. **Derm:** STEVENS-JOHNSON SYNDROME, TOXIC EPIDERMAL NECROLYSIS, rashes (↑ in cystic fibrosis patients), urticaria. **Hemat:** bleeding, leukopenia, neutropenia, thrombocytopenia. **Local:** pain, phlebitis at IV site. **Misc:** hypersensitivity reactions, including ANAPHYLAXIS and SERUM SICKNESS, fever (↑ in cystic fibrosis patients), superinfection.

Interactions

Drug-Drug: Probenecid ↓ renal excretion and ↑ blood levels. May alter excretion of **lithium**. **Potassium-losing diuretics**, **corticosteroids**, or **amphotericin B** may ↑ risk of hypokalemia. ↑ risk of hepatotoxicity with other **hepatotoxic agents**. May ↓ levels/effects of **aminoglycosides** in patients with renal impairment. May ↑ levels and risk of toxicity from **methotrexate**.

Route/Dosage

Contains 2.79 mEq (64 mg) sodium/g of piperacillin; adult doses below expressed as combined piperacillin/tazobactam content.

IV (Adults): *Most infections*—3.375 g q 6 hr. *Nosocomial pneumonia*—4.5 g q 6 hr.
IV (Adults): *Nosocomial pneumonia*—4.5 g q 6 hr.
IV (Adults and Children >40 kg): *Appendicitis and/or peritonitis*—3.375 g q 6 hr.
IV (Children ≥9 mo and ≤40 kg): *Appendicitis and/or peritonitis*—300 mg piperacillin component/kg/day divided q 8 hr.
IV (Infants 2–9 mo): *Appendicitis and/or peritonitis*—240 mg piperacillin component/kg/day divided q 8 hr.
IV (Infants and Children ≥6 mo): 240–400 mg/piperacillin component/kg/day divided q 6–8 hr (higher end of dosing range for serious pseudomonal infections); Max dose: 16 g piperacillin/day.
IV (Infants <6 mo): 150–300 mg/piperacillin component/kg/day divided q 6–8 hr.

Renal Impairment

IV (Adults): *CCr 20–40 mL/min*—2.25 g q 6 hr (3.375 g q 6 hr for nosocomial pneumonia); *CCr <20 mL/min*—2.25 g q 8 hr (2.25 g q 6 hr for nosocomial pneumonia); *Hemodialysis*—2.25 g q 12 h (2.25 g q 8 hr for nosocomial pneumonia).

Availability (generic available)

Powder for injection: 2-g piperacillin/0.25-g tazobactam vials and 50-mL premixed frozen containers, 3-g piperacillin/0.375-g tazobactam vials and 50-mL premixed frozen containers, 4-g piperacillin/0.5-g tazobactam vials and 50-mL premixed frozen containers, 36-g piperacillin/4.5-g tazobactam bulk vials.

NURSING IMPLICATIONS

Assessment

- Assess patient for infection (vital signs; appearance of wound, sputum, urine, and stool; WBC) at beginning of and during therapy.
- Obtain a history before initiating therapy to determine previous use of and reactions to penicillins or cephalosporins. Persons with a negative history of penicillin sensitivity may still have an allergic response.
- Obtain specimens for culture and sensitivity prior to initiating therapy. First dose may be given before receiving results.
- Observe patient for signs and symptoms of anaphylaxis (rash, pruritus, laryngeal edema, wheezing). Discontinue the drug and notify health care professional immediately if these occur. Keep epinephrine, an antihistamine, and resuscitation equipment close by in the event of an anaphylactic reaction.
- Monitor bowel function. Diarrhea, abdominal cramping, fever, and bloody stools should be reported to health care professional promptly as a sign of Clostridium difficile-associated diarrhea (CDAD). May begin up to several weeks following cessation of therapy.
- Assess for skin reactions (rash, fever, edema, mucosal erosions or ulcerations, red or inflamed eyes). Monitor patient with mild to moderate rash for progression. If rash becomes severe or systemic symptoms occur, discontinue piperacillin/tazobactam.
- ***Lab Test Considerations:*** Evaluate renal and hepatic function, CBC, serum potassium, and bleeding times prior to and routinely during therapy.
- May cause positive direct Coombs' test result.
- May cause ↑ BUN, creatinine, AST, ALT, serum bilirubin, alkaline phosphatase, and LDH.
- May cause leukopenia and neutropenia, especially with prolonged therapy or hepatic impairment.
- May cause prolonged prothrombin and partial thromboplastin time.
- May cause ↓ hemoglobin and hematocrit and thrombocytopenia, eosinophilia, leukopenia, and neutropenia. It also may cause proteinuria; hematuria; pyuria; hyperglycemia; ↓ total protein or albumin; and abnormalities in sodium, potassium, and calcium levels.

P

Potential Nursing Diagnoses

Risk for infection (Indications, Side Effects)
Deficient knowledge, related to medication regimen (Patient/Family Teaching)

Implementation

IV Administration

- **Intermittent Infusion:** Reconstitute each 1 g of piperacillin with at least 5 mL of 0.9% NaCl, sterile water for injection, or D5W. ***Diluent:*** Dilute further in 50–100 mL of 0.9% NaCl, D5W, D5/0.9% NaCl, or LR. Reconstituted vials stable for 24 hr at room temperature or 48 hr if refrigerated. Infusion stable for 24 hr at room temperature or 7 days if refrigerated. ***Rate:*** Infuse over 30 min.
- **Y-Site Compatibility:** alfentanil, allopurinol, amifostine, aminocaproic acid, aminophylline, amphotericin B lipid complex, amphotericin B liposome, anidulafungin, argatroban, aztreonam, bivalirudin, bleomycin, bumetanide, buprenorphine, busulfan, butorphanol, calcium acetate, calcium chloride, calcium gluconate, carboplatin, carmustine, cefepime, chloramphenicol , clindamycin, cyclophosphamide, cyclosporine, cytarabine, dactinomycin, daptomycin, dexamethasone, dexmedetomidine, dexrazoxane, diazepam, digoxin, diphenhydramine, docetaxel, dopamine, doxacurium, enalaprilat, ephedrine, epi-

nephrine, eptifibatide, erythromycin, esmolol, etoposide, etoposide phosphate, fenoldopam, fentanyl, floxuridine, fluconazole, fludarabine, fluorouracil, foscarnet, fosphenytoin, furosemide, granisetron, heparin, hetastarch, hydrocortisone, hydromorphone, ifosfamide, isoproterenol, ketamine, ketorolac, leucovorin calcium, lidocaine, linezolid, lorazepam, magnesium sulfate, mannitol, mechlorethamine, melphalan, meperidine, mesna, metaraminol, methotrexate, methylprednisolone, metoclopramide, metoprolol, metronidazole, milrinone, morphine, naloxone, nitroglycerin, nitroprusside, norepinephrine, octreotide, ondansetron, oxytocin, paclitaxel, palonosetron, pancuronium, pantoprazole, pemetrexed, pentobarbital, phenobarbital, phentolamine, phenylephrine, potassium acetate, potassium chloride, potassium phosphates, procainamide, ranitidine, remifentanil, rituximab, sargramostim, sodium acetate, sodium bicarbonate, sodium phosphates, succinylcholine, sufentanil, tacrolimus, telavancin, teniposide, theophylline, thiotepa, tigecycline, tirofiban, trimethoprim/sulfamethoxazole, vasopressin, vinblastine, vincristine, voriconazole, zidovudine, zoledronic acid.

- **Y-Site Incompatibility:** acyclovir, alemtuzumab, amiodarone, amphotericin B cholesteryl, amphotericin B colloidal, azithromycin, caspofungin, chlorpromazine, ciprofloxacin, cisplatin, dacarbazine, dantrolene, daunorubicin, diltiazem, dobutamine, doxorubicin, doxorubicin liposome, doxycycline, droperidol, epirubicin, famotidine, ganciclovir, gemcitabine, glycopyrrolate, haloperidol, hydralazine, hydroxyzine, idarubicin, insulin, irinotecan, labetalol, levofloxacin, methyldopate, midazolam, mitomycin, mitoxantrone, nalbuphine, nesiritide, nicardipine, pentamidine, pentazocine, phenytoin, prochlorperazine, promethazine, propranolol, quinupristin/dalfopristin, rocuronium, streptozocin, thiopental, tobramycin, tranexamic acid, trastuzumab, vecuronium, verapamil, vinorelbine.

Patient/Family Teaching

- Advise patient to report rash and signs of superinfection (black furry overgrowth on tongue, vaginal itching or discharge, loose or foul-smelling stools) and allergy.
- Caution patient to notify health care professional if fever and diarrhea occur, especially if stool contains blood, pus, or mucus. Advise patient not to treat diarrhea without consulting health care professional. May occur up to several weeks after discontinuation of medication.

Evaluation/Desired Outcomes

- Resolution of the signs and symptoms of infection. Length of time for complete resolution depends on the organism and site of infection.

pitavastatin, See HMG-CoA REDUCTASE INHIBITORS (statins).

polyethylene glycol

(po-lee-**eth**-e-leen **glye**-kole)

✤ClearLax, GlycoLax, ✤Lax-a-Day, MiraLax, ✤PegaLax, ✤PolyLax, ✤Relaxa, ✤RestoraLax

Classification
Therapeutic: laxatives
Pharmacologic: osmotics

Pregnancy Category C

Indications

Treatment of occasional constipation.

Action

Polyethylene glycol (PEG) in solution acts as an osmotic agent, drawing water into the lumen of the GI tract. **Therapeutic Effects:** Evacuation of the GI tract without water or electrolyte imbalance.

Pharmacokinetics

Absorption: Nonabsorbable.
Distribution: Unknown.
Metabolism and Excretion: Excreted in fecal contents.
Half-life: Unknown.

TIME/ACTION PROFILE (bowel movement)

ROUTE	ONSET	PEAK	DURATION
PO	unknown	1–3 days	unknown

Contraindications/Precautions

Contraindicated in: GI obstruction; Gastric retention; Toxic colitis; Megacolon; Bowel perforation.
Use Cautiously in: Abdominal pain of uncertain cause, particularly if accompanied by fever; OB, Pedi: Safety not established.

Adverse Reactions/Side Effects

Derm: urticaria. **GI:** abdominal bloating, cramping, flatulence, nausea.

Interactions

Drug-Drug: None significant.

Route/Dosage

PO (Adults): 17 g (heaping tablespoon) in 8 oz of water; may be used for up to 2 wk.
PO (Children >6 mo): 0.5–1.5 g/kg daily, titrate to effect (maximum: 17 g/day).

Availability (generic available)

Powder: 14-oz, 24-oz, and 26-oz containers.

NURSING IMPLICATIONS

Assessment

- Assess patient for abdominal distention, presence of bowel sounds, and usual pattern of bowel function.
- Assess color, consistency, and amount of stool produced.

Potential Nursing Diagnoses

Constipation (Indications)
Diarrhea (Side Effects)

Implementation

- Do not confuse Miralax (polyethylene glycol) with Mirapex (pramipexole).
- **PO:** Dissolve powder in 8 oz of water prior to administration.

Patient/Family Teaching

- Inform patient that 2–4 days may be required to produce a bowel movement. PEG should not be used for more than 2 wk. Prolonged, frequent, or excessive use may result in electrolyte imbalance and laxative dependence.
- Advise patient to notify health care professional if unusual cramps, bloating, or diarrhea occurs.

Evaluation/Desired Outcomes

- A soft, formed bowel movement.

polyethylene glycol/electrolyte

(po-lee-**eth**-e-leen **glye**-kole/e-**lek**-troe-lite)

Colyte, GoLYTELY, ✱Klean-Prep, MoviPrep, NuLytely, Suclear, TriLyte

Classification
Therapeutic: laxatives
Pharmacologic: osmotics

Pregnancy Category C

Indications

Bowel cleansing in preparation for GI examination. **Unlabeled Use:** Treatment of acute iron overdose in children.

Action

Polyethylene glycol (PEG) in solution acts as an osmotic agent, drawing water into the lumen of the GI tract. **Therapeutic Effects:** Evacuation of the GI tract without water or electrolyte imbalance.

Pharmacokinetics

Absorption: Ions in the solution are nonabsorbable.
Distribution: Unknown.
Metabolism and Excretion: Solution is excreted in fecal contents.
Half-life: Unknown.

TIME/ACTION PROFILE

ROUTE	ONSET	PEAK	DURATION
PO	1 hr	unknown	4 hr

Contraindications/Precautions

Contraindicated in: GI obstruction; Bowel perforation; Gastric retention; Toxic colitis; Toxic megacolon.
Use Cautiously in: Patients with absent or diminished gag reflex; Unconscious or semicomatose states, in which administration is via NG tube; History of ulcerative colitis (↑ risk of hypoglycemia, dehydration, and hypokalemia); Barium enema using double-contrast technique (may not allow proper barium coating of mucosa); Seizure disorders; Abdominal pain of uncertain cause, particularly if accompanied by fever; Geri: May be more sensitive to effects; Pedi: Children (safety not established; children <2 yr more prone to hypoglycemia, dehydration, and hypokalemia).

Adverse Reactions/Side Effects

GI: abdominal fullness, diarrhea, bloating, cramps, ischemic colitis, nausea, vomiting. **F and E:** fluid and electrolyte abnormalities. **Misc:** allergic reactions (rare).

Interactions

Drug-Drug: Interferes with the absorption of **orally administered medications** by decreasing transit time (do not administer within 1 hr of start of therapy).

Route/Dosage

PO (Adults): 240 mL q 10 min (up to 4 L) until fecal discharge appears clear and has no solid material; may be given through NG tube at 20–30 mL/min (up to 4 L); *Moviprep*—On evening before colonoscopy, give 240 mL q 15 min for 1 hr followed by 480 mL of clear liquid before going to bed; on morning of colonoscopy, give 240 mL q 15 min for 1 hr, followed by 480 mL of clear liquid at least 2 hr before test (alternative regimen is 240 mL q 15 min for 1 hr at least 3 hr before bedtime on evening before colonscopy, then 1.5 hr later, give 240 mL q 15 min for 1 hr; may drink clear fluids up to 2 hr before test); *Suclear*—On evening before colonoscopy, dilute 6–oz oral solution by pouring entire contents into 16–oz mixing container and then filling container with cool water to fill line. Drink entire container within 20 min. Refill container with 480 mL of water and drink over next 2 hr. Refill container with 480 mL of water and finish drinking before going to bed. On morning of colonoscopy (≥3.5 hr before exam), dissolve powder of Dose 2 by adding water to

fill line. Drink 480 mL every 20 min completing the dose ≥2 hr before test.
PO (Children ≥6 mo): 25 mL/kg/hr until fecal discharge is clear and has no solid material; may also be given through an NG tube (unlabeled).

Availability (generic available)

Powder for oral solution (regular, pineapple, citrus berry, lemon lime, orange, cherry flavor): CoLyte, NuLytely, TriLyte—powder in bottles for reconstitution, GoLYTLEY—powder in packets and bottles for reconstitution, MoviPrep—powder in pouches for reconstitution, Suclear—oral solution in bottle and powder for reconstitution in bottle.

NURSING IMPLICATIONS

Assessment

- Assess color, consistency, and amount of stool produced.
- Monitor semiconscious or unconscious patients closely for regurgitation when administering via NG tube.

Potential Nursing Diagnoses

Diarrhea (Side Effects)

Implementation

- Do not add extra flavorings or additional ingredients to solution prior to administration.
- Avoid solid food and milk within 1–2 hr of administration, but should be adequately hydrated prior to, during, and after administration.
- Patient should be allowed only clear liquids after administration.
- May be administered on the morning of the examination as long as time is allotted to drink solution (3 hr) and evacuate bowel (1 additional hr). For barium enema, administer solution early evening (6 PM) prior to exam to allow proper mucosal coating by barium.
- **PO:** Solution may be reconstituted with tap water. Shake vigorously until powder is dissolved.
- Follow 2 dose regimen for *Suclear*.
- May be administered via NG tube at a rate of 20–30 mL/min.

Patient/Family Teaching

- Instruct patient to drink 240 mL every 10 min until 4 L have been consumed or fecal discharge is clear and free of solid matter. Rapidly drinking each 240 mL is preferred over drinking small amounts continuously.
- Advise patient to avoid alcohol during prep.

Evaluation/Desired Outcomes

- Diarrhea, which cleanses the bowel within 4 hr. The first bowel movement usually occurs within 1 hr of administration.

posaconazole

(po-sa-**kon**-a-zole)
Noxafil, ✱Posanol

Classification
Therapeutic: antifungals
Pharmacologic: triazoles

Pregnancy Category C

Indications

Prevention of invasive aspergillus and candida infections in severely immunocompromised patients. Treatment of oropharyngeal candidiasis (including candidiasis unresponsive to itraconazole or fluconazole).

Action

Blocks ergosterol synthesis, a major component of fungal plasma membrane. **Therapeutic Effects:** Fungistatic/fungicidal action against susceptible fungi.

Pharmacokinetics

Absorption: Well absorbed following oral administration; absorption is optimized by food; IV administration results in complete bioavailability.
Distribution: Extensive extravascular distribution and penetration into body tissues.
Protein Binding: >98%.
Metabolism and Excretion: Some metabolism via UDP glucuronidation; 66% eliminated unchanged in feces, 13% in urine (mostly as metabolites).
Half-life: 35 hr.

TIME/ACTION PROFILE (blood levels)

ROUTE	ONSET	PEAK	DURATION
PO (suspension)	unknown	3–5 hr	8 hr
PO-ER	unknown	4–5 hr	24 hr
IV	unknown	2 hr	24 hr

Contraindications/Precautions

Contraindicated in: Hypersensitivity to posaconazole or other azole antifungals; Concurrent use of pimozide, quinidine, ergot alkaloids, sirolimus, simvastatin, atorvastatin, or lovastatin.
Use Cautiously in: History of/predisposition to QTc prolongation including congenital QTc prolongation, concurrent medications that prolong QTc, high cumulative anthracycline history or electrolyte abnormalities (hypokalemia, hypomagnesemia); correct pre-existing abnormalities prior to administration; Moderate-severe renal impairment (CCr <50 mL/min); use only if justified by risk/benefit assessment (IV form should be avoided, use oral form only); Severe diarrhea, vomiting, or renal impairment (monitor for breakthrough fungal infections); OB, Lactation: Use only if maternal benefit outweighs risk to child; Pedi: Children <18 yr (IV) or <13 yr (oral) (safety not established).

Adverse Reactions/Side Effects

CNS: headache. **CV:** TORSADES DE POINTES, QT interval prolongation. **GI:** HEPATOCELLULAR DAMAGE, diarrhea, nausea, vomiting. **Endo:** adrenal insufficiency. **Resp:** cough. **Metab:** ALLERGIC REACTIONS. **Misc:** fever.

Interactions

Drug-Drug: Posaconazole inhibits the CYP3A4 enzyme systems and should be expected to interact with other drugs affected by this system. ↑ **cyclosporine**, **sirolimus**, and **tacrolimus** levels and risk of toxicity; use with sirolimus contraindicated; for cyclosporine and tacrolimus, ↓ dose initially and monitor levels frequently. May ↑ **quinidine** and **pimozide** levels and the risk for arrhythmias; concurrent use contraindicated. May ↑ levels and risk of toxicity from **ergot alkaloids**, including **ergotamine** and **dihydroergotamine**; concurrent use contraindicated. May ↑ levels of **simvastatin**, **atorvastatin**, or **lovastatin** and the risk for rhabdomyolysis; concurrent use contraindicated. **Rifabutin**, **phenytoin**, **cimetidine**, and **efavirenz** ↓ levels and may ↓ antifungal effectiveness; avoid concurrent use. **Fos** ↓ levels and may ↓ antifungal effectiveness; monitor for breakthrough antifungal infections. **Esomeprazole** and **metoclopramide** may ↓ levels and may ↓ antifungal effectiveness. ↑ **rifabutin** levels; avoid concurrent use. May ↑ **digoxin** levels; monitor levels frequently. ↑ **phenytoin**, **midazolam**, **ritonavir**, and **atazanavir** levels; monitor for excess clinical effect. ↑ levels and risk of neurotoxicity of **vinca alkaloids**, including **vincristine** and **vinblastine**; consider dose adjustment. ↑ levels and risk of toxicity of **HMG CoA reductase inhibitors (statins)**; consider ↓ statin dose. May ↑ levels and risk of adverse cardiovascular reactions to **calcium channel blockers**; consider dosage reduction.

Route/Dosage

Prophylaxis of Invasive Fungal Infections

IV (Adults): 300 mg twice daily on day 1, then 300 mg once daily starting on day 2.

PO (Adults and Children ≥13 yr): *Delayed-release tablets*—300 mg twice daily on day 1, then 300 mg once daily starting on day 2; *Oral suspension*—200 mg 3 times daily.

Oropharyngeal Candidiasis

PO (Adults and Children ≥13 yr): *Oral suspension*—100 mg twice daily on day 1, then 100 mg once daily for next 13 days; for refractory oropharyngeal candidiasis, give 400 mg twice daily.

Availability

Oral suspension (cherry-flavor): 40 mg/mL. **Delayed-release tablets:** 100 mg. **Injection:** 18 mg/mL.

NURSING IMPLICATIONS

Assessment

- Assess for signs and symptoms of fungal infection.
- ***Lab Test Considerations:*** Monitor liver function tests prior to and periodically during therapy. May cause ↑ ALT, ↑ AST, ↑ alkaline phosphatase and ↑ total bilirubin levels; generally reversible on discontinuation. Discontinue posaconazole if clinical signs and symptoms of liver disease develop.

Potential Nursing Diagnoses

Risk for infection (Indications)

Implementation

- Delayed-release table and oral suspension are not interchangeable.
- **PO:** Shake suspension well before use. Administer with a full meal, liquid nutritional supplement or an acidic carbonated beverage (ginger ale) to enhance absorption. Rinse spoon for administration with water after each use. Alternative therapy or close monitoring for breakthrough fungal infections should be considered for patients unable to eat a full meal or tolerate a nutritional supplement.
- Administer delay-release tablets with food. Swallow tablets whole; do not divide, crush, or chew.

IV Administration

- **Intermittent Infusion:** Allow solution to reach room temperature before administering. ***Diluent:*** Dilute 167 mg of posaconazole in 150 mL of D5W or 0.9% NaCl. Do not dilute with other solutions.Use immediately; stable for 24 hrs if refrigerated. Discard unused solution. Solution is clear, colorless to yellow; do not administer solutions that are discolored or contain particulate matter. Administer through a 0.22 micron polyethersulfone (PES) or polyvinylidene difluoride (PVDF) filter via central venous line, including a central venous catheter or peripherally inserted central catheter (PICC) line. If no central catheter available, may be administered through a peripheral venous catheter by slow intravenous infusion over 30 minutes only as a single dose in advance of central venous line placement or to bridge the period during which a central venous line is replaced or is in use for other intravenous treatment. ***Rate:*** Infuse slowly over 90 min. Do not give as a bolus.
- **Y-Site Compatibility:** amikacin, caspofungin, ciprofloxacin, daptomycin, dobutamine, famotidine, filgrastim, gentamicin, hydromorphone, levofloxacin, lorazepam, meropenem, micafungin, morphine, norepinephrine, potassium chloride, vancomycin.

Patient/Family Teaching

- Instruct patient to take posaconazole during or immediately (within 20 min) following a full meal or

P

liquid nutritional supplement in order to enhance absorption. Take missed doses as soon as remembered. Instruct patient to read the *Patient Information* before taking posaconazole and with each Rx refill; may be new information.

- Advise patient to notify health care professional if severe diarrhea or vomiting occur; may decrease posaconazole blood levels and allow breakthrough fungal infections or if signs and symptoms of liver injury (itching, yellow eyes or skin, fatigue, flu-like symptoms) occur.
- Instruct patient to notify health care professional of all Rx or OTC medications, vitamins, or herbal products being taken and consult health care professional before taking any new medications.
- Advise patient to notify health care professional if pregnancy is planned or suspected or if breast feeding.

Evaluation/Desired Outcomes

- Resolution of clinical and laboratory indications of fungal infections. Duration of therapy is based on recovery from infection or neutropenia or immunosuppression.

potassium and sodium phosphates

(po-**tas**-e-um/**soe**-dee-um **foss**-fates)

K-Phos M.F, K-Phos Neutral, K-Phos No. 2, Neutra-Phos, Uro-KP Neutral

Classification

Therapeutic: antiurolithics, mineral and electrolyte replacements/supplements

Pregnancy Category C

Indications

Treatment and prevention of phosphate depletion in patients who are unable to ingest adequate dietary phosphate. Adjunct therapy of urinary tract infections with methenamine hippurate or mandelate. Prevention of calcium urinary stones. Phosphate salts of potassium may be used in hypokalemic patients with metabolic acidosis or coexisting phosphorus deficiency.

Action

Phosphate is present in bone and is involved in energy transfer and carbohydrate metabolism. Serves as a buffer for the excretion of hydrogen ions by the kidneys. Dibasic potassium phosphate is converted in renal tubule to monobasic salt, resulting in urinary acidification, which is required for methenamine hippurate or mandelate to be active as urinary anti-infectives. Acidification of urine increases solubility of calcium, decreasing calcium stone formation. **Therapeutic Effects:** Replacement of phosphorus in deficiency states. Urinary acidification. Increased efficacy of methenamine. Decreased formation of calcium urinary tract stones.

Pharmacokinetics

Absorption: Well absorbed following oral administration. Vitamin D promotes GI absorption of phosphates.
Distribution: Phosphates enter extracellular fluids and are then actively transported to sites of action.
Metabolism and Excretion: Excreted mainly (>90%) by the kidneys.
Half-life: Unknown.

TIME/ACTION PROFILE (effects on serum phosphate levels)

ROUTE	ONSET	PEAK	DURATION
PO	unknown	unknown	unknown

Contraindications/Precautions

Contraindicated in: Hyperkalemia (potassium salts); Hyperphosphatemia; Hypocalcemia; Severe renal impairment; Untreated Addison's disease (potassium salts).
Use Cautiously in: Hyperparathyroidism; Cardiac disease; Hypernatremia (sodium phosphate only); Hypertension (sodium phosphate only); Renal impairment.

Adverse Reactions/Side Effects

Related to hyperphosphatemia, unless otherwise indicated.
CNS: confusion, dizziness, headache, weakness. **CV:** ARRHYTHMIAS, CARDIAC ARREST, bradycardia, ECG changes (absent P waves, widening of the QRS complex with biphasic curve, peaked T waves), edema. **GI:** diarrhea, abdominal pain, nausea, vomiting. **F and E:** hyperkalemia, hypernatremia, hyperphosphatemia, hypocalcemia, hypomagnesemia. **MS:** *hypocalcemia, hyperkalemia*—muscle cramps. **Neuro:** flaccid paralysis, heaviness of legs, paresthesias, tremors.

Interactions

Drug-Drug: Concurrent use of **potassium-sparing, diuretics, ACE inhibitors**, or **angiotensin II receptor blockers** with potassium phosphates may result in hyperkalemia. Concurrent use of **corticosteroids** with sodium phosphate may result in hypernatremia. Concurrent administration of **calcium-, magnesium-**, or **aluminum-containing compounds** ↓ absorption of phosphates by formation of insoluble complexes. **Vitamin D** enhances the absorption of phosphates.
Drug-Food: Oxalates (in spinach and rhubarb) and **phytates** (in bran and whole grains) may ↓ absorption of phosphates by binding them in the GI tract.

Route/Dosage

Phosphorous Supplementation

PO (Adults and Children >4 yr): 250–500 mg (8–16 mmol) phosphorus (1–2 packets) 4 times daily.

PO (Children <4 yr): 250 mg (8 mmol) phosphorus (1 packet) 4 times daily.

Urinary Acidification

PO (Adults): 2 tablets 4 times/day.

Maintenance Phosphorus

PO (Adults): 50–150 mmol/day in divided doses.
PO (Children): 2–3 mmol/kg/day in divided doses.

Availability

Potassium and Sodium Phosphates

Tablets (K-Phos MF): elemental phosphorus 125.6 mg (4 mmol), sodium 67 mg (2.9 mEq), and potassium 44.5 mg (1.1 mEq). **Tablets (K-Phos Neutral):** elemental phosphorus 250 mg (8 mmol), sodium 298 mg (13 mEq), and potassium 45 mg (1.1 mEq). **Tablets (K-Phos No.2):** elemental phosphorus 250 mg (8 mmol), sodium 134 mg (5.8 mEq), and potassium 88 mg (2.3 mEq). **Tablets (Uro-KP Neutral):** elemental phosphorus 258 mg, sodium 262.4 mg (10.8 mEq), and potassium 49.4 mg (1.3 mEq). **Powder for oral solution (Neutra-Phos):** elemental phosphorus 250 mg (8 mmol), sodium 164 mg (7.1 mEq), and potassium 278 mg (7.1 mEq)/packet.

NURSING IMPLICATIONS

Assessment

- Assess patient for signs and symptoms of hypokalemia (weakness, fatigue, arrhythmias, presence of U waves on ECG, polyuria, polydipsia) and hypophosphatemia (anorexia, weakness, decreased reflexes, bone pain, confusion, blood dyscrasias) throughout therapy.
- Monitor intake and output ratios and daily weight. Report significant discrepancies.
- ***Lab Test Considerations:*** Monitor serum phosphate, potassium, sodium, and calcium levels prior to and periodically throughout therapy. Increased phosphate may cause hypocalcemia.
- Monitor renal function studies prior to and periodically throughout therapy.
- Monitor urinary pH in patients receiving potassium and sodium phosphate as a urinary acidifier.

Potential Nursing Diagnoses

Imbalanced nutrition: less than body requirements (Indications)

Implementation

- **PO:** Tablets should be dissolved in a full glass of water. Allow mixture to stand for 2–5 min to ensure it is fully dissolved. Solutions prepared by pharmacy should not be further diluted.
- Medication should be administered after meals to minimize gastric irritation and laxative effect.
- Do not administer simultaneously with antacids containing aluminum, magnesium, or calcium.

Patient/Family Teaching

- Explain to the patient the purpose of the medication and the need to take as directed. Take missed doses as soon as remembered unless within 1 or 2 hr of the next dose. Explain that the tablets should not be swallowed whole. Tablets should be dissolved in water.
- Instruct patients in low-sodium diet (see Appendix J).
- Advise patient of the importance of maintaining a high fluid intake (drinking at least one 8-oz glass of water each hr) to prevent kidney stones.
- Instruct the patient to promptly report diarrhea, weakness, fatigue, muscle cramps, unexplained weight gain, swelling of lower extremities, shortness of breath, unusual thirst, or tremors.

Evaluation/Desired Outcomes

- Prevention and correction of serum phosphate and potassium deficiencies.
- Maintenance of acid urine.
- Decreased urine calcium, which prevents formation of renal calculi.

P

---

potassium iodide, See IODINE, IODIDE.

HIGH ALERT

POTASSIUM SUPPLEMENTS

(poe-**tass**-ee-um)

potassium acetate

potassium bicarbonate/potassium chloride

potassium bicarbonate/potassium citrate

Effer-K, K-Lyte DS

potassium chloride

Klor-Con, Klor-Con M10, Klor-Con M15, Klor-Con M20, K-Tab, Micro-K, Micro-K 10

potassium gluconate

Classification

Therapeutic: mineral and electrolyte replacements/supplements

Pregnancy Category C

Indications

PO, IV: Treatment/prevention of potassium depletion.
IV: Arrhythmias due to digoxin toxicity.

Action

Maintain acid-base balance, isotonicity, and electrophysiologic balance of the cell. Activator in many enzymatic reactions; essential to transmission of nerve impulses; contraction of cardiac, skeletal, and smooth muscle; gastric secretion; renal function; tissue synthesis; and carbohydrate metabolism. **Therapeutic Effects:** Replacement. Prevention of deficiency.

Pharmacokinetics

Absorption: Well absorbed following oral administration.
Distribution: Enters extracellular fluid; then actively transported into cells.
Metabolism and Excretion: Excreted by the kidneys.
Half-life: Unknown.

TIME/ACTION PROFILE (↑ in serum potassium levels)

ROUTE	ONSET	PEAK	DURATION
PO	unknown	1–2 hr	unknown
IV	rapid	end of infusion	unknown

Contraindications/Precautions

Contraindicated in: Hyperkalemia; Severe renal impairment; Untreated Addison's disease; Severe tissue trauma; Hyperkalemic familial periodic paralysis; Some products may contain tartrazine (FDC yellow dye #5) or alcohol; avoid using in patients with known hypersensitivity or intolerance; Potassium acetate injection contains aluminum, which may become toxic with prolonged use to high risk groups (renal impairment, premature neonates).
Use Cautiously in: Cardiac disease; Renal impairment; Diabetes mellitus (liquids may contain sugar); Hypomagnesemia (may make correction of hypokalemia more difficult); GI hypomotility including dysphagia or esophageal compression from left atrial enlargement (tablets, capsules); Patients receiving potassium-sparing drugs.

Adverse Reactions/Side Effects

CNS: confusion, restlessness, weakness. **CV:** ARRHYTHMIAS, ECG changes. **GI:** abdominal pain, diarrhea, flatulence, nausea, vomiting; *tablets, capsules only*, GI ulceration, stenotic lesions. **Local:** irritation at IV site. **Neuro:** paralysis, paresthesia.

Interactions

Drug-Drug: Use with **potassium-sparing diuretics** or **ACE inhibitors** or **angiotensin II receptor antagonists** may lead to hyperkalemia. **Anticholinergics** may ↑ GI mucosal lesions in patients taking wax-matrix potassium chloride preparations.

Route/Dosage

Expressed as mEq of potassium. Potassium acetate contains 10.2 mEq/g; potassium bicarbonate contains 10 mEq potassium/g; potassium chloride contains 13.4 mEq potassium/g; potassium gluconate contains 4.3 mEq/g.

Normal Daily Requirements

PO, IV (Adults): 40–80 mEq/day.
PO, IV (Children): 2–3 mEq/kg/day.
PO, IV (Neonates): 2–6 mEq/kg/day.

Prevention of Hypokalemia during Diuretic Therapy

PO (Adults): 20–40 mEq/day in 1–2 divided doses; single dose should not exceed 20 mEq.
PO (Neonates , Infants, and Children): 1–2 mEq/kg/day in 1–2 divided doses.

Treatment of Hypokalemia

PO (Adults): 40–100 mEq/day in divided doses.
PO (Neonates , Infants, and Children): 2–5 mEq/kg/day in divided doses.
IV (Adults): *Serum potassium >2.5 mEq/L*—Up to 20 mEq/day as an infusion (not to exceed 10 mEq/hr) or a concentration of 40 mEq/L via peripheral line (up to 100 mEq/L have been used via central line [unlabeled]). *Serum potassium <2 mEq/L with symptoms*—Up to 40 mEq/day as an infusion (rate should generally not exceed 20 mEq/hr).
IV (Neonates , Infants, and Children): 0.5–1 mEq/kg/dose (maximum 30 mEq/dose) as an infusion to infuse at 0.3–0.5 mEq/kg/hr (maximum infusion rate 1 mEq/kg/hr).

Availability

Potassium Acetate (generic available)

Concentrate for injection (contains aluminum): 2 mEq/mL, 4 mEq/mL.

Potassium Bicarbonate/Potassium Chloride (generic available)

Tablets for effervescent oral solution: ✱12 mEq, 25 mEq.

Potassium Bicarbonate/Potassium Citrate (generic available)

Tablets for effervescent oral solution: 10 mEq, 20 mEq, 25 mEq, 50 mEq.

Potassium Chloride (generic available)

Extended-release tablets: 8 mEq, 10 mEq, 15 mEq, 20 mEq. **Cost:** *Generic*—8 mEq $53.64/100, 10 mEq $45.97/100, 20 mEq $45.97/100. **Extended-release capsules:** 8 mEq, 10 mEq. **Cost:** *Generic*—8 mEq $70.40/100, 10 mEq $72.62/100. **Oral solution:** 20 mEq/15 mL, 40 mEq/15 mL. **Cost:** *Generic*—20 mEq/15 mL $14.51/473 mL, 40 mEq/15 mL $27.11/473 mL.

Powder/packets for oral solution: 20-mEq/packet, 25-mEq/packet. **Cost:** 20 mEq $58.21/30 pkts, 25 mEq $69.20/30 pkts. **Concentrate for injection:** 0.1 mEq/mL in 10-mEq ampules and vials, 0.2 mEq/mL in 10- and 20-mEq ampules and vials, 0.3 mEq/mL in 30-mEq ampules and vials, 0.4 mEq/mL in 20- and 40-mEq ampules and vials, 1.5 mEq/mL, 2 mEq/mL, 3 mEq/mL. **Solution for IV infusion:** 10 mEq/L in various dextrose and saline solutions in 250-, 500-, and 100-mL containers, 20 mEq/L in dextrose/saline/LRs in 250-, 500-, and 100-mL containers, 30 mEq/L in various dextrose and saline solutions in 250-, 500-, and 100-mL containers, 40 mEq/L in various dextrose and saline solutions in 250-, 500-, and 100-mL containers.

Potassium Gluconate (generic available)
Tablets: 2 mEq, 5 mEq. **Elixir:** 20 mEq/15 mL.

NURSING IMPLICATIONS

Assessment
- Assess for signs and symptoms of hypokalemia (weakness, fatigue, U wave on ECG, arrhythmias, polyuria, polydipsia) and hyperkalemia (see Toxicity and Overdose).
- Monitor pulse, BP, and ECG periodically during IV therapy.
- ***Lab Test Considerations:*** Monitor serum potassium before and periodically during therapy. Monitor renal function, serum bicarbonate, and pH. Determine serum magnesium level if patient has refractory hypokalemia; hypomagnesemia should be corrected to facilitate effectiveness of potassium replacement. Monitor serum chloride because hypochloremia may occur if replacing potassium without concurrent chloride.
- ***Toxicity and Overdose:*** Symptoms of toxicity are those of hyperkalemia (slow, irregular heartbeat; fatigue; muscle weakness; paresthesia; confusion; dyspnea; peaked T waves; depressed ST segments; prolonged QT segments; widened QRS complexes; loss of P waves; and cardiac arrhythmias).
- Treatment includes discontinuation of potassium, administration of sodium bicarbonate to correct acidosis, dextrose and insulin to facilitate passage of potassium into cells, calcium salts to reverse ECG effects (in patients who are not receiving digoxin), sodium polystyrene used as an exchange resin, and/or dialysis for patient with impaired renal function.

Potential Nursing Diagnoses
Imbalanced nutrition: less than body requirements (Indications)

Implementation
- ***High Alert:*** Medication errors involving too rapid infusion or bolus IV administration of potassium chloride have resulted in fatalities. See IV administration guidelines below.
- For most purposes, potassium chloride should be used, except for renal tubular acidoses (hyperchloremic acidosis), in which other salts are more appropriate (potassium bicarbonate, potassium citrate, or potassium gluconate).
- If hypokalemia is secondary to diuretic therapy, consideration should be given to decreasing the dose of diuretic, unless there is a history of significant arrhythmias or concurrent digitalis glycoside therapy.
- **PO:** Administer with or after meals to decrease GI irritation.
- Use of tablets and capsules should be reserved for patients who cannot tolerate liquid preparations.
- Dissolve effervescent tablets in 3–8 oz of cold water. Ensure that effervescent tablet is fully dissolved. Powders and solutions should be diluted in 3–8 oz of cold water or juice (do not use tomato juice if patient is on sodium restriction). Instruct patient to drink slowly over 5–10 min.
- Tablets and capsules should be taken with a meal and full glass of water. Do not chew or crush enteric-coated or extended-release tablets or capsules. Micro-K ExtenCaps capsules can be opened and sprinkled on soft food (pudding, applesauce) and swallowed immediately with a glass of cool water or juice.
- **IV:** Assess for extravasation; severe pain and tissue necrosis may occur. ***High Alert:*** Never administer potassium IV push or bolus.

Potassium Acetate
- **Continuous Infusion:** ***High Alert:*** Do not administer undiluted. Each single dose *must* be diluted and thoroughly mixed in 100–1000 mL of dextrose, saline, Ringer's or LR, dextrose/saline, dextrose/Ringer's, or LR combinations. Usually limited to 80 mEq/L via peripheral line (200 mEq/L via central line).
- ***Rate: High Alert:*** Infuse slowly, at a rate up to 10 mEq/hr in adults or 0.5 mEq/kg/hr in children on general care areas. Check hospital policy for maximum infusion rates (maximum rate in monitored setting 40 mEq/hr in adults or 1 mEq/kg/hr in children).
- **Y-Site Compatibility:** ciprofloxacin.

Potassium Chloride
- **Continuous Infusion:** ***High Alert:*** Do not administer concentrations of ≥1.5 mEq/mL undiluted; fatalities have occurred. Concentrated products have black caps on vials or black stripes above constriction on ampules and are labeled with a warning about dilution requirement. Each single dose must be diluted and thoroughly mixed in 100–1000 mL

P

of IV solution. Usually limited to 80 mEq/L via peripheral line (200 mEq/L via central line).
- Concentrations of 0.1 and 0.4 mEq/mL are intended for administration via calibrated infusion device and do not require dilution.
- ***Rate: High Alert:*** Infuse slowly, at a rate up to 10 mEq/hr in adults or 0.5 mEq/kg/hr in children in general care areas. Check hospital policy for maximum infusion rates (maximum rate in monitored setting 40 mEq/hr in adults or 1 mEq/kg/hr in children). Use an infusion pump.
- **Solution Compatibility:** May be diluted in dextrose, saline, Ringer's solution, LR, dextrose/saline, dextrose/Ringer's solution, and dextrose/LR combinations. Commercially available premixed with many of the above IV solutions.
- **Y-Site Compatibility:** acyclovir, alemtuzumab, alfentanil, allopurinol, alprostadil, amifostine, amikacin, aminophylline, amiodarone, amphotericin B liposome, anidulafungin, argatroban, ascorbic acid, atropine, aztreonam, benztropine, betamethasone, bivalirudin, bleomycin, bumetanide, buprenorphine, butorphanol, calcium chloride, calcium gluconate, carboplatin, carmustine, caspofungin, cefazolin, cefotaxime, cefotetan, cefoxitin, ceftaroline, ceftazidime, ceftriaxone, cefuroxime, chloramphenicol, chlorpromazine, ciprofloxacin, cisatracurium, cisplatin, cladribine, clindamycin, cyanocobalamin, cyclophosphamide, cyclosporine, cytarabine, dactinomycin, daptomycin, dexamethasone sodium phosphate, dexmedetomidine, digoxin, diltiazem, diphenhydramine, dobutamine, docetaxel, dopamine, doripenem, doxorubicin hydrochloride, doxorubicin liposome, doxycycline, droperidol, edrophonium, enalaprilat, ephedrine, epinephrine, epirubicin, epoetin alfa, eptifibatide, ertapenem, esmolol, conjugated estrogens, etoposide, etoposide phosphate, famotidine, fenoldopam, fentanyl, filgrastim, fluconazole, fludarabine, fluorouracil, folic acid, furosemide, ganciclovir, gemcitabine, gentamicin, granisetron, heparin, hydrocortisone, hydromorphone, idarubicin , ifosfamide, imipenem/cilastatin, indomethacin, insulin, irinotecan, isoproterenol, ketamine, ketorolac, labetalol, levofloxacin, lidocaine, linezolid, lorazepam, magnesium sulfate, mannitol, mechlorethamine, melphalan, meperidine, meropenem, methotrexate, methoxamine, methyldopate, methylergonovine, meticlopramide, metoprolol, metronidazole, micafungin, midazolam, milrinone, mitoxantrone, morphine, multivitamine, mycophenolate, nafcillin, nalbuphine, naloxone, neostigmine, nesiritide, nicardipine, nitroglycerin, nitroprusside, norepinephrine, octreotide, ondansetron, oxacillin, oxaliplatin, oxytocin, paclitaxel, palonosetron, pamidronate, pancuronium, pantoprazole, papaverine, pemetrexed, penicillin G, pentazocine, pentobarbital, phenobarbital, phentolamine, phenylephrine, phytonadione, piperacillin/tazobactam, procainamide, prochlorperazine, propofol, propranolol, protamine, pyridostigmine, pyridoxime, quinupristin/dalfopristin, ranitidine, remifentanil, rituximab, rocuronium, sargramostim, scopolamine, sodium acetate, sodium bicarbonate, streptokinase, succinylcholine, tacrolimus, telavancin, teniposide, theophylline, thiamine, thiotepa, tirofiban, tobramycin, tolazoline, trastuzumab, trimetaphan, vancomycin, vasopressin, verapamil, vincristine, vinorelbine, voriconazole, warfarin, zidovudine, zoledronic acid.
- **Y-Site Incompatibility:** amphotericin B cholesteryl, amphotericin B colloidal, azithromycin, dantrolene, diazepam, diazoxide, haloperidol, hydralazine, pentamidine, phenytoin, trimethoprim/sulfamethoxazole.

Patient/Family Teaching

- Explain to patient purpose of the medication and the need to take as directed, especially when concurrent digoxin or diuretics are taken. Take missed doses as soon as remembered within 2 hr; if not, return to regular dose schedule. Do not double dose.
- Emphasize correct method of administration. GI irritation or ulceration may result from chewing enteric-coated tablets or insufficient dilution of liquid or powder forms.
- Some extended-release tablets are contained in a wax matrix that may be expelled in the stool. This occurrence is not significant.
- Instruct patient to avoid salt substitutes or low-salt milk or food unless approved by health care professional. Patient should be advised to read all labels to prevent excess potassium intake.
- Advise patient regarding sources of dietary potassium (see Appendix J). Encourage compliance with recommended diet.
- Instruct patient to report dark, tarry, or bloody stools; weakness; unusual fatigue; or tingling of extremities. Notify health care professional if nausea, vomiting, diarrhea, or stomach discomfort persists. Dosage may require adjustment.
- Emphasize the importance of regular follow-up exams to monitor serum levels and progress.

Evaluation/Desired Outcomes

- Prevention and correction of serum potassium depletion.
- Cessation of arrhythmias caused by digoxin toxicity.

pramipexole (pra-mi-**pex**-ole)

Mirapex, Mirapex ER

Classification

Therapeutic: antiparkinson agents

Pharmacologic: dopamine agonists

Pregnancy Category C

Indications

Management of Parkinson's disease. Restless leg syndrome (immediate-release only).

Action

Stimulates dopamine receptors in the striatum of the brain. **Therapeutic Effects:** Decreased tremor and rigidity in Parkinson's disease. Decreased leg restlessness.

Pharmacokinetics

Absorption: >90% absorbed following oral administration.

Distribution: Widely distributed.

Metabolism and Excretion: 90% excreted unchanged in urine.

Half-life: 8 hr (↑ in geriatric patients and patients with renal impairment).

TIME/ACTION PROFILE (blood levels)

ROUTE	ONSET	PEAK	DURATION
PO	unknown	2 hr	8 hr
PO-ER	unknown	6 hr	24 hr

Contraindications/Precautions

Contraindicated in: Hypersensitivity; Major psychotic disorder.

Use Cautiously in: Renal impairment (↑ dosing interval recommended if CCr <60 mL/min [immediate-release] or CCr <50 mL/min [extended-release]); OB, Lactation, Pedi: Safety not established; Geri: ↑ risk of hallucinations.

Adverse Reactions/Side Effects

CNS: SLEEP ATTACKS, amnesia, dizziness, drowsiness, hallucinations, weakness, abnormal dreams, aggressive behavior, agitation, confusion, delirium, delusions, disorientation, dyskinesia, extrapyramidal syndrome, headache, insomnia, paranoid ideation, psychotic-like behavior, urges (gambling, sexual). **CV:** orthostatic hypotension. **Derm:** melanoma, pruritis. **Endo:** SIADH. **GI:** constipation, dry mouth, dyspepsia, nausea, tooth disease. **GU:** urinary frequency. **MS:** leg cramps. **Neuro:** hypertonia, unsteadiness/falling.

Interactions

Drug-Drug: Concurrent **levodopa** ↑ risk of hallucinations and dyskinesia. **Cimetidine**, **ranitidine**, **diltiazem**, **triamterene**, **verapamil**, **quinidine**, **quinine**, and **cisplatin** may ↑ levels. Effectiveness may be ↓ by **dopamine antagonists**, including **butyrophenones**, **metoclopramide**, **phenothiazines**, or **thioxanthenes**.

Route/Dosage

When switching from immediate-release to extended-release product, the same total daily dose can be used.

Parkinson's Disease

PO (Adults): *Immediate-release*—0.125 mg 3 times daily initially; may be ↑ q 5–7 days (range 1.5–4.5 mg/day in 3 divided doses); *Extended-release*—0.375 mg once daily; may be ↑ to 0.75 mg once daily in 5–7 days, and then ↑ q 5–7 days by 0.75 mg/day (max dose = 4.5 mg/day).

Renal Impairment

PO (Adults Immediate-release): *CCr 35–59 mL/min*—0.125 mg twice daily initially, may be ↑ q 5–7 days up to 1.5 mg twice daily; *CCr 15–34 mL/min*—0.125 mg daily initially, may be ↑ q 5–7 days up to 1.5 mg daily.

Renal Impairment

PO (Adults Extended-release): *CCr 30–50 mL/min*—0.375 mg every other day; may consider ↑ dose to 0.375 mg once daily after 1 wk based on response and tolerability; may ↑ in 0.375 mg increments after 1 wk (max dose = 2.25 mg/day).

Restless Leg Syndrome

PO (Adults): 0.125 mg daily 1–3 hr before bedtime. May be ↑ at 4–7 day intervals to 0.25 mg daily, then up to 0.5 mg daily.

Renal Impairment

PO (Adults Immediate-release): *CCr 20–60 mL/min*—0.125 mg daily 1–3 hr before bedtime. May be ↑ at 14-day intervals to 0.25 mg daily, then up to 0.5 mg daily.

Availability (generic available)

Immediate-release tablets: 0.125 mg, 0.25 mg, 0.5 mg, 0.75 mg, 1 mg, 1.5 mg. **Cost:** *Generic*—0.125 mg $265.47/90, 0.25 mg $277.55/90, 0.5 mg $265.47/90, 0.75 mg $265.47/90, 1 mg $277.55/90, 1.5 mg $277.55/90. **Extended-release tablets:** 0.375 mg, 0.75 mg, 1.5 mg, 2.25 mg, 3 mg, 3.75 mg, 4.5 mg. **Cost:** 0.375 mg $103.92/7, 0.75 mg $103.92/7, 1.5 mg $103.92/7, 2.25 mg $445.40/30, 3 mg $445.40/30, 3.75 mg $445.40/30, 4.5 mg $445.40/30.

NURSING IMPLICATIONS

Assessment

- Assess patient for signs and symptoms of psychotic-like behavior (confusion, paranoid ideation, delusions, hallucinations, psychotic-like behavior, disorientation, aggressive behavior, agitation, delirium, hallucinations). Risk of symptoms increases with age. Notify health care professional if these occur.
- Monitor ECG and BP frequently during dose adjustment and periodically throughout therapy.
- Assess patient for drowsiness and sleep attacks. Drowsiness is a common side effect of pramipexole, but sleep attacks or episodes of falling asleep during

activities that require active participation may occur without warning. Assess patient for concomitant medications that have sedating effects or may increase serum pramipexole levels (see Interactions). May require discontinuation of therapy.
- **Parkinson's Disease:** Assess patient for signs and symptoms of Parkinson's disease (tremor, muscle weakness and rigidity, ataxia) before and throughout therapy.
- **Restless Leg Syndrome:** Assess sleep patterns and frequency of restless leg disturbances.

Potential Nursing Diagnoses
Impaired physical mobility (Indications)
Risk for injury (Indications, Side Effects)

Implementation
- Do not confuse Mirapex (pramipexole) with Miralax (polyethylene glycol).
- An attempt to reduce the dose of levodopa/carbidopa may be made cautiously during pramipexole therapy.
- **PO:** Administer with meals to minimize nausea; usually resolves with continued therapy. Swallow extended-release tablets whole; do not crush, break, or chew.

Patient/Family Teaching
- Instruct patient to take medication as directed. Take missed doses or immediate-release product as soon as remembered if it is not almost time for next dose. If extended release tablets are missed, skip dose and take next regular dose. Do not double doses. Consult health care professional before reducing dose or discontinuing medication; may cause fever, confusion, or severe muscle stiffness. Advise patient to read the *Patient Information* sheet before taking and with each Rx refill, changes may occur.
- May cause drowsiness and unexpected episodes of falling asleep. Caution patient to avoid driving or other activities requiring alertness until response to medication is known. Advise patient to notify health care professional if episodes of falling asleep occur.
- Advise patient to change position slowly to minimize orthostatic hypotension. May occur more frequently during initial therapy.
- Instruct patient to notify health care professional of all Rx or OTC medications, vitamins, or herbal products being taken and consult health care professional before taking any new medications.
- Advise patient to have periodic skin exams to check for lesions that may be melanoma.
- Advise patient to notify health care professional if new or increased gambling, sexual, or other intense urges or psychotic-like behaviors occur.
- Advise female patient to notify health care professional if pregnancy is planned or suspected or if breast feeding or planning to breast feed.

Evaluation/Desired Outcomes
- Decreased tremor and rigidity in Parkinson's disease.
- Decrease in restless legs and improved sleep.

prasugrel (pra-soo-**grel**)
Effient

Classification
Therapeutic: antiplatelet agents
Pharmacologic: thienopyridines

Pregnancy Category B

Indications
Reduction of thrombotic cardiovascular events (including stent thrombosis) in patients with acute coronary syndrome who will be managed with PCI including patients with unstable angina or non-ST-elevation myocardial infarction (NSTEMI). Reduction of thrombotic cardiovascular events (including stent thrombosis) in patients with ST-elevation myocardial infarciotn (STEMI) when managed with either primary/delayed percutaneous coronary intervention (PCI).

Action
Acts by irreversibly binding its active metabolite to the $P2Y_{12}$ class of ADP receptors on platelets; inhibiting platelet activation and aggregation. **Therapeutic Effects:** Decreased thrombotic events including cardiovascular death, nonfatal myocardial infarction (MI) and nonfatal stroke.

Pharmacokinetics
Absorption: Well absorbed following oral administration (79%), then rapidly converted to an active metabolite.
Distribution: Unknown.
Protein Binding: *Active metabolite*—98%.
Metabolism and Excretion: Active metabolite is metabolized to two inactive compounds; 68% excreted in the urine and 27% in feces as inactive metabolites.
Half-life: *Active metabolite*—7 hr (range 2–15 hr).

TIME/ACTION PROFILE (effect on platelet function)

ROUTE	ONSET	PEAK	DURATION
PO	within 1 hr	2 hr	5–9 days†

† Following discontinuation.

Contraindications/Precautions
Contraindicated in: Hypersensitivity; Active pathological bleeding; History of transient ischemic attack or stroke.
Use Cautiously in: Patients about to undergo coronary artery bypass grafting (CABG) (↑ risk of bleeding; discontinue at least 7 days prior to surgery); Premature

discontinuation (↑ risk of stent thrombosis, MI, and death); Body weight <60 kg, propensity to bleed, severe hepatic impairment, concurrent use of medications that ↑ the risk of bleeding (↑ risk of bleeding); Hypotension in the setting of recent coronary angiography, PCI, CABG, or other surgical procedure (suspect bleeding but do not discontinue prasugrel); Geri: Use in patients ≥75 yr of age generally not recommended (↑ risk of fatal/intracranial bleeding and questionable benefit, except in high-risk patients such as diabetes or prior MI); OB: Use only if potential benefit to mother justifies potential risk to fetus; Lactation: Use only if potential benefit to the mother justifies potential risk to nursing infant; Pedi: Safety and effectiveness not established.

Adverse Reactions/Side Effects

CNS: dizziness, fatigue, headache. **Resp:** cough, dyspnea. **CV:** atrial fibrillation, bradycardia, hypertension, hypotension, peripheral edema. **GI:** diarrhea, nausea. **Derm:** rash. **Hemat:** BLEEDING, THROMBOTIC THROMBOCYTOPENIC PURPURA, leukopenia. **Metab:** hyperlipidemia. **MS:** back pain, extremity pain. **Misc:** allergic reactions including ANGIOEDEMA, fever, non-cardiac chest pain.

Interactions

Drug-Drug: ↑ risk of bleeding with **warfarin** and **NSAIDs.**

Route/Dosage

Aspirin 75–325 mg/daily should be taken concurrently.

PO (Adults ≥60 kg): 60 mg initially as a loading dose, then 10 mg once daily.

PO (Adults < 60 kg): Consider maintenance dose of 5 mg once daily.

Availability

Tablets: 5 mg, 10 mg.

NURSING IMPLICATIONS

Assessment

- Assess patient for symptoms of stroke, peripheral vascular disease, or MI periodically during therapy.
- Monitor patient for signs of thrombotic thrombocytic purpura (thrombocytopenia, microangiopathic hemolytic anemia, neurologic findings, renal dysfunction, fever). May rarely occur, even after short exposure (<2 wk). Requires prompt treatment.
- ***Lab Test Considerations:*** Monitor bleeding time during therapy. Prolonged bleeding time, which is time- and dose-dependent, is expected.
- Monitor CBC with differential and platelet count periodically during therapy. Thrombocytopenia and anemia may rarely occur.

Potential Nursing Diagnoses

Risk for injury (Indications, Side Effects)

Implementation

- Discontinue prasugrel 7 days before planned surgical procedures.
- Patients should take aspirin 75–325 mg daily with prasugrel.
- *In patients with UA or NSTEMI,* dose is usually administered at time of diagnosis or at time of PCI.
- *In patients with STEMI* presenting within 12 hours of symptom onset, loading dose is usually administered at time of diagnosis or at time of PCI.
- **PO:** Administer once daily without regard to food.

Patient/Family Teaching

- Instruct patient to take medication as directed. Take missed doses as soon as possible unless almost time for next dose; do not double doses. Do not discontinue without consulting health care professional. Advise patient to read *Medication Guide* before taking and with each Rx refill; in case of changes.
- Advise patient to notify health care professional promptly if fever, weakness, skin paleness, purple skin patches, yellowing of skin or eyes, chills, sore throat, neurological changes, or unusual bleeding or bruising, swelling of lips, difficulty breathing, rash, or hives occurs.
- Advise patient to notify health care professional of medication regimen prior to treatment or surgery.
- Instruct patient to notify health care professional of all Rx or OTC medications, vitamins, or herbal products being taken and consult health care professional before taking any new medications, especially NSAIDs.
- Advise female patient to notify health care professional if pregnancy is planned or suspected or if breast feeding.

Evaluation/Desired Outcomes

- Prevention of stroke, MI, and vascular death in patients at risk.

pravastatin, See HMG-CoA REDUCTASE INHIBITORS (statins).

prazosin (pra-zoe-sin)

Minipress

Classification

Therapeutic: antihypertensives

Pharmacologic: peripherally acting antiadrenergics

Pregnancy Category C

P

Indications

Mild to moderate hypertension. **Unlabeled Use:** Management of urinary outflow obstruction in patients with benign prostatic hyperplasia.

Action

Dilates both arteries and veins by blocking postsynaptic alpha$_1$-adrenergic receptors. Decreases contractions in smooth muscle of prostatic capsule. **Therapeutic Effects:** Lowering of BP. Decreased cardiac preload and afterload. Decreased symptoms of prostatic hyperplasia (urinary urgency, urinary hesitancy, nocturia).

Pharmacokinetics

Absorption: 60% absorbed following oral administration.
Distribution: Widely distributed.
Protein Binding: 97%.
Metabolism and Excretion: Extensively metabolized by the liver. Minimal (5–10%) renal excretion of unchanged drug.
Half-life: 2–3 hr.

TIME/ACTION PROFILE (antihypertensive effects)

ROUTE	ONSET	PEAK	DURATION
PO	2 hr	2–4 hr†	10 hr

†Following single dose; maximal antihypertensive effects occur after 3–4 wk of chronic dosing.

Contraindications/Precautions

Contraindicated in: Hypersensitivity.
Use Cautiously in: Renal insufficiency (↑ sensitivity to effects; dose ↓ may be required); OB, Lactation, Pedi: Safety not established; Angina pectoris; When adding diuretics (↓ dose of prazosin); Patients undergoing cataract surgery (↑ risk of intraoperative floppy iris syndrome).

Adverse Reactions/Side Effects

CNS: dizziness, headache, weakness, drowsiness, mental depression, syncope. **EENT:** blurred vision, intraoperative floppy iris syndrome. **CV:** first-dose orthostatic hypotension, palpitations, angina, edema. **GI:** abdominal cramps, diarrhea, dry mouth, nausea, vomiting. **GU:** erectile dysfunction, priapism.

Interactions

Drug-Drug: Additive hypotension with acute ingestion of **alcohol**, other **antihypertensives**, or **nitrates**. Antihypertensive effects may be ↓ by **NSAIDs**.

Route/Dosage

Hypertension

PO (Adults): 1 mg 2–3 times daily (give first dose at bedtime) for initial 3 days of therapy, then ↑ gradually to maintenance dose of 6–15 mg/day in 2–3 divided doses (not to exceed 20–40 mg/day).
PO (Children): 50–400 mcg (0.05–0.4 mg)/kg/day in 2–3 divided doses (not to exceed 7 mg/dose or 15 mg/day).

Benign Prostatic Hyperplasia

PO (Adults): 1–5 mg twice daily.

Availability (generic available)

Capsules: 1 mg, 2 mg, 5 mg. **Tablets:** ✱ 1 mg, ✱ 2 mg, ✱ 5 mg.

NURSING IMPLICATIONS

Assessment

- Assess for first-dose orthostatic reaction (dizziness, weakness) and syncope. May occur 30 min–2 hr after initial dose and occasionally thereafter. Incidence may be dose related. Volume-depleted or sodium-restricted patients may be more sensitive. Observe patient closely during this period; take precautions to prevent injury. First dose may be given at bedtime to minimize this reaction.
- Monitor intake and output ratios and daily weight; assess for edema daily, especially at beginning of therapy.
- **Hypertension:** Monitor BP and pulse frequently during initial dosage adjustment and periodically throughout therapy. Report significant changes.
- Monitor frequency of prescription refills to determine adherence.
- **Benign Prostatic Hyperplasia:** Assess patient for symptoms of prostatic hyperplasia (urinary hesitancy, feeling of incomplete bladder emptying, interruption of urinary stream, impairment of size and force of urinary stream, terminal urinary dribbling, straining to start flow, dysuria, urgency) before and periodically during therapy.
- Rule out prostatic carcinoma before therapy; symptoms are similar.

Potential Nursing Diagnoses

Risk for injury (Side Effects)
Noncompliance (Patient/Family Teaching)

Implementation

- May be used in combination with diuretics or beta blockers to minimize sodium and water retention. If these are added to prazosin therapy, reduce dose of prazosin initially and titrate to effect.
- **PO:** Administer daily dose at bedtime. If necessary, dose may be increased to twice daily.

Patient/Family Teaching

- Instruct patient to take medication at the same time each day. Take missed doses as soon as remembered. If not remembered until next day, omit; do not double doses.
- Advise patient to weigh self twice weekly and assess feet and ankles for fluid retention.
- May cause dizziness or drowsiness. Advise patient to avoid driving or other activities requiring alertness until response to the medication is known.

- Caution patient to avoid sudden changes in position to decrease orthostatic hypotension. Alcohol, CNS depressants, standing for long periods, hot showers, and exercising in hot weather should be avoided because of enhanced orthostatic effects.
- Advise patient to notify health care professional of all Rx or OTC medications, vitamins, or herbal products being taken and to consult with health care professional before taking other medications, especially NSAIDs and cough, cold, or allergy remedies.
- Instruct patient to notify health care professional of medication regimen before any surgery.
- Advise patient to notify health care professional if immediately if erection last for 4 hrs or longer or if frequent dizziness, fainting, or swelling of feet or lower legs occurs.
- Advise female patient to notify health care professional if pregnancy is planned or suspected or if breast feeding.
- Emphasize the importance of follow-up exams to evaluate effectiveness of medication.
- **Hypertension:** Emphasize the importance of continuing to take this medication as directed, even if feeling well. Medication controls but does not cure hypertension.
- Encourage patient to comply with additional interventions for hypertension (weight reduction, low-sodium diet, smoking cessation, moderation of alcohol consumption, regular exercise, and stress management).
- Instruct patient and family on proper technique for BP monitoring. Advise them to check BP at least weekly and to report significant changes.

Evaluation/Desired Outcomes

- Decrease in BP without appearance of side effects.
- Decrease in symptoms of prostatic hyperplasia.

prednicarbate, See CORTICOSTEROIDS (TOPICAL/LOCAL).

prednisoLONE, See CORTICOSTEROIDS (SYSTEMIC).

predniSONE, See CORTICOSTEROIDS (SYSTEMIC).

pregabalin (pre-gab-a-lin)

Lyrica

Classification

Therapeutic: analgesics, anticonvulsants

Pharmacologic: gamma aminobutyric acid (GABA) analogues, nonopioid analgesics

Schedule V

Pregnancy Category C

Indications

Neuropathic pain associated with diabetic peripheral neuropathy. Postherpetic neuralgia. Fibromyalgia. Neuropathic pain associated with spinal cord injury. Adjunctive therapy of partial-onset seizures in adults.

Action

Binds to calcium channels in CNS tissues which regulate neurotransmitter release. Does not bind to opioid receptors. **Therapeutic Effects:** Decreased neuropathic or post-herpetic pain. Decreased partial-onset seizures.

Pharmacokinetics

Absorption: Well absorbed (90%) following oral administration.

Distribution: Probably crosses the blood-brain barrier.

Metabolism and Excretion: Minimally metabolized, 90% excreted unchanged in urine.

Half-life: 6 hr.

TIME/ACTION PROFILE (↓ post–herpetic pain)

ROUTE	ONSET	PEAK	DURATION
PO	unknown	2–4 wk	unknown

Contraindications/Precautions

Contraindicated in: Myopathy (known/suspected); Lactation: Lactation.

Use Cautiously in: All patients (may ↑ risk of suicidal thoughts/behaviors); Renal impairment (dose alteration recommended for CCr <60 mL/min); HF; History of drug dependence/drug-seeking behavior; OB: Use only if maternal benefit outweighs fetal risk; may ↑ risk of male-mediated teratogenicity; Pedi: Safety not established; Geri: Consider age-related ↓ in renal function when determining dose.

Adverse Reactions/Side Effects

CNS: SUICIDAL THOUGHTS, dizziness, drowsiness, impaired attention/concentration/thinking. **CV:** edema. **EENT:** blurred vision. **GI:** dry mouth, abdominal pain, constipation, ↑ appetite, vomiting. **Hemat:**

thrombocytopenia. **Metab:** weight gain. **Misc:** allergic reactions, fever.

Interactions

Drug-Drug: Concurrent use with **thiazolidinediones (pioglitazone, rosiglitazone)** may ↑ risk of fluid retention. ↑ risk of CNS depression with other **CNS depressants** including **opioids**, **alcohol**, **benzodiazepines**, or other **sedatives/hypnotics**.

Route/Dosage

Diabetic Neuropathic Pain

PO (Adults): 50 mg 3 times daily, ↑ over 7 days up to 100 mg 3 times daily.

Postherpetic Neuralgia

PO (Adults): 75 mg twice daily or 50 mg 3 times daily initially, may be ↑ over 7 days to 300 mg/day in 2–3 divided doses; after 2–4 wk may be ↑ to 600 mg/day in 2–3 divided doses.

Fibromyalgia

PO (Adults): 75 mg twice daily initially, may be ↑ to 150 mg twice daily within 1 wk based on efficacy and tolerability. May be ↑ to 225 twice daily.

Spinal Cord Injury Neuropathic Pain

PO (Adults): 75 mg twice daily initially, may be ↑ to 150 mg twice daily within 1 wk based on efficacy and tolerability; if insufficient pain relief after 2–3 wk, may ↑ to 300 twice daily.

Partial Onset Seizures

PO (Adults): 75 mg twice daily or 50 mg 3 times daily initially; may be gradually ↑ to 600 mg/day.

Renal Impairment

PO (Adults): *CCr 30–60 mL/min*—75–300 mg/day in 2–3 divided doses; *CCr 15–30 mL/min*—25–150 mg/day in 1–2 divided doses; *CCr < 15 mL/min*—25–75 mg/day as a single daily dose.

Availability (generic available)

Capsules: 25 mg, 50 mg, 75 mg, 100 mg, 150 mg, 200 mg, 225 mg, 300 mg. **Cost:** 25 mg $411.71/100, 50 mg $409.80/100, 75 mg $409.80/100, 100 mg $409.80/100, 150 mg $409.80/100, 200 mg $411.71/100, 225 mg $411.71/100. **Oral solution:** 20 mg/mL. **Cost:** $553.82/473 mL.

NURSING IMPLICATIONS

Assessment

- Monitor closely for notable changes in behavior that could indicate the emergence or worsening of suicidal thoughts or behavior or depression.
- **Diabetic Peripheral Neuropathy, Postherpetic Neuralgia, Fibromyalgia, and Spinal Cord Injury Pain:** Assess location, characteristics, and intensity of pain periodically during therapy.
- **Seizures:** Assess location, duration, and characteristics of seizure activity.
- ***Lab Test Considerations:*** May cause ↑ creatine kinase levels.
- May cause ↓ platelet count.

Potential Nursing Diagnoses

Risk for injury (Adverse Reactions)

Implementation

- Do not confuse Lyrica (pregabalin) with Lopressor (metoprolol). Do not confuse Lyrica with Hydrea (hydroxyurea).
- Pregabalin should be discontinued gradually over at least 1 wk. Abrupt discontinuation may cause insomnia, nausea, headache, anxiety, sweating, and diarrhea when used for pain and may cause increase in seizure frequency when treating seizures.
- **PO:** May be administered without regard to meals. Oral solution may be stored at room temperature.

Patient/Family Teaching

- Instruct patient to take medication as directed. If a dose is missed take as soon as remembered unless almost time for next dose; do not double doses. Do not discontinue abruptly; may cause insomnia, nausea, headache, or diarrhea or increase in frequency of seizures. Advise patient to read the *Patient Information Leaflet* prior to taking pregabalin and with each Rx refill in case of changes.
- May cause dizziness, drowsiness, and blurred vision. Caution patient to avoid driving or activities requiring alertness until response to medication is known. Advise patient to notify health care professional if changes in vision occur. Patients with seizures should not resume driving until health care professional gives clearance based on control of seizure disorder.
- Instruct patient to promptly report unexplained muscle pain, tenderness, or weakness, especially if accompanied by malaise or fever. Discontinue therapy if myopathy is diagnosed or suspected or if markedly elevated creatine kinase levels occur.
- Advise patient and family to notify health care professional if thoughts about suicide or dying, attempts to commit suicide; new or worse depression; new or worse anxiety; feeling very agitated or restless; panic attacks; trouble sleeping; new or worse irritability; acting aggressive; being angry or violent; acting on dangerous impulses; an extreme increase in activity and talking, other unusual changes in behavior or mood occur.
- Inform patient that pregabalin may cause edema and weight gain.
- Caution patient to avoid alcohol or other CNS depressants with pregabalin.
- Instruct patient to notify health care professional of medication regimen before treatment or surgery.
- Rep: Advise female patient to notify health care professional if pregnancy is planned or suspected or if

breast feeding. Inform male patients who plan to father a child of the potential risk of male-mediated teratogenicity. Encourage patients who become pregnant to enroll in the NAAED Pregnancy Registry by calling 1–800–233–2334.

- Advise patient to carry identification describing disease process and medication regimen at all times.

Evaluation/Desired Outcomes

- Decrease in intensity of chronic pain.
- Decrease in the frequency or cessation of seizures.

procaine penicillin G, See PENICILLINS.

procarbazine

(proe-**kar**-ba-zeen)

Matulane, ✱Natulan

Classification

Therapeutic: antineoplastics

Pharmacologic: alkylating agents

Pregnancy Category D

Indications

Hodgkin's disease (with other treatment modalities). **Unlabeled Use:** Other lymphomas. Brain and lung tumors. Multiple myeloma. Malignant melanoma. Polycythemia vera.

Action

Appears to inhibit DNA, RNA, and protein synthesis (cell-cycle S-phase–specific). **Therapeutic Effects:** Death of rapidly replicating cells, particularly malignant ones.

Pharmacokinetics

Absorption: Well absorbed following oral administration.

Distribution: Widely distributed; crosses the blood-brain barrier.

Metabolism and Excretion: Metabolized by the liver; <5% excreted unchanged by the kidneys; some respiratory elimination as methane and carbon dioxide.

Half-life: 1 hr.

TIME/ACTION PROFILE (effects on blood counts)

ROUTE	ONSET	PEAK	DURATION
PO	14 days	2–8 wk	28 days or more (up to 6 wk)

Contraindications/Precautions

Contraindicated in: Hypersensitivity; Alcoholism; Severe renal or liver impairment; Pheochromocytoma; HF; OB, Lactation: Pregnancy or lactation.

Use Cautiously in: Infection; ↓ bone marrow reserve; Headache; Psychiatric illness; Liver impairment; Cardiovascular disease; OB: Women with childbearing potential should be advised to avoid pregnancy; Pedi: Very close clinical monitoring required due to potential for toxicity.

Adverse Reactions/Side Effects

CNS: SEIZURES, confusion, dizziness, drowsiness, hallucinations, headache, mania, mental depression, nightmares, psychosis, syncope, tremor. **EENT:** nystagmus, photophobia, retinal hemorrhage. **Resp:** cough, pleural effusions. **CV:** edema, hypotension, tachycardia. **GI:** nausea, vomiting, anorexia, diarrhea, dry mouth, dysphagia, hepatic dysfunction, stomatitis. **GU:** gonadal suppression. **Derm:** alopecia, photosensitivity, pruritus, rashes. **Endo:** gynecomastia. **Hemat:** anemia, leukopenia, thrombocytopenia. **Neuro:** neuropathy, paresthesia. **Misc:** ascites, secondary malignancy.

Interactions

Drug-Drug: Concurrent use with **sympathomimetics** including **methylphenidate** may produce life-threatening hypertension (avoid concurrent use during and for 14 days following procarbazine). Deep coma and death may result from concurrent use of **opioid analgesics**; avoid **meperidine**. Use small incremental doses of other agents and titrate to effect. ↑ bone marrow depression may occur with other **antineoplastics** or **radiation therapy**. Seizures and hyperpyrexia may occur with concurrent use of **MAO inhibitors**, **tricyclic antidepressants**, **SSRI antidepressants** (should not be used within 5 wk of **fluoxetine**), or **carbamazepine**. May ↓ serum **digoxin** levels. Concurrent use with **levodopa** may result in flushing and hypertension. ↑ CNS depression with other **CNS depressants**, including **alcohol**, **antidepressants**, **antihistamines**, **opioid analgesics**, **phenothiazines**, and **sedative/hypnotics**. Disulfiram-like reaction may occur with **alcohol**. **Cigarette smoking** may ↑ the risk of secondary lung cancer.

Drug-Food: Ingestion of foods high in **tyramine** content (see Appendix J) may result in hypertension.

Ingestion of foods high in **caffeine** content may result in arrhythmias.

Route/Dosage

PO (Adults): 2–4 mg/kg/day as a single dose or in divided doses for 1 wk, then 4–6 mg/kg/day until response is obtained; then maintenance dose of 1–2 mg/kg/day. Dosage should be rounded off to the nearest 50 mg.

PO (Children): 50 mg/m^2/day for 7 days, then 100 mg/m^2/day, maintenance dose of 50 mg/m^2/day.

Availability

Capsules: 50 mg.

NURSING IMPLICATIONS

Assessment

- Monitor BP, pulse, and respiratory rate periodically during therapy. Report significant changes to health care professional.
- Assess nutritional status (appetite, intake and output ratios, weight, frequency and amount of emesis). Anorexia and weight loss can be decreased by feeding light, frequent meals. Nausea and vomiting can be minimized by administering an antiemetic at least 1 hr prior to receiving medication. Phenothiazine antiemetics should be avoided.
- Monitor for bone marrow depression. Assess for bleeding (bleeding gums, bruising, petechiae, guaiac stools, urine, and emesis) and avoid IM injections and taking rectal temperatures if platelet count is low. Apply pressure to venipuncture sites for 10 min. Assess for signs of infection during neutropenia. Anemia may occur. Monitor for increased fatigue, dyspnea, and orthostatic hypotension.
- Concurrent ingestion of tyramine-rich foods and many medications may result in life-threatening hypertensive crisis. Signs and symptoms of hypertensive crisis include chest pain, severe headache, nausea and vomiting, photosensitivity, and enlarged pupils. Treatment includes IV phentolamine.
- Procarbazine should be discontinued until side effects clear and then resumed at a lower dose if leukopenia, thrombocytopenia, hypersensitivity reaction, stomatitis (first small ulceration or persistent soreness), diarrhea, hemorrhage, or bleeding tendencies occur.
- ***Lab Test Considerations:*** Monitor hemoglobin, hematocrit, WBC, differential, reticulocytes, and platelet count prior to and every 3–4 days during therapy. Notify physician if WBC $<4000/mm^3$ or platelet count $<100,000/mm^3$. Therapy should be discontinued and resumed at a lower dose when counts improve. The nadir of leukopenia and thrombocytopenia occurs in approximately 2–8 wk, and recovery usually occurs in about 6 wk. Anemia also may occur.
- Assess hepatic and renal function prior to therapy. Monitor urinalysis, AST, ALT, alkaline phosphatase, and BUN at least weekly during therapy.
- Closely monitor serum glucose in diabetic patients. Oral hypoglycemics or insulin dosage may need to be reduced, because hypoglycemic effects are enhanced.
- Bone marrow aspiration studies are recommended prior to initiation of therapy and at time of maximum hematologic response to ensure adequate bone marrow reserve.

Potential Nursing Diagnoses

Risk for infection (Adverse Reactions)
Imbalanced nutrition: less than body requirements (Adverse Reactions)

Implementation

- **PO:** Administer with food or fluids if GI irritation occurs. Confer with pharmacist regarding opening of capsules if patient has difficulty swallowing.

Patient/Family Teaching

- Emphasize the need to take medication as directed. Take missed doses as soon as remembered within a few hours but not if several hours have passed or if almost time for next dose. Health care professional should be consulted if vomiting occurs shortly after a dose is taken.
- Instruct patient to notify health care professional promptly if signs of infection (fever, sore throat, chills, cough, thickened bronchial secretions, hoarseness, pain in lower back or side, difficult or painful urination); bleeding gums; bruising; petechiae; or blood in stool, urine, or emesis occurs. Caution patient to avoid crowds and persons with known infections. Instruct patient to use soft toothbrush and electric razor and to avoid falls. Patient should not receive IM injections or rectal temperatures. Caution patient not to drink alcoholic beverages or take medication containing aspirin or NSAIDs; may precipitate gastric bleeding.
- Caution patient to avoid alcohol, caffeinated beverages, CNS depressants, OTC drugs, and foods or beverages containing tyramine (see Appendix J for foods included) during therapy and for at least 2 wk after therapy has been discontinued, because they may precipitate a hypertensive crisis.
- Advise patient that an additional interaction of alcohol with procarbazine is a disulfiram-like reaction (flushing, nausea, vomiting, headache, abdominal cramps).
- Instruct patient to inspect oral mucosa for erythema and ulceration. If ulceration occurs, advise patient to notify health care professional and to use sponge brush and rinse mouth with water after eating and drinking. Topical agents may be used if mouth pain interferes with eating. Stomatitis pain may require treatment with opioid analgesics.
- May cause drowsiness or dizziness. Caution patient to avoid driving or other activities that require alertness until response to medication is known.

- Advise patient that this medication may have teratogenic effects. Contraception should be practiced during therapy and for at least 4 mo after therapy is concluded.
- Discuss the possibility of hair loss with patient. Explore methods of coping.
- Caution patient to use sunscreen and protective clothing to prevent photosensitivity reactions.
- Instruct patient not to receive any vaccinations without advice of health care professional.
- Advise patient to notify health care professional of medication regimen prior to treatment or surgery. This therapy usually should be withdrawn at least 2 wk prior to surgery.
- Instruct patient to inform health care professional if muscle or joint pain, nausea, vomiting, sweating, tiredness, weakness, constipation, headache, difficulty swallowing, or loss of appetite becomes pronounced.
- Advise patient to carry identification describing medication regimen at all times.
- Emphasize the need for periodic lab tests to monitor for side effects.

Evaluation/Desired Outcomes

- Decrease in size and spread of malignant tissue in Hodgkin's disease.

prochlorperazine

(proe-klor-**pair**-a-zeen)

~~Compazine~~, Compro, ✱Prochlorazine

Classification

Therapeutic: antiemetics, antipsychotics

Pharmacologic: phenothiazines

Pregnancy Category C

Indications

Management of nausea and vomiting. Treatment of psychoses. Treatment of anxiety.

Action

Alters the effects of dopamine in the CNS. Possesses significant anticholinergic and alpha-adrenergic blocking activity. Depresses the chemoreceptor trigger zone (CTZ) in the CNS. **Therapeutic Effects:** Diminished nausea and vomiting. Diminished signs and symptoms of psychoses or anxiety.

Pharmacokinetics

Absorption: Absorption from tablet is variable; may be better with oral liquid formulations. Well absorbed after IM administration.

Distribution: Widely distributed, high concentrations in the CNS. Crosses the placenta and probably enters breast milk.

Protein Binding: ≥90%.

Metabolism and Excretion: Highly metabolized by the liver and GI mucosa. Converted to some compounds with antipsychotic activity.

Half-life: Unknown.

TIME/ACTION PROFILE (antiemetic effect)

ROUTE	ONSET	PEAK	DURATION
PO	30–40 min	unknown	3–4 hr
Rect	60 min	unknown	3–4 hr
IM	10–20 min	10–30 min	3–4 hr
IV	rapid (min)	10–30 min	3–4 hr

Contraindications/Precautions

Contraindicated in: Hypersensitivity; Cross-sensitivity with other phenothiazines may exist; Angle-closure glaucoma; Bone marrow depression; Severe liver or cardiovascular disease; Hypersensitivity to bisulfites or benzyl alcohol (some parenteral products); Pedi: Children <2 yr or <9.1 kg.

Use Cautiously in: Diabetes mellitus; Respiratory disease; Prostatic hypertrophy; CNS tumors; Epilepsy; Intestinal obstruction; OB, Lactation: Safety not established; Geri: Dose ↓ recommended; ↑ risk of mortality in elderly patients treated for dementia-related psychosis.

Adverse Reactions/Side Effects

CNS: NEUROLEPTIC MALIGNANT SYNDROME, <u>extrapyramidal reactions</u>, sedation, tardive dyskinesia. **EENT:** <u>blurred vision</u>, <u>dry eyes</u>, lens opacities. **CV:** ECG changes, hypotension, tachycardia. **GI:** <u>constipation</u>, <u>dry mouth</u>, anorexia, drug-induced hepatitis, ileus. **GU:** pink or reddish-brown discoloration of urine, urinary retention. **Derm:** photosensitivity, pigment changes, rashes. **Endo:** galactorrhea. **Hemat:** AGRANULOCYTOSIS, leukopenia. **Metab:** hyperthermia. **Misc:** allergic reactions.

Interactions

Drug-Drug: Additive hypotension with **antihypertensives**, **nitrates**, or acute ingestion of **alcohol**. Additive CNS depression with other **CNS depressants**, including **alcohol**, **antidepressants**, **antihistamines**, **opioid analgesics**, **sedative/hypnotics**, or **general anesthetics**. Additive anticholinergic effects with other **drugs possessing anticholinergic properties**, including **antihistamines**, some **antidepressants**, **atropine**, **haloperidol**, and other **phenothiazines**. **Lithium** ↑ risk of extrapyramidal reactions. May mask early signs of **lithium** toxicity. ↑ risk of agranulocytosis with **antithyroid agents**. ↓ beneficial effects of **levodopa**. **Antacids** may ↓ absorption.

Drug-Natural Products: Concomitant use of **kava-kava**, **valerian**, **chamomile**, or **hops** can ↑

P

CNS depression. ↑ anticholinergic effects with **angel's trumpet, jimson weed**, and **scopolia**.

Route/Dosage

Pediatric dose should not exceed 10 mg on the 1st day and then should not exceed 20 mg/day in children 2–5 yr or 25 mg/day in children 6–12 yr.

Antiemetic

PO (Adults and Children ≥12 yr): 5–10 mg 3–4 times daily (not to exceed 40 mg/day).
PO (Children 18–39 kg): 2.5 mg 3 times daily *or* 5 mg twice daily (not to exceed 15 mg/day).
PO (Children 14–17 kg): 2.5 mg 2–3 times daily (not to exceed 10 mg/day).
PO (Children 9–13 kg): 2.5 mg 1–2 times daily (not to exceed 7.5 mg/day).
IM (Adults and Children ≥12 yr): 5–10 mg q 3–4 hr as needed. *Nausea/vomiting associated with surgery*—5–10 mg; may be repeated once.
IM (Children 2–12 yr): 132 mcg (0.132 mg)/kg; usually only 1 dose is required.
IV (Adults and Children ≥12 yr): 2.5–10 mg (not to exceed 40 mg/day). *Nausea/vomiting associated with surgery*—5–10 mg; may be repeated once.
Rect (Adults): 25 mg twice daily.
Rect (Children 18–39 kg): 2.5 mg 3 times daily or 5 mg twice daily (not to exceed 15 mg/day).
Rect (Children 14–17 kg): 2.5 mg 2–3 times daily (not to exceed 10 mg/day).
Rect (Children 9–13 kg): 2.5 mg 1–2 times daily (not to exceed 7.5 mg/day).

Antipsychotic

PO (Adults and Children ≥12 yr): 5–10 mg 3–4 times daily; may be ↑ q 2–3 days (up to 150 mg/day).
PO (Children 2–12 yr): 2.5 mg 2–3 times daily.
IM (Adults): 10–20 mg q 2–4 hr for up to 4 doses, then 10–20 mg q 4–6 hr (up to 200 mg/day).
IM (Children 2–12 yr): 132 mcg (0.132 mg)/kg (not to exceed 10 mg/dose).
IV (Adults and Children ≥12 yr): 2.5–10 mg (up to 40 mg/day).
Rect (Adults): 10 mg 3–4 times daily; may be ↑ by 5–10 mg q 2–3 days as needed.

Antianxiety

PO (Adults and Children ≥12 yr): 5 mg 3–4 times daily (not to exceed 20 mg/day or longer than 12 wk).
IM (Adults and Children ≥12 yr): 5–10 mg q 3–4 hr as needed (up to 40 mg/day).
IM (Children 2–12 yr): 132 mcg (0.132 mg)/kg.
IV (Adults): 2.5–10 mg (up to 40 mg/day).

Availability (generic available)

Tablets: 5 mg, 10 mg. **Cost:** *Generic*—5 mg $59.35/100, 10 mg $89.25/100. **Solution for injection:** 5 mg/mL (edisylate), 🍁5 mg/mL (mesylate). **Suppositories:** 🍁10 mg, 25 mg. **Cost:** *Generic*—$160.77/12.

NURSING IMPLICATIONS

Assessment

- Monitor BP (sitting, standing, lying down), ECG, pulse, and respiratory rate before and frequently during the period of dosage adjustment. May cause Q-wave and T-wave changes in ECG.
- Assess patient for level of sedation after administration.
- Monitor patient for onset of akathisia (restlessness or desire to keep moving) and extrapyramidal side effects (*parkinsonian*—difficulty speaking or swallowing, loss of balance control, pill rolling, mask-like face, shuffling gait, rigidity, tremors; and *dystonic*—muscle spasms, twisting motions, twitching, inability to move eyes, weakness of arms or legs) every 2 mo during therapy and 8–12 wk after therapy has been discontinued. Report these symptoms; reduction in dose or discontinuation may be necessary. Trihexyphenidyl or diphenhydramine may be used to control these symptoms.
- Monitor for tardive dyskinesia (uncontrolled rhythmic movement of mouth, face, and extremities; lip smacking or puckering; puffing of cheeks; uncontrolled chewing; rapid or worm-like movements of tongue). Report immediately; may be irreversible.
- Monitor for development of neuroleptic malignant syndrome (fever, respiratory distress, tachycardia, seizures, diaphoresis, hypertension or hypotension, pallor, tiredness, severe muscle stiffness, loss of bladder control). Notify health care professional immediately if these symptoms occur.
- **Antiemetic:** Assess patient for nausea and vomiting before and 30–60 min after administration.
- **Antipsychotic:** Monitor patient's mental status (orientation to reality and behavior) before and periodically during therapy.
- Observe patient carefully when administering oral medication to ensure that medication is actually taken and not hoarded.
- Assess fluid intake and bowel function. Increased bulk and fluids in the diet may help minimize constipation.
- **Anxiety:** Assess degree and manifestations of anxiety and mental status before and periodically during therapy.
- ***Lab Test Considerations:*** CBC and liver function tests should be evaluated periodically during therapy. May cause blood dyscrasias, especially between wk 4 and 10 of therapy. Hepatotoxicity is more likely to occur between wk 2 and 4 of therapy. May recur if medication is restarted. Liver function abnormalities may require discontinuation of therapy.
- May cause false-positive or false-negative pregnancy test results and false-positive urine bilirubin test results.
- May cause ↑ serum prolactin levels.

Potential Nursing Diagnoses

Deficient fluid volume (Indications)
Disturbed thought process (Indications)

Implementation

- To prevent contact dermatitis, avoid getting solution on hands.
- Phenothiazines should be discontinued 48 hr before and not resumed for 24 hr after myelography; they lower seizure threshold.
- **PO:** Administer with food, milk, or a full glass of water to minimize gastric irritation.
- **IM:** Do not inject subcut. Inject slowly, deep into well-developed muscle. Keep patient recumbent for at least 30 min after injection to minimize hypotensive effects. Slight yellow color will not alter potency. Do not administer solution that is markedly discolored or that contains a precipitate.

IV Administration

- **IV Push:** ***Concentration:*** Dilute to a concentration of 1 mg/mL. ***Rate:*** Administer at a rate of 1 mg/min; not to exceed 5 mg/min.
- **Intermittent Infusion:** ***Diluent:*** Dilute 20 mg in up to 1 L dextrose, saline, Ringer's or LR, dextrose/saline, dextrose/Ringer's, or lactated Ringer's combinations.
- **Continuous Infusion:** Has been used as infusion with 20 mg/L of compatible solution.
- **Y-Site Compatibility:** acetaminophen, alemtuzumab, alfentanil, amikacin, amsacrine, anidulafungin, argatroban, ascorbic acid, atracurium, atropine, benztropine, bleomycin, bumetanide, buprenorphine, butorphanol, carboplatin, carmustine, caspofungin, chlorpromazine, cisatracurium, cisplatin, cladribine, cyanocobalamin, cyclophosphamide, cyclosporine, cytarabine, dactinomycin, daptomycin, dexmedetomidine, dexrazoxane, digoxin, diltiazem, diphenhydramine, dobutamine, docetaxel, dolasetron, dopamine, doxacurium, doxorubicin hydrochloride, doxorubicin liposome, doxycycline, enalaprilat, ephedrine, epinephrine, epirubicin, eptifibatide, erythromycin, esmolol, etoposide, famotidine, fentanyl, fluconazole, gentamicin, glycopyrrolate, granisetron, hetastarch, hydrocortisone sodium succinate, hydromorphone, idarubicin, ifosfamide, irinotecan, isoproterenol, labetalol, leucovorin calcium, lidocaine, linezolid, magnesium sulfate, mannitol, mechlorethamine, melphalan, meperidine, methotrexate, methyldopate, methylprednisolone, metoclopramide, metoprolol, metronidazole, milrinone, morphine, moxifloxacin, multivitamins, mycophenolate, nafcillin, nalbuphine, naloxone, nicardipine, nesiritide, nitroglycerin, norepinephrine, octreotide, ondansetron, oxacillin, oxaliplatin, oxytocin, paclitaxel, palonosetron, pamidronate, pancuronium, papaverine, penicillin G, pentazocine, phentolamine, phenylephrine, phytonadione, potassium acetate, potassium chloride, procainamide, promethazine, propofol, propranolol, protamine, pyridoxime, quinupristin/dalfopristin, ranitidine, remifentanil, rituximab, rocuronium, sargramostim, sodium acetate, succinylcholine, sufentanil, tacrolimus, teniposide, theophylline, thiamine, thiotepa, tigecycline, tirofiban, tobramycin, tolazoline, topotecan, trastuzumab, vancomycin, vasopressin, vecuronium, verapamil, vinblastine, vincristine, vinorelbine, vitamin B complex with C, zoledronic acid.
- **Y-Site Incompatibility:** acyclovir, aldesleukin, allopurinol, amifostine, aminophylline, amphotericin B cholesteryl, amphotericin B colloidal, amphotericin B lipid complex, amphotericin B liposome, ampicillin, ampicillin/sulbactam, azathioprine, aztreonam, bivalirudin, calcium chloride, cefazolin, cefepime, cefotaxime, cefotetan, cefoxitin, ceftazidime, ceftriaxone, cefuroxime, chloramphenicol, clindamycin, dantrolene, dexamethasone, diazoxide, epoetin alfa, ertapenem, etoposide phosphate, fenoldopam, filgrastim, fludarabine, fluorouracil, folic acid, foscarnet, furosemide, ganciclovir, gemcitabine, imipenem/cilastatin, indomethacin, insulin, ketorolac, levofloxacin, midazolam, nitroprusside, pantoprazole, pemetrexed, pentamidine, pentobarbital, phenobarbital, phenytoin, piperacillin/tazobactam, sodium bicarbonate, streptokinase, trimethoprim/sulfamethoxazole.

Patient/Family Teaching

- Instruct patient to take medication as directed, not to skip doses or double up on missed doses. Take missed doses as soon as remembered unless almost time for next dose. If more than 2 doses are scheduled each day, missed dose should be taken within about 1 hr of the ordered time. Abrupt withdrawal may lead to gastritis, nausea, vomiting, dizziness, headache, tachycardia, and insomnia.
- Inform patient of possibility of extrapyramidal symptoms and tardive dyskinesia. Instruct patient to report these symptoms immediately to health care professional.
- Advise patient to change positions slowly to minimize orthostatic hypotension.
- May cause drowsiness. Caution patient to avoid driving or other activities requiring alertness until response to medication is known.
- Caution patient to avoid alcohol and CNS depressants. Advise patient to notify health care professional of all Rx or OTC medications, vitamins, or herbal products being taken and to consult with health care professional before taking other medications and alcohol.

P

- Advise patient to use sunscreen and protective clothing when exposed to the sun to prevent photosensitivity reactions. Extremes in temperature should also be avoided, because this drug impairs body temperature regulation.
- Instruct patient to use frequent mouth rinses, good oral hygiene, and sugarless gum or candy to minimize dry mouth. Consult health care professional if dry mouth continues for >2 wk.
- Advise patient not to take prochlorperazine within 2 hr of antacids or antidiarrheal medication.
- Advise patient that increasing bulk and fluids in the diet and exercise may help minimize the constipating effects of this medication.
- Inform patient that this medication may turn urine pink to reddish-brown.
- Advise patient to notify health care professional of medication regimen before treatment or surgery.
- Instruct patient to notify health care professional promptly if sore throat, fever, unusual bleeding or bruising, skin rashes, weakness, tremors, visual disturbances, dark-colored urine, or clay-colored stools are noted.
- Advise female patients to notify health care professional if pregnancy is planned or suspected or if breast feeding.
- Emphasize the importance of routine follow-up exams to monitor response to medication and detect side effects. Periodic ocular exams are indicated. Encourage continued participation in psychotherapy as ordered by health care professional.

Evaluation/Desired Outcomes

- Relief of nausea and vomiting.
- Decrease in excitable, paranoic, or withdrawn behavior when used as an antipsychotic.
- Decrease in feelings of anxiety.

progesterone

(proe-**jess**-te-rone)

Crinone, Endometrin, Prochieve, Prometrium

Classification

Therapeutic: hormones

Pharmacologic: progestins

Pregnancy Category D

Indications

Secondary amenorrhea and abnormal uterine bleeding due to hormonal imbalance. **Prometrium:** Prevention of cell overgrowth in the uterine lining in postmenopausal women who have not had a hysterectomy (with estrogen). Part of assisted reproductive technology (ART) in the management of infertility (4% and 8% vaginal gel). **Endometrin:** Support of embryo implantation and early pregnancy. **Unlabeled Use:** Corpus luteum dysfunction.

Action

Produces: Secretory changes in the endometrium, Increase in basal body temperature, Histologic changes in vaginal epithelium, Relaxation of uterine smooth muscle, Mammary alveolar tissue growth, Pituitary inhibition, Withdrawal bleeding in the presence of estrogen. **Therapeutic Effects:** Restoration of hormonal balance with control of uterine bleeding. Successful outcome in assisted reproduction.

Pharmacokinetics

Absorption: Micronization increases oral and vaginal absorption.

Distribution: Enters breast milk.

Protein Binding: ≥90%.

Metabolism and Excretion: Metabolized by the liver; 50–60% eliminated by kidneys; 10% eliminated in feces.

Half-life: Several minutes.

TIME/ACTION PROFILE (blood levels)

ROUTE	ONSET	PEAK	DURATION
PO	unknown	2–4 hr	unknown
Vaginal	unknown	34.8–55 hr	unknown
IM	unknown	19.6–28 hr	unknown

Contraindications/Precautions

Contraindicated in: Hypersensitivity; Hypersensitivity to parabens or sesame oil (IM suspension only); Hypersensitivity to peanuts (Prometrium only); Thromboembolic disease; Cerebrovascular disease; Severe liver disease; Breast or genital cancer; Porphyria; Missed abortion; OB: Contraindicated except in corpus luteum dysfunction.

Use Cautiously in: History of liver disease; Renal disease; Cardiovascular disease; Seizure disorders; Mental depression.

Adverse Reactions/Side Effects

CNS: depression. **EENT:** retinal thrombosis. **CV:** PULMONARY EMBOLISM, THROMBOEMBOLISM, thrombophlebitis. **GI:** gingival bleeding, hepatitis. **GU:** cervical erosions. **Derm:** chloasma, melasma, rashes. **Endo:** amenorrhea, breakthrough bleeding, breast tenderness, changes in menstrual flow, galactorrhea, spotting. **F and E:** edema. **Local:** irritation or pain at IM injection site. **Misc:** allergic reactions including ANAPHYLAXIS and ANGIOEDEMA, weight gain, weight loss.

Interactions

Drug-Drug: May ↓ effectiveness of **bromocriptine** when used concurrently for galactorrhea and amenorrhea.

Route/Dosage

PO (Adults): *Secondary amenorrhea*—400 mg once daily in the evening for 10 days; *prevention of post-*

menopausal estrogen-induced endometrial hyperplasia—200 mg once daily at bedtime for 14 days on days 8–21 of a 28-day cycle or on days 12–25 of a 30-day cycle; if patient currently receives ≥1.25 mg/day of estrogen, then a daily of dose of 300 mg of progesterone as 100 mg 2 hr after breakfast and 200 mg at bedtime is used; further adjustments may be required.
Vag (Adults): *Secondary amenorrhea*—45 mg (1 applicatorful of 4% gel) once every other day for up to 6 doses, may be ↑ to 90 mg (1 applicatorful of 8% gel) once every other day for up to 6 doses; *Corpus luteum insufficiency or assisted reproduction technology*—For luteal phase support: 90 mg (1 applicatorful of 8% gel) once daily; for *in vitro* fertilization: 90 mg (1 applicatorful of 8% gel) once daily beginning within 24 hr of embryo transfer and continued through day 30 post-transfer (if pregnancy occurs, treatment may be continued for up to 10–12 wk); *partial or complete ovarian failure*—90 mg (1 applicatorful of 8% gel) twice daily while undergoing donor oocyte transfer (if pregnancy occurs, treatment may be continued for up to 10–12 wk) *Support of embryo implantation and early pregnancy*—100 mg insert 2 or 3 times daily for up to 10 wk.
IM (Adults): *Secondary amenorrhea*—100–150 mg (single dose) or 5–10 mg daily for 6–8 days given 8–10 days before expected menstrual period. *Dysfunctional uterine bleeding*—5–10 mg daily for 6 days. *Corpus luteum insufficiency*—12.5 mg/day at onset of ovulation for 2 wk; may continue until 11th wk of gestation (unlabeled).

Availability (generic available)

Micronized capsules (Prometrium): 100 mg, 200 mg. **Bioadhesive vaginal gel (Crinone, Prochieve):** 4%, 8%. **Vaginal tablets (Endometrin):** 100 mg. **Injection:** 50 mg/mL.

NURSING IMPLICATIONS

Assessment

- BP be monitored periodically during therapy.
- Monitor intake and output ratios and weekly weight. Report significant discrepancies or steady weight gain.
- **Amenorrhea:** Assess patient's usual menstrual history. Administration of drug usually begins 8–10 days before anticipated menstruation. Withdrawal bleeding usually occurs 48–72 hr after course of therapy. Therapy should be discontinued if menses occur during injection series.
- **Dysfunctional Bleeding:** Monitor pattern and amount of vaginal bleeding (pad count). Bleeding should end by 6th day of therapy. Therapy should be discontinued if menses occur during injection series.
- ***Lab Test Considerations:*** Monitor hepatic function before and periodically during therapy.
- May cause ↑ plasma amino acid and alkaline phosphatase levels.
- May ↓ pregnanediol excretion concentrations.
- May cause ↑ serum concentrations of LDL and ↓ concentrations of HDL.
- High doses may ↑ sodium and chloride excretion.
- May alter thyroid function test results.

Potential Nursing Diagnoses

Sexual dysfunction (Indications)

Implementation

- **IM:** Shake vial before preparing IM dose. Administer deep IM. Rotate sites.
- **Vag:** Vaginal gel and insert are administered with disposable applicator provided by manufacturer.
- If dose increase is required from 4% gel to 8% gel, doubling the volume of the 4% gel will not accomplish dose increase; changing to 8% gel is required.

P

Patient/Family Teaching

- Advise patient to report signs and symptoms of fluid retention (swelling of ankles and feet, weight gain), thromboembolic disorders (pain, swelling, tenderness in extremities, headache, chest pain, blurred vision), mental depression, or hepatic dysfunction (yellowed skin or eyes, pruritus, dark urine, light-colored stools) to health care professional.
- Instruct patient to notify health care professional if change in vaginal bleeding pattern or spotting occurs.
- Instruct patient to stop taking medication and notify health care professional if pregnancy is suspected.
- Caution patient to use sunscreen and protective clothing to prevent photosensitivity reactions.
- Advise patient to notify health care professional of medication regimen before treatment or surgery.
- Emphasize the importance of routine follow-up physical exams, including BP; breast, abdomen, and pelvic examinations; and Pap smears.
- **Vag:** Instruct patient not to use vaginal gel concurrently with other vaginal agents. If these agents must be used concurrently, administer at least 6 hr before or after vaginal gel. Small, white globules may appear as a vaginal discharge possibly due to gel accumulation, even several days after use.

Evaluation/Desired Outcomes

- Development of normal cyclic menses.
- Successful outcome in assisted reproduction.

HIGH ALERT

promethazine
(proe-**meth**-a-zeen)
✱Histantil, ~~Phenergan~~

Classification
Therapeutic: antiemetics, antihistamines, sedative/hypnotics
Pharmacologic: phenothiazines

Pregnancy Category C

Indications
Treatment of various allergic conditions and motion sickness. Preoperative sedation. Treatment and prevention of nausea and vomiting. Adjunct to anesthesia and analgesia.

Action
Blocks the effects of histamine. Has inhibitory effect on the chemoreceptor trigger zone in the medulla, resulting in antiemetic properties. Alters the effects of dopamine in the CNS. Possesses significant anticholinergic activity. Produces CNS depression by indirectly decreased stimulation of the CNS reticular system. **Therapeutic Effects:** Relief of symptoms of histamine excess usually seen in allergic conditions. Diminished nausea or vomiting. Sedation.

Pharmacokinetics
Absorption: Well absorbed after oral (88%) and IM administration; rectal administration may be less reliable.
Distribution: Widely distributed; crosses the blood-brain barrier and the placenta.
Protein Binding: 65–90%.
Metabolism and Excretion: Metabolized by the liver.
Half-life: 9–16 hr.

TIME/ACTION PROFILE (noted as antihistaminic effects; sedative effects last 2–8 hr)

ROUTE	ONSET	PEAK	DURATION
PO, IM	20 min	unknown	4–12 hr
Rectal	20 min	unknown	4–12 hr
IV	3–5 min	unknown	4–12 hr

Contraindications/Precautions
Contraindicated in: Hypersensitivity; Comatose patients; Prostatic hypertrophy; Bladder neck obstruction; Some products contain alcohol or bisulfites and should be avoided in patients with known intolerance; Angle-closure glaucoma; Pedi: May cause fatal respiratory depression in children <2 yr.
Use Cautiously in: IV administration may cause severe injury to tissue; Hypertension; Cardiovascular disease; Impaired liver function; Prostatic hypertrophy; Glaucoma; Asthma; Sleep apnea; Epilepsy; Underlying bone marrow depression; Pedi: For children >2 yr, use lowest effective dose, avoid concurrent respiratory depressants; OB: Has been used safely during labor; avoid chronic use during pregnancy; Lactation: Safety not established; may cause drowsiness in infant; Geri: Appears on Beers list. Sensitive to anticholinergic effects and have ↑ risk for side effects.

Adverse Reactions/Side Effects
CNS: NEUROLEPTIC MALIGNANT SYNDROME, confusion, disorientation, sedation, dizziness, extrapyramidal reactions, fatigue, insomnia, nervousness. **EENT:** blurred vision, diplopia, tinnitus. **CV:** bradycardia, hypertension, hypotension, tachycardia. **GI:** constipation, drug-induced hepatitis, dry mouth. **Derm:** photosensitivity, severe tissue necrosis upon infiltration at IV site, rashes. **Hemat:** blood dyscrasias.

Interactions
Drug-Drug: Additive CNS depression with other **CNS depressants**, including **alcohol**, other **antihistamines**, **opioid analgesics**, and other **sedative/hypnotics**. Neuroleptic malignant syndrome can occur when used concurrently with **antipsychotics**. Additive anticholinergic effects with other **drugs possessing anticholinergic properties**, including other **antihistamines**, **antidepressants**, **atropine**, **haloperidol**, other **phenothiazines**, **quinidine**, and **disopyramide**. May precipitate seizures when used with **drugs that lower seizure threshold**. Concurrent use with **MAO inhibitors** may result in ↑ sedation and anticholinergic side effects.

Route/Dosage
Antihistamine
PO (Adults): 6.25–12.5 mg 3 times/day and 25 mg at bedtime.
PO (Children ≥2 yr): 0.1 mg/kg/dose (not to exceed 12.5 mg) q 6 hr during the day and 0.5 mg/kg/dose (not to exceed 25 mg) at bedtime.
IM, IV, Rect (Adults): 25 mg; may repeat in 2 hr.
Rect (Children ≥2 yr): 0.125 mg/kg q 4–6 hr *or* 0.5 mg/kg at bedtime.

Antivertigo (Motion Sickness)
PO (Adults): 25 mg 30–60 min before departure; may be repeated in 8–12 hr.
PO, Rect (Children ≥2 yr): 0.5 mg/kg (not to exceed 25 mg) 30–60 min before departure; may be given q 12 hr as needed.

Sedation
PO, Rect, IM, IV (Adults): 25–50 mg; may repeat q 4–6 hr if needed.
PO, Rect, IM (Children >2 yr): 0.5–1 mg/kg (not to exceed 50 mg) q 6 hr as needed.

Sedation during Labor
IM, IV (Adults): 50 mg in early labor; when labor is established, additional doses of 25–75 mg may be

given 1–2 times at 4-hr intervals (should not exceed 100 mg/24 hr).

Antiemetic

PO, Rect, IM, IV (Adults): 12.5–25 mg q 4 hr as needed; initial PO dose should be 25 mg.
PO, Rect, IM, IV (Children ≥2 yr): 0.25–1 mg/kg (not to exceed 25 mg) q 4–6 hr.

Availability (generic available)

Tablets: 12.5 mg, 25 mg, ✱ 25 mg[OTC], 50 mg, ✱ 50 mg[OTC]. **Cost:** *Generic*—12.5 mg $49.00/100, 25 mg $50.64/100, 50 mg $77.62/100. **Syrup (cherry flavor):** 6.25 mg/5 mL, ✱ 10 mg/5 mL[OTC]. **Cost:** *Generic*—$22.19/473 mL. **Injection:** 25 mg/mL, 50 mg/mL. **Suppositories:** 12.5 mg, 25 mg, 50 mg. **Cost:** *Generic*—12.5 mg $212.46/12, 25 mg $212.46/12, 50 mg $231.99/12. ***In combination with:*** codeine, dextromethorphan, and/or phenylephrine in a variety of cough and cold preparations.

NURSING IMPLICATIONS

Assessment

- Monitor BP, pulse, and respiratory rate frequently in patients receiving IV doses.
- Assess level of sedation after administration. Risk of sedation and respiratory depression are increased when administered concurrently with other drugs that cause CNS depression.
- Monitor patient for onset of extrapyramidal side effects (*akathisia*—restlessness; *dystonia*—muscle spasms and twisting motions; *pseudoparkinsonism*—mask-like face, rigidity, tremors, drooling, shuffling gait, dysphagia). Notify health care professional if these symptoms occur.
- Monitor for development of neuroleptic malignant syndrome (fever, respiratory distress, tachycardia, seizures, diaphoresis, hypertension or hypotension, pallor, tiredness, severe muscle stiffness, loss of bladder control). Notify health care professional immediately if these symptoms occur.
- Geri: Assess for adverse anticholinergic effects (delirium, acute confusion, dizziness, dry mouth, blurred vision, urinary retention, constipation, tachycardia).
- **Allergy:** Assess allergy symptoms (rhinitis, conjunctivitis, hives) before and periodically throughout course of therapy.
- **Antiemetic:** Assess patient for nausea and vomiting before and after administration.
- **IV:** ***High Alert:*** If administered IV, assess for burning and pain at IV site; may cause severe tissue injury. Avoid IV administration, if possible. If pain occurs, discontinue administration immediately.
- ***Lab Test Considerations:*** May cause false-positive or false-negative pregnancy test results.
- Evaluate CBC periodically during chronic therapy; blood dyscrasias may occur.
- May cause ↑ serum glucose.
- May cause false-negative results in skin tests using allergen extracts. Promethazine should be discontinued 72 hr before the test.

Potential Nursing Diagnoses

Deficient fluid volume (Indications)
Risk for injury (Side Effects)

Implementation

- When administering promethazine concurrently with opioid analgesics, supervise ambulation closely to prevent injury from increased sedation.
- **PO:** Administer with food, water, or milk to minimize GI irritation. Tablets may be crushed and mixed with food or fluids for patients with difficulty swallowing.
- **IM:** Administer deep into well-developed muscle. Subcut or inadvertent intra-arterial administration may cause severe tissue necrosis.

IV Administration

- **IV Push:** ***Diluent:*** Dilute with 0.9% NaCl or D5W. ***Concentration:*** Doses should not exceed a concentration of 25 mg/mL. Administer through a large-bore vein through a running IV line into the most distal port. Slight yellow color does not alter potency. Do not use if precipitate is present. ***Rate:*** Administer each 25 mg slowly, over at least 10–15 min (maximum rate = 25 mg/min). Rapid administration may produce a transient fall in BP.
- **Y-Site Compatibility:** alemtuzumab, alfentanil, amifostine, amikacin, amsacrine, anidulafungin, ascorbic acid, atropine, benztropine, bivalirudin, bumetanide, buprenorphine, butorphanol, calcium chloride, calcium gluconate, carboplatin, caspofungin, ceftaroline, ciprofloxacin, cisatracurium, cisplatin, cladribine, cyanocobalamin, cyclophosphamide, cyclosporine, cytarabine, dactinomycin, daptomycin, dexmedetomidine, digoxin, diltiazem, diphenhydramine, dobutamine, docetaxel, dopamine, doxorubicin, doxycycline, enalaprilat, ephedrine, epinephrine, epirubicin, epoetin alfa, eptifibatide, erythromycin, esmolol, etoposide, etoposide phosphate, famotidine, fenoldopam, fentanyl, filgrastim, fluconazole, fludarabine, gemcitabine, gentamicin, glycopyrrolate, granisetron, hydromorphone, ifosfamide, insulin, irinotecan, isoproterenol, ketamine, labetalol, levofloxacin, lidocaine, linezolid, lorazepam, magnesium sulfate, mannitol, mechlorethamine, melphalan, meperidine, methyldopate, metoclopramide, metoprolol, metronidazole, midazolam, milrinone, mitoxantrone, morphine, mycophenolate, nalbuphine, naloxone, nitroglycerin, norepi-

P

nephrine, octreotide, ondansetron, oxaliplatin, oxytocin, paclitaxel, palonosetron, pamidronate, pancuronium, pemetrexed, pentamidine, pentazocine, phentolamine, phenylephrine, procainamide, prochlorperazine, propranolol, protamine, pyridoxime, quinupristin/dalfopristin, ranitidine, remifentanil, rituximab, rocuronium, sargramostim, sodium acetate, succinylcholine, sufentanil, tacrolimus, teniposide, theophylline, thiamine, thiotepa, tigecycline, tirofiban, tobramycin, tolazoline, trastuzumab, trimetaphan, vancomycin, vasopressin, vecuronium, verapamil, vincristine, vinorelbine, voriconazole, zoledronic acid.

- **Y-Site Incompatibility:** acyclovir, aldesleukin, allopurinol, aminophylline, amphotericin B cholesteryl, amphotericin B colloidal, amphotericin B lipid complex, amphotericin B liposome, ampicillin, ampicillin/sulbactam, azathioprine, cefazolin, cefepime, cefotaxime, cefotetan, cefoxitin, ceftazidime, ceftriaxone, cefuroxime, chloramphenicol, clindamycin, dantrolene, dexamethasone, diazepam, diazoxide, doxorubicin liposome, ertapenem, fluorouracil, folic acid, foscarnet, furosemide, ganciclovir, heparin, indomethacin, ketorolac, methylprednisolone, nafcillin, nitroprusside, oxacillin, pantoprazole, penicillin G, pentobarbital, phenobarbital, phenytoin, piperacillin/tazobactam, sodium bicarbonate, streptokinase, trimethoprim/sulfamethoxazole.

Patient/Family Teaching

- Review dose schedule with patient. If medication is ordered regularly and a dose is missed, take as soon as remembered unless time for next dose. Pedi: Caution caregivers to use only the measuring device accompanying the liquid medication and not to use household measuring devices.
- May cause drowsiness. Caution patient to avoid driving or other activities requiring alertness until response to medication is known.
- Advise patient that frequent mouth rinses, good oral hygiene, and sugarless gum or candy may decrease dry mouth. Health care professional should be notified if dry mouth persists >2 wk.
- Caution patient to use sunscreen and protective clothing to prevent photosensitivity reactions.
- Advise patient to change positions slowly to minimize orthostatic hypotension. Geri: Geriatric patients are at increased risk.
- Caution patient to avoid concurrent use of alcohol and other CNS depressants with this medication.
- Instruct patient to notify health care professional if sore throat, fever, jaundice, or uncontrolled movements are noted.
- **Motion Sickness:** When used as prophylaxis for motion sickness, advise patient to take medication at least 30 min and preferably 1–2 hr before exposure to conditions that may cause motion sickness.

Evaluation/Desired Outcomes

- Relief from allergic symptoms.
- Prevention of motion sickness.
- Sedation.
- Relief from nausea and vomiting.

HIGH ALERT

propofol (proe-poe-fol)

Diprivan

Classification
Therapeutic: general anesthetics

Pregnancy Category B

Indications

Induction of general anesthesia in children >3 yr and adults. Maintenance of balanced anesthesia when used with other agents in children >2 mo and adults. Initiation and maintenance of monitored anesthesia care (MAC). Sedation of intubated, mechanically ventilated patients in intensive care units (ICUs).

Action

Short-acting hypnotic. Mechanism of action is unknown. Produces amnesia. Has no analgesic properties. **Therapeutic Effects:** Induction and maintenance of anesthesia.

Pharmacokinetics

Absorption: Administered IV only, resulting in complete absorption.
Distribution: Rapidly and widely distributed. Crosses the blood-brain barrier well; rapidly redistributed to other tissues. Crosses the placenta and enters breast milk.
Protein Binding: 95–99%.
Metabolism and Excretion: Rapidly metabolized by the liver.
Half-life: 3–12 hr (blood-brain equilibration half-life 2.9 min).

TIME/ACTION PROFILE (loss of consciousness)

ROUTE	ONSET	PEAK	DURATION†
IV	40 sec	unknown	3–5 min

†Time to recovery is 8 min (up to 19 min if opioid analgesics have been used).

Contraindications/Precautions

Contraindicated in: Hypersensitivity to propofol, soybean oil, egg lecithin, or glycerol; OB: Crosses placenta; may cause neonatal depression; Lactation: Enters breast milk; effects on newborn unknown.
Use Cautiously in: Cardiovascular disease; Lipid disorders (emulsion may have detrimental effect); ↑ intracranial pressure; Cerebrovascular disorders; Hypovolemic patients (lower induction and maintenance

dosage reduction recommended); Pedi: Not recommended for induction of anesthesia in children <3 yr, or for maintenance of anesthesia in infants <2 mo; not for ICU or pre-procedure sedation; Geri: Lower induction and maintenance dose reduction recommended.

Adverse Reactions/Side Effects

CNS: dizziness, headache. **Resp:** APNEA, cough. **CV:** bradycardia, hypotension, hypertension. **GI:** abdominal cramping, hiccups, nausea, vomiting. **Derm:** flushing. **Local:** burning, pain, stinging, coldness, numbness, tingling at IV site. **MS:** involuntary muscle movements, perioperative myoclonia. **GU:** discoloration of urine (green). **Misc:** PROPOFOL INFUSION SYNDROME, fever.

Interactions

Drug-Drug: Additive CNS and respiratory depression with **alcohol**, **antihistamines**, **opioid analgesics**, and **sedative/hypnotics** (dose ↓ may be required). **Theophylline** may antagonize the CNS effects of propofol. Propofol may ↑ levels of **alfentanil**. Cardiorespiratory instability can occur when used with **acetazolamide**. Serious bradycardia can occur with concurrent use of **fentanyl** in children. ↑ risk of hypertriglyceridemia with **intravenous fat emulsion**.

Route/Dosage

General Anesthesia

IV (Adults <55 yr): *Induction*—40 mg q 10 sec until induction achieved (2–2.5 mg/kg total). *Maintenance*—100–200 mcg/kg/min. Rates of 150–200 mcg/kg/min are usually required during first 10–15 min after induction, then ↓ by 30–50% during first 30 min of maintenance. Rates of 50–100 mcg/kg/min are associated with optimal recovery time. May also be given intermittently in increments of 25–50 mg.

IV (Geriatric Patients , Cardiac patients, Debilitated Patients, or Hypovolemic Patients): *Induction*—20 mg q 10 sec until induction achieved (1–1.5 mg/kg total). *Maintenance*—50–100 mcg/kg/min (dose in cardiac anesthesia ranges from 50–150 mcg/kg/min depending on concurrent use of opioid).

IV (Adults Undergoing Neurosurgical Procedures): *Induction*—20 mg q 10 sec until induction achieved (1–2 mg/kg total). *Maintenance*—100–200 mcg/kg/min.

IV (Children ≥3 yr–16 yr): *Induction*—2.5–3.5 mg/kg, use lower dose for children ASA III or IV.

IV (Children 2 mo–16 yr): *Maintenance*—125–300 mcg/kg/min (following first 30 min of maintenance, rate should be ↓ if possible), younger children may require larger infusion rates compared to older children.

Monitored Anesthesia Care (MAC) Sedation

IV (Adults <55 yr): *Initiation*—100–150 mcg/kg/min infusion *or* 0.5 mg/kg as slow injection. *Maintenance*—25–75 mcg/kg/min infusion or incremental boluses of 10–20 mg.

IV (Geriatric Patients, Debilitated Patients, or ASA III/IV Patients): *Initiation*—Use slower infusion or injection rates. *Maintenance*—20% less than the usual adult infusion dose; rapid/repeated bolus dosing should be avoided.

ICU Sedation

IV (Adults): 5 mcg/kg/min for a minimum of 5 min. Additional increments of 5–10 mcg/kg/min over 5–10 min may be given until desired response is obtained. (Range 5–50 mcg/kg/min.) Dose should be reassessed every 24 hr.

Availability (generic available)

Injection: 10 mg/mL.

NURSING IMPLICATIONS

Assessment

- Assess respiratory status, pulse, and BP continuously throughout propofol therapy. Frequently causes apnea lasting ≥60 sec. Maintain patent airway and adequate ventilation. Propofol should be used only by individuals experienced in endotracheal intubation, and equipment for this procedure should be readily available.
- Assess level of sedation and level of consciousness throughout and following administration.
- When using for ICU sedation, wake-up and assessment of CNS function should be done daily during maintenance to determine minimum dose required for sedation. Maintain a light level of sedation during these assessments; do not discontinue. Abrupt discontinuation may cause rapid awakening with anxiety, agitation, and resistance to mechanical ventilation.
- Monitor for propofol infusion syndrome (severe metabolic acidosis, hyperkalemia, lipemia, rhabdomyolysis, hepatomegaly, cardiac and renal failure). Most frequent with prolonged, high-dose infusions (>5 mg/kg/hr for >48 hr) but has also been reported following large-dose, short-term infusions during surgical anesthesia. If prolonged sedation or increasing dose is required, or metabolic acidosis occurs, consider alternative means of sedation.
- ***Toxicity and Overdose:*** If overdose occurs, monitor pulse, respiration, and BP continuously. Maintain patent airway and assist ventilation as needed. If hypotension occurs, treatment includes IV fluids, repositioning, and vasopressors.

Potential Nursing Diagnoses

Ineffective breathing pattern (Adverse Reactions)
Risk for injury (Side Effects)

Implementation

- Do not confuse Diprivan (propofol) with Diflucan (fluconazole) or Ditropan (oxybutynin).
- Dose is titrated to patient response.
- Propofol has no effect on the pain threshold. Adequate analgesia should *always* be used when propofol is used as an adjunct to surgical procedures.

IV Administration

- **IV Push:** ***Diluent:*** Usually administered undiluted. If dilution is necessary, use only D5W. Shake well before use. Solution is opaque, making detection of contaminants difficult. Do not use if separation of the emulsion is evident. Contains no preservatives; maintain sterile technique and administer immediately after preparation. ***Concentration:*** Undiluted: 10 mg/mL. If dilution is necessary, dilute to concentration ≥2 mg/mL.
- Discard unused portions and IV lines at the end of anesthetic procedure or within 6 hr. For ICU sedation, discard after 12 hr if administered directly from vial or after 6 hr if transferred to a syringe or other container. Do not administer via filter <5–micron pore size.
- Aseptic technique is essential. Solution is capable of rapid growth of bacterial contaminants. Infections and subsequent deaths have been reported. ***Rate:*** Administer over 3–5 min. Titrate to desired level of sedation. Frequently causes pain, burning, and stinging at injection site; use larger veins of the forearm, antecubital fossa, or a dedicated IV catheter. Lidocaine 10–20 mg IV may be administered prior to injection to minimize pain. Pedi: Induction doses may be administered over 20–30 seconds.
- **Intermittent/Continuous Infusion:** ***Diluent:*** Administer undiluted. Allow 3 to 5 min between dose adjustments to allow for and assess the clinical effects. ***Concentration:*** 10 mg/mL. ***Rate:*** Based on patient's weight (see Route/Dosage section).
- **Solution Compatibility:** D5W, LR, D5/LR, D5/0.45% NaCl, D5/0.2% NaCl.
- **Y-Site Compatibility:** acyclovir, alfentanil, aminophylline, ampicillin, aztreonam, bumetanide, buprenorphine, butorphanol, calcium gluconate, carboplatin, cefazolin, cefepime, cefotaxime, cefoxitin, ceftriaxone, cefuroxime, chlorpromazine, cisplatin, clindamycin, cyclophosphamide, cyclosporine, cytarabine, dexamethasone, dexmedetomidine, diphenhydramine, dobutamine, dopamine, doxycycline, droperidol, enalaprilat, epinephrine, esmolol, famotidine, fenoldopam, fentanyl, fluconazole, fluorouracil, furosemide, ganciclovir, glycopyrrolate, granisetron, haloperidol, heparin, hydrocortisone sodium succinate, hydromorphone, ifosfamide, imipenem/cilastatin, insulin, isoproterenol, ketamine, labetalol, levorphanol, lidocaine, lorazepam, magnesium sulfate, mannitol, meperidine, milrinone, nafcillin, nalbuphine, naloxone, nitroglycerin, nitroprusside, norepinephrine, paclitaxel, pentobarbital, phenobarbital, potassium chloride, prochlorperazine, propranolol, ranitidine, scopolamine, sodium bicarbonate, succinylcholine, sufentanil, thiopental, vecuronium.
- **Y-Site Incompatibility:** amikacin, amphotericin B colloidal, calcium chloride, ciprofloxacin, diazepam, digoxin, doripenem, doxorubicin, gentamicin, levofloxacin, methotrexate, methylpredisolone sodium succinate, metoclopramide, mitoxantrone, phenytoin, tobramycin, verapamil.

Patient/Family Teaching

- Inform patient that this medication will decrease mental recall of the procedure.
- May cause drowsiness or dizziness. Advise patient to request assistance prior to ambulation and transfer and to avoid driving or other activities requiring alertness for 24 hr following administration.
- Advise patient to avoid alcohol or other CNS depressants without the advice of a health care professional for 24 hr following administration.

Evaluation/Desired Outcomes

- Induction and maintenance of anesthesia.
- Amnesia.
- Sedation in mechanically ventilated patients in an intensive care setting.

HIGH ALERT

propranolol

(proe-**pran**-oh-lole)
Hemangeol, Inderal, Inderal LA, InnoPran XL

Classification
Therapeutic: antianginals, antiarrhythmics (Class II), antihypertensives, vascular headache suppressants
Pharmacologic: beta blockers

Pregnancy Category C

Indications

Management of hypertension, angina, arrhythmias, hypertrophic cardiomyopathy, thyrotoxicosis, essential tremors, pheochromocytoma (all but Hemangeol). Also used in the prevention and management of MI, and the prevention of vascular headaches (all but Hemangeol). Proliferating infantile hemangioma requiring systemic therapy (Hemangeol only). **Unlabeled Use:** Also used to manage alcohol withdrawal, aggressive behavior, antipsychotic-associated akathisia, situational anxiety, and esophageal varices. Post-traumatic stress disorder (PTSD) (ongoing clinical trials at National Institute for Mental Health [NIMH]).

Action

Blocks stimulation of $beta_1$ (myocardial) and $beta_2$ (pulmonary, vascular, and uterine)-adrenergic receptor sites; it's mechanism for the treatment of infantile hemangiomas is unknown. **Therapeutic Effects:** Decreased heart rate and BP. Suppression of arrhythmias. Prevention of MI. Hemangioma resolution.

Pharmacokinetics

Absorption: Well absorbed but undergoes extensive first-pass hepatic metabolism.
Distribution: Moderate CNS penetration. Crosses the placenta; enters breast milk.
Protein Binding: 93%.
Metabolism and Excretion: Almost completely metabolized by the liver (primarily for CYP2D6 isoenzyme) ⧖ (the CYP2D6 enzyme system exhibits genetic polymorphism; ~7% of population may be poor metabolizers and may have significantly ↑ propranolol concentrations and an ↑ risk of adverse effects).
Half-life: 3.4–6 hr.

TIME/ACTION PROFILE (cardiovascular effects)

ROUTE	ONSET	PEAK	DURATION
PO	30 min	60–90 min†	6–12 hr
PO–ER	unknown	6 hr	24 hr
IV	immediate	1 min	4–6 hr

†Following single dose, full effect not seen until several weeks of therapy.

Contraindications/Precautions

Contraindicated in: Hypersensitivity; Uncompensated HF; Pulmonary edema; Cardiogenic shock; Bradycardia, sick sinus syndrome, or heart block (unless pacemaker present); Premature infants with corrected age <5 wk (Hemangeol only); Infants <2 kg (Hemangeol only); Asthma or history of bronchospasm (Hemangeol only); BP <50/30 mmHg (Hemageol only); Pheochromocytoma (Hemangeol only).
Use Cautiously in: Renal or hepatic impairment; Pulmonary disease (including asthma); Diabetes mellitus (may mask signs of hypoglycemia); Thyrotoxicosis (may mask symptoms); History of severe allergic reactions (may ↑ intensity of response); Skeletal muscle disease (may exacerbate myopathy); OB: Crosses the placenta and may cause fetal/neonatal bradycardia, hypotension, hypoglycemia, or respiratory depression. May also ↓ blood supply to the placenta, ↑ the risk for premature birth or fetal death, and cause intrauterine growth retardation. May ↑ risk of cardiac and pulmonary complications in the infant during the neonatal time frame. Lactation: Appears in breast milk; use formula if propranolol must be taken; Pedi: ↑ risk of hypoglycemia, especially during periods of fasting such as before surgery, during prolonged exertion, or with coexisting renal insufficiency; Geri: ↑ sensitivity to all beta blockers; initial dose reduction and careful titration recommended.

Adverse Reactions/Side Effects

CNS: fatigue, weakness, anxiety, dizziness, drowsiness, insomnia, memory loss, mental depression, mental status changes, nervousness, nightmares. **EENT:** blurred vision, dry eyes, nasal stuffiness. **Resp:** bronchospasm, wheezing. **CV:** ARRHYTHMIAS, BRADYCARDIA, HF, PULMONARY EDEMA, orthostatic hypotension, peripheral vasoconstriction. **GI:** constipation, diarrhea, nausea. **GU:** erectile dysfunction, ↓ libido. **Derm:** ERYTHEMA MULTIFORME, EXFOLIATIVE DERMATITIS, STEVENS-JOHNSON SYNDROME, TOXIC EPIDERMAL NECROLYSIS, itching, rash. **Endo:** hyperglycemia, hypoglycemia (↑ in children). **MS:** arthralgia, back pain, muscle cramps, myopathy. **Neuro:** paresthesia. **Misc:** ANAPHYLAXIS, drug-induced lupus syndrome.

Interactions

Drug-Drug: General anesthesia, **IV phenytoin**, and **verapamil** may cause additive myocardial depression. Additive bradycardia may occur with **digoxin**. Additive hypotension may occur with other **antihypertensives**, acute ingestion of **alcohol**, or **nitrates**. Levels may be ↓ with chronic **alcohol** use. Concurrent use with **amphetamines**, **cocaine**, **ephedrine**, **epinephrine**, **norepinephrine**, **phenylephrine**, or **pseudoephedrine** may result in unopposed alpha-adrenergic stimulation (excessive hypertension, bradycardia). Concurrent **thyroid** administration may ↓ effectiveness. May alter the effectiveness of **insulin** or **oral hypoglycemics** (dose adjustments may be necessary). May ↓ effectiveness of **beta-adrenergic bronchodilators** and **theophylline**. May ↓ beneficial beta cardiovascular effects of **dopamine** or **dobutamine**. Use cautiously within 14 days of **MAO inhibitor** therapy (may result in hypertension). **Cimetidine** may ↑ blood levels and toxicity. Concurrent **NSAIDs** may ↓ antihypertensive action. **Smoking** ↑ metabolism and ↓ effects; smoking cessation may ↑ effects. May ↑ levels of **lidocaine** and **bupivacaine**.

Route/Dosage

PO (Adults): *Antianginal*—80–320 mg/day in 2–4 divided doses or once daily as extended/sustained-release capsules. *Antihypertensive*—40 mg twice daily initially; may be ↑ as needed (usual range 120–240 mg/day; doses up to 1 g/day have been used); *or* 80 mg once daily as extended/sustained-release capsules, ↑ as needed up to 120 mg. *InnoPran XL* dosing form is designed to be given once daily at bedtime. *Antiarrhythmic*—10–30 mg 3–4 times daily. *Prevention of MI*—180–240 mg/day in divided doses. *Hypertrophic*

P

cardiomyopathy—20–40 mg 3–4 times daily. *Adjunct therapy of pheochromocytoma*—20 mg 3 times daily to 40 mg 3–4 times daily concurrently with alpha-blocking therapy, started 3 days before surgery is planned. *Vascular headache prevention*—20 mg 4 times daily *or* 80 mg/day as extended/sustained-release capsules; may be ↑ as needed up to 240 mg/day. *Management of tremor*—40 mg twice daily; may be ↑ up to 120 mg/day (up to 320 mg have been used).
PO (Children): *Antihypertensive/antiarrhythmic*—0.5–1 mg/kg/day in 2–4 divided doses; may be ↑ as needed (usual range for maintenance dose is 2–4 mg/kg/day in 2 divided doses).
PO (Children 5 wk–5 mo): *Infantile hemangioma*—0.6 mg/kg twice daily (at least 9 hr apart); after 1 wk, ↑ to 1.1 mg/kg twice daily; after another wk, ↑ to 1.7 mg/kg twice daily and maintain for 6 mo.
IV (Adults): *Antiarrhythmic*—1–3 mg; may be repeated after 2 min and again in 4 hr if needed.
IV (Children): *Antiarrhythmic*—10–100 mcg (0.01–0.1 mg)/kg (up to 1 mg/dose); may be repeated q 6–8 hr if needed.

Availability (generic available)

Oral solution: 4 mg/mL, 8 mg/mL. **Oral solution (Hemangeol):** 4.28 mg/mL. **Tablets:** 10 mg, 20 mg, 40 mg, 60 mg, 80 mg. **Extended-release capsules:** 60 mg, 80 mg, 120 mg, 160 mg. **Injection:** 1 mg/mL. ***In combination with:*** hydrochlorothiazide (Inderide). See Appendix B.

NURSING IMPLICATIONS

Assessment

- Monitor BP and pulse frequently during dose adjustment period and periodically during therapy.
- Abrupt withdrawal of propranolol may precipitate life-threatening arrhythmias, hypertension, or myocardial ischemia. Drug should be tapered over a 2-wk period before discontinuation. Assess patient carefully during tapering and after medication is discontinued. Consider that patients taking propranolol for non-cardiac indications may have undiagnosed cardiac disease. Abrupt discontinuation or withdrawal over too-short a period of time (less than 9 days) should be avoided.
- Pedi: Assess pediatric patients for signs and symptoms of hypoglycemia, particularly when oral foods and fluids are restricted.
- Patients receiving **propranolol IV** must have continuous ECG monitoring and may have pulmonary capillary wedge pressure (PCWP) or central venous pressure (CVP) monitoring during and for several hours after administration.
- Assess for orthostatic hypotension when assisting patient up from supine position.
- Monitor intake and output ratios and daily weight. Assess patient routinely for evidence of fluid overload (peripheral edema, dyspnea, rales/crackles, fatigue, weight gain, jugular venous distention).
- Assess for rash periodically during therapy. May cause Stevens-Johnson syndrome. Discontinue therapy if severe or if accompanied with fever, general malaise, fatigue, muscle or joint aches, blisters, oral lesions, conjunctivitis, hepatitis and/or eosinophilia.
- **Angina:** Assess frequency and characteristics of anginal attacks periodically during therapy.
- **Vascular Headache Prophylaxis:** Assess frequency, severity, characteristics, and location of vascular headaches periodically during therapy.
- **PTSD:** Assess frequency of symptoms (flashbacks, nightmares, efforts to avoid thoughts or activities that may trigger memories of the trauma, and hypervigilance) periodically throughout therapy.
- **Infantile Hemangioma:** Monitor heart rate and BP for 2 hrs after propranolol initiation or dose increases. May worsen bradycardia or hypotension. Discontinue if severe (<80 beats per minute) or symptomatic bradycardia or hypotension (systolic BP <50 mmHg) occurs.
- ***Lab Test Considerations:*** May cause ↑ BUN, serum lipoprotein, potassium, triglyceride, and uric acid levels.
- May cause ↑ ANA titers.
- May cause ↓ or ↑ in blood glucose levels. In labile diabetic patients, hypoglycemia may be accompanied by precipitous ↑ of BP.
- ***Toxicity and Overdose:*** Monitor patients receiving beta blockers for signs of overdose (bradycardia, severe dizziness or fainting, severe drowsiness, dyspnea, bluish fingernails or palms, seizures). Notify health care professional immediately if these signs occur.
- Hypotension may be treated with modified Trendelenburg position and IV fluids unless contraindicated. Vasopressors (epinephrine, norepinephrine, dopamine, dobutamine) may also be used. Hypotension does not respond to beta agonists.
- Glucagon has been used to treat bradycardia and hypotension.

Potential Nursing Diagnoses

Decreased cardiac output (Side Effects)
Noncompliance (Patient/Family Teaching)

Implementation

- ***High Alert:*** IV vasoactive medications are inherently dangerous. Before administering intravenously, have second practitioner independently check the original order, dose calculations, and infusion pump settings. Also, patient harm or fatalities have occurred when switching from oral to IV *propranolol*; oral and parenteral doses are not interchangeable. IV dose is 1/10 of the oral dose. Change to oral therapy as soon as possible.
- ***High Alert:*** Do not confuse propranolol with Pravachol. Do not confuse Inderal (propranolol) with Adderall (an amphetamine/dextroamphetamine combination drug).

- **PO:** Take apical pulse prior to administering. If <50 bpm or if arrhythmia occurs, withhold medication and notify physician or other health care professional.
- Administer with meals or directly after eating to enhance absorption.
- Swallow extended release tablets whole; do not crush, break, or chew. *Propranolol tablets* may be crushed and mixed with food.
- Mix propranolol oral solution with liquid or semi-solid food (water, juices, applesauce, puddings). To ensure entire dose is taken, rinse glass with more liquid or have patient consume all of the applesauce or pudding. Do not store after mixing.
- Administer *Hemangeol* during or right after a feeding to prevent hypoglycemia. Skip dose is child is not eating or vomiting. Administer using oral syringe provided; if necessary may be diluted in small amount of milk or fruit juice and given in baby's bottle.

IV Administration

- **IV Push:** ***Diluent:*** Administer undiluted or dilute each 1 mg in 10 mL of D5W for injection. ***Concentration:*** Undiluted: 1 mg/mL. Diluted in 10 mL of D5W: 0.1 mg/mL. ***Rate:*** Administer at 0.5 mg/ min for adults to avoid hypotension and cardiac arrest; do not exceed 1 mg/min. Pedi: Administer over 10 min.
- **Intermittent Infusion:** ***Diluent:*** May be diluted in 50 mL of 0.9% NaCl, D5W, D5/0.45% NaCl, D5/0.9% NaCl, or lactated Ringer's injection. ***Concentration:*** Depends on dose. ***Rate:*** Infuse over 10–15 min.
- **Y-Site Compatibility:** acyclovir, alemtuzumab, alfentanil, alteplase, amikacin, aminocaproic acid, aminophylline, amiodarone, anidulafungin, argatroban, ascorbic acid, atropine, azathioprine, aztreonam, benztropine, bivalirudin, bleomycin, bumetanide, buprenorphine, butorphanol, calcium chloride, calcium gluconate, carboplatin, carmustine, caspofungin, cefazolin, cefotetan, ceftazidime, ceftriaxone, cefuroxime, chloramphenicol, chlorpromazine, cisplatin, clindamycin, cyanocobalamin, cyclophosphamide, cyclosporine, cytarabine, dactinomycin, daptomycin, daptomycin, daunorubicin, dexamethasone, dexmedetomidine, dexrazoxane, digoxin, diltiazem, diphenhydramine, dobutamine, docetaxel, dolasetron, dopamine, doxorubicin, doxorubicin liposomal, doxycycline, enalaprilat, ephedrine, epinephrine, epirubicin, epoetin alfa, eptifibatide, ertapenem, erythromycin, esmolol, etoposide, etoposide phosphate, famotidine, fenoldopam, fentanyl, fluconazole, fludarabine, fluorouracil, folic acid, foscarnet, fosphenytoin, furosemide, ganciclovir, gemcitabine, gentamicin, glycopyrrolate, granisetron, heparin, hydrocortisone, hydromorphone, idarubicin, ifosfamide, imipenem/cilastatin, isoproterenol, ketorolac, labetalol, leucovorin, levofloxacin, lidocaine, linezolid, lorazepam, magnesium sulfate, mannitol, mechlorethamine, meperidine, mesna, methotrexate, methylprednisolone, metoclopramide, metoprolol, metronidazole, midazolam, milrinone, mitoxantrone, morphine, moxifloxacin, multivitamins, mycophenolate, nafcillin, nalbuphine, naloxone, nesiritide, nicardipine, nitroglycerin, nitroprusside, norepinephrine, octreotide, ondansetron, oxacillin, oxaliplatin, oxytocin, palonosetron, pamidronate, pancuronium, papaverine, pemetrexed, penicillin G, pentamidine, pentazocine, pentobarbital, phenobarbital, phenylephrine, phytonadione, potassium acetate, potassium chloride, procainamide, prochlorperazine, promazine, promethazine, propofol, protamine, pyridoxine, quinupristin/dalfopristin, ranitidine, rocuronium, sodium acetate, sodium bicarbonate, streptokinase, succinylcholine, sufentanil, tacrolimus, teniposide, theophylline, thiamine, thiotepa, tigecycline, tirofiban, tobramycin, topotecan, vancomycin, vasopressin, vecuronium, verapamil, vinblastine, vincristine, vinorelbine, vitamin B complex with C, voriconazole, zoledronic acid.
- **Y-Site Incompatibility:** amphotericin B colloidal, amphotericin B lipid complex, amphotericin B liposome, dantrolene, diazepam, diazoxide, indomethacin, insulin, mitomycin, paclitaxel, pantoprazole, phenytoin, piperacillin/tazobactam, trimethoprim/sulfamethoxazole.

Patient/Family Teaching

- Instruct patient to take medication as directed, at the same time each day, even if feeling well; do not skip or double up on missed doses. Take missed doses as soon as possible up to 4 hr before next dose (8 hr with extended-release propranolol). Inform patient that abrupt withdrawal can cause life-threatening arrhythmias, hypertension, or myocardial ischemia. Advise parent to read medication guide prior to starting and with each Rx refill in case of changes in *Hemangeol*.
- Advise patient to make sure enough medication is available for weekends, holidays, and vacations. A written prescription may be kept in wallet in case of emergency.
- Teach patient and family how to check pulse daily and BP biweekly. Advise patient to hold dose and contact health care professional if pulse is <50 bpm or BP changes significantly.
- May cause drowsiness or dizziness. Caution patients to avoid driving or other activities that require alertness until response to the drug is known.

P

- Advise patients to change positions slowly to minimize orthostatic hypotension, especially during initiation of therapy or when dose is increased.
- Caution patient that this medication may increase sensitivity to cold.
- Instruct patient to notify health care professional of all Rx or OTC medications, vitamins, or herbal products being taken and to consult health care professional before taking other Rx, OTC, or herbal products, especially NSAIDs and cold preparations, concurrently with this medication.
- Advise diabetic patients to closely monitor blood sugar, especially if weakness, malaise, irritability, or fatigue occurs. Medication may mask some signs of hypoglycemia, but dizziness and sweating may still occur. Acute hypertension may occur following insulin-induced hypoglycemia in patients receiving propranolol. Instruct parents/caregivers of children receiving *Hemangeol* how to recognize signs of hypoglycemia, and to notify health care professional and take child to nearest emergency department if hypoglycemia is suspected.
- Advise patient to notify health care professional if slow pulse, difficulty breathing, wheezing, cold hands and feet, dizziness, light-headedness, confusion, depression, rash, fever, sore throat, unusual bleeding, or bruising occurs.
- Instruct patient to inform health care professional of medication regimen prior to treatment or surgery.
- Advise patient to carry identification describing disease process and medication regimen at all times.
- **Hypertension:** Reinforce the need to continue additional therapies for hypertension (weight loss, sodium restriction, stress reduction, regular exercise, moderation of alcohol consumption, and smoking cessation). Medication controls but does not cure hypertension.
- **Angina:** Caution patient to avoid overexertion with decrease in chest pain.
- **Vascular Headache Prophylaxis:** Caution patient that sharing this medication may be dangerous.
- **PTSD:** Advise patient that medication may relieve distressing symptoms but that psychotherapy is the primary treatment for the disorder. Refer patient and family to a PTSD support group.

Evaluation/Desired Outcomes

- Decrease in BP.
- Control of arrhythmias without appearance of detrimental side effects.
- Reduction in frequency of anginal attacks.
- Increase in activity tolerance.
- Prevention of MI.
- Prevention of vascular headaches.
- Management of thyrotoxicosis.
- Management of pheochromocytoma.
- Decrease in tremors.
- Management of hypertrophic cardiomyopathy.
- Decrease in symptoms associated with PTSD.
- Resolution of Infantile hemangioma (propranolol only).

propylthiouracil

(proe-pill-thye-oh-**yoor**-a-sill)

✱Propyl-Thyracil

Classification
Therapeutic: antithyroid agents
Pharmacologic: thioamides

Pregnancy Category D

Indications

Patients with Graves' disease with hyperthyroidism or toxic multinodular goiter who are intolerant to methimazole and for whom surgery or radioactive iodine therapy is not appropriate. Adjunct in the control of hyperthyroidism in preparation for thyroidectomy or radioactive iodine therapy in patients who are intolerant to methimazole.

Action

Inhibits the synthesis of thyroid hormones. **Therapeutic Effects:** Decreased signs and symptoms of hyperthyroidism.

Pharmacokinetics

Absorption: Rapidly absorbed from the GI tract.
Distribution: Concentrates in the thyroid gland; crosses the placenta and enters breast milk in low concentrations.
Metabolism and Excretion: Metabolized by the liver.
Half-life: 1–2 hr.

TIME/ACTION PROFILE (effects on clinical thyroid status)

ROUTE	ONSET	PEAK	DURATION
PO	10–21 days†	6–10 wk	wk

†Effects on serum thyroid hormone concentration may occur within 60 min of a single dose.

Contraindications/Precautions

Contraindicated in: Hypersensitivity.
Use Cautiously in: ↓ bone marrow reserve; OB: May be used safely; however, fetus may develop thyroid problems; mother and fetus may be at ↑ risk for hepatotoxicity; Lactation: Safety not established; Geri: May have ↑ sensitivity; should initiate therapy with lowest dose; Pedi: Children <6 yr (safety not established); not recommended unless methimazole not tolerated or surgery or radioactive iodine therapy not appropriate.

Adverse Reactions/Side Effects

CNS: drowsiness, headache, paresthesia, vertigo. **CV:** edema, vasculitis. **GI:** HEPATOTOXICITY, <u>nausea</u>, <u>vomit-</u>

ing, diarrhea, loss of taste. **Derm:** STEVENS-JOHNSON SYNDROME, TOXIC EPIDERMAL NECROLYSIS, rash, exfoliative dermatitis, hair loss, skin discoloration, urticaria. **Endo:** hypothyroidism. **GU:** glomerulonephritis. **Hemat:** AGRANULOCYTOSIS, APLASTIC ANEMIA, BLEEDING, leukopenia, thrombocytopenia. **MS:** arthralgia, myalgia. **Resp:** interstitial pneumonitis. **Misc:** fever, lymphadenopathy, parotitis, splenomegaly.

Interactions

Drug-Drug: Additive bone marrow depression with **antineoplastics** or **radiation therapy**. Additive antithyroid effects with **lithium**, or **potassium iodide**. ↑ risk of agranulocytosis with **phenothiazines**.

Route/Dosage

PO (Adults): 100 mg q 8 hr; may be ↑ to 400 mg/day (occasional patient may require 600–900 mg/day); usual maintenance dose = 100–150 mg/day.

PO (Children >10 yr): 50–300 mg/day given once daily or in 2–4 divided doses.

PO (Children 6–10 yr): 50–150 mg/day given once daily or in 2–4 divided doses.

Availability (generic available)

Tablets: 50 mg, ✤100 mg.

NURSING IMPLICATIONS

Assessment

- Monitor response of symptoms of hyperthyroidism or thyrotoxicosis (tachycardia, palpitations, nervousness, insomnia, fever, diaphoresis, heat intolerance, tremors, weight loss, diarrhea).
- Assess patient for development of hypothyroidism (intolerance to cold, constipation, dry skin, headache, listlessness, tiredness, or weakness). Dose adjustment may be required.
- Assess patient for skin rash or swelling of cervical lymph nodes. Treatment may be discontinued if this occurs.
- ***Lab Test Considerations:*** Thyroid function studies should be monitored prior to therapy, monthly during initial therapy, and every 2–3 mo throughout therapy.
- WBC and differential counts should be monitored periodically throughout therapy. Agranulocytosis may develop rapidly and usually occurs during first 2 mo. This necessitates discontinuation of therapy.
- May cause increased AST, ALT, LDH, alkaline phosphatase, serum bilirubin, and prothrombin time.

Potential Nursing Diagnoses

Deficient knowledge, related to medication regimen (Patient/Family Teaching)

Noncompliance (Patient/Family Teaching)

Implementation

- Do not confuse propylthiouracil with Purinethol (mercaptopurine).
- Can be compounded by pharmacist into enema or suppository.
- **PO:** Administer at same time in relation to meals every day. Food may either increase or decrease absorption.

Patient/Family Teaching

- Instruct patient to take medication exactly as directed, around the clock. If a dose is missed, take as soon as remembered; take both doses together if almost time for next dose; check with health care professional if more than 1 dose is missed. Consult health care professional prior to discontinuing medication.
- Instruct patient to monitor weight 2–3 times weekly. Report significant changes.
- May cause drowsiness. Caution patient to avoid driving or other activities requiring alertness until response to medication is known.
- Advise patient to consult health care professional regarding dietary sources of iodine (iodized salt, shellfish).
- Advise patient to report sore throat, fever, chills, headache, malaise, weakness, yellowing of eyes or skin, unusual bleeding or bruising, symptoms of hyperthyroidism or hypothyroidism, or rash to health care professional promptly.
- Advise patient to notify health care professional of all Rx or OTC medications, vitamins, or herbal products being taken and to consult with health care professional before taking other medications.
- Advise patient to carry identification describing medication regimen at all times and to notify health care professional of medication regimen prior to treatment or surgery.
- Advise female patient to notify health care professional if pregnancy is planned or suspected or if breast feeding.
- Emphasize the importance of routine exams to monitor progress and to check for side effects.

Evaluation/Desired Outcomes

- Decrease in severity of symptoms of hyperthyroidism (lowered pulse rate and weight gain).
- Return of thyroid function studies to normal.
- May be used as short-term adjunctive therapy to prepare patient for thyroidectomy or radiation therapy or may be used in treatment of hyperthyroidism. Treatment of 6 mo to several yr may be necessary, usually averaging 1 yr.

P

protamine sulfate
(proe-ta-meen)

Classification
Therapeutic: antidotes
Pharmacologic: antiheparins

Pregnancy Category C

Indications
Acute management of severe heparin overdosage. Used to neutralize heparin received during dialysis, cardiopulmonary bypass, and other procedures. **Unlabeled Use:** Management of overdose of heparin-like compounds.

Action
A strong base that forms a complex with heparin (an acid). **Therapeutic Effects:** Inactivation of heparin.

Pharmacokinetics
Absorption: Administered IV only, resulting in complete bioavailability.
Distribution: Unknown.
Metabolism and Excretion: Metabolic fate not known. Protamine-heparin complex eventually degrades.
Half-life: Unknown.

TIME/ACTION PROFILE (reversal of heparin effect)

ROUTE	ONSET	PEAK	DURATION
IV	30 sec–1 min	unknown	2 hr†

†Depends on body temperature.

Contraindications/Precautions
Contraindicated in: Hypersensitivity to protamine or fish.
Use Cautiously in: Patients who have received previous protamine-containing insulin or vasectomized men (↑ risk of hypersensitivity reactions); OB, Lactation, Pedi: Safety not established.

Adverse Reactions/Side Effects
Resp: dyspnea. **CV:** bradycardia, hypertension, hypotension, pulmonary hypertension. **GI:** nausea, vomiting. **Derm:** flushing, warmth. **Hemat:** bleeding. **MS:** back pain. **Misc:** hypersensitivity reactions, including ANAPHYLAXIS, ANGIOEDEMA, and PULMONARY EDEMA.

Interactions
Drug-Drug: None significant.

Route/Dosage
IV (Adults and Children): *Heparin overdose*—1 mg/100 units of heparin. If given >30 min after heparin, give 0.5 mg/100 units of heparin (not to exceed 100 mg/2 hr). Further doses should be determined by coagulation tests. If heparin was administered subcutaneously, use 1–1.5 mg protamine per 100 units of heparin, give 25–50 mg of the protamine dose slowly followed by a continuous infusion over 8–16 hr.
Enoxaparin overdose—1 mg/each mg of enoxaparin to be neutralized (unlabeled). *Dalteparin overdose*—1 mg/100 anti-Xa IU of dalteparin. If required, a second dose of 0.5 mg/100 anti-Xa IU of dalteparin may be given 2–4 hr later if laboratory assessment indicates need (unlabeled).

Availability (generic available)
Injection: 10 mg/mL.

NURSING IMPLICATIONS

Assessment
- Assess for bleeding and hemorrhage throughout therapy. Hemorrhage may recur 8–9 hr after therapy because of rebound effects of heparin. Rebound may occur as late as 18 hr after therapy in patients heparinized for cardiopulmonary bypass.
- Assess for allergy to fish (salmon), previous reaction to or use of protamine insulin or protamine sulfate. Vasectomized and infertile men also have higher risk of hypersensitivity reaction.
- Observe patient for signs and symptoms of hypersensitivity reaction (hives, edema, coughing, wheezing). Keep epinephrine, an antihistamine, and resuscitative equipment close by in the event of anaphylaxis.
- Assess for hypovolemia before initiation of therapy. Failure to correct hypovolemia may result in cardiovascular collapse from peripheral vasodilating effects of protamine sulfate.
- ***Lab Test Considerations:*** Monitor clotting factors, activated clotting time (ACT), activated partial thromboplastin time (aPTT), and thrombin time (TT) 5–15 min after therapy and again as necessary.

Potential Nursing Diagnoses
Risk for injury (Indications)
Ineffective tissue perfusion (Indications)

Implementation
- Do not confuse protamine with Protonix (pantoprazole).
- Discontinue heparin infusion. In milder cases, overdosage may be treated by heparin withdrawal alone.
- In severe cases, fresh frozen plasma or whole blood may also be required to control bleeding.
- Dose varies with type of heparin, route of heparin therapy, and amount of time elapsed since discontinuation of heparin.
- Do not administer >100 mg in 2 hr without rechecking clotting studies, as protamine sulfate has its own anticoagulant properties.

IV Administration

- **IV Push: *Diluent:*** May be administered undiluted. If further dilution is desired, D5W or 0.9% NaCl may be used. ***Concentration:*** 10 mg/mL. ***Rate:*** Administer by slow IV push over 1–3 min. Rapid infusion rate may result in hypotension, bradycardia, flushing, or feeling of warmth. If these symptoms occur, stop infusion and notify physician. No more than 50 mg should be administered within a 10-min period.

- **Y-Site Compatibility:** alfentanil, amikacin, aminophylline, ascorbic acid, atropine, azathioprine, aztreonam, benztropine, bumetanide, buprenorphine, butorphanol, calcium chloride, calcium gluconate, ceftazidime, chlorpromazine, clindamycin, cyanocobalamin, cyclosporine, digoxin, diphenhydramine, dobutamine, dopamine, doxycycline, enalaprilat, ephedrine, epinephrine, epoetin alfa, erythromycin, esmolol, famotidine, fentanyl, fluconazole, ganciclovir, gentamicin, glycopyrrolate, imipenem/cilastatin, isoproterenol, labetalol, lidocaine, magnesium sulfate, mannitol, meperidine, metaraminol, methoxamine, methyldopate, metoclopramide, metoprolol, midazolam, morphine, multivitamins, nalbuphine, naloxone, nitroglycerin, nitroprusside, norepinephrine, ondansetron, oxytocin, papaverine, pentazocine, phentolamine, phenylephrine, potassium chloride, procainamide, prochlorperazine, promethazine, propranolol, pyridoxime, ranitidine, sodium bicarbonate, succinylcholine, sufentanil, tobramycin, tolazoline, trimetaphan, vancomycin, vasopressin, verapamil.
- **Y-Site Incompatibility:** amphotericin B colloidal, ampicillin, ampicillin/sulbactam, cefazolin, cefotaxime, cefoxitin, ceftazidime, cefuroxime, chloramphenicol, dantrolene, dexamethasone sodium phosphate, diazepam, diazoxide, folic acid, furosemide, heparin, hydrocortisone sodium succinate, indomethacin, insulin, ketorolac, methylprednisolone sodium succinate, nafcillin, oxacillin, penicillin G, pentamidine, pentobarbital, phenobarbital, phenytoin, trimethoprim/sulfamethoxazole.

Patient/Family Teaching

- Explain purpose of the medication to patient. Instruct patient to report recurrent bleeding immediately.
- Advise patient to avoid activities that may result in bleeding (shaving, brushing teeth, receiving injections or rectal temperatures, or ambulating) until risk of hemorrhage has passed.

Evaluation/Desired Outcomes

- Control of bleeding.
- Normalization of clotting factors in heparinized patients.

pseudoephedrine

(soo-doe-e-**fed**-rin)

Silfedrine Children's, Sudafed 12 Hour, Sudafed 24 Hour, Sudafed Children's, SudoGest, SudoGest 12 Hour

Classification

Therapeutic: allergy, cold, and cough remedies, nasal drying agents/decongestants

Pharmacologic: adrenergics, alpha adrenergic agonists

Pregnancy Category B

Indications

Symptomatic management of nasal congestion associated with acute viral upper respiratory tract infections. Used in combination with antihistamines in the management of allergic conditions. Used to open obstructed eustachian tubes in chronic otic inflammation or infection.

Action

Stimulates alpha- and beta-adrenergic receptors. Produces vasoconstriction in the respiratory tract mucosa (alpha-adrenergic stimulation) and possibly bronchodilation ($beta_2$-adrenergic stimulation). **Therapeutic Effects:** Reduction of nasal congestion, hyperemia, and swelling in nasal passages.

Pharmacokinetics

Absorption: Well absorbed after oral administration.

Distribution: Appears to enter the CSF; probably crosses the placenta and enters breast milk.

Metabolism and Excretion: Partially metabolized by the liver. 55–75% excreted unchanged by the kidneys (depends on urine pH).

Half-life: Children: 3.1 hr; Adults: 9–16 hr (depends on urine pH).

TIME/ACTION PROFILE (decongestant effects)

ROUTE	ONSET	PEAK	DURATION
PO	15–30 min	unknown	4–6 hr
PO-ER	60 min	unknown	12 hr

Contraindications/Precautions

Contraindicated in: Hypersensitivity to sympathomimetic amines; Hypertension, severe coronary artery disease; Concurrent MAO inhibitor therapy; Known alcohol intolerance (some liquid products).

Use Cautiously in: Hyperthyroidism; Diabetes mellitus; Prostatic hyperplasia; Ischemic heart disease; Glaucoma; OB, Lactation: Safety not established; Pedi: Avoid OTC cough and cold products containing this medication in children <4 yr.

P

Adverse Reactions/Side Effects

CNS: SEIZURES, anxiety, nervousness, dizziness, drowsiness, excitability, fear, hallucinations, headache, insomnia, restlessness, weakness. **Resp:** respiratory difficulty. **CV:** CARDIOVASCULAR COLLAPSE, palpitations, hypertension, tachycardia. **GI:** anorexia, dry mouth. **GU:** dysuria. **Misc:** diaphoresis.

Interactions

Drug-Drug: Concurrent use with **MAO inhibitors** may cause hypertensive crisis. Additive adrenergic effects with other **adrenergics**. Concurrent use with **beta blockers** may result in hypertension or bradycardia. **Drugs that acidify the urine** may ↓ effectiveness. **Phenothiazines** and **tricyclic antidepressants** potentiate pressor effects. **Drugs that alkalinize the urine (sodium bicarbonate, high-dose antacid therapy)** may intensify effectiveness.
Drug-Food: Foods that acidify the urine may ↓ effectiveness. **Foods that alkalinize the urine** may intensify effectiveness (see lists in Appendix J).

Route/Dosage

PO (Adults and Children >12 yr): 60 mg q 6 hr as needed (not to exceed 240 mg/day) *or* 120 mg extended-release preparation q 12 hr *or* 240 mg extended-release preparation q 24 hr.
PO (Children 6–12 yr): 30 mg q 6 hr as needed (not to exceed 120 mg/day).
PO (Children 4–5 yr): 15 mg q 6 hr (not to exceed 60 mg/day).

Availability (generic available)

Tablets: 30 mg[OTC], 60 mg[OTC]. **Extended-release tablets:** 120 mg[OTC], 240 mg[OTC]. **Capsules:** ✱ 60 mg[OTC]. **Extended-release capsules:** ✱ 240 mg[OTC]. **Liquid (grape and others):** 15 mg/5 mL[OTC], 30 mg/5 mL[OTC]. ***In combination with:*** antihistamines, acetaminophen, cough suppressants, and expectorants[OTC]. See Appendix B.

NURSING IMPLICATIONS

Assessment

- Assess congestion (nasal, sinus, eustachian tube) before and periodically during therapy.
- Monitor pulse and BP before beginning therapy and periodically during therapy.
- Assess lung sounds and character of bronchial secretions. Maintain fluid intake of 1500–2000 mL/day to decrease viscosity of secretions.

Potential Nursing Diagnoses

Ineffective airway clearance (Indications)

Implementation

- Do not confuse Sudafed with sotalol or Sudafed PE. Do not confuse Sudafed 12 Hour with Sudafed 12 Hour Pressure + Pain.
- Administer pseudoephedrine at least 2 hr before bedtime to minimize insomnia.
- **PO:** Extended-release tablets and capsules should be swallowed whole; do not crush, break, or chew. Contents of the capsule can be mixed with jam or jelly and swallowed without chewing for patients with difficulty swallowing.

Patient/Family Teaching

- Instruct patient to take medication as directed and not to take more than recommended. Take missed doses within 1 hr; if remembered later, omit. Do not double doses. Caution parents to avoid OTC cough and cold products while breast feeding or to children <4 yr.
- Instruct patient to notify health care professional if nervousness, slow or fast heart rate, breathing difficulties, hallucinations, or seizures occur, because these symptoms may indicate overdose.
- Instruct patient to contact health care professional if symptoms do not improve within 7 days or if fever is present.

Evaluation/Desired Outcomes

- Decreased nasal, sinus, or eustachian tube congestion.

psyllium (sill-i-yum)

Alramucil, Cillium, Effer-Syllium, Fiberall, Fibrepur, Hydrocil, ✱Karacil, Konsyl, Metamucil, Modane Bulk, Mylanta Natural Fiber Supplement, Naturacil Caramels,
✱Natural Source Fibre Laxative, Perdiem, ✱Prodiem, Pro-Lax, Reguloid Natural, Serutan, Siblin, Syllact, Vitalax, V-Lax

Classification
Therapeutic: laxatives
Pharmacologic: bulk-forming agents

Pregnancy Category UK

Indications

Management of simple or chronic constipation, particularly if associated with a low-fiber diet. Useful in situations in which straining should be avoided (after MI, rectal surgery, prolonged bed rest). Used in the management of chronic watery diarrhea.

Action

Combines with water in the intestinal contents to form an emollient gel or viscous solution that promotes peristalsis and reduces transit time. **Therapeutic Effects:** Relief and prevention of constipation.

Pharmacokinetics

Absorption: Not absorbed from the GI tract.
Distribution: No distribution occurs.
Metabolism and Excretion: Excreted in feces.

Half-life: Unknown.

TIME/ACTION PROFILE (laxative effect)

ROUTE	ONSET	PEAK	DURATION
PO	12–24 hr	2–3 days	unknown

Contraindications/Precautions

Contraindicated in: Hypersensitivity; Abdominal pain, nausea, or vomiting (especially when associated with fever); Serious adhesions; Dysphagia.

Use Cautiously in: Some dosage forms contain sugar, aspartame, or excessive sodium and should be avoided in patients on restricted diets; OB: Lactation: Has been used safely.

Adverse Reactions/Side Effects

Resp: bronchospasm. **GI:** cramps, intestinal or esophageal obstruction, nausea, vomiting.

Interactions

Drug-Drug: May ↓ absorption of **warfarin**, **salicylates**, or **digoxin**.

Route/Dosage

PO (Adults): 1–2 tsp/packet/wafer (3–6 g psyllium) in or with a full glass of liquid 2–3 times daily. Up to 30 g daily in divided doses.

PO (Children >6 yr): 1 tsp/packet/wafer (1.5–3 g psyllium) in or with 4–8 oz glass of liquid 2–3 times daily. Up to 15 g daily in divided doses.

Availability (generic available)

Powder: 3.3–3.5 g/dose or packet^{OTC}. **Effervescent powder:** 3–3.5 g/dose or packet^{OTC}. **Granules:** 2.5 g/dose^{OTC}. **Wafers:** 3.4 g/dose^{OTC}.

NURSING IMPLICATIONS

Assessment

- Assess patient for abdominal distention, presence of bowel sounds, and usual pattern of bowel function.
- Assess color, consistency, and amount of stool produced.
- ***Lab Test Considerations:*** May cause elevated blood glucose levels with prolonged use of preparations containing sugar.

Potential Nursing Diagnoses

Constipation (Indications)

Implementation

- Packets are not standardized for volume, but each contains 3–3.5 g of psyllium.
- **PO:** Administer with a full glass of water or juice, followed by an additional glass of liquid. Solution should be taken immediately after mixing; it will congeal. Do not administer without sufficient fluid and do not chew granules.

Patient/Family Teaching

- Encourage patient to use other forms of bowel regulation, such as increasing bulk in the diet, increasing fluid intake, and increasing mobility. Normal bowel habits are individualized and may vary from 3 times/day to 3 times/wk.
- May be used for long-term management of chronic constipation.
- Instruct patients with cardiac disease to avoid straining during bowel movements (Valsalva maneuver).
- Advise patient not to use laxatives when abdominal pain, nausea, vomiting, or fever is present.

Evaluation/Desired Outcomes

- A soft, formed bowel movement, usually within 12–24 hr. May require 3 days of therapy for results.

pyrazinamide

(peer-a-**zin**-a-mide)

✱Tebrazid

Classification

Therapeutic: antituberculars

Pregnancy Category C

P

Indications

Used in combination with other agents in the treatment of active tuberculosis.

Action

Converted to pyrazinoic acid in susceptible strains of Mycobacterium which lowers the pH of the environment. **Therapeutic Effects:** Bacteriostatic action against susceptible mycobacteria. **Spectrum:** Active against mycobacteria only.

Pharmacokinetics

Absorption: Well absorbed after oral administration.

Distribution: Widely distributed. Reaches high concentrations in the CNS (same as plasma). Excreted in breast milk.

Protein Binding: 50%.

Metabolism and Excretion: Mostly metabolized by the liver. Metabolite (pyrazinoic acid) has antimycobacterial activity; 3–4% excreted unchanged by the kidneys.

Half-life: *Pyrazinamide*—9.5 hr. *Pyrazinoic acid*—12 hr. Both are ↑ in renal impairment.

TIME/ACTION PROFILE (blood levels)

ROUTE	ONSET	PEAK	DURATION
PO	unknown	1–2 hr (4–5 hr†)	24 hr

†For pyrazinoic acid.

Contraindications/Precautions

Contraindicated in: Hypersensitivity; Cross-sensitivity with ethionamide, isoniazid, niacin, or nicotinic acid may exist; Severe liver impairment.

Use Cautiously in: Gout; Renal failure; Diabetes mellitus; Acute intermittent porphyria; OB: Safety not established.

Adverse Reactions/Side Effects

GI: HEPATOTOXICITY, anorexia, diarrhea, nausea, vomiting. **GU:** dysuria. **Derm:** acne, itching, photosensitivity, rash. **Hemat:** anemia, thrombocytopenia. **Metab:** hyperuricemia. **MS:** arthralgia, gouty arthritis.

Interactions

Drug-Drug: Concurrent use with **rifampin** may result in life-threatening hepatoxicity and should be avoided. May ↓ blood levels and effectiveness of **cyclosporine**. May ↓ effectiveness of **antigout agents**.

Route/Dosage

PO (Adults and Children): 15–30 mg/kg/day as a single dose. Up to 60 mg/kg/day has been used in isoniazid-resistant tuberculosis (not to exceed 2 g/day as a single dose or 3 g/day in divided doses). May also be given as 50–70 mg/kg 2–3 times weekly (not to exceed 2 g/dose on daily regimen, 3 g/dose for 3-times-weekly regimen, or 4 g/dose for twice-weekly regimen). *Patients with HIV*—20–40 mg/kg/day for first 2 mo of therapy (maximum: 2 g/day); further dosing depends on regimen employed.

Availability (generic available)

Tablets: 500 mg. ***In combination with:*** rifampin and isoniazid (Rifater). See Appendix B.

NURSING IMPLICATIONS

Assessment

- Perform mycobacterial studies and susceptibility tests before and periodically during therapy to detect possible resistance.
- ***Lab Test Considerations:*** Evaluate hepatic function before and every 2–4 wk during therapy. Increased AST and ALT may not be predictive of clinical hepatitis and may return to normal levels during treatment. Patients with impaired liver function should receive pyrazinamide therapy only if crucial to treatment.
- Monitor serum uric acid concentrations during therapy. May cause ↑ resulting in precipitation of acute gout.
- May interfere with urine ketone determinations.

Potential Nursing Diagnoses

Risk for infection (Indications)
Noncompliance (Patient/Family Teaching)

Implementation

- **PO:** May be given concurrently with isoniazid.

Patient/Family Teaching

- Advise patient to take medication as directed and not to skip doses or double up on missed doses. Take missed doses as soon as remembered unless almost time for next dose. Emphasize the importance of continuing therapy even after symptoms have subsided. Length of therapy depends on regimen being used and underlying disease states.
- Inform diabetic patients that pyrazinamide may interfere with urine ketone measurements.
- Advise patients to notify health care professional if no improvement is noticed after 2–3 wk of therapy or if fever, anorexia, malaise, nausea, vomiting, darkened urine, yellowish discoloration of the skin and eyes, pain, or swelling of the joints occurs.
- Advise patients to use sunscreen and protective clothing to prevent photosensitivity reactions.
- Advise female patient to notify health care professional if pregnancy is planned or suspected or if breast feeding.
- Emphasize the importance of regular follow-up exams to monitor progress and check for side effects.

Evaluation/Desired Outcomes

- Resolution of signs and symptoms of tuberculosis.
- Negative sputum cultures.

pyridostigmine

(peer-id-oh-**stig**-meen)

Mestinon, ✤Mestinon SR, Mestinon Timespan, Regonol

Classification

Therapeutic: antimyasthenics

Pharmacologic: cholinergics

Pregnancy Category C

Indications

Used to increase muscle strength in the symptomatic treatment of myasthenia gravis. Reversal of nondepolarizing neuromuscular blocking agents. Prophylaxis of lethal effects of poisoning with the nerve agent soman.

Action

Inhibits the breakdown of acetylcholine and prolongs its effects (anticholinesterase). Effects include: Miosis, Increased intestinal and skeletal muscle tone, Bronchial and ureteral constriction, Bradycardia, Increased salivation, Lacrimation, Sweating. **Therapeutic Effects:** Improved muscular function in patients with myasthenia gravis. Reversal of paralysis from nondepolarizing neuromuscular blocking agents. Prevention of Soman nerve gas toxicity.

Pharmacokinetics

Absorption: Poorly absorbed after oral administration, necessitating large oral doses compared with parenteral doses.

Distribution: Appears to cross the placenta.
Metabolism and Excretion: Metabolized by plasma cholinesterases and the liver.
Half-life: *PO*—3.7 hr; *IV*—1.9 hr.

TIME/ACTION PROFILE (cholinergic effects)

ROUTE	ONSET	PEAK	DURATION
PO	30–35 min	unknown	3–6 hr
PO-SR	30–60 min	unknown	6–12 hr
IM	15 min	unknown	2–4 hr
IV	2–5 min	unknown	2–3 hr

Contraindications/Precautions

Contraindicated in: Hypersensitivity to pyridostigmine or bromides; Mechanical obstruction of the GI or GU tract; Known alcohol intolerance (syrup only).
Use Cautiously in: History of asthma; Ulcer disease; Cardiovascular disease; Epilepsy; Hyperthyroidism; OB: May cause uterine irritability after IV administration near term; 20% of newborns display transient muscle weakness; Lactation: Pedi: Safety not established.

Adverse Reactions/Side Effects

CNS: SEIZURES, dizziness, weakness. **EENT:** lacrimation, miosis. **Resp:** bronchospasm, excessive secretions. **CV:** bradycardia, hypotension. **GI:** abdominal cramps, diarrhea, excessive salivation, nausea, vomiting. **Derm:** sweating, rashes.

Interactions

Drug-Drug: Cholinergic effects may be antagonized by other **drugs possessing anticholinergic properties**, including **antihistamines, antidepressants, atropine, haloperidol, phenothiazines, procainamide, quinidine**, or **disopyramide**. Prolongs the action of **depolarizing muscle-relaxing agents** and **cholinesterase inhibitors (succinylcholine, decamethonium)**. ↑ toxicity with other **cholinesterase inhibitors**, including **echothiophate**.

Route/Dosage

Myasthenia Gravis

PO (Adults): *Tablets/syrup*—30–60 mg q 3–4 hr initially; then adjusted as required; usual maintenance dose is 600 mg/day in divided doses (range 60–1500 mg/day). *Extended-release tablets*—180–540 mg 1–2 times daily (dosing interval should be at least 6 hr; may be associated with increased risk of cholinergic crisis; concurrent immediate-release products may be required).
PO (Children): 7 mg/kg (200 mg/m^2)/day in 5–6 divided doses.
IM, IV (Adults): 2 mg (1/30 of oral dose); may be repeated q 2–3 hr. *During labor/delivery*—1 mg before second stage of labor is complete.
IM (Neonates Born to Myasthenic Mothers): 50–150 mcg/kg q 4–6 hr.

Antidote for Nondepolarizing Neuromuscular Blocking Agents

IV (Adults): 10–20 mg; pretreat with 0.6–1.2 mg atropine IV.

Prevention of Soman Nerve Gas Effects

PO (Adults): 30 mg every 8 hr before exposure, stopped on exposure to gas.

Availability (generic available)

Tablets: 60 mg. **Extended-release tablets:** 180 mg. **Syrup:** 60 mg/5 mL. **Injection:** 5 mg/mL.

NURSING IMPLICATIONS

Assessment

- Assess pulse, respiratory rate, and BP before administration. Report significant changes in heart rate.
- **Myasthenia Gravis:** Assess neuromuscular status, including vital capacity, ptosis, diplopia, chewing, swallowing, hand grasp, and gait before administering and at peak effect. Patients with myasthenia gravis may be advised to keep a daily record of their condition and the effects of this medication.
- Assess patient for overdose, underdose, or resistance. Both have similar symptoms (muscle weakness, dyspnea, dysphagia), but symptoms of overdosage usually occur within 1 hr of administration, whereas symptoms of underdose occur ≥3 hr after administration. Overdose (cholinergic crisis) symptoms may also include increased respiratory secretions and saliva, bradycardia, nausea, vomiting, cramping, diarrhea, and diaphoresis. A Tensilon test (edrophonium chloride) may be used to differentiate between overdosage and underdosage.
- **Antidote to Nondepolarizing Neuromuscular Blocking Agents:** Monitor reversal of effect of neuromuscular blocking agents with a peripheral nerve stimulator. Recovery usually occurs consecutively in the following muscles: diaphragm, intercostal muscles, muscles of the glottis, abdominal muscles, limb muscles, muscles of mastication, and levator muscles of eyelids. Closely observe patient for residual muscle weakness and respiratory distress throughout the recovery period. Maintain airway patency and ventilation until recovery of normal respirations occurs.
- ***Toxicity and Overdose:*** Atropine is the antidote.

Potential Nursing Diagnoses

Impaired physical mobility (Indications)
Ineffective breathing pattern (Indications)

Implementation

- For patients who have difficulty chewing, pyridostigmine may be administered 30 min before meals.

P

- Oral dose is not interchangeable with IV dose. Parenteral form is 30 times more potent.
- When used as an antidote to nondepolarizing neuromuscular blocking agents, atropine may be ordered before or currently with large doses of pyridostigmine to prevent or to treat bradycardia and other side effects.
- **PO:** Administer with food or milk to minimize side effects. Extended-release tablets should be swallowed whole; do not crush, break, or chew. Regular tablets or syrup may be administered with extended-release tablets for optimum control of symptoms. Mottled appearance of sustained-release tablet does not affect potency.

IV Administration

- **IV Push:** Administer undiluted. Do not add to IV solutions. May be given through Y-site of infusion of D5W, 0.9% NaCl, LR, D5/Ringer's solution, or D5/LR. ***Concentration:*** 5 mg/mL. ***Rate:*** For myasthenia gravis, administer each 0.5 mg over 1 min. For reversal of nondepolarizing neuromuscular blocking agents, administer each 5 mg over 1 min.
- **Syringe Compatibility:** glycopyrrolate.
- **Y-Site Compatibility:** heparin, hydrocortisone sodium succinate, potassium chloride, vitamin B complex with C.

Patient/Family Teaching

- Instruct patient to take medication as directed. Do not skip or double up on missed doses. Patients with a history of dysphagia should have a nonelectric or battery-operated back-up alarm clock to remind them of exact dose time. Patients with dysphagia may not be able to swallow medication if the dose is not taken exactly on time. Taking dose late may result in myasthenic crisis. Taking dose early may result in cholinergic crisis. Patients with myasthenia gravis must continue this regimen as a life-long therapy.
- Advise patient to carry identification describing disease and medication regimen at all times.
- Instruct patient to space activities to avoid fatigue.

Evaluation/Desired Outcomes

- Relief of ptosis and diplopia; improved chewing, swallowing, extremity strength, and breathing without the appearance of cholinergic symptoms.
- Reversal of nondepolarizing neuromuscular blocking agents in general anesthesia.
- Prevention of Soman nerve gas toxicity.

pyridoxine (peer-i-**dox**-een)

Neuro-K–250 TD, Neuro-K-250 Vitamin B6, Neuro-K-50, Neuro-K-500, Pyri 500, vitamin B_6

Classification
Therapeutic: vitamins
Pharmacologic: water soluble vitamins

Pregnancy Category A

Indications

Treatment and prevention of pyridoxine deficiency (may be associated with poor nutritional status or chronic debilitating illnesses). Treatment of pyridoxine-dependent seizures in infants. Treatment and prevention of neuropathy, which may develop from isoniazid, penicillamine, or hydralazine therapy. Management of isoniazid overdose >10 g.

Action

Required for amino acid, carbohydrate, and lipid metabolism. Used in the transport of amino acids, formation of neurotransmitters, and synthesis of heme. **Therapeutic Effects:** Prevention of pyridoxine deficiency. Prevention or reversal of neuropathy associated with hydralazine, penicillamine, or isoniazid therapy.

Pharmacokinetics

Absorption: Well absorbed from the GI tract.
Distribution: Stored in liver, muscle, and brain. Crosses the placenta and enters breast milk.
Metabolism and Excretion: Converted in RBCs to pyridoxal phosphate and another active metabolite. Amounts in excess of requirements are excreted unchanged by the kidneys.
Half-life: 15–20 days.

TIME/ACTION PROFILE

ROUTE	ONSET	PEAK	DURATION
PO, IM, IV	unknown	unknown	unknown

Contraindications/Precautions

Contraindicated in: Hypersensitivity to pyridoxine or any component.
Use Cautiously in: Parkinson's disease (treatment with levodopa only); OB: Chronic ingestion of large doses may produce pyridoxine-dependency syndrome in newborn.

Adverse Reactions/Side Effects

Adverse reactions listed are seen with excessive doses only.
Neuro: sensory neuropathy, paresthesia. **Misc:** pyridoxine-dependency syndrome.

Interactions

Drug-Drug: Interferes with the therapeutic response to **levodopa** when used without carbidopa. Requirements are increased by **isoniazid, hydralazine, chloramphenicol, penicillamine, estrogens**, and **immunosuppressants**. Decreases serum levels of **phenobarbital** and **phenytoin**.

Route/Dosage

Prevention of Deficiency (Recommended Daily Allowance)

PO (Adults and Children >14 yr): 1.2–1.7 mg/day (larger doses required with cycloserine, ethionamide, hydralazine, immunosuppressants, isoniazid, penicillamine, and estrogen-containing oral contraceptives).
PO (Children 9–13 yr): 1 mg/day (larger doses required with cycloserine, ethionamide, hydralazine, immunosuppressants, isoniazid, and penicillamine).
PO (Children 1–8 yr): 0.5–0.6 mg/day (larger doses required with cycloserine, ethionamide, hydralazine, immunosuppressants, isoniazid, and penicillamine).
PO (Infants 6–12 mo): 0.3 mg/day.
PO (Infants <6 mo): 0.1 mg/day.

Treatment of Deficiency

PO (Adults): 2.5–10 mg/day until clinical signs are corrected, then 2–5 mg/day.
PO (Children): 5–25 mg/day for 3 weeks, then 1.5–2.5 mg/day.

Pyridoxine-Dependent Seizures

PO, IM, IV (Neonates and Infants): 10–100 mg initially then 50–100 mg/day orally.

Drug-Induced Neuritis

PO (Adults): Treatment—100–300 mg/day; Prophylaxis—25–100 mg/day.
PO (Children): Treatment—10–50 mg/day; Prophylaxis—1–2 mg/kg/day.

Isoniazid Overdose (>10 g)

IM, IV (Adults and Children): Amount in mg equal to amount of isoniazid ingested given as 1–4 g IV, then 1 g IM q 30 min.

Availability (generic available)

Capsules: 250 mg^{OTC}. **Tablets:** 25 mg^{OTC}, 50 mg^{OTC}, 100 mg^{OTC}, 250 mg^{OTC}, 500 mg^{OTC}. **Extended-release tablets:** 200 mg^{OTC}, 500 mg^{OTC}. **Injection:** 100 mg/mL. ***In combination with:*** vitamins, minerals, and trace elements in a variety of multivitamin preparations^{OTC}.

NURSING IMPLICATIONS

Assessment

- Assess patient for signs of vitamin B_6 deficiency (anemia, dermatitis, cheilosis, irritability, seizures, nausea, and vomiting) before and periodically throughout therapy. Institute seizure precautions in pyridoxine-dependent infants.
- ***Lab Test Considerations:*** May cause false elevations in urobilinogen concentrations.

Potential Nursing Diagnoses

Imbalanced nutrition: less than body requirements (Indications)

Implementation

- ***High Alert:*** Do not confuse pyridoxine with Pyridium (phenazopyridine).
- Because of infrequency of single B-vitamin deficiencies, combinations are commonly administered.
- Administration of parenteral vitamin B_6 is limited to patients who are NPO or who have nausea and vomiting or malabsorption syndromes.
- Protect parenteral solution from light; decomposition will occur.
- **PO:** Extended-release capsules and tablets should be swallowed whole, without crushing, breaking, or chewing. For patients unable to swallow capsule, contents of capsules may be mixed with jam or jelly.
- **IM:** Rotate sites; burning or stinging at site may occur.
- **IV:** May be administered slowly by IV push or as infusion in standard IV solutions. Monitor respiratory rate, heart rate, and BP when administering large IV doses.
- Pyridoxine-dependent seizures should cease within 2–3 min of IV administration.
- ***Rate:*** Infusion rates of 15–30 min and up to 3 hr have been used.
- **Additive Incompatibility:** alkaline solutions, riboflavin.

Patient/Family Teaching

- Instruct patient to take medication as directed. If a dose is missed, it may be omitted because an extended period of time is required to become deficient in vitamin B_6.
- Encourage patient to comply with diet recommended by health care professional. Explain that the best source of vitamins is a well-balanced diet with foods from the four basic food groups. Foods high in vitamin B_6 include bananas, whole-grain cereals, potatoes, lima beans, and meats.
- Patients self-medicating with vitamin supplements should be cautioned not to exceed RDA. The effectiveness of megadoses for treatment of various medical conditions is unproved and may cause side effects, such as unsteady gait, numbness in feet, and difficulty with hand coordination.
- Advise female patient to notify health care professional if pregnancy is planned or suspected or if breast feeding.
- Emphasize the importance of follow-up exams to evaluate progress.

Evaluation/Desired Outcomes

- Decrease in the symptoms of vitamin B_6 deficiency.

P

QUEtiapine (kwet-eye-a-peen)
SEROquel, SEROquel XR

Classification
Therapeutic: antipsychotics, mood stabilizers

Pregnancy Category C

Indications
Schizophrenia. Depressive episodes with bipolar disorder. Acute manic episodes associated with bipolar I disorder (as monotherapy [for adults or adolescents] or with lithium or divalproex [adults only]). Maintenance treatment of bipolar I disorder (with lithium or divalproex). Adjunctive treatment of depression.

Action
Probably acts by serving as an antagonist of dopamine and serotonin. Also antagonizes histamine H_1 receptors and alpha$_1$-adrenergic receptors. **Therapeutic Effects:** Decreased manifestations of psychoses, depression, or acute mania.

Pharmacokinetics
Absorption: Well absorbed after oral administration.
Distribution: Widely distributed.
Metabolism and Excretion: Extensively metabolized by the liver (mostly by P450 CYP3A4 enyzme system); <1% excreted unchanged in the urine.
Half-life: 6 hr.

TIME/ACTION PROFILE (antipsychotic effects)

ROUTE	ONSET	PEAK	DURATION
PO	unknown	unknown	8–12 hr
PO-XR	unknown	unknown	unknown

Contraindications/Precautions
Contraindicated in: Hypersensitivity; Lactation: Lactation; Concurrent use of agents that prolong the QT interval, including dofetilide, sotalol, quinidine, disopyramide, amiodarone, dronedarone, thioridazine, chlorpromazine, droperidol, moxifloxacin, mefloquine, pentamidine, arsenic trioxide, dolasetron, tacrolimus, ziprasidone, erythromycin, citalopram, escitalopram, and clarithromycin (↑ risk of serious arrhythmias); History of arrhythmias, including bradycardia; Hypokalemia or hypomagnesemia (↑ risk of serious arrhythmias); Congenital long QT syndrome (↑ risk of serious arrhythmias).
Use Cautiously in: Cardiovascular disease, cerebrovascular disease, dehydration or hypovolemia (↑ risk of hypotension); History of seizures, Alzheimer's dementia; Diabetes (may ↑ risk of hyperglycemia); Patients at risk for aspiration pneumonia; Hepatic impairment (dose ↓ may be necessary); Hypothyroidism (may be exacerbated); History of suicide attempt; OB: Neonates at ↑ risk for extrapyramidal symptoms and withdrawal after delivery when exposed during the 3rd trimester; use only if maternal benefit outweighs risk to fetus; Pedi: May ↑ risk of suicide attempt/ideation especially during early treatment or dose adjustment; risk may be greater in children or adolescents; Geri: May require ↓ doses; ↑ risk of mortality and stroke in elderly patients treated for dementia-related psychosis.

Adverse Reactions/Side Effects
CNS: NEUROLEPTIC MALIGNANT SYNDROME, SEIZURES, dizziness, cognitive impairment, extrapyramidal symptoms, sedation, tardive dyskinesia. **EENT:** ear pain, rhinitis, pharyngitis. **Resp:** cough, dyspnea. **CV:** ↑ BP (children), palpitations, peripheral edema, postural hypotension. **GI:** PANCREATITIS, anorexia, constipation, dry mouth, dyspepsia. **Derm:** STEVENS-JOHNSON SYNDROME, sweating. **Hemat:** ↓ hemoglobin, leukopenia. **Endo:** weight gain, hyperglycemia, hyperlipidemia, hyperprolactinemia, hypertriglyceridemia, hypothyroidism. **MS:** rhabdomyolysis. **Misc:** flu-like syndrome.

Interactions
Drug-Drug: Concurrent use of **macrolide anti-infectives (erythromycin, clarithromycin), dofetilide, sotalol, quinidine, disopyramide, procainamide thioridazine, chlorpromazine, droperidol, gemifloxacin, moxifloxacin, mefloquine, pentamidine, arsenic trioxide, dolasetron, citalopram, escitalopram tacrolimus,** and **ziprasidone** ↑ the risk of serious ventricular arrhythmias and should be avoided. ↑ CNS depression may occur with **alcohol, antihistamines, opioid analgesics,** and **sedative/hypnotics**. ↑ risk of hypotension with acute ingestion of **alcohol** or **antihypertensives**. **Phenytoin** and **thioridazine** ↑ clearance and ↓ effectiveness of quetiapine (dose change may be necessary); similar effects may occur with **carbamazepine, barbiturates, rifampin,** or **corticosteroids**. Effects may be ↑ by **ketoconazole, itraconazole, fluconazole, protease inhibitors,** or **erythromycin**, as well as by other **agents that inhibit the cytochrome P450 CYP3A4 enzyme**.

Route/Dosage

Schizophrenia
PO (Adults): *Immediate-release*—25 mg twice daily on Day 1, ↑ by 25–50 mg 2–3 times daily on Days 2 and 3, up to 300–400 mg/day in 2–3 divided doses by Day 4 (not to exceed 800 mg/day); *Extended-release*—300 mg once daily, ↑ by 300 mg/day (not to exceed 800 mg/day); elderly patients or patients with hepatic impairment should be started on immediate-release product and converted to extended-release product once effective dose is reached.

PO (Children 13–17 yr): *Immediate-release*—25 mg twice daily on Day 1, ↑ to 50 mg twice daily on Day 2, then ↑ to 100 mg twice daily on Day 3, then ↑ to 150 mg twice daily on Day 4, then ↑ to 200 mg twice daily on Day 5; may then ↑ by no more than 100 mg/day (not to exceed 800 mg/day).

Acute Manic Episodes Associated with Bipolar I Disorder

PO (Adults): *Immediate-release*—50 mg twice daily on Day 1, then ↑ to 100 mg twice daily on Day 2, then ↑ to 150 mg twice daily on Day 3, then ↑ to 200 mg twice daily on Day 4; may then ↑ by no more than 200 mg/day up to 400 mg twice daily on Day 6 if needed; *Extended-release*—300 mg once daily on Day 1, then 600 mg once daily on Day 2, then 400–800 mg once daily starting on Day 3.
PO (Children 10–17 yr): *Immediate-release*—25 mg twice daily on Day 1, then ↑ to 50 mg twice daily on Day 2, then ↑ to 100 mg twice daily on Day 3, then ↑ to 150 mg twice daily on Day 4, then ↑ to 200 mg twice daily on Day 5; may then ↑ by no more than 100 mg/day (not to exceed 600 mg/day).

Acute Depressive Episodes Associated with Bipolar Disorder

PO (Adults): *Immediate-release or extended-release*—50 mg once daily at bedtime on Day 1, then ↑ to 100 mg daily at bedtime on Day 2, then ↑ to 200 mg daily at bedtime on Day 3, then ↑ to 300 mg daily at bedtime thereafter.

Maintenance Treatment of Bipolar I Disorder

PO (Adults): Continue at the dose required to maintain symptom remission (usual dosage: 400–800 mg/day given as once daily dose [extended-release] or in two divided doses [immediate-release]).
PO (Children 10–17 yr): Continue at the lowest dose required to maintain symptom remission.

Depression

PO (Adults): *Extended-release*—50 mg once daily on Days 1 and 2, then ↑ to 150 mg once daily starting on Day 3 (not to exceed 300 mg/day).

Availability (generic available)

Tablets: 25 mg, 50 mg, 100 mg, 200 mg, 300 mg, 400 mg. **Cost:** *Generic*—25 mg $17.59/100, 100 mg $26.94/100, 200 mg $39.30/100. **Extended-release Tablets:** 50 mg, 150 mg, 200 mg, 300 mg, 400 mg. **Cost:** 50 mg $460.84/60, 150 mg $827.50/60, 200 mg $910.78/60, 300 mg $1,194.14/60, 400 mg $1,403.42/60.

NURSING IMPLICATIONS

Assessment

- Monitor mental status (mood, orientation, behavior) before and periodically during therapy.
- Assess for suicidal tendencies, especially during early therapy. Restrict amount of drug available to patient. Risk may be increased in children, adolescents, and adults ≤24 yr.
- Assess weight and BMI initially and throughout therapy.
- Monitor BP (sitting, standing, lying) and pulse before and frequently during initial dose titration. If hypotension occurs during dose titration, return to the previous dose.
- Observe patient carefully when administering to ensure medication is swallowed and not hoarded or cheeked.
- Monitor for onset of extrapyramidal side effects (*akathisia*—restlessness; *dystonia*—muscle spasms and twisting motions; or *pseudoparkinsonism*—mask-like faces, rigidity, tremors, drooling, shuffling gait, dysphagia). Report these symptoms; reduction of dose or discontinuation may be necessary. Trihexyphenidyl or benztropine may be used to control these symptoms.
- Monitor for tardive dyskinesia (involuntary rhythmic movement of mouth, face, and extremities). Report immediately; may be irreversible.
- Monitor for development of neuroleptic malignant syndrome (fever, respiratory distress, tachycardia, seizures, diaphoresis, hypertension or hypotension, pallor, tiredness). Notify health care professional immediately if these symptoms occur.
- Assess for rash periodically during therapy. May cause Stevens-Johnson syndrome. Discontinue therapy if severe or if accompanied with fever, general malaise, fatigue, muscle or joint aches, blisters, oral lesions, conjunctivitis, hepatitis, and/or eosinophilia.
- Monitor for signs of pancreatitis (nausea, vomiting, anorexia, persistent severe abdominal pain, sometimes radiating to the back) during therapy.
- Monitor for symptoms related to hyperprolactinemia (menstrual abnormalities, galactorrhea, sexual dysfunction).
- ***Lab Test Considerations:*** May cause asymptomatic ↑ in AST and ALT.
- May also cause anemia, thrombocytopenia, leukocytosis, and leukopenia.
- May cause ↑ total cholesterol and triglycerides.
- Obtain fasting blood glucose and cholesterol levels initially and throughout therapy.
- Monitor serum prolactin prior to and periodically during therapy. May cause ↑ serum prolactin levels.

Potential Nursing Diagnoses

Risk for self-directed violence (Indications)
Disturbed thought process (Indications)
Imbalanced nutrition: risk for more than body requirements (Side Effects)

Implementation

- Do not confuse quetiapine with olanzapine. Do not confuse Seroquel with Seroquel XR, Serzone (nefazodone), or Sinequan (doxepin).

- If therapy is reinstituted after an interval of ≥1 wk off, follow initial titration schedule.
- **PO:** May be administered without regard to food. Extended-release tablets should be swallowed whole, do not break, crush, or chew.

Patient/Family Teaching

- Instruct patient to take medication as directed. Take missed doses as soon as remembered unless almost time for next dose; do not double doses. Consult health care professional prior to stopping quetiapine; should be discontinued gradually. Stopping abruptly may cause insomnia, nausea, and vomiting.
- Advise patient and caregiver that quetiapine should not be given to elderly patients with dementia-related psychosis; may ↑ risk of death.
- Inform patient of the possibility of extrapyramidal symptoms. Instruct patient to report symptoms immediately to health care professional.
- Advise patient to change positions slowly to minimize orthostatic hypotension.
- May cause drowsiness. Caution patient to avoid driving or other activities requiring alertness until response to medication is known.
- Advise patient to avoid extremes in temperature; this drug impairs body temperature regulation.
- Advise patient to notify health care professional of all Rx or OTC medications, vitamins, or herbal products being taken and to consult with health care professional before taking other medications and alcohol, especially other CNS depressants.
- Advise patient and family to notify health care professional if thoughts about suicide or dying, attempts to commit suicide; new or worse depression; new or worse anxiety; feeling very agitated or restless; panic attacks; trouble sleeping; new or worse irritability; acting aggressive; being angry or violent; acting on dangerous impulses; an extreme increase in activity and talking; other unusual changes in behavior or mood occur.
- Refer patient for nutritional, weight, or medical management of dyslipidemia as indicated.
- Advise patient to notify health care professional of medication regimen before treatment or surgery.
- Instruct patient to notify health care professional promptly of sore throat, fever, unusual bleeding or bruising, or rash.
- Advise female patients to notify health care professional if pregnancy is planned or suspected or if they are breast feeding or planning to breast feed.
- Emphasize importance of routine follow-up exams to monitor side effects and continued participation in psychotherapy as indicated to improve coping skills. Ophthalmologic exams should be performed before and every 6 mo during therapy.

Evaluation/Desired Outcomes

- Decrease in excited, manic, behavior.
- Decrease in signs of depression in patients with bipolar disorder.
- Decrease in manic episodes in patients with bipolar I disorder.
- Decrease in positive symptoms (delusions, hallucinations) of schizophrenia.
- Decrease in negative symptoms (social withdrawal, flat, blunt affect) of schizophrenia.

quinapril, See ANGIOTENSIN-CONVERTING ENZYME (ACE) INHIBITORS.

quinupristin/dalfopristin

(kwin-oo-**pris**-tin/dal-foe-**pris**-tin)

Synercid

Classification

Therapeutic: anti-infectives

Pharmacologic: streptogramins

Pregnancy Category B

Indications

Complicated skin/skin structure infections caused by *Staphylococcus aureus* (methicillin, susceptible) or *Streptococcus pyogenes*.

Action

Quinupristin inhibits the late phase of protein synthesis at the level of the bacterial ribosome; dalfopristin inhibits the early phase. **Therapeutic Effects:** Bacteriostatic effect against susceptible organisms. **Spectrum:** Active against, *S. aureus* (methicillin-susceptible) and *S. pyogenes*. Not active against *Enterococcus faecalis* or *Enterococcus faecium*.

Pharmacokinetics

Absorption: IV administration results in complete bioavailability.

Distribution: Unknown.

Protein Binding: Moderate.

Metabolism and Excretion: Both are converted to compounds with additional anti-infective activity; parent drugs and metabolites are mostly excreted in feces (75–77%); 15% of quinupristin and 17% of dalfopristin excreted in urine.

Half-life: *Quinupristin*—0.85 hr; *dalfopristin*—0.7 hr.

TIME/ACTION PROFILE

ROUTE	ONSET	PEAK	DURATION
IV	rapid	end of infusion	8–12 hr

Contraindications/Precautions

Contraindicated in: Hypersensitivity.

Use Cautiously in: Concurrent use of other drugs metabolized by the cytochrome P450 3A4 enzyme system (serious interactions may occur); Hepatic impairment (dose adjustment may be necessary); Patients with a history of GI disease, especially colitis; OB, Lactation, Pedi: Pregnancy, lactation, or children <12 yr (safety not established).

Adverse Reactions/Side Effects

CNS: headache. **CV:** thrombophlebitis. **GI:** CLOSTRIDIUM DIFFICILE-ASSOCIATED DIARRHEA (CDAD), diarrhea, nausea, vomiting. **Derm:** pruritus, rash. **Local:** edema/inflammation/pain at infusion site, infusion site reactions. **Misc:** allergic reactions including ANAPHYLAXIS, pain.

Interactions

Drug-Drug: Inhibits the cytochrome P450 3A4 drug metabolizing enzyme system; inhibits metabolism of **cyclosporine**, **midazolam**, and **nifedipine** and ↑ risk of toxicity (careful monitoring required). Similar effects may be expected with concurrent use of **delavirdine**, **nevirapine**, **indinavir**, **ritonavir**, **vinca alkaloids**, **docetaxel**, **paclitaxel**, **diazepam**, **verapamil**, **diltiazem**, **HMG CoA reductase inhibitors**, **tacrolimus**, **methylprednisolone**, **carbamazepine**, **quinidine**, **lidocaine**, and **disopyramide**.

Route/Dosage

IV (Adults and Children 12–17 yr): 7.5 mg/kg q 12 hr for at least 7 days.

Availability

Powder for injection: 500 mg/vial (150 mg quinupristin and 350 mg dalfopristin), 600 /vial (180 mg quinupristin and 420 mg dalfopristin).

NURSING IMPLICATIONS

Assessment

- Assess patient for infection (vital signs; appearance of wound, sputum, urine, and stool; WBC) at beginning of and throughout therapy.
- Obtain specimens for culture and sensitivity before initiating therapy. First dose may be given before receiving results.
- Monitor patient for pain or inflammation at the infusion site frequently throughout infusion. Increasing the volume of diluent from 250 mL to 500 mL or 750 mL or infusing via a peripherally inserted central catheter or central venous catheter may be required.
- Observe patient for signs and symptoms of anaphylaxis (rash, pruritus, laryngeal edema, wheezing). Discontinue drug and notify physician or other health care professional immediately if these problems occur. Keep epinephrine, an antihistamine, and resuscitation equipment close by in case of an anaphylactic reaction.
- Assess patient for myalgia and arthralgia after infusion. May be severe. Reducing dose frequency to every 12 hr may decrease pain. Symptoms usually resolve upon discontinuation of medication.
- ***Lab Test Considerations:*** May cause ↑ serum total bilirubin concentrations.

Potential Nursing Diagnoses

Risk for infection (Indications, Side Effects)
Diarrhea (Adverse Reactions)

Implementation

IV Administration

- **Intermittent Infusion:** Reconstitute the 500-mg vial with 5 mL and the 600-mg vial with 6 mL of D5W or sterile water for injection, respectively, for a concentration of 100 mg/mL. Avoid shaking to prevent foam formation. Allow solution to sit until all foam has disappeared. ***Diluent:*** Dilute further with 250 mL of D5W (100 mL can be used for central line administration). May dilute in 500 mL or 750 mL of D5W if severe venous irritation occurs after peripheral administration. Reconstituted vials should be used within 30 min. Infusion is stable for 5 hr at room temperature or 54 hr if refrigerated. ***Rate:*** Infuse over 60 min. Flush line before and after infusion with D5W.
- **Y-Site Compatibility:** alemtuzumab, alfentanil, amikacin, amiodarone, anidulafungin, argatroban, aztreonam, bleomycin, buprenorphine, busulfan, butorphanol, carboplatin, carmustine, caspofungin, chlorpromazine, ciprofloxacin, cisatracurium, cisplatin, cyclophosphamide, cyclosporine, cytarabine, dacarbazine, daptomycin, daunorubicin, dexmedetomidine, dexrazoxane, diltiazem, diphenhydramine, docetaxel, dolasetron, doxacurium, doxarubicin, doxycycline, droperidol, enalaprilat, ephedrine, epinephrine, epirubicin, esmolol, etoposide, etoposide phosphate, fenoldopam, fentanyl, fluconazole, gemcitabine, granisetron, haloperidol, hydromorphone, idarubicin, ifosfamide, isoproterenol, labetalol, levofloxacin, levorphanol, lidocaine, linezolid, lorazepam, magnesium sulfate, mannitol, mechlorethamine, meperidine, metoclopramide, metoprolol, midazolam, milrinone, mitomycin, mitoxantrone, morphine, mycophenolate, nalbuphine, naloxone, nesiritide, nicardipine, nitroglycerin, octreotide, ondansetron, oxaliplatin, oxytocin, paclitaxel, palonosetron, pamidronate, pancuronium, pentamidine, phenylephrine, potassium chloride, procainamide, prochlorperazine, promethazine, propranolol, rocuronium, sodium phosphates, succinylcholine, sufentanil, tacrolimus, teniposide, theophylline, thiotepa, tirofiban, tobramycin, vasopressin, vecuronium, verapamil, vinblastine, vincristine, vinorelbine, voriconazole, zidovudine, zoledronic acid.

- **Y-Site Incompatibility:** acyclovir, amifostine, aminophylline, amphotericin B colloidal, amphotericin B lipid complex, amphotericin B liposome, ampicillin, ampicillin/sulbactam, azithromycin, bivalirudin, bumetanide, calcium chloride, calcium gluconate, cefazolin, cefepime, cefotaxime, cefotetan, cefoxitin, ceftazidime, ceftriaxone, cefuroxime, clindamycin, dexamethasone sodium phosphate, diazepam, digoxin, ertapenem, fludarabine, fluorouracil, fosphenytoin, furosemide, ganciclovir, heparin, hydrocortisone, imipenem/cilastatin, insulin, ketorolac, leucovorin, meropenem, mesna, methotrexate, methylprednisolone sodium succinate, metronidazole, nitroprusside, pantoprazole, pemetrexed, pentobarbital, phenobarbital, phenytoin, piperacillin/tazobactam, potassium acetate, potassium phosphates, ranitidine, rituximab, sodium acetate, sodium bicarbonate, thiopental, tigecycline, trimethoprim/sulfamethoxazole.
- **Solution Incompatibility:** 0.9% NaCl.

Patient/Family Teaching

- Instruct patient to notify health care professional if signs and symptoms of anaphylaxis, fever, and diarrhea develop, especially if stool contains blood, pus, or mucus. Advise patient not to treat diarrhea without consulting health care professional.

Evaluation/Desired Outcomes

- Resolution of signs and symptoms of infection. Length of time for complete resolution depends on the organism and site of infection.

Q

RABEprazole (ra-bep-ra-zole)

Aciphex, Aciphex Sprinkle, ✱Pariet

Classification
Therapeutic: antiulcer agents
Pharmacologic: proton-pump inhibitors

Pregnancy Category C

Indications

Gastroesophageal reflux disease (GERD). Duodenal ulcers (including combination therapy with clarithromycin and amoxicillin to erradicate *Helicobacter pylori* and prevent recurrence). Pathological hypersecretory conditions, including Zollinger-Ellison syndrome.

Action

Binds to an enzyme in the presence of acidic gastric pH, preventing the final transport of hydrogen ions into the gastric lumen. **Therapeutic Effects:** Diminished accumulation of acid in the gastric lumen, with lessened acid reflux. Healing of duodenal ulcers and esophagitis. Decreased acid secretion in hypersecretory conditions.

Pharmacokinetics

Absorption: Delayed-release tablet is designed to allow rabeprazole, which is not stable in gastric acid, to pass through the stomach intact. Subsequently 52% is absorbed after oral administration.
Distribution: Unknown.
Protein Binding: 96.3%.
Metabolism and Excretion: Mostly metabolized by the liver (hepatic cytochrome P450 3A and 2C19 enzyme systems) (the CYP2C19 enzyme system exhibits genetic polymorphism; 15–20% of Asian patients and 3–5% of Caucasian and Black patients may be poor metabolizers and may have significantly ↑ rabeprazole concentrations and an ↑ risk of adverse effects); 10% excreted in feces; remainder excreted in urine as inactive metabolites.
Half-life: 1–2 hr.

TIME/ACTION PROFILE (acid suppression)

ROUTE	ONSET	PEAK	DURATION
PO	within 1 hr	unknown	24 hr†

†Suppression continues to increase over the first week of therapy.

Contraindications/Precautions

Contraindicated in: Hypersensitivity to rabeprazole or related drugs (benzimidazoles).
Use Cautiously in: Severe hepatic impairment (dose reduction may be necessary); Patients using high-doses for >1 yr (↑ risk of hip, wrist, or spine fractures); Patients using therapy for >3 yr (↑ risk of vitamin B_{12} deficiency; OB, Lactation, Pedi: Pregnancy, lactation, or children <12 yr (breast feeding not recommended; use in pregnancy only if needed; safety not established).

Adverse Reactions/Side Effects

CNS: dizziness, headache, malaise. **GI:** CLOSTRIDIUM DIFFICILE-ASSOCIATED DIARRHEA (CDAD), abdominal pain, constipation, diarrhea, nausea. **Derm:** photosensitivity, rash. **F and E:** hypomagnesemia (especially if treatment duration ≥3 mo). **GU:** acute interstitial nephritis. **MS:** bone fracture, neck pain. **Hemat:** vitamin B_{12} deficiency. **Misc:** allergic reactions, chills, fever.

Interactions

Drug-Drug: Rabeprazole is metabolized by the CYP450 enzyme system and may interact with other drugs metabolized by this sytem. May ↓ absorption of drugs requiring acid pH, including **ketoconazole**, **itraconazole**, **atazanavir**, **ampicillin esters**, **iron salts**, **erlotinib**, and **mycophenolate mofetil**; concomitant use with **atazanavir** not recommended. May ↑ levels of **digoxin** and **methotrexate**. Hypomagnesemia ↑ risk of **digoxin** toxicity. May ↑ the risk of bleeding with **warfarin** (monitor INR/PT).

Route/Dosage

Gastroesophageal Reflux Disease

PO (Adults): *Healing of erosive or ulcerative GERD*—20 mg once daily for 4–8 wk; *Maintenance of healing of erosive or ulcerative GERD*—20 mg once daily; *Symptomatic GERD*—20 mg once daily for 4 wk (additional 4 wk may be considered for non-responders).
PO (Children ≥12 yr): *Short-term treatment of symptomatic GERD*—20 mg once daily for up to 8 wk.
PO (Children 1–11 yr): *≥15 kg*—10 mg once daily for up to 12 wk (given as sprinkle); *<15 kg*—5 mg once daily for up to 12 wk (given as sprinkle); may ↑ up to 10 mg once daily if inadequate response.

Duodenal Ulcers

PO (Adults): *Healing of duodenal ulcers*—20 mg once daily for up to 4 wk.

H. pylori Eradication to Reduce the Risk of Duodenal Ulcer Recurrence (Triple Therapy)

PO (Adults): 20 mg twice daily for 7 days with amoxicillin 1000 mg twice daily for 7 days and clarithromycin 500 mg twice daily for 7 days.

R

Pathological Hypersecretory Conditions Including Zollinger-Ellison Syndrome

PO (Adults): 60 mg once daily initially, may be adjusted as needed and continued as necessary; doses up to 100 mg daily or 60 mg twice daily have been used.

Availability (generic available)

Delayed-release capsules (Sprinkle): 5 mg, 10 mg. **Delayed-release tablets:** ✤ 10 mg, 20 mg.

NURSING IMPLICATIONS

Assessment

- Assess routinely for epigastric or abdominal pain and frank or occult blood in the stool, emesis, or gastric aspirate.
- Monitor bowel function. Diarrhea, abdominal cramping, fever, and bloody stools should be reported to health care professional promptly as a sign of Clostridium difficile-associated diarrhea (CDAD). May begin up to several weeks following cessation of therapy.
- ***Lab Test Considerations:*** Monitor CBC with differential periodically during therapy.
- May cause hypomagnesemia. Monitor serum magnesium prior to and periodically during therapy.

Potential Nursing Diagnoses

Acute pain (Indications)

Implementation

- ***High Alert:*** Do not confuse rabeprazole with aripiprazole. Do not confuse Aciphex with Accupril or Aricept.
- **PO:** Administer doses before meals, preferably in the morning. Tablets should be swallowed whole; do not break, crush, or chew.
- *Aciphex Sprinkle:* open capsule and sprinkle granule contents on a small amount of soft food (apple sauce, fruit, or vegetable-based baby food, yogurt) or empty contents into small amount of liquid (infant formula, apple juice, pediatric electrolyte solution). Food or liquid should be at or below room temperature. Whole dose should be taken within 15 min of being sprinkled. Granules should not be chewed or crushed. Dose should be taken 30 min before a meal. Do not store mixture for future use.

Patient/Family Teaching

- Instruct patient to take medication as directed for the full course of therapy, even if feeling better. Take missed doses as soon as remembered but not if almost time for next dose. Do not double doses.
- May cause occasional drowsiness or dizziness. Caution patient to avoid driving or other activities requiring alertness until response to medication is known.
- Advise patient to avoid alcohol, products containing aspirin or NSAIDs, and foods that may cause an increase in GI irritation.
- Caution patients to wear sunscreen and protective clothing to prevent photosensitivity reactions.
- Advise patient to report onset of black, tarry stools; diarrhea; abdominal pain; or persistent headache to health care professional promptly.
- Instruct patient to notify health care professional of all Rx or OTC medications, vitamins, or herbal products being taken and consult health care professional before taking any new medications.
- Instruct patient to notify health care professional of onset of black, tarry stools; diarrhea; abdominal pain; or persistent headache or if fever and diarrhea develop, especially if stool contains blood, pus, or mucus. Advise patient not to treat diarrhea without consulting health care professional.
- Advise female patients to notify health care professional if pregnancy is planned or suspected or if breast feeding.

Evaluation/Desired Outcomes

- Decrease in abdominal pain or prevention of gastric irritation and bleeding. Healing of duodenal ulcers can be seen on x-ray examination or endoscopy.
- Decrease in symptoms of GERD. Therapy is continued for 4–8 wk after initial episode.

raloxifene (ra-**lox**-i-feen)

Evista

Classification
Therapeutic: bone resorption inhibitors
Pharmacologic: selective estrogen receptor modulators

Pregnancy Category X

Indications

Treatment and prevention of osteoporosis in postmenopausal women. Reduction of the risk of breast cancer in postmenopausal women with osteoporosis and those at high risk for invasive breast cancer.

Action

Binds to estrogen receptors, producing estrogen-like effects on bone, resulting in reduced resorption of bone and decreased bone turnover. **Therapeutic Effects:** Prevention of osteoporosis in patients at risk. Decreased risk of breast cancer.

Pharmacokinetics

Absorption: Although well absorbed (>60%), after oral administration, extensive first-pass metabolism results in 2% bioavailability.

Distribution: Highly bound to plasma proteins; remainder of distribution unknown.

Protein Binding: Highly bound to plasma proteins.

Metabolism and Excretion: Extensively metabolized by the liver; undergoes enterohepatic cycling; excreted primarily in feces.

Half-life: 27.7 hr.

TIME/ACTION PROFILE (effects on bone turnover)

ROUTE	ONSET	PEAK	DURATION
PO	unknown	3 mo	unknown

Contraindications/Precautions

Contraindicated in: Hypersensitivity; History of thromboembolic events; OB, Lactation: Not indicated for women with childbearing potential or who are breast feeding; Pedi: Safety not established.

Use Cautiously in: Potential immobilization (↑ risk of thromboembolic events); History of stroke or transient ischemic attack; Atrial fibrillation; Hypertension; Cigarette smoking.

Adverse Reactions/Side Effects

CNS: STROKE. **CV:** THROMBOEMBOLISM. **EENT:** retinal vein thrombosis. **MS:** leg cramps. **Misc:** hot flashes.

Interactions

Drug-Drug: Cholestyramine ↓ absorption (avoid concurrent use). May alter effects of **warfarin** and other **highly protein-bound drugs**. Concurrent systemic **estrogen** therapy is not recommended.

Route/Dosage

PO (Adults): 60 mg once daily.

Availability (generic available)

Tablets: 60 mg. **Cost:** $630.76/100.

NURSING IMPLICATIONS

Assessment

- Assess patient for bone mineral density with x-ray, serum, and urine bone turnover markers (bone-specific alkaline phosphatase, osteocalcin, and collagen breakdown products) before and periodically during therapy.
- ***Lab Test Considerations:*** May cause ↑ apolipoprotein A-I and reduced serum total cholesterol, LDL cholesterol, fibrinogen, apolipoprotein B, and lipoprotein.
- May cause ↑ hormone-binding globulin (sex steroid-binding globulin, thyroxine-binding globulin, corticosteroid-binding globulin) with ↑ total hormone concentrations.
- May cause small ↓ in serum total calcium, inorganic phosphate, total protein, and albumin.
- May also cause slight decrease in platelet count.

Potential Nursing Diagnoses

Risk for injury (Indications)

Implementation

- **PO:** May be administered without regard to meals.
- Calcium supplementation should be added to diet if daily intake is inadequate.

Patient/Family Teaching

- Instruct patient to take raloxifene as directed. Discuss the importance of adequate calcium and vitamin D intake or supplementation. Instruct patient to read the *Medication Guide* when initiating therapy and again with each prescription refill in case of changes.
- Advise patient to discontinue smoking and alcohol consumption.
- Emphasize the importance of regular weight-bearing exercise. Advise patient that raloxifene should be discontinued at least 72 hr before and during prolonged immobilization (recovery from surgery, prolonged bedrest). Instruct patient to avoid prolonged restrictions of movement during travel because of the increased risk of venous thrombosis.
- Advise patient that raloxifene will not reduce hot flashes or flushes associated with estrogen deficiency and may cause hot flashes.
- Instruct patient to notify health care professional immediately if leg pain or a feeling of warmth in the lower leg (calf); swelling of the legs, hands, or feet; sudden chest pain; shortness of breath or coughing up blood; or sudden change in vision, such as loss of vision or blurred vision occur. Being still for a long time (sitting still during a long car or airplane trip, being in bed after surgery) can increase risk of blood clots.
- Advise patient that raloxifene may have teratogenic effects. Instruct patient to notify health care provider immediately if pregnancy is planned or suspected or if breast feeding.

Evaluation/Desired Outcomes

- Prevention of osteoporosis in postmenopausal women.
- Reduced risk of breast cancer in postmenopausal women with osteoporosis and those at high risk for invasive breast cancer.

raltegravir (ral-teg-ra-veer)

Isentress

Classification

Therapeutic: antiretrovirals

Pharmacologic: integrase strand transfer inhibitors (INSTIs)

Pregnancy Category C

Indications

HIV-1 infection (with other antiretrovirals) in treatment-experienced or treatment-naïve patients.

Action

Inhibits HIV-1 integrase, which is required for viral replication. **Therapeutic Effects:** Evidence of de-

R

creased viral replication and reduced viral load with slowed progression of HIV and its sequelae.

Pharmacokinetics

Absorption: Well absorbed following oral administration.

Distribution: Unknown.

Metabolism and Excretion: Mostly metabolized by the uridine diphosphate glucuronosyltransferase (UGT) A1A enzyme system; 23% excreted in urine as parent drug and metabolite.

Half-life: 9 hr.

TIME/ACTION PROFILE (blood levels)

ROUTE	ONSET	PEAK	DURATION
PO	unknown	3 hr	12 hr

Contraindications/Precautions

Contraindicated in: Lactation: Breast feeding not recommended in HIV-infected patients.

Use Cautiously in: Concurrent use of medications associated with rhabdomyolysis/myopathy (may ↑ risk); Phenylketonuria (chewable tablets contain phenylalanine); Geri: Choose dose carefully, considering concurrent disease states, drug therapy, and age-related ↓ in hepatic and renal function; OB: Use in pregnancy only if maternal benefit outweighs fetal risk; Pedi: Children <4 wk (safety and effectiveness not established).

Adverse Reactions/Side Effects

CNS: SUICIDAL THOUGHTS, headache, depression, dizziness, fatigue, insomnia, weakness. **CV:** MYOCARDIAL INFARCTION. **GI:** diarrhea, abdominal pain, gastritis, hepatitis, nausea, vomiting. **GU:** renal failure/impairment. **Hemat:** anemia, neutropenia. **Metab:** lipodystrophy. **Derm:** STEVENS JOHNSON SYNDROME, TOXIC EPIDERMAL NECROLYSIS, rash. **MS:** RHABDOMYOLYSIS, ↑ creatine kinase, myopathy. **Misc:** hypersensitivity reactions, immune reconstitution syndrome, fever.

Interactions

Drug-Drug: Concurrent use with **strong inducers of the UGT A1A enzyme system** including **rifampin** may ↓ blood levels and effectiveness. Concurrent use with **strong inhibitors of the UGT A1A enzyme system** including **atazanavir** may ↑ blood levels. ↑ risk of rhabomyolysis/myopathy **HMG-CoA reductase inhibitors**. **Proton pump inhibitors** may ↑ levels. **Efavirenz, etravirine**, and **tipranavir/ritonavir** may ↓ levels. Administration with **antacids**, containing **magnesium** or **aluminum** ↓ absorption of raltegravir; separate administration of raltegravir and magnesium- or aluminum-containing antacids by ≥6 hr.

Route/Dosage

PO (Adults): 400 mg twice daily; ↑ dose to 800 mg twice daily when used with rifampin.

PO (Children ≥4 wk and ≥25 kg): *Tablet*—400 mg twice daily; *Chewable tablets (if unable to swallow tablet)*—25–28 kg: 150 mg twice daily; 28–39.9 kg: 200 mg twice daily; ≥40 kg: 300 mg twice daily.

PO (Children ≥4 wk and 20–<25 kg): *Chewable tablets*—150 mg twice daily.

PO (Children ≥4 wk and 14–<20 kg): *Oral suspension*—100 mg twice daily; *Chewable tablets*—100 mg twice daily.

PO (Children ≥4 wk and 11–<14 kg): *Oral suspension*—80 mg twice daily; *Chewable tablets*—75 mg twice daily.

PO (Children ≥4 wk and 8–<11 kg): *Oral suspension*—60 mg twice daily.

PO (Children ≥4 wk and 6–<8 kg): *Oral suspension*—40 mg twice daily.

PO (Children ≥4 wk and 4–<6 kg): *Oral suspension*—30 mg twice daily.

PO (Children ≥4 wk and 3–<4 kg): *Oral suspension*—20 mg twice daily.

Availability

Tablets: 400 mg. **Chewable tablets (orange-banana):** 25 mg, 100 mg. **Packet for oral suspension:** 100 mg.

NURSING IMPLICATIONS

Assessment

- Assess patient for change in severity of HIV symptoms and for symptoms of opportunistic infections during therapy.
- Monitor for anxiety, depression (especially in patients with a history of psychiatric illness), suicidal ideation, and paranoia during therapy.
- Assess for rash periodically during therapy. May cause Stevens-Johnson syndrome. Discontinue therapy if severe or if accompanied with fever, general malaise, fatigue, muscle or joint aches, blisters, oral lesions, conjunctivitis, hepatitis, and/or eosinophilia.
- ***Lab Test Considerations:*** Monitor viral load and CD4 counts regularly during therapy.
- May casue ↓ ANC, hemoglobin, and platelet counts.
- May cause ↑ serum glucose, AST, ALT, GGT, total bilirubin, alkaline phosphatase, pancreatic amylase, serum lipase, and creatinine kinase concentrations.

Potential Nursing Diagnoses

Risk for infection (Indications)
Noncompliance (Patient/Family Teaching)

Implementation

- Tablets are not interchangeable with chewable tablets or packets for oral suspension.
- **PO:** May be administered without regard to meals.
- Swallow tablets whole; do not break, crush, or chew.
- Chewable tablets may be chewed or swallowed.
- Pour packet for oral solution into 5 mL of water and mix. Once mixed, administer with syringe orally within 30 min of mixing. Discard unused solution.

Patient/Family Teaching

- Emphasize the importance of taking raltegravir as directed, at evenly spaced times throughout day. Do not take more than prescribed amount and do not stop taking without consulting health care professional. Take missed doses as soon as remembered unless almost time for next dose. Do not double doses. Advise patient to read *Patient Information* sheet before starting therapy and with each Rx renewal in case of changes.

- Instruct patient that raltegravir should not be shared with others.
- Instruct patient to notify health care professional of all Rx or OTC medications, vitamins, or herbal products being taken and consult health care professional before taking any new medications.
- Inform patient that raltegravir does not cure AIDS or prevent associated or opportunistic infections. Raltegravir does not reduce the risk of transmission of HIV to others through sexual contact or blood contamination. Caution patient to use a condom during sexual contact and to avoid sharing needles or donating blood to prevent spreading the AIDS virus to others. Advise patient that the long-term effects of raltegravir are unknown at this time.
- Advise patient to notify health care professional if they develop any unusual symptoms, if any known symptom persists or worsen, or if signs and symptoms of rhabdomyolysis (unexplained muscle pain, tenderness, weakness), rash, or depression or suicidal thoughts occur.
- Immune reconstitution syndrome may trigger opportunistic infections or autoimmune disorders. Notify health care professional if symptoms occur.
- Advise patients to notify health care professional if pregnancy is planned or suspected and to avoid breast feeding.
- Emphasize the importance of regular follow-up exams and blood counts to determine progress and monitor for side effects.

Evaluation/Desired Outcomes

- Delayed progression of AIDS and decreased opportunistic infections in patients with HIV.
- Decrease in viral load and improvement in CD4 cell counts.

ramelteon (ra-mel-tee-on)

Rozerem

Classification

Therapeutic: sedative/hypnotics

Pharmacologic: melatonin receptor agonists

Pregnancy Category C

Indications

Treatment of insomnia characterized by difficult sleep onset.

Action

Activates melatonin receptors, which promotes maintenance of circadian rhythm, a part of the sleep-wake cycle. **Therapeutic Effects:** Easier onset of sleep.

Pharmacokinetics

Absorption: Well absorbed (84%), but bioavailability is low (1.8%) due to extensive first pass liver metabolism. Absorption ↑ by a high fat meal.

Distribution: Widely distributed to body tissues.

Metabolism and Excretion: Extensively metabolized by the liver; mainly by CYP1A2 enzyme system. Metabolites are excreted mostly in urine (88%); 4% excreted in feces.

Half-life: 1–2.6 hr.

TIME/ACTION PROFILE (blood levels)

ROUTE	ONSET	PEAK	DURATION
PO	rapid	30–90 min	unknown

Contraindications/Precautions

Contraindicated in: Hypersensitivity; History of angioedema with previous use; Severe hepatic impairment; Concurrent use of fluvoxamine; Lactation: Lactation; Pedi: Safety not established.

Use Cautiously in: Depression or history of suicidal ideation; Moderate hepatic impairment; Concurrent use of CYP3A4 inhibitors, such as ketoconazole; Concurrent use of CYP2C9 inhibitors, such as fluconazole; OB: Use only if maternal benefit outweighs fetal risk.

Adverse Reactions/Side Effects

CNS: abnormal thinking, behavior changes, dizziness, fatigue, hallucinations, headache, insomnia (worsened), sleep—driving. **GI:** nausea. **Endo:** ↑ prolactin levels, ↓ testosterone levels. **Misc:** ANGIOEDEMA.

Interactions

Drug-Drug: Blood levels and effects are ↑ by **fluvoxamine**; concurrent use is contraindicated. Levels and effects may be ↓ by **rifampin**. Concurrent use of CYP3A4 inhibitors, such as **ketoconazole**, may ↑ levels and effects; use cautiously. Concurrent use of CYP2C9 inhibitors, such as **fluconazole**, may ↑ levels and effects; use cautiously. **Donepezil** and **doxepin** may ↑ levels. ↑ risk of excessive CNS depression with other CNS depressants including **alcohol**, **benzodiazepines**, **opioids**, and other **sedative/hypnotics**.

Route/Dosage

PO (Adults): 8 mg within 30 min of going to bed.

Availability (generic available)

Tablets: 8 mg.

R

NURSING IMPLICATIONS

Assessment

- Assess sleep patterns before and periodically throughout therapy.

Potential Nursing Diagnoses

Insomnia (Indications)
Risk for injury (Side Effects)

Implementation

- Do not confuse Rozerem (ramelteon) with Razadyne (galantamine).
- Do not administer with or immediately after a high-fat meal.
- Before administering, reduce external stimuli and provide comfort measures to increase effectiveness of medication.
- **PO:** Administer 30 min prior to going to bed.

Patient/Family Teaching

- Instruct patient to take ramelteon as directed, within 30 min of going to bed and to confine activities to those necessary to prepare for bed. Instruct patient to read the *Medication Guide* before starting and with each Rx refill; changes may occur.
- Causes drowsiness. Caution patient to avoid driving and other activities requiring alertness until response to medication is known.
- Caution patient that complex sleep-related behaviors (sleep-driving, making phone calls, preparing and eating food, having sex, sleep walking) may occur while asleep. Inform patient to notify health care professional if sleep-related behaviors (may include sleep-driving—driving while not fully awake after ingestion of a sedative-hypnotic product, with no memory of the event) occur.
- Advise patient to notify health care professional immediately if signs of anaphylaxis (swelling of the tongue or throat, trouble breathing, and nausea and vomiting) or angioedema (severe facial swelling) occur; may occur as early as the first time the product is taken.
- Caution patient to avoid concurrent use of alcohol or other CNS depressants.
- Advise female patients to notify health care professional if pregnancy is planned or suspected or if breast feeding.

Evaluation/Desired Outcomes

- Relief of insomnia.

ramipril, See ANGIOTENSIN-CONVERTING ENZYME (ACE) INHIBITORS.

ramucirumab

(ra-mue-**sir**-ue-mab)
Cyramza

Classification
Therapeutic: antineoplastics
Pharmacologic: vascular endothelial growth factor antagonists

Pregnancy Category C

Indications

Treatment of advanced gastric cancer or gastro-esophageal junction adenocarcinoma following unsuccessful combination treatment that included a fluoropyrimidine or platinum compound (as monotherapy or in combination with paclitaxel). Treatment of metastatic non-small cell lung cancer (NSCLC) with disease progression on or after platinum-based chemotherapy (in combination with docetaxel). Treatment of metastatic colorectal cancer with disease progression on or after treatment with bevacizumab, oxaliplatin, and a fluoropyrimidine (in combination with irinotecan, folinic acid, and 5–fluorouracil [FOLFIRI]).

Action

A monoclonal antibody that binds to vascular endothelial growth factor receptor 2 (VEGFR 2), antagonizing its effects, resulting in decreased angiogenesis. **Therapeutic Effects:** Decreased growth and spread of gastric cancer, gastro-esophageal junction adenocarcinoma, NSCLC, and colorectal cancer.

Pharmacokinetics

Absorption: IV administration results in complete bioavailability.
Distribution: Unknown.
Metabolism and Excretion: Unknown.
Half-life: Unknown.

TIME/ACTION PROFILE (improved survival)

ROUTE	ONSET	PEAK	DURATION
IV	within 1 mo	7–8 mos	24 mos

Contraindications/Precautions

Contraindicated in: OB: May cause fetal harm; Lactation: Discontinue ramucirumab or discontinue breast feeding.
Use Cautiously in: Child-Pugh Class B or C cirrhosis (use only if benefits outweigh risk of further deterioration); Surgery (discontinue prior to surgery, reinstate when healing is complete); Hypertension (must be controlled prior to treatment); OB: Patients with reproductive potential (effective contraception should be practiced during and for at least 3 mo following treatment); Pedi: Safety and effectiveness not established.

Adverse Reactions/Side Effects

CNS: REVERSIBLE POSTERIOR LEUKOENCEPHALOPATHY SYNDROME, headache. **CV:** ARTERIAL THROMBOTIC

EVENTS, hypertension. **Endo:** hypothyroidism. **GI:** GASTROINTESTINAL OBSTRUCTION/PERFORATION, diarrhea, worsened cirrhosis/hepatorenal syndrome, diarrhea. **GU:** impaired female fertility, nephrotic syndrome, proteinuria. **F and E:** hyponatremia. **Hemat:** BLEEDING, neutropenia. **Misc:** infusion-related reactions, impaired wound healing.

Interactions

Drug-Drug: ↑ risk of bleeding with **anticoagulants, antiplatelet agents** and **NSAIDs.**

Route/Dosage

Gastric Cancer

IV (Adults): 8 mg/kg every 2 wk continued until disease progression or intolerance; dose adjustment/interruption/discontinuation required for drug-related toxicities.

NSCLC

IV (Adults): 10 mg/kg on Day 1 of a 21–day cycle prior to docetaxel; continued until disease progression or intolerance; dose adjustment/interruption/discontinuation required for drug-related toxicities.

Colorectal Cancer

IV (Adults): 8 mg/kg every 2 wk prior to FOLFIRI administrated; continued until disease progression or intolerance; dose adjustment/interruption/discontinuation required for drug-related toxicities.

Availability

Solution for intravenous infusion (requires further dilution): 10 mg/mL.

NURSING IMPLICATIONS

Assessment

- Monitor for infusion-related reactions (rigors/tremors, back pain/spasms, chest pain and/or tightness, chills, flushing, dyspnea, wheezing, hypoxia, paresthesia, bronchospasm, supraventricular tachycardia, hypotension) during infusion. Reduce infusion rate by 50% for Grade 1 or 2 reactions, and immediately and permanently discontinue ramucirumab if Grade 3 or 4 reactions occur.
- Monitor BP prior to and at least every 2 wks during therapy. Interrupt therapy for severe hypertension until BP is under control. Permanently discontinue if unable to control hypertension.
- Avoid administration prior to surgery or until wound is healed.
- If arterial thromboembolic events (myocardial infarction, cardiac arrest, cerebrovascular accident, cerebral ischemia), GI perforation, or Grade 3 or 4 bleeding occur, permanently discontinue.
- ***Lab Test Considerations:*** Monitor urinary protein periodically during therapy. Interrupt ramucirumab for urine protein ≥2 g/24 hrs. Reinitiate therapy at reduced dose of 6 mg/kg every 2 wks once urinary protein levels <2 g/24 hrs. If protein level returns to ≥2 g/24 hrs interrupt therapy and reduce dose to 5 mg/kg every 2 wks once urinary protein levels return to <2 g/24 hrs. Discontinue therapy permanently if urine protein level >3 g/24 hrs or if nephrotic syndrome occurs.

Potential Nursing Diagnoses

Deficient knowledge, related to medication regimen (Patient/Family Teaching)

Implementation

- Prior to each dose, premedicate all patients with IV histamine H_1 antagonist (diphenhydramine). Premedicate patients who have experienced a Grade 1 or 2 infusion reaction with dexamethasone and acetaminophen prior to each infusion.

IV Administration

- **Intermittent Infusion:** Withdraw required volume from vial. ***Diluent:*** Dilute with 0.9% NaCl for a final volume of 250 mL. Do not use dextrose-containing solutions. Gently invert to ensure adequate mixing. Solution is clear to slightly opalescent and colorless to slightly yellow; do not administer solutions that are discolored or contain particulate material. Solution is stable for 24 hr if refrigerated or 4 hrs at room temperature. Discard unused solution. ***Rate:*** Infuse over 60 min via infusion pump through a separate infusion line using a 0.22 micron filter; do not administer as IV push or bolus. Flush line with 0.9% NaCl at end of infusion.
- **Y-Site Incompatibility:** Do not dilute with other solutions or infuse with other electrolyte solutions or medications.

Patient/Family Teaching

- Explain purpose of ramucirumab to patient.
- Advise patient to notify health care professional if bleeding or lightheadedness occur.
- Instruct patient in self BP monitoring and advise patient to notify health care professional if signs and symptoms of hypertension (elevated BP, severe headache, lightheadedness, neurologic symptoms) or if severe diarrhea, vomiting, or severe abdominal pain occur.
- Advise to notify health care professional of medication regimen prior to surgery; may impair wound healing.
- Advise female patient that ramucirumab may impair fertility and to use effective contraception during and for at least 3 mo after last dose. Notify health care professional if pregnancy is suspected and avoid breast feeding during therapy.

R

Evaluation/Desired Outcomes

- Decreased growth and spread of cancer.

ranitidine, See HISTAMINE H_2 ANTAGONISTS.

ranolazine (ra-nole-a-zeen)

Ranexa

Classification
Therapeutic: antianginals

Pregnancy Category C

Indications

Chronic angina pectoris.

Action

Does not ↓ BP or heart rate; remainder of mechanism is not known. **Therapeutic Effects:** Decreased frequency of angina.

Pharmacokinetics

Absorption: Highly variable.

Distribution: Unknown.

Metabolism and Excretion: Metabolized in the gut (P-glycoprotein) and by the liver (primarily CYP3A and less by CYP2D6); <5% excreted unchanged in urine and feces.

Half-life: 7 hr.

TIME/ACTION PROFILE (blood levels)

ROUTE	ONSET	PEAK	DURATION
PO	unknown	2–5 hr	12 hr

Contraindications/Precautions

Contraindicated in: Hypersensitivity; Concurrent use of potent inhibitors of CYP3A; Concurrent use of inducers of CYP3A; Hepatic impairment; Lactation: Lactation.

Use Cautiously in: Renal impairment; OB: Use only when potential benefit outweighs risk to fetus; Pedi: Safety not established; Geri: ↑ risk of adverse reactions in patients >75 yr.

Adverse Reactions/Side Effects

CNS: dizziness, headache. **EENT:** tinnitus. **CV:** TORSADES DE POINTES, palpitations, QTc prolongation. **GI:** abdominal pain, constipation, dry mouth, nausea, vomiting. **GU:** acute renal failure.

Interactions

Drug-Drug: Ketoconazole, **itraconazole**, **clarithromycin**, **nefazodone**, **nelfinavir**, **ritonavir**, **indinavir**, and **saquinavir** significantly ↑ levels; concurrent use contraindicated. **Rifampin**, **rifabutin**, **rifapentin**, **phenobarbital**, **phenytoin**, and **carbamazepine** significantly ↓ levels; concurrent use contraindicated. **Verapamil**, **diltiazem**, **aprepitant**, **erythromycin**, and **fluconazole** ↑ levels (do not exceed ranolazine dose of 500 mg twice daily). **Cyclosporine** may ↑ levels. **Paroxetine** may ↑ levels. May ↑ levels of **simvastatin**. May ↓ metabolism and ↑ effects of **metoprolol**, **tricyclic antidepressants**, and **antipsychotics**; dosage adjustments may be necessary. May ↑ **digoxin** levels; dose adjustment may be required.

Drug-Natural Products: St. John's wort significantly ↓ levels (contraindicated).

Drug-Food: Grapefruit juice↑ levels (do not exceed ranolazine dose of 500 mg twice daily).

Route/Dosage

PO (Adults): 500 mg twice daily initially, may be ↑ to 1000 mg twice daily.

Availability (generic available)

Extended-release tablet: 500 mg.

NURSING IMPLICATIONS

Assessment

- Assess location, duration, intensity, and precipitating factors of anginal pain.
- Monitor ECG at baseline and periodically during therapy to evaluate effects on QT interval.
- ***Lab Test Considerations:*** Monitor renal function after starting and periodically during therapy in patients with moderate to severe renal impairment (CCr < 60 mL/min) for ↑ serum creatinine accompanied by ↑ BUN. Usually has a rapid onset, but does not progress during therapy and is reversible with discontinuation of ranolazine. If acute renal failure develops, discontinue ranolazine.
- May cause transient eosinophilia.
- May cause small mean ↓ in hematocrit.

Potential Nursing Diagnoses

Ineffective tissue perfusion (Indications)
Activity intolerance (Indications)

Implementation

- Ranolazine should be used in combination with amlodipine, beta blockers, or nitrates.
- Do not administer with grapefruit juice or grapefruit products.
- **PO:** May be administered without regard to food. Tablets should be swallowed whole; do not break, crush, or chew.

Patient/Family Teaching

- Instruct patient to take ranolazine as directed. If a dose is missed, take the usual dose at the next scheduled time; do not double doses. Explain to patient that ranolazine is used for chronic therapy and will not help an acute angina episode.
- Advise patient to avoid grapefruit juice and grapefruit products when taking ranolazine.
- May cause dizziness and light-headedness. Caution patient to avoid driving and other activities requiring alertness until response to medication is known.

- Advise patient to notify health care professional if fainting occurs.
- Inform patient that ranolazine may cause changes in the ECG. Patient should inform health care professional if they have a personal or family history of QTc prolongation, congenital long QT syndrome, or proarrhythmic conditions such as hypokalemia.
- Instruct patient to notify health care professional of all Rx or OTC medications, vitamins, or herbal products being taken and consult health care professional before taking any new medications.

Evaluation/Desired Outcomes

- Decrease in frequency of angina attacks.

rasagiline (ra-za-ji-leen)

Azilect

Classification

Therapeutic: antiparkinson agents
Pharmacologic: monoamine oxidase type B inhibitors

Pregnancy Category C

Indications

Parkinson's disease.

Action

Irreversibly inactivates monoamine oxidase (MAO) by binding to it at type B (brain sites); inactivation of MAO leads to increased amounts of dopamine available in the CNS. Differs from selegiline by its nonamphetamine characteristics. **Therapeutic Effects:** Improvement in symptoms of Parkinson's disease, allowing increase in function.

Pharmacokinetics

Absorption: 36% absorbed following oral administration.

Distribution: Readily crosses the blood-brain barrier.

Metabolism and Excretion: Extensively metabolized by the liver (CYP1A2 enzyme) to an inactive metabolite; less than 1% excreted in urine.

Half-life: 1.3 hr; does not correlate with duration of MAO-B inhibition.

TIME/ACTION PROFILE

ROUTE	ONSET	PEAK	DURATION
PO	rapid	1 hr	40 days*

*Recovery of MAO-B function.

Contraindications/Precautions

Contraindicated in: Hypersensitivity; Concurrent meperidine, tramadol, methadone, sympathomimetic amines, dextromethorphan, mirtazapine, cyclobenzaprine, cocaine, St. John's wort, or another MAO inhibitor; Moderate to severe hepatic impairment; Elective surgery requiring general anesthesia; allow 14 days after discontinuation; Pheochromocytoma; Psychotic disorder.

Use Cautiously in: Mild hepatic impairment (↑ blood levels); OB: Use only if maternal benefit outweighs fetal risk; Lactation: May inhibit lactation; Pedi: Safety not established.

Adverse Reactions/Side Effects

CNS: depression, dizziness, drowsiness, hallucinations, impulse control disorders (gambling, sexual), malaise, sleep driving, vertigo. **EENT:** conjunctivitis, rhinitis. **Resp:** asthma. **CV:** orthostatic hypotension (may ↑ levodopa-induced hypotension), ↑ BP, chest pain, syncope. **GI:** anorexia, dizziness, dyspepsia, gastroenteritis, vomiting. **GU:** albuminuria, ↓ libido. **Derm:** alopecia, ecchymosis, ↑ melanoma risk, rash. **Endo:** weight loss. **Hemat:** leukopenia. **MS:** arthralgia, arthritis, neck pain. **Neuro:** dyskinesia (may ↑ levodopa-induced dyskinesia), paresthesia. **Misc:** allergic reactions, flu-like syndrome, ↑ fall risk, fever.

Interactions

Drug-Drug: Concurrent use of **meperidine, tramadol, methadone**, or other **MAO inhibitors** may ↑ risk of serotonin syndrome; concurrent use contraindicated. **Ciprofloxacin** and other **inhibitors of the CYP1A2 enzyme** ↑ rasagiline levels; dose adjustment is recommended. Concurrent use with **dextromethorphan** may result in psychosis/bizarre behavior and should be avoided. ↑ risk of adverse reactions with **mirtazapine** and **cyclobenzapine**; concurrent use should be avoided. Hypertensive crisis may occur with **sympathomimetic amines** including **amphetamines, cold products**, and some **weight loss products** containing **vasoconstrictors** such as **pseudoephedrine, phenylephrine**, or **ephedrine**; avoid concurrent use. ↑ risk of serotonin syndrome with **tricyclic antidepressants, SSRI antidepressants**, and **SNRI antidepressants**; rasagiline should be discontinued ≥14 days prior to initiation of antidepressants (**fluoxetine** should be discontinued ≥5 wk prior to rasagiline therapy).

Drug-Natural Products: Risk of toxicity is ↑ with **St. John's wort**.

Drug-Food: Ingestion of foods containing high amounts of **tyramine** (>150 mg) (e.g., cheese) may result in life-threatening hypertensive crisis.

Route/Dosage

PO (Adults): *Monotherapy or as adjunct therapy in patients not taking levodopa*—1 mg once daily; *Concurrent levodopa therapy*—0.5 mg once daily, may ↑ to 1 mg once daily; *Concurrent ciprofloxacin or other CYP1A2 inhibitors*—0.5 mg once daily.

Hepatic Impairment

PO (Adults): *Mild hepatic impairment*—0.5 mg daily.

Availability (generic available)

Tablets: 0.5 mg, 1 mg.

NURSING IMPLICATIONS

Assessment

- Assess signs and symptoms of Parkinson's disease (tremor, muscle weakness and rigidity, ataxic gait) prior to and during therapy.
- Monitor BP periodically during therapy.
- Assess skin for melanomas periodically during therapy.
- Assess for serotonin syndrome (mental changes [agitation, hallucinations, coma], autonomic instability [tachycardia, labile BP, hyperthermia], neuromuscular aberrations [hyperreflexia, incoordination], and/or GI symptoms [nausea, vomiting, diarrhea]), especially in patients taking other serotonergic drugs (SSRIs, SNRIs, triptans).
- ***Lab Test Considerations:*** May cause albuminuria, leukopenia, and abnormal liver function tests.
- ***Toxicity and Overdose:*** Concurrent ingestion of tyramine-rich foods and many medications may result in a life-threatening hypertensive crisis. Signs and symptoms of hypertensive crisis include chest pain, tachycardia or bradycardia, severe headache, neck stiffness or soreness, nausea and vomiting, sweating, photosensitivity, and enlarged pupils.

Potential Nursing Diagnoses

Impaired physical mobility (Indications)
Risk for injury (Indications, Side Effects)

Implementation

- Do not confuse Azilect (rasagiline) with Aricept (donepezil).
- If used in combination with levodopa, a reduction in levodopa dose may be considered based on individual results.
- **PO:** Administer once daily.

Patient/Family Teaching

- Instruct patient to take rasagiline as directed. Missed doses should be omitted and next dose taken at usual time the following day. Do not double doses. Do not discontinue abruptly; may cause elevated temperature, muscular rigidity, altered consciousness, and autonomic instability.
- Caution patient to avoid alcohol, CNS depressants, and foods or beverages containing tyramine (see Appendix J) during and for at least 2 wk after therapy has been discontinued; they may precipitate a hypertensive crisis. Contact health care professional immediately if symptoms of hypertensive crisis or serotonin syndrome develop.
- Instruct patient to notify health care professional of all Rx or OTC medications, vitamins, or herbal products being taken and consult health care professional before taking any new medications. Caution patient to avoid use of St. John's wort and analgesics meperidine, tramadol, or methadone during therapy.
- Caution patient to avoid elective surgery requiring general anesthesia, cocaine, or local anesthesia containing sympathomimetic vasoconstrictors within 14 days of discontinuing rasagiline. If surgery is necessary sooner, benzodiazepines, rapacuronium, fentanyl, morphine, and codeine may be used cautiously.
- May cause dizziness or drowsiness. Caution patient to avoid driving and other activities requiring alertness until response to medication is known.
- Caution patient to change positions slowly to minimize orthostatic hypotension. Geriatric patients are at increased risk for this side effect.
- Advise patient to monitor for melanomas frequently and on a regular basis.
- Caution patient to notify health care professional if new skin lesions, agitation, aggression, delirium, hallucinations, sleep driving or new or increased gambling, sexual, or other intense urges occur.
- Advise patient to notify health care professional immediately if severe headache, neck stiffness, heart racing, or palpitations, occur.
- Advise female patients to notify health care professionals if pregnancy is planned or suspected or if breast feeding.

Evaluation/Desired Outcomes

- Improvement in symptoms of Parkinson's disease, allowing increase in function.

rasburicase

(ras-**byoor**-i-case)
Elitek, ✱Fasturtec

Classification
Therapeutic: antigout agents, antihyperuricemics
Pharmacologic: enzymes

Pregnancy Category C

Indications

Initial management of increased uric acid levels in patients with leukemia, lymphoma, or other malignancies who are being treated with antineoplastics, which are expected to produce hyperuricemia.

Action

An enzyme that promotes the conversion of uric acid to allantoin, an inactive, water-soluble compound. Produced by recombinant DNA technology. **Therapeutic Effects:** Decreased sequelae of hyperuricemia (nephropathy, arthropathy).

Pharmacokinetics

Absorption: IV administration results in complete bioavailability.
Distribution: Unknown.
Metabolism and Excretion: Unknown.
Half-life: 18 hr.

TIME/ACTION PROFILE (↓ in uric acid)

ROUTE	ONSET	PEAK	DURATION
IV	rapid	unknown	4–24 hr

Contraindications/Precautions

Contraindicated in: G6PD deficiency (↑ risk of severe hemolysis); Previous allergic reaction, hemolysis, or methemoglobinemia from rasburicase; Lactation: Lactation.

Use Cautiously in: OB: Pregnancy (use only if clearly needed).

Adverse Reactions/Side Effects

CNS: headache. **Resp:** respiratory distress. **GI:** abdominal pain, constipation, diarrhea, nausea, vomiting, mucositis. **Derm:** rash. **Hemat:** HEMOLYSIS, METHEMOGLOBINEMIA, neutropenia. **Misc:** hypersensitivity reactions including ANAPHYLAXIS, fever, sepsis.

Interactions

Drug-Drug: None known.

Route/Dosage

IV (Adults and Children): 0.2 mg/kg daily as a single dose for 5 days.

Availability

Lyophilized powder for reconstitution: 1.5 mg/vial.

NURSING IMPLICATIONS

Assessment

- Monitor patients for signs of allergic reactions and anaphylaxis (chest pain, dyspnea, hypotension, urticaria). If these signs occur, rasburicase should be immediately and permanently discontinued.
- ***Lab Test Considerations:*** Monitor patients for hemolysis. Screen patients at higher risk for G6PD deficiency (patients of African American or Mediterranean ancestry) prior to therapy. If hemolysis occurs, discontinue and do not restart rasburicase.
- Monitor patients for methemoglobinemia. Discontinue rasburicase and do not restart in patients who develop methemoglobinemia.
- May cause spuriously low uric acid levels in blood samples left at room temperature. Collect blood for uric acid levels in pre-chilled tubes containing heparin and immediately immerse and maintain in an ice water bath. Uric acid must be analyzed in plasma. Plasma samples must be assayed within 4 hr of collection.

Potential Nursing Diagnoses

Deficient knowledge, related to medication regimen (Patient/Family Teaching)

Implementation

- Chemotherapy is initiated 4–24 hr after first dose of rasburicase.

IV Administration

- **Intermittent Infusion:** Determine number of vials of rasburicase needed based on patient's weight and dose/kg. Reconstitute in diluent provided. Add 1 mL of diluent provided to each vial and mix by swirling very gently. Do not shake or vortex. Solution should be clear and colorless. Do not use solutions that are discolored or contain particulate matter. ***Diluent:*** Remove dose from reconstituted vials and inject into infusion bag of 0.9% NaCl for a final total volume of 50 mL. Administer within 24 hr of reconstitution. Store reconstituted or diluted solution in refrigerator for up to 24 hr. ***Rate:*** Administer over 30 min. Do not administer as a bolus.
- **Y-Site Incompatibility:** Infuse through a separate line. Do not use a filter with infusion. If separate line is not possible, flush line with at least 15 mL of 0.9% NaCl prior to rasburicase infusion.

Patient/Family Teaching

- Inform patient and family of purpose of rasburicase infusion.

Evaluation/Desired Outcomes

- Decrease in plasma uric acid levels in pediatric patients receiving antineoplastics expected to result in tumor lysis and subsequent elevation of plasma uric acid levels. More than 1 course of therapy or administration beyond 5 days is not recommended.

R

regorafenib (re-goe-**raf**-e-nib)

Stivarga

Classification
Therapeutic: antineoplastics
Pharmacologic: kinase inhibitors

Pregnancy Category D

Indications

Metastatic colorectal cancer (CRC) that has failed previous treatment that included a fluoropyrimidine, oxiplatin, irinotecan, an anti-VEGF therapy, and additional anti-EGFR therapy if tumor is of the KRAS wild type.

Action

Inhibits kinases, which are responsible for many phases of cell function and proliferation. **Therapeutic Effects:** Decreased progression of metastatic CRC with improved survival.

Pharmacokinetics

Absorption: Well absorbed following oral administration (69–83%).

Distribution: Unknown.

Protein Binding: *Regorafenib*— >99.5%, *M-2 metabolite*—99.8%, *M-5 metabolite*—99.95%.

Metabolism and Excretion: Highly metabolized (by CYP3A4 and UGT1A9), 2 metabolites (M-2 and M-5) have antineoplastic activity. Undergoes enterohepatic circulation.

Half-life: *Regorafenib*—28 hr (range 14–58 hr), *M-2 metabolite*—25 hr (range 14–32 hr), *M-5 metabolite*—51 hr (range 32–70 hr). 47% excreted in feces as parent compound, 24% as metabolites; 19% excreted in urine (mostly as inactive metabolites).

TIME/ACTION PROFILE (improved survival)

ROUTE	ONSET	PEAK	DURATION
PO	3 mo	3 mo	up to 10 mo

Contraindications/Precautions

Contraindicated in: Avoid strong inducers/inhibitors of CYP3A4; Lactation: Breast feeding should be avoided; OB: May cause fetal harm; Severe hepatic impairment (Child-Pugh Class C).

Use Cautiously in: History of hypertension/cardiovascular disease (BP should be controlled prior to treatment); Elective surgical procedures (discontinue 2 wk prior to surgery); OB: Patients with reproductive potential (effective contraception should be practiced during and for 2 mo following treatment); Pedi: Safety and effectiveness not established.

Adverse Reactions/Side Effects

CNS: REVERSIBLE POSTERIOR LEUKOENCEPHALOPATHY, fatigue, headache. **EENT:** dysphonia. **CV:** CARDIAC ISCHEMIA/INFARCTION, HYPERTENSION. **GI:** GASTROINTESTINAL FISTULA/PERFORATION, HEPATOTOXICITY, ↓ appetite, diarrhea, mucositis, altered taste, dry mouth, gastrointestinal reflux, ↑ transaminases. **Derm:** PLANTAR ERYTHRODYSTHESIA, alopecia, impaired wound healing, rash. **Endo:** hypothyroidism. **F and E:** hypocalcemia, hypokalemia, hypophosphatemia, hyponatremia. **GU:** proteinuria. **Hemat:** BLEEDING, THROMBOCYTOPENIA, anemia, lymphopenia. **Metab:** weight loss, ↑ lipase, ↑ amylase. **MS:** pain, musculoskeletal stiffness. **Neuro:** tremor. **Misc:** HYPERSENSITIVITY REACTIONS, INFECTION, fever.

Interactions

Drug-Drug: **Strong inhibitors of CYP3A4** including **clarithromycin**, **itraconazole**, **ketoconazole**, **posaconazole**, **telithromycin**, and **voriconazole** ↑ blood levels and the risk of toxicity, avoid concurrent use. **Strong inducers of CYP3A4** including **carbamazepine**, **phenobarbital**, **phenytoin**, and **rifampin** ↓ blood levels and effectiveness, avoid concurrent use. May ↑ risk of bleeding with **warfarin**.

Drug-Natural Products: **St. John's wort** ↓ blood levels and effectiveness, avoid concurrent use.

Drug-Food: **Grapefruit juice** ↑ blood levels and the risk of toxicity, avoid concurrent use.

Route/Dosage

PO (Adults): 160 mg daily on days 1–21 of a 28-day cycle. Dose modifications required for hematologic toxicity, dermatologic toxicity, or hypertension. Discontinuation may be necessary for life-threatening toxicities.

Availability

Tablets: 40 mg.

NURSING IMPLICATIONS

Assessment

- Monitor BP prior to and weekly during the first 6 wk, then every cycle of therapy. Do not initiate regorafenib until BP is well controlled.
- Assess for cardiac ischemia or infarction during therapy.
- Assess for bleeding during therapy. Interrupt therapy if severe hemorrhage occurs.
- ***Lab Test Considerations:*** Obtain liver function test (ALT, AST, bilirubin) before starting, at least every 2 wk during first 2 mo of therapy, and monthly thereafter. Monitor liver function tests weekly in patients with ↑ liver function tests until improvement to <3 × the upper limit of normal or baseline.
- May cause anemia, thrombocytopenia, neutropenia, and lymphopenia.
- May cause hypocalcemia, hypokalemia, hyponatremia, and hypophosphatemia.
- May cause proteinuria, ↑ serum lipase, and ↑ serum amylase.
- May cause ↑ INR. Monitor INR levels more frequently in patients receiving warfarin.

Potential Nursing Diagnoses

Risk for impaired skin integrity
Deficient knowledge, related to medication regimen (Patient/Family Teaching)

Implementation

- ***High Alert:*** Fatalities have occurred with incorrect administration of chemotherapeutic agents. Before administering, clarify all ambiguous orders; double check single, daily, and course-of-therapy dose limits; have second practitioner independently double check original order and dose calculations. Therapy should be initiated by physician experienced in the treatment of patients with colorectal cancer.
- **PO:** Administer four 40 mg tablets once daily at same time of day with a whole glass of water for the first 21 days of the of each 28-day cycle. Swallow tablets whole with a low-fat meal that contains <30% fat and <600 calories.
- **Dose modifications:** *Interrupt therapy for* Grade 2 hand-foot skin reaction (HFSR) that is recurrent or does not improve in 7 days despite dose reduc-

tion; interrupt therapy for a minimum of 7 days for Grade 3 (HFSR), symptomatic Grade 2 hypertension, any Grade 3 or 4 adverse reactions.

- *Reduce dose to 120 mg daily for* first occurrence of Grade 2 HFSR of any duration, after first recovery of any Grade 3 or 4 adverse reaction, for Grade 3 ↑ AST or ALT; only resume if potential benefit outweighs risk of hepatotoxicity.
- *Reduce dose to 80 mg daily for* re-occuuence of Grade 2 HFSR at 120 mg dose, after recovery of any Grade 3 or 4 adverse reaction at 120 mg dose (except hepatotoxicity).
- *Discontinue regorafenib permanently for* failure to tolerate 80 mg dose, any occurrence of ↑ AST or ALT >20 × upper limit of normal, any occurrence of ↑ AST or ALT >3 × upper limit of normal with concurrent bilirubin >2 × upper limit of normal, re-occurrence of ↑ AST or ALT >5 × upper limit of normal despite reduction to 120 mg dose, any Grade 4 adverse reaction; only resume if the potential benefits outweigh the risks.

Patient/Family Teaching

- Instruct patient to take tablets at the same time each day with a low-fat meal. Take missed doses on the same day as soon as remembered; do not take 2 doses on the same day to make up for a missed dose. Store medicine in original container; do not place in daily or weekly pill boxes. Discard remaining tablets 28 days after opening bottle. Tightly close bottle after each opening and keep desiccant in bottle.
- Advise patient to avoid drinking grapefruit juice or eating grapefruit during regorafenib therapy.
- Advise patient to notify health care professional immediately if signs and symptoms of liver problems (yellowing of skin or white part of eyes, nausea, vomiting, dark tea-colored urine, change in sleep pattern), bleeding, skin changes (redness, pain, blisters, bleeding, swelling), hypertension (severe headache, lightheadedness, neurologic symptoms), myocardial ischemia or infarction (chest pain, shortness of breath, dizziness, fainting), or GI perforation or fistula (severe abdominal pain, persistent swelling of abdomen, high fever, chills, nausea, vomiting, severe diarrhea, dehydration) occur.
- Advise patient to notify health care provider of therapy prior to surgery or if had recent surgery.
- Advise patient to maintain adequate hydration to minimize risk and to notify health care professional promptly if signs and symptoms of reversible posterior leukoencephalopathy syndrome (RPLS) (headache, seizures, weakness, confusion, high BP, blindness or change in vision, problems thinking) occur.
- Instruct patient to notify health care professional of all Rx or OTC medications, vitamins, or herbal products being taken and consult health care professional before taking any new medications, especially St. John's wort.
- Inform female patient that regorafenib can cause fetal harm. Advise women with reproductive potential and men of the need for effective contraception during and for at least 2 mo after completion of therapy. Notify health care provider immediately if pregnancy is planned or suspected or if breast feeding.
- Emphasize importance of monitoring lab values to monitor for adverse reactions.

Evaluation/Desired Outcomes

- Decreased progression of metastatic CRC.

reteplase, See THROMBOLYTIC AGENTS.

Rh_0(D) IMMUNE GLOBULIN
(arr aych oh dee im-**yoon glob**-yoo-lin)

Rh_0(D) immune globulin standard dose IM
HyperRHO S/D Full Dose, RhoGAM

Rh_0(D) immune globulin microdose IM
HyperRHO S/D Mini-Dose, MICRhoGAM, Mini-Gamulin R

Rh_0(D) immune globulin IV
WinRho SDF

Rh_0(D) immune globulin microdose IM, IV
Rhophylac

Classification
Therapeutic: vaccines/immunizing agents
Pharmacologic: immune globulins

Pregnancy Category C

Indications

IM, IV: Administered to Rh_0(D)-negative patients who have been exposed to Rh_0(D)-positive blood by: Pregnancy or delivery of a Rh_0(D)-positive infant, Abortion of a Rh_0(D)-positive fetus, Fetal-maternal hemorrhage due to amniocentesis, other obstetrical manipulative procedure, or intra-abdominal trauma while carrying a Rh_0(D)-positive fetus, Transfusion of Rh_0(D)-positive blood or blood products to a Rh_0(D)-negative patient. **IV:** Management of immune thrombocytopenic purpura (ITP).

Action

Prevent production of anti-Rh_0(D) antibodies in Rh_0(D)-negative patients who were exposed to Rh_0(D)-positive blood. Increase platelet counts in patients with ITP. **Therapeutic Effects:** Prevention of antibody response and hemolytic disease of the newborn (erythroblastosis fetalis) in future pregnancies of women who have conceived a Rh_0(D)-positive fetus. Prevention of Rh_0(D) sensitization following transfusion accident. Decreased bleeding in patients with ITP.

Pharmacokinetics

Absorption: Completely absorbed with IV administration. Well absorbed from IM sites.
Distribution: Unknown.
Metabolism and Excretion: Unknown.
Half-life: approximately 25–30 days.

TIME/ACTION PROFILE (blood levels)

ROUTE	ONSET	PEAK	DURATION
IM	rapid	5–10 days	unknown
IV†	unknown	2 hr	unknown

†When given for ITP, platelet counts start to rise in 1–2 days, peak after 5–7 days, and last for 30 days.

Contraindications/Precautions

Contraindicated in: Prior hypersensitivity reaction to human immune globulin; Rh_0(D)- or Du-positive patients.
Use Cautiously in: ITP patients with pre-existing anemia (decrease dose if Hgb <10 g/dL). May also cause disseminated intravascular coagulation in ITP patients.

Adverse Reactions/Side Effects

CNS: dizziness, headache. **CV:** hypertension, hypotension. **Derm:** rash. **GI:** diarrhea, nausea, vomiting. **GU:** acute renal failure. **Hemat:** *ITP*— DISSEMINATED INTRAVASCULAR COAGULATION, INTRAVASCULAR HEMOLYSIS, anemia. **MS:** arthralgia, myalgia. **Local:** pain at injection site. **Misc:** fever.

Interactions

Drug-Drug: May ↓ antibody response to some **live-virus vaccines (measles, mumps, rubella)**.

Route/Dosage

Rh_0(D) Immune Globulin (for IM use only)

Following Delivery

IM (Adults): *HyperRHO S/D Full Dose, RhoGAM*— 1 vial standard dose (300 mcg) within 72 hr of delivery.

Before Delivery

IM (Adults): *HyperRHO S/D Full Dose, RhoGAM*— 1 vial standard dose (300 mcg) at 26–28 wk.

Termination of Pregnancy (<13 wk Gestation)

IM (Adults): *HyperRHO S/D Mini-Dose, MICRhoGAM*— 1 vial of microdose (50 mcg) within 72 hr.

Termination of Pregnancy (>13 wk Gestation)

IM (Adults): *RhoGAM*— 1 vial standard dose (300 mcg) within 72 hr.

Large Fetal-Maternal Hemorrhage (>15 mL)

IM (Adults): *RhoGAM*— 20 mcg/mL of Rh_0(D)-positive fetal RBCs.

Transfusion Accident

IM (Adults): *HyperRHO S/D Full Dose, RhoGAM*— (Volume of Rh-positive blood administered × Hct of donor blood)/15 = number of vials of standard dose (300 mcg) preparation (round to next whole number of vials).

Rh_0(D) Immune Globulin IV (for IM or IV Use)

Following Delivery

IM, IV (Adults): *WinRho SDF*— 600 IU (120 mcg) within 72 hr of delivery. *Rhophylac*— 1500 IU (300 mcg) within 72 hr of delivery.

Prior to Delivery

IM, IV (Adults): *WinRho SDF, Rhophylac*— 1500 IU (300 mcg) at 28 wk; if initiated earlier in pregnancy, repeat q 12 wk.

Following Amniocentesis or Chorionic Villus Sampling

IM, IV (Adults): *WinRho SDF (before 34 wk gestation)*— 1500 IU (300 mcg) immediately; repeat q 12 wk during pregnancy. *Rhophylac*— 1500 IU (300 mcg) within 72 hr of procedure.

Termination of Pregnancy, Amniocentesis, or Any Other Manipulation

IM, IV (Adults): *WinRho SDF*— 600 IU (120 mcg) within 72 hr after event.

Large Fetal-Maternal Hemorrhage/Transfusion Accident

IM (Adults): *WinRho SDF*— 6000 IU (1200 mcg) q 12 hr until total dose is given (total dose determined by amount of blood loss/hemorrhage).
IV (Adults): 3000 IU (600 mcg) q 8 hr until total dose is given (total dose determined by amount of blood loss/hemorrhage).

Immune Thrombocytopenic Purpura

IV (Adults and Children): *WinRho SDF, Rhophylac*— 50 mcg (250 IU)/kg initially (if Hgb <10 g/dL, ↓ dose to 25–40 mcg [125–200 IU]/kg); further dosing/frequency determined by clinical response (range 25–60 mcg [125–300 IU]/kg). Each dose may be given as a single dose or in 2 divided doses on separate days.

Availability

Rh_0(D) Immune Globulin (for IM Use)

Injection: 50 mcg/vial (microdose—MICRhoGAM, HyperRHO S/D Mini-Dose), 300 mcg/vial (standard dose—RhoGAM, HyperRHO S/D Full Dose).

Rh_0(D) Immune Globulin Intravenous (for IM or IV Use)

Injection: 600 IU (120 mcg)/vial, 1500 IU (300 mcg)/vial, 2500 IU (500 mcg)/vial, 5000 IU (1000 mcg)/vial, 15,000 IU (3000 mcg)/vial. **Prefilled syringes:** 1500 IU (300 mcg/2 mL).

NURSING IMPLICATIONS

Assessment

- **IV:** Assess vital signs periodically during therapy in patients receiving IV Rh_0(D) immune globulin.
- **ITP:** Monitor patient for signs and symptoms of intravascular hemolysis (IVH) (back pain, shaking chills, fever, hemoglobinuria), anemia, and renal insufficiency. If transfusions are required, use Rh_0(D)-negative packed red blood cells to prevent exacerbation of IVH.
- ***Lab Test Considerations:*** *Pregnancy:* Type and crossmatch of mother and newborn's cord blood must be performed to determine need for medication. Mother must be Rh_0(D)-negative and Du-negative. Infant must be Rh_0(D)-positive. If there is doubt regarding infant's blood type or if father is Rh_0(D)-positive, medication should be given.
- An infant born to a woman treated with Rh_0(D) immune globulin antepartum may have a weakly positive direct Coombs' test result on cord or infant blood.
- *ITP:* Monitor platelet counts, RBC counts, hemoglobin, and reticulocyte levels to determine effectiveness of therapy.

Potential Nursing Diagnoses

Deficient knowledge, related to medication regimen (Patient/Family Teaching)

Implementation

- Do not give to infant, to Rh_0(D)-positive individual, or to Rh_0(D)-negative individual previously sensitized to the Rh_0(D) antigen. However, there is no more risk than when given to a woman who is not sensitized. When in doubt, administer Rh_0(D) immune globulin.
- Do not confuse IM and IV formulations. Rh immune globulin for IV administration is labelled "Rh Immune Globulin Intravenous." Rh Immune Globulin Intravenous may be given IM; however, Rh Immune Globulin (microdose and standard dose) is for IM use only and cannot be given IV.
- When using prefilled syringes, allow solution to reach room temperature before administration.
- **IM:** Reconstitute Rh_0(D) immune globulin IV for IM use immediately before use with 1.25 mL of 0.9% NaCl. Inject diluent onto inside wall of vial and wet pellet by gently swirling until dissolved. Do not shake.
- Administer into the deltoid muscle. Dose should be given within 3 hr but may be given up to 72 hr after delivery, miscarriage, abortion, or transfusion.

IV Administration

- **IV Push:** Reconstitute Rh_0(D) immune globulin IV for IV administration immediately before use with 2.5 mL of 0.9% NaCl. Inject diluent onto inside wall of vial and wet pellet by gently swirling until dissolved. Do not shake. ***Rate:*** Administer over 3–5 min.

Patient/Family Teaching

- **Pregnancy:** Explain to patient that the purpose of this medication is to protect future Rh_0(D)-positive infants.
- **ITP:** Explain purpose of medication to patient.

Evaluation/Desired Outcomes

- Prevention of erythroblastosis fetalis in future Rh_0(D)-positive infants.
- Prevention of Rh_0(D) sensitization following incompatible transfusion.
- Decreased bleeding episodes in patients with ITP.

R

ribavirin (rye-ba-**vye**-rin)

Copegus, Ribasphere, Virazole

Classification
Therapeutic: antivirals
Pharmacologic: nucleoside analogues

Pregnancy Category X

Indications

Inhaln: Treatment of severe lower respiratory tract infections caused by the respiratory syncytial virus (RSV) in infants and young children. **PO:** *Copegus and Ribasphere*—with peginterferon alfa-2a (Pegasys) in the treatment of chronic hepatitis C in patients with compensated liver disease who have not previously been treated with interferon alfa. **Unlabeled Use:** Early (within 24 hr of symptoms) secondary treatment of influenza A or B in young adults.

Action

Inhibits viral DNA and RNA synthesis and subsequent replication. Must be phosphorylated intracellularly to be active. **Therapeutic Effects: Inhaln:** Virustatic action. **PO:** Decreased progression and sequelae of chronic hepatitis C.

Pharmacokinetics

Absorption: Systemic absorption occurs following nasal and oral inhalation. Rapidly and extensively absorbed following oral administration, but undergoes first-pass hepatic metabolism (64% bioavailability).
Distribution: 70% of inhaled drug is deposited in the respiratory tract. Appears to concentrate in the respiratory tract and red blood cells. Enters breast milk.
Metabolism and Excretion: Eliminated from the respiratory tract by distribution across membranes, macrophages, and ciliary motion. Metabolized primarily by the liver; metabolites are renally excreted.
Half-life: *Inhaln*—9.5 hr (40 days in RBCs); *oral*—43.6 hr (single dose); 12 days (multiple dose).

TIME/ACTION PROFILE (blood levels)

ROUTE	ONSET	PEAK	DURATION
Inhaln	unknown	end of inhaln	unknown
PO	unknown	1.7–3 hr	12 hr

Contraindications/Precautions

Contraindicated in: Hypersensitivity; Patients receiving mechanically assisted ventilation; OB, Lactation: Pregnancy or lactation; OB: Male partners of pregnant patients; CCr <50 mL/min; Significant/unstable cardiovascular disease; Hemoglobinopathies; Autoimmune hepatitis or hepatic decompensation before/during treatment (for combined therapy with interferon alfa-2b or peginterferon alfa-2a); Concurrent use of didanosine, stavudine, or zidovudine.
Use Cautiously in: Sarcoidosis (may exacerbate condition); Anemia (dose reduction/discontinuation may be required); Any pre-existing cardiac disease; Rep: Women with childbearing potential; Pedi: May result in ↓ growth.

Adverse Reactions/Side Effects

Inhalation.
CNS: dizziness, faintness. **EENT:** blurred vision, conjunctivitis, erythema of the eyelids, ocular irritation, photosensitivity. **CV:** CARDIAC ARREST, hypotension. **Derm:** rash. **Hemat:** hemolytic anemia (with interferon alpha 2b), reticulocytosis.

Oral (may reflect combination with interferon)

CNS: HOMICIDAL IDEATION, SUICIDAL IDEATION/ATTEMPTS, depression, aggressive behavior, emotional lability (↑ in children), fatigue (↓ in children), impaired concentration (↓ in children), insomnia (↓ in children), irritability (↓ in children). **EENT:** dry mouth, optic neuritis, papilledema, retinal artery/vein thrombosis, retinal detachment, retinal hemorrhage, retinopathy (with macular edema), visual abnormalities. **Resp:** dyspnea (↓ in children). **GI:** anorexia (↑ in children), dyspepsia (↓ in children), vomiting (↑ in children). **Hemat:** hemolytic anemia. **Derm:** STEVENS-JOHNSON SYNDROME, pruritus (↓ in children). **MS:** arthralgia (↓ in children). **Misc:** fever (↑ in children).

Interactions

Drug-Drug: Oral: May ↓ the antiretroviral action of **stavudine** and **zidovudine**. May ↑ hematologic toxicity of **zidovudine**. May ↑ risk of pancytopenia when used with **azathioprine**. May ↑ blood levels and risk of toxicity of **didanosine**. Although used together in the management of hepatitis, concurrent use with **interferon alpha 2b** ↑ risk of hemolytic anemia.

Route/Dosage

Inhaln (Infants and Young Children): 300 mL of 20 mg/mL solution delivered via mist for 12–18 hr/day.

Copegus or Ribasphere—viral genotype 1 or 4 (with peginterferon alfa-2a)

PO (Adults ≥75 kg): 600 mg twice daily for 48 wk.
PO (Adults <75 kg): 500 mg twice daily for 48 wk.
PO (Children ≥5 yr and ≥75 kg): 600 mg in the morning, then 600 mg in the evening for 48 wk.
PO (Children ≥5 yr and 60–74 kg): 400 mg in the morning, then 600 mg in the evening for 48 wk.
PO (Children ≥5 yr and 47–59 kg): 400 mg in the morning, then 400 mg in the evening for 48 wk.
PO (Children ≥5 yr and 34–46 kg): 200 mg in the morning, then 400 mg in the evening for 48 wk.
PO (Children ≥5 yr and 23–33 kg): 200 mg in the morning, then 200 mg in the evening for 48 wk.

Renal Impairment

PO (Adults): *CCr 30–50 mL/min*—200 mg/day alternating with 400 mg/day every other day for 48 wk; *CCr <30 mL/min or Hemodialysis*—200 mg once daily for 48 wk.

Copegus or Ribasphere—viral genotype 2 or 3 (with peginterferon alfa-2a)

PO (Adults): 400 mg twice daily for 24 wk.
PO (Children ≥5 yr and ≥75 kg): 600 mg in the morning, then 600 mg in the evening for 24 wk.
PO (Children ≥5 yr and 60–74 kg): 400 mg in the morning, then 600 mg in the evening for 24 wk.
PO (Children ≥5 yr and 47–59 kg): 400 mg in the morning, then 400 mg in the evening for 24 wk.
PO (Children ≥5 yr and 34–46 kg): 200 mg in the morning, then 400 mg in the evening for 24 wk.
PO (Children ≥5 yr and 23–33 kg): 200 mg in the morning, then 200 mg in the evening for 24 wk.

Renal Impairment

PO (Adults): *CCr 30–50 mL/min*—200 mg/day alternating with 400 mg/day every other day for 24 wk; *CCr <30 mL/min or Hemodialysis*—200 mg once daily for 24 wk.

Copegus—with HIV coinfection (regardless of viral genotype) (with peginterferon alfa-2a)

PO (Adults): 800 mg daily for 48 wk.

Availability (generic available)

Powder for reconstitution for aerosol use (Virazole): 6 g/vial. **Tablets (Copegus):** 200 mg. **Tablets (Ribasphere):** 200 mg, 400 mg, 600 mg.

NURSING IMPLICATIONS

Assessment

- **RSV:** Assess patient for infection (vital signs, sputum, WBC) at beginning and during therapy.
- Obtain specimens for culture and sensitivity prior to initiating therapy. First dose may be given before receiving results.
- Assess respiratory (lung sounds, quality and rate of respirations) and fluid status prior to and frequently throughout therapy.
- **Chronic Hepatitis C:** Monitor symptoms of hepatitis during therapy.
- Assess for signs of neuropsychiatric disorders (irritability, anxiety, depression, suicidal ideation, aggressive behavior). May require discontinuation of ribavirin.
- Obtain ECG prior to therapy in patients with pre-existing cardiac disease. Assess patient for cardiovascular disorders (pulse, BP, chest pain). Reduce dose or discontinue therapy if cardiac disorders occur. May cause myocardial infarction.
- Assess for signs of colitis (abdominal pain, bloody diarrhea, fever) and pancreatitis (nausea, vomiting, abdominal pain) during therapy. Discontinue therapy if these occur; may be fatal.
- Assess pulmonary status (lung sounds, respirations) periodically during therapy. May require discontinuation.
- Monitor for hypersensitivity reactions (urticaria, angioedema, bronchoconstriction, anaphylaxis). Discontinue immediately and institute supportive therapy.
- ***Lab Test Considerations:*** **Chronic Hepatitis C:** Monitor CBC with differential and platelet count prior to initiation, at week 2, and week 4, and regularly during therapy. If hemoglobin <10 g/dL in patients with no history of cardiac disease or ↓ more than 2 g/dL in any 4-wk treatment period in patients with history of stable cardiac disease, ↓ ribavirin dose to 600 mg (200 mg in AM and 400 mg in PM). If hemoglobin <8.5 g/dL in patients with no history of cardiac disease or <12 g/dL despite dose reduction in patients with history of stable cardiac disease, discontinue combination therapy permanently. If dose withheld in children, may restart with 1/2 original dose.
- Monitor biochemical tests and electrolytes prior to, after 4 wk, and periodically during therapy.
- Monitor liver function tests and thyroid stimulating hormone prior to and periodically during therapy.
- Monitor pregnancy tests prior to, monthly during, and for 6 mo following discontinuation of therapy in women of childbearing age. Ribavarin should be started following a negative pregnancy test.
- May cause ↑ serum bilirubin and uric acid levels.

Potential Nursing Diagnoses

Risk for infection (Indications, Side Effects)
Impaired gas exchange (Indications)

Implementation

- **Inhaln:** Infants requiring assisted ventilation should be suctioned every 1–2 hr and pulmonary pressures monitored every 2–4 hr.
- Ribavirin treatment should begin within the first 3 days of RSV infection to be effective.
- Ribavirin aerosol should be administered using the Viratek SPAG model SPAG-2 only. Do not administer via other aerosol-generating devices. Usually administered using an infant oxygen hood attached to the SPAG-2 aerosol generator. Administration by face mask may be used if the oxygen hood cannot be used.
- Reconstitute ribavirin 6-g vial with preservative-free sterile water for injection or inhalation. Transfer to clean, sterilized Erlenmeyer flask of the SPAG-2 reservoir and dilute to a final volume of 300 mL. This recommended concentration (20 mg/mL) in the reservoir provides a concentration of aerosol ribavirin of 190 mcg/L of air over a 12-hr period. Solution should be discarded and replaced every 24 hr.
- Aerosol treatments should be administered continuously 12–18 hr/day for 3–7 days.
- **PO:** Administer with food.
- For children, determine if child is able to swallow 200-mg tablet.

Patient/Family Teaching

- **RSV:** Explain the purpose and route of treatment to the patient and parents.
- Inform patient and parents that ribavirin may cause blurred vision and photosensitivity.
- **Chronic Hepatitis C:** Instruct patient to take ribavirin at the same time each day for the full course of therapy. Take missed doses as soon as remembered. If total day dose is missed, notify health care professional; do not double doses. Emphasize the importance of routine lab test to monitor for side effects.
- Advise patient to brush teeth twice daily, have regular dental examinations, and rinse mouth thoroughly after vomiting to prevent dental and periodontal disorders.
- May cause dizziness, confusion, fatigue, and drowsiness. Caution patient to avoid driving or other activities requiring alertness until response to medication is known.

R

- Inform patient that ribavirin may not reduce the risk of transmission of HCV to others or prevent cirrhosis, liver failure, or liver cancer.
- Advise patient to consult health care professional before taking any other Rx, OTC, or herbal products.
- Advise patient to stop taking ribavirin and notify health care professional immediately if rash with fever; blisters or sores in mouth, nose, or eyes; or conjunctivitis occurs and to notify health care professional if trouble breathing, hives or swelling, chest pain, severe stomach pain or low back pain, bloody diarrhea or bloody or black stools, bruising or unusual bleeding, change in vision, fever >100.5°F, worsening psoriasis, worsening depression, or suicidal thoughts occur.
- Rep: Inform patient about teratogenic effects of ribavirin. Instruct women with childbearing potential, and men, to use 2 forms of effective contraception during and for at least 6 mo following conclusion of therapy. Men must use a condom. Avoid breast feeding during use.

Evaluation/Desired Outcomes

- Resolution of the signs and symptoms of RSV.
- Decreased progression and sequelae of chronic hepatitis C. Therapy with peginterferon alfa-2a and ribavirin should be discontinued if at least a 2-log 10 reduction from baseline in HCV RNA by 12 wk of therapy, or undetectable HCV RNA levels after 24 wk of therapy.

rifabutin (riff-a-byoo-tin)

Mycobutin

Classification

Therapeutic: agents for atypical mycobacterium

Pregnancy Category B

Indications

Prevention of disseminated *Mycobacterium avium* complex (MAC) disease in patients with advanced HIV infection.

Action

Appears to inhibit DNA-dependent RNA polymerase in susceptible organisms. **Therapeutic Effects:** Antimycobacterial action against susceptible organisms. **Spectrum:** Active against *M. avium* and most strains of *M. tuberculosis*.

Pharmacokinetics

Absorption: Well absorbed following oral administration (50–85%). Absorption ↓ in HIV-positive patients (20%).

Distribution: Widely distributed to body tissues and fluids.

Metabolism and Excretion: Mostly metabolized by the liver; <5% excreted unchanged by the kidneys.

Half-life: 45 hr.

TIME/ACTION PROFILE (blood levels)

ROUTE	ONSET	PEAK	DURATION
PO	rapid	2–4 hr	24 hr

Contraindications/Precautions

Contraindicated in: Hypersensitivity. Cross-sensitivity with other rifamycins (rifampin) may occur; Active tuberculosis; Concurrent ritonavir or delavirdine. **Use Cautiously in:** OB, Lactation, Pedi: Safety not established. Use in pregnancy only if potential benefit justifies potential risk to fetus.

Adverse Reactions/Side Effects

EENT: ocular disturbances. **Resp:** dyspnea. **CV:** chest pain, chest pressure. **GI:** CLOSTRIDIUM DIFFICILE-ASSOCIATED DIARRHEA (CDAD), altered taste, drug-induced hepatitis. **Derm:** rash, skin discoloration. **Hemat:** hemolysis, neutropenia, thrombocytopenia. **MS:** arthralgia, myositis. **Misc:** brown-orange discoloration of body fluids (urine, tears, saliva), flu-like syndrome.

Interactions

Drug-Drug: May ↓ levels and effectiveness of **efavirenz**, **indinavir**, **nelfinavir**, **nevirapine**, **saquinavir** (dosage adjustment may be necessary), **delavirdine** (concurrent use should be avoided), **corticosteroids**, **disopyramide**, **quinidine**, **opioid analgesics**, **oral hypoglycemic agents**, **warfarin**, **estrogens**, **estrogen-containing contraceptives**, **phenytoin**, **verapamil**, **fluconazole**, **quinidine**, **theophylline**, **zidovudine**, and **chloramphenicol**. **Ritonavir** ↑ levels; (concurrent use contraindicated), similar effects occur with **efavirenz** and **nevirapine**.

Route/Dosage

PO (Adults): 300 mg once daily. If GI upset occurs, may give as 150 mg twice daily with food.

Availability (generic available)

Capsules: 150 mg.

NURSING IMPLICATIONS

Assessment

- Monitor patient for signs of active tuberculosis (purified protein derivative [PPD], chest x-ray, sputum culture, blood culture, urine culture, biopsy of suspicious lymph nodes) prior to and throughout therapy. Rifabutin must not be administered to patients with active tuberculosis.
- Monitor bowel function. Diarrhea, abdominal cramping, fever, and bloody stools should be reported to health care professional promptly as a sign of Clostridium difficile-associated diarrhea (CDAD). May begin up to several weeks following cessation of therapy.
- ***Lab Test Considerations:*** Monitor CBC periodically during therapy. May cause neutropenia and thrombocytopenia.

Potential Nursing Diagnoses

Risk for infection (Indications)
Noncompliance (Patient/Family Teaching)

Implementation

- Do not confuse rifabutin with rifampin.
- **PO:** May be administered without regard to meals. High-fat meals slow rate but not extent of absorption. May be mixed with foods such as applesauce. If GI upset occurs, administer with food.

Patient/Family Teaching

- Advise patient to take medication as directed. Do not skip doses or double up on missed doses. Emphasize the importance of continuing therapy even if asymptomatic.
- Advise patient to notify health care professional promptly if signs and symptoms of neutropenia (sore throat, fever, signs of infection), thrombocytopenia (unusual bleeding or bruising), or hepatitis (yellow eyes and skin, nausea, vomiting, anorexia, unusual tiredness, weakness) occur.
- Caution patient to avoid the use of alcohol during this therapy, because this may increase the risk of hepatotoxicity.
- Instruct patient to notify health care professional immediately if diarrhea, abdominal cramping, fever, or bloody stools occur and not to treat with antidiarrheals without consulting health care professionals.
- Instruct patient to report symptoms of myositis (myalgia, arthralgia) or uveitis (intraocular inflammation) to health care professional promptly.
- Inform patient that skin, saliva, sputum, sweat, tears, urine, and feces may become brown-orange and that soft contact lenses may become permanently discolored.
- Rep: Advise patient that this medication has teratogenic properties and may decrease the effectiveness of oral contraceptives. Counsel patient to use a nonhormonal form of contraception throughout therapy.
- Emphasize the importance of regular follow-up exams to monitor progress and to check for side effects.

Evaluation/Desired Outcomes

- Prevention of disseminated MAC in patients with advanced HIV infection.

rifampin (rif-**am**-pin)

Rifadin, ✱Rofact

Classification
Therapeutic: antituberculars
Pharmacologic: rifamycins

Pregnancy Category C

Indications

Active tuberculosis (with other agents). Elimination of meningococcal carriers. **Unlabeled Use:** Prevention of disease caused by *Haemophilus influenzae* type B in close contacts. Synergy with other antimicrobial agents for *S. aureus* infections.

Action

Inhibits RNA synthesis by blocking RNA transcription in susceptible organisms. **Therapeutic Effects:** Bactericidal action against susceptible organisms. **Spectrum:** Broad spectrum notable for activity against: *Mycobacterium* spp., *Staphylococcus aureus*, *H. influenzae*, *Legionella pneumophila*, *Neisseria meningitidis*.

Pharmacokinetics

Absorption: Well absorbed following oral administration.
Distribution: Widely distributed; enters CSF. Crosses placenta; enters breast milk.
Protein Binding: 80%.
Metabolism and Excretion: Mostly metabolized by the liver; 60% eliminated in feces via biliary elimination.
Half-life: 3 hr.

TIME/ACTION PROFILE (blood levels)

ROUTE	ONSET	PEAK	DURATION
PO	rapid	2–4 hr	12–24 hr
IV	rapid	end of infusion	12–24 hr

Contraindications/Precautions

Contraindicated in: Hypersensitivity; Concurrent use of atazanavir, darunavir, fosamprenavir, saquinavir, tipranavir, or ritonavir-boosted saquinavir.
Use Cautiously in: History of liver disease; Diabetes; Concurrent use of other hepatotoxic agents; OB, Lactation: Pregnancy or lactation.

Adverse Reactions/Side Effects

CNS: ataxia, confusion, drowsiness, fatigue, headache, weakness. **Derm:** rash, pruritus. **EENT:** red discoloration of tears. **GI:** abdominal pain, diarrhea, flatulence, heartburn, nausea, vomiting, ↑ liver enzymes, red discoloration of saliva. **GU:** red discoloration of urine. **Hemat:** hemolytic anemia, thrombocytopenia. **MS:** arthralgia, muscle weakness, myalgia. **Misc:** flu-like syndrome.

Interactions

Drug-Drug: ↑ risk of hepatotoxicity with ritonavir-boosted **saquinavir**; concurrent use contraindicated. Significantly ↓ blood levels of **atazanavir**, **darunavir**, **fosamprenavir**, **saquinavir**, and **tipranavir**; concurrent use contraindicated. ↑ risk of hepatotoxicity with other **hepatotoxic agents**, including **alcohol**, **ketoconazole**, **isoniazid**, **pyrazinamide** (concurrent use with **pyrazinamide** may result in potentially fatal hepatotoxicity and should be avoided). Significantly ↓ blood levels of **delavirdine**, **indinavir**, and **nelfinavir**. Rifampin stimulates liver enzymes, which may ↑ metabolism and ↓ effectiveness of other drugs, including **ritonavir**, **nevirapine**, and **efavirenz** (dose adjustment may be necessary), **ciprofloxacin**, **clarithromycin**, **corticosteroids**, **cyclosporine**, **diazepam**, **diltiazem**, **disopyramide**, **doxycycline**, **levothyroxine**, **methadone**, **nifedipine**, **quinidine**, **opioid analgesics**, **oral hypoglycemic agents**, **warfarin**, **estrogens**, **phenytoin**, **phenobarbital**, **tacrolimus**, **verapamil**, **fluconazole**, **ketoconazole**, **itraconazole**, **quinidine**, **theophylline**, **zidovudine**, **chloramphenicol**, and **hormonal contraceptive agents**.

Route/Dosage

Tuberculosis

PO, IV (Adults): 600 mg/day or 10 mg/kg/day (up to 600 mg/day) single dose; may also be given twice weekly.

PO, IV (Children and Infants): 10–20 mg/kg/day single dose or divided q 12 h (not to exceed 600 mg/day); may also be given twice weekly.

Asymptomatic Carriers of Meningococcus

PO, IV (Adults): 600 mg q 12 hr for 2 days.

PO, IV (Children ≥1 mo): 10 mg/kg q 12 hr for 2 days (max: 600 mg/dose).

PO (Infants <1 mo): 5 mg/kg q 12 hr for 2 days.

H. influenzae Prophylaxis

PO (Adults): 600 mg/day for 4 days.

PO (Children): 20 mg/kg/day for 4 days (max: 600 mg/dose).

PO (Neonates): 10 mg/kg/day for 4 days.

Synergy for *S. aureus* infections

PO (Adults): 300–600 mg BID.

PO (Children and Neonates): 5–20 mg/kg/day divided q 12 h (max: 600 mg/dose).

Availability (generic available)

Capsules: 150 mg, 300 mg. **Powder for injection:** 600 mg/vial. ***In combination with:*** isoniazid (IsonaRif, Rifamate); isoniazid and pyrazinamide (Rifater). See Appendix B.

NURSING IMPLICATIONS

Assessment

- Perform mycobacterial studies and susceptibility tests prior to and periodically during therapy to detect possible resistance.
- Assess lung sounds and character and amount of sputum periodically during therapy.
- ***Lab Test Considerations:*** Evaluate renal function, CBC, and urinalysis periodically and during therapy.
- Monitor hepatic function at least monthly during therapy. May cause ↑ BUN, AST, ALT, and serum alkaline phosphatase, bilirubin, and uric acid concentrations.
- May cause false-positive direct Coombs' test results. May interfere with folic acid and vitamin B assays.
- May interfere with dexamethasone suppression test results; discontinue rifampin 15 days prior to test.
- May interfere with methods for determining serum folate and vitamin B levels and with urine tests based on color reaction.
- May delay hepatic uptake and excretion of sulfobromophthalein (SBP) during SBP uptake and excretion tests; perform test prior to daily dose of rifampin.

Potential Nursing Diagnoses

Risk for infection (Indications)
Noncompliance (Patient/Family Teaching)

Implementation

- Do not confuse rifampin with rifabutin.
- **PO:** Administer medication on an empty stomach at least 1 hr before or 2 hr after meals with a full glass (240 mL) of water. If GI irritation becomes a problem, may be administered with food. Antacids may also be taken 1 hr prior to administration. Capsules may be opened and contents mixed with applesauce or jelly for patients with difficulty swallowing.
- Pharmacist can compound a syrup for patients unable to swallow solids.

IV Administration

- **Intermittent Infusion:** Reconstitute each 600-mg vial with 10 mL of sterile water for injection for a concentration of 60 mg/mL. ***Diluent:*** Dilute further in 100 mL or 500 mL of D5W or 0.9% NaCl. Reconstituted vials are stable for 24 hr at room temperature. Infusion is stable at room temperature for 4 hr (in D5W) or 24 hr (in 0.9% NaCl). ***Concentration:*** Not to exceed 6 mg/mL. ***Rate:*** Administer solutions diluted in 100 mL over 30 min and solutions diluted in 500 mL over 3 hr.
- **Y-Site Compatibility:** amiodarone, bumetanide, midazolam, pantoprazole, vancomycin.
- **Y-Site Incompatibility:** diltiazem.

Patient/Family Teaching

- Advise patient to take medication once daily (unless biweekly regimens are used), as directed, and not to skip doses or double up on missed doses. Emphasize the importance of continuing therapy even after symptoms have subsided. Length of therapy for tuberculosis depends on regimen being used and underlying disease states. Patients on short-term prophylactic therapy should also be advised of the importance of compliance with therapy.

- Advise patient to notify health care professional promptly if signs and symptoms of hepatitis (yellow eyes and skin, nausea, vomiting, anorexia, unusual tiredness, weakness) or of thrombocytopenia (unusual bleeding or bruising) occur.
- Caution patient to avoid the use of alcohol during this therapy, because this may increase the risk of hepatotoxicity.
- Instruct patient to report the occurrence of flu-like symptoms (fever, chills, myalgia, headache) promptly.
- Rifampin may occasionally cause drowsiness. Caution patient to avoid driving or other activities requiring alertness until response to medication is known.
- Inform patient that saliva, sputum, sweat, tears, urine, and feces may become red-orange to red-brown and that soft contact lenses may become permanently discolored.
- Advise patient that this medication has teratogenic properties and may decrease the effectiveness of oral contraceptives. Counsel patient to use a nonhormonal form of contraception throughout therapy.
- Emphasize the importance of regular follow-up exams to monitor progress and to check for side effects.

Evaluation/Desired Outcomes

- Decreased fever and night sweats.
- Diminished cough and sputum production.
- Negative sputum cultures.
- Increased appetite.
- Weight gain.
- Reduced fatigue.
- Sense of well-being in patients with tuberculosis.
- Prevention of meningococcal meningitis.
- Prevention of *H. influenzae* type B infection. Prophylactic course is usually short term.

rifaximin (ri-fax-i-min)

Xifaxan

Classification
Therapeutic: anti-infectives
Pharmacologic: rifamycins

Pregnancy Category C

Indications

Travelers' diarrhea due to noninvasive strains of *Escherichia coli*. Reduction in risk of overt hepatic encephalopathy recurrence. Treatment of irritable bowel syndrome (IBS) with diarrhea.

Action

Inhibits bacterial RNA synthesis by binding to bacterial DNA-dependent RNA polymerase. **Therapeutic Effects:** Decreased severity of travelers' diarrhea. Decreased episodes of overt hepatic encephalopathy. Decreased signs/symptoms of IBS. **Spectrum:** *Escherichia coli* (enterotoxigenic and enteroaggregative strains).

Pharmacokinetics

Absorption: Poorly absorbed (<0.4%), action is primarily in GI tract.
Distribution: 80–90% concentrated in gut.
Metabolism and Excretion: Almost exclusively excreted unchanged in feces.
Half-life: 6 hr.

TIME/ACTION PROFILE

ROUTE	ONSET	PEAK	DURATION
PO	unknown	unknown	unknown

Contraindications/Precautions

Contraindicated in: Hypersensitivity to rifaximin or other rifamycins; Diarrhea with fever or bloody stools; Diarrhea caused by other infections agents; Lactation: Potential for adverse effects in the infant. Switch to formula for duration of treatment.
Use Cautiously in: OB: Use only if benefit to mother outweighs risk to fetus; Pedi: Safety not established in children <18 yr (hepatic encephalopathy) or <12 yr (travelers' diarrhea).

Adverse Reactions/Side Effects

CNS: dizziness. **CV:** peripheral edema. **GI:** CLOSTRIDIUM DIFFICILE-ASSOCIATED DIARRHEA (CDAD).

Interactions

Drug-Drug: P-glycoprotein inhibitors, including **cyclosporine** may ↑ levels.

Route/Dosage

Travelers' Diarrhea

PO (Adults and Children ≥12 yr): 200 mg 3 times daily for 3 days.

Hepatic Encephalopathy

PO (Adults): 550 mg twice daily.

IBS with Diarrhea

PO (Adults): 550 mg 3 times daily for 14 days; if recurrence of symptoms, may treat up to an additional 2 times.

Availability

Tablets: 200 mg, 550 mg.

NURSING IMPLICATIONS

Assessment

- **Traveler's Diarrhea:** Assess frequency and consistency of stools and bowel sounds prior to and during therapy.

- Assess fluid and electrolyte balance and skin turgor for dehydration.
- **Hepatic Encephalopathy:** Assess mental status periodically during therapy.
- **IBS with Diarrhea:** Assess frequency and consistency of stools and other IBS symptoms (bloating, cramping) daily.
- Monitor bowel function. Diarrhea, abdominal cramping, fever, and bloody stools should be reported to health care professional promptly as a sign of Clostridium difficile-associated diarrhea (CDAD). May begin up to several weeks following cessation of therapy.
- ***Lab Test Considerations:*** May cause lymphocytosis, monocytosis, and neutropenia.

Potential Nursing Diagnoses

Diarrhea (Indications)
Risk for deficient fluid volume (Indications)

Implementation

- Do not confuse rifaximin with rifampin.
- **PO:** Administer with or without food.

Patient/Family Teaching

- Instruct patient to take rifaximin as directed and to complete therapy, even if feeling better. Caution patient to stop taking rifaximin if diarrhea symptoms get worse, persist more than 24–48 hr, or are accompanied by fever or blood in the stool. Consult health care professional if these occur. Advise patient not to treat diarrhea without consulting health care professional. May occur up to several weeks after discontinuation of medication.
- May cause dizziness. Caution patient to avoid driving and other activities requiring alertness until response to medication is known.
- Advise female patients to notify health care professional if pregnant or if pregnancy is suspected, or if breast feeding.

Evaluation/Desired Outcomes

- Decreased severity of travelers' diarrhea.
- Reduction in risk of overt hepatic encephalopathy recurrence.
- Reduction in symptoms of IBS with diarrhea.

rilpivirine (ril-pi-vir-een)

Edurant

Classification

Therapeutic: antiretrovirals
Pharmacologic: non-nucleoside reverse transcriptase inhibitors

Pregnancy Category B

Indications

Treatment-naïve adult patients with HIV infection with HIV-1 RNA ≤100,000 copies/mL at start of therapy.

Action

Inhibits HIV-replication by non-competitively inhibiting HIV reverse transcriptase. **Therapeutic Effects:** Slowed progression of HIV infection and decreased occurrence of sequelae. Increases CD4 cell counts and decreases viral load.

Pharmacokinetics

Absorption: Well absorbed following oral administration.
Distribution: Unknown.
Protein Binding: 99.7%.
Metabolism and Excretion: Mostly metabolized by the liver (CYP3A enzyme system); 25% excreted in feces unchanged, <1% excreted unchanged in urine.
Half-life: 50 hr.

TIME/ACTION PROFILE (blood levels)

ROUTE	ONSET	PEAK	DURATION
PO	unknown	4–5 hr	24 hr

Contraindications/Precautions

Contraindicated in: Concurrent use of drugs that induce the CYP3A enzyme system or ↑ gastric pH (↓ blood levels and effectiveness, ↑ resistance); Lactation: Breast feeding should be avoided due to possible transmission of virus in breast milk.
Use Cautiously in: Concurrent use of drugs that ↑ risk of torsades de pointes (may ↑ risk of arrhythmias); History of depression or suicide attempt; Hepatitis B or C; Concurrent use of antacids or H_2 antagonists (↓ levels and effectiveness); Geri: Consider ↓ hepatic/renal/cardiac function, concurrent diseases, and drug therapy; OB: Use only if potential maternal benefit justifies potential risk to fetus; Pedi: Children <12 yr (safety and effectiveness not established).

Adverse Reactions/Side Effects

CNS: <u>depression (↑ in children)</u>, dizziness, headache, insomnia. **Derm:** DRUG REACTION WITH EOSINOPHILIA AND SYSTEMIC SYMPTOMS (DRESS), rash. **Endo:** fat redistribution. **GI:** hepatotoxicity. **Misc:** immune reconstitution syndrome.

Interactions

Drug-Drug: Drugs that induce the CYP3A enzyme system including **carbamazepine**, **dexamethasone** (more than a single dose), **oxcarbazepine**, **phenobarbital**, **phenytoin**, **rifampin**, or, **rifapentine** ↓ levels and effectiveness and promote of virologic resistance; concurrent use contraindicated. **Proton pump inhibitors** including **esomeprazole**, **lansoprazole**, **omeprazole**, **pantoprazole**, and **rabeprazole** ↓ levels and effectiveness and may ↑ resistance; concurrent use contraindicated. Concurrent use with **antacids** may ↓ levels and effectiveness; use with caution, administer at least 2 hr before or 4 hr after rilpivirine. Concurrent use with **H_2 antagonists** may ↓ levels and effectiveness; use with caution, administer at least

12 hr before or 4 hr after rilpivirine. **Rifabutin** may ↓ levels; ↑ rilpivirine dose during concurrent use. **Delavirdine** may ↑ levels; avoid concurrent use. **Efavirenz**, **etravirine**, and **nevirapine** may ↓ levels; avoid concurrent use. **Darunavir/ritonavir**, **lopinavir/ritonavir**, **atazanavir/ritonavir**, **fosamprenavir/ritonavir**, **saquinavir/ritonavir**, **tipranavir/ritonavir**, **atazanavir**, **fosamprenavir**, **indinavir**, and **nelfinavir** may ↑ levels. **Clarithromyin**, **erythromycin**, or **troleandomycin** may ↑ levels; consider azithromycin. **Fluconazole**, **itraconazole**, **ketoconazole**, **posaconazole**, and **voriconazole** may ↑ levels; rilpivirine may ↓ **ketoconazole** levels. Concurrent use with **drugs that ↑ risk of torsades de pointes** may ↑ risk of serious arrhythmias. May ↓ levels of **methadone**; monitor clinical effects.

Drug-Natural Products: Concurrent use of **St. John's wort** ↓ blood levels and effectiveness, ↑ resistance; concurrent use contraindicated.

Route/Dosage

PO (Adults and Children ≥12 yr and ≥35 kg): 25 mg once daily; *Concurrent rifabutin therapy*—50 mg once daily (↓ dose to 25 mg once daily when rifabutin discontinued).

Availability

Tablets: 25 mg. ***In combination with:*** emtricitabine and tenofovir (Complera). See Appendix B.

NURSING IMPLICATIONS

Assessment

- Assess for change in severity of HIV symptoms and for symptoms of opportunistic infections during therapy.
- Monitor closely for notable changes in behavior that could indicate the emergence or worsening of suicidal thoughts or behavior or depression.
- Assess for rash periodically during therapy. May cause Stevens-Johnson syndrome. Discontinue therapy if severe or if accompanied with fever, general malaise, fatigue, muscle or joint aches, blisters, oral lesions, conjunctivitis, hepatitis, and/or eosinophilia.
- ***Lab Test Considerations:*** Monitor viral load and CD4 cell count regularly during therapy.
- Monitor liver function tests before and periodically during therapy in patients with underlying liver disease, hepatitis B or C, or marked ↑ transaminase. May cause ↑ serum creatinine, AST, ALT, total bilirubin, total cholesterol, LDL, and triglycerides.

Potential Nursing Diagnoses

Risk for infection (Indications)
Noncompliance (Patient/Family Teaching)

Implementation

- **PO:** Administer once daily with a meal.

Patient/Family Teaching

- Emphasize the importance of taking rilpivirine as directed, at the same time each day. It must always be used in combination with other antiretroviral drugs. Do not take more than prescribed amount and do not stop taking without consulting health care professional. Take missed doses with a meal if remembered <12 hr of the time it is usually taken, then return to regular schedule. If more than 12 hr from time dose is usually taken, omit dose and resume dosing schedule; do not double doses. Advise patient to read *Patient Information* prior to starting therapy and with each Rx refill in case of changes.
- Advise patient to take antacids 2 hr before or 4 hr after and H_2 antagonists 12 hr before or 4 hr after rilpivirine.
- Instruct patient that rilpivirine should not be shared with others.
- Inform patient that rilpivirine does not cure AIDS or prevent associated or opportunistic infections. Rilpivirine does not reduce the risk of transmission of HIV to others through sexual contact or blood contamination. Caution patient to use a condom and to avoid sharing needles or donating blood to prevent spreading the AIDS virus to others. Advise patient that the long-term effects of rilpivirine are unknown at this time.
- Inform patients and families of risk of suicidal thoughts and behavior and advise that behavioral changes, emergency or worsening signs and symptoms of depression, unusual changes in mood, or emergence of suicidal thoughts, behavior, or thoughts of self-harm should be reported to health care professional immediately.
- Immune reconstitution syndrome may trigger opportunistic infections or autoimmune disorders. Notify health care professional if symptoms or rash occur.
- May cause dizziness. Caution patient to avoid driving or other activities requiring alertness until response to medication is known.
- Advise patient to notify health care professional of all Rx or OTC medications, vitamins, or herbal products being taken and to consult with health care professional before taking other medications, especially St. John's wort.
- Inform patient that changes in body fat (increased fat in upper back and neck, breast, and around back, chest, and stomach area; loss of fats from legs, arms, and face) may occur.
- Rep: Advise patient taking oral contraceptives to use a nonhormonal method of birth control during nelfinavir therapy. If pregnancy is suspected notify health care professional promptly. Encourage pregnant women to enroll in the Antiretroviral Pregnancy

R

Registry by calling 1–800–258–4263. Advise female patient to avoid breast feeding during therapy.
- Emphasize the importance of regular follow-up exams and blood counts to determine progress and monitor for side effects.

Evaluation/Desired Outcomes
- Delayed progression of AIDS and decreased opportunistic infections in patients with HIV.
- Decrease in viral load and increase in CD4 cell counts.

risedronate (riss-**ed**-roe-nate)
Actonel, ✱Actonel DR, Atelvia

Classification
Therapeutic: bone resorption inhibitors
Pharmacologic: biphosphonates

Pregnancy Category C

Indications
Prevention and treatment of postmenopausal and corticosteroid-induced osteoporosis. Treatment of Paget's disease in men and women. Treatment of osteoporosis in men.

Action
Inhibits bone resorption by binding to bone hydroxyapatite, which inhibits osteoclast activity. **Therapeutic Effects:** Reversal of the progression of osteoporosis with decreased fractures and other sequelae. Reduced bone turnover and resorption; normalization of serum alkaline phosphatase with reduced complications of Paget's disease.

Pharmacokinetics
Absorption: Rapidly but poorly absorbed following oral administration (0.63% bioavailability).
Distribution: 60% of absorbed dose distributes to bone.
Metabolism and Excretion: 40% of absorbed dose is excreted unchanged by kidneys; unabsorbed drug is excreted in feces.
Half-life: *Initial*—1.5 hr; *terminal*—220 hr (reflects dissociation from bone).

TIME/ACTION PROFILE (effects on serum alkaline phosphatase)

ROUTE	ONSET	PEAK	DURATION
PO	within days	30 days	up to 16 mo

Contraindications/Precautions
Contraindicated in: Hypersensitivity; Hypocalcemia; Abnormalities of the esophagus, which delay esophageal emptying (i.e., strictures, achalasia); Inability to stand/sit upright for at least 30 min; Lactation: Lactation; Severe renal impairment (CCr <30 mL/min).
Use Cautiously in: History of upper GI disorders; Other disturbances of bone or mineral metabolism (correct abnormalities before initiating therapy); Dietary deficiencies (supplemental vitamin D and calcium may be required); Invasive dental procedures, cancer, receiving chemotherapy, corticosteroids, or angiogenesis inhibitors, poor oral hygeine, periodontal disease, dental disease, anemia, coagulopathy, infection, or poorly fitting dentures (may ↑ risk of jaw osteonecrosis); OB, Pedi: Safety not established; use in pregnancy only if potential benefit justifies potential risks.

Adverse Reactions/Side Effects
CNS: weakness. **EENT:** amblyopia, conjunctivitis, dry eyes, eye pain/inflammation, tinnitus. **CV:** chest pain, edema. **GI:** abdominal pain, diarrhea, belching, colitis, constipation, dysphagia, esophagitis, esophageal cancer, esophageal ulcer, gastric ulcer, nausea. **Derm:** STEVENS-JOHNSON SYNDROME, TOXIC EPIDERMAL NECROLYSIS, rash. **MS:** arthralgia, musculoskeletal pain, femur fractures, osteonecrosis (primarily of jaw). **Resp:** asthma exacerbation. **Misc:** flu-like syndrome.

Interactions
Drug-Drug: Concurrent use with **NSAIDs** or **aspirin** ↑ risk of GI irritation. Absorption is ↓ by **calcium supplements** or **antacids**. **Proton pump inhibitors** and **H2 antagonists** may cause a faster release of drug from the delayed-release product that can ↑ drug levels; concurrent use not recommended.
Drug-Food: Food ↓ absorption (administer at least 30 min before breakfast).

Route/Dosage
PO (Adults): *Postmenopausal osteoporosis*—5 mg daily; *or* 35 mg once weekly (immediate- or delayed-release); *or* 75 mg taken on 2 consecutive days for a total of 2 tablets each month; *or* 150 mg once monthly. *Osteoporosis in men*—35 mg once weekly (immediate-release); *Glucocorticoid-induced osteoporosis*—5 mg daily; *Paget's disease*—30 mg daily for 2 mo; retreatment may be considered after 2 mo off therapy.

Availability (generic available)
Tablets: 5 mg, 30 mg, 35 mg, 150 mg. **Delayed-release tablets (Atelvia):** 35 mg.

NURSING IMPLICATIONS
Assessment
- Perform a routine oral exam prior to initiation of therapy. Dental exam with appropriate preventative dentistry should be considered prior to therapy. Patients with history of tooth extraction, poor oral hygiene, gingival infections, diabetes, or use of a dental appliance or those taking immunosuppressive therapy, angiogenesis inhibitors, or systemic corticosteroids are at greater risk for osteonecrosis of the jaw.
- **Osteoporosis:** Assess patients via bone density study for low bone mass before and periodically during therapy.
- **Paget's disease:** Assess for symptoms of Paget's disease (bone pain, headache, decreased visual and auditory acuity, increased skull size).

- ***Lab Test Considerations:*** *Osteoporosis:* Assess serum calcium before and periodically during therapy. Hypocalcemia and vitamin D deficiency should be treated before initiating alendronate therapy. May cause mild, transient ↑ of calcium and phosphate.
- *Paget's disease:* Monitor alkaline phosphatase prior to and periodically during therapy to monitor effectiveness of therapy.

Potential Nursing Diagnoses
Risk for injury (Indications)

Implementation
- **PO:** Administer *Actonel* first thing in the morning with 6–8 oz of water, 30 min prior to other medications, beverages, or food. Waiting longer than 30 min will improve absorption. Administer *Atelvia* right after breakfast with 4 ounces of water. Tablet should be swallowed whole; do not crush, break, or chew.
- Calcium-, magnesium-, or aluminum-containing agents may interfere with absorption of risedronate and should be taken at a different time of day with food.
- Avoid administering delayed-release product with proton pump inhibitors or H_2 antagonists; may allow a faster release and increased drug level.

Patient/Family Teaching
- Instruct patient on the importance of taking as directed. Risedronate should be taken with 6–8 oz of water (mineral water, orange juice, coffee, and other beverages decrease absorption). *If a dose of Actonel 35 is missed,* take 1 tablet the morning remembered, then return to the 1 tablet/wk on the originally scheduled day; do not take 2 pills at once. *If 1 or both tablets of Actonel 75 are missed and the next month's scheduled doses are more than 7 days away:* if both Actonel 75 are missed take 1 the morning remembered and 1 the next morning. If only 1 Actonel 75 tablet is missed: take the missed tablet on the morning of the day after you remember, then return to original schedule. Do not take more than two 75 mg tablets within 7 days. *If 1 or both tablets of Actonel 75 are missed and the next month's scheduled doses are within 7 days,* omit and return to schedule next month. *If 1 or both tablets of Actonel 150 are missed and the next month's scheduled doses are more than 7 days away,* take the missed tablet on the morning of the day after you remember, then return to original schedule. Do not take more than two 150-mg tablets within 7 days. *If 1 or both tablets of Actonel 75 are missed and the next month's scheduled doses are within 7 days,* omit and return to schedule next month. Encourage patient to read the *Medication Guide* before starting therapy and with each Rx refill in case of changes.
- Caution patients to remain upright for 30 min following dose to facilitate passage to stomach and minimize risk of esophageal irritation.
- Advise patient to eat a balanced diet and consult health care professional about the need for supplemental calcium and vitamin D (see Appendix J).
- Inform patient that severe musculoskeletal pain may occur within days, months, or years after starting risendronate. Symptoms my resolve completely after discontinuation or slow or incomplete resolution may occur. Notify health care professional if severe pain occurs.
- Encourage patient to participate in regular exercise and to modify behaviors that increase the risk of osteoporosis (stop smoking, reduce alcohol consumption).
- Advise patient to inform health care professional of risedronate therapy prior to dental surgery.
- Advise female patients to notify health care professional if pregnancy is planned or suspected or if breast feeding.

Evaluation/Desired Outcomes
- Reversal of the progression of osteoporosis with decreased fractures and other sequelae. For patients at low risk of fracture, discontinue after 3 to 5 yr of use.
- Decrease in serum alkaline phosphatase and the progression of Paget's disease.

🧬 **risperidone** (riss-**per**-i-done)
Risperdal, Risperdal M-TAB, Risperdal Consta

Classification
Therapeutic: antipsychotics, mood stabilizers
Pharmacologic: benzisoxazoles

Pregnancy Category C

Indications
Schizophrenia in adults and adolescents aged 13–17 yr. Short-term treatment of acute manic or mixed episodes associated with Bipolar I Disorder (oral only) in adults, and children and adolescents aged 10–17 yr, maintenance treatment of Bipolar I Disorder (IM only) in adults only; can be used with lithium or valproate (adults only). Irritability associated with autistic disorder in children.

Action
May act by antagonizing dopamine and serotonin in the CNS. **Therapeutic Effects:** Decreased symptoms of psychoses, bipolar mania, or autism.

Pharmacokinetics

Absorption: 70% after administration of tablets, solution, or orally disintegrating tablets. Following IM administration, small initial release of drug, followed by 3-wk lag; the rest of release starts at 3 wk and lasts 4–6 wk.

Distribution: Unknown.

Metabolism and Excretion: Extensively metabolized by the liver. Metabolism is genetically determined; extensive metabolizers (most patients) convert risperidone to 9-hydroxyrisperidone rapidly. Poor metabolizers (6–8% of Whites) convert it more slowly. The 9-hydroxyrisperidone is an antipsychotic compound. Risperidone and its active metabolite are renally eliminated.

Half-life: *Extensive metabolizers*—3 hr for risperidone, 21 hr for 9-hydroxyrisperidone. *Poor metabolizers*—20 hr for risperidone and 30 hr for 9-hydroxyrisperidone.

TIME/ACTION PROFILE (clinical effects)

ROUTE	ONSET	PEAK	DURATION
PO	1–2 wk	unknown	up to 6 wk†
IM	3 wk	4–6 wk	up to 6 wk†

†After discontinuation.

Contraindications/Precautions

Contraindicated in: Hypersensitivity; Lactation: Discontinue drug or bottle feed.

Use Cautiously in: Debilitated patients, patients with renal or hepatic impairment (initial dose reduction recommended); Underlying cardiovascular disease (↑ risk of arrhythmias and hypotension); History of seizures; History of suicide attempt or drug abuse; Diabetes or risk factors for diabetes (may worsen glucose control); Patients at risk for aspiration; OB, Pedi: Safety not established; Geri: Initial dose ↓ recommended. ↑ risk of mortality in elderly patients treated for dementia-related psychosis.

Adverse Reactions/Side Effects

CNS: NEUROLEPTIC MALIGNANT SYNDROME, SUICIDAL THOUGHTS, aggressive behavior, dizziness, extrapyramidal reactions, headache, ↑ dreams, ↑ sleep duration, insomnia, sedation, fatigue, impaired temperature regulation, nervousness, tardive dyskinesia. **EENT:** pharyngitis, rhinitis, visual disturbances. **Resp:** cough, dyspnea. **CV:** arrhythmias, orthostatic hypotension, tachycardia. **GI:** constipation, diarrhea, dry mouth, nausea, weight gain, abdominal pain, anorexia, dyspepsia, polydipsia, ↑ salivation, vomiting, weight loss. **GU:** ↓ libido, dysmenorrhea/menorrhagia, difficulty urinating, polyuria, priapism. **Derm:** itching/skin rash, dry skin, ↑ pigmentation, sweating, photosensitivity, seborrhea. **Endo:** dyslipidemia, galactorrhea, hyperglycemia. **Hemat:** AGRANULOCYTOSIS, leukopenia, neutropenia. **MS:** arthralgia, back pain.

Interactions

Drug-Drug: May ↓ the antiparkinsonian effects of **levodopa** or other **dopamine agonists**. **Carbamazepine**, **phenytoin**, **rifampin**, **phenobarbital**, and other **enzyme inducers** ↑ metabolism and may ↓ effectiveness; dose adjustments may be necessary. **Fluoxetine** and **paroxetine** ↑ blood levels and may ↑ effects; dose adjustments may be necessary. **Clozapine** ↓ metabolism and may ↑ effects of risperidone. ↑ CNS depression may occur with other **CNS depressants**, including **alcohol**, **antihistamines**, **sedative/hypnotics**, or **opioid analgesics**.

Drug-Natural Products: Kava, valerian, or chamomile can ↑ CNS depression.

Route/Dosage

Schizophrenia

PO (Adults): 1 mg twice daily, ↑ by 1–2 mg/day no more frequently than every 24 hr to 4–8 mg daily.

PO (Children 13–17 yr): 0.5 mg once daily, ↑ by 0.5–1.0 mg no more frequently than every 24 hr to 3 mg daily. May administer half the daily dose twice daily if drowsiness persists.

IM (Adults): 25 mg every 2 wk; some patients may benefit from a higher dose of 37.5 or 50 mg every 2 wk.

Acute Manic or Mixed Episodes Associated with Bipolar I Disorder

PO (Adults): 2–3 mg/day as a single daily dose, dose may be ↑ at 24-hr intervals by 1 mg (range 1–5 mg/day).

PO (Children 13–17 yr): 0.5 mg once daily, ↑ by 0.5–1 mg no more frequently than every 24 hr to 2.5 mg daily. May administer half the daily dose twice daily if drowsiness persists.

PO (Geriatric Patients or Debilitated Patients): Start with 0.5 mg twice daily; ↑ by 0.5 mg twice daily, up to 1.5 mg twice daily; then ↑ at weekly intervals if necessary. May also be given as a single daily dose after initial titration.

Maintenance Treatment of Bipolar I Disorder

IM (Adults): 25 mg every 2 wk; some patients may benefit from a higher dose of 37.5 or 50 mg every 2 wk.

Irritability Associated with Autistic Disorder

PO (Children 5–16 yr weighing <20 kg): 0.25 mg/day initially. After at least 4 days of therapy, may ↑ to 0.5 mg/day. Dose ↑ in increments of 0.25 mg/day may be considered at 2-wk or longer intervals. May be as a single or divided dose.

PO (Children 5–16 yr weighing >20 kg): 0.5 mg/day initially. After at least 4 days of therapy, may ↑ to 1 mg/day. Dose ↑ in increments of 0.5 mg/day may be considered at 2-wk or longer intervals. May be as a single or divided dose.

Renal Impairment

Hepatic Impairment

PO (Adults): Start with 0.5 mg twice daily; ↑ by 0.5 mg twice daily, up to 1.5 mg twice daily; then ↑ at weekly intervals if necessary. May also be given as a single daily dose after initial titration.

Availability (generic available)

Tablets: 0.25 mg, 0.5 mg, 1 mg, 2 mg, 3 mg, 4 mg. **Cost:** *Generic*—0.25 mg $18.40/180, 0.5 mg $22.58/180, 1 mg $24.13/180, 2 mg $28.94/180, 3 mg $34.94/180, 4 mg $38.30/180. **Orally disintegrating tablets (Risperdal M-Tabs):** 0.25 mg, 0.5 mg, 1 mg, 2 mg, 3 mg, 4 mg. **Cost:** *Generic*—0.5 mg $131.86/28, 1 mg $154.07/28, 2 mg $250.49/28, 3 mg $316.12/28, 4 mg $424.45/28. **Oral solution:** 1 mg/mL. **Cost:** *Generic*—$152.56/30 mL. **Extended-release microspheres for injection (Risperdal Consta):** 12.5 mg/vial kit, 25 mg/vial kit, 37.5 mg/vial kit, 50 mg/vial kit.

NURSING IMPLICATIONS

Assessment

- Monitor patient's mental status (orientation, mood, behavior) and mood before and periodically during therapy. Monitor closely for notable changes in behavior that could indicate the emergence or worsening of suicidal thoughts or behavior or depression, especially during early therapy. Restrict amount of drug available to patient.
- Assess weight and BMI initially and throughout therapy. Monitor for symptoms of hyperglycemia polydipsia, polyuria, polyphagia,weakness) periodically during therapy.
- Monitor BP (sitting, standing, lying down) and pulse before and frequently during initial dose titration. May cause prolonged QT interval, tachycardia, and orthostatic hypotension. If hypotension occurs, dose may need to be decreased.
- Observe patient when administering medication to ensure medication is swallowed and not hoarded or cheeked.
- Monitor patient for onset of extrapyramidal side effects (*akathisia*—restlessness; *dystonia*—muscle spasms and twisting motions; or *pseudoparkinsonism*—mask-like face, rigidity, tremors, drooling, shuffling gait, dysphagia). Report these symptoms; reduction of dose or discontinuation may be necessary. Trihexyphenidyl or benztropine may be used to control symptoms.
- Monitor for tardive dyskinesia (involuntary rhythmic movement of mouth, face, and extremities). Report immediately; may be irreversible.
- Monitor for development of neuroleptic malignant syndrome (fever, respiratory distress, tachycardia, seizures, diaphoresis, hypertension or hypotension, pallor, tiredness). Notify health care professional immediately if these symptoms occur.
- ***Lab Test Considerations:*** May cause ↑ serum prolactin levels.
- May cause ↑ AST and ALT.
- May also cause anemia, thrombocytopenia, leukocytosis, and leukopenia.
- Obtain fasting blood glucose and cholesterol levels initially and periodically during therapy.
- Monitor CBC frequently during initial months of therapy in patients with pre-existing or history of low WBC. May cause leukopenia, neutropenia, or agranulocytosis. Discontinue therapy if this occurs.

Potential Nursing Diagnoses

Risk for self-directed violence (Indications)
Disturbed thought process (Indications)
Risk for injury (Side Effects)

Implementation

- Do not confuse risperidone with reserpine.
- When switching from other antipsychotics, discontinue previous agents when starting risperidone and minimize the period of overlapping antipsychotic agents.
- If therapy is reinstituted after an interval off risperidone, follow initial titration schedule.
- For IM use, establish tolerance with oral dosing before IM use and continue oral dosing for 3 wk following initial IM injection. Do not increase dose more frequently than every 4 wk.
- **PO:** Daily doses can be taken in the morning or evening.
- For orally disintegrating tablets, open blister pack by pealing back foil to expose tablet; do not try to push tablet through foil. Use dry hands to remove tablet from blister and immediately place entire tablet on tongue. Tablets disintegrate in mouth within seconds and can be swallowed with or without liquid. Do not attempt to split or chew tablet. Do not try to store tablets once removed from blister.
- Oral solution can be mixed with water, coffee, orange juice, or low-fat milk; do not mix with cola or tea.
- **IM:** Reconstitute with 2 mL of diluent provided by manufacturer. Administer via deep deltoid (1-inch needle) or gluteal (2-inch needle) injection using enclosed safety needle; alternate arms or buttocks with each injection. Allow solution to warm to room temperature prior to injection. Administer immediately after mixed with diluent; shake well to mix suspension. Must be administered within 6 hr of reconstitution. Store dose pack in refrigerator.
- Do not combine dose strengths in a single injection.

R

Patient/Family Teaching

- Instruct patient to take medication as directed.
- Inform patient of the possibility of extrapyramidal symptoms. Instruct patient to report these symptoms immediately to health care professional.
- Advise patient to change positions slowly to minimize orthostatic hypotension.
- May cause drowsiness. Caution patient to avoid driving or other activities requiring alertness until response to medication is known.
- Advise patient and family to notify health care professional if thoughts about suicide or dying, attempts to commit suicide; new or worse depression; new or worse anxiety; feeling very agitated or restless; panic attacks; trouble sleeping; new or worse irritability; acting aggressive; being angry or violent; acting on dangerous impulses; an extreme increase in activity and talking; other unusual changes in behavior or mood occur.
- Advise patient to use sunscreen and protective clothing when exposed to the sun to prevent photosensitivity reactions. Extremes in temperature should also be avoided; this drug impairs body temperature regulation.
- Instruct patient to notify health care professional of all Rx or OTC medications, vitamins, or herbal products being taken and consult health care professional before taking any new medications. Caution patient to avoid concurrent use of alcohol and other CNS depressants.
- Advise female patients to notify health care professional if pregnancy is planned or suspected, or if breast feeding or planning to breast feed.
- Advise patient to notify health care professional of medication regimen before treatment or surgery.
- Instruct patient to notify health care professional promptly if sore throat, fever, unusual bleeding or bruising, rash, tremors, or symptoms of hyperglycemia occur.
- Emphasize the importance of routine follow-up exams to monitor side effects and continued participation in psychotherapy to improve coping skills.

Evaluation/Desired Outcomes

- Decrease in excited, manic behavior.
- Decrease in positive symptoms (delusions, hallucinations) of schizophrenia.
- Decreased aggression toward others, deliberate self-injury, temper tantrums, and mood changes in children with autism.
- Decrease in negative symptoms (social withdrawal, flat, blunted affects) of schizophrenia.
- Decrease in autism symptoms.

ritonavir (ri-toe-na-veer)

Norvir

Classification
Therapeutic: antiretrovirals
Pharmacologic: protease inhibitors

Pregnancy Category B

Indications

HIV infection (with other antiretrovirals).

Action

Inhibits the action of HIV protease and prevents the cleavage of viral polyproteins. **Therapeutic Effects:** Increased CD4 cell counts and decreased viral load with subsequent slowed progression of HIV infection and its sequelae.

Pharmacokinetics

Absorption: Appears to be well absorbed after oral administration.
Distribution: Poor CNS penetration.
Protein Binding: 98–99%.
Metabolism and Excretion: Highly metabolized by the liver (by P450 CYP3A and CYP2D6 enzymes); 1 metabolite has antiretroviral activity; 3.5% excreted unchanged in urine.
Half-life: 3–5 hr.

TIME/ACTION PROFILE (blood levels)

ROUTE	ONSET	PEAK	DURATION
PO	rapid	4 hr*	12 hr

*Nonfasting.

Contraindications/Precautions

Contraindicated in: Hypersensitivity; Concurrent use of alfuzosin, amiodarone, dihydroergotamine, ergotamine, flecainide, fluticasone, lovastatin, meperidine, methylergonovine, midazolam (PO), pimozide, propafenone, quinidine, simvastatin, sildenafil (Revatio), St. John's wort, triazolam, or voriconazole; Hypersensitivity or intolerance to alcohol or castor oil (present in capsules and liquid).
Use Cautiously in: Impaired hepatic function, history of hepatitis; Diabetes mellitus; Hemophilia (↑ risk of bleeding); Structural heart disease, conduction abnormalities, ischemic heart disease, or heart failure (↑ risk of heart block); OB, Pedi: Pregnancy or children <12 yr (safety not established); Lactation: Breast feeding not recommended in HIV-infected patients.

Adverse Reactions/Side Effects

CNS: SEIZURES, abnormal thinking, weakness, dizziness, headache, malaise, somnolence, syncope. **EENT:** pharyngitis, throat irritation. **Resp:** ANGIOEDEMA, bronchospasm. **CV:** heart block, orthostatic hypotension, vasodilation. **GI:** abdominal pain, altered taste, anorexia, diarrhea, nausea, vomiting, constipation, dyspepsia, flatulence. **GU:** renal insufficiency. **Derm:** STEVENS-JOHNSON SYNDROME, TOXIC EPIDERMAL NECROLYSIS, rash, skin eruptions, sweating, urticaria. **Endo:** hyperglycemia. **F and E:** dehydration. **Metab:** hyperlipidemia. **MS:** ↑ creatine phosphokinase, myalgia. **Neuro:** circumoral paresthesia, peripheral paresthesia. **Misc:** hypersensitivity reactions including ANAPHYLAXIS, fat redistribution, fever, immune reconstitution syndrome.

Interactions

Drug-Drug: ↑ blood levels and risk of toxicity from some **antiarrhythmics (amiodarone, flecainide, pimozide, propafenone, quinidine)**, **ergot derivatives (dihydroergotamine, ergotamine, methylergonovine)**, **fluticasone (inhalation)**, **meperidine**, **sildenafil (Revatio)**, **alfuzosin**, **lovastatin**, **simvastatin**, **voriconazole**, **midazolam (oral)**, and **triazolam**; concurrent use contraindicated. ↑ levels of **maraviroc**; ↓ maraviroc dose to 150 mg twice daily. ↑ levels of **clarithromycin**; ↓ clarithromycin dose if CCr <60 mL/min. ↑ levels of **rifabutin**; ↓ rifabutin dose to 150 mg every other day or 3 times weekly. May also ↑ levels and effects of some **opioid analgesics (alfentanil, fentanyl, hydrocodone, oxycodone)**, **tramadol**; some **NSAIDs (diclofenac, ibuprofen, indomethacin)**; some **antiarrhythmics (disopyramide, lidocaine, mexiletine)**; many **antidepressants (amitriptyline, clomipramine, desipramine, imipramine, nortriptyline, nefazodone, sertraline, trazodone, fluoxetine, paroxetine, venlafaxine)**; some **antiemetics (dronabinol, ondansetron)**; some **beta blockers (metoprolol, pindolol, propranolol, timolol)**; many **calcium channel blockers (amlodipine, diltiazem, felodipine, isradipine, nicardipine, nifedipine, nimodipine, nisoldipine, verapamil)**; some **antineoplastics (etoposides, paclitaxel, tamoxifen, vinblastine, vincristine, dasatinib, nilotinib)**; some **corticosteroids (dexamethasone, prednisone)**; some **immunosuppressants (cyclosporine, tacrolimus)**; some **antipsychotics (chlorpromazine, haloperidol, perphenazine, risperidone, thioridazine)**; and also **quinidine**, **saquinavir**, **methamphetamine**, and **warfarin**. Dosage ↓ may be necessary. ↓ levels and effects of **hormonal contraceptives**, **zidovudine**, **bupropion**, and **theophylline**; dose alteration or alternative therapy may be necessary. Levels may be ↑ by **clarithromycin** or **fluoxetine**. ↑ risk of heart block with **beta blockers**, **verapamil**, **diltiazem**, **digoxin**, or **atazanavir**. May ↑ concentrations of phosphodiesterase type 5 inhibitors (PDE5) causing hypotension, visual changes, priapism; ↓ starting doses not to exceed 25 mg within 48 hr for **sildenafil** (Viagra), 2.5 mg q 72 hr for **vardenafil** and 10 mg q 72 hr for **tadalafil**. May ↑ risk of adverse effects with **salmeterol**; concurrent use not recommended. ↑ risk of myopathy with **atorvastatin** or **rosuvastatin**; use lowest possible dose of statin. May ↑ **bosentan** levels; initiate bosentan at 62.5 mg once daily or every other day; if patient already receiving bosentan, discontinue bosentan at least 36 hr before initiation of tipranavir and then restart bosentan at least 10 days later at 62.5 mg once daily or every other day. May ↑ **tadalafil (Adcirca)** levels; initiate tadalafil (Adcirca) at 20 mg once daily; if patient already receiving tadalfil (Adcirca), discontinue tadalafil (Adcirca) at least 24 hr before initiation of tipranavir and then restart tadalafil (Adcirca) at least 7 days later at 20 mg once daily. May ↑ **colchicine** levels; ↓ dose of colchicine; do not administer colchicine if patients have renal or hepatic impairment. May ↑ **simeprevir** levels; avoid concomitant use. May ↑ **quetiapine** levels; ↓ quetiapine dose to 1/6 of current dose.

Drug-Natural Products: St. John's wort ↓ levels and may promote resistance; avoid concomitant use.

Drug-Food: Food ↑ absorption.

Route/Dosage

PO (Adults): 300 mg twice daily for 1 day, then 400 mg twice daily for 3 days, then 500 mg twice daily for 1 day, then 600 mg twice daily as maintenance.

PO (Children >1 mo): 250 mg/m^2 twice daily initially; ↑ by 50 mg/m^2 twice daily q 2–3 days up to 400 mg/m^2 twice daily (if unable to get up to 400 mg/m^2 twice daily, additional antiretroviral therapy is required).

Availability

Capsules: 100 mg. **Tablets:** 100 mg. **Oral solution:** 80 mg/mL.

NURSING IMPLICATIONS

Assessment

- Assess patient for change in severity of HIV symptoms and for symptoms of opportunistic infections during therapy.
- Assess patient for rash (mild to moderate rash usually occurs in the 2nd wk of therapy and resolves within 1–2 wk of continued therapy). If rash is severe (extensive erythematous or maculopapular rash with moist desquamation or angioedema) or accompanied by systemic symptoms (serum sickness-like reaction, Stevens-Johnson syndrome, toxic epidermal necrolysis), therapy must be discontinued immediately.
- ***Lab Test Considerations:*** Monitor viral load and CD4 counts regularly during therapy.
- May cause hyperglycemia.
- Monitor serum triglycerides and total cholesterol prior to and periodically during therapy. May cause ↑ serum AST, ALT, GGT, total bilirubin, CPK, triglycerides, and uric acid concentrations.

R

Potential Nursing Diagnoses

Risk for infection (Indications)
Noncompliance (Patient/Family Teaching)

Implementation

- Do not confuse ritonavir with Retrovir (zidovudine).
- **PO:** Administer with a meal or light snack.
- Oral powder may be mixed with chocolate milk, *Ensure*, or *Advera* within 1 hr of dosing to improve taste. Use calibrated oral dosing syringe for oral solution. Oral solution does not require refrigeration if used within 30 days and stored below 77°F in the original container. Keep cap tightly closed. Tablets should be swallowed whole; do not crush, break, or chew. Store tablets at room temperature. Capsules should be stored in the refrigerator and protected from light.
- If nausea occurs on dose of 600 mg twice daily, may titrate by 300 mg twice daily for 1 day, then 400 mg twice daily for 2 days, then 500 mg twice daily for 1 day, then 600 mg twice daily thereafter.
- Patients initiating concurrent therapy with nucleoside analogues may have less GI intolerance by initiating ritonavir for 2 wk and then adding the nucleoside analogue.

Patient/Family Teaching

- Emphasize the importance of taking ritonavir as directed, at evenly spaced times throughout day. Do not take more than prescribed amount and do not stop taking without consulting health care professional. Take missed doses as soon as remembered; do not double doses.
- Instruct patient that ritonavir should not be shared with others.
- Advise patient to notify health care professional of all Rx or OTC medications, vitamins, or herbal products being taken and consult health care professional before taking any new medications, especially St. John's wort.
- Inform patient that ritonavir does not cure AIDS or prevent associated or opportunistic infections. Ritonavir does not reduce the risk of transmission of HIV to others through sexual contact or blood contamination. Caution patient to use a condom during sexual contact and to avoid sharing needles or donating blood to prevent spreading the AIDS virus to others. Advise patient that the long-term effects of ritonavir are unknown at this time.
- Inform patient that ritonavir may cause hyperglycemia. Advise patient to notify health care professional if increased thirst or hunger; unexplained weight loss; increased urination; fatigue; or dry, itchy skin occurs.
- Instruct patient to notify health care professional immediately if rash occurs.
- Inform patient that redistribution and accumulation of body fat may occur, causing central obesity, dorsocervical fat enlargement (buffalo hump), peripheral wasting, breast enlargement, and cushingoid appearance. The cause and long-term effects are not known.
- **Rep:** Advise patient taking oral contraceptives to use a nonhormonal method of birth control during nelfinavir therapy. If pregnancy is suspected notify health care professional promptly. Encourage pregnant women to enroll in the Antiretroviral Pregnancy Registry by calling 1–800–258–4263. Advise female patient to avoid breast feeding during therapy.
- Emphasize the importance of regular follow-up exams and blood counts to determine progress and monitor for side effects.

Evaluation/Desired Outcomes

- Delayed progression of AIDS and decreased opportunistic infections in patients with HIV.
- Decrease in viral load and improvement in CD4 cell counts.

riTUXimab (ri-tux-i-mab)

Rituxan

Classification
Therapeutic: antineoplastics
Pharmacologic: monoclonal antibodies

Pregnancy Category C

Indications

Relapsed or refractory, low-grade or follicular, CD20-positive, B-cell non-Hodgkin's lymphoma (NHL) as a single agent. Previously untreated follicular, CD20-positive, B-cell NHL in combination with first-line chemotherapy and, in patients achieving a complete or partial response to rituximab in combination with chemotherapy, as single-agent maintenance therapy. Non-progressing, low-grade, CD20-positive, B-cell NHL as monotherapy following treatment with cyclophosphamide, vincristine, and prednisolone (CVP). Previously untreated diffuse large B-cell, CD20–positive, NHL in combination with CHOP or another anthracycline-based chemotherapy regimen. CD-20 positive chronic lymphocytic leukemia (CLL) in combination with fludarabine and cyclophosphamide (FC). Moderately-to-severely active rheumatoid arthritis with methotrexate in patients who have had an inadequate response to one of more TNF antagonist therapies. Granulomatosis with polyangiitis (GPA) and microscopic polyangiitis (MPA) in combination with glucocorticoids.

Action

Binds to the CD20 antigen on the surface of lymphoma cells, preventing the activation process for cell cycle initiation and differentiation. **Therapeutic Effects:** Death of lymphoma cells. Prolonged progression-free survival in CLL. Reduced signs and symptoms of rheumatoid arthritis. Achievement of complete remission in GPA and MPA.

Pharmacokinetics

Absorption: IV administration results in complete bioavailability.

Distribution: Binds specifically to CD20 binding sites on lymphoma cells.

Metabolism and Excretion: Unknown.

Half-life: 59.8–174 hr (depending on tumor burden).

TIME/ACTION PROFILE (B-cell depletion)

ROUTE	ONSET	PEAK	DURATION
IV	within 14 days	3–4 wk	6–9 mo†

†Duration of depletion after 4 wk of treatment.

Contraindications/Precautions

Contraindicated in: Hypersensitivity to murine (mouse) proteins; OB: Can pass placental barrier potentially causing fetal B-cell depletion. Give only if clearly needed; Lactation: Potential for immunosuppresion in infant. Discontinue nursing.

Use Cautiously in: Pre-existing bone marrow depression; Hepatitis B infection (may reactivate infection during and for several months after treatment); Systemic lupus erythematosus (may cause fatal progressive multifocal leukoencephalopathy); HIV infection (may increase risk of HIV-associated lymphoma); Pedi: Safety not established.

Adverse Reactions/Side Effects

CNS: PROGRESSIVE MULTIFOCAL LEUKOENCEPHALOPATHY, headache. **Resp:** bronchospasm, cough, dyspnea. **CV:** ARRHYTHMIAS, hypotension, peripheral edema. **GI:** abdominal pain, altered taste, dyspepsia. **GU:** renal failure. **Derm:** MUCOCUTANEOUS SKIN REACTIONS, flushing, urticaria. **Endo:** hyperglycemia. **F and E:** hypocalcemia. **Hemat:** ANEMIA, NEUTROPENIA, THROMBOCYTOPENIA. **MS:** arthralgia, back pain. **Misc:** allergic reactions including ANAPHYLAXIS and ANGIOEDEMA, HEPATITIS B REACTIVATION, INFUSION REACTIONS, TUMOR LYSIS SYNDROME, fever/chills/rigors (infusion related), infections.

Interactions

Drug-Drug: None known.

Route/Dosage

Relapsed or Refractory, Low-Grade or Follicular, CD20-Positive, B-Cell NHL

IV (Adults): 375 mg/m² once weekly for 4 or 8 doses; may retreat with 375 mg/m² once weekly for 4 doses.

Previously Untreated Follicular, CD20–Positive, B-Cell NHL

IV (Adults): 375 mg/m² given on Day 1 of each cycle of CVP for up to 8 doses; if patients experience complete or partial response, give 375 mg/m² (as monotherapy) every 8 wk for 12 doses (initiate this maintenance therapy 8 wk after completion of rituximab + CVP regimen).

Non-Progressing Low-Grade, CD20-Positive, B-Cell NHL

IV (Adults): For patients who have not progressed following 6–8 cycles of CVP chemotherapy, 375 mg/m² given once weekly for 4 doses given every 6 mo for up to 16 doses.

Diffuse Large B-Cell NHL

IV (Adults): 375 mg/m² given on Day 1 of each cycle of chemotherapy for up to 8 infusions.

CLL

IV (Adults): 375 mg/m² given on the day before initiating FC chemotherapy, then 500 mg/m² on Day 1 of cycles 2–6 (every 28 days).

Rheumatoid Arthritis

IV (Adults): Two 1000 mg infusions separated by 2 wk.

GPA and MPA

IV (Adults): 375 mg/m² once weekly for 4 wk.

Availability

Solution for injection (requires dilution): 10 mg/mL.

R

NURSING IMPLICATIONS

Assessment

- Monitor patient for fever, chills/rigors, nausea, urticaria, fatigue, headache, pruritus, bronchospasm, dyspnea, sensation of tongue or throat swelling, rhinitis, vomiting, hypotension, flushing, and pain at disease sites. Infusion-related events occur frequently within 30 min–2 hr of beginning first infusion and may resolve with slowing or discontinuing infusion and treatment with IV saline, diphenhydramine, and acetaminophen. Patients with increased risk (females, patients with pulmonary infiltrates, chronic lymphocytic leukemia, or mantle cell leukemia) may have more severe reactions, which may be fatal. Signs of severe reactions include hypotension, angioedema, hypoxia, or bronchospasm and may require interruption of infusion. May result in pulmonary infiltrates, adult respiratory distress syndrome, MI, ventricular fibrillation, and cardiogenic shock. Monitor closely. Incidence decreases with subsequent infusions.
- Monitor patient for tumor lysis syndrome due to rapid reduction in tumor volume (acute renal failure, hyperkalemia, hypocalcemia, hyperuricemia, or hypophosphatemia) usually occurring 12–24 hr after first infusion. Risks are higher in patients with

greater tumor burden; may be fatal. Correct electrolyte abnormalities, monitor renal function and fluid balance, and administer supportive care, including dialysis, as indicated.

- Assess patient for hypersensitivity reactions (hypotension, bronchospasm, angioedema) during administration. May respond to decrease in infusion rate. Premedication with diphenhydramine and acetaminophen is recommended. Treatment includes diphenhydramine, acetaminophen, bronchodilators, or IV saline as indicated. Epinephrine, antihistamines, and corticosteroids should be readily available in the event of a severe reaction. If severe reactions occur, discontinue infusion; may be resumed at 50% of the rate when symptoms have resolved completely.
- Monitor ECG during and immediately after infusion in patients with pre-existing cardiac conditions (arrhythmias, angina) or patients who have developed arrhythmias during previous infusions of rituximab. Life-threatening arrhythmias may occur.
- Assess for signs of progressive multifocal leukoencephalopathy (hemiparesis, apathy, confusion, cognitive deficiencies, and ataxia) periodically during therapy.
- Assess for infection during and for 1 yr after therapy. Bacterial, fungal, and new or reactivated viral infections may occur. Screen patient for hepatitis B infection prior to therapy. Discontinue rituximab and any concomitant chemotherapy in patients who develop viral hepatitis or other serious infections, and institute appropriate treatment.
- Assess for mucocutaneous reactions periodically during therapy. May cause Stevens-Johnson syndrome and toxic epidermal necrolysis. Discontinue therapy if severe or if accompanied with fever, general malaise, fatigue, muscle or joint aches, blisters, oral lesions, conjunctivitis, hepatitis, and/or eosinophilia.
- ***Lab Test Considerations:*** Monitor CBC and platelet count regularly during therapy and frequently in patients with blood dyscrasias. May cause anemia, thrombocytopenia, or neutropenia.
- Frequently causes B-cell depletion with an associated ↓ in serum immunoglobulins in a minority of patients; does not appear to cause an increased incidence of infection.
- Obtain HBsAg and anti-HBc to screen patient for HBV infection before initiating therapy. May cause reactivation of hepatitis B up to 24 mo after therapy.

Potential Nursing Diagnoses

Risk for infection (Side Effects)

Implementation

- Do not confuse rituximab with infliximab.
- Transient hypotension may occur during infusion; antihypertensive medications may be held for 12 hr before infusion.
- **Rheumatoid Arthritis:** Administer 100 mg methylprednisolone IV or equivalent 30 min prior to each infusion to minimize infusion reactions.
- **GPA and MPA:** Administer methylprednisolone 1000 mg IV per day for 1 to 3 days followed by oral prednisone 1 mg/kg/day (not to exceed 80 mg/day and tapered per clinical need) to treat severe vasculitis symptoms. Begin regimen within 14 days prior to or with the initiation of rituximab and may continue during and after the 4 wk course of rituximab treatment.
- Prophylaxis against *Pneumocystis jiroveci* pneumonia and herpes virus recommended during treatment and for up to 12 mo following treatment as appropriate for patients with CLL, and during and for at least 6 mo following last rituximab infusion for patients with WG and MPA.

IV Administration

- **Intermittent Infusion:** ***Diluent:*** Dilute with 0.9% NaCl or D5W. ***Concentration:*** 1–4 mg/mL. Gently invert bag to mix. Solution is clear and colorless; do not administer solutions that are discolored or contain particulate matter. Discard unused portion remaining in vial. Solution is stable for 12 hr at room temperature and for 24 hr if refrigerated. ***Rate:*** Do not administer as an IV push or bolus.
- *First infusion:* Administer at an initial rate of 50 mg/hr. If hypersensitivity or infusion-related events do not occur, rate may be escalated in 50-mg/hr increments every 30 min to a maximum of 400 mg/hr.
- *Subsequent infusions:* May be administered at an initial rate of 100 mg/hr and increased by 100-mg/hr increments at 30-min intervals to a maximum of 400 mg/hr.
- For previously untreated non-Hodgkins lymphoma and B-cell non-Hodgkin's lymphoma, if no Grade 3 or 4 infusion-related reactions occurred in Cycle 1, may administer via 90-min infusion using glucocorticoids. Begin at rate of 20% of dose over 30 min, with remaining 80% dose over 60 min. If tolerated, then can be used for remainder of therapy.
- **Y-Site Compatibility:** acyclovir, amifostine, amikacin, aminophylline, ampicillin, ampicillin/sulbactam, aztreonam, bleomycin, bumetanide, buprenorphine, busulfan, butorphanol, calcium gluconate, carboplatin, carmustine, cefazolin, cefotaxime, cefotetan, cefoxitin, ceftazidime, ceftriaxone, cefuroxime, chlorpromazine, cisplatin, clindamycin, cyclophosphamide, cytarabine, dactinomycin, daunorubicin hydrochloride, dexamethasone sodium phosphate, dexrazoxane, digoxin, diphenhydramine, dobutamine, docetaxel, dopamine, doxorubicin liposome, doxycycline, droperidol, enalaprilat, etoposide phosphate, famotidine, fentanyl, filgrastim, floxuridine, fluconazole, fludarabine, fluorouracil, ganciclovir, gemcitabine, gentamicin, granisetron, haloperidol, heparin, hydrocortisone, hydromorphone, idarubicin, ifosfamide, imipenem/cilastatin, irinote-

can, leucovorin, levorphanol, lorazepam, magnesium sulfate, mannitol, meperidine, mesna, methotrexate, methylprednisolone, metoclopramide, metronidazole, mitomycin, mitoxantrone, morphine, nalbuphine, paclitaxel, pentamidine, piperacillin/tazobactam, potassium chloride, prochlorperazine, promethazine, ranitidine, sargramostim, streptozocin, teniposide, theophylline, thiotepa, tobramycin, trimethoprim/sulfamethoxazole, vinblastine, vincristine, vinorelbine, zidovudine.
- **Y-Site Incompatibility:** aldesleukin, amphotericin B colloidal, ciprofloxacin, cyclosporine, daunorubicin liposome, doxorubicin hydrochloride, furosemide, levofloxacin, minocycline, ondansetron, quinapristin/dalfopristin, sodium bicarbonate, topotecan, vancomycin.
- **Additive Incompatibility:** Do not admix with other medications.

Patient/Family Teaching

- Inform patient of the purpose of the medication. Advise patient to read the *Medication Guide* prior to starting therapy and before each infusion in case of changes.
- Advise patient to report infusion-related events or symptoms of hypersensitivity reactions immediately.
- Instruct patient to notify health care professional promptly if fever; chills; cough; hoarseness; sore throat; signs of infection; lower back or side pain; painful or difficult urination; bleeding gums; bruising; petechiae; blood in stools, urine, or emesis; increased fatigue; dyspnea; orthostatic hypotension; or painful ulcers or sores on your skin, lips, or in mouth, blisters, peeling skin, rash, pustule occurs. Caution patient to avoid crowds and persons with known infections. Instruct patient to use soft toothbrush and electric razor and to avoid falls. Caution patient not to drink alcoholic beverages or take medication containing aspirin or NSAIDs; may precipitate gastric bleeding.
- Advise patient to consult health care professional prior to receiving any vaccinations.
- Instruct patient to use effective contraception during therapy and for 12 mo following therapy, and to avoid breast feeding.

Evaluation/Desired Outcomes

- Decrease in spread of malignancy.
- Reduced signs and symptoms of rheumatoid arthritis.
- Achievement of complete remission in GPA and MPA.

rivaroxaban (ri-va-rox-a-ban)

Xarelto

Classification

Therapeutic: anticoagulants

Pharmacologic: antithrombotics, factor Xa inhibitors

Pregnancy Category C

Indications

Prevention of deep vein thrombosis that may lead to pulmonary embolism following knee or hip replacement surgery. Reduction in risk of stroke/systemic embolism in patients with nonvalvular atrial fibrillation. Treatment of and reduction in risk of recurrence of deep vein thrombosis or pulmonary embolism.

Action

Acts as selective factor X inhibitor that blocks the active site of factor Xa, inactivating the cascade of coagulation. **Therapeutic Effects:** Prevention of thromboembolic events.

Pharmacokinetics

Absorption: Well absorbed (80%) following oral administration; absorption occurs in the stomach and decreases as it enters the small intestine.

Distribution: Unknown.

Metabolism and Excretion: 51% metabolized by the liver; 36% excreted unchanged in urine. Metabolites do not have anticoagulant activity.

Half-life: 5–9 hr.

TIME/ACTION PROFILE (anticoagulant effect)

ROUTE	ONSET	PEAK	DURATION
PO	unknown	2–4 hr†	24 hr

† Blood levels.

Contraindications/Precautions

Contraindicated in: Hypersensitivity; Active major bleeding; Severe renal impairment [CCr <30 mL/min (deep vein thrombosis/pulmonary embolism treatment or prevention); CCr <15 mL/min (atrial fibrillation)] Prosthetic heart valves; Moderate to severe hepatic impairment (Child-Pugh B or C) or any liver pathology resulting in altered coagulation; Pulmonary embolism with hemodynamic instability or requiring thrombolysis or pulmonary embolectomy; Concurrent use of drugs that are combined P-gp inducers/CYP3A4 inducers or combined P-gp inhibitors/CYP3A4 inhibitors; Lactation: Avoid breast feeding.

Use Cautiously in: Neuroaxial spinal anesthesia or spinal puncture, especially if concurrent with an indwelling epidural catheter, drugs affecting hemostasis, history of traumatic/repeated spinal puncture or spinal

R

deformity (↑ risk of spinal hematoma); Use of feeding tube (proper placement of tube must be documented to ensure absorption); OB: Use only if potential benefit outweighs potential risk.

Adverse Reactions/Side Effects

CNS: syncope. **Derm:** blister, prutitus. **Hemat:** BLEEDING. **Local:** wound secretion. **MS:** extremity pain, muscle spasm.

Interactions

Drug-Drug: Rivaroxaban acts as a substrate of these subsets of the CYP450 enzyme system: CYP3A4/5, CYP2J2, and ATP-binding cassette G2 (ABCG2). Drugs that inhibit or induce these systems may alter effectiveness. Concurrent use of drugs that are combined P-gp inhibitors/strong CYP3A4 inhibitors, including **ketoconazole**, **itraconazole**, **lopinavir/ritonavir**, **ritonavir**, **indinavir**, and **conivaptan** may ↑ levels; avoid concomitant use. Concurrent use of drugs that are combined P-gp inducers/strong CYP3A4 inducers, including **carbamazepine**, **phenytoin**, or **rifampin** may ↓ levels; avoid concomitant use. Concurrent use with **aspirin** or **NSAIDs** may ↑ the risk of bleeding. Concurrent use of **clopidogrel** or other **anticoagulants** may ↑ risk of bleeding and should be avoided. **Drug-Natural Products: St. John's wort** may ↓ levels; avoid concomitant use.

Route/Dosage

Prevention of Deep Vein Thrombosis Following Knee or Hip Replacement Surgery

PO (Adults): 10 mg once daily, initiated 6–10 hr post-operatively (when hemostasis is achieved) continued for 35 days after hip replacement or 12 days after knee replacement.

Reduction in Risk of Stroke/Systemic Embolism in Nonvalvular Atrial Fibrillation

PO (Adults): 20 mg once daily with evening meal.

Renal Impairment

PO (Adults): *CCr 15–50 mL/min*—15 mg once daily with evening meal.

Treatment of and Reduction in Risk of Recurrence of Deep Vein Thrombosis or Pulmonary Embolism

PO (Adults): 15 mg twice daily for 21 days, then 20 mg once daily for remainder of treatment period.

Availability

Tablets: 10 mg, 15 mg, 20 mg.

NURSING IMPLICATIONS

Assessment

- Assess for signs of bleeding and hemorrhage (bleeding gums; nosebleed; unusual bruising; black, tarry stools; hematuria; fall in hematocrit or BP; guaiac-positive stools); bleeding from surgical site. Notify health care professional if these occur. May use prothrombin concentrate complex to reverse life-threatening bleeding.
- Monitor patients with epidural catheters frequently for signs and symptoms of neurologic impairment (midline back pain, sensory and motor deficits [numbness, tingling, weakness in lower limbs], bowel and/or bladder dysfunction). Epidural catheter should not be removed earlier than 18 hr after last administration of rivaroxaban; next dose should be at least 6 hr after catheter removal.
- ***Lab Test Considerations:*** May cause ↑ serum AST, ALT, total bilirubin, and GGT levels.

Potential Nursing Diagnoses

Ineffective tissue perfusion (Indications)
Risk for injury (Side Effects)

Implementation

- *When switching from warfarin to rivaroxaban,* discontinue warfarin and start rivaroxaban as soon as INR <3.0 to avoid periods of inadequate anticoagulation. *When switching from anticoagulants other than warfarin to rivaroxaban,* start rivaroxaban 0 to 2 hr prior to next scheduled evening dose and omit dose of other anticoagulant. For continuous heparin, discontinue heparin and administer rivaroxaban at same time. *When switching from rivaroxaban to warfarin or other anticoagulants,* no data is available. May discontinue rivaroxaban and begin both parenteral anticoagulant and warfarin at time of next rivaroxaban dose.
- Discontinue at least 24 hr prior to surgery and other interventions. Restart as soon as hemostasis has been restablished.
- If rivaroxaban must be discontinued for other than bleeding, consider replacing with another anticoagulant; discontinuation increases risk of thrombotic events.
- **PO:** Administer first dose 6–10 hr after surgery, once hemostasis has been established. 10-mg tablet may be administered without regard to food; 15-mg and 20-mg tablet should be taken with food.
- If unable to swallow tablet, 15-mg and 20-mg tablets may be crushed, mixed with applesauce, and administered immediately after mixing. Follow dose immediately with food. Tablets are stable in applesauce for up to 4 hr.
- If administering crushed tablet via GI feeding tube, check placement of tube. Rivaroxaban is absorbed from the GI tract, not the small intestine. Suspend crushed tablet in 50 mL water and administer. Follow administration of 15-mg or 20-mg tablet immediately with food.

Patient/Family Teaching

- Instruct patient to take medication as directed. Take missed doses as soon as remembered that day. If taking 15 mg twice daily, may take two 15-mg tablets to achieve 30 mg daily dose, then return to regular schedule. If taking 10 mg, 15 mg, or 20 mg once daily, take missed dose immediately. Inform health care professional of missed doses at time of checkup or lab tests. Inform patients that anticoagulant effect may persist for 2–5 days following discontinuation. Advise patient to read *Medication Guide* before starting therapy and with each Rx refill in case of changes. Caution patients not to discontinue medication early without consulting health care professional.

- Advise patient to report any symptoms of unusual bleeding or bruising (bleeding gums; nosebleed; black, tarry stools; hematuria; excessive menstrual flow) and symptoms of spinal or epidural hematoma (tingling; numbness, especially in lower extremities; muscular weakness) to health care professional immediately.
- Instruct patient not to drink alcohol or take other Rx, OTC, or herbal products, especially those containing aspirin, NSAIDs or St. John's wort, or to start or stop any new medications during rivaroxaban therapy without advice of health care professional.
- Advise female patients to notify health care professional if pregnancy is planned or suspected or if breast feeding.

Evaluation/Desired Outcomes

- Prevention of blood clots and subsequent pulmonary emboli following knee/hip replacement surgery. Duration of treatment is 35 days for patients with hip replacement and 12 days for patients with knee replacement surgery.

rivastigmine (rye-va-**stig**-meen)

Exelon

Classification

Therapeutic: anti-Alzheimer's agents

Pharmacologic: cholinergics (cholinesterase inhibitors)

Pregnancy Category B

Indications

PO: Mild to moderate dementia associated with Alzheimer's disease. **Transdermal:** Treatment of mild, moderate, or severe dementia associated with Alzheimer's disease and mild to moderate dementia associated with Parkinson's disease.

Action

Enhances cholinergic function by reversible inhibition of cholinesterase. Does not cure the disease. **Therapeutic Effects:** Decreased dementia (temporary) associated with Alzheimer's disease and Parkinson's disease. Enhanced cognitive ability.

Pharmacokinetics

Absorption: Well absorbed following oral administration. Transdermal patch is slowly absorbed over 8 hr.

Distribution: Widely distributed.

Metabolism and Excretion: Rapidly and extensively metabolized by the liver; metabolites are excreted by the kidneys.

Half-life: *PO*—1.5 hr; *Transdermal*—24 hr.

TIME/ACTION PROFILE (improvement in dementia)

ROUTE	ONSET	PEAK	DURATION
PO	within 2 wk	up to 12 wk	unknown
Transdermal	unknown	unknown	unknown

Contraindications/Precautions

Contraindicated in: Hypersensitivity to rivastigmine or other carbamates; History of application site reactions with transdermal product suggestive of allergic contact dermatitis.

Use Cautiously in: History of asthma or obstructive pulmonary disease; History of GI bleeding; Sick sinus syndrome or other supraventricular cardiac conduction abnormalities; Moderate or severe renal impairment (dose ↓ may be needed); Mild or moderate hepatic impairment (dose ↓ may be needed); Patients weighing <50 kg; at risk for ↑ adverse reactions (dose ↓ may be needed); OB, Lactation, Pedi: Safety not established.

Adverse Reactions/Side Effects

CNS: weakness, dizziness, drowsiness, headache, sedation (unusual). **CV:** edema, heart failure, hypotension. **GI:** anorexia, dyspepsia, nausea, vomiting, abdominal pain, diarrhea, flatulence, weight gain (unusual). **Derm:** allergic dermatitis. **Neuro:** tremor. **Misc:** fever, weight loss, application reactions (for transdermal patch only).

Interactions

Drug-Drug: Nicotine may ↑ metabolism and ↓ levels.

Route/Dosage

PO (Adults): 1.5 mg twice daily initially; after at least 2 wk, dose may be ↑ to 3 mg twice daily. Further increments may be made at 2-wk intervals up to 6 mg twice daily.

Transdermal (Adults): *Initial Dose*—4.6 mg/24-hr transdermal patch intially; ↑ to 9.5 mg/24-hr transdermal patch after at least 4 wk; may ↑ to 13.3 mg/24-hr transdermal patch if needed (is recommended effective dose for patients with severe Alzheimer's disease).

Hepatic Impairment

Transdermal (Adults): *Mild-Moderate Hepatic Impairment*—Do not exceed dose of 4.6 mg/24 hr.

R

Availability (generic available)

Capsules: 1.5 mg, 3 mg, 4.5 mg, 6 mg. **Transdermal patch:** 4.6 mg/24 hr, 9.5 mg/24 hr, 13.3 mg/24 hr.

NURSING IMPLICATIONS

Assessment

- Assess cognitive function (memory, attention, reasoning, language, ability to perform simple tasks) periodically throughout therapy.
- Monitor patient for nausea, vomiting, anorexia, and weight loss. Notify health care professional if these side effects occur.
- Monitor for hypersensitivity skin reactions; may occur after oral or transdermal administration. If allergic contact dermatitis is suspected after transdermal use, may switch to oral rivastigmine after negative allergy testing. If disseminated hypersensitivity reaction of the skin occurs, discontinue therapy.

Potential Nursing Diagnoses

Disturbed thought process (Indications)

Impaired environmental interpretation syndrome (Indications)

Imbalanced nutrition: less than body requirements (Side Effects)

Implementation

- Patients switching from oral doses of <6 mg to transdermal doses should use 4.6 mg/24 hr patch. Patients taking oral doses of 6 mg–12 mg may be converted directly to 9.5 mg/24 hr patch. Apply patch on the day following the last oral dose.
- **PO:** Administer in the morning and evening with food.
- **Transdermal:** Apply patch to clean, dry, hairless area that will not be rubbed by tight clothing. Upper or lower back is recommended, may also use upper arm or chest. Do not apply to red, irritated, or cut skin. Rotate sites to prevent irritation, do not use same site within 14 days. Remove adhesive liner and apply by pressing patch firmly until edges stick well. May be worn during bathing and hot weather. Each 24 hr, remove old patch and discard by folding in half and apply new patch to a new area.

Patient/Family Teaching

- **PO:** Emphasize the importance of taking rivastigmine at regular intervals as directed.
- Caution patient and caregiver that rivastigmine may cause dizziness. Caution patient to avoid driving or other activities requiring alertness until response to medication is known.
- Advise patient and caregiver to notify health care professional if nausea, vomiting, anorexia, or weight loss occur. If adverse effects become intolerable during treatment with *transdermal patch,* instruct patient to discontinue patches for several days and then restart at same or next lower dose level. If treatment is interrupted for more than several days, lowest dose level should be used when restarting and titrate according to Route and Dosage section.
- Advise patient and caregiver to notify health care professional of medication regimen prior to treatment or surgery.
- Inform patient and caregiver that improvement in cognitive functioning may take weeks to months and that the degenerative process is not reversed.
- Advise patient to notify health care professional if pregnancy is planned or suspected or if breast feeding.
- **Transdermal:** Instruct patient and caregiver on the correct application, rotation, and discarding of patch. Patch should be folded in half and discarded out of reach of children and pets; medication remains in discarded patch. Replace missed doses immediately and apply next patch at usual time. Advise patient and caregiver to avoid contact with eyes and to wash hands after applying patch. Avoid exposure to heat sources (excessive sunlight, saunas, heating pads) for long periods.
- Advise patient and caregiver to notify health care professional if skin reactions occur.
- Advise patient referred for MRI test to discuss patch with referring health care professional and MRI facility to determine if removal of patch is necessary prior to test and for directions for replacing patch.

Evaluation/Desired Outcomes

- Temporary improvement in cognitive function (memory, attention, reasoning, language, ability to perform simple tasks) in patients with Alzheimer's disease.
- Improvement in cognitive function and overall functioning in patients with Parkinson's disease.

rizatriptan (riz-a-**trip**-tan)

Maxalt, Maxalt-MLT

Classification

Therapeutic: vascular headache suppressants

Pharmacologic: 5-HT_1 agonists

Pregnancy Category C

Indications

Acute treatment of migraine with or without aura.

Action

Acts as an agonist at specific 5-HT_1 receptor sites in intracranial blood vessels and sensory trigeminal nerves. **Therapeutic Effects:** Cranial vessel vasoconstriction with associated decrease in release of neuropeptides and resultant decrease in migraine headache.

Pharmacokinetics

Absorption: Completely absorbed after oral administration, but first-pass metabolism results in 45% bioavailability.

Distribution: Unknown.
Metabolism and Excretion: Primarily metabolized by monoamine oxidase-A (MAO-A); minor conversion to an active compound; 14% excreted unchanged in urine.
Half-life: 2–3 hr.

TIME/ACTION PROFILE (blood levels)

ROUTE	ONSET	PEAK	DURATION
PO	30 min	1–1.5 hr	unknown

Contraindications/Precautions

Contraindicated in: Hypersensitivity; Ischemic or vasospastic cardiovascular, cerebrovascular, or peripheral vascular syndromes; History of significant cardiovascular disease; Uncontrolled hypertension; Should not be used within 24 hr of other 5-HT_1 agonists or ergot-type compounds (dihydroergotamine); Basilar or hemiplegic migraine; Concurrent MAO-A inhibitor therapy or within 2 wk of discontinuing MAO-A inhibitor therapy; Phenylketonuria (orally disintegrating tablet contains aspartame).
Use Cautiously in: Severe renal impairment, especially in patients on dialysis; Moderate hepatic impairment; OB, Lactation, Pedi: Pregnancy, lactation, or children <6 yr (safety not established).
Exercise Extreme Caution in: Cardiovascular risk factors (hypertension, hypercholesterolemia, cigarette smoking, obesity, diabetes, strong family history, menopausal women or men >40 yr); use only if cardiovascular status has been evaluated and determined to be safe and first dose is administered under supervision.

Adverse Reactions/Side Effects

CNS: dizziness, drowsiness, weakness. **CV:** CORONARY ARTERY VASOSPASM, MI, VENTRICULAR ARRHYTHMIAS, chest pain, myocardial ischemia. **GI:** dry mouth, nausea. **Misc:** hypersensitivity reactions including ANGIOEDEMA, toxic epidermal necrolysis, pain.

Interactions

Drug-Drug: Concurrent use with **MAO-A inhibitors** ↑ levels and adverse reactions (concurrent use or use within 2 wk of MAO inhibitor is contraindicated). Concurrent use with other **5-HT agonists** or **ergot-type compounds (dihydroergotamine)** may result in ↑ vasoactive properties (avoid use within 24 hr of each other). **Propranolol** ↑ levels and risk of adverse reactions (↓ dose of rizatriptan; rizatriptan not recommended in children <40 kg). ↑ risk of serotonin syndrome when used with **SSRI or SNRI antidepressants.**
Drug-Natural Products: ↑ risk of serotinergic side effects including serotonin syndrome with **St. John's wort** and **SAMe.**

Route/Dosage

PO (Adults): 5–10 mg (use 5-mg dose in patients receiving propranolol); may be repeated in 2 hr; not to exceed 3 doses/24 hr.
PO (Children 6–17 yr): ≥*40 kg*—10 mg single dose (use 5-mg dose in patients receiving propranolol); *<40 kg*—5 mg single dose (do NOT use in patients receiving propranolol).

Availability (generic available)

Tablets: 5 mg, 10 mg. **Orally disintegrating tablets (Maxalt-MLT) (peppermint flavor):** 5 mg, 10 mg.

NURSING IMPLICATIONS

Assessment

- Assess pain location, character, intensity, and duration and associated symptoms (photophobia, phonophobia, nausea, vomiting) during migraine attack.
- Assess for serotonin syndrome (mental changes [agitation, hallucinations, coma], autonomic instability [tachycardia, labile BP, hyperthermia], neuromuscular aberations [hyper reflexia, incoordination], and/or GI symptoms [nausea, vomiting, diarrhea]), especially in patients taking other serotonergic drugs (SSRIs, SNRIs).

Potential Nursing Diagnoses

Acute pain (Indications)

Implementation

- **PO:** Tablets should be swallowed whole with liquid.
- Orally disintegrating tablets should be left in the package until use. Remove from the blister pouch. Do not push tablet through the blister; peel open the blister pack with dry hands and place tablet on tongue. Tablet will dissolve rapidly and be swallowed with saliva. No liquid is needed to take the orally disintegrating tablet.

Patient/Family Teaching

- Inform patient that rizatriptan should be used only during a migraine attack. It is meant to be used for relief of migraine attacks but not to prevent or reduce the number of attacks.
- Instruct patient to administer rizatriptan as soon as symptoms of a migraine attack appear, but it may be administered at any time during an attack. If migraine symptoms return, a second dose may be used. Allow at least 2 hr between doses, and do not use more than 30 mg in any 24-hr period.
- If first dose does not relieve headache, additional rizatriptan doses are not likely to be effective; notify health care professional.
- Caution patient not to take rizatriptan within 24 hr of other vascular headache suppressants.
- Advise patient that lying down in a darkened room after rizatriptan administration may further help relieve headache.

R

- Advise patient that overuse (use more than 10 days/mo) may lead to exacerbation of headache (migraine-like daily headaches, or as a marked increase in frequency of migraine attacks). May require gradual withdrawal of rizatriptan and treatment of symptoms (transient worsening of headache).
- Advise patient to notify health care professional before next dose of rizatriptan if pain or tightness in the chest occurs during use. If pain is severe or does not subside, notify health care professional immediately. If feelings of tingling, heat, flushing, heaviness, pressure, drowsiness, dizziness, tiredness, or sickness develop, discuss with health care professional at next visit.
- May cause dizziness or drowsiness. Caution patient to avoid driving or other activities requiring alertness until response to medication is known.
- Advise patient to avoid alcohol, which aggravates headaches, during rizatriptan use.
- Advise patient to notify health care professional immediately if signs or symptoms of serotonin syndrome occur.
- Caution female patient to avoid rizatriptan if pregnant or breast feeding, or if pregnancy is suspected or planned. Adequate contraception should be used during therapy.

Evaluation/Desired Outcomes

- Relief of migraine attack.

rolapitant (rol-**ap**-i-tant)

Varubi

Classification
Therapeutic: antiemetics
Pharmacologic: neurokinin antagonists

Indications

With other antiemetic agents in adults to prevent delayed nausea and vomiting associated with initial/repeat courses of emetogenic cancer chemotherapy.

Action

Acts as a selective antagonist at substance P/neurokinin 1 (NK_1) receptors in the brain. **Therapeutic Effects:** Decreased nausea and vomiting associated with chemotherapy. Augments the antiemetic effects of dexamethasone and 5-HT_3 antagonists.

Pharmacokinetics

Absorption: Well absorbed following oral administration.
Distribution: Unk.
Protein Binding: 99.8%.
Metabolism and Excretion: Mostly metabolized, primarily by CYP3A4; one metabolite, C4–pyrrolidine-hydroxylated rolapitant (M19) has antiemetic activity. Excretion is mainly via hepato/biliary elimination. 14% excreted in urine (8% as metabolites), 73% in feces (38% as unchanged drug).
Half-life: *Rolapitant*—7 days; *M19*—7 days.

TIME/ACTION PROFILE (blood levels)

ROUTE	ONSET	PEAK	DURATION
PO	within 30 min	4 hr	7 days

Contraindications/Precautions

Contraindicated in: Concurrent use of thioridazine or pimozide.
Use Cautiously in: Concurrent use of other substrates of CYP2D6 with narrow therapeutic indeces (avoid concurrent use if possible, if necessary monitor carefully); Severe hepatic impairment (avoid if possible, if unavoidable monitor carefully); Severe renal impairment (effect on pharmacokinetics not known; Geri: Elderly patients may be more sensitive to drug effects; OB: Effects in pregnancy are unknown; Lactation: Weigh maternal benefits against risks to the infant; Pedi: Safe and effective use in children has not been established.

Adverse Reactions/Side Effects

CV: dizziness (↑ with anthracycline/cyclophosphamide regimens). **GI:** ↓ appetite (↑ with anthracycline/cyclophosphamide regimens), hiccups (↑ with cisplatin regimens). **Hemat:** neutropenia.

Interactions

Drug-Drug: ↑ levels and risk of serious cardiac toxicity with **thioridazine** and **pimozide**; thioridazine is contraindicated, pimozide should be avoided. ↑ levels effects and risk of toxicity from **irinotecan**, **methotrexate**, **rosuvastatin** and **topotecan**, may have a similar effect on other**drugs that are handled by Breast-Cancer-Resistance protein** (BCRP) transporter; dose reduction may be necessary. ↑ levels, effects and risk of toxicity from **digoxin** and other**drugs that are metabolized by P-glycoprotein** (P-gp) transporter, especially those with narrow therapeutic indeces, careful monitoring is recommended. **Strong CYP3A4 inducers** including **rifampin** ↓ blood levels and effectiveness.

Route/Dosage

PO (Adults): 180 mg 1–2 hour prior to start of chemotherapy; with dexamethasone and a 5-HT_3 antagonist.

Availability

Tablets: 90 mg.

NURSING IMPLICATIONS

Assessment

- Assess nausea, vomiting, appetite, bowel sounds, and abdominal pain prior to and following administration.
- ***Lab Test Considerations:*** May cause ↓ WBC.

Potential Nursing Diagnoses

Risk for deficient fluid volume (Indications)
Imbalanced nutrition: less than body requirements (Indications)

Implementation

- **PO:** Administer 1–2 hrs before chemotherapy without regard to food. Due to long action, administered no more frequently than onceevery 14 days. Given with dexamethasone and a 5-HT_3 antagonist.

Patient/Family Teaching

- Instruct patient to take rolapitant as directed. Direct patient to read the *Patient Package Insert* before starting therapy and each time Rx renewed in case of changes.
- Instruct patient to notify health care professional of all Rx or OTC medications, vitamins, or herbal products being taken and consult health care professional before taking any new medications.
- Advise patient and family to use general measures to decrease nausea (begin with sips of liquids and small, nongreasy meals; provide oral hygiene; remove noxious stimuli from environment).
- Advise patient to notify health care professional if pregnancy is planned or suspected or if breast feeding.

Evaluation/Desired Outcomes

- Decreased delayed nausea and vomiting associated with emetogenic chemotherapy.

rOPINIRole (roe-pin-i-role)

Requip, Requip XL

Classification
Therapeutic: antiparkinson agents
Pharmacologic: dopamine agonists

Pregnancy Category C

Indications

Management of signs and symptoms of idiopathic Parkinson's disease. Restless leg syndrome (immediate-release only).

Action

Stimulates dopamine receptors in the brain. **Therapeutic Effects:** Decreased tremor and rigidity in Parkinson's disease. Decreased leg restlessness.

Pharmacokinetics

Absorption: 55% absorbed following oral administration.
Distribution: Widely distributed.
Metabolism and Excretion: Extensively metabolized by the liver (by cytochrome P450 CYP1A2 enzyme system); <10% excreted unchanged in urine.
Half-life: 6 hr.

TIME/ACTION PROFILE

ROUTE	ONSET	PEAK	DURATION
PO	unknown	unknown	8 hr

Contraindications/Precautions

Contraindicated in: Hypersensitivity.
Use Cautiously in: Hepatic impairment (slower titration may be required); Severe cardiovascular disease; **OB, Lactation, Pedi:** Safety not established; may inhibit lactation; **Geri:** ↑ risk of hallucinations.

Adverse Reactions/Side Effects

CNS: SLEEP ATTACKS, dizziness, syncope, agitation, aggression, confusion, delirium, delusions, disorientation, drowsiness, dyskinesia, fatigue, hallucinations, headache, impulse control disorders (gambling, sexual), paranoid ideation, psychosis, weakness. **EENT:** abnormal vision. **CV:** orthostatic hypotension, peripheral edema. **GI:** constipation, dry mouth, dyspepsia, nausea, vomiting. **Derm:** sweating, melanoma.

Interactions

Drug-Drug: Drugs that alter the activity of cytochrome P450 CYP1A2 enzyme system may affect the activity of ropinirole. Effects may be ↑ by **estrogens**. Effects may be ↓ by **phenothiazines**, **butyrophenones**, **thioxanthenes**, or **metoclopramide**. May ↑ effects of **levodopa** (may allow dose ↓ of levodopa).

Route/Dosage

Parkinson's Disease

PO (Adults): *Immediate–release*0.25 mg 3 times daily for 1 wk, then 0.5 mg 3 times daily for 1 wk, then 0.75 mg 3 times daily for 1 wk, then 1 mg 3 times daily for 1 wk; then may ↑ by 1.5 mg/day every wk up to 9 mg/day; then may ↑ by up to 3 mg/day every wk up to 24 mg/day; *Extended–release*2 mg once daily for 1–2 wk; may ↑ by 2 mg/day every wk up to 24 mg/day.

Renal Impairment

PO (Adults): *Hemodialysis*—0.25 mg 3 times daily; may ↑ dose as needed based on response and tolerability (not to exceed 18 mg/day).

Restless Leg Syndrome

PO (Adults): *Immediate–release*0.25 mg once daily initially, 1–3 hr before bedtime. After 2 days, ↑ to 0.5 mg once daily and to 1 mg once daily by the end of first week of dosing, then ↑ by 0.5 mg weekly, up to 4 mg/day as needed/tolerated.

Renal Impairment

PO (Adults): *Hemodialysis*—0.25 mg once daily; may ↑ dose as needed based on response and tolerability (not to exceed 3 mg/day).

R

Availability (generic available)

Tablets: 0.25 mg, 0.5 mg, 1 mg, 2 mg, 3 mg, 4 mg, 5 mg. **Cost:** *Generic*—0.25 mg $250.21/100, 0.5 mg $250.21/100, 1 mg $250.21/100, 2 mg $250.21/100, 3 mg $259.54/100, 4 mg $259.85/100, 5 mg $259.85/100. **Extended-release tablets:** 2 mg, 4 mg, 6 mg, 8 mg, 12 mg. **Cost:** *Generic*—2 mg $82.05/30, 4 mg $164.10/30, 6 mg $246.16/30, 8 mg $246.16/30, 12 mg $410.47/30.

NURSING IMPLICATIONS

Assessment

- Assess BP periodically during therapy.
- Assess patient for drowsiness and sleep attacks. Drowsiness is a common side effect of ropinirole, but sleep attacks or episodes of falling asleep during activities that require active participation may occur without warning. Assess patient for concomitant medications that have sedating effects or may increase serum ropinirole levels (see Interactions). May require discontinuation of therapy.
- Assess patient for signs and symptoms of psychotic-like behavior (confusion, paranoid ideation, delusions, hallucinations, psychotic-like behavior, disorientation, aggressive behavior, agitation, delirium, hallucinations). Risk of symptoms increases with age. Notify health care professional if these occur.
- **Parkinson's Disease:** Assess patient for signs and symptoms of Parkinson's disease (tremor, muscle weakness and rigidity, ataxic gait) prior to and during therapy.
- **Restless Leg Syndrome:** Assess sleep patterns and frequency of restless leg disturbances.
- Monitor for *augmentation* (earlier onset of symptoms in the evening or afternoon), increase in symptoms, and spread of symptoms to involve other extremities) and *rebound* (new onset of symptoms in the early morning hours). If symptoms occur, consider dose adjustment or discontinuation of therapy.
- ***Lab Test Considerations:*** May cause ↑ BUN.

Potential Nursing Diagnoses

Impaired physical mobility (Indications)
Risk for injury (Indications, Side Effects)

Implementation

- Do not confuse ropinirole with Risperdal (risperidone) or risperidone.
- **PO:** May be administered with or without food. Administration with food may decrease nausea. Extended-release tablets should be swallowed whole; do not break, crush, or chew.

Patient/Family Teaching

- Instruct patient to take medication exactly as directed. Missed doses should be taken as soon as possible, but not if almost time for next dose. Do not double doses.
- Caution patient to change positions slowly to minimize orthostatic hypotension.
- May cause drowsiness and unexpected episodes of falling asleep. Caution patient to avoid driving or other activities requiring alertness until response to medication is known. Advise patient to notify health care professional if episodes of falling asleep occur.
- Advise patient to avoid alcohol and other CNS depressants concurrently with ropinirole.
- Advise patient that increasing fluids, sugarless gum or candy, ice, or saliva substitutes may help minimize dry mouth. Consult health care professional if dry mouth continues for >2 wk.
- Advise patient to have periodic skin exams to check for lesions that may be melanoma.
- Advise patient to notify health care professional if new or increased gambling, sexual, or other impulse control disorders or psychotic-like behaviors occur.

Evaluation/Desired Outcomes

- Decreased tremor and rigidity in Parkinson's disease.
- Decrease in restless legs and improved sleep.

---

ropivacaine, See EPIDURAL LOCAL ANESTHETICS.

---

rosuvastatin, See HMG-CoA REDUCTASE INHIBITORS (statins).

sacubitril/valsartan
(sa-**ku**-bi-tril/val-**sar**-tan)
Entresto

Classification
Therapeutic: vasodilators, antihypertensives
Pharmacologic: angiotensin II receptor antagonistsneprilysin inhibitors

Indications
To ↓ risk of cardiovascular death and hospitalization for chronic heart failure patients (NYHA Class II-IV and ↓ ejection fraction).

Action
sacubitril—a pro-drug converted to LBQ657, its active moeity. LBQ657 inhibits the enzyme neprilysin. Neprilysin degrades vasoactive peptides, including natriuretic peptides, bradykinin, and adrenomedullin resulting in ↑ levels of these peptides, causing vasodilation and ↓ ECF volume via sodium excretion. *Valsartan*—Blocks vasoconstrictor and aldosterone-producing effects of angiotensin II at receptor sites, including vascular smooth muscle and the adrenal glands. **Therapeutic Effects:** Reduced cardiovascular death and hospitalizations due to HF.

Pharmacokinetics
Absorption: *sacubitril*—≥60% absorbed following oral administration; rapidly converted to LBQ657, its active form. *Valsartan*—Absorption in combinations with sacubitril is greater than 10–35% absorbed following oral administration of single-entity formulation.
Distribution: *Sacubitril*—small amounts cross the blood-brain barrier. *Valsartan*—crosses the placenta.
Protein Binding: *sacubitril, valsartan*—94–97%.
Metabolism and Excretion: *sacubitril*—following conversion to LBQ657 metabolism is minimal; 52–68% excreted in urine. *Valsartan*—Minor metabolism by the liver; 13% excreted in urine, 83% in feces.
Half-life: *sacubitril*—1.4 hr. *LBQ657*—11.5 hr. *Valsartan*—9.9hr.

TIME/ACTION PROFILE (blood levels)

ROUTE	ONSET	PEAK	DURATION
sacubitril	unknown	0.5 hr	12 hr
LBQ657	unknown	2 hr	12 hr
Valsartan	unknown	1.5 hr	12 hr

Contraindications/Precautions
Contraindicated in: Hypersensitivity or history of angioedema from previous ACE inhibitors or ARBs; Concurrent use of ACE inhibitors during or for 36 hr before or after; Concurrent use with aliskiren in patients with diabetes or moderate-to-severe renal impairment (CCr <60 mL/min); Severe hepatic impairment; OB: Can cause injury or death of fetus—if pregnancy occurs, discontinue immediately; Lactation: Discontinue drug or use formula.
Use Cautiously in: HF (may result in azotemia, oliguria, acute renal failure and/or death); Volume- or salt-depleted patients or patients receiving high doses of diuretics (correct deficits before initiating therapy or initiate at lower doses); Black patients (may not be effective); Impaired renal function due to primary renal disease or HF (may worsen renal function); OB: Women of childbearing potential; Pedi: Safety not established in children.

Adverse Reactions/Side Effects
CNS: dizziness. **Resp:** cough. **CV:** hypotension. **F and E:** hyperkalemia. **Misc:** ANGIOEDEMA.

Interactions
Drug-Drug: NSAIDs and selective **COX-2 inhibitors** may ↑ the risk of renal dysfunction. ↑ risk of hypotension with other **antihypertensives** and **diuretics**. Concurrent use of **potassium-sparing diuretics, potassium-containing salt substitutes** or **potassium supplements** may ↑ risk of hyperkalemia. ↑ risk of hyperkalemia, renal dysfunction, hypotension, and syncope with concurrent use of **ACE inhibitors** or **aliskiren**; avoid concurrent use with aliskiren in patients with diabetes or CCr <60 mL/min; avoid concurrent use with ACE inhibitors. May ↑ **lithium** levels.

Route/Dosage
PO (Adults): Initial dose—sacubitril 49 mg/valsartan 51 mg twice daily, dose may be doubled every 2–4 wk to target dose of 97 mg/valsartan 103 mg as tolerated. *Patients not currently receiving angiotensin-converting enzyme inhibitors (ACEis) or angiotensin receptor blockers (ARBs) or receiving low doses*—initial dose sacubitril 24 mg/valsartan 26 mg twice daily dose may be doubled every 2–4 wk to target dose of 97 mg/valsartan 103 mg as tolerated.

Hepatic/Renal Impairment
PO (Adults): *Severe renal impairment (CCr <30 mL/min/1.73 m² or moderate hepatic impairment (Child-Pugh class B)*—initial dose sacubitril 24 mg/valsartan 26 mg twice daily dose may be doubled every 2–4 wk to target dose of 97 mg/valsartan 103 mg as tolerated.

Availability
Tablets: sacubitril 24 mg/valsartan 26 mg, sacubitril 49 mg/valsartan 52 mg, sacubitril 97 mg/valsartan 103 mg.

NURSING IMPLICATIONS
Assessment
- Assess BP (lying, sitting, standing) and pulse frequently during initial dose adjustment and periodi-

cally throughout therapy. Correct volume or salt depletion prior to administration of therapy. If hypotension occurs, consider reducing dose of diuretics, concomitant antihypertensive agents, and treatment of other causes of hypotension (hypovolemia). If hypotension persist, reduce the dose or temporarily discontinue therapy. Permanent discontinuation of therapy is usually not required.

- Monitor daily weight and assess patient routinely for resolution of fluid overload (peripheral edema, rales/crackles, dyspnea, weight gain, jugular venous distention).
- Monitor frequency of prescription refills to determine compliance.
- Assess patients for signs of angioedema (dyspnea, orofacial swelling); may occur more frequently in Black patients. If signs occur, discontinue therapy, provide supportive therapy, and monitor for airway compromise.
- ***Lab Test Considerations:*** Monitor renal function. May cause increase in BUN and serum creatinine. May require ↓ dose.
- May cause hyperkalemia. May require ↓ dose.
- May cause ↓ in hemoglobin and hematocrit.

Potential Nursing Diagnoses

Decreased cardiac output (Indications)

Implementation

- **PO:** Administer twice daily.
- If switching from an ACE inhibitor to *Entresto*, allow 36 hrs between last ACE inhibitor dose and starting *Entresto*.

Patient/Family Teaching

- Instruct patient to take *Entresto*as directed, at the same time each day, even if feeling well. Take missed doses as soon as remembered if not almost time for next dose; do not double doses. Warn patient not to discontinue therapy unless directed by health care professional. Advise patient to read *Patient Information* before starting therapy and with each Rx refill in case of changes.
- Caution patient to avoid salt substitutes containing potassium or foods containing high levels of potassium or sodium unless directed by health care professional. See Appendix J.
- Instruct patient to notify health care professional if swelling of face, eyes, lips, or tongue or if difficulty swallowing or breathing occur.
- May cause dizziness. Caution patient to avoid driving or other activities requiring alertness until response to medication is known.
- Instruct patient to notify health care professional of all Rx or OTC medications, vitamins, or herbal products being taken and to avoid concurrent use of Rx, OTC, and herbal products, especially NSAIDs, potassium supplements or salt substitute, ACE inhibitors, ARBs, lithium or aliskiren, without consulting health care professional.
- Instruct patient to notify health care professional of medication regimen before treatment or surgery.
- Advise women of childbearing age to use contraception and notify health care professional if pregnancy is planned or suspected, or if breast feeding. *Entresto* should be discontinued as soon as possible when pregnancy is detected.
- Emphasize the importance of follow-up exams to evaluate effectiveness of medication.

Evaluation/Desired Outcomes

- Decreased heart-failure-related hospitalizations in patients with heart failure.

SALICYLATES

aspirin (**as**-pir-in)
✽Arthrinol, ✽Arthrisin, ✽Artria S.R, ASA, ✽Asaphen, Ascriptin, Aspercin, Aspergum, Aspirtab, ✽Astrin, Bayer Aspirin, Bufferin, ✽Coryphen, Easprin, Ecotrin, ✽Entrophen, Genacote, Halfprin, ✽Headache Tablets, Healthprin, ✽Novasen, ✽Rivasa, St. Joseph Adult Chewable Aspirin, ZORprin

choline and magnesium salicylates
(**koe**-leen mag-**nee**-zhum sal-**i**-sil-ates)
~~Trilisate~~

magnesium salicylate
(mag-**nee**-zhum sal-**i**-sil-ate)
✽Doan's Backache Pills, Doan's Extra Strength, Keygesic, Momentum

salsalate (**sal**-sa-late)
~~Disalcid~~

Classification
Therapeutic: antipyretics, nonopioid analgesics
Pharmacologic: salicylates

Pregnancy Category D (aspirin—first trimester), C (magnesium salicylate, salsalate—first trimester)

Indications

Inflammatory disorders including: Rheumatoid arthritis, Osteoarthritis. Mild to moderate pain. Fever. **Aspirin:** Prophylaxis of transient ischemic attacks and MI.

Action

Produce analgesia and reduce inflammation and fever by inhibiting the production of prostaglandins. **Aspirin Only:** Decreases platelet aggregation. **Therapeutic Effects:** Analgesia. Reduction of inflammation. Reduction of fever. **Aspirin:** Decreased incidence of transient ischemic attacks and MI.

Pharmacokinetics

Absorption: *Aspirin*—Well absorbed from the upper small intestine; absorption from enteric-coated preparations may be unreliable; rectal absorption is slow and variable. *Choline and magnesium salicylates*—Well absorbed after oral administration. *Salsalate*—Splits into 2 molecules of salicylic acid after oral administration; absorbed in the small intestine.
Distribution: All salicylates are rapidly and widely distributed; cross the placenta and enter breast milk.
Metabolism and Excretion: Extensively metabolized by the liver; inactive metabolites excreted by the kidneys. Amount excreted unchanged by the kidneys depends on urine pH; as pH increases, amount excreted unchanged increases from 2–3% up to 80%.
Half-life: 2–3 hr for low doses; up to 15–30 hr with larger doses because of saturation of liver metabolism.

TIME/ACTION PROFILE (analgesia/fever reduction†)

ROUTE	ONSET	PEAK	DURATION
Aspirin–PO	5–30 min	1–3 hr	3–6 hr
Aspirin–PO-ER	5–30 min	2–4 hr	8–12 hr
Aspirin–Rect	1–2 hr	4–5 hr	7 hr
All other salicylates–PO	5–30 min	1–3 hr	3–6 hr

†Antirheumatic effect may take 2–3 wk of chronic dosing.

Contraindications/Precautions

Contraindicated in: Hypersensitivity to aspirin, tartrazine (FDC yellow dye #5), or other salicylates; Cross-sensitivity with other NSAIDs may exist (less with nonaspirin salicylates); Bleeding disorders or thrombocytopenia (more important with aspirin); Children or adolescents with viral infections (may increase the risk of Reye's syndrome); Peri-operative pain from coronary artery bypass graft (CABG) surgery.
Use Cautiously in: History of GI bleeding or ulcer disease; Chronic alcohol use/abuse; Severe renal disease (magnesium toxicity may occur with magnesium salicylate); Severe hepatic disease; Cardiovascular disease or risk factors for cardiovascular disease (may ↑ risk of serious cardiovascular thrombotic events, myocardial infarction, and stroke, especially with prolonged use); OB: Salicylates may have adverse effects on fetus and mother and, in general, should be avoided during pregnancy, especially during the 3rd trimester; Lactation: Safety not established; Geri: ↑ risk of adverse reactions especially GI bleeding; more sensitive to toxic levels.

Adverse Reactions/Side Effects

EENT: tinnitus. **GI:** GI BLEEDING, dyspepsia, epigastric distress, nausea, abdominal pain, anorexia, hepatotoxicity, vomiting. **Derm:** *salsalate*—EXFOLIATIVE DERMATITIS, STEVENS-JOHNSON SYNDROME, TOXIC EPIDERMAL NECROLYSIS. **Hemat:** *aspirin*—anemia, hemolysis, increased bleeding time. **Misc:** allergic reactions including ANAPHYLAXIS and LARYNGEAL EDEMA.

Interactions

Drug-Drug: Aspirin may ↑ the risk of bleeding with **warfarin**, **heparin**, **heparin-like agents**, **thrombolytic agents**, **clopidogrel**, **abciximab**, **tirofiban**, or **eptifibatide**, although these agents are frequently used safely in combination and in sequence. Ibuprofen may negate the cardioprotective antiplatelet effects of low-dose aspirin. Aspirin may ↑ risk of bleeding with **cefotetan**, and **valproic acid**. May ↑ activity of **penicillins**, **phenytoin**, **methotrexate**, **valproic acid**, **oral hypoglycemic agents**, and **sulfonamides**. May ↓ beneficial effects of **probenecid**. **Corticosteroids** may ↓ serum salicylate levels. **Urinary acidification** ↑ reabsorption and may ↑ serum salicylate levels. **Alkalinization of the urine** or the ingestion of large amounts of **antacids** ↑ excretion and ↓ serum salicylate level. May blunt the therapeutic response to **diuretics**, and **antihypertensives**. ↑ risk of GI irritation with **NSAIDs**.
Drug-Natural Products: ↑ anticoagulant effect and bleeding risk when using aspirin with **arnica**, **chamomile**, **clove**, **feverfew**, **garlic**, **ginger**, **ginkgo**, **Panax ginseng**, and others.
Drug-Food: Foods capable of acidifying the urine (see Appendix J) may ↑ serum salicylate levels.

S

Route/Dosage

Aspirin

Pain/Fever

PO, Rect (Adults): 325–1000 mg q 4–6 hr (not to exceed 4 g/day). *Extended-release tablets*—650 mg q 8 hr or 800 mg q 12 hr.
PO, Rect (Children 2–11 yr): 10–15 mg/kg q 4–6 hr (not to exceed 4 g/day).

Inflammation

PO (Adults): 2.4 g/day initially; increased to maintenance dose of 3.6–5.4 g/day in divided doses (up to 7.8 g/day for acute rheumatic fever).
PO (Children): 60–100 mg/kg/day in divided doses (up to 130 mg/kg/day for acute rheumatic fever).

Prevention of Transient Ischemic Attacks

PO (Adults): 50–325 mg once daily.

Prevention of Myocardial Infarction

PO (Adults): 80–325 mg once daily.
PO (Children): 3–10 mg/kg once daily (round dose to a convenient amount).

Kawasaki Disease

PO (Children): 80–100 mg/kg/day in 4 divided doses until fever resolves; may be followed by maintenance dose of 3–5 mg/kg/day as a single dose for up to 8 wk.

Magnesium Salicylate

PO (Adults): 304 mg q 4 hr or 467 mg q 6 hr.

Choline and Magnesium Salicylates

5 mL of liquid equivalent to 500 mg salicylate or 650 mg of aspirin. Tablet strength expressed in mg of salicylate: 500-mg tablet equivalent to 650 mg of aspirin, 750-mg tablet equivalent to 975 mg of aspirin, 1000-mg tablet equivalent to 1.3 g of aspirin.
PO (Adults): *Anti-inflammatory*—3 g/day of salicylate at bedtime or in 2–3 divided doses (not to exceed 4.5 g/day).
PO (Children >37 kg): 2.25 g of salicylate/day in 2 divided doses.
PO (Children <37 kg): 50 mg of salicylate/kg/day in 2 divided doses.

Salsalate

PO (Adults): 1 g 3 times daily initially; further titration may be required.

Availability

Aspirin (generic available)

Tablets: 81 mg^{OTC}, 162.5 mg^{OTC}, 325 mg^{OTC}, 500 mg^{OTC}, 650 mg^{OTC}, 🍁975 mg^{OTC}. **Chewable tablets:** 🍁80 mg^{OTC}, 81 mg^{OTC}. **Chewing gum:** 227 mg^{OTC}. **Dispersible tablets:** 325 mg^{OTC}, 500 mg^{OTC}. **Enteric-coated (delayed-release) tablets:** 80 mg^{OTC}, 165 mg^{OTC}, 🍁300 mg^{OTC}, 325 mg^{OTC}, 500 mg^{OTC}, 🍁600 mg^{OTC}, 650 mg^{OTC}, 975 mg^{OTC}. **Extended-release tablets:** 🍁325 mg^{OTC}, 650 mg^{OTC}, 800 mg. **Delayed-release capsules:** 🍁325 mg^{OTC}, 🍁500 mg^{OTC}. **Suppositories:** 60 mg^{OTC}, 120 mg^{OTC}, 125 mg^{OTC}, 130 mg^{OTC}, 🍁150 mg^{OTC}, 🍁160 mg^{OTC}, 195 mg^{OTC}, 200 mg^{OTC}, 300 mg^{OTC}, 🍁320 mg^{OTC}, 325 mg^{OTC}, 600 mg^{OTC}, 🍁640 mg^{OTC}, 650 mg^{OTC}, 1.2 g^{OTC}. ***In combination with:*** antihistamines, decongestants, cough suppressants^{OTC}, and opioids. See Appendix B.

Choline and Magnesium Salicylates (listed as salicylate content)

Liquid: 500 mg/5 mL.

Magnesium Salicylate (generic available)

Tablets: 580 mg^{OTC}, 600 mg, 650 mg^{OTC}.

Salsalate (generic available)

Tablets: 500 mg, 750 mg.

NURSING IMPLICATIONS

Assessment

- Patients who have asthma, allergies, and nasal polyps or who are allergic to tartrazine are at an increased risk for developing hypersensitivity reactions.
- Assess for rash periodically during therapy. May cause Stevens-Johnson syndrome or toxic epidermal necrolysis. Discontinue therapy if severe or if accompanied with fever, general malaise, fatigue, muscle or joint aches, blisters, oral lesions, conjunctivitis, hepatitis, and/or eosinophilia.
- **Pain:** Assess pain and limitation of movement; note type, location, and intensity before and at the peak (see Time/Action Profile) after administration.
- **Fever:** Assess fever and note associated signs (diaphoresis, tachycardia, malaise, chills).
- ***Lab Test Considerations:*** Monitor hepatic function before antirheumatic therapy and if symptoms of hepatotoxicity occur; more likely in patients, especially children, with rheumatic fever, systemic lupus erythematosus, juvenile arthritis, or pre-existing hepatic disease. May cause ↑ serum AST, ALT, and alkaline phosphatase, especially when plasma concentrations exceed 25 mg/100 mL. May return to normal despite continued use or dose reduction. If severe abnormalities or active liver disease occurs, discontinue and use with caution in future.
- Monitor serum salicylate levels periodically with prolonged high-dose therapy to determine dose, safety, and efficacy, especially in children with Kawasaki disease.
- *Aspirin:* Prolongs bleeding time for 4–7 days and, in large doses, may cause prolonged prothrombin time. Monitor hematocrit periodically in prolonged high-dose therapy to assess for GI blood loss.
- ***Toxicity and Overdose:*** Monitor patient for the onset of tinnitus, headache, hyperventilation, agitation, mental confusion, lethargy, diarrhea, and sweating. If these symptoms appear, withhold medication and notify health care professional immediately.

Potential Nursing Diagnoses

Acute pain (Indications)
Impaired physical mobility (Indications)

Implementation

- Use lowest effective dose for shortest period of time.
- **PO:** Administer after meals or with food or an antacid to minimize gastric irritation. Food slows but does not alter the total amount absorbed.
- Do not crush or chew enteric-coated tablets. Do not take antacids within 1–2 hr of enteric-coated tablets. Chewable tablets may be chewed, dissolved in liquid, or swallowed whole. Some extended-release tablets may be broken or crumbled but must not be ground up before swallowing. See manufacturer's prescribing information for individual products.

Patient/Family Teaching

- Instruct patient to take salicylates with a full glass of water and to remain in an upright position for 15–30 min after administration.
- Advise patient to report tinnitus; unusual bleeding of gums; bruising; black, tarry stools; or fever lasting longer than 3 days.
- Caution patient to avoid concurrent use of alcohol with this medication to minimize possible gastric irritation; 3 or more glasses of alcohol per day may increase the risk of GI bleeding. Caution patient to avoid taking concurrently with acetaminophen or NSAIDs for more than a few days, unless directed by health care professional to prevent analgesic nephropathy.
- Teach patients on a sodium-restricted diet to avoid effervescent tablets or buffered-aspirin preparations.
- Tablets with an acetic (vinegar-like) odor should be discarded.
- Instruct patient to notify health care professional if rash or signs and symptoms of hypersensitivity reaction occurs.
- Advise patients on long-term therapy to inform health care professional of medication regimen before surgery. Aspirin may need to be withheld for 1 wk before surgery.
- Pedi: Centers for Disease Control and Prevention warns against giving aspirin to children or adolescents with varicella (chickenpox) or influenza-like or viral illnesses because of a possible association with Reye's syndrome.
- **Transient Ischemic Attacks or MI:** Advise patients receiving aspirin prophylactically to take only prescribed dose. Increasing the dose has not been found to provide additional benefits.

Evaluation/Desired Outcomes

- Relief of mild to moderate discomfort.
- Increased ease of joint movement. May take 2–3 wk for maximum effectiveness.
- Reduction of fever.
- Prevention of transient ischemic attacks.
- Prevention of MI.

salmeterol (sal-me-te-role)

Serevent Diskus

Classification

Therapeutic: bronchodilators

Pharmacologic: adrenergics

Pregnancy Category C

Indications

As concomitant therapy for the treatment of asthma and the prevention of bronchospasm in patients who are currently taking but are inadequately controlled on a long-term asthma-control medication (e.g., inhaled corticosteroid). Prevention of exercise-induced bronchospasm. Maintenance treatment to prevent bronchospasm in chronic obstructive pulmonary disease (COPD) including chronic bronchitis and emphysema.

Action

Produces accumulation of cyclic adenosine monophosphate (cAMP) at $beta_2$-adrenergic receptors. Relatively specific for beta (pulmonary) receptors. **Therapeutic Effects:** Bronchodilation.

Pharmacokinetics

Absorption: Minimal systemic absorption follows inhalation.

Distribution: Action is primarily local.

Metabolism and Excretion: Unknown.

Half-life: 3–4 hr.

TIME/ACTION PROFILE (bronchodilation)

ROUTE	ONSET	PEAK	DURATION
Inhalation	10–25 min	3–4 hr	12 hr†

†9 hr in adolescents.

Contraindications/Precautions

Contraindicated in: Hypersensitivity; Acute attack of asthma (onset of action is delayed); Patients not receiving a long-term asthma-control medication (e.g., inhaled corticosteroid); Patients whose asthma is currently controlled on low- or medium-dose inhaled corticosteroid therapy.

Use Cautiously in: Cardiovascular disease (including angina and hypertension); Seizure disorders; Diabetes; Glaucoma; Hyperthyroidism; Pheochromocytoma; Excessive use (may lead to tolerance and paradoxical bronchospasm); OB: Use only if potential benefit justifies potential risk to fetus; may inhibit contractions during labor; Lactation: Use only if potential benefit justifies potential risk to infant. Consider discontinuing breast feeding while on salmeterol; Pedi: Children <4 yr (safety not estalished); a fixed-dose combination product containing salmeterol and an inhaled corticosteroid should be strongly considered to ensure adherence.

Adverse Reactions/Side Effects

CNS: headache, nervousness. **CV:** palpitations, tachycardia. **GI:** abdominal pain, diarrhea, nausea. **MS:** muscle cramps/soreness. **Neuro:** trembling. **Resp:** ASTHMA-RELATED DEATH, paradoxical bronchospasm, cough.

Interactions

Drug-Drug: Beta blockers may ↓ therapeutic effects. **MAO inhibitors** and **tricyclic antidepressants** potentiate cardiovascular effects. ↑ levels and ↑ risk of cardiovascular effects when used with potent CYP3A4 inhibitors (e.g., **ketoconazole**, **itraconazole**, **ritonavir**, **atazanavir**, **clarithromycin**, **indinavir**, **nefazodone**, **nelfinavir**, or **saquinavir**); concurrent use is not recommended.

Drug-Natural Products: Use with caffeine-containing herbs (**cola nut**, **guarana**, **mate**, **tea**, **coffee**) ↑ stimulant effect.

Route/Dosage

Asthma

Inhaln (Adults and Children ≥4 yr): 50 mcg (1 inhalation) twice daily (approximately 12 hr apart).

Prevention of Exercise-Induced Bronchospasm

Inhaln (Adults and Children ≥4 yr): 50 mcg (1 inhalation) at least 30 min before exercise; additional doses should not be used for at least 12 hr.

COPD

Inhaln (Adults): 50 mcg (1 inhalation) twice daily (approximately 12 hr apart).

Availability

Powder for oral inhalation (Serevent Diskus): 50 mcg/blister. ***In combination with:*** fluticasone (Advair Diskus, Advair HFA, see Appendix B).

NURSING IMPLICATIONS

Assessment

- Assess lung sounds, pulse, and BP before administration and periodically during therapy.
- Monitor pulmonary function tests before initiating therapy and periodically during therapy.
- Observe for paradoxical bronchospasm (wheezing, dyspnea, tightness in chest) and hypersensitivity reaction (rash; urticaria; swelling of the face, lips, or eyelids). Frequently occurs with first use of new canister or vial. If condition occurs, withhold medication and notify physician or other health care professional immediately.
- ***Lab Test Considerations:*** May cause ↑ serum glucose concentrations; occurs rarely with recommended doses and is more pronounced with frequent use of high doses.
- May cause ↓ serum potassium concentrations, which are usually transient and dose related; rarely occurs at recommended doses and is more pronounced with frequent use of high doses.
- ***Toxicity and Overdose:*** Symptoms of overdose include persistent agitation, chest pain or discomfort, decreased BP, dizziness, hyperglycemia, hypokalemia, seizures, tachyarrhythmias, persistent trembling, and vomiting.
- Treatment includes discontinuing salmeterol and other beta-adrenergic agonists and providing symptomatic, supportive therapy. Cardioselective beta blockers are used cautiously because they may induce bronchospasm.

Potential Nursing Diagnoses

Ineffective airway clearance (Indications)

Implementation

- Salmeterol should be used along with an inhaled corticosteroid, not as monotherapy. Patients taking salmeterol twice daily should not use additional doses for exercise-induced bronchospasm.
- **Inhaln:** Once removed from foil overwrap, discard diskus when every blister has been used or 6 wk have passed, whichever comes first.
- Do not use a spacer with powder for inhalation.

Patient/Family Teaching

- Advise patient to take salmeterol as directed. Do not use more than the prescribed dose. If a regularly scheduled dose is missed, use as soon as possible and resume regular schedule. Do not double doses. If symptoms occur before next dose is due, use a rapid-acting inhaled bronchodilator.
- Instruct patient using *powder for inhalation* never to exhale into diskus device and always to hold device in a level horizontal position. Mouthpiece should be kept dry; never wash.
- Caution patient not to use salmeterol to treat acute symptoms. A rapid-acting inhaled beta-adrenergic bronchodilator should be used for relief of acute asthma attacks.
- Advise patients on chronic therapy not to use additional salmeterol to prevent exercise-induced bronchospasm. Patients using salmeterol for prevention of exercise-induced bronchospasm should not use additional doses of salmeterol for 12 hr after prophylactic administration.
- Advise patient to notify health care professional immediately if difficulty in breathing persists after use of salmeterol, if condition worsens, if more inhalations of rapid-acting bronchodilator than usual are needed to relieve an acute attack, or if using 4 or more inhalations of a rapid-acting bronchodilator for 2 or more consecutive days or more than 1 canister in an 8-wk period.
- Salmeterol is often used with inhaled corticosteroids and is not a substitute for corticosteroids or adrenergic bronchodilators. Advise patients using inhalation or systemic corticosteroids to consult health care professional before stopping or reducing therapy.
- Emphasize the importance of regular follow-up exams to determine progress during therapy.

Evaluation/Desired Outcomes

- Prevention of bronchospasm or reduction of frequency of acute asthma attacks in patients with chronic asthma.
- Prevention of exercise-induced asthma.

salsalate, See SALICYLATES.

sargramostim
(sar-**gram**-oh-stim)
Leukine, rHu GM-CSF (recombinant human granulocyte/macrophage colony-stimulating factor)

Classification
Therapeutic: colony-stimulating factors
Pharmacologic: biologic response modifiers

Pregnancy Category C

Indications
Acceleration of bone marrow recovery after: Autologous bone marrow transplantation in patients with non-Hodgkin's lymphoma, acute lymphoblastic leukemia, or Hodgkin's disease; Allogenic bone marrow transplantation from HLA-matched donors. Management of bone marrow transplant failure or engraftment delay. After induction chemotherapy for acute myelogenous leukemia (AML) in patients ≥55 yr. Mobilization and after transplant of autologous peripheral blood progenitor cells (PBPCs); increases harvest by leukapheresis.

Action
Consists of a glycoprotein produced by recombinant DNA technique that is capable of binding to and stimulating the production, division, differentiation, and activation of granulocytes and macrophages. **Therapeutic Effects:** Accelerated recovery of bone marrow after autologous bone marrow transplantation, resulting in decreased risk of infection and other complications.

Pharmacokinetics
Absorption: After IV administration, absorption is essentially complete. Well absorbed after subcut administration.
Distribution: Unknown.
Metabolism and Excretion: Unknown.
Half-life: Unknown.

TIME/ACTION PROFILE (noted as effects on blood counts)

ROUTE	ONSET	PEAK	DURATION
Subcut, IV	rapid	unknown	3–7 days

Contraindications/Precautions
Contraindicated in: Presence of ≥10% leukemic myeloid blast cells in bone marrow or peripheral blood; Hypersensitivity to granulocyte macrophage colony-stimulating factor (GM-CSF), yeast products, or additives (mannitol, tromethamine, or sucrose); Pedi: Products containing benzyl alcohol should not be used in newborns.
Use Cautiously in: Pre-existing fluid retention, HF, or pulmonary infiltrates; Pre-existing cardiac disease; Myeloid malignancies; Previous extensive radiation or chemotherapy (response may be limited); OB: Use only if clearly needed; Lactation, Pedi: Safety not established.

Adverse Reactions/Side Effects
CNS: headache, malaise, weakness. **Resp:** dyspnea. **CV:** pericardial effusion, peripheral edema, transient supraventricular tachycardia. **GI:** diarrhea. **Derm:** itching, rash. **MS:** arthralgia, bone pain, myalgia. **Misc:** chills, fever, first-dose reaction.

Interactions
Drug-Drug: Lithium or **corticosteroids** may potentiate myeloproliferative effects of sargramostim (concurrent use should be undertaken cautiously).

Route/Dosage
After Bone Marrow Transplantation
IV (Adults): 250 mcg/m²/day for 21 days.

Failure/Delay of Engraftment after Bone Marrow Transplantation
IV (Adults): 250 mcg/m²/day for 14 days; may be repeated after a 7-day rest between courses; if results are inadequate, a 3rd course at 500 mcg/m²/day for 14 days may be given after a 7-day rest.

After Chemotherapy for AML
IV (Adults): 250 mcg/m²/day started around day 11 or 4 days after induction if day 10 bone marrow is hypoplastic with <5% blast cells and continued until absolute neutrophil count (ANC) >1500 cells/mm³ for 3 consecutive days (not to exceed 42 days); if adverse reactions occur, decrease dose by 50% or temporarily discontinue.

Mobilization of PBPCs
IV, Subcut (Adults): 250 mcg/m²/day continued throughout collection of PBPCs.

After PBPC Transplantation
IV, Subcut (Adults): 250 mcg/m²/day continued until ANC >1500 cells/mm³ for 3 consecutive days.

Availability
Powder for injection: 250 mcg/vial. **Solution for injection:** 500 mcg/vial.

NURSING IMPLICATIONS
Assessment
- Monitor heart rate, BP, and respiratory status during and immediately after infusion. If dyspnea develops, slow infusion rate by half. Reassess; medication may need to be discontinued. Assess for peripheral edema daily throughout therapy. Capillary leak syndrome (swelling of feet or lower legs, sudden weight

S

gain, dyspnea) and pleural or pericardial effusion may occur, usually at doses >32 mcg/kg/day.

- Monitor for first-dose reaction (flushing, hypotension, syncope, weakness). Does not recur with first dose of each course but may occur with first dose of more than 1 course.
- Assess for fever daily during therapy. Usually mild and dose-related and resolves with discontinuation or administration of antipyretics.
- Assess for arthralgias and myalgias, usually in lower extremities, which tend to occur when granulocyte counts are returning to normal. May also cause mild to moderate bone pain, possibly from bone marrow expansion. Usually occurs over 1–3 days before myeloid recovery and occurs in the sternum, spine, pelvis, and long bones. Treat with analgesics.
- ***Lab Test Considerations:*** Obtain a CBC with differential and platelet count before chemotherapy and twice weekly during therapy to avoid leukocytosis. Monitor ANC; may increase rapidly. If ANC >20,000/mm^3 or 10,000/mm^3 after the nadir has occurred or if platelet count >500,000/mm^3, interrupt administration and reduce dose by half or discontinue. Excessive blood levels usually return to baseline 3–7 days after discontinuation of therapy. If blast cells appear, sargramostim should be discontinued.
- Monitor renal and hepatic function before and biweekly throughout therapy in patients with renal or hepatic dysfunction. May cause ↑ BUN, creatinine, and hepatic enzymes.
- May cause ↓ serum albumin concentrations.

Potential Nursing Diagnoses

Risk for infection (Indications)

Implementation

- Administer 2–4 hr after bone marrow transplant and no earlier than 24 hr after cytotoxic chemotherapy or 12 hr after last dose of radiotherapy.
- Refrigerate but do not freeze powder, reconstituted solution, or diluted solution. Reconstitute with 1 mL of sterile water without preservatives injected toward side of vial. Swirl gently to avoid foaming. Do not shake. Solution should be clear and colorless. Discard if left at room temperature for >6 hr. Vial is for 1-time use only.
- **Subcut:** Administer reconstituted solution without further dilution.

IV Administration

- **Intermittent Infusion:** ***Diluent:*** Dilute in 0.9% NaCl. ***Concentration:*** If final concentration is <10 mcg/mL, add 1 mg human albumin per 1 mL of 0.9% NaCl before addition of sargramostim to prevent absorption of the components of the drug delivery system. Do not administer with an in-line filter. ***Rate:*** Usually infused over 2–4 hr. Has been administered over 30–60 min, over 5–12 hr, and as a continuous infusion over 24 hr.
- *After bone marrow transplantation or failure of engraftment:* Administer over 2 hr.
- *Chemotherapy for AML:* Administer over 4 hr.
- *Mobilization of PBPCs or PBPC transplant:* Administer as a continuous infusion over 24 hr.
- **Y-Site Compatibility:** amikacin, aminocaproic acid, aminophylline, aztreonam, bleomycin, butorphanol, calcium gluconate, carboplatin, carmustine, cefazolin, cefepime, cefotaxime, cefotetan, ceftriaxone, cefuroxime, cisplatin, clindamycin, cyclophosphamide, cyclosporine, cytarabine, dacarbazine, dactinomycin, dexamethasone sodium phosphate, diphenhydramine, dopamine, doxorubicin hydrochloride, doxycycline, droperidol, etoposide, famotidine, fentanyl, floxuridine, fluconazole, fluorouracil, furosemide, gentamicin, granisetron, heparin, idarubicin, ifosfamide, immune globulin, levofloxacin, magnesium sulfate, mannitol, mechlorethamine, meperidine, mesna, methotrexate, metoclopramide, metronidazole, mitoxantrone, pentostatin, piperacillin/tazobactam, potassium chloride, prochlorperazine, promethazine, ranitidine, rituximab, sodium acetate, teniposide, trastuzumab, trimethoprim/sulfamethoxazole, vinblastine, vincristine, zidovudine.
- **Y-Site Incompatibility:** acyclovir, ampicillin, ampicillin/sulbactam, chlorpromazine, ganciclovir, haloperidol, hydrocortisone, hydromorphone, hydroxyzine, imipenem/cilastatin, lorazepam, methylprednisolone sodium succinate, mitomycin, morphine, nalbuphine, nesiritide, ondansetron, sodium bicarbonate, tobramycin.
- **Additive Incompatibility:** Do not admix with other medications.

Patient/Family Teaching

- Explain purpose of sargramostim to patient.
- Instruct patient to notify health care professional if dyspnea or palpitations occur.

Evaluation/Desired Outcomes

- Acceleration of bone marrow recovery and decreased incidence of infection in patients after autologous and allogenic bone marrow transplantation, bone marrow transplant failure or engraftment delay, chemotherapy for AML, and PBPC transplantation.

saxagliptin (sax-a-**glip**-tin)

Onglyza

Classification

Therapeutic: antidiabetics

Pharmacologic: dipeptidyl peptidase-4 (DDP-4) inhibitors

Pregnancy Category B

Indications

Adjunct with diet and exercise to improve glycemic control in adults with type 2 diabetes mellitus.

Action

Acts as a competitive inhibitor of dipeptidyl peptidase-4 (DPP4), which slows inactivation of incretin hormones, thereby increasing their concentrations and reducing fasting and postprandial glucose concentrations.

Therapeutic Effects: Improved control of blood glucose.

Pharmacokinetics

Absorption: Well absorbed following oral administration.

Distribution: Unknown.

Metabolism and Excretion: Metabolized by the liver via the P450 3A4/5 (CYP3A4/5) enzyme system, with conversion to 5–hydroxysaxagliptin, a pharmacologically active metabolite; 24% of saxagliptin is excreted unchanged in urine, 36% of hydroxysaxagliptin is excreted unchanged in urine, 22% is eliminated in feces as unabsorbed drug/metabolites excreted in bile.

Half-life: *Saxagliptin*—2.5 hr; *5–hydroxysaxagliptin*—3.1 hr.

TIME/ACTION PROFILE (DDP-4 inhibition)

ROUTE	ONSET	PEAK	DURATION
PO	unknown	2 hr (4 hr for 5–hydroxysaxagliptin)†	24 hr

† Blood levels.

Contraindications/Precautions

Contraindicated in: Type 1 diabetes; Diabetic ketoacidosis; History of hypersensitivity reaction.

Use Cautiously in: Geri: May be more sensitive to effects; consider age-related ↓ in renal function; OB: Use only if clearly needed; Lactation: Use cautiously; Pedi: Safety and effectiveness not established.

Adverse Reactions/Side Effects

CNS: headache. **CV:** peripheral edema (↑ with thiazolidinediones). **GI:** PANCREATITIS, abdominal pain, vomiting. **Hemat:** ↓ lymphocyte count. **Endo:** hypoglycemia (↑ with sulfonylureas). **MS:** arthralgia. **Misc:** HYPERSENSITIVITY REACTIONS (ANAPHYLAXIS, ANGIOEDEMA, EXFOLIATIVE SKIN DISORDERS).

Interactions

Drug-Drug: Strong **CYP3A4/5 inhibitors**, including **ketoconazole**, **atazanavir**, **clarithromycin**, **indinavir**, **itraconazole**, **nefazodone**, **nelfinavir**, **ritonavir**, **saquinavir**, and **telithromycin** ↑ blood levels; daily dose should not exceed 2.5 mg. ↑ risk of hypoglycemia with **sulfonylureas** or **insulin**; may need to ↓ dose of sulfonylureas or insulin.

Route/Dosage

PO (Adults): 2.5–5 mg once daily; *Strong CYP3A4/5 inhibitors*—2.5 mg once daily.

Renal Impairment

PO (Adults): *CCr ≤50 mL/min*—2.5 mg once daily.

Availability

Tablets: 2.5 mg, 5 mg. ***In combination with:*** metformin XR (Kombiglyze XR); See Appendix B.

NURSING IMPLICATIONS

Assessment

- Observe patient for signs and symptoms of hypoglycemic reactions (abdominal pain, sweating, hunger, weakness, dizziness, headache, tremor, tachycardia, anxiety).
- Monitor for signs of pancreatitis (nausea, vomiting, anorexia, persistent severe abdominal pain, sometimes radiating to the back) during therapy. If pancreatitis occurs, discontinue saxagliptin and monitor serum and urine amylase, amylase/creatinine clearance ratio, electrolytes, serum calcium, glucose, and lipase.
- ***Lab Test Considerations:*** Monitor hemoglobin A1C prior to and periodically during therapy.
- Monitor renal function prior to and periodically during therapy.
- May cause ↓ absolute lymphocyte count.

Potential Nursing Diagnoses

Imbalanced nutrition: more than body requirements (Indications)

Noncompliance (Patient/Family Teaching)

Implementation

- Patients stabilized on a diabetic regimen who are exposed to stress, fever, trauma, infection, or surgery may require administration of insulin.
- **PO:** May be administered without regard to food. Swallow tablet whole, do not cut or split.

Patient/Family Teaching

- Instruct patient to take saxagliptin as directed. If a dose is missed, take the next dose as prescribed; do not double doses. Advise patient to read the *Patient Package Insert* before starting and with each Rx refill; new information may be available.
- Explain to patient that saxagliptin helps control hyperglycemia but does not cure diabetes. Therapy is usually long term.
- Instruct patient not to share this medication with others, even if they have the same symptoms; it may harm them.
- Encourage patient to follow prescribed diet, medication, and exercise regimen to prevent hyperglycemic or hypoglycemic episodes.
- Review signs of hypoglycemia and hyperglycemia with patient. If hypoglycemia occurs, advise patient to take a glass of orange juice or 2–3 tsp of sugar, honey, or corn syrup dissolved in water, and notify health care professional.

S

- Instruct patient in proper testing of blood glucose and urine ketones. These tests should be monitored closely during periods of stress or illness and health care professional notified if significant changes occur.
- Advise patient to notify health care professional promptly if swelling of hands, feet, or ankles; rash; hives; or swelling of face, lips, or throat occur.
- Instruct patient to notify health care professional of all Rx or OTC medications, vitamins, or herbal products being taken and consult health care professional before taking any new medications.
- Advise patient to notify health care professional if pregnancy is planned or suspected or if breast feeding.

Evaluation/Desired Outcomes

- Improved hemoglobin A1C, fasting plasma glucose and 2-hr post-prandial glucose levels.

scopolamine (scoe-**pol**-a-meen)

Transderm-Scop

Classification
Therapeutic: antiemetics
Pharmacologic: anticholinergics

Pregnancy Category C

Indications

Transdermal: Prevention of motion sickness. Prevention of postoperative nausea and vomiting. **PO:** Symptomatic treatment of postencephalitis parkinsonism and paralysis agitans. Treatment of spasticity. Inhibits excessive motility and hypertonus of GI tract in irritable colon syndrome, mild dysentery, diverticulitis, and pylorospasm. Prevention of motion sickness.

Action

Inhibits the muscarinic activity of acetylcholine. Corrects the imbalance of acetylcholine and norepinephrine in the CNS, which may be responsible for motion sickness. **Therapeutic Effects:** Reduction of postoperative nausea and vomiting. Reduction of spasms.

Pharmacokinetics

Absorption: Well absorbed following transdermal administration.
Distribution: Crosses the placenta and blood-brain barrier.
Metabolism and Excretion: Mostly metabolized by the liver.
Half-life: 8 hr.

TIME/ACTION PROFILE (antiemetic, sedative properties)

ROUTE	ONSET	PEAK	DURATION
PO	30 min	1 hr	4–6 hr
Transdermal	4 hr	unknown	72 hr

Contraindications/Precautions

Contraindicated in: Hypersensitivity; Angle-closure glaucoma; Acute hemorrhage; Prostatic hyperplasia (oral only); Pyloric obstruction (oral only); Tachycardia secondary to cardiac insufficiency or thyrotoxicosis.
Use Cautiously in: Possible intestinal obstruction; Prostatic hyperplasia; Chronic renal, hepatic, pulmonary, or cardiac disease; OB, Lactation: Safety not established; to minimize exposure to fetus, apply 1 hr prior to cesarean section; Pedi, Geri: ↑ risk of adverse reactions.

Adverse Reactions/Side Effects

CNS: drowsiness, confusion. **EENT:** blurred vision, mydriasis, photophobia. **CV:** tachycardia, palpitations. **GI:** dry mouth, constipation. **GU:** urinary hesitancy, urinary retention. **Derm:** ↓ sweating.

Interactions

Drug-Drug: ↑ anticholinergic effects with **antihistamines**, **antidepressants**, **quinidine**, or **disopyramide**. ↑ CNS depression with **alcohol**, **antidepressants**, **antihistamines**, **opioid analgesics**, or **sedative/hypnotics**. May alter the absorption of other **orally administered drugs** by slowing motility of the GI tract. May ↑ GI mucosal lesions in patients taking oral **wax-matrix potassium chloride preparations**.
Drug-Natural Products: ↑ anticholinergic effects with **jimson weed** and **scopolia**.

Route/Dosage

Transdermal (Adults): *Motion sickness*—Apply 1 patch 4 hr prior to travel and then every 3 days (as needed); *Preoperative*—Apply 1 patch the evening before surgery or 1 hr prior to cesarean section (remove 24 hr after surgery).
PO (Adults): 0.4–0.8 mg; may repeat every 8–12 hr as needed (dose may be ↑ in parkinsonism and spastic states); for motion sickness, give at least 1 hr before exposure to motion.

Availability (generic available)

Transdermal therapeutic system: Transderm-Scop— 1.5 mg scopolamine/patch releases 0.5 mg scopolamine over 3 days. **Tablets:** 0.4 mg.

NURSING IMPLICATIONS

Assessment

- Assess patient for signs of urinary retention periodically during therapy.
- Monitor heart rate periodically during parenteral therapy.
- Assess patient for pain prior to administration. Scopolamine may act as a stimulant in the presence of pain, producing delirium if used without opioid analgesics.
- **Antiemetic:** Assess patient for nausea and vomiting periodically during therapy.

Potential Nursing Diagnoses
Impaired oral mucous membrane (Indications, Side Effects)
Risk for injury (Side Effects)

Implementation
- **PO:** Administer at least 1 hr prior to exposure to travel for motion sickness. Tablets may be crushed or dissolved in water to decrease onset.

Patient/Family Teaching
- Instruct patient to take medication as directed. Take missed doses as soon as remembered. Do not double doses.
- May cause drowsiness or blurred vision. Caution patient to avoid driving or other activities requiring alertness until response to medication is known.
- Patient should use caution when exercising and in hot weather; overheating may result in heatstroke.
- Advise patient to avoid concurrent use of alcohol and other CNS depressants with this medication.
- Inform patient that frequent mouth rinses, good oral hygiene, and sugarless gum or candy may minimize dry mouth.
- **Transdermal:** Instruct patient on application of transdermal patches. Apply at least 4 hr (US product) before exposure to travel to prevent motion sickness. Wash hands and dry thoroughly before and after application. Apply to hairless, clean, dry area behind ear; avoid areas with cuts or irritation. Apply pressure over system to ensure contact with skin. System is effective for 3 days. If system becomes dislodged, replace with a new system on another site behind the ear. System is waterproof and not affected by bathing or showering.
- Instruct patient to remove patch and notify health care professional immediately if symptoms of acute angle-closure glaucoma (pain or reddening of the eyes with pupil dilation) occur.
- Caution patients engaging in underwater sports of potentially distorting effects of scopolamine.
- For *perioperative nausea and vomiting*, apply patch the night before surgery, or 1 hr prior to cesarean section to minimize exposure to infant. Keep patch in place for 24 hr, then remove and discard.
- Advise patient referred for MRI test to discuss patch with referring health care professional and MRI facility to determine if removal of patch is necessary prior to test and for directions for replacing patch.

Evaluation/Desired Outcomes
- Prevention of motion sickness.
- Prevention of postoperative nausea and vomiting.
- Reduction in spasms.
- Reduction in excessive GI motility.

selegiline (se-le-ji-leen)
Eldepryl, Zelapar

Classification
Therapeutic: antiparkinson agents
Pharmacologic: monoamine oxidase type B inhibitors

Pregnancy Category C

Indications
Management of Parkinson's disease (with levodopa or levodopa/carbidopa) in patients who fail to respond to levodopa/carbidopa alone.

Action
Following conversion by MAO to its active form, selegiline inactivates MAO by irreversibly binding to it at type B (brain) sites. Inactivation of MAO leads to increased amounts of dopamine available in the CNS. **Therapeutic Effects:** Increased response to levodopa/dopamine therapy in Parkinson's disease.

Pharmacokinetics
Absorption: Appears to be well absorbed following oral administration.
Distribution: Widely distributed.
Metabolism and Excretion: Metabolism involves some conversion to amphetamine and methamphetamine. 45% excreted in urine as metabolites.
Half-life: Unknown; orally disintegrating tablets 1.3 hr.

TIME/ACTION PROFILE (onset of beneficial effects in Parkinson's disease)

ROUTE	ONSET	PEAK	DURATION
PO	2–3 days	40–90 min	unknown
Orally disintegrating	5 min	10–15 min	unknown

Contraindications/Precautions
Contraindicated in: Hypersensitivity; Concurrent meperidine or opioid analgesic therapy (possible fatal reactions); Concurrent use of SSRIs or tricyclic antidepressants.
Use Cautiously in: Doses >10 m g/day (↑ risk of hypertensive reactions with tyramine-containing foods and some medications); History of peptic ulcer disease; Geri: ↑ risk of sedation.

Adverse Reactions/Side Effects
CNS: SEROTONIN SYNDROME, confusion, dizziness, fainting, hallucinations, insomnia, sedation, urges (gambling, sexual), vivid dreams. **Derm:** melanoma. **GI:** nausea, abdominal pain, dry mouth.

S

Interactions

Drug-Drug: Concurrent use with **meperidine** or other **opioid analgesics** may possibly result in a potentially fatal reaction (excitation, sweating, rigidity, and hypertension; or hypotension and coma). Serotonin syndrome (confusion, agitation, hyperpyrexia, hypertension, seizures) may occur with concurrent use of **nefazodone** or **SSRI antidepressants** (fluoxetine should be discontinued 5 wk prior to selegiline, **venlafaxine** should be discontinued 7 days before selegiline, other agents should be discontinued 2 wk before selegiline). Selegiline should be discontinued 2 wk before **SSRIs** are initiated. Concurrent use with **tricyclic antidepressants** may result in asystole, diaphoresis, hypertension, syncope, behavioral changes, altered consciousness, hyperpyrexia, tremors, muscle rigidity, and seizures (avoid concurrent use; discontinue selegiline 2 wk before initiating tricyclic antidepressant therapy). May initially ↑ risk of side effects of **levodopa/carbidopa** (dose of levodopa/carbidopa may need to be ↓ by 10–30%).

Drug-Food: Doses >10 m g/day may produce hypertensive reactions with **tyramine-containing foods** (see Appendix J).

Route/Dosage

PO (Adults): 5 mg twice daily, with breakfast and lunch (some patients may require further dividing of doses—2.5 mg 4 times daily).

PO (Adults): *Orally disintegrating tablets*—1.25 mg once daily for at least 6 wk. After 6 wk, may increase to 2.5 mg if effect not achieved and patient is tolerating medication.

Availability (generic available)

Capsules: 5 mg. **Tablets:** 5 mg. **Orally disintegrating tablets:** 1.25 mg.

NURSING IMPLICATIONS

Assessment

- Assess patient for signs and symptoms of Parkinson's disease (tremor, muscle weakness and rigidity, ataxic gait) prior to and during therapy.
- Assess BP periodically during therapy.

Potential Nursing Diagnoses

Impaired physical mobility (Indications)
Risk for injury (Indications, Side Effects)

Implementation

- Do not confuse selegiline with Salagen (pilocarpine). Do not confuse Zelapar (selegiline) with Zyprexa (olanzapine).
- An attempt to reduce the dose of levodopa/carbidopa by 10–30% may be made after 2–3 days of selegiline therapy.
- **PO:** Administer 5-mg tablet with breakfast and lunch.
- Administer *orally disintegrating tablets* in the morning, before breakfast and without liquid. Remove tablet gently from blister pack with clean, dry hands immediately before administering. Do not attempt to push tablet through backing. Tablet will disintegrate within seconds when placed on tongue. Avoid food or liquid within 5 min of administering orally disintegrating tablets.

Patient/Family Teaching

- Instruct patient to take medication as directed. Take missed doses as soon as possible, but not if late afternoon or evening or almost time for next dose. Do not double doses. Caution patient that taking more than the prescribed dose may increase side effects and place patient at risk for hypertensive crisis if foods containing tyramine are consumed (see Appendix J).
- Advise patients taking selegiline ≥20 mg/day to avoid large amounts of tyramine-containing foods (see Appendix J), alcoholic beverages, large quantities of caffeine-containing beverages, or OTC or herbal cough or cold medications.
- Caution patient and caregiver that selegiline may cause drowsiness and dizziness. Monitor and assist with ambulation and caution patient to avoid driving and other activities requiring alertness until response to medication is known.
- Inform patient and family of the signs and symptoms of MAO inhibitor–induced hypertensive crisis (severe headache, chest pain, nausea, vomiting, photosensitivity, enlarged pupils). Advise patient to notify health care professional immediately if severe headache or any other unusual symptoms occur.
- Caution patient to change positions slowly to minimize orthostatic hypotension.
- Advise patient to notify health care professional of signs and symptoms of serotonin syndrome (mental status changes [agitation, hallucinations, delirium, and coma], autonomic instability [tachycardia, labile BP, dizziness, diaphoresis, flushing, hyperthermia], neuromuscular changes [tremor, rigidity, myoclonus, hyperreflexia, incoordination], seizures, and/or gastrointestinal symptoms [nausea, vomiting, diarrhea]).
- Instruct patient to notify health care professional of all Rx or OTC medications, vitamins, or herbal products being taken and to consult with health care professional before taking other medications.
- Advise patient to have periodic skin exams to check for lesions that may be melanoma.
- Advise patient to notify health care professional if agitation, aggression, delirium, hallucinations, new or increased gambling, sexual, or other intense urges occur.
- Advise patient that increasing fluids, sugarless gum or candy, ice, or saliva substitutes may help minimize dry mouth. Consult health care professional if dry mouth continues for >2 wk.

Evaluation/Desired Outcomes

- Improved response to levodopa/carbidopa in patients with Parkinson's disease.

selegiline transdermal

(se-**le**-ji-leen)

Emsam

Classification

Therapeutic: antidepressants

Pharmacologic: monoamine oxidase type B inhibitors

Pregnancy Category C

Indications

Major depressive disorder.

Action

Following conversion by MAO to its active form, selegiline inactivates MAO by irreversibly binding to it at type B (brain) sites; this results in higher levels of monoamine neurotransmitters in the brain (dopamine, serotonin, norepinephrine). **Therapeutic Effects:** Decreased symptoms of depression.

Pharmacokinetics

Absorption: 25–30% of patch content is transdermally absorbed, blood levels are higher than those following oral administration because there is less first-pass hepatic metabolism.

Distribution: Rapidly distributes to all body tissues; crosses the blood-brain barrier.

Metabolism and Excretion: Mostly metabolized by the liver, primarily by the CYP2A6, CYP2C9, and CYP3A4/5 enzyme systems. 10% excreted in urine as metabolites, 2% in feces; negligible renal excretion of unchanged drug.

Half-life: 18–25 hr.

TIME/ACTION PROFILE

ROUTE	ONSET	PEAK	DURATION
transdermal	unknown	2 or more wk	2 wk (after discontinuation)

Contraindications/Precautions

Contraindicated in: Hypersensitivity; Pheochromocytoma; Concurrent selective serotonin reuptake inhibitors (fluoxetine, paroxetine citalopram, escitalopram, and others), nonselective serotonin re-uptake inhibitors (venlafaxine, duloxetine), tricyclic antidepressants (amitriptyline, imipramine, and others), carbamazepine, oxcarbazepine, amphetamines, vasoconstrictors (ephedrine, pseudoephedrine), bupropion, meperidine, tramadol, methadone, dextromethorphan, mirtazapine cyclobenzaprine, other MAO inhibitors (isocarboxazid, phenelzine, tranylcypromine), oral selegiline, sympathomimetic amines, amphetamines, cocaine, local anesthetics with vasoconstrictors, or St. John's wort; Alcohol; Pedi: Children <12 yr (↑ risk of hypertensive crises).

Use Cautiously in: Elective surgery within 10 days; benzodiazepines, rapacuronium, fentanyl, morphine, and codeine may be used cautiously; May ↑ risk of suicide attempt/ideation especially during early treatment or dose adjustment; risk may be greater in children or adolescents (safe use in children <12 yr not established); History of mania; Dosing at 9 mg/24 hr or 12 mg/24 hr requires dietary modification (avoid foods containing large amounts of tyramine); Geri: May be more susceptible to orthostatic hypotension; OB: Use only if benefit outweighs risk to the fetus; Lactation: Safety not established; Pedi: Children 12–17 yr (safety and effectiveness not established).

Adverse Reactions/Side Effects

CNS: SEROTONIN SYNDROME, insomnia, abnormal thinking, agitation, amnesia, worsening of mania/hypomania. **EENT:** tinnitus. **Resp:** ↑ cough. **CV:** HYPERTENSIVE CRISIS, chest pain, orthostatic hypotension, peripheral edema. **GI:** diarrhea, altered taste, anorexia, constipation, flatulence, gastroenteritis, vomiting. **GU:** dysmenorrhea, metrorrhagia, urinary frequency. **Derm:** application site reactions, acne, ecchymoses, pruritus, sweating. **MS:** mylagia, neck pain, pathologic fracture. **Neuro:** paresthesia.

Interactions

Drug-Drug: Concurrent **selective serotonin reuptake inhibitors (fluoxetine, paroxetine, citalopram, escitalopram**, and others), **nonselective serotonin re-uptake inhibitors (venlafaxine, duloxetine**), **tricyclic antidepressants (amitriptyline, imipramine**, and others), **carbamazepine, oxcarbazepine, amphetamines, vasoconstrictors (ephedrine, pseudoephedrine, phenylpropanolamine**), **bupropion, meperidine, tramadol, methadone, dextromethorphan, mirtazapine, cyclobenzaprine**, other MAO inhibitors (**isocarboxazid, phenelzine, tranylcypromine**), oral **selegiline, sympathomimetic amines, amphetamines, cocaine**, or **local anesthetics with vasoconstrictors**; these may all ↑ risk of hypertensive crisis. (**Fluoxetine** should not be used within 2 wk of initiating therapy.)

Drug-Natural Products: St. John's wort may ↑ risk of hypertensive crisis.

Route/Dosage

Transdermal (Adults): 6 mg/24 hr, if necessary, may be increased at 2-wk intervals in increments of 3 mg, up to 12 mg/24 hr.

Availability

Transdermal patch: 6 mg/24 hr, 9 mg/24 hr, 12 mg/24 hr.

NURSING IMPLICATIONS

Assessment

- Assess mental status, mood changes, and anxiety level frequently. Assess for suicidal tendencies, agitation, irritability, and unusual changes in behavior especially during early therapy. Monitor pediatric patients face-to-face weekly during first 4 wk, every other week for 4 wk, at 12 wk, and as clinically indicated during therapy. Restrict amount of drug available to patient.
- Monitor BP and pulse rate before and frequently during therapy. Report significant changes promptly.
- ***Toxicity and Overdose:*** Concurrent ingestion of tyramine-rich foods and many medications may result in a life-threatening hypertensive crisis. Signs and symptoms of hypertensive crisis include chest pain, tachycardia or bradycardia, severe headache, neck stiffness or soreness, nausea and vomiting, sweating, photosensitivity, and enlarged pupils. If hypertensive crisis occurs, discontinue selegiline transdermal and administer labetalol 20 mg slowly IV to control hypertension. Manage fever with external cooling. Monitor patient closely until symptoms have stabilized.

Potential Nursing Diagnoses

Ineffective coping (Indications)
Noncompliance (Patient/Family Teaching)

Implementation

- **Transdermal:** Apply system to dry, intact skin on the upper torso such as chest, back, upper thigh, or outer surface of the upper arm once every 24 hr at the same time each day. Avoid areas that are hairy, oily, irritated, broken, scarred, or calloused. Wash area gently with soap and warm water, rinse thoroughly. Allow skin to dry completely before application. Apply immediately after removing from package. Do not alter the system (i.e., cut) in any way before application. Remove liner from adhesive layer and press firmly in place with palm of hand for 30 sec, especially around the edges, to make sure contact is complete. Remove used system and fold so that adhesive edges are together. Only 1 selegiline patch should be worn at a time. Dispose away from children and pets. Apply new system to a different site. Wash hands thoroughly with soap and water to remove any medicine that may have gotten on them.

Patient/Family Teaching

- Instruct patient to apply patch as directed. Advise patients and caregivers to read the *Medication Guide about Using Antidepressants in Children and Teenagers*. Inform patient that improvement may be noticed after 1 to several weeks of therapy. Advise patient not to discontinue therapy without consulting health care professional.
- Caution patient to avoid alcohol and CNS depressants during and for at least 2 wk after therapy has been discontinued; they may precipitate a hypertensive crisis. Contact health care professional immediately if symptoms of hypertensive crisis develop. Patients taking 9 mg/24 hr or 12 mg/24 hr must avoid foods or beverages containing tyramine (see Appendix J) from the first day of the increased dose through 2 wk after discontinuation of selegiline transdermal therapy.
- Advise patient to avoid exposing application site to external sources of direct heat such as heating pads, electric blankets, heat lamps, saunas, hot tubs, heated water beds, and prolonged direct sunlight.
- May cause dizziness or drowsiness. Caution patient to avoid driving and other activities requiring alertness until response to medication is known.
- Caution patient to change positions slowly to minimize orthostatic hypotension. Geriatric patients are at increased risk for this side effect.
- Advise patient to notify health care professional of signs and symptoms of serotonin syndrome (mental status changes [agitation, hallucinations, delirium, and coma], autonomic instability [tachycardia, labile BP, dizziness, diaphoresis, flushing, hyperthermia], neuromuscular changes [tremor, rigidity, myoclonus, hyperreflexia, incoordination], seizures, and/or gastrointestinal symptoms [nausea, vomiting, diarrhea]).
- Advise patient referred for MRI test to discuss patch with referring health care professional and MRI facility to determine if removal of patch is necessary prior to test and for directions for replacing patch.
- Advise patients and caregivers to notify health care professional if severe headache, neck stiffness, heart racing or palpitations, anxiety, agitation, panic attacks, insomnia, irritability, hostility, aggressiveness, impulsivity, akathisia, hypomania, mania, change in behavior, worsening of depression, or suicidal ideation occur, especially during initial therapy or during changes in dose.
- Instruct patient to consult health care professional before taking any Rx, OTC, or herbal products. Caution patient to avoid use of St. John's wort and the analgesics meperidine, tramadol, or methadone during therapy.
- Advise patient to notify health care professional of medication regimen before treatment or surgery. If possible, therapy should be discontinued at least 2 wk before surgery.
- Advise patient to notify health care professional if pregnancy is planned or suspected or if breast feeding.

Evaluation/Desired Outcomes

- Improved mood in depressed patients.
- Decreased anxiety.

- Increased appetite.
- Improved energy level.
- Improved sleep. Evaluate effectiveness of therapy periodically.

sennosides (sen-oh-sides)
Black-Draught, Ex-Lax, Ex-Lax Chocolated, Fletchers' Castoria, Maximum Relief Ex-Lax, Sena-Gen, Senexon, Senokot, SenokotXTRA

Classification
Therapeutic: laxatives
Pharmacologic: stimulant laxatives

Pregnancy Category C

Indications
Treatment of constipation, particularly when associated with: Slow transit time, Constipating drugs, Irritable or spastic bowel syndrome, Neurologic constipation.

Action
Active components of senna (sennosides) alter water and electrolyte transport in the large intestine, resulting in accumulation of water and increased peristalsis.
Therapeutic Effects: Laxative action.

Pharmacokinetics
Absorption: Minimally absorbed following oral administration.
Distribution: Unknown.
Metabolism and Excretion: Unknown.
Half-life: Unknown.

TIME/ACTION PROFILE (laxative effect)

ROUTE	ONSET	PEAK	DURATION
PO	6–12 hr†	unknown	3–4 days

†May take as long as 24 hr.

Contraindications/Precautions
Contraindicated in: Hypersensitivity; Abdominal pain of unknown cause, especially if associated with fever; Rectal fissures; Ulcerated hemorrhoids; Known alcohol intolerance (some liquid products).
Use Cautiously in: Chronic use (may lead to laxative dependence); Possible intestinal obstruction; OB, Lactation: Safety not established.

Adverse Reactions/Side Effects
GI: cramping, diarrhea, nausea. **GU:** pink-red or brown-black discoloration of urine. **F and E:** electrolyte abnormalities (chronic use or dependence). **Misc:** laxative dependence.

Interactions
Drug-Drug: May ↓ absorption of other **orally administered drugs** because of ↓ transit time.

Route/Dosage
Larger doses have been used to treat/prevent opioid-induced constipation. Consult labeling of individual OTC products for more speceific dosing information.
PO (Adults and Children >12 yr): 12–50 mg 1–2 times daily.
PO (Children 6–12 yr): 6–25 mg 1–2 times daily.
PO (Children 2–6 yr): 3–12.5 mg 1–2 times daily.

Availability (generic available)

Noted as sennoside content
Tablets: 6 mg[OTC], 8.6 mg[OTC], 15 mg [OTC], 17 mg[OTC], 25 mg[OTC]. **Granules:** 15 mg/5 mL[OTC], 20 mg/5 mL[OTC]. **Syrup:** 8.8 mg/5 mL[OTC]. **Liquid:** 25 mg/15 mL[OTC], 33.3 mg/mL senna concentrate[OTC]. ***In combination with:*** psyllium and docusate[OTC]. See Appendix B.

NURSING IMPLICATIONS

Assessment
- Assess patient for abdominal distention, presence of bowel sounds, and usual pattern of bowel function.
- Assess color, consistency, and amount of stool produced.

Potential Nursing Diagnoses
Constipation (Indications)
Diarrhea (Side Effects)

Implementation
- **PO:** Take with a full glass of water. Administer at bedtime for evacuation 6–12 hr later. Administer on an empty stomach for more rapid results.
- Shake oral solution well before administering.
- Granules should be dissolved or mixed in water or other liquid before administration.

Patient/Family Teaching
- Advise patient that laxatives should be used only for short-term therapy. Long-term therapy may cause electrolyte imbalance and dependence.
- Encourage patient to use other forms of bowel regulation, such as increasing bulk in the diet, increasing fluid intake, and increasing mobility. Normal bowel habits are individualized and may vary from 3 times/day to 3 times/wk.
- Inform patient that this medication may cause a change in urine color to pink, red, violet, yellow, or brown.
- Instruct patients with cardiac disease to avoid straining during bowel movements (Valsalva maneuver).
- Advise patient not to use laxatives when abdominal pain, nausea, vomiting, or fever is present.

Evaluation/Desired Outcomes
- A soft, formed bowel movement.

S

sertraline (ser-tra-leen)
Zoloft

Classification
Therapeutic: antidepressants
Pharmacologic: selective serotonin reuptake inhibitors (SSRIs)

Pregnancy Category C

Indications

Major depressive disorder. Panic disorder. Obsessive-compulsive disorder (OCD). Post-traumatic stress disorder (PTSD). Social anxiety disorder (social phobia). Premenstrual dysphoric disorder (PMDD). **Unlabeled Use:** Generalized anxiety disorder (GAD).

Action

Inhibits neuronal uptake of serotonin in the CNS, thus potentiating the activity of serotonin. Has little effect on norepinephrine or dopamine. **Therapeutic Effects:** Antidepressant action. Decreased incidence of panic attacks. Decreased obsessive and compulsive behavior. Decreased feelings of intense fear, helplessness, or horror. Decreased social anxiety. Decrease in premenstrual dysphoria.

Pharmacokinetics

Absorption: Appears to be well absorbed after oral administration.
Distribution: Extensively distributed throughout body tissues.
Protein Binding: 98%.
Metabolism and Excretion: Extensively metabolized by the liver; 1 metabolite has some antidepressant activity; 14% excreted unchanged in feces.
Half-life: 24 hr.

TIME/ACTION PROFILE (antidepressant effect)

ROUTE	ONSET	PEAK	DURATION
PO	within 2–4 wk	unknown	unknown

Contraindications/Precautions

Contraindicated in: Hypersensitivity; Concurrent use of MAO inhibitors or MAO-like drugs (linezolid or methylene blue); Concurrent use of pimozide; Oral concentrate contains alcohol; avoid in patients with known intolerance.
Use Cautiously in: Severe hepatic or renal impairment; Patients with a history of mania; History of suicide attempt; Angle-closure glaucoma; OB: Use during third trimester may result in neonatal serotonin syndrome requiring prolonged hospitalization, respiratory and nutritional support. Use only if potential benefit justifies potential risk to fetus; Lactation: May cause sedation in infant; discontinue drug or bottle-feed; Pedi: May ↑ risk of suicide attempt/ideation especially during early treatment or dose adjustment; risk may be greater in children or adolescents.

Adverse Reactions/Side Effects

CNS: NEUROLEPTIC MALIGNANT SYNDROME, SUICIDAL THOUGHTS, dizziness, drowsiness, fatigue, headache, insomnia, agitation, anxiety, confusion, emotional lability, impaired concentration, manic reaction, nervousness, weakness, yawning. **EENT:** pharyngitis, rhinitis, tinnitus, visual abnormalities. **CV:** chest pain, palpitations. **GI:** diarrhea, dry mouth, nausea, abdominal pain, altered taste, anorexia, constipation, dyspepsia, flatulence, ↑ appetite, vomiting. **GU:** sexual dysfunction, menstrual disorders, urinary disorders, urinary frequency. **Derm:** ↑ sweating, hot flashes, rash. **Endo:** diabetes. **F and E:** hyponatremia. **MS:** back pain, myalgia. **Neuro:** tremor, hypertonia, hypoesthesia, paresthesia, twitching. **Misc:** SEROTONIN SYNDROME, fever, thirst.

Interactions

Drug-Drug: Serious, potentially fatal reactions (hyperthermia, rigidity, myoclonus, autonomic instability, with fluctuating vital signs and extreme agitation, which may proceed to delirium and coma) may occur with concurrent **MAO inhibitors**. MAO inhibitors should be stopped at least 14 days before sertraline therapy. Sertraline should be stopped at least 14 days before MAO inhibitor therapy. Concurrent use with **MAO-inhibitor–like drugs**, such as **linezolid** or **methylene blue** may ↑ risk of serotonin syndrome; concurrent use contraindicated; do not start therapy in patients receiving **linezolid** or **methylene blue**; if **linezolid** or **methylene blue** need to be started in a patient receiving sertraline, immediately discontinue sertraline and monitor for signs/symptoms of serotonin syndrome for 2 wk or until 24 hr after last dose of linezolid or methylene blue, whichever comes first (may resume sertraline therapy 24 hr after last dose of linezolid or methylene blue). May ↑ **pimozide** levels and the risk of potentially life-threatening cardiovascular reactions; concurrent use contraindicated. Drugs that affect serotonergic neurotransmitter systems, including **tricyclic antidepressants**, **SNRIs**, **fentanyl**, **buspirone**, **tramadol**, and **triptans** ↑ risk of serotonin syndrome. May ↑ sensitivity to **adrenergics** and ↑ the risk of serotonin syndrome. Concurrent use with **alcohol** is not recommended. May ↑ levels/effects of **warfarin**, **phenytoin**, **tricyclic antidepressants**, some **benzodiazepines (alprazolam)**, **cloazapine**, or **tolbutamide**. ↑ risk of bleeding with **NSAIDS**, **aspirin**, **clopidogrel**, or **warfarin**. **Cimetidine** ↑ blood levels and effects.
Drug-Natural Products: ↑ risk of serotinergic side effects including serotonin syndrome with **St. John's wort** and **SAMe**.

Route/Dosage

Depression/OCD

PO (Adults): 50 mg/day as a single dose in the morning or evening initially; after several weeks may be ↑ at

weekly intervals up to 200 mg/day, depending on response.
PO (Children 13–17 yr): *OCD*—50 mg once daily.
PO (Children 6–12 yr): *OCD*—25 mg once daily.

Panic Disorder

PO (Adults): 25 mg/day initially, may ↑ after 1 wk to 50 mg/day.

PTSD

PO (Adults): 25 mg once daily for 7 days, then ↑ to 50 mg once daily; may then be ↑ if needed at intervals of at least 7 days (range 50–200 mg once daily).

Social Anxiety Disorder

PO (Adults): 25 mg once daily initially, then 50 mg once daily; may be ↑ at weekly intervals up to 200 mg/day.

PMDD

PO (Adults): 50 mg/day initially either daily or daily during luteal phase of cycle. Daily dosing may be titrated upward in 50-mg increments at the beginning of a cycle. In luteal phase–only dosing a 50 mg/day titration step for 3 days at the beginning of each luteal phase dosing period should be used (range 50–150 mg/day).

Availability (generic available)

Tablets: 25 mg, 50 mg, 100 mg. **Cost:** *Generic*—25 mg $17.68/90, 50 mg $22.22/90, 100 mg $19.73/90. **Capsules:** ✤25 mg, ✤50 mg, ✤100 mg. **Oral concentrate (12% alcohol):** 20 mg/mL. **Cost:** *Generic*—$64.28/60 mL.

NURSING IMPLICATIONS

Assessment

- Assess for suicidal tendencies, especially during early therapy. Restrict amount of drug available to patient. Risk may be increased in children, adolescents, and adults ≤24 yr. After starting therapy, children, adolescents, and young adults should be seen by health care professional at least weekly for 4 wk, every 3 wk for next 4 wk, and on advice of health care professional thereafter.
- Monitor appetite and nutritional intake. Weigh weekly. Notify health care professional of continued weight loss. Adjust diet as tolerated to support nutritional status.
- Assess for serotonin syndrome (mental changes [agitation, hallucinations, coma], autonomic instability [tachycardia, labile BP, hyperthermia], neuromuscular aberrations [hyper-reflexia, incoordination], and/or GI symptoms [nausea, vomiting, diarrhea]), especially in patients taking other serotonergic drugs (SSRIs, SNRIs, triptans).
- **Depression:** Monitor mood changes. Inform health care professional if patient demonstrates significant increase in anxiety, nervousness, or insomnia.
- Assess for suicidal tendencies, especially during early therapy. Restrict amount of drug available to patient.
- **OCD:** Assess patient for frequency of obsessive-compulsive behaviors. Note degree to which these thoughts and behaviors interfere with daily functioning.
- **Panic Attacks:** Assess frequency and severity of panic attacks.
- **PTSD:** Assess patient for feelings of fear, helplessness, and horror. Determine effect on social and occupational functioning.
- **Social Anxiety Disorder:** Assess patient for symptoms of social anxiety disorder (blushing, sweating, trembling, tachycardia during interactions with new people, people in authority, or groups) periodically during therapy.
- **Premenstrual Dysphoric Disorder:** Assess patient for symptoms of premenstrual dysphoric disorder (feeling angry, tense, or tired; crying easily, feeling sad or hopeless; arguing with family or friends for no reason; difficulty sleeping or paying attention; feeling out of control or unable to cope; having cramping, bloating, food craving, or breast tenderness) periodically during therapy.
- ***Lab Test Considerations:*** May cause false-positive urine screening tests for benzodiazepines.
- May cause hyperglycemia and diabetes mellitus; monitor serum glucose if clinical symptoms occur.

Potential Nursing Diagnoses

Ineffective coping (Indications)
Risk for injury (Side Effects)
Sexual dysfunction (Side Effects)

Implementation

- Do not confuse sertraline with cetirizine or Soriatane (acitretin).
- Periodically reassess dose and continued need for therapy.
- **PO:** Administer as a single dose in the morning or evening.
- For oral concentrate, use dropper provided to remove oral concentrate and mix with 4 oz (1/2 cup) of water, ginger ale, lemon/lime soda, lemonade or orange juice ONLY. Do not mix with other liquids. Take immediately after mixing. Do not mix in advance. Slight haze may appear after mixing; this is normal. Dropper dispenser contains dry natural rubber, advise patient with latex allergy.

Patient/Family Teaching

- Instruct patient to take sertraline as directed. Take missed doses as soon as possible and return to regu-

S

lar dosing schedule. Do not double doses. Do not stop abruptly; may cause dysphoric mood, irritability, agitation, dizziness, sensory disturbances (paresthesias such as electric shock sensations), anxiety, confusion, headache, lethargy, emotional lability, insomnia, and hypomania.

- May cause drowsiness or dizziness. Caution patient to avoid driving and other activities requiring alertness until response to the drug is known.
- Advise patient, family, and caregivers to look for suicidality, especially during early therapy or dose changes. Notify health care professional immediately if thoughts about suicide or dying, attempts to commit suicide; new or worse depression or anxiety; agitation or restlessness; panic attacks; insomnia; new or worse irritability, aggressiveness, acting on dangerous impulses, mania, or other changes in mood or behavior or if symptoms of serotonin syndrome occur.
- Advise patient to avoid alcohol or other CNS depressant drugs during therapy and to consult with health care professional before taking other medications and to avoid alcohol or other CNS depressant drugs during therapy.
- Instruct patient to notify health care professional of all Rx or OTC medications, vitamins, or herbal products being taken and consult health care professional before taking any new medications, especially St. John's wort or SAMe.
- Inform patient that frequent mouth rinses, good oral hygiene, and sugarless gum or candy may minimize dry mouth. If dry mouth persists for more than 2 wk, consult health care professional regarding use of saliva substitute.
- Advise patient to wear sunscreen and protective clothing to prevent photosensitivity reactions.
- Advise patient to notify health care professional if headache, weakness, nausea, anorexia, anxiety, or insomnia persists.
- Instruct female patient to inform health care professional if pregnancy is planned or suspected or if breast feeding.
- Emphasize the importance of follow-up exams to monitor progress. Encourage patient participation in psychotherapy to improve coping skills.

Evaluation/Desired Outcomes

- Increased sense of well-being.
- Renewed interest in surroundings. May require 1–4 wk of therapy to obtain antidepressant effects.
- Decrease in obsessive-compulsive behaviors.
- Decrease in frequency and severity of panic attacks.
- Decrease in symptoms of PTSD.
- Decrease in social anxiety disorder.
- Decrease in symptoms of premenstrual dysphoric disorder.

sevelamer (se-vel-a-mer)

Renagel, Renvela

Classification

Therapeutic: electrolyte modifiers
Pharmacologic: phosphate binders

Pregnancy Category C

Indications

Reduction of serum phosphate levels in patients with hyperphosphatemia associated with end-stage renal disease.

Action

A polymer that binds phosphate in the GI tract, preventing its absorption. **Therapeutic Effects:** Decreased serum phosphate levels and reduction in the consequences of hyperphosphatemia (ectopic calcification, secondary hyperparathyroidism with osteitis fibrosa).

Pharmacokinetics

Absorption: Not absorbed; action is local (in GI tract).
Distribution: Unknown.
Metabolism and Excretion: Eliminated in feces.
Half-life: Unknown.

TIME/ACTION PROFILE (↓ in serum phosphate levels)

ROUTE	ONSET	PEAK	DURATION
PO	5 days	2 wk	unknown

Contraindications/Precautions

Contraindicated in: Hypersensitivity; Hypophosphatemia; Bowel obstruction.
Use Cautiously in: Dysphagia, swallowing disorders, severe GI motility disorders, or major GI tract surgery; OB, Lactation, Pedi: Safety not established.

Adverse Reactions/Side Effects

GI: BOWEL OBSTRUCTION/PERFORATION, ESOPHAGEAL OBSTRUCTION (tablet), diarrhea, dyspepsia, vomiting, choking (tablet), constipation, dysphagia (tablet), flatulence, nausea.

Interactions

Drug-Drug: May ↓ absorption of other drugs and ↓ effectiveness, especially **drugs whose efficacy is dependent on tightly controlled blood levels.** ↓ absorption of **ciprofloxacin.**

Route/Dosage

PO (Adults): 800–1600 mg with each meal; may titrate by 800 mg every 2 wk to achieve target serum phosphorus levels.

Availability

Tablets: 400 mg, 800 mg. **Powder for oral suspension:** 800 mg/packet, 2400 mg/packet.

NURSING IMPLICATIONS

Assessment

- Assess patient for GI side effects periodically during therapy.
- ***Lab Test Considerations:*** Monitor serum phosphorous, calcium, bicarbonate, and chloride levels periodically during therapy.

Potential Nursing Diagnoses

Deficient knowledge, related to medication regimen (Patient/Family Teaching)

Implementation

- Do not confuse Renagel with Renvela.
- Doses of concurrent medications, especially antiarrhythmics, should be spaced at least 1 hr before or 3 hr after sevelamer.
- **PO:** Administer with meals. Do not break, chew, or crush tablets; contents expand in water.
- Place contents of powder packet in a cup and mix thoroughly with at least 1 ounce of water for the 0.8-g dose or 2 ounces of water for the 2.4-g dose packet. Stir mixture vigorously (it does not dissolve) and drink entire preparation within 30 min or resuspend the preparation right before drinking.

Patient/Family Teaching

- Instruct patient to take sevelamer with meals as directed and to adhere to prescribed diet.
- Caution patient to space concurrent medications at least 1 hr before or 3 hr after sevelamer.
- Advise patient to notify health care professional if GI effects are severe or prolonged.

Evaluation/Desired Outcomes

- Decrease in serum phosphorous concentration to ≤6 mg/dL. Dose adjustment is based on serum phosphorous concentrations.

sildenafil (sil-den-a-fil)

Revatio, Viagra

Classification

Therapeutic: erectile dysfunction agents, vasodilators

Pharmacologic: phosphodiesterase type 5 inhibitors

Pregnancy Category B

Indications

Viagra: Erectile dysfunction. *Revatio:* Pulmonary arterial hypertension (WHO Group I).

Action

Viagra: Enhances effects of nitric oxide released during sexual stimulation. Nitric oxide activates guanylate cyclase, which produces increased levels of cyclic guanosine monophosphate (cGMP). cGMP produces smooth muscle relaxation of the corpus cavernosum, which promotes increased blood flow and subsequent erection. cGMP also leads to vasodilation of the pulmonary vasculature. Sildenafil inhibits the enzyme phosphodiesterase type 5 (PDE5), PDE5 inactivates cGMP. *Revatio:* Produces vasodilation of the pulmonary vascular bed. **Therapeutic Effects:** *Viagra:* Enhanced blood flow to the corpus cavernosum and erection sufficient to allow sexual intercourse. Requires sexual stimulation. *Revatio:* Improved exercise tolerance and delay worsening of disease.

Pharmacokinetics

Absorption: Rapidly absorbed (41%) after oral administration; IV administration results in complete bioavailability.

Distribution: Widely distributed to tissues; negligible amount in semen.

Protein Binding: 96%.

Metabolism and Excretion: Mostly metabolized by the liver (by P450 3A4 enzyme system); 1 metabolite is active and accounts for 20% or more of drug effect. Metabolites excreted mostly (80%) in feces; 13% excreted in urine.

Half-life: 4 hr (for sildenafil and active metabolite).

TIME/ACTION PROFILE (vasodilation, ability to produce erection)

ROUTE	ONSET	PEAK	DURATION
PO	within 1 hr	30–120 min	up to 4 hr

Contraindications/Precautions

Contraindicated in: Hypersensitivity; Concurrent use of nitrates or riociguat; Pulmonary veno-occlusive disease; OB, Pedi: Newborns, women, children; Pedi: *Revatio*: Chronic use not recommended for pulmonary hypertension due to lack of efficacy and ↑ risk of death.

Use Cautiously in: Serious underlying cardiovascular disease (including history of MI, stroke, or serious arrhythmia within 6 mo), cardiac failure, or coronary artery disease with unstable angina; History of HF, coronary artery disease, uncontrolled hypertension (BP >170/110 mm Hg) or hypotension (BP <90/50 mm Hg), dehydration, autonomic dysfunction, or severe left ventricular outflow obstruction; Pulmonary hypertension secondary to sickle cell anemia (may ↑ risk of vaso-occlusive crises); Concurrent treatment with antihypertensives or glipizide; Renal impairment (CCr <30 mL/min, hepatic impairment; all result in ↑ blood levels; ↓ dose required with Viagra); Anatomic penile deformity (angulation, cavernosal fibrosis, Peyronie disease); Conditions associated with priapism (sickle cell anemia, multiple myeloma, leukemia); Bleeding disorders or active peptic ulceration; History of sudden severe vision loss or at risk for non-arteritic ischemic op-

S

tic neuropathy (NAION); may ↑ risk of recurrence; Retinitis pigmentosa; Alpha adrenergic blockers (patients should be on stable dose of alpha blockers before starting sildenafil); Geri: ↑ blood levels and may require lower doses; consider age-related decrease in cardiac, hepatic, and renal function as well as concurrent drug therapy and chronic disease states; Lactation: Lactation.

Adverse Reactions/Side Effects

CNS: headache, dizziness, insomnia. **EENT:** epistaxis, hearing loss, nasal congestion, vision loss. **CV:** MYOCARDIAL INFARCTION, SUDDEN DEATH, hypotension, vaso-occlusive crises. **GI:** dyspepsia, diarrhea. **GU:** priapism, urinary tract infection. **Derm:** flushing, rash. **MS:** mylagia. **Neuro:** paresthesias.

Interactions

Drug-Drug: Concurrent use of **nitrates** may cause serious, life-threatening hypotension and is contraindicated. Concurrent use of **riociguat** may result in severe hypotension; concurrent use contraindicated. Blood levels and effects, including the risk of hypotension may be ↑ by **CYP3A4 inhibitors** including **cimetidine**, **erythromycin**, **tacrolimus**, **ketoconazole**, **itraconazole**, and **protease inhibitor antiretrovirals** including **nelfinavir**, **indinavir**, **ritonavir**, and **saquinavir** (initial dose of sildenafil for erectile dysfunction should be ↓ to 25 mg) (concurrent use of potent CYP3A inhibitors not recommended with oral Revatio). ↑ risk of hypotension with **alpha adrenergic blockers** and acute ingestion of **alcohol**. **CYP3A4 inducers**, including **rifampin**, **bosentan**, **barbiturates**, **carbamazepine**, **phenytoin**, **efavirenz**, **nevirapine**, **rifampin**, or **rifabutin** may ↓ blood levels and effects; dose adjustments may be necessary in the treatment of pulmonary arterial hypertension. ↑ levels of **bosentan**. Use cautiously with **glipizide**. May ↑ risk of bleeding with **warfarin**.

Route/Dosage

Viagra (for erectile dysfunction)

PO (Adults): 50 mg taken 1 hr before sexual activity (range 25–100 mg taken 30 min–4 hr before sexual activity); not more than once daily; *Concurrent use with alpha-blocker antihypertensives*—do not use 50–100 mg dose within 4 hr of alpha blocker, 25-mg dose may be taken anytime.
PO (Geriatric Patients ≥65 yr or with concurrent enzyme inhibitors): 25 mg taken 1 hr before sexual activity (range 25–100 mg taken 30 min–4 hr before sexual activity); not more than once daily.

Hepatic/Renal Impairment

PO (Adults): 25 mg taken 1 hr before sexual activity (range 25–100 mg taken 30 min–4 hr before sexual activity); not more than once daily.

Revatio (for pulmonary arterial hypertension)

IV therapy is indicated for patients unable to take PO therapy

PO (Adults): 5 mg or 20 mg 3 times daily; dose adjustments may be necessary for concurrent bosentan, barbiturates, carbamazepine, phenytoin, efavirenz, nevirapine, rifampin, or rifabutin.
IV (Adults): 2.5 mg or 10 mg 3 times daily.

Availability (generic available)

Tablets (Viagra): 25 mg, 50 mg, 100 mg. **Tablets (Revatio):** 20 mg. **Powder for oral suspension (Revatio):** 10 mg/mL. **Solution for injection (Revatio):** 0.8 mg/mL.

NURSING IMPLICATIONS

Assessment

- **Viagra:** Determine erectile dysfunction before administration. Sildenafil has no effect in the absence of sexual stimulation.
- **Revatio:** Monitor hemodynamic parameters and exercise tolerance prior to and periodically during therapy.

Potential Nursing Diagnoses

Sexual dysfunction (Indications)
Risk for activity intolerance (Indications)

Implementation

- Do not confuse Viagra (sildenafil) with Allegra (fexofenadine).
- **PO:** Dose for *erectile dysfunction* is usually administered 1 hr before sexual activity. May be administered 30 min–4 hr before sexual activity.
- Dose for *pulmonary arterial hypertension* is administered 3 times daily without regard to food. Doses should be spaced 4–6 hr apart.
- Use syringe provided for accurate dosing of oral suspension. Shake well before using. Solution is stable for 60 days from date of reconstitution.

IV Administration

- **IV Push:** Administer undiluted. Solution is clear and colorless; do not administer solutions that are discolored or contain a precipitate. ***Rate:*** Administer as a bolus three times daily.

Patient/Family Teaching

- Instruct patient to take sildenafil as directed. For *erectile dysfunction*, take approximately 1 hr before sexual activity and not more than once per day. If taking sildenafil for *pulmonary arterial hypertension*, take missed doses as soon as remembered unless almost time for next dose; do not double doses.
- Advise patient that *Viagra* is not indicated for use in women.
- Caution patient not to take sildenafil concurrently with alpha-adrenergic blockers (unless on a stable

dose) or nitrates. If chest pain occurs after taking sildenafil, instruct patient to seek immediate medical attention. Advise patient taking sildenafil for *pulmonary arterial hypertension* to notify health care professional of all Rx or OTC medications, vitamins, or herbal products being taken and to consult with health care professional before taking other medications.

- Instruct patient to notify health care professional promptly if erection lasts longer than 4 hr or if experience sudden or decreased vision loss in 1 or both eyes or loss or decrease in hearing, ringing in the ears, or dizziness.
- Inform patient that sildenafil offers no protection against sexually transmitted diseases. Counsel patient that protection against sexually transmitted diseases and HIV infection should be considered.

Evaluation/Desired Outcomes

- Male erection sufficient to allow intercourse.
- Increased exercise tolerance.

silodosin (si-lo-do-sin)

Rapaflo

Classification

Therapeutic: benign prostatic hyperplasia (BPH) agents

Pharmacologic: alpha-adrenergic blockers

Pregnancy Category B

Indications

Treatment of the signs/symptoms or benign prostatic hyperplasia (BPH).

Action

Blocks post synaptic alpha$_1$-adrenergic receptors. Decreases contractions in the smooth muscle of the prostatic capsule. **Therapeutic Effects:** Decreased signs and symptoms of BPH (urinary urgency, hesitancy, nocturia).

Pharmacokinetics

Absorption: 32% absorbed following oral administration.

Distribution: Unknown.

Protein Binding: 97%.

Metabolism and Excretion: Extensively metabolized (CYP3A4, UGT2B7, and other metabolic pathways involved); 33.5% excreted in urine and 54.9% in feces.

Half-life: 13.3 hr.

TIME/ACTION PROFILE (effect on symptoms of BPH)

ROUTE	ONSET	PEAK	DURATION
PO	rapid	24 hr	24 hr*

*Following discontinuation.

Contraindications/Precautions

Contraindicated in: Hypersensitivity; Not indicated for use in women or children; Severe renal impairment (CrCl less than 30 mL/min); Severe hepatic impairment (Child-Pugh score of ≥10); Concurrent use of strong CYP3A4 inhibitors or P-gp inhibitors.

Use Cautiously in: Moderate inhibitors of the CYP3A4 enzyme system; Cataract surgery (may cause intraoperative floppy iris syndrome); Moderate renal impairment (lower dose recommended); Geri: ↑ risk of orthostatic hypotention; Pedi: Safety and effectiveness not been established.

Adverse Reactions/Side Effects

CNS: dizziness, headache. **CV:** orthostatic hypotension. **GI:** diarrhea. **GU:** retrograde ejaculation. **Derm:** pruritis, rash, urticaria. **Misc:** allergic reactions.

Interactions

Drug-Drug: Strong inhibitors of CYP3A4 (including **ketoconazole**, **clarithromycin**, **itraconazole**, and **ritonavir**) ↓ metabolism, ↑ blood levels and risk of toxicity; concurrent use is contraindicated. Concurrent use with **moderate CYP3A4 inhibitors** (including **diltiazem**, **erythromycin**, and **verapamil**) may ↑ levels; use cautiously. Concurrent use with **antihypertensives** (including **calcium channel blockers** and **thiazides**), other **alpha blockers** and **phosphodiesterase type 5 inhibitors** (including **sildenafil**, **tadalafil**, and **vardenafil**) ↑ the risk of dizziness and orthostatic hypotension. **P-glycoprotein (P-gp) inhibitors** including **cyclosporine**) may ↑ levels; concurrent use not recommended.

Route/Dosage

PO (Adults): 8 mg once daily.

Renal Impairment

PO (Adults): *CCr 30–50 mL/min*—4 mg once daily.

Availability

Capsules: 4 mg, 8 mg.

NURSING IMPLICATIONS

Assessment

- Assess patient for symptoms of benign prostatic hyperplasia (urinary hesitancy, feeling of incomplete bladder emptying, interruption of urinary stream, impairment of size and force of urinary stream, terminal urinary dribbling, straining to start flow, fre-

S

quency, dysuria, nocturia, urgency) before and periodically during therapy.
- Assess patient for orthostatic reaction and syncope. Monitor BP (lying and standing) and during initial therapy and periodically thereafter.
- Rule out prostatic carcinoma before therapy; symptoms are similar.

Potential Nursing Diagnoses
Risk for injury (Side Effects)
Noncompliance (Patient/Family Teaching)

Implementation
- ***High Alert:*** Do not confuse Rapaflo with Rapamune (sirolimus). Do not confuse silodosin with sirolimus.
- **PO:** Administer with food at the same meal each day.
- If unable to swallow capsule, may open capsule and sprinkle powder inside on a tablespoonful of applesauce. Swallow immediately, within 5 min, without chewing; follow with 8 oz of cool water to ensure complete dose is swallowed. Use cool applesauce, soft enough to be swallowed without chewing. Do not store for future use or subdivide capsule contents.

Patient/Family Teaching
- Instruct patient to take medication with the same meal each day.
- May cause dizziness. Caution patient to avoid driving or other activities requiring alertness until response to the medication is known.
- Caution patient to avoid sudden changes in position to decrease orthostatic hypotension, especially patients with low BP or concurrently taking antihypertensives. Geri: Assess risk for falls; instruct patient and family in preventing falls at home.
- Instruct patient to notify health care professional of all Rx or OTC medications, vitamins, or herbal products being taken and consult health care professional before taking any new medications, especially cough, cold, or allergy remedies.
- Instruct patient to notify health care professional of medication regimen before any surgery. Patients planning cataract surgery should notify ophthalmologist of silodosin therapy prior to surgery.
- Inform patient that silodosin may cause retrograde ejaculation (orgasm with reduced or no semen). This does not pose a safety concern and is reversible with discontinuation.
- Emphasize the importance of follow-up exams to evaluate effectiveness of medication.

Evaluation/Desired Outcomes
- Decreased symptoms of benign prostatic hyperplasia.

simeprevir (sim-e-pre-vir)
Galexos, Olysio

Classification
Therapeutic: antivirals
Pharmacologic: protease inhibitors

Pregnancy Category C (alone), X (for combination with ribavarin and peginterferon alfa)

Indications
Treatment of hepatitis C in combination with other agents (peginterferon alfa and ribavirin; sofosbuvir) as a total regimen in patients with infection caused by the hepatitis C virus (HCV) genotype 1 (other genotypes may not respond). Not to be used as monotherapy.

Action
Inhibits viral replication; a direct-acting antiviral (DAA). **Therapeutic Effects:** Clearing of infection with decreased severity and sequelae of HCV.

Pharmacokinetics
Absorption: Well absorbed following oral administration, food ↑ and delays absorption (blood levels are ↑ in HCV-infected patients as compared to non-HCV-infected patients).
Distribution: Unknown.
Protein Binding: >99.9%.
Metabolism and Excretion: Highly metabolized (primarily by CYP3A), eliminated primarily via biliary excretion, 31% excreted unchanged in feces, <1% in urine.
Half-life: *HCV-infected patients*—41 hr; *HCV-uninfected patients* —10–13 hr.

TIME/ACTION PROFILE (blood levels)

ROUTE	ONSET	PEAK	DURATION
PO	unknown	6–8 hr	24 hr

Contraindications/Precautions
Contraindicated in: Patients with NS3 Q80K polymorphism (↓ efficacy of simeprevir + peginterferon alfa + ribavirin); Moderate-to-severe hepatic impairment; Previous failure to simeprevir or another HCV protease inhibitor; Any condition in which peginterferon alpha or ribavirin is contraindicated; Concurrent use of moderate or strong inhibitors or inducers of the CYP3A system (may significantly change blood levels, effectiveness and risk of toxicity/adverse reactions); OB: Pregnant women and men whose female partners are pregnant (ribavirin contraindication).
Use Cautiously in: History of sulfonamide hypersensitivity (cross sensitivity may occur); East Asian ancestry (high blood levels, ↑ risk of adverse reactions including rash and photosensitivity); Severe renal impairment/dialysis.

Adverse Reactions/Side Effects

Reflects combination use with peginterferon alfa and ribavirin.

Resp: dyspnea. **GI:** HEPATOTOXICITY, hyperbilirubinemia, nausea. **Derm:** photosensitivity, pruritus, rash. **MS:** myalgia.

Interactions

Drug-Drug: Blood levels and the risk of toxicity may be ↑ **moderate or strong inhibitors CYP3A** including **clarithromycin**, **cobicistat-containing products**, **darunavir/ritonavir**, **erythromycin**, **fluconazole**, **itraconazole**, **posiconazole**, **ritonavir**, **telithromycin** and **voriconazole**, concurrent use is not recommended. May ↑ levels and risk of toxicity of **digoxin** due to inhibition of P-gp (blood level monitoring recommended). Blood levels and therapeutic effects may be ↓ by inducers of CYP3A and CYP3A4 including **carbamazepine**, **dexamethasone**, **efavirenz**, **oxcarbazepine**, **phenobarbital**, **phenytoin**, **rifabutin**, **rifampin**, **rifapentine**; concurrent use is not recommended. Blood levels may be altered (↑ or ↓) by **atazanavir**, **delavirdine**, **etravirine**, **fosamprenavir**, **lopinavir**, **indinavir**, **nelfinavir**, **nevirapine**, **saquinavir**, or **tipranavir** (concurrent use is not recommended). May ↑ blood levels and risk of toxicity with **amlodipine**, **atorvastatin** (atorvastatin dose should not exceed 40 mg daily), **diltiazem**, **disopyramide**, **felodipine**, **flecainide**, **lovastatin** (use lowest effective dose), **mexiletine**, **nicardipine**, **nifendipine**, **nisoldipine**, **pitavastatin** (use lowest effective dose), **pravastatin** (use lowest effective dose), **propafenone**, **quinidine**, **rosuvastatin** (rosuvastatin dose should not exceed 10 mg daily), **simvastatin** (use lowest effective dose), and **verapamil**(clinical and/or blood level monitoring recommended). May alter blood levels of **sirolimus** (monitor sirolimus levels). May ↑ blood levels and risk of adverse reactions/toxicity of **sildenfil**, **tadalafil** and **vardenafil** (no adjustments needed when used for erectile dysfunction, when sildenafil or tadalafil are used for pulmonary arterial hypertension, use lowest effective dose and monitor clinically). May ↑ blood levels and the risk of sedation with **midazolam** or **triazolam**, use cautiously. Concomitant use with **tacrolimus** may ↓ tacrolimus levels and ↑ simeprevir levels. Concomitant use with **cyclosporine** may ↑ cyclosporine and simeprevir levels; concomitant use not recommended. **Amiodarone** may ↑ risk of symptomatic bradycardia when used with simeprevir and sofosbuvir; concurrent use not recommended; if amiodarone necessary, monitor patients in inpatient setting for first 48 hr of concomitant use and then monitor heart rate on outpatient basis for at least the first 2 wk of treatment (follow same monitoring procedure if discontinuing amiodarone immediately before initiation of sofosbuvir and simeprevir therapy).

Drug-Natural Products: Blood levels and risk of toxicity may be ↑ by **milk thistle** (concurrent use is not recommended). Blood levels and effectiveness may be ↓ by **St. John's wort**, concurrent use is not recommended.

Route/Dosage

PO (Adults): *With peginterferon alfa and ribavirin*— 150 mg once daily for 12 wk. Treatment with peginterferon alfa and ribavirin may continue for an additional 12 wk (for treatment-naïve patients and prior relapsers or 36 wk (for prior non-responders); *With sofosbuvir*— 150 mg once daily for 12 wk (patients without cirrhosis) or 24 wk (patients with cirrhosis).

Availability

Capsules: 150 mg.

NURSING IMPLICATIONS

Assessment

- Monitor for signs and symptoms of chronic hepatitis C.
- Assess for rash, especially during first 4 wk of therapy. Monitor mild to moderate rashes for progression, including mucosal signs (oral lesions, conjunctivitis). If rash becomes severe, discontinue simeprevir and monitor until rash resolved.
- ***Lab Test Considerations:*** Use a sensitive assay with a lower limit of quantification of at least 25 IU/mL for monitoring HCV RNA levels during treatment. *In treatment wk 4, if HCV RNA ≥25 IU/mL,* discontinue simeprevir, peginterferon alfa, and ribavirin. *In treatment wk 12, if HCV RNA ≥25 IU/mL,*, discontinue peginterferon alfa and ribavirin; simeprevir is completed at wk 12. *In treatment wk 24, if HCV RNA ≥25 IU/mL,* discontinue peginterferon alfa and ribavirin.
- 🧬 Prior to starting therapy with simprevir + peginterferon + ribavirin, screen patient with HCV genotype 1a infection for the presence of virus with the NS3 Q80K polymorphism. Consider alternative therapy for patients infected with HCV genotype 1a containing the Q80K polymorphism. May be considered before starting therapy with simeprevir + sobosuvir.
- A negative pregnancy test must be obtained immediately before beginning therapy and monthly thereafter.
- Monitor liver function tests prior to and periodically during therapy, as clinically indicated. May cause ↑ alkaline phosphatase and bilirubin. Monitor closely if serum bilirubin ↑ 2.5 x upper limit of normal. If accompanied by liver transaminase ↑ or clinical signs and symptoms of hepatic decompensation, discontinue therapy.

S

Potential Nursing Diagnoses
Risk for infection (Indications)

Implementation
- Must be administered in conjunction with ribavirin and peginterferon alfa. If ribavirin and peginterferon alfa are discontinued, simeprevir must be discontinued. If simeprevir is discontinued due to adverse reactions or inadequate response, do not restart simprevir.
- **PO:** Administer once daily with food.

Patient/Family Teaching
- Instruct patient to take simeprevir with ribavirin and pegainterferon alfa as directed. Take missed doses within 12 hr with food or skip dose and take next scheduled dose; do not double doses. Advise patient to read *Patient Information* before starting and with each refill in case of changes.
- Caution patient to wear sunscreen and protective clothing and avoid tanning devices to prevent photosensitivity reaction.
- Advise patient to notify health care professional if rash, signs and symptoms of hepatotoxicity (fatigue, weakness, lack of appetite, nausea and vomiting, jaundice, discolored feces) or photosensitivity reaction (burning, redness, swelling or blisters on skin; mouth sores or ulcers; red or inflamed eyes like pink eye or conjunctivitis) occurs.
- Instruct patient to notify health care professional of all Rx or OTC medications, vitamins, or herbal products being taken and consult health care professional before taking any new medications, especially St. Johns wort.
- Rep: Advise female patients and male patients with female partners who are pregnant or may become pregnant to use effective contraception due to risks for birth defects and fetal death and avoid breast feeding. Women and male partners must use 2 forms of non-hormonal contraception during and for at least 6 mo after discontinuation of therapy. Advise women who become pregnant to enroll in the Ribavirin Pregnancy Registry by calling 1-800-593-2214.

Evaluation/Desired Outcomes
- Decreased severity and sequelae of HCV following treatment with simeprevir, ribavirin, and peginterferon alfa for 12 wk.
- Patients who are treatment-naïve and prior relapser, including those with cirrhosis, should receive an additional 12 wk of peginterferon alfa and ribavirin for a total of 24 wk.
- Prior non-responders should receive an additional 36 wk of peginterferon alfa and ribavirin for a total of 48 wk.

simvastatin, See HMG-CoA REDUCTASE INHIBITORS (statins).

sipuleucel (si-pu-loo-sel)
Provenge

Classification
Therapeutic: antineoplastics
Pharmacologic: autologous cellular immunotherapies

Indications
Asymptomatic/minimally symptomatic metastatic castrate resistant (hormone refractory) prostate cancer.

Action
Autologous immunotherapy produced by collecting peripheral mononuclear cells during leukapheresis. Cells include antigen presenting cells (APCs), which are activated during a culture period with prostatic acid phosphatase (PAP, an antigen found in prostatic cancer tissue) linked to granulocyte-macrophage colony-stimulating factor (GM-CSF, which activates immune cells). Induces an immune response against prostatic acid phosphatase. **Therapeutic Effects:** ↓ spread of prostate cancer.

Pharmacokinetics
Absorption: IV administration results in complete bioavailability.
Distribution: Unknown.
Metabolism and Excretion: Unknown.
Half-life: Unknown.

TIME/ACTION PROFILE

ROUTE	ONSET	PEAK	DURATION
IV	unknown	unknown	unknown

Contraindications/Precautions
Contraindicated in: None noted.
Use Cautiously in: Intended for autologous use only.

Adverse Reactions/Side Effects
CNS: fatigue, headache, dizziness, insomnia. **Resp:** dyspnea. **CV:** hypertension, peripheral edema. **GI:** constipation, diarrhea, nausea, vomiting. **GU:** hematuria. **Derm:** flushing, rash, sweating. **Hemat:** anemia. **MS:** back pain, joint pain, extremity pain, muscle spasms, musculoskeletal pain. **Neuro:** paresthesia, tremor. **Misc:** chills, fever, acute infusion reactions, citrate toxicity.

Interactions
Drug-Drug: Concurrent use of **immunosuppressants** may alter safety/efficacy.

Route/Dosage
IV (Adults): One dose every 2 wk for a total of 3 doses.

Availability

Suspension for IV infusion: minimum of 50 million autologous CD54+ cells activated with PAP-GM-CSF suspended in 250 mL lactated ringer's injection.

NURSING IMPLICATIONS

Assessment

- Monitor for signs of acute infusion reaction (fever, chills, dyspnea, hypoxia, bronchospasm, dizziness, nausea, vomiting, fatigue, headache, muscle aches, hypertension, tachycardia), especially patients with cardiac or pulmonary conditions. If signs occur, infusion may be slowed or interrupted, depending on severity of reaction. If infusion must be interrupted, do not resume if infusion bag will be at room temperature for >3 hr. Monitor patient for at least 30 min following each infusion.

Potential Nursing Diagnoses

Deficient knowledge, related to medication regimen (Patient/Family Teaching)

Implementation

IV Administration

- Each infusion must be preceded by a leukaphresis procedure approximately 3 days prior. If patient is unable to receive an infusion, patient will need to undergo an additional leukaphresis procedure.
- Medication is not routinely tested for transmissible infectious diseases. Employ universal precautions in handling leukapheresis material or sipuleucel.
- Premedicate patient with acetaminophen and an antihistamine (diphenhydramine) 30 min prior to administration to minimize acute infusion reactions.
- Upon receipt of sipuleucel from manufacturer, open outer cardboard shipping box to verify product and patient-specific labels. Do not remove insulated container from shipping box or open lid of insulated container until patient is ready for infusion. Do not infuse until confirmation of product release has been received from manufacturer.
- Infusion must begin prior to expiration date and time. Do not infuse expired sipuleucel. Once infusion bag is removed from insulated container, infuse within 3 hr; do not return to shipping container.
- **Intermittent Infusion:** Once patient is prepared for infusion and Cell Product Disposition Form has been received, remove infusion bag from insulated container, and inspect bag for leakage. Contents will be slightly cloudy, with cream-to-pink color. Gently mix and re-suspend contents of bag, inspecting for clumps and clots. Small clumps should disperse with gentle manual mixing; do not administer if bag leaks or if clumps remain.
- Sipuleucel is solely for autologous use. Match patient's identity with the patient identifiers on the Cell Product Disposition Form and infusion bag. ***Rate:*** Infuse the entire volume of the bag over 60 min. Do not use a cell filter.

Patient/Family Teaching

- Explain the purpose of sipuleucel and the importance of maintaining all scheduled appointments, adhering to preparation instructions for leukaphresis procedure to patient.
- Inform patient that a central venous catheter may be required if adequate peripheral venous access is not available.
- Advise patient to notify health care professional if fever over 100°F, swelling or redness around catheter site, pain at infusion or collection sites, symptoms of cardiac arrhythmia (chest pains, racing heart, irregular heartbeats), signs of acute infusion reaction, or persistent side effects occur.
- Instruct patient to notify health care professional of all Rx or OTC medications, vitamins, or herbal products, especially immunosuppressive agents, being taken and consult health care professional before taking any new medications.

Evaluation/Desired Outcomes

- ↓ in the spread of prostate cancer.

sirolimus (sir-**oh**-li-mus)

Rapamune

Classification

Therapeutic: immunosuppressants

Pregnancy Category C

Indications

Prevention of organ rejection in allogenic kidney transplantation (with corticosteroids and cyclosporine). Treatment of lymphangioleiomyomatosis (LAM).

Action

Inhibits T-lymphocyte activation/proliferation, which occurs as a response to antigenic and cytokine stimulation; antibody production is also inhibited. **Therapeutic Effects:** Decreased incidence and severity of organ rejection. Improvement in pulmonary function.

Pharmacokinetics

Absorption: Rapidly absorbed following oral administration (14% bioavailability).

Distribution: Concentrates in erythrocytes; distributes to heart, intestines, kidneys, liver, lungs, muscle, spleen, and testes in high concentrations.

Protein Binding: 92%.

Metabolism and Excretion: Extensively metabolized (some metabolism by P450 3A4 system); 91% excreted in feces.

S

Half-life: 62 hr.

TIME/ACTION PROFILE (blood levels)

ROUTE	ONSET	PEAK	DURATION
PO	rapid	1–2 hr	24 hr

Contraindications/Precautions

Contraindicated in: Hypersensitivity; Alcohol intolerance/sensitivity (solution contains ethanol); Concurrent ketoconazole, voriconazole, itraconazole, erythromycin, telithromycin, clarithromycin, rifampin, rifabutin, or grapefruit juice; Severe hepatic impairment; OB, Lactation: Pregnancy and lactation.

Use Cautiously in: Mild to moderate hepatic impairment; Rep: Women with childbearing potential; Pedi: Children <13 yr (safety not established).

Adverse Reactions/Side Effects

Reflects combined therapy with corticosteroids and cyclosporine.

CNS: PROGRESSIVE MULTIFOCAL LEUKOENCEPHALOPATHY (PML), insomnia. **Resp:** interstitial lung disease. **CV:** edema, hypotension, pericardial effusion. **GI:** ascites, hepatotoxicity. **GU:** amenorrhea, menorrhagia, ovarian cysts, renal impairment. **Derm:** acne, rash, thrombocytopenic purpura. **F and E:** hypokalemia. **Hemat:** leukopenia, thrombocytopenia, anemia. **Endo:** diabetes, hyperglycemia. **Metab:** hypercholesterolemia, hypertriglyceridemia. **MS:** arthralgias. **Neuro:** tremor. **Misc:** infection (including activation of latent viral infections such as BK virus-associated nephropathy, Clostridium difficile-associated diarrhea (CDAD)), lymphocele, lymphoma, ↓ wound healing.

Interactions

Drug-Drug: **Cyclosporine (modified)** greatly ↑ blood levels (administer sirolimus 4 hr after cyclosporine). Drugs that inhibit the CYP3A4 enzyme system may be expected to ↑ blood levels and the risk of adverse reactions. **Ketoconazole**, **voriconazole**, **itraconazole**, **clarithromycin**, **erythromycin**, **telithromycin** significantly ↑ blood levels (concurrent use is contraindicated). Blood levels are also ↑ by **diltiazem** and **verapamil** (monitor sirolimus levels and adjust dose as necessary) and may be ↑ by **nicardipine**, **verapamil**, **clotrimazole**, **fluconazole**, **troleandomycin**, **metoclopramide**, **cimetidine**, **danazol**, and **protease inhibitors**. **Rifampin** and **rifabutin**↑ metabolism by stimulating the CYP3A4 enzyme system and significantly ↓ blood levels. Blood levels may also be ↓ by **carbamazepine**, **phenobarbital**, **phenytoin**, and **rifapentine**. Risk of renal impairment may be ↑ by concurrent use of other **nephrotoxic agents**. Concurrent use with **tacrolimus** and **corticosteroids** in lung transplantation may ↑ risk of anastamotic dehiscence; fatalites have been reported (not approved for this use). Concurrent use with **tacrolimus** and **corticosteroids** in liver transplantation may ↑ risk of hepatic artery thrombosis; fatalites have been reported (not approved for this use). May ↓ antibody response to and ↑ risk of adverse reactions to **live-virus vaccines** (avoid vaccination).

Drug-Natural Products: Concomitant use with **echinacea** and **melatonin** may interfere with immunosuppression. **St. John's wort** may ↑ blood levels and the risk of toxicity.

Drug-Food: Grapefruit juice ↓ CYP3A4 metabolism and ↑ levels; do not use as a diluent and avoid concurrent ingestion.

Route/Dosage

Kidney Transplantation

PO (Adults and Children ≥13 yr): 6-mg loading dose, followed by 2 mg/day maintenance dose. *Dosing following cyclosporine withdrawal*—Patients at low to moderate risk for rejection after transplantation may be withdrawn from cyclosporine over 4–8 wk beginning 2–4 mo after transplant. Thereafter, sirolimus dose should be titrated upward to maintain a whole blood trough level of 12–14 ng/mL. Clinical assessment should also be used to gauge dose. Dose changes can be made at 7–14 day intervals. The following formula may also be used: sirolimus maintenance dose = current dose × (target concentration/current concentration). If a large ↑ is needed, a loading dose may be given and blood levels reassessed 3–4 days later. Loading dose may be calculated by the following formula: sirolimus loading dose = 3 × (new maintenance dose-current maintenance dose). Loading doses >40 m g should be spread over 2 days.

PO (Adults and Children ≥13 yr and <40 kg): 3 mg/m^2 loading dose, followed by 1 mg/m^2/day maintenance dose. *See adjustments above for doses following cyclosporine withdrawal.*

Hepatic Impairment

PO (Adults and Children): *Mild or moderate hepatic impairment*—↓ maintenance dose by 33%; loading dose is unchanged; *Severe hepatic impairment*—↓ maintenance dose by 50%; loading dose is unchanged.

Lymphangioleiomyomatosis

PO (Adults): 2 mg once daily. Monitor whole blood trough level in 10–20 days and titrate dose to maintain level of 5–15 ng/mL. The following formula may also be used to adjust dose: sirolimus maintenance dose = current dose × (target concentration/current concentration). Further dose changes can be made at 7–14 day intervals. Once stable dose achieved, should monitor whole blood trough levels at least q 3 mo.

Hepatic Impairment

(Adults): *Mild or moderate hepatic impairment*—↓ dose by 33%: *Severe hepatic impairment*—↓ dose by 50%.

Availability (generic available)

Tablet: 0.5 mg, 1 mg, 2 mg. **Oral solution:** 1 mg/mL.

NURSING IMPLICATIONS

Assessment

- Monitor BP closely during therapy. Hypertension is a common complication of sirolimus therapy and should be treated.
- Assess for any new signs or symptoms that may be suggestive of PML, an opportunistic infection of the brain that leads to death or severe disability; withhold dose and notify health care professional promptly. Symptoms of PML may include hemiparesis, apathy, confusion, cognitive deficiencies, and ataxia. Consider decreasing the amount of immunosuppression in these patients.
- **Lymphangioleiomyomatosis:** Monitor for signs and symptoms of LAM (wheezing; cough, which may be bloody; shortness of breath; chest pain; pneumothorax) periodically during therapy.
- ***Lab Test Considerations:*** Monitor sirolimus blood levels when dose forms are changed and in patients likely to have altered drug metabolism, patients ≥13 yr who weigh <40 kg, patients with hepatic impairment, and during concurrent administration of drugs that may interact with sirolimus. Trough concentrations of ≥15 ng/mL are associated with an ↑ in adverse effects.
- Monitor patients for hyperlipidemia. May require additional interventions to treat hyperlipidemia.
- May cause anemia, leukopenia, thrombocytopenia, and hypokalemia.
- May cause ↑ AST, ↑ ALT, hypophosphatemia, and hyperglycemia.

Potential Nursing Diagnoses

Risk for infection (Adverse Reactions)

Implementation

- Therapy with sirolimus should be started as soon as possible post-transplant. Concurrent therapy with cyclosporine and corticosteroids is recommended. Sirolimus should be taken 4 hr after cyclosporine (MODIFIED, Neoral).
- Sirolimus should be ordered only by physicians skilled in immunosuppressive therapy, with the staff and facilities to manage renal transplant patients.
- Antimicrobial prophylaxis for *Pneumocystis jirovecii* pneumonia for 1 yr and for cytomegalovirus protection for 3 mo post-transplant are recommended.
- **PO:** Administer consistently with or without food. Swallow tablet whole; do not crush, break, or chew. Do not administer with or mix with grapefruit juice.
- To dilute from bottle, use amber oral dose syringe to withdraw prescribed amount. Empty sirolimus from syringe into a glass or plastic container holding at least 2 oz (60 mL) of water or orange juice; do not use other liquids. Stir vigorously and drink at once. Refill container with at least 4 oz of additional liquid, stir vigorously, and drink at once.
- If using the pouch, empty entire contents of pouch into at least 2 oz of water or orange juice; do not use other liquids. Stir vigorously and drink at once. Refill container with at least 4 oz of additional liquid, stir vigorously, and drink at once.
- Store bottles and pouches in refrigerator. Protect from light. Solution may develop a slight haze when refrigerated; allow to stand at room temperature and shake gently until haze disappears. Sirolimus may remain in syringe at room temperature or refrigerated for up to 24 hr. Discard syringe after 1 use. Oral solution must be used within 1 mo of opening bottle.

Patient/Family Teaching

- Instruct patient to take sirolimus at the same time each day, as directed. Advise patient to avoid taking with or diluting with grapefruit juice. Do not skip or double up on missed doses. Do not discontinue medication without advice of health care professional.
- Advise patient to avoid grapefruit and grapefruit juice during therapy.
- Reinforce the need for lifelong therapy to prevent transplant rejection. Review symptoms of rejection for transplanted organ and stress need to notify health care professional immediately if they occur.
- Advise patient to notify health care professional if swelling of your face, eyes, or mouth; trouble breathing or wheezing; throat tightness; chest pain or tightness; feeling dizzy or faint; rash or peeling of skin; swelling of hands or feet; or symptoms of PML occur.
- Advise patient to wear sunscreen and protective clothing and limit time in sunlight and UV light due to increased risk of skin cancer.
- Caution patient to notify health care professional if signs of infection occur.
- Advise patient to avoid vaccinations with a live virus during therapy.
- Rep: Advise patient of the risk of taking sirolimus during pregnancy. Caution women of childbearing age to use effective contraception prior to, during, and for 12 wk following therapy.
- Emphasize the importance of repeated lab tests during sirolimus therapy.

Evaluation/Desired Outcomes

- Prevention of transplanted kidney rejection.
- Reduction in symptoms of lymphangioleiomyomatosis (LAM).

S

sitaGLIPtin (sit-a-glip-tin)

Januvia

Classification

Therapeutic: antidiabetics

Pharmacologic: enzyme inhibitors

Pregnancy Category B

Indications

Adjunct to diet and exercise to improve glycemic control in patients with type 2 diabetes mellitus; may be used as monotherapy or combination therapy with metformin, a thiazolidinedione, a sulfonylurea, or insulin.

Action

Inhibits the enzyme dipeptidyl peptidase-4 (DPP-4), which slows the inactivation of incretin hormones, resulting in increased levels of active incretin hormones. These hormones are released by the intestine throughout the day and are involved in regulation of glucose homeostasis. Increased/prolonged incretin levels result in an increase in insulin release and decrease in glucagon levels. **Therapeutic Effects:** Improved control of blood glucose.

Pharmacokinetics

Absorption: 87% absorbed following oral administration.

Distribution: Unknown.

Metabolism and Excretion: 79% excreted unchanged in urine, minor metabolism.

Half-life: 12.4 hr.

TIME/ACTION PROFILE

ROUTE	ONSET	PEAK	DURATION
PO	rapid	1–4 hr	24 hr

Contraindications/Precautions

Contraindicated in: Type 1 diabetes mellitus; Diabetic ketoacidosis; Hypersensitivity.

Use Cautiously in: Renal impairment (dose ↓ required for CCr <50 mL/min); History of pancreatitis; History of angioedema to another DPP-4 inhibitor; OB: Use only if clearly needed. Lactation: Excretion into breast milk unknown; Pedi: Safety not established; Geri: Consider age-related ↓ in renal function when determining dose.

Adverse Reactions/Side Effects

CNS: headache. **GI:** PANCREATITIS, nausea, diarrhea. **GU:** acute renal failure. **Resp:** upper respiratory tract infection, nasopharyngitis. **MS:** arthralgia, back pain, myalgia. **Misc:** allergic reactions including ANAPHYLAXIS, ANGIOEDEMA, EXFOLIATIVE SKIN CONDITIONS (STEVENS-JOHNSON SYNDROME), rash, urticaria.

Interactions

Drug-Drug: May slightly ↑ serum digoxin levels; monitoring recommended. ↑ risk of hypoglycemia when used with **insulin, glyburide, glipizide,** or **glimepiride** (may need to ↓ dose of insulin or sulfonylurea).

Route/Dosage

PO (Adults): 100 mg once daily.

Renal Impairment

PO (Adults): *CCr 30–<50 mL/min*—50 mg once daily; *CCr <30 mL/min*—25 mg once daily.

Availability

Tablets: 25 mg, 50 mg, 100 mg. **Cost:** 25 mg $801.18/90, 50 mg $816.93/90, 100 mg $816.93/90. ***In combination with:*** metformin (Janumet), metformin XR (Janumet XR). See Appendix B.

NURSING IMPLICATIONS

Assessment

- Observe patient for signs and symptoms of hypoglycemic reactions (abdominal pain, sweating, hunger, weakness, dizziness, headache, tremor, tachycardia, anxiety).
- Monitor for signs of pancreatitis (nausea, vomiting, anorexia, persistent severe abdominal pain, sometimes radiating to the back) during therapy. If pancreatitis occurs, discontinue sitagliptin and monitor serum and urine amylase, amylase/creatinine clearance ratio, electrolytes, serum calcium, glucose, and lipase.
- Assess for rash periodically during therapy. May cause Stevens-Johnson syndrome. Discontinue therapy if severe or if accompanied with fever, general malaise, fatigue, muscle or joint aches, blisters, oral lesions, conjunctivitis, hepatitis, and/or eosinophilia.
- ***Lab Test Considerations:*** Monitor hemoglobin A1C prior to and periodically during therapy.
- Monitor renal function prior to and periodically during therapy.

Potential Nursing Diagnoses

Imbalanced nutrition: more than body requirements (Indications)

Noncompliance (Patient/Family Teaching)

Implementation

- Do not confuse sitagliptin with sumatriptan. Do not confuse Januvia (sitagliptin) with Enjuvia (estrogens, conjugated B), Jantoven (warfarin), or Janumet (sitagliptin/metformin).
- Patients stabilized on a diabetic regimen who are exposed to stress, fever, trauma, infection, or surgery may require administration of insulin.
- **PO:** May be administered without regard to food.

Patient/Family Teaching

- Instruct patient to take sitagliptin as directed. Take missed doses as soon as remembered, unless it is almost time for next dose; do not double doses. Advise patient to read *Medication Guide* before starting and with each Rx refill in case of changes.

- Explain to patient that sitagliptin helps control hyperglycemia but does not cure diabetes. Therapy is usually long term.
- Instruct patient not to share this medication with others, even if they have the same symptoms; it may harm them.
- Encourage patient to follow prescribed diet, medication, and exercise regimen to prevent hyperglycemic or hypoglycemic episodes.
- Review signs of hypoglycemia and hyperglycemia with patient. If hypoglycemia occurs, advise patient to take a glass of orange juice or 2–3 tsp of sugar, honey, or corn syrup dissolved in water, and notify health care professional.
- Instruct patient in proper testing of blood glucose and urine ketones. These tests should be monitored closely during periods of stress or illness and health care professional notified if significant changes occur.
- Advise patient to stop taking sitagliptin and notify health care professional promptly if symptoms of hypersensitivity reactions (rash; hives; swelling of face, lips, tongue, and throat; difficulty in breathing or swallowing) or pancreatitis occur.
- Advise patient to notify health care professional of all Rx or OTC medications, vitamins, or herbal products being taken and to consult with health care professional before taking other medications.
- Advise patient to notify health care professional if pregnancy is planned or suspected or if breast feeding. Encourage patients who become pregnant while taking sitagliptin to join the pregnancy registry by calling 1-800-986-8999.

Evaluation/Desired Outcomes

- Improved hemoglobin A1C, fasting plasma glucose and 2-hr post-prandial glucose levels.

sodium bicarbonate

(**soe**-dee-um bye-**kar**-boe-nate)

Baking Soda, Bell-Ans, Citrocarbonate, Neut, Soda Mint

Classification

Therapeutic: antiulcer agents

Pharmacologic: alkalinizing agents

Pregnancy Category C

Indications

PO, IV: Management of metabolic acidosis. **PO, IV:** Used to alkalinize urine and promote excretion of certain drugs in overdosage situations (phenobarbital, aspirin). **PO:** Antacid. **Unlabeled Use:** Stabilization of acid-base status in cardiac arrest and treatment of life-threatening hyperkalemia.

Action

Acts as an alkalinizing agent by releasing bicarbonate ions. Following oral administration, releases bicarbonate, which is capable of neutralizing gastric acid. **Therapeutic Effects:** Alkalinization. Neutralization of gastric acid.

Pharmacokinetics

Absorption: Following oral administration, excess bicarbonate is absorbed and results in metabolic alkalosis and alkaline urine.

Distribution: Widely distributed into extracellular fluid.

Metabolism and Excretion: Sodium and bicarbonate are excreted by the kidneys.

Half-life: Unknown.

TIME/ACTION PROFILE (PO = antacid effect; IV = alkalinization)

ROUTE	ONSET	PEAK	DURATION
PO	immediate	30 min	1–3 hr
IV	immediate	rapid	unknown

Contraindications/Precautions

Contraindicated in: Metabolic or respiratory alkalosis; Hypocalcemia; Hypernatremia; Excessive chloride loss; As an antidote following ingestion of strong mineral acids; Patients on sodium-restricted diets (oral use as an antacid only); Renal failure (oral use as an antacid only); Severe abdominal pain of unknown cause, especially if associated with fever (oral use as an antacid only).

Use Cautiously in: HF; Renal insufficiency; Concurrent corticosteroid therapy; Chronic use as an antacid (may cause metabolic alkalosis and possible sodium overload); Pedi: May ↑ risk of cerebral edema in children with diabetic ketoacidosis.

Adverse Reactions/Side Effects

CV: edema. **GI:** *PO*—flatulence, gastric distention. **F and E:** metabolic alkalosis, hypernatremia, hypocalcemia, hypokalemia, sodium and water retention. **Local:** irritation at IV site. **Neuro:** tetany, cerebral hemorrhage (with rapid injection in infants).

Interactions

Drug-Drug: Following oral administration, may ↓ absorption of **ketoconazole**. Concurrent use with **calcium-containing antacids** may lead to milk-alkali syndrome. Urinary alkalinization may result in ↓ **salicylate** or **barbiturate** blood levels; ↑ blood levels of **quinidine**, **mexiletine**, **flecainide**, or **amphetamines**; ↑ risk of crystalluria from **fluoroquinolones**; ↓ effectiveness of **methenamine**. May negate the protective effects of **enteric-coated products** (do not administer within 1–2 hr of each other).

S

Route/Dosage

Contains 12 mEq of sodium/g.

Alkalinization of Urine

PO (Adults): 48 mEq (4 g) initially. Then 12–24 mEq (1–2 g) q 4 hr (up to 48 mEq q 4 hr) or 1 tsp of powder q 4 hr as needed.
PO (Children): 1–10 mEq/kg (84–840 mg/kg) per day in divided doses.
IV (Adults and Children): 2–5 mEq/kg as a 4–8 hr infusion.

Antacid

PO (Adults): *Tablets/powder*—325 mg–2 g 1–4 times daily or ½ tsp q 2 hr as needed. *Effervescent powder*—3.9–10 g in water after meals; patients >60 yr should receive 1.9–3.9 g after meals.

Systemic Alkalinization/Cardiac Arrest

IV (Adults and Children and Infants): *Cardiac arrest/urgent situations*—1 mEq/kg; may repeat 0.5 mEq/kg q 10 min. *Less urgent situations*—2–5 mEq/kg as a 4–8 hr infusion.

Renal Tubular Acidosis

PO (Adults): 0.5–2 mEq/kg/day in 4–5 divided doses.
PO (Children): 2–3 mEq/kg/day in 3–4 divided doses.

Availability (generic available)

Oral powder: (20.9 mEq Na/½ tsp) in 120-, 240-, 480-, and 2400-g containers^OTC^. **Tablets:** 325 mg (3.9 mEq Na/tablet)^OTC^, ✤500 mg (6.0 mEq Na/tablet^OTC^, 520 mg (6.2 mEq Na/tablet)^OTC^, 650 mg (7.7 mEq Na/tablet)^OTC^. **Solution for injection:** 4.2% (0.5 mEq/mL) in 2.5-, 5-, and 10-mL prefilled syringes, 5% (0.6 mEq/mL) in 500-mL containers, 7.5% (0.9 mEq/mL) in 50-mL vials and prefilled syringes and 200-mL vials, 8.4% (1 mEq/mL) in 10- and 50-mL vials and prefilled syringes. **Neutralizing additive solution for injection:** 4% (0.48 mEq/mL) in 5-mL vials, 4.2% (0.5 mEq/mL) in 6-mL vials.

NURSING IMPLICATIONS

Assessment

- **IV:** Assess fluid balance (intake and output, daily weight, edema, lung sounds) throughout therapy. Report symptoms of fluid overload (hypertension, edema, dyspnea, rales/crackles, frothy sputum) if they occur.
- Assess patient for signs of acidosis (disorientation, headache, weakness, dyspnea, hyperventilation), alkalosis (confusion, irritability, paresthesia, tetany, altered breathing pattern), hypernatremia (edema, weight gain, hypertension, tachycardia, fever, flushed skin, mental irritability), or hypokalemia (weakness, fatigue, U wave on ECG, arrhythmias, polyuria, polydipsia) throughout therapy.
- Observe IV site closely. Avoid extravasation, as tissue irritation or cellulitis may occur. If infiltration occurs, confer with physician or other health care professional regarding warm compresses and infiltration of site with lidocaine or hyaluronidase.
- **Antacid:** Assess patient for epigastric or abdominal pain and frank or occult blood in the stool, emesis, or gastric aspirate.
- ***Lab Test Considerations:*** Monitor serum sodium, potassium, calcium, bicarbonate concentrations, serum osmolarity, acid-base balance, and renal function prior to and periodically throughout therapy.
- Obtain arterial blood gases (ABGs) frequently in emergency situations and during parenteral therapy.
- Monitor urine pH frequently when used for urinary alkalinization.
- Antagonizes effects of pentagastrin and histamine during gastric acid secretion test. Avoid administration during the 24 hr preceding the test.

Potential Nursing Diagnoses

Impaired gas exchange (Indications)
Excess fluid volume (Side Effects)

Implementation

- This medication may cause premature dissolution of enteric-coated tablets in the stomach.
- **PO:** Tablets must be taken with a full glass of water.
- When used in treatment of peptic ulcers, may be administered 1 and 3 hr after meals and at bedtime.

IV Administration

- **IV Push:** Used in cardiac arrest or urgent situations. ***Diluent:*** Use premeasured ampules or prefilled syringes to ensure accurate dose. ***Rate:*** Administer by rapid bolus. Flush IV line before and after administration to prevent incompatible medications used in arrest management from precipitating.
- **Continuous Infusion:** ***Diluent:*** May be diluted in dextrose, saline, and dextrose/saline combinations. Premixed infusions are already diluted and ready to use. ***Rate:*** May be administered over 4–8 hr.
- **Y-Site Compatibility:** acyclovir, amifostine, amikacin, aminophylline, asparaginase, atropine, aztreonam, bivalirudin, bumetanide, cefazolin, cefepime, ceftazidime, ceftriaxone, chloramphenicol, cimetidine, cladribine, clindamycin, cyclophosphamide, cyclosporine, cytarabine, daptomycin, daunorubicin, dexamethasone sodium phosphatedexmedetomidine, digoxin, docetaxel, doxorubicin, enalaprilat, ertapenem, erythromycin, esmolol, etoposide, etoposide phosphate, famotidine, fentanyl, filgrastim, fluconazole, fludarabine, furosemide, gemcitabine, gentamicin, granisetron, heparin, hydrocortisone sodium succinate, ifosfamide, indomethacin, insulin, ketorolac, labetalol, levofloxacin, lidocaine, linezolid, lorazepam, magnesium sulfate, melphalan, mesna, methylprednisolone sodium succinate, metoclopramide, metoprolol, metronidazole, milrinone, morphine, nafcillin, nitroglycerin, nitroprusside, paclitaxel, palonosetron, pantoprazole,

pemetrexed, penicillin G potassium, phenylephrine, phytonadione, piperacillin/tazobactam, potassium chloride, procainamide, propranolol, propofol, protamine, ranitidine, remifentanil, tacrolimus, teniposide, thiotepa, tirofiban, tobramycin, tolazoline, vasopressin, vitamin B complex with C, voriconazole.

- **Y-Site Incompatibility:** allopurinol, amiodarone, amphotericin B, amphotericin B cholesteryl sulfate complex, ampicillin, anidulafungin, calcium chloride, calcium gluconate, caspofungin, cefotaxime, cefoxitin, cefuroxime, diazepam, diphenhydramine, dobutamine, doxorubicin liposome, doxycycline, epinephrine, fenoldopam, ganciclovir, haloperidol, hydroxyzine, idarubicin, imipenem/cilastatin, isoproterenol, lansoprazole, leucovorin, meperidine, midazolam, nalbuphine, norepinephrine, ondansetron, phenytoin, prochlorperazine, promethazine, quinupristin/dalfopristin, sargramostim, trimethoprim/sulfamethoxazole, verapamil, vincristine, vinorelbine.
- **Solution Incompatibility:** Do not add to Ringer's solution, LR, or Ionosol products, as compatibility varies with concentration.

Patient/Family Teaching

- Instruct patient to take medication as directed. Take missed doses as soon as remembered unless almost time for next dose.
- Review symptoms of electrolyte imbalance with patients on chronic therapy; instruct patient to notify health care professional if these symptoms occur.
- Advise patient not to take milk products concurrently with this medication. Renal calculi or hypercalcemia (milk-alkali syndrome) may result.
- Emphasize the importance of regular follow-up examinations to monitor serum electrolyte levels and acid-base balance and to monitor progress.
- **Antacid:** Advise patient to avoid routine use of sodium bicarbonate for indigestion. Dyspepsia that persists >2 wk should be evaluated by a health care professional.
- Advise patient on sodium-restricted diet to avoid use of baking soda as a home remedy for indigestion.
- Instruct patient to notify health care professional if indigestion is accompanied by chest pain, difficulty breathing, or diaphoresis or if stools become dark and tarry.

Evaluation/Desired Outcomes

- Increase in urinary pH.
- Clinical improvement of acidosis.
- Enhanced excretion of selected overdoses and poisonings.
- Decreased gastric discomfort.

sodium citrate and citric acid

(**soe**-dee-um **sye**-trate and **sit**-rik **as**-id)

Bicitra, Oracit, ✱PMS-Dicitrate, Shohl's Solution modified

Classification

Therapeutic: antiurolithics, mineral and electrolyte replacements/supplements

Pharmacologic: alkalinizing agents

Pregnancy Category C

Indications

Management of chronic metabolic acidosis associated with chronic renal insufficiency or renal tubular acidosis. Alkalinization of urine. Prevention of cystine and urate urinary calculi. Prevention of aspiration pneumonitis during surgical procedures. Used as a neutralizing buffer.

Action

Converted to bicarbonate in the body, resulting in increased blood pH. As bicarbonate is renally excreted, urine is also alkalinized, increasing the solubility of cystine and uric acid. Neutralizes gastric acid. **Therapeutic Effects:** Provision of bicarbonate in metabolic acidosis. Alkalinization of the urine. Prevention of cystine and urate urinary calculi. Prevention of aspiration pneumonitis.

Pharmacokinetics

Absorption: Well absorbed following oral administration.

Distribution: Rapidly and widely distributed.

Metabolism and Excretion: Rapidly oxidized to bicarbonate, which is excreted primarily by the kidneys. Small amounts (<5%) excreted unchanged by the lungs.

Half-life: Unknown.

TIME/ACTION PROFILE (effects on serum pH)

ROUTE	ONSET	PEAK	DURATION
PO	rapid (min–hr)	unknown	4–6 hr

Contraindications/Precautions

Contraindicated in: Severe renal insufficiency; Severe sodium restriction; HF, untreated hypertension, edema, or toxemia of pregnancy.

Use Cautiously in: OB, Lactation: Safety not established.

Adverse Reactions/Side Effects

GI: diarrhea. **F and E:** fluid overload, hypernatremia (severe renal impairment), hypocalcemia, metabolic alkalosis (large doses only). **MS:** tetany.

Interactions

Drug-Drug: May partially antagonize the effects of **antihypertensives**. Urinary alkalinization may result in ↓ **salicylate** or **barbiturate** levels or ↑ levels of **quinidine**, **flecainide**, or **amphetamines**.

Route/Dosage

Adjust dosage according to urine pH. Contains 1 mEq sodium and 1 mEq bicarbonate/mL solution.

Alkalinizer

PO (Adults): 10–30 mL solution diluted in water 4 times daily.

PO (Children): 5–15 mL solution diluted in water 4 times daily.

Antiurolithic

PO (Adults): 10–30 mL solution diluted in water 4 times daily.

Neutralizing Buffer

PO (Adults): 15–30 mL solution diluted in 15–30 mL of water.

Availability

Oral solution: 500 mg sodium citrate/334 mg citric acid/5 mL (Bicitra, PMS-Dicitrate), 490 mg sodium citrate/640 mg citric acid/5 mL (Oracit).

NURSING IMPLICATIONS

Assessment

- Assess patient for signs of alkalosis (confusion, irritability, paresthesia, tetany, altered breathing pattern) or hypernatremia (edema, weight gain, hypertension, tachycardia, fever, flushed skin, mental irritability) throughout therapy.
- Monitor patients with renal dysfunction for fluid overload (discrepancy in intake and output, weight gain, edema, rales/crackles, and hypertension).
- ***Lab Test Considerations:*** Prior to and every 4 mo throughout chronic therapy, monitor hematocrit, hemoglobin, electrolytes, pH, creatinine, urinalysis, and 24-hr urine for citrate.
- Monitor urine pH if used to alkalinize urine.

Potential Nursing Diagnoses

Deficient knowledge, related to medication regimen (Patient/Family Teaching)

Implementation

- **PO:** Solution is more palatable if chilled. Administer with 30–90 mL of chilled water. Administer 30 min after meals or as bedtime snack to minimize saline laxative effect.
- When used as preanesthetic, administer 15–30 mL of sodium citrate with 15–30 mL of chilled water.

Patient/Family Teaching

- Instruct patient to take as directed. Missed doses should be taken within 2 hr. Do not double doses.
- Instruct patients receiving chronic sodium citrate on correct method of monitoring urine pH, maintenance of alkaline urine, and the need to increase fluid intake to 3000 mL/day. When treatment is discontinued, pH begins to fall toward pretreatment levels.
- Advise patients receiving long-term therapy on need to avoid salty foods.

Evaluation/Desired Outcomes

- Correction of metabolic acidosis.
- Maintenance of alkaline urine with resulting decreased stone formation.
- Buffering the pH of gastric secretions, thereby preventing aspiration pneumonitis associated with intubation and anesthesia.

---

sodium ferric gluconate complex, **See IRON SUPPLEMENTS.**

---

sodium polystyrene sulfonate

(**soe**-dee-um po-lee-**stye**-reen **sul**-fon-ate)

Kalexate, Kayexalate, ✱K-Exit, Kionex, SPS

Classification

Therapeutic: hypokalemic, electrolyte modifiers

Pharmacologic: cationic exchange resins

Pregnancy Category C

Indications

Mild to moderate hyperkalemia (if severe, more immediate measures such as sodium bicarbonate IV, calcium, or glucose/insulin infusion should be instituted).

Action

Exchanges sodium ions for potassium ions in the intestine (each 1 g is exchanged for 1 mEq potassium).

Therapeutic Effects: Reduction of serum potassium levels.

Pharmacokinetics

Absorption: Distributed throughout the intestine but is nonabsorbable.

Distribution: Not distributed.

Metabolism and Excretion: Eliminated in the feces.

Half-life: Unknown.

TIME/ACTION PROFILE (decrease in serum potassium)

ROUTE	ONSET	PEAK	DURATION
PO	2–12 hr	unknown	6–24 hr
Rectal	2–12 hr	unknown	4–6 hr

Contraindications/Precautions

Contraindicated in: Life-threatening hyperkalemia (other, more immediate measures should be instituted); Hypersensitivity to saccharin or parabens (some products); Ileus; Abnormal bowel function (↑ risk for intestinal necrosis); Postoperative patients with no bowel movement (↑ risk for intestinal necrosis); History of impaction, chronic constipation, inflammatory bowel disease, ischemic colitis, vascular intestinal atherosclerosis, previous bowel resection, or bowel obstruction (↑ risk for intestinal necrosis); Known alcohol intolerance (suspension only).

Use Cautiously in: Geri: Geriatric patients; Heart failure; Hypertension; Edema; Sodium restriction; Constipation.

Adverse Reactions/Side Effects

GI: INTESTINAL NECROSIS, <u>constipation</u>, <u>fecal impaction</u>, anorexia, gastric irritation, ischemic colitis, nausea, vomiting. **F and E:** hypocalcemia, hypokalemia, sodium retention, hypomagnesemia.

Interactions

Drug-Drug: Administration with **calcium** or **magnesium-containing antacids** may ↓ resin-exchanging ability and ↑ risk of systemic alkalosis. Hypokalemia may enhance **digoxin** toxicity. Use with **sorbitol** may ↑ risk of colonic necrosis (concomitant use not recommended).

Route/Dosage

4 level tsp = 15 g (4.1 mEq sodium/g).

PO (Adults): 15 g 1–4 times daily in water (up to 40 g 4 times daily).

Rect (Adults): 30–50 g as a retention enema; repeat as needed q 6 hr.

PO, Rect (Children): 1 g/kg/dose q 6 hr.

Availability (generic available)

Suspension: 15 g sodium polystyrene sulfonate with 20 g sorbitol/60 mL, 15 g sodium polystyrene sulfonate with 14.1 g sorbitol/60 mL. **Powder:** 15 g/4 level tsp.

NURSING IMPLICATIONS

Assessment

- Monitor response of symptoms of hyperkalemia (fatigue, muscle weakness, paresthesia, confusion, dyspnea, peaked T waves, depressed ST segments, prolonged QT segments, widened QRS complexes, loss of P waves, and cardiac arrhythmias). Assess for development of hypokalemia (weakness, fatigue, arrhythmias, flat or inverted T waves, prominent U waves).
- Monitor intake and output ratios and daily weight. Assess for symptoms of fluid overload (dyspnea, rales/crackles, jugular venous distention, peripheral edema). Concurrent low-sodium diet may be ordered for patients with HF (see Appendix J).
- In patients receiving concurrent digoxin, assess for symptoms of digoxin toxicity (anorexia, nausea, vomiting, visual disturbances, arrhythmias).
- Assess abdomen and note character and frequency of stools. Discontinue sodium polystyrene sulfonate if patient becomes constipated. Concurrent sorbitol or laxatives may be ordered to prevent constipation or impaction. Some products contain sorbitol to prevent constipation. Patient should ideally have 1–2 watery stools each day during therapy. Monitor for intestinal necrosis if sorbitol is added.
- ***Lab Test Considerations:*** Monitor serum potassium daily during therapy. Notify health care professional when potassium ↓ to 4–5 mEq/L.
- Monitor renal function and electrolytes (especially sodium, calcium, bicarbonate, and magnesium) prior to and periodically throughout therapy.

Potential Nursing Diagnoses

Constipation (Side Effects)

Implementation

- Solution is stable for 24 hr when refrigerated.
- Consult health care professional regarding discontinuation of medications that may increase serum potassium (angiotensin-converting enzyme inhibitors, potassium-sparing diuretics, potassium supplements, salt substitutes).
- An osmotic laxative (sorbitol) is usually administered concurrently to prevent constipation.
- **PO:** For oral administration, shake commercially available suspension well before use. When using powder, add prescribed amount to 3–4 mL water/g of powder. Shake well. Syrup may be ordered to improve palatability. Resin cookie or candy recipes are available; discuss with pharmacist or dietitian.
- **Retention Enema:** Precede retention enema with cleansing enema. Administer solution via rectal tube or 28-French Foley catheter with 30-mL balloon. Insert tube at least 20 cm and tape in place.
- For retention enema, add powder to 100 mL of prescribed solution (usually sorbitol or 20% dextrose in water). Shake well to dissolve powder thoroughly; should be of liquid consistency. Position patient on left side and elevate hips on pillow if solution begins to leak. Follow administration of medication with additional 50–100 mL of diluent to ensure administration of complete dose. Encourage patient to retain enema as long as possible, at least 30–60 min.

S

- After retention period, irrigate colon with 1–2 L of non–sodium-containing solution. Y-connector with tubing may be attached to Foley or rectal tube; cleansing solution is administered through 1 port of the Y and allowed to drain by gravity through the other port.

Patient/Family Teaching

- Explain purpose and method of administration of medication to patient.
- Advise patient to avoid taking antacids or laxatives during therapy, unless approved by health care professional; may cause systemic alkalosis.
- Advise female patient to notify health care professional if pregnant or breast feeding.
- Inform patient of need for frequent lab tests to monitor effectiveness.

Evaluation/Desired Outcomes

- Normalization of serum potassium levels.

solifenacin (so-li-fen-a-sin)

VESIcare

Classification

Therapeutic: urinary tract antispasmodics
Pharmacologic: anticholinergics

Pregnancy Category C

Indications

Overactive bladder with symptoms (urge incontinence, urgency, frequency).

Action

Acts as a muscarinic (cholinergic) receptor antagonist; antagonizes bladder smooth muscle contraction.
Therapeutic Effects: Decreased symptoms of overactive bladder.

Pharmacokinetics

Absorption: Well absorbed (90%).
Distribution: Unknown.
Protein Binding: 98%.
Metabolism and Excretion: Extensively metabolized by the CYP3A4 enzyme system. 69% excreted in urine as metabolites, 22% in feces.
Half-life: 45–68 hr.

TIME/ACTION PROFILE

ROUTE	ONSET	PEAK	DURATION
Oral	unknown	3–8 hr	24 hr

Contraindications/Precautions

Contraindicated in: Hypersensitivity; Urinary retention; Gastric retention; Uncontrolled angle-closure glaucoma; Severe hepatic impairment; Lactation: Lactation.
Use Cautiously in: Concurrent use of CYP3A4 inhibitors (use lower dose/clinical monitoring may be necessary); Moderate hepatic impairment (lower dose recommended); Renal impairment (dose should not exceed 5 mg/day if CCr <30 mL/min); Bladder outflow obstruction; GI obstructive disorders, severe constipation, or ulcerative colitis; Myasthenia gravis; Angle-closure glaucoma; OB: Use only if maternal benefit outweighs fetal risk; Pedi: Safety not established.

Adverse Reactions/Side Effects

CNS: confusion, drowsiness, hallucinations, headache. **CV:** palpitations, tachycardia. **EENT:** blurred vision. **GI:** constipation, dry mouth, dyspepsia, nausea. **MS:** muscle weakness. **Misc:** ANGIOEDEMA.

Interactions

Drug-Drug: Drugs that induce or inhibit the CYP3A4 enzyme system may significantly alter levels; **ketoconazole** ↑ levels and risk of toxicity (do not exceed 5 mg/day).

Route/Dosage

PO (Adults): 5 mg once daily, may be ↑ to 10 mg once daily; *Concurrent use of ketoconazole or other potent CYP3A4 inhibitors*—Dose should not exceed 5 mg/day.

Renal Impairment

(Adults): *CCr <30 mL/min*—Dose should not exceed 5 mg/day.

Hepatic Impairment

(Adults): *Moderate hepatic impairment*—Dose should not exceed 5 mg/day.

Availability (generic available)

Tablets: 5 mg, 10 mg. **Cost:** All strengths $703.66/90.

NURSING IMPLICATIONS

Assessment

- Monitor voiding pattern and assess symptoms of overactive bladder (urinary urgency, urinary incontinence, urinary frequency) to and periodically during therapy.

Potential Nursing Diagnoses

Impaired urinary elimination (Indications)

Implementation

- Do not confuse Vesicare (solifenacin) with Vesanoid (oral tretinoin).
- **PO:** Administer once daily without regard to food. Tablets must be swallowed whole; do not break, crush, or chew.

Patient/Family Teaching

- Instruct patient to take solifenacin as directed. Advise patient to read the *Patient Information* before starting therapy and with each prescription refill. If a dose is missed, skip dose and take next day; do not take 2 doses in same day.
- Do not share solifenacin with others; may be dangerous.

- May cause dizziness and blurred vision. Caution patient to avoid driving and other activities that require alertness until response to medication is known.
- Advise patient to notify health care professional immediately if hives; rash; swelling or lips, face, tongue, or throat; trouble breathing occurs.
- Inform patient of potential anticholinergic side effects (constipation, urinary retention, blurred vision, heat prostration in a hot environment).
- Instruct patient to notify health care professional of all Rx or OTC medications, vitamins, or herbal products being taken and consult health care professional before taking any new medications.

Evaluation/Desired Outcomes

- Decrease in symptoms of overactive bladder (urge urinary incontinence, urgency, frequency).

somatropin (recombinant), See GROWTH HORMONES.

sotalol (soe-ta-lole)

Betapace, Betapace AF, ♣Rylosol, Sorine, Sotylize

Classification

Therapeutic: antiarrhythmics (class III)

Pregnancy Category B

Indications

Management of life-threatening ventricular arrhythmias. **Betapace AF and Sotylize:** Maintenance of normal sinus rhythm in patients with highly symptomatic atrial fibrillation/atrial flutter (AF/AFL) who are currently in sinus rhythm.

Action

Blocks stimulation of $beta_1$ (myocardial) and $beta_2$ (pulmonary, vascular, and uterine) -adrenergic receptor sites. **Therapeutic Effects:** Suppression of arrhythmias.

Pharmacokinetics

Absorption: Well absorbed following oral administration (bioavailability 90–100%).

Distribution: Crosses the placenta; enters breast milk.

Metabolism and Excretion: Elimination is mostly renal.

Half-life: 12 hr (↑ in renal impairment).

TIME/ACTION PROFILE (antiarrhythmic effects)

ROUTE	ONSET	PEAK	DURATION
PO	hr	2–3 days	8–12 hr

Contraindications/Precautions

Contraindicated in: Hypersensitivity; Uncompensated HF; Pulmonary edema; Asthma; Cardiogenic shock; Congenital or acquired long QT syndromes; Sinus bradycardia, 2nd- and 3rd-degree AV block (unless a functioning pacemaker is present); CCr <40 mL/min in patients who are being treated with Betapace AF or Sotylize.

Use Cautiously in: Renal impairment (↑ dosing interval recommended if CCr ≤60 mL/min for patients with ventricular arrhythmias); Hepatic impairment; Hypokalemia (↑ risk of arrhythmias); Geri: ↑ sensitivity to beta blockers; Diabetes mellitus (may mask signs of hypoglycemia); Thyrotoxicosis (may mask symptoms); Patients with a history of severe allergic reactions (intensity of reactions may be increased); OB, Lactation, Pedi: Safety not established; may cause fetal/neonatal bradycardia, hypotension, hypoglycemia, or respiratory depression.

Adverse Reactions/Side Effects

CNS: fatigue, weakness, anxiety, dizziness, drowsiness, insomnia, memory loss, mental depression, mental status changes, nervousness, nightmares. **EENT:** blurred vision, dry eyes, nasal stuffiness. **Resp:** bronchospasm, wheezing. **CV:** ARRHYTHMIAS, BRADYCARDIA, HF, PULMONARY EDEMA, orthostatic hypotension, peripheral vasoconstriction. **GI:** constipation, diarrhea, nausea. **GU:** erectile dysfunction, ↓ libido. **Derm:** itching, rash. **Endo:** hyperglycemia, hypoglycemia. **MS:** arthralgia, back pain, muscle cramps. **Neuro:** paresthesia. **Misc:** drug-induced lupus syndrome.

Interactions

Drug-Drug: Concurrent use with other **class 1A antiarrhythmics** is not recommended due to ↑ risk of arrhythmias. **General anesthesia**, **IV phenytoin**, and **verapamil** may cause additive myocardial depression. Additive bradycardia may occur with **digoxin**, **beta-blockers**, **verapamil**, and **diltiazem**. Additive hypotension may occur with other **antihypertensives**, acute ingestion of **alcohol**, or **nitrates**. Concurrent use with **amphetamines**, **cocaine**, **ephedrine**, **epinephrine**, **norepinephrine**, **phenylephrine**, or **pseudoephedrine** may result in unopposed alpha-adrenergic stimulation (excessive hypertension, bradycardia). Concurrent **thyroid hormone** administration may ↓ effectiveness. May alter the effectiveness of **insulin** or **oral hypoglycemic agents** (dose adjustments may be necessary). May ↓ the effectiveness of **beta-adrenergic bronchodilators** and **theophylline**. May

↓ the beneficial $beta_1$ cardiovascular effects of **dopamine** or **dobutamine**. Discontinuation of **clonidine** in patients receiving sotalol may result in excessive rebound hypertension. Use cautiously within 14 days of **MAO inhibitors** (may result in hypertension).

Route/Dosage

Ventricular Arrhythmias

PO (Adults): 80 mg twice daily; may be gradually ↑ (usual maintenance dose is 160–320 mg/day in 2–3 divided doses; some patients may require up to 480–640 mg/day).

Renal Impairment

PO (Adults): *CCr 30–59 mL/min*—initial dose of 80 mg, with subsequent doses given q 24 hr; *CCr 10–29 mL/min*—initial dose of 80 mg, with subsequent doses given q 36–48 hr.

Atrial Fibrillation/Atrial Flutter

PO (Adults): 80 mg twice daily, may be ↑ during careful monitoring to 120 mg twice daily if necessary.

Renal Impairment

PO (Adults): *CCr 40–60 mL/min*—Administer q 24 hr.

Availability (generic available)

Tablets : 80 mg, 120 mg, 160 mg, 240 mg. **Tablets (Betapace AF):** 80 mg, 120 mg, 160 mg. **Oral solution (Sotylize) (grape flavor):** 5 mg/mL.

NURSING IMPLICATIONS

Assessment

- Monitor ECG prior to and periodically during therapy. May cause life-threatening ventricular tachycardia associated with QT interval prolongation. Do not initiate sotalol therapy if baseline QTc is longer than 450 ms. If QT interval becomes ≥500 ms, reduce dose, prolong duration of infusion, or discontinue therapy.
- Monitor BP and pulse frequently during dose adjustment period and periodically during therapy. Assess for orthostatic hypotension when assisting patient up from supine position.
- Monitor intake and output ratios and daily weight. Assess patient routinely for evidence of fluid overload (peripheral edema, dyspnea, rales/crackles, fatigue, weight gain, jugular venous distention).
- ***Lab Test Considerations:*** Calculate creatinine clearance prior to dosing.
- May cause ↑ BUN, serum lipoprotein, potassium, triglyceride, and uric acid levels.
- May cause increased ANA titers.
- May cause increase in blood glucose levels.
- ***Toxicity and Overdose:*** Monitor patients receiving beta blockers for signs of overdose (bradycardia, severe dizziness or fainting, severe drowsiness, dyspnea, bluish fingernails or palms, seizures). Notify health care professional immediately if these signs occur.
- Glucagon has been used to treat bradycardia and hypotension.

Potential Nursing Diagnoses

Decreased cardiac output (Side Effects)
Noncompliance (Patient/Family Teaching)

Implementation

- Do not confuse sotalol with Sudafed (pseudoephedrine).
- Patients should be hospitalized and monitored for arrhythmias for at least 3 days during initiation of therapy and dose increases.
- Do not substitute Betapace for Betapace AF. Make sure patients transferred from Betapace to Betapace AF have enough Betapace AF upon leaving the hospital to allow for uninterrupted therapy until Betapace AF prescription can be filled.
- **PO:** Take apical pulse prior to administering. If <50 bpm or if arrhythmia occurs, withhold medication and notify health care professional.
- Administer on an empty stomach, 1 hr before or 2 hr after meals. Administration with food, especially milk or milk products, reduces absorption by approximately 20%.
- Avoid administering antacids containing aluminum or magnesium within 2 hr before administration of sotalol.
- For patients unable to swallow pills, pharmacist can convert tablets to a solution.

Patient/Family Teaching

- Instruct patient to take medication as directed, at the same time each day, even if feeling well; do not skip or double up on missed doses. Take missed doses as soon as possible up to 8 hr before next dose. Abrupt withdrawal may precipitate life-threatening arrhythmias, hypertension, or myocardial ischemia. Advise patients taking *Betapace AF* to read *Medication Guide* before starting and with each Rx refill in case of changes.
- Advise patient to make sure enough medication is available for weekends, holidays, and vacations. A written prescription may be kept in wallet in case of emergency.
- Teach patient and family how to check pulse and BP. Instruct them to check pulse daily and BP biweekly. Advise patient to hold dose and contact physician or other health care professional if pulse is <50 bpm or if BP changes significantly.
- May cause drowsiness or dizziness. Caution patients to avoid driving or other activities that require alertness until response to the drug is known.
- Advise patients to change positions slowly to minimize orthostatic hypotension, especially during initiation of therapy or when dose is increased.
- Caution patient that this medication may increase sensitivity to cold.

- Advise patient to notify health care professional of all Rx or OTC medications, vitamins, or herbal products being taken and to consult with health care professional before taking other medications, especially cold preparations.
- Diabetic patients should closely monitor blood glucose, especially if weakness, malaise, irritability, or fatigue occurs. Medication may mask tachycardia and increased BP as signs of hypoglycemia, but dizziness and sweating may still occur.
- Advise patient to notify health care professional immediately if new fast heartbeats with lightheadedness and fainting occurs, or if slow pulse, difficulty breathing, wheezing, cold hands and feet, dizziness, confusion, depression, rash, fever, sore throat, unusual bleeding, bruising, or if pain or swelling at the infusion site occurs.
- Instruct patient to inform health care professional of medication regimen prior to treatment or surgery.
- Advise patient to carry identification describing disease process and medication regimen at all times.

Evaluation/Desired Outcomes

- Control of arrhythmias without appearance of detrimental side effects.

spironolactone, See DIURETICS (POTASSIUM-SPARING).

streptokinase, See THROMBOLYTIC AGENTS.

streptomycin, See AMINOGLYCOSIDES.

strong iodine solution, See IODINE, IODIDE.

sucralfate (soo-**kral**-fate)

Carafate, ✤Sulcrate

Classification
Therapeutic: antiulcer agents
Pharmacologic: GI protectants

Pregnancy Category B

Indications

Short-term management of duodenal ulcers. Maintenance (preventive) therapy of duodenal ulcers. **Unlabeled Use:** Management of gastric ulcer or gastroesophageal reflux. Prevention of gastric mucosal injury caused by high-dose aspirin or other NSAIDs in patients with rheumatoid arthritis or in high-stress situations (e.g., intensive care unit). **Suspension:** Mucositis/stomatitis/rectal or oral ulcerations from various etiologies.

Action

Aluminum salt of sulfated sucrose reacts with gastric acid to form a thick paste, which selectively adheres to the ulcer surface. **Therapeutic Effects:** Protection of ulcers, with subsequent healing.

Pharmacokinetics

Absorption: Systemic absorption is minimal (<5%).
Distribution: Unknown.
Metabolism and Excretion: >90% is eliminated in the feces.
Half-life: 6–20 hr.

TIME/ACTION PROFILE (mucosal protectant effect)

ROUTE	ONSET	PEAK	DURATION
PO	1–2 hr	unknown	6 hr

Contraindications/Precautions

Contraindicated in: Hypersensitivity.
Use Cautiously in: Renal failure (accumulation of aluminum can occur); Diabetes (↑ risk of hyperglycemia with suspension); Impaired swallowing (↑ risk of tablet aspiration).

Adverse Reactions/Side Effects

CNS: dizziness, drowsiness. **GI:** constipation, diarrhea, dry mouth, gastric discomfort, indigestion, nausea. **Derm:** pruritus, rashes. **Endo:** hyperglycemia (with suspension). **Misc:** ANAPHYLAXIS.

Interactions

Drug-Drug: May ↓ absorption of **phenytoin**, **fat-soluble vitamins**, or **tetracycline**. ↓ effectiveness when used with **antacids**, **cimetidine**, or **ranitidine**. ↓ absorption of **fluoroquinolones** (separate administration by 2 hr).

Route/Dosage

Treatment of Ulcers

PO (Adults): 1 g 4 times daily, given 1 hr before meals and at bedtime; or 2 g twice daily, on waking and at bedtime.

Prevention of Ulcers

PO (Adults): 1 g twice daily, given 1 hr before a meal.

Gastroesophageal Reflux

PO (Adults): 1 g 4 times daily, given 1 hr before meals and at bedtime (unlabeled).

S

PO (Children): 40–80 mg/kg/day divided q 6 hr, given 1 hr before meals and at bedtime (unlabeled).

Stomatitis

PO (Adults and Children): 5–10 mL of suspension swish and spit or swish and swallow 4 times daily.

Proctitis

Rect (Adults): 2 g of suspension given as an enema once or twice daily.

Availability (generic available)

Tablets: 1 g. **Cost:** *Generic*—$23.86/100. **Oral suspension:** 1 g/10 mL. **Cost:** $122.42/420 mL.

NURSING IMPLICATIONS

Assessment

- Assess patient routinely for abdominal pain and frank or occult blood in the stool.

Potential Nursing Diagnoses

Acute pain (Indications)
Constipation (Side Effects)
Deficient knowledge, related to medication regimen (Patient/Family Teaching)

Implementation

- **PO:** Administer on an empty stomach, 1 hr before meals and at bedtime. Tablet may be broken or dissolved in water before ingestion. Shake suspension well before administration.
- If nasogastric or feeding tube administration is required, consult pharmacist; protein-binding properties of sucralfate have resulted in formation of a bezoar when administered with enteral feedings and other medications.
- If antacids are also required for pain, administer 30 min before or after sucralfate dosage.

Patient/Family Teaching

- Advise patient to continue with course of therapy for 4–8 wk, even if feeling better, to ensure ulcer healing. If a dose is missed, take as soon as remembered unless almost time for next dose; do not double doses.
- Advise patient that increase in fluid intake, dietary bulk, and exercise may prevent drug-induced constipation.
- Emphasize the importance of routine examinations to monitor progress.

Evaluation/Desired Outcomes

- Decrease in abdominal pain.
- Prevention and healing of duodenal ulcers, seen by x-ray examination and endoscopy.

sulconazole, See ANTIFUNGALS (TOPICAL).

sulfaSALAzine

(sul-fa-**sal**-a-zeen)
Azulfidine, Azulfidine EN-tabs, ✱Salazopyrin

Classification
Therapeutic: antirheumatics (DMARD), gastrointestinal anti-inflammatories

Pregnancy Category B

Indications

Mild-to-moderate ulcerative colitis or as adjunctive therapy in severe ulcerative colitis. Rheumatoid arthritis unresponsive or intolerant tosalicylates and/or NSAIDs.

Action

Locally acting anti-inflammatory action in the colon, where activity is probably a result of inhibition of prostaglandin synthesis. **Therapeutic Effects:** Reduction in the symptoms of ulcerative colitis or rheumatoid arthritis.

Pharmacokinetics

Absorption: 10–15% absorbed after oral administration.
Distribution: Widely distributed; crosses the placenta and enters breast milk.
Protein Binding: 99%.
Metabolism and Excretion: Split by intestinal bacteria into sulfapyridine and 5-aminosalicylic acid. Some absorbed sulfasalazine is excreted by bile back into intestines; 15% excreted unchanged by the kidneys. Sulfapyridine also excreted mostly by the kidneys.
Half-life: 6 hr.

TIME/ACTION PROFILE (blood levels)

ROUTE	ONSET	PEAK	DURATION
PO	1 hr	1.5–6 hr	6–12 hr

Contraindications/Precautions

Contraindicated in: Hypersensitivity reactions to sulfonamides, salicylates, or sulfasalazine; Cross-sensitivity with furosemide, sulfonylurea hypoglycemic agents, or carbonic anhydrase inhibitors may exist; Glucose-6–phosphate dehydrogenase (G6PD) deficiency; Hypersensitivity to bisulfites (mesalamine enema only); Urinary tract or intestinal obstruction; Porphyria; Pedi: Children <2 yr (safety not established).
Use Cautiously in: Severe hepatic or renal impairment; History of porphyria; Blood dyscrasias; OB: Neural tube defects have been reported; Lactation: Safety not established; may compete with bilirubin for binding sites on plasma proteins in the newborn and cause kernicterus; bloody stools or diarrhea reported in breast-fed infants.

Adverse Reactions/Side Effects

CNS: headache. **Resp:** pneumonitis. **GI:** anorexia, diarrhea, nausea, vomiting, drug-induced hepatitis.

GU: crystalluria, infertility, oligospermia, orange-yellow discoloration of urine. **Derm:** EXFOLIATIVE DERMATITIS, STEVENS-JOHNSON SYNDROME, TOXIC EPIDERMAL NECROLYSIS, rash, photosensitivity, yellow discoloration. **Hemat:** AGRANULOCYTOSIS, APLASTIC ANEMIA, blood dyscrasias, eosinophilia, hemolytic anemia, megaloblastic anemia, thrombocytopenia. **Neuro:** peripheral neuropathy. **Misc:** ANGIOEDEMA; *hypersensitivity reactions including*, ANAPHYLAXIS, fever.

Interactions

Drug-Drug: May ↑ action/risk of toxicity from **oral hypoglycemic agents**, **phenytoin**, **methotrexate**, **zidovudine**, or **warfarin**. ↑ risk of drug-induced hepatitis with other **hepatotoxic agents**. ↑ risk of crystalluria with **methenamine**. May ↓ metabolism and increase effects/toxicity of **mercaptopurine** or **thioguanine**.

Drug-Food: May ↓ **iron** and **folic acid** absorption.

Route/Dosage

Ulcerative Colitis

PO (Adults): 1 g q 6–8 hr (may start with 500 mg q 6–12 hr), followed by maintenance dose of 500 mg q 6 hr.

PO (Children >2 yr): *Initial*—6.7–10 mg/kg q 4 hr *or* 10–15 mg/kg q 6 hr *or* 13.3–20 mg/kg q 8 hr. *Maintenance*—7.5 mg/kg q 6 hr (not to exceed 2 g/day).

Rheumatoid arthritis

PO (Adults): 500 mg–1 g/day (as delayed-release tablets) for 1 wk, then ↑ by 500 mg/day q wk up to 2 g/day in 2 divided doses; if no benefit seen after 12 wk, ↑ to 3 g/day in 2 divided doses.

PO (Children ≥6 yr): 30–50 mg/kg/day in 2 divided doses (as delayed-release tablets); initiate therapy at ¼–⅓ of planned maintenance dose and ↑ q 7 days until maintenance dose is reached (not to exceed 2 g/day).

Availability (generic available)

Tablets: 500 mg. **Delayed-release (enteric-coated) tablets (Azulfidine EN-tabs):** 500 mg.

NURSING IMPLICATIONS

Assessment

- Assess patient for allergy to sulfonamides and salicylates. Therapy should be discontinued if rash, difficulty breathing, swelling of face or lips, or fever occur.
- Monitor intake and output ratios. Fluid intake should be sufficient to maintain a urine output of at least 1200–1500 mL daily to prevent crystalluria and stone formation.
- Assess for rash periodically during therapy. May cause Stevens-Johnson syndrome. Discontinue therapy if severe or if accompanied with fever, general malaise, fatigue, muscle or joint aches, blisters, oral lesions, conjunctivitis, hepatitis, and/or eosinophilia.
- **Ulcerative Colitis:** Assess abdominal pain and frequency, quantity, and consistency of stools at the beginning of and during therapy.
- **Rheumatoid Arthritis:** Assess range of motion and degree of swelling and pain in affected joints before and periodically during therapy.
- ***Lab Test Considerations:*** Monitor urinalysis, BUN, and serum creatinine before and periodically during therapy. May cause crystalluria and urinary cell calculi formation.
- ***Lab Test Considerations:*** Monitor CBC with differential and liver function tests before and every second wk during first 3 mo of therapy, monthly during the second 3 mo, and every 3 mo thereafter of as clinically indicated Discontinue sulfasalazine if blood dyscrasias occur.
- ***Lab Test Considerations:*** Serum sulfapyridine levels may be monitored; concentrations >50 μg/mL may be associated with increased incidence of adverse reactions.

Potential Nursing Diagnoses

Acute pain (Indications)
Diarrhea (Indications)

Implementation

- Do not confuse sulfasalazine with sulfadiazine.
- Varying dosing regimens of sulfasalazine may be used to minimize GI side effects.
- **PO:** Administer after meals or with food to minimize GI irritation, with a full glass of water. Do not crush or chew enteric-coated tablets.

Patient/Family Teaching

- Instruct patient on the correct method of administration. Advise patient to take medication as directed, even if feeling better. Take missed doses as soon as remembered unless almost time for next dose.
- May cause dizziness. Caution patient to avoid driving or other activities that require alertness until response to medication is known.
- Advise patient to notify health care professional if skin rash, sore throat, fever, mouth sores, unusual bleeding or bruising, wheezing, fever, or hives occur.
- Caution patient to use sunscreen and protective clothing to prevent photosensitivity reactions.
- Inform patient that this medication may cause orange-yellow discoloration of urine and skin, which is not significant. May permanently stain contact lenses yellow.
- Instruct patient to notify health care professional if symptoms worsen or do not improve. If symptoms of acute intolerance (cramping, acute abdominal pain,

S

bloody diarrhea, fever, headache, rash) occur, discontinue therapy and notify health care professional immediately.
- Inform male patient that sulfasalazine may cause infertility.
- Instruct patient to notify health care professional if symptoms do not improve after 1–2 mo of therapy.

Evaluation/Desired Outcomes
- Decrease in diarrhea and abdominal pain.
- Return to normal bowel pattern in patients with ulcerative colitis. Effects may be seen within 3–21 days. The usual course of therapy is 3–6 wk.
- Maintenance of remission in patients with ulcerative colitis.
- Decrease in pain and inflammation and increase in mobility in patients with rheumatoid arthritis.

HIGH ALERT

SULFONYLUREAS

glimepiride (glye-**me**-pye-ride)
Amaryl

glipiZIDE (**glip**-i-zide)
Glucotrol, Glucotrol XL

glyBURIDE (**glye**-byoo-ride)
DiaBeta, ✱Euglucon, Glynase PresTab

Classification
Therapeutic: antidiabetics
Pharmacologic: sulfonylureas

Pregnancy Category B (glyburide [Glynase PresTab]), C (glimepiride, glipizide, and glyburide [Diabeta])

Indications
Control of blood glucose in type 2 diabetes mellitus when diet therapy fails. Require some pancreatic function.

Action
Lower blood glucose by stimulating the release of insulin from the pancreas and increasing the sensitivity to insulin at receptor sites. May also decrease hepatic glucose production. **Therapeutic Effects:** Lowering of blood glucose in diabetic patients.

Pharmacokinetics
Absorption: All agents are well absorbed after oral administration.
Distribution: *Glyburide*—reaches high concentrations in bile and crosses the placenta.
Protein Binding: *Glimepiride*—99.5%, *glipizide*—99%, *glyburide*—99%.
Metabolism and Excretion: All agents are mostly metabolized by the liver. *Glimepiride*—converted to a metabolite with some hypoglycemic activity; *Glyburide*—Primarily metabolized by CYP2C9.
Half-life: *Glimepiride*—5–9.2; *glipizide*—2.1–2.6 hr; *glyburide*—10 hr.

TIME/ACTION PROFILE (hypoglycemic activity)

ROUTE	ONSET	PEAK	DURATION
Glimepiride	unknown	2–3 hr	24 hr
Glipizide	15–30 min	1–2 hr	up to 24 hr
Glyburide	45–60 min	1.5–3 hr	24 hr

Contraindications/Precautions
Contraindicated in: Hypersensitivity; Hypersensitivity with sulfonamides (cross-sensitivity may occur); Type 1 diabetes; Diabetic coma or ketoacidosis; Concurrent use of bosentan (glyburide only).
Use Cautiously in: Geri: ↑ sensitivity; dose reduction may be required; Glucose 6-phosphate dehydrogenase deficiency (↑ risk of hemolytic anemia); Renal or hepatic dysfunction (↑ risk of hypoglycemia); Infection, trauma, or surgery (may alter requirements for control of blood glucose); Impaired pituitary or adrenal function; Prolonged nausea or vomiting; Debilitated or malnourished patients (↑ risk of hypoglycemia); OB, Lactation: Safety not established; insulin recommended during pregnancy; Pedi: Safety and effectiveness not established.

Adverse Reactions/Side Effects
CNS: dizziness, drowsiness, headache, weakness. **GI:** constipation, cramps, diarrhea, drug-induced hepatitis, heartburn, ↑ appetite, nausea, vomiting. **Derm:** photosensitivity, rashes. **Endo:** hypoglycemia. **F and E:** hyponatremia. **Hemat:** APLASTIC ANEMIA, agranulocytosis, hemolytic anemia, leukopenia, pancytopenia, thrombocytopenia.

Interactions
Drug-Drug: ↑ risk of elevated liver enzymes when **bosentan** used with glyburide (avoid concurrent use). Effectiveness may be ↓ by concurrent use of **diuretics, corticosteroids, phenothiazines, oral contraceptives, estrogens, thyroid preparations, phenytoin, niacin, sympathomimetics**, and **isoniazid. Alcohol, androgens (testosterone), chloramphenicol, clarithromycin, fluoroquinolones, MAO inhibitors, NSAIDs, salicylates, sulfonamides**, and **warfarin** may ↑ risk of hypoglycemia. Concurrent use with **warfarin** may alter the response to both agents (↑ effects of both initially, then ↓ activity); close monitoring recommended during any changes in dose. **Beta blockers** may mask the signs and symptoms of hypoglycemia. May ↑**cyclosporine** levels. **Colesevelam** may ↓ effects; administer glyburide, glipizide, and glimepiride ≥4 hr before colesevelam. **Topiramate** may ↓ levels and ↓ effects of glyburide.

Route/Dosage

Glimepiride

PO (Adults): 1–2 mg once daily initially; may ↑ q 1–2 wk up to 8 mg/day (usual range 1–4 mg/day).
PO (Geriatric Patients): 1 mg/day initially.

Glipizide

PO (Adults): 5 mg/day initially, may be ↑ by 2.5–5 mg/day at weekly intervals as needed (maximum dose = 40 mg/day immediate-release), 20 mg/day (XL); XL dose form is given once daily. Doses >15 mg/day should be given as 2 divided doses of immediate-release tablets (not XL).
PO (Geriatric Patients): 2.5 mg/day initially.

Glyburide

The nonmicronized formulation (Diabeta) cannot be used interchangeably with the micronized formulation (Glynase PresTab)

PO (Adults): *DiaBeta (nonmicronized)*—2.5–5 mg once daily initially; may be ↑ by 2.5–5 mg/day at weekly intervals (range 1.25–20 mg/day). *Glynase PresTab (micronized)*—1.5–3 mg/day initially; may be ↑ by 1.5 mg/day at weekly intervals (range 0.75–12 mg/day; doses >6 mg/day should be given as divided doses).
PO (Geriatric Patients): *DiaBeta (nonmicronized)*—1.25 mg/day initially; may be ↑ by 2.5 mg/day at weekly intervals. *Glynase PresTab (micronized)*—0.75 mg/day; may be ↑ by 1.5 mg/day at weekly intervals.

Availability

Glimepiride (generic available)

Tablets: 1 mg, 2 mg, 4 mg. **Cost:** *Generic*—1 mg $9.83/100, 2 mg $10.83/100, 4 mg $10.83/100. ***In combination with:*** pioglitazone (Duetact); rosiglitazone (Avandaryl); see Appendix B.

Glipizide (generic available)

Tablets: 5 mg, 10 mg. **Cost:** *Generic*—5 mg $10.83/100, 10 mg $7.18/100. **Extended-release tablets:** 2.5 mg, 5 mg, 10 mg. **Cost:** *Generic*—2.5 mg $23.76/90, 5 mg $22.86/90. ***In combination with:*** Metformin (Metaglip); see Appendix B.

Glyburide (generic available)

Tablets: 1.25 mg, 2.5 mg, 5 mg. **Cost:** *Generic*—All strengths $10.83/100. **Micronized tablets:** 1.5 mg, 3 mg, 6 mg. **Cost:** *Generic*—1.5 mg $37.50/100, 3 mg $60.50/100, 6 mg $107.32/100. ***In combination with:*** metformin (Glucovance); see Appendix B.

NURSING IMPLICATIONS

Assessment

- Observe for signs and symptoms of hypoglycemic reactions (sweating, hunger, weakness, dizziness, tremor, tachycardia, anxiety).
- Assess patient for allergy to sulfonamides.
- Patients on concurrent beta-blocker therapy may have very subtle signs of hypoglycemia.
- ***Lab Test Considerations:*** Monitor serum glucose and glycosylated hemoglobin (HbA1C) periodically during therapy to evaluate effectiveness of treatment.
- Monitor CBC periodically during therapy. Report ↓ in blood counts promptly.
- May cause an ↑ in AST, LDH, BUN, and serum creatinine.
- ***Toxicity and Overdose:*** Overdose is manifested by symptoms of hypoglycemia. Mild hypoglycemia may be treated with administration of oral glucose. Severe hypoglycemia should be treated with IV D50W followed by continuous IV infusion of more dilute dextrose solution at a rate sufficient to keep serum glucose at approximately 100 mg/dL.

Potential Nursing Diagnoses

Imbalanced nutrition: more than body requirements (Indications)
Noncompliance (Patient/Family Teaching)

Implementation

- ***High Alert:*** Accidental administration of oral hypoglycemic agents to non-diabetic adults and children has resulted in serious harm or death. Before administering, confirm that patient has type 2 diabetes.
- ***High Alert:*** Do not confuse Diabeta (glyburide) with Zebeta (bisoprolol). Do not confuse Amaryl with Reminyl (Canadian brand name for galantamine).
- Patients stabilized on a diabetic regimen who are exposed to stress, fever, trauma, infection, or surgery may require administration of insulin.
- To convert from other oral hypoglycemic agents, gradual conversion is not required. For insulin dosage of less than 20 units/day, change to oral hypoglycemic agents can be made without gradual dose adjustment. Patients taking 20 or more units/day should convert gradually by receiving oral agent and a 25–30% reduction in insulin dose every day or every 2nd day with gradual insulin dose reduction as tolerated. Monitor serum or urine glucose and ketones at least 3 times/day during conversion.
- **PO:** May be administered once in the morning with breakfast or divided into 2 doses.
- Administer *glipizide* 30 min before a meal.
- Do not administer *nonmicronized glyburide* with a meal high in fat. *Micronized glyburide* cannot be

substituted for *nonmicronized glyburide*. These preparations are not equivalent.

Patient/Family Teaching

- Instruct patient to take medication at same time each day. Take missed doses as soon as remembered unless almost time for next dose. Do not take if unable to eat.
- Explain to patient that this medication controls hyperglycemia but does not cure diabetes. Therapy is long term.
- Review signs of hypoglycemia and hyperglycemia with patient. If hypoglycemia occurs, advise patient to take a glass of orange juice or 2–3 tsp of sugar, honey, or corn syrup dissolved in water or an appropriate number of glucose tablets and notify health care professional.
- Encourage patient to follow prescribed diet, medication, and exercise regimen to prevent hypoglycemic or hyperglycemic episodes.
- Instruct patient in proper testing of serum glucose and ketones. These tests should be closely monitored during periods of stress or illness and health care professional notified if significant changes occur.
- Concurrent use of alcohol may cause a disulfiram-like reaction (abdominal cramps, nausea, flushing, headaches, and hypoglycemia).
- May occasionally cause dizziness or drowsiness. Caution patient to avoid driving or other activities requiring alertness until response to medication is known.
- Caution patient to avoid other medications, especially alcohol, while on this therapy without consulting health care professional.
- Caution patient to use sunscreen and protective clothing to prevent photosensitivity reactions.
- Advise patient to inform health care professional of medication regimen before treatment or surgery.
- Advise patient to carry a form of sugar (sugar packets, candy) and identification describing disease process and medication regimen at all times.
- Advise patient to notify health care professional promptly if unusual weight gain, swelling of ankles, drowsiness, shortness of breath, muscle cramps, weakness, sore throat, rash, or unusual bleeding or bruising occurs.
- Insulin is the recommended method of controlling blood glucose during pregnancy. Counsel female patients to use a form of contraception other than oral contraceptives and to notify health care professional promptly if pregnancy is planned or suspected or if breast feeding.
- Emphasize the importance of routine follow-up exams.

Evaluation/Desired Outcomes

- Control of blood glucose levels without the appearance of hypoglycemic or hyperglycemic episodes.

SUMAtriptan (soo-ma-**trip**-tan)

Alsuma, Imitrex, ✱Imitrex DF, Imitrex STATdose, Sumavel DosePro, Zecuity

Classification

Therapeutic: vascular headache suppressants

Pharmacologic: 5-HT_1 agonists

Pregnancy Category C

Indications

Subcut, PO, Intranasal, Transdermal: Acute treatment of migraine attacks. **Subcut:** Acute treatment of cluster headache episodes.

Action

Acts as a selective agonist of 5-HT_1 at specific vascular serotonin receptor sites, causing vasoconstriction in large intracranial arteries. **Therapeutic Effects:** Relief of acute attacks of migraine.

Pharmacokinetics

Absorption: Well absorbed (97%) after subcut administration. Absorption after oral administration is incomplete and significant amounts undergo substantial hepatic metabolism, resulting in poor bioavailability (14%). Well absorbed after intranasal and transdermal administration.

Distribution: Does not cross the blood-brain barrier. Remainder of distribution not known.

Metabolism and Excretion: Mostly metabolized (80%) by the liver.

Half-life: 2 hr.

TIME/ACTION PROFILE (relief of migraine)

ROUTE	ONSET	PEAK	DURATION
PO	within 30 min	2–4 hr	up to 24 hr
Subcut	30 min	up to 2 hr	up to 24 hr
Nasal	within 60 min	2 hr	unknown
TD	unknown	2 hr	unknown

Contraindications/Precautions

Contraindicated in: Hypersensitivity; Ischemic heart disease or signs and symptoms of ischemic heart disease, Prinzmetal's angina, or uncontrolled hypertension; Stroke or transient ischemic attack; Peripheral vascular disease (including, but not limited to, ischemic bowel disease); Concurrent MAO inhibitor therapy; Hemiplegic or basilar migraine; Concurrent use of (within 24 hr) ergotamine-containing or ergot-type drugs or other 5HT_1 agonists; Severe hepatic impairment; Geri: Excessive risk of cardiovascular complications.

Use Cautiously in: Patients with childbearing potential; OB, Lactation, Pedi: Safety not established; excreted in breast milk (avoid breast feeding for ≥12 hr after treatment).

Exercise Extreme Caution in: Cardiovascular risk factors (hypertension, hypercholesterolemia, smoking, obesity, diabetes, family history, menopausal women or men >40 yr); use only if cardiovascular status has been evaluated and determined to be safe and 1st dose is administered under supervision.

Adverse Reactions/Side Effects

All adverse reactions are less common after oral administration.

CNS: dizziness, vertigo, anxiety, drowsiness, fatigue, feeling of heaviness, feeling of tightness, headache, malaise, strange feeling, tight feeling in head, weakness. **EENT:** alterations in vision, nasal sinus discomfort, throat discomfort. **CV:** MI, angina, chest pressure, chest tightness, coronary vasospasm, ECG changes, transient hypertension. **GI:** abdominal discomfort, dysphagia. **Derm:** tingling, warm sensation, burning sensation, contact dermatitis (patch only), cool sensation, flushing. **Local:** injection site reaction. **MS:** jaw discomfort, muscle cramps, myalgia, neck pain, neck stiffness. **Neuro:** numbness.

Interactions

Drug-Drug: The risk of vasospastic reactions may be ↑ by concurrent use of **ergotamine** or **dihydroergotamine** (avoid within 24 hr of each other). Avoid concurrent use with other **$5HT_1$ agonists**. **MAO inhibitors** may ↑ levels (do not use within 2 wk of discontinuing MAO inhibitor). ↑ risk of serotonin syndrome when used with **SSRI or SNRI antidepressants**.

Drug-Natural Products: ↑ risk of serotonergic side effects including serotonin syndrome with **St. John's wort** and **SAMe**.

Route/Dosage

PO (Adults): 25 mg initially; if response is inadequate at 2 hr, up to 100 mg may be given (initial doses of 25–50 mg may be more effective than 25 mg). If headache recurs, doses may be repeated q 2 hr (not to exceed 300 mg/day). If PO therapy is to follow subcut injection, additional PO sumatriptan may be taken q 2 hr (not to exceed 200 mg/day).

Subcut (Adults): 6 mg; may repeat after 1 hr (not to exceed 12 mg in 24 hr).

Intranasal (Adults): Single dose of 5, 10, or 20 mg in 1 nostril; may be repeated in 2 hr, not to exceed 40 mg/24 hr or treatment of >5 episodes/mo.

Transdermal (Adults): Apply 1 patch; may be repeated in 2 hr, not to exceed 2 patches/24 hr.

Hepatic Impairment

PO (Adults): 25 mg initially; if response is inadequate at 2 hr, up to 50 mg may be given (initial doses of 25–50 mg may be more effective than 25 mg). If headache recurs, doses may be repeated q 2 hr (not to exceed 300 mg/day). If PO therapy is to follow subcut injection, additional PO sumatriptan may be taken q 2 hr (not to exceed 200 mg/day); no single oral dose should exceed 50 mg.

Availability (generic available)

Tablets: 25 mg, 50 mg, 100 mg. **Cost:** *Generic*—25 mg $243.47/9, 50 mg $226.26/9, 100 mg $226.26/9. **Solution for subcutanous injection:** 4 mg/0.5-mL prefilled syringes or needle-free delivery system, 6 mg/0.5-mL prefilled syringes, vials, or needle-free delivery system. **Cost:** *Generic*—4 mg/0.5 mL $60.56/0.5 mL, 6 mg/0.5 mL $31.20/0.5 mL. **Nasal spray:** 5 mg/spray, 20 mg/spray. **Cost:** *Generic*—All strengths $49.26/device. **Transdermal patch:** delivers 6.5 mg/4 hr. ***In combination with:*** naproxen (Treximet); see Appendix B.

NURSING IMPLICATIONS

Assessment

- Assess pain location, intensity, duration, and associated symptoms (photophobia, phonophobia, nausea, vomiting) during migraine attack.
- Give initial subcut dose under observation to patients with potential for coronary artery disease including postmenopausal women, men >40 yr, patients with risk factors for coronary artery disease such as hypertension, hypercholesterolemia, obesity, diabetes, smoking, or family history. Monitor BP before and for 1 hr after initial injection. If angina occurs, monitor ECG for ischemic changes.
- Monitor for serotonin syndrome in patients taking SSRIs or SNRIs concurrently with sumatriptan.

S

Potential Nursing Diagnoses

Acute pain (Indications)

Implementation

- Do not confuse sumatriptan with sitagliptin or zolmitriptan.
- **PO:** Tablets should be swallowed whole; do not crush, break, or chew. Tablets are film-coated to prevent contact with tablet contents, which have an unpleasant taste and may cause nausea and vomiting.
- **Subcut:** Administer as a single injection. Solution is clear and colorless or pale yellow; do not use if dark-colored or cloudy or if beyond expiration date.
- *Sumavel DosePro*: The snap-off tip should sit firmly on the end of the clear medication chamber; do not use if tip tilted or broken off upon removal from packaging. Administer only in abdomen or thigh.
- **Intranasal:** 10-mg dose may be administered as 2 sprays of 5 mg in 1 nostril or 1 spray in each nostril.
- **Transdermal:** Apply to dry, non-irritated, intact skin of upper arm or thigh. Site must be relatively free of hair and without scars, tattoos, abrasions, eczema, psoriasis, melanoma, or contact dermatitis. After application, push activation button within 15

min and red light emitting diode (LED) will turn on. Secure patch with medical tape if needed. System stops operating when dosing complete; activation light turns off signaling system can be removed. System cannot be reactivated when completed. If light turns off before 4 hr, dosing has stopped and patch can be removed. Fold patch so adhesive sides stick together and discard away from children and pets; contains lithium-manganese dioxide batteries; dispose in accordance with state and local regulations.

- If headache is not completely relieved, may retreat no sooner than 2 hr in a different site; use no more than 2 patches in 24 hr. Rotate sites; do not apply to a previous site until site is free from erythema for at least 3 days.

Patient/Family Teaching

- Inform patient that sumatriptan should be used only *during* a migraine attack. It is meant to be used for relief of migraine attacks but not to prevent or reduce the number of attacks.
- Instruct patient to administer sumatriptan as soon as symptoms of a migraine attack appear, but it may be administered at any time during an attack. If migraine symptoms return, a second injection may be used. Allow at least 1 hr between doses, and do not use more than 2 injections in any 24-hr period. Additional sumatriptan doses are not likely to be effective, and alternative medications may be used. If no relief from 1st dose, unlikely 2nd dose will provide relief. Advise patient to read *Patient Information* prior to using and with each Rx refill; new information may be available.
- Advise patient that lying down in a darkened room after sumatriptan administration may further help relieve headache.
- Advise patient that overuse (use more than 10 days/mo) may lead to exacerbation of headache (migraine-like daily headaches, or as a marked increase in frequency of migraine attacks). May require gradual withdrawal of sumatriptan and treatment of symptoms (transient worsening of headache).
- Advise patient to notify health care professional before next dose of sumatriptan if pain or tightness in chest occurs during use. If pain is severe or does not subside, notify health care professional immediately. If wheezing; heart throbbing; swelling of eyelids, face, or lips; skin rash; skin lumps; or hives occur, notify health care professional immediately, and do not take more sumatriptan without approval of health care professional. If usual dose fails to relieve 3 consecutive headaches, or if frequency and/or severity increases, notify health care professional. If feelings of tingling, heat, flushing, heaviness, pressure, drowsiness, dizziness, tiredness, or sickness develop, discuss with health care professional at next visit.
- Sumatriptan may cause dizziness or drowsiness. Caution patient to avoid driving or other activities requiring alertness until response to medication is known.
- Advise patient to avoid alcohol, which aggravates headaches, during sumatriptan use.
- Instruct patient to notify health care professional of all Rx or OTC medications, vitamins, or herbal products being taken and consult health care professional before taking any new medications. Patients concurrently taking SSRI or SNRI antidepressants should notify health care professional promptly if signs of serotonin syndrome (mental status changes: agitation, hallucinations, coma; autonomic instability: tachycardia, labile BP, hyperthermia; neuromuscular aberrations: hyper-reflexia, incoordination; and/or gastrointestinal symptoms: nausea, vomiting, diarrhea) occur.
- Caution patient not to use sumatriptan if pregnancy is planned or suspected or if breast feeding. Adequate contraception should be used during therapy.
- **Subcut:** Instruct patient on the proper technique for loading, administering, and discarding the *Imitrex STATdose pen* autoinjector or for using *Sumavel DosePro*. Patient information pamphlet is provided. Instructional video is available from the manufacturer.
- Inform patient that pain or redness at the injection site usually lasts less than 1 hr.
- **Intranasal:** Instruct patient in proper technique for intranasal administration. Usual dose is a single spray in 1 nostril. If headache returns, a 2nd dose may be administered in ≥2 hr. Do not administer 2nd dose if no relief was provided by 1st dose without consulting health care professional.
- **Transdermal:** Instruct patient to read *Patient Information and Instructions for Use* before starting and with each Rx refill, in case of changes.
- Advise patient not to bathe, shower, or swim while wearing patch.
- Inform patient that skin redness under patch site that disappears within 24 hr is common. If signs and symptoms of allergic contact dermatitis (itching, redness, irritation, blistering or peeling, warmth or tenderness of skin, blisters that ooze, drain, or crust over) occur, stop using sumatriptan transdermal and notify health care professional.
- Advise patient referred for MRI test to discuss patch with referring health care professional and MRI facility to determine if removal of patch is necessary prior to test and for directions for replacing patch.
- Advise patient not to use more than 4 times/mo without consulting health care professional.

Evaluation/Desired Outcomes

- Relief of migraine attack.

SUNItinib (su-ni-ti-nib)
Sutent

Classification
Therapeutic: antineoplastics
Pharmacologic: kinase inhibitors

Pregnancy Category D

Indications
Gastrointestinal stromal tumor (GIST) that has progressed or intolerance to imatinib. Advanced renal cell carcinoma (RCC). Advanced pancreatic neuroendocrine tumors (pNET).

Action
Inhibits multiple receptor tyrosine kinases, which are enzymes implicated in tumor growth, abnormal vascular growth, and tumor metastases. **Therapeutic Effects:** Decreased tumor spread.

Pharmacokinetics
Absorption: Well absorbed following oral administration.
Distribution: Unknown.
Protein Binding: *Sunitinib*—95%; *primary active metabolite*—90%.
Metabolism and Excretion: Metabolized by the CYP3A4 enzyme system to its primary active metabolite. This metabolite is further metabolized by CYP3A4. Excretion is primarily fecal.
Half-life: *Sunitinib*—40–60 hr; *primary active metabolite*—80–110 hr.

TIME/ACTION PROFILE (blood levels)

ROUTE	ONSET	PEAK	DURATION
PO	unknown	6–12 hr	24 hr

Contraindications/Precautions
Contraindicated in: Hypersensitivity; NYHA class II-IV HF; OB, Lactation: Pregnancy, lactation; Concurrent use of ketoconazole or St. John's wort.
Use Cautiously in: Hepatic/renal impairment; Concurrent use of bisphosphonates or a history of dental disease (may ↑ risk of jaw osteonecrosis); History of myocardial ischemia or MI; LVEF <50% and >20% below baseline with no signs/symptoms of HF (need to interrupt therapy or ↓ dose); Diabetes (↑ risk of hypoglycemia); OB: Childbearing potential; Pedi: Safety not established.

Adverse Reactions/Side Effects
CNS: REVERSIBLE POSTERIOR LEUKOENCEPHALOPATHY SYNDROME (RPLS), fatigue, dizziness, headache. **CV:** HF, MI, hypertension, peripheral edema, QT interval prolongation, thromboembolic events. **EENT:** epistaxis. **GI:** HEPATOTOXICITY, diarrhea, dyspepsia, nausea, stomatitis, vomiting, altered taste, anorexia, cholecystitis, constipation, esophagitis, ↑ lipase/amylase, ↑ liver enzymes, oral pain. **Derm:** ERYTHEMA MULTIFORME, NECROTIZING FASCIITIS, STEVENS-JOHNSON SYNDROME, TOXIC EPIDERMAL NECROLYSIS, alopecia, hand-foot syndrome, hair color change, impaired wound healing, rash, skin discoloration. **Endo:** hypoglycemia, hypothyroidism, adrenal insufficiency, hyperthyroidism. **F and E:** dehydration, hypophosphatemia. **GU:** HEMOLYTIC UREMIC SYNDROME, nephrotic syndrome, proteinuria, renal failure. **Hemat:** HEMORRHAGE, THROMBOTIC THROMBOCYTOPENIC PURPURA, anemia, lymphopenia, neutropenia, thrombocytopenia. **Metab:** hyperuricemia. **MS:** arthralgia, back pain, limb pain, myalgia, osteonecrosis (primarily of jaw). **Misc:** TUMOR LYSIS SYNDROME, fever.

Interactions
Drug-Drug: Ketoconazole and other **inhibitors of the CYP3A4 enzyme system** may ↑ levels and the risk of toxicity; ↓ dose to 37.5 mg daily (for GIST and RCC) or 25 mg daily (for pNET); avoid these strong inhibitors, if possible. **Rifampin** and other **inducers of the CYP3A4 enzyme system** may ↓ levels and effectiveness; ↑ dose to 87.5 mg daily (for GIST and RCC) or 62.5 mg daily (for pNET); avoid these strong inducers, if possible. Concurrent use with **alendronate**, **etidronate**, **ibandronate**, **pamidronate**, **risedronate**, **tiludronate**, or **zoledronic acid** may ↑ risk of jaw osteonecrosis. ↑ risk of microangiopathic hemolytic anemia when used with **bevacizumab** (concurrent use not recommended).
Drug-Natural Products: St. John's wort may ↓ levels and effectiveness; avoid concurrent use.
Drug-Food: Blood levels and effects are ↑ by **grapefruit juice**; concurrent use should be avoided.

Route/Dosage
GIST and RCC
PO (Adults): 50 mg once daily for 4 wk, followed by 2-wk rest; alteration of dose is based on safety/tolerability and is made in 12.5-mg increments/decrements.

pNET
PO (Adults): 37.5 mg once daily.

Availability (generic available)
Capsules: 12.5 mg, 25 mg, 37.5 mg, 50 mg.

NURSING IMPLICATIONS
Assessment
- Monitor for signs of HF (dyspnea, edema, jugular venous distention) during therapy. Assess left ventricular ejection fraction (LVEF) at baseline and periodically during therapy in patients with cardiac events

S

in the previous 12 mo and a baseline ejection fraction in patients without cardiovascular risk factors. Discontinue sunitinib if signs of HF occur.

- **Monitor for hypertension and treat with standard antihypertensive therapy. If severe hypertension occurs, may discontinue sunitinib until controlled.**
- Monitor ECG and electrolytes periodically during therapy; may cause QT prolongation and torsades de pointes.
- Monitor for rash. If progressive skin rash with blisters or mucosal lesions occurs discontinue and do not restart sunitinib.
- ***Lab Test Considerations:*** Monitor CBC with platelet count and serum chemistries including phosphate at the beginning of each treatment cycle. May cause neutropenia, lymphopenia, anemia, and thrombocytopenia. May cause ↑ creatinine, hypokalemia, hyperuricemia, and ↑ uric acid.
- Monitor ALT, AST, and bilirubin before starting therapy, during each cycle of treatment, and as clinically indicated. Stop therapy if Grade 3 or 4 drug-related hepatic adverse events occur and discontinue if there is no resolution. Do not restart sunitinib if patients subsequently experience severe changes in liver function tests or have other signs and symptoms of liver failure. May cause ↑ AST, ALT, alkaline phosphatase, total and indirect bilirubin, amylase, and lipase.
- Monitor thyroid function at baseline and in patients with symptoms of hypothyroidism or hyperthyroidism. May be treated with standard medical practice.
- Monitor urinalysis for urine protein at baseline and periodically during therapy. Follow up with 24-hr urine protein as clinically indicated. Interrupt sunitinib and reduce dose if 24-hr urine protein ≥3 grams. Discontinue for patients with nephrotic syndrome or repeat episodes of urine protein ≥3 grams despite dose reductions.
- Monitor blood glucose levels periodically during and after therapy. Assess if antidiabetic drug dose needs to be adjusted to minimize the risk of hypoglycemia.

Potential Nursing Diagnoses

Diarrhea (Adverse Reactions)
Nausea (Adverse Reactions)

Implementation

- Do not confuse sunitinib with sorafenib.
- **PO:** Administer once daily with or without food.

Patient/Family Teaching

- Instruct patient to take sunitinib as directed. Take missed doses as soon as remembered, but not just before next dose. Take next dose at regular time. Do not take more than 1 dose at a time. Tell your health care professional about the missed dose.
- Advise patient to avoid grapefruit juice and grapefruit products during therapy.
- Instruct patient to notify health care professional promptly if signs of liver failure (itching, yellow eyes or skin, dark urine, pain or discomfort in the right upper stomach area), rash, or tumor lysis syndrome (nausea, shortness of breath, irregular heartbeat, clouding of urine, tiredness) occur.
- **Advise patient that GI disorders (diarrhea, nausea, stomatitis, dyspepsia, vomiting) are common and may require antiemetic and antidiarrheal medications.**
- **Inform patient that sunitinib may cause discoloration (yellow) of skin and depigmentation of hair or skin.**
- **Instruct patient to notify health care professional of all Rx or OTC medications, vitamins, or herbal products being taken and consult health care professional before taking any new medications, especially St. John's wort.**
- Advise patient to notify health care professional if bleeding or swelling occur.
- Advise women of childbearing potential to avoid becoming pregnant while receiving sunitinib.

Evaluation/Desired Outcomes

- Decrease in tumor spread.

suvorexant (soo-voe-**rex**-ant)

Belsomra

Classification
Therapeutic: sedative/hypnotics
Pharmacologic: orexin receptor antagonists

Schedule IV

Pregnancy Category C

Indications

Treatment of insomnia associated with difficulty in sleep onset and/or maintenance.

Action

Antagonizes the effects of orexins A and B, naturally occurring neuropeptides that promote wakefulness, by binding to their receptors. **Therapeutic Effects:** Improved sleep.

Pharmacokinetics

Absorption: 82% absorbed following oral administration; a high fat meal will delay absorption and sleep onset. ↑ absorption in obese females.
Distribution: Does not distribute into RBCs.
Protein Binding: >99%.
Metabolism and Excretion: Extensively metabolized by CYP3A (minor metabolism by CYP2C19; metabolites are not active). 66% excreted in feces, 23% in urine, mostly as metabolites.
Half-life: 12 hr (↑ in hepatic impairment).

TIME/ACTION PROFILE (sleep)

ROUTE	ONSET	PEAK	DURATION
PO	30 min (delayed by food)	unknown	7 hr†

†Excess sedation may persist for several days after discontinuation.

Contraindications/Precautions

Contraindicated in: Narcolepsy; Concurrent use of strong inhibitors of CYP3A; Severe hepatic impairment.
Use Cautiously in: History of substance abuse or drug dependence; Concurrent use of moderate inhibitors of CYP3A (dose ↓ recommended); Obese patients (↑ levels, especially in women, dose ↓ may be warranted); History of or concurrent psychiatric diagnoses; Underlying pulmonary disease; OB: Use during pregnancy only if potential benefit justifies potential fetal risk; Lactation: Use cautiously if breast feeding; Pedi: Safe and effective use in children has not been established.

Adverse Reactions/Side Effects

Adverse reactions, especially related to CNS depression are dose-related, especially at the 20 mg dose.
CNS: drowsiness, cataplexy, daytime drowsiness, hallucinations, worsening of depression/suicidal ideation, sleep paralysis.

Interactions

Drug-Drug: Concurrent use of **strong inhibitors of CYP3A** including **boceprevir**, **clarithromycin**, **conivaptan**, **indinavir**, **itraconazole**, **ketoconazole**, **nefazodone**, **nelfinavir**, **posaconazole**, **ritonavir**, **saquinavir**, and **telithromycin** risk of excessive sedation and should be avoided. Concurrent use of **moderate inhibitors of CYP3A** including **aprepitant**, **atazanavir**, **ciprofloxacin**, **diltiazem**, **erythromycin**, **fluconazole**, **fosamprenavir**, **imatinib**, and **verapamil** may result in ↑ sedation (↓ dose recommended). Risk of CNS depression, next-day impairment, "sleep-driving" and other complex behaviors while not fully awake ↑ with other **CNS depressants** including **alcohol**, some **antihistamines**, **opioids**, other **sedative/hypnotics** (including **benzodiazepines**) and **tricyclic antidepressants**; dose adjustments may be necessary). Concurrent use of **CYP3A inducers** including **carbamazepine**, **phenytoin** and **rifampin** may ↓ effectiveness. May alter **digoxin** levels (blood level monitoring recommended).
Drug-Food: **Grapefruit juice** may result in ↑ blood levels and excess sedation (↓ dose recommended).

Route/Dosage

PO (Adults): 10 mg within 30 minutes of going to bed, if well tolerated but not optimally effective, dose may be increased next night, not to exceed 20 mg (dose may not be repeated on a single night and should be when at least 7 hr of sleep time is anticipated before planned awakening). *Concurrent use of moderate inhibitors of CYP3A* —5 mg initially, dose may be ↑ to 10 mg if lower dose is tolerated but not optimally effective. Lowest effective dose should be used.

Availability

Tablets: 5 mg, 10 mg, 15 mg, 20 mg.

NURSING IMPLICATIONS

Assessment

- Assess mental status, sleep patterns, and potential for abuse prior to administration. Prolonged use of >7–10 days may lead to physical and psychological dependence. Limit amount of drug available to the patient.
- Assess alertness at time of peak effect. Notify health care professional if desired sedation does not occur.

Potential Nursing Diagnoses

Insomnia (Indications)
Risk for injury (Side Effects)

Implementation

- Before administering, reduce external stimuli and provide comfort measures to increase effectiveness of medication.
- Protect patient from injury. Raise bed side rails. Assist with ambulation. Remove patient's cigarettes.
- Use lowest effective dose.
- **PO:** Tablets should be swallowed whole with full glass of water. Take no more than once/night and within 30 min of going to bed. Take only if at least 7 hr remaining before awaking. For faster onset of sleep, do not administer with or immediately after a meal.

Patient/Family Teaching

- Instruct patient to take suvorexant as directed. Advise patient not to take suvorexant unless able to stay in bed a full night (7 hr) before being active again. Do not take more than the amount prescribed because of the habit-forming potential. Not recommended for use longer than 7–10 days. Instruct patient to read *Medication Guide* for correct product before taking and with each Rx refill, changes may occur.
- Because of rapid onset, advise patient to go to bed immediately after taking suvorexant.

S

- May cause daytime drowsiness or dizziness. Advise patient to avoid driving or other activities requiring alertness until response to this medication is known.
- Caution patient that complex sleep-related behaviors (sleep-driving) may occur while asleep. Inform families and advise to notify health care professional if these behaviors occur.
- Instruct patient to notify health care professional of all Rx or OTC medications, vitamins, or herbal products being taken and to avoid concurrent use of Rx, OTC, and herbal products without consulting health care professional.
- Caution patient to avoid concurrent use of alcohol or other CNS depressants.
- Advise patient to notify health care professional if depression worsens or suicidal thoughts occur.
- Advise patient to notify health care professional immediately if signs of anaphylaxis (swelling of the tongue or throat, trouble breathing, and nausea and vomiting) occur.
- Advise female patient to notify health care professional if pregnancy is planned or suspected or if breast feeding.

Evaluation/Desired Outcomes

- Relief of insomnia.

TACROLIMUS

tacrolimus (oral, IV)

(ta-**kroe**-li-mus)

✱Advagraf, Astagraf XL, Envarsus XR, Prograf

tacrolimus (topical)

Protopic

Classification

Therapeutic: immunosuppressants

Pregnancy Category C

Indications

PO, IV: Prevention of organ rejection in patients who have undergone allogenic liver, kidney, or heart transplantation (used concurrently with corticosteroids) (used concurrently with azathioprine or mycophenolate mofetil in kidney or heart transplants) (extended-release only indicated for kidney transplant). **Topical:** Moderate to severe atopic dermatitis in patients who do not respond to or cannot tolerate alternative, conventional therapies.

Action

Inhibit T-lymphocyte activation. **Therapeutic Effects:** Prevention of transplanted organ rejection. Improvement in signs/symptoms of atopic dermatitis.

Pharmacokinetics

Absorption: Absorption following oral administration is erratic and incomplete (bioavailability ranges 5–67%); minimal amounts absorbed following topical use.

Distribution: Crosses the placenta and enters breast milk.

Protein Binding: 99%.

Metabolism and Excretion: 99% metabolized by the liver; <1% excreted unchanged in the urine.

Half-life: *Liver transplant patients*—11.7 hr; *healthy volunteers*—21.2 hr.

TIME/ACTION PROFILE (immunosuppression)

ROUTE	ONSET	PEAK	DURATION
PO	rapid	1.3–3.2 hr*	12 hr
PO-ER	unknown	unknown	24 hr
IV	rapid	unknown	8–12 hr
Topical†	unknown	1–2 wk	unknown

*Blood level.

†Improvement in atopic dermatitis.

Contraindications/Precautions

Contraindicated in: Hypersensitivity to tacrolimus or to castor oil (a component in the injection); Concurrent use with cyclosporine or sirolimus should be avoided; Congenital long QT syndrome; Lactation: Breast feeding should be avoided; Weakened/compromised immune system; Malignant or premalignant skin condition; Pedi: Children <2 yr (safety not established).

Use Cautiously in: Heart failure, bradycardia, or electrolyte disorders (hypokalemia, hypomagnesemia, hypocalcemia); Concurrent use of other drugs known to prolong the QT interval; Renal or hepatic impairment (dose ↓ may be required; if oliguria occurs, wait 48 hr before initiating tacrolimus); Exposure to sunlight/UV light (may ↑ risk of malignant skin changes); OB: Hyperkalemia and renal impairment may occur in the newborn; use only if benefit to mother justifies risk to the fetus; Pedi: Higher end of dosing range required to maintain adequate blood levels; Superficial skin infections.

Adverse Reactions/Side Effects

Noted primarily for PO and IV use.

CNS: POSTERIOR REVERSIBLE ENCEPHALOPATHY SYNDROME (PRES), SEIZURES, dizziness, headache, insomnia, tremor, abnormal dreams, agitation, anxiety, confusion, depression, emotional lability, hallucinations, psychoses, somnolence. **EENT:** abnormal vision, amblyopia, sinusitis, tinnitus. **Resp:** cough, pleural effusion, asthma, bronchitis, pharyngitis, pneumonia, pulmonary edema. **CV:** hypertension, peripheral edema, QTc interval prolongation. **GI:** GI BLEEDING, GI PERFORATION, abdominal pain, anorexia, ascites, constipation, diarrhea, dyspepsia, ↑ liver enzymes, nausea, vomiting, cholangitis, cholestatic jaundice, dysphagia, flatulence, ↑ appetite, oral thrush, peritonitis. **GU:** nephrotoxicity, urinary tract infection. **Derm:** pruritus, rash, alopecia, herpes simplex, hirsutism, photosensitivity, sweating. **Endo:** hyperglycemia, hyperlipidemia. **F and E:** hyperkalemia, hypomagnesemia, hyperphosphatemia, hypocalcemia, hyponatremia, hypophosphatemia, metabolic acidosis, metabolic alkalosis. **Hemat:** anemia, leukocytosis, leukopenia, thrombocytopenia, coagulation defects, pure red cell aplasia. **Local:** *topical*—burning, stinging. **MS:** arthralgia, hypertonia, leg cramps, muscle spasm, myalgia, myasthenia, osteoporosis. **Neuro:** paresthesia, neuropathy. **Misc:** allergic reactions including ANAPHYLAXIS, generalized pain, abnormal healing, chills, fever, infection (including activation of latent viral infections such as BK virus-associated nephropathy), ↑ risk of lymphoma/skin cancer.

Interactions

Noted primarily for PO and IV use, but should be considered for topical use.

Drug-Drug: Risk of nephrotoxicity is ↑ by concurrent use of **aminoglycosides**, **amphotericin B**, **cisplatin**, or **cyclosporine** (allow 24 hr to pass after stopping cyclosporine before starting tacrolimus). Concurrent use of **potassium-sparing diuretics**, **ACE inhibitors**, or **angiotensin II receptor blockers** ↑ risk of hyperkalemia. **Strong CYP3A4 inhibitors**, including **ketoconazole**, **itraconazole**, **voriconazole**, **ritonavir**, **clarithromycin**, and **boceprevir** may significantly ↑ levels; closely monitor tacrolimus whole blood trough concentrations. **Bromocriptine**, **calcium channel blockers**, **chloramphenicol**, **cimetidine**, **lansoprazole**, **cyclosporine**, **amiodarone**, **danazol**, **ethinyl estradiol**, **erythromycin**, **magnesium/aluminum hydroxide methylprednisolone**, **omeprazole**, **nefazodone**, and **metoclopramide**, and **protease inhibitors** may ↑ levels; avoid concurrent use with **nelfinavir**. Concurrent use with **CYP3A4 substrates** or **CYP3A4 inhibitors** that also prolong the QT interval may ↑ the risk of QT interval prolongation. **Strong CYP3A4 inducers**, including **rifampin** and **rifabutin** may significantly ↓ levels; closely monitor tacrolimus whole blood trough concentrations. **Phenobarbital**, **phenytoin**, **caspofungin**, **sirolimus** and **carbamazepine** may ↓ levels; closely monitor tacrolimus whole blood trough concentrations. **Vaccinations** may be less effective if given concurrently with tacrolimus (avoid use of live-virus vaccines). May ↑ levels of **mycophenolate mofetil** or **mycophenolic acid**.

Drug-Natural Products: Concomitant use with **astragalus**, **echinacea**, and **melatonin** may interfere with immunosuppression. **St. John's wort** may ↓ tacrolimus blood levels.

Drug-Food: Food ↓ the rate and extent of GI absorption. **Grapefruit juice** ↑ absorption.

Route/Dosage

Because of the potential risk for anaphylaxis, the IV route of administration should be reserved for those patients unable to take the drug orally. Extended-release capsules are not interchangeable with immediate-release capsules or other extended-release products. Black patients may require a higher dose to achieve desired tacrolimus trough concentrations.

Kidney Transplantation

PO (Adults): *Initial dose of immediate-release capsules (with azathioprine)*—0.2 mg/kg/day in 2 divided doses; titrate to achieve recommended whole blood trough concentration; *Initial dose of immediate-release capsules (with mycophenolate mofetil and IL-2 antagonist)*—0.1 mg/kg/day in 2 divided doses; titrate to achieve recommended whole blood trough concentration; *Extended-release capsules (Astagraf XL) (with basiliximab induction)*—0.15 mg/kg once daily (to be started either before or within 48 hr of completion of transplant); *Extended-release capsules (Astagraf XL) (without basiliximab induction)*—0.1 mg/kg given as single dose preoperatively within 12 hr prior to reperfusion, followed by 0.2 mg/kg once daily started postoperatively at least 4 hr after preoperative dose and within 12 hr after reperfusion; *Conversion from immediate-release capsules to extended-release capsules (Envarsus XR)*—Initiate extended-release treatment with a once daily dose that is 80% of the total daily dose of the immediate-release product.

PO (Children): *Immediate-release capsules*—0.15–0.4 mg/kg/day in 2 divided doses; titrate to achieve recommended whole blood trough concentration.

IV (Adults): *Initial dose*—0.03–0.1 mg/kg/day as a continuous infusion; titrate to achieve recommended whole blood trough concentration.

IV (Children): 0.03–0.15 mg/kg/day.

Liver Transplantation

PO (Adults): *Initial dose of immediate–release capsules*—0.1–0.15 mg/kg/day in two divided doses; titrate to achieve recommended whole blood trough concentration.

PO (Children): *Initial dose of immediate–release capsules*—0.15–0.2 mg/kg/day in 2 divided doses; titrate to achieve recommended whole blood trough concentration.

IV (Adults and Children): Same as for kidney transplant.

Heart Transplantation

PO (Adults): *Initial dose of immediate-release capsules*—0.075 mg/kg/day in two divided doses; titrate to achieve recommended whole blood trough concentration.

IV (Adults): *Initial dose*—0.01 mg/kg/day as a continuous infusion; titrate to achieve recommended whole blood trough concentration.

Atopic Dermatitis

Topical (Adults): Apply 0.03% or 0.1% ointment twice daily. Discontinue when signs/symptoms of atopic dermatitis resolve.

Topical (Children ≥2–15 yr): Apply 0.03% ointment twice daily. Discontinue when signs/symptoms of atopic dermatitis resolve.

Availability (generic available)

Immediate-release capsules: 0.5 mg, 1 mg, 5 mg. **Extended-release capsules (Astagraf XL):** 0.5 mg, 1 mg, ✱3 mg, 5 mg. **Extended-release tablets (Envarsus XR):** 0.75 mg, 1 mg, 4 mg. **Injection:** 5 mg/mL. **Ointment:** 0.03%, 0.1%.

NURSING IMPLICATIONS

Assessment

- Assess for symptoms of PRES (headache, altered mental status, seizures, visual disturbances, hypertension) periodically during therapy. Confirm diagnosis by radiologic procedure. If PRES is suspected or diagnosed, maintain BP control and immediately reduce immunosuppression. Symptoms are usually reversed on reduction or discontinuation of immunosuppression.

- **Prevention of Organ Rejection:** Monitor BP closely during therapy. Hypertension is a common complication of tacrolimus therapy and should be treated.
- Observe patients receiving IV tacrolimus for the development of anaphylaxis (rash, pruritus, laryngeal edema, wheezing) for at least 30 min and frequently thereafter. If signs develop, stop infusion and initiate treatment.
- **Atopic Dermatitis:** Assess skin lesions prior to and periodically during therapy.
- Use only for short time, not continuously, and in the minimum dose possible to decrease risk of developing skin cancer.
- ***Lab Test Considerations:*** Tacrolimus blood level monitoring may be helpful in the evaluation of rejection and toxicity, dose adjustments, and assessment of compliance. *For kidney transplantation*, during the first 3 mo, most patients maintained tacrolimus whole blood concentrations between 7–20 ng/mL and then between 5–15 ng/mL through 1 yr. *For heart transplantation*, from wk 1 to 3 mo, most patients maintained tacrolimus trough whole blood concentrations between 8–20 ng/mL and then between 6–18 ng/mL from 3–18 mo post-transplant.
- Monitor serum creatinine, potassium, and glucose closely. ↑ serum creatinine and ↓ urine output may indicate nephrotoxicity. May also cause insulin-dependent post-transplant diabetes mellitus (incidence is higher in African American and Hispanic patients).
- May also cause hyperuricemia, hypokalemia, hyperkalemia, hypomagnesemia, metabolic acidosis, metabolic alkalosis, hyperlipidemia, hyperphosphatemia, hypophosphatemia, hypocalcemia, and hyponatremia.
- Monitor CBC. May cause anemia, leukocytosis, and thrombocytopenia.

Potential Nursing Diagnoses

Risk for infection (Adverse Reactions)

Implementation

- Do not confuse Prograf (tacrolimus) with Prozac (fluoxetine).
- Do not confuse immediate-release tacrolimus with extended-release tacrolimus.
- Should only be prescribed by health care professionals experienced with immunosuppressive therapy and organ transplant patients.
- Begin therapy with tacrolimus no sooner than 6 hr post-transplantation. Concurrent therapy with corticosteroids is recommended in the early postoperative period.
- Tacrolimus should not be used concomitantly with cyclosporine. Tacrolimus or cyclosporine should be discontinued at least 24 hr before starting the other.
- Oral therapy is preferred because of the risk of anaphylactic reactions with IV tacrolimus. IV therapy should be replaced with oral therapy as soon as possible.
- Adults should be started at the lower end of the dose range; children require a higher doses to maintain blood trough concentrations similar to adults.
- Immediate and extended-release capsules are not interchangeable.
- **PO:** Oral doses can be initiated 8–12 hr after discontinuation of IV doses. May be taken without regard to food, but should be consistent, with or without food and at same time each day.
- Take extended-release capsules at the same time each day, preferably in the morning, on an empty stomach at least 1 hr before or 2 hrs after breakfast. Swallow capsules whole; do not chew, divide, or crush.
- **Topical:** Do not use continuously for a long time.
- **Topical:** Wash hands before applying. Apply a thin layer of ointment twice daily to affected skin. Use smallest amount of ointment needed to control signs and symptoms of eczema. Do not cover treated area with bandages, dressings or wraps. If not treating areas on hands, wash hands with soap and water after applying to remove any ointment on hands.

IV Administration

- **Continuous Infusion:** ***Diluent:*** Dilute in 0.9% NaCl or D5W. ***Concentration:*** 0.004–0.02 mg/mL. May be stored in polyethylene or glass containers for 24 hr following dilution. Do not store in PVC containers. Do not administer solutions that are discolored or contain particulate matter. ***Rate:*** Administer daily dose as a continuous infusion over 24 hr.
- **Y-Site Compatibility:** alemtuzumab, alfentanil, amifostine, amikacin, aminocaproic acid, aminophylline, amiodarone, amphotericin B colloidal, amphotericin B lipid complex, amphotericin B liposome, anidulafungin, argatroban, azithromycin, aztreonam, benztropine, bivalirudin, bleomycin, bumetanide, buprenorphine, busulfan, butorphanol, calcium acetate, calcium chloride, calcium gluconate, carboplatin, carmustine, caspofungin, cefazolin, cefotaxime, cefotetan, cefoxitin, ceftazidime, ceftriaxone, cefuroxime, chloramphenicol, chlorpromazine, ciprofloxacin, cisatracurium, cisplatin, clindamycin, cyclophosphamide, cyclosporine, cytarabine, dacarbazine, dactinomycin, daptomycin, daunorubicin hydrochloride, dexamethasone, dexmedetomidine, dexrazoxane, digoxin, diltiazem, diphenhydramine, dobutamine, docetaxel, dolasetron, dopamine, doripenem, doxorubicin hydrochloride, doxorubicin liposomal, doxycycline, droperidol, enalaprilat, ephedrine, epinephrine, epirubicin, ertapenem, erythromycin, es-

molol, etoposide, etoposide phosphate, famotidine, fenoldopam, fentanyl, fluconazole, fludarabine, foscarnet, fosphenytoin, gemcitabine, gentamicin, glycopyrrolate, granisetron, haloperidol, heparin, hetastarch, hydralazine, hydrocortisone, hydromorphone, idarubicin, ifosfamide, imipenem/cilastatin, insulin, irinotecan, isoproterenol, ketorolac, labetalol, leucovorin, levofloxacin, levorphanol, lidocaine, linezolid, lorazepam, magnesium sulfate, mannitol, mechlorethamine, meperidine, meropenem, mesna, methotrexate, methyldopate, methylprednisolone, metoclopramide, metoprolol, metronidazole, micafungin, midazolam, milrinone, mitomycin, mitoxantrone, morphine, moxifloxacin, multivitamins, mycophenolate, nafcillin, nalbuphine, naloxone, nesiritide, nicardipine, nitroglycerin, nitroprusside, norepinephrine, octreotide, ondansetron, oxacillin, oxaliplatin, oxytocin, paclitaxel, palonosetron, pamidronate, pancuronium, pemetrexed, penicillin G potassium, pentamidine, pentazocine, phenylephrine, piperacillin/tazobactam, potassium acetate, potassium chloride, potassium phosphates, procainamide, prochlorperazine, promethazine, propranolol, quinupristin/dalfopristin, ranitidine, remifentanil, rocuronium, sodium acetate, sodium bicarbonate, sodium phosphates, streptozocin, succinylcholine, sufentanil, teniposide, theophylline, thiotepa, tigecycline, tirofiban, tobramycin, topotecan, vancomycin, vasopressin, vecuronium, verapamil, vinblastine, vincristine, vinorelbine, voriconazole, zidovudine, zoledronic acid.

- **Y-Site Incompatibility:** acyclovir, allopurinol, azathioprine, cefepime, dantrolene, diazepam, esomeprazole, folic acid, ganciclovir, iron sucrose, levothyroxine, phenytoin, thiopental.

Patient/Family Teaching

- Instruct patient to take tacrolimus at the same time each day, with or without food, as directed. Do not skip or double up on missed doses. Do not discontinue medication without advice of health care professional. Take missed doses of extended-release capsule as soon as remembered unless more than 14 hrs after scheduled dose; do not double doses. Advise patient to read the *Patient Information* before starting tacrolimus and with each refill in case of changes. Instruct patient to inspect capsules with each new Rx, before taking. Contact health care professional if appearance of capsules or dose has changed.
- Advise patient to avoid grapefruit and grapefruit juice and alcohol during therapy.
- Reinforce the need for lifelong therapy to prevent transplant rejection. Review symptoms of rejection for transplanted organ and stress need to notify health care professional immediately if they occur.
- Advise patient to avoid eating raw oysters or other shellfish; make sure they are fully cooked before eating.
- Instruct patient to notify health care professional if signs of diabetes mellitus (frequent urination, increased thirst or hunger), infection (fever, sweats, chills, cough or flu-like symptoms, muscle aches, warm, red, painful areas on skin), neurotoxicity (vision changes, deliriums, or tremors), or PRES occur.
- Advise patient to wear protective clothing and sunscreen to avoid photosensitivity reactions.
- Instruct patient to avoid exposure to chicken pox, measles, mumps, and rubella. If exposed, see health care professional for prophylactic therapy.
- Instruct patient to notify health care professional of all Rx or OTC medications, vitamins, or herbal products being taken and consult health care professional before taking any new medications.
- Inform patient of the risk of lymphoma or skin cancer with tacrolimus therapy.
- Advise patient of the risk of taking tacrolimus during pregnancy or breast feeding. Caution female patient to notify health care professional if pregnancy is planned or suspected or if breast feeding.
- Emphasize the importance of repeated lab tests during tacrolimus therapy.
- **Topical:** Instruct apply ointment as directed. Advise patient to read the *Medication Guide* prior to starting and with each Rx renewal; new information may be available.
- Advise patient not to bathe, shower, or swim right after applying; may wash off ointment. May use moisturizers with ointment. Instruct patient to check with health care professional first about products to use. If moisturizers are used, apply them after application of ointment.
- Advise patients to contact health care professional if their symptoms do not improve after 6 wk of therapy, if their symptoms worsen, or they develop a skin infection.
- Instruct patient to use ointment only on areas of skin with atopic dermatitis.
- Advise patient to stop using the ointment when the signs/symptoms of atopic dermatitis go away.
- Advise patient to limit sun exposure during treatment.
- Advise patient of the risk of using topical tacrolimus during pregnancy.
- Inform patient of the risk of lymphoma or skin cancer with topical tacrolimus therapy.

Evaluation/Desired Outcomes

- Prevention of transplanted organ rejection.
- Management of atopic dermatitis.

tadalafil (ta-da-la-fil)

Adcirca, Cialis

Classification

Therapeutic: erectile dysfunction agents, vasodilators

Pharmacologic: phosphodiesterase type 5 inhibitors

Pregnancy Category B

Indications

Cialis: Treatment of: Erectile dysfunction (ED), Benign prostatic hyperplasia (BPH), ED and BPH. *Adcirca:* Pulmonary arterial hypertension.

Action

Increases cyclic guanosine monophosphate (cGMP) levels by inhibiting phosphodiesterase type 5 (PDE5) an enzyme responsible for the breakdown of cGMP. cGMP produces smooth muscle relaxation of the corpus cavernosum, which in turn promotes increased blood flow and subsequent erection. cGMP also leads to vasodilation of the pulmonary vasculature. **Therapeutic Effects:** *Cialis:* Enhanced blood flow to the corpus cavernosum and erection sufficient to allow sexual intercourse. Improved signs and symptoms of BPH. *Adcirca:* Improved exercise tolerance.

Pharmacokinetics

Absorption: Well absorbed following oral administration.

Distribution: Extensive tissue distribution; penetrates semen.

Protein Binding: 94%.

Metabolism and Excretion: Mostly metabolized by the liver (mainly CYP3A4 enzyme system); metabolites are excreted in feces (61%) and urine (36%).

Half-life: 17.5 hr.

TIME/ACTION PROFILE (vasodilation, improved erectile function)

ROUTE	ONSET	PEAK	DURATION
PO	rapid	0.5–6 hr	36

Contraindications/Precautions

Contraindicated in: Hypersensitivity; Concurrent use of nitrates or riociguat; Unstable angina, recent history of stroke, life-threatening heart failure within 6 mo, uncontrolled hypertension, arrhythmias, stroke within 6 mo or MI within 90 days; Any other cardiovascular pathology precluding sexual activity; Known hereditary degenerative retinal disorders; Severe hepatic impairment; Severe renal impairment (Adcirca only); Severe renal impairment (CCr <30 mL/min) (Cialis once daily dosing); Congenital or acquired QT interval prolongation or concurrent use of Class IA or III antiarrhythmics; Concurrent use of ketoconazole, itraconazole, or rifampin (Adcirca only); Alpha adrenergic blockers (when tadalafil used for BPH); Women; Pedi: Children or newborns.

Use Cautiously in: Left ventricular outflow obstruction; Penile deformity; Renal impairment; Underlying conditions predisposing to priapism including sickle cell anemia, multiple myeloma, or leukemia; Bleeding disorders or active peptic ulcer disease; Strong inhibitors of the CYP3A4 enzyme system; Alpha adrenergic blockers (patients should be on stable dose of alpha blockers before starting tadalafil for ED); History of sudden severe vision loss or non arteritic ischemic optic neuropathy (NAION); may ↑ risk of recurrence; Low cup to disk ratio, age >50 yr, diabetes, hypertension, coronary artery disease, hyperlipidemia, or smoking (↑ risk of NAION); Geri: May experience more side effects.

Adverse Reactions/Side Effects

CNS: headache. **EENT:** hearing loss, nasal congestion, vision loss. **CV:** hypotension. **GI:** dyspepsia. **GU:** priapism. **Derm:** flushing. **MS:** back pain, limb pain, myalgia.

Interactions

Drug-Drug: Concurrent use of **nitrates** may cause serious, life threatening hypotension and is contraindicated. Concurrent use of **riociguat** may result in severe hypotension; concurrent use contraindicated. ↑ risk of hypotension with **alpha adrenergic blockers** and acute ingestion of **alcohol**; discontinue alpha-adrenergic blocker therapy ≥1 day before starting Cialis for BPH. Strong inhibitors of CYP3A4 including **ritonavir**, **ketoconazole**, **itraconazole** ↑ effects and the risk of adverse reactions (dose adjustments recommended; ketoconazole and itraconazole contraindicated with Adcirca). Similar effects may be expected of other **inhibitors of CY3A4**. **CYP3A4 inducers** may ↓ effects (**rifampin** contraindicated with Adcirca).

Route/Dosage

Cialis (for ED)

PO (Adults): 10 mg prior to sexual activity (range 5–20 mg; not to exceed one dose/24 hr) *or* 2.5 mg once daily (max: 5 mg/day); *Concurrent use of CYP3A4 inhibitors including itraconazole, ketoconazole and ritonavir*—single dose should not exceed 10 mg in any 72 hour period; for once daily dose regimen, should not exceed 2.5 mg/day.

Renal Impairment

PO (Adults): *CCr 30–50 mL/min (as needed dosing)*—Initial dose should not exceed 5 mg/day; maximum dose should not exceed 10 mg in 48 hr; *CCr <30 mL/min (as needed dosing)*—Maximum dose should not exceed 5 mg in 72 hr; *CCr <30 mL/min (once daily dosing)*—Not recommended for use.

Hepatic Impairment

PO (Adults): *Mild or moderate hepatic impairment (Child–Pugh class A or B)*—Daily dose should not exceed 10 mg (once daily dose regimen not recommended) *Severe hepatic impairment (Child–Pugh class C)*—Not recommended for use.

Cialis (for BPH or ED/BPH)

PO (Adults): 5 mg once daily; *Concurrent use of CYP3A4 inhibitors including itraconazole, ketoconazole and ritonavir*—Should not exceed 2.5 mg/day.

Renal Impairment

PO (Adults): *CCr 30–50 mL/min*—Initial dose should not exceed 2.5 mg/day; maximum dose should not exceed 5 mg/day; *CCr <30 mL/min*—Not recommended for use.

Hepatic Impairment

PO (Adults): Not recommended for use.

Adcirca (for pulmonary arterial hypertension)

PO (Adults): 40 mg once daily; *If receiving ritonavir for ≥1 wk*—start 20 mg once daily; may then ↑ to 40 mg once daily based on tolerability; *If initiating ritonavir while on Adcirca*—stop Adcirca ≥24 hr before starting ritonavir; may reinitiate Adcirca at 20 mg once daily after ≥1 wk of therapy with ritonavir; may then ↑ to 40 mg once daily based on tolerability.

Renal Impairment

(Adults): *CCr 31–80 mL/min*—Start 20 mg once daily; may then ↑ to 40 mg once daily based on tolerability.

Hepatic Impairment

PO (Adults): *Mild or moderate hepatic impairment (Child–Pugh class A or B)*—Start with 20 mg once daily.

Availability

Tablets (Cialis): 2.5 mg, 5 mg, 10 mg, 20 mg. **Tablets (Adcirca):** 20 mg.

NURSING IMPLICATIONS

Assessment

- *Cialis: for ED*: Determine ED before administration. Tadalafil has no effect in the absence of sexual stimulation.
- *Cialis for BPH*: Assess for symptoms of prostatic hyperplasia (urinary hesitancy, feeling of incomplete bladder emptying, interruption of urinary stream, impairment of size and force of urinary stream, terminal urinary dribbling, straining to start flow, dysuria, urgency) before and periodically during therapy.
- Digital rectal examinations should be performed before and periodically during therapy for BPH.
- *Adcirca*: Monitor hemodynamic parameters and exercise tolerance prior to and periodically during therapy.

Potential Nursing Diagnoses

Sexual dysfunction (Indications)
Impaired urinary elimination (Indications)
Risk for activity intolerance (Indications)

Implementation

- **PO:** Administer dose *as needed for ED* at least 30 min prior to sexual activity; effectiveness may continue for 36 hr.
- Administer dose for *pulmonary hypertension, BPH, ED/BPH, or daily for ED* once daily at the same time each day.
- May be administered without regard to food. Swallow tablets whole; do not crush, break, or chew.

Patient/Family Teaching

- Instruct patient to take tadalafil as needed for ED at least 30 min before sexual activity and not more than once per day. Inform patient that sexual stimulation is required for an erection to occur after taking tadalafil.
- Advise patient that tadalafil is not indicated for use in women.
- Caution patient not to take tadalafil concurrently with alpha adrenergic blockers (unless on a stable dose) or nitrates. If chest pain occurs after taking tadalafil, instruct patient to seek immediate medical attention.
- Advise patient to avoid excess alcohol intake (≥5 units) in combination with tadalafil; may increase risk of orthostatic hypotension, increased heart rate, decreased standing BP, dizziness, headache.
- Instruct patient to notify health care professional promptly if erection lasts longer than 4 hr, if they are not satisfied with their sexual performance or develop unwanted side effects or if they experience sudden or decreased vision loss in one or both eyes or loss or decrease in hearing, ringing in the ears, or dizziness.
- Advise patient to notify health care professional of all Rx or OTC medications, vitamins, or herbal products being taken and to consult with health care professional before taking other medications.
- Inform patient that tadalafil offers no protection against sexually transmitted diseases. Counsel patient that protection against sexually transmitted diseases and HIV infection should be considered.

Evaluation/Desired Outcomes

- Male erection sufficient to allow intercourse.
- Decrease in urinary symptoms of benign prostatic hyperplasia.
- Increased exercise tolerance.

tamoxifen (ta-mox-i-fen)

~~Nolvadex~~, ✱Nolvadex-D, ✱Tamofen, ✱Tamone, ✱Tamoplex

Classification
Therapeutic: antineoplastics
Pharmacologic: antiestrogens

Pregnancy Category D

Indications

Adjuvant therapy of breast cancer after surgery and radiation (delays recurrence). Palliative or adjunctive treatment of advanced breast cancer. Prevention of breast cancer in high-risk patients. Treatment of ductal carcinoma *in situ* following breast surgery and radiation.

Action

Competes with estrogen for binding sites in breast and other tissues. Reduces DNA synthesis and estrogen response. **Therapeutic Effects:** Suppression of tumor growth. Reduced incidence of breast cancer in high-risk patients.

Pharmacokinetics

Absorption: Absorbed after oral administration.
Distribution: Widely distributed.
Metabolism and Excretion: Mostly metabolized by the liver. Slowly eliminated in the feces. Minimal amounts excreted in the urine.
Half-life: 7 days.

TIME/ACTION PROFILE (tumor response)

ROUTE	ONSET	PEAK	DURATION
PO	4–10 wk	several mo	several wk

Contraindications/Precautions

Contraindicated in: Hypersensitivity; Concurrent warfarin therapy with history of deep vein thrombosis (patients at high risk for breast cancer only); OB, Lactation: Pregnancy or lactation.
Use Cautiously in: ↓ bone marrow reserve; Women with childbearing potential.

Adverse Reactions/Side Effects

CNS: STROKE, confusion, depression, headache, weakness. **EENT:** blurred vision. **CV:** THROMBOEMBOLISM, edema. **GI:** nausea, vomiting. **GU:** UTERINE MALIGNANCIES, vaginal bleeding. **F and E:** hypercalcemia. **Hemat:** leukopenia, thrombocytopenia. **Metab:** hot flashes. **MS:** bone pain. **Misc:** tumor flare.

Interactions

Drug-Drug: Estrogens may ↓ effectiveness of concurrently administered tamoxifen. Blood levels are ↑ by **bromocriptine**. May ↑ the anticoagulant effect of **warfarin**. Risk of thromboembolic events is ↑ by concurrent use of other **antineoplastics**.

Route/Dosage

Treatment of Breast Cancer

PO (Adults): 10–20 mg twice daily; doses of 20 mg/day may be taken as a single dose.

Prevention of Breast Cancer/Ductal Carcinoma *in situ*

PO (Adults): 20 mg once daily for 5 yr.

Availability (generic available)

Tablets: 10 mg, 20 mg. **Enteric-coated tablets:** ✱20 mg.

NURSING IMPLICATIONS

Assessment

- Assess for an increase in bone or tumor pain. Confer with health care professional regarding analgesics. This transient pain usually resolves despite continued therapy.
- ***Lab Test Considerations:*** Monitor CBC, platelets, and calcium levels before and during therapy. May cause transient hypercalcemia in patients with metastases to the bone. An estrogen receptor assay should be assessed before initiation of therapy.
- Monitor serum cholesterol and triglyceride concentrations in patients with pre-existing hyperlipidemia. May cause ↑ concentrations.
- Monitor hepatic function tests and thyroxine (T_4) periodically during therapy. May cause ↑ serum hepatic enzyme and thyroxine concentrations.
- Gynecologic examinations should be performed regularly; may cause variations in Papanicolaou and vaginal smears.

Potential Nursing Diagnoses

Deficient knowledge, related to medication regimen (Patient/Family Teaching)

Implementation

- **PO:** Administer with food or fluids if GI irritation becomes a problem. Consult health care professional if patient vomits shortly after administration of medication to determine need for repeat dose.
- Do not crush, break, chew, or administer an antacid within 1–2 hr of enteric-coated tablet.

Patient/Family Teaching

- Instruct patient to take medication as directed. If a dose is missed, it should be omitted.
- If skin lesions are present, inform patient that lesions may temporarily increase in size and number and may have increased erythema.
- Advise patient to report bone pain to health care professional promptly. This pain may be severe. Analgesics should be ordered to control pain. Inform

T

patient that this may be an indication of the drug's effectiveness and will resolve over time.

- Instruct patient to monitor weight weekly. Weight gain or peripheral edema should be reported to health care professional.
- Advise patient that medication may cause hot flashes. Notify health care professional if these become bothersome.
- Instruct patient to notify health care professional promptly if pain or swelling of legs, shortness of breath, weakness, sleepiness, confusion, nausea, vomiting, weight gain, dizziness, headache, loss of appetite, or blurred vision occurs. Patient should also report menstrual irregularities, vaginal bleeding, pelvic pain or pressure.
- This medication may induce ovulation and may have teratogenic properties. Advise patient to use a nonhormonal method of contraception during and for 1 mo after the therapy.

Evaluation/Desired Outcomes

- Decrease in the size or spread of breast cancer. Observable effects of therapy may not be seen for 4–10 wk after initiation.

tamsulosin (tam-soo-loe-sin)

Flomax

Classification

Therapeutic: none assigned

Pharmacologic: peripherally acting antiadrenergics

Pregnancy Category B

Indications

Management of signs/symptoms of benign prostatic hyperplasia (BPH).

Action

Decreases contractions in smooth muscle of the prostatic capsule by preferentially binding to alpha$_1$-adrenergic receptors. **Therapeutic Effects:** Decreased symptoms of prostatic hyperplasia (urinary urgency, hesitancy, nocturia).

Pharmacokinetics

Absorption: Slowly absorbed after oral administration.

Distribution: Widely distributed.

Protein Binding: 94–99%.

Metabolism and Excretion: Extensively metabolized by the liver; <10% excreted unchanged in urine.

Half-life: 14 hr.

TIME/ACTION PROFILE (↑ in urine flow)

ROUTE	ONSET	PEAK	DURATION
PO	unknown	2 wk	unknown

Contraindications/Precautions

Contraindicated in: Hypersensitivity.

Use Cautiously in: Patients at risk for prostate carcinoma (symptoms may be similar); Patients undergoing cataract surgery (↑ risk of intraoperative floppy iris syndrome); Sulfa allergy.

Adverse Reactions/Side Effects

CNS: dizziness, headache. **EENT:** intraoperative floppy iris syndrome, rhinitis. **CV:** orthostatic hypotension. **GU:** priapism, retrograde/diminished ejaculation.

Interactions

Drug-Drug: Cimetidine may ↑ blood levels and the risk of toxicity. ↑ risk of hypotension with other peripherally acting anti-adrenergics (**doxazosin**, **prazosin**, **terazosin**); concurrent use should be avoided. ↑ risk of hypotension with **sildenafil**, **tadalafil**, and **vardenafil**. Strong **CYP3A4 inhibitors** and **CYP2D6 inhibitors** may ↑ blood levels (concurrent use should be avoided.

Route/Dosage

PO (Adults): 0.4 mg once daily after a meal; may be ↑ after 2–4 wk to 0.8 mg/day.

Availability (generic available)

Capsules: 0.4 mg. **Cost:** *Generic*—$26.89/100. ***In combination with:*** dutasteride (Jalyn); see Appendix B.

NURSING IMPLICATIONS

Assessment

- Assess patient for symptoms of BPH (urinary hesitancy, feeling of incomplete bladder emptying, interruption of urinary stream, impairment of size and force of urinary stream, terminal urinary dribbling, straining to start flow, dysuria, urgency) before and periodically during therapy.
- Assess patient for first-dose orthostatic hypotension and syncope. Incidence may be dose related. Observe patient closely during this period and take precautions to prevent injury.
- Monitor intake and output ratios and daily weight, and assess for edema daily, especially at beginning of therapy. Report weight gain or edema.
- Rectal exams prior to and periodically throughout therapy to assess prostate size are recommended.

Potential Nursing Diagnoses

Risk for injury (Side Effects)

Impaired urinary elimination (Indications)

Implementation

- **PO:** Administer daily dose 30 min after the same meal each day. Swallow capsules whole; do not open, crush, or chew.
- If dose is interrupted for several days at either the 0.4-mg or 0.8-mg dose, restart therapy with the 0.4-mg/day dose.

Patient/Family Teaching

- Emphasize the importance of continuing to take this medication, even if feeling well. Instruct patient to take medication at the same time each day. If a dose is missed, take as soon as remembered unless almost time for next dose. Do not double doses.
- May cause dizziness. Advise patient to avoid driving or other activities requiring alertness until response to medication is known.
- Caution patient to change positions slowly to minimize orthostatic hypotension.
- Instruct patient to notify health care professional of all Rx or OTC medications, vitamins, or herbal products being taken and consult health care professional before taking any new medications, especially cough, cold, or allergy remedies.
- Emphasize the importance of follow-up visits to determine effectiveness of therapy.

Evaluation/Desired Outcomes

- Decrease in urinary symptoms of BPH.

REMS

tapentadol (ta-pen-ta-dol)

Nucynta, ✱Nucynta IR, Nucynta ER

Classification

Therapeutic: analgesics (centrally acting), opioid analgesics

Pharmacologic: opioid agonists

Schedule II

Pregnancy Category C

Indications

Management of moderate to severe pain. Moderate to severe chronic pain in opioid-tolerant patients requiring use of daily, around-the-clock long-term opioid treatment and for which alternative treatment options are inadequate (extended-release). Diabetic pain associated with diabetic peripheral neuropathy in patients requiring around-the-clock opioid analgesia for an extended time.

Action

Acts as μ-opioid receptor agonist. Also inhibits the reuptake of norepinephrine. **Therapeutic Effects:** Decrease in pain severity.

Pharmacokinetics

Absorption: 32% absorbed following oral administration.

Distribution: Widely distributed.

Metabolism and Excretion: Undergoes extensive first-pass hepatic metabolism (97%); metabolites have no analgesic activity; metabolized drug is 99% renally excreted.

Half-life: 4 hr.

TIME/ACTION PROFILE (analgesic effect)

ROUTE	ONSET	PEAK	DURATION
PO	unknown	1 hr	4–6 hr

Contraindications/Precautions

Contraindicated in: Hypersensitivity; Significant respiratory depression in unmonitored settings or where resuscitative equipment is not readily available; Paralytic ileus; Severe hepatic or renal impairment; Concurrent MAO inhibitors or use of MAO inhibitors in the preceding 2 wk; Acute or severe bronchial asthma; Acute, mild, intermittent, or postoperative pain (extended-release only); Pedi: Safety not established.

Use Cautiously in: Conditions associated with hypoxia, hypercapnea, or ↓ respiratory reserve including asthma, chronic obstructive pulmonary disease, cor pulmonale, extreme obesity, sleep apnea syndrome, myxedema, kyphoscoliosis, CNS depression, use of other CNS depressants or coma (↑ risk of further respiratory depression); use smallest effective dose; History of substance abuse or addiction disorder; Seizure disorders; Moderate hepatic impairment; Geri: Geriatric or debilitated patients (↑ risk of respiratory depression; dose ↓ suggested); OB, Lactation: Avoid chronic use; prolonged use of extended-release tapentadol during pregnancy can result in neonatal opioid withdrawal syndrome.

Adverse Reactions/Side Effects

CNS: SEIZURES, dizziness, headache, somnolence. **Resp:** RESPIRATORY DEPRESSION. **CV:** hypotension. **GI:** diarrhea, nausea, vomiting. **Misc:** ANAPHYLAXIS, ANGIOEDEMA.

Interactions

Drug-Drug: Concurrent **MAO inhibitors** or use of MAO inhibitors in the preceding 2 wk can result in potentially life-threatening adverse cardiovascular reactions due to additive effects on norepinephrine levels. Concurrent use of other **CNS depressants** including **sedative/hypnotics**, **alcohol**, **antihistamines**, **antidepressants**, **phenothiazines**, and other **opioids** ↑ risk of further CNS depression; consider dose ↓ of one or both agents. **Alcohol** may ↑ levels and ↑ the risk of toxicity. ↑ risk of serotonin syndrome with **SNRIs**, **SSRIs**, **triptans**, **tricyclic antidepressants**, and **MAO inihibitors**.

Route/Dosage

When switching from immediate-release to extended-release product, the same total daily dose can be used.

PO (Adults): *Immediate-release or oral solution*—50 mg, 75 mg, or 100 mg initially, then every 4–6 hr as

T

needed and tolerated. If pain control is not achieved within first hour of first dose, additional dose may be given. Doses should not exceed 700 mg on the first day or 600 mg/day thereafter; *Extended-release*—50 twice daily; titrate dose up to 100–250 mg twice daily (not to exceed dose of 500 mg/day).

Hepatic Impairment

PO (Adults): *Moderate hepatic impairment*—Immediate release or oral solution: 50 mg every 8 hr initially, then titrate to maintain analgesia without intolerable side effects; Extended-release: 50 mg once daily; may titrate up to maximum dose of 100 mg once daily, if needed.

Availability

Immediate-release tablets: 50 mg, 75 mg, 100 mg. **Extended-release tablets:** 50 mg, 100 mg, 150 mg, 200 mg, 250 mg. **Oral solution:** 20 mg/mL.

NURSING IMPLICATIONS

Assessment

- Assess type, location, and intensity of pain before and 1 hr (peak) after administration.
- Assess BP and respiratory rate before and periodically during administration. Monitor for respiratory depression especially during initial dosing and with patients at increased risk.
- Assess bowel function routinely. Prevention of constipation should be instituted with increased intake of fluids and bulk and with laxatives to minimize constipating effects. Administer stimulant laxatives routinely if opioid use exceeds 2–3 days, unless contraindicated.
- Prolonged use may lead to physical and psychological dependence and tolerance, although these may be milder than with opioids. This should not prevent patient from receiving adequate analgesia. Most patients who receive tapentadol for pain do not develop psychological dependence.
- Monitor patient for seizures. May occur within recommended dose range. Risk is increased in patients with a history of seizures and in patients taking antidepressants (SSRIs, SNRIs, tricyclics) or other drugs that decrease the seizure threshold.
- Monitor for serotonin syndrome (mental-status changes [agitation, hallucinations, coma]), autonomic instability [tachycardia, labile BP, hyperthermia], neuromuscular aberrations [hyperreflexia, incoordination] and/or gastrointestinal symptoms [nausea, vomiting, diarrhea] in patients taking SSRIs, SNRIs, triptans, tricyclic antidepressants, or MAO inhibitors concurrently with tapentadol.
- Assess risk for opioid addiction, abuse, or misuse prior to administration. Abuse or misuse of extended-release preparations by crushing, chewing, snorting, or injecting dissolved product will result in uncontrolled delivery of tapentatol and can result in overdose and death.
- ***Toxicity and Overdose:*** Overdose may cause respiratory depression. Naloxone (Narcan) may reverse some, but not all, of the symptoms of overdose. Treatment should be symptomatic and supportive. Maintain adequate respiratory exchange.

Potential Nursing Diagnoses

Acute pain (Indications)
Chronic pain (Indications)
Risk for injury (Side Effects)

Implementation

- Initial immediate-release dose of 50 mg, 75 mg, or 100 mg is individualized based on pain severity, previous experience with similar drugs, and ability to monitor patient. Second dose may be administered as soon as 1 hr after first dose if adequate pain relief is not obtained with first dose.
- **PO:** Tapentadol may be administered without regard to meals.
- Swallow extended-release tablets whole; do not crush, break or chew.
- Use calibrated syringe to administer correct dose of oral solution.

Patient/Family Teaching

- Instruct patient on how and when to ask for and take pain medication and to take tapentadol as directed; do not adjust dose without consulting health care professional. Report breakthrough pain and adverse reactions to health care professional. Do not take tapentadol if pain is mild or can be controlled with other pain medications such as NSAIDs or acetaminophen. Do not stop abruptly; may cause withdrawal symptoms (anxiety, sweating, insomina, rigors, pain, nausea, tremors, diarrhea, upper respiratory symptoms, hallucinations). Decrease dose gradually. Advise patient to read the *Medication Guide* prior to taking tapentadol and with each Rx refill, in case of changes.
- Advise patient that tapentadol is a drug with known abuse potential. Protect it from theft, and never give to anyone other than the individual for whom it was prescribed; may be dangerous.
- May cause dizziness and drowsiness. Caution patient to avoid driving or other activities requiring alertness until response to medication is known.
- Inform patient that tapentadol may cause seizures. Stop taking tapentadol and notify health care professional immediately if seizures occur.
- Advise patient to change positions slowly to minimize orthostatic hypotension.
- Caution patient to avoid concurrent use of alcohol or other CNS depressants with this medication.
- Instruct patient to notify health care professional of all Rx or OTC medications, vitamins, or herbal products being taken and consult health care professional before taking any new medications.
- Advise patient to notify health care professional if signs of serotonin syndrome occur.

- Encourage patient to turn, cough, and breathe deeply every 2 hr to prevent atelectasis.
- Advise female patients to notify health care professional if pregnancy is planned or suspected, or if breast feeding.

Evaluation/Desired Outcomes

- Decrease in severity of pain without a significant alteration in level of consciousness or respiratory status.

tedizolid (ted-eye-**zoe**-lid)

Sivextro

Classification
Therapeutic: anti-infectives
Pharmacologic: oxazolidinones

Pregnancy Category C

Indications

Treatment of acute bacterial skin and skin structure infections (ABSSSI).

Action

Inhibits bacterial protein synthesis at the level of the 23S ribosome of the 50S subunit. **Therapeutic Effects:** Bacteriostatic action against enterococci, staphylococci and streptococci, resulting is resolution of infection. **Spectrum:** Active against *Staphylococcus aureus* including methicillin-resistant strains (MRSA), *Streptococcus pyogens*, *Streptococcus agalactiae*, *Streptococcus anginosus* Group (including *Streptococcus anginosus*, *Streptococcus intermedius*, *Streptococcus constellatus*) and *Enterococcus faecalis*.

Pharmacokinetics

Absorption: IV administration results in complete bioavailability; well absorbed (91%) following oral administration, rapidly converted by phosphatases to its active form.

Distribution: Penetrates interstitial fluid space of adipose and skeletal muscle resulting in similar levels to plasma.

Metabolism and Excretion: Eliminated via liver with inactive metabolites excreted in feces (82%) and urine (18%); <3% excreted unchanged in urine or feces.

Half-life: 12 hr.

TIME/ACTION PROFILE (blood levels)

ROUTE	ONSET	PEAK	DURATION
PO	unknown	2.5 hr	24 hr
IV	rapid	end of infusion	24 hr

Contraindications/Precautions

Contraindicated in: Uncontrolled HTN, pheochromocytoma, thyrotoxicosis, or concurrent use of sympathomimetic agents, vasopressors, or dopaminergic agents (↑ risk of hypertensive response); Concurrent or recent (<2 wk) use of monoamine oxidase (MAO) inhibitors (↑ risk of hypertensive response); Carcinoid syndrome or concurrent use of SSRIs, TCAs, triptans, meperidine, or buspirone (↑ risk of serotonin syndrome).

Use Cautiously in: Neutropenia (safety and efficacy not established if WBC <1000 cells/mm^3); OB: Use in pregnancy only in potential maternal benefit justifies potential risk to fetus; Lactation: Use cautiously if breast feeding; Pedi: Safe and effective use in children <18 yr has not been established.

Adverse Reactions/Side Effects

CNS: dizziness, headache. **GI:** CLOSTRIDIUM DIFFICILE-ASSOCIATED DIARRHEA (CDAD), nausea, diarrhea, vomiting.

Interactions

Drug-Drug: ↑ risk of hypertensive response with **MAO inhibitors**, **sympathomimetics** (e.g., **pseudoephedrine**), **vasopressors** (e.g., **epinephrine**, **norepinephrine**), and **dopaminergic agents** (e.g., **dopamine**, **dobutamine**); concurrent or recent use should be avoided. ↑ risk of serotonin syndrome with **SSRIs**, **TCAs**, **triptans**, **meperidine**, **bupropion**, or **buspirone**; avoid concurrent use.

Route/Dosage

PO, IV (Adults): 200 mg once daily for six days.

Availability

Tablets: 200 mg. **Lyophilized powder for intravenous injection (requires reconstitution):** 200 mg/vial.

NURSING IMPLICATIONS

Assessment

- Assess for infection (vital signs; appearance of wound, sputum, urine, and stool; WBC) at beginning of and during therapy.
- Obtain specimens for culture and sensitivity prior to initiating therapy. First dose may be given before receiving.
- Monitor bowel function. Diarrhea, abdominal cramping, fever, and bloody stools should be reported to health care professional promptly as a sign of Clostridium difficile-associated diarrhea (CDAD). May begin up to several mo following cessation of therapy.

T

- ***Lab Test Considerations:*** Consider alternate therapies in patients with neutrophil counts <1000 cells/mm^3.
- May cause anemia.

Potential Nursing Diagnoses

Risk for infection (Indications)
Diarrhea (Adverse Reactions)

Implementation

- Dose adjustment is not necessary when switching from IV to oral dose.
- **PO:** May be administered with or without food.

IV Administration

- **Intermittent Infusion:** Reconstitute each vial with 4 mL of Sterile Water for Injection. Gently swirl and let vial stand until completely dissolved; avoid shaking. ***Diluent:*** Dilute further with 250 mL of 0.9% NaCl by slowing injecting reconstituted solution into 250 mL bag. Gently invert bag to mix; avoid shaking to minimize foaming. Solution is clear and colorless to pale yellow; do not administer solutions that are discolored or contain particulate material. Must be used within 24 hrs of reconstitution at room temperature or under refrigeration. ***Rate:*** Infuse over 1 hr.
- **Y-Site Incompatibility:** solutions containing calcium or magnesium, Lactated Ringer's, Hartmann's solution.

Patient/Family Teaching

- Advise patients taking oral tedizolid to take as directed, for full course of therapy, even if feeling better. Take missed doses as soon as remembered up to 8 hrs before next dose; if less than 8 hrs before next dose, wait until next scheduled dose. Do not double dose.
- Advise patient to notify health care professional of all Rx or OTC medications, vitamins, or herbal products being taken and to consult with health care professional before taking other medications.
- Instruct patient to notify health care professional if changes in vision occur or immediately if diarrhea, abdominal cramping, fever, or bloody stools occur and not to treat with antidiarrheals without consulting health care professionals.
- Advise female patient to notify health care professional if pregnancy is planned or suspected or if breast feeding.
- Advise patient to notify health care professional if no improvement is seen in a few days.

Evaluation/Desired Outcomes

- Resolution of signs and symptoms of infection. Length of time for complete resolution depends on organism and site of infection.

REMS

telavancin (tel-a-van-sin)

Vibativ

Classification
Therapeutic: anti-infectives
Pharmacologic: lipoglycopeptides

Pregnancy Category C

Indications

Treatment of complicated skin/skin structure infections caused by susceptible bacteria. Hospital-acquired and ventilator-associated bacterial pneumonia caused by *Staphylococcus aureus*.

Action

Inhibits bacterial cell wall synthesis by interfering with the polymerization and cross-linking of peptidoglycan. **Therapeutic Effects:** Bactericidal action against susceptible organisms. **Spectrum:** Active against *Staphylococcus aureus* (including methicillin-susceptible and -resistant strains), *Streptococcus pyogenes*, *Streptococcus agalactiae*, *Streptococcus anginosus* (including *S. anginosus*, *S. intermedius*, and *S. constellatus*), and *Enterococcus faecalis* (vancomycin-susceptible strains only).

Pharmacokinetics

Absorption: IV administration results in complete bioavailability.
Distribution: Penetrates blister fluid.
Metabolism and Excretion: Metabolism is not known; 76% excreted unchanged in urine <1% in feces.
Half-life: 8 hr.

TIME/ACTION PROFILE

ROUTE	ONSET	PEAK	DURATION
IV	unknown	end of infusion	24 hr

Contraindications/Precautions

Contraindicated in: Hypersensitivity; Congenital long QT syndrome, known prolongation of the QT interval, uncompensated HF, or severe left ventricular hypertrophy (risk of fatal arrhythmias); Concurrent use of unfractionated heparin (aPTT may be falsely ↑ for up to 18 hr after telavancin therapy); OB: Do not use unless potential maternal benefit outweighs potential risk to fetus.
Use Cautiously in: Renal impairment (efficacy may be ↓ dose ↓ recommended for CCr ≤50 mL/min) (↑ risk of mortality in patients with CCr ≤50 mL/min; use only if benefit outweighs risk) (↑ risk of renal impairment); Diabetes, HF, hypertension (↑ risk of renal impairment); Geri: Consider age-related ↓ in renal function, adjust dose accordingly (↑ risk of adverse renal reactions); Lactation: Use cautiously; Pedi: Safety and effectiveness not established.

Adverse Reactions/Side Effects

CNS: dizziness. **CV:** QT interval prolongation. **GI:** CLOSTRIDIUM DIFFICILE-ASSOCIATED DIARRHEA (CDAD), taste disturbance, nausea, vomiting, abdominal pain. **GU:** foamy urine, nephrotoxicity. **Misc:** ANAPHYLAXIS, infusion reactions.

Interactions

Drug-Drug: Concurrent use of other **medications known to prolong QT interval** may ↑ risk of arrhythmias. Concurrent use of **NSAIDs, ACE inhibitors**, and **loop diuretics** may ↑ risk of adverse renal effects.

Route/Dosage

Complicated Skin/Skin Structure Infections

IV (Adults): 10 mg/kg ever 24 hr for 7–14 days.

Hospital-Acquired/Ventilator-Associated Bacterial Pneumonia

IV (Adults): 10 mg/kg ever 24 hr for 7–21 days.

Renal Impairment

IV (Adults): *CCr 30–50 mL/min*—7.5 mg/kg every 24 hr; *CCr 10–≤30 mL/min*—10 mg/kg every 48 hr.

Availability

Sterile lyophilized powder for IV use (requires reconstitution): 250 mg/vial, 750 mg/vial.

NURSING IMPLICATIONS

Assessment

- Assess for infection (vital signs; appearance of wound, sputum, urine, and stool; WBC) at beginning of and throughout therapy.
- Obtain specimens for culture and sensitivity prior to therapy. First dose may be given before receiving results.
- Rep: Assess women of child bearing age for pregnancy. Women should have a negative serum pregnancy test before starting telavancin.
- Monitor bowel function. Diarrhea, abdominal cramping, fever, and bloody stools should be reported to health care professional promptly as a sign of Clostridium difficile-associated diarrhea (CDAD). May begin up to several weeks following cessation of therapy.
- Monitor for infusion reactions (Red-man syndrome—flushing of upper body, urticaria, pruritus, rash). May resolve with stopping or slowing infusion.
- Observe patient for signs and symptoms of anaphylaxis (rash, pruritus, laryngeal edema, wheezing). Discontinue drug and notify health care professional immediately if symptoms occur. Keep epinephrine, an antihistamine, and resuscitation equipment close by in case of anaphylactic reaction.
- ***Lab Test Considerations:*** Monitor renal function (serum creatinine, creatinine clearance) prior to, every 48–72 hrs during, and at the end of therapy. May cause nephrotoxicity. If renal function decreases, reassess need for telavancin.
- May interfere with prothrombin time, INR, aPTT, activated clotting time, and coagulation based factor Xa tests. Collect blood samples for theses tests as close to next dose of telavancin as possible.
- Interferes with urine qualitative dipstick protein assays and quantitative dye methods; may use microalbumin assays.

Potential Nursing Diagnoses

Risk for infection (Indications)
Diarrhea (Adverse Reactions)

Implementation

IV Administration

- **Intermittent Infusion:** Reconstitute the 250 mg vial with 15 mL and the 750 mg vial with 45 mL of D5W, sterile water for injection, or 0.9% NaCl for concentrations of 15 mg/mL. Reconstitution time is usually under 2 min but may require up to 20 min. Mix thoroughly with contents dissolved completely. Do not administer solution that is discolored or contains particulate matter. Discard vial if vacuum did not pull diluent into vial. Time in vial plus time in bag should not exceed 4 hr at room temperature or 72 hr if refrigerated. ***Diluent:*** For doses of 150–800 mg dilute further with 100–250 mL of D5W, 0.9% NaCl, or LR. ***Concentration:*** For doses <150 mg or >800 mg dilute for a final concentration of 0.6–8 mg/mL. ***Rate:*** Administer over at least 60 min to minimize infusion reactions. Flush line with D5W, 0.9% NaCl, or LR before and after administration.
- **Y-Site Compatibility:** amphotericin B lipid complex, ampicillin/sulbactam, azithromycin, calcium gluconate, caspofungin, cefepime, ceftazidime, ceftriaxone, ciprofloxacin, dexamethasone, diltiazem, dobutamine, dopamine, doripenem, doxycycline, ertapenem, famotidine, fluconazole, gentamicin, hydrocortisone, labetalol, magnesium sulfate, mannitol, meropenem, metoclopramide, milrinone, norepinephrine, ondansetron, pantoprazole, phenylephrine, piperacillin/tazobactam, potassium chloride, potassium phosphates, ranitidine, sodium bicarbonate, sodium phosphates, tigecycline, tobramycin, vasopressin.
- **Y-Site Incompatibility:** amphotericin B colloidal, amphotericin B liposome, digoxin, esomeprazole, furosemide, levofloxacin, micafungin.

T

Patient/Family Teaching

- Instruct patient to notify health care professional immediately if diarrhea, abdominal cramping, fever, or bloody stools occur and not to treat with antidiarrheals without consulting health care professionals.
- Inform patient that common side effects include taste disturbance, nausea, vomiting, headache and foamy urine. Notify health care professional if signs of infusion reaction occur.
- Instruct patient to notify health care professional of all Rx or OTC medications, vitamins, or herbal products being taken and consult health care professional before taking any new medications.
- Rep: Advise female patients to use effective contraception during therapy and to notify health care professional if pregnancy is suspected. Encourage pregnant patients to enroll in the VIBATIV pregnancy registry by calling 1-855-633-8479.
- Instruct the patient to notify health care professional if symptoms do not improve.

Evaluation/Desired Outcomes

- Resolution of the signs and symptoms of infection. Length of time for complete resolution depends on the organism and site of infection.

---

telmisartan, See ANGIOTENSIN II RECEPTOR ANTAGONISTS.

---

temazepam (tem-az-a-pam)

Restoril

Classification

Therapeutic: sedative/hypnotics

Pharmacologic: benzodiazepines

Schedule IV

Pregnancy Category X

Indications

Short-term management of insomnia (<4 weeks).

Action

Acts at many levels in the CNS, producing generalized depression. Effects may be mediated by GABA, an inhibitory neurotransmitter. **Therapeutic Effects:** Relief of insomnia.

Pharmacokinetics

Absorption: Well absorbed after oral administration.

Distribution: Widely distributed; crosses blood-brain barrier. Probably crosses the placenta and enters breast milk. Accumulation of drug occurs with chronic dosing.

Protein Binding: 96%.

Metabolism and Excretion: Metabolized by the liver.

Half-life: 10–20 hr.

TIME/ACTION PROFILE (sedation)

ROUTE	ONSET	PEAK	DURATION
PO	30 min	2–3 hr	6–8 hr

Contraindications/Precautions

Contraindicated in: Hypersensitivity; Cross-sensitivity with other benzodiazepines may exist; Pre-existing CNS depression; Severe uncontrolled pain; Angle-closure glaucoma; Impaired respiratory function; Sleep apnea; OB: Neonates born to mothers taking temazepam may experience withdrawal effects; Lactation: Infants may become sedated. Discontinue drug or bottle feed.

Use Cautiously in: Pre-existing hepatic dysfunction; History of suicide attempt or drug addiction; Geri: Elderly patients have increased sensitivity to benzodiazepines. Appears on Beers list and is associated with increased risk of falls (↓ dose required).

Adverse Reactions/Side Effects

CNS: abnormal thinking, behavior changes, hangover, dizziness, drowsiness, hallucinations, lethargy, paradoxic excitation, sleep—driving. **EENT:** blurred vision. **GI:** constipation, diarrhea, nausea, vomiting. **Derm:** rash. **Misc:** physical dependence, psychological dependence, tolerance.

Interactions

Drug-Drug: ↑ CNS depression with **alcohol**, **antidepressants**, **antihistamines**, **opioid analgesics**, and other **sedative/hypnotics**. May ↓ efficacy of **levodopa**. **Rifampin** or **smoking** ↑ metabolism and may ↓ effectiveness of temazepam. **Probenecid** may prolong effects of temazepam. Sedative effects may be ↓ by **theophylline**.

Drug-Natural Products: Concomitant use of **kava-kava**, **valerian**, **skullcap**, **chamomile**, or **hops** can ↑ CNS depression.

Route/Dosage

PO (Adults): 15–30 mg at bedtime initially if needed; some patients may require only 7.5 mg.

PO (Geriatric Patients or Debilitated Patients): 7.5 mg at bedtime.

Availability (generic available)

Capsules: 7.5 mg, 15 mg, 22.5 mg, 30 mg. **Cost:** *Generic*—7.5 mg $995.03/100, 15 mg $73.45/100, 22.5 mg $298.21/30, 30 mg $88.45/100.

NURSING IMPLICATIONS

Assessment

- Assess mental status (orientation, mood, behavior) and potential for abuse prior to administering medication.
- Assess sleep patterns before and periodically throughout therapy.
- Prolonged high-dose therapy may lead to psychological or physical dependence. Restrict amount of

drug available to patient, especially if patient is depressed or suicidal or has a history of addiction.

- Geri: Assess CNS effects and risk of falls. Institute falls prevention strategies.

Potential Nursing Diagnoses

Insomnia (Indications)
Risk for falls (Side Effects)

Implementation

- Do not confuse Restoril (temazepam) with Risperdal (risperidone).
- Supervise ambulation and transfer of patients after administration. Remove cigarettes. Side rails should be raised and call bell within reach at all times.
- **PO:** Administer with food if GI irritation becomes a problem.

Patient/Family Teaching

- Instruct patient to take temazepam as directed. Teach sleep hygiene techniques (dark room, quiet, bedtime ritual, limit daytime napping, avoidance of nicotine and caffeine). If less effective after a few weeks, consult health care professional; do not increase dose.
- May cause daytime drowsiness or dizziness. Caution patient to avoid driving or other activities requiring alertness until response to medication is known. Geri: Instruct patient and family how to reduce falls risk at home.
- Advise patient to avoid the use of alcohol and other CNS depressants and to consult health care professional before using OTC preparations that contain antihistamines or alcohol.
- Caution patient that complex sleep-related behaviors (sleep-driving, making phone calls, preparing and eating food, having sex, sleep walking) may occur while asleep. Inform patient to notify health care professional if sleep-related behaviors, (may include sleep-driving—driving while not fully awake after ingestion of a sedative-hypnotic product, with no memory of the event) occur.
- Emphasize the importance of follow-up appointments to monitor progress.
- Refer for psychotherapy if ineffective coping is basis for sleep pattern disturbance.
- Advise patient to take temazepam only if able to devote 8 hr to sleep.
- Advise patient to inform health care professional if pregnancy is planned or suspected and to avoid breast feeding while taking temazepam.

Evaluation/Desired Outcomes

- Improvement in sleep pattern with decreased number of nighttime awakenings, improved sleep onset, and increased total sleep time, which may not be noticeable until the 3rd day of therapy.

tenecteplase, See THROMBOLYTIC AGENTS.

tenofovir (te-noe-fo-veer)

Viread

Classification
Therapeutic: antiretrovirals
Pharmacologic: nucleoside reverse transcriptase inhibitors

Pregnancy Category B

Indications

HIV infection (with other antiretrovirals). Chronic hepatitis B.

Action

Active drug (tenofovir) is phosphorylated intracellularly; tenofovir diphosphate inhibits HIV reverse transcriptase resulting in disruption of DNA synthesis. **Therapeutic Effects:** Slowed progression of HIV infection and decreased occurrence of sequelae. Increased CD4 cell count and decreased viral load. Decreased progression/sequelae of chronic hepatitis B infection.

Pharmacokinetics

Absorption: Tenofovir disoproxil fumarate is a prodrug, which is split into tenofovir, the active component.
Distribution: Absorption is enhanced by food.
Metabolism and Excretion: 70–80% excreted unchanged in urine by glomerular filtration and active tubular secretion.
Half-life: Unknown.

TIME/ACTION PROFILE (blood levels)

ROUTE	ONSET	PEAK	DURATION
PO	unknown	2 hr*	24 hr

*When taken with food.

Contraindications/Precautions

Contraindicated in: Hypersensitivity; Concurrent use of antiretroviral combination products containing tenofovir; Concurrent or recent use of NSAIDs (↑ risk of acute renal failure); Lactation: HIV-infected women should not breast feed.
Use Cautiously in: Co-infection with HIV and chronic hepatitis B; Obesity, women, prolonged nucleoside exposure (may be risk factors for lactic acidosis/hepatomegaly); Renal impairment (↑ dosing interval if CCr <50 mL/min); History of pathologic bone fractures or at risk for osteopenia; OB: Has been used safely; Pedi: Children <2 yr (safety not established).

T

Adverse Reactions/Side Effects

CNS: depression, headache, weakness. **Endo:** fat redistibution. **GI:** HEPATOMEGALY, (with steatosis), diarrhea, nausea, abdominal pain, anorexia, vomiting, flatulence. **GU:** ACUTE RENAL FAILURE/FANCONI SYNDROME, proximal renal tubulopathy, renal impairment. **F and E:** LACTIC ACIDOSIS, hypophosphatemia. **Derm:** rash. **MS:** bone pain, ↓ bone mineral density, muscle pain, osteomalacia. **Misc:** immune reconstitution syndrome.

Interactions

Drug-Drug: May ↑ **didanosine** levels; ↓ didanosine dose. Blood levels may be ↑ by **cidofovir, acyclovir, ganciclovir**, or **valganciclovir**. Risk of renal toxicity ↑ by other **nephrotoxic agents**. Combination therapy with **atazanavir** may lead to ↓ virologic response and possible resistance to atazanavir (small amounts of **ritonavir** may be added to boost blood levels); may also ↑ tenofovir levels. **Lopinavir/ritonavir** may ↑ levels. Concurrent use with **adefovir** for chronic hepatitis B infection should be avoided. Concurrent use with **NSAIDs** may ↑ risk of acute renal failure.

Route/Dosage

HIV

PO (Adults and Children ≥12 yr and ≥35 kg): 300 mg once daily.

Renal Impairment

PO (Adults): *CCr 30–49 mL/min*—300 mg every 48 hr; *CCr 10–29 mL/min*—300 mg every 72–96 hr; *Hemodialysis*—300 mg every 7 days following dialysis.

PO (Children 2–11 yr and ≥17 kg): Tablets: *≥35 kg*—300 mg once daily; *28–34.9 kg*—250 mg once daily; *22–27.9 kg*—200 mg once daily; *17–21.9 kg*—150 mg once daily;.

PO (Children 2–11 yr): Oral Powder: *≥35 kg*—7.5 scoops (300 mg) once daily; *34–34.9 kg*—7 scoops (280 mg) once daily; *32–33.9 kg*—6.5 scoops (260 mg) once daily; *29–31.9 kg*—6 scoops (240 mg) once daily; *27–28.9 kg*—5.5 scoops (220 mg) once daily; *24–26.9 kg*—5 scoops (200 mg) once daily; *22–23.9 kg*—4.5 scoops (180 mg) once daily; *19–21.9 kg*—4 scoops (160 mg) once daily; *17–18.9 kg*—3.5 scoops (140 mg) once daily; *14–16.9 kg*—3 scoops (120 mg) once daily; *12–13.9 kg*—2.5 scoops (100 mg) once daily; *10–11.9 kg*—2 scoops (80 mg) once daily;.

Chronic Hepatitis B

PO (Adults and Children ≥12 yr and ≥35 kg): 300 mg once daily.

Renal Impairment

PO (Adults): *CCr 30–49 mL/min*—300 mg every 48 hr; *CCr 10–29 mL/min*—300 mg every 72–96 hr; *Hemodialysis*—300 mg every 7 days following dialysis.

Availability

Tablets: 150 mg, 200 mg, 250 mg, 300 mg. **Oral powder:** 40 mg/scoop. ***In combination with:*** emtricitabine (Truvada); emtricitabine and rilpivirine (Complera); efavirenz and emtricitabine (Atripla); elvitegravir, cobicistat, and emtricitabine (Stribild). See Appendix B.

NURSING IMPLICATIONS

Assessment

- Monitor for change in severity of HIV symptoms and for symptoms of opportunistic infection before and during therapy.
- Monitor bone mineral density in patients who have a history of pathologic bone fracture or are at risk for osteoporosis or bone loss.
- ***Lab Test Considerations:*** Monitor viral load and CD4 count before and routinely during therapy to determine response.
- Monitor liver function tests and hepatitis B virus levels throughout and following therapy. If therapy is discontinued, may cause severe exacerbation of hepatitis B. May cause ↑ AST, ALT, alkaline phosphatase, creatine kinase, amylase, and triglyceride concentrations. Lactic acidosis may occur with hepatic toxicity causing hepatic steatosis; may be fatal, especially in women.
- Calculate creatinine clearance prior to and periodically during therapy and when clinically indicated. In patients at risk of renal dysfunction, assess creatinine clearance, serum phosphorus, urine glucose, and urine protein prior to and periodically during therapy.
- Monitor serum phosphate periodically during therapy in patients at risk for renal impairment. May cause hypophosphatemia in patients with renal impairment.
- May cause hyperglycemia and glucosuria.

Potential Nursing Diagnoses

Risk for infection (Indications, Side Effects)
Risk for injury (Side Effects)

Implementation

- When tenofovir is administered concomitantly with didanosine, administer tenofovir 2 hr before or 1 hr after didanosine.
- **PO:** Administer once daily with or without food.
- Patients unable to swallow tablets can use oral powder. Using only dosing scoop, mix in soft food (applesauce, baby food, yogurt). Do not mix in liquid; powder floats to top even after stirring. Ingest entire mixture immediately to avoid bitter taste.

Patient/Family Teaching

- Instruct patient on the importance of taking tenofovir as directed, even if feeling better. Do not take more than prescribed amount and do not stop taking without consulting health care professional. Discontinuing therapy may lead to severe exacerbations. Take missed doses as soon as remembered unless almost time for next dose; do not double doses. Caution patient not to share or trade this medication with others.

- Inform patient that tenofovir may cause hyperglycemia. Advise patient to notify health care professional if increased thirst or hunger; unexplained weight loss; increased urination; fatigue; or dry, itchy skin occurs.
- Instruct patient to notify health care professional of all Rx or OTC medications, vitamins, or herbal products being taken and consult health care professional before taking any new medications.
- Caution patient to avoid crowds and persons with known infections.
- Inform patient that tenofovir does not cure AIDS and does not reduce the risk of transmission of HIV to others through sexual contact or blood contamination. Caution patient to use a condom and avoid sharing needles or donating blood to prevent spreading HIV to others.
- Advise patient to notify health care professional immediately if symptoms of lactic acidosis (nausea, vomiting, unusual or unexpected stomach discomfort, and weakness) or signs of Immune Reconstitution Syndrome (signs and symptoms of an infection) occur.
- Inform patient that changes in body fat distribution (increased fat in upper back and neck, breast, and trunk, and loss of fat from legs, arms, and face) may occur, but may not be related to drug therapy.
- Rep: Advise patient taking oral contraceptives to use a nonhormonal method of birth control during tenofovir therapy. If pregnancy is suspected notify health care professional promptly. Encourage pregnant women to enroll in the Antiretroviral Pregnancy Registry by calling 1–800–258–4263. Advise female patient to avoid breast feeding during therapy.
- Emphasize the importance of regular exams to monitor for side effects.

Evaluation/Desired Outcomes

- Decreased incidence of opportunistic infection and slowed progression of HIV infection.
- Slowed progression of chronic hepatitis B infection.

terazosin (ter-ay-zoe-sin)

♣Hytrin, ~~Hytrin~~

Classification

Therapeutic: antihypertensives

Pharmacologic: peripherally acting antiadrenergics

Pregnancy Category C

Indications

Mild to moderate hypertension (alone or with other agents). Treatment of signs/symptoms of benign prostatic hyperplasia (BPH).

Action

Dilates both arteries and veins by blocking postsynaptic $alpha_1$-adrenergic receptors. Decreases contractions in smooth muscle of the prostatic capsule. **Therapeutic Effects:** Lowering of BP. Decreased symptoms of prostatic hyperplasia (urinary urgency, hesitancy, nocturia).

Pharmacokinetics

Absorption: Well absorbed after oral administration.

Distribution: Unknown.

Metabolism and Excretion: 50% metabolized by the liver. 10% excreted unchanged by the kidneys. 20% excreted unchanged in feces. 40% eliminated in bile.

Half-life: 12 hr.

TIME/ACTION PROFILE

ROUTE	ONSET†	PEAK‡	DURATION†
PO-hypertension	15 min	6–8 wk	24 hr
PO-BPH	2–6 wk	unknown	unknown

†After single dose.

‡After multiple oral dosing.

Contraindications/Precautions

Contraindicated in: Hypersensitivity.

Use Cautiously in: Deyhdration, volume or sodium depletion (↑ risk of hypotension); Patients undergoing cataract surgery (↑ risk of intraoperative floppy iris syndrome); OB, Lactation, Pedi: Safety not established.

Adverse Reactions/Side Effects

CNS: dizziness, headache, weakness, drowsiness, nervousness. **EENT:** nasal congestion, blurred vision, conjunctivitis, intraoperative floppy iris syndrome, sinusitis. **Resp:** dyspnea. **CV:** first-dose orthostatic hypotension, arrhythmias, chest pain, palpitations, peripheral edema, tachycardia. **GI:** nausea, abdominal pain, diarrhea, dry mouth, vomiting. **GU:** erectile dysfunction, urinary frequency. **Derm:** pruritus. **Metab:** weight gain. **MS:** arthralgia, back pain, extremity pain. **Neuro:** paresthesia. **Misc:** fever.

Interactions

Drug-Drug: ↑ risk of hypotension with **sildenafil**, **tadalafil**, **vardenafil**, other **antihypertensives**, **nitrates**, or acute ingestion of **alcohol**. **NSAIDs**, **sympathomimetics**, or **estrogens** may ↓ effects of antihypertensive therapy.

Route/Dosage

The first dose should be taken at bedtime.

T

Hypertension

PO (Adults): 1 mg initially, then slowly ↑ up to 5 mg/day (usual range 1–5 mg/day); may be given as single dose or in 2 divided doses (not to exceed 20 mg/day).

Benign Prostatic Hyperplasia

PO (Adults): 1 mg at bedtime; gradually may be ↑ up to 5–10 mg/day.

Availability (generic available)

Capsules: 1 mg, 2 mg, 5 mg, 10 mg. **Tablets:** ✽1 mg, ✽2 mg, ✽5 mg, ✽10 mg. **Cost:** *Generic*—All strengths $160.38/100.

NURSING IMPLICATIONS

Assessment

- Assess for first-dose orthostatic reaction (dizziness, weakness) and syncope. May occur 30 min–2 hr after initial dose and occasionally thereafter. Incidence may be dose related. Volume-depleted or sodium-restricted patients may be more sensitive. Observe patient closely during this period; take precautions to prevent injury. First dose may be given at bedtime to minimize this reaction.
- Monitor intake and output ratios and daily weight; assess for edema daily, especially at beginning of therapy.
- **Hypertension:** Monitor BP and pulse frequently during initial dosage adjustment and periodically throughout therapy. Report significant changes.
- Monitor frequency of prescription refills to determine adherence.
- **BPH:** Assess patient for symptoms of BPH (urinary hesitancy, feeling of incomplete bladder emptying, interruption of urinary stream, impairment of size and force of urinary stream, terminal urinary dribbling, straining to start flow, dysuria, urgency) before and periodically during therapy.
- Rule out prostatic carcinoma before therapy; symptoms are similar.

Potential Nursing Diagnoses

Risk for injury (Side Effects)
Noncompliance (Patient/Family Teaching)

Implementation

- May be used in combination with diuretics or beta blockers to minimize sodium and water retention. If these are added to terazosin therapy, reduce dose of terazosin initially and titrate to effect.
- **PO:** Administer daily dose at bedtime. If necessary, dose may be increased to twice daily.

Patient/Family Teaching

- Instruct patient to take medication at the same time each day. Take missed doses as soon as remembered. If not remembered until next day, omit; do not double doses.
- Advise patient to weigh self twice weekly and assess feet and ankles for fluid retention.
- May cause dizziness or drowsiness. Advise patient to avoid driving or other activities requiring alertness until response to the medication is known.
- Caution patient to avoid sudden changes in position to decrease orthostatic hypotension. Alcohol, CNS depressants, standing for long periods, hot showers, and exercising in hot weather should be avoided because of enhanced orthostatic effects.
- Advise patient to notify health care professional of all Rx or OTC medications, vitamins, or herbal products being taken and to consult with health care professional before taking other medications, especially NSAIDs, cough, cold, or allergy remedies.
- Instruct patient to notify health care professional of medication regimen before any surgery.
- Advise patient to notify health care professional if frequent dizziness, fainting, or swelling of feet or lower legs occurs.
- Emphasize the importance of follow-up exams to evaluate effectiveness of medication.
- **Hypertension:** Emphasize the importance of continuing to take this medication as directed, even if feeling well. Medication controls but does not cure hypertension.
- Encourage patient to comply with additional interventions for hypertension (weight reduction, low-sodium diet, smoking cessation, moderation of alcohol consumption, regular exercise, and stress management).
- Instruct patient and family on proper technique for BP monitoring. Advise them to check BP at least weekly and to report significant changes.

Evaluation/Desired Outcomes

- Decrease in BP without appearance of side effects.
- Decreased symptoms of BPH. May require 2–6 wk of therapy before effects are noticeable.

terbinafine (ter-**bi**-na-feen)

LamISIL

Classification
Therapeutic: antifungals (systemic)

Pregnancy Category B

For topical use, refer to Antifungals, Topical monograph

Indications

Onychomycosis (fungal nail infection). Tinea capitis.

Action

Interferes with fungal cell wall synthesis (ergosterol biosynthesis) by inhibiting the enzyme squalene epoxidase. **Therapeutic Effects:** Fungal cell death. **Spectrum:** Active against dermatophytes and other fungi.

Pharmacokinetics

Absorption: 70–80% absorbed after oral administration.

Distribution: Extensively distributed; penetrates dermis and epidermis; concentrates in stratum corneum, hair, scalp, and nails. Enters breast milk.
Protein Binding: 99%.
Metabolism and Excretion: Extensively metabolized by the liver by CYP isoenzymes 1A2, 2C9, 2C19, and 3A4.
Half-life: *Plasma*—22 days; longer from skin and nails.

TIME/ACTION PROFILE (antifungal tissue levels)

ROUTE	ONSET	PEAK	DURATION
PO	several days	days–wk	several wk

Contraindications/Precautions

Contraindicated in: Hypersensitivity; Chronic or active liver disease; Heart failure or left ventricular dysfunction.
Use Cautiously in: History of alcoholism; Renal impairment (dose ↓ recommended for CCr <50 mL/min); OB, Lactation: Safety not established.

Adverse Reactions/Side Effects

CNS: depression, headache. **Resp:** cough, nasopharyngitis. **CV:** heart failure. **GI:** HEPATOTOXICITY, anorexia, diarrhea, nausea, stomach pain, vomiting, drug-induced hepatitis, smell disturbance, taste disturbance. **Derm:** DRUG REACTION WITH EOSINOPHILIA AND SYSTEMIC SYMPTOMS SYNDROME, STEVENS-JOHNSON SYNDROME, TOXIC EPIDERMAL NECROLYSIS, itching, rash. **Hemat:** neutropenia, pancytopenia. **Misc:** pyrexia.

Interactions

Drug-Drug: **Alcohol** or other **hepatotoxic agents** may ↑ risk of hepatotoxicity. **Rifampin** may ↓ effectiveness. **Fluconazole** and **cimetidine** may ↑ levels. May ↑ effects of CYP2D6 substrates including **tricyclic antidepressants, selective serotonin reuptake inhibitors, beta-blockers, flecainide**, and **propafenone**.
Drug-Natural Products: ↑ **caffeine** levels and side effects with caffeine-containing herbs (**cola nut, guarana, mate, tea, coffee**).

Route/Dosage

PO (Adults): 250 mg once daily for 6 wk for fingernail infection or 12 wk for toenail infection.
PO (Children ≥4 yr—≥35 kg): 250 mg/day for 6 wk.
PO (Children ≥4 yr—25–35 kg): 187.5 mg/day for 6 wk.
PO (Children ≥4 yr—<25 kg): 125 mg/day for 6 wk.

Availability (generic available)

Tablets: 250 mg. **Oral granules:** 125 mg/packet, 187.5 mg/packet.

NURSING IMPLICATIONS

Assessment

- Assess for signs and symptoms of infection (nail beds, scalp) before and periodically throughout therapy.
- Specimens for culture should be taken before instituting therapy. Therapy may be started before results are obtained.
- Monitor for depression periodically during therapy.
- Assess for rash periodically during therapy. May cause Stevens-Johnson syndrome. Discontinue therapy if severe or if accompanied with fever, general malaise, fatigue, muscle or joint aches, blisters, oral lesions, conjunctivitis, hepatitis and/or eosinophilia.
- ***Lab Test Considerations:*** CBC should be monitored in patients receiving therapy for >6 wk. Discontinue if abnormal values occur.
- Monitor AST and ALT prior to, and periodically throughout, therapy. Terbinafine should be discontinued if symptomatic elevations occur.
- If signs of secondary infection occur, monitor neutrophil count. If <1000/mm³, discontinue treatment.
- May cause ↓ absolute lymphocyte count.
- Monitor serum potassium. May cause hypokalemia.

Potential Nursing Diagnoses

Risk for infection (Indications)
Noncompliance (Patient/Family Teaching)

Implementation

- Do not confuse Lamisil (terbinafine) with Lamictal (lamotrigine).
- **PO:** May be administered without regard to food.
- *Oral granules* should be taken with food and may be sprinkled on a spoonful of pudding or other soft, nonacidic food, such as mashed potatoes and swallowed in entirety. Applesauce or fruit-based foods should not be used.

Patient/Family Teaching

- Instruct patient to take medication as directed, for the full course of therapy, even if feeling better. Doses should be taken at the same time each day.
- Instruct patient to notify health care professional immediately if signs and symptoms of liver dysfunction (unusual fatigue, anorexia, nausea, vomiting, upper right abdominal pain, jaundice, dark urine, or pale stools) depression, or rash occur. Terbinafine should be discontinued.
- May cause disturbance in smell. Advise patient to notify health care professional if this occurs.
- Advise patient to notify health care professional of all Rx or OTC medications, vitamins, or herbal products being taken and to consult with health care professional before taking other medications.

Evaluation/Desired Outcomes

- Resolution of clinical and laboratory indications of fungal nail infections. Inadequate period of treatment may lead to recurrence of active infection.
- Resolution of tinea capitis infection.

terbinafine, See ANTIFUNGALS (TOPICAL).

terbutaline (ter-byoo-ta-leen)

~~Bricanyl~~

Classification
Therapeutic: bronchodilators
Pharmacologic: adrenergics

Pregnancy Category B

Indications

Management of reversible airway disease due to asthma or COPD; inhalation and subcut used for short-term control and oral agent as long-term control. **Unlabeled Use:** Management of preterm labor (tocolytic) (the FDA has recommended that injectable terbutaline should not be used in pregnancy for the prevention or prolonged treatment [>48–72 hr] of preterm labor in either the inpatient or outpatient settings because of the potential for serious maternal heart problems and death; oral terbutaline should not be used for the prevention or any treatment of preterm labor because of a lack of efficacy and the potential for serious material heart problems and death).

Action

Results in the accumulation of cyclic adenosine monophosphate (cAMP) at beta-adrenergic receptors. Produces bronchodilation. Inhibits the release of mediators of immediate hypersensitivity reactions from mast cells. Relatively selective for $beta_2$ (pulmonary)-adrenergic receptor sites, with less effect on $beta_1$ (cardiac)-adrenergic receptors. **Therapeutic Effects:** Bronchodilation.

Pharmacokinetics

Absorption: 35–50% absorbed following oral administration but rapidly undergoes first-pass metabolism. Well absorbed following subcut administration.
Distribution: Enters breast milk.
Metabolism and Excretion: Partially metabolized by the liver; 60% excreted unchanged by the kidneys following subcut administration.
Half-life: Unknown.

TIME/ACTION PROFILE (bronchodilation)

ROUTE	ONSET	PEAK	DURATION
PO	within 60–120 min	within 2–3 hr	4–8 hr
Subcut	within 15 min	within 0.5–1 hr	1.5–4 hr

Contraindications/Precautions

Contraindicated in: Hypersensitivity to adrenergic amines.
Use Cautiously in: Cardiac disease; Hypertension; Hyperthyroidism; Diabetes; Glaucoma; Geri: More susceptible to adverse reactions; may require dose ↓ Excessive use may lead to tolerance and paradoxical bronchospasm (inhaler); OB, Lactation: Pregnancy (near term) and lactation.

Adverse Reactions/Side Effects

CNS: nervousness, restlessness, tremor, headache, insomnia. **Resp:** pulmonary edema. **CV:** angina, arrhythmias, hypertension, myocardial ischemia, tachycardia. **GI:** nausea, vomiting. **Endo:** hyperglycemia. **F and E:** hypokalemia.

Interactions

Drug-Drug: Concurrent use with other **adrenergics** (sympathomimetic) will have additive adrenergic side effects. Use with **MAO inhibitors** may lead to hypertensive crisis. **Beta blockers** may negate therapeutic effect.
Drug-Natural Products: Use with caffeine-containing herbs (**cola nut, guarana, mate, tea, coffee**) ↑ stimulant effect.

Route/Dosage

PO (Adults and Children >15 yr): *Bronchodilation*—2.5–5 mg 3 times daily, given q 6 hr (not to exceed 15 mg/24 hr).
PO (Children 12–15 yr): *Bronchodilation*—2.5 mg 3 times daily (given q 6 hr) (not to exceed 7.5 mg/24 hr).
PO (Children <12 yr): *Bronchodilation*—0.05 mg/kg 3 times daily; may ↑ gradually (not to exceed 0.15 mg/kg 3–4 times daily or 5 mg/24 hr).
Subcut (Adults and Children ≥12 yr): *Bronchodilation*—250 mcg; may repeat in 15–30 min (not to exceed 500 mcg/4 hr).
Subcut (Children <12 yr): *Bronchodilation*—0.005–0.01 mg/kg; may repeat in 15–20 min.
IV (Adults): *Tocolysis*—2.5–10 mcg/min infusion; ↑ by 5 mcg/min q 10 min until contractions stop (not to exceed 30 mcg/min). After contractions have stopped for 30 min, ↓ infusion rate to lowest effective amount and maintain for 4–8 hr (unlabeled).

Availability (generic available)

Tablets: 2.5 mg, 5 mg. **Injection:** 1 mg/mL.

NURSING IMPLICATIONS

Assessment

- **Bronchodilator:** Assess lung sounds, respiratory pattern, pulse, and BP before administration and during peak of medication. Note amount, color, and character of sputum produced, and notify health care professional of abnormal findings.
- Monitor pulmonary function tests before initiating therapy and periodically throughout therapy to determine effectiveness of medication.
- **Preterm Labor:** Monitor maternal pulse and BP, frequency and duration of contractions, and fetal heart rate. Notify health care professional if contractions persist or increase in frequency or duration or if symptoms of maternal or fetal distress occur. Maternal side effects include tachycardia, palpitations, tremor, anxiety, and headache.
- Assess maternal respiratory status for symptoms of pulmonary edema (increased rate, dyspnea, rales/crackles, frothy sputum).
- Monitor mother and neonate for symptoms of hypoglycemia (anxiety; chills; cold sweats; confusion; cool, pale skin; difficulty in concentration; drowsiness; excessive hunger; headache; irritability; nausea; nervousness; rapid pulse; shakiness; unusual tiredness; or weakness) and mother for hypokalemia (weakness, fatigue, U wave on ECG, arrhythmias).
- ***Lab Test Considerations:*** May cause transient ↓ in serum potassium concentrations with higher than recommended doses.
- Monitor maternal serum glucose and electrolytes. May cause hypokalemia and hypoglycemia. Monitor neonate's serum glucose, because hypoglycemia may also occur in neonates.
- ***Toxicity and Overdose:*** Symptoms of overdose include persistent agitation, chest pain or discomfort, decreased BP, dizziness, hyperglycemia, hypokalemia, seizures, tachyarrhythmias, persistent trembling, and vomiting.
- Treatment includes discontinuing beta-adrenergic agonists and symptomatic, supportive therapy. Cardioselective beta blockers are used cautiously, because they may induce bronchospasm.

Potential Nursing Diagnoses

Ineffective airway clearance (Indications)

Implementation

- Do not confuse Brethine (terbutaline) with Methergine (methylergonovine).
- **PO:** Administer with meals to minimize gastric irritation.
- Tablet may be crushed and mixed with food or fluids for patients with difficulty swallowing.
- **Subcut:** Administer subcut injections in lateral deltoid area. Do not use solution if discolored.

IV Administration

- **Continuous Infusion:** ***Diluent:*** May be diluted in D5W, 0.9% NaCl, or 0.45% NaCl. ***Concentration:*** 1 mg/mL (undiluted). ***Rate:*** Use infusion pump to ensure accurate dose. Begin infusion at 10 mcg/min. Increase dosage by 5 mcg every 10 min until contractions cease. Maximum dose is 80 mcg/min. Begin to taper dose in 5-mcg decrements after a 30–60 min contraction-free period is attained. Switch to oral dose form after patient is contraction-free 4–8 hr on the lowest effective dose.
- **Y-Site Compatibility:** insulin.

Patient/Family Teaching

- Instruct patient to take medication as directed. If on a scheduled dosing regimen, take a missed dose as soon as possible; space remaining doses at regular intervals. Do not double doses. Caution patient not to exceed recommended dose; may cause adverse effects, paradoxical bronchospasm, or loss of effectiveness of medication.
- Instruct patient to contact health care professional immediately if shortness of breath is not relieved by medication or is accompanied by diaphoresis, dizziness, palpitations, or chest pain.
- Advise patient to consult health care professional before taking any OTC medications or alcoholic beverages concurrently with this therapy. Caution patient also to avoid smoking and other respiratory irritants.
- **Preterm Labor:** Notify health care professional immediately if labor resumes or if significant side effects occur.

Evaluation/Desired Outcomes

- Prevention or relief of bronchospasm.
- Increase in ease of breathing.
- Control of preterm labor in a fetus of 20–36 wk gestational age.

terconazole, See ANTIFUNGALS (VAGINAL).

teriflunomide

(ter-i-**floo**-noe-mide)

Aubagio

Classification

Therapeutic: anti-multiple sclerosis agents

Pharmacologic: immune response modifiers, pyrimidine synthesis inhibitors

Pregnancy Category X

Indications

Management of relapsing forms of multiple sclerosis (MS).

Action

Inhibits an enzyme required for pyrimidine synthesis; has antiproliferative and anti-inflammatory effects. **Therapeutic Effects:** ↓ incidence and severity of relapses in MS, with a decrease in disability progression.

Pharmacokinetics

Absorption: Well absorbed following oral administration.
Distribution: Unknown.
Protein Binding: >99%.
Metabolism and Excretion: Eliminated via biliary excretion of unchanged drug with renal excretion of metabolites (37.5 in feces and 22.6% in urine), some metabolism occurs.
Half-life: 18–19 days.

TIME/ACTION PROFILE (decrease in disability progression)

ROUTE	ONSET	PEAK	DURATION
PO	3–6 mo	unknown	unknown

Contraindications/Precautions

Contraindicated in: Severe hepatic impairment; Concurrent leflunomide treatment; Live virus vaccinations; Active acute or chronic infection; Severe immunodeficiency, bone marrow disease or severe uncontrolled infection; Lactation: Discontinue teriflunomide or discontinue breast feeding; OB: Pregnancy or woman with childbearing potential using unreliable contraception (may cause fetal harm).
Use Cautiously in: Pre-existing liver disease; Severe immunodeficiency, bone marrow disease or severe uncontrolled infection; Hypertension (treat appropriately prior); Geri: Age >60 yr, concurrent neurotoxic medications or diabetes mellitus (↑ risk of peripheral neuropathy); OB: Women with child-bearing potential; Pedi: Safe and effective use in children has not been established.

Adverse Reactions/Side Effects

CV: hypertension. **Resp:** INTERSTITIAL LUNG DISEASE (rare). **GI:** HEPATOTOXICITY, diarrhea, ↑ transaminases, nausea. **GU:** acute renal failure (urate nephropathy). **Derm:** severe skin reactions including STEVENS-JOHNSON SYNDROME and TOXIC EPIDERMAL NECROLYSIS, alopecia. **F and E:** hyperkalemia, hypophosphatemia. **Hemat:** leukopenia, neutropenia, thrombocytopenia. **Neuro:** paresthesia, peripheral neuropathy. **Misc:** ATYPICAL INFECTIONS, INCLUDING LATENT TUBERCULOSIS, influenza.

Interactions

Drug-Drug: May ↑ levels and effects of **drugs metabolized by the CYP2C8 enzyme system** including **paclitaxel**, **pioglitazone**, **repaglinide**, and **rosiglitazone**. May ↓ levels and effectiveness of **drugs metabolized by the CYP1A2 enzyme system** including **alosetron**, **duloxetine**, **thoephylline**, and **tizanidine**. May ↓ response to and ↑ risk of adverse reactions from **live vaccines** (avoid live vaccinations and consider long half-life of teriflunomide before administering). May ↑ levels and effects of **ethinylestradiol** and **levonorgestrel**. May ↑ risk of bleeding with **warfarin**. ↑ risk of additive immunosuppression with other **immunosuppressants** or **antineoplastics** (consider long half-life of teriflunomide). Levels and effects may be ↑ by breast cancer resistant protein (BCRP) inhibitors including **cyclosporine**, **eltrombopag**, and **gefitinib**. May alter response to **warfarin**. May ↑ risk of adverse reactions and ↓ antibody response to **live virus vaccines**.

Route/Dosage

PO (Adults): 7 or 14 mg once daily.

Availability

Film-coated tablets: 7 mg, 14 mg.

NURSING IMPLICATIONS

Assessment

- Assess BP before starting and periodically during therapy. Treat hypertension as needed.
- ***Lab Test Considerations:*** Monitor liver function tests (transaminases, bilirubin) within 6 months of starting therapy and monthly after teriflunomide therapy begins. Do not administer if ALT >2 × upper limit of normal. Consider discontinuing therapy if serum transaminase ↑ >3 × upper limit of normal is confirmed. Monitor serum transaminase and bilirubin in patients with symptoms of liver dysfunction. If liver injury is suspected, discontinue teriflunomide, begin accelerated elimination procedure, and monitor liver function tests weekly until normal.
- Obtain a pregnancy test from female patients prior to beginning therapy.
- Monitor CBC with platelet count within 6 months prior to starting and periodically during therapy based on signs and symptoms of infection. Mean decrease in WBC occurs during first 6 wks and remains low during therapy.
- Monitor INR closely in patients taking warfarin, a decrease in warfarin peak may occur.

Potential Nursing Diagnoses

Impaired physical mobility (Indications)

Implementation

- Administer a tuberculin skin test prior to administration of teriflunomide. Patients with active latent TB should be treated for TB prior to therapy.
- **PO:** Administer once daily without regard to food.
- **Drug Elimination Procedure:** Either of the following procedures is recommended to achieve nondetectable plasma levels <0.02 mg/L after stopping treatment with teriflunomide. 1) Administer cholestyramine 8 g 3 times daily (every 8 hrs) for 11 days. If cholestyramine 8 g is not well tolerated, cholestyramine 4 g 3 times/day can be used. *or* 2) Administration of 50 g oral activated charcoal powder every

12 hr for 11 days. (Days do not need to be consecutive unless rapid lowering of levels is desired.) Verify plasma levels <0.02 mg/L by 2 separate tests at least 14 days apart. Plasma levels may take up to 2 yr to reach nondetectable levels without drug elimination procedure.

Patient/Family Teaching

- Instruct patient to take teriflunomide as directed. Advise patient to read *Medication Guide* before starting therapy and with each Rx refill in case of changes.
- Advise patient to notify health care professional promptly if symptoms of liver problems (nausea, vomiting, stomach pain, loss of appetite, tiredness, skin or whites of eyes yellowing, dark urine), serious skin problems (redness or peeling), infection (fever, tiredness, body aches, chills, nausea, vomiting), or interstitial lung disease (cough, dyspnea, with or without fever) occur.
- Instruct patient to notify health care professional if symptoms of peripheral neuropathy (numbness and tingling in hands and feet different from symptoms of MS), kidney problems (flank pain), high potassium level (nausea or racing heartbeat), or high BP occur.
- Instruct patient to notify health care professional of all Rx or OTC medications, vitamins, or herbal products being taken and consult health care professional before taking any new medications.
- Instruct patient to avoid vaccinations with live vaccines during and following therapy without consulting health care professional.
- Discuss the possibility of hair loss with patient. Explore methods of coping.
- Advise patient that teriflunomide is teratogenic. Effective birth control should be used during therapy and until blood levels of teriflunomide are low enough. If pregnancy is planned or suspected, or if breast feeding notify health care professional immediately, accelerated eliminated procedure may be used to decrease blood levels more rapidly. Male patients with female partner who plans to become pregnant may also use this method. If female partner does not plan to become pregnant, use effective birth control until blood levels are low enough; may require 2 years. Females of childbearing potential are recommended to undergo accelerated elimination procedure upon discontinuation of teriflunomide. Patients who become pregnant should be encouraged to enroll in the Aubagio Pregnancy Registry at 1-800-745-4447 to collect information about mother and baby's health.

Evaluation/Desired Outcomes

- Decrease in the number of MS flares (relapses) and slowing of physical problems caused by MS.

tesamorelin (tess-a-**moe**-rel-in)
Egrifta

Classification
Therapeutic: none assigned
Pharmacologic: growth hormone-releasing factor analogues

Pregnancy Category X

Indications

Reduction of excess abdominal fat (lipodystrophy) seen in HIV-infected patients.

Action

Acts as an analog of human growth hormone-releasing factor (GRF, GHRH), resulting in endogenous production of growth hormone (GH), which has anabolic and lipolytic properties. **Therapeutic Effects:** Reduction of abdominal adipose tissue in HIV-infected patients.

Pharmacokinetics

Absorption: <4% absorbed following subcutaneous administration.
Distribution: Unknown.
Metabolism and Excretion: Unknown.
Half-life: 26–38 min.

TIME/ACTION PROFILE (effect on visceral adipose tissue)

ROUTE	ONSET	PEAK	DURATION
Subcut	within 3 mos	10–12 mos	3 mos†

†Following discontinuation.

Contraindications/Precautions

Contraindicated in: Hypersensitivity to tesamorelin or mannitol; Any pathology that alters the hypothalamic-pituitary axis, including hypophysectomy, hypopituitarism, pituitary surgery/tumor, cranial irradiation/trauma; OB: may cause fetal harm; Lactation: Breast feeding should be avoided by HIV-infected patients.
Use Cautiously in: Acute critical illness (may ↑ risk of serious complications; consider discontinuation); Pre-existing malignancy (disease should be inactive or treatment completed); Non-malignant neoplasms (carefully consider benefit); Persistently elevated Insulin-like Growth Factor (IGF-1; may require discontinuation); Diabetes mellitus (may cause glucose intolerance); Pedi: Safe and effective use in children not established.

Adverse Reactions/Side Effects

CV: peripheral edema. **Endo:** glucose intolerance. **Local:** erythema, hemorrhage, irritation, pain, pruritus. **MS:** arthralgia, carpal tunnel syndrome, extremity pain, myalgia. **Misc:** hypersensitivity reactions.

T

Interactions

Drug-Drug: May alter the clearance and actions of drugs known to be metabolized by the CYPP450 enzyme system including **corticosteroids**, **androgens**, **estrogens** and **progestins** (including **hormonal contraceptives**), **anticonvulsants**, and **cyclosporine**, careful monitoring for efficacy and/or toxicity recommended. Inhibits the conversion of **cortisone acetate** and **prednisone** to active forms; patients on replacement therapy may need ↑ maintenance/stress doses.

Route/Dosage

Subcut (Adults): 2 mg once daily.

Availability

Lyophilized powder for subcutaneous administration (requires reconstitution): 1 mg/vial.

NURSING IMPLICATIONS

Assessment

- Assess for fluid retention which manifests as ↑ tissue turgor and musculoskeletal discomfort (edema, arthralgia, extremity pain, carpal tunnel syndrome). May be transient or resolve with discontinuation of treatment.
- ***Lab Test Considerations:*** Monitor serum IGF-I closely during therapy; tesamorelin stimulates growth hormone production and the effect on progression of malignancies is unknown. Consider discontinuing tesamorelin in patients with persistent elevations of IGF-I levels, especially if efficacy response is not strong.
- May cause glucose intolerance and ↑ risk of developing diabetes. Monitor serum glucose prior to starting and periodically during therapy. Monitor diabetic patients closely for worsening of retinopathy.

Potential Nursing Diagnoses

Disturbed body image (Indications)

Implementation

- **Subcut:** Sterile Water for Injection 10 mL diluent is provided. Inject 2.2 mL of Sterile Water into tesamorelin, angled so that water goes down inside wall to prevent foaming. Roll vial gently between hands for 30 seconds to mix; do not shake. Change needle. Withdraw solution and inject into 2nd tesamorelin vial with solution against wall of vial. Mix between hands for 30 seconds. Withdraw all solution (2 mg/ 2.2 mL). Solution is clear and colorless; do not administer solution that is discolored or contains particulate matter. Use solution immediately upon reconstitution or discard; do not refrigerate or freeze. Change needle to 1/2 inch 27 gauge needle. Pinch skin and inject at right angle into abdomen below navel; rotate sites. Remove hand from pinched area and inject slowly. Do not inject into scar, bruises, or the navel. Prior to reconstitution, vials must be refrigerated and protected from light.

Patient/Family Teaching

- Instruct patient on correct technique for administration of tesamorelin. Caution patient never to share needles with others.
- Inform patient that tesamorelin may cause symptoms of fluid retention (edema, arthralgia, carpal tunnel syndrome); usually transient or resolve with discontinuation of therapy.
- Advise patient to discontinue tesamorelin and notify health care professional promptly if signs and symptoms of hypersensitivity (rash, urticaria, hives, swelling of face or throat, shortness of breath, fast heartbeat, fainting) occur.
- Advise female patients to notify health care professional if pregnancy is planned or suspected or if breast feeding.

Evaluation/Desired Outcomes

- Reduction of excess abdominal fat in HIV-infected patients with lipodystrophy.

REMS

TESTOSTERONE

(tess-**toss**-te-rone)

testosterone buccal system, mucoadhesive
Striant

testosterone cypionate
Depo-Testosterone

testosterone enanthate
Delatestryl

testosterone nasal gel
Natesto

testosterone pellets
Testopel

testosterone topical gel
Androgel, Fortesta, Testim, Vogelxo

testosterone topical solution
Axiron

testosterone transdermal
Androderm

testosterone undecanoate
Aveed

Classification
Therapeutic: hormones
Pharmacologic: androgens

Schedule III

Pregnancy Category X

Indications
Hypogonadism in men with low testosterone serum concentrations. Delayed puberty in men (enanthate and pellets). Androgen-responsive breast cancer in postmenopausal women (palliative) (enanthate).

Action
Responsible for the normal growth and development of male sex organs. Maintenance of male secondary sex characteristics: Growth and maturation of the prostate, seminal vesicles, penis, scrotum, Development of male hair distribution, Vocal cord thickening, Alterations in body musculature and fat distribution. **Therapeutic Effects:** Correction of hormone deficiency in male hypogonadism: Initiation of male puberty. Suppression of tumor growth in some forms of breast cancer.

Pharmacokinetics
Absorption: Well absorbed from IM sites, through buccal mucosa, through skin, or through nasal mucosa. Cypionate, enanthate, and undecanoate salts are absorbed slowly. Skin serves as reservoir for sustained release of testosterone into systemic circulation; 10% absorbed into systemic circulation during 24–hr period.
Distribution: Crosses the placenta.
Protein Binding: 98%.
Metabolism and Excretion: Metabolized by the liver. Absorption from buccal mucosa bypasses initial liver metabolism. 90% eliminated in urine as metabolites.
Half-life: *Buccal, enanthate, nasal gel, pellets, topical gel, topical solution, undecanoate*—10–100 min; *transdermal*—70 min; *cypionate*—8 days.

TIME/ACTION PROFILE (androgenic effects†)

ROUTE	ONSET	PEAK	DURATION
IM—cypionate, enanthate	unknown	unknown	2–4 wk
IM—undecanoate	unknown	unknown	10 wk
Buccal	unknown	10–12 hr	12 hr
Nasal gel	unknown	unknown	3 mo
Pellets	unknown	unknown	3–6 mo
Topicalsolution	unknown	14 days	7–10 days
Transdermal (gel)	30 min	unknown	24 hr
Transdermal (patch)	unknown	6–8 hr‡	24 hr§

†Response is highly variable among individuals; may take months.
‡Plasma testosterone levels following applications of patch.
§Following patch removal.

Contraindications/Precautions
Contraindicated in: Hypersensitivity; Male patients with breast or prostate cancer; Severe liver, renal, or cardiac disease (propionate); Some products contain benzyl alcohol and should be avoided in patients with known hypersensitivity; Women (buccal, pellets, nasal gel, patch, topical gel, topical solution); OB, Lactation: Pregnancy or lactation.
Use Cautiously in: Diabetes mellitus; Coronary artery disease (enanthate); Pre-existing cardiac, renal, or liver disease; Benign prostatic hyperplasia; Hypercalcemia; Sleep apnea; Obesity (buccal); Chronic lung disease; Polycythemia; Nasal disorders, nasal/sinus surgery, nasal fracture in previous 6 mo, nasal fracture that caused deviated anterior nasal septum, mucosal inflammatory disorders (e.g. Sjogren's syndrome), or sinus disorders (nasal gel); Pedi: Prepubertal males exposed to testosterone may experience premature development of secondary sexual characteristics, aggression, and other side effects; Geri: ↑ risk of prostatic hyperplasia/carcinoma.

Adverse Reactions/Side Effects
CNS: anxiety, confusion, depression, fatigue, headache, vertigo. **EENT:** deepening of voice; *nasal gel,* epistaxis, nasal scabbing, nasopharyngitis, rhinorrhea. **CV:** MI, STROKE, VENOUS THROMBOEMBOLISM, edema. **GI:** abdominal cramps, changes in appetite, ↑ liver enzymes, nausea, vomiting; *buccal*—bitter taste, ginigivitis, gum edema, gum tenderness. **GU:** ↓ fertility, menstrual irregularities, nocturia, priapism, prostatic enlargement, urinary hesitancy, urinary incontinence. **Endo:** *women*—change in libido, clitoral enlargement, ↓ breast size; *men*—acne, facial hair, gynecomastia, erectile dysfunction, oligospermia, priapism. **F and E:** hypercalcemia, hyperkalemia, hyperphosphatemia. **Derm:** male pattern baldness. **Resp:** sleep apnea. **Local:** ANAPHYLAXIS, chronic skin irritation (transdermal), pain at injection/implantation site, pulmonary oil microembolism reactions (IM).

Interactions
Drug-Drug: May ↑ action of **warfarin**, **oral hypoglycemic agents**, and **insulin**. Concurrent use with **corticosteroids** may ↑ risk of edema formation.

Route/Dosage
Replacement Therapy
IM (Adults): 50–400 mg q 2–4 wk (enanthate or cypionate); 750 mg initially, then at wk 4, then q 10 wk.
Intranasal (Adults): 1 actuation (5.5 mg) in each nostril 3 times daily.
Transdermal(patch) (Adults): One 4–mg/day system applied q 24 hr in the evening; adjust dose based on serum testosterone concentrations (dosing range = 2–6 mg/day).

Transdermal (Adults): *Androgel 1% or Testim*—5 g (contains 50 mg of testosterone; 5 mg systemically absorbed) applied once daily (morning preferable), if needed may be ↑ to maximum of 10 g (contains 100 mg of testosterone; 10 mg systemically absorbed); *Androgel 1.62%*—40.5 mg of testosterone (2 pump actuations) applied once daily (morning preferable); dose may be adjusted down to a minimum of 20.25 mg or up to a maximum of 81 mg of testosterone, if needed (dose based on serum testosterone levels) *Fortesta*—40 mg of testosterone (4 pump actuations) applied once daily (morning preferable); dose may be adjusted down to a minimum of 10 mg or up to a maximum of 70 mg of testosterone, if needed (dose based on serum testosterone levels); *Vogelxo*—50 mg of testosterone (1 tube, 1 packet, or 4 pump actuations) applied once daily; dose may be adjusted up to a maximum of 100 mg of testosterone, if needed (dose based on serum testosterone levels).
Buccal (Adults): 30 mg (one system) applied to gum region twice daily (in the morning and evening, spaced 12 hr apart).
Subcut(for subcutaneous implantation) (pellets) (Adults): 150–450 mg q 3–6 mo.
Topical (Adults): 60 mg (2 pump actuations) applied once daily; may be ↑ up to 120 mg (4 pump actuations) based on serum testosterone concentrations.

Delayed Male Puberty

IM (Children): 50–200 mg q 2–4 wk for up to 6 mo (enanthate).
Subcut(for subcutaneous implantation) (pellets) (Children): 150–450 mg q 3–6 mo.

Palliative Management of Breast Cancer

IM (Adults): 200–400 mg q 2–4 wk (enanthate).

Availability (generic available)

Testosterone cypionate injection (in oil): 100 mg/mL, 200 mg/mL. **Testosterone enanthate injection (in oil):** 200 mg/mL. **Testosterone undeanoate injection (in oil):** 250 mg/mL. **Transdermal patch:** 2 mg/24 hr, 4 mg/24 hr. **1% topical gel (Androgel):** 25 mg/packet, 50 mg/packet, 75–g metered dose pump (each pump dispenses 60 metered 12.5–mg doses). **1% topical gel (Testim):** 50 mg/unit–dose tube. **1% topical gel (Vogelxo):** 50 mg/unit–dose tube, 50 mg/packet, 75–g metered dose pump (each pump dispenses 60 metered 12.5–mg doses). **1.62% topical gel (Androgel):** 20.25 mg/packet, 40.5 mg/packet, 88–g metered dose pump (each pump dispenses 60 metered 20.25–mg doses). **2% topical gel (Fortesta):** 60–g metered dose pump (each pump dispenses 120 metered 10–mg doses). **Buccal, mucoadhesive:** 30 mg/system. **Pellets:** 75 mg. **Topical solution:** 30 mg/pump actuation. **Nasal gel:** 5.5 mg/pump actuation.

NURSING IMPLICATIONS

Assessment

- Monitor intake and output ratios, weigh patient twice weekly, and assess patient for edema. Report significant changes indicative of fluid retention.
- **Men:** Monitor for precocious puberty in boys (acne, darkening of skin, development of male secondary sex characteristics—increase in penis size, frequent erections, growth of body hair). Bone age determinations should be measured every 6 mo to determine rate of bone maturation and effects on epiphyseal closure.
- Monitor for breast enlargement, persistent erections, and increased urge to urinate in men. Monitor for difficulty urinating in elderly men, because prostate enlargement may occur.
- **Women:** Assess for virilism (deepening of voice, unusual hair growth or loss, clitoral enlargement, acne, menstrual irregularity).
- In women with metastatic breast cancer, monitor for symptoms of hypercalcemia (nausea, vomiting, constipation, lethargy, loss of muscle tone, thirst, polyuria).
- ***Lab Test Considerations:*** Prior to therapy, measure serum testosterone in the morning on at least two separate days. Normal range (300 to 1050 ng/dL). Monitor serum testosterone concentrations 4–12 wk after starting therapy. Discontinue therapy is concentrations are consistently outside of normal range.
- Monitor hemoglobin and hematocrit periodically during therapy; may cause polycythemia.
- Monitor hepatic function tests, prostate specific antigen and serum cholesterol levels periodically during therapy. May cause ↑ serum AST, ALT, and bilirubin, ↑ cholesterol levels, and suppress clotting factors II, V, VII, and X.
- Monitor serum and urine calcium levels and serum alkaline phosphatase concentrations in women with metastatic breast cancer.
- Monitor serum sodium, chloride, potassium, and phosphate concentrations (may be ↑).
- Monitor blood glucose closely in patients with diabetes who are receiving oral hypoglycemic agents or insulin.
- *Transdermal:* Monitor serum testosterone concentrations 2 weeks after starting therapy; these concentrations should be obtained in the morning (following application of patch during the previous evening). Serum testosterone concentrations measured in the early morning outside range of 400 – 930 ng/dL require increasing daily dose to 6 mg (one 4 mg/day and one 2 mg/day system) or decreasing daily dose to 2 mg (one 2 mg/day system), maintaining nightly application.
- *Buccal:* Monitor serum testosterone concentrations 4–12 wk after starting therapy. Discontinue therapy is concentrations are consistently outside of normal range.

- *Topical Solution:* Measure serum testosterone concentrations after initiation of therapy to ensure desired concentrations (300 ng/dL–1050 ng/dL) are achieved. Adjust dose based on serum testosterone concentration from a single blood draw 2–8 hours after applying and at least 14 days after starting treatment or following dose adjustment. If concentration is below 300 ng/dL, daily dose may be increased from 60 mg (2 pump actuations) to 90 mg (3 pump actuations) or from 90 mg to 120 mg (4 pump actuations). If concentration exceeds 1050 ng/dL, the daily testosterone dose should be decreased from 60 mg (2 pump actuations) to 30 mg (1 pump actuation) as instructed by health care professional. If concentration consistently exceeds 1050 ng/dL at lowest daily dose of 30 mg (1 pump actuation), discontinue therapy.
- *Nasal gel:* Monitor serum testosterone concentrations after 1 month and periodically during therapy. If total testosterone concentrations consistently exceed 1050 ng/dL, discontinue therapy. If total testosterone concentrations are consistently below 300 ng/dL, consider alternative therapy.

Potential Nursing Diagnoses

Sexual dysfunction (Indications, Side Effects)

Implementation

- Range-of-motion exercises should be done with all bedridden patients to prevent mobilization of calcium from the bone.
- **IM:** Administer IM deep into gluteal muscle. Crystals may form when vials are stored at low temperatures; warming and shaking vial will redissolve crystals. Use of a wet syringe or needle may cause solution to become cloudy but will not affect its potency.
- **Subcut:** Pellets are to be implanted subcutaneously by a health care professional.
- **Transdermal:** Apply patch to clean, dry, hairless skin on the back, abdomen, upper arms, or thighs. Do not apply to the scrotum. Avoid application over bony prominences or a part of the body that may be subject to prolonged pressure during sleep or sitting. The patch does not need to be removed while swimming or taking a shower or bath.
- The sites of application should be rotated; once a patch is removed, the same site should not be used again for at least 1 wk.
- If skin irritation occurs, apply a small amount of OTC topical hydrocortisone cream after system removal or a small amount of 0.1% triamcinolone cream may be applied to the skin under the central drug reservoir of the *Androderm* system without affecting the absorption of testosterone. Ointment formulations should not be used for pretreatment because they may significantly reduce testosterone absorption.
- Patch should be removed if undergoing a magnetic resonance imaging (MRI) scan. The system contains aluminum and may predispose the patient to skin burns during the test.
- **Buccal:** Apply to gum region twice daily (about 12 hr apart), rotating sides with each dose.
- **Topical: Solution:** Apply *Axiron* to axilla using applicator at the same time each morning, to clean, dry, intact skin. Do not apply to other parts of the body including to the scrotum, penis, abdomen, shoulders or upper arms. Prime pump when using for first time by depressing pump 3 times, discard any product dispensed directly into a basin, sink, or toilet and then wash liquid away thoroughly. Prime only prior to first use of each pump. After priming, completely depress pump once with nozzle over applicator cup to dispense 30 mg of testosterone. Apply in 30 mg (1 pump actuation) increments. Place actuator into the axilla and wipe steadily down and up into the axilla. If solution drips or runs, wipe back up with applicator cup. Do not rub into skin with fingers or hand. Repeat process for each 30 mg dose needed. When repeat application to same axilla, allow axilla to dry completely before more is applied. Rinse applicator under room temperature, running water and pat dry with a tissue. Allow axilla to dry completely prior to dressing. Solution has an alcohol based and is flammable until dry. Apply deodorant prior to application of testosterone solution. Avoid swimming or washing for 2 hrs after application. Wash hands immediately with soap and water after application.
- **Topical: Gel:** Apply gel once daily, preferably in the morning, to clean dry intact skin of shoulders and upper arms (*Androgel*, *Testim*, and *Vogelxo*) or abdomen (Androgel only) or front or inner thighs (Fortesta). Gel should not be applied to scrotum (5–30 x more permeable than other sites). Refer to the chart on the pump label to determine how many full pump depressions are required for the daily prescribed dose.
- The dose of Fortesta should be titrated based on the serum testosterone concentration from a single blood draw 2 hours after applying Fortesta and at approximately 14 days and 35 days after starting treatment or following dose adjustment.
- **Intranasal:** Prime pump by inverting, depressing pump 10 times, and discarding any amount dispensed directly into a sink and washing gel away thoroughly with warm water. Wipe tip with a clean, dry tissue. If gel gets on hands, wash hands with warm water and soap. Priming should be done only prior to first use of each dispenser. Blow nose. Place right index finger on pump of actuator and while in front of a mirror, slowly advance tip of actuator into left nostril upwards until finger on the pump reaches

the base of the nose. Tilt the actuator so that the opening on the tip of the actuator is in contact with the lateral wall of the nostril to ensure that the gel is applied to the nasal wall. Slowly depress the pump until it stops. Remove the actuator from the nose while wiping the tip along the inside of the lateral nostril wall to fully transfer the gel. Repeat with right nostril. Press on the nostrils at a point just below bridge of the nose and lightly massage. Refrain from blowing nose or sniffing for 1 hour after administration.

Patient/Family Teaching

- Advise patient to report the following signs and symptoms promptly: *in male patients,* priapism (sustained and often painful erections) difficulty urinating, or gynecomastia; *in female patients,* virilism (which may be reversible if medication is stopped as soon as changes are noticed), or hypercalcemia (nausea, vomiting, constipation, and weakness); *in male or female patients,* edema (unexpected weight gain, swelling of feet), hepatitis (yellowing of skin or eyes and abdominal pain), or unusual bleeding or bruising.
- Explain rationale for prohibiting use of testosterone for increasing athletic performance. Testosterone is neither safe nor effective for this use and has a potential risk of serious side effects.
- Advise diabetic patients to monitor blood closely for alterations in blood glucose concentrations.
- Emphasize the importance of regular follow-up physical exams, lab tests, and x-ray exams to monitor progress.
- Radiologic bone age determinations should be evaluated every 6 mo in prepubertal children to determine rate of bone maturation and effects on epiphyseal centers.
- Instruct females to notify health care professional immediately if pregnancy is planned or suspected or if breast feeding.
- **Transdermal:** Advise patient to notify health care professional if their female sexual partner develops signs/symptoms of virilization (e.g. change in body hair distribution, significant increase in acne, deepening of voice, menstrual irregularities).
- Instruct patient that the protective plastic liner must be removed before applying the patch.
- Instruct patient to apply patch to a clean, dry area of skin on back, abdomen, upper arms, or thighs. The patch should not be applied to their genitals or over bony areas (e.g., upper shoulders or upper hip).
- Instruct patient to rotate the sites of application. Once a patch is removed, the site should not be used again for at least 1 week.
- Advise patient that the patch does not need to be removed while showering, bathing, or swimming.
- Avoid contact of patch with women and children.
- Advise patient that the patch should be removed prior to undergoing an MRI scan.
- If a patch falls off before noon, advise patient to replace it with a fresh patch which should be worn until a new patch is applied in the evening. If a patch falls off after noon, advise patient that it does not need to be replaced until a fresh patch is applied in the evening.
- **Buccal:** Instruct patient to place the rounded side surface of the buccal system in a comfortable position against the gum just above incisor tooth. Hold the system firmly in place with a finger over the lip and against the product for 30 seconds to ensure adhesion. Buccal system is designed to stay in position until removed; if it fails to adhere to the gum or falls off within the first 8 hr after application, remove original system and apply a new one (this counts as replacing the first dose; apply the next system ~12 hr after the original system was applied). If the buccal system falls off after 8 hr but before 12 hr, replace the original system (this replacement can serve as the second dose for that day).
- Advise patient to avoid dislodging buccal system and to check on placement after toothbrushing, use of mouthwash, eating or drinking. Do not chew or swallow buccal system. To remove, slide system downwards from gum toward tooth to avoid scratching the gum.
- **Topical:** Explain application to patient.
- Advise patient that women and children should avoid contact with unclothed or unwashed application site. Patients should cover the application site(s) with clothing (T-shirt) after solution has dried. For direct skin-to-skin contact, patient should wash application site thoroughly with soap and water to remove any testosterone residue. If unwashed or unclothed skin with testosterone solution comes in direct contact with skin of another person, wash area of contact with soap and water as soon as possible.
- **Intranasal:** Advise patient to notify health care professional if nasal signs or symptoms (nasopharyngitis, rhinorrhea, epistaxis, nasal discomfort, nasal scabbing) occur.

Evaluation/Desired Outcomes

- Resolution of the signs of androgen deficiency without side effects. Therapy is usually limited to 3–6 mo followed by bone growth or maturation determinations.
- Decrease in the size and spread of breast malignancy in postmenopausal women. In antineoplastic therapy, response may require 3 mo of therapy; if signs of disease progression appear, therapy should be discontinued.

TETRACYCLINES

doxycycline (dox-i-**sye**-kleen)
Acticlate, ✤Apprilon, ✤Atridox, Doryx, Doxteric, Doxy, ✤Doxycin, ✤Doxytab, ✤Doxytab, Monodox,

Oracea, Periostat, Vibramycin, ✱Vibra-Tabs

minocycline (min-oh-**sye**-kleen)
Dynacin, Minocin, Solodyn

tetracycline (te-tra-**sye**-kleen)
~~Sumycin~~

Classification
Therapeutic: anti-infectives
Pharmacologic: tetracyclines

Pregnancy Category D

Indications

Treatment of various infections caused by unusual organisms, including: *Mycoplasma*, *Chlamydia*, *Rickettsia*, *Borellia burgdorferi*. Treatment of gonorrhea and syphilis in penicillin-allergic patients. Prevention of exacerbations of chronic bronchitis. Treatment of inhalational anthrax (postexposure) and cutaneous anthrax (doxycycline only). Treatment of acne. Malaria prophylaxis (doxycycline only). Inflammatory lesions of nonnodular acne vulgaris (Solodyn).

Action

Inhibits bacterial protein synthesis at the level of the 30S bacterial ribosome. **Therapeutic Effects:** Bacteriostatic action against susceptible bacteria. **Spectrum:** Includes activity against some gram-positive pathogens: *Bacillus anthracis*, *Clostridium perfringens*, *Clostridium tetani*, *Listeria monocytogenes*, *Nocardia*, *Propionibacterium acnes*, *Actinomyces israelii*. Active against some gram-negative pathogens: *Haemophilus influenzae*, *Legionella pneumophila*, *Yersinia enterocolitica*, *Yersinia pestis*, *Neisseria gonorrhoeae*, *Neisseria meningitidis*. Also active against several other pathogens, including: *Mycoplasma*, *Treponema pallidum*, *Chlamydia*, *Rickettsia*, *B. burgdorferi*.

Pharmacokinetics

Absorption: *Tetracycline*—60–80% absorbed following oral administration. *Doxycycline, minocycline*—well absorbed from the GI tract.
Distribution: Widely distributed, some penetration into CSF; crosses the placenta and enters breast milk.
Metabolism and Excretion: *Doxycycline*—20–40% excreted unchanged by the urine; some inactivation in the intestine and some enterohepatic circulation with excretion in bile and feces. *Minocycline*—5–20% excreted unchanged by the urine; some metabolism by the liver with enterohepatic circulation and excretion in bile and feces. *Tetracycline*—Excreted mostly unchanged by the kidneys.
Half-life: *Doxycycline*—14–17 hr (↑ in severe renal impairment). *Minocycline*—11–26 hr. *Tetracycline*—6–12 hr.

TIME/ACTION PROFILE (blood levels)

ROUTE	ONSET	PEAK	DURATION
Doxycycline-PO	1–2 hr	1.5–4 hr	12 hr
Doxycycline-IV	rapid	end of infusion	12 hr
Minocycline-PO	rapid	2–3 hr	6–12 hr
Minocycline-PO—ER	unknown	3.5–4 hr	24 hr
Tetracycline-PO	1–2 hr	2–4 hr	6–12 hr

Contraindications/Precautions

Contraindicated in: Hypersensitivity; Some products contain alcohol or bisulfites; avoid in patients with known hypersensitivity or intolerance; OB: Risk of permanent staining of teeth in infant if used during last half of pregnancy (doxycycline may be used to treat anthrax in pregnant women due to the seriousness of the disease); Lactation: Lactation; Pedi: Children <8 yr (permanent staining of teeth) (unless used for anthrax; doxycycline may be used to treat anthrax in children due to the seriousness of the disease).
Use Cautiously in: Renal impairment; Hepatic impairment (minocycline); Nephrogenic diabetes insipidus; OB: Women of childbearing age.

Adverse Reactions/Side Effects

CNS: intracranial hypertension; *minocycline*, dizziness. **EENT:** *minocycline*, vestibular reactions. **GI:** HEPATOTOXICITY, CLOSTRIDIUM DIFFICILE-ASSOCIATED DIARRHEA (CDAD), diarrhea, nausea, vomiting, esophagitis, pancreatitis. **Derm:** DRUG RASH WITH EOSINOPHILIA AND SYSTEMIC SYMPTOMS, ERYTHEMA MULTIFORME, STEVENS-JOHNSON SYNDROME, TOXIC EPIDERMAL NECROLYSIS, photosensitivity, rashes; *minocycline*, pigmentation of skin and mucous membranes. **Hemat:** blood dyscrasias. **Endo:** *minocycline*—thyroid disorders. **MS:** *minocycline*—lupus-like syndrome. **Local:** *doxycycline, minocycline*—phlebitis at IV site. **Misc:** hypersensitivity reactions, superinfection.

Interactions

Drug-Drug: May ↑ effect of **warfarin**. May ↓ effectiveness of **estrogen-containing hormonal contraceptives**. **Antacids**, **calcium**, **iron**, **zinc**, **aluminum**, and **magnesium** form insoluble compounds (chelates) and ↓absorption of tetracyclines. **Sucralfate** may bind to tetracycline and ↓ its absorption from the GI tract. **Cholestyramine** or **colestipol** ↓ oral absorption of tetracyclines. **Adsorbent antidiarrheals** may ↓ absorption of tetracyclines. **Barbiturates**, **carba-**

mazepine, or **phenytoin** may ↓ activity of doxycycline. **Isotretinoin** may ↑ risk of intracranial hypertension with doxycycline; avoid concomitant use.
Drug-Food: Calcium in foods or **dairy products** ↓ absorption by forming insoluble compounds (chelates).

Route/Dosage

Doxycycline

PO (Adults and Children >8 yr and >45 k g): *Most infections*—100 mg q 12 hr on the 1st day, then 100–200 mg once daily or 50–100 mg q 12 hr; *Gonorrhea*—100 mg q 12 hr for 7 days or 200 mg once daily for 7 days (delayed-release tablets) or 300 mg followed 1 hr later by another 300-mg dose; *Uncomplicated urethral, endocervical, or rectal infection caused by Chlamydia trachomatis*—100 mg q 12 hr for 7 days; *Syphilis (early)*—100 mg q 12 hr for 14 days; *Syphilis (>1 yr duration)*—100 mg q 12 hr for 4 wk; *Malaria prophylaxis*—100 mg once daily (2 mg/kg once daily for children >85 k yr); *Lyme disease*—100 mg twice daily; *Periodontitis*—20 mg twice daily; *Rosacea*—40 mg once daily in morning.
PO (Children >8 yr and ≤45 kr): *Most infections*—2.2 mg/kg q 12 hr on the 1st day, then 2.2–4.4 mg/kg once daily or 1.1–2.2 mg/kg q 12 hr.
PO, IV (Adults and Children >45 kg): *Inhalational anthrax (post–exposure)*—100 mg IV q 12 hr; change to 100 mg PO q 12 hr when clinically appropriate for a total of 60 days; one or two other anti-infectives may be added initially, depending on clinical situation; *Cutaneous anthrax*—100 mg PO q 12 hr for 60 days; some patients may require IV therapy initially depending on clinical situation.
PO, IV (Children ≤45 kg): *Inhalational anthrax (post–exposure)*—2.2 mg/kg IV q 12 hr; change to 2.2 mg/kg PO q 12 hr when clinically appropriate for a total of 60 days; one or two other anti-infectives may be added initially, depending on clinical situation; *Cutaneous anthrax*—2.2 mg/kg q 12 hr for 60 days; some patients may require IV therapy initially depending on clinical situation.

Minocycline

PO (Adults): 100–200 mg initially, then 100 mg q 12 hr or 50 mg q 6 hr.
PO, IV (Children ≥8 yr): 4 mg/kg initially, then 2 mg/kg q 12 hr.
PO (Adults and Children ≥12 yrs [Solodyn]): *126–136 kg*135 mg once daily for 12 wks; *111–125 kg*—115 mg once daily for 12 wks; *97–110 kg*—105 mg once daily for 12 wks; *85–96 kg*—90 mg once daily for 12 wks; *72–84 kg*—80 mg once daily for 12 wks; *60–71 kg*—65 mg once daily for 12 wks; *50–59 kg*—55 mg once daily for 12 wks; *45–49 kg*—45 mg once daily for 12 wks.
IV (Adults): 200 mg initially, then 100 mg q 12 hr (not to exceed 400 mg/day).

Tetracycline

PO (Adults): 250–500 mg q 6 hr or 500 mg–1 g q 12 hr. *Chronic treatment of acne*—500 mg–2 g/day for 3 wk, then ↓ to 125 mg–1 g/day.
PO (Children ≥8 yr): 6.25–12.5 mg/kg q 6 hr or 12.5–25 mg/kg q 12 hr.

Availability

Doxycycline (generic available)

Tablets: 20 mg, 50 mg, 75 mg, 100 mg, 150 mg. **Cost:** *Generic*—20 mg $118.90/100, 50 mg $335.71/100, 75 mg $498.35/100, 100 mg $246.02/50, 150 mg $274.17/30. **Delayed-release tablets:** 50 mg, 75 mg, 100 mg, 150 mg, 200 mg. **Cost:** *Generic*—75 mg $613.45/60, 100 mg $1,314.83/100, 150 mg $1,759.94/100. **Capsules:** 50 mg, 75 mg, 100 mg, 150 mg. **Cost:** *Generic*—50 mg $118.74/100, 75 mg $1,639.77/100, 100 mg $96.92/50, 150 mg $1,479.01/60. **Delayed-release capsules:** 40 mg. **Cost:** $501.12/30. **Oral suspension (raspberry flavor):** 25 mg/5 mL. **Cost:** *Generic*—$22.77/60 mL. **Syrup (apple-raspberry flavor):** 50 mg/5 mL. **Cost:** $339.47/473 mL. **Powder for injection:** 100 mg/vial, 200 mg/vial.

Minocycline (generic available)

Capsules: 50 mg, 75 mg, 100 mg. **Cost:** *Generic*—50 mg $169.87/100, 75 mg $197.96/100, 100 mg $169.87/50. **Tablets:** 50 mg, 75 mg, 100 mg. **Cost:** *Generic*—50 mg $343.47/100, 75 mg $504.25/100, 100 mg $300.98/50. **Extended-release tablets:** 45 mg, 55 mg, 65 mg, 80 mg, 90 mg, 105 mg, 115 mg, 135 mg. **Cost:** *Generic*—45 mg $605.01/30, 90 mg $605.01/30, 135 mg $605.01/30; *Solodyn*—55 mg $1,044.22/30, 65 mg $1,044.22/30, 80 mg $1,044.22/30, 105 mg $1,044.22/30, 115 mg $1,044.22/30. **Lyophilized powder for injection (requires reconstitution):** 100 mg/vial.

Tetracycline (generic available)

Capsules: 250 mg, 500 mg. **Cost:** *Generic*—250 mg $6.88/100, 500 mg $11.80/100.

NURSING IMPLICATIONS

Assessment

- Assess for infection (vital signs; appearance of wound, sputum, urine, and stool; WBC) at beginning of and throughout therapy.
- Obtain specimens for culture and sensitivity before initiating therapy. First dose may be given before receiving results.
- Monitor bowel function. Diarrhea, abdominal cramping, fever, and bloody stools should be reported to health care professional promptly as a sign of Clostridium difficile-associated diarrhea (CDAD). May begin up to several weeks following cessation of therapy.
- Assess for rash periodically during therapy. May cause Stevens-Johnson syndrome or toxic epidermal

necrolysis. Discontinue therapy if severe or if accompanied with fever, general malaise, fatigue, muscle or joint aches, blisters, oral lesions, conjunctivitis, hepatitis and/or eosinophilia.

- **IV:** Assess IV site frequently; may cause thrombophlebitis.
- ***Lab Test Considerations:*** Monitor renal and hepatic function and CBC periodically during long-term therapy.
- May cause ↑ AST, ALT, serum alkaline phosphatase, bilirubin, and amylase concentrations. Tetracyclines, except doxycycline, may cause ↑ serum BUN.

Potential Nursing Diagnoses

Risk for infection (Indications, Side Effects)
Noncompliance (Patient/Family Teaching)

Implementation

- Do not confuse Oracea with Orencia (abatacept). Do not confuse Dynacin with Dynacirc (isradipine).
- May cause yellow-brown discoloration and softening of teeth and bones if administered prenatally or during early childhood. Not recommended for children under 8 yr of age or during pregnancy or lactation unless used for the treatment of anthrax.
- **PO:** Administer around the clock. Administer at least 1 hr before or 2 hr after meals. *Doxycycline and minocycline* may be taken with food or milk if GI irritation occurs. Administer with a full glass of liquid and at least 1 hr before going to bed to avoid esophageal ulceration. Use calibrated measuring device for liquid preparations. Shake liquid preparations well. Do not administer within 1–3 hr of other medications.
- Do not open, break, crush or chew extended release capsules and tablets.
- Avoid administration of calcium, zinc, antacids, magnesium- or aluminum-containing medications, sodium bicarbonate, or iron supplements within 1–3 hr of oral tetracyclines.

Doxycycline

- The *Oracea* product is only indicated for rosacea, not for infections.
- **PO: Public Health Emergency —Exposure to Anthrax**: To prepare doses for infants and children exposed to anthrax, place one 100 mg tablet in a small bowl and crush to a fine powder with a metal spoon, leaving no large pieces. Add 4 level teaspoons of lowfat milk, lowfat chocolate milk, regular chocolate milk, chocolate pudding, or apple juice. Mix food or drink and doxycycline powder until powder dissolves. Mixture is stable in a covered container for 24 hr if refrigerated (if made with milk or pudding) or at room temperature (if made with juice). Number of teaspoons to administer/dose is based on child's weight (0–12.5 lb—1/2 tsp; 12.5–25 lb—1 tsp; 25–37.5 lb—1 1/2 tsp; 37.5–50 lb—2 tsp; 50–62.5 lb—2 1/2 tsp; 62.5–75 lb—3 tsp; 75–87.5 lb—3 1/2 tsp; 87.5–100 lb—4 tsp).
- Capsules may also be administered by carefully opening and sprinkling capsule contents on a spoonful of applesauce. The applesauce should be swallowed immediately without chewing and followed with a cool 8-ounce glass of water to ensure complete swallowing of the capsule contents. The applesauce should not be hot, and it should be soft enough to be swallowed without chewing. If mixture cannot be taken immediately, discard; do not store for later use.

IV Administration

- **Intermittent Infusion:** Reconstitute each 100 mg with 10 mL of sterile water or 0.9% NaCl for injection. ***Diluent:*** Dilute further in 100–1000 mL of 0.9% NaCl, D5W, D5/LR, Ringer's, or lactated Ringer's solution. Solution is stable for 12 hr at room temperature and 72 hr if refrigerated. If diluted with D5/LR or lactated Ringer's solution, administer within 6 hr. Protect solution from direct sunlight. ***Concentration:*** Concentrations of less than 1 mcg/mL or greater than 1 mg/mL are not recommended. ***Rate:*** Administer over a minimum of 1–4 hr. Avoid rapid administration. Avoid extravasation.
- **Y-Site Compatibility:** acyclovir , alemtuzumab, alfentanyl, amifostine, amikacin, aminophylline, amiodarone, anidulafungin, argatroban, ascorbic acid, atropine, azithromycin, aztreonam, benztropine, bivalirudin, bleomycin, bumetanide, buprenorphine, butorphanol, calcium chloride, calcium gluconate, cangrelor, carboplatin, carmustine, caspofungin, cefotaxime, ceftriaxone, chlorpromazine, cisatracurium, cisplatin, clindamycin, cyanocobalamin, cyclophosphamide, cyclosporine, cytarabine, dacarbazine, dactinomycin, daptomycin, daunorubicin hydrochloride, dexmedetomidine, dexrazoxane, digoxin, diltiazem, diphenhydramine, dobutamine, docetaxel, dolasetron, dopamine, doxorubicin hydrochloride, enalaprilat, ephedrine, epinephrine, epirubicin, epoetin alfa, eptifibatide, ertapenem, esmolol, etoposide, etoposide phosphate, famotidine, fenoldopam, fentanyl, filgrastim, fluconazole, fludarabine, fosphenytoin, gemcitabine, gentamicin, glycopyrrolate, granisetron, hetastarch, hydromorphone, idarubicin, ifosfamide, imipenem/cilastatin, insulin, irinotecan, isoproterenol, labetalol, leucovorin, levofloxacin, lidocaine, linezolid, lorazepam, magnesium sulfate, mannitol, mechlorethamine, melphalan, meperidine, mesna, methyldopate, metoclopramide, metoprolol, metronidazole, midazolam, milrinone, mitoxantrone, morphine, multi-

T

vitamins, mycophenolate, nalbuphine, naloxone, nesiritide, nicardipine, nitroglycerin, nitroprusside, norepinephrine, octreotide, ondansetron, oxaliplatin, oxytocin, paclitaxel, pamidronate, pancuronium, pantoprazole, papaverine, pentamidine, pentazocine, phenylephrine, phytonadione, potassium chloride, procainamide, prochlorperazine, promethazine, propofol, propranolol, protamine, pyridoxine, quinupristin/dalfopristin, ranitidine, remifentanil, rituximab, rocuronium, sargramostim, sodium acetate, streptokinase, succinylcholine, sufentanil, tacrolimus, telavancin, teniposide, theophylline, thiamine, thiotepa, tirofiban, tobramycin, topotecan, trastuzumab, vancomycin, vasopressin, vecuronium, verapamil, vinblastine, vincristine, vinorelbine, voriconazole, zoledronic acid.

- **Y-Site Incompatibility:** allopurinol, aminocaproic acid, amphotericin B colloidal, amphotericin B lipid complex, amphotericin B liposome, ampicillin, ampicillin/sulbactam, cefazolin, cefotetan, cefoxitin, ceftazidime, cefuroxime, chloramphenicol, dantrolene, dexamethasone, diazepam, erythromycin, fluorouracil, folic acid, furosemide, ganciclovir, heparin, hydrocortisone, indomethacin, ketorolac, methotrexate, methylprednisolone, nafcillin, oxacillin, palonosetron, pemetrexed, penicillin G, pentobarbital, phenobarbital, phenytoin, piperacillin/tazobactam, potassium acetate, sodium bicarbonate, trimethoprim/sulfamethoxazole.

Minocycline

IV Administration

- IV doses are indicated only when oral therapy is not adequate or tolerated. Resume oral doses as soon as possible.
- **Intermittent Infusion:** Reconstitute vial with 5 mL of Sterile Water for injection. ***Diluent:*** 100 mL to 1,000 mL 0.9% NaCl, D5W, or D5/0.9% NaCl, or in 250 mL to 1000 mL LR, but not with other solutions containing calcium; precipitate may form especially in neutral and alkaline solutions. Solutions are stable for 4 hrs at room temperature or 24 hrs if refrigerated. ***Rate:*** Infuse over 60 min. Do not infuse rapidly.
- **Y-Site Incompatibility:** Do not administer with other medications or solutions. Flush line between doses.

Patient/Family Teaching

- Instruct patient to take medication around the clock and to finish the drug completely as directed, even if feeling better. Take missed doses as soon as possible unless it is almost time for next dose; do not double doses. Advise patient that sharing of this medication may be dangerous.
- Advise patient to avoid taking milk or other dairy products concurrently with oral tetracyclines. Also avoid taking antacids, zinc, calcium, magnesium- or aluminum-containing medications, sodium bicarbonate, and iron supplements within 1–3 hr of oral tetracyclines.
- Instruct patient to notify health care professional immediately if rash, diarrhea, abdominal cramping, fever, or bloody stools occur and not to treat with antidiarrheals without consulting health care professionals.
- *Minocycline* commonly causes dizziness or unsteadiness. Caution patient to avoid driving or other activities requiring alertness until response to medication is known. Notify health care professional if these symptoms occur.
- Caution patient to use sunscreen and protective clothing to prevent photosensitivity reactions.
- Advise patient to report the signs of superinfection (black, furry overgrowth on the tongue; vaginal itching or discharge; loose or foul-smelling stools) or intracranial hypertension (headache, blurred vision, diplopia, vision loss). Women who are overweight, of childbearing age or have a history of IH are at greater risk for developing tetracyclines—associated IH. Skin rash, pruritus, and urticaria should also be reported.
- Advise patient to notify health care professional of all Rx or OTC medications, vitamins, or herbal products being taken and to consult with health care professional before taking other medications.
- Instruct patient to notify health care professional of medication regimen before treatment or surgery.
- Rep: Advise female patient to use a nonhormonal method of contraception while taking tetracyclines and until next menstrual period. Men attempting to father a child should not take minocycline.
- Instruct patient to notify health care professional if symptoms do not improve within a few days for systemic preparations.
- Caution patient to discard outdated or decomposed tetracyclines; they may be toxic.
- **Malaria Prophylaxis:** Advise patient to avoid being bitten by mosquitoes by using protective measures, especially from dusk to dawn (e.g., staying in well-screened areas, using mosquito nets, covering the body with clothing, and using an effective insect repellant). Doxycycline prophylaxis should begin 1–2 days before travel to the malarious area, continued daily while in the malarious area and after leaving the malarious area, should be continued for 4 more weeks to avoid development of malaria. Do not exceed 4 mo.

Evaluation/Desired Outcomes

- Resolution of the signs and symptoms of infection. Length of time for complete resolution depends on the organism and site of infection.
- Decrease in acne lesions.
- Treatment of inhalation anthrax (post exposure) or treatment of cutaneous anthrax (doxycycline).
- Prevention of malaria.
- Reduction in inflammatory lesions associated with rosacea.

REMS

thalidomide (tha-lid-oh-mide)

Thalomid

Classification

Therapeutic: immunosuppressants

Pregnancy Category X

Indications

Cutaneous manifestations of moderate to severe erythema nodosum leprosum (ENL). Prevention (maintenance) and suppression of recurrent ENL. Newly diagnosed multiple myeloma (with dexamethasone). **Unlabeled Use:** Bechet's syndrome. HIV-associated wasting syndrome. Aphthous stomatitis (including HIV associated). Crohn's disease.

Action

May suppress excess levels of tumor necrosis factor-alpha (TNF-alpha) in patients with ENL and alter leukocyte migration by altering characteristics of cell surfaces. **Therapeutic Effects:** Decreased skin lesions in ENL and prevention of recurrence.

Pharmacokinetics

Absorption: 67–93% absorbed following oral administration.

Distribution: Crosses the placenta; highly protein bound.

Protein Binding: Highly bound.

Metabolism and Excretion: Hydrolyzed in plasma to multiple metabolites.

Half-life: 5–7 hr.

TIME/ACTION PROFILE (dermatologic effects)

ROUTE	ONSET	PEAK	DURATION
PO	48 hr	1–2 mo	unknown

Contraindications/Precautions

Contraindicated in: Hypersensitivity; Seizure disorders; Rep: Women with childbearing potential (unless specific conditions are met); Rep: Sexually mature men (unless specific conditions are met); OB: Pregnancy (can cause fetal harm); Lactation: Potential for serious adverse reactions in the infant.

Use Cautiously in: Pedi: Children <12 yr (safety not established).

Adverse Reactions/Side Effects

CNS: SEIZURES, dizziness, drowsiness. **CV:** bradycardia, edema, orthostatic hypotension, thromboembolic events (↑ risk with dexamethasone in multiple myeloma). **GI:** constipation. **Derm:** STEVENS-JOHNSON SYNDROME, TOXIC EPIDERMAL NECROLYSIS, rash, photosensitivity. **Hemat:** neutropenia, thrombocytopenia. **Neuro:** peripheral neuropathy. **Misc:** SEVERE BIRTH DEFECTS, hypersensitivity reactions, ↑ HIV viral load, tumor lysis syndrome.

Interactions

Drug-Drug: ↑ CNS depression with concurrent use of **barbiturates**, **sedative/hypnotics**, **alcohol**, **chlorpromazine**, **reserpine**, or other **CNS depressants**. Concurrent use of **agents that may cause peripheral neuropathy** ↑ risk of peripheral neuropathy.

Drug-Natural Products: Concommitant use with **echinacea**, and **melatonin** may interfere with immunosuppression.

Route/Dosage

ENL

PO (Adults ≥50 kg): 100–300 mg/day initially; up to 400 mg/day has been used, depending on previous response. Every 3–6 mo, attempts should be made to taper and discontinue in decrements of 50 mg q 2–4 wk.

PO (Adults <50 kg): 100 mg/day initially; up to 400 mg/day has been used, depending on previous response. Every 3–6 mo, attempts should be made to taper and discontinue in decrements of 50 mg q 2–4 wk.

Multiple Myeloma

PO (Adults): 200 mg daily in 28-day treatment cycles. Dexamethasone 40 mg is administered on Days 1–4, 9–12, 17–20.

Availability

Capsules: 50 mg, 100 mg, 150 mg, 200 mg.

NURSING IMPLICATIONS

Assessment

- Assess monthly for initial 3 mo and periodically during therapy to detect early signs of peripheral neuropathy (numbness, tingling, or pain in hands and feet). Commonly occurs with prolonged therapy, but has occurred following short-term use or following completion of therapy. May be severe and irreversible. Electrophysiologic testing may be done at baseline and every 6 mo to detect asymptomatic peripheral neuropathy. If symptoms occur, discontinue thalidomide immediately to limit further damage. Reinstate therapy only if neuropathy returns to baseline.
- Monitor for signs of hypersensitivity reaction (erythematous macular rash, fever, tachycardia, hypotension). May require discontinuation of therapy if severe. If reaction recurs when dosing is resumed, discontinue thalidomide.
- Monitor for signs and symptoms of bleeding (petechiae, epistaxis, gastrointestinal bleeding) during therapy. May require dose interruption, reduction, or discontinuation.

T

- Monitor for side effects (constipation, oversedation, peripheral neuropathy); may require discontinuation or dose reduction until side effects resolve.
- **Multiple Myeloma:** Assess for venous thromboembolism (dyspnea, chest pain, arm or leg swelling) periodically during therapy, especially in patients concurrently taking dexamethasone. Consider prophylaxis depending on patient risk factors.
- ***Lab Test Considerations:*** Monitor WBC with differential and platelet count during therapy. May cause ↓ WBC. Do not initiate therapy with an ANC ≤750/mm³. If ANC ↓ to ≤750/mm³ during therapy, re-evaluate medication regimen; if neutropenia persists, consider discontinuing therapy. May cause thrombocytopenia.
- May cause ↑ viral load levels in patients with HIV.

Potential Nursing Diagnoses

Impaired skin integrity (Indications)
Risk for injury (Adverse Reactions)

Implementation

- Do not confuse Thalomid (thalidomide) with thiamine.
- Rep: Due to teratogenic effects, thalidomide may be prescribed only by prescribers registered in the *System for Thalidomide Education and Prescribing Safety (STEPS)* program. Thalidomide is started within 24 hr of a negative pregnancy test with a sensitivity of at least 50 mIU/mL. Pregnancy testing must occur weekly during first month of therapy, then monthly thereafter in women with a regular menstrual cycle. For women with irregular menses, pregnancy testing should occur every 2 wk. If pregnancy occurs, thalidomide should be discontinued immediately. Any suspected fetal exposure must be reported to the FDA and the manufacturer, and patient should be referred to an obstetrician/gynecologist experienced in reproductive toxicity.
- If health care professionals or other caregivers are exposed to body fluids from patients receiving thalidomide, use appropriate precautions, such as wearing gloves to prevent the potential cutaneous exposure to thalidomide or washing the exposed area with soap and water.
- Corticosteroids may be used concurrently with thalidomide for patients with moderate to severe neuritis associated with a severe ENL reaction. Use of corticosteroids can be tapered and discontinued when neuritis resolves.
- **PO:** Administer once daily with water, preferably at bedtime and at least 1 hr after the evening meal. If divided doses are used, administer at least 1 hr after meals.

Patient/Family Teaching

- Instruct patient to take thalidomide as directed. Do not discontinue without notifying health care professional; dose should be tapered gradually. Explain *STEPS* program to patient.
- Advise patient that thalidomide should not be shared with others.
- Frequently causes drowsiness or dizziness. Caution patient to avoid driving or other activities requiring alertness until response to medication is known.
- Advise patient to change positions slowly to minimize orthostatic hypotension.
- Caution patient to use sunscreen and protective clothing to prevent photosensitivity reactions.
- Instruct patient not to donate blood and male patients not to donate sperm while taking thalidomide and for 1 month following discontinuation.
- Advise patient to notify health care professional immediately if pain, numbness, tingling, or burning in hands or feet or shortness of breath, chest pain, swelling of arms or legs occur.
- Rep: Caution patient on the extreme importance of maintaining contraception for 1 mo prior to, during, and for 1 mo following discontinuation of therapy. *For women of childbearing age,* two methods of reliable contraception must be used unless complete abstinence is used. *For men,* a latex condom must be used, even if a successful vasectomy has been performed. Patients must meet *ALL* of the STEPS conditions: Understands and can follow instructions and is capable of complying with contraceptive measures, pregnancy testing, patient registration, and patient survey. Patients must receive verbal and written warnings of the potential teratogenicity of thalidomide and must acknowledge in writing their understanding and acceptance of these conditions.
- Advise patient to notify health care professional of all Rx or OTC medications, vitamins, or herbal products being taken and to consult with health care professional before taking other medications. Concomitant use of HIV-protease inhibitors, modafinil, penicillins, rifampin, rifabutin, phenytoin, carbamazepine, or certain herbal supplements such as St. John's wort with hormonal contraceptive agents may reduce the effectiveness of contraception during and for up to one month after discontinuation of these concomitant therapies. Therefore, women requiring treatment with one or more of these drugs must use two other effective or highly effective methods of contraception or abstain from heterosexual sexual contact while taking thalidomide.

Evaluation/Desired Outcomes

- Resolution of the signs and symptoms of active ENL reaction. Usually requires at least 2 wk of therapy; then taper medication in 50 mg decrements every 2–4 wk.
- Prevention of recurrent ENL. Tapering off medication should be attempted every 3–6 mo in decrements of 50 mg every 2–4 wk.
- Decrease in serum and urine paraprotein measurements in patients with multiple myeloma.

thiamine (thye-a-min)

Betaxin, vitamin B1

Classification
Therapeutic: vitamins
Pharmacologic: water soluble vitamins

Pregnancy Category A

Indications

Treatment of thiamine deficiencies (beriberi). Prevention of Wernicke's encephalopathy. Dietary supplement in patients with GI disease, alcoholism, or cirrhosis.

Action

Required for carbohydrate metabolism. **Therapeutic Effects:** Replacement in deficiency states.

Pharmacokinetics

Absorption: Well absorbed from the GI tract by an active process. Excessive amounts are not absorbed completely. Also well absorbed from IM sites.
Distribution: Widely distributed. Enters breast milk.
Metabolism and Excretion: Metabolized by the liver. Excess amounts are excreted unchanged by the kidneys.
Half-life: Unknown.

TIME/ACTION PROFILE (time for symptoms of deficiency—edema and heart failure—to resolve†)

ROUTE	ONSET	PEAK	DURATION
PO, IM, IV	hr	days	days–wk

†Confusion and psychosis take longer to respond.

Contraindications/Precautions

Contraindicated in: Hypersensitivity; Known alcohol intolerance or bisulfite hypersensitivity (elixir only).
Use Cautiously in: Wernicke's encephalopathy (condition may be worsened unless thiamine is administered before glucose).

Adverse Reactions/Side Effects

Adverse reactions and side effects are extremely rare and are usually associated with IV administration or extremely large doses.
CNS: restlessness, weakness. **EENT:** tightness of the throat. **Resp:** pulmonary edema, respiratory distress. **CV:** VASCULAR COLLAPSE, hypotension, vasodilation. **GI:** GI bleeding, nausea. **Derm:** cyanosis, pruritus, sweating, tingling, urticaria, warmth. **Misc:** ANGIOEDEMA.

Interactions

Drug-Drug: None significant.

Route/Dosage

Thiamine Deficiency (Beriberi)

PO (Adults): 5–10 mg 3 times daily.
PO (Children): 10–50 mg/day in divided doses.
IM, IV (Adults): 5–100 mg 3 times daily.
IM, IV (Children): 10–25 mg/day.

Dietary Supplement

PO (Adults): 1–1.6 mg/day.
PO (Children 4–10 yr): 0.9–1 mg/day.
PO (Children birth–3 yr): 0.3–0.7 mg/day.

Availability (generic available)

Tablets: 5 mg[OTC], 10 mg[OTC], 25 mg[OTC], 50 mg[OTC], 100 mg[OTC], 250 mg[OTC], 500 mg[OTC]. **Injection:** 100 mg/mL. ***In combination with:*** other vitamins, minerals, and trace elements in multi-vitamin preparations[OTC].

NURSING IMPLICATIONS

Assessment

- Assess for signs and symptoms of thiamine deficiency (anorexia, GI distress, irritability, palpitations, tachycardia, edema, paresthesia, muscle weakness and pain, depression, memory loss, confusion, psychosis, visual disturbances, elevated serum pyruvic acid levels).
- Assess patient's nutritional status (diet, weight) prior to and throughout therapy.
- Monitor patients receiving IV thiamine for anaphylaxis (wheezing, urticaria, edema).
- ***Lab Test Considerations:*** May interfere with certain methods of testing serum theophylline, uric acid, and urobilinogen concentrations.

Potential Nursing Diagnoses

Imbalanced nutrition: less than body requirements (Indications)

Implementation

- Do not confuse thiamine with Thalomid (thalidomide).
- Because of infrequency of single B-vitamin deficiencies, combinations are commonly administered.
- **IM, IV:** Parenteral administration is reserved for patients in whom oral administration is not feasible.
- **IM:** Administration may cause tenderness and induration at injection site. Cool compresses may decrease discomfort.

IV Administration

- **IV:** Sensitivity reactions and death have occurred from IV administration. An intradermal test dose is recommended in patients with suspected sensitivity. Monitor site for erythema and induration.
- **IV Push:** ***Concentration:*** Administer undiluted at 100 mg/mL. ***Rate:*** Administer at a rate of 100 mg over 5 min.

T

- **Continuous Infusion:** ***Diluent:*** May be diluted in dextrose/Ringer's or LR combinations, dextrose/saline combinations, D5W, D10W, Ringer's and LR injection, 0.9% NaCl, or 0.45% NaCl. Usually administered with other vitamins.
- **Y-Site Compatibility:** alfentanil, amikacin, ascorbic acid, atracurium, atropine, aztreonam, benztropine, bumetanide, buprenorphine, butorphanol, calcium chloride, calcium gluconate, cefazolin, cefonocid, cefotaxime, cefotetan, cefoxitin, ceftriaxone, cefuroxime, chlorpromazine, clindamycin, cyanocobalamin, cyclosporine, dexamethasone, digoxin, diphenhydramine, dobutamine, dopamine, doxycycline, enalaprilat, ephedrine, epinephrine, erythromycin, esmolol, famotidine, fentanyl, gentamicin, glycopyrrolate, heparin, insulin, isoproterenol, labetalol, lidocaine, magnesium sulfate, mannitol, meperidine, metaraminol, methoxamine, methyldopate, metoclopramide, metoprolol, morphine, multivitamins, nafcillin, nalbuphine, naloxone, nitroglycerin, nitroprusside, norepinephrine, oxacillin, oxytocin, papaverine, penicillin G, pentamidine, pentazocine, phentolamine, phenylephrine, phytonadione, potassium chloride, procainamide, prochlorperazine, promethazine, propranolol, protamine, pyridoxime, ranitidine, streptokinase, succinylcholine, sufentanil, theophylline, tobramycin, tolazoline, trimetaphan, vancomycin, vasopressin, verapamil.
- **Y-Site Incompatibility:** aminophylline, amphotericin B colloidal, azathioprine, ceftazidime, chloramphenicol, dantrolene, diazepam, diazoxide, folic acid, furosemide, ganciclovir, hydrocortisone, imipenem/cilastatin, indomethacin, methylprednisolone, pentobarbital, phenobarbital, phenytoin, sodium bicarbonate, trimethoprim/sulfamethoxazole.
- **Additive Incompatibility:** Solutions with neutral or alkaline pH, such as carbonates, bicarbonates, citrates, and acetates.

Patient/Family Teaching

- Encourage patient to comply with dietary recommendations of health care professional. Explain that the best source of vitamins is a well-balanced diet with foods from the four basic food groups.
- Teach patient that foods high in thiamine include cereals (whole grain and enriched), meats (especially pork), and fresh vegetables; loss is variable during cooking.
- Caution patients self-medicating with vitamin supplements not to exceed RDA. The effectiveness of megadoses of vitamins for treatment of various medical conditions is unproved and may cause side effects.

Evaluation/Desired Outcomes

- Prevention of or decrease in the signs and symptoms of vitamin B deficiency.
- Decrease in the symptoms of neuritis, ocular signs, ataxia, edema, and heart failure may be seen within hours of administration and may disappear within a few days.
- Confusion and psychosis may take longer to respond and may persist if nerve damage has occurred.

HIGH ALERT

THROMBOLYTIC AGENTS

alteplase (**al**-te-plase)
Activase, ✦Activase rt-PA, Cathflo Activase, tissue plasminogen activator, t-PA

reteplase (**re**-te-plase)
Retavase

streptokinase (strep-toe-**kye**-nase)
Streptase

tenecteplase (te-**nek**-te-plase)
TNKase

Classification
Therapeutic: thrombolytics
Pharmacologic: plasminogen activators

Pregnancy Category C

Indications

Alteplase, reteplase, streptokinase, tenecteplase: Acute myocardial infarction (MI). **Alteplase, streptokinase:** Acute massive pulmonary emboli. **Alteplase:** Acute ischemic stroke. **Streptokinase:** Acute deep vein thrombosis. **Streptokinase:** Acute arterial thrombi. **Streptokinase:** Occluded arteriovenous cannulae. **Alteplase:** Occluded central venous access devices.

Action

Convert plasminogen to plasmin, which is then able to degrade fibrin present in clots. Alteplase, reteplase, and tenecteplase directly activate plasminogen. Streptokinase combines with plasminogen to form activator complexes, which then converts plasminogen to plasmin. **Therapeutic Effects:** Lysis of thrombi in coronary arteries, with preservation of ventricular function or improvement of ventricular function (and ↓ risk of HF or death). Lysis of pulmonary emboli or deep vein thrombosis. Lysis of thrombi causing ischemic stroke, reducing risk of neurologic sequelae. Restoration of cannula or catheter patency and function.

Pharmacokinetics

Absorption: Complete after IV administration. Intracoronary administration or administration into occluded catheters or cannulae has a more localized effect.

Distribution: Streptokinase appears to cross the placenta minimally, if at all. Remainder of distribution for streptokinase or other agents is not known.

Metabolism and Excretion: *Alteplase, tenecteplase*—Rapidly metabolized by the liver. *Reteplase*—Cleared primarily by the liver and kidneys. *Streptokinase*—Rapidly cleared from circulation by antibodies and other unknown mechanism.

Half-life: *Alteplase*—35 min; *reteplase*—13–16 min; *streptokinase*—initially 18 min (due to clearance by antibodies), then 83 min; *Tenecteplase*—20–24 min (initial phase), 90–130 min (terminal phase).

TIME/ACTION PROFILE (fibrinolysis)

ROUTE	ONSET	PEAK	DURATION
Alteplase IV	30 min	60 min	unknown
Reteplase IV	30 min	30–90 min	48 hr
Streptokinase IV	immediate	rapid	4 hr (up to 12 hr)
Tenecteplase IV	rapid	unknown	unknown

Contraindications/Precautions

Contraindicated in: Active internal bleeding; History of cerebrovascular accident; Recent (within 2 mo) intracranial or intraspinal injury or trauma; Intracranial neoplasm, AV malformation, or aneurysm; Severe uncontrolled hypertension; Known bleeding tendencies; Hypersensitivity; cross-sensitivity with other thrombolytics may occur.

Use Cautiously in: Recent (within 10 days) major surgery, trauma, GI, or GU bleeding; Left heart thrombus; Severe hepatic or renal disease; Hemorrhagic ophthalmic conditions; Septic phlebitis; Previous puncture of a noncompressible vessel; Subacute bacterial endocarditis or acute pericarditis; Recent streptococcal infection or previous therapy with streptokinase (from 5 days–6 mo); may produce resistance because of antibody formation; ↑ dosage requirements may be encountered (streptokinase only); Geri: >75 yr; ↑ risk of intracranial bleeding; OB, Lactation, Pedi: Safety not established.

Exercise Extreme Caution in: Patients receiving concurrent anticoagulant therapy (↑ risk of intracranial bleeding).

Adverse Reactions/Side Effects

CNS: INTRACRANIAL HEMORRHAGE. **EENT:** epistaxis, gingival bleeding. **Resp:** bronchospasm, hemoptysis. **CV:** hypotension, reperfusion arrhythmias. **GI:** GI BLEEDING, RETROPERITONEAL BLEEDING, nausea, vomiting. **GU:** GU TRACT BLEEDING. **Derm:** ecchymoses, flushing, urticaria. **Hemat:** BLEEDING. **Local:** hemorrhage at injection sites, phlebitis at IV site. **MS:** musculoskeletal pain. **Misc:** allergic reactions including ANAPHYLAXIS, fever.

Interactions

Drug-Drug: Concurrent use of **aspirin**, other **NSAIDs**, **warfarin**, **heparin**, **low-molecular-weight heparins**, **direct thrombin inhibitors**, **abciximab**, **eptifibatide**, **tirofiban**, **clopidogrel**, or **dipyridamole** may ↑ risk of bleeding, although these agents are frequently used together or in sequence. Effects may be ↓ by **antifibrinolytic agents**, including **aminocaproic acid** or **tranexamic acid**.

Drug-Natural Products: ↑ anticoagulant effect and bleeding risk with **anise**, **arnica**, **chamomile**, **clove**, **dong quai**, **fenugreek**, **feverfew**, **garlic**, **ginger**, **ginkgo**, **Panax ginseng**, **licorice**, and others.

Route/Dosage

Alteplase

Myocardial Infarction (Accelerated or Front-Loading Infusion)

IV (Adults): 15 mg bolus, then 0.75 mg/kg (up to 50 mg) over 30 min, then 0.5 mg/kg (up to 35 mg) over next 60 min; usually accompanied by heparin therapy.

Myocardial Infarction (3-Hour Infusion)

IV (Adults >65 kg): 60 mg over 1st hr (6–10 mg given as a bolus over first 1–2 min), 20 mg over the 2nd hr, and 20 mg over the 3rd hr for a total dose of 100 mg.

IV (Adults <65 kg): 0.75 mg/kg over 1st hr (0.075–0.125 mg/kg given as a bolus over first 1–2 min), 0.25 mg/kg over the 2nd hr, and 0.25 mg/kg over the 3rd hr for a total dose of 1.25 mg/kg (not to exceed 100 mg total).

Pulmonary Embolism

IV (Adults): 100 mg over 2 hr; follow with heparin.

Acute Ischemic Stroke

IV (Adults): 0.9 mg/kg (not to exceed 90 mg), given as an infusion over 1 hr, with 10% of the dose given as a bolus over the 1st min.

Occluded Venous Access Devices

IV (Adults and Children >30 kg): 2 mg/2 mL instilled into occluded catheter; if unsuccessful, may repeat once after 2 hr.

IV (Adults and Children <30 kg): 110% of the lumen volume (not to exceed 2 mg in 2 mL) instilled into occluded catheter; if unsuccessful, may repeat once after 2 hr.

Reteplase

IV (Adults): 10 units, followed 30 min later by an additional 10 units.

Streptokinase

Myocardial Infarction

IV (Adults): 1.5 million units given as a continuous infusion over up to 60 min.

Intracoronary (Adults): 20,000 unit bolus followed by 2000–4000 units/min infusion for 30–90 min.

Deep Vein Thrombosis, Pulmonary Emboli, Arterial Emboli, or Arterial Thromboses

IV (Adults): 250,000 unit loading dose over 30 min, followed by 100,000 unit/hr for 24 hr for pulmonary emboli or arterial thrombosis/embolism, 72 hr for deep vein thrombosis.

Tenecteplase

IV (Adults <60 kg): 30 mg.
IV (Adults ≥60 kg and <70 kg): 35 mg.
IV (Adults ≥70 kg and <80 kg): 40 mg.
IV (Adults ≥80 kg and <90 kg): 45 mg.
IV (Adults ≥90 kg): 50 mg.

Availability

Alteplase

Powder for injection: 2 mg/vial, 50 mg/vial, 100 mg/vial.

Reteplase

Powder for injection: 10.8 units/vial.

Streptokinase

Powder for injection: 250,000 units/vial, 750,000 units/vial, 1,500,000 units/vial.

Tenecteplase

Powder for injection: 50 mg/vial.

NURSING IMPLICATIONS

Assessment

- Begin therapy as soon as possible after the onset of symptoms.
- Monitor vital signs, including temperature, continuously for coronary thrombosis and at least every 4 hr during therapy for other indications. Do not use lower extremities to monitor BP. Notify health care professional if systolic BP >180 mm Hg or diastolic BP >110 mm Hg. Should not be given if hypertension is uncontrolled. Inform health care professional if hypotension occurs. Hypotension may result from the drug, hemorrhage, or cardiogenic shock.
- Assess patient carefully for bleeding every 15 min during the 1st hr of therapy, every 15–30 min during the next 8 hr, and at least every 4 hr for the duration of therapy. Frank bleeding may occur from sites of invasive procedures or from body orifices. Internal bleeding may also occur (decreased neurologic status; abdominal pain with coffee-grounds emesis or black, tarry stools; hematuria; joint pain). If uncontrolled bleeding occurs, stop medication and notify health care professional immediately.
- Inquire about previous reaction to streptokinase therapy. Assess patient for hypersensitivity reaction (rash, dyspnea, fever, changes in facial color, swelling around the eyes, wheezing). If these occur, inform health care professional promptly. Keep epinephrine, an antihistamine, and resuscitation equipment close by in the event of an anaphylactic reaction.
- Inquire about recent streptococcal infection. *Streptokinase* may be less effective if administered between 5 days and 6 mo of a streptococcal infection.
- Assess neurologic status throughout therapy. Altered sensorium or neurologic changes may be indicative of intracranial bleeding.
- **Myocardial Infarction:** Monitor ECG continuously. Notify health care professional if significant arrhythmias occur. Monitor cardiac enzymes. Radionuclide myocardial scanning and/or coronary angiography may be ordered 7–10 days after therapy to monitor effectiveness of therapy.
- Assess intensity, character, location, and radiation of chest pain. Note presence of associated symptoms (nausea, vomiting, diaphoresis). Notify health care professional if chest pain is unrelieved or recurs.
- Monitor heart sounds and breath sounds frequently. Inform health care professional if signs of HF occur (rales/crackles, dyspnea, S_3 heart sound, jugular venous distention).
- **Acute Ischemic Stroke:** Assess neurologic status. Determine time of onset of stroke symptoms. Alteplase must be administered within 3–4.5 hr of onset (within 3 hr in patients older than 80 yr, those taking oral anticoagulants, those with a baseline National Institutes of Health Stroke Scale score 25, or those with both a history of stroke and diabetes).
- **Pulmonary Embolism:** Monitor pulse, BP, hemodynamics, and respiratory status (rate, degree of dyspnea, ABGs).
- **Deep Vein Thrombosis/Acute Arterial Thrombosis:** Observe extremities and palpate pulses of affected extremities every hour. Notify health care professional immediately if circulatory impairment occurs. Computerized tomography, impedance plethysmography, quantitative Doppler effect determination, and/or angiography or venography may be used to determine restoration of blood flow and duration of therapy; however, repeated venograms are not recommended.
- **Cannula/Catheter Occlusion:** Monitor ability to aspirate blood as indicator of patency. Ensure that patient exhales and holds breath when connecting and disconnecting IV syringe to prevent air embolism.
- ***Lab Test Considerations:*** Hematocrit, hemoglobin, platelet count, fibrin/fibrin degradation product (FDP) titer, fibrinogen concentration, prothrombin time, thrombin time, and activated partial thromboplastin time (aPTT) may be evaluated before and frequently during therapy. Bleeding time may be assessed before therapy if patient has received platelet inhibitors.
- Obtain type and crossmatch and have blood available at all times in case of hemorrhage.
- Stools should be tested for occult blood loss and urine for hematuria periodically during therapy.

- ***Toxicity and Overdose: High Alert:*** If local bleeding occurs, apply pressure to site. If severe or internal bleeding occurs, discontinue infusion. Clotting factors and/or blood volume may be restored through infusions of whole blood, packed RBCs, fresh frozen plasma, or cryoprecipitate. Do not administer dextran; it has antiplatelet activity. Aminocaproic acid (Amicar) may be used as an antidote.

Potential Nursing Diagnoses

Ineffective tissue perfusion (Indications)
Risk for injury (Side Effects)

Implementation

- ***High Alert:*** Overdose and underdose of thrombolytic medications have resulted in patient harm or death. Have second practitioner independently check original order, dosage calculations, and infusion pump settings. Do not confuse the abbreviation *t-PA* for alteplase (Activase) with the abbreviation *TNK t-PA* for tenecteplase (TNKase) and *r-PA* for reteplase (Retavase). Clarify orders that contain either of these abbreviations.
- Thrombolytic agents should be used only in settings in which hematologic function and clinical response can be adequately monitored.
- Starting two IV lines before therapy is recommended: one for the thrombolytic agent, the other for any additional infusions.
- Avoid invasive procedures, such as IM injections or arterial punctures, with this therapy. If such procedures must be performed, apply pressure to all arterial and venous puncture sites for at least 30 min. Avoid venipunctures at noncompressible sites (jugular vein, subclavian site).
- Acetaminophen may be ordered to control fever.

Alteplase

IV Administration

- **Intermittent Infusion:** Vials are packaged with sterile water for injection (without preservatives) to be used as diluent. Do not use bacteriostatic water for injection. Reconstitute 20-mg vials with 20-mL and 50-mg vials with 50 mL using an 18-gauge needle. Avoid excess agitation during dilution; swirl or invert gently to mix. Solution may foam upon reconstitution. Bubbles will resolve upon standing a few min. Solution will be clear to pale yellow. Stable for 8 hr at room temperature. ***Concentration:*** May be administered as reconstituted (1 mg/mL). ***Diluent:*** May be further diluted immediately before use in an equal amount of 0.9% NaCl or D5W. ***Rate:*** Flush line with 20–30 mL of saline at completion of infusion to ensure entire dose is received. See Route and Dosage section for specific rates.
- **Y-Site Compatibility:** eptifibatide, lidocaine, metoprolol, propranolol.
- **Y-Site Incompatibility:** bivalirudin, dobutamine, dopamine, heparin, nitroglycerin.
- **Cathflo Activase:** Reconstitute by withdrawing 2.2 mL of sterile water (provided) and injecting into Cathflo Activase vial, directing diluent into powder for a concentration of 1 mg/mL. Allow slight foaming to dissipate by letting vial stand undisturbed. Do not use bacteriostatic water. Mix by gently swirling to dissolve; complete dissolution should occur within 3 min. Do not shake. Solution should be colorless to pale yellow. Use solution within 8 hr.
- Withdraw 2.0 mL of reconstituted solution and instill into occluded catheter. After 30 min dwell time, attempt to aspirate blood. If catheter remains occluded, allow 120 min dwell time. If catheter function is not restored after one dose, second dose may be instilled. If catheter function is restored, aspirate 4–5 mL of blood to remove Cathflo Activase and residual clot. Gently irrigate catheter with 0.9% NaCl.

Reteplase

IV Administration

- **IV Push:** Reconstitute using diluent, needle, syringe, and dispensing pin provided. Reconstitute only with sterile water for injection without preservatives. Solution is colorless. Do not administer solutions that are discolored or contain a precipitate. Slight foaming may occur; allow vial to stand undisturbed for several min to dissipate bubbles. Reconstitute immediately before use. Stable for 4 hr at room temperature. ***Concentration:*** Administer undiluted. ***Rate:*** Administer each bolus over 2 min into an IV line containing D5W; flush line before and after bolus.
- **Y-Site Incompatibility:** bivalirudin, heparin. No other medication should be infused or injected into line used for reteplase.

Streptokinase

IV Administration

- **Intracoronary:** Dilute 250,000 IU vial to a total volume of 125 mL with 0.9% NaCl or D5W. Administer 20,000 IU (10 mL) via bolus injection.
- ***Rate:*** Intracoronary bolus is administered over 15 sec–2 min.
- **Intermittent Infusion:** Reconstitute with 5 mL of 0.9% NaCl or D5W (direct to sides of vial) and swirl gently; do not shake. ***Diluent:*** Dilute further with 0.9% NaCl for a total volume of 45–500 mL (45 mL for MI, 90 mL for deep vein thrombosis or pulmonary embolism). Solution is slightly yellow in color. Administer through 0.8-micron pore–size filter. Use reconstituted solution within 24 hr. ***Rate:*** Administer dose for MI within 60 min.
- Intracoronary bolus should be followed by an intracoronary maintenance infusion of 2000 IU/min for 60 min.

T

- Loading dose for *deep vein thrombosis* or *pulmonary embolism* is administered over 30 min, followed by an infusion of 100,000 IU/hr.
- Use infusion pump to ensure accurate dose.
- **Y-Site Compatibility:** alfentanil, amikacin, aminophylline, ascorbic acid, atracurium, atropine, aztreonam, benztropine, bumetanide, buprenorphine, butorphanol, calcium chloride, calcium gluconate, cefazolin, cefonocid, cefotaxime, cefotetan, cefoxitin, ceftazidime, ceftriaxone, cefuroxime, chloramphenicol, clindamycin, cyanocobalamin, cyclosporine, dexamethasone, digoxin, diphenhydramine, dobutamine, dopamine, doxycycline, enalaprilat, ephedrine, epinephrine, epoetin alfa, erythromycin, esmolol, famotidine, fentanyl, fluconazole, folic acid, furosemide, gentamicin, glycopyrrolate, heparin, hydrocortisone, imipenem/cilastatin, indomethacin, insulin, isoproterenol, ketorolac, labetalol, lidocaine, magnesium sulfate, mannitol, meperidine, methoxamine, methyldopate, methylprednisolone, metoclopramide, metoprolol, midazolam, morphine, multivitamins, nafcillin, naloxone, nitroglycerin, nitroprusside, norepinephrine, ondansetron, oxacillin, oxytocin, penicillin G, pentazocine, pentobarbital, phenobarbital, phentolamine, phenylephrine, phytonadione, potassium chloride, procainamide, propranolol, pyridoxime, ranitidine, sodium bicarbonate, succinylcholine, sufentanil, theophylline, thiamine, tobramycin, trimetaphan, verapamil.
- **Y-Site Incompatibility:** azathioprine, bivalirudin, chlorpromazine, dantrolene, diazepam, diazoxide, ganciclovir, hydroxyzine, nalbuphine, pentamidine, phenytoin, prochlorperazine, promethazine, trimethoprim/sulfamethoxazole, vancomycin.
- **Additive Incompatibility:** Do not admix with any other medication.
- **Cannula/Catheter Clearance:** Dilute 250,000 IU in 2 mL of 0.9% NaCl or D5W.
- ***Rate:*** Administer slowly, over 25–35 min, into each occluded limb of cannula, and then clamp for at least 2 hr. Aspirate contents carefully and flush lines with 0.9% NaCl.

Tenecteplase

IV Administration

- **Intermittent Infusion:** Vials are packaged with sterile water for injection (without preservatives) to be used as diluent. Do not use bacteriostatic water for injection. Do not discard shield assembly. To reconstitute aseptically withdraw 10 mL of diluent and inject into the tenectplase vial, directing the stream into the powder. Slight foaming may occur; large bubbles will dissipate if left standing undisturbed for several minutes. Swirl gently until contents are completely dissolved; do not shake. ***Concentration:*** Solution containing 5 mg/mL is clear and colorless to pale yellow. Withdraw dose from reconstituted vial with the syringe and discard unused portion. Once dose is in syringe, stand the shield vertically on a flat surface (with green side down) and passively recap the red hub cannula. Remove the entire shield assembly, including the red hub cannula, by twisting counter clockwise. Shield assembly also contains the clear-ended blunt plastic cannula; retain for split septum IV access. Reconstitute immediately before use. May be refrigerated and administered within 8 hr. ***Rate:*** Administer as a single IV bolus over 5 seconds.
- **Y-Site Incompatibility:** Precipate forms in line when administered with dextrose-containing solutions. Flush line with saline-containing solution prior to and following administration of tenecteplase.
- **Additive Incompatibility:** Do not admix.

Patient/Family Teaching

- Explain purpose of medication and the need for close monitoring to patient and family. Instruct patient to report hypersensitivity reactions (rash, dyspnea) and bleeding or bruising.
- Explain need for bedrest and minimal handling during therapy to avoid injury. Avoid all unnecessary procedures such as shaving and vigorous tooth brushing.

Evaluation/Desired Outcomes

- Lysis of thrombi and restoration of blood flow.
- Prevention of neurologic sequelae in acute ischemic stroke.
- Cannula or catheter patency.

tiagabine (tye-a-ga-been)

Gabitril

Classification

Therapeutic: anticonvulsants

Pregnancy Category C

Indications

Adjunctive treatment of partial seizures.

Action

Enhances the activity of gamma-aminobutyric acid, an inhibitory neurotransmitter. **Therapeutic Effects:** Decreased frequency of seizures.

Pharmacokinetics

Absorption: 90% absorbed following oral administration.

Distribution: Unknown.

Protein Binding: 96%.

Metabolism and Excretion: Mostly metabolized by the liver; 2% excreted unchanged in urine.

Half-life: *Without enzyme-inducing antiepileptic drugs*—7–9 hr; *with enzyme-inducing antiepileptic drugs*—4–7 hr.

TIME/ACTION PROFILE (blood levels)

ROUTE	ONSET	PEAK	DURATION
PO	unknown	45 min	unknown

Contraindications/Precautions

Contraindicated in: Hypersensitivity.

Use Cautiously in: All patients (may ↑ risk of suicidal thoughts/behaviors); Hepatic impairment (↓ dose/increased interval may be necessary); Patients receiving concurrent non–enzyme-inducing antiepileptic drug therapy such as valproates (may require lower doses and/or slower titration); Using tiagabine for off-label uses or other conditions leading to ↑ levels (may ↑ risk of new onset seizures); OB, Lactation, Pedi: Pregnancy, lactation, or children <12 yr (safety not established).

Adverse Reactions/Side Effects

CNS: SUICIDAL THOUGHTS, dizziness, drowsiness, nervousness, weakness, cognitive impairment, confusion, difficulty concentrating, hallucinations, headache, mental depression, personality disorder. **EENT:** abnormal vision, ear pain, tinnitus. **Resp:** dyspnea, epistaxis. **CV:** chest pain, edema, hypertension, palpitations, syncope, tachycardia. **GI:** abdominal pain, gingivitis, nausea, stomatitis. **GU:** dysmenorrhea, dysuria, metrorrhagia, urinary incontinence. **Derm:** alopecia, dry skin, rash, sweating. **Metab:** weight gain, weight loss. **MS:** arthralgia, neck pain. **Neuro:** ataxia, tremors. **Misc:** allergic reactions, chills, lymphadenopathy.

Interactions

Drug-Drug: Carbamazepine, **phenytoin**, **primidone**, and **phenobarbital** induce metabolism and ↓ blood levels; although concurrent therapy is usually necessary, adjustments may be required when altering regimens.

Route/Dosage

PO (Adults >18 yr): 4 mg once daily initially for 1 wk; may ↑ by 4–8 mg/day at weekly intervals, up to 56 mg/day in 2–4 divided doses.

PO (Children 12–18 yr): 4 mg once daily initially for 1 wk; may ↑ by 4 mg/day after 1 wk, then may ↑ by 4–8 mg/day at weekly intervals, up to 32 mg/day in 2–4 divided doses.

Availability (generic available)

Tablets: 2 mg, 4 mg, 12 mg, 16 mg.

NURSING IMPLICATIONS

Assessment

- Assess location, duration, and characteristics of seizure activity.
- Assess mental status. May cause impaired concentration, speech or language problems, confusion, fatigue, and drowsiness. Symptoms may decrease with dose reduction or discontinuation.
- Monitor closely for notable changes in behavior that could indicate the emergence or worsening of suicidal thoughts or behavior or depression.
- ***Toxicity and Overdose:*** Therapeutic serum levels have not been determined. However, levels may be monitored prior to and following changes in the therapeutic regimen.

Potential Nursing Diagnoses

Risk for injury (Side Effects)

Implementation

- Do not confuse tiagabine with tizanidine.
- **PO:** Administer with food.
- Discontinue tiagabine gradually. Abrupt discontinuation may cause increase in seizure frequency.

Patient/Family Teaching

- Instruct patient to take medication as directed. Take missed doses as soon as possible unless almost time for next dose. Do not double doses. Do not discontinue abruptly; may cause increase in frequency of seizures. Instruct patient to read the *Medication Guide* before starting and with each Rx refill, changes may occur.
- Advise patient to notify health care professional immediately if frequency of seizures increases.
- May cause dizziness. Caution patient to avoid driving or activities requiring alertness until response to medication is known. Do not resume driving until physician gives clearance based on control of seizure disorder.
- Advise patient and family to notify health care professional if thoughts about suicide or dying, attempts to commit suicide; new or worse depression; new or worse anxiety; feeling very agitated or restless; panic attacks; trouble sleeping; new or worse irritability; acting aggressive; being angry or violent; acting on dangerous impulses; an extreme increase in activity and talking, other unusual changes in behavior or mood occur.
- Advise patient to notify health care professional of all Rx or OTC medications, vitamins, or herbal products being taken and to consult with health care professional before taking other medications.
- Instruct patient to notify health care professional of medication regimen prior to treatment or surgery.
- Advise patient to carry identification describing disease process and medication regimen at all times.
- Advise patient to notify health care professional if pregnancy is planned or suspected or if breast feeding.

Evaluation/Desired Outcomes

- Decrease in the frequency or cessation of seizures.

T

ticagrelor (tye-ka-**grel**-or)
Brilinta

Classification
Therapeutic: antiplatelet agents
Pharmacologic: platelet aggregation inhibitors

Pregnancy Category C

Indications

To decrease the incidence of thrombotic cardiovascular events associated with acute coronary syndrome (ACS). Also reduces the incidence of stent thrombosis in patients who have received an intracoronary stent for ACS.

Action

Both parent drug and its active metabolite inhibit platelet aggregation by reversibly interacting with platelet $P2Y_{12}$ADP-receptors, preventing signal transduction and platelet activation. **Therapeutic Effects:** Reduced sequelae of ACS including cardiovascular death, MI and stroke. Reduction in stent thrombosis.

Pharmacokinetics

Absorption: 36% absorbed following oral administration.
Distribution: Unknown.
Protein Binding: 99% for ticagrelor and its active metabolite.
Metabolism and Excretion: Mostly metabolized in the liver (CYP3A4 enzyme system, some metabolism by CYP3A5) with conversion to an active metabolite (AR-C124910XX); excretion primarily via biliary secretion; <1% excreted unchanged or as active metabolite in urine.
Half-life: *Ticagrelor*—7 hr; *Active metabolite*—9 hr.

TIME/ACTION PROFILE (inhibition of platelet aggregation)

ROUTE	ONSET	PEAK	DURATION
PO	within 30 min	4 hr	5 days†

† Following discontinuation.

Contraindications/Precautions

Contraindicated in: Hypersensitivity; Active bleeding; History of intracranial bleeding; Severe hepatic impairment (increased risk of bleeding); Impending coronary artery bypass graft (CABG) surgery or other surgery (discontinue 5 days prior); Lactation: Avoid breast feeding; Strong inhibitors/inducers of CYP3A enzyme system (avoid concurrent use if possible).
Use Cautiously in: Moderate hepatic impairment (consider risks of increased levels); Hypotension following recent CABG or percutaneous coronary intervention (PCI) in patients receiving ticagrelor (consider bleeding as a cause); Geri: Some elderly patients may be more sensitive to effects; OB: Use only during pregnancy if potential maternal benefit justifies potential risk to fetus; Pedi: Safety and effectiveness not established.

Adverse Reactions/Side Effects

CV: bradycardia. **Resp:** dyspnea. **Endo:** gynecomastia. **Hemat:** BLEEDING. **Misc:** hypersensitivity reactions including ANGIOEDEMA.

Interactions

Drug-Drug: Strong inhibitors of CYP3A4/5 including **atazanavir**, **clarithromycin**, **indinavir**, **itraconazole**, **ketoconazole**, **nefazodone**, **nelfinavir**, **ritonavir**, **saquinavir**, **telithromycin** and **voriconazole**↑ levels and the risk of bleeding and should be avoided. **Potent inducers of CYP3A** including **carbamazepine**, **dexamethasone**, **phenobarbital**, **phenytoin**, **rifampin** may ↓ levels and effectiveness and should be avoided. **P-glycoprotein inhibitors** including **cyclosporine** may ↑ levels and the risk of bleeding. Concurrent use of **lovastatin** or **simvastatin** in doses >40 m g/day ↑ risk of statin-related adverse reactions. Effectiveness is ↓ by **aspirin** >100 mg/day (maintain aspirin at 75–100 mg/day). May alter **digoxin** levels (monitoring recommended). Risk of bleeding ↑ by **anticoagulants**, **fibrinolytics** and chronic **NSAIDs**.

Route/Dosage

PO (Adults): *Loading dose*—180 mg; followed by *maintenance dose*—90 mg twice daily for 1 yr, then 60 mg twice daily.

Availability

Tablets: 60 mg, 90 mg.

NURSING IMPLICATIONS

Assessment

- Assess patient for symptoms of stroke, peripheral vascular disease, or MI periodically during therapy.
- Observe patient for signs and symptoms of hypersensitivity reactions (rash, facial swelling, pruritus, laryngeal edema, wheezing). Discontinue drug and notify health care professional immediately if symptoms occur. Keep epinephrine, an antihistamine, and resuscitation equipment close by in case of anaphylactic reaction.
- ***Lab Test Considerations:*** May cause ↑ serum uric acid and ↑ serum creatinine.

Potential Nursing Diagnoses

Risk for injury (Adverse Reactions)

Implementation

- ***High Alert:*** Do not confuse Brilinta (ticagrelor) with Brintellix (vortioxetine).
- **PO:** Administer ticagrelor 180 mg (two 90 mg tablets) as a loading dose, followed by 90 mg twice daily for 1 yr, then 60 mg twice daily. After initial 325 mg loading dose of aspirin, administer mainte-

nance dose of 75–100 mg daily. Administer without regard for food.

- For patients unable to swallow, tablets can be crushed and mixed with water. Mixture can also be administered via a nasogastric tube.
- Patients who have received a loading dose of clopidogrel may be started on ticagrelor.
- Discontinue ticagrelor 5 days before planned surgical procedures. If ticagrelor must be temporarily discontinued, restart as soon as possible. Premature discontinuation of therapy may increase risk of myocardial infarction, stent thrombosis, and death.

Patient/Family Teaching

- Instruct patient to take ticagrelor exactly as directed. Take missed doses as soon as possible unless almost time for next dose; do not double doses. Do not discontinue ticagrelor without consulting health care professional; may increase risk of cardiovascular events. Advise patient to read the *Medication Guide* before starting therapy and with each Rx refill in case of changes.
- Advise patient that daily aspirin should not exceed 100 mg and to avoid taking other medications that contain aspirin.
- Inform patient that they will bleed and bruise more easily and it will take longer to stop bleeding. Advise patient to notify health care professional promptly if unusual, prolonged, or excessive bleeding or blood in stool or urine occurs.
- Inform patient that ticagrelor may cause shortness of breath which usually resolved during therapy. Advise patient to notify health care professional if unexpected or severe shortness of breath or symptoms of hypersensitivity reactions occur.
- Advise patient to notify health care professional of medication regimen prior to treatment or surgery or dental procedure. Prescriber should be consulted before stopping ticagrelor.
- Instruct patient to notify health care professional of all Rx or OTC medications, vitamins, or herbal products being taken and consult health care professional before taking any new medications, especially aspirin or NSAIDs.
- Advise patient to notify health care professional if pregnancy is planned or suspected or if breast feeding.

Evaluation/Desired Outcomes

- Decreased thrombotic cardiovascular events in patients with ACS.

tigecycline (tye-gi-**sye**-kleen)

Tygacil

Classification
Therapeutic: anti-infectives
Pharmacologic: glycylcyclines

Pregnancy Category D

Indications

Complicated skin/skin structure infections, complicated intra-abdominal infections, or community-acquired bacterial pneumonia caused by susceptible bacteria (Should only be used when alternative treatments are not suitable; should NOT be used for diabetic foot infections).

Action

Inhibits bacterial protein synthesis by binding to the 30S ribosomal subunit. **Therapeutic Effects:** Resolution of infection. **Spectrum:** Active against the following Gram-positive bacteria: *Enterococcus faecalis* (vancomycin-susceptible strains only), *Staphylococcus aureus* (methicillin-sensitive and methicillin-resistant strains), *Streptococcus agalactiae*, *Streptococcus anginosus*, *Streptococcus pneumoniae*, and *Streptococcus pyogenes*. Also active against these Gram-positive organisms: *Citrobacter freundii*, *Enterobacter cloacae*, *Escherichia coli*, *Haemophilus influenzae* (beta-lactamase negative strains only), *Legionella pneumophila*, *Klebsiella oxytoca*, and *Klebsiella pneumoniae*. Additionally active against the following anaerobes: *Bacteroides fragilis*, *Bacteroides thetaiotaomicron*, *Bacteroides uniformis*, *Bacteroides vulgatus*, *Clostridium perfringens*, and *Peptostreptococcus micros*.

Pharmacokinetics

Absorption: IV administration results in complete bioavailability.

Distribution: Widely distributed with good penetration into gall bladder, lung, and colon; crosses the placenta.

Metabolism and Excretion: Minimal metabolism; primary route of elimination is biliary/fecal excretion of unchanged drug and metabolites (59%), 33% renal (22% unchanged).

Half-life: 27.1 hr (after 1 dose); 42.4 hr after multiple doses.

TIME/ACTION PROFILE (blood levels)

ROUTE	ONSET	PEAK	DURATION
IV	rapid	end of infusion	12 hr

T

Contraindications/Precautions

Contraindicated in: Hypersensitivity; Diabetic foot infections; Hospital-acquired or ventilator-associated pneumonia; Pedi: Children.

Use Cautiously in: Complicated intra-abdominal infections due to perforation; Severe hepatic impairment (↓ maintenance dose recommended); Geri: May be more sensitive to adverse effects; OB, Lactation: Use in pregnancy only when potential maternal benefit outweighs fetal risk; use cautiously during lactation.

Adverse Reactions/Side Effects

CNS: somnolence. **Derm:** STEVENS-JOHNSON SYNDROME. **GI:** PANCREATITIS, CLOSTRIDIUM DIFFICILE-ASSOCIATED DIARRHEA (CDAD), nausea, vomiting, altered taste, anorexia, dry mouth, hepatotoxicity, jaundice. **GU:** ↑ serum creatinine. **Endo:** hyperglycemia, hypoglycemia. **F and E:** hypocalcemia, hyponatremia. **Resp:** pneumonia. **Local:** injection site reactions. **Misc:** DEATH, allergic reactions.

Interactions

Drug-Drug: May ↓ the effectiveness of **hormonal contraceptives**. Effects on **warfarin** are unknown (monitoring recommended).

Route/Dosage

IV (Adults >18 yr): 100 mg initially, then 50 mg every 12 hr for 5–14 days (skin/skin structure infections and intra-abdominal infections) or 7–14 days (pneumonia).

Hepatic Impairment

IV (Adults >18 yr): *Child-Pugh C*—100 mg initially, then 25 mg every 12 hr.

Availability

Lyophilized powder for reconstitution: 50 mg/vial.

NURSING IMPLICATIONS

Assessment

- Assess for infection (vital signs; appearance of wound, sputum, urine, and stool; WBC) at beginning of and throughout therapy.
- Obtain specimens for culture and sensitivity before initiating therapy. 1st dose may be given before receiving results.
- Before initiating therapy, obtain a history of tetracycline hypersensitivity; may also have an allergic response to tigecycline.
- Monitor bowel function. Diarrhea, abdominal cramping, fever, and bloody stools should be reported to health care professional promptly as a sign of Clostridium difficile-associated diarrhea (CDAD). May begin up to several weeks following cessation of therapy.
- Assess patient for signs of pancreatitis (nausea, vomiting, abdominal pain, increased serum lipase or amylase) periodically during therapy. May require discontinuation of therapy.
- Assess for rash periodically during therapy. May cause Stevens-Johnson syndrome. Discontinue therapy if severe or if accompanied with fever, general malaise, fatigue, muscle or joint aches, blisters, oral lesions, conjunctivitis, hepatitis and/or eosinophilia.
- ***Lab Test Considerations:*** May cause anemia, leukocytosis, and thrombocythemia.
- May cause ↑ serum alkaline phosphatase, amylase, bilirubin, LDH, AST, and ALT.
- May cause hyperglycemia, hypokalemia, hypoproteinemia, hypocalcemia, hyponatremia, and ↑ BUN level.

Potential Nursing Diagnoses

Risk for infection (Indications)

Implementation

- May cause yellow-brown discoloration and softening of teeth and bones if administered prenatally or during early childhood. Not recommended for children under 8 yr of age or during pregnancy or lactation unless used for the treatment of anthrax.

IV Administration

- **Intermittent Infusion:** Reconstitute each vial with 5.3 mL of 0.9% NaCl or D5W to achieve a concentration of 10 mg/mL. ***Diluent:*** Dilute further in 100 mL of D5W, LR, or 0.9% NaCl. Reconstituted solution should be yellow to orange in color. Do not administer solutions that are discolored or contain particulate matter. Infusion is stable for up to 24 hr at room temperature or for up to 48 hr if refrigerated. ***Concentration:*** Final concentration of infusion should be ≤1 mg/mL. ***Rate:*** Infuse over 30–60 min. Flush line before and after infusion with 0.9% NaCl or D5W.
- **Y-Site Compatibility:** acyclovir, alfentanil, allopurinol, amifostine, amikacin, aminocaproic acid, aminophylline, amphotericin B liposome, ampicillin, ampicillin/sulbactam, argatroban, azithromycin, aztreonam, bivalirudin, bumetanide, buprenorphine, busulfan, butorphanol, calcium chloride, calcium gluconate, carboplatin, carmustine, caspofungin, cefazolin, cefepime, cefotaxime, cefotetan, cefoxitin, ceftazidime, ceftriaxone, cefuroxime, ciprofloxacin, cisatracurium, cisplatin, clindamycin, cyclophosphamide, cyclosporine, cytarabine, dacarbazine, dactinomycin, daptomycin, daunorubicin hydrochloride, dexamethasone, dexmedetomidine, dexrazoxane, digoxin, diltiazem, diphenhydramine, dobutamine, docetaxel, dolasetron, dopamine, doripenem, doxorubicin hydrochloride, doxorubicin liposome, droperidol, enalaprilat, epinephrine, eptifibatide, ertapenem, erythromycin, esmolol, etoposide, etoposide phosphate, famotidine, fenoldopam, fentanyl, fluconazole, fludarabine, fluorouracil, foscarnet, fosphenytoin, furosemide, ganciclovir, gemcitabine, gentamicin, glycopyrrolate, granisetron, haloperidol, heparin, hydrocortisone, hydromorphone, ifosfamide, imipenem/cilastatin, insulin,

irinotecan, isoproterenol, ketorolac, labetalol, lansoprazole, leucovorin, levofloxacin, lidocaine, linezolid, lorazepam, magnesium sulfate, mannitol, mechlorethamine, melphalan, meperidine, meropenem, mesna, methohexital, methotrexate, methyldopate, metoclopramide, metoprolol, metronidazole, midazolam, milrinone, mitomycin, mitoxantrone, morphine, moxifloxacin, mycophenolate, nafcillin, nalbuphine, naloxone, nesiritide, nitroglycerin, nitroprusside, norepinephrine, octreotide, ondansetron, oxaliplatin, oxytocin, paclitaxel, palonosetron, pamidronate, pancuronium, pantoprazole, pemetrexed, pemtamidine, pentazocine, pentobarbital, phenobarbital, phenylephrine, piperacillin/tazobactam, potassium acetate, potassium chloride, potassium phosphates, procainamide, prochlorperazine, promethazine, propofol, propranolol, ranitidine, remifentanil, rocuronium, sodium acetate, sodium bicarbonate, sodium phosphates, streptozocin, succinylcholine, sufentanil, tacrolimus, telavancin, teniposide, theophylline, thiopental, thiotepa, tirofiban, tobramycin, topotecan, trimethoprim/sulfamethoxazole, vancomycin, vasopressin, vecuronium, vinblastine, vincristine, vinorelbine, zidovudine, zoledronic acid.
- **Y-Site Incompatibility:** amiodarone, amphotericin B colloidal, amphotericin B lipid complex, bleomycin, chloramphenicol, chlorpromazine, dantrolene, diazepam, epirubicin, esomeprazole, hydralazine, idarubicin, nicardipine, phenytoin, quinupristin/dalfopristin, verapamil.

Patient/Family Teaching
- Advise patient that full course of therapy should be completed, even if feeling better. Skipping doses or not completing full course of therapy may result in decreased effectiveness and increased risk of bacterial resistance.
- Instruct patient to notify health care professional if fever and diarrhea develop, especially if stool contains blood, pus, or mucus. Advise patient not to treat diarrhea without consulting health care professional.
- Advise patient to report the signs of superinfection (black, furry overgrowth on the tongue, vaginal itching or discharge, loose or foul-smelling stools). Skin rash, pruritus, and urticaria should also be reported.
- Advise female patient to use a nonhormonal method of contraception while taking tigecycline and until next menstrual period.

Evaluation/Desired Outcomes
- Resolution of signs and symptoms of infection.

tioconazole, See ANTIFUNGALS (VAGINAL).

tiotropium (tye-o-**trope**-ee-yum)

✱Spiriva, Spiriva Handihaler, Spiriva Respimat

Classification
Therapeutic: bronchodilators
Pharmacologic: anticholinergics

Pregnancy Category C

Indications
Long-term maintenance treatment of bronchospasm due to COPD. Reduce exacerbations in patients with COPD. Long-term maintenance treatment of asthma.

Action
Acts as anticholinergic by selectively and reversibly inhibiting M_3 receptors in smooth muscle of airways. **Therapeutic Effects:** Decreased incidence and severity of bronchospasm in COPD and asthma.

Pharmacokinetics
Absorption: *Handihaler*—19% absorbed following inhalation; *Respimat*—33% absorbed following inhalation.

Distribution: Extensive tissue distribution; due to route of administration ↑ concentrations occur in lung.

Metabolism and Excretion: 74% excreted unchanged in urine; 25% of absorbed drug is metabolized.

Half-life: 5–6 days.

TIME/ACTION PROFILE (bronchodilation)

ROUTE	ONSET	PEAK	DURATION
inhaln	rapid	5 min	24 hr

Contraindications/Precautions
Contraindicated in: Hypersensitivity to tiotropium or ipratropium; Concurrent ipratropium.

Use Cautiously in: Hypersensitivity to atropine or milk proteins; Narrow-angle glaucoma, prostatic hyperplasia, bladder neck obstruction (may worsen condition); CCr ≤60 mL/min (monitor closely); OB, Lactation, Pedi: Safety not established.

Adverse Reactions/Side Effects
EENT: glaucoma. **Resp:** paradoxical bronchospasm. **CV:** tachycardia. **GI:** dry mouth, constipation. **GU:** urinary difficulty, urinary retention. **Derm:** rash. **Misc:** hypersensitivity reactions including ANGIOEDEMA.

Interactions

Drug-Drug: Should not be used concurrently with **ipratropium** due to risk of additive anticholinergic effects.

Route/Dosage

Inhaln (Adults): *Handihaler*—18 mcg once daily; *Respimat*—2 inhalations of 2.5 mcg once daily.
Inhaln (Adults and Children ≥12 yr): *Respimat*—2 inhalations of 1.25 mcg once daily.

Availability

Dry powder capsules for inhalation (Handihaler): 18 mcg. **Cost:** $317.33/30 capsules. **Inhalation spray (Respimat):** 1.25 mcg/metered inhalation in cartridge (delivers 28 or 60 metered inhalations), 2.5 mcg/metered inhalation in cartridge (delivers 28 or 60 metered inhalations).

NURSING IMPLICATIONS

Assessment

- **Inhaln:** Assess respiratory status (rate, breath sounds, degree of dyspnea, pulse) before administration and at peak of medication. Consult health care professional about alternative medication if severe bronchospasm is present; onset of action is too slow for patients in acute distress. If paradoxical bronchospasm (wheezing) occurs, withhold medication and notify health care professional immediately.

Potential Nursing Diagnoses

Ineffective airway clearance (Indications)
Risk for activity intolerance (Indications)

Implementation

- Do not confuse Spiriva (tiotropium) with Inspra (eplerenone).
- **Inhaln:** See Appendix D for administration of inhalation medications.

Patient/Family Teaching

- Instruct patient to take medication as directed. Capsules are for inhalation only and must not be swallowed. Take missed doses as soon as remembered unless almost time for the next dose; space remaining doses evenly during day. Do not double doses.
- Advise patient that tiotropium is not to be used for acute bronchospasm attacks, but may be continued during an acute exacerbation.
- Advise patient to notify health care professional immediately if signs and symptoms of angioedema (swelling of the lips, tongue, or throat, itching, rash) or signs of glaucoma (eye pain or discomfort, blurred vision, visual halos or colored images in association with red eyes from conjunctival congestion and corneal edema) occur.
- Caution patient to avoid spraying medication in eyes; may cause blurring of vision and pupil dilation.
- Advise patient that rinsing mouth after using inhaler, good oral hygiene, and sugarless gum or candy may minimize dry mouth; usually resolves with continued treatment.
- Instruct patient to notify health care professional of all Rx or OTC medications, vitamins, or herbal products being taken and consult health care professional before taking any new medications, including eye drops.
- Advise patient to inform health care professional if pregnancy is planned or suspected or if breast feeding.
- **Handihaler:** Instruct patient in proper use and cleaning of the Handihaler inhaler. Review the *Patient's Instructions for Use* guide with patient. Capsules should be stored in sealed blisters; remove immediately before use or effectiveness of capsules is reduced. Tear blister strip carefully to expose only one capsule at a time. Discard capsules that are inadvertently exposed to air. *Spiriva* should be administered only via the Handihaler and the Handihaler should not be used with other medications. When disposing of capsule, tiny amount of powder left in capsule is normal.
- **Respimat:** Advise patient to prime inhaler by actuating inhaler toward the ground until an aerosol cloud is visible, then repeat process 3 more times. If not used for >3 days, actuate inhaler once to prepare inhaler for use. If not used for >21 days, actuate inhaler until an aerosol cloud is visible, then repeat 3 more times to prepare inhaler for use. Discard 3 months from 1st use.

Evaluation/Desired Outcomes

- Decreased dyspnea.
- Improved breath sounds.
- Fewer exacerbations in patients with COPD and asthma.

HIGH ALERT

tirofiban (tye-roe-**fye**-ban)

Aggrastat

Classification
Therapeutic: antiplatelet agents
Pharmacologic: glycoprotein IIb/IIIa inhibitors

Pregnancy Category B

Indications

To reduce the incidence of thrombotic cardiovascular events (death, MI, or refractory ischemia/repeat cardiac procedure in patients with non-ST elevation acute coronary syndrome (unstable angina/non–Q-wave MI).

Action

Decreases platelet aggregation by reversibly antagonizing the binding of fibrinogen to the glycoprotein IIb/IIIa binding site on platelet surfaces. **Therapeutic Effects:** Inhibition of platelet aggregation resulting in decreased incidence of new MI, death, or refractory ischemia with the need for repeat cardiac procedures.

Pharmacokinetics

Absorption: IV administration results in complete bioavailability.

Distribution: Unknown.

Metabolism and Excretion: Excreted mostly unchanged by the kidneys (65%); 25% excreted unchanged in feces.

Half-life: 2 hr.

TIME/ACTION PROFILE (effects on platelet function)

ROUTE	ONSET	PEAK	DURATION
IV	rapid	30 min†	brief‡

†>90% inhibition of platelet aggregation at end of initial 30-min infusion.

‡Inhibition is reversible following cessation of infusion.

Contraindications/Precautions

Contraindicated in: Hypersensitivity; Active internal bleeding or history of bleeding within previous 30 days; History of intracranial hemorrhage, intracranial neoplasm, arteriovenous malformation or aneurysm; History of thrombocytopenia during previous tirofiban therapy; History of hemorrhagic stroke or other stroke within 30 days; Major surgical procedure or severe physical trauma within 30 days; History, symptoms, or other findings associated with aortic aneurysm; Severe hypertension (systolic BP >180 mm Hg and/or diastolic BP >110 mm Hg); Concurrent use of other glycoprotein IIb/IIIa receptor antagonists; Acute pericarditis; Lactation: Lactation.

Use Cautiously in: Platelet count <150,000/mm³; Hemorrhagic retinopathy; Female patients (↑ risk of bleeding); Severe renal insufficiency (↓ rate of infusion by 50% if CCr <30 mL/min); OB, Pedi: Safety not established; use in pregnancy only if clearly needed; Geri: ↑ risk of bleeding.

Adverse Reactions/Side Effects

Noted for patients receiving heparin and aspirin in addition to tirofiban.

CNS: dizziness, headache. **CV:** bradycardia, coronary dissection, edema, vasovagal reaction. **GI:** nausea. **Derm:** hives, rash. **Hemat:** bleeding, thrombocytopenia. **MS:** leg pain. **Misc:** fever, hypersensitivity reactions, pelvic pain, sweating.

Interactions

Drug-Drug: Concurrent use of **aspirin**, **NSAIDs**, **warfarin**, **heparin**, **heparin-like agents**, **abciximab**, **eptifibatide**, **clopidogrel**, or **dipyridamole** may ↑ risk of bleeding, although these agents are frequently used together or in sequence. Risk of bleeding may be ↑ by concurrent use of **cefotetan valproic acid**.

Drug-Natural Products: ↑ anticoagulant effect and bleeding risk with **anise**, **arnica**, **chamomile**, **clove**, **dong quai**, **fenugreek**, **feverfew**, **garlic**, **ginger**, **ginkgo**, **Panax ginseng**, **licorice**, and others.

Route/Dosage

IV (Adults): 25 mcg/kg within 5 min, then 0.15 mcg/kg/min for up to 18 hr.

Renal Impairment

IV (Adults): *CCr ≤60 mL/min*—25 mcg/kg within 5 min then 0.075 mcg/kg/min for up to 18 hr.

Availability

Premixed solution for infusion: 5 mg/100 mL (50 mcg/mL), 12.5 mg/250 mL (50 mcg/mL).

NURSING IMPLICATIONS

Assessment

- Assess for bleeding. Most common is oozing from the arterial access site for cardiac catheterization. Arterial and venous punctures, IM injections, and use of urinary catheters, nasotracheal intubation, and nasogastric tubes should be minimized. Noncompressible sites for IV access should be avoided. If bleeding cannot be controlled with pressure, discontinue tirofiban and heparin immediately.
- During vascular access, avoid puncturing posterior wall of femoral artery. Maintain bedrest with head of bed elevated 30° and affected limb restrained in a straight position while the vascular sheath is in place. Heparin should be discontinued for 3–4 hr and activated clotting time (ACT) <180 sec or activated partial thromboplastin time (aPTT) <45 sec prior to pulling the sheath. Use compressive techniques to obtain hemostasis and monitor closely. Sheath hemostasis should be maintained for >4 hr before discharge from the hospital.
- Monitor for signs of thrombocytopenia (chills, low-grade fever) during therapy.
- ***Lab Test Considerations:*** Assess hemoglobin, hematocrit, and platelet count prior to tirofiban therapy, within 6 hr following loading infusion, and at least daily during therapy (more frequently if evidence of significant decline). May cause ↓ hemoglobin and hematocrit.
- If platelet count ↓ to <90,000/mm³, perform additional platelet counts to rule out pseudothrombocytopenia. If thrombocytopenia is confirmed, tirofiban and heparin should be discontinued and condition monitored and treated.
- To monitor unfractionated heparin, assess aPTT 6 hr after the start of heparin infusion. Adjust heparin to maintain aPTT at approximately 2 times control.
- May cause presence of urine and fecal occult blood.

T

Potential Nursing Diagnoses

Ineffective tissue perfusion (Indications)

Implementation

- Do not confuse Aggrastat (tirofiban) with argatroban.
- ***High Alert:*** Use of antiplatelet medications has resulted in patient harm and/or death from internal hemorrhage or intracranial bleeding. Have second practitioner independently check original order, dosage calculations, and infusion pump settings.
- Most patients receive heparin and aspirin concurrently with tirofiban.
- Do not administer solutions that are discolored or contain particulate matter. Discard unused portion.

IV Administration

- **Intermittent Infusion:** ***Diluent:*** Tirofiban injection premix is ready for administration and dose not require any further dilution. ***Concentration:*** 50 mcg/mL. ***Rate:*** Based on patient's weight (see Route/Dosage section).
- **Y-Site Compatibility:** acyclovir, alfentanil, allopurinol, amifostine, amikacin, aminocaproic acid, aminophylline, amiodarone, ampicillin, ampicillin/sulbactam, anidulafungin, argatroban, arsenic trioxide, atropine, azithromycin, aztreonam, bivalirudin, bleomycin, bumetanide, buprenorphine, busulfan, butorphanol, calcium chloride, calcium gluconate, cangrelor, capreomycin, carboplatin, carmustine, caspofungin, cefazolin, cefepime, cefotaxime, cefotetan, cefoxitin, ceftazidime, ceftriaxone, cefuroxime, chloramphenicol, chlorpromazine, ciprofloxacin, cisatracurium, cisplatin, clindamycin, cyclophosphamide, cyclosporine, cytarabine, dacarbazine, dactinomycin, daptomycin, dexamethasone, dexmedetomidine, dexrazoxane, digoxin, diltiazem, diphenhydramine, dobutamine, docetaxel, dolasetron, dopamine, doxorubicin hydrochloride, doxorubicin liposomal, doxycycline, droperidol, enalaprilat, ephedrine, epinephrine, epirubicin, ertapenem, erythromycin, esmolol, etoposide, etoposide phosphate, famotidine, fenoldopam, fentanyl, fluconazole, fludarabine, fluorouracil, foscarnet, fosphenytoin, furosemide, ganciclovir, gemcitabine, gentamicin, glycopyrrolate, granisetron, haloperidol, heparin, hydralazine, hydrocortisone, hydromorphone, idarubicin, ifosfamide, imipenem/cilastatin, insulin, irinotecan, isoproterenol, ketorolac, labetalol, leucovorin, levofloxacin, lidocaine, linezolid, lorazepam, magnesium sulfate, mannitol, mechlorethamine, melphalan, meperidine, meropenem, mesna, methotrexate, methyldopate, methylprednisolone, metoclopramide, metoprolol, metronidazole, midazolam, milrinone, mitomycin, mitoxantrone, morphine, moxifloxacin, mycophenolate, nafcillin, nalbuphine, naloxone, nesiritide, nicardipine, nitroglycerin, nitroprusside, norepinephrine, octreotide, ondansetron, oxaliplatin, oxytocin, paclitaxel, palonosetron, pamidronate, pancuronium, pantoprazole, pemetrexed, pentobarbital, phenobarbital, phenylephrine, piperacillin/tazobactam, potassium acetate, potassium chloride, potassium phosphates, procainamide, prochlorperazine, promethazine, propranolol, quinupristin/dalfopristin, ranitidine, remifentanil, rocuronium, sodium acetate, sodium bicarbonate, sodium phosphates, streptozocin, succinylcholine, sufentanil, tacrolimus, teniposide, theophylline, thiopental, thiotepa, tigecycline, tobramycin, topotecan, vancomycin, vasopressin, vecuronium, verapamil, vinblastine, vincristine, vinorelbine, voriconazole, zidovudine, zoledronic acid.
- **Y-Site Incompatibility:** amphotericin B colloidal, amphotericin B lipid complex, dantrolene, diazepam, phenytoin.

Patient/Family Teaching

- Inform patient of the purpose of tirofiban.
- Instruct patient to notify health care professional immediately if any bleeding is noted.

Evaluation/Desired Outcomes

- Inhibition of platelet aggregation resulting in decreased incidence of new MI, death, or refractory ischemia with the need for repeat cardiac procedures.

tiZANidine (tye-**zan**-i-deen)

Zanaflex

Classification

Therapeutic: antispasticity agents (centrally acting)

Pharmacologic: adrenergics

Pregnancy Category C

Indications

Increased muscle tone associated with spasticity due to multiple sclerosis or spinal cord injury.

Action

Acts as an agonist at central alpha-adrenergic receptor sites. Reduces spasticity by increasing presynaptic inhibition of motor neurons. **Therapeutic Effects:** Decreased spasticity, allowing better function.

Pharmacokinetics

Absorption: Completely absorbed after oral administration but rapidly metabolized, resulting in 40% bioavailability.

Distribution: Widely distributed.

Metabolism and Excretion: 95% metabolized by the liver.

Half-life: 2.5 hr.

TIME/ACTION PROFILE (reduced muscle tone)

ROUTE	ONSET	PEAK	DURATION
PO	unknown	1–2 hr	3–6 hr

Contraindications/Precautions

Contraindicated in: Hypersensitivity.

Use Cautiously in: Renal impairment; Concurrent antihypertensive therapy; OB, Lactation, Pedi: Safety not established; Geri: Dose ↓ may be necessary due to ↓ clearance.

Exercise Extreme Caution in: Impaired hepatic function.

Adverse Reactions/Side Effects

CNS: anxiety, depression, dizziness, sedation, weakness, dyskinesia, hallucinations, nervousness. **EENT:** blurred vision, pharyngitis, rhinitis. **CV:** hypotension, bradycardia. **GI:** abdominal pain, diarrhea, dry mouth, dyspepsia, constipation, hepatocellular injury, ↑ liver enzymes, vomiting. **GU:** urinary frequency. **Derm:** rash, skin ulcers, sweating. **MS:** back pain, myasthenia, paresthesia. **Misc:** fever, speech disorder.

Interactions

Drug-Drug: Levels and effects ↑ by concurrent use of **hormonal contraceptives** or **alcohol**. ↑ risk of hypotension with **alpha$_2$-adrenergic agonist antihypertensives** (avoid concurrent use). ↑ CNS depression may occur with **alcohol** or other **CNS depressants** including some **antidepressants, sedative/hypnotics, antihistamines**, and **opioid analgesics**. Concurrent **CYP1A2 inhibitors (ciprofloxacin, fluvoxamine** and others) may ↑ levels and risk of hypotension and excessive sedation.

Route/Dosage

Tablets are not interchangeable with capsules

PO (Adults): 4 mg q 6–8 hr initially (no more than 3 doses/24 hr); ↑ by 2–4 mg/dose up to 8 mg/dose or 24 mg/day (not to exceed 36 mg/day). Some patients may tolerate twice-daily dosing.

Availability (generic available)

Tablets: 2 mg, 4 mg. **Cost:** *Generic*—2 mg $35.39/100, 4 mg $47.93/100. **Capsules:** 2 mg, 4 mg, 6 mg. **Cost:** *Generic*—2 mg $406.72/150, 4 mg $515.53/150, 6 mg $773.24/150.

NURSING IMPLICATIONS

Assessment

- Assess muscle spasticity before and periodically during therapy.
- Monitor BP and pulse, especially during dose titration. May cause orthostatic hypotension, bradycardia, dizziness, and, rarely, syncope. Effects are usually dose related.
- Observe patient for drowsiness, dizziness, and asthenia. A change in dose may alleviate these problems.
- ***Lab Test Considerations:*** Monitor liver function tests before and at 1, 3, and 6 mo of therapy. May cause ↑ in serum glucose, alkaline phosphatase, AST, and ALT levels.

Potential Nursing Diagnoses

Impaired physical mobility (Indications)
Risk for injury (Adverse Reactions)

Implementation

- Do not confuse tizanidine with tiagabine.
- Doses should be titrated carefully to prevent side effects.
- **PO:** May be taken without regard to meals.

Patient/Family Teaching

- Instruct patient to take tizanidine as directed. Tizanidine may need to be discontinued gradually.
- May cause dizziness and drowsiness. Advise patient to avoid driving or other activities requiring alertness until response to drug is known.
- Instruct patient to change positions slowly to minimize orthostatic hypotension.
- Advise patient to avoid concurrent use of alcohol or other CNS depressants while taking this medication.

Evaluation/Desired Outcomes

- Decrease in muscle spasticity with an increased ability to perform activities of daily living.

T

tobramycin, See AMINOGLYCOSIDES.

REMS

tocilizumab (toe-si-**liz**-oo-mab)

Actemra

Classification

Therapeutic: antirheumatics, immunosuppressants

Pharmacologic: interleukin antagonists

Pregnancy Category C

Indications

Treatment of adults with moderately- to severely-active rheumatoid arthritis who have not responded to one or more disease-modifying antirheumatic drugs [DMARDs]) (as monotherapy or with methotrexate or other non-biologic DMARDs). Active systemic juvenile idiopathic arthritis (as monotherapy or with methotrexate). Active polyarticular juvenile idiopathic arthritis (as monotherapy or with methotrexate).

Action

Acts as in inhibitor of interleukin-6 (IL-6) receptors by binding to them. IL-6 is a mediator of various inflammatory processes. **Therapeutic Effects:** Slowed progression of rheumatoid arthritis or systemic/polyarticular juvenile idiopathic arthritis.

Pharmacokinetics

Absorption: IV administration results in complete bioavailability.
Distribution: Unknown.
Metabolism and Excretion: Unknown.
Half-life: *4 mg/kg dose*—up to 11 days; *8 mg/kg*—up to 13 days.

TIME/ACTION PROFILE (improvement)

ROUTE	ONSET	PEAK	DURATION
IV	within 1 mo	4 mo	unknown
Subcut	unknown	unknown	unknown

Contraindications/Precautions

Contraindicated in: Hypersensitivity; Serious infections; Active hepatic disease/impairment; Absolute neutrophil count (ANC) <2000/mm³ (<500/mm³ while on therapy) or platelet count below 100,000/mm³ (<50,000/mm³ while on therapy); Lactation: Not recommended.
Use Cautiously in: Patients at risk for GI perforation, including patients with diverticulitis; Renal or hepatic impairment; Patients with tuberculosis risk factors; Geri: ↑ risk of adverse reactions; OB: Use only if potential benefit justifies potential risk to fetus; Pedi: Children <2 yr (safety not established).

Adverse Reactions/Side Effects

CNS: headache, dizziness. **EENT:** nasopharyngitis. **Resp:** upper respiratory tract infections. **CV:** hypertension. **GI:** GASTROINTESTINAL PERFORATION, ↑ liver enzymes. **Derm:** STEVENS-JOHNSON SYNDROME, rash. **Hemat:** NEUTROPENIA, THROMBOCYTOPENIA. **Metab:** ↑ lipids. **Misc:** ANAPHYLAXIS, SERIOUS INFECTIONS INCLUDING TUBERCULOSIS, DISSEMINATED FUNGAL INFECTIONS AND INFECTIONS WITH OPPORTUNISTIC PATHOGENS, hypersensitivity reactions including ANAPHYLAXIS, infusion reactions.

Interactions

Drug-Drug: May alter the activity of CYP450 enzymes; the effects of the following drugs should be monitored: **cyclosporine**, **theophylline**, **warfarin**, **hormonal contraceptives**, **atorvastatin** and **lovastatin**. Other drugs which are substrates for this system should also be monitored; effect may persist for several weeks after discontinuation. May ↓ antibody response to and ↑ risk of adverse reactions to **live virus vaccines**; do not administer concurrently.

Route/Dosage

Rheumatoid Arthritis

IV (Adults): 4 mg/kg every 4 wk; may be ↑ to 8 mg/kg given every 4 wk based on clinical response.
Subcut (Adults <100 kg): 162 mg every 2 wk, may ↑ to every wk based on clinical response.
Subcut (Adults ≥100 kg): 162 mg every wk.

Systemic Juvenile Idiopathic Arthritis

IV (Children ≥2 yr and <30 kg): 12 mg/kg every 2 wk.
IV (Children ≥2 yr and ≥30 kg): 8 mg/kg every 2 wk.

Polyarticular Juvenile Idiopathic Arthritis

IV (Children ≥2 yr and <30 kg): 10 mg/kg every 4 wk.
IV (Children ≥2 yr and ≥30 kg): 8 mg/kg every 4 wk.

Availability

Solution for IV infusion (requires dilution): 20 mg/mL. **Prefilled syringes:** 162 mg/0.9 mL.

NURSING IMPLICATIONS

Assessment

- Assess pain and range of motion before and periodically during therapy.
- Assess for signs of infection (fever, dyspnea, flu-like symptoms, frequent or painful urination, redness or swelling at the site of a wound), including tuberculosis, prior to injection. Tocilizumab is contraindicated in patients with active infection. Monitor new infections closely; most common are upper respiratory tract infections, bronchitis, and urinary tract infections. Signs and symptoms of inflammation may be lessened due to suppression from tocilizumab. Infections may be fatal, especially in patients taking immunosuppressive therapy. If patient develops a serious infection, discontinue tocilizumab until infection is controlled.
- Monitor for injection site reactions (redness and/or itching, rash, hemorrhage, bruising, pain, or swelling). Rash will usually disappear within a few days. Application of a towel soaked in cold water may relieve pain or swelling.
- Monitor patient for signs of anaphylaxis (urticaria, dyspnea, facial edema) following injection. Medications (antihistamines, corticosteroids, epinephrine) and equipment should be readily available in the event of a severe reaction. Discontinue tocilizumab immediately if anaphylaxis or other severe allergic reaction occurs.
- Assess patient for latent tuberculosis with a tuberculin skin test prior to initiation of therapy. Treatment of latent tuberculosis should be started before therapy with tocilizumab.
- Assess for signs and symptoms of systemic fungal infections (fever, malaise, weight loss, sweats, cough,

dypsnea, pulmonary infiltrates, serious systemic illness with or without concomitant shock). Ascertain if patient lives in or has traveled to areas of endemic mycoses. Consider empiric antifungal treatment for patients at risk of histoplasmosis and other invasive fungal infections until the pathogens are identified. Consult with an infectious diseases specialist. Consider stopping tocilizumab until the infection has been diagnosed and adequately treated.

- ***Lab Test Considerations:*** Assess CBC with platelet count and liver function prior to initiating therapy and after 4–8 wks, then every 3 months during therapy. Do not administer tocilizumab to patients with an ANC <2000/mm^3, platelet count <100,000/mm^3, or ALT or AST above 1.5 times the upper limit of normal (ULN).
- *If ANC > 1000/mm^3*, maintain dose. *If ANC 500–1000/mm^3*, interrupt IV tocilizumab until ANC >1000/mm^3, then resume at 4 mg/kg and ↑ to 8 mg/kg as clinically appropriate or reduce subcut tocilizumab to every other week and increase frequency to every week as clinically appropriate. *If ANC <500/mm^3*, discontinue tocilizumab.
- *If platelet count 50,000–100,000/mm^3*, interrupt dosing until platelet count is >100,000/mm^3 then resume IV dosing at 4 mg/kg and ↑ to 8 mg/kg as clinically appropriate or reduce subcut tocilizumab to every other week and increase frequency to every week as clinically appropriate. *If platelet count is <50,000/mm^3*, discontinue tocilizumab.
- *If liver enzymes persistently ↑ >1–3x ULN,* reduce IV tocilizumab dose to 4 mg/kg and reduce subcut injection to every other week or interrupt until AST/ALT have normalized. *If >3–5x ULN* (confirmed by repeat testing), interrupt tocilizumab until <3x ULN and follow recommendations for ↑ >1–3x ULN. *If persistent ↑ >1–3x ULN or >5x ULN*, discontinue tocilizumab.
- Monitor lipid levels every 4–8 wks following initiation of therapy, then at 6 month intervals. May cause ↑ total cholesterol, triglycerides, LDL cholesterol, and/or HDL cholesterol.

Potential Nursing Diagnoses

Chronic pain (Indications)
Risk for infection (Adverse Reactions)

Implementation

- Administer a tuberculin skin test prior to administration of tocilizumab. Patients with latent TB should be treated for TB prior to therapy.
- Immunizations should be current prior to initiating therapy. Patients on tocilizumab may receive concurrent vaccinations, except for live vaccines.
- Do not administer solutions that are discolored or contain particulate matter. Discard unused solution.
- Other DMARDs should be continued during tocilizumab therapy.
- **Children:** Do not change dose based on single visit weight; weight fluctuates.
- To switch from IV to Subcut, administer next dose Subcut instead of IV.
- **Subcut:** Only for adult patients with RA. Solution is clear and colorless to pale yellow; do not administer solutions that are discolored or contain particulate matter. Rotate injection sites; avoid sites with moles, scars, areas where skin is tender, bruised, red, hard, or not intact.

IV Administration

- **Intermittent Infusion:** ***Diluent:*** Withdraw volume of 0.9% NaCl from a 100 mL bag (50 mL bag for children <30 kg) equal to volume of solution required for patient's dose. Slowly add tocilizumab from each vial to infusion bag. Invert slowly to mix; avoid foaming. Do not infuse solutions that are discolored or contain particulate matter. Diluted solution is stable for 24 hr if refrigerated or at room temperature; protect from light. Allow solution to reach room temperature before infusing. ***Rate:*** Infuse over 60 min. Do not administer via IV push or bolus.
- **Y-Site Incompatibility:** Do not infuse concomitantly in the same line with other drugs.

Patient/Family Teaching

- Instruct patient on the purpose for tocilizumab. If a dose is missed, contact health care professional to schedule next infusion. Instruct patient and caregiver in correct technique for subcut injections and care and disposal of equipment.
- Caution patient to notify health care professional immediately if signs of infection (fever, sweating, chills, muscle aches, cough, shortness of breath, blood in phlegm, weight loss, warm, red or painful skin or sores, diarrhea or stomach pain, burning on urination, urinary frequency, feeling tired), fever and stomach-area pain that does not go away, change bowel habits, severe rash, swollen face, or difficulty breathing occurs while taking. If signs and symptoms of anaphylaxis occur, discontinue injections and notify health care professional immediately.
- Instruct patient to notify health care professional of all Rx or OTC medications, vitamins, or herbal products being taken and consult health care professional before taking any new medications.
- Instruct patient to notify health care professional of medication regimen prior to treatment or surgery.
- Advise female patients to notify health care professional if pregnancy is planned or suspected or if breast feeding, Pregnant women should be encouraged to participate in the pregnancy registry by calling 1-877-311-8972.

T

Evaluation/Desired Outcomes

- Decreased pain and swelling with decreased rate of joint destruction in patients with rheumatoid arthritis, systemic idiopathic juvenile arthritis, or polyarticular juvenile idiopathic arthritis.

REMS

tofacitinib (toe-fa-**sye**-ti-nib)

Xeljanz

Classification

Therapeutic: antirheumatics
Pharmacologic: kinase inhibitors

Pregnancy Category C

Indications

Treatment of adults with moderately to severely active rheumatoid arthritis who have had an inadequate response/intolerance to methotrexate. Can be used as monotherapy or with methotrexate or other nonbiologic disease-modifying antirheumatic drugs (DMARDs). Not to be used with biologic DMARDs or potent immunosuppressants including azathioprine and cyclosporine.

Action

Acts as a Janus kinase (JAK) inhibitor. Some results of inhibition include decreased hematopoiesis and immune cell function. Decreases circulating killer cells, increases in B cell count and decreases serum C-reactive protein (CRP). **Therapeutic Effects:** Improvement in clinical and symptomatic parameters of rheumatoid arthritis.

Pharmacokinetics

Absorption: Well absorbed following oral administration (74%).
Distribution: Distributes equally between red blood cells and plasma.
Metabolism and Excretion: 70% metabolized by the liver (primarily CYP3A4 with some contribution from CYP2C19). 30% renal excretion of the parent drug.
Half-life: 3 hr.

TIME/ACTION PROFILE (clinical improvement)

ROUTE	ONSET	PEAK	DURATION
PO	within 2 wk	3 mo	unknown

Contraindications/Precautions

Contraindicated in: Active infection; Administration of live vaccines; Severe hepatic impairment; Lymphocyte count <500 cells/mm^3, absolute neutrophil count (ANC) <1000 cells/mm^3, or hemoglobin levels <9 g/dL; Lactation: Should not be used in nursing mothers.
Use Cautiously in: Patients with risk of gastric perforation; Japanese patients (↑ risk of herpes zoster); Geri: Infection risk may be ↑ OB: Use during pregnancy only if potential benefit justifies potential fetal risk; Pedi: Safety and effectiveness not established.

Adverse Reactions/Side Effects

CNS: fatigue, headache, insomnia. **CV:** peripheral edema. **GI:** GASTRIC PERFORATION, abdominal pain, diarrhea, dyspepsia, gastritis, ↑ liver enzymes, vomiting. **GU:** ↑ serum creatinine. **Derm:** erythema, pruritus, rash. **F and E:** dehydration. **Hemat:** anemia, neutropenia. **Metab:** ↑ lipids. **MS:** arthralgia, joint swelling, musculoskeletal pain, tendonitis. **Neuro:** paresthesia. **Misc:** MALIGNANCY, SERIOUS INFECTIONS including tuberculosis, invasive fungal infections, bacterial, viral, and other infections due to opportunistic pathogens, fever.

Interactions

Drug-Drug: May ↑ risk of adverse reactions and ↓ antibody response to **live vaccines**; avoid concurrent use. Blood levels and effects may be ↑ by **strong CYP3A4 inhibitors** including **ketoconazole** or **moderate CYP3A4 inhibitors/strong CYP2C19 inhibitors** including **fluconazole**; dose ↓ recommended. Blood levels and effectiveness may be ↓ **strong CYP3A4 inducers** including **rifampin**; avoid concurrent use. ↑ risk of immunosuppression when used concurrently with other potent **immunosuppressants** including **azathioprine**, **cyclosporine**, **tacrolimus**, **antineoplastics**, or **radiation therapy**.

Route/Dosage

PO (Adults): 5 mg twice daily; *Concurrent use of strong CYP3A4 inhibitors or moderate CYP3A4 inhibitors/strong CYP2C19 inhibitors*—5 mg once daily; dosage adjustments recommended for neutropenia, anemia or infection.

Renal Impairment

PO (Adults): *Moderate to severe renal impairment*—5 mg once daily.

Hepatic Impairment

PO (Adults): *Moderate hepatic impairment*—5 mg once daily.

Availability

Tablets: 5 mg.

NURSING IMPLICATIONS

Assessment

- Assess pain and range of motion before and periodically during therapy.
- Assess for signs of infection (fever, dyspnea, flu-like symptoms, frequent or painful urination, redness or swelling at the site of a wound), including tuberculosis, prior to and periodically during therapy. Tofacitinib is contraindicated in patients with active infection. New infections should be monitored closely; most common are upper respiratory tract infections, bronchitis, and urinary tract infections. Infections

may be fatal, especially in patients taking immunosuppressive therapy.

- Assess for signs and symptoms of systemic fungal infections (fever, malaise, weight loss, sweats, cough, dypsnea, pulmonary infiltrates, serious systemic illness with or without concomitant shock). Ascertain if patient lives in or has traveled to areas of endemic mycoses. Consider empiric antifungal treatment for patients at risk of histoplasmosis and other invasive fungal infections until the pathogens are identified. Consult with an infectious diseases specialist. Consider stopping tofacitinib until the infection has been diagnosed and adequately treated.
- ***Lab Test Considerations:*** Monitor CBC prior to and periodically during therapy. Do not initiate tofacitinib in patients with lymphocyte count <500 cells/mm³, an ANC <1000 cells/mm³, or who have hemoglobin level <9 g/dL.
- Monitor lymphocyte count at baseline and every 3 mo thereafter. *If lymphocyte count ≥500 cells/mm³* maintain dose. *If lymphocyte count <500 cells/mm³ and confirmed by repeat testing,* discontinue tofacitinib.
- Monitor neutrophil count at baseline, after 4–8 wk of therapy, and every 3 mo thereafter. *If ANC >1000 cells/mm³*, maintain dose. *If ANC 500–1000 cells/mm³*, for persistent decreases in this range, interrupt dosing until ANC is >1000 cells/mm³. *If ANC <500 cells/mm³ and confirmed by repeat testing,* discontinue tofacitinib.
- Monitor hemoglobin at baseline, after 4–8 wk of therapy, and every 3 mo thereafter. *If hemoglobin ≤2 g/dL decrease and ≥9.0 g/dL and confirmed by repeat testing,* maintain dose. *If hemoglobin >2 dL decrease and <8.0 g/dL,* interrupt administration of tofacitinib until hemoglobin values have normalized.
- Monitor liver enzymes prior to and periodically during therapy.
- Monitor total cholesterol, LDL cholesterol, HDL cholesterol 4–8 wk following initiation of therapy.

Potential Nursing Diagnoses

Impaired physical mobility (Indications)
Risk for infection (Adverse Reactions)

Implementation

- Administer a tuberculin skin test prior to administration of tofacitinib. Patients with active latent TB should be treated for TB prior to therapy.
- Immunizations should be current prior to initiating therapy. Patients on tofacitinib should not receive live vaccines.
- Screen patient for viral hepatitis before starting therapy.
- **PO:** Administer twice daily without regard to food.

Patient/Family Teaching

- Instruct patient to take tofacitinib as directed. Advise patient to read Medication Guide before starting and with each Rx refill in case of changes.
- Caution patient to notify health care professional immediately if signs of infection (fever, sweating, chills, muscle aches, cough, shortness of breath, blood in phlegm, weight loss, warm, red, or painful skin or sores, diarrhea or stomach pain, burning on urination or urinating more often than normal, feeling very tired) or stomach or intestinal perforation (fever, stomach-area pain that does not go away, change in bowel habits) occur.
- Advise patient to notify health care professional of all Rx or OTC medications, vitamins, or herbal products being taken and to consult with health care professional before taking other medications.
- Instruct patient to notify health care professional of medication regimen prior to treatment or surgery.
- Inform patient of increased risk of lymphoma and other cancers. Advise patient to have periodic skin exams for new lesions of skin cancer.
- Rep: Advise female patients to notify health care professional if pregnancy is planned or suspected or if breast feeding. Encourage patient to contact the pregnancy registry by calling 1-877-311-8972 if pregnant.
- Emphasize the importance of follow-up lab tests to monitor for adverse reactions.

Evaluation/Desired Outcomes

- Decreased pain and swelling with improved physical functioning and decreased rate of joint destruction in patients with rheumatoid arthritis.

tolcapone (tole-ka-pone)

Tasmar

Classification

Therapeutic: antiparkinson agents
Pharmacologic: catechol-*O*-methyltransferase inhibitors

Pregnancy Category C

Indications

Management of Parkinson's disease with carbidopa/levodopa in patients without severe movement abnormalities who do not respond to other treatment.

Action

Acts as a selective and reversible inhibitor of the enzyme catechol-*O*-methyltransferase. Inhibition of this enzyme prevents the breakdown of levodopa, greatly increasing its availability to the CNS. **Therapeutic Effects:** Prolongs duration of response to levodopa with-

T

out end-of-dose motor fluctuations. Decreased signs and symptoms of Parkinson's disease.

Pharmacokinetics

Absorption: Rapidly absorbed following oral administration with 65% bioavailability.
Distribution: Unknown.
Protein Binding: >99% bound to plasma proteins.
Metabolism and Excretion: Mostly metabolized by the liver; <0.5% excreted unchanged in urine.
Half-life: 2–3 hr.

TIME/ACTION PROFILE (blood levels)

ROUTE	ONSET	PEAK	DURATION
PO	unknown	1.7 hr	8 hr

Contraindications/Precautions

Contraindicated in: Hypersensitivity; Concurrent MAO inhibitor therapy; Clinical evidence of liver disease.
Use Cautiously in: Severe renal impairment (safety not established if CCr <25 mL/min); OB: Lactation: Safety not established.

Adverse Reactions/Side Effects

CNS: headache, sleep disorder, hallucinations, syncope, urges (gambling, sexual). **CV:** orthostatic hypotension. **GI:** HEPATOTOXICITY, constipation, diarrhea, anorexia, ↑ liver enzymes, nausea, vomiting. **GU:** hematuria, yellow discoloration of urine. **Derm:** ↑ sweating, melanoma. **Neuro:** dyskinesia, dystonia.

Interactions

Drug-Drug: Concurrent use with **MAO inhibitors** is not recommended; both agents inhibit the metabolic pathways of catecholamines. May ↑ the effects of **methyldopa**, **apomorphine**, **dobutamine**, or **isoproterenol**; dose reduction may be necessary. ↑ the bioavailability of **levodopa** by two-fold; this is a desired effect.

Route/Dosage

PO (Adults): 100 mg 3 times daily; may cautiously ↑ to 200 mg 3 times daily if benefit is justified.

Availability (generic available)

Tablets: 100 mg.

NURSING IMPLICATIONS

Assessment

- Assess patient for signs and symptoms of Parkinson's disease (tremor, muscle weakness and rigidity, ataxic gait) prior to and throughout therapy.
- Assess BP periodically during therapy.
- Monitor for signs and symptoms of liver dysfunction (persistent nausea, fatigue, lethargy, anorexia, jaundice, dark urine, pruritus, right upper quadrant tenderness) periodically during therapy.
- ***Lab Test Considerations:*** Monitor liver function tests before every 2–4 wk for the first 6 mo following initiation or dose increase and periodically thereafter. Discontinue tolcapone if liver function tests reach two times the upper limit of normal or if jaundice occurs; do not reinstate.

Potential Nursing Diagnoses

Impaired physical mobility (Indications)
Risk for injury (Indications, Side Effects)

Implementation

- **PO:** Administer 1st dose of the day of tolcapone together with carbidopa/levodopa. Administer subsequent doses 6 and 12 hr later.
- May be administered without regard to food.

Patient/Family Teaching

- Instruct patient to take medication as directed. Caution patient not to discontinue tolcapone without consulting health care professional. Abrupt discontinuation or rapid dose reduction may result in neuroleptic malignant syndrome (↑ temperature, muscular rigidity, altered consciousness).
- Caution patient to make position changes slowly to minimize orthostatic hypotension, especially at the beginning of therapy.
- May affect mental and/or motor performance. Caution patient to avoid driving or other activities requiring alertness until response to medication is known.
- Advise patient to avoid taking alcohol or other CNS depressants concurrently with tolcapone.
- Inform patient and caregiver that hallucinations, nausea, dyskinesia, or dystonia may occur during tolcapone therapy.
- Instruct patient to notify health care professional if persistent diarrhea occurs.
- Advise patient to notify health care professional if symptoms of liver failure (clay-colored stools, jaundice, fatigue, loss of appetite, lethargy), suspicious or unusual skin changes, hallucinations, or new or increased gambling, sexual, or other intense urges occur.
- Advise patient to notify health care professional if pregnancy is planned or suspected.
- Emphasize the importance of routine follow-up exams.

Evaluation/Desired Outcomes

- Decrease in signs and symptoms of Parkinson's disease.

tolnaftate, See ANTIFUNGALS (TOPICAL).

tolterodine (tol-ter-oh-deen)

Detrol, Detrol LA

Classification

Therapeutic: urinary tract antispasmodics
Pharmacologic: anticholinergics

Pregnancy Category C

Indications

Treatment of overactive bladder function that results in urinary frequency, urgency, or urge incontinence.

Action

Acts as a competitive muscarinic receptor antagonist resulting in inhibition of cholinergically mediated bladder contraction. **Therapeutic Effects:** Decreased urinary frequency, urgency, and urge incontinence.

Pharmacokinetics

Absorption: Well absorbed (77%) following oral administration.

Distribution: Unknown.

Protein Binding: 96.3%.

Metabolism and Excretion: Extensively metabolized by the liver (primarily by CYP2D6 isoenzyme) (the CYP2D6 enzyme system exhibits genetic polymorphism; ~7% of population may be poor metabolizers and may have significantly ↑ tolterodine concentrations and an ↑ risk of adverse effects); one metabolite (5-hydroxymethyltolterodine) is active; other metabolites are excreted in urine.

Half-life: *Tolterodine*—1.9–3.7 hr; *5-hydroxymethyltolterodine*—2.9–3.1 hr.

TIME/ACTION PROFILE (effects on bladder function)

ROUTE	ONSET	PEAK	DURATION
PO	unknown	unknown	12 hr

Contraindications/Precautions

Contraindicated in: Hypersensitivty to tolterodine or fesoterodine; Urinary retention; Gastric retention; Uncontrolled angle-closure glaucoma; Lactation: Lactation.

Use Cautiously in: GI obstructive disorders, including pyloric stenosis (↑ risk of gastric retention); Significant bladder outflow obstruction (↑ risk of urinary retention); Controlled angle-closure glaucoma; Myasthenia gravis; Significant hepatic impairment (lower doses recommended); Impaired renal function; OB: Safety not established; use only if potential maternal benefit justifies potential risk to fetus; Pedi: Safety not established.

Adverse Reactions/Side Effects

CNS: headache, dizziness, sedation. **EENT:** blurred vision, dry eyes. **GI:** dry mouth, constipation, dyspepsia. **Derm:** STEVENS-JOHNSON SYNDROME. **Misc:** ANAPHYLAXIS, ANGIOEDEMA.

Interactions

Drug-Drug: Erythromycin, clarithromycin, ketoconazole, itraconazole, and **miconazole** may inhibit metabolism and ↑ effects.

Route/Dosage

PO (Adults): 2 mg twice daily as tablets; may be lowered depending on response *or* 2–4 mg once daily as extended-release capsules.

PO (Adults with impaired hepatic function or concurrent enzyme inhibitors): 1 mg twice daily.

Availability (generic available)

Tablets: 1 mg, 2 mg. **Cost:** *Generic*—1 mg $198.55/60, 2 mg $203.79/60. **Extended-release capsules:** 2 mg, 4 mg. **Cost:** 2 mg $458.03/60, 4 mg $447.85/60.

NURSING IMPLICATIONS

Assessment

- Assess patient for urinary urgency, frequency, and urge incontinence periodically during therapy.
- Monitor for signs and symptoms of anaphylaxis and angioedema (difficulty breathing, upper airway obstruction, fall in BP, rash, swelling of face or neck). Have emergency equipment readily available.
- Assess for rash periodically during therapy. May cause Stevens-Johnson syndrome or toxic epidermal necrolysis. Discontinue therapy if severe or if accompanied with fever, general malaise, fatigue, muscle or joint aches, blisters, oral lesions, conjunctivitis, hepatitis and/or eosinophilia.

Potential Nursing Diagnoses

Impaired urinary elimination (Indications)
Urinary retention (Indications)

Implementation

- **PO:** Administer without regard to food.
- Extended-release capsules should be swallowed whole; do not open, crush, dissolve, or chew.

Patient/Family Teaching

- Instruct patient to take tolterodine as directed.
- May cause dizziness and blurred vision. Caution patient to avoid driving or other activities requiring alertness until response to medication is known.
- Instruct patient to notify health care professional immediately if rash or signs and symptoms of anaphylaxis or angioedema occur.

Evaluation/Desired Outcomes

- Decreased urinary frequency, urgency, and urge incontinence.

T

tolvaptan (tol-vap-tan)

✱Jinarc, Samsca

Classification
Therapeutic: electrolyte modifiers
Pharmacologic: vasopressin antagonists

Pregnancy Category C

Indications

Treatment of significant hypervolemic and euvolemic hyponatremia (serum sodium <125 mEq/L or less marked symptomatic hyponatremia that has resisted correction by fluid restriction), including patients with heart failure and syndrome of inappropriate antidiuretic hormone (SIADH).

Action

Acts as a selective vasopressin V2-receptor antagonist, resulting in increased renal water excretion and increased serum sodium. **Therapeutic Effects:** Correction of hyponatremia.

Pharmacokinetics

Absorption: 40% absorbed following oral administration.
Distribution: >99%.
Metabolism and Excretion: Extensively metabolized primarily by the CYP3A4 enzyme system; no renal elimination.
Half-life: 12 hr.

TIME/ACTION PROFILE

ROUTE	ONSET	PEAK	DURATION
PO	within 8 hr	2–4 hr†	7 days

† Blood level.

Contraindications/Precautions

Contraindicated in: Hypersensitivity; Urgent need to acutely raise serum sodium; Patients who cannot appropriately sense/respond to thirst; Hypovolemic hyponatremia; Concurrent use of strong or moderate CYP3A inhibitors; Anuria; Liver disease; Lactation: Avoid use.
Use Cautiously in: Severe malnutrition, alcoholism or advanced liver disease (↑ risk of osmotic demyelination; correct electrolyte abnormalities at a slower rates); Cirrhosis (↑ risk of GI bleeding, use only when the need to treat outweighs risk); Geri: May have ↑ sensitivity to effects; OB: Use only if the potential benefit justifies the potential risk to the fetus; Pedi: Safety and effectiveness not established.

Adverse Reactions/Side Effects

CNS: weakness. **GI:** HEPATOTOXICITY, constipation, dry mouth. **GU:** polyuria. **F and E:** thirst. **Metab:** hyperglycemia. **Neuro:** osmotic demyelination. **Misc:** ANAPHYLAXIS.

Interactions

Drug-Drug: Strong inhibitors of the CYP3A enzyme system including **ketoconazole, clarithromycin, itraconazole, telithromycin, saquinavir, nelfinavir, ritonavir**, and **nefazodone** ↑ levels and may ↑ effects and risk of toxicity; concurrent use should be avoided. **Moderate CYP 3A inhibitors** including **erythromycin, fluconazole, aprepitant, diltiazem**, and **verapamil** may have a similar effect and should also be avoided. **Inducers of the CYP3A enzyme system** including **rifampin** can ↓ blood levels and effectiveness; dosage adjustments may be necessary. Levels and risk of toxicity are also ↑ **P-gp inhibitors** including **cyclosporine**; dosage adjustments may be necessary. May ↑ **digoxin** levels; monitor carefully. May ↑ risk of hyperkalemia with **angiotensin receptor blockers, ACE inhibitors**, and **potassium-sparing diuretics**.
Drug-Food: Grapefruit juice ↑ levels and the risk of toxicity; avoid concurrent use.

Route/Dosage

PO (Adults): 15 mg once daily initially; may be ↑ at intervals of at least one day to 30 mg once daily, up to a maximum of 60 mg once daily. Do not use for longer than 30 days.

Availability

Tablets: 15 mg, 30 mg, ✱45 mg, ✱60 mg, ✱90 mg.

NURSING IMPLICATIONS

Assessment

- Monitor neurologic status and assess for signs and symptoms of osmotic demyelination syndrome (trouble speaking, dysphagia, drowsiness, confusion, mood changes, involuntary movements, weakness, seizures), especially during initiation and after titration. If a rapid ↑ in sodium or symptoms occur, discontinue tolvaptan and consider administration of hypotonic fluid.
- Monitor fluid balance. If hypovolemia occurs interrupt or discontinue tolvaptan and provide supportive care (monitor vital signs, balance fluid and electrolytes).
- Monitor for signs and symptoms of liver injury (fatigue, anorexia, right upper abdominal discomfort, dark urine, jaundice) periodically during therapy. If symptoms occur, discontinue therapy.
- ***Lab Test Considerations:*** Monitor serum sodium levels frequently during initiation and dose titration and periodically during therapy. Too rapid correction of hyponatremia (>12 mEq/L/24 hr) can cause osmotic demyelination syndrome.
- Monitor serum potassium in patients with serum potassium >5 mEq/L or taking medication known to ↑ potassium.

Potential Nursing Diagnoses

Risk for imbalanced fluid volume (Indications)

Implementation

- Initiate and re-initiate therapy in a hospital.
- Avoid fluid restriction during first 24 hr of therapy.
- **PO:** Administer once daily without regard to meals.

Patient/Family Teaching

- Instruct patient to take tolvaptan as directed. Avoid drinking grapefruit juice during therapy; may cause ↑ levels. Take missed doses as soon as remembered, but not if just before next dose; do not double doses. Do not stop and restart therapy. Restarting therapy may require hospitalization.
- Inform patients they can continue fluid ingestion in response to thirst during therapy and should have water available to drink at all times during therapy. Following discontinuation of therapy, resume fluid restriction.
- Advise patient to notify health care professional of all Rx or OTC medications, vitamins, or herbal products being taken and to consult with health care professional before taking other medications.
- Advise patient to notify health care professional if signs of dehydration (vomiting, diarrhea, inability to drink normally, dizziness, feeling faint) or bleeding (vomiting bright red blood, dark blood clots, or coffee-ground-like material; black, tarry stools; bloody stools).
- Advise female patients to notify health care professional if pregnancy is planned or suspected or if breast feeding.

Evaluation/Desired Outcomes

- Normalization of serum sodium levels. Therapy should be limited to 30 days.

topiramate (toe-peer-i-mate)

Qudexy XR, Topamax, Topamax Sprinkle, Trokendi XR

Classification

Therapeutic: anticonvulsants, mood stabilizers

Pregnancy Category D

Indications

Seizures including: partial-onset, primary generalized tonic-clonic, seizures due to Lennox-Gastaut syndrome. Prevention of migraine headache (immediate-release only). **Unlabeled Use:** Adjunct in treatment of bipolar disorder. Infantile spasms.

Action

Action may be due to: Blockade of sodium channels in neurons, Enhancement of gamma-aminobutyrate (GABA), an inhibitory neurotransmitter, Prevention of activation of excitatory receptors. **Therapeutic Effects:** Decreased incidence of seizures. Decreased incidence/severity of migraine headache.

Pharmacokinetics

Absorption: Well absorbed (80%) after oral administration.

Distribution: Unknown.

Metabolism and Excretion: 70% excreted unchanged in urine.

Half-life: 21 hr; *Extended-release*—31 hr.

TIME/ACTION PROFILE (blood levels†)

ROUTE	ONSET	PEAK	DURATION
PO	unknown	2 hr	12 hr
PO-ER	unknown	24 hr	unknown

†After single dose.

Contraindications/Precautions

Contraindicated in: Hypersensitivity; Recent alcohol use (within 6 hr before and after use of extended-release product); Metabolic acidosis (on metformin) (with extended-release product only); Lactation: Lactation.

Use Cautiously in: All patients (may ↑ risk of suicidal thoughts/behaviors); Renal impairment (dose reduction recommended if CCr <70 mL/min/1.73 m²); Hepatic impairment; Dehydration; Patients predisposed to metabolic acidosis; Patients allergic to sulfa; OB: May ↑ risk for cleft palate and/or cleft lip in infants exposed during pregnancy; use only if maternal benefit outweighs fetal risk; Pedi: Children are more prone to oligohydrosis and hyperthermia; safety in children <2 yr (immediate-release) and <6 yr (extended-release) not established; Geri: Consider age-related ↓ in renal/hepatic impairment, concurrent disease states and drug therapy.

T

Adverse Reactions/Side Effects

CNS: ↑ SEIZURES, SUICIDAL THOUGHTS, dizziness, drowsiness, fatigue, impaired concentration/memory, nervousness, psychomotor slowing, speech problems, sedation, aggressive reaction, agitation, anxiety, cognitive disorders, confusion, depression, malaise, mood problems. **EENT:** abnormal vision, diplopia, nystagmus, acute myopia/secondary angle closure glaucoma, visual field defects. **GI:** nausea, abdominal pain, anorexia, constipation, dry mouth, encephalopathy, hyperammonemia. **GU:** kidney stones. **Derm:** oligohydrosis (↑ in children). **F and E:** hyperchloremic metabolic acidosis. **Hemat:** BLEEDING, leukopenia. **Metab:** weight loss, hyperthermia (↑ in children). **Neuro:** ataxia, paresthesia, tremor. **Misc:** fever.

Interactions

Drug-Drug: Alcohol use within 6 hr before or after use of Trokendi XR may significantly alter topiramate levels; use during this time frame contraindicated. Levels and effects may be ↓ by **phenytoin**, **carbamazepine**, or **valproic acid**. May ↑ levels and effects of **phenytoin**, **amitriptyline**, or **lithium**. May ↓ levels and effects of **hormonal contraceptives**, **risperidone**, or **valproic acid**. ↑ risk of CNS depression with

alcohol or other **CNS depressants. Carbonic anhydrase inhibitors** (e.g. **acetazolamide** or **zonisamide**) may ↑ risk of metabolic acidosis and kidney stones. Concurrent use with **valproic acid** may ↑ risk of hyperammonemia, encephalopathy, and hypothermia. ↑ risk of bleeding with **aspirin, clopidogrel, ticagrelor, prasugrel, warfarin, dabigatran, rivaroxaban, apixaban, edoxaban, NSAIDs**, or **SSRIs**.

Route/Dosage

Epilepsy (monotherapy)

PO (Adults and children ≥10 yr): *Immediate-release*—25 mg twice daily initially, gradually ↑ at weekly intervals to 200 mg twice daily over a 6–wk period; *Extended-release*—50 mg once daily initially, gradually ↑ at weekly intervals to 400 mg once daily over a 6–wk period.
PO (Children 2–<10 yr and ≤11 kg): *Immediate-release*—25 mg once daily in the evening initially, gradually ↑ at weekly intervals to 75 mg twice daily over a 5–7-wk period; if needed may continue to titrate dose on a weekly basis up to 125 mg twice daily; *Extended-release*—25 mg once daily for 1 wk, then ↑ to 50 mg once daily for 1 wk, then ↑ by 25–50 mg/day at weekly intervals over a 5–7-wk period to target dose of 150–250 mg once daily.
PO (Children 2–<10 yr and 12–22 kg): *Immediate-release*—25 mg once daily in the evening initially, gradually ↑ at weekly intervals to 100 mg twice daily over a 5–7-wk period; if needed may continue to titrate dose on a weekly basis up to 150 mg twice daily; *Extended-release*—25 mg once daily for 1 wk, then ↑ to 50 mg once daily for 1 wk, then ↑ by 25–50 mg/day at weekly intervals over a 5–7-wk period to target dose of 200–300 mg once daily.
PO (Children 2–<10 yr and 23–31 kg): *Immediate-release*—25 mg once daily in the evening initially, gradually ↑ at weekly intervals to 100 mg twice daily over a 5–7-wk period; if needed may continue to titrate dose on a weekly basis up to 175 mg twice daily; *Extended-release*—25 mg once daily for 1 wk, then ↑ to 50 mg once daily for 1 wk, then ↑ by 25–50 mg/day at weekly intervals over a 5–7-wk period to target dose of 200–350 mg once daily.
PO (Children 2–<10 yr and 32–38 kg): *Immediate-release*—25 mg once daily in the evening initially, gradually ↑ at weekly intervals to 125 mg twice daily over a 5–7-wk period; if needed may continue to titrate dose on a weekly basis up to 175 mg twice daily; *Extended-release*—25 mg once daily for 1 wk, then ↑ to 50 mg once daily for 1 wk, then ↑ by 25–50 mg/day at weekly intervals over a 5–7-wk period to target dose of 250–350 mg once daily.
PO (Children 2–<10 yr and >38 k g): *Immediate-release*—25 mg once daily in the evening initially, gradually ↑ at weekly intervals to 125 mg twice daily over a 5–7-wk period; if needed may continue to titrate dose on a weekly basis up to 200 mg twice daily; *Extended-release*—25 mg once daily for 1 wk, then ↑ to 50 mg once daily for 1 wk, then ↑ by 25–50 mg/day at weekly intervals over a 5–7-wk period to target dose of 250–400 mg once daily.

Renal Impairment

PO (Adults): *CCr <70 mL/min*—↓ dose by 50%.

Epilepsy (adjunctive therapy)

PO (Adults and Children ≥17 yr): *Immediate-release*—25–50 mg/day initially, ↑ by 25–50 mg/day at weekly intervals up to 200–400 mg/day in 2 divided doses (200–400 mg/day in 2 divided doses for partial seizures or Lennox-Gastaut syndrome and 400 mg/day in 2 divided doses for primary generalized tonic-clonic seizures); *Extended-release*—25–50 mg once daily initially, ↑ by 25–50 mg/day at weekly intervals up to 200–400 mg once daily (for partial seizures or Lennox-Gastaut syndrome) and 400 mg once daily (for primary generalized tonic-clonic seizures).
PO (Children 2–16 yr): *Immediate–release and extended–release (Qudexy XR)* 25 mg once daily at night initially for first wk, ↑ at 1–2 wk intervals by 1–3 mg/kg/day up to 5–9 mg/kg/day in 2 divided doses.
PO (Children 6–16 yr): *Extended–release (Trokendi XR)*—25 mg once daily at night initially for first wk, ↑ at 1–2 wk intervals by 1–3 mg/kg/day up to 5–9 mg/kg/day given once daily at night.

Renal Impairment

PO (Adults): *CCr <70 mL/min*—↓ dose by 50%.

Migraine Prevention

PO (Adults and Children ≥12 yr): 25 mg at night initially, ↑ by 25 mg/day at weekly intervals up to target dose of 100 mg/day in 2 divided doses.

Renal Impairment

PO (Adults): *CCr <70 mL/min*—↓ dose by 50%.

Availability (generic available)

Sprinkle capsules: 15 mg, 25 mg. **Cost:** *Generic*—15 mg $144.97/60, 25 mg $175.26/60. **Extended-release capsules (Trokendi XR):** 25 mg, 50 mg, 100 mg, 200 mg. **Extended-release capsules (Qudexy XR):** 25 mg, 50 mg, 100 mg, 150 mg, 200 mg. **Tablets:** 25 mg, 50 mg, 100 mg, 200 mg. **Cost:** *Generic*—25 mg $21.85/180, 50 mg $33.03/180, 100 mg $41.48/180, 200 mg $54.38/180. ***In combination with:*** phentermine (Qsymia). See Appendix B.

NURSING IMPLICATIONS

Assessment

- Monitor closely for notable changes in behavior that could indicate the emergence or worsening of suicidal thoughts or behavior or depression.
- **Seizures:** Assess location, duration, and characteristics of seizure activity.
- **Migraines:** Assess pain location, intensity, duration, and associated symptoms (photophobia, phonopho-

bia, nausea, vomiting) during migraine attack. Monitor frequency and intensity of pain on pain scale.

- **Bipolar Disorder:** Assess mental status (mood, orientation, behavior) and cognitive abilities before and periodically during therapy.
- ***Lab Test Considerations:*** Monitor CBC with differential and platelet count before therapy to determine baseline levels and periodically during therapy. Frequently causes anemia.
- Hepatic function should be monitored periodically throughout therapy. May cause ↑ AST and ALT levels.
- Evaluate serum bicarbonate prior to and periodically during therapy. Monitor for signs and symptoms of metabolic acidosis (hyperventilation, fatigue, anorexia, cardiac arrhythmias, stupor). If metabolic acidosis occurs, dosing taper or discontinuation may be necessary.

Potential Nursing Diagnoses

Risk for injury (Indications, Side Effects)
Disturbed thought process (Indications)

Implementation

- Implement seizure precautions.
- Do not confuse Topamax (topiramate) with Toprol XL (metoprolol).
- **PO:** May be administered without regard to meals.
- Do not break/crush tablets because of bitter taste.
- Contents of the sprinkle capsules can be sprinkled on a small amount (teaspoon) of soft food, such as applesauce, custard, ice cream, oatmeal, pudding, or yogurt. To open, hold the capsule upright so that you can read the word "TOP." Carefully twist off the clear portion of the capsule. It may be best to do this over the small portion of the food onto which you will be pouring the sprinkles. Sprinkle the entire contents of the capsule onto the food. Be sure the patient swallows the entire spoonful of the sprinkle/food mixture immediately without chewing. Follow with fluids immediately to make sure all of the mixture is swallowed. Never store a sprinkle/food mixture for use at another time.
- A 6 mg/mL oral suspension may be compounded by pharmacy for pediatric patients.
- Swallow extended-release capsules *(Trokendi XR)* whole; do not sprinkle on food, or break, crush, dissolve, or chew.
- Swallow extended-release capsules *(Qudexy XR)* whole; may be opened and sprinkled on soft food; do not crush or chew. Swallow immediately, do not save for later.

Patient/Family Teaching

- Instruct patient to take topiramate exactly as directed. Take missed doses as soon as possible but not just before next dose; do not double doses. Notify health care professional if more than 1 dose is missed. Medication should be gradually discontinued to prevent seizures and status epilepticus. Instruct patient to read the *Medication Guide* before starting and with each Rx refill in case of changes.
- May cause decreased sweating and increased body temperature. Advise patients, especially parents of pediatric patients, to provide adequate hydration and monitoring, especially during hot weather.
- May cause dizziness, drowsiness, confusion, and difficulty concentrating. Caution patients to avoid driving or other activities requiring alertness until response to medication is known.
- Advise patient to maintain a fluid intake of 2000–3000 mL of fluid/day to prevent the formation of kidney stones.
- Instruct patient to notify health care professional immediately if periorbital pain or blurred vision occur. Medication should be discontinued if ocular symptoms occur. May lead to permanent loss of vision.
- Advise patient and family to notify health care professional if thoughts about suicide or dying, attempts to commit suicide; new or worse depression; new or worse anxiety; feeling very agitated or restless; panic attacks; trouble sleeping; new or worse irritability; acting aggressive; being angry or violent; acting on dangerous impulses; an extreme increase in activity and talking, other unusual changes in behavior or mood occur.
- Inform patients that topiramate may cause encephalopathy. If signs and symptoms (unexplained lethargy, vomiting, changes in mental status) occur, notify health care professional.
- Caution patient to make position changes slowly to minimize orthostatic hypotension.
- Instruct patient to notify health care professional of all Rx or OTC medications, vitamins, or herbal products being taken and consult health care professional before taking any new medications.
- Advise patient not to take alcohol or other CNS depressants concurrently with this medication. Avoid alcohol 6 hrs before and 6 hrs after taking *Trokendi XR*.
- Instruct patient to notify health care professional of medication regimen before treatment or surgery.
- Advise patient to use sunscreen and wear protective clothing to prevent photosensitivity reactions.
- Rep: Advise patient to use a nonhormonal form of contraception while taking topiramate; may make hormonal contraceptives less effective. Notify health care professional if pregnancy is planned or suspected or if breast feeding. If pregnancy occurs, encourage patient to enroll in the North American Drug Pregnancy Registry by calling 1-877-376-3872.
- Advise patient to carry identification describing disease and medication regimen at all times.

T

Evaluation/Desired Outcomes

- Absence or reduction of seizure activity.
- Decrease in incidence and severity of migraine headaches.
- Remission of manic symptoms.

HIGH ALERT

topotecan (toe-poe-**tee**-kan)
Hycamtin

Classification
Therapeutic: antineoplastics
Pharmacologic: enzyme inhibitors

Pregnancy Category D

Indications

IV: Metastatic ovarian cancer that has not responded to previous chemotherapy. Small cell lung cancer unresponsive to first line therapy. Stage IV-B persistent or recurrent cervical cancer not amenable to treatment with surgery or radiation (with cisplatin). **PO:** Relapsed small cell lung cancer in patients with a complete or partial prior response and who are at least 45 days from the end of first-line chemotherapy.

Action

Interferes with DNA synthesis by inhibiting the enzyme topoisomerase. **Therapeutic Effects:** Death of rapidly replicating cells, particularly malignant ones.

Pharmacokinetics

Absorption: IV administration results in complete bioavailability.
Distribution: Unknown.
Metabolism and Excretion: 30% excreted in urine; small amounts metabolized by the liver.
Half-life: *PO*—3–6 hr; *IV*—2–3 hr.

TIME/ACTION PROFILE (effects on WBCs)

ROUTE	ONSET	PEAK	DURATION
PO	unknown	1–2 hr	24 hr
IV	within days	11 days	7 days

Contraindications/Precautions

Contraindicated in: Hypersensitivity; OB, Lactation: Pregnancy or lactation.
Use Cautiously in: Impaired renal function (↓ dose if CCr <40 mL/min); Platelet count <25,000 cells/mm³ (↓ dose); History of interstitial lung disease, pulmonary fibrosis, lung cancer, thoracic radiation, or use of pneumotoxic drugs or colony stimulating factors; Rep: Patients with childbearing potential; Geri: May require dose ↓ due to age-related ↓ in renal function.

Adverse Reactions/Side Effects

CNS: headache, fatigue, weakness. **Resp:** INTERSTITIAL LUNG DISEASE, dyspnea. **GI:** abdominal pain, diarrhea, nausea, vomiting, anorexia, constipation, ↑ liver enzymes, stomatitis. **Derm:** alopecia. **Hemat:** anemia, leukopenia, thrombocytopenia. **MS:** arthralgia.

Interactions

Drug-Drug: P-glycoprotein inhibitors, including **amiodarone, azithromycin, captopril, carvedilol, clarithromycin, conivaptan, cyclosporine, diltiazem, dronedarone, erythromycin, felodipine, itraconazole, ketoconazole, lopinavir, ritonavir, quinidine, ranolazine, ticagrelort**, or **verapamil** may ↑ levels; avoid concurrent use. Neutropenia is prolonged by concurrent use of **filgrastim** (do not use until day 6; 24 hr following completion of topotecan). ↑ myelosuppression with other **antineoplastics** (especially **cisplatin**) or **radiation therapy**. May ↓ antibody response to and ↑ risk of adverse reactions from **live virus vaccines**.

Route/Dosage

PO (Adults): 2.3 mg/m²/day for 5 days starting on day 1 of a 21–day course (round calculated oral dose to nearest 0.25 mg and prescribe the minimum number of 1 mg and 0.25 mg capsules with the same number of capsules prescribed for each of the 5 days).
IV (Adults): *Ovarian and Small Cell Lung Cancer*—1.5 mg/m²/day for 5 days starting on day 1 of a 21-day course; *Cervical Cancer*—75 mg/m² on Days 1, 2, and 3 followed by cisplatin on Day 1 and repeated every 21 days.

Renal Impairment

PO (Adults): *CCr 30–49 mL/min*—1.5 mg/m²/day for 5 days starting on day 1 of a 21-day course; dose may be ↑after first course by 0.4 mg/m²/day if no severe hematologic or GI toxicities occur; *CCr <30 mL/min*—0.6 mg/m²/day for 5 days starting on day 1 of a 21-day course; dose may be ↑after first course by 0.4 mg/m²/day if no severe hematologic or GI toxicities occur.

Renal Impairment

IV (Adults): *CCr 20–39 mL/min*—0.75 mg/m²/day for 5 days starting on day 1 of a 21-day course. *Cervical Cancer*—Administer at standard doses only if serum creatinine is ≤1.5 mg/dL. Do not administer if serum creatinine >1.5 m g/dL.

Availability (generic available)

Capsules: 0.25 mg, 1 mg. **Powder for injection:** 4 mg/vial. **Solution for injection:** 1 mg/mL.

NURSING IMPLICATIONS

Assessment

- Monitor vital signs frequently during administration.
- Monitor for bone marrow depression. Assess for bleeding (bleeding gums, bruising, petechiae; guaiac stools, urine, and emesis) and avoid IM injections and taking rectal temperatures if platelet count is low. Apply pressure to venipuncture sites for 10 min. Assess for signs of infection during neu-

tropenia. Anemia may occur. Monitor for increased fatigue, dyspnea, and orthostatic hypotension.

- Nausea and vomiting are common. Pretreatment with antiemetics should be considered.
- Assess IV site frequently for extravasation, which causes mild local erythema and bruising.
- Monitor for signs and symptoms of interstitial lung disease (cough, fever, dyspnea, hypoxia). Discontinue topotecan if interstitial lung disease is confirmed.
- ***Lab Test Considerations:*** Monitor CBC with differential and platelet count prior to administration and frequently during therapy. Baseline neutrophil count of ≥1500 cells/mm³ and platelet count of ≥100,000 cells/mm³ are required before first dose. The nadir of neutropenia occurs in 11 days, with a duration of 7 days. The nadir of thrombocytopenia occurs in 15 days, with a duration of 5 days. The nadir of anemia occurs in 15 days. Subsequent doses should not be administered until neutrophils recover to >1000 cells/mm³, platelets recover to >100,000 cells/mm³, and hemoglobin levels recover to 9.0 mg/dL. **When topotecan used as a single-agent,** ↓ dose to 1.25 mg/m² if *neutrophil <500 cells/mm³*, or administer granulocyte-colony stimulating factor (G-CSF) starting no sooner than 24 hrs following the last dose or *platelet counts less than 25,000 cells/mm³* during previous cycle. **When topotecan used with cisplatin,** ↓ dose to 0.60 mg/m² (and to 0.45 mg/m² if necessary) for febrile neutropenia (***neutrophil counts <1,000 cells/mm³ with temperature of ≥38.0°C (100.4°F)***, or administer G-CSF starting no sooner than 24 hrs following the last dose or *platelet counts less than 25,000 cells/mm³* during previous cycle.
- Monitor liver function. May cause transient ↑ in AST, ALT, and bilirubin concentrations.

Potential Nursing Diagnoses

Risk for infection (Adverse Reactions)

Implementation

- ***High Alert:*** Fatalities have occurred with chemotherapeutic agents. Before administering, clarify all ambiguous orders; double check single, daily, and course-of-therapy dose limits; have second practitioner independently double check original order, dose calculations and infusion pump settings.
- **PO:** May be taken without regard to food. Capsules must be swallowed whole; do not open, crush, or chew. If patient vomits after taking dose, do not replace dose.
- Do not administer capsules to patients with Grade 3 or 4 diarrhea. When recovered to ≤Grade 1, resume with dose decreased by 0.4 mg/m²/day for subsequent courses.

IV Administration

- Solution should be prepared in a biologic cabinet. Wear gloves, gown, and mask while handling IV medication. Discard IV equipment in specially designated containers.
- **Intermittent Infusion:** Reconstitute each vial with 4 mL of sterile water for injection. ***Diluent:*** Dilute further in D5W or 0.9% NaCl. Infusion is stable for 24 hr at room temperature or up to 7 days if refrigerated. Solution is yellow to yellow-green. ***Concentration:*** 10–50 mcg/mL. ***Rate:*** Infuse over 30 min.
- **Y-Site Compatibility:** alemtuzumab, alfentanil, amikacin, amiodarone, anidulafungin, argatroban, aztreonam, bivalirudin, buprenorphine, butorphanol, calcium chloride, carboplatin, caspofungin, cefazolin, cefotaxime, cefotetan, cefoxitin, ceftriaxone, cefuroxime, chloramphenicol, chlorpromazine, ciprofloxacin, cisatracurium, cisplatin, cyclophosphamide, cyclosporine, dacarbazine, dactinomycin, daptomycin, daunorubicin hydrochloride, dexmedetomidine, dexrazoxane, diltiazem, diphenhydramine, dobutamine, docetaxel, dopamine, doxorubicin hydrochloride, doxorubicin liposomal, doxycycline, droperidol, enalaprilat, ephedrine, epinephrine, erythromycin, esmolol, etoposide, etoposide phosphate, famotidine, fenoldopam, fentanyl, fluconazole, fludarabine, furosemide, gemcitabine, gentamicin, glycopyrrolate, granisetron, haloperidol, heparin, hetastarch, hydralazine, hydrocortisone, hydromorphone, idarubicin, ifosfamide, insulin, isoproterenol, labetalol, leucovorin, levofloxacin, lidocaine, linezolid, lorazepam, magnesium sulfate, mannitol, meperidine, methyldopate, methylprednisolone, metoclopramide, metoprolol, metronidazole, midazolam, milrinone, mitoxantrone, morphine, moxifloxacin, nalbuphine, naloxone, nesiritide, nitroglycerin, nitroprusside, norepinephrine, octreotide, ondansetron, oxaliplatin, paclitaxel, palonosetron, pamidronate, pancuronium, pentamidine, pentazocine, phenylephrine, potassium chloride, procainamide, prochlorperazine, promethazine, propranolol, ranitidine, remifentanil, succinylcholine, sufentanil, tacrolimus, teniposide, theophylline, thiotepa, tigecycline, tirofiban, tobramycin, vancomycin, vasopressin, vecuronium, verapamil, vinblastine, vincristine, vinorelbine, voriconazole, zidovudine, zoledronic acid.
- **Y-Site Incompatibility:** acyclovir, allopurinol, amifostine, aminophylline, amphotericin B colloidal, amphotericin B lipid complex, ampicillin, ampicillin/sulbactam, bumetanide, calcium gluconate, cefepime, ceftazidime, clindamycin, dantrolene, dexamethasone, diazepam, digoxin, ertapenem, fluorouracil, foscarnet, fosphenytoin, ganciclovir, hydrocortisone, imipenem/cilastatin, ketorolac,

T

meropenem, mitomycin, nafcillin, pantoprazole, pemetrexed, pentobarbital, phenobarbital, phenytoin, piperacillin/tazobactam, potassium acetate, potassium phosphates, rituximab, sodium bicarbonate, sodium phosphates, thiopental, trastuzumab, trimethoprim/sulfamethoxazole.

Patient/Family Teaching

- Instruct patient to take as directed. If patient vomits after taking, do not replace dose; notify health care professional. Do not take missed doses; take next scheduled dose and notify health care professional. If any capsules are broken or leaking, do not touch with bare hands; dispose of capsules and wash hands with soap and water. Patient should be instructed to read the *Patient Information* guide prior to first dose and with each Rx refillin case of changes.
- May cause drowsiness or sleepiness during and for several days after therapy. Caution patient to avoid driving and other activities requiring alertness until response to medication is known.
- Instruct patient to notify health care professional if fever; chills; sore throat; signs of infection; bleeding gums; bruising; petechiae; blood in urine, stool, emesis or signs and symptoms of interstitial lung disease occur. Caution patient to avoid crowds and persons with known infections. Instruct patient to use soft toothbrush and electric razor. Patient should be cautioned not to drink alcoholic beverages or take products containing aspirin or NSAIDs.
- May cause diarrhea. Advise patient to notify health care professional if diarrhea with fever or stomach pain or cramps or diarrhea that occurs more than 3 times/day.
- Advise patient to notify health care professional of all Rx or OTC medications, vitamins, or herbal products being taken and to consult with health care professional before taking other medications.
- Discuss with patient the possibility of hair loss. Explore methods of coping.
- Instruct patient not to receive any vaccinations without advice of health care professional.
- Rep: Advise male and female patient that topotecan may cause infertility and may have teratogenic effects. Contraception should be used during therapy and for at least 1 month after last dose; and breast feeding avoided.
- Emphasize the need for periodic lab tests to monitor for side effects.

Evaluation/Desired Outcomes

- Decrease in size and spread of malignancy.

torsemide (tore-se-mide)

Demadex

Classification

Therapeutic: antihypertensives

Pharmacologic: loop diuretics

Pregnancy Category B

Indications

Edema due to: HF, Hepatic or renal disease. Hypertension.

Action

Inhibits the reabsorption of sodium and chloride from the loop of Henle and distal renal tubule. Increases renal excretion of water, sodium, chloride, magnesium, hydrogen, and calcium. Effectiveness persists in impaired renal function. **Therapeutic Effects:** Diuresis and subsequent mobilization of excess fluid (edema, pleural effusions). Decreased BP.

Pharmacokinetics

Absorption: 80% absorbed after oral administration.

Distribution: Widely distributed.

Protein Binding: ≥99%.

Metabolism and Excretion: 80% metabolized by liver, 20% excreted in urine.

Half-life: 3.5 hr.

TIME/ACTION PROFILE (diuretic effect)

ROUTE	ONSET	PEAK	DURATION
PO	within 60 min	60–120 min	6–8 hr

Contraindications/Precautions

Contraindicated in: Hypersensitivity; Cross-sensitivity with thiazides and sulfonamides may occur; Hepatic coma or anuria.

Use Cautiously in: Severe liver disease (may precipitate hepatic coma; concurrent use with potassium-sparing diuretics may be necessary); Electrolyte depletion; Diabetes mellitus; Increasing azotemia; Geri: May have ↑ risk of side effects, especially hypotension and electrolyte imbalance, at usual doses; OB, Lactation, Pedi: Safety not established.

Adverse Reactions/Side Effects

CNS: dizziness, headache, nervousness. **EENT:** hearing loss, tinnitus. **CV:** hypotension. **GI:** constipation, diarrhea, dry mouth, dyspepsia, nausea, vomiting. **GU:** ↑ BUN, excessive urination. **Derm:** STEVENS-JOHNSON SYNDROME, TOXIC EPIDERMAL NECROLYSIS, photosensitivity, rash. **Endo:** hyperglycemia, hyperuricemia. **F and E:** dehydration, hypocalcemia, hypochloremia, hypokalemia, hypomagnesemia, hyponatremia, hypovolemia, metabolic alkalosis. **MS:** arthralgia, muscle cramps, myalgia.

Interactions

Drug-Drug: ↑ hypotension with **antihypertensives**, **nitrates**, or acute ingestion of **alcohol**. ↑ risk of hypokalemia with other **diuretics**, **amphotericin B**, **stimulant laxatives**, and **corticosteroids**. Hypokalemia may ↑ risk of **digoxin** toxicity and ↑ risk of arrhythmia in patients taking drugs that prolong the QT interval. May ↑ risk of **lithium** toxicity. ↑ risk of ototoxicity with **aminoglycosides**. **NSAIDS** may ↓ effects. ↑ risk of **salicylate** toxicity (with use of high-dose **salicylate** therapy). **Cholestyramine** may ↓ absorption.

Route/Dosage

HF

PO (Adults): 10–20 mg once daily; dose may be doubled until desired effect is obtained (maximum daily dose = 200 mg).

Chronic Renal Failure

PO (Adults): 20 mg once daily; dose may be doubled until desired effect is obtained (maximum daily dose = 200 mg).

Hepatic Cirrhosis

PO (Adults): 5–10 mg once daily (with aldosterone antagonist or potassium-sparing diuretic); dose may be doubled until desired effect is obtained (maximum daily dose = 40 mg).

Hypertension

PO (Adults): 2.5–5 mg once daily, may be ↑ to 10 mg once daily after 4–6 wk (if still not effective, add another agent).

Availability (generic available)

Tablets: 5 mg, 10 mg, 20 mg, 100 mg. **Cost:** *Generic*—5 mg $63.42/100, 10 mg $70.27/100, 20 mg $82.08/100, 100 mg $304.00/100.

NURSING IMPLICATIONS

Assessment

- Assess fluid status during therapy. Monitor daily weight, intake and output ratios, amount and location of edema, lung sounds, skin turgor, and mucous membranes. Notify health care provider if thirst, dry mouth, lethargy, weakness, hypotension, or oliguria occurs.
- Monitor BP and pulse before and during administration. Monitor frequency of prescription refills to determine adherence in patients treated for hypertension.
- Assess patients receiving digoxin for anorexia, nausea, vomiting, muscle cramps, paresthesia, and confusion. Patients taking digoxin are at increased risk of digoxin toxicity due to potassium-depleting effect of the diuretic. Potassium supplements or potassium-sparing diuretics may be used concurrently to prevent hypokalemia.
- Assess patient for tinnitus and hearing loss. Audiometry is recommended for patients receiving prolonged high-dose IV therapy. Hearing loss is most common following rapid or high-dose IV administration in patients with decreased renal function or those taking other ototoxic drugs.
- Assess for allergy to sulfonamides.
- Assess patient for skin rash frequently during therapy. Discontinue torsemide at first sign of rash; may be life-threatening. Stevens-Johnson syndrome or toxic epidermal necrolysis may develop. Treat symptomatically; may recur once treatment is stopped.
- Geri: Diuretic use is associated with increased risk for falls in older adults. Assess falls risk and implement fall prevention strategies.
- ***Lab Test Considerations:*** Monitor electrolytes, renal and hepatic function, serum glucose, and uric acid levels before and periodically during therapy. May cause ↓ serum sodium, potassium, calcium, and magnesium concentrations. May also cause ↑ BUN, serum glucose, creatinine, and uric acid levels.

Potential Nursing Diagnoses

Excess fluid volume (Indications)
Risk for deficient fluid volume (Side Effects)

Implementation

- Administer medication in the morning to prevent disruption of sleep cycle.
- **PO:** May be taken with food or milk to minimize gastric irritation.

Patient/Family Teaching

- Instruct patient to take torsemide as directed. Take missed doses as soon as possible; do not double doses.
- Caution patient to change positions slowly to minimize orthostatic hypotension. Caution patient that the use of alcohol, exercise during hot weather, or standing for long periods during therapy may enhance orthostatic hypotension.
- Instruct patient to consult health care professional regarding a diet high in potassium (see Appendix J).
- Advise patient to contact health care professional if they gain more than 2–3 lb/day.
- Instruct patient to notify health care professional of all Rx or OTC medications, vitamins, or herbal products being taken and to consult health care professional before taking any OTC medications concurrently with this therapy.
- Instruct patient to notify health care professional of medication regimen prior to treatment or surgery.
- Caution patient to use sunscreen and protective clothing to prevent photosensitivity reactions.
- Advise patient to contact health care professional immediately if rash muscle weakness, cramps, nausea, dizziness, numbness, or tingling of extremities occurs.

T

- Advise diabetic patients to monitor blood glucose closely; may cause increased blood glucose levels.
- Emphasize the importance of routine follow-up examinations.
- **Hypertension:** Advise patients on antihypertensive regimen to continue taking medication even if feeling better. Torsemide controls but does not cure hypertension.
- Reinforce the need to continue additional therapies for hypertension (weight loss, exercise, restricted sodium intake, stress reduction, regular exercise, moderation of alcohol consumption, cessation of smoking).

Evaluation/Desired Outcomes

- Decrease in edema.
- Decrease in abdominal girth and weight.
- Increase in urinary output.
- Decrease in BP.

traMADol (tra-ma-dol)

ConZip, ✱Durela, ✱Ralivia, ✱Tridural, Ultram, Ultram ER, ✱Zytram XL

Classification

Therapeutic: analgesics (centrally acting)

Schedule IV

Pregnancy Category C

Indications

Moderate to moderately severe pain (extended-release formulations indicated for patients who require around-the-clock pain management).

Action

Binds to μ-opioid receptors. Inhibits reuptake of serotonin and norepinephrine in the CNS. **Therapeutic Effects:** Decreased pain.

Pharmacokinetics

Absorption: *Immediate-release*—75% absorbed after oral administration; *Extended-release (Ultram)*—85–90% (compared with immediate-release).

Distribution: Crosses the placenta; enters breast milk.

Metabolism and Excretion: Mostly metabolized by the liver; one metabolite has analgesic activity; 30% is excreted unchanged in urine.

Half-life: *Tramadol*—6–8 hr, *ER*—7.9 hr; *active metabolite*—7–9 hr; both are ↑ in renal or hepatic impairment.

TIME/ACTION PROFILE (analgesia)

ROUTE	ONSET	PEAK	DURATION
PO	1 hr	2–3 hr	4–6 hr
ER	unknown	12 hr	24 hr

Contraindications/Precautions

Contraindicated in: Hypersensitivity; Cross-sensitivity with opioids may occur; Patients who are acutely intoxicated with alcohol, sedatives/hypnotics, centrally acting analgesics, opioid analgesics, or psychotropic agents; Patients who are physically dependent on opioid analgesics (may precipitate withdrawal); OB, Lactation: Pregnancy or lactation; *ER only*—CCr <30 mL/min or hepatic impairment.

Use Cautiously in: Geri: *Immediate-release*—Not to exceed 300 mg/day in patients >75 yr; *ER*—Use with extreme caution in patients >75 yr; Patients with a history of epilepsy or risk factors for seizures; Renal impairment (↑ dosing interval recommended if CCr <30 mL/min); Hepatic impairment (↑ dosing interval recommended in patients with cirrhosis); Patients receiving MAO inhibitors, neuroleptics, SSRIs, or TCAs, or other CNS depressants; Patients who are suicidal or prone to addiction (↑ risk of suicide); Excessive use of alcohol (↑ risk of suicide); ↑ intracranial pressure or head trauma; Patients with a history of opioid dependence or who have recently received large doses of opioids; Pedi: Children <16 yr (safety not established).

Adverse Reactions/Side Effects

CNS: SEIZURES, dizziness, headache, somnolence, anxiety, CNS stimulation, confusion, coordination disturbance, euphoria, malaise, nervousness, sleep disorder, weakness. **EENT:** visual disturbances. **CV:** vasodilation. **GI:** constipation, nausea, abdominal pain, anorexia, diarrhea, dry mouth, dyspepsia, flatulence, vomiting. **GU:** menopausal symptoms, urinary retention/frequency. **Derm:** pruritus, sweating. **Neuro:** hypertonia. **Misc:** SEROTONIN SYNDROME, physical dependence, psychological dependence, tolerance.

Interactions

Drug-Drug: ↑ risk of CNS depression when used concurrently with other **CNS depressants**, including **alcohol**, **antihistamines**, **sedative/hypnotics**, **opioid analgesics**, **anesthetics**, or **psychotropic agents**. ↑ risk of seizures with high doses of **penicillins**, **cephalosporins**, **phenothiazines**, **opioid analgesics**, or **antidepressants**. **Carbamazepine** ↑ metabolism and ↓ effectiveness of tramadol (increased doses may be required). Use cautiously in patients who are receiving **MAO inhibitors** (↑ risk of adverse reactions). **Quinidine**, **fluoxetine**, **paroxetine**, **amitriptyline**, **ketoconazole**, and **erythromycin** may ↑ levels. ↑ risk of serotonin syndrome when used with **SSRI and SNRI antidepressants**, **TCAs**, **MAO inhibitors**, **$5HT_1$ agonists**, **CYP2D6 inhibitors**, and **CYP3A4 inhibitors**.

Drug-Natural Products: Concomitant use of **kava-kava, valerian**, or **chamomile** can ↑ CNS depression. ↑ risk of serotonin syndrome when used with **St. John's wort**.

Route/Dosage

Immediate-release

PO (Adults ≥18 yr): *Rapid titration*—50–100 mg q 4–6 hr (not to exceed 400 mg/day [300 mg in patients >75 yr]). *Gradual titration*—25 mg/day initially, ↑ by 25 mg/day q 3 days to reach dose of 25 mg 4 times daily, then ↑ by 50 mg/day q 3 days to reach dose of 50 mg 4 times daily; may then use 50–100 mg q 4–6 hr (maximum dose = 400 mg/day).

Renal Impairment

PO (Adults): *CCr <30 mL/min*—↑ dosing interval to q 12 hr (not to exceed 200 mg/day).

Hepatic Impairment

PO (Adults): 50 mg q 12 hr.

Extended-release

PO (Adults): *Ultram ER and Conzip (not currently receiving immediate-release)*—100 mg once daily initially, may then titrate q 5 days up to 300 mg/day; *Ultram ER and Conzip (currently receiving immediate-release)*—calculate 24-hr total dose of immediate-release product and give same dose (rounded down to next lowest 100-mg increment) of ER once daily (maximum dose = 300 mg/day).

Availability (generic available)

Tablets: 50 mg. **Cost:** *Generic*—$83.40/100. **Extended-release capsules (Conzip):** 100 mg, 200 mg, 300 mg. **Cost:** 100 mg $232.19/30, 200 mg $289.79/30, 300 mg $365.98/30. **Extended-release tablets (Ultram ER):** 100 mg, 200 mg, 300 mg. **Cost:** *Generic*—100 mg $126.95/30, 200 mg $209.95/30, 300 mg $292.93/30. ***In combination with:*** acetaminophen (Ultracet). See Appendix B.

NURSING IMPLICATIONS

Assessment

- Assess type, location, and intensity of pain before and 2–3 hr (peak) after administration.
- Assess BP and respiratory rate before and periodically during administration. Respiratory depression has not occurred with recommended doses.
- Assess bowel function routinely. Prevention of constipation should be instituted with increased intake of fluids and bulk and with laxatives to minimize constipating effects.
- Prolonged use may lead to physical and psychological dependence and tolerance, although these may be milder than with opioids. This should not prevent patient from receiving adequate analgesia. Most patients who receive tramadol for pain do not develop psychological dependence. If tolerance develops, changing to an opioid agonist may be required to relieve pain.
- Monitor patient for seizures. May occur within recommended dose range. Risk is increased with higher doses and in patients taking antidepressants (SSRIs, SNRIs, tricyclics, or MAO inhibitors), opioid analgesics, or other drugs that decrease the seizure threshold. Also monitor for serotonin syndrome (mental-status changes (e.g., agitation, hallucinations, coma), autonomic instability (e.g., tachycardia, labile BP, hyperthermia), neuromuscular aberrations (e.g., hyperreflexia, incoordination) and/or gastrointestinal symptoms (e.g., nausea, vomiting, diarrhea) in patients taking these drugs concurrently).
- ***Lab Test Considerations:*** May cause ↑ serum creatinine, ↑ liver enzymes, ↓ hemoglobin, and proteinuria.
- ***Toxicity and Overdose:*** Overdose may cause respiratory depression and seizures. Naloxone may reverse some, but not all, of the symptoms of overdose. Treatment should be symptomatic and supportive. Maintain adequate respiratory exchange. Hemodialysis is not helpful because it removes only a small portion of administered dose. Seizures may be managed with barbiturates or benzodiazepines; naloxone increases risk of seizures.

Potential Nursing Diagnoses

Acute pain (Indications)
Risk for injury (Side Effects)

Implementation

- ***High Alert:*** Do not confuse tramadol with trazodone. Do not confuse Ultram with lithium.
- Tramadol is considered to provide more analgesia than codeine 60 mg but less than combined aspirin 650 mg/codeine 60 mg for acute postoperative pain.
- For chronic pain, daily doses of 250 mg of tramadol provide pain relief similar to that of 5 doses/day of acetaminophen 300 mg/codeine 30 mg, 5 doses/day of aspirin 325 mg/codeine 30 mg, or 2–3 doses/day of acetaminophen 500 mg/oxycodone 5 mg.
- Explain therapeutic value of medication before administration to enhance the analgesic effect.
- Regularly administered doses may be more effective than prn administration. Analgesic is more effective if given before pain becomes severe.
- Tramadol should be discontinued gradually after long-term use to prevent withdrawal symptoms.
- **PO:** Tramadol may be administered without regard to meals. Swallow extended-release tablets and capsules whole; do not crush, break, dissolve, or chew.

T

Patient/Family Teaching

- Instruct patient on how and when to ask for pain medication.
- May cause dizziness and drowsiness. Caution patient to avoid driving or other activities requiring alertness until response to medication is known.
- Advise patient to change positions slowly to minimize orthostatic hypotension.
- Caution patient to avoid concurrent use of alcohol or other CNS depressants with this medication. Advise patient to notify health care professional before taking other RX, OTC, or herbal products concurrently.
- Advise patient to notify health care professional if seizures or if symptoms of serotonin syndrome occur.
- Encourage patient to turn, cough, and breathe deeply every 2 hr to prevent atelectasis.
- Advise female patients to notify health care professional if pregnancy is planned or suspected, or if breast feeding.

Evaluation/Desired Outcomes

- Decrease in severity of pain without a significant alteration in level of consciousness or respiratory status.

trandolapril, See ANGIOTENSIN-CONVERTING ENZYME (ACE) INHIBITORS.

tranylcypromine, See MONOAMINE OXIDASE (MAO) INHIBITORS.

HIGH ALERT

trastuzumab

(traz-**too**-zoo-mab)

Herceptin

Classification

Therapeutic: antineoplastics

Pharmacologic: monoclonal antibodies

Pregnancy Category D

Indications

First-line treatment of metastatic breast cancer (with paclitaxel) that displays overexpression of the human epidermal growth factor receptor 2 (HER2) protein. Treatment of HER2–overexpressing metastatic breast cancer (as monotherapy) in patients who have already received other chemotherapy regimens. Adjuvant treatment of HER2–overexpressing node positive or node negative breast cancer (to be used alone after multimodality anthracycline-based therapy or as part of one of the following regimens: doxorubicin, cyclophosphamide, and either paclitaxel or docetaxel; with docetaxel and carboplatin). Treatment of HER2–overexpressing metastatic gastric or gastroesophageal adenocarcinoma (with cisplatin and capecitabine or 5–fluorouracil) in patients who have not received prior treatment for metastatic disease.

Action

A monoclonal antibody that binds to HER2 sites in breast cancer tissue and inhibits proliferation of cells that overexpress HER2 protein. **Therapeutic Effects:** Regression of breast, gastric, or gastroesophageal cancer and metastases.

Pharmacokinetics

Absorption: IV administration results in complete bioavailability.

Distribution: Binds to HER2 proteins.

Metabolism and Excretion: Unknown.

Half-life: 10-mg dose—1.7 days; 500-mg dose—12 days.

TIME/ACTION PROFILE (blood levels)

ROUTE	ONSET	PEAK	DURATION
IV	unknown	unknown	unknown

Contraindications/Precautions

Contraindicated in: OB: Avoid use during pregnancy; Lactation: Discontinue drug or discontinue breast feeding.

Use Cautiously in: Pre-existing pulmonary conditions; Hypersensitivity to trastuzumab, Chinese hamster ovary cell proteins, or other components of the product; Hypersensitivity to benzyl alcohol (use sterile water for injection instead of bacteriostatic water, which accompanies the vial); Geri: May have ↑ risk of cardiac dysfunction; Rep: Women with reproductive potential; Pedi: Safety not established.

Exercise Extreme Caution in: Patients with pre-existing cardiac dysfunction.

Adverse Reactions/Side Effects

CNS: dizziness, headache, insomnia, weakness, depression. **Resp:** INTERSTITIAL PNEUMONITIS, PULMONARY EDEMA, PULMONARY FIBROSIS, dyspnea, increased cough, pharyngitis, rhinitis, sinusitis. **CV:** ARRHYTHMIAS, HF, hypertension, tachycardia. **GI:** abdominal pain, anorexia, diarrhea, nausea, vomiting. **Derm:** rash, acne, herpes simplex. **F and E:** edema. **Hemat:** anemia, leukopenia. **MS:** back pain, arthralgia, bone pain. **Neuro:** neuropathy, paresthesia, peripheral neuritis. **Misc:** HYPERSENSITIVITY REACTIONS, chills, fever, infection, pain, allergic reactions, flu-like syndrome.

Interactions

Drug-Drug: Concurrent **anthracycline (daunorubicin, doxorubicin**, or **idarubicin)** therapy may ↑ risk of cardiotoxicity. Blood levels are ↑ by concurrent **paclitaxel**.

Route/Dosage

Adjuvant Treatment of Breast Cancer

IV (Adults): *During and following paclitaxel, docetaxel, or docetaxel/carboplatin*—4 mg/kg initially, then 2 mg/kg weekly during chemotherapy for the first 12 wk (paclitaxel or docetaxel) or 18 wk (docetaxel/carboplatin); one wk after the last weekly dose, give 6 mg/kg q 3 wk. Do not exceed treatment duration of 1 yr; *As single agent within 3 wk following completion of multi-modality, anthracycline-based chemotherapy regimens*—8 mg/kg initially, then 6 mg/kg q 3 wk. Do not exceed treatment duration of 1 yr.

Metastatic Breast Cancer

IV (Adults): 4 mg/kg initially, then 2 mg/kg weekly until disease progresses.

Metastatic Gastric Cancer

IV (Adults): 8 mg/kg initially, then 6 mg/kg q 3 wk until disease progresses.

Availability

Lyophilized powder for injection: 440 mg/vial with 20 mL bacteriostatic water for injection (contains benzyl alcohol).

NURSING IMPLICATIONS

Assessment

- Assess for infusion-related symptoms (chills, fever, nausea, vomiting, pain [in some cases at tumor sites], headache, dizziness, dyspnea, hypotension, rash, and asthenia) following initial infusion. Severe reactions (bronchospasm, anaphylaxis, angioedema, hypoxia, severe hypotension) may occur during or immediately following the initial infusion. May be treated with epinephrine, corticosteroids, diphenhydramine, bronchodilators, and oxygen. Discontinue if dyspnea or severe hypotension occurs and discontinue permanently if severe reaction occurs.
- Assess for signs and symptoms of HF (dyspnea, increased cough, paroxysmal nocturnal dyspnea, peripheral edema, S_3 gallop, reduced ejection fraction) prior to and frequently during therapy. Baseline cardiac assessment of history, physical exam, and left ventricular ejection fraction (LVEF) with ECG or multiple gated acquisition (MUGA) scan. Monitor LVEF every 3 mo and at completion of therapy, every 6 mo for 2 yr. Withhold trastuzumab for ≥16% absolute decrease in LVEF from pre-treatment values or an LVEF value below institutional limits of normal and ≥10% absolute decrease in LVEF from pretreatment values. Repeat LVEF measures every 4 wk if dose is withheld. HF associated with trastuzumab may be severe, resulting in cardiac failure, death, and stroke. Trastuzumab should be discontinued upon the development of significant HF.
- Monitor patient for signs of pulmonary hypersensitivity reactions (dyspnea, pulmonary infiltrates, pleural effusion, noncardiogenic pulmonary edema, pulmonary insufficiency, hypoxia, acute respiratory distress syndrome). Patients with symptomatic pulmonary disease or extensive lung tumor involvement are at increased risk. Infusion should be discontinued if severe symptoms occur.
- ***Lab Test Considerations:*** HER2 protein overexpression is used to determine whether treatment with trastuzumab is indicated. HER2 protein overexpression is detected by HercepTest (IHC assay) and PathVysion (FISH assay).
- May cause anemia and leukopenia.

Potential Nursing Diagnoses

Diarrhea (Adverse Reactions)
Risk for infection (Adverse Reactions)

Implementation

- ***High Alert:*** Do not confuse trastuzumab (Herceptin) with ado-trastuzumab (Kadcyla).
- ***High Alert:*** Fatalities have occurred with chemotherapeutic agents. Before administering, clarify all ambiguous orders; double check single, daily, and course-of-therapy dose limits; have second practitioner independently double check original order, dose calculations and infusion pump settings.
- May be administered in the outpatient setting.
- *If a dose is missed by ≤1 wk,* administer usual maintenance dose as soon as possible. Do not wait until next planned cycle. Administer subsequent maintenance doses 7 days or 21 days later according to the weekly or three-weekly schedules, respectively. *If a dose is missed by >1 wk,* administer a re-loading dose as soon as possible. Administer subsequent maintenance doses 7 days or 21 days later according to weekly or three-weekly schedules, respectively.

IV Administration

- **Intermittent Infusion:** Reconstitute each vial with 20 mL of bacteriostatic water for injection, directing the stream of diluent into lyophilized cake of trastuzumab. ***Concentration:*** 21 mg/mL. Swirl the vial gently; do not shake. May foam slightly; allow the vial to stand undisturbed for 5 min. Solution should be clear to slightly opalescent and colorless to pale yellow, without particulate matter. Label vial immediately in the area marked "Do not use after" with the date 28 days from the date of reconstitution. Stable for 24 hr at room temperature or 28 days if refrigerated. If patient is allergic to benzyl alcohol, use sterile water for injection for reconstitution. Use immediately and discard any unused portion ***Diluent:***

T

Calculate to volume required for the desired dose, withdraw, and add it to an infusion containing 250 mL of 0.9% NaCl. Invert bag gently to mix. ***Rate:*** Infuse the 4 mg/kg loading dose over 90 min and the weekly 2 mg/kg dose over 30 min or 6 mg/kg over 90 min every 3 wk if the loading dose was well tolerated. Do not administer as an IV push or bolus.

- **Y-Site Compatibility:** acyclovir, amifostine, aminophylline, ampicillin, ampicillin/sulbactam, bleomycin, bumetanide, buprenorphine, busulfan, butorphanol, calcium gluconate, carboplatin, carmustine, cefazolin, ceftazidime, ceftriaxone, cefuroxime, ciprofloxacin, cisplatin, cyclophosphamide, cytarabine, dactinomycin, daunorubicin hydrochloride, dexamethasone, digoxin, diphenhydramine, dobutamine, docetaxel, dopamine, doxorubicin hydrochloride, doxorubicin liposomal, doxycycline, droperidol, enalaprilat, etoposide phosphate, famotidine, fentanyl, filgrastim, fluconazole, fluorouracil, ganciclovir, gemcitabine, gentamicin, granisetron, haloperidol, heparin, hydrocortisone, hydromorphone, ifosfamide, imipenem/cilastatin, leucovorin, lorazepam, magnesium sulfate, mannitol, meperidine, mesna, methotrexate, methylprednisolone, metoclopramide, metronidazole, mitomycin, mitoxantrone, paclitaxel, pentamidine, potassium chloride, prochlorperazine, promethazine, ranitidine, remifentanil, sargramostim, sodium bicarbonate, teniposide, theophylline, thiotepa, tobramycin, trimethoprim/sulfamethoxazole, vancomycin, vinblastine, vincristine, vinorelbine, zidovudine.
- **Y-Site Incompatibility:** aldesleukin, amikacin, amphotericin B colloidal, aztreonam, cefotaxime, cefotetan, cefoxitin, chlorpromazine, clindamycin, cyclosporine, fludarabine, furosemide, idarubicin, irinotecan, levofloxacin, levorphanol, morphine, nalbuphine, ondansetron, piperacillin/tazobactam, streptozocin, topotecan.
- **Additive Incompatibility:** Do not dilute trastuzumab with or add to solutions containing dextrose. Do not mix or dilute with other drugs.

Patient/Family Teaching

- Instruct patient to notify health care professional promptly if new onset or worsening shortness of breath, cough, swelling of the ankles/legs, swelling of the face, palpitations, weight gain of more than 5 pounds in 24 hours, dizziness or loss of consciousness occur. Caution patient to avoid crowds and persons with known infections.
- Rep: Advise female patient that trastuzumab is teratogenic and to notify health care professional immediately if pregnancy is planned or suspected or if breast feeding. Caution patient to use effective contraception during and for 7 mo following last dose. Women who are breast feeding should be advised to discontinue nursing or discontinue trastuzumab. Encourage women who may be exposed during pregnancy to enroll in the MotHER Pregnancy Registry by contacting 1-800-690-6720 and report exposure to the Genentech Adverse Event Line at 1-888-835-2555. Monitor patients who become pregnant for oligohydramnios.
- Advise patient not to receive any vaccinations without advice of health care professional.

Evaluation/Desired Outcomes

- Regression of breast, gastric, or gastroesophageal cancer and metastases.

traZODone (traz-oh-done)

~~Desyrel~~, ✤Oleptro, ✤Trazorel

Classification

Therapeutic: antidepressants

Pregnancy Category C

Indications

Major depression. **Unlabeled Use:** Insomnia, chronic pain syndromes, including diabetic neuropathy, and anxiety.

Action

Alters the effects of serotonin in the CNS. **Therapeutic Effects:** Antidepressant action, which may develop only over several weeks.

Pharmacokinetics

Absorption: Well absorbed after oral administration.
Distribution: Widely distributed.
Protein Binding: 89–95%.
Metabolism and Excretion: Extensively metabolized by the liver (CYP3A4 enzyme system); minimal excretion of unchanged drug by the kidneys.
Half-life: 5–9 hr (immediate-release).

TIME/ACTION PROFILE (antidepressant effect)

ROUTE	ONSET	PEAK	DURATION
PO	1–2 wk	2–4 wk	wks

Contraindications/Precautions

Contraindicated in: Hypersensitivity; Recovery period after MI; Concurrent electroconvulsive therapy; Concurrent use of MAO inhibitors or MAO-like drugs (linezolid or methylene blue); Angle-closure glaucoma.
Use Cautiously in: Cardiovascular disease; Suicidal behavior; May ↑ risk of suicide attempt/ideation especially during early treatment or dose adjustment; Severe hepatic or renal disease (dose ↓ recommended); Lactation: Discontinue drug or bottle feed; Pedi: Suicide risk may be greater in children and adolescents; safety not established; Geri: Initial dose ↓ recommended.

Adverse Reactions/Side Effects

CNS: SUICIDAL THOUGHTS, drowsiness, confusion, dizziness, fatigue, hallucinations, headache, insomnia, nightmares, slurred speech, syncope, weakness. **EENT:** blurred vision, tinnitus. **CV:** hypotension, arrhythmias, chest pain, hypertension, palpitations, QT interval prolongation, tachycardia. **GI:** dry mouth, altered taste, constipation, diarrhea, excess salivation, flatulence, nausea, vomiting. **GU:** hematuria, erectile dysfunction, priapism, urinary frequency. **Derm:** rash. **Hemat:** anemia, leukopenia. **MS:** myalgia. **Neuro:** tremor.

Interactions

Drug-Drug: Serious, potentially fatal reactions (hyperthermia, rigidity, myoclonus, autonomic instability, with fluctuating vital signs and extreme agitation, which may proceed to delirium and coma) may occur with concurrent **MAO inhibitors**. MAO inhibitors should be stopped at least 14 days before trazodone therapy. Trazodone should be stopped at least 14 days before MAO inhibitor therapy. Concurrent use with **MAO-inhibitor like drugs**, such as **linezolid** or **methylene blue** may ↑ risk of serotonin syndrome; concurrent use contraindicated; do not start therapy in patients receiving **linezolid** or **methylene blue**; if **linezolid** or **methylene blue** need to be started in a patient receiving trazodone, immediately discontinue trazodone and monitor for signs/symptoms of serotonin syndrome for 2 wk or until 24 hr after last dose of linezolid or methylene blue, whichever comes first (may resume trazodone therapy 24 hr after last dose of linezolid or methylene blue). May ↑ **digoxin** or **phenytoin** serum levels. ↑ CNS depression with other **CNS depressants**, including **alcohol**, **opioid analgesics**, and **sedative/hypnotics**. ↑ hypotension with **antihypertensives**, acute ingestion of **alcohol**, or **nitrates**. Concurrent use with **fluoxetine** ↑ levels and risk of toxicity from trazodone. **Drugs that inhibit the CYP3A4 enzyme system**, including **ritonavir indinavir** and **ketoconazole**↑ levels and the risk of toxicity. **Drugs that induce the CYP3A4 enzyme system**, including **carbamazepine** ↓ levels and may decrease effectiveness. Drugs that affect serotonergic neurotransmitter systems, including **tricyclic antidepressants**, **fentanyl**, **buspirone**, **tramadol** and **triptans** ↑ risk of serotonin syndrome. ↑ risk of bleeding with **NSAIDS**, **aspirin**, **clopidogrel**, or **warfarin**.
Drug-Natural Products: Concomitant use of **kava-kava**, **valerian**, or **chamomile** can ↑ CNS depression. ↑ risk of serotinergic side effects including serotonin syndrome with **St. John's wort** and **SAMe**.

Route/Dosage

Depression

PO (Adults): 150 mg/day in 3 divided doses; ↑ by 50 mg/day q 3–4 days until desired response (not to exceed 400 mg/day in outpatients or 600 mg/day in hospitalized patients).
PO (Geriatric Patients): 75 mg/day in divided doses initially; may be ↑ q 3–4 days.

Insomnia

PO (Adults): 25–100 mg at bedtime.

Availability (generic available)

Tablets (immediate-release): 50 mg, 100 mg, 150 mg, 300 mg. **Cost:** *Generic*—All strengths $10.83/100. **Tablets (extended-release) (Oleptro):** ✱150 mg, ✱300 mg.

NURSING IMPLICATIONS

Assessment

- Monitor BP and pulse rate before and during initial therapy. Monitor ECGs in patients with pre-existing cardiac disease before and periodically during therapy to detect arrhythmias.
- Assess for possible sexual dysfunction.
- Assess for serotonin syndrome (mental changes [agitation, hallucinations, coma], autonomic instability [tachycardia, labile BP, hyperthermia], neuromuscular aberrations [hyper-reflexia, incoordination], and/or GI symptoms [nausea, vomiting, diarrhea]), especially in patients taking other serotonergic drugs (SSRIs, SNRIs, triptans).
- **Depression:** Assess mental status (orientation, mood, and behavior) frequently.
- Assess for suicidal tendencies, especially during early therapy. Restrict amount of drug available to patient. Risk may be increased in children, adolescents, and adults ≤24 yr. After starting therapy, children, adolescents, and young adults should be seen by health care professional at least weekly for 4 wk, every 3 wk for next 4 wk, and on advice of health care professional thereafter.
- **Pain:** Assess location, duration, intensity, and characteristics of pain before and periodically during therapy. Use pain scale to assess effectiveness of medicine.
- ***Lab Test Considerations:*** Assess CBC and renal and hepatic function before and periodically during therapy. Slight, clinically insignificant ↓ in leukocyte and neutrophil counts may occur.

Potential Nursing Diagnoses

Ineffective coping (Indications)
Sexual dysfunction (Side Effects)

Implementation

- Do not confuse trazodone with tramadol.
- **PO:** Administer with or immediately after meals to minimize side effects (nausea, dizziness) and allow maximum absorption of trazodone. A larger portion of the total daily dose may be given at bedtime to decrease daytime drowsiness and dizziness.

Patient/Family Teaching

- Instruct patient to take medication as directed. If a dose is missed, take as soon as remembered. Do not

T

take if within 4 hr of next scheduled dose; do not double doses. Consult health care professional before discontinuing medication; gradual dose reduction is necessary to prevent aggravation of condition. Advise patient to read *Medication Guide* prior starting therapy and with each Rx refill in case of changes.

- May cause drowsiness and blurred vision. Caution patient to avoid driving and other activities requiring alertness until response to drug is known.
- Caution patient to change positions slowly to minimize orthostatic hypotension.
- Advise patient to avoid concurrent use of alcohol or other CNS depressant drugs.
- Advise patient, family, and caregivers to look for suicidality, especially during early therapy or dose changes. Notify health care professional immediately if thoughts about suicide or dying, attempts to commit suicide, new or worse depression or anxiety, agitation or restlessness, panic attacks, insomnia, new or worse irritability, aggressiveness, acting on dangerous impulses, mania, or other changes in mood or behavior or if symptoms of serotonin syndrome occur.
- Advise patient to notify health care professional of all Rx or OTC medications, vitamins, or herbal products being taken and to consult with health care professional before taking other medications, especially aspirin and NSAIDs.
- Inform patient that frequent rinses, good oral hygiene, and sugarless candy or gum may diminish dry mouth. Health care professional should be notified if this persists >2 wk. An increase in fluid intake, fiber, and exercise may prevent constipation.
- Advise patient to notify health care professional of medication regimen before treatment or surgery.
- Instruct patient to notify health care professional if priapism, irregular heartbeat, fainting, confusion, skin rash, or tremors occur or if dry mouth, nausea and vomiting, dizziness, headache, muscle aches, constipation, or diarrhea becomes pronounced.
- Instruct patient to notify health care professional if signs of serotonin syndrome (mental status changes: agitation, hallucinations, coma; autonomic instability: tachycardia, labile BP, hyperthermia; neuromuscular aberrations: hyperreflexia, incoordination; and/or gastrointestinal symptoms: nausea, vomiting, diarrhea) occur.
- Advise female patients to notify health care professional if pregnancy is planned or suspected or if breast feeding.
- Emphasize the importance of follow-up exams to evaluate progress.

Evaluation/Desired Outcomes

- Resolution of depression.
- Increased sense of well-being.
- Renewed interest in surroundings.
- Increased appetite.
- Improved energy level.
- Improved sleep.
- Decrease in severity of pain in chronic pain syndromes. Therapeutic effects are usually seen within 1 wk, although 4 wk may be required to obtain significant therapeutic results.

triamcinolone, See CORTICOSTEROIDS (NASAL), CORTICOSTEROIDS (SYSTEMIC), and CORTICOSTEROIDS (TOPICAL/LOCAL).

triamterene, See DIURETICS (POTASSIUM-SPARING).

triazolam (trye-az-oh-lam)

Halcion

Classification

Therapeutic: sedative/hypnotics

Pharmacologic: benzodiazepines

Schedule IV

Pregnancy Category X

Indications

Short-term management of insomnia.

Action

Acts at many levels in the CNS, producing generalized depression. Effects may be mediated by GABA, an inhibitory neurotransmitter. **Therapeutic Effects:** Relief of insomnia.

Pharmacokinetics

Absorption: Well absorbed following oral administration.

Distribution: Widely distributed, crosses blood-brain barrier. Probably crosses the placenta and enters breast milk.

Protein Binding: 89%.

Metabolism and Excretion: Metabolized by the liver.

Half-life: 1.6–5.4 hr.

TIME/ACTION PROFILE (sedation)

ROUTE	ONSET	PEAK	DURATION
PO	15–30 min	6–8 hr	unknown

Contraindications/Precautions

Contraindicated in: Hypersensitivity; Cross-sensitivity with other benzodiazepines may occur; Pre-existing CNS depression; Uncontrolled severe pain; Concomitant use of potent CYP3A4 inhibitors; OB, Lactation: Pedi: Safety not established.

Use Cautiously in: Pre-existing hepatic dysfunction (dose ↓ recommended); History of suicide attempt or drug addiction; Geri: Appears on Beers list and is associated with ↑ risk of falls (↓ dose required); ↑sensitivity to benzodiazepines.

Adverse Reactions/Side Effects

CNS: abnormal thinking, behavior changes, dizziness, excessive sedation, hangover, headache, anterograde amnesia, confusion, hallucinations, sleep-driving, lethargy, mental depression, paradoxical excitation. **EENT:** blurred vision. **GI:** constipation, diarrhea, nausea, vomiting. **Derm:** rashes. **Misc:** physical dependence, psychological dependence, tolerance.

Interactions

Drug-Drug: Concomitant use of potent CYP3A4 inhibitors, including, **itraconazole**, **ketoconazole**, **nefazodone**, **indinavir**, **nelfinavir**, **ritonavir**, **saquinavir**, and **lopinavir** may ↓ metabolism and ↑ levels; concurrent use contraindicated. **Erythromycin**, **clarithromycin**, and **cimetidine** may ↑ levels; consider ↓ triazolam dose. Additive CNS depression with **alcohol**, **antidepressants**, **antihistamines**, and **opioid analgesics**. May ↓ effectiveness of **levodopa**. May ↑ toxicity of **zidovudine**. **Isoniazid** may ↓ excretion and ↑ effects of triazolam. Sedative effects may be ↓ by **theophylline**.
Drug-Natural Products: Concomitant use of **kava-kava**, **valerian**, **chamomile**, or **hops** can ↑ CNS depression.
Drug-Food: **Grapefruit juice** significantly ↑ blood levels and effects.

Route/Dosage

PO (Adults): 0.125–0.25 mg (up to 0.5 mg) at bedtime.
PO (Geriatric Patients or Debilitated Patients): 0.125 mg at bedtime initially; may be ↑ as needed.

Availability (generic available)

Tablets: 0.125 mg, 0.25 mg.

NURSING IMPLICATIONS

Assessment

- Assess sleep patterns prior to and periodically throughout therapy.
- Assess CNS effects and risk of falls. Institute falls prevention strategies.
- Prolonged high-dose therapy may lead to psychological or physical dependence. Restrict the amount of drug available to patient, especially if patient is depressed, suicidal, or has a history of substance use disorder.

Potential Nursing Diagnoses

Insomnia (Indications)
Risk for injury (Side Effects)

Implementation

- Supervise ambulation and transfer of patients following administration. Remove cigarettes. Side rails should be raised and call bell within reach at all times.
- **PO:** Administer right before going to bed. Do not take with or right after a meal.

Patient/Family Teaching

- Instruct patient to take triazolam as directed. Discuss the importance of preparing environment for sleep (dark room, quiet, avoidance of nicotine and caffeine). If less effective after a few weeks, consult health care professional; do not increase dose.
- Advise patient to avoid grapefruit and grapefruit juice during therapy.
- May cause daytime drowsiness or dizziness. Caution patient to avoid driving or other activities requiring alertness until response to medication is known. Instruct patient and family how to reduce falls risk at home.
- Inform patient that after taking triazolam patient may get out of bed and perform activities (driving a car ("sleep-driving"), making and eating food, talking on the phone, having sex, sleep-walking) while unaware. You may not remember anything done during the night; increased risk with alcohol or other CNS depressants.
- Advise patient to avoid the use of alcohol and other CNS depressants and to consult health care professional prior to using OTC preparations that contain antihistamines or alcohol.
- Instruct patient to notify health care professional if an increase in daytime anxiety occurs. May occur after as few as 10 days of therapy. May require discontinuation of triazolam.
- Advise patient to inform health care professional if confusion, depression, or persistent headaches occur. Instruct family or caregiver to notify health care professional if personality changes occur.
- Advise female patient to notify health care professional if pregnancy is planned or suspected or if breast feeding.
- Emphasize the importance of follow-up appointments to monitor progress.

Evaluation/Desired Outcomes

- Improvement in sleep patterns, which may not be noticeable until the 3rd day of therapy.

T

tricalcium phosphate, See CALCIUM SALTS.

trimethoprim/ sulfamethoxazole

(trye-**meth**-oh-prim/sul-fa-meth-**ox**-a-zole)

Bactrim, Bactrim DS, ✱Protrin DF, Septra, Septra DS, Sulfatrim, TMP/SMX, TMP/SMZ, ✱Trisulfa DS, ✱Trisulfa S

Classification

Therapeutic: anti-infectives, antiprotozoals

Pharmacologic: folate antagonists, sulfonamides

Pregnancy Category C

Indications

Treatment of: Bronchitis, *Shigella* enteritis, Otitis media, *Pneumocystis jirovecii* pneumonia (PCP), Urinary tract infections, Traveler's diarrhea. Prevention of PCP in HIV-positive patients. **Unlabeled Use:** Biliary tract infections, osteomyelitis, burn and wound infections, chlamydial infections, endocarditis, gonorrhea, intra-abdominal infections, nocardiosis, rheumatic fever prophylaxis, sinusitis, eradication of meningococcal carriers, prophylaxis of urinary tract infections, and an alternative agent in the treatment of chancroid. Prevention of bacterial infections in immunosuppressed patients.

Action

Combination inhibits the metabolism of folic acid in bacteria at two different points. **Therapeutic Effects:** Bactericidal action against susceptible bacteria. **Spectrum:** Active against many strains of gram-positive aerobic pathogens including: *Streptococcus pneumoniae*, *Staphylococcus aureus*, Group A beta-hemolytic streptococci, *Nocardia*, *Enterococcus*. Has activity against many aerobic gram-negative pathogens, such as: *Acinetobacter*, *Enterobacter*, *Klebsiella pneumoniae*, *Escherichia coli*, *Proteus mirabilis*, *Shigella*, *Xanthomonas maltophilia*, *Haemophilus influenzae*, including ampicillin-resistant strains. *P. jirovecii*. Not active against *Pseudomonas aeruginosa*.

Pharmacokinetics

Absorption: Well absorbed from the GI tract.

Distribution: Widely distributed. Crosses the blood-brain barrier and placenta and enters breast milk.

Protein Binding: TMP: 45%; SMX: 68%.

Metabolism and Excretion: Some metabolism by the liver (20%); remainder excreted unchanged by the kidneys.

Half-life: *Trimethoprim*—6–11 hr; *sulfamethoxazole*—9–12 hr, both prolonged in renal failure.

TIME/ACTION PROFILE (blood levels)

ROUTE	ONSET	PEAK	DURATION
PO	rapid	2–4 hr	6–12 hr
IV	rapid	end of infusion	6–12 hr

Contraindications/Precautions

Contraindicated in: Hypersensitivity to sulfonamides or trimethoprim; History of drug-induced immune thrombocytopenia due to sulfonamides or trimethoprim; Megaloblastic anemia secondary to folate deficiency; Severe hepatic or renal impairment; OB, Lactation, Pedi: Pregnancy, lactation, or children <2 mo (can cause kernicterus in neonates). Exception: neonates born to HIV-infected mothers (prophylaxis should be initiated at 4–6 weeks of age).

Use Cautiously in: Mild to moderate hepatic or renal impairment (dose ↓ required if CCr <30 mL/min); Glucose–6–phosphate dehydrogenase deficiency (↑ risk hemolysis); HIV-positive patients (↑ incidence of adverse reactions).

Adverse Reactions/Side Effects

CV: hypotension. **CNS:** fatigue, hallucinations, headache, insomnia, mental depression, kernicterus in neonates. **F and E:** hyperkalemia, hyponatremia. **GI:** CLOSTRIDIUM DIFFICILE-ASSOCIATED DIARRHEA (CDAD), HEPATIC NECROSIS, nausea, vomiting, diarrhea, stomatitis, hepatitis, cholestatic jaundice, pancreatitis. **GU:** crystalluria. **Derm:** ERYTHEMA MULTIFORME, STEVENS-JOHNSON SYNDROME, TOXIC EPIDERMAL NECROLYSIS, rash, photosensitivity. **Endo:** hypoglycemia. **Hemat:** AGRANULOCYTOSIS, APLASTIC ANEMIA, hemolytic anemia, leukopenia, megaloblastic anemia, thrombocytopenia. **Local:** phlebitis at IV site. **Misc:** fever.

Interactions

Drug-Drug: May ↑ half-life, ↓ clearance, and exaggerate folic acid deficiency caused by **phenytoin**. May ↑ effects of **sulfonylureas**, **pioglitazone**, **rosiglitazone**, **repaglinide**, **phenytoin**, **digoxin**, and **warfarin**. May ↑ toxicity of **methotrexate**. ↑ risk of thrombocytopenia from **thiazide diuretics** (↑ in geriatric patients). ↓ levels of and ↑ risk of nephrotoxicity with **cyclosporine**. Concurrent use with **ACE inhibitors** may ↑ risk of hyperkalemia. May ↓ the effects of **tricyclic antidepressants**. Concurrent use with **leucovorin** may result in treatment failure and ↑ risk of death (avoid concurrent use).

Route/Dosage

(TMP = trimethoprim; SMX = sulfamethoxazole). Dosing based on TMP content.

Bacterial Infections

PO, IV (Adults and Children >2 mo): *Mild-moderate infections*—6–12 mg TMP/kg/day divided q 12 hr; *Serious infection/Pneumocystis*—15–20 mg TMP/kg /day/divided q 6–8 hr.

PO (Adults): *Urinary tract infection/chronic bronchitis*—1 double strength tablet (160 mg TMP/800 mg SMX) q 12 hr for 10–14 days.

Urinary Tract Infection Prophylaxis

PO, IV (Adults and Children >2 mo): 2 mg TMP/kg/dose daily or 5 mg TMP/kg/dose twice weekly.

P. jirovecii Pneumonia (Prevention)

PO (Adults): 1 double strength tablet (160 mg TMP/800 mg SMX) daily (may also be given 3 times weekly). **PO (Children >1 mo):** 150 mg TMP/m²/day divided q 12 hr or given as a single dose on 3 consecutive days/wk (not to exceed 320 mg TMP/1600 mg SMX per day).

Availability (generic available)

Tablets: ✤ 20 mg TMP/100 mg SMX, 80 mg TMP/400 mg SMX, double strength– 160 mg TMP/800 mg SMX. **Cost:** *Generic*—80 mg TMP/400 mg SMX $6.99/30, 160 mg TMP/800 mg SMX $6.70/30. **Oral suspension (cherry, grape flavors):** 40 mg TMP/200 mg SMX per 5 mL. **Cost:** *Generic*—$58.10/473 mL. **Injection:** 16 mg TMP/80 mg SMX per mL.

NURSING IMPLICATIONS

Assessment

- Assess for infection (vital signs; appearance of wound, sputum, urine, and stool; WBC) at beginning of and during therapy.
- Obtain specimens for culture and sensitivity before initiating therapy. First dose may be given before receiving results.
- Inspect IV site frequently. Phlebitis is common.
- Assess patient for allergy to sulfonamides.
- Monitor intake and output ratios. Fluid intake should be sufficient to maintain a urine output of at least 1200–1500 mL daily to prevent crystalluria and stone formation.
- Monitor bowel function. Diarrhea, abdominal cramping, fever, and bloody stools should be reported to health care professional promptly as a sign of Clostridium difficile-associated diarrhea (CDAD). May begin up to several weeks following cessation of therapy.
- Assess for rash periodically during therapy. May cause Stevens-Johnson syndrome. Discontinue therapy if severe or if accompanied with fever, general malaise, fatigue, muscle or joint aches, blisters, oral lesions, conjunctivitis, hepatitis and/or eosinophilia.
- ***Lab Test Considerations:*** Monitor CBC and urinalysis periodically during therapy.
- May produce ↑ serum bilirubin, ↑ potassium, creatinine, and alkaline phosphatase.
- May cause hypoglycemia.

Potential Nursing Diagnoses

Risk for infection (Indications, Side Effects)
Noncompliance (Patient/Family Teaching)

Implementation

- Do not confuse DS (double-strength) formulations with single-strength formulations.
- Do not administer medication IM.
- **PO:** Administer around the clock with a full glass of water. Use calibrated measuring device for liquid preparations.

IV Administration

- **Intermittent Infusion:** ***Diluent:*** Dilute each 5-mL of trimethoprim/sulfamethoxazole with 125 mL of D5W (stable for 24 hr at room temperature). May also dilute each 5-mL of drug with 75 mL of D5W if fluid restriction is required (stable for 6 hr at room temperature). Do not refrigerate. ***Concentration:*** Should not exceed 1.06 mg/mL. ***Rate:*** Infuse over 60–90 min.
- **Y-Site Compatibility:** acyclovir, aldesleukin, alemtuzumab, allopurinol, amifostine, aminocaproic acid, amphotericin B cholesteryl, amphotericin B liposome, anidulafungin, argatroban, azithromycin, bivalirudin, bleomycin, carboplatin, carmustine, cefepime, ceftaroline, cisplatin, cyclophosphamide, cytarabine, dactinomycin, daptomycin, dexmedetomidine, diltiazem, docetaxel, doxorubicin liposome, eptifibatide, ertapenem, etoposide, etoposide phosphate, fenoldopam, filgrastim, fludarabine, fluorouracil, gemcitabine, granisetron, hetastarch, hydromorphone, ifosfamide, irinotecan, levofloxacin, linezolid, lorazepam, melphalan, methotrexate, metronidazole, milrinone, mitoxantrone, nicardipine, octreotide, oxaliplatin, paclitaxel, palonosetron, pamidronate, pancuronium, pantoprazole, pemetrexed, perphenazine, piperacillin/tazobactam, potassium acetate, remifentanil, rituximab, sargramostim, sodium acetate, teniposide, thiotepa, tigecycline, tirofiban, trastuzumab, vecuronium, vinblastine, vincristine, voriconazole, zidovudine, zoledronic acid.
- **Y-Site Incompatibility:** alfentanil, amikacin, aminophylline, amphotericin B colloidal, amphotericin B lipid complex, ampicillin, ampicillin/sulbactam, ascorbic acid, atropine, azathioprine, benztropine, bumetanide, buprenorphine, butorphanol, calcium chloride, calcium gluconate, caspofungin, cefazolin, cefotaxime, cefoxitin, ceftazidime, ceftriaxone, cefuroxime, chloramphenicol, chlorpromazine, clindamycin, cyanocobalamin, cyclosporine, dantrolene, dexamethasone, dexrazoxane, diazepam, diazoxide, digoxin, diphenhydramine, dobutamine, dolasetron, dopamine, doxorubicin, doxycycline, ephedrine, epinephrine, epirubicin, epoetin alfa, erythromycin, famotidine, fentanyl, fluconazole, folic acid, furosemide, ganciclovir, gentamicin, glycopyrrolate, haloperidol, heparin, hydralazine, hydrocortisone, hydroxyzine, idarubicin, imipenem/cilastatin,

T

indomethacin, insulin, isoproterenol, ketamine, ketorolac, lidocaine, mannitol, mechlorethamine, metaraminol, methyldopate, methylprednisolone, metoclopramide, metoprolol, midazolam, multivitamins, mycophenolate, nafcillin, nalbuphine, naloxone, nitroglycerin, nitroprusside, norepinephrine, ondansetron, oxacillin, oxytocin, papaverine, penicillin G, pentamidine, pentazocine, pentobarbital, phenobarbital, phentolamine, phenylephrine, phenytoin, phytonadione, potassium chloride, procainamide, prochlorperazine, promethazine, propranolol, protamine, pyridoxime, quinupristin/dalfopristin, ranitidine, sodium bicarbonate, streptokinase, succinylcholine, sufentanil, theophylline, thiamine, tobramycin, tolazoline, vancomycin, verapamil, vinorelbine.

Patient/Family Teaching

- Instruct patient to take medication around the clock and to finish drug completely as directed, even if feeling well. Take missed doses as soon as remembered unless almost time for next dose. Advise patient that sharing of this medication may be dangerous.
- Instruct patient to notify health care professional if rash, or fever and diarrhea develop, especially if diarrhea contains blood, mucus, or pus. Advise patient not to treat diarrhea without consulting health care professional.
- Caution patient to use sunscreen and protective clothing to prevent photosensitivity reactions.
- Advise patient to notify health care professional if skin rash, sore throat, fever, mouth sores, or unusual bleeding or bruising occurs.
- Instruct patient to notify health care professional if symptoms do not improve within a few days.
- Emphasize importance of regular follow-up exams to monitor blood counts in patients on prolonged therapy.
- **Home Care Issues:** Instruct family or caregiver on dilution, rate, and administration of drug and proper care of IV equipment.

Evaluation/Desired Outcomes

- Resolution of the signs and symptoms of infection. Length of time for complete resolution depends on organism and site of infection.
- Resolution of symptoms of traveler's diarrhea.
- Prevention of *Pneumocystis jirovecii* pneumonia in patients with HIV.

trospium (tros-pee-yum)

Sanctura, Sanctura XR, ✤Trosec

Classification

Therapeutic: urinary tract antispasmodics

Pharmacologic: antimuscarinics

Pregnancy Category C

Indications

Overactive bladder with symptoms of urge urinary incontinence, urgency and urinary frequency.

Action

Antagonizes the effect of acetylcholine at muscarinic receptors in the bladder; this parasympatholytic action reduces bladder smooth muscle tone. **Therapeutic Effects:** Increased bladder capacity and decreased symptoms of overactive bladder.

Pharmacokinetics

Absorption: Less than 10% absorbed following oral administration; food significantly ↓ absorption.

Distribution: Mostly distributed to plasma.

Metabolism and Excretion: Of the 10% absorbed, 40% is metabolized. Unabsorbed drug is mainly excreted in feces. Of absorbed drug, 60% is eliminated in urine as unchanged drug via active tubular secretion.

Half-life: 20 hr.

TIME/ACTION PROFILE (anticholinergic effects)

ROUTE	ONSET	PEAK	DURATION
PO	unknown	5–6 hr	24 hr

Contraindications/Precautions

Contraindicated in: Hypersensitivity; Gastric or urinary retention, uncontrolled angle-closure glaucoma or risk for these conditions.

Use Cautiously in: Bladder outflow obstruction; Gastrointestinal obstructive disorders (ulcerative colitis, intestinal atony, myasthenia gravis); Controlled angle-closure glaucoma (use only if necessary and with careful monitoring); CCr <30 mL/min (dose ↓ recommended); Moderate to severe hepatic impairment; OB, Lactation: Use only if benefit justifies risks to fetus/newborn; Pedi: Safety not established; Geri: May have ↑ sensitivity to anticholinergic effects; ↓ dose may be required.

Adverse Reactions/Side Effects

CNS: headache, confusion, dizziness, drowsiness, fatigue, hallucinations. **EENT:** blurred vision. **GI:** constipation, dry mouth, dyspepsia. **GU:** urinary retention, urinary tract infection. **Misc:** ANGIOEDEMA, fever, heat stroke.

Interactions

Drug-Drug: May interact with other **drugs that compete for tubular secretion**. **Metformin** may ↓ levels. ↑ risk of anticholinergic effects with other **drugs having anticholinergic properties**.

Route/Dosage

PO (Adults): 20 mg twice daily or 60 mg once daily (XR dose form).

PO (Adults ≥75 yr): Based on tolerability, dose may be ↓ to 20 mg once daily.

Renal Impairment

PO (Adults): *CCr <30 mL/min*—20 mg once daily at bedtime.

Availability (generic available)

Tablets: 20 mg. **Extended release tablets:** 60 mg.

NURSING IMPLICATIONS

Assessment

- Monitor voiding pattern and intake and output ratios.

Potential Nursing Diagnoses

Impaired urinary elimination (Indications)

Implementation

- **PO:** Administer 1 hr prior to meals or on an empty stomach.

Patient/Family Teaching

- Instruct patient to take as directed. If a dose is skipped, take next dose 1 hr prior to next meal.
- May cause drowsiness, dizziness, and blurred vision. Caution patient to avoid driving and other activities requiring alertness until response to medication is known. Advise patient to avoid alcohol; may increase drowsiness.
- Advise patient to notify health care professional immediately of signs and symptoms of angioedema (edema of the tongue or laryngopharynx, difficulty breathing) occur.
- Caution patient that heat prostration (fever and heat stroke due to decreased sweating) may occur when trospium is taken in a hot environment.
- Instruct patient to notify health care professional of all Rx or OTC medications, vitamins, or herbal products being taken and consult health care professional before taking any new medications.
- Advise female patient to notify health care professional if pregnancy is planned or suspected, or if breast feeding.

Evaluation/Desired Outcomes

- Increased bladder capacity and decreased symptoms of overactive bladder.

T

ulipristal, See CONTRACEPTIVES, HORMONAL.

umeclidinium

(ue-mek-li-**din**-ee-um)

Incruse Ellipta

Classification

Therapeutic: bronchodilators

Pharmacologic: anticholinergics

Pregnancy Category C

Indications

Maintenance management of airflow obstruction in patients with COPD.

Action

Acts as an anticholinergic by inhibiting M3 muscarinic receptors in bronchial smooth muscle resulting in bronchodilation. **Therapeutic Effects:** Bronchodilation with decreased airflow obstruction.

Pharmacokinetics

Absorption: Minimal oral absorption; remainder of absorption occurs in lungs.

Distribution: Unknown.

Metabolism and Excretion: Primarily metabolized by CYP2D6, metabolites do not contribute to bronchodilation.

Half-life: 11 hr.

TIME/ACTION PROFILE (bronchodilation)

ROUTE	ONSET	PEAK	DURATION
inhaln	1 hr	2–12 hr	24 hr

Contraindications/Precautions

Contraindicated in: Severe/acute symptoms of airflow obstruction; Severe hypersensitivity to milk proteins or other ingredients; Concurrent use with other anticholinergics; Lactation: Discontinue drug or discontinue breast feeding.

Use Cautiously in: Narrow-angle glaucoma (may cause acute angle closure); Urinary retention, prostatic hyperplasia, bladder-neck obstruction; Severe hepatic impairment; Geri: May be more sensitive to drug effects; OB: Use only if potential benefit justifies potential fetal risk; Pedi: Safety and effectiveness not established.

Adverse Reactions/Side Effects

EENT: acute narrow-angle glaucoma, cough, nasopharyngitis. **Resp:** PARADOXICAL BRONCHOSPASM. **CV:** chest pain. **GU:** urinary retention. **MS:** arthralgia.

Interactions

Drug-Drug: ↑ risk of adverse anticholinergic adverse reactions when used concurrently with other **anticholinergics** (avoid concurrent use).

Route/Dosage

Inhaln (Adults): One inhalation (62.5 mcg) once daily.

Availability

Powder for inhalation in blister strips (contains lactose): 62.5 mcg/blister. ***In combination with:*** vilanterol (Anoro Ellipta). See Appendix B.

NURSING IMPLICATIONS

Assessment

- Assess respiratory status (rate, breath sounds, degree of dyspnea, pulse) before administration and at peak of medication. Consult health care professional about alternative medication if severe bronchospasm is present; onset of action is too slow for patients in acute distress. If paradoxical bronchospasm (wheezing) occurs, withhold medication and notify health care professional immediately.

Potential Nursing Diagnoses

Ineffective airway clearance (Indications)

Risk for activity intolerance (Indications)

Implementation

- **Inhaln:** Follow manufacturer's instructions for use of inhaler. Breathe out; do not blow into mouthpiece. Close lips around mouthpiece. Breathe in a long, steady deep breath. Continue to hold breath as long as possible while removing inhaler from mouth. Slide cover over mouthpiece.

Patient/Family Teaching

- Instruct patient in the correct use of inhaler. Advise patient not to discontinue without consulting health care professional; symptoms may recur.
- Inform patient that umeclidinium should not be used for treating sudden breathing problems.
- Advise patient to notify health care professional if worsening symptoms; decreasing effectiveness of inhaled, short-acting $beta_2$–agonists; need for more inhalations than usual of inhaled, short-acting $beta_2$–agonists; or significant decrease in lung function occur.

U

- Instruct patient to notify health care professional of all Rx or OTC medications, vitamins, or herbal products being taken and to avoid concurrent use of Rx, OTC, and herbal products without consulting health care professional.
- Advise patient to notify health care professional if signs and symptoms of worsening narrow-angle glaucoma (eye pain or discomfort, blurred vision, visual halos, colored images associated with red dyes from conjunctival congestion, corneal edema) or worsening urinary retention (difficulty passing urine, painful urination) occur.
- Advise female patient to notify health care professional if pregnancy is planned or suspected or if breast feeding.

Evaluation/Desired Outcomes

- Decrease in the number of flare-ups or the worsening of COPD symptoms (exacerbations).

valACYclovir
(val-ay-**sye**-kloe-veer)
Valtrex

Classification
Therapeutic: antivirals

Pregnancy Category B

Indications
Treatment of herpes zoster (shingles). Treatment/suppression of genital herpes. Reduction of transmission of genital herpes. Treatment of chickenpox. Treatment of herpes labialis (cold sores).

Action
Rapidly converted to acyclovir. Acyclovir interferes with viral DNA synthesis. **Therapeutic Effects:** Inhibited viral replication, decreased viral shedding, reduced time to healing of lesions. Reduced transmission of genital herpes.

Pharmacokinetics
Absorption: 54% bioavailable as acyclovir after oral administration of valacyclovir.

Distribution: CSF concentrations of acyclovir are 50% of plasma concentrations. Acyclovir crosses placenta; enters breast milk.

Metabolism and Excretion: Rapidly converted to acyclovir via intestinal/hepatic metabolism.

Half-life: 2.5–3.3 hr; up to 14 hr in renal impairment (acyclovir).

TIME/ACTION PROFILE (blood levels†)

ROUTE	ONSET	PEAK	DURATION
PO	unknown	1.5–2.5 hr	8–24 hr

†Acyclovir.

Contraindications/Precautions
Contraindicated in: Hypersensitivity to valacyclovir or acyclovir.

Use Cautiously in: Renal impairment (↓ dose/↑ dosing interval recommended if CCr <50 mL/min); OB, Lactation, Pedi: Pregnancy, lactation, or children <2 yr (safety not established); Geri: Dose ↓ may be necessary due to ↑ risk of acute renal failure and CNS side effects.

Adverse Reactions/Side Effects
CNS: headache, agitation, confusion, delirium, dizziness, encephalopathy, hallucinations, seizures, weakness. **GI:** nausea, abdominal pain, anorexia, constipation, diarrhea. **GU:** RENAL FAILURE, crystalluria.

Hemat: THROMBOTIC THROMBOCYTOPENIC PURPURA/HEMOLYTIC UREMIC SYNDROME (very high doses in immunosuppressed patients).

Interactions
Drug-Drug: Probenecid and **cimetidine** ↑ blood levels; significant only in renal impairment. Concurrent use of other **nephrotoxic drugs** ↑ risk of adverse renal effects.

Route/Dosage
Herpes Zoster
PO (Adults): 1 g 3 times daily for 7 days.

Genital Herpes
PO (Adults): *Initial treatment*—1 g twice daily for 10 days. *Recurrence*—500 mg twice daily for 3 days. *Suppression of recurrence*—1 g once daily or 500 mg once daily in patients experiencing <10 recurrences/yr. *Suppression of recurrence in HIV-infected patients*—500 mg q 12 hr. *Reduction of transmission*—500 mg once daily for source partner.

Herpes Labialis
PO (Adults and Children ≥12 yr): 2 g then 2 g 12 hr later.

Chickenpox
PO (Children ≥2 yr): 20 mg/kg 3 times daily for 5 days (not to exceed 1 g 3 times daily).

Renal Impairment
PO (Adults): *CCr 30–49 mL/min*—1 g q 12 hr for herpes zoster treatment, no ↓ required for treatment of genital herpes; 1 g then 1 g 12 hr later for herpes labialis. *CCr 10–29 mL/min*—1 g q 24 hr for initial treatment of genital herpes, 500 mg q 24 hr for treatment of recurrent episodes of genital herpes, 500 mg q 48 hr for suppression of genital herpes in patients with 9 or fewer recurrences/yr, 500 mg q 24 hr for suppression of genital herpes in patients with ≥10 recurrences/yr or HIV-infected patients, 1 g q 24 hr for treatment of herpes zoster; 500 mg then 500 mg 12 hr later for herpes labialis. *CCr <10 mL/min*—500 mg q 24 hr for initial treatment of genital herpes, 500 mg q 24 hr for treatment of recurrent episodes of genital herpes, 500 mg q 48 hr for suppression of genital herpes in patients with 9 or fewer recurrences/yr, 500 mg q 24 hr for suppression of genital herpes in patients with ≥10 recurrences/yr or HIV-infected patients, 500 mg q 24 hr for treatment of herpes zoster; single 500 mg dose for herpes labialis.

Availability (generic available)
Tablets: 500 mg, 1 g. **Cost:** *Generic*—500 mg $31.44/30, 1 g $53.34/30.

NURSING IMPLICATIONS
Assessment
- Assess lesions before and daily during therapy.
- Monitor patient for signs of thrombotic thrombocytic purpura/hemolytic uremic syndrome (throm-

V

bocytopenia, microangiopathic hemolytic anemia, neurologic findings, renal dysfunction, fever). Requires prompt treatment; may be fatal.

Potential Nursing Diagnoses

Risk for impaired skin integrity (Indications)
Risk for infection (Indications, Patient/Family Teaching)

Implementation

- ***High Alert:*** Do not confuse valacyclovir with valganciclovir. Do not confuse Valtrex (valacyclovir) with Valcyte (valganciclovir).
- **PO:** May be administered without regard to meals.
- **Herpes Zoster:** Implement valacyclovir therapy as soon as possible after the onset of signs or symptoms of herpes zoster; most effective if started within 48 hr of the onset of zoster rash. Efficacy of treatment started >72 hr after rash onset is unknown.
- **Genital Herpes and Herpes Labialis:** Implement treatment for genital herpes as soon as possible after onset of symptoms (tingling, itching, burning).
- **Chicken Pox:** Initiate therapy at the earliest sign or symptom; preferably within 24 hr of onset of rash.

Patient/Family Teaching

- Instruct patient to take valacyclovir exactly as directed for the full course of therapy. Take missed doses as soon as remembered if not just before next dose; do not double doses. Advise patient to read the *Patient Information* before starting therapy.
- Advise patient to maintain adequate hydration during therapy.
- Advise patient to notify health care professional promptly if nervous system symptoms (aggressive behavior, unsteady movement, shaky movements, confusion, speech problems, hallucinations, seizures, coma) occur.
- Instruct patient to notify health care professional of all Rx or OTC medications, vitamins, or herbal products being taken and consult health care professional before taking any new medications.
- Instruct female patients to notify health care professional if pregnancy is planned or suspected, or if breast feeding.
- **Herpes Zoster:** Inform patient that valacyclovir does not prevent the spread of infection to others. Precautions should be taken around others who have not had chickenpox or varicella vaccine, or are immunosuppressed, until all lesions have crusted.
- **Genital Herpes and Herpes Labialis:** Inform patient that valacyclovir does not prevent the spread of herpes labialis to others. Advise patient to avoid contact with lesions while lesions or symptoms are present. Valacyclovir reduces transmission of genital herpes to others. Advise patient to practice safe sex (avoid sexual intercourse when lesions are present and wear a condom made of latex or polyurethane during sexual contact).

Evaluation/Desired Outcomes

- Decrease in time to full crusting, loss of vesicles, loss of ulcers, and development of crusts in patients with acute herpes zoster (shingles).
- Decrease in time to full crusting, loss of vesicles, loss of ulcers, and development of crusts in patients with genital herpes.
- Decrease in frequency of outbreaks in patients with genital herpes.
- Decrease in time to full crusting, loss of vesicles, loss of ulcers, and development of crusts in patients with herpes labialis. Decrease in transmission of genital herpes.
- Treatment of chickenpox.

valGANciclovir

(val-gan-**sye**-kloe-veer)
Valcyte

Classification
Therapeutic: antivirals

Pregnancy Category C

Indications

Treatment of cytomegalovirus (CMV) retinitis in patients with AIDS. Prevention of CMV disease in kidney, kidney/pancreas and heart transplant patients at risk.

Action

Valganciclovir is a prodrug which is rapidly converted to ganciclovir by intestinal and hepatic enzymes. CMV virus converts ganciclovir to its active form (ganciclovir phosphate) inside host cell, where it inhibits viral DNA polymerase. **Therapeutic Effects:** Antiviral effect directed preferentially against CMV-infected cells.

Pharmacokinetics

Absorption: 59.4% absorbed following oral administration, rapidly converted to ganciclovir.
Distribution: Unknown.
Metabolism and Excretion: Rapidly converted to ganciclovir; ganciclovir is mostly excreted by the kidneys.
Half-life: 4.1 hr (intracellular half-life of ganciclovir phosphate is 18 hr).

TIME/ACTION PROFILE (ganciclovir blood levels)

ROUTE	ONSET	PEAK	DURATION
PO	rapid	2 hr	12–24 hr

Contraindications/Precautions

Contraindicated in: Hypersensitivity to valganciclovir or ganciclovir; Hemodialysis; Patients undergoing liver transplantation; OB: Pregnancy or planned pregnancy; Lactation: Lactation.
Use Cautiously in: Renal impairment (dosage ↓ recommended if CCr <60 mL/min); Pre-existing bone

marrow depression; Previous or concurrent myelosuppressive drug therapy or radiation therapy; Geri: Age-related ↓ in renal function requires dosage reduction; Pedi: Children <4 mo (safety not established).

Adverse Reactions/Side Effects

CNS: SEIZURES, headache, insomnia, agitation, confusion, dizziness, hallucinations, psychosis, sedation. **GI:** abdominal pain, diarrhea, nausea, vomiting. **GU:** renal impairment. **Hemat:** NEUTROPENIA, THROMBOCYTOPENIA, anemia, aplastic anemia, bone marrow depression, pancytopenia. **Neuro:** ataxia, paresthesia, peripheral neuropathy. **Misc:** fever, hypersensitivity reactions, infections.

Interactions

Drug-Drug: ↑ risk of hematologic toxicity with **zidovudine**. Blood levels and effects may be ↑ by **probenecid**. Patients with renal impairment may experience accumulation of metabolites of **mycophenolate** and valganciclovir. ↑ blood levels and risk of toxicity from **didanosine**.
Drug-Food: Food ↑ absorption.

Route/Dosage

Treatment of CMV Disease

PO (Adults): *Induction*—900 mg twice daily for 21 days; *Maintenance treatment or patients with inactive CMV retinitis*—900 mg once daily.

Renal Impairment

CCr 40–59 mL/min (Adults): *Induction*—450 mg twice daily for 21 days; *Maintenance treatment or patients with inactive CMV retinitis*—450 mg once daily.

Renal Impairment

CCr 25–39 mL/min (Adults): *Induction*—450 mg once daily for 21 days; *Maintenance treatment or patients with inactive CMV retinitis*—450 mg every 2 days.

Renal Impairment

CCr 10–24 mL/min (Adults): *Induction*—450 mg every 2 days for 21 days; *Maintenance treatment or patients with inactive CMV retinitis*—450 mg twice weekly.

Prevention of CMV Disease in Transplant Patients

PO (Adults): *Kidney/pancreas, or heart transplant*—900 mg once daily, starting 10 days prior to transplant and continued for 100 days after; *Kidney transplant*—900 mg once daily, starting 10 days prior to transplant and continued for 200 days after.

Renal Impairment

PO (Adults): *CCr 40–59 mL/min*—450 mg once daily; *CCr 25–39 mL/min*—450 mg every 2 days; *CCr 12–24 mL/min*—450 mg twice weekly.
PO (Children 4 mo-16 yr): *Kidney transplant*—Dose is based on body surface area (BSA) and CCr. Dose = 7 × BSA × CCr (see prescribing information for equations used for BSA and CCr); all calculated doses should be rounded to nearest 10 mg (max = 900 mg) and administered as oral solution; should be started 10 days prior to transplant and continued for 200 days after.
PO (Children 4 mo-16 yr): *Heart transplant*—Dose is based on BSAand CCr. Dose = 7 × BSA × CCr (see prescribing information for equations used for BSA and CCr); all calculated doses should be rounded to nearest 10 mg (max = 900 mg) and administered as oral solution; should be started 10 days prior to transplant and continued for 100 days after.

Renal Impairment

PO (Adults): *CCr 40–59 mL/min*—450 mg once daily; *CCr 25–39 mL/min*—450 mg every 2 days; *CCr 12–24 mL/min*—450 mg twice weekly.

Availability (generic available)

Tablets: 450 mg. **Oral solution (tutti-frutti flavor):** 50 mg/mL.

NURSING IMPLICATIONS

Assessment

- Diagnosis of CMV retinitis should be determined by ophthalmoscopy prior to treatment with valganciclovir.
- Culture for CMV (urine, blood, throat) may be taken prior to administration. However, a negative CMV culture does not rule out CMV retinitis. If symptoms do not respond after several weeks, resistance to valganciclovir may have occurred. Ophthalmologic exams should be performed weekly during induction and every 2 wk during maintenance or more frequently if the macula or optic nerve is threatened. Progression of CMV retinitis may occur during or following ganciclovir treatment.
- Assess for signs of infection (fever, chills, cough, hoarseness, lower back or side pain, sore throat, difficult or painful urination). Notify health care professional if these symptoms occur.
- Assess for bleeding (bleeding gums, bruising, petechiae, or guaiac stools, urine, and emesis). Avoid IM injections and taking rectal temperatures. Apply pressure to venipuncture sites for 10 min.
- ***Lab Test Considerations:*** May cause granulocytopenia, anemia, and thrombocytopenia. Monitor neutrophil and platelet count closely throughout therapy. Do not administer if ANC <500/mm³, platelet count <25,000/mm³, or hemoglobin <8 g/dL.

V

Recovery begins within 3–7 days of discontinuation of therapy.

- Monitor BUN and serum creatinine at least once every 2 wk throughout therapy. May cause ↑ in serum creatinine.

Potential Nursing Diagnoses

Risk for infection (Indications, Patient/Family Teaching)

Implementation

- Do not confuse valganciclovir with valacyclovir. Do not confuse Valcyte (valganciclovir) with Valtrex (valacyclovir).
- **PO:** Administer tablets and oral solution with food. Adults should take tablets, not oral solution. Handle valganciclovir tablets carefully. Do not break or crush. May be potentially teratogenic; avoid direct contact with broken or crushed tablets. If contact with the skin or mucous membranes occurs, wash thoroughly with soap and water and rinse eyes thoroughly with plain water.
- Oral solution (50 mg/mL) must be prepared by the pharmacist prior to dispensing to the patient. Shake well prior to use. Use oral dispenser provided for accurate dose. Store oral solution in refrigerator for no longer than 49 days.

Patient/Family Teaching

- Instruct patient to take valganciclovir with food, as directed. Take missed doses as soon as remembered, unless almost time for next dose; do not double doses. Advise patient to read *Patient Information* before starting therapy and with each Rx refill in case of changes.
- Inform patient that valganciclovir is not a cure for CMV retinitis. Progression of retinitis may continue in immunocompromised patients during and following therapy. Advise patients to have regular ophthalmic exams at least every 4–6 wk. Duration of therapy for CMV prevention is based on the duration and degree of immunosuppression.
- May cause seizures, sedation, dizziness, ataxia, and/or confusion. Caution patient not to drive or do other activities requiring alertness until response to medication is known.
- Advise patient to notify health care professional if fever; chills; sore throat; other signs of infection; bleeding gums; bruising; petechiae; or blood in urine, stool, or emesis occurs. Caution patient to avoid crowds and persons with known infections. Instruct patient to use soft toothbrush and electric razor. Patient should be cautioned not to drink alcoholic beverages or take products containing aspirin or NSAIDs.
- Advise patient that valganciclovir may have teratogenic effects. Women should use a nonhormonal during and for at least 30 days following therapy. If their female sexual partner can become pregnant, men should use a barrier method of contraception during and for at least 90 days following therapy. Advise male patient that valganciclovir may lower the amount of sperm in a man's body and cause fertility problems.
- Caution patient to use sunscreen and protective clothing to prevent photosensitivity reactions.
- Emphasize the importance of frequent follow-up exams to monitor blood counts.

Evaluation/Desired Outcomes

- Management of the symptoms of CMV retinitis in patients with AIDS.
- Prevention of CMV disease in kidney, kidney/pancreas and heart transplant patients at risk.

VALPROATES

divalproex sodium
(dye-val-**proe**-ex **soe**-dee-um)
Depakote, Depakote ER, Depakote Sprinkle, ✤Epival

valproate sodium
(val-**proe**-ate **soe**-dee-um)
Depacon

valproic acid (val-**proe**-ik **as**-id)
Depakene

Classification
Therapeutic: anticonvulsants, vascular headache suppressants

Pregnancy Category D, X (migraines)

Indications

Monotherapy and adjunctive therapy for simple and complex absence seizures. Monotherapy and adjunctive therapy for complex partial seizures. Adjunctive therapy for patients with multiple seizure types, including absence seizures. **Divalproex sodium only**. Manic episodes associated with bipolar disorder. Prevention of migraine headache.

Action

Increase levels of GABA, an inhibitory neurotransmitter in the CNS. **Therapeutic Effects:** Suppression of seizure activity. Decreased manic episodes. Decreased frequency of migraine headaches.

Pharmacokinetics

Absorption: Well absorbed following oral administration; divalproex is enteric-coated, and absorption is delayed. ER form produces lower blood levels. IV administration results in complete bioavailability.
Distribution: Rapidly distributed into plasma and extracellular water. Cross blood-brain barrier and placenta; enters breast milk.
Protein Binding: 80–90%, decreased in neonates, elderly, renal impairment, or chronic hepatic disease.

Metabolism and Excretion: Mostly metabolized by the liver; minimal amounts excreted unchanged in urine.
Half-life: Adults: 9–16 hr.

TIME/ACTION PROFILE (onset = anticonvulsant effect; peak = blood levels)

ROUTE	ONSET	PEAK	DURATION
PO—liquid	2–4 days	15–120 min	6–24 hr
PO—capsules	2–4 days	1–4 hr	6–24 hr
PO—delayed-release products	2–4 days	3–5 hr	12–24 hr
PO—extended-release products	2–4 days	7–14 hr	24 hr
IV	2–4 days	end of infusion	6–24 hr

Contraindications/Precautions

Contraindicated in: Hypersensitivity; Hepatic impairment; 🧬 Known/suspected urea cycle disorders (may result in fatal hyperammonemic encephalopathy); Mitochondrial disorders caused by mutations in mitochondrial DNA polymerase gamma (↑ risk for potentially fatal hepatotoxicity); Pedi: Children <2 yr with suspected mitochondrial disorder caused by mutations in mitochondrial DNA polymerase gamma (↑ risk for potentially fatal hepatotoxicity); OB: Pregnancy (for migraines only).
Use Cautiously in: All patients (may ↑ risk of suicidal thoughts/behaviors); Bleeding disorders; History of liver disease; Organic brain disease; Bone marrow depression; Renal impairment; Women of childbearing potential; Geri: ↑ risk of adverse effects; Rep: Women with childbearing potential; Lactation: Passes into breast milk. Consider discontinuing nursing when valproates are administered to the nursing mother.

Adverse Reactions/Side Effects

CNS: SUICIDAL THOUGHTS, agitation, dizziness, headache, insomnia, sedation, confusion, depression. **CV:** peripheral edema. **EENT:** visual disturbances. **GI:** HEPATOTOXICITY, PANCREATITIS, abdominal pain, anorexia, diarrhea, indigestion, nausea, vomiting, constipation, ↑ appetite. **Derm:** DRUG REACTION WITH EOSINOPHILIA AND SYSTEMIC SYMPTOMS (DRESS), alopecia, rashes. **Endo:** weight gain. **Hemat:** thrombocytopenia, leukopenia. **Metab:** HYPERAMMONEMIA. **Neuro:** HYPOTHERMIA, tremor, ataxia.

Interactions

Drug-Drug: ↑ risk of bleeding with **warfarin**. Blood levels and toxicity may be ↑ by **aspirin, carbamazepine, chlorpromazine, cimetidine, erythromycin,** or **felbamate**. ↑ CNS depression with other **CNS depressants**, including **alcohol, antihistamines, antidepressants, opioid analgesics, MAO inhibitors,** and **sedative/hypnotics**. **MAO inhibitors** and other **antidepressants** may ↓ seizure threshold and ↓ effectiveness of valproate. **Carbamazepine, meropenem, phenobarbital, phenytoin,** or **rifampin** may ↓ valproate blood levels. Valproate may ↑ toxicity of **carbamazepine, diazepam, amitriptyline, nortriptyline, ethosuximide, lamotrigine, phenobarbital, phenytoin, topiramate,** or **zidovudine**. Concurrent use with **topiramate** may ↑ risk of hypothermia and hyperammonemia with or without encephalopathy. **Ertapenem, imipenem,** or **meropenem** may ↓ valproate blood levels.

Route/Dosage

Regular-release and delayed-release formulations usually given in 2–4 divided doses daily; extended-release formulation (Depakote ER) usually given once daily.

Anticonvulsant

PO (Adults and Children >10 yr): *Single-agent therapy (complex partial seizures)*—Initial dose of 10–15 mg/kg/day in 1–4 divided doses; ↑ by 5–10 mg/kg/day weekly until therapeutic response achieved (not to exceed 60 mg/kg/day); when daily dose exceeds 250 mg, give in divided doses. *Polytherapy (complex partial seizures)*—Initial dose of 10–15 mg/kg/day; ↑ by 5–10 mg/kg/day weekly until therapeutic response achieved (not to exceed 60 mg/kg/day); when daily dosage exceeds 250 mg, give in divided doses.
PO (Adults and Children >2 yr [>10 yr for Depakote ER]): *Simple and complex absence seizures*—Initial dose of 15 mg/kg/day in 1–4 divided doses; ↑ by 5–10 mg/kg/day weekly until therapeutic response achieved (not to exceed 60 mg/kg/day); when daily dose exceeds 250 mg, give in divided doses.
IV (Adults and Children): Give same daily dose and at same frequency as was given orally; switch to oral formulation as soon as possible.
Rect (Adults and Children): Dilute syrup 1:1 with water for use as a retention enema. Give 17–20 mg/kg load, maintenance 10–15 mg/kg/dose q 8 hr.

Mood Stabilizer

PO (Adults): *Depakote*—Initial dose of 750 mg/day in divided doses initially, titrated rapidly to desired clinical effect or trough plasma levels of 50–125 mcg/mL (not to exceed 60 mg/kg/day). *Depakote ER*—Initial dose of 25 mg/kg once daily; titrated rapidly to desired clinical effect of trough plasma levels of 85–125 mcg/mL (not to exceed 60 mg/kg/day).

Migraine Prevention

PO (Adults and Children ≥16 yr): *Depakote*—250 mg twice daily (up to 1000 mg/day). *Depakote ER*—

500 mg once daily for 1 wk, then ↑ to 1000 mg once daily.

Availability

Valproic Acid (generic available)

Capsules: 250 mg, ✤500 mg. **Cost:** *Generic*—$37.90/100. **Syrup:** 250 mg/5 mL.

Valproate Sodium (generic available)

Injection: 100 mg/mL.

Divalproex Sodium (generic available)

Delayed-release tablets (Depakote): 125 mg, 250 mg, 500 mg. **Cost:** 125 mg $89.72/100, 250 mg $176.23/100, 500 mg $324.97/100. **Capsules-sprinkle:** 125 mg. **Cost:** $137.53/100. **Extended-release tablets (Depakote ER):** 250 mg, 500 mg. **Cost:** 250 mg $167.91/100, 500 mg $295.36/100.

NURSING IMPLICATIONS

Assessment

- **Seizures:** Assess location, duration, and characteristics of seizure activity. Institute seizure precautions.
- **Bipolar Disorder:** Assess mood, ideation, and behavior frequently.
- **Migraine Prophylaxis:** Monitor frequency and intensity of migraine headaches.
- Geri: Assess geriatric patients for excessive somnolence.
- Assess for suicidal tendencies, especially during early therapy. Restrict amount of drug available to patient. Risk may be increased in children, adolescents, and adults ≤24 yr.
- Monitor for signs and symptoms of pancreatitis (abdominal pain, nausea, vomiting, anorexia). If pancreatitis occurs, valproates should be discontinued and alternate therapy initiated.
- Monitor for signs and symptoms of DRESS (fever, rash, lymphadenopathy, hepatitis, nephritis, hematological abnormalities, myocarditis, myositis, eosinophilia). If symptoms occur and DRESS is confirmed, discontinue valproate and do not restart.
- ***Lab Test Considerations:*** Monitor CBC, platelet count, and bleeding time prior to and periodically during therapy. May cause leukopenia and thrombocytopenia.
- Monitor hepatic function (LDH, AST, ALT, and bilirubin) and serum ammonia concentrations prior to and periodically during therapy. May cause hepatotoxicity; monitor closely, especially during initial 6 mo of therapy; fatalities have occurred. Therapy should be discontinued if hyperammonemia occurs.
- May interfere with accuracy of thyroid function tests.
- May cause false-positive results in urine ketone tests.
- ***Toxicity and Overdose:*** Therapeutic serum levels range from 50–100 mcg/mL (50–125 mcg/mL for mania). Doses are gradually ↑ until a pre-dose serum concentration of at least 50 mcg/mL is reached. However, a good correlation among daily dose, serum level, and therapeutic effects has not been established. Monitor patients receiving near the maximum recommended 60 mg/kg/day for toxicity.

Potential Nursing Diagnoses

Risk for injury (Indications)

Implementation

- Do not confuse *Depakote ER* and regular dose forms. *Depakote ER* produces lower blood levels than *Depakote* dosing forms. If switching from *Depakote* to *Depakote ER*, increase dose by 8-20%.
- Single daily doses are usually administered at bedtime because of sedation.
- **PO:** Administer with or immediately after meals to minimize GI irritation. Extended-release and delayed-release tablets and capsules should be swallowed whole, do not open, break, or chew; will cause mouth or throat irritation and destroy extended release mechanism. Do not administer tablets with milk or carbonated beverages (may cause premature dissolution). Delayed-release divalproex sodium may cause less GI irritation than valproic acid capsules.
- Shake liquid preparations well before pouring. Use calibrated measuring device to ensure accurate dose. Syrup may be mixed with food or other liquids to improve taste.
- Sprinkle capsules may be swallowed whole or opened and entire capsule contents sprinkled on a teaspoonful of soft, cool food (applesauce, pudding). Do not chew mixture. Administer immediately; do not store for future use.
- To convert from valproic acid to divalproex sodium, initiate divalproex sodium at same total daily dose and dosing schedule as valproic acid. Once patient is stabilized on divalproex sodium, attempt administration 2–3 times daily.
- **Rect:** Dilute syrup 1:1 with water for use as a retention enema.

IV Administration

- **Intermittent Infusion:** ***Diluent:*** May be diluted in at least 50 mL of D5W, 0.9% NaCl, or LR. Solution is stable for 24 hr at room temperature. ***Concentration:*** 2 mg/mL. ***Rate:*** Infuse over 60 min (≤20 mg/min). Rapid infusion may cause increased side effects. Has been given as a one-time infusion of 1000 mg over 5–10 min @ 3 mg/kg/min up to 15 mg/kg in patients with no detectable valproate levels.
- **Y-Site Compatibility:** cefepime, ceftazidime, naloxone.
- **Y-Site Incompatibility:** vancomycin.

Patient/Family Teaching

- Instruct patient to take medication as directed. If a dose is missed on a once-a-day schedule, take as soon as remembered that day. If on a multiple-dose schedule, take it within 6 hr of the scheduled time, then space remaining doses throughout the remainder of the day. Abrupt withdrawal may lead to status epilepticus.

- May cause drowsiness or dizziness. Caution patient to avoid driving or other activities requiring alertness until effects of medication are known. Tell patient not to resume driving until physician gives clearance based on control of seizure disorder.
- Instruct patient to notify health care professional of all Rx or OTC medications, vitamins, or herbal products being taken and consult health care professional before taking any new medications, especially CNS depressants. Caution patient to avoid alcohol during therapy.
- Advise patient and family to notify health care professional if thoughts about suicide or dying, attempts to commit suicide; new or worse depression; new or worse anxiety; feeling very agitated or restless; panic attacks; trouble sleeping; new or worse irritability; acting aggressive; being angry or violent; acting on dangerous impulses; an extreme increase in activity and talking, other unusual changes in behavior or mood occur.
- Instruct patient to notify health care professional of medication regimen prior to treatment or surgery.
- Advise patient to notify health care professional if anorexia, abdominal pain, severe nausea and vomiting, yellow skin or eyes, fever, sore throat, malaise, weakness, facial edema, lethargy, unusual bleeding or bruising, pregnancy, or loss of seizure control occurs. Children <2 yr of age are especially at risk for fatal hepatotoxicity.
- Rep: May cause teratogenic effects. Instruct female patients to notify health care professional immediately if pregnancy is planned or suspected or if breast feeding. Advise pregnant patients taking valproates to enroll in the NAAED Pregnancy Registry by calling 1-888-233-2334; call must be made by patient. Registry Web site is www.aedpregnancyregistry.org.
- Advise patient to carry identification at all times describing medication regimen.
- Emphasize the importance of routine exams to monitor progress.

Evaluation/Desired Outcomes

- Decreased seizure activity.
- Decreased incidence of manic episodes in patients with bipolar disorders.
- Decreased frequency of migraine headaches.

valsartan, See ANGIOTENSIN II RECEPTOR ANTAGONISTS.

vancomycin (van-koe-mye-sin)

Vancocin

Classification
Therapeutic: anti-infectives

Pregnancy Category C

Indications

IV: Treatment of potentially life-threatening infections when less toxic anti-infectives are contraindicated. Particularly useful in staphylococcal infections, including: Endocarditis, Meningitis, Osteomyelitis, Pneumonia, Septicemia, Soft-tissue infections in patients who have allergies to penicillin or its derivatives or when sensitivity testing demonstrates resistance to methicillin. **PO:** Treatment of staphylococcal enterocolitis or diarrhea due to *Clostridium difficile*. **IV:** Part of endocarditis prophylaxis in high-risk patients who are allergic to penicillin.

Action

Binds to bacterial cell wall, resulting in cell death. **Therapeutic Effects:** Bactericidal action against susceptible organisms. **Spectrum:** Active against gram-positive pathogens, including: Staphylococci (including methicillin-resistant strains of *Staphylococcus aureus*), Group A beta-hemolytic streptococci, *Streptococcus pneumoniae*, *Corynebacterium*, *Clostridium difficile*, *Enterococcus faecalis*, *Enterococcus faecium*.

Pharmacokinetics

Absorption: Poorly absorbed from the GI tract.
Distribution: Widely distributed. Some penetration (20–30%) of CSF; crosses placenta.
Metabolism and Excretion: Oral doses excreted primarily in the feces; IV vancomycin eliminated almost entirely by the kidneys.
Half-life: Neonates: 6–10 hr; Children 3 mo–3 yr: 4 hr; Children >3 yr: 2–2.3 hr; Adults: 5–8 hr (↑ in renal impairment).

TIME/ACTION PROFILE (blood levels)

ROUTE	ONSET	PEAK	DURATION
IV	rapid	end of infusion	12–24 hr

Contraindications/Precautions

Contraindicated in: Hypersensitivity.
Use Cautiously in: Renal impairment (dosage reduction required if CCr ≤80 mL/min); Hearing impairment; Intestinal obstruction or inflammation (↑ systemic absorption when given orally); OB, Lactation: Safety not established.

Adverse Reactions/Side Effects

EENT: ototoxicity. **CV:** hypotension. **GI:** nausea, vomiting. **GU:** nephrotoxicity. **Derm:** rashes. **Hemat:** eosinophilia, leukopenia. **Local:** phlebitis. **MS:** back and neck pain. **Misc:** hypersensitivity reactions including ANAPHYLAXIS, chills, fever, "red man" syndrome (with rapid infusion), superinfection.

Interactions

Drug-Drug: May cause additive ototoxicity and nephrotoxicity with other **ototoxic** and **nephrotoxic drugs** (**aspirin**, **aminoglycosides**, **cyclosporine**, **cisplatin**, **loop diuretics**). May enhance neuromuscular blockade from **nondepolarizing neuromuscular blocking agents.** ↑ risk of histamine flush when used with **general anesthetics** in children.

Route/Dosage

Serious Systemic Infections

IV (Adults): 500 mg q 6 hr *or* 1 g q 12 hr (up to 4 g/day).
IV (Children >1 mo): 40 mg/kg/day divided q 6–8 hr *Staphylococcal CNS infection*—60 mg/kg/day divided q 6 hr, maximum dose: 1 g/dose.
IV (Neonates 1 wk–1 mo): <1200 g: 15 mg/kg/day q 24 hr. 1200–2000 g: 10–15 mg/kg/dose q 8–12 hr. >2000 g: 15–20 mg/kg/dose q 8 hr.
IV (Neonates <1 wk): <1200 g: 15 mg/kg/day q 24 hr. 1200–2000 g: 10–15 mg/kg/dose q 12–18 hr. >2000 g: 10–15 mg/kg/dose q 8–12 hr.
IT (Adults): 20 mg/day.
IT (Children): 5–20 mg/day.
IT (Neonates): 5–10 mg/day.

Endocarditis Prophylaxis in Penicillin-Allergic Patients

IV (Adults and Adolescents): 1-g single dose 1-hr preprocedure.
IV (Children): 20-mg/kg single dose 1-hr preprocedure.

Diarrhea Due to *C. difficile*

PO (Adults): 125 mg q 6 hr for 10 days.
PO (Children): 40 mg/kg/day divided into 3 or 4 doses for 7–10 days (not to exceed 2 g/day).

Staphylococcal Enterocolitis

PO (Adults): 500–2000 mg/day in 3–4 divided doses for 7–10 days.
PO (Children): 40 mg/kg/day in 3–4 divided doses for 7–10 days (not to exceed 2 g/day).

Renal Impairment

IV (Adults): An initial loading dose of 750 mg–1 g (not less than 15 mg/kg); serum level monitoring is optimal for choosing maintenance dose in patients with renal impairment; these guidelines may be helpful. *CCr 50–80 mL/min*—1 g q 1–3 days; *CCr 10–50 mL/min*—1 g q 3–7 days; *CCr <10 mL/min*—1 g q 7–14 days.

Availability (generic available)

Capsules: 125 mg, 250 mg. **Injection:** 500-mg, 750-mg, 1-, 5-, 10-g vials.

NURSING IMPLICATIONS

Assessment

- Assess patient for infection (vital signs; appearance of wound, sputum, urine, and stool; WBC) at beginning of and throughout therapy.
- Obtain specimens for culture and sensitivity prior to initiating therapy. First dose may be given before receiving results.
- Monitor IV site closely. Vancomycin is irritating to tissues and causes necrosis and severe pain with extravasation. Rotate infusion site.
- Monitor BP throughout IV infusion.
- Evaluate eighth cranial nerve function by audiometry and serum vancomycin levels prior to and throughout therapy in patients with borderline renal function or those >60 yr of age. Prompt recognition and intervention are essential in preventing permanent damage.
- Monitor intake and output ratios and daily weight. Cloudy or pink urine may be a sign of nephrotoxicity.
- Assess patient for signs of superinfection (black, furry overgrowth on tongue; vaginal itching or discharge; loose or foul-smelling stools). Report occurrence.
- Observe patient for signs and symptoms of anaphylaxis (rash, pruritus, laryngeal edema, wheezing). Discontinue drug and notify health care professional immediately if these problems occur. Keep epinephrine, an antihistamine, and resuscitation equipment close by in case of an anaphylactic reaction.
- **Pseudomembranous Colitis:** Assess bowel status (bowel sounds, frequency and consistency of stools, presence of blood in stools) throughout therapy.
- ***Lab Test Considerations:*** Monitor for casts, albumin, or cells in the urine or decreased specific gravity, CBC, and renal function periodically during therapy.
- May cause increased BUN levels.
- ***Toxicity and Overdose:*** Trough concentrations should not exceed 10 mcg/mL (mild-moderate infections) or 15–20 mcg/mL (for severe infections).

Potential Nursing Diagnoses

Risk for infection (Indications)
Disturbed sensory perception (auditory) (Side Effects)

Implementation

- Vancomicin must be given orally for treatment of staphylococcal enterocolitis and *C. difficile*-associated diarrhea. Orally administered vancomycin is not effective for other types of infections.
- **PO:** Use calibrated measuring device for liquid preparations. IV dose form may be diluted in 30 mL of water for oral or nasogastric tube administration.

Resulting solution has bitter, unpleasant taste. May mix with a flavoring syrup to mask taste. Stable for 14 days if refrigerated.

IV Administration

- **Intermittent Infusion:** ***Diluent:*** To reconstitute, add 10 mL of sterile water for injection to 500-mg vial or 20 mL of sterile water for injection to 1-g vial for a concentration of 50 mg/mL. Dilute further with at least 100 mL of 0.9% NaCl, D5W, D5/0.9% NaCl, or LR for every 500 mg of vancomycin being administered. Reconstituted vials stable for 14 days if refrigerated. Infusion is stable for 96 hr if refrigerated. ***Concentration:*** ≤5 mg/mL. ***Rate:*** Infuse over at least 60 min (90 min for doses >10 g). Do not administer rapidly or as a bolus, to minimize risk of thrombophlebitis, hypotension, and "red-man (neck)" syndrome (sudden, severe hypotension; flushing and/or maculopapular rash of face, neck, chest, and upper extremities). May need to slow infusion further to 1.5–2 hr if red-man syndrome occurs.
- **IT:** ***Diluent:*** Dilute with preservative-free NS. ***Concentration:*** 1–5 mg/mL. ***Rate:*** Directly instill into ventricular cerebrospinal fluid.
- **Y-Site Compatibility:** acetylcysteine, acyclovir, aldesleukin, alemtuzumab, alfentanil, allopurinol, alprostadil, amifostine, amikacin, amiodarone, amsacrine, anidulafungin, argatroban, ascorbic acid, atracurium, atropine, azithromycin, benztropine, bleomycin, bumetanide, buprenorphine, butorphanol, calcium chloride, calcium gluconate, carboplatin, carmustine, caspofungin, chlorpromazine, ciprofloxacin, cisatracurium, cisplatin, clindamycin, cyanocobalamin, cyclophosphamide, cyclosporine, cytarabine, dactinomycin, dexamethasone, dexmedetomidine, dexrazoxane, digoxin, diltiazem, diphenhydramine, dobutamine, docetaxel, dolasetron, dopamine, doripenem, doxacurium, doxapram, doxorubicin hydrochloride, doxorubicin liposome, doxycycline, enalaprilat, ephedrine, epinephrine, epirubicin, eptifibatide, ertapenem, erythromycin, esmolol, etoposide, etoposide phosphate, famotidine, fenoldopam, fentanyl, filgrastim, fluconazole, fludarabine, folic acid, gemcitabine, gentamicin, glycopyrrolate, granisetron, hetastarch, hydromorphone, ifosfamide, insulin, irinotecan, isoproterenol, ketamine, labetalol, levofloxacin, lidocaine, linezolid, lorazepam, magnesium sulfate, mannitol, mechlorethamine, melphalan, meperidine, meropenem, metaraminol, methyldopate, metoclopramide, metoprolol, metronidazole, midazolam, milrinone, mitoxantrone, morphine, multivitamins, mycophenolate, nalbuphine, naloxone, nesiritide, nicardipine, nitroglycerin, nitroprusside, norepinephrine, octreotide, ondansetron, oxacillin, oxaliplatin, oxytocin, paclitaxel, palonosetron, pamidronate, pancuronium, papaverine, pemetrexed, penicillin G, pentamidine, pentazocine, pentobarbital, perphenazine, phenobarbital, phentolamine, phenylephrine, phytonadione, potassium acetate, potassium chloride, procainamide, prochlorperazine, promethazine, propranolol, protamine, pyridoxime, ranitidine, remifentanil, rifampin, sodium acetate, sodium bicarbonate, sodium citrate, succinylcholine, sufentanil, tacrolimus, teniposide, thiamine, thiotepa, tigecycline, tirofiban, tobramycin, tolazoline, trastuzumab, vasopressin, vecuronium, verapamil, vinblastine, vincristine, vinorelbine, voriconazole, zidovudine, zoledronic acid.
- **Y-Site Incompatibility:** albumin, aminophylline, amphotericin B cholesteryl, amphotericin B colloidal, amphotericin lipid complex, amphotericin B liposome, azathioprine, bivalirudin, chloramphenicol, dantrolene, daptomycin, diazepam, diazoxide, epoetin alfa, fluorouracil, furosemide, ganciclovir, heparin, ibuprofen, idarubicin, indomethacin, ketorolac, leucovorin calcium, methylprednisolone, mitomycin, moxifloxacin, phenytoin, rituximab, streptokinase, trimethoprim/sulfamethoxazole, valproate sodium.

Patient/Family Teaching

- Advise patients on oral vancomycin to take as directed. Take missed doses as soon as remembered unless almost time for next dose; do not double dose.
- Instruct patient to report signs of hypersensitivity, tinnitus, vertigo, or hearing loss.
- Advise patient to notify health care professional if no improvement is seen in a few days.
- Patients with a history of rheumatic heart disease or valve replacement need to be taught importance of using antimicrobial prophylaxis prior to invasive dental or medical procedures.
- Advise female patient to notify health care professional if pregnancy is planned or suspected or if breast feeding.

Evaluation/Desired Outcomes

- Resolution of signs and symptoms of infection. Length of time for complete resolution depends on organism and site of infection.
- Endocarditis prophylaxis.

REMS

vandetanib (van-det-a-nib)

Caprelsa

Classification
Therapeutic: antineoplastics
Pharmacologic: kinase inhibitors

Pregnancy Category D

Indications

Treatment of symptomatic/progressive medullary thyroid cancer in patients with unresectable, locally advanced, or metastatic disease.

Action

Inhibits tyrosine kinase; results in inhibited action of epidermal growth factor (EGFR), vascular endothelial cell growth factor (VEGF) and other kinase based actions. Inhibits endothelial cell migration/proliferation/survival and new blood vessel formation. Also inhibits EGFR-dependent cell survival. **Therapeutic Effects:** Decreased spread of thyroid cancer.

Pharmacokinetics

Absorption: Well absorbed following oral administration.

Distribution: Unknown.

Metabolism and Excretion: Mostly metabolized by the liver; 44% excreted in feces, 25% in urine.

Half-life: 19 days.

TIME/ACTION PROFILE (blood levels)

ROUTE	ONSET	PEAK	DURATION
PO	unknown	4–10 hr	24 hr

Contraindications/Precautions

Contraindicated in: Congenital long QT syndrome or QTcF interval >450 msec; Hypocalcemia (serum calcium should be within normal range), hypokalemia (serum potassium should >4.0 mEq/L and within normal range), or hypomagnesemia (serum magnesium should be within normal range); Concurrent use of strong inducers of the CYP3A4 enzyme system; OB: Can cause fetal harm; Lactation: Avoid breast feeding.

Use Cautiously in: Diarrhea (↑ risk of electrolyte abnormalities and risk of arrhythmias); Renal impairment (dose ↓ recommended for CCr <50 mL/min with close monitoring of QT interval); Moderate to severe hepatic impairment (Child-Pugh Class B or C; safety and effectiveness not established); OB: Women with childbearing potential; Pedi: Safety and effectiveness not established.

Exercise Extreme Caution in: Concurrent use of other drugs know to prolong QT interval (avoid if possible; if medically necessary, monitoring is required).

Adverse Reactions/Side Effects

CNS: REVERSIBLE POSTERIOR LEUKOENCEPHALOPATHY SYNDROME, fatigue, headache, depression, insomnia, reversible posterior leukoencephalopathy. **Resp:** INTERSTITIAL LUNG DISEASE, upper respiratory tract infection. **CV:** HEART FAILURE, ISCHEMIC CEREBROVASCULAR EVENTS, TORSADE DE POINTES, hypertension, QT interval prolongation. **GI:** abdominal pain, ↓ appetite, diarrhea, nausea, dyspepsia, intestinal perforation, vomiting. **GU:** proteinuria. **Derm:** STEVENS-JOHNSON SYNDROME, acne, photosensitivity reaction, rash, skin reactions, pruritus. **Endo:** hypothyroidism. **F and E:** hypocalcemia. **Hemat:** BLEEDING.

Interactions

Drug-Drug: Strong CYP3A4 inducers including **carbamazepine**, **dexamethasone**, **phenobarbital**, **phenytoin**, **rifabutin**, **rifampin**, **rifapentine**, and **phenobartital**; may ↓ levels and effectiveness; concurrent use should be avoided. Concurrent use with other drugs that prolong the QT interval should be including some **antiarrhythmics (amiodarone**, **disopyramide**, **procainamide**, **sotalol**, **dofetilide)**, **chloroquine**, **clarithromycin**, **dolasetreon**, **granisetron**, **haloperidol**, **methadone**, **moxifloxacin**, and **pimozide**. May ↑ **metformin** and **digoxin** levels.

Drug-Natural Products: St. John's wort may ↓ levels and effectiveness and should be avoided.

Route/Dosage

PO (Adults): 300 mg once daily.

Renal Impairment

PO (Adults): *CCr <50 mL/min*—200 mg once daily.

Availability

Tablets: 100 mg, 300 mg.

NURSING IMPLICATIONS

Assessment

- May prolong QT intervals. Obtain ECG at baseline, at 2–4 wks, at 8–12 wks after starting therapy and every 3 mo there after. Use these parameters to assess QT interval following dose reduction for QT prolongation or dose interruption >2 wks. May require more frequent monitoring if diarrhea occurs.
- Assess patient for rash periodically during therapy. Mild to moderate skin reactions may include rash, acne, dry skin, dermatitis, and pruritus and may be treated with topical or systemic corticosteroids, oral antihistamines, and topical and systemic antibiotics. Treatment of severe rash (Grade 3 or greater) may include systemic corticosteroids and discontinuation of treatment until improved. Upon improvement, may be restarted at a reduced dose.
- Assess for signs and symptoms of interstitial lung disease (hypoxia, pleural effusion, cough, dyspnea). If radiological changes occur with few or no symptoms, therapy may continue. If symptoms are moderate, consider interrupting therapy until symptoms improve. If symptoms are severe, discontinue therapy; permanent discontinuation should be considered. Treat with antibiotics and corticosteroids.

- Assess for signs and symptoms of heart failure (intake and output rations, daily weight, peripheral edema, rales and crackles upon lung auscultation, dyspnea) periodically during therapy.
- Monitor BP during therapy. Control hypertension during therapy.
- Monitor for diarrhea. If severe diarrhea develops, hold therapy until resolved.
- Monitor for signs and symptoms of reversible posterior leukoencephalopathy syndrome (seizures, headache, visual disturbances, confusion, altered mental status); may require discontinuation of therapy.
- ***Lab Test Considerations:*** Monitor serum calcium, potassium, and magnesium periodically during therapy. Maintain serum potassium at ≥4 mEq/L. Maintain serum calcium and magnesium within normal limits. May require more frequent monitoring if diarrhea occurs.
- Monitor TSH at baseline, at 2–4 wks, at 8–12 wks, and every 3 mo thereafter in patients with thyroidectomy. If symptoms of hypothyroidism occur, check TSH levels and adjust thyroid replacement.
- May cause ↓ serum glucose, WBC, hemoglobin, neutrophils, and platelets.
- May cause ↑ serum ALT, creatinine, bilirubin, and glucose.

Potential Nursing Diagnoses

Activity intolerance

Implementation

- Only prescribers and pharmacies certified with the Caprelsa REMS program are able to prescribe and dispense vandetanib.
- Correct hypocalcemia, hypokalemia, and hypomagnesemia prior to therapy.
- **PO:** May be administered daily without regard to food. Swallow tablets whole, do not crush, break or chew. If unable to swallow tablet, tablet may be dispersed in a class containing 2 ounces of non-carbonated water and stirred for approximately 10 min until tablet is dispersed (will not completely dissolve). No other liquids should be used. Swallow dispersion immediately, then mix any residue with 4 ounces of non-carbonated water and swallow. Dispersion may also be administered through nasogastric or gastrostomy tubes. Avoid direct contact with crushed tablets with skin or mucous membranes. Wash thoroughly to avoid exposure.

Patient/Family Teaching

- Instruct patient to take vandetanib as directed. Take missed doses as soon as remembered unless within 12 hrs of next dose. Instruct patient to read *Medication Guide* prior to starting therapy and with each Rx refill in case of changes.
- Advise patients to notify health care professional if rash or signs and symptoms of interstitial lung disease or reversible posterior leukoencephalopathy syndrome. If diarrhea occurs, instruct patient to treat with antidiarrheal medications and notify health care professional if diarrhea becomes severe or persistent.
- May cause tiredness, weakness, or blurred vision. Caution patients to avoid driving or other activities requiring alertness until response to medication is known.
- Caution patient to wear sunscreen and protective clothing during and for 4 mo after therapy is discontinued to prevent photosensitivity reactions.
- Advise patient to notify health care professional of all Rx or OTC medications, vitamins, or herbal products being taken and to consult with health care professional before taking other medications, especially St. John's wort.
- Advise female patients to use effective contraception during and for 4 mo after therapy and to avoid breast feeding.
- Emphasize the importance of regular follow-up exams, ECGs, and blood counts to determine progress and monitor for side effects.

Evaluation/Desired Outcomes

- Decreased spread of thyroid cancer.

vardenafil (var-**den**-a-fil)

Staxyn, Levitra

Classification

Therapeutic: erectile dysfunction agents

Pharmacologic: phosphodiesterase type 5 inhibitors

Pregnancy Category B

Indications

Erectile dysfunction.

Action

Increases cyclic guanosine monophosphate (cGMP) levels by inhibiting phosphodiesterase type 5 (PDE5) an enzyme responsible for the breakdown of cGMP. cGMP produces smooth muscle relaxation of the corpus cavernosum, which in turn promotes increased blood flow and subsequent erection. **Therapeutic Effects:** Enhanced blood flow to the corpus cavernosum and erection sufficient to allow sexual intercourse. Requires sexual stimulation.

Pharmacokinetics

Absorption: 15% absorbed following oral administration; absorption is rapid.

Distribution: Extensive tissue distribution; penetrates semen.

Protein Binding: 95%.
Metabolism and Excretion: Mostly metabolized by the liver (mainly CYP3A4 enzyme system, minor metabolism by CYP2C). M1 metabolite has anti-erectile dysfunction activity. Parent drug and metabolites are mostly excreted in feces. 2–6% renally eliminated.
Half-life: 4–6 hr.

TIME/ACTION PROFILE

ROUTE	ONSET	PEAK	DURATION
PO	rapid	0.5–2 hr	4 hr

Contraindications/Precautions

Contraindicated in: Hypersensitivity; Concurrent use of nitrates or nitric oxide donors; Unstable angina, recent history of stroke, life-threatening arrhythmias, HF or MI within 6 mo; End-stage renal disease requiring dialysis; Known hereditary degenerative retinal disorders; Moderate hepatic impairment (Child-Pugh B) (Staxyn only); Severe hepatic impairment (Child-Pugh C); Congenital or acquired QT prolongation or concurrent use of Class IA or III antiarrhythmics; Moderate or potent inhibitors of the CYP3A4 enzyme system (e.g. ketoconazole, itraconazole, ritonavir, indinavir, saquinavir, atazanavir, clarithromycin erythromycin) (Staxyn only); Pedi: Women, children or newborns.
Use Cautiously in: Other serious underlying cardiovascular disease or left ventricular outflow obstruction; Penile deformity; Underlying conditions predisposing to priapism including sickle cell anemia, multiple myeloma or leukemia; Bleeding disorders or active peptic ulcer diseases; History of sudden severe vision loss or non arteritic ischemic optic neuropathy (NAION); may ↑ risk of recurrence; Low cup to disk ratio, age >50 yr, diabetes, hypertension, coronary artery disease, hyperlipidemia, or smoking (↑ risk of NAION); Moderate or potent inhibitors of the CYP3A4 enzyme system (ketoconazole, itraconazole, ritonavir, indinavir, saquinavir, atazanavir, clarithromycin, erythromycin); need to ↓ dose of Levitra; Alpha adrenergic blockers (patients should be on stable dose of alpha blockers before starting vardenafil; should start therapy with tablets (Staxyn should not be used)); Geri: Have ↑ blood levels; ↓ dose required.

Adverse Reactions/Side Effects

CNS: headache, amnesia, dizziness. **EENT:** HEARING LOSS, VISION LOSS, rhinitis, sinusitis. **GI:** dyspepsia, nausea. **GU:** priapism. **Derm:** flushing. **Misc:** flu syndrome.

Interactions

Drug-Drug: Concurrent use of **nitrates** may cause serious, life-threatening hypotension and is contraindicated. Concurrent use of Class IA antiarrhythmics (such as **quinidine** or **procainamide**) or **Class III antiarrhythmics** (such as **amiodarone** or **sotalol**) ↑ risk of serious arrhythmias and should be avoided. Concurrent use of alpha-adrenergic blockers may cause serious hypotension, lowest doses of each should be used initially. Strong inhibitors of CYP3A4 including **ritonavir**, **saquinavir**, **indinavir**, **atazanavir**, **ketoconazole**, **itraconazole**, and **clarithromycin** ↑ levels and the risk of adverse reactions; concurrent use of moderate inhibitors of CYP3A4 including **erythromycin** may also ↑ effects; concurrent use of any of these drugs is contraindicated with Staxyn; dose of Levitra must be ↓. ↑ risk of hypotension with **alpha adrenergic blockers** and acute ingestion of **alcohol**.

Route/Dosage

The tablets and orally disintegrating tablets are not interchangeable; the orally disintegrating tablets provide a higher level of systemic exposure compared to the tablets.

Levitra

PO (Adults): 10 mg taken 1 hr prior to sexual activity (range 5–20 mg; not to exceed one dose/24 hr); *Concurrent use of ritonavir*—single dose should not exceed 2.5 mg in any 72-hour period; *Concurrent use of indinavir, saquinavir, atazanavir, clarithromycin, ketoconazole 400 mg daily, or itraconazole 400 mg daily*—single dose should not exceed 2.5 mg/24 hr; *Concurrent use of ketoconazole 200 mg daily, itraconazole 200 mg daily, or erythromycin*—single dose should not exceed 5 mg/24 hr; *Concurrent use of stable alpha-blocker therapy (not on potent CYP3A4 inhibitor)*—5 mg initial dose; titrate as tolerated; *Concurrent use of stable alpha-blocker and potent CYP3A4 inhibitor therapy*—2.5 mg initial dose; titrate as tolerated.
PO (Geriatric Patients ≥65 yr): 5 mg initial dose; titrate as tolerated.

Hepatic Impairment

PO (Adults): *Moderate hepatic impairment (Child-Pugh B)*—May start with 5 mg dose (not to exceed 10 mg).

Staxyn

PO (Adults): 10 mg taken 1 hr prior to sexual activity (not to exceed one dose/24 hr).

Availability (generic available)

Tablets: 2.5 mg, 5 mg, 10 mg, 20 mg. **Orally disintegrating tablets (Staxyn):** 10 mg.

NURSING IMPLICATIONS

Assessment

- Determine erectile dysfunction before administration. Vardenafil has no effect in the absence of sexual stimulation.

Potential Nursing Diagnoses

Sexual dysfunction (Indications)

Implementation

- *Levitra* and *Staxyn* are not interchangeable.
- **PO:** *Levitra* is usually administered 1 hr before sexual activity. May be administered 30 min to 4 hr before sexual activity.
- Administer *Staxyn* 1 hr before sexual activity. Orally disintegrating tablets should be left in the package until use. Remove from the blister pouch. Do not push tablet through the blister; peel open the blister pack with dry hands and place tablet on tongue. Tablet will dissolve rapidly and be swallowed with saliva. No liquid is needed to take the orally disintegrating tablet.
- May be administered without regard to food.

Patient/Family Teaching

- Instruct patient to take vardenafil approximately 30 min–1 hr before sexual activity and not more than once per day. Inform patient that sexual stimulation is required for an erection to occur after taking vardenafil.
- Advise patient that vardenafil is not indicated for use in women.
- Caution patient not to take vardenafil concurrently with alpha adrenergic blockers (unless on a stable dose) or nitrates. If chest pain occurs after taking vardenafil, instruct patient to seek immediate medical attention.
- Instruct patient to notify health care professional promptly if erection lasts longer than 4 hr or if sudden or decreased vision loss in one or both eyes, or loss or decrease in hearing, ringing in the ears, or dizziness occurs.
- Instruct patient to notify health care professional of all Rx or OTC medications, vitamins, or herbal products being taken and consult health care professional before taking any new medications.
- Inform patient that vardenafil offers no protection against sexually transmitted diseases. Counsel patient that protection against sexually transmitted diseases and HIV infection should be considered.

Evaluation/Desired Outcomes

- Male erection sufficient to allow intercourse.

REMS

varenicline (ver-**en**-i-cline)

✱Champix, Chantix

Classification

Therapeutic: smoking deterrents

Pharmacologic: nicotine agonists

Pregnancy Category C

Indications

Treatment of smoking cessation; in conjunction with nonpharmacologic support (educational materials/counseling).

Action

Selectively binds to alpha$_4$, beta$_2$ nicotinic acetylcholine receptors, acting as a nicotine agonist; prevents the binding of nicotine to receptors. **Therapeutic Effects:** Decreased desire to smoke.

Pharmacokinetics

Absorption: 100% absorbed following oral administration.

Distribution: 24 hr.

Metabolism and Excretion: Minimally metabolized; 92% excreted in urine unchanged.

Half-life: 24 hr.

TIME/ACTION PROFILE

ROUTE	ONSET	PEAK	DURATION
PO	unknown	3–4 hr	24 hr

Contraindications/Precautions

Contraindicated in: Hypersensitivity; Lactation: Lactation; Pedi: Safety not established.

Use Cautiously in: Severe renal impairment (↓ dose recommended if CCr <30 mL/min); Stable cardiovascular disease (may ↑ risk of cardiovascular events); Psychiatric illness; Seizure disorders; Geri: Consider age-related ↓ in renal function; OB: Use only if maternal benefit outweighs fetal risk.

Adverse Reactions/Side Effects

CNS: HOMICIDAL THOUGHTS/BEHAVIOR, SEIZURES, STROKE, SUICIDAL THOUGHTS/BEHAVIOR, ↓ attention span, anxiety, depression, insomnia, irritability, dizziness, restlessness, abnormal dreams, agitation, aggression, amnesia, anxiety, delusions, disorientation, dissociation, hallucinations, hostility, mania, mood changes, migraine, panic, paranoia, psychosis. **EENT:** blurred vision, visual disturbances. **CV:** MYOCARDIAL INFARCTION, syncope. **GI:** diarrhea, gingivitis, nausea, ↑ appetite, constipation, dyspepsia, dysphagia, enterocolitis, eructation, flatulence, gallbladder disorder, GI bleeding, ↑ liver enzymes, vomiting. **Derm:** STEVENS-JOHNSON SYNDROME, flushing, hyperhydrosis, acne, dermatitis, dry skin. **Hemat:** anemia. **MS:** arthralgia, back pain, musculoskeletal pain, muscle cramps, myalgia, restless legs. **Misc:** ANGIOEDEMA, accidental injury, chills, fever, hypersensitivity, mild physical dependence.

Interactions

Drug-Drug: Smoking cessation may ↓ metabolism of **theophylline**, **warfarin**, and **insulin** resulting in ↑ effects; careful monitoring is recommended. Risk of adverse reactions (nausea, vomiting, dizziness, fatigue, headache) may be ↑ with **nicotine** replacement therapy (nicotine transdermal patches). Concomitant use with **alcohol** may ↑ risk of worsening neuropsychiatric events.

Route/Dosage

PO (Adults): Treatment is started one week prior to planned smoking cessation (may also begin dosing and then quit smoking between days 8 and 35 of treatment); 0.5 mg once daily on the first three days, then 0.5 mg twice daily for the next 4 days, then 1 mg twice daily.

Renal Impairment

PO (Adults): *CCr <30 mL/min*—0.5 mg daily, may ↑ to 0.5 mg twice daily.

Availability

Tablets: 0.5 mg, 1 mg. **Cost:** All strengths $237.71/56.

NURSING IMPLICATIONS

Assessment

- Assess for desire to stop smoking.
- Assess for nausea. Usually dose-dependent. May require dose reduction.
- Assess mental status and mood changes, especially during initial few months of therapy and during dose changes. Risk may be increased in children, adolescents, and adults ≤24 yr. Inform health care professional if patient demonstrates significant increase in signs of depression (depressed mood, loss of interest in usual activities, significant change in weight and/or appetite, insomnia or hypersomnia, psychomotor agitation or retardation, increased fatigue, feelings of guilt or worthlessness, slowed thinking or impaired concentration, suicide attempt or suicidal or homicidal ideation). Restrict amount of drug available to patient.
- Assess for rash periodically during therapy. May cause Stevens-Johnson syndrome. Discontinue therapy if severe or if accompanied with fever, general malaise, fatigue, muscle or joint aches, blisters, oral lesions, conjunctivitis, hepatitis and/or eosinophilia.
- ***Lab Test Considerations:*** May cause anemia.

Potential Nursing Diagnoses

Ineffective coping (Indications)

Implementation

- **PO:** Administer after eating with a full glass of water.

Patient/Family Teaching

- Instruct patient to take varenicline as directed. Set a date to stop smoking. Start taking varenicline 1 wk before quit date. Begin with 0.5 mg/day for the first 3 days, then for the next 4 days take one 0.5 mg tablet in the morning and in the evening. After first 7 days, increase to 1 mg tablet in the morning and evening. Advise patient to read *Medication Guide* before starting therapy.
- Encourage patient to attempt to quit, even if they had early lapses after quit day.
- Advise patient to stop taking varenicline and contact health care professional promptly if agitation, depressed mood, any changes in behavior that are not typical of nicotine withdrawal, or if suicidal thoughts or behavior; rash with mucosal lesions or skin reaction, or chest pain, pressure, or dyspnea occur. Encourage patient to reduce amount of alcohol consumed until effects of medication are known.
- Provide patient with educational materials and counseling to support attempts to quit smoking.
- Caution patient not to share varenicline with others. May be harmful.
- May cause blurred vision, dizziness, and disturbance in attention. Caution patient to avoid driving and other activities requiring alertness until response to medication is known.
- Inform patient that nausea, insomnia, and vivid, unusual, or strange dreams may occur and are usually transient. Advise patient to notify health care professional if these symptoms are persistent and bothersome; dose reduction may be considered.
- Instruct patient to notify health care professional of all Rx or OTC medications, vitamins, or herbal products being taken and consult health care professional before taking any new medications. Inform patient that some medications may require dose adjustments after quitting smoking.
- Advise patient to notify health care professional if pregnancy is planned or suspected or if breast feeding.

Evaluation/Desired Outcomes

- Smoking cessation. Patients who have successfully stopped smoking at the end of 12 wk, should take an additional 12 wk course to increase the likelihood of long-term abstinence. Patients who do not succeed in stopping smoking during 12 wk of initial therapy or who relapse after treatment, should be encouraged to make another attempt once factors contributing to the failed attempt have been identified and addressed.

vasopressin (vay-soe-**press**-in)

~~Pitressin~~, ✱ Pressyn, Vasostrict

Classification

Therapeutic: hormones

Pharmacologic: antidiuretic hormones, vasopressors

Pregnancy Category C

Indications

Central diabetes insipidus due to deficient antidiuretic hormone. Vasodilatory shock. **Unlabeled Use:** Management of pulseless VT/VF unresponsive to initial shocks, asystole, or pulseless electrical activity (PEA) (ACLS guidlines). Gastrointestinal hemorrhage.

Action

Alters the permeability of the renal collecting ducts, allowing reabsorption of water. Directly stimulates musculature of GI tract. In high doses acts as a nonadrenergic peripheral vasoconstrictor. **Therapeutic Effects:** Decreased urine output and increased urine osmolality in diabetes insipidus. Increased BP.

Pharmacokinetics

Absorption: IM absorption may be unpredictable.
Distribution: Widely distributed throughout extracellular fluid.
Metabolism and Excretion: Rapidly degraded by the liver and kidneys; <5% excreted unchanged by the kidneys.
Half-life: <10 min.

TIME/ACTION PROFILE (antidiuretic effect)

ROUTE	ONSET	PEAK	DURATION
IM, subcut	unknown	unknown	2–8 hr
IV	unknown	unknown	30–60 min

Contraindications/Precautions

Contraindicated in: Chronic renal failure with ↑ BUN; Hypersensitivity to 8-L arginine vasopressin or chlorobutanol.
Use Cautiously in: Perioperative polyuria (increased sensitivity to vasopressin); Comatose patients; Seizures; Migraine headaches; Asthma; Heart failure; Cardiovascular disease; Renal impairment; OB: Higher doses (0.07 units/min) for vasodilatory shock may be needed in 2nd and 3rd trimesters; Geri: ↑ sensitivity to vasopressin effects; Pedi: Safety not established.

Adverse Reactions/Side Effects

CNS: dizziness, "pounding" sensation in head. **CV:** MI, angina, chest pain. **GI:** abdominal cramps, belching, diarrhea, flatulence, heartburn, nausea, vomiting. **Derm:** paleness, perioral blanching, sweating. **Neuro:** trembling. **Misc:** allergic reactions, fever, water intoxication (higher doses).

Interactions

Drug-Drug: Antidiuretic effect may be ↓ by concurrent administration of **clozapine**, **lithium**, **demeclocycline**, **foscarnet**. Antidiuretic effect may be ↑ by concurrent administration of **chlorpropamide**, **cyclophosphamide**, **enalapril**, **felbamate**, **haloperidol**, **ifosfamide**, **methyldopa**, **pentamidine**, **tricyclic antidepressants**, **SSRIs**, or **vincristine**. Vasopressor effect may be ↑ by concurrent administration of **ganglionic blocking agents**, **indomethacin**, or **catecholamines**. **Furosemide** ↑ urine flow.

Route/Dosage

Diabetes insipidus

IM, Subcut (Adults): 5–10 units 2–4 times daily.
IM, Subcut (Children): 2.5–10 units 2–4 times daily.
IV (Adults and Children): 0.0005 units/kg/hr, double dose q 30 min as needed to a maximum of 0.01 units/kg/hr.

Pulseless VT/VF, Asystole, or PEA (ACLS guidelines)

IV (Adults): 40 units as a single dose (unlabeled).
IV (Children): 0.4 units/kg after resuscitation and at least 2 doses of epinephrine.

Vasodilatory shock

IV (Adults): 0.01 units/min, titrate by 0.005 units/min q 10–15 min until target BP achieved; (max dose = 0.07 units/min).
IV (Infants and Children): 0.0003–0.002 units/kg/min, titrate to effect.

GI Hemorrhage

IV (Adults): 0.2–0.4 units/min then titrate to maximum dose of 0.9 units/min; if bleeding stops continue same dose for 12 hr then taper off over 24–48 hr.
IV (Children): 0.002–0.005 units/kg/min then titrate to maximum dose of 0.01 units/kg/min; if bleeding stops continue same dose for 12 hr then taper off over 24–48 hr.

Availability (generic available)

Solution for injection: 20 units/mL.

NURSING IMPLICATIONS

V

Assessment

- Monitor BP, HR, and ECG periodically throughout therapy and continuously throughout cardiopulmonary resuscitation.
- **Diabetes Insipidus:** Monitor urine osmolality and urine volume frequently to determine effects of medication. Assess patient for symptoms of dehydration (excessive thirst, dry skin and mucous membranes, tachycardia, poor skin turgor). Weigh patient daily, monitor intake and output, and assess for edema.
- ***Lab Test Considerations:*** Monitor urine specific gravity throughout therapy.
- Monitor serum electrolyte concentrations periodically during therapy.
- ***Toxicity and Overdose:*** Signs and symptoms of water intoxication include confusion, drowsiness, headache, weight gain, difficulty urinating, seizures, and coma.
- Treatment of overdose includes water restriction and temporary discontinuation of vasopressin until polyuria occurs. If symptoms are severe, administra-

tion of mannitol, hypertonic dextrose, urea, and/or furosemide may be used.

Potential Nursing Diagnoses

Deficient fluid volume (Indications)
Excess fluid volume (Adverse Reactions)

Implementation

- Aqueous vasopressin injection may be administered subcut or IM for diabetes insipidus.
- Administer 1–2 glasses of water at the time of administration to minimize side effects (blanching of skin, abdominal cramps, nausea).

IV Administration

- **IV Push:** ***Diluent:*** Administer undiluted. ***Concentration:*** 20 units/mL. ***Rate:*** Administer over 1–2 sec during pulseless VT/VF, asystole, or PEA.
- **Continuous Infusion:** ***Diluent:*** Dilute 2.5 mg or 5 mg of vasopresssin in 500 mL or 100 mL respectively of 0.9% NaCl or D5W. ***Concentration:*** 0.1 units/mL or 1 unit/mL. Solution is stable for 18 hrs at room temperature or 24 hr if refrigerated. ***Rate:*** See Route/Dosage section.
- **Y-Site Compatibility:** acyclovir, alemtuzumab, alfentanil, allopurinol, amifostine, amikacin, aminocaproic acid, aminophylline, amiodarone, amphotericin B liposome, anidulafungin, argatroban, ascorbic acid, asparaginase, atracurium , atropine, azathioprine, azithromycin, aztreonam, benztropine, bivalirudin, bleomycin, bumetanide, buprenorphine, busulfan, butorphanol, calcium chloride, calcium gluconate, carboplatin, carmustine, caspofungin, cefazolin, cefepime, cefotaxime, cefotetan, cefoxitin, ceftaroline, ceftazidime, ceftriaxone, cefuroxime, chloramphenicol, chlorpromazine, ciprofloxacin, cisatracurium, cisplatin, clindamycin, cyanocobalamin, cyclophosphamide, cyclosporine, cytarabine, dacarbazine, dactinomycin, daptomycin, dexamethasone, dexmedetomidine, dexrazoxane, digoxin, diltiazem, diphenhydramine, dobutamine, docetaxel, dopamine, doxorubicin hydrochloride, doxycycline, droperidol, enalaprilat, ephedrine, epinephrine, epirubicin, epoetin alfa, ertapenem, erythromycin, esmolol, etoposide, etoposide phosphate, famotidine, fenoldopam, fentanyl, fluconazole, fludarabine, fluorouracil, folic acid, foscarnet, fosphenytoin, ganciclovir, gemcitabine, gentamicin, glycopyrrolate, granisetron, heparin, hetastarch, hydrocortisone, hydromorphone, idarubicin, ifosfamide, imipenem/cilastatin, irinotecan, isoproterenol, ketorolac, labetalol, levofloxacin, lidocaine, linezolid, lorazepam, magnesium sulfate, mannitol, mechlorethamine, melphalan, meperidine, meropenem, mesna, metaraminol, methohexital, methotrexate, methylprednisolone, metoclopramide, metoprolol, metronidazole, micafungin, midazolam, milrinone, mitomycin, mitoxantrone, morphine, moxifloxacin, multivitamins, mycophenolate, nafcillin, nalbuphine, naloxone, nesiritide, nicardipine, nitroglycerin, nitroprusside, norepinephrine, octreotide, ondansetron, oxacillin, oxaliplatin, oxytocin, paclitaxel, palonosetron, pamidronate, pantoprazole, papaverine, penicillin G, pentamidine, pentazocine, phenobarbital, phenylephrine, phytonadione, piperacillin/tazobactam, potassium acetate, potassium chloride, potassium phosphates, procainamide, prochlorperazine, promethazine, propranolol, protamine, pyridoxime, quinupristin/dalfopristin, ranitidine, remifentanil, rocuronium, sodium acetate, sodium bicarbonate, sodium phosphates, streptozocin, succinylcholine, sufentanil, tacrolimus, telavancin, teniposide, theophylline, thiamine, thiopental, thiotepa, tigecycline, tirofiban, tobramycin, tolazoline, topotecan, vancomycin, vecuronium, verapamil, vinblastine, vincristine, vinorelbine, voriconazole, zidovudine, zoledronic acid.
- **Y-Site Incompatibility:** amphotericin B colloidal, amphotericin B lipid complex, dantrolene, diazepam, diazoxide, indomethacin, pemetrexed, phenytoin.

Patient/Family Teaching

- Instruct patient to take medication as directed. Caution patient not to use more than prescribed amount. Take missed doses as soon as remembered, unless almost time for next dose.
- Advise patient to drink 1–2 glasses of water at time of administration to minimize side effects (blanching of skin, abdominal cramps, nausea). Inform patient that these side effects are not serious and usually disappear in a few minutes.
- Caution patient to avoid concurrent use of alcohol while taking vasopressin.
- Patients with diabetes insipidus should carry identification at all times describing disease process and medication regimen.

Evaluation/Desired Outcomes

- Decrease in urine volume.
- Relief of polydipsia.
- Increased urine osmolality in patients with central diabetes insipidus.
- Increase in BP.
- Resolution of VT/VF.

vedolizumab

(ve-doe-**liz**-yoo-mab)
Entyvio

Classification

Therapeutic: gastrointestinal anti-inflammatories
Pharmacologic: monoclonal antibodies, integrin receptor antagonists

Pregnancy Category B

Indications

Moderately to severely active ulcerative colitis or Crohn's disease that has not responded adequately to/lost response to/become intolerant to tumor necrosis factor (TNF) blockers or immunomodulators; or has become intolerant to/dependant on corticosteroids and failed to induce/maintain beneficial response/remission, improved endoscopic appearance (ulcerative colitis) or achieved corticosteroid-free remission.

Action

A monoclonal antibody that binds to certain integrins, blocking their interaction with substances involved in mucosal cell adhesion, also inhibits migration of memory T-lymphocytes across endothelium into inflamed GI tissue. **Therapeutic Effects:** Decreased chronic GI inflammation and symptomatology associated with ulcerative colitis and Crohn's disease.

Pharmacokinetics

Absorption: IV administration results in complete bioavailability.
Distribution: Unknown.
Metabolism and Excretion: Unknown.
Half-life: 25 days.

TIME/ACTION PROFILE (clinical improvement)

ROUTE	ONSET	PEAK	DURATION
IV	within 6 wk	unknown	up to 8 wk

Contraindications/Precautions

Contraindicated in: Hypersensitivity; Active severe infection; Live-virus vaccinations; Concurrent use of natalizumab; Concurrent use of TNF blockers.
Use Cautiously in: OB: Use during pregnancy if maternal benefits outweigh risk to the unborn child; Lactation: Use cautiously if breast feeding; Pedi: Safe and effective use in children has not been established.

Adverse Reactions/Side Effects

CNS: headache, fatigue. **Resp:** cough. **GI:** oropharyngeal pain, ↑ transaminases. **Derm:** pruritus, rash. **MS:** arthralgia, back pain, extremity pain. **Misc:** fever, hypersensitivity reactions including ANAPHYLAXIS, ↑ risk of infection.

Interactions

Drug-Drug: May ↓ antibody response to and ↑ risk of adverse reactions from **live-virus vaccines** (complete immunizations prior to treatment). Concurrent use with **natalizumab** may ↑ risk of infections and Progressive Multifocal Leukoencephalopathy and should be avoided. Concurrent use with **TNF blockers** may ↑ risk of infections and should be avoided.

Route/Dosage

IV (Adults): 300 mg wk zero, two and six, then every 8 wk; treatment may be continued if beneficial response is obtained by wk 14.

Availability

Lyophilized powder for injection (requires reconstitution and further dilution): 300 mg in 20 mL single-use vial.

NURSING IMPLICATIONS

Assessment

- Assess abdominal pain and frequency, quantity, and consistency of stools at beginning and during therapy.
- Assess for signs of hypersensitivity or infusion-related reactions (dyspnea, bronchospasm, urticaria, flushing, rash, swelling of lips, tongue, throat, or face, wheezing, hypertension, tachycardia). If anaphylaxis or serious allergic reactions occur, discontinue vedolizumab and treat symptoms.
- Assess for new signs or symptoms suggestive of progressive multifocal leukoencephalopathy (PML), an opportunistic infection of the brain caused by the JC virus, leading to death or severe disability; withhold dose and notify health care professional promptly. Monitor during therapy and for at least 6 mo following discontinuation. PML symptoms may begin gradually but usually over days to wk and leads to death or severe disability over wk to mo. Symptoms include progressive weakness on one side of body or clumsiness of limbs, disturbance of vision, changes in thinking, memory and orientation leading to confusion and personality changes. Diagnosis is usually made via gadolinium-enhanced MRI and CSF analysis. Withhold vedolizumab at first sign of PML.
- ***Lab Test Considerations:*** May cause ↑ AST, ALT, and serum bilirubin. Discontinue in patients with jaundice or other evidence of liver injury.

Potential Nursing Diagnoses

Risk for infection (Adverse Reactions)

Implementation

- Perform test for latent TB. If positive, begin treatment for TB prior to starting vedolizumab therapy. Monitor for TB throughout therapy, even if latent TB test is negative.

IV Administration

- **Intermittent Infusion:** Reconstitute with 4.8 mL Sterile Water for Injection using 21 to 25 gauge needle. Direct stream to wall of vial to prevent excessive foaming. Gently swirl vial for at least 15 seconds to dissolve; do not invert of shake vigorously. Allow to sit for up to 20 min at room temperature for reconstitution and settling of foam. If not fully dissolved after 20 min, allow another 10 min. Do not use vial if not dissolved within 30 min. Solution is clear or opalescent, colorless to light brownish yellow; do not administer solutions that are discolored or contain particulate matter. Swirl gently and invert vial 3 times prior to withdrawing. Withdraw 5 mL (300 mg) using 21 to 25 gauge needle. Discard unused portion. ***Diluent:*** 250 mL 0.9% NaCl. Gently mix bag. Use as soon as possible. Stable up to 4 hrs if refrigerated; do not freeze. Flush line with 30 mL of 0.9% NaCl after infusion. ***Rate:*** Infuse over 30 min; do not administer as IV push or bolus.

- **Y-Site Incompatibility:** Do not administer with other solutions or medications.

Patient/Family Teaching

- Explain purpose of vedolizumab to patient. Advise patient to read *Medication Guide* prior to therapy.
- Instruct patient to report symptoms of PML (progressive weakness on one side of the body or clumsiness of limbs; disturbance of vision; changes in thinking, memory, and orientation leading to confusion and personality changes), hypersensitivity reactions, hepatotoxicity (yellowing of the skin and eyes, unusual darkening of the urine, anorexia, nausea, feeling tired or weak, vomiting, right upper abdominal pain), or worsening of symptoms (new or sudden change in your thinking, eyesight, balance, or strength or other problems) that persist over several days to health care professional immediately.
- Inform patient of risk of infection. Advise patient to notify health care professional if symptoms of infection (fever, chills, muscle aches, shortness of breath, runny nose, cough, sore throat, red or painful skin or open cuts or sores, tiredness, pain during urination) occur.
- Advise patient to notify health care professional of all Rx or OTC medications, vitamins, or herbal products being taken and to consult with health care professional before taking other medications.
- Advise female patient to notify health care professional if pregnancy is planned or suspected or if breast feeding. Encourage pregnant women to join Entyvio Pregnancy Registry by calling 1-877-825-3327. Registry monitors pregnancy outcomes in women exposed to vedolizumab during pregnancy.

Evaluation/Desired Outcomes

- Decreased chronic GI inflammation and symptomatology associated with ulcerative colitis and Crohn's disease. Discontinue therapy if no improvement by Week 14.

vemurafenib

(vem-u-**raf**-e-nib)

Zelboraf

Classification

Therapeutic: antineoplastics

Pharmacologic: kinase inhibitors

Pregnancy Category D

Indications

Treatment of unresectable or metastatic melanoma with BRAF ^{V600E} mutation.

Action

Inhibits mutated forms of the enzyme kinase. Inhibits proliferation that occurs in conjunction with activated BRAF proteins. **Therapeutic Effects:** Decreased spread of melanoma.

Pharmacokinetics

Absorption: Some absorption follows oral administration, bioavailability is not known.

Distribution: Unknown.

Protein Binding: >99%.

Metabolism and Excretion: Mostly metabolized by the liver (mostly by the CYP3A4 enzyme system), 1% eliminated in urine.

Half-life: 57 hr (range 30–120 hr).

TIME/ACTION PROFILE (blood levels)

ROUTE	ONSET	PEAK	DURATION
PO	unknown	3 hr	12 hr

Contraindications/Precautions

Contraindicated in: Underlying electrolyte abnormalities (↑ risk of serious arrhythmias; correct prior to administration); Congenital or acquired prolonged QT syndromes; Baseline QTc interval >500 msec; Concurrent use of QT-interval prolonging drugs; OB: Should not be used during pregnancy, may cause fetal harm; Lactation: Breast feeding should be avoided.

Use Cautiously in: Pre-existing severe hepatic or renal impairment; Geri: ↑ risk of cutaneous squamous cell carcinoma, nausea, ↓ appetite, peripheral edema, keratoacanthoma and atrial fibrillation; Concurrent use of strong CYP3A4 inducers/inhibitors or drugs that are substrates of CYP3A4, CYP1A2 or CYP2D6 enzyme systems; monitoring of effects and necessary dose adjustments may be necessary; Receiving radiation therapy prior to, during, or after therapy (↑ risk of radiation sensitization/recall); Rep: Patients with childbearing potential; Pedi: Safety and effectiveness not established.

Adverse Reactions/Side Effects

CNS: fatigue, weakness, headache. **EENT:** iritis, retinal vein occlusion, uveitis. **Resp:** cough. **CV:** QTc prolongation, TORSADE DE POINTES, peripheral edema. **GI:** HEPATOTOXICITY, ↓ appetite, dysgeusia, nausea. **Derm:**

MALIGNANCY, STEVENS-JOHNSON SYNDROME, TOXIC EPIDERMAL NECROLYSIS, alopecia, dry skin, rash(↑ in females), pruritus, rash, photosensitivity (↑ in females), skin papilloma, keratocanthoma (↑ in males). **GU:** ↑ creatinine (↑ in females). **MS:** arthralgia(↑ in females), myalgia, back pain, musculoskeletal pain. **Misc:** DRUG REACTION WITH EOSINOPHILIA AND SYSTEMIC SYMPTOMS (DRESS), hypersensitivity reactions including ANAPHYLAXIS, fever, radiation sensitization/recall.

Interactions

Drug-Drug: QT interval prolonging drugs may ↑ the risk of QT interval prolongation with arrhythmias; concurrent use contraindicated. Concurrent use with **agents with narrow therapeutic indices that are metabolized by the CYP1A2 enzyme systems** not recommended. Consider dose ↓ of substrates. Strong CYP3A inhibitors, including **atazanavir**, **clarithromycin**, **indinavir**, **itraconazole**, **ketoconazole**, **nefazodone**, **nelfinavir**, **ritonavir**, **saquinavir**, **telithromycin** and **voriconazole** may ↑ levels and effects; avoid concurrent use. Strong inducers of CYP3A4 including **carbamazepine**, **phenobarbital**, **phenytoin**, **rifabutin**, **rifampin**, **rifapentine** may ↓ levels and effectiveness; avoid concurrent use. May ↑ risk of bleeding with **warfarin**. Concurrent use with **ipilimumab** may ↑ risk of hepatotoxicity. May ↑ **digoxin** levels and lead to toxicity.

Route/Dosage

PO (Adults): 960 mg twice daily. Treatment should continue until unacceptable toxicity or disease progression occurs.

Availability

Tablets: 240 mg.

NURSING IMPLICATIONS

Assessment

- Perform dermatologic evaluation prior to initiation and every 2 mo during therapy. Excise any suspicious lesions, send for dermapathologic evaluation, and treat with standard care. Continue monitoring for 6 mo following discontinuation of therapy.
- Monitor ECG 15 days after initiation of therapy, monthly during first 3 mo, every 3 mo thereafter, and more often if clinically indicated.
- Monitor for hypersensitivity reactions (rash, erythema, hypotension). Permanently discontinue therapy if severe reaction occurs.
- Monitor for signs and symptoms of uveitis periodically during therapy. May require treatment with steroid and mydriatic ophthalmic drops.
- Assess patient for rash (mild to moderate rash usually occurs in the 2nd wk of therapy and resolves within 1–2 wk of continued therapy). If rash is severe (extensive erythematous or maculopapular rash with moist desquamation or angioedema) or accompanied by systemic symptoms (serum sickness-like reaction, Stevens-Johnson syndrome, toxic epidermal necrolysis), therapy must be discontinued immediately.
- ***Lab Test Considerations:*** Monitor serum potassium, magnesium, and calcium before starting therapy and after dose modification.
- Monitor AST, ALT, alkaline phosphatase, and bilirubin before starting therapy, monthly during therapy, and as clinically indicated. May require dose reduction, treatment interruption or discontinuation.

Potential Nursing Diagnoses

Impaired skin integrity (Indications)

Implementation

- **PO:** Administer (four 240 mg tablets) twice daily, without regard to food. Take first dose in the morning with second dose about 12 hrs later. Swallow tablets whole, do not crush or chew.
- Adverse reactions or QTc prolongation may occur requiring dose modification. *If Grade 1 or 2 (tolerable) occur,* maintain dose at 960 mg twice daily. *If Grade 2 (Intolerable) or Grade 3, 1st appearance occurs,* interrupt therapy until Grade 0–1. Resume dosing at 720 mg twice daily. *If 2nd appearance,* interrupt therapy until Grade 0–1. Resume dosing at 480 mg twice daily. *If 3rd appearance,* discontinue permanently. *If Grade 4, 1st appearance occurs,* discontinue permanently or interrupt therapy until Grade 0–1. Resume dosing at 480 twice daily. *If 2nd appearance,* discontinue permanently. Doses below 480 mg twice daily are not recommended.

Patient/Family Teaching

- Instruct patient to take venurafenib as directed. If vomiting occurs, do not an additional dose, take next dose as scheduled. Take missed doses as soon as remembered up to 4 hrs before next dose; do not double dose.
- 🧬 Inform patient that assessment of BRAF mutation is required for selection of patients.
- Instruct patient to stop taking vemurafenib and notify health care professional immediately if signs and symptoms of allergic reaction (rash or redness all over body; feeling faint; difficulty breathing or swallowing; throat tightness or hoarseness; fast heartbeat; swelling of face, lips, or tongue) or severe skin reactions (blisters on skin; blisters or sores in mouth; peeling of skin, fever, redness or swelling of face, hands, or soles of feet) occur.
- Advise patient to wear broad spectrum UVA/UVB sunscreen, lip balm (SPF ≥30) and protective clothing, and to avoid sun exposure to prevent photosensitivity reactions. Severe photosensitivity reactions may require dose modifications.

- Advise patient to notify health care professional if signs and symptoms of liver dysfunction (yellow skin or whites of eyes; feeling tired; urine turns dark or brown; nausea or vomiting; loss of appetite; pain on right side of stomach) or eye problems (eye pain, swelling, or redness; blurred vision; vision changes) occur.
- Instruct patient to notify health care professional of all Rx or OTC medications, vitamins, or herbal products being taken and consult health care professional before taking any new medications.
- Inform patient that regular assessments of skin and assessments for signs and symptoms of other malignancies must be done during and for up to 6 mo after therapy. Advise patient to notify health care professional immediately if any changes in skin occur.
- Rep: Advise women of childbearing potential and men to use appropriate contraceptive measures during and for at least 2 mo after discontinuation of vemurafenib, and to avoid breast feeding.

Evaluation/Desired Outcomes

- Decreased spread of melanoma.

venlafaxine (ven-la-**fax**-een)

~~Effexor~~, Effexor XR

Classification

Therapeutic: antidepressants, antianxiety agents

Pharmacologic: selective serotonin/norepinephrine reuptake inhibitors

Pregnancy Category C

Indications

Major depressive disorder. Generalized anxiety disorder (Effexor XR only). Social anxiety disorder (Effexor XR only). Panic disorder (Effexor XR only). **Unlabeled Use:** Premenstrual dysphoric disorder.

Action

Inhibits serotonin and norepinephrine reuptake in the CNS. **Therapeutic Effects:** Decrease in depressive symptomatology, with fewer relapses/recurrences. Decreased anxiety. Decrease in panic attacks.

Pharmacokinetics

Absorption: 92–100% absorbed after oral administration.

Distribution: Extensive distribution into body tissues.

Metabolism and Excretion: Extensively metabolized on first pass through the liver (primarily through CYP2D6 enzyme pathway). A small percentage of the population are poor metabolizers and will have higher blood levels with ↑ effects. One metabolite, O-desmethylvenlafaxine (ODV), has antidepressant activity; 5% of venlafaxine is excreted unchanged in urine; 30% of the active metabolite is excreted in urine.

Half-life: *Venlafaxine*—3–5 hr; *ODV*—9–11 hr (both are ↑ in hepatic/renal impairment).

TIME/ACTION PROFILE (antidepressant action)

ROUTE	ONSET	PEAK	DURATION
PO	within 2 wk	2–4 wk	unknown

Contraindications/Precautions

Contraindicated in: Hypersensitivity; Concurrent use of MAO inhibitors or MAO-like drugs (linezolid or methylene blue).

Use Cautiously in: Cardiovascular disease, including hypertension; Hepatic impairment (↓ dose recommended); Impaired renal function (↓ dose recommended); History of seizures or neurologic impairment; History of mania; History of drug abuse; Angle-closure glaucoma; OB: Use only if clearly required, weighing benefit to mother versus potential harm to fetus (potential for discontinuation syndrome or toxicity in the neonate when venlafaxine is taken during the 3rd trimester); Lactation: Potential for serious adverse reactions in infant; discontinue drug or discontinue breast feeding; Pedi: ↑ risk of suicidal thinking and behavior (suicidality) in children and adolescents with major depressive disorder and other psychiatric disorders. Observe closely for suicidality and behavior changes.

Adverse Reactions/Side Effects

CNS: NEUROLEPTIC MALIGNANT SYNDROME, SEIZURES, SUICIDAL THOUGHTS, abnormal dreams, anxiety, dizziness, headache, insomnia, nervousness, weakness, abnormal thinking, agitation, confusion, depersonalization, drowsiness, emotional lability, worsening depression. **EENT:** rhinitis, visual disturbances, epistaxis, tinnitus. **CV:** chest pain, hypertension, palpitations, tachycardia. **GI:** abdominal pain, altered taste, anorexia, constipation, diarrhea, dry mouth, dyspepsia, nausea, vomiting, weight loss. **GU:** sexual dysfunction, urinary frequency, urinary retention. **Derm:** ecchymoses, itching, photosensitivity, skin rash. **Neuro:** paresthesia, twitching. **Misc:** SEROTONIN SYNDROME, chills, bleeding, yawning.

Interactions

Drug-Drug: Concurrent use with **MAO inhibitors** may result in serious, potentially fatal reactions (wait at least 2 wk after stopping MAO inhibitor before initiating venlafaxine; wait at least 1 wk after stopping venlafaxine before starting MAO inhibitors). Concurrent use with **MAO-inhibitor like drugs**, such as **linezolid** or **methylene blue** may ↑ risk of serotonin syndrome; concurrent use contraindicated; do not start therapy in patients receiving **linezolid** or **methylene blue**; if **linezolid** or **methylene blue** need to be started in a patient receiving venlafaxine, immediately discontinue venlafaxine and monitor for signs/symptoms of serotonin syndrome for 2 wk or until 24 hr after last dose of linezolid or methylene blue, whichever comes first (may resume venlafaxine therapy 24 hr after last dose of linezolid or methylene blue). Concurrent use with **alcohol** or other **CNS depressants**, including **sedatives/hypnotics**, **antihistamines**, and **opioid analgesics** in depressed patients is not recommended. Drugs that affect serotonergic neurotransmitter systems, including **tricyclic antidepressants**, **SNRIs**, **fentanyl**, **buspirone**, **tramadol** and **triptans** ↑ risk of serotonin syndrome. **Lithium** may have ↑ serotonergic effects with venlafaxine; use cautiously in patients receiving venlafaxine. ↑ blood levels and may ↑ effects of **desipramine** and **haloperidol**. **Cimetidine** may ↑ the effects of venlafaxine (may be more pronounced in geriatric patients, those with hepatic or renal impairment, or those with pre-existing hypertension). **Ketoconazole** may ↑ the effects of venlafaxine. ↑ risk of bleeding with **NSAIDS**, **aspirin**, **clopidogrel**, or **warfarin**.

Drug-Natural Products: Concomitant use of **kava-kava**, **valerian**, **chamomile**, or **hops** can ↑ CNS depression. ↑ risk of serotinergic side effects including serotonin syndrome with **St. John's wort** and **SAMe**.

Route/Dosage

Major Depressive Disorder

PO (Adults): *Tablets*—75 mg/day in 2–3 divided doses; may ↑ by up to 75 mg/day every 4 days, up to 225 mg/day (not to exceed 375 mg/day in 3 divided doses); *Extended-release (XR) capsules*—75 mg once daily (some patients may be started at 37.5 mg once daily) for 4–7 days; may ↑ by up to 75 mg/day at intervals of not less than 4 days (not to exceed 225 mg/day).

General Anxiety Disorder

PO (Adults): *Extended-release (XR) capsules*—75 mg once daily (some patients may be started at 37.5 mg once daily) for 4–7 days; may ↑ by up to 75 mg/day at intervals of not less than 4 days (not to exceed 225 mg/day).

Social Anxiety Disorder

PO (Adults): *Extended-release (XR) capsules*—75 mg once daily.

Panic Disorder

PO (Adults): *Extended-release (XR) capsules*—37.5 mg once daily for 7 days; may then ↑ to 75 mg once daily; may then ↑ by 75 mg/day every 7 days (not to exceed 225 mg/day).

Hepatic Impairment

PO (Adults): ↓ daily dose by 50% in patients with mild-to-moderate hepatic impairment.

Renal Impairment

PO (Adults): *CCr 10–70 mL/min*—↓ daily dose by 25–50%; *Hemodialysis*—↓ daily dose by 50%.

Availability (generic available)

Tablets: 25 mg, 37.5 mg, 50 mg, 75 mg, 100 mg. **Cost:** *Generic*—25 mg $32.24/100, 37.5 mg $39.41/100, 75 mg $38.00/100. **Extended-release capsules:** 37.5 mg, 75 mg, 150 mg, 225 mg. **Cost:** *Generic*—37.5 mg $32.14/90, 75 mg $271.37/100, 150 mg $29.94/100.

NURSING IMPLICATIONS

Assessment

- Assess mental status and mood changes. Inform health care professional if patient demonstrates significant increase in anxiety, nervousness, or insomnia.
- Assess suicidal tendencies, especially in early therapy. Restrict amount of drug available to patient. Risk may be increased in children, adolescents, and adults ≤24 yr.
- Monitor BP before and periodically during therapy. Sustained hypertension may be dose-related; decrease dose or discontinue therapy if this occurs.
- Monitor appetite and nutritional intake. Weigh weekly. Report continued weight loss. Adjust diet as tolerated to support nutritional status.
- Assess for serotonin syndrome (mental changes [agitation, hallucinations, coma], autonomic instability [tachycardia, labile BP, hyperthermia], neuromuscular aberrations [hyper-reflexia, incoordination], and/or GI symptoms [nausea, vomiting, diarrhea]), especially in patients taking other serotonergic drugs (SSRIs, SNRIs, triptans).
- ***Lab Test Considerations:*** Monitor CBC with differential and platelet count periodically during therapy. May cause anemia, leukocytosis, leukopenia, thrombocytopenia, basophilia, and eosinophilia.
- May cause an ↑ in serum alkaline phosphatase, bilirubin, AST, ALT, BUN, and creatinine.
- May also cause ↑ serum cholesterol.
- May cause electrolyte abnormalities (hyperglycemia or hypoglycemia, hyperkalemia or hypokalemia, hyperuricemia, hyperphosphatemia or hypophosphatemia, and hyponatremia).
- May cause false-positive immunoassay screening tests for phencyclidine (PCP) and amphetamine.

Potential Nursing Diagnoses

Ineffective coping (Indications)
Risk for injury (Side Effects)

Implementation

- **PO:** Administer venlafaxine with food.
- Extended-release capsules should be swallowed whole; do not crush, break, or chew.

V

- Extended-release capsules may be opened and contents sprinkled on a spoonful of applesauce. Take immediately and follow with a glass of water. Do not store mixture for later use.

Patient/Family Teaching

- Instruct patient to take venlafaxine as directed at the same time each day. Take missed doses as soon as possible unless almost time for next dose. Do not double doses or discontinue abruptly. Patients taking venlafaxine for >6 wk should have dose gradually decreased before discontinuation.
- Advise patient, family, and caregivers to look for suicidality, especially during early therapy or dose changes. Notify health care professional immediately if thoughts about suicide or dying, attempts to commit suicide; new or worse depression or anxiety; agitation or restlessness; panic attacks; insomnia; new or worse irritability; aggressiveness; acting on dangerous impulses, mania, or other changes in mood or behavior or if symptoms of serotonin syndrome occur.
- May cause drowsiness or dizziness. Caution patient to avoid driving or other activities requiring alertness until response to the drug is known.
- Instruct patient to notify health care professional of all Rx or OTC medications, vitamins, or herbal products being taken and consult health care professional before taking any new medications. Caution patient to avoid taking alcohol or other CNS-depressant drugs during therapy.
- Instruct patient to notify health care professional if signs of allergy (rash, hives) occur.
- Instruct female patients to inform health care professional if pregnancy is planned or suspected or if breast feeding.
- Emphasize the importance of follow-up exams to monitor progress. Encourage patient participation in psychotherapy.

Evaluation/Desired Outcomes

- Increased sense of well-being.
- Renewed interest in surroundings. Need for therapy should be periodically reassessed. Therapy is usually continued for several months.
- Decreased anxiety.

verapamil (ver-ap-a-mil)

Calan, Calan SR, Isoptin SR, Verelan, Verelan PM

Classification

Therapeutic: antianginals, antiarrhythmics (class IV), antihypertensives, vascular headache suppressants
Pharmacologic: calcium channel blockers

Pregnancy Category C

Indications

Management of hypertension, angina pectoris, and/or vasospastic (Prinzmetal's) angina. Management of supraventricular arrhythmias and rapid ventricular rates in atrial flutter or fibrillation. **Unlabeled Use:** Prevention of migraine headache.

Action

Inhibits the transport of calcium into myocardial and vascular smooth muscle cells, resulting in inhibition of excitation-contraction coupling and subsequent contraction. Decreases SA and AV conduction and prolongs AV node refractory period in conduction tissue. **Therapeutic Effects:** Systemic vasodilation resulting in decreased BP. Coronary vasodilation resulting in decreased frequency and severity of attacks of angina. Reduction of ventricular rate during atrial fibrillation or flutter.

Pharmacokinetics

Absorption: 90% absorbed after oral administration, but much is rapidly metabolized, resulting in bioavailability of 20–25%.
Distribution: Small amounts enter breast milk.
Protein Binding: 90%.
Metabolism and Excretion: Mostly metabolized by the liver (primarily by CYP3A4).
Half-life: 4.5–12 hr.

TIME/ACTION PROFILE (cardiovascular effects)

ROUTE	ONSET	PEAK	DURATION
PO	1–2 hr	30–90 min†	3–7 hr
PO-ER	unknown	5–7 hr	24 hr
IV	1–5 min‡	3–5 min	2 hr‡

†Single dose; effects from multiple doses may not be evident for 24–48 hr.
‡Antiarrhythmic effects; hemodynamic effects begin 3–5 min after injection and persist for 10–20 min.

Contraindications/Precautions

Contraindicated in: Hypersensitivity; Sick sinus syndrome; 2nd- or 3rd-degree AV block (unless an artificial pacemaker is in place); Systolic BP <90 mm Hg; HF, severe ventricular dysfunction, or cardiogenic shock, unless associated with supraventricular tachyarrhythmias; Concurrent IV beta blocker therapy.
Use Cautiously in: Severe hepatic impairment (dose ↓ recommended); History of serious ventricular arrhythmias or HF; Geri: Dose ↓/slower IV infusion rates recommended (↑ risk of hypotension); OB, Lactation: Safety not established.

Adverse Reactions/Side Effects

CNS: abnormal dreams, anxiety, confusion, dizziness/lightheadedness, drowsiness, extrapyramidal reactions, headache, jitteriness, nervousness, psychiatric disturbances, weakness. **EENT:** blurred vision, disturbed equilibrium, epistaxis, tinnitus. **Resp:** cough, dyspnea, shortness of breath. **CV:** ARRHYTHMIAS, HF, bradycardia, chest pain, hypotension, palpitations, peripheral edema, syncope, tachycardia. **GI:** ↑ liver enzymes, anorexia, constipation, diarrhea, dry mouth, dysgeusia, dyspepsia, nausea, vomiting. **GU:** dysuria, nocturia, polyuria, sexual dysfunction, urinary frequency. **Derm:** STEVENS-JOHNSON SYNDROME, dermatitis, erythema multiforme, flushing, photosensitivity, pruritus/urticaria, rash, sweating. **Endo:** gynecomastia, hyperglycemia. **Hemat:** anemia, leukopenia, thrombocytopenia. **Metab:** weight gain. **MS:** joint stiffness, muscle cramps. **Neuro:** paresthesia, tremor. **Misc:** gingival hyperplasia.

Interactions

Drug-Drug: Additive hypotension may occur when used concurrently with **fentanyl**, other **antihypertensives**, **nitrates**, acute ingestion of **alcohol**, or **quinidine**. Antihypertensive effects may be ↓ by concurrent use of **NSAIDs**. Serum **digoxin** levels may be ↑. Concurrent use with **beta blockers**, **digoxin**, **disopyramide**, **clonidine**, or **phenytoin** may result in bradycardia, conduction defects, or HF. ↑ risk of hypotension and bradycardia with **erythromycin**, **clarithromycin**, **telithromycin**, or **ritonavir**. May ↓ metabolism of and ↑ risk of toxicity from **cyclosporine**, **prazosin**, **quinidine**, or **carbamazepine**. May ↓ effectiveness of **rifampin**. ↑ the muscle-paralyzing effects of **nondepolarizing neuromuscular-blocking agents**. Effectiveness may be ↓ by coadministration with **vitamin D compounds** and **calcium**. May alter serum **lithium** levels. May ↑ **doxorubicin** and **paclitaxel** levels. May ↑ risk of bleeding with **aspirin**.
Drug-Natural Products: ↑ **caffeine** levels with caffeine-containing herbs (**cola nut**, **guarana**, **mate**, **tea**, **coffee**).
Drug-Food: Grapefruit juice ↑ serum levels and effect.

Route/Dosage

PO (Adults): 80–120 mg 3 times daily, ↑ as needed. *Patients with hepatic impairment or geriatric patients*—40 mg 3 times daily initially. *Extended-release preparations*—120–240 mg/day as a single dose; may be ↑ as needed (range 240–480 mg/day).
PO (Children up to 15 yr): 4–8 mg/kg/day in divided doses.
IV (Adults): 5–10 mg (75–150 mcg/kg); may repeat with 10 mg (150 mcg/kg) after 15–30 min.
IV (Children 1–15 yr): 2–5 mg (100–300 mcg/kg); may repeat after 30 min (initial dose not to exceed 5 mg; repeat dose not to exceed 10 mg).
IV (Children <1 yr): 0.75–2 mg (100–200 mcg/kg); may repeat after 30 min.

Availability (generic available)

Tablets: 40 mg, 80 mg, 120 mg. **Cost:** *Generic*—40 mg $21.85/100, 80 mg $10.83/100. **Extended-release tablets (Isoptin SR):** 120 mg, 180 mg, 240 mg. **Cost:** *Generic*—120 mg $31.44/100, 180 mg $35.98/100, 240 mg $27.80/100. **Extended-release capsules (Verelan PM):** 100 mg, 200 mg, 300 mg. **Cost:** *Generic*—100 mg $195.84/100, 200 mg $252.23/100, 300 mg $366.98/100. **Extended-release capsules (Verelan):** 120 mg, 180 mg, 240 mg, 360 mg. **Cost:** *Generic*—120 mg $130.25/100, 180 mg $135.16/100, 240 mg $152.54/100, 360 mg $209.94/100. **Solution for injection:** 2.5 mg/mL. ***In combination with:*** trandolapril (Tarka); see Appendix B.

NURSING IMPLICATIONS

Assessment

- Monitor BP and pulse before therapy, during dosage titration, and periodically throughout therapy. Monitor ECG periodically during prolonged therapy. Verapamil may cause prolonged PR interval.
- Monitor intake and output ratios and daily weight. Assess for signs of HF (peripheral edema, rales/crackles, dyspnea, weight gain, jugular venous distention).
- Patients receiving digoxin concurrently with calcium channel blockers should have routine serum digoxin levels and be monitored for signs and symptoms of digoxin toxicity.
- Assess for rash periodically during therapy. May cause Stevens-Johnson syndrome. Discontinue therapy if severe or if accompanied with fever, general malaise, fatigue, muscle or joint aches, blisters, oral lesions, conjunctivitis, hepatitis and/or eosinophilia.
- **Angina:** Assess location, duration, intensity, and precipitating factors of patient's anginal pain.
- **Arrhythmias:** Monitor ECG continuously during administration. Notify health care professional promptly if bradycardia or prolonged hypotension occurs. Emergency equipment and medication should be available. Monitor BP and pulse before and frequently during administration.
- ***Lab Test Considerations:*** Total serum calcium concentrations are not affected by calcium channel blockers.
- Monitor serum potassium periodically. Hypokalemia ↑ risk of arrhythmias and should be corrected.
- Monitor renal and hepatic functions periodically during long-term therapy. May cause ↑ hepatic enzymes after several days of therapy, which return to normal on discontinuation of therapy.

Potential Nursing Diagnoses

Decreased cardiac output (Indications)
Acute pain (Indications)

Implementation

- **PO:** Administer verapamil with meals or milk to minimize gastric irritation.

V

- Do not open, crush, break, or chew sustained-release capsules or tablets. Empty tablets that appear in stool are not significant.

IV Administration

- **IV:** Patients should remain recumbent for at least 1 hr after IV administration to minimize hypotensive effects.
- **IV Push:** ***Diluent:*** Administer undiluted. ***Concentration:*** 2.5 mg/mL. ***Rate:*** Administer over 2 min. Geri: Administer over 3 min.
- **Y-Site Compatibility:** alemtuzumab, alfentanil, amikacin, aminocaproic acid, amphotericin B lipid complex, anidulafungin, argatroban, ascorbic acid, atracurium, atropine, aztreonam, benztropine, bivalirudin, bleomycin, bumetanide, buprenorphine, butorphanol, calcium chloride, calcium gluconate, carboplatin, carmustine, caspofungin, cefazolin, cefotaxime, cefotetan, cefoxitin, ceftriaxone, cefuroxime, chlorpromazine, ciprofloxacin, cisplatin, clindamycin, cyanocobalamin, cyclophosphamide, cyclosporine, cytarabine, dactinomycin, daptomycin, dexamethasone, dexmedetomidine, dexrazoxane, digoxin, diltiazem, diphenhydramine, dobutamine, docetaxel, dolasetron, dopamine, doxorubicin hydrochloride, doxorubicin liposomal, doxycycline, enalaprilat, ephedrine, epinephrine, epirubicin, epotein alfa, eptifibatide, erythromycin, esmolol, etoposide, etoposide phosphate, famotidine, fenoldopam, fentanyl, fluconazole, fludarabine, gemcitabine, gentamicin, glycopyrrolate, granisetron, heparin, hydrocortisone sodium succinate, hydromorphone, idarubicin, ifosfamide, imipenem/cilastatin, insulin, irinotecan, isoproterenol, ketorolac, labetalol, leucovorin calcium, levofloxacin, lidocaine, linezolid, lorazepam, magnesium sulfate, mannitol, mechlorethamine, meperidine, metaraminol, methotrexate, methyldopate, methylprednisolone sodium succinate, metoclopramide, metoprolol, metronidazole, midazolam, milrinone, mitoxantrone, morphine, moxifloxacin, multivitamins, mycophenolate, nalbuphine, naloxone, nesiritide, nitroglycerin, nitroprusside, norepinephrine, octreotide, ondansetron, oxaliplatin, oxytocin, paclitaxel, palonosetron, pamidronate, pancuronium, papaverine, pemetrexed, penicillin G, pentamidine, pentazocine, phentolamine, phenylephrine, phytonadione, potassium acetate, potassium chloride, procainamide, prochlorperazine, promethazine, propranolol, protamine, pyridoxime, quinupristin/dalfopristin, ranitidine, rocuronium, sodium acetate, streptokinase, succinylcholine, sufentanil, tacrolimus, teniposide, theophylline, thiamine, tirofiban, tobramycin, tolazoline, vancomycin, vasopressin, vecuronium, vinblastine, vincristine, vinorelbine, voriconazole, zoledronic acid.
- **Y-Site Incompatibility:** acyclovir, albumin, aminophylline, amphotericin B cholesteryl, amphotericin B colloidal, amphotericin B liposome, ampicillin, ampicillin/sulbactam, azathioprine, ceftazidime, chloramphenicol, dantrolene, diazepam, diazoxide, ertapenem, fluorouracil, folic acid, foscarnet, furosemide, ganciclovir, indomethacin, pantoprazole, pentobarbital, phenobarbital, phenytoin, piperacillin/tazobactam, propofol, sodium bicarbonate, thiotepa, tigecycline, trimethoprim/sulfamethoxazole.

Patient/Family Teaching

- Advise patient to take medication as directed, even if feeling well. Take missed doses as soon as possible unless almost time for next dose; do not double doses. May need to be discontinued gradually.
- Advise patient to avoid large amounts (6–8 glasses of grapefruit juice/day) during therapy.
- Instruct patient on correct technique for monitoring pulse. Instruct patient to contact health care professional if heart rate is <50 bpm.
- Caution patient to change positions slowly to minimize orthostatic hypotension.
- May cause drowsiness or dizziness. Advise patient to avoid driving or other activities requiring alertness until response to the medication is known.
- Instruct patient on importance of maintaining good dental hygiene and seeing dentist frequently for teeth cleaning to prevent tenderness, bleeding, and gingival hyperplasia (gum enlargement).
- Instruct patient to notify health care professional of all Rx or OTC medications, vitamins, or herbal products being taken and consult health care professional before taking any new medications, especially cold preparations.
- Advise patient to notify health care professional if irregular heartbeats, rash, dyspnea, swelling of hands and feet, pronounced dizziness, nausea, constipation, or hypotension occurs or if headache is severe or persistent.
- Caution patient to wear protective clothing and use sunscreen to prevent photosensitivity reactions.
- **Angina:** Instruct patient on concurrent nitrate or beta-blocker therapy to continue taking both medications as directed and use SL nitroglycerin as needed for anginal attacks.
- Advise patient to contact health care professional if chest pain does not improve, worsens after therapy, or occurs with diaphoresis; if shortness of breath occurs; or if severe, persistent headache occurs.
- Caution patient to discuss exercise restrictions with health care professional before exertion.
- **Hypertension:** Encourage patient to comply with other interventions for hypertension (weight reduction, low-sodium diet, smoking cessation, moderation of alcohol consumption, regular exercise, and stress management). Medication controls but does not cure hypertension.
- Instruct patient and family in proper technique for monitoring BP. Advise patient to take BP weekly and to report significant changes to health care professional.

Evaluation/Desired Outcomes

- Decrease in BP.
- Decrease in frequency and severity of anginal attacks.
- Decrease in need for nitrate therapy.
- Increase in activity tolerance and sense of well-being.
- Suppression and prevention of atrial tachyarrhythmias.

REMS

vigabatrin (vye-gah-bat-rin)

Sabril

Classification
Therapeutic: anticonvulsants

Pregnancy Category C

Indications

Management (adjunctive) of refractory complex partial seizures in patients who have responded inadequately to several alternative treatments (and where potential benefit outweighs risk of vision loss); not a first-line treatment. Management of infantile spasms (IS).

Action

Acts an irreversible inhibitor of γ-aminobutyric acid transaminase (GABA-T), the enzyme responsible for the metabolism of the inhibitory neurotransmitter GABA. This action results in increased levels of GABA in the central nervous system. **Therapeutic Effects:** Decreased incidence and severity of refractory complex partial seizures.

Pharmacokinetics

Absorption: Completely absorbed following oral administration.
Distribution: Enters breast milk, remainder of distribution unknown.
Protein Binding: None.
Metabolism and Excretion: Minimal metabolism, mostly eliminated unchanged in urine.
Half-life: 7.5 hr.

TIME/ACTION PROFILE (anticonvulsant effect)

ROUTE	ONSET	PEAK	DURATION
PO	unknown	1 hr†	12 hr‡

†blood level.
‡clinical benefit should be seen in 2–4 week for IS or within 3 mo for complex partial seizures.

Contraindications/Precautions

Contraindicated in: History or high risk of other types of irreversible vision loss unless benefits of treatment clearly outweigh risks; OB: Use only if the potential benefit justifies the potential risk to the fetus (may cause fetal harm); Lactation: Enters breast milk; breast feeding should be avoided.
Use Cautiously in: Renal impairment (dose modification recommended for CCr <50 mL/min); History of suicidal ideation; Geri: Consider age-related ↓ in renal function adjust dose accordingly (↑ risk of sedation/confusion); Pedi: Abnormal MRI signal changes have been seen in infants.

Adverse Reactions/Side Effects

CNS: SUICIDAL THOUGHTS, confusional state, memory impairment, drowsiness, fatigue. **CV:** edema. **Derm:** STEVENS-JOHNSON SYNDROME, TOXIC EPIDERMAL NECROLYSIS. **EENT:** blurred vision, nystagmus, vision loss. **Hemat:** anemia. **Metab:** weight gain. **MS:** arthralgia. **Neuro:** abnormal coordination, tremor, peripheral neuropathy.

Interactions

Drug-Drug: Should not be used concurrently with other **drugs having adverse ocular effects**; ↑ risk of additive toxicity. May ↓ **phenytoin** levels and effectiveness.

Route/Dosage

Refractory Complex Partial Seizures

PO (Adults and Children >16 yr): 500 mg twice daily initially, may be ↑ in 500 mg increments every 7 days depending on response up to 1500 mg twice daily.
PO (Children 10–16 yr and >60 kg): 500 mg twice daily initially, may be ↑ in 500 mg increments every 7 days depending on response up to 1500 mg twice daily.
PO (Children 10–16 yr and 25–60 kg): 250 mg twice daily initially, may be ↑ every 7 days depending on response up to 1000 mg twice daily.

V

Renal Impairment

PO (Adults and Children ≥10 yr and ≥25 kg): *CCr >50–80 mL/min*—↓ dose by 25%; *CCr >30–50 mL/min*—↓ dose by 50%; *CCr >10–30 mL/min*—↓ dose by 75%.

Infantile Spasms

PO (Children 1 mo–2 yr): 50 mg/kg/day given in 2 divided doses initially, ↑ by 25-50 mg/kg/day increments every 3 days up to a maximum of 150 mg/kg/day; dosage adjustments are necessary for renal impairment.

Availability

Tablets: 500 mg. **Powder packets for oral solution:** 500 mg/packet.

NURSING IMPLICATIONS

Assessment

- Assess location, duration, and characteristics of seizure activity. Institute seizure precautions. Assess response to and continued need for vigabatrin periodically during therapy.

- Monitor closely for notable changes in behavior that could indicate the emergence or worsening of suicidal thoughts or behavior or depression.
- Test vision at baseline (no later than 4 wks after starting), at least every 3 months during, and 3–6 months after discontinuation of therapy.
- Assess for signs and symptoms of peripheral neuropathy (numbness or tingling or toes or feet, reduced lower limb vibration or position sensation, progressive loss of reflexes, starting at ankles).
- Assess for rash periodically during therapy. May cause Stevens-Johnson syndrome. Discontinue therapy if severe or if accompanied with fever, general malaise, fatigue, muscle or joint aches, blisters, oral lesions, conjunctivitis, hepatitis and/or eosinophilia.
- ***Lab Test Considerations:*** Monitor CBC periodically during therapy. May cause anemia.
- May cause ↓ AST and ALT levels precluding use to detect hepatic injury.
- May ↑ amino acids in urine causing false positive results of genetic metabolic diseases.

Potential Nursing Diagnoses

Risk for injury (Indications)
Disturbed sensory perception (Adverse Reactions)

Implementation

- Available only through *SHARE* program of restricted distribution. Only prescribers and pharmacies registered in the program and patients enrolled in the program have access. Patients receive vigabatrin from a specialty pharmacy. Contact *SHARE* program at 1-888-45-SHARE.
- **PO:** Administer twice daily without regard to food.
- Mix oral solution for babies by mixing the powder in each packet with 10 mL of water; may be cold or room temperature. Follow manufacturer's instruction for mixing oral solution. Oral solution may be administered at the same time as food, but should only be mixed with water.

Patient/Family Teaching

- Enroll patient in *SHARE* Program. Instruct patient to take vigabatrin around the clock, as directed. Discuss with health care professional what to do if a dose is missed. Medication should be gradually discontinued to prevent seizures. Advise patient to read the *Medication Guide* before starting therapy and with each Rx refill in case of changes.
- Educate patient on risks of vigabatrin. Inform patient of the risk of permanent vision loss, particularly loss of peripheral vision, and that vision loss may not be detected before it is severe and is irreversible. Emphasize the importance of monitoring vision every 3 months. Advise patient to notify health care professional immediately if changes in vision (not seeing as well as before starting therapy, tripping, bumping into things, more clumsy than usual, surprised by people or things coming in front of you that seem to come out of nowhere) or changes in infant's vision are suspected.
- May cause drowsiness, ataxia, fatigue and confusion. Caution patient to avoid driving or other activities requiring alertness until response to medication is known. Tell patient not to resume driving until physician gives clearance based on control of seizure disorder.
- Inform patients and families of risk of suicidal thoughts and behavior and advise that behavioral changes, emergency or worsening signs and symptoms of depression, unusual changes in mood, or emergence of suicidal thoughts, behavior, or thoughts of self-harm or rash should be reported to health care professional immediately.
- Advise patient to notify health care professional if an increase in seizures, weight gain, or edema occurs or if sleepiness, ear infection, or irritability occurs in an infant.
- Instruct patient to notify health care professional of all Rx or OTC medications, vitamins, or herbal products being taken, to consult health care professional before taking any new medications and to avoid taking alcohol or other CNS depressants concurrently with lacosamide.
- Advise female patients to notify health care professional if pregnancy is planned or suspected or if breast feeding. Encourage pregnant patients to enroll in the North American Antiepileptic Drug (NAAED) Pregnancy Registry by calling 1-888-233-2334; information is available at www.aedpregnancyregistry.org.

Evaluation/Desired Outcomes

- Decreased seizure activity. If no substantial clinical benefit within 3 months of initiation, discontinue vigabatrin.
- Decreased in infantile spasms. If no substantial clinical benefit within 2–4 wk of initiation, discontinue vigabatrin.

vilazodone (vil-az-oh-done)

Viibryd

Classification

Therapeutic: antidepressants
Pharmacologic: selective serotonin reuptake inhibitors (SSRIs), benzofurans

Pregnancy Category C

Indications

Treatment of major depressive disorder.

Action

Increases serotonin activity in the CNS by inhibiting serotonin reuptake. Also binds selectively with high affinity to 5-HT_{1A} receptors and is a 5-HT_{1A} receptor partial agonist. **Therapeutic Effects:** Improvement in symptoms of depression.

Pharmacokinetics

Absorption: 72% absorbed following oral administration with food.

Distribution: Unknown.

Protein Binding: 96–99%.

Metabolism and Excretion: Mostly metabolized by the liver, primarily by the CYP3A4 enzyme system; 1% excreted unchanged in urine.

Half-life: 25 hr.

TIME/ACTION PROFILE (blood levels)

ROUTE	ONSET	PEAK	DURATION
PO	unknown	4–5 hr	unknown

Contraindications/Precautions

Contraindicated in: Concurrent use of MAO inhibitors or MAO-like drugs (linezolid or methylene blue).

Use Cautiously in: History of seizure disorder; History of suicide attempt/suicidal ideation; Bipolar disorder; may ↑ risk of mania/hypomania; Angle-closure glaucoma; OB: Use only if maternal benefit outweighs fetal risk; use during third trimester may result in need for prolonged hospitalization, respiratory support and tube feeding; Lactation: Breast feed only if maternal benefit outweighs newborn risk; Pedi: Safety and effectiveness not established; ↑ risk of suicidal thinking/behavior in children, adolescents and young adults.

Adverse Reactions/Side Effects

CNS: NEUROLEPTIC MALIGNANT-LIKE SYNDROME, SEIZURES, SUICIDAL THOUGHTS, insomnia, abnormal dreams, dizziness. **GI:** diarrhea, nausea, dry mouth, restlessness, vomiting. **Endo:** ↓ libido, sexual dysfunction, syndrome of inappropriate antidiuretic hormone (SIADH). **F and E:** hyponatremia. **Hemat:** bleeding. **Misc:** SEROTONIN SYNDROME.

Interactions

Drug-Drug: Concurrent use with, or use within 14 days of starting or stopping **MAOIs** may ↑ risk of neuroleptic malignant syndrome or serotonin syndrome and should be avoided. Concurrent use with **MAO-inhibitor like drugs**, such as **linezolid** or **methylene blue** may ↑ risk of serotonin syndrome; concurrent use contraindicated; do not start therapy in patients receiving **linezolid** or **methylene blue**; if **linezolid** or **methylene blue** need to be started in a patient receiving vilazodone, immediately discontinue vilazodone and monitor for signs/symptoms of serotonin syndrome for 2 wk or until 24 hr after last dose of linezolid or methylene blue, whichever comes first (may resume vilazodone therapy 24 hr after last dose of linezolid or methylene blue). Drugs that affect serotonergic neurotransmitter systems, including **tricyclic antidepressants**, **SNRIs**, **fentanyl**, **buspirone**, **tramadol** and **triptans** ↑ risk of serotonin syndrome. Concurrent use with **NSAIDs**, **aspirin**, **antiplatelet drugs**, or other **drugs that affect coagulation** may ↑ risk of bleeding. Concurrent use of **strong inhibitors of CYP3A4**, including **ketoconazole** ↑ blood levels and the risk of adverse reactions/toxicity; daily dose should not exceed 20 mg. Concurrent use of **moderate inhibitors of CYP3A4**, including **erythromycin** may require dose ↓ to 20 mg daily if adverse reactions/toxicity occurs. Concurrent use of **strong inducers of CYP3A4**, including **carbamazepine** for >14 days may require ↑ dose up to 2–fold (do not exceed dose of 80 mg/day). Use cautiously with other **CNS-active drugs**.

Drug-Natural Products: ↑ risk of serotonin syndrome with **St. John's wort**.

Route/Dosage

PO (Adults): 10 mg once daily for one week, then 20 mg once daily for one week; dose may be ↑ to 40 mg once daily (recommended dose = 20–40 mg/day). *Concurrent use of strong inhibitors of CYP3A4*—daily dose should not exceed 20 mg; *Concurrent use of strong inducers of CYP3A4 (if used for >14 days)*—may need to ↑ dose up to 2–fold (daily dose should not exceed 80 mg).

Availability

Tablets: 10 mg, 20 mg, 40 mg.

NURSING IMPLICATIONS

Assessment

- Assess mental status and mood changes. Inform health care professional if patient demonstrates significant ↑ in anxiety, nervousness, or insomnia.
- Prior to starting therapy, screen patient for bipolar disorder (detailed psychiatric history, including family/personal history of suicide, bipolar disorder, depression). Use cautiously in patients with a positive history.
- Assess suicidal tendencies, especially in early therapy. Restrict amount of drug available to patient. Risk may be ↑ in children, adolescents, and adults ≤24 yr.
- Assess for signs and symptoms of hyponatremia (headache, difficulty concentrating, memory impairment, confusion, weakness, unsteadiness). May require discontinuation of therapy.
- Assess for serotonin syndrome (mental changes [agitation, hallucinations, coma], autonomic instability [tachycardia, labile BP, hyperthermia], neuromuscular aberrations [hyper-reflexia, incoordination], and/or GI symptoms [nausea, vomiting, diarrhea]), especially in patients taking other serotonergic drugs (SSRIs, SNRIs, triptans).
- Monitor for development of neuroleptic malignant syndrome (fever, muscle rigidity, altered mental

V

status, respiratory distress, tachycardia, seizures, diaphoresis, hypertension or hypotension, pallor, tiredness, loss of bladder control). Discontinue vilazodone and notify health care professional immediately if these symptoms occur.

- ***Lab Test Considerations:*** Monitor serum sodium concentrations periodically during therapy. May cause hyponatremia potentially as a result of syndrome of inappropriate antidiuretic hormone secretion (SIADH).
- May cause altered anticoagulant effects. Monitor patients receiving warfarin, NSAIDs, or aspirin concurrently.

Potential Nursing Diagnoses

Ineffective coping (Indications)
Risk for injury (Side Effects)

Implementation

- **PO:** Administer vilazodone with food; administration without food can result in inadequate drug concentrations and may ↓ effectiveness.
- When discontinuing therapy, decrease dose gradually; 40 mg once daily to 20 mg once daily for 4 days, followed by 10 mg once daily for 3 days. Taper patients taking 20 mg once daily dose to 10 mg once daily for 7 days. Stopping abruptly may cause flu-like symptoms (headache, sweating, and nausea), anxiety, high or low mood, irritability, feeling restless or sleepy, dizziness, electric shock-like sensations, tremor, and confusion.

Patient/Family Teaching

- Instruct patient to take vilazodone as directed at the same time each day. Take missed doses as soon as possible unless almost time for next dose. Do not double doses or discontinue abruptly. Gradually ↓ dose before discontinuation. Advise patient to read *Medication Guide* before starting therapy and with each Rx refill; new information may be available.
- Advise patient, family, and caregivers to look for activation of maina/hypomania and suicidality, especially during early therapy or dose changes. Notify health care professional immediately if thoughts about suicide or dying, attempts to commit suicide; new or worse depression or anxiety; agitation or restlessness; panic attacks; insomnia; new or worse irritability; aggressiveness; acting on dangerous impulses, mania, or other changes in mood or behavior or if symptoms of serotonin syndrome occur.
- Caution patient of the risk of serotonin syndrome and neuroleptic malignant syndrome, especially when taking triptans, tramadol, tryptophan supplements and other serotonergic or antipsychotic agents.
- May cause dizziness. Caution patient to avoid driving or other activities requiring alertness until response to the drug is known.
- Instruct patient to notify health care professional of all Rx or OTC medications, vitamins, or herbal products being taken and to avoid concurrent use of Rx, OTC, and herbal products, especially NSAIDs, aspirin, and warfarin, without consulting health care professional.
- Caution patient to avoid taking alcohol or other CNS-depressant drugs during therapy.
- Instruct female patients to inform health care professional if pregnancy is planned or suspected or if breast feeding.
- Emphasize the importance of follow-up exams to monitor progress. Encourage patient participation in psychotherapy.

Evaluation/Desired Outcomes

- ↑ sense of well-being.
- Renewed interest in surroundings. Need for therapy should be periodically reassessed. Therapy is usually continued for several months.
- ↓ anxiety.

HIGH ALERT

vinBLAStine (vin-**blass**-teen)

Classification
Therapeutic: antineoplastics
Pharmacologic: vinca alkaloids

Pregnancy Category D

Indications

Combination chemotherapy of: Lymphomas, Nonseminomatous testicular carcinoma, Advanced breast cancer, Other tumors.

Action

Binds to proteins of mitotic spindle, causing metaphase arrest. Cell replication is stopped as a result (cell cycle–specific for M phase). **Therapeutic Effects:** Death of rapidly replicating cells, particularly malignant ones. Has immunosuppressive properties.

Pharmacokinetics

Absorption: Administered IV only, resulting in complete bioavailability.
Distribution: Does not cross the blood-brain barrier well.
Metabolism and Excretion: Converted by the liver to an active antineoplastic compound; excreted in the feces via biliary excretion, some renal elimination.
Half-life: 24 hr.

TIME/ACTION PROFILE (effects on white blood cell counts)

ROUTE	ONSET	PEAK	DURATION
IV	5–7 days	10 days	7–14 days

Contraindications/Precautions

Contraindicated in: Hypersensitivity; OB, Lactation: Pregnancy or lactation.

Use Cautiously in: Infection; ↓ bone marrow reserve; Patients with impaired hepatic function (↓ dose by 50% if serum bilirubin >3 m g/dL); Rep: Women with childbearing potential.

Adverse Reactions/Side Effects

CNS: SEIZURES, mental depression, neurotoxicity, weakness. **Resp:** BRONCHOSPASM. **GI:** nausea, vomiting, anorexia, constipation, diarrhea, stomatitis. **GU:** gonadal suppression. **Derm:** alopecia, dermatitis, vesiculation. **Endo:** syndrome of inappropriate antidiuretic hormone (SIADH). **Hemat:** anemia, leukopenia, thrombocytopenia. **Local:** phlebitis at IV site. **Metab:** hyperuricemia. **Neuro:** neuritis, paresthesia, peripheral neuropathy.

Interactions

Drug-Drug: Additive bone marrow depression with other **antineoplastics** or **radiation therapy**. Bronchospasm may occur in patients who have been previously treated with **mitomycin**. May ↓ antibody response to **live-virus vaccines** and ↑ risk of adverse reactions. May ↓ **phenytoin** levels.

Route/Dosage

Doses may vary greatly, depending on tumor, schedule, condition of patient, and blood counts.

IV (Adults): *Initial*—3.7 mg/m^2 (100 mcg/kg), single dose; ↑ weekly as tolerated by 1.8 mg/m^2 (50 mcg/kg) to maximum of 18.5 mg/m^2 (usual dose is 5.5–7.4 mg/m^2). *Maintenance*—10 mg 1–2 times/mo or one increment less than last dose q 7–14 days.

IV (Children): *Initial*—2.5 mg/m^2, single dose; ↑ weekly as tolerated by 1.25 mg/m^2 to maximum of 7.5 mg/m^2. *Maintenance*—one increment less than last dose q 7 days.

Availability (generic available)

Solution for injection: 1 mg/mL. **Powder for injection (requires reconstitution):** 10 mg/vial.

NURSING IMPLICATIONS

Assessment

- Monitor BP, pulse, and respiratory rate during therapy. Bronchospasm can be life-threatening and may occur at time of infusion or several hours to weeks later.
- Monitor for bone marrow depression. Assess for bleeding (bleeding gums, bruising, petechiae, guaiac stools, urine, and emesis) and avoid IM injections and taking rectal temperatures if platelet count is low. Apply pressure to venipuncture sites for 10 min. Assess for signs of infection during neutropenia. Anemia may occur. Monitor for increased fatigue, dyspnea, and orthostatic hypotension.
- May cause nausea and vomiting. Monitor intake and output, appetite, and nutritional intake. Prophylactic antiemetics may be used. Adjust diet as tolerated.
- Assess injection site frequently for redness, irritation, or inflammation. If extravasation occurs, infusion must be stopped and restarted elsewhere to avoid damage to subcut tissue. Standard treatment includes infiltration with hyaluronidase and application of heat.
- Monitor for symptoms of gout (increased uric acid, joint pain, edema). Encourage patient to drink at least 2 L of fluid per day. Allopurinol or alkalinization of urine may be used to decrease uric acid levels.
- ***Lab Test Considerations:*** Monitor CBC prior to and routinely throughout therapy. If WBC <2000, subsequent doses are usually withheld until WBC is ≥4000. The nadir of leukopenia occurs in 5–10 days and recovery usually occurs 7–14 days later. Thrombocytopenia may also occur in patients who have received radiation or other chemotherapy agents.
- Monitor liver function studies (AST, ALT, LDH, bilirubin) and renal function studies (BUN, creatinine) prior to and periodically throughout therapy.
- May cause ↑ uric acid. Monitor periodically during therapy.

Potential Nursing Diagnoses

Risk for infection (Adverse Reactions)
Imbalanced nutrition: less than body requirements (Adverse Reactions)

Implementation

- ***High Alert:*** Fatalities have occurred with chemotherapeutic agents. Before administering, clarify all ambiguous orders; double check single, daily, and course-of-therapy dose limits; have second practitioner independently double check original order, dose calculations, and infusion pump settings. Do not administer subcut, IM, or intrathecally (IT). IT administration is fatal. Vinblastine must be dispensed in an overwrap stating, "For IV use only." Overwrap should remain in place until immediately before administration.
- ***High Alert:*** Do not confuse vinblastine with vincristine.
- Solution should be prepared in a biologic cabinet. Wear gloves, gown, and mask while handling medication. Discard IV equipment in specially designated containers.
- Do not inject into extremities with impaired circulation; may cause thrombophlebitis.

IV Administration

- **IV Push:** ***Diluent:*** Dilute each 10 mg with 10 mL of 0.9% NaCl for injection with phenol or benzyl alcohol. Solution is clear. Reconstituted medication is stable for 28 days if refrigerated. ***Concentration:*** 1 mg/mL. ***Rate:*** Administer each single dose over 1 min through Y-site injection of a free-flowing infusion of 0.9% NaCl or D5W.

- **Intermittent Infusion:** Dilution in large volumes (100–250 mL) or prolonged infusion (≥30 min) increases chance of vein irritation and extravasation.
- **Y-Site Compatibility:** acyclovir, alemtuzumab, alfentanil, allopurinol, amifostine, amikacin, aminophylline , amiodarone, amphotericin B lipid complex, ampicillin, ampicillin/sulbactam, anidulafungin, argatroban, aztreonam, bivalirudin, bleomycin, bumetanide, buprenorphine, busulfan, butorphanol, calcium chloride, calcium gluconate, carboplatin, carmustine, caspofungin, cefazolin, cefotaxime, cefotetan, cefoxitin, ceftazidime, ceftriaxone, cefuroxime, chloramphenicol, chlorpromazine, ciprofloxacin, cisatracurium, cisplatin, clindamycin, cyclophosphamide, cyclosporine, dacarbazine, dactinomycin, daptomycin, daunorubicin hydrochloride, dexamethasone, dexmedetomidine, dexrazoxane, digoxin, diltiazem, diphenhydramine, dobutamine, docetaxel, dolasetron, dopamine, doxorubicin hydrochloride, doxorubicin liposomal, doxycycline, droperidol, enalaprilat, ephedrine, epinephrine, epirubicin, ertapenem, erythromycin, esmolol, etoposide, etoposide phosphate, famotidine, fenoldopam, fentanyl, filgrastim, fluconazole, fludarabine, fluorouracil, foscarnet, fosphenytoin, ganciclovir, gemcitabine, gentamicin, glycopyrrolate, granisetron, haloperidol, heparin, hetastarch, hydralazine, hydrocortisone, hydromorphone, idarubicin, ifosfamide, imipenem/cilastatin, insulin, irinotecan, isoproterenol, ketorolac, labetalol, leucovorin calcium, levofloxacin, lidocaine, linezolid, lorazepam, magnesium sulfate, mannitol, mechlorethamine, melphalan, meperidine, meropenem, mesna, methotrexate, methyldopate, metoclopramide, metoprolol, metronidazole, midazolam, milrinone, mitomycin, mitoxantrone, morphine, moxifloxacin, nafcillin, nalbuphine, naloxone, nesiritide, nitroglycerin, nitroprusside, norepinephrine, octreotide, ondansetron, oxaliplatin, paclitaxel, palonosetron, pamidronate, pancuronium, pemetrexed, pentamidine, pentazocine, pentobarbital, phenobarbital, phenylephrine, piperacillin/tazobactam, potassium chloride, potassium phosphates, procainamide, prochlorperazine, promethazine, propranolol, quinupristin/dalfopristin, ranitidine, remifentanil, rituximab, sargramostim, sodium acetate, sodium bicarbonate, sodium phosphates, succinylcholine, sufentanil, tacrolimus, teniposide, theophylline, thiopental, thiotepa, tigecycline, tirofiban, tobramycin, topotecan, trastuzumab, tripmethoprim/sulfamethoxazole, vancomycin, vasopressin, vecuronium, verapamil, vincristine, vinorelbine, voriconazole, zidovudine, zoledronic acid.
- **Y-Site Incompatibility:** amphotericin B colloidal, amphotericin B liposome, cefepime, dantrolene, diazepam, furosemide, pantoprazole, phenytoin.

Patient/Family Teaching

- Advise patient to notify health care professional if fever; chills; sore throat; signs of infection; bleeding gums; bruising; petechiae; or blood in urine, stool, or emesis occurs. Caution patient to avoid crowds and persons with known infections. Instruct patient to use soft toothbrush and electric razor. Caution patient not to drink alcoholic beverages or take products containing aspirin or NSAIDs.
- Instruct patient to inspect oral mucosa for redness and ulceration. Advise patient that, if ulceration occurs, to avoid spicy foods, use sponge brush, and rinse mouth with water after eating and drinking. Topical agents may be used if mouth pain interferes with eating. Stomatitis pain may require treatment with opioid analgesics.
- Instruct patient to report symptoms of neurotoxicity (paresthesia, pain, difficulty walking, persistent constipation).
- Advise patient that jaw pain, pain in organs containing tumor tissue, nausea, and vomiting may occur. Avoid constipation and report other adverse reactions.
- Discuss with patient the possibility of hair loss. Explore coping strategies.
- Instruct patient not to receive any vaccinations without advice of health care professional.
- Rep: Advise patient that this medication may have teratogenic effects. Contraception should be used during and for at least 2 mo after therapy is concluded.
- Emphasize need for periodic lab tests to monitor for side effects.

Evaluation/Desired Outcomes

- Regression of malignancy without the appearance of detrimental side effects.

HIGH ALERT

vinCRIStine (vin-**kriss**-teen)

~~Vincasar PFS~~

Classification
Therapeutic: antineoplastics
Pharmacologic: vinca alkaloids

Pregnancy Category D

Indications

Used alone and in combination with other treatment modalities (antineoplastics, surgery, or radiation therapy) in treatment of: Hodgkin's disease, Leukemias, Neuroblastoma, Malignant lymphomas, Rhabdomyosarcoma, Wilms' tumor, Other tumors.

Action

Binds to proteins of mitotic spindle, causing metaphase arrest. Cell replication is stopped as a result (cell cycle–specific for M phase). Has little or no effect on bone marrow. **Therapeutic Effects:** Death of rapidly replicating cells, particularly malignant ones. Has immunosuppressive properties.

Pharmacokinetics

Absorption: Administered IV only, resulting in complete bioavailability.

Distribution: Rapidly and widely distributed; extensively bound to tissues.

Metabolism and Excretion: Metabolized by the liver and eliminated in the feces via biliary excretion.

Half-life: 10.5–37.5 hr.

TIME/ACTION PROFILE (effects on blood counts†)

ROUTE	ONSET	PEAK	DURATION
IV	unknown	4 days	7 days

†Usually mild.

Contraindications/Precautions

Contraindicated in: Hypersensitivity; OB, Lactation: Pregnancy or lactation.

Use Cautiously in: Infection; ↓ bone marrow reserve; Hepatic impairment (50% dose ↓ recommended if serum bilirubin >3 m g/dL); Rep: Women with child-bearing potential.

Adverse Reactions/Side Effects

CNS: agitation, insomnia, mental depression, mental status changes. **EENT:** cortical blindness, diplopia. **Resp:** bronchospasm. **GI:** nausea, vomiting, abdominal cramps, anorexia, constipation, ileus, stomatitis. **GU:** gonadal suppression, nocturia, oliguria, urinary retention. **Derm:** alopecia. **Endo:** syndrome of inappropriate antidiuretic hormone (SIADH). **Hemat:** anemia, leukopenia, thrombocytopenia (mild and brief). **Local:** phlebitis at IV site, tissue necrosis (from extravasation). **Metab:** hyperuricemia. **Neuro:** ascending peripheral neuropathy.

Interactions

Drug-Drug: Bronchospasm may occur in patients who have been previously treated with **mitomycin**. **L-asparaginase** may ↓ hepatic metabolism of vincristine (give vincristine 12–24 hr prior to asparaginase). May ↓ antibody response to **live-virus vaccines** and ↑ risk of adverse reactions.

Route/Dosage

Many other protocols are used.

IV (Adults): 10–30 mcg/kg (0.4–1.4 mg/m^2); may repeat weekly (not to exceed 2 mg/dose).

IV (Children >10 kg): 1.5–2 mg/m^2 single dose; may repeat weekly.

IV (Children <10 kg): 50 mcg/kg single dose; may repeat weekly.

Availability (generic available)

Solution for injection: 1 mg/mL.

NURSING IMPLICATIONS

Assessment

- Monitor BP, pulse, and respiratory rate during therapy. Report significant changes.
- Monitor neurologic status. Assess for paresthesia (numbness, tingling, pain), loss of deep tendon reflexes (Achilles reflex is usually first involved), weakness (wrist drop or footdrop, gait disturbances), cranial nerve palsies (jaw pain, hoarseness, ptosis, visual changes), autonomic dysfunction (ileus, difficulty voiding, orthostatic hypotension, impaired sweating), and CNS dysfunction (decreased level of consciousness, agitation, hallucinations). Notify physician if these symptoms develop, as they may persist for months.
- Monitor intake and output ratios and daily weight; report significant discrepancies. Decreased urine output with concurrent hyponatremia may indicate SIADH, which usually responds to fluid restriction.
- Assess infusion site frequently for redness, irritation, or inflammation. If extravasation occurs, infusion must be stopped and restarted elsewhere to avoid damage to subcut tissue. Cellulitis and discomfort may be minimized by infiltration with hyaluronidase and application of moderate heat or by application of cold compresses.
- Assess nutritional status. An antiemetic may be used to minimize nausea and vomiting.
- Monitor for symptoms of gout (increased uric acid, joint pain, edema). Encourage patient to drink at least 2 liters of fluid per day. Allopurinol or alkalinization of urine may be used to decrease uric acid levels.
- ***Lab Test Considerations:*** Monitor CBC prior to and periodically throughout therapy. May cause slight leukopenia 4 days after therapy, which resolves within 7 days. Platelet count may ↑ or ↓.
- Monitor liver function studies (AST, ALT, LDH, bilirubin) and renal function studies (BUN, creatinine) prior to and periodically throughout therapy.
- May cause ↑ uric acid. Monitor periodically during therapy.

Potential Nursing Diagnoses

Risk for injury (Adverse Reactions)

Imbalanced nutrition: less than body requirements (Adverse Reactions)

Implementation

- ***High Alert:*** Fatalities have occurred with chemotherapeutic agents. Before administering, clarify all ambiguous orders; double check single, daily, and course-of-therapy dose limits; have second practitioner independently double check original order, dose calculations, and infusion pump settings. Do not administer subcut, IM, or intrathecally (IT). IT

V

administration is fatal. Vincristine must be dispensed in an overwrap stating "For IV use only." Overwrap should remain in place until immediately before administration.

- ***High Alert:*** Do not confuse vincristine with vinblastine.
- Solution should be prepared in a biologic cabinet. Wear gloves, gown, and mask while handling medication. Discard IV equipment in specially designated containers.

IV Administration

- **IV Push:** ***Diluent:*** Does not need to be reconstituted. ***Concentration:*** Administer undiluted at 1 mg/mL. ***Rate:*** Administer each dose IV push over 1 min through Y-site injection of a free-flowing infusion of 0.9% NaCl or D5W.
- **Y-Site Compatibility:** acyclovir, alemtuzumab, alfentanil, allopurinol, amifostine, amikacin, aminophylline, amiodarone, amphotericin B lipid complex, amphotericin B liposome, ampicillin, ampicillin/sulbactam, anidulafungin, argatroban, azithromycin, aztreonam, bivalirudin, bleomycin, bumetanide, buprenorphine, butorphanol, calcium chloride, calcium gluconate, carboplatin, carmustine, caspofungin, cefazolin, cefotetan, cefoxitin, ceftazidime, ceftriaxone, cefuroxime, chlorpromazine, ciprofloxacin, cisatracurium, cladribine, cisplatin, cladribine, clindamycin, cyclophosphamide, cyclosporine, cytarabine, dactinomycin, daptomycin, daunorubicin hydrochloride, dexamethasone, dexmedetomidine, dexrazoxane, digoxin, diltiazem, diphenhydramine, dobutamine, docetaxel, dolasetron, dopamine, doxorubicin hydrochloride, doxorubicin liposomal, doxycycline, droperidol, enalaprilat, ephedrine, epinephrine, epirubicin, ertapenem, erythromycin, esmolol, etoposide, etoposide phosphate, famotidine, fenoldopam, fentanyl, filgrastim, fluconazole, fludarabine, fluorouracil, foscarnet, fosphenytoin, fosphenytoin, ganciclovir, gemcitabine, gentamicin, granisetron, haloperidol, heparin, hetastarch, hydrocortisone, hydromorphone, ifosfamide, imipenem/cilastatin, insulin, isoproterenol, ketorolac, labetalol, leucovorin calcium, levofloxacin, levorphanol, lidocaine, linezolid, lorazepam, magnesium sulfate, mannitol, mechlorethamine, melphalan, meperidine, meropenem, mesna, methotrexate, methoprednisolone, metoclopramide, metoprolol, metronidazole, midazolam, milrinone, mitomycin, mitoxantrone, morphine, moxifloxacin, nalbuphine, naloxone, nesiritide, nicardipine, nitroglycerin, nitroprusside, norepinephrine, octreotide, ondansetron, oxaliplatin, paclitaxel, palonosetron, pancuronium, pemetrexed, pentamidine, pentazocine, pentobarbital, phenobarbital, phenylephrine, piperacillin/tazobactam, potassium acetate, potassium chloride, potassium phosphates, procainamide, prochlorperazine, promethazine, propranolol, quinupristin/dalfopristin, ranitidine, remifentanil, rituximab, rocuronium, sargramostim, sodium acetate, sodium phosphates, succinylcholine, sufentanil, tacrolimus, teniposide, theophylline, thiopental, thiotepa, tigecycline, tirofiban, tobramycin, topotecan, trastuzumab, trimethoprim/sulfamethoxazole, vancomycin, vasopressin, vecuronium, verapamil, vinblastine, vinorelbine, voriconazole, zidovudine, zoledronic acid.
- **Y-Site Incompatibility:** amphotericin B colloidal, cefepime, diazepam, idarubicin, nafcillin, pantoprazole, phenytoin.

Patient/Family Teaching

- Instruct patient to notify health care professional immediately if redness, swelling, or pain at injection site occurs.
- Instruct patient to report symptoms of neurotoxicity (paresthesia, pain, difficulty walking, persistent constipation). Inform patient that increased fluid intake, dietary fiber, and exercise may minimize constipation. Stool softeners or laxatives may be used. Patient should inform health care professional if severe constipation or abdominal discomfort occurs, as this may be a sign of neuropathy.
- Advise patient to notify health care professional if fever; chills; sore throat; signs of infection; bleeding gums; bruising; petechiae; blood in urine, stool, or emesis; or mouth sores occur. Caution patient to avoid crowds and persons with known infections.
- Discuss with patient the possibility of hair loss. Explore coping strategies.
- Instruct patient not to receive any vaccinations without advice of health care professional.
- Rep: Advise patient that this medication may have teratogenic effects. Contraception should be used during and for at least 2 mo after therapy is concluded.
- Emphasize need for periodic lab tests to monitor for side effects.

Evaluation/Desired Outcomes

- Regression of malignancy without the appearance of detrimental side effects.

HIGH ALERT

vinorelbine (vine-oh-**rel**-been)

Navelbine

Classification

Therapeutic: antineoplastics

Pharmacologic: vinca alkaloids

Pregnancy Category D

Indications

Inoperable non–small-cell cancer of the lung in ambulatory patients (alone or with cisplatin).

Action

Binds to a protein (tubulin) of cellular microtubules, where it interferes with microtubule assembly. Cell replication is stopped as a result (cell cycle–specific for M phase). **Therapeutic Effects:** Death of rapidly replicating cells, particularly malignant ones.

Pharmacokinetics

Absorption: IV administration results in complete bioavailability.

Distribution: Highly bound to platelets and lymphocytes.

Metabolism and Excretion: Mostly metabolized by the liver. At least one metabolite is active. Large amounts eliminated in feces; 11% excreted unchanged by the kidneys.

Half-life: 28–44 hr.

TIME/ACTION PROFILE (effect on WBCs)

ROUTE	ONSET	PEAK	DURATION
IV	unknown	7–10 days	7–15 days

Contraindications/Precautions

Contraindicated in: Hypersensitivity; Active infections; ↓ bone marrow reserve; OB, Lactation: Pregnancy or lactation.

Use Cautiously in: Impaired hepatic function (dose ↓ recommended if total bilirubin >2 m g/dL); Debilitated patients (↑ risk of hyponatremia); Granulocytopenic patients (temporarily discontinue or reduce dose); Pedi: Safety not established; OB: Instruct women of childbearing potential to avoid pregnancy during treatment.

Adverse Reactions/Side Effects

CNS: fatigue. **Resp:** shortness of breath. **CV:** chest pain. **GI:** constipation, nausea, abdominal pain, anorexia, diarrhea, transient ↑ in liver enzymes, vomiting. **Derm:** alopecia, rashes. **F and E:** hyponatremia. **Hemat:** anemia, neutropenia, thrombocytopenia. **Local:** irritation at IV site, skin reactions, phlebitis. **MS:** arthralgia, back pain, jaw pain, myalgia. **Neuro:** neurotoxicity. **Misc:** pain in tumor-containing tissue.

Interactions

Drug-Drug: ↑ bone marrow depression with other **antineoplastics** or **radiation therapy**. Concurrent use with **cisplatin** ↑ risk and severity of bone marrow depression. Concurrent use with **mitomycin** or **chest radiation** ↑ risk of pulmonary reactions.

Route/Dosage

IV (Adults): 30 mg/m^2 once weekly.

Hepatic Impairment

IV (Adults): *Total bilirubin 2.1–3 mg/dL*—15 mg/m^2 once weekly; *total bilirubin ≥3 mg/dL*—7.5 mg/m^2 once weekly.

Availability (generic available)

Solution for injection: 10 mg/mL.

NURSING IMPLICATIONS

Assessment

- Monitor BP, pulse, and respiratory rate during therapy. Note significant changes. Acute shortness of breath and severe bronchospasm may occur infrequently shortly after administration. Treatment with corticosteroids, bronchodilators, and supplemental oxygen may be required, especially in patients with a history of pulmonary disease.
- Assess frequently for signs of infection (sore throat, temperature, cough, mental status changes), especially when nadir of granulocytopenia is expected.
- Monitor neurologic status. Assess for paresthesia (numbness, tingling, pain), loss of deep tendon reflexes (Achilles reflex is usually first involved), weakness (wrist drop or footdrop, gait disturbances), cranial nerve palsies (jaw pain, hoarseness, ptosis, visual changes), autonomic dysfunction (constipation, ileus, difficulty voiding, orthostatic hypotension, impaired sweating), and CNS dysfunction (decreased level of consciousness, agitation, hallucinations). These symptoms may persist for months. The incidence of neurotoxicity associated with vinorelbine is less than that of other vinca alkaloids.
- Monitor intake and output and daily weight for significant discrepancies.
- Assess nutritional status. Mild to moderate nausea is common. An antiemetic may be used to minimize nausea and vomiting.
- Monitor for symptoms of gout (increased uric acid, joint pain, edema). Encourage patient to drink at least 2 L of fluid/day. Allopurinol and alkalinization of urine may decrease uric acid levels.
- ***Lab Test Considerations:*** Monitor CBC prior to each dose and routinely during therapy. The nadir of granulocytopenia usually occurs 7–10 days after vinorelbine administration and recovery usually follows within 7–15 days. If granulocyte count is <1500/mm^3, dose reduction or temporary interruption of vinorelbine may be warranted. If repeated episodes of fever and/or sepsis occur during granulocytopenia, future dose of vinorelbine should be modified. May also cause mild to moderate anemia. Thrombocytopenia rarely occurs.
- Monitor liver function studies (AST, ALT, LDH, bilirubin) and renal function studies (BUN, creatinine) prior to and periodically during therapy. May cause ↑ uric acid; monitor periodically during therapy.

Potential Nursing Diagnoses

Risk for injury (Adverse Reactions)
Risk for infection (Adverse Reactions)

Implementation

- ***High Alert:*** Fatalities have occurred with chemotherapeutic agents. Before administering, clarify all ambiguous orders; double check single, daily, and course-of-therapy dose limits; have second practitioner independently double check original order, dose calculations, and infusion pump settings.

- Solution should be prepared in a biologic cabinet. Wear gloves, gown, and mask while handling medication. Discard IV equipment in specially designated containers.
- Assess infusion site frequently for redness, irritation, or inflammation. Vinorelbine is a vesicant. If extravasation occurs, infusion must be stopped and restarted elsewhere to avoid damage to subcut tissue. Treatment of extravasation includes application of warm compresses applied over the area immediately for 30–60 min, then alternating on/off every 15 min for 1 day to increase systemic absorption of the drug. Hyaluronidase 150 units diluted in 1–2 mL of 0.9% NaCl, 1 mL for each mL extravasated, should be injected through existing IV cannula or subcut if the needle has been removed to enhance absorption and dispersion of the extravasated drug.

IV Administration

- **IV Push:** ***Diluent:*** Dilute vinorelbine with 0.9% NaCl or D5W. ***Concentration:*** 1.5–3 mg/mL. ***Rate:*** Infuse over 6–10 min into Y-site closest to bag of a free-flowing IV or into a central line.
- Flush vein with at least 75–125 mL of 0.9% NaCl or D5W administered over 10 min or more following administration of vinorelbine.
- **Intermittent Infusion:** ***Diluent:*** Dilute vinorelbine with 0.9% NaCl, D5W, 0.45% NaCl, D5/0.45% NaCl, Ringer's or lactated Ringer's injection. Solution should be colorless to pale yellow. Do not administer solutions that are discolored or contain particulate matter. Diluted solution is stable for 24 hr at room temperature. ***Concentration:*** 0.5–2 mg/mL. ***Rate:*** Infuse over 6–10 min (up to 30 min) into Y-site closest to bag of a free-flowing IV or into a central line.
- Flush vein with at least 75–125 mL of 0.9% NaCl or D5W administered over 10 min or more following administration of vinorelbine.
- **Y-Site Compatibility:** amikacin, aztreonam, bleomycin, bumetanide, buprenorphine, butorphanol, calcium gluconate, carboplatin, carmustine, cefotaxime, ceftazidime, chlorpromazine, cimetidine, cisplatin, clindamycin, cyclophosphamide, cytarabine, dacarbazine, dactinomycin, daunorubicin, dexamethasone sodium phosphate, diphenhydramine, doxorubicin, doxorubicin liposome, doxycycline, droperidol, enalaprilat, etoposide, famotidine, filgrastim, floxuridine, fluconazole, fludarabine, gemcitabine, gentamicin, granisetron, haloperidol, hydrocortisone, hydromorphone, idarubicin, ifosfamide, imipenem/cilastatin, lorazepam, mannitol, mechlorethamine, melphalan, meperidine, mesna, methotrexate, metoclopramide, metronidazole, mitoxantrone, morphine, nalbuphine, ondansetron, oxaliplatin, potassium chloride, prochlorperazine, promethazine, ranitidine, streptozocin, teniposide, tobramycin, vancomycin, vinblastine, vincristine, zidovudine.
- **Y-Site Incompatibility:** acyclovir, allopurinol, aminophylline, amphotericin B, amphotericin B cholesteryl sulfate, ampicillin, cefazolin, ceftriaxone, cefuroxime, fluorouracil, furosemide, ganciclovir, lansoprazole, methylprednisolone, mitomycin, sodium bicarbonate, thiotepa, trimethoprim/sulfamethoxazole.

Patient/Family Teaching

- Instruct patient to report symptoms of neurotoxicity (paresthesia, pain, difficulty walking, persistent constipation).
- Inform patient that increased fluid intake, dietary fiber, and exercise may minimize constipation. Stool softeners or laxatives may be necessary. Patient should be advised to report severe constipation or abdominal discomfort, as this may be a sign of ileus, which may occur as a consequence of neuropathy.
- Advise patient to notify health care professional if fever; chills; sore throat; signs of infection; bleeding gums; bruising; petechiae; blood in urine, stool, or emesis; or mouth sores occur.
- Caution patient to avoid crowds and persons with known infections.
- Advise patient that this medication may have teratogenic effects. Contraception should be used during and for at least 2 mo after therapy is concluded.
- Discuss with patient the possibility of hair loss and explore coping strategies.
- Instruct patient not to receive any vaccinations without advice of health care professional.
- Emphasize the need for periodic lab tests to monitor for side effects.

Evaluation/Desired Outcomes

- Decrease in the size or spread of malignancy without detrimental side effects.

VITAMIN B_{12} PREPARATIONS

cyanocobalamin
(sye-an-oh-koe-**bal**-a-min)
Nascobal, Rubramin PC

hydroxocobalamin
(hye-drox-oh-koe-**bal**-a-min)
Cyanokit

Classification
Therapeutic: antianemics, vitamins
Pharmacologic: water soluble vitamins

Pregnancy Category C

Indications

Vitamin B_{12} deficiency (parenteral product or nasal spray should be used when deficiency is due to malabsorption). Pernicious anemia (only parenteral products should be used for initial therapy; nasal or oral products are not indicated until patients have achieved hematologic remission following parenteral therapy and have no signs of CNS involvement). Part of the Schilling test (vitamin B_{12} absorption test) (diagnostic). Cyanide poisoning (Cyanokit only).

Action

Necessary coenzyme for metabolic processes, including fat and carbohydrate metabolism and protein synthesis. Required for cell production and hematopoiesis.
Therapeutic Effects: Corrects manifestations of pernicious anemia (megaloblastic indices, GI lesions, and neurologic damage). Corrects vitamin B_{12} deficiency. Reverses symptoms of cyanide toxicity (Cyanokit only).

Pharmacokinetics

Absorption: Oral absorption in GI tract requires intrinsic factor and calcium; well absorbed after IM, subcut and nasal administration.
Distribution: Stored in the liver and bone marrow; crosses placenta, enters breast milk.
Metabolism and Excretion: Primarily excreted unchanged in urine.
Half-life: *Cyanocobalamin*—6 days (400 days in liver); *Hydroxocobalamin*—26–31 hr.

TIME/ACTION PROFILE (reticulocytosis)

ROUTE	ONSET	PEAK	DURATION
Cyanocobalamin IM, subcut, nasal	unknown	3–10 days	unknown
Hydroxocobalamin IM	unknown	unknown	unknown

Contraindications/Precautions

Contraindicated in: Hypersensitivity; Pedi: Avoid using preparations containing benzyl alcohol in premature infants (associated with fatal "gasping syndrome").
Use Cautiously in: Hereditary optic nerve atrophy (accelerates nerve damage); Uremia, folic acid deficiency, concurrent infection, iron deficiency (response to B_{12} will be impaired); Renal dysfunction (when using aluminum-containing products); Pedi: *Cyanokit*—Safety and effectiveness not established; OB: *Cyanokit*—Use only if potential benefit justifies potential risk to fetus.

Adverse Reactions/Side Effects

CNS: headache; *Cyanokit*, dizziness, memory impairment, restlessness. **CV:** heart failure; *Cyanokit*, hypertension, chest pain, tachycardia. **EENT:** *Cyanokit*—dry throat, eye redness, eye swelling. **GI:** diarrhea; *Cyanokit*, abdominal discomfort, dyspepsia, dysphagia, hematochezia, nausea, vomiting. **Derm:** itching; *Cyanokit*, erythema, rash. **F and E:** hypokalemia. **GU:** *Cyanokit*—red urine. **Hemat:** thrombocytosis. **Resp:** pulmonary edema; *Cyanokit*, dyspnea. **Local:** pain at IM site. **Misc:** hypersensitivity reactions including ANAPHYLAXIS.

Interactions

Drug-Drug: Chloramphenicol and **antineoplastics** may ↓ hematologic response to vitamin B_{12}. **Colchicine**, **aminosalicylic acid**, **cimetidine**, and excess intake of **alcohol**, or **vitamin C** may ↓ oral absorption/effectiveness of vitamin B_{12}.

Route/Dosage

Cyanocobalamin (oral products are usually not recommended due to poor absorption and should be used only if patient refuses the IM, deep subcutaneous, or intranasal route of administration)

PO (Adults and Children): *Vitamin B_{12} deficiency*—amount depends on deficiency (up to 1000 mcg/day have been used).
PO (Adults): *Pernicious anemia (for hematologic remission only)*—1000–2000 mcg/day.
IM, Subcut (Adults): *Vitamin B_{12} deficiency*—30 mcg/day for 5–10 days, then 100–200 mcg/month. *Pernicious anemia*—100 mcg/day for 6–7 days; if improvement, give same dose every other day for 7 doses, then every 3–4 days for 2–3 wk; once hematologic values return to normal (remission), can give maintenance dose of 100 mcg/month (doses up to 1000 mcg have been used for maintenance) (could alternatively use oral or intranasal formulations below for maintenance at specified doses). *Schilling test*—Flushing dose is 1000 mcg.
IM, Subcut (Children): *Vitamin B_{12} deficiency*—0.2 mcg/kg for 2 days, then 1000 mcg/day for 2–7 days, then 100 mcg/week for 1 mo. *Pernicious anemia*—30–50 mcg/day for 2 or more weeks (to a total dose of 1000–5000 mcg), then give maintenance dose of 100 mcg/month (doses up to 1000 mcg have been used for maintenance).
Intranasal (Adults): *Vitamin B_{12} deficiency*—500 mcg (one spray) in one nostril once weekly. *Pernicious anemia (for hematologic remission only)*—500 mcg (one spray) in one nostril once weekly.

V

Hydroxocobalamin

IM (Adults): *Vitamin B_{12} deficiency*—30 mcg/day for 5–10 days, then 100–200 mcg/month. *Pernicious anemia*—100 mcg/day for 6–7 days; if improvement, give same dose every other day for 7 doses, then every 3–4 days for 2–3 wk; once hematologic values return to normal (remission), give maintenance dose of 100 mcg/month. *Schilling test*—Flushing dose is 1000 mcg.
IM (Children): *Vitamin B_{12} deficiency*—100 mcg/day for 2 or more weeks (to achieve total dose of 1000–5000 mcg), then 30–50 mcg/month. *Pernicious anemia*—30–50 mcg/day for 2 or more weeks (to achieve total dose of 1000–5000 mcg), then 100 mcg/month.
IV (Adults): *Cyanide poisoning (Cyanokit only)*—5 g over 15 min; another 5 g dose may be infused over 15–120 min depending upon severity of poisoning (maximum cumulative dose = 10 g).

Availability

Cyanocobalamin (generic available)

Tablets: 50 mcg^{OTC}, 100 mcg^{OTC}, 250 mcg^{OTC}, 500 mcg^{OTC}, 1000 mcg^{OTC}, 5000 mcg^{OTC}. **Extended-release tablets:** 1000 mcg^{OTC}, 1500 mcg^{OTC}. **Sublingual tablets:** 2500 mcg^{OTC}. **Lozenges:** 100 mcg^{OTC}, 250 mcg^{OTC}, 500 mcg^{OTC}. **Nasal spray:** 500 mcg/0.1 mL actuation (8 sprays/bottle). **Injection:** 1000 mcg/mL.

Hydroxocobalamin (generic available)

Injection: 1000 mcg/mL. **Powder for injection (Cyanokit):** 5 g/vial.

NURSING IMPLICATIONS

Assessment

- Assess patient for signs of vitamin B_{12} deficiency (pallor; neuropathy; psychosis; red, inflamed tongue) before and periodically during therapy.
- ***Lab Test Considerations:*** Monitor plasma folic acid, vitamin B_{12}, and iron levels, hemoglobin, hematocrit, and reticulocyte count before treatment, 1 mo after the start of therapy, and then every 3–6 mo. Evaluate serum potassium level in patients receiving vitamin B_{12} for pernicious anemia for hypokalemia during the first 48 hr of treatment. Serum potassium and platelet counts should be monitored routinely during the course of therapy.
- **Cyanokit: :** Management of cyanide poisoning should also include establishment of airway, ensuring adequate oxygenation and hydration, cardiovascular support, and seizure management. Monitor BP and heart rate continuously during and after infusion and immediately report significant changes. The maximal ↑ in BP usually occurs toward the end of the infusion. BP usually returns to baseline within 4 hr of drug administration.

Potential Nursing Diagnoses

Imbalanced nutrition: less than body requirements (Indications)
Activity intolerance (Indications)

Implementation

- Usually administered in combination with other vitamins; solitary vitamin B_{12} deficiencies are rare.
- Administration of vitamin B_{12} by the oral route is useful only for nutritional deficiencies. Patients with small-bowel disease, malabsorption syndrome, or gastric or ileal resections require parenteral administration.
- **PO:** Administer with meals to increase absorption.
- May be mixed with fruit juices. Administer immediately after mixing; ascorbic acid alters stability.
- **Intranasal:** Dose should not be administered within 1 hr of hot food or liquids (these substances may result in the formation of nasal secretions which may result in ↓ effectiveness of nasal spray).
- **IM, Subcut:** Vials should be protected from light.
- If subcutaneous route used, deep subcutaneous administration is preferred.

IV Administration

- **IV:** IV route should only be used with Cyanokit.
- **Intermittent Infusion:** ***Diluent:*** Dilute each Cyanokit vial with 200 mL of 0.9% NaCl, D5W, or LR. Gently invert the vial for at least 60 sec prior to infusion. Reconstituted vial can be hung for infusion and is stable for 6 hr at room temperature. Discard any unused solution after 6 hr. ***Rate:*** Administer initial 5-g dose over 15 min. Administer additional 5-g dose over 15–120 min.
- **Y-Site Incompatibility:** ascorbic acid, blood products, diazepam, dobutamine, dopamine, fentanyl, nitroglycerin, pentobarbital, propofol, sodium thiosulfate, thiopental.

Patient/Family Teaching

- Encourage patient to comply with diet recommendations of health care professional. Explain that the best source of vitamins is a well-balanced diet with foods from the four basic food groups.
- Foods high in vitamin B_{12} include meats, seafood, egg yolk, and fermented cheeses; few vitamins are lost with ordinary cooking.
- Patients self-medicating with vitamin supplements should be cautioned not to exceed RDA. Effectiveness of megadoses for treatment of various medical conditions is unproved and may cause side effects.
- Inform patients with pernicious anemia of the lifelong need for vitamin B_{12} replacement.
- Emphasize the importance of follow-up exams to evaluate progress.
- **Intranasal:** Instruct patient in proper administration technique. Review *Patient Information Sheet* and demonstrate use of actuator. Unit must be primed with 3 strokes upon using for the first time. Unit must be primed with 1 stroke before each of the remaining doses. Advise patient to clear nose, then place tip approximately 1 inch into nostril and press pump once, firmly and quickly. After dose, remove

unit from nose and massage dosed nostril gently for a few seconds. Vial delivers 8 doses. Unit should be stored at room temperature and protected from light.

- **Intermittent Infusion:** Advise patient that skin redness may last up to 2 wk and that their urine may remain red for up to 5 wk after drug administration. Instruct patient to avoid sun exposure while their skin is red. Advise patient to contact health care professional if skin or urine redness persist after these time periods. Advise patient that a rash may develop from 7–28 days after drug administration. It will usually resolve without treatment within a few weeks. Advise patient to contact health care professional if rash persists after this time period.

Evaluation/Desired Outcomes

- Resolution of the symptoms of vitamin B_{12} deficiency.
- Increase in reticulocyte count.
- Improvement in manifestations of pernicious anemia.
- Resolution of symptoms of cyanide poisoning.

VITAMIN D COMPOUNDS

calcitriol (kal-si-**trye**-ole)
1,25-dihydroxycholecalciferol, ~~Calcijex~~, ✽Calcijex, Rocaltrol, vitamin D_3 (active)

cholecalciferol (kol-e-kal-**sif**-e-role)
Delta-D, vitamin D_3 (inactive)

doxercalciferol (**dox**-er-kal-**sif**-e-role)
Hectorol, vitamin D_2

ergocalciferol (**er**-goe-kal-**sif**-e-role)
Drisdol, vitamin D_2

paricalcitol (par-i-**kal**-si-tole)
Zemplar

Classification
Therapeutic: vitamins
Pharmacologic: fat-soluble vitamins

Pregnancy Category B (doxercalciferol), C (calcitriol, cholecalciferol, ergocalciferol, paricalcitol)

Indications

Calcitriol: Management of hypocalcemia in chronic renal dialysis (IV and PO). Treatment of hypocalcemia in patients with hypoparathyroidism or pseudohypoparathyroidism (PO only). Management of secondary hyperparathyroidism and resulting metabolic bone disease in predialysis patients with moderate to severe renal insufficiency (CCr 15–55 mL/min) (PO only). **Cholecalciferol:** Treatment or prevention of vitamin D deficiency. **Doxercaliciferol:** Treatment of secondary hyperparathyroidism in patients undergoing chronic renal dialysis (IV and PO). Treatment of secondary hyperparathyroidism in patients with Stage 3 or 4 chronic kidney disease (PO only). **Ergocalciferol:** Treatment of familial hypophosphatemia. Treatment of hypoparathyroidism. Treatment of vitamin D-resistant rickets. **Paricalcitol:** Prevention and treatment of secondary hyperparathyroidism in patients with Stage 3 or 4 (PO) or Stage 5 (PO and IV) chronic kidney disease.

Action

Cholecalciferol requires activation in the liver and kidneys to create the active form of vitamin D_3 (calcitriol). Doxercalciferol and ergocalciferol require activation in the liver to create the active form of vitamin D_2. Paricalcitol is a synthetic analogue of calcitriol. Vitamin D: Promotes the absorption of calcium and ↓ parathyroid hormone concentration. **Therapeutic Effects:** Treatment and prevention of deficiency states, particularly bone manifestations. Improved calcium and phosphorous homeostasis in patients with chronic kidney disease.

Pharmacokinetics

Absorption: *Calcitriol, doxercalciferol, ergocalciferol, paricalcitol*—Well absorbed following oral administration. *Calcitriol, doxercalciferol, paricalcitol*—IV administration results in complete bioavailability.
Distribution: Calcitriol and paricalcitol cross the placenta; calcitriol also enters breast milk.
Protein Binding: *Calcitriol and paricalcitol*—99.9%.
Metabolism and Excretion: *Calcitriol*—Undergoes enterohepatic recycling and is excreted mostly in bile. *Cholecalciferol*—Converted by the liver and kidneys to calcitriol (active form of vitamin D_3). *Ergocalciferol*—Converted to active form of vitamin D_2 by sunlight, the liver, and the kidneys. *Doxercalciferol*—Converted by the liver to the active form of vitamin D_2. *Paricalcitol*—mostly metabolized by the liver and excreted via hepatobiliary elimination.
Half-life: *Calcitriol*—5–8 hr. *Cholecalciferol*—14 hr. *Doxercalciferol*—32–37 hr (up to 96 hr). *Paricalcitol*—14–20 hr.

V

TIME/ACTION PROFILE (effects on serum calcium)

ROUTE	ONSET	PEAK	DURATION
Calcitriol-PO	2–6 hr	2–6 hr	3–5 days
Calcitriol-IV	unknown	unknown	unknown
Cholecalciferol-PO	unknown	unknown	unknown
Doxercalciferol PO	unknown	8 wk	1 wk
Doxercalciferol-IV	unknown	8 wk	1 wk
Ergocalciferol-PO	12–24 hr	unknown	up to 6 mo
Paricalcitol-PO	unknown	2–4 wk	unknown
Paricalitol IV	unknown	up to 2 wk	unknown

Contraindications/Precautions

Contraindicated in: Hypersensitivity; Hypercalcemia; Vitamin D toxicity; Lactation: Potential for serious adverse reactions in infant; Concurrent use of magnesium-containing antacids or other vitamin D supplements; **Ergocalciferol**: Known intolerance to tartrazine; **Cholecalciferol and ergocalciferol**: Malabsorption problems.

Use Cautiously in: Calcitriol, doxercalciferol, paricalcitol: Patients receiving digoxin; OB: Safety not established.

Adverse Reactions/Side Effects

Seen primarily as manifestations of toxicity (hypercalcemia).

CNS: headache, somnolence, weakness; *doxercalciferol*, dizziness, malaise. **EENT:** conjunctivitis, photophobia, rhinorrhea. **Resp:** *doxercalciferol and ergocalciferol*—dyspnea. **CV:** arrhythmias, edema, hypertension; *doxercalciferol*, bradycardia; *paricalcitol*, palpitations. **GI:** PANCREATITIS, abdominal pain, anorexia, constipation, dry mouth, ↑ liver enzymes, metallic taste, nausea, polydipsia, vomiting, weight loss. **GU:** albuminuria, azotemia, ↓ libido, nocturia, polyuria. **Derm:** pruritus. **F and E:** hypercalcemia. **Metab:** hyperthermia. **MS:** bone pain, muscle pain; *doxercalciferol*, arthralgia; *paricalcitol*, metastatic calcification. **Local:** pain at injection site. **Misc:** *calcitriol*—allergic reactions, chills, fever.

Interactions

Drug-Drug: Cholestyramine, **colestipol**, or **mineral oil** ↓ absorption of vitamin D analogues. Use with **thiazide diuretics** may result in hypercalcemia. **Corticosteroids** ↓ effectiveness of vitamin D analogues. Using calcitriol, doxercalciferol, or paricalcitol with **digoxin** may ↑ risk of arrhythmias. Vitamin D requirements ↓ by **phenytoin** and other **hydantoin anticonvulsants**, **sucralfate**, **barbiturates**, and **primidone**. Concurrent use with **magnesium-containing drugs** may lead to hypermagnesemia. Concurrent use of **calcium-containing drugs** may ↑ risk of hypercalcemia. Concurrent use of other **vitamin D supplements** may ↑ risk of hypercalcemia. **Agents that induce liver enzymes (phenobarbital, rifampin)** and **agents that inhibit liver enzymes (atazanavir, clarithromycin, erythromycin, indinavir, itraconazole, ketoconazole, nefazodone, nelfinavir, ritonavir, saquinavir, verapamil, voriconazole)** may alter requirements for doxercalciferol and paricalcitol (monitoring of calcium and phosphorus recommended).

Drug-Food: Ingestion of **foods high in calcium content** (see Appendix J) may lead to hypercalcemia.

Route/Dosage

Calcitriol

PO (Adults): *Hypocalcemia during dialysis*—0.25 mcg/day or every other day; if needed, may ↑ by 0.25 mcg/day at 4–8 wk intervals (typical dosage = 0.5–1 mcg/day). *Hypoparathyroidism*—0.25 mcg/day initially; if needed, may ↑ dose by 0.25 mcg/day at 2–4 wk intervals (typical dosage = 0.5–2 mcg/day). *Predialysis patients*—0.25 mcg/day (up to 0.5 mcg/day).

PO (Children): *Hypocalcemia during dialysis*—0.25–2 mcg/day. *Hypoparathyroidism (children ≥6 yr)*—0.25 mcg/day initially; if needed, may ↑ dose by 0.25 mcg/day at 2–4 wk intervals (typical dosage = 0.5–2 mcg/day). *Hypoparathyroidism (children 1–5 yr)*—0.25–0.75 mcg/day. *Hypoparathyroidism (children <1 yr)*—0.04–0.08 mcg/kg/day. *Predialysis patients (children ≥3 yr)*—0.25 mcg/day (up to 0.5 mcg/day). *Predialysis patients (children <3 yr)*—10–15 ng/kg/day.

IV (Adults): *Hypocalcemia during dialysis*—0.5 mcg (0.01 mcg/kg) 3 times weekly. May be increased by 0.25–0.5 mcg/dose at 2–4 wk intervals (typical maintenance dose = 0.5–3.0 mcg 3 times weekly [0.01–0.05 mcg/kg 3 times weekly]).

IV (Children): *Hypocalcemia during dialysis*—0.01–0.05 mcg/kg 3 times weekly.

Cholecalciferol

PO (Adults): 400–1000 units daily.

PO (Infants): *Exclusively or partially breast fed*—400 IU daily.

Doxercalciferol

PO (Adults): *Dialysis patients*—10 mcg 3 times weekly (at dialysis); dose may be adjusted by 2.5 mcg at 8-wk intervals based on intact PTH concentrations (maximum dose = 20 mcg 3 times weekly). *Non-dialysis patients*—1 mcg/day; dose may be adjusted by 0.5 mcg at 2 wk intervals based on intact PTH concentrations (maximum dose = 3.5 mcg/day).

IV (Adults): 4 mcg 3 times weekly at the end of dialysis; dose may be adjusted by 1–2 mcg at 8-wk intervals based on intact PTH concentrations (maximum dose = 6 mcg 3 times weekly).

Ergocalciferol

PO (Adults): *Vitamin D–resistant rickets*—12,000–500,000 units/day (to be used with phosphate

supplement). *Familial hypophosphatemia*—10,000–80,000 units/day (with phosphorus 1–2 g/day). *Hypoparathyroidism*—50,000–200,000 units/day (to be used with calcium supplement).
PO (Children): *Vitamin D–resistant rickets*—40,000–80,000 units/day (to be used with phosphate supplement). *Familial hypophosphatemia*—10,000–80,000 units/day (with phosphorus 1–2 g/day). *Hypoparathyroidism*—50,000–200,000 units/day (to be used with calcium supplement).
PO (Infants): *Exclusively or partially breast fed*—400 IU daily.

Paricalcitol

Stage 3 or 4 Chronic Kidney Disease

PO (Adults): *Baseline intact PTH concentration ≤500 pg/mL*—Initiate with 1 mcg/day or 2 mcg 3 times weekly; dose can be adjusted at 2–4 wk intervals based on intact PTH, calcium, and phosphate concentrations. *Baseline intact PTH concentration >500 p g/mL*—Initiate with 2 mcg/day or 4 mcg 3 times weekly; dose can be adjusted at 2–4 wk intervals based on intact PTH, calcium, and phosphate concentrations.

Stage 5 Chronic Kidney Disease

PO (Adults): Initial dose (in mcg) is based on following equation: baseline intact PTH concentration (pg/mL)/80; dose should be given 3 times weekly; dose can be adjusted at 2–4 wk intervals based on intact PTH, calcium, and phosphate concentrations.
IV (Adults and Children ≥5 yr): 0.04–0.1 mcg/kg 3 times weekly during dialysis; dose can be adjusted by 2–4 mcg at 2–4 wk intervals based on intact PTH, calcium, and phosphate concentrations (doses up to 0.24 mcg/kg have been used).

Availability

Calcitriol (generic available)

Capsules: 0.25 mcg, 0.5 mcg. **Oral solution:** 1 mcg/mL. **Solution for injection:** 1 mcg/mL.

Cholecalciferol

Tablets: 400 units[OTC], 1000 units[OTC]. **Oral solution:** 400 IU/drop[OTC]. ***In combination with:*** alendronate (Fosamax Plus D), see Appendix B.

Doxercalciferol (generic available)

Capsules: 0.5 mcg, 1 mcg, 2.5 mcg. **Solution for injection:** 2 mcg/mL.

Ergocalciferol (generic available)

Liquid: 8000 units/mL[Rx, OTC]. **Capsules:** 50,000 units. **Tablets:** 400 IU.

Paricalcitol (generic available)

Capsules: 1 mcg, 2 mcg, 4 mcg. **Solution for injection:** 2 mcg/mL, 5 mcg/mL.

NURSING IMPLICATIONS

Assessment

- Assess for symptoms of vitamin deficiency prior to and periodically during therapy.
- Assess patient for bone pain and weakness prior to and during therapy.
- Observe patient carefully for evidence of hypocalcemia (paresthesia, muscle twitching, laryngospasm, colic, cardiac arrhythmias, and Chvostek's or Trousseau's sign). Protect symptomatic patient by raising and padding side rails; keep bed in low position.
- Pedi: Monitor height and weight; growth arrest may occur in prolonged high-dose therapy.
- **Rickets/Osteomalacia:** Assess patient for bone pain and weakness prior to and during therapy.
- ***Lab Test Considerations:*** During *calcitriol* therapy, serum calcium and phosphate concentrations should be drawn twice weekly initially. Serum calcium, magnesium, alkaline phosphatase, and intact PTH should then be monitored at least monthly. During *cholecalciferol* therapy, serum calcium, phosphate, and alkaline phosphatase concentrations should be monitored periodically. During *doxercalciferol* therapy, serum ionized calcium, phosphate, and intact PTH concentrations should be monitored prior to initiation of therapy, and then weekly during the first 12 wk of therapy, then periodically. Alkaline phosphatase should be monitored periodically. During *ergocalciferol* therapy, serum calcium and phosphate concentrations should be monitored every 2 wk. During oral *paricalcitol* therapy, serum calcium, phosphate, and intact PTH concentrations should be monitored at least every 2 wk for the first 3 mo of therapy or after any dosage adjustment, then monthly for 3 mo, then every 3 mo. During IV *paricalcitol* therapy, serum calcium and phosphate concentrations should be monitored twice weekly initially until dosage stabilized, and then at least monthly. Serum intact PTH concentrations should be monitored every 3 mo.
- The serum calcium × phosphate product (Ca × P) should not exceed 70 mg^2/dL^2 (55 mg^2/dL^2 for doxercalciferol) (patients may be at ↑ risk of calcification).
- Calcitriol may cause false ↑ cholesterol levels.
- ***Toxicity and Overdose:*** Toxicity is manifested as hypercalcemia, hypercalciuria, and hyperphosphatemia. Assess patient for appearance of nausea, vomiting, anorexia, weakness, constipation, headache, bone pain, and metallic taste. Later symptoms include polyuria, polydipsia, photophobia, rhinorrhea, pruritus, and cardiac arrhythmias. Notify health care professional immediately if these signs of hypervitaminosis D occur. Treatment usually consists of discontinuation of calcitriol, a low-calcium diet, use of low-calcium dialysate in peritoneal dialy-

V

sis patients, and administration of a laxative. IV hydration and loop diuretics may be ordered to increase urinary excretion of calcium. Hemodialysis may also be used.

Potential Nursing Diagnoses

Imbalanced nutrition: less than body requirements (Indications)

Implementation

- **PO:** May be administered without regard to meals. Measure solution accurately with calibrated dropper provided by manufacturer. May be mixed with juice, cereal, or food, or dropped directly into mouth. Calcitriol capsules or solution should be protected from light.

IV Administration

- **IV Push:** Administer *calcitriol, doxercalciferol, and paracalcitol* undiluted by rapid injection through the catheter at the end of a hemodialysis period.

Patient/Family Teaching

- Advise patient to take medication as directed. Take missed doses as soon as remembered that day, unless almost time for next dose; do not double up on doses.
- Review diet modifications with patient. See Appendix J for foods high in calcium and vitamin D. Renal patients must still consider renal failure diet in food selection. Health care professional may order concurrent calcium supplement.
- Encourage patient to comply with dietary recommendations of health care professional. Explain that the best source of vitamins is a well-balanced diet with foods from the 4 basic food groups and the importance of sunlight exposure. See Appendix J for foods high in vitamin D.
- Patients self-medicating with vitamin supplements should be cautioned not to exceed RDA. The effectiveness of megadoses for treatment of various medical conditions is unproved and may cause side effects.
- Advise patient to avoid concurrent use of antacids containing magnesium.
- Review symptoms of overdosage and instruct patient to report these promptly to health care professional.
- Emphasize the importance of follow-up exams to evaluate progress.

Evaluation/Desired Outcomes

- Normalization of serum calcium and parathyroid hormone levels.
- Resolution or prevention of vitamin D deficiency.
- Improvement in symptoms of vitamin D–resistant rickets.

vorapaxar (vor-a-pax-ar)

Zontivity

Classification
Therapeutic: antiplatelet agents
Pharmacologic: protease-activated receptor-1 (PAR-1) antagonists

Pregnancy Category B

Indications

To reduce thrombotic cardiovascular events in patients who have a history of MI or peripheral arterial disease (PAD); can be used with aspirin and/or clopidogrel.

Action

Acts as an antagonist of the protease-activated receptor-1 (PAR-1) on platelet surfaces. Inhibits platelet aggregation. **Therapeutic Effects:** Decreased cardiovascular events.

Pharmacokinetics

Absorption: Completely absorbed (100%) following oral administration.
Distribution: Unknown.
Protein Binding: >99%.
Metabolism and Excretion: Extensively metabolized (CYP3A4 and CYP2J2); one metabolite (M20) has antiplatelet activity (20% of parent compound). Excreted mostly in feces (58%) and some in urine (25%) as metabolites.
Half-life: *Effective half-life*—3–4 days, *terminal elimination half-life*—8 days (range 5–13 days, similar for M20).

TIME/ACTION PROFILE (antiplatelet effect)

ROUTE	ONSET	PEAK	DURATION
PO	within 1 wk	unknown	4 wk

Contraindications/Precautions

Contraindicated in: History of stroke, transient ischemic attack or intracranial hemorrhage; Active pathologic bleeding; Concurrent use of anticoagulants including warfarin; Concurrent use of strong inhibitors or inducers or CYP3A should be avoided; Severe hepatic impairment (↑ risk of bleeding); Lactation: Discontinue vorapaxar or discontinue breast feeding.
Use Cautiously in: Existing risk factors for bleeding including ↑ age, ↓ body weight, ↓ renal/hepatic function, concurrent chronic NSAIDs, other antiplatelet agents or history of bleeding disorders; Geri: Elderly patients may be at ↑ risk of bleeding; OB: use during pregnancy only if potential matenral benefit to justifies potential risk to the fetus; Pedi: Safe and effective use in children has not been established.

Adverse Reactions/Side Effects

Hemat: BLEEDING.

Interactions

Drug-Drug: Blood levels and risk of bleeding may be ↑ by strong **inhibitors of CYP3A** including **boceprevir, clarithromycin, conivaptan, indinavir, itraconazole, ketoconazole, nefazodone, nelfinavir, posaconazole, ritonavir, saquinavir, telapravir** or **telithromycin**; concurrent use should be avoided. Blood levels and effectiveness may be ↓ by **strong inducers of CYP3A** including **carbamazepine, phenytoin** or **rifampin**; concurrent use should be avoided. ↑ risk of bleeding with **anticoagulants**, other **antiplatelet agents, fibrinolytics**, chronic **NSAID** use, **SSRIs** or **SNRIs**; avoid concurrent use of **warfarin** or other **anticoagulants**.

Drug-Natural Products: Blood levels and effectiveness may be ↓ by **St. John's wort**; concurrent use should be avoided.

Route/Dosage

PO (Adults): 2.08 mg (one tablet) once daily.

Availability

Tablets: 2.08 mg.

NURSING IMPLICATIONS

Assessment

- Assess for signs and symptoms of bleeding periodically during therapy.

Potential Nursing Diagnoses

Decreased cardiac output (Indications)

Implementation

- **PO:** Administer once daily without regard to food.
- Administer with aspirin or clopidogrel according to directions.

Patient/Family Teaching

- Instruct patient to take vorapaxar as directed. Do not stop therapy without consulting health care professional. Advise patient to read *Medication Guide* before starting therapy and with each Rx refill in case of changes.
- Caution patient to notify health care professional immediately if signs and symptoms of bleeding (bleeding that is severe or cannot be controlled, pink, red, or brown urine, vomiting blood or coffee ground-like vomit, red or black, tar-like stools, coughing up blood or blood clots) occur.
- Advise patient to notify health care professional of medication regimen before treatment or surgery.
- Advise patient to notify health care professional of all Rx or OTC medications, vitamins, or herbal products being taken and to consult with health care professional before taking other medications.
- Advise female patient to notify health care professional if pregnancy is planned or suspected or if breast feeding.

Evaluation/Desired Outcomes

- Decrease in cardiac events.

⚕ voriconazole

(vor-i-**kon**-a-zole)

Vfend

Classification

Therapeutic: antifungals

Pregnancy Category D

Indications

Serious systemic fungal infections including candidemia, esophageal candidiasis, candidal deep tissue and skin infections, abdominal, kidney, bladder wall and wound infections, and aspergillosis.

Action

Inhibits fungal ergosterol synthesis leading to production of abnormal fungal plasma membrane. **Therapeutic Effects:** Antifungal activity.

Pharmacokinetics

Absorption: Well absorbed following oral administration (96%); IV administration results in complete bioavailability.

Distribution: Extensive tissue distribution.

Protein Binding: 58%.

Metabolism and Excretion: Highly metabolized by the hepatic P450 enzymes (CYP2C19, CYP2C9, CYP3A4); <2% excreted unchanged in urine. Much individual variation in metabolism; metabolites are inactive. ⚕ The CYP2C19 enzyme system exhibits genetic polymorphism; 15–20% of Asian patients and 3–5% of Caucasian and Black patients may be poor metabolizers and may have significantly ↑ voriconazole concentrations and an ↑ risk of adverse effects.

Half-life: Dose-dependent (adults 6–9 hrs); ↑ in hepatic impairment.

TIME/ACTION PROFILE (blood levels)

ROUTE	ONSET	PEAK	DURATION
PO	rapid	1–2 hr	12 hr
IV	rapid	end of infusion	12 hr

Contraindications/Precautions

Contraindicated in: Concurrent use of ritonavir, rifampin, rifabutin, St. John's wort, carbamazepine, and phenobarbital (↓ antifungal activity); Concurrent use of sirolimus, pimozide, quinidine, ergotamine, and dihydroergotamine (↑ risk of toxicity of these agents); Concurrent use of efavirenz at doses ≥400 mg/day; Tablets contain lactose and should be avoided in patients with galactose intolerance, Lapp lactase deficiency, or glucose-galactose malabsorption.

V

Use Cautiously in: Mild to moderate liver disease (Child-Pugh Class A and B); maintenance dose reduction recommended; Renal impairment (CCr <50 mL/min); use only if justified by risk/benefit assessment (IV form should be avoided, use oral form only); Congenital/acquired QT interval prolongation, HF, sinus bradycardia, hypokalemia, hypomagnesemia, or symptomatic arrhythmias; Concurrent use of drugs that prolong the QTc interval; Hematologic malignancy (↑ risk of hepatotoxicity); OB, Lactation: Use only if benefits justify risk; Pedi: Children <12 yr (limited dosing information); suspension contains benzyl alcohol which may cause potentially fatal "gasping syndrome" in neonates; ↑ risk of photosensitivity reactions.

Adverse Reactions/Side Effects

CNS: dizziness, hallucinations, headache. **EENT:** visual disturbances, eye hemorrhage. **CV:** QT INTERVAL PROLONGATION, changes in BP, peripheral edema, tachycardia. **GI:** HEPATOTOXICITY, abdominal pain, diarrhea, nausea, pancreatitis, vomiting. **Derm:** MELANOMA, SQUAMOUS CELL CARCINOMA, STEVENS-JOHNSON SYNDROME, photosensitivity, rash. **F and E:** hypokalemia, hypomagnesemia, hyperglycemia. **MS:** fluorosis, periostitis. **Misc:** chills, fever, infusion reactions.

Interactions

Drug-Drug: Voriconazole is a substrate and inhibitor of the **CYP3A4**, **CYP2C9**, and **CYP2C19** enzyme systems. **Carbamazepine**, **ritonavir**, **phenobarbital**, **St. John's wort**, **rifabutin**, and **rifampin** may ↓ levels and effectiveness; concurrent use contraindicated. May ↑ levels of **dihydroergotamine**, **ergotamine**, **pimozide**, **quinidine**, **rifabutin**, and **sirolimus**; concurrent use contraindicated. Concurrent use with **efavirenz** at doses of ≥400 mg q 24 hr is contraindicated since it may ↑ efavirenz levels and ↓ voriconazole levels; if used together, ↑ dose of voriconazole to 400 mg q 12 hr and ↓ dose of efavirenz to 300 mg daily. **Fluconazole** may ↑ levels of voriconazole; avoid concurrent use. May ↑ levels of **cyclosporine**; ↓ cyclosporine dose by 50%. May ↑ levels of **tacrolimus**; ↓ tacrolimus dose to 1/3 of the starting dose. May ↑ levels of **HMG-CoA reductase inhibitors**, some **benzodiazepines (alprazolam, midazolam, triazolam)**, **fentanyl**, **oxycodone**, **NSAIDs (ibuprofen, diclofenac)**, some **calcium channel blockers**, **sulfonylureas (glipizide, glyburide)**, **phenytoin**, **alfentanil**, **warfarin**, and **vinca alkaloids (vincristine, vinblastine)**; dose ↓ may be needed and careful monitoring required during concurrent use. May ↑ **methadone** levels and ↑ risk of QT interval prolongation. Concurrent use with **hormonal contraceptives** containing **ethinyl estadiol** and **norethindone** may ↑ voriconazole, ethinyl estradiol and norethindrone levels. May ↑ levels of **everolimus**; concurrent use not recommended. ↑ blood levels of **omeprazole**; if patient receiving ≥40 mg/day of omeprazole, ↓ omeprazole dose by 50%. Similar effects may occur with other **proton-pump inhibitors**. May ↓ metabolism and ↑ blood levels and effects of **protease-inhibitor antiretrovirals** and **non-nucleoside reverse transcriptase inhibitor antiretrovirals**; frequent monitoring recommended. **Non-nucleoside reverse transcriptase inhibitor antiretrovirals**; may induce or inhibit the metabolism of voriconazole; frequent monitoring recommended.

Drug-Natural Products: **St. John's wort** ↑ metabolism and may ↓ effectiveness; concurrent use contraindicated.

Route/Dosage

IV (Adults and children >12 yr): *Loading dose*—6 mg/kg every 12 hour for 2 doses, followed by *maintenance dosing*—3–4 mg/kg every 12 hours. IV then switched to oral dosing when possible. If intolerance occurs, dose may be ↓ to 3 mg/kg every 12 hr. If phenytoin is coadministered, ↑ maintenance dose to 5 mg/kg every 12 hr.

IV (Children 2–11 yrs): *Loading dose*—6–8 mg/kg (maximum: 400 mg/dose) every 12 hour for 2 doses, followed by *Maintenance dosing*—7 mg/kg (maximum: 200 mg/dose) every 12 hours. *Invasive aspergillosis*—5–7 mg/kg every 12 hr.

PO (Adults and children >12 yr and >40 k g): *Most infections*— (following IV loading dose) 200 mg every 12 hr; may be increased to 300 mg every 12 hr if response if inadequate. If phenytoin is coadministered, ↑ maintenance dose to 400 mg every 12 hr; *Esophageal candidiasis*—200 mg every 12 hr for 14 days or 7 days following symptom resolution.

PO (Adults and children >12 yr and <40 kg): *Most infections*— (following IV loading dose) 100 mg every 12 hr; may be increased to 150 mg every 12 hr if response is inadequate. If phenytoin is coadministered, ↑ maintenance dose to 200 mg every 12 hr; *Esophageal candidiasis*—100 mg every 12 hr for 14 days or 7 days following symptom resolution.

PO (Children <12 yrs or <25 kg): *Invasive aspergillosis*—8 mg/kg/dose (maximum: 400 mg/dose) q 12 hr x 2 doses then *Maintenance dosing*—7 mg/kg (maximum: 200 mg/dose) every 12 hrs.

Hepatic Impairment

IV (Adults and Children >12 yr): *Child-Pugh Class A and B*—Use standard loading dose, ↓ maintenance dose by 50%; *Child-Pugh Class C*—Not recommended.

Availability (generic available)

Tablets: 50 mg, 200 mg. **Oral suspension (orange):** 40 mg/mL. **Powder for injection (requires reconstitution):** 200 mg/vial.

NURSING IMPLICATIONS

Assessment

- Monitor for signs and symptoms of fungal infections prior to and during therapy.

- Obtain specimens for culture and histopathology prior to therapy to isolate and identify organism. Therapy may be started before results are received.
- Monitor visual function including visual acuity, visual field, and color perception in patients receiving more than 28 days of therapy. Vision usually returns to normal within 14 days after discontinuation of therapy.
- Monitor for allergic reactions during infusion of voriconazole (flushing, fever, sweating, tachycardia, chest tightness, dyspnea, faintness, nausea, pruritus, rash). Symptoms occur immediately upon start of infusion. May require discontinuation.
- Monitor patients with risk factors for acute pancreatitis (recent chemotherapy, hematopoietic stem cell transplantation [HSCT]) for the signs of pancreatitis (abdominal pain, ↑ serum amylase and lipase).
- Assess for rash periodically during therapy. May cause Stevens-Johnson syndrome. Discontinue therapy if severe or if accompanied with fever, general malaise, fatigue, muscle or joint aches, blisters, oral lesions, conjunctivitis, hepatitis and/or eosinophilia.
- ***Lab Test Considerations:*** Monitor liver function tests (AST, ALT, and bilirubin) prior to, weekly during first month and monthly during therapy. If abnormal liver function tests occur, monitor for development of severe hepatic injury. Discontinue therapy if markedly ↑ or clinical signs and symptoms of liver disease develop.
- Monitor renal function (serum creatinine) during therapy.

Potential Nursing Diagnoses

Risk for infection (Indications)

Implementation

- Once patient can tolerate oral medication, PO voriconazole may be used.
- Correct electrolyte disturbances (hypokalemia, hypomagnesemia, hypocalcemia) prior to initiation and during therapy.
- **PO:** Administer 1 hr before or 1 hr after a meal.
- Shake suspension well (approximately 10 seconds) before measuring suspension. Do not mix suspension with other medicine, flavored liquid, or syrup.

IV Administration

- Do not administer voriconazole with blood products or concentrated electrolytes, even in separate lines. Non-concentrated electrolytes can be infused at same time, but separate lines must be used. TPN can be administered simultaneously but must be via separate line or via a different port in a multi-lumen catheter.
- **Intermittent Infusion:** Reconstitute each 200-mg vial with 19 mL of sterile water for injection to achieve concentration of 10 mg/mL. Calculate volume of 10 mg/mL solution required for patient dose. ***Diluent:*** Withdraw and discard equal volume of diluent from infusion bag or bottle to be used. Withdraw required volume of voriconazole solution from vial(s) and add to appropriate volume of 0.9% NaCl, LR, D5/LR, D5/0.45% NaCl, D5W, 0.45% NaCl, or D5/0.9% NaCl. Reconstituted solution stable for 24 hr if refrigerated. Discard partially used vials. ***Concentration:*** Final concentration of infusion should be 0.5–5 mg/mL. ***Rate:*** Infuse over 1–2 hr at a rate not to exceed 3 mg/kg/hr.
- **Y-Site Compatibility:** acyclovir, alemtuzumab, alfentanil, allopurinol, amifostine, amikacin, aminophylline, amiodarone, amphotericin B liposome, ampicillin, ampicillin/sulbactam, anidulafungin, argatroban, azithromycin, aztreonam, bivalirudin, bleomycin, buprenorphine, butorphanol, bumetanide, buprenorphine, butorphanol, calcium acetate, calcium chloride, calcium gluconate, cangrelor, carboplatin, carmustine, caspofungin, cefazolin, cefotaxime, cefotetan, cefoxitin, ceftaroline, ceftazidime, ceftriaxone, chloramphenicol, chlorpromazine, ciprofloxacin, cisatracurium, cisplatin, clindamycin, cyclophosphamide, cytarabine, dacarbazine, dactinomycin, daptomycin, daunorubicin hydrochloride, dexamethasone, dexmedetomidine, dexrazoxane, digoxin, diltiazem, diphenhydramine, dobutamine, docetaxel, dolasetron, dopamine, doripenem, doxycycline, droperidol, enalaprilat, ephedrine, epinephrine, epirubicin, ertapenem, erythromycin, esmolol, etoposide, etoposide phosphate, famotidine, fenoldopam, fentanyl, fluconazole, fludarabine, fluorouracil, foscarnet, fosphenytoin, furosemide, ganciclovir, gemcitabine, gentamicin, glycopyrrolate, granisetron, haloperidol, heparin, hydralazine, hydrocortisone, ifosfamide, imipenem/cilastatin, insulin, irinotecan, isoproterenol, ketorolac, labetalol, leucovorin, levofloxacin, lidocaine, linezolid, lorazepam, magnesium sulfate, mannitol, mechlorethamine, melphalan, meperidine, meropenem, mesna, methohexital, methotrexate, methyldopate, methylprednisolone, metoclopramide, metoprolol, metronidazole, midazolam, milrinone, mitomycin, morphine, mycophenolate, nafcillin, nalbuphine, naloxone, nicardipine, nitroglycerin, norepinephrine, octreotide, ondansetron, oxaliplatin, oxytocin, paclitaxel, pamidronate, pancuronium, pentamidine, pentazocine, pentobarbital, phenobarbital, phenylephrine, piperacillin/tazobactam, potassium acetate, potassium chloride, potassium phosphates, procainamide, promethazine, propranolol, quinupristin/dalfopristin, remifentanil, rocuronium, sodium acetate, sodium bicarbonate, sodium phosphates, streptozocin, succinylcholine, sufentanil, tacrolimus, teniposide, theophylline, thiotepa, tirofiban, tobramycin, topotecan, trimethoprim/sulfamethox-

V

azole, vancomycin, vasopressin, vecuronium, verapamil, vinblastine, vincristine, vinorelbine, zidovudine, zoledronic acid.

- **Y-Site Incompatibility:** amphotericin B colloidal, amphotericin B lipid complex, busulfan, cefepime, cyclosporine, dantrolene, diazepam, doxorubicin hydrochloride, idarubicin, mitoxantrone, moxifloxacin, nitroprusside, pantoprazole, phenytoin, thiopental.

Patient/Family Teaching

- Advise patient to take voriconazole as directed, on an empty stomach.
- May cause blurred vision, photophobia, and dizziness. Caution patient to avoid driving and other activities requiring alertness until response to medication is known. Also advise patient to avoid driving at night during voriconazole therapy.
- Advise patient to avoid direct sunlight, sunlamps and tanning beds during voriconazole therapy. Use sunscreen and protective clothing to prevent severe sunburn. Advise patient to have dermatologic evaluation regular basis to allow early detection and management of premalignant lesions; squamous cell carcinoma of the skin and melanoma have been reported during long-term therapy.
- Instruct patient to notify health care professional of all Rx or OTC medications, vitamins, or herbal products being taken and consult health care professional before taking any new medications.
- Advise patient to notify health care professional if rash or signs and symptoms of allergic reaction occur.
- Advise women of childbearing age to use contraception and notify health care professional if pregnancy is planned or suspected or if breast feeding. If pregnancy is detected, discontinue medication as soon as possible.

Evaluation/Desired Outcomes

- Resolution of fungal infections.

HIGH ALERT

warfarin (war-fa-rin)

Coumadin, Jantoven

Classification

Therapeutic: anticoagulants

Pharmacologic: coumarins

Pregnancy Category X

Indications

Prophylaxis and treatment of: Venous thrombosis, Pulmonary embolism, Atrial fibrillation with embolization. Management of myocardial infarction: Decreases risk of death, Decreases risk of subsequent MI, Decreases risk of future thromboembolic events. Prevention of thrombus formation and embolization after prosthetic valve placement.

Action

Interferes with hepatic synthesis of vitamin K-dependent clotting factors (II, VII, IX, and X). **Therapeutic Effects:** Prevention of thromboembolic events.

Pharmacokinetics

Absorption: Well absorbed from the GI tract after oral administration.

Distribution: Crosses the placenta but does not enter breast milk.

Protein Binding: 99%.

Metabolism and Excretion: Metabolized by the liver.

Half-life: 42 hr.

TIME/ACTION PROFILE (effects on coagulation tests)

ROUTE	ONSET	PEAK	DURATION
PO	36–72 hr	5–7 days†	2–5 days‡

† At a constant dose

‡ After discontinuation

Contraindications/Precautions

Contraindicated in: Uncontrolled bleeding; Open wounds; Active ulcer disease; Recent brain, eye, or spinal cord injury or surgery; Severe liver or kidney disease; Uncontrolled hypertension; OB: Crosses placenta and may cause fatal hemorrhage in the fetus. May also cause congenital malformation.

Use Cautiously in: Malignancy; Patients with history of ulcer or liver disease; History of poor compliance; Women with childbearing potential; Asian patients or those who carry the CYP2C9*2 allele and/or the CYP2C9*3 allele, or with the VKORC1 AA genotype (↑ risk of bleeding with standard dosing; lower initial doses should be considered); Pedi: Has been used safely but may require more frequent PT/INR assessments; Geri: Due to greater than expected anticoagulant response, initiate and maintain at lower doses.

Adverse Reactions/Side Effects

GI: cramps, nausea. **Derm:** dermal necrosis. **Hemat:** BLEEDING. **Misc:** fever.

Interactions

Drug-Drug: Abciximab, **androgens**, **capecitabine**, **cefotetan**, **chloramphenicol**, **clopidogrel**, **disulfiram**, **fluconazole**, **fluoroquinolones**, **itraconazole**, **metronidazole** (including vaginal use), **thrombolytics**, **eptifibatide**, **tirofiban**, **sulfonamides**, **quinidine**, **quinine**, **NSAIDs**, **valproates**, and **aspirin** may ↑ the response to warfarin and ↑ the risk of bleeding. Chronic use of **acetaminophen** may ↑ the risk of bleeding. Chronic **alcohol** ingestion may ↓ action of warfarin; if chronic **alcohol** abuse results in significant liver damage, action of warfarin may be ↑ due to ↓ production of clotting factor. Acute **alcohol** ingestion may ↑ action of warfarin. **Barbiturates**, **carbamazepine**, **rifampin**, and **hormonal contraceptives containing estrogen** may ↓ the anticoagulant response to warfarin. **Many other drugs** may affect the activity of warfarin.

Drug-Natural Products: St. John's wort ↓ effect. ↑ bleeding risk with **anise**, **arnica**, **chamomile**, **clove**, **dong quai**, **fenugreek**, **feverfew**, **garlic**, **ginger**, **ginkgo**, **Panax ginseng**, **licorice**, and others.

Drug-Food: Ingestion of large quantities of **foods high in vitamin K content** (see list in Appendix J) may antagonize the anticoagulant effect of warfarin.

Route/Dosage

PO (Adults): 2–5 mg/day for 2–4 days; then adjust daily dose by results of INR. Initiate therapy with lower doses in geriatric or debilitated patients or in Asian patients or those with CYP2C9*2 and/or CYP2C9*3 alleles or VKORC1 AA genotype.

PO (Children >1 mo): *Initial loading dose*—0.2 mg/kg (maximum dose: 10 mg) for 2–4 days then adjust daily dose by results of INR, use 0.1 mg/kg if liver dysfunction is present. *Maintenance dose range*—0.05–0.34 mg/kg/day.

Availability (generic available)

Tablets: 1 mg, 2 mg, 2.5 mg, 3 mg, 4 mg, 5 mg, 6 mg, 7.5 mg, 10 mg. **Cost:** *Generic*—1 mg $10.83/100, 2 mg $10.83/100, 2.5 mg $10.83/100, 3 mg $10.83/100, 4 mg $10.83/100, 5 mg $8.52/100, 6 mg $10.64/100, 7.5 mg $10.83/100, 10 mg $10.83/100.

NURSING IMPLICATIONS

Assessment

- Assess for signs of bleeding and hemorrhage (bleeding gums; nosebleed; unusual bruising; tarry, black stools; hematuria; fall in hematocrit or BP; guaiac-positive stools, urine, or nasogastric aspirate).

W

- Assess for evidence of additional or increased thrombosis. Symptoms depend on area of involvement.
- ***Lab Test Considerations:*** Monitor PT, INR and other clotting factors frequently during therapy. Therapeutic PT ranges 1.3–1.5 times greater than control; however, the INR, a standardized system that provides a common basis for communicating and interpreting PT results, is usually referenced. Normal INR (not on anticoagulants) is 0.8–1.2. An INR of 2.5–3.5 is recommended for patients at very high risk of embolization (for example, patients with mitral valve replacement and ventricular hypertrophy). Lower levels are acceptable when risk is lower. Heparin may affect the PT/INR; draw blood for PT/INR in patients receiving both heparin and warfarin at least 5 hr after the IV bolus dose, 4 hr after cessation of IV infusion, or 24 hr after subcut heparin injection. Asian patients and those who carry the CYP2C9*2 allele and/or the CYP2C9*3 allele, or those with VKORC1 AA genotype may require more frequent monitoring and lower doses.
- Geri: Patients over 60 yr exhibit greater than expected PT/INR response. Monitor for side effects at lower therapeutic ranges.
- Pedi: Achieving and maintaining therapeutic PT/INR ranges may be more difficult in pediatric patients. Assess PT/INR levels more frequently.
- Monitor hepatic function and CBC before and periodically throughout therapy.
- Monitor stool and urine for occult blood before and periodically during therapy.
- ***Toxicity and Overdose:*** Withholding 1 or more doses of warfarin is usually sufficient if INR is excessively elevated or if minor bleeding occurs. If overdose occurs or anticoagulation needs to be immediately reversed, the antidote is vitamin K (phytonadione, AquaMEPHYTON). Administration of whole blood or plasma also may be required in severe bleeding because of the delayed onset of vitamin K.

Potential Nursing Diagnoses

Ineffective tissue perfusion (Indications)
Risk for injury (Side Effects)

Implementation

- ***High Alert:*** Do not confuse Coumadin (warfarin) with Avandia (rosiglitazone) or Cardura (doxazosin). Do not confuse Jantoven (warfarin) with Janumet (sitagliptin/metformin) or Januvia (sitagliptin).
- Because of the large number of medications capable of significantly altering warfarin's effects, careful monitoring is recommended when new agents are started or other agents are discontinued. Interactive potential should be evaluated for all new medications (Rx, OTC, and herbal products).
- **PO:** Administer medication at same time each day. Medication requires 3–5 days to reach effective levels; usually begun while patient is still on heparin.
- Do not interchange brands; potencies may not be equivalent.

Patient/Family Teaching

- Instruct patient to take medication as directed. Take missed doses as soon as remembered that day; do not double doses. Inform health care professional of missed doses at time of checkup or lab tests. Inform patients that anticoagulant effect may persist for 2–5 days following discontinuation. Advise patient to read *Medication Guide* before starting therapy and with each Rx refill in case of changes.
- Review foods high in vitamin K (see Appendix J). Patient should have consistent limited intake of these foods, as vitamin K is the antidote for warfarin, and alternating intake of these foods will cause PT levels to fluctuate. Advise patient to avoid cranberry juice or products during therapy.
- Caution patient to avoid IM injections and activities leading to injury. Instruct patient to use a soft toothbrush, not to floss, and to shave with an electric razor during warfarin therapy. Advise patient that venipunctures and injection sites require application of pressure to prevent bleeding or hematoma formation.
- Advise patient to report any symptoms of unusual bleeding or bruising (bleeding gums; nosebleed; black, tarry stools; hematuria; excessive menstrual flow) and pain, color, or temperature change to any area of your body to health care professional immediately. Patients with a deficiency in protein C and/or S mediated anticoagulant response may be at greater risk for tissue necrosis.
- Instruct patient not to drink alcohol or take other Rx, OTC, or herbal products, especially those containing aspirin or NSAIDs, or to start or stop any new medications during warfarin therapy without advice of health care professional.
- Advise patient to notify health care professional if pregnancy is planned or suspected or if breast feeding.
- Instruct patient to carry identification describing medication regimen at all times and to inform all health care personnel caring for patient on anticoagulant therapy before lab tests, treatment, or surgery.
- Emphasize the importance of frequent lab tests to monitor coagulation factors.

Evaluation/Desired Outcomes

- Prolonged PT (1.3–2.0 times the control; may vary with indication) or INR of 2–4.5 without signs of hemorrhage.

zaleplon (za-lep-lon)
Sonata

Classification
Therapeutic: sedative/hypnotics

Schedule IV

Pregnancy Category C

Indications
Short-term management of insomnia in patients unable to get at least 4 hr of sleep; especially useful in sleep initiation disorders.

Action
Produces CNS depression by binding to GABA receptors in the CNS. Has no analgesic properties. **Therapeutic Effects:** Induction of sleep.

Pharmacokinetics
Absorption: Rapidly absorbed following oral administration.
Distribution: Enters breast milk.
Metabolism and Excretion: Extensively metabolized in the liver (mostly by aldehyde oxidase and some by CYP 450 3A4 enzymes).
Half-life: Unknown.

TIME/ACTION PROFILE

ROUTE	ONSET	PEAK	DURATION
PO	within min	unknown	3–4 hr

Contraindications/Precautions
Contraindicated in: Hypersensitivity; Severe hepatic impairment; OB, Lactation: Pregnancy or lactation.
Use Cautiously in: Mild to moderate hepatic impairment, weight ≤50 kg, or concurrent cimetidine therapy (initiate therapy at lowest dose); Impaired respiratory function; History of suicide attempt; Pedi: Safety not established; Geri: ↑ risk of cognitive impairment. If used, start at lowest dose.

Adverse Reactions/Side Effects
CNS: abnormal thinking, amnesia, anxiety, behavior changes, depersonalization, dizziness, drowsiness, hallucinations, headache, impaired memory (briefly following dose), impaired psychomotor function (briefly following dose), malaise, nightmares, sleep-driving, vertigo, weakness. **EENT:** abnormal vision, ear pain, epistaxis, hearing sensitivity, ocular pain, altered sense of smell. **CV:** peripheral edema. **GI:** abdominal pain, anorexia, colitis, dyspepsia, nausea. **GU:** dysmenorrhea. **Derm:** photosensitivity. **Neuro:** hyperesthesia, paresthesia, tremor. **Misc:** fever.

Interactions
Drug-Drug: Cimetidine ↓ metabolism and ↑ effects (initiate therapy at a lower dose). Additive CNS depression with other **CNS depressants** including **alcohol**, **antihistamines**, **opioid analgesics**, other **sedative/hypnotics**, **phenothiazines**, and **tricyclic antidepressants**. Effects may be ↓ by drugs that induce the CYP 450 3A4 enzyme system including **rifampin**, **phenytoin**, **carbamazepine**, and **phenobarbital**.
Drug-Natural Products: Concomitant use of **kava-kava**, **valerian**, **chamomile**, or **hops** can ↑ CNS depression.
Drug-Food: Concurrent ingestion of a **high-fat meal** slows the rate of absorption.

Route/Dosage
PO (Adults <65 yr): 10 mg (range 5–20 mg) at bedtime.
PO (Geriatric Patients or Patients <50 kg): Initiate therapy at 5 mg at bedtime (not to exceed 10 mg at bedtime).

Hepatic Impairment
PO (Adults): Initiate therapy at 5 mg at bedtime (not to exceed 10 mg at bedtime).

Availability (generic available)
Capsules: 5 mg, 10 mg.

NURSING IMPLICATIONS

Assessment
- Assess mental status, sleep patterns, and potential for abuse prior to administering this medication. Zaleplon is used to treat short-term difficulty in falling asleep; decreases time to sleep onset. May not increase total sleep time or decrease number of wakenings after falling asleep. Prolonged use of >7–10 days may lead to physical and psychological dependence. Limit amount of drug available to the patient.
- Assess alertness at time of peak effect. Notify health care professional if desired sedation does not occur.
- Assess patient for pain. Medicate as needed. Untreated pain decreases sedative effects.

Potential Nursing Diagnoses
Insomnia (Indications)
Risk for injury (Side Effects)

Implementation
- Do not confuse Sonata with Soriatane.
- Before administering, reduce external stimuli and provide comfort measures to increase effectiveness of medication.
- Protect patient from injury. Supervise ambulation and transfer of patients after administration. Remove cigarettes. Side rails should be raised and call bell within reach at all times.

- **PO:** Tablets should be swallowed whole with full glass of water immediately before bedtime or after going to bed and experiencing difficulty falling asleep. Do not administer with or immediately after a high-fat or heavy meal.

Patient/Family Teaching

- Instruct patient to take zaleplon as directed. Do not take more than the amount prescribed because of the habit-forming potential. Not recommended for use longer than 7–10 days. Rebound insomnia (1–2 nights) may occur when stopped. If used for 2 wk or longer, abrupt withdrawal may result in dysphoria, insomnia, abdominal or muscle cramps, vomiting, sweating, tremors, and seizures.
- Because of rapid onset, advise patient to go to bed immediately after taking zaleplon.
- May cause daytime drowsiness or dizziness. Advise patient to avoid driving or other activities requiring alertness until response to this medication is known.
- Inform patient that amnesia may occur, but can be avoided if zaleplon is only taken when patient is able to get >4 hr sleep.
- Caution patient that complex sleep-related behaviors (sleep-driving, making phone calls, preparing and eating food, having sex, sleep walking) may occur while asleep. Inform patient to notify health care professional if sleep-related behaviors, (may include sleep-driving—driving while not fully awake after ingestion of a sedative-hypnotic product, with no memory of the event) occur.
- Caution patient to avoid concurrent use of alcohol or other CNS depressants.
- Advise female patient to notify health care professional if pregnancy is planned or suspected or if breast feeding.

Evaluation/Desired Outcomes

- Improved ability to fall asleep; decreased time to sleep onset.

zanamivir (za-**na**-mi-veer)

Relenza

Classification

Therapeutic: antivirals

Pharmacologic: neuraminidase inhibitors

Pregnancy Category C

Indications

Treatment of uncomplicated acute illness caused by influenza virus in patients ≥7 yr who have been symptomatic ≤2 days. Prevention of influenza in patients ≥5 yr.

Action

Inhibits the enzyme neuramidase, which may alter virus particle aggregation and release. **Therapeutic Effects:** Reduced duration or prevention of flu-related symptoms.

Pharmacokinetics

Absorption: 4–17% of inhaled dose is systemically absorbed.

Distribution: Unknown.

Protein Binding: <10%.

Metabolism and Excretion: Mainly excreted by kidneys as unchanged drug; unabsorbed drug is excreted in feces.

Half-life: 2.5–5.1 hr.

TIME/ACTION PROFILE (blood levels)

ROUTE	ONSET	PEAK	DURATION
Inhalation	rapid	1–2 hr	12 hr

Contraindications/Precautions

Contraindicated in: Hypersensitivity to zanamivir or lactose.

Use Cautiously in: Chronic obstructive pulmonary disease or asthma (↑ risk of decreased lung function and/or bronchospasm); OB, Lactation: Safety not established; Pedi: Children <7 yr (for treatment) or <5 yr (for prophylaxis) (safety not established; may be at ↑ risk for neuropsychiatric events).

Adverse Reactions/Side Effects

CNS: SEIZURES, abnormal behavior, agitation, delirium, hallucinations, nightmares. **Resp:** bronchospasm. **Misc:** allergic reactions.

Interactions

Drug-Drug: None noted.

Route/Dosage

Treatment

Inhaln (Adults and children ≥7 yr): 10 mg (given as 2 inhalations of 5 mg each) twice daily for 5 days.

Prophylaxis

Inhaln (Adults and children ≥5 yr): 10 mg (given as 2 inhalations of 5 mg each) daily for 10 days (for household setting) (28 days for community outbreaks).

Availability

Powder for inhalation: 5 mg/blister.

NURSING IMPLICATIONS

Assessment

- Assess patient for signs and symptoms of influenza (fever, headache, myalgia, cough, sore throat) before administration. Determine duration of symptoms. Indicated for patients who have been symptomatic for up to 2 days.
- Determine if patient is lactose intolerant; may cause allergic reaction.

Potential Nursing Diagnoses

Risk for infection (Indications)

Implementation

- Consider available information on influenza drug susceptibility patterns and treatment effects before using zanamivir for prophylaxis.
- **Inhaln:** Administer 2 doses on the first day of treatment whenever possible; must have at least 2 hours between doses. Doses should be administered 12 hr apart on subsequent days. Zanamivir is only for oral inhalation via DISKHALER; do not attempt via nebulization or mechanical ventilation.

Patient/Family Teaching

- Instruct patient to use zanamivir exactly as directed and to finish entire course, even if feeling better.
- Instruct patient in the use of the DISKHALER. Patient should read the accompanying *Patient Instructions for Use*.
- Advise patients that zanamivir is not a substitute for a flu shot. Patients should receive annual flu shot according to immunization guidelines.
- Patients with a history of asthma should be advised to have a fast-acting inhaled bronchodilator available in case of bronchospasm following zanamivir administration. If using bronchodilator and zanamivir concurrently, administer bronchodilator first.
- Advise patients to report behavioral changes (hallucinations, delirium, and abnormal behavior) to health care professional immediately.
- Inform patient that zanamivir does not replace flu shot. Flu shot should be taken according to instructions of health care professional.
- Advise female patient to avoid zanamivir if pregnant or breast feeding.

Evaluation/Desired Outcomes

- Reduced duration or prevention of flu-related symptoms.

zidovudine (zye-**doe**-vue-deen)

AZT, Retrovir

Classification

Therapeutic: antiretrovirals

Pharmacologic: nucleoside reverse transcriptase inhibitors

Pregnancy Category C

Indications

HIV infection (with other antiretrovirals). Reduction of maternal/fetal transmission of HIV. **Unlabeled Use:** Chemoprophylaxis after occupational exposure to HIV.

Action

Following intracellular conversion to its active form, inhibits viral RNA synthesis by inhibiting the enzyme DNA polymerase (reverse transcriptase). Prevents viral replication. **Therapeutic Effects:** Virustatic action against selected retroviruses. Slowed progression and decreased sequelae of HIV infection. Decreased viral load and improved CD4 cell counts. Decreased transmission of HIV to infants born to HIV-infected mothers.

Pharmacokinetics

Absorption: Well absorbed following oral administration.

Distribution: Widely distributed; enters the CNS. Crosses the placenta.

Metabolism and Excretion: Mostly (75%) metabolized by the liver; 15–20% excreted unchanged by the kidneys.

Half-life: 1 hr.

TIME/ACTION PROFILE (blood levels)

ROUTE	ONSET	PEAK	DURATION
PO	unknown	0.5–1.5 hr	4 hr
IV	rapid	end of infusion	4 hr

Contraindications/Precautions

Contraindicated in: Hypersensitivity; Lactation: Breast feeding not recommended in HIV-infected patients.

Use Cautiously in: ↓ bone marrow reserve (dose ↓ required for anemia or granulocytopenia); Severe hepatic or renal disease (dose modification may be required); Geri: Select dose carefully due to potential for age-related ↓ in hepatic, renal, or cardiac function.

Adverse Reactions/Side Effects

CNS: SEIZURES, headache, weakness, anxiety, confusion, ↓ mental acuity, dizziness, insomnia, mental depression, restlessness, syncope. **GI:** HEPATOMEGALY (with steatosis), PANCREATITIS, abdominal pain, diarrhea, nausea, anorexia, drug-induced hepatitis, dyspepsia, oral mucosa pigmentation, vomiting. **F and E:** LACTIC ACIDOSIS. **Derm:** nail pigmentation. **Endo:** fat redistribution, gynecomastia. **Hemat:** anemia, granulocytopenia, pure red-cell aplasia, thrombocytosis. **MS:** back pain, myopathy. **Neuro:** tremor. **Misc:** immune reconstitution syndrome.

Interactions

Drug-Drug: ↑ bone marrow depression with other **agents having bone marrow–depressing properties, antineoplastics, radiation therapy**, or **ganciclovir**. ↑ neurotoxicity may occur with **acyclovir**. Toxicity may be ↑ by concurrent administration of **probenecid** or **fluconazole**. Levels are ↓ by **clarithromycin**.

Z

Route/Dosage

Management of HIV Infection

PO (Adults): 100 mg q 4 hr while awake or 200 mg 3 times daily or 300 mg twice daily (depends on combination and clinical situation).

PO (Children 4 wk–<18 yr): *4–8.9 kg*–12 mg/kg twice daily or 8 mg/kg 3 times daily; *9–29.9 kg*–9 mg/kg twice daily or 6 mg/kg 3 times daily; *≥30 kg*–300 mg twice daily or 200 mg 3 times daily.

IV (Adults and Children >12 yr): 1 mg/kg infused over 1 hr q 4 hr. Change to oral therapy as soon as possible.

IV (Children): 120 mg/m^2 q 6 hr (not to exceed 160 mg/dose) or 20 mg/m^2/hr as a continuous infusion.

Prevention of Maternal/Fetal Transmission of HIV Infection

PO (Adults >14 wk Pregnant): 100 mg 5 times daily until onset of labor.

IV (Adults during Labor and Delivery): 2 mg/kg over 1 hr, then continuous infusion of 1 mg/kg/hr until umbilical cord is clamped.

IV (Infants): 1.5 mg/kg q 6 hr until able to take PO.

PO (Infants): 2 mg/kg q 6 hr, started within 12 hr of birth and continued for 6 wk.

PO (Neonates premature <30 wk gestational age at birth): 2 mg/kg q 12 hr then ↑ to q 8 hr at 4 wk of age.

PO (Neonates premature ≥30 wk gestational age at birth): 2 mg/kg q 12 hr then ↑ to q 8 hr at 2 wk of age.

IV (Neonates premature <30 wk gestational age at birth): 1.5 mg/kg q 12 hr then ↑ to q 8 hr at 4 wk of age.

IV (Neonates premature ≥30 wk gestational age at birth): 1.5 mg/kg q 12 hr then ↑ to q 8 hr at 2 wk of age.

Availability (generic available)

Capsules: 100 mg. **Tablets:** 300 mg. **Oral syrup:** 50 mg/5 mL. **Solution for injection:** 10 mg/mL. ***In combination with:*** lamivudine (Combivir); abacavir and lamivudine (Trizivir); see Appendix B.

NURSING IMPLICATIONS

Assessment

- Assess patient for change in severity of symptoms of HIV and for symptoms of opportunistic infections during therapy.
- ***Lab Test Considerations:*** Monitor viral load and CD4 counts prior to and periodically during therapy.
- Monitor CBC every 2 wk during the first 8 wk of therapy in patients with advanced HIV disease, and decrease to every 4 wk after the first 2 mo if zidovudine is well tolerated or monthly during the first 3 mo and every 3 mo thereafter unless indicated in patients who are asymptomatic or have early symptoms. Commonly causes granulocytopenia and anemia. Anemia may occur 2–4 wk after initiation of therapy. Anemia may respond to epoetin administration (see epoetin monograph). Granulocytopenia usually occurs after 6–8 wk of therapy. Consider dose reduction, discontinuation of therapy, or blood transfusions if hemoglobin is <7.5 g/dL or reduction of >25% from baseline and/or granulocyte count is <750/mm^3 or reduction of >50% from baseline. Therapy may be gradually resumed when bone marrow recovery is evident.
- May cause ↑ serum AST, ALT, and alkaline phosphatase levels. Lactic acidosis may occur with hepatic toxicity, causing hepatic steatosis; may be fatal, especially in women.
- Monitor serum amylase, lipase, and triglycerides periodically during therapy. Elevated serum levels may indicate pancreatitis and require discontinuation.

Potential Nursing Diagnoses

Risk for infection (Indications, Side Effects)

Implementation

- Do not confuse Retrovir (zidovudine) with ritonavir.
- **PO:** Administer doses around the clock.
- **IV:** Patient should receive the IV infusion only until oral therapy can be administered.

IV Administration

- **Intermittent Infusion:** ***Diluent:*** Remove calculated dose from the vial and dilute with D5W or 0.9% NaCl. Do not use solutions that are discolored. Stable for 8 hr at room temperature or 24 hr if refrigerated. ***Concentration:*** Not to exceed 4 mg/mL. ***Rate:*** Infuse at a constant rate over 1 hr or over 30 min in neonates. Avoid rapid infusion or bolus injection.
- **Continuous Infusion:** Has also been administered via continuous infusion.
- **Y-Site Compatibility:** acyclovir, alemtuzumab, allopurinol, amifostine, amikacin, amphotericin B cholesteryl, amphotericin B colloidal, amphotericin B lipid complex, amphotericin B liposome, anidulafungin, argatroban, azithromycin, aztreonam, bivalirudin, bleomycin, carboplatin, carmustine, caspofungin, cefepime, ceftazidime, ceftriaxone, cisatracurium, cisplatin, clindamycin, cyclophosphamide, cytarabine, dactinomycin, daptomycin, dexamethasone sodium phosphate, dexmedetomidine, diltiazem, dobutamine, docetaxel, dolasetron, dopamine, doripenem, doxacurium, doxorubicin hydrochloride, doxorubicin liposome, epirubicin, eptifibatide, ertapenem, erythromycin lactobionate, etoposide, etoposide phosphate, fenoldopam, filgrastim, fluconazole, fludarabine, fluorouracil, foscarnet, gemcitabine, gentamicin, granisetron, heparin, hydromorphone, idarubicin, ifosfamide, imipenem/cilastatin, irinotecan, leucovorin, levofloxacin, linezolid, lorazepam, mechlorethamine, melphalan, meperidine, methotrexate, metoclopramide, metronidazole, milrinone, mitoxantrone, mor-

phine, mycophenolate, nafcillin, nesiritide, nicardipine, octreotide, ondansetron, oxacillin, oxaliplatin, oxytocin, paclitaxel, palonosetron, pamidronate, pancuronium, pantoprazole, pemetrexed, pentamidine, phenylephrine, piperacillin/tazobactam, potassium acetate, potassium chloride, quinapristin/dalfopristin, ranitidine, remifentanil, rituxumab, rocuronium, sargramostim, sodium acetate, tacrolimus, teniposide, thiotepa, tigecycline, tirofiban, tobramycin, trastuzumab, trimethoprim/sulfamethoxazole, trastuzumab, vancomycin, vasopressin, vecuronium, vinblastine, vincristine, vinorelbine, voriconazole, zoledronic acid.

- **Additive Incompatibility:** blood products or protein solutions, dexrazoxane.

Patient/Family Teaching

- Instruct patient to take zidovudine as directed, around the clock, even if sleep is interrupted. Emphasize the importance of compliance with therapy, not taking more than prescribed amount, and not discontinuing without consulting health care professional. Take missed doses as soon as remembered unless almost time for next dose; do not double doses. Inform patient that long-term effects of zidovudine are unknown at this time.
- Instruct patient that zidovudine should not be shared with others.
- Zidovudine may cause dizziness or fainting. Caution patient to avoid driving or other activities requiring alertness until response to medication is known.
- Inform patient that zidovudine does not cure HIV and does not reduce the risk of transmission of HIV to others through sexual contact or blood contamination. Caution patient to use a condom during sexual contact and avoid sharing needles or donating blood to prevent spreading the AIDS virus to others.
- Instruct patient to notify health care professional promptly if fever, sore throat, signs of infection, muscle weakness, or shortness of breath occurs. Caution patient to avoid crowds and persons with known infections. Instruct patient to use soft toothbrush, to use caution when using toothpicks or dental floss, and to have dental work done prior to therapy or deferred until blood counts return to normal. Patient should also notify health care professional immediately if shortness of breath, muscle weakness, muscle aches, symptoms of hepatitis or pancreatitis, or other unexpected reactions occur.
- Advise patient to notify health care professional of all Rx or OTC medications, vitamins, or herbal products being taken and to consult with health care professional before taking other medications.
- Inform patient that redistribution and accumulation of body fat may occur, causing central obesity, dorsocervical fat enlargement (buffalo hump), peripheral wasting, breast enlargement, and cushingoid appearance. The cause and long-term effects are not known.
- Advise patients not to breast feed during therapy.
- Emphasize the importance of regular follow-up exams and blood counts to determine progress and monitor for side effects.

Evaluation/Desired Outcomes

- Decrease in viral load and increase in CD4 counts in patients with HIV.
- Delayed progression of AIDS and decreased opportunistic infections in patients with HIV.
- Reduction of maternal/fetal transmission of HIV.

zinc sulfate (zink **sul**-fate)

Orazinc, ✱PMS Egozinc, Verazinc, Zinc 220, Zincate, Zinkaps

Classification

Therapeutic: mineral and electrolyte replacements/supplements

Pharmacologic: trace metals

Pregnancy Category C (parenteral)

Indications

Replacement and supplementation therapy in patients who are at risk for zinc deficiency, including patients on long-term parenteral nutrition. **Unlabeled Use:** Management of impaired wound healing due to zinc deficiency.

Action

Serves as a cofactor for many enzymatic reactions. Required for normal growth and tissue repair, wound healing, and senses of taste and smell. **Therapeutic Effects:** Replacement in deficiency states.

Pharmacokinetics

Absorption: Poorly absorbed from the GI tract (20–30%).

Distribution: Widely distributed. Concentrates in muscle, bone, skin, kidney, liver, pancreas, retina, prostate, RBCs, and WBCs.

Metabolism and Excretion: 90% excreted in feces, remainder lost in urine and sweat.

Half-life: Unknown.

TIME/ACTION PROFILE (blood levels)

ROUTE	ONSET	PEAK	DURATION
PO	unknown	2 hr	unknown
IV	unknown	unknown	unknown

Contraindications/Precautions

Contraindicated in: Hypersensitivity or allergy to any components in formulation; Pregnancy or lactation

Z

(supplemental amounts >RDA for pregnant or lactating patients); Preparations containing benzyl alcohol should not be used in neonates.
Use Cautiously in: Renal failure.

Adverse Reactions/Side Effects

GI: gastric irritation (oral use only), nausea, vomiting.

Interactions

Drug-Drug: Oral zinc may ↓ absorption of **tetracyclines** or **fluoroquinolones**.
Drug-Food: Caffeine, **dairy products**, and **bran** may ↓ absorption of orally administered zinc.

Route/Dosage

RDA = 15 mg. Doses expressed in mg of elemental zinc unless otherwise noted. Zinc sulfate contains 23% zinc.

Deficiency

PO (Adults): *Prevention of deficiency*—15–19 mg/day; *treatment of deficiency*—must be individualized; based on degree of deficiency.

IV Nutritional Supplementation—Metabolically Stable Patients

IV (Adults): 2.5–4 mg/day; up to 12 mg/day in patients with excessive losses.
IV (Infants and Children ≤5 yr): 100 mcg/kg/day.
IV (Infants up to 3 kg): 300 mcg/kg/day.

Availability (generic available)

Tablets: 66 mg^{OTC}, 110 mg^{OTC}. **Capsules:** 220 mg^{OTC}. **Injection:** 1 mg/mL in 10- and 30-mL vials, 5 mg/mL in 5- and 10-mL vials.

NURSING IMPLICATIONS

Assessment

- Monitor progression of zinc deficiency symptoms (impaired wound healing, growth retardation, decreased sense of taste, decreased sense of smell) during therapy.
- ***Lab Test Considerations:*** Serum zinc levels may not accurately reflect zinc deficiency.
- Long-term high-dose zinc therapy may cause ↓ serum copper concentrations.
- Monitor serum alkaline phosphatase concentrations monthly; may ↑ with zinc therapy.
- Monitor HDL concentrations monthly in patients on long-term high-dose zinc therapy. Serum concentrations may be ↓.

Potential Nursing Diagnoses

Imbalanced nutrition: less than body requirements (Indications)

Implementation

- **PO:** Administer oral doses with food to decrease gastric irritation. Administration with caffeine, dairy products, or bran may impair absorption.
- **IV:** Zinc is often included as a trace mineral in total parenteral nutrition solution prepared by pharmacist.

Patient/Family Teaching

- Encourage patient to comply with diet recommendations of health care professional. Explain that the best source of vitamins is a well-balanced diet with foods from the four basic food groups. Foods high in zinc include seafood, organ meats, and wheat germ.
- Patients self-medicating with vitamin supplements should be cautioned not to exceed RDA. The effectiveness of megadoses for treatment of various medical conditions is unproved and may cause side effects.
- Instruct patients receiving oral zinc to notify health care professional if severe nausea or vomiting, abdominal pain, or tarry stools occur.
- Emphasize the importance of follow-up exams to evaluate progress.

Evaluation/Desired Outcomes

- Improved wound healing.
- Improved senses of taste or smell. 6–8 wk of therapy may be required before full effect is seen.

ziprasidone (zi-pra-si-done)

Geodon, ✦Zeldox

Classification
Therapeutic: antipsychotics, mood stabilizers
Pharmacologic: piperazine derivatives

Pregnancy Category C

Indications

Schizophrenia; IM form is reserved for control of acutely agitated patients. Treatment of acute manic or mixed episodes associated with Bipolar I Disorder (oral only). Maintenance treatment of Bipolar I Disorder (as adjunct to lithium or valproate) (oral only).

Action

Effects probably mediated by antagonism of dopamine type 2 (D2) and serotonin type 2 (5-HT_2). Also antagonizes α_2 adrenergic receptors. **Therapeutic Effects:** Diminished schizophrenic behavior.

Pharmacokinetics

Absorption: 60% absorbed following oral administration; 100% absorbed from IM sites.
Distribution: Unknown.
Protein Binding: 99%; potential for drug interactions due to drug displacement is minimal.
Metabolism and Excretion: 99% metabolized by the liver; <1% excreted unchanged in urine.
Half-life: *PO*—7 hr; *IM*—2–5 hr.

TIME/ACTION PROFILE (blood levels)

ROUTE	ONSET	PEAK	DURATION
PO	within hours	1–3 days†	unknown
IM	rapid	60 min	unknown

†Steady state achieved following continuous use.

Contraindications/Precautions

Contraindicated in: Hypersensitivity; History of QT prolongation (persistent QTc measurements >500 msec), arrhythmias, recent MI or uncompensated heart failure; Concurrent use of other drugs known to prolong the QT interval including quinidine, dofetilide, sotalol, other class Ia and III antiarrhythmics, pimozide, sotalol, thioridazine, chlorpromazine, pentamidine, arsenic trioxide, mefloquine, dolasetron, tacrolimus, droperidol, and moxifloxacin; Hypokalemia or hypomagnesemia; Lactation: Discontinue drug or bottle feed.

Use Cautiously in: Concurrent diuretic therapy or diarrhea (may ↑ the risk of hypotension, hypokalemia, or hypomagnesemia); Significant hepatic impairment; History of cardiovascular or cerebrovascular disease; Hypotension, concurrent antihypertensive therapy, dehydration, or hypovolemia (may ↑ risk of orthostatic hypotension); Patients at risk for aspiration pneumonia; History of suicide attempt; OB: Neonates at ↑ risk for extrapyramidal symptoms and withdrawal after delivery when exposed during the 3rd trimester; use only if maternal benefit outweighs risk to fetus; Pedi: Safety not established; Geri: Alzheimer's dementia or age >65 yr (may ↑ risk of seizures). Geriatric patients (may require ↓ doses; ↑ risk of mortality in elderly patients treated for dementia-related psychosis).

Adverse Reactions/Side Effects

CNS: NEUROLEPTIC MALIGNANT SYNDROME, seizures, dizziness, drowsiness, restlessness, extrapyramidal reactions, syncope, tardive dyskinesia. **Derm:** DRUG REACTION WITH EOSINOPHILIA AND SYSTEMIC SYMPTOMS (DRESS), STEVENS-JOHNSON SYNDROME. **Resp:** cough/runny nose. **CV:** PROLONGED QT INTERVAL, orthostatic hypotension. **GI:** constipation, diarrhea, nausea, dysphagia. **GU:** amenorrhea, impotence. **Hemat:** AGRANULOCYTOSIS, leukopenia, neutropenia. **Endo:** galactorrhea, hyperglycemia, hyperlipidemia, weight gain. **Derm:** rash, urticaria.

Interactions

Drug-Drug: Concurrent use of **quinidine**, **dofetilide**, **other class Ia and III antiarrhythmics**, **pimozide**, **sotalol**, **thioridazine**, **chlorpromazine**, **pentamidine**, **arsenic trioxide**, **mefloquine**, **dolasetron**, **tacrolimus**, **droperidol**, **moxifloxacin**, or other agents that prolong the QT interval may result in potentially life-threatening adverse drug reactions (concurrent use contraindicated). Additive CNS depression may occur with **alcohol**, **antidepressants**, **antihistamines**, **opioid analgesics**, or **sedative/hypnotics**. Blood levels and effectiveness may be ↓ by **carbamazepine**. Blood levels and effects may be ↑ by **ketoconazole**.

Route/Dosage

Schizophrenia

PO (Adults): 20 mg twice daily initially; dose increments may be made at 2-day intervals up to 80 mg twice daily.

IM (Adults): 10–20 mg as needed up to 40 mg/day; may be given as 10 mg every 2 hr or 20 mg every 4 hr.

Acute Manic or Mixed Episodes Associated with Bipolar I Disorder

PO (Adults): 40 mg twice on first day, then 60 or 80 mg twice daily on second day, then 40–80 mg twice daily.

Maintenance Treatment of Bipolar I Disorder (as adjunct to lithium or valproate)

PO (Adults): Continue same dose on which patient was initially stabilized (range: 40–80 mg twice daily).

Availability (generic available)

Capsules: 20 mg, 40 mg, 60 mg, 80 mg. **Cost:** *Generic*—20 mg $380.02/180, 40 mg $544.16/180, 60 mg $451.99/180, 80 mg $451.99/180. **Lyophilized powder for injection (requires reconstitution):** 20 mg/vial.

NURSING IMPLICATIONS

Assessment

- Monitor patient's mental status (orientation, mood, behavior) prior to and periodically during therapy.
- Assess weight and BMI initially and periodically during therapy.
- Monitor BP (sitting, standing, lying) and pulse rate prior to and frequently during initial dose titration. Patients found to have persistent QTc measurements of >500 msec should have ziprasidone discontinued. Patients who experience dizziness, palpitations, or syncope may require further evaluation (i.e., Holter monitoring).
- Assess for rash during therapy. May be treated with antihistamines or corticosteroids. Usually resolves upon discontinuation of ziprasidone. Medication should be discontinued if no alternative etiology for rash is found. May cause Stevens-Johnson syndrome or DRESS. Discontinue therapy if severe or if accompanied with fever, general malaise, fatigue, muscle or joint aches, blisters, oral lesions, conjunctivitis, hepatitis and/or eosinophilia.
- Observe carefully when administering medication to ensure medication is actually taken and not hoarded or cheeked.
- Monitor for onset of akathisia (restlessness or desire to keep moving) and extrapyramidal side effects (*parkinsonian*—difficulty speaking or swallowing, loss of balance control, pill rolling of hands, mask-like face, shuffling gait, rigidity, tremors and dys-

Z

tonic muscle spasms, twisting motions, twitching, inability to move eyes, weakness of arms or legs) every 2 mo during therapy and 8–12 wk after therapy has been discontinued. Notify health care professional if these symptoms occur, as reduction in dose or discontinuation of medication may be necessary. Trihexyphenidyl or benztropine may be used to control these symptoms.
- Although not yet reported for ziprasidone, monitor for possible tardive dyskinesia (uncontrolled rhythmic movement of mouth, face, and extremities, lip smacking or puckering, puffing of cheeks, uncontrolled chewing, rapid or worm-like movements of tongue). Report these symptoms immediately; may be irreversible.
- Monitor frequency and consistency of bowel movements. Increasing bulk and fluids in the diet may help to minimize constipation.
- Ziprasidone lowers the seizure threshold. Institute seizure precautions for patients with history of seizure disorder.
- Monitor for development of neuroleptic malignant syndrome (fever, respiratory distress, tachycardia, seizures, diaphoresis, hypertension or hypotension, pallor, tiredness). Notify health care professional immediately if these symptoms occur.
- Monitor for symptoms related to hyperprolactinemia (menstrual abnormalities, galactorrhea, sexual dysfunction).
- ***Lab Test Considerations:*** Monitor serum potassium and magnesium prior to and periodically during therapy. Patients with low potassium or magnesium should have levels treated and checked prior to resuming therapy. Obtain fasting blood glucose and cholesterol levels initially and periodically during therapy.
- Monitor CBC frequently during initial months of therapy in patients with pre-existing or history of low WBC. May cause leukopenia, neutropenia, or agranulocytosis. Discontinue therapy if this occurs.
- Monitor serum prolactin prior to and periodically during therapy. May cause ↑ serum prolactin levels.

Potential Nursing Diagnoses

Risk for other-directed violence (Indications)
Disturbed thought process (Indications)
Imbalanced nutrition: risk for more than body requirements (Side Effects)

Implementation

- Dose adjustments should be made at intervals of no less than 2 days. Usually patients should be observed for several weeks before dose titration.
- Patients on parenteral therapy should be converted to oral doses as soon as possible.
- **PO:** Administer capsules with food or milk to decrease gastric irritation. Swallow capsules whole; do not open.
- **IM:** Add 1.2 mL of Sterile Water for Injection to the vial; shake vigorously until all drug is dissolved for a concentration of 20 mg/mL. Discard unused portion. Do not mix with other products or solutions. Do not administer solutions that are discolored or contain particulate matter.

Patient/Family Teaching

- Instruct patient to take medication as directed, at the same time each day. Do not discontinue medication without discussing with health care professional, even if feeling well. Patients on long-term therapy may need to discontinue gradually.
- Inform patient of possibility of extrapyramidal symptoms. Instruct patient to report these symptoms immediately.
- Advise patient to change positions slowly to minimize orthostatic hypotension.
- May cause seizures and drowsiness. Caution patient to avoid driving or other activities requiring alertness until response to medication is known.
- Advise patient to notify health care professional of all Rx or OTC medications, vitamins, or herbal products being taken and to consult with health care professional before taking other medications. Caution patient to avoid concurrent use of alcohol and other CNS depressants.
- Advise patient to notify health care professional of medication regimen prior to treatment or surgery.
- Instruct patient to notify health care professional promptly if dizziness, loss of consciousness, palpitations, menstrual abnormalities, galactorrhea or sexual dysfunction occur.
- Advise female patients to notify health care professional if pregnancy is planned or suspected, or if breast feeding or planning to breast feed.
- Advise patient of need for continued medical follow-up for psychotherapy, eye exams, and laboratory tests.

Evaluation/Desired Outcomes

- Decrease in acute excited, manic behavior.
- Decrease in positive (delusions, hallucinations) and negative symptoms (social withdrawal, flat, blunted affect) of schizophrenia.
- Management of signs and symptoms of Bipolar I Disorder.

ziv-aflibercept

(ziv a-**flib**-er-sept)
Zaltrap

Classification
Therapeutic: antineoplastics
Pharmacologic: fusion proteins

Pregnancy Category C

Indications

Used in combination with 5-fluorouracil, leucovorin and irinotecan-(FOLFIRI), for metastatic colorectal cancer (mCRC) that is resistant to/progressed after an oxaliplatin-containing regimen.

Action

Binds to human Vascular Endothelial Growth Factor (VEGF-A), resulting in decreased neovascularization and decreased vascular permeability. Also inhibits proliferation of endothelial cells, decreasing growth of new blood vessels. **Therapeutic Effects:** Decreased spread of mCRC.

Pharmacokinetics

Absorption: IV administration results in complete bioavailability.
Distribution: Unknown.
Metabolism and Excretion: Unknown.
Half-life: 6 days (range 4–7 days).

TIME/ACTION PROFILE (improved survival)

ROUTE	ONSET	PEAK	DURATION
IV	4–6	unknown	unknown

Contraindications/Precautions

Contraindicated in: OB: Pregnancy (may cause fetal harm); Lactation: Should not be used in nursing mothers.
Use Cautiously in: Elective surgery; Geri: ↑ risk of adverse effects especially diarrhea/dehydration; Females/males with reproductive potential; Pedi: Safety and effectivenessnot established.

Adverse Reactions/Side Effects

CNS: REVERSIBLE POSTERIOR LEUKOENCEPHALOPATHY SYNDROME, fatigue, headache. **EENT:** dysphonia. **CV:** ARTERIAL THROMBOTIC EVENTS, hypertension. **GI:** GI PERFORATION, abdominal pain, anorexia, diarrhea, fistula formation, ↑ liver enzymes, stomatitis. **GU:** NEPHROTIC SYNDROME, ↑serum creatinine, proteinuria. **Derm:** impaired wound healing, Palmar-Plantar Erythrodysesthesia Syndrome, skin hyperpigmentation. **F and E:** dehydration. **Hemat:** BLEEDING, NEUTROPENIA, THROMBOTIC MICROANGIOPATHY, leukopenia, thrombocytopenia. **Metab:** weight loss.

Interactions

Drug-Drug: ↑ risk of bone marrow depression with other **antineoplastics** or **radiation therapy**.

Route/Dosage

IV (Adults): 4 mg/kg every 2 wk continued until disease progression or unacceptable toxicity.

Availability

Solution for intravenous administration (requires dilution): 25 mg/mL.

NURSING IMPLICATIONS

Assessment

- Monitor for signs and symptoms of bleeding. Do not initiate ziv-aflibercept in patients with severe hemorrhage. Discontinue in patients who develop severe hemorrhage.
- Monitor for signs and symptoms of GI perforation. Discontinue therapy in patients with GI perforation or who develop a fistula.
- Monitor BP every 2 wk or more frequently as needed during therapy. Treat with antihypertensive agents. Temporarily suspend ziv-aflibercept in patients with uncontrolled hypertnesion until controlled, and permanently reduce dose to 2 mg/kg for subsequent cycles. Discontinue in hypertensive crisis or with hypertensive encephalopathy.
- Monitor for arterial thrombotic events (TIA, CVA, angina). Discontinue therapy in patients with an arterial thrombotic event.
- Assess for diarrhea during therapy. Geri: Incidence is greater with elderly patients.
- ***Lab Test Considerations:*** Monitor proteinuria by urine dipstick and urinary protein creatinine ratio (UPCR) for development or worsening proteinuria. Obtain 24–hr urine collection in patients with ≥2+ for protein or UPCR >1. Suspend therapy for proteinuria ≥2 g/24 hr and resume when proteinuria is <2 g/24 hr. If recurrent, suspend until proteinuria <2 g/24 hr and then permanently reduce ziv-aflibercept dose to 2 mg/kg. Discontinue therapy in patients who develop nephrotic syndrome.
- Monitor CBC with differential at baseline and before each cycle. Delay therapy until neutrophil count is $\geq 1.5 \times 10^9$/L.
- May cause ↑ serum AST and ALT.

Potential Nursing Diagnoses

Diarrhea (Adverse Reactions)
Risk for impaired skin integrity (Adverse Reactions)

Implementation

- Administer ziv-aflibercept prior to other components of the FOLFIRI regimen on the day of treatment.
- ***High Alert:*** Fatalities have occurred with chemotherapeutic agents. Before administering, clarify all ambiguous orders; double check single, daily, and course-of-therapy dose limits; have second practitioner independently double check original order, dose calculations and infusion pump settings.

IV Administration

- **Intermittent Infusion:** Solution should be clear and colorless to pale yellow; do not administer solutions that are discolored or contain particulate matter. Do not re-enter vial after initial puncture; discard unused portion. ***Diluent:*** Withdraw prescribed dose and dilute with 0.9% NaCl or D5W.

Z

Concentration: 0.6–8 mg/mL. Use polyvinyl chloride (PVC) infusion bags containing bis (2–ethylhexyl) phthalate (DEHP) or polyolefin infusion bags. Store infusion bags for up to 4 hr; discard unused portion. ***Rate:*** Infuse over 1 hr through a 0.2 micron polyethersulfone filter. Do not use filters made of polyvinylidene fluoride (PVDF) or nylon every 2 wk. Do not administer as IV push or bolus. Use infusion set made of PVC containing DEHP, DEHP free PVC containing trioctyl-trimellitate (TOTM), polypropylene, polypropylene lined PVC, or polyurethane.

- **Y-Site Incompatibility:** Do not combine with other drugs in same infusion bag or IV line.

Patient/Family Teaching

- Explain purpose of therapy and potential adverse effects to patient.
- Advise patient to notify health care professional immediately if signs of bleeding (lightheadedness), hypertension (severe headache, lightheadedness, neurologic symptoms), severe diarrhea, vomiting, severe abdominal pain, fever or other signs of infection, or symptoms of arterial thromboembolic events occur.
- Advise patient to maintain adequate hydration to minimize risk and to notify health care professional promptly if signs and symptoms of reversible posterior leukoencephalopathy syndrome (RPLS) (headache, seizures, weakness, confusion, high BP, blindness or change in vision, problems thinking) occur. Symptoms usually resolve within days.
- Advise patient to notify health care provider of therapy prior to surgery or if had recent surgery. Ziv-aflibercept should be suspended for at least 4 wk prior to major surgery and until surgical wounds fully healed. For minor surgery, such as central venous access port placement, biopsy, and tooth extraction ziv-aflibercept may be initiated/resumed once wound is fully healed. Discontinuation is needed in patients with compromised wound healing.
- Inform female patient that ziv-aflibercept can cause fetal harm. Advise women with reproductive potential and men of the need for effective contraception during and for at least 3 mo after completion of therapy. Notify health care provider immediately if pregnancy is planned or suspected or if breast feeding.
- Emphasize importance of monitoring lab values to monitor for adverse reactions.

Evaluation/Desired Outcomes

- Decrease in spread of metastatic colorectal cancer.

zoledronic acid

(zoe-led-**dron**-ic **as**-id)

✱Aclasta, Reclast, Zometa

Classification
Therapeutic: bone resorption inhibitors, electrolyte modifiers, hypocalcemics
Pharmacologic: biphosphonates

Pregnancy Category C

Indications

Hypercalcemia of malignancy (Zometa only). Multiple myeloma and metastatic bone lesions from solid tumors (Zometa only). Paget's disease (Reclast only). Treatment of osteoporosis in men (Reclast only). Treatment and prevention of osteoporosis in postmenopausal women (Reclast only). Treatment and prevention of glucocorticoid-induced osteoporosis in patients expected to be on glucocorticoids for at least 12 mo (Reclast only).

Action

Inhibits bone resorption. Inhibits increased osteoclast activity and skeletal calcium release induced by tumors. **Therapeutic Effects:** Decreased serum calcium. Decreased serum alkaline phosphatase. Decreased fractures, radiation/surgery to bone, or spinal cord compression in patients with multiple myeloma or metastatic bone lesions. Decreased hip, vertebral, or non-vertebral osteoporosis-related fractures in postmenopausal women. Increased bone mass in men, postmenopausal women, and patients on prolonged corticosteroid therapy.

Pharmacokinetics

Absorption: IV administration results in complete bioavailability.
Distribution: Unknown.
Metabolism and Excretion: Mostly excreted unchanged by the kidneys.
Half-life: 167 hr.

TIME/ACTION PROFILE (effect on serum calcium)

ROUTE	ONSET	PEAK	DURATION
IV	within 4 days	4–7 days	30 days

Contraindications/Precautions

Contraindicated in: Hypersensitivity to zoledronic acid or other bisphosphonates; Severe renal impairment (CCr <35 mL/min) or acute renal failure; Hypocalcemia (correct before administering); adequate supplemental calcium and vitamin D required.
Use Cautiously in: History of aspirin-induced asthma; Chronic renal impairment; Chronic renal impairment, concurrent use of diuretics or nephrotoxic drugs, or dehydration (↑ risk of renal impairment; correct deficits prior to use); Concurrent use of nephrotoxic drugs; Invasive dental procedures, cancer, receiving chemotherapy, corticosteroids, or angiogenesis inhibitors, undergoing radiation, poor oral hygiene, periodontal disease, dental disease, anemia, coagulop-

athy, infection, or poorly-fitting dentures (may ↑ risk of jaw osteonecrosis); Geri: ↑ risk of renal impairment; OB, Lactation, Pedi: Safety not established.

Adverse Reactions/Side Effects

CNS: agitation, anxiety, confusion, insomnia. **EENT:** conjunctivitis. **CV:** hypotension, chest pain, leg edema. **GI:** abdominal pain, constipation, diarrhea, nausea, vomiting, dysphagia. **GU:** renal impairment/failure. **Derm:** STEVENS-JOHNSON SYNDROME, TOXIC EPIDERMAL NECROLYSIS, pruritus, rash. **F and E:** hypophosphatemia, hypocalcemia, hypokalemia, hypomagnesemia. **Hemat:** anemia. **MS:** musculoskeletal pain, femur fractures, osteonecrosis (primarily of jaw). **Resp:** asthma exacerbation. **Misc:** fever, flu-like syndrome.

Interactions

Drug-Drug: Concurrent use of **loop diuretics**, **calcitonin**, or **aminoglycosides** ↑ risk of hypocalcemia. Concurrent use of **NSAIDs** may ↑ risk of nephrotoxicity.

Route/Dosage

Reclast

IV (Adults): *Paget's disease*— 5 mg as a single dose (information regarding retreatment unknown); *Treatment of osteoporosis in men or postmenopausal women, treatment/prevention of glucocorticoid-induced osteoporosis*— 5 mg once early; *Prevention of osteoporosis in postmenopausal women*— 5 mg every 2 yr.

Zometa

IV (Adults): *Hypercalcemia of malignancy*— 4 mg; may be repeated after 7 days; *Multiple myeloma and bone metastases from solid tumors*— 4 mg q 3–4 wk (has been used for up to 15 mo).

Availability (generic available)

Solution for IV infusion (Zometa): 4 mg/5–mL vial. **Solution for IV infusion (premixed) (Zometa):** 4 mg/100 mL. **Solution for IV infusion (premixed) (Reclast):** 5 mg/100 mL.

NURSING IMPLICATIONS

Assessment

- Monitor intake and output ratios. Initiate a vigorous saline hydration promptly and maintain a urine output of 2 L/day during therapy. Patients should be adequately hydrated, but avoid overhydration. Do not use diuretics prior to treatment of hypovolemia.
- Assess for acute-phase reaction (fever, mylagia, flu-like symptoms, headache, arthralgia). Usually occur within 3 days of dose and resolve within 3 days of onset, but may take 7–14 days to resolve; incidence decreases with repeat dosing.
- Perform a routine oral exam prior to initiation of therapy. Dental exam with appropriate preventative dentistry should be considered prior to therapy. Patients with history of tooth extraction, poor oral hygiene, gingival infections, diabetes, cancer, receiving radiation, anemia, coagulopathy, or use of a dental appliance or those taking immunosuppressive therapy, angiogenesis inhibitors, or systemic corticosteroids are at greater risk for osteonecrosis of the jaw.
- **Hypercalcemia:** Monitor symptoms of hypercalcemia (nausea, vomiting, anorexia, weakness, constipation, thirst, cardiac arrhythmias).
- Observe for evidence of hypocalcemia (paresthesia, muscle twitching, laryngospasm, Chvostek's or Trousseau's sign).
- **Paget's Disease:** Assess for symptoms of Paget's disease (bone pain, headache, decreased visual and auditory acuity, increased skull size) periodically during therapy.
- **Osteoporosis:** Assess patients via bone density study for low bone mass before and periodically during therapy.
- ***Lab Test Considerations:*** Monitor serum creatinine, calculated based on actual body weight using the Cockcroft-Gault formula, prior to each treatment. Patients with a normal serum creatinine prior to treatment, who develop an increase of 0.5 mg/dL within 2 wk of next dose should have next dose withheld until serum creatinine is within 10% of baseline value. Patients with an abnormal serum creatinine prior to treatment who have an increase of 1.0 mg/dL within 2 wk of next dose should have next dose withheld until serum creatinine is within 10% of baseline value.
- Assess serum calcium, phosphate, and magnesium before and periodically during therapy. If hypocalcemia, hypophosphatemia, or hypomagnesemia occur, temporary supplementation may be required. Hypocalcemia and vitamin D deficiency should be treated before initiating zoledronic acid therapy.
- Monitor CBC with differential and hemoglobin and hematocrit closely during therapy.
- *Paget's Disease:* Monitor serum alkaline phosphatase prior to and periodically during therapy to monitor effectiveness.

Potential Nursing Diagnoses

Risk for injury (Indications)

Implementation

- Vigorous saline hydration alone may be sufficient to treat mild, asymptomatic hypercalcemia. Adequate rehydration is required prior to administration.
- Patients on long-term therapy should have 1200 mg of oral calcium and 800–1000 units of Vitamin D each day.
- Patients treated for *Paget's disease* should receive 1500 mg elemental calcium and 800 IU of vitamin D daily, particularly during the 2 wk after dosing. Pa-

tients with osteoporosis should take 1200 mg of calcium and 800–1000 IU of Vitamin D daily. Patients with multiple myeloma and bone metastasis of solid tumors take an oral calcium supplement of 500 mg and a multiple vitamin containing 400 international units of vitamin D daily.

- Administration of acetaminophen or ibuprofen following administration may reduce the incidence of acute-phase reaction symptoms.

IV Administration

- **Intermittent Infusion:** ***Diluent:*** Reconstitute *Zometa* by adding 5 mL of sterile water for injection to each vial for a solution containing 4 mg of zoledronic acid. Medication must be completely dissolved prior to withdrawal of solution. Dilute 4-mg dose further with 100 mL of 0.9% NaCl or D5W. If not used immediately, may be refrigerated for up to 24 hr. *Reclast* comes ready to use 5 mg in 100-mL solution. If refrigerated, allow solution to reach room temperature prior to administration. Do not administer solution that is discolored or contains particulate matter. ***Rate:*** Administer as a single infusion over at least 15 min. Rapid infusions increase risk of renal deterioration and renal failure.
- **Y-Site Compatibility:** acyclovir, alfentanil, allopurinol, amifostine, amikacin, aminophylline, amiodarone, amphotericin B colloidal, amphotericin B lipid complex, amphotericin B liposome, ampicillin, ampicillin/sulbactam, anidulafungin, argatroban, azithromycin, aztreonam, bivalirudin, bleomycin, bumetanide, buprenorphine, busulfan, butorphanol, carboplatin, carmustine, caspofungin, cefazolin, cefepime, cefotaxime, cefotetan, cefoxitin, ceftazidime, ceftriaxone, cefuroxime, chloramphenicol, chlorpromazine, ciprofloxacin, cisatracurium, cisplatin, clindamycin, cyclophosphamide, cyclosporine, cytarabine, dacarbazine, dactinomycin, daptomycin, daunorubicin hydrochloride, dexamethasone, dexmedetomidine, dexrazoxane, digoxin, diltiazem, diphenhydramine, dobutamine, docetaxel, dolasetron, dopamine, doxorubicin hydrochloride, doxorubicin liposomal, doxycycline, droperidol, enalaprilat, ephedrine, epinephrine, epirubicin, eptifibatide, ertapenem, erythromycin, esmolol, etoposide, etoposide phosphate, famotidine, fenoldopam, fentanyl, fluconazole, fludarabine, fluorouracil, foscarnet, fosphenytoin, furosemide, ganciclovir, gemcitabine, gentamicin, glycopyrrolate, granisetron, haloperidol, heparin, hydralazine, hydrocortisone, hydromorphone, idarubicin, ifosfamide, imipenem/cilastatin, insulin, irinotecan, isoproterenol, ketorolac, labetalol, levofloxacin, lidocaine, linezolid, lorazepam, magnesium sulfate, mannitol, mechlorethamine, melphalan, meperidine, meropenem, mesna, methotrexate, methyldopate, methylprednisolone, metoclopramide, metoprolol, metronidazole, midazolam, milrinone, mitomycin, mitoxantrone, morphine, moxifloxacin, mycophenolate, nafcillin, nalbuphine, naloxone, nesiritide, nicardipine, nitroglycerin, nitroprusside, norepinephrine, octreotide, ondansetron, oxaliplatin, oxytocin, paclitaxel, pancuronium, pantoprazole, pemetrexed, pentamidine, pentazocine, pentobarbital, phenobarbital, phenylephrine, piperacillin/tazobactam, potassium acetate, potassium chloride, potassium phosphates, procainamide, prochlorperazine, promethazine, propranolol, quinupristin/dalfopristin, ranitidine, remifentanil, rocuronium, sodium acetate, sodium bicarbonate, sodium phosphates, streptozocin, succinylcholine, sufentanil, tacrolimus, teniposide, theophylline, thiopental, thiotepa, tigecycline, tirofiban, tobramycin, topotecan, trimethoprim/sulfamethoxazole, vancomycin, vecuronium, verapamil, vinblastine, vincristine, vinorelbine, voriconazole, zidovudine.
- **Y-Site Incompatibility:** alemtuzumab, calcium-containing solutions, dantrolene, diazepam, phenytoin. Manufacturer recommends administration as a single infusion in a line separate from all other drugs.
- **Additive Incompatibility:** Do not mix with solutions containing calcium, such as Lactated Ringer's solution.

Patient/Family Teaching

- Explain the purpose of zoledronic acid to patient. Advise patient to read *Medication Guide* prior to each administration in case of changes.
- Advise patients of the importance of adequate hydration. Patient should be instructed to drink at least two glasses of water prior to receiving dose.
- Advise patient to notify health care professional of all Rx or OTC medications, vitamins, or herbal products being taken and to consult with health care professional before taking other medications.
- Advise patient to eat a balanced diet and consult health care professional about the need for supplemental calcium and vitamin D.
- Inform patient that severe musculoskeletal pain may occur within days, months, or yr after starting zoledronic acid. Symptoms may resolve completely after discontinuation or slow or incomplete resolution may occur. Notify health care professional if severe pain occurs.
- Encourage patient to participate in regular exercise and to modify behaviors that increase the risk of osteoporosis (stop smoking, reduce alcohol consumption).
- Advise patient to notify health care professional if signs and symptoms if osteonecrosis of the jaw (pain, numbness, swelling of or drainage from the jaw, mouth, or teeth) or hypocalcemia (spasms, twitches, or cramps in muscles; numbness or tingling in fingers, toes, or around mouth) or thigh, hip, or groin pain occur.
- Advise patient to inform health care professional of zoledronic acid therapy prior to dental surgery.

- Advise patient to notify health care professional if pregnancy is planned or suspected or if breast feeding.
- Emphasize the importance of lab tests to monitor progress.

Evaluation/Desired Outcomes

- Decrease in serum calcium.
- Decrease in serum alkaline phosphatase and the progression of Paget's disease.
- Reversal of the progression of osteoporosis with decreased fractures and other sequelae. Discontinuation after 3–5 years should be considered for postmenopausal women with low risk for fractures.

ZOLMitriptan (zole-mi-trip-tan)

Zomig, Zomig-ZMT

Classification

Therapeutic: vascular headache suppressants

Pharmacologic: 5-HT_1 agonists

Pregnancy Category C

Indications

Acute treatment of migraine headache.

Action

Acts as an agonist at specific 5-HT_1 receptor sites in intracranial blood vessels and sensory trigeminal nerves.
Therapeutic Effects: Cranial vessel vasoconstriction with resultant decrease in migraine headache.

Pharmacokinetics

Absorption: Well absorbed (40%) following oral and intranasal administration.
Distribution: Unknown.
Metabolism and Excretion: Mostly metabolized by the liver; some conversion to metabolites that are more active than zolmitriptan. 8% excreted unchanged in urine.
Half-life: 3 hr (for zolmitriptan and active metabolite).

TIME/ACTION PROFILE (relief of headache)

ROUTE	ONSET	PEAK	DURATION
PO	unknown	1.5 hr*	unknown
Intranasal	unknown	3 hr	unknown

*3 hr for orally disintegrating tablets.

Contraindications/Precautions

Contraindicated in: Hypersensitivity; Significant underlying heart disease (including ischemic heart disease, history of MI, coronary artery vasospasm, uncontrolled hypertension); Stroke or transient ischemic attack; Peripheral vascular disease (including, but not limited to ischemic bowel disease); Concurrent (or within 24 hr) use of other 5-HT agonists, ergotamine, or ergot-type medications; Concurrent (or within 2 wk) use of MAO inhibitors; Hemiplegic or basilar migraine; Symptomatic Wolff-Parkinson-White syndrome or other arrhythmias; Moderate-severe hepatic impairment (nasal spray only).
Use Cautiously in: Cardiovascular risk factors (hypertension, hypercholesterolemia, cigarette smoking, obesity, diabetes, strong family history, menopausal females or males >40 yr [use only if cardiovascular status has been evaluated and determined to be safe and 1st dose is administered under supervision]); Hepatic impairment (use lower doses of oral); OB, Lactation, Pedi: Children <18 yr (safety and effectiveness not established for PO); children <12 yr (safety and effectiveness not established for intranasal).

Adverse Reactions/Side Effects

CNS: dizziness, drowsiness, vertigo, weakness. **EENT:** throat pain/tightness/pressure. **CV:** MI, angina, chest pain/pressure/tightness/heaviness, hypertension, palpitations. **GI:** dry mouth, dyspepsia, dysphagia, nausea. **Derm:** sweating, warm/cold sensation. **MS:** myalgia, myasthenia. **Neuro:** hypesthesia, paresthesia. **Misc:** feeling of heaviness, pain.

Interactions

Drug-Drug: Because of ↑ risk of cerebral vasospasm, avoid concurrent use of other **5-HT agonists** (**naratriptan**, **sumatriptan**, **rizatriptan**) and/or **ergot-type preparations** (**dihydroergotamine**). Concurrent use of **MAO inhibitors** ↑ blood levels and risk of toxicity (avoid use within 2 wk of MAO inhibitors). Blood levels may be ↑ by **hormonal contraceptives**. **Cimetidine** ↑ half-life of zolmitriptan and its active metabolite. ↑ risk of serotonin syndrome when used with **SSRI or SNRI antidepressants**.
Drug-Natural Products: ↑ risk of serotinergic side effects including serotonin syndrome with **St. John's wort** and **SAMe**.

Route/Dosage

PO (Adults): 1.25–2.5 mg initially; if headache returns, dose may be repeated after 2 hr (not to exceed 10 mg/24 hr); *Concurrent cimetidine therapy*—Single dose not to exceed 2.5 mg (not to exceed 5 mg/24 hr).

Hepatic Impairment

PO (Adults): *Moderate-severe hepatic impairment (oral tablets only)*—1.25 mg initially; if headache returns, dose may be repeated after 2 hr (not to exceed 5 mg/24 hr).
Intranasal (Adults and Children ≥12 yr): Single 2.5-mg dose (maximum single dose = 5 mg); may be repeated after 2 hr (not to exceed 10 mg/24 hr); *Con-*

Z

current cimetidine therapy—Single dose not to exceed 2.5 mg (not to exceed 5 mg/24 hr).

Availability (generic available)

Tablets: 2.5 mg, 5 mg. **Orally disintegrating tablets:** 2.5 mg, 5 mg. **Nasal spray:** 2.5 mg/100 mcL unit-dose spray device (package of 6), 5 mg/100 mcL unit-dose spray device (package of 6).

NURSING IMPLICATIONS

Assessment

- Assess pain location, intensity, duration, and associated symptoms (photophobia, phonophobia, nausea, vomiting) during migraine attack.
- Monitor for serotonin syndrome in patients taking SSRIs or SNRIs concurrently with zolmitriptan.

Potential Nursing Diagnoses

Acute pain (Indications)

Implementation

- Do not confuse zolmitriptan with sumatriptan.
- **PO:** Initial dose is 2.5 mg. Lower doses can be achieved by breaking 2.5-mg tablet.
- Orally disintegrating tablets should be left in the package until use. Remove from the blister pouch. Do not push tablet through the blister; peel open the blister pack with dry hands and place tablet on tongue. Do not break orally disintegrating tablet. Tablet will dissolve rapidly and be swallowed with saliva. No liquid is needed to take the orally disintegrating tablet.
- **Intranasal:** Remove cap from nasal spray. Hold upright and block one nostril. Tilt head slightly back, insert device into opposite nostril, and depress plunger. May repeat in 2 hr.

Patient/Family Teaching

- Inform patient that zolmitriptan should be used only during a migraine attack. It is meant to be used to relieve migraine attack but not to prevent or reduce the number of attacks.
- Instruct patient to administer zolmitriptan as soon as symptoms appear, but it may be administered any time during an attack. If migraine symptoms return, a 2nd dose may be used. Allow at least 2 hr between doses, and do not use more than 10 mg in any 24-hr period.
- If dose does not relieve headache, additional zolmitriptan doses are not likely to be effective; notify health care professional.
- Advise patient that lying down in a darkened room following zolmitriptan administration may further help relieve headache.
- May cause dizziness or drowsiness. Caution patient to avoid driving or other activities requiring alertness until response to medication is known.
- Advise patient to notify health care professional prior to next dose of zolmitriptan if pain or tightness in the chest occurs during use. If pain is severe or does not subside, notify health care professional immediately. If wheezing; heart throbbing; swelling of eyelids, face, or lips; skin rash; skin lumps; or hives occur, notify health care professional immediately and do not take more zolmitriptan without approval of health care professional. If feelings of tingling, heat, flushing, heaviness, pressure, drowsiness, dizziness, tiredness, or sickness develop, discuss with health care professional at next visit.
- Advise patient to avoid alcohol, which aggravates headaches, during zolmitriptan use.
- Advise patient that overuse (use more than 10 days/month) may lead to exacerbation of headache (migraine-like daily headaches, or as a marked increase in frequency of migraine attacks). May require gradual withdrawal of zolmitriptan and treatment of symptoms (transient worsening of headache).
- Advise patient to notify health care professional of all Rx or OTC medications, vitamins, or herbal products being taken and to consult with health care professional before taking other medications. Patients concurrently taking SSRI or SNRI antidepressants should notify health care professional promptly if signs of serotonin syndrome (mental status changes: agitation, hallucinations, coma; autonomic instability: tachycardia, labile BP, hyperthermia; neuromuscular aberrations: hyper-reflexia, incoordination; and/or gastrointestinal symptoms: nausea, vomiting, diarrhea) occur.
- Caution patient not to use zolmitriptan if pregnancy is planned or suspected or if breast feeding. Adequate contraception should be used during therapy.

Evaluation/Desired Outcomes

- Relief of migraine attack.

zolpidem (zole-pi-dem)

Ambien, Ambien CR, Edluar, Intermezzo, ✽Sublinox, Zolpimist

Classification

Therapeutic: sedative/hypnotics

Schedule IV

Pregnancy Category C

Indications

Insomnia with difficulties in sleep initiation (Intermezzo is indicated for insomnia when a middle-of-the-night awakening is followed by difficulty returning to sleep).

Action

Produces CNS depression by binding to GABA receptors. Has no analgesic properties. **Therapeutic Effects:** Sedation and induction of sleep.

Pharmacokinetics

Absorption: Rapidly absorbed following oral administration. Controlled-release formulation releases 10 mg immediately, then another 2.5 mg later.

Distribution: Minimal amounts enter breast milk; remainder of distribution not known.

Metabolism and Excretion: Converted to inactive metabolites, which are excreted by the kidneys; clearance of Intermezzo lower in women than in men.

Half-life: 2.5–3 hr (↑ in geriatric patients and patients with hepatic impairment).

TIME/ACTION PROFILE (sedation)

ROUTE	ONSET	PEAK*	DURATION
PO	rapid	30 min–2 hr	6–8 hr
PO-ER	rapid	2–4 hr	6–8 hr
PO-Spray	rapid	unknown	unknown
SL	rapid	unknown	unknown

*Food delays peak levels and effects.

Contraindications/Precautions

Contraindicated in: Hypersensitivity; Sleep apnea.

Use Cautiously in: History of previous psychiatric illness, suicide attempt, drug or alcohol abuse; Hepatic impairment (initial dose ↓ recommended); Pulmonary disease; Sleep apnea; Myasthenia gravis; Geri: Initial dose ↓ recommended; OB, Lactation, Pedi: Safety not established.

Adverse Reactions/Side Effects

CNS: daytime drowsiness, dizziness, abnormal thinking, agitation, amnesia, behavior changes, "drugged" feeling, hallucinations, sleep-driving. **GI:** diarrhea, nausea, vomiting. **Misc:** ANAPHYLAXIS, hypersensitivity reactions, physical dependence, psychological dependence, tolerance.

Interactions

Drug-Drug: CNS depression may ↑ with **sedatives/hypnotics**, **alcohol**, **phenothiazines**, **tricyclic antidepressants**, **opioid analgesics**, or **antihistamines**.

Drug-Natural Products: Concomitant use of **kava-kava**, **valerian**, or **chamomile** can ↑ CNS depression.

Drug-Food: **Food** ↓ and delays absorption.

Route/Dosage

PO, SL (Adults): *Tablets, spray, or SL tablets (Edluar)*—5 mg (for women) and 5–10 mg (for men) at bedtime; may ↑ to 10 mg at bedtime if 5–mg dose not effective; *SL tablets (Intermezzo)*—1.75 mg (for women) or 3.5 mg (for men) once upon awakening in the middle-of-the-night; *Extended-release tablets*—6.25 mg (for women) and 6.25–12.5 mg (for men) at bedtime; may ↑ to 12.5 mg at bedtime if 6.25–mg dose not effective.

PO, SL (Geriatric Patients , Debilitated Patients, or Patients with Hepatic Impairment): *Tablets, spray or SL tablets (Edluar)*—Do not exceed dose of 5 mg at bedtime; *Extended-release tablets*—Do not exceed dose of 6.25 mg at bedtime.

SL (Geriatric Patients , Patients taking concomitant CNS depressants, or Patients with Hepatic Impairment): *SL tablets (Intermezzo)*—Do not exceed dose of 1.75 mg at bedtime (in either men or women).

Availability (generic available)

Tablets: 5 mg, 10 mg. **Cost:** *Generic*—5 mg $7.81/30. **Extended-release tablets:** 6.25 mg, 12.5 mg. **Cost:** *Generic*—6.25 mg $42.14/30, 12.5 mg $37.39/30. **Sublingual tablets (Edluar):** 5 mg, 10 mg. **Cost:** All strengths $235.19/30. **Sublingual tablets (Intermezzo):** 1.75 mg, 3.5 mg. **Cost:** All strengths $248.46/30. **Oral spray (Zolpimist):** 5 mg/spray (60 sprays/container). **Cost:** $79.20/7.7 mL.

NURSING IMPLICATIONS

Assessment

- Assess mental status, sleep patterns, and potential for abuse prior to administration. Prolonged use of >7–10 days may lead to physical and psychological dependence. Limit amount of drug available to the patient.
- Assess alertness at time of peak effect. Notify health care professional if desired sedation does not occur.
- Assess patient for pain. Medicate as needed. Untreated pain decreases sedative effects.

Potential Nursing Diagnoses

Insomnia (Indications)
Risk for injury (Side Effects)

Implementation

- ***High Alert:*** Do not confuse zolpidem with Zyloprim (allopurinol).
- Before administering, reduce external stimuli and provide comfort measures to increase effectiveness of medication.
- Protect patient from injury. Raise bed side rails. Assist with ambulation. Remove patient's cigarettes.
- Use lowest effective dose.
- **PO:** Tablets should be swallowed whole with full glass of water. For faster onset of sleep, do not administer with or immediately after a meal.
- Swallow extended-release tablets whole; do not crush, break, or chew.
- **SL:** To open the blister pack, separate the individual blisters at the perforations. Peel off top layer of paper and push tablet through foil. Place the tablet under the tongue, allow to disintegrate; do not swallow or take with water.
- *Intermezzo*—Only take if at least 4 hr left prior to time to awakening.

Z

- **Oral Spray:** Do not take with or immediately after a meal; may slow effect. Spray is a clear, colorless, and cherry-flavor solution.

Patient/Family Teaching

- Instruct patient to take zolpidem as directed. Advise patient not to take zolpidem unless able to stay in bed a full night (7–8 hours) before being active again. Do not take more than the amount prescribed because of the habit-forming potential. Not recommended for use longer than 7–10 days. If used for 2 wk or longer, abrupt withdrawal may result in fatigue, nausea, flushing, light-headedness, uncontrolled crying, vomiting, GI upset, panic attack, or nervousness. Instruct patient to read *Patient Information* for correct product before taking and with each Rx refill in case of changes.
- Because of rapid onset, advise patient to go to bed immediately after taking zolpidem.
- May cause daytime drowsiness or dizziness. Advise patient to avoid driving or other activities requiring alertness until response to this medication is known.
- Caution patient that complex sleep-related behaviors (sleep-driving) may occur while asleep.
- Advise patient to notify health care professional immediately if signs of anaphylaxis (swelling of the tongue or throat, trouble breathing, and nausea and vomiting) occur.
- Caution patient to avoid concurrent use of alcohol or other CNS depressants.
- **Oral Spray:** To prime, patients should be told to point the black spray opening away from their face and other people and spray 5 times. For administration, hold container upright with the black spray opening pointed directly into the mouth. Press down fully on pump to make sure a full dose (5 mg) is sprayed directly into mouth over tongue. For 10-mg dose, a second spray should be administered. If not used for 14 days, re-prime with 1 spray.

Evaluation/Desired Outcomes

- Relief of insomnia.
- Re-evaluate insomnia after 7–10 days of *Intermezzo*.

zonisamide (zoe-**niss**-a-mide)

Zonegran

Classification

Therapeutic: anticonvulsants

Pharmacologic: sulfonamides

Pregnancy Category C

Indications

Partial seizures in adults.

Action

Raises the threshold for seizures and reduces duration of seizures probably by action on sodium and calcium channels. **Therapeutic Effects:** Decreased frequency of partial seizures.

Pharmacokinetics

Absorption: Well absorbed following oral administration.

Distribution: Binds extensively to red blood cells.

Protein Binding: 40%.

Metabolism and Excretion: Mostly metabolized by the liver; 35% excreted unchanged in urine. Some metabolism occurs via CYP3A4 enzyme system.

Half-life: 63 hr (plasma).

TIME/ACTION PROFILE (blood levels†)

ROUTE	ONSET	PEAK	DURATION
PO	unknown	2–6 hr	24 hr

†Requires 2 weeks of dosing to achieve steady-state blood levels.

Contraindications/Precautions

Contraindicated in: Hypersensitivity to zonisamide or sulfonamides.

Use Cautiously in: All patients (may ↑ risk of suicidal thoughts/behaviors); Hepatic or renal disease (may require slower titration/more frequent monitoring; ↑ risk of metabolic acidosis with renal impairment); Patients with respiratory disorders, diarrhea, or undergoing surgery (↑ risk of metabolic acidosis); OB, Lactation: Use only if potential benefit justifies risk to fetus/infant; Pedi: Children ≤16 yr (safety not established; ↑ risk of oligohydrosis, hyperthermia, and/or metabolic acidosis).

Adverse Reactions/Side Effects

CNS: SUICIDAL THOUGHTS, drowsiness, fatigue, agitation/irritability, depression, dizziness, psychomotor slowing, psychosis, weakness. **EENT:** amblyopia, tinnitus. **Resp:** cough, pharyngitis. **GI:** anorexia, nausea, vomiting. **F and E:** metabolic acidosis. **GU:** kidney stones. **Derm:** STEVENS-JOHNSON SYNDROME, oligohydrosis (↑ in children), rash. **Metab:** hyperthermia (↑ in children). **Neuro:** abnormal gait, hyperasthesia, incoordination, tremor.

Interactions

Drug-Drug: Drugs that induce or inhibit CYP3A4 may alter blood levels and effects of zonisamide. Blood levels and effects may be ↓ by **phenytoin**, **carbamazepine**, **phenobarbital**, or **valproate**. May enhance the adverse/toxic effect of **carbonic anhydrase inhibitors**, avoid combination.

Route/Dosage

PO (Adults and Children >16 yr): 100 mg once daily initially for 2 wk, then ↑ to 200 mg daily for 2 wk; with subsequent increments of 100 mg made at 2-wk intervals as required (range 100–600 mg/day). Can be given as a single daily dose or in 2 divided doses.

PO (Infants and Children): Initial: 1–2 mg/kg/day given in two divided doses/day; increase dose in increments of 0.5–1 mg/kg/day every 2 weeks (maximum dose: 12 mg/kg/day).

Availability (generic available)

Capsules: 25 mg, 50 mg, 100 mg. **Cost:** *Generic*—25 mg $54.80/100, 50 mg $109.60/100, 100 mg $219.20/100.

NURSING IMPLICATIONS

Assessment

- Monitor closely for notable changes in behavior that could indicate the emergence or worsening of suicidal thoughts or behavior or depression.
- Monitor frequency, duration, and characteristics of seizures.
- Monitor patient frequently for development of skin rash. Unexplained rash may require discontinuation of therapy.
- Assess patient for allergy to sulfa drugs.
- ***Lab Test Considerations:*** Monitor renal function periodically during therapy. May cause ↑ creatinine and BUN.
- Measure serum bicarbonate before starting and periodically during therapy. Metabolic acidosis may be more frequent and severe in younger patients.
- May cause ↑ in serum alkaline phosphatase.

Potential Nursing Diagnoses

Risk for injury (Adverse Reactions)

Implementation

- **PO:** May be administered with or without meals. Capsules should be swallowed whole.

Patient/Family Teaching

- Instruct patient to take zonisamide as directed, even if feeling well. Consult health care professional if a dose is missed. Do not discontinue abruptly without consulting health care professional; may cause seizures. Instruct patient to read the *Medication Guide* before starting and with each Rx refill, changes may occur.
- Instruct patient to contact health care professional immediately if skin rash occurs or seizures worsen. Patient should also contact health care professional if a child taking zonisamide is not sweating as usual, with or without a fever, or if they develop fever, sore throat, oral ulcers, easy bruising, depression, unusual thoughts, speech or language problems.
- May cause drowsiness. Caution patient to avoid driving or other activities requiring alertness until cleared by health care professional and effects of medication is known.
- Advise patient to increase fluid intake to at least 6–8 glasses of water/day to minimize risk of kidney stones. Instruct patient to contact health care professional if symptoms of kidney stones (sudden back pain, abdominal pain, blood in urine) occur.
- Advise patient and family to notify health care professional if thoughts about suicide or dying, attempts to commit suicide; new or worse depression; new or worse anxiety; feeling very agitated or restless; panic attacks; trouble sleeping; new or worse irritability; acting aggressive; being angry or violent; acting on dangerous impulses; an extreme increase in activity and talking, other unusual changes in behavior or mood occur.
- Advise patient to notify health care professional of all Rx or OTC medications, vitamins, or herbal products being taken and to consult with health care professional before taking other medications.
- May have teratogenic effects. Advise women of childbearing age to use effective contraception throughout therapy. Instruct patient to notify health care professional if pregnancy is planned or suspected or if planning to breast feed.

Evaluation/Desired Outcomes

- Decrease in frequency and duration of partial seizures.

Drugs Approved in Canada

These monographs describe medications approved for use in Canada by the Therapeutic Products Directorate, a division of Health Canada's Health Products and Food Branch. The medications are not approved by the United States Food and Drug Administration; however, similar formulations carrying different generic or brand names might be available in the US.

alfacalcidol (al-fa kal-si-dol)

✱One-Alpha

Classification

Therapeutic: vitamins

Pharmacologic: vitamin D analogues

Indications

Management of hypocalcemia, secondary hyperparathyroidism and osteodystrophy associated with chronic renal failure.

Action

Stimulates intestinal absorption of calcium and phosphorus, reabsorption of calcium from bone and renal reabsorption of calcium. Does not require renal activation.

Therapeutic Effects: Improved calcium and phosphorus homeostasis in patients with chronic kidney disease.

Pharmacokinetics

Absorption: Completely absorbed following oral administration.

Distribution: Unknown.

Protein Binding: Extensively protein bound.

Metabolism and Excretion: Following absorption, 50 % is rapidly converted by liver to active metabolite (1.25–$(OH)_2D$; 13% renally excreted.

Half-life: 3 hr.

TIME/ACTION PROFILE (levels of active metabolite)

ROUTE	ONSET†	PEAK	DURATION‡
PO	6 hr	12 hr	few days–1wk
IV	unknown	4 hr	few days–1 wk

†Effect on intestinal calcium absorption, bone pain and muscle weakness improve within 2 wk–3 mo.

‡Effect on serum calcium levels following discontinuation.

Contraindications/Precautions

Contraindicated in: Lactation: Breast feeding should be avoided; Concurrent use of other Vitamin D analogues or magnesium-containing antacids.

Use Cautiously in: OB: potential benefits should be weighed against hazards to fetus and mother; Pedi: safe and effective use in children has not been established.

Adverse Reactions/Side Effects

CNS: headache, drowsiness, weakness. **CV:** ARRHYTHMIAS, hypertension. **EENT:** conjunctivitis, photophobia. **GI:** constipation, nausea, anorexia, dry mouth, metallic taste, pancreatitis, polydipsia, vomiting. **Derm:** pruritus. **F and E:** HYPERCALCEMIA, hyperphosphatemia, hyperthermia, ↑ thirst. **GU:** albuminuria, hypercalcuria, ↓ libido, nocturia, polyuria. **Metab:** ectopic calcification, hypercholesterolemia, hyperthermia. **MS:** bone pain, muscle pain.

Interactions

Drug-Drug: Hypercalcemia ↑ risk of toxicity from **digitalis glycosides**, including **digoxin**. ↑ risk of toxicity and adverse reactions with concurrent use of other **vitamin D analogues**. Concurrent use of **bile acid sequestrants** including **cholestyramine** or **mineral oil** ↓ absorption and effectiveness. Concurrent use of **barbiturates** and other **anticonvulsants** may ↓ effectiveness, larger doses of alfacalcidol may be required.

Route/Dosage

PO (Adults): *Pre-dialysis patients*—0.25 mcg/day for 2 mo initially, if necessary dose increments of 0.25 mg/day may be made at 2 mo intervals (usual range 0.5–1.0 mcg/day); *dialysis patients* —1 mcg/day, if necessary dose increments of 0.5 mcg/day may be made at 2–4 wk intervals (usual range 1–2 mcg/day, up to 3 mcg/day). When normalization occurs, dose should be ↓ to minimum amount required to maintain normal serum calcium levels.

IV (Adults): *Dialysis patients*—1 mcg during each dialysis (2–3 times weekly), if necessary dose may be increased weekly by 1 mcg per dialysis up to 12 mcg/wk (range 1.5–12 mcg/wk). When normalization occurs, dose should be ↓ to minimum amount required to maintain normal serum calcium levels.

Availability

Soft gel capsules: 0.25 mcg, 1 mcg; Oral drops: 2 mcg/mL; Solution for intravenous injection (contains ethanol and propylene glycol): 2 mcg/mL.

NURSING IMPLICATIONS

Assessment

- Assess for signs of vitamin D deficiency prior to and during treatment.
- Assess patient for bone pain and weakness during therapy; usually decreases within 2 wk to 3 mo.
- ***Lab Test Considerations:*** *For pre-dialysis patients:* Monitor serum calcium and phosphate levels monthly and electrolytes periodically during treatment. *For dialysis patients:* Monitor serum calcium at least twice weekly during dose titration. If hypercalcemia occurs decrease dose of alfacalcidol by 50% and stop all calcium supplements until calcium levels return to normal. May cause ↑ plasma phosphorous

levels. Maintain serum phosphate levels <2.0 mmol/L. Monitor inorganic phosphorus, magnesium, alkaline phosphatase, creatinine, BUN, 24-hour urinary calcium and protein as needed.

- ***Toxicity and Overdose:*** Toxicity is manifested as hypercalcemia, hypercalciuria, and hyperphosphatemia. Assess patient for appearance of nausea, vomiting, anorexia, weakness, constipation, headache, bone pain, and metallic taste. Later symptoms include polyuria, polydipsia, photophobia, rhinorrhea, pruritus, and cardiac arrhythmias. Notify health care professional immediately if these signs of hypervitaminosis D occur. Treatment usually consists of discontinuation of alfacalcidol, a low-calcium diet, stopping calcium supplements. Persistent or markedly elevated serum calcium levels in hemodialysis patients may be corrected by dialysis against a calcium-free dialysate.

Potential Nursing Diagnoses

Imbalanced nutrition: less than body requirements

Implementation

- **PO:** Administer with food. Use calibrated dropper with oral for accurate dose. Oral solution may be mixed with water or milk.
- **IV:** Administer IV during hemodialysis. Shake well before use. Keep refrigerated. Single use vials; discard unused portion.

Patient/Family Teaching

- Advise patient to take medication as directed. Do not stop taking without consulting with health care professional.
- Advise patient and family to notify health care professional if signs and symptoms of hypercalcemia occur.
- Review diet modifications with patient. See Appendix J for foods high in calcium and vitamin D. Renal patients must still consider renal failure diet in food selection. Health care professional may order concurrent calcium supplement.
- Encourage patient to comply with dietary recommendations. Explain that best source of vitamins is a well-balanced diet with foods from all 4 basic food groups, and sunlight exposure for Vitamin D.
- Advise patient to avoid concurrent use of antacids containing magnesium during therapy.
- Instruct patient to notify health care professional of all Rx or OTC medications, vitamins, or herbal products being taken and to consult health care professional before taking any other Rx, OTC, or herbal products.
- Advise female patient to notify health care professional if pregnancy is planned or suspected or if breast feeding.
- Emphasize the importance of follow-up exams to evaluate progress.

Evaluation

- Improved levels of calcium and phosphorous in patients with kidney disease.

bezafibrate (bezz-uh-**fibe**-rate)

✱Bezalip SR

Classification

Therapeutic: lipid-lowering agents

Pharmacologic: fibric acid derivatives

Indications

Use in conjunction with diet and other modalities in the treatment of hypercholesterolemia (Type IIa and IIb mixed hyperlipidemia, to decrease serum TG, LDL cholesterol and apolipoprotein B and increase HDL cholesterol and apolipoprotein A). Treatment of adults with hypertriglyceridemia (Type IV and V hyperlipidemias) at risk pancreatitis and other sequelae.

Action

Inhibits triglyceride synthesis. **Therapeutic Effects:** Lowered cholesterol and triglycerides, increased HDL, with decreased risk of pancreatitis and other sequelae.

Pharmacokinetics

Absorption: Well absorbed (100%) following oral admininistration.

Distribution: Unknown.

Metabolism and Excretion: 50% metabolized, 50% excreted unchanged in urine, remainder as metabolites. 3% excreted in feces.

Half-life: 1–2 hr.

TIME/ACTION PROFILE (blood levels)

ROUTE	ONSET	PEAK	DURATION
PO	unknown	3–4 hr	24 hr

Contraindications/Precautions

Contraindicated in: Hypersensitivity/photosensitivity to bezafibrate or other fibric acid or fibrate derivatives; Severe liver or kidney impairment (CCr <60 mL/min), primary biliary cirrhosis, gallstone or gallbladder disease or hypoalbuminemia; OB: Avoid use during pregnancy (discontinue several mo prior to conception); Lactation: Discontinue breast feeding.

Use Cautiously in: History of liver disease; Doses >400 m g/day in conjuction with HMG coA reductase inhibitors (statins) with any risk factors (renal impairment, infection, trauma, surgery, hormonal or electrolyte imbalance) ↑ risk for rhabdomyolysis; Geri: Consider age-related decrease in renal function, avoid in patients >70 yr; Pedi: limited experience in children at a dose of 10–20 mg/kg/day, use cautiously.

Adverse Reactions/Side Effects

CNS: dizziness, headache. **GI:** dyspepsia, flatulence, gastritis, abdominal distension, abdominal pain, ↓ appetite, cholestasis, constipation, diarrhea, nausea. **GU:** erectile dysfunction, renal failure. **Derm:** alopecia, pruritus, urticaria, photosensitivity reaction, alopecia, rash. **MS:** muscle cramps, muscular weakness, myalgia, RHABDOMYOLYSIS. **Misc:** hypersensitivity reactions including ANAPHYLAXIS.

Interactions

Drug-Drug: ↑ risk of bleeding with **oral anticoagulants**; dose of anticoagulant should be ↓ by 50% with frequent monitoring. **Cyclosporine** ↑ risk of severe myositis/rhabdomyolysis, risk of combined therapy should be undertaken with caution. Concurrent use of **immunosuppressants** may ↑ risk of reversible renal impairment. ↑ risk of myopathy **HMG CoA reductase inhibitors (statins)**, combination therapy should be undertaken with extreme caution and must be discontinued at the first signs of myopathy and should not be undertaken in the presence of predisposing factors including impaired renal function, severe infection, trauma, surgery, hormonal /electrolyte imbalance or ↑ alcohol intake. ↑ risk of serious hypoglycemia with **insulin** or **sulphonylureas**. Concurrent use with **MAO inhibitors** may ↑ risk of hepatotoxicity. **Cholestyramine** and other **bile-acid sequestrants** may ↓ absorption, separate administration by ≥2 hr. Effectiveness may be ↓ by concurrent **estrogen**.

Route/Dosage
PO (Adults): 400 mg once daily.

Availability
Sustained-release tablet: 400 mg.

NURSING IMPLICATIONS

Assessment
- Obtain a diet history with regard to fat consumption. Before starting benzafibrate, every attempt should be made to obtain a normal triglyceride level with diet, exercise and weight loss.
- Assess patient for cholelithiasis. If gallbladder studies are indicated, and gallstones are found, discontinue therapy.
- ***Lab Test Considerations:*** Monitor serum lipids prior to and periodically during therapy.
- ***Lab Test Considerations:*** Monitor AST and ALT serums periodically during therapy to assess for increased levels. Discontinue therapy if levels rise >3 times normal value.
- ***Lab Test Considerations:*** If patient develops muscle tenderness during therapy, monitor CPK levels. If CPK levels are markedly ↑ or myopathy occurs, discontinue therapy.

Potential Nursing Diagnoses
Noncompliance

Implementation
- **PO:** Administer without regards to meals. Swallow sustained-release tablets whole; do not crush, break, or chew.

Patient/Family Teaching
- Instruct the patient to take the medication as directed, and to not share medication. Missed doses should be taken as soon as remembered. Do not double dose. Medication helps control but does not cure elevated serum triglyceride levels.
- Advise patient that medication should be taken in conjunction with diet restrictions of fat, cholesterol, carbohydrates, and alcohol, as well as an exercise regimen, and cessation of smoking.
- Instruct patient to notify health care professional of unexplained muscle pain or weakness, tiredness, fever, nausea, vomiting, abdominal pain.
- Instruct patient to notify health care professional of all Rx or OTC medications, vitamins, or herbal products being taken and to consult health care professional before taking any other Rx, OTC, or herbal products.
- Instruct female patients to immediately notify health care professional if pregnancy is planned or suspected.
- Emphasize importance of follow-up appointments, and lab tests to evaluate effectiveness.

Evaluation
- A decrease in serum triglyceride and LDL cholesterol levels.
- An increase in HDL levels.

buserelin (bue-se-**rel**-in)
✱Suprefact

Classification
Therapeutic: antineoplastics, hormones
Pharmacologic: luteinizing hormone-releasing hormone (LHRH) analogues

Indications
Subcutaneous injection—Initial and maintenance palliative treatment of advanced hormone-dependent prostate cancer (usually given with an anti-androgen). *Nasal solution*—Maintenance palliative treatment of advanced hormone-dependent prostate cancer (usually given with an anti-androgen). *Nasal solution*—Non-surgical treatment of endometriosis (course of treatment 6–9 mo).

Action
Acts as a synthetic analog of endogenous gonadotropin-releasing hormone (GnRH/LHRH). Chronic use results in inhibited secretion of gonadotropin release and gonadal steroid production. The overall effect is due to down-regulation of pituitary LHRH receptors. In males, testosterone synthesis and release is decreased. In females, secretion of estrogen in decreased. **Therapeutic Effects:** Decreased spread of advanced prostate cancer. Decreased sequelae of endometriosis (pain, dysmenorrhea).

Pharmacokinetics
Absorption: *Subcut*—70%; *intranasal*—1–3%; *implant*—drug is slowly absorbed over 2–3 mo.
Distribution: Accumulates in liver, kidneys and anterior pituitary lobe; enters breast milk in small amounts.
Metabolism and Excretion: Metabolized in liver, kidneys and by enzymes on membranes in the pituitary gland.
Half-life: *Subcut*—80 min; *intranasal*—1–2 hr; *implant*—20–30 days.

TIME/ACTION PROFILE

ROUTE	ONSET	PEAK	DURATION
prostate cancer †	7 days	4 mos	until discontinuation
endometriosis ‡(intranasal)	unknown	unknown	duration of treatment

†Decrease in testosterone levels.
‡Symptom improvement.

Contraindications/Precautions

Contraindicated in: Hypersensitivity; Non-hormonal-dependent prostate cancer or previous orchiectomy; Females with undiagnosed vaginal bleeding; OB: Pregnancy (avoid use); Lactation: Breast feeding is contraindicated (small amounts enter breast milk; injection contains benzyl alcohol).

Use Cautiously in: Prostate cancer with urinary tract obstruction or spinal lesions; Pedi: Safe and effective use in children had not been established (injection contains benzyl alcohol).

Adverse Reactions/Side Effects

CNS: depression, dizziness. **CV:** hypertension. **Endo:** glucose intolerance. **Hemat:** anemia. **Local:** injection site reactions. **MS:** osteoporosis (long-term use. **Misc:** transient exacerbation of metastatic prostate cancer or endometriosis.

Prostate cancer

CNS: headache (nasal solution). **EENT:** nasal irritation (nasal spray). **GU:** ↓ libido, impotence. **Derm:** hot flushes. **Endo:** gynecomastia, testosterone flair. **MS:** bone pain.

Endometriosis

CNS: headache, weakness, insomnia. **CV:** edema. **GI:** constipation, gastrointestinal disorders, nausea. **GU:** ↓ libido, vaginal dryness, menorrhagia. **Derm:** hot flushes, acne. **Endo:** supression of ovulation. **MS:** back pain.

Interactions

Drug-Drug: Risk of serious arrhythmias may be↑ by concurrent **amiodarone**, **disopyramide**, **dofetilide**, **flecainide ibutilide**, **propafenone quinidine**, **sotalol**, **antipsychotics** (including **chlorpromazine)** **antidepressants** (including **amitrypline** and **nortriptyline**), **opioids** (including **methadone**), **macrolide anti-infectives**(including **azithromycin**, **erythromycin** and **clarithromycin**), **quinolone anti-infectives** (including **moxifloxacin**), **azole antifungals**, **5-HT3 antagonists** (including **ondansetron**), **beta-2 receptor agonists** (including **salbutamol**), **pentamidine**, and **quinine**.

Route/Dosage

Prostate cancer

Subcut (Adults): *Initial treatment*— 500 mcg every 8 hr for 7 days, *maintenance treatment*— 200 mcg daily.
Intranasal (Adults): *maintenance treatment*— 400 mcg (200 mcg in each nostril) three times daily.
Implant (Adults): 6.3 mg every 2 mo or 9.45 mg every 3 mo.

Endometriosis

Intranasal (Adults): 400 mcg (200 mcg in each nostril) three times daily. Treatment is usually continued for 6 mo, not to exceed 9 mo.

Availability

Solution for subcutaneous injection (contains benzyl alcohol): 1000 mcg/mL; Intranasal Solution : 1 mg/mL (delivers 100 mcg per actuation); Implant (depot): 6.3 mg (2 mo implant), 9.45 mg (3 mo implant).

NURSING IMPLICATIONS

Assessment

- **Cancer:** Monitor patients with vertebral metastases for increased back pain and decreased sensory/motor function.
- Monitor intake and output ratios and assess for bladder distention in patients with urinary tract obstruction during initiation of therapy.
- **Endometriosis:** Assess patient for signs and symptoms of endometriosis before and periodically during therapy. Amenorrhea usually occurs within 8 wk of initial administration and menses usually resume 8 wk after completion.
- ***Lab Test Considerations:*** During treatment male patients should have blood tests every 3 mo to measure testosterone levels. When treatment begins, testosterone levels can temporarily markedly increase and patients may need another medication to decrease levels.
- Monitor blood glucose in patients with diabetes frequently; may affect blood glucose levels.
- Women should have a negative pregnancy test result prior to starting treatment.

Potential Nursing Diagnoses

Sexual dysfunction

Potential Nursing Diagnoses

Disturbed body image

Implementation

Prostate Cancer

- **Subcut:** Only use syringes that come with kit for accurate dose. Inject into fatty tissue of abdomen, arm, or leg 3 times a day for 7 days; then daily during maintenance.
- **Intranasal:** When used as maintenance, begin nasal spray in each nostril 3 times daily. If patient also receives decongestant nasal spray, wait 30 minutes to give buserelin spray before or after the decongestant.
- **Implant:** Implant is inserted in subcut tissue of upper abdominal wall every 28 days. Local anesthesia may be used before injection.
- If the implant needs to be removed for any reason, it can be located by ultrasound.

Endometriosis

- **Intranasal:** One spray in each nostril 3 times daily for 6–9 mo.

Patient/Family Teaching

- Men may experience breast swelling and tenderness, decreased libido, hot flashes and sweats, impotence and weight gain. Notify health care professional if these symptoms occur.
- Women may experience decreased libido, constipation, painful sexual intercourse, menopausal symptoms, changes in hair growth. Notify health care professional if these symptoms occur.
- Caution both male and female patients to use contraception while taking this drug. Advise female patient to inform health care professional if pregnancy is suspected. Buserelin can be harmful to a fetus.
- **Subcut:** Instruct patient in proper technique for self-injection, care and disposal of equipment. Use only sy-

ringes included in kit. Instruct patients that syringes may only be used once, and then discarded.

- **Intranasal:** Instruct patient on proper nasal spray technique. Prime pump before use.
- Advise patients that the nasal spray can cause nose bleeds, and may change smell and taste senses.

Evaluation

- Decrease in the spread of prostate cancer.
- Decrease in lesions and pain in endometriosis.

cannabidiol (ka-**na**-bi-dye-ole)

delta-9–tetrahydrocannabinol (THC)

(**del**-ta nine tet-re-hye-dro-ka-**na**-bi-nole)

✱Sativex

Classification

Therapeutic: analgesic adjuncts, therapeutic, antispasticity agents

Pharmacologic: cannabinoids

Indications

Adjunct treatment of spasticity in adults with multiple sclerosis (MS) who have not responded to other therapies. Analgesic adjunct in the management of neuropathic pain in patients with MS or advanced cancer who have not responded to opioids or other analgesics for severe pain.

Action

Acts on cannabinoid receptors located in pain pathways in the brain, spinal cord and peripheral nerve terminals. Has analgesic and muscle relaxant properties. **Therapeutic Effects:** Decreased pain and spasticity.

Pharmacokinetics

Absorption: Buccal absorption is slower than inhalation.
Distribution: Highly lipid soluble, distributes and accumulates in fatty tissues. Cannabinoids enter breast milk in considerable amounts.
Metabolism and Excretion: Some first-pass hepatic metabolism occurs; highly metabolized by the CYP450 enzyme system. Metabolites can be stored in fatty tissues and re-released over time (up to weeks); one metabolite of THC is pharmacologically active (11–hydroxy-THC). Further metabolism occurs in renal and biliary systems.
Half-life: Bi-exponential half-lives with short initial phases of *Cannabidiol*—1.4–1.8 hr; *THC*—1.3–1.7 hr *11–hydroxy-THC*—1.9–2.1 hr; terminal elimination half-life of *cannabinoids*—24–26 hr or more.

TIME/ACTION PROFILE (analgesic and antispasticity effects)

ROUTE	ONSET	PEAK†	DURATION
cannabidiol	unknown	1.6–2.8 hr	up to 12 hr
THC	unknown	1.6–2.4 hr	up to 12 hr

†Blood levels peak more quickly when administered under the tongue.

Contraindications/Precautions

Contraindicated in: Allergy/hypersensitivity to cannabinoids, propylene glycol or peppermint oil; Serious cardiovascular disease, including ischemic heart disease, arrhythmias, poorly controlled hypertension or severe heart failure; History of schizophrenia/psychoses; Patients with child-bearing potential who are not using reliable contraception; Sore/inflamed mucosa (may alter absorption); OB: Pregnancy (avoid use); Lactation: Avoid breast-feeding (Cannabinoids enter breast milk in considerable amounts); Pedi: Safe and effective use in children <18 yr has not been established; avoid use.
Use Cautiously in: History of epilepsy/recurrent seizures; History of substance abuse; Perioperative state (consider possible changes in cardiovascular status); History of depression/suicide attempt or ideation; Significant hepatic/renal impairment; Patients with child-bearing potential (reliable contraception must be ensured); Cancer patients with urinary tract pathology (↑ risk of urinary tract adverse reactions); Geri: should used cautiously in this population.

Adverse Reactions/Side Effects

CNS: dizziness, fatigue, confusion, depression, disorientation, drowsiness, euphoria, hallucinations, psychotic reactions, suicidal ideation, weakness. **CV:** hypertension, palpitations, tachycardia, postural hypotension. **GI:** appetite change, constipation, dry mouth, dysgeusia, mucosal/teeth discoloration, nausea (↑ in cancer patients), stomatitis. **GU:** urinary retention (↑ in cancer patients). **Local:** application site irritation. **Misc:** physical dependence, psychological dependence.

Interactions

Drug-Drug: ↑ risk of CNS depression with other **CNS depressants** including **alcohol**, some **antidepressants**, some **antihistamines**, **benzodiazepines**, **GABA inhibitors**, **sedative/hypnotics**, **opioids** and **psychotropics/antipsychotics**. Cannabidiol inhibits the CYP450 enzyme system; may ↑ effects of **amitriptyline**, **alfentanil**, **fentanyl** and **sufentanil**.
Drug-Natural Products: ↑ risk of intoxication with other forms of **cannibis**.

Route/Dosage

Buccal (Adults): *Day 1*—One spray in the morning and one in the evening; *subsequent days*—Increase by one spray/day. Wait at least 15 min between sprays. Spread out sprays used per day. If unacceptable effects occur temporarily discontinue and re-institute at a lower amount sprays/day or longer intervals between sprays. Titrate to optimal maintenance dose (usual range 4–8 sprays/day, usually not more than 12 spray/day; higher doses have been used/tolerated). Adjust dose to changes in patient condition.

Availability

Buccal spray contains ethanol (50% v/v), propylene glycol and peppermint oil: Each ml contains *Cannabidiol*—25 mg and *THC*—27 mg/ml. Delivers 100 microliter/spray, each spray provides cannabidiol 2.5 mg and THC 2.7 mg.

DRUGS APPROVED IN CANADA

NURSING IMPLICATIONS

Assessment

- Assess patient's pain level before and after cannabidiol.

Potential Nursing Diagnoses

Acute pain
Chronic pain

Implementation

- Administer one spray 2 times a day, in morning and in evening, on first day. Administer under tongue or in buccal area. Rotate sites in mouth to avoid irritation. Effects should be noticed in about 30 minutes. Do not spray the back of throat or into nose. After first day, increase dose by 1 spray every 24 hours, spacing doses evenly. No more than 12 doses should be used over a 24 hour period. Space each spray by at least 15 min.
- Prime pump before first use. Shake vial gently and remove protective cap. Hold vial in an upright position and press firmly and quickly on the actuator 2 or 3 times, until a fine spray appears. Point spray into a tissue, away from patient.

Patient/Family Teaching

- Caution patient to use medication as directed.
- Instruct patient on correct spray technique. Instruct patient to rotate sites in the mouth between under the tongue and buccal locations.
- Instruct patient to store unopened bottles in refrigerator. Do not freeze. Keep away from sources of heat such as direct sunlight or flames (product is flammable). Opened bottles may be stored at room temperature. Keep out of reach of children.
- Inform patient that any unused contents should be discarded after 28 days. Do not dispose of medications in wastewater (e.g. down the sink or in the toilet) or in household garbage. Consult pharmacist how to dispose of expired or unneeded medication.
- Caution patient to avoid alcohol while taking cannabidiol.

Evaluation

- Decrease in pain.
- Decrease in muscle spasticity.

cilazapril (sye-**lay**-za-pril)

✱Inhibace

Classification
Therapeutic: antihypertensives
Pharmacologic: ACE inhibitors

Indications

Alone or with other agents in the management of hypertension. Management of HF.

Action

ACE inhibitors block the conversion of angiotensin I to the vasoconstrictor angiotensin II. ACE inhibitors also prevent the degradation of bradykinin and other vasodilatory prostaglandins. ACE inhibitors also ↑ plasma renin levels and ↓ aldosterone levels. Net result is systemic vasodilation. **Therapeutic Effects:** Lowering of BP in hypertensive patients. Improved symptoms in patients with HF.

Pharmacokinetics

Absorption: Well absorbed following oral administration, rapidly converted to active metabolite, cilazaprilat (57% bioavailability for cilazaprilat).

Distribution: Enters breast milk.

Metabolism and Excretion: Cilazaprilat is eliminated unchanged by the kidneys (91%).

Half-life: *Early elimination phase*—0.9 hr; *terminal elimination phase (enzyme–bound cilazaprilat)* 36–49 hr.

TIME/ACTION PROFILE (effects on hemodynamics)

ROUTE	ONSET	PEAK	DURATION
PO (hypertension)	within 1 hr	3–7 hr	12–24 hr
PO (heart failure)	1–2 hr	2–4 hr	24 hr

Contraindications/Precautions

Contraindicated in: Hypersensitivity; History of angioedema with previous use of ACE inhibitors; Concurrent use with aliskiren in patients with diabetes or moderate-to-severe renal impairment (CCr <60 mL/min); OB: Can cause injury or death of fetus—if pregnancy occurs, discontinue immediately; Lactation: Discontinue drug or use formula.

Use Cautiously in: Renal impairment, hepatic impairment, hypovolemia, hyponatremia, concurrent diuretic therapy; Black patients with hypertension (monotherapy less effective, may require additional therapy; ↑ risk of angioedema); Women of childbearing potential; Surgery/anesthesia (hypotension may be exagerated); Geri: Initial dose ↓ recommended for most agents due to age-related ↓ in renal function; Pedi: Safe use in children has not been established.

Exercise Extreme Caution in: Family history of angioedema.

Adverse Reactions/Side Effects

CNS: dizziness, drowsiness, fatigue, headache, insomnia, vertigo, weakness. **Resp:** <u>cough</u>, dyspnea. **CV:** <u>hypotension</u>, chest pain, edema, tachycardia. **Endo:** hyperuricemia. **GI:** <u>taste disturbances</u>, abdominal pain, anorexia, constipation, diarrhea, nausea, vomiting. **GU:** erectile dysfunction, proteinuria, renal dysfunction, renal failure. **Derm:** flushing, pruritis, rashes. **F and E:** hyperkalemia. **Hemat:** AGRANULOCYTOSIS. **MS:** back pain, muscle cramps, myalgia. **Misc:** ANGIOEDEMA, fever.

Interactions

Drug-Drug: Excessive hypotension may occur with concurrent use of **diuretics** or other **antihypertensives** or **alcohol**. ↑ risk of hyperkalemia with concurrent use of **potassium supplements**, **potassium-sparing diuretics**, or **potassium-containing salt substitutes**. ↑ risk of hyperkalemia, renal dysfunction, hypotension, and syncope with concurrent use of **angiotensin II receptor antagonists** or **aliskiren**; avoid concurrent use with aliskiren in patients with diabetes or CCr <60 mL/min. **NSAIDs** and selective **COX-2 inhibitors** may blunt the antihypertensive effect and ↑ the risk of renal dysfunction. ↑ levels and may ↑ risk of **lithium** toxicity.

Route/Dosage

Hypertension

PO (Adults ≤65 yr): *Hypertension (monotherapy)*—2.5 mg once daily initially, may be increased every 2 wk by 2.5 mg/day; usual dose 2.5–5 mg once daily, not to exceed 10 mg/day. Twice daily administration may be necessary in some patients; *hypertension (concurrent diuretics)*—0.5 mg once daily initially, titrate carefully.

PO (Adults >65 yr): *Hypertension (monotherapy)*—1.25 mg once daily initially, titrate carefully.

Renal Impairment

PO (Adults): *CCr >40 mL/min*—1 mg once daily initially, titrate carefully, not to exceed 5 mg once daily; *CCr 10–40 mL/min*—0.5 mg once daily initially, titrate carefully, not to exceed 2.5 mg once daily; *CCr <10 mL/min*—0.25–0.5 mg once or twice weekly depending on blood pressure response.

Hepatic Impairment

PO (Adults): 0.5 mg once daily or less.

Heart Failure

PO (Adults): After considering concurrent diuretic therapy/salt/volume depletion, ***Initial dose***—0.5 mg/day with careful monitoring, after 5 days dose may be ↑ to 1 mg/day, dose may then be carefully titrated as needed/tolerated up to 2.5 mg/day, rarely patients may require 5 mg/day.

Renal Impairment/hyponatremia

PO (Adults): *CCr 10–40 mL/min*—0.25–0.5 mg once daily; *CCr <10 mL/min*—0.25–0.5 mg once or twice weekly depending on response.

Availability

Tablets: 1 mg, 2.5 mg, 5 mg. ***In combination with:*** hydrochlorothiazide 12.5 mg (Inhibace Plus).

NURSING IMPLICATIONS

Assessment

- Assess patient for signs of angioedema; dyspnea and facial swelling.
- **Hypertension:** Monitor BP and pulse frequently during initial dose adjustment and periodically during therapy. Notify health care professional of significant changes.
- **Heart Failure:** Monitor daily weight and assess frequently for fluid overload (dyspnea, rales/crackles, weight gain, jugular venous distention).
- ***Lab Test Considerations:*** Monitor BUN, creatinine, and serum electrolyte levels periodically during therapy.
- Monitor CBC periodically. May cause agranulocytosis.
- May cause ↑ AST, ALT, alkaline phosphatase, serum bilirubin, uric acid, and glucose.

Potential Nursing Diagnoses

Decreased cardiac output
Noncompliance

Implementation

- Tablets may be taken before or after meals.

Patient/Family Teaching

- Instruct patient to take cilazapril as directed. Take missed dose as soon as remembered. If not until the following day, skip missed dose. Do not double doses.
- Caution patient to change positions slowly to minimize hypotension. Use of alcohol, standing for long periods, exercising, and hot weather may ↑ orthostatic hypotension.
- May cause dizziness. Caution patient to avoid driving and other activities requiring alertness until response to medication is known.
- Instruct patient on proper technique for monitoring blood pressure. Advise patient to check BP and weight weekly and record and report results to health care professional.
- Provide patient with additional interventions for hypertension control (weight reduction, low sodium diet, cessation of smoking, exercise regimen, stress management, and moderation of alcohol consumption). Medication controls but does not cure hypertension.
- Instruct patient to notify health care professional of all Rx or OTC medications, vitamins, or herbal products being taken and consult health care professional before taking any new medications, especially cough, cold, or allergy remedies.
- Advise women of childbearing age to use contraception and to notify health care professional if planning or suspecting pregnancy. Discontinue medication immediately if pregnancy is confirmed.

Evaluation

- Decrease in blood pressure.
- Decrease in signs and symptoms of heart failure.

cloxacillin (klox-a-**sill**-in)

♣Apo Cloxi, ♣ Novo-Cloxin, ♣ Nu-Cloxi

Classification
Therapeutic: anti-infectives
Pharmacologic: penicillinase resistant penicillins

Indications

Treatment of the following infections due to penicillinase-producing staphylococci: respiratory tract infections, sinusitis, septicemia, endocarditis, osteomyelitis, skin and skin structure infections.

Action

Bind to bacterial cell wall, leading to cell death. Not inactivated by penicillinase enzymes. **Therapeutic Effects:** Bactericidal action. **Spectrum:** Active against most gram-positive aerobic cocci. Spectrum is notable for activity against: Penicillinase-producing strains of *Staphylococcus aureus*, *Staphylococcus epidermidis*. Not active against methicillin-resistant bacteria (MRSA).

Pharmacokinetics

Absorption: IV administration results in complete bioavailability. Moderately absorbed (50%) following oral administration.

Distribution: Widely distributed; penetration into CSF is minimal but sufficient in the presence of inflamed meninges; crosses the placenta and enters breast milk.
Metabolism and Excretion: Some metabolism by the liver (9–22%) and some renal excretion of unchanged drug (20 %).
Half-life: 0.5–1.1 hr (increased in severe hepatic, renal dysfunction and in neonates).

TIME/ACTION PROFILE

ROUTE	ONSET	PEAK	DURATION
PO	30 min	30–120 min	6 hr
IM	unknown	unknown	6 hr
IV	rapid	end of injection/infusion	6 hr

Contraindications/Precautions
Contraindicated in: Previous hypersensitivity to penicillins (cross-sensitivity exists with cephalosporins and other beta-lactam antibiotics).
Use Cautiously in: Severe renal or hepatic impairment; OB: Safe use in pregnancy has not been established; Pedi: Safe use in premature and newborn infants has not been established.

Adverse Reactions/Side Effects
CNS: SEIZURES. **GI:** CLOSTRIDIUM DIFFICILE-ASSOCIATED DIARRHEA (CDAD), diarrhea, epigastric distress, nausea, vomiting. **GU:** interstitial nephritis. **Derm:** rash, urticaria. **Hemat:** eosinophilia, leukopenia. **Misc:** allergic reactions including ANAPHYLAXIS and SERUM SICKNESS, superinfection.

Interactions
Drug-Drug: Cloxacillin may ↓ effectiveness of **oral contraceptive agents**. **Probenecid** ↓ renal excretion and ↑ blood levels of cloxacillin (therapy may be combined for this purpose). **Neomycin** may ↓ absorption of cloxacillin. Concurrent use with **methotrexate** ↓ methotrexate elimination and ↑ risk of serious toxicity.
Drug-Food: Food ↓ oral absorption by 50%.

Route/Dosage
PO (Adults): 250–500 mg q 6 hr.
PO (Children >1 mo): 50–100 mg/kg/day divided q 6 hr up to a maximum of 4 g/day.
IM, IV (Adults): 250–500 mg every 6 hr, maximum dose 6 g/day.
IM, IV (Children up to 20 kg): 25–50 mg/kg/day in 4 equally divided doses every 6 hr.

Availability
Capsules: ✱ 250 mg, ✱ 500 mg; Oral solution: ✱ 125 mg/5 mL; Powder for injection (requires reconstitution/dilution: ✱ 250-mg, ✱ 500-mg, ✱ 2-g vials.

NURSING IMPLICATIONS

Assessment
- Assess for infection (vital signs; appearance of wound, sputum, urine, and stool; WBC) at beginning of and throughout therapy.
- Obtain a history before initiating therapy to determine previous use of and reactions to cephalosporins or other beta-lactam antibiotics. Persons with no history of penicillin sensitivity may still have an allergic response.
- Obtain specimens for culture and sensitivity prior to initiating therapy. First dose may be given before receiving results.
- Observe patient for signs and symptoms of anaphylaxis (rash, pruritus, laryngeal edema, wheezing, abdominal pain). Discontinue drug and notify health care professional immediately if these occur. Keep epinephrine, an antihistamine, and resuscitation equipment close by in event of an anaphylactic reaction.
- Monitor bowel function. Diarrhea, abdominal cramping, fever, and bloody stools should be reported to health care professional promptly as a sign of Clostridium difficile-associated diarrhea (CDAD). May begin up to several wk following cessation of therapy.
- ***Lab Test Considerations:*** May cause leukopenia and neutropenia, especially with prolonged therapy or hepatic impairment.
- May cause positive direct Coombs' test result.
- May cause ↑ AST, ALT, LDH, and serum alkaline phosphatase concentrations.

Potential Nursing Diagnoses
Risk for infection (Indications) (Side Effects)
Noncompliance (Patient/Family Teaching)

Implementation
- **PO:** Administer around the clock on an empty stomach at least 1 hr before or 2 hr after meals. Take with a full glass of water; acidic juices may decrease absorption of penicillins. Swallow capsules whole; do not crush, chew, or open capsules.
- Use calibrated measuring device for liquid preparations. Shake well. Solution is stable for 14 days if refrigerated.
- **IM:** Reconstitute by adding 1.9 mL and 1.7 mL Sterile Water to 250 mg and 500 mg respectively, for concentrations of 125 mg/mL and 250 mg/mL. Shake well to dissolve. Stable for 24 hr at room temperature or 48 hr if refrigerated.
- **IV:** For IV use, reconstitute 250 mg vial with 4.9 mL, 500 mg vial with 4.8 mL, and 1000 mg vial with 9.6 mL Sterile Water for concentrations of 50 mg/mL, 100 mg/mL, and 100 mg/mL respectively. Shake well. Use reconstituted solution immediately. Infuse over 2-4 min.
- **IV:** Reconstitute for infusion with Sterile Water for injection using 3.4 mL for 1000 mg, 6.8 mL for 2000 mg, and 34 mL for 10,000 mg, resulting in 250 mg/mL. Add to an appropriate infusion fluid in amount calculated to give desired dose. Shake well to dissolve. Use solution immediately. Infuse over 30-40 min.
- **Y-Site Compatibility:** epinephrine, ketamine.
- **Y-Site Incompatibility:** pantoprazole, rocuronium.

Patient/Family Teaching
- Instruct patient to take medication around the clock and to finish the drug completely as directed, even if feeling better. Missed doses should be taken as soon as remembered. Advise patient that sharing of this medication may be dangerous.
- Advise patient to report signs of superinfection (black, furry overgrowth on the tongue; vaginal itching or discharge; loose or foul-smelling stools) and allergy.

- Instruct patient to notify health care professional if fever and diarrhea develop, especially if stool contains blood, pus, or mucus. Advise patient not to treat diarrhea without consulting health care professional.
- Instruct patient to notify health care professional if symptoms do not improve.

Evaluation

- Resolution of the signs and symptoms of infection. Length of time for complete resolution depends on the organism and site of infection.

cyproterone (sy-**proe**te-rone)

✱Androcur

Classification

Therapeutic: antineoplastics, hormones

Pharmacologic: antiandrogens

Indications

Palliative treatment of advanced prostate cancer.

Action

Has antiandrogenic and progestogenic/antigonadotropic properties, resulting in blocked binding of the active metabolite of testosterone on the surface of prostatic cancer cells and decreased production of testicular testosterone. **Therapeutic Effects:** Decreased spread of prostate cancer.

Pharmacokinetics

Absorption: Completely absorbed following oral administration. Absorption after IM depot injection is delayed and prolonged.

Distribution: Unknown.

Metabolism and Excretion: Metabolized by the CYP3A enzyme system; excreted in feces (60%) and urine (33%), as unchanged drug and metabolites.

Half-life: *PO*—38 hr; *IM*—4 days.

TIME/ACTION PROFILE (blood levels)

ROUTE	ONSET	PEAK	DURATION
PO	unknown	3–4 hr	8–12 hr
IM (depot)	unknown	3.4 days	1–2 wk

Contraindications/Precautions

Contraindicated in: Hypersensitivity; Liver disease/hepatic dysfunction/liver tumors (not due to prostate cancer); Dubin Johnson syndrome; Rotor syndrome; History of meningioma; Wasting diseases (not related to prostate cancer); Severe depression; Thromboembolism; OB: Not indicated for use in women ; Pedi: Not recommended for use in children <18 yr.

Use Cautiously in: History of cardiovascular disease; Renal impairment.

Adverse Reactions/Side Effects

CNS: MENINGIOMAS, fatigue, weakness, depression. **Resp:** cough, dyspnea, pulmonary microembolism. **CV:** THROMBOEMBOLISM, edema, heart failure, myocardial infarction, hypotension, syncope, tachycardia, vasovagal reactions. **GI:** HEPATOTOXICITY, LIVER TUMORS, anorexia, constipation, diarrhea, nausea, vomiting. **Derm:** dry skin, hot flashes, ↑ sweating, patchy hair loss. **Endo:** adrenal suppression, antiandrogen withdrawal syndrome, gynecomastia. **F and E:** hypercalcemia. **GU:** infertility, impotence. **Hemat:** anemia, thrombocytopenia. **Metab:** glucose intolerance, hyperlipidemia. **MS:** osteoporosis (long term use). **Misc:** allergic reactions.

Interactions

Drug-Drug: Antiandrogenic effect may be ↓ by **alcohol**. Effectiveness/long-term survival may be ↓ by concurrent **GnRH agonist** treatment. ↑ risk of myopathy with **HMG CoA reductase inhibitors (statins)**. Blood levels and effects may be ↑ by **strong inhibitors of CYP3A4** including **clotrimazole**, **itraconazole**, **ketoconazole** and **ritonavir**. Blood levels and effectiveness may be ↓ by **inducers of CYP3A4** including **phenytoin** and **rifampicin**. Use cautiously with other **drugs that are substrates of the P450 enzymes**.

Drug-Natural Products: Blood levels and effectiveness may be ↓ by **St. John's wort**.

Route/Dosage

PO (Adults): 200–300 mg/day in 2–3 divided doses, not to exceed 300 mg/day; *after orchiectomy*—100–200 mg/day.

IM (Adults): 300 mg once weekly; *after orchiectomy*—300 mg every 2 wk.

Availability

Tablets: 50 mg; Depot injection: 100 mg/mL in 3–mL ampules. ***In combination with:*** Ethinyl estradiol (Diane-35, Cyestra-35).

NURSING IMPLICATIONS

Assessment

- Assess patient for signs and symptoms of thromboembolism (chest pain, dyspnea, vital signs, level of consciousness). Discontinue therapy if symptoms occur.
- Monitor mood changes, especially during first 6-8 wk. Note degree to which these thoughts and behaviors interfere with daily functioning. Inform health care professional if patient demonstrates significant increase in anxiety, nervousness, or insomnia.
- ***Lab Test Considerations:*** Monitor PSA during therapy. May cause increase in PSA. If PSA increase occurs discontinue therapy and monitor for 6–8 wk for withdrawal response prior to any decision to proceed with other prostate cancer therapy.
- ***Lab Test Considerations:*** May impair carbohydrate metabolism. Monitor fasting blood glucose and glucose tolerance tests periodically during therapy, especially in patients with diabetes. May require dose changes in insulin or oral antidiabetic agents.
- ***Lab Test Considerations:*** Monitor CBC and platelet count periodically during therapy.
- ***Lab Test Considerations:*** Monitor liver function tests prior to and periodically during therapy and if symptoms of hepatotoxicity occur. May develop several wk to mo after therapy starts. Discontinue therapy if hepatotoxicity occurs.

- ***Lab Test Considerations:*** Monitor adrenocortical function tests by serum cortisol assay periodically during therapy.

Potential Nursing Diagnoses

Disturbed body image

Implementation

- **PO:** Take by mouth two or three times a day with or just after meals as directed. Dose is usually lower after orchiectomy.

Patient/Family Teaching

- Instruct patient to take cyproterone as directed. Take missed doses as soon as remembered, unless almost time for next dose, then skip missed dose and resume usual dosing schedule. Do not double dose.
- Inform patient that benign breast lumps may occur; they generally subside 1–3 mo after discontinuation of therapy and/or after dose reduction. Dose reduction should be weighed against the risk of inadequate tumor control.
- Advise patient to avoid alcohol during therapy.
- May cause fatigue and lassitude during first few wk of therapy; then diminishes. Caution patient to avoid driving and other activities requiring alertness until response to medication is known.
- Inform patient that sperm count and volume of ejaculate decrease with therapy. Infertility is common but is reversible when therapy is discontinued.
- Discuss with patient potential for patchy hair loss. Explore methods of coping.
- Emphasize the importance of follow-up appointments and blood tests to monitor progression of treatment.

Evaluation

- Decreased spread of prostate cancer.

danaparoid (da-nap-a-roid)

✷Organ

Classification

Therapeutic: anticoagulants

Pharmacologic: heparins (low molecular weight)

Indications

Prevention of thromboembolic phenomena including deep vein thrombosis and pulmonary emboli after surgical procedures known to increase the risk of such complications (knee/hip replacement, abdominal surgery). Management of non-hemorrhagic stroke. Treatment/prevention of thromboembolic phenomena in patients with a history of heparin-induced thrombocytopenia (HIT). Maintenance of catheter patency.

Action

Potentiates the inhibitory effect of antithrombin on factor Xa and thrombin. Danaparoid is a heparinoid. **Therapeutic Effects:** Prevention of thrombus formation.

Pharmacokinetics

Absorption: 100% absorbed after subcut administration; IV administration results in complete bioavailability.
Distribution: Unknown.
Metabolism and Excretion: Excreted mostly by the kidneys.
Half-life: 24 hr.

TIME/ACTION PROFILE (anticoagulant effect)

ROUTE	ONSET	PEAK	DURATION
Subcut	unknown	2–5 hr	12 hr

Contraindications/Precautions

Contraindicated in: Hypersensitivity to danaparoid, pork products, or sulfites; Uncontrolled bleeding; Imminent/threatened abortion; Lactation: Breast feeding should be avoided.
Use Cautiously in: Severe liver or kidney disease (dosage ↓ may be necessary in severe renal impairment); Retinopathy (hypertensive or diabetic); Untreated hypertension; Recent history of ulcer disease; Spinal/epidural anesthesia; History of congenital or acquired bleeding disorder; Geriatric patients; Malignancy; History of thrombocytopenia related to heparin (HIT), has been used successfully; OB: Safe use in pregnancy has not been established; Pedi: Use with caution.
Exercise Extreme Caution in: Severe uncontrolled hypertension; Bacterial endocarditis, bleeding disorders; GI bleeding/ulceration/pathology; Hemorrhagic stroke; Recent CNS or ophthalmologic surgery; Active GI bleeding/ulceration.

Adverse Reactions/Side Effects

CNS: dizziness, headache, insomnia. **CV:** edema. **GI:** constipation, nausea, reversible increase in liver enzymes, vomiting. **GU:** urinary retention. **Derm:** ecchymoses, pruritus, rash, urticaria. **Hemat:** <u>BLEEDING, anemia, thrombocytopenia</u>. **Local:** erythema at injection site, <u>hematoma</u>, irritation, pain. **Misc:** fever.

Interactions

Drug-Drug: Risk of bleeding may be ↑ by concurrent use of other **anticoagulants** including **warfarin** or **drugs that affect platelet function**, including **aspirin, NSAIDs, dipyridamole**, some **penicillins, clopidogrel, ticlopidine**, and **dextran**.

Route/Dosage

Prophylaxis of DVT (non HIT patients)

Subcut (Adults): 750 anti-factor Xa IU q 12 hr starting 1–4 hr preop and at least 2 hr postop for 7–10 days or until ambulatory (up to 14 days). *Prophylaxis of DVT following Orthopedic, Major Abdominal Surgery and Thoracic Surgery*—750 anti-factor Xa units, twice daily up to 14 days, initiate 1–4 hr preop.
IV, Subcut (Adults): *Prophylaxis of Deep Vein Thrombosis in Non-hemorrhagic Stroke Patients*—up to 1000 anti-Xa units IV, followed by 750 anti-Xa units subcutaneously, twice daily for 7–14 days.
IV (Children): *Acute Thrombosis (arterial and/or venous)*—30 anti-Xa units/kg iv bolus injection, then 1.2-4.0 anti-Xa units kg/hr.
Subcut (Children): *Prophylaxis*—10 anti-Xa units/kg twice daily.

Renal Impairment

IV (Children <10 yr): *Renal Dialysis*—(for the first two dialyses)—30 anti-Xa units/kg + 1000 anti-Xa units (if pre-dialysis plasma anti-Xa level >500 U/L, then

no danaparoid is required for next dialysis, if level is 300–500 U/L then decrease total dose by 250 anti-Xa units, <300 anti-Xa units/L then give previous dialysis dose).
IV (Children 10–17 years): *Renal Dialysis*—30 anti-Xa units/kg + 1500U (3rd and subsequent dialyses) (if pre-dialysis plasma anti-Xa level > 500 U/L, then no danaparoid is required for next dialysis, if level is 300–500 U/L then decrease total dose by 250 anti-Xa units, <300 *DVT prophylaxis*/L then give previous dialysis dose).
IV (Adults and Children): *Catheter patency*—750 anti-Xa units diluted in 50 mL saline; 5–10 mL of this solution is used to flush each line/port.

HIT patients

IV, Subcut (Adults): *DVT prophylaxis, current HIT, ≤90 kg*—750 anti-Xa units SC two or three times daily for 7–10 days (initial bolus of 1250 anti-Xa units IV may be used); *DVT prophylaxis, current HIT, >90 kg*—1250 anti-Xa units SC two or three times daily for 7–10 days (initial bolus of 1250 anti-Xa units IV may be used); *DVT prophylaxis, past (>3 mos) HIT, ≤90 kg*—750 anti-Xa units SC two or three times daily for 7–10 days; *DVT prophylaxis, past (>3 mos) HIT, >90 kg*—750 anti-Xa units SC three times daily or 1250 anti-Xa units SC twice daily for 7–10 days; ***Established pulmonary embolism or DVT, thrombus <5 days, >90 kg***—3750 anti-Xa units IV bolus, then 400 anti-Xa units/hr for 4 hr, then 300 anti-Xa units/hr for 4 hr, then 150–200 anti-Xa units/hr for 5–7 days or 1750 anti-Xa units SC twice daily for 4–7 days; ***Established pulmonary embolism or DVT, thrombus <5 days, 55–90 kg***—2250–2500 anti-Xa units IV bolus, then 400 anti-Xa units/hr for 4 hr, then 300 anti-Xa units/hr for 4 hr, then 150–200 anti-Xa units/hr for 5–7 days or 2000 anti-Xa units SC twice daily for 4–7 days; ***Established pulmonary embolism or DVT, thrombus <5 days, <55 kg***—1250–1500 anti-Xa units IV bolus, then 400 anti-Xa units/hr for 4 hr, then 300 anti-Xa units/hr for 4 hr, then 150–200 anti-Xa units/hr for 5–7 days or 1500 anti-Xa units SC twice daily for 4–7 days; ***Established pulmonary embolism or DVT, thrombus ≥5 days, >90 kg***—1250 anti-Xa units IV bolus, then 750 anti-Xa units SC three times daily or 1250 anti-Xa units twice daily; ***Established pulmonary embolism or DVT, thrombus ≥5 days, ≤90 kg***—1250 anti-Xa units IV bolus, then 750 anti-Xa units SC two to three times daily; *Surgical prophylaxis, nonvascular surgery, >90 kg*—750 anti-Xa units SC, repeat ≥6 hr after procedure, then 1250 anti-Xa units SC twice daily for 7–10 days; *Surgical prophylaxis, nonvascular surgery, ≤90 kg*—750 anti-Xa units SC, repeat ≥6 hr after procedure, then 750 anti-Xa units SC twice daily for 7–10 days; *Surgical prophylaxis, embolectomy, >90 kg*—2250–2500 anti-Xa units IV bolus before procedure, then 150–200 anti-Xa units/hr IVstarting ≥6 hr after procedure for 5–7 days or 750 anti-Xa units two to three times daily or change to oral anticoagulants after several days; *Surgical prophylaxis, embolectomy, 55–90 kg*—2250–2500 anti-Xa units IV bolus before procedure, then 1250 anti-Xa units SC twice daily starting ≥6 hr after procedure, then 750 anti-Xa units two to three times daily or change to oral anticoagulants after several days; *Cardiac catheterization >90 k g*—3750 anti-Xa units IV bolus prior to procedure; *Cardiac catheterization <90 kg*—2500 anti-Xa units IV bolus prior to procedure; *Percutaneous transluminal coronary angioplasty*—2500 anti-Xa units IV prior to procedure, then 150–200 anti-Xa units/hr IV for 1–2 days after procedure, may be followed by 750 anti-Xa units SC for several several days; *Intra-aortic balloon pump catherization, >90 kg*—3750 anti-Xa units IV bolus before procedure, then 150–200 anti-Xa units/hr IV or a second bolus of 1250 anti-Xa units IV or 750 anti-Xa units SC two or three times daily or 1250 anti-Xa units SC twice daily; *Intra-aortic balloon pump catherization, <90 kg*—2500 anti-Xa units IV bolus before procedure, then 150–200 anti-Xa units/hr IV or a second bolus of 1250 anti-Xa units IV or 750 anti-Xa units SC two or three times daily or 1250 anti-Xa units SC twice daily; *Peripheral vascular bypass*—2250–2500 anti-Xa units IV bolus before procedure, then 150–200 anti-Xa units/hr IV started ≥6 hr after procedure for 5–7 days or 750 anti-Xa units SC two or three times daily or change to oral anticoagulants.

Availability

Solution for injection (contains sulfites): 750 anti-factor Xa units/0.6 mL ampule.

NURSING IMPLICATIONS

Assessment

- Assess patient for signs of bleeding and hemorrhage (bleeding gums; nosebleed; unusual bruising; black, tarry stools; hematuria; fall in hematocrit or BP; guaiac-positive stools); bleeding from surgical site. Notify health care professional if these occur.
- Assess patient for evidence of additional or increased thrombosis. Symptoms will depend on area of involvement. Monitor neurological status frequently for signs of neurological impairment. May require urgent treatment.
- Monitor patient for hypersensitivity reactions (chills, fever, urticaria).
- Monitor patients with epidural catheters frequently for signs and symptoms of neurologic impairment.
- **Subcut:** Observe injection sites for hematomas, ecchymosis, or inflammation.
- ***Lab Test Considerations:*** Monitor CBC, and stools for occult blood periodically throughout therapy. Monitor platelet count every other day for first wk, twice weekly for next 2 wks, and weekly thereafter. If thrombocytopenia occurs, monitor closely. If hematocrit decreases unexpectedly, assess patient for potential bleeding sites.
- Special monitoring of clotting times (aPTT) is not necessary.
- May cause increases in AST, ALT, and alkaline phosphatase levels.
- ***Toxicity and Overdose:*** Danaparoid is not reversed with protamine sulfate. If overdose occurs, discontinue danaparoid. Transfusion with fresh frozen plasma and plasmapheresis has been used if bleeding is uncontrollable.

Potential Nursing Diagnoses

Ineffective tissue perfusion (Indications)
Risk for injury (Side Effects)
Deficient knowledge, related to medication regimen (Patient/Family Teaching)

Implementation

- Cannot be used interchangeably (unit for unit) with unfractionated heparin or other low-molecular-weight heparins.
- Conversion to oral anticogulant therapy (unless it is contraindicated) should not be started until adequate anti-thrombotic control with parenteral danaparoid has been achieved; conversion may take up to 5 days.
- **Subcut:** Administer deep into subcut tissue. Alternate injection sites daily between the left and right anterolateral and left and right posterolateral abdominal wall. Inject entire length of needle at a 45° or 90° angle into a skin fold held between thumb and forefinger; hold skin fold throughout injection. Do not aspirate or massage. Rotate sites frequently. Do not administer IM because of danger of hematoma formation. Solution should be clear; do not inject solution containing particulate matter.
- If excessive bruising occurs, ice cube massage of site before injection may lessen bruising.

IV Administration

- **Catheter Patency:** May be used intermittently to maintain patency of iv lines/catheters, and/or access ports, if saline flushes do not work adequately. 1 ampoule, 750 U (0.6 mL) can be diluted in 50 mL 0.9% NaCl. Use 5-10 mL to flush each line/port as required.
- **IV Push:** Subcut is preferred route. ***Diluent:*** If administered IV, give as a bolus. May dilute with 0.9% NaCl, D5/0.9% NaCl, Ringer's, LR, and mannitol. Stable for up to 48 hr at room temperature.
- **Y-Site Incompatibility:** Administer separately; do not mix with other drugs.

Patient/Family Teaching

- Instruct patient in correct technique for self injection, care and disposal of equipment.
- Advise patient to report any symptoms of unusual bleeding or bruising, dizziness, itching, rash, fever, swelling, or difficulty breathing to health care professional immediately.
- Instruct patient not to take aspirin, naproxen, or ibuprofen without consulting health care professional while on danaparoid therapy.
- Advise female patient to notify health care professional if pregnancy is planned or suspected or if breast feeding.

Evaluation

- Prevention of deep vein thrombosis and pulmonary emboli.
- Maintenance of catheter patency.

domperidone (dom-per-i-done)

Motilium

Classification

Therapeutic: gastric stimulant
Pharmacologic: butyrophenones, dopamine antagonists

Indications

Management of symptoms associated with GI motility disorders including subacute/chronic gastritis and diabetic gastroparesis. Treatment of nausea/vomiting associated with dopamine agonist antiparkinson therapy. **Unlabeled Use:** To stimulate lactation.

Action

Acts as a peripheral dopamine receptor blocker. Increases GI motility, peristalsis and lower esophageal sphincter pressure. Facilitates gastric emptying and decreases small bowel transit time. Also increases prolactin levels. **Therapeutic Effects:** Improved GI motility. Decreased nausea/vomiting associated with dopamine agonist antiparkinson therapy.

Pharmacokinetics

Absorption: Well absorbed following oral administration.
Distribution: Does not cross the blood-brain barrier; enters breast milk in low concentrations.
Metabolism and Excretion: Undergoes extensive first-pass hepatic metabolism; much via the CYP3A4 enzyme system. 31% excreted in urine, 66% in feces.
Half-life: 7 hr.

TIME/ACTION PROFILE

ROUTE	ONSET	PEAK	DURATION
PO	unknown	30 min (blood levels)	6–8 hr

Contraindications/Precautions

Contraindicated in: Known hypersensitivity/intolerance; Concurrent use of ketoconazole; Prolactinoma; Conditions where GI stimulation is dangerous including GI hemorrhage/mechanical obstruction/perforation; Lactation: Breast feeding is not recommended unless potential benefits outweigh potential risks.
Use Cautiously in: History of breast cancer; Hepatic impairment; Severe renal impairment (dose adjustment may be necessary during chronic therapy); OB: Use only if expected benefit outweighs potential hazard; Pedi: Safe and effective use in children has not been established.

Adverse Reactions/Side Effects

CNS: headache, insomnia. **GI:** dry mouth. **GU:** amenorrhea, impotence. **Derm:** hot flushes, rash. **Endo:** galactorrhea, gynecomastia, hyperprolactinemia.

Interactions

Drug-Drug: Ketoconazole↑ blood levels and the risk of cardiovascular toxicity and is contraindicated; other **azole antifungals**, **macrolide anti-infectives** and **protease inhibitors** may have similar effects. Risk of adverse cardiovascular reactions may be ↑ by concurrent use of **drugs known to ↑ QT interval** including other **anti-arrhythmics**, some **fluoroquinolones**, **antipsychotics**, **beta-2 adrenergic agonists**, **antimalarials**, **SSRIs**, **tri/tetracyclic antidepressants** and **nefazodone** and should be undertaken cautiously, especially if other risk factors for *torsade de pointes* exists. Effectiveness may be ↓ by concurrent use of **anticholingerics**. Due to effects on gastric motility, absorption of drugs from the small intestine may be accelerated, while absorption of drugs from the stomach may be slowed, especially **sustained-release** or **enteric-coated** formulations. Concurrent use with **MAOIs** should be undertaken with caution.

Drug-Food: Grapefruit juice may ↑ blood levels.

Route/Dosage

PO (Adults): *Upper GI motility disorders*—10 mg 3 to 4 times daily; may be increased to 20 mg 3 to 4 times daily; *nausea/vomiting due to dopamine agonist antiparkinson agents*—20 mg 3 to 4 times daily, higher doses may be required during dose titration.

Renal Impairment

PO (Adults): Depending on degree of impairment, dosing during chronic therapy should be reduced to once or twice daily.

Availability

Tablets: 10 mg.

NURSING IMPLICATIONS

Assessment

- Assess for nausea, vomiting, abdominal distention, and bowel sounds before and after administration.
- Monitor BP (sitting, standing, lying down) and pulse before and periodically during therapy. May cause prolonged QT interval, tachycardia, and orthostatic hypotension, especially in patients older than 60 yrs or taking >30 m g/day.
- Monitor for symptoms related to hyperprolactinemia (menstrual abnormalities, galactorrhea, sexual dysfunction).
- ***Lab Test Considerations:*** May cause ↑ serum ALT, AST, and cholesterol.
- Monitor serum prolactin prior to and periodically during therapy. May cause ↑ serum prolactin levels.

Potential Nursing Diagnoses

Imbalanced nutrition: less than body requirements
Risk for injury (side effects)

Implementation

- Use lowest effective dose.
- Administer 3–4 times daily, 15–30 min before meals and at bedtime.

Patient/Family Teaching

- Instruct patient to take as directed. Advise patient to avoid grapefruit juice during therapy.
- Advise patient to notify health care professional if galactorrhea (excessive or spontaneous flow of breast milk), gynecomastia (excessive development of male mammary gland), menstrual irregularities (spotting or delayed periods), palpitations, irregular heart beat (arrhythmia), dizziness, or fainting occur.
- Advise female patient to notify health care professional if pregnancy is planned or suspected or if breast feeding.

Evaluation

- Prevention or relief of nausea and vomiting.
- Decreased symptoms of gastric stasis.

flupentixol (floo-pen-tiks-ol)

🍁Fluanxol

Classification
Therapeutic: antipsychotics
Pharmacologic: thioxanthenes

Indications

Maintenance treatment of schizophrenia in patients whose symptomatology does not include excitement, agitation of hyperactivity. Not indicated for the treatment of dementia in the elderly.

Action

Alters the effects of dopamine in the CNS. Has some anticholinergic and alpha-adrenergic blocking activity.
Therapeutic Effects: Diminished signs and symptoms of schizophrenia.

Pharmacokinetics

Absorption: *Flupentixol dihydrochloride*—40% absorbed following oral administration; *Flupentixol decanoate*—slowly released from IM injection sites.
Distribution: Distributes to lungs, liver and spleen, enter CNS; extensive tissue distribution.
Protein Binding: 99%.
Metabolism and Excretion: Mostly metabolized, metabolites do not have antipsychotic activity. Most metabolites are excreted in feces, some renal elimination.
Half-life: *Flupentixol dihydrochloride*—35 hr; *Flupentixol decanoate*—3 wk.

TIME/ACTION PROFILE (antipsychotic effect)

ROUTE	ONSET	PEAK	DURATION
PO	within 2–3 days	3–8 hr (blood level)	8 hr
IM (depot)	24–72 hr	4–7 days (blood level)	2–4 wk

Contraindications/Precautions

Contraindicated in: Hypersensitivity to flupentixol or other thioxanthines (cross sensitivity with phenothiazines may occur); CNS depression due to any cause, including comatose states, cortical brain damage (known or suspected), or circulatory collapse; Opiate, alcohol or barbiturate intoxication; Liver impairment, cerebrovascular insufficiency or severe cardiovascular pathology; Concurrent use of other drugs known to prolong QT interval; Pedi: Safe and effective use in children <18 yr has not been established, not recommended.
Use Cautiously in: Brain tumors or intestinal obstruction (may mask symptoms); Patients exposed to extreme heat or organophosphorous insecticides; Risk factors for/history of stroke; Any risk factors for QT prolongation including hypokalmia, hypomagnesemia, genetic predisposition, cardiovascular disease history (including bradycardia), recent MI, HF or arrhythmias; Known/suspected glaucoma; History of seizures (may ↓ seizure

threshold); Parkinson's Disease (may worsen symptoms); Geri: Use cautiously in patients >65 yr, consider age-related decreases in renal, cardiac and hepatic function; OB: Safe use in pregnancy has not been established, use only if expected benefit outweighs potential risks to infant; Lactation: Safe use not established, low levels in breast milk are not expected to affect infant if therapeutic doses are used.

Adverse Reactions/Side Effects

CNS: NEUROLEPTIC MALIGNANT SYNDROME, dizziness. **EENT:** blurred vision. **CV:** QT PROLONGATION, THROMBOEMBOLISM, extrapyramidal symptoms, tachycardia, hypotension, sedation, tardive dyskinesia. **GI:** constipation, dry mouth, excess salivation, hepatotoxicity. **GU:** ↓ libido, urinary retention. **Derm:** photosensitivity reactions, rash, sweating. **Endo:** glucose intolerance, hyperprolactinemia, menstrual irregularity. **Hemat:** agranulocytosis, granulocytopenia, neutropenia. **Metab:** weight change. **MS:** osteoporosis (long term use).

Interactions

Drug-Drug: ↑ CNS depression with other **CNS depressants** including **alcohol**, some **antidepressants**, some **antihistamines**, **anxiolytics**, **benzodiazepines** and **sedative/hypnotics**. ↑ risk of QT prolongation and serious arrhythmias with **Class Ia and III antiarrhythmics** (including **quinidine**, **amiodarone** and **sotalol**), some **antipsychotics** (including **thioridazine**), some **macrolide anti-infectives** (including **erythromycin**) and some **quinolone anti-infectives** (including **moxifloxacin**); concurrent use should be avoided. Concurrent use of **diuretics** and other **drugs affecting electrolytes** may ↑ risk of QT prolongation and serious arrthythmias. ↑ risk of anticholinergic adverse reactions, including paralytic ileus when used concurrently with other **anticholinergics** or **drugs with anticholinergic side effects**. May ↓ metabolism and ↑ effects of **tricyclic antidepressants**. ↑ risk of extrapyramidal symptoms with **metoclopramide**. May ↓ effectiveness of **levodopa** and **dopamine agonists**. May ↓ antihypertensive effectiveness of **guanethidine** and similar drugs; concurrent use should be avoided.

Route/Dosage

PO (Adults): 1 mg three times daily initially, increase by 1 mg every 2–3 days until desired response, usual effective dose is 3–6 mg/day in divided doses (up to 12 mg/day has been used); if insomnia occurs, evening dose may be decreased.

IM (Adults): Initiate with a 5–20 mg test dose (use 5 mg dose in elderly/frail/cachectic patients) as the 2% injection. Patients previously treated with long-acting neuroleptic injections may tolerate initial doses of 20 mg. A second 20 mg dose may be given 4–10 days later and then 20–40 mg every 2–3 wk depending on response. Oral flupentixol should be continued, but gradually decreased in the first week following depot injection. Guidelines for conversion from PO to depot IM injection: daily oral dose (mg) x 4 = dose of depot injection (mg) given every 2 wk *or* daily oral dose (mg) x 8 = depot injection (mg) given every 4 wk.

Availability

Tablets (flupentixol dihydrochloride): 0.5 mg, 3 mg, 5 mg; Depot injection (flupentixol decanoate—contains medium-chain triglycerides [coconut oil]): 20 mg/mL (2%) in 10 mL vials, 100 mg/mL (10%) in 2 mL vials.

NURSING IMPLICATIONS

Assessment

- Assess mental status (orientation, mood, behavior) before and periodically during therapy.
- Monitor BP (sitting, standing, lying), ECG, pulse, and respiratory rate before and frequently during the period of dose adjustment. May cause Q-T prolongation.
- Observe carefully when administering oral medication to ensure that medication is actually taken and not hoarded.
- Assess weight and BMI initially and throughout therapy.
- Assess fluid intake and bowel function. Increased bulk and fluids in the diet help minimize constipation.
- Monitor for onset of akathisia (restlessness or desire to keep moving) and extrapyramidal side effects (*parkinsonian*—difficulty speaking or swallowing, loss of balance control, pill rolling, mask-like face, shuffling gait, rigidity, tremors; *dystonic*—muscle spasms, twisting motions, twitching, inability to move eyes, weakness of arms or legs) every 2 mo during therapy and 8–12 wk after therapy has been discontinued. Reduction in dose or discontinuation of medication may be necessary. Benztropine or diphenhydramine may be used to control these symptoms.
- Monitor for tardive dyskinesia (uncontrolled rhythmic movement of mouth, face, and extremities; lip smacking or puckering; puffing of cheeks; uncontrolled chewing; rapid or worm-like movements of tongue). Report immediately; may be irreversible.
- Monitor for development of neuroleptic malignant syndrome (fever, respiratory distress, tachycardia, seizures, diaphoresis, arrhythmias, hypertension or hypotension, pallor, tiredness, severe muscle stiffness, loss of bladder control). Report immediately.
- Monitor for symptoms related to hyperprolactinemia (menstrual abnormalities, galactorrhea, sexual dysfunction).
- ***Lab Test Considerations:*** Monitor CBC and liver function tests periodically during treatment. May cause ↑ AST, ALT, and alkaline phosphatase.
- Monitor blood glucose prior to and periodically during therapy. May cause hyperglycemia.
- Monitor serum prolactin prior to and periodically during therapy. May cause ↑ serum prolactin levels.
- May cause false-positive pregnancy tests.

Potential Nursing Diagnoses

Disturbed thought process
Risk for injury

Implementation

- **PO:** Initially, take tablets 3 times daily, without regard to food. Dose will increase for first few days until desired results. Maintenance dose is usually taken in morning.
- When converting to IM doses, PO dose is usually continued in decreasing doses for first wk.
- **IM:** Inject deep IM preferably into gluteus maximus. Solution is a yellow viscous oil, aspirate prior to injection to ensure dose is not injected IV. Do not adminis-

ter solutions that are discolored, hazy, or contain particulate matter.

- For large doses or pain with large volume, flupentizol decanoate BP 10% (100 mg/mL) may be used instead of flupentixol decanoate BP 2% (20 mg/mL).

Patient/Family Teaching

- Instruct patient to take as directed. If a dose is missed, omit and take next dose as scheduled. Discontinuation should be gradual; abrupt discontinuation may cause withdrawal symptoms (nausea, vomiting, anorexia, diarrhoea, rhinorrhoea, sweating, myalgias, paraesthesias, insomnia, restlessness, anxiety, agitation, vertigo, feelings of warmth and coldness, tremor). Symptoms begin within 1 to 4 days of withdrawal and abate within 7 to 14 days. Advise patient to read *Patient Information* leaflet prior to starting therapy and with each Rx refill in case of changes.
- Inform patient of possibility of extrapyramidal symptoms and tardive dyskinesia. Caution patient to report these symptoms immediately to health care professional.
- Advise patient to change positions slowly to minimize orthostatic hypotension.
- Medication may cause drowsiness. Caution patient to avoid driving or other activities requiring alertness until response to medication is known.
- Advise patient to notify health care professional of all Rx or OTC medications, vitamins, or herbal products being taken and to consult with health care professional before taking other medications.
- Caution patient to avoid concurrent use of alcohol and other CNS depressants.
- Instruct patient to notify health care professional promptly if sore throat, fever, unusual bleeding or bruising, rash, weakness, tremors, visual disturbances, dark-colored urine, or clay-colored stools occur.
- Instruct patient to avoid sun exposure and to wear protective clothing and sunscreen when outdoors.
- Advise patient to notify health care professional of medication regimen before treatment or surgery.
- Advise female patients to notify health care professional if pregnancy is planned or suspected or if breast feeding or planning to breast feed.

Evaluation

- Decreased symptoms of schizophrenia (delusions, hallucinations, social withdrawal, flat, blunt affect).

framycetin (fray-mye-**see**-tin)

✦Soframycin

Classification

Therapeutic: anti-infectives

Pharmacologic: aminoglycosides

Indications

Local treatment of ocular infections due to susceptible organisms including blepharitis, conjunctivitis, corneal injuries, corneal ulcers, meibomianitis, ocular infections, following foreign body removal (prevention of infection).

Action

Inhibits protein synthesis in susceptible bacteria by binding to ribosomal subunits; not active against fungi, viruses, and most anaerobic bacteria. Active against *Staphylococcus aureus*, the proteus group of bacteria, coliforms, and *Pseudomonas aeruginosa*. **Therapeutic Effects:** Erradication/prevention of infection.

Pharmacokinetics

Absorption: Poorly absorbed following oral administration. Minimal systemic absorption following ophthalmic use.

Distribution: Unknown.

Metabolism and Excretion: Unknown.

Half-life: Unknown.

TIME/ACTION PROFILE

ROUTE	ONSET	PEAK	DURATION
ophth	rapid	unknown	1–6 hr (longer for opth ointment)

Contraindications/Precautions

Contraindicated in: Hypersensitivity (cross-sensitivity with other aminoglycosides may occur).

Use Cautiously in: OB: has been used safely; Lactation: has been used safely; Pedi: Safe and effective use not established.

Adverse Reactions/Side Effects

Local: allergic cutaneous reactions. **Misc:** overgrowth of nonsusceptible organisms (prolonged use).

Interactions

Drug-Drug: None noted.

Route/Dosage

Ophth (Adults): *Ophthalmic solution*— 1–2 drops every 1–2 hr acutely for 2–3 days, then 1–2 drops 3–4 times daily; *ophthalmic ointment*— apply 2–3 times daily or use at bedtime if solution has been used during the day.

Availability

Ophthalmic solution: 5 mg/ml in 8-mL bottles; Ophthalmic ointment: 5 mg/g in 5-g tubes. ***In combination with:*** phenylephrine (Soframycin Nasal Spray), gramicidin (Soframycin Skin Ointment).

NURSING IMPLICATIONS

Assessment

- Assess the degree of pain and visual impairment.

Potential Nursing Diagnoses

Acute pain (Indications)

Implementation

- When administering avoid touching any part of eye. Wash hands and wear gloves to administer ophthalmic medication. See Appendix D for administration instructions.

DRUGS APPROVED IN CANADA

- **Ophth:** *Drops:* Apply 1 or 2 drops to affected eye every 1–2 hrs for first 2–3 days. Dose may then decrease to 1 or 2 drops to affected eye 3 or 4 times daily.
- **Ophth:** *Ointment:* Apply ointment to affected eye 2 or 3 times per day, or at bedtime if solution has been used during day.

Patient/Family Teaching
- Instruct patient on proper technique for applying drops or ointment.

Evaluation
- Resolution of signs and symptoms of eye infection.

fusidic acid (fyoo-**sid**-ik **as**-id)
✱Fucidin, ✱ Fucithalmic

Classification
Therapeutic: anti-infectives

Indications
Topical —Local treatment of primary and secondary bacterial skin infections including impetigo contagiosa, erythrasma and secondary skin infections such as infected wounds/burns. *Ophthalmic*— Treatment of superficial eye infections.

Action
Inhibits bacterial protein synthesis. **Therapeutic Effects:** Resolution of localized bacterial infections. Not active against Gram-negative organisms; active against Staphylococci, Streptococci and Corynebacterium.

Pharmacokinetics
Absorption: Unknown.
Distribution: Systemically absorbed drug crosses the placenta and enters breast milk.
Metabolism and Excretion: Absorbed drug is extensively metabolized.
Half-life: 5–6 hr.

TIME/ACTION PROFILE

ROUTE	ONSET	PEAK	DURATION
Top	unknown	unknown	6–8 hr
ophth	unknown	unknown	12 hr

Contraindications/Precautions
Contraindicated in: Hypersensitivity to fusidic acid or other components of the formulation (topical ointment contains lanolin).
Use Cautiously in: OB: Safe use during pregnancy has not been established, potential benefits should be weighed against the possible hazards to the fetus (crosses the placenta); Lactation: Safe use during breast feeding has not been established (enters breast milk).

Adverse Reactions/Side Effects
Derm: mild local irritation.

Interactions
Drug-Drug: None noted for topical use.

Route/Dosage
Topical (Adults and Children): Apply to affected area 3–4 times daily.
Ophth (Adults and Children): One drop into conjunctival sac of both eyes every 12 hr for 7 days.

Availability
Topical cream: 2% (20 mg/g); Topical ointment (contains lanolin): 2% (20 mg/g); Ophthalmic Viscous Drops (microcrystalline suspension): 1%. ***In combination with:*** hydrocortisone (Fucidin H).

NURSING IMPLICATIONS

Assessment
- Inspect involved areas of skin and mucous membranes before and frequently during therapy. Increased skin irritation may indicate need to discontinue medication.

Potential Nursing Diagnoses
Risk for infection (Indications)
Acute pain (Indications)

Implementation
- Do not confuse topical product with ophthalmic product.
- **Topical:** Consult health care professional for proper cleansing technique before applying medication. Apply small amount to cover affected area completely. Avoid the use of occlusive wrappings or dressings unless directed by health care professional.
- **Ophth:** Administer 1 drop into conjunctival sac of both eyes every 12 hr for 7 days. See Appendix D for instructions.

Patient/Family Teaching
- Instruct patient to apply medication as directed for full course of therapy, even if feeling better. Emphasize the importance of avoiding the eyes.
- Advise patient to report increased skin irritation or lack of response to therapy to health care professional.

Evaluation
- Resolution of skin or eye infection.

gliclazide (**glik**-la-zide)
✱Diamicron MR

Classification
Therapeutic: antidiabetics
Pharmacologic: sulfonylureas

Indications
Control of blood sugar in type 2 diabetes mellitus when control of diet and exercise fails or when insulin is not an option. Requires some pancreatic function.

Action
Lowers blood glucose by stimulating the release of insulin from the pancreas and increasing sensitivity to insulin at receptor sites. **Therapeutic Effects:** Lowering of blood glucose in diabetic patients.

Pharmacokinetics
Absorption: Well absorbed following oral administration (97%).
Distribution: Unknown.
Protein Binding: 95%.

Metabolism and Excretion: Extensively metabolized, metabolites are mostly eliminated (60–70%) in urine, 10–20% in feces; <1% excreted unchanged in urine.
Half-life: *Tablets*— 10.4 hr; *modified-release tablets*— 16 hr.

TIME/ACTION PROFILE (effect on blood sugar)

ROUTE	ONSET	PEAK	DURATION
PO	unknown	4–6 hr (blood levels)	12–24 hr

Contraindications/Precautions

Contraindicated in: Hypersensitivity; cross sensitivity with other sulfonylureas may occur; Unstable diabetes, type 1 diabetes mellitus, diabetic ketoacidosis, diabetic coma or pre-coma; Severe hepatic or renal disease; Concurrent use of oral/oromucosal miconazole, alcohol or alcohol-containing medications, or systemic phenylbutazone; OB: Should not be used during pregnancy, insulin is preferred; Lactation: Should not be used during lactation, insulin is perferred.
Use Cautiously in: Glucose 6-phosphate dehydrogenase deficiency (↑ risk of hemolytic anemia); Infection, stress, or changes in diet may alter requirements for control of blood sugar or require use of insulin; Impaired thyroid, pituitary, or adrenal function; Malnutrition, high fever, prolonged nausea, or vomiting; Pedi: Safe and effective use in children <18 yr has not been established.

Adverse Reactions/Side Effects

Endo: hypoglycemia. **GI:** abdominal pain, diarrhea, dyspepsia, ↑ liver enzymes, nausea, vomiting. **Derm:** photosensitivity, rashes.

Interactions

Drug-Drug: Concurrent use of **chlorpromazine**, **corticosteroids**, **ritodrine**, **salbutamol**, **terbutaline** or **anticoagulants** should be undertaken with caution due to alteration of effects. Concurrent use of **alcohol**, **angiotensin converting-enzyme inhibitors**, **antituberculars**, **azole antifungals**, **beta-blockers**, **clarithromycin**, **clofibrate**, **dispyramide**, **H2–receptor antagonists**, **MAO inhibitors**, **NSAIDs**, **phenylbutazone**, **salicylates**, long-acting **sulfonamides**, **warfarin**, may ↑ risk of hypoglycemia. ↑ risk of hypoglycemia with other **antidiabetic agents** including **alpha glucosidase inhibitors**, **biguanides**, and **insulin**. Concurrent use of **chlorpromazine**, **corticosteroids**, **danazol**, **diuretics**, (including **thiazides**, and **furosemide**), **hormonal contraceptives** (**estrogen** and **progestogen**), **nicotinic acid** (pharmacologic doses), **ritodrine**, **salbutamol**, **terbutaline**, or **tetracosactrin** may ↑ risk of hyperglycemia and lead to loss of diabetic control. May ↑ risk of bleeding with **warfarin**. Concurrent use with **alcohol** may result in a disulfiram-like reaction and should be avoided. **Beta-blockers** may ↓ some symptoms of hyperglycemia.

Route/Dosage

PO (Adults): *Tablets*— 80–320 mg/day, doses >160 m g/day should be divided and given twice daily; *modified-release tablets*— 30 mg daily, may be increased in 30 mg increments every 2 wk until blood sugar is controlled up to 120 mg/day.

Availability

Tablets (contain lactose): 80 mg; Modified-release tablets: 30 mg, 60 mg.

NURSING IMPLICATIONS

Assessment

- Observe for signs and symptoms of hypoglycemia (hunger, weakness, sweating, dizziness, tachycardia, anxiety).
- Assess patient for allergy to sulfonyureas.
- ***Lab Test Considerations:*** Monitor serum glucose and glycosylated hemoglobin periodically during therapy to evaluate effectiveness of treatment.
- Monitor liver function periodically in patients with mild to moderate liver dysfunction. May cause ↑ AST, ALT, alkaline phosphatase and LDH.
- Monitor renal function periodically in patients with mild to moderate renal dysfunction. May cause ↑ creatinine and hyponatremia.
- ***Toxicity and Overdose:*** Overdose is manifested by symptoms of hypoglycemia. Mild hypoglycemia may be treated with administration of oral glucose. Treat severe hypoglycemia with IV D50W followed by continuous IV infusion of more dilute dextrose solution at a rate sufficient to keep serum glucose at approximately 100 mg/dL.

Potential Nursing Diagnoses

Imbalanced nutrition: more than body requirements (indications)
Noncompliance

Implementation

- Patients on a diabetic regimen exposed to stress, fever, infection, trauma, or surgery may require administration of insulin.
- **PO:** Administer with meals at the same time every day.

Patient/Family Teaching

- Instruct patient to take gliclazides as directed at the same time every day.
- Explain to patient that this medication does not cure diabetes and must be used in conjunction with a prescribed diet, exercise regimen, to prevent hypoglycemic and hyperglycemic events.
- Instruct patient on proper technique for home glucose monitoring. Monitor closely during periods of stress or illness and health care professional notified if significant changes occur.
- Review signs of hypoglycemia and hyperglycemia with patient. If hypoglycemia occurs, advise patient to drink a glass of orange juice or ingest 2–3 tsp of sugar, honey, or corn syrup dissolved in water or an appropriate number of glucose tablets and notify health care professional.

- Encourage patient to follow prescribed diet, medication, and exercise regimen to prevent hypoglycemic or hyperglycemic episodes.
- Concurrent use of alcohol may cause a disulfiram-like reaction (abdominal cramps, nausea, flushing, headaches, and hypoglycemia).
- Instruct patient to avoid sun exposure and to wear protective clothing and sunscreen when outdoors.
- Caution patient to avoid other medications, especially aspirin and alcohol, while on this therapy without consulting health care professional.
- Advise patient to notify health care professional promptly if unusual weight gain, swelling of ankles, drowsiness, shortness of breath, muscle cramps, weakness, sore throat, rash, or unusual bleeding or bruising occurs.
- Advise patient to inform health care professional of medication regimen prior to treatment or surgery.
- Advise patient to carry sugar packets or candy, and identification describing diabetes diagnosis and medication regimen.
- Insulin is the recommended method of controlling blood sugar during pregnancy. Counsel female patients to use a form of contraception other than oral contraceptives and to notify health care professional promptly if pregnancy is planned or suspected.
- Emphasize the importance of routine follow-up exams.

Evaluation

- Control of blood glucose levels to avoid episodes of hypoglycemia and hyperglycemia.

methotrimeprazine

(meth-oh-try-**mep**-ra-zeen)

✱Meprazine, ✱ Methoprazine, ✱ Nozinan

Classification

Therapeutic: antipsychotics, nonopioid analgesics

Pharmacologic: phenothiazines

Indications

Management of psychotic disturbances. Management of conditions associated with anxiety/tension. As an analgesic and adjunct in pain due to cancer, zona, trigeminal neuralgia, intercostal neuralgia, phantom limb pain, and muscular discomforts. Used as a preoperative sedative. As an antiemetic. As a sedative in the treatment of insomnia.

Action

Sedation. **Therapeutic Effects:** Reduction in severity of pain.

Pharmacokinetics

Absorption: Well absorbed after PO/IM administration. IV administration results in complete bioavailability.

Distribution: Enters CSF and crosses the placenta. Minimal amounts enter breast milk.

Metabolism and Excretion: Mostly metabolized by the liver. Some metabolites are active; 1% excreted unchanged by the kidneys.

Half-life: *PO*—10.3–10.8 hr; *IM*—15–30 hr.

TIME/ACTION PROFILE

ROUTE	ONSET	PEAK	DURATION
PO (blood levels)	unknown	2.7–2.9 hr	8–12 hr
IM (analgesia)	unknown	20–40 min	8 hr (up to 24 hr in children)

Contraindications/Precautions

Contraindicated in: Blood dyscrasias; Hepatic impairment; Hypersensitivity to methotrimeprazine, phenothiazines or sulfites; Comatose patients or those who have overdosed on CNS depressants including alcohol, analgesics, opioids or sedative/hypnotics; OB: Third-trimester use may result in agitation, hypotonia, tremor, somnolence, respiratory distress and feeding disturbances in newborn and should be avoided.

Use Cautiously in: History of seizures; History of glaucoma or prostatic hypertrophy (↑ risk of anticholinergic adverse reactions); Bradycardia, electrolyte abnormalities, congenital/acquired prolonged QT interval or concurrent use of drugs that may prolong QT interval (↑ risk of serious arrhythmias); Underlying cardiovascular disease including stroke, arteriosclerosis, or thromboembolism (↑ risk of adverse cardiovascular effects); Geri: Geriatric or debilitated patients (initial dosage ↓ recommended, ↑ risk of death in elderly patients with dementia); Lactation: Safety not established; Pedi: Safe use in children not established.

Adverse Reactions/Side Effects

CNS: NEUROLEPTIC MALIGNANT SYNDROME, SEIZURES, amnesia, drowsiness, excess sedation, disorientation, euphoria, extrapyramidal reactions, headache, slurred speech, tardive dyskinesia, weakness. **EENT:** nasal congestion. **CV:** orthostatic hypotension, bradycardia, palpitations, tachycardia. **GI:** constipation, abdominal discomfort, dry mouth, nausea, vomiting. **GU:** difficulty in urination. **Endo:** hyperglycemia, hyperprolactinemia. **Hemat:** blood dyscrasias. **Local:** pain at injection site. **Misc:** chills.

Interactions

Drug-Drug: ↑ CNS depression with other **CNS depressants**, including **alcohol**, **antihistamines**, **antidepressants**, **opioids**, or **sedative/hypnotics**; decrease dose of these agents by 50% initially. ↑ anticholinergic effects with **antihistamines**, **antidepressants**, **phenothiazines**, **quinidine**, **disopyramide**, **atropine**, or **scopolamine** (reduce doses of concurrent atropine or scopolamine). Reverses vasopressor effects of **epinephrine** (avoid concurrent use—if vasopressor required, use phenylephrine, methoxamine, or norepinephrine). ↑ risk of hypotension with acute ingestion of **alcohol**, **nitrates**, **MAO inhibitors**, or **antihypertensives**. Concurrent use with **succinylcholine** may result in tachycardia, hypotension, CNS stimulation, delirium, and ↑ extrapyramidal symptoms.

Drug-Natural Products: Concomitant use of **kava**, **valerian**, **skullcap**, **chamomile**, or **hops** ↑ risk of CNS depression.

Route/Dosage

PO (Adults): *Minor conditions*—6–25 mg/day in three divided doses (if sedation occurs, use smaller daytime doses and a larger dose at bedtime); *Night time sedative*—10–25 mg as a single bedtime dose; *Psychoses/intense pain*—50–75 mg/day in two to three divided doses, dose may be titrated upward to desired effect (doses of 1 g/day have been used, if daily dose exceeds 100–200 mg, administer in divided doses and keep patient at bedrest).
PO (Children): 0.25 mg/kg/day in two to three divided doses (not to exceed 40 mg/day in children <12 yr).
IM (Adults): *Post-operative analgesic adjunct*—10–25 mg q 8 hr, if given with opioids/decrease opioid dose by 50%.
IM (Children): *Analgesia*—62.5–125 mcg (0.0625–0.125 mg)/kg/day single dose or divided doses, change to oral medication as soon as possible.
IV (Children): *Palliative care setting*—62.5 mcg (0.0625 mg)/kg/day in 250 mL of 5% dextrose solution as a slow infusion (20–40 drops/min).

Availability

Tablets: 2 mg, 5 mg, 25 mg, 50 mg; Solution for injection (requires further dilution for IV use): 25 mg/mL in 1-mL ampules.

NURSING IMPLICATIONS

Assessment

- Assess type, location, and intensity of pain before and 30 min after administration.
- Monitor BP frequently after injection. Orthostatic hypotension, fainting, syncope, and weakness frequently occur from 10 min to 12 hr after administration. Patient should remain supine for 6–12 hr after injection.
- Assess weight and BMI initially and throughout therapy.
- Observe patient carefully for extrapyramidal side effects (*parkinsonian*—difficulty speaking or swallowing, loss of balance control, pill rolling, mask-like face, shuffling gait, rigidity, tremors; *dystonic*—muscle spasms, twisting motions, twitching, inability to move eyes, weakness of arms or legs). Usually occur only after prolonged or high-dose therapy. Usually resolve with dose decrease or administration of antiparkinsonian agent.
- Monitor for tardive dyskinesia (involuntary rhythmic movement of mouth, face, and extremities). Report immediately and discontinue therapy; may be irreversible.
- Monitor for development of neuroleptic malignant syndrome (fever, respiratory distress, tachycardia, seizures, diaphoresis, hypertension or hypotension, pallor, tiredness). Discontinue methotrimeprazine and notify health care professional immediately if these symptoms occur.
- Methotrimeprazine potentiates the action of other CNS depressants but can be given in conjunction with modified doses of opioid analgesics for management of severe pain. This medication does not significantly depress respiratory status and can be useful where pulmonary reserve is low.
- Monitor for symptoms related to hyperprolactinemia (menstrual abnormalities, galactorrhea, sexual dysfunction).
- ***Lab Test Considerations:*** Monitor CBC prior to and periodically during therapy and liver function tests should be evaluated periodically throughout long-term (>30 days) therapy.
- Monitor blood glucose prior to and periodically during therapy may therapy. May cause hyperglycemia.
- Monitor serum prolactin prior to and periodically during therapy. May cause ↑ serum prolactin levels.

Potential Nursing Diagnoses

Acute pain (Indications)
Risk for injury (Side Effects)

Implementation

- **PO:** May be administered during day or only at night depending on indication,.
- **IM:** Do not inject subcut. Inject slowly into deep, well-developed muscle. Rotate injection sites.
- **Intermittent Infusion:** For patients in palliative care, may be infused as 0.0625 mg/kg/day in 250 mL of D5W. ***Rate:*** Infuse slowly 20–40 drops per minute.
- **Y-Site Compatibility:** fentanyl hydromorphone, methadone, morphine, sufentanil.
- **Y-Site Incompatibility:** heparin.

Patient/Family Teaching

- Instruct patient on how and when to ask for pain medication.
- Instruct patient to take medication as directed. Take missed doses as soon as remembered unless almost time for next dose; do not double dose. Advise patient to read *Patient Information* leaflet prior to starting therapy and with each Rx refill in case of changes.
- Advise patients to make position changes slowly and to remain recumbent for 6–12 hr after administration to minimize orthostatic hypotension.
- May cause drowsiness. Caution patient to request assistance with ambulation and transfer and to avoid driving or other activities requiring alertness until response to the medication is known.
- Advise patient to notify health care professional of all Rx or OTC medications, vitamins, or herbal products being taken and to consult with health care professional before taking other medications, especially cold medications.
- Caution patient to avoid taking alcohol or other CNS depressants concurrently with this medication.
- Advise patient to use sunscreen and protective clothing when exposed to the sun. Extremes of temperature should also be avoided because this drug impairs body temperature regulation.
- Instruct patient to use frequent mouth rinses, good oral hygiene, and sugarless gum or candy to minimize dry mouth.

- Instruct patient to notify health care professional promptly if sore throat, fever, unusual bleeding or bruising, rash, weakness, tremors, dark-colored urine, or clay-colored stools or signs of blood clots (swelling, pain and redness in an arm or leg that can be warm to touch, sudden chest pain, difficulty breathing, heart palpitations) occur.

Evaluation

- Decrease in severity of pain.
- Sedation.

moclobemide

(moe-**kloe**-be-mide)

✱Manerix

Classification

Therapeutic: antidepressants

Pharmacologic: monamine oxidase (MAO) inhibitors, benzamides

Indications

Treatment of depression.

Action

Short-acting, Reversible Inhibitor of Monoamine oxidase type A (RIMA). Increases concentrations of serotonin, norepinephrine, and dopamine. **Therapeutic Effects:** Decreased symptoms of depression, with improved mood and quality of life.

Pharmacokinetics

Absorption: 98% absorbed following oral administration, but undergoes first-pass hepatic metabolism resulting in 90% bioavailability.

Distribution: Unknown.

Metabolism and Excretion: Extensively metabolized (partially by CYP2C19 and CYP2D6), very small amounts are pharmacologically active, less than 1% excreted unchanged in urine.

Half-life: 1.5 hr (increases with dose).

TIME/ACTION PROFILE

ROUTE	ONSET	PEAK	DURATION
PO	days–several wk (antidepressant effect)	0.5–3.5 hr (blood levels)	24 hr (MAO-A inhibition)

Contraindications/Precautions

Contraindicated in: Known hypersensitivity; Acute confusional states; Pedi: Safe use in children <18 yr has not been established, use is not recommended; Concurrent use of tricyclic antidepressants; Concurrent use of SSRIs or other MAO inhibitors; Concurrent use of dextromethorphan, meperidine, selegiline or thioridazine.

Use Cautiously in: History of suicide attempt or ideation; History of thyrotoxicosis or pheochromocytoma (possible risk of hypertensive reaction); Severe hepatic impairment (↓ dose required); Renal impairment; OB: Safe use in pregnancy has not been established, should not be used unless anticipated benefits justify potential harm to fetus; Lactation: Not recommended unless anticipated benefits justify potential harm to infant.

Adverse Reactions/Side Effects

CNS: SUICIDAL IDEATION, agitation, insomnia, restlessness, tremor. **CV:** hypotension.

Interactions

Drug-Drug: ↑ levels and risk of QT prolongation with **thioridazine**, avoid concurrent use. Concurrent use with **selegiline** greatly ↑ sensitivity to tyramine and is contraindicated. Concurrent use with **tricyclic antidepressants** may result in severe adverse reactions and is contraindicated. Should not be used with **SSRIs** or other **MAO inhibitors**; when making a switch allow 4–5 half-lives of previous drug; for **fluoxetine** wait at least 5 wk. Exessive **alcohol** should be avoided. **Cimetidine** ↓ metabolism and ↑ blood levels, ↓ moclobemide dose by 50%. Because of the potential for interactions with **anesthetics**, especially local anesthetics containing **epinephrine**, moclobemide should be discontinued at least 2 days prior to procedures. Concurrent use with **opioids** should be avoided; dosage adjustments may be necessary. Concurrent use of **sympathomimetics** including **ephedrine** and **amphetamines** may ↑ blood pressure and should be avoided. Concurrent use with **dextromethorphan** may result in vertigo, tremor, nausea and vomiting and should be avoided. Concurrent use with **antihypertensives** should be carefully monitored.

Drug-Food: Ingestion of large amounts of **tyramine-containing foods** including some cheeses and **Marmite yeast extract** may result in hypertension and arrhythmias and should be undertaken with caution.

Route/Dosage

PO (Adults): 150 mg twice daily initially, increased gradually after one week as needed/tolerated up to 600 mg/day.

Hepatic Impairment

PO (Adults): *Severe hepatic impairment or concurrent enzyme inhibitor (cimetidine)*—Decrease daily dose to 1/3 to 1/2 of standard dose.

Availability

Tablets: 100 mg, 150 mg, 300 mg.

NURSING IMPLICATIONS

Assessment

- Assess mental status for orientation, mood, behavior and anxiety. Assess for suicidal tendencies. Restrict amount of drug available to patient.
- Monitor BP and pulse before and frequently during therapy. Report significant changes promptly.
- Monitor mood changes. Assess for suicidal tendencies, especially during early therapy. Restrict amount of drug available to patient.
- Monitor intake and output ratios and daily weight. Assess patient for peripheral edema and urinary retention.
- ***Lab Test Considerations:*** Monitor liver and kidney function periodically during treatment.
- Monitor serum glucose closely in diabetic patients; hypoglycemia may occur.
- ***Toxicity and Overdose:*** Concurrent ingestion of tyramine-rich foods and many medications may result in a life-threatening hypertensive crisis. Signs and symptoms of hypertensive crisis include chest pain,

tachycardia, severe headache, nausea and vomiting, photosensitivity, and enlarged pupils. Treatment includes IV phentolamine.

- Symptoms of overdose include anxiety, irritability, tachycardia, hypertension or hypotension, respiratory distress, dizziness, drowsiness, hallucinations, confusion, seizures, fever, and diaphoresis. Treatment includes induction of vomiting or gastric lavage and supportive therapy as symptoms arise.

Potential Nursing Diagnoses
Ineffective coping
Noncompliance (Patient/Family Teaching)

Implementation
- Administer after meals. Swallow tablet whole; do not crush, break, or chew. Dose may be adjusted gradually during the first wk of therapy.

Patient/Family Teaching
- Instruct patient to take medication as directed. Take missed doses if remembered unless almost time for next dose; do not double doses. Do not discontinue abruptly; withdrawal symptoms (nausea, vomiting, malaise, nightmares, agitation, psychosis, seizures) may occur. Advise patient to read *Patient Information* leaflet prior to starting and with each Rx refill in case of changes.
- Caution patient to avoid alcohol, CNS depressants, OTC drugs, and foods or beverages containing tyramine (see Appendix J) during and for at least 2 wk after therapy has been discontinued; they may precipitate a hypertensive crisis. Contact health care professional immediately if symptoms of hypertensive crisis develop.
- Caution patient to notify health care professional if neck stiffness, changes in vision, diarrhea, constipation, rapid/pounding heart beat, sudden and severe headache, stiff neck, confusion, disorientation, slurred speech, behavioral changes, seizures.
- Advise patient and family to notify health care professional if thoughts about suicide or dying, attempts to commit suicide; new or worse depression; new or worse anxiety; feeling very agitated or restless; panic attacks; trouble sleeping; new or worse irritability; acting aggressive; being angry or violent; acting on dangerous impulses; an extreme increase in activity and talking; other unusual changes in behavior or mood occur.
- Instruct patient to carry identification describing medication regimen.
- Advise female patients to notify health care professional if pregnancy is planned or suspected or if breast feeding or planning to breast feed.
- Encourage patient to participate in psychotherapy in conjunction with taking medication.

Evaluation
- Improved mood in depressed patients.
- Decreased anxiety.

pinaverium
(pin-ah-**veer**-ee-um)
✱Dicetel

Classification
Therapeutic: anti-irritable bowel syndrome agents
Pharmacologic: calcium channel blockers

Indications
Management of symptoms of Irritable Bowel Syndrome (IBS) including abdominal pain, bowel disturbances and discomfort. Treatment of symptoms related to biliary tract disorders.

Action
Acts as a calcium channel blocker with specific selectivity for intestinal smooth muscle. Relaxes gastrointestinal (mainly colon) and biliary tracts, inhibits colonic motor response to food/pharmacologic stimulation. **Therapeutic Effects:** Decreased symptoms of IBS.

Pharmacokinetics
Absorption: Poorly absorbed (1–10%).
Distribution: Distributes selectively to digestive tract.
Protein Binding: 97%.
Metabolism and Excretion: Minimal enterohepatic cycling, eliminated almost entirely in feces. Some metabolism.
Half-life: 1.5 hr.

TIME/ACTION PROFILE (blood levels)

ROUTE	ONSET	PEAK	DURATION
PO	unknown	1 hr	unknown

Contraindications/Precautions
Contraindicated in: Known hypersensitivity; Galactose intolerance/Lapp lactase deficiency/glucose-galactose malabsorption (tablets contain lactose); Lactation: May enter breast milk, avoid use if breast-feeding; Pedi: Safe and effective use in children has not been established, use is not recommended.
Use Cautiously in: Pre-existing eosphageal lesions/hiatal hernia (glass of water and snack should be taken with each dose); OB: Safe use in pregnancy has not been established, should be used only if essential to welfare of patient.

Adverse Reactions/Side Effects
All less than 1%. **CNS:** drowsiness, headache, vertigo. **GI:** constipation, diarrhea, distention, dry mouth, epigastric pain/fullness, esophageal irritation, nausea. **Derm:** rash.

Interactions
Drug-Drug: Concurrent use of **anticholinergics** may ↑ spasmolytic effects.

Route/Dosage
PO (Adults): 50 mg three times daily, may be increased as needed/tolerated up to 100 mg three times daily.

Availability
Tablets (contain lactose): 50 mg, 100 mg.

NURSING IMPLICATIONS

Assessment

- Assess patient for symptoms of IBS (abdominal pain or discomfort, bloating, constipation).
- Assess patient for lactose intolerance; product contains lactose.

Potential Nursing Diagnoses

Acute pain
Diarrhea

Implementation

- **PO:** Administer tablet with a glass of water and food. Swallow tablet whole, do not crush, chew or suck. If >3 tablets/day prescribed, take additional tablets with glass of water and a snack. May be irritating to esophagus. Do not take the tablet while lying down or just before bedtime.

Patient/Family Teaching

- Instruct patient to take pinaverium as directed. Take missed doses as soon as remembered unless almost time for next dose; do not double doses.
- Caution patient to inform health care professional if the following side effects persist or worsen; stomach pain or fullness, nausea, constipation or diarrhea, heartburn, headache, dry mouth, dizziness, skin rash.
- Instruct patient to avoid alcohol intake while taking this medication.
- Advise female patient to inform health care professional if pregnancy is planned or suspected or if breast feeding.

Evaluation

- A decrease in symptoms of irritable bowel syndrome. The length of treatment depends on the condition being treated.

prucalopride

(proo-**kal**-o-pride)

✱Resotran

Classification

Therapeutic: prokinetic agents

Pharmacologic: dihydrobenzofurancarboxamides

Indications

Treatment of chronic idiopathic constipation in adult females who do not respond to laxatives.

Action

Acts as a serotonin (5–HT_4) receptor agonist with prokinetic properties. Enhances peristalsis and gastrointestinal propulsion. **Therapeutic Effects:** Laxative effect.

Pharmacokinetics

Absorption: Rapidly absorbed (90%) following oral administration.

Distribution: Rapidly and extensively distributed, enters breast milk.

Metabolism and Excretion: 60% excreted unchanged in urine, 3–8% unchanged in feces, minor amounts are extensively metabolized.

Half-life: 24 hr.

TIME/ACTION PROFILE (normalization of bowel movements)

ROUTE	ONSET	PEAK	DURATION
PO	3–4 days	1–4 wk	unknown

Contraindications/Precautions

Contraindicated in: Hypersensitivity; Renal impairment requiring dialysis; Intestinal obstruction/perforation (structural or function), obstructive ileus, severe gastrointestinal inflammatory disease, including Crohn's disease, ulcerative colitis, toxic megacolon/megarectum; Galactose intolerance, Lapp lactase deficiency or glucose/galactose malabsorption (tablets contain lactose); OB: Not recommended for use during pregnancy (effective contraception should be used); Lactation: Not recommended for use while breast feeding (enters breast milk); Pedi: Not recommended for use in children <18 yr.

Use Cautiously in: Severe/clinically stable concurrent chronic diseases including liver, cardiovascular or lung disease, neurological or psychiatric disorders, cancer, AIDS or other disorders or insulin-dependent diabetes mellitus; History of arrhythmias or cardiovascular disease, ischemic heart disease, pre-excitation syndromes (including Wolff-Parksinson-White syndrome, Lown-Ganong-Levine syndrome or AV nodal disorders (↑ risk of arrhythmias); Severe renal impairment (↓ dose recommended); Geri: Due to age-related ↓ in renal function, ↓ dose is recommended.

Adverse Reactions/Side Effects

CNS: headache, dizziness, fatigue. **CV:** palpitations, ↓ PR interval, tachycardia. **GI:** abdominal pain, diarrhea, nausea, vomiting.

Interactions

Drug-Drug: Severe diarrhea may ↓ effectiveness of **oral hormonal contraceptives** (additional method of contraception recommended). Blood levels and effects are ↑ by concurrent CYP3A4 and P-gp inhibitors including **ketoconazole**, **verapamil**, **cyclosporine** and **quinidine**. Beneficial effects may be ↓ by concurrent use of **anticholinergics**.

Route/Dosage

PO (Adults): 2 mg once daily. If no bowel movement occurs in 3–4 days, add-on laxatives should be considered. If benefit is not obtained after 4 wk, prucalopride should be discontinued.

PO (Adults >65 yr): 1 mg once daily.

Renal Impairment

PO (Adults): *GFR <30 mL/min/1.73m²*— 1 mg once daily.

Availability

Tablets (contain lactose): 1 mg, 2 mg.

NURSING IMPLICATIONS

Assessment

- Assess patient for symptoms of chronic constipation (abdominal pain or discomfort, bloating, constipation).

Potential Nursing Diagnoses

Constipation

Implementation

- **PO:** Medication should be taken with food or on an empty stomach at the same time each day.

Patient/Family Teaching

- Instruct patient to take prucalopride as directed.
- Caution the patient to discontinue the medication and notify health care professional with occurrence of severe diarrhea, signs of heart attack, black tarry stools, vomiting of blood or material that looks like coffee grounds.
- Advise patient on a nutritional regimen and hydration, and exercise to decrease constipation.
- Inform patient that if no bowel movement within 3 days of treatment, a "rescue" laxative may be added occasionally while taking prucalopride.
- Advise women of childbearing age who are taking prucalopride to use an effective method of birth control during treatment. If pregnant occurs while taking this medication, contact health care professional immediately.

Evaluation

- A soft formed bowel movement.

trimebutine (try-meh-boo-teen)

✱Modulon

Classification

Therapeutic: lower gastrointestinal tract motility regulators, spasmolytics

Indications

Symptomatic treatment of irritable bowel syndrome (IBS). Treatment of postoperative paralytic ileus.

Action

Acts as a spasmolytic. **Therapeutic Effects:** ↓ symptoms of IBS. Resumption of intestinal transit following abdominal surgical procedures.

Pharmacokinetics

Absorption: Rapidly absorbed following oral administration.

Distribution: Unknown.

Metabolism and Excretion: Extensively metabolized, <2.4% excreted unchanged in urine.

Half-life: 2.7–3.1 hr.

TIME/ACTION PROFILE (symptom relief)

ROUTE	ONSET	PEAK	DURATION
PO	within 3 days–2 wk	1 hr (blood level)	>1 wk (following discontinuation)

Contraindications/Precautions

Contraindicated in: Hypersensitivity.

Use Cautiously in: OB: Safety and effective use in pregnancy has not been esatablished, not recommended for use during pregnancy; Pedi: Safe and effective use in children has not been established, not recommended for use in children <12 yr.

Adverse Reactions/Side Effects

CNS: dizziness, drowsiness, fatigue, headache. **GI:** diarrhea, dry mouth, dysguesia, dyspepsia, epigastric pain, nausea. **Derm:** hot/cold sensation, rash.

Interactions

Drug-Drug: May ↑ duration of **d-tubocurarine**-induced curarization.

Route/Dosage

PO (Adults): 200 mg three times daily.

Availability

Tablets: 100 mg, 200 mg.

NURSING IMPLICATIONS

Assessment

- Assess for symptoms of irritable bowel syndrome (cramping, constipation and diarrhea, mucus in stools).
- Assess for abdominal distention and assess bowel sounds.
- Monitor intake and output and record.

Potential Nursing Diagnoses

Acute pain
Diarrhea

Implementation

- **PO:** Administer three times daily before meals.

Patient/Family Teaching

- Instruct patient to take trimebutine as directed.
- Advise female patient to inform health care professional if pregnancy is planned or suspected or if breast feeding.

Evaluation

- Decrease signs and symptoms of irritable bowel disease.

zopiclone (zoe-pi-clone)

✱Imovane

Classification

Therapeutic: sedative/hypnotics
Pharmacologic: cyclopyrrolones

Indications

Short-term treatment of insomnia characterized by difficulty falling asleep and frequent/early awakenings.

Action

Interacts with GABA-receptor complexes; not a benzodiazepine. **Therapeutic Effects:** Improved sleep with decrease latency and increased maintenance of sleep.

Pharmacokinetics

Absorption: Rapidly absorbed (75%) following oral administration.

Distribution: Rapidly distributed from extravascular compartment. Enters breast milk in concentrations that are 50% of plasma levels.

Metabolism and Excretion: Extensively metabolized (mostly by the CYP3A4 enzyme system), metabolites have minimal sedative/hypnotic activity; 4–5% excreted unchanged in urine.
Half-life: 5 hr.

TIME/ACTION PROFILE

ROUTE	ONSET	PEAK	DURATION
PO	rapid	2 hr	6 hr

Contraindications/Precautions

Contraindicated in: Hypersensitivity; Myasthenia gravis; Severe hepatic impairment; Severe respiratory impairment (including sleep apnea); OB: May cause fetal harm, neonatal CNS depression or withdrawal; Lactation: Breast feeding is not recommended; Galactose intolerance (5 mg tablet contains lactose).
Use Cautiously in: Renal, hepatic or pulmonary impairment (dosage reduction may be recommended); Past history of paradoxical reactions to sedative/hypnotics or alcohol or violent behavior; History of depression or suicidal ideation; Geri: Increased sensitivity may increase the risk of falls, confusion or anterograde amnesia (use lowest effective dose); Pedi: Safe and effective use in children <18 yr has not been established.
Exercise Extreme Caution in: History of substance/alcohol abuse.

Adverse Reactions/Side Effects

CV: abnormal thinking, behavioral changes, sleep-driving. **GI:** bitter taste, anorexia, constipation, dry mouth, dyspepsia. **Misc:** allergic reactions including ANAPHYLAXIS, ANAPHYLACTOID REACTIONS and ANGIOEDEMA.

Interactions

Drug-Drug: ↑ risk of CNS depression with other **CNS depressants** including **antihistamines**, **antidepressants**, **opioids**, **sedative/hypnotics**, and **antipsychotics**. ↑ levels and risk of CNS depression with **drugs that inhibit the CYP3A4 enzyme system**, including **erythromycin ketoconazole**, **itraconazole**, **clarithromycin**, **nefazodone**, **ritonavir**, and **nelfinavir**; ↓ dose may be necessary. Levels and effectiveness may be ↓ by **drugs that induce the CYP3A4 enzyme system**, including **carbamazepine**, **phenobarbital**, **phenytoin**, **rifampicin**, and **rifampin**; dose increase may be necessary.

Route/Dosage

PO (Adults): 5–7.5 mg taken immediately before bedtime; not to exceed 7.5 mg or 7–10 days use. Geri: 3.75 mg initially taken immediately before bedtime; may be increased up to 7.5 mg if needed..

Hepatic Impairment

Renal Impairment

PO (Adults): 3.75 mg initially taken immediately before bedtime; may be increased up to 7.5 mg if needed.

Availability

Tablets: 5 mg, 7.5 mg.

NURSING IMPLICATIONS

Assessment

- Assess mental status, sleep patterns, and previous use of sedative/hypnotics. Prolonged use of >7–10 days may lead to physical and psychological dependence.
- Assess alertness at time of peak of drug. Notify health care professional if desired sedation does not occur.
- Assess patient for pain. Medicate as needed. Untreated pain decreases sedative effects.

Potential Nursing Diagnoses

Insomnia
Risk for injury

Implementation

- Before administering, reduce external stimuli and provide comfort measures to increase effectiveness of medication.
- Protect patient from injury. Raise bed side rails. Assist with ambulation. Remove patient's cigarettes.
- Use lowest effective dose.
- **PO:** Tablets should be swallowed with full glass of water. For faster onset of sleep, do not administer with or immediately after a meal.

Patient/Family Teaching

- Instruct patient to take zopiclone as directed. Advise patient not to take zopiclone unless able to stay in bed a full night (7–8 hours) before being active again. Do not take more than the amount prescribed because of the habit-forming potential. Not recommended for use longer than 7–10 days. If used for 2 wk or longer, abrupt withdrawal may result in fatigue, nausea, flushing, light-headedness, uncontrolled crying, vomiting, GI upset, panic attack, or nervousness. Instruct patient to read *Patient Information* for correct product before taking and with each Rx refill, changes may occur.
- Because of rapid onset, advise patient to go to bed immediately after taking zopiclone.
- May cause daytime drowsiness or dizziness. Advise patient to avoid driving or other activities requiring alertness until response to this medication is known.
- Caution patient that complex sleep-related behaviors (sleep-driving) may occur while asleep.
- Advise patient to notify health care professional immediately if signs of anaphylaxis (swelling of the tongue or throat, trouble breathing, and nausea and vomiting) occur.
- Caution patient to avoid concurrent use of alcohol or other CNS depressants.

Evaluation

- Relief of insomnia by improved falling asleep and decreased frequency of nocturnal and early morning awakenings.

zuclopenthixol

(zoo-kloe-pen-**thix**-ole)
✱Clopixol, ✱Clopixol-Acuphase, ✱Clopixol Depot

Classification
Therapeutic: antipsychotics
Pharmacologic: thioxanthenes

Indications

Management of schizophrenia; *oral*— initial and maintenance management; *IM (acuphase)* — initial treatment of acute psychotic episodes or exacerbation of psychosis due to schizophrenia; *IM (depot)* — maintenance management of schizophrenia.

Action

Has high affinity for dopamine D_1 and D_2 receptors, α_1–adrenergic and 5–HT_2 receptors. Dopaminergic blockade produces neuroleptic activity. **Therapeutic Effects:** Decreases psychoses due to schizophrenia.

Pharmacokinetics

Absorption: *PO*— well absorbed following oral administration; *IM (depot and acuphase)* — slowly absorbed from IM sites.
Distribution: Enters breast milk.
Metabolism and Excretion: Mostly metabolized (partially by the CYP2D6 enzyme system), metabolites do not have antipsychotic activity; minimal amounts excreted unchanged in urine.
Half-life: *PO*— 20 hr.

TIME/ACTION PROFILE (antipsychotic effect))

ROUTE	ONSET	PEAK	DURATION
PO	within hrs	4 hr (blood level)	8–24 hr
IM (acetae [Acuphase])	2–4 hr	8 hr (sedation)	2–3 days
IM (decanoiate [Depot])	within 3 days	3–7 days (blood level)	2–4 wk

Contraindications/Precautions

Contraindicated in: Treatment of dementia; Narrow angle glaucoma; Pedi: Safe and effective use in children <18 yr has not been established and is not recommended.
Use Cautiously in: Impaired hepatic or renal function; Electrolyte abnormalities, including hypokalemia, hypomagnesemia, concurrent diuretic therapy or drugs affecting QT interval or cardiovascular disease/history (↑ risk of serious arrhythmias); Intestinal pathology or brain lesions (anti-emetic effect may mask symptoms); History of seizures (may ↓ threshold); Parkinson's disease (may cause deterioration); Risk factors/history of stroke; Abrupt discontinuation (should be tapered); Geri: Consider age-related decrease in renal, hepatic and cardiovascular function, concurrent disease states and drug therapies in patients >65 yr; OB: Infants exposed in the third trimester may exhibit extrapyramidal and withdrawal reactions including agitation, hyertonia, hypotonia, tremor, somnolence, respiratory distress and feeding disorders, do not use in pregnancy unless expected benefit to the mother outweighs potential fetal risks; Lactation: Enters breast milk, safe use has not been established.

Adverse Reactions/Side Effects

CNS: NEUROLEPTIC MALIGNANT SYNDROME, dizziness, extrapyramidal symptoms, fatigue, sedation, tardive dyskinesia, weakness, syncope. **EENT:** abnormal vision accommodation. **CV:** THROMBOEMBOLISM, arrhythmias, hypotension, tachycardia. **GI:** constipation, dry mouth, diarrhea, thirst, vomiting. **Derm:** photosensitivity reactions, ↑ sweating. **Endo:** hyperprolactinemia, hyperglycemia. **GU:** ↓ libido, abnormal urination. **Hemat:** anemia, granulocytopenia. **Metab:** weight change. **MS:** myalgia.

Interactions

Drug-Drug: ↑ risk of CNS depression with other **CNS depressants** including **alcohol**, some **antihistamines**, some **antidepressants**, **anxiolytics**, **barbiturates**, **benzodiazepines**, and **sedative/hypnotics**. ↑ blood levels and risk of toxicity with **drugs that inhibit the CYP2D6 enzyme system**. Concurrent use of **diuretics**, **lithium**, **Class Ia and III antiarrhythmics** including **amiodarone**, **sotalol**, and **quinidine**; some **antipsychotics** including **thioridazine**, some **macrolide anti-infectives** including **erythromycin**; and some **quinolone anti-infectives** including **moxifloxacin** ↑ risk of QT prolongation and serious arrhythmias; concurrent use should be avoided. ↑ risk of anticholinergic adverse reactions with other **anticholingeric drugs**. ↑ risk of hypotension with **antihypertensives** and **diuretics**. May ↓ antihypertensive effects of **guanthidine** and similar drugs. Concurrent use with **tricyclic antidepressants** may result in altered metabolism and effects of both. ↑ risk of extrapyramidal symptoms with **metoclopramide**. May ↓ beneficial effects of **levodopa** and **dopamine agonists**.

Route/Dosage

PO (Adults): *Acute psychoses*— 10–50 mg/day in 2–3 divided doses initially, may be increased by 10–20 mg/day every 2–3 days, titrate according to response. Usual dose range is 20–60 mg/day; doses >100 m g/day are not recommended. Dose should be reduced to lowest dose needed to control symptoms (usual range 20–40 mg/day). Once maintenance dose is established, may be given as a single daily dose.
IM (Adults): *Zuclopenthixol acetate [Acuphase]*— 50–150 mg, may be repeated every 2–3 days if necessary, some patients may need an additional dose 1–2 days after first injection only; care must be taken to avoid over-medicating due to delay in absorption and antipsychotic effects. Maximum cumulative dose should not exceed 400 mg or four injections. *Zuclopenthixol acetate (Acuphase)* dose form is not meant for long-term use, duration should not exceed 2 wk. If injection volume exceeds 2 mL, dose should be divided and given in two sites. If oral maintenance is to be used, treatment with tablets should be initiated 2–3 days following the last dose of the *Zuclopenthixol acetate (Acuphase)* dose form; if *Zucopenthixol decanoate (Depot)* dose form is to be used for maintenance, may be given concurrently with the last injection of *Zuclopenthixol acetate (Acuphase)* dose form. *Suggested transfer regimen to oral*

dosing—If *Zuclopenthixol acetate (Acuphase)* dose was 50 mg, then daily oral dose could be 20 mg; if *Zuclopenthixol acetate (Acuphase)* dose was 100 mg, then daily oral dose could be 40 mg; if *Zuclopenthixol acetate (Acuphase)* dose was 150 mg, then daily oral dose could be 60 mg. *Suggested transfer regimen to Zuclopenthixol decanoate (Depot) dosing*—If *Zuclopenthixol acetate (Acuphase)* dose was 50 mg, then IM dose of *Zuclopenthixol decanoate (Depot)* could be 100 mg every 2 wk; if *Zuclopenthixol acetate (Acuphase)* dose was 100 mg, then IM dose of *Zuclopenthixol decanoate (Depot)* could be 200 mg every 2 wk; if *Zuclopenthixol acetate (Acuphase)* dose was 150 mg, then IM dose of *Zuclopenthixol decanoate (Depot)* could be 300 mg every 2 wk.

IM (Adults): *Zuclopenthixol decanoate [depot]*—Usual maintenance dose is 150–300 mg every 2–4 wk, regimens should be individualized according to response, care must be taken not to over-medicate due to delayed/prolonged absorption and effects. If injection volume exceeds 2 mL, dose should be divided and given in two sites.

Availability

Zuclopenthixol hydrochloride tablets —contain castor oil: 10 mg, 25 mg; zuclopenthixol acetate injection (Acuphase)—contains medium-chain triglycerides: 50 mg/mL in 1– and 2–mL ampules; zuclopenthixol decanoate injection (Depot) —contains medium-chain triglycerides: 200 mg/mL in 1–mL ampules and 10–mL vials.

NURSING IMPLICATIONS

Assessment

- Assess mental status (orientation, mood, behavior) before and periodically during therapy.
- Observe carefully when administering oral medication to ensure that medication is actually taken and not hoarded.
- Assess weight and BMI initially and throughout therapy.
- Assess fluid intake and bowel function. Increased bulk and fluids in the diet help minimize constipation.
- Monitor for onset of akathisia (restlessness or desire to keep moving) and extrapyramidal side effects (*parkinsonian*—difficulty speaking or swallowing, loss of balance control, pill rolling, mask-like face, shuffling gait, rigidity, tremors; *dystonic*—muscle spasms, twisting motions, twitching, inability to move eyes, weakness of arms or legs) every 2 mo during therapy and 8–12 wk after therapy has been discontinued. Reduction in dose or discontinuation of medication may be necessary. Benztropine or diphenhydramine may be used to control these symptoms.
- Monitor for tardive dyskinesia (uncontrolled rhythmic movement of mouth, face, and extremities; lip smacking or puckering; puffing of cheeks; uncontrolled chewing; rapid or worm-like movements of tongue). Report immediately; may be irreversible.
- Monitor for development of neuroleptic malignant syndrome (fever, respiratory distress, tachycardia, seizures, diaphoresis, arrhythmias, hypertension or hypotension, pallor, tiredness, severe muscle stiffness, loss of bladder control). Report immediately.
- Monitor for symptoms related to hyperprolactinemia (menstrual abnormalities, galactorrhea, sexual dysfunction).
- ***Lab Test Considerations:*** Monitor CBC and liver function tests every 6 mo and periodically as needed during treatment. May cause ↑ AST, ALT, and alkaline phosphatase.
- Monitor blood glucose prior to and periodically during therapy. May cause hyperglycemia.
- Monitor serum prolactin prior to and periodically during therapy. May cause ↑ serum prolactin levels.

Potential Nursing Diagnoses

Risk for injury
Disturbed thought process

Implementation

- **PO:** Administer tablets before or after meals.
- **IM:** Administer deep in large muscle. A test dose may be ordered for first administration.

Patient/Family Teaching

- Instruct patient to take as directed. If a dose is missed, omit and take next dose as scheduled. Discontinuation should be gradual.
- Inform patient of possibility of extrapyramidal symptoms and tardive dyskinesia. Caution patient to report these symptoms immediately to health care professional.
- Advise patient to change positions slowly to minimize orthostatic hypotension.
- Medication may cause drowsiness. Caution patient to avoid driving or other activities requiring alertness until response to medication is known.
- Advise patient to notify health care professional of all Rx or OTC medications, vitamins, or herbal products being taken and to consult with health care professional before taking other medications.
- Instruct patient to notify health care professional promptly if sore throat, fever, unusual bleeding or bruising, rash, weakness, tremors, visual disturbances, dark-colored urine, or clay-colored stools occur.
- Instruct patient to avoid sun exposure and to wear protective clothing and sunscreen when outdoors.
- Advise patient to notify health care professional of medication regimen before treatment or surgery.
- Advise female patients to notify health care professional if pregnancy is planned or suspected or if breast feeding or planning to breast feed.

Evaluation

- Decreased symptoms of schizophrenia (delusions, hallucinations, social withdrawal, flat, blunt affect).

Natural/Herbal Products

The following monographs introduce some commonly used natural products. Because the amounts of active ingredients in these agents are not standardized or currently subject to FDA guidelines for medicines, *Davis's Drug Guide for Nurses*, although respectful of patients' right to choose from a variety of therapeutic options, does not endorse their routine use unless supervised by a knowledgeable health care professional. Users should take into account the possibility of adverse reactions and interactions and consider the relative lack of data supporting widespread use of these products. Doses are poorly standardized, and individuals are advised to read package labels carefully to ensure safe and efficacious use.

aloe (al-oh)

Other Name(s):
Aloe vera, Cape aloe, Aloe latex, Burn plant, Curacao aloe

Classification
Therapeutic: laxatives, wound/ulcer/decubiti healing agent

Common Uses

PO: Cathartic laxative. **Topical:** Use on burns/sunburns, wounds, irritated skin, psoriasis; topical anti-infective.

Action

PO: Exerts a laxative effect by increasing colonic motility, reducing water absorption from the bowel and stimulating bowel, chloride secretion, and water content. **Topical:** May help accelerate wound healing through inhibition of thromboxane A2 and increased microcirculation, although the evidence is inconsistent. May have some activity against gram-positive, gram-negative bacteria and yeast. **Therapeutic Effects:** Relief of constipation. Improved wound healing.

Pharmacokinetics

Absorption: Unknown.
Distribution: Unknown.
Metabolism and Excretion: Unknown.
Half-life: Unknown.

TIME/ACTION PROFILE

ROUTE	ONSET	PEAK	DURATION
PO, Topical	unknown	unknown	unknown

Contraindications/Precautions

Contraindicated in: Intestinal obstruction; Inflammatory intestinal diseases (including Crohn's disease); Appendicitis and abdominal pain of unknown origin; OB: Safety not established; Pedi: Oral aloe not appropriate for children <12 yr.
Use Cautiously in: Renal disease; Fluid or electrolyte abnormalities; Diabetes; Alcohol containing products should be used cautiously in patients with known intolerance or liver disease; Pedi: Cautious use in children >12 yr.

Adverse Reactions/Side Effects

Derm: Contact dermatitis, skin irritation. **Endo:** hypoglycemia. **F and E:** HYPOKALEMIA, dehydration. **GI:** Cramping, diarrhea, laxative dependence (chronic use). **GU:** hematuria.

Interactions

Natural Product-Drug: Combining oral aloe with potassium-wasting drugs (e.g., **diuretics**, other **laxatives**, **corticosteroids**, **cisplatin**, **amphotericin B**) may worsen hypokalemia. Hypokalemia may ↑ risk of toxicity from **digoxin** and some **antiarrhythmics**. May have additive effects with **antidiabetic** agents. May ↑ bleeding risk with **warfarin**. **Alcohol**-containing preparations may interact with **disulfiram** and **metronidazole**.
Natural-Natural: ↑ hypokalemia risk with **licorice** and **horsetail**. Additive effects with stimulant laxative herbs and herbs with hypoglycemic potential.

Route/Commonly Used Doses

PO (Adults): *Constipation*— 100–200 mg aloe or 50 mg of aloe extract taken in the evening. Do not use for >1–2 wk without medical advice; *Juice*— 1 teaspoonful tid after meals.
Topical (Adults): Aloe gel can be applied liberally to affected areas 3–5 times daily.

Availability

Alone or in combination with other herbal medicinals^{OTC}; Capsules^{OTC}; Juice^{OTC}; Tincture (1:10 in 50% alcohol)^{OTC}; Topical or gel or applied directly from cut plant.

NURSING IMPLICATIONS

Assessment

- **Constipation:** Assess for abdominal distention, presence of bowel sounds, and usual pattern of elimination.
- Assess color, consistency, and amount of stool produced.
- **Topical:** Perform baseline skin assessment prior to applying aloe to minor wounds, burns, and abrasions. Observe the size, character, and location of the affected area prior to the application of aloe.
- Note topical response assessing for increased inflammation, drainage, pain, warmth, and/or pruritus.
- ***Lab Test Considerations:*** Monitor serum potassium in patients with chronic use and CBC in patients who self-medicate and experience bloody diarrhea or have ulcerative colitis or Crohn's disease.

Potential Nursing Diagnoses

Constipation (Indications)
Risk for impaired skin integrity
Deficient knowledge, related to medication regimen

Implementation

- **PO:** Administer laxative at bedtime to induce a bowel movement in the morning.
- **Topical:** Wash hands and then apply liberally to affected area of skin. Cover broken areas of skin with a light nonadhering dressing (e.g., band-aid dressing with *Telfa* lining) to facilitate keeping area clean. Do not apply an occlusive dressing over site of application.

Patient/Family Teaching

- **Constipation:** Instruct patients with pre-existing intestinal disorders (e.g., ulcerative colitis, Crohn's disease, irritable bowel syndrome) not to take aloe juice without the advice of a health care professional.
- Counsel patients that the oral juice should not be taken if they are experiencing abdominal pain, nausea, vomiting, or fever.
- Inform patients that occasional constipation may not be an issue but persistent constipation may represent a more serious health problem and to consult their health care professional.
- Advise patients to expect laxative response to the oral juice in 8–12 hr.
- Caution patients that the cathartic effects may be dramatic and that accompanying dehydration and electrolyte imbalances may occur. If severe diarrhea occurs or persists, seek out treatment from their health care professional.
- Advise patients other than those with spinal cord injury that laxatives should only be used for short-term therapy. Although this is considered by some to be a natural way of correcting constipation it still carries the risk of electrolyte imbalance and dependency with chronic use.
- Encourage patients to use other forms of bowel regulation: increasing bulk in the diet, increasing fluid intake, and increasing mobility, as appropriate. Normal bowel habits are individualized and may vary from 3 times/day to 3 times/wk.
- Advise patients to consume 1500–2000 mL/day of fluids during therapy to prevent dehydration.
- Direct patients with a known cardiac history not to take this herbal supplement without the advice of their health care professional because of the risk of hypokalemia worsening arrhythmias.
- Caution patients with cardiac history to avoid straining during bowel movements (Valsalva maneuver).
- **Topical:** Advise patients that topical applications should only be used for minor burns, abrasions, or wounds. Wounds of larger size or more serious burns should be treated by a health care professional.
- Instruct patients using topical application on a nonintact skin surface about signs and symptoms of infection (milky or discolored drainage, redness, warmth, swelling, pain) and to promptly seek out treatment of a health care professional if this occurs.
- Counsel patients that if improvement in the wound is not occurring or it worsens, stop treatment with aloe vera and seek the advice of a health care professional.
- Warn patients with risk factors for delayed wound healing (e.g., diabetic patients, vascular disease) not to self-medicate with aloe vera without the approval of their health care professional.

Evaluation

- A soft, formed bowel movement.
- Evacuation of the colon.
- Relief of sunburn pain.
- Wound healing in small localized burns or abrasions.

arnica (ar-ni-cuh)

Other Name(s):
Arnica montana, leopard's bane, mountain tobacco, mountain snuff, wolf's bane

Classification
Therapeutic: immune stimulant, anti-inflammatory

Common Uses
Topical treatment of insect bites, bruises, acne, boils, sprains, muscle, and joint pain.

Action
Polysaccharides in arnica may produce a slight anti-inflammatory and analgesic effect. Some antibacterial effects are seen, in addition to a counterirritant effect, which may aid in wound healing. **Therapeutic Effects:** Decreased inflammation. Pain relief.

Pharmacokinetics
Absorption: Systemic absorption may occur following topical application to broken skin.
Distribution: Unknown.
Metabolism and Excretion: Unknown.
Half-life: Unknown.

TIME/ACTION PROFILE

ROUTE	ONSET	PEAK	DURATION
Topical	unknown	unknown	unknown

Contraindications/Precautions
Contraindicated in: Not for oral use (except in highly diluted homeopathic preparations); Arnica allergy; Avoid use on broken skin; Infectious or inflammatory GI conditions; OB: Pregnancy and lactation.
Use Cautiously in: Infectious or inflammatory GI conditions; Surgery (discontinue use 2 wk prior to procedure due to antiplatelet effects).

Adverse Reactions/Side Effects
GI: abdominal pain, vomiting, diarrhea (if taken orally). **Derm:** edematous dermatitis with pustules (chronic treatment of damaged skin), eczema (prolonged use). **Misc:** local allergic reactions.

Interactions
Natural Product-Drug: Alcohol-containing preparations may interact with **disulfuram** and **metronidazole**. Potential for reduced effectiveness of **antihypertensives** has been noted. May potentiate the effects of **anticoagulants** and **antiplatelet agents**, increasing the risk of bleeding.
Natural-Natural: May increase risk of bleeding with **clove**, **garlic**, **ginger**, **ginkgo**, and **ginseng**.

Route/Commonly Used Doses
Topical (Adults): *Topical*—rub or massage arnica tincture, cream, or gel onto injured area. Do not apply to broken skin; *Compress*—dilute 1 tablespoon of arnica tincture in 1/2 L water. Wet a gauze pad with solution and apply to affected area for 15 minutes. For use in poultices, dilute tincture 3 to 10 times with water.

Availability
Cream, tincture, salve, ointment, gel, and oil[OTC]; Topical (preparations should contain not more than 20–25% arnica tincture or 15% arnica oil)[OTC]; Homeopathic preparations[OTC].

NURSING IMPLICATIONS

Assessment
- Inspect skin for breaks prior to application to ensure arnica is applied only to an intact surface. Note the size, character, and location of affected area prior to application of arnica.
- After application, assess the affected area for signs of allergic response.
- ***Toxicity and Overdose:*** Systemic absorption may result in nausea, vomiting, organ damage, hypertension, cardiotoxicity, arrhythmias, muscular weakness, collapse, vertigo, renal dysfunction, coma, and death. If ingested orally, induce emesis and gastric lavage to remove undigested contents. Supportive care may be necessary. Do not take orally or apply to nonintact skin to avoid systemic absorption.

Potential Nursing Diagnoses
Acute pain (Indications)

Implementation
- Clean skin with a nonalcohol containing cleanser prior to applying arnica. Apply topically to affected area, or site of injury, ensuring skin is intact.
- Do not take orally or apply to an open wound because of potential for systemic absorption with toxicity.

Patient/Family Teaching
- Teach patients to inspect the affected area for breaks in the skin and not to apply arnica to any areas where the skin is broken.
- Warn patients that use on nonintact skin and oral ingestion may cause life-threatening toxicity.
- Advise patients that arnica should only be used for short period of time in the treatment of minor aches and pains associated with local muscle, joint, or skin pain. Prolonged use may cause allergic/hypersensitivity reactions to develop.

- Instruct patients taking antihypertensive agents to avoid concurrent use of arnica.
- Advise female patients to notify health care professional if pregnancy is planned or suspected. Arnica should be avoided during pregnancy.

Evaluation
- Relief of, or improvement in, minor aches and pains associated with muscle or joint overuse, or sprains and/or local skin irritation from insect bites, bruises, boils, or acne.

bilberry (bill-beh-ree)

Other Name(s):
Vaccinium myrtillus

Classification
Therapeutic: ocular agents

Common Uses
Visual acuity improvement, atherosclerosis, venous insufficiency, varicose veins, diabetes mellitus, diarrhea, hemorrhoids, peptic ulcer disease, osteoarthritis, and chronic fatigue syndrome.

Action
Anthocyanidins in bilberry have a variety of effects including increased glycosaminoglycans synthesis, decreasing vascular permeability, reducing membrane thickness, redistribution of microvascular blood flow, and formation of interstitial fluid. **Therapeutic Effects:** Decreased inflammation. Decreased edema. Decreased blood glucose. Improved circulation.

Pharmacokinetics
Absorption: Unknown.
Distribution: Unknown.
Metabolism and Excretion: Eliminated by the kidneys.
Half-life: Unknown.

TIME/ACTION PROFILE

ROUTE	ONSET	PEAK	DURATION
PO	Unknown	Unknown	Unknown

Contraindications/Precautions
Contraindicated in: Hypersensitivity or allergy to bilberry; Leaves are potentially toxic with chronic use of 1.5 g/kg/day.
Use Cautiously in: Diabetic patients; Patients at risk for bleeding; OB: Avoid use in pregnancy due to lack of safety data.

Adverse Reactions/Side Effects
Endo: low blood sugar. **GI:** diarrhea, upset stomach. **Hemat:** bleeding, bruising.

Interactions
Natural Product-Drug: May ↑ effects of **anticoagulants and antiplatelet drugs** and ↓ platelet activity. May ↑ effects of **antidiabetic agents** and cause hypoglycemia.
Natural-Natural: Avoid use with chromium-containing herbs and supplements (bilberry contains chromium). Avoid use with herbs with hypoglycemic properties.

Route/Commonly Used Doses
PO (Adults): 80–480 mg of bilberry extract daily in 2–3 divided doses.

Availability
Liquid extract; Tablets; Softgel capsules.

NURSING IMPLICATIONS

Assessment
- Monitor BP periodically during therapy, coagulation panel, blood glucose.
- ***Lab Test Considerations:*** Monitor coagulation studies in patients on anticoagulants and antiplatelet agents.
- Monitor blood glucose periodically during therapy. May cause hypoglycemia.

Potential Nursing Diagnoses
Activity intolerance (Indications)
Diarrhea (Indications)

Implementation
- Administer without regard to food.

Patient/Family Teaching
- Instruct patient to take bilberry as directed.

Evaluation
- Improvement in vascular insufficiency.
- Decrease in diarrhea.

black cohosh (blak coe-hosh)
Remifemin

Other Name(s):
baneberry, black snakeroot, bugbane, phytoestrogen, rattle root, rattleweed, rattle top, squawroot

Classification
Therapeutic: none assigned

Do not confuse black cohosh with blue or white cohosh

Common Uses
Management of menopausal symptoms. Premenstrual discomfort. Dysmenorrhea. Mild sedative. Rheumatism.

Action

Therapeutic effects are produced by glycosides isolated from the fresh or dried rhizome with attached roots. Mechanism of action is unclear. **Therapeutic Effects:** May decrease symptoms of menopause, including hot flashes, sweating, sleep disturbance, and anxiety. Has no effect on vaginal epithelium.

Pharmacokinetics

Absorption: Unknown.
Distribution: Unknown.
Metabolism and Excretion: Unknown.
Half-life: Unknown.

TIME/ACTION PROFILE

ROUTE	ONSET	PEAK	DURATION
PO	unknown	unknown	unknown

Contraindications/Precautions

Contraindicated in: OB: Pregnancy and lactation.
Use Cautiously in: Breast cancer (may increase risk of metastasis); Hormone-sensitive cancers; Protein S deficiency (increased risk for thrombosis); Liver disease.

Adverse Reactions/Side Effects

Neuro: SEIZURES (in combination with evening primrose and chasteberry), headache, dizziness. **GI:** GI upset, hepatotoxicity. **Derm:** rash. **Misc:** weight gain, cramping, breast tenderness, vaginal spotting/bleeding.

Interactions

Natural Product-Drug: Unknown effects when combined with hormone replacement therapy and **antiestrogens** (e.g., **tamoxifen**). Concurrent use with **hepatotoxic drugs** may ↑ risk of liver damage. **Alcohol-containing preparations** may interact with **disulfiram** and **metronidazole**. May ↓ cytotoxic effects of **cisplatin**. May precipitate hypotension when used in combination with **antihypertensives**.
Natural-Natural: May ↑ risk of hepatotoxicity when used with **chaparral**, **comfrey**, **kava-kava**, and **niacin**.

Route/Commonly Used Doses

PO (Adults): *Tablets (Remifemin®)*—20 mg bid. *Liquid extract*—0.3–2 mL bid-tid. *Tincture*—2–4 mL bid–tid. *Dried rhizome*—0.3–2 g tid. Do not use for more than 6 mo.

Availability

Alone or in combination with other herbal medicinals^OTC; Tablets (Remifemin® 20 mg [best studied black cohosh product])^OTC; Liquid extract (1:1 in 90% alcohol)^OTC; Tincture (1:10 in 60% alcohol)^OTC; Dried rhizome.

NURSING IMPLICATIONS

Assessment

- Assess frequency and severity of menopausal symptoms.
- Monitor BP for patients on antihypertensive drugs; may increase effects and cause hypotension.
- Assess for history of seizures or liver disease.

Potential Nursing Diagnoses

Sleep deprivation (Indications)

Implementation

- Administration with food may help to minimize nausea.

Patient/Family Teaching

- Advise patient to notify health care professional if pregnancy is planned or suspected. Avoid use during pregnancy; may induce a miscarriage.
- Patients with seizures, liver dysfunction, excessive alcohol intake, cancer, or other medical problems should be advised to consult their health care professional prior to initiating self-therapy with this herb.
- Advise patient to consult health care professional before taking with other estrogen replacements.
- Emphasize the importance of continued medical supervision for Pap smears, mammograms, pelvic examinations, and BP monitoring at the intervals indicated by health care professional.

Evaluation

- Resolution of menopausal vasomotor symptoms.

chondroitin (konn-**droy**-tinn)

Other Name(s):
chondroitin polysulfate, CPS, CDS

Classification
Therapeutic: nonopioid analgesics

Common Uses

Osteoarthritis. Ischemic heart disease. Hyperlipidemia. Osteoporosis. **Ophth:** In combination with sodium hyaluronate, for use as a surgical aid in cataract extraction or lens implantation, and as a lubricant.

Action

May serve as a building block of articular cartilage. May protect cartilage against degradation. May have antiatherogenic properties. **Therapeutic Effects:** Improvement in osteoarthritis symptoms.

Pharmacokinetics

Absorption: 8–18% is absorbed orally.
Distribution: Unknown.

Metabolism and Excretion: Unknown.
Half-life: Unknown.

TIME/ACTION PROFILE

ROUTE	ONSET	PEAK	DURATION
PO	unknown	unknown	unknown

Contraindications/Precautions
Contraindicated in: OB: Pregnancy and lactation.
Use Cautiously in: Asthma (may exacerbate symptoms); Clotting disorders (may ↑ risk of bleeding); Prostate cancer (may ↑ risk of metastasis or recurrence).

Adverse Reactions/Side Effects
GI: heartburn, nausea, diarrhea. **Hemat:** bleeding (antiplatelet effect). **Misc:** allergic reactions, edema, hair loss.

Interactions
Natural Product-Drug: Use of chondroitin with **anticoagulant** and **antiplatelet** drugs, **thrombolytics**, **NSAIDs**, some **cephalosporins**, and **valproates** may ↑ risk of bleeding.
Natural-Natural: Herbs with anticoagulant or antiplatelet properties may ↑ bleeding risk when combined with chondroitin, including: **anise**, **arnica**, **chamomile**, **clove**, **dong quai**, **fenugreek**, **feverfew**, **ginger**, **ginkgo**, **Panax ginseng**, **licorice**, and others.

Route/Commonly Used Doses
PO (Adults): *Osteoarthritis*—200–400 mg 2–3 times daily or 1000–1200 mg once daily. *Prevention of recurrent myocardial infarction*—10 grams daily in 3 divided doses for 3 mo followed by 1.5 grams daily in 3 divided doses as maintenance therapy.
IM (Adults): *Osteoarthritis*—50 mg twice weekly for 8 wk every 4 mo.

Availability
Tablets[OTC]; **Capsules**[OTC]; **Injection (not available in US)**; Ophthalmic Drops Rx in combination with sodium hyaluronate (Viscoat).

NURSING IMPLICATIONS

Assessment
- Evaluate drug profile before starting therapy with this herbal supplement. If the patient is taking anticoagulants or antiplatelet drugs, avoid use of this herb.
- Monitor pain (type, location, and intensity) and range of motion on an ongoing basis as an indicator of drug efficacy.
- Evaluate gastric discomfort and instruct patient to seek out the advice of a health care professional if persistent gastric discomfort occurs.
- Assess for signs of bleeding and discontinue herbal supplement promptly and seek out health care professional for follow-up.

Potential Nursing Diagnoses
Chronic pain (Indications)
Impaired physical mobility (Indications)

Implementation
- Administer with food.

Patient/Family Teaching
- Advise patients that this herbal supplement is usually taken with glucosamine.
- Caution patients who take aspirin or NSAIDs or other non-prescription medications not to take this herbal supplement without conferring with their health care professional.
- Advise female patients to notify health care professional if pregnancy is planned or suspected or if breast feeding; avoid use.
- Instruct patients that this medication works by building up cartilage and that this requires that the medication be taken consistently over a period of time. It is not recommended as a supplemental pain medication.

Evaluation
- Improvement in pain and range of motion.
- Reduced need for supplemental or breakthrough pain medication.

Crataegus Species, see **hawthorne**.

dong quai (don kwi)

Other Name(s):
Angelica sinensis, Chinese Angelica, Dang Gui, Danggui, Don Quai, Ligustilides, Phytoestrogen, *Radix angelicae gigantis*, Tang Kuei, Tan Kue Bai Zhi

Classification
Therapeutic: none assigned

Common Uses
Premenstrual syndrome. Various uses as a blood purifier. Topically in combination with other ingredients for premature ejaculation.

Action
May have vasodilating and antispasmodic properties. Binds to estrogen receptors. **Therapeutic Effects:** Improved ejaculatory latency.

Pharmacokinetics
Absorption: Unknown.
Distribution: Unknown.

Metabolism and Excretion: Unknown.
Half-life: Unknown.

TIME/ACTION PROFILE

ROUTE	ONSET	PEAK	DURATION
PO	unknown	unknown	unknown

Contraindications/Precautions
Contraindicated in: Allergy to carrot, celery, mugwort, or other members of the Apiaceae family; OB: Pregnancy and lactation.
Use Cautiously in: Hormone sensitive cancers and conditions (may exacerbate effects or stimulate growth of cancer cells); Protein S deficiency (↑ risk for thrombosis); Surgery (discontinue 2 wk prior to procedure).

Adverse Reactions/Side Effects
Derm: photosensitivity. **GI:** diarrhea. **Misc:** Some constituents are carcinogenic and mutagenic.

Interactions
Natural Product-Drug: Alcohol-containing preparations may interact with **disulfiram** and **metronidazole**. Use of dong quai with **anticoagulant** and **antiplatelet** drugs, **thrombolytics**, **NSAIDs**, some **cephalosporins**, and **valproates** may increase risk of bleeding.
Natural-Natural: Herbs with antiplatelet or anticoagulant properties may increase bleeding risk when combined with dong quai including: **angelica**, **clove**, **danshen**, **garlic**, **ginger**, **ginkgo**, ***Panax ginseng***, and **willow**.

Route/Commonly Used Doses
PO (Adults): *Bulk herb*—3–4.5 g per day in divided doses with meals; *Extract*—1 ml (20–40 drops) three times daily.

Availability
Bulk herb[OTC]**; Extract**[OTC]**.**

NURSING IMPLICATIONS

Assessment
- Assess pain and menstrual patterns prior to and following menstrual cycle to determine effectiveness of this herbal supplement.
- Assess for pregnancy prior to recommending use of the herbal supplement and warn women not to take this herb if pregnancy is planned or suspected.
- Assess for history of hormone sensitive cancers or conditions and warn against use.
- Assess medication profile including prescription and over-the-counter use of products such as aspirin- and ibuprofen-based products to treat menstrual pain.

Potential Nursing Diagnoses
Acute pain (Indications)
Deficient knowledge, related to medication regimen (Patient/Family Teaching)

Implementation
- Take with meals.

Patient/Family Teaching
- Warn patients not to take this medication if pregnant or breast feeding.
- Inform patients to avoid use of aspirin or other NSAIDs concurrently because of the risk of bleeding.
- Notify patients that there are no studies supporting the use of this herbal supplement for treatment of menopausal symptoms.
- Tell patients to consult their health care professional if taking prescription medications before taking dong quai.
- Discontinue the herbal supplement if diarrhea or excessive bleeding occurs and contact a health care provider if symptoms do not resolve.
- Instruct patients that photosensitivity may occur and to wear sunscreen and protective clothing if sun exposure is anticipated.

Evaluation
- Reduction in menstrual pain and cramping and regular periods with normal flow.

echinacea (*Echinacea purpurea*) (ek-i-**nay**-sha)

Other Name(s):
American coneflower, black sampson, black susan, *brauneria angustifolia*, kansas snakeroot, purple coneflower, red sunflower, *rudbeckia*, sampson root, scurvy root

Classification
Therapeutic: immune stimulants

Common Uses
Bacterial and viral infections. Prevention and treatment of colds, coughs, flu, and bronchitis. Fevers. Wounds and burns. Inflammation of the mouth and pharynx. Urinary tract infections. Vaginal candidiasis.

Action
Medicinal parts derived from the roots, leaves, or whole plant of perennial herb (Echinacea). *Echinacea purpurea herba* has been reported to promote wound healing, which may be due to an increase in white blood cells, spleen cells, and increased activity

NATURAL/HERBAL PRODUCTS

of granulocytes, as well as an increase in helper T cells and cytokines. *E. purpurea radix* has been shown to have antibacterial, antiviral, anti-inflammatory, and immune-modulating effects. **Therapeutic Effects:** Resolution of respiratory and urinary tract infections. Decreased duration and intensity of common cold. Improved wound healing. Stimulates phagocytosis; inhibits action of hyaluronidase (secreted by bacteria), which helps bacteria gain access to healthy cells. Externally, has antifungal and bacteriostatic properties.

Pharmacokinetics

Absorption: Unknown.
Distribution: Unknown.
Metabolism and Excretion: Unknown.
Half-life: Unknown.

TIME/ACTION PROFILE

ROUTE	ONSET	PEAK	DURATION
PO	unknown	unknown	unknown

Contraindications/Precautions

Contraindicated in: Multiple sclerosis, leukosis, collagenoses, AIDS, tuberculosis, autoimmune diseases; Hypersensitivity and cross-sensitivity in patients allergic to plants in *Asteraceae/Compositae* plant family (daisies, chrysanthemums, marigolds, etc.); OB: Pregnancy and lactation.
Use Cautiously in: Diabetes; Pedi: May increase risk of rash in children; Tinctures should be used cautiously in alcoholics or patients with liver disease; Do not take longer than 8 wk—may suppress immune function.

Adverse Reactions/Side Effects

CNS: dizziness, fatigue, headache, somnolence. **EENT:** tingling sensation on tongue, sore throat. **GI:** nausea, vomiting, heartburn, constipation, abdominal pain, diarrhea. **Derm:** allergic reaction, rash (more common in children). **Misc:** fever.

Interactions

Natural Product-Drug: May possibly interfere with **immunosuppressants** because of its immunostimulant activity. May ↑ risk for hepatotoxicity from **anabolic steroids**, **methotrexate**, or **ketoconazole** when taken with echinacea. May ↑ **midazolam** availability.
Natural-Natural: May ↑ risk for hepatotoxicity when taken with **kava**.

Route/Commonly Used Doses

PO (Adults): *Tablets*—6.78 mg tablets, take 2 tabs 3 times daily. *Capsules*—500–1000 mg 3 times a day for 5–7 days. *Fluid extract*—1–2 mL tid; solid form (6.5:1)—150–300 mg tid. Should not be used for more than 8 wk at a time. *Tea*—1/2 tsp comminuted drug, steeped and strained after 10 min, 1 cup 5–6 times daily on the first day, titrating down to 1 cup daily over the next 5 days. *Echinacea purpuren herb juice*—6–9 mL/day. *Liquid*—20 drops every 2 hr for the first day of symptoms, then 3 times daily for up to 10 days.
Topical (Adults): *Ointment, lotion, tincture used externally*—1.5–7.5 mL tincture, 2–5 g dried root.

Availability

Capsules[OTC]; **Tablets** ; Dried Root[OTC]; **The dried root can be steeped and strained in boiling water and taken as a tea**; Liquid extract[OTC]; **1:1 in 45% alcohol**; Tincture[OTC]; **1:5 in 45% alcohol**; Blended teas[OTC]; ***Echinacea purpuren* herb juice**[OTC].

NURSING IMPLICATIONS

Assessment

- Assess wound for size, appearance, and drainage prior to the start of and periodically during therapy.
- Assess frequency of common mild illnesses (such as a cold) in response to use.

Potential Nursing Diagnoses

Risk for impaired skin integrity (Indications)

Implementation

- Tinctures may contain significant concentrations of alcohol and may not be suitable for children, alcoholics, patients with liver disease, or those taking disulfiram, metronidazole, some cephalosporins, or sulfonylurea oral antidiabetic agents.
- Prolonged use of this agent may cause overstimulation of the immune system, and use beyond 8 wk is not recommended. Therapy of 10–14 days is usually considered sufficient.
- May be taken without regard to food.

Patient/Family Teaching

- Herb is more effective for treatment than prevention of colds. Take at first sign of symptoms.
- Advise patient to seek immediate treatment for an illness that does not improve after taking this herb.
- Instruct patient that the usual course of therapy is 10–14 days and 8 wk is the maximum.
- Inform patient that use of this herb is not recommended in severe illnesses (e.g., AIDS, tuberculosis) or autoimmune diseases (e.g., multiple sclerosis, collagen diseases, etc.).
- Caution patient that prolonged use of this herb may result in overstimulation of the immune system, possibly with subsequent immunosuppression.

- Warn pregnant or breast feeding women not to use this herb.
- Instruct patient to consult health care professional before taking any prescription or OTC medications concurrently with echinacea.
- Keep tincture in a dark bottle away from sunlight. Should be taken several times a day.
- Store herb in airtight container away from sunlight.

Evaluation

- Improved wound healing.
- Infrequent common illnesses.
- Illnesses of shorter duration and less severity.

feverfew (fee-vurr-fyoo)

Other Name(s):

Altamisa, Bachelor's Button, *Chrysanthemum parethenium*, Featerfoiul, Featherfew, Featherfoil, Flirtwort Midsummer Daisy, *Pyrethrum parthenium*, Santa Maria, *Tanaceti parthenii*, Wild chamomile, Wild quinine

Classification

Therapeutic: vascular headache suppressants

Common Uses

PO: Migraine headache prophylaxis. **Topical:** Toothaches and as an antiseptic.

Action

The sesquiterpene lactone, parthenolide, may provide feverfew's migraine prophylaxis effects. Feverfew may also have antiplatelet and vasodilatory effects and block prostaglandin synthesis.
Therapeutic Effects: May reduce the symptoms and frequency of migraine headaches.

Pharmacokinetics

Absorption: Unknown.
Distribution: Unknown.
Metabolism and Excretion: Unknown.
Half-life: Unknown.

TIME/ACTION PROFILE

ROUTE	ONSET	PEAK	DURATION
PO	2–4 mo	unknown	unknown

Contraindications/Precautions

Contraindicated in: OB: Pregnancy and lactation; Feverfew hypersensitivity or allergy to *Asteraceae/ Compositae* family plants, including ragweed, chrysanthemums, daisies, and marigolds.
Use Cautiously in: Use >4 mo (safety and efficacy not established).

Adverse Reactions/Side Effects

CNS: "Post-Feverfew Syndrome" (anxiety, headache, insomnia, muscle and joint aches). **CV:** *with long-term use*—tachycardia. **GI:** nausea, vomiting, diarrhea, heartburn, mouth ulceration and soreness (from chewing fresh leaves). **Derm:** contact dermatitis (when used topically).

Interactions

Natural Product-Drug: Use of feverfew with **anticoagulant** and **antiplatelet** drugs, **thrombolytics**, **NSAIDs**, some **cephalosporins**, and **valproates** may increase risk of bleeding. Concomitant use with **NSAIDs** may also reduce feverfew effectiveness.
Natural-Natural: Use with **anise**, **arnica**, **chamomile**, **clove**, **dong quai**, **fenugreek**, **garlic**, **ginger**, **gingko**, **licorice**, and ***Panax ginseng*** may increase anticoagulant potential of feverfew.

Route/Commonly Used Doses

PO (Adults): 50–100 mg feverfew extract daily (standardized to 0.2–0.35% parthenolide) or 50–125 mg freeze-dried leaf daily with or after food.

Availability

Feverfew extractstandardized to 0.2-0.35% parthenolide**OTC**; **Freash leaf**OTC; **Freeze-dried leaf**OTC.

NURSING IMPLICATIONS

Assessment

- Monitor frequency, intensity, and duration of migraine headaches prior to and during ongoing therapy.
- Assess for mouth ulcers or skin ulcerations during therapy.

Potential Nursing Diagnoses

Acute pain (Indications)
Deficient knowledge, related to medication regimen (Patient/Family Teaching)

Implementation

- Take with food or on a full stomach.

Patient/Family Teaching

- Instruct patients to take this medication on a consistent basis to prevent migraine headaches. This herbal supplement is not for treatment of migraines.
- Warn patients about mouth ulcers and sores and that if this occurs to seek the advice of a health care professional. Encourage proper oral hygiene.
- Advise patients not to abruptly stop this product because of the possibility of post- feverfew syndrome. Tell patients that anxiety, headache, in-

*CAPITALS indicates life-threatening; underlines indicate most frequent.

NATURAL/HERBAL PRODUCTS

somnia, and muscle aches may indicate withdrawal. Feverfew should be gradually tapered.

- Review dietary and medication profile of patient to identify potential interactions. Instruct patient about other herbs that may interact with feverfew.
- Counsel patients on anticoagulants not to take feverfew except as directed by their health care provider.
- Advise patients to avoid using NSAIDs as this may reduce the effectiveness of feverfew.
- Instruct patients to look for signs of bleeding such as unusual bruising or inability to clot after a cut and to seek the advice of a health care professional if this occurs.
- Inform patients that feverfew should reduce the number of migraines and severity of symptoms but that duration of the migraine may not be affected.

Evaluation

- Reduction in the frequency and severity of migraine headaches.

garlic (gar-lik)

Other Name(s):
Alli sativa bulbus, *Allium sativum*

Classification
Therapeutic: lipid-lowering agents

Common Uses

PO: Hypertension, hyperlipidemia, cardiovascular disease prevention, colorectal and gastric cancer prevention. **Topical:** Dermal fungal infections including tinea corporis, cruris, and pedis.

Action

May have HMG-CoA inhibitor properties in lowering cholesterol, but less effectively than statin drugs; vasodilatory and antiplatelet properties. **Therapeutic Effects:** Decreased cholesterol levels. Decreased platelet aggregation.

Pharmacokinetics

Absorption: Garlic oil is well absorbed.
Distribution: Unknown.
Metabolism and Excretion: Kidney and lungs.
Half-life: Unknown.

TIME/ACTION PROFILE

ROUTE	ONSET	PEAK	DURATION
PO	4–25 wk	unknown	unknown

Contraindications/Precautions

Contraindicated in: Bleeding disorders. Discontinue use 1–2 weeks prior to surgery.
Use Cautiously in: Diabetes, gastrointestinal infection or inflammation.

Adverse Reactions/Side Effects

CNS: dizziness. **GI:** Irritation of the mouth, esophagus, and stomach, nausea, bad breath, vomiting, flatulence, diarrhea. **Derm:** Contact dermatitis and other allergic reactions (asthma, rash, anaphylaxis [rare]), Diaphoresis. **Hemat:** Chronic use or excessive dose may lead to ↓ hemoglobin production and lysis of RBCs, platelet dysfunction, prolonged bleeding time. **Misc:** body odor.

Interactions

Natural Product-Drug: Use of garlic with **anticoagulants**, **antiplatelet agents**, and **thrombolytics** may ↑ risk of bleeding. May ↓ the effectiveness of **contraceptive drugs** and **cyclosporine**. May ↓ plasma concentrations of **saquinavir**, **nevirapine**, **delavirdine**, and **efavirenz**. May ↓ **isoniazid** levels by 65%.
Natural-Natural: Herbs with anticoagulant or antiplatelet properties may increase bleeding risk when combined with garlic, including: **angelica**, **anise**, **asafoetida**, **bogbean**, **boldo**, **capsicum**, **celery**, **chamomile**, **clove**, **danshen**, **dong quai**, **fenugreek**, **feverfew**, **ginger**, **ginkgo**, ***Panax ginseng***, **horse chestnut**, **horseradish**, **licorice**, **meadowsweet**, **prickly ash**, **onion**, **papain**, **passionflower**, **poplar**, **quassia**, **red clover**, **turmeric**, **wild carrot**, **wild lettuce**, **willow**, and others.

Route/Commonly Used Doses

PO (Adults): 200–400 mg tid of standardized garlic powder extract with 1.3% allin. *Fresh garlic*—1–7 cloves per day. One clove contains approximately 4 grams of garlic.
Topical (Adults): *Tinea infections*—0.4% cream, 0.6% gel, or 1% gel applied bid x 7 days.

Availability

Capsules[OTC]; **Tablets**[OTC]; **Topical cream**; Topical gel; Fresh garlic[OTC].

NURSING IMPLICATIONS

Assessment

- Elicit from patients their usual dietary intake especially in regard to fat consumption.
- Assess patient's reason for using this herbal remedy and knowledge about hyperlipidemia.
- Ascertain the amount of garlic the patient consumes on a regular basis.

Potential Nursing Diagnoses

Deficient knowledge, related to medication regimen (Patient/Family Teaching)
Noncompliance (Patient/Family Teaching)

Implementation
- Take orally as fresh clove, capsule, or tablet.
- Do not exceed recommended dose.

Patient/Family Teaching
- Instruct patients about the need to follow a healthy diet (low in fat and high in vegetables and fruits) in conjunction with garlic. Other lipid-reducing strategies, such as exercise and smoking cessation, should also be employed.
- Inform patients that there are other more effective agents for lipid reduction available.
- Emphasize the need for follow-up exams with a healthcare professional to assess effectiveness of the regimen.
- Warn patients about the potential for bleeding and not to take this herbal remedy without notifying their health care provider if they are on other medications. Instruct patients undergoing elective surgery to stop using garlic 2 wk prior to surgery and to notify the surgeon that they are taking garlic in the event of emergent surgery.
- Notify patients that allergies may occur and to discontinue use if symptoms develop.

Evaluation
- Normalization of lipid profile.
- Prevention of cardiac disease.

ginger (*Zingiber officinale*) (jin-jer)

Other Name(s):
Calicut, cochin, gengibre, ginger root, imber, ingwerwurzel, ingwer, Jamaica ginger, jenjibre, kankyo, jiang, zingiber

Classification
Therapeutic: antianemics

Common Uses
Prevention and treatment of nausea and vomiting associated with motion sickness, loss of appetite, pregnancy, surgery, and chemotherapy. Prevention of postoperative nausea and vomiting. May be used for dyspepsia, flatulence, relief of joint pain in rheumatoid arthritis, cramping, and diarrhea. Migraine headache. Tonic (toning/strengthening agent) in gout, gas, respiratory infections, anti-inflammatory, stimulant (tones the gut, increases saliva and gastric juices, acts as anticoagulant, decreases blood cholesterol).

Action
Antiemetic effect due to increasing GI motility and transport; may act on serotonin receptors. Shown to be hypoglycemic, hypotensive, or hypertensive, and positive inotropic agent. Inhibits prostaglandins and platelets, lowers cholesterol, and improves appetite and digestion. **Therapeutic Effects:** ↓ nausea and vomiting due to motion sickness, surgery, and chemotherapy. ↓ joint pain and improvement of joint motion in rheumatoid arthritis. Antioxidant.

Pharmacokinetics
Absorption: Unknown.
Distribution: Unknown.
Metabolism and Excretion: Unknown.
Half-life: Unknown.

TIME/ACTION PROFILE

ROUTE	ONSET	PEAK	DURATION
PO	unknown	unknown	unknown

Contraindications/Precautions
Contraindicated in: Lactation (if using large amounts); Gallstones.
Use Cautiously in: Pregnancy (preliminary evidence that ginger might affect fetal sex hormones); Patients with ↑ risk of bleeding; Diabetes; Anticoagulant therapy; Cardiovascular disease.

Adverse Reactions/Side Effects
GI: minor heartburn. **Derm:** dermatitis (when used topically).

Interactions
Natural Product-Drug: May ↑ risk of bleeding when used with **anticoagulants**, **antiplatelet agents**, and **thrombolytics**. May have additive effects with **antidiabetic agents** (causing hypoglycemia) and **calcium channel blockers** (causing hypotension).
Natural-Natural: May theoretically ↑ risk of bleeding when used with other **herbs** that have anticoagulant or antiplatelet activities.

Route/Commonly Used Doses
PO (Adults): *Motion sickness*— 1000 mg dried ginger root taken 30 min–4 hr before travel or 250 mg qid. *Postoperative nausea prevention*— 1000 mg ginger taken 1 hr before induction or anesthesia. *Chemotherapy-induced nausea*— 2–4 g/day. Up to 2 g freshly powdered drug has been used as an antiemetic (not to exceed 4 g/day). *Migraine headache*— 500 mg at onset then 500 mg every 4 hrs up to 1.5–2 g/day for 3–4 days. *Osteoarthritis*— 170 mg tid or 255 mg bid of ginger extract. *Whole root rhizome*— 0.25–1 g for other illnesses. *Tea*— pour 150 mL boiling water over 0.5–1 g of ginger and strain after 5 min. *Tinture*— 0.25-3 mL.

Availability
Alone or in combination with other herbal medicinals[OTC]**; Dried powdered root**[OTC]**;**

Syrup[OTC]; Tincture[OTC]; Tablets[OTC]; Capsules (≥550 mg)[OTC]; Spice[OTC]; Tea[OTC].

NURSING IMPLICATIONS

Assessment

- Assess patient for nausea, vomiting, abdominal distention, and pain prior to and after administration of the herb when used as an antiemetic agent.
- Assess pain location, duration, intensity, and associated symptoms (photophobia, phonophobia, nausea, vomiting) during migraine attack.
- Assess pain, swelling, and range of motion in affected joints prior to and after administration when used in the treatment of arthritis.
- Assess patient for epigastric pain prior to and after administration when used as a gastroprotective agent.
- Monitor BP and heart rate in patients with cardiovascular disease including hypertension.
- ***Lab Test Considerations:*** Monitor blood glucose and coagulation panels periodically during therapy.

Potential Nursing Diagnoses

Acute pain (Indications)
Deficient knowledge, related to medication regimen (Patient/Family Teaching)

Implementation

- Administer ginger prior to situations where nausea or vomiting is anticipated (e.g., motion sickness).
- Dosage form and strengths vary with each disease state. Ensure that proper formulation and dose are administered for the indicated use.

Patient/Family Teaching

- Instruct patients receiving anticoagulants not to take this herb without the advice of health care professional (increased risk of bleeding).
- Tell patient to stop the herb immediately if palpitations occur and notify health care professional.
- Advise patient to observe for easy bruising or other signs of bleeding. If they occur, stop the herb immediately and notify health care professional.
- Warn patients with a history of gallbladder disease to use this herb only under the supervision of health care professional.
- Instruct patient to consult health care professional before taking any Rx, OTC, or other herbal products concurrently with ginger.
- Herb is meant to be used as a tonic, not for long-term use.

Evaluation

- Prevention of nausea and vomiting.
- Relief of epigastric pain.
- Improved joint mobility and relief of pain.
- Relief of migraine headache.

ginkgo (ging-ko)

Other Name(s):
Bai guo ye, fossil tree, ginkgo folium, Japanese silver apricot, kew tree, maidenhair-tree, *salisburia adiantifolia*, yinhsing

Classification
Therapeutic: antiplatelet agents, central nervous system stimulants

Common Uses

Symptomatic relief of organic brain dysfunction (dementia syndromes, short-term memory deficits, inability to concentrate, depression). Intermittent claudication. Vertigo and tinnitus of vascular origin. Improvement of peripheral circulation. Premenstrual syndrome.

Action

Improves tolerance to hypoxemia, especially in cerebral tissue. Inhibits development of cerebral edema and accelerates its regression. Improves memory, blood flow (microcirculation), compensation of disequilibrium, and rheological properties of blood. Inactivates toxic oxygen radicals. Antagonizes platelet-activating factor. Interferes with bronchoconstriction and phagocyte chemotaxis. **Therapeutic Effects:** Symptomatic relief of dementia syndromes. Inhibits arterial spasm, decreases capillary fragility and blood viscosity. Improves venous tone, relaxes vascular smooth muscle.

Pharmacokinetics

Absorption: 70–100% absorption.
Distribution: Unknown.
Metabolism and Excretion: Unknown.
Half-life: Unknown.

TIME/ACTION PROFILE

ROUTE	ONSET	PEAK	DURATION
PO	unknown	unknown	unknown

Contraindications/Precautions

Contraindicated in: Hypersensitivity; Pregnancy and lactation.
Use Cautiously in: Bleeding disorders; Children (fresh seeds have caused seizures and death); Diabetes; Epilepsy; Surgery (discontinue use 2 wk prior).

Adverse Reactions/Side Effects
CNS: CEREBRAL BLEEDING, dizziness, headache, vertigo, seizure. **CV:** palpitations. **GI:** flatulence, stomach upset. **Derm:** allergic skin reaction. **Hemat:** bleeding. **Misc:** hypersensitivity reactions.

Interactions
Natural Product-Drug: Theoretically may potentiate effects of **anticoagulants**, **thrombolytics**, **antiplatelet agents**, and **MAO inhibitors**. May also ↑ risk of bleeding with some **cephalosporins**, **valproic acid**, and **NSAIDs**. May ↓ effectiveness of **anticonvulsants**. May alter **insulin** metabolism requiring dose adjustments of antidiabetic drugs.
Natural-Natural: May ↑ risk of bleeding when used with other **herbs** with antiplatelet effects (including **angelica**, **arnica**, **chamomile**, **feverfew**, **garlic**, **ginger**, and **licorice**).

Route/Commonly Used Doses

Organic Brain Syndromes
PO (Adults): 120–240 mg ginkgo leaf extract daily in 2 or 3 doses.

Intermittent Claudication
PO (Adults): 120–240 mg ginkgo leaf extract daily in 2 or 3 doses.

Vertigo and Tinnitus
PO (Adults): 120–160 mg ginkgo leaf extract daily in 2 or 3 doses.

Cognitive Function Improvement
PO (Adults): 120–600 mg per day.

Premenstrual Syndrome
PO (Adults): 80 mg BID starting on the 16th day of the menstrual cycle until the 5th day of the next cycle.

Availability
Ginkgo leaf extract (acetone/water): 22–27% flavonoid glycosides, 5–7% terpene lactones, 2.6–3.2% bilobalide, <5 ppm of ginkgolic acids.

NURSING IMPLICATIONS

Assessment
- Exclude other treatable causes of dementia prior to instituting treatment with ginkgo.
- Assess cognitive function (memory, attention, reasoning, language, ability to perform simple tasks) periodically throughout therapy.
- Assess frequency, duration, and severity of muscle cramps (claudication) experienced by the patient prior to and periodically throughout therapy.
- Assess for headache and neurosystem changes (thromboembolism).

Potential Nursing Diagnoses
Disturbed thought process (Indications)
Acute pain (Indications)
Deficient knowledge, related to medication regimen (Patient/Family Teaching)

Implementation
- Start dose at 120 mg per day and increase as needed to minimize side effects.
- Administration for a minimum of 6–8 wk of 80 mg (tid) (not <6 wk) is required to determine response.
- May be administered without regard to food.
- Use of dried leaf preparations in the form of a tea is not recommended because of insufficient quantity of active ingredients.
- Advise patients to avoid crude ginkgo plant parts which can cause severe allergic reactions.
- Take this herb at the same time daily.
- Keep this herb out of the reach of children as seizures may occur with increased doses of ginkgo seeds.

Patient/Family Teaching
- Advise patient to observe for easy bruising and other signs of bleeding and report to health care professional if they occur.
- Caution patient to keep this herb out of the reach of children because ingestion has been associated with seizures.
- Warn patient to avoid handling the pulp or seed coats because of the risk of contact dermatitis. Wash skin under free-flowing water promptly if contact does occur.
- Instruct patient not to exceed recommended doses because large doses may result in toxicity (restlessness, diarrhea, nausea and vomiting, headache).
- Notify patients receiving anticoagulant or antiplatelet therapy not to take this medication without approval of health care professional and frequent monitoring.
- Instruct patient to consult health care professional before taking any prescription or OTC medications concurrently with ginkgo.

Evaluation
- Improvement in walking distances pain-free.
- Improvement in tinnitus and vertigo.
- Improvement in short-term memory, attention span, and ability to perform simple tasks.
- Improvement in sexual function.
- Decreased symptoms of premenstrual syndrome.

ginseng (*Panax ginseng*)
(jin-seng)

Other Name(s):
Asian ginseng, Chinese ginseng, hong shen, Japanese ginseng, Korean ginseng, red ginseng, renshen, white ginseng

Classification
Therapeutic: none assigned

Common Uses
Improving physical and mental stamina. General tonic to energize during times of fatigue and inability to concentrate. Sedative, sleep aid, antidepressant. Diabetes. Enhanced sexual performance/aphrodisiac. Increased longevity. Adjunctive treatment of cancer. Increased immune response. Increased appetite.

Action
Main active ingredient is ginsenoside from the dried root. Serves as CNS stimulant and depressant. Enhances immune function. Interferes with platelet aggregation and coagulation. Has analgesic, anti-inflammatory, and estrogen-like effects. **Therapeutic Effects:** Improves mental and physical ability. May improve appetite, memory, sleep pattern. May reduce fasting blood glucose level in diabetic patients.

Pharmacokinetics
Absorption: Unknown.
Distribution: Unknown.
Metabolism and Excretion: Unknown.
Half-life: Unknown.

TIME/ACTION PROFILE

ROUTE	ONSET	PEAK	DURATION
PO	unknown	unknown	unknown

Contraindications/Precautions
Contraindicated in: Pregnancy (androgenization of fetus); Lactation; Children; Manic-depressive disorders and psychosis; Hypertension; Asthma; Infection; Organ transplant recipients (can interfere with immunosuppressive therapy); Hormone-sensitive cancers.
Use Cautiously in: Autoimmune diseases; Cardiovascular disease; Diabetics (may have hypoglycemic effects); Patients receiving anticoagulants; Bleeding disorders; Schizophrenia (may cause agitation).

Adverse Reactions/Side Effects
CNS: agitation, depression, dizziness, euphoria, headaches, insomnia, nervousness. **CV:** hypertension, tachycardia. **GI:** diarrhea. **GU:** amenorrhea, vaginal bleeding. **Derm:** skin eruptions. **Endo:** estrogen-like effects. **Misc:** fever, mastalgia, STEVENS-JOHNSON SYNDROME.

Interactions
Natural Product-Drug: May ↓ anticoagulant activity of **warfarin**. May interfere with **MAO inhibitors** treatment and cause headache, tremulousness, and manic episodes. May enhance blood glucose lowering effects of **oral hypoglycemics** and **insulin**. May interfere with **immunosuppressant** therapy. Use with caution when taking **estrogens**.
Natural-Natural: May ↑ risk of bleeding when used with **herbs** that have antiplatelet or anticoagulant activities. May prolong the QT interval when used with **bitter orange**, **country mallow**, and **ephedra** and ↑ risk of life-threatening arrhythmias. May ↑ risk of hypoglycemia when used with herbs with hypoglycemic potential.
Natural-Food: May potentiate effects of **caffeine** in **coffee** or **tea** and CNS stimulant effects of **mate**.

Route/Commonly Used Doses
PO (Adults): *Capsule*—200–600 mg/day; *extract*—100–300 mg 3 times daily; *crude root*—1–2g/day; *infusion—tea*—1–2g root daily (1/2 tbsp/cup water) up to 3 times daily (*P. ginseng* tea bag usually contains 1500 mg of ginseng root). Do not use for longer than 3 mo. *Cold/flu prevention*—100 mg daily 4 wk prior to influenza vaccination and continued for 8 wk; *Chronic bronchitis*—100 mg BID for 9 days combined with antibiotic therapy; *Erectile dysfunction*—900 mg TID; *Type 2 diabetes*—200 mg daily.

Availability (generic available)
Root powder[OTC]**; Extract in alcohol**[OTC]**; Capsules**[OTC]**; Tea bags**[OTC]**.**

NURSING IMPLICATIONS

Assessment
- Assess level of energy, attention span, and fatigue person is experiencing prior to initiating and periodically during therapy.
- Assess appetite; sleep duration; and perceived quality, emotional lability, and work efficiency prior to and during therapy.
- Patients with chronic medical problems should not use this herb without the advice of health care professional.
- Assess for ginseng toxicity (nervousness, insomnia, palpitations, and diarrhea).
- Monitor patients with diabetes more frequently for hypoglycemia until response to the agent is ascertained.
- Assess for the development of ginseng abuse syndrome (occurs when large doses of the herb are

*CAPITALS indicates life-threatening; underlines indicate most frequent.

taken concomitantly with other psychomotor stimulants such as coffee and tea. May present as diarrhea, hypertension, restlessness, insomnia, skin eruptions, depression, appetite suppression, euphoria, and edema).

Potential Nursing Diagnoses

Energy field disturbance (Indications)
Insomnia (Indications)

Implementation

- May be taken without regard to food.
- Take at the same time daily and do not increase dose above the recommended amount because of potential toxic effects.

Patient/Family Teaching

- Warn patients with cardiovascular disease, hypertension or hypotension, or on steroid therapy to avoid the use of this herb.
- Caution pregnant or breast-feeding women not to use this herb.
- Instruct patient in the symptoms of ginseng toxicity and to reduce dose or stop use of the herb if they occur.
- Inform patient to limit the amount of caffeine consumed.
- Advise patients with diabetes to monitor blood sugar levels until response to this agent is known.
- Inform patient that the recommended course of therapy is 3 wk. A repeated course is feasible. Do not use for longer than 3 mo.
- Teach patient about the signs and symptoms of hepatitis (yellow skin or whites of eyes, dark urine, light-colored stools, lack of appetite for several days or longer, nausea, abdominal pain) and to stop use of the herb and promptly contact health care professional if they occur. (This herb is hepatoprotectant at low doses, but hepatodestructive at high doses.).
- Caution patient not to exceed recommended doses because of potential side effects and toxicity.
- If diarrhea develops, stop herb.
- Instruct patient to consult health care professional before taking any Rx or OTC medications concurrently with ginseng.

Evaluation

- Improved energy level and sense of well-being.
- Improved quality of sleep.
- Improved concentration and work efficiency.
- Improved appetite.
- May need to take for several weeks before seeing results.

glucosamine
(glew-**kos**-ah-meen)

Other Name(s):
2-amino-2-deoxyglucose sulfate, chitosamine

Classification
Therapeutic: antirheumatics

Common Uses

Osteoarthritis. Temporomandibular joint (TMJ) arthritis. Glaucoma.

Action

May stop or slow osteoarthritis progression by stimulating cartilage and synovial tissue metabolism.
Therapeutic Effects: Decreased pain and improved joint function.

Pharmacokinetics

Absorption: 0.9% absorbed.
Distribution: Unknown.
Metabolism and Excretion: 74% eliminated via first-pass metabolism.
Half-life: Unknown.

TIME/ACTION PROFILE

ROUTE	ONSET	PEAK	DURATION
PO	unknown	unknown	unknown

Contraindications/Precautions

Contraindicated in: Shellfish allergy (glucosamine is often derived from marine exoskeletons); Pregnancy and lactation.
Use Cautiously in: Diabetes (may worsen glycemic control); Asthma (may exacerbate symptoms).

Adverse Reactions/Side Effects

GI: nausea, heartburn, diarrhea, constipation. **CNS:** headache, drowsiness. **Derm:** skin reactions.

Interactions

Natural Product-Drug: May antagonize the effects of **antidiabetics**. May induce resistance to some chemotherapy drugs such as **etoposide**, **teniposide**, and **doxorubicin**.
Natural-Natural: None known.

Route/Commonly Used Doses

PO (Adults): 500 mg three times daily.
Topical (Adults): Use cream as needed for up to 8 wk.

Availability

Tablets[OTC]; **Capsules**[OTC]; **Topical cream:** 30 mg/g in combination with other ingredients[OTC].

NURSING IMPLICATIONS

Assessment

- Evaluate for shellfish allergy prior to initiating therapy.
- Monitor pain (type, location, and intensity) and range of motion on an ongoing basis as an indicator of drug efficacy.
- Assess glucose levels via home-monitoring device for patients with diabetes until response is ascertained.
- Evaluate gastric discomfort and instruct patient to seek out the advice of a health care provider if persistent gastric discomfort occurs.
- Assess bowel function and symptomatically treat constipation with improved fluid intake and bulk in diet and bulk laxatives if necessary.

Potential Nursing Diagnoses

Acute pain (Indications)
Impaired physical mobility (Indications)

Implementation

- Take prior to meals.

Patient/Family Teaching

- Warn patients with a shellfish allergy that this herbal supplement should not be used.
- Instruct patients that the effects of this drug come from stimulating cartilage and synovial tissue metabolism and that the supplement must be taken on a regular basis to achieve benefit. It should not be used as an intermittent pain medication.
- Contact a health care provider if gastric discomfort develops and persists.
- Caution diabetics to monitor glucose values to ascertain impact on glycemic control.

Evaluation

- Improvement in pain and range of motion.

grape seed extract

(grayp seed **ex**-trakt)

Other Name(s):
Vitis vinifera, Vitis coignetiae, Oligomeric Proanthocyanidins (OPCs)

Classification
Therapeutic: cardioprotective agents

Common Uses

Chronic venous insufficiency, edema, diabetic retinopathy, varicose veins, cancer prevention, atherosclerosis, cirrhosis, prevention of collagen breakdown, vision problems, constipation, antioxidant, wound healing.

Action

Grape flavonoids have a wide range of effects including antioxidant, vasodilatory, antiplatelet, decreased superoxide production, free-radical removal, and inhibition of collagenase. **Therapeutic Effects:** Reduced risk of coronary disease. Decreased skin and vasculature breakdown.

Pharmacokinetics

Absorption: unknown.
Distribution: unknown.
Metabolism and Excretion: unknown.
Half-life: unknown.

TIME/ACTION PROFILE

	ONSET	PEAK	DURATION
PO	Unknown	Unknown	Unknown

Contraindications/Precautions

Contraindicated in: Hypersensitivity or allergy to grape seed extract; Patients with bleeding disorders or receiving anticoagulant therapy.
Use Cautiously in: OB: Avoid use in pregnancy due to lack of safety data.

Adverse Reactions/Side Effects

CV: hypertension. **CNS:** dizziness, headache. **Derm:** dry skin. **EENT:** sore throat, cough. **GI:** nausea, diarrhea. **Hemat:** ↑ risk of bleeding.

Interactions

Natural Product-Drug: May ↑ anticoagulant effects of **warfarin**. May ↓ plasma levels of CYP1A2 substrates.
Natural-Natural: May inhibit the growth of **lactobacillus acidophilus**. May ↑ BP in hypertensive patients also taking**vitamin c**.

Route/Commonly Used Doses

PO (Adults): 75–300 mg daily.

Availability

Tablets; Capsules.

NURSING IMPLICATIONS

Assessment

- Monitor BP periodically during therapy.
- ***Lab Test Considerations:*** Monitor serum cholesterol levels periodically during therapy.

Potential Nursing Diagnoses

Activity intolerance (Indications)

Implementation

- Administer as directed. Doses may vary.

Patient/Family Teaching

- Advise patient not to take grape seed extract with vitamin C; may cause increase in BP.
- Advise female patients to notify health care professional if pregnancy is planned or suspected.

Evaluation
- Decrease in cholesterol.
- Decrease in BP.

green tea (green tee)

Other Name(s):
Camellia sinensis

Classification
Therapeutic: central nervous system stimulants

Common Uses
Bladder, esophageal, ovarian, and pancreatic cancer risk reduction, mental alertness, hypotension, cervical dysplasia associated with human papillomavirus infection, hyperlipidemia, weight loss, protection of the skin from sun damage, genital warts, dental caries, Parkinson's disease.

Action
Caffeine in green tea stimulates the CNS and cardiovascular system through adenosine receptor blockade and phosphodiesterase inhibition. **Therapeutic Effects:** Improved cognitive performance and mental alertness.

Pharmacokinetics
Absorption: Unknown.
Distribution: Unknown.
Metabolism and Excretion: Unknown.
Half-life: Unknown.

TIME/ACTION PROFILE

ROUTE	ONSET	PEAK	DURATION
PO	Unknown	Unknown	Unknown

Contraindications/Precautions
Contraindicated in: Allergy/hypersensitivity; Pregnancy and lactation (doses >200 m g/day due to caffeine content).
Use Cautiously in: Patients with caffeine sensitivity. Long-term use of doses >250 m g/day may produce tolerance, psychological dependence, tachyarrhythmias, and sleep disturbances; Iron deficiency anemia (may worsen); Diabetes (may impair glucose control); Cardiac conditions (may induce arrhythmias in sensitive individuals); Bleeding disorders.

Adverse Reactions/Side Effects
CV: arrhythmia, tachycardia. **CNS:** agitation, dizziness, excitement, insomnia, tremors. **GI:** nausea, vomiting, diarrhea, hepatotoxicity, abdominal pain. **F and E:** hypokalemia. **Endo:** hyperglycemia. **Hemat:** prolonged bleeding time.

Interactions
Natural Product-Drug: Green tea may ↓ effects of **adenosine**. ↑ risk of bleeding with **anticoagulants** or **antiplatelet** agents. ↑ effects of **CNS stimulants**. May impair glucose control from **antidiabetic** agents. Abrupt withdrawal can ↑ **lithium** levels. May ↓ **dipyridamole**—induced vasodilation. **Verapamil** can ↑ caffeine concentrations by 25%. Additive effects with **methylxanthines**. **Natural-Natural:** ↑ risk of adverse cardiovascular effects with **bitter orange**. ↑ risk of hepatotoxicity with hepatotoxic herbs or supplements. ↑ risk of seizures, hypertension, or stroke with **ephedra** and **creatine**.

Route/Commonly Used Doses
PO (Adults): Range: 1–10 cups/day. One cup provides approximately 60 mg of caffeine.

Availability
Tea leaves.

NURSING IMPLICATIONS

Assessment
- Monitor BP and heart rate periodically during therapy.
- ***Lab Test Considerations:*** Monitor serum glucose, homocysteine, and uric acid levels periodically during therapy.
- Monitor liver and kidney function periodically during therapy.

Potential Nursing Diagnoses
Impaired memory (Indications)

Implementation
- May be taken as tea or as an extract in capsules.

Patient/Family Teaching
- Advise women who may be pregnant or who are breast feeding to limit green tea due to the caffeine content.

Evaluation
- Improvement in memory.

hawthorne (Crataegus Species) (haw-thorn)

Other Name(s):
aubepine, cum flore, hagedorn, maybush, whitehorn

Classification
Therapeutic: antihypertensives, inotropics

Common Uses
Hypertension. Mild to moderate HF. Angina. Spasmolytic. Sedative.

Action
Active compounds in hawthorne include flavonoids and procyanidins. Increase coronary blood flow.

Positive inotropic and chronotropic effects because of increased permeability to calcium and inhibition of phosphodiesterase. **Therapeutic Effects:** Increased cardiac output. Decreased BP, myocardial workload, and oxygen consumption.

Pharmacokinetics

Absorption: Unknown.
Distribution: Unknown.
Metabolism and Excretion: Unknown.
Half-life: Unknown.

TIME/ACTION PROFILE

ROUTE	ONSET	PEAK	DURATION
PO	unknown	6–8 wk	unknown

Contraindications/Precautions

Contraindicated in: Pregnancy (potential uterine activity); Lactation.
Use Cautiously in: Concurrent use with ACE inhibitors and digoxin; Do not discontinue use abruptly.

Adverse Reactions/Side Effects

CNS: agitation, dizziness, fatigue, vertigo, headache, sedation (high dose), sleeplessness, sweating. **CV:** hypotension (high dose), palpitations. **Derm:** rash. **GI:** nausea.

Interactions

Natural Product-Drug: May potentiate effects of **digoxin**, **calcium channel blockers**, and **beta blockers**. Concurrent use with **phosphodiesterase-5 inhibitors (sildenafil, tadalafil, vardenafil)** and **nitrates** may potentiate vasodilatory effects. May cause additive CNS depression when used with other **CNS depressants**.
Natural-Natural: Additive effect with other cardiac glycoside–containing **herbs (digitalis leaf, black hellebore, oleander leaf**, and others). Additive hypotensive effects with herbs than lower BP such as **ginger**, ***Panax ginseng***, **coenzyme Q-10** and **valerian**. Additive effect with other cardioactive herbs **(devil's claw, fenugreek**, and others).

Route/Commonly Used Doses

PO (Adults): *Heart failure*— 160–1800 mg standardized hawthorne leaf with flower extract in 2–3 divided doses daily. *Hawthorne fluid extract (1:1 in 25% alcohol)*—0.5–1 mL tid; *hawthorne fruit tincture (1:5 in 45% alcohol)*—1–2 mL tid; *dried hawthorne berries*—300–1000 mg tid.

Availability (generic available)

Dried fruit[OTC]; Liquid extract of the fruit or leaf[OTC]; Tincture of the fruit or leaf[OTC].

NURSING IMPLICATIONS

Assessment

- Monitor intake and output rations and daily weight. Assess for peripheral edema, auscultate lungs for rales and crackles during therapy.
- Assess BP and pulse periodically during therapy.

Potential Nursing Diagnoses

Decreased cardiac output (Indications)
Deficient knowledge, related to medication regimen (Patient/Family Teaching)

Implementation

- Administered as 2–3 divided doses daily at the same time.
- May be taken without regard to food.

Patient/Family Teaching

- Advise patients that there are other proven therapies available for treatment of heart failure. These therapies should be employed prior to initiating treatment with hawthorne.
- Tell patient not to take hawthorne without the advice of health care professional.
- Instruct patients in the symptoms of a heart attack (pain in the region of the heart, jaw, arm, or upper abdomen; sweating; chest tightness) and heart failure (shortness of breath, chest tightness, dizziness, sweating) and to promptly contact health care professional if they occur.
- Advise patient to report weight gain or persistent swelling of the feet to health care professional.
- May cause dizziness and fatigue. Patients should avoid driving or other activities that require mental alertness until response to herb is known.
- Avoid alcohol and other CNS depressants while taking hawthorne without consulting health care professional.
- Profuse sweating and dehydration under extreme heat may increase the BP-lowering properties of hawthorne, leading to severe hypotension. Warn patients to avoid exertion in hot weather to minimize the risk of side effects.
- Instruct patients that hawthorne helps control the symptoms of heart failure but does not cure the disease. Lifestyle changes (salt restriction, weight management, exercise as tolerated, adherence to medication regimens) still need to be followed.
- Instruct patient to consult health care professional before taking Rx, OTC, or other herbal products concurrently with hawthorne.
- Advise female patients to use contraception during therapy and to notify health care professional if pregnancy is planned or suspected or if breast feeding.

Evaluation

- Decrease in symptoms of HF. Effects may not be seen for 6 wks.
- Improved cardiac output as evidenced by improved activity tolerance.

Hypericum perforatum, see **St. John's wort**

kava-kava (*Piper methysticum*) (ka-va ka-va)

Other Name(s):

Ava pepper, intoxicating pepper, kao, kew, tonga, wurzelstock, yagona

Classification

Therapeutic: antianxiety agents, sedative/hypnotics

Common Uses

Anxiety, stress, restlessness, insomnia, benzodiazepine withdrawal. Mild muscle aches and pains. Menstrual cramps and PMS.

Action

Alters the limbic system modulation of emotional processes. Shown to have centrally acting skeletal muscle relaxant properties activated. **Therapeutic Effects:** Relief of anxiety. Sedation.

Pharmacokinetics

Absorption: Peak plasma level occurs about 1.8 hr after an oral dose.
Distribution: Enters breast milk.
Metabolism and Excretion: Elimination occurs primarily by renal excretion (both unchanged and metabolites) and in the feces. Metabolized by the liver (reduction or demethylation).
Half-life: Approximately 9 hr.

TIME/ACTION PROFILE

ROUTE	ONSET	PEAK	DURATION
PO	1.8 hr	unknown	8 hr

Contraindications/Precautions

Contraindicated in: Pregnancy (may affect uterine tone) and lactation; Patients with endogenous depression (may ↑ risk of suicide); Children under 12 yr of age; Hepatitis or other liver disease.
Use Cautiously in: Concurrent use of other hepatotoxic agents; Depression and Parkinson's disease (may worsen symptoms); Should not be used for >3 mo to prevent psychological addiction.

Adverse Reactions/Side Effects

CNS: dizziness, headache, drowsiness, sensory disturbances, extrapyramidal effects. **EENT:** Pupil dilation, red eyes, visual accommodation disorders. **GI:** HEPATIC TOXICITY, gastrointestinal complaints. **Derm:** allergic skin reactions, yellow discoloration of skin, pellagroid dermopathy. **Hemat:** decreased lymphocytes, decreased platelets. **Metab:** weight loss (long term, high dose). **Neuro:** ataxia, muscle weakness.

Interactions

Natural Product-Drug: Additive effect when used with **alprazolam**. Potentiates effect of **CNS depressants** (**ethanol**, **barbiturates**, **benzodiazepines**, **opioid analgesics**). Has ↓ effectiveness of **levodopa** in few cases. May have additive effects with **antiplatelet agents**. May ↑ risk of liver damage with other **hepatotoxic agents**.
Natural-Natural: Concurrent use with other hepatotoxic products such as **DHEA**, **coenzyme Q-10** (high doses), and **niacin** can ↑ risk of liver damage. May have additive sedative effects when used with other **herbs** with sedative properties.

Route/Commonly Used Doses

PO (Adults): *Antianxiety*— 100 mg (70 mg kavalactones) 3 times daily; *Benzodiazepine withdrawal*— 50–300 mg/day over 1 wk while tapering benzodiazepine over 2 wk (use 70% kavalactone extract). *Insomnia*— 180–210 mg kavalactones. Typically taken as a tea by simmering the root in boiling water and then straining.

Availability (generic available)

Dried root extracts (alcohol or acetone based) containing 30–70% kavapyrones.

NURSING IMPLICATIONS

Assessment

- Assess muscle spasm, associated pain, and limitations of movement prior to and periodically during therapy.
- Assess degree of anxiety and level of sedation (visual disturbances and changes in motor reflexes are side effects) prior to and periodically during therapy.
- Assess sleep patterns and level of sedation upon arising.
- Prolonged use may lead to ↓ of platelet and lymphocyte counts and ↑ liver function tests.

Potential Nursing Diagnoses

Anxiety (Indications)
Impaired physical mobility (Adverse Reactions)
Risk for injury (Side Effects)

Implementation

- Prepared as a drink from pulverized roots, tablets, capsules, or extract.

Patient/Family Teaching

- Inform patient that significant, serious side effects may occur with prolonged use. Use for longer than 1 mo is not recommended without supervision of health care professional.
- Caution patient to avoid alcohol or other CNS depressants while taking this herb; may increase sedative effect.
- May cause drowsiness. Caution patient to avoid driving or other activities requiring alertness until response to herb is known.
- Warn patients to stop use of the herb immediately if shortness of breath or signs of liver disease (yellowing of the skin or whites of the eyes, brown urine, nausea, vomiting, light-colored stools, unusual tiredness, weakness, stomach or abdominal pain, loss of appetite) occur and contact health care professional.
- Advise patients who have liver disease or liver problems, or persons who are taking drug products that can affect the liver, to consult health care professional before using kava-containing supplements.
- Inform patient that although there is no evidence of physiological dependence, the risk of psychological dependence still exists.
- Advise female patients to use contraception during therapy and to notify health care professional immediately if pregnancy is planned or suspected or if breast feeding.
- Instruct patient to consult health care professional before taking any Rx, OTC, or other herbal products concurrently with kava-kava.
- Kava has been banned in other countries due to hepatotoxicity.

Evaluation

- Decrease in anxiety level.
- Decrease in muscle spasms.
- Relief of insomnia.

milk thistle (milk this-ul)

Other Name(s):
Holy thistle, Lady's thistle, Mary Thistle, Silybin, Silymarin

Classification
Therapeutic: antidotes

Common Uses

Cirrhosis, chronic hepatitis, gallstones, psoriasis, liver cleansing and detoxification, treatment of liver toxicity due to Amanita mushroom poisoning (European IV formulation), and chemicals. Dyspepsia (in combination with other herbs). Diabetes.

Action

The active component, silymarin, has antioxidant and hepatoprotectant actions. Silymarin helps prevent toxin penetration and stimulates hepatocyte regeneration. **Therapeutic Effects:** Liver detoxification. Improved dyspepsia symptoms. Decreased fasting blood glucose.

Pharmacokinetics

Absorption: 23–47% absorbed after oral administration.
Distribution: Unknown.
Metabolism and Excretion: Hepatic metabolism by cytochrome P450 3A4.
Half-life: 6 hr.

TIME/ACTION PROFILE

ROUTE	ONSET	PEAK	DURATION
PO	5–30 days or more	unknown	unknown

Contraindications/Precautions

Contraindicated in: Pregnancy and lactation (insufficient information available); Allergy to chamomile, ragweed, asters, chrysanthemums, and other members of the family *Asteraceae/Compositae*.
Use Cautiously in: Hormone sensitive cancers/conditions (milk thistle plant parts may have estrogenic effects).

Adverse Reactions/Side Effects

GI: Laxative effect, nausea, bloating, anorexia. **Misc:** Allergic reactions.

Interactions

Natural Product-Drug: In vitro, milk thistle extract inhibited the drug-metabolizing enzyme **cytochrome P450 3A4**. Interactions have not been reported in humans, but milk thistle should be used cautiously with other drugs metabolized by 3A4, such as **cyclosporine**, **carbamazepine**, **HMG-CoA inhibitors**, **ketoconazole**, and **alprazolam**.
Natural-Natural: None known.

Route/Commonly Used Doses

PO (Adults): *Hepatic cirrhosis*—420 mg/day of extract containing 70–80% silymarin; *Chronic active hepatitis*—240 mg bid of silibinin; *Diabetes*—200 mg tid of silymarin; *Tea*—3–4 times daily 30 minutes before meals. Tea is not recommended as silymarin is not sufficiently water soluble.
IV (Adults): 20–50 mg/kg over 24 hr, 48 hr post mushroom ingestion (IV formulation not available in US).

Availability

Capsules^{OTC}; Tablets^{OTC}; Crude drug^{OTC}; Tea^{OTC}; Extract^{OTC}.

NURSING IMPLICATIONS

Assessment

- Assess patients for signs of liver failure (jaundice, mental status changes, abdominal distention, ascites, generalized edema).
- Evaluate consistency and frequency of bowel movements.
- ***Lab Test Considerations:*** Monitor liver function, lipid profile, and blood glucose periodically during therapy.

Potential Nursing Diagnoses

Deficient knowledge, related to medication regimen (Patient/Family Teaching)

Implementation

- Orally as an extract, capsule, tablets, or as a dried fruit as a single daily dose or divided into three doses.
- Tea is not recommended as milk thistle is not water-soluble.

Patient/Family Teaching

- Inform patient of the symptoms of liver failure; advise patient to report worsening symptomotolgy promptly to health care professional.
- Emphasize the need for blood tests to monitor liver function tests.
- Advise patients to avoid alcohol and follow diet for liver or gall bladder disease being treated.

Evaluation

- Normalization of liver function tests.
- Reduction in jaundice, abdominal distention, fatigue and other symptoms associated with liver disease.

Panax ginseng, see **ginseng**.

Piper methysticum, see **kava-kava**.

SAMe (sam-ee)

Other Name(s):
Ademetionine, S-adenosylmethionine,

Classification
Therapeutic: antidepressants

Pregnancy Category UK

Common Uses

Treatment of depression. Has also been used to manage: osteoarthritis, fibromyalgia, liver disease, migraine headaches.

Action

May aid in the production, activation, and metabolism of various amines, phospholipids, hormones, and neurotransmitters. May stimulate articular cartilage growth and repair. **Therapeutic Effects:** Decreased depression. Anti-inflammatory and analgesic effects improve symptoms of osteoarthritis.

Pharmacokinetics

Absorption: Rapidly and extensively metabolized following oral administration.
Distribution: Unknown.
Metabolism and Excretion: Actively metabolized by the liver.
Half-life: 100 min.

TIME/ACTION PROFILE (antidepressant action)

ROUTE	ONSET	PEAK	DURATION
PO (depression)	1–2 wk	unknown	unknown
PO (osteoarthritis)	30 days	unknown	unknown

Contraindications/Precautions

Contraindicated in: Hypersensitivity; Bipolar disorder.
Use Cautiously in: Pregnancy, lactation, or children (safety not established); Bipolar disorder (can induce mania); Parkinson's disease (may worsen symptoms); Surgery (discontinue 2 wk prior to elective procedures).

Adverse Reactions/Side Effects

CNS: agitation, dizziness, mild insomnia, manic reactions (in patients with bipolar disorder). **GI:** vomiting, diarrhea, flatulence.

Interactions

Natural Product-Drug: Avoid use with **antidepressants**, **meperidine**, **pentazocine**, **tramadol**, and **dextromethorphan** (additive serotinergic effects may occur). May ↓ effectiveness of **levodopa** and worsen Parkinsonian symptoms. Should not be used concurrently with **MAO inhibitors**. Avoid use of SAMe within 2 wk of using a **MAO inhibitor**.
Natural-Natural: Avoid use with natural products that increase serotonin levels such as **l-tryptophan** and **St. John's wort**.

Route/Commonly Used Doses

PO (Adults): *Depression*— 200 mg once or twice daily, adjusted upward over 2 wk (range 400–1600 mg/day); *Liver disorders*— 1200–1600 mg/day;

Osteoarthritis—200 mg tid; *Fibromyalgia*—800 mg/day.

Availability

Tablets: 100 mg, 200 mg, 400 mg[OTC].

NURSING IMPLICATIONS

Assessment

- Assess mental status for symptoms of depression prior to and periodically during therapy; advise patients with depression to be evaluated by a health care professional.
- Assess symptoms of pain and fatigue prior to and periodically during therapy.

Potential Nursing Diagnoses

Ineffective coping (Indications)
Deficient knowledge, related to medication regimen (Patient/Family Teaching)

Implementation

- **PO:** Administer on an empty stomach. Initial dose should be 200 mg once or twice daily to minimize GI disturbances. Dose may be adjusted upward over 1–2 wk depending on response and tolerance.

Patient/Family Teaching

- Instruct patient to take SAMe as directed.
- Advise patients to discontinue 2 wk prior to elective surgical procedures.
- Advise women to consult health care professional if pregnancy is planned or suspected or if breast feeding.

Evaluation

- Decrease in symptoms of depression.
- Improvement in osteoarthritis symptoms.

saw palmetto
(saw pal-**met**-toe)

Other Name(s):
American Dwarf Palm Tree, Cabbage Palm, Ju-Zhong, Palmier Nain, Sabal, Sabal Fructus, Saw Palmetto Berry, *Serenoa repens*

Classification
Therapeutic: benign prostatic hyperplasia (BPH) agents

Common Uses

Benign prostatic hyperplasia.

Action

Exerts antiandrogenic, anti-inflammatory, and antiproliferative properties in prostate tissue resulting in improvement in BPH symptoms such as frequent urination, hesitancy, urgency, and nocturia. Comparable in efficacy to finasteride but may be less effective than prazosin. **Therapeutic Effects:** Decreased urinary symptoms of BPH.

Pharmacokinetics

Absorption: Unknown.
Distribution: Unknown.
Metabolism and Excretion: Unknown.
Half-life: Unknown.

TIME/ACTION PROFILE

ROUTE	ONSET	PEAK	DURATION
PO	1–2 mo	unknown	48 wk (longest studied treatment duration)

Contraindications/Precautions

Contraindicated in: Pregnancy and lactation.
Use Cautiously in: Prior to surgery (discontinue 2 wk before to prevent bleeding).

Adverse Reactions/Side Effects

CNS: dizziness, headache. **GI:** nausea, vomiting, constipation, and diarrhea.

Interactions

Natural Product-Drug: Hormonal action may interfere with other hormonal therapies (**testosterone**, **hormonal contraceptives**). Avoid use with **antiplatelet** or **anticoagulant drugs** (may ↑ bleeding risk).
Natural-Natural: Concomitant use with herbs that affect platelet aggregation such as **ginger**, **garlic**, **gingko**, and **ginseng** may ↑ bleeding risk.

Route/Commonly Used Doses

PO (Adults): *Lipophilic extract (80–90% fatty acids)*—160 mg twice daily or 320 mg once daliy. *Whole berries*—1–2 grams daily. *Liquid extract from berry pulp*—1–2 mL three times daily. *Tea (efficacy is questionable due to lipophilicity of active constituents)*—1 cup three times daily. Tea is prepared by steeping 0.5–1 gram dried berry in 150 mL boiling water for 5–10 minutes.

Availability

Lipophilic extract (80-90% fatty acids)[OTC]; Whole berries[OTC]; Liquid extract[OTC].

NURSING IMPLICATIONS

Assessment

- Assess patient for symptoms of benign prostatic hypertrophy (BPH) (urinary hesitancy, feeling of incomplete bladder emptying, interruption in urinary stream, impairment in size and force of urinary stream, terminal urinary dribbling, straining to start flow, dysuria, urgency) before and periodically during therapy.

- Rectal exams prior to and periodically throughout therapy to assess prostate size are recommended.

Potential Nursing Diagnoses

Impaired urinary elimination (Indications)
Deficient knowledge, related to medication regimen (Patient/Family Teaching)

Implementation

- Take on a full stomach to minimize GI effects.

Patient/Family Teaching

- Advise patients to start therapy with this herbal supplement only after evaluation by a health care professional who will provide continued follow-up care.
- Inform patients that saw palmetto does not alter the size of the prostate but still should relieve the symptoms associated with BPH.
- Tell patients that taking this herbal supplement with food should reduce the GI effects and make it easier to tolerate.

Evaluation

- Decrease in urinary symptoms of BPH.

St. John's wort (*Hypericum perforatum*)

(saynt **jonz** wort)

Other Name(s):
Amber, Demon chaser, Goatweed, Hardhay, Klamath weed, Rosin rose, Tipton weed

Classification
Therapeutic: antidepressants

Common Uses

PO: Management of mild to moderate depression and obsessive compulsive disorder (OCD). (Not effective for major depression.). **Topical:** Inflammation of the skin, blunt injury, wounds, and burns. Other uses are for capillary strengthening, decreasing uterine bleeding, and reducing tumor size.

Action

Derived from *Hypericum perforatum*; the active component is *hypericin*. **PO:** Antidepressant action my be due to ability to inhibit reuptake of serotonin and other neurotransmitters. **Topical:** Anti-inflammatory, antifungal, antiviral, and antibacterial properties. **Therapeutic Effects: PO:** Decreased signs and symptoms of depression. **Topical:** Decreased inflammation of burns or other wounds.

Pharmacokinetics

Absorption: Unknown.
Distribution: Unknown.
Metabolism and Excretion: Unknown.
Half-life: *Hypericum constituents*—24.8–26.5 hr.

TIME/ACTION PROFILE

ROUTE	ONSET	PEAK	DURATION
PO	10–14 days	within 4–6 wk	unknown

Contraindications/Precautions

Contraindicated in: Pregnancy, lactation, or children.
Use Cautiously in: History of phototoxicity; Surgery (discontinue 2 wk prior to surgical procedures); Alzheimer's disease (may induce psychosis); Patients undergoing general anesthesia (may cause cardiovascular collapse); History of suicide attempt, severe depression, schizophrenia, or bipolar disorder (can induce hypomania or psychosis).

Adverse Reactions/Side Effects

CNS: dizziness, restlessness, sleep disturbances. **CV:** hypertension. **Endo:** hypoglycemia. **GI:** abdominal pain, bloating, diarrhea, dry mouth, feeling of fullness, flatulence, nausea, vomiting. **Neuro:** neuropathy. **Derm:** allergic skin reactions (hives, itching, skin rash), phototoxicity. **Misc:** serotonin syndrome.

Interactions

Natural Product-Drug: Concurrent use with **alcohol** or other **antidepressants** (including **SSRIs** and **MAO inhibitors**) may ↑ risk of adverse CNS reactions. May ↓ the effectiveness and serum concentrations of **digoxin**, **alprazolam**, **amitriptyline**, **imatinib**, **irinotecan**, **warfarin**, and **protease inhibitors**. Use with **MAO Inhibitors**, **tramadol**, **pentazocine**, and **selective serotonin agonists** could result in serotonin syndrome. May ↓ effectiveness of **oral contraceptives**. May ↓ plasma **cyclosporine** and **tacrolimus** levels by 30–70% and cause acute transplant rejection. May ↑ metabolism of **phenytoin** and **phenobarbital** and cause loss of seizure control. Avoid use of St. John's Wort and **MAO Inhibitors** within 2 wk of each other.
Natural-Natural: May ↑ risk of serotonin syndrome when taken with **tryptophan**and **SAM-e**.

Route/Commonly Used Doses

PO (Adults): *Mild Depression*—300 mg of St. John's Wort (standardized to 0.3% hypericin) 3 times daily or 250 mg twice daily of 0.2% hypericin extract. *OCD*-450 mg twice daily of extended release preparation.
Topical (Adults): 0.2–1 mg total hypericin daily.

Availability

Preparations for Oral Use

Dried herb[OTC]; **Dried (hydroalcoholic) extract**[OTC]; **Oil**[OTC]; **Tincture**[OTC].

Preparations for Topical Application

Liquid[OTC]; **Semisolid**[OTC].

NURSING IMPLICATIONS

Assessment

- **Depression:** Assess patient for depression periodically during therapy.
- **Inflammation:** Assess skin or skin lesions periodically during therapy.

Potential Nursing Diagnoses

Ineffective coping (Indications)
Anxiety (Indications)
Deficient knowledge, related to medication regimen (Patient/Family Teaching)

Implementation

- **PO:** Tea can be prepared by mixing 2–4 dried herbs in 150 mL of boiling water and steeping for 10 min.

Patient/Family Teaching

- Instruct patient to take St. John's wort as directed.
- Patients with depression should be evaluated by health care professional. Standard therapy may be of greater benefit for moderate to severe depression.
- Advise patient to notify health care professional of medication regimen prior to treatment or surgery.
- Caution patients to avoid sun exposure and use protective sunscreen to reduce the risk of photosensitivity reactions.
- Inform patient to purchase herbs from a reputable source and that products and their contents vary among different manufacturers.
- Caution patient not to use alcohol while taking St. John's wort.
- Warn patients that St. John's Wort may reduce the therapeutic effectiveness of several drugs.
- May potentiate effect of sedatives and side effects of other antidepressants. Do not take within 2 wk of MAO Inhibitor therapy.
- Instruct patient to consult health care professional before taking other Rx, OTC, or herbal products concurrently with St. John's wort.
- Inform patient that St. John's wort is usually taken for a period of 4–6 wk. If no improvement is seen, another therapy should be considered.

Evaluation

- Decrease in signs and symptoms of depression or anxiety.
- Improvement in skin inflammation.

valerian (vuh-lare-ee-en)

Other Name(s):

Amantilla, All-Heal, Baldrian, Baldrianwurzel, Belgium Valerian, Common Valerian, Fragrant Valerian, Garden Heliotrope, Garden Valerian, Indian Valerian, Mexican Valerian, Pacific Valerian, Tagara, Valeriana, *Valeriana officinalis, Valerianae radix*, Valeriana rhizome, Valeriane

Classification

Therapeutic: antianxiety agents, sedative/hypnotics

Common Uses

Insomnia. Anxiety.

Action

May increase concentrations of the inhibitory CNS transmitter GABA. **Therapeutic Effects:** Improvement in sleep quality.

Pharmacokinetics

Absorption: Unknown.
Distribution: Unknown.
Metabolism and Excretion: Unknown.
Half-life: Unknown.

TIME/ACTION PROFILE

ROUTE	ONSET	PEAK	DURATION
PO	30–60 min	2 hr	unknown

Contraindications/Precautions

Contraindicated in: Pregnancy and lactation.
Use Cautiously in: Alcohol use (may have additive sedative effects); Surgery (discontinue use 2 wk prior to elective procedures).

Adverse Reactions/Side Effects

CNS: drowsiness, headache. **GI:** dry mouth. **Misc:** Benzodiazepine-like withdrawal symptoms with discontinuation after long-term use.

Interactions

Natural Product-Drug: Additive CNS depression with **alcohol**, **antihistamines**, **anesthetic agents**, **sedative hypnotics**, and other **CNS depressants**. Alcohol-containing preparations may interact with **disulfiram** and **metronidazole**.
Natural-Natural: Additive sedative effects can occur when used with herbal supplements with seda-

tive properties such as **kava**, **l-tryptophan**, **melatonin**, **SAMe**, and **St. John's wort**.

Route/Commonly Used Doses

PO (Adults): *Tea*—1 cup tea 1–5 times daily. Tea is made by steeping 2–3 g root in 150 mL boiling water for 5–10 min then straining. *Tincture*—1–3 mL 1–5 times daily. *Extract*—400–900 mg up to 2 hours before bedtime or 300–450 mg divided tid.

Availability

Capsules[OTC]; **Extract**[OTC]; **Tea**[OTC]; **Tincture**[OTC].

NURSING IMPLICATIONS

Assessment

- Assess degree of anxiety and level of sedation prior to and periodically throughout therapy.
- Assess sleep patterns.
- Assess response in the elderly population where drowsiness and loss of balance may pose a significant risk for injury.

Potential Nursing Diagnoses

Anxiety (Indications)
Risk for injury (Side Effects)

Implementation

- Take 1–2 hr before bedtime if used for nighttime hypnotic.
- Administer orally three to five times daily to control anxiety.

Patient/Family Teaching

- Encourage patients to avoid stimulants such as caffeine and to provide an environment that promotes restful sleep.
- May cause drowsiness. Caution patient to avoid driving or other activities requiring alertness until response to drug is known.
- Caution patient to avoid use of alcohol and other medications or herbals that have a sedative effect; may increase drowsiness.
- Advise patients to discontinue 2 wk prior to elective surgical procedures.
- Inform patients not to take this herbal supplement if pregnant or breast-feeding.
- Notify patients that dependence with withdrawal symptoms may develop with prolonged use.

Evaluation

- Decreased anxiety level.
- Improvement in sleep with a feeling of restfulness without drowsiness upon awakening.

Zingiber officinale, see **ginger**.

*CAPITALS indicates life-threatening; underlines indicate most frequent.

PEDIATRIC INTRAVENOUS MEDICATION QUICK REFERENCE CHART

Risk of fluid overload in infants and children is always a consideration when administering IV medications. The following table provides maximum concentrations—the smallest amount of fluid necessary for diluting specific medications—and the maximum rate at which the medications be given.

Drug	Maximum Concentration	Maximum Rate
acetaminophen	10 mg/ml	Give over 15 min
acetazolamide	100 mg/ml	500 mg/min[2]
acyclovir	7 mg/ml	Give over 1 hr
adenosine	3 mg/ml	Give over 1–2 sec
allopurinol	6 mg/ml	Give over 30 min
amikacin	10 mg/ml	Give over 30–60 min
aminocaproic acid	20 mg/ml	Give over 1 hr
aminophylline	25 mg/ml	25 mg/min
amphotericin B conventional	0.1 mg/ml (peripherally) 0.5 mg/ml (centrally)	Give over 2–6 hr Give over 2–6 hr
amphotericin B liposomal	2 mg/ml	Give over 2 hr
amphotericin B colloidal	0.83 mg/ml	Give over 2 hr
ampicillin	100 mg/ml	100 mg/min
ampicillin/sulbactam	30 mg/ml (ampicillin)	Give over 15–30 min
anidulafungin	0.77 mg/ml	1.1 mg/min
atropine	1 mg/ml	Give over 1 min
azithromycin	2 mg/ml	Give over 1 hr
aztreonam	20 mg/ml	Give over 20–60 min
bumetanide	0.25 mg/ml	Give over 1–2 min
caffeine citrate	20 mg/ml	Give over 10–20 min
calcitriol	2 mcg/ml	Give over 15 sec
calcium chloride	100 mg/ml	100 mg/min
calcium gluconate	100 mg/ml	100 mg/min[2]
caspofungin	0.5 mg/ml	Give over 1 hr
cefazolin	138 mg/ml (IVP) 20 mg/ml (Intermittent infusion)	Give over 3–5 min Give over 10–60 min
cefepime	160 mg/ml	Give over 30 min
cefotaxime	200 mg/ml (IVP) 60 mg/ml (Intermittent infusion)	Give over 3–5 min Give over 10–30 min
cefoxitin	200 mg/ml (IVP) 40 mg/ml (Intermittent infusion)	Give over 3–5 min Give over 10–60 min
ceftazidime	180 mg/ml (IVP) 40 mg/ml (Intermittent infusion)	Give over 3–5 min Give over 10–30 min
ceftriaxone	40 mg/ml	Give over 10–30 min
cefuroxime	100 mg/ml (IVP) 137 mg/ml (Intermittent infusion)[2]	Give over 3–5 min Give over 15–30 min
chlorothiazide	28 mg/ml	3–5 min
chlorpromazine	1 mg/ml	0.5 mg/min
ciprofloxacin	2 mg/ml	Give over 60 min
clindamycin	18 mg/ml	30 mg/min
cyclosporine	2.5 mg/ml	Give over 2–6 hr
dexamethasone	10 mg/ml	Doses ≤ 10 mg: Give over 1–4 min Doses > 10 mg: Give over 15–30 min
dexmedetomidine	4 mcg/ml	Give bolus over 5–10 min
diazepam	5 mg/ml	2 mg/min
digoxin	100 mcg/ml	Give over 5 min
diphenhydramine	25 mg/ml	25 mg/min
doxycycline	1 mg/ml	Give over 1 hr
enalaprilat	1.25 mg/ml	Give over 5 min
erythromycin	5 mg/ml	Give over 20–120 min
esomeprazole	8 mg/ml	Give over 10–30 min
ethacrynic acid	2 mg/ml	Give over 5–30 min
famotidine	4 mg/ml (IVP) 0.2 mg/ml (Intermittent infusion)	10 mg/min Give over 15–30 min
fentanyl	50 mcg/ml	Give over 1–3 min
fluconazole	2 mg/ml	Give over 1–2 hr
flumazenil	0.1 mg/ml	0.2 mg/min
foscarnet	12 mg/ml (peripherally) 24 mg/ml (centrally)	60 mg/kg/hr
fosphenytoin	25 mg/ml	3 mg/kg/min
furosemide	10 mg/ml	0.5 mg/kg/min
ganciclovir	10 mg/ml	Give over 1 hr
gentamicin	10 mg/ml	Give over 30 min
glycopyrrolate	0.2 mg/ml	20 mcg/min
granisetron	1 mg/ml (IVP) 50 mcg/ml (Intermittent infusion)	Give over 30 sec Give over 30–60 min
hydralazine	20 mg/ml	0.2 mg/kg/min
hydrocortisone sodium succinate	50 mg/ml (IVP) 5 mg/ml (Intermittent infusion)	Give over 30 sec Give over 10–30 min

PEDIATRIC INTRAVENOUS MEDICATION QUICK REFERENCE CHART

Drug	Maximum Concentration	Maximum Rate
ibuprofen	10 mg/ml	Give over 15 min
imipenem/cilastatin[2]	7 mg/ml	Give over 15–60 min
inamrinone	5 mg/ml	Give bolus over 2–3 min
indomethacin	1 mg/ml	Give over 20–30 min
kanamycin	5 mg/ml	Give over 30–60 min
ketamine	50 mg/ml (IVP) 2 mg/ml (Intermittent infusion)	0.5 mg/kg/min 0.5 mg/kg/min
ketorolac	30 mg/ml	Give over 1–5 min
labetalol	5 mg/ml (IVP)	2 mg/min
lacosamide	10 mg/ml	Give over 30–60 min
levetiracetam	15 mg/ml	Give over 5–15 min
levocarnitine	200 mg/ml	Give over 2–3 min
levothyroxine	100 mcg/ml	Give over 2–3 min
linezolid	2 mg/ml	Give over 30–120 min
lorazepam	4 mg/ml	2 mg/min or 0.05 mg/kg over 2–5 min
magnesium sulfate	200 mg/ml	10–20 min
meperidine[2]	10 mg/ml	Give over 5 min
meropenem	50 mg/ml (Intermittent infusion) 20 mg/ml (Intermittent infusion)	Give over 3–5 min Give over 15–30 min
methylprednisolone	125 mg/ml (IVP) 2.5 mg/ml (Intermittent infusion)	Give over 1–30 min Give over 20–60 min
metoclopramide	5 mg/ml	5 mg/min
metronidazole	8 mg/ml	Give over 1 hr
micafungin	1.5 mg/ml	Give over 1 hr
midazolam	5 mg/ml	Give over 20–30 sec (5 min in neonates)
milrinone	1 mg/ml	Give over 10 min
morphine[2]	5 mg/ml	Give over 5–30 min
nafcillin[2]	125 mg/ml	Give over 15–60 min
naloxone	1 mg/ml	Give over 30 sec
ondansetron	2 mg/ml	Give over 2–15 min
oxacillin	100 mg/ml (IVP) 40 mg/ml (Intermittent infusion)	Give over 10 min Give over 15–30 min
pancuronium	2 mg/ml (IVP)	Give over 3–5 seconds
pantoprazole	4 mg/ml	Give over 2–15 min
penicillin g[2]	100,000 units/ml	Give over 15–30 min
pentamidine	6 mg/ml	Give over 1–2 hr
pentobarbital	50 mg/ml	50 mg/min
phenobarbital	130 mg/ml	30 mg/min
phenytoin	10 mg/ml	1 mg/kg/min (neonates) 3 mg/kg/min (children)
phytonadione	10 mg/ml	1 mg/min
piperacillin	200 mg/ml (IVP) 20 mg/ml (Intermittent infusion)	Give over 3–5 min Give over 20–60 min
piperacillin/tazobactam	200 mg/ml	Give over 30 min
potassium chloride	80 mEq/L (peripherally) 200 mEq/L (centrally)	1 mEq/kg/hr
promethazine	25 mg/ml	25 mg/min
propranolol	1 mg/ml	1 mg/min
protamine	10 mg/ml	5 mg/min
ranitidine	2.5 mg/ml	10 mg/min
rifampin	6 mg/ml	Give over 30 min
tacrolimus	0.02 mg/ml	Give over 4–24 hr
terbutaline	1 mg/ml	Give over 5–10 min
ticarcillin/clavulanate	100 mg/ml	Give over 30 min
tobramycin	10 mg/ml	Give over 30 min
trimethoprim/sulfamethoxazole	1 ml drug per 10 ml diluent[2]	Give over 1–1.5 hr
valproate sodium	50 mg/ml	3 mg/kg/min
vancomycin	5 mg/ml	Give over 60 min
vasopressin	1 unit/ml	Give over 5–30 min
verapamil	2.5 mg/ml (IVP)	Give over 2–3 min
voriconazole	5 mg/ml	3 mg/kg/hr
zidovudine	4 mg/ml	Give over 60 min

1. Phelps SJ, Hagemann TM, Lee KR, Thompson AJ: Pediatric Injectable Drugs, 10th Edition. American Society of Health-System Pharmacists, Bethesda, MD 2013.
2. Taketomo CK, Hodding JH, Kraus DM: Pediatric and Neonatal Dosage Handbook, 20th Edition, Lexi-Comp, Hudson, OH 2013.

BEERS CRITERIA

The Beers criteria for potentially inappropriate medication use in adults 65 and older in the United States is a compilation of drugs and drug classes found to increase the risk of adverse events in older adults. Frequently, older adults are more sensitive to the medications or their side effects. These adverse events have significant economic and quality of life costs for society and individuals and can result in more frequent hospitalizations, permanent injury, or death. Often, the potential for adverse events can be minimized by prescribing safer alternatives or prescribing at the lowest effective dose. The list of medications below represents an update to the list previously published in 2012.

alprazolam (Xanax)	ketorolac
amobarbital (Amytal Sodium)	lansoprazole (Prevacid)
amiodarone (Cordarone, Pacerone)	lorazepam (Ativan)
amitriptyline	loxapine (Adasuve)
amoxapine	lurasidone (Latuda)
aripiprazole (Abilify)	meclizine
asenapine (Saphris)	meclofenamate
aspirin (>325 mg/day)	mefenamicacid (Ponstel)
atropine (Atropen)	megestrol (Megace, Megace ES)
belladonna alkaloids (Donnatal)	meloxicam (Mobic)
benztropine (Cogentin)	meperidine (Demerol)
brexipiprazole (Rexulti)	meprobamate
brompheniramine	metaxalone (Skelaxin)
butabarbital (Butisol Sodium)	methocarbamol (Robaxin)
carbinoxamine (Karbinal ER)	methyldopa
cariprazine (Vraylar)	methyldopa-hydrochlorothiazide
carisoprodol (Soma)	methyltestosterone (Android, Testred)
chlordiazepoxide (Librium)	metoclopramide (Metozolv ODT, Reglan)
chlordiazepoxide-amitriptyline	mineral oil
chlorpheniramine (Chlor-Trimeton)	nabumetone
chlorpromazine	naproxen (Aleve, Anaprox, Naprelan, Naprosyn)
chlorpropamide (Diabinese)	nifedipine (short-acting) (Procardia)
chlorzoxazone (Parafon Forte DSC)	nitrofurantoin (Furadantin, Macrobid, Microdantin)
clidinium-chlordiazepoxide (Librax)	nortriptyline (Pamelor)
clomipramine (Anafranil)	olanzapine (Zyprexa)
clonazepam (Klonopin)	olanzapine-fluoxetine (Symbyax)
clonidine (Catapres, Duraclon, Kapvay)	omeprazole
clorazepate (Tranxene)	orphenadrine
clozapine (Clozaril, FazaClo, Versacloz)	oxaprozin (Daypro)
cyclobenzaprine (Amrix, Fexmid)	oxazepam
cyproheptadine	paliperidone (Invega)
desipramine (Norpramin)	pantoprazole (Protonix)
desmopressin (DDAVP, Stimate)	paroxetine (Brisdelle, Paxil, Paxil CR, Pexeva)
dessicatedthyroid (Armour Thyroid)	pentazocine (Talwin)
dexchlorpheniramine	pentobarbital (Nembutal Sodium)
dexlansoprazole (Dexilant)	perphenazine
diazepam (Valium)	perphenazine-amitriptyline
diclofenac (Cambia, Cataflam, Dyloject, Voltaren XR, Zipsor, Zorvolex)	phenobarbital
dicyclomine (Bentyl)	pimozide (Orap)
diflunisal	piroxicam (Feldene)
digoxin (>0.125 mg/day) (Lanoxin)	prazosin (Minipress)
dimenhydrinate (Dramamine)	procainamide
diphenhydramine (Benadryl)	promethazine
dipyridamole (short-acting) (Persantine)	propafenone (Rythmol, Rythmol SR)
disopyramide (Norpace)	propantheline
dofetilide (Tikosyn)	protriptyline (Vivactil)
doxylamine	quazepam (Doral)
doxazosin (Cardura)	quetiapine (Seroquel)
doxepin (>6 mg/day) (Silenor)	quinidine
dronedarone (Multaq)	rabeprazole (Aciphex)
ergoloidmesylates (Hydergine)	reserpine (>0.1 mg/day)
esomeprazole (Nexium)	risperidone (Risperdal)
estazolam	scopolamine (Transderm-Scop)
estrogens	secobarbital (Seconal Sodium)
eszopiclone (Lunesta)	sotalol (Betapace, Betapace AF, Sorine)
etodolac	spironolactone (>25 mg/day) (Aldactone)
fenoprofen (Nalfon)	sulindac (Clinoril)
flecainide	temazepam (Restoril)
fluoxetine (Prozac)	terazosin
fluphenazine	testosterone (Androderm, Androgel, Aveed, Axiron, Delatestryl, Fortesta, Natesto, Striant, Testim, Vogelxo)
flurazepam	thioridazine
glyburide (Diabeta, Glynase)	thiothixene
growth hormone	ticlopidine
guanfacine (Intuniv, Tenex)	tolmetin
haloperidol (Haldol)	triazolam (Halcion)
hydroxyzine (Vistaril)	trifluoperazine
hyoscyamine (Anaspaz, Levsin)	trihexyphenidyl
ibuprofen (Advil, Motrin)	trimethobenzamide (Tigan)
ibutilide (Corvert)	trimipramine (Surmontil)
iloperidone (Fanapt)	zaleplon (Sonata)
imipramine (Tofranil)	ziprasidone (Geodon)
indomethacin (Indocin, Tivorbex)	zolpidem (Ambien, Ambien CR, Edluar, Intermezzo, Zolpimist)
insulin (sliding scale)	
isoxsuprine	
ketoprofen	

The American Geriatrics Society 2015 Beers Criteria Update Expert Panel. American Geriatrics Society 2015 updated Beers criteria for potentially inappropriate medication use in older adults. J Am Geriatr Soc. 2015 Oct 8 [Epub ahead of print].

DRUGS ASSOCIATED WITH INCREASED RISK OF FALLS IN THE ELDERLY

Many factors are associated with falls in the elderly, including frailty, disease, vision, polypharmacy, and certain medications. Below is a list of drugs associated with falls. Assess geriatric patients on these medications for fall risk and implement fall reduction strategies.

ACE Inhibitors

benazepril (Lotensin)
captopril
enalapril (Vasotec)
fosinopril
lisinopril (Prinivil, Zestril)
moexipril (Univasc)
perindopril (Aceon)
quinapril (Accupril)
ramipril (Altace)
trandolapril (Mavik)

Angiotensin II Receptor Antagonists

azilsartan (Edarbi)
candesartan (Atacand)
eprosartan (Teveten)
irbesartan (Avapro)
losartan (Cozaar)
olmesartan (Benicar)
telmisartan (Micardis)
valsartan (Diovan)

Antiarrhythmics

digoxin (Lanoxin)
disopyramide (Norpace)

Anticonvulsants

carbamazepine (Carbatrol, Epitol, Equetro, Tegretol)
ethosuximide (Zarontin)
felbamate (Felbatol)
gabapentin (Gralise, Neurontin)
lamotrigine (Lamictal)
levetiracetam (Keppra)
methsuximide (Celontin)
phenobarbital (Luminal)
phenytoin (Dilantin, Phenytek)
pregabalin (Lyrica)
primidone (Mysoline)
tiagabine (Gabatril)
topiramate (Qudexy XR, Topamax, Trokendi XR)
valproate (Depakene, Depakote, Stavzor)
zonisamide (Zonegran)

Antidepressants

amitriptyline
amoxapine
bupropion (Aplenzin, Wellbutrin)
citalopram (Celexa)
clomipramine (Anafranil)
desipramine (Norpramin)
doxepin
duloxetine (Cymbalta)
escitalopram (Lexapro)
fluoxetine (Prozac)
fluvoxamine (Luvox CR)
imipramine (Tofranil)
isocarboxazid (Marplan)
maprotiline
mirtazapine (Remeron)
nefazodone
paroxetine (Paxil, Pexeva)
phenelzine (Nardil)
protriptyline (Vivactil)
sertraline (Zoloft)
tranylcypromine (Parnate)
trazodone
trimipramine (Surmontil)
venlafaxine (Effexor XR)

Antihistamines/Antinauseants

dimenhydrinate (Dramamine)
diphenhydramine (Benadryl)
hydroxyzine (Vistaril)
meclizine (Bonine)
metoclopramide (Metozolv ODT, Reglan)
prochlorperazine (Compro)
promethazine
scopolamine patch (Transderm, Scop)

Antiparkinsonian Agents

amantadine
bromocriptine (Parlodel)
entacapone (Comtan)
levodopa/carbidopa (Duopa, Rytary, Sinemet)
pramipexole (Mirapex)
selegiline (Eldepryl, Zelapar)

Antipsychotics (Atypical)

aripiprazole (Abilify)
clozapine (Clozaril, FazaClo, Versacloz)
olanzapine (Zyprexa)
paliperidone (Invega)
quetiapine (Seroquel)
risperidone (Risperdal)
ziprasidone (Geodon)

Antipsychotics (Neuroleptics)

chlorpromazine
fluphenazine
haloperidol (Haldol)
loxapine (Adasuve)
perphenazine
pimozide (Orap)
thioridazine
thiothixine (Navane)
trifluoperazine

Anxiolytics

buspirone
meprobamate

Benzodiazepines (Long Acting)

chlordiazepoxide (Librium)
clonazepam (Klonopin)
clorazepate (Tranxene)
diazepam (Valium)
flurazepam

Benzodiazepines (Intermediate Acting)

alprazolam (Niravam, Xanax)
estazolam
lorazepam (Ativan)
oxazepam
temazepam (Restoril)

Benzodiazepines (Short Acting)

triazolam (Halcion)

Beta Blockers

acebutolol (Sectral)
atenolol (Tenormin)
bisoprolol (Zebeta)
carvedilol (Coreg)
labetalol (Trandate)
metoprolol (Lopressor, Toprol XL)
propranolol (Inderal, InnoPran XL)
timolol

Calcium Channel Blockers

amlodipine (Norvasc)
diltiazem (Cardizem, Cartia XT, Taztia XT, Tiazac)
felodipine
isradipine
nicardipine (Cardene)
nifedipine (Adalat CC, Afeditab CC, Procardia XL)
nisoldipine (Sular)
verapamil (Calan, Isoptin SR, Verelan)

Diuretics

amiloride/HCTZ
bumetanide
furosemide (Lasix)
hydrochlorothiazide (Microzide)
triamterene/HCTZ (Dyazide, Maxzide)

Opioid Analgesics

codeine
fentanyl (Abstral, Actiq, Duragesic, Fentora, Ionsys, Lazanda, Sublimaze, Subsys)
hydrocodone (Hysingla ER, Zohydro ER)
hydromorphone (Dilaudid, Exalgo)
levorphanol
meperidine (Demerol)
methadone (Dolophine)
morphine (Astramorph, Duramorph, Infumorph, Kadian, MS Contin)
oxycodone (Oxaydo, OxyContin, Roxicodone)
oxymorphone (Opana)
pentazocine (Talwin)

Skeletal Muscle Relaxants

baclofen (Gablofen, Lioresal)

Vasodilators

doxazosin (Cardura)
hydralazine
Isosorbide dinitrate/mononitrate (Dilatrate SR, Isordil, Monoket)
nitroglycerin (Minitran, Nitro-Dur, Nitrolingual, Nitromist, Nitrostat)
prazosin (Minipress)
terazosin

American Geriatrics Society (AGS) Panel on Falls in Older Persons, Guideline for the Prevention of Falls in Older Persons JAGS 49:664–672, 2001.
Keys PA. Preventing Falls in the Elderly: The Role of the Pharmacist. J Pharm Pract. 17(2):149–152, 2004.
Cooper JW, Burfield AH. Medication Interventions for Fall Prevention in the Older Adult. J Am Pharm Assoc. 49:e70-84, 2009.

LIST OF CONFUSED DRUG NAMES

Drug Name	Confused Drug Name
Abelcet	amphotericin B
Accupril	Aciphex
aceta**ZOLAMIDE**	aceto**HEXAMIDE**
acetic acid for irrigation	glacial acetic acid
aceto**HEXAMIDE**	aceta**ZOLAMIDE**
Aciphex	Accupril
Aciphex	Aricept
Activase	Cathflo Activase
Activase	TNKase
Actonel	Actos
Actos	Actonel
Adacel (Tdap)	Daptacel (DTaP)
Adderall	Inderal
Adderall	Adderall XR
Adderall XR	Adderall
Ado-trastuzumab emtansine	trastuzumab
Advair	Advicor
Advicor	Advair
Advicor	Altocor
Afrin (oxymetazoline)	Afrin (saline)
Afrin (saline)	Afrin (oxymetazoline)
Aggrastat	argatroban
Aldara	Alora
Alkeran	Leukeran
Alkeran	Myleran
Allegra	Allegra Anti-Itch Cream (diphenhydramine/ allantoin)
Allegra	Viagra
Allegra Anti-Itch Cream (diphenhydramine/ allantoin)	Allegra
Alora	Aldara
ALPRAZolam	**LOR**azepam
Altocor	Advicor
amantadine	amiodarone
Amaryl	Reminyl
Ambisome	amphotericin B
Amicar	Omacor
Amikin	Kineret
a**MIL**oride	am**LODIP**ine
amiodarone	amantadine
am**LODIP**ine	a**MIL**oride
amphotericin B	Abelcet
amphotericin B	Ambisome
Anacin	Anacin-3
Anacin-3	Anacin
antacid	Atacand
Anticoagulant Citrate Dextrose Solution	Anticoagulant Sodium Citrate Solution Formula A
Anticoagulant Sodium Citrate Solution	Anticoagulant Citrate Dextrose Solution Formula A
Antivert	Axert
Anzemet	Avandamet
Apresoline	Priscoline
argatroban	Aggrastat
argatroban	Orgaran

Drug Name	Confused Drug Name
Aricept	Aciphex
Aricept	Azilect
ARIPiprazole	proton pump inhibitors
ARIPiprazole	**RABE**prazole
Arista AH (absorbable hemostatic agent)	Arixtra
Arixtra	Arista AH (absorbable hemostatic agent)
Asacol	Os-Cal
Atacand	Antacid
Atomoxetine	Atorvastatin
Atorvastatin	Atomoxetine
Atrovent	Natru-Vent
Avandamet	Anzemet
Avandia	Prandin
Avandia	Coumadin
AVINza	**INV**anz
AVINza	Evista
Axert	Antivert
aza**CITID**ine	aza**THIO**prine
aza**THIO**prine	aza**CITID**ine
Azilect	Aricept
B & O (belladonna and opium)	Beano
BabyBIG	HBIG (hepatitis B immune globulin)
Bayhep-B	Bayrab
Bayhep-B	Bayrho-D
Bayrab	Bayhep-B
Bayrab	Bayrho-D
Bayrho-D	Bayhep-B
Bayrho-D	Bayhep-B
Beano	B & O (belladonna and opium)
Benadryl	benazepril
benazepril	Benadryl
Benicar	Mevacor
Betadine (with povidone-iodine)	Betadine (without povidone-iodine)
Betadine (without povidone-iodine)	Betadine (with povidone-iodine)
Bextra	Zetia
Bicillin C-R	Bicillin L-A
Bicillin L-A	Bicillin C-R
Bicitra	Polycitra
Bidex	Videx
Bio-T-Gel	T-Gel
Brethine	Methergine
Brevibloc	Brevital
Brevital	Brevibloc
Brilinta	Brintellix
Brintellix	Brilinta
bu**PROP**ion	bus**PIR**one
bus**PIR**one	bupropion
Capadex [non-US product]	Kapidex
Capex	Kapidex
Carac	Kuric
captopril	carvedilol

Brand names always start with an upper case letter. Some brand names incorporate tall man letters in initial characters and may not be readily recognized as brand names. Brand name products appear in black; generic/other products appear in red.

LIST OF CONFUSED DRUG NAMES continued

Drug Name	Confused Drug Name
carBAMazepine	OXcarbazepine
CARBOplatin	CISplatin
Cardura	Coumadin
carvedilol	captopril
Casodex	Kapidex
Cathflo Activase	Activase
Cedax	Cidex
ceFAZolin	cefTRIAXone
cefTRIAXone	ceFAZolin
CeleBREX	CeleXA
CeleBREX	Cerebyx
CeleXA	ZyPREXA
CeleXA	CeleBREX
CeleXA	Cerebyx
Cerebyx	CeleBREX
Cerebyx	CeleXA
cetirizine	sertraline
cetirizine	stavudine
chlordiazePOXIDE	chlorproMAZINE
chlorproMAZINE	chlordiazePOXIDE
chlorproMAZINE	chlorproPAMIDE
chlorproPAMIDE	chlorproMAZINE
Cidex	Cedax
CISplatin	CARBOplatin
Claritin (loratadine)	Claritin Eye (ketotifen fumarate)
Claritin-D	Claritin-D 24
Claritin-D 24	Claritin-D 24 Claritin-D
Claritin Eye (ketotifen fumarate)	Claritin (loratadine)
Clindesse	Clindets
Clindets	Clindesse
Clobazam	clonazePAM
clomiPHENE	clomiPRAMINE
clomiPRAMINE	clomiPHENE
clonazePAM	cloNIDine
clonazePAM	LORazepam
cloNIDine	clonazePAM
cloNIDine	KlonoPIN
Clozaril	Colazal
coagulation factor IX (recombinant)	factor IX complex, vapor heated
codeine	Lodine
Colace	Cozaar
Colazal	Clozaril
colchicine	Cortrosyn
Comvax	Recombivax HB
Cortrosyn	colchicine
Coumadin	Avandia
Coumadin	Cardura
Covaryx HS	Covera HS
Covera HS	Covaryx HS
Cozaar	Colace
Cozaar	Zocor
cyclophosphamide	cycloSPORINE
cycloSERINE	cycloSPORINE
cycloSPORINE	cyclophosphamide

Drug Name	Confused Drug Name
cycloSPORINE	cycloSERINE
Cymbalta	Symbyax
DACTINomycin	DAPTOmycin
Daptacel (DTaP)	Adacel (Tdap)
DAPTOmycin	DACTINomycin
Darvocet	Percocet
Darvon	Diovan
DAUNOrubicin	DAUNOrubicin citrate liposomal
DAUNOrubicin	DOXOrubicin
DAUNOrubicin	IDArubicin
DAUNOrubicin citrate liposomal	DAUNOrubicin
Denavir	indinavir
Depakote	Depakote ER
Depakote ER	Depakote
Depo-Medrol	Solu-MEDROL
Depo-Provera	Depo-subQ provera 104
Depo-subQ provera 104	Depo-Provera
desipramine	disopyramide
Desyrel	SEROquel
dexmethylphenidate	methadone
Diabinese	Diamox
Diabeta	Zebeta
Diamox	Diabinese
Diflucan	Diprivan
Dilacor XR	Pilocar
Dilaudid	Dilaudid-5
Dilaudid-5	Dilaudid
dimenhyDRINATE	diphenhydrAMINE
diphenhydrAMINE	dimenhyDRINATE
Dioval	Diovan
Diovan	Dioval
Diovan	Zyban
Diovan	Darvon
Diprivan	Diflucan
Diprivan	Ditropan
disopyramide	desipramine
Ditropan	Diprivan
DOBUTamine	DOPamine
DOPamine	DOBUTamine
Doribax	Zovirax
Doxil	Paxil
DOXOrubicin	DAUNOrubicin
DOXOrubicin	DOXOrubicin liposomal
DOXOrubicin	IDArubicin
DOXOrubicin liposomal	DOXOrubicin
Dulcolax (bisacodyl)	Dulcolax (docusate sodium)
Dulcolax (docusate sodium)	Dulcolax (bisacodyl)
DULoxetine	FLUoxetine
Durasal	Durezol
Durezol	Durasal
Duricef	Ultracet
Dynacin	Dynacirc
Dynacirc	Dynacin

Brand names always start with an upper case letter. Some brand names incorporate tall man letters in initial characters and may not be readily recognized as brand names. Brand name products appear in black; generic/other products appear in red.

LIST OF CONFUSED DRUG NAMES continued

Drug Name	Confused Drug Name
edetate calcium disodium	edetate disodium
edetate disodium	edetate calcium disodium
Effexor	Effexor XR
Effexor XR	Effexor
Effexor XR	Enablex
Enablex	Effexor XR
Enbrel	Levbid
Engerix-B adult	Engerix-B pediatric/ adolescent
Engerix-B pediatric/ adolescent	Engerix-B adult
Enjuvia	Januvia
e**PHED**rine	EPINEPHrine
EPINEPHrine	e**PHED**rine
Epirubicin	eribulin
eribulin	Epirubicin
Estratest	Estratest HS
Estratest HS	Estratest
ethambutol	Ethmozine
Ethaverine [non-US product]	etravirine
Ethmozine	ethambutol
etravirine	Ethaverine [non-US product]
Evista	**AVIN**za
factor IX complex, vapor heated	coagulation factor IX (recombinant)
Fanapt	Xanax
Farxiga	Fetzima
Femara	Femhrt
Femhrt	Femara
fenta**NYL**	**SUF**entanil
Fetzima	Farxiga
Fioricet	Fiorinal
Fiorinal	Fioricet
flavox**ATE**	fluvoxa**MINE**
Flonase	Flovent
Floranex	Florinef
Florastor	Florinef
Florinef	Floranex
Flovent	Flonase
flumazenil	influenza virus vaccine
FLUoxetine	**PAR**oxetine
FLUoxetine	**DUL**oxetine
FLUoxetine	Loxitane
fluvoxa**MINE**	flavox**ATE**
Focalgin B	Focalin
Focalin	Focalgin B
Folex	Foltx
folic acid	folinic acid (leucovorin calcium)
folinic acid (leucovorin calcium)	folic acid
Foltx	Folex
fomepizole	omeprazole
Foradil	Fortical
Foradil	Toradol
Fortical	Foradil
gentamicin	gentian violet
gentian violet	gentamicin
glacial acetic acid	acetic acid for irrigation
glipi**ZIDE**	gly**BURIDE**
Glucotrol	Glycotrol
gly**BURIDE**	glipi**ZIDE**
Glycotrol	Glucotrol
Granulex	Regranex
guai**FEN**esin	guan**FACINE**
guan**FACINE**	guai**FEN**esin
HBIG (hepatitis B immune globulin)	BabyBIG
Healon	Hyalgan
heparin	Hespan
Hespan	heparin
HMG-CoA reductase inhibitors ("statins")	nystatin
Huma**LOG**	Humu**LIN**
Huma**LOG**	Novo**LOG**
Huma**LOG** Mix 75/25	Humu**LIN** 70/30
Humapen Memoir (for use with Huma**LOG**)	Humira Pen
Humira Pen	Humapen Memoir (for use with Huma**LOG**)
Humu**LIN**	Novo**LIN**
Humu**LIN**	Huma**LOG**
Humu**LIN** 70/30	Huma**LOG** Mix 75/25
Humu**LIN** R U-100	Humu**LIN** R U-500
Humu**LIN** R U-500	Humu**LIN** R U-100
Hyalgan	Healon
hydr**ALAZINE**	hydr**OXY**zine
Hydrea	Lyrica
HYDROcodone	oxy**CODONE**
Hydrogesic	hydr**OXY**zine
HYDROmorphone	morphine
hydr**OXY**zine	Hydrogesic
hydr**OXY**zine	hydr**ALAZINE**
IDArubicin	**DAUNO**rubicin
IDArubicin	**DOXO**rubicin
Inderal	Adderall
indinavir	Denavir
in**FLIX**imab	ri**TUX**imab
influenza virus vaccine	flumazenil
influenza virus vaccine	perflutren lipid microspheres
influenza virus vaccine	tuberculin purified protein derivative (PPD)
Inspra	Spiriva
Intuniv	Invega
INVanz	**AVIN**za
Invega	Intuniv
iodine	Lodine
Isordil	Plendil
ISOtretinoin	tretinoin
Jantoven	Janumet
Jantoven	Januvia
Janumet	Jantoven
Janumet	Januvia
Janumet	Sinemet

Brand names always start with an upper case letter. Some brand names incorporate tall man letters in initial characters and may not be readily recognized as brand names. Brand name products appear in black; generic/other products appear in red.

LIST OF CONFUSED DRUG NAMES continued

Drug Name	Confused Drug Name
Januvia	Enjuvia
Januvia	Jantoven
Januvia	Janumet
K-Phos Neutral	Neutra-Phos-K
Kadian	Kapidex
Kaletra	Keppra
Kaopectate (bismuth subsalicylate)	Kaopectate (docusate calcium)
Kaopectate (docusate calcium)	Kaopectate (bismuth subsalicylate)
Kapidex	Capadex [non-US product]
Kapidex	Capex
Kapidex	Casodex
Kapidex	Kadian
Keflex	Keppra
Keppra	Kaletra
Keppra	Keflex
Ketalar	ketorolac
ketorolac	Ketalar
ketorolac	methadone
Kineret	Amikin
Klono**PIN**	clo**NID**ine
Kuric	Carac
Kwell	Qwell
La**MIC**tal	Lami**SIL**
Lami**SIL**	La**MIC**tal
lami**VUD**ine	lamo**TRI**gine
lamo**TRI**gine	lami**VUD**ine
lamo**TRI**gine	lev**ETIRA**cetam
lamo**TRI**gine	levothyroxine
Lanoxin	levothyroxine
Lanoxin	naloxone
lanthanum carbonate	lithium carbonate
Lantus	Latuda
Lantus	Lente
Lariam	Levaquin
Lasix	Luvox
Latuda	Lantus
Lente	Lantus
leucovorin calcium	Leukeran
leucovorin calcium	Levoleucovorin
Leukeran	Alkeran
Leukeran	Myleran
Leukeran	leucovorin calcium
Levaquin	Lariam
Levbid	Enbrel
Levemir	Lovenox
lev**ETIRA**cetam	lamo**TRI**gine
lev**ETIRA**cetam	lev**OCARN**itine
lev**ETIRA**cetam	levofloxacin
lev**OCARN**itine	lev**ETIRA**cetam
levofloxacin	lev**ETIRA**cetam
Levoleucovorin	Leucovorin calcium
levothyroxine	lamo**TRI**gine
levothyroxine	Lanoxin
levothyroxine	liothyronine
Lexapro	Loxitane
Lexiva	Pexeva
liothyronine	levothyroxine
Lipitor	Loniten
Lipitor	Zyr**TEC**
lithium	Ultram
lithium carbonate	lanthanum carbonate
Lodine	codeine
Lodine	iodine
Loniten	Lipitor
Lopressor	Lyrica
LORazepam	**ALPRAZ**olam
LORazepam	clonaze**PAM**
LORazepam	Lovaza
Lotronex	Protonix
Lovaza	**LOR**azepam
Lovenox	Levemir
Loxitane	Lexapro
Loxitane	**FLU**oxetine
Loxitane	Soriatane
Lunesta	Neulasta
Lupron Depot-3 Month	Lupron Depot-Ped
Lupron Depot-Ped	Lupron Depot-3 Month
Luvox	Lasix
Lyrica	Hydrea
Lyrica	Lopressor
Maalox	Maalox Total Stomach Relief
Maalox Total Stomach Relief	Maalox
Matulane	Materna
Materna	Matulane
Maxzide	Microzide
Menactra	Menomune
Menomune	Menactra
Mephyton	methadone
Metadate	methadone
Metadate CD	Metadate ER
Metadate ER	Metadate CD
Metadate ER	methadone
met**FORMIN**	metro**NIDAZOLE**
methadone	dexmethylphenidate
methadone	ketorolac
methadone	Mephyton
methadone	Metadate
methadone	Metadate ER
methadone	methylphenidate
methadone	metolazone
Methergine	Brethine
methimazole	metolazone
methimazole	Metolazone
methylene blue	VisionBlue
methylphenidate	methadone
metolazone	methadone
metolazone	methimazole
metoprolol succina	metoprolol tartrate
metoprolol tartrate	metoprolol succinate

Brand names always start with an upper case letter. Some brand names incorporate tall man letters in initial characters and may not be readily recognized as brand names. Brand name products appear in black; generic/other products appear in red.

LIST OF CONFUSED DRUG NAMES continued

Drug Name	Confused Drug Name
metro**NIDAZOLE**	met**FORMIN**
Mevacor	Benicar
Micronase	Microzide
Microzide	Maxzide
Microzide	Micronase
midodrine	Midrin
Midrin	midodrine
mifepristone	misoprostol
Miralax	Mirapex
Mirapex	Miralax
misoprostol	mifepristone
mito**MY**cin	mito**XAN**trone
mito**XAN**trone	mito**MY**cin
morphine	**HYDRO**morphone
morphine - non-concentrated oral liquid	morphine - oral liquid concentrate
morphine - oral liquid concentrate	morphine - non-concentrated oral liquid
Motrin	Neurontin
MS Contin	Oxy**CONTIN**
Mucinex	Mucinex Allergy
Mucinex	Mucomyst
Mucinex Allergy	Mucinex
Mucinex D	Mucinex DM
Mucinex DM	Mucinex D
Mucomyst	Mucinex
Myleran	Alkeran
Myleran	Leukeran
nalbuphine	naloxone
naloxone	Lanoxin
naloxone	nalbuphine
Narcan	Norcuron
Natru-Vent	Atrovent
Navane	Norvasc
Neo-Synephrine (oxymetazoline)	Neo-Synephrine (phenylephrine)
Neo-Synephrine (phenylephrine)	Neo-Synephrine (oxymetazoline)
Neulasta	Lunesta
Neulasta	Neumega
Neulasta	Nuedexta
Neumega	Neupogen
Neumega	Neulasta
Neupogen	Neumega
Neurontin	Motrin
Neurontin	Noroxin
Neutra-Phos-K	K-Phos Neutral
Nex**AVAR**	Nex**IUM**
Nex**IUM**	Nex**AVAR**
ni**CAR**dipine	**NIFE**dipine
NIFEdipine	ni**CAR**dipine
NIFEdipine	ni**MOD**ipine
ni**MOD**ipine	**NIFE**dipine
Norcuron	Narcan
Normodyne	Norpramin
Noroxin	Neurontin
Norpramin	Normodyne
Norvasc	Navane
Novo**LIN**	Humu**LIN**
Novo**LIN**	Novo**LOG**
Novo**LIN** 70/30	Novo**LOG** Mix 70/30
Novo**LOG**	Huma**LOG**
Novo**LOG**	Novo**LIN**
Novo**LOG** FLEXPEN	Novo**LOG** Mix 70/30 FLEXPEN
Novo**LOG** Mix 70/30 FLEXPEN	Novo**LOG** FLEXPEN
Novo**LOG** Mix 70/30	Novo**LIN** 70/30
Nuedexta	Neulasta
nystatin	HMG-CoA reductase inhibitors (ÒstatinsÓ)
Occlusal-HP	Ocuflox
Ocuflox	Occlusal-HP
OLANZapine	**QUE**tiapine
Omacor	Amicar
omeprazole	fomepizole
opium tincture	paregoric (camphorated tincture of opium)
Oracea	Orencia
Orencia	Oracea
Orgaran	argatroban
OrthoTri-Cyclen	Ortho Tri-Cyclen LO
Ortho Tri-Cyclen LO	OrthoTri-Cyclen
Os-Cal	Asacol
oxaprozin	**OX**carbazepine
OXcarbazepine	car**BAM**azepine
OXcarebazepine	oxaprozin
oxy**CODONE**	**HYDRO**codone
oxy**CODONE**	Oxy**CONTIN**
Oxy**CONTIN**	MS Contin
Oxy**CONTIN**	oxy**CODONE**
PACLitaxel	**PACL**itaxel protein-bound particles
PACLitaxel protein-bound particles	**PACL**itaxel
Pamelor	Panlor DC
Pamelor	Tambocor
Panlor DC	Pamelor
paregoric (camphorated tincture of opium)	opium tincture
PARoxetine	**FLU**oxetine
PARoxetine	piroxicam
Patanol	Platinol
Pavulon	Peptavlon
Paxil	Doxil
Paxil	Taxol
Paxil	Plavix
PAZOPanib	**PONAT**inib
PEMEtrexed	**PRALA**trexate
penicill**AMINE**	penicillin
penicillin	penicill**AMINE**
Peptavlon	Pavulon
Percocet	Darvocet
Percocet	Procet
perflutren lipid microspheres	influenza virus vaccine

Brand names always start with an upper case letter. Some brand names incorporate tall man letters in initial characters and may not be readily recognized as brand names. Brand name products appear in black; generic/other products appear in red.

LIST OF CONFUSED DRUG NAMES continued

Drug Name	Confused Drug Name
Pexeva	Lexiva
PENTobarbital	**PHEN**obarbital
PHENobarbital	**PENT**obarbital
Pilocar	Dilacor XR
piroxicam	**PAR**oxetine
Platinol	Patanol
Plavix	Paxil
Plavix	Pradax [non-US product]
Plavix	Pradaxa
Plendil	Isordil
pneumococcal 7-valent vaccine	pneumococcal polyvalent vaccine
pneumococcal polyvalent vaccine	pneumococcal 7-valent vaccine
Polycitra	Bicitra
PONATinib	**PAZOP**anib
Potassium acetate	sodium acetate
Pradax [non-US product]	Plavix
Pradaxa	Plavix
PRALAtrexate	**PEME**trexed
Prandin	Avandia
Precare	Precose
Precose	Precare
predniso**LONE**	predni**SONE**
predni**SONE**	predniso**LONE**
Prenexa	Ranexa
Pri**LOSEC**	Pristiq
Pri**LOSEC**	**PRO**zac
Priscoline	Apresoline
Pristiq	Pri**LOSEC**
probenecid	Procanbid
Procan SR	Procanbid
Procanbid	probenecid
Procanbid	Procan SR
Procardia XL	Protain XL
Procet	Percocet
Prograf	**PRO**zac
propylthiouracil	Purinethol
Proscar	Provera
Protain XL	Procardia XL
protamine	Protonix
proton pump inhibitors	**ARIP**iprazole
Protonix	Lotronex
Protonix	protamine
Provera	Proscar
Provera	**PRO**zac
PROzac	Prograf
PROzac	Pri**LOSEC**
PROzac	Provera
Purinethol	propylthiouracil
Pyridium	pyridoxine
pyridoxine	Pyridium
QUEtiapine	**OLANZ**apine
qui**NID**ine	qui**NINE**
qui**NINE**	qui**NID**ine
Qwell	Kwell
RABEprazole	**ARIP**iprazole

Drug Name	Confused Drug Name
Ranexa	Prenexa
Rapaflo	Rapamune
Rapamune	Rapaflo
Razadyne	Rozerem
Recombivax HB	Comvax
Regranex	Granulex
Reminyl	Robinul
Reminyl	Amaryl
Renagel	Renvela
Renvela	Renagel
Reprexain	Zy**PREXA**
Restoril	Risper**DAL**
Retrovir	ritonavir
Rifadin	Rifater
Rifamate	rifampin
rifampin	Rifamate
rifampin	rifaximin
Rifater	Rifadin
rifaximin	rifampin
RisperDAL	Restoril
risperi**DONE**	r**OPINIR**ole
Ritalin	ritodrine
Ritalin LA	Ritalin SR
Ritalin SR	Ritalin LA
ritodrine	Ritalin
ritonavir	Retrovir
ri**TUX**imab	in**FLIX**imab
Robinul	Reminyl
r**OPINIR**ole	risperi**DONE**
Roxanol	Roxicodone Intensol
Roxanol	Roxicet
Roxicet	Roxanol
Roxicodone Intensol	Roxanol
Rozerem	Razadyne
Salagen	selegiline
Sand**IMMUNE**	Sando**STATIN**
Sando**STATIN**	Sand**IMMUNE**
saquinavir	**SINE**quan
saquinavir (free base)	saquinavir mesylate
saquinavir mesylate	saquinavir (free base)
Sarafem	Serophene
selegiline	Salagen
Serophene	Sarafem
SEROquel	Desyrel
SEROquel	**SERO**quel XR
SEROquel	Serzone
SEROquel	**SINE**quan
SEROquel XR	**SERO**quel
sertraline	cetirizine
sertraline	Soriatane
Serzone	**SERO**quel
silodosin	sirolimus
Sinemet	Janumet
SINEquan	saquinavir
SINEquan	**SERO**quel
SINEquan	Singulair
SINEquan	Zonegran

Brand names always start with an upper case letter. Some brand names incorporate tall man letters in initial characters and may not be readily recognized as brand names. Brand name products appear in black; generic/other products appear in red.

LIST OF CONFUSED DRUG NAMES continued

Drug Name	Confused Drug Name
Singulair	**SINE**quan
sita**GLIP**tin	**SUMA**triptan
Sodium acetate	Potassium acetate
Solu-**CORTEF**	Solu-**MEDROL**
Solu-**MEDROL**	Depo-Medrol
Solu-**MEDROL**	Solu-**CORTEF**
Sonata	Sonata Soriatane
Soriatane	Loxitane
Soriatane	sertraline
Soriatane	Sonata
sotalol	Sudafed
Spiriva	Apidra
Spiriva	Inspra
stavudine	cetirizine
Sudafed	sotalol
Sudafed	Sudafed PE
Sudafed 12 Hour	Sudafed 12 Hour Pressure + Pain
Sudafed 12 Hour Pressure + Pain	Sudafed 12 Hour
Sudafed PE	Sudafed
SUFentanil	fenta**NYL**
sulf**ADIAZINE**	sulfa**SALA**zine
sulf**ADIAZINE**	sulfi**SOXAZOLE**
sulfa**SALA**zine	sulf**ADIAZINE**
sulfi**SOXAZOLE**	sulf**ADIAZINE**
SUMAtriptan	sita**GLIP**tin
SUMAtriptan	**ZOLM**itriptan
Symbyax	Cymbalta
T-Gel	Bio-T-Gel
Tambocor	Pamelor
Taxol	Taxotere
Taxol	Paxil
Taxotere	Taxol
TEGretol	**TEG**retol XR
TEGretol	Tequin
TEGretol	**TREN**tal
TEGretol XR	**TEG**retol
Tenex	Xanax
Tequin	**TEG**retol
Tequin	Ticlid
Testoderm TTS	Testoderm
Testoderm TTS	Testoderm with Adhesive
Testoderm with Adhesive	Testoderm
Testoderm with Adhesive	Testoderm TTS
Testoderm	Testoderm TTS
Testoderm	Testoderm with Adhesive
tetanus diphtheria toxoid (Td)	tuberculin purified protein derivative (PPD)
Thalomid	Thiamine
Thiamine	Thalomid
tia**GAB**ine	ti**ZAN**idine
Tiazac	Ziac
Ticlid	Tequin
ti**ZAN**idine	tia**GAB**ine
TNKase	Activase
TNKase	t-PA
Tobradex	Tobrex
Tobrex	Tobradex
TOLAZamide	**TOLBUT**amide
TOLBUTamide	**TOLAZ**amide
Topamax	Toprol-XL
Toprol-XL	Topamax
Toradol	Foradil
t-PA	TNKase
Tracleer	Tricor
tra**MAD**ol	tra**ZOD**one
trastuzumab	ado-trastuzumab emtansine
tra**ZOD**one	tra**MAD**ol
TRENtal	**TEG**retol
tretinoin	**ISO**tretinoin
Tricor	Tracleer
tromethamine	Trophamine
Trophamine	tromethamine
tuberculin purified protein derivative (PPD)	influenza virus vaccine
tuberculin purified protein derivative (PPD)	tetanus diphtheria toxoid (Td)
Tylenol	Tylenol PM
Tylenol PM	Tylenol
Ultracet	Duricef
Ultram	lithium
val**ACY**clovir	val**GAN**ciclovir
Valcyte	Valtrex
val**GAN**ciclovir	val**ACY**clovir
Valtrex	Valcyte
Varivax	VZIG (varicella-zoster immune globulin)
Vesanoid	Vesicare
Vesicare	Vesanoid
Vexol	Vosol
Viagra	Allegra
Videx	Bidex
vin**BLAS**tine	vin**CRIS**tine
vin**CRIS**tine	vin**BLAS**tine
Viokase	Viokase 8
Viokase 8	Viokase
Vioxx	Zyvox
Viracept	Viramune
Viramune	Viracept
VisionBlue	methylene blue
Vosol	Vexol
VZIG (varicella-zoster immune globulin)	Varivax
Wellbutrin SR	Wellbutrin XL
Wellbutrin XL	Wellbutrin SR
Xanax	Fanapt
Xanax	Tenex
Xanax	Zantac
Xeloda	Xenical
Xenical	Xeloda
Yasmin	Yaz
Yaz	Yasmin

Brand names always start with an upper case letter. Some brand names incorporate tall man letters in initial characters and may not be readily recognized as brand names. Brand name products appear in black; generic/other products appear in red.

LIST OF CONFUSED DRUG NAMES continued

Drug Name	Confused Drug Name
Zantac	Xanax
Zantac	ZyrTEC
Zavesca (escitalopram) [non-US product]	Zavesca (miglustat)
Zavesca (miglustat)	Zavesca (escitalopram) [non-US product]
Zebeta	Diabeta
Zebeta	Zetia
Zegerid	Zestril
Zelapar (Zydis formulation)	Zy**PREXA** Zydis
Zerit	Zyr**TEC**
Zestril	Zegerid
Zestril	Zetia
Zestril	Zy**PREXA**
Zetia	Bextra
Zetia	Zebeta
Zetia	Zestril
Ziac	Tiazac
Zocor	Cozaar
Zocor	Zyr**TEC**
ZOLMitriptan	**SUMA**triptan
zolpidem	Zyloprim
Zonegran	**SINE**quan
Zostrix	Zovirax

Drug Name	Confused Drug Name
Zovirax	Doribax
Zovirax	Zyvox
Zovirax	Zostrix
Zyban	Diovan
Zyloprim	zolpidem
Zy**PREXA**	Cele**XA**
Zy**PREXA**	Reprexain
Zy**PREXA**	Zestril
Zy**PREXA**	Zyr**TEC**
Zy**PREXA** Zydis	Zelapar (Zydis formulation)
Zyr**TEC**	Lipitor
Zyr**TEC**	Zantac
Zyr**TEC**	Zerit
Zyr**TEC**	Zocor
Zyr**TEC**	Zy**PREXA**
Zyr**TEC**	Zyr**TEC**-D
Zyr**TEC** (cetirizine)	Zyr**TEC** Itchy Eye Drops (ketotifen fumarate)
Zyr**TEC**-D	Zyr**TEC**
Zyr**TEC** Itchy Eye Drops (ketotifen fumarate)	Zyr**TEC** (cetirizine)
Zyvox	Vioxx
Zyvox	Zovirax

Brand names always start with an upper case letter. Some brand names incorporate tall man letters in initial characters and may not be readily recognized as brand names. Brand name products appear in black; generic/other products appear in red.

DO NOT CRUSH!

Do not crush any oral medication that is labeled as:

Delayed Release
Enteric-Coated **(EC)**
Extended Release
Effervescent Tablet **(EVT)**
Mucous Membrane Irritant **(MMI)**
Orally Disintegrating Tablets **(ODT)**
Slow-Release **(SR)**
Sublingual forms of drugs
Sustained-Release

Do not crush any oral medication that ends in the following letters:

CD CR ER LA SR XL XR XT

MEDICATIONS THAT SHOULD NOT BE CRUSHED:

Abosrbica Capsule **(MMI)**
Aciphex Tablet **(SR)**
Acticlate Tablet (film-coated)—see code **"B"**
Actiq Lozenge **(SR)**
Actonel Tablet **(MMI)**
Adalat CC Tablet **(SR)**
Adderall XR Capsule **(SR)**—see code "**C**"
Afeditab CR Tablet **(SR)**
Afinitor Tablet **(MMI)**
Aggrenox Capsule **(SR)**
Alavert Allergy Sinus 12-Hour Tablet **(SR)**
Allegra-D Tablet **(SR)**
Alprazolam ER Tablet **(SR)**
Altoprev Tablet **(SR)**
Ambien CR Tablet **(SR)**
Amitiza Capsule **(SR)**
Amnesteem Capsule **(MM)**
Ampyra Tablet **(SR)**
Amrix Capsule **(SR)**
Aplenzin Tablet **(SR)**
Apriso Capsule **(SR)**—see code "**C**"
Aptivus Capsule
Aricept 23-mg Tablet **(crushing may ↑ rate of absorption)**
Arthrotec Tablet **(EC)**
Asacol Tablet **(SR)**
Aspirin Regimen Bayer Regular Dose Caplet **(EC)**
Atelvia Tablet **(SR, MMI)**
Augmentin XR Tablet—see codes **"A," "B"**
Avinza Capsule **(SR)**—see code "**C**"
Avodart Capsule—see code **"F"**
Azulfidine EN-Tablet **(SR, EC)**
Bayer Low Dose Aspirin Tablet **(EC)**
Bayer Women's Low Dose Aspirin Caplet **(EC)**
Belsomra Tablet
Biaxin-XL Tablet **(SR)**
Biltricide Tablet **(crushing, breaking or chewing tablet can leave bitter taste)**—see code **"B"**
Bisa-lax Tablet **(EC)**—see code "**D**"
Bisac-Evac Tablet **(EC)**—see code **"D"**
Bisacodyl Tablet **(EC)**—see code **"D"**
Boniva Tablet **(MMI)**
Budeprion SR Tablet **(SR)**
Bunavail Buccal Film **(chewing or swallowing may ↓ bioavailability)**
Calan SR Tablet **(SR)**—see code "**B**"
Carbatrol Capsule **(SR)**—see code **"C"**
Cardizem Tablet
Cardizem CD Capsule **(SR)**
Cardizem LA Tablet **(SR)**
Cardura XL Tablet **(SR)**
Cartia XT Capsule **(SR)**
Cefaclor ER Tablet **(SR)**—see code **"A"**
Ceftin Tablet—see code **"A"**
Cefuroxime Tablet—see code **"A"**
CellCept Capsule, Tablet—see code **"I"**
Cerdegla Capsule **(preferably taken with water)**
Chlor-Trimeton 12-Hour Tablet **(SR)**
Cipro XR Tablet **(SR)**—see code **"A"**
Claravis Capsule **(MMI)**
Claritin-D 12 Hour Tablet **(SR)**
Claritin-D 24 Hour Tablet **(SR)**
Colace Capsule
Colestid Tablet **(SR)**
Commit Lozenge **(integrity compromised by chewing or crushing)**
Concerta Tablet **(SR)**
Creon Capsule—see code "**C**"
Crixivan Capsule—see code "**C**"
Cymbalta Capsule **(SR)**—see code **"C"**
Cytovene Capsule **(MMI)**
Cytoxan Tablet
Depakene Capsule **(SR, MMI)**—see code **"A"**
Depakote Tablet **(SR)**
Depakote ER Tablet **(SR)**
Depakote Sprinkle Capsule (SR)—see code **"C"**
Detrol LA Capsule **(SR)**
Dexilant Capsule **(SR)**—see code **"C"**
Diclegis Tablet **(SR)**
Dilatrate-SR Capsule **(SR)**
Dilt—CD Capsule **(SR)**
Diltiazem CD Capsule **(SR)**
Ditropan XL Tablet **(SR)**
Divalproex ER Tablet **(SR)**
Doxidan Tablet **(EC)**—see code **"D"**
Drisdol Capsule
Droxia Capsule **(wear gloves to administer)**
Dulcolax Tablet, Capsule **(EC)**—see code "**D**"
EC-Naprosyn Tablet **(SR, EC)**
Ecotrin Tablet **(EC)**
E.E.S. 400 Tablet **(EC)**
Effer-K Tablet **(EVT)**
Effexor XR Capsule **(SR)**
Embeda Capsule **(SR)**—see code **"C"**
Enablex Tablet **(SR)**
Entocort EC Capsule **(EC)**
Equetro Capsule **(SR)**—see code **"C"**
Epanova Capsule **(do not put contents in styrofoam or plastic container)**
Ergomar Sublingual Tablet—see code **"E"**
Erivedge Capsule—see code **"I"**
Ery-Tab Tablet **(SR, EC)**
Erythromycin Base Tablet **(EC)**
Erythomycin Delayed-Release Capsule **(SR) (contains pellets)**—see code **"C"**
Evista Tablet—see code **"I"**
Exalgo Tablet **(SR) (crushing, chewing, or dissolving tablet could cause overdose)**
Exjade Tablet—**(tablets must be dispersed in liquid)**
Feldene Capsule **(MMI)**
Fentanyl Lozenge **(SR)**
Fentora Buccal Tablet **(crushing could ↓ effectiveness)**
Feosol Tablet **(EC)**—see code **"A"**
Feratab Tablet **(EC)**—see code **"A"**
Fergon Tablet **(EC)**
Flagyl ER Tablet **(SR)**
Fleet Laxative Tablet **(EC)**—see code **"D"**
Flomax Capsule **(SR)**
Focalin XR Capsule **(SR)**—see code **"C"**
Fortamet Tablet **(SR)**
Fosamax Tablet **(MMI)**
Gleevec Tablet—see code **"B"**
Glipizide XR Tablet **(SR)**
Glucophage XR Tablet **(SR)**
Glucotrol XL Tablet **(SR)**
Glumetza Tablet **(SR)**
Gralise Tablet **(SR)**
Halfprin Tablet **(EC)**
Hetlioz Capsule
Horizant Tablet **(SR)**
Hydrea Capsule **(wear gloves to administer)**
Hysingla ER Tablet **(SR) (crushing, chewing, or dissolving tablet could cause overdose)**
Imbruvica Capsule
Imdur Tablet **(SR)**—see code "**B**"
Impavido Capsule
Inderal LA Capsule **(SR)**
Indomethacin SR Capsule **(SR)**—see codes **"A," "C"**
InnoPran XL Capsule **(SR)**
Intelence Tablet **(may disperse in water)**
Intermezzo Sublingual Tablet—see code **"E"**
Intuniv Tablet **(SR)**
Invega Tablet **(SR)**
Isoptin SR Tablet **(SR)**—see code **"B"**
Isosorbide SR Tablet **(SR)**
Jakafi Tablet **(may disperse in water)**
Jalyn Capsule **(MMI)**—see code **"F"**
Janumet XR Tablet **(SR)**
Kadian Capsule **(SR) (do not give via NG tube)**—see code **"C"**
Kaletra Tablet **(film-coated)**—see code **"A"**
Kapvay Tablet **(SR)**
Kazano Tablet
Keppra Tablet—see code "A"
Keppra XR Tablet (SR)—see code **"A"**
Ketek Tablet **(SR)**
Khedezla Tablet **(SR)**
Klor-Con Tablet **(SR)**—see codes **"A," "B"**
Klor-Con M Tablet **(SR)**
Kombiglyze XR Tablet **(SR)**
K-Tab Tablet **(SR)**—see code **"A"**
Lamictal XR Tablet **(SR)**
Lescol XL Tablet **(SR)**
Letairis Tablet **(SR)**
Levbid Tablet **(SR)**—see code **"B"**
Lialda Tablet **(SR)**
Lithobid Tablet **(SR)**
Lovaza Capsule **(do not put contents in styrofoam or plastic container)**
Luvox CR Capsule **(SR)**

DO NOT CRUSH!

MEDICATIONS THAT SHOULD NOT BE CRUSHED:

Mestinon Timespan Tablet **(SR)**—see code **"A"**
Metadate CD Capsule **(SR)**—see code **"C"**
Metadate ER Tablet **(SR)**
Methylin ER Tablet **(SR)**
Metoprolol Succinate Tablet **(SR)**
Micro K Capsule **(SR)** see codes **"A," "C"**
Mirapex ER Tablet **(SR)**
Morphine Sulfate ER Tablet **(SR)**
Motrin Tablet—see code **"A"**
Movantik Tablet **(film-coated)**
Moxatag Tablet **(SR)**
MS Contin Tablet **(SR)** see code **"A"**
Mucinex Tablet **(SR)**
Mucinex DM Tablet **(SR)**
Myfortic Tablet **(SR)**
Myrbetriq Tablet—**(ER)**
Myorisan Capsule **(MMI)**
Namenda XR Capsule **(SR)**—see code **"C"**
Neprelan Tablet **(SR)**
Nexium Capsule **(SR)**—see code **"C"**
Niaspan Tablet **(SR)**
Nicotinic Acid Capsule, Tablet **(SR)**—see code **"B"**
Nifediac CC Tablet **(SR)**
Nifedical XL Tablet **(SR)**
Nitrostat Sublingual Tablet—see code **"E"**
Norpace CR Capsule **(SR)**
Northera Capsule
Norvir Tablet **(crushing—crushing reduces ↓ bioavailability)**—see code **"A"**
Nucynta ER Tablet **(SR) (crushing, chewing, or dissolving tablet could cause overdose)**
OFEV Capsule **(crushing or chewing capsule can leave bitter taste)**
Omtryg Capsule **(do not put contents in styrofoam or plastic container)**
Opana ER Tablet **(SR) (crushing, chewing, or dissolving tablet could cause overdose)**
Oracea Capsule **(SR)**
Orphenadrine citrate ER Tablet **(SR)**
Otezla Tablet **(film-coated)**
OxyContin Tablet **(SR) (crushing could cause overdose)
Oxymorphone ER Tablet **(SR) (crushing, chewing or dissolving tablet could cause overdose)**
Pancrelipase Capsule **(EC)**—see code **"C"**
Paxil CR Tablet **(SR)**
Pentasa Capsule **(SR)**—see code **"C"**
Pertyze Capsule **(SR)**—see code **"C"**
Plendil Tablet **(SR)**
Pradaxa Capsule **(breaking, chewing, or emptying capsule ↑ bioavailability)**
Prevacid Capsule **(SR)**
Prevacid SoluTab Tablet **(ODT) (may dissolve in water to administer via NG tube)**
Prilosec Capsule **(SR)**—see code **"A"**
Prilosec OTC Tablet **(SR)**
Pristiq Tablet **(SR)**
Procardia XL Tablet Capsule **(SR)**
Propecia Tablet—see code **"F"**
Proquin XR Tablet **(SR)**
Proscar Tablet—see code **"F"**
Protonix Tablet **(SR)**
Prozac Weekly Tablet **(EC)**
Qudexy XR Capsule **(SR)**—see code **"C"**
Ranexa Tablet **(SR)**
Rapamune Tablet—see code **"A"**
Rayos Tablet **(SR)**
Razadyne ER Capsule **(SR)**
Renagel Tablet **(expands in liquid when crushed or broken)**
Renvela Tablet **(expands in liquid when crushed or broken)**—see code **"A"**
Requip XL Tablet **(SR)**
Revlimid Capsule—see code **"F"**
Reyataz Capsule **(oral powder available)**
Risperdal M-Tablet **(ODT)**
Ritalin LA Capsule **(SR)**—see code **"C"**
Ritalin SR Tablet **(SR)**
Rythmol SR Capsule **(SR)**
Sensipar Tablet
Seroquel XR Tablet **(SR)**
Sinemet CR Tablet **(SR)**—see code **"B"**
Slo-Niacin Tablet **(SR)**—see code **"B"**
Solodyn Tablet **(SR)**
Sprycel Tablet—see code **"F"**
Straterra Capsule **(contents can cause ocular irritation)**
Sudafed 12-Hour Tablet Capsule **(SR)**
Sudafed 24-Hour Capsule **(SR)**
Sular Tablet **(SR)**
Symax Duotab Tablet **(SR)**
Symax SR Tablet **(SR)**
Tasigna Capsule **(Altering tablet may cause ↑ toxicity)**
Taztia XT Capsule **(SR)**—see code **"C"**
Tecfidera Capsule
Tegretol-XR Tablet **(SR)**—see code **"A"**
Temodar Capsule **(MMI)**
Tessalon Perles Capsule **(chewing or crushing may cause local anesthesia of mucous membranes which could lead to choking)**
Theo-24 Capsule **(SR)**
Theochron Tablet **(SR)**
Tiazac Capsule **(SR)**—see code **"C"**
Topamax Tablet, Capsule **(crushing, breaking or chewing tablet can leave bitter taste)**—see code **"C"**
Toprol XL Tablet **(SR)**—see code **"B"**
Toviaz Tablet **(SR)**
Traceleer Tablet—see code **"F"**
Trental Tablet **(SR)**
Treximet Tablet **(chewing, crushing, or breaking may cause rapid absorption)**
Trilipix Capsule **(SR)**
Tylenol Arthritis Tablet **(SR)**
Uceris Tablet **(SR)**
Ultram ER Tablet **(SR) (crushing could cause overdose)**
Ultresa Capsule **(SR)**—see code **"C"**
Uniphyl Tablet **(SR)**
Urocit-K Tablet **(wax coated to prevent upper GI disease)**
Uroxatral Tablet **(SR)**
Valcyte Tablet—see codes **"A," "F"**
Verapamil SR Tablet **(SR)**—see code **"B"**
Verelan Capsule **(SR)**—see code **"C"**
Verelan PM Capsule **(SR)**—see code **"C"**
Vesicare Tablet **(film-coated)**
Videx EC Capsule **(SR)**
Vimovo Tablet **(SR)**
Viokace Tablet **(MMI)**
Viramune XR Tablet **(SR)**—see code **"A"**
Voltaren XR Tablet **(SR)**
VoSpire ER Tablet **(SR)**
Votrient Tablet **(crushing ↑ bioavailability)**
Wellbutrin SR, XL Tablet **(SR)**
Xanax XR Tablet **(SR)**
Xarelto Tablet **(crushed tablet must be given within 4 hr)**
Xartemis XR Tablet **(SR) (crushing, chewing, or dissolving tablet could cause overdose)**
Xigduo XR Tablet **(SR)**
Zegerid OTC Capsule **(SR)**—see code **"A"**
Zenatane Capsule **(MMI)**
Zenpen Capsule **(SR)**—see code **"A"**
Zohydro ER Capsule **(SR) (crushing, chewing, or dissolving capsule could cause overdose)**
Zolinza Capsule **(MMI)**
Zortress Tablet **(MMI)**
Zyban Tablet **(SR)**
Zydelig Tablet **(film-coated)**
Zyflo CR Tablet **(SR)**

CODES:

A: Liquid forms are available
B: Tablets that are scored may be broken in half
C: Capsule can be opened—contents may be used in pudding or applesauce
D: Do not take with antacids or milk products
E: Disintegrate under the tongue—do not chew
F: Women who are of childbearing age should not handle crushed or broken tablets

TERATOGENIC REACTION:

An adverse effect to normal cellular development of an embryo or fetus.

FDA-APPROVED LIST OF GENERIC DRUG NAMES WITH TALL MAN LETTERS

Drug Name with Tall Man Letters	Confused with
acetaZOLAMIDE	acetoHEXAMIDE
acetoHEXAMIDE	acetaZOLAMIDE
buPROPion	busPIRone
busPIRone	buPROPion
chlorproMAZINE	chlorproPAMIDE
chlorproPAMIDE	chlorproMAZINE
clomiPHENE	clomiPRAMINE
clomiPRAMINE	clomiPHENE
cycloSERINE	cycloSPORINE
cycloSPORINE	cycloSERINE
DAUNOrubicin	DOXOrubicin
dimenhyDRINATE	diphenhydrAMINE
diphenhydrAMINE	dimenhyDRINATE
DOBUTamine	DOPamine
DOPamine	DOBUTamine
DOXOrubicin	DAUNOrubicin
glipiZIDE	glyBURIDE
glyBURIDE	glipiZIDE

Drug Name with Tall Man Letters	Confused with
hydrALAZINE	hydrOXYzine
hydrOXYzine	hydrALAZINE
medroxPROGESTERone	methylPREDNISolone—methylTESTOSTERone
methylPREDNISolone	medroxyPROGESTERone—methylPREDNISolone
methylTESTOSTERone	medroxyPROGESTERone—methylPREDNISolone
niCARdipine	NIFEdipine
NIFEdipine	niCARdipine
prednisoLONE	predniSONE
predniSONE	prednisoLONE
sulfADIAZINE	sulfi SOXAZOLE
sulfiSOXAZOLE	sulfADIAZINE
TOLAZamide	TOLBUTamide
TOLBUTamide	TOLAZamide
vinBLAStine	vinCRIStine
vinCRIStine	vinBLAStine

ISMP LIST OF ADDITIONAL DRUG NAMES WITH TALL MAN LETTERS

Drug Name with Tall Man Letters	Confused with
ALPRAZolam	LORazepam
aMILoride	amLODIPine
amLODIPine	aMILoride
ARIPiprazole	RABEprazole
AVINza*	INVanz*
azaCITIDine	azaTHIOprine
azaTHIOprine	azaCITIDine
carBAMazepine	OXcarbazepine
CARBOplatin	CISplatin
ceFAZolin	cefoTEtan—cefOXitin—cefTAZidime—cefTRIAXone
cefoTEtan	ceFAZolin—cefOXitin—cefTAZidime—cefTRIAXone
cefOXitin	ceFAZolin—cefoTEtan—cefTAZidime—cefTRIAXone
cefTAZidime	ceFAZolin—cefoTEtan—cefOXitin—cefTRIAXone
cefTRIAXone	ceFAZolin—cefoTEtan—cefOXitin—cefTAZidime
CeleBREX*	CeleXA*
CeleXA*	CeleBREX*
chlordiazePOXIDE	chlorproMAZINE
chlorproMAZINE	chlordiazePOXIDE
CISplatin	CARBOplatin

Drug Name with Tall Man Letters	Confused with
clonazePAM	cloNIDine—cloZAPine—LORazepam
cloNIDine	clonazePAM—cloZAPine—KlonoPIN*
cloZAPine	clonazePAM —cloNIDine
DACTINomycin	DAPTOmycin
DAPTOmycin	DACTINomycin
DOCEtaxel	PACLitaxel
DOXOrubicin	IDArubicin
DULoxetine	FLUoxetine—PARoxetine
ePHEDrine	EPINEPHrine
EPINEPHrine	ePHEDrine
fentaNYL	SUFentanil
flavoxATE	fluvoxaMINE
FLUoxetine	DULoxetine—PARoxetine
fluPHENAZine	fluvoxaMINE
fluvoxaMINE	fluPHENAZine—flavoxATE
guaiFENesin	guanFACINE
guanFACINE	guaiFENesin
HumaLOG*	HumuLIN*
HumuLIN*	HumaLOG*
HYDROcodone	oxyCODONE
HYDROmorphone	morphine

*Brand names always start with an upper case letter. Some brand names incorporate tall man letters in initial characters and may not be readily recognized as brand names. An asterisk follows all brand names in IMSP List of Additional Drug Names with Tall Man Letters.

 Report actual and potential medication errors to the Medication Errors Reporting Program (MERP) via the Web at www.ismp.org or by calling 1 -800- FAIL- SAF(E).

ISMP LIST OF ADDITIONAL DRUG NAMES WITH TALL MAN LETTERS continued

Drug Name with Tall Man Letters	Confused with
IDArubicin	**DOXO**rubicin
in**FLIX**imab	ri**TUX**imab
INVanz*	**AVIN**za*
ISOtretinoin	tretinoin
Klono**PIN***	clo**NID**ine
La**MIC**tal*	Lam**ISIL***
Lam**ISIL***	La**MIC**tal*
lami**VUD**ine	lamo**TRI**gine
lamo**TRI**gine	lami**VUD**ine
lev**ETIRA**cetam	lev**OCARN**itine
lev**OCARN**itine	lev**ETIRA**cetam
LORazepam	**ALPRAZ**olam—clonaze**PAM**
met**FORMIN**	metro**NIDAZOLE**
metro**NIDAZOLE**	met**FORMIN**
mito**MY**cin	mito**XAN**trone
mito**XAN**trone	mito**MY**cin
Nex**AVAR***	Nex**IUM***
Nex**IUM***	Nex**AVAR***
ni**CAR**dipine	ni**MOD**ipine—**NIFE**dipine
NIFEdipine	ni**MOD**ipine—ni**CAR**dipine
ni**MOD**ipine	**NIFE**dipine—ni**CAR**dipine
Novo**LIN***	Novo**LOG***
Novo**LOG***	Novo**LIN***
OLANZapine	**QUE**tiapine
OXcarbazepine	car**BAM**azepine
oxy**CODONE**	**HYDRO**codone—Oxy**CONTIN***
Oxy**CONTIN***	oxy**CODONE**
PACLitaxel	**DOCE**taxel
PARoxetine	**FLU**oxetine — **DUL**oxetine
PEMEtrexed	**PRALA**trexate
PENTobarbital	**PHEN**obarbital
PHENobarbital	**PENT**obarbital
PRALAtrexate	**PEME**trexed
Pri**LOSEC***	**PRO**zac*

Drug Name with Tall Man Letters	Confused with
PROzac*	Pri**LOSEC***
QUEtiapine	**OLANZ**apine
qui**NID**ine	qui**NINE**
qui**NINE**	qui**NID**ine
RABEprazole	**ARIP**iprazole
Risper**DAL***	r**OPINIR**ole
risperi**DONE**	r**OPINIR**ole
ri**TUX**imab	in**FLIX**imab
romi**DEP**sin	romi**PLOS**tim
romi**PLOS**tim	romi**DEP**sin
r**OPINIR**ole	Risper**DAL***— risperi**DONE**
Sand**IMMUNE***	Sando**STATIN***
Sando**STATIN***	Sand**IMMUNE***
SEROquel*	**SINE**quan*
SINEquan*	**SERO**quel*
sita**GLIP**tin	**SUMA**triptan
Solu—**CORTEF***	Solu—**MEDROL***
Solu—**MEDROL***	Solu—**CORTEF***
SORAfenib	**SUNI**tinib
SUFentanil	fenta**NYL**
sulf**ADIAZINE**	sulfa**SALA**zine
sulfa**SALA**zine	sulf**ADIAZINE**
SUMAtriptan	sita**GLIP**tin—**ZOLM**itriptan
SUNItinib	**SORA**fenib
TEGretol*	**TREN**tal*
tia**GAB**ine	ti**ZAN**idine
ti**ZAN**idine	tia**GAB**ine
tra**MAD**ol	tra**ZOD**one
tra**ZOD**one	tra**MAD**ol
TRENtal*	**TEG**retol*
val**ACY**clovir	val**GAN**ciclovir
val**GAN**ciclovir	val**ACY**clovir
ZOLMitriptan	**SUMA**triptan
Zy**PREXA***	Zyr**TEC***
Zyr**TEC***	Zy**PREXA***

*Brand names always start with an upper case letter. Some brand names incorporate tall man letters in initial characters and may not be readily recognized as brand names. An asterisk follows all brand names in IMSP List of Additional Drug Names with Tall Man Letters.

APPENDICES

APPENDIX A

Recent Drug Approvals

To view full-text monographs of drugs that have been recently released from the FDA or to learn about changes to dosage forms, please visit www.DrugGuide.com.

alectinib (al-ek-ti-nib)

Alecensa

Classification
Therapeutic: antineoplastics
Pharmacologic: kinase inhibitors

Indications

Patients with metastatic non-small cell lung cancer (NSCLC) that is positive for anaplastic lymphoma kinase (ALK) who have progressed on or are intolerant to crizotinib.

Contraindications/Precautions

Contraindicated in: OB: May cause fetal harm; Lactation: Breast feeding should be avoided during treatment and for 1 wk after therapy.
Use Cautiously in: Severe renal impairment (CCr <30 mL/min); Moderate or severe hepatic impairment; Rep: Patients with childbearing potential; Pedi: Safety and effectiveness not established.

Adverse Reactions/Side Effects

CNS: fatigue, headache. **CV:** bradycardia, edema. **Derm:** photosensitivity, rash. **EENT:** blurred vision, diplopia. **Endo:** hyperglycemia. **F and E:** hypocalcemia, hypokalemia, hyponatremia, hypophosphatemia. **GI:** HEPATOTOXICITY, constipation, diarrhea, hyperbilirubinemia, nausea, vomiting, vomiting. **GU:** ↑ serum creatinine. **Hemat:** HEMORRHAGE, anemia, lymphopenia. **Metab:** ↑ weight. **MS:** ↑ creatine kinase, back pain, myalgia. **Resp:** INTERSTITIAL LUNG DISEASE, PULMONARY EMBOLISM, cough, dyspnea.

Route/Dosage

PO (Adults): 600 mg twice daily with food; dose adjusted according to tolerance, toxicity or adverse effects.

cobimetinib (koe-bi-me-ti-nib)

Cotellic

Classification
Therapeutic: antineoplastics
Pharmacologic: kinase inhibitors

Indications

Treatment of metastatic/unresectable melanoma with the BRAF V600E or V600K mutation (in combination with vemurafenib).

Contraindications/Precautions

Contraindicated in: Concurrent use of strong or moderate CYP3A4 inhibitors or inducers; OB: May cause fetal harm; Lactation: Breast feeding should be avoided during treatment and for 2 wk after therapy.
Use Cautiously in: Left ventricular ejection fraction <50%; Severe renal impairment (CCr <30 mL/min); Moderate or severe hepatic impairment; Rep: Patients with childbearing potential; Pedi: Safety and effectiveness not established.

Adverse Reactions/Side Effects

CV: CARDIOMYOPATHY, hypertension. **Derm:** alopecia, erythema, photosensitivity, rash. **EENT:** retinopathy. **F and E:** hyperkalemia, hypocalcemia, hypokalemia, hyponatremia, hypophosphatemia. **GI:** HEPATOTOXICITY, diarrhea, hypoalbuminemia, nausea, stomatitis, vomiting. **GU:** ↑ serum creatinine. **Hemat:** HEMORRHAGE, anemia, lymphopenia, thrombocytopenia. **MS:** RHABDOMYOLYSIS. **Misc:** MALIGNANCY, fever.

Route/Dosage

PO (Adults): 60 mg once daily for days 1–21 of each 28-day cycle; continue until disease progression or unacceptable toxic; *Concurrent short-term use of moderate CYP3A4 inhibitor*—20 mg once daily; resume 60 mg once daily once 3A4 inhibitor discontinued (avoid use of strong or moderate CYP3A4 inhibitor if patient already taking reduced dose of 20–40 mg once daily).

ivacaftor/lumacaftor

(**eye**-va-**kaf**-tor/loo-ma-**kaf**-tor)
Orkambi

Classification
Therapeutic: cystic fibrosis therapy adjuncts
Pharmacologic: transmembrane conductance regulator potentiators

Indications

Treatment of cystic fibrosis (CF) in patients ≥12 yr who are homozygous for the *F508del* mutation in the *CFTR* gene.

Contraindications/Precautions

Contraindicated in: Concurrent use of strong CYP3A inducers; Concurrent use of sensitive CYP3A substrates or those with a narrow therapeutic index.
Use Cautiously in: Concurrent use of CYP3A inhibitors; Moderate or severe hepatic impairment (dose ↓ recommended); Severe renal impairment (CCr <30 mL/min) or end stage renal disease; OB: Use in pregnancy only if clearly needed; Lactation: Use cautiously during breast feeding; Pedi: Children <12 yr (safety and effectiveness not established).

Adverse Reactions/Side Effects

CNS: fatigue. **Derm:** rash. **EENT:** cataracts, rhinorrhea. **GI:** diarrhea, nausea, flatulence, ↑ bilirubin, ↑ liver enzymes. **GU:** amenorrhea, dysmenorrhea, menorrhagia. **MS:** ↑ creatine kinase. **Resp:** dyspnea, chest discomfort.

Route/Dosage

PO (Adults and Children ≥12 yr): 2 tablets q 12 h with fat-containing food; *Initiation of therapy in patients receiving strong CYP3A inhibitor*—1 tablet once daily for 1 wk, then ↑ to 2 tablets q12h.

Hepatic Impairment

PO (Adults and Children ≥12 yr): *Moderate hepatic impairment (Child-Pugh Class B)*—2 tablets in AM and 1 tablet in PM; *Severe hepatic impairment (Child-Pugh Class C)*—1 tablet in AM and 1 tablet in PM.

ixazomib (ix-**az**-oh-mib)

Ninlaro

Classification
Therapeutic: antineoplastics
Pharmacologic: proteasome inhibitors

Indications

Treatment of multiple myeloma in patients whose disease has relapsed despite receiving ≥1 previous drug therapy (in combination with lenalidomide and dexamethasone).

Contraindications/Precautions

Contraindicated in: Concurrent use of strong CYP3A inducers; OB: Pregnancy (may cause fetal harm); Lactation: Breast feeding should be avoided.
Use Cautiously in: Moderate or severe hepatic impairment (↓ dose recommended); Severe renal impairment or end stage renal disease (↓ dose recommended); Rep: Patients with childbearing potential; Pedi: Safety and effectiveness not established.

Adverse Reactions/Side Effects

CV: edema. **Derm:** rash. **EENT:** blurred vision, conjunctivitis, dry eye. **GI:** HEPATOTOXICITY, constipation, diarrhea, nausea, vomiting. **Hemat:** NEUTROPENIA, THROMBOCYTOPENIA. **MS:** back pain. **Neuro:** peripheral neuropathy.

Route/Dosage

PO (Adults): 4 mg once per wk on Days 1, 8, and 15 of a 28-day treatment cycle.

Renal Impairment

(Adults): *CCr <30 mL/min or requiring dialysis*—3 mg once per wk on Days 1, 8, and 15 of a 28-day treatment cycle.

Hepatic Impairment

(Adults): *Moderate or severe hepatic impairment (total bilirubin >1.5xULN)*—3 mg once per wk on Days 1, 8, and 15 of a 28-day treatment cycle.

necitumumab

(ne-si-**toom**-oo-mab)
Portrazza

Classification
Therapeutic: antineoplastics
Pharmacologic: epidermal growth factor receptor (EGFR) inhibitors monoclonal antibodies

Indications

First-line treatment of metastatic, squamous non-small cell lung cancer (NSCLC) (in combination with gemcitabine and cisplatin).

Contraindications/Precautions

Contraindicated in: Non-squamous NSCLC (↑ mortality and ↑ toxicity); OB: May cause fetal harm; Lactation: Breast feeding should be avoided during treatment and for 3 mo after therapy.
Use Cautiously in: History of thromboembolism; Electrolyte abnormalities (correct before initiating therapy); Rep: Patients with childbearing potential; Pedi: Safety not established.

Adverse Reactions/Side Effects

CNS: headache. **CV:** SUDDEN CARDIAC DEATH, THROMBOEMBOLIC EVENTS. **Derm:** dermatitis acneiform, rash, acne, dry skin, erythema, pruritis, skin fissures. **F and E:** hypocalcemia, hypokalemia, hypomagnesemia, hypophosphatemia. **GI:** diarrhea, stomatitis, vomiting, dysphagia. **Metab:** ↓ weight. **MS:** muscle spasms. **Resp:** hemoptysis. **Misc:** INFUSION REACTIONS.

Route/Dosage

IV (Adults): 800 mg as a 60-min infusion on Days 1 and 8 of each 3-wk cycle prior to gemcitabine and cisplatin infusion; continue until disease progression or unacceptable toxicity.

osimertinib

(oh-si-**mer**-ti-nib)
Tagrisso

Classification
Therapeutic: antineoplastics
Pharmacologic: epidermal growth factor receptor (EGFR) inhibitors

Indications

Treatment of metastatic epidermal growth factor receptor (EGFR) T790M mutation-positive non–small-cell lung cancer (NSCLC) in patients who have progressed on or after EGFR tyrosine kinase inhibitor therapy.

Contraindications/Precautions

Contraindicated in: Concurrent use of strong CYP3A4 inhibitors or inducers; OB: May cause fetal harm; Lactation: Breast feeding should be avoided during treatment and for 2 wk after therapy.
Use Cautiously in: Congenital long QT syndrome, HF, electrolyte abnormalities, or taking QT interval prolonging medications; Severe renal impairment or end-stage renal disease; Moderate or severe hepatic impairment; Rep: Patients with childbearing potential; Pedi: Safety and effectiveness not established.

Adverse Reactions/Side Effects

CNS: STROKE, fatigue, headache. **CV:** CARDIOMYOPATHY, QT INTERVAL PROLONGATION, VENOUS THROMBOEMBOLISM. **Derm:** dry skin, nail disorders, pruritis, rash. **EENT:** blepharitis, blurred vision, cataracts, dry eye, eye pain, ↑ lacrimation, keratitis. **F and E:** hypermagnesemia, hyponatremia. **GI:** constipation, ↓ appetite, diarrhea, nausea, stomatitis. **Hemat:** NEUTROPENIA, THROMBOCYTOPENIA, anemia, lymphopenia. **MS:** back pain. **Resp:** INTERSTITIAL LUNG DISEASE, cough.

Route/Dosage

PO (Adults): 80 mg once daily; continued until disease progression or unacceptable toxicity.

sonidegib (soe-ni-**deg**-ib)
Odomzo

Classification
Therapeutic: antineoplastics
Pharmacologic: hedgehog pathway inhibitors

Indications
Treatment of locally advanced basal cell carcinoma (BCC) that had recurred despite surgery or radiation therapy or for use in those who are not candidates for surgery or radiation.

Contraindications/Precautions
Contraindicated in: Patients with reproductive potential (females are required to have negative pregnancy testing and use effective contraception during and for 20 mo after; males must use condoms during and for 8 mo following treatment); Blood donation should be avoided during and for 20 mo following treatment; Concurrent strong CYP3A inhibitors or prolonged (>14 days) use of moderate inhibitors; Concurrent use of strong or moderate CYP3A inducers; OB: Pregnancy (sonidegib is a embryotoxic, fetotoxic and teratogenic); Lactation: Breast feeding should be avoided during and for 20 mo following treatment.
Use Cautiously in: Moderate to severe hepatic impairment; Geri: ↑ risk of adverse reactions in patients ≥65 years; Pedi: Safe and effective use in children has not been established.

Adverse Reactions/Side Effects
CNS: fatigue, headache. **GI:** abdominal pain, ↓ appetite, diarrhea, dysgeusia, ↑ liver enzymes, nausea, vomiting. **GU:** ↑ creatinine. **Derm:** alopecia, pruritus. **Endo:** hyperglycemia, amenorrhea. **Hemat:** anemia, lymphopenia. **Metab:** ↓ weight. **MS:** ↑ CK, muscle spasms, musculoskeletal pain, myalgia, rhabdomyolysis. **Misc:** generalized pain.

Route/Dosage
PO (Adults): 200 mg once daily; alteration in dose required for adverse musculoskeletal reactions and ↑ creatine kinase (CK).

sugammadex (soo-**gam**-ma-dex)
Bridion

Classification
Therapeutic: antidotes

Indications
Reversal of neuromuscular blockade induced by rocuronium or vecuronium in adults undergoing surgery.

Contraindications/Precautions
Contraindicated in: Hypersensitivity; Severe renal impairment or end-stage renal disease.
Use Cautiously in: Patients with coagulopathies or being treated with anticoagulants; OB, Lactation: Pregnancy or lactation; Rep: Patients with childbearing potential (may ↓ efficacy of hormonal contraception); Pedi: Safety and effectiveness not established.

Adverse Reactions/Side Effects
CNS: headache. **CV:** bradycardia, hypotension. **GI:** nausea, vomiting. **Hemat:** ↑ activated partial thromboplastin time (aPTT), ↑ prothrombin time (PT)/international normalized ratio (INR). **Misc:** ANAPHYLAXIS.

Route/Dosage
Following sugammadex use, wait 24 hr before readministering rocuronium or vecuronium. If more immediate neuromuscular blockade is needed, a nonsteroidal neuromuscular-blocking agent (e.g. succinylcholine) may be required.

Routine Reversal of Rocuronium- or Vecuronium-Induced Blockade
IV (Adults): *Deep block (if spontaneous recovery of twitch response has reached 1–2 post-tetanic counts and there are no twitch responses to train-of-four [TOF] stimulation)*—4 mg/kg as single dose; *Moderate block (if spontaneous recovery has reached the reappearance of the 2nd twitch [T2] in response to TOF stimulation)*—2 mg/kg as single dose.

Immediate Reversal of Rocuronium-Induced Blockade
IV (Adults): 16 mg/kg as single dose administered soon (3 min) after administration of a single dose of 1.2 mg/kg of rocuronium.

trifluridine/tipiracil

(tri-**floo**-ri-deen/ti-**peer**-a-sil)
Lonsurf

Classification
Therapeutic: antineoplastics
Pharmacologic: nucleoside metabolic inhibitorsthymidine phosphorylase inhibitors

Indications

Metastatic colorectal cancer in patients previously treated with fluoropyrmidine-, oxalplatin- or irinotecan-based chemotherapies, an anti-VEGF based biological and an anti-EGFR agent (if RAS wild-type positive).

Contraindications/Precautions

Contraindicated in: Initial ANC <1500/mm³ or platelets <75,000/mm³, resolution of grade 3 or 4 non-hematologic toxicity to grade 0 or 1; During treatment ANC <500 mm³ or febrile neutropenia, platelets <50,000/mm³ or grade 3 or 4 non-hematologic toxicity; OB: Pregnancy should be avoided, may cause fetal harm; Lactation: Breast feeding should be avoided.

Use Cautiously in: Moderate to severe hepatic impairment/severe renal impairment (effects of drug are not known); Moderate renal impairment ↑ risk of toxicity, dose alteration may be required; Females with reproductive potential (effective contraception required); Males with female partners with reproductive potential (condom use required); Geri: ↑ risk and severity of myelosuppression in patients ≥65 yr.

Adverse Reactions/Side Effects

CNS: asthenia. **GI:** abdominal pain, ↓ appetite, diarrhea, nausea, vomiting, stomatitis. **Derm:** alopecia. **Hemat:** MYELOSUPRESSION. **Misc:** fever.

Route/Dosage

PO (Adults): 35 mg/m²/dose (based on trifluridine content rounded to the nearest 5 mg) twice daily on days 1–5 and 8–12 of each 28 day cycle (single dose should not exceed 80 mg). Dose reduction by 5 mg/dose required for hematologic and grade 3 or 4 non-hematologic toxicity.

uridine triacetate

(**ure**-i-deen trye-**as**-e-tate)
Vistogard

Classification
Therapeutic: antidotes

Indications

Emergency treatment of fluorouracil or capecitabine overdose regardless of the presence of symptoms. Emergency treatment of patients who exhibit early-onset, severe, or life-threatening cardiovascular or central nervous system toxicity, and/or early-onset, unusually severe adverse reactions within 96 hr following the end of fluorouracil or capecitabine administration.

Contraindications/Precautions

Contraindicated in: None.

Use Cautiously in: OB, Lactation: Pregnancy or lactation; Pedi: Children <1 yr (safety not established).

Adverse Reactions/Side Effects

GI: vomiting, diarrhea, nausea.

Route/Dosage

PO (Adults): 10 g every 6 hr for a total of 20 doses.

PO (Children ≥1 yr): 6.2 g/m² body surface area (max = 10 g/dose) every 6 hr for total of 20 doses.

NEW DOSAGE FORMS

Generic Name (Brand Name)	New Dosage Form
amphetamine (Dyanavel XR)	Extended-release oral suspension for the treatment of Attention Deficit Hyperactivity Disorder (ADHD).
antihemophilic factor (recombinant) pegylated (Adynovate)	Control/prevention of bleeding associated with hemophilia A (pegylation increases half-life of the factor).
aripiprazole (Aristada)	Extended-release injectable for schizophrenia.
buprenorphine (Belbuca)	Buccal film for the management of chronic pain.
glycopyrrolate (Seebri)	Long-term maintenance inhaler treatment of airflow obstruction in patients with chronic obstructive pulmonary disease (COPD).
influenza vaccine, adjuvanted (Fluad)	Contains an adjuvant to improve immune response in elderly.
irinotecan (Onivyde)	Liposomal Injection for the treatment of post-gemcitabine metastatic adenocarcinoma of the pancreas.
levetiracetam, Elepsia XR	Higher strength tablet for partial onset seizures.
levetiracetam (Spritam)	Tablets manufactured by 3D printing.
meloxicam (Vivlodex)	Low dose once daily capsules for the management of osteoarthritis pain.
methylphenidate (Aptensio XR)	Extended-release capsule formulation for ADHD.
methylphenidate (QuilliChew ER)	Extended-release chewable formulation for ADHD.
morphine (MorphaBond)	Extended-release, abuse-deterrent dose form for treatment of severe pain requiring daily, around-the-clock, long-term opioids.

New Combinations

Generic Name (Brand Name)	Indications
betamethasone/calcipotriene (Enstilar)	Topical foam formulation for treatment of psoriasis vulgaris.
empagliflozin/metformin (Synjardy)	Combination SLGT2 and metformin tablet for type 2 diabetes.
indacaterol/glycopyrrolate (Utibron)	Long-term maintenance inhaler treatment of airflow obstruction due to COPD.
perindopril/amlodipine (Prestalia)	Combination ACEi and calcium channel blocker tablet for hypertension.

RECENT LABELING CHANGES (New Warnings/Indications)

Generic Name (Brand Name)	Labeling Change
ambrisentan (Letairis)	Can be used in combination with tadalafil for Pulmonary Arterial Hypertension (WHO Group 1).
adalimumab (Humira)	Expanded indication for moderate to severe Hidradenitis Suppurativa.
clozaril (Clozaril, FazaClo, Versacloz)	Changes in monitoring, prescribing, dispensing, and receiving related to risk of severe neutropenia.
DPP-4 INHIBITORS alogliptin (Nisena), **linagliptin** (Tradjenta), **saxagliptin** (Onglyza), **sitagliptin**, (Januvia)	May cause severe/disabling joint pain.
eltrombopag (Promacta)	Expanded indication for children 2–5 yr.
interferon beta-1b (Betaseron)	New dosage regimen using Betaconnect Electronic Autoinjector.
ipilimumab (Yervoy)	Indication expanded to include ↓ risk of melanoma recurrence following surgery.
nivolumab (Opdivo)	Warnings expanded to include autoimmune encephalitis, toxic-epidermal necrolysis and Stevens-Johnson syndrome; New dosage regimen with ipilimumab in BRAF V600 Wild-Type Melanoma; Expanded indication to include advanced lung cancer.
ombitasvir/paritaprevir/ ritonavir (Technivie)	Risk of serious liver toxicity.
ombitasvir/paritaprevir/ ritonavir/dasabuvir (Viekira Pak)	Risk of serious liver toxicity.
oxycodone (Oxycontin)	Management of severe pain requiring daily, around-the-clock, long-term opioids.
pembrolizumab (Keytruda)	Expanded indication includes advanced Non-Small Cell Lung Cancer (NSCLC).
ticagrelor (Brilinta) MIM	Expanded indication includes long-term use in patients with a history of MI.
tiotropium (Spiriva Respimat)	Expanded indication for maintenance treatment of asthma in adults and adolescents.
tramadol (Ultram)	Rare ↑ risk of respiratory depression in children especially after tonsillectomy/ adenoidectomy.

OTHER NEW DRUGS

Generic Name (Brand Name)	Indication(s)
alectinib (Alcensa)	Treatment of ALK-positive, locally advanced/metastatic/progressive non-small cell lung cancer (NSCLC) despite treatment with/intolerance to crizotinib.
asfotase alfa (Strensiq)	Perinatal/infantile- and juvenile-onset hypophosphatasia (HPP).
coagulation factor X (human) (Coagadex)	Treatment of hereditary factor X deficiency.
cobimetinib (Cotellic)	With vemurafenib for the treatment of advanced melanoma with a BRAF V600E or V600K mutation.
dichlorphenamide (Keveyis)	Primary hyperkalemic periodic paralysis, primary hypokalemic periodic paralysis and variants.
deoxycholic acid (Kybella)	Improve appearance of submental fat in adults.

OTHER NEW DRUGS (continued)

Generic Name (Brand Name)	Indication(s)
daratumumab (Darzalex)	Multiple myeloma.
elotuzumab (Empliciti)	Multiple myeloma (in combination with two other therapies).
irinotecan liposome (Onivyde)	Metastatic pancreatic cancer (in combination with two other therapies) following disease progression despite gemcitabine-based therapy.
ixazomib (Ninlaro)	Multiple myeloma (in combination with lenalidomide and dexamethasone) in patients who have had at least one prior therapy.
lesinurad (Zurampic)	Combination treatment of hyperuricemia associated with gout.
lumacaftor/ivacaftor (Orkambi)	Cystic fibrosis patients >12 yr homozygous for F508del mutation.
mepolizumab (Nucala)	Add-on maintenance treatment of severe asthma in patients ≥12 years with an eosinophilic phenotype.
necitumumab (Portrazza)	With gemcitabine and cisplatin for the treatment of patients with metastatic squamous non-small cell lung cancer.
osimertinib (Tagrisso)	Metastatic EGFR T790M mutation-positive non-small cell lung cancer with progression on or after EGFR-TKI therapy.
patiromer (Veltassa)	Chronic hyperkalemia.
sebelipase alfa (Kanuma)	Lysosomal lipase deficiency.
selexipag (Uptravi)	Pulmonary hypertension.
sonidegib (Odomzo)	Locally advanced basal cell carcinoma.
sugammadex (Bridion)	Reversal of non-depolarizing muscle relaxants.
talimogene laherparepvec (Imlygic)	Melanoma in skin and lymph nodes.
trabectedin (Yondelis)	Unresectable/metastatic liposarcoma or leiomyosarcoma.
trifluridine/tipiracil (Lonsurf)	Metastatic colorectal cancer.
uridine triacetate (Xuridan)	Hereditary orotic aciduria.
von willebrand factor (recombinant) (Vonvendi)	Immediate treatment/control of bleeding in adults with von Willebrand disease.

DISCONTINUED DRUGS

Generic Name (Brand Name)	Reason for Discontinuation
acetohexamide (Dymelor)	Discontinued by manufacturer.
biperidin (Akineton)	Discontinued by manufacturer.
cefoperazone (Cefobid)	Discontinued by manufacturer.
denileukin deftitox (Ontak)	Discontinued by manufacturer.
ergonovine	Discontinued by manufacturer.
gemtuzumab ozogamicin (Mylotarg)	Discontinued by manufacturer.
hydroxyprogesterone (Delalutin) (Makena)	Discontinued by manufacturer.
interferon alfacon1 (Infergen)	Discontinued by manufacturer.

DISCONTINUED DRUGS (continued)

Generic Name (Brand Name)	Reason for Discontinuation
norfloxacin (Chibroxin) (Noroxin)	Discontinued by manufacturer.
peginesatide (Omontys)	Hypersensitivity reactions.
penbutolol (Levatol)	Discontinued by manufacturer.
phentolamine (Oraverse)	Discontinued by manufacturer.
quazepam (Doral)	Discontinued by manufacturer.
telaprevir (Incivek)	Discontinued by manufacturer.
ticarcillin clavulanate (Timentin)	Discontinued by manufacturer.
ticlopidine (Ticlid)	Discontinued by manufacturer.
tositumomab (Bexxar)	Discontinued by manufacturer.

APPENDIX B

Combination Drugs

Note: The drugs listed in this section are in alphabetical order according to trade names. If the trade name does not specify dose form, the dose form is either a tablet or capsule. Following each trade name are the generic names and doses of the active ingredients contained in each preparation. For information on these drugs, look up each generic name in the combination. For inert ingredients, see drug label. **(OTC)** signifies "over-the-counter" or nonprescription medication.

Acanya Topical Gel—1.2% clindamycin + 2.5% benzoyl peroxide
Accuretic 10/12.5—quinapril 10 mg + hydrochlorothiazide 12.5 mg
Accuretic 20/12.5—quinapril 20 mg + hydrochlorothiazide 12.5 mg
Accuretic 20/25—quinapril 20 mg + hydrochlorothiazide 25 mg
Activella 0.5/0.1—estradiol 0.5 mg + norethindrone 0.1 mg
Activella 1/0.5—estradiol 1 mg + norethindrone 0.5 mg
Actoplus Met 15/500—pioglitazone 15 mg + metformin 500 mg
Actoplus Met 15/850—pioglitazone 15 mg+ metformin 850 mg
Actoplus Met XR 15/1000—pioglitazone 15 mg + metformin extended-release 1000 mg
Actoplus Met XR 30/1000—pioglitazone 30 mg + metformin extended-release 1000 mg
Adderall XR 5 mg—dextroamphetamine saccharate 1.25 mg + dextroamphetamine sulfate 1.25 mg + amphetamine aspartate monohydrate 1.25 mg + amphetamine sulfate 1.25 mg
Adderall XR 10 mg—dextroamphetamine saccharate 2.5 mg + dextroamphetamine sulfate 2.5 mg + amphetamine aspartate monohydrate 2.5 mg + amphetamine sulfate 2.5 mg
Adderall XR 15 mg—dextroamphetamine saccharate 3.75 mg + dextroamphetamine sulfate 3.75 mg + amphetamine aspartate monohydrate 3.75 mg + amphetamine sulfate 3.75 mg
Adderall XR 20 mg—dextroamphetamine saccharate 5 mg + dextroamphetamine sulfate 5 mg + amphetamine aspartate monohydrate 5 mg + amphetamine sulfate 5 mg
Adderall XR 25 mg—dextroamphetamine saccharate 6.25 mg + dextroamphetamine sulfate 6.25 mg + amphetamine aspartate monohydrate 6.25 mg + amphetamine sulfate 6.25 mg
Adderall XR 30 mg—dextroamphetamine saccharate 7.5 mg + dextroamphetamine sulfate 7.5 mg + amphetamine aspartate monohydrate 7.5 mg + amphetamine sulfate 7.5 mg
Advair Diskus 100—(per actuation) fluticasone 100 mcg + salmeterol 50 mcg
Advair Diskus 250—(per actuation) fluticasone 250 mcg + salmeterol 50 mcg
Advair Diskus 500—(per actuation) fluticasone 500 mcg + salmeterol 50 mcg
Advair HFA 45—(per actuation) fluticasone 45 mcg + salmeterol 21 mcg
Advair HFA 115—(per actuation) fluticasone 115 mcg + salmeterol 21 mcg
Advair HFA 230—(per actuation) fluticasone 230 mcg + salmeterol 21 mcg
Advicor 500/20—extended-release niacin 500 mg + lovastatin 20 mg
Advicor 750/20—extended-release niacin 750 mg + lovastatin 20 mg
Advicor 1000/20—extended-release niacin 1000 mg + lovastatin 20 mg
Advicor 1000/40—extended-release niacin 1000 mg + lovastatin 40 mg
Advil Allergy & Congestion Relief—phenylephrine 10 mg + ibuprofen 200 mg + chlorpheniramine 4 mg **(OTC)**
Advil Allergy Sinus—pseudoephedrine 30 mg + ibuprofen 200 mg + chlorpheniramine 2 mg **(OTC)**
Advil Cold & Sinus—pseudoephedrine 30 mg + ibuprofen 200 mg **(OTC)**
Advil PM—diphenhydramine citrate 38 mg + ibuprofen 200 mg **(OTC)**
Advil PM Liquigels—diphenhydramine 25 mg + ibuprofen 200 mg **(OTC)**
Advil Sinus Congestion & Pain—phenylephrine 10 mg + ibuprofen 200 mg **(OTC)**
Aggrenox—aspirin 25 mg + extended-release dipyridamole 200 mg
Alavert Allergy and Sinus D-12—loratadine 5 mg + pseudoephedrine 120 mg **(OTC)**
Aldactazide 25/25—hydrochlorothiazide 25 mg + spironolactone 25 mg
Aldactazide 50/50—hydrochlorothiazide 50 mg + spironolactone 50 mg

Aleve-D Sinus & Cold—naproxen 220 mg + extended-release pseudoephedrine 120 mg **(OTC)**
Aleve-D Sinus & Headache—naproxen 220 mg + extended-release pseudoephedrine 120 mg **(OTC)**
Alka-Seltzer Effervescent, Original—citric acid 1000 mg + sodium bicarbonate 1916 mg + aspirin 325 mg **(OTC)**
Alka-Seltzer Effervescent, Xtra-Strength—citric acid 1000 mg + sodium bicarbonate 1985 mg + aspirin 500 mg **(OTC)**
Alka-Seltzer Plus Cold & Cough Formula Effervescent Tablets—dextromethorphan 10 mg + phenylephrine 7.8 mg + chlorpheniramine 2 mg + aspirin 325 mg **(OTC)**
Alka-Seltzer Plus Cold & Cough Liquid Gels—dextromethorphan 10 mg + phenylephrine 5 mg + chlorpheniramine 2 mg + acetaminophen 325 mg **(OTC)**
Alka-Seltzer Plus Cold Formula Effervescent Tablets—phenylephrine 7.8 mg + chlorpheniramine 2 mg + aspirin 325 mg **(OTC)**
Alka-Seltzer Plus Night Cold Formula Effervescent Tablets—dextromethorphan 10 mg + phenylephrine 7.8 mg + doxylamine 6.25 mg + aspirin 500 mg **(OTC)**
Alka-Seltzer Plus-D Multi-Symptom Sinus & Cold Liquid Gels—dextromethorphan 10 mg + pseudoephedrine 30 mg + chlorpheniramine 2 mg + acetaminophen 325 mg **(OTC)**
Alka-Seltzer Plus Day Non-Drowsy Cold & Flu Formula Liquid Gels—dextromethorphan 10 mg + phenylephrine 5 mg + acetaminophen 325 mg **(OTC)**
Alka-Seltzer Plus Day Severe Cold & Flu—dextromethorphan 20 mg + phenylephrine 10 mg + acetaminophen 500 mg + guaifenesin 400 mg **(OTC)**
Alka-Seltzer Plus Night Cold & Flu Formula Liquid Gels—acetaminophen 325 mg + doxylamine 6.25 mg + dextromethorphan 10 mg + phenylephrine 5 mg **(OTC)**
Alka-Seltzer Plus Severe Cold & Cough Night Liquid—(per 30 mL) dextromethorphan 30 mg + doxylamine 12.5 mg + acetaminophen 650 mg **(OTC)**
Alka-Seltzer Plus Severe Cold & Flu Formula Effervescent Tablets—dextromethorphan 10 mg + phenylephrine 5 mg + chlorpheniramine 2 mg + acetaminophen 250 mg **(OTC)**
Alka-Seltzer Plus Severe Cough, Mucus, & Congestion Liquid Gels—dextromethorphan 10 mg + phenylephrine 5 mg + acetaminophen 250 mg + guaifenesin 200 mg **(OTC)**
Alka-Seltzer Plus Severe Sinus Cold & Cough Liquid Gels—dextromethorphan 10 mg + phenylephrine 5 mg + acetaminophen 250 mg + guaifenesin 200 mg **(OTC)**
Alka-Seltzer Plus Severe Sinus Congestion, Allergy, & Cough Liquid Gels—acetaminophen 325 mg + doxylamine 6.25 mg + dextromethorphan 10 mg + phenylephrine 5 mg **(OTC)**
Alka-Seltzer Plus Severe Sinus Congestion & Cough Liquid Gels—acetaminophen 325 mg + dextromethorphan 10 mg + phenylephrine 5 mg **(OTC)**
Allegra-D 12 Hour—fexofenadine 60 mg + extended-release pseudoephedrine 120 mg
Allegra-D 24 Hour—fexofenadine 180 mg + extended-release pseudoephedrine 240 mg
Altavera—levonorgestrel 0.15 mg + ethinyl estradiol 30 mcg
Alyacen 1/35—norethindrone 1 mg + ethinyl estradiol 35 mcg
Alyacen 7/7/7
  Phase I—norethindrone 0.5 mg + ethinyl estradiol 35 mcg
  Phase II—norethindrone 0.75 mg + ethinyl estradiol 35 mcg
  Phase III—norethindrone 1 mg + ethinyl estradiol 35 mcg
Amethia—levonorgestrel 0.15 mg + ethinyl estradiol 30 mcg
Amethia Lo—levonorgestrel 0.1 mg + ethinyl estradiol 20 mcg
Amethyst—levonorgestrel 0.09 mg + ethinyl estradiol 20 mcg
Amturnide 150/5/12.5—aliskiren 150 mg + amlodipine 5 mg + hydrochlorothiazide 12.5 mg
Amturnide 300/5/12.5—aliskiren 300 mg + amlodipine 5 mg + hydrochlorothiazide 12.5 mg
Amturnide 300/5/25—aliskiren 300 mg + amlodipine 5 mg + hydrochlorothiazide 25 mg
Amturnide 300/10/12.5—aliskiren 300 mg + amlodipine 10 mg + hydrochlorothiazide 12.5 mg
Amturnide 300/10/25—aliskiren 300 mg + amlodipine 10 mg + hydrochlorothiazide 25 mg
Anacin—aspirin 400 mg + caffeine 32 mg **(OTC)**
Anacin Max Strength—aspirin 500 mg + caffeine 32 mg **(OTC)**
Analpram HC Topical Cream 1/1—1% hydrocortisone + 1% pramoxine
Analpram HC Topical Cream/Lotion 2.5/1—2.5% hydrocortisone + 1% pramoxine
Anexsia 5/325—hydrocodone 5 mg + acetaminophen 325 mg
Anexsia 7.5/325—hydrocodone 7.5 mg + acetaminophen 325 mg
Angeliq 0.25/0.5—drospirenone 0.25 mg + estradiol 0.5 mg
Angeliq 0.5/1—drospirenone 0.5 mg + estradiol 1 mg
Apri-28—desogestrel 0.15 mg + ethinyl estradiol 30 mcg

Aranelle

Phase I—norethindrone 0.5 mg + ethinyl estradiol 35 mcg
Phase II—norethindrone 1 mg + ethinyl estradiol 35 mcg
Phase III—norethindrone 0.5 mg + ethinyl estradiol 35 mcg

Arthrotec 50/200—diclofenac 50 mg + misoprostol 200 mcg
Arthrotec 75/200—diclofenac 75 mg + misoprostol 200 mcg
Ashlyna—levonorgestrel 0.15 mg + ethinyl estradiol 30 mcg/10 mcg
Atacand HCT 16/12.5—candesartan 16 mg + hydrochlorothiazide 12.5 mg
Atacand HCT 32/12.5—candesartan 32 mg + hydrochlorothiazide 12.5 mg
Atacand HCT 32/25—candesartan 32 mg + hydrochlorothiazide 25 mg
🍁 **Atacand Plus**—candesartan 16 mg + hydrochlorothiazide 12.5 mg
🍁 **Atacand Plus**—candesartan 32 mg + hydrochlorothiazide 12.5 mg
🍁 **Atacand Plus**—candesartan 32 mg + hydrochlorothiazide 25 mg
Atripla—efavirenz 600 mg + emtricitabine 200 mg + tenofovir 300 mg
Aubra—levonorgestrel 0.1 mg + ethinyl estradiol 20 mcg
Avalide 150/12.5—irbesartan 150 mg + hydrochlorothiazide 12.5 mg
Avalide 300/12.5—irbesartan 300 mg + hydrochlorothiazide 12.5 mg
Aviane-28—levonorgestrel 0.1 mg + ethinyl estradiol 20 mcg
Azor 5/20—amlodipine 5 mg + olmesartan 20 mg
Azor 5/40—amlodipine 5 mg + olmesartan 40 mg
Azor 10/20—amlodipine 10 mg + olmesartan 20 mg
Azor 10/40—amlodipine 10 mg + olmesartan 40 mg
Azurette—desogestrel 0.15 mg + ethinyl estradiol 20 mcg/10 mcg
Balziva-28—norethindrone 0.4 mg + ethinyl estradiol 35 mcg
Bayer Back & Body—aspirin 500 mg + caffeine 32.5 mg **(OTC)**
Bekyree—desogestrel 0.15 mg + ethinyl estradiol 20 mcg/10 mcg
Benicar HCT 20/12.5—olmesartan 20 mg + hydrochlorothiazide 12.5 mg
Benicar HCT 40/12.5—olmesartan 40 mg + hydrochlorothiazide 12.5 mg
Benicar HCT 40/25—olmesartan 40 mg + hydrochlorothiazide 25 mg
BenzaClin Topical Gel—1% clindamycin + 5% benzoyl peroxide
Benzamycin Topical Gel—5% benzoyl peroxide + 3% erythromycin

Beyaz

Phase I—drospirenone 3 mg + ethinyl estradiol 20 mcg + levomefolate 0.451 mg
Phase II—levomefolate 0.451 mg

Bicitra Solution—(per 5 ml) sodium citrate 500 mg + citric acid 334 mg
Bidil—isosorbide dinitrate 20 mg + hydralazine 37.5 mg
Blephamide Ophthalmic Suspension/Ointment—0.2% prednisolone + 10% sodium sulfacetamide
Breo Ellipta—(per blister for inhalation) fluticasone 100 mcg + vilanterol 25 mcg
Brevicon-28—norethindrone 0.5 mg + ethinyl estradiol 35 mcg
Briellyn—norethindrone 0.4 mg + ethinyl estradiol 35 mcg
Bromfed DM Liquid—(per 5 mL) brompheniramine 2 mg + dextromethorphan 10 mg + pseudoephedrine 30 mg
Bronkaid Dual Action—ephedrine 25 mg + guaifenesin 400 mg **(OTC)**
Bufferin—aspirin 325 mg + calcium carbonate 158 mg + magnesium oxide 63 mg + magnesium carbonate 34 mg **(OTC)**
Bunavail 2.1/0.3—buprenorphine 2.1 mg + naloxone 0.3 mg
Bunavail 4.2/0.7—buprenorphine 4.2 mg + naloxone 0.7 mg
Bunavail 6.3/1—buprenorphine 6.3 mg + naloxone 1 mg
Caduet 2.5/10—amlodipine 2.5 mg + atorvastatin 10 mg
Caduet 2.5/20—amlodipine 2.5 mg + atorvastatin 20 mg
Caduet 2.5/40—amlodipine 2.5 mg + atorvastatin 40 mg
Caduet 5/10—amlodipine 5 mg + atorvastatin 10 mg
Caduet 5/20—amlodipine 5 mg + atorvastatin 20 mg
Caduet 5/40—amlodipine 5 mg + atorvastatin 40 mg
Caduet 5/80—amlodipine 5 mg + atorvastatin 80 mg
Caduet 10/10—amlodipine 10 mg + atorvastatin 10 mg
Caduet 10/20—amlodipine 10 mg + atorvastatin 20 mg
Caduet 10/40—amlodipine 10 mg + atorvastatin 40 mg
Caduet 10/80—amlodipine 10 mg + atorvastatin 80 mg
Cafergot—ergotamine 1 mg + caffeine 100 mg

Caltrate 600+D$_3$—vitamin D 800 IU + calcium 600 mg **(OTC)**
Camrese—levonorgestrel 0.15 mg + ethinyl estradiol 30 mcg/10 mcg
Camrese Lo—levonorgestrel 0.1 mg + ethinyl estradiol 20 mcg
Caziant
Phase I—desogestrel 0.1 mg + ethinyl estradiol 25 mcg
Phase II—desogestrel 0.125 mg + ethinyl estradiol 25 mcg
Phase III—desogestrel 0.15 mg + ethinyl estradiol 25 mcg
Cetacaine Topical Spray—14% benzocaine + 2% tetracaine + 2% butamben + 0.005% cetyl dimethyl ethyl ammonium bromide
Chateal—levonorgestrel 0.15 mg + ethinyl estradiol 30 mcg
Ciprodex Otic Suspension—0.3% ciprofloxacin + 0.1% dexamethasone
Cipro HC Otic Suspension—0.2% ciprofloxacin + 1% hydrocortisone
Clarinex-D 12 Hour—desloratadine 2.5 mg + pseudoephedrine 120 mg
Clarinex-D 24 Hour—desloratadine 5 mg + pseudoephedrine 240 mg
Claritin-D 12 Hour—loratadine 5 mg + pseudoephedrine 120 mg **(OTC)**
Claritin-D 24-Hour—loratadine 10 mg + pseudoephedrine 240 mg **(OTC)**
Climara Pro Transdermal Patch (release per day)—estradiol 0.045 mg + levonorgestrel 0.015 mg
Clorpres 15/0.1—chlorthalidone 15 mg + clonidine 0.1 mg
Clorpres 15/0.2—chlorthalidone 15 mg + clonidine 0.2 mg
Clorpres 15/0.3—chlorthalidone 15 mg + clonidine 0.3 mg
Col-Probenecid—probenecid 500 mg + colchicine 0.5 mg
Coly-Mycin S Otic Suspension—1% hydrocortisone + 0.33% neomycin base + 0.3% colistin + 0.05% thonzonium bromide
Colyte—PEG 3350 240 g + sodium sulfate 22.72 g + sodium bicarbonate 6.72 g + sodium chloride 5.84 g + potassium chloride 2.98 g
Combigan Ophthalmic Solution—0.2% brimonidine + 0.5% timolol
CombiPatch 0.05/0.14—estradiol 0.05 mg/day + norethindrone 0.14 mg/day
CombiPatch 0.05/0.25—estradiol 0.05 mg/day + norethindrone 0.25 mg/day
Combivent Respimat—(per actuation) ipratropium bromide 20 mcg + albuterol 100 mcg
Combivir—lamivudine 150 mg + zidovudine 300 mg
Complera—emtricitabine 200 mg + rilpivirine 25 mg + tenofovir 300 mg
Congestac—guaifenesin 400 mg + pseudoephedrine 60 mg **(OTC)**
Contac Cold & Flu Day Non-Drowsy Maximum Strength Caplets—phenylephrine 5 mg + acetaminophen 500 mg **(OTC)**
Contac Cold & Flu Night Maximum Strength Caplets—chlorpheniramine 2 mg + phenylephrine 5 mg + acetaminophen 500 mg **(OTC)**
Coricidin HBP Chest Congestion and Cough—dextromethorphan 10 mg + guaifenesin 200 mg **(OTC)**
Coricidin HBP Cold and Flu—acetaminophen 325 mg + chlorpheniramine 2 mg **(OTC)**
Coricidin HBP Cough and Cold—chlorpheniramine 4 mg + dextromethorphan 30 mg **(OTC)**
Coricidin HBP Maximum Strength Flu—acetaminophen 500 mg + chlorpheniramine 2 mg + dextromethorphan 15 mg **(OTC)**
Coricidin HBP Nighttime Multi-Symptom Cold—(per 15 mL) acetaminophen 325 mg + doxylamine 6.25 mg + dextromethorphan 15 mg **(OTC)**
Cortisporin Otic Solution/Suspension—(per mL) neomycin 3.5 mg + polymyxin B 10,000 units + hydrocortisone 10 mg
Cortisporin Topical Cream—(per g) neomycin 3.5 mg + polymyxin B 10,000 units + hydrocortisone 5 mg
Corzide 40/5—nadolol 40 mg + bendroflumethiazide 5 mg
Corzide 80/5—nadolol 80 mg + bendroflumethiazide 5 mg
Cosopt Ophthalmic Solution—2% dorzolamide + 0.5% timolol
🍁 **Coversyl Plus**—perindopril 4 mg + indapamide 1.25 mg
🍁 **Coversyl Plus HD**—perindopril 8 mg + indapamide 2.5 mg
🍁 **Coversyl Plus LD**—perindopril 2 mg + indapamide 0.625 mg
Creon—lipase 3000 units + amylase 15,000 units + protease 9,500 units
Creon—lipase 6000 units + amylase 30,000 units + protease 19,000 units
Creon—lipase 12,000 units + amylase 60,000 units + protease 38,000 units
Creon—lipase 24,000 units + amylase 120,00 units + protease 76,000 units
Creon—lipase 36,000 units + amylase 180,000 units + protease 114,000 units
Cryselle—norgestrel 0.3 mg + ethinyl estradiol 30 mcg
Cyclafem 1/35—norethindrone 1 mg + ethinyl estradiol 35 mcg

Cyclafem 7/7/7
Phase I—norethindrone 0.5 mg + ethinyl estradiol 35 mcg
Phase II—norethindrone 0.75 mg + ethinyl estradiol 35 mcg
Phase III—norethindrone 1 mg + ethinyl estradiol 35 mcg
Cyclessa
Phase I—desogestrel 0.1 mg + ethinyl estradiol 25 mcg
Phase II—desogestrel 0.125 mg + ethinyl estradiol 25 mcg
Phase III—desogestrel 0.15 mg + ethinyl estradiol 25 mcg
Cyclomydril Ophthalmic Solution—0.2% cyclopentolate + 1% phenylephrine
Dasetta 1/35—norethindrone 1 mg + ethinyl estradiol 35 mcg
Dasetta 7/7/7
Phase I—norethindrone 0.5 mg + ethinyl estradiol 35 mcg
Phase II—norethindrone 0.75 mg + ethinyl estradiol 35 mcg
Phase III—norethindrone 1 mg + ethinyl estradiol 35 mcg
Dayquil Cold & Flu Relief Liquid—(per 15 mL) acetaminophen 325 mg + dextromethorphan 10 mg + phenylephrine 5 mg **(OTC)**
Dayquil Cough & Congestion Liquid—(per 15 mL) dextromethorphan 10 mg + guaifenesin 200 mg **(OTC)**
Dayquil Severe Cold & Flu Relief Liquid—(per 15 mL) acetaminophen 325 mg + dextromethorphan 10 mg + guaifenesin 200 mg + phenylephrine 5 mg **(OTC)**
Daysee—levonorgestrel 0.15 mg + ethinyl estradiol 30 mcg/10 mcg
Desogen—ethinyl estradiol 30 mcg + desogestrel 0.15 mg
Dimetapp Cold & Allergy Syrup—(per 10 mL) phenylephrine 5 mg + brompheniramine 2 mg **(OTC)**
Dimetapp Cold & Cough Syrup—(per 10 mL) phenylephrine 5 mg + brompheniramine 2 mg + dextromethorphan 10 mg **(OTC)**
Dimetapp Long-Acting Cough Plus Cold Syrup—(per 10 mL) chlorpheniramine 2 mg + dextromethorphan 15 mg **(OTC)**
Dimetapp Multi-Symptom Cold & Flu Syrup—(per 10 mL) acetaminophen 320 mg + diphenhydramine 12.5 mg + phenylephrine 5 mg **(OTC)**
Dimetapp Nighttime Cold & Congestion Syrup—(per 10 mL) diphenhydramine 12.5 mg + phenylephrine 5 mg **(OTC)**
Diovan HCT 80/12.5—valsartan 80 mg + hydrochlorothiazide 12.5 mg
Diovan HCT 160/12.5—valsartan 160 mg + hydrochlorothiazide 12.5 mg
Diovan HCT 160/25—valsartan 160 mg + hydrochlorothiazide 25 mg
Diovan HCT 320/12.5—valsartan 320 mg + hydrochlorothiazide 12.5 mg
Diovan HCT 320/25—valsartan 320 mg + hydrochlorothiazide 25 mg
Donnatal Elixir—(per 5 mL) phenobarbital 16.2 mg + hyoscyamine 0.1037 mg + atropine 0.0194 mg + scopolamine 0.0065 mg + 23% alcohol
Donnatal Tablets—phenobarbital 16.2 mg + hyoscyamine 0.1037 mg + atropine 0.0194 mg + scopolamine 0.0065 mg
Dristan Cold Multi-Symptom Formula—acetaminophen 325 mg + phenylephrine 5 mg + chlorpheniramine 2 mg **(OTC)**
Duac Topical Gel—1.2% clindamycin + 5% benzoyl peroxide
Duavee—conjugated estrogens 0.45 mg + bazedoxifene 20 mg
Duetact 2/30—glimepiride 2 mg + pioglitazone 30 mg
Duetact 4/30—glimepiride 4 mg + pioglitazone 30 mg
Duexis—ibuprofen 800 mg + famotidine 26.6 mg
Dulera 100/5—(per actuation) mometasone 100 mcg + formoterol 5 mcg
Dulera 200/5—(per actuation) mometasone 200 mcg + formoterol 5 mcg
DuoNeb—(per 3 mL) albuterol sulfate 2.5 mg + ipratropium bromide 0.5 mg inhalation solution
Dutoprol 12.5/25—hydrochlorothiazide 12.5 mg + metoprolol succinate 25 mg
Dutoprol 12.5/50—hydrochlorothiazide 12.5 mg + metoprolol succinate 50 mg
Dutoprol 12.5/100—hydrochlorothiazide 12.5 mg + metoprolol succinate 100 mg
Dyazide—hydrochlorothiazide 25 mg + triamterene 37.5 mg
Dymista—(per actuation) azelastine 0.125 mg + fluticasone 50 mcg
Edarbyclor 40/12.5—azilsartan 40 mg + chlorthalidone 12.5 mg
Edarbyclor 40/25—azilsartan 40 mg + chlorthalidone 25 mg
Elinest—norgestrel 0.3 mg + ethinyl estradiol 30 mcg
Embeda 20/0.8—morphine sulfate 20 mg + naltrexone 0.8 mg
Embeda 30/1.2—morphine sulfate 30 mg + naltrexone 1.2 mg

Embeda 50/2—morphine sulfate 50 mg + naltrexone 2 mg
Embeda 60/2.4—morphine sulfate 60 mg + naltrexone 2.4 mg
Embeda 80/3.2—morphine sulfate 80 mg + naltrexone 3.2 mg
Embeda 100/4—morphine sulfate 100 mg + naltrexone 4 mg
EMLA Topical Cream—2.5% lidocaine + 2.5% prilocaine
Emoquette—ethinyl estradiol 30 mcg + desogestrel 0.15 mg
Endocet 2.5/325—oxycodone 2.5 mg + acetaminophen 325 mg
Endocet 5/325—oxycodone 5 mg + acetaminophen 325 mg
Endocet 7.5/325—oxycodone 7.5 mg + acetaminophen 325 mg
Endocet 10/325—oxycodone 10 mg + acetaminophen 325 mg
Endodan—oxycodone 4.84 mg + aspirin 325 mg
Enpresse-28
 Phase I—levonorgestrel 0.05 mg + ethinyl estradiol 30 mcg
 Phase II—levonorgestrel 0.075 mg + ethinyl estradiol 40 mcg
 Phase III—levonorgestrel 0.125 mg + ethinyl estradiol 30 mcg
Enskyce—desogestrel 0.15 mg + ethinyl estradiol 30 mcg
Epiduo Topical Gel—0.1% adapalene + 2.5% benzoyl peroxide
Epiduo Forte Topical Gel—0.3% adapalene + 2.5% benzoyl peroxide
Epifoam Aerosol Foam—1% hydrocortisone + 1% pramoxine
Epzicom—abacavir 600 mg + lamivudine 300 mg
Estarylla—norgestimate 0.25 mg + ethinyl estradiol 35 mcg
Estrostep Fe
 Phase I—norethindrone 1 mg + ethinyl estradiol 20 mcg
 Phase II—norethindrone 1 mg + ethinyl estradiol 30 mcg
 Phase III—norethindrone 1 mg + ethinyl estradiol 35 mcg
 Phase IV—ferrous fumarate 75 mg
Excedrin Extra Strength Caplets—acetaminophen 250 mg + aspirin 250 mg + caffeine 65 mg **(OTC)**
Excedrin Migraine Caplets—aspirin 250 mg + acetaminophen 250 mg + caffeine 65 mg **(OTC)**
Excedrin P.M. Headache Caplets—acetaminophen 250 mg + aspirin 250 mg + diphenhydramine citrate 38 mg **(OTC)**
Excedrin Tension Headache Caplets—acetaminophen 500 mg + caffeine 65 mg **(OTC)**
Exforge 5/160—amlodipine 5 mg + valsartan 160 mg
Exforge 5/320—amlodipine 5 mg + valsartan 320 mg
Exforge 10/160—amlodipine 10 mg + valsartan 160 mg
Exforge 10/320—amlodipine 10 mg + valsartan 320 mg
Exforge HCT 5/160/12.5—amlodipine 5 mg + valsartan 160 mg + hydrochlorothiazide 12.5 mg
Exforge HCT 5/160/25—amlodipine 5 mg + valsartan 160 mg + hydrochlorothiazide 25 mg
Exforge HCT 10/160/12.5—amlodipine 10 mg + valsartan 160 mg + hydrochlorothiazide 12.5 mg
Exforge HCT 10/160/25—amlodipine 10 mg + valsartan 160 mg + hydrochlorothiazide 25 mg
Exforge HCT 10/320/25—amlodipine 10 mg + valsartan 320 mg + hydrochlorothiazide 25 mg
Falmina—levonorgestrel 0.1 mg + ethinyl estradiol 20 mcg
Femcon Fe—norethindrone 0.4 mg + ethinyl estradiol 35 mcg + ferrous fumarate 75 mg
Femhrt 0.5/2.5—norethindrone 0.5 mg + ethinyl estradiol 2.5 mcg
Femhrt 1/5—norethindrone 1 mg + ethinyl estradiol 5 mcg
Ferro-Sequels—docusate sodium 100 mg + ferrous fumarate 150 mg **(OTC)**
Fioricet—acetaminophen 325 mg + caffeine 40 mg + butalbital 50 mg
Fioricet with Codeine—acetaminophen 300 mg + caffeine 40 mg + butalbital 50 mg + codeine 30 mg
Fiorinal—aspirin 325 mg + caffeine 40 mg + butalbital 50 mg
Fiorinal with Codeine—aspirin 325 mg + caffeine 40 mg + butalbital 50 mg + codeine 30 mg
Fosamax Plus D 70/2800—alendronate 70 mg + cholecalciferol 2800 IU
Fosamax Plus D 70/5600—alendronate 70 mg + cholecalciferol 5600 IU
Gaviscon Extra Strength Liquid—(per 5 mL) aluminum hydroxide 254 mg + magnesium carbonate 237.5 mg **(OTC)**
Gaviscon Extra Strength Tablets—magnesium carbonate 105 mg + aluminum hydroxide 160 mg **(OTC)**
Gaviscon Regular Strength Liquid—(per 15 mL) aluminum hydroxide 95 mg + magnesium carbonate 358 mg **(OTC)**
Gaviscon Regular Strength Tablets—magnesium trisilicate 14.2 mg + aluminum hydroxide 80 mg **(OTC)**
Gelusil—aluminum hydroxide 200 mg + magnesium hydroxide 200 mg + simethicone 25 mg **(OTC)**
Generess Fe—norethindrone 0.8 mg + ethinyl estradiol 25 mcg + ferrous fumarate 75 mg

Gianvi—drospirenone 3 mg + ethinyl estradiol 20 mcg
Gildagia—norethindrone 0.4 mg + ethinyl estradiol 35 mcg
Gildess 1/20—norethindrone 1 mg + ethinyl estradiol 20 mcg
Gildess Fe 1/20—norethindrone 1 mg + ethinyl estradiol 20 mcg + ferrous fumarate 75 mg
Gildess 1.5/30—norethindrone 1.5 mg + ethinyl estradiol 30 mcg
Gildess Fe 1.5/30—norethindrone 1.5 mg + ethinyl estradiol 30 mcg + ferrous fumarate 75 mg
Glucovance 1.25/250—glyburide 1.25 mg + metformin 250 mg
Glucovance 2.5/500—glyburide 2.5 mg + metformin 500 mg
Glucovance 5/500—glyburide 5 mg + metformin 500 mg
Glyxambi 10/5—empagliflozin 10 mg + linagliptin 5 mg
Glyxambi 25/5—empagliflozin 25 mg + linagliptin 5 mg
Golytely—PEG 3350 236 g + sodium sulfate 22.74 g + sodium bicarbonate 6.74 g + sodium chloride 5.86 g + potassium chloride 2.97 g
Golytely Packets—PEG 3350 227.1 g + sodium sulfate 21.5 g + sodium bicarbonate 6.36 g + sodium chloride 5.53 g + potassium chloride 2.82 g
Granulex Topical Aerosol—(per 0.8 mL) trypsin 0.12 mg + Balsam Peru 87 mg + castor oil 788 mg
Hycofenix Oral Solution—(per 5 mL) hydrocodone 2.5 mg + pseudoephedrine 30 mg + guaifenesin 200 mg
Hyzaar 50/12.5—losartan 50 mg + hydrochlorothiazide 12.5 mg
Hyzaar 100/12.5—losartan 100 mg + hydrochlorothiazide 12.5 mg
Hyzaar 100/25—losartan 100 mg + hydrochlorothiazide 25 mg
Imodium Multi-Symptom Relief—loperamide 2 mg + simethicone 125 mg **(OTC)**
Inderide 40/25—propranolol 40 mg + hydrochlorothiazide 25 mg
Introvale—levonorgestrel 0.15 mg + ethinyl estradiol 30 mcg
Invokamet 50/500—canagliflozin 50 mg + metformin 500 mg
Invokamet 50/1000—canagliflozin 50 mg + metformin 1000 mg
Invokamet 150/500—canagliflozin 150 mg + metformin 500 mg
Invokamet 150/1000—canagliflozin 150 mg + metformin 1000 mg
Isibloom—desogestrel 0.15 mg + ethinyl estradiol 30 mcg
IsonaRif—isoniazid 150 mg + rifampin 300 mg
Jalyn—dutasteride 0.5 mg + tamsulosin 0.4 mg
Janumet 50/500—sitagliptin 50 mg + metformin 500 mg
Janumet 50/1000—sitagliptin 50 mg + metformin 1000 mg
Janumet XR 50/500—sitagliptin 50 mg + metformin extended-release 500 mg
Janumet XR 50/1000—sitagliptin 50 mg + metformin extended-release 1000 mg
Janumet XR 100/1000—sitagliptin 100 mg + metformin extended-release 500 mg
Jentadueto 2.5/500—linagliptin 2.5 mg + metformin 500 mg
Jentadueto 2.5/850—linagliptin 2.5 mg + metformin 850 mg
Jentadueto 2.5/1000—linagliptin 2.5 mg + metformin 1000 mg
Jinteli—norethindrone 1 mg + ethinyl estradiol 5 mcg
Jolessa—levonorgestrel 0.15 mg + ethinyl estradiol 30 mcg
Junel 1/20—norethindrone 1 mg + ethinyl estradiol 20 mcg
Junel 1.5/30—norethindrone 1.5 mg + ethinyl estradiol 30 mcg
Junel Fe 1/20—norethindrone 1 mg + ethinyl estradiol 20 mcg + ferrous fumarate 75 mg
Junel Fe 1.5/30—norethindrone 1.5 mg + ethinyl estradiol 30 mcg + ferrous fumarate 75 mg
Kariva—desogestrel 0.15 mg + ethinyl estradiol 20 mcg/10 mcg
Kazano 12.5/500—alogliptin 12.5 mg + metformin 500 mg
Kazano 12.5/1000—alogliptin 12.5 mg + metformin 1000 mg
Kelnor—ethynodiol 1 mg + ethinyl estradiol 35 mcg
Kimidess—desogestrel 0.15 mg + ethinyl estradiol 20 mcg/10 mcg
Kombiglyze XR 2.5/1000—saxagliptin 2.5 mg + metformin extended-release 1000 mg
Kombiglyze XR 5/500—saxagliptin 5 mg + metformin extended-release 500 mg
Kombiglyze XR 5/1000—saxagliptin 5 mg + metformin extended-release 1000 mg
Kurvelo—levonorgestrel 0.15 mg + ethinyl estradiol 30 mcg
Lactinex—mixed culture of *Lactobacillus acidophilus* and *L. bulgaricus* **(OTC)**
Larin 1/20—norethindrone 1 mg + ethinyl estradiol 20 mcg
Larin Fe 1/20—norethindrone 1 mg + ethinyl estradiol 20 mcg + ferrous fumarate 75 mg
Larin 1.5/30—norethindrone 1.5 mg + ethinyl estradiol 30 mcg
Larin Fe 1.5/30—norethindrone 1.5 mg + ethinyl estradiol 30 mcg + ferrous fumarate 75 mg

Leena

Phase I—norethindrone 0.5 mg + ethinyl estradiol 35 mcg

Phase II—norethindrone 1 mg + ethinyl estradiol 35 mcg

Phase III—norethindrone 0.5 mg + ethinyl estradiol 35 mcg

Lessina-28—levonorgestrel 0.1 mg + ethinyl estradiol 20 mcg

Levonest

Phase I—levonorgestrel 0.05 mg + ethinyl estradiol 30 mcg

Phase II—levonorgestrel 0.075 mg + ethinyl estradiol 40 mcg

Phase III—levonorgestrel 0.125 mg + ethinyl estradiol 30 mcg

Levora-28—levonorgestrel 0.15 mg + ethinyl estradiol 30 mcg

Lida-Mantle-HC Topical Cream—0.5% hydrocortisone + 3% lidocaine

Loestrin 21 1/20—norethindrone 1 mg + ethinyl estradiol 20 mcg

Loestrin 21 1.5/30—norethindrone 1.5 mg + ethinyl estradiol 30 mcg

Loestrin Fe 1/20—norethindrone 1 mg + ethinyl estradiol 20 mcg with 7 tablets of ferrous fumarate 75 mg per container

Loestrin Fe 1.5/30—norethindrone 1.5 mg + ethinyl estradiol 30 mcg with 7 tablets of ferrous fumarate 75 mg per container

Lo Loestrin Fe

Phase I—norethindrone 1 mg + ethinyl estradiol 10 mcg

Phase II—ethinyl estradiol 10 mcg

Phase III—ferrous fumarate 75 mg

Lo Minastrin Fe—norethindrone 1 mg + ethinyl estradiol 10 mcg + ferrous fumarate 75 mcg

Lo/Ovral-28—ethinyl estradiol 30 mcg + norgestrel 0.3 mg

Lopressor HCT 50/25—metoprolol tartrate 50 mg + hydrochlorothiazide 25 mg

Lopressor HCT 100/25—metoprolol tartrate 100 mg + hydrochlorothiazide 25 mg

Loryna—drospirenone 3 mg + ethinyl estradiol 20 mcg

LoSeasonique—levonorgestrel 0.1 mg + ethinyl estradiol 20 mcg

Lotensin HCT 5/6.25—benazepril 5 mg + hydrochlorothiazide 6.25 mg

Lotensin HCT 10/12.5—benazepril 10 mg + hydrochlorothiazide 12.5 mg

Lotensin HCT 20/12.5—benazepril 20 mg + hydrochlorothiazide 12.5 mg

Lotensin HCT 20/25—benazepril 20 mg + hydrochlorothiazide 25 mg

Lotrel 2.5/10—amlodipine 2.5 mg + benazepril 10 mg

Lotrel 5/10—amlodipine 5 mg + benazepril 10 mg

Lotrel 5/20—amlodipine 5 mg + benazepril 20 mg

Lotrel 5/40—amlodipine 5 mg + benazepril 40 mg

Lotrel 10/20—amlodipine 10 mg + benazepril 20 mg

Lotrel 10/40—amlodipine 10 mg + benazepril 40 mg

Lotrisone Topical Cream/Lotion—0.05% betamethasone + 1% clotrimazole

Low-Ogestrel-28—norgestrel 0.3 mg + ethinyl estradiol 30 mcg

Lutera—levonorgestrel 0.1 mg + ethinyl estradiol 20 mcg

Maalox Advanced Maximum Strength Chewables—calcium carbonate 1000 mg + simethicone 60 mg **(OTC)**

Maalox Advanced Maximum Strength Liquid—(per 5 mL) aluminum hydroxide 400 mg + magnesium hydroxide 400 mg + simethicone 40 mg **(OTC)**

Maalox Advanced Regular Strength Liquid—(per 5 mL) aluminum hydroxide 200 mg + magnesium hydroxide 200 mg + simethicone 20 mg **(OTC)**

Malarone—atovaquone 250 mg + proguanil 100 mg

Malarone Pediatric—atovaquone 62.5 mg + proguanil 25 mg

Marlissa—levonorgestrel 0.15 mg + ethinyl estradiol 30 mcg

Maxitrol Ophthalmic Suspension/Ointment—(per g) neomycin 3.5 mg + 0.1% dexamethasone + polymyxin B 10,000 units

Maxzide—hydrochlorothiazide 50 mg + triamterene 75 mg

Maxzide-25—hydrochlorothiazide 25 mg + triamterene 37.5 mg

Micardis HCT 40/12.5—telmisartan 40 mg + hydrochlorothiazide 12.5 mg

Micardis HCT 80/12.5—telmisartan 80 mg + hydrochlorothiazide 12.5 mg

Micardis HCT 80/25—telmisartan 80 mg + hydrochlorothiazide 25 mg

Microgestin 1/20—norethindrone 1 mg + ethinyl estradiol 20 mcg

Microgestin 1.5/30—norethindrone 1.5 mg + ethinyl estradiol 30 mcg

Microgestin Fe 1/20—norethindrone 1 mg + ethinyl estradiol 20 mcg + ferrous fumarate 75 mg

Microgestin Fe 1.5/30—norethindrone 1.5 mg + ethinyl estradiol 30 mcg + ferrous fumarate 75 mg

Midol Complete Caplets—acetaminophen 500 mg + caffeine 60 mg + pyrilamine 15 mg **(OTC)**
Midol Teen Caplets—acetaminophen 500 mg + pamabrom 25 mg **(OTC)**
Migergot Suppositories—ergotamine 2 mg + caffeine 100 mg
Minastrin 24 Fe—norethindrone 1 mg + ethinyl estradiol 20 mcg + ferrous fumarate 75 mg
Modicon-28—norethindrone 0.5 mg + ethinyl estradiol 35 mcg
Mono-Linyah—norgestimate 0.25 mg + ethinyl estradiol 35 mcg
Mononessa—norgestimate 0.25 mg + ethinyl estradiol 35 mcg
Motrin PM—ibuprofen 200 mg + diphenhydramine 38 mg **(OTC)**
Moviprep—PEG 3350 100 g + sodium sulfate 7.5 g + sodium chloride 2.69 g + potassium chloride 1.02 g
Mucinex Cold, Cough, & Sore Throat Liquid for Children—(per 10 mL) acetaminophen 325 mg + guaifenesin 200 mg + dextromethorphan 10 mg + phenylephrine 5 mg **(OTC)**
Mucinex Congestion & Cough Liquid for Children—(per 5 mL) guaifenesin 100 mg + dextromethorphan 5 mg + phenylephrine 2.5 mg **(OTC)**
Mucinex Cough Liquid for Children—(per 5 mL) guaifenesin 100 mg + dextromethorphan 5 mg **(OTC)**
Mucinex Cough Mini-Melts—guaifenesin 100 mg + dextromethorphan 5 mg **(OTC)**
Mucinex D Maximum Strength Tablets—guaifenesin 1200 mg + pseudoephedrine 120 mg **(OTC)**
Mucinex D Tablets—guaifenesin 600 mg + pseudoephedrine 60 mg **(OTC)**
Mucinex DM Maximum Strength Tablets—guaifenesin 1200 mg + dextromethorphan 60 mg **(OTC)**
Mucinex DM Tablets—guaifenesin 600 mg + dextromethorphan 30 mg **(OTC)**
Mucinex Maximum Strength Fast-Max Cold & Sinus Caplets—acetaminophen 325 mg + guaifenesin 200 mg + phenylephrine 5 mg **(OTC)**
Mucinex Maximum Strength Fast-Max Cold & Sinus Liquid—(per 20 mL) acetaminophen 650 mg + guaifenesin 400 mg + phenylephrine 10 mg **(OTC)**
Mucinex Maximum Strength Fast-Max Cold, Flu, & Sore Throat Caplets—acetaminophen 325 mg + guaifenesin 200 mg + dextromethorphan 10 mg + phenylephrine 5 mg **(OTC)**
Mucinex Maximum Strength Fast-Max Cold, Flu, & Sore Throat Liquid—(per 20 mL) acetaminophen 650 mg + guaifenesin 400 mg + dextromethorphan 20 mg + phenylephrine 10 mg **(OTC)**
Mucinex Maximum Strength Fast-Max DM Max Liquid—(per 20 mL) guaifenesin 400 mg + dextromethorphan 20 mg **(OTC)**
Mucinex Maximum Strength Fast-Max Night Time Cold & Flu Caplets—acetaminophen 325 mg + diphenhydramine 25 mg + phenylephrine 5 mg **(OTC)**
Mucinex Maximum Strength Fast-Max Night Time Cold & Flu Liquid—(per 20 mL) acetaminophen 650 mg + diphenhydramine 25 mg + phenylephrine 10 mg **(OTC)**
Mucinex Maximum Strength Fast-Max Severe Cold Caplets—acetaminophen 325 mg + guaifenesin 200 mg + dextromethorphan 10 mg + phenylephrine 5 mg **(OTC)**
Mucinex Maximum Strength Fast-Max Severe Cold Liquid—(per 20 mL) acetaminophen 650 mg + guaifenesin 400 mg + dextromethorphan 20 mg + phenylephrine 10 mg **(OTC)**
Mucinex Maximum Strength Fast-Max Severe Congestion & Cough Caplets—guaifenesin 200 mg + dextromethorphan 10 mg + phenylephrine 5 mg **(OTC)**
Mucinex Maximum Strength Fast-Max Severe Congestion & Cough Liquid—(per 20 mL) guaifenesin 400 mg + dextromethorphan 20 mg + phenylephrine 10 mg **(OTC)**
Mucinex Maximum Strength Sinus-Max Night Time Congestion Liquid—(per 20 mL) acetaminophen 650 mg + diphenhydramine 25 mg + phenylephrine 10 mg **(OTC)**
Mucinex Maximum Strength Sinus-Max Pressure & Pain Caplets—acetaminophen 325 mg + guaifenesin 200 mg + phenylephrine 5 mg **(OTC)**
Mucinex Maximum Strength Sinus-Max Pressure & Pain Liquid—(per 20 mL) acetaminophen 650 mg + guaifenesin 400 mg + phenylephrine 10 mg **(OTC)**
Mucinex Maximum Strength Sinus-Max Severe Congestion Relief Caplets—acetaminophen 325 mg + guaifenesin 200 mg + phenylephrine 5 mg **(OTC)**
Mucinex Maximum Strength Sinus-Max Severe Congestion Relief Liquid—(per 20 mL) acetaminophen 650 mg + guaifenesin 400 mg + phenylephrine 10 mg **(OTC)**
Mucinex Multi-Symptom Cold & Fever Liquid for Children—(per 10 mL) acetaminophen 325 mg + guaifenesin 200 mg + dextromethorphan 10 mg + phenylephrine 5 mg **(OTC)**
Mucinex Multi-Symptom Cold Liquid for Children—(per 5 mL) guaifenesin 100 mg + dextromethorphan 5 mg + phenylephrine 2.5 mg **(OTC)**
Mucinex Night Time Multi-Symptom Cold Liquid for Children—(per 10 mL) acetaminophen 325 mg + diphenhydramine 12.5 mg + phenylephrine 5 mg **(OTC)**
Mucinex Stuffy Nose & Cold Liquid for Children—(per 5 mL) guaifenesin 100 mg +phenylephrine 2.5 mg **(OTC)**

Myzilra
  Phase I—levonorgestrel 0.05 mg + ethinyl estradiol 30 mcg
  Phase II—levonorgestrel 0.075 mg + ethinyl estradiol 40 mcg
  Phase III—levonorgestrel 0.125 mg + ethinyl estradiol 30 mcg
Natazia
  Phase I—estradiol valerate 3 mg
  Phase II—estradiol valerate 2 mg + dienogest 2 mg
  Phase III—estradiol valerate 2 mg + dienogest 3 mg
  Phase IV—estradiol valerate 1 mg
Necon 0.5/35—norethindrone 0.5 mg + ethinyl estradiol 35 mcg
Necon 1/35—norethindrone 1 mg + ethinyl estradiol 35 mcg
Necon 1/50—norethindrone 1 mg + mestranol 50 mcg
Necon 7/7/7
  Phase I—norethindrone 0.5 mg + ethinyl estradiol 35 mcg
  Phase II—norethindrone 0.75 mg + ethinyl estradiol 35 mcg
  Phase III—norethindrone 1 mg + ethinyl estradiol 35 mcg
Necon 10/11
  Phase I—norethindrone 0.5 mg + ethinyl estradiol 35 mcg
  Phase II—norethindrone 1 mg + ethinyl estradiol 35 mcg
Neosporin Antibiotic Topical Ointment—(per g) neomycin 3.5 mg + bacitracin 400 units + polymyxin B 5000 units **(OTC)**
Neosporin G.U. Irrigant—(per mL) neomycin 40 mg + polymyxin B 200,000 units
Neosporin Ophthalmic Solution—(per mL) polymyxin B 10,000 units + neomycin 1.75 mg + gramicidin 0.025 mg
Neosporin + Pain Relief Antibiotic Topical Cream—(per g) neomycin 3.5 mg + polymyxin B 10,000 units + pramoxine 10 mg **(OTC)**
Neosporin + Pain Relief Antibiotic Topical Ointment—(per g) neomycin 3.5 mg + polymyxin B 10,000 units + bacitracin 500 units + pramoxine 10 mg **(OTC)**
Nikki—drospirenone 3 mg + ethinyl estradiol 20 mcg
Norco 5/325—hydrocodone 5 mg + acetaminophen 325 mg
Norco 7.5/325—hydrocodone 7.5 mg + acetaminophen 325 mg
Norco 10/325—hydrocodone 10 mg + acetaminophen 325 mg
Norinyl 1/35—norethindrone 1 mg + ethinyl estradiol 35 mcg
Norinyl 1/50—norethindrone 1 mg + mestranol 50 mcg
Nortrel 0.5/35—norethindrone 0.5 mg + ethinyl estradiol 35 mcg
Nortrel 1/35—norethindrone 1 mg + ethinyl estradiol 35 mcg
Nortrel 7/7/7
  Phase I—norethindrone 0.5 mg + ethinyl estradiol 35 mcg
  Phase II—norethindrone 0.75 mg + ethinyl estradiol 35 mcg
  Phase III—norethindrone 1 mg + ethinyl estradiol 35 mcg
Nuedextra—dextromethorphan 20 mg + quinidine sulfate 10 mg
NuLytely—PEG 3350 420 g + sodium bicarbonate 5.72 g + sodium chloride 11.2 g + potassium chloride 1.48 g
Nuvaring—etonogestrel 0.12 mg/day + ethinyl estradiol 15 mcg/day
Nyquil Children's Cold & Cough Liquid—(per 15 mL) dextromethorphan 15 mg + chlorpheniramine 2 mg **(OTC)**
Nyquil Cold & Flu Nighttime Relief Liquicaps—acetaminophen 325 mg + dextromethorphan 15 mg + doxylamine 6.25 mg **(OTC)**
Nyquil Cold & Flu Nighttime Relief Liquid—(per 30 mL) acetaminophen 650 mg + dextromethorphan 30 mg + doxylamine 12.5 mg **(OTC)**
Nyquil Cough Suppressant Liquid—(per 30 mL) dextromethorphan 30 mg + doxylamine 12.5 mg **(OTC)**
Nyquil Severe Cold & Flu Relief Liquid—(per 30 mL) acetaminophen 650 mg + dextromethorphan 20 mg + doxylamine 12.5 mg + phenylephrine 10 mg **(OTC)**
Obredon Solution—(per 5 mL) hydrocodone 2.5 mg + guaifenesin 200 mg
Ocella—drospirenone 3 mg + ethinyl estradiol 30 mcg
Ogestrel-28—norgestrel 0.5 mg + ethinyl estradiol 50 mcg
Onexton Topical Gel—1.2% clindamycin + 3.75% benzoyl peroxide
Opcon-A Ophthalmic Solution—0.027% naphazoline + 0.3% pheniramine **(OTC)**
Oraqix Periodontal Gel—2.5% lidocaine + 2.5% prilocaine
Orsythia—levonorgestrel 0.1 mg + ethinyl estradiol 20 mcg

Ortho-Cept—ethinyl estradiol 30 mcg + desogestrel 0.15 mg
Ortho-Cyclen-28—ethinyl estradiol 35 mcg + norgestimate 0.25 mg
Ortho-Novum 1/35—norethindrone 1 mg + ethinyl estradiol 35 mcg
Ortho-Novum 7/7/7
  Phase I—norethindrone 0.5 mg + ethinyl estradiol 35 mcg
  Phase II—norethindrone 0.75 mg + ethinyl estradiol 35 mcg
  Phase III—norethindrone 1 mg + ethinyl estradiol 35 mcg
Ortho Tri-Cyclen-28
  Phase I—norgestimate 0.18 mg + ethinyl estradiol 35 mcg
  Phase II—norgestimate 0.215 mg + ethinyl estradiol 35 mcg
  Phase III—norgestimate 0.25 mg + ethinyl estradiol 35 mcg
Ortho Tri-Cyclen Lo
  Phase I—norgestimate 0.18 mg + ethinyl estradiol 25 mcg
  Phase II—norgestimate 0.215 mg + ethinyl estradiol 25 mcg
  Phase III—norgestimate 0.25 mg + ethinyl estradiol 25 mcg
Oseni 12.5/15—alogliptin 12.5 mg + pioglitazone 15 mg
Oseni 12.5/30—alogliptin 12.5 mg + pioglitazone 30 mg
Oseni 12.5/45—alogliptin 12.5 mg + pioglitazone 45 mg
Oseni 25/15—alogliptin 25 mg + pioglitazone 15 mg
Oseni 25/30—alogliptin 25 mg + pioglitazone 30 mg
Oseni 25/45—alogliptin 25 mg + pioglitazone 45 mg
Oxycet—oxycodone 5 mg + acetaminophen 325 mg
Pamprin Maximum Strength Max—acetaminophen 250 mg + aspirin 250 mg + caffeine 65 mg **(OTC)**
Pamprin Maximum Strength Multi-Symptom—acetaminophen 500 mg + pamabrom 25 mg + pyrilamine 15 mg **(OTC)**
Pancreaze—lipase 2600 units + amylase 10,850 units + protease 6200 units
Pancreaze—lipase 4200 units + amylase 17,500 units + protease 10,000 units
Pancreaze—lipase 10,500 units + amylase 43,750 units + protease 25,000 units
Pancreaze—lipase 16,800 units + amylase 70,000 units + protease 40,000 units
Pancreaze—lipase 21,000 units + amylase 61,000 units + protease 37,000 units
Pediacare Children's Cough & Congestion Liquid—(per 5 mL) dextromethorphan 5 mg + guaifenesin 100 mg **(OTC)**
Pediacare Children's Cough & Runny Nose Plus Acetaminophen Liquid—(per 5 mL) acetaminophen 160 mg + chlorpheniramine 1 mg + dextromethorphan 5 mg **(OTC)**
Pediacare Children's Daytime Multi-Symptom Cold Liquid—(per 5 mL) phenylephrine 2.5 mg + dextromethorphan 5 mg **(OTC)**
Pediacare Children's Flu Plus Acetaminophen Liquid—(per 5 mL) acetaminophen 160 mg + chlorpheniramine 1 mg + phenylephrine 2.5 mg + dextromethorphan 5 mg **(OTC)**
Pediacare Children's Multi-Symptom Cold Plus Acetaminophen Liquid—(per 5 mL) acetaminophen 160 mg + chlorpheniramine 1 mg + phenylephrine 2.5 mg + dextromethorphan 5 mg **(OTC)**
Pediacare Children's Nighttime Multi-Symptom Cold Liquid—(per 5 mL) diphenhydramine 6.25 mg + phenylephrine 2.5 mg **(OTC)**
Pepcid Complete—calcium carbonate 800 mg + magnesium hydroxide 165 mg + famotidine 10 mg **(OTC)**
Percocet 2.5/325—oxycodone 2.5 mg + acetaminophen 325 mg
Percocet 5/325—oxycodone 5 mg + acetaminophen 325 mg
Percocet 7.5/325—oxycodone 7.5 mg + acetaminophen 325 mg
Percocet 10/325—oxycodone 10 mg + acetaminophen 325 mg
Percodan—oxycodone 4.84 mg + aspirin 325 mg
Peri-Colace—docusate sodium 50 mg + sennosides 8.6 mg **(OTC)**
Pertyze—lipase 8000 units + amylase 30,250 units +protease 28,750 units
Pertyze—lipase 16,000 units + amylase 60,500 units +protease 57,500 units
Philith—norethindrone 0.4 mg + ethinyl estradiol 35 mcg
Phrenilin Forte—butalbital 50 mg + acetaminophen 650 mg
Pimtrea—desogestrel 0.15 mg + ethinyl estradiol 20 mcg/10 mcg
Pirmella 1/35—norethindrone 1 mg + ethinyl estradiol 35 mcg
Pirmella 7/7/7
  Phase I—norethindrone 0.5 mg + ethinyl estradiol 35 mcg
  Phase II—norethindrone 0.75 mg + ethinyl estradiol 35 mcg
  Phase III—norethindrone 1 mg + ethinyl estradiol 35 mcg
Pliaglis Topical Cream—7% lidocaine + 7% tetracaine

Polysporin Topical Ointment/Powder—(per g) polymyxin B 10,000 units + bacitracin 500 units (OTC)
Polytrim Ophthalmic Solution—(per mL) polymyxin B 10,000 units + trimethoprim 1 mg
Portia-28—levonorgestrel 0.15 mg + ethinyl estradiol 30 mcg
Pramosone Topical Cream 1/0.5—1% pramoxine + 0.5% hydrocortisone
Pramosone Topical Cream/Lotion 1/1—1% pramoxine + 1% hydrocortisone
Pramosone Topical Cream/Lotion 1/2.5—1% pramoxine + 2.5% hydrocortisone
PrandiMet 1/500—repaglinide 1 mg + metformin 500 mg
PrandiMet 2/500—repaglinide 2 mg + metformin 500 mg
Premphase—conjugated estrogens 0.625 mg + medroxyprogesterone 5 mg (14 tablets) plus conjugated estrogens 0.625 mg (14 tablets) in a compliance package
❋ **Premplus 0.625/2.5**—conjugated estrogens 0.625 mg + medroxyprogesterone 2.5 mg
❋ **Premplus 0.625/5**—conjugated estrogens 0.625 mg + medroxyprogesterone 5 mg
Prempro 0.3/1.5—conjugated estrogens 0.3 mg + medroxyprogesterone 1.5 mg
Prempro 0.45/1.5—conjugated estrogens 0.45 mg + medroxyprogesterone 1.5 mg
Prempro 0.625/2.5—conjugated estrogens 0.625 mg + medroxyprogesterone 2.5 mg
Prempro 0.625/5—conjugated estrogens 0.625 mg + medroxyprogesterone 5 mg
Prestalia 3.5/2.5—perindopril 3.5 mg + amlodipine 2.5 mg
Prestalia 7.5/5—perindopril 7.5 mg + amlodipine 5 mg
Prestalia 14/10—perindopril 14 mg + amlodipine 10 mg
Previfem—norgestimate 0.25 mg + ethinyl estradiol 35 mcg
Prevpac—amoxicillin 500-mg capsules + clarithromycin 500-mg tablets + lansoprazole 30-mg capsules in a compliance package
Primatene Tablets—ephedrine 12.5 mg + guaifenesin 200 mg (OTC)
Primlev 5/300—oxycodone 5 mg + acetaminophen 300 mg
Primlev 7.5/300—oxycodone 7.5 mg + acetaminophen 300 mg
Primlev 10/300—oxycodone 10 mg + acetaminophen 300 mg
Prinzide 10/12.5—lisinopril 10 mg + hydrochlorothiazide 12.5 mg
Prinzide 20/12.5—lisinopril 20 mg + hydrochlorothiazide 12.5 mg
Proctofoam-HC Rectal Foam—1% hydrocortisone + 1% pramoxine
Pylera—bismuth subcitrate potassium 140 mg + metronidazole 125 mg + tetracycline 125 mg
Qsymia 3.75/23—phentermine 3.75 mg + extended-release topiramate 23 mg
Qsymia 7.5/46—phentermine 7.5 mg + extended-release topiramate 46 mg
Qsymia 11.25/69—phentermine 11.25 mg + extended-release topiramate 69 mg
Qsymia 15/92—phentermine 15 mg + extended-release topiramate 92 mg
Quartette
Phase I—levonorgestrel 0.15 mg + ethinyl estradiol 20 mcg
Phase II—levonorgestrel 0.15 mg + ethinyl estradiol 25 mcg
Phase III—levonorgestrel 0.15 mg + ethinyl estradiol 30 mcg
Phase IV—ethinyl estradiol 10 mcg
Quasense—levonorgestrel 0.15 mg + ethinyl estradiol 30 mcg
Quinaretic 10/12.5—quinapril 10 mg + hydrochlorothiazide 12.5 mg
Quinaretic 20/12.5—quinapril 20 mg + hydrochlorothiazide 12.5 mg
Quinaretic 20/25—quinapril 20 mg + hydrochlorothiazide 25 mg
Reclipsen—desogestrel 0.15 mg + ethinyl estradiol 30 mcg
Reprexain 2.5/200—hydrocodone 2.5 mg + ibuprofen 200 mg
Reprexain 5/200—hydrocodone 5 mg + ibuprofen 200 mg
Reprexain 10/200—hydrocodone 10 mg + ibuprofen 200 mg
Rezira Solution—(per 5 mL) hydrocodone 5 mg + pseudoephedrine 60 mg
RID Lice Killing Shampoo—0.33% pyrethrins + 4% piperonyl butoxide (OTC)
Rifamate—isoniazid 150 mg + rifampin 300 mg
Rifater—rifampin 120 mg + isoniazid 50 mg + pyrazinamide 300 mg
❋ **Robaxacet**—methocarbamol 400 mg + acetaminophen 325 mg
❋ **Robaxacet-8**—methocarbamol 400 mg + acetaminophen 325 mg + codeine 8 mg
❋ **Robaxacet Extra Strength**—methocarbamol 400 mg + acetaminophen 500 mg
❋ **Robitussin AC Liquid**—(per 5 mL) guaifenesin 100 mg + codeine 10 mg + pheniramine 7.5 mg (OTC)
Robitussin Children's Cough & Chest Congestion DM Liquid—(per 5 mL) guaifenesin 100 mg + dextromethorphan 5 mg (OTC)
Robitussin Children's Cough & Cold CF Liquid—(per 10 mL) guaifenesin 100 mg + phenylephrine 5 mg + dextromethorphan 10 mg (OTC)

Robitussin Children's Cough & Cold Long-Acting Liquid—(per 10 mL) chlorpheniramine 2 mg + dextromethorphan 15 mg **(OTC)**

Robitussin Children's Nighttime Cough Long-Acting DM Liquid—(per 10 mL) chlorpheniramine 2 mg + dextromethorphan 15 mg **(OTC)**

Robitussin Maximum Strength Cough + Chest Congestion DM Capsules—guaifenesin 200 mg + dextromethorphan 10 mg **(OTC)**

Robitussin Maximum Strength Cough + Chest Congestion DM Liquid—(per 10 mL) guaifenesin 400 mg + dextromethorphan 20 mg **(OTC)**

Robitussin Maximum Strength Nighttime Cough DM Liquid—(per 10 mL) dextromethorphan 30 mg + doxylamine 12.5 mg **(OTC)**

Robitussin Peak Cold Cough + Chest Congestion DM Liquid—(per 10 mL) guaifenesin 200 mg + dextromethorphan 20 mg **(OTC)**

Robitussin Peak Cold Maximum Strength Multi-Symptom Cold Liquid—(per 10 mL) guaifenesin 400 mg + phenylephrine 10 mg + dextromethorphan 20 mg **(OTC)**

Robitussin Peak Cold Multi-Symptom Cold Liquid—(per 10 mL) guaifenesin 200 mg + phenylephrine 10 mg + dextromethorphan 20 mg **(OTC)**

Robitussin Peak Cold Nighttime Multi-Symptom Cold Liquid—(per 20 mL) acetaminophen 640 mg + phenylephrine 10 mg + diphenhydramine 25 mg **(OTC)**

Robitussin Severe Multi-Symptom Cough Cold & Flu Liquid—(per 20 mL) acetaminophen 650 mg + guaifenesin 400 mg + phenylephrine 10 mg + dextromethorphan 20 mg **(OTC)**

Robitussin Severe Multi-Symptom Cough Cold & Flu Nighttime Liquid—(per 20 mL) acetaminophen 650 mg + phenylephrine 10 mg + diphenhydramine 25 mg **(OTC)**

Rolaids Advanced Tablets—calcium carbonate 1000 mg + magnesium hydroxide 200 mg + simethicone 40 mg **(OTC)**

Rolaids Extra Strength Tablets—calcium carbonate 675 mg + magnesium hydroxide 135 mg **(OTC)**

Rolaids Regular Strength Tablets—calcium carbonate 550 mg + magnesium hydroxide 110 mg **(OTC)**

Rolaids Softchews—calcium carbonate 1330 mg + magnesium hydroxide 235 mg **(OTC)**

Rolaids Ultra Strength Liquid—(per 5 mL) calcium carbonate 1000 mg + magnesium hydroxide 200 mg **(OTC)**

Rolaids Ultra Strength Tablets—calcium carbonate 1000 mg + magnesium hydroxide 200 mg **(OTC)**

Roxicet 5/325—oxycodone 5 mg + acetaminophen 325 mg

Roxicet Solution—(per 5 mL) oxycodone 5 mg + acetaminophen 325 mg

Safyral

Phase I—drospirenone 3 mg + ethinyl estradiol 30 mcg + levomefolate 0.451 mg

Phase II—levomefolate 0.451 mg

Scot-Tussin DM Maximum Strength Cough Suppressant & Cold Relief Liquid—(per 5 mL) chlorpheniramine 2 mg + dextromethorphan 15 mg **(OTC)**

Scot-Tussin Original Multi-Symptom Cold & Allergy Relief Liquid—(per 5 mL) acetaminophen 160 mg + pheniramine 4 mg + phenylephrine 4 mg **(OTC)**

Scot-Tussin Senior Maximum Strength Cough Suppressant & Expectorant Liquid—(per 5 mL) guaifenesin 200 mg + dextromethorphan 15 mg **(OTC)**

Seasonale—levonorgestrel 0.15 mg + ethinyl estradiol 30 mcg

Seasonique—levonorgestrel 0.15 mg + ethinyl estradiol 30 mcg/10 mcg

Semprex-D—acrivastine 8 mg + pseudoephedrine 60 mg

Senokot-S—sennosides 8.6 mg + docusate sodium 50 mg **(OTC)**

Setlakin—levonorgestrel 0.15 mg + ethinyl estradiol 30 mcg

Silafed Syrup—(per 5 mL) pseudoephedrine 30 mg + triprolidine 1.25 mg **(OTC)**

Simbrinza Ophthalmic Suspension—0.2% brimonidine + 1% brinzolamide

Simcor 500/20—niacin 500 mg + simvastatin 20 mg

Simcor 500/40—niacin 500 mg + simvastatin 40 mg

Simcor 750/20—niacin 750 mg + simvastatin 20 mg

Simcor 1000/20—niacin 1000 mg + simvastatin 20 mg

Simcor 1000/40—niacin 1000 mg + simvastatin 40 mg

Solia—desogestrel 0.15 mg + ethinyl estradiol 30 mcg

Soma Compound—aspirin 325 mg + carisoprodol 200 mg

Soma Compound with Codeine—aspirin 325 mg + carisoprodol 200 mg + codeine 16 mg

Sprintec—norgestimate 0.25 mg + ethinyl estradiol 35 mcg

Sronyx—levonorgestrel 0.1 mg + ethinyl estradiol 20 mcg

Stalevo 50—carbidopa 12.5 mg + entacapone 200 mg + levodopa 50 mg

Stalevo 75—carbidopa 18.75 mg + entacapone 200 mg + levodopa 75 mg

Stalevo 100—carbidopa 25 mg + entacapone 200 mg + levodopa 100 mg
Stalevo 125—carbidopa 31.25 mg + entacapone 200 mg + levodopa 125 mg
Stalevo 150—carbidopa 37.5 mg + entacapone 200 mg + levodopa 150 mg
Stalevo 200—carbidopa 50 mg + entacapone 200 mg + levodopa 200 mg
Stribild—cobicistat 150 mg + elvitegravir 150 mg + tenofovir 300 mg + emtricitabine 200 mg
Suboxone 2/0.5—buprenorphine 2 mg + naloxone 0.5 mg
Suboxone 4/1—buprenorphine 4 mg + naloxone 1 mg
Suboxone 8/2—buprenorphine 8 mg + naloxone 2 mg
Suboxone 12/3—buprenorphine 12 mg + naloxone 3 mg
Sudafed 12 Hour Pressure + Pain Caplets—naproxen 220 mg + extended-release pseudoephedrine 120 mg **(OTC)**
Sudafed PE Pressure + Pain Caplets—acetaminophen 325 mg + phenylephrine 5 mg **(OTC)**
Sudafed PE Pressure + Pain + Cold Caplets—acetaminophen 325 mg + phenylephrine 5 mg + guaifenesin 100 mg + dextromethorphan 10 mg **(OTC)**
Sudafed PE Pressure + Pain + Cough Caplets—acetaminophen 325 mg + phenylephrine 5 mg + dextromethorphan 10 mg **(OTC)**
Sudafed PE Pressure + Pain + Mucus Caplets—phenylephrine 5 mg + guaifenesin 200 mg + acetaminophen 325 mg **(OTC)**
Syeda—drospirenone 3 mg + ethinyl estradiol 30 mcg
Symbicort 80/4.5—(per actuation) budesonide 80 mcg + formoterol 4.5 mcg
Symbicort 160/4.5—(per actuation) budesonide 160 mcg + formoterol 4.5 mcg
Symbyax 3/25—olanzapine 3 mg + fluoxetine 25 mg
Symbyax 6/25—olanzapine 6 mg + fluoxetine 25 mg
Symbyax 6/50—olanzapine 6 mg + fluoxetine 50 mg
Symbyax 12/25—olanzapine 12 mg + fluoxetine 25 mg
Symbyax 12/50—olanzapine 12 mg + fluoxetine 50 mg
Synalgos-DC—aspirin 356.4 mg + caffeine 30 mg + dihydrocodeine 16 mg
Synera Transdermal Patch—lidocaine 70 mg + tetracaine 70 mg
Synjardy 5/500—empagliflozin 5 mg + metformin 500 mg
Synjardy 5/1000—empagliflozin 5 mg + metformin 1000 mg
Synjardy 12.5/500—empagliflozin 12.5 mg + metformin 500 mg
Synjardy 12.5/1000—empagliflozin 12.5 mg + metformin 1000 mg
Taclonex Topical Ointment/Suspension—0.005% calcipotriene + 0.064% betamethasone
Tarka 1/240—trandolapril 1 mg + sustained-release verapamil 240 mg
Tarka 2/180—trandolapril 2 mg + sustained-release verapamil 180 mg
Tarka 2/240—trandolapril 2 mg + sustained-release verapamil 240 mg
Tarka 4/240—trandolapril 4 mg + sustained-release verapamil 240 mg
Tekturna HCT 150/12.5—aliskiren 150 mg + hydrochlorothiazide 12.5 mg
Tekturna HCT 150/25—aliskiren 150 mg + hydrochlorothiazide 25 mg
Tekturna HCT 300/12.5—aliskiren 300 mg + hydrochlorothiazide 12.5 mg
Tekturna HCT 300/25—aliskiren 300 mg + hydrochlorothiazide 25 mg
Tenoretic 50—chlorthalidone 25 mg + atenolol 50 mg
Tenoretic 100—chlorthalidone 25 mg + atenolol 100 mg
Terramycin with Polymyxin B Sulfate Ophthalmic Ointment—(per g) polymyxin B 10,000 units + oxytetracycline 5 mg
Teveten HCT 600/12.5—eprosartan 600 mg + hydrochlorothiazide 12.5 mg
Teveten HCT 600/25—eprosartan 600 mg + hydrochlorothiazide 25 mg
TheraFlu Daytime Severe Cold & Cough—(per packet) acetaminophen 650 mg + phenylephrine 10 mg + dextromethorphan 20 mg **(OTC)**
TheraFlu Expressmax Daytime Severe Cold & Cough Liquid—(per 30 mL) acetaminophen 650 mg + phenylephrine 10 mg + dextromethorphan 20 mg **(OTC)**
TheraFlu Expressmax Flu, Cough & Sore Throat Liquid—(per 30 mL) acetaminophen 650 mg + phenylephrine 10 mg + diphenhydramine 25 mg **(OTC)**
TheraFlu Expressmax Nighttime Severe Cold & Cough Liquid—(per 30 mL) acetaminophen 650 mg + phenylephrine 10 mg + diphenhydramine 25 mg **(OTC)**
TheraFlu Flu & Sore Throat—(per packet) acetaminophen 650 mg + phenylephrine 10 mg + pheniramine 20 mg **(OTC)**
TheraFlu Multi-Symptom Severe Cold—(per packet) acetaminophen 500 mg + phenylephrine 10 mg + dextromethorphan 20 mg **(OTC)**

TheraFlu Nighttime Multi-Symptom Severe Cold—(per packet) acetaminophen 500 mg + phenylephrine 10 mg + diphenhydramine 25 mg **(OTC)**
TheraFlu Nighttime Severe Cold & Cough—(per packet) acetaminophen 650 mg + phenylephrine 10 mg + diphenhydramine 25 mg **(OTC)**
Tilia Fe
Phase I—norethindrone 1 mg + ethinyl estradiol 20 mcg
Phase II—norethindrone 1 mg + ethinyl estradiol 30 mcg
Phase III—norethindrone 1 mg + ethinyl estradiol 35 mcg
Phase IV—ferrous fumarate 75 mg
TobraDex Ophthalmic Suspension/Ointment—0.1% dexamethasone + 0.3% tobramycin
TobraDex ST Ophthalmic Suspension—0.05% dexamethasone + 0.3% tobramycin
Treximet 10/60—sumatriptan 10 mg + naproxen 60 mg
Treximet 85/500—sumatriptan 85 mg + naproxen 500 mg
Tri—Estarylla
Phase I—norgestimate 0.18 mg + ethinyl estradiol 35 mcg
Phase II—norgestimate 0.215 mg + ethinyl estradiol 35 mcg
Phase III—norgestimate 0.25 mg + ethinyl estradiol 35 mcg
Tri—Legest–21
Phase I—norethindrone 1 mg + ethinyl estradiol 20 mcg
Phase II—norethindrone 1 mg + ethinyl estradiol 30 mcg
Phase III—norethindrone 1 mg + ethinyl estradiol 35 mcg
Tri—Legest Fe
Phase I—norethindrone 1 mg + ethinyl estradiol 20 mcg
Phase II—norethindrone 1 mg + ethinyl estradiol 30 mcg
Phase III—norethindrone 1 mg + ethinyl estradiol 35 mcg
Phase IV—ferrous fumarate 75 mg
Tri—Linyah
Phase I—norgestimate 0.18 mg + ethinyl estradiol 35 mcg
Phase II—norgestimate 0.215 mg + ethinyl estradiol 35 mcg
Phase III—norgestimate 0.25 mg + ethinyl estradiol 35 mcg
Tri-Lo-Estarylla
Phase I—norgestimate 0.18 mg + ethinyl estradiol 25 mcg
Phase II—norgestimate 0.215 mg + ethinyl estradiol 25 mcg
Phase III—norgestimate 0.25 mg + ethinyl estradiol 25 mcg
Tri-Luma Topical Cream—0.01% fluocinolone + 4% hydroquinone + 0.05% tretinoin
Tri-Norinyl
Phase I—norethindrone 0.5 mg + ethinyl estradiol 35 mcg
Phase II—norethindrone 1 mg + ethinyl estradiol 35 mcg
Phase III—norethindrone 0.5 mg + ethinyl estradiol 35 mcg
Tri-Previfem
Phase I—norgestimate 0.18 mg + ethinyl estradiol 35 mcg
Phase II—norgestimate 0.215 mg + ethinyl estradiol 35 mcg
Phase III—norgestimate 0.25 mg + ethinyl estradiol 35 mcg
Tri-Sprintec
Phase I—norgestimate 0.18 mg + ethinyl estradiol 35 mcg
Phase II—norgestimate 0.215 mg + ethinyl estradiol 35 mcg
Phase III—norgestimate 0.25 mg + ethinyl estradiol 35 mcg
Triacin-C Cough Syrup—(per 5 mL) codeine 10 mg + pseudoephedrine 30 mg + triprolidine 1.25 mg
Triaminic Cough & Congestion Liquid—(per 5 mL) guaifenesin 100 mg + dextromethorphan 5 mg **(OTC)**
Triaminic Cough & Sore Throat Liquid—(per 5 mL) acetaminophen 160 mg + dextromethorphan 5 mg **(OTC)**
Triaminic Day Time Cold & Cough Liquid—(per 5 mL) phenylephrine 2.5 mg + dextromethorphan 5 mg **(OTC)**
Triaminic Multi-Symptom Fever & Cold Liquid—(per 5 mL) acetaminophen 160 mg + dextromethorphan 5 mg + chlorpheniramine 1 mg + phenylephrine 2.5 mg **(OTC)**
Triaminic Night Time Cold & Cough Liquid—(per 5 mL) phenylephrine 2.5 mg + diphenhydramine 6.25 mg **(OTC)**
Tribenzor 20/5/12.5—olmesartan 20 mg + amlodipine 5 mg + hydrochlorothiazide 12.5 mg
Tribenzor 40/5/12.5—olmesartan 40 mg + amlodipine 5 mg + hydrochlorothiazide 12.5 mg
Tribenzor 40/5/25—olmesartan 40 mg + amlodipine 5 mg + hydrochlorothiazide 25 mg

Tribenzor 40/10/12.5—olmesartan 40 mg + amlodipine 10 mg + hydrochlorothiazide 12.5 mg
Tribenzor 40/10/25—olmesartan 40 mg + amlodipine 10 mg + hydrochlorothiazide 25 mg
TriLyte—PEG 3350 420 g + sodium bicarbonate 5.72 g + sodium chloride 11.2 g + potassium chloride 1.48 g
TriNessa
Phase I—norgestimate 0.18 mg + ethinyl estradiol 35 mcg
Phase II—norgestimate 0.215 mg + ethinyl estradiol 35 mcg
Phase III—norgestimate 0.25 mg + ethinyl estradiol 35 mcg
Triumeq—abacavir 600 mg + dolutegravir 50 mg + lamivudine 300 mg
Trivora-28
Phase I—levonorgestrel 0.05 mg + ethinyl estradiol 30 mcg
Phase II—levonorgestrel 0.075 mg + ethinyl estradiol 40 mcg
Phase III—levonorgestrel 0.125 mg + ethinyl estradiol 30 mcg
Trizivir—abacavir 300 mg + lamivudine 150 mg + zidovudine 300 mg
Truvada—emtricitabine 200 mg + tenofovir 300 mg
TussiCaps 5/4—hydrocodone 5 mg + chlorpheniramine 4 mg
TussiCaps 10/8—hydrocodone 10 mg + chlorpheniramine 8 mg
Tussigon—hydrocodone 5 mg + homatropine 1.5 mg
Tussionex Suspension—(per 5 mL) chlorpheniramine 8 mg + hydrocodone 10 mg
Twynsta 40/5—telmisartan 40 mg + amlodipine 5 mg
Twynsta 40/10—telmisartan 40 mg + amlodipine 10 mg
Twynsta 80/5—telmisartan 80 mg + amlodipine 5 mg
Twynsta 80/10—telmisartan 80 mg + amlodipine 10 mg
Tylenol Cold & Flu Severe Caplets—acetaminophen 325 mg + phenylephrine 5 mg + dextromethorphan 10 mg + guaifenesin 200 mg **(OTC)**
Tylenol Cold & Flu Severe Warming Liquid—(per 15 mL) acetaminophen 325 mg + phenylephrine 5 mg + dextromethorphan 10 mg + guaifenesin 200 mg **(OTC)**
Tylenol Cold Head Congestion Severe Caplets—acetaminophen 325 mg + phenylephrine 5 mg + guaifenesin 200 mg **(OTC)**
Tylenol Cold Multi-Symptom Daytime Caplets—acetaminophen 325 mg + phenylephrine 5 mg + dextromethorphan 10 mg **(OTC)**
Tylenol Cold Multi-Symptom Daytime Liquid—(per 15 mL) acetaminophen 325 mg + phenylephrine 5 mg + dextromethorphan 10 mg **(OTC)**
Tylenol Cold Multi-Symptom Nighttime Liquid—(per 15 mL) acetaminophen 325 mg + phenylephrine 5 mg + dextromethorphan 10 mg + doxylamine 6.25 mg **(OTC)**
Tylenol Cold Multi-Symptom Severe Liquid—(per 15 mL) acetaminophen 325 mg + guaifenesin 200 mg + phenylephrine 5 mg + dextromethorphan 10 mg **(OTC)**
Tylenol PM Caplets—acetaminophen 500 mg + diphenhydramine 25 mg **(OTC)**
Tylenol Sinus Congestion & Pain Daytime Caplets—acetaminophen 325 mg + phenylephrine 5 mg **(OTC)**
🍁 **Tylenol with Codeine No. 1**—acetaminophen 300 mg + codeine 8 mg + caffeine 15 mg **(OTC)**
Tylenol with Codeine No. 3—acetaminophen 300 mg + codeine 30 mg
Tylenol with Codeine No. 4—acetaminophen 300 mg + codeine 60 mg
Ultracet—tramadol 37.5 mg + acetaminophen 325 mg
Ultresa—lipase 13,800 units + amylase 27,600 units + protease 27,600 units
Ultresa—lipase 20,700 units + amylase 41,400 units + protease 41,400 units
Ultresa—lipase 23,000 units + amylase 46,000 units + protease 46,000 units
Uniretic 7.5/12.5—moexipril 7.5 mg + hydrochlorothiazide 12.5 mg
Uniretic 15/12.5—moexipril 15 mg + hydrochlorothiazide 12.5 mg
Uniretic 15/25—moexipril 15 mg + hydrochlorothiazide 25 mg
Vanoxide HC Topical Lotion—0.5% hydrocortisone + 5% benzoyl peroxide
Vanquish Extra Strength Pain Reliever—aspirin 227 mg + acetaminophen 194 mg + caffeine 33 mg **(OTC)**
Vaseretic 5/12.5—enalapril 5 mg + hydrochlorothiazide 12.5 mg
Vaseretic 10/25—enalapril 10 mg + hydrochlorothiazide 25 mg
Velivet
Phase I—desogestrel 0.1 mg + ethinyl estradiol 25 mcg
Phase II—desogestrel 0.125 mg + ethinyl estradiol 25 mcg
Phase III—desogestrel 0.15 mg + ethinyl estradiol 25 mcg
Veltin Topical Gel—1.2% clindamycin + 0.025% tretinoin

Vestura—drospirenone 3 mg + ethinyl estradiol 20 mcg
Vicoprofen—hydrocodone 7.5 mg + ibuprofen 200 mg
Vienva—levonorgestrel 0.1 mg + ethinyl estradiol 20 mcg
Vimovo 375/20—naproxen 375 mg + esomeprazole 20 mg
Vimovo 500/20—naproxen 500 mg + esomeprazole 20 mg
Viokace—lipase 10,440 units + amylase 39,150 units + protease 39,150 units
Viokace—lipase 20,880 units + amylase 78,300 units + protease 78,300 units
Viorele—desogestrel 0.15 mg + ethinyl estradiol 20 mcg/10 mcg
Visine-A Eye Allergy Relief Ophthalmic Solution—0.025% naphazoline + 0.3% pheniramine **(OTC)**
Vituz Solution—(per 5 mL) hydrocodone 5 mg + chlorpheniramine 4 mg
Vusion Topical Ointment—0.25% miconazole + 15% zinc oxide
Vyfemla—norethindrone 0.4 mg + ethinyl estradiol 35 mcg
Vytorin 10/10—ezetimibe 10 mg + simvastatin 10 mg
Vytorin 10/20—ezetimibe 10 mg + simvastatin 20 mg
Vytorin 10/40—ezetimibe 10 mg + simvastatin 40 mg
Vytorin 10/80—ezetimibe 10 mg + simvastatin 80 mg
Wera—norethindrone 0.5 mg + ethinyl estradiol 35 mcg
Wymzya Fe—norethindrone 0.4 mg + ethinyl estradiol 35 mcg + ferrous fumarate 75 mg
Xartemis XR—oxycodone 7.5 mg + acetaminophen 325 mg
Xenaderm Topical Ointment—(per g) trypsin 90 USP units + Balsam Peru 87 mg + castor oil 788 mg
Xerese Topical Cream—5% acyclovir + 1% hydrocortisone
Xigduo XR 5/500—dapagliflozin 5 mg + metformin 500 mg
Xigduo XR 5/1000—dapagliflozin 5 mg + metformin 1000 mg
Xigduo XR 10/500—dapagliflozin 10 mg + metformin 500 mg
Xigduo XR 10/1000—dapagliflozin 10 mg + metformin 1000 mg
Xulane—norelgestromin 150 mcg/day + ethinyl estradiol 35 mcg/day
Xylocaine with Epinephrine Injection 0.5/0.0005—0.5% lidocaine + 0.0005% epinephrine
Xylocaine with Epinephrine Injection 1/0.001—1% lidocaine + 0.001% epinephrine
Xylocaine with Epinephrine Injection 2/0.001—2% lidocaine + 0.001% epinephrine
Yaela—drospirenone 3 mg + ethinyl estradiol 30 mcg
Yasmin—drospirenone 3 mg + ethinyl estradiol 30 mcg
Yaz—drospirenone 3 mg + ethinyl estradiol 20 mcg
Zarah—drospirenone 3 mg + ethinyl estradiol 30 mcg
Zegerid Capsules 20/1100—omeprazole 20 mg + sodium bicarbonate 1100 mg
Zegerid Capsules 40/1100—omeprazole 40 mg + sodium bicarbonate 1100 mg
Zegerid OTC Capsules—omeprazole 20 mg + sodium bicarbonate 1100 mg **(OTC)**
Zegerid Powder for Oral Suspension 20/1680—(per pkt) omeprazole 20 mg + sodium bicarbonate 1680 mg **(OTC)**
Zegerid Powder for Oral Suspension 40/1680—(per pkt) omeprazole 40 mg + sodium bicarbonate 1680 mg
Zenchent—norethindrone 0.4 mg + ethinyl estradiol 35 mcg
Zenchent Fe—norethindrone 0.4 mg + ethinyl estradiol 35 mcg + ferrous fumarate 75 mg
Zenpep—lipase 3000 units + amylase 16,000 units + protease 10,000 units
Zenpep—lipase 5000 units + amylase 27,000 units + protease 17,000 units
Zenpep—lipase 10,000 units + amylase 55,000 units + protease 34,000 units
Zenpep—lipase 15,000 units + amylase 82,000 units + protease 51,000 units
Zenpep—lipase 20,000 units + amylase 109,000 units + protease 68,000 units
Zenpep—lipase 25,000 units + amylase 136,000 units + protease 85,000 units
Zenpep—lipase 40,000 units + amylase 218,000 units + protease 136,000 units
Zestoretic 10/12.5—lisinopril 10 mg + hydrochlorothiazide 12.5 mg
Zestoretic 20/12.5—lisinopril 20 mg + hydrochlorothiazide 12.5 mg
Zestoretic 20/25—lisinopril 20 mg + hydrochlorothiazide 25 mg
Ziac 2.5/6.25—bisoprolol 2.5 mg + hydrochlorothiazide 6.25 mg
Ziac 5/6.25—bisoprolol 5 mg + hydrochlorothiazide 6.25 mg
Ziac 10/6.25—bisoprolol 10 mg + hydrochlorothiazide 6.25 mg
Ziana Topical Gel—1.2% clindamycin + 0.025% tretinoin
Zovia 1/35—ethynodiol 1 mg + ethinyl estradiol 35 mcg
Zovia 1/50—ethynodiol 1 mg + ethinyl estradiol 50 mcg
Zubsolv 1.4/0.36—buprenorphine 1.4 mg + naloxone 0.36 mg
Zubsolv 2.9/0.71—buprenorphine 2.9 mg + naloxone 0.71 mg

Zubsolv 5.7/1.4—buprenorphine 5.7 mg + naloxone 1.4 mg
Zubsolv 8.6/2.1—buprenorphine 8.6 mg + naloxone 2.1 mg
Zubsolv 11.4/2.9—buprenorphine 11.4 mg + naloxone 2.9 mg
Zutripro Solution—(per 5 mL) chlorpheniramine 4 mg + pseudoephedrine 60 mg + hydrocodone 5 mg
Zylet Ophthalmic Suspension—0.5% loteprednol + 0.3% tobramycin
Zyrtec-D Allergy & Congestion—cetirizine 5 mg + pseudoephedrine 120 mg **(OTC)**

APPENDIX C

Ophthalmic Medications

General Info: See Appendix D for administration techniques for ophthalmic agents.
Consult health care professional regarding:
Concurrent use of contact lenses (medication or additives may be absorbed by the lens).
Concurrent administration of other ophthalmic agents (order and spacing may be important).
ADRs = adverse reactions.

DRUG NAME	DOSE	NOTES
Anesthetics		
Uses: Provide brief local anesthesia to allow measurement of intraocular pressure, removal of foreign bodies, or other superficial procedures. **CAUTIONS:** Repeated use may result in ↑ risk of CNS and cardiovascular toxicity; cross-sensitivity with some local anesthetics may occur.		
lidocaine (Akten)	**Adults and children:** 2 drops of 3.5% gel (single dose).	• Does not interact with ophthalmic cholinesterase inhibitors • ADRs: ophthalmic—irritation; systemic—irregular heartbeat, CNS depression
proparacaine (Alcaine)	**Adults and children:** 1–2 drops of 0.5% solution (single dose).	• Does not interact with ophthalmic cholinesterase inhibitors • ADRs: ophthalmic—irritation; systemic—irregular heartbeat, CNS depression
tetracaine (Altacaine, 🍁 Pontocaine, Tetcaine)	**Adults:** 1–2 drops of 0.5% solution (single dose).	• May interact with ophthalmic cholinesterase inhibitors, resulting in ↑ duration of action and risk of toxicity • ADRs: ophthalmic—irritation; systemic—irregular heartbeat, CNS depression
Antihistamines		
Uses: Various forms of allergic conjunctivitis.		
alcaftadine (Lastacaft)	**Adults and children ≥2 yr:** 1 drop of 0.25% solution once daily.	• ADRs: transient burning/stinging, headache
azelastine (Optivar)	**Adults and children ≥3 yr:** 1 drop of 0.05% solution twice daily.	• ADRs: transient burning/stinging, headache, bitter taste
bepotastine (Bepreve)	**Adults and children ≥2 yr:** 1 drop of 1.5% solution twice daily.	• ADRs: taste disturbance, headache, local irritation
emedastine (Emadine)	**Adults and children ≥3 yr:** 1 drop of 0.05% solution up to 4 times daily.	• ADRs: headache, drowsiness, malaise, local irritation
epinastine (Elestat)	**Adults and children ≥2 yr:** 1 drop of 0.05% solution twice daily.	• ADRs: headache, local irritation
ketotifen (Alaway, Claritin Eye, Zaditor, Zyrtec Itchy Eye)	**Adults and children ≥3 yr:** 1 drop of 0.025% solution twice daily (given 8–12 hr apart).	• OTC • ADRs: local irritation
olopatadine (Pataday, Patanol, Pazeo)	**Adults and children ≥2 yr (Pataday, Patanol; ≥3 yr (Pazeo):** *Patanol*—1 drop of 0.1% solution twice daily (given 6–8 hr apart); *Pataday*—1 drop of 0.2% solution once daily; *Pazeo*—1 drop of 0.7% solution once daily.	• Small amounts are absorbed; excreted in urine • ADRs: headache, conjunctival irritation
Anti-infectives/Antifungals/Antivirals		
Uses: Localized superficial ophthalmic infections (e.g., bacterial conjunctivitis). **CAUTIONS:** Small amounts may be absorbed and result in hypersensitivity reactions.		

DRUG NAME	DOSE	NOTES
azithromycin (AzaSite)	**Adults and children ≥1 yr:** 1 drop of 1% solution twice daily (given 8–12 hr apart) for 2 days, then once daily for 5 more days.	• When used to treat ocular chlamydial infections, concurrent systemic therapy is required • ADRs: eye irritation
bacitracin	**Adults and children:** ¼–½-in. strip q 3–4 hr for acute infections or 2–3 times daily for mild-moderate infections.	• ADRs: eye irritation
besifloxacin (Besivance)	**Adults and children ≥1 yr:** 1 drop of 0.6% suspension 3 times daily (given 4–12 hr apart) for 7 days.	• ADRs: headache, eye irritation
ciprofloxacin (Ciloxan)	**Adults and children >1 yr (solution) or >2 yr (ointment):** *Bacterial conjunctivitis*—Solution: 1–2 drops of 0.3% solution q 2 hr while awake for 2 days, then q 4 hr while awake for 5 more days; Ointment: ½-in. strip 3 times daily for 2 days, then twice daily for 5 more days; *Corneal ulcers*—Solution: 2 drops of 0.3% solution q 15 min for 6 hr, then q 30 min while awake for rest of day, then q 1 hr while awake for next 24 hr, then q 4 hr while awake for next 12 days or longer if re-epithelialization does not occur.	• May cause harmless white crystalline precipitate that resolves over time • ADRs: altered taste, systemic allergic reactions, photophobia, discomfort
erythromycin (🍁 Diomycin)	**Adults and children:** *Treatment of infections*—½-in. strip 2–6 times daily. Infants: *Prophylaxis of ophthalmia neonatorum*—thin strip in each eye as a single dose.	• ADRs: irritation
fusidic acid (🍁 Fucithalmic)	**Adults and children ≥2 yr:** 1 drop of 1% solution twice daily for 7 days.	• ADRs: irritation
gatifloxacin (🍁 Zymar, Zymaxid)	**Adults and children ≥1 yr:** 1 drop of 0.5% solution q 2 hr while awake (up to 8 times/day) for 1 day, then 2–4 times daily while awake for 6 more days.	• ADRs: irritation, headache, ↓ visual acuity, taste disturbance
gentamicin (🍁 Diogent, Genoptic, Gentak)	**Adults and children:** *Solution*—1–2 drops of 0.3% solution q 2–4 hr; *Ointment*—½-in. strip q 8–12 hr.	• ADRs: irritation, burning, stinging, blurred vision (ointment)
levofloxacin	**Adults and children ≥6 yr:** *Bacterial conjunctivitis*—1–2 drops of 0.5% solution q 2 hr while awake for 2 days (up to 8 times/day); then every 4 hr while awake for 5 more days (up to 4 times/day).	• ADRs: altered taste, systemic allergic reactions, photophobia
moxifloxacin (Moxeza, Vigamox)	**Adults and children ≥1 yr (Vigamox) or ≥4 mo (Moxeza):** *Moxeza*—1 drop of 0.5% solution twice daily for 7 days; *Vigamox*—1 drop of 0.5% solution 3 times daily for 7 days.	• ADRs: irritation, ↓ visual acuity
ofloxacin (Ocuflox)	**Adults and children ≥1 yr:** *Bacterial conjunctivitis*—1–2 drops of 0.3% solution q 2–4 hr while awake for 2 days, then 4 times daily for 5 more days; *Corneal ulcer*—1–2 drops of 0.3% solution q 30 min while awake and q 4–6 hr while sleeping for 2 days, then q hr while awake for 4–6 more days, then 4 times daily until cured.	• ADRs: altered taste, systemic allergic reactions, photophobia

DRUG NAME	DOSE	NOTES
sulfacetamide (AK Sulf Liq, Bleph-10, ✱ Diosulf, ✱ Sodium Sulamyd)	**Adults and children ≥2 mo:** *Solution*—1–2 drops of 10% solution q 2–3 hr while awake (less frequently at night) for 7–10 days; *Ointment*—½-in. strip q 3–4 hr and at bedtime for 7–10 days.	• Cross-sensitivity with other sulfonamides (including thiazides) may occur • ADRs: local irritation
tobramycin (AK-Tob, Tobrex)	**Adults and children ≥2 mo:** *Solution*—1–2 drops of 0.3% solution q 2–4 hr depending on severity of infection; *Ointment*—½-in. strip q 8–12 hr.	• Ointment may retard corneal wound healing • ADRs: irritation, burning, stinging, blurred vision (ointment)
Antifungal		
natamycin (Natacyn)	**Adults:** *Fungal keratitis*—1 drop of 5% suspension q 1–2 hr for 3–4 days, then 6–8 times/day for 2–3 wk; *Fungal blepharitis or conjunctivitis*—1 drop of 5% suspension q 4–6 hr for for 2–3 wk.	• ADRs: irritation, swelling
Antivirals		
ganciclovir (Zirgan)	**Adults and children ≥2 yr:** 1 drop of 0.15% gel 5 times daily (q 3 hr while awake) until corneal ulcer heals, then 3 times daily for 7 days.	• ADRs: blurred vision, irritation, keratopathy
trifluridine (Viroptic)	**Adults and children ≥6 yr:** 1 drop of 1% solution q 2 hr while awake (up to 9 drops/day) until re-epithelialization occurs, then q 4 hr while awake for 7 more days (not to exceed 21 days).	• ADRs: burning, stinging, keratopathy
Artificial Tears/Ocular Lubricants (sterile buffered isotonic solutions/ointments) **Uses:** Artificial tears—keep the eyes moist with isotonic solutions and wetting agents in the management of dry eyes due to lack of tears; also provide lubrication for artificial eyes. Ocular lubricants—provide lubrication and protection in a variety of conditions including exposure keratitis, ↓ corneal sensitivity, corneal erosions, keratitis sicca, during/following ocular surgery or removal of a foreign body.		
Artificial tears (Akwa Tears, Bion Tears, Blink, Cellufresh, Celluvisc, ✱ Duolube, ✱ Duratears Lubricant Eye Gel, Duratears Naturale, Genteal Lubricant Eye Gel, ✱ Hylo, HypoTears, HypoTears PF, ✱ Isopto Tears, Just Tears, Lacri-Lube NP, Lacri-Lube S.O.P., Liquifilm Forte, Liquifilm Tears, Murine Tears, Nature's Tears, Nu-Tears, Nu-Tears II, Nutra Tear, Refresh, Refresh PM, Soothe, Systane, Teargen, Tearisol, Tears Naturale, Tears Naturale Free, Tears Naturale II, Tears Plus, Tears Renewed, Ultra Tears, Viva-Drops)	**Adults and children:** *Artificial tears*—Solution: 1–2 drops 3–4 times daily; Insert: 1 insert 1–2 times daily; *Ocular lubricants*—small amount instilled into conjunctiva several times daily.	• May alter effects of other concurrently administered ophthalmic medications • ADRs: photophobia, lid edema stinging (insert only), transient blurred vision, eye discomfort
Beta Blockers **Uses:** Treatment of open-angle glaucoma and other forms of ocular hypertension (↓ formation of aqueous humor). **CAUTIONS:** Systemic absorption is minimal but may occur. Systemic absorption may result in additive adverse cardiovascular effects (bradycardia, hypotension), especially when used with other cardiovascular agents (antihypertensives, antiarrhythmics). Other systemic adverse reactions may occur, including bronchospasm or delirium (geriatric patients). Concurrent use with ophthalmic epinephrine may ↓ effectiveness.		
betaxolol (Betoptic, Betoptic S)	**Adults:** *Betoptic*—1–2 drops of 0.5% solution twice daily; *Betoptic S*—1 drop of 0.25% suspension twice daily.	• ADRs: conjunctivitis, ↓ visual acuity, ocular burning, rash (may be less likely than others to cause bronchospasm if systemically absorbed)
carteolol	**Adults:** 1 drop of 1% solution twice daily.	• ADRs: ocular burning, ↓ visual acuity

DRUG NAME	DOSE	NOTES
levobunolol (AKBeta, Betagan)	**Adults:** 1–2 drops of 0.25% solution twice daily or 1–2 drops of 0.5% solution once daily.	• ADRs: conjunctivitis, ↓ visual acuity, ocular burning, rash
metipranolol (OptiPranolol)	**Adults:** 1 drop of 0.3% solution twice daily.	• Lasts up to 24 hr • ADRs: conjunctivitis, ↓ visual acuity, ocular burning, rash
timolol (Betimol, Istalol, Timoptic, Timoptic-XE)	**Adults:** *Solution*—1 drop of 0.25–0.5% solution 1–2 times daily; *Gel-forming solution*—1 drop of 0.25–0.5% solution once daily.	• Lasts up to 24 hr • ADRs: conjunctivitis, ↓ visual acuity, ocular burning, rash

Carbonic Anhydrase Inhibitors

Uses: Treatment of open-angle glaucoma and other forms of ocular hypertension (↓ formation of aqueous humor).
CAUTIONS: May exacerbate kidney stones; should not be used in patients with CCr <30 mL/min; may have cross-sensitivity with sulfonamides.

DRUG NAME	DOSE	NOTES
brinzolamide (Azopt)	**Adults:** 1 drop of 1% suspension 3 times daily.	• ADRs: burning, stinging, unusual taste
dorzolamide (Trusopt)	**Adults and Children:** 1 drop of 2% solution 3 times daily.	• ADRs: bitter taste, ocular irritation, or allergy

Cholinergics (direct-acting)

Uses: Treatment of open-angle glaucoma (facilitates the outflow of aqueous humor); also used to facilitate miosis after ophthalmic surgery or before examination (to counteract mydriatics).
CAUTIONS: Conditions in which pupillary constriction occurs should be avoided. If significant systemic absorption occurs, bronchospasm, sweating, and ↑ urination and salivation may occur.

DRUG NAME	DOSE	NOTES
acetylcholine (Miochol-E)	**Adults:** 0.5–2 mL instilled into anterior chamber before or after securing one or more sutures.	• ADRs: corneal edema, corneal clouding
carbachol (Isopto Carbachol, Miostat)	**Adults:** *Glaucoma*—1–2 drops of 0.01–3% solution 1–3 times daily; *To facilitate miosis*—0.5 mL instilled into anterior chamber before or after securing sutures.	• ADRs: blurred vision, altered vision, stinging, eye pain
pilocarpine (🍁 Diocarpine, Isopto Carpine)	**Adults:** *Glaucoma*—Solution: 1–2 drops of 0.5–4% solution up to 6 times daily; *Counteracting mydriatic sympathomimetics*—1 drop of 1% solution (may be repeated prior to surgery).	• ADRs: blurred vision, altered vision, stinging, eye pain, headache

Cholinergics (cholinesterase inhibitors)

Uses: Treatment of open-angle glaucoma not controlled with short-acting miotics or other agents; also used in varying doses for accommodative esotropia (diagnosis and treatment).
CAUTIONS: Enhance neuromuscular blockade from succinylcholine; intensify the actions of cocaine and some other local anesthetics; additive toxicity with antimyasthenics, anticholinergics, and cholinesterase inhibitors (including some pesticides). Use cautiously in patients with history or risk of retinal detachment.

DRUG NAME	DOSE	NOTES
echothiophate (Phospholine Iodide)	**Adults:** 1 drop of 0.125% solution 1–2 times daily.	• Irreversible cholinesterase inhibitor • May cause hyperactivity in patients with Down syndrome • ADRs: blurred vision, change in vision, brow ache, miosis, eyelid twitching, watering eyes

Corticosteroids

Uses: Management of inflammatory eye conditions including allergic conjunctivitis, nonspecific superficial keratitis, anterior endogenous uveitis; infectious conjunctivitis (with anti-infectives); management of corneal injury; suppression of graft rejection following keratoplasty; prevention of postoperative inflammation.
CAUTIONS: Use cautiously in patients with infectious ocular processes (avoid in herpes simplex keratitis), especially fungal and viral ocular infections (may mask symptoms); diabetes, glaucoma, or epithelial compromise.

DRUG NAME	DOSE	NOTES
dexamethasone (✱ Diodex, Maxidex)	**Adults:** *Solution*—1–2 drops of 0.1% solution q hr during the day and q 2 hr during the night, gradually ↓ the dose to 1 drop q 4 hr, then to 3–4 times daily; *Suspension*—1–2 drops of 0.1% suspension up to 4–6 times daily.	• As condition improves, ↓ frequency of administration • ADRs: corneal thinning, ↑ intraocular pressure, irritation
difluprednate (Durezol)	**Adults and children:** *Postoperative inflammation*—1 drop of 0.05% emulsion 4 times daily beginning 24 hr after surgery and continued for 2 wk, then 2 times daily for 1 wk, then taper; *Uveitis*—1 drops of 0.05% emulsion 4 times daily for 14 days, then taper.	• As condition improves, ↓ frequency of administration • ADRs: blepharitis, photophobia, ↓ visual acuity
fluorometholone (Flarex, FML, FML Forte)	**Adults and children ≥2 yr:** *Suspension*—1–2 drops of 0.1% suspension 4 times daily (up to 2 drops q 2 hr during initial 24–48 hr) or 1 drop of 0.25% suspension 2–4 times daily (up to 1 drop q 4 hr during initial 24–48 hr); *Ointment*—½-in. strip 1–3 times daily (up to q 4 hr during initial 24–48 hr).	• As condition improves, ↓ frequency of administration • ADRs: blurred vision (ointment), corneal thinning, ↑ intraocular pressure, irritation
loteprednol (Alrex, Lotemax)	**Adults:** *Allergic conjunctivitis*—Alrex: 1 drop of 0.2% suspension 4 times daily; *Inflammatory conditions*—Lotemax: 1–2 drops of 0.5% suspension 4 times daily (up to 1 drop q hr may be used in first wk); *Postoperative inflammation*—Lotemax gel/suspension: 1–2 drops of 0.5% gel/suspension 4 times daily beginning 24 hr after surgery and continued for 2 wk; Lotemax ointment: ½-in. strip 4 times daily beginning 24 hr after surgery and continued for 2 wk.	• ADRs: corneal thinning, ↑ intraocular pressure, irritation
prednisolone (✱ Diopred, Omnipred, Pred Forte, Pred Mild)	**Adults and children:** 1–2 drops of 0.12–1% solution/suspension 2–4 times daily.	• As condition improves, ↓ frequency of administration • ADRs: corneal thinning, ↑ intraocular pressure, irritation
rimexolone (Vexol)	**Adults:** *Postoperative inflammation*—1–2 drops of 1% suspension 4 times daily beginning 24 hr after surgery and continued for 2 wk; *Uveitis*—1–2 drops of 1% suspension q hr while awake for 1 wk, then 1 drop q 2 hr while awake for 1 wk, then taper.	• As condition improves, ↓ frequency of administration • ADRs: corneal thinning, ↑ intraocular pressure, irritation

Cycloplegic Mydriatics

Uses: Preparation for cycloplegic refraction; management of uveitis (not tropicamide).

CAUTIONS: Use cautiously in patients with a history of glaucoma; systemic absorption may cause anticholinergic effects such as confusion, unusual behavior, flushing, hallucinations, slurred speech, drowsiness, swollen stomach (infants), tachycardia, or dry mouth.

DRUG NAME	DOSE	NOTES
atropine (✱ Isopto Atropine)	**Adults:** *Cycloplegic refraction*—1–2 drops of 1% solution 1 hr before procedure; *Uveitis*—Solution: 1–2 drops of 1% solution 4 times daily; Ointment: 0.3–0.5-cm strip up to 3 times daily.	• Effects on accommodation may last 6 days; mydriasis may last 12 days • ADRs: irritation, blurred vision, photophobia

DRUG NAME	DOSE	NOTES
cyclopentolate (Cyclogyl, 🍁 Diopentolate, Pentolair)	**Adults:** 1–2 drops of 0.5–2% solution; may repeat in 5–10 min. **Children:** 1 drop of 0.5–2% solution; may be followed 5–10 min later by 1 drop of 0.5–1% solution.	• Peak of cycloplegia is within 25–75 min and lasts 6–24 hr • Peak of mydriasis is within 30–60 min and may last several days • 2% solution used for heavily pigmented iris • ADRs: irritation, blurred vision, photophobia
homatropine (Isopto Homatropine)	**Adults:** *Cycloplegic refraction*—1–2 drops of 2–5% solution, may repeat in 5–10 min for 2 more doses; *Uveitis*—1–2 drops of 2–5% solution 2–3 times daily (up to q 4 hr). **Children:** *Cycloplegic refraction*—1–2 drops of 2% solution, may repeat in 10–15 min if needed; *Uveitis*—1–2 drops of 2% solution 2–3 times daily (up to q 4 hr).	• Cycloplegia and mydriasis may last for 24–72 hr • ADRs: irritation, blurred vision, photophobia
scopolamine (Isopto Hyoscine)	**Adults:** *Cycloplegic refraction*—1–2 drops of 0.25% solution 1 hr before procedure; *Uveitis*—1–2 drops of 0.25% solution up to 4 times daily.	• Shorter duration than atropine, but mydriasis and cycloplegia may last for 3–7 days • ADRs: irritation, blurred vision, photophobia
tropicamide (🍁 Diotrope, Mydriacyl, Tropicacyl)	**Adults and children:** 1–2 drops of 0.5–1% solution.	• Stronger solution/repeated dosing may be required in patients with dark irides • Peak effect occurs in 20–40 min • Cycloplegia lasts 2–6 hr; mydriasis lasts up to 7 hr • ADRs: irritation, blurred vision, photophobia

Immunomodulators

Uses: ↑ tear production when the cause of dry eye is inflammation secondary to keratoconjunctivitis sicca.
CAUTIONS: Tear production is not ↑ during concurrent use of ophthalmic NSAIDs or punctal plugs.

DRUG NAME	DOSE	NOTES
cyclosporine (Restasis)	**Adults and Children ≥16 yr:** 1 drop of 0.05% emulsion q 12 hr.	• Emulsion should be inverted to obtain uniform opaque appearance prior to use. • ADRs: irritation, blurred vision

Mast Cell Stabilizers

Uses: Vernal keratoconjunctivitis.
CAUTIONS: Require several days of treatment before effects are seen.

DRUG NAME	DOSE	NOTES
cromolyn (Opticrom)	**Adults and children >4 yr:** 1–2 drops of 4% solution 4–6 times daily.	• ADRs: irritation
lodoxamide (Alomide)	**Adults and children >2 yr:** 1–2 drops of 0.1% solution 4 times daily for up to 3 mo.	• ADRs: blurred vision, foreign body sensation, irritation
nedocromil (Alocril)	**Adults and children ≥3 yr:** 1–2 drops of 2% solution twice daily throughout period of exposure to allergen.	• ADRs: headache, ocular burning, unpleasant taste, nasal congestion

Nonsteroidal Anti-inflammatory Drugs

Uses: Management of pain/inflammation following surgery (bromfenac, diclofenac, ketorolac, nepafenac), allergic conjunctivitis (ketorolac), inhibition of perioperative miosis (flurbiprofen).
CAUTIONS: Cross-sensitivity with systemic NSAIDs may occur; concurrent use of anticoagulants, other NSAIDs, thrombolytics, some cephalosporins, and valproates may ↑ the risk of bleeding. May slow/delay healing. Avoid contact lens use.

DRUG NAME	DOSE	NOTES
bromfenac (Bromday, Prolensa)	**Adults:** *Bromday*—1 drop of 0.09% solution once daily starting 1 day before surgery and continued on day of surgery and for 2 wk after surgery; *Prolensa*—1 drop of 0.07% solution once daily starting 1 day before surgery and continued on day of surgery and for 2 wk after surgery.	• Contains sulfites • ADRs: irritation, headache
diclofenac (Voltaren Ophthalmic)	**Adults:** *Cataract surgery*—1 drop of 0.1% solution 4 times daily starting 24 hr after surgery and for 2 wk after surgery; *Corneal refractive surgery*—1–2 drops of 0.1% solution within hr before surgery, within 15 min after surgery, then continue 4 times daily for up to 3 days.	• ADRs: irritation, allergic reactions
flurbiprofen (Ocufen)	**Adults:** 1 drop of 0.03% solution q 30 min, beginning 2 hr prior to surgery (4 drops total in each eye).	• ADRs: irritation, allergic reactions
ketorolac (Acular, Acular LS, Acuvail)	**Adults and children ≥2 yr:** *Allergic conjunctivitis*—Acular: 1 drop of 0.5% solution 4 times daily; *Postoperative pain/inflammation*—Acular: 1 drop of 0.5% solution 4 times daily starting 24 hr after cataract surgery and for 2 wk after surgery; Acular LS: 1 drop of 0.4% solution 4 times daily for up to 4 days after corneal refractive surgery; Acuvail: 1 drop of 0.45% solution twice daily starting 1 day before cataract surgery and continued for 2 wk after surgery.	• ADRs: irritation, allergic reactions
nepafenac (Ilevro, Nevanac)	**Adults and children ≥10 yr:** *Ilevro*—1 drop of 0.3% suspension once daily starting one day before cataract surgery and continued for 2 wk after surgery; instill 1 additional drop 30–120 min before surgery; *Nevanac*—1 drop of 0.1% suspension 3 times daily starting one day before cataract surgery and continued for 2 wk after surgery.	• ADRs: irritation, photophobia, headache, hypertension, nausea/vomiting

Ocular Decongestants/Vasoconstrictors

Uses: ↓ ocular congestion due to irritation by vasoconstricting conjunctival blood vessels; stronger solutions have mydriatic effects. **CAUTIONS:** Systemic absorption may result in adverse cardiovascular effects; excessive/prolonged use may produce rebound hyperemia; use caution in patients at risk for acute angle-closure glaucoma; cardiovascular effects may be exaggerated by MAO inhibitors and dose adjustment may be required within 21 days of MAO inhibitors; ↑ risk of arrhythmias with inhalation anesthetics.

DRUG NAME	DOSE	NOTES
naphazoline (Albalon, Clear Eyes Redness Relief, Comfort Eye Drops, 🍁 Diopticon, Naphcon Forte, VasoClear)	**Adults:** 1–2 drops of 0.012–0.025% solution up to 4 times daily (for up to 3 days) or 1–2 drops of 0.1% solution q 3–4 hr as needed.	• ADRs: ophthalmic-rebound hyperemia; systemic-dizziness, headache, nausea, sweating, weakness
oxymetazoline (Visine LR)	**Adults and children ≥6 yr:** 1–2 drops of 0.025% solution q 6 hr as needed (for up to 3 days).	• ADRs: ophthalmic-rebound hyperemia; systemic-headache, insomnia, nervousness, tachycardia
phenylephrine (🍁 AK Dilate, 🍁 Dionephrine, 🍁 Mydfrin)	**Adults:** *Decongestant*—1–2 drops of 0.12% solution up to 4 times daily as needed (for up to 3 days); *Mydriasis*—1 drop of 2.5–10% solution, may repeat in 10–60 min as needed. **Children ≥1 yr:** *Mydriasis*—1 drop of 2.5–10% solution, may repeat in 10–60 min as needed.	• ADRs: ophthalmic-blurred vision, irritation; systemic-dizziness, tachycardia, hypertension, paleness, sweating, trembling

DRUG NAME	DOSE	NOTES
tetrahydrozoline (Visine)	**Adults:** 1–2 drops of 0.05% solution 2–4 times daily.	• ADRs: ophthalmic—irritation; systemic—tachycardia, hypertension

Prostaglandin Agonists

Uses: Treatment of open-angle glaucoma (↑ outflow of aqueous humor).

CAUTIONS: May change eye color to brown; will form precipitate with thimerosal-containing products; can be used with other agents to ↓ intraocular pressure.

DRUG NAME	DOSE	NOTES
bimatoprost (Lumigan)	**Adults:** 1 drop of 0.01–0.03% solution once daily in the evening.	• ADRs: local irritation, foreign body sensation, ↑ eyelash growth, ↑ brown pigmentation in iris
latanoprost (Xalatan)	**Adults:** 1 drop of 0.005% solution once daily in the evening.	• ADRs: local irritation, foreign body sensation, ↑ eyelash growth, ↑ brown pigmentation in iris
tafluprost (Zioptan)	**Adults:** 1 drop of 0.0015% solution once daily in the evening.	• ADRs: local irritation, foreign body sensation, ↑ eyelash growth, ↑ brown pigmentation in iris
travoprost (Travatan Z)	**Adults and Children ≥16 yr:** 1 drop of 0.004% solution once daily in the evening.	• ADRs: local irritation, foreign body sensation, ↑ eyelash growth, ↑ brown pigmentation in iris

Sympathomimetics

Uses: Treatment of open-angle glaucoma and other forms of intraocular hypertension (↓ formation of aqueous humor).

CAUTIONS: Systemic absorption may result in adverse cardiovascular and CNS reactions (especially in patients with cardiovascular disease); avoid use in patients predisposed to acute angle-closure glaucoma.

DRUG NAME	DOSE	NOTES
apraclonidine (Iopidine)	**Adults:** *Postoperative reduction of intraocular pressure*—1–2 drops of 0.5% solution 3 times daily or 1 drop of 1% solution 1 hr before surgery and upon completion of surgery.	• Used to ↓ intraocular pressure after surgery • A selective alpha-adrenergic agonist • Monitor pulse and blood pressure • Avoid concurrent use with MAO inhibitors • ADRs: ophthalmic-irritation, mydriasis; systemic-allergic reactions, arrhythmias, bradycardia, drowsiness, dry nose, fainting, headache, nervousness, weakness
brimonidine (Alphagan P)	**Adults and children ≥2 yr:** 1 drop of 0.1–0.15% solution 3 times daily (8 hr apart).	• A selective alpha-adrenergic agonist • Avoid concurrent use with MAO inhibitors • Tricyclic antidepressants may ↓ effectiveness; additive CNS depression may occur with other CNS depressants, additive adverse cardiovascular effects with other cardiovascular agents • ADRs: ophthalmic—irritation; systemic—drowsiness, dizziness, dry mouth, headache, weakness, muscular pain

APPENDIX D

Medication Administration Techniques

Subcutaneous Injection Sites

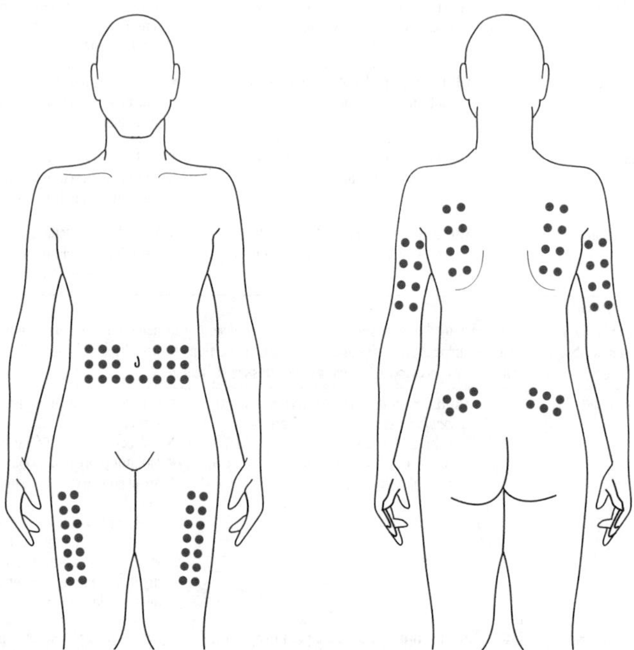

Administration of Ophthalmic Medications

For instillation of ophthalmic solutions, instruct patient to lie down or tilt head back and look at ceiling. Pull down on lower lid, creating a small pocket, and instill solution into pocket. With systemically acting drugs, apply pressure to the inner canthus for 1–2 min to minimize systemic absorption. Instruct patient to gently close eye. Wait 5 min before instilling second drop or any other ophthalmic solutions.

For instillation of ophthalmic ointment, instruct patient to hold tube in hand for several minutes to warm. Squeeze a small amount of ointment (¼–½ in.) inside lower lid. Instruct patient to close eye gently and roll eyeball around in all directions with eye closed. Wait 10 min before instilling any other ophthalmic ointments.

Do not touch cap or tip of container to eye, fingers, or any surface.

Administration of Medications with Metered-Dose Inhalers

Instruct patient on the proper use of the metered-dose inhaler. There are 3 methods of using a metered-dose inhaler. Shake inhaler well. (1) Take a drink of water to moisten the throat; place the inhaler mouthpiece 2 finger-widths away from mouth; tilt head back slightly. While activating the inhaler, take a slow, deep breath for 3–5 sec; hold the breath for 10 sec; and breathe out slowly. (2) Exhale and close lips firmly around mouthpiece. Administer during second half of inhalation, and hold breath for as long as possible to ensure deep instillation of medication. (3) Use of spacer. Consult health care professional to determine method desired prior to instruction. Allow 1–2 min between inhalations. Rinse mouth with water or mouthwash after each use to minimize dry mouth and hoarseness. Wash inhalation assembly at least daily in warm running water.

For use of dry powder inhalers, turn head away from inhaler and exhale (do not blow into inhaler). Do not shake. Close mouth tightly around the mouthpiece of the inhaler and inhale rapidly.

Steps for Using Your Inhaler*

1. Remove the cap and hold inhaler upright.
2. Shake the inhaler.
3. Tilt your head back slightly and breathe out slowly.
4. Position the inhaler in one of the following ways (A or B is optimal, but C is acceptable for those who have difficulty with A or B. C is required for breath-activated inhalers):

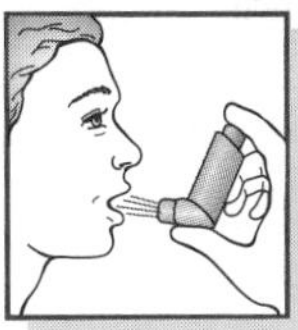

A. Open mouth with inhaler 1 to 2 inches away.

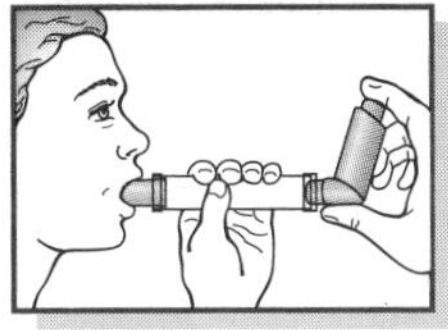

B. Use space/holding chamber (this is recommended especially for young children and for people using corticosteroids).

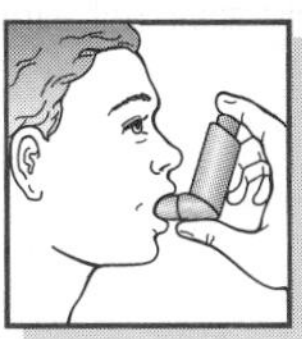

C. In the mouth. Do not use for corticosteroids.

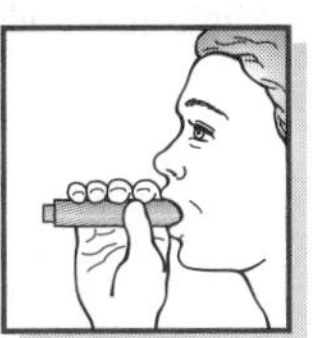

D. NOTE: Inhaled dry powder capsules require a different inhalation technique. To use a dry powder inhaler, it is important to close the mouth tightly around the mouthpiece of the inhaler and to inhale rapidly.

5. Press down on the inhaler to release medication as you start to breathe in slowly.
6. Breathe in slowly (3–5 sec).
7. Hold your breath for 10 sec to allow the medicine to reach deeply into your lungs.
8. Repeat puff as directed. Waiting 1 minute between puffs may permit second puff to penetrate your lungs better.
9. Spacers/holding chambers are useful for all patients. They are particularly recommended for young children and older adults and for use with **inhaled corticosteroids**. Avoid common inhaler mistakes. Follow these inhaler tips:
   - Breathe out before pressing your inhaler.
   - Inhale slowly.
   - Breathe in through your mouth, not your nose.
   - Press down on your inhaler at the start of inhalation (or within the first second of inhalation).
   - Keep inhaling as you press down on inhaler.
   - Press your inhaler only once while you are inhaling (one breath for each puff).
   - Make sure you breathe in evenly and deeply.
   - If you are using a short-acting bronchodilator inhaler and a corticosteroid inhaler, use the bronchodilator first, and allow 5 min to elapse before using the corticosteroid.

Other inhalers have become available in addition to the one illustrated here. Different types of inhalers may require different techniques.

Administration of Medications by Nebulizer

Administer in a location where patient can sit comfortably for 10–15 min. Plug in compressor. Mix medication as directed, or empty unit-dose vials into nebulizer. Do not mix different types of medications

*Source: Expert Panel Report 2: Guidelines for the Diagnosis and Management of Asthma. National Asthma Education and Prevention Program, National Heart, Lung, and Blood Institute, 1997.

without checking with health care professional. Assemble mask or mouthpiece and connect tubing to port on compressor. Have patient sit in a comfortable upright position. Make sure that mask fits properly over nose and mouth and that mist does not flow into eyes, or put mouthpiece into mouth. Turn on compressor. Instruct patient to take slow deep breaths. If possible, patient should hold breath for 10 sec before slowly exhaling. Continue this process until medication chamber is empty. Wash mask in hot soapy water; rinse well and allow to air dry before next use.

Administration of Nasal Sprays

Clear nasal passages of secretions prior to use. If nasal passages are blocked, use a decongestant immediately prior to use to ensure adequate penetration of the spray. Keep head upright. Breathe in through nose during administration. Sniff hard for a few minutes after administration.

APPENDIX E

Formulas Helpful for Calculating Doses

Ratio and Proportion

A ratio is the same as a fraction and can be expressed as a fraction (½) or in the algebraic form (1:2). This relationship is stated as *one is to two*.

A proportion is an equation of equal fractions or ratios.

$$\frac{1}{2} = \frac{4}{8}$$

To calculate doses, begin each proportion with the two known values, for example 15 grains = 1 gram (known equivalent) or 10 milligrams = 2 milliliters (dosage available) on one side of the equation. Next, make certain that the units of measure on the opposite side of the equation are the same as the units of the known values and are placed on the same level of the equation.

Problem A: $$\frac{15 \text{ gr}}{1 \text{ g}} = \frac{10 \text{ gr}}{x \text{ g}}$$

Problem B: $$\frac{10 \text{ mg}}{2 \text{ mL}} = \frac{5 \text{ mg}}{x \text{ mL}}$$

Once the proportion is set up correctly, cross-multiply the opposing values of the proportion.

Problem A: $$\frac{15 \text{ gr}}{1 \text{ g}} \times \frac{10 \text{ gr}}{x \text{ g}}$$

$$15x = 10$$

Problem B: $$\frac{10 \text{ mg}}{2 \text{ mL}} \times \frac{5 \text{ mg}}{x \text{ mL}}$$

$$10x = 10$$

Next, divide each side of the equation by the number with the x to determine the answer. Then, add the unit of measure corresponding to x in the original equation.

Problem A: $$\frac{15x}{15} = \frac{10}{15}$$

$$x = \frac{2}{3} \text{ or } 0.6 \text{ g}$$

Problem B: $$\frac{10x}{10} = \frac{10}{10}$$

$$x = 1 \text{ mL}$$

Calculation of IV Drip Rate

To calculate the drip rate for an intravenous infusion, 3 values are needed:

I. The amount of solution and corresponding time for infusion. May be ordered as:

1000 mL over 8 hr

or

125 mL/hr

II. The equivalent in time to convert hr to min.

$$1 \text{ hr} = 60 \text{ min}$$

III. The drop factor or number of drops that equal 1 mL of fluid. (This information can be found on the IV tubing box.)

$$10 \text{ gtt} = 1 \text{ mL}$$

Set up the problem by placing each of the 3 values in a proportion.

$$\frac{125 \text{ mL}}{1 \text{ hr}} \times \frac{1 \text{ hr}}{60 \text{ min}} \times \frac{10 \text{ gtt}}{1 \text{ mL}}$$

Units of measure can be canceled out from the upper and lower levels of the equation. The units cancel, leaving:

$$\frac{125}{1} \times \frac{1}{60 \text{ min}} \times \frac{10 \text{ gtt}}{1}$$

Next, multiply each level across and divide the numerator by the denominator for the answer.

$$\frac{125}{1} \times \frac{1}{6 \text{ min}} \times \frac{1 \text{ gtt}}{1}$$

$$125/6 = 20.8 \text{ or } 21 \text{ gtt/min}$$

Calculation of Creatinine Clearance (CCr) in Adults from Serum Creatinine

$$\text{Men: CCr} = \frac{\text{ideal body weight (kg)} \times (140 - \text{age})}{72 \times \text{serum creatinine (mg/dL)}}$$

$$\text{Women: CCr} = 0.85 \times \text{calculation for men}$$

Calculation of Body Surface Area (BSA) in Adults and Children

Dubois method:

$\text{SA (cm}^2) = \text{wt (kg)}^{0.425} \times 71.84$

$\text{SA (m}^2)\ K \times \sqrt[3]{\text{wt}^2 \text{ (kg)}}$ (common K value 0.1 for toddlers, 0.103 for neonates)

Simplified method:

$$\text{BSA (m}^2) = \sqrt{\frac{\text{ht (cm)} \times \text{wt (kg)}}{3600}}$$

Body Mass Index

$$\text{BMI} = \text{wt (kg)/ht (m}^2)$$

APPENDIX F

Normal Values of Common Laboratory Tests

SERUM TESTS

HEMATOLOGIC	MEN	WOMEN
Hemoglobin	13.5–18 g/dL	12–16 g/dL
Hematocrit	40–54%	38–47%
Red blood cells (RBC)	4.6–6.2 million/mm^3	4.2–5.4 million/mm^3
Mean corpuscular volume (MCV)	76–100 (micrometer)^3	76–100 (micrometer)^3
Mean corpuscular hemoglobin (MCH)	27–33 picogram	27–33 picogram
Mean corpuscular hemoglobin concentration (MCHC)	33–37 g/dL	33–37 g/dL
Erythrocyte sedimentation rate (ESR)	≤20 mm/hr	≤30 mm/hr
Leukocytes (WBC)	5000–10,000/mm^3	5000–10,000/mm^3
Neutrophils	54–75% (3000–7500/mm^3)	54–75% (3000–7500/mm^3)
Bands	3–8% (150–700/mm^3)	3–8% (150–700/mm^3)
Eosinophils	1–4% (50–400/mm^3)	1–4% (50–400/mm^3)
Basophils	0–1% (25–100/mm^3)	0–1% (25–100/mm^3)
Monocytes	2–8% (100–500/mm^3)	2–8% (100–500/mm^3)
Lymphocytes	25–40% (1500–4500/mm^3)	25–40% (1500–4500/mm^3)
T lymphocytes	60–80% of lymphocytes	60–80% of lymphocytes
B lymphocytes	10–20% of lymphocytes	10–20% of lymphocytes
Platelets	150,000–450,000/mm^3	150,000–450,000/mm^3
Prothrombin time (PT)	9.6–11.8 sec	9.5–11.3 sec
Partial thromboplastin time (PTT)	30–45 sec	30–45 sec
Bleeding time (duke)	1–3 min	1–3 min
(ivy)	3–6 min	3–6 min
(template)	3–6 min	3–6 min

CHEMISTRY	MEN	WOMEN
Sodium	135–145 mEq/L	135–145 mEq/L
Potassium	3.5–5.0 mEq/L	3.5–5.0 mEq/L
Chloride	95–105 mEq/L	95–105 mEq/L
Bicarbonate (HCO_3)	19–25 mEq/L	19–25 mEq/L
Total calcium	9–11 mg/dL or 4.5–5.5 mEq/L	9–11 mg/dL or 4.5–5.5 mEq/L
Ionized calcium	4.2–5.4 mg/dL or 2.1–2.6 mEq/L	4.2–5.4 mg/dL or 2.1–2.6 mEq/L
Phosphorus/phosphate	2.4–4.7 mg/dL	2.4–4.7 mg/dL
Magnesium	1.8–3.0 mg/dL or 1.5–2.5 mEq/L	1.8–3.0 mg/dL or 1.5–2.5 mEq/L
Glucose	65–99 mg/dL	65–99 mg/dL
Osmolality	285–310 mOsm/kg	285–310 mOsm/kg
Ammonia (NH_3)	10–80 mcg/dL	10–80 mcg/dL
Amylase	≤130 U/L	≤130 U/L
Creatine phosphokinase total (CK, CPK)	<150 U/L	<150 U/L
Creatine kinase isoenzymes, MB fraction	>5% in MI	>5% in MI
Lactic dehydrogenase (LDH)	50–150 U/L	50–150 U/L
Protein, total	6–8 g/d	6–8 g/d
Albumin	4–6 g/dL	4–6 g/dL

HEPATIC	MEN	WOMEN
AST	8–46 U/L	7–34 U/L
ALT	10–30 IU/mL	10–30 IU/mL
Total bilirubin	0.3–1.2 mg/dL	0.3–1.2 mg/dL
Conjugated bilirubin	0.0–0.2 mg/dL	0.0–0.2 mg/dL
Unconjugated (indirect) bilirubin	0.2–0.8 mg/dL	0.2–0.8 mg/dL
Alkaline phosphatase	20–90 U/L	20–90 U/L

RENAL	MEN	WOMEN
BUN	6–20 mg/dL	6–20 mg/dL
Creatinine	0.6–1.3 mg/dL	0.5–1.0 mg/dL
Uric acid	4.0–8.5 mg/dL	2.7–7.3 mg/dL

ARTERIAL BLOOD GASES	MEN	WOMEN
pH	7.35–7.45	7.35–7.45
Po_2	80–100 mm Hg	80–100 mm Hg
Pco_2	35–45 mm Hg	35–45 mm Hg
O_2 saturation	95–97%	95–97%
Base excess	+2–(−2)	+2–(−2)
Bicarbonate (HCO_3^-)	22–26 mEq/L	22–26 mEq/L

URINE TESTS

URINE	MEN	WOMEN
pH	4.5–8.0	4.5–8.0
Specific gravity	1.010–1.025	1.010–1.025

DRUG LEVELS, THERAPEUTIC AND TOXIC CONVENTIONAL (US SYSTEM OF MEASUREMENTS)

DRUG	THERAPEUTIC LEVEL	TOXIC LEVEL
acetaminophen	10–30 mcg/mL	>200 mcg/mL at 4 hr or 50 mcg/mL at 12 hr after ingestion
amikacin	peak: 20–30 mcg/mL trough: <8 mcg/mL	peak: >40 mcg/mL trough: >10 mcg/mL
amiodarone	0.5–2.5 mg/L	>2.5 mg/L
amitriptyline	0.5–2.5 mcg/mL	>2.5 mcg/mL
amoxapine	120–150 ng/mL	>500 ng/mL
carbamazepine	4–12 mcg/mL	>15 mcg/mL
chloramphenicol	peak: 10–25 mcg/mL trough: 5–15 mcg/mL	peak: >40 mcg/mL trough: >15 mcg/mL
chlordiazepoxide	0.1–3 mcg/mL	>25 mcg/mL
chlorpromazine	50–300 ng/mL	>750 ng/mL
clonazepam	20–80 ng/mL	>80 ng/mL
cyclosporine	100–400 ng/mL	>400 ng/mL
desipramine	50–300 ng/mL	>300 ng/mL
diazepam	0.2–1.5 mcg/mL	>1.5 mcg/mL
digoxin	0.5–2 ng/mL	>2.5 ng/mL
disopyramide	2.8–7.5 mcg/mL	>7.5 mcg/mL
doxepin	110–250 ng/mL	>500 ng/mL
ethosuximide	40–100 mcg/mL	>100 mcg/mL
flecainide	0.2–1 mcg/mL	>1 mcg/mL
gentamicin	peak: 6–10 mcg/mL trough: <1 mcg/mL	trough: >1 mcg/mL
haloperidol	5–20 ng/mL	>42 ng/mL
imipramine	150–250 ng/mL	>500 ng/mL
kanamycin	peak: 15–30 mcg/mL trough: 5–10 mcg/mL	peak: >35 mcg/mL trough: >10 mcg/mL
lidocaine	1.5–5 mcg/mL	>6 mcg/mL
lithium	0.6–1.2 mEq/L	>1.5 mEq/L
meperidine	70–500 ng/mL	>1000 ng/mL
mexiletine	0.5–2 mcg/mL	>2 mcg/mL
morphine	65–80 ng/mL	>200 ng/mL
nortriptyline	50–150 ng/mL	>500 ng/mL
phenobarbital	15–40 mcg/mL	>40 mcg/mL
phenytoin	10–20 mcg/mL	>30 mcg/mL
primidone	5–12 mcg/mL	>15 mcg/mL
procainamide	procainamide: 4–10 mcg/mL	procainamide: >10 mcg/mL

	N-acetylprocainamide (NAPA): 15–25 mcg/mL	
propranolol	50–100 ng/mL	>150 ng/mL
quinidine	2–5 mcg/mL	>6 mcg/mL
salicylate	100–400 mcg/mL	>400 mcg/mL
theophylline	10–20 mcg/mL	>20 mcg/mL
tobramycin	peak: 6–10 mcg/mL trough: <1 mcg/mL	trough: >1 mcg/mL
trazadone	0.5–2.5 mcg/mL	>2.5 mcg/mL
valproic acid	50–125 mcg/mL	>125 mcg/mL
vancomycin	trough: 10–20 mcg/mL	trough: >20 mcg/mL

APPENDIX G

Pregnancy Categories

Category A

Adequate, well-controlled studies in pregnant women have not shown an increased risk of fetal abnormalities.

Category B

Animal studies have revealed no evidence of harm to the fetus; however, there are no adequate and well-controlled studies in pregnant women. **or** Animal studies have shown an adverse effect, but adequate and well-controlled studies in pregnant women have failed to demonstrate a risk to the fetus.

Category C

Animal studies have shown an adverse effect and there are no adequate and well-controlled studies in pregnant women. **or** No animal studies have been conducted and there are no adequate and well-controlled studies in pregnant women.

Category D

Studies, adequate well-controlled or observational, in pregnant women have demonstrated a risk to the fetus. However, the benefits of therapy may outweigh the potential risk.

Category X

Studies, adequate well-controlled or observational, in animals or pregnant women have demonstrated positive evidence of fetal abnormalities. The use of the product is contraindicated in women who are or may become pregnant.

Note: The designation UK is used when the pregnancy category is unknown.

APPENDIX H

Controlled Substances Schedules

General

A controlled substance is any type of drug that the federal government has categorized as having significant potential for abuse or addiction. While controlled substances are regulated in both the United States (U.S.) and Canada, differences exist between the two countries with respect to scheduling and enforcement.

In the United States:

The Drug Enforcement Agency (DEA), an arm of the United States Justice Department, classifies controlled substances according to five schedules, based on the potential for abuse and dependence liability (physical and psychological) of the medication. Some states may have stricter prescription regulations. Physicians, dentists, podiatrists, and veterinarians may prescribe controlled substances. Nurse practitioners and physician assistants may also prescribe controlled substances with limitations that vary from state to state.

Schedule I (C-I)

Potential for abuse is so high as to be unacceptable. May be used for research with appropriate limitations. Examples are LSD and heroin.

Schedule II (C-II)

High potential for abuse and extreme liability for physical and psychological dependence (amphetamines, opioid analgesics, dronabinol, certain barbiturates). Outpatient prescriptions must be in writing. In emergencies, telephone orders may be acceptable if a written prescription is provided within 72 hr. No refills are allowed.

Schedule III (C-III)

Intermediate potential for abuse (less than C-II) and intermediate liability for physical and psychological dependence (certain nonbarbiturate sedatives, certain nonamphetamine CNS stimulants, and certain opioid analgesics). Outpatient prescriptions can be refilled 5 times within 6 mo from date of issue if authorized by prescriber. Telephone orders are acceptable.

Schedule IV (C-IV)

Less abuse potential than Schedule III with minimal liability for physical or psychological dependence (certain sedative/hypnotics, certain antianxiety agents, some barbiturates, benzodiazepines, chloral hydrate, pentazocine, and propoxyphene). Outpatient prescriptions can be refilled 6 times within 6 mo from date of issue if authorized by prescriber. Telephone orders are acceptable.

Schedule V (C-V)

Minimal abuse potential. Number of outpatient refills determined by prescriber. Some products (cough suppressants with small amounts of codeine, antidiarrheals containing paregoric) may be available without prescription to patients >18 yr of age.

In Canada:

The federal *Controlled Drugs and Substances Act (CDSA)* along with the *Narcotic Control Regulations*, Part G of the *Food and Drug Regulations*, and the *Benzodiazepines and Other Targeted Substances Regulations* regulate narcotics, controlled drugs, and targeted substances.

The CDSA classifies controlled substances according to eight schedules and three classes of precursors. While a few examples are listed below, a complete list of drugs scheduled in Canada's Controlled Drugs and Substances act can be accessed at: http://laws-lois.justice.gc.ca/eng/acts/C%2D38.8/

Schedule I

—opioids and derivatives and related drugs (e.g., morphine, oxycodone, heroin)

Schedule II

—cannabis (marihuana) and derivatives

Schedule III

—amphetamines and related drugs and substances (e.g., methylphenidate, LSD)

Schedule IV

—barbiturates and derivatives, anabolic steroids and related drugs, and benzodiazepines (e.g., diazepam)

Schedule V

—propylhexedrine

Schedule VI

—precursors Class A (e.g., pseudoephedrine and salts)
—precursors Class B (e.g., acetone, toluene)
—precursors Class C mixtures of the above

Schedules VII & VIII

—cannabis and its resins in varying amounts

(Note: In Canada marihuana may be used for medical purposes. It is regulated by the Marihuana for Medical Purposes Regulations.)

The CDSA federally regulates conditions of sale, distribution, and accountability relating to controlled substances. Provincial legislation compliments how patients access controlled substances from regulated health professionals. As such, it is imperative for an individual to become familiar with legislation pertaining to the specific province he/she is working in. Some federal regulations are as follows:

Narcotic drug—Two subcategories of prescription narcotics—"Straight" Narcotics and Verbal Prescription Narcotics

(e.g., codeine, morphine, fentanyl, oxycodone)

Straight Narcotics

- All single active ingredient products containing a narcotic, along with all narcotics for parenteral use and narcotic compounds containing more than one narcotic entity or less than two non-narcotic ingredients.
- Prescription can be written or faxed and must be signed and dated by prescriber.
- Refills are not permitted, but a prescription may be dispensed in divided portions. Prescription transfers from one pharmacist to another are not permitted.

Verbal Prescription Narcotic

(e.g., Tylenol No.2 and Tylenol No.3)

- Refers to oral combination products containing only one narcotic and two or more non-narcotic ingredients in a therapeutic dose. (Excluding diacetylmorphine, oxycodone, hydrocodone, methadone, or pentazocine. This means that an oral combination product that contains these drugs cannot be classified as a Verbal Prescription Narcotic.)
- Similar rules as above but prescriptions may be verbal.

Exempted Codeine Preparations

(e.g., Tylenol No.1)

- Under federal regulations, products containing codeine (meaning codeine phosphate or its equivalent) may be purchased over the counter, without a prescription, provided they have two other medicinal ingredients and a **maximum** of 8 mg of codeine per solid oral dosage unit or 20 mg per 30 mL of liquid.
- The product may not be supplied if there are reasonable grounds to suspect the product will be used for other than recognized medical or dental purposes.

Controlled Drugs—Part 1

(e.g., Dexedrine, Ritalin, pentobarbital, secobarbital)

- Refers to drugs listed in Part I of the Schedule to Part G of the Food and Drug Regulations.
- Prescription may be written or verbal; no refills allowed if prescription is verbal.
- Refills are permitted if the number of repeats and the frequency or interval between refills is specified. Prescription transfers are not permitted.

Controlled Drugs—Parts 2 and 3

(e.g., other barbiturates and anabolic steroids)

- Refers to drugs listed in Parts II and III of the Schedule to Part G of the Food and Drug Regulations.
- Prescription may be written or verbal.
- Refills are permitted if prescribed in writing or verbally and the number of repeats and frequency or interval between refills is specified. Prescription transfers are not permitted.

Benzodiazepines and Other Targeted Substances

(e.g., lorazepam, diazepam)

- Refers to all benzodiazepines except flunitrazepam, which is listed in Schedule III of the Act as an illicit substance.
- Prescriptions may be written or verbal. Refills are permitted if the prescription is less than 1 year old and the prescriber specifies the number of times it can be refilled. If the prescriber indicated the interval between refills, the pharmacist cannot refill the prescription if that interval has expired. Prescription transfers are permitted, but only once.

References:

Government of Canada. Canada Gazette Vol. 146 No.24(2012). http://gazette.gc.ca/rp-pr/p2/2012/2012-11-21/html/sor-dors230-eng.html (accessed 16 July 2013).

Controlled Drugs and Substances Act (S.C. 1996, c. 19). Available at http://laws-lois.justice.gc.ca/eng/acts/C-38.8/index.html (accessed 17 July 2013).

National Association of Pharmacy Regulatory Authorities (www.napra.org)

APPENDIX I

Equianalgesic Dosing Guidelines

OPIOID ANALGESICS STARTING ORAL DOSE COMMONLY USED FOR SEVERE PAIN

	EQUIANALGESIC DOSE		STARTING ORAL DOSE			
NAME	ORAL*	PARENTERAL†	ADULTS	CHILDREN	COMMENTS	PRECAUTIONS AND CONTRAINDICATIONS
a. Morphine-like agonists (mu agonists)						
morphine	30 mg	10 mg	15–30 mg	0.3 mg/kg	Standard of comparison for opioid analgesics. Sustained release preparations (MS Contin, OramorphSR) release over 8–12 hr. Other formulations (Kadian and Avinza) last 12–24 hr. Generic sustained release morphine preparations are now available.	For all opioids, caution in patients with impaired ventilation, bronchial asthma, increased intracranial pressure, liver failure.
hydromorphone (Dilaudid)	7.5 mg	1.5 mg	4–8 mg	0.06 mg/kg	Slightly shorter duration than morphine.	
fentanyl		0.1 mg				
oxycodone	20 mg	—	10–20 mg	0.3 mg/kg		
methadone	10 mg	5 mg	5–10 mg	0.2 mg/kg	Good oral potency, long plasma half-life (24–36 hr).	Accumulates with repeated dosing, requiring decreases in dose size and frequency, especially on days 2–5. Use with caution in older adults.
levorphanol (Levodromoran)	4 mg (acute), 1 mg (chronic)	2 mg (acute), 1 mg (chronic)	2–4 mg	0.04 mg/kg	Long plasma half-life (12–16 hr, but may be as long as 90–120 hr after one wk of dosing).	Accumulates on days 2 and 3. Use with caution in older adults.
oxymorphone (Opana)	10 mg	1 mg	—	—	5 mg rectal suppository ~5 mg morphine parenteral.	Like parenteral morphine.

NAME	EQUIANALGESIC DOSE		STARTING ORAL DOSE		COMMENTS	PRECAUTIONS AND CONTRAINDICATIONS
	ORAL*	PARENTERAL†	ADULTS	CHILDREN		
meperidine (Demerol)	Not recommended	Not recommended	Not Recommended		Slightly shorter acting than morphine accumulates with repetitive dosing causing CNS excitation; avoid in children with impaired renal function or who are receiving monoamine oxidase inhibitors.‡	Use with caution. Normeperidine (toxic metabolite) accumulates with repetitive dosing causing CNS excitation and a high risk of seizure. Avoid in children, renal impairment, and patients on monoamine oxidase inhibitors.‡
b. Mixed agonists–antagonists (kappa agonists)						
nalbuphine (Nubain)	—	10 mg	—	—	Not available orally, not scheduled under Controlled Substances Act.	Incidence of psychotomimetic effects lower than with pentazocine; may precipitate withdrawal in opioid-dependent patients.
butorphanol (Stadol)	—	2 mg	—	—	Like nalbuphine. Also available in nasal spray.	Like nalbuphine.
pentazocine (Talwin)	50 mg	30 mg	—	—		
c. Partial agonist						
buprenorphine (Buprenex)	—	0.4 mg	—	—	Lower abuse liability than morphine; does not produce psychotomimetic effects. Sublingual tablets now available both plain and with naloxone for opioid-dependent patient management for specially certified physicians. These tablets are not approved as analgesics.	May precipitate withdrawal in narcotic-dependent patients; not readily reversed by naloxone; avoid in labor.

*Starting dose should be lower for older adults.

†These are standard parenteral doses for acute pain in adults and can also be used to convert doses for IV infusions and repeated small IV boluses. For single IV boluses, use half the IM dose. IV doses for children >6 mo. = parenteral equianalgesic dose times weight (kg)/100.

‡Irritating to tissues with repeated IM injections.

Modified from *American Pain Society, Principles of Analgesic Use in the Treatment of Acute Pain and Cancer Pain*, ed.6. American Pain Society, 2008.

GUIDELINES FOR PATIENT-CONTROLLED INTRAVENOUS OPIOID ADMINISTRATION FOR ADULTS WITH ACUTE PAIN

DRUG	USUAL STARTING DOSE AFTER LOADING	USUAL DOSE RANGE	USUAL LOCKOUT (MIN)	USUAL LOCKOUT RANGE (MIN)
Morphine (1 mg/mL)	1 mg	0.5–2.5 mg	8	5–10
Hydromorphone (0.2 mg/mL)	0.2 mg	0.05–0.4 mg	8	5–10
Fentanyl (50 mcg/mL)	20 mcg	10–50 mcg	6	5–8

*Standard concentrations for most PCA machines are listed in parentheses.
Modified from *American Pain Society, Principles of Analgesic Use in the Treatment of Acute Pain and Cancer Pain*, ed.6. American Pain Society, 2008.

FENTANYL TRANSDERMAL DOSE BASED ON DAILY MORPHINE DOSE

ORAL 24-HR MORPHINE (mg/day)	TRANSDERMAL FENTANYL (mg/day)	FENTANYL TRANSDERMAL (mcg/hr)
30–90	0.6	25
91–150	1.2	50
151–210	1.8	75
211–270	2.4	100
271–330	3.0	125
331–390	3.6	150
391–450	4.2	175
451–510	4.8	200
511–570	5.4	225
571–630	6.0	250
631–690	6.6	275
691–750	7.2	300
For each additional 60 mg/day	+0.6	+25

*A 10-mg IM or 60-mg oral dose of morphine every 4 hr for 24 hr (total of 60 mg/day IM or 360 mg/day oral) was considered approximately equivalent to fentanyl transdermal 100 mcg/hr.

APPENDIX J

Food Sources for Specific Nutrients

Potassium-Rich Foods

artichoke
avocados
bananas
cantaloupe
cassava
dried fruits
grapefruit
honey dew
jack fruit
kiwi
kohlrabi
lima beans
mango
meats
milk
dried peas and beans
nuts
oranges/orange juice
papaya
peaches
pears
plantains
pomegranate
potatoes (white and sweet)
prunes/prune juice
pumpkin
rhubarb
salt substitute
spinach
sunflower seeds
Swiss chard
tomatoes/tomato juice
vegetable juice
winter squash

Sodium-Rich Foods

baking mixes (pancakes, muffins)
barbecue sauce
buttermilk
butter/margarine
canned chili
canned seafood
canned soups
canned spaghetti sauce
cured meats
dry onion soup mix
"fast" foods
frozen dinners
macaroni and cheese
microwave dinners
Parmesan cheese
pickles
potato salad
pretzels, potato chips
salad dressings (prepared)
salt
sauerkraut
tomato ketchup

Calcium-Rich Foods

almond (milk/nuts)
calcium fortified foods
canned salmon/sardines
cheese
cream soups (with milk)
greens: collard/ mustard/ turnip
kale
milk
soy (beans/milk)
spinach
tofu
yogurt

Vitamin K-Rich Foods

asparagus
beet greens
broccoli
brussel sprouts
cabbage
collard greens
dandelion leaves
garden cress
green tea leaves
kale
mustard greens
parsley
spinach
swiss chard
turnip greens

Low-Sodium Foods

baked or broiled poultry
canned pumpkin
cooked turnips
egg yolk
fresh vegetables
fruit
grits (not instant)
honey
jams and jellies
lean meats
low-calorie mayonnaise
macaroons
potatoes
puffed wheat and rice
red kidney and lima beans
sherbet
unsalted nuts
whiskey

Foods That Acidify Urine

cheeses
corn
cranberries
eggs
fish
grains (breads and cereals)
lentils
meats
nuts (Brazil, filberts, walnuts)
pasta
plums
poultry
prunes
rice

Foods That Alkalinize Urine

all fruits except cranberries, prunes, plums
all vegetables (except corn)
milk
nuts (almonds, chesnuts)

Foods Containing Tyramine

aged cheeses (blue, Boursault, brick, Brie, Camembert, cheddar, Emmenthaler, Gruyère, mozzarella, Parmesan, Romano, Roquefort, Stilton, Swiss)
American processed cheese
avocados (especially over-ripe)
bananas
bean curd
beer and ale
caffeine-containing beverages (coffee, tea, colas)
caviar
chocolate
distilled spirits
fermented sausage (bologna, salami, pepperoni, summer sausage)
liver
meats prepared with tenderizer
miso soup
over-ripe fruit
peanuts
raisins
raspberries
red wine (especially Chianti)
sauerkraut
sherry
shrimp paste
smoked or pickled fish
soy sauce
vermouth
yeasts
yogurt

Iron-Rich Foods

cereals
clams
dried beans and peas
dried fruit
leafy green vegetables
lean red meats
molasses (blackstrap)
organ meats

Vitamin D-Rich Foods

canned salmon, sardines, tuna
cereals
fish
fish liver oils
fortified milk
nonfat dry milk

APPENDIX K

Insulins and Insulin Therapy

The goal of therapy for diabetic patients is to provide insulin coverage that most closely resembles endogenous insulin production and results in the best glycemic control without hypoglycemia. Although daytime control of hyperglycemia may be accomplished with bolus doses of rapid-acting insulin analogs, elevations in fasting glucose may remain a problem. If fasting blood glucose levels remain elevated, the basal insulin dose (intermediate or long-acting) may have to be adjusted.

Most insulins used today are recombinant DNA human insulins. Produced through genetic engineering, synthetic human insulin is "manufactured" by yeast or nonpathogenic *E. coli*. In recent years, pharmaceutical companies have developed several new types and formulations of insulin.

Different insulins are distinguished by how quickly they are absorbed, the time and length of peak activity, and overall duration of action. Onset, peak, and duration of action times are approximate and vary according to individual factors such as injection site, blood supply, concurrent illnesses, lifestyle, and exercise level. These factors can vary from patient to patient and can vary in any patient from day to day.

There are 5 kinds of insulins: rapid-acting, short-acting, intermediate-acting, long-acting, and combination insulins.

Rapid-Acting Insulins

Rapid-acting insulins are analogs of regular insulin. An analog is a chemical structure very similar to another but differing in one component. Humalog (lispro), Apidra (glulisine), and Novolog (aspart) are rapid-acting insulin analogs. The amino acid sequences of these analogs are nearly identical to human insulin. They differ in the positioning of certain proteins, which allow them to enter the bloodstream rapidly—within 15 min of subcutaneous injection. This closely mimics the body's own insulin response and allows greater flexibility in eating schedules for diabetic patients. Also, because these insulins leave the bloodstream quickly, the risk of hypoglycemic episodes several hours after the meal is lessened. The peak time for rapid-acting insulins is 1–2 hr and the duration is 3–4 hr. Rapid-acting insulin solutions are clear. Both insulin aspart and insulin glulisine can be given intravenously in selected situations under medical supervision.

Short-Acting Insulin

Regular insulin is short-acting insulin and is available commercially as Humulin R or Novolin R. The onset of regular insulin is 0.5–1 hr; its peak activity occurs 2–4 hr after subcutaneous injection and its duration of action is 5–7 hr. This time/action profile makes rigid meal scheduling necessary, as the patient must estimate that a meal will occur within 45 min of injection. Short-acting insulin solutions are clear. Regular insulin can be given intravenously.

Intermediate-Acting Insulins

Intermediate-acting insulin contains protamine, which delays onset, peak, and duration of action to provide basal insulin coverage. Basal insulins are given to control blood glucose levels throughout the day when not eating. Commercially, intermediate-acting insulins are available as Humulin N or Novolin N. (The "N" stands for NPH.) Action starts between 2 and 4 hr after injecting. Peak activity occurs between 4 and 10 hr. Duration of action lasts 10–16 hr. The addition of protamine causes the cloudy appearance of intermediate-acting insulins and results in the formulation being a suspension rather than a solution. This is why these insulins must be gently mixed before administering. Intermediate-acting insulins can be mixed with short- or rapid-acting insulins to provide both basal and bolus coverage.

Long-Acting Insulins

Long-acting insulins have the most delayed onset and the longest duration of all insulins. Products include Lantus (insulin glargine) and Levemir (insulin detemir). Peaks are not as prominent in long-acting insulins. In fact, insulin glargine has no real peak action because it forms slowly dissolving crystals in the subcutaneous tissue. The onset of action of insulin glargine is 3–4 hr after subcutaneous injection. Full activity occurs within 4 to 5 hr and remains constant for 24 hr. Even though insulin glargine and insulin detemir are clear solutions, neither can be diluted or mixed with any other insulin or solution. Mixing insulin glargine or insulin detemir with other insulin products can alter the onset of action and time to peak effect. If bolus insulin is to be given at the same time as insulin glargine or insulin detemir, two separate syringes and injection sites must be used.

Combination Insulins

Various combinations of premixed insulins are available, containing fixed proportions of two different insulins, usually a short- and an intermediate-acting insulin. Typically the intermediate-acting insulin makes up 70–75% of the mixture, with rapid- or short- acting insulin making up the remainder. Onset, peak, and duration vary according to each specific product. Brand names of these products include Humulin 70/30 (70% NPH, 30% regular), Humalog Mix 75/25 (75% insulin lispro protamine suspension and 25% insulin lispro), Humalog Mix 50/50 (50% insulin lispro protamine suspension and 50% insulin lispro), and Novolin 70/30 (70% NPH, 30% regular), or Novolog 70/30 (70% insulin aspart protamine suspension and 30% insulin aspart).

BRAND NAME	GENERIC NAME	TYPE OF INSULIN	ONSET/PEAK/DURATION
Humalog Mix 75/25 Humalog Mix 50/50	insulin lispro protamine suspension & insulin lispro injection mixtures	Combination Insulins	15–30 min/2.8 hr/24 hr
Novolog Mix 70/30	insulin aspart protamine suspension insulin & aspart injection mixtures	Combination Insulins	15 min/1–4 hr/18–24 hr
Humulin 70/30 Novolin 70/30	NPH/regular insulin mixture	Combination Insulins	15 min/2–12 hr/24 hr
Apidra	insulin glulisine	Rapid-Acting	Within 15 min/1–2 hr/3–4 hr
Humalog	insulin lispro	Rapid-Acting	Within 15 min/1–2 hr/3–4 hr
Novolog	insulin aspart	Rapid-Acting	Within 15 min/1–2 hr/3–4 hr
Humulin R	regular insulin (subcut)	Short-Acting	½–1 hr/2–4 hr/5–7 hr
Novolin R	regular insulin (IV)	Short-Acting	10–30 min/15–30 min/30–60 min
Humulin N Novolin N	NPH	Intermediate-Acting	2–4 hr/4–10 hr/10–16 hr
Levemir	insulin detemir	Long-Acting	3–4 hr/3–14 hr/6–24 hr
Lantus	insulin glargine	Long-Acting	3–4 hr/No Peak/24 hr

APPENDIX L

Canadian and U.S. Pharmaceutical Practices

In the United States (U.S.) and Canada, most drugs are prescribed and used similarly. However, certain processes and actions of the U.S. and Canadian pharmaceutical industries differ in significant ways, affecting both consumers and health care providers. Safety, marketing, and availability are three of these issues.

Safety

Controversy related to the importation of medications from Canada by U.S. consumers has sometimes raised concerns about the safety of these drugs. These fears are unfounded; in fact, the Canadian approval and manufacturing processes are very similar to U.S. processes. Both countries have pharmaceutical-related standards, laws, and policies to ensure that chemical entities marketed for human diseases and conditions are safe and effective. The process of taking a new drug from the laboratory to the pharmacy shelves includes:

Scientific development. The process begins with research. Scientists develop a new molecular entity targeted at a specific disease, symptom, or condition.

Patenting. A manufacturer applies for a patent, which prevents other drug companies from manufacturing a chemically identical drug. Patent protection lasts 17 years in the U.S. and 20 years in Canada. After a patent expires, any manufacturer can make generic versions of the chemical; generic drugs typically cost much less than the brand-name drugs.

Preclinical testing. Before a drug is taken by human subjects, preclinical testing of the chemical is performed first on animals. Testing helps identify drug action, toxicity effects, side effects, adverse reactions, dosage amounts and routes, and administration procedures. This phase can last anywhere from 3–5 years.

Permission to begin clinical testing. Once a drug is found to have demonstrable positive health effects and is safe for animal consumption, a manufacturer seeks permission to begin clinical studies with human subjects. In the U.S., this process is called New Drug Application (NDA) and is administered by the Food and Drug Administration (FDA). In Canada, the process is referred to as a Clinical Trial Application (CTA) and is administered by Health Canada.

Clinical trials. Clinical trials are initiated to establish the potential benefits and risks for humans. Several sub-phases are required in the clinical trials phase whereby increasingly larger sample sizes are necessary.

Phase 0: A new designation for first-in-human trials, which are designed to assess whether the drug affects humans in a manner that is expected.

Phase 1: Between 20 and 80 healthy volunteers are recruited to assess safety, tolerance, dosage ranges, pharmacokinetics, and pharmacodynamics.

Phase 2: Up to 300 patients with the drug-targeted disease are enrolled to assess efficacy and toxicity. Variables from Phase I trials may also be assessed.

Phase 3: Between 1000 and 3000 patients are entered into a randomized, double-blinded study designed to confirm drug effectiveness, comparability with existing treatments, and further exploration of potential and real side effects.

Ongoing surveillance of a drug for rare or long-term effects continues after approval is received and marketing begun.

Approval. The results of the clinical studies are reviewed by Health Canada in Canada and by the FDA in the U.S. These regulatory bodies assess all aspects of a drug, including the labeling. The approval process is often deemed excessively long by physicians and patients who are anxious to try new remedies for refractory or terminal diseases. Efforts are ongoing to shorten the process in both countries.[1]

Marketing. Once a drug has been approved, it can be prescribed to consumers or, if it does not require a prescription, purchased by them.

Postmarketing Surveillance. More clinical data become available when a drug is marketed and used by many people for longer periods of time. Pharmacovigilance is the term used to refer to the process of ongoing assessment of a drug's safety and effectiveness during this phase.

Differences Between Canadian and U.S. Drug Pricing and Marketing

One major difference between Canadian and U.S drug regulatory processes is pricing. In Canada, the Patented Medicine Prices Review Board (PMPRB) regulates the prices that manufacturers can charge for prescription and nonprescription medicines. This is to ensure that prices are not excessive. No such control exists in the U.S., which is why many citizens purchase their medications from Canadian online pharmacies. One study identified that U.S. citizens can save approximately 24% if they buy their medications from Canadian pharmacies rather than from a U.S. chain pharmacies.[2]

Another difference is in advertising. In the U.S., manufacturers can market drugs directly, and forcefully, to consumers, a controversial privilege that has resulted in consumers requesting specific medications despite not necessarily understanding all of the risks and benefits. In Canada, such advertising is limited and subject to the approval of the Advertising Standards Canada (ASC) agency and the Pharmaceutical Advertising Advisory Board (PAAB). To address this issue in the U.S., the Institute of Medicine (IOM) has recommended that the FDA ban direct-to-consumer advertising during the first 2 years after a drug is marketed. Such a delay may help to prevent large numbers of people experiencing side effects not observed in the clinical trials, such as occurred with sildenafil (Viagra) when several patients died or developed vision problems in the first months after marketing began.

Natural Health Products

In Canada, Natural Health Products (NHPs) are regulated by Health Canada. A Natural Product Number (NPN) or Homeopathic Medicine Number (DIN-HM) is issued for the product only after it has been determined to be safe, effective and of high quality. The term "Natural Product" refers to vitamins and mineral supplements, herbal products, traditional and homeopathic medicines, probiotics and enzymes or personal care items for consumption that contain natural ingredients.

In the U.S., the FDA classifies natural products as food products under the Dietary Supplements Health Education Act, so claims about the ability of a supplement to diagnose, prevent, treat or cure a disease is prohibited. It is not necessary, however, for natural products to undergo review or approval, or for testing to be done for identity, purity of active ingredients.

Drug Schedule, Availability, and Pregnancy Category Differences

In Canada, drug schedules are used to classify medication according to accessibility. The Canadian drug schedules as defined by NAPRA (the National Pharmacy Regulatory Authorities) are:

- **Schedule I:** Available only by prescription and provided by a pharmacist.
- **Schedule II:** Available only from a pharmacist; must be kept in an area with no public access.
- **Schedule III:** Available via open access in a pharmacy (over-the-counter).
- **Unscheduled:** Can be sold in any store without professional supervision.

(note: The province of Québec has not adopted this national model.)

The U.S., in contrast, categorizes medications according to two general classes:

- **Prescription Only:** Available only by prescription and provided by a pharmacist.
- **Over-the-Counter (OTC):** Available via open access in the pharmacy.

As a result of these differences in accessibility some potentially dangerous drugs (such as heparin, insulin, and codeine-containing cough medicines) are available only with a prescription in the U.S. and available without a prescription but in consultation with a pharmacist in Canada. Similarly, some Canadian drugs are available in combinations not found in the U.S. (see Appendix B for new Canadian combination drugs). Other differences also exist with respect to drug availability between the two countries.

Canada currently does not have pregnancy categories as those established by the U.S. Canadian prescribers practice under the premise that no drug should be given to a pregnant woman unless benefits to the mother clearly outweigh potential risks to the fetus. Canadian health care providers may refer to a drug's FDA pregnancy category for guidance (see Appendix G).

SOURCES CITED

1. Rawson, Nigel, S.B. "New Drug Approval Times and Safety Warnings in the United States and Canada, 1992-2011." J Popul Ther Clin Pharmacol Vol 20(2):e67-e81; April 22, 2013.
2. Quon B., Firszt R., Eisenberg M. "A Comparison of Brand-Name Drug Prices Between Canadian-Based Internet Pharmacies and Major U.S. Drug Chain Pharmacies. Ann Intern Med. 143(6):397–403, 2005. http://www.annals.org/cgi/content/abstract/143/6/397 (accessed 10 December 2007).

ADDITIONAL REFERENCES

Canadian Pharmacists Association. "From Research Lab to Pharmacy Shelf." http://www.pharmacists.ca/content/hcp/resource_centre/drug_therapeutic_info/pdf/DrugApprovalProcess.pdf (accessed 15 December 2007).

Health Canada. http://www.hc-sc.gc.ca/ahc-asc/index_e.html (accessed 15 December 2007).

Tomalin A. "Drugs Used in Pregnancy: The Regulatory Process." Can J Clin Pharmacol. 14(1):e5–e9, 2007. http://www.cjcp.ca/pdf/CJCP2007_e5_e9.pdf (accessed 10 December 2007).

U.S. Food and Drug Administration. http://www.fda.gov (accessed 15 December 2007).

APPENDIX M

Routine Pediatric and Adult Immunizations

Immunization recommendations change frequently. For the latest recommendations see http://www.cdc.gov/vaccines/schedules/hcp/index.html.
For Canadian recommendations see the Canadian Immunization Guide (Public Health Agency of Canada) http://www.phac-aspc.gc.ca/publicat/cig-gci/index-eng.php

ROUTINE PEDIATRIC IMMUNIZATIONS (0–18 yr)

GENERIC NAME (BRAND NAMES)	ROUTE/DOSAGE	CONTRAINDICATIONS	ADVERSE REACTIONS/ SIDE EFFECTS	NOTES
Diphtheria toxoid,tetanus toxoid, andacellular pertussis vaccine (DTaP, Daptacel, Infanrix)	0.5 mL IM at 2, 4, 6, 15–18 mo and 4–6 yr (1st dose may be given as early as age 6 wk; 4th dose may be given as early as age 12 mo).	Anaphylactic reaction after a previous dose or to vaccine component; encephalopathy within 7 days of administration of previous dose of Tdap, DTP, or DTaP vaccines.	Crying, ↓ appetite, fever, irritability, malaise, redness, tenderness, vomiting.	Individual components may be given as separate injections if unusual reactions occur. The same product should be used for all doses when possible. Do not give to children ≥7 yr.
Haemophilus b conjugate vaccine (Hib, ActHIB, Hiberix, PedvaxHIB)	*ActHIB*—0.5 mL IM at 2, 4, and 6 mo, with a booster at 12–15 mo (1st dose may be given as early as age 6 wk); *PedvaxHIB*—0.5 mL IM at 2 and 4 mo, with a booster dose at 12–15 mo (1st dose may be given as early as age 6 wk); *Hiberix*—0.5 mL IM; can only be used for the booster dose (any of the products can be used for the booster dose).	Anaphylactic reaction after a previous dose or to vaccine component.	Anorexia, crying, diarrhea, fever, irritability, malaise, tenderness, vomiting, weakness.	If different brands of vaccine are used for 1st and 2nd doses, need to administer 3rd dose followed by a booster afer 12 mo. Give only one dose to unvaccinated children 5–18 yr with HIV. Give only one dose to unvaccinated children 15–59 mo.
Hepatitis A vaccine (HepA, Havrix, Vaqta)	0.5 mL IM of pediatric formulation initiated at 12–23 mo, followed by 0.5 mL IM of pediatric formulation 6–18 mo later.	Anaphylactic reaction after a previous dose or to vaccine component.	↓ appetite, drowsiness, fever, headache, irritability, pain at injection site, weakness.	Also recommended in children ≥2 yr who live in areas with high rates of hepatitis A or are in other high-risk groups (e.g., chronic liver disease, clotting factor disorders, illicit drug users, adolescent males who have sex with other males, close personal contact within first 60 days of arrival of international adoptee from country where hepatitis A is endemic).

GENERIC NAME (BRAND NAMES)	ROUTE/DOSAGE	CONTRAINDICATIONS/ PRECAUTIONS	ADVERSE REACTIONS/ SIDE EFFECTS	NOTES
Hepatitis B vaccine (HepB, Engerix-B, Recombivax HB)	0.5 mL IM at 0, 1–2, and 6–18 mo; if mother's HBsAg status is unknown, administer hepatitis B vaccine within 12 hr of birth. *Infants born to HBsAg-positive mothers:* Administer 0.5 mL of hepatitis B immune globulin IM and 1st dose of hepatitis B vaccine within 12 hr of birth; give 2nd and 3rd doses of hepatitis B vaccine at 1–2 mo and 6 mo, respectively.	Anaphylactic reaction after a previous dose or to vaccine component (including yeast).	Injection site reactions.	A 2-dose series (separated by ≥4 mo) of the adult formulation (Recombivax HB) can be used in children 11–15 yr.
Human papillomavirus vaccine, bivalent (HPV2, Cervarix)	0.5 mL IM in females age 11–26 yr (1st dose may be given as early as age 9 yr), repeat at 1–2 mo and 6 mo after 1st dose.	Anaphylactic reaction after a previous dose or to vaccine component (including yeast).	Arthralgia, fatigue, itching, myalgia, pain at injection site, myalgia.	Used to prevent cervical cancer caused by HPV types 16 and 18 in females. HPV series should be completed with same product, when possible.
Human papillomavirus vaccine, quadrivalent (HPV4, Gardasil)	0.5 mL IM in males and females age 11–26 yr (1st dose may be given as early as age 9 yr), repeat at 1–2 mo and 6 mo after 1st dose.	Anaphylactic reaction after a previous dose or to vaccine component (including yeast).	Diarrhea, dizziness, fever, headache, nausea, pain at injection site, syncope.	Used to prevent cervical, vulvar, and vaginal cancer caused by HPV types 16 and 18 in females and to prevent genital warts caused by HPV types 6 and 11 and anal cancer caused by HPV types 16 and 18 in males and females. HPV series should be completed with same product, when possible.
Human papillomavirus vaccine, 9–valent (HPV9, Gardasil 9)	0.5 mL IM in males and females age 11–26 yr (1st dose may be given as early as age 9 yr), repeat at 1–2 mo and 6 mo after 1st dose.	Anaphylactic reaction after a previous dose or to vaccine component (including yeast).	Dizziness, fever, headache, pain at injection site, syncope.	Used to prevent cervical, vulvar, and vaginal cancer caused by HPV types 16, 18, 31, 33, 45, 52, and 58 in females and to prevent genital warts caused by HPV types 6 and 11 and anal cancer caused by HPV types 16, 18, 31, 33, 45, 52, and 58 in males and females. HPV series should be completed with same product, when possible.
Influenza vaccine *Injection (inactivated):* (Afluria, Fluarix, FluLaval, Fluvirin, Fluzone); *Intranasal (live attenuated):* (FluMist)	*Injection: Age 6–35 mo:* 2 doses of 0.25 mL IM given 4 wk apart for initial season, then one dose annually. *Age 3–8 yr:* 2 doses of 0.5 mL IM given 4 wk apart for initial season, then one dose annually. *Age ≥9 yr:* 0.5 mL IM single dose annually. *Intranasal: Age 2–8 yr:* If not previously vaccinated with influenza vaccine—2 doses of 0.2 mL (given as 0.1 mL in each nostril) 4 wk apart, then one dose annually. If previously vaccinated with influenza vaccine—1 dose of 0.2 mL (given as 0.1 mL in each nostril) annually. *Age ≥9 yr:* 1 dose of 0.2 mL (given as 0.1 mL dose in each nostril) annually.	Anaphylactic reaction after a previous dose or to vaccine component, including eggs/egg products and thimerosal (injection only). Avoid use in patients with acute neurologic compromise. FluMist should be avoided in children <2 yr; egg allergy; pregnancy; chronic pulmonary (including asthma), cardiovascular (not hypertension), renal, hepatic, neurological, hematologic, or metabolic (including diabetes) disorders; immunosuppression (including HIV); children <5 yr with wheezing in past 12 mo; chronic salicylate therapy (children 2 –17 yr); taken influenza antiviral medication in previous 48 hr.	*Injection:* local soreness, fever, myalgia, possible neurologic toxicity. *Intranasal:* upper respiratory congestion, malaise.	Immunosuppression may ↓ antibody response and ↑ the risk of viral transmission with intranasal route. Afluria should only be used in children ≥9 yr (because of ↑ risk of fever and febrile seizures in children 5–8 yr). Fluvirin should only be used in children ≥4 yr. Fluarix and FluLaval should only be used in children ≥3 yr. Flublok and Flucelvak should only be used in patients ≥18 yr. If patient experiences anaphylactic reaction to eggs or egg-containing foods, inactivated influenza vaccine should be administered by health care professional with experience in recognition and management of severe allergic conditions and patient should be closely monitored for ≥30 min after vaccination.

GENERIC NAME (BRAND NAMES)	ROUTE/DOSAGE	CONTRAINDICATIONS/ PRECAUTIONS	ADVERSE REACTIONS/ SIDE EFFECTS	NOTES
Measles, mumps, and rubella vaccine (MMR, M-M-R II)	0.5 mL subcut at 12–15 mo and at 4–6 yr (2nd dose may be given earlier if ≥4 wk have elapsed since the 1st dose).	Anaphylactic reaction after a previous dose or to vaccine component (including, eggs, neomycin, or gelatin); severe immunosuppression (in the absence of severe immunosuppression, HIV is not a contraindication); pregnancy.	Arthralgia, encephalitis, fever, pain at injection site.	If unusual reactions occur, individual components may be given as separate injections. Immunosuppression may ↓ antibody response to injection and ↑ the risk of viral transmission.
Meningococcal conjugate vaccine (MCV4, Menactra, Menveo)	0.5 mL IM single dose at 11–12 yr with a booster dose at age 16 yr; single dose can be given at age 13–18 yr if not previously vaccinated (if received 1st dose at age 13–15 yr, should receive booster dose at age 16–18 yr [with an interval of ≥8 wk between doses] if received 1st dose at age ≥16 yr, no booster dose needed). Single dose should be given to previously unvaccinated college freshmen (19–21 yr) living in dormitories.	Anaphylactic reaction after a previous dose or to vaccine component.	Anorexia, arthralgia, diarrhea, fatigue, fever, headache, myalgia, nausea, irritability, malaise, pain at injection site, vomiting.	Routine vaccination with meningococcal vaccine also is recommended for certain children (≥2 mo) who are at high risk (anatomic or functional asplenia; persistent complement component deficiency; travel or reside in areas in which meningococcal disease is epidemic).Vaccinate children 11–18 yr with HIV with 2 doses administered ≥8 wk apart.
Pneumococcal conjugate vaccine (13–valent) (PCV13, Prevnar 13)	0.5 mL IM at 2, 4, 6, and 12–15 mo (1st dose may be given as early as age 6 wk). If previously received 4 doses of Prevnar 7 (and age 14–59 mo), give single dose of Prevnar 13 ≥2 mo after most recent dose. If previously received 4 doses of Prevnar 7 (and high-risk children age 24–71 mo), give single dose of Prevnar 13 ≥2 mo after most recent dose of Prevnar 7.	Anaphylactic reaction after a previous dose or to vaccine component (including diphtheria toxoid).	Arthralgia, chills, ↓ appetite, fatigue, fever, headache, insomnia, irritability, myalgia, pain at injection site, rash.	One dose may also be given to previously unvaccinated healthy children age 24–59 mo. For high-risk children (e.g., sickle cell disease; anatomic or functional asplenia; chronic cardiac, pulmonary, or renal disease; diabetes; HIV; immunosuppression; cerebrospinal fluid leaks; cochlear implant) age 24–71 mo, give 2 doses (≥8 wk apart, with 1st dose being given ≥8 wk after most recent dose) if previously unvaccinated or received <3 doses (if previously received 3 doses, give 1 dose ≥8 wk after most recent dose).
Pneumococcal polysaccharide vaccine (PPSV23, Pneumovax 23)	0.5 mL IM or subcut ≥8 wk after final dose of PCV in high-risk children ≥2 yr (see Notes section for pneumococcal conjugate vaccine for definition of high risk).	Anaphylactic reaction after a previous dose or to vaccine component.	Chills, fever, injection site reactions.	A 2nd dose may be given 5 yr later in children with immunosuppression, sickle cell disease, or anatomic/functional asplenia.
Polio vaccine, inactivated (IPV, IPOL)	0.5 mL IM or subcut at 2, 4, and 6–18 mo and at 4–6 yr (1st dose may be given as early as age 6 wk).	Anaphylactic reaction after a previous dose or to vaccine component (including neomycin, streptomycin, or polymyxin B).	Anorexia, fatigue, fever, Irritability, pain at injection site, vomiting.	Oral polio vaccine (OPV) is no longer recommended for use in the United States.

GENERIC NAME (BRAND NAMES)	ROUTE/DOSAGE	CONTRAINDICATIONS/ PRECAUTIONS	ADVERSE REACTIONS/ SIDE EFFECTS	NOTES
Rotavirus vaccine (RV, Rotarix [RV1], RotaTeq [RV5])	*Rotarix*—1 mL PO at 2 and 4 mo; *RotaTeq*—2 mL PO at 2, 4, and 6 mo. First dose of either product may be given as early as age 6 wk; final dose should be given no later than age 8 mo.	Anaphylactic reaction after a previous dose or to vaccine component (if allergic to latex, do not use Rotarix); history of uncorrected congenital malformation of GI tract (Rotarix only); history of intussusception; severe combined immunodeficiency disease.	Diarrhea, fever, irritability, vomiting.	Series should not be started in infants ≥15 wk. Series should be completed with same product, when possible. If RotaTeq used in any of the doses, a total of 3 doses should be given.
Tetanus toxoid, **reduced** diphtheria toxoid, and acellular pertussis vaccine absorbed (Tdap, Adacel, Boostrix)	0.5 mL IM given at age 11–12 yr if previously completed DTaP series, then followed by booster doses of Td every 10 yr; one-time dose (in place of single Td booster) may be given to all adolescents who have not received previous Tdap at age 11 or 12.	Anaphylactic reaction after a previous dose or to vaccine component; encephalopathy within 7 days of administration of previous dose of Tdap, DTP, or DTaP vaccines.	Abdominal pain, arthralgia, chills, diarrhea, fatigue, headache, myalgia, nausea, pain at injection site, vomiting.	Should also be given to pregnant adolescents during each pregnancy (preferably during 27–36 wk gestation) regardless of interval since prior Td or Tdap.
Varicella vaccine (Var, Varivax)	0.5 mL subcut at 12–15 mo and at 4–6 yr (2nd dose may be given earlier if ≥3 mo have elapsed since the 1st dose); for persons 7–18 yr who do not have evidence of immunity, 2 doses should be given (≥3 mo apart if 7–12 yr or ≥4 wk apart if ≥13 yr).	Anaphylactic reaction after a previous dose or to vaccine component (including gelatin or neomycin); severe immunosuppression (in the absence of severe immunosuppression, HIV is not a contraindication); pregnancy.	Anorexia, chills, diarrhea, fatigue, fever, headache, injection site reaction, irritability, nausea, vomiting.	Immunosuppression may ↓ antibody response to injection and ↑ the risk of viral transmission.

Nursing Implications:

Assessment

Assess previous immunization history and history of hypersensitivity.

Assess for history of latex allergy. Some prefilled syringes may use latex components and should be avoided in those with hypersensitivity.

Potential Nursing Diagnoses

Infection, risk for (Indications).

Knowledge, deficient, related to medication regimen (Patient/Family Teaching).

Implementation

Measles, mumps, and rubella vaccine and diphtheria toxoid, tetanus toxoid, and pertussis vaccine may be given concomitantly.

Do not administer FluMist concurrently with other vaccines, or in patients who have received a live virus vaccine within 1 mo or an inactivated vaccine within 2 wk of vaccination.

Administer each immunization by appropriate route:

PO: Rotavirus.

Subcut: measles, mumps, rubella, polio, varicella, pneumococcal polysaccharide.

IM: diphtheria, tetanus toxoid, pertussis, polio, Haemophilus b, hepatitis B, meningococcal conjugate, hepatitis A, pneumococcal conjugate, pneumococcal polysaccharide, influenza injection, human papillomavirus.

Intranasal: FluMist.

Patient/Family Teaching

Inform parent of potential and reportable side effects of immunization. Notify health care professional if patient develops fever higher than 39.4° C (103° F); difficulty breathing; hives; itching; swelling of eyes, face, or inside of nose; sudden, severe tiredness or weakness; or convulsions.

Review next scheduled immunization with parent.

Evaluation

Prevention of diseases through active immunity.

ROUTINE ADULT IMMUNIZATIONS

GENERIC NAME (BRAND NAMES)	INDICATIONS	DOSAGE/ROUTE	CONTRAINDICATIONS	ADVERSE REACTIONS/SIDE EFFECTS
Hepatitis A vaccine (HepA, Havrix, Vaqta)	High-risk groups (e.g., chronic liver disease, receive clotting factor concentrates, users of injection/noninjection illicit drugs, men who have sex with men, working with infected primates or with hepatitis A virus in a research laboratory setting); travel to endemic areas; unvaccinated individuals who anticipate close personal contact with an international adoptee during the initial 60 days after their arrival in the U.S. from a country with intermediate or high endemicity.	1 mL IM, followed by 1 mL IM 6–12 mo (for Havrix) or 6–18 mo (for Vaqta) later.	Anaphylactic reaction after a previous dose or to vaccine component.	↓ appetite, drowsiness, fever, injection site reactions, irritability, headache.
Hepatitis B vaccine (HepB, Engerix-B, Recombivax HB)	High-risk patients (e.g., household contacts or sex partners of persons with chronic hepatitis B virus infection, injection drug users, sexually active persons not in a long-term monogamous relationship [having >1 sex partner in past 6 mo], men who have sex with men, HIV, STDs, end-stage renal disease, hemodialysis, health care workers, chronic liver disease; clients and staff of institutions for those with developmental disabilities; adults in STD treatment facilities, HIV testing/treatment facilities, drug abuse prevention/treatment facilities, facilities providing services to injection drug users or men who have sex with men, correctional facilities, end-stage renal disease programs, hemodialysis facilities, or facilities for those with developmental disabilities); travel to endemic areas; unvaccinated adults (19–59 yr) with diabetes (may also be administered at prescriber's discretion to adults ≥60 yr with diabetes).	Immunocompetent: 1 mL IM, given at 0, 1 and 6 mo. Immunosuppressed: 1 mL (Recombivax HB) or 2 mL (Engerix-B) IM at 0, 1, and 6 mo.	Anaphylactic reaction after a previous dose or to vaccine component.	Injection site reactions.
Human papillomavirus vaccine, bivalent (HPV2, Cervarix)	All previously unvaccinated women through age 26 yr. Not indicated for males.	0.5 mL IM, repeat at 1–2 and 6 mo after initial dose.	Anaphylactic reaction after a previous dose or to vaccine component; pregnancy.	Arthralgia, fatigue, injection site reactions, myalgia.
Human papillomavirus vaccine, quadrivalent (HPV4, Gardasil)	All previously unvaccinated females and males through age 26 yr.	0.5 mL IM, repeat at 1–2 and 6 mo after initial dose.	Anaphylactic reaction after a previous dose or to vaccine component; pregnancy.	Dizziness, fever, headache, injection site reactions, syncope.

GENERIC NAME (BRAND NAMES)	INDICATIONS	DOSAGE/ROUTE	CONTRAINDICATIONS	ADVERSE REACTIONS/SIDE EFFECTS
Influenza vaccine *Injection (inactivated):* (Afluria, Fluarix, Flublok, Flucelvax, FluLaval, Fluvirin, Fluzone); *Intranasal (live attenuated):* FluMist)	All adults.	*Injection:* 0.5 mL IM annually. *Intranasal (for healthy, nonpregnant adults <50 yr):* 0.2 mL (given as 0.1 mL in each nostril) intranasally annually.	Anaphylactic reaction after a previous dose or to vaccine component, including eggs/egg products (recommend product that does not contain egg protein [Flublok]) and thimerosal (injection only). FluMist should be avoided in pregnancy; chronic pulmonary, cardiovascular (not hypertension), renal, hepatic, neurological, hematologic, or metabolic (including diabetes) disorders; immunosuppression (including HIV); age ≥50 yr; egg allergy of any severity; use of influenza antiviral medications (e.g. amantadine, rimantadine, oseltamivir, zanamivir) with previous 48 hr or 14 days after vaccination.	*Injection:* fever, injection site reactions, myalgia. *Intranasal:* abdominal pain, cough, ↓ appetite, headache, irritability, lethargy, nasal congestion, myalgia, rhinorrhea, sore throat.
Measles, mumps, and rubella vaccine (MMR, M-M-R II)	Adults born in or after 1957 with unreliable documentation of previous vaccination (unless have laboratory evidence of immunity to all 3 diseases); health care workers born before 1957 who do not have laboratory evidence of immunity to all measles, mumps, and/or rubella.	Adults born in or after 1957 with unreliable history: 1 or 2 doses of 0.5 mL subcut (with ≥28 days between doses); high-risk groups should receive a total of 2 doses (with ≥28 days between doses).	Allergy to egg, gelatin, or neomycin; severe immunosuppression (in the absence of severe immunosuppression, HIV is not a contraindication); pregnancy (also avoid becoming pregnant for 4 wk after immunization).	Burning, stinging, pain at injection site; arthritis/arthralgia; fever; encephalitis; allergic reactions. Immunosuppression may ↓ antibody response to injection and ↑ the risk of viral transmission (live vaccine).
Meningococcal conjugate vaccine *Conjugate:* (Menactra (MCV4 or MenACWY-D), Menveo (MenACWY-CRM) *Polysaccharide:* , Menomune-A/C/Y/W-135 (MPSV4))	College freshmen (up to age 21) living in dormitories if they have not previously received a dose on or after their 16th birthday; military recruits; anatomic or functional asplenia; persistent complement component deficiency; travel or reside in areas in which meningococcal disease is hyperendemic or epidemic; persons at risk during an outbreak due to a vaccine serogroup.	Age ≤55 yr: 0.5 mL IM single dose; Age ≤55 yr with anatomic or functional asplenia, persistent complement component deficiency, or HIV: 0.5 mL IM, repeat at least 2 mo after initial dose. Revaccination with MenACWY every 5 yr is indicated in patients previously vaccinated with MenACWY or MPSV4 and who also remain at ↑ risk for infection (anatomic or functional asplenia or persistent complement component deficiency); MenACWY is preferred for adults ≥56 yr who previously received MenACWY and need to be revaccinated or for whom multiple doses are needed; MPSV4 is preferred for adults ≥56 yr who have not previously received MenACWY and who only require a single dose.	Anaphylactic reaction after a previous dose or to vaccine component.	Anorexia, arthralgia, diarrhea, fatigue, fever, headache, myalgia, nausea, irritability, malaise, pain at injection site, vomiting.
Pneumococcal conjugate vaccine (13–valent) (PCV13, Prevnar 13)	All adults ≥65 yr; adults ≤64 yr with chronic renal failure, anatomic or functional asplenia, sickle cell disease, cerebrospinal fluid leaks, cochlear implants, or immunsuppression.	0.5 mL IM single dose followed by single dose of PPSV23 ≥8 wk later; if already received PPSV23, give PCV13 single dose (0.5 mL IM) ≥1 yr after dose of PPSV23.	Anaphylactic reaction after a previous dose or to vaccine component including diphtheria toxoid.	Arthralgia, chills, ↓ appetite, fatigue, fever, headache, insomnia, irritability, myalgia, pain at injection site, rash.

GENERIC NAME (BRAND NAMES)	INDICATIONS	DOSAGE/ROUTE	CONTRAINDICATIONS	ADVERSE REACTIONS/SIDE EFFECTS
Pneumococcal polysaccharide vaccine (PPSV23, Pneumovax 23)	All adults ≥65 yr; high-risk adults ≤64 yr (e.g., chronic cardiac [excluding hypertension] or pulmonary disease [including COPD and asthma], chronic liver disease, alcoholism, diabetes, cigarette smoker, anatomic or functional asplenia, sickle cell disease; immunosuppression (including HIV), chronic renal failure, cochlear implants, cerebrospinal fluid leaks, residents of long-term care facilities).	0.5 mL IM or subcut; one-time revaccination should also be given ≥5 yr after 1st dose to those ≥65 yr (if 1st dose was given ≥5 yr ago and before age 65) and to high-risk patients age 19–64 yr (chronic renal failure, anatomic or functional asplenia, sickle cell disease, immunosuppression).	Anaphylactic reaction after a previous dose or to vaccine component.	Chills, fever, injection site reactions.
Tetanus toxoid, **reduced** diphtheria toxoid and acellular pertussis vaccine absorbed (Tdap, Adacel, Boostrix)	Single dose should be given to replace one of the 10-yr Td boosters in all adults who did not previously receive a dose of Tdap or if their vaccine status is unknown. Single dose should also be given as soon as feasible to all pregnant women (preferred during 27–36 weeks' gestation), close contacts of infants <12 mo, and health care workers with direct patient contact.	0.5 mL IM single dose.	Anaphylactic reaction after a previous dose or to vaccine component; encephalopathy within 7 days of administration of previous dose of Tdap, DTP, or DTaP vaccines.	Abdominal pain, arthralgia, chills, diarrhea, fatigue, headache, myalgia, nausea, pain at injection site, vomiting.
Tetanus-diphtheria (Td, Tenivac)	All adults who lack written documentation of a primary series consisting of ≥3 doses of tetanus– and diphtheria–toxoid-containing vaccine; booster dose should be given to all adults every 10 yr (see info above regarding use of Tdap to replace one dose of Td in booster series).	*Unimmunized:* 2 doses of 0.5 mL IM ≥4 wk apart, then a 3rd dose 6–12 mo later; *Immunized:* 0.5 mL IM booster every 10 yr.	Anaphylactic reaction after a previous dose or to vaccine component.	Arthralgia, chills, diarrhea, fatigue, headache, myalgia, nausea, pain at injection site.
Varicella vaccine (Var, Varivax)	Any adult without a history of chickenpox or herpes zoster (shingles), a history of receiving 2 doses of varicella vaccine ≥4 wk apart, or laboratory evidence of immunity. Health care workers and pregnant women born in U.S. before 1980 who do not meet the above criteria should be tested for immunity.	0.5 mL subcut; repeated 4–8 wk later.	Anaphylactic reaction after a previous dose or to vaccine component (including gelatin or neomycin); severe immunosuppression (in the absence of severe immunosuppression, HIV is not a contraindication); pregnancy (also avoid becoming pregnant for 4 wk after immunization).	Fever, pain at injection site. Immunosuppression may ↓ antibody response to injection and ↑ the risk of viral transmission (live vaccine).
Zoster vaccine (Zos, Zostavax)	All adults ≥60 yr (regardless of previous history of chickenpox or herpes zoster).	0.65 mL subcut single dose.	Anaphylactic reaction after a previous dose or to vaccine component (including gelatin or neomycin); severe immunosuppression (in the absence of severe immunosuppression, HIV is not a contraindication); pregnancy.	Fever, pain at injection site. Immunosuppression may ↓ antibody response to injection and ↑ the risk of viral transmission (live vaccine).

SOURCE: Adapted from the recommendations of the Department of Health and Human Services, Centers for Disease Control and Prevention: http://www.cdc.gov/vaccines/schedules/hcp/index.html.

APPENDIX N
Administering Medications to Children

General Guidelines

Medication administration to a pediatric patient can be challenging. Prescribers should order dosage forms that are age appropriate for their patients. If a child is unable to take a particular dosage form, ask the pharmacist if another form is available or for other options.

Oral Liquids

Pediatric liquid medicines may be given with plastic medicine cups, oral syringes, oral droppers, or cylindrical dosing spoons. Parents should be taught to use these calibrated devices rather than using household utensils. If a medicine comes with a particular measuring device, do not use it with another product. For young children, it is best to squirt a little of the dose at a time into the side of the cheek away from the bitter taste buds at the back of the tongue.

Eye Drops/Ointments

Tilt the child's head back and gently press the skin under the lower eyelid and pull the lower lid away slightly until a small pouch is visible. Insert the ointment or drop (1 at a time) and close the eye for a few minutes to keep the medicine in the eye.

Ear Drops

Shake otic suspensions well before administration. For children <3 yr, pull the outer ear outward and downward before instilling drops. For children ≥3 yr, pull the outer ear outward and upward. Keep child on side for 2 min and instill a cotton plug into ear.

Nose Drops

Clear nose of secretions prior to use. A nasal aspirator (bulb syringe) or a cotton swab may be used in infants and young children. Ask older children to blow their nose. Tilt child's head back over a pillow and squeeze dropper without touching the nostril. Keep child's head back for 2 min.

Suppositories

Keep refrigerated for easier administration. Wearing gloves, moisten the rounded end with water or petroleum jelly prior to insertion. Using your pinky finger for children <3 yr and your index finger for those ≥3 yr, insert the suppository into the rectum about ½ to 1 inch beyond the sphincter. If the suppository slides out, insert it a little farther than before. Hold the buttocks together for a few minutes and have the child hold their position for about 20 min, if possible.

Topicals

Clean affected area and dry well prior to application. Apply a thin layer to the skin and rub in gently. Do not apply coverings over the area unless instructed to do so by the prescriber.

Metered-Dose Inhalers

Generally the same principles apply in children as in adults, except the use of spacers is recommended for young children (see Appendix D).

APPENDIX O

Pediatric Dosage Calculations

Most drugs in children are dosed according to body weight (mg/kg) or body surface area (BSA) (mg/m^2). Care must be taken to properly convert body weight from pounds to kilograms (1 kg= 2.2 lb) before calculating doses based on body weight. Doses are often expressed as mg/kg/day or mg/kg/dose, therefore orders written "mg/kg/d," which is confusing, *require further clarification from the prescriber.*

Chemotherapeutic drugs are commonly dosed according to body surface area, which requires an extra verification step (BSA calculation) prior to dosing. Medications are available in multiple concentrations, therefore *orders written in "mL" rather than "mg" are not acceptable and require further clarification.*

Dosing also varies by indication, therefore diagnostic information is helpful when calculating doses. The following examples are typically encountered when dosing medication in children.

Example 1.

Calculate the dose of amoxicillin suspension in mLs for otitis media for a 1-yr-old child weighing 22 lb. The dose required is 40 mg/kg/day divided BID and the suspension comes in a concentration of 400 mg/5 mL.

Step 1. Convert pounds to kg:	22 lb × 1 kg/2.2 lb = 10 kg
Step 2. Calculate the dose in mg:	10 kg × 40 mg/kg/day = 400 mg/day
Step 3. Divide the dose by the frequency:	400 mg/day ÷ 2 (BID) = 200 mg/dose BID
Step 4. Convert the mg dose to mL:	200 mg/dose ÷ 400 mg/5 mL = **2.5 mL BID**

Example 2.

Calculate the dose of ceftriaxone in mLs for meningitis for a 5-yr-old weighing 18 kg. The dose required is 100 mg/kg/day given IV once daily and the drug comes prediluted in a concentration of 40 mg/mL.

Step 1. Calculate the dose in mg:	18 kg × 100 mg/kg/day = 1800 mg/day
Step 2. Divide the dose by the frequency:	1800 mg/day ÷ 1 (daily) = 1800 mg/dose
Step 3. Convert the mg dose to mL:	1800 mg/dose ÷ 40 mg/mL = **45 mL once daily**

Example 3.

Calculate the dose of vincristine in mLs for a 4-yr-old with leukemia weighing 37 lb and is 97 cm tall. The dose required in 2 mg/m^2 and the drug comes in 1 mg/mL concentration.

Step 1. Convert pounds to kg:	37 lb × 1 kg/2.2 lb = 16.8 kg
Step 2. Calculate BSA:	$\sqrt{16.8 \text{ kg} \times 97 \text{ cm}/3600} = 0.67 \text{ m}^2$
Step 3. Calculate the dose in mg:	2 mg/m^2 × 0.67 m^2 = 1.34 mg
Step 4. Calculate the dose in mL:	1.34 mg ÷ 1 mg/mL = **1.34 mL**

APPENDIX P

Pediatric Fluid and Electrolyte Requirements

How to calculate maintenance fluid requirements in children:

1. **Body Surface Area Method** (commonly used in children >10 kg):

$$1500\text{–}2000 \text{ mL/m}^2\text{/day} \div 24 = \text{fluid rate in mL/hr}$$

Example: Calculate maintenance fluids in mL/hr for a child with a BSA = 0.8 m^2.

Answer: $1500 \text{ mL/m}^2\text{/day} \times 0.8 \text{ m}^2 = 1200 \text{ mL/day} \div 24 \text{ hr} = 50 \text{ mL/hr}$
$2000 \text{ mL/m}^2\text{/day} \times 0.8 \text{ m}^2 = 1600 \text{ mL/day} \div 24 \text{ hr} = 66.6 \text{ mL/hr}$

Range: 50–66.6 mL/hr.

2. **Body Weight Method**

<10 kg	100 mL/kg/day
11–20 kg	1000 mL + 50 mL/kg for each kg >10
>20 kg	1500 mL + 20 mL/kg for each kg >20

Example: Calculate maintenance fluids in mL/hr for a child weighing 25 kg.

Answer: $1500 \text{ mL} + 20 \text{ mL/kg} \times 5 \text{ kg} = 1500 \text{ mL} + 100 \text{ mL} = 1600 \text{ mL}$
$1600 \text{ mL} \div 24 \text{ hr} = 66.6 \text{ mL/hr}$

Daily Electrolyte Requirements in Children

Sodium	2–6 mEq/kg/day
Potassium	2–4 mEq/kg/day
Calcium	1–4 mEq/kg/day*
Magnesium	0.3–0.5 mEq/kg/day
Phosphorous	0.5–2 mmol/kg/day*

*Neonates may require the higher end of the calcium and phosphorous dosage range due to rapid bone development.

Conditions That May Alter Fluid Requirements in Children

Fever
Hyperventilation
Sweating
Hyperthyroidism
Renal failure
Diarrhea
Congential heart disease
Chronic lung disease

Oral Rehydration Therapy (ORT)

ORT is as effective as IV therapy in managing fluid and electrolytes in children with mild to moderate dehydration due to diarrhea. Commercially available premixed ORT solutions typically contain low concentrations of glucose (2–3%), 45–75 mEq/L sodium, 20–25 mEq/L potassium, 30–35 mEq/L of citrate (bicarbonate source). Low sugar content provides little caloric support but facilitates intestinal sodium and water absorption. All commercially available ORT solutions are equally safe and effective, and are preferred over household remedies (e.g., colas, juices, chicken broth) that are not formulated based on the physiology of acute diarrhea.

BIBLIOGRAPHY

AHFS Drug Information BOOK ONLINE. Jackson, WY: Teton Data Systems, 2007. Based on: Gerald K. McEvoy, editor. AHFS Drug Information (2011). Bethesda, MD: American Society of Health-System Pharmacists, Inc.; 2007. STAT!Ref Medical Reference Library.

American Hospital Formulary Service: Drug Information 2011. American Society of Hospital Pharmacists, Bethesda, MD, 2011.

American Pain Society: Principles of Analgesic Use in the Treatment of Acute Pain and Cancer Pain, ed 6. American Pain Society, Skokie, IL, 2008.

Blumenthal, M, et al: The Complete German Commission E Monographs: Therapeutic Guide to Herbal Medicines. Integrative Medical Communications, Boston, 1998.

DRUGDEX® System [intranet database]. Version 5.1. Greenwood Village, Colo: Thomson Healthcare.

Drug Facts and Comparisons On-line, version 4.0. Facts and Comparisons, a Wolters Kluwer Company, St. Louis, 2011.

Fetrow, CW, and Avila, JR: Professional's Handbook of Complementary & Alternative Medicines, ed. 3. Lippincott Williams & Wilkins, Philadelphia, PA, 2004.

IV INDEX® System [intranet database]. Version 5.1. Greenwood Village, Colo: Thomson Healthcare.

Jonas, WB, and Levin, JS (eds): Essentials of Complementary and Alternative Medicine. Lippincott Williams & Wilkins, a Wolters Kluwer Company, Baltimore and Philadelphia, 1999.

Kemp, SF, and deShazo, RD: Prevention and treatment of anaphylaxis. Clin Allergy Immunol 2008;21:477–498.

Kuhn, MA, and Winston, D: Herbal Therapy and Supplements: A Scientific and Traditional Approach. Lippincott Williams & Wilkins, Philadelphia, 2001.

Van Leeuwen, AM, Kranpitz, T, and Smith, L: Davis's Comprehensive Handbook of Laboratory and Diagnostic Tests with Nursing Implications, ed 2. FA Davis Company, Philadelphia, PA, 2006.

Lexi-Comp, Inc: (Lexi-Drugs [Comp + Specialties]). Lexi-Comp, Inc., Hudson, Ohio.

McCaffery, M, and Pasero, C: Pain: Clinical Manual, ed 2. Mosby-Yearbook, St Louis, 1999.

MICROMEDEX® 2.0 and MICROMEDEX® 1.0 (Healthcare Series).

National Institutes of Health Warren Grant Magnuson Clinical Center: Drug—Nutrient Interactions, Bethesda, MD, 2005. http://www.cc.nih.gov/ccc/supplements/intro.html.

National Kidney Foundation: A-Z Guide for High Potassium Foods, National Kidney Foundation, 2005.

PDR for Herbal Medicines, ed 4. Thomson Healthcare, New York, NY, 2011.

Pennington, JAT, and Douglass, JS: Bowes and Church's Food Values of Portions Commonly Used, ed 18. Philadelphia: Lippincott Williams & Wilkins, 2004. 1–496.

Phelps, SJ, Hak, EB, and Crill, CM: Pediatric Injectable Drugs, ed. 8. American Society of Health-System Pharmacists, Bethesda, MD, 2007.

Physicians' Desk Reference (PDR): Thomson Healthcare, Montvale, NJ, 2011.

Polovich, M, White, JM, and Kelleher, LO: Chemotherapy and Biotherapy Guidelines and Recommendations for Practice, ed. 2. Oncology Nursing Society, Pittsburgh, 2005.

Taketomo, CK, Hodding, JH, and Kraus, DM: Pediatric Dosage Handbook, ed 14. Lexi-Comp, Hudson, Ohio, 2007–2008.

http://www.fda.gov/cder/index.html.

http://www.ons.org/news.shtml.

http://www.accessdata.fda.gov/scripts/cder/drugsatfda/.

COMPREHENSIVE INDEX*

*Entries for **generic** names appear in **boldface type.** Trade names appear in regular type, with Canadian names preceded by a maple leaf icon (🍁). **CLASSIFICATIONS** appear in **BOLDFACE SMALL CAPS.** *Combination Drugs* appear in *italics,* herbal products are preceded by a yin-yang icon (☯), and drugs with genetic implications are preceded by a double-helix icon (🧬).

*Entries for **generic** names appear in **boldface type.** Trade names appear in regular type, with Canadian names preceded by a maple leaf icon (🍁). **CLASSIFICATIONS** appear in **BOLDFACE SMALL CAPS.** *Combination Drugs* appear in *italics,* herbal products are preceded by a yin-yang icon (☯), and drugs with genetic implications are preceded by a double-helix icon (🧬).

*Entries for **generic** names appear in **boldface type.** Trade names appear in regular type, with Canadian names preceded by a maple leaf icon. CLASSIFICATIONS appear in BOLDFACE SMALL CAPS. *Combination Drugs* appear in *italics*, herbal products are preceded by a yin-yang icon, and drugs with genetic implications are preceded by a double-helix icon.

*Entries for **generic** names appear in **boldface type.** Trade names appear in regular type, with Canadian names preceded by a maple leaf icon (🍁). **CLASSIFICATIONS** appear in **BOLDFACE SMALL CAPS.** *Combination Drugs* appear in *italics,* herbal products are preceded by a yin-yang icon (☯), and drugs with genetic implications are preceded by a double-helix icon (🧬).

*Entries for **generic** names appear in **boldface type.** Trade names appear in regular type, with Canadian names preceded by a maple leaf icon (🍁). **CLASSIFICATIONS** appear in **BOLDFACE SMALL CAPS.** *Combination Drugs* appear in *italics,* herbal products are preceded by a yin-yang icon (☯), and drugs with genetic implications are preceded by a double-helix icon (🧬).

*Entries for **generic** names appear in **boldface type.** Trade names appear in regular type, with Canadian names preceded by a maple leaf icon (🍁). **CLASSIFICATIONS** appear in **BOLDFACE SMALL CAPS.** *Combination Drugs* appear in *italics,* herbal products are preceded by a yin-yang icon (☯), and drugs with genetic implications are preceded by a double-helix icon (🧬).

*Entries for **generic** names appear in **boldface type.** Trade names appear in regular type, with Canadian names preceded by a maple leaf icon (🍁). **CLASSIFICATIONS** appear in **BOLDFACE SMALL CAPS.** *Combination Drugs* appear in *italics,* herbal products are preceded by a yin-yang icon (☯), and drugs with genetic implications are preceded by a double-helix icon (🧬).

D

*Entries for **generic** names appear in **boldface type.** Trade names appear in regular type, with Canadian names preceded by a maple leaf icon (🍁). **CLASSIFICATIONS** appear in **BOLDFACE SMALL CAPS.** *Combination Drugs* appear in *italics,* herbal products are preceded by a yin-yang icon (☯), and drugs with genetic implications are preceded by a double-helix icon (🧬).

E

*Entries for **generic** names appear in **boldface type.** Trade names appear in regular type, with Canadian names preceded by a maple leaf icon (🍁). **CLASSIFICATIONS** appear in **BOLDFACE SMALL CAPS.** *Combination Drugs* appear in *italics,* herbal products are preceded by a yin-yang icon (☯), and drugs with genetic implications are preceded by a double-helix icon (🧬).

F

*Entries for **generic** names appear in **boldface type.** Trade names appear in regular type, with Canadian names preceded by a maple leaf icon (🍁). **CLASSIFICATIONS** appear in **BOLDFACE SMALL CAPS.** *Combination Drugs* appear in *italics,* herbal products are preceded by a yin-yang icon (☯), and drugs with genetic implications are preceded by a double-helix icon (🧬).

H

*Entries for **generic** names appear in **boldface type.** Trade names appear in regular type, with Canadian names preceded by a maple leaf icon (🍁). **CLASSIFICATIONS** appear in **BOLDFACE SMALL CAPS.** *Combination Drugs* appear in *italics,* herbal products are preceded by a yin-yang icon (☯), and drugs with genetic implications are preceded by a double-helix icon (🧬).

J

*Entries for **generic** names appear in **boldface type.** Trade names appear in regular type, with Canadian names preceded by a maple leaf icon (🍁). **CLASSIFICATIONS** appear in **BOLDFACE SMALL CAPS.** *Combination Drugs* appear in *italics,* herbal products are preceded by a yin-yang icon (☯), and drugs with genetic implications are preceded by a double-helix icon (🧬).

*Entries for **generic** names appear in **boldface type.** Trade names appear in regular type, with Canadian names preceded by a maple leaf icon (🍁). **CLASSIFICATIONS** appear in **BOLDFACE SMALL CAPS.** *Combination Drugs* appear in *italics,* herbal products are preceded by a yin-yang icon (☯), and drugs with genetic implications are preceded by a double-helix icon (🧬).

*Entries for **generic** names appear in **boldface type.** Trade names appear in regular type, with Canadian names preceded by a maple leaf icon (✽). **CLASSIFICATIONS** appear in **BOLDFACE SMALL CAPS.** *Combination Drugs* appear in *italics,* herbal products are preceded by a yin-yang icon (☯), and drugs with genetic implications are preceded by a double-helix icon (§).

N

*Entries for **generic** names appear in **boldface type.** Trade names appear in regular type, with Canadian names preceded by a maple leaf icon (🍁). **CLASSIFICATIONS** appear in **BOLDFACE SMALL CAPS.** *Combination Drugs* appear in *italics,* herbal products are preceded by a yin-yang icon (☯), and drugs with genetic implications are preceded by a double-helix icon (🧬).

COMPREHENSIVE INDEX

*Entries for **generic** names appear in **boldface type.** Trade names appear in regular type, with Canadian names preceded by a maple leaf icon (🍁). **CLASSIFICATIONS** appear in **BOLDFACE SMALL CAPS.** *Combination Drugs* appear in *italics,* herbal products are preceded by a yin-yang icon (☯), and drugs with genetic implications are preceded by a double-helix icon (🧬).

P

*Entries for **generic** names appear in **boldface type.** Trade names appear in regular type, with Canadian names preceded by a maple leaf icon (🍁). **CLASSIFICATIONS** appear in **BOLDFACE SMALL CAPS.** *Combination Drugs* appear in *italics,* herbal products are preceded by a yin-yang icon (☯), and drugs with genetic implications are preceded by a double-helix icon (🧬).

Q

R

*Entries for **generic** names appear in **boldface type.** Trade names appear in regular type, with Canadian names preceded by a maple leaf icon (🍁). CLASSIFICATIONS appear in BOLDFACE SMALL CAPS. *Combination Drugs* appear in *italics,* herbal products are preceded by a yin-yang icon (☯), and drugs with genetic implications are preceded by a double-helix icon (ꕤ).

COMPREHENSIVE INDEX

S

*Entries for **generic** names appear in **boldface type.** Trade names appear in regular type, with Canadian names preceded by a maple leaf icon (🍁). **CLASSIFICATIONS** appear in **BOLDFACE SMALL CAPS.** *Combination Drugs* appear in *italics,* herbal products are preceded by a yin-yang icon (☯), and drugs with genetic implications are preceded by a double-helix icon (🧬).

*Entries for **generic** names appear in **boldface type.** Trade names appear in regular type, with Canadian names preceded by a maple leaf icon (🍁). **CLASSIFICATIONS** appear in **BOLDFACE SMALL CAPS.** *Combination Drugs* appear in *italics,* herbal products are preceded by a yin-yang icon (☯), and drugs with genetic implications are preceded by a double-helix icon (🧬).

*Entries for **generic** names appear in **boldface type.** Trade names appear in regular type, with Canadian names preceded by a maple leaf icon (✤). **CLASSIFICATIONS** appear in **BOLDFACE SMALL CAPS.** *Combination Drugs* appear in *italics,* herbal products are preceded by a yin-yang icon (☯), and drugs with genetic implications are preceded by a double-helix icon (🧬).

W

*Entries for **generic** names appear in **boldface type.** Trade names appear in regular type, with Canadian names preceded by a maple leaf icon. **CLASSIFICATIONS** appear in **BOLDFACE SMALL CAPS.** *Combination Drugs* appear in *italics*, herbal products are preceded by a yin-yang icon, and drugs with genetic implications are preceded by a double-helix icon.

Measurement Conversion Table

Metric System Equivalents

1 gram (g) = 1000 milligrams (mg)
1000 grams = 1 kilogram (kg)
.001 milligram = 1 microgram (mcg)
1 liter (L) = 1000 milliliters (ml)
1 milliliter = 1 cubic centimeter (cc)
1 meter = 100 centimeters (cm)
1 meter = 1000 millimeters (mm)

Conversion Equivalents

Volume

1 milliliter = 15 minims (M) = 15 drops (gtt)

5 milliliters = 1 fluidram = 1 teaspoon (tsp)

15 milliliters = 4 fluidrams = 1 tablespoon (T)

30 milliliters = 1 ounce (oz) = 2 tablespoons

500 milliliters = 1 pint (pt)

1000 milliliters = 1 quart (qt)

Weight

1 kilogram = 2.2 pounds (lb)
1 gram (g) = 1000 milligrams = 15 grains (gr)
0.6 gram = 600 milligrams = 10 grains
0.5 gram = 500 milligrams = 7.5 grains
0.3 gram = 300 milligrams = 5 grains
0.06 gram = 60 milligrams = 1 grain

Length

2.5 centimeters = 1 inch

Centigrade/Fahrenheit Conversions

$C = (F - 32) \times {}^{5}/_{9}$

$F = (C \times {}^{9}/_{5}) + 32$

(cm)
1
2
3
4
5
6
7
8
9
10
11
12
13
14
15

PUPIL SCALE mm	1	2	3	4	5	6	7	8

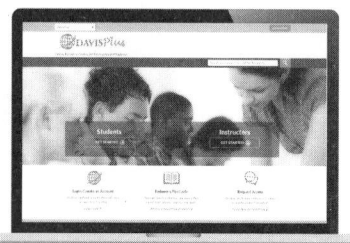